Important Message

No Official Addenda to ICD-9-CM Volumes 1 & 2 for 2014

Because the National Center for Health Statistics (NCHS) did not release official ICD-9-CM addenda for volumes 1 & 2 for fiscal 2014, there will be no ICD-9-CM code changes. As a result, the "Summary of Code Changes" and the "ICD-9-CM Code Changes: An Insider's View" (Expert editions only) are not included in this manual. There are no official changes to the Alphabetic Index or Tabular List sections, including instructional notes, title revisions, or other content, though there are changes to other parts of the manual that keep the book up-to-date (see "What is NEW for the 2014 ICD-9-CM Volumes 1, 2, & 3," below).

The Official ICD-9-CM Guidelines for Coding and Reporting included in this manual were effective October 1, 2011. This set of guidelines was approved by the Cooperating Parties and the Editorial Advisory Board for *Coding Clinic for ICD-9-CM*. The Health Insurance Portability and Accountability Act (HIPAA) requires adherence to these guidelines when ICD-9-CM diagnosis codes are being assigned. Since no official ICD-9-CM addendum to the guidelines was released in 2013, the guidelines included in this book stand as the official version effective October 1, 2013, through September 30, 2014. ICD-9-CM is under a "limited update" or "code set freeze" as we prepare for the transition to and implementation of ICD-10-CM on October 1, 2014.

Official Addenda to ICD-9-CM Volume 3 for 2014 Includes Four New Procedure Codes

The Centers for Medicare and Medicaid Services did release official ICD-9-CM addenda for volume 3 that included new procedure codes that meet the criteria for new technology. This code will go into effect on October 1, 2013.

Four new codes were added to Volume 3, procedures. These four procedures represent new technologies and therefore meet the criteria for inclusion in this limited update to ICD-9-CM.

- 00.96 Infusion of 4-Factor Prothrombin Complex Concentrate
- 14.81 Implantation of epiretinal visual prosthesis
- 14.82 Removal of epiretinal visual prosthesis
- 14.83 Revision or replacement of epiretinal visual prosthesis

What Is NEW for the 2014 ICD-9-CM Volumes 1, 2, & 3

Remember: ICD-9-CM remains the valid code set for reporting until October 1, 2014. Optum is committed to keeping users up-to-date and will continue to update the code books during the code set freeze.

- HIPAA compliance is ma[...] code set for reporting u[...]
- There is no freeze on the [...] systems—our hallmark c[...] updated.

Your 2014 ICD-9-CM code book includes a new feature plus updated content:

- ICD-10-CM Coding Proficiency and Documentation Self-Assessment Test with Answers — How ready are you for ICD-10-CM? This is a self-assessment tool for identifying the areas that may require additional coding training or documentation improvement.
- Updated official coding tips
- Updated Medicare Code Edits (color-coding and symbols) for facility specific prospective payment systems
- Updated American Hospital Association's *Coding Clinic for ICD-9-CM* references
- Updated AHA's *Coding Clinic for ICD-9-CM* topic summaries (Expert edition *only*)
- Monthly "Inside Track" eZine: See "Product Alerts and Regulatory Updates" below

Binder Expert Editions Have Been Discontinued. Please Read This Notice

ICD-9-CM is under a "code freeze" until the implementation of ICD-10-CM/PCS on October 1, 2014, with no new codes expected to be released. In addition, *AHA Coding Clinic* has already begun transitioning to the *ICD-10-CM/PCS Coding Clinic*, and the ICD-9-CM Coordination & Maintenance Committee has begun its transition to becoming the ICD-10-CM/PCS Coordination & Maintenance Committee. Plus, changes to the existing edits under the Medicare Code Editor have been minimal.

With no significant changes expected to either the code set or the reimbursement system (represented by our hallmark color-coding representing the Medicare code edits), Optum has decided to discontinue the updateable ICD-9-CM editions as of November 2012.

All current subscriptions will be honored and fulfill as follows:

- September 2013—Copy of the 2014 ICD-9-CM Expert spiral-bound edition, including the "Summary of AHA Coding Clinic Topics"
- February 2014 through end of subscription—Newsletter updates

If you have any questions or comments concerning your subscription and what this decision means to you, please do not hesitate to call our customer service department at 1.800.464.3649, option 1.

ICD-10 Implementation Date Delayed One Year

Due to previous rulemaking, the ICD-10 code set was to be implemented on October 1, 2013, as described in the final rule, "Health Insurance Portability and Accountability Act (HIPAA) Administrative Simplification: Modifications to Medical Data Code Sets Standards to Adopt ICD-10-CM and ICD-10-PCS" (74 FR 3328–3362, January 16, 2009). However, on April 17, 2012, a proposed rule was released (45 CFR Part 162) that would delay for one year implementation of the ICD-10-CM and ICD-10-PCS data sets until October 1, 2014. The Centers for Medicare and Medicaid Services believes this change will give covered entities the additional time needed to synchronize system and business process preparation and to make the necessary changes to accommodate the updated medical data code sets.

In addition, the ICD-10 final rule analyzed the compliance date, emphasizing the interdependency between implementation of ICD-10 and version 5010 of the transaction standards under HIPAA and the need to balance the benefits of ICD-10 with the need to ensure adequate time for preparation and testing before implementation. The original version 5010 standards compliance date was set for January 1, 2012, but due to a number of issues, the full compliance date was delayed until January 2013. It was recognized that any delay in attaining compliance with version 5010 would negatively impact ICD-10 implementation and compliance. Based on the National Committee on Vital and Health Statistics (NCVHS) recommendations and industry feedback, it was determined that 24 months is the minimum amount of time the industry needs to comply with ICD-10 once version 5010 has moved into external (level 2) testing.

While considering a number of alternatives for the delay, CMS determined that a one-year delay would provide sufficient time for small providers and small hospitals to become ICD-10 compliant and would be the least financially burdensome to those who had planned to be compliant on October 1, 2013. In its March 2, 2012, letter to the Health and Human Services secretary on a possible delay of the ICD-10 compliance date, the NCVHS urged that any delay should be announced as soon as possible and should not be for more than one year. Among the alternatives ruled out were setting different implementation dates for ICD-10-CM and ICD-10-PCS, moving directly to ICD-11, and implementing a delay of two years. The one-year delay, with a compliance date of October 1, 2014, best meets the objectives for all covered entities.

Effect on Code Set Freeze

A code set freeze is a suspension of updates to ICD-9-CM and ICD-10 code sets. The ICD-9-CM Coordination and Maintenance Committee implemented a partial code set freeze of the ICD-9-CM and ICD-10 codes before the October 1, 2013, ICD-10 compliance deadline. As a result, on October 1, 2012, there were only limited code updates to both the ICD-9-CM and the ICD-10 code sets to capture new technologies and diseases as required by section 503(a) of Pub. L. 108-173. With the one-year delay in the compliance and implementation date, the same limited code set freeze is in effect for October 1, 2013.

Please note that while the code set freeze limits the number of new codes, it does not limit any necessary corrections or adjustments to the existing classification systems. This means that until ICD-10-CM and PCS are implemented (October 1, 2014), changes may be made to the draft indexes, tabular lists, and coding guidelines. It is essential at this time to stay updated on all the changes to the code sets. Effective training requires using the most current code set version.

Also note that while the ICD-9-CM code set may be under the freeze, regulatory issues continue to evolve that may affect coding guidance and coding edits in the code books.

ICD-10 Readiness Recommendations

Most industry experts recommend that providers and others remain HIPAA compliant by continuing to submit claims using current ICD-9-CM coding resources until the compliance date of October 1, 2014, and to continue to aggressively prepare for the new ICD-10 implementation date by fully assessing the impact of ICD-10, working with software and systems vendors to ensure all systems are fully compliant, and training staff well in advance to help mitigate any loss of productivity or revenue.

Product Alerts and Regulatory Updates

Optum is committed to providing customers with the latest information to code accurately and remain HIPAA compliant. Log on to www.optumcoding.com/productalerts to view, download, and print special reports and announcements regarding official changes to the ICD-9-CM code set or guidelines, as well as regulatory changes affecting coding and reimbursement.

In addition, the purchase of this ICD-9-CM code book automatically entitles the user to receive the complimentary *Inside Track to ICD-10*, a monthly eNewsletter that will help readers stay current on all regulatory changes to ICD-9-CM and transition more smoothly to ICD-10-CM.

September 2013

Dear Optum Customer:

The codes contained in this book are the official code set issued by the U.S. Department of Health and Human Services, effective October 1, 2013, through September 30, 2014.

NOTE: The official coding guidelines included in your *ICD-9-CM for Hospitals, Volumes 1, 2 & 3* were effective October 1, 2011. This set of guidelines was approved by the Cooperating Parties and the Editorial Advisory Board for *Coding Clinic for ICD-9-CM*. The Health Insurance Portability and Accountability Act (HIPAA) requires adherence to these guidelines when ICD-9-CM diagnosis codes are assigned. No official ICD-9-CM addendum to the guidelines has been released since 2011. The guidelines included in this book stand as the official version effective October 1, 2013, through September 30, 2014.

Your new *ICD-9-CM for Hospitals, Volumes 1, 2 & 3*, Professional and Expert editions features:

- **ICD-10-CM Coding Proficiency and Documentation Self-Assessment:** A self-assessment tool for identifying the areas that may require additional coding training or documentation improvement.
- **I-10 Spotlight.** Preview ICD-10-CM codes with the most frequently reported ICD-9-CM codes to learn as you work.
- **Coding Tips.** Coding tips from the official coding guidelines and AHA's *Coding Clinic* are presented throughout the tabular section to provide instant coding guidance.
- **Coding Instruction Alerts.** Instructional notes are presented in red type as a visual alert to critical coding instruction.
- **Hospital Acquired Condition (HAC) Alerts:** HAC diagnoses are identified by our signature color coding.
- **Exclusive color coding and symbols for all major Medicare code edits**
  Note: Not all Medicare edits for the new 2014 ICD-9-CM codes were released in time to be published in this edition. Once these edits are released we will post them on our website. Please visit www.optumcoding.com/productalerts to view these edits.
- **Optum Edge** — Integration of the MCC and CC condition alerts and principal diagnosis exclusion lists that are critical to the MS-DRG classification system.
- **Exclusive** — Present on Admission Indicator Tutorial with case scenarios and a table of official guidelines regarding the use of information documented in the medical record.
- Updated MS-DRG system CC principal diagnosis exclusion list with each MCC and CC condition for fiscal year 2014 official ICD-9-CM codes
- Updated AHA's *Coding Clinic for ICD-9-CM* references
- Clinically oriented illustrations and comprehensive definitions
- Check fourth- and fifth-digit symbols in the index and tabular sections
- Color coding to identify adjunct codes, which are assigned only in addition to a major procedure to provide supplemental information about the primary procedure performed
- HIV major related condition notations

In addition to the features listed above, the *ICD-9-CM Expert for Hospitals, Volumes 1, 2 & 3*, includes:

- Summary of the most recent topics covered in the AHA's *Coding Clinic for ICD-9-CM*
- Email alerts of special reports and regulatory information posted on our website
- Completely updated Dx/MDC/DRG list for the MS-DRG system
- Listing of the common drugs and pharmacology considerations to link treatment with disease
- A complete listing of all major complications and comorbidities (MCC) and complications and comorbidities (CC) that affect MS-DRG assignment
- Valid three-digit code list as a quick reference to speed auditing of claims
- The "10 Steps to Correct Coding" tutorial

We appreciate your choosing Optum to meet your coding needs. If you have any questions or comments concerning your *ICD-9-CM for Hospitals, Volumes 1, 2 & 3*, please do not hesitate to call our customer service department. The toll-free number is 1-800-464-3649, option 1.

Optum has decided to discontinue (see Important Message page) the updateable ICD-9-CM editions.

All current subscriptions will be honored and fullfill as follows:

- Sept 2013 – Copy of the 2014 ICD-9-CM Expert edition spiral including the "Summary of AHA Coding Clinic Topics"
- Feb 2014 through end of subscription – Newsletter updates

If you have any questions or comments concerning your subscription and what this decision means to you, please do not hesitate to call our customer service department at 1.800.464.3649, option 1.

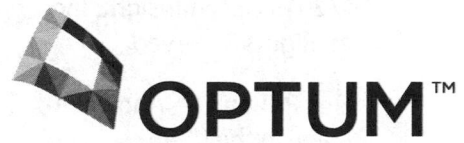

ICD-9-CM

for Hospitals and Payers – Volumes 1, 2, & 3

2014 | Expert

International Classification of Diseases
9th Revision
Clinical Modification
Sixth Edition

Edited by:
Anita C. Hart, RHIA, CCS, CCS-P

Codes Valid October 1, 2013, through September 30, 2014

Publisher's Notice

All codes, indexes, and other material in the ICD-9-CM are compiled from official ICD-9-CM codes and instructions as well as the Medicare regulations and manuals issued or authorized by the Centers for Medicare and Medicaid Services. The code book is designed to provide accurate and authoritative information in regard to the subject covered, and every reasonable effort has been made to ensure the accuracy of the information within these pages. However, the ultimate responsibility for correct coding lies with the provider of services.

Optum, its employees, agents and staff make no representation, warranty or guarantee that this compilation of codes and narratives is error-free or that the use of this code book will prevent differences of opinion or disputes with Medicare or other third-party payers as to the codes that are accepted or the amounts that will be paid to providers for services, and will bear no responsibility or liability for the results or consequences of the use of this code book.

Our Commitment to Accuracy

Optum is committed to producing accurate and reliable materials. To report corrections, please visit www.optumcoding.com/accuracy or email accuracy@optum.com. You can also reach customer service by calling 1.800.464.3649, option 1.

Special Reports and Announcements

Purchase of this publication entitles you to Special Reports and announcements via email. Please call customer service at 800-464-3649 or contact your bookstore to take advantage of this exciting free service that will keep you abreast of important code changes and regulatory developments.

Review, download, and print the Special Reports in .pdf format. Log on to www.optumcoding.com/productalerts

Preface

Since the federal government implemented diagnosis-related groups (DRGs) on October 1, 1983, medical record professionals and others have had to refer to many sources for ICD-9-CM codes and coding and reimbursement principles.

ICD-9-CM for Hospitals, Volumes 1, 2 & 3, has been designed with the health information professional in mind. All three volumes of the most recent official government version of ICD-9-CM have been combined into one book.

Our technical experts have drawn upon their extensive hands-on experience to enhance the government's book with valuable features essential to correct coding and reimbursement. Without these enhancements, health information management departments would spend hours locating the information required to code each record accurately. Because of the thoroughness, accuracy, timeliness and ease of use of *ICD-9-CM for Hospitals,* health information departments nationwide have turned to them for their coding needs.

ICD-9-CM for Hospitals includes many of the enhancements described below in direct response to requests from our subscribers. As you review the content, you'll find the following:

- The complete ICD-9-CM official guidelines for coding and reporting, published by the U.S. Department of Health and Human Services and approved by the cooperating parties (American Hospital Association, American Health Information Management Association, Centers for Medicare and Medicaid Services and National Center for Health Statistics)
- All the official ICD-9-CM codes, indexes, notes, footnotes and symbols
- Color-highlighted illustrations and clearly worded definitions integrated in the tabular, provide important clinical information
- Exclusive color coding, symbols, and footnotes that alert coders to coding and reimbursement issues, including the majority of the Medicare code edits and identification of conditions that significantly affect DRG assignment.
- The complication and comorbidity (CC) exclusion list, integrated beneath the applicable codes makes it easier to determine complications and comorbidities excluded with a particular principal diagnosis
- The American Hospital Association (AHA's) *Coding Clinic for ICD-9-CM* references, integrated beneath the applicable codes to provide easy reference to official coding advice as designated by the four cooperating parties (AHA, AHIMA, CMS, and NCHS)
- Check fourth- and fifth-digit symbols identify codes that require the addition of a fourth or fifth digit for code specificity and validity
- Symbols identify new codes and text revisions and pages are dated to indicate when the changes were made
- Synopsis of the code changes for the current year
- Color coding and symbol legend at the bottom of each page
- Exclusive QuickFlip Color Tabs for quick, easy location of terms and codes in the index and Tabular List

Please review "How to Use *ICD-9-CM for Hospitals (Volumes 1, 2 & 3)*" in this section to learn about the features that will help you assign and report correct codes, ensuring appropriate reimbursement.

Use of Official Sources

The *ICD-9-CM for Hospitals* contains the official U.S. Department of Health and Human Services, Ninth Revision, Sixth Edition ICD-9-CM codes, effective for the current year.

The color-coding, footnotes and symbols, which identify coding and reimbursement issues, are derived from official federal government sources, including the Medicare Code Edits (MCE), Version 30.0.

The American Hospital Association's (AHA) *Coding Clinic for ICD-9-CM* references are used with permission of the AHA.

Technical Editors

Anita C. Hart, RHIA, CCS, CCS-P, *Product Manager, Optum*
Ms. Hart's experience includes 15 years conducting and publishing research in clinical medicine and human genetics for Yale University, Massachusetts General Hospital, and Massachusetts Institute of Technology. Her research conclusions have been published in several peer-reviewed journals. In addition, Ms. Hart has supervised medical records management, health information management, coding and reimbursement, and workers' compensation issues as the office manager for a physical therapy rehabilitation clinic. Ms. Hart is an expert in physician and facility coding, reimbursement systems, and compliance issues. She is also the author of several Optum publications and has served as subject matter advisor on numerous other publications for hospital and physician practices. Ms. Hart is the ICD-9-CM and ICD-10-CM/PCS subject matter expert for Optum, has served as product manager for that product line for 15 years, and has presented at numerous national conferences. Ms. Hart is a member of the American Academy of Professional Coders (AAPC) and is a fully credentialed active member of the American Health Information Management Association (AHIMA). Ms. Hart is a current AHIMA Approved ICD-10-CM/PCS Trainer and leads the training initiatives within Optum Coding Solutions business unit.

In addition to the editors, the following people have contributed to this book:

Stacy Perry, *Manager, Desktop Publishing*
Tracy Betzler, *Senior Desktop Publishing Specialist*
Hope M. Dunn, *Senior Desktop Publishing Specialist*
Katie Russell, *Desktop Publishing Specialist*
Kate Holden, *Editor*

What to Do If You Have Questions

If you have any questions call our customer service department toll-free at 800-464-3649, option 1.

If you have comments on the content of this book, please email them to customerservice@ingenix.com or fax to 801-982-4033.

Additional Copies

Contact the customer service order department toll-free at 800-464-3649, option 1.

Introduction

History and Future of ICD-9-CM

The International Classification of Diseases, Ninth Revision, Clinical Modification (ICD-9-CM) is based on the official version of the World Health Organization's Ninth Revision, International Classification of Diseases (ICD-9). ICD-9 classifies morbidity and mortality information for statistical purposes, and for the indexing of hospital records by disease and operations, for data storage and retrieval.

This modification of ICD-9 supplants the Eighth Revision International Classification of Diseases, Adapted for Use in the United States (ICDA-8) and the Hospital Adaptation of ICDA (H-ICDA).

The concept of extending the International Classification of Diseases for use in hospital indexing was originally developed in response to a need for a more efficient basis for storage and retrieval of diagnostic data. In 1950, the U.S. Public Health Service and the Veterans Administration began independent tests of the International Classification of Diseases for hospital indexing purposes. The following year, the Columbia Presbyterian Medical Center in New York City adopted the International Classification of Diseases, Sixth Revision, with some modifications for use in its medical record department. A few years later, the Commission on Professional and Hospital Activities (CPHA) in Ann Arbor, Mich., adopted the International Classification of Diseases with similar modifications for use in hospitals participating in the Professional Activity Study.

The problem of adapting ICD for indexing hospital records was taken up by the U.S. National Committee on Vital and Health Statistics through its subcommittee on hospital statistics. The subcommittee reviewed the modifications made by the various users of ICD and proposed that uniform changes be made. This was done by a small working party.

In view of the growing interest in the use of the International Classification of Diseases for hospital indexing, a study was undertaken in 1956 by the American Hospital Association and the American Medical Record Association (then the American Association of Medical Record Librarians) of the relative efficiencies of coding systems for diagnostic indexing. This study indicated the International Classification of Diseases provided a suitable and efficient framework for indexing hospital records. The major users of the International Classification of Diseases for hospital indexing purposes then consolidated their experiences, and an adaptation was first published in December 1959. A revision was issued in 1962 and the first "Classification of Operations and Treatments" was included.

In 1966, the international conference for revising the International Classification of Diseases noted the eighth revision of ICD had been constructed with hospital indexing in mind and considered the revised classification suitable, in itself, for hospital use in some countries. However, it was recognized that the basic classification might provide inadequate detail for diagnostic indexing in other countries. A group of consultants was asked to study the eighth revision of ICD (ICD-8) for applicability to various users in the United States. This group recommended that further detail be provided for coding of hospital and morbidity data. The American Hospital Association was requested to develop the needed adaptation proposals. This was done by an advisory committee (the Advisory Committee to the Central Office on ICDA). In 1968 the United States Public Health Service published the product, Eighth Revision International Classification of Diseases, Adapted for Use in the United States. This became commonly known as ICDA-8, and beginning in 1968 it served as the basis for coding diagnostic data for both official morbidity and mortality statistics in the United States.

In 1968, the CPHA published the Hospital Adaptation of ICDA (H-ICDA) based on both the original ICD-8 and ICDA-8. In 1973, CPHA published a revision of H-ICDA, referred to as H-ICDA-2. Hospitals throughout the United States were divided in their use of these classifications until January 1979, when ICD-9-CM was made the single classification intended primarily for use in the United States, replacing these earlier related, but somewhat dissimilar, classifications.

Physicians have been required by law to submit diagnosis codes for Medicare reimbursement since the passage of the Medicare Catastrophic Coverage Act of 1988. This act requires physician offices to include the appropriate diagnosis codes when billing for services provided to Medicare beneficiaries on or after April 1, 1989. The Centers for Medicare and Medicaid Services (formerly known as Health Care Financing Administration) designated ICD-9-CM as the coding system physicians must use.

The ICD-10-CM classification system was developed by the National Center for Health Statistics (NCHS) as a clinical modification to the ICD-10 system developed by the World Health Organization (WHO), primarily as a unique system for use in the United States for morbidity and mortality reporting. Although ICD-10-CM has not yet been implemented for use in the United States, ICD-10 has been adopted for use in the coding and classification of mortality data from death certificates. ICD-10 replaced ICD-9 for this purpose as of January 1, 1999. The Department of Health and Human Services (HHS) published the final rule regarding the adoption of both ICD-10-CM and ICD-10-PCS in the January 16, 2009 *Federal Register* (45 CFR part 162[CMS—0013—F]). On April 17, 2012, the Department of Health and Human Services released a notice postponing the date by which certain health care entities must comply with diagnosis and procedure codes from the International Classification of Diseases, 10th edition (ICD-10). The compliance date for implementing ICD-10-CM and ICD-10-PCS as a replacement for ICD-9-CM is October 1, 2014.

ICD-9-CM Background

In February 1977, a steering committee was convened by the National Center for Health Statistics to provide advice and counsel in developing a clinical modification of ICD-9. The organizations represented on the steering committee included the following:

- American Association of Health Data Systems
- American Hospital Association
- American Medical Record Association
- Association for Health Records
- Council on Clinical Classifications
- Centers for Medicare and Medicaid Services, Department of Health and Human Services
- WHO Center for Classification of Diseases for North America, sponsored by the National Center for Health Statistics, Department of Health and Human Services

The Council on Clinical Classifications was sponsored by the following:

- American Academy of Pediatrics
- American College of Obstetricians and Gynecologists
- American College of Physicians
- American College of Surgeons
- American Psychiatric Association
- Commission on Professional and Hospital Activities

The steering committee met periodically in 1977. Clinical guidance and technical input were provided by task forces on classification from the Council on Clinical Classification's sponsoring organizations.

ICD-9-CM is a clinical modification of the World Health Organization's ICD-9. The term "clinical" is used to emphasize the modification's intent: to serve as a useful tool to classify morbidity data for indexing medical records, medical care review, and ambulatory and other medical care programs, as well as for basic health statistics. To describe the clinical picture of the patient, the codes must be more precise than those needed only for statistical groupings and trend analysis.

Characteristics of ICD-9-CM

ICD-9-CM far exceeds its predecessors in the number of codes provided. The disease classification has been expanded to include health-related conditions and to provide greater specificity at the fifth-digit level of detail. These fifth digits are not optional; they are intended for use in recording the information substantiated in the clinical record.

Volume I (Tabular List) of ICD-9-CM contains four appendixes:

Appendix A:	Morphology of Neoplasms
Appendix B:	Deleted Effective October 1, 2004
Appendix C:	Classification of Drugs by American Hospital Formulary Service List Number and Their ICD-9-CM Equivalents
Appendix D:	Classification of Industrial Accidents According to Agency
Appendix E:	List of Three-Digit Categories

These appendixes are included as a reference to provide further information about the patient's clinical picture, to further define a diagnostic statement, to aid in classifying new drugs or to reference three-digit categories.

Volume 2 (Alphabetic Index) of ICD-9-CM contains many diagnostic terms that do not appear in Volume I since the index includes most diagnostic terms currently in use.

Volume 3 (Procedure Index and Procedure Tabular) of ICD-9-CM contains codes for operations and procedures. The format for the tabular is the same as Volume 1 disease tabular, except the codes consist of two digits with one or two digits following the decimal point. Conventions in the index follow Volume 2 conventions except some subterms appear immediately below the main term rather than following alphabetizing rules.

The Disease Classification

ICD-9-CM is totally compatible with its parent system, ICD-9, thus meeting the need for comparability of morbidity and mortality statistics at the international level. A few fourth-digit codes were created in existing three-digit rubrics only when the necessary detail could not be accommodated by the use of a fifth-digit subclassification. To ensure that each rubric of ICD-9-CM collapses back to its ICD-9 counterpart the following specifications governed the ICD-9-CM disease classification:

Specifications for the Tabular List:

1. Three-digit rubrics and their contents are unchanged from ICD-9.

2. The sequence of three-digit rubrics is unchanged from ICD-9.

3. Three-digit rubrics are not added to the main body of the classification.

4. Unsubdivided three-digit rubrics are subdivided where necessary to

    • add clinical detail

    • isolate terms for clinical accuracy.

5. The modification in ICD-9-CM is accomplished by adding a fifth digit to existing ICD-9 rubrics, except as noted under #7.

6. The optional dual classification in ICD-9 is modified.

    • Duplicate rubrics are deleted:

        – four-digit manifestation categories duplicating etiology entries

        – manifestation inclusion terms duplicating etiology entries

    • Manifestations of disease are identified, to the extent possible, by creating five-digit codes in the etiology rubrics.

    • When the manifestation of a disease cannot be included in the etiology rubrics, provision for its identification is made by retaining the ICD-9 rubrics used for classifying manifestations of disease.

7. The format of ICD-9-CM is revised from that used in ICD-9.

    • American spelling of medical terms is used.

    • Inclusion terms are indented beneath the titles of codes.

    • Codes not to be used for primary tabulation of disease are printed in italics with the notation, "code first underlying disease."

Specifications for the Alphabetic Index:

1. The format of the Alphabetic Index follows that of ICD-9.

2. When two codes are required to indicate etiology and manifestation, the manifestation code appears in brackets (e.g., diabetic cataract 250.5 [366.41]).

The ICD-9-CM Coordination and Maintenance Committee

The ICD-9-CM Coordination and Maintenance Committee, a federal committee, was created as a forum for proposals to update International Classification of Diseases, Ninth Revision, Clinical Modification, Sixth Edition (ICD-9-CM). A representative from the National Center for Health Statistics (NCHS) and one from the Centers for Medicare and Medicaid Services (CMS) co-chair the ICD-9-CM Coordination and Maintenance Committee meetings. Responsibility for maintaining ICD-9-CM is divided between the two agencies, with NCHS classifying diagnoses (volumes 1 and 2) and CMS classifying procedures (volume 3).

Proposals for changes to the ICD-9-CM classification system are submitted and discussed in open forum meetings held in March and September of each year at the headquarters of CMS in Baltimore. Comments received during or after the meetings are then reviewed and evaluated. All final decisions are made by the director of NCHS and the administrator of CMS. The complete official document of changes to the classification system is released as the Addenda for the International Classification of Disease, Ninth Revision, Clinical Modification, Sixth Edition, Volume 1, 2 & 3.

The *ICD-9-CM for Hospitals, Volume 1, 2 & 3* is based on the official version of the International Classification of Diseases, Ninth Revision, Clinical Modification, Sixth Edition, issued by the U.S. Department of Health and Human Services. Annual code changes are implemented by the government and are effective October 1 and valid through September 30 of the following year. If a convincing case is made that requires a new code to capture new technology or an emerging disease, this new code may be implemented on April 1 of the following year.

How to Use the ICD-9-CM for Hospitals (Volumes 1, 2 & 3)

ICD-9-CM for Hospitals is based on the official version of the International Classification of Diseases, Ninth Revision, Clinical Modification, Sixth Edition, issued by the U.S. Department of Health and Human Services. Annual code changes are implemented by the government and are effective Oct. 1 and valid through Sept. 30 of the following year.

The code book is totally compatible with its parent system, ICD-9, thus meeting the need for comparability of morbidity and mortality statistics at the international level.

This book is consistent with the content of the government's version of ICD-9-CM. However, to accommodate the coder's approach to coding, the Alphabetic Index has been placed before the Tabular List in both the disease and procedure classifications. This allows the user to locate the correct codes in a logical, natural manner by locating the term in the index, then confirming the accuracy of the code in the Tabular List.

Steps to Correct Coding

1. Look up the main term in the Alphabetic Index and scan the subterm entries as appropriate. Follow any cross-references such as *"see"* and *"see also."* Do not code from the Alphabetic Index without verifying the accuracy of the code in the Tabular List.

2. Locate the code in the numerically arranged Tabular List.

3. Observe the punctuation, footnotes, cross-references, color-coded prompts and other conventions described in the 'Conventions' section.

4. To determine the appropriateness of the code selection, read all instructional material:

   • "includes" and *"excludes"* notes

   • *"see," "see also"* and *"see category"* cross-references

   • "use additional code" and *"code first underlying disease"* instructions

   • "code also" and *"omit code"* notes

   • fourth- and fifth-digit requirements

   • CC exclusions

5. Consult definitions, relevant illustrations, CC exclusions, color coding and reimbursement prompts, the check fourth- and fifth-digit, age and sex symbols. Refer to the color/symbol legend at the bottom of each page for symbols. Refer to the list of footnotes that is included in the "Additional Conventions" section of this book for a full explanation of a footnote associated with a code.

6. Consult the official ICD-9-CM guidelines for coding and reporting, and refer to the AHA's *Coding Clinic for ICD-9-CM* for coding guidelines governing the use of specific codes.

7. Confirm and transcribe the correct code.

Organization

Introduction
The introductory material in this book includes the history and future of ICD-9-CM as well as an overview of the classification system.

Official ICD-9-CM Conventions
This section provides a full explanation of all the official footnotes, symbols, instructional notes, and conventions found in the official government version.

Additional Conventions
Exclusive color-coding, symbols, and notations have been included in the *ICD-9-CM for Hospitals, Volumes 1, 2 & 3* to alert coders to important coding and reimbursement issues. This section provides a full explanation of the additional conventions used throughout this book.

ICD-10-CM Coding Proficiency and Documentation Self-Assessment
Use this self-assessment to identify the areas that may require additional coding training or documentation improvement before ICD-10-CM is implemented on October 1, 2014.

Summary of AHA's *Coding Clinic for ICD-9-CM* Topics
This is a brief summary of the official advice concerning coding topics covered in the latest issues of AHA's *Coding Clinic for ICD-9-CM* and is found **only** in the *ICD-9-CM Expert for Hospitals*.

Coding Guidelines
Included in this book are the official ICD-9-CM coding guidelines as approved by the four cooperating parties of the ICD-9-CM Coordination and Maintenance Committee. Failure to comply with the official coding guidelines may result in denied or delayed claims.

Disease Classification: Alphabetic Index to Diseases
The Alphabetic Index to Diseases is separated by tabs labeled with the letters of the alphabet, contains diagnostic terms for illnesses, injuries and reasons for encounters with health care professionals. The Table of Drugs and Chemicals is easily located with the tab in this section.

The warning statement at the bottom of every page of the index, ▽ Subterms under main terms may continue to next column or page, is a reminder to always check for additional subterms before making final selection.

Disease Classification: Tabular List of Diseases
The Tabular List of Diseases arranges the ICD-9-CM codes and descriptors numerically. QuickFlip color tabs divide this section into chapters, identified by the code range on the tab.

The Tabular List includes two supplementary classifications:

• V Codes—Supplementary Classification of Factors Influencing Health Status and Contact with Health Services (V01–V91)

• E Codes—Supplementary Classification of External Causes of Injury and Poisoning (E000–E999)

ICD-9-CM includes four official appendixes.

• Appendix A   Morphology of Neoplasms
• Appendix B: Deleted Effective October 1, 2004
• Appendix C   Classification of Drugs by AHFS List
• Appendix D   Classification of Industrial Accidents According to Agency
• Appendix E   List of Three-digit Categories

These appendixes are included as a reference to provide further information about the patient's circumstances, help further define a diagnostic statement, maintain a tumor registry and aid in classifying new drugs.

Procedure Classification: Alphabetic Index to Procedures
The Alphabetic Index to Procedures lists common surgical and procedural terminology.

The warning statement at the bottom of every page of the index, ▽ Subterms under main terms may continue to next column or page, is a reminder to always check for additional subterms before making a final selection.

Procedure Classification: Tabular List of Procedures
The Tabular List of Procedures numerically arranges the procedure codes and their descriptors.

Resources
Listed below are the exclusive resources found **ONLY** in the *ICD-9-CM Expert for Hospitals, Volumes 1, 2 & 3* books.

Dx/MDC/DRG List

Provides the complete list of principal diagnosis codes and the MDC and medical MS-DRG to which they group, with the exception of a combination of principal and secondary diagnosis affecting DRG assignment.

MCC Condition List

A complete list of all codes considered MCC (Major Complications and Comorbidities) that will affect DRG assignment. This is an essential auditing tool for assigning the most appropriate DRG.

CC Condition List

A complete list of all codes considered CC (Complications and Comorbidities) that will affect DRG assignment. This an essential auditing tool for assigning the most appropriate DRG.

Pharmacological Listings

The most common generic and brand names of drugs are linked with the disease processes to assist in the identification of CC, thereby improving DRG assignment practices.

Valid Three-digit Code Table

ICD-9-CM is composed of codes with either 3, 4, or 5 digits. A code is invalid if it has not been coded to the full number of digits required for that code. There are a certain number codes that are valid for reporting as three digit codes. A list of the valid three-digit code is included as a convenient reference when auditing claims.

Present on Admission (POA) Indicator Tutorial

This resource presents an in-depth explanation of guidelines for assigning the present on admission (POA) indicators with case scenarios and exemptions. A table of official guidelines is included for quick reference regarding the use of information documented in the medical record.

10 Steps to Correct Coding

This is a valuable resource that takes the coder step by step through the coding process with detailed explanations accompanied by coding examples that demonstrate the practical application of ICD-9-CM conventions and coding guidelines in 10 steps.

ICD-9-CM Official Conventions

ICD-9-CM Footnotes, Symbols, Instructional Notes and Conventions

This *ICD-9-CM for Hospitals* preserves all the footnotes, symbols, instructional notes and conventions found in the government's official version. Accurate coding depends upon understanding the meaning of these elements.

The following appear in the disease Tabular List, unless otherwise noted.

Official Government Symbols

§   The section mark preceding a code denotes a footnote on the page. This symbol is used in the Tabular List of Diseases and in the Tabular List of Procedures.

ICD-9-CM Conventions Used in the Tabular List

In addition to the symbols and footnotes above, the ICD-9-CM disease tabular has certain abbreviations, punctuation, symbols and other conventions. Our *ICD-9-CM for Hospitals* preserves these conventions. Proper use of the conventions will lead to efficient and accurate coding.

Abbreviations

NEC   Not elsewhere classifiable
This abbreviation is used when the ICD-9-CM system does not provide a code specific for the patient's condition.

NOS   Not otherwise specified
This abbreviation is the equivalent of "unspecified" and is used only when the coder lacks the information necessary to code to a more specific four-digit subcategory.

[ ]   Brackets enclose synonyms, alternative terminology or explanatory phrases:

> **482.2** **Pneumonia due to Hemophilus influenzae [H. influenzae]**

Brackets that appear beneath a code indicate the fifth digits that are considered valid fifth digits for the code. This convention is applied for those instances in ICD-9-CM where not all common fifth digits are considered valid for each subcategory within a category.

> **715.0** **Osteoarthrosis, generalized**
> [0,4,9]

Generalized arthrosis can only be assigned in cases for which the degenerative joint disease involves multiple joints. Therefore, this code is considered for arthrosis in the sites described as unspecified, hand (which consists of multiple joints), or multiple sites. Therefore, only fifth digits 0, 4, and 9 are valid with subcategory 715.0.

[]   Slanted brackets that appear in the Alphabetic Indexes indicate mandatory multiple coding. Both codes must be assigned to fully describe the condition and are sequenced in the order listed.

> **Tachycardia**
>   ventricular (paroxysmal)
>   psychogenic 316 *[427.1]*

Psychogenic paroxysmal tachycardia is reported using both 316, Psychogenic factors associated with diseases classified elsewhere, and 427.1, Paroxysmal ventricular tachycardia.

> **Diversion**
>   biliopancreatic (BPD) 43.7 *[45.51] [45.91]*

Code assignment of biliopancreatic diversion is reported using all three codes 43.7, Partial gastrectomy with anastomosis to jejunum, 45.51, Isolation of segment of small intestine, and 45.91, Small-to-small intestinal anastomosis.

( )   Parentheses enclose supplementary words, called nonessential modifiers, that may be present in the narrative description of a disease without affecting the code assignment:

> **198.4** **Other parts of nervous system**
>   Meninges (cerebral) (spinal)

:   Colons are used in the Tabular List after an incomplete term that needs one or more of the modifiers that follow in order to make it assignable to a given category:

> **021.1** **Enteric tularemia**
>   Tularemia:
>   cryptogenic
>   intestinal
>   typhoidal

}   Braces enclose a series of terms, each of which is modified by the statement appearing to the right of the brace:

> **560.2** **Volvulus**
>   Knotting
>   Strangulation   } of intestine, bowel, or
>   Torsion   colon
>   Twist

Other Conventions

Boldface Boldface type is used for all codes and titles in the Tabular List.

Italicized Italicized type is used for all exclusion notes and to identify codes that should not be used for describing the principal or first-listed diagnosis.

General Notes Used in the Tabular

These notes appear only in the Tabular List of Diseases:

Includes: An includes note further defines or clarifies the content of the chapter, subchapter, category, subcategory or subclassification. The includes note in the example below applies only to category 461.

Excludes: Terms following the word "Excludes" are not classified to the chapter, subchapter, category, subcategory or specific subclassification code under which it is found. The note also may provide the location of the excluded diagnosis. Excludes notes are italicized.

> **461 Acute sinusitis**
>   `INCLUDES` abscess
>   empyema   } acute, of sinus
>   infection   (accessory)
>   inflammation   (nasal)
>   suppuration
>   `EXCLUDES` *chronic or unspecified sinusitis (473.0-473.9)*

Instructional Notes

The following official instructional notes are critical to correct coding practices. The instructional notes appear in red type in the Tabular List.

Use additional code:
This instruction signals the coder that an additional code should be used if the information is available to provide a more complete picture of that diagnosis.

For emphasis this instructional note appears in red type in the tabular section.

362.13 Changes in vascular appearance
Vascular sheathing of retina
Use additional code for any associated atherosclerosis (440.8)

There are coding circumstances outside of the etiology/ manifestation convention when multiple coding for a single condition is required. The "Use additional code" note will be found under the associated condition code in the tabular. In the index, the multiple coding requirement is indicated by the use of the slanted bracket. The two codes are to be sequenced as listed in the index. For example, retinal arteriosclerosis must be coded using two codes sequenced as listed in the index.

Arteriosclerosis, arteriosclerotic
retinal (vascular) 440.8 *[362.13]*

Code first underlying disease:

The *"Code first underlying disease"* instructional note found under certain codes is a sequencing rule. Most often this sequencing rule applies to the etiology/manifestation convention and is found under the manifestation code. The manifestation code may never be used alone or as a principal or first-listed diagnosis (i.e., sequenced first). The instructional note, the code and its descriptor appear in italics in the Tabular List.

590.81 *Pyelitis or pyelonephritis in diseases classified elsewhere*
Code first underlying disease as:
tuberculosis (016.0)

Not all codes with a "Code first underlying disease" instructional note are part of the etiology/manifestation convention. The "Code first" note will appear, but the title of the code and the instructional note are not in italics. These codes may be reported alone or as the secondary diagnosis. For example, disseminated chorioretinitis may be reported as a principal diagnosis. However, if the underlying condition that caused disseminated chorioretinitis is known, such as tuberculous disseminated chorioretinitis, two codes are required and sequenced as listed in the index.

363.13 Disseminated choroiditis and chorioretinitis, generalized
Code first underlying disease as:
tuberculosis (017.3)

For emphasis this instructional note appears in red type in the tabular section.

Code, if applicable, any causal condition first:

A code with this note indicates that this code may be assigned as a principal diagnosis when the causal condition is unknown or not applicable. If a causal condition is known, then the code for that condition should be sequenced as the principal or first-listed diagnosis.

590.0 Chronic pyelonephritis
Chronic pyelitis
Chronic pyonephrosis
Code, if applicable, any causal condition first

For emphasis this instructional note appears in red type in the tabular section.

Instructional Notes Used in the Index

Omit code:

"Omit code" is used to instruct the coder that no code is to be assigned. When this instruction is found in the Alphabetic Index to Diseases the medical term should not be coded as a diagnosis.

Metaplasia
cervix — *omit code*

When used in Volume 3, *omit code* is meant to indicate procedures that do not merit separate code assignments, such as minor procedures preformed in conjunction with more extensive procedures or procedures that represent an operative approach.

Arthrotomy 80.10
as operative approach — *omit code*

See Condition:

The *"see condition"* note found in the Alphabetic Index to Disease instructs the coder to refer to a main term for the condition. This note will follow index terms that are nouns for anatomical sites or adjectival forms of disease term. In the example below, the index terms "Cervix" and "Diffuse" are followed by the — *see* condition. Coders should search the index using a condition term such as atrophy or prolapse.

Cervix — *see* condition
Diffuse — *see* condition

Morphology Codes

For each neoplastic disease listed in the index, a morphology code is provided that identifies histological type and behavior.

Example:

Myelolipoma (M8870/0) — *see* Neoplasm, by site, benign

The histology is identified by the first four digits and the behavior is identified by the digit following the slash. Appendix A of Volume 1 contains a listing of morphology codes. This appendix is helpful when the pathology report identifies the neoplasm by using an M code. The coder may refer to Appendix A to determine the nomenclature of the neoplasm that will be the main term to search in the Index. The behavior classification is as follows:

- 0 Benign
- 1 Uncertain whether benign or malignant
  Borderline malignancy
- 2 Carcinoma in situ
  Intraepithelial
  Noninfiltrating
  Noninvasive
- 3 Malignant, primary site
- 6 Malignant, metastatic site
  Secondary site
- 9 Malignant, uncertain whether primary or metastatic site

Additional Conventions

New and Revised Text Symbols

● A bullet at a code or line of text indicates that that the entry is new.

▲ A triangle in the Tabular List indicates that the code title is revised. In the Alphabetic Index the triangle indicates that a code has changed.

►◄ These symbols appear at the beginning and at the end of a section of new or revised text.

When these symbols appear on a page there will be a date on the lower outside corner of the page indicating the date of the change (e.g., October 2013).

Additional Digits Required

√3ʳ This symbol indicates that the code requires a third digit.

√4ᵗ This symbol indicates that the code requires a fourth digit.

√5ᵗ This symbol indicates that a code requires a fifth digit.

☑ This symbol found only in the Alphabetic Index sections and the Table of Drugs and Chemicals indicates that an additional digit is required. Referring to the tabular section is essential to locate the appropriate additional digit.

Definitions

DEF: This symbol indicates a definition of disease or procedure term. The definition will appear in blue type in the Disease and Procedure Tabular Lists.

AHA's *Coding Clinic for ICD-9-CM* References

The four cooperating parties have designated the AHA's *Coding Clinic for ICD-9-CM* as the official publication for coding guidelines. The references are identified by the notation **AHA:** followed by the issue, year and page number.

In the example below, AHA's *Coding Clinic for ICD-9-CM*, third quarter 1991, page 15, contains a discussion on code assignment for vitreous hemorrhage:

> **379.23 Vitreous hemorrhage**
> **AHA:** 3Q, '91, 15

The table below explains the abbreviations in the Coding Clinic references:

J-F	January/February
M-A	March/April
M-J	May/June
J-A	July/August
S-O	September/October
N-D	November/December
1Q	First quarter
2Q	Second quarter
3Q	Third quarter
4Q	Fourth quarter

AHA's *Coding Clinic for ICD-9-CM* references appear in blue type in the Tabular List.

Medicare Code Edits

Note: The Medicare Code Edit updates dated October 2013 are based upon the proposed rule for the inpatient prospective payment system (IPPS) published in the *Federal Register* on May 10, 2013. Should any changes be made in these designations in the final rule that is expected to be published in August, Optum will post the changes on the website http://www.optumcoding.com/Product/Announcements/.

Fiscal intermediaries use Medicare code edits (MCE) to check the coding accuracy on claims. The Medicare code edits are listed below:

- Invalid diagnosis or procedure code
- E-code as principal diagnosis
- Duplicate of principal diagnosis (PDx) (as applied to a secondary diagnosis)
- *Age conflict
- *Sex conflict
- *Manifestation code as principal diagnosis
- *Questionable admission
- *Unacceptable principal diagnosis
- *Noncovered procedure
- *Bilateral procedure
- Invalid age
- Invalid sex
- Invalid discharge status
- *Limited coverage procedure
- *Wrong surgery
- Length of stay less than four (4) days for mechanical ventilation

Starred edits are identified by colors, symbols or footnotes as described below.

Age and Sex Edit Symbols

The age edits below address MCE edit 4 and are used to detect inconsistencies between the patient's age and diagnosis. The following edit symbols appear in the Tabular List of Diseases to the right of the code description.

Newborn Age: 0 ⓝ
These diagnoses are intended for newborns and neonates and the patient's age must be 0 years.

Pediatric Age: 0-17 ⓟ
These diagnoses are intended for children and the patient's age must between 0 and 17 years.

Maternity Age: 12-55 ⓜ
These diagnoses are intended for the patients between the age of 12 and 55 years.

Adult Age: 15-124 ⓐ
These diagnoses are intended for the patients between the age of 15 and 124 years.

The sex symbols below address MCE edit 5 and are used to detect inconsistencies between the patient's sex and diagnosis or procedure. These symbols appear in the Tabular Lists to the right of the code description:

♂ **Male diagnosis or procedure only**
This symbol appears to the right of the code description. This reference appears in the disease and procedure Tabular List.

♀ **Female diagnosis or procedure only**
This symbol appears to the right of the code description. This reference appears in the disease and procedure Tabular List.

Color Coding

For a quick reference to the color codes and their meaning, refer to the color/symbol legend located at the bottom of each page.

To alert the coder to important reimbursement issues affected by the code assignment, color bars have been added. The colors represent Medicare code edits as well as other reimbursement issues.

Color coding appears in both Tabular Lists. Some codes carry more than one color. Please note that the same color may appear in the disease and procedure Tabular Lists, but with different meanings.

Disease Tabular List

Manifestation Code

These codes will appear in italic type as well as with a blue color bar over the code title. A manifestation code is not allowed to be reported as a principal or first-listed diagnosis because each describes a manifestation of some other underlying disease, not the disease process itself. In the Alphabetic Index these codes are listed as the secondary code in slanted brackets with the code for the underlying disease listed first.

Unacceptable PDx

These codes will appear with a gray color bar over the code title. These codes do not describe a current illness or injury, but a circumstance which influences a patient's health status. These are considered an unacceptable principal diagnosis for inpatient admission.

Questionable Admission

These codes will also appear with a gray color bar over the code title. These codes identify a condition that usually is insufficient justification for hospital admission. Since these codes are considered an unacceptable principal diagnoses for inpatient admission, they are color coded in the same manner as the "Unacceptable PDx" codes.

Nonspecific PDx

Effective October 1, 2007 the Medicare code edit for Non-Specific Diagnoses was deactivated. Therefore, these codes will no longer be identified by a yellow color bar over the code title.

Hospital Acquired Condition (HAC)

These codes will appear with a yellow color bar over the code title. These codes identify conditions that are high cost or high volume or both, a complication or comorbidity (CC) or major complication or comorbidity (MCC) that as a secondary diagnosis would result in assignment of a case to a higher-paying MS-DRG, and reasonably preventable through the application of evidence-based guidelines. If the condition is not present on admission, the case would not group to the higher-paying MS-DRG based solely upon the reporting of the HAC.

Procedure Tabular List

Nonspecific OR Procedure

Effective October 1, 2007 the Medicare code edit for Non-Specific OR was deactivated. Therefore, these codes will no longer be identified by a yellow color bar over the code title.

Valid OR

A procedure that triggers a change in DRG assignment and is designated by a gray color bar over the code title.

Non-OR Procedure

A non-operating room procedure that affects DRG assignment and is designated by a blue color bar over the code title.

Adjunct Codes

These codes are not to be reported alone and are indicated by the red color bar over the code title. Adjunct codes are assigned only in addition to a principal procedure. Their purpose is to provide supplemental information about the principal procedure performed. Adjunct codes are not procedure codes, but serve to provide additional detail about the principal procedure.

> *Example:*
>
> PTCA balloon inflation of two vessels, with insertion of one intravascular coronary stent.
>
> Code assignment:
>
> **00.66 Percutaneous transluminal coronary angioplasty [PTCA] or coronary atherectomy**
>
> **00.41 Procedure on two vessels**
>
> **00.45 Insertion of one vascular stent**
>
> In the above example, codes 00.41 and 00.45 are adjunct codes that provide specific detail about the PTCA procedure performed.

Footnotes

All footnotes are identified by a numerical superscript that appears to the upper left of the code:

[1] 427.41 Ventricular fibrillation

The footnote 1 indicates "MCC = Only if patient is discharged alive." This means that ventricular fibrillation is considered a major complication or comorbidity that may affect DRG assignment only if the patient is discharged alive. Otherwise ventricular fibrillation is assigned as a non CC condition.

The following list identifies the meaning of each footnote number and the classification in which the footnote appears:

Disease Tabular

1   Major complication or comorbidity (MCC) that may affect DRG assignment only if the patient is discharged alive.

2   These V codes may be used as principal diagnosis on Medicare patients.

3   This V code, with the fourth digit of 1 or 2, is unacceptable as a principal diagnosis.

4   These codes, with the fourth digit of 0, may be used as a principal diagnosis for Medicare patients.

5   Rehabilitation codes acceptable as a principal diagnosis when accompanied by a secondary diagnosis reflecting the condition treated.

6   These V codes are acceptable as principal diagnosis when accompanied by a diagnosis of personal history of malignancy. These codes group to MS-DRG 949-950.

7   Diagnosis code with fifth digit of 0 is considered a "Questionable Admission" diagnosis when used as a principal diagnosis.

8   These codes are considered CC/MCC conditions that affect DRG assignment, except when reported in combination with diagnosis code 996.64 and the condition is not present on admission.

9   This condition is designated as a hospital acquired condition (HAC) that when reported as not present upon admission and when in combination with a procedure code from 36.10-36.19 will not solely group the case to a higher-paying MS-DRG.

10 The codes within the category or subcategory qualify as hospital acquired conditions when not present upon admission and only for the valid CC and MCC codes within that range.

11 This condition is designated as a hospital acquired condition (HAC) when reported as a secondary condition with procedure codes 00.85–00.87, or 81.51, 81.52, or 81.54 and the condition is not present on admission.

12 This condition is designated as a hospital acquired condition (HAC) when reported as a secondary condition with procedure codes 81.01–81.08, 81.23–81.24, 81.31–81.38, 81.83, or 81.85 and the condition is not present on admission.

13 This condition is designated as a hospital acquired condition (HAC) when reported as a secondary condition with procedure codes 81.01–81.08, 81.23–81.24, 81.31–81.38, 81.83, 81.85, or procedure code 44.38, 44.39, or 44.95 with principal diagnosis code 278.01 and the condition is not present on admission.

14 This condition is designated as a hospital acquired condition (HAC) when reported with principal diagnosis 278.01 and with procedure code 44.38, 44.39, or 44.95 and the condition is not present on admission.

15 This condition is designated as a hospital acquired condition (HAC) when reported with procedure(s) 00.50-00.54, 37.74-37.77, 37.79, 37.80-37.89, 37.94, 37.96, or 37.98 and the condition is not present on admission.

16 This condition is designated as a hospital acquired condition (HAC) when reported with procedure 38.93 and the condition is not present on admission.

*   Wrong Surgery edit applies to the E code which when reported will trigger the Wrong Surgery edit and the claim will be denied and returned to the provider.

Procedure Tabular

1   Valid OR procedure code if accompanied by one of the following codes: 37.80, 37.81, 37.82, 37.85, 37.86, 37.87.

2   Valid OR procedure code if accompanied by one of the following codes: 37.80, 37.83.

3   Valid OR procedure code if accompanied by one of the following codes: 37.80, 37.85, 37.86, 37.87.

4   Valid OR procedure code if accompanied by any one of the following codes: 37.80, 37.81, 37.82, 37.83, 37.85, 37.86, 37.87.

5   Valid OR procedure code if accompanied by any one of the following codes: 37.70, 37.71, 37.73, 37.74.

6   Valid OR procedure code if accompanied by one of the following codes: 37.72, 37.74.

7   Non-covered except when reported with procedure code 00.65, Percutaneous insertion of intracranial vascular stent(s).

8   Non-covered procedure only when the following diagnoses are present as either a principal or secondary diagnosis: 204.00, 205.00, 205.10, 205.11, 206.00, 207.00, 208.00.

9   Non-covered procedure only when the following diagnoses are present as either a principal or secondary diagnosis: 203.00, 203.01.

10 Non-covered procedure unless reported with code 55.69 or a diagnosis code from 250.x1 or 250.x3 or 251.3.

11 Non-covered except when the patient is 60 years old or less.

12 Limited coverage for the procedure is provided only when reported in combination with diagnosis code V70.7. Medicare limits the coverage to a portion of the costs and only when certain criteria are met such as participation in a clinical study.

13 When the code representing mechanical ventilation for 96 or more consecutive hours (96.72) is assigned, the length of stay must be equal to or greater than four (4) days.

Other Notations

Alphabetic Indexes

▽ **Subterms under main terms may continue to next column or page.** This warning statement is a reminder to always check for additional subterms and information that may continue onto the next page or column before making a final selection.

Disease Tabular

TIPS:

This symbol precedes official coding advice found in the official coding guidelines and AHA's *Coding Clinic for ICD-9-CM*. Coding tips appear in blue type in the Tabular List.

I-10

In preparation for the transition to coding using the ICD-10-CM classification system, examples of ICD-10-CM codes have been provided for selected ICD-9-CM diagnosis codes. This symbol indicates that the code provided is an ICD-10-CM code to which the selected ICD-9-CM code is mapped.

Note: Coding professionals should keep in mind the following points when referring to the ICD-10-CM codes provided:

- ICD-10-CM codes are not currently valid for reporting purposes.

- The ICD-10-CM code may represent only one possible coding option. Since mappings between ICD-9-CM and ICD-10-CM are not always straightforward one-to-one correspondences due to the differences in terminology and clinical concepts, the mapping may result in a one-to-many code option. Not all code options for a particular ICD-9-CM code are provided. For cases in which many code alternatives are possible in ICD-10-CM, only one example is provided.

- The ICD-10-CM code examples are provided only for the most frequently reported ICD-9-CM codes in each chapter.

- The ICD-10-CM codes are examples only and are provided to ease the transition to the new classification system.

CC **CC Condition**

This symbol designates a complication or comorbidity diagnosis that may affect DRG assignment. A complication or comorbidity diagnosis, CC condition, is defined as a significant acute disease, a significant acute manifestation of a chronic disease, an advanced or end stage chronic disease, or a chronic disease associated with systemic physiological decompensation and debility that have consistently greater impact on hospital resources.

A CC listed with a digit or range of digits indicates that only the fifth-digit assignments stated for that code are to be considered CC conditions. For example, code 642.1 has a CC 3-4 which means that only codes 642.13 and 642.14 are considered CC conditions. Codes 642.11 and 642.12 are considered major complications or comorbidity (MCC) conditions. Code 642.10 is not designated as CC or MCC.

MCC **MCC Condition**

This symbol designates a complication or comorbidity diagnosis that meets the criteria established for the revised CC list and was an AP-DRG major CC and was an APR-DRG default severity level 3 (major) or level 4 (extensive) with the exception of the newborn, maternity, and congenital anomalies which are APR-DRG default severity level 3 (major) or level 4 (extensive) only.

An MCC listed with a digit or range of digits indicates that only the fifth-digit assignments stated for that code are to be considered MCC conditions. For example; code 642.1 has a CC 3-4 which means that only codes 642.13 and 642.14 are considered CC conditions. Codes 642.11 and 642.12 are considered major complications or comorbidity (MCC) conditions and code 642.1 also has an MCC 1-2 designation. Code 642.10 is not designated as CC or MCC.

CC Exclusion List

An exclusive feature of *ICD-9-CM for Hospitals* is the integration of the government's CC exclusion list with each affected code.

The CC exclusion list indicates secondary diagnosis codes that are excluded as CC or MCC conditions with certain principal diagnoses. This exclusion occurs because the cited conditions are inherent to the disease process of the principal diagnosis, conditions that could not coexist, nonspecific codes for the principal diagnosis, or conditions affecting proximal anatomical sites.

Listed below each code that is considered a complication or comorbidity (CC) or a major complication or comorbidity (MCC) are the codes or code ranges representing principal diagnoses for which the CC or MCC will not be recognized as such for DRG assignment.

In the example below, code 254.1 is considered a CC condition. However, the CC exclusion (CC Excl:) notation indicates that if a code from the listed code ranges is assigned as the principal diagnosis, the secondary diagnosis of 254.1 will not be recognized as a CC condition in DRG assignment.

> **254.1   Abscess of thymus**   **CC**
> **CC Excl:** 254.0-254.9, 259.50-259.9

Please note that the same notation, CC Exclusion (**CC Excl:**), is used for both the MCC and CC conditions. Both MCC and CC are considered complication and comorbidity conditions. And for both, the same criteria are applied in determining which principal diagnosis for which the designated CC or MCC will not affect DRG assignment.

HIV **HIV**

This symbol indicates that the condition is considered a major HIV related diagnosis. When the condition is coded in combination with a diagnosis of human immunodeficiency virus (HIV), code 042, the case will move from MS-DRG 977 to MS-DRGs 974–976.

Wrong Surgery Edit

The Wrong Surgery edit was created to identify cases in which wrong surgeries occurred. Any claim submitted with a code from the

E876.5-E876.7 code range, whether they are in the principal or secondary diagnosis position, will trigger the Wrong Surgery edit. The claim will be denied and returned to the provider. A surgical or other invasive procedure is considered to be a wrong procedure if:

- The procedure was performed on the wrong site
- The procedure was performed on the wrong patient, or
- The incorrect procedure was performed on a patient

V Code That May Be Principal or First-Listed Diagnosis

The instructions for V code use contained in the new official coding guidelines only identify those V codes that can only be used as a PDx. All other V codes may either be SDx or PDx depending upon circumstances of the encounter, by meeting the definition of first-listed or principal diagnosis, and by following any specific V code guidelines in section I.C.18 a-e. With the elimination of the V Code Table, the responsibility of those assigning the V codes as PDx is to make sure the circumstances of the encounter meet the definition of first-listed or principal diagnosis, follow all coding instructions, and follow the V code specific guidelines.

Note: Please note that while the official guidelines [Section 1. C.18.e.] include the V codes that may be principal or first-listed diagnoses, the reporting designations indicated by this section are often in conflict with the Medicare code edits (MCE) for the inpatient prospective payment system (IPPS). Therefore, only the inpatient prospective payment system code edits are represented in this edition.

Procedure Tabular

ᴺᶜ Noncovered Procedure

A procedure not covered by Medicare. In some instances this procedure may also be identified as a valid operating room (OR) procedure that may trigger a DRG assignment. Even if a DRG assignment is made, Medicare may not reimburse for the noncovered procedure.

ᴸᶜ Limited Coverage Procedure

A procedure whose medical complexity and serious nature incur associated costs that are deemed extraordinary and Medicare limits coverage to a portion of the cost.

ᴮᴵ Bilateral Edit

Due to the lack of laterality in ICD-9-CM, there are certain lower extremity joint procedure codes that do not accurately reflect procedures that are performed in one admission on two different bilateral joints. To group to MS-DRG 461 or 462, Bilateral or Multiple Joint Procedures of Lower Extremity with or without MCC, a case must be coded with a combination of two or more different major lower extremity joint procedures. The bilateral procedure symbol identifies those procedure codes that when coded twice represent the same procedure performed on both of the same bilateral joints of the lower extremity. Otherwise, a code edit will instruct the fiscal intermediary to verify that the two different procedures were performed on two different bilateral joints.

ICD-10-CM Coding and Documentation Proficiency Self-Assessment

Introduction

This self-assessment covers ICD-10-CM coding guidance and the required level of detail for clinical documentation of heart disease, diabetes, and pneumonia. These high-volume diagnoses have numerous coding guidelines and documentation requirements. The assessment also covers ICD-10-CM conventions that are new or problematic. Use this self-assessment to identify the areas that may require additional coding training or documentation improvement before ICD-10-CM is implemented on October 1, 2014.

Instructions

Code assignments are based upon the 2012 ICD-10-CM diagnosis code set for all reportable diagnoses, including external causes of morbidity (V00–Y99), as appropriate, according to the instructions in ICD-10-CM conventions and the 2012 *ICD-10-CM Draft Official Guidelines for Coding and Reporting*. Answer each question based on the information provided. Note that for some questions, the codes in the answer are not based upon the information provided, requiring that the provider be queried for specific information because the documentation is insufficient to assign codes correctly.

The answers to the questions can be found immediately following the assessment.

Self-Assessment Questions

1. There are two classifications of pneumonia by anatomical site rather than cause. What are the anatomical classifications and which site of the lung does each affect?

   _____ pneumonia affecting _____ (sites) of lung

   _____ pneumonia affecting _____ (sites) of lung

2. The attending physician's final diagnosis on the progress note on the day of discharge: atypical pneumonia. Sputum results: normal flora. Chest x-ray: bilateral lower lobe consolidation.

   A Assign J18.9 Pneumonia, unspecified organism.

   B Documentation does not follow guidelines and/or the physician must be queried to determine the following:

   • Clinical significance of the sputum results

   • Clinical significance of the chest x-ray

3. What is the appropriate diagnosis code assignment(s) for ESRD due to type I diabetes on chronic dialysis via right arm AV shunt and hypertension as documented by the provider?

   Code assignment:_____

4. Attending admission note: Patient is a 42-year-old female who presents with diabetes with hypoglycemia.

   A Assign E11.649 Type II diabetes mellitus with hypoglycemia without coma.

   B Documentation does not follow guidelines and/or the physician must be queried to determine the following:

   • Type of diabetes mellitus

   • Cause of the hypoglycemia

5. Assign the appropriate code(s) for a diagnosis by the provider of ischemic heart disease and coronary artery disease without history of coronary bypass and current smoker.

   Code assignment:_____

6. Assign the appropriate code(s) for a patient diagnosed by the provider with community-acquired pneumonia who presented with hemoptysis, productive cough, fever, and an increased respiratory rate with sputum culture stain showing gram-negative bacilli.

   Code assignment:_____

7. Discharge summary: 1. VAP, with sputum stain identifying *Klebsiella pneumoniae*, sensitivity performed and Keflex administered. 2. Vent-dependent patient.

   A Assign J95.851 Ventilator associated pneumonia, B96.1 Klebsiella pneumoniae [K. pneumoniae] as the cause of diseases classified elsewhere, and Z99.11 Dependence on respirator [ventilator] status.

   B Documentation does not follow guidelines and/or the physician must be queried to determine the following:

   • Clinical significance of the sputum results

   • Pneumonia: present on admission or post admission

8. Assign the appropriate diagnosis code(s) for diabetes II with Charcôt joint, left hallux with ulcer, with dry gangrene and with chronic osteomyelitis. The patient is admitted for amputation due to osteomyelitis documented in the surgeon's admission note.

   Code assignment:_____

9. What is the appropriate code assignment for a diagnosis of ischemic cardiomyopathy and coronary artery disease, as documented by the provider?

   Code assignment:_____

10. Discharge summary: Patient was admitted from the ED for work-up of precordial chest pain, elevated troponin; history of CABG, congestive heart failure, hypertension. Final diagnosis: ASCAD with USA, s/p CABG, CHF. Most recent diagnostic left heart catheterization showed clean vein and mammary grafts with 90% atherosclerotic stenosis of the native LAD portion. Plans are for future coronary angioplasty as an outpatient. Continue Lasix, Norvasc, and Nitrolingual.

   A Assign I25.110 Atherosclerotic heart disease of native coronary artery with unstable angina, I11.9 Hypertensive heart disease without heart failure, I50.9 Heart failure, unspecified, Z95.1 Presence of aortocoronary bypass graft.

   B Documentation does not follow guidelines and/or the physician must be queried to determine the following:

   • Description of relationship between the hypertension and congestive heart failure

   • Type of congestive heart failure

11. What is the appropriate diagnosis code assignment for the postobstructive pneumonia, right middle lobe, due to hilar lung cancer right lobe when the treatment is directed only toward the pneumonia as documented in the admission note by the resident?

    Code assignment:_____

12. Discharge summary: RSV pneumonia with acute bronchiolitis in one-month-old, high-risk due to being ex-35-week preemie.

    A   Assign J12.1 Respiratory syncytial virus pneumonia, J21.Ø Acute bronchiolitis due to RSV, PØ7.38 Preterm newborn, gestational age 35 completed weeks.

    B   Documentation does not follow guidelines and/or the physician must be queried to determine the following:

        • Clinical significance of the history of prematurity

        • Identification of the causal organism of the bronchiolitis

13. Assign the appropriate diagnosis code(s) for a subsequent encounter for a patient on prescribed steroids with steroid-induced diabetes mellitus, requiring insulin regimen, determined to be inadequately controlled due to dietary noncompliance as documented by the provider.

    Code assignment:_____

14. What is the appropriate code assignment for a diagnosis of unstable angina in a patient who is a nonsmoker with coronary artery disease due to second-hand smoke, as documented by the provider?

    Code assignment:_____

15. Order for outpatient pre-op labs via telephone by office manager of surgeon's office; registrar sends a fax-back form that confirms the order with physician signature. Both office and lab enter note into medical record of phone order. Reason for the surgery and history are furnished by the patient at registration: angioplasty of AV fistula, right arm due to stenosis, end-stage kidney disease, hypertension, on weekly dialysis.

    A   Assign ZØ1.812 Encounter for preprocedural laboratory examination, T82.858A Stenosis of vascular prosthetic devices, implants and grafts, initial encounter, I12.Ø Hypertensive chronic kidney disease with stage 5 chronic kidney disease or end-stage renal disease, N18.6 End-stage renal disease, and Z99.2 Dependence on renal dialysis.

    B   Documentation does not follow guidelines and/or the physician must be queried to determine the following:

        • Etiology of the end-stage renal failure

        • Hypertension, further qualified

16. What is the appropriate code assignment for the diagnosis of mixed bacterial pneumonia due to *Streptococcus pneumoniae* and *Hemophilus influenzae* identified on sputum culture stain and confirmed by the attending physician in the discharge summary?

    Code assignment:_____

17. Discharge summary: Atypical pneumonia, based on presentation clinical indicators and chest CT showing bronchial wall thickening. Last progress note: Awaiting immunoassay results. Addendum to last progress note by PA: Change antibiotic to Azithromycin. At the time of coding, the immunoassay report is posted to the chart and indicates mycoplasma pneumonia. Upon review of the sensitivity test post discharge, the provider's PA ordered a different antibiotic after consulting the attending by phone.

    A   Assign J18.9 Pneumonia, unspecified organism.

    B   Documentation does not follow guidelines and/or the physician must be queried to determine the following:

        • Clinical significance of the immunoassay results and treatment re-evaluation

        • Provide an addendum if the type of pneumonia can be further specified

18. What is the appropriate diagnosis code assignment for physician documentation of a 15-year-old with diabetes on insulin regimen?

    Code assignment:_____

19. Discharge summary signed by attending: A diagnosis of borderline diabetes is listed and body of summary notes FPG test of 124 mg/dl and indicates a need for follow-up testing in three months with diabetic counseling on next office visit recommended.

    Code assignment:_____

20. What is the appropriate diagnosis code assignment for an admission documented by the resident as due to decompensated congestive heart failure with chronic diastolic heart failure, due to patient not refilling her prescription for Lanoxin because she cannot afford the medication this month?

    Code assignment:_____

21. Order for outpatient echocardiogram. Reason: O9Ø.3, with stamped signature of treating physician. Patient presents to testing facility with order. States order is for monitoring since she is being treated for congestive heart failure and is two months post delivery.

    A   Assign O9Ø.3 Peripartum cardiomyopathy, I5Ø.9 Heart failure.

    B   Documentation does not follow guidelines and/or the physician must be queried to determine the following:

        • Provide signed/dated order

        • Provide a written diagnostic statement

22. Which code is appropriate for the diagnosis of gram-positive pneumonia: J15.8 Pneumonia due to other specified bacteria, or J15.9 Unspecified bacterial pneumonia?

    Code assignment:_____

23. What is the appropriate diagnosis code to reflect physician documentation of an office visit of a 14-year-old female G1PØ for evaluation of diet-controlled gestational diabetes, second trimester at 26 weeks?

    Code assignment:_____

24. Progress note: Patient with chronic deep ulcer on right heel. Schedule surgery to debride and consult wound care. Monitor glucose levels for patient's diabetes 2.

    A Assign E11.621 Type 2 diabetes mellitus with foot ulcer, and L97.419 Non-pressure chronic ulcer of right heel and midfoot with unspecified severity.

    B Documentation does not follow guidelines and/or the physician must be queried to determine the following:

    • Etiology of the ulcer

    • Stage or severity of the ulcer

25. What is the appropriate diagnosis code when the PA documents a history of congestive heart failure and combined diastolic and systolic dysfunction under treatment?

    Code assignment:_____

26. Office note by provider: Patient presents today for prenatal visit. Patient is 36-year-old G1P2, at 32 weeks, with history of essential hypertension, currently treated and monitored for signs of pre-eclampsia, asymptomatic mitral valve prolapse, history of smoking that ceased prior to pregnancy.

    A Assign O09.523 Supervision of elderly multigravida, third trimester, O10.013 Pre-existing essential hypertension complicating pregnancy, third trimester, I34.1 Nonrheumatic mitral (valve) prolapse, Z3A.32 32 weeks gestation of pregnancy.

    B Documentation does not follow guidelines and/or the physician must be queried to determine the following:

    • Type of hypertension

    • Significance of patient's age affecting the pregnancy

27. Which of these two coding conventions means the information is insufficient to assign a more specific code; for example, for the diagnosis of bacterial pneumonia?

    A NOS

    B NEC

28. Discharge summary: CMV pneumonia right lung, s/p right lung transplant in 2010 for end-stage emphysema. History of smoking. Continue outpatient pulmonary rehab.

    A Assign T86.812 Lung transplant infection, B25.0 Cytomegaloviral pneumonitis, J43.9 Emphysema, unspecified.

    B Documentation does not follow guidelines and/or the physician must be queried to determine the following:

    • Whether the CMV infection of the right lung transplant is a complication of the transplant or unrelated to the transplant

    • Whether the emphysema is a current diagnosis or by history only

    • History of smoking: former history of use or dependence

29. What is the appropriate diagnosis code for an emergency department visit for an 89-year-old patient with bleeding of a left calf ulcer due to diabetes 2 with diabetic peripheral angiopathy, exacerbated by Coumadin use for chronic atrial fibrillation. The bleeding could not be controlled by pressure at nursing home as documented by the ED physician.

    Code assignment:_____

30. Physician office visit note by provider: Weekly obstetric visit. 27-year-old G4P2A1, now at 30 weeks with history of miscarriage, current gestational diabetes, being treated with insulin.

    A Assign O09.293 Supervision of pregnancy with other poor reproductive or obstetric history, third trimester, O24.414 Gestational diabetes mellitus in pregnancy, insulin controlled, Z3A.30 30 weeks gestation of pregnancy.

    B Documentation does not follow guidelines and/or the physician must be queried to determine the following:

    • Insulin as a long-term medication

    • Clinical significance of previous miscarriage

31. What is the appropriate code assignment for a diagnosis of hypertensive heart disease with congestive heart failure, as documented by the emergency department physician?

    Code assignment:_____

32. Observation record final diagnosis by nephrologist: Admitted to observation from emergency department due to fluid overload from missing weekly dialysis, acute renal failure, end-stage renal failure, hypertension, history of congestive heart failure on Lasix (compensated). Treated with dialysis.

    A Assign E87.70 Fluid overload unspecified, N17.9 Acute kidney failure, I50.9 heart failure, I12.0 Hypertensive chronic kidney disease with stage 5 chronic kidney disease or end-stage renal disease, N18.6 End-stage renal disease, Z91.15 Patient's noncompliance with renal dialysis.

    B Documentation does not follow guidelines and/or the physician must be queried to determine the following:

    • End-stage renal failure relationship to hypertension

    • Etiology of the fluid overload

33. Which of these two coding conventions means the information provides detail for which a specific code does not exist. An example of when the convention is used is for the diagnosis *Moraxella catarrhalis* pneumonia.

    A NOS

    B NEC

34. Admitting note LTCH: 1. Gram-negative pneumonia, resolving: Admit to continue antibiotics three days more to complete regimen ordered during acute inpatient admission, then repeat chest x-ray to evaluate for presence of previously seen consolidation.

    A Assign J15.9 Unspecified bacterial pneumonia.

    B Documentation does not follow guidelines and/or the physician must be queried to determine the following:

    • Whether the diagnosis of pneumonia is current (acute phase) for this encounter or resolved on admission and sequela of illness is under treatment (specify residual)

    • Clinical significance of the repeat chest x-ray (results)

35. What are the appropriate diagnosis codes for admission to the ASC, as documented by the procedure physician, for pancreatic transplant biopsy to evaluate ongoing rejection. The patient has diabetes type 1 with severe nonproliferative retinopathy and gastroparesis and is on the transplant list awaiting a second pancreas transplant. The patient has a functioning kidney allograft with CKD stage 1, due to diabetic renal disease.

    Code assignment:_____

36. Wound care note by wound care nurse: 32-year-old male with diabetes 1 (poly)neuropathic ulcer, 2cmx1cm improvement from last week of 2cmx2xm, right lateral 5th toe, Grade 2 subcutaneous tissue involvement, presented with dry, clean dressing, no drainage present, no odor, granular tissue present, no signs of infection, will continue enzymatic debridement. Note: patient is status post kidney/pancreas transplants, which are functioning.

   A   Assign E10.621 Type 1 diabetes mellitus with foot ulcer, E10.42 Type 1 diabetes mellitus with diabetic polyneuropathy, L97.512 Non-pressure chronic ulcer of other part of right foot with fat layer exposed, Z94.0 Kidney transplant status, Z94.83 Pancreas transplant status.

   B   Documentation does not follow guidelines and/or the physician must be queried to determine the following:
   - Physician must co-sign wound care note
   - Diabetes current diagnosis

37. What is the appropriate diagnosis code for Hospital B for a transfer for therapeutic intervention due to an acute STEMI inferior wall myocardial infarction where the patient suffered an acute subendocardial myocardial infarction prior to discharge, as the physician documented in the discharge summary?

   Code assignment:_____

38. Script written by PCP for outpatient chest x-ray: Productive cough, increased respiratory rate, crackles on inspiration, fever, rule out pneumonia. Script written by PCP for outpatient urinalysis and culture: Fever, tachypnea, history of recurrent urinary tract infections. Radiologist final reading: Pneumonia, COPD. Lab results: Urinalysis was abnormal, culture showed *E. coli*. Sensitivity test results were also performed.

   A   Radiology: Assign J18.9 Pneumonia, unspecified organism. Lab: Assign R50.9 Fever, unspecified, R06.82 Tachypnea, not elsewhere classified, Z87.440 Personal history of urinary (tract) infections.

   B   Documentation does not follow guidelines and/or the physician must be queried to determine the following:
   - PCP: Etiology for the presenting symptoms identified
   - PCP: Clinical significance of the finding of COPD

39. What is the appropriate diagnosis code for a patient with diabetes 1, inadequately controlled, with an insulin pump who is admitted as an outpatient to evaluate insulin pump function. Insulin pump was found to be functioning. The insulin dosage and titration were changed, as documented by the procedure physician.

   Code assignment:_____

40. What is the appropriate diagnosis code for an encounter the emergency department physician documents as for cardiac arrest due to ventricular fibrillation with cardiogenic shock?

   Code assignment:_____

41. ED record, signed by ED attending: Cardiac arrest, history of coronary artery disease, s/p CABG in 2011, hypertension, history of myocardial infarction in 2011. Patient admitted in cardiac arrest, CPR and defibrillation in the ED, resuscitation was unsuccessful and patient expired. Labs: CK-MB: 12.6, troponin I: 5.0. EKG: ST segment elevation and ventricular fibrillation.

   A   Assign I46.9 Cardiac arrest, cause unspecified, I25.10 Atherosclerotic heart disease of native coronary artery without angina pectoris, I10 Essential (primary) hypertension, Z95.1 Presence of aortocoronary bypass graft, I25.2 Old myocardial infarction.

   B   Documentation does not follow guidelines and/or the physician must be queried to determine the following:
   - Etiology of cardiac arrest
   - Clinical significance of the lab results and EKG reading

42. What is the appropriate diagnosis code for the second episode in six months of *Pneumocystis jiroveci* pneumonia in a patient who is noted to be HIV positive, as documented by the provider?

   Code assignment:_____

43. Office visit note: Follow-up for recent pneumonia, course of antibiotics completed last week. Patient without complaint. Repeat chest x-ray is negative.

   A   Assign Z09 Encounter for follow-up examination after completed treatment for conditions other than malignant neoplasm, Z87.01 Personal history of pneumonia (recurrent).

   B   Documentation does not follow guidelines and/or the physician must be queried to determine the following:
   - Type of pneumonia be further specified
   - Pneumonia current or by history only

44. Emergency department record, signed by ED attending: Fractured nose, right black eye of eyelid/ocular area, due to battery assault by boyfriend during domestic abuse incident; apartment residence. Patient is 20-year-old female, G3P2 at 35 weeks with diabetes 1, on insulin, with poor control due to noncompliance and financial difficulties. Admit to labor and delivery observation.

   A   Assign O9A.313 Physical abuse complicating pregnancy, third trimester, S02.2XXA Fracture of nasal bones, initial encounter for closed fracture, S00.11XA Contusion of right eyelid and periocular area, initial encounter, O24.013 Pre-existing diabetes mellitus, type 1, in pregnancy, third trimester, E10.65 Type 1 diabetes mellitus with hyperglycemia, T38.3X6A Underdosing of insulin and oral hypoglycemic [antidiabetic] drugs, initial encounter, Z3A.35 35 weeks gestation of pregnancy, Y04.0XXA Assault by unarmed brawl or fight, Y07.03 Male partner, perpetrator of maltreatment and neglect, Z91.14 Patient's other noncompliance with medication regimen, Z91.120 Patient's intentional underdosing of medication regimen due to financial hardship, Z79.4 Long-term (current) use of insulin, Y92.039 Unspecified place in apartment as the place of occurrence of the external cause.

   B   Documentation does not follow guidelines and/or the physician must be queried to determine the following:
   - Medical significance of noncompliance
   - Effects of trauma on pregnancy

45. Progress note by critical care physician: Code blue called after patient arrived on floor after cardiac catheterization with stent placement for coronary artery disease stenosis, history of recent myocardial infarction, no intraop complications noted. Nurse found patient in cardiac arrest; responding team initiated CPR, defibrillation, endotrachial intubation, epinephrine administered. Patient was resuscitated successfully; admit to inpatient status.

   A   Assign I46.9 Cardiac arrest cause unspecified.

   B   Documentation does not follow guidelines and/or the physician must be queried to determine the following:

   - Cause of cardiac arrest

   - Whether the cardiac arrest was a complication of the procedure

46. What is the correct code if the resident documents the diagnosis of pneumonia due to mechanical ventilation and the lab record shows vent cultures growing yeast?

   Code assignment:_____

47. What is the appropriate diagnosis code when a surgeon documents that a newborn infant was delivered by cesarean on this encounter with macrosomia and the newborn has a diagnosis of syndrome of infant of a diabetic mother?

   Code assignment:_____

48. Visit to endocrinologist: Progress note, signed by provider: diabetes 2; 4 months postpartum who had developed gestational diabetes, now with peripartum diabetes 2, under treatment with metaformin.

   A   Assign E11.9 Type 2 diabetes mellitus without complications, Z86.32 Personal history of gestational diabetes, and O94 Sequela of complication of pregnancy, childbirth, and the puerperium.

   B   Documentation does not follow guidelines and/or the physician must be queried to determine the following:

   - Risk factors for diabetes

   - Diabetic complications

49. What is the appropriate diagnosis code assignment as documented by the emergency department physician for an encounter with a woman who had acute chest pain on inspiration while surveying the damage in the yard of her former home, with acute emotional stress reaction due to surviving a tornado and losing her home to it today?

   Code assignment:_____

50. Admit note by resident: PMH: h/o cardiac arrest due to acute myocardial infarction in 2010, treated by thrombolysis. Admit note: Found to have coronary artery disease, treated medically until now. Admitted today for CABG due to progressive angina. What past history would be appropriate to assign?

   A   Assign Z86.74 Personal history of sudden cardiac arrest, and I25.2 Old myocardial infarction.

   B   Documentation does not follow guidelines and/or the physician must be queried to determine the following:

   - Type of angina

   - Significance of history of myocardial infarction treatment

Coding and Documentation Review Answers

1. *Answer:* **Lobar pneumonia affects an area of a lobe of the lung; Bronch(o)(ial) pneumonia affects the walls of the bronchioles.**

   Rationale: Under the ICD-10-CM Alphabetic Index entry for pneumonia, the subterms that indicate anatomical areas, such as alveolar, apex, confluent, diffuse, etc., index to *"see"* references. The two *"see"* references are *"see* Pneumonia, lobar*"* or *"see* Pneumonia, broncho." These two terms are anatomical classifications of pneumonia that indicate the sites in the lung where clinical indicators of consolidation can be seen on radiologic displays. Since these types of pneumonia are identified by radiological findings rather than causal organism, they are classified as pneumonia caused by unspecified organism. Lobar affects an area of the lung lobe. Bronch(o)(ial)pneumonia or lobular pneumonia affects the walls of the bronchioles with multiple foci of isolated consolidation in one or more basal lobes of the lung.

2. *Answer:* **A** **Assign J18.9 Pneumonia, unspecified organism.**

   Rationale: The type of pneumonia is identified only as "atypical," and no specific organism is attributable; the Alphabetic Index entry for "Pneumonia, atypical" lists J18.9 Pneumonia, unspecified organism. Normal flora identified in a culture indicates a mixture of bacteria normally found at specific body sites and does not represent pathogens and is not clinically significant. The chest x-ray shows bilateral lower lobe consolidation, which can also be seen in congestive heart failure and empyema, among other causes. OCG.I.C.18.b states that signs or symptoms routinely associated with a disease process should not be identified with additional codes unless the physician instructs otherwise.

3. *Answer:* **E10.22 Type 1 diabetes mellitus with diabetic chronic kidney disease, I12.0 Hypertensive chronic kidney disease with stage 5 chronic kidney disease or end-stage renal disease, N18.6 End-stage renal disease, Z99.2 Dependence on renal dialysis**

   Rationale: The type of diabetes is stated as type I, and the chronic kidney disease is due to the diabetes; therefore, assign a code from category E10. ICD-10-CM assumes a cause-and-effect relationship when both hypertension and chronic kidney disease are present (*Official Coding Guidelines* [OCG], section I.C.9.a.2); consequently a code from category I12 is assigned. The tabular "code also" note indicates that the coder should assign an additional code to identify the stage of chronic kidney disease, in this case, end-stage renal disease, N18.6. An instructional note under code N18.6 instructs the coder to use an additional code to identify dialysis status, which is Z99.2 Dependence on renal dialysis.

4. *Answer:* **A** **E11.649 Type II diabetes mellitus with hypoglycemia without coma**

   Rationale: ICD-10-CM OCG section I.C.4.a.2 states that E11- Type 2 diabetes mellitus, is assigned as the default when the type is not specified. Guideline section I.A.15 indicates that the word "with" means "due to" in the Alphabetic Index; therefore, the documentation links the diabetes and hypoglycemia. Diabetes mellitus codes are combination codes, and the Alphabetic Index entry for diabetes with hypoglycemia, Type 2, refers to E11.649 Type II diabetes mellitus with hypoglycemia without coma.

5. *Answer:* **I25.10 Atherosclerotic heart disease of native coronary artery without angina pectoris, Z72.0 Tobacco use**

   Rationale: The ICD-10-CM Alphabetic Index main term "Disease, coronary (artery)" directs the coder to *"see"* Disease, heart, ischemic, atherosclerotic. Under "Disease/heart/ischemic/atherosclerotic," the code default is I25.10. Both stated conditions are classified to the single code I25.10 Atherosclerotic heart disease of native coronary artery without angina pectoris. When there is no history or documentation of a previous coronary artery bypass graft (CABG) or heart transplant, a code

   for atherosclerosis of native artery should be assigned. The Alphabetic Index lists code Z72.0 under "Tobacco, use."

6. *Answer:* **J18.9 Pneumonia, unspecified organism, R04.2 Hemoptysis**

   Rationale: The ICD-10-CM Alphabetic Index does not list the nonessential modifier "hemorrhagic" after the term "pneumonia." Therefore, unless documentation links this symptom to the pneumonia, the hemoptysis would be assigned as an additional code. The provider/documentation does not confirm that the sputum culture stain showing gram-negative bacilli is clinically significant. See OCG 1.C.18.b, "Use of a symptom code with a definitive diagnosis," and OCG III, "Reporting Additional Findings, B. Abnormal findings."

7. *Answer:* **A** **Assign J95.851 Ventilator associated pneumonia, B96.1 Klebsiella pneumoniae [K. pneumoniae] as the cause of diseases classified elsewhere, Z99.11 Dependence on respirator [ventilator] status.**

   Rationale: The ICD-10-CM OCG section I.C.10.d.1 states that the assignment of a complication code is based on the provider's documentation of the relationship between the pneumonia and the mechanical ventilation. In this case, the documentation describes the pneumonia as due to the ventilator. An additional code is assigned if an identified organism is attributed to the VAP, but not a pneumonia code from J12–J18.

8. *Answer:* **E11.610 Type 2 diabetes mellitus with diabetic neuropathic arthropathy, E11.621 Type 2 diabetes mellitus with foot ulcer, E11.52 Type 2 diabetes mellitus with diabetic peripheral angiopathy with gangrene, L97.524 Non-pressure chronic ulcer of other part of left foot with necrosis of bone**

   Rationale: ICD-10-CM OCG section I.A.15 states that the use of the term "with" is to be interpreted to mean "associated with" or "due to" when it appears in a code title, the Alphabetic Index, or an instructional note in the Tabular List. Therefore, the listed conditions are coded as diabetic complications. Guideline section I.C.4.a states that as many codes within a particular category should be assigned as describe all the complications, with sequencing based on the reason for a particular encounter. E11.610 Type 2 diabetes mellitus with diabetic neuropathic arthropathy is sequenced first since this describes the osteomyelitis.

9. *Answer:* **I25.5 Ischemic cardiomyopathy and I25.10 Atherosclerotic heart disease of native coronary artery without angina pectoris**

   Rationale: Ischemic cardiomyopathy is an extrinsic cardiomyopathy due to reduced blood flow to the heart muscle. The ICD-10-CM Alphabetic Index lists I25.5 Ischemic cardiomyopathy under the term "Cardiomyopathy, ischemic to." The "excludes2" note under I25.5 indicates that coronary atherosclerosis (I25.1-, I25.7-) is not included; therefore, these two conditions can be coded together when documented.

10. *Answer:* **B** **Documentation does not follow guidelines and/or the physician must be queried to determine the following: description of relationship between the hypertension and congestive heart failure, and specify type of the congestive heart failure.**

    Rationale: The relationship between hypertension and congestive heart failure is not assumed in ICD-10-CM and must be documented. Second, if the type of heart failure can be further specified as diastolic, systolic, or both, a more accurate code can be assigned from category I50 Heart failure. Heart disease without a stated causal relationship to hypertension is coded separately.

11. *Answer:* J18.9 Pneumonia, unspecified organism, and C34.Ø1 Malignant neoplasm of right main bronchus or lung

    Rationale: There is no specific entry in the Alphabetic Index for postobstructive pneumonia; therefore, only the term "Pneumonia" is listed. When a specified type of pneumonia is not documented, J18.9 Pneumonia, unspecified organism, is the default code and should be assigned. The malignancy is sequenced as an additional code according to OCG section C.2.I.4.

12. *Answer:* <u>A</u> Assign J12.1 Respiratory syncytial virus pneumonia, J21.Ø Acute bronchiolitis due to RSV, PØ7.38 Preterm newborn, gestational age 35 completed weeks.

    Rationale: The ICD-1Ø-CM Alphabetic Index entry for "Pneumonia, respiratory syncytial virus" lists J12.1. Respiratory syncytial virus is a common community-acquired infection in children. OCG section I.C.16.a.5 states that if a newborn condition is community-acquired, a code from chapter 16, "Certain Conditions Originating in the Perinatal Period," is not assigned. RSV bronchiolitis is also documented and is also assigned. Both are acute conditions, and when the patient is admitted for both and both are equal in work-up, focus, and treatment, either can be sequenced as the principal diagnosis, following OCG section II.B. The additional information that the patient is a former preemie is coded as its clinical significance is documented and OCG section I.C.16.e states that prematurity is coded when it affects the patient's current health status.

13. *Answer:* EØ9.65 Drug or chemical induced diabetes mellitus with hyperglycemia, T38.ØX5D Adverse effect of glucocorticoids and synthetic analogues subsequent encounter, Z79.4 Long term (current) use of insulin, Z91.11 Patient's noncompliance with dietary regimen

    Rationale: Since the steroid use is prescribed and there is no indication of incorrect usage, this is considered an adverse effect and not a poisoning. The diabetes is drug-induced, and according to OCG section I.C.4.a.6.b, sequencing is to "code first" EØ9 Drug or chemical induced diabetes mellitus, followed by an additional code for the adverse effect to identify the drug T36–T5Ø with a fifth/sixth character of 5. ICD-1Ø-CM does not use the terms "uncontrolled," "inadequately controlled," or "out of control, poorly controlled." The index instructs the user to "code Diabetes, by type, with hyperglycemia." Therefore, the first-listed code is EØ9.65 Drug or chemical induced diabetes mellitus with hyperglycemia. This is followed by T38.ØX5- Adverse effect of glucocorticoids and synthetic analogues, which is located in the Table of Drugs and Chemicals under the main term "Steroid" with the appropriate additional character requirement, which in this case is a character for a subsequent encounter (D). The patient is maintained on insulin, Z79.4, which OCG section I.C.4.a.6.a, indicates is coded when documented. The diabetes is inadequately controlled due to dietary noncompliance, Z91.11, which is located in the Alphabetic Index under "Noncompliance, with, dietary regimen."

14. *Answer:* I25.11Ø Atherosclerotic heart disease of native coronary artery with unstable angina pectoris, Z77.22 Contact with and (suspected) exposure to environmental tobacco smoke (acute) (chronic)

    Rationale: OCG section I.C.9.b states that ICD-1Ø-CM provides combination codes that link coronary artery disease with angina since the relationship between them is to be assumed unless otherwise documented. No separate code is assigned from category I2Ø Angina pectoris. Code Z77.22 Contact with and (suspected) exposure to environmental tobacco smoke (acute) (chronic) is assigned as a secondary code when the provider documents that the second-hand smoke is the external cause of the patient's condition. Locate the code in the Alphabetic Index under the term "Exposure, second hand tobacco smoke (acute) (chronic)." When there is no history or documentation of a previous coronary artery bypass graft (CABG) or heart transplant, a code for atherosclerosis of native artery is assigned.

15. *Answer:* <u>A</u> Assign ZØ1.812 Encounter for preprocedural laboratory examination, T82.858A Stenosis of vascular prosthetic devices, implants and grafts, initial encounter, I12.Ø Hypertensive chronic kidney disease with stage 5 chronic kidney disease or end-stage renal disease, N18.6 End-stage renal disease, and Z99.2 Dependence on renal dialysis.

    Rationale: A telephone call from the treating physician's office to the testing facility to order a diagnostic outpatient service is acceptable if, as required by the Centers for Medicare and Medicaid Services, payer, state, conditions of participation bylaws, Joint Commission and Office of Inspector General requirements, both the treating physician/office and the testing facility document the phone call in their copies of the patient's medical record. This information may be obtained from the patient or the medical record, but the coder should attempt to confirm this information with the physician, and it is recommended to have a "fax-back" policy in place for the registration sites. In the example, the reason for the order is to have pre-op lab testing performed; "Examination, pre-procedural (pre-operative), laboratory" in the Alphabetic Index lists ZØ1.812 Encounter for preprocedural laboratory examination. OCG section I.C.21.c.16 indicates that category ZØ1 is a "first-listed" diagnosis and therefore should be sequenced first followed by the reason for the surgery/procedure.

16. *Answer:* J13 Pneumonia due to Streptococcus pneumoniae, and J14 Pneumonia due to Haemophilus influenzae

    Rationale: Since the attending physician confirmed both identified infective organisms, both individual codes are assigned. If the organisms were not identified, then only pneumonia, bacterial (unspecified organism) would be assigned, not the "bacterial, specified" code, since the terms "mixed bacterial" do not identify specified organisms not elsewhere classified.

17. *Answer:* <u>B</u> Documentation does not follow guidelines and/or the physician must be queried to determine the following: the clinical significance of the immunoassay results and treatment re-evaluation and provide an addendum if the type of pneumonia can be further specified.

    Rationale: After the documentation is reviewed, a query is warranted to further specify the type of pneumonia. The physician assistant documented a change in treatment based upon the results of the immunoassay test. Although the test results are posted to the chart, the coder should ask about their clinical significance and the reason behind the change in medication. Additionally, the findings on chest x-ray further support a more specific pneumonia as due to the identified organism. Coders are responsible for querying when the clinical documentation as a whole suggests a higher level of specificity.

18. *Answer:* E11.9 Type 2 diabetes mellitus without complications, and Z79.4 Long-term (current) use of insulin

    Rationale: According to OCG section I.C.4.a.2.3, the type of diabetes mellitus cannot be determined by patient age or the use of insulin. The guideline further states that when the type of diabetes is not documented, the default is diabetes mellitus type 2 and that insulin documented as a maintenance drug is assigned as an additional code.

19. *Answer:* Assign R73.Ø9 Other abnormal glucose.

    Rationale: Without further documentation of a diagnosis of diabetes, the attending's attestation to the discharge summary confirming the lab findings and the indication of clinical significance, only a code from subcategory "abnormal glucose" can be assigned. This can be found in the Alphabetic Index under the main term "Findings, abnormal, inconclusive, without findings, glucose" or by the documentation of borderline diabetes mellitus or diabetes, latent. Code R73.Ø9 Other abnormal glucose, lists "prediabetes" and "latent diabetes" as inclusion terms.

20. *Answer:* I50.33 Acute on chronic diastolic (congestive) heart failure, T46.0X6A Underdosing of cardiac-stimulant glycosides and drugs of similar action initial encounter, and Z91.120 Patient's intentional underdosing of medication regimen due to financial hardship

    Rationale: The code for "chronic on acute (i.e., acute on chronic)" is assigned because the acute exacerbation of a chronic condition is coded as acute on chronic, and when a combination code is available, only a single code is assigned. The exacerbation of the congestive heart failure was due to the lack of Lanoxin and is sequenced before the code for the underdosing, according to OCG section I.C.19.e.5.c. The seventh-character assignment of A, indicating the initial encounter, is required to complete code T46.0X6. An additional code to represent noncompliance and the reason and intent is assigned: Z91.120 Patient's intentional underdosing of medication regimen due to financial hardship. The ICD-10-CM Alphabetic Index and Tabular List now provide the nonessential modifier "congestive" in the descriptor of the diastolic and systolic types of heart failure. Therefore an additional code for "congestive heart failure" is not assigned.

21. *Answer:* **B** Documentation does not follow guidelines and/or the physician must be queried to determine the following: provide signed/dated order and provide a written diagnostic statement.

    Rationale: A valid order must follow CMS, payer, state, conditions of participation, bylaws and Joint Commission and OIG requirements. Signatures are required for certain diagnostic tests, and CMS Transmittal 327 states that stamped signatures are not acceptable. The introduction to the OCG states that ICD-10-CM is a morbidity classification for classifying diagnoses and reason for health care visits. Codes are not diagnoses—they may not be used as a substitute for a written diagnostic statement within the medical record.

22. *Answer:* J15.9 Unspecified bacterial pneumonia

    Rationale: Since the term "gram-positive" is nonspecific and does not identify a specific organism, assign J15.9 Unspecified bacterial pneumonia. When a specific bacterial organism is identified but has no specific entry in the Alphabetic Index or a corresponding ICD-10-CM diagnosis code, the default is J15.8 Pneumonia due to other specified bacteria. The same applies to viral pneumonia coding.

23. *Answer:* O09.612 Supervision of young primigravida, second trimester, O24.410 Gestational diabetes mellitus in pregnancy, diet controlled, Z3A.26, 26 weeks gestation of pregnancy

    Rationale: OCG section I.C.15.i covers gestational diabetes. Since the patient is 14 years old and this is her first pregnancy (identified by "G1P0"), the coder would look in the index under "Pregnancy, supervision of, young mother, primigravida." The sixth character "2" specifies second trimester as defined by the note at the introduction to chapter 15. The Alphabetic Index lists the main term "Diabetes" with the subterm "gestational, diet controlled," which references code O24.410. Follow the instructional note for chapter 15 and use an additional code from category Z3A to describe the number of weeks of gestation.

24. *Answer:* **B** Documentation does not follow guidelines and/or the physician must be queried to determine the following: etiology of the ulcer and stage or severity of the ulcer.

    Rationale: If the ulcer is of diabetic origin, the link to diabetes must be stated before the ulcer can be coded. The term "deep" does not indicate the tissues involved, and the tissues need to be documented to further classify the stage or level of necrosis for code severity specificity.

25. *Answer:* I50.42 Chronic combined systolic (congestive) and diastolic (congestive) heart failure

    Rationale: The ICD-10-CM Alphabetic Index does not have entries for diastolic or systolic under the main term "Dysfunction." Diastolic dysfunction is the decline in performance of one or both ventricles of the heart during the time phase of diastole; left/systemic/body and right/pulmonary/lungs. Dysfunction has a subterm "ventricular/with congestive heart failure," which references I50.9 Heart failure unspecified. However, when there is diastolic or systolic dysfunction in the presence of heart failure, the relationship is assumed. In this example, the heart failure is specified as combined diastolic and systolic. Code I50.42 is the appropriate code. If diastolic or systolic dysfunction is documented without documentation of heart failure, assign I51.9 Heart disease, unspecified. In this case, however, because of the known history of heart failure, the case is coded as chronic.

26. *Answer:* **A** Assign O09.523 Supervision of elderly multigravida, third trimester, O10.013 Pre-existing essential hypertension complicating pregnancy third trimester, I34.1 Nonrheumatic mitral (valve) prolapse, Z3A.32 32 weeks gestation of pregnancy.

    Rationale: For this scenario, OCG section I.C.15.b.2 states that the principal diagnosis should be a code from category O09 for supervision of a high-risk (elderly) pregnancy. The patient is 36 years old and has delivered once (G1P2). Assign code O09.523 as the first-listed diagnosis. The sixth character indicates the third trimester, as defined by the note in the introduction to chapter 15. Code Z3A.32 32 weeks gestation of pregnancy, is assigned according to the instructional note for chapter 15. Code O10.013 Pre-existing essential hypertension complicating pregnancy, third trimester, would be assigned as a secondary diagnosis code. Mitral valve prolapse, although asymptomatic, is coded because it is medically significant during pregnancy.

27. *Answer:* **A** NOS

    Rationale: The coding convention NOS, or not otherwise specified, is the equivalent of "unspecified" and is assigned when the documentation does not provide more specific information about the condition. In the example, the term bacterial pneumonia means that the specified bacterial organism causing the pneumonia is unknown, or cannot be determined. What is known is that the causal organism is bacterial as opposed to viral. The Alphabetic Index lists the terms "Pneumonia, bacterial"; therefore, the default is J15.9 Unspecified bacterial pneumonia.

28. *Answer:* **A** Assign T86.812 Lung transplant infection, B25.0 Cytomegaloviral pneumonitis, J43.9 Emphysema, unspecified.

    Rationale: According to OCG section I.C.19.g.3.a, the code for transplant complications is assigned only if the complication affects the function of the transplanted organ. The complication requires two codes, one from category T86 to identify the type of complication and a second to identify the manifestation. Cytomegaloviral pneumonitis, or CMV, is an opportunistic pneumonia. Since the pneumonitis is in the allograft, it is coded as a lung transplant complication, specifically as an infection. The transplant was performed only on the right, so the emphysema is not "cured" and is still present. Therefore, the emphysema is assigned as an additional diagnosis. Only history of tobacco dependence, not history of smoking or tobacco use, has an index entry. Therefore, the history of smoking is not coded.

29. *Answer:* E11.622 Type 2 diabetes mellitus with other skin ulcer, T45.515A Adverse effect of anticoagulants, E11.51 Type 2 diabetes mellitus with diabetic peripheral angiopathy without gangrene, L97.229 Non-pressure chronic ulcer of left calf with unspecified severity, I48.2 Chronic atrial fibrillation

Rationale: As the bleeding from the ulcer is an adverse effect of the prescribed Coumadin, follow the guidelines in OCG section I.C.19.e.5.a and sequence the nature of the adverse effect first, which in this case is also a diabetic complication, E11.622 Type 2 diabetes mellitus with other skin ulcer. This is followed by the code identifying the drug and adverse effect, T45.515A Adverse effect of anticoagulants, found in the Table of Drugs and Chemicals. Code also all other diabetic complications, E11.51 Type 2 diabetes mellitus with diabetic peripheral angiopathy without gangrene. Also list code L97.229 Non-pressure chronic ulcer of left calf with unspecified severity to identify the site and severity of the ulcer per the "use additional code" instruction note under E11.622. Code I48.2 Chronic atrial fibrillation, indicates the condition for which the Coumadin is taken.

30. *Answer:* A Assign O09.293 Supervision of pregnancy with other poor reproductive or obstetric history, third trimester, O24.414 Gestational diabetes mellitus in pregnancy, insulin controlled, Z3A.30, 30 weeks gestation of pregnancy.

Rationale: The provider's documentation indicates this is a routine prenatal visit for a high-risk pregnancy due to a history of miscarriage with current gestational diabetes. OCG section I.C.15.b.2 states that a code from category O09 Supervision of high-risk pregnancy, should be assigned as the first-listed diagnosis, followed by any other applicable chapter 15 codes to describe comorbid conditions affecting the pregnancy. The code for gestational diabetes does not indicate trimester, but the fourth character does represent "in pregnancy." From the instructional note "use additional code from category Z3A" for chapter 15, code Z3A.30 30 weeks gestation of pregnancy, is assigned. OCG section I.C.15.i notes that additional code Z79.4 Long-term (current) use of insulin, should not be assigned with codes from subcategory O24.4.

31. *Answer:* I11.0 Hypertensive heart disease with heart failure, I50.9 Heart failure, unspecified

Rationale: According to OCG section I.C.9.1, when a causal relationship between hypertension and heart failure (I50.-) or heart disease (I51.4.-I51.9) is stated (due to) or implied (hypertensive), assign a code from category I11 Hypertensive heart disease. Also the OCG section I.A.15 states that in the Alphabetic Index, the subentry term "with" means "associated with" or "due to." Therefore, a diagnostic statement of "with" provides the link between two conditions. The tabular note instructs the coder to "use additional code to identify type of heart failure I50.-." In the example, the type is not documented; therefore an additional code for heart failure, unspecified is assigned.

32. *Answer:* A Assign E87.70 Fluid overload unspecified, N17.9 Acute kidney failure, I50.9 Heart failure, I12.0 Hypertensive chronic kidney disease with stage 5 chronic kidney disease or end-stage renal disease, N18.6 End-stage renal disease, Z91.15 Patient's noncompliance with renal dialysis.

Rationale: The acute conditions necessitating admission were the fluid overload and the acute renal failure. Since the dialysis is treatment for both conditions, according to OCG section II.C either may be sequenced as the principal diagnosis unless one is considered the more significant problem. As long as the admission is clearly documented as to treat the fluid overload and as not related to the history of congestive heart failure, the fluid overload can be coded separately. The congestive heart failure is noted to be "compensated," meaning it is not in acute

exacerbation; note that unspecified heart failure I50.9 makes no distinction between acute or decompensated and compensated. If the record indicates that the type of heart failure can be specified further, the coder should query the physician for the type as well as a possible relationship between the heart failure and hypertension. Acute renal failure can be coded in the presence of end-stage kidney disease as there are no excludes or includes notes or instructional notes that indicate otherwise. The cause of the fluid overload was the noncompliance with dialysis, which is in the Alphabetic Index as "Noncompliance, with, dialysis," Z91.15. The dialysis status code is not assigned when the noncompliance is coded, Z91.15, as indicated by the "excludes1" note under Z99.2 Dependence on renal dialysis.

33. *Answer:* B NEC

Rationale: The coding convention NEC, or not elsewhere classified, is the equivalent of "specified (other, other specified)" and applies when the documentation specifies a condition but there is no individual code for that condition. In the example, the type of bacteria causing the pneumonia is identified (specified), but the ICD-10-CM Alphabetic Index does not list an individual code for that particular organism. Therefore, the user would look in the index under "Pneumonia, specified, bacterium NEC," leading to J15.8 Pneumonia due to other specified bacteria.

34. *Answer:* B Documentation does not follow guidelines and/or the physician must be queried to determine the following: diagnosis of pneumonia current (acute phase) for this encounter or resolved on admission and sequela of illness is under treatment (specify residual); and clinical significance of the repeat chest x-ray (results).

Rationale: Long-term care hospitals may assign codes for acute unresolved conditions, sequelae, or rehab. The selection of principal diagnosis follows the guidelines in OCG section II. When the patient is admitted for continuation of treatment of an acute condition, OCG section I.B.10 may apply if the acute phase has resolved and it is the sequela that is being treated. This provider must document that the residual condition is being treated and is the reason for admission. If the patient no longer has the clinical indicators of the acute disease, the coder should query the physician for clarification as to whether the acute condition is present or if a sequela is receiving the continuation of care and treatment. As long as an acute condition is the target of treatment, it is coded. For this example, the facility must decide how to address the issue of acute condition versus sequela for "resolving" conditions that may or may not have clinical indicators.

35. *Answer:* T86.890 Other transplanted tissue rejection, E10.349 Type 1 diabetes mellitus with severe nonproliferative diabetic retinopathy without macular edema, E10.43 Type 1 diabetes mellitus with diabetic autonomic (poly)neuropathy (gastroparesis), E10.22 Type 1 diabetes mellitus with diabetic chronic kidney disease, N18.1 Chronic kidney disease, stage 1, Z94.0 Kidney transplant status, and Z76.82 Awaiting organ transplant status

Rationale: Rejection affects the transplanted pancreas and is a complication of the pancreas transplant. As the reason for the encounter, the transplant rejection is sequenced first. The patient has ongoing complications of retinopathy and gastroparesis due to diabetes 1, which must also be coded. The patient is also status post kidney transplant due to diabetic renal disease, and the transplanted kidney is functioning with mild CKD stage 1, which is not documented as a complication but is residual renal disease. OCG section I.C.14.a.2 indicates that the CKD stage with kidney transplant status should be assigned. Also indicate that the patient is awaiting transplant by looking in the index under "Transplant, awaiting organ," code Z76.82.

36. *Answer:* <u>A</u> Assign E10.621 Type 1 diabetes mellitus with foot ulcer, E10.42 Type 1 diabetes mellitus with diabetic polyneuropathy, L97.512 Non-pressure chronic ulcer of other part of right foot with fat layer exposed, Z94.0 Kidney transplant status, Z94.83 Pancreas transplant status.

    Rationale: The term provider is used throughout the *Official Coding Guidelines* to indicate a physician or any qualified health care practitioner who is legally accountable for establishing the patient's diagnosis. State laws define the scope of practice and, for health care entities, regulatory laws establish who may provide documentation; wound care nursing documentation is recognized as valid. Although the patient has a functioning pancreas transplant, diabetes is coded since there are related complications. The diabetes 1 is linked to the ulcer by its description as diabetes 1 neuropathic ulcer. Because the Wagner non-pressure foot ulcer classification grade 2 is penetration through the subcutaneous tissue, the severity chosen is "with fat layer exposed." The ulcer is sequenced first before the neuropathy because it is the reason for the encounter.

37. *Answer:* **I21.19 ST elevation (STEMI) myocardial infarction involving other coronary artery of inferior wall, and I22.2 Subsequent non-ST elevation (NSTEMI) myocardial infarction**

    Rationale: OCG section I.C.9.e.1 states that a code for the site is assigned for an acute STEMI myocardial infarction for encounters occurring when the MI is equal to or less than four weeks old, including transfers during this timeframe. New for ICD-10-CM, OCG section I.C.9.e.4 states that after an initial myocardial infarction, a subsequent or new acute myocardial infarction during the same four-week timeframe is coded to category I22 Subsequent ST elevation (STEMI) and non-ST elevation (NSTEMI) myocardial infarction. When there are both an initial and subsequent acute myocardial infarction, codes from both I21 and I22 are assigned, sequenced based on the circumstances of the encounter.

38. *Answer:* <u>A</u> Radiology: Assign J18.9 Pneumonia, unspecified organism. Lab: Assign R50.9 Fever, unspecified, R06.82 Tachypnea, not elsewhere classified, Z87.440 Personal history of urinary (tract) infections.

    Rationale: In the outpatient setting, uncertain diagnoses cannot be assigned (OCG section IV.H). The referring provider should document signs, symptoms, and abnormal findings that prompt the outpatient encounter. If a physician has interpreted a diagnostic test and the results are available, the confirmed or definitive diagnosis is coded; the related or integral signs and symptoms are not coded, according to OCG section IV.K.. The second script lists signs and symptoms and history, but the test results are by lab only. Therefore, the signs and symptoms and history codes are assigned. When possible, the coder should ask the PCP to clarify the lab results. Until the PCP confirms the test results for the scripts, only the codes for the symptoms for which the tests were ordered are assigned.

39. *Answer:* **E10.65 Type 1 diabetes mellitus with hyperglycemia and Z46.81 Encounter for fitting and adjustment of insulin pump**

    Rationale: The ICD-10-CM Alphabetic Index lists the terms inadequately controlled, out of control, and poorly controlled to represent diabetes mellitus uncontrolled, with the instruction to assign diabetes, by type, with hyperglycemia. Therefore, assign E10.65 Type 1 diabetes mellitus with hyperglycemia as the first diagnosis as the diabetes was symptomatic and the reason for the encounter, not just an evaluation of the insulin pump or for titration adjustment. Add Z46.81 Encounter for fitting and adjustment of insulin pump, since titration adjustment was performed. The status code Z96.41 Presence of insulin pump (external) (internal) is not assigned since the reason for encounter code indicates the type of status according to OCG section I.C.21.c.3.

40. *Answer:* I49.01 Ventricular fibrillation, I46.2 Cardiac arrest due to underlying cardiac condition, and R57.0 Cardiogenic shock

    Rationale: The ICD-10-CM Alphabetic Index now provides separate codes for cardiac arrest due to underlying cardiac condition, due to (other) specified underlying condition (trauma, overdose, etc.) or unspecified cause. Codes for both the cardiac arrest and the underlying condition should be assigned, when the condition is known. In the example for the ED encounter, the ventricular fibrillation is known and should be sequenced first, followed by the code for the cardiac arrest as instructed by the tabular "code first" note under category I46 Cardiac arrest. If further work-up determines the cause of the ventricular fibrillation, such as cardiac ischemia or coronary artery disease, cardiomyopathy, acute myocardial infarction, trauma, overdose, etc., that condition is the principal diagnosis and the appropriate code from category I46 Cardiac arrest, is secondary, along with I49.01 Ventricular fibrillation. Since the cardiogenic shock is not integral to the ventricular fibrillation or the cardiac arrest, the code for shock is assigned even though it is not a chapter 18 code (OCG section I.C.18.b). Review and apply the guidelines in the OCG section II introduction for the UHDDS definition of principal diagnosis for inpatient, and in OCG section IV.G, IV.k and IV.l for the reason of the outpatient encounter. Keep in mind that, according to OCG section IV.A, the coding conventions and the general and disease-specific guidelines take precedence over the outpatient guidelines.

41. *Answer:* <u>A</u> Assign I46.9 Cardiac arrest, cause unspecified, I25.10 Atherosclerotic heart disease of native coronary artery without angina pectoris, I10 Essential (primary) hypertension, Z95.1 Presence of aortocoronary bypass graft, I25.2 Old myocardial infarction.

    Rationale: When an emergency department patient dies before the cause of a cardiac arrest is known, the code for the cardiac arrest is the first-listed diagnosis. When the underlying condition is known, the code for the condition is sequenced first, with the code for cardiac arrest as an additional diagnosis. In ICD-10-CM, cardiac arrest now has three subcategories based on whether the underlying condition is known or not and whether it is cardiac or other specified condition. Since there is no documentation of recent cardiac catheterization, the coronary artery disease post CABG is assumed to be of native vessel without angina pectoris.

42. *Answer:* B20 Human immunodeficiency virus [HIV] disease and B59 Pneumocystosis

    Rationale: ICD-10-CM OCG section I.C.1.a.1 instructs that confirmation of HIV status can be made by the provider's statement that the patient has an HIV-related illness. Also, section I.C.1.a.2.f states that cases involving patients with any known prior diagnosis of an HIV-related illness are assigned code B20 Human immunodeficiency virus [HIV] disease. The Centers for Disease Control (CDC) classifies *Pneumocystis jiroveci* pneumonia, an opportunistic pneumonia, as an AIDS-defining condition and one of the clinical criteria for HIV stage 3 or AIDS. Another clinical criterion is an HIV-positive patient having bacterial pneumonia twice within one year.

43. *Answer:* <u>A</u> Assign Z09 Encounter for follow-up examination after completed treatment for conditions other than malignant neoplasm, Z87.01 Personal history of pneumonia (recurrent).

    Rationale: OCG section I.C.21.c.8 states that follow-up codes are assigned when the encounter is for surveillance following completed treatment and the condition no longer exists. Follow-up codes are not used for sequelae or ongoing care of a condition that is healing or resolving. A history code representing the healed/resolved condition is assigned as a secondary code to fully explain the reason for the encounter. The follow-up code is not assigned if the condition is found to have recurred on the follow-up encounter, and instead the code for the condition is listed first.

44. *Answer:* <u>A</u> Assign O9A.313 Physical abuse complicating pregnancy, third trimester, S02.2XXA Fracture of nasal bones, initial encounter for closed fracture, S00.11XA Contusion of right eyelid and periocular area, initial encounter, O24.013 Pre-existing diabetes mellitus, type 1, in pregnancy, third trimester, E10.65 Type 1 diabetes mellitus with hyperglycemia, T38.3X6A Underdosing of insulin and oral hypoglycemic [antidiabetic] drugs, initial encounter, Z3A.35 35 weeks gestation of pregnancy, Y04.0XXA Assault by unarmed brawl or fight, Y07.03 Male partner, perpetrator of maltreatment and neglect, Z91.120 Patient's intentional underdosing of medication regimen due to financial hardship, Z79.4 Long term (current) use of insulin, Y92.039 Unspecified place in apartment as the place of occurrence of the external cause

Rationale: The ED provider documentation that is attested by signature confirms the injuries are due to physical abuse. The *Official Coding Guidelines* section I.C.15.r states that abuse in a pregnant patient is sequenced first and coded to category O9A Physical abuse complicating pregnancy, childbirth, and the puerperium, when suspected or confirmed; associated injuries are coded as additional diagnoses. Pre-existing diabetes 1 with poor control is assigned to category O24 Diabetes mellitus in pregnancy, childbirth, and the puerperium, with an additional code from category E10 Type 1 diabetes mellitus, to further identify manifestation of hyperglycemia, indicated in the Alphabetic Index as poor control. Underdosing of medication is covered in OCG section I.C.19.e.5.c and is assigned from category T38 with the sixth character of 6. Sequencing of multiple codes from chapter 20, "External Causes of Morbidity," is explained in OCG section I.C.20.f.

45. *Answer:* <u>B</u> Documentation does not follow guidelines and/or the physician must be queried to determine the following: cause of cardiac arrest and whether the cardiac arrest a complication of the procedure.

Rationale: When a cardiac arrest occurs during an inpatient hospitalization and the patient is resuscitated, a code from category I46 Cardiac arrest, is assigned as an additional diagnosis. It would be appropriate to ask the physician the cause or contributing cause if it is not stated when there is clinical evidence to support the query. When a cardiac arrest is the reason for an inpatient death (the patient is not resuscitated) and the cause or contributing cause is known, the code for cardiac arrest is not assigned.

46. *Answer:* J95.851 Ventilator associated pneumonia

Rationale: ICD-10-CM OCG section I.C.10.d.1 states that the code for a complication is based on the provider's documentation of the relationship between the complication and the cause, in this case, the pneumonia and the mechanical ventilation. Therefore, code J95.851 Ventilator associated pneumonia, is assigned only when the link is expressly stated and not merely when a patient on a mechanical ventilator has pneumonia. An additional code is assigned if an identified organism is attributed to the VAP, but not a code from J12–J18. In the example, since the yeast cultures are identified only as a lab value and are not documented by the provider as related to the VAP, a code for the yeast organism is not assigned. The coder should ask the provider to state the clinical significance of the lab results; if the results are related to the VAP, B37.9 Candidiasis, unspecified, would be assigned.

47. *Answer:* Z38.01 Single liveborn infant, delivered by cesarean, P70.1 Syndrome of infant of a diabetic mother

Rationale: The code for a newborn delivered by cesarean on this admission is found by looking in the Alphabetic Index under "Newborn, born in hospital, by cesarean," code Z38.01. Macrosomia is not listed in the ICD-10-CM Alphabetic Index but is synonymous with "large for gestational age," or LGA, which the index entry for "Large, baby" indicates is coded with P08.1. This is not assigned, however, because subcategory E08.1 has an "excludes1" note indicating that LGA in "syndrome of diabetic mother" is to be included in P70.1.

48. *Answer:* <u>A</u> Assign E11.9 Type 2 diabetes mellitus without complications, Z86.32 Personal history of gestational diabetes, and O94 Sequela of complication of pregnancy, childbirth, and the puerperium.

Rationale: When diagnosed with gestational diabetes mellitus, patients have a high risk of developing diabetes 2 post delivery, which is why clinical guidelines recommend the patients return for postpartum glucose testing. When the postpartum impaired glucose regulation indicates diabetes, the case is coded as diabetes and no longer abnormal glucose finding. OCG section I.C.15.o.3 states that if the provider documents a condition as related to pregnancy, codes from chapter 15 may be assigned. OCG section I.C.15.p states that when an initial complication of a pregnancy develops a sequela requiring care or treatment, code O94 is assigned and sequenced after the code identifying the sequela condition. The documented personal history of gestational diabetes is also coded.

49. *Answer:* R07.1 Chest pain on breathing, F43.0 Acute stress reaction, X37.1XXA Tornado, and Y92.017 Garden or yard in a single-family (private) house as the place of occurrence of the external cause

Rationale: The ICD-10-CM Alphabetic Index no longer provides a separate code for other acute pain for use with a specified site of pain. Instead, only the pain of the site is coded when stated as acute of a specified site. The index entry for "Pain, acute" shows R52 Pain, unspecified, which has an "excludes1" note instructing the user to code to pain by site for localized pain of unspecified type. The chest pain is described as "on inspiration"; the Alphabetic Index lists "Pain, chest, on breathing or pleurodynia," R07.1. Always review the entire record for a description of the chest pain and assign a code of the highest level of specificity based on physician documentation; query when appropriate. Since the chest pain is not linked to the stress the patient is experiencing, code F43.9 Acute stress reaction is assigned. To describe the situation related to the diagnoses, assign X37.1XXA Tornado, and Y92.017 Garden or yard in a single-family (private) house, as the place of occurrence of the external cause, for this initial encounter, according to OCG section I.C.20.b.

50. *Answer:* <u>A</u> Assign Z86.74 Personal history of sudden cardiac arrest, and I25.2 Old myocardial infarction.

Rationale: The past medical history documents a past cardiac arrest and myocardial infarction. Since the patient presents for CABG due to progressive angina for which the history of cardiac arrest and myocardial infarction would be relevant, assign the personal history code for both. The Alphabetic Index lists "History, personal, cardiac arrest (death) successfully resuscitated," code Z86.74. The index entry for history of myocardial infarction is "History, personal, myocardial infarction (old)," code I25.2. History codes are appropriate for an encounter when facility policy requires them or when the history is significant to the encounter based on medical significance or in relationship to other diagnoses or conditions. OCG section III.A states that previous conditions may be coded as additional diagnoses when they affect current care or treatment.

Summary of AHA's *Coding Clinic for ICD-9-CM* Topics

The following overview briefly summarizes the topics presented in AHA's *Coding Clinic for ICD-9-CM*, first quarter of 2013. Please refer to the *Coding Clinic* for the full discussion, including the coding question, coding scenarios, and official advice.

First Quarter 2013

Bifurcated Endurant Graft

Report the appropriate code for the type of graft device deployed according to the documentation in the record concerning the device configuration (e.g., bifurcated, contralateral, tapered, straight). The use of limb extensions is included in the procedure code and is not coded separately. An endovascular graft placement procedure for abdominal aortic aneurysm (AAA) repair by deployment of graft to seal off the aneurysm with bilateral iliac extensions does not represent the use of a fenestrated or branching graft. Report an additional code to indicate that the procedure is performed on a vessel bifurcation.

Bilateral Peripheral Neuropathy

Report a bilateral neuropathy as polyneuropathy since the disease affects multiple nerves, even if the neuropathy affects the same nerve in both limbs.

Bladder Stretch Injury Secondary to Urinary Retention

Chronic bladder distension or dilation due to urinary retention may result in a "stretch injury" of the bladder. Report this diagnosis as other specified disorder of bladder. Assign a separate code for urinary retention as the cause of injury.

Cardiac Arrest With and Without Underlying Condition

Sequence cardiac arrest first when the condition meets the definition of principal diagnosis but the underlying cause of the event is unknown or established before the patient expires. Cardiac arrest is a reportable secondary diagnosis when the cause is known (sequencing underlying cause first), regardless of the success of resuscitation attempts. Report also resuscitative and life support procedures.

Catheter/Snare Retrieval of Broken Guide Wire

Report the appropriate complication of surgical and medical care with a code from category 996 when a guide wire breaks during a heart catheterization procedure. Also assign an external cause code indicating mechanical instrument failure during a procedure. Report any associated arterial catheterization procedure performed to retrieve retained or broken instrumentation.

Central Nervous System Lymphoma

ICD-9-CM classifies central nervous system lymphoma as a primary neoplasm. In the case of CNS lymphoma, the term "Primary" does not have to appear in the medical record for the primary neoplasm code to be assigned.

Congenital Sacral Nevus

Congenital nevi and other anomalies are reportable diagnoses when documented by the provider even in the absence of documented clinical evaluation or treatment. Such conditions may have implications for future health care needs. This guidance is consistent with *ICD-10-CM Official Guidelines for Coding and Reporting* section I.C.14.

Elderly Multigravida

ICD-9-CM category 659 is to be used to indicate reasons for intervention related to labor and delivery, such as delivery by cesarean section due to elderly multigravida status.

Emaciated/Emaciation Without Documented Malnutrition

Documentation of emaciation (e.g., wasting) is a descriptive term rather than a definitive diagnosis such as malnutrition. The physician must document a diagnosis of malnutrition to support a malnutrition code, regardless of type or degree of the condition. Instead, report the code for "cachexia" for conditions documented as "emaciation" or "emaciated" status.

Implantation of Vertical Expandable Prosthetic Titanium Rib

Report the implantation of a vertical expandable prosthetic titanium rib (VEPTR) device as a repair or plastic operation of the scapula/clavicle/thorax (ribs/sternum). This device consists of an expandable, curved metal rod that straightens the spine and corrects the shape of thoracic insufficiency anomalies when placed between the ribs or the ribs and spine/pelvis.

Intermittent (Nocturnal) Ventilation

For coding purposes, include the total hours of intermittent (nocturnal) ventilation, which include actual ventilation time and the weaning period, until ventilation is discontinued (i.e., turned off).

Medium and Large Vein Disease

Documentation of "medium and large vein disease" is nonspecific for coding and reporting purposes, requiring clarification by the provider. If a more precise diagnosis cannot be obtained, report the condition as an unspecified circulatory disorder.

Multifocal Motor Neuropathy

Multifocal motor neuropathy (MMN) is a rare, chronic, acquired, immune-mediated disease characterized by progressive muscle weakness, wasting, cramping, and involuntary contractions due to multifocal motor nerve conduction blocks. Treatment may include immunosupressants and immunoglobin. Report this condition as other inflammatory and toxic neuropathy.

Nonexcisional Versus Excisional Debridement

Excisional debridement must be clearly and specifically documented by the provider. Otherwise, assign the nonexcisional procedure code, regardless of site of debridement (e.g., skin, muscle, fascia, bone). For example, an open wound or fracture may require either type of debridement—the coder cannot assume debridement by excisional procedure. Coders should query for clarification as necessary.

Pipeline Embolization Device for Treatment of Carotid Artery Aneurysm

The Pipeline Embolization Device (PED) is a mesh cylinder implanted within a large brain artery to divert blood flow from the aneurysm, thus promoting therapeutic clot formation with resultant shrinkage of aneurysm. Report this procedure as an endovascular (total) embolization or occlusion of head and neck vessels.

POA for Chronic Kidney Disease, Stage 3, Progressing to End-Stage Renal Disease

Assign POA indicator "Y" for a patient with chronic kidney disease who experiences worsening or deterioration of the renal status, which occurred during admission to the hospital. Report only one code for the highest level of disease severity in accordance with previous advice.

Postsurgical Cardiac Arrest

Report cardiac arrest that occurs during or following surgery with the appropriate code from category 997 for the complication affecting the body system, in this case cardiac. Assign an additional code to report the cardiac arrest. The outcome of resuscitation procedures does not affect code assignment.

Prophylactic Cranial Irradiation Therapy for Small-Cell Lung Cancer

Prophylactic cranial irradiation (PCI) destroys quiescent malignant cells to mitigate risk of brain metastasis in high-risk neoplasm. Assign the appropriate category V58 code as the first-listed diagnosis for neoplasm therapy encounters. Indicate prophylactic therapies with the appropriate V07 code. Report a neoplastic disease in remission as a personal history of neoplasm, by anatomic site.

Pulseless Electrical Activity

Documentation of pulseless electrical activity (PEA) indicates the presence of electrical cardiac activity, although insufficient to coordinate myocardial contractions to produce a detectable pulse. Underlying causes include hypovolemia or respiratory failure with hypoxia. Report documented PEA as a cardiac arrest.

Rib Fracture due to Cardiopulmonary Resuscitation

Rib fracture is a common risk associated with cardiopulmonary resuscitation (CPR) and is not considered a complication of the procedure. Assign the appropriate rib fracture and external cause codes.

Sacral Dimple in a Newborn

Sacral dimple is a congenital condition sometimes associated with an underlying spinal cord anomaly. When documented by the provider, this condition should be reported as other specified anomaly of the skin.

Self-Extubation and Mechanical Ventilation

Report total hours of mechanical ventilation, whether or not the patient self-extubates or requires re-intubation. Clinical indicators and a physician's order determine discontinuation time for ventilation.

Tracheostomy

Assign temporary tracheostomy, not other permanent tracheostomy, as the default procedure code when tracheostomy is not further specified.

Transsphenoidal Resection of Pituitary Tumor with Placement of Fat Graft

Pituitary tumor resection may require multiple codes. Assign the appropriate hypophysectomy code according to the surgical approach. Also assign additional codes for fat graft harvested from abdomen to fill the surgical defect and any lumbar drain placement to treat cerebrospinal fluid (CSF) leak.

Ventilator Weaning

Continuous invasive mechanical ventilation time ends when the ventilator is turned off. Subsequent patient monitoring and evaluation time is not included in the total hours reported.

Official ICD-9-CM Guidelines for Coding and Reporting

Effective October 1, 2011
Note: Since no official ICD-9-CM addendum to the guidelines was released since 2011, the guidelines included in this book stand as the official guidelines effective October 1, 2013, through September 30, 2014.

The Centers for Medicare and Medicaid Services (CMS) and the National Center for Health Statistics (NCHS), two departments within the U.S. Federal Government's Department of Health and Human Services (DHHS) provide the following guidelines for coding and reporting using the International Classification of Diseases, 9th Revision, Clinical Modification (ICD-9-CM). These guidelines should be used as a companion document to the official version of the ICD-9-CM as published on CD-ROM by the U.S. Government Printing Office (GPO).

These guidelines have been approved by the four organizations that make up the Cooperating Parties for the ICD-9-CM: the American Hospital Association (AHA), the American Health Information Management Association (AHIMA), CMS, and NCHS. These guidelines are included on the official government version of the ICD-9-CM, and also appear in *"Coding Clinic for ICD-9-CM"* published by the AHA.

These guidelines are a set of rules that have been developed to accompany and complement the official conventions and instructions provided within the ICD-9-CM itself. The instructions and conventions of the classification take precedence over guidelines. These guidelines are based on the coding and sequencing instructions in Volumes I, II and III of ICD-9-CM, but provide additional instruction. Adherence to these guidelines when assigning ICD-9-CM diagnosis and procedure codes is required under the Health Insurance Portability and Accountability Act (HIPAA). The diagnosis codes (Volumes 1-2) have been adopted under HIPAA for all healthcare settings. Volume 3 procedure codes have been adopted for inpatient procedures reported by hospitals. A joint effort between the healthcare provider and the coder is essential to achieve complete and accurate documentation, code assignment, and reporting of diagnoses and procedures. These guidelines have been developed to assist both the healthcare provider and the coder in identifying those diagnoses and procedures that are to be reported. The importance of consistent, complete documentation in the medical record cannot be overemphasized. Without such documentation accurate coding cannot be achieved. The entire record should be reviewed to determine the specific reason for the encounter and the conditions treated.

The term encounter is used for all settings, including hospital admissions. In the context of these guidelines, the term provider is used throughout the guidelines to mean physician or any qualified health care practitioner who is legally accountable for establishing the patient's diagnosis. Only this set of guidelines, approved by the Cooperating Parties, is official.

The guidelines are organized into sections. Section I includes the structure and conventions of the classification and general guidelines that apply to the entire classification, and chapter-specific guidelines that correspond to the chapters as they are arranged in the classification. Section II includes guidelines for selection of principal diagnosis for non-outpatient settings. Section III includes guidelines for reporting additional diagnoses in non-outpatient settings. Section IV is for outpatient coding and reporting.

Section I. Conventions, general coding guidelines and chapter specific guidelines

A. Conventions for the ICD-9-CM
  1. Format:
  2. Abbreviations
      a. Index abbreviations
      b. Tabular abbreviations
  3. Punctuation
  4. Includes and Excludes Notes and Inclusion terms
  5. Other and Unspecified codes
      a. "Other" codes
      b. "Unspecified" codes
  6. Etiology/manifestation convention ("code first", "use additional code" and "in diseases classified elsewhere" notes)
  7. "And"

8. "With"
9. "See" and "See Also"

B. General Coding Guidelines
  1. Use of Both Alphabetic Index and Tabular List
  2. Locate each term in the Alphabetic Index
  3. Level of Detail in Coding
  4. Code or codes from 001.0 through V91.99
  5. Selection of codes 001.0 through 999.9
  6. Signs and symptoms
  7. Conditions that are an integral part of a disease process
  8. Conditions that are not an integral part of a disease process
  9. Multiple coding for a single condition
  10. Acute and Chronic Conditions
  11. Combination Code
  12. Late Effects
  13. Impending or Threatened Condition
  14. Reporting Same Diagnosis Code More than Once
  15. Admissions/Encounters for Rehabilitation
  16. Documentation for BMI and Pressure Ulcer Stages
  17. Syndromes
  18. Documentation of Complications of Care

C. Chapter-Specific Coding Guidelines
  1. Chapter 1: Infectious and Parasitic Diseases (001-139)
      a. Human Immunodeficiency Virus (HIV) Infections
      b. Septicemia, Systemic Inflammatory Response Syndrome (SIRS), Sepsis, Severe Sepsis and Septic Shock
      c. Methicillin Resistant *Staphylococcus aureus* (MRSA) Conditions
  2. Chapter 2: Neoplasms (140-239)
      a. Treatment directed at the malignancy
      b. Treatment of secondary site
      c. Coding and sequencing of complications
      d. Primary malignancy previously excised
      e. Admissions/Encounters involving chemotherapy, immunotherapy and radiation therapy
      f. Admission/encounter to determine extent of malignancy
      g. Symptoms, signs, and ill-defined conditions listed in Chapter 16 associated with neoplasms
      h. Admission/encounter for pain control/management
      i. Malignant neoplasm associated with transplanted organ
  3. Chapter 3: Endocrine, Nutritional, and Metabolic Diseases and Immunity Disorders (240-279)
      a. Diabetes mellitus
  4. Chapter 4: Diseases of Blood and Blood Forming Organs (280-289)
      a. Anemia of chronic disease
  5. Chapter 5: Mental Disorders (290-319)
      Reserved for future guideline expansion
  6. Chapter 6: Diseases of Nervous System and Sense Organs (320-389)
      a. Pain - Category 338
      b. Glaucoma
  7. Chapter 7: Diseases of Circulatory System (390-459)
      a. Hypertension
      b. Cerebral infarction/stroke/ from cerebrovascular accident (CVA)
      c. Postoperative cerebrovascular accident
      d. Late Effects of Cerebrovascular Disease
      e. Acute myocardial infarction (AMI)

Section II. Selection of Principal Diagnosis

Section III. Reporting Additional Diagnoses

Section IV. Diagnostic Coding and Reporting Guidelines for Outpatient Services

Appendix I: Present on Admission Reporting Guidelines

Section I. Conventions, general coding guidelines and chapter specific guidelines

The conventions, general guidelines and chapter-specific guidelines are applicable to all health care settings unless otherwise indicated. The conventions and instructions of the classification take precedence over guidelines.

A. Conventions for the ICD-9-CM

The conventions for the ICD-9-CM are the general rules for use of the classification independent of the guidelines. These conventions are incorporated within the index and tabular of the ICD-9-CM as instructional notes. The conventions are as follows:

1. Format:

The ICD-9-CM uses an indented format for ease in reference

2. Abbreviations

a. Index abbreviations

NEC "Not elsewhere classifiable"

This abbreviation in the index represents "other specified" when a specific code is not available for a condition the index directs the coder to the "other specified" code in the tabular.

b. Tabular abbreviations

NEC "Not elsewhere classifiable"

This abbreviation in the tabular represents "other specified". When a specific code is not available for a condition the tabular includes an NEC entry under a code to identify the code as the "other specified" code.
(See Section I.A.5.a. "Other" codes").

NOS "Not otherwise specified"

This abbreviation is the equivalent of unspecified.
(See Section I.A.5.b., "Unspecified" codes)

3. Punctuation

[ ]   Brackets are used in the tabular list to enclose synonyms, alternative wording or explanatory phrases. Brackets are used in the index to identify manifestation codes.
(See Section I.A.6. "Etiology/manifestations")

( )   Parentheses are used in both the index and tabular to enclose supplementary words that may be present or absent in the statement of a disease or procedure without affecting the code number to which it is assigned. The terms within the parentheses are referred to as nonessential modifiers.

:   Colons are used in the Tabular list after an incomplete term which needs one or more of the modifiers following the colon to make it assignable to a given category.

4. Includes and Excludes Notes and Inclusion terms

Includes: This note appears immediately under a three-digit code title to further define, or give examples of, the content of the category.

Excludes: An excludes note under a code indicates that the terms excluded from the code are to be coded elsewhere. In some cases the codes for the excluded terms should not be used in conjunction with the code from which it is excluded. An example of this is a congenital condition excluded from an acquired form of the same condition. The congenital and acquired codes should not be used together. In other cases, the excluded terms may be used together with an excluded code. An example of this is when fractures of different bones are coded to different codes. Both codes may be used together if both types of fractures are present.

Inclusion terms: List of terms is included under certain four and five digit codes. These terms are the conditions for which that code number is to be used. The terms may be synonyms of the code title, or, in the case of "other specified" codes, the terms are a list of the various conditions assigned to that code. The inclusion terms are not necessarily exhaustive. Additional terms found only in the index may also be assigned to a code.

5. Other and Unspecified codes

a. "Other" codes

Codes titled "other" or "other specified" (usually a code with a 4th digit 8 or fifth-digit 9 for diagnosis codes) are for use when the information in the medical record provides detail for which a specific code does not exist. Index entries with NEC in the line designate "other" codes in the tabular. These index entries represent specific disease entities for which no specific code exists so the term is included within an "other" code.

b. "Unspecified" codes

Codes (usually a code with a 4th digit 9 or 5th digit 0 for diagnosis codes) titled "unspecified" are for use when the information in the medical record is insufficient to assign a more specific code.

6. Etiology/manifestation convention ("code first", "use additional code" and "in diseases classified elsewhere" notes)

Certain conditions have both an underlying etiology and multiple body system manifestations due to the underlying etiology. For such conditions, the ICD-9-CM has a coding convention that requires the underlying condition be sequenced first followed by the manifestation. Wherever such a combination exists, there is a "use additional code" note at the etiology code, and a "code first" note at the manifestation code. These instructional notes indicate the proper sequencing order of the codes, etiology followed by manifestation.

In most cases the manifestation codes will have in the code title, "in diseases classified elsewhere." Codes with this title are a component of the etiology/ manifestation convention. The code title indicates that it is a manifestation code. "In diseases classified elsewhere" codes are never permitted to be used as first listed or principal diagnosis codes. They must be used in conjunction with an underlying condition code and they must be listed following the underlying condition.

There are manifestation codes that do not have "in diseases classified elsewhere" in the title. For such codes a "use additional code" note will still be present and the rules for sequencing apply.

In addition to the notes in the tabular, these conditions also have a specific index entry structure. In the index both conditions are listed together with the etiology code first followed by the manifestation codes in brackets. The code in brackets is always to be sequenced second.

The most commonly used etiology/manifestation combinations are the codes for Diabetes mellitus, category 250. For each code under category 250 there is a use additional code note for the manifestation that is specific for that particular diabetic manifestation. Should a patient have more than one manifestation of diabetes, more than one code from category 250 may be used with as many manifestation codes as are needed to fully describe the patient's complete diabetic condition. The category 250 diabetes codes should be sequenced first, followed by the manifestation codes.

"Code first" and "Use additional code" notes are also used as sequencing rules in the classification for certain codes that are not part of an etiology/ manifestation combination.
See - Section I.B.9. "Multiple coding for a single condition".

7. "And"

The word "and" should be interpreted to mean either "and" or "or" when it appears in a title.

8. "With"

The word "with" should be interpreted to mean "associated with" or "due to" when it appears in a code title, the Alphabetic Index, or an instructional note in the Tabular List.

The word "with" in the alphabetic index is sequenced immediately following the main term, not in alphabetical order.

9. "See" and "See Also"

The "see" instruction following a main term in the index indicates that another term should be referenced. It is necessary to go to the main term referenced with the "see" note to locate the correct code.

A "see also" instruction following a main term in the index instructs that there is another main term that may also be referenced that may provide additional index entries that may be useful. It is not necessary to follow the "see also" note when the original main term provides the necessary code.

B. General Coding Guidelines

1. Use of Both Alphabetic Index and Tabular List

Use both the Alphabetic Index and the Tabular List when locating and assigning a code. Reliance on only the Alphabetic Index or the Tabular List leads to errors in code assignments and less specificity in code selection.

2. Locate each term in the Alphabetic Index

Locate each term in the Alphabetic Index and verify the code selected in the Tabular List. Read and be guided by instructional notations that appear in both the Alphabetic Index and the Tabular List.

3. Level of Detail in Coding

Diagnosis and procedure codes are to be used at their highest number of digits available.

ICD-9-CM diagnosis codes are composed of codes with 3, 4, or 5 digits. Codes with three digits are included in ICD-9-CM as the heading of a category of codes that may be further subdivided by the use of fourth and/or fifth digits, which provide greater detail.

A three-digit code is to be used only if it is not further subdivided. Where fourth-digit subcategories and/or fifth-digit subclassifications are provided, they must be assigned. A code is invalid if it has not been coded to the full number of digits required for that code. For example, Acute myocardial infarction, code 410, has fourth digits that describe the location of the infarction (e.g., 410.2, Of inferolateral wall), and fifth digits that identify the episode of care. It would be incorrect to report a code in category 410 without a fourth and fifth digit.

ICD-9-CM Volume 3 procedure codes are composed of codes with either 3 or 4 digits. Codes with two digits are included in ICD-9-CM as the heading of a category of codes that may be further subdivided by the use of third and/or fourth digits, which provide greater detail.

4. Code or codes from 001.0 through V91.99

The appropriate code or codes from 001.0 through V91.99 must be used to identify diagnoses, symptoms, conditions, problems, complaints or other reason(s) for the encounter/visit.

5. Selection of codes 001.0 through 999.9

The selection of codes 001.0 through 999.9 will frequently be used to describe the reason for the admission/encounter. These codes are from the section of ICD-9-CM for the classification of diseases and injuries (e.g., infectious and parasitic diseases; neoplasms; symptoms, signs, and ill-defined conditions, etc.).

6. Signs and symptoms

Codes that describe symptoms and signs, as opposed to diagnoses, are acceptable for reporting purposes when a related definitive diagnosis has not been established (confirmed) by the provider. Chapter 16 of ICD-9-CM, Symptoms, Signs, and Ill-defined conditions (codes 780.0 - 799.9) contain many, but not all codes for symptoms.

7. Conditions that are an integral part of a disease process

Signs and symptoms that are associated routinely with a disease process should not be assigned as additional codes, unless otherwise instructed by the classification.

8. Conditions that are not an integral part of a disease process

Additional signs and symptoms that may not be associated routinely with a disease process should be coded when present.

9. Multiple coding for a single condition

In addition to the etiology/manifestation convention that requires two codes to fully describe a single condition that affects multiple body systems, there are other single conditions that also require more than one code. "Use additional code" notes are found in the tabular at codes that are not part of an etiology/manifestation pair where a secondary code is useful to fully describe a condition. The sequencing rule is the same as the etiology/manifestation pair - "use additional code" indicates that a secondary code should be added.

For example, for infections that are not included in chapter 1, a secondary code from category 041, Bacterial infection in conditions classified elsewhere and of unspecified site, may be required to identify the bacterial organism causing the infection. A "use additional code" note will normally be found at the infectious disease code, indicating a need for the organism code to be added as a secondary code.

"Code first" notes are also under certain codes that are not specifically manifestation codes but may be due to an underlying cause. When a "code first" note is present and an underlying condition is present the underlying condition should be sequenced first.

"Code, if applicable, any causal condition first", notes indicate that this code may be assigned as a principal diagnosis when the causal condition is unknown or not applicable. If a causal condition is known, then the code for that condition should be sequenced as the principal or first-listed diagnosis.

Multiple codes may be needed for late effects, complication codes and obstetric codes to more fully describe a condition. See the specific guidelines for these conditions for further instruction.

10. Acute and Chronic Conditions

If the same condition is described as both acute (subacute) and chronic, and separate subentries exist in the Alphabetic Index at the same indentation level, code both and sequence the acute (subacute) code first.

11. Combination Code

A combination code is a single code used to classify:

- Two diagnoses, or
- A diagnosis with an associated secondary process (manifestation)
- A diagnosis with an associated complication

Combination codes are identified by referring to subterm entries in the Alphabetic Index and by reading the inclusion and exclusion notes in the Tabular List.

Assign only the combination code when that code fully identifies the diagnostic conditions involved or when the Alphabetic Index so directs. Multiple coding should not be used when the classification provides a combination code that clearly identifies all of the elements documented in the diagnosis. When the combination code lacks necessary specificity in describing the manifestation or complication, an additional code should be used as a secondary code.

12. Late Effects

A late effect is the residual effect (condition produced) after the acute phase of an illness or injury has terminated. There is no time limit on when a late effect code can be used. The residual may be apparent early, such as in cerebrovascular accident cases, or it may occur months or years later, such as that due to a previous injury. Coding of late effects generally requires two codes sequenced in the following order: The condition or nature of the late effect is sequenced first. The late effect code is sequenced second.

Exceptions to the above guidelines are those instances the late effect code has been expanded (at the fourth and fifth-digit levels) to include the manifestation(s) or the classification instructs otherwise. The code for the acute phase of an illness or injury that led to the late effect is never used with a code for the late effect.

13. Impending or Threatened Condition

Code any condition described at the time of discharge as "impending" or "threatened" as follows:

If it did occur, code as confirmed diagnosis.
If it did not occur, reference the Alphabetic Index to determine if the condition has a subentry term for "impending" or "threatened" and also reference main term entries for "Impending" and for "Threatened."
If the subterms are listed, assign the given code.
If the subterms are not listed, code the existing underlying condition(s) and not the condition described as impending or threatened.

14. Reporting Same Diagnosis Code More than Once

Each unique ICD-9-CM diagnosis code may be reported only once for an encounter. This applies to bilateral conditions or two different conditions classified to the same ICD-9-CM diagnosis code.

15. Admissions/Encounters for Rehabilitation

When the purpose for the admission/encounter is rehabilitation, sequence the appropriate V code from category V57, Care involving use of rehabilitation procedures, as the principal/first-listed diagnosis. The code for the condition for which the service is being performed should be reported as an additional diagnosis.

Only one code from category V57 is required. Code V57.89, Other specified rehabilitation procedures, should be assigned if more than one type of rehabilitation is performed during a single encounter. A procedure code should be reported to identify each type of rehabilitation therapy actually performed.

16. Documentation for BMI and Pressure Ulcer Stages

For the Body Mass Index (BMI) and pressure ulcer stage codes, code assignment may be based on medical record documentation from clinicians who are not the patient's provider (i.e., physician or other qualified healthcare practitioner legally accountable for establishing the patient's diagnosis), since this information is typically documented by other clinicians involved in the care of the patient (e.g., a dietitian often documents the BMI and nurses often documents the pressure ulcer stages). However, the associated diagnosis (such as overweight, obesity, or pressure ulcer) must be documented by the patient's provider. If there is conflicting medical record documentation, either from the same clinician or different clinicians, the patient's attending provider should be queried for clarification.

The BMI and pressure ulcer stage codes should only be reported as secondary diagnoses. As with all other secondary diagnosis codes, the BMI and pressure ulcer stage codes should only be assigned when they meet the definition of a reportable additional diagnosis (see Section III, Reporting Additional Diagnoses).

17. Syndromes

Follow the Alphabetic Index guidance when coding syndromes. In the absence of index guidance, assign codes for the documented manifestations of the syndrome.

18. Documentation of complications of care

Code assignment is based on the provider's documentation of the relationship between the condition and the care or procedure. The guideline extends to any complications of care, regardless of the chapter the code is located in. It is important to note that not all conditions that occur during or following medical care or surgery are classified as complications. There must be a cause-and-effect relationship between the care provided and the condition, and an indication in the documentation that it is a complication. Query the provider for clarification, if the complication is not clearly documented.

C. Chapter-Specific Coding Guidelines

In addition to general coding guidelines, there are guidelines for specific diagnoses and/or conditions in the classification. Unless otherwise indicated, these guidelines apply to all health care settings. Please refer to Section II for guidelines on the selection of principal diagnosis.

1. Chapter 1: Infectious and Parasitic Diseases (001-139)

a. Human Immunodeficiency Virus (HIV) Infections

1) Code only confirmed cases

Code only confirmed cases of HIV infection/illness. This is an exception to the hospital inpatient guideline Section II, H.

In this context, "confirmation" does not require documentation of positive serology or culture for HIV; the provider's diagnostic statement that the patient is HIV positive, or has an HIV-related illness is sufficient.

2) Selection and sequencing of HIV codes

(a) Patient admitted for HIV-related condition

If a patient is admitted for an HIV-related condition, the principal diagnosis should be 042, followed by additional diagnosis codes for all reported HIV-related conditions.

(b) Patient with HIV disease admitted for unrelated condition

If a patient with HIV disease is admitted for an unrelated condition (such as a traumatic injury), the code for the unrelated condition (e.g., the nature of injury code) should be the principal diagnosis. Other diagnoses would be 042 followed by additional diagnosis codes for all reported HIV-related conditions.

(c) Whether the patient is newly diagnosed

Whether the patient is newly diagnosed or has had previous admissions/encounters for HIV conditions is irrelevant to the sequencing decision.

(d) Asymptomatic human immunodeficiency virus

V08 Asymptomatic human immunodeficiency virus [HIV] infection, is to be applied when the patient without any documentation of symptoms is listed as being "HIV positive," "known HIV," "HIV test positive," or similar terminology. Do not use this code if the term "AIDS" is used or if the patient is treated for any HIV-related illness or is described as having any condition(s) resulting from his/her HIV positive status; use 042 in these cases.

(e) Patients with inconclusive HIV serology

Patients with inconclusive HIV serology, but no definitive diagnosis or manifestations of the illness, may be assigned code 795.71, Inconclusive serologic test for Human Immunodeficiency Virus [HIV].

(f) Previously diagnosed HIV-related illness

Patients with any known prior diagnosis of an HIV-related illness should be coded to 042. Once a patient has developed an HIV-related illness, the patient should always be assigned code 042 on every subsequent admission/encounter. Patients previously diagnosed with any HIV illness (042) should never be assigned to 795.71 or V08.

(g) HIV Infection in Pregnancy, Childbirth and the Puerperium

During pregnancy, childbirth or the puerperium, a patient admitted (or presenting for a health care encounter) because of an HIV-related illness should receive a principal diagnosis code of 647.6x, Other specified infectious and parasitic diseases in the mother classifiable elsewhere, but complicating the pregnancy, childbirth or the puerperium, followed by 042 and the code(s) for the HIV-related illness(es). Codes from Chapter 15 always take sequencing priority.

Patients with asymptomatic HIV infection status admitted (or presenting for a health care encounter) during pregnancy, childbirth, or the puerperium should receive codes of 647.6x and V08.

(h) Encounters for testing for HIV

If a patient is being seen to determine his/her HIV status, use code V73.89, Screening for other specified viral disease. Use code V69.8, Other problems related to lifestyle, as a secondary code if an asymptomatic patient is in a known high risk group for HIV. Should a patient with signs or symptoms or illness, or a confirmed HIV related diagnosis be tested for HIV, code the signs and symptoms or the diagnosis. An additional counseling code V65.44 may be used if counseling is provided during the encounter for the test.

When a patient returns to be informed of his/her HIV test results use code V65.44, HIV counseling, if the results of the test are negative.

If the results are positive but the patient is asymptomatic use code V08, Asymptomatic HIV infection. If the results are positive and the patient is symptomatic use code 042, HIV infection, with codes for the HIV related symptoms or diagnosis. The HIV counseling code may also be used if counseling is provided for patients with positive test results.

b. Septicemia, Systemic Inflammatory Response Syndrome (SIRS), Sepsis, Severe Sepsis, and Septic Shock

1) SIRS, Septicemia, and Sepsis

(a) The terms *septicemia* and *sepsis* are often used interchangeably by providers, however they are not considered synonymous terms. The following descriptions are provided for reference but do not preclude querying the provider for clarification about terms used in the documentation:

(i) Septicemia generally refers to a systemic disease associated with the presence of pathological microorganisms or toxins in the blood, which can include bacteria, viruses, fungi or other organisms.

(ii) Systemic inflammatory response syndrome (SIRS) generally refers to the systemic response to infection, trauma/burns, or other insult (such as cancer) with symptoms including fever, tachycardia, tachypnea, and leukocytosis.

(iii) Sepsis generally refers to SIRS due to infection.

(iv) Severe sepsis generally refers to sepsis with associated acute organ dysfunction.

(b) The Coding of SIRS, sepsis and severe sepsis

The coding of SIRS, sepsis and severe sepsis requires a minimum of 2 codes: a code for the underlying cause (such as infection or trauma) and a code from subcategory 995.9 Systemic inflammatory response syndrome (SIRS).

(i) The code for the underlying cause (such as infection or trauma) must be sequenced before the code from subcategory 995.9 Systemic inflammatory response syndrome (SIRS).

(ii) Sepsis and severe sepsis require a code for the systemic infection (038.xx, 112.5, etc.) and either code 995.91, Sepsis, or 995.92, Severe sepsis. If the causal organism is not documented, assign code 038.9, Unspecified septicemia.

(iii) Severe sepsis requires additional code(s) for the associated acute organ dysfunction(s).

(iv) If a patient has sepsis with multiple organ dysfunctions, follow the instructions for coding severe sepsis.

(v) Either the term sepsis or SIRS must be documented to assign a code from subcategory 995.9.

(vi) See Section I.C.17.g), Injury and poisoning, for information regarding systemic inflammatory response syndrome (SIRS) due to trauma/burns and other non-infectious processes.

(c) Due to the complex nature of sepsis and severe sepsis, some cases may require querying the provider prior to assignment of the codes.

2) Sequencing sepsis and severe sepsis

(a) Sepsis and severe sepsis as principal diagnosis

If sepsis or severe sepsis is present on admission, and meets the definition of principal diagnosis, the systemic infection code (e.g., 038.xx, 112.5, etc) should be assigned as the principal diagnosis, followed by code 995.91, Sepsis, or 995.92, Severe sepsis, as required by the sequencing rules in the Tabular List. Codes from subcategory 995.9 can never be assigned as a principal diagnosis. A code should also be assigned for any localized infection, if present.

If the sepsis or severe sepsis is due to a postprocedural infection, see Section I.C.1.b.10 for guidelines related to sepsis due to postprocedural infection.

(b) Sepsis and severe sepsis as secondary diagnoses

When sepsis or severe sepsis develops during the encounter (it was not present on admission), the systemic infection code and code 995.91 or 995.92 should be assigned as secondary diagnoses.

(c) Documentation unclear as to whether sepsis or severe sepsis is present on admission

Sepsis or severe sepsis may be present on admission but the diagnosis may not be confirmed until sometime after admission. If the documentation is not clear whether the sepsis or severe sepsis was present on admission, the provider should be queried.

3) Sepsis/SIRS with Localized Infection

If the reason for admission is both sepsis, severe sepsis, or SIRS and a localized infection, such as pneumonia or cellulitis, a code for the systemic infection (038.xx, 112.5, etc) should be assigned first, then code 995.91 or 995.92, followed by the code for the localized infection. If the patient is admitted with a localized infection, such as pneumonia, and sepsis/SIRS doesn't develop until after admission, see guideline I.C.1.b.2.b).

If the localized infection is postprocedural, *see Section I.C.1.b.10 for guidelines related to sepsis due to postprocedural infection.*

Note: The term urosepsis is a nonspecific term. If that is the only term documented then only code 599.0 should be assigned based on the default for the term in the ICD-9-CM index, in addition to the code for the causal organism if known.

4) Bacterial Sepsis and Septicemia

In most cases, it will be a code from category 038, Septicemia, that will be used in conjunction with a code from subcategory 995.9 such as the following:

(a) Streptococcal sepsis

If the documentation in the record states streptococcal sepsis, codes 038.0, Streptococcal septicemia, and code 995.91 should be used, in that sequence.

(b) Streptococcal septicemia

If the documentation states streptococcal septicemia, only code 038.0 should be assigned, however, the provider should be queried whether the patient has sepsis, an infection with SIRS.

5) Acute organ dysfunction that is not clearly associated with the sepsis

If a patient has sepsis and an acute organ dysfunction, but the medical record documentation indicates that the acute organ dysfunction is related to a medical condition other than the sepsis, do not assign code 995.92, Severe sepsis. An acute organ dysfunction must be associated with the sepsis in order to assign the severe sepsis code. If the documentation is not clear as to whether an acute organ dysfunction is related to the sepsis or another medical condition, query the provider.

6) Septic shock

(a) Sequencing of septic shock

Septic shock generally refers to circulatory failure associated with severe sepsis, and, therefore, it represents a type of acute organ dysfunction.

For cases of septic shock, the code for the systemic infection should be sequenced first, followed by codes 995.92, Severe sepsis and 785.52, Septic shock or 998.02, Postoperative septic shock. Any additional codes for other acute organ dysfunctions should also be assigned. As noted in the sequencing instructions in the Tabular List, the code for septic shock cannot be assigned as a principal diagnosis.

(b) Septic Shock without documentation of severe sepsis

Since septic shock indicates the presence of severe sepsis, code 995.92, Severe sepsis, can be assigned with code 785.52, Septic shock, or code 998.02 Postoperative shock, septic, even if the term severe sepsis is not documented in the record.

7) Sepsis and septic shock complicating abortion and pregnancy

Sepsis and septic shock complicating abortion, ectopic pregnancy, and molar pregnancy are classified to category codes in Chapter 11 (630-639).

See section I.C.11.i.7. for information on the coding of puerperal sepsis.

8) Negative or inconclusive blood cultures

Negative or inconclusive blood cultures do not preclude a diagnosis of septicemia or sepsis in patients with clinical evidence of the condition, however, the provider should be queried.

9) Newborn sepsis

See Section I.C.15.j for information on the coding of newborn sepsis.

10) Sepsis due to a Postprocedural Infection

(a) Documentation of causal relationship

As with all postprocedural complications, code assignment is based on the provider's documentation of the relationship between the infection and the procedure.

(b) Sepsis due to postprocedural infection

In cases of postprocedural sepsis, the complication code, such as code 998.59, Other postoperative infection, or 674.3x, Other complications of obstetrical surgical wounds should be coded first followed by the appropriate sepsis codes (systemic infection code and either code 995.91 or 995.92). An additional code(s) for any acute organ dysfunction should also be assigned for cases of severe sepsis.

See Section see Section I.C.1.b.6 if the sepsis or severe sepsis results in postprocedural septic shock.

(c) Postprocedural infection and postprocedural septic shock

In cases where a postprocedural infection has occurred and has resulted in severe sepsis and postprocedural septic shock, the code for the precipitating complication such as code 998.59, Other postoperative infection, or 674.3x, Other complications of obstetrical surgical wounds should be coded first followed by the appropriate sepsis codes (systemic infection code and code 995.92). Code 998.02, Postoperative septic shock, should be assigned as an additional code. In cases of severe sepsis, an additional code(s) for any acute organ dysfunction should also be assigned.

11) External cause of injury codes with SIRS

Refer to Section I.C.19.a.7 for instruction on the use of external cause of injury codes with codes for SIRS resulting from trauma.

12) Sepsis and Severe Sepsis Associated with Non-infectious Process

In some cases, a non-infectious process, such as trauma, may lead to an infection which can result in sepsis or severe sepsis. If sepsis or severe sepsis is documented as associated with a non-infectious condition, such as a burn or serious injury, and this condition meets the definition for principal diagnosis, the code for the non-infectious condition should be sequenced first, followed by the code for the systemic infection and either code 995.91, Sepsis, or 995.92, Severe sepsis. Additional codes for any associated acute organ dysfunction(s) should also be assigned for cases of severe sepsis. If the sepsis or severe sepsis meets the definition of principal diagnosis, the systemic infection and sepsis codes should be sequenced before the non-infectious condition. When both the associated non-infectious condition and the sepsis or severe sepsis meet the definition of principal diagnosis, either may be assigned as principal diagnosis.

See Section I.C.1.b.2.a. for guidelines pertaining to sepsis or severe sepsis as the principal diagnosis.

Only one code from subcategory 995.9 should be assigned. Therefore, when a non-infectious condition leads to an infection resulting in sepsis or severe sepsis, assign either code 995.91 or 995.92. Do not additionally assign code 995.93, Systemic inflammatory response syndrome due to non-infectious process without acute organ dysfunction, or 995.94, Systemic inflammatory response syndrome with acute organ dysfunction.

See Section I.C.17.g for information on the coding of SIRS due to trauma/burns or other non-infectious disease processes.

c. Methicillin Resistant Staphylococcus aureus (MRSA) Conditions

1) Selection and sequencing of MRSA codes

(a) Combination codes for MRSA infection

When a patient is diagnosed with an infection that is due to methicillin resistant *Staphylococcus aureus* (MRSA), and that infection has a combination code that includes the causal organism (e.g., septicemia, pneumonia) assign the appropriate code for the condition (e.g., code 038.12, Methicillin resistant Staphylococcus aureus septicemia or code 482.42, Methicillin resistant pneumonia due to Staphylococcus aureus). Do not assign code 041.12, Methicillin resistant Staphylococcus aureus, as an additional code because the code includes the type of infection and the MRSA organism. Do not assign a code from subcategory V09.0, Infection with microorganisms resistant to penicillins, as an additional diagnosis.

See Section C.1.b.1 for instructions on coding and sequencing of septicemia.

(b) Other codes for MRSA infection

When there is documentation of a current infection (e.g., wound infection, stitch abscess, urinary tract infection) due to MRSA, and that infection does not have a combination code that includes the causal organism, select the appropriate code to identify the condition along with code 041.12, Methicillin resistant Staphylococcus aureus, for the MRSA infection. Do not assign a code from subcategory V09.0, Infection with microorganisms resistant to penicillins.

(c) Methicillin susceptible Staphylococcus aureus (MSSA) and MRSA colonization

The condition or state of being colonized or carrying MSSA or MRSA is called colonization or carriage, while an individual person is described as being colonized or being a carrier. Colonization means that MSSA or MSRA is present on or in the body without necessarily causing illness. A positive MRSA colonization test might be documented by the provider as "MRSA screen positive" or "MRSA nasal swab positive".

Assign code V02.54, Carrier or suspected carrier, Methicillin resistant Staphylococcus aureus, for patients documented as having MRSA colonization. Assign code V02.53, Carrier or suspected carrier, Methicillin susceptible Staphylococcus aureus, for patient documented as having MSSA colonization. Colonization is not necessarily indicative of a disease process or as the cause of a specific condition the patient may have unless documented as such by the provider.

Code V02.59, Other specified bacterial diseases, should be assigned for other types of staphylococcal colonization (e.g., S. *epidermidis*, S. *saprophyticus*). Code

V02.59 should not be assigned for colonization with any type of *Staphylococcus aureus* (MRSA, MSSA).

(d) MRSA colonization and infection

If a patient is documented as having both MRSA colonization and infection during a hospital admission, code V02.54, Carrier or suspected carrier, Methicillin resistant *Staphylococcus aureus*, and a code for the MRSA infection may both be assigned.

2. **Chapter 2: Neoplasms (140-239)**

General guidelines

Chapter 2 of the ICD-9-CM contains the codes for most benign and all malignant neoplasms. Certain benign neoplasms, such as prostatic adenomas, may be found in the specific body system chapters. To properly code a neoplasm it is necessary to determine from the record if the neoplasm is benign, in-situ, malignant, or of uncertain histologic behavior. If malignant, any secondary (metastatic) sites should also be determined.

The neoplasm table in the Alphabetic Index should be referenced first. However, if the histological term is documented, that term should be referenced first, rather than going immediately to the Neoplasm Table, in order to determine which column in the Neoplasm Table is appropriate. For example, if the documentation indicates "adenoma," refer to the term in the Alphabetic Index to review the entries under this term and the instructional note to "see also neoplasm, by site, benign." The table provides the proper code based on the type of neoplasm and the site. It is important to select the proper column in the table that corresponds to the type of neoplasm. The tabular should then be referenced to verify that the correct code has been selected from the table and that a more specific site code does not exist.

See Section I. C. 18.d.4. for information regarding V codes for genetic susceptibility to cancer.

a. Treatment directed at the malignancy

If the treatment is directed at the malignancy, designate the malignancy as the principal diagnosis.

The only exception to this guideline is if a patient admission/encounter is solely for the administration of chemotherapy, immunotherapy or radiation therapy, assign the appropriate V58.x code as the first-listed or principal diagnosis, and the diagnosis or problem for which the service is being performed as a secondary diagnosis.

b. Treatment of secondary site

When a patient is admitted because of a primary neoplasm with metastasis and treatment is directed toward the secondary site only, the secondary neoplasm is designated as the principal diagnosis even though the primary malignancy is still present.

c. Coding and sequencing of complications

Coding and sequencing of complications associated with the malignancies or with the therapy thereof are subject to the following guidelines:

1) Anemia associated with malignancy

When admission/encounter is for management of an anemia associated with the malignancy, and the treatment is only for anemia, the appropriate anemia code (such as code 285.22, Anemia in neoplastic disease) is designated as the principal diagnosis and is followed by the appropriate code(s) for the malignancy.

Code 285.22 may also be used as a secondary code if the patient suffers from anemia and is being treated for the malignancy.

If anemia in neoplastic disease and anemia due to antineoplastic chemotherapy are both documented, assign codes for both conditions.

2) Anemia associated with chemotherapy, immunotherapy and radiation therapy

When the admission/encounter is for management of an anemia associated with chemotherapy, immunotherapy or radiotherapy and the only treatment is for the anemia, the

anemia is sequenced first. The appropriate neoplasm code should be assigned as an additional code.

3) Management of dehydration due to the malignancy

When the admission/encounter is for management of dehydration due to the malignancy or the therapy, or a combination of both, and only the dehydration is being treated (intravenous rehydration), the dehydration is sequenced first, followed by the code(s) for the malignancy.

4) Treatment of a complication resulting from a surgical procedure

When the admission/encounter is for treatment of a complication resulting from a surgical procedure, designate the complication as the principal or first-listed diagnosis if treatment is directed at resolving the complication.

d. Primary malignancy previously excised

When a primary malignancy has been previously excised or eradicated from its site and there is no further treatment directed to that site and there is no evidence of any existing primary malignancy, a code from category V10, Personal history of malignant neoplasm, should be used to indicate the former site of the malignancy. Any mention of extension, invasion, or metastasis to another site is coded as a secondary malignant neoplasm to that site. The secondary site may be the principal or first-listed with the V10 code used as a secondary code.

e. Admissions/Encounters involving chemotherapy, immunotherapy and radiation therapy

1) Episode of care involves surgical removal of neoplasm

When an episode of care involves the surgical removal of a neoplasm, primary or secondary site, followed by adjunct chemotherapy or radiation treatment during the same episode of care, the neoplasm code should be assigned as principal or first-listed diagnosis, using codes in the 140-198 series or where appropriate in the 200-203 series.

2) Patient admission/encounter solely for administration of chemotherapy, immunotherapy and radiation therapy

If a patient admission/encounter is solely for the administration of chemotherapy, immunotherapy or radiation therapy assign code V58.0, Encounter for radiation therapy, or V58.11, Encounter for antineoplastic chemotherapy, or V58.12, Encounter for antineoplastic immunotherapy as the first-listed or principal diagnosis. If a patient receives more than one of these therapies during the same admission more than one of these codes may be assigned, in any sequence.

The malignancy for which the therapy is being administered should be assigned as a secondary diagnosis.

3) Patient admitted for radiotherapy/chemotherapy and immunotherapy and develops complications

When a patient is admitted for the purpose of radiotherapy, immunotherapy or chemotherapy and develops complications such as uncontrolled nausea and vomiting or dehydration, the principal or first-listed diagnosis is V58.0, Encounter for radiotherapy, or V58.11, Encounter for antineoplastic chemotherapy, or V58.12, Encounter for antineoplastic immunotherapy followed by any codes for the complications.

f. Admission/encounter to determine extent of malignancy

When the reason for admission/encounter is to determine the extent of the malignancy, or for a procedure such as paracentesis or thoracentesis, the primary malignancy or appropriate metastatic site is designated as the principal or first-listed diagnosis, even though chemotherapy or radiotherapy is administered.

g. Symptoms, signs, and ill-defined conditions listed in Chapter 16 associated with neoplasms

Symptoms, signs, and ill-defined conditions listed in Chapter 16 characteristic of, or associated with, an existing primary or secondary site malignancy cannot be used to replace the malignancy as principal or first-listed diagnosis, regardless of the number of admissions or encounters for treatment and care of the neoplasm.

h. Admission/encounter for pain control/management

See Section I.C.6.a.5 for information on coding admission/encounter for pain control/management.

i. Malignant neoplasm associated with transplanted organ

A malignant neoplasm of a transplanted organ should be coded as a transplant complication. Assign first the appropriate code from subcategory 996.8, Complications of transplanted organ, followed by code 199.2, Malignant neoplasm associated with transplanted organ. Use an additional code for the specific malignancy.

3. Chapter 3: Endocrine, Nutritional, and Metabolic Diseases and Immunity Disorders (240-279)

a. Diabetes mellitus

Codes under category 250, Diabetes mellitus, identify complications/manifestations associated with diabetes mellitus. A fifth-digit is required for all category 250 codes to identify the type of diabetes mellitus and whether the diabetes is controlled or uncontrolled.

See I.C.3.a.7 for secondary diabetes

1) Fifth-digits for category 250:

The following are the fifth-digits for the codes under category 250:

0   type II or unspecified type, not stated as uncontrolled

1   type I, [juvenile type], not stated as uncontrolled

2   type II or unspecified type, uncontrolled

3   type I, [juvenile type], uncontrolled

The age of a patient is not the sole determining factor, though most type I diabetics develop the condition before reaching puberty. For this reason type I diabetes mellitus is also referred to as juvenile diabetes.

2) Type of diabetes mellitus not documented

If the type of diabetes mellitus is not documented in the medical record the default is type II.

3) Diabetes mellitus and the use of insulin

All type I diabetics must use insulin to replace what their bodies do not produce. However, the use of insulin does not mean that a patient is a type I diabetic. Some patients with type II diabetes mellitus are unable to control their blood sugar through diet and oral medication alone and do require insulin.   If the documentation in a medical record does not indicate the type of diabetes but does indicate that the patient uses insulin, the appropriate fifth-digit for type II must be used. For type II patients who routinely use insulin, code V58.67, Long-term (current) use of insulin, should also be assigned to indicate that the patient uses insulin. Code V58.67 should not be assigned if insulin is given temporarily to bring a type II patient's blood sugar under control during an encounter.

4) Assigning and sequencing diabetes codes and associated conditions

When assigning codes for diabetes and its associated conditions, the code(s) from category 250 must be sequenced before the codes for the associated conditions. The diabetes codes and the secondary codes that correspond to them are paired codes that follow the etiology/manifestation convention of the classification *(See Section I.A.6., Etiology/manifestation convention)*. Assign as many codes from category 250 as needed to identify all of the associated conditions that the patient has. The corresponding secondary codes are listed under each of the diabetes codes.

(a) Diabetic retinopathy/diabetic macular edema

Diabetic macular edema, code 362.07, is only present with diabetic retinopathy. Another code from subcategory 362.0, Diabetic retinopathy, must be used with code 362.07. Codes under subcategory 362.0 are diabetes manifestation codes, so they must be used following the appropriate diabetes code.

5) Diabetes mellitus in pregnancy and gestational diabetes

(a) For diabetes mellitus complicating pregnancy, *see Section I.C.11.f., Diabetes mellitus in pregnancy.*

(b) For gestational diabetes, *see Section I.C.11, g., Gestational diabetes.*

6) Insulin pump malfunction

(a) Underdose of insulin due insulin pump failure

An underdose of insulin due to an insulin pump failure should be assigned 996.57, Mechanical complication due to insulin pump, as the principal or first listed code, followed by the appropriate diabetes mellitus code based on documentation.

(b) Overdose of insulin due to insulin pump failure

The principal or first listed code for an encounter due to an insulin pump malfunction resulting in an overdose of insulin, should also be 996.57, Mechanical complication due to insulin pump, followed by code 962.3, Poisoning by insulins and antidiabetic agents, and the appropriate diabetes mellitus code based on documentation.

7) Secondary Diabetes Mellitus

Codes under category 249, Secondary diabetes mellitus, identify complications/manifestations associated with secondary diabetes mellitus. Secondary diabetes is always caused by another condition or event (e.g., cystic fibrosis, malignant neoplasm of pancreas, pancreatectomy, adverse effect of drug, or poisoning).

(a) Fifth-digits for category 249:

A fifth-digit is required for all category 249 codes to identify whether the diabetes is controlled or uncontrolled.

(b) Secondary diabetes mellitus and the use of insulin

For patients who routinely use insulin, code V58.67, Long-term (current) use of insulin, should also be assigned. Code V58.67 should not be assigned if insulin is given temporarily to bring a patient's blood sugar under control during an encounter.

(c) Assigning and sequencing secondary diabetes codes and associated conditions

When assigning codes for secondary diabetes and its associated conditions (e.g. renal manifestations), the code(s) from category 249 must be sequenced before the codes for the associated conditions. The secondary diabetes codes and the diabetic manifestation codes that correspond to them are paired codes that follow the etiology/manifestation convention of the classification. Assign as many codes from category 249 as needed to identify all of the associated conditions that the patient has. The corresponding codes for the associated conditions are listed under each of the secondary diabetes codes. For example, secondary diabetes with diabetic nephrosis is assigned to code 249.40, followed by 581.81.

(d) Assigning and sequencing secondary diabetes codes and its causes

The sequencing of the secondary diabetes codes in relationship to codes for the cause of the diabetes is based on the reason for the encounter, applicable

ICD-9-CM sequencing conventions, and chapter-specific guidelines.

If a patient is seen for treatment of the secondary diabetes or one of its associated conditions, a code from category 249 is sequenced as the principal or first-listed diagnosis, with the cause of the secondary diabetes (e.g. cystic fibrosis) sequenced as an additional diagnosis.

If, however, the patient is seen for the treatment of the condition causing the secondary diabetes (e.g., malignant neoplasm of pancreas), the code for the cause of the secondary diabetes should be sequenced as the principal or first-listed diagnosis followed by a code from category 249.

(i)Secondary diabetes mellitus due to pancreatectomy

For postpancreatectomy diabetes mellitus (lack of insulin due to the surgical removal of all or part of the pancreas), assign code 251.3, Postsurgical hypoinsulinemia. Assign a code from subcategory 249, Secondary diabetes mellitus and a code from subcategory V88.1, Acquired absence of pancreas as additional codes. Code also any diabetic manifestations (e.g. diabetic nephrosis 581.81).

(ii)Secondary diabetes due to drugs

Secondary diabetes may be caused by an adverse effect of correctly administered medications, poisoning or late effect of poisoning.

See section I.C.17.e for coding of adverse effects and poisoning, and section I.C.19 for E code reporting.

4. **Chapter 4: Diseases of Blood and Blood Forming Organs (280-289)**

   a. **Anemia of chronic disease**

   Subcategory 285.2, Anemia in chronic illness, has codes for anemia in chronic kidney disease, code 285.21; anemia in neoplastic disease, code 285.22; and anemia in other chronic illness, code 285.29. These codes can be used as the principal/first listed code if the reason for the encounter is to treat the anemia. They may also be used as secondary codes if treatment of the anemia is a component of an encounter, but not the primary reason for the encounter. When using a code from subcategory 285 it is also necessary to use the code for the chronic condition causing the anemia.

   1) **Anemia in chronic kidney disease**

      When assigning code 285.21, Anemia in chronic kidney disease, it is also necessary to assign a code from category 585, Chronic kidney disease, to indicate the stage of chronic kidney disease.

      See I.C.10.a. Chronic kidney disease (CKD).

   2) **Anemia in neoplastic disease**

      When assigning code 285.22, Anemia in neoplastic disease, it is also necessary to assign the neoplasm code that is responsible for the anemia. Code 285.22 is for use for anemia that is due to the malignancy, not for anemia due to antineoplastic chemotherapy drugs. Assign the appropriate code for anemia due to antineoplastic chemotherapy.

      See I.C.2.c.1 Anemia associated with malignancy.

      See I.C.2.c.2 Anemia associated with chemotherapy, immunotherapy and radiation therapy.

5. **Chapter 5: Mental Disorders (290-319)**

   Reserved for future guideline expansion

6. **Chapter 6: Diseases of Nervous System and Sense Organs (320-389)**

   a. **Pain - Category 338**

      1) **General coding information**

         Codes in category 338 may be used in conjunction with codes from other categories and chapters to provide more detail about acute or chronic pain and neoplasm-related pain, unless otherwise indicated below.

         If the pain is not specified as acute or chronic, do not assign codes from category 338, except for post-thoracotomy pain, postoperative pain, neoplasm related pain, or central pain syndrome.

         A code from subcategories 338.1 and 338.2 should not be assigned if the underlying (definitive) diagnosis is known, unless the reason for the encounter is pain control/management and not management of the underlying condition.

         (a) **Category 338 Codes as Principal or First-Listed Diagnosis**

             Category 338 codes are acceptable as principal diagnosis or the first-listed code:

             - When pain control or pain management is the reason for the admission/encounter (e.g., a patient with displaced intervertebral disc, nerve impingement and severe back pain presents for injection of steroid into the spinal canal). The underlying cause of the pain should be reported as an additional diagnosis, if known.

             - When an admission or encounter is for a procedure aimed at treating the underlying condition (e.g., spinal fusion, kyphoplasty), a code for the underlying condition (e.g., vertebral fracture, spinal stenosis) should be assigned as the principal diagnosis. No code from category 338 should be assigned.

             - When a patient is admitted for the insertion of a neurostimulator for pain control, assign the appropriate pain code as the principal or first listed diagnosis. When an admission or encounter is for a procedure aimed at treating the underlying condition and a neurostimulator is inserted for pain control during the same admission/encounter, a code for the underlying condition should be assigned as the principal diagnosis and the appropriate pain code should be assigned as a secondary diagnosis.

         (b) **Use of Category 338 Codes in Conjunction with Site Specific Pain Codes**

             (i) **Assigning Category 338 Codes and Site-Specific Pain Codes**

                 Codes from category 338 may be used in conjunction with codes that identify the site of pain (including codes from chapter 16) if the category 338 code provides additional information. For example, if the code describes the site of the pain, but does not fully describe whether the pain is acute or chronic, then both codes should be assigned.

             (ii) **Sequencing of Category 338 Codes with Site-Specific Pain Codes**

                  The sequencing of category 338 codes with site-specific pain codes (including chapter 16 codes), is dependent on the circumstances of the encounter/admission as follows:

                  - If the encounter is for pain control or pain management, assign the code from category 338 followed by the code identifying the specific site of pain (e.g., encounter for pain management for acute neck pain from trauma is assigned code 338.11, Acute pain due to trauma, followed by code 723.1, Cervicalgia, to identify the site of pain).

- If the encounter is for any other reason except pain control or pain management, and a related definitive diagnosis has not been established (confirmed) by the provider, assign the code for the specific site of pain first, followed by the appropriate code from category 338.

2) Pain due to devices, implants and grafts

Pain associated with devices, implants or grafts left in a surgical site (for example painful hip prosthesis) is assigned to the appropriate code(s) found in Chapter 17, Injury and Poisoning. Use additional code(s) from category 338 to identify acute or chronic pain due to presence of the device, implant or graft (338.18-338.19 or 338.28-338.29).

3) Postoperative Pain

Post-thoracotomy pain and other postoperative pain are classified to subcategories 338.1 and 338.2, depending on whether the pain is acute or chronic. The default for post-thoracotomy and other postoperative pain not specified as acute or chronic is the code for the acute form.

Routine or expected postoperative pain immediately after surgery should not be coded.

(a) Postoperative pain not associated with specific postoperative complication

Postoperative pain not associated with a specific postoperative complication is assigned to the appropriate postoperative pain code in category 338.

(b) Postoperative pain associated with specific postoperative complication

Postoperative pain associated with a specific postoperative complication (such as painful wire sutures) is assigned to the appropriate code(s) found in Chapter 17, Injury and Poisoning. If appropriate, use additional code(s) from category 338 to identify acute or chronic pain (338.18 or 338.28). If pain control/management is the reason for the encounter, a code from category 338 should be assigned as the principal or first-listed diagnosis in accordance with *Section I.C.6.a.1.a above.*

(c) Postoperative pain as principal or first-listed diagnosis

Postoperative pain may be reported as the principal or first-listed diagnosis when the stated reason for the admission/encounter is documented as postoperative pain control/ management.

(d) Postoperative pain as secondary diagnosis

Postoperative pain may be reported as a secondary diagnosis code when a patient presents for outpatient surgery and develops an unusual or inordinate amount of postoperative pain.

The provider's documentation should be used to guide the coding of postoperative pain, as well as *Section III. Reporting Additional Diagnoses and Section IV. Diagnostic Coding and Reporting in the Outpatient Setting.*

See Section II.I.2 for information on sequencing of diagnoses for patients admitted to hospital inpatient care following post-operative observation.

See Section II.J for information on sequencing of diagnoses for patients admitted to hospital inpatient care from outpatient surgery.

See Section IV.A.2 for information on sequencing of diagnoses for patients admitted for observation.

4) Chronic pain

Chronic pain is classified to subcategory 338.2. There is no time frame defining when pain becomes chronic pain. The provider's documentation should be used to guide use of these codes.

5) Neoplasm Related Pain

Code 338.3 is assigned to pain documented as being related, associated or due to cancer, primary or secondary malignancy, or tumor. This code is assigned regardless of whether the pain is acute or chronic.

This code may be assigned as the principal or first-listed code when the stated reason for the admission/encounter is documented as pain control/pain management. The underlying neoplasm should be reported as an additional diagnosis.

When the reason for the admission/encounter is management of the neoplasm and the pain associated with the neoplasm is also documented, code 338.3 may be assigned as an additional diagnosis.

See Section I.C.2 for instructions on the sequencing of neoplasms for all other stated reasons for the admission/encounter (except for pain control/pain management).

6) Chronic pain syndrome

This condition is different than the term "chronic pain," and therefore this code should only be used when the provider has specifically documented this condition.

b. Glaucoma

1) Glaucoma

For types of glaucoma classified to subcategories 365.1-365.6, an additional code should be assigned from subcategory 365.7, Glaucoma stage, to identify the glaucoma stage. Codes from 365.7, Glaucoma stage, may not be assigned as a principal or first-listed diagnosis.

2) Bilateral glaucoma with same stage

When a patient has bilateral glaucoma and both are documented as being the same type and stage, report only the code for the type of glaucoma and one code for the stage.

3) Bilateral glaucoma stage with different stages

When a patient has bilateral glaucoma and each eye is documented as having a different stage, assign one code for the type of glaucoma and one code for the highest glaucoma stage.

4) Bilateral glaucoma with different types and different stages

When a patient has bilateral glaucoma and each eye is documented as having a different type and a different stage, assign one code for each type of glaucoma and one code for the highest glaucoma stage.

5) Patient admitted with glaucoma and stage evolves during the admission

If a patient is admitted with glaucoma and the stage progresses during the admission, assign the code for highest stage documented.

6) Indeterminate stage glaucoma

Assignment of code 365.74, Indeterminate stage glaucoma, should be based on the clinical documentation. Code 365.74 is used for glaucoma whose stage cannot be clinically determined. This code should not be confused with code 365.70, Glaucoma stage, unspecified. Code 365.70 should be assigned when there is no documentation regarding the stage of the glaucoma.

7. Chapter 7: Diseases of Circulatory System (390-459)

a. Hypertension

Hypertension Table

The Hypertension Table, found under the main term, "Hypertension", in the Alphabetic Index, contains a complete listing of all conditions due to or associated with hypertension and classifies them according to malignant, benign, and unspecified.

1) Hypertension, Essential, or NOS

Assign hypertension (arterial) (essential) (primary) (systemic) (NOS) to category code 401 with the appropriate fourth digit to indicate malignant (.0), benign (.1), or unspecified (.9). Do not use either .0 malignant or .1 benign unless medical record documentation supports such a designation.

2) Hypertension with Heart Disease

Heart conditions (425.8, 429.0-429.3, 429.8, 429.9) are assigned to a code from category 402 when a causal relationship is stated (due to hypertension) or implied (hypertensive). Use an additional code from category 428 to identify the type of heart failure in those patients with heart failure. More than one code from category 428 may be assigned if the patient has systolic or diastolic failure and congestive heart failure.

The same heart conditions (425.8, 429.0-429.3, 429.8, 429.9) with hypertension, but without a stated causal relationship, are coded separately. Sequence according to the circumstances of the admission/encounter.

3) Hypertensive Chronic Kidney Disease

Assign codes from category 403, Hypertensive chronic kidney disease, when conditions classified to category 585 or code 587 are present with hypertension. Unlike hypertension with heart disease, ICD-9-CM presumes a cause-and-effect relationship and classifies chronic kidney disease (CKD) with hypertension as hypertensive chronic kidney disease.

Fifth digits for category 403 should be assigned as follows:

- 0 with CKD stage I through stage IV, or unspecified.
- 1 with CKD stage V or end stage renal disease.

The appropriate code from category 585, Chronic kidney disease, should be used as a secondary code with a code from category 403 to identify the stage of chronic kidney disease.

See Section I.C.10.a for information on the coding of chronic kidney disease.

4) Hypertensive Heart and Chronic Kidney Disease

Assign codes from combination category 404, Hypertensive heart and chronic kidney disease, when both hypertensive kidney disease and hypertensive heart disease are stated in the diagnosis. Assume a relationship between the hypertension and the chronic kidney disease, whether or not the condition is so designated. Assign an additional code from category 428, to identify the type of heart failure. More than one code from category 428 may be assigned if the patient has systolic or diastolic failure and congestive heart failure.

Fifth digits for category 404 should be assigned as follows:

- 0 without heart failure and with chronic kidney disease (CKD) stage I through stage IV, or unspecified
- 1 with heart failure and with CKD stage I through stage IV, or unspecified
- 2 without heart failure and with CKD stage V or end stage renal disease
- 3 with heart failure and with CKD stage V or end stage renal disease

The appropriate code from category 585, Chronic kidney disease, should be used as a secondary code with a code from category 404 to identify the stage of kidney disease.

See Section I.C.10.a for information on the coding of chronic kidney disease.

5) Hypertensive Cerebrovascular Disease

First assign codes from 430-438, Cerebrovascular disease, then the appropriate hypertension code from categories 401-405.

6) Hypertensive Retinopathy

Two codes are necessary to identify the condition. First assign the code from subcategory 362.11, Hypertensive retinopathy, then the appropriate code from categories 401-405 to indicate the type of hypertension.

7) Hypertension, Secondary

Two codes are required: one to identify the underlying etiology and one from category 405 to identify the hypertension. Sequencing of codes is determined by the reason for admission/encounter.

8) Hypertension, Transient

Assign code 796.2, Elevated blood pressure reading without diagnosis of hypertension, unless patient has an established diagnosis of hypertension. Assign code 642.3x for transient hypertension of pregnancy.

9) Hypertension, Controlled

Assign appropriate code from categories 401-405. This diagnostic statement usually refers to an existing state of hypertension under control by therapy.

10) Hypertension, Uncontrolled

Uncontrolled hypertension may refer to untreated hypertension or hypertension not responding to current therapeutic regimen. In either case, assign the appropriate code from categories 401-405 to designate the stage and type of hypertension. Code to the type of hypertension.

11) Elevated Blood Pressure

For a statement of elevated blood pressure without further specificity, assign code 796.2, Elevated blood pressure reading without diagnosis of hypertension, rather than a code from category 401.

b. Cerebral infarction/stroke/cerebrovascular accident (CVA)

The terms stroke and CVA are often used interchangeably to refer to a cerebral infarction. The terms stroke, CVA, and cerebral infarction NOS are all indexed to the default code 434.91, Cerebral artery occlusion, unspecified, with infarction.

Additional code(s) should be assigned for any neurologic deficits associated with the acute CVA, regardless of whether or not the neurologic deficit resolves prior to discharge.

See Section I.C.18.d.3 for information on coding status post administration of tPA in a different facility within the last 24 hours.

c. Postoperative cerebrovascular accident

A cerebrovascular hemorrhage or infarction that occurs as a result of medical intervention is coded to 997.02, Iatrogenic cerebrovascular infarction or hemorrhage. Medical record documentation should clearly specify the cause- and-effect relationship between the medical intervention and the cerebrovascular accident in order to assign this code. A secondary code from the code range 430-432 or from a code from subcategories 433 or 434 with a fifth digit of "1" should also be used to identify the type of hemorrhage or infarct.

This guideline conforms to the use additional code note instruction at category 997. Code 436, Acute, but ill-defined, cerebrovascular disease, should not be used as a secondary code with code 997.02.

d. Late Effects of Cerebrovascular Disease

1) Category 438, Late Effects of Cerebrovascular disease

Category 438 is used to indicate conditions classifiable to categories 430-437 as the causes of late effects (neurologic deficits), themselves classified elsewhere. These "late effects" include neurologic deficits that persist after initial onset of conditions classifiable to 430-437. The neurologic deficits caused by cerebrovascular disease may be present from the onset or may arise at any time after the onset of the condition classifiable to 430-437.

Codes in category 438 are only for use for late effects of cerebrovascular disease, not for neurologic deficits associated with an acute CVA.

2) Codes from category 438 with codes from 430-437

Codes from category 438 may be assigned on a health care record with codes from 430-437, if the patient has a current cerebrovascular accident (CVA) and deficits from an old CVA.

3) **Code V12.54**

Assign code V12.54, Transient ischemic attack (TIA), and cerebral infarction without residual deficits (and not a code from category 438) as an additional code for history of cerebrovascular disease when no neurologic deficits are present.

e. **Acute myocardial infarction (AMI)**

1) **ST elevation myocardial infarction (STEMI) and non ST elevation myocardial infarction (NSTEMI)**

The ICD-9-CM codes for acute myocardial infarction (AMI) identify the site, such as anterolateral wall or true posterior wall. Subcategories 410.0-410.6 and 410.8 are used for ST elevation myocardial infarction (STEMI). Subcategory 410.7, Subendocardial infarction, is used for non ST elevation myocardial infarction (NSTEMI) and nontransmural MIs.

2) **Acute myocardial infarction, unspecified**

Subcategory 410.9 is the default for the unspecified term acute myocardial infarction. If only STEMI or transmural MI without the site is documented, query the provider as to the site, or assign a code from subcategory 410.9.

3) **AMI documented as nontransmural or subendocardial but site provided**

If an AMI is documented as nontransmural or subendocardial, but the site is provided, it is still coded as a subendocardial AMI. If NSTEMI evolves to STEMI, assign the STEMI code. If STEMI converts to NSTEMI due to thrombolytic therapy, it is still coded as STEMI.

See Section I.C.18.d.3 for information on coding status post administration of tPA in a different facility within the last 24 hours.

8. **Chapter 8: Diseases of Respiratory System (460-519)**

See I.C.17.f. for ventilator-associated pneumonia.

a. **Chronic Obstructive Pulmonary Disease [COPD] and Asthma**

1) **Conditions that comprise COPD and Asthma**

The conditions that comprise COPD are obstructive chronic bronchitis, subcategory 491.2, and emphysema, category 492. All asthma codes are under category 493, Asthma. Code 496, Chronic airway obstruction, not elsewhere classified, is a nonspecific code that should only be used when the documentation in a medical record does not specify the type of COPD being treated.

2) **Acute exacerbation of chronic obstructive bronchitis and asthma**

The codes for chronic obstructive bronchitis and asthma distinguish between uncomplicated cases and those in acute exacerbation. An acute exacerbation is a worsening or a decompensation of a chronic condition. An acute exacerbation is not equivalent to an infection superimposed on a chronic condition, though an exacerbation may be triggered by an infection.

3) **Overlapping nature of the conditions that comprise COPD and asthma**

Due to the overlapping nature of the conditions that make up COPD and asthma, there are many variations in the way these conditions are documented. Code selection must be based on the terms as documented. When selecting the correct code for the documented type of COPD and asthma, it is essential to first review the index, and then verify the code in the tabular list. There are many instructional notes under the different COPD subcategories and codes. It is important that all such notes be reviewed to assure correct code assignment.

4) **Acute exacerbation of asthma and status asthmaticus**

An acute exacerbation of asthma is an increased severity of the asthma symptoms, such as wheezing and shortness of breath. Status asthmaticus refers to a patient's failure to respond to therapy administered during an asthmatic episode and is a life threatening complication that requires

emergency care. If status asthmaticus is documented by the provider with any type of COPD or with acute bronchitis, the status asthmaticus should be sequenced first. It supersedes any type of COPD including that with acute exacerbation or acute bronchitis. It is inappropriate to assign an asthma code with 5th digit 2, with acute exacerbation, together with an asthma code with 5th digit 1, with status asthmatics. Only the 5th digit 1 should be assigned.

b. **Chronic Obstructive Pulmonary Disease [COPD] and Bronchitis**

1) **Acute bronchitis with COPD**

Acute bronchitis, code 466.0, is due to an infectious organism. When acute bronchitis is documented with COPD, code 491.22, Obstructive chronic bronchitis with acute bronchitis, should be assigned. It is not necessary to also assign code 466.0. If a medical record documents acute bronchitis with COPD with acute exacerbation, only code 491.22 should be assigned. The acute bronchitis included in code 491.22 supersedes the acute exacerbation. If a medical record documents COPD with acute exacerbation without mention of acute bronchitis, only code 491.21 should be assigned.

c. **Acute Respiratory Failure**

1) **Acute respiratory failure as principal diagnosis**

Code 518.81, Acute respiratory failure, may be assigned as a principal diagnosis when it is the condition established after study to be chiefly responsible for occasioning the admission to the hospital, and the selection is supported by the Alphabetic Index and Tabular List. However, chapter-specific coding guidelines (such as obstetrics, poisoning, HIV, newborn) that provide sequencing direction take precedence.

2) **Acute respiratory failure as secondary diagnosis**

Respiratory failure may be listed as a secondary diagnosis if it occurs after admission, or if it is present on admission, but does not meet the definition of principal diagnosis.

3) **Sequencing of acute respiratory failure and another acute condition**

When a patient is admitted with respiratory failure and another acute condition, (e.g., myocardial infarction, cerebrovascular accident, aspiration pneumonia), the principal diagnosis will not be the same in every situation. This applies whether the other acute condition is a respiratory or nonrespiratory condition. Selection of the principal diagnosis will be dependent on the circumstances of admission. If both the respiratory failure and the other acute condition are equally responsible for occasioning the admission to the hospital, and there are no chapter-specific sequencing rules, the guideline regarding two or more diagnoses that equally meet the definition for principal diagnosis *(Section II, C.)* may be applied in these situations.

If the documentation is not clear as to whether acute respiratory failure and another condition are equally responsible for occasioning the admission, query the provider for clarification.

d. **Influenza due to certain identified viruses**

Code only confirmed cases of avian influenza (codes 488.01-488.02, 488.09, Influenza due to identified avian influenza virus), 2009 H1N1 influenza virus (codes 488.11-488.12, 488.19), or novel influenza A (codes 488.81-488.82, 488.89, Influenza due to identified novel influenza A virus). This is an exception to the hospital inpatient guideline Section II, H. (Uncertain Diagnosis).

In this context, "confirmation" does not require documentation of positive laboratory testing specific for avian, 2009 H1N1 or novel influenza A virus. However, coding should be based on the provider's diagnostic statement that the patient has avian influenza, 2009 H1N1 influenza, or novel influenza A.

If the provider records "suspected" or "possible" or "probable" avian, 2009 H1N1, or novel influenza A, the appropriate influenza code from category 487, Influenza should be assigned. A code from category 488, Influenza due to certain identified influenza viruses, should not be assigned.

9. **Chapter 9: Diseases of Digestive System (520-579)**

    Reserved for future guideline expansion

10. **Chapter 10: Diseases of Genitourinary System (580-629)**

    a. **Chronic kidney disease**

        1) **Stages of chronic kidney disease (CKD)**

            The ICD-9-CM classifies CKD based on severity. The severity of CKD is designated by stages I-V. Stage II, code 585.2, equates to mild CKD; stage III, code 585.3, equates to moderate CKD; and stage IV, code 585.4, equates to severe CKD. Code 585.6, End stage renal disease (ESRD), is assigned when the provider has documented end-stage-renal disease (ESRD).

            If both a stage of CKD and ESRD are documented, assign code 585.6 only.

        2) **Chronic kidney disease and kidney transplant status**

            Patients who have undergone kidney transplant may still have some form of CKD, because the kidney transplant may not fully restore kidney function. Therefore, the presence of CKD alone does not constitute a transplant complication. Assign the appropriate 585 code for the patient's stage of CKD and code V42.0. If a transplant complication such as failure or rejection is documented, see section I.C.17.f.2.b for information on coding complications of a kidney transplant. If the documentation is unclear as to whether the patient has a complication of the transplant, query the provider.

        3) **Chronic kidney disease with other conditions**

            Patients with CKD may also suffer from other serious conditions, most commonly diabetes mellitus and hypertension. The sequencing of the CKD code in relationship to codes for other contributing conditions is based on the conventions in the tabular list.

            See I.C.3.a.4 for sequencing instructions for diabetes.
            See I.C.4.a.1 for anemia in CKD.
            See I.C.7.a.3 for hypertensive chronic kidney disease.
            See I.C.17.f.2.b, Kidney transplant complications, for instructions on coding of documented rejection or failure.

11. **Chapter 11: Complications of Pregnancy, Childbirth, and the Puerperium (630-679)**

    a. **General Rules for Obstetric Cases**

        1) **Codes from chapter 11 and sequencing priority**

            Obstetric cases require codes from chapter 11, codes in the range 630-679, Complications of Pregnancy, Childbirth, and the Puerperium. Chapter 11 codes have sequencing priority over codes from other chapters. Additional codes from other chapters may be used in conjunction with chapter 11 codes to further specify conditions. Should the provider document that the pregnancy is incidental to the encounter, then code V22.2 should be used in place of any chapter 11 codes. It is the provider's responsibility to state that the condition being treated is not affecting the pregnancy.

        2) **Chapter 11 codes used only on the maternal record**

            Chapter 11 codes are to be used only on the maternal record, never on the record of the newborn.

        3) **Chapter 11 fifth-digits**

            Categories 640-648, 651-676 have required fifth-digits, which indicate whether the encounter is antepartum, postpartum and whether a delivery has also occurred.

        4) **Fifth-digits, appropriate for each code**

            The fifth-digits, which are appropriate for each code number, are listed in brackets under each code. The fifth-digits on each code should all be consistent with each other. That is, should a delivery occur all of the fifth-digits should indicate the delivery.

    b. **Selection of OB Principal or First-listed Diagnosis**

        1) **Routine outpatient prenatal visits**

            For routine outpatient prenatal visits when no complications are present codes V22.0, Supervision of normal first pregnancy, and V22.1, Supervision of other normal pregnancy, should be used as the first-listed diagnoses. These codes should not be used in conjunction with chapter 11 codes.

        2) **Prenatal outpatient visits for high-risk patients**

            For routine prenatal outpatient visits for patients with high-risk pregnancies, a code from category V23, Supervision of high-risk pregnancy, should be used as the first-listed diagnosis. Secondary chapter 11 codes may be used in conjunction with these codes if appropriate.

        3) **Episodes when no delivery occurs**

            In episodes when no delivery occurs, the principal diagnosis should correspond to the principal complication of the pregnancy, which necessitated the encounter. Should more than one complication exist, all of which are treated or monitored, any of the complications codes may be sequenced first.

        4) **When a delivery occurs**

            When a delivery occurs, the principal diagnosis should correspond to the main circumstances or complication of the delivery. In cases of cesarean delivery, the selection of the principal diagnosis should be the condition established after study that was responsible for the patient's admission. If the patient was admitted with a condition that resulted in the performance of a cesarean procedure, that condition should be selected as the principal diagnosis. If the reason for the admission/encounter was unrelated to the condition resulting in the cesarean delivery, the condition related to the reason for the admission/encounter should be selected as the principal diagnosis, even if a cesarean was performed.

        5) **Outcome of delivery**

            An outcome of delivery code, V27.0-V27.9, should be included on every maternal record when a delivery has occurred. These codes are not to be used on subsequent records or on the newborn record.

    c. **Fetal Conditions Affecting the Management of the Mother**

        1) **Codes from categories 655 and 656**

            Codes from categories 655, Known or suspected fetal abnormality affecting management of the mother, and 656, Other known or suspected fetal and placental problems affecting the management of the mother, are assigned only when the fetal condition is actually responsible for modifying the management of the mother, i.e., by requiring diagnostic studies, additional observation, special care, or termination of pregnancy. The fact that the fetal condition exists does not justify assigning a code from this series to the mother's record.

            See I.C.18.d. for suspected maternal and fetal conditions not found

        2) **In utero surgery**

            In cases when surgery is performed on the fetus, a diagnosis code from category 655, Known or suspected fetal abnormalities affecting management of the mother, should be assigned identifying the fetal condition. Procedure code 75.36, Correction of fetal defect, should be assigned on the hospital inpatient record.

            No code from Chapter 15, the perinatal codes, should be used on the mother's record to identify fetal conditions. Surgery performed in utero on a fetus is still to be coded as an obstetric encounter.

    d. **HIV Infection in Pregnancy, Childbirth and the Puerperium**

        During pregnancy, childbirth or the puerperium, a patient admitted because of an HIV-related illness should receive a principal diagnosis of 647.6x, Other specified infectious and parasitic diseases in the mother classifiable elsewhere, but complicating the pregnancy, childbirth or the puerperium, followed by 042 and the code(s) for the HIV-related illness(es).

Patients with asymptomatic HIV infection status admitted during pregnancy, childbirth, or the puerperium should receive codes of 647.6x and V08.

e. Current Conditions Complicating Pregnancy

Assign a code from subcategory 648.x for patients that have current conditions when the condition affects the management of the pregnancy, childbirth, or the puerperium. Use additional secondary codes from other chapters to identify the conditions, as appropriate.

f. Diabetes mellitus in pregnancy

Diabetes mellitus is a significant complicating factor in pregnancy. Pregnant women who are diabetic should be assigned code 648.0x, Diabetes mellitus complicating pregnancy, and a secondary code from category 250, Diabetes mellitus, or category 249, Secondary diabetes to identify the type of diabetes.

Code V58.67, Long-term (current) use of insulin, should also be assigned if the diabetes mellitus is being treated with insulin.

g. Gestational diabetes

Gestational diabetes can occur during the second and third trimester of pregnancy in women who were not diabetic prior to pregnancy. Gestational diabetes can cause complications in the pregnancy similar to those of pre-existing diabetes mellitus. It also puts the woman at greater risk of developing diabetes after the pregnancy. Gestational diabetes is coded to 648.8x, Abnormal glucose tolerance. Codes 648.0x and 648.8x should never be used together on the same record.

Code V58.67, Long-term (current) use of insulin, should also be assigned if the gestational diabetes is being treated with insulin.

h. Normal Delivery, Code 650

1) **Normal delivery**

Code 650 is for use in cases when a woman is admitted for a full-term normal delivery and delivers a single, healthy infant without any complications antepartum, during the delivery, or postpartum during the delivery episode. Code 650 is always a principal diagnosis. It is not to be used if any other code from chapter 11 is needed to describe a current complication of the antenatal, delivery, or perinatal period. Additional codes from other chapters may be used with code 650 if they are not related to or are in any way complicating the pregnancy.

2) **Normal delivery with resolved antepartum complication**

Code 650 may be used if the patient had a complication at some point during her pregnancy, but the complication is not present at the time of the admission for delivery.

3) **V27.0, Single liveborn, outcome of delivery**

V27.0, Single liveborn, is the only outcome of delivery code appropriate for use with 650.

i. The Postpartum and Peripartum Periods

1) **Postpartum and peripartum periods**

The postpartum period begins immediately after delivery and continues for six weeks following delivery. The peripartum period is defined as the last month of pregnancy to five months postpartum.

2) **Postpartum complication**

A postpartum complication is any complication occurring within the six-week period.

3) **Pregnancy-related complications after 6 week period**

Chapter 11 codes may also be used to describe pregnancy-related complications after the six-week period should the provider document that a condition is pregnancy related.

4) **Postpartum complications occurring during the same admission as delivery**

Postpartum complications that occur during the same admission as the delivery are identified with a fifth digit of "2." Subsequent admissions/encounters for postpartum complications should be identified with a fifth digit of "4."

5) **Admission for routine postpartum care following delivery outside hospital**

When the mother delivers outside the hospital prior to admission and is admitted for routine postpartum care and no complications are noted, code V24.0, Postpartum care and examination immediately after delivery, should be assigned as the principal diagnosis.

6) **Admission following delivery outside hospital with postpartum conditions**

A delivery diagnosis code should not be used for a woman who has delivered prior to admission to the hospital. Any postpartum conditions and/or postpartum procedures should be coded.

7) **Puerperal sepsis**

Code 670.2x, Puerperal sepsis, should be assigned with a secondary code to identify the causal organism (e.g., for a bacterial infection, assign a code from category 041, Bacterial infections in conditions classified elsewhere and of unspecified site). A code from category 038, Septicemia, should not be used for puerperal sepsis. Do not assign code 995.91, Sepsis, as code 670.2x describes the sepsis. If applicable, use additional codes to identify severe sepsis (995.92) and any associated acute organ dysfunction.

j. Code 677, Late effect of complication of pregnancy

1) **Code 677**

Code 677, Late effect of complication of pregnancy, childbirth, and the puerperium is for use in those cases when an initial complication of a pregnancy develops a sequelae requiring care or treatment at a future date.

2) **After the initial postpartum period**

This code may be used at any time after the initial postpartum period.

3) **Sequencing of Code 677**

This code, like all late effect codes, is to be sequenced following the code describing the sequelae of the complication.

k. Abortions

1) **Fifth-digits required for abortion categories**

Fifth-digits are required for abortion categories 634-637. Fifth digit assignment is based on the status of the patient at the beginning (or start) of the encounter. Fifth-digit 1, incomplete, indicates that all of the products of conception have not been expelled from the uterus. Fifth-digit 2, complete, indicates that all products of conception have been expelled from the uterus.

2) **Code from categories 640-648 and 651-659**

A code from categories 640-648 and 651-659 may be used as additional codes with an abortion code to indicate the complication leading to the abortion.

Fifth digit 3 is assigned with codes from these categories when used with an abortion code because the other fifth digits will not apply. Codes from the 660-669 series are not to be used for complications of abortion.

3) **Code 639 for complications**

Code 639 is to be used for all complications following abortion. Code 639 cannot be assigned with codes from categories 634-638.

4) **Abortion with Liveborn Fetus**

When an attempted termination of pregnancy results in a liveborn fetus assign code 644.21, Early onset of delivery, with an appropriate code from category V27, Outcome of Delivery. The procedure code for the attempted termination of pregnancy should also be assigned.

5) Retained Products of Conception following an abortion

Subsequent admissions for retained products of conception following a spontaneous or legally induced abortion are assigned the appropriate code from category 634, Spontaneous abortion, or 635 Legally induced abortion, with a fifth digit of "1" (incomplete). This advice is appropriate even when the patient was discharged previously with a discharge diagnosis of complete abortion.

12. Chapter 12: Diseases Skin and Subcutaneous Tissue (680-709)

a. Pressure ulcer stage codes

1) Pressure ulcer stages

Two codes are needed to completely describe a pressure ulcer: A code from subcategory 707.0, Pressure ulcer, to identify the site of the pressure ulcer and a code from subcategory 707.2, Pressure ulcer stages.

The codes in subcategory 707.2, Pressure ulcer stages, are to be used as an additional diagnosis with a code(s) from subcategory 707.0, Pressure Ulcer. Codes from 707.2, Pressure ulcer stages, may not be assigned as a principal or first-listed diagnosis. The pressure ulcer stage codes should only be used with pressure ulcers and not with other types of ulcers (e.g., stasis ulcer).

The ICD-9-CM classifies pressure ulcer stages based on severity, which is designated by stages I-IV and unstageable.

2) Unstageable pressure ulcers

Assignment of code 707.25, Pressure ulcer, unstageable, should be based on the clinical documentation. Code 707.25 is used for pressure ulcers whose stage cannot be clinically determined (e.g., the ulcer is covered by eschar or has been treated with a skin or muscle graft) and pressure ulcers that are documented as deep tissue injury but not documented as due to trauma. This code should not be confused with code 707.20, Pressure ulcer, stage unspecified. Code 707.20 should be assigned when there is no documentation regarding the stage of the pressure ulcer.

3) Documented pressure ulcer stage

Assignment of the pressure ulcer stage code should be guided by clinical documentation of the stage or documentation of the terms found in the index. For clinical terms describing the stage that are not found in the index, and there is no documentation of the stage, the provider should be queried.

4) Bilateral pressure ulcers with same stage

When a patient has bilateral pressure ulcers (e.g., both buttocks) and both pressure ulcers are documented as being the same stage, only the code for the site and one code for the stage should be reported.

5) Bilateral pressure ulcers with different stages

When a patient has bilateral pressure ulcers at the same site (e.g., both buttocks) and each pressure ulcer is documented as being at a different stage, assign one code for the site and the appropriate codes for the pressure ulcer stage.

6) Multiple pressure ulcers of different sites and stages

When a patient has multiple pressure ulcers at different sites (e.g., buttock, heel, shoulder) and each pressure ulcer is documented as being at different stages (e.g., stage 3 and stage 4), assign the appropriate codes for each different site and a code for each different pressure ulcer stage.

7) Patients admitted with pressure ulcers documented as healed

No code is assigned if the documentation states that the pressure ulcer is completely healed.

8) Patients admitted with pressure ulcers documented as healing

Pressure ulcers described as healing should be assigned the appropriate pressure ulcer stage code based on the documentation in the medical record. If the documentation does not provide information about the stage of the healing pressure ulcer, assign code 707.20, Pressure ulcer stage, unspecified.

If the documentation is unclear as to whether the patient has a current (new) pressure ulcer or if the patient is being treated for a healing pressure ulcer, query the provider.

9) Patient admitted with pressure ulcer evolving into another stage during the admission

If a patient is admitted with a pressure ulcer at one stage and it progresses to a higher stage, assign the code for highest stage reported for that site.

13. Chapter 13: Diseases of Musculoskeletal and Connective Tissue (710-739)

a. Coding of Pathologic Fractures

1) Acute Fractures vs. Aftercare

Pathologic fractures are reported using subcategory 733.1, when the fracture is newly diagnosed. Subcategory 733.1 may be used while the patient is receiving active treatment for the fracture. Examples of active treatment are: surgical treatment, emergency department encounter, evaluation and treatment by a new physician.

Fractures are coded using the aftercare codes (subcategories V54.0, V54.2, V54.8 or V54.9) for encounters after the patient has completed active treatment of the fracture and is receiving routine care for the fracture during the healing or recovery phase. Examples of fracture aftercare are: cast change or removal, removal of external or internal fixation device, medication adjustment, and follow up visits following fracture treatment.

Care for complications of surgical treatment for fracture repairs during the healing or recovery phase should be coded with the appropriate complication codes.

Care of complications of fractures, such as malunion and nonunion, should be reported with the appropriate codes.

See Section I. C. 17.b for information on the coding of traumatic fractures.

14. Chapter 14: Congenital Anomalies (740-759)

a. Codes in categories 740-759, Congenital Anomalies

Assign an appropriate code(s) from categories 740-759, Congenital Anomalies, when an anomaly is documented. A congenital anomaly may be the principal/first listed diagnosis on a record or a secondary diagnosis.

When a congenital anomaly does not have a unique code assignment, assign additional code(s) for any manifestations that may be present.

When the code assignment specifically identifies the congenital anomaly, manifestations that are an inherent component of the anomaly should not be coded separately. Additional codes should be assigned for manifestations that are not an inherent component.

Codes from Chapter 14 may be used throughout the life of the patient. If a congenital anomaly has been corrected, a personal history code should be used to identify the history of the anomaly. Although present at birth, a congenital anomaly may not be identified until later in life. Whenever the condition is diagnosed by the physician, it is appropriate to assign a code from codes 740-759.

For the birth admission, the appropriate code from category V30, Liveborn infants, according to type of birth should be sequenced as the principal diagnosis, followed by any congenital anomaly codes, 740-759.

15. Chapter 15: Newborn (Perinatal) Guidelines (760-779)

For coding and reporting purposes the perinatal period is defined as before birth through the 28th day following birth. The following guidelines are provided for reporting purposes. Hospitals may record other diagnoses as needed for internal data use.

a. General Perinatal Rules

1) Chapter 15 Codes

They are never for use on the maternal record. Codes from Chapter 11, the obstetric chapter, are never permitted on the newborn record. Chapter 15 code may be used throughout the life of the patient if the condition is still present.

2) Sequencing of perinatal codes

Generally, codes from Chapter 15 should be sequenced as the principal/first-listed diagnosis on the newborn record, with the exception of the appropriate V30 code for the birth episode, followed by codes from any other chapter that provide additional detail. The "use additional code" note at the beginning of the chapter supports this guideline. If the index does not provide a specific code for a perinatal condition, assign code 779.89, Other specified conditions originating in the perinatal period, followed by the code from another chapter that specifies the condition. Codes for signs and symptoms may be assigned when a definitive diagnosis has not been established.

3) Birth process or community acquired conditions

If a newborn has a condition that may be either due to the birth process or community acquired and the documentation does not indicate which it is, the default is due to the birth process and the code from Chapter 15 should be used. If the condition is community-acquired, a code from Chapter 15 should not be assigned.

4) Code all clinically significant conditions

All clinically significant conditions noted on routine newborn examination should be coded. A condition is clinically significant if it requires:

- clinical evaluation; or
- therapeutic treatment; or
- diagnostic procedures; or
- extended length of hospital stay; or
- increased nursing care and/or monitoring; or
- has implications for future health care needs

Note: The perinatal guidelines listed above are the same as the general coding guidelines for "additional diagnoses", except for the final point regarding implications for future health care needs. Codes should be assigned for conditions that have been specified by the provider as having implications for future health care needs. Codes from the perinatal chapter should not be assigned unless the provider has established a definitive diagnosis.

b. Use of codes V30-V39

When coding the birth of an infant, assign a code from categories V30-V39, according to the type of birth. A code from this series is assigned as a principal diagnosis, and assigned only once to a newborn at the time of birth.

c. Newborn transfers

If the newborn is transferred to another institution, the V30 series is not used at the receiving hospital.

d. Use of category V29

1) Assigning a code from category V29

Assign a code from category V29, Observation and evaluation of newborns and infants for suspected conditions not found, to identify those instances when a healthy newborn is evaluated for a suspected condition that is determined after study not to be present. Do not use a code from category V29 when the patient has identified signs or symptoms of a suspected problem; in such cases, code the sign or symptom.

A code from category V29 may also be assigned as a principal code for readmissions or encounters when the V30 code no longer applies. Codes from category V29 are for use only for healthy newborns and infants for which no condition after study is found to be present.

2) V29 code on a birth record

A V29 code is to be used as a secondary code after the V30, Outcome of delivery, code.

e. Use of other V codes on perinatal records

V codes other than V30 and V29 may be assigned on a perinatal or newborn record code. The codes may be used as a principal or first-listed diagnosis for specific types of encounters or for readmissions or encounters when the V30 code no longer applies.

See Section I.C.18 for information regarding the assignment of V codes.

f. Maternal Causes of Perinatal Morbidity

Codes from categories 760-763, Maternal causes of perinatal morbidity and mortality, are assigned only when the maternal condition has actually affected the fetus or newborn. The fact that the mother has an associated medical condition or experiences some complication of pregnancy, labor or delivery does not justify the routine assignment of codes from these categories to the newborn record.

g. Congenital Anomalies in Newborns

For the birth admission, the appropriate code from category V30, Liveborn infants according to type of birth, should be used, followed by any congenital anomaly codes, categories 740-759. Use additional secondary codes from other chapters to specify conditions associated with the anomaly, if applicable.

Also, see Section I.C.14 for information on the coding of congenital anomalies.

h. Coding Additional Perinatal Diagnoses

1) Assigning codes for conditions that require treatment

Assign codes for conditions that require treatment or further investigation, prolong the length of stay, or require resource utilization.

2) Codes for conditions specified as having implications for future health care needs

Assign codes for conditions that have been specified by the provider as having implications for future health care needs.

Note: This guideline should not be used for adult patients.

3) Codes for newborn conditions originating in the perinatal period

Assign a code for newborn conditions originating in the perinatal period (categories 760-779), as well as complications arising during the current episode of care classified in other chapters, only if the diagnoses have been documented by the responsible provider at the time of transfer or discharge as having affected the fetus or newborn.

i. Prematurity and Fetal Growth Retardation

Providers utilize different criteria in determining prematurity. A code for prematurity should not be assigned unless it is documented. The 5th digit assignment for codes from category 764 and subcategories 765.0 and 765.1 should be based on the recorded birth weight and estimated gestational age.

A code from subcategory 765.2, Weeks of gestation, should be assigned as an additional code with category 764 and codes from 765.0 and 765.1 to specify weeks of gestation as documented by the provider in the record.

j. Newborn sepsis

Code 771.81, Septicemia [sepsis] of newborn, should be assigned with a secondary code from category 041, Bacterial infections in conditions classified elsewhere and of unspecified site, to identify the organism. A code from category 038, Septicemia, should not be used on a newborn record. Do not assign code 995.91, Sepsis, as code 771.81 describes the sepsis. If applicable, use additional codes to identify severe sepsis (995.92) and any associated acute organ dysfunction.

16. **Chapter 16: Signs, Symptoms and Ill-Defined Conditions (780-799)**

    Reserved for future guideline expansion

17. **Chapter 17: Injury and Poisoning (800-999)**

    a. **Coding of Injuries**

    When coding injuries, assign separate codes for each injury unless a combination code is provided, in which case the combination code is assigned. Multiple injury codes are provided in ICD-9-CM, but should not be assigned unless information for a more specific code is not available. These traumatic injury codes are not to be used for normal, healing surgical wounds or to identify complications of surgical wounds.

    The code for the most serious injury, as determined by the provider and the focus of treatment, is sequenced first.

    1) **Superficial injuries**

        Superficial injuries such as abrasions or contusions are not coded when associated with more severe injuries of the same site.

    2) **Primary injury with damage to nerves/blood vessels**

        When a primary injury results in minor damage to peripheral nerves or blood vessels, the primary injury is sequenced first with additional code(s) from categories 950-957, Injury to nerves and spinal cord, and/or 900-904, Injury to blood vessels. When the primary injury is to the blood vessels or nerves, that injury should be sequenced first.

    b. **Coding of Traumatic Fractures**

    The principles of multiple coding of injuries should be followed in coding fractures. Fractures of specified sites are coded individually by site in accordance with both the provisions within categories 800-829 and the level of detail furnished by medical record content. Combination categories for multiple fractures are provided for use when there is insufficient detail in the medical record (such as trauma cases transferred to another hospital), when the reporting form limits the number of codes that can be used in reporting pertinent clinical data, or when there is insufficient specificity at the fourth-digit or fifth-digit level. More specific guidelines are as follows:

    1) **Acute Fractures vs. Aftercare**

        Traumatic fractures are coded using the acute fracture codes (800-829) while the patient is receiving active treatment for the fracture.   Examples of active treatment are: surgical treatment, emergency department encounter, and evaluation and treatment by a new physician.

        Fractures are coded using the aftercare codes (subcategories V54.0, V54.1, V54.8, or V54.9) for encounters after the patient has completed active treatment of the fracture and is receiving routine care for the fracture during the healing or recovery phase. Examples of fracture aftercare are: cast change or removal, removal of external or internal fixation device, medication adjustment, and follow up visits following fracture treatment.

        Care for complications of surgical treatment for fracture repairs during the healing or recovery phase should be coded with the appropriate complication codes.

        Care of complications of fractures, such as malunion and nonunion, should be reported with the appropriate codes.

        Pathologic fractures are not coded in the 800-829 range, but instead are assigned to subcategory 733.1. *See Section I.C.13.a for additional information.*

    2) **Multiple fractures of same limb**

        Multiple fractures of same limb classifiable to the same three-digit or four-digit category are coded to that category.

    3) **Multiple unilateral or bilateral fractures of same bone**

        Multiple unilateral or bilateral fractures of same bone(s) but classified to different fourth-digit subdivisions (bone part) within the same three-digit category are coded individually by site.

    4) **Multiple fracture categories 819 and 828**

        Multiple fracture categories 819 and 828 classify bilateral fractures of both upper limbs (819) and both lower limbs (828), but without any detail at the fourth-digit level other than open and closed type of fractures.

    5) **Multiple fractures sequencing**

        Multiple fractures are sequenced in accordance with the severity of the fracture. The provider should be asked to list the fracture diagnoses in the order of severity.

    c. **Coding of Burns**

    Current burns (940-948) are classified by depth, extent and by agent (E code). Burns are classified by depth as first degree (erythema), second degree (blistering), and third degree (full-thickness involvement).

    1) **Sequencing of burn and related condition codes**

        Sequence first the code that reflects the highest degree of burn when more than one burn is present.

        a. When the reason for the admission or encounter is for treatment of external multiple burns, sequence first the code that reflects the burn of the highest degree.

        b. When a patient has both internal and external burns, the circumstances of admission govern the selection of the principal diagnosis or first-listed diagnosis.

        c. When a patient is admitted for burn injuries and other related conditions such as smoke inhalation and/or respiratory failure, the circumstances of admission govern the selection of the principal or first-listed diagnosis.

    2) **Burns of the same local site**

        Classify burns of the same local site (three-digit category level, 940-947) but of different degrees to the subcategory identifying the highest degree recorded in the diagnosis.

    3) **Non-healing burns**

        Non-healing burns are coded as acute burns.

        Necrosis of burned skin should be coded as a non-healed burn.

    4) **Code 958.3, Posttraumatic wound infection**

        Assign code 958.3, Posttraumatic wound infection, not elsewhere classified, as an additional code for any documented infected burn site.

    5) **Assign separate codes for each burn site**

        When coding burns, assign separate codes for each burn site. Category 946 Burns of Multiple specified sites, should only be used if the location of the burns are not documented.

        Category 949, Burn, unspecified, is extremely vague and should rarely be used.

    6) **Assign codes from category 948, Burns**

        Burns classified according to extent of body surface involved, when the site of the burn is not specified or when there is a need for additional data. It is advisable to use category 948 as additional coding when needed to provide data for evaluating burn mortality, such as that needed by burn units. It is also advisable to use category 948 as an additional code for reporting purposes when there is mention of a third-degree burn involving 20 percent or more of the body surface.

        In assigning a code from category 948:

            Fourth-digit codes are used to identify the percentage of total body surface involved in a burn (all degree).

Fifth-digits are assigned to identify the percentage of body surface involved in third-degree burn.

Fifth-digit zero (0) is assigned when less than 10 percent or when no body surface is involved in a third-degree burn.

Category 948 is based on the classic "rule of nines" in estimating body surface involved: head and neck are assigned nine percent, each arm nine percent, each leg 18 percent, the anterior trunk 18 percent, posterior trunk 18 percent, and genitalia one percent. Providers may change these percentage assignments where necessary to accommodate infants and children who have proportionally larger heads than adults and patients who have large buttocks, thighs, or abdomen that involve burns.

7) Encounters for treatment of late effects of burns

Encounters for the treatment of the late effects of burns (i.e., scars or joint contractures) should be coded to the residual condition (sequelae) followed by the appropriate late effect code (906.5-906.9). A late effect E code may also be used, if desired.

8) Sequelae with a late effect code and current burn

When appropriate, both a sequelae with a late effect code, and a current burn code may be assigned on the same record (when both a current burn and sequelae of an old burn exist).

d. Coding of Debridement of Wound, Infection, or Burn

Excisional debridement involves surgical removal or cutting away, as opposed to a mechanical (brushing, scrubbing, washing) debridement.

For coding purposes, excisional debridement is assigned to code 86.22.

Nonexcisional debridement is assigned to code 86.28.

e. Adverse Effects, Poisoning and Toxic Effects

The properties of certain drugs, medicinal and biological substances or combinations of such substances, may cause toxic reactions. The occurrence of drug toxicity is classified in ICD-9-CM as follows:

1) Adverse Effect

When the drug was correctly prescribed and properly administered, code the reaction plus the appropriate code from the E930-E949 series. Codes from the E930-E949 series must be used to identify the causative substance for an adverse effect of drug, medicinal and biological substances, correctly prescribed and properly administered. The effect, such as tachycardia, delirium, gastrointestinal hemorrhaging, vomiting, hypokalemia, hepatitis, renal failure, or respiratory failure, is coded and followed by the appropriate code from the E930-E949 series.

Adverse effects of therapeutic substances correctly prescribed and properly administered (toxicity, synergistic reaction, side effect, and idiosyncratic reaction) may be due to (1) differences among patients, such as age, sex, disease, and genetic factors, and (2) drug-related factors, such as type of drug, route of administration, duration of therapy, dosage, and bioavailability.

2) Poisoning

(a) Error was made in drug prescription

Errors made in drug prescription or in the administration of the drug by provider, nurse, patient, or other person, use the appropriate poisoning code from the 960-979 series.

(b) Overdose of a drug intentionally taken

If an overdose of a drug was intentionally taken or administered and resulted in drug toxicity, it would be coded as a poisoning (960-979 series).

(c) Nonprescribed drug taken with correctly prescribed and properly administered drug

If a nonprescribed drug or medicinal agent was taken in combination with a correctly prescribed and properly administered drug, any drug toxicity or other reaction resulting from the interaction of the two drugs would be classified as a poisoning.

(d) Interaction of drug(s) and alcohol

When a reaction results from the interaction of a drug(s) and alcohol, this would be classified as poisoning.

(e) Sequencing of poisoning

When coding a poisoning or reaction to the improper use of a medication (e.g., wrong dose, wrong substance, wrong route of administration) the poisoning code is sequenced first, followed by a code for the manifestation. If there is also a diagnosis of drug abuse or dependence to the substance, the abuse or dependence is coded as an additional code.

See Section I.C.3.a.6.b. if poisoning is the result of insulin pump malfunctions and Section I.C.19 for general use of E-codes.

3) Toxic Effects

(a) Toxic effect codes

When a harmful substance is ingested or comes in contact with a person, this is classified as a toxic effect. The toxic effect codes are in categories 980-989.

(b) Sequencing toxic effect codes

A toxic effect code should be sequenced first, followed by the code(s) that identify the result of the toxic effect.

(c) External cause codes for toxic effects

An external cause code from categories E860-E869 for accidental exposure, codes E950.6 or E950.7 for intentional self-harm, category E962 for assault, or categories E980-E982, for undetermined, should also be assigned to indicate intent.

f. Complications of care

1) Complications of care

(a) Documentation of complications of care

See Section I.B.18. for information on documentation of complications of care.

(b) Use additional code to identify nature of complication

An additional code identifying the complication should be assigned with codes in categories 996-999, Complications of Surgical and Medical Care NEC, when the additional code provides greater specificity as to the nature of the condition. If the complication code fully describes the condition, no additional code is necessary.

2) Transplant complications

(a) Transplant complications other than kidney

Codes under subcategory 996.8, Complications of transplanted organ, are for use for both complications and rejection of transplanted organs. A transplant complication code is only assigned if the complication affects the function of the transplanted organ. Two codes are required to fully describe a transplant complication, the appropriate code from subcategory 996.8 and a secondary code that identifies the complication.

Pre-existing conditions or conditions that develop after the transplant are not coded as complications unless they affect the function of the transplanted organs.

See I.C.18.d.3 for transplant organ removal status

See I.C.2.i for malignant neoplasm associated with transplanted organ.

(b) Chronic kidney disease and kidney transplant complications

Patients who have undergone kidney transplant may still have some form of chronic kidney disease (CKD) because the kidney transplant may not fully restore kidney function. Code 996.81 should be assigned for documented complications of a kidney transplant, such as transplant failure or rejection or other transplant complication. Code 996.81 should not be assigned for post kidney transplant patients who have chronic kidney (CKD) unless a transplant complication such as transplant failure or rejection is documented. If the documentation is unclear as to whether the patient has a complication of the transplant, query the provider.

Conditions that affect the function of the transplanted kidney, other than CKD, should be assigned code 996.81, Complications of transplanted organ, Kidney, and a secondary code that identifies the complication.

For patients with CKD following a kidney transplant, but who do not have a complication such as failure or rejection, *see section I.C.10.a.2, Chronic kidney disease and kidney transplant status.*

3) Ventilator associated pneumonia

(a) Documentation of Ventilator associated Pneumonia

As with all procedural or postprocedural complications, code assignment is based on the provider's documentation of the relationship between the condition and the procedure.

Code 997.31, Ventilator associated pneumonia, should be assigned only when the provider has documented ventilator associated pneumonia (VAP). An additional code to identify the organism (e.g., Pseudomonas aeruginosa, code 041.7) should also be assigned. Do not assign an additional code from categories 480-484 to identify the type of pneumonia.

Code 997.31 should not be assigned for cases where the patient has pneumonia and is on a mechanical ventilator but the provider has not specifically stated that the pneumonia is ventilator-associated pneumonia.

If the documentation is unclear as to whether the patient has a pneumonia that is a complication attributable to the mechanical ventilator, query the provider.

(b) Patient admitted with pneumonia and develops VAP

A patient may be admitted with one type of pneumonia (e.g., code 481, Pneumococcal pneumonia) and subsequently develop VAP. In this instance, the principal diagnosis would be the appropriate code from categories 480-484 for the pneumonia diagnosed at the time of admission. Code 997.31, Ventilator associated pneumonia, would be assigned as an additional diagnosis when the provider has also documented the presence of ventilator associated pneumonia.

g. SIRS due to Non-infectious Process

The systemic inflammatory response syndrome (SIRS) can develop as a result of certain non-infectious disease processes, such as trauma, malignant neoplasm, or pancreatitis. When SIRS is documented with a noninfectious condition, and no subsequent infection is documented, the code for the underlying condition, such as an injury, should be assigned, followed by code 995.93, Systemic inflammatory response syndrome due to noninfectious process without acute organ dysfunction, or 995.94, Systemic inflammatory response syndrome due to non-infectious process with acute organ dysfunction. If an acute organ dysfunction is documented, the appropriate code(s) for the associated acute organ dysfunction(s) should be assigned in addition to code 995.94. If acute organ dysfunction is documented, but it cannot be determined if the acute organ

dysfunction is associated with SIRS or due to another condition (e.g., directly due to the trauma), the provider should be queried.

When the non-infectious condition has led to an infection that results in SIRS, *see Section I.C.1.b.12 for the guideline for sepsis and severe sepsis associated with a non-infectious process.*

18. Classification of Factors Influencing Health Status and Contact with Health Service (Supplemental V01-V91)

Note: The chapter specific guidelines provide additional information about the use of V codes for specified encounters.

a. Introduction

ICD-9-CM provides codes to deal with encounters for circumstances other than a disease or injury. The Supplementary Classification of Factors Influencing Health Status and Contact with Health Services (V01.0 - V91.99) is provided to deal with occasions when circumstances other than a disease or injury (codes 001-999) are recorded as a diagnosis or problem.

There are four primary circumstances for the use of V codes:

1) A person who is not currently sick encounters the health services for some specific reason, such as to act as an organ donor, to receive prophylactic care, such as inoculations or health screenings, or to receive counseling on health related issues.

2) A person with a resolving disease or injury, or a chronic, long-term condition requiring continuous care, encounters the health care system for specific aftercare of that disease or injury (e.g., dialysis for renal disease; chemotherapy for malignancy; cast change). A diagnosis/symptom code should be used whenever a current, acute, diagnosis is being treated or a sign or symptom is being studied.

3) Circumstances or problems influence a person's health status but are not in themselves a current illness or injury.

4) Newborns, to indicate birth status

b. V codes use in any healthcare setting

V codes are for use in any healthcare setting. V codes may be used as either a first listed (principal diagnosis code in the inpatient setting) or secondary code, depending on the circumstances of the encounter. Certain V codes may only be used as first listed, others only as secondary codes.

See Section I.C.18.e, V Codes That May Only be Principal/First-Listed Diagnosis.

c. V Codes indicate a reason for an encounter

They are not procedure codes. A corresponding procedure code must accompany a V code to describe the procedure performed.

d. Categories of V Codes

1) Contact/Exposure

Category V01 indicates contact with or exposure to communicable diseases. These codes are for patients who do not show any sign or symptom of a disease but have been exposed to it by close personal contact with an infected individual or are in an area where a disease is epidemic. These codes may be used as a first listed code to explain an encounter for testing, or, more commonly, as a secondary code to identify a potential risk.

Codes V15.84 – V15.86 describe contact with or (suspected) exposure to asbestos, potentially hazardous body fluids, and lead.

Subcategories V87.0 – V87.3 describe contact with or (suspected) exposure to hazardous metals, aromatic compounds, other potentially hazardous chemicals, and other potentially hazardous substances.

2) Inoculations and vaccinations

Categories V03-V06 are for encounters for inoculations and vaccinations. They indicate that a patient is being seen to receive a prophylactic inoculation against a disease. The injection itself must be represented by the appropriate procedure code. A code from V03-V06 may be used as a secondary code if the inoculation is given as a routine part of preventive health care, such as a well-baby visit.

3) Status

Status codes indicate that a patient is a carrier of a disease, has the sequelae or residual of a past disease or condition, or has another factor influencing a person's health status. This includes such things as the presence of prosthetic or mechanical devices resulting from past treatment. A status code is informative, because the status may affect the course of treatment and its outcome. A status code is distinct from a history code. The history code indicates that the patient no longer has the condition.

A status code should not be used with a diagnosis code from one of the body system chapters, if the diagnosis code includes the information provided by the status code. For example, code V42.1, Heart transplant status, should not be used with code 996.83, Complications of transplanted heart. The status code does not provide additional information. The complication code indicates that the patient is a heart transplant patient.

The status V codes/categories are:

V02   Carrier or suspected carrier of infectious diseases

Carrier status indicates that a person harbors the specific organisms of a disease without manifest symptoms and is capable of transmitting the infection.

V07.5x Use of agents affecting estrogen receptors and estrogen level

This code indicates when a patient is receiving a drug that affects estrogen receptors and estrogen levels for prevention of cancer.

V08   Asymptomatic HIV infection status

This code indicates that a patient has tested positive for HIV but has manifested no signs or symptoms of the disease.

V09   Infection with drug-resistant microorganisms

This category indicates that a patient has an infection that is resistant to drug treatment. Sequence the infection code first.

V21   Constitutional states in development

V22.2   Pregnant state, incidental

This code is a secondary code only for use when the pregnancy is in no way complicating the reason for visit. Otherwise, a code from the obstetric chapter is required.

V26.5x Sterilization status

V42   Organ or tissue replaced by transplant

V43   Organ or tissue replaced by other means

V44   Artificial opening status

V45   Other postsurgical states

Assign code V45.87, Transplant organ removal status, to indicate that a transplanted organ has been previously removed. This code should not be assigned for the encounter in which the transplanted organ is removed. The complication necessitating removal of the transplant organ should be assigned for that encounter.

See section I.C17.f.2. for information on the coding of organ transplant complications.

Assign code V45.88, Status post administration of tPA (rtPA) in a different facility within the last 24 hours prior to admission to the current facility, as a secondary diagnosis when a patient is received by transfer into a facility and documentation indicates they were administered tissue plasminogen activator (tPA) within the last 24 hours prior to admission to the current facility.

This guideline applies even if the patient is still receiving the tPA at the time they are received into the current facility.

The appropriate code for the condition for which the tPA was administered (such as cerebrovascular disease or myocardial infarction) should be assigned first.

Code V45.88 is only applicable to the receiving facility record and not to the transferring facility record.

V46   Other dependence on machines

V49.6   Upper limb amputation status

V49.7   Lower limb amputation status

Note: Categories V42-V46, and subcategories V49.6, V49.7 are for use only if there are no complications or malfunctions of the organ or tissue replaced, the amputation site or the equipment on which the patient is dependent.

V49.81 Asymptomatic postmenopausal status (age-related) (natural)

V49.82 Dental sealant status

V49.83 Awaiting organ transplant status

V49.86 Do not resuscitate status

This code may be used when it is documented by the provider that a patient is on do not resuscitate status at any time during the stay.

V49.87 Physical restraint status

This code may be used when it is documented by the provider that a patient has been put in restraints during the current encounter. Please note that this code should not be reported when it is documented by the provider that a patient is temporarily restrained during a procedure.

V58.6x Long-term (current) drug use

Codes from this subcategory indicate a patient's continuous use of a prescribed drug (including such things as aspirin therapy) for the long-term treatment of a condition or for prophylactic use. It is not for use for patients who have addictions to drugs. This subcategory is not for use of medications for detoxification or maintenance programs to prevent withdrawal symptoms in patients with drug dependence (e.g., methadone maintenance for opiate dependence). Assign the appropriate code for the drug dependence instead.

Assign a code from subcategory V58.6, Long-term (current) drug use, if the patient is receiving a medication for an extended period as a prophylactic measure (such as for the prevention of deep vein thrombosis) or as treatment of a chronic condition (such as arthritis) or a disease requiring a lengthy course of treatment (such as cancer). Do not assign a code from subcategory V58.6 for medication being administered for a brief period of time to treat an acute illness or injury (such as a course of antibiotics to treat acute bronchitis).

V83   Genetic carrier status

Genetic carrier status indicates that a person carries a gene, associated with a particular disease, which may be passed to offspring who may develop that disease. The person does not have the disease and is not at risk of developing the disease.

V84   Genetic susceptibility status

Genetic susceptibility indicates that a person has a gene that increases the risk of that person developing the disease.

Codes from category V84, Genetic susceptibility to disease, should not be used as principal or first-listed codes. If the patient has the condition to which he/she is susceptible, and that condition is the reason for the encounter, the code for the current condition should be sequenced first. If the patient is being seen for follow-up after completed treatment for this condition, and the condition no longer exists, a follow-up code should be sequenced first, followed by the appropriate personal history and genetic susceptibility codes. If the purpose of the encounter is genetic counseling associated with procreative management, a code from subcategory V26.3, Genetic counseling and testing, should be assigned as the first-listed code, followed by a code from category V84. Additional codes should be assigned for any applicable family or personal history.

See Section I.C. 18.d.14 for information on prophylactic organ removal due to a genetic susceptibility.

V85	Body Mass Index (BMI)
V86	Estrogen receptor status
V88	Acquired absence of other organs and tissue
V90	Retained foreign body

4) History (of)

There are two types of history V codes, personal and family. Personal history codes explain a patient's past medical condition that no longer exists and is not receiving any treatment, but that has the potential for recurrence, and therefore may require continued monitoring. The exceptions to this general rule are category V14, Personal history of allergy to medicinal agents, and subcategory V15.0, Allergy, other than to medicinal agents. A person who has had an allergic episode to a substance or food in the past should always be considered allergic to the substance.

Family history codes are for use when a patient has a family member(s) who has had a particular disease that causes the patient to be at higher risk of also contracting the disease.

Personal history codes may be used in conjunction with follow-up codes and family history codes may be used in conjunction with screening codes to explain the need for a test or procedure. History codes are also acceptable on any medical record regardless of the reason for visit. A history of an illness, even if no longer present, is important information that may alter the type of treatment ordered.

The history V code categories are:

V10	Personal history of malignant neoplasm
V12	Personal history of certain other diseases
V13	Personal history of other diseases
	Except: V13.4, Personal history of arthritis, and subcategory V13.6, Personal history of congenital (corrected) malformations. These conditions are life-long so are not true history codes.
V14	Personal history of allergy to medicinal agents
V15	Other personal history presenting hazards to health
	Except: Codes V15.7, Personal history of contraception; V15.84, Contact with and (suspected) exposure to asbestos; V15.85, Contact with and (suspected) exposure to potentially hazardous body fluids; V15.86, Contact with and (suspected) exposure to lead.
V16	Family history of malignant neoplasm
V17	Family history of certain chronic disabling diseases
V18	Family history of certain other specific diseases
V19	Family history of other conditions
V87	Other specified personal exposures and history presenting hazards to health
	Except: Subcategories V87.0, Contact with and (suspected) exposure to hazardous metals; V87.1, Contact with and (suspected) exposure to hazardous aromatic compounds; V87.2, Contact with and (suspected) exposure to other potentially

hazardous chemicals; and V87.3, Contact with and (suspected) exposure to other potentially hazardous substances.

5) Screening

Screening is the testing for disease or disease precursors in seemingly well individuals so that early detection and treatment can be provided for those who test positive for the disease. Screenings that are recommended for many subgroups in a population include: routine mammograms for women over 40, a fecal occult blood test for everyone over 50, an amniocentesis to rule out a fetal anomaly for pregnant women over 35, because the incidence of breast cancer and colon cancer in these subgroups is higher than in the general population, as is the incidence of Down's syndrome in older mothers.

The testing of a person to rule out or confirm a suspected diagnosis because the patient has some sign or symptom is a diagnostic examination, not a screening. In these cases, the sign or symptom is used to explain the reason for the test.

A screening code may be a first listed code if the reason for the visit is specifically the screening exam. It may also be used as an additional code if the screening is done during an office visit for other health problems. A screening code is not necessary if the screening is inherent to a routine examination, such as a pap smear done during a routine pelvic examination.

Should a condition be discovered during the screening then the code for the condition may be assigned as an additional diagnosis.

The V code indicates that a screening exam is planned. A procedure code is required to confirm that the screening was performed.

The screening V code categories:

V28	Antenatal screening
V73-V82	Special screening examinations

6) Observation

There are three observation V code categories. They are for use in very limited circumstances when a person is being observed for a suspected condition that is ruled out. The observation codes are not for use if an injury or illness or any signs or symptoms related to the suspected condition are present. In such cases the diagnosis/symptom code is used with the corresponding E code to identify any external cause. The observation codes are to be used as principal diagnosis only. The only exception to this is when the principal diagnosis is required to be a code from the V30, Live born infant, category. Then the V29 observation code is sequenced after the V30 code. Additional codes may be used in addition to the observation code but only if they are unrelated to the suspected condition being observed.

Codes from subcategory V89.0, Suspected maternal and fetal conditions not found, may either be used as a first listed or as an additional code assignment depending on the case. They are for use in very limited circumstances on a maternal record when an encounter is for a suspected maternal or fetal condition that is ruled out during that encounter (for example, a maternal or fetal condition may be suspected due to an abnormal test result). These codes should not be used when the condition is confirmed. In those cases, the confirmed condition should be coded. In addition, these codes are not for use if an illness or any signs or symptoms related to the suspected condition or problem are present. In such cases the diagnosis/symptom code is used.

Additional codes may be used in addition to the code from subcategory V89.0, but only if they are unrelated to the suspected condition being evaluated.

Codes from subcategory V89.0 may not be used for encounters for antenatal screening of mother. *See Section I.C.18.d., Screening.*

For encounters for suspected fetal condition that are inconclusive following testing and evaluation, assign the appropriate code from category 655, 656, 657 or 658.

The observation V code categories:

V29   Observation and evaluation of newborns for suspected condition not found

> For the birth encounter, a code from category V30 should be sequenced before the V29 code.

V71   Observation and evaluation for suspected condition not found

V89   Suspected maternal and fetal conditions not found

7) Aftercare

Aftercare visit codes cover situations when the initial treatment of a disease or injury has been performed and the patient requires continued care during the healing or recovery phase, or for the long-term consequences of the disease. The aftercare V code should not be used if treatment is directed at a current, acute disease or injury. The diagnosis code is to be used in these cases. Exceptions to this rule are codes V58.0, Radiotherapy, and codes from subcategory V58.1, Encounter for chemotherapy and immunotherapy for neoplastic conditions. These codes are to be first listed, followed by the diagnosis code when a patient's encounter is solely to receive radiation therapy or chemotherapy for the treatment of a neoplasm. Should a patient receive both chemotherapy and radiation therapy during the same encounter code V58.0 and V58.1 may be used together on a record with either one being sequenced first.

The aftercare codes are generally first listed to explain the specific reason for the encounter. An aftercare code may be used as an additional code when some type of aftercare is provided in addition to the reason for admission and no diagnosis code is applicable. An example of this would be the closure of a colostomy during an encounter for treatment of another condition.

Aftercare codes should be used in conjunction with any other aftercare codes or other diagnosis codes to provide better detail on the specifics of an aftercare encounter visit, unless otherwise directed by the classification. The sequencing of multiple aftercare codes is discretionary.

Certain aftercare V code categories need a secondary diagnosis code to describe the resolving condition or sequelae, for others, the condition is inherent in the code title.

Additional V code aftercare category terms include fitting and adjustment, and attention to artificial openings.

Status V codes may be used with aftercare V codes to indicate the nature of the aftercare. For example code V45.81, Aortocoronary bypass status, may be used with code V58.73, Aftercare following surgery of the circulatory system, NEC, to indicate the surgery for which the aftercare is being performed. Also, a transplant status code may be used following code V58.44, Aftercare following organ transplant, to identify the organ transplanted. A status code should not be used when the aftercare code indicates the type of status, such as using V55.0, Attention to tracheostomy with V44.0, Tracheostomy status.

See Section I. B.16 Admissions/Encounter for Rehabilitation

The aftercare V category/codes:

V51.0   Encounter for breast reconstruction following mastectomy

V52   Fitting and adjustment of prosthetic device and implant

V53   Fitting and adjustment of other device

V54   Other orthopedic aftercare

V55   Attention to artificial openings

V56   Encounter for dialysis and dialysis catheter care

V57   Care involving the use of rehabilitation procedures

V58.0   Radiotherapy

V58.11   Encounter for antineoplastic chemotherapy

V58.12   Encounter for antineoplastic immunotherapy

V58.3x   Attention to dressings and sutures

V58.41   Encounter for planned post-operative wound closure

V58.42   Aftercare, surgery, neoplasm

V58.43   Aftercare, surgery, trauma

V58.44   Aftercare involving organ transplant

V58.49   Other specified aftercare following surgery

V58.7x   Aftercare following surgery

V58.81   Fitting and adjustment of vascular catheter

V58.82   Fitting and adjustment of non-vascular catheter

V58.83   Monitoring therapeutic drug

V58.89   Other specified aftercare

8) Follow-up

The follow-up codes are used to explain continuing surveillance following completed treatment of a disease, condition, or injury. They imply that the condition has been fully treated and no longer exists. They should not be confused with aftercare codes that explain current treatment for a healing condition or its sequelae. Follow-up codes may be used in conjunction with history codes to provide the full picture of the healed condition and its treatment. The follow-up code is sequenced first, followed by the history code.

A follow-up code may be used to explain repeated visits. Should a condition be found to have recurred on the follow-up visit, then the diagnosis code should be used in place of the follow-up code.

The follow-up V code categories:

V24   Postpartum care and evaluation

V67   Follow-up examination

9) Donor

Category V59 is the donor codes. They are used for living individuals who are donating blood or other body tissue. These codes are only for individuals donating for others, not for self donations. They are not for use to identify cadaveric donations.

10) Counseling

Counseling V codes are used when a patient or family member receives assistance in the aftermath of an illness or injury, or when support is required in coping with family or social problems. They are not necessary for use in conjunction with a diagnosis code when the counseling component of care is considered integral to standard treatment.

The counseling V categories/codes:

V25.0   General counseling and advice for contraceptive management

V26.3   Genetic counseling

V26.4   General counseling and advice for procreative management

V61.x   Other family circumstances

V65.1   Person consulted on behalf of another person

V65.3   Dietary surveillance and counseling

V65.4   Other counseling, not elsewhere classified

11) Obstetrics and related conditions

See Section I.C.11., the Obstetrics guidelines for further instruction on the use of these codes.

V codes for pregnancy are for use in those circumstances when none of the problems or complications included in the codes from the Obstetrics chapter exist (a routine prenatal visit or postpartum care). Codes V22.0, Supervision of normal first pregnancy, and V22.1, Supervision of other normal pregnancy, are always first listed and are not to be used with any other code from the OB chapter.

The outcome of delivery, category V27, should be included on all maternal delivery records. It is always a secondary code.

V codes for family planning (contraceptive) or procreative management and counseling should be included on an obstetric record either during the pregnancy or the postpartum stage, if applicable.

Obstetrics and related conditions V code categories:

V22	Normal pregnancy
V23	Supervision of high-risk pregnancy
	Except: V23.2, Pregnancy with history of abortion. Code 646.3, Recurrent pregnancy loss, from the OB chapter is required to indicate a history of abortion during a pregnancy.
V24	Postpartum care and evaluation
V25	Encounter for contraceptive management
	Except V25.0x
	(See Section I.C.18.d.11, Counseling)
V26	Procreative management
	Except: V26.5x, Sterilization status, V26.3 and V26.4
	(See Section I.C.18.d.11., Counseling)
V27	Outcome of delivery
V28	Antenatal screening
	(See Section I.C.18.d.6., Screening)
V91	Multiple gestation placenta status

12) Newborn, infant and child

See Section I.C.15, the Newborn guidelines for further instruction on the use of these codes.

Newborn V code categories:

V20	Health supervision of infant or child
V29	Observation and evaluation of newborns for suspected condition not found
	(See Section I.C.18.d.7, Observation)
V30-V39	Liveborn infant according to type of birth

13) Routine and administrative examinations

The V codes allow for the description of encounters for routine examinations, such as, a general check-up, or examinations for administrative purposes, such as a pre-employment physical. The codes are not to be used if the examination is for diagnosis of a suspected condition or for treatment purposes. In such cases the diagnosis code is used. During a routine exam, should a diagnosis or condition be discovered, it should be coded as an additional code. Pre-existing and chronic conditions and history codes may also be included as additional codes as long as the examination is for administrative purposes and not focused on any particular condition.

Pre-operative examination and pre-procedural laboratory examination V codes are for use only in those situations when a patient is being cleared for a procedure or surgery and no treatment is given.

The V codes categories/code for routine and administrative examinations:

V20.2	Routine infant or child health check
	Any injections given should have a corresponding procedure code.
V70	General medical examination
V72	Special investigations and examinations
	Codes V72.5 and V72.62 may be used if the reason for the patient encounter is for routine laboratory/radiology testing in the absence of any signs, symptoms, or associated diagnosis. If routine testing is performed during the same encounter as

a test to evaluate a sign, symptom, or diagnosis, it is appropriate to assign both the V code and the code describing the reason for the non-routine test.

14) Miscellaneous V codes

The miscellaneous V codes capture a number of other health care encounters that do not fall into one of the other categories. Certain of these codes identify the reason for the encounter, others are for use as additional codes that provide useful information on circumstances that may affect a patient's care and treatment.

Prophylactic Organ Removal

For encounters specifically for prophylactic removal of breasts, ovaries, or another organ due to a genetic susceptibility to cancer or a family history of cancer, the principal or first listed code should be a code from subcategory V50.4, Prophylactic organ removal, followed by the appropriate genetic susceptibility code and the appropriate family history code.

If the patient has a malignancy of one site and is having prophylactic removal at another site to prevent either a new primary malignancy or metastatic disease, a code for the malignancy should also be assigned in addition to a code from subcategory V50.4. A V50.4 code should not be assigned if the patient is having organ removal for treatment of a malignancy, such as the removal of the testes for the treatment of prostate cancer.

Miscellaneous V code categories/codes:

V07	Need for isolation and other prophylactic or treatment measures
	Except V07.5X, Use of agents affecting estrogen receptors and estrogen levels
V40.31	Wandering in diseases classified elsewhere
V50	Elective surgery for purposes other than remedying health states
V58.5	Orthodontics
V60	Housing, household, and economic circumstances
V62	Other psychosocial circumstances
V63	Unavailability of other medical facilities for care
V64	Persons encountering health services for specific procedures, not carried out
V66	Convalescence and Palliative Care
V68	Encounters for administrative purposes
V69	Problems related to lifestyle

15) Nonspecific V codes

Certain V codes are so non-specific, or potentially redundant with other codes in the classification, that there can be little justification for their use in the inpatient setting. Their use in the outpatient setting should be limited to those instances when there is no further documentation to permit more precise coding. Otherwise, any sign or symptom or any other reason for visit that is captured in another code should be used.

Nonspecific V code categories/codes:

V11	Personal history of mental disorder
	A code from the mental disorders chapter, with an in remission fifth-digit, should be used.
V13.4	Personal history of arthritis
V13.6	Personal history of congenital malformations
V15.7	Personal history of contraception
V23.2	Pregnancy with history of abortion
V40	Mental and behavioral problems
	Exception: V40.31 Wandering in diseases classified elsewhere
V41	Problems with special senses and other special functions
V47	Other problems with internal organs

| V48 | Problems with head, neck, and trunk |
| V49 | Problems with limbs and other problems |

Exceptions:

V49.6	Upper limb amputation status
V49.7	Lower limb amputation status
V49.81	Asymptomatic postmenopausal status (age-related) (natural)
V49.82	Dental sealant status
V49.83	Awaiting organ transplant status
V49.86	Do not resuscitate status
V49.87	Physical restraints status

V51.8	Other aftercare involving the use of plastic surgery
V58.2	Blood transfusion, without reported diagnosis
V58.9	Unspecified aftercare

See Section IV.K. and Section IV.L. of the Outpatient guidelines.

e.   V Codes That May Only be Principal/First-Listed Diagnosis

The list of V codes/categories below may only be reported as the principal/first-listed diagnosis, except when there are multiple encounters on the same day and the medical records for the encounters are combined or when there is more than one V code that meets the definition of principal diagnosis (e.g., a patient is admitted to home healthcare for both aftercare and rehabilitation and they equally meet the definition of principal diagnosis). These codes should not be reported if they do not meet the definition of principal or first-listed diagnosis.

See Section II and Section IV.A for information on selection of principal and first-listed diagnosis.

See Section II.C for information on two or more diagnoses that equally meet the definition for principal diagnosis.

V20.x	Health supervision of infant or child
V22.0	Supervision of normal first pregnancy
V22.1	Supervision of other normal pregnancy
V24.x	Postpartum care and examination
V26.81	Encounter for assisted reproductive fertility procedure cycle
V26.82	Encounter for fertility preservation procedure
V30.x	Single liveborn
V31.x	Twin, mate liveborn
V32.x	Twin, mate stillborn
V33.x	Twin, unspecified
V34.x	Other multiple, mates all liveborn
V35.x	Other multiple, mates all stillborn
V36.x	Other multiple, mates live- and stillborn
V37.x	Other multiple, unspecified
V39.x	Unspecified
V46.12	Encounter for respirator dependence during power failure
V46.13	Encounter for weaning from respirator [ventilator]
V51.0	Encounter for breast reconstruction following mastectomy
V56.0	Extracorporeal dialysis
V57.x	Care involving use of rehabilitation procedures
V58.0	Radiotherapy
V58.11	Encounter for antineoplastic chemotherapy
V58.12	Encounter for antineoplastic immunotherapy
V59.x	Donors
V66.0	Convalescence and palliative care following surgery
V66.1	Convalescence and palliative care following radiotherapy
V66.2	Convalescence and palliative care following chemotherapy
V66.3	Convalescence and palliative care following psychotherapy and other treatment for mental disorder
V66.4	Convalescence and palliative care following treatment of fracture
V66.5	Convalescence and palliative care following other treatment
V66.6	Convalescence and palliative care following combined treatment
V66.9	Unspecified convalescence
V68.x	Encounters for administrative purposes
V70.0	Routine general medical examination at a health care facility
V70.1	General psychiatric examination, requested by the authority
V70.2	General psychiatric examination, other and unspecified
V70.3	Other medical examination for administrative purposes
V70.4	Examination for medicolegal reasons
V70.5	Health examination of defined subpopulations
V70.6	Health examination in population surveys
V70.8	Other specified general medical examinations
V70.9	Unspecified general medical examination
V71.x	Observation and evaluation for suspected conditions not found

19. Supplemental Classification of External Causes of Injury and Poisoning (E-codes, E000-E999)

Introduction: These guidelines are provided for those who are currently collecting E codes in order that there will be standardization in the process. If your institution plans to begin collecting E codes, these guidelines are to be applied. The use of E codes is supplemental to the application of ICD-9-CM diagnosis codes.

External causes of injury and poisoning codes (categories E000 and E800-E999) are intended to provide data for injury research and evaluation of injury prevention strategies. Activity codes (categories E001-E030) are intended to be used to describe the activity of a person seeking care for injuries as well as other health conditions, when the injury or other health condition resulted from an activity or the activity contributed to a condition. E codes capture how the injury, poisoning, or adverse effect happened (cause), the intent (unintentional or accidental; or intentional, such as suicide or assault), the person's status (e.g. civilian, military), the associated activity and the place where the event occurred.

Some major categories of E codes include:

transport accidents

poisoning and adverse effects of drugs, medicinal substances and biologicals

accidental falls

accidents caused by fire and flames

accidents due to natural and environmental factors

late effects of accidents, assaults or self injury

assaults or purposely inflicted injury

suicide or self inflicted injury

These guidelines apply for the coding and collection of E codes from records in hospitals, outpatient clinics, emergency departments, other ambulatory care settings and provider offices, and nonacute care settings, except when other specific guidelines apply.

a.   General E Code Coding Guidelines

1)   Used with any code in the range of 001-V91

An E code from categories E800-E999 may be used with any code in the range of 001-V91, which indicates an injury, poisoning, or adverse effect due to an external cause.

An activity E code (categories E001-E030) may be used with any code in the range of 001-V91 that indicates an injury, or other health condition that resulted from an activity, or the activity contributed to a condition.

2) Assign the appropriate E code for all initial treatments

Assign the appropriate E code for the initial encounter of an injury, poisoning, or adverse effect of drugs, not for subsequent treatment.

External cause of injury codes (E-codes) may be assigned while the acute fracture codes are still applicable.

See Section I.C.17.b.1 for coding of acute fractures.

3) Use the full range of E codes

Use the full range of E codes (E800 – E999) to completely describe the cause, the intent and the place of occurrence, if applicable, for all injuries, poisonings, and adverse effects of drugs.

See a.1.), j.), and k.) in this section for information on the use of status and activity E codes.

4) Assign as many E codes as necessary

Assign as many E codes as necessary to fully explain each cause.

5) The selection of the appropriate E code

The selection of the appropriate E code is guided by the Index to External Causes, which is located after the alphabetical index to diseases and by Inclusion and Exclusion notes in the Tabular List.

6) E code can never be a principal diagnosis

An E code can never be a principal (first listed) diagnosis.

7) External cause code(s) with systemic inflammatory response syndrome (SIRS)

An external cause code is not appropriate with a code from subcategory 995.9, unless the patient also has another condition for which an E code would be appropriate (such as an injury, poisoning, or adverse effect of drugs.

8) Multiple Cause E Code Coding Guidelines

More than one E-code is required to fully describe the external cause of an illness, injury or poisoning. The assignment of E-codes should be sequenced in the following priority:

If two or more events cause separate injuries, an E code should be assigned for each cause. The first listed E code will be selected in the following order:

E codes for child and adult abuse take priority over all other E codes.

See Section I.C.19.e., Child and Adult abuse guidelines.

E codes for terrorism events take priority over all other E codes except child and adult abuse.

E codes for cataclysmic events take priority over all other E codes except child and adult abuse and terrorism.

E codes for transport accidents take priority over all other E codes except cataclysmic events, child and adult abuse and terrorism.

Activity and external cause status codes are assigned following all causal (intent) E codes.

The first-listed E code should correspond to the cause of the most serious diagnosis due to an assault, accident, or self-harm, following the order of hierarchy listed above.

9) If the reporting format limits the number of E codes

If the reporting format limits the number of E codes that can be used in reporting clinical data, report the code for the cause/intent most related to the principal diagnosis. If the format permits capture of additional E codes, the cause/intent, including medical misadventures, of the additional events should be reported rather than the codes for place, activity or external status.

b. Place of Occurrence Guideline

Use an additional code from category E849 to indicate the Place of Occurrence. The Place of Occurrence describes the place where the event occurred and not the patient's activity at the time of the event.

Do not use E849.9 if the place of occurrence is not stated.

c. Adverse Effects of Drugs, Medicinal and Biological Substances Guidelines

1) Do not code directly from the Table of Drugs

Do not code directly from the Table of Drugs and Chemicals. Always refer back to the Tabular List.

2) Use as many codes as necessary to describe

Use as many codes as necessary to describe completely all drugs, medicinal or biological substances.

If the reporting format limits the number of E codes, and there are different fourth digit codes in the same three digit category, use the code for "Other specified" of that category of drugs, medicinal or biological substances. If there is no "Other specified" code in that category, use the appropriate "Unspecified" code in that category.

If the reporting format limits the number of E codes, and the codes are in different three digit categories, assign the appropriate E code for other multiple drugs and medicinal substances.

3) If the same E code would describe the causative agent

If the same E code would describe the causative agent for more than one adverse reaction, assign the code only once.

4) If two or more drugs, medicinal or biological substances

If two or more drugs, medicinal or biological substances are reported, code each individually unless the combination code is listed in the Table of Drugs and Chemicals. In that case, assign the E code for the combination.

5) When a reaction results from the interaction of a drug(s)

When a reaction results from the interaction of a drug(s) and alcohol, use poisoning codes and E codes for both.

6) Codes from the E930-E949 series

Codes from the E930-E949 series must be used to identify the causative substance for an adverse effect of drug, medicinal and biological substances, correctly prescribed and properly administered. The effect, such as tachycardia, delirium, gastrointestinal hemorrhaging, vomiting, hypokalemia, hepatitis, renal failure, or respiratory failure, is coded and followed by the appropriate code from the E930-E949 series.

d. Child and Adult Abuse Guideline

1) Intentional injury

When the cause of an injury or neglect is intentional child or adult abuse, the first listed E code should be assigned from categories E960-E968, Homicide and injury purposely inflicted by other persons, (except category E967). An E code from category E967, Child and adult battering and other maltreatment, should be added as an additional code to identify the perpetrator, if known.

2) Accidental intent

In cases of neglect when the intent is determined to be accidental E code E904.0, Abandonment or neglect of infant and helpless person, should be the first listed E code.

e. Unknown or Suspected Intent Guideline

1) If the intent (accident, self-harm, assault) of the cause of an injury or poisoning is unknown

If the intent (accident, self-harm, assault) of the cause of an injury or poisoning is unknown or unspecified, code the intent as undetermined E980-E989.

2) If the intent (accident, self-harm, assault) of the cause of an injury or poisoning is questionable

If the intent (accident, self-harm, assault) of the cause of an injury or poisoning is questionable, probable or suspected, code the intent as undetermined E980-E989.

f.   Undetermined Cause

When the intent of an injury or poisoning is known, but the cause is unknown, use codes: E928.9, Unspecified accident, E958.9, Suicide and self-inflicted injury by unspecified means, and E968.9, Assault by unspecified means.

These E codes should rarely be used, as the documentation in the medical record, in both the inpatient outpatient and other settings, should normally provide sufficient detail to determine the cause of the injury.

g.   Late Effects of External Cause Guidelines

1)   Late effect E codes

Late effect E codes exist for injuries and poisonings but not for adverse effects of drugs, misadventures and surgical complications.

2)   Late effect E codes (E929, E959, E969, E977, E989, or E999.1)

A late effect E code (E929, E959, E969, E977, E989, or E999.1) should be used with any report of a late effect or sequela resulting from a previous injury or poisoning (905-909).

3)   Late effect E code with a related current injury

A late effect E code should never be used with a related current nature of injury code.

4)   Use of late effect E codes for subsequent visits

Use a late effect E code for subsequent visits when a late effect of the initial injury or poisoning is being treated. There is no late effect E code for adverse effects of drugs.

Do not use a late effect E code for subsequent visits for follow-up care (e.g., to assess healing, to receive rehabilitative therapy) of the injury or poisoning when no late effect of the injury has been documented.

h.   Misadventures and Complications of Care Guidelines

1)   Code range E870-E876

Assign a code in the range of E870-E876 if misadventures are stated by the provider. When applying the E code guidelines pertaining to sequencing, these E codes are considered causal codes.

2)   Code range E878-E879

Assign a code in the range of E878-E879 if the provider attributes an abnormal reaction or later complication to a surgical or medical procedure, but does not mention misadventure at the time of the procedure as the cause of the reaction.

i.   Terrorism Guidelines

1)   Cause of injury identified by the Federal Government (FBI) as terrorism

When the cause of an injury is identified by the Federal Government (FBI) as terrorism, the first-listed E-code should be a code from category E979, Terrorism. The definition of terrorism employed by the FBI is found at the inclusion note at E979. The terrorism E-code is the only E-code that should be assigned. Additional E codes from the assault categories should not be assigned.

2)   Cause of an injury is suspected to be the result of terrorism

When the cause of an injury is suspected to be the result of terrorism a code from category E979 should not be assigned. Assign a code in the range of E codes based circumstances on the documentation of intent and mechanism.

3)   Code E979.9, Terrorism, secondary effects

Assign code E979.9, Terrorism, secondary effects, for conditions occurring subsequent to the terrorist event. This code should not be assigned for conditions that are due to the initial terrorist act.

4)   Statistical tabulation of terrorism codes

For statistical purposes these codes will be tabulated within the category for assault, expanding the current category from E960-E969 to include E979 and E999.1.

j.   Activity Code Guidelines

Assign a code from category E001-E030 to describe the activity that caused or contributed to the injury or other health condition.

Unlike other E codes, activity E codes may be assigned to indicate a health condition (not just injuries) resulted from an activity, or the activity contributed to the condition.

The activity codes are not applicable to poisonings, adverse effects, misadventures or late effects.

Do not assign E030, Unspecified activity, if the activity is not stated.

k.   External cause status

A code from category E000, External cause status, should be assigned whenever any other E code is assigned for an encounter, including an Activity E code, except for the events noted below. Assign a code from category E000, External cause status, to indicate the work status of the person at the time the event occurred. The status code indicates whether the event occurred during military activity, whether a non-military person was at work, whether an individual including a student or volunteer was involved in a non-work activity at the time of the causal event.

A code from E000, External cause status, should be assigned, when applicable, with other external cause codes, such as transport accidents and falls. The external cause status codes are not applicable to poisonings, adverse effects, misadventures or late effects.

Do not assign a code from category E000 if no other E codes (cause, activity) are applicable for the encounter.

Do not assign code E000.9, Unspecified external cause status, if the status is not stated.

Section II. Selection of Principal Diagnosis

The circumstances of inpatient admission always govern the selection of principal diagnosis. The principal diagnosis is defined in the Uniform Hospital Discharge Data Set (UHDDS) as "that condition established after study to be chiefly responsible for occasioning the admission of the patient to the hospital for care."

The UHDDS definitions are used by hospitals to report inpatient data elements in a standardized manner. These data elements and their definitions can be found in the July 31, 1985, Federal Register (Vol. 50, No, 147), pp. 31038-40.

Since that time the application of the UHDDS definitions has been expanded to include all non-outpatient settings (acute care, short term, long term care and psychiatric hospitals; home health agencies; rehab facilities; nursing homes, etc).

In determining principal diagnosis the coding conventions in the ICD-9-CM, Volumes I and II take precedence over these official coding guidelines.

(See Section I.A., Conventions for the ICD-9-CM)

The importance of consistent, complete documentation in the medical record cannot be overemphasized. Without such documentation the application of all coding guidelines is a difficult, if not impossible, task.

A.   Codes for symptoms, signs, and ill-defined conditions

Codes for symptoms, signs, and ill-defined conditions from Chapter 16 are not to be used as principal diagnosis when a related definitive diagnosis has been established.

B.   Two or more interrelated conditions, each potentially meeting the definition for principal diagnosis.

When there are two or more interrelated conditions (such as diseases in the same ICD-9-CM chapter or manifestations characteristically associated with a certain disease) potentially meeting the definition of principal diagnosis, either condition may be sequenced first, unless the circumstances of the admission, the therapy provided, the Tabular List, or the Alphabetic Index indicate otherwise.

C. Two or more diagnoses that equally meet the definition for principal diagnosis

In the unusual instance when two or more diagnoses equally meet the criteria for principal diagnosis as determined by the circumstances of admission, diagnostic workup and/or therapy provided, and the Alphabetic Index, Tabular List, or another coding guidelines does not provide sequencing direction, any one of the diagnoses may be sequenced first.

D. Two or more comparative or contrasting conditions.

In those rare instances when two or more contrasting or comparative diagnoses are documented as "either/or" (or similar terminology), they are coded as if the diagnoses were confirmed and the diagnoses are sequenced according to the circumstances of the admission. If no further determination can be made as to which diagnosis should be principal, either diagnosis may be sequenced first.

E. A symptom(s) followed by contrasting/comparative diagnoses

When a symptom(s) is followed by contrasting/comparative diagnoses, the symptom code is sequenced first. All the contrasting/comparative diagnoses should be coded as additional diagnoses.

F. Original treatment plan not carried out

Sequence as the principal diagnosis the condition, which after study occasioned the admission to the hospital, even though treatment may not have been carried out due to unforeseen circumstances.

G. Complications of surgery and other medical care

When the admission is for treatment of a complication resulting from surgery or other medical care, the complication code is sequenced as the principal diagnosis. If the complication is classified to the 996-999 series and the code lacks the necessary specificity in describing the complication, an additional code for the specific complication should be assigned.

H. Uncertain Diagnosis

If the diagnosis documented at the time of discharge is qualified as "probable", "suspected", "likely", "questionable", "possible", or "still to be ruled out", or other similar terms indicating uncertainty, code the condition as if it existed or was established. The bases for these guidelines are the diagnostic workup, arrangements for further workup or observation, and initial therapeutic approach that correspond most closely with the established diagnosis.

Note: This guideline is applicable only to inpatient admissions to short-term, acute, long-term care and psychiatric hospitals.

I. Admission from Observation Unit

1. Admission Following Medical Observation

When a patient is admitted to an observation unit for a medical condition, which either worsens or does not improve, and is subsequently admitted as an inpatient of the same hospital for this same medical condition, the principal diagnosis would be the medical condition which led to the hospital admission.

2. Admission Following Post-Operative Observation

When a patient is admitted to an observation unit to monitor a condition (or complication) that develops following outpatient surgery, and then is subsequently admitted as an inpatient of the same hospital, hospitals should apply the Uniform Hospital Discharge Data Set (UHDDS) definition of principal diagnosis as "that condition established after study to be chiefly responsible for occasioning the admission of the patient to the hospital for care."

J. Admission from Outpatient Surgery

When a patient receives surgery in the hospital's outpatient surgery department and is subsequently admitted for continuing inpatient care at the same hospital, the following guidelines should be followed in selecting the principal diagnosis for the inpatient admission:

- If the reason for the inpatient admission is a complication, assign the complication as the principal diagnosis.
- If no complication, or other condition, is documented as the reason for the inpatient admission, assign the reason for the outpatient surgery as the principal diagnosis.
- If the reason for the inpatient admission is another condition unrelated to the surgery, assign the unrelated condition as the principal diagnosis.

Section III. Reporting Additional Diagnoses
GENERAL RULES FOR OTHER (ADDITIONAL) DIAGNOSES

For reporting purposes the definition for "other diagnoses" is interpreted as additional conditions that affect patient care in terms of requiring:

clinical evaluation; or

therapeutic treatment; or

diagnostic procedures; or

extended length of hospital stay; or

increased nursing care and/or monitoring.

The UHDDS item #11-b defines Other Diagnoses as "all conditions that coexist at the time of admission, that develop subsequently, or that affect the treatment received and/or the length of stay. Diagnoses that relate to an earlier episode which have no bearing on the current hospital stay are to be excluded." UHDDS definitions apply to inpatients in acute care, short-term, long term care and psychiatric hospital setting. The UHDDS definitions are used by acute care short-term hospitals to report inpatient data elements in a standardized manner. These data elements and their definitions can be found in the July 31, 1985, Federal Register (Vol. 50, No, 147), pp. 31038-40.

Since that time the application of the UHDDS definitions has been expanded to include all non-outpatient settings (acute care, short term, long term care and psychiatric hospitals; home health agencies; rehab facilities; nursing homes, etc).

The following guidelines are to be applied in designating "other diagnoses" when neither the Alphabetic Index nor the Tabular List in ICD-9-CM provide direction. The listing of the diagnoses in the patient record is the responsibility of the attending provider.

A. Previous conditions

If the provider has included a diagnosis in the final diagnostic statement, such as the discharge summary or the face sheet, it should ordinarily be coded. Some providers include in the diagnostic statement resolved conditions or diagnoses and status-post procedures from previous admission that have no bearing on the current stay. Such conditions are not to be reported and are coded only if required by hospital policy.

However, history codes (V10-V19) may be used as secondary codes if the historical condition or family history has an impact on current care or influences treatment.

B. Abnormal findings

Abnormal findings (laboratory, x-ray, pathologic, and other diagnostic results) are not coded and reported unless the provider indicates their clinical significance. If the findings are outside the normal range and the attending provider has ordered other tests to evaluate the condition or prescribed treatment, it is appropriate to ask the provider whether the abnormal finding should be added.

Please note: This differs from the coding practices in the outpatient setting for coding encounters for diagnostic tests that have been interpreted by a provider.

C. Uncertain Diagnosis

If the diagnosis documented at the time of discharge is qualified as "probable", "suspected", "likely", "questionable", "possible", or "still to be ruled out" or other similar terms indicating uncertainty, code the condition as if it existed or was established. The bases for these guidelines are the diagnostic workup, arrangements for further workup or observation, and initial therapeutic approach that correspond most closely with the established diagnosis.

Note: This guideline is applicable only to inpatient admissions to short-term, acute, long-term care and psychiatric hospitals.

Section IV. Diagnostic Coding and Reporting Guidelines for Outpatient Services

These coding guidelines for outpatient diagnoses have been approved for use by hospitals/ providers in coding and reporting hospital-based outpatient services and provider-based office visits.

Information about the use of certain abbreviations, punctuation, symbols, and other conventions used in the ICD-9-CM Tabular List (code numbers and titles), can be found in Section IA of these guidelines, under "Conventions Used in the Tabular List." Information about the correct sequence to use in finding a code is also described in Section I.

The terms encounter and visit are often used interchangeably in describing outpatient service contacts and, therefore, appear together in these guidelines without distinguishing one from the other.

Though the conventions and general guidelines apply to all settings, coding guidelines for outpatient and provider reporting of diagnoses will vary in a number of instances from those for inpatient diagnoses, recognizing that:

> The Uniform Hospital Discharge Data Set (UHDDS) definition of principal diagnosis applies only to inpatients in acute, short-term, long-term care and psychiatric hospitals.

> Coding guidelines for inconclusive diagnoses (probable, suspected, rule out, etc.) were developed for inpatient reporting and do not apply to outpatients.

A. Selection of first-listed condition

In the outpatient setting, the term first-listed diagnosis is used in lieu of principal diagnosis.

In determining the first-listed diagnosis the coding conventions of ICD-9-CM, as well as the general and disease specific guidelines take precedence over the outpatient guidelines.

Diagnoses often are not established at the time of the initial encounter /visit. It may take two or more visits before the diagnosis is confirmed.

The most critical rule involves beginning the search for the correct code assignment through the Alphabetic Index. Never begin searching initially in the Tabular List as this will lead to coding errors.

1. Outpatient Surgery

When a patient presents for outpatient surgery, code the reason for the surgery as the first-listed diagnosis (reason for the encounter), even if the surgery is not performed due to a contraindication.

2. Observation Stay

When a patient is admitted for observation for a medical condition, assign a code for the medical condition as the first-listed diagnosis.

When a patient presents for outpatient surgery and develops complications requiring admission to observation, code the reason for the surgery as the first reported diagnosis (reason for the encounter), followed by codes for the complications as secondary diagnoses.

B. Codes from 001.0 through V91.99

The appropriate code or codes from 001.0 through V91.99 must be used to identify diagnoses, symptoms, conditions, problems, complaints, or other reason(s) for the encounter/visit.

C. Accurate reporting of ICD-9-CM diagnosis codes

For accurate reporting of ICD-9-CM diagnosis codes, the documentation should describe the patient's condition, using terminology which includes specific diagnoses as well as symptoms, problems, or reasons for the encounter. There are ICD-9-CM codes to describe all of these.

D. Selection of codes 001.0 through 999.9

The selection of codes 001.0 through 999.9 will frequently be used to describe the reason for the encounter. These codes are from the section of ICD-9-CM for the classification of diseases and injuries (e.g. infectious and parasitic diseases; neoplasms; symptoms, signs, and ill-defined conditions, etc.).

E. Codes that describe symptoms and signs

Codes that describe symptoms and signs, as opposed to diagnoses, are acceptable for reporting purposes when a diagnosis has not been established (confirmed) by the provider. Chapter 16 of ICD-9-CM, Symptoms, Signs, and Ill-defined conditions (codes 780.0 - 799.9) contain many, but not all codes for symptoms.

F. Encounters for circumstances other than a disease or injury

ICD-9-CM provides codes to deal with encounters for circumstances other than a disease or injury. The Supplementary Classification of factors Influencing Health Status and Contact with Health Services (V01.0- V91.99) is provided to deal with occasions when circumstances other than a disease or injury are recorded as diagnosis or problems. *See Section I.C. 18 for information on V-codes.*

G. Level of Detail in Coding

1. ICD-9-CM codes with 3, 4, or 5 digits

ICD-9-CM is composed of codes with either 3, 4, or 5 digits. Codes with three digits are included in ICD-9-CM as the heading of a category of codes that may be further subdivided by the use of fourth and/or fifth digits, which provide greater specificity.

2. Use of full number of digits required for a code

A three-digit code is to be used only if it is not further subdivided. Where fourth-digit subcategories and/or fifth-digit subclassifications are provided, they must be assigned. A code is invalid if it has not been coded to the full number of digits required for that code.

See also discussion under Section I.b.3., General Coding Guidelines, Level of Detail in Coding.

H. ICD-9-CM code for the diagnosis, condition, problem, or other reason for encounter/visit

List first the ICD-9-CM code for the diagnosis, condition, problem, or other reason for encounter/visit shown in the medical record to be chiefly responsible for the services provided. List additional codes that describe any coexisting conditions. In some cases the first-listed diagnosis may be a symptom when a diagnosis has not been established (confirmed) by the physician.

I. Uncertain diagnosis

Do not code diagnoses documented as "probable", "suspected," "questionable," "rule out," or "working diagnosis" or other similar terms indicating uncertainty. Rather, code the condition(s) to the highest degree of certainty for that encounter/visit, such as symptoms, signs, abnormal test results, or other reason for the visit.

Please note: This differs from the coding practices used by short-term, acute care, long-term care and psychiatric hospitals.

J. Chronic diseases

Chronic diseases treated on an ongoing basis may be coded and reported as many times as the patient receives treatment and care for the condition(s)

K. Code all documented conditions that coexist

Code all documented conditions that coexist at the time of the encounter/visit, and require or affect patient care treatment or management. Do not code conditions that were previously treated and no longer exist. However, history codes (V10-V19) may be used as secondary codes if the historical condition or family history has an impact on current care or influences treatment.

L. Patients receiving diagnostic services only

For patients receiving diagnostic services only during an encounter/visit, sequence first the diagnosis, condition, problem, or other reason for encounter/visit shown in the medical record to be chiefly responsible for the outpatient services provided during the encounter/visit. Codes for other diagnoses (e.g., chronic conditions) may be sequenced as additional diagnoses.

For encounters for routine laboratory/radiology testing in the absence of any signs, symptoms, or associated diagnosis, assign V72.5 and/or a code from subcategory V72.6. If routine testing is performed during the same encounter as a test to evaluate a sign, symptom, or diagnosis, it is appropriate to assign both the V code and the code describing the reason for the non-routine test.

For outpatient encounters for diagnostic tests that have been interpreted by a physician, and the final report is available at the time of coding, code any confirmed or definitive diagnosis(es) documented in the interpretation. Do not code related signs and symptoms as additional diagnoses.

Please note: This differs from the coding practice in the hospital inpatient setting regarding abnormal findings on test results.

M. Patients receiving therapeutic services only

For patients receiving therapeutic services only during an encounter/visit, sequence first the diagnosis, condition, problem, or other reason for encounter/visit shown in the medical record to be chiefly responsible for the outpatient services provided during the encounter/visit. Codes for other diagnoses (e.g., chronic conditions) may be sequenced as additional diagnoses.

The only exception to this rule is that when the primary reason for the admission/encounter is chemotherapy, radiation therapy, or rehabilitation, the appropriate V code for the service is listed first, and the diagnosis or problem for which the service is being performed listed second.

N. Patients receiving preoperative evaluations only

For patients receiving preoperative evaluations only, sequence first a code from category V72.8, Other specified examinations, to describe the pre-op consultations. Assign a code for the condition to describe the reason for the surgery as an additional diagnosis. Code also any findings related to the pre-op evaluation.

O. Ambulatory surgery

For ambulatory surgery, code the diagnosis for which the surgery was performed. If the postoperative diagnosis is known to be different from the preoperative diagnosis at the time the diagnosis is confirmed, select the postoperative diagnosis for coding, since it is the most definitive.

P. Routine outpatient prenatal visits

For routine outpatient prenatal visits when no complications are present, codes V22.0, Supervision of normal first pregnancy, or V22.1, Supervision of other normal pregnancy, should be used as the principal diagnosis. These codes should not be used in conjunction with chapter 11 codes.

APPENDIX I. PRESENT ON ADMISSION REPORTING GUIDELINES

Introduction

These guidelines are to be used as a supplement to the *ICD-9-CM Official Guidelines for Coding and Reporting* to facilitate the assignment of the Present on Admission (POA) indicator for each diagnosis and external cause of injury code reported on claim forms (UB-04 and 837 Institutional).

These guidelines are not intended to replace any guidelines in the main body of the *ICD-9-CM Official Guidelines for Coding and Reporting*. The POA guidelines are not intended to provide guidance on when a condition should be coded, but rather, how to apply the POA indicator to the final set of diagnosis codes that have been assigned in accordance with Sections I, II, and III of the official coding guidelines. Subsequent to the assignment of the ICD-9-CM codes, the POA indicator should then be assigned to those conditions that have been coded.

As stated in the Introduction to the ICD-9-CM Official Guidelines for Coding and Reporting, a joint effort between the healthcare provider and the coder is essential to achieve complete and accurate documentation, code assignment, and reporting of diagnoses and procedures. The importance of consistent, complete documentation in the medical record cannot be overemphasized. Medical record documentation from any provider involved in the care and treatment of the patient may be used to support the determination of whether a condition was present on admission or not. In the context of the official coding guidelines, the term "provider" means a physician or any qualified healthcare practitioner who is legally accountable for establishing the patient's diagnosis.

These guidelines are not a substitute for the provider's clinical judgment as to the determination of whether a condition was/was not present on admission. The provider should be queried regarding issues related to the linking of signs/symptoms, timing of test results, and the timing of findings.

General Reporting Requirements

All claims involving inpatient admissions to general acute care hospitals or other facilities that are subject to a law or regulation mandating collection of present on admission information.

Present on admission is defined as present at the time the order for inpatient admission occurs -- conditions that develop during an outpatient encounter, including emergency department, observation, or outpatient surgery, are considered as present on admission.

POA indicator is assigned to principal and secondary diagnoses (as defined in Section II of the Official Guidelines for Coding and Reporting) and the external cause of injury codes.

Issues related to inconsistent, missing, conflicting or unclear documentation must still be resolved by the provider.

If a condition would not be coded and reported based on UHDDS definitions and current official coding guidelines, then the POA indicator would not be reported.

Reporting Options

Y - Yes

N - No

U - Unknown

W – Clinically undetermined

Unreported/Not used (or "1" for Medicare usage) – (Exempt from POA reporting)

Reporting Definitions

Y = present at the time of inpatient admission

N = not present at the time of inpatient admission

U = documentation is insufficient to determine if condition is present on admission

W = provider is unable to clinically determine whether condition was present on admission or not

Timeframe for POA Identification and Documentation

There is no required timeframe as to when a provider (per the definition of "provider" used in these guidelines) must identify or document a condition to be present on admission. In some clinical situations, it may not be possible for a provider to make a definitive diagnosis (or a condition may not be recognized or reported by the patient) for a period of time after admission. In some cases it may be several days before the provider arrives at a definitive diagnosis. This does not mean that the condition was not present on admission. Determination of whether the condition was present on admission or not will be based on the applicable POA guideline as identified in this document, or on the provider's best clinical judgment.

If at the time of code assignment the documentation is unclear as to whether a condition was present on admission or not, it is appropriate to query the provider for clarification.

ASSIGNING THE POA INDICATOR

Condition is on the "Exempt from Reporting" list

Leave the "present on admission" field blank if the condition is on the list of ICD-9-CM codes for which this field is not applicable. This is the only circumstance in which the field maybe left blank.

POA explicitly documented

Assign Y for any condition the provider explicitly documents as being present on admission.

Assign N for any condition the provider explicitly documents as not present at the time of admission.

Conditions diagnosed prior to inpatient admission

Assign "Y" for conditions that were diagnosed prior to admission (example: hypertension, diabetes mellitus, asthma)

Conditions diagnosed during the admission but clearly present before admission

Assign "Y" for conditions diagnosed during the admission that were clearly present but not diagnosed until after admission occurred.

Diagnoses subsequently confirmed after admission are considered present on admission if at the time of admission they are documented as suspected, possible, rule out, differential diagnosis, or constitute an underlying cause of a symptom that is present at the time of admission.

Condition develops during outpatient encounter prior to inpatient admission

Assign Y for any condition that develops during an outpatient encounter prior to a written order for inpatient admission.

Documentation does not indicate whether condition was present on admission

Assign "U" when the medical record documentation is unclear as to whether the condition was present on admission. "U" should not be routinely assigned and used only in very limited circumstances. Coders are encouraged to query the providers when the documentation is unclear.

Documentation states that it cannot be determined whether the condition was or was not present on admission

Assign "W" when the medical record documentation indicates that it cannot be clinically determined whether or not the condition was present on admission.

Chronic condition with acute exacerbation during the admission

If the code is a combination code that identifies both the chronic condition and the acute exacerbation, see POA guidelines pertaining to combination codes.

If the combination code only identifies the chronic condition and not the acute exacerbation (e.g., acute exacerbation of chronic leukemia), assign "Y".

Conditions documented as possible, probable, suspected, or rule out at the time of discharge

If the final diagnosis contains a possible, probable, suspected, or rule out diagnosis, and this diagnosis was based on signs, symptoms or clinical findings suspected at the time of inpatient admission, assign "Y".

If the final diagnosis contains a possible, probable, suspected, or rule out diagnosis, and this diagnosis was based on signs, symptoms or clinical findings that were not present on admission, assign "N".

Conditions documented as impending or threatened at the time of discharge

If the final diagnosis contains an impending or threatened diagnosis, and this diagnosis is based on symptoms or clinical findings that were present on admission, assign "Y".

If the final diagnosis contains an impending or threatened diagnosis, and this diagnosis is based on symptoms or clinical findings that were not present on admission, assign "N".

Acute and chronic conditions

Assign "Y" for acute conditions that are present at time of admission and N for acute conditions that are not present at time of admission.

Assign "Y" for chronic conditions, even though the condition may not be diagnosed until after admission.

If a single code identifies both an acute and chronic condition, see the POA guidelines for combination codes.

Combination codes

Assign "N" if any part of the combination code was not present on admission (e.g., obstructive chronic bronchitis with acute exacerbation and the exacerbation was not present on admission; gastric ulcer that does not start bleeding until after admission; asthma patient develops status asthmaticus after admission)

Assign "Y" if all parts of the combination code were present on admission (e.g., patient with diabetic nephropathy is admitted with uncontrolled diabetes).

If the final diagnosis includes comparative or contrasting diagnoses, and both were present, or suspected, at the time of admission, assign "Y".

For infection codes that include the causal organism, assign "Y" if the infection (or signs of the infection) was present on admission, even though the culture results may not be known until after admission (e.g., patient is admitted with pneumonia and the provider documents pseudomonas as the causal organism a few days later).

Same diagnosis code for two or more conditions

When the same ICD-9-CM diagnosis code applies to two or more conditions during the same encounter (e.g. bilateral condition, or two separate conditions classified to the same ICD-9-CM diagnosis code):

Assign "Y" if all conditions represented by the single ICD-9-CM code were present on admission (e.g. bilateral fracture of the same bone, same site, and both fractures were present on admission)

Assign "N" if any of the conditions represented by the single ICD-9-CM code was not present on admission (e.g. dehydration with hyponatremia is assigned to code 276.1, but only one of these conditions was present on admission).

Obstetrical conditions

Whether or not the patient delivers during the current hospitalization does not affect assignment of the POA indicator. The determining factor for POA assignment is whether the pregnancy complication or obstetrical condition described by the code was present at the time of admission or not.

If the pregnancy complication or obstetrical condition was present on admission (e.g., patient admitted in preterm labor), assign "Y".

If the pregnancy complication or obstetrical condition was not present on admission (e.g., 2nd degree laceration during delivery, postpartum hemorrhage that occurred during current hospitalization, fetal distress develops after admission), assign "N".

If the obstetrical code includes more than one diagnosis and any of the diagnoses identified by the code were not present on admission assign "N". (e.g., Code 642.7, Pre-eclampsia or eclampsia superimposed on pre-existing hypertension).

If the obstetrical code includes information that is not a diagnosis, do not consider that information in the POA determination. (e.g. Code 652.1x, Breech or other malpresentation successfully converted to cephalic presentation should be reported as present on admission if the fetus was breech on admission but was converted to cephalic presentation after admission (since the conversion to cephalic presentation does not represent a diagnosis, the fact that the conversion occurred after admission has no bearing on the POA determination).

Perinatal conditions

Newborns are not considered to be admitted until after birth. Therefore, any condition present at birth or that developed in utero is considered present at admission and should be assigned "Y". This includes conditions that occur during delivery (e.g., injury during delivery, meconium aspiration, exposure to streptococcus B in the vaginal canal).

Congenital conditions and anomalies

Assign "Y" for congenital conditions and anomalies, **except for categories 740-759, Congenital anomalies, which are on the exempt list.** Congenital conditions are always considered present on admission.

External cause of injury codes

Assign "Y" for any E code representing an external cause of injury or poisoning that occurred prior to inpatient admission (e.g., patient fell out of bed at home, patient fell out of bed in emergency room prior to admission)

Assign "N" for any E code representing an external cause of injury or poisoning that occurred during inpatient hospitalization (e.g., patient fell out of hospital bed during hospital stay, patient experienced an adverse reaction to a medication administered after inpatient admission)

CATEGORIES AND CODES EXEMPT FROM DIAGNOSIS PRESENT ON ADMISSION REQUIREMENT

Note: *"Diagnosis present on admission" for these code categories are exempt because they represent circumstances regarding the healthcare encounter or factors influencing health status that do not represent a current disease or injury or are always present on admission.*

Categories or subcategories listed are inclusive of all codes within those categories or subcategories, unless otherwise indicated. In order to streamline the POA exempt list and make it easier to read, where all of the codes in a code range are POA exempt, only the code range is shown, rather than listing each of the individual codes in the range.

137-139	Late effects of infectious and parasitic diseases
268.1	Rickets, late effect
326	Late effects of intracranial abscess or pyogenic infection
412	Old myocardial infarction
438	Late effects of cerebrovascular disease
650	Normal delivery
660.7	Failed forceps or vacuum extractor, unspecified
677	Late effect of complication of pregnancy, childbirth, and the puerperium
740-759	Congenital anomalies
905-909	Late effects of injuries, poisonings, toxic effects, and other external causes
V02	Carrier or suspected carrier of infectious diseases
V03	Need for prophylactic vaccination and inoculation against bacterial diseases
V04	Need for prophylactic vaccination and inoculation against certain viral diseases
V05	Need for other prophylactic vaccination and inoculation against single diseases
V06	Need for prophylactic vaccination and inoculation against combinations of diseases
V07	Need for isolation and other prophylactic or treatment measures

V10	Personal history of malignant neoplasm	V88	Acquired absence of other organs and tissue
V11	Personal history of mental disorder	V89	Suspected maternal and fetal conditions not found
V12	Personal history of certain other diseases	V90	Retained foreign body
V13	Personal history of other diseases	V91	Multiple gestation placenta status
V14	Personal history of allergy to medicinal agents	E000	External cause status
V15	Other personal history presenting hazards to health	E001-E030	Activity
V16	Family history of malignant neoplasm	E800-E807	Railway accidents
V17	Family history of certain chronic disabling diseases	E810-E819	Motor vehicle traffic accidents
V18	Family history of certain other specific conditions	E820-E825	Motor vehicle nontraffic accidents
V19	Family history of other conditions	E826-E829	Other road vehicle accidents
V20	Health supervision of infant or child	E830-E838	Water transport accidents
V21	Constitutional states in development	E840-E845	Air and space transport accidents
V22	Normal pregnancy	E846-E848	Vehicle accidents not elsewhere classifiable
V23	Supervision of high-risk pregnancy	E849	Place of occurrence (Except E849.7)
V24	Postpartum care and examination	E883.1	Accidental fall into well
V25	Encounter for contraceptive management	E883.2	Accidental fall into storm drain or manhole
V26	Procreative management	E884.0	Fall from playground equipment
V27	Outcome of delivery	E884.1	Fall from cliff
V28	Antenatal screening	E885.0	Fall from (nonmotorized) scooter
V29	Observation and evaluation of newborns for suspected condition not found	E885.1	Fall from roller skates
V30-V39	Liveborn infants according to type of birth	E885.2	Fall from skateboard
V42	Organ or tissue replaced by transplant	E885.3	Fall from skis
V43	Organ or tissue replaced by other means	E885.4	Fall from snowboard
V44	Artificial opening status	E886.0	Fall on same level from collision, pushing, or shoving, by or with other person, In sports
V45	Other postprocedural states	E890.0-E890.9	Conflagration in private dwelling
V46	Other dependence on machines and devices	E893.0	Accident caused by ignition of clothing, from controlled fire in private dwelling
V49.60-V49.77	Upper and lower limb amputation status	E893.2	Accident caused by ignition of clothing, from controlled fire not in building or structure
V49.81-V49.85	Other specified conditions influencing health status	E894	Ignition of highly inflammable material
V50	Elective surgery for purposes other than remedying health states	E895	Accident caused by controlled fire in private dwelling
V51	Aftercare involving the use of plastic surgery	E897	Accident caused by controlled fire not in building or structure
V52	Fitting and adjustment of prosthetic device and implant	E917.0	Striking against or struck accidentally by objects or persons, in sports without subsequent fall
V53	Fitting and adjustment of other device	E917.1	Striking against or struck accidentally by objects or persons, caused by a crowd, by collective fear or panic without subsequent fall
V54	Other orthopedic aftercare		
V55	Attention to artificial openings		
V56	Encounter for dialysis and dialysis catheter care	E917.2	Striking against or struck accidentally by objects or persons, in running water without subsequent fall
V57	Care involving use of rehabilitation procedures		
V58	Encounter for other and unspecified procedures and aftercare	E917.5	Striking against or struck accidentally by objects or persons, object in sports with subsequent fall
V59	Donors		
V60	Housing, household, and economic circumstances	E917.6	Striking against or struck accidentally by objects or persons, caused by a crowd, by collective fear or panic with subsequent fall
V61	Other family circumstances		
V62	Other psychosocial circumstances		
V64	Persons encountering health services for specific procedures, not carried out	E919	Accident caused by machinery (Except E919.2)
V65	Other persons seeking consultation	E921	Accident caused by explosion of pressure vessel
V66	Convalescence and palliative care	E922	Accident caused by firearm and air gun missile
V67	Follow-up examination	E926.2	Visible and ultraviolet light sources
V68	Encounters for administrative purposes	E928.0-E928.8	Other and unspecified environmental and accidental causes
V69	Problems related to lifestyle	E929.0-E929.9	Late effects of accidental injury
V70	General medical examination	E959	Late effects of self-inflicted injury
V71	Observation and evaluation for suspected condition not found	E970-E978	Legal intervention
V72	Special investigations and examinations	E979	Terrorism
V73	Special screening examination for viral and chlamydial diseases	E981	Poisoning by gases in domestic use, undetermined whether accidentally or purposely inflicted
V74	Special screening examination for bacterial and spirochetal diseases	E982	Poisoning by other gases, undetermined whether accidentally or purposely inflicted
V75	Special screening examination for other infectious diseases	E985	Injury by firearms, air guns and explosives, undetermined whether accidentally or purposely inflicted
V76	Special screening for malignant neoplasms		
V77	Special screening for endocrine, nutritional, metabolic, and immunity disorders	E987.0	Falling from high place, undetermined whether accidentally or purposely inflicted, residential premises
V78	Special screening for disorders of blood and blood-forming organs	E987.2	Falling from high place, undetermined whether accidentally or purposely inflicted, natural sites
V79	Special screening for mental disorders and developmental handicaps	E989	Late effects of injury, undetermined whether accidentally or purposely inflicted
V80	Special screening for neurological, eye, and ear diseases	E990-E999	Injury resulting from operations of war
V81	Special screening for cardiovascular, respiratory, and genitourinary diseases		
V82	Special screening for other conditions		
V83	Genetic carrier status		
V84	Genetic susceptibility to disease		
V85	Body Mass Index		
V86	Estrogen receptor status		
V87.32	Contact with and (suspected) exposure to algae bloom		
V87.4	Personal history of drug therapy		

A

AAT (alpha-1 antitrypsin) deficiency 273.4
AAV (disease) (illness) (infection) — *see* Human immunodeficiency virus (disease) (illness) (infection)
Abactio — *see* Abortion, induced
Abactus venter — *see* Abortion, induced
Abarognosis 781.99
Abasia (-astasia) 307.9
  atactica 781.3
  choreic 781.3
  hysterical 300.11
  paroxysmal trepidant 781.3
  spastic 781.3
  trembling 781.3
  trepidans 781.3
Abderhalden-Kaufmann-Lignac syndrome (cystinosis) 270.0
Abdomen, abdominal — *see also* condition
  accordion 306.4
  acute 789.0 ☑
  angina 557.1
  burst 868.00
  convulsive equivalent (*see also* Epilepsy) 345.5 ☑
  heart 746.87
  muscle deficiency syndrome 756.79
  obstipum 756.79
Abdominalgia 789.0 ☑
  periodic 277.31
Abduction contracture, hip or other joint — *see* Contraction, joint
Abercrombie's syndrome (amyloid degeneration) 277.39
Aberrant (congenital) — *see also* Malposition, congenital
  adrenal gland 759.1
  blood vessel NEC 747.60
    arteriovenous NEC 747.60
    cerebrovascular 747.81
    gastrointestinal 747.61
    lower limb 747.64
    renal 747.62
    spinal 747.82
    upper limb 747.63
  breast 757.6
  endocrine gland NEC 759.2
  gastrointestinal vessel (peripheral) 747.61
  hepatic duct 751.69
  lower limb vessel (peripheral) 747.64
  pancreas 751.7
  parathyroid gland 759.2
  peripheral vascular vessel NEC 747.60
  pituitary gland (pharyngeal) 759.2
  renal blood vessel 747.62
  sebaceous glands, mucous membrane, mouth 750.26
  spinal vessel 747.82
  spleen 759.0
  testis (descent) 752.51
  thymus gland 759.2
  thyroid gland 759.2
  upper limb vessel (peripheral) 747.63
Aberratio
  lactis 757.6
  testis 752.51
Aberration — *see also* Anomaly
  chromosome — *see* Anomaly, chromosome(s)
  distantial 368.9
  mental (*see also* Disorder, mental, nonpsychotic) 300.9
Abetalipoproteinemia 272.5
Abionarce 780.79
Abiotrophy 799.89
Ablatio
  placentae — *see* Placenta, ablatio
  retinae (*see also* Detachment, retina) 361.9
Ablation
  pituitary (gland) (with hypofunction) 253.7
  placenta — *see* Placenta, ablatio
  uterus 621.8
Ablepharia, ablepharon, ablephary 743.62
Ablepsia — *see* Blindness
Ablepsy — *see* Blindness

Ablutomania 300.3
Abnormal, abnormality, abnormalities — *see also* Anomaly
acid base balance 276.4
  fetus or newborn — *see* Distress, fetal
adaptation curve, dark 368.63
alveolar ridge 525.9
amnion 658.9 ☑
  affecting fetus or newborn 762.9
anatomical relationship NEC 759.9
apertures, congenital, diaphragm 756.6
auditory perception NEC 388.40
autosomes NEC 758.5
  13 758.1
  18 758.2
  21 or 22 758.0
  D_1 758.1
  E_3 758.2
  G 758.0
ballistocardiogram 794.39
basal metabolic rate (BMR) 794.7
biosynthesis, testicular androgen 257.2
blood level (of)
  cobalt 790.6
  copper 790.6
  iron 790.6
  lead 790.6
  lithium 790.6
  magnesium 790.6
  mineral 790.6
  zinc 790.6
blood pressure
  elevated (without diagnosis of hypertension) 796.2
  low (*see also* Hypotension) 458.9
    reading (incidental) (isolated) (nonspecific) 796.3
blood sugar 790.29
bowel sounds 787.5
breathing behavior — *see* Respiration
caloric test 794.19
cervix (acquired) NEC 622.9
  congenital 752.40
  in pregnancy or childbirth 654.6 ☑
    causing obstructed labor 660.2 ☑
      affecting fetus or newborn 763.1
chemistry, blood NEC 790.6
chest sounds 786.7
chorion 658.9 ☑
  affecting fetus or newborn 762.9
chromosomal NEC 758.89
  analysis, nonspecific result 795.2
  autosomes (*see also* Abnormal, autosomes NEC) 758.5
  fetal, (suspected) affecting management of pregnancy 655.1 ☑
  sex 758.81
clinical findings NEC 796.4
communication — *see* Fistula
configuration of pupils 379.49
coronary
  artery 746.85
  vein 746.9
cortisol-binding globulin 255.8
course, Eustachian tube 744.24
creatinine clearance 794.4
dentofacial NEC 524.9
  functional 524.50
  specified type NEC 524.89
development, developmental NEC 759.9
  bone 756.9
  central nervous system 742.9
direction, teeth 524.30
Dynia (*see also* Defect, coagulation) 286.9
Ebstein 746.2
echocardiogram 793.2
echoencephalogram 794.01
echogram NEC — *see* Findings, abnormal, structure
electro-oculogram (EOG) 794.12
electrocardiogram (ECG) (EKG) 794.31
electroencephalogram (EEG) 794.02
electromyogram (EMG) 794.17
  ocular 794.14
electroretinogram (ERG) 794.11
erythrocytes 289.9

Abnormal, abnormality, abnormalities — *see also* Anomaly — *continued*
erythrocytes — *continued*
  congenital, with perinatal jaundice 282.9 *[774.0]*
Eustachian valve 746.9
excitability under minor stress 301.9
fat distribution 782.9
feces 787.7
fetal heart rate — *see* Distress, fetal
fetus NEC
  affecting management of pregnancy — *see* Pregnancy, management affected by, fetal
  causing disproportion 653.7 ☑
    affecting fetus or newborn 763.1
    causing obstructed labor 660.1 ☑
      affecting fetus or newborn 763.1
findings without manifest disease — *see* Findings, abnormal
fluid
  amniotic 792.3
  cerebrospinal 792.0
  peritoneal 792.9
  pleural 792.9
  synovial 792.9
  vaginal 792.9
forces of labor NEC 661.9 ☑
  affecting fetus or newborn 763.7
form, teeth 520.2
function studies
  auditory 794.15
  bladder 794.9
  brain 794.00
  cardiovascular 794.30
  endocrine NEC 794.6
  kidney 794.4
  liver 794.8
  nervous system
    central 794.00
    peripheral 794.19
  oculomotor 794.14
  pancreas 794.9
  placenta 794.9
  pulmonary 794.2
  retina 794.11
  special senses 794.19
  spleen 794.9
  thyroid 794.5
  vestibular 794.16
gait 781.2
  hysterical 300.11
gastrin secretion 251.5
globulin
  cortisol-binding 255.8
  thyroid-binding 246.8
glucagon secretion 251.4
glucose 790.29
  in pregnancy, childbirth, or puerperium 648.8 ☑
  fetus or newborn 775.0
  non-fasting 790.29
gravitational (G) forces or states 994.9
hair NEC 704.2
hard tissue formation in pulp 522.3
head movement 781.0
heart
  rate
    fetus, affecting liveborn infant
      before the onset of labor 763.81
      during labor 763.82
      unspecified as to time of onset 763.83
    intrauterine
      before the onset of labor 763.81
      during labor 763.82
      unspecified as to time of onset 763.83
    newborn
      before the onset of labor 763.81
      during labor 763.82
      unspecified as to time of onset 763.83
  shadow 793.2
  sounds NEC 785.3

Abnormal, abnormality, abnormalities — *see also* Anomaly — *continued*
hemoglobin (*see also* Disease, hemoglobin) 282.7
  trait — *see* Trait, hemoglobin, abnormal
hemorrhage, uterus — *see* Hemorrhage, uterus
histology NEC 795.4
increase
  in
    appetite 783.6
    development 783.9
involuntary movement 781.0
jaw closure 524.51
karyotype 795.2
knee jerk 796.1
laboratory findings — *see* Findings, abnormal
labor NEC 661.9 ☑
  affecting fetus or newborn 763.7
length, organ or site, congenital — *see* Distortion
liver function test 790.6
loss of height 781.91
loss of weight 783.21
lung shadow 793.19
mammogram 793.80
  calcification 793.89
  calculus 793.89
  microcalcification 793.81
Mantoux test 795.51
membranes (fetal)
  affecting fetus or newborn 762.9
  complicating pregnancy 658.8 ☑
menstruation — *see* Menstruation
metabolism (*see also* condition) 783.9
movement 781.0
  disorder NEC 333.90
    sleep related, unspecified 780.58
    specified NEC 333.99
  head 781.0
  involuntary 781.0
  specified type NEC 333.99
muscle contraction, localized 728.85
myoglobin (Aberdeen) (Annapolis) 289.9
narrowness, eyelid 743.62
optokinetic response 379.57
organs or tissues of pelvis NEC
  in pregnancy or childbirth 654.9 ☑
    affecting fetus or newborn 763.89
    causing obstructed labor 660.2 ☑
      affecting fetus or newborn 763.1
origin — *see* Malposition, congenital
palmar creases 757.2
Papanicolaou (smear)
  anus 796.70
    with
      atypical squamous cells
        cannot exclude high grade squamous intraepithelial lesion (ASC-H) 796.72
        of undetermined significance (ASC-US) 796.71
      cytologic evidence of malignancy 796.76
      high grade squamous intraepithelial lesion (HGSIL) 796.74
      low grade squamous intraepithelial lesion (LGSIL) 796.73
    glandular 796.70
    specified finding NEC 796.79
  cervix 795.00
    with
      atypical squamous cells
        cannot exclude high grade squamous intraepithelial lesion (ASC-H) 795.02
        of undetermined significance (ASC-US) 795.01
      cytologic evidence of malignancy 795.06
      high grade squamous intraepithelial lesion (HGSIL) 795.04

☑ **Additional Digit Required** — Refer to the Tabular List for Digit Selection   ⬃ **Subterms under main terms may continue to next column or page**

2014 ICD-9-CM   ▶◀ **Revised Text**   ● **New Line**   ▲ **Revised Code**   **Volume 2 — 1**

AAT — Abnormal, abnormality, abnormalities

Abnormal, abnormality, abnormalities —
see also Anomaly — *continued*
Papanicolaou — *continued*
  cervix — *continued*
    with — *continued*
      low grade squamous intraepithe-
        lial lesion (LGSIL) 795.03
      nonspecific finding NEC 795.09
  other site 796.9
  vagina 795.10
    with
      atypical squamous cells
        cannot exclude high grade
          squamous intraepithe-
          lial lesion (ASC-H)
          795.12
        of undetermined significance
          (ASC-US) 795.11
      cytologic evidence of malignancy
        795.16
      high grade squamous intraepithe-
        lial lesion (HGSIL) 795.14
      low grade squamous intraepithe-
        lial lesion (LGSIL) 795.13
    glandular 795.10
    specified finding NEC 795.19
parturition
  affecting fetus or newborn 763.9
  mother — *see* Delivery, complicated
pelvis (bony) — *see* Deformity, pelvis
percussion, chest 786.7
periods (grossly) (*see also* Menstruation)
  626.9
phonocardiogram 794.39
placenta — *see* Placenta, abnormal
plantar reflex 796.1
plasma protein — *see* Deficiency, plasma,
  protein
pleural folds 748.8
position (*see also* Malposition)
  gravid uterus 654.4 ☑
    causing obstructed labor 660.2 ☑
      affecting fetus or newborn 763.1
posture NEC 781.92
presentation (fetus) — *see* Presentation,
  fetus, abnormal
product of conception NEC 631.8
puberty — *see* Puberty
pulmonary
  artery 747.39
  function, newborn 770.89
  test results 794.2
  ventilation, newborn 770.89
    hyperventilation 786.01
pulsations in neck 785.1
pupil reflexes 379.40
quality of milk 676.8 ☑
radiological examination 793.99
  abdomen NEC 793.6
  biliary tract 793.3
  breast 793.89
    mammogram NOS 793.80
    mammographic
      calcification 793.89
      calculus 793.89
      microcalcification 793.81
  gastrointestinal tract 793.4
  genitourinary organs 793.5
  head 793.0
  image test inconclusive due to excess
    body fat 793.91
  intrathoracic organ NEC 793.2
  lung (field) 793.19
  musculoskeletal system 793.7
  retroperitoneum 793.6
  skin and subcutaneous tissue 793.99
  skull 793.0
red blood cells 790.09
  morphology 790.09
  volume 790.09
reflex NEC 796.1
renal function test 794.4
respiration signs — *see* Respiration
response to nerve stimulation 794.10
retinal correspondence 368.34
rhythm, heart (*see also* Arrhythmia)

Abnormal, abnormality, abnormalities —
see also Anomaly — *continued*
rhythm, heart (*see also* Arrhythmia) — *continued*
  fetus — *see* Distress, fetal
saliva 792.4
scan
  brain 794.09
  kidney 794.4
  liver 794.8
  lung 794.2
  thyroid 794.5
secretion
  gastrin 251.5
  glucagon 251.4
semen 792.2
serum level (of)
  acid phosphatase 790.5
  alkaline phosphatase 790.5
  amylase 790.5
  enzymes NEC 790.5
  lipase 790.5
shape
  cornea 743.41
  gallbladder 751.69
  gravid uterus 654.4 ☑
    affecting fetus or newborn 763.89
    causing obstructed labor 660.2 ☑
      affecting fetus or newborn 763.1
  head (*see also* Anomaly, skull) 756.0
  organ or site, congenital NEC — *see*
    Distortion
sinus venosus 747.40
size
  fetus, complicating delivery 653.5 ☑
    causing obstructed labor 660.1 ☑
  gallbladder 751.69
  head (*see also* Anomaly, skull) 756.0
  organ or site, congenital NEC — *see*
    Distortion
  teeth 520.2
skin and appendages, congenital NEC 757.9
soft parts of pelvis — *see* Abnormal, organs
  or tissues of pelvis
spermatozoa 792.2
sputum (amount) (color) (excessive) (odor)
  (purulent) 786.4
stool NEC 787.7
  bloody 578.1
    occult 792.1
  bulky 787.7
  color (dark) (light) 792.1
  content (fat) (mucus) (pus) 792.1
  occult blood 792.1
synchondrosis 756.9
test results without manifest disease — *see*
  Findings, abnormal
thebesian valve 746.9
thermography — *see* Findings, abnormal,
  structure
threshold, cones or rods (eye) 368.63
thyroid-binding globulin 246.8
thyroid product 246.8
toxicology (findings) NEC 796.0
tracheal cartilage (congenital) 748.3
transport protein 273.8
ultrasound results — *see* Findings, abnormal, structure
umbilical cord
  affecting fetus or newborn 762.6
  complicating delivery 663.9 ☑
  specified NEC 663.8 ☑
union
  cricoid cartilage and thyroid cartilage
    748.3
  larynx and trachea 748.3
  thyroid cartilage and hyoid bone 748.3
urination NEC 788.69
  psychogenic 306.53
  stream
    intermittent 788.61
    slowing 788.62
    splitting 788.61
    weak 788.62
  urgency 788.63
urine (constituents) NEC 791.9

Abnormal, abnormality, abnormalities —
see also Anomaly — *continued*
uterine hemorrhage (*see also* Hemorrhage,
  uterus) 626.9
  climacteric 627.0
  postmenopausal 627.1
vagina (acquired) (congenital)
  in pregnancy or childbirth 654.7 ☑
    affecting fetus or newborn 763.89
    causing obstructed labor 660.2 ☑
      affecting fetus or newborn 763.1
vascular sounds 785.9
vectorcardiogram 794.39
visually evoked potential (VEP) 794.13
vulva (acquired) (congenital)
  in pregnancy or childbirth 654.8 ☑
    affecting fetus or newborn 763.89
    causing obstructed labor 660.2 ☑
      affecting fetus or newborn 763.1
weight
  gain 783.1
    of pregnancy 646.1 ☑
      with hypertension — *see* Tox-
        emia, of pregnancy
  loss 783.21
x-ray examination — *see* Abnormal, radiological examination
Abnormally formed uterus — *see* Anomaly,
uterus
Abnormity (any organ or part) — *see* Anomaly
ABO
hemolytic disease 773.1
incompatibility (due to transfusion of blood
  or blood products)
  with hemolytic transfusion reaction
    (HTR) (not specified as acute or
    delayed) 999.61
    24 hours or more after transfusion
      999.63
    acute 999.62
    delayed 999.63
    less than 24 hours after transfusion
      999.62
    unspecified time after transfusion
      999.61
  reaction 999.60
    specified NEC 999.69
Abocclusion 524.20
Abolition, language 784.69
Aborter, habitual or recurrent NEC
without current pregnancy 629.81
current abortion (*see also* Abortion, spontaneous) 634.9 ☑
  affecting fetus or newborn 761.8
observation in current pregnancy 646.3 ☑
Abortion (complete) (incomplete) (inevitable)
(with retained products of conception)
637.9 ☑

> *Note* — Use the following fifth-digit
> subclassification with categories
> 634–637:
>
> 0   unspecified
>
> 1   incomplete
>
> 2   complete

with
  complication(s) (any) following previous
    abortion — *see* category 639 ☑
  damage to pelvic organ (laceration)
    (rupture) (tear) 637.2 ☑
  embolism (air) (amniotic fluid) (blood
    clot) (pulmonary) (pyemic) (sep-
    tic) (soap) 637.6 ☑
  genital tract and pelvic infection
    637.0 ☑
  hemorrhage, delayed or excessive
    637.1 ☑
  metabolic disorder 637.4 ☑
  renal failure (acute) 637.3 ☑
  sepsis (genital tract) (pelvic organ)
    637.0 ☑
    urinary tract 637.7 ☑
  shock (postoperative) (septic) 637.5 ☑
  specified complication NEC 637.7 ☑

Abortion — *continued*
with — *continued*
  toxemia 637.3 ☑
  unspecified complication(s) 637.8 ☑
  urinary tract infection 637.7 ☑
accidental — *see* Abortion, spontaneous
artificial — *see* Abortion, induced
attempted (failed) — *see* Abortion, failed
criminal — *see* Abortion, illegal
early — *see* Abortion, spontaneous
elective — *see* Abortion, legal
failed (legal) 638.9
  with
    damage to pelvic organ (laceration)
      (rupture) (tear) 638.2
    embolism (air) (amniotic fluid) (blood
      clot) (pulmonary) (pyemic)
      (septic) (soap) 638.6
    genital tract and pelvic infection
      638.0
    hemorrhage, delayed or excessive
      638.1
    metabolic disorder 638.4
    renal failure (acute) 638.3
    sepsis (genital tract) (pelvic organ)
      638.0
    urinary tract 638.7
    shock (postoperative) (septic) 638.5
    specified complication NEC 638.7
    toxemia 638.3
    unspecified complication(s) 638.8
    urinary tract infection 638.7
fetal indication — *see* Abortion, legal
fetus 779.6
following threatened abortion — *see* Abortion, by type
habitual or recurrent (care during pregnancy) 646.3 ☑
  with current abortion (*see also* Abortion,
    spontaneous) 634.9 ☑
    affecting fetus or newborn 761.8
  without current pregnancy 629.81
homicidal — *see* Abortion, illegal
illegal 636.9 ☑
  with
    damage to pelvic organ (laceration)
      (rupture) (tear) 636.2 ☑
    embolism (air) (amniotic fluid) (blood
      clot) (pulmonary) (pyemic)
      (septic) (soap) 636.6 ☑
    genital tract and pelvic infection
      636.0 ☑
    hemorrhage, delayed or excessive
      636.1 ☑
    metabolic disorder 636.4 ☑
    renal failure 636.3 ☑
    sepsis (genital tract) (pelvic organ)
      636.0 ☑
      urinary tract 636.7 ☑
    shock (postoperative) (septic)
      636.5 ☑
    specified complication NEC 636.7 ☑
    toxemia 636.3 ☑
    unspecified complication(s) 636.8 ☑
    urinary tract infection 636.7 ☑
  fetus 779.6
induced 637.9 ☑
  illegal — *see* Abortion, illegal
  legal indications — *see* Abortion, legal
  medical indications — *see* Abortion, le-
    gal
  therapeutic — *see* Abortion, legal
late — *see* Abortion, spontaneous
legal (legal indication) (medical indication)
  (under medical supervision) 635.9 ☑
  with
    damage to pelvic organ (laceration)
      (rupture) (tear) 635.2 ☑
    embolism (air) (amniotic fluid) (blood
      clot) (pulmonary) (pyemic)
      (septic) (soap) 635.6 ☑
    genital tract and pelvic infection
      635.0 ☑
    hemorrhage, delayed or excessive
      635.1 ☑

☑ **Additional Digit Required** — Refer to the Tabular List for Digit Selection   ▽ **Subterms under main terms may continue to next column or page**

2 — Volume 2   ▶◀ **Revised Text**   ● **New Line**   ▲ **Revised Code**   **2014 ICD-9-CM**

Abortion — *continued*
  legal — *continued*
    with — *continued*
      metabolic disorder 635.4 ☑
      renal failure (acute) 635.3 ☑
      sepsis (genital tract) (pelvic organ)
        635.0 ☑
        urinary tract 635.7 ☑
      shock (postoperative) (septic)
        635.5 ☑
      specified complication NEC 635.7 ☑
      toxemia 635.3 ☑
      unspecified complication(s) 635.8 ☑
      urinary tract infection 635.7 ☑
    fetus 779.6
  medical indication — *see* Abortion, legal
  mental hygiene problem — *see* Abortion, legal
  missed 632
  operative — *see* Abortion, legal
  psychiatric indication — *see* Abortion, legal
  recurrent — *see* Abortion, spontaneous
  self-induced — *see* Abortion, illegal
  septic — *see* Abortion, by type, with sepsis
  spontaneous 634.9 ☑
    with
      damage to pelvic organ (laceration)
        (rupture) (tear) 634.2 ☑
      embolism (air) (amniotic fluid) (blood
        clot) (pulmonary) (pyemic)
        (septic) (soap) 634.6 ☑
      genital tract and pelvic infection
        634.0 ☑
      hemorrhage, delayed or excessive
        634.1 ☑
      metabolic disorder 634.4 ☑
      renal failure 634.3 ☑
      sepsis (genital tract) (pelvic organ)
        634.0 ☑
        urinary tract 634.7 ☑
      shock (postoperative) (septic)
        634.5 ☑
      specified complication NEC 634.7 ☑
      toxemia 634.3 ☑
      unspecified complication(s) 634.8 ☑
      urinary tract infection 634.7 ☑
    fetus 761.8
    threatened 640.0 ☑
      affecting fetus or newborn 762.1
  surgical — *see* Abortion, legal
  therapeutic — *see* Abortion, legal
  threatened 640.0 ☑
    affecting fetus or newborn 762.1
  tubal — *see* Pregnancy, tubal
  voluntary — *see* Abortion, legal
Abortus fever 023.9
Aboulomania 301.6
Abrachia 755.20
Abrachiatism 755.20
Abrachiocephalia 759.89
Abrachiocephalus 759.89
Abrami's disease (acquired hemolytic jaundice) 283.9
Abramov-Fiedler myocarditis (acute isolated myocarditis) 422.91
Abrasion — *see also* Injury, superficial, by site
  cornea 918.1
  dental 521.20
    extending into
      dentine 521.22
      pulp 521.23
    generalized 521.25
    limited to enamel 521.21
    localized 521.24
  teeth, tooth (dentifrice) (habitual) (hard tissues) (occupational) (ritual) (traditional) (wedge defect) (*see also* Abrasion, dental) 521.20
Abrikossov's tumor (M9580/0) — *see also* Neoplasm, connective tissue, benign
  malignant (M9580/3) — *see* Neoplasm, connective tissue, malignant
Abrism 988.8
Abruption, placenta — *see* Placenta, abruptio
Abruptio placentae — *see* Placenta, abruptio

Abscess (acute) (chronic) (infectional) (lymphangitic) (metastatic) (multiple) (pyogenic) (septic) (with lymphangitis) — *see also* Cellulitis 682.9
  abdomen, abdominal
    cavity 567.22
    wall 682.2
  abdominopelvic 567.22
  accessory sinus (chronic) (*see also* Sinusitis) 473.9
  adrenal (capsule) (gland) 255.8
  alveolar 522.5
    with sinus 522.7
  ambic 006.3
    bladder 006.8
    brain (with liver or lung abscess) 006.5
    liver (without mention of brain or lung
      abscess) 006.3
      with
        brain abscess (and lung abscess)
          006.5
        lung abscess 006.4
    lung (with liver abscess) 006.4
      with brain abscess 006.5
    seminal vesicle 006.8
    specified site NEC 006.8
    spleen 006.8
  anaerobic 040.0
  ankle 682.6
  anorectal 566
  antecubital space 682.3
  antrum (chronic) (Highmore) (*see also* Sinusitis, maxillary) 473.0
  anus 566
  apical (tooth) 522.5
    with sinus (alveolar) 522.7
  appendix 540.1
  areola (acute) (chronic) (nonpuerperal) 611.0
    puerperal, postpartum 675.1 ☑
  arm (any part, above wrist) 682.3
  artery (wall) 447.2
  atheromatous 447.2
  auditory canal (external) 380.10
  auricle (ear) (staphylococcal) (streptococcal) 380.10
  axilla, axillary (region) 682.3
    lymph gland or node 683
  back (any part) 682.2
  Bartholin's gland 616.3
    with
      abortion — *see* Abortion, by type, with sepsis
      ectopic pregnancy (*see also* categories 633.0–633.9) 639.0
      molar pregnancy (*see also* categories 630–632) 639.0
    complicating pregnancy or puerperium 646.6 ☑
    following
      abortion 639.0
      ectopic or molar pregnancy 639.0
  bartholinian 616.3
  Bezold's 383.01
  bile, biliary, duct or tract (*see also* Cholecystitis) 576.8
  bilharziasis 120.1
  bladder (wall) 595.89
    amebic 006.8
  bone (subperiosteal) (*see also* Osteomyelitis) 730.0
    accessory sinus (chronic) (*see also* Sinusitis) 473.9
    acute 730.0 ☑
    chronic or old 730.1 ☑
    jaw (lower) (upper) 526.4
    mastoid — *see* Mastoiditis, acute
    petrous (*see also* Petrositis) 383.20
    spinal (tuberculous) (*see also* Tuberculosis) 015.0 ☑ *[730.88]*
      nontuberculous 730.08
  bowel 569.5
  brain (any part) 324.0
    amebic (with liver or lung abscess) 006.5
    cystic 324.0
    late effect — *see* category 326

Abscess — *see also* Cellulitis — *continued*
  brain — *continued*
    otogenic 324.0
    tuberculous (*see also* Tuberculosis) 013.3 ☑
  breast (acute) (chronic) (nonpuerperal) 611.0
    newborn 771.5
    puerperal, postpartum 675.1 ☑
    tuberculous (*see also* Tuberculosis) 017.9 ☑
  broad ligament (chronic) (*see also* Disease, pelvis, inflammatory) 614.4
    acute 614.3
  Brodie's (chronic) (localized) (*see also* Osteomyelitis) 730.1 ☑
  bronchus 519.19
  buccal cavity 528.3
  bulbourethral gland 597.0
  bursa 727.89
    pharyngeal 478.29
  buttock 682.5
  canaliculus, breast 611.0
  canthus 372.20
  cartilage 733.99
  cecum 569.5
    with appendicitis 540.1
  cerebellum, cerebellar 324.0
    late effect — *see* category 326
  cerebral (embolic) 324.0
    late effect — *see* category 326
  cervical (neck region) 682.1
    lymph gland or node 683
    stump (*see also* Cervicitis) 616.0
  cervix (stump) (uteri) (*see also* Cervicitis) 616.0
  cheek, external 682.0
    inner 528.3
  chest 510.9
    with fistula 510.0
    wall 682.2
  chin 682.0
  choroid 363.00
  ciliary body 364.3
  circumtonsillar 475
  cold (tuberculous) (*see also* Tuberculosis, abscess)
    articular — *see* Tuberculosis, joint
  colon (wall) 569.5
  colostomy or enterostomy 569.61
  conjunctiva 372.00
  connective tissue NEC 682.9
  cornea 370.55
    with ulcer 370.00
  corpus
    cavernosum 607.2
    luteum (*see also* Salpingo-oophoritis) 614.2
  Cowper's gland 597.0
  cranium 324.0
  cul-de-sac (Douglas') (posterior) (*see also* Disease, pelvis, inflammatory) 614.4
    acute 614.3
  dental 522.5
    with sinus (alveolar) 522.7
  dentoalveolar 522.5
    with sinus (alveolar) 522.7
  diaphragm, diaphragmatic 567.22
  digit NEC 681.9
  Douglas' cul-de-sac or pouch (*see also* Disease, pelvis, inflammatory) 614.4
    acute 614.3
  Dubois' 090.5
  ductless gland 259.8
  ear
    acute 382.00
    external 380.10
    inner 386.30
    middle — *see* Otitis media
  elbow 682.3
  endamebic — *see* Abscess, amebic
  entamebic — *see* Abscess, amebic
  enterostomy 569.61
  epididymis 604.0
  epidural 324.9
    brain 324.0

Abscess — *see also* Cellulitis — *continued*
  epidural — *continued*
    late effect — *see* category 326
    spinal cord 324.1
  epiglottis 478.79
  epiploon, epiploic 567.22
  erysipelatous (*see also* Erysipelas) 035
  esophagostomy 530.86
  esophagus 530.19
  ethmoid (bone) (chronic) (sinus) (*see also* Sinusitis, ethmoidal) 473.2
  external auditory canal 380.10
  extradural 324.9
    brain 324.0
    late effect — *see* category 326
    spinal cord 324.1
  extraperitoneal — *see* Abscess, peritoneum
  eye 360.00
  eyelid 373.13
  face (any part, except eye) 682.0
  fallopian tube (*see also* Salpingo-oophoritis) 614.2
  fascia 728.89
  fauces 478.29
  fecal 569.5
  femoral (region) 682.6
  filaria, filarial (*see also* Infestation, filarial) 125.9
  finger (any) (intrathecal) (periosteal) (subcutaneous) (subcuticular) 681.00
  fistulous NEC 682.9
  flank 682.2
  foot (except toe) 682.7
  forearm 682.3
  forehead 682.0
  frontal (sinus) (chronic) (*see also* Sinusitis, frontal) 473.1
  gallbladder (*see also* Cholecystitis, acute) 575.0
  gastric 535.0 ☑
  genital organ or tract NEC
    female 616.9
      with
        abortion — *see* Abortion, by type, with sepsis
        ectopic pregnancy (*see also* categories 633.0–633.9) 639.0
        molar pregnancy (*see also* categories 630–632) 639.0
      following
        abortion 639.0
        ectopic or molar pregnancy 639.0
        puerperal, postpartum, childbirth 670.8 ☑
    male 608.4
  genitourinary system, tuberculous (*see also* Tuberculosis) 016.9 ☑
  gingival 523.30
  gland, glandular (lymph) (acute) NEC 683
  glottis 478.79
  gluteal (region) 682.5
  gonorrheal NEC (*see also* Gonococcus) 098.0
  groin 682.2
  gum 523.30
  hand (except finger or thumb) 682.4
  head (except face) 682.8
  heart 429.89
  heel 682.7
  helminthic (*see also* Infestation, by specific parasite) 128.9
  hepatic 572.0
    amebic (*see also* Abscess, liver, amebic) 006.3
    duct 576.8
  hip 682.6
    tuberculous (active) (*see also* Tuberculosis) 015.1 ☑
  ileocecal 540.1
  ileostomy (bud) 569.61
  iliac (region) 682.2
    fossa 540.1
  iliopsoas 567.31
    nontuberculous 728.89
    tuberculous (*see also* Tuberculosis) 015.0 ☑ *[730.88]*
  infraclavicular (fossa) 682.3

☑ **Additional Digit Required** — Refer to the Tabular List for Digit Selection   ▽ **Subterms under main terms may continue to next column or page**

2014 ICD-9-CM   ▶◀ Revised Text   ● New Line   ▲ Revised Code   Volume 2 — 3

Abscess — *see also* Cellulitis — *continued*
inguinal (region) 682.2
  lymph gland or node 683
intersphincteric (anus) 566
intestine, intestinal 569.5
  rectal 566
intra-abdominal (*see also* Abscess, peritoneum) 567.22
  postoperative 998.59
intracranial 324.0
  late effect — *see* category 326
intramammary — *see* Abscess, breast
intramastoid (*see also* Mastoiditis, acute) 383.00
intraorbital 376.01
intraperitoneal 567.22
intraspinal 324.1
  late effect — *see* category 326
intratonsillar 475
iris 364.3
ischiorectal 566
jaw (bone) (lower) (upper) 526.4
  skin 682.0
joint (*see also* Arthritis, pyogenic) 711.0 ☑
  vertebral (tuberculous) (*see also* Tuberculosis) 015.0 ☑ *[730.88]*
    nontuberculous 724.8
kidney 590.2
  with
    abortion — *see* Abortion, by type, with urinary tract infection
    calculus 592.0
    ectopic pregnancy (*see also* categories 633.0–633.9) 639.8
    molar pregnancy (*see also* categories 630–632) 639.8
    complicating pregnancy or puerperium 646.6 ☑
      affecting fetus or newborn 760.1
  following
    abortion 639.8
    ectopic or molar pregnancy 639.8
knee 682.6
  joint 711.06
  tuberculous (active) (*see also* Tuberculosis) 015.2 ☑
labium (majus) (minus) 616.4
  complicating pregnancy, childbirth, or puerperium 646.6 ☑
lacrimal (passages) (sac) (*see also* Dacryocystitis) 375.30
  caruncle 375.30
  gland (*see also* Dacryoadenitis) 375.00
lacunar 597.0
larynx 478.79
lateral (alveolar) 522.5
  with sinus 522.7
leg, except foot 682.6
lens 360.00
lid 373.13
lingual 529.0
  tonsil 475
lip 528.5
Littre's gland 597.0
liver 572.0
  amebic 006.3
    with
      brain abscess (and lung abscess) 006.5
      lung abscess 006.4
  due to Entamoeba histolytica 006.3
  dysenteric (*see also* Abscess, liver, amebic) 006.3
  pyogenic 572.0
  tropical (*see also* Abscess, liver, amebic) 006.3
loin (region) 682.2
lumbar (tuberculous) (*see also* Tuberculosis) 015.0 ☑ *[730.88]*
  nontuberculous 682.2
lung (miliary) (putrid) 513.0
  amebic (with liver abscess) 006.4
    with brain abscess 006.5
lymphangitic, acute — *see* Cellulitis
lymph, lymphatic, gland or node (acute) 683
  any site, except mesenteric 683

Abscess — *see also* Cellulitis — *continued*
lymph, lymphatic, gland or node — *continued*
  mesentery 289.2
malar 526.4
mammary gland — *see* Abscess, breast
marginal (anus) 566
mastoid (process) (*see also* Mastoiditis, acute) 383.00
  subperiosteal 383.01
maxilla, maxillary 526.4
  molar (tooth) 522.5
    with sinus 522.7
  premolar 522.5
  sinus (chronic) (*see also* Sinusitis, maxillary) 473.0
mediastinum 513.1
meibomian gland 373.12
meninges (*see also* Meningitis) 320.9
mesentery, mesenteric 567.22
mesosalpinx (*see also* Salpingo-oophoritis) 614.2
milk 675.1 ☑
Monro's (psoriasis) 696.1
mons pubis 682.2
mouth (floor) 528.3
multiple sites NEC 682.9
mural 682.2
muscle 728.89
  psoas 567.31
myocardium 422.92
nabothian (follicle) (*see also* Cervicitis) 616.0
nail (chronic) (with lymphangitis) 681.9
  finger 681.02
  toe 681.11
nasal (fossa) (septum) 478.19
  sinus (chronic) (*see also* Sinusitis) 473.9
nasopharyngeal 478.29
nates 682.5
navel 682.2
  newborn NEC 771.4
neck (region) 682.1
  lymph gland or node 683
nephritic (*see also* Abscess, kidney) 590.2
nipple 611.0
  puerperal, postpartum 675.0 ☑
nose (septum) 478.19
  external 682.0
omentum 567.22
operative wound 998.59
orbit, orbital 376.01
ossifluent — *see* Abscess, bone
ovary, ovarian (corpus luteum) (*see also* Salpingo-oophoritis) 614.2
oviduct (*see also* Salpingo-oophoritis) 614.2
palate (soft) 528.3
  hard 526.4
palmar (space) 682.4
pancreas (duct) 577.0
paradontal 523.30
parafrenal 607.2
parametric, parametrium (chronic) (*see also* Disease, pelvis, inflammatory) 614.4
  acute 614.3
paranephric 590.2
parapancreatic 577.0
parapharyngeal 478.22
pararectal 566
parasinus (*see also* Sinusitis) 473.9
parauterine (*see also* Disease, pelvis, inflammatory) 614.4
  acute 614.3
paravaginal (*see also* Vaginitis) 616.10
parietal region 682.8
parodontal 523.30
parotid (duct) (gland) 527.3
  region 528.3
parumbilical 682.2
  newborn 771.4
pectoral (region) 682.2
pelvirectal 567.22
pelvis, pelvic
  female (chronic) (*see also* Disease, pelvis, inflammatory) 614.4
    acute 614.3

Abscess — *see also* Cellulitis — *continued*
pelvis, pelvic — *continued*
  male, peritoneal (cellular tissue) — *see* Abscess, peritoneum
  tuberculous (*see also* Tuberculosis) 016.9 ☑
penis 607.2
  gonococcal (acute) 098.0
    chronic or duration of 2 months or over 098.2
perianal 566
periapical 522.5
  with sinus (alveolar) 522.7
periappendiceal 540.1
pericardial 420.99
pericecal 540.1
pericemental 523.30
pericholecystic (*see also* Cholecystitis, acute) 575.0
pericoronal 523.30
peridental 523.30
perigastric 535.0 ☑
perimetric (*see also* Disease, pelvis, inflammatory) 614.4
  acute 614.3
perinephric, perinephritic (*see also* Abscess, kidney) 590.2
perineum, perineal (superficial) 682.2
  deep (with urethral involvement) 597.0
  urethra 597.0
periodontal (parietal) 523.31
  apical 522.5
periosteum, periosteal (*see also* Periostitis) 730.3 ☑
  with osteomyelitis (*see also* Osteomyelitis) 730.2 ☑
    acute or subacute 730.0 ☑
    chronic or old 730.1 ☑
peripleuritic 510.9
  with fistula 510.0
periproctic 566
periprostatic 601.2
perirectal (staphylococcal) 566
perirenal (tissue) (*see also* Abscess, kidney) 590.2
perisinuous (nose) (*see also* Sinusitis) 473.9
peritoneum, peritoneal (perforated) (ruptured) 567.22
  with
    abortion — *see* Abortion, by type, with sepsis
    appendicitis 540.1
    ectopic pregnancy (*see also* categories 633.0–633.9) 639.0
    molar pregnancy (*see also* categories 630–632) 639.0
  following
    abortion 639.0
    ectopic or molar pregnancy 639.0
  pelvic, female (*see also* Disease, pelvis, inflammatory) 614.4
    acute 614.3
  postoperative 998.59
  puerperal, postpartum, childbirth 670.8 ☑
  tuberculous (*see also* Tuberculosis) 014.0 ☑
peritonsillar 475
perityphlic 540.1
periureteral 593.89
periurethral 597.0
  gonococcal (acute) 098.0
    chronic or duration of 2 months or over 098.2
periuterine (*see also* Disease, pelvis, inflammatory) 614.4
  acute 614.3
perivesical 595.89
pernicious NEC 682.9
petrous bone — *see* Petrositis
phagedenic NEC 682.9
  chancroid 099.0
pharynx, pharyngeal (lateral) 478.29
phlegmonous NEC 682.9
pilonidal 685.0
pituitary (gland) 253.8

Abscess — *see also* Cellulitis — *continued*
pleura 510.9
  with fistula 510.0
popliteal 682.6
postanal 566
postcecal 540.1
postlaryngeal 478.79
postnasal 478.19
postpharyngeal 478.24
posttonsillar 475
posttyphoid 002.0
Pott's (*see also* Tuberculosis) 015.0 ☑ *[730.88]*
pouch of Douglas (chronic) (*see also* Disease, pelvis, inflammatory) 614.4
premammary — *see* Abscess, breast
prepatellar 682.6
prostate (*see also* Prostatitis) 601.2
  gonococcal (acute) 098.12
    chronic or duration of 2 months or over 098.32
psoas 567.31
  nontuberculous 728.89
  tuberculous (*see also* Tuberculosis) 015.0 ☑ *[730.88]*
pterygopalatine fossa 682.8
pubis 682.2
puerperal — *see* Puerperal, abscess, by site
pulmonary — *see* Abscess, lung
pulp, pulpal (dental) 522.0
  finger 681.01
  toe 681.10
pyemic — *see* Septicemia
pyloric valve 535.0 ☑
rectovaginal septum 569.5
rectovesical 595.89
rectum 566
regional NEC 682.9
renal (*see also* Abscess, kidney) 590.2
retina 363.00
retrobulbar 376.01
retrocecal 567.22
retrolaryngeal 478.79
retromammary — *see* Abscess, breast
retroperineal 682.2
retroperitoneal 567.38
  postprocedural 998.59
retropharyngeal 478.24
  tuberculous (*see also* Tuberculosis) 012.8 ☑
retrorectal 566
retrouterine (*see also* Disease, pelvis, inflammatory) 614.4
  acute 614.3
retrovesical 595.89
root, tooth 522.5
  with sinus (alveolar) 522.7
round ligament (*see also* Disease, pelvis, inflammatory) 614.4
  acute 614.3
rupture (spontaneous) NEC 682.9
sacrum (tuberculous) (*see also* Tuberculosis) 015.0 ☑ *[730.88]*
  nontuberculous 730.08
salivary duct or gland 527.3
scalp (any part) 682.8
scapular 730.01
sclera 379.09
scrofulous (*see also* Tuberculosis) 017.2 ☑
scrotum 608.4
seminal vesicle 608.0
  amebic 006.8
septal, dental 522.5
  with sinus (alveolar) 522.7
septum (nasal) 478.19
serous (*see also* Periostitis) 730.3 ☑
shoulder 682.3
side 682.2
sigmoid 569.5
sinus (accessory) (chronic) (nasal) (*see also* Sinusitis) 473.9
  intracranial venous (any) 324.0
    late effect — *see* category 326
Skene's duct or gland 597.0
skin NEC 682.9

☑ **Additional Digit Required** — Refer to the Tabular List for Digit Selection

☝ **Subterms under main terms may continue to next column or page**

Abscess — *see also* Cellulitis — *continued*
skin — *continued*
tuberculous (primary) (*see also* Tuberculosis) 017.0 ☑
sloughing NEC 682.9
specified site NEC 682.8
amebic 006.8
spermatic cord 608.4
sphenoidal (sinus) (*see also* Sinusitis, sphenoidal) 473.3
spinal
cord (any part) (staphylococcal) 324.1
tuberculous (*see also* Tuberculosis) 013.5 ☑
epidural 324.1
spine (column) (tuberculous) (*see also* Tuberculosis) 015.0 ☑ [730.88]
nontuberculous 730.08
spleen 289.59
amebic 006.8
staphylococcal NEC 682.9
stitch 998.59
stomach (wall) 535.0 ☑
strumous (tuberculous) (*see also* Tuberculosis) 017.2 ☑
subarachnoid 324.9
brain 324.0
cerebral 324.0
late effect — *see* category 326
spinal cord 324.1
subareolar (*see also* Abscess, breast)
puerperal, postpartum 675.1 ☑
subcecal 540.1
subcutaneous NEC 682.9
subdiaphragmatic 567.22
subdorsal 682.2
subdural 324.9
brain 324.0
late effect — *see* category 326
spinal cord 324.1
subgaleal 682.8
subhepatic 567.22
sublingual 528.3
gland 527.3
submammary — *see* Abscess, breast
submandibular (region) (space) (triangle) 682.0
gland 527.3
submaxillary (region) 682.0
gland 527.3
submental (pyogenic) 682.0
gland 527.3
subpectoral 682.2
subperiosteal — *see* Abscess, bone
subperitoneal 567.22
subphrenic (*see also* Abscess, peritoneum) 567.22
postoperative 998.59
subscapular 682.2
subungual 681.9
suburethral 597.0
sudoriparous 705.89
suppurative NEC 682.9
supraclavicular (fossa) 682.3
suprahepatic 567.22
suprapelvic (*see also* Disease, pelvis, inflammatory) 614.4
acute 614.3
suprapubic 682.2
suprarenal (capsule) (gland) 255.8
sweat gland 705.89
syphilitic 095.8
teeth, tooth (root) 522.5
with sinus (alveolar) 522.7
supporting structures NEC 523.30
temple 682.0
temporal region 682.0
temporosphenoidal 324.0
late effect — *see* category 326
tendon (sheath) 727.89
testicle — *see* Orchitis
thecal 728.89
thigh (acquired) 682.6
thorax 510.9
with fistula 510.0
throat 478.29

Abscess — *see also* Cellulitis — *continued*
thumb (intrathecal) (periosteal) (subcutaneous) (subcuticular) 681.00
thymus (gland) 254.1
thyroid (gland) 245.0
toe (any) (intrathecal) (periosteal) (subcutaneous) (subcuticular) 681.10
tongue (staphylococcal) 529.0
tonsil(s) (lingual) 475
tonsillopharyngeal 475
tooth, teeth (root) 522.5
with sinus (alveolar) 522.7
supporting structure NEC 523.30
trachea 478.9
trunk 682.2
tubal (*see also* Salpingo-oophoritis) 614.2
tuberculous — *see* Tuberculosis, abscess
tubo-ovarian (*see also* Salpingo-oophoritis) 614.2
tunica vaginalis 608.4
umbilicus NEC 682.2
newborn 771.4
upper arm 682.3
upper respiratory 478.9
urachus 682.2
urethra (gland) 597.0
urinary 597.0
uterus, uterine (wall) (*see also* Endometritis) 615.9
ligament (*see also* Disease, pelvis, inflammatory) 614.4
acute 614.3
neck (*see also* Cervicitis) 616.0
uvula 528.3
vagina (wall) (*see also* Vaginitis) 616.10
vaginorectal (*see also* Vaginitis) 616.10
vas deferens 608.4
vermiform appendix 540.1
vertebra (column) (tuberculous) (*see also* Tuberculosis) 015.0 ☑ [730.88]
nontuberculous 730.0 ☑
vesical 595.89
vesicouterine pouch (*see also* Disease, pelvis, inflammatory) 614.4
vitreous (humor) (pneumococcal) 360.04
vocal cord 478.5
von Bezold's 383.01
vulva 616.4
complicating pregnancy, childbirth, or puerperium 646.6 ☑
vulvovaginal gland (*see also* Vaginitis) 616.3
web-space 682.4
wrist 682.4
Absence (organ or part) (complete or partial)
acoustic nerve 742.8
adrenal (gland) (congenital) 759.1
acquired V45.79
albumin (blood) 273.8
alimentary tract (complete) (congenital) (partial) 751.8
lower 751.5
upper 750.8
alpha-fucosidase 271.8
alveolar process (acquired) 525.8
congenital 750.26
anus, anal (canal) (congenital) 751.2
aorta (congenital) 747.22
aortic valve (congenital) 746.89
appendix, congenital 751.2
arm (acquired) V49.60
above elbow V49.66
below elbow V49.65
congenital (*see also* Deformity, reduction, upper limb) 755.20
lower — *see* Absence, forearm, congenital
upper (complete) (partial) (with absence of distal elements, incomplete) 755.24
with
complete absence of distal elements 755.21
forearm (incomplete) 755.23
artery (congenital) (peripheral) NEC (*see also* Anomaly, peripheral vascular system) 747.60

Absence — *continued*
artery (*see also* Anomaly, peripheral vascular system) — *continued*
brain 747.81
cerebral 747.81
coronary 746.85
pulmonary 747.31
umbilical 747.5
atrial septum 745.69
auditory canal (congenital) (external) 744.01
auricle (ear) (with stenosis or atresia of auditory canal), congenital 744.01
bile, biliary duct (common) or passage (congenital) 751.61
bladder (acquired) V45.74
congenital 753.8
bone (congenital) NEC 756.9
marrow 284.9
acquired (secondary) 284.89
congenital 284.09
hereditary 284.09
idiopathic 284.9
skull 756.0
bowel sounds 787.5
brain 740.0
specified part 742.2
breast(s) (acquired) V45.71
congenital 757.6
broad ligament (congenital) 752.19
bronchus (congenital) 748.3
calvarium, calvaria (skull) 756.0
canaliculus lacrimalis, congenital 743.65
carpal(s) (congenital) (complete) (partial) (with absence of distal elements, incomplete) (*see also* Deformity, reduction, upper limb) 755.28
with complete absence of distal elements 755.21
cartilage 756.9
caudal spine 756.13
cecum (acquired) (postoperative) (posttraumatic) V45.72
congenital 751.2
cementum 520.4
cerebellum (congenital) (vermis) 742.2
cervix (acquired) (uteri) V88.01
with remaining uterus V88.03
and uterus V88.01
congenital 752.43
chin, congenital 744.89
cilia (congenital) 743.63
acquired 374.89
circulatory system, part NEC 747.89
clavicle 755.51
clitoris (congenital) 752.49
coccyx, congenital 756.13
cold sense (*see also* Disturbance, sensation) 782.0
colon (acquired) (postoperative) V45.72
congenital 751.2
congenital
lumen — *see* Atresia
organ or site NEC — *see* Agenesis
septum — *see* Imperfect, closure
corpus callosum (congenital) 742.2
cricoid cartilage 748.3
diaphragm (congenital) (with hernia) 756.6
with obstruction 756.6
digestive organ(s) or tract, congenital (complete) (partial) 751.8
acquired V45.79
lower 751.5
upper 750.8
ductus arteriosus 747.89
duodenum (acquired) (postoperative) V45.72
congenital 751.1
ear, congenital 744.09
acquired V45.79
auricle 744.01
external 744.01
inner 744.05
lobe, lobule 744.21
middle, except ossicles 744.03
ossicles 744.04
ossicles 744.04

Absence — *continued*
ejaculatory duct (congenital) 752.89
endocrine gland NEC (congenital) 759.2
epididymis (congenital) 752.89
acquired V45.77
epiglottis, congenital 748.3
epileptic (atonic) (typical) (*see also* Epilepsy) 345.0 ☑
erythrocyte 284.9
erythropoiesis 284.9
congenital 284.01
esophagus (congenital) 750.3
Eustachian tube (congenital) 744.24
extremity (acquired)
congenital (*see also* Deformity, reduction) 755.4
lower V49.70
upper V49.60
extrinsic muscle, eye 743.69
eye (acquired) V45.78
adnexa (congenital) 743.69
congenital 743.00
muscle (congenital) 743.69
eyelid (fold), congenital 743.62
acquired 374.89
face
bones NEC 756.0
specified part NEC 744.89
fallopian tube(s) (acquired) V45.77
congenital 752.19
femur, congenital (complete) (partial) (with absence of distal elements, incomplete) (*see also* Deformity, reduction, lower limb) 755.34
with
complete absence of distal elements 755.31
tibia and fibula (incomplete) 755.33
fibrin 790.92
fibrinogen (congenital) 286.3
acquired 286.6
fibula, congenital (complete) (partial) (with absence of distal elements, incomplete) (*see also* Deformity, reduction, lower limb) 755.37
with
complete absence of distal elements 755.31
tibia 755.35
with
complete absence of distal elements 755.31
femur (incomplete) 755.33
with complete absence of distal elements 755.31
finger (acquired) V49.62
congenital (complete) (partial) (*see also* Deformity, reduction, upper limb) 755.29
meaning all fingers (complete) (partial) 755.21
transverse 755.21
fissures of lungs (congenital) 748.5
foot (acquired) V49.73
congenital (complete) 755.31
forearm (acquired) V49.65
congenital (complete) (partial) (with absence of distal elements, incomplete) (*see also* Deformity, reduction, upper limb) 755.25
with
complete absence of distal elements (hand and fingers) 755.21
humerus (incomplete) 755.23
fovea centralis 743.55
fucosidase 271.8
gallbladder (acquired) V45.79
congenital 751.69
gamma globulin (blood) 279.00
genital organs
acquired V45.77
congenital
female 752.89
external 752.49

☑ **Additional Digit Required — Refer to the Tabular List for Digit Selection**   ⩒ **Subterms under main terms may continue to next column or page**

2014 ICD-9-CM   ▶◀ **Revised Text**   ● **New Line**   ▲ **Revised Code**   **Volume 2 — 5**

Absence — *continued*
  genital organs — *continued*
    congenital — *continued*
      female — *continued*
        internal NEC 752.89
      male 752.89
        penis 752.69
  genitourinary organs, congenital NEC 752.89
  glottis 748.3
  gonadal, congenital NEC 758.6
  hair (congenital) 757.4
    acquired — *see* Alopecia
  hand (acquired) V49.63
    congenital (complete) (*see also* Deformity, reduction, upper limb) 755.21
  heart (congenital) 759.89
    acquired — *see* Status, organ replacement
  heat sense (*see also* Disturbance, sensation) 782.0
  humerus, congenital (complete) (partial) (with absence of distal elements, incomplete) (*see also* Deformity, reduction, upper limb) 755.24
    with
      complete absence of distal elements 755.21
      radius and ulna (incomplete) 755.23
  hymen (congenital) 752.49
  ileum (acquired) (postoperative) (posttraumatic) V45.72
    congenital 751.1
  immunoglobulin, isolated NEC 279.03
    IgA 279.01
    IgG 279.03
    IgM 279.02
  incus (acquired) 385.24
    congenital 744.04
  internal ear (congenital) 744.05
  intestine (acquired) (small) V45.72
    congenital 751.1
      large 751.2
    large V45.72
      congenital 751.2
  iris (congenital) 743.45
  jaw — *see* Absence, mandible
  jejunum (acquired) V45.72
    congenital 751.1
  joint (acquired) (following prior explantation of joint prosthesis) (with or without presence of antibiotic-impregnated cement spacer) NEC V88.29
    congenital NEC 755.8
    hip V88.21
    knee V88.22
  kidney(s) (acquired) V45.73
    congenital 753.0
  labium (congenital) (majus) (minus) 752.49
  labyrinth, membranous 744.05
  lacrimal apparatus (congenital) 743.65
  larynx (congenital) 748.3
  leg (acquired) V49.70
    above knee V49.76
    below knee V49.75
    congenital (partial) (unilateral) (*see also* Deformity, reduction, lower limb) 755.31
      lower (complete) (partial) (with absence of distal elements, incomplete) 755.35
        with
          complete absence of distal elements (foot and toes) 755.31
          thigh (incomplete) 755.33
            with complete absence of distal elements 755.31
      upper — *see* Absence, femur
  lens (congenital) 743.35
    acquired 379.31
  ligament, broad (congenital) 752.19
  limb (acquired)
    congenital (complete) (partial) (*see also* Deformity, reduction) 755.4
      lower 755.30

Absence — *continued*
  limb — *continued*
    congenital (*see also* Deformity, reduction) — *continued*
      lower — *continued*
        complete 755.31
        incomplete 755.32
        longitudinal — *see* Deficiency, lower limb, longitudinal
        transverse 755.31
      upper 755.20
        complete 755.21
        incomplete 755.22
        longitudinal — *see* Deficiency, upper limb, longitudinal
        transverse 755.21
    lower NEC V49.70
    upper NEC V49.60
  lip 750.26
  liver (congenital) (lobe) 751.69
  lumbar (congenital) (vertebra) 756.13
    isthmus 756.11
    pars articularis 756.11
  lumen — *see* Atresia
  lung (bilateral) (congenital) (fissure) (lobe) (unilateral) 748.5
    acquired (any part) V45.76
  mandible (congenital) 524.09
  maxilla (congenital) 524.09
  menstruation 626.0
  metacarpal(s), congenital (complete) (partial) (with absence of distal elements, incomplete) (*see also* Deformity, reduction, upper limb) 755.28
    with all fingers, complete 755.21
  metatarsal(s), congenital (complete) (partial) (with absence of distal elements, incomplete) (*see also* Deformity, reduction, lower limb) 755.38
    with complete absence of distal elements 755.31
  muscle (congenital) (pectoral) 756.81
    ocular 743.69
  musculoskeletal system (congenital) NEC 756.9
  nail(s) (congenital) 757.5
  neck, part 744.89
  nerve 742.8
  nervous system, part NEC 742.8
  neutrophil 288.00
  nipple (congenital) 757.6
    acquired V45.71
  nose (congenital) 748.1
    acquired 738.0
  nuclear 742.8
  ocular muscle (congenital) 743.69
  organ
    of Corti (congenital) 744.05
    or site
      acquired V45.79
      congenital NEC 759.89
  osseous meatus (ear) 744.03
  ovary (acquired) V45.77
    congenital 752.0
  oviduct (acquired) V45.77
    congenital 752.19
  pancreas (congenital) 751.7
    acquired (postoperative) (posttraumatic) V88.11
      partial V88.12
      total V88.11
  parathyroid gland (congenital) 759.2
  parotid gland(s) (congenital) 750.21
  patella, congenital 755.64
  pelvic girdle (congenital) 755.69
  penis (congenital) 752.69
    acquired V45.77
  pericardium (congenital) 746.89
  perineal body (congenital) 756.81
  phalange(s), congenital 755.4
    lower limb (complete) (intercalary) (partial) (terminal) (*see also* Deformity, reduction, lower limb) 755.39
      meaning all toes (complete) (partial) 755.31

Absence — *continued*
  phalange(s), congenital — *continued*
    lower limb (*see also* Deformity, reduction, lower limb) — *continued*
      transverse 755.31
    upper limb (complete) (intercalary) (partial) (terminal) (*see also* Deformity, reduction, upper limb) 755.29
      meaning all digits (complete) (partial) 755.21
      transverse 755.21
  pituitary gland (congenital) 759.2
  postoperative — *see* Absence, by site, acquired
  prostate (congenital) 752.89
    acquired V45.77
  pulmonary
    artery 747.31
    trunk 747.31
    valve (congenital) 746.01
    vein 747.49
  punctum lacrimale (congenital) 743.65
  radius, congenital (complete) (partial) (with absence of distal elements, incomplete) 755.26
    with
      complete absence of distal elements 755.21
      ulna 755.25
        with
          complete absence of distal elements 755.21
          humerus (incomplete) 755.23
  ray, congenital 755.4
    lower limb (complete) (partial) (*see also* Deformity, reduction, lower limb) 755.38
      meaning all rays 755.31
      transverse 755.31
    upper limb (complete) (partial) (*see also* Deformity, reduction, upper limb) 755.28
      meaning all rays 755.21
      transverse 755.21
  rectum (congenital) 751.2
    acquired V45.79
  red cell 284.9
    acquired (secondary) 284.81
    congenital 284.01
    hereditary 284.01
    idiopathic 284.9
  respiratory organ (congenital) NEC 748.9
  rib (acquired) 738.3
    congenital 756.3
  roof of orbit (congenital) 742.0
  round ligament (congenital) 752.89
  sacrum, congenital 756.13
  salivary gland(s) (congenital) 750.21
  scapula 755.59
  scrotum, congenital 752.89
  seminal tract or duct (congenital) 752.89
    acquired V45.77
  septum (congenital) (*see also* Imperfect, closure, septum)
    atrial 745.69
      and ventricular 745.7
    between aorta and pulmonary artery 745.0
    ventricular 745.3
      and atrial 745.7
  sex chromosomes 758.81
  shoulder girdle, congenital (complete) (partial) 755.59
  skin (congenital) 757.39
  skull bone 756.0
    with
      anencephalus 740.0
      encephalocele 742.0
      hydrocephalus 742.3
        with spina bifida (*see also* Spina bifida) 741.0 ☑
      microcephalus 742.1
  spermatic cord (congenital) 752.89
  spinal cord 742.59
  spine, congenital 756.13

Absence — *continued*
  spleen (congenital) 759.0
    acquired V45.79
  sternum, congenital 756.3
  stomach (acquired) (partial) (postoperative) V45.75
    with postgastric surgery syndrome 564.2
    congenital 750.7
  submaxillary gland(s) (congenital) 750.21
  superior vena cava (congenital) 747.49
  tarsal(s), congenital (complete) (partial) (with absence of distal elements, incomplete) (*see also* Deformity, reduction, lower limb) 755.38
  teeth, tooth (congenital) 520.0
    with abnormal spacing 524.30
    acquired 525.10
      with malocclusion 524.30
      due to
        caries 525.13
        extraction 525.10
        periodontal disease 525.12
        trauma 525.11
  tendon (congenital) 756.81
  testis (congenital) 752.89
    acquired V45.77
  thigh (acquired) 736.89
  thumb (acquired) V49.61
    congenital 755.29
  thymus gland (congenital) 759.2
  thyroid (gland) (surgical) 246.8
    with hypothyroidism 244.0
    cartilage, congenital 748.3
    congenital 243
  tibia, congenital (complete) (partial) (with absence of distal elements, incomplete) (*see also* Deformity, reduction, lower limb) 755.36
    with
      complete absence of distal elements 755.31
      fibula 755.35
        with
          complete absence of distal elements 755.31
          femur (incomplete) 755.33
            with complete absence of distal elements 755.31
  toe (acquired) V49.72
    congenital (complete) (partial) 755.39
      meaning all toes 755.31
      transverse 755.31
    great V49.71
  tongue (congenital) 750.11
  tooth, teeth (congenital) 520.0
    with abnormal spacing 524.30
    acquired 525.10
      with malocclusion 524.30
      due to
        caries 525.13
        extraction 525.10
        periodontal disease 525.12
        trauma 525.11
  trachea (cartilage) (congenital) (rings) 748.3
  transverse aortic arch (congenital) 747.21
  tricuspid valve 746.1
  ulna, congenital (complete) (partial) (with absence of distal elements, incomplete) (*see also* Deformity, reduction, upper limb) 755.27
    with
      complete absence of distal elements 755.21
      radius 755.25
        with
          complete absence of distal elements 755.21
          humerus (incomplete) 755.23
  umbilical artery (congenital) 747.5
  ureter (congenital) 753.4
    acquired V45.74
  urethra, congenital 753.8
    acquired V45.74
  urinary system, part NEC, congenital 753.8
    acquired V45.74

☑ Additional Digit Required — Refer to the Tabular List for Digit Selection   ▽ Subterms under main terms may continue to next column or page

6 — Volume 2   ▶◀ Revised Text   ● New Line   ▲ Revised Code   2014 ICD-9-CM

Absence — *continued*
  uterus (acquired) V88.01
    with remaining cervical stump V88.02
    and cervix V88.01
    congenital 752.31
  uvula (congenital) 750.26
  vagina, congenital 752.45
    acquired V45.77
  vas deferens (congenital) 752.89
    acquired V45.77
  vein (congenital) (peripheral) NEC (*see also* Anomaly, peripheral vascular system) 747.60
    brain 747.81
    great 747.49
    portal 747.49
    pulmonary 747.49
  vena cava (congenital) (inferior) (superior) 747.49
  ventral horn cell 742.59
  ventricular septum 745.3
  vermis of cerebellum 742.2
  vertebra, congenital 756.13
  vulva, congenital 752.49
Absentia epileptica — *see also* Epilepsy 345.0 ☑
Absinthemia — *see also* Dependence 304.6 ☑
Absinthism — *see also* Dependence 304.6 ☑
Absorbent system disease 459.89
Absorption
  alcohol, through placenta or breast milk 760.71
  anti-infective, through placenta or breast milk 760.74
  antibiotics, through placenta or breast milk 760.74
  anticonvulsants, through placenta or breast milk 760.77
  antifungals, through placenta or breast milk 760.74
  antimetabolics, through placenta or breast milk 760.78
  chemical NEC 989.9
    specified chemical or substance — *see* Table of Drugs and Chemicals
    through placenta or breast milk (fetus or newborn) 760.70
      alcohol 760.71
      anti-infective agents 760.74
      anticonvulsants 760.77
      antifungals 760.74
      antimetabolics 760.78
      cocaine 760.75
      "crack" 760.75
      diethylstilbestrol [DES] 760.76
      hallucinogenic agents 760.73
      medicinal agents NEC 760.79
      narcotics 760.72
      obstetric anesthetic or analgesic drug 763.5
      specified agent NEC 760.79
      suspected, affecting management of pregnancy 655.5 ☑
  cocaine, through placenta or breast milk 760.75
  drug NEC (*see also* Reaction, drug)
    through placenta or breast milk (fetus or newborn) 760.70
      alcohol 760.71
      anti-infective agents 760.74
      anticonvulsants 760.77
      antifungals 760.74
      antimetabolics 760.78
      cocaine 760.75
      "crack" 760.75
      diethylstilbestrol [DES] 760.76
      hallucinogenic agents 760.73
      medicinal agents NEC 760.79
      narcotics 760.72
      obstetric anesthetic or analgesic drug 763.5
      specified agent NEC 760.79
      suspected, affecting management of pregnancy 655.5 ☑
  fat, disturbance 579.8

Absorption — *continued*
  hallucinogenic agents, through placenta or breast milk 760.73
  immune sera, through placenta or breast milk 760.79
  lactose defect 271.3
  medicinal agents NEC, through placenta or breast milk 760.79
  narcotics, through placenta or breast milk 760.72
  noxious substance — *see* Absorption, chemical
  protein, disturbance 579.8
  pus or septic, general — *see* Septicemia
  quinine, through placenta or breast milk 760.74
  toxic substance — *see* Absorption, chemical
  uremic — *see* Uremia
Abstinence symptoms or syndrome
  alcohol 291.81
  drug 292.0
  neonatal 779.5
Abt-Letterer-Siwe syndrome (acute histiocytosis X) (M9722/3) 202.5 ☑
Abulia 799.89
Abulomania 301.6
Abuse
  adult 995.80
    emotional 995.82
    multiple forms 995.85
    neglect (nutritional) 995.84
    physical 995.81
    psychological 995.82
    sexual 995.83
  alcohol — *see also* Alcoholism 305.0 ☑
    dependent 303.9 ☑
    non-dependent 305.0 ☑
  child 995.50
    counseling
      perpetrator
        non-parent V62.83
        parent V61.22
      victim V61.21
    emotional 995.51
    multiple forms 995.59
    neglect (nutritional) 995.52
    physical 995.54
      shaken infant syndrome 995.55
    psychological 995.51
    sexual 995.53
  drugs, nondependent 305.9 ☑

Note — Use the following fifth-digit subclassification with the following codes: 305.0, 305.2–305.9:

0   unspecified
1   continuous
2   episodic
3   in remission

    amphetamine type 305.7 ☑
    antidepressants 305.8 ☑
    anxiolytic 305.4 ☑
    barbiturates 305.4 ☑
    caffeine 305.9 ☑
    cannabis 305.2 ☑
    cocaine type 305.6 ☑
    hallucinogens 305.3 ☑
    hashish 305.2 ☑
    hypnotic 305.4 ☑
    inhalant 305.9 ☑
    LSD 305.3 ☑
    marijuana 305.2 ☑
    mixed 305.9 ☑
    morphine type 305.5 ☑
    opioid type 305.5 ☑
    phencyclidine (PCP) 305.9 ☑
    sedative 305.4 ☑
    specified NEC 305.9 ☑
    tranquilizers 305.4 ☑
  spouse 995.80
  tobacco 305.1
Acalcerosis 275.40
Acalcicosis 275.40
Acalculia 784.69

Acalculia — *continued*
  developmental 315.1
Acanthocheilonemiasis 125.4
Acanthocytosis 272.5
Acanthokeratodermia 701.1
Acantholysis 701.8
  bullosa 757.39
Acanthoma (benign) (M8070/0) — *see also* Neoplasm, by site, benign
  malignant (M8070/3) — *see* Neoplasm, by site, malignant
Acanthosis (acquired) (nigricans) 701.2
  adult 701.2
  benign (congenital) 757.39
  congenital 757.39
  glycogenic
    esophagus 530.89
  juvenile 701.2
  tongue 529.8
Acanthrocytosis 272.5
Acapnia 276.3
Acarbia 276.2
Acardia 759.89
Acardiacus amorphus 759.89
Acardiotrophia 429.1
Acardius 759.89
Acariasis 133.9
  sarcoptic 133.0
Acaridiasis 133.9
Acarinosis 133.9
Acariosis 133.9
Acarodermatitis 133.9
  urticarioides 133.9
Acarophobia 300.29
Acatalasemia 277.89
Acatalasia 277.89
Acatamathesia 784.69
Acataphasia 784.59
Acathisia 781.0
  due to drugs 333.99
Acceleration, accelerated
  atrioventricular conduction 426.7
  idioventricular rhythm 427.89
Accessory (congenital)
  adrenal gland 759.1
  anus 751.5
  appendix 751.5
  atrioventricular conduction 426.7
  auditory ossicles 744.04
  auricle (ear) 744.1
  autosome(s) NEC 758.5
    21 or 22 758.0
  biliary duct or passage 751.69
  bladder 753.8
  blood vessels (peripheral) (congenital) NEC (*see also* Anomaly, peripheral vascular system) 747.60
    cerebral 747.81
    coronary 746.85
  bone NEC 756.9
    foot 755.67
  breast tissue, axilla 757.6
  carpal bones 755.56
  cecum 751.5
  cervix 752.44
  chromosome(s) NEC 758.5
    13-15 758.1
    16-18 758.2
    21 or 22 758.0
    autosome(s) NEC 758.5
    D_1 758.1
    E_3 758.2
    G 758.0
    sex 758.81
  coronary artery 746.85
  cusp(s), heart valve NEC 746.89
    pulmonary 746.09
  cystic duct 751.69
  digits 755.00
  ear (auricle) (lobe) 744.1
  endocrine gland NEC 759.2
  external os 752.44
  eyelid 743.62
  eye muscle 743.69
  face bone(s) 756.0
  fallopian tube (fimbria) (ostium) 752.19

Accessory — *continued*
  fingers 755.01
  foreskin 605
  frontonasal process 756.0
  gallbladder 751.69
  genital organ(s)
    female 752.89
      external 752.49
      internal NEC 752.89
    male NEC 752.89
      penis 752.69
  genitourinary organs NEC 752.89
  heart 746.89
    valve NEC 746.89
      pulmonary 746.09
  hepatic ducts 751.69
  hymen 752.49
  intestine (large) (small) 751.5
  kidney 753.3
  lacrimal canal 743.65
  leaflet, heart valve NEC 746.89
    pulmonary 746.09
  ligament, broad 752.19
  liver (duct) 751.69
  lobule (ear) 744.1
  lung (lobe) 748.69
  muscle 756.82
  navicular of carpus 755.56
  nervous system, part NEC 742.8
  nipple 757.6
  nose 748.1
  organ or site NEC — *see* Anomaly, specified type NEC
  ovary 752.0
  oviduct 752.19
  pancreas 751.7
  parathyroid gland 759.2
  parotid gland (and duct) 750.22
  pituitary gland 759.2
  placental lobe — *see* Placenta, abnormal
  preauricular appendage 744.1
  prepuce 605
  renal arteries (multiple) 747.62
  rib 756.3
    cervical 756.2
  roots (teeth) 520.2
  salivary gland 750.22
  sesamoids 755.8
  sinus — *see* condition
  skin tags 757.39
  spleen 759.0
  sternum 756.3
  submaxillary gland 750.22
  tarsal bones 755.67
  teeth, tooth 520.1
    causing crowding 524.31
  tendon 756.89
  thumb 755.01
  thymus gland 759.2
  thyroid gland 759.2
  toes 755.02
  tongue 750.13
  tragus 744.1
  ureter 753.4
  urethra 753.8
  urinary organ or tract NEC 753.8
  uterus 752.2
  vagina 752.49
  valve, heart NEC 746.89
    pulmonary 746.09
  vertebra 756.19
  vocal cords 748.3
  vulva 752.49
Accident, accidental — *see also* condition
  birth NEC 767.9
  cardiovascular (*see also* Disease, cardiovascular) 429.2
  cerebral (*see also* Disease, cerebrovascular, acute) 434.91
  cerebrovascular (current) (CVA) (*see also* Disease, cerebrovascular, acute) 434.91
    aborted 434.91
    embolic 434.11
    healed or old V12.54
    hemorrhagic — *see* Hemorrhage, brain

Absence — Accident, accidental

☑ **Additional Digit Required** — Refer to the Tabular List for Digit Selection   ᵂ **Subterms under main terms may continue to next column or page**

2014 ICD-9-CM   ▶◀ **Revised Text**   ● **New Line**   ▲ **Revised Code**   Volume 2 — 7

Accident, accidental — see also condition — continued
  cerebrovascular (see also Disease, cerebrovascular, acute) — continued
    impending 435.9
    ischemic 434.91
    late effect — see Late effect(s) (of) cerebrovascular disease
    postoperative 997.02
    thrombotic 434.01
  coronary (see also Infarct, myocardium) 410.9 ☑
  craniovascular (see also Disease, cerebrovascular, acute) 436
  during pregnancy, to mother, affecting fetus or newborn 760.5
  heart, cardiac (see also Infarct, myocardium) 410.9 ☑
  intrauterine 779.89
  vascular — see Disease, cerebrovascular, acute
Accommodation
  disorder of 367.51
    drug-induced 367.89
    toxic 367.89
  insufficiency of 367.4
  paralysis of 367.51
    hysterical 300.11
  spasm of 367.53
Accouchement — see Delivery
Accreta placenta (without hemorrhage) 667.0 ☑
  with hemorrhage 666.0 ☑
Accretio cordis (nonrheumatic) 423.1
Accretions on teeth 523.6
Accumulation secretion, prostate 602.8
Acephalia, acephalism, acephaly 740.0
Acephalic 740.0
Acephalobrachia 759.89
Acephalocardia 759.89
Acephalocardius 759.89
Acephalochiria 759.89
Acephalochirus 759.89
Acephalogaster 759.89
Acephalostomus 759.89
Acephalothorax 759.89
Acephalus 740.0
Acetonemia 790.6
  diabetic 250.1 ☑
    due to secondary diabetes 249.1 ☑
Acetonglycosuria 982.8
Acetonuria 791.6
Achalasia 530.0
  cardia 530.0
  digestive organs congenital NEC 751.8
  esophagus 530.0
  pelvirectal 751.3
  psychogenic 306.4
  pylorus 750.5
  sphincteral NEC 564.89
Achard-Thiers syndrome (adrenogenital) 255.2
Ache(s) — see Pain
Acheilia 750.26
Acheiria 755.21
Achillobursitis 726.71
Achillodynia 726.71
Achlorhydria, achlorhydric 536.0
  anemia 280.9
  diarrhea 536.0
  neurogenic 536.0
  postvagotomy 564.2
  psychogenic 306.4
  secondary to vagotomy 564.2
Achloroblepsia 368.52
Achloropsia 368.52
Acholia 575.8
Acholuric jaundice (familial) (splenomegalic) — see also Spherocytosis 282.0
  acquired 283.9
Achondroplasia 756.4
Achrestic anemia 281.8
Achroacytosis, lacrimal gland 375.00
  tuberculous (see also Tuberculosis) 017.3 ☑
Achroma, cutis 709.00
Achromate (congenital) 368.54

Achromatopia 368.54
Achromatopsia (congenital) 368.54
Achromia
  congenital 270.2
  parasitica 111.0
  unguium 703.8
Achylia
  gastrica 536.8
    neurogenic 536.3
    psychogenic 306.4
  pancreatica 577.1
Achylosis 536.8
Acid
  burn (see also Burn, by site)
    from swallowing acid — see Burn, internal organs
  deficiency
    amide nicotinic 265.2
    amino 270.9
    ascorbic 267
    folic 266.2
    nicotinic (amide) 265.2
    pantothenic 266.2
  intoxication 276.2
  peptic disease 536.8
  stomach 536.8
    psychogenic 306.4
Acidemia 276.2
  arginosuccinic 270.6
  fetal
    affecting management of pregnancy 656.3 ☑
    before onset of labor, in liveborn infant 768.2
    during labor and delivery in liveborn infant 768.3
    intrauterine 656.3 ☑
    unspecified as to time of onset, in liveborn infant 768.4
  newborn 775.81
  pipecolic 270.7
Acidity, gastric (high) (low) 536.8
  psychogenic 306.4
Acidocytopenia 288.59
Acidocytosis 288.3
Acidopenia 288.59
Acidosis 276.2
  diabetic 250.1 ☑
    due to secondary diabetes 249.1 ☑
  fetal, affecting management of pregnancy 656.8 ☑
  fetal, affecting newborn 775.81
  kidney tubular 588.89
    newborn 775.81
  lactic 276.2
  metabolic NEC 276.2
    with respiratory acidosis 276.4
      of newborn 775.81
    late, of newborn 775.7
  newborn 775.81
  renal
    hyperchloremic 588.89
    tubular (distal) (proximal) 588.89
  respiratory 276.2
    complicated by
      metabolic acidosis 276.4
        of newborn 775.81
      metabolic alkalosis 276.4
Aciduria 791.9
  arginosuccinic 270.6
  beta-aminoisobutyric (BAIB) 277.2
  glutaric
    type I 270.7
    type II (type IIA, IIB, IIC) 277.85
    type III 277.86
  glycolic 270.7
  methylmalonic 270.3
    with glycinemia 270.7
  organic 270.9
  orotic (congenital) (hereditary) (pyrimidine deficiency) 281.4
Acladiosis 111.8
  skin 111.8
Aclasis
  diaphyseal 756.4
  tarsoepiphyseal 756.59

Acleistocardia 745.5
Aclusion 524.4
Acmesthesia 782.0
Acne (pustular) (vulgaris) 706.1
  agminata (see also Tuberculosis) 017.0 ☑
  artificialis 706.1
  atrophica 706.0
  cachecticorum (Hebra) 706.1
  conglobata 706.1
  conjunctiva 706.1
  cystic 706.1
  decalvans 704.09
  erythematosa 695.3
  eyelid 706.1
  frontalis 706.0
  indurata 706.1
  keloid 706.1
  lupoid 706.0
  necrotic, necrotica 706.0
    miliaris 704.8
  neonatal 706.1
  nodular 706.1
  occupational 706.1
  papulosa 706.1
  rodens 706.0
  rosacea 695.3
  scorbutica 267
  scrofulosorum (Bazin) (see also Tuberculosis) 017.0 ☑
  summer 692.72
  tropical 706.1
  varioliformis 706.0
Acneiform drug eruptions 692.3
Acnitis (primary) — see also Tuberculosis 017.0 ☑
Acomia 704.00
Acontractile bladder 344.61
Aconuresis — see also Incontinence 788.30
Acosta's disease 993.2
Acousma 780.1
Acoustic — see condition
Acousticophobia 300.29
Acquired — see condition
Acquired immune deficiency syndrome — see Human immunodeficiency virus (disease) (illness) (infection)
Acquired immunodeficiency syndrome — see Human immunodeficiency virus (disease) (illness) (infection)
Acragnosis 781.99
Acrania 740.0
Acroagnosis 781.99
Acroangiodermatitis 448.9
Acroasphyxia, chronic 443.89
Acrobrachycephaly 756.0
Acrobystiolith 608.89
Acrobystitis 607.2
Acrocephalopolysyndactyly 755.55
Acrocephalosyndactyly 755.55
Acrocephaly 756.0
Acrochondrohyperplasia 759.82
Acrocyanosis 443.89
  newborn 770.83
    meaning transient blue hands and feet — omit code
Acrodermatitis 686.8
  atrophicans (chronica) 701.8
  continua (Hallopeau) 696.1
  enteropathica 686.8
  Hallopeau's 696.1
  perstans 696.1
  pustulosa continua 696.1
  recalcitrant pustular 696.1
Acrodynia 985.0
Acrodysplasia 755.55
Acrohyperhidrosis — see also Hyperhidrosis 780.8
Acrokeratosis verruciformis 757.39
Acromastitis 611.0
Acromegaly, acromegalia (skin) 253.0
Acromelalgia 443.82
Acromicria, acromikria 756.59
Acronyx 703.0
Acropachyderma 757.39
Acropachy, thyroid — see also Thyrotoxicosis 242.9 ☑

Acroparesthesia 443.89
  simple (Schultz's type) 443.89
  vasomotor (Nothnagel's type) 443.89
Acropathy thyroid — see also Thyrotoxicosis 242.9 ☑
Acrophobia 300.29
Acroposthitis 607.2
Acroscleriasis — see also Scleroderma 710.1
Acroscleroderma — see also Scleroderma 710.1
Acrosclerosis — see also Scleroderma 710.1
Acrosphacelus 785.4
Acrosphenosyndactylia 755.55
Acrospiroma, eccrine (M8402/0) — see Neoplasm, skin, benign
Acrostealgia 732.9
Acrosyndactyly — see also Syndactylism 755.10
Acrotrophodynia 991.4
Actinic — see also condition
  cheilitis (due to sun) 692.72
    chronic NEC 692.74
    due to radiation, except from sun 692.82
  conjunctivitis 370.24
  dermatitis (due to sun) (see also Dermatitis, actinic) 692.70
    due to
      roentgen rays or radioactive substance 692.82
      ultraviolet radiation, except from sun 692.82
      sun NEC 692.70
  elastosis solare 692.74
  granuloma 692.73
  keratitis 370.24
  ophthalmia 370.24
  reticuloid 692.73
Actinobacillosis, general 027.8
Actinobacillus
  lignieresii 027.8
  mallei 024
  muris 026.1
Actinocutitis NEC — see also Dermatitis, actinic 692.70
Actinodermatitis NEC — see also Dermatitis, actinic 692.70
Actinomyces
  israelii (infection) — see Actinomycosis
  muris-ratti (infection) 026.1
Actinomycosis, actinomycotic 039.9
  with
    pneumonia 039.1
  abdominal 039.2
  cervicofacial 039.3
  cutaneous 039.0
  pulmonary 039.1
  specified site NEC 039.8
  thoracic 039.1
Actinoneuritis 357.89
Action, heart
  disorder 427.9
    postoperative 997.1
  irregular 427.9
    postoperative 997.1
    psychogenic 306.2
Active — see condition
Activity decrease, functional 780.99
Acute — see also condition
  abdomen NEC 789.0 ☑
  gallbladder (see also Cholecystitis, acute) 575.0
Acyanoblepsia 368.53
Acyanopsia 368.53
Acystia 753.8
Acystinervia — see Neurogenic, bladder
Acystineuria — see Neurogenic, bladder
Adactylia, adactyly (congenital) 755.4
  lower limb (complete) (intercalary) (partial) (terminal) (see also Deformity, reduction, lower limb) 755.39
    meaning all digits (complete) (partial) 755.31
    transverse (complete) (partial) 755.31
  upper limb (complete) (intercalary) (partial) (terminal) (see also Deformity, reduction, upper limb) 755.29

☑ **Additional Digit Required** — Refer to the Tabular List for Digit Selection   ▽ **Subterms under main terms may continue to next column or page**

8 — Volume 2   ▶◀ Revised Text   ● New Line   ▲ Revised Code   2014 ICD-9-CM

Adactylia, adactyly — *continued*
  upper limb (*see also* Deformity, reduction, upper limb) — *continued*
    meaning all digits (complete) (partial) 755.21
    transverse (complete) (partial) 755.21
Adair-Dighton syndrome (brittle bones and blue sclera, deafness) 756.51
Adamantinoblastoma (M9310/0) — *see* Ameloblastoma
Adamantinoma (M9310/0) — *see* Ameloblastoma
Adamantoblastoma (M9310/0) — *see* Ameloblastoma
Adams-Stokes (-Morgagni) disease or syndrome (syncope with heart block) 426.9
Adaptation reaction — *see also* Reaction, adjustment 309.9
Addiction — *see also* Dependence
  absinthe 304.6 ☑
  alcoholic (ethyl) (methyl) (wood) 303.9 ☑
    complicating pregnancy, childbirth, or puerperium 648.4 ☑
      affecting fetus or newborn 760.71
      suspected damage to fetus affecting management of pregnancy 655.4 ☑
  drug (*see also* Dependence) 304.9 ☑
  ethyl alcohol 303.9 ☑
  heroin 304.0 ☑
  hospital 301.51
  methyl alcohol 303.9 ☑
  methylated spirit 303.9 ☑
  morphine (-like substances) 304.0 ☑
  nicotine 305.1
  opium 304.0 ☑
  tobacco 305.1
  wine 303.9 ☑
Addison-Biermer anemia (pernicious) 281.0
Addison-Gull disease — *see* Xanthoma
Addison's
  anemia (pernicious) 281.0
  disease (bronze) (primary adrenal insufficiency) 255.41
    tuberculous (*see also* Tuberculosis) 017.6 ☑
  keloid (morphea) 701.0
  melanoderma (adrenal cortical hypofunction) 255.41
Addisonian crisis or melanosis (acute adrenocortical insufficiency) 255.41
Additional — *see also* Accessory
  chromosome(s) 758.5
    13-15 758.1
    16-18 758.2
    21 758.0
    autosome(s) NEC 758.5
    sex 758.81
Adduction contracture, hip or other joint — *see* Contraction, joint
ADEM (acute disseminated encephalomyelitis) (postinfectious) 136.9 *[323.61]*
  infectious 136.9 *[323.61]*
  noninfectious 323.81
Adenasthenia gastrica 536.0
Aden fever 061
Adenitis — *see also* Lymphadenitis 289.3
  acute, unspecified site 683
    epidemic infectious 075
  axillary 289.3
    acute 683
    chronic or subacute 289.1
  Bartholin's gland 616.89
  bulbourethral gland (*see also* Urethritis) 597.89
  cervical 289.3
    acute 683
    chronic or subacute 289.1
  chancroid (Ducrey's bacillus) 099.0
  chronic (any lymph node, except mesenteric) 289.1
    mesenteric 289.2
  Cowper's gland (*see also* Urethritis) 597.89
  epidemic, acute 075
  gangrenous 683
  gonorrheal NEC 098.89

Adenitis — *see also* Lymphadenitis — *continued*
  groin 289.3
    acute 683
    chronic or subacute 289.1
  infectious 075
  inguinal (region) 289.3
    acute 683
    chronic or subacute 289.1
  lymph gland or node, except mesenteric 289.3
    acute 683
    chronic or subacute 289.1
    mesenteric (acute) (chronic) (nonspecific) (subacute) 289.2
  mesenteric (acute) (chronic) (nonspecific) (subacute) 289.2
    due to Pasteurella multocida (P. septica) 027.2
  parotid gland (suppurative) 527.2
  phlegmonous 683
  salivary duct or gland (any) (recurring) (suppurative) 527.2
  scrofulous (*see also* Tuberculosis) 017.2 ☑
  septic 289.3
  Skene's duct or gland (*see also* Urethritis) 597.89
  strumous, tuberculous (*see also* Tuberculosis) 017.2 ☑
  subacute, unspecified site 289.1
  sublingual gland (suppurative) 527.2
  submandibular gland (suppurative) 527.2
  submaxillary gland (suppurative) 527.2
  suppurative 683
  tuberculous — *see* Tuberculosis, lymph gland
  urethral gland (*see also* Urethritis) 597.89
  venereal NEC 099.8
  Wharton's duct (suppurative) 527.2
Adenoacanthoma (M8570/3) — *see* Neoplasm, by site, malignant
Adenoameloblastoma (M9300/0) 213.1
  upper jaw (bone) 213.0
Adenocarcinoma (M8140/3) — *see also* Neoplasm, by site, malignant

> *Note* — The list of adjectival modifiers below is not exhaustive. A description of adenocarcinoma that does not appear in this list should be coded in the same manner as carcinoma with that description. Thus, "mixed acidophil-basophil adenocarcinoma," should be coded in the same manner as "mixed acidophil-basophil carcinoma," which appears in the list under "Carcinoma."
>
> Except where otherwise indicated, the morphological varieties of adenocarcinoma in the list below should be coded by site as for "Neoplasm, malignant."

  with
    apocrine metaplasia (M8573/3)
    cartilaginous (and osseous) metaplasia (M8571/3)
    osseous (and cartilaginous) metaplasia (M8571/3)
    spindle cell metaplasia (M8572/3)
    squamous metaplasia (M8570/3)
  acidophil (M8280/3)
    specified site — *see* Neoplasm, by site, malignant
    unspecified site 194.3
  acinar (M8550/3)
  acinic cell (M8550/3)
  adrenal cortical (M8370/3) 194.0
  alveolar (M8251/3)
    and
      epidermoid carcinoma, mixed (M8560/3)
      squamous cell carcinoma, mixed (M8560/3)
  apocrine (M8401/3)
    breast — *see* Neoplasm, breast, malignant
    specified site NEC — *see* Neoplasm, skin, malignant

Adenocarcinoma — *see also* Neoplasm, by site, malignant — *continued*
  apocrine — *continued*
    unspecified site 173.99
  basophil (M8300/3)
    specified site — *see* Neoplasm, by site, malignant
    unspecified site 194.3
  bile duct type (M8160/3)
    liver 155.1
    specified site NEC — *see* Neoplasm, by site, malignant
    unspecified site 155.1
  bronchiolar (M8250/3) — *see* Neoplasm, lung, malignant
  ceruminous (M8420/3) 173.29
  chromophobe (M8270/3)
    specified site — *see* Neoplasm, by site, malignant
    unspecified site 194.3
  clear cell (mesonephroid type) (M8310/3)
  colloid (M8480/3)
  cylindroid type (M8200/3)
  diffuse type (M8145/3)
    specified site — *see* Neoplasm, by site, malignant
    unspecified site 151.9
  duct (infiltrating) (M8500/3)
    with Paget's disease (M8541/3) — *see* Neoplasm, breast, malignant
    specified site — *see* Neoplasm, by site, malignant
    unspecified site 174.9
  embryonal (M9070/3)
  endometrioid (M8380/3) — *see* Neoplasm, by site, malignant
  eosinophil (M8280/3)
    specified site — *see* Neoplasm, by site, malignant
    unspecified site 194.3
  follicular (M8330/3)
    and papillary (M8340/3) 193
    moderately differentiated type (M8332/3) 193
    pure follicle type (M8331/3) 193
    specified site — *see* Neoplasm, by site, malignant
    trabecular type (M8332/3) 193
    unspecified type 193
    well differentiated type (M8331/3) 193
  gelatinous (M8480/3)
  granular cell (M8320/3)
  Hürthle cell (M8290/3) 193
  in
    adenomatous
      polyp (M8210/3)
      polyposis coli (M8220/3) 153.9
    polypoid adenoma (M8210/3)
    tubular adenoma (M8210/3)
    villous adenoma (M8261/3)
  infiltrating duct (M8500/3)
    with Paget's disease (M8541/3) — *see* Neoplasm, breast, malignant
    specified site — *see* Neoplasm, by site, malignant
    unspecified site 174.9
  inflammatory (M8530/3)
    specified site — *see* Neoplasm, by site, malignant
    unspecified site 174.9
  in situ (M8140/2) — *see* Neoplasm, by site, in situ
  intestinal type (M8144/3)
    specified site — *see* Neoplasm, by site, malignant
    unspecified site 151.9
  intraductal (noninfiltrating) (M8500/2)
    papillary (M8503/2)
      specified site — *see* Neoplasm, by site, in situ
      unspecified site 233.0
    specified site — *see* Neoplasm, by site, in situ
    unspecified site 233.0

Adenocarcinoma — *see also* Neoplasm, by site, malignant — *continued*
  islet cell (M8150/3)
    and exocrine, mixed (M8154/3)
      specified site — *see* Neoplasm, by site, malignant
      unspecified site 157.9
    pancreas 157.4
      specified site NEC — *see* Neoplasm, by site, malignant
      unspecified site 157.4
  lobular (M8520/3)
    specified site — *see* Neoplasm, by site, malignant
    unspecified site 174.9
  medullary (M8510/3)
  mesonephric (M9110/3)
  mixed cell (M8323/3)
  mucin-producing (M8481/3)
  mucinous (M8480/3)
  mucoid (M8480/3) (*see also* Neoplasm, by site, malignant)
    cell (M8300/3)
      specified site — *see* Neoplasm, by site, malignant
      unspecified site 194.3
  nonencapsulated sclerosing (M8350/3) 193
  oncocytic (M8290/3)
  oxyphilic (M8290/3)
  papillary (M8260/3)
    and follicular (M8340/3) 193
    intraductal (noninfiltrating) (M8503/2)
      specified site — *see* Neoplasm, by site, in situ
      unspecified site 233.0
    serous (M8460/3)
      specified site — *see* Neoplasm, by site, malignant
      unspecified site 183.0
  papillocystic (M8450/3)
    specified site — *see* Neoplasm, by site, malignant
    unspecified site 183.0
  pseudomucinous (M8470/3)
    specified site — *see* Neoplasm, by site, malignant
    unspecified site 183.0
  renal cell (M8312/3) 189.0
  sebaceous (M8410/3)
  serous (M8441/3) (*see also* Neoplasm, by site, malignant)
    papillary
      specified site — *see* Neoplasm, by site, malignant
      unspecified site 183.0
  signet ring cell (M8490/3)
  superficial spreading (M8143/3)
  sweat gland (M8400/3) — *see* Neoplasm, skin, malignant
  trabecular (M8190/3)
  tubular (M8211/3)
  villous (M8262/3)
  water-clear cell (M8322/3) 194.1
Adenofibroma (M9013/0)
  clear cell (M8313/0) — *see* Neoplasm, by site, benign
  endometrioid (M8381/0) 220
    borderline malignancy (M8381/1) 236.2
    malignant (M8381/3) 183.0
  mucinous (M9015/0)
    specified site — *see* Neoplasm, by site, benign
    unspecified site 220
  prostate
    with
      other lower urinary tract symptoms (LUTS) 600.21
      urinary
        obstruction 600.21
        retention 600.21
  serous (M9014/0)
    specified site — *see* Neoplasm, by site, benign
    unspecified site 220
  specified site — *see* Neoplasm, by site, benign

☑ **Additional Digit Required** — Refer to the Tabular List for Digit Selection   ▽ **Subterms under main terms may continue to next column or page**

2014 ICD-9-CM   ▶◀ **Revised Text**   ● **New Line**   ▲ **Revised Code**   **Volume 2 — 9**

Adenofibroma — *continued*
  unspecified site 220
Adenofibrosis
  breast 610.2
  endometrioid 617.0
Adenoiditis 474.01
  acute 463
  chronic 474.01
    with chronic tonsillitis 474.02
Adenoids (congenital) (of nasal fossa) 474.9
  hypertrophy 474.12
  vegetations 474.2
Adenolipomatosis (symmetrical) 272.8
Adenolymphoma (M8561/0)
  specified site — *see* Neoplasm, by site, benign
  unspecified 210.2
Adenomatosis (M8220/0)
  endocrine (multiple) (M8360/1)
    single specified site — *see* Neoplasm, by site, uncertain behavior
    two or more specified sites 237.4
    unspecified site 237.4
  erosive of nipple (M8506/0) 217
  pluriendocrine — *see* Adenomatosis, endocrine
  pulmonary (M8250/1) 235.7
    malignant (M8250/3) — *see* Neoplasm, lung, malignant
  specified site — *see* Neoplasm, by site, benign
  unspecified site 211.3
Adenomatous
  cyst, thyroid (gland) — *see* Goiter, nodular
  goiter (nontoxic) (*see also* Goiter, nodular) 241.9
    toxic or with hyperthyroidism 242.3 ☑
Adenoma (sessile) (M8140/0) — *see also* Neoplasm, by site, benign

Note — Except where otherwise indicated, the morphological varieties of adenoma in the list below should be coded by site as for "Neoplasm, benign."

  acidophil (M8280/0)
    specified site — *see* Neoplasm, by site, benign
    unspecified site 227.3
  acinar (cell) (M8550/0)
  acinic cell (M8550/0)
  adrenal (cortex) (cortical) (functioning) (M8370/0) 227.0
    clear cell type (M8373/0) 227.0
    compact cell type (M8371/0) 227.0
    glomerulosa cell type (M8374/0) 227.0
    heavily pigmented variant (M8372/0) 227.0
    mixed cell type (M8375/0) 227.0
  alpha cell (M8152/0)
    pancreas 211.7
    specified site NEC — *see* Neoplasm, by site, benign
    unspecified site 211.7
  alveolar (M8251/0)
  apocrine (M8401/0)
    breast 217
    specified site NEC — *see* Neoplasm, skin, benign
    unspecified site 216.9
  basal cell (M8147/0)
  basophil (M8300/0)
    specified site — *see* Neoplasm, by site, benign
    unspecified site 227.3
  beta cell (M8151/0)
    pancreas 211.7
    specified site NEC — *see* Neoplasm, by site, benign
    unspecified site 211.7
  bile duct (M8160/0) 211.5
  black (M8372/0) 227.0
  bronchial (M8140/1) 235.7
    carcinoid type (M8240/3) — *see* Neoplasm, lung, malignant
    cylindroid type (M8200/3) — *see* Neoplasm, lung, malignant
  ceruminous (M8420/0) 216.2

Adenoma — *see also* Neoplasm, by site, benign — *continued*
  chief cell (M8321/0) 227.1
  chromophobe (M8270/0)
    specified site — *see* Neoplasm, by site, benign
    unspecified site 227.3
  clear cell (M8310/0)
  colloid (M8334/0)
    specified site — *see* Neoplasm, by site, benign
    unspecified site 226
  cylindroid type, bronchus (M8200/3) — *see* Neoplasm, lung, malignant
  duct (M8503/0)
  embryonal (M8191/0)
  endocrine, multiple (M8360/1)
    single specified site — *see* Neoplasm, by site, uncertain behavior
    two or more specified sites 237.4
    unspecified site 237.4
  endometrioid (M8380/0) (*see also* Neoplasm, by site, benign)
    borderline malignancy (M8380/1) — *see* Neoplasm, by site, uncertain behavior
  eosinophil (M8280/0)
    specified site — *see* Neoplasm, by site, benign
    unspecified site 227.3
  fetal (M8333/0)
    specified site — *see* Neoplasm, by site, benign
    unspecified site 226
  follicular (M8330/0)
    specified site — *see* Neoplasm, by site, benign
    unspecified site 226
  hepatocellular (M8170/0) 211.5
  Hürthle cell (M8290/0) 226
  intracystic papillary (M8504/0)
  islet cell (functioning) (M8150/0)
    pancreas 211.7
    specified site NEC — *see* Neoplasm, by site, benign
    unspecified site 211.7
  liver cell (M8170/0) 211.5
  macrofollicular (M8334/0)
    specified site NEC — *see* Neoplasm, by site, benign
    unspecified site 226
  malignant, malignum (M8140/3) — *see* Neoplasm, by site, malignant
  mesonephric (M9110/0)
  microfollicular (M8333/0)
    specified site — *see* Neoplasm, by site, benign
    unspecified site 226
  mixed cell (M8323/0)
  monomorphic (M8146/0)
  mucinous (M8480/0)
  mucoid cell (M8300/0)
    specified site — *see* Neoplasm, by site, benign
    unspecified site 227.3
  multiple endocrine (M8360/1)
    single specified site — *see* Neoplasm, by site, uncertain behavior
    two or more specified sites 237.4
    unspecified site 237.4
  nipple (M8506/0) 217
  oncocytic (M8290/0)
  oxyphilic (M8290/0)
  papillary (M8260/0) (*see also* Neoplasm, by site, benign)
    intracystic (M8504/0)
  papillotubular (M8263/0)
  Pick's tubular (M8640/0)
    specified site — *see* Neoplasm, by site, benign
    unspecified site
      female 220
      male 222.0
  pleomorphic (M8940/0)
  polypoid (M8210/0)
  prostate (benign) 600.20

Adenoma — *see also* Neoplasm, by site, benign — *continued*
  prostate — *continued*
    with
      other lower urinary tract symptoms (LUTS) 600.21
      urinary
        obstruction 600.21
        retention 600.21
  rete cell 222.0
  sebaceous, sebaceum (gland) (senile) (M8410/0) (*see also* Neoplasm, skin, benign)
    disseminata 759.5
  Sertoli cell (M8640/0)
    specified site — *see* Neoplasm, by site, benign
    unspecified site
      female 220
      male 222.0
  skin appendage (M8390/0) — *see* Neoplasm, skin, benign
  sudoriferous gland (M8400/0) — *see* Neoplasm, skin, benign
  sweat gland or duct (M8400/0) — *see* Neoplasm, skin, benign
  testicular (M8640/0)
    specified site — *see* Neoplasm, by site, benign
    unspecified site
      female 220
      male 222.0
  thyroid 226
  trabecular (M8190/0)
  tubular (M8211/0) (*see also* Neoplasm, by site, benign)
    papillary (M8460/3)
    Pick's (M8640/0)
      specified site — *see* Neoplasm, by site, benign
      unspecified site
        female 220
        male 222.0
  tubulovillous (M8263/0)
  villoglandular (M8263/0)
  villous (M8261/1) — *see* Neoplasm, by site, uncertain behavior
  water-clear cell (M8322/0) 227.1
  wolffian duct (M9110/0)
Adenomyoma (M8932/0) — *see also* Neoplasm, by site, benign
  prostate 600.20
    with
      other lower urinary tract symptoms (LUTS) 600.21
      urinary
        obstruction 600.21
        retention 600.21
Adenomyometritis 617.0
Adenomyosis (uterus) (internal) 617.0
Adenopathy (lymph gland) 785.6
  inguinal 785.6
  mediastinal 785.6
  mesentery 785.6
  syphilitic (secondary) 091.4
  tracheobronchial 785.6
    tuberculous (*see also* Tuberculosis) 012.1 ☑
      primary, progressive 010.8 ☑
  tuberculous (*see also* Tuberculosis, lymph gland) 017.2 ☑
    tracheobronchial 012.1 ☑
      primary, progressive 010.8 ☑
Adenopharyngitis 462
Adenophlegmon 683
Adenosalpingitis 614.1
Adenosarcoma (M8960/3) 189.0
Adenosclerosis 289.3
Adenosis
  breast (sclerosing) 610.2
  vagina, congenital 752.49
Adentia (complete) (partial) — *see also* Absence, teeth 520.0
Adherent
  labium (minus) 624.4
  pericardium (nonrheumatic) 423.1

Adherent — *continued*
  pericardium — *continued*
    rheumatic 393
  placenta 667.0 ☑
    with hemorrhage 666.0 ☑
  prepuce 605
  scar (skin) NEC 709.2
  tendon in scar 709.2
Adhesion(s), adhesive (postinfectional) (postoperative)
  abdominal (wall) (*see also* Adhesions, peritoneum) 568.0
  amnion to fetus 658.8 ☑
    affecting fetus or newborn 762.8
  appendix 543.9
  arachnoiditis — *see* Meningitis
  auditory tube (Eustachian) 381.89
  bands (*see also* Adhesions, peritoneum)
    cervix 622.3
    uterus 621.5
  bile duct (any) 576.8
  bladder (sphincter) 596.89
  bowel (*see also* Adhesions, peritoneum) 568.0
  cardiac 423.1
    rheumatic 398.99
  cecum (*see also* Adhesions, peritoneum) 568.0
  cervicovaginal 622.3
    congenital 752.49
    postpartal 674.8 ☑
      old 622.3
  cervix 622.3
  clitoris 624.4
  colon (*see also* Adhesions, peritoneum) 568.0
  common duct 576.8
  congenital (*see also* Anomaly, specified type NEC)
    fingers (*see also* Syndactylism, fingers) 755.11
    labium (majus) (minus) 752.49
    omental, anomalous 751.4
    ovary 752.0
    peritoneal 751.4
    toes (*see also* Syndactylism, toes) 755.13
    tongue (to gum or roof of mouth) 750.12
  conjunctiva (acquired) (localized) 372.62
    congenital 743.63
    extensive 372.63
  cornea — *see* Opacity, cornea
  cystic duct 575.8
  diaphragm (*see also* Adhesions, peritoneum) 568.0
  due to foreign body — *see* Foreign body
  duodenum (*see also* Adhesions, peritoneum) 568.0
    with obstruction 537.3
  ear, middle — *see* Adhesions, middle ear
  epididymis 608.89
  epidural — *see* Adhesions, meninges
  epiglottis 478.79
  Eustachian tube 381.89
  eyelid 374.46
    postoperative 997.99
      surgically created V45.69
  gallbladder (*see also* Disease, gallbladder) 575.8
  globe 360.89
  heart 423.1
    rheumatic 398.99
  ileocecal (coil) (*see also* Adhesions, peritoneum) 568.0
  ileum (*see also* Adhesions, peritoneum) 568.0
  intestine (postoperative) (*see also* Adhesions, peritoneum) 568.0
    with obstruction 560.81
      with hernia (*see also* Hernia, by site, with obstruction)
        gangrenous — *see* Hernia, by site, with gangrene
  intra-abdominal (*see also* Adhesions, peritoneum) 568.0
  iris 364.70
    to corneal graft 996.79

☑ **Additional Digit Required** — Refer to the Tabular List for Digit Selection   ▽ **Subterms under main terms may continue to next column or page**

10 — Volume 2   ▶◀ Revised Text   ● New Line   ▲ Revised Code   2014 ICD-9-CM

Adhesion(s), adhesive — *continued*
  joint (*see also* Ankylosis) 718.5 ☑
  kidney 593.89
  labium (majus) (minus), congenital 752.49
  liver 572.8
  lung 511.0
  mediastinum 519.3
  meninges 349.2
    cerebral (any) 349.2
      congenital 742.4
    congenital 742.8
    spinal (any) 349.2
      congenital 742.59
    tuberculous (cerebral) (spinal) (*see also*
      Tuberculosis, meninges) 013.0 ☑
  mesenteric (*see also* Adhesions, peritoneum)
    568.0
  middle ear (fibrous) 385.10
    drum head 385.19
      to
        incus 385.11
        promontorium 385.13
        stapes 385.12
    specified NEC 385.19
  nasal (septum) (to turbinates) 478.19
  nerve NEC 355.9
    spinal 355.9
      root 724.9
        cervical NEC 723.4
        lumbar NEC 724.4
        lumbosacral 724.4
        thoracic 724.4
  ocular muscle 378.60
  omentum (*see also* Adhesions, peritoneum)
    568.0
  organ or site, congenital NEC — *see*
    Anomaly, specified type NEC
  ovary 614.6
    congenital (to cecum, kidney, or omen-
      tum) 752.0
  parauterine 614.6
  parovarian 614.6
  pelvic (peritoneal)
    female (postoperative) (postinfection)
      614.6
    male (postoperative) (postinfection) (*see*
      also Adhesions, peritoneum)
      568.0
    postpartal (old) 614.6
    tuberculous (*see also* Tuberculosis)
      016.9 ☑
  penis to scrotum (congenital) 752.69
  periappendiceal (*see also* Adhesions, peri-
    toneum) 568.0
  pericardium (nonrheumatic) 423.1
    rheumatic 393
    tuberculous (*see also* Tuberculosis)
      017.9 ☑ [420.0]
  pericholecystic 575.8
  perigastric (*see also* Adhesions, peritoneum)
    568.0
  periovarian 614.6
  periprostatic 602.8
  perirectal (*see also* Adhesions, peritoneum)
    568.0
  perirenal 593.89
  peritoneum, peritoneal (fibrous) (postoper-
    ative) 568.0
    with obstruction (intestinal) 560.81
      with hernia (*see also* Hernia, by site,
        with obstruction)
        gangrenous — *see* Hernia, by site,
          with gangrene
      duodenum 537.3
    congenital 751.4
    female (postoperative) (postinfective)
      614.6
    pelvic, female 614.6
    pelvic, male 568.0
    postpartal, pelvic 614.6
    to uterus 614.6
  peritubal 614.6
  periureteral 593.89
  periuterine 621.5
  perivesical 596.89
  perivesicular (seminal vesicle) 608.89

Adhesion(s), adhesive — *continued*
  pleura, pleuritic 511.0
    tuberculous (*see also* Tuberculosis,
      pleura) 012.0 ☑
  pleuropericardial 511.0
  postoperative (gastrointestinal tract) (*see
    also* Adhesions, peritoneum) 568.0
    eyelid 997.99
      surgically created V45.69
    pelvic female 614.9
    pelvic male 568.0
    urethra 598.2
  postpartal, old 624.4
  preputial, prepuce 605
  pulmonary 511.0
  pylorus (*see also* Adhesions, peritoneum)
    568.0
  Rosenmüller's fossa 478.29
  sciatic nerve 355.0
  seminal vesicle 608.89
  shoulder (joint) 726.0
  sigmoid flexure (*see also* Adhesions, peri-
    toneum) 568.0
  spermatic cord (acquired) 608.89
    congenital 752.89
  spinal canal 349.2
    nerve 355.9
      root 724.9
        cervical NEC 723.4
        lumbar NEC 724.4
        lumbosacral 724.4
        thoracic 724.4
  stomach (*see also* Adhesions, peritoneum)
    568.0
  subscapular 726.2
  tendonitis 726.90
    shoulder 726.0
  testicle 608.89
  tongue (congenital) (to gum or roof of
    mouth) 750.12
    acquired 529.8
  trachea 519.19
  tubo-ovarian 614.6
  tunica vaginalis 608.89
  ureter 593.89
  uterus 621.5
    to abdominal wall 614.6
      in pregnancy or childbirth 654.4 ☑
        affecting fetus or newborn 763.89
  vagina (chronic) (postoperative) (postradia-
    tion) 623.2
  vaginitis (congenital) 752.49
  vesical 596.89
  vitreomacular adhesion 379.27
  vitreous 379.29
Adie (-Holmes) syndrome (tonic pupillary reaction) 379.46
Adiponecrosis neonatorum 778.1
Adiposa dolorosa 272.8
Adiposalgia 272.8
Adiposis
  cerebralis 253.8
  dolorosa 272.8
  tuberosa simplex 272.8
Adiposity 278.02
  heart (*see also* Degeneration, myocardial)
    429.1
  localized 278.1
Adiposogenital dystrophy 253.8
Adjustment
  prosthesis or other device — *see* Fitting of
  reaction — *see* Reaction, adjustment
Administration, prophylactic
  antibiotics, long-term V58.62
    short-term use — *omit code*
  antitoxin, any V07.2
  antivenin V07.2
  chemotherapeutic agent NEC V07.39
  chemotherapy NEC V07.39
  diphtheria antitoxin V07.2
  fluoride V07.31
  gamma globulin V07.2
  immune sera (gamma globulin) V07.2
  passive immunization agent V07.2
  RhoGAM V07.2

Admission (encounter)
  as organ donor — *see* Donor
  by mistake V68.9
  for
    adequacy testing (for)
      hemodialysis V56.31
      peritoneal dialysis V56.32
    adjustment (of)
      artificial
        arm (complete) (partial) V52.0
        eye V52.2
        leg (complete) (partial) V52.1
      brain neuropacemaker V53.02
      breast
        implant V52.4
          exchange (different material)
            (different size) V52.4
        prosthesis V52.4
      cardiac device V53.39
        defibrillator, automatic im-
          plantable (with syn-
          chronous cardiac pacemak-
          er) V53.32
        pacemaker V53.31
          carotid sinus V53.39
      catheter
        non-vascular V58.82
        vascular V58.81
      cerebral ventricle (communicating)
        shunt V53.01
      colostomy belt V55.3
      contact lenses V53.1
      cystostomy device V53.6
      dental prosthesis V52.3
      device, unspecified type V53.90
        abdominal V53.59
        cardiac V53.39
          defibrillator, automatic im-
            plantable (with syn-
            chronous cardiac pace-
            maker V53.32
          pacemaker V53.31
        carotid sinus V53.39
        cerebral ventricle (communicat-
          ing) shunt V53.01
        gastrointestinal NEC V53.59
        insulin pump V53.91
        intestinal V53.50
        nervous system V53.09
        orthodontic V53.4
        other device V53.99
        prosthetic V52.9
          breast V52.4
          dental V52.3
          eye V52.2
          specified type NEC V52.8
        special senses V53.09
        substitution
          auditory V53.09
          nervous system V53.09
          visual V53.09
        urinary V53.6
      dialysis catheter
        extracorporeal V56.1
        peritoneal V56.2
      diaphragm (contraceptive) V25.02
      gastric lap band V53.51
      gastrointestinal appliance and device
        NEC V53.59
      growth rod V54.02
      hearing aid V53.2
      ileostomy device V55.2
      intestinal appliance and device
        V53.50
      neuropacemaker (brain) (peripheral
        nerve) (spinal cord) V53.02
      orthodontic device V53.4
      orthopedic (device) V53.7
        brace V53.7
        cast V53.7
        shoes V53.7
      pacemaker
        brain V53.02
        cardiac V53.31
        carotid sinus V53.39
        peripheral nerve V53.02

Admission — *continued*
  for — *continued*
    adjustment — *continued*
      pacemaker — *continued*
        spinal cord V53.02
      prosthesis V52.9
        arm (complete) (partial) V52.0
        breast V52.4
        dental V52.3
        eye V52.2
        leg (complete) (partial) V52.1
        specified type NEC V52.8
      spectacles V53.1
      wheelchair V53.8
    adoption referral or proceedings V68.89
    aftercare (*see also* Aftercare) V58.9
      cardiac pacemaker V53.31
      chemotherapy (oral) (intravenous)
        V58.11
      dialysis
        extracorporeal (renal) V56.0
        peritoneal V56.8
        renal V56.0
      fracture (*see also* Aftercare, fracture)
        V54.9
      medical NEC V58.89
      organ transplant V58.44
      orthopedic V54.9
        following explanation of joint
          prosthesis (for joint pros-
          thesis insertion) (staged
          procedure) V54.82
        specified care NEC V54.89
      pacemaker device
        brain V53.02
        cardiac V53.31
        carotid sinus V53.39
        nervous system V53.02
        spinal cord V53.02
      postoperative NEC V58.49
        wound closure, planned V58.41
      postpartum
        immediately after delivery V24.0
        routine follow-up V24.2
      postradiation V58.0
      radiation therapy V58.0
      removal of
        non-vascular catheter V58.82
        vascular catheter V58.81
      specified NEC V58.89
      surgical NEC V58.49
        wound closure, planned V58.41
    antineoplastic
      chemotherapy (oral) (intravenous)
        V58.11
      immunotherapy V58.12
    artificial insemination V26.1
    assisted reproductive fertility procedure
      cycle V26.81
    attention to artificial opening (of) V55.9
      artificial vagina V55.7
      colostomy V55.3
      cystostomy V55.5
      enterostomy V55.4
      gastrostomy V55.1
      ileostomy V55.2
      jejunostomy V55.4
      nephrostomy V55.6
      specified site NEC V55.8
        intestinal tract V55.4
        urinary tract V55.6
      tracheostomy V55.0
      ureterostomy V55.6
      urethrostomy V55.6
    battery replacement
      cardiac pacemaker V53.31
    blood typing V72.86
      Rh typing V72.86
    boarding V65.0
    breast
      augmentation or reduction V50.1
      implant exchange (different material)
        (different size) V52.4
      reconstruction following mastectomy
        V51.0

☑ **Additional Digit Required** — Refer to the Tabular List for Digit Selection   ▽ **Subterms under main terms may continue to next column or page**

Admission — *continued*
for — *continued*
breast — *continued*
removal
prophylactic V50.41
tissue expander without synchronous insertion of permanent implant V52.4
change of
cardiac pacemaker (battery) V53.31
carotid sinus pacemaker V53.39
catheter in artificial opening — *see* Attention to, artificial, opening
drains V58.49
dressing
wound V58.30
nonsurgical V58.30
surgical V58.31
fixation device
external V54.89
internal V54.01
Kirschner wire V54.89
neuropacemaker device (brain) (peripheral nerve) (spinal cord) V53.02
nonsurgical wound dressing V58.30
pacemaker device
brain V53.02
cardiac V53.31
carotid sinus V53.39
nervous system V53.02
plaster cast V54.89
splint, external V54.89
Steinmann pin V54.89
surgical wound dressing V58.31
traction device V54.89
wound packing V58.30
nonsurgical V58.30
surgical V58.31
checkup only V70.0
chemotherapy, (oral) (intravenous) antineoplastic V58.11
circumcision, ritual or routine (in absence of medical indication) V50.2
clinical research investigation (control) (normal comparison) (participant) V70.7
closure of artificial opening — *see* Attention to, artificial, opening
contraceptive
counseling V25.09
emergency V25.03
postcoital V25.03
management V25.9
specified type NEC V25.8
convalescence following V66.9
chemotherapy V66.2
psychotherapy V66.3
radiotherapy V66.1
surgery V66.0
treatment (for) V66.5
combined V66.6
fracture V66.4
mental disorder NEC V66.3
specified condition NEC V66.5
cosmetic surgery NEC V50.1
breast reconstruction following mastectomy V51.0
following healed injury or operation V51.8
counseling (*see also* Counseling) V65.40
without complaint or sickness V65.49
contraceptive management V25.09
emergency V25.03
postcoital V25.03
dietary V65.3
exercise V65.41
fertility preservation (prior to cancer therapy) (prior to surgical removal of gonads) V26.42
for
nonattending third party V65.19

Admission — *continued*
for — *continued*
counseling (*see also* Counseling) — *continued*
for — *continued*
pediatric
pre-adoption visit for adoptive parent(s) V65.11
pre-birth visit for expectant parent(s) V65.11
victim of abuse
child V61.21
partner or spouse V61.11
genetic V26.33
gonorrhea V65.45
HIV V65.44
human immunodeficiency virus V65.44
injury prevention V65.43
insulin pump training V65.46
natural family planning
procreative V26.41
to avoid pregnancy V25.04
procreative management V26.49
using natural family planning V26.41
sexually transmitted disease NEC V65.45
HIV V65.44
specified reason NEC V65.49
substance use and abuse V65.42
syphilis V65.45
victim of abuse
child V61.21
partner or spouse V61.11
desensitization to allergens V07.1
dialysis V56.0
catheter
fitting and adjustment
extracorporeal V56.1
peritoneal V56.2
removal or replacement
extracorporeal V56.1
peritoneal V56.2
extracorporeal (renal) V56.0
peritoneal V56.8
renal V56.0
dietary surveillance and counseling V65.3
drug monitoring, therapeutic V58.83
ear piercing V50.3
elective surgery V50.9
breast
augmentation or reduction V50.1
reconstruction following mastectomy V51.0
removal, prophylactic V50.41
circumcision, ritual or routine (in absence of medical indication) V50.2
cosmetic NEC V50.1
breast reconstruction following mastectomy V51.0
following healed injury or operation V51.8
ear piercing V50.3
face-lift V50.1
hair transplant V50.0
plastic
breast reconstruction following mastectomy V51.0
cosmetic NEC V50.1
following healed injury or operation V51.8
prophylactic organ removal V50.49
breast V50.41
ovary V50.42
repair of scarred tissue (following healed injury or operation) V51.8
specified type NEC V50.8
end-of-life care V66.7
examination (*see also* Examination) V70.9
administrative purpose NEC V70.3
adoption V70.3

Admission — *continued*
for — *continued*
examination (*see also* Examination) — *continued*
allergy V72.7
antibody response V72.61
at health care facility V70.0
athletic team V70.3
camp V70.3
cardiovascular, preoperative V72.81
clinical research investigation (control) (participant) V70.7
dental V72.2
developmental testing (child) (infant) V20.2
donor (potential) V70.8
driver's license V70.3
ear V72.19
employment V70.5
eye V72.0
fertility preservation (prior to cancer therapy) (prior to surgical removal of gonads) V26.82
follow-up (routine) — *see* Examination, follow-up
for admission to
old age home V70.3
school V70.3
general V70.9
specified reason NEC V70.8
gynecological V72.31
health supervision
child (over 28 days old) V20.2
infant (over 28 days old) V20.2
newborn
8 to 28 days old V20.32
under 8 days old V20.31
hearing V72.19
following failed hearing screening V72.11
immigration V70.3
infant
8 to 28 days old V20.32
over 28 days old, routine V20.2
under 8 days old V20.31
insurance certification V70.3
laboratory V72.60
ordered as part of a routine general medical examination V72.62
pre-operative V72.63
pre-procedural V72.63
specified NEC V72.69
marriage license V70.3
medical (general) (*see also* Examination, medical) V70.9
medicolegal reasons V70.4
naturalization V70.3
pelvic (annual) (periodic) V72.31
postpartum checkup V24.2
pregnancy (possible) (unconfirmed) V72.40
negative result V72.41
positive result V72.42
preoperative V72.84
cardiovascular V72.81
respiratory V72.82
specified NEC V72.83
preprocedural V72.84
cardiovascular V72.81
general physical V72.83
respiratory V72.82
specified NEC V72.83
prior to chemotherapy V72.83
prison V70.3
psychiatric (general) V70.2
requested by authority V70.1
radiological NEC V72.5
respiratory, preoperative V72.82
school V70.3
screening — *see* Screening
skin hypersensitivity V72.7
specified type NEC V72.85
sport competition V70.3
vision V72.0
well baby and child care V20.2

Admission — *continued*
for — *continued*
exercise therapy V57.1
face-lift, cosmetic reason V50.1
fertility preservation (prior to cancer therapy) (prior to surgical removal of gonads) V26.82
fitting (of)
artificial
arm (complete) (partial) V52.0
eye V52.2
leg (complete) (partial) V52.1
biliary drainage tube V58.82
brain neuropacemaker V53.02
breast V52.4
implant V52.4
prosthesis V52.4
cardiac pacemaker V53.31
catheter
non-vascular V58.82
vascular V58.81
cerebral ventricle (communicating) shunt V53.01
chest tube V58.82
colostomy belt V55.2
contact lenses V53.1
cystostomy device V53.6
dental prosthesis V52.3
device, unspecified type V53.90
abdominal V53.59
cerebral ventricle (communicating) shunt V53.01
gastrointestinal NEC V53.59
insulin pump V53.91
intestinal V53.50
intrauterine contraceptive
insertion V25.11
removal V25.12
and reinsertion V25.13
replacement V25.13
nervous system V53.09
orthodontic V53.4
other device V53.99
prosthetic V52.9
breast V52.4
dental V52.3
eye V52.2
special senses V53.09
substitution
auditory V53.09
nervous system V53.09
visual V53.09
diaphragm (contraceptive) V25.02
fistula (sinus tract) drainage tube V58.82
gastric lap band V53.51
gastrointestinal appliance and device NEC V53.59
growth rod V54.02
hearing aid V53.2
ileostomy device V55.2
intestinal appliance and device V53.50
intrauterine contraceptive device
insertion V25.11
removal V25.12
and reinsertion V25.13
replacement V25.13
neuropacemaker (brain) (peripheral nerve) (spinal cord) V53.02
orthodontic device V53.4
orthopedic (device) V53.7
brace V53.7
cast V53.7
shoes V53.7
pacemaker
brain V53.02
cardiac V53.31
carotid sinus V53.39
spinal cord V53.02
pleural drainage tube V58.82
portacath V58.81
prosthesis V52.9
arm (complete) (partial) V52.0
breast V52.4
dental V52.3

☑ **Additional Digit Required — Refer to the Tabular List for Digit Selection** ▽ **Subterms under main terms may continue to next column or page**

12 — Volume 2 ▶◀ **Revised Text** ● **New Line** ▲ **Revised Code** **2014 ICD-9-CM**

Admission — continued
  for — continued
    fitting — continued
      prosthesis — continued
        eye V52.2
        leg (complete) (partial) V52.1
        specified type NEC V52.8
      spectacles V53.1
      wheelchair V53.8
    follow-up examination (routine) (following) V67.9
      cancer chemotherapy V67.2
      chemotherapy V67.2
      high-risk medication NEC V67.51
      injury NEC V67.59
      psychiatric V67.3
      psychotherapy V67.3
      radiotherapy V67.1
      specified surgery NEC V67.09
      surgery V67.00
        vaginal pap smear V67.01
      treatment (for) V67.9
        combined V67.6
        fracture V67.4
        involving high-risk medication NEC V67.51
        mental disorder V67.3
        specified NEC V67.59
    hair transplant, for cosmetic reason V50.0
    health advice, education, or instruction V65.4 ☑
    hearing conservation and treatment V72.12
    hormone replacement therapy (postmenopausal) V07.4
    hospice care V66.7
    immunizations (childhood) appropriate for age V20.2
    immunotherapy, antineoplastic V58.12
    insertion (of)
      intrauterine contraceptive device V25.11
      subdermal implantable contraceptive V25.5
    insulin pump titration V53.91
    insulin pump training V65.46
    intrauterine device
      insertion V25.11
      management V25.42
      removal V25.12
        and reinsertion V25.13
      replacement V25.13
    investigation to determine further disposition V63.8
    in vitro fertilization cycle V26.81
    isolation V07.0
    issue of
      disability examination certificate V68.01
      medical certificate NEC V68.09
      repeat prescription NEC V68.1
        contraceptive device NEC V25.49
    kidney dialysis V56.0
    lengthening of growth rod V54.02
    mental health evaluation V70.2
      requested by authority V70.1
    natural family planning counseling and advice
      procreative V26.41
      to avoid pregnancy V25.04
    nonmedical reason NEC V68.89
    nursing care evaluation V63.8
    observation (without need for further medical care) (see also Observation) V71.9
      accident V71.4
      alleged rape or seduction V71.5
      criminal assault V71.6
      following accident V71.4
        at work V71.3
      foreign body ingestion V71.89
      growth and development variations, childhood V21.0
      inflicted injury NEC V71.6

Admission — continued
  for — continued
    observation (see also Observation) — continued
      ingestion of deleterious agent or foreign body V71.89
      injury V71.6
      malignant neoplasm V71.1
      mental disorder V71.09
      newborn — see Observation, suspected, condition, newborn
      rape V71.5
      specified NEC V71.89
      suspected
        abuse V71.81
        accident V71.4
          at work V71.3
        benign neoplasm V71.89
        cardiovascular V71.7
        disorder V71.9
        exposure
          anthrax V71.82
          biological agent NEC V71.83
          SARS V71.83
        heart V71.7
        inflicted injury NEC V71.6
        malignant neoplasm V71.1
        maternal and fetal problem not found
          amniotic cavity and membrane V89.01
          cervical shortening V89.05
          fetal anomaly V89.03
          fetal growth V89.04
          oligohydramnios V89.01
          other specified NEC V89.09
          placenta V89.02
          polyhydramnios V89.01
        mental NEC V71.09
        neglect V71.81
        specified condition NEC V71.89
        tuberculosis V71.2
      tuberculosis V71.2
    occupational therapy V57.21
    organ transplant, donor — see Donor
    ovary, ovarian removal, prophylactic V50.42
    palliative care V66.7
    Papanicolaou smear
      cervix V76.2
        for suspected malignant neoplasm V76.2
        no disease found V71.1
        routine, as part of gynecological examination V72.31
        to confirm findings of recent normal smear following initial abnormal smear V72.32
      vaginal V76.47
        following hysterectomy for malignant condition V67.01
    passage of sounds or bougie in artificial opening — see Attention to, artificial, opening
    paternity testing V70.4
    peritoneal dialysis V56.32
    physical therapy NEC V57.1
    plastic surgery
      breast reconstruction following mastectomy V51.0
      cosmetic NEC V50.1
      following healed injury or operation V51.8
    postmenopausal hormone replacement therapy V07.4
    postpartum observation
      immediately after delivery V24.0
      routine follow-up V24.2
    poststerilization (for restoration) V26.0
    procreative management V26.9
      assisted reproductive fertility procedure cycle V26.81
      in vitro fertilization cycle V26.81
      specified type NEC V26.89

Admission — continued
  for — continued
    prophylactic
      administration of
        antibiotics, long-term V58.62
          short-term use — omit code
        antitoxin, any V07.2
        antivenin V07.2
        chemotherapeutic agent NEC V07.39
        chemotherapy NEC V07.39
        diphtheria antitoxin V07.2
        fluoride V07.31
        gamma globulin V07.2
        immune sera (gamma globulin) V07.2
        RhoGAM V07.2
        tetanus antitoxin V07.2
      breathing exercises V57.0
      chemotherapy NEC V07.39
        fluoride V07.31
      measure V07.9
        specified type NEC V07.8
      organ removal V50.49
        breast V50.41
        ovary V50.42
    psychiatric examination (general) V70.2
      requested by authority V70.1
    radiation management V58.0
    radiotherapy V58.0
    reconstruction following mastectomy V51.0
    reforming of artificial opening — see Attention to, artificial, opening
    rehabilitation V57.9
      multiple types V57.89
      occupational V57.21
      orthoptic V57.4
      orthotic V57.81
      physical NEC V57.1
      specified type NEC V57.89
      speech (-language) V57.3
      vocational V57.22
    removal of
      breast tissue expander without synchronous insertion of permanent implant V52.4
      cardiac pacemaker V53.31
      cast (plaster) V54.89
      catheter from artificial opening — see Attention to, artificial, opening
      cerebral ventricle (communicating) shunt V53.01
      cystostomy catheter V55.5
      device
        cerebral ventricle (communicating) shunt V53.01
        fixation
          external V54.89
          internal V54.01
        intrauterine contraceptive V25.12
        traction, external V54.89
      drains V58.49
      dressing
        wound V58.30
          nonsurgical V58.30
          surgical V58.31
      fixation device
        external V54.89
        internal V54.01
      intrauterine contraceptive device V25.12
      Kirschner wire V54.89
      neuropacemaker (brain) (peripheral nerve) (spinal cord) V53.02
      nonsurgical wound dressing V58.30
      orthopedic fixation device
        external V54.89
        internal V54.01
      pacemaker device
        brain V53.02
        cardiac V53.31
        carotid sinus V53.39
        nervous system V53.02
      plaster cast V54.89

Admission — continued
  for — continued
    removal of — continued
      plate (fracture) V54.01
      rod V54.01
      screw (fracture) V54.01
      splint, traction V54.89
      staples V58.32
      Steinmann pin V54.89
      subdermal implantable contraceptive V25.43
      surgical wound dressing V58.31
      sutures V58.32
      traction device, external V54.89
      ureteral stent V53.6
      wound packing V58.30
        nonsurgical V58.30
        surgical V58.31
    repair of scarred tissue (following healed injury or operation) V51.8
    replacement of intrauterine contraceptive device V25.13
    reprogramming of cardiac pacemaker V53.31
    respirator [ventilator] dependence during
      mechanical failure V46.14
      power failure V46.12
      for weaning V46.13
    restoration of organ continuity (poststerilization) (tuboplasty) (vasoplasty) V26.0
    Rh typing V72.86
    routine infant and child vision and hearing testing V20.2
    sensitivity test (see also Test, skin)
      allergy NEC V72.7
      bacterial disease NEC V74.9
      Dick V74.8
      Kveim V82.89
      Mantoux V74.1
      mycotic infection NEC V75.4
      parasitic disease NEC V75.8
      Schick V74.3
      Schultz-Charlton V74.8
    social service (agency) referral or evaluation V63.8
    speech (-language) therapy V57.3
    sterilization V25.2
    suspected disorder (ruled out) (without need for further care) — see Observation
    terminal care V66.7
    tests only — see Test
    therapeutic drug monitoring V58.83
    therapy
      blood transfusion, without reported diagnosis V58.2
      breathing exercises V57.0
      chemotherapy, antineoplastic V58.11
        prophylactic NEC V07.39
          fluoride V07.31
      dialysis (intermittent) (treatment)
        extracorporeal V56.0
        peritoneal V56.8
        renal V56.0
        specified type NEC V56.8
      exercise (remedial) NEC V57.1
        breathing V57.0
      immunotherapy, antineoplastic V58.12
      long-term (current) (prophylactic) drug use NEC V58.69
        anti-inflammatories, nonsteroidal (NSAID) V58.64
        antibiotics V58.62
          short-term use — omit code
        anticoagulants V58.61
        antiplatelets V58.63
        antithrombotics V58.63
        aspirin V58.66
        bisphosphonates V58.68
        high-risk medications NEC V58.69
        insulin V58.67
        methadone for pain control V58.69

Admission — Aftercare

Admission — *continued*
for — *continued*
  therapy — *continued*
    long-term drug use — *continued*
      opiate analgesic V58.69
      steroids V58.65
    occupational V57.21
    orthoptic V57.4
    physical NEC V57.1
    radiation V58.0
    speech (-language) V57.3
    vocational V57.22
  toilet or cleaning
    of artificial opening — *see* Attention
      to, artificial, opening
    of non-vascular catheter V58.82
    of vascular catheter V58.81
  treatment
    measure V07.9
      specified type NEC V07.8
  tubal ligation V25.2
  tuboplasty for previous sterilization V26.0
  ultrasound, routine fetal V28.3
  vaccination, prophylactic (against)
    arthropod-borne virus, viral NEC V05.1
      disease NEC V05.1
      encephalitis V05.0
    Bacille Calmette Guérin (BCG) V03.2
    BCG V03.2
    chickenpox V05.4
    cholera alone V03.0
      with typhoid-paratyphoid (cholera + TAB) V06.0
    common cold V04.7
    dengue V05.1
    diphtheria-tetanus-pertussis (DTP) (DTaP) V06.1
      with
        poliomyelitis (DTP + polio) V06.3
        typhoid-paratyphoid (DTP + TAB) V06.2
    diphtheria-tetanus [Td] [DT] without pertussis V06.5
    diphtheria alone V03.5
    disease (single) NEC V05.9
      bacterial NEC V03.9
        specified type NEC V03.89
      combinations NEC V06.9
        specified type NEC V06.8
      specified type NEC V05.8
      viral NEC V04.89
    encephalitis, viral, arthropod-borne V05.0
    Hemophilus influenzae, type B [Hib] V03.81
    hepatitis, viral V05.3
    human papillomavirus (HPV) V04.89
    immune sera (gamma globulin) V07.2
    influenza V04.81
      with
        Streptococcus pneumoniae [pneumococcus] V06.6
    Leishmaniasis V05.2
    measles-mumps-rubella (MMR) V06.4
    measles alone V04.2
    mumps alone V04.6
      with measles and rubella (MMR) V06.4
    not done because of contraindication V64.09
    pertussis alone V03.6
    plague V03.3
    pneumonia V03.82
    poliomyelitis V04.0
      with diphtheria-tetanus-pertussis (DTP+ polio) V06.3
    rabies V04.5
    respiratory syncytial virus (RSV) V04.82
    rubella alone V04.3
      with measles and mumps (MMR) V06.4

Admission — *continued*
for — *continued*
  vaccination, prophylactic — *continued*
    smallpox V04.1
    specified type NEC V05.8
    Streptococcus pneumoniae [pneumococcus] V03.82
      with
        influenza V06.6
    tetanus toxoid alone V03.7
      with diphtheria [Td] [DT] V06.5
        and pertussis (DTP) (DTaP) V06.1
    tuberculosis (BCG) V03.2
    tularemia V03.4
    typhoid-paratyphoid alone (TAB) V03.1
    typhoid alone V03.1
      with diphtheria-tetanus-pertussis (TAB + DTP) V06.2
    typhus V05.8
    varicella (chicken pox) V05.4
    viral encephalitis, arthropod-borne V05.0
    viral hepatitis V05.3
    yellow fever V04.4
  vasectomy V25.2
  vasoplasty for previous sterilization V26.0
  vision examination V72.0
  vocational therapy V57.22
  waiting period for admission to other facility V63.2
    undergoing social agency investigation V63.8
  well baby and child care V20.2
  x-ray of chest
    for suspected tuberculosis V71.2
    routine V72.5

Adnexitis (suppurative) — *see also* Salpingo-oophoritis 614.2
Adolescence NEC V21.2
Adoption
  agency referral V68.89
  examination V70.3
  held for V68.89
Adrenal gland — *see* condition
Adrenalism 255.9
  tuberculous (*see also* Tuberculosis) 017.6 ☑
Adrenalitis, adrenitis 255.8
  meningococcal hemorrhagic 036.3
Adrenarche, precocious 259.1
Adrenocortical syndrome 255.2
Adrenogenital syndrome (acquired) (congenital) 255.2
  iatrogenic, fetus or newborn 760.79
Adrenoleukodystrophy 277.86
  neonatal 277.86
  x-linked 277.86
Adrenomyeloneuropathy 277.86
Adventitious bursa — *see* Bursitis
Adynamia (episodica) (hereditary) (periodic) 359.3
Adynamic
  ileus or intestine (*see also* Ileus) 560.1
  ureter 753.22
Aeration lung, imperfect, newborn 770.5
Aero-otitis media 993.0
Aerobullosis 993.3
Aerocele — *see* Embolism, air
Aerodermectasia
  subcutaneous (traumatic) 958.7
    surgical 998.81
  surgical 998.81
Aerodontalgia 993.2
Aeroembolism 993.3
Aerogenes capsulatus infection — *see also* Gangrene, gas 040.0
Aerophagy, aerophagia 306.4
  psychogenic 306.4
Aerosinusitis 993.1
Aerotitis 993.0
Affection, affections — *see also* Disease
  sacroiliac (joint), old 724.6
  shoulder region NEC 726.2

Afibrinogenemia 286.3
  acquired 286.6
  congenital 286.3
  postpartum 666.3 ☑
African
  sleeping sickness 086.5
  tick fever 087.1
  trypanosomiasis 086.5
    Gambian 086.3
    Rhodesian 086.4
After-cataract 366.50
  obscuring vision 366.53
  specified type, not obscuring vision 366.52
Aftercare V58.9
  amputation stump V54.89
  artificial openings — *see* Attention to, artificial, opening
  blood transfusion without reported diagnosis V58.2
  breathing exercise V57.0
  cardiac device V53.39
    defibrillator, automatic implantable (with synchronous cardiac pacemaker) V53.32
    pacemaker V53.31
      carotid sinus V53.39
  carotid sinus pacemaker V53.39
  cerebral ventricle (communicating) shunt V53.01
  chemotherapy (oral) (intravenous) session (adjunctive) (maintenance) V58.11
  defibrillator, automatic implantable cardiac (with synchronous cardiac pacemaker) V53.32
  exercise (remedial) (therapeutic) V57.1
    breathing V57.0
  extracorporeal dialysis (intermittent) (treatment) V56.0
  following surgery NEC V58.49
    for
      injury V58.43
      neoplasm V58.42
      organ transplant V58.44
      trauma V58.43
    joint
      explantation of prosthesis (staged procedure) V54.82
      replacement V54.81
    of
      circulatory system V58.73
      digestive system V58.75
      genital organs V58.76
      genitourinary system V58.76
      musculoskeletal system V58.78
      nervous system V58.72
      oral cavity V58.75
      respiratory system V58.74
      sense organs V58.71
      skin V58.77
      subcutaneous tissue V58.77
      teeth V58.75
      urinary system V58.76
    spinal — *see* Aftercare, following surgery, of, specified body system
    wound closure, planned V58.41
  fracture V54.9
    healing V54.89
      pathologic
        ankle V54.29
        arm V54.20
          lower V54.22
          upper V54.21
        finger V54.29
        foot V54.29
        hand V54.29
        hip V54.23
        leg V54.24
          lower V54.26
          upper V54.25
        pelvis V54.29
        specified site NEC V54.29
        toe(s) V54.29
        vertebrae V54.27
        wrist V54.29
      traumatic
        ankle V54.19

Aftercare — *continued*
  fracture — *continued*
    healing — *continued*
      traumatic — *continued*
        arm V54.10
          lower V54.12
          upper V54.11
        finger V54.19
        foot V54.19
        hand V54.19
        hip V54.13
        leg V54.14
          lower V54.16
          upper V54.15
        pelvis V54.19
        specified site NEC V54.19
        toe(s) V54.19
        vertebrae V54.17
        wrist V54.19
    removal of
      external fixation device V54.89
      internal fixation device V54.01
    specified care NEC V54.89
  gait training V57.1
    for use of artificial limb(s) V57.81
  internal fixation device V54.09
  involving
    dialysis (intermittent) (treatment)
      extracorporeal V56.0
      peritoneal V56.8
      renal V56.0
    gait training V57.1
      for use of artificial limb(s) V57.81
    growth rod
      adjustment V54.02
      lengthening V54.02
    internal fixation device V54.09
    orthoptic training V57.4
    orthotic training V57.81
    radiotherapy session V58.0
    removal of
      drains V58.49
      dressings
        wound V58.30
          nonsurgical V58.30
          surgical V58.31
      fixation device
        external V54.89
        internal V54.01
      fracture plate V54.01
      nonsurgical wound dressing V58.30
      pins V54.01
      plaster cast V54.89
      rods V54.01
      screws V58.32
      staples V58.32
      surgical wound dressings V58.31
      sutures V58.32
      traction device, external V54.89
      wound packing V58.30
        nonsurgical V58.30
        surgical V58.31
  neuropacemaker (brain) (peripheral nerve) (spinal cord) V53.02
  occupational therapy V57.21
  orthodontic V58.5
  orthopedic V54.9
    change of external fixation or traction device V54.89
    following joint
      explantation of prosthesis (staged procedure) V54.82
      replacement V54.81
    internal fixation device V54.09
    removal of fixation device
      external V54.89
      internal V54.01
    specified care NEC V54.89
  orthoptic training V57.4
  orthotic training V57.81
  pacemaker
    brain V53.02
    cardiac V53.31
    carotid sinus V53.39
    peripheral nerve V53.02
    spinal cord V53.02

☑ Additional Digit Required — Refer to the Tabular List for Digit Selection

▽ Subterms under main terms may continue to next column or page

Aftercare — *continued*
    peritoneal dialysis (intermittent) (treatment) V56.8
    physical therapy NEC V57.1
      breathing exercises V57.0
    radiotherapy session V58.0
    rehabilitation procedure V57.9
      breathing exercises V57.0
      multiple types V57.89
      occupational V57.21
      orthoptic V57.4
      orthotic V57.81
      physical therapy NEC V57.1
      remedial exercises V57.1
      specified type NEC V57.89
      speech (-language) V57.3
      therapeutic exercises V57.1
      vocational V57.22
    renal dialysis (intermittent) (treatment) V56.0
    specified type NEC V58.89
      removal of non-vascular catheter V58.82
      removal of vascular catheter V58.81
    speech (-language) V57.3
    stump, amputation V54.89
    vocational rehabilitation V57.22
Agalactia 676.4 ☑
Agammaglobulinemia 279.00
    with lymphopenia 279.2
    acquired (primary) (secondary) 279.06
    Bruton's X-linked 279.04
    infantile sex-linked (Bruton's) (congenital) 279.04
    Swiss-type 279.2
Aganglionosis (bowel) (colon) 751.3
Age (old) — *see also* Senile 797
Agenesis — *see also* Absence, by site, congenital
    acoustic nerve 742.8
    adrenal (gland) 759.1
    alimentary tract (complete) (partial) NEC 751.8
      lower 751.2
      upper 750.8
    anus, anal (canal) 751.2
    aorta 747.22
    appendix 751.2
    arm (complete) (partial) (*see also* Deformity, reduction, upper limb) 755.20
    artery (peripheral) NEC (*see also* Anomaly, peripheral vascular system) 747.60
      brain 747.81
      coronary 746.85
      pulmonary 747.31
      umbilical 747.5
    auditory (canal) (external) 744.01
    auricle (ear) 744.01
    bile, biliary duct or passage 751.61
    bone NEC 756.9
    brain 740.0
      specified part 742.2
    breast 757.6
    bronchus 748.3
    canaliculus lacrimalis 743.65
    carpus NEC (*see also* Deformity, reduction, upper limb) 755.28
    cartilage 756.9
    cecum 751.2
    cerebellum 742.2
    cervix 752.43
    chin 744.89
    cilia 743.63
    circulatory system, part NEC 747.89
    clavicle 755.51
    clitoris 752.49
    coccyx 756.13
    colon 751.2
    corpus callosum 742.2
    cricoid cartilage 748.3
    diaphragm (with hernia) 756.6
    digestive organ(s) or tract (complete) (partial) NEC 751.8
      lower 751.2
      upper 750.8
    ductus arteriosus 747.89
    duodenum 751.1

Agenesis — *see also* Absence, by site, congenital — *continued*
    ear NEC 744.09
      auricle 744.01
      lobe 744.21
    ejaculatory duct 752.89
    endocrine (gland) NEC 759.2
    epiglottis 748.3
    esophagus 750.3
    Eustachian tube 744.24
    extrinsic muscle, eye 743.69
    eye 743.00
      adnexa 743.69
    eyelid (fold) 743.62
    face
      bones NEC 756.0
      specified part NEC 744.89
    fallopian tube 752.19
    femur NEC (*see also* Absence, femur, congenital) 755.34
    fibula NEC (*see also* Absence, fibula, congenital) 755.37
    finger NEC (*see also* Absence, finger, congenital) 755.29
    foot (complete) (*see also* Deformity, reduction, lower limb) 755.31
    gallbladder 751.69
    gastric 750.8
    genitalia, genital (organ)
      female 752.89
        external 752.49
        internal NEC 752.89
      male 752.89
        penis 752.69
    glottis 748.3
    gonadal 758.6
    hair 757.4
    hand (complete) (*see also* Deformity, reduction, upper limb) 755.21
    heart 746.89
      valve NEC 746.89
        aortic 746.89
        mitral 746.89
        pulmonary 746.01
    hepatic 751.69
    humerus NEC (*see also* Absence, humerus, congenital) 755.24
    hymen 752.49
    ileum 751.1
    incus 744.04
    intestine (small) 751.1
      large 751.2
    iris (dilator fibers) 743.45
    jaw 524.09
    jejunum 751.1
    kidney(s) (partial) (unilateral) 753.0
    labium (majus) (minus) 752.49
    labyrinth, membranous 744.05
    lacrimal apparatus (congenital) 743.65
    larynx 748.3
    leg NEC (*see also* Deformity, reduction, lower limb) 755.30
    lens 743.35
    limb (complete) (partial) (*see also* Deformity, reduction) 755.4
      lower NEC 755.30
      upper 755.20
    lip 750.26
    liver 751.69
    lung (bilateral) (fissures) (lobe) (unilateral) 748.5
    mandible 524.09
    maxilla 524.09
    metacarpus NEC 755.28
    metatarsus NEC 755.38
    muscle (any) 756.81
    musculoskeletal system NEC 756.9
    nail(s) 757.5
    neck, part 744.89
    nerve 742.8
    nervous system, part NEC 742.8
    nipple 757.6
    nose 748.1
    nuclear 742.8
    organ
      of Corti 744.05

Agenesis — *see also* Absence, by site, congenital — *continued*
    organ — *continued*
      or site not listed — *see* Anomaly, specified type NEC
    osseous meatus (ear) 744.03
    ovary 752.0
    oviduct 752.19
    pancreas 751.7
    parathyroid (gland) 759.2
    patella 755.64
    pelvic girdle (complete) (partial) 755.69
    penis 752.69
    pericardium 746.89
    perineal body 756.81
    pituitary (gland) 759.2
    prostate 752.89
    pulmonary
      artery 747.31
      trunk 747.31
      vein 747.49
    punctum lacrimale 743.65
    radioulnar NEC (*see also* Absence, forearm, congenital) 755.25
    radius NEC (*see also* Absence, radius, congenital) 755.26
    rectum 751.2
    renal 753.0
    respiratory organ NEC 748.9
    rib 756.3
    roof of orbit 742.0
    round ligament 752.89
    sacrum 756.13
    salivary gland 750.21
    scapula 755.59
    scrotum 752.89
    seminal duct or tract 752.89
    septum
      atrial 745.69
      between aorta and pulmonary artery 745.0
      ventricular 745.3
    shoulder girdle (complete) (partial) 755.59
    skull (bone) 756.0
      with
        anencephalus 740.0
        encephalocele 742.0
        hydrocephalus 742.3
          with spina bifida (*see also* Spina bifida) 741.0 ☑
        microcephalus 742.1
    spermatic cord 752.89
    spinal cord 742.59
    spine 756.13
      lumbar 756.13
        isthmus 756.11
        pars articularis 756.11
    spleen 759.0
    sternum 756.3
    stomach 750.7
    tarsus NEC 755.38
    tendon 756.81
    testicular 752.89
    testis 752.89
    thymus (gland) 759.2
    thyroid (gland) 243
      cartilage 748.3
    tibia NEC (*see also* Absence, tibia, congenital) 755.36
    tibiofibular NEC 755.35
    toe (complete) (partial) (*see also* Absence, toe, congenital) 755.39
    tongue 750.11
    trachea (cartilage) 748.3
    ulna NEC (*see also* Absence, ulna, congenital) 755.27
    ureter 753.4
    urethra 753.8
    urinary tract NEC 753.8
    uterus 752.31
    uvula 750.26
    vagina (total) (partial) 752.45
    vas deferens 752.89
    vein(s) (peripheral) NEC (*see also* Anomaly, peripheral vascular system) 747.60
      brain 747.81

Agenesis — *see also* Absence, by site, congenital — *continued*
    vein(s) (*see also* Anomaly, peripheral vascular system) — *continued*
      great 747.49
      portal 747.49
      pulmonary 747.49
      vena cava (inferior) (superior) 747.49
    vermis of cerebellum 742.2
    vertebra 756.13
      lumbar 756.13
        isthmus 756.11
        pars articularis 756.11
    vulva 752.49
Ageusia — *see also* Disturbance, sensation 781.1
Aggressiveness 301.3
Aggressive outburst — *see also* Disturbance, conduct 312.0 ☑
    in children or adolescents 313.9
Aging skin 701.8
Agitated — *see* condition
Agitation 307.9
    catatonic (*see also* Schizophrenia) 295.2 ☑
Aglossia (congenital) 750.11
Aglycogenosis 271.0
Agnail (finger) (with lymphangitis) 681.02
Agnosia (body image) (tactile) 784.69
    verbal 784.69
      auditory 784.69
        secondary to organic lesion 784.69
      developmental 315.8
      secondary to organic lesion 784.69
    visual 368.16
      object 368.16
Agoraphobia 300.22
    with panic disorder 300.21
Agrammatism 784.69
Agranulocytopenia — *see also* Agranulocytosis 288.09
Agranulocytosis — *see also* Neutropenia 288.09
    chronic 288.09
    cyclical 288.02
    due to infection 288.04
    genetic 288.01
    infantile 288.01
    periodic 288.02
    pernicious 288.09
Agraphia (absolute) 784.69
    with alexia 784.61
    developmental 315.39
Agrypnia — *see also* Insomnia 780.52
Ague — *see also* Malaria 084.6
    brass-founders' 985.8
    dumb 084.6
    tertian 084.1
Agyria 742.2
AHTR (acute hemolytic transfusion reaction) — *see* Complications, transfusion
Ahumada-del Castillo syndrome (nonpuerperal galactorrhea and amenorrhea) 253.1
AIDS-associated retrovirus (disease) (illness) 042
    infection — *see* Human immunodeficiency virus, infection
AIDS-associated virus (disease) (illness) 042
    infection — *see* Human immunodeficiency virus, infection
AIDS-like disease (illness) (syndrome) 042
AIDS-related complex 042
AIDS-related conditions 042
AIDS-related virus (disease) (illness) 042
    infection — *see* Human immunodeficiency virus, infection
AIDS 042
AIDS virus (disease) (illness) 042
    infection — *see* Human immunodeficiency virus, infection
Ailment, heart — *see* Disease, heart
Ailurophobia 300.29
Ainhum (disease) 136.0
AIN I (anal intraepithelial neoplasia I) (histologically confirmed) 569.44

☑ Additional Digit Required — Refer to the Tabular List for Digit Selection   ▽ Subterms under main terms may continue to next column or page

AIN II (anal intraepithelial neoplasia II) (histologically confirmed) 569.44
AIN III (anal intraepithelial neoplasia III) 230.6
    anal canal 230.5
AIPHI (acute idiopathic pulmonary hemorrhage in infants (over 28 days old)) 786.31
Air
    anterior mediastinum 518.1
    compressed, disease 993.3
    embolism (any site) (artery) (cerebral) 958.0
        with
            abortion — see Abortion, by type, with embolism
            ectopic pregnancy (see also categories 633.0–633.9) 639.6
            molar pregnancy (see also categories 630–632) 639.6
        due to implanted device — see Complications, due to (presence of) any device, implant, or graft classified to 996.0–996.5 NEC
        following
            abortion 639.6
            ectopic or molar pregnancy 639.6
        infusion, perfusion, or transfusion 999.1
        in pregnancy, childbirth, or puerperium 673.0 ☑
        traumatic 958.0
    hunger 786.09
        psychogenic 306.1
    leak (lung) (pulmonary) (thorax) 512.84
        iatrogenic 512.1
        persistent 512.84
        postoperative 512.2
    rarefied, effects of — see Effect, adverse, high altitude
    sickness 994.6
Airplane sickness 994.6
Akathisia, acathisia 781.0
    due to drugs 333.99
    neuroleptic-induced acute 333.99
Akinesia algeria 352.6
Akiyami 100.89
Akureyri disease (epidemic neuromyasthenia) 049.8
Alacrima (congenital) 743.65
Alactasia (hereditary) 271.3
Alagille syndrome 759.89
Alalia 784.3
    developmental 315.31
        receptive-expressive 315.32
    secondary to organic lesion 784.3
Alaninemia 270.8
Alastrim 050.1
Albarrán's disease (colibacilluria) 791.9
Albers-Schönberg's disease (marble bones) 756.52
Albert's disease 726.71
Albinism, albino (choroid) (cutaneous) (eye) (generalized) (isolated) (ocular) (oculocutaneous) (partial) 270.2
Albinismus 270.2
Albright (-Martin) (-Bantam) disease (pseudohypoparathyroidism) 275.49
Albright (-McCune) (-Sternberg) syndrome (osteitis fibrosa disseminata) 756.59
Albuminous — see condition
Albuminuria, albuminuric (acute) (chronic) (subacute) 791.0
    Bence-Jones 791.0
    cardiac 785.9
    complicating pregnancy, childbirth, or puerperium 646.2 ☑
        with hypertension — see Toxemia, of pregnancy
        affecting fetus or newborn 760.1
    cyclic 593.6
    gestational 646.2 ☑
    gravidarum 646.2 ☑
        with hypertension — see Toxemia, of pregnancy
        affecting fetus or newborn 760.1
    heart 785.9
    idiopathic 593.6
    orthostatic 593.6

Albuminuria, albuminuric — continued
    postural 593.6
    pre-eclamptic (mild) 642.4 ☑
        affecting fetus or newborn 760.0
        severe 642.5 ☑
            affecting fetus or newborn 760.0
    recurrent physiologic 593.6
    scarlatinal 034.1
Albumosuria 791.0
    Bence-Jones 791.0
    myelopathic (M9730/3) 203.0 ☑
Alcaptonuria 270.2
Alcohol, alcoholic
    abstinence 291.81
    acute intoxication 305.0 ☑
        with dependence 303.0 ☑
    addiction (see also Alcoholism) 303.9 ☑
        maternal
            with suspected fetal damage affecting management of pregnancy 655.4 ☑
            affecting fetus or newborn 760.71
    amnestic disorder, persisting 291.1
    anxiety 291.89
    brain syndrome, chronic 291.2
    cardiopathy 425.5
    chronic (see also Alcoholism) 303.9 ☑
    cirrhosis (liver) 571.2
    delirium 291.0
        acute 291.0
        chronic 291.1
        tremens 291.0
        withdrawal 291.0
    dementia NEC 291.2
    deterioration 291.2
    drunkenness (simple) 305.0 ☑
    hallucinosis (acute) 291.3
    induced
        circadian rhythm sleep disorder 291.82
        hypersomnia 291.82
        insomnia 291.82
        mental disorder 291.9
            anxiety 291.89
            mood 291.89
            sexual 291.89
            sleep 291.82
            specified type 291.89
        parasomnia 291.82
        persisting
            amnestic disorder 291.1
            dementia 291.2
        psychotic disorder
            with
                delusions 291.5
                hallucinations 291.3
        sleep disorder 291.82
    insanity 291.9
    intoxication (acute) 305.0 ☑
        with dependence 303.0 ☑
        pathological 291.4
    jealousy 291.5
    Korsakoff's, Korsakov's, Korsakow's 291.1
    liver NEC 571.3
        acute 571.1
        chronic 571.2
    mania (acute) (chronic) 291.9
    mood 291.89
    paranoia 291.5
    paranoid (type) psychosis 291.5
    pellagra 265.2
    poisoning, accidental (acute) NEC 980.9
        specified type of alcohol — see Table of Drugs and Chemicals
    psychosis (see also Psychosis, alcoholic) 291.9
        Korsakoff's, Korsakov's, Korsakow's 291.1
    polyneuritic 291.1
        with
            delusions 291.5
            hallucinations 291.3
    related disorder 291.9
    withdrawal symptoms, syndrome NEC 291.81
        delirium 291.0
        hallucinosis 291.3

Alcoholism 303.9 ☑

> Note — Use the following fifth-digit subclassification with category 303:
>
> 0   unspecified
> 1   continuous
> 2   episodic
> 3   in remission

    with psychosis (see also Psychosis, alcoholic) 291.9
    acute 303.0 ☑
    chronic 303.9 ☑
        with psychosis 291.9
    complicating pregnancy, childbirth, or puerperium 648.4 ☑
        affecting fetus or newborn 760.71
    history V11.3
    Korsakoff's, Korsakov's, Korsakow's 291.1
    suspected damage to fetus affecting management of pregnancy 655.4 ☑
Alder-Reilly anomaly (leukocyte granulation) 288.2
Alder's anomaly or syndrome (leukocyte granulation anomaly) 288.2
Aldosteronism (primary) 255.10
    congenital 255.10
    familial type I 255.11
    glucocorticoid-remediable 255.11
    secondary 255.14
Aldosteronoma (M8370/1) 237.2
Aldrich (-Wiskott) syndrome (eczema-thrombocytopenia) 279.12
Aleppo boil 085.1
Aleukemic — see condition
Aleukia
    congenital 288.09
    hemorrhagica 284.9
        acquired (secondary) 284.89
        congenital 284.09
        idiopathic 284.9
    splenica 289.4
Alexia (congenital) (developmental) 315.01
    secondary to organic lesion 784.61
Algoneurodystrophy 733.7
Algophobia 300.29
Alibert-Bazin disease (M9700/3) 202.1 ☑
Alibert's disease (mycosis fungoides) (M9700/3) 202.1 ☑
Alice in Wonderland syndrome 293.89
Alienation, mental — see also Psychosis 298.9
Alkalemia 276.3
Alkalosis 276.3
    metabolic 276.3
        with respiratory acidosis 276.4
    respiratory 276.3
Alkaptonuria 270.2
Allen-Masters syndrome 620.6
Allergic bronchopulmonary aspergillosis 518.6
Allergy, allergic (reaction) 995.3
    air-borne substance — see also Fever, hay 477.9
        specified allergen NEC 477.8
    alveolitis (extrinsic) 495.9
        due to
            Aspergillus clavatus 495.4
            cryptostroma corticale 495.6
            organisms (fungal, thermophilic actinomycete, other) growing in ventilation (air conditioning systems) 495.7
        specified type NEC 495.8
    anaphylactic reaction or shock 995.0
        due to food — see Anaphylactic reaction or shock, due to, food
    angioderma 995.1
    angioneurotic edema 995.1
    animal (cat) (dog) (epidermal) 477.8
        dander 477.2
        hair 477.2
    arthritis (see also Arthritis, allergic) 716.2 ☑
    asthma — see Asthma
    bee sting (anaphylactic shock) 989.5
    biological — see Allergy, drug

Allergy, allergic — continued
    bronchial asthma — see Asthma
    conjunctivitis (eczematous) 372.14
    dander, animal (cat) (dog) 477.2
    dandruff 477.8
    dermatitis (venenata) — see Dermatitis
    diathesis V15.09
    drug, medicinal substance, and biological (any) (correct medicinal substance properly administered) (external) (internal) 995.27
        wrong substance given or taken NEC 977.9
        specified drug or substance — see Table of Drugs and Chemicals
    dust (house) (stock) 477.8
    eczema — see Eczema
    endophthalmitis 360.19
    epidermal (animal) 477.8
    existing dental restorative material
    feathers 477.8
    food (any) (ingested) 693.1
        atopic 691.8
        in contact with skin 692.5
    gastritis 535.4 ☑
    gastroenteritis 558.3
    gastrointestinal 558.3
    grain 477.0
    grass (pollen) 477.0
        asthma (see also Asthma) 493.0 ☑
        hay fever 477.0
    hair, animal (cat) (dog) 477.2
    hay fever (grass) (pollen) (ragweed) (tree) (see also Fever, hay) 477.9
    history (of) V15.09
        to
            arachnid bite V15.06
            eggs V15.03
            food additives V15.05
            insect bite V15.06
            latex V15.07
            milk products V15.02
            nuts V15.05
                peanuts V15.01
            radiographic dye V15.08
            seafood V15.04
            specified food NEC V15.05
            spider bite V15.06
    horse serum — see Allergy, serum
    inhalant 477.9
        dust 477.8
        pollen 477.0
        specified allergen other than pollen 477.8
    kapok 477.8
    medicine — see Allergy, drug
    migraine 339.00
    milk protein 558.3
    pannus 370.62
    pneumonia 518.3
    pollen (any) (hay fever) 477.0
        asthma (see also Asthma) 493.0 ☑
    primrose 477.0
    primula 477.0
    purpura 287.0
    ragweed (pollen) (Senecio jacobae) 477.0
        asthma (see also Asthma) 493.0 ☑
        hay fever 477.0
    respiratory (see also Allergy, inhalant) 477.9
        due to
            drug — see Allergy, drug
            food — see Allergy, food
    rhinitis (see also Fever, hay) 477.9
        due to food 477.1
    rose 477.0
    Senecio jacobae 477.0
    serum (prophylactic) (therapeutic) 999.59
        anaphylactic reaction or shock 999.49
    shock (anaphylactic) (due to adverse effect of correct medicinal substance properly administered) 995.0
        food — see Anaphylactic reaction or shock, due to, food
        from
            administration of blood and blood products 999.41

Allergy, allergic — continued
  shock — continued
    from — continued
      immunization 999.42
      serum NEC 999.49
  sinusitis (see also Fever, hay) 477.9
  skin reaction 692.9
    specified substance — see Dermatitis, due to
  tree (any) (hay fever) (pollen) 477.0
    asthma (see also Asthma) 493.0 ☑
  upper respiratory (see also Fever, hay) 477.9
  urethritis 597.89
  urticaria 708.0
  vaccine — see Allergy, serum
Allescheriosis 117.6
Alligator skin disease (ichthyosis congenita) 757.1
  acquired 701.1
Allocheiria, allochiria — see also Disturbance, sensation 782.0
Almeida's disease (Brazilian blastomycosis) 116.1
Alopecia (atrophicans) (pregnancy) (premature) (senile) 704.00
  adnata 757.4
  areata 704.01
  celsi 704.01
  cicatrisata 704.09
  circumscripta 704.01
  congenital, congenitalis 757.4
  disseminata 704.01
  effluvium (telogen) 704.02
  febrile 704.09
  generalisata 704.09
  hereditaria 704.09
  marginalis 704.01
  mucinosa 704.09
  postinfectional 704.09
  seborrheica 704.09
  specific 091.82
  syphilitic (secondary) 091.82
  telogen effluvium 704.02
  totalis 704.09
  toxica 704.09
  universalis 704.09
  x-ray 704.09
Alpers' disease 330.8
Alpha-lipoproteinemia 272.4
Alpha thalassemia 282.43
Alphos 696.1
Alpine sickness 993.2
Alport's syndrome (hereditary hematuri-anephropathy-deafness) 759.89
ALPS (autoimmune lymphoproliferative syndrome) 279.41
ALTE (apparent life threatening event) **in newborn and infant** 799.82
Alteration (of), altered
  awareness 780.09
    transient 780.02
  consciousness 780.09
    persistent vegetative state 780.03
    transient 780.02
  mental status 780.97
    amnesia (retrograde) 780.93
    memory loss 780.93
Alternaria (infection) 118
Alternating — see condition
Altitude, high (effects) — see Effect, adverse, high altitude
Aluminosis (of lung) 503
Alvarez syndrome (transient cerebral ischemia) 435.9
Alveolar capillary block syndrome 516.64
Alveolus, alveolar — see condition
Alymphocytosis (pure) 279.2
Alymphoplasia, thymic 279.2
Alzheimer's
  dementia (senile)
    with behavioral disturbance 331.0 [294.11]
    without behavioral disturbance 331.0 [294.10]
  disease or sclerosis 331.0

Alzheimer's — continued
  disease or sclerosis — continued
    with dementia — see Alzheimer's, dementia
Amastia — see also Absence, breast 611.89
Amaurosis (acquired) (congenital) — see also Blindness 369.00
  fugax 362.34
  hysterical 300.11
  Leber's (congenital) 362.76
  tobacco 377.34
  uremic — see Uremia
Amaurotic familial idiocy (infantile) (juvenile) (late) 330.1
Ambisexual 752.7
Amblyopia (acquired) (congenital) (partial) 368.00
  color 368.59
    acquired 368.55
  deprivation 368.02
  ex anopsia 368.00
  hysterical 300.11
  nocturnal 368.60
    vitamin A deficiency 264.5
  refractive 368.03
  strabismic 368.01
  suppression 368.01
  tobacco 377.34
  toxic NEC 377.34
  uremic — see Uremia
Ameba, amebic (histolytica) — see also Amebiasis
  abscess 006.3
    bladder 006.8
    brain (with liver and lung abscess) 006.5
    liver 006.3
      with
        brain abscess (and lung abscess) 006.5
        lung abscess 006.4
    lung (with liver abscess) 006.4
      with brain abscess 006.5
    seminal vesicle 006.8
    spleen 006.8
  carrier (suspected of) V02.2
  meningoencephalitis
    due to Naegleria (gruberi) 136.29
    primary 136.29
Amebiasis NEC 006.9
  with
    brain abscess (with liver or lung abscess) 006.5
    liver abscess (without mention of brain or lung abscess) 006.3
    lung abscess (with liver abscess) 006.4
      with brain abscess 006.5
  acute 006.0
  bladder 006.8
  chronic 006.1
  cutaneous 006.6
  cutis 006.6
  due to organism other than Entamoeba histolytica 007.8
  hepatic (see also Abscess, liver, amebic) 006.3
  nondysenteric 006.2
  seminal vesicle 006.8
  specified
    organism NEC 007.8
    site NEC 006.8
Ameboma 006.8
Amelia 755.4
  lower limb 755.31
  upper limb 755.21
Ameloblastoma (M9310/0) 213.1
  jaw (bone) (lower) 213.1
    upper 213.0
  long bones (M9261/3) — see Neoplasm, bone, malignant
  malignant (M9310/3) 170.1
    jaw (bone) (lower) 170.1
      upper 170.0
  mandible 213.1
  tibial (M9261/3) 170.7
Amelogenesis imperfecta 520.5
  nonhereditaria (segmentalis) 520.4

Amenorrhea (primary) (secondary) 626.0
  due to ovarian dysfunction 256.8
  hyperhormonal 256.8
Amentia — see also Disability, intellectual 319
  Meynert's (nonalcoholic) 294.0
    alcoholic 291.1
  nevoid 759.6
American
  leishmaniasis 085.5
  mountain tick fever 066.1
  trypanosomiasis — see Trypanosomiasis, American
Ametropia — see also Disorder, accommodation 367.9
Amianthosis 501
Amimia 784.69
Amino acid
  deficiency 270.9
    anemia 281.4
  metabolic disorder (see also Disorder, amino acid) 270.9
Aminoaciduria 270.9
  imidazole 270.5
Amnesia (retrograde) 780.93
  auditory 784.69
    developmental 315.31
    secondary to organic lesion 784.69
  dissociative 300.12
  hysterical or dissociative type 300.12
  psychogenic 300.12
  transient global 437.7
Amnestic (confabulatory) **syndrome** 294.0
  alcohol-induced persisting 291.1
  drug-induced persisting 292.83
  posttraumatic 294.0
Amniocentesis screening (for) V28.2
  alphafetoprotein level, raised V28.1
  chromosomal anomalies V28.0
Amnion, amniotic — see also condition
  nodosum 658.8 ☑
Amnionitis (complicating pregnancy) 658.4 ☑
  affecting fetus or newborn 762.7
Amoral trends 301.7
Amotio retinae — see also Detachment, retina 361.9
Ampulla
  lower esophagus 530.89
  phrenic 530.89
Amputation
  any part of fetus, to facilitate delivery 763.89
  cervix (supravaginal) (uteri) 622.8
    in pregnancy or childbirth 654.6 ☑
      affecting fetus or newborn 763.89
  clitoris — see Wound, open, clitoris
  congenital
    lower limb 755.31
    upper limb 755.21
  neuroma (traumatic) (see also Injury, nerve, by site)
    surgical complication (late) 997.61
  penis — see Amputation, traumatic, penis
  status (without complication) — see Absence, by site, acquired
  stump (surgical) (posttraumatic)
    abnormal, painful, or with complication (late) 997.60
    healed or old NEC (see also Absence, by site, acquired)
      lower V49.70
      upper V49.60
  traumatic (complete) (partial)

Note — "Complicated" includes traumatic amputation with delayed healing, delayed treatment, foreign body, or infection.

---

    arm 887.4
      at or above elbow 887.2
        complicated 887.3
      below elbow 887.0
        complicated 887.1
      both (bilateral) (any level(s)) 887.6
        complicated 887.7
      complicated 887.5
    finger(s) (one or both hands) 886.0
      with thumb(s) 885.0
        complicated 885.1

Amputation — continued
  traumatic — continued
    finger(s) — continued
      complicated 886.1
    foot (except toe(s) only) 896.0
      and other leg 897.6
        complicated 897.7
      both (bilateral) 896.2
        complicated 896.3
      complicated 896.1
    toe(s) only (one or both feet) 895.0
      complicated 895.1
    genital organ(s) (external) NEC 878.8
      complicated 878.9
    hand (except finger(s) only) 887.0
      and other arm 887.6
        complicated 887.7
      both (bilateral) 887.6
        complicated 887.7
      complicated 887.1
    finger(s) (one or both hands) 886.0
      with thumb(s) 885.0
        complicated 885.1
      complicated 886.1
    thumb(s) (with fingers of either hand) 885.0
      complicated 885.1
    head 874.9
    late effect — see Late, effects (of), amputation
    leg 897.4
      and other foot 897.6
        complicated 897.7
      at or above knee 897.2
        complicated 897.3
      below knee 897.0
        complicated 897.1
      both (bilateral) 897.6
        complicated 897.7
      complicated 897.5
    lower limb(s) except toe(s) — see Amputation, traumatic, leg
    nose — see Wound, open, nose
    penis 878.0
      complicated 878.1
    sites other than limbs — see Wound, open, by site
    thumb(s) (with finger(s) of either hand) 885.0
      complicated 885.1
    toe(s) (one or both feet) 895.0
      complicated 895.1
    upper limb(s) — see Amputation, traumatic, arm
Amputee (bilateral) (old) — see also Absence, by site, acquired V49.70
Amusia 784.69
  developmental 315.39
  secondary to organic lesion 784.69
Amyelencephalus 740.0
Amyelia 742.59
Amygdalitis — see Tonsillitis
Amygdalolith 474.8
Amyloid disease or degeneration 277.30
  heart 277.39 [425.7]
Amyloidosis (familial) (general) (generalized) (genetic) (primary) 277.30
  with lung involvement 277.39 [517.8]
  cardiac, hereditary 277.39
  heart 277.39 [425.7]
  nephropathic 277.39 [583.81]
  neuropathic (Portuguese) (Swiss) 277.39 [357.4]
  pulmonary 277.39 [517.8]
  secondary 277.39
  systemic, inherited 277.39
Amylopectinosis (brancher enzyme deficiency) 271.0
Amylophagia 307.52
Amyoplasia, congenita 756.89
Amyotonia 728.2
  congenita 358.8
Amyotrophia, amyotrophy, amyotrophic 728.2
  congenita 756.89
  diabetic 250.6 ☑ [353.5]

☑ **Additional Digit Required** — Refer to the Tabular List for Digit Selection   ▽ **Subterms under main terms may continue to next column or page**

2014 ICD-9-CM   ▶◀ **Revised Text**   ● **New Line**   ▲ **Revised Code**   Volume 2 — 17

Amyotrophia, amyotrophy, amyotrophic —
continued
  diabetic — *continued*
    due to secondary diabetes
      249.6 ☑ *[353.5]*
  lateral sclerosis (syndrome) 335.20
  neuralgic 353.5
  sclerosis (lateral) 335.20
  spinal progressive 335.21
Anacidity, gastric 536.0
  psychogenic 306.4
Anaerosis of newborn 770.88
Analbuminemia 273.8
Analgesia — *see also* Anesthesia 782.0
Analphalipoproteinemia 272.5
Anaphylactic reaction or shock (correct
  substance properly administered) 995.0
  due to
    administration of blood and blood
      products 999.41
    chemical — *see* Table of Drugs and
      Chemicals
    correct medicinal substance properly
      administered 995.0
    drug or medicinal substance
      correct substance properly adminis-
        tered 995.0
      overdose or wrong substance given
        or taken 977.9
        specified drug — *see* Table of
          Drugs and Chemicals
    following sting(s) 989.5
    food 995.60
      additives 995.66
      crustaceans 995.62
      eggs 995.68
      fish 995.65
      fruits 995.63
      milk products 995.67
      nuts (tree) 995.64
      peanuts 995.61
      seeds 995.64
      specified NEC 995.69
      tree nuts 995.64
      vegetables 995.63
    immunization 999.42
    overdose or wrong substance given or
      taken 977.9
      specified drug — *see* Table of Drugs
        and Chemicals
    serum NEC 999.49
  following sting(s) 989.5
  purpura 287.0
  serum NEC 999.49
Anaphylactoid reaction or shock — *see*
  Anaphylactic reaction or shock
Anaphylaxis — *see* Anaphylactic reaction or
  shock
Anaplasia, cervix 622.10
Anaplasmosis, human 082.49
Anarthria 784.51
Anarthritic rheumatoid disease 446.5
Anasarca 782.3
  cardiac (*see also* Failure, heart) 428.0
  fetus or newborn 778.0
  lung 514
  nutritional 262
  pulmonary 514
  renal (*see also* Nephrosis) 581.9
Anaspadias 752.62
Anastomosis
  aneurysmal — *see* Aneurysm
  arteriovenous, congenital NEC (*see also*
    Anomaly, arteriovenous) 747.60
    ruptured, of brain (*see also* Hemorrhage,
      subarachnoid) 430
  intestinal 569.89
    complicated NEC 997.49
      involving urinary tract 997.5
  retinal and choroidal vessels 743.58
    acquired 362.17
Anatomical narrow angle (glaucoma) 365.02
Ancylostoma (infection) (infestation) 126.9
  americanus 126.1
  braziliense 126.2
  caninum 126.8

Ancylostoma — *continued*
  ceylanicum 126.3
  duodenale 126.0
  Necator americanus 126.1
Ancylostomiasis (intestinal) 126.9
  ancylostoma
    americanus 126.1
    caninum 126.8
    ceylanicum 126.3
    duodenale 126.0
  braziliense 126.2
  Necator americanus 126.1
Anders' disease or syndrome (adiposis
  tuberosa simplex) 272.8
Andersen's glycogen storage disease 271.0
Anderson's disease 272.7
Andes disease 993.2
Andrews' disease (bacterid) 686.8
Androblastoma (M8630/1)
  benign (M8630/0)
    specified site — *see* Neoplasm, by site,
      benign
    unspecified site
      female 220
      male 222.0
  malignant (M8630/3)
    specified site — *see* Neoplasm, by site,
      malignant
    unspecified site
      female 183.0
      male 186.9
  specified site — *see* Neoplasm, by site, un-
    certain behavior
  tubular (M8640/0)
    with lipid storage (M8641/0)
      specified site — *see* Neoplasm, by
        site, benign
      unspecified site
        female 220
        male 222.0
    specified site — *see* Neoplasm, by site,
      benign
    unspecified site
      female 220
      male 222.0
  unspecified site
    female 236.2
    male 236.4
Android pelvis 755.69
  with disproportion (fetopelvic) 653.3 ☑
    affecting fetus or newborn 763.1
    causing obstructed labor 660.1 ☑
      affecting fetus or newborn 763.1
Anectasis, pulmonary (newborn or fetus)
  770.5
Anemia 285.9
  with
    disorder of
      anaerobic glycolysis 282.3
      pentose phosphate pathway 282.2
    koilonychia 280.9
  6-phosphogluconic dehydrogenase deficien-
    cy 282.2
  achlorhydric 280.9
  achrestic 281.8
  Addison-Biermer (pernicious) 281.0
  Addison's (pernicious) 281.0
  agranulocytic 288.09
  amino acid deficiency 281.4
  antineoplastic chemotherapy induced 285.3
  aplastic 284.9
    acquired (secondary) 284.89
    congenital 284.01
    constitutional 284.01
    due to
      antineoplastic chemotherapy 284.89
      chronic systemic disease 284.89
      drugs 284.89
      infection 284.89
      radiation 284.89
    idiopathic 284.9
    myxedema 244.9
    of or complicating pregnancy 648.2 ☑
    red cell (acquired) (adult) (with thymo-
      ma) 284.81
      congenital 284.01

Anemia — *continued*
  aplastic — *continued*
    red cell — *continued*
      pure 284.01
      specified type NEC 284.89
      toxic (paralytic) 284.89
  aregenerative 284.9
    congenital 284.01
  asiderotic 280.9
  atypical (primary) 285.9
  autohemolysis of Selwyn and Dacie (type I)
    282.2
  autoimmune hemolytic 283.0
  Baghdad Spring 282.2
  Balantidium coli 007.0
  Biermer's (pernicious) 281.0
  blood loss (chronic) 280.0
    acute 285.1
  bothriocephalus 123.4
  brickmakers' (*see also* Ancylostomiasis)
    126.9
  cerebral 437.8
  childhood 282.9
  chlorotic 280.9
  chronic 285.9
    blood loss 280.0
    hemolytic 282.9
      idiopathic 283.9
    simple 281.9
  chronica congenita aregenerativa 284.01
  combined system disease NEC 281.0 *[336.2]*
    due to dietary deficiency 281.1 *[336.2]*
  complicating pregnancy or childbirth
    648.2 ☑
  congenital (following fetal blood loss) 776.5
    aplastic 284.01
    due to isoimmunization NEC 773.2
    Heinz-body 282.7
    hereditary hemolytic NEC 282.9
    nonspherocytic
      Type I 282.2
      Type II 282.3
    pernicious 281.0
    spherocytic (*see also* Spherocytosis)
      282.0
  Cooley's (erythroblastic) 282.44
  crescent — *see* Disease, sickle-cell
  cytogenic 281.0
  Dacie's (nonspherocytic)
    type I 282.2
    type II 282.3
  Davidson's (refractory) 284.9
  deficiency 281.9
    2, 3 diphosphoglycurate mutase 282.3
    2, 3 PG 282.3
    6-PGD 282.2
    6-phosphogluronic dehydrogenase
      282.2
    amino acid 281.4
    combined B_{12} and folate 281.3
    enzyme, drug-induced (hemolytic) 282.2
    erythrocytic glutathione 282.2
    folate 281.2
      dietary 281.2
      drug-induced 281.2
    folic acid 281.2
      dietary 281.2
      drug-induced 281.2
    G-6-PD 282.2
    GGS-R 282.2
    glucose-6-phosphate dehydrogenase
      (G-6-PD) 282.2
    glucose-phosphate isomerase 282.3
    glutathione peroxidase 282.2
    glutathione reductase 282.2
    glyceraldehyde phosphate dehydroge-
      nase 282.3
    GPI 282.3
    G SH 282.2
    hexokinase 282.3
    iron (Fe) 280.9
      specified NEC 280.8
    nutritional 281.9
      with
        poor iron absorption 280.9
        specified deficiency NEC 281.8

Anemia — *continued*
  deficiency — *continued*
    nutritional — *continued*
      due to inadequate dietary iron intake
        280.1
      specified type NEC 281.8
    of or complicating pregnancy 648.2 ☑
    pentose phosphate pathway 282.2
    PFK 282.3
    phosphofructo-aldolase 282.3
    phosphofructokinase 282.3
    phosphoglycerate kinase 282.3
    PK 282.3
    protein 281.4
    pyruvate kinase (PK) 282.3
    TPI 282.3
    triosephosphate isomerase 282.3
    vitamin B_{12} NEC 281.1
      dietary 281.1
      pernicious 281.0
  Diamond-Blackfan (congenital hypoplastic)
    284.01
  dibothriocephalus 123.4
  dimorphic 281.9
  diphasic 281.8
  diphtheritic 032.89
  Diphyllobothrium 123.4
  drepanocytic (*see also* Disease, sickle-cell)
    282.60
  due to
    antineoplastic chemotherapy 285.3
    blood loss (chronic) 280.0
      acute 285.1
    chemotherapy, antineoplastic 285.3
    defect of Embden-Meyerhof pathway
      glycolysis 282.3
    disorder of glutathione metabolism
      282.2
    drug — *see* Anemia, by type (*see also*
      Table of Drugs and Chemicals)
      chemotherapy, antineoplastic 285.3
    fetal blood loss 776.5
    fish tapeworm (D. latum) infestation
      123.4
    glutathione metabolism disorder 282.2
    hemorrhage (chronic) 280.0
      acute 285.1
    hexose monophosphate (HMP) shunt
      deficiency 282.2
    impaired absorption 280.9
    loss of blood (chronic) 280.0
      acute 285.1
    myxedema 244.9
    Necator americanus 126.1
    prematurity 776.6
    selective vitamin B_{12} malabsorption with
      proteinuria 281.1
  Dyke-Young type (secondary)
    (symptomatic) 283.9
  dyserythropoietic (congenital) (types I, II,
    III) 285.8
  dyshemopoietic (congenital) 285.8
  Egypt (*see also* Ancylostomiasis) 126.9
  elliptocytosis (*see also* Elliptocytosis) 282.1
  enzyme deficiency, drug-induced 282.2
  epidemic (*see also* Ancylostomiasis) 126.9
  EPO resistant 285.21
  erythroblastic
    familial 282.44
    fetus or newborn (*see also* Disease,
      hemolytic) 773.2
    late 773.5
  erythrocytic glutathione deficiency 282.2
  erythropoietin-resistant (EPO resistant ane-
    mia) 285.21
  essential 285.9
  Faber's (achlorhydric anemia) 280.9
  factitious (self-induced blood letting) 280.0
  familial erythroblastic (microcytic) 282.44
  Fanconi's (congenital pancytopenia) 284.09
  favism 282.2
  fetal 678.0 ☑
    following blood loss, affecting newborn
      776.5

☑ **Additional Digit Required** — Refer to the Tabular List for Digit Selection   ▽ **Subterms under main terms may continue to next column or page**

18 — Volume 2   ▶◀ **Revised Text**   ● **New Line**   ▲ **Revised Code**   **2014 ICD-9-CM**

Anemia — *continued*

fetus or newborn

due to

ABO

antibodies 773.1

incompatibility, maternal/fetal 773.1

isoimmunization 773.1

Rh

antibodies 773.0

incompatibility, maternal/fetal 773.0

isoimmunization 773.0

following fetal blood loss 776.5

fish tapeworm (D. latum) infestation 123.4

folate (folic acid) deficiency 281.2

dietary 281.2

drug-induced 281.2

folate malabsorption, congenital 281.2

folic acid deficiency 281.2

dietary 281.2

drug-induced 281.2

G-6-PD 282.2

general 285.9

glucose-6-phosphate dehydrogenase deficiency 282.2

glutathione-reductase deficiency 282.2

goat's milk 281.2

granulocytic 288.09

Heinz-body, congenital 282.7

hemoglobin deficiency 285.9

hemolytic 283.9

acquired 283.9

with hemoglobinuria NEC 283.2

autoimmune (cold type) (idiopathic) (primary) (secondary) (symptomatic) (warm type) 283.0

due to

cold reactive antibodies 283.0

drug exposure 283.0

warm reactive antibodies 283.0

fragmentation 283.19

idiopathic (chronic) 283.9

infectious 283.19

autoimmune 283.0

non-autoimmune 283.10

toxic 283.19

traumatic cardiac 283.19

acute 283.9

due to enzyme deficiency NEC 282.3

fetus or newborn (*see also* Disease, hemolytic) 773.2

late 773.5

Lederer's (acquired infectious hemolytic anemia) 283.19

autoimmune (acquired) 283.0

chronic 282.9

idiopathic 283.9

cold type (secondary) (symptomatic) 283.0

congenital (spherocytic) (*see also* Spherocytosis) 282.0

nonspherocytic — *see* Anemia, hemolytic, nonspherocytic, congenital

drug-induced 283.0

enzyme deficiency 282.2

due to

cardiac conditions 283.19

drugs 283.0

enzyme deficiency NEC 282.3

drug-induced 282.2

presence of shunt or other internal prosthetic device 283.19

thrombotic thrombocytopenic purpura 446.6

elliptocytotic (*see also* Elliptocytosis) 282.1

familial 282.9

hereditary 282.9

due to enzyme deficiency NEC 282.3

specified NEC 282.8

idiopathic (chronic) 283.9

infectious (acquired) 283.19

mechanical 283.19

microangiopathic 283.19

Anemia — *continued*

hemolytic — *continued*

non-autoimmune NEC 283.10

nonspherocytic

congenital or hereditary NEC 282.3

glucose-6-phosphate dehydrogenase deficiency 282.2

pyruvate kinase (PK) deficiency 282.3

type I 282.2

type II 282.3

type I 282.2

type II 282.3

of or complicating pregnancy 648.2 ☑

resulting from presence of shunt or other internal prosthetic device 283.19

secondary 283.19

autoimmune 283.0

sickle-cell — *see* Disease, sickle-cell

Stransky-Regala type (Hb-E) (*see also* Disease, hemoglobin) 282.7

symptomatic 283.19

autoimmune 283.0

toxic (acquired) 283.19

uremic (adult) (child) 283.11

warm type (secondary) (symptomatic) 283.0

hemorrhagic (chronic) 280.0

acute 285.1

HEMPAS 285.8

hereditary erythroblast multinuclearity-positive acidified serum test 285.8

Herrick's (hemoglobin S disease) 282.61

hexokinase deficiency 282.3

high A$_2$ 282.46

hookworm (*see also* Ancylostomiasis) 126.9

hypochromic (idiopathic) (microcytic) (normoblastic) 280.9

with iron loading 285.0

due to blood loss (chronic) 280.0

acute 285.1

familial sex linked 285.0

pyridoxine-responsive 285.0

hypoplasia, red blood cells 284.81

congenital or familial 284.01

hypoplastic (idiopathic) 284.9

congenital 284.01

familial 284.01

of childhood 284.09

idiopathic 285.9

hemolytic, chronic 283.9

in (due to) (with)

chronic illness NEC 285.29

chronic kidney disease 285.21

end-stage renal disease 285.21

neoplastic disease 285.22

infantile 285.9

infective, infectional 285.9

intertropical (*see also* Ancylostomiasis) 126.9

iron (Fe) deficiency 280.9

due to blood loss (chronic) 280.0

acute 285.1

of or complicating pregnancy 648.2 ☑

specified NEC 280.8

Jaksch's (pseudoleukemia infantum) 285.8

Joseph-Diamond-Blackfan (congenital hypoplastic) 284.01

labyrinth 386.50

Lederer's (acquired infectious hemolytic anemia) 283.19

leptocytosis (hereditary) 282.40

leukoerythroblastic 284.2

macrocytic 281.9

nutritional 281.2

of or complicating pregnancy 648.2 ☑

tropical 281.2

malabsorption (familial), selective B$_{12}$ with proteinuria 281.1

malarial (*see also* Malaria) 084.6

malignant (progressive) 281.0

malnutrition 281.9

marsh (*see also* Malaria) 084.6

Mediterranean 282.40

with hemoglobinopathy 282.49

megaloblastic 281.9

Anemia — *continued*

megaloblastic — *continued*

combined B$_{12}$ and folate deficiency 281.3

nutritional (of infancy) 281.2

of infancy 281.2

of or complicating pregnancy 648.2 ☑

refractory 281.3

specified NEC 281.3

megalocytic 281.9

microangiopathic hemolytic 283.19

microcytic (hypochromic) 280.9

due to blood loss (chronic) 280.0

acute 285.1

familial 282.49

hypochromic 280.9

microdrepanocytosis 282.41

miners' (*see also* Ancylostomiasis) 126.9

myelopathic 285.8

myelophthisic (normocytic) 284.2

newborn (*see also* Disease, hemolytic) 773.2

due to isoimmunization (*see also* Disease, hemolytic) 773.2

late, due to isoimmunization 773.5

posthemorrhagic 776.5

nonregenerative 284.9

nonspherocytic hemolytic — *see* Anemia, hemolytic, nonspherocytic

normocytic (infectional) (not due to blood loss) 285.9

due to blood loss (chronic) 280.0

acute 285.1

myelophthisic 284.2

nutritional (deficiency) 281.9

with

poor iron absorption 280.9

specified deficiency NEC 281.8

due to inadequate dietary iron intake 280.1

megaloblastic (of infancy) 281.2

of childhood 282.9

of chronic

disease NEC 285.29

illness NEC 285.29

of or complicating pregnancy 648.2 ☑

affecting fetus or newborn 760.8

of prematurity 776.6

orotic aciduric (congenital) (hereditary) 281.4

osteosclerotic 289.89

ovalocytosis (hereditary) (*see also* Elliptocytosis) 282.1

paludal (*see also* Malaria) 084.6

pentose phosphate pathway deficiency 282.2

pernicious (combined system disease) (congenital) (dorsolateral spinal degeneration) (juvenile) (myelopathy) (neuropathy) (posterior sclerosis) (primary) (progressive) (spleen) 281.0

of or complicating pregnancy 648.2 ☑

pleochromic 285.9

of sprue 281.8

portal 285.8

posthemorrhagic (chronic) 280.0

acute 285.1

newborn 776.5

postoperative

due to (acute) blood loss 285.1

chronic blood loss 280.0

other 285.9

postpartum 648.2 ☑

pressure 285.9

primary 285.9

profound 285.9

progressive 285.9

malignant 281.0

pernicious 281.0

protein-deficiency 281.4

pseudoleukemica infantum 285.8

puerperal 648.2 ☑

pure red cell 284.81

congenital 284.01

pyridoxine-responsive (hypochromic) 285.0

pyruvate kinase (PK) deficiency 282.3

refractoria sideroblastica 238.72

Anemia — *continued*

refractory (primary) 238.72

with

excess

blasts-1 (RAEB-1) 238.72

blasts-2 (RAEB-2) 238.73

hemochromatosis 238.72

ringed sideroblasts (RARS) 238.72

due to

drug 285.0

myelodysplastic syndrome 238.72

toxin 285.0

hereditary 285.0

idiopathic 238.72

megaloblastic 281.3

sideroblastic 238.72

hereditary 285.0

sideropenic 280.9

Rietti-Greppi-Micheli (thalassemia minor) 282.46

scorbutic 281.8

secondary (to) 285.9

blood loss (chronic) 280.0

acute 285.1

hemorrhage 280.0

acute 285.1

inadequate dietary iron intake 280.1

semiplastic 284.9

septic 285.9

sickle-cell (*see also* Disease, sickle-cell) 282.60

sideroachrestic 285.0

sideroblastic (acquired) (any type) (congenital) (drug-induced) (due to disease) (hereditary) (primary) (secondary) (sex-linked hypochromic) (vitamin B$_6$ responsive) 285.0

refractory 238.72

congenital 285.0

drug-induced 285.0

hereditary 285.0

sex-linked hypochromic 285.0

vitamin B$_6$-responsive 285.0

sideropenic (refractory) 280.9

due to blood loss (chronic) 280.0

acute 285.1

simple chronic 281.9

specified type NEC 285.8

spherocytic (hereditary) (*see also* Spherocytosis) 282.0

splenic 285.8

familial (Gaucher's) 272.7

splenomegalic 285.8

stomatocytosis 282.8

syphilitic 095.8

target cell (oval) 285.8

with thalassemia — *see* Thalassemia

thalassemia 282.40

thrombocytopenic (*see also* Thrombocytopenia) 287.5

toxic 284.89

triosephosphate isomerase deficiency 282.3

tropical, macrocytic 281.2

tuberculous (*see also* Tuberculosis) 017.9 ☑

vegan's 281.1

vitamin

B$_6$-responsive 285.0

B$_{12}$ deficiency (dietary) 281.1

pernicious 281.0

von Jaksch's (pseudoleukemia infantum) 285.8

Witts' (achlorhydric anemia) 280.9

Zuelzer (-Ogden) [nutritional megaloblastic anemia] 281.2

Anencephalus, anencephaly 740.0

fetal, affecting management of pregnancy 655.0 ☑

Anergasia — *see also* Psychosis, organic 294.9

senile 290.0

Anesthesia, anesthetic 782.0

complication or reaction NEC 995.22

due to

correct substance properly administered 995.22

☑ **Additional Digit Required** — Refer to the Tabular List for Digit Selection   ▽ **Subterms under main terms may continue to next column or page**

2014 ICD-9-CM   ▶◀ **Revised Text**   ● **New Line**   ▲ **Revised Code**   Volume 2 — 19

Anesthesia, anesthetic — *continued*
  complication or reaction — *continued*
    due to — *continued*
      overdose or wrong substance given 968.4
      specified anesthetic — *see* Table of Drugs and Chemicals
  cornea 371.81
  death from
    correct substance properly administered 995.4
    during delivery 668.9 ☑
    overdose or wrong substance given 968.4
    specified anesthetic — *see* Table of Drugs and Chemicals
  eye 371.81
  functional 300.11
  hyperesthetic, thalamic 338.0
  hysterical 300.11
  local skin lesion 782.0
  olfactory 781.1
  sexual (psychogenic) 302.72
  shock
    due to
      correct substance properly administered 995.4
      overdose or wrong substance given 968.4
      specified anesthetic — *see* Table of Drugs and Chemicals
  skin 782.0
  tactile 782.0
  testicular 608.9
  thermal 782.0
Anetoderma (maculosum) 701.3
Aneuploidy NEC 758.5
Aneurin deficiency 265.1
Aneurysm (anastomotic) (artery) (cirsoid) (diffuse) (false) (fusiform) (multiple) (ruptured) (saccular) (varicose) 442.9
  abdominal (aorta) 441.4
    ruptured 441.3
    syphilitic 093.0
  aorta, aortic (nonsyphilitic) 441.9
    abdominal 441.4
      dissecting 441.02
      ruptured 441.3
      syphilitic 093.0
    arch 441.2
      ruptured 441.1
    arteriosclerotic NEC 441.9
      ruptured 441.5
    ascending 441.2
      ruptured 441.1
    congenital 747.29
    descending 441.9
      abdominal 441.4
        ruptured 441.3
      ruptured 441.5
      thoracic 441.2
        ruptured 441.1
    dissecting 441.00
      abdominal 441.02
      thoracic 441.01
      thoracoabdominal 441.03
    due to coarctation (aorta) 747.10
    ruptured 441.5
    sinus, right 747.29
    syphilitic 093.0
    thoracoabdominal 441.7
      ruptured 441.6
    thorax, thoracic (arch) (nonsyphilitic) 441.2
      dissecting 441.01
      ruptured 441.1
      syphilitic 093.0
    transverse 441.2
      ruptured 441.1
    valve (heart) (*see also* Endocarditis, aortic) 424.1
  arteriosclerotic NEC 442.9
    cerebral 437.3
      ruptured (*see also* Hemorrhage, subarachnoid) 430

Aneurysm — *continued*
  arteriovenous (congenital) (peripheral) NEC (*see also* Anomaly, arteriovenous) 747.60
    acquired NEC 447.0
      brain 437.3
        ruptured (*see also* Hemorrhage, subarachnoid) 430
      coronary 414.11
      pulmonary 417.0
    brain (cerebral) 747.81
      ruptured (*see also* Hemorrhage, subarachnoid) 430
    coronary 746.85
    pulmonary 747.32
    retina 743.58
    specified site NEC 747.89
      acquired 447.0
    traumatic (*see also* Injury, blood vessel, by site) 904.9
  basal — *see* Aneurysm, brain
  berry (congenital) (ruptured) (*see also* Hemorrhage, subarachnoid) 430
    nonruptured 437.3
  brain 437.3
    arteriosclerotic 437.3
      ruptured (*see also* Hemorrhage, subarachnoid) 430
    arteriovenous 747.81
      acquired 437.3
        ruptured (*see also* Hemorrhage, subarachnoid) 430
      ruptured (*see also* Hemorrhage, subarachnoid) 430
    berry (congenital) (ruptured) (*see also* Hemorrhage, subarachnoid) 430
      nonruptured 437.3
    congenital 747.81
      ruptured (*see also* Hemorrhage, subarachnoid) 430
    meninges 437.3
      ruptured (*see also* Hemorrhage, subarachnoid) 430
    miliary (congenital) (ruptured) (*see also* Hemorrhage, subarachnoid) 430
    mycotic 421.0
      ruptured (*see also* Hemorrhage, subarachnoid) 430
      nonruptured 437.3
    ruptured (*see also* Hemorrhage, subarachnoid) 430
    syphilitic 094.87
    syphilitic (hemorrhage) 094.87
    traumatic — *see* Injury, intracranial
  cardiac (false) (*see also* Aneurysm, heart) 414.10
  carotid artery (common) (external) 442.81
    internal (intracranial portion) 437.3
      extracranial portion 442.81
      ruptured into brain (*see also* Hemorrhage, subarachnoid) 430
    syphilitic 093.89
      intracranial 094.87
  cavernous sinus (*see also* Aneurysm, brain) 437.3
    arteriovenous 747.81
      ruptured (*see also* Hemorrhage, subarachnoid) 430
    congenital 747.81
      ruptured (*see also* Hemorrhage, subarachnoid) 430
  celiac 442.84
  central nervous system, syphilitic 094.89
  cerebral — *see* Aneurysm, brain
  chest — *see* Aneurysm, thorax
  circle of Willis (*see also* Aneurysm, brain) 437.3
    congenital 747.81
      ruptured (*see also* Hemorrhage, subarachnoid) 430
    ruptured (*see also* Hemorrhage, subarachnoid) 430
  common iliac artery 442.2
  congenital (peripheral) NEC 747.60
    brain 747.81

Aneurysm — *continued*
  congenital — *continued*
    brain — *continued*
      ruptured (*see also* Hemorrhage, subarachnoid) 430
    cerebral — *see* Aneurysm, brain, congenital
    coronary 746.85
    gastrointestinal 747.61
    lower limb 747.64
    pulmonary 747.32
    renal 747.62
    retina 743.58
    specified site NEC 747.89
    spinal 747.82
    upper limb 747.63
  conjunctiva 372.74
  conus arteriosus (*see also* Aneurysm, heart) 414.10
  coronary (arteriosclerotic) (artery) (vein) (*see also* Aneurysm, heart) 414.11
    arteriovenous 746.85
    congenital 746.85
    syphilitic 093.89
  cylindrical 441.9
    ruptured 441.5
    syphilitic 093.9
  dissecting 442.9
    aorta 441.00
      abdominal 441.02
      thoracic 441.01
      thoracoabdominal 441.03
    syphilitic 093.9
  ductus arteriosus 747.0
  embolic — *see* Embolism, artery
  endocardial, infective (any valve) 421.0
  femoral 442.3
  gastroduodenal 442.84
  gastroepiploic 442.84
  heart (chronic or with a stated duration of over 8 weeks) (infectional) (wall) 414.10
    acute or with a stated duration of 8 weeks or less (*see also* Infarct, myocardium) 410.9 ☑
    congenital 746.89
    valve — *see* Endocarditis
  hepatic 442.84
  iliac (common) 442.2
  infective (any valve) 421.0
  innominate (nonsyphilitic) 442.89
    syphilitic 093.89
  interauricular septum (*see also* Aneurysm, heart) 414.10
  interventricular septum (*see also* Aneurysm, heart) 414.10
  intracranial — *see* Aneurysm, brain
  intrathoracic (nonsyphilitic) 441.2
    ruptured 441.1
    syphilitic 093.0
  jugular vein (acute) 453.89
    chronic 453.76
  lower extremity 442.3
  lung (pulmonary artery) 417.1
  malignant 093.9
  mediastinal (nonsyphilitic) 442.89
    syphilitic 093.89
  miliary (congenital) (ruptured) (*see also* Hemorrhage, subarachnoid) 430
  mitral (heart) (valve) 424.0
  mural (arteriovenous) (heart) (*see also* Aneurysm, heart) 414.10
  mycotic, any site 421.0
    without endocarditis — *see* Aneurysm by site
    ruptured, brain (*see also* Hemorrhage, subarachnoid) 430
  myocardium (*see also* Aneurysm, heart) 414.10
  neck 442.81
  pancreaticoduodenal 442.84
  patent ductus arteriosus 747.0
  peripheral NEC 442.89
    congenital NEC (*see also* Aneurysm, congenital) 747.60
  popliteal 442.3

Aneurysm — *continued*
  pulmonary 417.1
    arteriovenous 747.32
      acquired 417.0
    syphilitic 093.89
    valve (heart) (*see also* Endocarditis, pulmonary) 424.3
  racemose 442.9
    congenital (peripheral) NEC 747.60
  radial 442.0
  Rasmussen's (*see also* Tuberculosis) 011.2 ☑
  renal 442.1
  retinal (acquired) 362.17
    congenital 743.58
    diabetic 250.5 ☑ [362.01]
      due to secondary diabetes 249.5 ☑ [362.01]
  sinus, aortic (of Valsalva) 747.29
  specified site NEC 442.89
  spinal (cord) 442.89
    congenital 747.82
    syphilitic (hemorrhage) 094.89
  spleen, splenic 442.83
  subclavian 442.82
    syphilitic 093.89
  superior mesenteric 442.84
  syphilitic 093.9
    aorta 093.0
    central nervous system 094.89
    congenital 090.5
    spine, spinal 094.89
  thoracoabdominal 441.7
    ruptured 441.6
  thorax, thoracic (arch) (nonsyphilitic) 441.2
    dissecting 441.01
    ruptured 441.1
    syphilitic 093.0
  traumatic (complication) (early) — *see* Injury, blood vessel, by site
  tricuspid (heart) (valve) — *see* Endocarditis, tricuspid
  ulnar 442.0
  upper extremity 442.0
  valve, valvular — *see* Endocarditis
  venous 456.8
    congenital NEC (*see also* Aneurysm, congenital) 747.60
  ventricle (arteriovenous) (*see also* Aneurysm, heart) 414.10
  visceral artery NEC 442.84
Angiectasis 459.89
Angiectopia 459.9
Angiitis 447.6
  allergic granulomatous 446.4
  hypersensitivity 446.20
    Goodpasture's syndrome 446.21
    specified NEC 446.29
  necrotizing 446.0
    Wegener's (necrotizing respiratory granulomatosis) 446.4
Angina (attack) (cardiac) (chest) (effort) (heart) (pectoris) (syndrome) (vasomotor) 413.9
  abdominal 557.1
  accelerated 411.1
  agranulocytic 288.03
  aphthous 074.0
  catarrhal 462
  crescendo 411.1
  croupous 464.4
  cruris 443.9
    due to atherosclerosis NEC (*see also* Arteriosclerosis, extremities) 440.20
  decubitus 413.0
  diphtheritic (membranous) 032.0
  equivalent 413.9
  erysipelatous 034.0
  erythematous 462
  exudative, chronic 476.0
  faucium 478.29
  gangrenous 462
    diphtheritic 032.0
  infectious 462
  initial 411.1
  intestinal 557.1
  ludovici 528.3
  Ludwig's 528.3

Angina — *continued*
  malignant 462
    diphtheritic 032.0
  membranous 464.4
    diphtheritic 032.0
  mesenteric 557.1
  monocytic 075
  nocturnal 413.0
  phlegmonous 475
    diphtheritic 032.0
  preinfarctional 411.1
  Prinzmetal's 413.1
  progressive 411.1
  pseudomembranous 101
  psychogenic 306.2
  pultaceous, diphtheritic 032.0
  scarlatinal 034.1
  septic 034.0
  simple 462
  stable NEC 413.9
  staphylococcal 462
  streptococcal 034.0
  stridulous, diphtheritic 032.3
  syphilitic 093.9
    congenital 090.5
  tonsil 475
  trachealis 464.4
  unstable 411.1
  variant 413.1
  Vincent's 101
Angioblastoma (M9161/1) — *see* Neoplasm, connective tissue, uncertain behavior
Angiocholecystitis — *see also* Cholecystitis, acute 575.0
Angiocholitis — *see also* Cholecystitis, acute 576.1
Angiodysgensis spinalis 336.1
Angiodysplasia (intestinalis) (intestine) 569.84
  with hemorrhage 569.85
  duodenum 537.82
    with hemorrhage 537.83
  stomach 537.82
    with hemorrhage 537.83
Angioedema (allergic) (any site) (with urticaria) 995.1
  hereditary 277.6
Angioendothelioma (M9130/1) — *see also* Neoplasm, by site, uncertain behavior
  benign (M9130/0) (*see also* Hemangioma, by site) 228.00
  bone (M9260/3) — *see* Neoplasm, bone, malignant
  Ewing's (M9260/3) — *see* Neoplasm, bone, malignant
  nervous system (M9130/0) 228.09
Angiofibroma (M9160/0) — *see also* Neoplasm, by site, benign
  juvenile (M9160/0) 210.7
    specified site — *see* Neoplasm, by site, benign
    unspecified site 210.7
Angiohemophilia (A) (B) 286.4
Angioid streaks (choroid) (retina) 363.43
Angiokeratoma (M9141/0) — *see also* Neoplasm, skin, benign
  corporis diffusum 272.7
Angiokeratosis
  diffuse 272.7
Angioleiomyoma (M8894/0) — *see* Neoplasm, connective tissue, benign
Angioleucitis 683
Angiolipoma (M8861/0) — *see also* Lipoma, by site 214.9
  infiltrating (M8861/1) — *see* Neoplasm, connective tissue, uncertain behavior
Angioma (M9120/0) — *see also* Hemangioma, by site 228.00
  capillary 448.1
  hemorrhagicum hereditaria 448.0
  malignant (M9120/3) — *see* Neoplasm, connective tissue, malignant
  pigmentosum et atrophicum 757.33
  placenta — *see* Placenta, abnormal
  plexiform (M9131/0) — *see* Hemangioma, by site
  senile 448.1

Angioma — *see also* Hemangioma, by site — *continued*
  serpiginosum 709.1
  spider 448.1
  stellate 448.1
Angiomatosis 757.32
  bacillary 083.8
  corporis diffusum universale 272.7
  cutaneocerebral 759.6
  encephalocutaneous 759.6
  encephalofacial 759.6
  encephalotrigeminal 759.6
  hemorrhagic familial 448.0
  hereditary familial 448.0
  heredofamilial 448.0
  meningo-oculofacial 759.6
  multiple sites 228.09
  neuro-oculocutaneous 759.6
  retina (Hippel's disease) 759.6
  retinocerebellosa 759.6
  retinocerebral 759.6
  systemic 228.09
Angiomyolipoma (M8860/0)
  specified site — *see* Neoplasm, connective tissue, benign
  unspecified site 223.0
Angiomyoliposarcoma (M8860/3) — *see* Neoplasm, connective tissue, malignant
Angiomyoma (M8894/0) — *see* Neoplasm, connective tissue, benign
Angiomyosarcoma (M8894/3) — *see* Neoplasm, connective tissue, malignant
Angioneurosis 306.2
Angioneurotic edema (allergic) (any site) (with urticaria) 995.1
  hereditary 277.6
Angiopathia, angiopathy 459.9
  diabetic (peripheral) 250.7 ☑ *[443.81]*
    due to secondary diabetes 249.7 ☑ *[443.81]*
  peripheral 443.9
    diabetic 250.7 ☑ *[443.81]*
      due to secondary diabetes 249.7 ☑ *[443.81]*
    specified type NEC 443.89
  retinae syphilitica 093.89
  retinalis (juvenilis) 362.18
    background 362.10
    diabetic 250.5 ☑ *[362.01]*
      due to secondary diabetes 249.5 ☑ *[362.01]*
    proliferative 362.29
    tuberculous (*see also* Tuberculosis) 017.3 ☑ *[362.18]*
Angiosarcoma (M9120/3) — *see* Neoplasm, connective tissue, malignant
Angiosclerosis — *see* Arteriosclerosis
Angioscotoma, enlarged 368.42
Angiospasm 443.9
  brachial plexus 353.0
  cerebral 435.9
  cervical plexus 353.2
  nerve
    arm 354.9
      axillary 353.0
      median 354.1
      ulnar 354.2
    autonomic (*see also* Neuropathy, peripheral, autonomic) 337.9
    axillary 353.0
    leg 355.8
      plantar 355.6
    lower extremity — *see* Angiospasm, nerve, leg
    median 354.1
    peripheral NEC 355.9
    spinal NEC 355.9
    sympathetic (*see also* Neuropathy, peripheral, autonomic) 337.9
    ulnar 354.2
    upper extremity — *see* Angiospasm, nerve, arm
  peripheral NEC 443.9
  traumatic 443.9
    foot 443.9
    leg 443.9

Angiospasm — *continued*
  vessel 443.9
Angiospastic disease or edema 443.9
Angle's
  class I 524.21
  class II 524.22
  class III 524.23
Anguillulosis 127.2
Angulation
  cecum (*see also* Obstruction, intestine) 560.9
  coccyx (acquired) 738.6
    congenital 756.19
  femur (acquired) 736.39
    congenital 755.69
  intestine (large) (small) (*see also* Obstruction, intestine) 560.9
  sacrum (acquired) 738.5
    congenital 756.19
  sigmoid (flexure) (*see also* Obstruction, intestine) 560.9
  spine (*see also* Curvature, spine) 737.9
  tibia (acquired) 736.89
    congenital 755.69
  ureter 593.3
  wrist (acquired) 736.09
    congenital 755.59
Angulus infectiosus 686.8
Anhedonia 780.99
Anhidrosis (lid) (neurogenic) (thermogenic) 705.0
Anhydration 276.51
  with
    hypernatremia 276.0
    hyponatremia 276.1
Anhydremia 276.52
  with
    hypernatremia 276.0
    hyponatremia 276.1
Anidrosis 705.0
Aniridia (congenital) 743.45
Anisakiasis (infection) (infestation) 127.1
Anisakis larva infestation 127.1
Aniseikonia 367.32
Anisocoria (pupil) 379.41
  congenital 743.46
Anisocytosis 790.09
Anisometropia (congenital) 367.31
Ankle — *see* condition
Ankyloblepharon (acquired) (eyelid) 374.46
  filiforme (adnatum) (congenital) 743.62
  total 743.62
Ankylodactly — *see also* Syndactylism 755.10
Ankyloglossia 750.0
Ankylosis (fibrous) (osseous) 718.50
  ankle 718.57
  any joint, produced by surgical fusion V45.4
  cricoarytenoid (cartilage) (joint) (larynx) 478.79
  dental 521.6
  ear ossicle NEC 385.22
    malleus 385.21
  elbow 718.52
  finger 718.54
  hip 718.55
  incostapedial joint (infectional) 385.22
  joint, produced by surgical fusion NEC V45.4
  knee 718.56
  lumbosacral (joint) 724.6
  malleus 385.21
  multiple sites 718.59
  postoperative (status) V45.4
  sacroiliac (joint) 724.6
  shoulder 718.51
  specified site NEC 718.58
  spine NEC 724.9
  surgical V45.4
  teeth, tooth (hard tissues) 521.6
  temporomandibular joint 524.61
  wrist 718.53
Ankylostoma — *see* Ancylostoma
Ankylostomiasis (intestinal) — *see* Ancylostomiasis
Ankylurethria — *see also* Stricture, urethra 598.9
Annular — *see also* condition
  detachment, cervix 622.8

Annular — *see also* condition — *continued*
  organ or site, congenital NEC — *see* Distortion
  pancreas (congenital) 751.7
Anodontia (complete) (partial) (vera) 520.0
  with abnormal spacing 524.30
  acquired 525.10
    causing malocclusion 524.30
    due to
      caries 525.13
      extraction 525.10
      periodontal disease 525.12
      trauma 525.11
Anomaly, anomalous (congenital) (unspecified type) 759.9
  abdomen 759.9
  abdominal wall 756.70
  acoustic nerve 742.9
  adrenal (gland) 759.1
  Alder (-Reilly) (leukocyte granulation) 288.2
  alimentary tract 751.9
    lower 751.5
      specified type NEC 751.8
    upper (any part, except tongue) 750.9
      tongue 750.10
        specified type NEC 750.19
  alveolar 524.70
    ridge (process) 525.8
    specified type NEC 524.79
  ankle (joint) 755.69
  anus, anal (canal) 751.5
  aorta, aortic 747.20
    arch 747.21
    coarctation (postductal) (preductal) 747.10
    cusp or valve NEC 746.9
    septum 745.0
    specified type NEC 747.29
  aorticopulmonary septum 745.0
  apertures, diaphragm 756.6
  appendix 751.5
  aqueduct of Sylvius 742.3
    with spina bifida (*see also* Spina bifida) 741.0 ☑
  arm 755.50
    reduction (*see also* Deformity, reduction, upper limb) 755.20
  arteriovenous (congenital) (peripheral) NEC 747.60
    brain 747.81
    cerebral 747.81
    coronary 746.85
    gastrointestinal 747.61
      acquired — *see* Angiodysplasia
    lower limb 747.64
    renal 747.62
    specified site NEC 747.69
    spinal 747.82
    upper limb 747.63
  artery (*see also* Anomaly, peripheral vascular system) NEC 747.60
    brain 747.81
    cerebral 747.81
    coronary 746.85
    eye 743.9
    pulmonary 747.39
    renal 747.62
    retina 743.9
    umbilical 747.5
  arytenoepiglottic folds 748.3
  atrial
    bands 746.9
    folds 746.9
    septa 745.5
  atrioventricular
    canal 745.69
    common 745.69
    conduction 426.7
    excitation 426.7
    septum 745.4
  atrium — *see* Anomaly, atrial
  auditory canal 744.3
    specified type NEC 744.29
      with hearing impairment 744.02
  auricle
    ear 744.3

☑ **Additional Digit Required** — Refer to the Tabular List for Digit Selection   ᵂ **Subterms under main terms may continue to next column or page**

2014 ICD-9-CM   ▶◀ **Revised Text**   ● **New Line**   ▲ **Revised Code**   **Volume 2 — 21**

Anomaly, anomalous — *continued*
auricle — *continued*
  ear — *continued*
    causing impairment of hearing 744.02
    heart 746.9
    septum 745.5
  autosomes, autosomal NEC 758.5
  Axenfeld's 743.44
  back 759.9
  band
    atrial 746.9
    heart 746.9
    ventricular 746.9
  Bartholin's duct 750.9
  biliary duct or passage 751.60
    atresia 751.61
  bladder (neck) (sphincter) (trigone) 753.9
    specified type NEC 753.8
  blood vessel 747.9
    artery — *see* Anomaly, artery
    peripheral vascular — *see* Anomaly, peripheral vascular system
    vein — *see* Anomaly, vein
  bone NEC 756.9
    ankle 755.69
    arm 755.50
    chest 756.3
    cranium 756.0
    face 756.0
    finger 755.50
    foot 755.67
    forearm 755.50
    frontal 756.0
    head 756.0
    hip 755.63
    leg 755.60
    lumbosacral 756.10
    nose 748.1
    pelvic girdle 755.60
    rachitic 756.4
    rib 756.3
    shoulder girdle 755.50
    skull 756.0
      with
        anencephalus 740.0
        encephalocele 742.0
        hydrocephalus 742.3
          with spina bifida (*see also* Spina bifida) 741.0 ☑
        microcephalus 742.1
    toe 755.66
  brain 742.9
    multiple 742.4
    reduction 742.2
    specified type NEC 742.4
    vessel 747.81
  branchial cleft NEC 744.49
    cyst 744.42
    fistula 744.41
    persistent 744.41
    sinus (external) (internal) 744.41
  breast 757.6
  broad ligament 752.10
    specified type NEC 752.19
  bronchus 748.3
  bulbar septum 745.0
  bulbus cordis 745.9
    persistent (in left ventricle) 745.8
  bursa 756.9
  canal of Nuck 752.9
  canthus 743.9
  capillary NEC (*see also* Anomaly, peripheral vascular system) 747.60
  cardiac 746.9
    septal closure 745.9
      acquired 429.71
    valve NEC 746.9
      pulmonary 746.00
      specified type NEC 746.89
  cardiovascular system 746.9
    complicating pregnancy, childbirth, or puerperium 648.5 ☑
  carpus 755.50
  cartilage, trachea 748.3
  cartilaginous 756.9

Anomaly, anomalous — *continued*
caruncle, lacrimal, lachrymal 743.9
cascade stomach 750.7
cauda equina 742.59
cecum 751.5
cerebral (*see also* Anomaly, brain vessels) 747.81
cerebrovascular system 747.81
cervix (uterus) 752.40
  with doubling of vagina and uterus 752.2
  in pregnancy or childbirth 654.6 ☑
    affecting fetus or newborn 763.89
    causing obstructed labor 660.2 ☑
      affecting fetus or newborn 763.1
Chédiak-Higashi (-Steinbrinck) (congenital gigantism of peroxidase granules) 288.2
cheek 744.9
chest (wall) 756.3
chin 744.9
  specified type NEC 744.89
chordae tendineae 746.9
choroid 743.9
  plexus 742.9
chromosomes, chromosomal 758.9
  13 (13-15) 758.1
  18 (16-18) 758.2
  21 or 22 758.0
  autosomes NEC (*see also* Abnormal, autosomes) 758.5
    deletion 758.39
    Christchurch 758.39
  D_1 758.1
  E_3 758.2
  G 758.0
  mitochondrial 758.9
  mosaics 758.89
  sex 758.81
    complement, XO 758.6
    complement, XXX 758.81
    complement, XXY 758.7
    complement, XYY 758.81
    gonadal dysgenesis 758.6
    Klinefelter's 758.7
    Turner's 758.6
  trisomy 21 758.0
cilia 743.9
circulatory system 747.9
  specified type NEC 747.89
clavicle 755.51
clitoris 752.40
coccyx 756.10
colon 751.5
common duct 751.60
communication
  coronary artery 746.85
  left ventricle with right atrium 745.4
concha (ear) 744.3
connection
  renal vessels with kidney 747.62
  total pulmonary venous 747.41
connective tissue 756.9
  specified type NEC 756.89
cornea 743.9
  shape 743.41
  size 743.41
  specified type NEC 743.49
coronary
  artery 746.85
  vein 746.89
cranium — *see* Anomaly, skull
cricoid cartilage 748.3
cushion, endocardial 745.60
  specified type NEC 745.69
cystic duct 751.60
dental arch 524.20
  specified NEC 524.29
dental arch relationship 524.20
  angle's class I 524.21
  angle's class II 524.22
  angle's class III 524.23
  articulation
    anterior 524.27
    posterior 524.27
    reverse 524.27

Anomaly, anomalous — *continued*
dental arch relationship — *continued*
  disto-occlusion 524.22
    division I 524.22
    division II 524.22
  excessive horizontal overlap 524.26
  interarch distance (excessive) (inadequate) 524.28
  mesio-occlusion 524.23
  neutro-occlusion 524.21
  open
    anterior occlusal relationship 524.24
    posterior occlusal relationship 524.25
  specified NEC 524.29
dentition 520.6
dentofacial NEC 524.9
  functional 524.50
  specified type NEC 524.89
dermatoglyphic 757.2
Descemet's membrane 743.9
  specified type NEC 743.49
development
  cervix 752.40
  vagina 752.40
  vulva 752.40
diaphragm, diaphragmatic (apertures) NEC 756.6
digestive organ(s) or system 751.9
  lower 751.5
  specified type NEC 751.8
  upper 750.9
distribution, coronary artery 746.85
ductus
  arteriosus 747.0
  Botalli 747.0
duodenum 751.5
dura 742.9
  brain 742.4
  spinal cord 742.59
ear 744.3
  causing impairment of hearing 744.00
    specified type NEC 744.09
  external 744.3
    causing impairment of hearing 744.02
    specified type NEC 744.29
  inner (causing impairment of hearing) 744.05
  middle, except ossicles (causing impairment of hearing) 744.03
    ossicles 744.04
  ossicles 744.04
  prominent auricle 744.29
  specified type NEC 744.29
    with hearing impairment 744.09
Ebstein's (heart) 746.2
  tricuspid valve 746.2
ectodermal 757.9
Eisenmenger's (ventricular septal defect) 745.4
ejaculatory duct 752.9
  specified type NEC 752.89
elbow (joint) 755.50
endocardial cushion 745.60
  specified type NEC 745.69
endocrine gland 759.2
epididymis 752.9
epiglottis 748.3
esophagus 750.9
  specified type NEC 750.4
Eustachian tube 744.3
  specified type NEC 744.24
eye (any part) 743.9
  adnexa 743.9
    specified type NEC 743.69
  anophthalmos 743.00
  anterior
    chamber and related structures 743.9
      angle 743.9
        specified type NEC 743.44
      specified type NEC 743.44
    segment 743.9
      combined 743.48
      multiple 743.48
      specified type NEC 743.49
  cataract (*see also* Cataract) 743.30

Anomaly, anomalous — *continued*
eye — *continued*
  glaucoma (*see also* Buphthalmia) 743.20
  lid 743.9
    specified type NEC 743.63
  microphthalmos (*see also* Microphthalmos) 743.10
  posterior segment 743.9
    specified type NEC 743.59
    vascular 743.58
    vitreous 743.9
      specified type NEC 743.51
  ptosis (eyelid) 743.61
  retina 743.9
    specified type NEC 743.59
  sclera 743.9
    specified type NEC 743.47
  specified type NEC 743.8
eyebrow 744.89
eyelid 743.9
  specified type NEC 743.63
face (any part) 744.9
  bone(s) 756.0
  specified type NEC 744.89
fallopian tube 752.10
  specified type NEC 752.19
fascia 756.9
  specified type NEC 756.89
femur 755.60
fibula 755.60
finger 755.50
  supernumerary 755.01
  webbed (*see also* Syndactylism, fingers) 755.11
fixation, intestine 751.4
flexion (joint) 755.9
  hip or thigh (*see also* Dislocation, hip, congenital) 754.30
folds, heart 746.9
foot 755.67
foramen
  Botalli 745.5
  ovale 745.5
forearm 755.50
forehead (*see also* Anomaly, skull) 756.0
form, teeth 520.2
fovea centralis 743.9
frontal bone (*see also* Anomaly, skull) 756.0
gallbladder 751.60
Gartner's duct 752.41
gastrointestinal tract 751.9
  specified type NEC 751.8
  vessel 747.61
genitalia, genital organ(s) or system
  female 752.9
    external 752.40
      specified type NEC 752.49
    internal NEC 752.9
  male (external and internal) 752.9
    epispadias 752.62
    hidden penis 752.65
    hydrocele, congenital 778.6
    hypospadias 752.61
    micropenis 752.64
    testis, undescended 752.51
      retractile 752.52
    specified type NEC 752.89
genitourinary NEC 752.9
Gerbode 745.4
globe (eye) 743.9
glottis 748.3
granulation or granulocyte, genetic 288.2
  constitutional 288.2
  leukocyte 288.2
gum 750.9
gyri 742.9
hair 757.9
  specified type NEC 757.4
hand 755.50
hard tissue formation in pulp 522.3
head (*see also* Anomaly, skull) 756.0
heart 746.9
  auricle 746.9
  bands 746.9
  fibroelastosis cordis 425.3
  folds 746.9

Anomaly, anomalous — *continued*
  heart — *continued*
    malposition 746.87
    maternal, affecting fetus or newborn
      760.3
    obstructive NEC 746.84
    patent ductus arteriosus (Botalli) 747.0
    septum 745.9
      acquired 429.71
      aortic 745.0
      aorticopulmonary 745.0
      atrial 745.5
      auricular 745.5
      between aorta and pulmonary artery
        745.0
      endocardial cushion type 745.60
        specified type NEC 745.69
      interatrial 745.5
      interventricular 745.4
        with pulmonary stenosis or atre-
          sia, dextraposition of aor-
          ta, and hypertrophy of
          right ventricle 745.2
        acquired 429.71
      specified type NEC 745.8
      ventricular 745.4
        with pulmonary stenosis or atre-
          sia, dextraposition of aor-
          ta, and hypertrophy of
          right ventricle 745.2
        acquired 429.71
    specified type NEC 746.89
    tetralogy of Fallot 745.2
    valve NEC 746.9
      aortic 746.9
        atresia 746.89
        bicuspid valve 746.4
        insufficiency 746.4
        specified type NEC 746.89
        stenosis 746.3
          subaortic 746.81
          supravalvular 747.22
      mitral 746.9
        atresia 746.89
        insufficiency 746.6
        specified type NEC 746.89
        stenosis 746.5
      pulmonary 746.00
        atresia 746.01
        insufficiency 746.09
        stenosis 746.02
          infundibular 746.83
          subvalvular 746.83
      tricuspid 746.9
        atresia 746.1
        stenosis 746.1
      ventricle 746.9
  heel 755.67
  Hegglin's 288.2
  hemianencephaly 740.0
  hemicephaly 740.0
  hemicrania 740.0
  hepatic duct 751.60
  hip (joint) 755.63
  hourglass
    bladder 753.8
    gallbladder 751.69
    stomach 750.7
  humerus 755.50
  hymen 752.40
  hypersegmentation of neutrophils, heredi-
    tary 288.2
  hypophyseal 759.2
  ileocecal (coil) (valve) 751.5
  ileum (intestine) 751.5
  ilium 755.60
  integument 757.9
    specified type NEC 757.8
  interarch distance (excessive) (inadequate)
    524.28
  intervertebral cartilage or disc 756.10
  intestine (large) (small) 751.5
    fixational type 751.4
  iris 743.9
    specified type NEC 743.46
  ischium 755.60

Anomaly, anomalous — *continued*
  jaw-cranial base relationship 524.10
    specified NEC 524.19
  jaw NEC 524.9
    closure 524.51
    size (major) NEC 524.00
    specified type NEC 524.89
  jejunum 751.5
  joint 755.9
    hip
      dislocation (*see also* Dislocation, hip,
        congenital) 754.30
      predislocation (*see also* Subluxation,
        congenital, hip) 754.32
      preluxation (*see also* Subluxation,
        congenital, hip) 754.32
      subluxation (*see also* Subluxation,
        congenital, hip) 754.32
    lumbosacral 756.10
      spondylolisthesis 756.12
      spondylosis 756.11
    multiple arthrogryposis 754.89
    sacroiliac 755.69
  Jordan's 288.2
  kidney(s) (calyx) (pelvis) 753.9
    vessel 747.62
  Klippel-Feil (brevicollis) 756.16
  knee (joint) 755.64
  labium (majus) (minus) 752.40
  labyrinth, membranous (causing impair-
    ment of hearing) 744.05
  lacrimal
    apparatus, duct or passage 743.9
      specified type NEC 743.65
    gland 743.9
      specified type NEC 743.64
  Langdon Down (mongolism) 758.0
  larynx, laryngeal (muscle) 748.3
    web, webbed 748.2
  leg (lower) (upper) 755.60
    reduction NEC (*see also* Deformity, reduc-
      tion, lower limb) 755.30
  lens 743.9
    shape 743.36
    specified type NEC 743.39
  leukocytes, genetic 288.2
    granulation (constitutional) 288.2
  lid (fold) 743.9
  ligament 756.9
    broad 752.10
    round 752.9
  limb, except reduction deformity 755.9
    lower 755.60
      reduction deformity (*see also* Defor-
        mity, reduction, lower limb)
        755.30
      specified type NEC 755.69
    upper 755.50
      reduction deformity (*see also* Defor-
        mity, reduction, upper limb)
        755.20
      specified type NEC 755.59
  lip 750.9
    harelip (*see also* Cleft, lip) 749.10
    specified type NEC 750.26
  liver (duct) 751.60
    atresia 751.69
  lower extremity 755.60
    vessel 747.64
  lumbosacral (joint) (region) 756.10
  lung (fissure) (lobe) NEC 748.60
    agenesis 748.5
    specified type NEC 748.69
  lymphatic system 759.9
  Madelung's (radius) 755.54
  mandible 524.9
    size NEC 524.00
  maxilla 524.9
    size NEC 524.00
  May (-Hegglin) 288.2
  meatus urinarius 753.9
    specified type NEC 753.8
  meningeal bands or folds, constriction of
    742.8
  meninges 742.9
    brain 742.4

Anomaly, anomalous — *continued*
  meninges — *continued*
    spinal 742.59
  meningocele (*see also* Spina bifida) 741.9 ☑
    acquired 349.2
  mesentery 751.9
  metacarpus 755.50
  metatarsus 755.67
  middle ear, except ossicles (causing impair-
    ment of hearing) 744.03
    ossicles 744.04
  mitral (leaflets) (valve) 746.9
    atresia 746.89
    insufficiency 746.6
    specified type NEC 746.89
    stenosis 746.5
  mouth 750.9
    specified type NEC 750.26
  multiple NEC 759.7
    specified type NEC 759.89
  muscle 756.9
    eye 743.9
      specified type NEC 743.69
    specified type NEC 756.89
  musculoskeletal system, except limbs 756.9
    specified type NEC 756.9
  nail 757.9
    specified type NEC 757.5
  narrowness, eyelid 743.62
  nasal sinus or septum 748.1
  neck (any part) 744.9
    specified type NEC 744.89
  nerve 742.9
    acoustic 742.9
      specified type NEC 742.8
    optic 742.9
      specified type NEC 742.8
    specified type NEC 742.8
  nervous system NEC 742.9
    brain 742.9
      specified type NEC 742.4
    specified type NEC 742.8
  neurological 742.9
  nipple 757.6
  nonteratogenic NEC 754.89
  nose, nasal (bone) (cartilage) (septum) (si-
    nus) 748.1
  ocular muscle 743.9
  omphalomesenteric duct 751.0
  opening, pulmonary veins 747.49
  optic
    disc 743.9
      specified type NEC 743.57
    nerve 742.9
  opticociliary vessels 743.9
  orbit (eye) 743.9
    specified type NEC 743.66
  organ
    of Corti (causing impairment of hearing)
      744.05
    or site 759.9
      specified type NEC 759.89
  origin
    both great arteries from same ventricle
      745.11
    coronary artery 746.85
    innominate artery 747.69
    left coronary artery from pulmonary
      artery 746.85
    pulmonary artery 747.39
    renal vessels 747.62
    subclavian artery (left) (right) 747.21
  osseous meatus (ear) 744.03
  ovary 752.0
  oviduct 752.10
  palate (hard) (soft) 750.9
    cleft (*see also* Cleft, palate) 749.00
  pancreas (duct) 751.7
  papillary muscles 746.9
  parathyroid gland 759.2
  paraurethral ducts 753.9
  parotid (gland) 750.9
  patella 755.64
  Pelger-Huët (hereditary hyposegmentation)
    288.2
  pelvic girdle 755.60

Anomaly, anomalous — *continued*
  pelvic girdle — *continued*
    specified type NEC 755.69
  pelvis (bony) 755.60
    complicating delivery 653.0 ☑
    rachitic 268.1
      fetal 756.4
  penis (glans) 752.69
  pericardium 746.89
  peripheral vascular system NEC 747.60
    gastrointestinal 747.61
    lower limb 747.64
    renal 747.62
    specified site NEC 747.69
    spinal 747.82
    upper limb 747.63
  Peter's 743.44
  pharynx 750.9
    branchial cleft 744.41
    specified type NEC 750.29
  Pierre Robin 756.0
  pigmentation 709.00
    congenital 757.33
    specified NEC 709.09
  pituitary (gland) 759.2
  pleural folds 748.8
  portal vein 747.40
  position tooth, teeth 524.30
    crowding 524.31
    displacement 524.30
      horizontal 524.33
      vertical 524.34
    distance
      interocclusal
        excessive 524.37
        insufficient 524.36
    excessive spacing 524.32
    rotation 524.35
    specified NEC 524.39
  preauricular sinus 744.46
  prepuce 752.9
  prostate 752.9
  pulmonary 748.60
    artery 747.39
    circulation 747.39
    specified type NEC 748.69
    valve 746.00
      atresia 746.01
      insufficiency 746.09
      specified type NEC 746.09
      stenosis 746.02
        infundibular 746.83
        subvalvular 746.83
    vein 747.40
    venous
      connection 747.49
        partial 747.42
        total 747.41
      return 747.49
        partial 747.42
        total (TAPVR) (complete) (subdi-
          aphragmatic) (supradi-
          aphragmatic) 747.41
  pupil 743.9
  pylorus 750.9
    hypertrophy 750.5
    stenosis 750.5
  rachitic, fetal 756.4
  radius 755.50
  rectovaginal (septum) 752.40
  rectum 751.5
  refraction 367.9
  renal 753.9
    vessel 747.62
  respiratory system 748.9
    specified type NEC 748.8
  rib 756.3
    cervical 756.2
  Rieger's 743.44
  rings, trachea 748.3
  rotation (*see also* Malrotation)
    hip or thigh (*see also* Subluxation, con-
      genital, hip) 754.32
  round ligament 752.9
  sacroiliac (joint) 755.69
  sacrum 756.10

☑ **Additional Digit Required** — Refer to the Tabular List for Digit Selection
▽ **Subterms under main terms may continue to next column or page**

2014 ICD-9-CM   ▶◀ **Revised Text**   ● **New Line**   ▲ **Revised Code**   Volume 2 — 23

Anomaly, anomalous — Anomaly, anomalous

Anomaly, anomalous — *continued*
saddle
    back 754.2
    nose 754.0
        syphilitic 090.5
salivary gland or duct 750.9
    specified type NEC 750.26
scapula 755.50
sclera 743.9
    specified type NEC 743.47
scrotum 752.9
sebaceous gland 757.9
seminal duct or tract 752.9
sense organs 742.9
    specified type NEC 742.8
septum
    heart — *see* Anomaly, heart, septum
    nasal 748.1
sex chromosomes NEC (*see also* Anomaly, chromosomes) 758.81
shoulder (girdle) (joint) 755.50
    specified type NEC 755.59
sigmoid (flexure) 751.5
sinus of Valsalva 747.29
site NEC 759.9
skeleton generalized NEC 756.50
skin (appendage) 757.9
    specified type NEC 757.39
skull (bone) 756.0
    with
        anencephalus 740.0
        encephalocele 742.0
        hydrocephalus 742.3
            with spina bifida (*see also* Spina bifida) 741.0 ☑
        microcephalus 742.1
specified type NEC
    adrenal (gland) 759.1
    alimentary tract (complete) (partial) 751.8
        lower 751.5
        upper 750.8
    ankle 755.69
    anus, anal (canal) 751.5
    aorta, aortic 747.29
        arch 747.21
    appendix 751.5
    arm 755.59
    artery (peripheral) NEC (*see also* Anomaly, peripheral vascular system) 747.60
        brain 747.81
        coronary 746.85
        eye 743.58
        pulmonary 747.39
        retinal 743.58
        umbilical 747.5
    auditory canal 744.29
        causing impairment of hearing 744.02
    bile duct or passage 751.69
    bladder 753.8
        neck 753.8
    bone(s) 756.9
        arm 755.59
        face 756.0
        leg 755.69
        pelvic girdle 755.69
        shoulder girdle 755.59
        skull 756.0
            with
                anencephalus 740.0
                encephalocele 742.0
                hydrocephalus 742.3
                    with spina bifida (*see also* Spina bifida) 741.0 ☑
                microcephalus 742.1
        brain 742.4
        breast 757.6
        broad ligament 752.19
        bronchus 748.3
        canal of Nuck 752.89
        cardiac septal closure 745.8
        carpus 755.59
        cartilaginous 756.9

Anomaly, anomalous — *continued*
specified type — *continued*
    cecum 751.5
    cervix 752.49
    chest (wall) 756.3
    chin 744.89
    ciliary body 743.46
    circulatory system 747.89
    clavicle 755.51
    clitoris 752.49
    coccyx 756.19
    colon 751.5
    common duct 751.69
    connective tissue 756.89
    cricoid cartilage 748.3
    cystic duct 751.69
    diaphragm 756.6
    digestive organ(s) or tract 751.8
        lower 751.5
        upper 750.8
    duodenum 751.5
    ear 744.29
        auricle 744.29
            causing impairment of hearing 744.02
        causing impairment of hearing 744.09
        inner (causing impairment of hearing) 744.05
        middle, except ossicles 744.03
            ossicles 744.04
    ejaculatory duct 752.89
    endocrine 759.2
    epiglottis 748.3
    esophagus 750.4
    Eustachian tube 744.24
    eye 743.8
        lid 743.63
        muscle 743.69
    face 744.89
        bone(s) 756.0
    fallopian tube 752.19
    fascia 756.89
    femur 755.69
    fibula 755.69
    finger 755.59
    foot 755.67
    fovea centralis 743.55
    gallbladder 751.69
    Gartner's duct 752.89
    gastrointestinal tract 751.8
    genitalia, genital organ(s)
        female 752.89
            external 752.49
            internal NEC 752.89
        male 752.89
            penis 752.69
            scrotal transposition 752.81
    genitourinary tract NEC 752.89
    glottis 748.3
    hair 757.4
    hand 755.59
    heart 746.89
        valve NEC 746.89
            pulmonary 746.09
    hepatic duct 751.69
    hydatid of Morgagni 752.89
    hymen 752.49
    integument 757.8
    intestine (large) (small) 751.5
        fixational type 751.4
    iris 743.46
    jejunum 751.5
    joint 755.8
    kidney 753.3
    knee 755.64
    labium (majus) (minus) 752.49
    labyrinth, membranous 744.05
    larynx 748.3
    leg 755.69
    lens 743.39
    limb, except reduction deformity 755.8
        lower 755.69
            reduction deformity (*see also* Deformity, reduction, lower limb) 755.30

Anomaly, anomalous — *continued*
specified type — *continued*
    limb, except reduction deformity — *continued*
        upper 755.59
            reduction deformity (*see also* Deformity, reduction, upper limb) 755.20
    lip 750.26
    liver 751.69
    lung (fissure) (lobe) 748.69
    meatus urinarius 753.8
    metacarpus 755.59
    mouth 750.26
    Müllerian
        cervix 752.49
        uterus 752.39
        vagina 752.49
    muscle 756.89
        eye 743.69
    musculoskeletal system, except limbs 756.9
    nail 757.5
    neck 744.89
    nerve 742.8
        acoustic 742.8
        optic 742.8
    nervous system 742.8
    nipple 757.6
    nose 748.1
    organ NEC 759.89
        of Corti 744.05
    osseous meatus (ear) 744.03
    ovary 752.0
    oviduct 752.19
    pancreas 751.7
    parathyroid 759.2
    patella 755.64
    pelvic girdle 755.69
    penis 752.69
    pericardium 746.89
    peripheral vascular system NEC (*see also* Anomaly, peripheral vascular system) 747.60
    pharynx 750.29
    pituitary 759.2
    prostate 752.89
    radius 755.59
    rectum 751.5
    respiratory system 748.8
    rib 756.3
    round ligament 752.89
    sacrum 756.19
    salivary duct or gland 750.26
    scapula 755.59
    sclera 743.47
    scrotum 752.89
        transposition 752.81
    seminal duct or tract 752.89
    shoulder girdle 755.59
    site NEC 759.89
    skin 757.39
    skull (bone(s)) 756.0
        with
            anencephalus 740.0
            encephalocele 742.0
            hydrocephalus 742.3
                with spina bifida (*see also* Spina bifida) 741.0 ☑
            microcephalus 742.1
    specified organ or site NEC 759.89
    spermatic cord 752.89
    spinal cord 742.59
    spine 756.19
    spleen 759.0
    sternum 756.3
    stomach 750.7
    tarsus 755.67
    tendon 756.89
    testis 752.89
    thorax (wall) 756.3
    thymus 759.2
    thyroid (gland) 759.2
        cartilage 748.3
    tibia 755.69
    toe 755.66

Anomaly, anomalous — *continued*
specified type — *continued*
    tongue 750.19
    trachea (cartilage) 748.3
    ulna 755.59
    urachus 753.7
    ureter 753.4
        obstructive 753.29
    urethra 753.8
        obstructive 753.6
    urinary tract 753.8
    uterus (Müllerian) 752.39
    uvula 750.26
    vagina 752.49
    vascular NEC (*see also* Anomaly, peripheral vascular system) 747.60
        brain 747.81
    vas deferens 752.89
    vein(s) (peripheral) NEC (*see also* Anomaly, peripheral vascular system) 747.60
        brain 747.81
        great 747.49
        portal 747.49
        pulmonary 747.49
    vena cava (inferior) (superior) 747.49
    vertebra 756.19
    vulva 752.49
spermatic cord 752.9
spine, spinal 756.10
    column 756.10
    cord 742.9
        meningocele (*see also* Spina bifida) 741.9 ☑
        specified type NEC 742.59
        spina bifida (*see also* Spina bifida) 741.9 ☑
        vessel 747.82
    meninges 742.59
    nerve root 742.9
spleen 759.0
Sprengel's 755.52
sternum 756.3
stomach 750.9
    specified type NEC 750.7
submaxillary gland 750.9
superior vena cava 747.40
talipes — *see* Talipes
tarsus 755.67
    with complete absence of distal elements 755.31
teeth, tooth NEC 520.9
    position 524.30
        crowding 524.31
        displacement 524.30
            horizontal 524.33
            vertical 524.34
        distance
            interocclusal
                excessive 524.37
                insufficient 524.36
        excessive spacing 524.32
        rotation 524.35
        specified NEC 524.39
    spacing 524.30
tendon 756.9
    specified type NEC 756.89
termination
    coronary artery 746.85
testis 752.9
thebesian valve 746.9
thigh 755.60
    flexion (*see also* Subluxation, congenital, hip) 754.32
thorax (wall) 756.3
throat 750.9
thumb 755.50
    supernumerary 755.01
thymus gland 759.2
thyroid (gland) 759.2
    cartilage 748.3
tibia 755.60
    saber 090.5
toe 755.66
    supernumerary 755.02

Anomaly, anomalous — *continued*
  toe — *continued*
    webbed (*see also* Syndactylism, toes) 755.13
  tongue 750.10
    specified type NEC 750.19
  trachea, tracheal 748.3
    cartilage 748.3
    rings 748.3
  tragus 744.3
  transverse aortic arch 747.21
  trichromata 368.59
  trichromatopsia 368.59
  tricuspid (leaflet) (valve) 746.9
    atresia 746.1
    Ebstein's 746.2
    specified type NEC 746.89
    stenosis 746.1
  trunk 759.9
  Uhl's (hypoplasia of myocardium, right ventricle) 746.84
  ulna 755.50
  umbilicus 759.9
    artery 747.5
  union, trachea with larynx 748.3
  unspecified site 759.9
  upper extremity 755.50
    vessel 747.63
  urachus 753.7
    specified type NEC 753.7
  ureter 753.9
    obstructive 753.20
    specified type NEC 753.4
      obstructive 753.29
  urethra (valve) 753.9
    obstructive 753.6
    specified type NEC 753.8
  urinary tract or system (any part, except urachus) 753.9
    specified type NEC 753.8
    urachus 753.7
  uterus 752.39
    with only one functioning horn 752.33
    in pregnancy or childbirth 654.0 ☑
      affecting fetus or newborn 763.89
      causing obstructed labor 660.2 ☑
        affecting fetus or newborn 763.1
  uvula 750.9
  vagina 752.40
  valleculae 748.3
  valve (heart) NEC 746.9
    formation, ureter 753.29
    pulmonary 746.00
    specified type NEC 746.89
  vascular NEC (*see also* Anomaly, peripheral vascular system) 747.60
    ring 747.21
  vas deferens 752.9
  vein(s) (peripheral) NEC (*see also* Anomaly, peripheral vascular system) 747.60
    brain 747.81
    cerebral 747.81
    coronary 746.89
    great 747.40
      specified type NEC 747.49
    portal 747.40
    pulmonary 747.40
    retina 743.9
  vena cava (inferior) (superior) 747.40
  venous — *see* Anomaly, vein
  venous return (pulmonary) 747.49
    partial 747.42
    total 747.41
  ventricle, ventricular (heart) 746.9
    bands 746.9
    folds 746.9
    septa 745.4
  vertebra 756.10
  vesicourethral orifice 753.9
  vessels NEC (*see also* Anomaly, peripheral vascular system) 747.60
    optic papilla 743.9
  vitelline duct 751.0
  vitreous humor 743.9
    specified type NEC 743.51
  vulva 752.40

Anomaly, anomalous — *continued*
  wrist (joint) 755.50
Anomia 784.69
Anonychia 757.5
  acquired 703.8
Anophthalmos, anophthalmus (clinical) (congenital) (globe) 743.00
  acquired V45.78
Anopsia (altitudinal) (quadrant) 368.46
Anorchia 752.89
Anorchism, anorchidism 752.89
Anorexia 783.0
  hysterical 300.11
  nervosa 307.1
Anosmia — *see also* Disturbance, sensation 781.1
  hysterical 300.11
  postinfectional 478.9
  psychogenic 306.7
  traumatic 951.8
Anosognosia 780.99
Anosphrasia 781.1
Anosteoplasia 756.50
Anotia 744.09
Anovulatory cycle 628.0
Anoxemia 799.02
  newborn 770.88
Anoxia 799.02
  altitude 993.2
  cerebral 348.1
    with
      abortion — *see* Abortion, by type, with specified complication NEC
      ectopic pregnancy (*see also* categories 633.0–633.9) 639.8
      molar pregnancy (*see also* categories 630–632) 639.8
    complicating
      delivery (cesarean) (instrumental) 669.4 ☑
      ectopic or molar pregnancy 639.8
      obstetric anesthesia or sedation 668.2 ☑
    during or resulting from a procedure 997.01
    following
      abortion 639.8
      ectopic or molar pregnancy 639.8
    newborn (*see also* Distress, fetal, liveborn infant) 770.88
  due to drowning 994.1
  fetal, affecting newborn 770.88
  heart — *see* Insufficiency, coronary
  high altitude 993.2
  intrauterine
    fetal death (before onset of labor) 768.0
      during labor 768.1
    liveborn infant — *see* Distress, fetal, liveborn infant
  myocardial — *see* Insufficiency, coronary
  newborn 768.9
    mild or moderate 768.6
    severe 768.5
  pathological 799.02
Anteflexion — *see* Anteversion
Antenatal
  care, normal pregnancy V22.1
    first V22.0
  sampling
    chorionic villus V28.89
  screening of mother (for) V28.9
    based on amniocentesis NEC V28.2
      chromosomal anomalies V28.0
      raised alphafetoprotein levels V28.1
    chromosomal anomalies V28.0
    fetal growth retardation using ulatrasonics V28.4
    genomic V28.89
    isoimmunization V28.5
    malformations using ulatrasonics V28.3
    proteomic V28.89
    raised alphafetoprotein levels in amniotic fluid V28.1
    risk
      pre-term labor V28.82

Antenatal — *continued*
  screening of mother — *continued*
    specified condition NEC V28.89
    Streptococcus B V28.6
  survey
    fetal anatomic V28.81
  testing
    nuchal translucency V28.89
Antepartum — *see* condition
Anterior — *see also* condition
  spinal artery compression syndrome 721.1
Antero-occlusion 524.24
Anteversion
  cervix — *see* Anteversion, uterus
  femur (neck), congenital 755.63
  uterus, uterine (cervix) (postinfectional) (postpartal, old) 621.6
    congenital 752.39
    in pregnancy or childbirth 654.4 ☑
      affecting fetus or newborn 763.89
      causing obstructed labor 660.2 ☑
        affecting fetus or newborn 763.1
Anthracosilicosis (occupational) 500
Anthracosis (lung) (occupational) 500
  lingua 529.3
Anthrax 022.9
  with pneumonia 022.1 [484.5]
  colitis 022.2
  cutaneous 022.0
  gastrointestinal 022.2
  intestinal 022.2
  pulmonary 022.1
  respiratory 022.1
  septicemia 022.3
  specified manifestation NEC 022.8
Anthropoid pelvis 755.69
  with disproportion (fetopelvic) 653.2 ☑
    affecting fetus or newborn 763.1
    causing obstructed labor 660.1 ☑
      affecting fetus or newborn 763.1
Anthropophobia 300.29
Antibioma, breast 611.0
Antibodies
  maternal (blood group) (*see also* Incompatibility) 656.2 ☑
    anti-D, cord blood 656.1 ☑
      fetus or newborn 773.0
Antibody
  anticardiolipin 795.79
    with
      hemorrhagic disorder 286.53
      hypercoagulable state 289.81
  antiphosphatidylglycerol 795.79
    with
      hemorrhagic disorder 286.53
      hypercoagulable state 289.81
  antiphosphatidylinositol 795.79
    with
      hemorrhagic disorder 286.53
      hypercoagulable state 289.81
  antiphosphatidylserine 795.79
    with
      hemorrhagic disorder 286.53
      hypercoagulable state 289.81
  antiphospholipid 795.79
    with
      hemorrhagic disorder 286.53
      hypercoagulable state 289.81
  deficiency syndrome
    agammaglobulinemic 279.00
    congenital 279.04
    hypogammaglobulinemic 279.00
Anticoagulant
  intrinsic, circulating, causing hemorrhagic disorder (*see also* Circulating, anticoagulants) 286.59
  lupus (LAC) 795.79
    with
      hemorrhagic disorder 286.53
      hypercoagulable state 289.81
Antimongolism syndrome 758.39
Antimonial cholera 985.4
Antisocial personality 301.7
Antithrombinemia — *see also* Circulating anticoagulants 286.59

Antithromboplastinemia — *see also* Circulating anticoagulants 286.59
Antithromboplastinogenemia — *see also* Circulating anticoagulants 286.59
Antitoxin complication or reaction — *see* Complications, vaccination
Anton (-Babinski) syndrome (hemiasomatognosia) 307.9
Antritis (chronic) 473.0
  maxilla 473.0
    acute 461.0
  stomach 535.4 ☑
Antrum, antral — *see* condition
Anuria 788.5
  with
    abortion — *see* Abortion, by type, with renal failure
    ectopic pregnancy (*see also* categories 633.0–633.9) 639.3
    molar pregnancy (*see also* categories 630–632) 639.3
  calculus (impacted) (recurrent) 592.9
    kidney 592.0
    ureter 592.1
  congenital 753.3
  due to a procedure 997.5
  following
    abortion 639.3
    ectopic or molar pregnancy 639.3
  newborn 753.3
  postrenal 593.4
  puerperal, postpartum, childbirth 669.3 ☑
  specified as due to a procedure 997.5
  sulfonamide
    correct substance properly administered 788.5
    overdose or wrong substance given or taken 961.0
  traumatic (following crushing) 958.5
Anus, anal — *see also* condition
  high risk human papillomavirus (HPV) DNA test positive 796.75
  low risk human papillomavirus (HPV) DNA test positive 796.79
Anusitis 569.49
Anxiety (neurosis) (reaction) (state) 300.00
  alcohol-induced 291.89
  depression 300.4
  drug-induced 292.89
  due to or associated with physical condition 293.84
  generalized 300.02
  hysteria 300.20
  in
    acute stress reaction 308.0
    transient adjustment reaction 309.24
  panic type 300.01
  separation, abnormal 309.21
  syndrome (organic) (transient) 293.84
Aorta, aortic — *see* condition
Aortectasia — *see also* Ectasia, aortic 447.70
  with aneurysm 441.9
Aortitis (nonsyphilitic) 447.6
  arteriosclerotic 440.0
  calcific 447.6
  Döhle-Heller 093.1
  luetic 093.1
  rheumatic (*see also* Endocarditis, acute, rheumatic) 391.1
  rheumatoid — *see* Arthritis, rheumatoid
  specific 093.1
  syphilitic 093.1
    congenital 090.5
Apathetic 799.25
  thyroid storm (*see also* Thyrotoxicosis) 242.9 ☑
Apathy 799.25
Apepsia 536.8
  achlorhydric 536.0
  psychogenic 306.4
Aperistalsis, esophagus 530.0
Apert-Gallais syndrome (adrenogenital) 255.2
Apertognathia 524.20
Apert's syndrome (acrocephalosyndactyly) 755.55
Aphagia 787.20

☑ **Additional Digit Required** — Refer to the Tabular List for Digit Selection   ▽ **Subterms under main terms may continue to next column or page**

Aphagia — continued
  psychogenic 307.1
Aphakia (acquired) (bilateral) (postoperative)
  (unilateral) 379.31
  congenital 743.35
Aphalangia (congenital) 755.4
  lower limb (complete) (intercalary) (partial)
    (terminal) 755.39
    meaning all digits (complete) (partial)
      755.31
    transverse 755.31
  upper limb (complete) (intercalary) (partial)
    (terminal) 755.29
    meaning all digits (complete) (partial)
      755.21
    transverse 755.21
Aphasia (amnestic) (ataxic) (auditory) (Broca's)
  (choreatic) (classic) (expressive) (global)
  (ideational) (ideokinetic) (ideomotor)
  (jargon) (motor) (nominal) (receptive)
  (semantic) (sensory) (syntactic) (verbal)
  (visual) (Wernicke's) 784.3
  developmental 315.31
  syphilis, tertiary 094.89
  uremic — see Uremia
Aphemia 784.3
  uremic — see Uremia
Aphonia 784.41
  clericorum 784.49
  hysterical 300.11
  organic 784.41
  psychogenic 306.1
Aphthae, aphthous — see also condition
  Bednar's 528.2
  cachectic 529.0
  epizootic 078.4
  fever 078.4
  oral 528.2
  stomatitis 528.2
  thrush 112.0
  ulcer (oral) (recurrent) 528.2
    genital organ(s) NEC
      female 616.50
      male 608.89
    larynx 478.79
Apical — see condition
Apical ballooning syndrome 429.83
Aplasia — see also Agenesis
  alveolar process (acquired) 525.8
    congenital 750.26
  aorta (congenital) 747.22
  aortic valve (congenital) 746.89
  axialis extracorticalis (congenital) 330.0
  bone marrow (myeloid) 284.9
    acquired (secondary) 284.89
    congenital 284.01
    idiopathic 284.9
  brain 740.0
    specified part 742.2
  breast 757.6
  bronchus 748.3
  cementum 520.4
  cerebellar 742.2
  congenital (pure) red cell 284.01
  corpus callosum 742.2
  erythrocyte 284.81
    congenital 284.01
  extracortical axial 330.0
  eye (congenital) 743.00
  fovea centralis (congenital) 743.55
  germinal (cell) 606.0
  iris 743.45
  labyrinth, membranous 744.05
  limb (congenital) 755.4
    lower NEC 755.30
    upper NEC 755.20
  lung (bilateral) (congenital) (unilateral)
    748.5
  nervous system NEC 742.8
  nuclear 742.8
  ovary 752.0
  Pelizaeus-Merzbacher 330.0
  prostate (congenital) 752.89
  red cell (with thymoma) 284.81
    acquired (secondary) 284.81
    due to drugs 284.81

Aplasia — see also Agenesis — continued
  red cell — continued
    adult 284.81
    congenital 284.01
    hereditary 284.01
    of infants 284.01
    primary 284.01
    pure 284.01
      due to drugs 284.81
  round ligament (congenital) 752.89
  salivary gland 750.21
  skin (congenital) 757.39
  spinal cord 742.59
  spleen 759.0
  testis (congenital) 752.89
  thymic, with immunodeficiency 279.2
  thyroid 243
  uterus 752.39
  ventral horn cell 742.59
Apleuria 756.3
Apnea, apneic (spells) 786.03
  newborn, neonatorum 770.81
    essential 770.81
    obstructive 770.82
    primary 770.81
    sleep 770.81
    specified NEC 770.82
  psychogenic 306.1
  sleep, unspecified 780.57
    with
      hypersomnia, unspecified 780.53
      hyposomnia, unspecified 780.51
      insomnia, unspecified 780.51
      sleep disturbance 780.57
    central, in conditions classified else-
      where 327.27
    obstructive (adult) (pediatric) 327.23
    organic 327.20
      other 327.29
    primary central 327.21
Apneumatosis newborn 770.4
Apodia 755.31
Aponeurosis 726.90
Apophysitis (bone) — see also Osteochondrosis 732.9
  calcaneus 732.5
  juvenile 732.6
Apoplectiform convulsions — see also Disease, cerebrovascular, acute 436
Apoplexy, apoplexy, apoplectic — see also
  Disease, cerebrovascular, acute 436
  abdominal 569.89
  adrenal 036.3
  attack 436
  basilar (see also Disease, cerebrovascular,
    acute) 436
  brain (see also Disease, cerebrovascular,
    acute) 436
  bulbar (see also Disease, cerebrovascular,
    acute) 436
  capillary (see also Disease, cerebrovascular,
    acute) 436
  cardiac (see also Infarct, myocardium)
    410.9 ☑
  cerebral (see also Disease, cerebrovascular,
    acute) 436
  chorea (see also Disease, cerebrovascular,
    acute) 436
  congestive (see also Disease, cerebrovascu-
    lar, acute) 436
    newborn 767.4
  embolic (see also Embolism, brain) 434.1 ☑
  fetus 767.0
  fit (see also Disease, cerebrovascular, acute)
    436
  healed or old V12.54
  heart (auricle) (ventricle) (see also Infarct,
    myocardium) 410.9 ☑
  heat 992.0
  hemiplegia (see also Disease, cerebrovascu-
    lar, acute) 436
  hemorrhagic (stroke) (see also Hemorrhage,
    brain) 432.9
  ingravescent (see also Disease, cerebrovas-
    cular, acute) 436

Apoplexia, apoplexy, apoplectic — see also
  Disease, cerebrovascular, acute —
  continued
  late effect — see Late effect(s) (of) cere-
    brovascular disease
  lung — see Embolism, pulmonary
  meninges, hemorrhagic (see also Hemor-
    rhage, subarachnoid) 430
  neonatorum 767.0
  newborn 767.0
  pancreatitis 577.0
  placenta 641.2 ☑
  progressive (see also Disease, cerebrovascu-
    lar, acute) 436
  pulmonary (artery) (vein) — see Embolism,
    pulmonary
  sanguineous (see also Disease, cerebrovas-
    cular, acute) 436
  seizure (see also Disease, cerebrovascular,
    acute) 436
  serous (see also Disease, cerebrovascular,
    acute) 436
  spleen 289.59
  stroke (see also Disease, cerebrovascular,
    acute) 436
  thrombotic (see also Thrombosis, brain)
    434.0 ☑
  uremic — see Uremia
  uteroplacental 641.2 ☑
Appendage
  fallopian tube (cyst of Morgagni) 752.11
  intestine (epiploic) 751.5
  preauricular 744.1
  testicular (organ of Morgagni) 752.89
Appendicitis 541
  with
    perforation, peritonitis (generalized), or
      rupture 540.0
      with peritoneal abscess 540.1
    peritoneal abscess 540.1
  acute (catarrhal) (fulminating) (gangrenous)
    (inflammatory) (obstructive) (retroce-
    cal) (suppurative) 540.9
    with
      perforation, peritonitis, or rupture
        540.0
        with peritoneal abscess 540.1
      peritoneal abscess 540.1
  amebic 006.8
  chronic (recurrent) 542
  exacerbation — see Appendicitis, acute
  fulminating — see Appendicitis, acute
  gangrenous — see Appendicitis, acute
  healed (obliterative) 542
  interval 542
  neurogenic 542
  obstructive 542
  pneumococcal 541
  recurrent 542
  relapsing 542
  retrocecal 541
  subacute (adhesive) 542
  subsiding 542
  suppurative — see Appendicitis, acute
  tuberculous (see also Tuberculosis) 014.8 ☑
Appendiclausis 543.9
Appendicolithiasis 543.9
Appendicopathia oxyurica 127.4
Appendix, appendicular — see also condition
  Morgagni (male) 752.89
    fallopian tube 752.11
Appetite
  depraved 307.52
  excessive 783.6
    psychogenic 307.51
  lack or loss (see also Anorexia) 783.0
    nonorganic origin 307.59
  perverted 307.52
    hysterical 300.11
Apprehension, apprehensiveness (abnormal)
  (state) 300.00
  specified type NEC 300.09
Approximal wear 521.10
Apraxia (classic) (ideational) (ideokinetic)
  (ideomotor) (motor) 784.69
  oculomotor, congenital 379.51

Apraxia — continued
  verbal 784.69
Aptyalism 527.7
Aqueous misdirection 365.83
Arabicum elephantiasis — see also Infesta-
  tion, filarial 125.9
Arachnidism 989.5
Arachnitis — see Meningitis
Arachnodactyly 759.82
Arachnoidism 989.5
Arachnoiditis (acute) (adhesive) (basic) (brain)
  (cerebrospinal) (chiasmal) (chronic)
  (spinal) — see also Meningitis 322.9
  meningococcal (chronic) 036.0
  syphilitic 094.2
  tuberculous (see also Tuberculosis,
    meninges) 013.0 ☑
Araneism 989.5
Arboencephalitis, Australian 062.4
Arborization block (heart) 426.6
Arbor virus, arbovirus (infection) NEC 066.9
Arc-welders' lung 503
Arc-welders' syndrome (photokeratitis) 370.24
ARC 042
Arches — see condition
Arcuate uterus 752.36
Arcuatus uterus 752.36
Arcus (cornea)
  juvenilis 743.43
    interfering with vision 743.42
  senilis 371.41
Areflexia 796.1
Areola — see condition
Argentaffinoma (M8241/1) — see also Neo-
  plasm, by site, uncertain behavior
  benign (M8241/0) — see Neoplasm, by site,
    benign
  malignant (M8241/3) — see Neoplasm, by
    site, malignant
  syndrome 259.2
Argentinian hemorrhagic fever 078.7
Arginosuccinicaciduria 270.6
Argonz-Del Castillo syndrome (nonpuerperal
  galactorrhea and amenorrhea) 253.1
Argyll-Robertson phenomenon, pupil, or
  syndrome (syphilitic) 094.89
  atypical 379.45
  nonluetic 379.45
  nonsyphilitic 379.45
  reversed 379.45
Argyria, argyriasis NEC 985.8
  conjunctiva 372.55
  cornea 371.16
  from drug or medicinal agent
    correct substance properly administered
      709.09
    overdose or wrong substance given or
      taken 961.2
Arhinencephaly 742.2
Arias-Stella phenomenon 621.30
Ariboflavinosis 266.0
Arizona enteritis 008.1
Arm — see condition
Armenian disease 277.31
Arnold-Chiari obstruction or syndrome —
  see also Spina bifida 741.0 ☑
  type I 348.4
  type II (see also Spina bifida) 741.0 ☑
  type III 742.0
  type IV 742.2
Arousals
  confusional 327.41
Arrest, arrested
  active phase of labor 661.1 ☑
    affecting fetus or newborn 763.7
  any plane in pelvis
    complicating delivery 660.1 ☑
      affecting fetus or newborn 763.1
  bone marrow (see also Anemia, aplastic)
    284.9
  cardiac 427.5
    with
      abortion — see Abortion, by type,
        with specified complication
        NEC

☑ Additional Digit Required — Refer to the Tabular List for Digit Selection   ⁽ᴺˢ⁾ Subterms under main terms may continue to next column or page

26 — Volume 2   ▶◀ Revised Text   ● New Line   ▲ Revised Code   2014 ICD-9-CM

Arrest, arrested — *continued*
  cardiac — *continued*
    with — *continued*
      ectopic pregnancy (*see also* categories 633.0–633.9) 639.8
      molar pregnancy (*see also* categories 630–632) 639.8
    complicating
      anesthesia
        correct substance properly administered 427.5
        obstetric 668.1 ☑
        overdose or wrong substance given 968.4
          specified anesthetic — *see* Table of Drugs and Chemicals
    delivery (cesarean) (instrumental) 669.4 ☑
    ectopic or molar pregnancy 639.8
    surgery (nontherapeutic) (therapeutic) 997.1
  fetus or newborn 779.85
  following
    abortion 639.8
    ectopic or molar pregnancy 639.8
  personal history, successfully resuscitated V12.53
  postoperative (immediate) 997.1
    long-term effect of cardiac surgery 429.4
  cardiorespiratory (*see also* Arrest, cardiac) 427.5
  deep transverse 660.3 ☑
    affecting fetus or newborn 763.1
  development or growth
    bone 733.91
    child 783.40
    fetus 764.9 ☑
      affecting management of pregnancy 656.5 ☑
    tracheal rings 748.3
  epiphyseal 733.91
  granulopoiesis 288.09
  heart — *see* Arrest, cardiac
  respiratory 799.1
    newborn 770.87
  sinus 426.6
  transverse (deep) 660.3 ☑
    affecting fetus or newborn 763.1
Arrhenoblastoma (M8630/1)
  benign (M8630/0)
    specified site — *see* Neoplasm, by site, benign
    unspecified site
      female 220
      male 222.0
  malignant (M8630/3)
    specified site — *see* Neoplasm, by site, malignant
    unspecified site
      female 183.0
      male 186.9
  specified site — *see* Neoplasm, by site, uncertain behavior
  unspecified site
    female 236.2
    male 236.4
Arrhinencephaly 742.2
  due to
    trisomy 13 (13-15) 758.1
    trisomy 18 (16-18) 758.2
Arrhythmia (auricle) (cardiac) (cordis) (gallop rhythm) (juvenile) (nodal) (reflex) (sinus) (supraventricular) (transitory) (ventricle) 427.9
  bigeminal rhythm 427.89
  block 426.9
  bradycardia 427.89
  contractions, premature 427.60
  coronary sinus 427.89
  ectopic 427.89
  extrasystolic 427.60
  postoperative 997.1
  psychogenic 306.2
  vagal 780.2

Arrillaga-Ayerza syndrome (pulmonary artery sclerosis with pulmonary hypertension) 416.0
Arsenical
  dermatitis 692.4
  keratosis 692.4
  pigmentation 985.1
    from drug or medicinal agent
      correct substance properly administered 709.09
      overdose or wrong substance given or taken 961.1
Arsenism 985.1
  from drug or medicinal agent
    correct substance properly administered 692.4
    overdose or wrong substance given or taken 961.1
Arterial — *see* condition
Arteriectasis 447.8
Arteriofibrosis — *see* Arteriosclerosis
Arteriolar sclerosis — *see* Arteriosclerosis
Arteriolith — *see* Arteriosclerosis
Arteriolitis 447.6
  necrotizing, kidney 447.5
  renal — *see* Hypertension, kidney
Arteriolosclerosis — *see* Arteriosclerosis
Arterionephrosclerosis — *see also* Hypertension, kidney 403.90
Arteriopathy 447.9
Arteriosclerosis, arteriosclerotic (artery) (deformans) (diffuse) (disease) (endarteritis) (general) (obliterans) (obliterative) (occlusive) (senile) (with calcification) 440.9
  with
    gangrene 440.24
    psychosis (*see also* Psychosis, arteriosclerotic) 290.40
    ulceration 440.23
  aorta 440.0
  arteries of extremities — *see* Arteriosclerosis, extremities
  basilar (artery) (*see also* Occlusion, artery, basilar) 433.0 ☑
  brain 437.0
  bypass graft
    coronary artery 414.05
      autologous artery (gastroepiploic) (internal mammary) 414.04
      autologous vein 414.02
      nonautologous biological 414.03
      of transplanted heart 414.07
    extremity 440.30
      autologous vein 440.31
      nonautologous biological 440.32
  cardiac — *see* Arteriosclerosis, coronary
  cardiopathy — *see* Arteriosclerosis, coronary
  cardiorenal (*see also* Hypertension, cardiorenal) 404.90
  cardiovascular (*see also* Disease, cardiovascular) 429.2
  carotid (artery) (common) (internal) (*see also* Occlusion, artery, carotid) 433.1 ☑
  central nervous system 437.0
  cerebral 437.0
    late effect — *see* Late effect(s) (of) cerebrovascular disease
  cerebrospinal 437.0
  cerebrovascular 437.0
  coronary (artery) 414.00
    due to
      calcified coronary lesion (severely) 414.4
      lipid rich plaque 414.3
    graft — *see* Arteriosclerosis, bypass graft
    native artery 414.01
    of transplanted heart 414.06
  extremities (native artery) NEC 440.20
    bypass graft 440.30
      autologous vein 440.31
      nonautologous biological 440.32
    claudication (intermittent) 440.21
      and
        gangrene 440.24
        rest pain 440.22

Arteriosclerosis, arteriosclerotic — *continued*
  extremities — *continued*
    claudication — *continued*
      and — *continued*
        rest pain — *continued*
          and
            gangrene 440.24
            ulceration 440.23
              and gangrene 440.24
      ulceration 440.23
        and gangrene 440.24
    gangrene 440.24
    rest pain 440.22
      and
        gangrene 440.24
        ulceration 440.23
          and gangrene 440.24
    specified site NEC 440.29
    ulceration 440.23
      and gangrene 440.24
  heart (disease) (*see also* Arteriosclerosis, coronary)
    valve 424.99
      aortic 424.1
      mitral 424.0
      pulmonary 424.3
      tricuspid 424.2
  iliac 440.8
  kidney (*see also* Hypertension, kidney) 403.90
  labyrinth, labyrinthine 388.00
  medial NEC (*see also* Arteriosclerosis, extremities) 440.20
  mesentery (artery) 557.1
  Mönckeberg's (*see also* Arteriosclerosis, extremities) 440.20
  myocarditis 429.0
  nephrosclerosis (*see also* Hypertension, kidney) 403.90
  peripheral (of extremities) — *see* Arteriosclerosis, extremities
  precerebral 433.9 ☑
    specified artery NEC 433.8 ☑
  pulmonary (idiopathic) 416.0
  renal (*see also* Hypertension, kidney) 403.90
    arterioles (*see also* Hypertension, kidney) 403.90
    artery 440.1
  retinal (vascular) 440.8 [362.13]
  specified artery NEC 440.8
    with gangrene 440.8 [785.4]
  spinal (cord) 437.0
  vertebral (artery) (*see also* Occlusion, artery, vertebral) 433.2 ☑
Arteriospasm 443.9
Arteriovenous — *see* condition
Arteritis 447.6
  allergic (*see also* Angiitis, hypersensitivity) 446.20
  aorta (nonsyphilitic) 447.6
    syphilitic 093.1
  aortic arch 446.7
  brachiocephalica 446.7
  brain 437.4
    syphilitic 094.89
  branchial 446.7
  cerebral 437.4
    late effect — *see* Late effect(s) (of) cerebrovascular disease
    syphilitic 094.89
  coronary (artery) (*see also* Arteriosclerosis, coronary)
    rheumatic 391.9
      chronic 398.99
    syphilitic 093.89
  cranial (left) (right) 446.5
  deformans — *see* Arteriosclerosis
  giant cell 446.5
  necrosing or necrotizing 446.0
  nodosa 446.0
  obliterans (*see also* Arteriosclerosis)
    subclaviocarotica 446.7
  pulmonary 417.8
  retina 362.18
  rheumatic — *see* Fever, rheumatic

Arteritis — *continued*
  senile — *see* Arteriosclerosis
  suppurative 447.2
  syphilitic (general) 093.89
    brain 094.89
    coronary 093.89
    spinal 094.89
  temporal 446.5
  young female, syndrome 446.7
Artery, arterial — *see* condition
Arthralgia — *see also* Pain, joint 719.4 ☑
  allergic (*see also* Pain, joint) 719.4 ☑
  in caisson disease 993.3
  psychogenic 307.89
  rubella 056.71
  Salmonella 003.23
  temporomandibular joint 524.62
Arthritis, arthritic (acute) (chronic) (subacute) 716.9 ☑
  meaning Osteoarthritis — *see* Osteoarthrosis

> *Note* — Use the following fifth-digit subclassification with categories 711–712, 715–716:
>
> 0   *site unspecified*
> 1   *shoulder region*
> 2   *upper arm*
> 3   *forearm*
> 4   *hand*
> 5   *pelvic region and thigh*
> 6   *lower leg*
> 7   *ankle and foot*
> 8   *other specified sites*
> 9   *multiple sites*

  allergic 716.2 ☑
  ankylosing (crippling) (spine) 720.0
    sites other than spine 716.9 ☑
  atrophic 714.0
    spine 720.9
  back (*see also* Arthritis, spine) 721.90
  Bechterew's (ankylosing spondylitis) 720.0
  blennorrhagic 098.50
  cervical, cervicodorsal (*see also* Spondylosis, cervical) 721.0
  Charcôt's 094.0 [713.5]
    diabetic 250.6 ☑ [713.5]
      due to secondary diabetes 249.6 ☑ [713.5]
    syringomyelic 336.0 [713.5]
    tabetic 094.0 [713.5]
  chylous (*see also* Filariasis) 125.9 [711.7] ☑
  climacteric NEC 716.3 ☑
  coccyx 721.8
  cricoarytenoid 478.79
  crystal (-induced) — *see* Arthritis, due to crystals
  deformans (*see also* Osteoarthrosis) 715.9 ☑
    spine 721.90
      with myelopathy 721.91
  degenerative (*see also* Osteoarthrosis) 715.9 ☑
    idiopathic 715.09
    polyarticular 715.09
    spine 721.90
      with myelopathy 721.91
  dermatoarthritis, lipoid 272.8 [713.0]
  due to or associated with
    acromegaly 253.0 [713.0]
    actinomycosis 039.8 [711.4] ☑
    amyloidosis 277.39 [713.7]
    bacterial disease NEC 040.89 [711.4] ☑
    Behçet's syndrome 136.1 [711.2] ☑
    blastomycosis 116.0 [711.6] ☑
    brucellosis (*see also* Brucellosis) 023.9 [711.4] ☑
    caisson disease 993.3
    coccidioidomycosis 114.3 [711.6] ☑
    coliform (Escherichia coli) 711.0 ☑
    colitis, ulcerative (*see also* Colitis, ulcerative) 556.9 [713.1]

☑ **Additional Digit Required** — Refer to the Tabular List for Digit Selection
⬚ **Subterms under main terms may continue to next column or page**

2014 ICD-9-CM   ▶◀ Revised Text   ● New Line   ▲ Revised Code   **Volume 2 — 27**

Arrest, arrested — Arthritis, arthritic

Arthritis, arthritic — *continued*
  due to or associated with — *continued*
    cowpox 051.01 *[711.5]* ☑
    crystals (*see also* Gout)
      dicalcium phosphate
        275.49 *[712.1]* ☑
      pyrophosphate 275.49 *[712.2]* ☑
      specified NEC 275.49 *[712.8]* ☑
    dermatoarthritis, lipoid 272.8 *[713.0]*
    dermatological disorder NEC
      709.9 *[713.3]*
    diabetes 250.6 *[713.5]*
      due to secondary diabetes
        249.6 *[713.5]*
    diphtheria 032.89 *[711.4]* ☑
    dracontiasis 125.7 *[711.7]* ☑
    dysentery 009.0 *[711.3]* ☑
    endocrine disorder NEC 259.9 *[713.0]*
    enteritis NEC 009.1 *[711.3]* ☑
      infectious (*see also* Enteritis, infectious) 009.0 *[711.3]* ☑
      specified organism NEC
        008.8 *[711.3]* ☑
      regional (*see also* Enteritis, regional)
        555.9 *[713.1]*
      specified organism NEC
        008.8 *[711.3]* ☑
    epiphyseal slip, nontraumatic (old)
      716.8 ☑
    erysipelas 035 *[711.4]* ☑
    erythema
      epidemic 026.1
      multiforme 695.10 *[713.3]*
      nodosum 695.2 *[713.3]*
    Escherichia coli 711.0 ☑
    filariasis NEC 125.9 *[711.7]* ☑
    gastrointestinal condition NEC
      569.9 *[713.1]*
    glanders 024 *[711.4]* ☑
    Gonococcus 098.50
    gout 274.00
    helminthiasis NEC 128.9 *[711.7]* ☑
    hematological disorder NEC 289.9 *[713.2]*
    hemochromatosis 275.03 *[713.0]*
    hemoglobinopathy NEC (*see also* Disease, hemoglobin) 282.7 *[713.2]*
    hemophilia (*see also* Hemophilia)
      286.0 *[713.2]*
    Hemophilus influenzae (H. influenzae)
      711.0 ☑
    Henoch (-Schönlein) purpura
      287.0 *[713.6]*
    H. influenzae 711.0 ☑
    histoplasmosis NEC (*see also* Histoplasmosis) 115.99 *[711.6]* ☑
    human parvovirus 079.83 *[711.5]* ☑
    hyperparathyroidism 252.00 *[713.0]*
    hypersensitivity reaction NEC
      995.3 *[713.6]*
    hypogammaglobulinemia (*see also* Hypogamma-globulinemia)
      279.00 *[713.0]*
    hypothyroidism NEC 244.9 *[713.0]*
    infection (*see also* Arthritis, infectious)
      711.9 ☑
    infectious disease NEC 136.9 *[711.8]* ☑
    leprosy (*see also* Leprosy)
      030.9 *[711.4]* ☑
    leukemia NEC (M9800/3) 208.9 *[713.2]*
    lipoid dermatoarthritis 272.8 *[713.0]*
    Lyme disease 088.81 *[711.8]* ☑
    Mediterranean fever, familial
      277.31 *[713.7]*
    meningococcal infection 036.82
    metabolic disorder NEC 277.9 *[713.0]*
    multiple myelomatosis (M9730/3) 203.0
      [713.2]
    mumps 072.79 *[711.5]* ☑
    mycobacteria 031.8 *[711.4]* ☑
    mycosis NEC 117.9 *[711.6]* ☑
    neurological disorder NEC 349.9 *[713.5]*
    ochronosis 270.2 *[713.0]*
    O'Nyong Nyong 066.3 *[711.5]* ☑
    parasitic disease NEC 136.9 *[711.8]* ☑

Arthritis, arthritic — *continued*
  due to or associated with — *continued*
    paratyphoid fever (*see also* Fever, paratyphoid) 002.9 *[711.3]* ☑
    parvovirus B19 079.83 *[711.5]* ☑
    Pneumococcus 711.0 ☑
    poliomyelitis (*see also* Poliomyelitis)
      045.9 *[711.5]* ☑
    Pseudomonas 711.0 ☑
    psoriasis 696.0
    pyogenic organism (E. coli) (H. influenzae) (Pseudomonas) (Streptococcus) 711.0 ☑
    rat-bite fever 026.1 *[711.4]* ☑
    regional enteritis (*see also* Enteritis, regional) 555.9 *[713.1]*
    Reiter's disease 099.3 *[711.1]* ☑
    respiratory disorder NEC 519.9 *[713.4]*
    reticulosis, malignant (M9720/3) 202.3
      [713.2]
    rubella 056.71
    salmonellosis 003.23
    sarcoidosis 135 *[713.7]*
    serum sickness 999.59 *[713.6]*
    Staphylococcus 711.0 ☑
    Streptococcus 711.0 ☑
    syphilis (*see also* Syphilis)
      094.0 *[711.4]* ☑
    syringomyelia 336.0 *[713.5]*
    thalassemia (*see also* Thalassemia)
      282.40 *[713.2]*
    tuberculosis (*see also* Tuberculosis, arthritis) 015.9 *[711.4]* ☑
    typhoid fever 002.0 *[711.3]* ☑
    ulcerative colitis (*see also* Colitis, ulcerative) 556.9 *[713.1]*
    urethritis
      nongonococcal (*see also* Urethritis, nongonococcal)
        099.40 *[711.1]* ☑
      nonspecific (*see also* Urethritis, nongonococcal) 099.40 *[711.1]* ☑
      Reiter's 099.3
    viral disease NEC 079.99 *[711.5]* ☑
  erythema epidemic 026.1
  gonococcal 098.50
  gouty 274.00
    acute 274.01
  hypertrophic (*see also* Osteoarthrosis)
    715.9 ☑
    spine 721.90
      with myelopathy 721.91
  idiopathic, blennorrheal 099.3
  in caisson disease 993.3 *[713.8]*
  infectious or infective (acute) (chronic)
    (subacute) NEC 711.9 ☑
    nonpyogenic 711.9 ☑
    spine 720.9
  inflammatory NEC 714.9
  juvenile rheumatoid (chronic) (polyarticular)
    714.30
    acute 714.31
    monoarticular 714.33
    pauciarticular 714.32
  lumbar (*see also* Spondylosis, lumbar) 721.3
  meningococcal 036.82
  menopausal NEC 716.3 ☑
  migratory — *see* Fever, rheumatic
  neuropathic (Charcôt's) 094.0 *[713.5]*
    diabetic 250.6 *[713.5]*
      due to secondary diabetes
        249.6 ☑ *[713.5]*
    nonsyphilitic NEC 349.9 *[713.5]*
    syringomyelic 336.0 *[713.5]*
    tabetic 094.0 *[713.5]*
  nodosa (*see also* Osteoarthrosis) 715.9 ☑
    spine 721.90
      with myelopathy 721.91
  nonpyogenic NEC 716.9 ☑
    spine 721.90
      with myelopathy 721.91
  ochronotic 270.2 *[713.0]*
  palindromic (*see also* Rheumatism, palindromic) 719.3
  pneumococcal 711.0 ☑

Arthritis, arthritic — *continued*
  postdysenteric 009.0 *[711.3]* ☑
  postrheumatic, chronic (Jaccoud's) 714.4
  primary progressive 714.0
    spine 720.9
  proliferative 714.0
    spine 720.0
  psoriatic 696.0
  purulent 711.0 ☑
  pyogenic or pyemic 711.0 ☑
  reactive 099.3
  rheumatic 714.0
    acute or subacute — *see* Fever, rheumatic
    chronic 714.0
    spine 720.9
  rheumatoid (nodular) 714.0
    with
      splenoadenomegaly and leukopenia
        714.1
      visceral or systemic involvement
        714.2
    aortitis 714.89
    carditis 714.2
    heart disease 714.2
    juvenile (chronic) (polyarticular) 714.30
      acute 714.31
      monoarticular 714.33
      pauciarticular 714.32
    spine 720.0
  rubella 056.71
  sacral, sacroiliac, sacrococcygeal (*see also* Spondylosis, sacral) 721.3
  scorbutic 267
  senile or senescent (*see also* Osteoarthrosis)
    715.9 ☑
    spine 721.90
      with myelopathy 721.91
  septic 711.0 ☑
  serum (nontherapeutic) (therapeutic)
    999.59 *[713.6]*
  specified form NEC 716.8 ☑
  spine 721.90
    with myelopathy 721.91
    atrophic 720.9
    degenerative 721.90
      with myelopathy 721.91
    hypertrophic (with deformity) 721.90
      with myelopathy 721.91
    infectious or infective NEC 720.9
    Marie-Strümpell 720.0
    nonpyogenic 721.90
      with myelopathy 721.91
    pyogenic 720.9
    rheumatoid 720.0
    traumatic (old) 721.7
    tuberculous (*see also* Tuberculosis)
      015.0 ☑ *[720.81]*
  staphylococcal 711.0 ☑
  streptococcal 711.0 ☑
  suppurative 711.0 ☑
  syphilitic 094.0 *[713.5]*
    congenital 090.49 *[713.5]*
  syphilitica deformans (Charcôt) 094.0 *[713.5]*
  temporomandibular joint 524.69
  thoracic (*see also* Spondylosis, thoracic)
    721.2
  toxic of menopause 716.3 ☑
  transient 716.4 ☑
  traumatic (chronic) (old) (post) 716.1 ☑
    current injury — *see* nature of injury
  tuberculous (*see also* Tuberculosis, arthritis)
    015.9 ☑ *[711.4]* ☑
  urethritica 099.3 *[711.1]* ☑
  urica, uratic 274.00
  venereal 099.3 *[711.1]* ☑
  vertebral (*see also* Arthritis, spine) 721.90
  villous 716.8 ☑
  von Bechterew's 720.0
Arthro-onychodysplasia 756.89
Arthro-osteo-onychodysplasia 756.89
Arthrocele — *see also* Effusion, joint 719.0 ☑
Arthrochondritis — *see* Arthritis
Arthrodesis status V45.4
Arthrodynia — *see also* Pain, joint 719.4 ☑
  psychogenic 307.89

Arthrodysplasia 755.9
Arthrofibrosis joint — *see also* Ankylosis
  718.5 ☑
Arthrogryposis 728.3
  multiplex, congenita 754.89
Arthrokatadysis 715.35
Arthrolithiasis 274.00
Arthropathy — *see also* Arthritis 716.9 ☑

Note — *Use the following fifth-digit subclassification with categories 711–712, 716:*

0   *site unspecified*

1   *shoulder region*

2   *upper arm*

3   *forearm*

4   *hand*

5   *pelvic region and thigh*

6   *lower leg*

7   *ankle and foot*

8   *other specified sites*

9   *multiple sites*

  Behçet's 136.1 *[711.2]* ☑
  Charcôt's 094.0 *[713.5]*
    diabetic 250.6 *[713.5]*
      due to secondary diabetes
        249.6 ☑ *[713.5]*
    syringomyelic 336.0 *[713.5]*
    tabetic 094.0 *[713.5]*
  crystal (-induced) — *see* Arthritis, due to crystals
  gouty 274.00
    acute 274.01
    chronic (without mention of tophus (tophi)) 274.02
      with tophus (tophi) 274.03
  neurogenic, neuropathic (Charcôt's) (tabetic) 094.0 *[713.5]*
    diabetic 250.6 *[713.5]*
      due to secondary diabetes
        249.6 *[713.5]*
    nonsyphilitic NEC 349.9 *[713.5]*
    syringomyelic 336.0 *[713.5]*
  postdysenteric NEC 009.0 *[711.3]* ☑
  postrheumatic, chronic (Jaccoud's) 714.4
  psoriatic 696.0
  pulmonary 731.2
  specified NEC 716.8 ☑
  syringomyelia 336.0 *[713.5]*
  tabes dorsalis 094.0 *[713.5]*
  tabetic 094.0 *[713.5]*
  transient 716.4 ☑
  traumatic 716.1 ☑
  uric acid 274.00
Arthrophyte — *see also* Loose, body, joint
  718.1 ☑
Arthrophytis 719.80
  ankle 719.87
  elbow 719.82
  foot 719.87
  hand 719.84
  hip 719.85
  knee 719.86
  multiple sites 719.89
  pelvic region 719.85
  shoulder (region) 719.81
  specified site NEC 719.88
  wrist 719.83
Arthropyosis — *see also* Arthritis, pyogenic
  711.0 ☑
Arthroscopic surgical procedure converted to open procedure V64.43
Arthrosis (deformans) (degenerative) — *see also* Osteoarthrosis 715.9 ☑
  Charcôt's 094.0 *[713.5]*
  polyarticular 715.09
  spine (*see also* Spondylosis) 721.90
Arthus phenomenon 995.21
  due to
    correct substance properly administered
      995.21

☑ Additional Digit Required — Refer to the Tabular List for Digit Selection   ▽ Subterms under main terms may continue to next column or page

28 — Volume 2   ►◄ Revised Text   ● New Line   ▲ Revised Code   2014 ICD-9-CM

Arthus phenomenon — *continued*
  due to — *continued*
    overdose or wrong substance given or taken 977.9
      specified drug — *see* Table of Drugs and Chemicals
    serum 999.59
Articular — *see also* condition
  disc disorder (reducing or non-reducing) 524.63
  spondylolisthesis 756.12
Articulation
  anterior 524.27
  posterior 524.27
  reverse 524.27
Artificial
  device (prosthetic) — *see* Fitting, device
  insemination V26.1
  menopause (states) (symptoms) (syndrome) 627.4
  opening status (functioning) (without complication) V44.9
    anus (colostomy) V44.3
    colostomy V44.3
    cystostomy V44.50
      appendico-vesicostomy V44.52
      cutaneous-vesicostomy V44.51
      specified type NEC V44.59
    enterostomy V44.4
    gastrostomy V44.1
    ileostomy V44.2
    intestinal tract NEC V44.4
    jejunostomy V44.4
    nephrostomy V44.6
    specified site NEC V44.8
    tracheostomy V44.0
    ureterostomy V44.6
    urethrostomy V44.6
    urinary tract NEC V44.6
    vagina V44.7
    vagina status V44.7
ARV (disease) (illness) (infection) — *see* Human immunodeficiency virus (disease) (illness) (infection)
Arytenoid — *see* condition
Asbestosis (occupational) 501
Asboe-Hansen's disease (incontinentia pigmenti) 757.33
ASC-H (atypical squamous cells cannot exclude high grade squamous intraepithelial lesion)
  anus 796.72
  cervix 795.02
  vagina 795.12
ASC-US (atypical squamous cells of undetermined significance)
  anus 796.71
  cervix 795.01
  vagina 795.11
Ascariasis (intestinal) (lung) 127.0
Ascaridiasis 127.0
Ascaridosis 127.0
Ascaris 127.0
  lumbricoides (infestation) 127.0
  pneumonia 127.0
Ascending — *see* condition
Aschoff's bodies — *see also* Myocarditis, rheumatic 398.0
Ascites 789.59
  abdominal NEC 789.59
  cancerous (M8000/6) 789.51
  cardiac 428.0
  chylous (nonfilarial) 457.8
    filarial (*see also* Infestation, filarial) 125.9
  congenital 778.0
  due to S. japonicum 120.2
  fetal, causing fetopelvic disproportion 653.7 ☑
  heart 428.0
  joint (*see also* Effusion, joint) 719.0 ☑
  malignant (M8000/6) 789.51
  pseudochylous 789.59
  syphilitic 095.2
  tuberculous (*see also* Tuberculosis) 014.0 ☑
Ascorbic acid (vitamin C) **deficiency** (scurvy) 267

ASCVD (arteriosclerotic cardiovascular disease) 429.2
Aseptic — *see* condition
Asherman's syndrome 621.5
Asialia 527.7
Asiatic cholera — *see also* Cholera 001.9
Asocial personality or trends 301.7
Asomatognosia 781.8
Aspergillosis 117.3
  with pneumonia 117.3 [484.6]
  allergic bronchopulmonary 518.6
  nonsyphilitic NEC 117.3
Aspergillus (flavus) (fumigatus) (infection) (terreus) 117.3
Aspermatogenesis 606.0
Aspermia (testis) 606.0
Asphyxia, asphyxiation (by) 799.01
  antenatal — *see* Distress, fetal
  bedclothes 994.7
  birth (*see also* Asphyxia, newborn) 768.9
  bunny bag 994.7
  carbon monoxide 986
  caul (*see also* Asphyxia, newborn) 768.9
  cave-in 994.7
    crushing — *see* Injury, internal, intrathoracic organs
  constriction 994.7
  crushing — *see* Injury, internal, intrathoracic organs
  drowning 994.1
  fetal, affecting newborn 768.9
  food or foreign body (in larynx) 933.1
    bronchioles 934.8
    bronchus (main) 934.1
    lung 934.8
    nasopharynx 933.0
    nose, nasal passages 932
    pharynx 933.0
    respiratory tract 934.9
      specified part NEC 934.8
    throat 933.0
    trachea 934.0
  gas, fumes, or vapor NEC 987.9
    specified — *see* Table of Drugs and Chemicals
  gravitational changes 994.7
  hanging 994.7
  inhalation — *see* Inhalation
  intrauterine
    fetal death (before onset of labor) 768.0
      during labor 768.1
    liveborn infant — *see* Distress, fetal, liveborn infant
  local 443.0
  mechanical 994.7
    during birth (*see also* Distress, fetal) 768.9
  mucus 933.1
    bronchus (main) 934.1
    larynx 933.1
    lung 934.8
    nasal passages 932
    newborn 770.18
    pharynx 933.0
    respiratory tract 934.9
      specified part NEC 934.8
    throat 933.0
    trachea 934.0
    vaginal (fetus or newborn) 770.18
  newborn 768.9
    with neurologic involvement 768.5
    blue 768.6
    livida 768.6
    mild or moderate 768.6
    pallida 768.5
    severe 768.5
    white 768.5
  pathological 799.01
  plastic bag 994.7
  postnatal (*see also* Asphyxia, newborn) 768.9
    mechanical 994.7
  pressure 994.7
  reticularis 782.61
  strangulation 994.7
  submersion 994.1

Asphyxia, asphyxiation — *continued*
  traumatic NEC — *see* Injury, internal, intrathoracic organs
  vomiting, vomitus — *see* Asphyxia, food or foreign body
Aspiration
  acid pulmonary (syndrome) 997.39
    obstetric 668.0 ☑
  amniotic fluid 770.13
    with respiratory symptoms 770.14
  bronchitis 507.0
  clear amniotic fluid 770.13
    with
      pneumonia 770.14
      pneumonitis 770.14
      respiratory symptoms 770.14
  contents of birth canal 770.17
    with respiratory symptoms 770.18
  fetal 770.10
    blood 770.15
      with
        pneumonia 770.16
        pneumonitis 770.16
      pneumonitis 770.18
  food, foreign body, or gasoline (with asphyxiation) — *see* Asphyxia, food or foreign body
  meconium 770.11
    with
      pneumonia 770.12
      pneumonitis 770.12
      respiratory symptoms 770.12
    below vocal cords 770.11
      with respiratory symptoms 770.12
  mucus 933.1
    into
      bronchus (main) 934.1
      lung 934.8
      respiratory tract 934.9
        specified part NEC 934.8
      trachea 934.0
    newborn 770.17
    vaginal (fetus or newborn) 770.17
  newborn 770.10
    with respiratory symptoms 770.18
    blood 770.15
      with
        pneumonia 770.16
        pneumonitis 770.16
        respiratory symptoms 770.16
  pneumonia 507.0
    fetus or newborn 770.18
    meconium 770.12
  pneumonitis 507.0
    fetus or newborn 770.18
    meconium 770.12
    obstetric 668.0 ☑
  postnatal stomach contents 770.85
    with
      pneumonia 770.86
      pneumonitis 770.86
      respiratory symptoms 770.86
  syndrome of newborn (massive) 770.18
    meconium 770.12
  vernix caseosa 770.12
Asplenia 759.0
  with mesocardia 746.87
Assam fever 085.0
Assimilation, pelvis
  with disproportion 653.2 ☑
    affecting fetus or newborn 763.1
    causing obstructed labor 660.1 ☑
      affecting fetus or newborn 763.1
Assmann's focus — *see also* Tuberculosis 011.0 ☑
Astasia (-abasia) 307.9
  hysterical 300.11
Asteatosis 706.8
  cutis 706.8
Astereognosis 780.99
Asterixis 781.3
  in liver disease 572.8
Asteroid hyalitis 379.22
Asthenia, asthenic 780.79
  cardiac (*see also* Failure, heart) 428.9
    psychogenic 306.2

Asthenia, asthenic — *continued*
  cardiovascular (*see also* Failure, heart) 428.9
    psychogenic 306.2
  heart (*see also* Failure, heart) 428.9
    psychogenic 306.2
  hysterical 300.11
  myocardial (*see also* Failure, heart) 428.9
    psychogenic 306.2
  nervous 300.5
  neurocirculatory 306.2
  neurotic 300.5
  psychogenic 300.5
  psychoneurotic 300.5
  psychophysiologic 300.5
  reaction, psychoneurotic 300.5
  senile 797
  Stiller's 780.79
  tropical anhidrotic 705.1
Asthenopia 368.13
  accommodative 367.4
  hysterical (muscular) 300.11
  psychogenic 306.7
Asthenospermia 792.2
Asthma, asthmatic (bronchial) (catarrh) (spasmodic) 493.9 ☑

> *Note* — Use the following fifth-digit subclassification with codes 493.0–493.2, 493.9:
>
> 0   without mention of status asthmaticus or acute exacerbation or unspecified
>
> 1   with status asthmaticus
>
> 2   with acute exacerbation

  with
    chronic obstructive pulmonary disease (COPD) 493.2 ☑
    hay fever 493.0 ☑
    rhinitis, allergic 493.0 ☑
  allergic 493.9 ☑
    stated cause (external allergen) 493.0 ☑
  atopic 493.0 ☑
  cardiac (*see also* Failure, ventricular, left) 428.1
  cardiobronchial (*see also* Failure, ventricular, left) 428.1
  cardiorenal (*see also* Hypertension, cardiorenal) 404.90
  childhood 493.0 ☑
  Colliers' 500
  cough variant 493.82
  croup 493.9 ☑
  detergent 507.8
  due to
    detergent 507.8
    inhalation of fumes 506.3
    internal immunological process 493.0 ☑
  endogenous (intrinsic) 493.1 ☑
  eosinophilic 518.3
  exercise induced bronchospasm 493.81
  exogenous (cosmetics) (dander or dust) (drugs) (dust) (feathers) (food) (hay) (platinum) (pollen) 493.0 ☑
  extrinsic 493.0 ☑
  grinders' 502
  hay 493.0 ☑
  heart (*see also* Failure, ventricular, left) 428.1
  IgE 493.0 ☑
  infective 493.1 ☑
  intrinsic 493.1 ☑
  Kopp's 254.8
  late-onset 493.1 ☑
  meat-wrappers' 506.9
  Millar's (laryngismus stridulus) 478.75
  millstone makers' 502
  miners' 500
  Monday morning 504
  New Orleans (epidemic) 493.0 ☑
  platinum 493.0 ☑
  pneumoconiotic (occupational) NEC 505
  potters' 502
  psychogenic 316 [493.9] ☑
  pulmonary eosinophilic 518.3
  red cedar 495.8

☑ Additional Digit Required — Refer to the Tabular List for Digit Selection   � Subterms under main terms may continue to next column or page

2014 ICD-9-CM   ▶◀ Revised Text   ● New Line   ▲ Revised Code   **Volume 2 — 29**

Asthma, asthmatic — continued
  Rostan's (see also Failure, ventricular, left) 428.1
  sandblasters' 502
  sequoiosis 495.8
  stonemasons' 502
  thymic 254.8
  tuberculous (see also Tuberculosis, pulmonary) 011.9 ☑
  Wichmann's (laryngismus stridulus) 478.75
  wood 495.8
Astigmatism (compound) (congenital) 367.20
  irregular 367.22
  regular 367.21
Astroblastoma (M9430/3)
  nose 748.1
  specified site — see Neoplasm, by site, malignant
  unspecified site 191.9
Astrocytoma (cystic) (M9400/3)
  anaplastic type (M9401/3)
    specified site — see Neoplasm, by site, malignant
    unspecified site 191.9
  fibrillary (M9420/3)
    specified site — see Neoplasm, by site, malignant
    unspecified site 191.9
  fibrous (M9420/3)
    specified site — see Neoplasm, by site, malignant
    unspecified site 191.9
  gemistocytic (M9411/3)
    specified site — see Neoplasm, by site, malignant
    unspecified site 191.9
  juvenile (M9421/3)
    specified site — see Neoplasm, by site, malignant
    unspecified site 191.9
  nose 748.1
  pilocytic (M9421/3)
    specified site — see Neoplasm, by site, malignant
    unspecified site 191.9
  piloid (M9421/3)
    specified site — see Neoplasm, by site, malignant
    unspecified site 191.9
  protoplasmic (M9410/3)
    specified site — see Neoplasm, by site, malignant
    unspecified site 191.9
  specified site — see Neoplasm, by site, malignant
  subependymal (M9383/1) 237.5
    giant cell (M9384/1) 237.5
  unspecified site 191.9
Astroglioma (M9400/3)
  nose 748.1
  specified site — see Neoplasm, by site, malignant
  unspecified site 191.9
Asymbolia 784.60
Asymmetrical breathing 786.09
Asymmetry — see also Distortion
  breast, between native and reconstructed 612.1
  chest 786.9
  face 754.0
  jaw NEC 524.12
    maxillary 524.11
  pelvis with disproportion 653.0 ☑
    affecting fetus or newborn 763.1
    causing obstructed labor 660.1 ☑
      affecting fetus or newborn 763.1
Asynergia 781.3
Asynergy 781.3
  ventricular 429.89
Asystole (heart) — see also Arrest, cardiac 427.5
Ataxia-telangiectasia 334.8
Ataxia, ataxy, ataxic 781.3
  acute 781.3
  brain 331.89
  cerebellar 334.3

Ataxia, ataxy, ataxic — continued
  cerebellar — continued
    hereditary (Marie's) 334.2
    in
      alcoholism 303.9 ☑ [334.4]
      myxedema (see also Myxedema) 244.9 [334.4]
      neoplastic disease NEC 239.9 [334.4]
  cerebral 331.89
  family, familial 334.2
    cerebral (Marie's) 334.2
    spinal (Friedreich's) 334.0
  Friedreich's (heredofamilial) (spinal) 334.0
  frontal lobe 781.3
  gait 781.2
    hysterical 300.11
  general 781.3
  hereditary NEC 334.2
    cerebellar 334.2
    spastic 334.1
    spinal 334.0
  heredofamilial (Marie's) 334.2
  hysterical 300.11
  locomotor (progressive) 094.0
    diabetic 250.6 ☑ [337.1]
      due to secondary diabetes 249.6 ☑ [337.1]
  Marie's (cerebellar) (heredofamilial) 334.2
  nonorganic origin 307.9
  partial 094.0
  postchickenpox 052.7
  progressive locomotor 094.0
  psychogenic 307.9
  Sanger-Brown's 334.2
  spastic 094.0
    hereditary 334.1
    syphilitic 094.0
  spinal
    hereditary 334.0
    progressive locomotor 094.0
  telangiectasia 334.8
Atelectasis (absorption collapse) (complete) (compression) (massive) (partial) (postinfective) (pressure collapse) (pulmonary) (relaxation) 518.0
  newborn (congenital) (partial) 770.5
    primary 770.4
  primary 770.4
  tuberculous (see also Tuberculosis, pulmonary) 011.9 ☑
Ateleiosis, ateliosis 253.3
Atelia — see Distortion
Ateliosis 253.3
Atelocardia 746.9
Atelomyelia 742.59
Athelia 757.6
Atheroembolism
  extremity
    lower 445.02
    upper 445.01
  kidney 445.81
  specified site NEC 445.89
Atheroma, atheromatous — see also Arteriosclerosis 440.9
  aorta, aortic 440.0
    valve (see also Endocarditis, aortic) 424.1
  artery — see Arteriosclerosis
  basilar (artery) (see also Occlusion, artery, basilar) 433.0 ☑
  carotid (artery) (common) (internal) (see also Occlusion, artery, carotid) 433.1 ☑
  cerebral (arteries) 437.0
  coronary (artery) — see Arteriosclerosis, coronary
  degeneration — see Arteriosclerosis
  heart, cardiac — see Arteriosclerosis, coronary
  mitral (valve) 424.0
  myocardium, myocardial — see Arteriosclerosis, coronary
  pulmonary valve (heart) (see also Endocarditis, pulmonary) 424.3
  skin 706.2
  tricuspid (heart) (valve) 424.2
  valve, valvular — see Endocarditis

Atheroma, atheromatous — see also Arteriosclerosis — continued
  vertebral (artery) (see also Occlusion, artery, vertebral) 433.2 ☑
Atheromatosis — see also Arteriosclerosis
  arterial, congenital 272.8
Atherosclerosis — see Arteriosclerosis
Athetosis (acquired) 781.0
  bilateral 333.79
  congenital (bilateral) 333.6
  double 333.71
  unilateral 781.0
Athlete's
  foot 110.4
  heart 429.3
Athletic team examination V70.3
Athrepsia 261
Athyrea (acquired) — see also Hypothyroidism 244.9
  congenital 243
Athyreosis (congenital) 243
  acquired — see Hypothyroidism
Athyroidism (acquired) — see also Hypothyroidism 244.9
  congenital 243
Atmospheric pyrexia 992.0
Atonia, atony, atonic
  abdominal wall 728.2
  bladder (sphincter) 596.4
    neurogenic NEC 596.54
      with cauda equina syndrome 344.61
  capillary 448.9
  cecum 564.89
    psychogenic 306.4
  colon 564.89
    psychogenic 306.4
  congenital 779.89
  dyspepsia 536.3
    psychogenic 306.4
  intestine 564.89
    psychogenic 306.4
  stomach 536.3
    neurotic or psychogenic 306.4
    psychogenic 306.4
  uterus 661.2 ☑
    with hemorrhage (postpartum) 666.1 ☑
    without hemorrhage
      intrapartum 661.2 ☑
      postpartum 669.8 ☑
  vesical 596.4
Atopy NEC V15.09
Atransferrinemia, congenital 273.8
Atresia, atretic (congenital) 759.89
  alimentary organ or tract NEC 751.8
    lower 751.2
    upper 750.8
  ani, anus, anal (canal) 751.2
  aorta 747.22
    with hypoplasia of ascending aorta and defective development of left ventricle (with mitral valve atresia) 746.7
    arch 747.11
    ring 747.21
  aortic (orifice) (valve) 746.89
    arch 747.11
  aqueduct of Sylvius 742.3
    with spina bifida (see also Spina bifida) 741.0 ☑
  artery NEC (see also Atresia, blood vessel) 747.60
    cerebral 747.81
    coronary 746.85
    eye 743.58
    pulmonary 747.31
    umbilical 747.5
  auditory canal (external) 744.02
  bile, biliary duct (common) or passage 751.61
    acquired (see also Obstruction, biliary) 576.2
  bladder (neck) 753.6
  blood vessel (peripheral) NEC 747.60
    cerebral 747.81
    gastrointestinal 747.61
    lower limb 747.64

Atresia, atretic — continued
  blood vessel — continued
    pulmonary artery 747.31
    renal 747.62
    spinal 747.82
    upper limb 747.63
  bronchus 748.3
  canal, ear 744.02
  cardiac
    valve 746.89
      aortic 746.89
      mitral 746.89
      pulmonary 746.01
      tricuspid 746.1
  cecum 751.2
  cervix (acquired) 622.4
    congenital 752.43
    in pregnancy or childbirth 654.6 ☑
      affecting fetus or newborn 763.89
      causing obstructed labor 660.2 ☑
        affecting fetus or newborn 763.1
  choana 748.0
  colon 751.2
  cystic duct 751.61
    acquired 575.8
      with obstruction (see also Obstruction, gallbladder) 575.2
  digestive organs NEC 751.8
  duodenum 751.1
  ear canal 744.02
  ejaculatory duct 752.89
  epiglottis 748.3
  esophagus 750.3
  Eustachian tube 744.24
  fallopian tube (acquired) 628.2
    congenital 752.19
  follicular cyst 620.0
  foramen of
    Luschka 742.3
      with spina bifida (see also Spina bifida) 741.0 ☑
    Magendie 742.3
      with spina bifida (see also Spina bifida) 741.0 ☑
  gallbladder 751.69
  genital organ
    external
      female 752.49
      male NEC 752.89
        penis 752.69
    internal
      female 752.89
      male 752.89
  glottis 748.3
  gullet 750.3
  heart
    valve NEC 746.89
      aortic 746.89
      mitral 746.89
      pulmonary 746.01
      tricuspid 746.1
  hymen 752.42
    acquired 623.3
    postinfective 623.3
  ileum 751.1
  intestine (small) 751.1
    large 751.2
  iris, filtration angle (see also Buphthalmia) 743.20
  jejunum 751.1
  kidney 753.3
  lacrimal, apparatus 743.65
    acquired — see Stenosis, lacrimal
  larynx 748.3
  ligament, broad 752.19
  lung 748.5
  meatus urinarius 753.6
  mitral valve 746.89
    with atresia or hypoplasia of aortic orifice or valve, with hypoplasia of ascending aorta and defective development of left ventricle 746.7
  nares (anterior) (posterior) 748.0
  nasolacrimal duct 743.65
  nasopharynx 748.8

☑ Additional Digit Required — Refer to the Tabular List for Digit Selection   Ⓥ Subterms under main terms may continue to next column or page

30 — Volume 2   ►◄ Revised Text   ● New Line   ▲ Revised Code   2014 ICD-9-CM

Atresia, atretic — *continued*
  nose, nostril 748.0
    acquired 738.0
  organ or site NEC — *see* Anomaly, specified type NEC
  osseous meatus (ear) 744.03
  oviduct (acquired) 628.2
    congenital 752.19
  parotid duct 750.23
    acquired 527.8
  pulmonary (artery) 747.31
    valve 746.01
    vein 747.49
  pulmonic 746.01
  pupil 743.46
  rectum 751.2
  salivary duct or gland 750.23
    acquired 527.8
  sublingual duct 750.23
    acquired 527.8
  submaxillary duct or gland 750.23
    acquired 527.8
  trachea 748.3
  tricuspid valve 746.1
  ureter 753.29
  ureteropelvic junction 753.21
  ureterovesical orifice 753.22
  urethra (valvular) 753.6
  urinary tract NEC 753.29
  uterus 752.31
    acquired 621.8
  vagina (acquired) 623.2
    congenital (total) (partial) 752.45
    postgonococcal (old) 098.2
    postinfectional 623.2
    senile 623.2
  vascular NEC (*see also* Atresia, blood vessel) 747.60
    cerebral 747.81
  vas deferens 752.89
  vein NEC (*see also* Atresia, blood vessel) 747.60
    cardiac 746.89
    great 747.49
    portal 747.49
    pulmonary 747.49
    vena cava (inferior) (superior) 747.49
  vesicourethral orifice 753.6
  vulva 752.49
    acquired 624.8
Atrichia, atrichosis 704.00
  congenital (universal) 757.4
Atrioventricularis commune 745.69
At risk for falling V15.88
Atrophia — *see also* Atrophy
  alba 709.09
  cutis 701.8
    idiopathica progressiva 701.8
    senilis 701.8
  dermatological, diffuse (idiopathic) 701.8
  flava hepatis (acuta) (subacuta) (*see also* Necrosis, liver) 570
  gyrata of choroid and retina (central) 363.54
    generalized 363.57
  senilis 797
    dermatological 701.8
  unguium 703.8
    congenita 757.5
Atrophoderma, atrophodermia 701.9
  diffusum (idiopathic) 701.8
  maculatum 701.3
    et striatum 701.3
      due to syphilis 095.8
    syphilitic 091.3
  neuriticum 701.8
  pigmentosum 757.33
  reticulatum symmetricum faciei 701.8
  senile 701.8
  symmetrical 701.8
  vermiculata 701.8
Atrophy, atrophic
  adrenal (autoimmune) (capsule) (cortex) (gland) 255.41
    with hypofunction 255.41
  alveolar process or ridge (edentulous) 525.20

Atrophy, atrophic — *continued*
  alveolar process or ridge — *continued*
    mandible 525.20
      minimal 525.21
      moderate 525.22
      severe 525.23
    maxilla 525.20
      minimal 525.24
      moderate 525.25
      severe 525.26
  appendix 543.9
  Aran-Duchenne muscular 335.21
  arm 728.2
  arteriosclerotic — *see* Arteriosclerosis
  arthritis 714.0
    spine 720.9
  bile duct (any) 576.8
  bladder 596.89
  blanche (of Milian) 701.3
  bone (senile) 733.99
    due to
      disuse 733.7
      infection 733.99
      tabes dorsalis (neurogenic) 094.0
    posttraumatic 733.99
  brain (cortex) (progressive) 331.9
    with dementia 290.10
    Alzheimer's 331.0
      with dementia — *see* Alzheimer's, dementia
    circumscribed (Pick's) 331.11
      with dementia
        with behavioral disturbance 331.11 [294.11]
        without behavioral disturbance 331.11 [294.10]
    congenital 742.4
    hereditary 331.9
    senile 331.2
  breast 611.4
    puerperal, postpartum 676.3 ☑
  buccal cavity 528.9
  cardiac (brown) (senile) (*see also* Degeneration, myocardial) 429.1
  cartilage (infectional) (joint) 733.99
  cast, plaster of Paris 728.2
  cerebellar — *see* Atrophy, brain
  cerebral — *see* Atrophy, brain
  cervix (endometrium) (mucosa) (myometrium) (senile) (uteri) 622.8
    menopausal 627.8
  Charcôt-Marie-Tooth 356.1
  choroid 363.40
    diffuse secondary 363.42
    hereditary (*see also* Dystrophy, choroid) 363.50
      gyrate
        central 363.54
        diffuse 363.57
        generalized 363.57
    senile 363.41
  ciliary body 364.57
  colloid, degenerative 701.3
  conjunctiva (senile) 372.89
  corpus cavernosum 607.89
  cortical (*see also* Atrophy, brain) 331.9
  Cruveilhier's 335.21
  cystic duct 576.8
  dacryosialadenopathy 710.2
  degenerative
    colloid 701.3
    senile 701.3
  Déjérine-Thomas 333.0
  diffuse idiopathic, dermatological 701.8
  disuse
    bone 733.7
    muscle 728.2
    pelvic muscles and anal sphincter 618.83
  Duchenne-Aran 335.21
  ear 388.9
  edentulous alveolar ridge 525.20
    mandible 525.20
      minimal 525.21
      moderate 525.22
      severe 525.23
    maxilla 525.20

Atrophy, atrophic — *continued*
  edentulous alveolar ridge — *continued*
    maxilla — *continued*
      minimal 525.24
      moderate 525.25
      severe 525.26
  emphysema, lung 492.8
  endometrium (senile) 621.8
    cervix 622.8
  enteric 569.89
  epididymis 608.3
  eyeball, cause unknown 360.41
  eyelid 374.50
  facial (skin) 701.9
  facioscapulohumeral (Landouzy-Déjérine) 359.1
  fallopian tube (senile), acquired 620.3
  fatty, thymus (gland) 254.8
  gallbladder 575.8
  gastric 537.89
  gastritis (chronic) 535.1 ☑
  gastrointestinal 569.89
  genital organ, male 608.89
  glandular 289.3
  globe (phthisis bulbi) 360.41
  gum (*see also* Recession, gingival) 523.20
  hair 704.2
  heart (brown) (senile) (*see also* Degeneration, myocardial) 429.1
  hemifacial 754.0
    Romberg 349.89
  hydronephrosis 591
  infantile 261
    paralysis, acute (*see also* Poliomyelitis, with paralysis) 045.1 ☑
  intestine 569.89
  iris (generalized) (postinfectional) (sector shaped) 364.59
    essential 364.51
    progressive 364.51
    sphincter 364.54
  kidney (senile) (*see also* Sclerosis, renal) 587
    with hypertension (*see also* Hypertension, kidney) 403.90
    congenital 753.0
    hydronephrotic 591
    infantile 753.0
  lacrimal apparatus (primary) 375.13
    secondary 375.14
  Landouzy-Déjérine 359.1
  laryngitis, infection 476.0
  larynx 478.79
  Leber's optic 377.16
  lip 528.5
  liver (acute) (subacute) (*see also* Necrosis, liver) 570
    chronic (yellow) 571.8
    yellow (congenital) 570
      with
        abortion — *see* Abortion, by type, with specified complication NEC
        ectopic pregnancy (*see also* categories 633.0–633.9) 639.8
        molar pregnancy (*see also* categories 630–632) 639.8
      chronic 571.8
      complicating pregnancy 646.7 ☑
      following
        abortion 639.8
        ectopic or molar pregnancy 639.8
      from injection, inoculation or transfusion (onset within 8 months after administration) — *see* Hepatitis, viral
      healed 571.5
      obstetric 646.7 ☑
      postabortal 639.8
      postimmunization — *see* Hepatitis, viral
      posttransfusion — *see* Hepatitis, viral
      puerperal, postpartum 674.8 ☑
  lung (senile) 518.89
    congenital 748.69
  macular (dermatological) 701.3
    syphilitic, skin 091.3

Atrophy, atrophic — *continued*
  macular — *continued*
    syphilitic, skin — *continued*
      striated 095.8
  muscle, muscular 728.2
    disuse 728.2
    Duchenne-Aran 335.21
    extremity (lower) (upper) 728.2
    familial spinal 335.11
    general 728.2
    idiopathic 728.2
    infantile spinal 335.0
    myelopathic (progressive) 335.10
    myotonic 359.21
    neuritic 356.1
    neuropathic (peroneal) (progressive) 356.1
    peroneal 356.1
    primary (idiopathic) 728.2
    progressive (familial) (hereditary) (pure) 335.21
      adult (spinal) 335.19
      infantile (spinal) 335.0
      juvenile (spinal) 335.11
      spinal 335.10
        adult 335.19
        hereditary or familial 335.11
        infantile 335.0
    pseudohypertrophic 359.1
    spinal (progressive) 335.10
      adult 335.19
      Aran-Duchenne 335.21
      familial 335.11
      hereditary 335.11
      infantile 335.0
      juvenile 335.11
    syphilitic 095.6
  myocardium (*see also* Degeneration, myocardial) 429.1
  myometrium (senile) 621.8
    cervix 622.8
  myotatic 728.2
  myotonia 359.21
  nail 703.8
    congenital 757.5
  nasopharynx 472.2
  nerve (*see also* Disorder, nerve)
    abducens 378.54
    accessory 352.4
    acoustic or auditory 388.5
    cranial 352.9
      first (olfactory) 352.0
      second (optic) (*see also* Atrophy, optic nerve) 377.10
      third (oculomotor) (partial) 378.51
        total 378.52
      fourth (trochlear) 378.53
      fifth (trigeminal) 350.8
      sixth (abducens) 378.54
      seventh (facial) 351.8
      eighth (auditory) 388.5
      ninth (glossopharyngeal) 352.2
      tenth (pneumogastric) (vagus) 352.3
      eleventh (accessory) 352.4
      twelfth (hypoglossal) 352.5
    facial 351.8
    glossopharyngeal 352.2
    hypoglossal 352.5
    oculomotor (partial) 378.51
      total 378.52
    olfactory 352.0
    peripheral 355.9
    pneumogastric 352.3
    trigeminal 350.8
    trochlear 378.53
    vagus (pneumogastric) 352.3
  nervous system, congenital 742.8
  neuritic (*see also* Disorder, nerve) 355.9
  neurogenic NEC 355.9
    bone
      tabetic 094.0
  nutritional 261
  old age 797
  olivopontocerebellar 333.0

Atrophy, atrophic — *continued*
  optic nerve (ascending) (descending) (infectional) (nonfamilial) (papillomacular bundle) (postretinal) (secondary NEC) (simple) 377.10
    associated with retinal dystrophy 377.13
    dominant hereditary 377.16
    glaucomatous 377.14
    hereditary (dominant) (Leber's) 377.16
    Leber's (hereditary) 377.16
    partial 377.15
    postinflammatory 377.12
    primary 377.11
    syphilitic 094.84
      congenital 090.49
      tabes dorsalis 094.0
  orbit 376.45
  ovary (senile), acquired 620.3
  oviduct (senile), acquired 620.3
  palsy, diffuse 335.20
  pancreas (duct) (senile) 577.8
  papillary muscle 429.81
  paralysis 355.9
  parotid gland 527.0
  patches skin 701.3
    senile 701.8
  penis 607.89
  pharyngitis 472.1
  pharynx 478.29
  pluriglandular 258.8
  polyarthritis 714.0
  prostate 602.2
  pseudohypertrophic 359.1
  renal (*see also* Sclerosis, renal) 587
  reticulata 701.8
  retina (*see also* Degeneration, retina) 362.60
    hereditary (*see also* Dystrophy, retina) 362.70
  rhinitis 472.0
  salivary duct or gland 527.0
  scar NEC 709.2
  sclerosis, lobar (of brain) 331.0
    with dementia
      with behavioral disturbance 331.0 *[294.11]*
      without behavioral disturbance 331.0 *[294.10]*
  scrotum 608.89
  seminal vesicle 608.89
  senile 797
    degenerative, of skin 701.3
  skin (patches) (senile) 701.8
  spermatic cord 608.89
  spinal (cord) 336.8
    acute 336.8
    muscular (chronic) 335.10
      adult 335.19
      familial 335.11
      juvenile 335.10
    paralysis 335.10
      acute (*see also* Poliomyelitis, with paralysis) 045.1 ☑
  spine (column) 733.99
  spleen (senile) 289.59
  spots (skin) 701.3
    senile 701.8
  stomach 537.89
  striate and macular 701.3
    syphilitic 095.8
  subcutaneous 701.9
    due to injection 999.9
  sublingual gland 527.0
  submaxillary gland 527.0
  Sudeck's 733.7
  suprarenal (autoimmune) (capsule) (gland) 255.41
    with hypofunction 255.41
  tarso-orbital fascia, congenital 743.66
  testis 608.3
  thenar, partial 354.0
  throat 478.29
  thymus (fat) 254.8
  thyroid (gland) 246.8
    with
      cretinism 243
      myxedema 244.9

Atrophy, atrophic — *continued*
  thyroid — *continued*
    congenital 243
  tongue (senile) 529.8
    papillae 529.4
    smooth 529.4
  trachea 519.19
  tunica vaginalis 608.89
  turbinate 733.99
  tympanic membrane (nonflaccid) 384.82
    flaccid 384.81
  ulcer (*see also* Ulcer, skin) 707.9
  upper respiratory tract 478.9
  uterus, uterine (acquired) (senile) 621.8
    cervix 622.8
    due to radiation (intended effect) 621.8
  vagina (senile) 627.3
  vascular 459.89
  vas deferens 608.89
  vertebra (senile) 733.99
  vulva (primary) (senile) 624.1
  Werdnig-Hoffmann 335.0
  yellow (acute) (congenital) (liver) (subacute) (*see also* Necrosis, liver) 570
    chronic 571.8
    resulting from administration of blood, plasma, serum, or other biological substance (within 8 months of administration) — *see* Hepatitis, viral

Attack
  akinetic (*see also* Epilepsy) 345.0 ☑
  angina — *see* Angina
  apoplectic (*see also* Disease, cerebrovascular, acute) 436
  benign shuddering 333.93
  bilious — *see* Vomiting
  cataleptic 300.11
  cerebral (*see also* Disease, cerebrovascular, acute) 436
  coronary (*see also* Infarct, myocardium) 410.9 ☑
  cyanotic, newborn 770.83
  epileptic (*see also* Epilepsy) 345.9 ☑
  epileptiform 780.39
  heart (*see also* Infarct, myocardium) 410.9 ☑
  hemiplegia (*see also* Disease, cerebrovascular, acute) 436
  hysterical 300.11
  jacksonian (*see also* Epilepsy) 345.5 ☑
  myocardium, myocardial (*see also* Infarct, myocardium) 410.9 ☑
  myoclonic (*see also* Epilepsy) 345.1 ☑
  panic 300.01
  paralysis (*see also* Disease, cerebrovascular, acute) 436
  paroxysmal 780.39
  psychomotor (*see also* Epilepsy) 345.4 ☑
  salaam (*see also* Epilepsy) 345.6 ☑
  schizophreniform (*see also* Schizophrenia) 295.4 ☑
  sensory and motor 780.39
  syncope 780.2
  toxic, cerebral 780.39
  transient ischemic (TIA) 435.9
  unconsciousness 780.2
    hysterical 300.11
  vasomotor 780.2
  vasovagal (idiopathic) (paroxysmal) 780.2

Attention to
  artificial opening (of) V55.9
    digestive tract NEC V55.4
    specified site NEC V55.8
    urinary tract NEC V55.6
    vagina V55.7
  colostomy V55.3
  cystostomy V55.5
  dressing
    wound V58.30
      nonsurgical V58.30
      surgical V58.31
  gastrostomy V55.1
  ileostomy V55.2
  jejunostomy V55.4
  nephrostomy V55.6

Attention to — *continued*
  surgical dressings V58.31
  sutures V58.32
  tracheostomy V55.0
  ureterostomy V55.6
  urethrostomy V55.6
Attrition
  gum (*see also* Recession, gingival) 523.20
  teeth (hard tissues) 521.10
    excessive 521.10
      extending into
        dentine 521.12
        pulp 521.13
      generalized 521.15
      limited to enamel 521.11
      localized 521.14
Atypical — *see also* condition
  cells
    endocervical 795.00
    endometrial 795.00
    glandular
      anus 796.70
      cervical 795.00
      vaginal 795.10
  distribution, vessel (congenital) (peripheral) NEC 747.60
  endometrium 621.9
  kidney 593.89
Atypism, cervix 622.10
Audible tinnitus — *see also* Tinnitus 388.30
Auditory — *see* condition
Audry's syndrome (acropachyderma) 757.39
Aujeszky's disease 078.89
Aura
  jacksonian (*see also* Epilepsy) 345.5 ☑
  persistent migraine 346.5 ☑
    with cerebral infarction 346.6 ☑
    without cerebral infarction 346.5 ☑
Aurantiasis, cutis 278.3
Auricle, auricular — *see* condition
Auriculotemporal syndrome 350.8
Australian
  Q fever 083.0
  X disease 062.4
Autism, autistic (child) (infantile) 299.0 ☑
Autodigestion 799.89
Autoerythrocyte sensitization 287.2
Autographism 708.3
Autoimmune
  cold sensitivity 283.0
  disease NEC 279.49
  hemolytic anemia 283.0
  inhibitors to clotting factors 286.52
  lymphoproliferative syndrome (ALPS) 279.41
  thyroiditis 245.2
Autoinfection, septic — *see* Septicemia
Autointoxication 799.89
Automatism 348.89
  with temporal sclerosis 348.81
  epileptic (*see also* Epilepsy) 345.4 ☑
  paroxysmal, idiopathic (*see also* Epilepsy) 345.4 ☑
Autonomic, autonomous
  bladder 596.54
    neurogenic 596.54
      with cauda equina 344.61
  dysreflexia 337.3
  faciocephalalgia (*see also* Neuropathy, peripheral, autonomic) 337.9
  hysterical seizure 300.11
  imbalance (*see also* Neuropathy, peripheral, autonomic) 337.9
Autophony 388.40
Autosensitivity, erythrocyte 287.2
Autotopagnosia 780.99
Autotoxemia 799.89
Autumn — *see* condition
Avellis' syndrome 344.89
Aversion
  oral 783.3
    newborn 779.31
    nonorganic origin 307.59
Aviators
  disease or sickness (*see also* Effect, adverse, high altitude) 993.2

Aviators — *continued*
  ear 993.0
  effort syndrome 306.2
Avitaminosis (multiple NEC) — *see also* Deficiency, vitamin 269.2
  A 264.9
  B 266.9
    with
      beriberi 265.0
      pellagra 265.2
  B_1 265.1
  B_2 266.0
  B_6 266.1
  B_{12} 266.2
  C (with scurvy) 267
  D 268.9
    with
      osteomalacia 268.2
      rickets 268.0
  E 269.1
  G 266.0
  H 269.1
  K 269.0
  multiple 269.2
  nicotinic acid 265.2
  P 269.1
Avulsion (traumatic) 879.8
  blood vessel — *see* Injury, blood vessel, by site
  cartilage (*see also* Dislocation, by site)
    knee, current (*see also* Tear, meniscus) 836.2
    symphyseal (inner), complicating delivery 665.6 ☑
  complicated 879.9
  diaphragm — *see* Injury, internal, diaphragm
  ear — *see* Wound, open, ear
  epiphysis of bone — *see* Fracture, by site
  external site other than limb — *see* Wound, open, by site
  eye 871.3
  fingernail — *see* Wound, open, finger
  fracture — *see* Fracture, by site
  genital organs, external — *see* Wound, open, genital organs
  head (intracranial) NEC (*see also* Injury, intracranial, with open intracranial wound)
    complete 874.9
    external site NEC 873.8
      complicated 873.9
  internal organ or site — *see* Injury, internal, by site
  joint (*see also* Dislocation, by site)
    capsule — *see* Sprain, by site
  ligament — *see* Sprain, by site
  limb (*see also* Amputation, traumatic, by site)
    skin and subcutaneous tissue — *see* Wound, open, by site
  muscle — *see* Sprain, by site
  nerve (root) — *see* Injury, nerve, by site
  scalp — *see* Wound, open, scalp
  skin and subcutaneous tissue — *see* Wound, open, by site
  symphyseal cartilage (inner), complicating delivery 665.6 ☑
  tendon (*see also* Sprain, by site)
    with open wound — *see* Wound, open, by site
  toenail — *see* Wound, open, toe(s)
  tooth 873.63
    complicated 873.73
Awaiting organ transplant status V49.83
Awareness of heart beat 785.1
Axe grinders' disease 502
Axenfeld's anomaly or syndrome 743.44
Axilla, axillary — *see also* condition
  breast 757.6
Axonotmesis — *see* Injury, nerve, by site
Ayala's disease 756.89
Ayerza's disease or syndrome (pulmonary artery sclerosis with pulmonary hypertension) 416.0

☑ **Additional Digit Required** — Refer to the Tabular List for Digit Selection   ▽ **Subterms under main terms may continue to next column or page**

2014 ICD-9-CM   ▶◀ Revised Text   ● New Line   ▲ Revised Code   **Volume 2 — 33**

Beigel's disease or morbus (white piedra) 111.2

Bejel 104.0

Bekhterev-Strümpell-Marie syndrome (ankylosing spondylitis) 720.0

Bekhterev's disease (ankylosing spondylitis) 720.0

Belching — see also Eructation 787.3

Bell's
  disease (see also Psychosis, affective) 296.0 ☑
  mania (see also Psychosis, affective) 296.0 ☑
  palsy, paralysis 351.0
    infant 767.5
    newborn 767.5
    syphilitic 094.89
  spasm 351.0

Bence-Jones albuminuria, albuminosuria, or proteinuria 791.0

Bends 993.3

Benedikt's syndrome (paralysis) 344.89

Benign — see also condition
  cellular changes, cervix 795.09
  prostate
    with
      other lower urinary tract symptoms (LUTS) 600.21
      urinary
        obstruction 600.21
        retention 600.21
    hyperplasia 600.20
    neoplasm 222.2

Bennett's
  disease (leukemia) 208.9 ☑
  fracture (closed) 815.01
    open 815.11

Benson's disease 379.22

Bent
  back (hysterical) 300.11
  nose 738.0
    congenital 754.0

Bereavement V62.82
  as adjustment reaction 309.0

Bergeron's disease (hysteroepilepsy) 300.11

Berger's paresthesia (lower limb) 782.0

Beriberi (acute) (atrophic) (chronic) (dry) (subacute) (wet) 265.0
  with polyneuropathy 265.0 [357.4]
  heart (disease) 265.0 [425.7]
  leprosy 030.1
  neuritis 265.0 [357.4]

Berlin's disease or edema (traumatic) 921.3

Berloque dermatitis 692.72

Bernard-Horner syndrome — see also Neuropathy, peripheral, autonomic 337.9

Bernard-Sergent syndrome (acute adrenocortical insufficiency) 255.41

Bernard-Soulier disease or thrombopathy 287.1

Bernhardt-Roth disease or syndrome (paresthesia) 355.1

Bernhardt's disease or paresthesia 355.1

Bernheim's syndrome — see also Failure, heart 428.0

Bertielliasis 123.8

Bertolotti's syndrome (sacralization of fifth lumbar vertebra) 756.15

Berylliosis (acute) (chronic) (lung) (occupational) 503

Besnier-Boeck-Schaumann disease (sarcoidosis) 135

Besnier-Boeck disease or sarcoid 135

Besnier's
  lupus pernio 135
  prurigo (atopic dermatitis) (infantile eczema) 691.8

Best's disease 362.76

Bestiality 302.1

Beta-adrenergic hyperdynamic circulatory state 429.82

Beta-aminoisobutyric aciduria 277.2

Beta-mercaptolactate-cysteine disulfiduria 270.0

Beta thalassemia (mixed) 282.44
  major 282.44
  minor 282.46

Beurmann's disease (sporotrichosis) 117.1

Bezoar 938
  intestine 936
  stomach 935.2

Bezold's abscess — see also Mastoiditis 383.01

Bianchi's syndrome (aphasia-apraxia-alexia) 784.69

Bicornuate or bicornis uterus (complete) (partial) 752.34
  in pregnancy or childbirth 654.0 ☑
    with obstructed labor 660.2 ☑
      affecting fetus or newborn 763.1
    affecting fetus or newborn 763.89

Bicuspid aortic valve 746.4

Biedl-Bardet syndrome 759.89

Bielschowsky-Jansky
  amaurotic familial idiocy 330.1
  disease 330.1

Bielschowsky's disease 330.1

Biemond's syndrome (obesity, polydactyly, and intellectual disabilities) 759.89

Biermer's anemia or disease (pernicious anemia) 281.0

Biett's disease 695.4

Bifid (congenital) — see also Imperfect, closure
  apex, heart 746.89
  clitoris 752.49
  epiglottis 748.3
  kidney 753.3
  nose 748.1
  patella 755.64
  scrotum 752.89
  toe 755.66
  tongue 750.13
  ureter 753.4
  uterus 752.34
  uvula 749.02
    with cleft lip (see also Cleft, palate, with cleft lip) 749.20

Biforis uterus (suprasimplex) 752.34

Bifurcation (congenital) — see also Imperfect, closure
  gallbladder 751.69
  kidney pelvis 753.3
  renal pelvis 753.3
  rib 756.3
  tongue 750.13
  trachea 748.3
  ureter 753.4
  urethra 753.8
  uvula 749.02
    with cleft lip (see also Cleft, palate, with cleft lip) 749.20
  vertebra 756.19

Bigeminal pulse 427.89

Bigeminy 427.89

Big spleen syndrome 289.4

Bilateral — see condition

Bile duct — see condition

Bile pigments in urine 791.4

Bilharziasis — see also Schistosomiasis 120.9
  chyluria 120.0
  cutaneous 120.3
  galacturia 120.0
  hematochyluria 120.0
  intestinal 120.1
  lipemia 120.9
  lipuria 120.0
  Oriental 120.2
  piarhemia 120.9
  pulmonary 120.2
  tropical hematuria 120.0
  vesical 120.0

Biliary — see condition

Bilious (attack) — see also Vomiting
  fever, hemoglobinuric 084.8

Bilirubinuria 791.4

Biliuria 791.4

Billroth's disease
  meningocele (see also Spina bifida) 741.9 ☑

Bilobate placenta — see Placenta, abnormal

Bilocular
  heart 745.7
  stomach 536.8

Bing-Horton syndrome (histamine cephalgia) 339.00

Binswanger's disease or dementia 290.12

Biörck (-Thorson) syndrome (malignant carcinoid) 259.2

Biparta, bipartite — see also Imperfect, closure
  carpal scaphoid 755.59
  patella 755.64
  placenta — see Placenta, abnormal
  vagina 752.49

Bird
  face 756.0
  fanciers' lung or disease 495.2
  flu — see also Influenza, avian 488.02

Bird's disease (oxaluria) 271.8

Birt-Hogg-Dube syndrome 759.89

Birth
  abnormal fetus or newborn 763.9
  accident, fetus or newborn — see Birth, injury
  complications in mother — see Delivery, complicated
  compression during NEC 767.9
  defect — see Anomaly
  delayed, fetus 763.9
  difficult NEC, affecting fetus or newborn 763.9
  dry, affecting fetus or newborn 761.1
  forced, NEC, affecting fetus or newborn 763.89
  forceps, affecting fetus or newborn 763.2
  hematoma of sternomastoid 767.8
  immature 765.1 ☑
    extremely 765.0 ☑
  inattention, after or at 995.52
  induced, affecting fetus or newborn 763.89
  infant — see Newborn
  injury NEC 767.9
    adrenal gland 767.8
    basal ganglia 767.0
    brachial plexus (paralysis) 767.6
    brain (compression) (pressure) 767.0
    cerebellum 767.0
    cerebral hemorrhage 767.0
    conjunctiva 767.8
    eye 767.8
    fracture
      bone, any except clavicle or spine 767.3
      clavicle 767.2
      femur 767.3
      humerus 767.3
      long bone 767.3
      radius and ulna 767.3
      skeleton NEC 767.3
      skull 767.3
      spine 767.4
      tibia and fibula 767.3
    hematoma 767.8
      liver (subcapsular) 767.8
      mastoid 767.8
      skull 767.19
      sternomastoid 767.8
      testes 767.8
      vulva 767.8
    intracranial (edema) 767.0
    laceration
      brain 767.0
      by scalpel 767.8
      peripheral nerve 767.7
    liver 767.8
    meninges
      brain 767.0
      spinal cord 767.4
    nerves (cranial, peripheral) 767.7
      brachial plexus 767.6
      facial 767.5
    paralysis 767.7
      brachial plexus 767.6
      Erb (-Duchenne) 767.6
      facial nerve 767.5
      Klumpke (-Déjérine) 767.6
      radial nerve 767.6
      spinal (cord) (hemorrhage) (laceration) (rupture) 767.4
    rupture
      intracranial 767.0

Birth — continued
  injury — continued
    rupture — continued
      liver 767.8
      spinal cord 767.4
      spleen 767.8
      viscera 767.8
    scalp 767.19
    scalpel wound 767.8
    skeleton NEC 767.3
    specified NEC 767.8
    spinal cord 767.4
    spleen 767.8
    subdural hemorrhage 767.0
    tentorial, tear 767.0
    testes 767.8
    vulva 767.8
  instrumental, NEC, affecting fetus or newborn 763.2
  lack of care, after or at 995.52
  multiple
    affected by maternal complications of pregnancy 761.5
    healthy liveborn — see Newborn, multiple
  neglect, after or at 995.52
  newborn — see Newborn
  palsy or paralysis NEC 767.7
  precipitate, fetus or newborn 763.6
  premature (infant) 765.1 ☑
  prolonged, affecting fetus or newborn 763.9
  retarded, fetus or newborn 763.9
  shock, newborn 779.89
  strangulation or suffocation
    due to aspiration of clear amniotic fluid 770.13
    with respiratory symptoms 770.14
    mechanical 767.8
  trauma NEC 767.9
  triplet
    affected by maternal complications of pregnancy 761.5
    healthy liveborn — see Newborn, multiple
  twin
    affected by maternal complications of pregnancy 761.5
    healthy liveborn — see Newborn, twin
  ventouse, affecting fetus or newborn 763.3

Birthmark 757.32

Bisalbuminemia 273.8

Biskra button 085.1

Bite(s)
  with intact skin surface — see Contusion
  animal — see Wound, open, by site
    intact skin surface — see Contusion
  bedbug — see Injury, superficial, by site
  centipede 989.5
  chigger 133.8
  fire ant 989.5
  flea — see Injury, superficial, by site
  human (open wound) (see also Wound, open, by site)
    intact skin surface — see Contusion
  insect
    nonvenomous — see Injury, superficial by site
    venomous 989.5
  mad dog (death from) 071
  open
    anterior 524.24
    posterior 524.25
  poisonous 989.5
  red bug 133.8
  reptile 989.5
    nonvenomous — see Wound, open, by site
  snake 989.5
    nonvenomous — see Wound, open, by site
  spider (venomous) 989.5
    nonvenomous — see Injury, superficial by site
  venomous 989.5

Biting
  cheek or lip 528.9

☑ Additional Digit Required — Refer to the Tabular List for Digit Selection   ▽ Subterms under main terms may continue to next column or page

34 — Volume 2   ▶◀ Revised Text   ● New Line   ▲ Revised Code   2014 ICD-9-CM

Biting — continued
nail 307.9
Black
death 020.9
eye NEC 921.0
hairy tongue 529.3
heel 924.20
lung disease 500
palm 923.20
Blackfan-Diamond anemia or syndrome
(congenital hypoplastic anemia) 284.01
Blackhead 706.1
Blackout 780.2
Blackwater fever 084.8
Bladder — see condition
Blast
blindness 921.3
concussion — see Blast, injury
injury 869.0
with open wound into cavity 869.1
abdomen or thorax — see Injury, internal, by site
brain (see also Concussion, brain) 850.9
with skull fracture — see Fracture, skull
ear (acoustic nerve trauma) 951.5
with perforation, tympanic membrane — see Wound, open, ear, drum
lung (see also Injury, internal, lung) 861.20
otitic (explosive) 388.11
Blastomycosis, blastomycotic (chronic) (cutaneous) (disseminated) (lung) (pulmonary) (systemic) 116.0
Brazilian 116.1
European 117.5
keloidal 116.2
North American 116.0
primary pulmonary 116.0
South American 116.1
Bleb(s) 709.8
emphysematous (bullous) (diffuse) (lung) (ruptured) (solitary) 492.0
filtering, eye (postglaucoma) (status) V45.69
with complication 997.99
postcataract extraction (complication) 997.99
lung (ruptured) 492.0
congenital 770.5
subpleural (emphysematous) 492.0
Bleeder (familial) (hereditary) — see Defect, coagulation 286.9
nonfamilial 286.9
Bleeding — see also Hemorrhage 459.0
anal 569.3
anovulatory 628.0
atonic, following delivery 666.1 ☑
capillary 448.9
due to subinvolution 621.1
puerperal 666.2 ☑
ear 388.69
excessive, associated with menopausal onset 627.0
familial (see also Defect, coagulation) 286.9
following intercourse 626.7
gastrointestinal 578.9
gums 523.8
hemorrhoids — see Hemorrhoids, bleeding
intermenstrual
irregular 626.6
regular 626.5
intraoperative 998.11
irregular NEC 626.4
menopausal 627.0
mouth 528.9
nipple 611.79
nose 784.7
ovulation 626.5
postclimacteric 627.1
postcoital 626.7
postmenopausal 627.1
following induced menopause 627.4
postoperative 998.11
preclimacteric 627.0
puberty 626.3

Bleeding — see also Hemorrhage — continued
puberty — continued
excessive, with onset of menstrual periods 626.3
rectum, rectal 569.3
tendencies (see also Defect, coagulation) 286.9
throat 784.8
umbilical stump 772.3
umbilicus 789.9
unrelated to menstrual cycle 626.6
uterus, uterine 626.9
climacteric 627.0
dysfunctional 626.8
functional 626.8
unrelated to menstrual cycle 626.6
vagina, vaginal 623.8
functional 626.8
vicarious 625.8
Blennorrhagia, blennorrhagic — see Blennorrhea
Blennorrhea (acute) 098.0
adultorum 098.40
alveolaris 523.40
chronic or duration of 2 months or over 098.2
gonococcal (neonatorum) 098.40
inclusion (neonatal) (newborn) 771.6
neonatorum 098.40
Blepharelosis — see also Entropion 374.00
Blepharitis (eyelid) 373.00
angularis 373.01
ciliaris 373.00
with ulcer 373.01
marginal 373.00
with ulcer 373.01
scrofulous (see also Tuberculosis)
017.3 ☑ [373.00]
squamous 373.02
ulcerative 373.01
Blepharochalasis 374.34
congenital 743.62
Blepharoclonus 333.81
Blepharoconjunctivitis — see also Conjunctivitis 372.20
angular 372.21
contact 372.22
Blepharophimosis (eyelid) 374.46
congenital 743.62
Blepharoplegia 374.89
Blepharoptosis 374.30
congenital 743.61
Blepharopyorrhea 098.49
Blepharospasm 333.81
due to drugs 333.85
Blessig's cyst 362.62
Blighted ovum 631.8
Blind
bronchus (congenital) 748.3
eye (see also Blindness)
hypertensive 360.42
hypotensive 360.41
loop syndrome (postoperative) 579.2
sac, fallopian tube (congenital) 752.19
spot, enlarged 368.42
tract or tube (congenital) NEC — see Atresia
Blindness (acquired) (congenital) (both eyes) 369.00
with deafness V49.85
blast 921.3
with nerve injury — see Injury, nerve, optic
Bright's — see Uremia
color (congenital) 368.59
acquired 368.55
blue 368.53
green 368.52
red 368.51
total 368.54
concussion 950.9
cortical 377.75
day 368.10
acquired 368.10
congenital 368.10
hereditary 368.10

Blindness — continued
day — continued
specified type NEC 368.10
due to
injury NEC 950.9
refractive error — see Error, refractive
eclipse (total) 363.31
emotional 300.11
face 368.16
hysterical 300.11
legal (both eyes) (USA definition) 369.4
with impairment of better (less impaired) eye
near-total 369.02
with
lesser eye impairment 369.02
near-total 369.04
total 369.03
profound 369.05
with
lesser eye impairment 369.05
near-total 369.07
profound 369.08
total 369.06
severe 369.21
with
lesser eye impairment 369.21
blind 369.11
near-total 369.13
profound 369.14
severe 369.22
total 369.12
total
with lesser eye impairment
total 369.01
mind 784.69
moderate
both eyes 369.25
with impairment of lesser eye (specified as)
blind, not further specified 369.15
low vision, not further specified 369.23
near-total 369.17
profound 369.18
severe 369.24
total 369.16
one eye 369.74
with vision of other eye (specified as)
near-normal 369.75
normal 369.76
near-total
both eyes 369.04
with impairment of lesser eye (specified as)
blind, not further specified 369.02
total 369.03
one eye 369.64
with vision of other eye (specified as)
near-normal 369.65
normal 369.66
night 368.60
acquired 368.62
congenital (Japanese) 368.61
hereditary 368.61
specified type NEC 368.69
vitamin A deficiency 264.5
nocturnal — see Blindness, night
one eye 369.60
with low vision of other eye 369.10
profound
both eyes 369.08
with impairment of lesser eye (specified as)
blind, not further specified 369.05
near-total 369.07
total 369.06
one eye 369.67
with vision of other eye (specified as)
near-normal 369.68
normal 369.69
psychic 784.69
severe
both eyes 369.22

Blindness — continued
severe — continued
both eyes — continued
with impairment of lesser eye (specified as)
blind, not further specified 369.11
low vision, not further specified 369.21
near-total 369.13
profound 369.14
total 369.12
one eye 369.71
with vision of other eye (specified as)
near-normal 369.72
normal 369.73
snow 370.24
sun 363.31
temporary 368.12
total
both eyes 369.01
one eye 369.61
with vision of other eye (specified as)
near-normal 369.62
normal 369.63
transient 368.12
traumatic NEC 950.9
word (developmental) 315.01
acquired 784.61
secondary to organic lesion 784.61
Blister — see also Injury, superficial, by site
beetle dermatitis 692.89
due to burn — see Burn, by site, second degree
fever 054.9
fracture — omit code
multiple, skin, nontraumatic 709.8
Bloating 787.3
Bloch-Siemens syndrome (incontinentia pigmenti) 757.33
Bloch-Stauffer dyshormonal dermatosis 757.33
Bloch-Sulzberger disease or syndrome (incontinentia pigmenti) (melanoblastosis) 757.33
Block
alveolar capillary 516.8
arborization (heart) 426.6
arrhythmic 426.9
atrioventricular (AV) (incomplete) (partial) 426.10
with
2:1 atrioventricular response block 426.13
atrioventricular dissociation 426.0
first degree (incomplete) 426.11
second degree (Mobitz type I) 426.13
Mobitz (type) II 426.12
third degree 426.0
complete 426.0
congenital 746.86
congenital 746.86
Mobitz (incomplete)
type I (Wenckebach's) 426.13
type II 426.12
partial 426.13
auriculoventricular (see also Block, atrioventricular) 426.10
complete 426.0
congenital 746.86
congenital 746.86
bifascicular (cardiac) 426.53
bundle branch (complete) (false) (incomplete) 426.50
bilateral 426.53
left (complete) (main stem) 426.3
with right bundle branch block 426.53
anterior fascicular 426.2
with
posterior fascicular block 426.3
right bundle branch block 426.52
hemiblock 426.2
incomplete 426.2

☑ **Additional Digit Required** — Refer to the Tabular List for Digit Selection

▽ **Subterms under main terms may continue to next column or page**

2014 ICD-9-CM

▶◀ Revised Text   ● New Line   ▲ Revised Code

Volume 2 — 35

Biting — Block

Block — *continued*
  bundle branch — *continued*
    left — *continued*
      incomplete — *continued*
        with right bundle branch block 426.53
      posterior fascicular 426.2
        with
          anterior fascicular block 426.3
          right bundle branch block 426.51
    right 426.4
      with
        left bundle branch block (incomplete) (main stem) 426.53
        left fascicular block 426.53
          anterior 426.52
          posterior 426.51
    Wilson's type 426.4
  cardiac 426.9
  conduction 426.9
    complete 426.0
  Eustachian tube (*see also* Obstruction, Eustachian tube) 381.60
  fascicular (left anterior) (left posterior) 426.2
  foramen Magendie (acquired) 331.3
    congenital 742.3
      with spina bifida (*see also* Spina bifida) 741.0 ☑
  heart 426.9
    first degree (atrioventricular) 426.11
    second degree (atrioventricular) 426.13
    third degree (atrioventricular) 426.0
    bundle branch (complete) (false) (incomplete) 426.50
      bilateral 426.53
      left (*see also* Block, bundle branch, left) 426.3
      right (*see also* Block, bundle branch, right) 426.4
    complete (atrioventricular) 426.0
    congenital 746.86
    incomplete 426.13
    intra-atrial 426.6
    intraventricular NEC 426.6
    sinoatrial 426.6
    specified type NEC 426.6
  hepatic vein 453.0
  intraventricular (diffuse) (myofibrillar) 426.6
    bundle branch (complete) (false) (incomplete) 426.50
      bilateral 426.53
      left (*see also* Block, bundle branch, left) 426.3
      right (*see also* Block, bundle branch, right) 426.4
  kidney (*see also* Disease, renal) 593.9
    postcystoscopic 997.5
  myocardial (*see also* Block, heart) 426.9
  nodal 426.10
  optic nerve 377.49
  organ or site (congenital) NEC — *see* Atresia
  parietal 426.6
  peri-infarction 426.6
  portal (vein) 452
  sinoatrial 426.6
  sinoauricular 426.6
  spinal cord 336.9
  trifascicular 426.54
  tubal 628.2
  vein NEC 453.9
Blocq's disease or syndrome (astasia-abasia) 307.9
Blood-forming organ disease 289.9
Blood
  constituents, abnormal NEC 790.6
  disease 289.9
    specified NEC 289.89
  donor V59.01
    other blood components V59.09
    stem cells V59.02
    whole blood V59.01
  dyscrasia 289.9

Blood — *continued*
  dyscrasia — *continued*
    with
      abortion — *see* Abortion, by type, with hemorrhage, delayed or excessive
      ectopic pregnancy (*see also* categories 633.0–633.9) 639.1
      molar pregnancy (*see also* categories 630–632) 639.1
    following
      abortion 639.1
      ectopic or molar pregnancy 639.1
    newborn NEC 776.9
    puerperal, postpartum 666.3 ☑
  flukes NEC (*see also* Infestation, Schistosoma) 120.9
  in
    feces (*see also* Melena) 578.1
      occult 792.1
    urine (*see also* Hematuria) 599.70
  mole 631.8
  occult 792.1
  poisoning (*see also* Septicemia) 038.9
  pressure
    decreased, due to shock following injury 958.4
    fluctuating 796.4
    high (*see also* Hypertension) 401.9
      borderline 796.2
      incidental reading (isolated) (nonspecific), without diagnosis of hypertension 796.2
    low (*see also* Hypotension) 458.9
      incidental reading (isolated) (nonspecific), without diagnosis of hypotension 796.3
  spitting (*see also* Hemoptysis) 786.30
  staining cornea 371.12
  transfusion
    without reported diagnosis V58.2
    donor V59.01
      stem cells V59.02
    reaction or complication — *see* Complications, transfusion
  tumor — *see* Hematoma
  vessel rupture — *see* Hemorrhage
  vomiting (*see also* Hematemesis) 578.0
Bloodgood's disease 610.1
Bloodshot eye 379.93
Bloom (-Machacek) (-Torre) syndrome 757.39
Blotch, palpebral 372.55
Blount-Barber syndrome (tibia vara) 732.4
Blount's disease (tibia vara) 732.4
Blue
  baby 746.9
  bloater 491.20
    with
      acute bronchitis 491.22
      exacerbation (acute) 491.21
  diaper syndrome 270.0
  disease 746.9
  dome cyst 610.0
  drum syndrome 381.02
  sclera 743.47
    with fragility of bone and deafness 756.51
  toe syndrome 445.02
Blueness — *see also* Cyanosis 782.5
Blurring, visual 368.8
Blushing (abnormal) (excessive) 782.62
BMI (body mass index)
  adult
    25.0-25.9 V85.21
    26.0-26.9 V85.22
    27.0-27.9 V85.23
    28.0-28.9 V85.24
    29.0-29.9 V85.25
    30.0-30.9 V85.30
    31.0-31.9 V85.31
    32.0-32.9 V85.32
    33.0-33.9 V85.33
    34.0-34.9 V85.34
    35.0-35.9 V85.35
    36.0-36.9 V85.36
    37.0-37.9 V85.37

BMI — *continued*
  adult — *continued*
    38.0-38.9 V85.38
    39.0-39.9 V85.39
    40.0-44.9 V85.41
    45.0-49.9 V85.42
    50.0-59.9 V85.43
    60.0-69.9 V85.44
    70 and over V85.45
    between 19-24 V85.1
    less than 19 V85.0
  pediatric
    5th percentile to less than 85th percentile for age V85.52
    85th percentile to less than 95th percentile for age V85.53
    greater than or equal to 95th percentile for age V85.54
    less than 5th percentile for age V85.51
Boarder, hospital V65.0
  infant V65.0
Bockhart's impetigo (superficial folliculitis) 704.8
Bodechtel-Guttmann disease (subacute sclerosing panencephalitis) 046.2
Boder-Sedgwick syndrome (ataxia-telangiectasia) 334.8
Body, bodies
  Aschoff (*see also* Myocarditis, rheumatic) 398.0
  asteroid, vitreous 379.22
  choroid, colloid (degenerative) 362.57
    hereditary 362.77
  cytoid (retina) 362.82
  drusen (retina) (*see also* Drusen) 362.57
    optic disc 377.21
  fibrin, pleura 511.0
  foreign — *see* Foreign body
  Hassall-Henle 371.41
  loose
    joint (*see also* Loose, body, joint) 718.1 ☑
      knee 717.6
    knee 717.6
    sheath, tendon 727.82
  Mallory's 034.1
  mass index (BMI)
    adult
      25.0-25.9 V85.21
      26.0-26.9 V85.22
      27.0-27.9 V85.23
      28.0-28.9 V85.24
      29.0-29.9 V85.25
      30.0-30.9 V85.30
      31.0-31.9 V85.31
      32.0-32.9 V85.32
      33.0-33.9 V85.33
      34.0-34.9 V85.34
      35.0-35.9 V85.35
      36.0-36.9 V85.36
      37.0-37.9 V85.37
      38.0-38.9 V85.38
      39.0-39.9 V85.39
      40.0-44.9 V85.41
      45.0-49.9 V85.42
      50.0-59.9 V85.43
      60.0-69.9 V85.44
      70 and over V85.45
      between 19-24 V85.1
      less than 19 V85.0
    pediatric
      5th percentile to less than 85th percentile for age V85.52
      85th percentile to less than 95th percentile for age V85.53
      greater than or equal to 95th percentile for age V85.54
      less than 5th percentile for age V85.51
  Mooser 081.0
  Negri 071
  rice (joint) (*see also* Loose, body, joint) 718.1 ☑
    knee 717.6
  rocking 307.3

Boeck's
  disease (sarcoidosis) 135
  lupoid (miliary) 135
  sarcoid 135
Boerhaave's syndrome (spontaneous esophageal rupture) 530.4
Boggy
  cervix 622.8
  uterus 621.8
Boil — *see also* Carbuncle 680.9
  abdominal wall 680.2
  Aleppo 085.1
  ankle 680.6
  anus 680.5
  arm (any part, above wrist) 680.3
  auditory canal, external 680.0
  axilla 680.3
  back (any part) 680.2
  Baghdad 085.1
  breast 680.2
  buttock 680.5
  chest wall 680.2
  corpus cavernosum 607.2
  Delhi 085.1
  ear (any part) 680.0
  eyelid 373.13
  face (any part, except eye) 680.0
  finger (any) 680.4
  flank 680.2
  foot (any part) 680.7
  forearm 680.3
  Gafsa 085.1
  genital organ, male 608.4
  gluteal (region) 680.5
  groin 680.2
  hand (any part) 680.4
  head (any part, except face) 680.8
  heel 680.7
  hip 680.6
  knee 680.6
  labia 616.4
  lacrimal (*see also* Dacryocystitis) 375.30
    gland (*see also* Dacryoadenitis) 375.00
    passages (duct) (sac) (*see also* Dacryocystitis) 375.30
  leg, any part, except foot 680.6
  multiple sites 680.9
  natal 085.1
  neck 680.1
  nose (external) (septum) 680.0
  orbit, orbital 376.01
  partes posteriores 680.5
  pectoral region 680.2
  penis 607.2
  perineum 680.2
  pinna 680.0
  scalp (any part) 680.8
  scrotum 608.4
  seminal vesicle 608.0
  shoulder 680.3
  skin NEC 680.9
  specified site NEC 680.8
  spermatic cord 608.4
  temple (region) 680.0
  testis 608.4
  thigh 680.6
  thumb 680.4
  toe (any) 680.7
  tropical 085.1
  trunk 680.2
  tunica vaginalis 608.4
  umbilicus 680.2
  upper arm 680.3
  vas deferens 608.4
  vulva 616.4
  wrist 680.4
Bold hives — *see also* Urticaria 708.9
Bolivian hemorrhagic fever 078.7
Bombé, iris 364.74
Bomford-Rhoads anemia (refractory) 238.7
Bone — *see* condition
Bonnevie-Ullrich syndrome 758.6
Bonnier's syndrome 386.19
Bonvale Dam fever 780.79
Bony block of joint 718.80
  ankle 718.87

☑ **Additional Digit Required** — Refer to the Tabular List for Digit Selection   ▽ **Subterms under main terms may continue to next column or page**

36 — Volume 2   ▶◀ **Revised Text**   ● **New Line**   ▲ **Revised Code**   **2014 ICD-9-CM**

Bony block of joint — *continued*
  elbow 718.82
  foot 718.87
  hand 718.84
  hip 718.85
  knee 718.86
  multiple sites 718.89
  pelvic region 718.85
  shoulder (region) 718.81
  specified site NEC 718.88
  wrist 718.83
BOOP (bronchiolitis obliterans organized
  pneumonia) 516.8
Borderline
  diabetes mellitus 790.29
  hypertension 796.2
  intellectual functioning V62.89
  osteopenia 733.90
  pelvis 653.1 ☑
    with obstruction during labor 660.1 ☑
      affecting fetus or newborn 763.1
  psychosis (*see also* Schizophrenia) 295.5 ☑
    of childhood (*see also* Psychosis, child-
      hood) 299.8 ☑
  schizophrenia (*see also* Schizophrenia)
      295.5 ☑
Borna disease 062.9
Bornholm disease (epidemic pleurodynia)
  074.1
Borrelia vincentii (mouth) (pharynx) (tonsils)
  101
Bostock's catarrh — *see also* Fever, hay 477.9
Boston exanthem 048
Botalli, ductus (patent) (persistent) 747.0
Bothriocephalus latus infestation 123.4
Botulism 005.1
  food poisoning 005.1
  infant 040.41
  non-foodborne 040.42
  wound 040.42
Bouba — *see also* Yaws 102.9
Bouffée délirante 298.3
Bouillaud's disease or syndrome (rheumatic
  heart disease) 391.9
Bourneville's disease (tuberous sclerosis)
  759.5
Boutonneuse fever 082.1
Boutonniere
  deformity (finger) 736.21
  hand (intrinsic) 736.21
Bouveret (-Hoffmann) disease or syndrome
  (paroxysmal tachycardia) 427.2
Bovine heart — *see* Hypertrophy, cardiac
Bowel — *see* condition
Bowen's
  dermatosis (precancerous) (M8081/2) —
    see Neoplasm, skin, in situ
  disease (M8081/2) — *see* Neoplasm, skin,
    in situ
  epithelioma (M8081/2) — *see* Neoplasm,
    skin, in situ
  type
    epidermoid carcinoma in situ (M8081/2)
      — *see* Neoplasm, skin, in situ
    intraepidermal squamous cell carcinoma
      (M8081/2) — *see* Neoplasm, skin,
      in situ
Bowing
  femur 736.89
    congenital 754.42
  fibula 736.89
    congenital 754.43
  forearm 736.09
    away from midline (cubitus valgus)
      736.01
    toward midline (cubitus varus) 736.02
  leg(s), long bones, congenital 754.44
  radius 736.09
    away from midline (cubitus valgus)
      736.01
    toward midline (cubitus varus) 736.02
  tibia 736.89
    congenital 754.43
Bowleg(s) 736.42
  congenital 754.44
  rachitic 268.1

Boyd's dysentery 004.2
Brachial — *see* condition
Brachman-de Lange syndrome (Amsterdam
  dwarf, intellectual disabilities, and
  brachycephaly) 759.89
Brachycardia 427.89
Brachycephaly 756.0
Brachymorphism and ectopia lentis 759.89
Bradley's disease (epidemic vomiting) 078.82
Bradycardia 427.89
  chronic (sinus) 427.81
  newborn 779.81
  nodal 427.89
  postoperative 997.1
  reflex 337.09
  sinoatrial 427.89
    with paroxysmal tachyarrhythmia or
      tachycardia 427.81
    chronic 427.81
  sinus 427.89
    with paroxysmal tachyarrhythmia or
      tachycardia 427.81
    chronic 427.81
    persistent 427.81
    severe 427.81
  tachycardia syndrome 427.81
  vagal 427.89
Bradykinesia 781.0
Bradypnea 786.09
Brailsford-Morquio disease or syndrome
  (mucopolysaccharidosis IV) 277.5
Brailsford's disease 732.3
  radial head 732.3
  tarsal scaphoid 732.5
Brain — *see also* condition
  death 348.82
  syndrome (acute) (chronic) (nonpsychotic)
    (organic) (with neurotic reaction)
    (with behavioral reaction) (*see also*
    Syndrome, brain) 310.9
    with
      presenile brain disease 290.10
      psychosis, psychotic reaction (*see al-
        so* Psychosis, organic) 294.9
    congenital (*see also* Disability, intellectu-
      al) 319
Branched-chain amino-acid disease 270.3
Branchial — *see* condition
Brandt's syndrome (acrodermatitis enteropath-
  ica) 686.8
Brash (water) 787.1
Brass-founders' ague 985.8
Bravais-Jacksonian epilepsy — *see also*
  Epilepsy 345.5 ☑
Braxton Hicks contractions 644.1 ☑
Braziers' disease 985.8
Brazilian
  blastomycosis 116.1
  leishmaniasis 085.5
BRBPR (bright red blood per rectum) 569.3
Break
  cardiorenal — *see* Hypertension, cardiorenal
  retina (*see also* Defect, retina) 361.30
Breakbone fever 061
Breakdown
  device, implant, or graft — *see* Complica-
    tions, mechanical
  nervous (*see also* Disorder, mental, nonpsy-
    chotic) 300.9
  perineum 674.2 ☑
Breast — *see also* condition
  buds 259.1
    in newborn 779.89
  dense 793.82
  nodule 793.89
Breast feeding difficulties 676.8 ☑
Breath
  foul 784.99
  holder, child 312.81
  holding spells 786.9
  shortness 786.05
Breathing
  asymmetrical 786.09
  bronchial 786.09
  exercises V57.0
  labored 786.09

Breathing — *continued*
  mouth 784.99
    causing malocclusion 524.59
  periodic 786.09
    high altitude 327.22
  tic 307.20
Breathlessness 786.09
Breda's disease — *see also* Yaws 102.9
Breech
  delivery, affecting fetus or newborn 763.0
  extraction, affecting fetus or newborn 763.0
  presentation (buttocks) (complete) (frank)
    652.2 ☑
    with successful version 652.1 ☑
    before labor, affecting fetus or newborn
      761.7
    during labor, affecting fetus or newborn
      763.0
Breisky's disease (kraurosis vulvae) 624.09
Brennemann's syndrome (acute mesenteric
  lymphadenitis) 289.2
Brenner's
  tumor (benign) (M9000/0) 220
    borderline malignancy (M9000/1) 236.2
    malignant (M9000/3) 183.0
    proliferating (M9000/1) 236.2
Bretonneau's disease (diphtheritic malignant
  angina) 032.0
Breus' mole 631.8
Brevicollis 756.16
Bricklayers' itch 692.89
Brickmakers' anemia 126.9
Bridge
  myocardial 746.85
Bright's
  blindness — *see* Uremia
  disease (*see also* Nephritis) 583.9
    arteriosclerotic (*see also* Hypertension,
      kidney) 403.90
Bright red blood per rectum (BRBPR) 569.3
Brill-Symmers disease (follicular lymphoma)
  (M9690/3) 202.0 ☑
Brill-Zinsser disease (recrudescent typhus)
  081.1
Brill's disease (recrudescent typhus) 081.1
  flea-borne 081.0
  louse-borne 081.1
Brinton's disease (linitis plastica) (M8142/3)
  151.9
Brion-Kayser disease — *see also* Fever,
  paratyphoid 002.9
Briquet's disorder or syndrome 300.81
Brissaud-Meige syndrome (infantile
  myxedema) 244.9
Brissaud's
  infantilism (infantile myxedema) 244.9
  motor-verbal tic 307.23
Brittle
  bones (congenital) 756.51
  nails 703.8
    congenital 757.5
Broad — *see also* condition
  beta disease 272.2
  ligament laceration syndrome 620.6
Brock's syndrome (atelectasis due to enlarged
  lymph nodes) 518.0
Brocq-Duhring disease (dermatitis herpetiformis) 694.0
Brocq's disease 691.8
  atopic (diffuse) neurodermatitis 691.8
  lichen simplex chronicus 698.3
  parakeratosis psoriasiformis 696.2
  parapsoriasis 696.2
Brodie's
  abscess (localized) (chronic) (*see also* Os-
    teomyelitis) 730.1 ☑
  disease (joint) (*see also* Osteomyelitis)
    730.1 ☑
Broken
  arches 734
    congenital 755.67
  back — *see* Fracture, vertebra, by site
  bone — *see* Fracture, by site
  compensation — *see* Disease, heart
  heart syndrome 429.83

Broken — *continued*
  implant or internal device — *see* listing un-
    der Complications, mechanical
  neck — *see* Fracture, vertebra, cervical
  nose 802.0
    open 802.1
  tooth, teeth 873.63
    complicated 873.73
Bromhidrosis 705.89
Bromidism, bromism
  acute 967.3
    correct substance properly administered
      349.82
    overdose or wrong substance given or
      taken 967.3
  chronic (*see also* Dependence) 304.1 ☑
Bromidrosiphobia 300.23
Bromidrosis 705.89
Bronchi, bronchial — *see* condition
Bronchiectasis (cylindrical) (diffuse) (fusiform)
  (localized) (moniliform) (postinfectious)
  (recurrent) (saccular) 494.0
  with acute exacerbation 494.1
  congenital 748.61
  tuberculous (*see also* Tuberculosis) 011.5 ☑
Bronchiolectasis — *see* Bronchiectasis
Bronchiolitis (acute) (infectious) (subacute)
  466.19
  with
    bronchospasm or obstruction 466.19
    influenza, flu, or grippe (*see also* Influen-
      za) 487.1
  catarrhal (acute) (subacute) 466.19
  chemical 506.0
    chronic 506.4
  chronic (obliterative) 491.8
  due to external agent — *see* Bronchitis,
    acute, due to
  fibrosa obliterans 491.8
  influenzal (*see also* Influenza) 487.1
  obliterans 491.8
    with organizing pneumonia (BOOP)
      516.8
    status post lung transplant 996.84
  obliterative (chronic) (diffuse) (subacute)
    491.8
    due to fumes or vapors 506.4
  respiratory syncytial virus 466.11
  vesicular — *see* Pneumonia, broncho-
Bronchitis (diffuse) (hypostatic) (infectious)
  (inflammatory) (simple) 490
  with
    emphysema — *see* Emphysema
    influenza, flu, or grippe (*see also* Influen-
      za) 487.1
    obstruction airway, chronic 491.20
      with
        acute bronchitis 491.22
        exacerbation (acute) 491.21
    tracheitis 490
      acute or subacute 466.0
        with bronchospasm or obstruc-
          tion 466.0
      chronic 491.8
  acute or subacute 466.0
    with
      bronchiectasis 494.1
      bronchospasm 466.0
      obstruction 466.0
      tracheitis 466.0
    chemical (due to fumes or vapors) 506.0
    due to
      fumes or vapors 506.0
      radiation 508.8
  allergic (acute) (*see also* Asthma) 493.9 ☑
  arachidic 934.1
  aspiration 507.0
    due to fumes or vapors 506.0
  asthmatic (acute) 493.90
    with
      acute exacerbation 493.92
      status asthmaticus 493.91
    chronic 493.2 ☑
  capillary 466.19
    with bronchospasm or obstruction
      466.19

☑ **Additional Digit Required** — **Refer to the Tabular List for Digit Selection**   🖜 **Subterms under main terms may continue to next column or page**

2014 ICD-9-CM   ▶◀ **Revised Text**   ● **New Line**   ▲ **Revised Code**   **Volume 2 — 37**

Bronchitis — *continued*
  capillary — *continued*
    chronic 491.8
    caseous (see also Tuberculosis) 011.3 ☑
  Castellani's 104.8
  catarrhal 490
    acute — *see* Bronchitis, acute
    chronic 491.0
  chemical (acute) (subacute) 506.0
    chronic 506.4
    due to fumes or vapors (acute) (subacute) 506.0
      chronic 506.4
  chronic 491.9
    with
      tracheitis (chronic) 491.8
    asthmatic 493.2 ☑
    catarrhal 491.0
    chemical (due to fumes and vapors) 506.4
    due to
      fumes or vapors (chemical) (inhalation) 506.4
      radiation 508.8
      tobacco smoking 491.0
    mucopurulent 491.1
    obstructive 491.20
      with
        acute bronchitis 491.22
        exacerbation (acute) 491.21
      purulent 491.1
    simple 491.0
    specified type NEC 491.8
  croupous 466.0
    with bronchospasm or obstruction 466.0
    due to fumes or vapors 506.0
  emphysematous 491.20
    with
      acute bronchitis 491.22
      exacerbation (acute) 491.21
  exudative 466.0
  fetid (chronic) (recurrent) 491.1
  fibrinous, acute or subacute 466.0
    with bronchospasm or obstruction 466.0
  grippal (see also Influenza) 487.1
  influenzal (see also Influenza) 487.1
  membranous, acute or subacute 466.0
    with bronchospasm or obstruction 466.0
  moulders' 502
  mucopurulent (chronic) (recurrent) 491.1
    acute or subacute 466.0
  obliterans 491.8
  obstructive (chronic) 491.20
    with
      acute bronchitis 491.22
      exacerbation (acute) 491.21
  pituitous 491.1
  plastic (inflammatory) 466.0
  pneumococcal, acute or subacute 466.0
    with bronchospasm or obstruction 466.0
  pseudomembranous 466.0
  purulent (chronic) (recurrent) 491.1
    acute or subacute 466.0
      with bronchospasm or obstruction 466.0
  putrid 491.1
  scrofulous (see also Tuberculosis) 011.3 ☑
  senile 491.9
  septic, acute or subacute 466.0
    with bronchospasm or obstruction 466.0
  smokers' 491.0
  spirochetal 104.8
  suffocative, acute or subacute 466.0
  summer (see also Asthma) 493.9 ☑
  suppurative (chronic) 491.1
    acute or subacute 466.0
  tuberculous (see also Tuberculosis) 011.3 ☑
  ulcerative 491.8
    Vincent's 101
  Vincent's 101
  viral, acute or subacute 466.0
Bronchoalveolitis 485
Bronchoaspergillosis 117.3
Bronchocele
  meaning
    dilatation of bronchus 519.19

Bronchocele — *continued*
  meaning — *continued*
    goiter 240.9
Bronchogenic carcinoma 162.9
Bronchohemisporosis 117.9
Broncholithiasis 518.89
  tuberculous (see also Tuberculosis) 011.3 ☑
Bronchomalacia 748.3
Bronchomoniliasis 112.89
Bronchomycosis 112.89
Bronchonocardiosis 039.1
Bronchopleuropneumonia — *see* Pneumonia, broncho-
Bronchopneumonia — *see* Pneumonia, broncho-
Bronchopneumonitis — *see* Pneumonia, broncho-
Bronchopulmonary — *see* condition
Bronchopulmonitis — *see* Pneumonia, broncho-
Bronchorrhagia 786.30
  newborn 770.3
  tuberculous (see also Tuberculosis) 011.3 ☑
Bronchorrhea (chronic) (purulent) 491.0
  acute 466.0
Bronchospasm 519.11
  with
    asthma — *see* Asthma
    bronchiolitis, acute 466.19
      due to respiratory syncytial virus 466.11
    bronchitis — *see* Bronchitis
    chronic obstructive pulmonary disease (COPD) 496
    emphysema — *see* Emphysema
      due to external agent — *see* Condition, respiratory, acute, due to
  acute 519.11
  exercise induced 493.81
Bronchospirochetosis 104.8
Bronchostenosis 519.19
Bronchus — *see* condition
Bronze, bronzed
  diabetes 275.01
  disease (Addison's) (skin) 255.41
    tuberculous (see also Tuberculosis) 017.6 ☑
Brooke's disease or tumor (M8100/0) — *see* Neoplasm, skin, benign
Brown-Séquard's paralysis (syndrome) 344.89
Brown enamel of teeth (hereditary) 520.5
Brown's tendon sheath syndrome 378.61
Brow presentation complicating delivery 652.4 ☑
Brucella, brucellosis (infection) 023.9
  abortus 023.1
  canis 023.3
  dermatitis, skin 023.9
  melitensis 023.0
  mixed 023.8
  suis 023.2
Bruck-de Lange disease or syndrome (Amsterdam dwarf, intellectual disabilities, and brachycephaly) 759.89
Bruck's disease 733.99
Brugada syndrome 746.89
Brug's filariasis 125.1
Brugsch's syndrome (acropachyderma) 757.39
Bruhl's disease (splenic anemia with fever) 285.8
Bruise (skin surface intact) — *see also* Contusion
  with
    fracture — *see* Fracture, by site
    open wound — *see* Wound, open, by site
    internal organ (abdomen, chest, or pelvis) — *see* Injury, internal, by site
    umbilical cord 663.6 ☑
      affecting fetus or newborn 762.6
Bruit 785.9
  arterial (abdominal) (carotid) 785.9
  supraclavicular 785.9
Brushburn — *see* Injury, superficial, by site
Bruton's X-linked agammaglobulinemia 279.04

Bruxism 306.8
  sleep related 327.53
Bubbly lung syndrome 770.7
Bubo 289.3
  blennorrhagic 098.89
  chancroidal 099.0
  climatic 099.1
  due to Hemophilus ducreyi 099.0
  gonococcal 098.89
  indolent NEC 099.8
  inguinal NEC 099.8
    chancroidal 099.0
    climatic 099.1
    due to H. ducreyi 099.0
  scrofulous (see also Tuberculosis) 017.2 ☑
  soft chancre 099.0
  suppurating 683
  syphilitic 091.0
    congenital 090.0
  tropical 099.1
  venereal NEC 099.8
  virulent 099.0
Bubonic plague 020.0
Bubonocele — *see* Hernia, inguinal
Buccal — *see* condition
Buchanan's disease (juvenile osteochondrosis of iliac crest) 732.1
Buchem's syndrome (hyperostosis corticalis) 733.3
Buchman's disease (osteochondrosis, juvenile) 732.1
Bucket handle fracture (semilunar cartilage) — *see also* Tear, meniscus 836.2
Budd-Chiari syndrome (hepatic vein thrombosis) 453.0
Budgerigar-fanciers' disease or lung 495.2
Büdinger-Ludloff-Läwen disease 717.89
Buds
  breast 259.1
  in newborn 779.89
Buerger's disease (thromboangiitis obliterans) 443.1
Bulbar — *see* condition
Bulbus cordis 745.9
  persistent (in left ventricle) 745.8
Bulging fontanels (congenital) 756.0
Bulimia 783.6
  nervosa 307.51
  nonorganic origin 307.51
Bulky uterus 621.2
Bulla(e) 709.8
  lung (emphysematous) (solitary) 492.0
Bullet wound — *see also* Wound, open, by site
  fracture — *see* Fracture, by site, open
  internal organ (abdomen, chest, or pelvis) — *see* Injury, internal, by site, with open wound
  intracranial — *see* Laceration, brain, with open wound
Bullis fever 082.8
Bullying — *see also* Disturbance, conduct 312.0 ☑
Bundle
  branch block (complete) (false) (incomplete) 426.50
    bilateral 426.53
    left (see also Block, bundle branch, left) 426.3
      hemiblock 426.2
    right (see also Block, bundle branch, right) 426.4
  of His — *see* condition
  of Kent syndrome (anomalous atrioventricular excitation) 426.7
Bungpagga 040.81
Bunion 727.1
Bunionette 727.1
Bunyamwera fever 066.3
Buphthalmia, buphthalmos (congenital) 743.20
  associated with
    keratoglobus, congenital 743.22
    megalocornea 743.22
    ocular anomalies NEC 743.22
  isolated 743.21

Buphthalmia, buphthalmos — *continued*
  simple 743.21
Bürger-Grütz disease or syndrome (essential familial hyperlipemia) 272.3
Buried roots 525.3
Burke's syndrome 577.8
Burkitt's
  tumor (M9750/3) 200.2 ☑
  type malignant, lymphoma, lymphoblastic, or undifferentiated (M9750/3) 200.2 ☑
Burn (acid) (cathode ray) (caustic) (chemical) (electric heating appliance) (electricity) (fire) (flame) (hot liquid or object) (irradiation) (lime) (radiation) (steam) (thermal) (x-ray) 949.0

> *Note — Use the following fifth-digit subclassification with category 948 to indicate the percent of body surface with third degree burn:*
>
> 0   *Less than 10% or unspecified*
> 1   *10–19%*
> 2   *20–29%*
> 3   *30–39%*
> 4   *40–49%*
> 5   *50–59%*
> 6   *60–69%*
> 7   *70–79%*
> 8   *80–89%*
> 9   *90% or more of body surface*

  with
    blisters — *see* Burn, by site, second degree
    erythema — *see* Burn, by site, first degree
    skin loss (epidermal) (see also Burn, by site, second degree)
    full thickness (see also Burn, by site, third degree)
      with necrosis of underlying tissues — *see* Burn, by site, third degree, deep
  first degree — *see* Burn, by site, first degree
  second degree — *see* Burn, by site, second degree
  third degree — *see* Burn, by site, third degree
    deep — *see* Burn, by site, third degree, deep
  abdomen, abdominal (muscle) (wall) 942.03
    with
      trunk — *see* Burn, trunk, multiple sites
    first degree 942.13
    second degree 942.23
    third degree 942.33
      deep 942.43
        with loss of body part 942.53
  ankle 945.03
    with
      lower limb(s) — *see* Burn, leg, multiple sites
    first degree 945.13
    second degree 945.23
    third degree 945.33
      deep 945.43
        with loss of body part 945.53
  anus — *see* Burn, trunk, specified site NEC
  arm(s) 943.00
    first degree 943.10
    second degree 943.20
    third degree 943.30
      deep 943.40
        with loss of body part 943.50
    lower — *see* Burn, forearm(s)
    multiple sites, except hand(s) or wrist(s) 943.09
      first degree 943.19
      second degree 943.29
      third degree 943.39
        deep 943.49

☑ **Additional Digit Required** — Refer to the Tabular List for Digit Selection   ▽ **Subterms under main terms may continue to next column or page**

38 — Volume 2   ▶◀ **Revised Text**   ● **New Line**   ▲ **Revised Code**   **2014 ICD-9-CM**

Burn — *continued*
  arm(s) — *continued*
    multiple sites, except hand(s) or wrist(s) — *continued*
      third degree — *continued*
        deep — *continued*
          with loss of body part 943.59
      upper 943.03
        first degree 943.13
        second degree 943.23
        third degree 943.33
          deep 943.43
            with loss of body part 943.53
    auditory canal (external) — *see* Burn, ear
    auricle (ear) — *see* Burn, ear
    axilla 943.04
      with
        upper limb(s), except hand(s) or wrist(s) — *see* Burn, arm(s), multiple sites
      first degree 943.14
      second degree 943.24
      third degree 943.34
        deep 943.44
          with loss of body part 943.54
  back 942.04
    with
      trunk — *see* Burn, trunk, multiple sites
    first degree 942.14
    second degree 942.24
    third degree 942.34
      deep 942.44
        with loss of body part 942.54
  biceps
    brachii — *see* Burn, arm(s), upper
    femoris — *see* Burn, thigh
  breast(s) 942.01
    with
      trunk — *see* Burn, trunk, multiple sites
    first degree 942.11
    second degree 942.21
    third degree 942.31
      deep 942.41
        with loss of body part 942.51
  brow — *see* Burn, forehead
  buttock(s) — *see* Burn, back
  canthus (eye) 940.1
    chemical 940.0
  cervix (uteri) 947.4
  cheek (cutaneous) 941.07
    with
      face or head — *see* Burn, head, multiple sites
    first degree 941.17
    second degree 941.27
    third degree 941.37
      deep 941.47
        with loss of body part 941.57
  chest wall (anterior) 942.02
    with
      trunk — *see* Burn, trunk, multiple sites
    first degree 942.12
    second degree 942.22
    third degree 942.32
      deep 942.42
        with loss of body part 942.52
  chin 941.04
    with
      face or head — *see* Burn, head, multiple sites
    first degree 941.14
    second degree 941.24
    third degree 941.34
      deep 941.44
        with loss of body part 941.54
  clitoris — *see* Burn, genitourinary organs, external
  colon 947.3
  conjunctiva (and cornea) 940.4
    chemical
      acid 940.3
      alkaline 940.2
  cornea (and conjunctiva) 940.4

Burn — *continued*
  cornea — *continued*
    chemical
      acid 940.3
      alkaline 940.2
  costal region — *see* Burn, chest wall
  due to ingested chemical agent — *see* Burn, internal organs
  ear (auricle) (canal) (drum) (external) 941.01
    with
      face or head — *see* Burn, head, multiple sites
    first degree 941.11
    second degree 941.21
    third degree 941.31
      deep 941.41
        with loss of a body part 941.51
  elbow 943.02
    with
      hand(s) and wrist(s) — *see* Burn, multiple specified sites
      upper limb(s), except hand(s) or wrist(s) (*see also* Burn, arm(s), multiple sites)
    first degree 943.12
    second degree 943.22
    third degree 943.32
      deep 943.42
        with loss of body part 943.52
  electricity, electric current — *see* Burn, by site
  entire body — *see* Burn, multiple, specified sites
  epididymis — *see* Burn, genitourinary organs, external
  epigastric region — *see* Burn, abdomen
  epiglottis 947.1
  esophagus 947.2
  extent (percent of body surface)
    less than 10 percent 948.0 ☑
    10-19 percent 948.1 ☑
    20-29 percent 948.2 ☑
    30-39 percent 948.3 ☑
    40-49 percent 948.4 ☑
    50-59 percent 948.5 ☑
    60-69 percent 948.6 ☑
    70-79 percent 948.7 ☑
    80-89 percent 948.8 ☑
    90 percent or more 948.9 ☑
  extremity
    lower — *see* Burn, leg
    upper — *see* Burn, arm(s)
  eye(s) (and adnexa) (only) 940.9
    with
      face, head, or neck 941.02
        first degree 941.12
        second degree 941.22
        third degree 941.32
          deep 941.42
            with loss of body part 941.52
      other sites (classifiable to more than one category in 940–945) — *see* Burn, multiple, specified sites
      resulting rupture and destruction of eyeball 940.5
    specified part — *see* Burn, by site
  eyeball (*see also* Burn, eye)
    with resulting rupture and destruction of eyeball 940.5
  eyelid(s) 940.1
    chemical 940.0
  face — *see* Burn, head
  finger (nail) (subungual) 944.01
    with
      hand(s) — *see* Burn, hand(s), multiple sites
      other sites — *see* Burn, multiple, specified sites
      thumb 944.04
        first degree 944.14
        second degree 944.24
        third degree 944.34
          deep 944.44

Burn — *continued*
  finger — *continued*
    with — *continued*
      thumb — *continued*
        third degree — *continued*
          deep — *continued*
            with loss of body part 944.54
    first degree 944.11
    second degree 944.21
    third degree 944.31
      deep 944.41
        with loss of body part 944.51
    multiple (digits) 944.03
      with thumb — *see* Burn, finger, with thumb
      first degree 944.13
      second degree 944.23
      third degree 944.33
        deep 944.43
          with loss of body part 944.53
  flank — *see* Burn, abdomen
  foot 945.02
    with
      lower limb(s) — *see* Burn, leg, multiple sites
    first degree 945.12
    second degree 945.22
    third degree 945.32
      deep 945.42
        with loss of body part 945.52
  forearm(s) 943.01
    with
      upper limb(s), except hand(s) or wrist(s) — *see* Burn, arm(s), multiple sites
    first degree 943.11
    second degree 943.21
    third degree 943.31
      deep 943.41
        with loss of body part 943.51
  forehead 941.07
    with
      face or head — *see* Burn, head, multiple sites
    first degree 941.17
    second degree 941.27
    third degree 941.37
      deep 941.47
        with loss of body part 941.57
  fourth degree — *see* Burn, by site, third degree, deep
  friction — *see* Injury, superficial, by site
  from swallowing caustic or corrosive substance NEC — *see* Burn, internal organs
  full thickness — *see* Burn, by site, third degree
  gastrointestinal tract 947.3
  genitourinary organs
    external 942.05
      with
        trunk — *see* Burn, trunk, multiple sites
      first degree 942.15
      second degree 942.25
      third degree 942.35
        deep 942.45
          with loss of body part 942.55
    internal 947.8
  globe (eye) — *see* Burn, eyeball
  groin — *see* Burn, abdomen
  gum 947.0
  hand(s) (phalanges) (and wrist) 944.00
    first degree 944.10
    second degree 944.20
    third degree 944.30
      deep 944.40
        with loss of body part 944.50
    back (dorsal surface) 944.06
      first degree 944.16
      second degree 944.26
      third degree 944.36
        deep 944.46
          with loss of body part 944.56
    multiple sites 944.08

Burn — *continued*
  hand(s) — *continued*
    multiple sites — *continued*
      first degree 944.18
      second degree 944.28
      third degree 944.38
        deep 944.48
          with loss of body part 944.58
  head (and face) 941.00
    first degree 941.10
    second degree 941.20
    third degree 941.30
      deep 941.40
        with loss of body part 941.50
    eye(s) only 940.9
    specified part — *see* Burn, by site
    multiple sites 941.09
      with eyes — *see* Burn, eyes, with face, head, or neck
      first degree 941.19
      second degree 941.29
      third degree 941.39
        deep 941.49
          with loss of body part 941.59
  heel — *see* Burn, foot
  hip — *see* Burn, trunk, specified site NEC
  iliac region — *see* Burn, trunk, specified site NEC
  infected 958.3
  inhalation (*see also* Burn, internal organs) 947.9
  internal organs 947.9
    from caustic or corrosive substance (swallowing) NEC 947.9
    specified NEC (*see also* Burn, by site) 947.8
  interscapular region — *see* Burn, back
  intestine (large) (small) 947.3
  iris — *see* Burn, eyeball
  knee 945.05
    with
      lower limb(s) — *see* Burn, leg, multiple sites
    first degree 945.15
    second degree 945.25
    third degree 945.35
      deep 945.45
        with loss of body part 945.55
  labium (majus) (minus) — *see* Burn, genitourinary organs, external
  lacrimal apparatus, duct, gland, or sac 940.1
    chemical 940.0
  larynx 947.1
  late effect — *see* Late, effects (of), burn
  leg 945.00
    first degree 945.10
    second degree 945.20
    third degree 945.30
      deep 945.40
        with loss of body part 945.50
    lower 945.04
      with other part(s) of lower limb(s) — *see* Burn, leg, multiple sites
      first degree 945.14
      second degree 945.24
      third degree 945.34
        deep 945.44
          with loss of body part 945.54
    multiple sites 945.09
      first degree 945.19
      second degree 945.29
      third degree 945.39
        deep 945.49
          with loss of body part 945.59
    upper — *see* Burn, thigh
  lightning — *see* Burn, by site
  limb(s)
    lower (including foot or toe(s)) — *see* Burn, leg
    upper (except wrist and hand) — *see* Burn, arm(s)
  lip(s) 941.03
    with
      face or head — *see* Burn, head, multiple sites
    first degree 941.13

☑ **Additional Digit Required — Refer to the Tabular List for Digit Selection**   ▽ **Subterms under main terms may continue to next column or page**

2014 ICD-9-CM   ▶◀ Revised Text   ● New Line   ▲ Revised Code   **Volume 2 — 39**

Index

Burn — Cake kidney

Burn — *continued*
lip(s) — *continued*
    second degree 941.23
    third degree 941.33
      deep 941.43
        with loss of body part 941.53
lumbar region — *see* Burn, back
lung 947.1
malar region — *see* Burn, cheek
mastoid region — *see* Burn, scalp
membrane, tympanic — *see* Burn, ear
midthoracic region — *see* Burn, chest wall
mouth 947.0
multiple (*see also* Burn, unspecified) 949.0
    specified sites classifiable to more than
      one category in
      940-945 ☑, 946.0
    first degree 946.1
    second degree 946.2
    third degree 946.3
      deep 946.4
        with loss of body part 946.5
muscle, abdominal — *see* Burn, abdomen
nasal (septum) — *see* Burn, nose
neck 941.08
    with
      face or head — *see* Burn, head, mul-
        tiple sites
    first degree 941.18
    second degree 941.28
    third degree 941.38
      deep 941.48
        with loss of body part 941.58
nose (septum) 941.05
    with
      face or head — *see* Burn, head, mul-
        tiple sites
    first degree 941.15
    second degree 941.25
    third degree 941.35
      deep 941.45
        with loss of body part 941.55
occipital region — *see* Burn, scalp
orbit region 940.1
    chemical 940.0
oronasopharynx 947.0
palate 947.0
palm(s) 944.05
    with
      hand(s) and wrist(s) — *see* Burn,
        hand(s), multiple sites
    first degree 944.15
    second degree 944.25
    third degree 944.35
      deep 944.45
        with loss of a body part 944.55
parietal region — *see* Burn, scalp
penis — *see* Burn, genitourinary organs,
    external
perineum — *see* Burn, genitourinary organs,
    external
periocular area 940.1
    chemical 940.0
pharynx 947.0
pleura 947.1
popliteal space — *see* Burn, knee
prepuce — *see* Burn, genitourinary organs,
    external
pubic region — *see* Burn, genitourinary or-
    gans, external
pudenda — *see* Burn, genitourinary organs,
    external
rectum 947.3
sac, lacrimal 940.1
    chemical 940.0
sacral region — *see* Burn, back
salivary (ducts) (glands) 947.0
scalp 941.06
    with
      face or neck — *see* Burn, head, multi-
        ple sites
    first degree 941.16
    second degree 941.26
    third degree 941.36
      deep 941.46
        with loss of body part 941.56

Burn — *continued*
scapular region 943.06
    with
      upper limb(s), except hand(s) or
        wrist(s) — *see* Burn, arm(s),
        multiple sites
    first degree 943.16
    second degree 943.26
    third degree 943.36
      deep 943.46
        with loss of body part 943.56
sclera — *see* Burn, eyeball
scrotum — *see* Burn, genitourinary organs,
    external
septum, nasal — *see* Burn, nose
shoulder(s) 943.05
    with
      hand(s) and wrist(s) — *see* Burn,
        multiple, specified sites
      upper limb(s), except hand(s) or
        wrist(s) — *see* Burn, arm(s),
        multiple sites
    first degree 943.15
    second degree 943.25
    third degree 943.35
      deep 943.45
        with loss of body part 943.55
skin NEC (*see also* Burn, unspecified) 949.0
skull — *see* Burn, head
small intestine 947.3
sternal region — *see* Burn, chest wall
stomach 947.3
subconjunctival — *see* Burn, conjunctiva
subcutaneous — *see* Burn, by site, third
    degree
submaxillary region — *see* Burn, head
submental region — *see* Burn, chin
sun — *see* Sunburn
supraclavicular fossa — *see* Burn, neck
supraorbital — *see* Burn, forehead
temple — *see* Burn, scalp
temporal region — *see* Burn, scalp
testicle — *see* Burn, genitourinary organs,
    external
testis — *see* Burn, genitourinary organs,
    external
thigh 945.06
    with
      lower limb(s) — *see* Burn, leg, multi-
        ple sites
    first degree 945.16
    second degree 945.26
    third degree 945.36
      deep 945.46
        with loss of body part 945.56
thorax (external) — *see* Burn, chest wall
throat 947.0
thumb(s) (nail) (subungual) 944.02
    with
      finger(s) — *see* Burn, finger, with
        other sites, thumb
      hand(s) and wrist(s) — *see* Burn,
        hand(s), multiple sites
    first degree 944.12
    second degree 944.22
    third degree 944.32
      deep 944.42
        with loss of body part 944.52
toe (nail) (subungual) 945.01
    with
      lower limb(s) — *see* Burn, leg, multi-
        ple sites
    first degree 945.11
    second degree 945.21
    third degree 945.31
      deep 945.41
        with loss of body part 945.51
tongue 947.0
tonsil 947.0
trachea 947.1
trunk 942.00
    first degree 942.10
    second degree 942.20
    third degree 942.30
      deep 942.40
        with loss of body part 942.50

Burn — *continued*
trunk — *continued*
    multiple sites 942.09
      first degree 942.19
      second degree 942.29
      third degree 942.39
        deep 942.49
          with loss of body part 942.59
    specified site NEC 942.09
      first degree 942.19
      second degree 942.29
      third degree 942.39
        deep 942.49
          with loss of body part 942.59
tunica vaginalis — *see* Burn, genitourinary
    organs, external
tympanic membrane — *see* Burn, ear
tympanum — *see* Burn, ear
ultraviolet 692.82
unspecified site (multiple) 949.0
    with extent of body surface involved
      specified
      less than 10 percent 948.0 ☑
      10-19 percent 948.1 ☑
      20-29 percent 948.2 ☑
      30-39 percent 948.3 ☑
      40-49 percent 948.4 ☑
      50-59 percent 948.5 ☑
      60-69 percent 948.6 ☑
      70-79 percent 948.7 ☑
      80-89 percent 948.8 ☑
      90 percent or more 948.9 ☑
    first degree 949.1
    second degree 949.2
    third degree 949.3
      deep 949.4
        with loss of body part 949.5
uterus 947.4
uvula 947.0
vagina 947.4
vulva — *see* Burn, genitourinary organs,
    external
wrist(s) 944.07
    with
      hand(s) — *see* Burn, hand(s), multi-
        ple sites
    first degree 944.17
    second degree 944.27
    third degree 944.37
      deep 944.47
        with loss of body part 944.57
Burnett's syndrome (milk-alkali) 275.42
Burnier's syndrome (hypophyseal dwarfism)
    253.3
Burning
    feet syndrome 266.2
    sensation (*see also* Disturbance, sensation)
      782.0
    tongue 529.6
Burns' disease (osteochondrosis, lower ulna)
    732.3
Bursa — *see also* condition
    pharynx 478.29
Bursitis NEC 727.3
    Achilles tendon 726.71
    adhesive 726.90
      shoulder 726.0
    ankle 726.79
    buttock 726.5
    calcaneal 726.79
    collateral ligament
      fibular 726.63
      tibial 726.62
    Duplay's 726.2
    elbow 726.33
    finger 726.8
    foot 726.79
    gonococcal 098.52
    hand 726.4
    hip 726.5
    infrapatellar 726.69
    ischiogluteal 726.5
    knee 726.60
    occupational NEC 727.2
    olecranon 726.33
    pes anserinus 726.61

Bursitis — *continued*
    pharyngeal 478.29
    popliteal 727.51
    prepatellar 726.65
    radiohumeral 727.3
    scapulohumeral 726.19
      adhesive 726.0
    shoulder 726.10
      adhesive 726.0
    subacromial 726.19
      adhesive 726.0
    subcoracoid 726.19
    subdeltoid 726.19
      adhesive 726.0
    subpatellar 726.69
    syphilitic 095.7
    Thornwaldt's, Tornwaldt's (pharyngeal)
      478.29
    toe 726.79
    trochanteric area 726.5
    wrist 726.4
Burst stitches or sutures (complication of
    surgery) (external) (*see also* Dehiscence)
    998.32
    internal 998.31
Buruli ulcer 031.1
Bury's disease (erythema elevatum diutinum)
    695.89
Buschke's disease or scleredema (adultorum)
    710.1
Busquet's disease (osteoperiostitis) — *see also*
    Osteomyelitis 730.1 ☑
Busse-Buschke disease (cryptococcosis) 117.5
Buttock — *see* condition
Button
    Biskra 085.1
    Delhi 085.1
    oriental 085.1
Buttonhole hand (intrinsic) 736.21
Bwamba fever (encephalitis) 066.3
Byssinosis (occupational) 504
Bywaters' syndrome 958.5

C

Cacergasia 300.9
Cachexia 799.4
    cancerous (*see also* Neoplasm, by site, ma-
      lignant) 799.4
    cardiac — *see* Disease, heart
    dehydration 276.51
      with
        hypernatremia 276.0
        hyponatremia 276.1
    due to malnutrition 799.4
    exophthalmic 242.0 ☑
    heart — *see* Disease, heart
    hypophyseal 253.2
    hypopituitary 253.2
    lead 984.9
      specified type of lead — *see* Table of
        Drugs and Chemicals
    malaria 084.9
    malignant (*see also* Neoplasm, by site, ma-
      lignant) 799.4
    marsh 084.9
    nervous 300.5
    old age 797
    pachydermic — *see* Hypothyroidism
    paludal 084.9
    pituitary (postpartum) 253.2
    renal (*see also* Disease, renal) 593.9
    saturnine 984.9
      specified type of lead — *see* Table of
        Drugs and Chemicals
    senile 797
    Simmonds' (pituitary cachexia) 253.2
    splenica 289.59
    strumipriva (*see also* Hypothyroidism) 244
    tuberculous NEC (*see also* Tuberculosis)
      011.9 ☑
Café au lait spots 709.09
Caffey's disease or syndrome (infantile corti-
    cal hyperostosis) 756.59
Caisson disease 993.3
Caked breast (puerperal, postpartum) 676.2
Cake kidney 753.3

☑ Additional Digit Required — Refer to the Tabular List for Digit Selection   ▽ Subterms under main terms may continue to next column or page

Calabar swelling 125.2
Calcaneal spur 726.73
Calcaneoapophysitis 732.5
Calcaneonavicular bar 755.67
Calcareous — *see* condition
Calcicosis (occupational) 502
Calciferol (vitamin D) **deficiency** 268.9
  with
    osteomalacia 268.2
    rickets (*see also* Rickets) 268.0
Calcification
  adrenal (capsule) (gland) 255.41
    tuberculous (*see also* Tuberculosis)
      017.6 ☑
  aorta 440.0
  artery (annular) — *see* Arteriosclerosis
  auricle (ear) 380.89
  bladder 596.89
    due to S. hematobium 120.0
  brain (cortex) — *see* Calcification, cerebral
  bronchus 519.19
  bursa 727.82
  cardiac (*see also* Degeneration, myocardial)
    429.1
  cartilage (postinfectional) 733.99
  cerebral (cortex) 348.89
    artery 437.0
  cervix (uteri) 622.8
  choroid plexus 349.2
  conjunctiva 372.54
  corpora cavernosa (penis) 607.89
  cortex (brain) — *see* Calcification, cerebral
  dental pulp (nodular) 522.2
  dentinal papilla 520.4
  disc, intervertebral 722.90
    cervical, cervicothoracic 722.91
    lumbar, lumbosacral 722.93
    thoracic, thoracolumbar 722.92
  fallopian tube 620.8
  falx cerebri — *see* Calcification, cerebral
  fascia 728.89
  gallbladder 575.8
  general 275.40
  heart (*see also* Degeneration, myocardial)
    429.1
    valve — *see* Endocarditis
  intervertebral cartilage or disc (postinfection-
    al) 722.90
    cervical, cervicothoracic 722.91
    lumbar, lumbosacral 722.93
    thoracic, thoracolumbar 722.92
  intracranial — *see* Calcification, cerebral
  intraspinal ligament 728.89
  joint 719.80
    ankle 719.87
    elbow 719.82
    foot 719.87
    hand 719.84
    hip 719.85
    knee 719.86
    multiple sites 719.89
    pelvic region 719.85
    shoulder (region) 719.81
    specified site NEC 719.88
    wrist 719.83
  kidney 593.89
    tuberculous (*see also* Tuberculosis)
      016.0 ☑
  larynx (senile) 478.79
  lens 366.8
  ligament 728.89
    intraspinal 728.89
    knee (medial collateral) 717.89
  lung 518.89
    active 518.89
    postinfectional 518.89
    tuberculous (*see also* Tuberculosis, pul-
      monary) 011.9 ☑
  lymph gland or node (postinfectional) 289.3
    tuberculous (*see also* Tuberculosis,
      lymph gland) 017.2 ☑
  mammographic 793.89
  massive (paraplegic) 728.10
  medial NEC (*see also* Arteriosclerosis, extrem-
    ities) 440.20
  meninges (cerebral) 349.2

Calcification — *continued*
  metastatic 275.40
  Mönckeberg's — *see* Arteriosclerosis
  muscle 728.10
    heterotopic, postoperative 728.13
  myocardium, myocardial (*see also* Degener-
    ation, myocardial) 429.1
  ovary 620.8
  pancreas 577.8
  penis 607.89
  periarticular 728.89
  pericardium (*see also* Pericarditis) 423.8
  pineal gland 259.8
  pleura 511.0
    postinfectional 518.89
    tuberculous (*see also* Tuberculosis,
      pleura) 012.0 ☑
  pulp (dental) (nodular) 522.2
  renal 593.89
  Rider's bone 733.99
  sclera 379.16
  semilunar cartilage 717.89
  spleen 289.59
  subcutaneous 709.3
  suprarenal (capsule) (gland) 255.41
  tendon (sheath) 727.82
    with bursitis, synovitis or tenosynovitis
      727.82
  trachea 519.19
  ureter 593.89
  uterus 621.8
  vitreous 379.29
Calcified — *see also* Calcification
  hematoma NEC 959.9
Calcinosis (generalized) (interstitial) (tumoral)
  (universalis) 275.49
  circumscripta 709.3
  cutis 709.3
  intervertebralis 275.49 [722.90]
  Raynaud's phenomenonsclerodactylytelang-
    iectasis (CRST) 710.1
Calciphylaxis — *see also* Calcification, by site
  275.49
Calcium
  blood
    high (*see also* Hypercalcemia) 275.42
    low (*see also* Hypocalcemia) 275.41
  deposits (*see also* Calcification, by site)
    in bursa 727.82
    in tendon (sheath) 727.82
      with bursitis, synovitis or tenosynovi-
        tis 727.82
  salts or soaps in vitreous 379.22
Calciuria 791.9
Calculi — *see* Calculus
Calculosis, intrahepatic — *see* Choledocholithiasis
Calculus, calculi, calculous 592.9
  ampulla of Vater — *see* Choledocholithiasis
  anuria (impacted) (recurrent) 592.0
  appendix 543.9
  bile duct (any) — *see* Choledocholithiasis
  biliary — *see* Cholelithiasis
  bilirubin, multiple — *see* Cholelithiasis
  bladder (encysted) (impacted) (urinary)
    594.1
    diverticulum 594.0
  bronchus 518.89
  calyx (kidney) (renal) 592.0
    congenital 753.3
  cholesterol (pure) (solitary) —
    Cholelithiasis
  common duct (bile) — *see* Choledocholithi-
    asis
  conjunctiva 372.54
  cystic 594.1
    duct — *see* Cholelithiasis
  dental 523.6
    subgingival 523.6
    supragingival 523.6
  epididymis 608.89
  gallbladder (*see also* Cholelithiasis)
    congenital 751.69
  hepatic (duct) — *see* Choledocholithiasis
  intestine (impaction) (obstruction) 560.39

Calculus, calculi, calculous — *continued*
  kidney (impacted) (multiple) (pelvis) (recur-
    rent) (staghorn) 592.0
    congenital 753.3
  lacrimal (passages) 375.57
  liver (impacted) — *see* Choledocholithiasis
  lung 518.89
  mammographic 793.89
  nephritic (impacted) (recurrent) 592.0
  nose 478.19
  pancreas (duct) 577.8
  parotid gland 527.5
  pelvis, encysted 592.0
  prostate 602.0
  pulmonary 518.89
  renal (impacted) (recurrent) 592.0
    congenital 753.3
  salivary (duct) (gland) 527.5
  seminal vesicle 608.89
  staghorn 592.0
  Stensen's duct 527.5
  sublingual duct or gland 527.5
    congenital 750.26
  submaxillary duct, gland, or region 527.5
  suburethral 594.8
  tonsil 474.8
  tooth, teeth 523.6
  tunica vaginalis 608.89
  ureter (impacted) (recurrent) 592.1
  urethra (impacted) 594.2
  urinary (duct) (impacted) (passage) (tract)
    592.9
    lower tract NEC 594.9
      specified site 594.8
    vagina 623.8
    vesical (impacted) 594.1
    Wharton's duct 527.5
Caliectasis 593.89
California
  disease 114.0
  encephalitis 062.5
Caligo cornea 371.03
Callositas, callosity (infected) 700
Callus (infected) 700
  bone 726.91
  excessive, following fracture (*see also* Late,
    effect (of), fracture)
Calvé (-Perthes) disease (osteochondrosis,
  femoral capital) 732.1
Calvities — *see also* Alopecia 704.00
Cameroon fever — *see also* Malaria 084.6
Camptocormia 300.11
Camptodactyly (congenital) 755.59
Camurati-Engelmann disease (diaphyseal
  sclerosis) 756.59
Canal — *see* condition
Canaliculitis (lacrimal) (acute) 375.31
  Actinomyces 039.8
  chronic 375.41
Canavan's disease 330.0
Cancer (M8000/3) — *see also* Neoplasm, by
  site, malignant

> *Note* — The term "cancer" when modi-
> *fied by an adjective or adjectival phrase*
> *indicating a morphological type should*
> *be coded in the same manner as "carci-*
> *noma" with that adjective or phrase.*
> *Thus, "squamous-cell cancer" should be*
> *coded in the same manner as "squa-*
> *mous-cell carcinoma," which appears in*
> *the list under "Carcinoma."*

  bile duct type (M8160/3), liver 155.1
  hepatocellular (M8170/3) 155.0
Cancerous (M8000/3) — *see* Neoplasm, by site,
  malignant
Cancerphobia 300.29
Cancrum oris 528.1
Candidiasis, candidal 112.9
  with pneumonia 112.4
  balanitis 112.2
  congenital 771.7
  disseminated 112.5
  endocarditis 112.81
  esophagus 112.84
  intertrigo 112.3
  intestine 112.85

Candidiasis, candidal — *continued*
  lung 112.4
  meningitis 112.83
  mouth 112.0
  nails 112.3
  neonatal 771.7
  onychia 112.3
  otitis externa 112.82
  otomycosis 112.82
  paronychia 112.3
  perionyxis 112.3
  pneumonia 112.4
  pneumonitis 112.4
  skin 112.3
  specified site NEC 112.89
  systemic 112.5
  urogenital site NEC 112.2
  vagina 112.1
  vulva 112.1
  vulvovaginitis 112.1
Candidiosis — *see* Candidiasis
Candiru infection or infestation 136.8
Canities (premature) 704.3
  congenital 757.4
Canker (mouth) (sore) 528.2
  rash 034.1
Cannabinosis 504
Canton fever 081.9
Cap
  cradle 690.11
Capillariasis 127.5
Capillary — *see* condition
Caplan-Colinet syndrome 714.81
Caplan's syndrome 714.81
Capsule — *see* condition
Capsulitis (joint) 726.90
  adhesive (shoulder) 726.0
  hip 726.5
  knee 726.60
  labyrinthine 387.8
  thyroid 245.9
  wrist 726.4
Caput
  crepitus 756.0
  medusae 456.8
  succedaneum 767.19
Carapata disease 087.1
Carate — *see* Pinta
**Carbohydrate-deficient glycoprotein syn-
  drome** (CGDS) 271.8
Carboxyhemoglobinemia 986
Carbuncle 680.9
  abdominal wall 680.2
  ankle 680.6
  anus 680.5
  arm (any part, above wrist) 680.3
  auditory canal, external 680.0
  axilla 680.3
  back (any part) 680.2
  breast 680.2
  buttock 680.5
  chest wall 680.2
  corpus cavernosum 607.2
  ear (any part) (external) 680.0
  eyelid 373.13
  face (any part, except eye) 680.0
  finger (any) 680.4
  flank 680.2
  foot (any part) 680.7
  forearm 680.3
  genital organ (male) 608.4
  gluteal (region) 680.5
  groin 680.2
  hand (any part) 680.4
  head (any part, except face) 680.8
  heel 680.7
  hip 680.6
  kidney (*see also* Abscess, kidney) 590.2
  knee 680.6
  labia 616.4
  lacrimal
    gland (*see also* Dacryoadenitis) 375.00
    passages (duct) (sac) (*see also* Dacryocys-
      titis) 375.30
  leg, any part except foot 680.6
  lower extremity, any part except foot 680.6

☑ **Additional Digit Required** — Refer to the Tabular List for Digit Selection   ⬇ **Subterms under main terms may continue to next column or page**

2014 ICD-9-CM   ▶◀ Revised Text   ● New Line   ▲ Revised Code   **Volume 2 — 41**

Carbuncle — *continued*
  malignant 022.0
  multiple sites 680.9
  neck 680.1
  nose (external) (septum) 680.0
  orbit, orbital 376.01
  partes posteriores 680.5
  pectoral region 680.2
  penis 607.2
  perineum 680.2
  pinna 680.0
  scalp (any part) 680.8
  scrotum 608.4
  seminal vesicle 608.0
  shoulder 680.3
  skin NEC 680.9
  specified site NEC 680.8
  spermatic cord 608.4
  temple (region) 680.0
  testis 608.4
  thigh 680.6
  thumb 680.4
  toe (any) 680.7
  trunk 680.2
  tunica vaginalis 608.4
  umbilicus 680.2
  upper arm 680.3
  urethra 597.0
  vas deferens 608.4
  vulva 616.4
  wrist 680.4
Carbunculus — *see also* Carbuncle 680.9
Carcinoid (tumor) (M8240/1) — *see* Tumor, carcinoid
Carcinoidosis 259.2
Carcinomaphobia 300.29
Carcinomatosis
  peritonei (M8010/6) 197.6
  specified site NEC (M8010/3) — *see* Neoplasm, by site, malignant
  unspecified site (M8010/6) 199.0
Carcinoma (M8010/3) — *see also* Neoplasm, by site, malignant

Note — Except where otherwise indicated, the morphological varieties of carcinoma in the list below should be coded by site as for "Neoplasm, malignant."

  with
    apocrine metaplasia (M8573/3)
    cartilaginous (and osseous) metaplasia (M8571/3)
    osseous (and cartilaginous) metaplasia (M8571/3)
    productive fibrosis (M8141/3)
    spindle cell metaplasia (M8572/3)
    squamous metaplasia (M8570/3)
  acidophil-basophil, mixed (M8281/3)
    specified site — *see* Neoplasm, by site, malignant
    unspecified site 194.3
  acidophil (M8280/3)
    specified site — *see* Neoplasm, by site, malignant
    unspecified site 194.3
  acinar (cell) (M8550/3)
  acinic cell (M8550/3)
  adenocystic (M8200/3)
  adenoid
    cystic (M8200/3)
    squamous cell (M8075/3)
  adenosquamous (M8560/3)
  adnexal (skin) (M8390/3) — *see* Neoplasm, skin, malignant
  adrenal cortical (M8370/3) 194.0
  alveolar (M8251/3)
    cell (M8250/3) — *see* Neoplasm, lung, malignant
  anaplastic type (M8021/3)
  apocrine (M8401/3)
    breast — *see* Neoplasm, breast, malignant
    specified site NEC — *see* Neoplasm, skin, malignant
    unspecified site 173.99
  basal-squamous cell, mixed (M8094/3) — *see* Neoplasm, skin, malignant

Carcinoma — *see also* Neoplasm, by site, malignant — *continued*
  basal cell (pigmented) (M8090/3) (*see also* Neoplasm, skin, malignant) 173.91
    fibro-epithelial type (M8093/3) — *see* Neoplasm, skin, malignant
    morphea type (M8092/3) — *see* Neoplasm, skin, malignant
    multicentric (M8091/3) — *see* Neoplasm, skin, malignant
  basaloid (M8123/3)
  basophil-acidophil, mixed (M8281/3)
    specified site — *see* Neoplasm, by site, malignant
    unspecified site 194.3
  basophil (M8300/3)
    specified site — *see* Neoplasm, by site, malignant
    unspecified site 194.3
  basosquamous (M8094/3) — *see* Neoplasm, skin, malignant
  bile duct type (M8160/3)
    and hepatocellular, mixed (M8180/3) 155.0
    liver 155.1
    specified site NEC — *see* Neoplasm, by site, malignant
    unspecified site 155.1
  branchial or branchiogenic 146.8
  bronchial or bronchogenic — *see* Neoplasm, lung, malignant
  bronchiolar (terminal) (M8250/3) — *see* Neoplasm, lung, malignant
  bronchiolo-alveolar (M8250/3) — *see* Neoplasm, lung, malignant
  bronchogenic (epidermoid) 162.9
  C cell (M8510/3)
    specified site — *see* Neoplasm, by site, malignant
    unspecified site 193
  ceruminous (M8420/3) 173.29
  chorionic (M9100/3)
    specified site — *see* Neoplasm, by site, malignant
    unspecified site
      female 181
      male 186.9
  chromophobe (M8270/3)
    specified site — *see* Neoplasm, by site, malignant
    unspecified site 194.3
  clear cell (mesonephroid type) (M8310/3)
  cloacogenic (M8124/3)
    specified site — *see* Neoplasm, by site, malignant
    unspecified site 154.8
  colloid (M8480/3)
  cribriform (M8201/3)
  cylindroid type (M8200/3)
  diffuse type (M8145/3)
    specified site — *see* Neoplasm, by site, malignant
    unspecified site 151.9
  duct (cell) (M8500/3)
    with Paget's disease (M8541/3) — *see* Neoplasm, breast, malignant
    infiltrating (M8500/3)
      specified site — *see* Neoplasm, by site, malignant
      unspecified site 174.9
  ductal (M8500/3)
  ductular, infiltrating (M8521/3)
  embryonal (M9070/3)
    and teratoma, mixed (M9081/3)
    combined with choriocarcinoma (M9101/3) — *see* Neoplasm, by site, malignant
    infantile type (M9071/3)
    liver 155.0
    polyembryonal type (M9072/3)
  endometrioid (M8380/3)
  eosinophil (M8280/3)
    specified site — *see* Neoplasm, by site, malignant
    unspecified site 194.3

Carcinoma — *see also* Neoplasm, by site, malignant — *continued*
  epidermoid (M8070/3) (*see also* Carcinoma, squamous cell)
    and adenocarcinoma, mixed (M8560/3)
    in situ, Bowen's type (M8081/2) — *see* Neoplasm, skin, in situ
    intradermal — *see* Neoplasm, skin, in situ
  fibroepithelial type basal cell (M8093/3) — *see* Neoplasm, skin, malignant
  follicular (M8330/3)
    and papillary (mixed) (M8340/3) 193
    moderately differentiated type (M8332/3) 193
    pure follicle type (M8331/3) 193
    specified site — *see* Neoplasm, by site, malignant
    trabecular type (M8332/3) 193
    unspecified site 193
    well differentiated type (M8331/3) 193
  gelatinous (M8480/3)
  giant cell (M8031/3)
    and spindle cell (M8030/3)
  granular cell (M8320/3)
  granulosa cell (M8620/3) 183.0
  hepatic cell (M8170/3) 155.0
  hepatocellular (M8170/3) 155.0
    and bile duct, mixed (M8180/3) 155.0
  hepatocholangiolitic (M8180/3) 155.0
  Hürthle cell (thyroid) 193
  hypernephroid (M8311/3)
  in
    adenomatous
      polyp (M8210/3)
      polyposis coli (M8220/3) 153.9
    pleomorphic adenoma (M8940/3)
    polypoid adenoma (M8210/3)
    situ (M8010/3) — *see* Carcinoma, in situ
    tubular adenoma (M8210/3)
    villous adenoma (M8261/3)
  infiltrating duct (M8500/3)
    with Paget's disease (M8541/3) — *see* Neoplasm, breast, malignant
    specified site — *see* Neoplasm, by site, malignant
    unspecified site 174.9
  inflammatory (M8530/3)
    specified site — *see* Neoplasm, by site, malignant
    unspecified site 174.9
  in situ (M8010/2) (*see also* Neoplasm, by site, in situ)
    epidermoid (M8070/2) (*see also* Neoplasm, by site, in situ)
      with questionable stromal invasion (M8076/2)
      specified site — *see* Neoplasm, by site, in situ
      unspecified site 233.1
    Bowen's type (M8081/2) — *see* Neoplasm, skin, in situ
    intraductal (M8500/2)
      specified site — *see* Neoplasm, by site, in situ
      unspecified site 233.0
    lobular (M8520/2)
      specified site — *see* Neoplasm, by site, in situ
      unspecified site 233.0
    papillary (M8050/2) — *see* Neoplasm, by site, in situ
    squamous cell (M8070/2) (*see also* Neoplasm, by site, in situ)
      with questionable stromal invasion (M8076/2)
      specified site — *see* Neoplasm, by site, in situ
      unspecified site 233.1
    transitional cell (M8120/2) — *see* Neoplasm, by site, in situ
  intestinal type (M8144/3)
    specified site — *see* Neoplasm, by site, malignant
    unspecified site 151.9

Carcinoma — *see also* Neoplasm, by site, malignant — *continued*
  intraductal (noninfiltrating) (M8500/2)
    papillary (M8503/2)
      specified site — *see* Neoplasm, by site, in situ
      unspecified site 233.0
    specified site — *see* Neoplasm, by site, in situ
    unspecified site 233.0
  intraepidermal (M8070/2) (*see also* Neoplasm, skin, in situ)
    squamous cell, Bowen's type (M8081/2) — *see* Neoplasm, skin, in situ
  intraepithelial (M8010/2) (*see also* Neoplasm, by site, in situ)
    squamous cell (M8072/2) — *see* Neoplasm, by site, in situ
  intraosseous (M9270/3) 170.1
    upper jaw (bone) 170.0
  islet cell (M8150/3)
    and exocrine, mixed (M8154/3)
      specified site — *see* Neoplasm, by site, malignant
      unspecified site 157.9
    pancreas 157.4
    specified site NEC — *see* Neoplasm, by site, malignant
    unspecified site 157.4
  juvenile, breast (M8502/3) — *see* Neoplasm, breast, malignant
  Kulchitsky's cell (carcinoid tumor of intestine) 259.2
  large cell (M8012/3)
    squamous cell, non-keratinizing type (M8072/3)
  Leydig cell (testis) (M8650/3)
    specified site — *see* Neoplasm, by site, malignant
    unspecified site 186.9
      female 183.0
      male 186.9
  liver cell (M8170/3) 155.0
  lobular (infiltrating) (M8520/3)
    non-infiltrating (M8520/3)
      specified site — *see* Neoplasm, by site, in situ
      unspecified site 233.0
    specified site — *see* Neoplasm, by site, malignant
    unspecified site 174.9
  lymphoepithelial (M8082/3)
  medullary (M8510/3)
    with
      amyloid stroma (M8511/3)
        specified site — *see* Neoplasm, by site, malignant
        unspecified site 193
      lymphoid stroma (M8512/3)
        specified site — *see* Neoplasm, by site, malignant
        unspecified site 174.9
  Merkel cell 209.36
    buttock 209.36
    ear 209.31
    eyelid, including canthus 209.31
    face 209.31
    genitals 209.36
    lip 209.31
    lower limb 209.34
    neck 209.32
    nodal presentation 209.75
    scalp 209.32
    secondary (any site) 209.75
    specified site NEC 209.36
    trunk 209.35
    unknown primary site 209.75
    upper limb 209.33
    visceral metastatic presentation 209.75
  mesometanephric (M9110/3)
  mesonephric (M9110/3)
  metastatic (M8010/6) — *see* Metastasis, cancer
  metatypical (M8095/3) — *see* Neoplasm, skin, malignant

☑ **Additional Digit Required** — Refer to the Tabular List for Digit Selection   ⬏ **Subterms under main terms may continue to next column or page**

42 — Volume 2   ▶◀ **Revised Text**   ● **New Line**   ▲ **Revised Code**   **2014 ICD-9-CM**

Carbuncle — Carcinoma

Carcinoma — *see also* Neoplasm, by site, malignant — *continued*
- morphea type basal cell (M8092/3) — *see* Neoplasm, skin, malignant
- mucin-producing (M8481/3)
- mucin-secreting (M8481/3)
- mucinous (M8480/3)
- mucoepidermoid (M8430/3)
- mucoid (M8480/3)
  - cell (M8300/3)
    - specified site — *see* Neoplasm, by site, malignant
    - unspecified site 194.3
- mucous (M8480/3)
- neuroendocrine
  - high grade (M8240/3) 209.30
  - malignant poorly differentiated (M8240/3) 209.30
- nonencapsulated sclerosing (M8350/3) 193
- noninfiltrating
  - intracystic (M8504/2) — *see* Neoplasm, by site, in situ
  - intraductal (M8500/2)
    - papillary (M8503/2)
      - specified site — *see* Neoplasm, by site, in situ
      - unspecified site 233.0
    - specified site — *see* Neoplasm, by site, in situ
    - unspecified site 233.0
  - lobular (M8520/2)
    - specified site — *see* Neoplasm, by site, in situ
    - unspecified site 233.0
- oat cell (M8042/3)
  - specified site — *see* Neoplasm, by site, malignant
  - unspecified site 162.9
- odontogenic (M9270/3) 170.1
  - upper jaw (bone) 170.0
- onocytic (M8290/3)
- oxyphilic (M8290/3)
- papillary (M8050/3)
  - and follicular (mixed) (M8340/3) 193
  - epidermoid (M8052/3)
  - intraductal (noninfiltrating) (M8503/2)
    - specified site — *see* Neoplasm, by site, in situ
    - unspecified site 233.0
  - serous (M8460/3)
    - specified site — *see* Neoplasm, by site, malignant
    - surface (M8461/3)
      - specified site — *see* Neoplasm, by site, malignant
      - unspecified site 183.0
    - unspecified site 183.0
  - squamous cell (M8052/3)
  - transitional cell (M8130/3)
- papillocystic (M8450/3)
  - specified site — *see* Neoplasm, by site, malignant
  - unspecified site 183.0
- parafollicular cell (M8510/3)
  - specified site — *see* Neoplasm, by site, malignant
  - unspecified site 193
- pleomorphic (M8022/3)
- polygonal cell (M8034/3)
- prickle cell (M8070/3)
- pseudoglandular, squamous cell (M8075/3)
- pseudomucinous (M8470/3)
  - specified site — *see* Neoplasm, by site, malignant
  - unspecified site 183.0
- pseudosarcomatous (M8033/3)
- regaud type (M8082/3) — *see* Neoplasm, nasopharynx, malignant
- renal cell (M8312/3) 189.0
- reserve cell (M8041/3)
- round cell (M8041/3)
- Schmincke (M8082/3) — *see* Neoplasm, nasopharynx, malignant
- Schneiderian (M8121/3)
  - specified site — *see* Neoplasm, by site, malignant

Carcinoma — *see also* Neoplasm, by site, malignant — *continued*
- Schneiderian — *continued*
  - unspecified site 160.0
- scirrhous (M8141/3)
- sebaceous (M8410/3) — *see* Neoplasm, skin, malignant
- secondary (M8010/6) — *see* Neoplasm, by site, malignant, secondary
- secretory, breast (M8502/3) — *see* Neoplasm, breast, malignant
- serous (M8441/3)
  - papillary (M8460/3)
    - specified site — *see* Neoplasm, by site, malignant
    - unspecified site 183.0
  - surface, papillary (M8461/3)
    - specified site — *see* Neoplasm, by site, malignant
    - unspecified site 183.0
- Sertoli cell (M8640/3)
  - specified site — *see* Neoplasm, by site, malignant
  - unspecified site 186.9
- signet ring cell (M8490/3)
  - metastatic (M8490/6) — *see* Neoplasm, by site, secondary
- simplex (M8231/3)
- skin appendage (M8390/3) — *see* Neoplasm, skin, malignant
- small cell (M8041/3)
  - fusiform cell type (M8043/3)
  - squamous cell, non-keratinizing type (M8073/3)
- solid (M8230/3)
  - with amyloid stroma (M8511/3)
    - specified site — *see* Neoplasm, by site, malignant
    - unspecified site 193
- spheroidal cell (M8035/3)
- spindle cell (M8032/3)
  - and giant cell (M8030/3)
- spinous cell (M8070/3)
- squamous (cell) (M8070/3)
  - adenoid type (M8075/3)
  - and adenocarcinoma, mixed (M8560/3)
  - intraepidermal, Bowen's type — *see* Neoplasm, skin, in situ
  - keratinizing type (large cell) (M8071/3)
  - large cell, non-keratinizing type (M8072/3)
  - microinvasive (M8076/3)
    - specified site — *see* Neoplasm, by site, malignant
    - unspecified site 180.9
  - non-keratinizing type (M8072/3)
  - papillary (M8052/3)
  - pseudoglandular (M8075/3)
  - skin (*see also* Neoplasm, skin, malignant) 173.92
  - small cell, non-keratinizing type (M8073/3)
  - spindle cell type (M8074/3)
  - verrucous (M8051/3)
- superficial spreading (M8143/3)
- sweat gland (M8400/3) — *see* Neoplasm, skin, malignant
- theca cell (M8600/3) 183.0
- thymic (M8580/3) 164.0
- trabecular (M8190/3)
- transitional (cell) (M8120/3)
  - papillary (M8130/3)
  - spindle cell type (M8122/3)
- tubular (M8211/3)
- undifferentiated type (M8020/3)
- urothelial (M8120/3)
- ventriculi 151.9
- verrucous (epidermoid) (squamous cell) (M8051/3)
- villous (M8262/3)
- water-clear cell (M8322/3) 194.1
- wolffian duct (M9110/3)

Carcinosarcoma (M8980/3) — *see also* Neoplasm, by site, malignant
- embryonal type (M8981/3) — *see* Neoplasm, by site, malignant

Cardiac — *see also* condition
- death — *see* Disease, heart
- device
  - defibrillator, automatic implantable (with synchronous cardiac pacemaker) V45.02
    - in situ NEC V45.00
  - pacemaker
    - cardiac
      - fitting or adjustment V53.31
      - in situ V45.01
    - carotid sinus
      - fitting or adjustment V53.39
      - in situ V45.09
  - pacemaker — *see* Cardiac, device, pacemaker
- tamponade 423.3

Cardia, cardial — *see* condition

Cardialgia — *see also* Pain, precordial 786.51

Cardiectasis — *see* Hypertrophy, cardiac

Cardiochalasia 530.81

Cardiomalacia — *see also* Degeneration, myocardial 429.1

Cardiomegalia glycogenica diffusa 271.0

Cardiomegaly — *see also* Hypertrophy, cardiac 429.3
- congenital 746.89
- glycogen 271.0
- hypertensive (*see also* Hypertension, heart) 402.90
- idiopathic 429.3

Cardiomyoliposis — *see also* Degeneration, myocardial 429.1

Cardiomyopathy (congestive) (constrictive) (familial) (infiltrative) (obstructive) (restrictive) (sporadic) 425.4
- alcoholic 425.5
- amyloid 277.39 *[425.7]*
- beriberi 265.0 *[425.7]*
- cobalt-beer 425.5
- congenital 425.3
- due to
  - amyloidosis 277.39 *[425.7]*
  - beriberi 265.0 *[425.7]*
  - cardiac glycogenosis 271.0 *[425.7]*
  - Chagas' disease 086.0
  - Friedreich's ataxia 334.0 *[425.8]*
  - hypertension — *see* Hypertension, with, heart involvement
  - mucopolysaccharidosis 277.5 *[425.7]*
  - myotonia atrophica 359.21 *[425.8]*
  - progressive muscular dystrophy 359.1 *[425.8]*
  - sarcoidosis 135 *[425.8]*
- glycogen storage 271.0 *[425.7]*
- hypertensive — *see* Hypertension, with, heart involvement
- hypertrophic 425.18
  - nonobstructive 425.18
  - obstructive 425.11
    - congenital 746.84
- idiopathic (concentric) 425.4
- in
  - Chagas' disease 086.0
  - sarcoidosis 135 *[425.8]*
- ischemic 414.8
- metabolic NEC 277.9 *[425.7]*
  - amyloid 277.39 *[425.7]*
  - thyrotoxic (*see also* Thyrotoxicosis) 242.9 ☑ *[425.7]*
  - thyrotoxicosis (*see also* Thyrotoxicosis) 242.9 ☑ *[425.7]*
- newborn 425.4
  - congenital 425.3
- nutritional 269.9 *[425.7]*
  - beriberi 265.0 *[425.7]*
- obscure of Africa 425.2
- peripartum 674.5 ☑
- postpartum 674.5 ☑
- primary 425.4
- secondary 425.9
- stress inuced 429.83
- takotsubo 429.83
- thyrotoxic (*see also* Thyrotoxicosis) 242.9 ☑ *[425.7]*
- toxic NEC 425.9

Cardiomyopathy — *continued*
- tuberculous (*see also* Tuberculosis) 017.9 ☑ *[425.8]*

Cardionephritis — *see* Hypertension, cardiorenal

Cardionephropathy — *see* Hypertension, cardiorenal

Cardionephrosis — *see* Hypertension, cardiorenal

Cardioneurosis 306.2

Cardiopathia nigra 416.0

Cardiopathy — *see also* Disease, heart 429.9
- hypertensive (*see also* Hypertension, heart) 402.90
- idiopathic 425.4
- mucopolysaccharidosis 277.5 *[425.7]*

Cardiopericarditis — *see also* Pericarditis 423.9

Cardiophobia 300.29

Cardioptosis 746.87

Cardiorenal — *see* condition

Cardiorrhexis — *see also* Infarct, myocardium 410.9 ☑

Cardiosclerosis — *see* Arteriosclerosis, coronary

Cardiosis — *see* Disease, heart

Cardiospasm (esophagus) (reflex) (stomach) 530.0
- congenital 750.7

Cardiostenosis — *see* Disease, heart

Cardiosymphysis 423.1

Cardiothyrotoxicosis — *see* Hyperthyroidism

Cardiovascular — *see* condition

Carditis (acute) (bacterial) (chronic) (subacute) 429.89
- Coxsackie 074.20
- hypertensive (*see also* Hypertension, heart) 402.90
- meningococcal 036.40
- rheumatic — *see* Disease, heart, rheumatic
- rheumatoid 714.2

Care (of)
- child (routine) V20.1
- convalescent following V66.9
  - chemotherapy V66.2
  - medical NEC V66.5
  - psychotherapy V66.3
  - radiotherapy V66.1
  - surgery V66.0
  - surgical NEC V66.0
  - treatment (for) V66.5
    - combined V66.6
    - fracture V66.4
    - mental disorder NEC V66.3
    - specified type NEC V66.5
- end-of-life V66.7
- family member (handicapped) (sick)
  - creating problem for family V61.49
  - provided away from home for holiday relief V60.5
  - unavailable, due to
    - absence (person rendering care) (sufferer) V60.4
    - inability (any reason) of person rendering care V60.4
- holiday relief V60.5
- hospice V66.7
- lack of (at or after birth) (infant) (child) 995.52
  - adult 995.84
- lactation of mother V24.1
- palliative V66.7
- postpartum
  - immediately after delivery V24.0
  - routine follow-up V24.2
- prenatal V22.1
  - first pregnancy V22.0
  - high-risk pregnancy V23.9
    - inconclusive fetal viability V23.87
    - specified problem NEC V23.89
- terminal V66.7
- unavailable, due to
  - absence of person rendering care V60.4
  - inability (any reason) of person rendering care V60.4
- well baby V20.1

☑ Additional Digit Required — Refer to the Tabular List for Digit Selection   ▽ Subterms under main terms may continue to next column or page

2014 ICD-9-CM   ▶◀ Revised Text   ● New Line   ▲ Revised Code   **Volume 2 — 43**

Caries (bone) — *see also* Tuberculosis, bone
   015.9 ☑ *[730.8]* ☑
  arrested 521.04
  cementum 521.03
  cerebrospinal (tuberculous)
    015.0 ☑ *[730.88]* ☑
  dental (acute) (chronic) (incipient) (infected)
    521.00
    with pulp exposure 521.03
    extending to
      dentine 521.02
      pulp 521.03
    other specified NEC 521.09
    pit and fissure 521.06
    primary
      pit and fissure origin 521.06
      root surface 521.08
      smooth surface origin 521.07
    root surface 521.08
    smooth surface 521.07
  dentin (acute) (chronic) 521.02
  enamel (acute) (chronic) (incipient) 521.01
  external meatus 380.89
  hip (*see also* Tuberculosis) 015.1 ☑ *[730.85]*
  initial 521.01
  knee 015.2 ☑ *[730.86]*
  labyrinth 386.8
  limb NEC 015.7 ☑ *[730.88]*
  mastoid (chronic) (process) 383.1
  middle ear 385.89
  nose 015.7 ☑ *[730.88]*
  orbit 015.7 ☑ *[730.88]*
  ossicle 385.24
  petrous bone 383.20
  sacrum (tuberculous) 015.0 ☑ *[730.88]*
  spine, spinal (column) (tuberculous)
    015.0 ☑ *[730.88]*
  syphilitic 095.5
    congenital 090.0 *[730.8]* ☑
  teeth (internal) 521.00
    initial 521.01
  vertebra (column) (tuberculous)
    015.0 ☑ *[730.88]*
Carini's syndrome (ichthyosis congenita) 757.1
Carious teeth 521.00
Carneous mole 631.8
Carnosinemia 270.5
Carotid body or sinus syndrome 337.01
Carotidynia 337.01
Carotinemia (dietary) 278.3
Carotinosis (cutis) (skin) 278.3
Carpal tunnel syndrome 354.0
Carpenter's syndrome 759.89
Carpopedal spasm — *see also* Tetany 781.7
Carpoptosis 736.05
Carrier (suspected) of
  amebiasis V02.2
  bacterial disease (meningococcal, staphylo-
    coccal) NEC V02.59
  cholera V02.0
  cystic fibrosis gene V83.81
  defective gene V83.89
  diphtheria V02.4
  dysentery (bacillary) V02.3
    amebic V02.2
  Endamoeba histolytica V02.2
  gastrointestinal pathogens NEC V02.3
  genetic defect V83.89
  gonorrhea V02.7
  group B streptococcus V02.51
  HAA (hepatitis Australian-antigen) V02.61
  hemophilia A (asymptomatic) V83.01
    symptomatic V83.02
  hepatitis V02.60
    Australian-antigen (HAA) V02.61
    B V02.61
    C V02.62
    serum V02.61
    specified type NEC V02.69
    viral V02.60
  infective organism NEC V02.9
  malaria V02.9
  paratyphoid V02.3
  Salmonella V02.3
    typhosa V02.1
  serum hepatitis V02.61

Carrier (suspected) **of** — *continued*
  Shigella V02.3
  Staphylococcus NEC V02.59
    methicillin
      resistant Staphylococcus aureus
        V02.54
      susceptible Staphylococcus aureus
        V02.53
  Streptococcus NEC V02.52
    group B V02.51
  typhoid V02.1
  venereal disease NEC V02.8
Carrión's disease (Bartonellosis) 088.0
Car sickness 994.6
Carter's
  relapsing fever (Asiatic) 087.0
Cartilage — *see* condition
Caruncle (inflamed)
  abscess, lacrimal (*see also* Dacryocystitis)
    375.30
  conjunctiva 372.00
    acute 372.00
  eyelid 373.00
  labium (majus) (minus) 616.89
  lacrimal 375.30
  urethra (benign) 599.3
  vagina (wall) 616.89
Cascade stomach 537.6
Caseation lymphatic gland — *see also* Tuberculosis 017.2 ☑
Caseous
  bronchitis — *see* Tuberculosis, pulmonary
  meningitis 013.0 ☑
  pneumonia — *see* Tuberculosis, pulmonary
Cassidy (-Scholte) syndrome (malignant carcinoid) 259.2
Castellani's bronchitis 104.8
Castleman's tumor or lymphoma (mediastinal lymph node hyperplasia) 785.6
Castration, traumatic 878.2
  complicated 878.3
Casts in urine 791.7
Cat-scratch — *see also* Injury, superficial
  disease or fever 078.3
Catalepsy 300.11
  catatonic (acute) (*see also* Schizophrenia)
    295.2 ☑
  hysterical 300.11
  schizophrenic (*see also* Schizophrenia)
    295.2 ☑
Cataphasia — *see also* Disorder, fluency 315.35
Cataplexy (idiopathic) — *see* Narcolepsy
Cataract (anterior cortical) (anterior polar)
  (black) (capsular) (central) (cortical) (hypermature) (immature) (incipient) (mature) 366.9
  anterior
    and posterior axial embryonal 743.33
    pyramidal 743.31
    subcapsular polar
      infantile, juvenile, or presenile 366.01
      senile 366.13
  associated with
    calcinosis 275.40 *[366.42]*
    craniofacial dysostosis 756.0 *[366.44]*
    galactosemia 271.1 *[366.44]*
    hypoparathyroidism 252.1 *[366.42]*
    myotonic disorders 359.21 *[366.43]*
    neovascularization 366.33
  blue dot 743.39
  cerulean 743.39
  complicated NEC 366.30
  congenital 743.30
    capsular or subcapsular 743.31
    cortical 743.32
    nuclear 743.33
    specified type NEC 743.39
    total or subtotal 743.34
    zonular 743.32
  coronary (congenital) 743.39
    acquired 366.12
  cupuliform 366.14
  diabetic 250.5 ☑ *[366.41]*
    due to secondary diabetes
      249.5 ☑ *[366.41]*
  drug-induced 366.45

Cataract — *continued*
  due to
    chalcosis 360.24 *[366.34]*
    chronic choroiditis (*see also* Choroiditis)
      363.20 *[366.32]*
    degenerative myopia 360.21 *[366.34]*
    glaucoma (*see also* Glaucoma)
      365.9 *[366.31]*
    infection, intraocular NEC 366.32
    inflammatory ocular disorder NEC 366.32
    iridocyclitis, chronic 364.10 *[366.33]*
    pigmentary retinal dystrophy
      362.74 *[366.34]*
    radiation 366.46
  electric 366.46
  glassblowers' 366.46
  heat ray 366.46
  heterochromic 366.33
  in eye disease NEC 366.30
  infantile (*see also* Cataract, juvenile) 366.00
  intumescent 366.12
  irradiational 366.46
  juvenile 366.00
    anterior subcapsular polar 366.01
    combined forms 366.09
    cortical 366.03
    lamellar 366.03
    nuclear 366.04
    posterior subcapsular polar 366.02
    specified NEC 366.09
    zonular 366.03
  lamellar 743.32
    infantile, juvenile, or presenile 366.03
  morgagnian 366.18
  myotonic 359.21 *[366.43]*
  myxedema 244.9 *[366.44]*
  nuclear 366.16
  posterior, polar (capsular) 743.31
    infantile, juvenile, or presenile 366.02
    senile 366.14
  presenile (*see also* Cataract, juvenile) 366.00
  punctate
    acquired 366.12
    congenital 743.39
  secondary (membrane) 366.50
    obscuring vision 366.53
    specified type, not obscuring vision
      366.52
  senile 366.10
    anterior subcapsular polar 366.13
    combined forms 366.19
    cortical 366.15
    hypermature 366.18
    immature 366.12
    incipient 366.12
    mature 366.17
    nuclear 366.16
    posterior subcapsular polar 366.14
    specified NEC 366.19
    total or subtotal 366.17
  snowflake 250.5 ☑ *[366.41]*
    due to secondary diabetes
      249.5 ☑ *[366.41]*
  specified NEC 366.8
  subtotal (senile) 366.17
    congenital 743.34
  sunflower 360.24 *[366.34]*
  tetanic NEC 252.1 *[366.42]*
  total (mature) (senile) 366.17
    congenital 743.34
    localized 366.21
    traumatic 366.22
  toxic 366.45
  traumatic 366.20
    partially resolved 366.23
    total 366.22
  zonular (perinuclear) 743.32
    infantile, juvenile, or presenile 366.03
Cataracta 366.10
  brunescens 366.16
  cerulea 743.39
  complicata 366.30
  congenita 743.30
  coralliformis 743.39
  coronaria (congenital) 743.39
    acquired 366.12

Cataracta — *continued*
  diabetic 250.5 ☑ *[366.41]*
    due to secondary diabetes
      249.5 ☑ *[366.41]*
  floriformis 360.24 *[366.34]*
  membranacea
    accreta 366.50
    congenita 743.39
  nigra 366.16
Catarrh, catarrhal (inflammation) — *see also*
  condition 460
  acute 460
  asthma, asthmatic (*see also* Asthma)
    493.9 ☑
  Bostock's (*see also* Fever, hay) 477.9
  bowel — *see* Enteritis
  bronchial 490
    acute 466.0
    chronic 491.0
    subacute 466.0
  cervix, cervical (canal) (uteri) — *see* Cervicitis
  chest (*see also* Bronchitis) 490
  chronic 472.0
  congestion 472.0
  conjunctivitis 372.03
  due to syphilis 095.9
    congenital 090.0
  enteric — *see* Enteritis
  epidemic (*see also* Influenza) 487.1
  Eustachian 381.50
  eye (acute) (vernal) 372.03
  fauces (*see also* Pharyngitis) 462
  febrile 460
  fibrinous acute 466.0
  gastroenteric — *see* Enteritis
  gastrointestinal — *see* Enteritis
  gingivitis 523.00
  hay (*see also* Fever, hay) 477.9
  infectious 460
  intestinal — *see* Enteritis
  larynx (*see also* Laryngitis, chronic) 476.0
  liver 070.1
    with hepatic coma 070.0
  lung (*see also* Bronchitis) 490
    acute 466.0
    chronic 491.0
  middle ear (chronic) — *see* Otitis media,
    chronic
  mouth 528.00
  nasal (chronic) (*see also* Rhinitis) 472.0
    acute 460
  nasobronchial 472.2
  nasopharyngeal (chronic) 472.2
    acute 460
  nose — *see* Catarrh, nasal
  ophthalmia 372.03
  pneumococcal, acute 466.0
  pulmonary (*see also* Bronchitis) 490
    acute 466.0
    chronic 491.0
  spring (eye) 372.13
  suffocating (*see also* Asthma) 493.9 ☑
  summer (hay) (*see also* Fever, hay) 477.9
  throat 472.1
  tracheitis 464.10
    with obstruction 464.11
  tubotympanal 381.4
    acute (*see also* Otitis media, acute, non-
      suppurative) 381.00
    chronic 381.10
  vasomotor (*see also* Fever, hay) 477.9
  vesical (bladder) — *see* Cystitis
Catarrhus aestivus — *see also* Fever, hay 477.9
Catastrophe, cerebral — *see also* Disease,
  cerebrovascular, acute 436
Catatonia, catatonic (acute) 781.99
  with
    affective psychosis — *see* Psychosis, af-
      fective
  agitation 295.2 ☑
  dementia (praecox) 295.2 ☑
  due to or associated with physical condition
    293.89
  excitation 295.2 ☑
  excited type 295.2 ☑
  in conditions classified elsewhere 293.89

☑ **Additional Digit Required** — Refer to the Tabular List for Digit Selection   ▽ **Subterms under main terms may continue to next column or page**

44 — Volume 2   ▶◀ **Revised Text**   ● **New Line**   ▲ **Revised Code**   **2014 ICD-9-CM**

Catatonia, catatonic — *continued*
  schizophrenia 295.2 ☑
  stupor 295.2 ☑
Cat's ear 744.29
Cauda equina — *see also* condition
  syndrome 344.60
Cauliflower ear 738.7
Caul over face 768.9
Causalgia 355.9
  lower limb 355.71
  upper limb 354.4
Cause
  external, general effects NEC 994.9
  not stated 799.9
  unknown 799.9
Caustic burn — *see also* Burn, by site
  from swallowing caustic or corrosive substance — *see* Burn, internal organs
Cavare's disease (familial periodic paralysis) 359.3
Cave-in, injury
  crushing (severe) (*see also* Crush, by site) 869.1
  suffocation 994.7
Cavernitis (penis) 607.2
  lymph vessel — *see* Lymphangioma
Cavernositis 607.2
Cavernous — *see* condition
Cavitation of lung — *see also* Tuberculosis 011.2 ☑
  nontuberculous 518.89
  primary, progressive 010.8 ☑
Cavity
  lung — *see* Cavitation of lung
  optic papilla 743.57
  pulmonary — *see* Cavitation of lung
  teeth 521.00
  vitreous (humor) 379.21
Cavovarus foot, congenital 754.59
Cavus foot (congenital) 754.71
  acquired 736.73
Cazenave's
  disease (pemphigus) NEC 694.4
  lupus (erythematosus) 695.4
CDGS (carbohydrate-deficient glycoprotein syndrome) 271.8
Cecitis — *see* Appendicitis
Cecocele — *see* Hernia
Cecum — *see* condition
Celiac
  artery compression syndrome 447.4
  disease 579.0
  infantilism 579.0
Cell, cellular — *see also* condition
  anterior chamber (eye) (positive aqueous ray) 364.04
Cellulitis (diffuse) (with lymphangitis) — *see also* Abscess 682.9
  abdominal wall 682.2
  anaerobic (*see also* Gas gangrene) 040.0
  ankle 682.6
  anus 566
  areola 611.0
  arm (any part, above wrist) 682.3
  auditory canal (external) 380.10
  axilla 682.3
  back (any part) 682.2
  breast 611.0
    postpartum 675.1 ☑
  broad ligament (*see also* Disease, pelvis, inflammatory) 614.4
    acute 614.3
  buttock 682.5
  cervical (neck region) 682.1
  cervix (uteri) (*see also* Cervicitis) 616.0
  cheek, external 682.0
    internal 528.3
  chest wall 682.2
  chronic NEC 682.9
  colostomy 569.61
  corpus cavernosum 607.2
  digit 681.9
  Douglas' cul-de-sac or pouch (chronic) (*see also* Disease, pelvis, inflammatory) 614.4
    acute 614.3

Cellulitis — *see also* Abscess — *continued*
  drainage site (following operation) 998.59
  ear, external 380.10
  enterostomy 569.61
  erysipelar (*see also* Erysipelas) 035
  esophagostomy 530.86
  eyelid 373.13
  face (any part, except eye) 682.0
  finger (intrathecal) (periosteal) (subcutaneous) (subcuticular) 681.00
  flank 682.2
  foot (except toe) 682.7
  forearm 682.3
  gangrenous (*see also* Gangrene) 785.4
  genital organ NEC
    female — *see* Abscess, genital organ, female
    male 608.4
  glottis 478.71
  gluteal (region) 682.5
  gonococcal NEC 098.0
  groin 682.2
  hand (except finger or thumb) 682.4
  head (except face) NEC 682.8
  heel 682.7
  hip 682.6
  jaw (region) 682.0
  knee 682.6
  labium (majus) (minus) (*see also* Vulvitis) 616.10
  larynx 478.71
  leg, except foot 682.6
  lip 528.5
  mammary gland 611.0
  mouth (floor) 528.3
  multiple sites NEC 682.9
  nasopharynx 478.21
  navel 682.2
    newborn NEC 771.4
  neck (region) 682.1
  nipple 611.0
  nose 478.19
    external 682.0
  orbit, orbital 376.01
  palate (soft) 528.3
  pectoral (region) 682.2
  pelvis, pelvic
    with
      abortion — *see* Abortion, by type, with sepsis
      ectopic pregnancy (*see also* categories 633.0–633.9) 639.0
      molar pregnancy (*see also* categories 630–632) 639.0
    female (*see also* Disease, pelvis, inflammatory) 614.4
      acute 614.3
    following
      abortion 639.0
      ectopic or molar pregnancy 639.0
    male 567.21
    puerperal, postpartum, childbirth 670.8 ☑
  penis 607.2
  perineal, perineum 682.2
  perirectal 566
  peritonsillar 475
  periurethral 597.0
  periuterine (*see also* Disease, pelvis, inflammatory) 614.4
    acute 614.3
  pharynx 478.21
  phlegmonous NEC 682.9
  rectum 566
  retromammary 611.0
  retroperitoneal (*see also* Peritonitis) 567.2 ☑, 567.38
  round ligament (*see also* Disease, pelvis, inflammatory) 614.4
    acute 614.3
  scalp (any part) 682.8
    dissecting 704.8
  scrotum 608.4
  seminal vesicle 608.0
  septic NEC 682.9
  shoulder 682.3

Cellulitis — *see also* Abscess — *continued*
  specified sites NEC 682.8
  spermatic cord 608.4
  submandibular (region) (space) (triangle) 682.0
    gland 527.3
  submaxillary 528.3
    gland 527.3
  submental (pyogenic) 682.0
    gland 527.3
  suppurative NEC 682.9
  testis 608.4
  thigh 682.6
  thumb (intrathecal) (periosteal) (subcutaneous) (subcuticular) 681.00
  toe (intrathecal) (periosteal) (subcutaneous) (subcuticular) 681.10
  tonsil 475
  trunk 682.2
  tuberculous (primary) (*see also* Tuberculosis) 017.0 ☑
  tunica vaginalis 608.4
  umbilical 682.2
    newborn NEC 771.4
  vaccinal 999.39
  vagina — *see* Vaginitis
  vas deferens 608.4
  vocal cords 478.5
  vulva (*see also* Vulvitis) 616.10
  wrist 682.4
Cementoblastoma, benign (M9273/0) 213.1
  upper jaw (bone) 213.0
Cementoma (M9273/0) 213.1
  gigantiform (M9275/0) 213.1
    upper jaw (bone) 213.0
  upper jaw (bone) 213.0
Cementoperiostitis 523.40
  acute 523.33
  apical 523.40
Cephalgia, cephalalgia — *see also* Headache 784.0
  histamine 339.00
  nonorganic origin 307.81
  other trigeminal autonomic (TACS) 339.09
  psychogenic 307.81
  tension 307.81
Cephalhematocele, cephalematocele
  due to birth injury 767.19
  fetus or newborn 767.19
  traumatic (*see also* Contusion, head) 920
Cephalhematoma, cephalematoma (calcified)
  due to birth injury 767.19
  fetus or newborn 767.19
  traumatic (*see also* Contusion, head) 920
Cephalic — *see* condition
Cephalitis — *see* Encephalitis
Cephalocele 742.0
Cephaloma — *see* Neoplasm, by site, malignant
Cephalomenia 625.8
Cephalopelvic — *see* condition
Cercomoniasis 007.3
Cerebellitis — *see* Encephalitis
Cerebellum (cerebellar) — *see* condition
Cerebral — *see* condition
Cerebritis — *see* Encephalitis
Cerebrohepatorenal syndrome 759.89
Cerebromacular degeneration 330.1
Cerebromalacia — *see also* Softening, brain 348.89
  due to cerebrovascular accident 438.89
Cerebrosidosis 272.7
Cerebrospasticity — *see* Palsy, cerebral
Cerebrospinal — *see* condition
Cerebrum — *see* condition
Ceroid storage disease 272.7
Cerumen (accumulation) (impacted) 380.4
Cervical — *see also* condition
  auricle 744.43
  high risk human papillomavirus (HPV) DNA test positive 795.05
  intraepithelial glandular neoplasia 233.1
  low risk human papillomavirus (HPV) DNA test positive 795.09
  rib 756.2

Cervical — *see also* condition — *continued*
  shortening — *see* Short, cervical
Cervicalgia 723.1
Cervicitis (acute) (chronic) (nonvenereal) (subacute) (with erosion or ectropion) 616.0
  with
    abortion — *see* Abortion, by type, with sepsis
    ectopic pregnancy (*see also* categories 633.0–633.9) 639.0
    molar pregnancy (*see also* categories 630–632) 639.0
    ulceration 616.0
  chlamydial 099.53
  complicating pregnancy or puerperium 646.6 ☑
    affecting fetus or newborn 760.8
  following
    abortion 639.0
    ectopic or molar pregnancy 639.0
  gonococcal (acute) 098.15
    chronic or duration of 2 months or more 098.35
  senile (atrophic) 616.0
  syphilitic 095.8
  trichomonal 131.09
  tuberculous (*see also* Tuberculosis) 016.7 ☑
Cervicoaural fistula 744.49
Cervicocolpitis (emphysematosa) — *see also* Cervicitis 616.0
Cervix — *see* condition
Cesarean delivery, operation or section NEC 669.7 ☑
  affecting fetus or newborn 763.4
  (planned) occurring after 37 completed weeks of gestation but before 39 completed weeks gestation due to (spontaneous) onset of labor 649.8 ☑
  post mortem, affecting fetus or newborn 761.6
  previous, affecting management of pregnancy 654.2 ☑
Céstan-Chenais paralysis 344.89
Céstan-Raymond syndrome 433.8 ☑
Céstan's syndrome 344.89
Cestode infestation NEC 123.9
  specified type NEC 123.8
Cestodiasis 123.9
CGF (congenital generalized fibromatosis) 759.89
Chabert's disease 022.9
Chacaleh 266.2
Chafing 709.8
Chagas' disease — *see also* Trypanosomiasis, American 086.2
  with heart involvement 086.0
Chagres fever 084.0
Chalasia (cardiac sphincter) 530.81
Chalazion 373.2
Chalazoderma 757.39
Chalcosis 360.24
  cornea 371.15
  crystalline lens 360.24 [366.34]
  retina 360.24
Chalicosis (occupational) (pulmonum) 502
Chancre (any genital site) (hard) (indurated) (infecting) (primary) (recurrent) 091.0
  congenital 090.0
  conjunctiva 091.2
  Ducrey's 099.0
  extragenital 091.2
  eyelid 091.2
  Hunterian 091.0
  lip (syphilis) 091.2
  mixed 099.8
  nipple 091.2
  Nisbet's 099.0
  of
    carate 103.0
    pinta 103.0
    yaws 102.0
  palate, soft 091.2
  phagedenic 099.0
  Ricord's 091.0

☑ **Additional Digit Required** — Refer to the Tabular List for Digit Selection   ⬇ **Subterms under main terms may continue to next column or page**

2014 ICD-9-CM   ▶◀ **Revised Text**   ● **New Line**   ▲ **Revised Code**   **Volume 2 — 45**

Chancre — *continued*
  Rollet's (syphilitic) 091.0
  seronegative 091.0
  seropositive 091.0
  simple 099.0
  soft 099.0
    bubo 099.0
  urethra 091.0
  yaws 102.0
Chancriform syndrome 114.1
Chancroid 099.0
  anus 099.0
  penis (Ducrey's bacillus) 099.0
  perineum 099.0
  rectum 099.0
  scrotum 099.0
  urethra 099.0
  vulva 099.0
Chandipura fever 066.8
Chandler's disease (osteochondritis dissecans, hip) 732.7
Change(s) (of) — *see also* Removal of —
  arteriosclerotic — *see* Arteriosclerosis
  battery
    cardiac pacemaker V53.31
  bone 733.90
    diabetic 250.8 ☑ *[731.8]*
      due to secondary diabetes 249.8 ☑ *[731.8]*
    in disease, unknown cause 733.90
  bowel habits 787.99
  cardiorenal (vascular) (*see also* Hypertension, cardiorenal) 404.90
  cardiovascular — *see* Disease, cardiovascular
  circulatory 459.9
  cognitive or personality change of other type, nonpsychotic 310.1
  color, teeth, tooth
    during formation 520.8
    extrinsic 523.6
    intrinsic posteruptive 521.7
  contraceptive device V25.42
  cornea, corneal
    degenerative NEC 371.40
    membrane NEC 371.30
    senile 371.41
  coronary (*see also* Ischemia, heart) 414.9
  degenerative
    chamber angle (anterior) (iris) 364.56
    ciliary body 364.57
    spine or vertebra (*see also* Spondylosis) 721.90
  dental pulp, regressive 522.2
  drains V58.49
  dressing
    wound V58.30
      nonsurgical V58.30
      surgical V58.31
  fixation device V54.89
    external V54.89
    internal V54.01
  heart (*see also* Disease, heart)
  hip joint 718.95
  hyperplastic larynx 478.79
  hypertrophic
    nasal sinus (*see also* Sinusitis) 473.9
    turbinate, nasal 478.0
    upper respiratory tract 478.9
  inflammatory — *see* Inflammation
  joint (*see also* Derangement, joint) 718.90
    sacroiliac 724.6
  Kirschner wire V54.89
  knee 717.9
  macular, congenital 743.55
  malignant (M — — /3) (*see also* Neoplasm, by site, malignant)

Note — for malignant change occurring in a neoplasm, use the appropriate M code with behavior digit /3 e.g., malignant change in uterine fibroid — M8890/3. For malignant change occurring in a nonneoplastic condition (e.g., gastric ulcer) use the M code M8000/3.

  mental (status) NEC 780.97

Change(s) — *see also* Removal of — *continued*
  mental — *continued*
    due to or associated with physical condition — *see* Syndrome, brain
  myocardium, myocardial — *see* Degeneration, myocardial
  of life (*see also* Menopause) 627.2
  pacemaker battery (cardiac) V53.31
  peripheral nerve 355.9
  personality (nonpsychotic) NEC 310.1
  plaster cast V54.89
  refractive, transient 367.81
  regressive, dental pulp 522.2
  retina 362.9
    myopic (degenerative) (malignant) 360.21
    vascular appearance 362.13
  sacroiliac joint 724.6
  scleral 379.19
    degenerative 379.16
  senile (*see also* Senility) 797
  sensory (*see also* Disturbance, sensation) 782.0
  skin texture 782.8
  spinal cord 336.9
  splint, external V54.89
  subdermal implantable contraceptive V25.5
  suture V58.32
  traction device V54.89
  trophic 355.9
    arm NEC 354.9
    leg NEC 355.8
    lower extremity NEC 355.8
    upper extremity NEC 354.9
  vascular 459.9
  vasomotor 443.9
  voice 784.49
    psychogenic 306.1
  wound packing V58.30
    nonsurgical V58.30
    surgical V58.31
Changing sleep-work schedule, affecting sleep 327.36
Changuinola fever 066.0
Chapping skin 709.8
Character
  depressive 301.12
Charcôt-Marie-Tooth disease, paralysis, or syndrome 356.1
Charcôt's
  arthropathy 094.0 *[713.5]*
  cirrhosis — *see* Cirrhosis, biliary
  disease 094.0
    spinal cord 094.0
  fever (biliary) (hepatic) (intermittent) — *see* Choledocholithiasis
  joint (disease) 094.0 *[713.5]*
    diabetic 250.6 ☑ *[713.5]*
      due to secondary diabetes 249.6 ☑ *[713.5]*
    syringomyelic 336.0 *[713.5]*
  syndrome (intermittent claudication) 443.9
    due to atherosclerosis 440.21
CHARGE association (syndrome) 759.89
Charleyhorse (quadriceps) 843.8
  muscle, except quadriceps — *see* Sprain, by site
Charlouis' disease — *see also* Yaws 102.9
Chauffeur's fracture — *see* Fracture, ulna, lower end
Cheadle (-Möller) (-Barlow) disease or syndrome (infantile scurvy) 267
Checking (of)
  contraceptive device (intrauterine) V25.42
  device
    fixation V54.89
      external V54.89
      internal V54.09
    traction V54.89
  Kirschner wire V54.89
  plaster cast V54.89
  splint, external V54.89
Checkup
  following treatment — *see* Examination
  health V70.0

Checkup — *continued*
  infant (over 28 days old) (not sick) V20.2
  newborn, routine
    8 to 28 days old V20.32
    over 28 days old, routine V20.2
    under 8 days old V20.31
    weight V20.32
  pregnancy (normal) V22.1
    first V22.0
    high-risk pregnancy V23.9
      inconclusive fetal viability V23.87
      specified problem NEC V23.89
Chédiak-Higashi (-Steinbrinck) anomaly, disease, or syndrome (congenital gigantism of peroxidase granules) 288.2
Cheek — *see also* condition
  biting 528.9
Cheese itch 133.8
Cheese washers' lung 495.8
Cheilitis 528.5
  actinic (due to sun) 692.72
    chronic NEC 692.74
    due to radiation, except from sun 692.82
    due to radiation, except from sun 692.82
  acute 528.5
  angular 528.5
  catarrhal 528.5
  chronic 528.5
  exfoliative 528.5
  gangrenous 528.5
  glandularis apostematosa 528.5
  granulomatosa 351.8
  infectional 528.5
  membranous 528.5
  Miescher's 351.8
  suppurative 528.5
  ulcerative 528.5
  vesicular 528.5
Cheilodynia 528.5
Cheilopalatoschisis — *see also* Cleft, palate, with cleft lip 749.20
Cheilophagia 528.9
Cheiloschisis — *see also* Cleft, lip 749.10
Cheilosis 528.5
  with pellagra 265.2
  angular 528.5
  due to
    dietary deficiency 266.0
    vitamin deficiency 266.0
Cheiromegaly 729.89
Cheiropompholyx 705.81
Cheloid — *see also* Keloid 701.4
Chemical burn — *see also* Burn, by site
  from swallowing chemical — *see* Burn, internal organs
Chemodectoma (M8693/1) — *see* Paraganglioma, nonchromaffin
Chemoprophylaxis NEC V07.39
Chemosis, conjunctiva 372.73
Chemotherapy
  convalescence V66.2
  encounter (for) (oral) (intravenous) V58.11
  maintenance (oral) (intravenous) V58.11
  prophylactic NEC V07.39
    fluoride V07.31
Cherubism 526.89
Chest — *see* condition
Cheyne-Stokes respiration (periodic) 786.04
Chiari-Frommel syndrome 676.6 ☑
Chiari's
  disease or syndrome (hepatic vein thrombosis) 453.0
  malformation
    type I 348.4
    type II (*see also* Spina bifida) 741.0 ☑
    type III 742.0
    type IV 742.2
    network 746.89
Chicago disease (North American blastomycosis) 116.0
Chickenpox — *see also* Varicella 052.9
  exposure to V01.71
  vaccination and inoculation (prophylactic) V05.4
Chiclero ulcer 085.4

Chiggers 133.8
Chignon 111.2
  fetus or newborn (from vacuum extraction) 767.19
Chigoe disease 134.1
Chikungunya fever 066.3
Chilaiditi's syndrome (subphrenic displacement, colon) 751.4
Chilblains 991.5
  lupus 991.5
Child
  behavior causing concern V61.20
    adopted child V61.24
    biological child V61.23
    foster child V61.25
Childbed fever 670.8 ☑
Childbirth — *see also* Delivery
  puerperal complications — *see* Puerperal
Childhood, period of rapid growth V21.0
Chill(s) 780.64
  with fever 780.60
  without fever 780.64
  congestive 780.99
    in malarial regions 084.6
  septic — *see* Septicemia
  urethral 599.84
Chilomastigiasis 007.8
Chin — *see* condition
Chinese dysentery 004.9
Chiropractic dislocation — *see also* Lesion, nonallopathic, by site 739.9
Chitral fever 066.0
Chlamydia, chlamydial — *see* condition
Chloasma 709.09
  cachecticorum 709.09
  eyelid 374.52
    congenital 757.33
    hyperthyroid 242.0 ☑
  gravidarum 646.8 ☑
  idiopathic 709.09
  skin 709.09
  symptomatic 709.09
Chloroma (M9930/3) 205.3 ☑
Chlorosis 280.9
  Egyptian (*see also* Ancylostomiasis) 126.9
  miners' (*see also* Ancylostomiasis) 126.9
Chlorotic anemia 280.9
Chocolate cyst (ovary) 617.1
Choked
  disk or disc — *see* Papilledema
  on food, phlegm, or vomitus NEC (*see also* Asphyxia, food) 933.1
  phlegm 933.1
  while vomiting NEC (*see also* Asphyxia, food) 933.1
Chokes (resulting from bends) 993.3
Choking sensation 784.99
Cholangiectasis — *see also* Disease, gallbladder 575.8
Cholangiocarcinoma (M8160/3)
  and hepatocellular carcinoma, combined (M8180/3) 155.0
  liver 155.1
  specified site NEC — *see* Neoplasm, by site, malignant
  unspecified site 155.1
Cholangiohepatitis 575.8
  due to fluke infestation 121.1
Cholangiohepatoma (M8180/3) 155.0
Cholangiolitis (acute) (chronic) (extrahepatic) (gangrenous) 576.1
  intrahepatic 575.8
  paratyphoidal (*see also* Fever, paratyphoid) 002.9
  typhoidal 002.0
Cholangioma (M8160/0) 211.5
  malignant — *see* Cholangiocarcinoma
Cholangitis (acute) (ascending) (catarrhal) (chronic) (infective) (malignant) (primary) (recurrent) (sclerosing) (secondary) (stenosing) (suppurative) 576.1
  chronic nonsuppurative destructive 571.6
  nonsuppurative destructive (chronic) 571.6
Cholecystdocholithiasis — *see* Choledocholithiasis
Cholecystitis 575.10

☑ Additional Digit Required — Refer to the Tabular List for Digit Selection   ⌐ Subterms under main terms may continue to next column or page

46 — Volume 2   ▶◀ Revised Text   ● New Line   ▲ Revised Code   2014 ICD-9-CM

Cholecystitis — *continued*
  with
    calculus, stones in
      bile duct (common) (hepatic) — *see* Choledocholithiasis
      gallbladder — *see* Cholelithiasis
    acute 575.0
    acute and chronic 575.12
    chronic 575.11
    emphysematous (acute) (*see also* Cholecystitis, acute) 575.0
    gangrenous (*see also* Cholecystitis, acute) 575.0
    paratyphoidal, current (*see also* Fever, paratyphoid) 002.9
    suppurative (*see also* Cholecystitis, acute) 575.0
    typhoidal 002.0
Choledochitis (suppurative) 576.1
Choledocholith — *see* Choledocholithiasis
Choledocholithiasis 574.5 ☑

> *Note* — Use the following fifth-digit subclassification with category 574:
>
> 0   without mention of obstruction
> 1   with obstruction

  with
    cholecystitis 574.4 ☑
      acute 574.3 ☑
      chronic 574.4 ☑
    cholelithiasis 574.9 ☑
      with
        cholecystitis 574.7 ☑
          acute 574.6 ☑
            and chronic 574.8 ☑
          chronic 574.7 ☑
Cholelithiasis (impacted) (multiple) 574.2 ☑

> *Note* — Use the following fifth-digit subclassification with category 574:
>
> 0   without mention of obstruction
> 1   with obstruction

  with
    cholecystitis 574.1 ☑
      acute 574.0 ☑
      chronic 574.1 ☑
    choledocholithiasis 574.9 ☑
      with
        cholecystitis 574.7 ☑
          acute 574.6 ☑
            and chronic 574.8 ☑
          chronic cholecystitis 574.7 ☑
Cholemia — *see also* Jaundice 782.4
  familial 277.4
  Gilbert's (familial nonhemolytic) 277.4
Cholemic gallstone — *see* Cholelithiasis
Choleperitoneum, choleperitonitis — *see also* Disease, gallbladder 567.81
Cholera (algid) (Asiatic) (asphyctic) (epidemic) (gravis) (Indian) (malignant) (morbus) (pestilential) (spasmodic) 001.9
  antimonial 985.4
  carrier (suspected) of V02.0
  classical 001.0
  contact V01.0
  due to
    Vibrio
      cholerae (Inaba, Ogawa, Hikojima serotypes) 001.0
      El Tor 001.1
  El Tor 001.1
  exposure to V01.0
  vaccination, prophylactic (against) V03.0
Cholerine — *see also* Cholera 001.9
Cholestasis 576.8
  due to total parenteral nutrition (TPN) 573.8
Cholesteatoma (ear) 385.30
  attic (primary) 385.31
  diffuse 385.35
  external ear (canal) 380.21
  marginal (middle ear) 385.32
    with involvement of mastoid cavity 385.33

Cholesteatoma — *continued*
  marginal — *continued*
    secondary (with middle ear involvement) 385.33
  mastoid cavity 385.30
  middle ear (secondary) 385.32
    with involvement of mastoid cavity 385.33
  postmastoidectomy cavity (recurrent) 383.32
  primary 385.31
  recurrent, postmastoidectomy cavity 383.32
  secondary (middle ear) 385.32
    with involvement of mastoid cavity 385.33
Cholesteatosis (middle ear) — *see also* Cholesteatoma 385.30
  diffuse 385.35
Cholesteremia 272.0
Cholesterin
  granuloma, middle ear 385.82
  in vitreous 379.22
Cholesterol
  deposit
    retina 362.82
    vitreous 379.22
  elevated (high) 272.0
    with elevated (high) triglycerides 272.2
  imbibition of gallbladder (*see also* Disease, gallbladder) 575.6
Cholesterolemia 272.0
  essential 272.0
  familial 272.0
  hereditary 272.0
Cholesterosis, cholesterolosis (gallbladder) 575.6
  with
    cholecystitis — *see* Cholecystitis
    cholelithiasis — *see* Cholelithiasis
  middle ear (*see also* Cholesteatoma) 385.30
Cholocolic fistula — *see also* Fistula, gallbladder 575.5
Choluria 791.4
Chondritis (purulent) 733.99
  auricle 380.03
  costal 733.6
    Tietze's 733.6
  patella, posttraumatic 717.7
  pinna 380.03
  posttraumatica patellae 717.7
  tuberculous (active) (*see also* Tuberculosis) 015.9 ☑
    intervertebral 015.0 ☑ [730.88]
Chondro-osteodysplasia (Morquio-Brailsford type) 277.5
Chondro-osteodystrophy 277.5
Chondro-osteoma (M9210/0) — *see* Neoplasm, bone, benign
Chondroangiopathia calcarea seu punctate 756.59
Chondroblastoma (M9230/0) — *see also* Neoplasm, bone, benign
  malignant (M9230/3) — *see* Neoplasm, bone, malignant
Chondrocalcinosis (articular) (crystal deposition) (dihydrate) — *see also* Arthritis, due to, crystals 275.49 [712.3] ☑
  due to
    calcium pyrophosphate 275.49 [712.2] ☑
    dicalcium phosphate crystals 275.49 [712.1] ☑
    pyrophosphate crystals 275.49 [712.2] ☑
Chondrodermatitis nodularis helicis 380.00
Chondrodysplasia 756.4
  angiomatose 756.4
  calcificans congenita 756.59
  epiphysialis punctata 756.59
  hereditary deforming 756.4
  rhizomelic punctata 277.86
Chondrodystrophia (fetalis) 756.4
  calcarea 756.4
  calcificans congenita 756.59
  fetalis hypoplastica 756.59
  hypoplastica calcinosa 756.59
  punctata 756.59

Chondrodystrophia — *continued*
  tarda 277.5
Chondrodystrophy (familial) (hypoplastic) 756.4
  myotonic (congenital) 359.23
Chondroectodermal dysplasia 756.55
Chondrolysis 733.99
Chondroma (M9220/0) — *see also* Neoplasm, cartilage, benign
  juxtacortical (M9221/0) — *see* Neoplasm, bone, benign
  periosteal (M9221/0) — *see* Neoplasm, bone, benign
Chondromalacia 733.92
  epiglottis (congenital) 748.3
  generalized 733.92
  knee 717.7
  larynx (congenital) 748.3
  localized, except patella 733.92
  patella, patellae 717.7
  systemic 733.92
  tibial plateau 733.92
  trachea (congenital) 748.3
Chondromatosis (M9220/1) — *see* Neoplasm, cartilage, uncertain behavior
Chondromyxosarcoma (M9220/3) — *see* Neoplasm, cartilage, malignant
Chondropathia tuberosa 733.6
Chondrosarcoma (M9220/3) — *see also* Neoplasm, cartilage, malignant
  juxtacortical (M9221/3) — *see* Neoplasm, bone, malignant
  mesenchymal (M9240/3) — *see* Neoplasm, connective tissue, malignant
Chordae tendineae rupture (chronic) 429.5
Chordee (nonvenereal) 607.89
  congenital 752.63
  gonococcal 098.2
Chorditis (fibrinous) (nodosa) (tuberosa) 478.5
Chordoma (M9370/3) — *see* Neoplasm, by site, malignant
Chorea (gravis) (minor) (spasmodic) 333.5
  with
    heart involvement — *see* Chorea with rheumatic heart disease
    rheumatic heart disease (chronic, inactive, or quiescent) (conditions classifiable to 393–398) (*see* rheumatic heart condition involved)
      active or acute (conditions classifiable to 391) 392.0
  acute — *see* Chorea, Sydenham's
  apoplectic (*see also* Disease, cerebrovascular, acute) 436
  chronic 333.4
  electric 049.8
  gravidarum — *see* Eclampsia, pregnancy
  habit 307.22
  hereditary 333.4
  Huntington's 333.4
  posthemiplegic 344.89
  pregnancy — *see* Eclampsia, pregnancy
  progressive 333.4
    chronic 333.4
    hereditary 333.4
  rheumatic (chronic) 392.9
    with heart disease or involvement — *see* Chorea, with rheumatic heart disease
  senile 333.5
  Sydenham's 392.9
    with heart involvement — *see* Chorea, with rheumatic heart disease
    nonrheumatic 333.5
  variabilis 307.23
Choreoathetosis (paroxysmal) 333.5
Chorioadenoma (destruens) (M9100/1) 236.1
Chorioamnionitis 658.4 ☑
  affecting fetus or newborn 762.7
Chorioangioma (M9120/0) 219.8
Choriocarcinoma (M9100/3)
  combined with
    embryonal carcinoma (M9101/3) — *see* Neoplasm, by site, malignant

Choriocarcinoma — *continued*
  combined with — *continued*
    teratoma (M9101/3) — *see* Neoplasm, by site, malignant
  specified site — *see* Neoplasm, by site, malignant
  unspecified site
    female 181
    male 186.9
Chorioencephalitis, lymphocytic (acute) (serous) 049.0
Chorioepithelioma (M9100/3) — *see* Choriocarcinoma
Choriomeningitis (acute) (benign) (lymphocytic) (serous) 049.0
Chorionepithelioma (M9100/3) — *see* Choriocarcinoma
Chorionitis — *see also* Scleroderma 710.1
Chorioretinitis 363.20
  disseminated 363.10
    generalized 363.13
    in
      neurosyphilis 094.83
      secondary syphilis 091.51
    peripheral 363.12
    posterior pole 363.11
    tuberculous (*see also* Tuberculosis) 017.3 ☑ [363.13]
  due to
    histoplasmosis (*see also* Histoplasmosis) 115.92
    toxoplasmosis (acquired) 130.2
      congenital (active) 771.2
  focal 363.00
    juxtapapillary 363.01
    peripheral 363.04
    posterior pole NEC 363.03
  juxtapapillaris, juxtapapillary 363.01
  progressive myopia (degeneration) 360.21
  syphilitic (secondary) 091.51
    congenital (early) 090.0 [363.13]
    late 090.5 [363.13]
    late 095.8 [363.13]
  tuberculous (*see also* Tuberculosis) 017.3 ☑ [363.13]
Choristoma — *see* Neoplasm, by site, benign
Choroid — *see* condition
Choroideremia, choroidermia (initial stage) (late stage) (partial or total atrophy) 363.55
Choroiditis — *see also* Chorioretinitis 363.20
  leprous 030.9 [363.13]
  senile guttate 363.41
  sympathetic 360.11
  syphilitic (secondary) 091.51
    congenital (early) 090.0 [363.13]
    late 090.5 [363.13]
    late 095.8 [363.13]
  Tay's 363.41
  tuberculous (*see also* Tuberculosis) 017.3 ☑ [363.13]
Choroidopathy NEC 363.9
  degenerative (*see also* Degeneration, choroid) 363.40
  hereditary (*see also* Dystrophy, choroid) 363.50
  specified type NEC 363.8
Choroidoretinitis — *see* Chorioretinitis
Choroidosis, central serous 362.41
Choroidretinopathy, serous 362.41
Christian-Weber disease (nodular nonsuppurative panniculitis) 729.30
Christian's syndrome (chronic histiocytosis X) 277.89
Christmas disease 286.1
Chromaffinoma (M8700/0) — *see also* Neoplasm, by site, benign
  malignant (M8700/3) — *see* Neoplasm, by site, malignant
Chromatopsia 368.59
Chromhidrosis, chromidrosis 705.89
Chromoblastomycosis 117.2
Chromomycosis 117.2
Chromophytosis 111.0
Chromotrichomycosis 111.8
Chronic — *see* condition

Churg-Strauss syndrome 446.4
Chyle cyst, mesentery 457.8
Chylocele (nonfilarial) 457.8
  filarial (*see also* Infestation, filarial) 125.9
  tunica vaginalis (nonfilarial) 608.84
    filarial (*see also* Infestation, filarial) 125.9
Chylomicronemia (fasting) (with hyperprebetalipoproteinemia) 272.3
Chylopericardium (acute) 420.90
Chylothorax (nonfilarial) 457.8
  filarial (*see also* Infestation, filarial) 125.9
Chylous
  ascites 457.8
  cyst of peritoneum 457.8
  hydrocele 603.9
  hydrothorax (nonfilarial) 457.8
    filarial (*see also* Infestation, filarial) 125.9
Chyluria 791.1
  bilharziasis 120.0
  due to
    Brugia (malayi) 125.1
    Wuchereria (bancrofti) 125.0
      malayi 125.1
  filarial (*see also* Infestation, filarial) 125.9
  filariasis (*see also* Infestation, filarial) 125.9
  nonfilarial 791.1
Cicatricial (deformity) — *see* Cicatrix
Cicatrix (adherent) (contracted) (painful) (vicious) 709.2
  adenoid 474.8
  alveolar process 525.8
  anus 569.49
  auricle 380.89
  bile duct (*see also* Disease, biliary) 576.8
  bladder 596.89
  bone 733.99
  brain 348.89
  cervix (postoperative) (postpartal) 622.3
    in pregnancy or childbirth 654.6 ☑
      causing obstructed labor 660.2 ☑
  chorioretinal 363.30
    disseminated 363.35
    macular 363.32
    peripheral 363.34
    posterior pole NEC 363.33
  choroid — *see* Cicatrix, chorioretinal
  common duct (*see also* Disease, biliary) 576.8
  congenital 757.39
  conjunctiva 372.64
  cornea 371.00
    tuberculous (*see also* Tuberculosis) 017.3 ☑ [371.05]
  duodenum (bulb) 537.3
  esophagus 530.3
  eyelid 374.46
    with
      ectropion — *see* Ectropion
      entropion — *see* Entropion
  hypopharynx 478.29
  knee, semilunar cartilage 717.5
  lacrimal
    canaliculi 375.53
    duct
      acquired 375.56
      neonatal 375.55
    punctum 375.52
    sac 375.54
  larynx 478.79
  limbus (cystoid) 372.64
  lung 518.89
  macular 363.32
    disseminated 363.35
    peripheral 363.34
  middle ear 385.89
  mouth 528.9
  muscle 728.89
  nasolacrimal duct
    acquired 375.56
    neonatal 375.55
  nasopharynx 478.29
  palate (soft) 528.9
  penis 607.89
  prostate 602.8
  rectum 569.49
  retina 363.30

Cicatrix — *continued*
  retina — *continued*
    disseminated 363.35
    macular 363.32
    peripheral 363.34
    posterior pole NEC 363.33
  semilunar cartilage — *see* Derangement, meniscus
  seminal vesicle 608.89
  skin 709.2
    infected 686.8
    postinfectional 709.2
    tuberculous (*see also* Tuberculosis) 017.0 ☑
  specified site NEC 709.2
  throat 478.29
  tongue 529.8
  tonsil (and adenoid) 474.8
  trachea 478.9
  tuberculous NEC (*see also* Tuberculosis) 011.9 ☑
  ureter 593.89
  urethra 599.84
  uterus 621.8
  vagina 623.4
    in pregnancy or childbirth 654.7 ☑
      causing obstructed labor 660.2 ☑
  vocal cord 478.5
  wrist, constricting (annular) 709.2
CIDP (chronic inflammatory demyelinating polyneuropathy) 357.81
CIN I (cervical intraepithelial neoplasia I) 622.11
CIN II (cervical intraepithelial neoplasia II) 622.12
CIN III (cervical intraepithelial neoplasia III) 233.1
Cinchonism
  correct substance properly administered 386.9
  overdose or wrong substance given or taken 961.4
Circine herpes 110.5
Circle of Willis — *see* condition
Circular — *see also* condition
  hymen 752.49
Circulating anticoagulants, antibodies, or inhibitors — *see also* Anticoagulants 286.59
  extrinsic 287.8
  following childbirth 666.3 ☑
  intrinsic, causing hemorrhagic disorder 286.59
    with
      acquired hemophilia 286.52
      antiphospholipid antibody 286.53
  postpartum 666.3 ☑
Circulation
  collateral (venous), any site 459.89
  defective 459.9
    congenital 747.9
    lower extremity 459.89
  embryonic 747.9
  failure 799.89
    fetus or newborn 779.89
    peripheral 785.59
  fetal, persistent 747.83
  heart, incomplete 747.9
Circulatory system — *see* condition
Circulus senilis 371.41
Circumcision
  in absence of medical indication V50.2
  ritual V50.2
  routine V50.2
  status (post), female 629.20
Circumscribed — *see* condition
Circumvallata placenta — *see* Placenta, abnormal
Cirrhosis, cirrhotic 571.5
  with alcoholism 571.2
  alcoholic (liver) 571.2
  atrophic (of liver) — *see* Cirrhosis, portal
  Baumgarten-Cruveilhier 571.5

Cirrhosis, cirrhotic — *continued*
  biliary (cholangiolitic) (cholangitic) (cholestatic) (extrahepatic) (hypertrophic) (intrahepatic) (nonobstructive) (obstructive) (pericholangiolitic) (posthepatic) (primary) (secondary) (xanthomatous) 571.6
    due to
      clonorchiasis 121.1
      flukes 121.3
  brain 331.9
  capsular — *see* Cirrhosis, portal
  cardiac 571.5
    alcoholic 571.2
  central (liver) — *see* Cirrhosis, liver
  Charcôt's 571.6
  cholangiolitic — *see* Cirrhosis, biliary
  cholangitic — *see* Cirrhosis, biliary
  cholestatic — *see* Cirrhosis, biliary
  clitoris (hypertrophic) 624.2
  coarsely nodular 571.5
  congestive (liver) — *see* Cirrhosis, cardiac
  Cruveilhier-Baumgarten 571.5
  cryptogenic (of liver) 571.5
    alcoholic 571.2
  dietary (*see also* Cirrhosis, portal) 571.5
  due to
    bronzed diabetes 275.01
    congestive hepatomegaly — *see* Cirrhosis, cardiac
    cystic fibrosis 277.00
    hemochromatosis (*see also* Hemochromatosis) 275.03
    hepatolenticular degeneration 275.1
    passive congestion (chronic) — *see* Cirrhosis, cardiac
    Wilson's disease 275.1
    xanthomatosis 272.2
  extrahepatic (obstructive) — *see* Cirrhosis, biliary
  fatty 571.8
    alcoholic 571.0
  florid 571.2
  Glisson's — *see* Cirrhosis, portal
  Hanot's (hypertrophic) — *see* Cirrhosis, biliary
  hepatic — *see* Cirrhosis, liver
  hepatolienal — *see* Cirrhosis, liver
  hobnail — *see* Cirrhosis, portal
  hypertrophic (*see also* Cirrhosis, liver)
    biliary — *see* Cirrhosis, biliary
    Hanot's — *see* Cirrhosis, biliary
  infectious NEC — *see* Cirrhosis, portal
  insular — *see* Cirrhosis, portal
  intrahepatic (obstructive) (primary) (secondary) — *see* Cirrhosis, biliary
  juvenile (*see also* Cirrhosis, portal) 571.5
  kidney (*see also* Sclerosis, renal) 587
  Laennec's (of liver) 571.2
    nonalcoholic 571.5
  liver (chronic) (hepatolienal) (hypertrophic) (nodular) (splenomegalic) (unilobar) 571.5
    with alcoholism 571.2
    alcoholic 571.2
    congenital (due to failure of obliteration of umbilical vein) 777.8
    cryptogenic 571.5
      alcoholic 571.2
    fatty 571.8
      alcoholic 571.0
    macronodular 571.5
      alcoholic 571.2
    micronodular 571.5
      alcoholic 571.2
    nodular, diffuse 571.5
      alcoholic 571.2
    pigmentary 275.01
    portal 571.5
      alcoholic 571.2
    postnecrotic 571.5
      alcoholic 571.2
    syphilitic 095.3
  lung (chronic) (*see also* Fibrosis, lung) 515
  macronodular (of liver) 571.5
    alcoholic 571.2

Cirrhosis, cirrhotic — *continued*
  malarial 084.9
  metabolic NEC 571.5
  micronodular (of liver) 571.5
    alcoholic 571.2
  monolobular — *see* Cirrhosis, portal
  multilobular — *see* Cirrhosis, portal
  nephritis (*see also* Sclerosis, renal) 587
  nodular — *see* Cirrhosis, liver
  nutritional (fatty) 571.5
  obstructive (biliary) (extrahepatic) (intrahepatic) — *see* Cirrhosis, biliary
  ovarian 620.8
  paludal 084.9
  pancreas (duct) 577.8
  pericholangiolitic — *see* Cirrhosis, biliary
  periportal — *see* Cirrhosis, portal
  pigment, pigmentary (of liver) 275.01
  portal (of liver) 571.5
    alcoholic 571.2
  posthepatitic (*see also* Cirrhosis, postnecrotic) 571.5
  postnecrotic (of liver) 571.5
    alcoholic 571.2
  primary (intrahepatic) — *see* Cirrhosis, biliary
  pulmonary (*see also* Fibrosis, lung) 515
  renal (*see also* Sclerosis, renal) 587
  septal (*see also* Cirrhosis, postnecrotic) 571.5
  spleen 289.51
  splenomegalic (of liver) — *see* Cirrhosis, liver
  stasis (liver) — *see* Cirrhosis, liver
  stomach 535.4 ☑
  Todd's (*see also* Cirrhosis, biliary) 571.6
  toxic (nodular) — *see* Cirrhosis, postnecrotic
  trabecular — *see* Cirrhosis, postnecrotic
  unilobar — *see* Cirrhosis, liver
  vascular (of liver) — *see* Cirrhosis, liver
  xanthomatous (biliary) (*see also* Cirrhosis, biliary) 571.6
    due to xanthomatosis (familial) (metabolic) (primary) 272.2
Cistern, subarachnoid 793.0
Citrullinemia 270.6
Citrullinuria 270.6
Ciuffini-Pancoast tumor (M8010/3) (carcinoma, pulmonary apex) 162.3
Civatte's disease or poikiloderma 709.09
CJD (Creutzfeldt-Jakob disease) 046.19
  variant (vCJD) 046.11
CLABSI (central line-associated bloodstream infection) 999.32
Clam diggers' itch 120.3
Clap — *see* Gonorrhea
Clarke-Hadfield syndrome (pancreatic infantilism) 577.8
Clark's paralysis 343.9
Clastothrix 704.2
Claude Bernard-Horner syndrome — *see also* Neuropathy, peripheral, autonomic 337.9
Claude's syndrome 352.6
Claudication, intermittent 443.9
  cerebral (artery) (*see also* Ischemia, cerebral, transient) 435.9
  due to atherosclerosis 440.21
  spinal cord (arteriosclerotic) 435.1
    syphilitic 094.89
  spinalis 435.1
  venous (axillary) 453.89
Claudicatio venosa intermittens 453.89
Claustrophobia 300.29
Clavus (infected) 700
Clawfoot (congenital) 754.71
  acquired 736.74
Clawhand (acquired) 736.06
  congenital 755.59
Clawtoe (congenital) 754.71
  acquired 735.5
Clay eating 307.52
Clay shovelers' fracture — *see* Fracture, vertebra, cervical
Cleansing of artificial opening — *see also* Attention to artificial opening V55.9
Cleft (congenital) — *see also* Imperfect, closure

☑ Additional Digit Required — Refer to the Tabular List for Digit Selection   ▽ Subterms under main terms may continue to next column or page

48 — Volume 2   ▶◀ Revised Text   ● New Line   ▲ Revised Code   2014 ICD-9-CM

Cleft — *see also* Imperfect, closure — *continued*
  alveolar process 525.8
  branchial (persistent) 744.41
    cyst 744.42
  clitoris 752.49
  cricoid cartilage, posterior 748.3
  facial (*see also* Cleft, lip) 749.10
  lip 749.10
    with cleft palate 749.20
      bilateral (lip and palate) 749.24
        with unilateral lip or palate 749.25
          complete 749.23
          incomplete 749.24
        unilateral (lip and palate) 749.22
          with bilateral lip or palate 749.25
            complete 749.21
            incomplete 749.22
      bilateral 749.14
        with cleft palate, unilateral 749.25
          complete 749.13
          incomplete 749.14
      unilateral 749.12
        with cleft palate, bilateral 749.25
          complete 749.11
          incomplete 749.12
  nose 748.1
  palate 749.00
    with cleft lip 749.20
      bilateral (lip and palate) 749.24
        with unilateral lip or palate 749.25
          complete 749.23
          incomplete 749.24
        unilateral (lip and palate) 749.22
          with bilateral lip or palate 749.25
            complete 749.21
            incomplete 749.22
      bilateral 749.04
        with cleft lip, unilateral 749.25
          complete 749.03
          incomplete 749.04
      unilateral 749.02
        with cleft lip, bilateral 749.25
          complete 749.01
          incomplete 749.02
  penis 752.69
  posterior, cricoid cartilage 748.3
  scrotum 752.89
  sternum (congenital) 756.3
  thyroid cartilage (congenital) 748.3
  tongue 750.13
  uvula 749.02
    with cleft lip (*see also* Cleft, lip, with cleft palate) 749.20
  water 366.12
Cleft hand (congenital) 755.58
Cleidocranial dysostosis 755.59
Cleidotomy, fetal 763.89
Cleptomania 312.32
Clérambault's syndrome 297.8
  erotomania 302.89
Clergyman's sore throat 784.49
Click, clicking
  systolic syndrome 785.2
Clifford's syndrome (postmaturity) 766.22
Climacteric — *see also* Menopause 627.2
  arthritis NEC (*see also* Arthritis, climacteric) 716.3 ☑
  depression (*see also* Psychosis, affective) 296.2 ☑
  disease 627.2
    recurrent episode 296.3 ☑
    single episode 296.2 ☑
  female (symptoms) 627.2
  male (symptoms) (syndrome) 608.89
  melancholia (*see also* Psychosis, affective) 296.2 ☑
    recurrent episode 296.3 ☑
    single episode 296.2 ☑
  paranoid state 297.2
  paraphrenia 297.2
  polyarthritis NEC 716.39
    male 608.89
  symptoms (female) 627.2

Clinical research investigation (control) (participant) V70.7
Clinodactyly 755.59
Clitoris — *see* condition
Cloaca, persistent 751.5
Clonorchiasis 121.1
Clonorchiosis 121.1
Clonorchis infection, liver 121.1
Clonus 781.0
Closed bite 524.20
Closed surgical procedure converted to open procedure
  arthroscopic V64.43
  laparoscopic V64.41
  thoracoscopic V64.42
Closure
  artificial opening (*see also* Attention to artificial opening) V55.9
  congenital, nose 748.0
  cranial sutures, premature 756.0
  defective or imperfect NEC — *see* Imperfect, closure
  fistula, delayed — *see* Fistula
  fontanelle, delayed 756.0
  foramen ovale, imperfect 745.5
  hymen 623.3
  interauricular septum, defective 745.5
  interventricular septum, defective 745.4
  lacrimal duct 375.56
    congenital 743.65
    neonatal 375.55
  nose (congenital) 748.0
    acquired 738.0
  primary angle without glaucoma damage 365.06
  vagina 623.2
  valve — *see* Endocarditis
  vulva 624.8
Clot (blood)
  artery (obstruction) (occlusion) (*see also* Embolism) 444.9
  atrial appendage 429.89
  bladder 596.7
  brain (extradural or intradural) (*see also* Thrombosis, brain) 434.0 ☑
    late effect — *see* Late effect(s) (of) cerebrovascular disease
  circulation 444.9
  heart (*see also* Infarct, myocardium) 410.9 ☑
    without myocardial infarction 429.89
  vein (*see also* Thrombosis) 453.9
Clotting defect NEC — *see also* Defect, coagulation 286.9
Clouded state 780.09
  epileptic (*see also* Epilepsy) 345.9 ☑
  paroxysmal (idiopathic) (*see also* Epilepsy) 345.9 ☑
Clouding
  corneal graft 996.51
Cloudy
  antrum, antra 473.0
  dialysis effluent 792.5
Clouston's (hidrotic) ectodermal dysplasia 757.31
Clubbing of fingers 781.5
Clubfinger 736.29
  acquired 736.29
  congenital 754.89
Clubfoot (congenital) 754.70
  acquired 736.71
  equinovarus 754.51
  paralytic 736.71
Club hand (congenital) 754.89
  acquired 736.07
Clubnail (acquired) 703.8
  congenital 757.5
Clump kidney 753.3
Clumsiness 781.3
  syndrome 315.4
Cluttering — *see also* Disorder, fluency 315.35
Clutton's joints 090.5
Coagulation, intravascular (diffuse) (disseminated) — *see also* Fibrinolysis 286.6
  newborn 776.2

Coagulopathy — *see also* Defect, coagulation 286.9
  consumption 286.6
  intravascular (disseminated) NEC 286.6
    newborn 776.2
Coalition
  calcaneoscaphoid 755.67
  calcaneus 755.67
  tarsal 755.67
Coal miners'
  elbow 727.2
  lung 500
Coal workers' lung or pneumoconiosis 500
Coarctation
  aorta (postductal) (preductal) 747.10
  pulmonary artery 747.31
Coated tongue 529.3
Coats' disease 362.12
Cocainism — *see also* Dependence 304.2 ☑
Coccidioidal granuloma 114.3
Coccidioidomycosis 114.9
  with pneumonia 114.0
  cutaneous (primary) 114.1
  disseminated 114.3
  extrapulmonary (primary) 114.1
  lung 114.5
    acute 114.0
    chronic 114.4
    primary 114.0
  meninges 114.2
  primary (pulmonary) 114.0
    acute 114.0
  prostate 114.3
  pulmonary 114.5
    acute 114.0
    chronic 114.4
    primary 114.0
  specified site NEC 114.3
Coccidioidosis 114.9
  lung 114.5
    acute 114.0
    chronic 114.4
    primary 114.0
  meninges 114.2
Coccidiosis (colitis) (diarrhea) (dysentery) 007.2
Cocciuria 791.9
Coccus in urine 791.9
Coccydynia 724.79
Coccygodynia 724.79
Coccyx — *see* condition
Cochin-China
  diarrhea 579.1
    anguilluliasis 127.2
  ulcer 085.1
Cockayne-Weber syndrome (epidermolysis bullosa) 757.39
Cockayne's disease or syndrome (microcephaly and dwarfism) 759.89
Cocked-up toe 735.2
Cock's peculiar tumor 706.2
Codman's tumor (benign chondroblastoma) (M9230/0) — *see* Neoplasm, bone, benign
Coenurosis 123.8
Coffee workers' lung 495.8
Cogan's syndrome 370.52
  congenital oculomotor apraxia 379.51
  nonsyphilitic interstitial keratitis 370.52
Coiling, umbilical cord — *see* Complications, umbilical cord
Coitus, painful (female) 625.0
  male 608.89
  psychogenic 302.76
Cold 460
  with influenza, flu, or grippe (*see also* Influenza) 487.1
  abscess (*see also* Tuberculosis, abscess)
    articular — *see* Tuberculosis, joint
  agglutinin
    disease (chronic) or syndrome 283.0
    hemoglobinuria 283.0
      paroxysmal (cold) (nocturnal) 283.2
  allergic (*see also* Fever, hay) 477.9
  bronchus or chest — *see* Bronchitis
    with grippe or influenza (*see also* Influenza) 487.1

Cold — *continued*
  common (head) 460
    vaccination, prophylactic (against) V04.7
  deep 464.10
  effects of 991.9
    specified effect NEC 991.8
  excessive 991.9
    specified effect NEC 991.8
  exhaustion from 991.8
  exposure to 991.9
    specified effect NEC 991.8
  grippy (*see also* Influenza) 487.1
  head 460
  injury syndrome (newborn) 778.2
  intolerance 780.99
  on lung — *see* Bronchitis
  rose 477.0
  sensitivity, autoimmune 283.0
  virus 460
Coldsore — *see also* Herpes, simplex 054.9
Colibacillosis 041.49
  generalized 038.42
Colibacilluria 791.9
Colic (recurrent) 789.7
  abdomen 789.7
    psychogenic 307.89
  appendicular 543.9
  appendix 543.9
  bile duct — *see* Choledocholithiasis
  biliary — *see* Cholelithiasis
  bilious — *see* Cholelithiasis
  common duct — *see* Choledocholithiasis
  Devonshire NEC 984.9
    specified type of lead — *see* Table of Drugs and Chemicals
  flatulent 787.3
  gallbladder or gallstone — *see* Cholelithiasis
  gastric 536.8
  hepatic (duct) — *see* Choledocholithiasis
  hysterical 300.11
  in
    adult 789.0 ☑
    child over 12 months old 789.0 ☑
    infant 789.7
  infantile 789.7
  intestinal 789.7
  kidney 788.0
  lead NEC 984.9
    specified type of lead — *see* Table of Drugs and Chemicals
  liver (duct) — *see* Choledocholithiasis
  mucous 564.9
    psychogenic 316 *[564.9]*
  nephritic 788.0
  painter's NEC 984.9
  pancreas 577.8
  psychogenic 306.4
  renal 788.0
  saturnine NEC 984.9
    specified type of lead — *see* Table of Drugs and Chemicals
  spasmodic 789.7
  ureter 788.0
  urethral 599.84
    due to calculus 594.2
  uterus 625.8
    menstrual 625.3
  vermicular 543.9
  virus 460
  worm NEC 128.9
Colicystitis — *see also* Cystitis 595.9
Colitis (acute) (catarrhal) (croupous) (cystica superficialis) (exudative) (hemorrhagic) (noninfectious) (phlegmonous) (presumed noninfectious) 558.9
  adaptive 564.9
  allergic 558.3
  amebic (*see also* Amebiasis) 006.9
    nondysenteric 006.2
  anthrax 022.2
  bacillary (*see also* Infection, Shigella) 004.9
  balantidial 007.0
  chronic 558.9
    ulcerative (*see also* Colitis, ulcerative) 556.9
  coccidial 007.2

☑ **Additional Digit Required** — Refer to the Tabular List for Digit Selection | ▼ **Subterms under main terms may continue to next column or page**

2014 ICD-9-CM | ▶◀ **Revised Text** | ● **New Line** | ▲ **Revised Code** | **Volume 2 — 49**

Colitis — *continued*
  dietetic 558.9
  due to radiation 558.1
  eosinophilic 558.42
  functional 558.9
  gangrenous 009.0
  giardial 007.1
  granulomatous 555.1
  gravis (*see also* Colitis, ulcerative) 556.9
  infectious (*see also* Enteritis, due to, specific organism) 009.0
    presumed 009.1
  ischemic 557.9
    acute 557.0
    chronic 557.1
    due to mesenteric artery insufficiency 557.1
  membranous 564.9
    psychogenic 316 [564.9]
  mucous 564.9
    psychogenic 316 [564.9]
  necrotic 009.0
  polyposa (*see also* Colitis, ulcerative) 556.9
  protozoal NEC 007.9
  pseudomembranous 008.45
  pseudomucinous 564.9
  regional 555.1
  segmental 555.1
  septic (*see also* Enteritis, due to, specific organism) 009.0
  spastic 564.9
    psychogenic 316 [564.9]
  Staphylococcus 008.41
    food 005.0
  thromboulcerative 557.0
  toxic 558.2
  transmural 555.1
  trichomonal 007.3
  tuberculous (ulcerative) 014.8 ☑
  ulcerative (chronic) (idiopathic) (nonspecific) 556.9
    entero- 556.0
    fulminant 557.0
    ileo- 556.1
    left-sided 556.5
    procto- 556.2
    proctosigmoid 556.3
    psychogenic 316 [556] ☑
    specified NEC 556.8
    universal 556.6
Collagen disease NEC 710.9
  nonvascular 710.9
  vascular (allergic) (*see also* Angiitis, hypersensitivity) 446.20
Collagenosis — *see also* Collagen disease 710.9
  cardiovascular 425.4
  mediastinal 519.3
Collapse 780.2
  adrenal 255.8
  cardiorenal (*see also* Hypertension, cardiorenal) 404.90
  cardiorespiratory 785.51
    fetus or newborn 779.85
  cardiovascular (*see also* Disease, heart) 785.51
    fetus or newborn 779.85
  circulatory (peripheral) 785.59
    with
      abortion — *see* Abortion, by type, with shock
      ectopic pregnancy (*see also* categories 633.0–633.9) 639.5
      molar pregnancy (*see also* categories 630–632) 639.5
    during or after labor and delivery 669.1 ☑
    fetus or newborn 779.85
    following
      abortion 639.5
      ectopic or molar pregnancy 639.5
  during or after labor and delivery 669.1 ☑
    fetus or newborn 779.89
  during or resulting from a surgical procedure 998.00
  external ear canal 380.50

Collapse — *continued*
  external ear canal — *continued*
    secondary to
      inflammation 380.53
      surgery 380.52
      trauma 380.51
  general 780.2
  heart — *see* Disease, heart
  heat 992.1
  hysterical 300.11
  labyrinth, membranous (congenital) 744.05
  lung (massive) (*see also* Atelectasis) 518.0
    pressure, during labor 668.0 ☑
  myocardial — *see* Disease, heart
  nervous (*see also* Disorder, mental, nonpsychotic) 300.9
  neurocirculatory 306.2
  nose 738.0
  postoperative (cardiovascular) 998.09
  pulmonary (see also Atelectasis) 518.0
    fetus or newborn 770.5
      partial 770.5
      primary 770.4
  thorax 512.89
    iatrogenic 512.1
    postoperative 512.1
  trachea 519.19
  valvular — *see* Endocarditis
  vascular (peripheral) 785.59
    with
      abortion — *see* Abortion, by type, with shock
      ectopic pregnancy (*see also* categories 633.0–633.9) 639.5
      molar pregnancy (*see also* categories 630–632) 639.5
    cerebral (*see also* Disease, cerebrovascular, acute) 436
    during or after labor and delivery 669.1 ☑
    fetus or newborn 779.89
    following
      abortion 639.5
      ectopic or molar pregnancy 639.5
  vasomotor 785.59
  vertebra 733.13
Collateral — *see also* condition
  circulation (venous) 459.89
  dilation, veins 459.89
Colles' fracture (closed) (reversed) (separation) 813.41
  open 813.51
Collet-Sicard syndrome 352.6
Collet's syndrome 352.6
Colliculitis urethralis — *see also* Urethritis 597.89
Colliers'
  asthma 500
  lung 500
  phthisis (*see also* Tuberculosis) 011.4 ☑
Collodion baby (ichthyosis congenita) 757.1
Colloid milium 709.3
Coloboma NEC 743.49
  choroid 743.59
  fundus 743.52
  iris 743.46
  lens 743.36
  lids 743.62
  optic disc (congenital) 743.57
    acquired 377.23
  retina 743.56
  sclera 743.47
Coloenteritis — *see* Enteritis
Colon — *see* condition
Colonization
  MRSA (methicillin resistant Staphylococcus aureus) V02.54
  MSSA (methicillin susceptible Staphylococcus aureus) V02.53
Coloptosis 569.89
Color
  amblyopia NEC 368.59
    acquired 368.55
  blindness NEC (congenital) 368.59
    acquired 368.55

Colostomy
  attention to V55.3
  fitting or adjustment V55.3
  malfunctioning 569.62
  status V44.3
Colpitis — *see also* Vaginitis 616.10
Colpocele 618.6
Colpocystitis — *see also* Vaginitis 616.10
Colporrhexis 665.4 ☑
Colpospasm 625.1
Column, spinal, vertebral — *see* condition
Coma 780.01
  apoplectic (*see also* Disease, cerebrovascular, acute) 436
  diabetic (with ketoacidosis) 250.3 ☑
    due to secondary diabetes 249.3 ☑
    hyperosmolar 250.2 ☑
      due to secondary diabetes 249.2 ☑
  eclamptic (*see also* Eclampsia) 780.39
  epileptic 345.3
  hepatic 572.2
  hyperglycemic 250.3 ☑
    due to secondary diabetes 249.3 ☑
  hyperosmolar (diabetic) (nonketotic) 250.2 ☑
    due to secondary diabetes 249.2 ☑
  hypoglycemic 251.0
    diabetic 250.3 ☑
      due to secondary diabetes 249.3 ☑
  insulin 250.3 ☑
    due to secondary diabetes 249.3 ☑
    hyperosmolar 250.2 ☑
      due to secondary diabetes 249.2 ☑
    non-diabetic 251.0
    organic hyperinsulinism 251.0
  Kussmaul's (diabetic) 250.3 ☑
    due to secondary diabetes 249.3 ☑
  liver 572.2
  newborn 779.2
  prediabetic 250.2 ☑
    due to secondary diabetes 249.2 ☑
  uremic — *see* Uremia
Combat fatigue — *see also* Reaction, stress, acute 308.9
Combined — *see* condition
Comedo 706.1
Comedocarcinoma (M8501/3) — *see also* Neoplasm, breast, malignant
  noninfiltrating (M8501/2)
    specified site — *see* Neoplasm, by site, in situ
    unspecified site 233.0
Comedomastitis 610.4
Comedones 706.1
  lanugo 757.4
Comma bacillus, carrier (suspected) of V02.3
Comminuted fracture — *see* Fracture, by site
Common
  aortopulmonary trunk 745.0
  atrioventricular canal (defect) 745.69
  atrium 745.69
  cold (head) 460
    vaccination, prophylactic (against) V04.7
  truncus (arteriosus) 745.0
  ventricle 745.3
Commotio (current)
  cerebri (*see also* Concussion, brain) 850.9
    with skull fracture — *see* Fracture, skull, by site
  retinae 921.3
  spinalis — *see* Injury, spinal, by site
Commotion (current)
  brain (without skull fracture) (*see also* Concussion, brain) 850.9
    with skull fracture — *see* Fracture, skull, by site
  spinal cord — *see* Injury, spinal, by site
Communication
  abnormal (*see also* Fistula)
    between
      base of aorta and pulmonary artery 745.0
      left ventricle and right atrium 745.4
      pericardial sac and pleural sac 748.8
      pulmonary artery and pulmonary vein 747.39

Communication — *continued*
  abnormal (*see also* Fistula) — *continued*
    congenital, between uterus and anterior abdominal wall 752.39
      bladder 752.39
      intestine 752.39
      rectum 752.39
    left ventricular — right atrial 745.4
    pulmonary artery-pulmonary vein 747.39
Compartment syndrome — *see* Syndrome, compartment
Compensation
  broken — *see* Failure, heart
  failure — *see* Failure, heart
  neurosis, psychoneurosis 300.11
Complaint — *see also* Disease
  bowel, functional 564.9
    psychogenic 306.4
  intestine, functional 564.9
    psychogenic 306.4
  kidney (*see also* Disease, renal) 593.9
  liver 573.9
  miners' 500
Complete — *see* condition
Complex
  cardiorenal (*see also* Hypertension, cardiorenal) 404.90
  castration 300.9
  Costen's 524.60
  ego-dystonic homosexuality 302.0
  Eisenmenger's (ventricular septal defect) 745.4
  homosexual, ego-dystonic 302.0
  hypersexual 302.89
  inferiority 301.9
  jumped process
    spine — *see* Dislocation, vertebra
  primary, tuberculosis (*see also* Tuberculosis) 010.0 ☑
  regional pain syndrome 355.9
    type I 337.20
      lower limb 337.22
      specified site NEC 337.29
      upper limb 337.21
    type II
      lower limb 355.71
      upper limb 354.4
  Taussig-Bing (transposition, aorta and overriding pulmonary artery) 745.11
Complications
  abortion NEC — *see* categories 634-639 ☑
  accidental puncture or laceration during a procedure 998.2
  amniocentesis, fetal 679.1 ☑
  amputation stump (late) (surgical) 997.60
    traumatic — *see* Amputation, traumatic
  anastomosis (and bypass) (*see also* Complications, due to (presence of) any device, implant, or graft classified to 996.0–996.5 NEC)
    hemorrhage NEC 998.11
    intestinal (internal) NEC 997.49
      involving urinary tract 997.5
    mechanical — *see* Complications, mechanical, graft
    urinary tract (involving intestinal tract) 997.5
  anesthesia, anesthetic NEC (*see also* Anesthesia, complication) 995.22
    in labor and delivery 668.9 ☑
      affecting fetus or newborn 763.5
      cardiac 668.1 ☑
      central nervous system 668.2 ☑
      pulmonary 668.0 ☑
      specified type NEC 668.8 ☑
  aortocoronary (bypass) graft 996.03
    atherosclerosis — *see* Arteriosclerosis, coronary
    embolism 996.72
    occlusion NEC 996.72
    thrombus 996.72
  arthroplasty (*see also* Complications, prosthetic joint) 996.49
  artificial opening
    cecostomy 569.60
    colostomy 569.60

☑ **Additional Digit Required** — Refer to the Tabular List for Digit Selection   ☷ **Subterms under main terms may continue to next column or page**

50 — Volume 2   ▶◀ Revised Text   ● New Line   ▲ Revised Code   **2014 ICD-9-CM**

Complications — *continued*
artificial opening — *continued*
cystostomy 596.83
infection 596.81
mechanical 596.82
specified complication NEC 596.83
enterostomy 569.60
esophagostomy 530.87
infection 530.86
mechanical 530.87
gastrostomy 536.40
ileostomy 569.60
jejunostomy 569.60
nephrostomy 997.5
tracheostomy 519.00
ureterostomy 997.5
urethrostomy 997.5
bariatric surgery
gastric band procedure 539.09
infection 539.01
specified procedure NEC 539.89
infection 539.81
bile duct implant (prosthetic) NEC 996.79
infection or inflammation 996.69
mechanical 996.59
bleeding (intraoperative) (postoperative)
998.11
blood vessel graft 996.1
aortocoronary 996.03
atherosclerosis — *see* Arteriosclerosis, coronary
embolism 996.72
occlusion NEC 996.72
thrombus 996.72
atherosclerosis — *see* Arteriosclerosis, extremities
embolism 996.74
occlusion NEC 996.74
thrombus 996.74
bone growth stimulator NEC 996.78
infection or inflammation 996.67
bone marrow transplant 996.85
breast implant (prosthetic) NEC 996.79
infection or inflammation 996.69
mechanical 996.54
bypass (*see also* Complications, anastomosis)
aortocoronary 996.03
atherosclerosis — *see* Arteriosclerosis, coronary
embolism 996.72
occlusion NEC 996.72
thrombus 996.72
carotid artery 996.1
atherosclerosis — *see* Arteriosclerosis, extremities
embolism 996.74
occlusion NEC 996.74
thrombus 996.74
cardiac (*see also* Disease, heart) 429.9
device, implant, or graft NEC 996.72
infection or inflammation 996.61
long-term effect 429.4
mechanical (*see also* Complications, mechanical, by type) 996.00
valve prosthesis 996.71
infection or inflammation 996.61
postoperative NEC 997.1
long-term effect 429.4
cardiorenal (*see also* Hypertension, cardiorenal) 404.90
carotid artery bypass graft 996.1
atherosclerosis — *see* Arteriosclerosis, extremities
embolism 996.74
occlusion NEC 996.74
thrombus 996.74
cataract fragments in eye 998.82
catheter device NEC (*see also* Complications, due to (presence of) any device, implant, or graft classified to 996.0–996.5 NEC)
mechanical — *see* Complications, mechanical, catheter
cecostomy 569.60
cesarean section wound 674.3 ☑

Complications — *continued*
chemotherapy (antineoplastic) 995.29
chin implant (prosthetic) NEC 996.79
infection or inflammation 996.69
mechanical 996.59
colostomy (enterostomy) 569.60
specified type NEC 569.69
contraceptive device, intrauterine NEC
996.76
infection 996.65
inflammation 996.65
mechanical 996.32
cord (umbilical) — *see* Complications, umbilical cord
cornea
due to
contact lens 371.82
coronary (artery) bypass (graft) NEC 996.03
atherosclerosis — *see* Arteriosclerosis, coronary
embolism 996.72
infection or inflammation 996.61
mechanical 996.03
occlusion NEC 996.72
specified type NEC 996.72
thrombus 996.72
cystostomy 596.83
infection 596.81
mechanical 596.82
specified complication NEC 596.83
delivery 669.9 ☑
procedure (instrumental) (manual) (surgical) 669.4 ☑
specified type NEC 669.8 ☑
dialysis (hemodialysis) (peritoneal) (renal)
NEC 999.9
catheter NEC (*see also* Complications, due to (presence of) any device, implant, or graft classified to 996.0–996.5 NEC)
infection or inflammation 996.62
peritoneal 996.68
mechanical 996.1
peritoneal 996.56
drug NEC 995.29
due to (presence of) any device, implant, or graft classified to 996.0–996.5 NEC 996.70
with infection or inflammation — *see* Complications, infection or inflammation, due to (presence of) any device, implant, or graft classified to 996.0–996.5 NEC
arterial NEC 996.74
coronary NEC 996.03
atherosclerosis — *see* Arteriosclerosis, coronary
embolism 996.72
occlusion NEC 996.72
specified type NEC 996.72
thrombus 996.72
renal dialysis 996.73
arteriovenous fistula or shunt NEC
996.74
bone growth stimulator 996.78
breast NEC 996.79
cardiac NEC 996.72
defibrillator 996.72
pacemaker 996.72
valve prosthesis 996.71
catheter NEC 996.79
spinal 996.75
urinary, indwelling 996.76
vascular NEC 996.74
renal dialysis 996.73
ventricular shunt 996.75
coronary (artery) bypass (graft) NEC
996.03
atherosclerosis — *see* Arteriosclerosis, coronary
embolism 996.72
occlusion NEC 996.72
thrombus 996.72
electrodes
brain 996.75
heart 996.72

Complications — *continued*
due to any device, implant, or graft classified to 996.0–996.5 — *continued*
esophagostomy 530.87
gastrointestinal NEC 996.79
genitourinary NEC 996.76
heart valve prosthesis NEC 996.71
infusion pump 996.74
insulin pump 996.57
internal
joint prosthesis 996.77
orthopedic NEC 996.78
specified type NEC 996.79
intrauterine contraceptive device NEC
996.76
joint prosthesis, internal NEC 996.77
mechanical — *see* Complications, mechanical
nervous system NEC 996.75
ocular lens NEC 996.79
orbital NEC 996.79
orthopedic NEC 996.78
joint, internal 996.77
renal dialysis 996.73
specified type NEC 996.79
urinary catheter, indwelling 996.76
vascular NEC 996.74
ventricular shunt 996.75
during dialysis NEC 999.9
ectopic or molar pregnancy NEC 639.9
electroshock therapy NEC 999.9
enterostomy 569.60
specified type NEC 569.69
esophagostomy 530.87
infection 530.86
mechanical 530.87
external (fixation) device with internal
component(s) NEC 996.78
infection or inflammation 996.67
mechanical 996.49
extracorporeal circulation NEC 999.9
eye implant (prosthetic) NEC 996.79
infection or inflammation 996.69
mechanical
ocular lens 996.53
orbital globe 996.59
fetal, from amniocentesis 679.1 ☑
gastrointestinal, postoperative NEC (*see also*
Complications, surgical procedures)
997.49
gastrostomy 536.40
specified type NEC 536.49
genitourinary device, implant or graft NEC
996.76
erosion of implanted vaginal mesh
629.31
exposure of implanted vaginal mesh
629.32
infection or inflammation 996.65
urinary catheter, indwelling 996.64
mechanical (*see also* Complications, mechanical, by type) 996.30
specified NEC 996.39
graft (bypass) (patch) (*see also* Complications, due to (presence of) any device, implant, or graft classified to 996.0–996.5 NEC)
bone marrow 996.85
corneal NEC 996.79
infection or inflammation 996.69
rejection or reaction 996.51
retroprosthetic membrane 996.51
mechanical — *see* Complications, mechanical, graft
organ (immune or nonimmune cause)
(partial) (total) 996.80
bone marrow 996.85
heart 996.83
intestines 996.87
kidney 996.81
liver 996.82
lung 996.84
pancreas 996.86
specified NEC 996.89
skin NEC 996.79
infection or inflammation 996.69

Complications — *continued*
graft (*see also* Complications, due to any device, implant, or graft classified to 996.0–996.5) — *continued*
skin — *continued*
rejection 996.52
artificial 996.55
decellularized allodermis 996.55
heart (*see also* Disease, heart transplant (immune or nonimmune cause))
996.83
hematoma (intraoperative) (postoperative)
998.12
hemorrhage (intraoperative) (postoperative)
998.11
hyperalimentation therapy NEC 999.9
immunization (procedure) — *see* Complications, vaccination
implant (*see also* Complications, due to (presence of) any device, implant, or graft classified to 996.0–996.5 NEC)
dental placement, hemorrhagic 525.71
mechanical — *see* Complications, mechanical, implant
infection and inflammation
due to (presence of) any device, implant or graft classified to 996.0–996.5
NEC 996.60
arterial NEC 996.62
coronary 996.61
renal dialysis 996.62
arteriovenous fistula or shunt 996.62
artificial heart 996.61
bone growth stimulator 996.67
breast 996.69
cardiac 996.61
catheter NEC 996.69
central venous 999.31
bloodstream 999.32
localized 999.33
Hickman 999.31
bloodstream 999.32
localized 999.33
peripherally inserted central
(PICC) 999.31
bloodstream 999.32
localized 999.33
peritoneal 996.68
portacath (port-a-cath) 999.31
bloodstream 999.32
localized 999.33
spinal 996.63
triple lumen 999.31
bloodstream 999.32
localized 999.33
umbilical venous 999.31
bloodstream 999.32
localized 999.33
urinary, indwelling 996.64
vascular (arterial) (dialysis) (peripheral venous) NEC
996.62
ventricular shunt 996.63
central venous catheter 999.31
bloodstream 999.32
localized 999.33
coronary artery bypass 996.61
electrodes
brain 996.63
heart 996.61
gastrointestinal NEC 996.69
genitourinary NEC 996.65
indwelling urinary catheter
996.64
heart assist device 996.61
heart valve 996.61
Hickman catheter 999.31
bloodstream 999.32
localized 999.33
infusion pump 996.62
insulin pump 996.69
intrauterine contraceptive device
996.65
joint prosthesis, internal 996.66
ocular lens 996.69
orbital (implant) 996.69

☑ **Additional Digit Required** — Refer to the Tabular List for Digit Selection   ⊠ **Subterms under main terms may continue to next column or page**

2014 ICD-9-CM   ▶◀ **Revised Text**   ● **New Line**   ▲ **Revised Code**   **Volume 2 — 51**

Complications — *continued*
infection and inflammation — *continued*
due to any device, implant or graft classified to 996.0–996.5 — *continued*
orthopedic NEC 996.67
joint, internal 996.66
peripherally inserted central catheter (PICC) 999.31
bloodstream 999.32
localized 999.33
portacath (port-a-cath) 999.31
bloodstream 999.32
localized 999.33
specified type NEC 996.69
triple lumen catheter 999.31
bloodstream 999.32
localized 999.33
umbilical venous catheter 999.31
bloodstream 999.32
localized 999.33
urinary catheter, indwelling 996.64
ventricular shunt 996.63
infusion (procedure) 999.88
blood — *see* Complications, transfusion
infection NEC 999.39
sepsis NEC 999.39
inhalation therapy NEC 999.9
injection (procedure) 999.9
drug reaction (*see also* Reaction, drug) 995.27
infection NEC 999.39
sepsis NEC 999.39
serum (prophylactic) (therapeutic) — *see* Complications, vaccination
vaccine (any) — *see* Complications, vaccination
inoculation (any) — *see* Complications, vaccination
insulin pump 996.57
internal device (catheter) (electronic) (fixation) (prosthetic) (*see also* Complications, due to (presence of) any device, implant, or graft classified to 996.0–996.5 NEC)
mechanical — *see* Complications, mechanical
intestinal pouch, specified NEC 569.79
intestinal transplant (immune or nonimmune cause) 996.87
intraoperative bleeding or hemorrhage 998.11
intrauterine contraceptive device (*see also* Complications, contraceptive device) 996.76
with fetal damage affecting management of pregnancy 655.8 ☑
infection or inflammation 996.65
in utero procedure
fetal 679.1 ☑
maternal 679.0 ☑
jejunostomy 569.60
kidney transplant (immune or nonimmune cause) 996.81
labor 669.9 ☑
specified condition NEC 669.8 ☑
liver transplant (immune or nonimmune cause) 996.82
lumbar puncture 349.0
mechanical
anastomosis — *see* Complications, mechanical, graft
artificial heart 996.09
bypass — *see* Complications, mechanical, graft
catheter NEC 996.59
cardiac 996.09
cystostomy 596.82
dialysis (hemodialysis) 996.1
peritoneal 996.56
during a procedure 998.2
urethral, indwelling 996.31
colostomy 569.62
device NEC 996.59

Complications — *continued*
mechanical — *continued*
device — *continued*
balloon (counterpulsation), intra-aortic 996.1
cardiac 996.00
automatic implantable defibrillator 996.04
long-term effect 429.4
specified NEC 996.09
contraceptive, intrauterine 996.32
counterpulsation, intra-aortic 996.1
fixation, external, with internal components 996.49
fixation, internal (nail, rod, plate) 996.40
genitourinary 996.30
specified NEC 996.39
insulin pump 996.57
nervous system 996.2
orthopedic, internal 996.40
prosthetic joint (*see also* Complications, mechanical, device, orthopedic, prosthetic, joint) 996.47
prosthetic NEC 996.59
joint 996.47
articular bearing surface wear 996.46
aseptic loosening 996.41
breakage 996.43
dislocation 996.42
failure 996.47
fracture 996.43
around prosthetic 996.44
peri-prosthetic 996.44
instability 996.42
loosening 996.41
peri-prosthetic osteolysis 996.45
subluxation 996.42
wear 996.46
umbrella, vena cava 996.1
vascular 996.1
dorsal column stimulator 996.2
electrode NEC 996.59
brain 996.2
cardiac 996.01
spinal column 996.2
enterostomy 569.62
esophagostomy 530.87
fistula, arteriovenous, surgically created 996.1
gastrostomy 536.42
graft NEC 996.52
aortic (bifurcation) 996.1
aortocoronary bypass 996.03
blood vessel NEC 996.1
bone 996.49
cardiac 996.00
carotid artery bypass 996.1
cartilage 996.49
corneal 996.51
coronary bypass 996.03
decellularized allodermis 996.55
genitourinary 996.30
specified NEC 996.39
muscle 996.49
nervous system 996.2
organ (immune or nonimmune cause) 996.80
heart 996.83
intestines 996.87
kidney 996.81
liver 996.82
lung 996.84
pancreas 996.86
specified NEC 996.89
orthopedic, internal 996.49
peripheral nerve 996.2
prosthetic NEC 996.59
skin 996.52
artificial 996.55
specified NEC 996.59
tendon 996.49
tissue NEC 996.52

Complications — *continued*
mechanical — *continued*
graft — *continued*
tooth 996.59
ureter, without mention of resection 996.39
vascular 996.1
heart valve prosthesis 996.02
long-term effect 429.4
implant NEC 996.59
cardiac 996.00
automatic implantable defibrillator 996.04
long-term effect 429.4
specified NEC 996.09
electrode NEC 996.59
brain 996.2
cardiac 996.01
spinal column 996.2
genitourinary 996.30
nervous system 996.2
orthopedic, internal 996.49
prosthetic NEC 996.59
in
bile duct 996.59
breast 996.54
chin 996.59
eye
ocular lens 996.53
orbital globe 996.59
vascular 996.1
insulin pump 996.57
nonabsorbable surgical material 996.59
pacemaker NEC 996.59
brain 996.2
cardiac 996.01
nerve (phrenic) 996.2
patch — *see* Complications, mechanical, graft
prosthesis NEC 996.59
bile duct 996.59
breast 996.54
chin 996.59
ocular lens 996.53
reconstruction, vas deferens 996.39
reimplant NEC 996.59
extremity (*see also* Complications, reattached, extremity) 996.90
organ (*see also* Complications, transplant, organ, by site) 996.80
repair — *see* Complications, mechanical, graft
respirator [ventilator] V46.14
shunt NEC 996.59
arteriovenous, surgically created 996.1
ventricular (communicating) 996.2
stent NEC 996.59
tracheostomy 519.02
vas deferens reconstruction 996.39
ventilator [respirator] V46.14
medical care NEC 999.9
cardiac NEC 997.1
gastrointestinal NEC 997.49
nervous system NEC 997.00
peripheral vascular NEC 997.2
respiratory NEC 997.39
urinary NEC 997.5
vascular
mesenteric artery 997.71
other vessels 997.79
peripheral vessels 997.2
renal artery 997.72
nephrostomy 997.5
nervous system
device, implant, or graft NEC 349.1
mechanical 996.2
postoperative NEC 997.00
obstetric 669.9 ☑
procedure (instrumental) (manual) (surgical) 669.4 ☑
specified NEC 669.8 ☑
surgical wound 674.3 ☑
ocular lens implant NEC 996.79
infection or inflammation 996.69
mechanical 996.53

Complications — *continued*
organ transplant — *see* Complications, transplant, organ, by site
orthopedic device, implant, or graft
internal (fixation) (nail) (plate) (rod) NEC 996.78
infection or inflammation 996.67
joint prosthesis 996.77
infection or inflammation 996.66
mechanical 996.40
pacemaker (cardiac) 996.72
infection or inflammation 996.61
mechanical 996.01
pancreas transplant (immune or nonimmune cause) 996.86
perfusion NEC 999.9
perineal repair (obstetrical) 674.3 ☑
disruption 674.2 ☑
pessary (uterus) (vagina) — *see* Complications, contraceptive device
phototherapy 990
postcystoscopic 997.5
postmastoidectomy NEC 383.30
postoperative — *see* Complications, surgical procedures
pregnancy NEC 646.9 ☑
affecting fetus or newborn 761.9
prosthetic device, internal (*see also* Complications, due to (presence of) any device, implant or graft classified to 996.0–996.5 NEC)
mechanical NEC (*see also* Complications, mechanical) 996.59
puerperium NEC (*see also* Puerperal) 674.9 ☑
puncture, spinal 349.0
pyelogram 997.5
radiation 990
radiotherapy 990
reattached
body part, except extremity 996.99
extremity (infection) (rejection) 996.90
arm(s) 996.94
digit(s) (hand) 996.93
foot 996.95
finger(s) 996.93
foot 996.95
forearm 996.91
hand 996.92
leg 996.96
lower NEC 996.96
toe(s) 996.95
upper NEC 996.94
reimplant NEC (*see also* Complications, due to (presence of) any device, implant, or graft classified to 996.0–996.5 NEC)
bone marrow 996.85
extremity (*see also* Complications, reattached, extremity) 996.90
due to infection 996.90
mechanical — *see* Complications, mechanical, reimplant
organ (immune or nonimmune cause) (partial) (total) (*see also* Complications, transplant, organ, by site) 996.80
renal allograft 996.81
renal dialysis — *see* Complications, dialysis
respirator [ventilator], mechanical V46.14
respiratory 519.9
device, implant or graft NEC 996.79
infection or inflammation 996.69
mechanical 996.59
distress syndrome, adult, following trauma and surgery 518.52
insufficiency, acute, postoperative 518.52
postoperative NEC 997.39
therapy NEC 999.9
sedation during labor and delivery 668.9 ☑
affecting fetus or newborn 763.5
cardiac 668.1 ☑
central nervous system 668.2 ☑
pulmonary 668.0 ☑
specified type NEC 668.8 ☑

☑ Additional Digit Required — Refer to the Tabular List for Digit Selection   ⚕ Subterms under main terms may continue to next column or page

52 — Volume 2   ▶◀ Revised Text   ● New Line   ▲ Revised Code   2014 ICD-9-CM

Complications — *continued*
- seroma (intraoperative) (postoperative) (noninfected) 998.13
  - infected 998.51
- shunt (*see also* Complications, due to (presence of) any device, implant, or graft classified to 996.0–996.5 NEC)
  - mechanical — *see* Complications, mechanical, shunt
- specified body system NEC
  - device, implant, or graft — *see* Complications, due to (presence of) any device, implant, or graft classified to 996.0–996.5 NEC
  - postoperative NEC 997.99
- spinal puncture or tap 349.0
- stoma, external
  - gastrointestinal tract
    - colostomy 569.60
    - enterostomy 569.60
    - esophagostomy 530.87
      - infection 530.86
      - mechanical 530.87
    - gastrostomy 536.40
  - urinary tract 997.5
- stomach banding 539.09
- stomach stapling 539.89
- surgical procedures 998.9
  - accidental puncture or laceration 998.2
  - amputation stump (late) 997.60
  - anastomosis — *see* Complications, anastomosis
  - burst stitches or sutures (external) (*see also* Dehiscence) 998.32
    - internal 998.31
  - cardiac 997.1
    - long-term effect following cardiac surgery 429.4
  - cataract fragments in eye 998.82
  - catheter device — *see* Complications, catheter device
  - cecostomy malfunction 569.62
  - colostomy malfunction 569.62
  - cystostomy malfunction 596.82
    - infection 596.81
    - mechanical 596.82
    - specified complication NEC 596.83
  - dehiscence (of incision) (external) (*see also* Dehiscence) 998.32
    - internal 998.31
  - dialysis NEC (*see also* Complications, dialysis) 999.9
  - disruption (*see also* Dehiscence)
    - anastomosis (internal) — *see* Complications, mechanical, graft
    - internal suture (line) 998.31
    - wound (external) 998.32
      - internal 998.31
  - dumping syndrome (postgastrectomy) 564.2
  - elephantiasis or lymphedema 997.99
    - postmastectomy 457.0
  - emphysema (surgical) 998.81
  - enterostomy malfunction 569.62
  - esophagostomy malfunction 530.87
  - evisceration 998.32
  - fistula (persistent postoperative) 998.6
  - foreign body inadvertently left in wound (sponge) (suture) (swab) 998.4
  - from nonabsorbable surgical material (Dacron) (mesh) (permanent suture) (reinforcing) (Teflon) — *see* Complications, due to (presence of) any device, implant, or graft classified to 996.0–996.5 NEC
  - gastrointestinal NEC 997.49
  - gastrostomy malfunction 536.42
  - hematoma 998.12
  - hemorrhage 998.11
  - ileostomy malfunction 569.62
  - internal prosthetic device NEC (*see also* Complications, internal device) 996.70
    - hemolytic anemia 283.19
    - infection or inflammation 996.60

Complications — *continued*
- surgical procedures — *continued*
  - internal prosthetic device (*see also* Complications, internal device) — *continued*
    - malfunction — *see* Complications, mechanical
    - mechanical complication — *see* Complications, mechanical
    - thrombus 996.70
  - jejunostomy malfunction 569.62
  - nervous system NEC 997.00
  - obstruction, internal anastomosis — *see* Complications, mechanical, graft
  - other body system NEC 997.99
  - peripheral vascular NEC 997.2
  - postcardiotomy syndrome 429.4
  - postcholecystectomy syndrome 576.0
  - postcommissurotomy syndrome 429.4
  - postgastrectomy dumping syndrome 564.2
  - postmastectomy lymphedema syndrome 457.0
  - postmastoidectomy 383.30
    - cholesteatoma, recurrent 383.32
    - cyst, mucosal 383.31
    - granulation 383.33
    - inflammation, chronic 383.33
  - postvagotomy syndrome 564.2
  - postvalvulotomy syndrome 429.4
  - reattached extremity (infection) (rejection) (*see also* Complications, reattached, extremity) 996.90
  - respiratory NEC 997.39
  - seroma 998.13
  - shock (endotoxic) (septic) 998.02
    - hypovolemic 998.09
  - shunt, prosthetic (thrombus) (*see also* Complications, due to (presence of) any device, implant, or graft classified to 996.0–996.5 NEC)
    - hemolytic anemia 283.19
    - specified complication NEC 596.83
    - specified complication NEC 998.89
  - stitch abscess 998.59
  - transplant — *see* Complications, graft
  - ureterostomy malfunction 997.5
  - urethrostomy malfunction 997.5
  - urinary NEC 997.5
  - vascular
    - mesenteric artery 997.71
    - other vessels 997.79
    - peripheral vessels 997.2
    - renal artery 997.72
  - wound infection 998.59
- therapeutic misadventure NEC 999.9
  - surgical treatment 998.9
- tracheostomy 519.00
- transfusion (blood) (lymphocytes) (plasma) 999.80
  - acute lung injury (TRALI) 518.7
  - atrophy, liver, yellow, subacute (within 8 months of administration) — *see* Hepatitis, viral
  - bone marrow 996.85
  - embolism
    - air 999.1
    - thrombus 999.2
  - febrile nonhemolytic reaction (FNHTR) 780.66
  - hemolysis NEC 999.89
    - bone marrow 996.85
  - hemolytic reaction, incompatibility unspecified 999.83
    - acute 999.84
    - delayed 999.85
  - hepatitis (serum) (type B) (within 8 months after administration) — *see* Hepatitis, viral
  - incompatibility reaction
    - ABO 999.60
      - with hemolytic transfusion reaction (HTR) (not specified as acute or delayed) 999.61
      - acute 999.62
      - delayed 999.63

Complications — *continued*
- transfusion — *continued*
  - incompatibility reaction — *continued*
    - ABO — *continued*
      - specified type NEC 999.69
    - minor blood group 999.89
    - non-ABO (minor antigens) (Duffy) (Kell) (Kidd) (Lewis) (M) (N) (P) (S) 999.75
      - with hemolytic transfusion reaction (HTR) (not specified as acute or delayed) 999.76
      - acute 999.77
      - delayed 999.78
      - specified type NEC 999.79
    - Rh antigen (C) (c) (D) (E) (e) (factor) 999.70
      - with hemolytic transfusion reaction (HTR) (not specified as acute or delayed) 999.71
      - acute 999.72
      - delayed 999.73
      - specified type NEC 999.74
  - infection 999.39
    - acute 999.34
  - jaundice (serum) (within 8 months after administration) — *see* Hepatitis, viral
  - sepsis 999.39
  - shock or reaction NEC 999.89
    - bone marrow 996.85
  - specified reaction NEC 999.89
  - subacute yellow atrophy of liver (within 8 months after administration) — *see* Hepatitis, viral
  - thromboembolism 999.2
- transplant NEC (*see also* Complications, due to (presence of) any device, implant, or graft classified to 996.0–996.5 NEC)
  - bone marrow 996.85
  - organ (immune or nonimmune cause) (partial) (total) 996.80
    - bone marrow 996.85
    - heart 996.83
    - intestines 996.87
    - kidney 996.81
    - liver 996.82
    - lung 996.84
    - pancreas 996.86
    - specified NEC 996.89
    - stem cell(s) 996.88
      - from
        - peripheral blood 996.88
        - umbilical cord 996.88
  - trauma NEC (early) 958.8
  - ultrasound therapy NEC 999.9
  - umbilical cord
    - affecting fetus or newborn 762.6
    - complicating delivery 663.9 ☑
      - affecting fetus or newborn 762.6
      - specified type NEC 663.8 ☑
  - urethral catheter NEC 996.76
    - infection or inflammation 996.64
    - mechanical 996.31
  - urinary, postoperative NEC 997.5
  - vaccination 999.9
    - anaphylaxis NEC 999.42
    - cellulitis 999.39
    - encephalitis or encephalomyelitis 323.51
    - hepatitis (serum) (type B) (within 8 months after administration) — *see* Hepatitis, viral
    - infection (general) (local) NEC 999.39
    - jaundice (serum) (within 8 months after administration) — *see* Hepatitis, viral
    - meningitis 997.09 [321.8]
    - myelitis 323.52
    - protein sickness 999.52
    - reaction (allergic) 999.52
      - serum 999.52
    - sepsis 999.39
    - serum intoxication, sickness, rash, or other serum reaction NEC 999.52

Complications — *continued*
- vaccination — *continued*
  - shock (allergic) (anaphylactic) 999.49
  - subacute yellow atrophy of liver (within 8 months after administration) — *see* Hepatitis, viral
  - vaccinia (generalized) 999.0
    - localized 999.39
- vascular
  - device, implant, or graft NEC 996.74
    - infection or inflammation 996.62
    - mechanical NEC 996.1
      - cardiac (*see also* Complications, mechanical, by type) 996.00
  - following infusion, perfusion, or transfusion 999.2
  - postoperative NEC 997.2
    - mesenteric artery 997.71
    - other vessels 997.79
    - peripheral vessels 997.2
    - renal artery 997.72
  - ventilation therapy NEC 999.9
- ventilator [respirator], mechanical V46.14

Compound presentation, complicating delivery 652.8 ☑
- causing obstructed labor 660.0 ☑

Compressed air disease 993.3

Compression
- with injury — *see* specific injury
- arm NEC 354.9
- artery 447.1
  - celiac, syndrome 447.4
- brachial plexus 353.0
- brain (stem) 348.4
  - due to
    - contusion, brain — *see* Contusion, brain
    - injury NEC (*see also* Hemorrhage, brain, traumatic)
    - birth — *see* Birth, injury, brain
    - laceration, brain — *see* Laceration, brain
  - osteopathic 739.0
- bronchus 519.19
- by cicatrix — *see* Cicatrix
- cardiac 423.9
- cauda equina 344.60
  - with neurogenic bladder 344.61
- celiac (artery) (axis) 447.4
- cerebral — *see* Compression, brain
- cervical plexus 353.2
- cord (umbilical) — *see* Compression, umbilical cord
- cranial nerve 352.9
  - second 377.49
  - third (partial) 378.51
    - total 378.52
  - fourth 378.53
  - fifth 350.8
  - sixth 378.54
  - seventh 351.8
- divers' squeeze 993.3
- duodenum (external) (*see also* Obstruction, duodenum) 537.3
- during birth 767.9
- esophagus 530.3
  - congenital, external 750.3
- Eustachian tube 381.63
- facies (congenital) 754.0
- fracture — *see* Fracture, by site
- heart — *see* Disease, heart
- intestine (*see also* Obstruction, intestine) 560.9
  - with hernia — *see* Hernia, by site, with obstruction
- laryngeal nerve, recurrent 478.79
- leg NEC 355.8
- lower extremity NEC 355.8
- lumbosacral plexus 353.1
- lung 518.89
- lymphatic vessel 457.1
- medulla — *see* Compression, brain
- nerve NEC (*see also* Disorder, nerve)
  - arm NEC 354.9

☑ **Additional Digit Required** — Refer to the Tabular List for Digit Selection   ▽ **Subterms under main terms may continue to next column or page**

2014 ICD-9-CM   ▶◀ **Revised Text**   ● **New Line**   ▲ **Revised Code**   **Volume 2 — 53**

Index · Compression — Congestion, congestive

Compression — *continued*
nerve (*see also* Disorder, nerve) — *continued*
  autonomic nervous system (*see also* Neuropathy, peripheral, autonomic) 337.9
  axillary 353.0
  cranial NEC 352.9
  due to displacement of intervertebral disc 722.2
    with myelopathy 722.70
    cervical 722.0
      with myelopathy 722.71
    lumbar, lumbosacral 722.10
      with myelopathy 722.73
    thoracic, thoracolumbar 722.11
      with myelopathy 722.72
  iliohypogastric 355.79
  ilioinguinal 355.79
  leg NEC 355.8
  lower extremity NEC 355.8
  median (in carpal tunnel) 354.0
  obturator 355.79
  optic 377.49
  plantar 355.6
  posterior tibial (in tarsal tunnel) 355.5
  root (by scar tissue) NEC 724.9
    cervical NEC 723.4
    lumbar NEC 724.4
    lumbosacral 724.4
    thoracic 724.4
  saphenous 355.79
  sciatic (acute) 355.0
  sympathetic 337.9
  traumatic — *see* Injury, nerve
  ulnar 354.2
  upper extremity NEC 354.9
peripheral — *see* Compression, nerve
spinal (cord) (old or nontraumatic) 336.9
  by displacement of intervertebral disc — *see* Displacement, intervertebral disc
  nerve
    root NEC 724.9
      postoperative 722.80
        cervical region 722.81
        lumbar region 722.83
        thoracic region 722.82
      traumatic — *see* Injury, nerve, spinal
    traumatic — *see* Injury, nerve, spinal
  spondylogenic 721.91
    cervical 721.1
    lumbar, lumbosacral 721.42
    thoracic 721.41
  traumatic (*see also* Injury, spinal, by site)
    with fracture, vertebra — *see* Fracture, vertebra, by site, with spinal cord injury
spondylogenic — *see* Compression, spinal cord, spondylogenic
subcostal nerve (syndrome) 354.8
sympathetic nerve NEC 337.9
syndrome 958.5
thorax 512.89
  iatrogenic 512.1
  postoperative 512.1
trachea 519.19
  congenital 748.3
ulnar nerve (by scar tissue) 354.2
umbilical cord
  affecting fetus or newborn 762.5
    cord prolapsed 762.4
  complicating delivery 663.2 ☑
    cord around neck 663.1 ☑
    cord prolapsed 663.0 ☑
upper extremity NEC 354.9
ureter 593.3
urethra — *see* Stricture, urethra
vein 459.2
vena cava (inferior) (superior) 459.2
vertebral NEC — *see* Compression, spinal (cord)

Compulsion, compulsive
eating 307.51
neurosis (obsessive) 300.3

Compulsion, compulsive — *continued*
personality 301.4
states (mixed) 300.3
swearing 300.3
  in Gilles de la Tourette's syndrome 307.23
tics and spasms 307.22
water drinking NEC (syndrome) 307.9
Concato's disease (pericardial polyserositis) 423.2
peritoneal 568.82
pleural — *see* Pleurisy
Concavity, chest wall 738.3
Concealed
hemorrhage NEC 459.0
penis 752.65
Concentric fading 368.12
Concern (normal) **about sick person in family** V61.49
Concrescence (teeth) 520.2
Concretio cordis 423.1
rheumatic 393
Concretion — *see also* Calculus
appendicular 543.9
canaliculus 375.57
clitoris 624.8
conjunctiva 372.54
eyelid 374.56
intestine (impaction) (obstruction) 560.39
lacrimal (passages) 375.57
prepuce (male) 605
  female (clitoris) 624.8
salivary gland (any) 527.5
seminal vesicle 608.89
stomach 537.89
tonsil 474.8
Concussion (current) 850.9
with
  loss of consciousness 850.5
    brief (less than one hour)
      30 minutes or less 850.11
      31-59 minutes 850.12
    moderate (1-24 hours) 850.2
    prolonged (more than 24 hours)
      (with complete recovery)
      (with return to pre-existing conscious level) 850.3
      without return to pre-existing conscious level 850.4
  mental confusion or disorientation (without loss of consciousness) 850.0
    with loss of consciousness — *see* Concussion, with, loss of consciousness
without loss of consciousness 850.0
blast (air) (hydraulic) (immersion) (underwater) 869.0
  with open wound into cavity 869.1
  abdomen or thorax — *see* Injury, internal, by site
  brain — *see* Concussion, brain
  ear (acoustic nerve trauma) 951.5
    with perforation, tympanic membrane — *see* Wound, open, ear drum
  thorax — *see* Injury, internal, intrathoracic organs NEC
brain or cerebral (without skull fracture) 850.9
with
  loss of consciousness 850.5
    brief (less than one hour)
      30 minutes or less 850.11
      31-59 minutes 850.12
    moderate (1-24 hours) 850.2
    prolonged (more than 24 hours)
      (with complete recovery)
      (with return to pre-existing conscious level) 850.3
      without return to pre-existing conscious level 850.4
  mental confusion or disorientation (without loss of consciousness) 850.0

Concussion — *continued*
brain or cerebral — *continued*
  with — *continued*
    mental confusion or disorientation — *continued*
      with loss of consciousness — *see* Concussion, brain, with, loss of consciousness
    skull fracture — *see* Fracture, skull, by site
  without loss of consciousness 850.0
cauda equina 952.4
cerebral — *see* Concussion, brain
conus medullaris (spine) 952.4
hydraulic — *see* Concussion, blast
internal organs — *see* Injury, internal, by site
labyrinth — *see* Injury, intracranial
ocular 921.3
osseous labyrinth — *see* Injury, intracranial
spinal (cord) (*see also* Injury, spinal, by site)
  due to
    broken
      back — *see* Fracture, vertebra, by site, with spinal cord injury
      neck — *see* Fracture, vertebra, cervical, with spinal cord injury
    fracture, fracture dislocation, or compression fracture of spine or vertebra — *see* Fracture, vertebra, by site, with spinal cord injury
syndrome 310.2
underwater blast — *see* Concussion, blast
Condition — *see also* Disease
fetal hematologic 678.0 ☑
psychiatric 298.9
respiratory NEC 519.9
  acute or subacute NEC 519.9
    due to
      external agent 508.9
        specified type NEC 508.8
      fumes or vapors (chemical) (inhalation) 506.3
      radiation 508.0
  chronic NEC 519.9
    due to
      external agent 508.9
        specified type NEC 508.8
      fumes or vapors (chemical) (inhalation) 506.4
      radiation 508.1
  due to
    external agent 508.9
      specified type NEC 508.8
    fumes or vapors (chemical) (inhalation) 506.9
    smoke inhalation 508.2
Conduct disturbance — *see also* Disturbance, conduct 312.9
adjustment reaction 309.3
hyperkinetic 314.2
Condyloma NEC 078.11
acuminatum 078.11
gonorrheal 098.0
latum 091.3
syphilitic 091.3
  congenital 090.0
venereal, syphilitic 091.3
Confinement — *see* Delivery
Conflagration — *see also* Burn, by site
asphyxia (by inhalation of gases, fumes, or vapors) 987.9
specified agent — *see* Table of Drugs and Chemicals
Conflict
family V61.9
  specified circumstance NEC V61.8
interpersonal NEC V62.81
marital V61.10
  involving
    divorce V61.03
    estrangement V61.09
parent (guardian)-child V61.20
  adopted child V61.24

Conflict — *continued*
parent-child — *continued*
  biological child V61.23
  foster child V61.25
partner V61.10
Confluent — *see* condition
Confusional arousals 327.41
Confusion, confused (mental) (state) — *see also* State, confusional 298.9
acute 293.0
epileptic 293.0
postoperative 293.9
psychogenic 298.2
reactive (from emotional stress, psychological trauma) 298.2
subacute 293.1
Congelation 991.9
Congenital — *see also* condition
aortic septum 747.29
generalized fibromatosis (CGF) 759.89
intrinsic factor deficiency 281.0
malformation — *see* Anomaly
Congestion, congestive
asphyxia, newborn 768.9
bladder 596.89
bowel 569.89
brain (*see also* Disease, cerebrovascular NEC) 437.8
  malarial 084.9
breast 611.79
bronchi 519.19
bronchial tube 519.19
catarrhal 472.0
cerebral — *see* Congestion, brain
cerebrospinal — *see* Congestion, brain
chest 786.9
chill 780.99
  malarial (*see also* Malaria) 084.6
circulatory NEC 459.9
conjunctiva 372.71
due to disturbance of circulation 459.9
duodenum 537.3
enteritis — *see* Enteritis
eye 372.71
fibrosis syndrome (pelvic) 625.5
gastroenteritis — *see* Enteritis
general 799.89
glottis 476.0
heart (*see also* Failure, heart) 428.0
hepatic 573.0
hypostatic (lung) 514
intestine 569.89
intracranial — *see* Congestion, brain
kidney 593.89
labyrinth 386.50
larynx 476.0
liver 573.0
lung 786.9
  active or acute (*see also* Pneumonia) 486
    congenital 770.0
  chronic 514
  hypostatic 514
  idiopathic, acute 518.52
  passive 514
malaria, malarial (brain) (fever) (*see also* Malaria) 084.6
medulla — *see* Congestion, brain
nasal 478.19
nose 478.19
orbit, orbital 376.33
  inflammatory (chronic) 376.10
    acute 376.00
ovary 620.8
pancreas 577.8
pelvic, female 625.5
pleural 511.0
prostate (active) 602.1
pulmonary — *see* Congestion, lung
renal 593.89
retina 362.89
seminal vesicle 608.89
spinal cord 336.1
spleen 289.51
  chronic 289.51
stomach 537.89
trachea 464.11

☑ **Additional Digit Required — Refer to the Tabular List for Digit Selection**

ᵂ **Subterms under main terms may continue to next column or page**

Congestion, congestive — *continued*
  urethra 599.84
  uterus 625.5
    with subinvolution 621.1
  viscera 799.89
Congestive — *see* Congestion
Conical
  cervix 622.6
  cornea 371.60
  teeth 520.2
Conjoined twins 759.4
  causing disproportion (fetopelvic) 678.1 ☑
  fetal 678.1 ☑
Conjugal maladjustment V61.10
  involving
    divorce V61.03
    estrangement V61.09
Conjunctiva — *see* condition
Conjunctivitis (exposure) (infectious)
  (nondiphtheritic) (pneumococcal) (pustular) (staphylococcal) (streptococcal)
  NEC 372.30
  actinic 370.24
  acute 372.00
    atopic 372.05
    chemical 372.06
    contagious 372.03
    follicular 372.02
    hemorrhagic (viral) 077.4
    toxic 372.06
  adenoviral (acute) 077.3
  allergic (chronic) 372.14
    with hay fever 372.05
  anaphylactic 372.05
  angular 372.03
  Apollo (viral) 077.4
  atopic 372.05
  blennorrhagic (neonatorum) 098.40
  catarrhal 372.03
  chemical 372.06
    allergic 372.05
    meaning corrosion — *see* Burn, conjunc-
    tiva
  chlamydial 077.98
    due to
      Chlamydia trachomatis — *see* Tra-
      choma
      paratrachoma 077.0
  chronic 372.10
    allergic 372.14
    follicular 372.12
    simple 372.11
    specified type NEC 372.14
    vernal 372.13
  diphtheritic 032.81
  due to
    dust 372.05
    enterovirus type 70 077.4
    erythema multiforme 695.10 *[372.33]*
    filariasis (*see also* Filariasis) 125.9 *[372.15]*
    mucocutaneous
      disease NEC 372.33
      leishmaniasis 085.5 *[372.15]*
    Reiter's disease 099.3 *[372.33]*
    syphilis 095.8 *[372.10]*
    toxoplasmosis (acquired) 130.1
      congenital (active) 771.2
    trachoma — *see* Trachoma
  dust 372.05
  eczematous 370.31
  epidemic 077.1
    hemorrhagic 077.4
  follicular (acute) 372.02
    adenoviral (acute) 077.3
    chronic 372.12
  glare 370.24
  gonococcal (neonatorum) 098.40
  granular (trachomatous) 076.1
    late effect 139.1
  hemorrhagic (acute) (epidemic) 077.4
  herpetic (simplex) 054.43
    zoster 053.21
  inclusion 077.0
  infantile 771.6
  influenzal 372.03
  Koch-Weeks 372.03

Conjunctivitis — *continued*
  light 372.05
  medicamentosa 372.05
  membranous 372.04
  meningococcic 036.89
  Morax-Axenfeld 372.02
  mucopurulent NEC 372.03
  neonatal 771.6
    gonococcal 098.40
  Newcastle's 077.8
  nodosa 360.14
  of Beal 077.3
  parasitic 372.15
    filariasis (*see also* Filariasis) 125.9 *[372.15]*
    mucocutaneous leishmaniasis
      085.5 *[372.15]*
  Parinaud's 372.02
  petrificans 372.39
  phlyctenular 370.31
  pseudomembranous 372.04
    diphtheritic 032.81
  purulent 372.03
  Reiter's 099.3 *[372.33]*
  rosacea 695.3 *[372.31]*
  serous 372.01
    viral 077.99
  simple chronic 372.11
  specified NEC 372.39
  sunlamp 372.04
  swimming pool 077.0
  toxic 372.06
  trachomatous (follicular) 076.1
    acute 076.0
    late effect 139.1
  traumatic NEC 372.39
  tuberculous (*see also* Tuberculosis)
    017.3 ☑ *[370.31]*
  tularemic 021.3
  tularensis 021.3
  vernal 372.13
    limbar 372.13 *[370.32]*
  viral 077.99
    acute hemorrhagic 077.4
    specified NEC 077.8
Conjunctivochalasis 372.81
Conjunctoblepharitis — *see* Conjunctivitis
Connective tissue — *see* condition
Conn (-Louis) syndrome (primary aldosteronism) 255.12
Conradi (-Hünermann) syndrome or disease
  (chondrodysplasia calcificans congenita)
  756.59
Consanguinity V19.7
Consecutive — *see* condition
Consolidated lung (base) — *see* Pneumonia,
  lobar
Constipation 564.00
  atonic 564.09
  drug induced
    correct substance properly administered
      564.09
    overdose or wrong substance given or
      taken 977.9
      specified drug — *see* Table of Drugs
      and Chemicals
  neurogenic 564.09
  other specified NEC 564.09
  outlet dysfunction 564.02
  psychogenic 306.4
  simple 564.00
  slow transit 564.01
  spastic 564.09
Constitutional — *see also* condition
  arterial hypotension (*see also* Hypotension)
    458.9
  obesity 278.00
    morbid 278.01
  psychopathic state 301.9
  short stature in childhood 783.43
  state, developmental V21.9
    specified development NEC V21.8
  substandard 301.6
Constitutionally substandard 301.6
Constriction
  anomalous, meningeal bands or folds 742.8
  aortic arch (congenital) 747.10

Constriction — *continued*
  asphyxiation or suffocation by 994.7
  bronchus 519.19
  canal, ear (*see also* Stricture, ear canal, ac-
    quired) 380.50
  duodenum 537.3
  gallbladder (*see also* Obstruction, gallblad-
    der) 575.2
    congenital 751.69
  intestine (*see also* Obstruction, intestine)
    560.9
  larynx 478.74
    congenital 748.3
  meningeal bands or folds, anomalous 742.8
  organ or site, congenital NEC — *see* Atresia
  prepuce (congenital) 605
  pylorus 537.0
    adult hypertrophic 537.0
    congenital or infantile 750.5
    newborn 750.5
  ring (uterus) 661.4 ☑
    affecting fetus or newborn 763.7
  spastic (*see also* Spasm)
    ureter 593.3
    urethra — *see* Stricture, urethra
  stomach 537.89
  ureter 593.3
  urethra — *see* Stricture, urethra
  visual field (functional) (peripheral) 368.45
Constrictive — *see* condition
Consultation
  without complaint or sickness V65.9
    feared complaint unfounded V65.5
    specified reason NEC V65.8
  medical (*see also* Counseling, medical)
    specified reason NEC V65.8
Consumption — *see* Tuberculosis
Contact — *see also* Exposure (suspected)
  with
    AIDS virus V01.79
    anthrax V01.81
    asbestos V15.84
    cholera V01.0
    communicable disease V01.9
      specified type NEC V01.89
      viral NEC V01.79
    Escherichia coli (E. coli) V01.83
    German measles V01.4
    gonorrhea V01.6
    HIV V01.79
    human immunodeficiency virus V01.79
    lead V15.86
    meningococcus V01.84
    parasitic disease NEC V01.89
    poliomyelitis V01.2
    potentially hazardous body fluids V15.85
    rabies V01.5
    rubella V01.4
    SARS-associated coronavirus V01.82
    smallpox V01.3
    syphilis V01.6
    tuberculosis V01.1
    varicella V01.71
    venereal disease V01.6
    viral disease NEC V01.79
  dermatitis — *see* Dermatitis
Contamination, food — *see also* Poisoning,
  food 005.9
Contraception, contraceptive
  advice NEC V25.09
    family planning V25.09
    fitting of diaphragm V25.02
    prescribing or use of
      oral contraceptive agent V25.01
      specified agent NEC V25.02
  counseling NEC V25.09
    emergency V25.03
    family planning V25.09
    fitting of diaphragm V25.02
    prescribing or use of
      oral contraceptive agent V25.01
      emergency V25.03
      postcoital V25.03
      specified agent NEC V25.02
  device (in situ) V45.59
    causing menorrhagia 996.76

Contraception, contraceptive —
  continued
  device — *continued*
    checking V25.42
    complications 996.32
    insertion V25.11
    intrauterine V45.51
    reinsertion V25.13
    removal V25.12
      and reinsertion V25.13
    replacement V25.13
    subdermal V45.52
  fitting of diaphragm V25.02
  insertion
    intrauterine contraceptive device V25.11
    subdermal implantable V25.5
  maintenance V25.40
    examination V25.40
      oral contraceptive V25.41
      specified method NEC V25.49
      subdermal implantable V25.43
        intrauterine device V25.42
    intrauterine device V25.42
    oral contraceptive V25.41
    specified method NEC V25.49
    subdermal implantable V25.43
  management NEC V25.49
  prescription
    oral contraceptive agent V25.01
      emergency V25.03
      postcoital V25.03
      repeat V25.41
    specified agent NEC V25.02
      repeat V25.49
  sterilization V25.2
  surveillance V25.40
    intrauterine device V25.42
    oral contraceptive agent V25.41
    subdermal implantable V25.43
    specified method NEC V25.49
Contraction, contracture, contracted
  Achilles tendon (*see also* Short, tendon,
    Achilles) 727.81
  anus 564.89
  axilla 729.90
  bile duct (*see also* Disease, biliary) 576.8
  bladder 596.89
    neck or sphincter 596.0
  bowel (*see also* Obstruction, intestine) 560.9
  Braxton Hicks 644.1 ☑
  breast implant, capsular 611.83
  bronchus 519.19
  burn (old) — *see* Cicatrix
  capsular, of breast implant 611.83
  cecum (*see also* Obstruction, intestine) 560.9
  cervix (*see also* Stricture, cervix) 622.4
    congenital 752.49
  cicatricial — *see* Cicatrix
  colon (*see also* Obstruction, intestine) 560.9
  conjunctiva trachomatous, active 076.1
    late effect 139.1
  Dupuytren's 728.6
  eyelid 374.41
  eye socket (after enucleation) 372.64
  face 729.90
  fascia (lata) (postural) 728.89
    Dupuytren's 728.6
    palmar 728.6
    plantar 728.71
  finger NEC 736.29
    congenital 755.59
    joint (*see also* Contraction, joint) 718.44
  flaccid, paralytic
    joint (*see also* Contraction, joint)
      718.4 ☑
    muscle 728.85
      ocular 378.50
  gallbladder (*see also* Obstruction, gallblad-
    der) 575.2
  hamstring 728.89
    tendon 727.81
  heart valve — *see* Endocarditis
  Hicks' 644.1 ☑
  hip (*see also* Contraction, joint) 718.4 ☑
  hourglass
    bladder 596.89

☑ **Additional Digit Required — Refer to the Tabular List for Digit Selection**   ▽ **Subterms under main terms may continue to next column or page**

2014 ICD-9-CM   ▶◀ **Revised Text**   ● **New Line**   ▲ **Revised Code**   **Volume 2 — 55**

Contraction, contracture, contracted — *continued*
　hourglass — *continued*
　　bladder — *continued*
　　　congenital 753.8
　　gallbladder (*see also* Obstruction, gall-
　　　bladder) 575.2
　　　congenital 751.69
　　stomach 536.8
　　　congenital 750.7
　　　psychogenic 306.4
　　uterus 661.4 ☑
　　　affecting fetus or newborn 763.7
　hysterical 300.11
　infantile (*see also* Epilepsy) 345.6 ☑
　internal os (*see also* Stricture, cervix) 622.4
　intestine (*see also* Obstruction, intestine)
　　560.9
　joint (abduction) (acquired) (adduction)
　　(flexion) (rotation) 718.40
　　ankle 718.47
　　congenital NEC 755.8
　　　generalized or multiple 754.89
　　　　lower limb joints 754.89
　　　hip (*see also* Subluxation, congenital,
　　　　hip) 754.32
　　　lower limb (including pelvic girdle)
　　　　not involving hip 754.89
　　　upper limb (including shoulder gir-
　　　　dle) 755.59
　　elbow 718.42
　　foot 718.47
　　hand 718.44
　　hip 718.45
　　hysterical 300.11
　　knee 718.46
　　multiple sites 718.49
　　pelvic region 718.45
　　shoulder (region) 718.41
　　specified site NEC 718.48
　　wrist 718.43
　kidney (granular) (secondary) (*see also*
　　Sclerosis, renal) 587
　　congenital 753.3
　　hydronephritic 591
　　pyelonephritic (*see also* Pyelitis, chronic)
　　　590.00
　　tuberculous (*see also* Tuberculosis)
　　　016.0 ☑
　ligament 728.89
　　congenital 756.89
　liver — *see* Cirrhosis, liver
　muscle (postinfectional) (postural) NEC
　　728.85
　　congenital 756.89
　　　sternocleidomastoid 754.1
　　extraocular 378.60
　　eye (extrinsic) (*see also* Strabismus) 378.9
　　　paralytic (*see also* Strabismus, paralyt-
　　　　ic) 378.50
　　flaccid 728.85
　　hysterical 300.11
　　ischemic (Volkmann's) 958.6
　　paralytic 728.85
　　posttraumatic 958.6
　　psychogenic 306.0
　　　specified as conversion reaction
　　　　300.11
　　myotonic 728.85
　neck (*see also* Torticollis) 723.5
　　congenital 754.1
　　psychogenic 306.0
　ocular muscle (*see also* Strabismus) 378.9
　　paralytic (*see also* Strabismus, paralytic)
　　　378.50
　organ or site, congenital NEC — *see* Atresia
　outlet (pelvis) — *see* Contraction, pelvis
　palmar fascia 728.6
　paralytic
　　joint (*see also* Contraction, joint)
　　　718.4 ☑
　　muscle 728.85
　　　ocular (*see also* Strabismus, paralytic)
　　　　378.50
　pelvis (acquired) (general) 738.6
　　affecting fetus or newborn 763.1

Contraction, contracture, contracted —
　continued
　pelvis — *continued*
　　complicating delivery 653.1 ☑
　　　causing obstructed labor 660.1 ☑
　　　generally contracted 653.1 ☑
　　　　causing obstructed labor
　　　　　660.1 ☑
　　　inlet 653.2 ☑
　　　　causing obstructed labor
　　　　　660.1 ☑
　　　midpelvic 653.8 ☑
　　　　causing obstructed labor
　　　　　660.1 ☑
　　　midplane 653.8 ☑
　　　　causing obstructed labor
　　　　　660.1 ☑
　　　outlet 653.3 ☑
　　　　causing obstructed labor
　　　　　660.1 ☑
　plantar fascia 728.71
　premature
　　atrial 427.61
　　auricular 427.61
　　auriculoventricular 427.61
　　heart (junctional) (nodal) 427.60
　　supraventricular 427.61
　　ventricular 427.69
　prostate 602.8
　pylorus (*see also* Pylorospasm) 537.81
　rectosigmoid (*see also* Obstruction, intes-
　　tine) 560.9
　rectum, rectal (sphincter) 564.89
　　psychogenic 306.4
　ring (Bandl's) 661.4 ☑
　　affecting fetus or newborn 763.7
　scar — *see* Cicatrix
　sigmoid (*see also* Obstruction, intestine)
　　560.9
　socket, eye 372.64
　spine (*see also* Curvature, spine) 737.9
　stomach 536.8
　　hourglass 536.8
　　　congenital 750.7
　　psychogenic 306.4
　tendon (sheath) (*see also* Short, tendon)
　　727.81
　toe 735.8
　ureterovesical orifice (postinfectional) 593.3
　urethra 599.84
　uterus 621.8
　　abnormal 661.9 ☑
　　　affecting fetus or newborn 763.7
　　clonic, hourglass or tetanic 661.4 ☑
　　　affecting fetus or newborn 763.7
　　dyscoordinate 661.4 ☑
　　　affecting fetus or newborn 763.7
　　hourglass 661.4 ☑
　　　affecting fetus or newborn 763.7
　　hypotonic NEC 661.2 ☑
　　　affecting fetus or newborn 763.7
　　incoordinate 661.4 ☑
　　　affecting fetus or newborn 763.7
　　inefficient or poor 661.2 ☑
　　　affecting fetus or newborn 763.7
　　irregular 661.2 ☑
　　　affecting fetus or newborn 763.7
　　tetanic 661.4 ☑
　　　affecting fetus or newborn 763.7
　vagina (outlet) 623.2
　vesical 596.89
　　neck or urethral orifice 596.0
　visual field, generalized 368.45
　Volkmann's (ischemic) 958.6
Contusion (skin surface intact) 924.9
　with
　　crush injury — *see* Crush
　　dislocation — *see* Dislocation, by site
　　fracture — *see* Fracture, by site
　　internal injury (*see also* Injury, internal,
　　　by site)
　　　heart — *see* Contusion, cardiac
　　　kidney — *see* Contusion, kidney
　　　liver — *see* Contusion, liver
　　　lung — *see* Contusion, lung
　　　spleen — *see* Contusion, spleen

Contusion — *continued*
　with — *continued*
　　intracranial injury — *see* Injury, intracra-
　　　nial
　　nerve injury — *see* Injury, nerve
　　open wound — *see* Wound, open, by
　　　site
　abdomen, abdominal (muscle) (wall) 922.2
　　organ(s) NEC 868.00
　adnexa, eye NEC 921.9
　ankle 924.21
　　with other parts of foot 924.20
　arm 923.9
　　lower (with elbow) 923.10
　　upper 923.03
　　　with shoulder or axillary region
　　　　923.09
　auditory canal (external) (meatus) (and
　　other part(s) of neck, scalp, or face,
　　except eye) 920
　auricle, ear (and other part(s) of neck, scalp,
　　or face except eye) 920
　axilla 923.02
　　with shoulder or upper arm 923.09
　back 922.31
　bone NEC 924.9
　brain (cerebral) (membrane) (with hemor-
　　rhage) 851.8 ☑

> **Note** — Use the following fifth–digit
> subclassification with categories
> 851–854:
>
> 0　unspecified state of consciousness
>
> 1　with no loss of consciousness
>
> 2　with brief [less than one hour]
> 　　loss of consciousness
>
> 3　with moderate [1–24 hours] loss
> 　　of consciousness
>
> 4　with prolonged [more than 24
> 　　hours] loss of consciousness and
> 　　return to pre–existing conscious
> 　　level
>
> 5　with prolonged [more than 24
> 　　hours] loss of consciousness,
> 　　without return to pre–existing
> 　　conscious level
>
> Use fifth–digit 5 to designate when a
> patient is unconscious and dies before
> regaining consciousness, regardless of
> the duration of the loss of consciousness
>
> 6　with loss of consciousness of un-
> 　　specified duration
>
> 9　with concussion, unspecified

　　with
　　　open intracranial wound 851.9 ☑
　　　skull fracture — *see* Fracture, skull,
　　　　by site
　　cerebellum 851.4 ☑
　　　with open intracranial wound
　　　　851.5 ☑
　　cortex 851.0 ☑
　　　with open intracranial wound
　　　　851.1 ☑
　　occipital lobe 851.4 ☑
　　　with open intracranial wound
　　　　851.5 ☑
　　stem 851.4 ☑
　　　with open intracranial wound
　　　　851.5 ☑
　breast 922.0
　brow (and other part(s) of neck, scalp, or
　　face, except eye) 920
　buttock 922.32
　canthus 921.1
　cardiac 861.01
　　with open wound into thorax 861.11
　cauda equina (spine) 952.4
　cerebellum — *see* Contusion, brain, cerebel-
　　lum
　cerebral — *see* Contusion, brain
　cheek(s) (and other part(s) of neck, scalp, or
　　face, except eye) 920

Contusion — *continued*
　chest (wall) 922.1
　chin (and other part(s) of neck, scalp, or face,
　　except eye) 920
　clitoris 922.4
　conjunctiva 921.1
　conus medullaris (spine) 952.4
　cornea 921.3
　corpus cavernosum 922.4
　cortex (brain) (cerebral) — *see* Contusion,
　　brain, cortex
　costal region 922.1
　ear (and other part(s) of neck, scalp, or face
　　except eye) 920
　elbow 923.11
　　with forearm 923.10
　epididymis 922.4
　epigastric region 922.2
　eyeball 921.3
　eyelid(s) (and periocular area) 921.1
　eye NEC 921.9
　face (and neck, or scalp, any part, except
　　eye) 920
　femoral triangle 922.2
　fetus or newborn 772.6
　finger(s) (nail) (subungual) 923.3
　flank 922.2
　foot (with ankle) (excluding toe(s)) 924.20
　forearm (and elbow) 923.10
　forehead (and other part(s) of neck, scalp,
　　or face, except eye) 920
　genital organs, external 922.4
　globe (eye) 921.3
　groin 922.2
　gum(s) (and other part(s) of neck, scalp, or
　　face, except eye) 920
　hand(s) (except fingers alone) 923.20
　head (any part, except eye) (and face) (and
　　neck) 920
　heart — *see* Contusion, cardiac
　heel 924.20
　hip 924.01
　　with thigh 924.00
　iliac region 922.2
　inguinal region 922.2
　internal organs (abdomen, chest, or pelvis)
　　NEC — *see* Injury, internal, by site
　interscapular region 922.33
　iris (eye) 921.3
　kidney 866.01
　　with open wound into cavity 866.11
　knee 924.11
　　with lower leg 924.10
　labium (majus) (minus) 922.4
　lacrimal apparatus, gland, or sac 921.1
　larynx (and other part(s) of neck, scalp, or
　　face, except eye) 920
　late effect — *see* Late, effects (of), contusion
　leg 924.5
　　lower (with knee) 924.10
　lens 921.3
　lingual (and other part(s) of neck, scalp, or
　　face, except eye) 920
　lip(s) (and other part(s) of neck, scalp, or
　　face, except eye) 920
　liver 864.01
　　with
　　　laceration — *see* Laceration, liver
　　　open wound into cavity 864.11
　lower extremity 924.5
　　multiple sites 924.4
　lumbar region 922.31
　lung 861.21
　　with open wound into thorax 861.31
　malar region (and other part(s) of neck,
　　scalp, or face, except eye) 920
　mandibular joint (and other part(s) of neck,
　　scalp, or face, except eye) 920
　mastoid region (and other part(s) of neck,
　　scalp, or face, except eye) 920
　membrane, brain — *see* Contusion, brain
　midthoracic region 922.1
　mouth (and other part(s) of neck, scalp, or
　　face, except eye) 920
　multiple sites (not classifiable to same three-
　　digit category) 924.8

☑ **Additional Digit Required** — Refer to the Tabular List for Digit Selection　　　　　　　　　ᵂ **Subterms under main terms may continue to next column or page**

56 — Volume 2　　　　　▶◀ Revised Text　　　　　● New Line　　　　　▲ Revised Code　　　　　**2014 ICD-9-CM**

Contusion — *continued*
  multiple sites — *continued*
    lower limb 924.4
    trunk 922.8
    upper limb 923.8
  muscle NEC 924.9
  myocardium — *see* Contusion, cardiac
  nasal (septum) (and other part(s) of neck,
    scalp, or face, except eye) 920
  neck (and scalp or face, any part, except eye)
    920
  nerve — *see* Injury, nerve, by site
  nose (and other part(s) of neck, scalp, or
    face, except eye) 920
  occipital region (scalp) (and neck or face,
    except eye) 920
    lobe — *see* Contusion, brain, occipital
      lobe
  orbit (region) (tissues) 921.2
  palate (soft) (and other part(s) of neck, scalp,
    or face, except eye) 920
  parietal region (scalp) (and neck or face,
    except eye) 920
    lobe — *see* Contusion, brain
  penis 922.4
  pericardium — *see* Contusion, cardiac
  perineum 922.4
  periocular area 921.1
  pharynx (and other part(s) of neck, scalp, or
    face, except eye) 920
  popliteal space (*see also* Contusion, knee)
    924.11
  prepuce 922.4
  pubic region 922.4
  pudenda 922.4
  pulmonary — *see* Contusion, lung
  quadriceps femoralis 924.00
  rib cage 922.1
  sacral region 922.32
  salivary ducts or glands (and other part(s)
    of neck, scalp, or face, except eye)
    920
  scalp (and neck, or face any part, except eye)
    920
  scapular region 923.01
    with shoulder or upper arm 923.09
  sclera (eye) 921.3
  scrotum 922.4
  shoulder 923.00
    with upper arm or axillar regions 923.09
  skin NEC 924.9
  skull 920
  spermatic cord 922.4
  spinal cord (*see also* Injury, spinal, by site)
    cauda equina 952.4
    conus medullaris 952.4
  spleen 865.01
    with open wound into cavity 865.11
  sternal region 922.1
  stomach — *see* Injury, internal, stomach
  subconjunctival 921.1
  subcutaneous NEC 924.9
  submaxillary region (and other part(s) of
    neck, scalp, or face, except eye) 920
  submental region (and other part(s) of neck,
    scalp, or face, except eye) 920
  subperiosteal NEC 924.9
  supraclavicular fossa (and other part(s) of
    neck, scalp, or face, except eye) 920
  supraorbital (and other part(s) of neck, scalp,
    or face, except eye) 920
  temple (region) (and other part(s) of neck,
    scalp, or face, except eye) 920
  testis 922.4
  thigh (and hip) 924.00
  thorax 922.1
    organ — *see* Injury, internal, intratho-
      racic
  throat (and other part(s) of neck, scalp, or
    face, except eye) 920
  thumb(s) (nail) (subungual) 923.3
  toe(s) (nail) (subungual) 924.3
  tongue (and other part(s) of neck, scalp, or
    face, except eye) 920
  trunk 922.9
    multiple sites 922.8

Contusion — *continued*
  trunk — *continued*
    specified site — *see* Contusion, by site
  tunica vaginalis 922.4
  tympanum (membrane) (and other part(s)
    of neck, scalp, or face, except eye)
    920
  upper extremity 923.9
    multiple sites 923.8
  uvula (and other part(s) of neck, scalp, or
    face, except eye) 920
  vagina 922.4
  vocal cord(s) (and other part(s) of neck,
    scalp, or face, except eye) 920
  vulva 922.4
  wrist 923.21
    with hand(s), except finger(s) alone
      923.20
Conus (any type) (congenital) 743.57
  acquired 371.60
  medullaris syndrome 336.8
Convalescence (following) V66.9
  chemotherapy V66.2
  medical NEC V66.5
  psychotherapy V66.3
  radiotherapy V66.1
  surgery NEC V66.0
  treatment (for) NEC V66.5
    combined V66.6
    fracture V66.4
    mental disorder NEC V66.3
    specified disorder NEC V66.5
Conversion
  closed surgical procedure to open proce-
    dure
    arthroscopic V64.43
    laparoscopic V64.41
    thoracoscopic V64.42
  hysteria, hysterical, any type 300.11
  neurosis, any 300.11
  reaction, any 300.11
Converter, tuberculosis (test reaction) 795.51
Convulsions (idiopathic) 780.39
  apoplectiform (*see also* Disease, cerebrovas-
    cular, acute) 436
  brain 780.39
  cerebral 780.39
  cerebrospinal 780.39
  due to trauma NEC — *see* Injury, intracranial
  eclamptic (*see also* Eclampsia) 780.39
  epileptic (*see also* Epilepsy) 345.9 ☑
  epileptiform (*see also* Seizure, epileptiform)
    780.39
  epileptoid (*see also* Seizure, epileptiform)
    780.39
  ether
    anesthetic
      correct substance properly adminis-
        tered 780.39
      overdose or wrong substance given
        968.2
    other specified type — *see* Table of
      Drugs and Chemicals
  febrile (simple) 780.31
    complex 780.32
  generalized 780.39
  hysterical 300.11
  infantile 780.39
    epilepsy — *see* Epilepsy
  internal 780.39
  jacksonian (*see also* Epilepsy) 345.5 ☑
  myoclonic 333.2
  newborn 779.0
  paretic 094.1
  pregnancy (nephritic) (uremic) — *see*
    Eclampsia, pregnancy
  psychomotor (*see also* Epilepsy) 345.4 ☑
  puerperal, postpartum — *see* Eclampsia,
    pregnancy
  recurrent 780.39
    epileptic — *see* Epilepsy
  reflex 781.0
  repetitive 780.39
    epileptic — *see* Epilepsy
  salaam (*see also* Epilepsy) 345.6 ☑
  scarlatinal 034.1

Convulsions — *continued*
  spasmodic 780.39
  tetanus, tetanic (*see also* Tetanus) 037
  thymic 254.8
  uncinate 780.39
  uremic 586
Convulsive — *see also* Convulsions
  disorder or state 780.39
    epileptic — *see* Epilepsy
    equivalent, abdominal (*see also* Epilepsy)
      345.5 ☑
Cooke-Apert-Gallais syndrome (adrenogeni-
    tal) 255.2
Cooley's anemia (erythroblastic) 282.44
Coolie itch 126.9
Cooper's
  disease 610.1
  hernia — *see* Hernia, Cooper's
Coordination disturbance 781.3
Copper wire arteries, retina 362.13
Copra itch 133.8
Coprolith 560.39
Coprophilia 302.89
Coproporphyria, hereditary 277.1
Coprostasis 560.32
  with hernia (*see also* Hernia, by site, with
    obstruction)
    gangrenous — *see* Hernia, by site, with
      gangrene
Cor
  biloculare 745.7
  bovinum — *see* Hypertrophy, cardiac
  bovis (*see also* Hypertrophy, cardiac)
  pulmonale (chronic) 416.9
    acute 415.0
  triatriatum, triatrium 746.82
  triloculare 745.8
    biatriatum 745.3
    biventriculare 745.69
Corbus' disease 607.1
Cord — *see also* condition
  around neck (tightly) (with compression)
    affecting fetus or newborn 762.5
    complicating delivery 663.1 ☑
      without compression 663.3 ☑
        affecting fetus or newborn 762.6
  bladder NEC 344.61
    tabetic 094.0
  prolapse
    affecting fetus or newborn 762.4
    complicating delivery 663.0 ☑
Cord's angiopathy — *see also* Tuberculosis
  017.3 ☑ [362.18]
Cordis ectopia 746.87
Corditis (spermatic) 608.4
Corectopia 743.46
Cori type glycogen storage disease — *see*
  Disease, glycogen storage
Cork-handlers' disease or lung 495.3
Corkscrew esophagus 530.5
Corlett's pyosis (impetigo) 684
Corn (infected) 700
Cornea — *see also* condition
  donor V59.5
  guttata (dystrophy) 371.57
  plana 743.41
Cornelia de Lange's syndrome (Amsterdam
    dwarf, intellectual disabilities, and
    brachycephaly) 759.89
Cornual gestation or pregnancy — *see*
  Pregnancy, cornual
Cornu cutaneum 702.8
Coronary (artery) — *see also* condition
  arising from aorta or pulmonary trunk
    746.85
Corpora — *see also* condition
  amylacea (prostate) 602.8
  cavernosa — *see* condition
Corpulence — *see* Obesity
Corpus — *see* condition
Corrigan's disease — *see* Insufficiency, aortic
Corrosive burn — *see* Burn, by site
Corsican fever — *see also* Malaria 084.6
Cortical — *see also* condition
  blindness 377.75
  necrosis, kidney (bilateral) 583.6

Corticoadrenal — *see* condition
Corticosexual syndrome 255.2
Coryza (acute) 460
  with grippe or influenza (*see also* Influenza)
    487.1
  syphilitic 095.8
    congenital (chronic) 090.0
Costen's syndrome or complex 524.60
Costiveness — *see also* Constipation 564.00
Costochondritis 733.6
Cotard's syndrome (paranoia) 297.1
Cot death 798.0
Cotia virus 059.8
Cotungo's disease 724.3
Cough 786.2
  with hemorrhage (*see also* Hemoptysis)
    786.39
  affected 786.2
  bronchial 786.2
    with grippe or influenza (*see also* Influen-
      za) 487.1
  chronic 786.2
  epidemic 786.2
  functional 306.1
  hemorrhagic 786.39
  hysterical 300.11
  laryngeal, spasmodic 786.2
  nervous 786.2
  psychogenic 306.1
  smokers' 491.0
  tea tasters' 112.89
Counseling NEC V65.40
  without complaint or sickness V65.49
  abuse victim NEC V62.89
    child V61.21
    partner V61.11
    spouse V61.11
  child abuse, maltreatment, or neglect
    V61.21
  contraceptive NEC V25.09
    device (intrauterine) V25.02
    maintenance V25.40
      intrauterine contraceptive device
        V25.42
      oral contraceptive (pill) V25.41
      specified type NEC V25.49
      subdermal implantable V25.43
    management NEC V25.9
    oral contraceptive (pill) V25.01
      emergency V25.03
      postcoital V25.03
    prescription NEC V25.02
      oral contraceptive (pill) V25.01
        emergency V25.03
        postcoital V25.03
      repeat prescription V25.41
    repeat prescription V25.40
    subdermal implantable V25.43
    surveillance NEC V25.40
  dietary V65.3
  exercise V65.41
  expectant parent(s)
    pediatric pre-adoption visit V65.11
    pediatric pre-birth visit V65.11
  explanation of
    investigation finding NEC V65.49
    medication NEC V65.49
  family planning V25.09
    natural
      procreative V26.41
      to avoid pregnancy V25.04
  for nonattending third party V65.19
  genetic V26.33
  gonorrhea V65.45
  health (advice) (education) (instruction) NEC
    V65.49
  HIV V65.44
  human immunodeficiency virus V65.44
  injury prevention V65.43
  insulin pump training V65.46
  marital V61.10
  medical (for) V65.9
    boarding school resident V60.6
    condition not demonstrated V65.5
    feared complaint and no disease found
      V65.5

☑ **Additional Digit Required — Refer to the Tabular List for Digit Selection**

🔻 **Subterms under main terms may continue to next column or page**

Counseling — *continued*
  medical — *continued*
    institutional resident V60.6
    on behalf of another V65.19
    person living alone V60.3
  natural family planning
    procreative V26.41
    to avoid pregnancy V25.04
  parent (guardian)-child conflict V61.20
    adopted child V61.24
    biological child V61.23
    foster child V61.25
    specified problem NEC V61.29
  partner abuse
    perpetrator V61.12
    victim V61.11
  pediatric
    pre-adoption visit for adoptive parent(s) V65.11
    pre-birth visit for expectant parents V65.11
  perpetrator of
    child abuse V62.83
      parental V61.22
    partner abuse V61.12
    spouse abuse V61.12
  procreative V65.49
  sex NEC V65.49
    transmitted disease NEC V65.45
      HIV V65.44
  specified reason NEC V65.49
  spousal abuse
    perpetrator V61.12
    victim V61.11
  substance use and abuse V65.42
  syphilis V65.45
  victim (of)
    abuse NEC V62.89
    child abuse V61.21
    partner abuse V61.11
    spousal abuse V61.11
Coupled rhythm 427.89
Couvelaire uterus (complicating delivery) — *see* Placenta, separation
Cowper's gland — *see* condition
Cowperitis — *see also* Urethritis 597.89
  gonorrheal (acute) 098.0
    chronic or duration of 2 months or over 098.2
Cowpox (abortive) 051.01
  due to vaccination 999.0
  eyelid 051.01 *[373.5]*
    postvaccination 999.0 *[373.5]*
Coxa
  plana 732.1
  valga (acquired) 736.31
    congenital 755.61
    late effect of rickets 268.1
  vara (acquired) 736.32
    congenital 755.62
    late effect of rickets 268.1
Coxae malum senilis 715.25
Coxalgia (nontuberculous) 719.45
  tuberculous (*see also* Tuberculosis) 015.1 ☑ *[730.85]*
Coxalgic pelvis 736.30
Coxitis 716.65
Coxsackie (infection) (virus) 079.2
  central nervous system NEC 048
  endocarditis 074.22
  enteritis 008.67
  meningitis (aseptic) 047.0
  myocarditis 074.23
  pericarditis 074.21
  pharyngitis 074.0
  pleurodynia 074.1
  specific disease NEC 074.8
Crabs, meaning pubic lice 132.2
Crack baby 760.75
Cracked
  nipple 611.2
    puerperal, postpartum 676.1 ☑
  tooth 521.81
Cradle cap 690.11
Craft neurosis 300.89
Craigiasis 007.8

Cramp(s) 729.82
  abdominal 789.0 ☑
  bathing 994.1
  colic 789.7
    infantile 789.7
    psychogenic 306.4
  due to immersion 994.1
  extremity (lower) (upper) NEC 729.82
  fireman 992.2
  heat 992.2
  hysterical 300.11
  immersion 994.1
  intestinal 789.0 ☑
    psychogenic 306.4
  linotypist's 300.89
    organic 333.84
  muscle (extremity) (general) 729.82
    due to immersion 994.1
    hysterical 300.11
  occupational (hand) 300.89
    organic 333.84
  psychogenic 307.89
  salt depletion 276.1
  sleep related leg 327.52
  stoker 992.2
  stomach 789.0 ☑
  telegraphers' 300.89
    organic 333.84
  typists' 300.89
    organic 333.84
  uterus 625.8
    menstrual 625.3
  writers' 333.84
    organic 333.84
    psychogenic 300.89
Cranial — *see* condition
Cranioclasis, fetal 763.89
Craniocleidodysostosis 755.59
Craniofenestria (skull) 756.0
Craniolacunia (skull) 756.0
Craniopagus 759.4
Craniopathy, metabolic 733.3
Craniopharyngeal — *see* condition
Craniopharyngioma (M9350/1) 237.0
Craniorachischisis (totalis) 740.1
Cranioschisis 756.0
Craniostenosis 756.0
Craniosynostosis 756.0
Craniotabes (cause unknown) 733.3
  rachitic 268.1
  syphilitic 090.5
Craniotomy, fetal 763.89
Cranium — *see* condition
Craw-craw 125.3
CRBSI (catheter-related bloodstream infection) 999.31
Creaking joint 719.60
  ankle 719.67
  elbow 719.62
  foot 719.67
  hand 719.64
  hip 719.65
  knee 719.66
  multiple sites 719.69
  pelvic region 719.65
  shoulder (region) 719.61
  specified site NEC 719.68
  wrist 719.63
Creeping
  eruption 126.9
  palsy 335.21
  paralysis 335.21
Crenated tongue 529.8
Creotoxism 005.9
Crepitus
  caput 756.0
  joint 719.60
    ankle 719.67
    elbow 719.62
    foot 719.67
    hand 719.64
    hip 719.65
    knee 719.66
    multiple sites 719.69
    pelvic region 719.65
    shoulder (region) 719.61

Crepitus — *continued*
  joint — *continued*
    specified site NEC 719.68
    wrist 719.63
Crescent or conus choroid, congenital 743.57
Cretin, cretinism (athyrotic) (congenital) (endemic) (metabolic) (nongoitrous) (sporadic) 243
  goitrous (sporadic) 246.1
  pelvis (dwarf type) (male type) 243
    with disproportion (fetopelvic) 653.1 ☑
      affecting fetus or newborn 763.1
      causing obstructed labor 660.1 ☑
        affecting fetus or newborn 763.1
  pituitary 253.3
Cretinoid degeneration 243
Creutzfeldt-Jakob disease (CJD) (syndrome) 046.19
  with dementia
    with behavioral disturbance 046.19 *[294.11]*
    without behavioral disturbance 046.19 *[294.10]*
  familial 046.19
  iatrogenic 046.19
  specified NEC 046.19
  sporadic 046.19
  variant (vCJD) 046.11
    with dementia
      with behavioral disturbance 046.11 *[294.11]*
      without behavioral disturbance 046.11 *[294.10]*
Cri-du-chat syndrome 758.31
Crib death 798.0
Cribriform hymen 752.49
Crigler-Najjar disease or syndrome (congenital hyperbilirubinemia) 277.4
Crimean hemorrhagic fever 065.0
Criminalism 301.7
Crisis
  abdomen 789.0 ☑
  addisonian (acute adrenocortical insufficiency) 255.41
  adrenal (cortical) 255.41
  asthmatic — *see* Asthma
  brain, cerebral (*see also* Disease, cerebrovascular, acute) 436
  celiac 579.0
  Dietl's 593.4
  emotional NEC 309.29
    acute reaction to stress 308.0
    adjustment reaction 309.9
    specific to childhood or adolescence 313.9
  gastric (tabetic) 094.0
  glaucomatocyclitic 364.22
  heart (*see also* Failure, heart) 428.9
  hypertensive — *see* Hypertension
  nitritoid
    correct substance properly administered 458.29
    overdose or wrong substance given or taken 961.1
  oculogyric 378.87
    psychogenic 306.7
  Pel's 094.0
  psychosexual identity 302.6
  rectum 094.0
  renal 593.81
  sickle cell 282.62
  stomach (tabetic) 094.0
  tabetic 094.0
  thyroid (*see also* Thyrotoxicosis) 242.9 ☑
  thyrotoxic (*see also* Thyrotoxicosis) 242.9 ☑
  vascular — *see* Disease, cerebrovascular, acute
Crocq's disease (acrocyanosis) 443.89
Crohn's disease — *see also* Enteritis, regional 555.9
Cronkhite-Canada syndrome 211.3
Crooked septum, nasal 470
Cross
  birth (of fetus) complicating delivery 652.3 ☑
    with successful version 652.1 ☑

Cross — *continued*
  birth complicating delivery — *continued*
    causing obstructed labor 660.0 ☑
  bite, anterior or posterior 524.27
  eye (*see also* Esotropia) 378.00
Crossed ectopia of kidney 753.3
Crossfoot 754.50
Croup, croupous (acute) (angina) (catarrhal) (infective) (inflammatory) (laryngeal) (membranous) (nondiphtheritic) (pseudomembranous) 464.4
  asthmatic (*see also* Asthma) 493.9 ☑
  bronchial 466.0
  diphtheritic (membranous) 032.3
  false 478.75
  spasmodic 478.75
    diphtheritic 032.3
  stridulous 478.75
    diphtheritic 032.3
Crouzon's disease (craniofacial dysostosis) 756.0
Crowding, teeth 524.31
CRST syndrome (cutaneous systemic sclerosis) 710.1
Cruchet's disease (encephalitis lethargica) 049.8
Cruelty in children — *see also* Disturbance, conduct 312.9
Crural ulcer — *see also* Ulcer, lower extremity 707.10
Crush, crushed, crushing (injury) 929.9
  abdomen 926.19
    internal — *see* Injury, internal, abdomen
  ankle 928.21
    with other parts of foot 928.20
  arm 927.9
    lower (and elbow) 927.10
    upper 927.03
      with shoulder or axillary region 927.09
  axilla 927.02
    with shoulder or upper arm 927.09
  back 926.11
  breast 926.19
  buttock 926.12
  cheek 925.1
  chest — *see* Injury, internal, chest
  ear 925.1
  elbow 927.11
    with forearm 927.10
  face 925.1
  finger(s) 927.3
    with hand(s) 927.20
      and wrist(s) 927.21
  flank 926.19
  foot, excluding toe(s) alone (with ankle) 928.20
  forearm (and elbow) 927.10
  genitalia, external (female) (male) 926.0
    internal — *see* Injury, internal, genital organ NEC
  hand, except finger(s) alone (and wrist) 927.20
  head — *see* Fracture, skull, by site
  heel 928.20
  hip 928.01
    with thigh 928.00
  internal organ (abdomen, chest, or pelvis) — *see* Injury, internal, by site
  knee 928.11
    with leg, lower 928.10
  labium (majus) (minus) 926.0
  larynx 925.2
  late effect — *see* Late, effects (of), crushing
  leg 928.9
    lower 928.10
      and knee 928.11
    upper 928.00
  limb
    lower 928.9
      multiple sites 928.8
    upper 927.9
      multiple sites 927.8
  multiple sites NEC 929.0
  neck 925.2
  nerve — *see* Injury, nerve, by site

☑ Additional Digit Required — Refer to the Tabular List for Digit Selection   ▽ Subterms under main terms may continue to next column or page

58 — Volume 2   ▶◀ Revised Text   ● New Line   ▲ Revised Code   2014 ICD-9-CM

Crush, crushed, crushing — *continued*
  nose 802.0
    open 802.1
  penis 926.0
  pharynx 925.2
  scalp 925.1
  scapular region 927.01
    with shoulder or upper arm 927.09
  scrotum 926.0
  shoulder 927.00
    with upper arm or axillary region 927.09
  skull or cranium — *see* Fracture, skull, by
    site
  spinal cord — *see* Injury, spinal, by site
  syndrome (complication of trauma) 958.5
  testis 926.0
  thigh (with hip) 928.00
  throat 925.2
  thumb(s) (and fingers) 927.3
  toe(s) 928.3
    with foot 928.20
      and ankle 928.21
  tonsil 925.2
  trunk 926.9
    chest — *see* Injury, internal, intrathoracic
      organs NEC
    internal organ — *see* Injury, internal, by
      site
    multiple sites 926.8
    specified site NEC 926.19
  vulva 926.0
  wrist 927.21
    with hand(s), except fingers alone 927.20
Crusta lactea 690.11
Crusts 782.8
Crutch paralysis 953.4
Cruveilhier-Baumgarten cirrhosis, disease,
  or syndrome 571.5
Cruveilhier's disease 335.21
Cruz-Chagas disease — *see also* Trypanosomi-
  asis 086.2
Crying
  constant, continuous
    adolescent 780.95
    adult 780.95
    baby 780.92
    child 780.95
    infant 780.92
    newborn 780.92
  excessive
    adolescent 780.95
    adult 780.95
    baby 780.92
    child 780.95
    infant 780.92
    newborn 780.92
Cryofibrinogenemia 273.2
Cryoglobulinemia (mixed) 273.2
Crypt (anal) (rectal) 569.49
Cryptitis (anal) (rectal) 569.49
Cryptococcosis (European) (pulmonary) (systemic) 117.5
Cryptococcus 117.5
  epidermicus 117.5
  neoformans, infection by 117.5
Cryptopapillitis (anus) 569.49
Cryptophthalmos (eyelid) 743.06
Cryptorchid, cryptorchism, cryptorchidism
  752.51
Cryptosporidiosis 007.4
  hepatobiliary 136.8
  respiratory 136.8
Cryptotia 744.29
Crystallopathy
  calcium pyrophosphate (*see also* Arthritis)
    275.49 *[712.2]* ☑
  dicalcium phosphate (*see also* Arthritis)
    275.49 *[712.1]* ☑
  gouty 274.00
  pyrophosphate NEC (*see also* Arthritis)
    275.49 *[712.2]* ☑
  uric acid 274.00
Crystalluria 791.9
Csillag's disease (lichen sclerosis et atrophicus)
  701.0
Cuban itch 050.1

Cubitus
  valgus (acquired) 736.01
    congenital 755.59
    late effect of rickets 268.1
  varus (acquired) 736.02
    congenital 755.59
    late effect of rickets 268.1
Cultural deprivation V62.4
Cupping of optic disc 377.14
Curling esophagus 530.5
Curling's ulcer — *see* Ulcer, duodenum
Curschmann (-Batten) (-Steinert) disease or
  syndrome 359.21
Curvature
  organ or site, congenital NEC — *see* Distor-
    tion
  penis (lateral) 752.69
  Pott's (spinal) (*see also* Tuberculosis)
    015.0 ☑ *[737.43]*
  radius, idiopathic, progressive (congenital)
    755.54
  spine (acquired) (angular) (idiopathic) (incor-
    rect) (postural) 737.9
    congenital 754.2
    due to or associated with
      Charcôt-Marie-Tooth disease
        356.1 *[737.40]*
      mucopolysaccharidosis
        277.5 *[737.40]*
      neurofibromatosis 237.71 *[737.40]*
      osteitis
        deformans 731.0 *[737.40]*
        fibrosa cystica 252.01 *[737.40]*
      osteoporosis (*see also* Osteoporosis)
        733.00 *[737.40]*
      poliomyelitis (*see also* Poliomyelitis)
        138 *[737.40]*
      tuberculosis (Pott's curvature) (*see*
        also Tuberculosis)
        015.0 ☑ *[737.43]*
    kyphoscoliotic (*see also* Kyphoscoliosis)
      737.30
    kyphotic (*see also* Kyphosis) 737.10
    late effect of rickets 268.1 *[737.40]*
    Pott's 015.0 ☑ *[737.40]*
    scoliotic (*see also* Scoliosis) 737.30
    specified NEC 737.8
    tuberculous 015.0 ☑ *[737.40]*
Cushing's
  basophilism, disease, or syndrome (iatro-
    genic) (idiopathic) (pituitary ba-
    sophilism) (pituitary dependent)
    255.0
  ulcer — *see* Ulcer, peptic
Cushingoid due to steroid therapy
  correct substance properly administered
    255.0
  overdose or wrong substance given or taken
    962.0
Cut (external) — *see* Wound, open, by site
Cutaneous — *see also* condition
  hemorrhage 782.7
  horn (cheek) (eyelid) (mouth) 702.8
  larva migrans 126.9
Cutis — *see also* condition
  hyperelastic 756.83
    acquired 701.8
  laxa 756.83
    senilis 701.8
  marmorata 782.61
  osteosis 709.3
  pendula 756.83
    acquired 701.8
  rhomboidalis nuchae 701.8
  verticis gyrata 757.39
    acquired 701.8
Cyanopathy, newborn 770.83
Cyanosis 782.5
  autotoxic 289.7
  common atrioventricular canal 745.69
  congenital 770.83
  conjunctiva 372.71
  due to
    endocardial cushion defect 745.60
    nonclosure, foramen botalli 745.5
    patent foramen botalli 745.5

Cyanosis — *continued*
  due to — *continued*
    persistent foramen ovale 745.5
    enterogenous 289.7
    fetus or newborn 770.83
    ostium primum defect 745.61
    paroxysmal digital 443.0
    retina, retinal 362.10
Cycle
  anovulatory 628.0
  menstrual, irregular 626.4
Cyclencephaly 759.89
Cyclical vomiting 536.2
  associated with migraine 346.2 ☑
  psychogenic 306.4
Cyclitic membrane 364.74
Cyclitis — *see also* Iridocyclitis 364.3
  acute 364.00
    primary 364.01
    recurrent 364.02
  chronic 364.10
    in
      sarcoidosis 135 *[364.11]*
      tuberculosis (*see also* Tuberculosis)
        017.3 ☑ *[364.11]*
  Fuchs' heterochromic 364.21
  granulomatous 364.10
  lens induced 364.23
  nongranulomatous 364.00
  posterior 363.21
  primary 364.01
  recurrent 364.02
  secondary (noninfectious) 364.04
    infectious 364.03
  subacute 364.00
    primary 364.01
    recurrent 364.02
Cyclokeratitis — *see* Keratitis
Cyclophoria 378.44
Cyclopia, cyclops 759.89
Cycloplegia 367.51
Cyclospasm 367.53
Cyclosporiasis 007.5
Cyclothymia 301.13
Cyclothymic personality 301.13
Cyclotropia 378.33
Cyesis — *see* Pregnancy
Cylindroma (M8200/3) — *see also* Neoplasm,
  by site, malignant
  eccrine dermal (M8200/0) — *see* Neoplasm,
    skin, benign
  skin (M8200/0) — *see* Neoplasm, skin, be-
    nign
Cylindruria 791.7
Cyllosoma 759.89
Cynanche
  diphtheritic 032.3
  tonsillaris 475
Cynorexia 783.6
Cyphosis — *see* Kyphosis
Cyprus fever — *see also* Brucellosis 023.9
Cyriax's syndrome (slipping rib) 733.99
Cyst (mucus) (retention) (serous) (simple)

> *Note* — *In general, cysts are not neo-*
> *plastic and are classified to the appro-*
> *priate category for disease of the speci-*
> *fied anatomical site. This generalization*
> *does not apply to certain types of cysts*
> *which are neoplastic in nature, for ex-*
> *ample, dermoid, nor does it apply to*
> *cysts of certain structures, for example,*
> *branchial cleft, which are classified as*
> *developmental anomalies.*
>
> *The following listing includes some of*
> *the most frequently reported sites of*
> *cysts as well as qualifiers which indicate*
> *the type of cyst. The latter qualifiers*
> *usually are not repeated under the*
> *anatomical sites. Since the code assign-*
> *ment for a given site may vary depend-*
> *ing upon the type of cyst, the coder*
> *should refer to the listings under the*
> *specified type of cyst before considera-*
> *tion is given to the site.*

  accessory, fallopian tube 752.11

Cyst — *continued*
  adenoid (infected) 474.8
  adrenal gland 255.8
    congenital 759.1
  air, lung 518.89
  allantoic 753.7
  alveolar process (jaw bone) 526.2
  amnion, amniotic 658.8 ☑
  anterior chamber (eye) 364.60
    exudative 364.62
    implantation (surgical) (traumatic)
      364.61
    parasitic 360.13
  anterior nasopalatine 526.1
  antrum 478.19
  anus 569.49
  apical (periodontal) (tooth) 522.8
  appendix 543.9
  arachnoid, brain 348.0
  arytenoid 478.79
  auricle 706.2
  Baker's (knee) 727.51
    tuberculous (*see also* Tuberculosis)
      015.2 ☑
  Bartholin's gland or duct 616.2
  bile duct (*see also* Disease, biliary) 576.8
  bladder (multiple) (trigone) 596.89
  Blessig's 362.62
  blood, endocardial (*see also* Endocarditis)
    424.90
  blue dome 610.0
  bone (local) 733.20
    aneurysmal 733.22
    jaw 526.2
      developmental (odontogenic) 526.0
      fissural 526.1
      latent 526.89
    solitary 733.21
    unicameral 733.21
  brain 348.0
    congenital 742.4
    hydatid (*see also* Echinococcus) 122.9
    third ventricle (colloid) 742.4
  branchial (cleft) 744.42
  branchiogenic 744.42
  breast (benign) (blue dome) (pedunculated)
    (solitary) (traumatic) 610.0
    involution 610.4
    sebaceous 610.8
  broad ligament (benign) 620.8
    embryonic 752.11
  bronchogenic (mediastinal) (sequestration)
    518.89
    congenital 748.4
  buccal 528.4
  bulbourethral gland (Cowper's) 599.89
  bursa, bursal 727.49
    pharyngeal 478.26
  calcifying odontogenic (M9301/0) 213.1
    upper jaw (bone) 213.0
  canal of Nuck (acquired) (serous) 629.1
    congenital 752.41
  canthus 372.75
  carcinomatous (M8010/3) — *see* Neoplasm,
    by site, malignant
  cartilage (joint) — *see* Derangement, joint
  cauda equina 336.8
  cavum septi pellucidi NEC 348.0
  celomic (pericardium) 746.89
  cerebellopontine (angle) — *see* Cyst, brain
  cerebellum — *see* Cyst, brain
  cerebral — *see* Cyst, brain
  cervical lateral 744.42
  cervix 622.8
    embryonal 752.41
    nabothian (gland) 616.0
  chamber, anterior (eye) 364.60
    exudative 364.62
    implantation (surgical) (traumatic)
      364.61
    parasitic 360.13
  chiasmal, optic NEC (*see also* Lesion, chias-
    mal) 377.54
  chocolate (ovary) 617.1
  choledochal (congenital) 751.69
    acquired 576.8

☑ **Additional Digit Required** — **Refer to the Tabular List for Digit Selection**   ◥ **Subterms under main terms may continue to next column or page**

2014 ICD-9-CM   ▶◀ Revised Text   ● New Line   ▲ Revised Code   Volume 2 — 59

Cyst — *continued*
choledochus 751.69
chorion 658.8 ☑
choroid plexus 348.0
chyle, mesentery 457.8
ciliary body 364.60
   exudative 364.64
   implantation 364.61
   primary 364.63
clitoris 624.8
coccyx (*see also* Cyst, bone) 733.20
colloid
   third ventricle (brain) 742.4
   thyroid gland — *see* Goiter
colon 569.89
common (bile) duct (*see also* Disease, biliary) 576.8
congenital NEC 759.89
   adrenal glands 759.1
   epiglottis 748.3
   esophagus 750.4
   fallopian tube 752.11
   kidney 753.10
      multiple 753.19
      single 753.11
   larynx 748.3
   liver 751.62
   lung 748.4
   mediastinum 748.8
   ovary 752.0
   oviduct 752.11
   pancreas 751.7
   periurethral (tissue) 753.8
   prepuce NEC 752.69
      penis 752.69
   sublingual 750.26
   submaxillary gland 750.26
   thymus (gland) 759.2
   tongue 750.19
   ureterovesical orifice 753.4
   vulva 752.41
conjunctiva 372.75
cornea 371.23
corpora quadrigemina 348.0
corpus
   albicans (ovary) 620.2
   luteum (ruptured) 620.1
Cowper's gland (benign) (infected) 599.89
cranial meninges 348.0
craniobuccal pouch 253.8
craniopharyngeal pouch 253.8
cystic duct (*see also* Disease, gallbladder) 575.8
Cysticercus (any site) 123.1
Dandy-Walker 742.3
   with spina bifida (*see also* Spina bifida) 741.0 ☑
dental 522.8
   developmental 526.0
   eruption 526.0
   lateral periodontal 526.0
   primordial (keratocyst) 526.0
   root 522.8
dentigerous 526.0
   mandible 526.0
   maxilla 526.0
dermoid (M9084/0) (*see also* Neoplasm, by site, benign)
   with malignant transformation (M9084/3) 183.0
   implantation
      external area or site (skin) NEC 709.8
      iris 364.61
      skin 709.8
      vagina 623.8
      vulva 624.8
   mouth 528.4
   oral soft tissue 528.4
   sacrococcygeal 685.1
      with abscess 685.0
developmental of ovary, ovarian 752.0
dura (cerebral) 348.0
   spinal 349.2
ear (external) 706.2
echinococcal (*see also* Echinococcus) 122.9

Cyst — *continued*
embryonal
   cervix uteri 752.41
   genitalia, female external 752.41
   uterus 752.39
   vagina 752.41
endometrial 621.8
   ectopic 617.9
endometrium (uterus) 621.8
   ectopic — *see* Endometriosis
enteric 751.5
enterogenous 751.5
epidermal (inclusion) (*see also* Cyst, skin) 706.2
epidermoid (inclusion) (*see also* Cyst, skin) 706.2
   mouth 528.4
   not of skin — *see* Cyst, by site
   oral soft tissue 528.4
epididymis 608.89
epiglottis 478.79
epiphysis cerebri 259.8
epithelial (inclusion) (*see also* Cyst, skin) 706.2
epoophoron 752.11
eruption 526.0
esophagus 530.89
ethmoid sinus 478.19
eye (retention) 379.8
   congenital 743.03
   posterior segment, congenital 743.54
eyebrow 706.2
eyelid (sebaceous) 374.84
   infected 373.13
   sweat glands or ducts 374.84
falciform ligament (inflammatory) 573.8
fallopian tube 620.8
   congenital 752.11
female genital organs NEC 629.89
fimbrial (congenital) 752.11
fissural (oral region) 526.1
follicle (atretic) (graafian) (ovarian) 620.0
   nabothian (gland) 616.0
follicular (atretic) (ovarian) 620.0
   dentigerous 526.0
frontal sinus 478.19
gallbladder or duct 575.8
ganglion 727.43
Gartner's duct 752.41
gas, of mesentery 568.89
gingiva 523.8
gland of moll 374.84
globulomaxillary 526.1
graafian follicle 620.0
granulosal lutein 620.2
hemangiomatous (M9121/0) (*see also* Hemangioma) 228.00
hydatid (*see also* Echinococcus) 122.9
   fallopian tube (Morgagni) 752.11
   liver NEC 122.8
   lung NEC 122.9
   Morgagni 752.89
      fallopian tube 752.11
   specified site NEC 122.9
hymen 623.8
   embryonal 752.41
hypopharynx 478.26
hypophysis, hypophyseal (duct) (recurrent) 253.8
   cerebri 253.8
implantation (dermoid)
   anterior chamber (eye) 364.61
   external area or site (skin) NEC 709.8
   iris 364.61
   vagina 623.8
   vulva 624.8
incisor, incisive canal 526.1
inclusion (epidermal) (epithelial) (epidermoid) (mucous) (squamous) (*see also* Cyst, skin) 706.2
   not of skin — *see* Neoplasm, by site, benign
intestine (large) (small) 569.89
intracranial — *see* Cyst, brain
intraligamentous 728.89
   knee 717.89

Cyst — *continued*
intrasellar 253.8
iris (idiopathic) 364.60
   exudative 364.62
   implantation (surgical) (traumatic) 364.61
   miotic pupillary 364.55
   parasitic 360.13
Iwanoff's 362.62
jaw (bone) (aneurysmal) (extravasation) (hemorrhagic) (traumatic) 526.2
   developmental (odontogenic) 526.0
   fissural 526.1
keratin 706.2
kidney (congenital) 753.10
   acquired 593.2
   calyceal (*see also* Hydronephrosis) 591
   multiple 753.19
   pyelogenic (*see also* Hydronephrosis) 591
   simple 593.2
   single 753.11
   solitary (not congenital) 593.2
labium (majus) (minus) 624.8
   sebaceous 624.8
lacrimal
   apparatus 375.43
   gland or sac 375.12
larynx 478.79
lens 379.39
   congenital 743.39
lip (gland) 528.5
liver 573.8
   congenital 751.62
   hydatid (*see also* Echinococcus) 122.8
      granulosis 122.0
      multilocularis 122.5
lung 518.89
   congenital 748.4
   giant bullous 492.0
lutein 620.1
lymphangiomatous (M9173/0) 228.1
lymphoepithelial
   mouth 528.4
   oral soft tissue 528.4
macula 362.54
malignant (M8000/3) — *see* Neoplasm, by site, malignant
mammary gland (sweat gland) (*see also* Cyst, breast) 610.0
mandible 526.2
   dentigerous 526.0
   radicular 522.8
maxilla 526.2
   dentigerous 526.0
   radicular 522.8
median
   anterior maxillary 526.1
   palatal 526.1
mediastinum (congenital) 748.8
meibomian (gland) (retention) 373.2
   infected 373.12
membrane, brain 348.0
meninges (cerebral) 348.0
   spinal 349.2
meniscus knee 717.5
mesentery, mesenteric (gas) 568.89
   chyle 457.8
   gas 568.89
mesonephric duct 752.89
mesothelial
   peritoneum 568.89
   pleura (peritoneal) 568.89
milk 611.5
miotic pupillary (iris) 364.55
Morgagni (hydatid) 752.89
   fallopian tube 752.11
mouth 528.4
Müllerian duct 752.89
   appendix testis 608.89
   cervix (embryonal) 752.41
   fallopian tube 752.11
   prostatic utricle 599.89
   vagina (embryonal) 752.41
multilocular (ovary) (M8000/1) 239.5
myometrium 621.8

Cyst — *continued*
nabothian (follicle) (ruptured) 616.0
nasal sinus 478.19
nasoalveolar 528.4
nasolabial 528.4
nasopalatine (duct) 526.1
   anterior 526.1
nasopharynx 478.26
neoplastic (M8000/1) (*see also* Neoplasm, by site, unspecified nature)
   benign (M8000/0) — *see* Neoplasm, by site, benign
   uterus 621.8
nervous system — *see* Cyst, brain
neuroenteric 742.59
neuroepithelial ventricle 348.0
nipple 610.0
nose 478.19
   skin of 706.2
odontogenic, developmental 526.0
omentum (lesser) 568.89
   congenital 751.8
oral soft tissue (dermoid) (epidermoid) (lymphoepithelial) 528.4
ora serrata 361.19
orbit 376.81
ovary, ovarian (twisted) 620.2
   adherent 620.2
   chocolate 617.1
   corpus
      albicans 620.2
      luteum 620.1
   dermoid (M9084/0) 220
   developmental 752.0
   due to failure of involution NEC 620.2
   endometrial 617.1
   follicular (atretic) (graafian) (hemorrhagic) 620.0
   hemorrhagic 620.2
   in pregnancy or childbirth 654.4 ☑
      affecting fetus or newborn 763.89
      causing obstructed labor 660.2 ☑
         affecting fetus or newborn 763.1
   multilocular (M8000/1) 239.5
   pseudomucinous (M8470/0) 220
   retention 620.2
   serous 620.2
   theca lutein 620.2
   tuberculous (*see also* Tuberculosis) 016.6 ☑
   unspecified 620.2
oviduct 620.8
palatal papilla (jaw) 526.1
palate 526.1
   fissural 526.1
   median (fissural) 526.1
palatine, of papilla 526.1
pancreas, pancreatic 577.2
   congenital 751.7
   false 577.2
   hemorrhagic 577.2
   true 577.2
paralabral
   hip 718.85
   shoulder 840.7
paramesonephric duct — *see* Cyst, Müllerian duct
paranephric 593.2
para ovarian 752.11
paraphysis, cerebri 742.4
parasitic NEC 136.9
parathyroid (gland) 252.8
paratubal (fallopian) 620.8
paraurethral duct 599.89
paroophoron 752.11
parotid gland 527.6
   mucous extravasation or retention 527.6
parovarian 752.11
pars planus 364.60
   exudative 364.64
   primary 364.63
pelvis, female
   in pregnancy or childbirth 654.4 ☑
      affecting fetus or newborn 763.89
      causing obstructed labor 660.2 ☑
         affecting fetus or newborn 763.1

Cyst — continued
- penis (sebaceous) 607.89
- periapical 522.8
- pericardial (congenital) 746.89
  - acquired (secondary) 423.8
- pericoronal 526.0
- perineural (Tarlov's) 355.9
- periodontal 522.8
  - lateral 526.0
- peripancreatic 577.2
- peripelvic (lymphatic) 593.2
- periodontal 522.8
- peritoneum 568.89
  - chylous 457.8
- pharynx (wall) 478.26
- pilar 704.41
- pilonidal (infected) (rectum) 685.1
  - with abscess 685.0
  - malignant (M9084/3) 173.59
- pituitary (duct) (gland) 253.8
- placenta (amniotic) — see Placenta, abnormal
- pleura 519.8
- popliteal 727.51
- porencephalic 742.4
  - acquired 348.0
- postanal (infected) 685.1
  - with abscess 685.0
- posterior segment of eye, congenital 743.54
- postmastoidectomy cavity 383.31
- preauricular 744.47
- prepuce 607.89
  - congenital 752.69
- primordial (jaw) 526.0
- prostate 600.3
- pseudomucinous (ovary) (M8470/0) 220
- pudenda (sweat glands) 624.8
- pupillary, miotic 364.55
  - sebaceous 624.8
- radicular (residual) 522.8
- radiculodental 522.8
- ranular 527.6
- Rathke's pouch 253.8
- rectum (epithelium) (mucous) 569.49
- renal — see Cyst, kidney
- residual (radicular) 522.8
- retention (ovary) 620.2
- retina 361.19
  - macular 362.54
  - parasitic 360.13
  - primary 361.13
  - secondary 361.14
- retroperitoneal 568.89
- sacrococcygeal (dermoid) 685.1
  - with abscess 685.0
- salivary gland or duct 527.6
  - mucous extravasation or retention 527.6
- Sampson's 617.1
- sclera 379.19
- scrotum (sebaceous) 706.2
  - sweat glands 706.2
- sebaceous (duct) (gland) 706.2
  - breast 610.8
  - eyelid 374.84
  - genital organ NEC
    - female 629.89
    - male 608.89
  - scrotum 706.2
- semilunar cartilage (knee) (multiple) 717.5
- seminal vesicle 608.89
- serous (ovary) 620.2
- sinus (antral) (ethmoidal) (frontal) (maxillary) (nasal) (sphenoidal) 478.19
- Skene's gland 599.89
- skin (epidermal) (epidermoid, inclusion) (epithelial) (inclusion) (retention) (sebaceous) 706.2
  - breast 610.8
  - eyelid 374.84
  - genital organ NEC
    - female 629.89
    - male 608.89
  - neoplastic 216.3
  - scrotum 706.2
  - sweat gland or duct 705.89
- solitary
  - bone 733.21

Cyst — continued
- solitary — continued
  - kidney 593.2
- spermatic cord 608.89
- sphenoid sinus 478.19
- spinal meninges 349.2
- spine (see also Cyst, bone) 733.20
- spleen NEC 289.59
  - congenital 759.0
  - hydatid (see also Echinococcus) 122.9
- spring water (pericardium) 746.89
- subarachnoid 348.0
  - intrasellar 793.0
- subdural (cerebral) 348.0
  - spinal cord 349.2
- sublingual gland 527.6
  - mucous extravasation or retention 527.6
- submaxillary gland 527.6
  - mucous extravasation or retention 527.6
- suburethral 599.89
- suprarenal gland 255.8
- suprasellar — see Cyst, brain
- sweat gland or duct 705.89
- sympathetic nervous system 337.9
- synovial 727.40
  - popliteal space 727.51
- Tarlov's 355.9
- tarsal 373.2
- tendon (sheath) 727.42
- testis 608.89
- theca-lutein (ovary) 620.2
- Thornwaldt's, Tornwaldt's 478.26
- thymus (gland) 254.8
- thyroglossal (duct) (infected) (persistent) 759.2
- thyroid (gland) 246.2
  - adenomatous — see Goiter, nodular
  - colloid (see also Goiter) 240.9
- thyrolingual duct (infected) (persistent) 759.2
- tongue (mucous) 529.8
- tonsil 474.8
- tooth (dental root) 522.8
- trichilemmal (proliferating) 704.42
- tubo-ovarian 620.8
  - inflammatory 614.1
- tunica vaginalis 608.89
- turbinate (nose) (see also Cyst, bone) 733.20
- Tyson's gland (benign) (infected) 607.89
- umbilicus 759.89
- urachus 753.7
- ureter 593.89
- ureterovesical orifice 593.89
  - congenital 753.4
- urethra 599.84
- urethral gland (Cowper's) 599.89
- uterine
  - ligament 620.8
    - embryonic 752.11
  - tube 620.8
- uterus (body) (corpus) (recurrent) 621.8
  - embryonal 752.39
- utricle (ear) 386.8
  - prostatic 599.89
- utriculus masculinus 599.89
- vagina, vaginal (squamous cell) (wall) 623.8
  - embryonal 752.41
  - implantation 623.8
  - inclusion 623.8
- vallecula, vallecular 478.79
- ventricle, neuroepithelial 348.0
- verumontanum 599.89
- vesical (orifice) 596.89
- vitreous humor 379.29
- vulva (sweat glands) 624.8
  - congenital 752.41
  - implantation 624.8
  - inclusion 624.8
  - sebaceous gland 624.8
- vulvovaginal gland 624.8
- wolffian 752.89

Cystadenocarcinoma (M8440/3) — see also Neoplasm, by site, malignant
- bile duct type (M8161/3) 155.1
- endometrioid (M8380/3) — see Neoplasm, by site, malignant

Cystadenocarcinoma — see also Neoplasm, by site, malignant — continued
- mucinous (M8470/3)
  - papillary (M8471/3)
    - specified site — see Neoplasm, by site, malignant
    - unspecified site 183.0
  - specified site — see Neoplasm, by site, malignant
  - unspecified site 183.0
- papillary (M8450/3)
  - mucinous (M8471/3)
    - specified site — see Neoplasm, by site, malignant
    - unspecified site 183.0
  - pseudomucinous (M8471/3)
    - specified site — see Neoplasm, by site, malignant
    - unspecified site 183.0
  - serous (M8460/3)
    - specified site — see Neoplasm, by site, malignant
    - unspecified site 183.0
  - specified site — see Neoplasm, by site, malignant
  - unspecified 183.0
- pseudomucinous (M8470/3)
  - papillary (M8471/3)
    - specified site — see Neoplasm, by site, malignant
    - unspecified site 183.0
  - specified site — see Neoplasm, by site, malignant
  - unspecified site 183.0
- serous (M8441/3)
  - papillary (M8460/3)
    - specified site — see Neoplasm, by site, malignant
    - unspecified site 183.0
  - specified site — see Neoplasm, by site, malignant
  - unspecified site 183.0

Cystadenofibroma (M9013/0)
- clear cell (M8313/0) — see Neoplasm, by site, benign
- endometrioid (M8381/0) 220
  - borderline malignancy (M8381/1) 236.2
  - malignant (M8381/3) 183.0
- mucinous (M9015/0)
  - specified site — see Neoplasm, by site, benign
  - unspecified site 220
- serous (M9014/0)
  - specified site — see Neoplasm, by site, benign
  - unspecified site 220
- specified site — see Neoplasm, by site, benign
- unspecified site 220

Cystadenoma (M8440/0) — see also Neoplasm, by site, benign
- bile duct (M8161/0) 211.5
- endometrioid (M8380/0) (see also Neoplasm, by site, benign)
  - borderline malignancy (M8380/1) — see Neoplasm, by site, uncertain behavior
  - malignant (M8440/3) — see Neoplasm, by site, malignant
- mucinous (M8470/0)
  - borderline malignancy (M8470/1)
    - specified site — see Neoplasm, uncertain behavior
    - unspecified site 236.2
  - papillary (M8471/0)
    - borderline malignancy (M8471/1)
      - specified site — see Neoplasm, by site, uncertain behavior
      - unspecified site 236.2
    - specified site — see Neoplasm, by site, benign
    - unspecified site 220
  - specified site — see Neoplasm, by site, benign
  - unspecified site 220

Cystadenoma — see also Neoplasm, by site, benign — continued
- papillary (M8450/0)
  - borderline malignancy (M8450/1)
    - specified site — see Neoplasm, by site, uncertain behavior
    - unspecified site 236.2
  - lymphomatosum (M8561/0) 210.2
  - mucinous (M8471/0)
    - borderline malignancy (M8471/1)
      - specified site — see Neoplasm, by site, uncertain behavior
      - unspecified site 236.2
    - specified site — see Neoplasm, by site, benign
    - unspecified site 220
  - pseudomucinous (M8471/0)
    - borderline malignancy (M8471/1)
      - specified site — see Neoplasm, by site, uncertain behavior
      - unspecified site 236.2
    - specified site — see Neoplasm, by site, benign
    - unspecified site 220
  - serous (M8460/0)
    - borderline malignancy (M8460/1)
      - specified site — see Neoplasm, by site, uncertain behavior
      - unspecified site 236.2
    - specified site — see Neoplasm, by site, benign
    - unspecified site 220
  - specified site — see Neoplasm, by site, benign
  - unspecified site 220
- pseudomucinous (M8470/0)
  - borderline malignancy (M8470/1)
    - specified site — see Neoplasm, by site, uncertain behavior
    - unspecified site 236.2
  - papillary (M8471/0)
    - borderline malignancy (M8471/1)
      - specified site — see Neoplasm, by site, uncertain behavior
      - unspecified site 236.2
    - specified site — see Neoplasm, by site, benign
    - unspecified site 220
  - specified site — see Neoplasm, by site, benign
  - unspecified site 220
- serous (M8441/0)
  - borderline malignancy (M8441/1)
    - specified site — see Neoplasm, by site, uncertain behavior
    - unspecified site 236.2
  - papillary (M8460/0)
    - borderline malignancy (M8460/1)
      - specified site — see Neoplasm, by site, uncertain behavior
      - unspecified site 236.2
    - specified site — see Neoplasm, by site, benign
    - unspecified site 220
  - specified site — see Neoplasm, by site, benign
  - unspecified site 220
- thyroid 226

Cystathioninemia 270.4
Cystathioninuria 270.4
Cystic — see also condition
- breast, chronic 610.1
- corpora lutea 620.1
- degeneration, congenital
  - brain 742.4
  - kidney (see also Cystic, disease, kidney) 753.10
- disease
  - breast, chronic 610.1
  - kidney, congenital 753.10
    - medullary 753.16
    - multiple 753.19
    - polycystic — see Polycystic, kidney
    - single 753.11
    - specified NEC 753.19
  - liver, congenital 751.62

☑ **Additional Digit Required** — Refer to the Tabular List for Digit Selection   ▽ **Subterms under main terms may continue to next column or page**

2014 ICD-9-CM   ▶◀ **Revised Text**   ● **New Line**   ▲ **Revised Code**   **Volume 2 — 61**

Cystic — see also condition — continued
  disease — continued
    lung 518.89
      congenital 748.4
    pancreas, congenital 751.7
    semilunar cartilage 717.5
  duct — see condition
  eyeball, congenital 743.03
  fibrosis (pancreas) 277.00
    with
      manifestations
        gastrointestinal 277.03
        pulmonary 277.02
        specified NEC 277.09
      meconium ileus 277.01
      pulmonary exacerbation 277.02
  hygroma (M9173/0) 228.1
  kidney, congenital 753.10
    medullary 753.16
    multiple 753.19
    polycystic — see Polycystic, kidney
    single 753.11
    specified NEC 753.19
  liver, congenital 751.62
  lung 518.89
    congenital 748.4
  mass — see Cyst
  mastitis, chronic 610.1
  ovary 620.2
  pancreas, congenital 751.7
Cysticerciasis 123.1
Cysticercosis (mammary) (subretinal) 123.1
Cysticercus 123.1
  cellulosae infestation 123.1
Cystinosis (malignant) 270.0
Cystinuria 270.0
Cystitis (bacillary) (colli) (diffuse) (exudative)
    (hemorrhagic) (purulent) (recurrent)
    (septic) (suppurative) (ulcerative) 595.9
  with
    abortion — see Abortion, by type, with
      urinary tract infection
    ectopic pregnancy (see also categories
      633.0–633.9) 639.8

Cystitis — continued
  with — continued
    fibrosis 595.1
    leukoplakia 595.1
    malakoplakia 595.1
    metaplasia 595.1
    molar pregnancy (see also categories
      630–632) 639.8
  actinomycotic 039.8 [595.4]
  acute 595.0
    of trigone 595.3
  allergic 595.89
  amebic 006.8 [595.4]
  bilharzial 120.9 [595.4]
  blennorrhagic (acute) 098.11
    chronic or duration of 2 months or more
      098.31
  bullous 595.89
  calculous 594.1
  chlamydial 099.53
  chronic 595.2
    interstitial 595.1
    of trigone 595.3
  complicating pregnancy, childbirth, or
    puerperium 646.6 ☑
    affecting fetus or newborn 760.1
  cystic(a) 595.81
  diphtheritic 032.84
  echinococcal
    granulosus 122.3 [595.4]
    multilocularis 122.6 [595.4]
  emphysematous 595.89
  encysted 595.81
  follicular 595.3
  following
    abortion 639.8
    ectopic or molar pregnancy 639.8
  gangrenous 595.89
  glandularis 595.89
  gonococcal (acute) 098.11
    chronic or duration of 2 months or more
      098.31
  incrusted 595.89
  interstitial 595.1

Cystitis — continued
  irradiation 595.82
  irritation 595.89
  malignant 595.89
  monilial 112.2
  of trigone 595.3
  panmural 595.1
  polyposa 595.89
  prostatic 601.3
  radiation 595.82
  Reiter's (abacterial) 099.3
  specified NEC 595.89
  subacute 595.2
  submucous 595.1
  syphilitic 095.8
  trichomoniasis 131.09
  tuberculous (see also Tuberculosis) 016.1 ☑
  ulcerative 595.1
Cystocele
  female (without uterine prolapse) 618.01
    with uterine prolapse 618.4
      complete 618.3
      incomplete 618.2
    lateral 618.02
    midline 618.01
    paravaginal 618.02
  in pregnancy or childbirth 654.4 ☑
    affecting fetus or newborn 763.89
    causing obstructed labor 660.2 ☑
      affecting fetus or newborn 763.1
  male 596.89
Cystoid
  cicatrix limbus 372.64
  degeneration macula 362.53
Cystolithiasis 594.1
Cystoma (M8440/0) — see also Neoplasm, by
    site, benign
  endometrial, ovary 617.1
  mucinous (M8470/0)
    specified site — see Neoplasm, by site,
      benign
    unspecified site 220

Cystoma — see also Neoplasm, by site, benign
  — continued
  serous (M8441/0)
    specified site — see Neoplasm, by site,
      benign
    unspecified site 220
  simple (ovary) 620.2
Cystoplegia 596.53
Cystoptosis 596.89
Cystopyelitis — see also Pyelitis 590.80
Cystorrhagia 596.89
Cystosarcoma phyllodes (M9020/1) 238.3
  benign (M9020/0) 217
  malignant (M9020/3) — see Neoplasm,
    breast, malignant
Cystostomy status V44.50
  with complication 596.83
    infection 596.81
    mechanical 596.82
    specified complication NEC 596.83
  appendico-vesicostomy V44.52
  cutaneous-vesicostomy V44.51
  specified type NEC V44.59
Cystourethritis — see also Urethritis 597.89
Cystourethrocele — see also Cystocele
  female (without uterine prolapse) 618.09
    with uterine prolapse 618.4
      complete 618.3
      incomplete 618.2
  male 596.89
Cytomegalic inclusion disease 078.5
  congenital 771.1
Cytomycosis, reticuloendothelial — see also
    Histoplasmosis, American 115.00
Cytopenia 289.9
  refractory
    with
      multilineage dysplasia (RCMD)
        238.72
        and ringed sideroblasts (RCMD-
          RS) 238.72

☑ **Additional Digit Required — Refer to the Tabular List for Digit Selection**

▽ **Subterms under main terms may continue to next column or page**

▶◀ **Revised Text**   ● **New Line**   ▲ **Revised Code**

D

Daae (-Finsen) disease (epidemic pleurodynia) 074.1
Dabney's grip 074.1
Da Costa's syndrome (neurocirculatory asthenia) 306.2
Dacryoadenitis, dacryadenitis 375.00
  acute 375.01
  chronic 375.02
Dacryocystitis 375.30
  acute 375.32
  chronic 375.42
  neonatal 771.6
  phlegmonous 375.33
  syphilitic 095.8
    congenital 090.0
  trachomatous, active 076.1
    late effect 139.1
  tuberculous (see also Tuberculosis) 017.3 ☑
Dacryocystoblenorrhea 375.42
Dacryocystocele 375.43
Dacryolith, dacryolithiasis 375.57
Dacryoma 375.43
Dacryopericystitis (acute) (subacute) 375.32
  chronic 375.42
Dacryops 375.11
Dacryosialadenopathy, atrophic 710.2
Dacryostenosis 375.56
  congenital 743.65
Dactylitis
  bone (see also Osteomyelitis) 730.2 ☑
  sickle-cell 282.62
    Hb-C 282.64
    Hb-SS 282.62
    specified NEC 282.69
  syphilitic 095.5
  tuberculous (see also Tuberculosis) 015.5 ☑
Dactylolysis spontanea 136.0
Dactylosymphysis — see also Syndactylism 755.10
Damage
  arteriosclerotic — see Arteriosclerosis
  brain 348.9
    anoxic, hypoxic 348.1
      during or resulting from a procedure 997.01
    ischemic, in newborn 768.70
      mild 768.71
      moderate 768.72
      severe 768.73
    child NEC 343.9
    due to birth injury 767.0
    minimal (child) (see also Hyperkinesia) 314.9
    newborn 767.0
  cardiac (see also Disease, heart)
  cardiorenal (vascular) (see also Hypertension, cardiorenal) 404.90
  central nervous system — see Damage, brain
  cerebral NEC — see Damage, brain
  coccyx, complicating delivery 665.6 ☑
  coronary (see also Ischemia, heart) 414.9
  eye, birth injury 767.8
  heart (see also Disease, heart)
    valve — see Endocarditis
  hypothalamus NEC 348.9
  liver 571.9
    alcoholic 571.3
  medication 995.20
  myocardium (see also Degeneration, myocardial) 429.1
  pelvic
    joint or ligament, during delivery 665.6 ☑
    organ NEC
      with
        abortion — see Abortion, by type, with damage to pelvic organs
        ectopic pregnancy (see also categories 633.0–633.9) 639.2
        molar pregnancy (see also categories 630–632) 639.2
      during delivery 665.5 ☑

Damage — continued
  pelvic — continued
    organ — continued
      following
        abortion 639.2
        ectopic or molar pregnancy 639.2
  renal (see also Disease, renal) 593.9
  skin, solar 692.79
    acute 692.72
    chronic 692.74
  subendocardium, subendocardial (see also Degeneration, myocardial) 429.1
  vascular 459.9
Dameshek's syndrome (erythroblastic anemia) 282.49
Dana-Putnam syndrome (subacute combined sclerosis with pernicious anemia) 281.0 [336.2]
Danbolt (-Closs) syndrome (acrodermatitis enteropathica) 686.8
Dandruff 690.18
Dandy-Walker deformity or syndrome (atresia, foramen of Magendie) 742.3
  with spina bifida (see also Spina bifida) 741.0 ☑
Dandy fever 061
Dangle foot 736.79
Danielssen's disease (anesthetic leprosy) 030.1
Danlos' syndrome 756.83
Darier-Roussy sarcoid 135
Darier's disease (congenital) (keratosis follicularis) 757.39
  due to vitamin A deficiency 264.8
  meaning erythema annulare centrifugum 695.0
Dark area on retina 239.81
Darling's
  disease (see also Histoplasmosis, American) 115.00
  histoplasmosis (see also Histoplasmosis, American) 115.00
Dartre 054.9
Darwin's tubercle 744.29
Davidson's anemia (refractory) 284.9
Davies-Colley syndrome (slipping rib) 733.99
Davies' disease 425.0
Dawson's encephalitis 046.2
Day blindness — see also Blindness, day 368.60
Dead
  fetus
    retained (in utero) 656.4 ☑
      early pregnancy (death before 22 completed weeks gestation) 632
      late (death after 22 completed weeks gestation) 656.4 ☑
    syndrome 641.3 ☑
  labyrinth 386.50
  ovum, retained 631.8
Deaf and dumb NEC 389.7
Deaf mutism (acquired) (congenital) NEC 389.7
  endemic 243
  hysterical 300.11
  syphilitic, congenital 090.0
Deafness (acquired) (complete) (congenital) (hereditary) (middle ear) (partial) 389.9
  with
    blindness V49.85
    blue sclera and fragility of bone 756.51
  auditory fatigue 389.9
  aviation 993.0
    nerve injury 951.5
  boilermakers' 951.5
  central 389.14
    with conductive hearing loss 389.20
      bilateral 389.22
      unilateral 389.21
  conductive (air) 389.00
    with sensorineural hearing loss 389.20
      bilateral 389.22
      unilateral 389.21
    bilateral 389.06
    combined types 389.08
    external ear 389.01

Deafness — continued
  conductive — continued
    inner ear 389.04
    middle ear 389.03
    multiple types 389.08
    tympanic membrane 389.02
    unilateral 389.05
  emotional (complete) 300.11
  functional (complete) 300.11
  high frequency 389.8
  hysterical (complete) 300.11
  injury 951.5
  low frequency 389.8
  mental 784.69
  mixed conductive and sensorineural 389.20
    bilateral 389.22
    unilateral 389.21
  nerve
    with conductive hearing loss 389.20
      bilateral 389.22
      unilateral 389.21
    bilateral 389.12
    unilateral 389.13
  neural
    with conductive hearing loss 389.20
      bilateral 389.22
      unilateral 389.21
    bilateral 389.12
    unilateral 389.13
  noise-induced 388.12
    nerve injury 951.5
  nonspeaking 389.7
  perceptive 389.10
    with conductive hearing loss 389.20
      bilateral 389.22
      unilateral 389.21
    central 389.14
    neural
      bilateral 389.12
      unilateral 389.13
    sensorineural 389.10
      asymmetrical 389.16
      bilateral 389.18
      unilateral 389.15
    sensory
      bilateral 389.11
      unilateral 389.17
  psychogenic (complete) 306.7
  sensorineural (see also Deafness, perceptive) 389.10
    asymmetrical 389.16
    bilateral 389.18
    unilateral 389.15
  sensory
    with conductive hearing loss 389.20
      bilateral 389.22
      unilateral 389.21
    bilateral 389.11
    unilateral 389.17
  specified type NEC 389.8
  sudden NEC 388.2
  syphilitic 094.89
  transient ischemic 388.02
  transmission — see Deafness, conductive
  traumatic 951.5
  word (secondary to organic lesion) 784.69
    developmental 315.31
Death
  after delivery (cause not stated) (sudden) 674.9 ☑
  anesthetic
    due to
      correct substance properly administered 995.4
      overdose or wrong substance given 968.4
      specified anesthetic — see Table of Drugs and Chemicals
    during delivery 668.9 ☑
  brain 348.82
  cardiac (sudden) (SCD) — code to underlying condition
    family history of V17.41
    personal history of, successfully resuscitated V12.53
  cause unknown 798.2

Death — continued
  cot (infant) 798.0
  crib (infant) 798.0
  fetus, fetal (cause not stated) (intrauterine) 779.9
    early, with retention (before 22 completed weeks gestation) 632
    from asphyxia or anoxia (before labor) 768.0
      during labor 768.1
    late, affecting management of pregnancy (after 22 completed weeks gestation) 656.4 ☑
  from pregnancy NEC 646.9 ☑
  instantaneous 798.1
  intrauterine (see also Death, fetus) 779.9
    complicating pregnancy 656.4 ☑
  maternal, affecting fetus or newborn 761.6
  neonatal NEC 779.9
  sudden (cause unknown) 798.1
    cardiac (SCD)
      family history of V17.41
      personal history of, successfully resuscitated V12.53
    during delivery 669.9 ☑
      under anesthesia NEC 668.9 ☑
    infant, syndrome (SIDS) 798.0
    puerperal, during puerperium 674.9 ☑
  unattended (cause unknown) 798.9
  under anesthesia NEC
    due to
      correct substance properly administered 995.4
      overdose or wrong substance given 968.4
      specified anesthetic — see Table of Drugs and Chemicals
    during delivery 668.9 ☑
  violent 798.1
de Beurmann-Gougerot disease (sporotrichosis) 117.1
Debility (general) (infantile) (postinfectional) 799.3
  with nutritional difficulty 269.9
  congenital or neonatal NEC 779.9
  nervous 300.5
  old age 797
  senile 797
Débove's disease (splenomegaly) 789.2
Decalcification
  bone (see also Osteoporosis) 733.00
  teeth 521.89
Decapitation 874.9
  fetal (to facilitate delivery) 763.89
Decapsulation, kidney 593.89
Decay
  dental 521.00
  senile 797
  tooth, teeth 521.00
Decensus, uterus — see Prolapse, uterus
Deciduitis (acute)
  with
    abortion — see Abortion, by type, with sepsis
    ectopic pregnancy (see also categories 633.0–633.9) 639.0
    molar pregnancy (see also categories 630–632) 639.0
  affecting fetus or newborn 760.8
  following
    abortion 639.0
    ectopic or molar pregnancy 639.0
  in pregnancy 646.6 ☑
  puerperal, postpartum 670.1 ☑
Deciduoma malignum (M9100/3) 181
Deciduous tooth (retained) 520.6
Decline (general) — see also Debility 799.3
Decompensation
  cardiac (acute) (chronic) (see also Disease, heart) 429.9
    failure — see Failure, heart
  cardiorenal (see also Hypertension, cardiorenal) 404.90
  cardiovascular (see also Disease, cardiovascular) 429.2
  heart (see also Disease, heart) 429.9

☑ Additional Digit Required — Refer to the Tabular List for Digit Selection   ▽ Subterms under main terms may continue to next column or page

2014 ICD-9-CM   ▶◀ Revised Text   ● New Line   ▲ Revised Code   Volume 2 — 63

Decompensation — *continued*
heart (*see also* Disease, heart) — *continued*
  failure — *see* Failure, heart
hepatic 572.2
myocardial (acute) (chronic) (*see also* Disease, heart) 429.9
  failure — *see* Failure, heart
respiratory 519.9
Decompression sickness 993.3
Decrease, decreased
blood
  platelets (*see also* Thrombocytopenia) 287.5
  pressure 796.3
    due to shock following
      injury 958.4
      operation 998.00
  white blood cell count 288.50
    specified NEC 288.59
cardiac reserve — *see* Disease, heart
estrogen 256.39
  postablative 256.2
fetal movements 655.7 ☑
fragility of erythrocytes 289.89
function
  adrenal (cortex) 255.41
    medulla 255.5
  ovary in hypopituitarism 253.4
  parenchyma of pancreas 577.8
  pituitary (gland) (lobe) (anterior) 253.2
    posterior (lobe) 253.8
functional activity 780.99
glucose 790.29
haptoglobin (serum) NEC 273.8
leukocytes 288.50
libido 799.81
lymphocytes 288.51
platelets (*see also* Thrombocytopenia) 287.5
pulse pressure 785.9
respiration due to shock following injury 958.4
sexual desire 799.81
tear secretion NEC 375.15
tolerance
  fat 579.8
  salt and water 276.9
vision NEC 369.9
white blood cell count 288.50
Decubital gangrene — *see also* Ulcer, pressure 707.00 *[785.4]*
Decubiti — *see also* Ulcer, pressure 707.00
Decubitus (ulcer) — *see also* Ulcer, pressure 707.00
with gangrene 707.00 *[785.4]*
ankle 707.06
back
  lower 707.03
  upper 707.02
buttock 707.05
coccyx 707.03
elbow 707.01
head 707.09
heel 707.07
hip 707.04
other site 707.09
sacrum 707.03
shoulder blades 707.02
Deepening acetabulum 718.85
Defect, defective 759.9
3-beta-hydroxysteroid dehydrogenase 255.2
11-hydroxylase 255.2
21-hydroxylase 255.2
abdominal wall, congenital 756.70
aorticopulmonary septum 745.0
aortic septal 745.0
atrial septal (ostium secundum type) 745.5
  acquired 429.71
  ostium primum type 745.61
  sinus venosus 745.8
atrioventricular
  canal 745.69
  septum 745.4
    acquired 429.71
atrium secundum 745.5
  acquired 429.71

Defect, defective — *continued*
auricular septal 745.5
  acquired 429.71
bilirubin excretion 277.4
biosynthesis, testicular androgen 257.2
bridge 525.60
bulbar septum 745.0
butanol-insoluble iodide 246.1
chromosome — *see* Anomaly, chromosome
circulation (acquired) 459.9
  congenital 747.9
  newborn 747.9
clotting NEC (*see also* Defect, coagulation) 286.9
coagulation (factor) (*see also* Deficiency, coagulation factor) 286.9
  with
    abortion — *see* Abortion, by type, with hemorrhage
    ectopic pregnancy (*see also* categories 634–638) 639.1
    molar pregnancy (*see also* categories 630–632) 639.1
  acquired (any) 286.7
  antepartum or intrapartum 641.3 ☑
    affecting fetus or newborn 762.1
  causing hemorrhage of pregnancy or delivery 641.3 ☑
  complicating pregnancy, childbirth, or puerperium 649.3 ☑
  due to
    liver disease 286.7
    vitamin K deficiency 286.7
  newborn, transient 776.3
  postpartum 666.3 ☑
  specified type NEC 286.9
conduction (heart) 426.9
  bone (*see also* Deafness, conductive) 389.00
congenital, organ or site NEC (*see also* Anomaly)
  circulation 747.9
  Descemet's membrane 743.9
    specified type NEC 743.49
  diaphragm 756.6
  ectodermal 757.9
  esophagus 750.9
  pulmonic cusps — *see* Anomaly, heart valve
  respiratory system 748.9
    specified type NEC 748.8
crown 525.60
cushion endocardial 745.60
dental restoration 525.60
dentin (hereditary) 520.5
Descemet's membrane (congenital) 743.9
  acquired 371.30
  specific type NEC 743.49
deutan 368.52
developmental (*see also* Anomaly, by site)
  cauda equina 742.59
  left ventricle 746.9
    with atresia or hypoplasia of aortic orifice or valve, with hypoplasia of ascending aorta 746.7
    in hypoplastic left heart syndrome 746.7
  testis 752.9
  vessel 747.9
diaphragm
  with elevation, eventration, or hernia — *see* Hernia, diaphragm
  congenital 756.6
    with elevation, eventration, or hernia 756.6
    gross (with elevation, eventration, or hernia) 756.6
ectodermal, congenital 757.9
Eisenmenger's (ventricular septal defect) 745.4
endocardial cushion 745.60
  specified type NEC 745.69
esophagus, congenital 750.9
extensor retinaculum 728.9
fibrin polymerization (*see also* Defect, coagulation) 286.3

Defect, defective — *continued*
filling
  biliary tract 793.3
  bladder 793.5
  dental 525.60
  gallbladder 793.3
  kidney 793.5
  stomach 793.4
  ureter 793.5
fossa ovalis 745.5
gene, carrier (suspected) of V83.89
Gerbode 745.4
glaucomatous, without elevated tension 365.89
Hageman (factor) (*see also* Defect, coagulation) 286.3
hearing (*see also* Deafness) 389.9
high grade 317
homogentisic acid 270.2
interatrial septal 745.5
  acquired 429.71
interauricular septal 745.5
  acquired 429.71
interventricular septal 745.4
  with pulmonary stenosis or atresia, dextraposition of aorta, and hypertrophy of right ventricle 745.2
  acquired 429.71
  in tetralogy of Fallot 745.2
iodide trapping 246.1
iodotyrosine dehalogenase 246.1
kynureninase 270.2
learning, specific 315.2
major osseous 731.3
mental (*see also* Disability, intellectual) 319
osseous, major 731.3
osteochondral NEC 738.8
ostium
  primum 745.61
  secundum 745.5
pericardium 746.89
peroxidase-binding 246.1
placental blood supply — *see* Placenta, insufficiency
platelet (qualitative) 287.1
  constitutional 286.4
postural, spine 737.9
protan 368.51
pulmonic cusps, congenital 746.00
renal pelvis 753.9
  obstructive 753.29
  specified type NEC 753.3
respiratory system, congenital 748.9
  specified type NEC 748.8
retina, retinal 361.30
  with detachment (*see also* Detachment, retina, with retinal defect) 361.00
  multiple 361.33
    with detachment 361.02
  nerve fiber bundle 362.85
  single 361.30
    with detachment 361.01
septal (closure) (heart) NEC 745.9
  acquired 429.71
  atrial 745.5
  specified type NEC 745.8
speech NEC 784.59
  developmental 315.39
  late effect of cerebrovascular disease — *see* Late effect(s) (of) cerebrovascular disease, speech and language deficit
  secondary to organic lesion 784.59
Taussig-Bing (transposition, aorta and overriding pulmonary artery) 745.11
teeth, wedge 521.20
thyroid hormone synthesis 246.1
tritan 368.53
ureter 753.9
  obstructive 753.29
vascular (acquired) (local) 459.9
  congenital (peripheral) NEC 747.60
    gastrointestinal 747.61
    lower limb 747.64
    renal 747.62
    specified NEC 747.69

Defect, defective — *continued*
vascular — *continued*
  congenital — *continued*
    spinal 747.82
    upper limb 747.63
ventricular septal 745.4
  with pulmonary stenosis or atresia, dextraposition of aorta, and hypertrophy of right ventricle 745.2
  acquired 429.71
  atrioventricular canal type 745.69
  between infundibulum and anterior portion 745.4
  in tetralogy of Fallot 745.2
  isolated anterior 745.4
vision NEC 369.9
visual field 368.40
  arcuate 368.43
  heteronymous, bilateral 368.47
  homonymous, bilateral 368.46
  localized NEC 368.44
  nasal step 368.44
  peripheral 368.44
  sector 368.43
voice and resonance 784.40
wedge, teeth (abrasion) 521.20
Defeminization syndrome 255.2
Deferentitis 608.4
gonorrheal (acute) 098.14
  chronic or duration of 2 months or over 098.34
Defibrination syndrome — *see also* Fibrinolysis 286.6
Deficiency, deficient
3-beta-hydroxysteroid dehydrogenase 255.2
6-phosphogluconic dehydrogenase (anemia) 282.2
11-beta-hydroxylase 255.2
17-alpha-hydroxylase 255.2
18-hydroxysteroid dehydrogenase 255.2
20-alpha-hydroxylase 255.2
21-hydroxylase 255.2
AAT (alpha-1 antitrypsin) 273.4
abdominal muscle syndrome 756.79
accelerator globulin (Ac G) (blood) (*see also* Defect, coagulation) 286.3
AC globulin (congenital) (*see also* Defect, coagulation) 286.3
  acquired 286.7
activating factor (blood) (*see also* Defect, coagulation) 286.3
adenohypophyseal 253.2
adenosine deaminase 277.2
aldolase (hereditary) 271.2
alpha-1-antitrypsin 273.4
alpha-1-trypsin inhibitor 273.4
alpha-fucosidase 271.8
alpha-lipoprotein 272.5
alpha-mannosidase 271.8
amino acid 270.9
anemia — *see* Anemia, deficiency
aneurin 265.1
  with beriberi 265.0
antibody NEC 279.00
antidiuretic hormone 253.5
antihemophilic
  factor (A) 286.0
    B 286.1
    C 286.2
  globulin (AHG) NEC 286.0
antithrombin III 289.81
antitrypsin 273.4
argininosuccinate synthetase or lyase 270.6
ascorbic acid (with scurvy) 267
autoprothrombin
  I (*see also* Defect, coagulation) 286.3
  II 286.1
  C (*see also* Defect, coagulation) 286.3
bile salt 579.8
biotin 266.2
biotinidase 277.6
bradykinase-1 277.6
brancher enzyme (amylopectinosis) 271.0
calciferol 268.9
  with
    osteomalacia 268.2

Deficiency, deficient — *continued*
 calciferol — *continued*
  with — *continued*
   rickets (*see also* Rickets) 268.0
 calcium 275.40
  dietary 269.3
 calorie, severe 261
 carbamyl phosphate synthetase 270.6
 cardiac (*see also* Insufficiency, myocardial) 428.0
 carnitine 277.81
  due to
   hemodialysis 277.83
   inborn errors of metabolism 277.82
   valproic acid therapy 277.83
  iatrogenic 277.83
  palmitoyltransferase (CPT1, CPT2) 277.85
  palmityl transferase (CPT1, CPT2) 277.85
  primary 277.81
  secondary 277.84
 carotene 264.9
 Carr factor (*see also* Defect, coagulation) 286.9
 central nervous system 349.9
 ceruloplasmin 275.1
 cevitamic acid (with scurvy) 267
 choline 266.2
 Christmas factor 286.1
 chromium 269.3
 citrin 269.1
 clotting (blood) (*see also* Defect, coagulation) 286.9
 coagulation factor NEC 286.9
  with
   abortion — *see* Abortion, by type, with hemorrhage
   ectopic pregnancy (*see also* categories 634–638) 639.1
   molar pregnancy (*see also* categories 630–632) 639.1
  acquired (any) 286.7
  antepartum or intrapartum 641.3 ☑
   affecting fetus or newborn 762.1
  complicating pregnancy, childbirth, or puerperium 649.3 ☑
  due to
   liver disease 286.7
   vitamin K deficiency 286.7
  newborn, transient 776.3
  postpartum 666.3 ☑
  specified type NEC 286.3
 color vision (congenital) 368.59
  acquired 368.55
 combined glucocorticoid and mineralocorticoid 255.41
 combined, two or more coagulation factors (*see also* Defect, coagulation) 286.9
 complement factor NEC 279.8
 contact factor (*see also* Defect, coagulation) 286.3
 copper NEC 275.1
 corticoadrenal 255.41
 craniofacial axis 756.0
 cyanocobalamin (vitamin B$_{12}$) 266.2
 debrancher enzyme (limit dextrinosis) 271.0
 desmolase 255.2
 diet 269.9
 dihydrofolate reductase 281.2
 dihydropteridine reductase 270.1
 dihydropyrimidine dehydrogenase (DPD) 277.6
 disaccharidase (intestinal) 271.3
 disease NEC 269.9
 ear(s) V48.8
 edema 262
 endocrine 259.9
 enzymes, circulating NEC (*see also* Deficiency, by specific enzyme) 277.6
 ergosterol 268.9
  with
   osteomalacia 268.2
   rickets (*see also* Rickets) 268.0
 erythrocytic glutathione (anemia) 282.2
 eyelid(s) V48.8
 factor (*see also* Defect, coagulation) 286.9
  I (congenital) (fibrinogen) 286.3

Deficiency, deficient — *continued*
 factor (*see also* Defect, coagulation) — *continued*
  I — *continued*
   antepartum or intrapartum 641.3 ☑
    affecting fetus or newborn 762.1
   newborn, transient 776.3
   postpartum 666.3 ☑
  II (congenital) (prothrombin) 286.3
  V (congenital) (labile) 286.3
  VII (congenital) (stable) 286.3
  VIII (congenital) (functional) 286.0
   with
    functional defect 286.0
    vascular defect 286.4
  IX (Christmas) (congenital) (functional) 286.1
  X (congenital) (Stuart-Prower) 286.3
  XI (congenital) (plasma thromboplastin antecedent) 286.2
  XII (congenital) (Hageman) 286.3
  XIII (congenital) (fibrin stabilizing) 286.3
  Hageman 286.3
  multiple (congenital) 286.9
   acquired 286.7
 fibrin-stabilizing factor (congenital) (*see also* Defect, coagulation) 286.3
 fibrinase (*see also* Defect, coagulation) 286.3
 fibrinogen (congenital) (*see also* Defect, coagulation) 286.3
  acquired 286.6
 finger — *see* Absence, finger
 fletcher factor (*see also* Defect, coagulation) 286.9
 fluorine 269.3
 folate, anemia 281.2
 folic acid (vitamin B$_c$) 266.2
  anemia 281.2
 follicle-stimulating hormone (FSH) 253.4
 fructokinase 271.2
 fructose-1-phosphate aldolase 271.2
 fructose-1, 6-diphosphate 271.2
 FSH (follicle-stimulating hormone) 253.4
 fucosidase 271.8
 galactokinase 271.1
 galactose-1-phosphate uridyl transferase 271.1
 gamma globulin in blood 279.00
 glass factor (*see also* Defect, coagulation) 286.3
 glucocorticoid 255.41
 glucose-6-phosphatase 271.0
 glucose-6-phosphate dehydrogenase anemia 282.2
 glucuronyl transferase 277.4
 glutathione-reductase (anemia) 282.2
 glycogen synthetase 271.0
 growth hormone 253.3
 Hageman factor (congenital) (*see also* Defect, coagulation) 286.3
 head V48.0
 hemoglobin (*see also* Anemia) 285.9
 hepatophosphorylase 271.0
 hexose monophosphate (HMP) shunt 282.2
 HG-PRT 277.2
 HGH (human growth hormone) 253.3
 homogentisic acid oxidase 270.2
 hormone (*see also* Deficiency, by specific hormone)
  anterior pituitary (isolated) (partial) NEC 253.4
   growth (human) 253.3
  follicle-stimulating 253.4
  growth (human) (isolated) 253.3
  human growth 253.3
  interstitial cell-stimulating 253.4
  luteinizing 253.4
  melanocyte-stimulating 253.4
  testicular 257.2
 human growth hormone 253.3
 humoral 279.00
  with
   hyper-IgM 279.05
    autosomal recessive 279.05
    X-linked 279.05
   increased IgM 279.05

Deficiency, deficient — *continued*
 humoral — *continued*
  congenital hypogammaglobulinemia 279.04
   non-sex-linked 279.06
  selective immunoglobulin NEC 279.03
   IgA 279.01
   IgG 279.03
   IgM 279.02
    increased 279.05
  specified NEC 279.09
 hydroxylase 255.2
 hypoxanthine-guanine phosphoribosyltransferase (HG-PRT) 277.2
 ICSH (interstitial cell-stimulating hormone) 253.4
 immunity NEC 279.3
  cell-mediated 279.10
   with
    hyperimmunoglobulinemia 279.2
    thrombocytopenia and eczema 279.12
   specified NEC 279.19
  combined (severe) 279.2
   syndrome 279.2
  common variable 279.06
  humoral NEC 279.00
  IgA (secretory) 279.01
  IgG 279.03
  IgM 279.02
 immunoglobulin, selective NEC 279.03
  IgA 279.01
  IgG 279.03
  IgM 279.02
 inositol (B complex) 266.2
 interferon 279.49
 internal organ V47.0
 interstitial cell-stimulating hormone (ICSH) 253.4
 intrinsic factor (Castle's) (congenital) 281.0
 intrinsic (urethral) sphincter (ISD) 599.82
 invertase 271.3
 iodine 269.3
 iron, anemia 280.9
 labile factor (congenital) (*see also* Defect, coagulation) 286.3
  acquired 286.7
 lacrimal fluid (acquired) 375.15
  congenital 743.64
 lactase 271.3
 Laki-Lorand factor (*see also* Defect, coagulation) 286.3
 lecithin-cholesterol acyltranferase 272.5
 LH (luteinizing hormone) 253.4
 limb V49.0
  lower V49.0
   congenital (*see also* Deficiency, lower limb, congenital) 755.30
  upper V49.0
   congenital (*see also* Deficiency, upper limb, congenital) 755.20
 lipocaic 577.8
 lipoid (high-density) 272.5
 lipoprotein (familial) (high density) 272.5
 liver phosphorylase 271.0
 long chain 3-hydroxyacyl CoA dehydrogenase (LCHAD) 277.85
 long chain/very long chain acyl CoA dehydrogenase (LCAD, VLCAD) 277.85
 lower limb V49.0
  congenital 755.30
   with complete absence of distal elements 755.31
   longitudinal (complete) (partial) (with distal deficiencies, Incomplete) 755.32
    with complete absence of distal elements 755.31
    combined femoral, tibial, fibular (incomplete) 755.33
    femoral 755.34
    fibular 755.37
    metatarsal(s) 755.38
    phalange(s) 755.39
     meaning all digits 755.31
    tarsal(s) 755.38

Deficiency, deficient — *continued*
 lower limb — *continued*
  congenital — *continued*
   longitudinal — *continued*
    tibia 755.36
    tibiofibular 755.35
    transverse 755.31
 luteinizing hormone (LH) 253.4
 lysosomal alpha-1, 4 glucosidase 271.0
 magnesium 275.2
 mannosidase 271.8
 medium chain acyl CoA dehydrogenase (MCAD) 277.85
 melanocyte-stimulating hormone (MSH) 253.4
 menadione (vitamin K) 269.0
  newborn 776.0
 mental (familial) (hereditary) (*see also* Disability, intellectual) 319
 methylenetetrahydrofolate reductase (MTHFR) 270.4
 mineralocorticoid 255.42
 mineral NEC 269.3
 molybdenum 269.3
 moral 301.7
 multiple, syndrome 260
 myocardial (*see also* Insufficiency, myocardial) 428.0
 myophosphorylase 271.0
 NADH-diaphorase or reductase (congenital) 289.7
 NADH (DPNH)-methemoglobin-reductase (congenital) 289.7
 neck V48.1
 niacin (amide) (-tryptophan) 265.2
 nicotinamide 265.2
 nicotinic acid (amide) 265.2
 nose V48.8
 number of teeth (*see also* Anodontia) 520.0
 nutrition, nutritional 269.9
  specified NEC 269.8
 ornithine transcarbamylase 270.6
 ovarian 256.39
 oxygen (*see also* Anoxia) 799.02
 pantothenic acid 266.2
 parathyroid (gland) 252.1
 phenylalanine hydroxylase 270.1
 phosphoenolpyruvate carboxykinase 271.8
 phosphofructokinase 271.2
 phosphoglucomutase 271.0
 phosphohexosisomerase 271.0
 phosphomannomutase 271.8
 phosphomannose isomerase 271.8
 phosphomannosyl mutase 271.8
 phosphorylase kinase, liver 271.0
 pituitary (anterior) 253.2
  posterior 253.5
 placenta — *see* Placenta, insufficiency
 plasma
  cell 279.00
  protein (paraproteinemia) (pyroglobulinemia) 273.8
  gamma globulin 279.00
  thromboplastin
   antecedent (PTA) 286.2
   component (PTC) 286.1
 platelet NEC 287.1
  constitutional 286.4
 polyglandular 258.9
 potassium (K) 276.8
 proaccelerin (congenital) (*see also* Defect, congenital) 286.3
  acquired 286.7
 proconvertin factor (congenital) (*see also* Defect, coagulation) 286.3
  acquired 286.7
 prolactin 253.4
 protein 260
  anemia 281.4
  C 289.81
  plasma — *see* Deficiency, plasma, protein
  S 289.81
 prothrombin (congenital) (*see also* Defect, coagulation) 286.3
  acquired 286.7

☑ **Additional Digit Required** — Refer to the Tabular List for Digit Selection   🔺 **Subterms under main terms may continue to next column or page**

2014 ICD-9-CM   ▶◀ **Revised Text**   ● **New Line**   ▲ **Revised Code**   **Volume 2 — 65**

Deficiency, deficient — *continued*
  Prower factor (*see also* Defect, coagulation) 286.3
  PRT 277.2
  pseudocholinesterase 289.89
  psychobiological 301.6
  PTA 286.2
  PTC 286.1
  purine nucleoside phosphorylase 277.2
  pyracin (alpha) (beta) 266.1
  pyridoxal 266.1
  pyridoxamine 266.1
  pyridoxine (derivatives) 266.1
  pyruvate carboxylase 271.8
  pyruvate dehydrogenase 271.8
  pyruvate kinase (PK) 282.3
  riboflavin (vitamin B_2) 266.0
  saccadic eye movements 379.57
  salivation 527.7
  salt 276.1
  secretion
    ovary 256.39
    salivary gland (any) 527.7
    urine 788.5
  selenium 269.3
  serum
    antitrypsin, familial 273.4
    protein (congenital) 273.8
  short chain acyl CoA dehydrogenase (SCAD) 277.85
  short stature homeobox gene (SHOX)
    with
      dyschondrosteosis 756.89
      short stature (idiopathic) 783.43
      Turner's syndrome 758.6
  smooth pursuit movements (eye) 379.58
  sodium (Na) 276.1
  SPCA (*see also* Defect, coagulation) 286.3
  specified NEC 269.8
  stable factor (congenital) (*see also* Defect, coagulation) 286.3
    acquired 286.7
  Stuart (-Prower) factor (*see also* Defect, coagulation) 286.3
  sucrase-isomaltase 271.3
  sucrase 271.3
  sulfite oxidase 270.0
  syndrome, multiple 260
  thiamine, thiaminic (chloride) 265.1
  thrombokinase (*see also* Defect, coagulation) 286.3
    newborn 776.0
  thrombopoieten 287.39
  thymolymphatic 279.2
  thyroid (gland) 244.9
  tocopherol 269.1
  toe — *see* Absence, toe
  tooth bud (*see also* Anodontia) 520.0
  trunk V48.1
  UDPG-glycogen transferase 271.0
  upper limb V49.0
    congenital 755.20
      with complete absence of distal elements 755.21
      longitudinal (complete) (partial) (with distal deficiencies, incomplete) 755.22
        carpal(s) 755.28
        combined humeral, radial, ulnar (incomplete) 755.23
        humeral 755.24
        metacarpal(s) 755.28
        phalange(s) 755.29
          meaning all digits 755.21
        radial 755.26
        radioulnar 755.25
        ulnar 755.27
      transverse (complete) (partial) 755.21
  vascular 459.9
  vasopressin 253.5
  viosterol (*see also* Deficiency, calciferol) 268.9
  vitamin (multiple) NEC 269.2
    A 264.9
      with
        Bitôt's spot 264.1

Deficiency, deficient — *continued*
  vitamin — *continued*
    A — *continued*
      with — *continued*
        Bitôt's spot — *continued*
          corneal 264.2
            with corneal ulceration 264.3
        keratomalacia 264.4
        keratosis, follicular 264.8
        night blindness 264.5
        scar of cornea, xerophthalmic 264.6
        specified manifestation NEC 264.8
          ocular 264.7
        xeroderma 264.8
        xerophthalmia 264.7
        xerosis
          conjunctival 264.0
            with Bitôt's spot 264.1
          corneal 264.2
            with corneal ulceration 264.3
    B_1 NEC 265.1
      beriberi 265.0
    B_2 266.0
    B_6 266.1
    B_{12} 266.2
    B_c (folic acid) 266.2
    B (complex) NEC 266.9
      with
        beriberi 265.0
        pellagra 265.2
      specified type NEC 266.2
    C (ascorbic acid) (with scurvy) 267
    D (calciferol) (ergosterol) 268.9
      with
        osteomalacia 268.2
        rickets (*see also* Rickets) 268.0
    E 269.1
    folic acid 266.2
    G 266.0
    H 266.2
    K 269.0
      of newborn 776.0
    nicotinic acid 265.2
    P 269.1
    PP 265.2
    specified NEC 269.1
  zinc 269.3

Deficient — *see also* Deficiency
  blink reflex 374.45
  craniofacial axis 756.0
  number of teeth (*see also* Anodontia) 520.0
  secretion of urine 788.5

Deficit
  attention 799.51
  cognitive communication 799.52
  concentration 799.51
  executive function 799.55
  frontal lobe 799.55
  neurologic NEC 781.99
    due to
      cerebrovascular lesion (*see also* Disease, cerebrovascular, acute) 436
      late effect — *see* Late effect(s) (of) cerebrovascular disease
      transient ischemic attack 435.9
      ischemic
        reversible (RIND) 434.91
          history of (personal) V12.54
          prolonged (PRIND) 434.91
            history of (personal) V12.54
  oxygen 799.02
  psychomotor 799.54
  visuospatial 799.53

Deflection
  radius 736.09
  septum (acquired) (nasal) (nose) 470
  spine — *see* Curvature, spine
  turbinate (nose) 470

Defluvium
  capillorum (*see also* Alopecia) 704.00
  ciliorum 374.55

Defluvium — *continued*
  unguium 703.8

Deformity 738.9
  abdomen, congenital 759.9
  abdominal wall
    acquired 738.8
    congenital 756.70
    muscle deficiency syndrome 756.79
  acquired (unspecified site) 738.9
    specified site NEC 738.8
  adrenal gland (congenital) 759.1
  alimentary tract, congenital 751.9
    lower 751.5
    specified type NEC 751.8
    upper (any part, except tongue) 750.9
      specified type NEC 750.8
      tongue 750.10
        specified type NEC 750.19
  ankle (joint) (acquired) 736.70
    abduction 718.47
    congenital 755.69
    contraction 718.47
    specified NEC 736.79
  anus (congenital) 751.5
    acquired 569.49
  aorta (congenital) 747.20
    acquired 447.8
    arch 747.21
      acquired 447.8
    coarctation 747.10
  aortic
    arch 747.21
      acquired 447.8
    cusp or valve (congenital) 746.9
      acquired (*see also* Endocarditis, aortic) 424.1
    ring 747.21
  appendix 751.5
  arm (acquired) 736.89
    congenital 755.50
  arteriovenous (congenital) (peripheral) NEC 747.60
    gastrointestinal 747.61
    lower limb 747.64
    renal 747.62
    specified NEC 747.69
    spinal 747.82
    upper limb 747.63
  artery (congenital) (peripheral) NEC (*see also* Deformity, vascular) 747.60
    acquired 447.8
    cerebral 747.81
    coronary (congenital) 746.85
      acquired (*see also* Ischemia, heart) 414.9
    retinal 743.9
    umbilical 747.5
  atrial septal (congenital) (heart) 745.5
  auditory canal (congenital) (external) (*see also* Deformity, ear) 744.3
    acquired 380.50
  auricle
    ear (congenital) (*see also* Deformity, ear) 744.3
      acquired 380.32
    heart (congenital) 746.9
  back (acquired) — *see* Deformity, spine
  Bartholin's duct (congenital) 750.9
  bile duct (congenital) 751.60
    acquired 576.8
      with calculus, choledocholithiasis, or stones — *see* Choledocholithiasis
  biliary duct or passage (congenital) 751.60
    acquired 576.8
      with calculus, choledocholithiasis, or stones — *see* Choledocholithiasis
  bladder (neck) (sphincter) (trigone) (acquired) 596.89
    congenital 753.9
  bone (acquired) NEC 738.9
    congenital 756.9
    turbinate 738.0
  boutonniere (finger) 736.21
  brain (congenital) 742.9

Deformity — *continued*
  brain — *continued*
    acquired 348.89
    multiple 742.4
    reduction 742.2
    vessel (congenital) 747.81
  breast (acquired) 611.89
    congenital 757.6
    reconstructed 612.0
  bronchus (congenital) 748.3
    acquired 519.19
  bursa, congenital 756.9
  canal of Nuck 752.9
  canthus (congenital) 743.9
    acquired 374.89
  capillary (acquired) 448.9
    congenital NEC (*see also* Deformity, vascular) 747.60
  cardiac — *see* Deformity, heart
  cardiovascular system (congenital) 746.9
  caruncle, lacrimal (congenital) 743.9
    acquired 375.69
  cascade, stomach 537.6
  cecum (congenital) 751.5
    acquired 569.89
  cerebral (congenital) 742.9
    acquired 348.89
  cervix (acquired) (uterus) 622.8
    congenital 752.40
  cheek (acquired) 738.19
    congenital 744.9
  chest (wall) (acquired) 738.3
    congenital 754.89
    late effect of rickets 268.1
  chin (acquired) 738.19
    congenital 744.9
  choroid (congenital) 743.9
    acquired 363.8
    plexus (congenital) 742.9
      acquired 349.2
  cicatricial — *see* Cicatrix
  cilia (congenital) 743.9
    acquired 374.89
  circulatory system (congenital) 747.9
  clavicle (acquired) 738.8
    congenital 755.51
  clitoris (congenital) 752.40
    acquired 624.8
  clubfoot — *see* Clubfoot
  coccyx (acquired) 738.6
    congenital 756.10
  colon (congenital) 751.5
    acquired 569.89
  concha (ear) (congenital) (*see also* Deformity, ear) 744.3
    acquired 380.32
  congenital, organ or site not listed (*see also* Anomaly) 759.9
  cornea (congenital) 743.9
    acquired 371.70
  coronary artery (congenital) 746.85
    acquired (*see also* Ischemia, heart) 414.9
  cranium (acquired) 738.19
    congenital (*see also* Deformity, skull, congenital) 756.0
  cricoid cartilage (congenital) 748.3
    acquired 478.79
  cystic duct (congenital) 751.60
    acquired 575.8
  Dandy-Walker 742.3
    with spina bifida (*see also* Spina bifida) 741.0 ☑
  diaphragm (congenital) 756.6
    acquired 738.8
  digestive organ(s) or system (congenital) NEC 751.9
    specified type NEC 751.8
  ductus arteriosus 747.0
  duodenal bulb 537.89
  duodenum (congenital) 751.5
    acquired 537.89
  dura (congenital) 742.9
    brain 742.4
      acquired 349.2
    spinal 742.59
      acquired 349.2

Deformity — continued
- ear (congenital) 744.3
  - acquired 380.32
  - auricle 744.3
    - causing impairment of hearing 744.02
  - causing impairment of hearing 744.00
  - external 744.3
    - causing impairment of hearing 744.02
  - internal 744.05
  - lobule 744.3
  - middle 744.03
    - ossicles 744.04
  - ossicles 744.04
- ectodermal (congenital) NEC 757.9
  - specified type NEC 757.8
- ejaculatory duct (congenital) 752.9
  - acquired 608.89
- elbow (joint) (acquired) 736.00
  - congenital 755.50
  - contraction 718.42
- endocrine gland NEC 759.2
- epididymis (congenital) 752.9
  - acquired 608.89
  - torsion 608.24
- epiglottis (congenital) 748.3
  - acquired 478.79
- esophagus (congenital) 750.9
  - acquired 530.89
- Eustachian tube (congenital) NEC 744.3
  - specified type NEC 744.24
- extremity (acquired) 736.9
  - congenital, except reduction deformity 755.9
    - lower 755.60
    - upper 755.50
  - reduction — see Deformity, reduction
- eye (congenital) 743.9
  - acquired 379.8
  - muscle 743.9
- eyebrow (congenital) 744.89
- eyelid (congenital) 743.9
  - acquired 374.89
  - specified type NEC 743.62
- face (acquired) 738.19
  - congenital (any part) 744.9
    - due to intrauterine malposition and pressure 754.0
- fallopian tube (congenital) 752.10
  - acquired 620.8
- femur (acquired) 736.89
  - congenital 755.60
- fetal
  - with fetopelvic disproportion 653.7 ☑
    - affecting fetus or newborn 763.1
  - causing obstructed labor 660.1 ☑
    - affecting fetus or newborn 763.1
  - known or suspected, affecting management of pregnancy 655.9 ☑
- finger (acquired) 736.20
  - boutonniere type 736.21
  - congenital 755.50
  - flexion contracture 718.44
  - swan neck 736.22
- flexion (joint) (acquired) 736.9
  - congenital NEC 755.9
  - hip or thigh (acquired) 736.39
    - congenital (see also Subluxation, congenital, hip) 754.32
- foot (acquired) 736.70
  - cavovarus 736.75
    - congenital 754.59
  - congenital NEC 754.70
    - specified type NEC 754.79
  - valgus (acquired) 736.79
    - congenital 754.60
      - specified type NEC 754.69
  - varus (acquired) 736.79
    - congenital 754.50
      - specified type NEC 754.59
- forearm (acquired) 736.00
  - congenital 755.50
- forehead (acquired) 738.19
  - congenital (see also Deformity, skull, congenital) 756.0

Deformity — continued
- frontal bone (acquired) 738.19
  - congenital (see also Deformity, skull, congenital) 756.0
- gallbladder (congenital) 751.60
  - acquired 575.8
- gastrointestinal tract (congenital) NEC 751.9
  - acquired 569.89
  - specified type NEC 751.8
- genitalia, genital organ(s) or system NEC
  - congenital 752.9
  - female (congenital) 752.9
    - acquired 629.89
    - external 752.40
    - internal 752.9
  - male (congenital) 752.9
    - acquired 608.89
- globe (eye) (congenital) 743.9
  - acquired 360.89
- gum (congenital) 750.9
  - acquired 523.9
- gunstock 736.02
- hand (acquired) 736.00
  - claw 736.06
  - congenital 755.50
  - minus (and plus) (intrinsic) 736.09
  - pill roller (intrinsic) 736.09
  - plus (and minus) (intrinsic) 736.09
  - swan neck (intrinsic) 736.09
- head (acquired) 738.10
  - congenital (see also Deformity, skull congenital) 756.0
  - specified NEC 738.19
- heart (congenital) 746.9
  - auricle (congenital) 746.9
  - septum 745.9
    - auricular 745.5
    - specified type NEC 745.8
    - ventricular 745.4
  - valve (congenital) NEC 746.9
    - acquired — see Endocarditis
    - pulmonary (congenital) 746.00
    - specified type NEC 746.89
  - ventricle (congenital) 746.9
- heel (acquired) 736.76
  - congenital 755.67
- hepatic duct (congenital) 751.60
  - acquired 576.8
    - with calculus, choledocholithiasis, or stones — see Choledocholithiasis
- hip (joint) (acquired) 736.30
  - congenital NEC 755.63
  - flexion 718.45
    - congenital (see also Subluxation, congenital, hip) 754.32
- hourglass — see Contraction, hourglass
- humerus (acquired) 736.89
  - congenital 755.50
- hymen (congenital) 752.40
- hypophyseal (congenital) 759.2
- ileocecal (coil) (valve) (congenital) 751.5
  - acquired 569.89
- ileum (intestine) (congenital) 751.5
  - acquired 569.89
- ilium (acquired) 738.6
  - congenital 755.60
- integument (congenital) 757.9
- intervertebral cartilage or disc (acquired) (see also Displacement, intervertebral disc)
  - congenital 756.10
- intestine (large) (small) (congenital) 751.5
  - acquired 569.89
- iris (acquired) 364.75
  - congenital 743.9
  - prolapse 364.89
- ischium (acquired) 738.6
  - congenital 755.60
- jaw (acquired) (congenital) NEC 524.9
  - due to intrauterine malposition and pressure 754.0
- joint (acquired) NEC 738.8
  - congenital 755.9

Deformity — continued
- joint — continued
  - contraction (abduction) (adduction) (extension) (flexion) — see Contraction, joint
  - kidney(s) (calyx) (pelvis) (congenital) 753.9
    - acquired 593.89
    - vessel 747.62
      - acquired 459.9
  - Klippel-Feil (brevicollis) 756.16
  - knee (acquired) NEC 736.6
    - congenital 755.64
  - labium (majus) (minus) (congenital) 752.40
    - acquired 624.8
  - lacrimal apparatus or duct (congenital) 743.9
    - acquired 375.69
  - larynx (muscle) (congenital) 748.3
    - acquired 478.79
    - web (glottic) (subglottic) 748.2
  - leg (lower) (upper) (acquired) NEC 736.89
    - congenital 755.60
      - reduction — see Deformity, reduction, lower limb
  - lens (congenital) 743.9
    - acquired 379.39
  - lid (fold) (congenital) 743.9
    - acquired 374.89
  - ligament (acquired) 728.9
    - congenital 756.9
  - limb (acquired) 736.9
    - congenital, except reduction deformity 755.9
      - lower 755.60
        - reduction (see also Deformity, reduction, lower limb) 755.30
      - upper 755.50
        - reduction (see also Deformity, reduction, upper limb) 755.20
    - specified NEC 736.89
  - lip (congenital) NEC 750.9
    - acquired 528.5
    - specified type NEC 750.26
  - liver (congenital) 751.60
    - acquired 573.8
    - duct (congenital) 751.60
      - acquired 576.8
        - with calculus, choledocholithiasis, or stones — see Choledocholithi-asis
  - lower extremity — see Deformity, leg
  - lumbosacral (joint) (region) (congenital) 756.10
    - acquired 738.5
  - lung (congenital) 748.60
    - acquired 518.89
    - specified type NEC 748.69
  - lymphatic system, congenital 759.9
  - Madelung's (radius) 755.54
  - maxilla (acquired) (congenital) 524.9
  - meninges or membrane (congenital) 742.9
    - brain 742.4
      - acquired 349.2
    - spinal (cord) 742.59
      - acquired 349.2
  - mesentery (congenital) 751.9
    - acquired 568.89
  - metacarpus (acquired) 736.00
    - congenital 755.50
  - metatarsus (acquired) 736.70
    - congenital 754.70
  - middle ear, except ossicles (congenital) 744.03
    - ossicles 744.04
  - mitral (leaflets) (valve) (congenital) 746.9
    - acquired — see Endocarditis, mitral
    - Ebstein's 746.89
    - parachute 746.5
    - specified type NEC 746.89
    - stenosis, congenital 746.5
  - mouth (acquired) 528.9
    - congenital NEC 750.9
      - specified type NEC 750.26
  - multiple, congenital NEC 759.7

Deformity — continued
- multiple, congenital — continued
  - specified type NEC 759.89
- muscle (acquired) 728.9
  - congenital 756.9
    - specified type NEC 756.89
    - sternocleidomastoid (due to intrauterine malposition and pressure) 754.1
- musculoskeletal system, congenital NEC 756.9
  - specified type NEC 756.9
- nail (acquired) 703.9
  - congenital 757.9
- nasal — see Deformity, nose
- neck (acquired) NEC 738.2
  - congenital (any part) 744.9
    - sternocleidomastoid 754.1
- nervous system (congenital) 742.9
- nipple (congenital) 757.6
  - acquired 611.89
- nose, nasal (cartilage) (acquired) 738.0
  - bone (turbinate) 738.0
  - congenital 748.1
    - bent 754.0
    - squashed 754.0
  - saddle 738.0
    - syphilitic 090.5
  - septum 470
    - congenital 748.1
  - sinus (wall) (congenital) 748.1
    - acquired 738.0
  - syphilitic (congenital) 090.5
    - late 095.8
- ocular muscle (congenital) 743.9
  - acquired 378.60
- opticociliary vessels (congenital) 743.9
- orbit (congenital) (eye) 743.9
  - acquired NEC 376.40
    - associated with craniofacial deformities 376.44
    - due to
      - bone disease 376.43
      - surgery 376.47
      - trauma 376.47
- organ of Corti (congenital) 744.05
- ovary (congenital) 752.0
  - acquired 620.8
- oviduct (congenital) 752.10
  - acquired 620.8
- palate (congenital) 750.9
  - acquired 526.89
  - cleft (congenital) (see also Cleft, palate) 749.00
  - hard, acquired 526.89
  - soft, acquired 528.9
- pancreas (congenital) 751.7
  - acquired 577.8
- parachute, mitral valve 746.5
- parathyroid (gland) 759.2
- parotid (gland) (congenital) 750.9
  - acquired 527.8
- patella (acquired) 736.6
  - congenital 755.64
- pelvis, pelvic (acquired) (bony) 738.6
  - with disproportion (fetopelvic) 653.0 ☑
    - affecting fetus or newborn 763.1
    - causing obstructed labor 660.1 ☑
      - affecting fetus or newborn 763.1
  - congenital 755.60
  - rachitic (late effect) 268.1
- penis (glans) (congenital) 752.9
  - acquired 607.89
- pericardium (congenital) 746.9
  - acquired — see Pericarditis
- pharynx (congenital) 750.9
  - acquired 478.29
- Pierre Robin (congenital) 756.0
- pinna (acquired) 380.32
  - congenital 744.3
- pituitary (congenital) 759.2
- pleural folds (congenital) 748.8
- portal vein (congenital) 747.40
- posture — see Curvature, spine
- prepuce (congenital) 752.9
  - acquired 607.89

☑ Additional Digit Required — Refer to the Tabular List for Digit Selection   ⌐ Subterms under main terms may continue to next column or page

2014 ICD-9-CM   ▶◀ Revised Text   ● New Line   ▲ Revised Code   Volume 2 — 67

Deformity — *continued*
prostate (congenital) 752.9
　acquired 602.8
pulmonary valve — *see* Endocarditis, pulmonary
pupil (congenital) 743.9
　acquired 364.75
pylorus (congenital) 750.9
　acquired 537.89
rachitic (acquired), healed or old 268.1
radius (acquired) 736.00
　congenital 755.50
　　reduction — *see* Deformity, reduction, upper limb
rectovaginal septum (congenital) 752.40
　acquired 623.8
rectum (congenital) 751.5
　acquired 569.49
reduction (extremity) (limb) 755.4
　brain 742.2
　lower limb 755.30
　　with complete absence of distal elements 755.31
　　longitudinal (complete) (partial) (with distal deficiencies, incomplete) 755.32
　　　with complete absence of distal elements 755.31
　　　combined femoral, tibial, fibular (incomplete) 755.33
　　　femoral 755.34
　　　fibular 755.37
　　　metatarsal(s) 755.38
　　　phalange(s) 755.39
　　　　meaning all digits 755.31
　　　tarsal(s) 755.38
　　　tibia 755.36
　　　tibiofibular 755.35
　　transverse 755.31
　upper limb 755.20
　　with complete absence of distal elements 755.21
　　longitudinal (complete) (partial) (with distal deficiencies, incomplete) 755.22
　　　with complete absence of distal elements 755.21
　　　carpal(s) 755.28
　　　combined humeral, radial, ulnar (incomplete) 755.23
　　　humeral 755.24
　　　metacarpal(s) 755.28
　　　phalange(s) 755.29
　　　　meaning all digits 755.21
　　　radial 755.26
　　　radioulnar 755.25
　　　ulnar 755.27
　　transverse (complete) (partial) 755.21
renal — *see* Deformity, kidney
respiratory system (congenital) 748.9
　specified type NEC 748.8
rib (acquired) 738.3
　congenital 756.3
　　cervical 756.2
rotation (joint) (acquired) 736.9
　congenital 755.9
　hip or thigh 736.39
　　congenital (*see also* Subluxation, congenital, hip) 754.32
sacroiliac joint (congenital) 755.69
　acquired 738.5
sacrum (acquired) 738.5
　congenital 756.10
saddle
　back 737.8
　nose 738.0
　　syphilitic 090.5
salivary gland or duct (congenital) 750.9
　acquired 527.8
scapula (acquired) 736.89
　congenital 755.50
scrotum (congenital) 752.9
　acquired 608.89
sebaceous gland, acquired 706.8
seminal tract or duct (congenital) 752.9
　acquired 608.89

Deformity — *continued*
septum (nasal) (acquired) 470
　congenital 748.1
shoulder (joint) (acquired) 736.89
　congenital 755.50
　　specified type NEC 755.59
　contraction 718.41
sigmoid (flexure) (congenital) 751.5
　acquired 569.89
sinus of Valsalva 747.29
skin (congenital) 757.9
　acquired NEC 709.8
skull (acquired) 738.19
　congenital 756.0
　　with
　　　anencephalus 740.0
　　　encephalocele 742.0
　　　hydrocephalus 742.3
　　　　with spina bifida (*see also* Spina bifida) 741.0 ☑
　　　microcephalus 742.1
　　due to intrauterine malposition and pressure 754.0
soft parts, organs or tissues (of pelvis)
　in pregnancy or childbirth NEC 654.9 ☑
　　affecting fetus or newborn 763.89
　　causing obstructed labor 660.2 ☑
　　　affecting fetus or newborn 763.1
spermatic cord (congenital) 752.9
　acquired 608.89
　　torsion 608.22
　　　extravaginal 608.21
　　　intravaginal 608.22
spinal
　column — *see* Deformity, spine
　cord (congenital) 742.9
　　acquired 336.8
　　vessel (congenital) 747.82
　nerve root (congenital) 742.9
　　acquired 724.9
spine (acquired) NEC 738.5
　congenital 756.10
　　due to intrauterine malposition and pressure 754.2
　kyphoscoliotic (*see also* Kyphoscoliosis) 737.30
　kyphotic (*see also* Kyphosis) 737.10
　lordotic (*see also* Lordosis) 737.20
　rachitic 268.1
　scoliotic (*see also* Scoliosis) 737.30
spleen
　acquired 289.59
　congenital 759.0
Sprengel's (congenital) 755.52
sternum (acquired) 738.3
　congenital 756.3
stomach (congenital) 750.9
　acquired 537.89
submaxillary gland (congenital) 750.9
　acquired 527.8
swan neck (acquired)
　finger 736.22
　hand 736.09
talipes — *see* Talipes
teeth, tooth NEC 520.9
testis (congenital) 752.9
　acquired 608.89
　torsion 608.20
thigh (acquired) 736.89
　congenital 755.60
thorax (acquired) (wall) 738.3
　congenital 754.89
　late effect of rickets 268.1
thumb (acquired) 736.20
　congenital 755.50
thymus (tissue) (congenital) 759.2
thyroid (gland) (congenital) 759.2
　cartilage 748.3
　　acquired 478.79
tibia (acquired) 736.89
　congenital 755.60
　saber 090.5
toe (acquired) 735.9
　congenital 755.66
　specified NEC 735.8
tongue (congenital) 750.10

Deformity — *continued*
tongue — *continued*
　acquired 529.8
tooth, teeth NEC 520.9
trachea (rings) (congenital) 748.3
　acquired 519.19
transverse aortic arch (congenital) 747.21
tricuspid (leaflets) (valve) (congenital) 746.9
　acquired — *see* Endocarditis, tricuspid
　atresia or stenosis 746.1
　specified type NEC 746.89
trunk (acquired) 738.3
　congenital 759.9
ulna (acquired) 736.00
　congenital 755.50
upper extremity — *see* Deformity, arm
urachus (congenital) 753.7
ureter (opening) (congenital) 753.9
　acquired 593.89
urethra (valve) (congenital) 753.9
　acquired 599.84
urinary tract or system (congenital) 753.9
　urachus 753.7
uterus (congenital) 752.39
　acquired 621.8
uvula (congenital) 750.9
　acquired 528.9
vagina (congenital) 752.40
　acquired 623.8
valve, valvular (heart) (congenital) 746.9
　acquired — *see* Endocarditis
　pulmonary 746.00
　specified type NEC 746.89
vascular (congenital) (peripheral) NEC 747.60
　acquired 459.9
　gastrointestinal 747.61
　lower limb 747.64
　renal 747.62
　specified site NEC 747.69
　spinal 747.82
　upper limb 747.63
vas deferens (congenital) 752.9
　acquired 608.89
vein (congenital) NEC (*see also* Deformity, vascular) 747.60
　brain 747.81
　coronary 746.9
　great 747.40
vena cava (inferior) (superior) (congenital) 747.40
vertebra — *see* Deformity, spine
vesicourethral orifice (acquired) 596.89
　congenital NEC 753.9
　　specified type NEC 753.8
vessels of optic papilla (congenital) 743.9
visual field (contraction) 368.45
vitreous humor (congenital) 743.9
　acquired 379.29
vulva (congenital) 752.40
　acquired 624.8
wrist (joint) (acquired) 736.00
　congenital 755.50
　contraction 718.43
　valgus 736.03
　　congenital 755.59
　varus 736.04
　　congenital 755.59

Degeneration, degenerative
adrenal (capsule) (gland) 255.8
　with hypofunction 255.41
　fatty 255.8
　hyaline 255.8
　infectional 255.8
　lardaceous 277.39
amyloid (any site) (general) 277.39
anterior cornua, spinal cord 336.8
anterior labral 840.8
aorta, aortic 440.0
　fatty 447.8
　valve (heart) (*see also* Endocarditis, aortic) 424.1
arteriovascular — *see* Arteriosclerosis
artery, arterial (atheromatous) (calcareous) (*see also* Arteriosclerosis)
　amyloid 277.39

Degeneration, degenerative — *continued*
artery, arterial (*see also* Arteriosclerosis) — *continued*
　lardaceous 277.39
　medial NEC (*see also* Arteriosclerosis, extremities) 440.20
articular cartilage NEC (*see also* Disorder, cartilage, articular) 718.0 ☑
　elbow 718.02
　knee 717.5
　patella 717.7
　shoulder 718.01
　spine (*see also* Spondylosis) 721.90
atheromatous — *see* Arteriosclerosis
bacony (any site) 277.39
basal nuclei or ganglia NEC 333.0
bone 733.90
brachial plexus 353.0
brain (cortical) (progressive) 331.9
　arteriosclerotic 437.0
　childhood 330.9
　　specified type NEC 330.8
　congenital 742.4
　cystic 348.0
　　congenital 742.4
　familial NEC 331.89
　grey matter 330.8
　heredofamilial NEC 331.89
　in
　　alcoholism 303.9 ☑ *[331.7]*
　　beriberi 265.0 *[331.7]*
　　cerebrovascular disease 437.9 *[331.7]*
　　congenital hydrocephalus 742.3 *[331.7]*
　　　with spina bifida (*see also* Spina bifida) 741.0 ☑ *[331.7]*
　　Fabry's disease 272.7 *[330.2]*
　　Gaucher's disease 272.7 *[330.2]*
　　Hunter's disease or syndrome 277.5 *[330.3]*
　　lipidosis
　　　cerebral 330.1
　　　generalized 272.7 *[330.2]*
　　mucopolysaccharidosis 277.5 *[330.3]*
　　myxedema (*see also* Myxedema) 244.9 *[331.7]*
　　neoplastic disease NEC (M8000/1) 239.9 *[331.7]*
　　Niemann-Pick disease 272.7 *[330.2]*
　　sphingolipidosis 272.7 *[330.2]*
　　vitamin B$_{12}$ deficiency 266.2 *[331.7]*
　motor centers 331.89
　senile 331.2
　specified type NEC 331.89
breast — *see* Disease, breast
Bruch's membrane 363.40
bundle of His 426.50
　left 426.3
　right 426.4
calcareous NEC 275.49
capillaries 448.9
　amyloid 277.39
　fatty 448.9
　lardaceous 277.39
cardiac (brown) (calcareous) (fatty) (fibrous) (hyaline) (mural) (muscular) (pigmentary) (senile) (with arteriosclerosis) (*see also* Degeneration, myocardial) 429.1
　valve, valvular — *see* Endocarditis
cardiorenal (*see also* Hypertension, cardiorenal) 404.90
cardiovascular (*see also* Disease, cardiovascular) 429.2
　renal (*see also* Hypertension, cardiorenal) 404.90
cartilage (joint) — *see* Derangement, joint
cerebellar NEC 334.9
　primary (hereditary) (sporadic) 334.2
cerebral — *see* Degeneration, brain
cerebromacular 330.1
cerebrovascular 437.1
　due to hypertension 437.2
　late effect — *see* Late effect(s) (of) cerebrovascular disease
cervical plexus 353.2

Degeneration, degenerative — *continued*
cervix 622.8
  due to radiation (intended effect) 622.8
    adverse effect or misadventure 622.8
changes, spine or vertebra (*see also* Spondylosis) 721.90
chitinous 277.39
chorioretinal 363.40
  congenital 743.53
  hereditary 363.50
choroid (colloid) (drusen) 363.40
  hereditary 363.50
  senile 363.41
    diffuse secondary 363.42
cochlear 386.8
collateral ligament (knee) (medial) 717.82
  lateral 717.81
combined (spinal cord) (subacute) 266.2 *[336.2]*
  with anemia (pernicious) 281.0 *[336.2]*
    due to dietary deficiency 281.1 *[336.2]*
    due to vitamin B$_{12}$ deficiency anemia (dietary) 281.1 *[336.2]*
conjunctiva 372.50
  amyloid 277.39 *[372.50]*
cornea 371.40
  calcerous 371.44
  familial (hereditary) (*see also* Dystrophy, cornea) 371.50
    macular 371.55
    reticular 371.54
  hyaline (of old scars) 371.41
  marginal (Terrien's) 371.48
  mosaic (shagreen) 371.41
  nodular 371.46
  peripheral 371.48
  senile 371.41
cortical (cerebellar) (parenchymatous) 334.2
  alcoholic 303.9 ☑ *[334.4]*
  diffuse, due to arteriopathy 437.0
corticobasal 331.6
corticostriatal-spinal 334.8
cretinoid 243
cruciate ligament (knee) (posterior) 717.84
  anterior 717.83
cutis 709.3
  amyloid 277.39
dental pulp 522.2
disc disease — *see* Degeneration, intervertebral disc
dorsolateral (spinal cord) — *see* Degeneration, combined
endocardial 424.90
extrapyramidal NEC 333.90
eye NEC 360.40
  macular (*see also* Degeneration, macula) 362.50
    congenital 362.75
    hereditary 362.76
fatty (diffuse) (general) 272.8
  liver 571.8
    alcoholic 571.0
  localized site — *see* Degeneration, by site, fatty
  placenta — *see* Placenta, abnormal
globe (eye) NEC 360.40
  macular — *see* Degeneration, macula
grey matter 330.8
heart (brown) (calcareous) (fatty) (fibrous) (hyaline) (mural) (muscular) (pigmentary) (senile) (with arteriosclerosis) (*see also* Degeneration, myocardial) 429.1
  amyloid 277.39 *[425.7]*
  atheromatous — *see* Arteriosclerosis, coronary
  gouty 274.82
  hypertensive (*see also* Hypertension, heart) 402.90
  ischemic 414.9
  valve, valvular — *see* Endocarditis
hepatolenticular (Wilson's) 275.1
hepatorenal 572.4
heredofamilial
  brain NEC 331.89

Degeneration, degenerative — *continued*
heredofamilial — *continued*
  spinal cord NEC 336.8
hyaline (diffuse) (generalized) 728.9
  localized (*see also* Degeneration, by site)
    cornea 371.41
    keratitis 371.41
hypertensive vascular — *see* Hypertension
infrapatellar fat pad 729.31
internal semilunar cartilage 717.3
intervertebral disc 722.6
  with myelopathy 722.70
  cervical, cervicothoracic 722.4
    with myelopathy 722.71
  lumbar, lumbosacral 722.52
    with myelopathy 722.73
  thoracic, thoracolumbar 722.51
    with myelopathy 722.72
intestine 569.89
  amyloid 277.39
  lardaceous 277.39
iris (generalized) (*see also* Atrophy, iris) 364.59
  pigmentary 364.53
  pupillary margin 364.54
ischemic — *see* Ischemia
joint disease (*see also* Osteoarthrosis) 715.9 ☑
  multiple sites 715.09
  spine (*see also* Spondylosis) 721.90
kidney (*see also* Sclerosis, renal) 587
  amyloid 277.39 *[583.81]*
  cyst, cystic (multiple) (solitary) 593.2
    congenital (*see also* Cystic, disease, kidney) 753.10
  fatty 593.89
  fibrocystic (congenital) 753.19
  lardaceous 277.39 *[583.81]*
  polycystic (congenital) 753.12
    adult type (APKD) 753.13
    autosomal dominant 753.13
    autosomal recessive 753.14
    childhood type (CPKD) 753.14
    infantile type 753.14
  waxy 277.39 *[583.81]*
Kuhnt-Junius (retina) 362.52
labyrinth, osseous 386.8
lacrimal passages, cystic 375.12
lardaceous (any site) 277.39
lateral column (posterior), spinal cord (*see also* Degeneration, combined) 266.2 *[336.2]*
lattice 362.63
lens 366.9
  infantile, juvenile, or presenile 366.00
  senile 366.10
lenticular (familial) (progressive) (Wilson's) (with cirrhosis of liver) 275.1
  striate artery 437.0
lethal ball, prosthetic heart valve 996.02
ligament
  collateral (knee) (medial) 717.82
    lateral 717.81
  cruciate (knee) (posterior) 717.84
    anterior 717.83
liver (diffuse) 572.8
  amyloid 277.39
  ▶congenital (cystic) 751.62◀
  cystic 572.8
    congenital 751.62
  fatty 571.8
    alcoholic 571.0
  hypertrophic 572.8
  lardaceous 277.39
  parenchymatous, acute or subacute (*see also* Necrosis, liver) 570
  pigmentary 572.8
  toxic (acute) 573.8
  waxy 277.39
lung 518.89
lymph gland 289.3
  hyaline 289.3
  lardaceous 277.39
macula (acquired) (senile) 362.50
  atrophic 362.51
  Best's 362.76

Degeneration, degenerative — *continued*
macula — *continued*
  congenital 362.75
  cystic 362.54
  cystoid 362.53
  disciform 362.52
  dry 362.51
  exudative 362.52
  familial pseudoinflammatory 362.77
  hereditary 362.76
  hole 362.54
  juvenile (Stargardt's) 362.75
  nonexudative 362.51
  pseudohole 362.54
  wet 362.52
medullary — *see* Degeneration, brain
membranous labyrinth, congenital (causing impairment of hearing) 744.05
meniscus — *see* Derangement, joint
microcystoid 362.62
mitral — *see* Insufficiency, mitral
Mönckeberg's (*see also* Arteriosclerosis, extremities) 440.20
moral 301.7
motor centers, senile 331.2
mural (*see also* Degeneration, myocardial) 429.1
  heart, cardiac (*see also* Degeneration, myocardial) 429.1
  myocardium, myocardial (*see also* Degeneration, myocardial) 429.1
muscle 728.9
  fatty 728.9
  fibrous 728.9
  heart (*see also* Degeneration, myocardial) 429.1
  hyaline 728.9
muscular progressive 728.2
myelin, central nervous system NEC 341.9
myocardium, myocardial (brown) (calcareous) (fatty) (fibrous) (hyaline) (mural) (muscular) (pigmentary) (senile) (with arteriosclerosis) 429.1
  with rheumatic fever (conditions classifiable to 390) 398.0
    active, acute, or subacute 391.2
      with chorea 392.0
    inactive or quiescent (with chorea) 398.0
  amyloid 277.39 *[425.7]*
  congenital 746.89
  fetus or newborn 779.89
  gouty 274.82
  hypertensive (*see also* Hypertension, heart) 402.90
  ischemic 414.8
  rheumatic (*see also* Degeneration, myocardium, with rheumatic fever) 398.0
  syphilitic 093.82
nasal sinus (mucosa) (*see also* Sinusitis) 473.9
  frontal 473.1
  maxillary 473.0
nerve — *see* Disorder, nerve
nervous system 349.89
  amyloid 277.39 *[357.4]*
  autonomic (*see also* Neuropathy, peripheral, autonomic) 337.9
  fatty 349.89
  peripheral autonomic NEC (*see also* Neuropathy, peripheral, autonomic) 337.9
nipple 611.9
nose 478.19
oculoacousticocerebral, congenital (progressive) 743.8
olivopontocerebellar (familial) (hereditary) 333.0
osseous labyrinth 386.8
ovary 620.8
  cystic 620.2
  microcystic 620.2
pallidal, pigmentary (progressive) 333.0
pancreas 577.8

Degeneration, degenerative — *continued*
pancreas — *continued*
  tuberculous (*see also* Tuberculosis) 017.9 ☑
papillary muscle 429.81
paving stone 362.61
penis 607.89
peritoneum 568.89
pigmentary (diffuse) (general)
  localized — *see* Degeneration, by site
  pallidal (progressive) 333.0
  secondary 362.65
pineal gland 259.8
pituitary (gland) 253.8
placenta (fatty) (fibrinoid) (fibroid) — *see* Placenta, abnormal
popliteal fat pad 729.31
posterolateral (spinal cord) (*see also* Degeneration, combined) 266.2 *[336.2]*
pulmonary valve (heart) (*see also* Endocarditis, pulmonary) 424.3
pulp (tooth) 522.2
pupillary margin 364.54
renal (*see also* Sclerosis, renal) 587
  fibrocystic 753.19
  polycystic 753.12
    adult type (APKD) 753.13
    autosomal dominant 753.13
    autosomal recessive 753.14
    childhood type (CPKD) 753.14
    infantile type 753.14
reticuloendothelial system 289.89
retina (peripheral) 362.60
  with retinal defect (*see also* Detachment, retina, with retinal defect) 361.00
  cystic (senile) 362.50
  cystoid 362.53
  hereditary (*see also* Dystrophy, retina) 362.70
    cerebroretinal 362.71
    congenital 362.75
    juvenile (Stargardt's) 362.75
    macula 362.76
  Kuhnt-Junius 362.52
  lattice 362.63
  macular (*see also* Degeneration, macula) 362.50
  microcystoid 362.62
  palisade 362.63
  paving stone 362.61
  pigmentary (primary) 362.74
    secondary 362.65
  posterior pole (*see also* Degeneration, macula) 362.50
  secondary 362.66
  senile 362.60
    cystic 362.53
    reticular 362.64
saccule, congenital (causing impairment of hearing) 744.05
sacculocochlear 386.8
senile 797
  brain 331.2
  cardiac, heart, or myocardium (*see also* Degeneration, myocardial) 429.1
  motor centers 331.2
  reticule 362.64
  retina, cystic 362.50
  vascular — *see* Arteriosclerosis
silicone rubber poppet (prosthetic valve) 996.02
sinus (cystic) (*see also* Sinusitis) 473.9
  polypoid 471.1
skin 709.3
  amyloid 277.39
  colloid 709.3
spinal (cord) 336.8
  amyloid 277.39
  column 733.90
  combined (subacute) (*see also* Degeneration, combined) 266.2 *[336.2]*
    with anemia (pernicious) 281.0 *[336.2]*
  dorsolateral (*see also* Degeneration, combined) 266.2 *[336.2]*
  familial NEC 336.8

Degeneration, degenerative — Degeneration, degenerative

Degeneration, degenerative — *continued*
  spinal — *continued*
    fatty 336.8
    funicular (*see also* Degeneration, combined) 266.2 *[336.2]*
    heredofamilial NEC 336.8
    posterolateral (*see also* Degeneration, combined) 266.2 *[336.2]*
    subacute combined — *see* Degeneration, combined
    tuberculous (*see also* Tuberculosis) 013.8 ☑
  spine 733.90
  spleen 289.59
    amyloid 277.39
    lardaceous 277.39
  stomach 537.89
    lardaceous 277.39
  strionigral 333.0
  sudoriparous (cystic) 705.89
  suprarenal (capsule) (gland) 255.8
    with hypofunction 255.41
  sweat gland 705.89
  synovial membrane (pulpy) 727.9
  tapetoretinal 362.74
    adult or presenile form 362.50
  testis (postinfectional) 608.89
  thymus (gland) 254.8
    fatty 254.8
    lardaceous 277.39
  thyroid (gland) 246.8
  tricuspid (heart) (valve) — *see* Endocarditis, tricuspid
  tuberculous NEC (*see also* Tuberculosis) 011.9 ☑
  turbinate 733.90
  uterus 621.8
    cystic 621.8
  vascular (senile) (*see also* Arteriosclerosis)
    hypertensive — *see* Hypertension
  vitreoretinal (primary) 362.73
    secondary 362.66
  vitreous humor (with infiltration) 379.21
  wallerian NEC — *see* Disorder, nerve
  waxy (any site) 277.39
  Wilson's hepatolenticular 275.1
Deglutition
  paralysis 784.99
    hysterical 300.11
  pneumonia 507.0
Degos' disease or syndrome 447.8
Degradation disorder, branched-chain amino acid 270.3
Dehiscence
  anastomosis — *see* Complications, anastomosis
  cesarean wound 674.1 ☑
  closure of
    cornea 998.32
    fascia, superficial or muscular 998.31
    internal organ 998.31
    mucosa 998.32
    muscle or muscle flap 998.31
    ribs or rib cage 998.31
    skin 998.32
    skull or craniotomy 998.31
    sternum or sternotomy 998.31
    subcutaneous tissue 998.32
    tendon or ligament 998.31
    traumatic laceration (external) (internal) 998.31
  episiotomy 674.2 ☑
  operation wound 998.32
    deep 998.31
    external 998.32
    internal 998.31
    superficial 998.32
  perineal wound (postpartum) 674.2 ☑
  postoperative 998.32
    abdomen 998.32
      internal 998.31
    internal 998.31
  traumatic injury wound repair 998.33
  uterine wound 674.1 ☑
Dehydration (cachexia) 276.51

Dehydration — *continued*
  with
    hypernatremia 276.0
    hyponatremia 276.1
  newborn 775.5
Deiters' nucleus syndrome 386.19
Déjérine-Klumpke paralysis 767.6
Déjérine-Roussy syndrome 338.0
Déjérine-Sottas disease or neuropathy (hypertrophic) 356.0
Déjérine-Thomas atrophy or syndrome 333.0
Déjérine's disease 356.0
de Lange's syndrome (Amsterdam dwarf, intellectual disabilities, and brachycephaly) 759.89
Delay, delayed
  adaptation, cones or rods 368.63
  any plane in pelvis
    affecting fetus or newborn 763.1
    complicating delivery 660.1 ☑
  birth or delivery NEC 662.1 ☑
    affecting fetus or newborn 763.89
    second twin, triplet, or multiple mate 662.3 ☑
  closure (*see also* Fistula)
    cranial suture 756.0
    fontanel 756.0
  coagulation NEC 790.92
  conduction (cardiac) (ventricular) 426.9
  delivery NEC 662.1 ☑
    second twin, triplet, etc. 662.3 ☑
      affecting fetus or newborn 763.89
  development
    in childhood 783.40
      physiological 783.40
    intellectual NEC 315.9
    learning NEC 315.2
    reading 315.00
    sexual 259.0
    speech 315.39
      and language due to hearing loss 315.34
      associated with hyperkinesis 314.1
    spelling 315.09
  gastric emptying 536.8
  menarche 256.39
    due to pituitary hypofunction 253.4
  menstruation (cause unknown) 626.8
  milestone in childhood 783.42
  motility — *see* Hypomotility
  passage of meconium (newborn) 777.1
  primary respiration 768.9
  puberty 259.0
  separation of umbilical cord 779.83
  sexual maturation, female 259.0
  vaccination V64.00
Del Castillo's syndrome (germinal aplasia) 606.0
Déleage's disease 359.89
Deletion syndrome
  5p 758.31
  22q11.2 758.32
  autosomal NEC 758.39
  constitutional 5q deletion 758.39
Delhi (boil) (button) (sore) 085.1
Delinquency (juvenile) 312.9
  group (*see also* Disturbance, conduct) 312.2 ☑
  neurotic 312.4
Delirium, delirious 780.09
  acute 780.09
    due to conditions classified elsewhere 293.0
  alcoholic 291.0
    acute 291.0
    chronic 291.1
  alcoholicum 291.0
  chronic (*see also* Psychosis) 293.89
    due to or associated with physical condition — *see* Psychosis, organic
  drug-induced 292.81
  due to conditions classified elsewhere 293.0
  eclamptic (*see also* Eclampsia) 780.39
  exhaustion (*see also* Reaction, stress, acute) 308.9
  hysterical 300.11

Delirium, delirious — *continued*
  in
    presenile dementia 290.11
    senile dementia 290.3
  induced by drug 292.81
  manic, maniacal (acute) (*see also* Psychosis, affective) 296.0 ☑
    recurrent episode 296.1 ☑
    single episode 296.0 ☑
  puerperal 293.9
  senile 290.3
  subacute (psychotic) 293.1
  thyroid (*see also* Thyrotoxicosis) 242.9 ☑
  traumatic (*see also* Injury, intracranial)
    with
      lesion, spinal cord — *see* Injury, spinal, by site
      shock, spinal — *see* Injury, spinal, by site
  tremens (impending) 291.0
  uremic — *see* Uremia
  withdrawal
    alcoholic (acute) 291.0
      chronic 291.1
    drug 292.0

Delivery

Note — Use the following fifth-digit subclassification with categories 640–649, 651–676:

0   unspecified as to episode of care

1   delivered, with or without mention of antepartum condition

2   delivered, with mention of postpartum complication

3   antepartum condition or complication

4   postpartum condition or complication

  breech (assisted) (buttocks) (complete) (frank) (spontaneous) 652.2 ☑
    affecting fetus or newborn 763.0
    extraction NEC 669.6 ☑
  cesarean (for) 669.7 ☑
    abnormal
      cervix 654.6 ☑
      pelvic organs or tissues 654.9 ☑
      pelvis (bony) (major) NEC 653.0 ☑
      presentation or position 652.9 ☑
        in multiple gestation 652.6 ☑
      size, fetus 653.5 ☑
      soft parts (of pelvis) 654.9 ☑
      uterus, congenital 654.0 ☑
      vagina 654.7 ☑
      vulva 654.8 ☑
    abruptio placentae 641.2 ☑
    acromion presentation 652.8 ☑
    affecting fetus or newborn 763.4
    anteversion, cervix or uterus 654.4 ☑
    atony, uterus 661.2 ☑
      with hemorrhage 666.1 ☑
    bicornis or bicornuate uterus 654.0 ☑
    breech presentation (buttocks) (complete) (frank) 652.2 ☑
    brow presentation 652.4 ☑
    cephalopelvic disproportion (normally formed fetus) 653.4 ☑
    chin presentation 652.4 ☑
    cicatrix of cervix 654.6 ☑
    contracted pelvis (general) 653.1 ☑
      inlet 653.2 ☑
      outlet 653.3 ☑
    cord presentation or prolapse 663.0 ☑
    cystocele 654.4 ☑
    deformity (acquired) (congenital)
      pelvic organs or tissues NEC 654.9 ☑
      pelvis (bony) NEC 653.0 ☑
    displacement, uterus NEC 654.4 ☑
    disproportion NEC 653.9 ☑
    distress
      fetal 656.8 ☑
      maternal 669.0 ☑
    eclampsia 642.6 ☑

Delivery — *continued*
  cesarean — *continued*
    face presentation 652.4 ☑
    failed
      forceps 660.7 ☑
      trial of labor NEC 660.6 ☑
      vacuum extraction 660.7 ☑
      ventouse 660.7 ☑
    fetal-maternal hemorrhage 656.0 ☑
    fetal deformity 653.7 ☑
    fetus, fetal
      distress 656.8 ☑
      prematurity 656.8 ☑
    fibroid (tumor) (uterus) 654.1 ☑
    footling 652.8 ☑
      with successful version 652.1 ☑
    hemorrhage (antepartum) (intrapartum) NEC 641.9 ☑
    hydrocephalic fetus 653.6 ☑
    incarceration of uterus 654.3 ☑
    incoordinate uterine action 661.4 ☑
    inertia, uterus 661.2 ☑
      primary 661.0 ☑
      secondary 661.1 ☑
    lateroversion, uterus or cervix 654.4 ☑
    mal lie 652.9 ☑
    malposition
      fetus 652.9 ☑
        in multiple gestation 652.6 ☑
      pelvic organs or tissues NEC 654.9 ☑
      uterus NEC or cervix 654.4 ☑
    malpresentation NEC 652.9 ☑
      in multiple gestation 652.6 ☑
    maternal
      diabetes mellitus (conditions classifiable to 249 and 250) 648.0 ☑
      heart disease NEC 648.6 ☑
    meconium in liquor 656.8 ☑
      staining only 792.3
    oblique presentation 652.3 ☑
    oversize fetus 653.5 ☑
    pelvic tumor NEC 654.9 ☑
    placental insufficiency 656.5 ☑
    placenta previa 641.0 ☑
      with hemorrhage 641.1 ☑
    (planned) occurring after 37 completed weeks of gestation but before 39 completed weeks gestation due to (spontaneous) onset of labor 649.8 ☑
    poor dilation, cervix 661.0 ☑
    pre-eclampsia 642.4 ☑
      severe 642.5 ☑
    previous
      cesarean delivery, section 654.2 ☑
      surgery (to)
        cervix 654.6 ☑
        gynecological NEC 654.9 ☑
        rectum 654.8 ☑
        uterus NEC 654.9 ☑
          previous cesarean delivery, section 654.2 ☑
        vagina 654.7 ☑
    prolapse
      arm or hand 652.7 ☑
      uterus 654.4 ☑
    prolonged labor 662.1 ☑
    rectocele 654.4 ☑
    retroversion, uterus or cervix 654.3 ☑
    rigid
      cervix 654.6 ☑
      pelvic floor 654.4 ☑
      perineum 654.8 ☑
      vagina 654.7 ☑
      vulva 654.8 ☑
    sacculation, pregnant uterus 654.4 ☑
    scar(s)
      cervix 654.6 ☑
      cesarean delivery, section 654.2 ☑
      uterus NEC 654.9 ☑
        due to previous cesarean delivery, section 654.2 ☑
    Shirodkar suture in situ 654.5 ☑
    shoulder presentation 652.8 ☑

☑ Additional Digit Required — Refer to the Tabular List for Digit Selection   ▽ Subterms under main terms may continue to next column or page

Delivery — continued
cesarean — continued
    stenosis or stricture, cervix 654.6
    transverse presentation or lie 652.3 ☑
    tumor, pelvic organs or tissues NEC
       654.4 ☑
    umbilical cord presentation or prolapse
       663.0 ☑
completely normal case — see category 650
complicated (by) NEC 669.9 ☑
  abdominal tumor, fetal 653.7 ☑
    causing obstructed labor 660.1 ☑
  abnormal, abnormality of
    cervix 654.6 ☑
      causing obstructed labor
        660.2 ☑
    forces of labor 661.9 ☑
    formation of uterus 654.0 ☑
    pelvic organs or tissues 654.9 ☑
      causing obstructed labor
        660.2 ☑
    pelvis (bony) (major) NEC 653.0 ☑
      causing obstructed labor
        660.1 ☑
    presentation or position NEC
      652.9 ☑
      causing obstructed labor
        660.0 ☑
    size, fetus 653.5 ☑
      causing obstructed labor
        660.1 ☑
    soft parts (of pelvis) 654.9 ☑
      causing obstructed labor
        660.2 ☑
    uterine contractions NEC 661.9 ☑
    uterus (formation) 654.0 ☑
      causing obstructed labor
        660.2 ☑
    vagina 654.7 ☑
      causing obstructed labor
        660.2 ☑
  abnormally formed uterus (any type)
    (congenital) 654.0 ☑
    causing obstructed labor 660.2 ☑
  acromion presentation 652.8 ☑
    causing obstructed labor 660.0 ☑
  adherent placenta 667.0 ☑
    with hemorrhage 666.0 ☑
  adhesions, uterus (to abdominal wall)
    654.4 ☑
  advanced maternal age NEC 659.6 ☑
    multigravida 659.6 ☑
    primigravida 659.5 ☑
  air embolism 673.0 ☑
  amnionitis 658.4 ☑
  amniotic fluid embolism 673.1 ☑
  anesthetic death 668.9 ☑
  annular detachment, cervix 665.3 ☑
  antepartum hemorrhage — see Delivery,
    complicated, hemorrhage
  anteversion, cervix or uterus 654.4 ☑
    causing obstructed labor 660.2 ☑
  apoplexy 674.0 ☑
    placenta 641.2 ☑
  arrested active phase 661.1 ☑
  asymmetrical pelvis bone 653.0 ☑
    causing obstructed labor 660.1 ☑
  atony, uterus with hemorrhage (hypo-
    tonic) (inertia) 666.1 ☑
    hypertonic 661.4 ☑
  Bandl's ring 661.4 ☑
  battledore placenta — see Placenta, ab-
    normal
  bicornis or bicornuate uterus 654.0 ☑
    causing obstructed labor 660.2 ☑
  birth injury to mother NEC 665.9 ☑
  bleeding (see also Delivery, complicated,
    hemorrhage) 641.9 ☑
  breech presentation (assisted) (buttocks)
    (complete) (frank) (spontaneous)
    652.2 ☑
    with successful version 652.1 ☑
  brow presentation 652.4 ☑

Delivery — continued
complicated — continued
  cephalopelvic disproportion (normally
    formed fetus) 653.4 ☑
    causing obstructed labor 660.1 ☑
  cerebral hemorrhage 674.0 ☑
  cervical dystocia 661.2 ☑
  chin presentation 652.4 ☑
    causing obstructed labor 660.0 ☑
  cicatrix
    cervix 654.6 ☑
      causing obstructed labor
        660.2 ☑
    vagina 654.7 ☑
      causing obstructed labor
        660.2 ☑
  coagulation defect 649.3 ☑
  colporrhexis 665.4 ☑
    with perineal laceration 664.0 ☑
  compound presentation 652.8 ☑
    causing obstructed labor 660.0 ☑
  compression of cord (umbilical) 663.2 ☑
    around neck 663.1 ☑
    cord prolapsed 663.0 ☑
  contraction, contracted pelvis 653.1 ☑
    causing obstructed labor 660.1 ☑
    general 653.1 ☑
      causing obstructed labor
        660.1 ☑
    inlet 653.2 ☑
      causing obstructed labor
        660.1 ☑
    midpelvic 653.8 ☑
      causing obstructed labor
        660.1 ☑
    midplane 653.8 ☑
      causing obstructed labor
        660.1 ☑
    outlet 653.3 ☑
      causing obstructed labor
        660.1 ☑
  contraction ring 661.4 ☑
  cord (umbilical) 663.9 ☑
    around neck, tightly or with compres-
      sion 663.1 ☑
      without compression 663.3 ☑
    bruising 663.6 ☑
    complication NEC 663.9 ☑
      specified type NEC 663.8 ☑
    compression NEC 663.2 ☑
    entanglement NEC 663.3 ☑
      with compression 663.2 ☑
    forelying 663.0 ☑
    hematoma 663.6 ☑
    marginal attachment 663.8 ☑
    presentation 663.0 ☑
    prolapse (complete) (occult) (partial)
      663.0 ☑
    short 663.4 ☑
    specified complication NEC 663.8 ☑
    thrombosis (vessels) 663.6 ☑
    vascular lesion 663.6 ☑
    velamentous insertion 663.8 ☑
  Couvelaire uterus 641.2 ☑
  cretin pelvis (dwarf type) (male type)
    653.1 ☑
    causing obstructed labor 660.1 ☑
  crossbirth 652.3 ☑
    with successful version 652.1 ☑
    causing obstructed labor 660.0 ☑
  cyst (Gartner's duct) 654.7 ☑
  cystocele 654.4 ☑
    causing obstructed labor 660.2 ☑
  death of fetus (near term) 656.4 ☑
    early (before 22 completed weeks
      gestation) 632
  deformity (acquired) (congenital)
    fetus 653.7 ☑
      causing obstructed labor
        660.1 ☑
    pelvic organs or tissues NEC 654.9 ☑
      causing obstructed labor
        660.2 ☑
    pelvis (bony) NEC 653.0 ☑

Delivery — continued
complicated — continued
  deformity — continued
    pelvis — continued
      causing obstructed labor
        660.1 ☑
  delay, delayed
    delivery in multiple pregnancy
      662.3 ☑
    due to locked mates 660.5 ☑
    following rupture of membranes
      (spontaneous) 658.2 ☑
      artificial 658.3 ☑
  depressed fetal heart tones 659.7 ☑
  diastasis recti 665.8 ☑
  dilatation
    bladder 654.4 ☑
      causing obstructed labor
        660.2 ☑
    cervix, incomplete, poor or slow
      661.0 ☑
  diseased placenta 656.7 ☑
  displacement uterus NEC 654.4 ☑
    causing obstructed labor 660.2 ☑
  disproportion NEC 653.9 ☑
    causing obstructed labor 660.1 ☑
  disruptio uteri — see Delivery, complicat-
    ed, rupture, uterus
  distress
    fetal 656.8 ☑
    maternal 669.0 ☑
  double uterus (congenital) 654.0 ☑
    causing obstructed labor 660.2 ☑
  dropsy amnion 657.0 ☑
  dysfunction, uterus 661.9 ☑
    hypertonic 661.4 ☑
    hypotonic 661.2 ☑
      primary 661.0 ☑
      secondary 661.1 ☑
    incoordinate 661.4 ☑
  dystocia
    cervical 661.2 ☑
    fetal — see Delivery, complicated,
      abnormal, presentation
    maternal — see Delivery, complicat-
      ed, prolonged labor
    pelvic — see Delivery, complicated,
      contraction pelvis
    positional 652.8 ☑
    shoulder girdle 660.4 ☑
  eclampsia 642.6 ☑
  ectopic kidney 654.4 ☑
    causing obstructed labor 660.2 ☑
  edema, cervix 654.6 ☑
    causing obstructed labor 660.2 ☑
  effusion, amniotic fluid 658.1 ☑
  elderly multigravida 659.6 ☑
  elderly primigravida 659.5 ☑
  embolism (pulmonary) 673.2 ☑
    air 673.0 ☑
    amniotic fluid 673.1 ☑
    blood clot 673.2 ☑
    cerebral 674.0 ☑
    fat 673.8 ☑
    pyemic 673.3 ☑
    septic 673.3 ☑
  entanglement, umbilical cord 663.3 ☑
    with compression 663.2 ☑
    around neck (with compression)
      663.1 ☑
  eversion, cervix or uterus 665.2 ☑
  excessive
    fetal growth 653.5 ☑
      causing obstructed labor
        660.1 ☑
    size of fetus 653.5 ☑
      causing obstructed labor
        660.1 ☑
  face presentation 652.4 ☑
    causing obstructed labor 660.0 ☑
    to pubes 660.3 ☑
  failure, fetal head to enter pelvic brim
    652.5 ☑
    causing obstructed labor 660.0 ☑

Delivery — continued
complicated — continued
  female genital mutilation 660.8 ☑
  fetal
    acid-base balance 656.8 ☑
    death (near term) NEC 656.4 ☑
      early (before 22 completed weeks
        gestation) 632
    deformity 653.7 ☑
      causing obstructed labor
        660.1 ☑
    distress 656.8 ☑
    heart rate or rhythm 659.7 ☑
    reduction of multiple fetuses reduced
      to single fetus 651.7 ☑
  fetopelvic disproportion 653.4 ☑
    causing obstructed labor 660.1 ☑
  fever during labor 659.2 ☑
  fibroid (tumor) (uterus) 654.1 ☑
    causing obstructed labor 660.2 ☑
  fibromyomata 654.1 ☑
    causing obstructed labor 660.2 ☑
  forelying umbilical cord 663.0 ☑
  fracture of coccyx 665.6 ☑
  hematoma 664.5 ☑
    broad ligament 665.7 ☑
    ischial spine 665.7 ☑
    pelvic 665.7 ☑
    perineum 664.5 ☑
    soft tissues 665.7 ☑
    subdural 674.0 ☑
    umbilical cord 663.6 ☑
    vagina 665.7 ☑
    vulva or perineum 664.5 ☑
  hemorrhage (uterine) (antepartum) (in-
    trapartum) (pregnancy) 641.9 ☑
    accidental 641.2 ☑
    associated with
      afibrinogenemia 641.3 ☑
      coagulation defect 641.3 ☑
        hyperfibrinolysis 641.3 ☑
        hypofibrinogenemia 641.3 ☑
    cerebral 674.0 ☑
    due to
      low-lying placenta 641.1 ☑
      placenta previa 641.1 ☑
      premature separation of placenta
        (normally implanted)
        641.2 ☑
      retained placenta 666.0 ☑
      trauma 641.8 ☑
      uterine leiomyoma 641.8 ☑
    marginal sinus rupture 641.2 ☑
    placenta NEC 641.9 ☑
    postpartum (atonic) (immediate)
      (within 24 hours) 666.1 ☑
      with retained or trapped placenta
        666.0 ☑
      delayed 666.2 ☑
      secondary 666.2 ☑
      third stage 666.0 ☑
  hourglass contraction, uterus 661.4 ☑
  hydramnios 657.0 ☑
  hydrocephalic fetus 653.6 ☑
    causing obstructed labor 660.1 ☑
  hydrops fetalis 653.7 ☑
    causing obstructed labor 660.1 ☑
  hypertension — see Hypertension,
    complicating pregnancy
  hypertonic uterine dysfunction 661.4 ☑
  hypotonic uterine dysfunction 661.2 ☑
  impacted shoulders 660.4 ☑
  incarceration, uterus 654.3 ☑
    causing obstructed labor 660.2 ☑
  incomplete dilation (cervix) 661.0 ☑
  incoordinate uterus 661.4 ☑
  indication NEC 659.9 ☑
    specified type NEC 659.8 ☑
  inertia, uterus 661.2 ☑
    hypertonic 661.4 ☑
    hypotonic 661.2 ☑
      primary 661.0 ☑
      secondary 661.1 ☑

☑ Additional Digit Required — Refer to the Tabular List for Digit Selection   ⱽ Subterms under main terms may continue to next column or page

2014 ICD-9-CM   ▶◀ Revised Text   ● New Line   ▲ Revised Code   Volume 2 — 71

Delivery — Delivery

Delivery — *continued*
  complicated — *continued*
    infantile
      genitalia 654.4 ✓
        causing obstructed labor
          660.2 ✓
      uterus (os) 654.4 ✓
        causing obstructed labor
          660.2 ✓
    injury (to mother) NEC 665.9 ✓
    intrauterine fetal death (near term) NEC
      656.4 ✓
      early (before 22 completed weeks
        gestation) 632
    inversion, uterus 665.2 ✓
    kidney, ectopic 654.4 ✓
      causing obstructed labor 660.2 ✓
    knot (true), umbilical cord 663.2 ✓
    labor
      onset (spontaneous) after 37 complet-
        ed weeks of gestation but be-
        fore 39 completed weeks
        gestation with delivery by
        (planned) cesarean section
        649.8 ✓
      premature (before 37 completed
        weeks gestation) 644.2 ✓
    laceration 664.9 ✓
      anus (sphincter) (healed) (old)
        654.8 ✓
        with mucosa 664.3 ✓
        not associated with third-degree
          perineal laceration
          664.6 ✓
      bladder (urinary) 665.5 ✓
      bowel 665.5 ✓
      central 664.4 ✓
      cervix (uteri) 665.3 ✓
      fourchette 664.0 ✓
      hymen 664.0 ✓
      labia (majora) (minora) 664.0 ✓
      pelvic
        floor 664.1 ✓
        organ NEC 665.5 ✓
      perineum, perineal 664.4 ✓
        first degree 664.0 ✓
        second degree 664.1 ✓
        third degree 664.2 ✓
        fourth degree 664.3 ✓
        central 664.4 ✓
        extensive NEC 664.4 ✓
        muscles 664.1 ✓
        skin 664.0 ✓
        slight 664.0 ✓
      peritoneum (pelvic) 665.5 ✓
      periurethral tissue 664.8 ✓
      rectovaginal (septum) (without per-
        ineal laceration) 665.4 ✓
        with perineum 664.2 ✓
          with anal or rectal mucosa
          664.3 ✓
      skin (perineum) 664.0 ✓
      specified site or type NEC 664.8 ✓
      sphincter ani (healed) (old) 654.8 ✓
        with mucosa 664.3 ✓
        not associated with third-degree
          perineal laceration
          664.6 ✓
      urethra 665.5 ✓
      uterus 665.1 ✓
        before labor 665.0 ✓
      vagina, vaginal (deep) (high) (sulcus)
        (wall) (without perineal lacer-
        ation) 665.4 ✓
        with perineum 664.0 ✓
        muscles, with perineum 664.1 ✓
      vulva 664.0 ✓
    lateroversion, uterus or cervix 654.4 ✓
      causing obstructed labor 660.2 ✓
    locked mates 660.5 ✓
    low implantation of placenta — *see* De-
      livery, complicated, placenta,
      previa
    mal lie 652.9 ✓

Delivery — *continued*
  complicated — *continued*
    malposition
      fetus NEC 652.9 ✓
        causing obstructed labor
          660.0 ✓
      pelvic organs or tissues NEC 654.9 ✓
        causing obstructed labor
          660.2 ✓
      placenta 641.1 ✓
        without hemorrhage 641.0 ✓
      uterus NEC or cervix 654.4 ✓
        causing obstructed labor
          660.2 ✓
    malpresentation 652.9 ✓
      causing obstructed labor 660.0 ✓
    marginal sinus (bleeding) (rupture)
      641.2 ✓
    maternal hypotension syndrome
      669.2 ✓
    meconium in liquor 656.8 ✓
    membranes, retained — *see* Delivery,
      complicated, placenta, retained
    mentum presentation 652.4 ✓
      causing obstructed labor 660.0 ✓
    metrorrhagia (myopathia) — *see* Deliv-
      ery, complicated, hemorrhage
    metrorrhexis — *see* Delivery, complicat-
      ed, rupture, uterus
    multiparity (grand) 659.4 ✓
    myelomeningocele, fetus 653.7 ✓
      causing obstructed labor 660.1 ✓
    Nägele's pelvis 653.0 ✓
      causing obstructed labor 660.1 ✓
    nonengagement, fetal head 652.5 ✓
      causing obstructed labor 660.0 ✓
    oblique presentation 652.3 ✓
      causing obstructed labor 660.0 ✓
    obstetric
      shock 669.1 ✓
      trauma NEC 665.9 ✓
    obstructed labor 660.9 ✓
      due to
        abnormality of pelvic organs or
          tissues (conditions classifi-
          able to 654.0–654.9)
          660.2 ✓
        deep transverse arrest 660.3 ✓
        impacted shoulders 660.4 ✓
        locked twins 660.5 ✓
        malposition and malpresentation
          of fetus (conditions classi-
          fiable to 652.0–652.9)
          660.0 ✓
        persistent occipitoposterior
          660.3 ✓
        shoulder dystocia 660.4 ✓
    occult prolapse of umbilical cord
      663.0 ✓
    oversize fetus 653.5 ✓
      causing obstructed labor 660.1 ✓
    pathological retraction ring, uterus
      661.4 ✓
    pelvic
      arrest (deep) (high) (of fetal head)
        (transverse) 660.3 ✓
      deformity (bone) (*see also* Deformity,
        pelvis, with disproportion)
      soft tissue 654.9 ✓
        causing obstructed labor
          660.2 ✓
      tumor NEC 654.9 ✓
        causing obstructed labor
          660.2 ✓
    penetration, pregnant uterus by instru-
      ment 665.1 ✓
    perforation — *see* Delivery, complicated,
      laceration
    persistent
      hymen 654.8 ✓
        causing obstructed labor
          660.2 ✓
      occipitoposterior 660.3 ✓

Delivery — *continued*
  complicated — *continued*
    placenta, placental
      ablatio 641.2 ✓
      abnormality 656.7 ✓
        with hemorrhage 641.2 ✓
      abruptio 641.2 ✓
      accreta 667.0 ✓
        with hemorrhage 666.0 ✓
      adherent (without hemorrhage)
        667.0 ✓
        with hemorrhage 666.0 ✓
      apoplexy 641.2 ✓
      battledore placenta — *see* Placenta,
        abnormal
      detachment (premature) 641.2 ✓
      disease 656.7 ✓
      hemorrhage NEC 641.9 ✓
      increta (without hemorrhage)
        667.0 ✓
        with hemorrhage 666.0 ✓
      low (implantation) 641.1 ✓
        without hemorrhage 641.0 ✓
      malformation 656.7 ✓
        with hemorrhage 641.2 ✓
      malposition 641.1 ✓
        without hemorrhage 641.0 ✓
      marginal sinus rupture 641.2 ✓
      percreta 667.0 ✓
        with hemorrhage 666.0 ✓
      premature separation 641.2 ✓
      previa (central) (lateral) (marginal)
        (partial) 641.1 ✓
        without hemorrhage 641.0 ✓
      retained (with hemorrhage) 666.0 ✓
        without hemorrhage 667.0 ✓
      rupture of marginal sinus 641.2 ✓
      separation (premature) 641.2 ✓
      trapped 666.0 ✓
        without hemorrhage 667.0 ✓
      vicious insertion 641.1 ✓
    polyhydramnios 657.0 ✓
    polyp, cervix 654.6 ✓
      causing obstructed labor 660.2 ✓
    precipitate labor 661.3 ✓
    premature
      labor (before 37 completed weeks
        gestation) 644.2 ✓
      rupture, membranes 658.1 ✓
        delayed delivery following
          658.2 ✓
    presenting umbilical cord 663.0 ✓
    previous
      cesarean delivery, section 654.2 ✓
      surgery
        cervix 654.6 ✓
          causing obstructed labor
            660.2 ✓
        gynecological NEC 654.9 ✓
          causing obstructed labor
            660.2 ✓
        perineum 654.8 ✓
        rectum 654.8 ✓
        uterus NEC 654.9 ✓
          due to previous cesarean de-
            livery, section 654.2 ✓
        vagina 654.7 ✓
          causing obstructed labor
            660.2 ✓
        vulva 654.8 ✓
    primary uterine inertia 661.0 ✓
    primipara, elderly or old 659.5 ✓
    prolapse
      arm or hand 652.7 ✓
        causing obstructed labor
          660.0 ✓
      cord (umbilical) 663.0 ✓
      fetal extremity 652.8 ✓
      foot or leg 652.8 ✓
        causing obstructed labor
          660.0 ✓
      umbilical cord (complete) (occult)
        (partial) 663.0 ✓
      uterus 654.4 ✓

Delivery — *continued*
  complicated — *continued*
    prolapse — *continued*
      uterus — *continued*
        causing obstructed labor
          660.2 ✓
    prolonged labor 662.1 ✓
      first stage 662.0 ✓
      second stage 662.2 ✓
      active phase 661.2 ✓
      due to
        cervical dystocia 661.2 ✓
        contraction ring 661.4 ✓
        tetanic uterus 661.4 ✓
        uterine inertia 661.2 ✓
          primary 661.0 ✓
          secondary 661.1 ✓
      latent phase 661.0 ✓
    pyrexia during labor 659.2 ✓
    rachitic pelvis 653.2 ✓
      causing obstructed labor 660.1 ✓
    rectocele 654.4 ✓
      causing obstructed labor 660.2 ✓
    retained membranes or portions of pla-
      centa 666.2 ✓
      without hemorrhage 667.1 ✓
    retarded (prolonged) birth 662.1 ✓
    retention secundines (with hemorrhage)
      666.2 ✓
      without hemorrhage 667.1 ✓
    retroversion, uterus or cervix 654.3 ✓
      causing obstructed labor 660.2 ✓
    rigid
      cervix 654.6 ✓
        causing obstructed labor
          660.2 ✓
      pelvic floor 654.4 ✓
        causing obstructed labor
          660.2 ✓
      perineum or vulva 654.8 ✓
        causing obstructed labor
          660.2 ✓
      vagina 654.7 ✓
        causing obstructed labor
          660.2 ✓
    Robert's pelvis 653.0 ✓
      causing obstructed labor 660.1 ✓
    rupture (*see also* Delivery, complicated,
      laceration)
      bladder (urinary) 665.5 ✓
      cervix 665.3 ✓
      marginal sinus 641.2 ✓
      membranes, premature 658.1 ✓
      pelvic organ NEC 665.5 ✓
      perineum (without mention of other
        laceration) — *see* Delivery,
        complicated, laceration, per-
        ineum
      peritoneum (pelvic) 665.5 ✓
      urethra 665.5 ✓
      uterus (during labor) 665.1 ✓
        before labor 665.0 ✓
    sacculation, pregnant uterus 654.4 ✓
    sacral teratomas, fetal 653.7 ✓
      causing obstructed labor 660.1 ✓
    scar(s)
      cervix 654.6 ✓
        causing obstructed labor
          660.2 ✓
      cesarean delivery, section 654.2 ✓
        causing obstructed labor
          660.2 ✓
      perineum 654.8 ✓
        causing obstructed labor
          660.2 ✓
      uterus NEC 654.9 ✓
        causing obstructed labor
          660.2 ✓
        due to previous cesarean delivery,
          section 654.2 ✓
      vagina 654.7 ✓
        causing obstructed labor
          660.2 ✓
      vulva 654.8 ✓

Delivery — *continued*
complicated — *continued*
scar(s) — *continued*
vulva — *continued*
causing obstructed labor 660.2 ✓
scoliotic pelvis 653.0 ✓
causing obstructed labor 660.1 ✓
secondary uterine inertia 661.1 ✓
secundines, retained — *see* Delivery, complicated, placenta, retained
separation
placenta (premature) 641.2 ✓
pubic bone 665.6 ✓
symphysis pubis 665.6 ✓
septate vagina 654.7 ✓
causing obstructed labor 660.2 ✓
shock (birth) (obstetric) (puerperal) 669.1 ✓
short cord syndrome 663.4 ✓
shoulder
girdle dystocia 660.4 ✓
presentation 652.8 ✓
causing obstructed labor 660.0 ✓
Siamese twins 678.1 ✓
slow slope active phase 661.2 ✓
spasm
cervix 661.4 ✓
uterus 661.4 ✓
spondylolisthesis, pelvis 653.3 ✓
causing obstructed labor 660.1 ✓
spondylolysis (lumbosacral) 653.3 ✓
causing obstructed labor 660.1 ✓
spondylosis 653.0 ✓
causing obstructed labor 660.1 ✓
stenosis or stricture
cervix 654.6 ✓
causing obstructed labor 660.2 ✓
vagina 654.7 ✓
causing obstructed labor 660.2 ✓
sudden death, unknown cause 669.9 ✓
tear (pelvic organ) (*see also* Delivery, complicated, laceration) 664.9 ✓
anal sphincter (healed) (old) 654.8 ✓
not associated with third-degree perineal laceration 664.6 ✓
teratomas, sacral, fetal 653.7 ✓
causing obstructed labor 660.1 ✓
tetanic uterus 661.4 ✓
tipping pelvis 653.0 ✓
causing obstructed labor 660.1 ✓
transverse
arrest (deep) 660.3 ✓
presentation or lie 652.3 ✓
with successful version 652.1 ✓
causing obstructed labor 660.0 ✓
trauma (obstetrical) NEC 665.9 ✓
periurethral 664.8 ✓
tumor
abdominal, fetal 653.7 ✓
causing obstructed labor 660.1 ✓
pelvic organs or tissues NEC 654.9 ✓
causing obstructed labor 660.2 ✓
umbilical cord (*see also* Delivery, complicated, cord) 663.9 ✓
around neck tightly, or with compression 663.1 ✓
entanglement NEC 663.3 ✓
with compression 663.2 ✓
prolapse (complete) (occult) (partial) 663.0 ✓
unstable lie 652.0 ✓
causing obstructed labor 660.0 ✓
uterine
inertia (*see also* Delivery, complicated, inertia, uterus) 661.2 ✓
spasm 661.4 ✓

Delivery — *continued*
complicated — *continued*
vasa previa 663.5 ✓
velamentous insertion of cord 663.8 ✓
young maternal age 659.8 ✓
delayed NEC 662.1 ✓
following rupture of membranes (spontaneous) 658.2 ✓
artificial 658.3 ✓
second twin, triplet, etc. 662.3 ✓
difficult NEC 669.9 ✓
previous, affecting management of pregnancy or childbirth V23.49
specified type NEC 669.8 ✓
early onset (spontaneous) 644.2 ✓
footling 652.8 ✓
with successful version 652.1 ✓
forceps NEC 669.5 ✓
affecting fetus or newborn 763.2
missed (at or near term) 656.4 ✓
multiple gestation NEC 651.9 ✓
with fetal loss and retention of one or more fetus(es) 651.6 ✓
following (elective) fetal reduction 651.7 ✓
specified type NEC 651.8 ✓
with fetal loss and retention of one or more fetus(es) 651.6 ✓
following (elective) fetal reduction 651.7 ✓
nonviable infant 656.4 ✓
normal — *see* category 650
precipitate 661.3 ✓
affecting fetus or newborn 763.6
premature NEC (before 37 completed weeks gestation) 644.2 ✓
previous, affecting management of pregnancy V23.41
quadruplet NEC 651.2 ✓
with fetal loss and retention of one or more fetus(es) 651.5 ✓
following (elective) fetal reduction 651.7 ✓
quintuplet NEC 651.8 ✓
with fetal loss and retention of one or more fetus(es) 651.6 ✓
following (elective) fetal reduction 651.7 ✓
sextuplet NEC 651.8 ✓
with fetal loss and retention of one or more fetus(es) 651.6 ✓
following (elective) fetal reduction 651.7 ✓
specified complication NEC 669.8 ✓
stillbirth (near term) NEC 656.4 ✓
early (before 22 completed weeks gestation) 632
term pregnancy (live birth) NEC — *see* category 650
stillbirth NEC 656.4 ✓
threatened premature 644.2 ✓
triplets NEC 651.1 ✓
with fetal loss and retention of one or more fetus(es) 651.4 ✓
delayed delivery (one or more mates) 662.3 ✓
following (elective) fetal reduction 651.7 ✓
locked mates 660.5 ✓
twins NEC 651.0 ✓
with fetal loss and retention of one fetus 651.3 ✓
delayed delivery (one or more mates) 662.3 ✓
following (elective) fetal reduction 651.7 ✓
locked mates 660.5 ✓
uncomplicated — *see* category 650
vacuum extractor NEC 669.5 ✓
affecting fetus or newborn 763.3
ventouse NEC 669.5 ✓
affecting fetus or newborn 763.3
Dellen, cornea 371.41
Delusions (paranoid) 297.9

Delusions — *continued*
grandiose 297.1
parasitosis 300.29
systematized 297.1
Dementia 294.20
with behavioral disturbance (aggressive) (combative) (violent) 294.21
alcohol-induced persisting (*see also* Psychosis, alcoholic) 291.2
Alzheimer's — *see* Alzheimer's, dementia
arteriosclerotic (simple type) (uncomplicated) 290.40
with
acute confusional state 290.41
delirium 290.41
delusions 290.42
depressed mood 290.43
depressed type 290.43
paranoid type 290.42
Binswanger's 290.12
catatonic (acute) (*see also* Schizophrenia) 295.2 ✓
congenital (*see also* Disability, intellectual) 319
degenerative 290.9
presenile-onset — *see* Dementia, presenile
senile-onset — *see* Dementia, senile
developmental (*see also* Schizophrenia) 295.9 ✓
dialysis 294.8
transient 293.9
drug-induced persisting (*see also* Psychosis, drug) 292.82
due to or associated with condition(s) classified elsewhere
Alzheimer's
with behavioral disturbance 331.0 [294.11]
without behavioral disturbance 331.0 [294.10]
cerebral lipidoses
with behavioral disturbance 330.1 [294.11]
without behavioral disturbance 330.1 [294.10]
epilepsy
with behavioral disturbance 345.9 ✓ [294.11]
without behavioral disturbance 345.9 ✓ [294.10]
hepatolenticular degeneration
with behavioral disturbance 275.1 [294.11]
without behavioral disturbance 275.1 [294.10]
HIV
with behavioral disturbance 042 [294.11]
without behavioral disturbance 042 [294.10]
Huntington's chorea
with behavioral disturbance 333.4 [294.11]
without behavioral disturbance 333.4 [294.10]
Jakob-Creutzfeldt disease (CJD)
with behavioral disturbance 046.19 [294.11]
without behavioral disturbance 046.19 [294.10]
variant (vCJD) 046.11
with dementia
with behavioral disturbance 046.11 [294.11]
without behavioral disturbance 046.11 [294.10]
Lewy bodies
with behavioral disturbance 331.82 [294.11]
without behavioral disturbance 331.82 [294.10]
multiple sclerosis
with behavioral disturbance 340 [294.11]

Dementia — *continued*
due to or associated with condition(s) classified elsewhere — *continued*
multiple sclerosis — *continued*
without behavioral disturbance 340 [294.10]
neurosyphilis
with behavioral disturbance 094.9 [294.11]
without behavioral disturbance 094.9 [294.10]
Parkinsonism
with behavioral disturbance 331.82 [294.11]
without behavioral disturbance 331.82 [294.10]
Parkinson's disease
with behavioral disturbance 332.0 [294.11]
without behavioral disturbance 332.0 [294.10]
Pelizaeus-Merzbacher disease
with behavioral disturbance 333.0 [294.11]
without behavioral disturbance 333.0 [294.10]
Pick's disease
with behavioral disturbance 331.11 [294.11]
without behavioral disturbance 331.11 [294.10]
polyarteritis nodosa
with behavioral disturbance 446.0 [294.11]
without behavioral disturbance 446.0 [294.10]
syphilis
with behavioral disturbance 094.1 [294.11]
without behavioral disturbance 094.1 [294.10]
Wilson's disease
with behavioral disturbance 275.1 [294.11]
without behavioral disturbance 275.1 [294.10]
frontal 331.19
with behavioral disturbance 331.19 [294.11]
without behavioral disturbance 331.19 [294.10]
frontotemporal 331.19
with behavioral disturbance 331.19 [294.11]
without behavioral disturbance 331.19 [294.10]
hebephrenic (acute) 295.1 ✓
Heller's (infantile psychosis) (*see also* Psychosis, childhood) 299.1 ✓
idiopathic 290.9
presenile-onset — *see* Dementia, presenile
senile-onset — *see* Dementia, senile
in
arteriosclerotic brain disease 290.40
senility 290.0
induced by drug 292.82
infantile, infantilia (*see also* Psychosis, childhood) 299.0 ✓
Lewy body 331.82
with behavioral disturbance 331.82 [294.11]
without behavioral disturbance 331.82 [294.10]
multi-infarct (cerebrovascular) (*see also* Dementia, arteriosclerotic) 290.40
old age 290.0
paralytica, paralytic 094.1
juvenilis 090.40
syphilitic 094.1
congenital 090.40
tabetic form 094.1
paranoid (*see also* Schizophrenia) 295.3 ✓
paraphrenic (*see also* Schizophrenia) 295.3 ✓
paretic 094.1

✓ Additional Digit Required — Refer to the Tabular List for Digit Selection   ⩊ Subterms under main terms may continue to next column or page

2014 ICD-9-CM   ▶◄ Revised Text   ● New Line   ▲ Revised Code   Volume 2 — 73

Dementia — continued
praecox (see also Schizophrenia) 295.9 ☑
presenile 290.10
with
acute confusional state 290.11
delirium 290.11
delusional features 290.12
depressive features 290.13
depressed type 290.13
paranoid type 290.12
simple type 290.10
uncomplicated 290.10
primary (acute) (see also Schizophrenia)
295.0 ☑
progressive, syphilitic 094.1
puerperal — see Psychosis, puerperal
schizophrenic (see also Schizophrenia)
295.9 ☑
senile 290.0
with
acute confusional state 290.3
delirium 290.3
delusional features 290.20
depressive features 290.21
depressed type 290.21
exhaustion 290.0
paranoid type 290.20
simple type (acute) (see also Schizophrenia)
295.0 ☑
simplex (acute) (see also Schizophrenia)
295.0 ☑
syphilitic 094.1
uremic — see Uremia
vascular 290.40
with
delirium 290.41
delusions 290.42
depressed mood 290.43
Demerol dependence — see also Dependence
304.0 ☑
Demineralization, ankle — see also Osteoporosis 733.00
Demodex folliculorum (infestation) 133.8
Demoralization 799.25
de Morgan's spots (senile angiomas) 448.1
Demyelinating
polyneuritis, chronic inflammatory 357.81
Demyelination, demyelinization
central nervous system 341.9
specified NEC 341.8
corpus callosum (central) 341.8
global 340
Dengue (fever) 061
sandfly 061
vaccination, prophylactic (against) V05.1
virus hemorrhagic fever 065.4
Dens
evaginatus 520.2
in dente 520.2
invaginatus 520.2
Dense
breast(s) 793.82
Density
increased, bone (disseminated) (generalized) (spotted) 733.99
lung (nodular) 518.89
Dental — see also condition
examination only V72.2
Dentia praecox 520.6
Denticles (in pulp) 522.2
Dentigerous cyst 526.0
Dentin
irregular (in pulp) 522.3
opalescent 520.5
secondary (in pulp) 522.3
sensitive 521.89
Dentinogenesis imperfecta 520.5
Dentinoma (M9271/0) 213.1
upper jaw (bone) 213.0
Dentition 520.7
abnormal 520.6
anomaly 520.6
delayed 520.6
difficult 520.7
disorder of 520.6
precocious 520.6

Dentition — continued
retarded 520.6
Denture sore (mouth) 528.9
Dependence

Note — Use the following fifth-digit
subclassification with category 304:

0   unspecified
1   continuous
2   episodic
3   in remission

with
withdrawal symptoms
alcohol 291.81
drug 292.0
14-hydroxy-dihydromorphinone 304.0 ☑
absinthe 304.6 ☑
acemorphan 304.0 ☑
acetanilid(e) 304.6 ☑
acetophenetidin 304.6 ☑
acetorphine 304.0 ☑
acetyldihydrocodeine 304.0 ☑
acetyldihydrocodeinone 304.0 ☑
Adalin 304.1 ☑
Afghanistan black 304.3 ☑
agrypnal 304.1 ☑
alcohol, alcoholic (ethyl) (methyl) (wood)
303.9 ☑
maternal, with suspected fetal damage
affecting management of pregnancy 655.4 ☑
allobarbitone 304.1 ☑
allonal 304.1 ☑
allylisopropylacetylurea 304.1 ☑
alphaprodine (hydrochloride) 304.0 ☑
Alurate 304.1 ☑
Alvodine 304.0 ☑
amethocaine 304.6 ☑
amidone 304.0 ☑
amidopyrine 304.6 ☑
aminopyrine 304.6 ☑
amobarbital 304.1 ☑
amphetamine(s) (type) (drugs classifiable
to 969.7) 304.4 ☑
amylene hydrate 304.6 ☑
amylobarbitone 304.1 ☑
amylocaine 304.6 ☑
Amytal (sodium) 304.1 ☑
analgesic (drug) NEC 304.6 ☑
synthetic with morphine-like effect
304.0 ☑
anesthetic (agent) (drug) (gas) (general)
(local) NEC 304.6 ☑
Angel dust 304.6 ☑
anileridine 304.0 ☑
antipyrine 304.6 ☑
anxiolytic 304.1 ☑
aprobarbital 304.1 ☑
aprobarbitone 304.1 ☑
atropine 304.6 ☑
Avertin (bromide) 304.6 ☑
barbenyl 304.1 ☑
barbital(s) 304.1 ☑
barbitone 304.1 ☑
barbiturate(s) (compounds) (drugs classifiable to 967.0) 304.1 ☑
barbituric acid (and compounds) 304.1 ☑
benzedrine 304.4 ☑
benzylmorphine 304.0 ☑
Beta-chlor 304.1 ☑
bhang 304.3 ☑
blue velvet 304.0 ☑
Brevital 304.1 ☑
bromal (hydrate) 304.1 ☑
bromide(s) NEC 304.1 ☑
bromine compounds NEC 304.1 ☑
bromisovalum 304.1 ☑
Bromo-seltzer 304.1 ☑
bromoform 304.1 ☑
bromural 304.1 ☑
butabarbital (sodium) 304.1 ☑
butabarpal 304.1 ☑

Dependence — continued
butallylonal 304.1 ☑
butethal 304.1 ☑
buthalitone (sodium) 304.1 ☑
Butisol 304.1 ☑
butobarbitone 304.1 ☑
butyl chloral (hydrate) 304.1 ☑
caffeine 304.4 ☑
cannabis (indica) (sativa) (resin) (derivatives)
(type) 304.3 ☑
carbamazepine 304.6 ☑
Carbrital 304.1 ☑
carbromal 304.1 ☑
carisoprodol 304.6 ☑
Catha (edulis) 304.4 ☑
chloral (betaine) (hydrate) 304.1 ☑
chloralamide 304.1 ☑
chloralformamide 304.1 ☑
chloralose 304.1 ☑
chlordiazepoxide 304.1 ☑
Chloretone 304.1 ☑
chlorobutanol 304.1 ☑
chlorodyne 304.1 ☑
chloroform 304.6 ☑
Cliradon 304.0 ☑
coca (leaf) and derivatives 304.2 ☑
cocaine 304.2 ☑
hydrochloride 304.2 ☑
salt (any) 304.2 ☑
codeine 304.0 ☑
combination of drugs (excluding morphine
or opioid type drug) NEC 304.8 ☑
morphine or opioid type drug with any
other drug 304.7 ☑
croton-chloral 304.1 ☑
cyclobarbital 304.1 ☑
cyclobarbitone 304.1 ☑
d-lysergic acid diethylamide 304.5 ☑
dagga 304.3 ☑
Delvinal 304.1 ☑
Demerol 304.0 ☑
desocodeine 304.0 ☑
desomorphine 304.0 ☑
desoxyephedrine 304.4 ☑
DET 304.5 ☑
dexamphetamine 304.4 ☑
dexedrine 304.4 ☑
dextromethorphan 304.0 ☑
dextromoramide 304.0 ☑
dextronorpseudoephedrine 304.4 ☑
dextrorphan 304.0 ☑
diacetylmorphine 304.0 ☑
Dial 304.1 ☑
diallylbarbituric acid 304.1 ☑
diamorphine 304.0 ☑
diazepam 304.1 ☑
dibucaine 304.6 ☑
dichloroethane 304.6 ☑
diethyl barbituric acid 304.1 ☑
diethylsulfone-diethylmethane 304.1 ☑
difencloxazine 304.0 ☑
dihydrocodeine 304.0 ☑
dihydrocodeinone 304.0 ☑
dihydrohydroxycodeinone 304.0 ☑
dihydroisocodeine 304.0 ☑
dihydromorphine 304.0 ☑
dihydromorphinone 304.0 ☑
dihydroxcodeinone 304.0 ☑
Dilaudid 304.0 ☑
dimenhydrinate 304.6 ☑
dimethylmeperidine 304.0 ☑
dimethyltriptamine 304.5 ☑
Dionin 304.0 ☑
diphenoxylate 304.6 ☑
dipipanone 304.0 ☑
DMT 304.5 ☑
Dolophine 304.0 ☑
DOM 304.2 ☑
Doriden 304.1 ☑
dormiral 304.1 ☑
Dormison 304.1 ☑
Dromoran 304.0 ☑
drug NEC 304.9 ☑

Dependence — continued
drug — continued
analgesic NEC 304.6 ☑
combination (excluding morphine or
opioid type drug) NEC 304.8 ☑
morphine or opioid type drug with
any other drug 304.7 ☑
complicating pregnancy, childbirth, or
puerperium 648.3 ☑
affecting fetus or newborn 779.5
hallucinogenic 304.5 ☑
hypnotic NEC 304.1 ☑
narcotic NEC 304.9 ☑
psychostimulant NEC 304.4 ☑
sedative 304.1 ☑
soporific NEC 304.1 ☑
specified type NEC 304.6 ☑
suspected damage to fetus affecting
management of pregnancy
655.5 ☑
synthetic, with morphine-like effect
304.0 ☑
tranquilizing 304.1 ☑
duboisine 304.6 ☑
ectylurea 304.1 ☑
Endocaine 304.6 ☑
Equanil 304.1 ☑
Eskabarb 304.1 ☑
ethchlorvynol 304.1 ☑
ether (ethyl) (liquid) (vapor) (vinyl) 304.6 ☑
ethidene 304.6 ☑
ethinamate 304.1 ☑
ethoheptazine 304.6 ☑
ethyl
alcohol 303.9 ☑
bromide 304.6 ☑
carbamate 304.6 ☑
chloride 304.6 ☑
morphine 304.0 ☑
ethylene (gas) 304.6 ☑
dichloride 304.6 ☑
ethylidene chloride 304.6 ☑
etilfen 304.1 ☑
etorphine 304.0 ☑
etoval 304.1 ☑
eucodal 304.0 ☑
euneryl 304.1 ☑
Evipal 304.1 ☑
Evipan 304.1 ☑
fentanyl 304.0 ☑
ganja 304.3 ☑
gardenal 304.1 ☑
gardenpanyl 304.1 ☑
gelsemine 304.6 ☑
Gelsemium 304.6 ☑
Gemonil 304.1 ☑
glucochloral 304.1 ☑
glue (airplane) (sniffing) 304.6 ☑
glutethimide 304.1 ☑
hallucinogenics 304.5 ☑
hashish 304.3 ☑
headache powder NEC 304.6 ☑
Heavenly Blue 304.5 ☑
hedonal 304.1 ☑
hemp 304.3 ☑
heptabarbital 304.1 ☑
Heptalgin 304.0 ☑
heptobarbitone 304.1 ☑
heroin 304.0 ☑
salt (any) 304.0 ☑
hexethal (sodium) 304.1 ☑
hexobarbital 304.1 ☑
Hycodan 304.0 ☑
hydrocodone 304.0 ☑
hydromorphinol 304.0 ☑
hydromorphinone 304.0 ☑
hydromorphone 304.0 ☑
hydroxycodeine 304.0 ☑
hypnotic NEC 304.1 ☑
Indian hemp 304.3 ☑
inhalant 304.6 ☑
intranarcon 304.1 ☑
Kemithal 304.1 ☑

☑ **Additional Digit Required** — Refer to the Tabular List for Digit Selection

⬝⬝ **Subterms under main terms may continue to next column or page**

Dependence — *continued*
- ketobemidone 304.0 ☑
- khat 304.4 ☑
- kif 304.3 ☑
- Lactuca (virosa) extract 304.1 ☑
- lactucarium 304.1 ☑
- laudanum 304.0 ☑
- Lebanese red 304.3 ☑
- Leritine 304.0 ☑
- lettuce opium 304.1 ☑
- Levanil 304.1 ☑
- Levo-Dromoran 304.0 ☑
- levo-iso-methadone 304.0 ☑
- levorphanol 304.0 ☑
- Librium 304.1 ☑
- Lomotil 304.6 ☑
- Lotusate 304.1 ☑
- LSD (-25) (and derivatives) 304.5 ☑
- Luminal 304.1 ☑
- lysergic acid 304.5 ☑
  - amide 304.5 ☑
- maconha 304.3 ☑
- magic mushroom 304.5 ☑
- marihuana 304.3 ☑
- MDA (methylene dioxyamphetamine) 304.4 ☑
- Mebaral 304.1 ☑
- Medinal 304.1 ☑
- Medomin 304.1 ☑
- megahallucinogenics 304.5 ☑
- meperidine 304.0 ☑
- mephobarbital 304.1 ☑
- meprobamate 304.1 ☑
- mescaline 304.5 ☑
- methadone 304.0 ☑
- methamphetamine(s) 304.4 ☑
- methaqualone 304.1 ☑
- metharbital 304.1 ☑
- methitural 304.1 ☑
- methobarbitone 304.1 ☑
- methohexital 304.1 ☑
- methopholine 304.6 ☑
- methyl
  - alcohol 303.9 ☑
  - bromide 304.6 ☑
  - morphine 304.0 ☑
  - sulfonal 304.1 ☑
- methylaparafynol 304.1 ☑
- methylated spirit 303.9 ☑
- methylbutinol 304.6 ☑
- methyldihydromorphinone 304.0 ☑
- methylene
  - chloride 304.6 ☑
  - dichloride 304.6 ☑
  - dioxyamphetamine (MDA) 304.4 ☑
- methylphenidate 304.4 ☑
- methyprylone 304.1 ☑
- metopon 304.0 ☑
- Miltown 304.1 ☑
- morning glory seeds 304.5 ☑
- morphinan(s) 304.0 ☑
- morphine (sulfate) (sulfite) (type) (drugs classifiable to 965.00–965.09) 304.0 ☑
- morphine or opioid type drug (drugs classifiable to 965.00–965.09) with any other drug 304.7 ☑
- morphinol(s) 304.0 ☑
- morphinon 304.0 ☑
- morpholinylethylmorphine 304.0 ☑
- mylomide 304.1 ☑
- myristicin 304.5 ☑
- narcotic (drug) NEC 304.9 ☑
- nealbarbital 304.1 ☑
- nealbarbitone 304.1 ☑
- Nembutal 304.1 ☑
- Neonal 304.1 ☑
- Neraval 304.1 ☑
- Neravan 304.1 ☑
- neurobarb 304.1 ☑
- nicotine 305.1
- Nisentil 304.0 ☑
- nitrous oxide 304.6 ☑

Dependence — *continued*
- Noctec 304.1 ☑
- Noludar 304.1 ☑
- nonbarbiturate sedatives and tranquilizers with similar effect 304.1 ☑
- noptil 304.1 ☑
- normorphine 304.0 ☑
- noscapine 304.0 ☑
- Novocaine 304.6 ☑
- Numorphan 304.0 ☑
- nunol 304.1 ☑
- Nupercaine 304.6 ☑
- Oblivon 304.1 ☑
- on
  - aspirator V46.0
  - hemodialysis V45.11
  - hyperbaric chamber V46.8
  - iron lung V46.11
  - machine (enabling) V46.9
    - specified type NEC V46.8
  - peritoneal dialysis V45.11
  - Possum (Patient-Operated-Selector-Mechanism) V46.8
  - renal dialysis machine V45.11
  - respirator [ventilator] V46.11
    - encounter
      - during
        - mechanical failure V46.14
        - power failure V46.12
      - for weaning V46.13
  - supplemental oxygen V46.2
  - wheelchair V46.3
- opiate 304.0 ☑
- opioids 304.0 ☑
- opioid type drug 304.0 ☑
  - with any other drug 304.7 ☑
- opium (alkaloids) (derivatives) (tincture) 304.0 ☑
- ortal 304.1 ☑
- Oxazepam 304.1 ☑
- oxycodone 304.0 ☑
- oxymorphone 304.0 ☑
- Palfium 304.0 ☑
- Panadol 304.6 ☑
- pantopium 304.0 ☑
- pantopon 304.0 ☑
- papaverine 304.0 ☑
- paracetamol 304.6 ☑
- paracodin 304.0 ☑
- paraldehyde 304.1 ☑
- paregoric 304.0 ☑
- Parzone 304.0 ☑
- PCP (phencyclidine) 304.6 ☑
- Pearly Gates 304.5 ☑
- pentazocine 304.0 ☑
- pentobarbital 304.1 ☑
- pentobarbitone (sodium) 304.1 ☑
- Pentothal 304.1 ☑
- Percaine 304.6 ☑
- Percodan 304.0 ☑
- Perichlor 304.1 ☑
- Pernocton 304.1 ☑
- Pernoston 304.1 ☑
- peronine 304.0 ☑
- pethidine (hydrochloride) 304.0 ☑
- petrichloral 304.1 ☑
- peyote 304.5 ☑
- Phanodron 304.1 ☑
- phenacetin 304.6 ☑
- phenadoxone 304.0 ☑
- phenaglycodol 304.1 ☑
- phenazocine 304.0 ☑
- phencyclidine 304.6 ☑
- phenmetrazine 304.4 ☑
- phenobal 304.1 ☑
- phenobarbital 304.1 ☑
- phenobarbitone 304.1 ☑
- phenomorphan 304.0 ☑
- phenonyl 304.1 ☑
- phenoperidine 304.0 ☑
- pholcodine 304.0 ☑
- piminodine 304.0 ☑
- Pipadone 304.0 ☑
- Pitkin's solution 304.6 ☑

Dependence — *continued*
- Placidyl 304.1 ☑
- polysubstance 304.8 ☑
- Pontocaine 304.6 ☑
- pot 304.3 ☑
- potassium bromide 304.1 ☑
- Preludin 304.4 ☑
- Prinadol 304.0 ☑
- probarbital 304.1 ☑
- procaine 304.6 ☑
- propanal 304.1 ☑
- propoxyphene 304.6 ☑
- psilocibin 304.5 ☑
- psilocin 304.5 ☑
- psilocybin 304.5 ☑
- psilocyline 304.5 ☑
- psilocyn 304.5 ☑
- psychedelic agents 304.5 ☑
- psychostimulant NEC 304.4 ☑
- psychotomimetic agents 304.5 ☑
- pyrahexyl 304.3 ☑
- Pyramidon 304.6 ☑
- quinalbarbitone 304.1 ☑
- racemoramide 304.0 ☑
- racemorphan 304.0 ☑
- Rela 304.6 ☑
- scopolamine 304.6 ☑
- secobarbital 304.1 ☑
- Seconal 304.1 ☑
- sedative NEC 304.1 ☑
  - nonbarbiturate with barbiturate effect 304.1 ☑
- Sedormid 304.1 ☑
- sernyl 304.1 ☑
- sodium bromide 304.1 ☑
- Soma 304.6 ☑
- Somnal 304.1 ☑
- Somnos 304.1 ☑
- Soneryl 304.1 ☑
- soporific (drug) NEC 304.1 ☑
- specified drug NEC 304.6 ☑
- speed 304.4 ☑
- spinocaine 304.6 ☑
- Stovaine 304.6 ☑
- STP 304.5 ☑
- stramonium 304.6 ☑
- Sulfonal 304.1 ☑
- sulfonethylmethane 304.1 ☑
- sulfonmethane 304.1 ☑
- Surital 304.1 ☑
- synthetic drug with morphine-like effect 304.0 ☑
- talbutal 304.1 ☑
- tetracaine 304.6 ☑
- tetrahydrocannabinol 304.3 ☑
- tetronal 304.1 ☑
- THC 304.3 ☑
- thebacon 304.0 ☑
- thebaine 304.0 ☑
- thiamil 304.1 ☑
- thiamylal 304.1 ☑
- thiopental 304.1 ☑
- tobacco 305.1
- toluene, toluol 304.6 ☑
- tranquilizer NEC 304.1 ☑
  - nonbarbiturate with barbiturate effect 304.1 ☑
- tribromacetaldehyde 304.6 ☑
- tribromethanol 304.6 ☑
- tribromomethane 304.6 ☑
- trichloroethanol 304.6 ☑
- trichoroethyl phosphate 304.1 ☑
- triclofos 304.1 ☑
- Trional 304.1 ☑
- Tuinal 304.1 ☑
- Turkish Green 304.3 ☑
- urethan(e) 304.6 ☑
- Valium 304.1 ☑
- Valmid 304.1 ☑
- veganin 304.0 ☑
- veramon 304.1 ☑
- Veronal 304.1 ☑
- versidyne 304.6 ☑

Dependence — *continued*
- vinbarbital 304.1 ☑
- vinbarbitone 304.1 ☑
- vinyl bitone 304.1 ☑
- vitamin B₆ 266.1
- wine 303.9 ☑
- Zactane 304.6 ☑

Dependency
- passive 301.6
- reactions 301.6

Depersonalization (episode, in neurotic state) (neurotic) (syndrome) 300.6

Depletion
- carbohydrates 271.9
- complement factor 279.8
- extracellular fluid 276.52
- plasma 276.52
- potassium 276.8
  - nephropathy 588.89
- salt or sodium 276.1
  - causing heat exhaustion or prostration 992.4
  - nephropathy 593.9
- volume 276.50
  - extracellular fluid 276.52
  - plasma 276.52

Deployment (military)
- personal history of V62.22
- returned from V62.22
- status V62.21

Deposit
- argentous, cornea 371.16
- bone, in Boeck's sarcoid 135
- calcareous, calcium — *see* Calcification
- cholesterol
  - retina 362.82
  - skin 709.3
  - vitreous (humor) 379.22
- conjunctival 372.56
- cornea, corneal NEC 371.10
  - argentous 371.16
  - in
    - cystinosis 270.0 *[371.15]*
    - mucopolysaccharidosis 277.5 *[371.15]*
- crystalline, vitreous (humor) 379.22
- hemosiderin, in old scars of cornea 371.11
- metallic, in lens 366.45
- skin 709.3
- teeth, tooth (betel) (black) (green) (materia alba) (orange) (soft) (tobacco) 523.6
- urate, in kidney (*see also* Disease, renal) 593.9

Depraved appetite 307.52

Depression 311
- acute (*see also* Psychosis, affective) 296.2 ☑
  - recurrent episode 296.3 ☑
  - single episode 296.2 ☑
- agitated (*see also* Psychosis, affective) 296.2 ☑
  - recurrent episode 296.3 ☑
  - single episode 296.2 ☑
- anaclitic 309.21
- anxiety 300.4
- arches 734
  - congenital 754.61
- autogenous (*see also* Psychosis, affective) 296.2 ☑
  - recurrent episode 296.3 ☑
  - single episode 296.2 ☑
- basal metabolic rate (BMR) 794.7
- bone marrow 289.9
- central nervous system 799.1
  - newborn 779.2
- cerebral 331.9
  - newborn 779.2
- cerebrovascular 437.8
  - newborn 779.2
- chest wall 738.3
- endogenous (*see also* Psychosis, affective) 296.2 ☑
  - recurrent episode 296.3 ☑
  - single episode 296.2 ☑
- functional activity 780.99
- hysterical 300.11

☑ Additional Digit Required — Refer to the Tabular List for Digit Selection   ▽ Subterms under main terms may continue to next column or page

2014 ICD-9-CM   ▶◀ Revised Text   ● New Line   ▲ Revised Code   Volume 2 — 75

Dependence — Depression

Depression — *continued*
  involutional, climacteric, or menopausal (*see also* Psychosis, affective) 296.2 ☑
    recurrent episode 296.3 ☑
    single episode 296.2 ☑
  major 296.2 ☑
    recurrent episode 296.3 ☑
    single episode 296.2 ☑
  manic (*see also* Psychosis, affective) 296.80
  medullary 348.89
    newborn 779.2
  mental 300.4
  metatarsal heads — *see* Depression, arches
  metatarsus — *see* Depression, arches
  monopolar (*see also* Psychosis, affective) 296.2 ☑
    recurrent episode 296.3 ☑
    single episode 296.2 ☑
  nervous 300.4
  neurotic 300.4
  nose 738.0
  postpartum 648.4 ☑
  psychogenic 300.4
    reactive 298.0
  psychoneurotic 300.4
  psychotic (*see also* Psychosis, affective) 296.2 ☑
    reactive 298.0
    recurrent episode 296.3 ☑
    single episode 296.2 ☑
  reactive 300.4
    neurotic 300.4
    psychogenic 298.0
    psychoneurotic 300.4
    psychotic 298.0
  recurrent 296.3 ☑
  respiratory center 348.89
    newborn 770.89
  scapula 736.89
  senile 290.21
  situational (acute) (brief) 309.0
    prolonged 309.1
  skull 754.0
  sternum 738.3
  visual field 368.40

Depressive reaction — *see also* Reaction, depressive
  acute (transient) 309.0
    with anxiety 309.28
  prolonged 309.1
  situational (acute) 309.0
    prolonged 309.1

Deprivation
  cultural V62.4
  emotional V62.89
    affecting
      adult 995.82
      infant or child 995.51
  food 994.2
    specific substance NEC 269.8
  protein (familial) (kwashiorkor) 260
  sleep V69.4
  social V62.4
    affecting
      adult 995.82
      infant or child 995.51
  symptoms, syndrome
    alcohol 291.81
    drug 292.0
  vitamins (*see also* Deficiency, vitamin) 269.2
  water 994.3

de Quervain's
  disease (tendon sheath) 727.04
  syndrome 259.51
  thyroiditis (subacute granulomatous thyroiditis) 245.1

Derangement
  ankle (internal) 718.97
    current injury (*see also* Dislocation, ankle) 837.0
    recurrent 718.37
  cartilage (articular) NEC (*see also* Disorder, cartilage, articular) 718.0 ☑
    knee 717.9
      recurrent 718.36
    recurrent 718.3 ☑

Derangement — *continued*
  collateral ligament (knee) (medial) (tibial) 717.82
    current injury 844.1
      lateral (fibular) 844.0
    lateral (fibular) 717.81
      current injury 844.0
  cruciate ligament (knee) (posterior) 717.84
    anterior 717.83
      current injury 844.2
    current injury 844.2
  elbow (internal) 718.92
    current injury (*see also* Dislocation, elbow) 832.00
    recurrent 718.32
  gastrointestinal 536.9
  heart — *see* Disease, heart
  hip (joint) (internal) (old) 718.95
    current injury (*see also* Dislocation, hip) 835.00
    recurrent 718.35
  intervertebral disc — *see* Displacement, intervertebral disc
  joint (internal) 718.90
    ankle 718.97
    current injury (*see also* Dislocation, by site)
      knee, meniscus or cartilage (*see also* Tear, meniscus) 836.2
    elbow 718.92
    foot 718.97
    hand 718.94
    hip 718.95
    knee 717.9
    multiple sites 718.99
    pelvic region 718.95
    recurrent 718.30
      ankle 718.37
      elbow 718.32
      foot 718.37
      hand 718.34
      hip 718.35
      knee 718.36
      multiple sites 718.39
      pelvic region 718.35
      shoulder (region) 718.31
      specified site NEC 718.38
      temporomandibular (old) 524.69
      wrist 718.33
    shoulder (region) 718.91
    specified site NEC 718.98
    spine NEC 724.9
    temporomandibular 524.69
    wrist 718.93
  knee (cartilage) (internal) 717.9
    current injury (*see also* Tear, meniscus) 836.2
    ligament 717.89
      capsular 717.85
      collateral — *see* Derangement, collateral ligament
      cruciate — *see* Derangement, cruciate ligament
      specified NEC 717.85
      recurrent 718.36
  low back NEC 724.9
  meniscus NEC (knee) 717.5
    current injury (*see also* Tear, meniscus) 836.2
    lateral 717.40
      anterior horn 717.42
      posterior horn 717.43
      specified NEC 717.49
    medial 717.3
      anterior horn 717.1
      posterior horn 717.2
    recurrent 718.3 ☑
    site other than knee — *see* Disorder, cartilage, articular
  mental (*see also* Psychosis) 298.9
  rotator cuff (recurrent) (tear) 726.10
    current 840.4
  sacroiliac (old) 724.6
    current — *see* Dislocation, sacroiliac
  semilunar cartilage (knee) 717.5
    current injury 836.2

Derangement — *continued*
  semilunar cartilage — *continued*
    current injury — *continued*
      lateral 836.1
      medial 836.0
    recurrent 718.3 ☑
  shoulder (internal) 718.91
    current injury (*see also* Dislocation, shoulder) 831.00
    recurrent 718.31
  spine (recurrent) NEC 724.9
    current — *see* Dislocation, spine
  temporomandibular (internal) (joint) (old) 524.69
    current — *see* Dislocation, jaw

Dercum's disease or syndrome (adiposis dolorosa) 272.8
Derealization (neurotic) 300.6
Dermal — *see* condition
Dermaphytid — *see* Dermatophytosis
Dermatergosis — *see* Dermatitis
Dermatitis (allergic) (contact) (occupational) (venenata) 692.9
  ab igne 692.82
  acneiform 692.9
  actinic (due to sun) 692.70
    acute 692.72
    chronic NEC 692.74
    other than from sun NEC 692.82
  ambustionis
    due to
      burn or scald — *see* Burn, by site
      sunburn (*see also* Sunburn) 692.71
  amebic 006.6
  ammonia 691.0
  anaphylactoid NEC 692.9
  arsenical 692.4
  artefacta 698.4
    psychogenic 316 *[698.4]*
  asthmatic 691.8
  atopic (allergic) (intrinsic) 691.8
    psychogenic 316 *[691.8]*
  atrophicans 701.8
    diffusa 701.8
    maculosa 701.3
  autoimmune progesterone 279.49
  berlock, berloque 692.72
  blastomycetic 116.0
  blister beetle 692.89
  Brucella NEC 023.9
  bullosa 694.9
    striata pratensis 692.6
  bullous 694.9
    mucosynechial, atrophic 694.60
      with ocular involvement 694.61
    seasonal 694.8
  calorica
    due to
      burn or scald — *see* Burn, by site
      cold 692.89
      sunburn (*see also* Sunburn) 692.71
  caterpillar 692.89
  cercarial 120.3
  combustionis
    due to
      burn or scald — *see* Burn, by site
      sunburn (*see also* Sunburn) 692.71
  congelationis 991.5
  contusiformis 695.2
  diabetic 250.8 ☑
  diaper 691.0
  diphtheritica 032.85
  due to
    acetone 692.2
    acids 692.4
    adhesive plaster 692.4
    alcohol (skin contact) (substances classifiable to 980.0–980.9) 692.4
      taken internally 693.8
    alkalis 692.4
    allergy NEC 692.9
    ammonia (household) (liquid) 692.4
    animal
      dander (cat) (dog) 692.84
      hair (cat) (dog) 692.84
    arnica 692.3

Dermatitis — *continued*
  due to — *continued*
    arsenic 692.4
      taken internally 693.8
    blister beetle 692.89
    cantharides 692.3
    carbon disulphide 692.2
    caterpillar 692.89
    caustics 692.4
    cereal (ingested) 693.1
      contact with skin 692.5
    chemical(s) NEC 692.4
      internal 693.8
      irritant NEC 692.4
      taken internally 693.8
    chlorocompounds 692.2
    coffee (ingested) 693.1
      contact with skin 692.5
    cold weather 692.89
    cosmetics 692.81
    cyclohexanes 692.2
    dander, animal (cat) (dog) 692.84
    deodorant 692.81
    detergents 692.0
    dichromate 692.4
    drugs and medicinals (correct substance properly administered) (internal use) 693.0
      external (in contact with skin) 692.3
        wrong substance given or taken 976.9
          specified substance — *see* Table of Drugs and Chemicals
      wrong substance given or taken 977.9
        specified substance — *see* Table of Drugs and Chemicals
    dyes 692.89
      hair 692.89
    epidermophytosis — *see* Dermatophytosis
    esters 692.2
    external irritant NEC 692.9
      specified agent NEC 692.89
    eye shadow 692.81
    fish (ingested) 693.1
      contact with skin 692.5
    flour (ingested) 693.1
      contact with skin 692.5
    food (ingested) 693.1
      in contact with skin 692.5
    fruit (ingested) 693.1
      contact with skin 692.5
    fungicides 692.3
    furs 692.84
    glycols 692.2
    greases NEC 692.1
    hair, animal (cat) (dog) 692.84
    hair dyes 692.89
    hot
      objects and materials — *see* Burn, by site
      weather or places 692.89
    hydrocarbons 692.2
    infrared rays, except from sun 692.82
      solar NEC (*see also* Dermatitis, due to, sun) 692.70
    ingested substance 693.9
      drugs and medicinals (*see also* Dermatitis, due to, drugs and medicinals) 693.0
      food 693.1
      specified substance NEC 693.8
    ingestion or injection of chemical 693.8
      drug (correct substance properly administered) 693.0
        wrong substance given or taken 977.9
          specified substance — *see* Table of Drugs and Chemicals
    insecticides 692.3
    internal agent 693.9
      drugs and medicinals (*see also* Dermatitis, due to, drugs and medicinals) 693.0

Dermatitis — continued
due to — continued
   internal agent — continued
      food (ingested) 693.1
         in contact with skin 692.5
         specified agent NEC 693.8
      iodine 692.3
      iodoform 692.3
      irradiation 692.82
      jewelry 692.83
      keratolytics 692.3
      ketones 692.2
      lacquer tree (Rhus verniciflua) 692.6
      light (sun) NEC (see also Dermatitis, due
        to, sun) 692.70
        other 692.82
      low temperature 692.89
      mascara 692.81
      meat (ingested) 693.1
        contact with skin 692.5
      mercury, mercurials 692.3
      metals 692.83
      milk (ingested) 693.1
        contact with skin 692.5
      Neomycin 692.3
      nylon 692.4
      oils NEC 692.1
      paint solvent 692.2
      pediculocides 692.3
      petroleum products (substances classifi-
        able to 981) 692.4
      phenol 692.3
      photosensitiveness, photosensitivity
        (sun) 692.72
        other light 692.82
      plants NEC 692.6
      plasters, medicated (any) 692.3
      plastic 692.4
      poison
        ivy (Rhus toxicodendron) 692.6
        oak (Rhus diversiloba) 692.6
        plant or vine 692.6
        sumac (Rhus venenata) 692.6
        vine (Rhus radicans) 692.6
      preservatives 692.89
      primrose (primula) 692.6
      primula 692.6
      radiation 692.82
        sun NEC (see also Dermatitis, due to,
         sun) 692.70
        tanning bed 692.82
      radioactive substance 692.82
      radium 692.82
      ragweed (Senecio jacobae) 692.6
      Rhus (diversiloba) (radicans) (toxicoden-
        dron) (venenata) (verniciflua)
        692.6
      rubber 692.4
      scabicides 692.3
      Senecio jacobae 692.6
      solar radiation — see Dermatitis, due to,
        sun
      solvents (any) (substances classifiable to
        982.0–982.8) 692.2
        chlorocompound group 692.2
        cyclohexane group 692.2
        ester group 692.2
        glycol group 692.2
        hydrocarbon group 692.2
        ketone group 692.2
        paint 692.2
      specified agent NEC 692.89
      sun 692.70
        acute 692.72
        chronic NEC 692.74
        specified NEC 692.79
      sunburn (see also Sunburn) 692.71
      sunshine NEC (see also Dermatitis, due
        to, sun) 692.70
      tanning bed 692.82
      tetrachlorethylene 692.2
      toluene 692.2
      topical medications 692.3
      turpentine 692.2
      ultraviolet rays, except from sun 692.82

Dermatitis — continued
due to — continued
   ultraviolet rays, except from sun — con-
      tinued
      sun NEC (see also Dermatitis, due to,
        sun) 692.70
   vaccine or vaccination (correct substance
      properly administered) 693.0
      wrong substance given or taken
        bacterial vaccine 978.8
          specified — see Table of
            Drugs and Chemicals
        other vaccines NEC 979.9
          specified — see Table of
            Drugs and Chemicals
   varicose veins (see also Varicose, vein,
      inflamed or infected) 454.1
   x-rays 692.82
dyshydrotic 705.81
dysmenorrheica 625.8
eczematoid NEC 692.9
   infectious 690.8
eczematous NEC 692.9
epidemica 695.89
erysipelatosa 695.81
escharotica — see Burn, by site
exfoliativa, exfoliative 695.89
   generalized 695.89
   infantum 695.81
   neonatorum 695.81
eyelid 373.31
   allergic 373.32
   contact 373.32
   eczematous 373.31
   herpes (zoster) 053.20
      simplex 054.41
   infective 373.5
      due to
        actinomycosis 039.3 [373.5]
        herpes
          simplex 054.41
          zoster 053.20
        impetigo 684 [373.5]
        leprosy (see also Leprosy)
          030.0 [373.4]
        lupus vulgaris (tuberculous) (see
          also Tuberculosis)
          017.0 ☑ [373.4]
        mycotic dermatitis (see also Der-
          matomycosis)
          111.9 [373.5]
        vaccinia 051.02 [373.5]
          postvaccination 999.0 [373.5]
        yaws (see also Yaws) 102.9 [373.4]
facta, factitia 698.4
   psychogenic 316 [698.4]
ficta 698.4
   psychogenic 316 [698.4]
flexural 691.8
follicularis 704.8
friction 709.8
fungus 111.9
   specified type NEC 111.8
gangrenosa, gangrenous (infantum) (see
      also Gangrene) 785.4
gestationis 646.8 ☑
gonococcal 098.89
gouty 274.89
harvest mite 133.8
heat 692.89
herpetiformis (bullous) (erythematous)
      (pustular) (vesicular) 694.0
   juvenile 694.2
   senile 694.5
hiemalis 692.89
hypostatic, hypostatica 454.1
   with ulcer 454.2
impetiginosa 684
infantile (acute) (chronic) (intertriginous)
      (intrinsic) (seborrheic) 690.12
infectiosa eczematoides 690.8
infectious (staphylococcal) (streptococcal)
      686.9
   eczematoid 690.8
infective eczematoid 690.8
Jacquet's (diaper dermatitis) 691.0

Dermatitis — continued
due to — continued
leptus 133.8
lichenified NEC 692.9
lichenoid, chronic 701.0
lichenoides purpurica pigmentosa 709.1
meadow 692.6
medicamentosa (correct substance properly
      administered) (internal use) (see also
      Dermatitis, due to, drugs or medici-
      nals) 693.0
   due to contact with skin 692.3
mite 133.8
multiformis 694.0
   juvenile 694.2
   senile 694.5
napkin 691.0
neuro 698.3
neurotica 694.0
nummular NEC 692.9
osteatosis, osteatotic 706.8
papillaris capillitii 706.1
pellagrous 265.2
perioral 695.3
perstans 696.1
photosensitivity (sun) 692.72
   other light 692.82
pigmented purpuric lichenoid 709.1
polymorpha dolorosa 694.0
primary irritant 692.9
pruriginosa 694.0
pruritic NEC 692.9
psoriasiform nodularis 696.2
psychogenic 316
purulent 686.00
pustular contagious 051.2
pyococcal 686.00
pyocyaneus 686.09
pyogenica 686.00
radiation 692.82
repens 696.1
Ritter's (exfoliativa) 695.81
Schamberg's (progressive pigmentary der-
      matosis) 709.09
schistosome 120.3
seasonal bullous 694.8
seborrheic 690.10
   infantile 690.12
sensitization NEC 692.9
septic (see also Septicemia) 686.00
   gonococcal 098.89
solar, solare NEC (see also Dermatitis, due
      to, sun) 692.70
stasis 454.1
   due to
      postphlebitic syndrome 459.12
        with ulcer 459.13
      varicose veins — see Varicose
   ulcerated or with ulcer (varicose) 454.2
sunburn (see also Sunburn) 692.71
suppurative 686.00
traumatic NEC 709.8
trophoneurotica 694.0
ultraviolet, except from sun 692.82
   due to sun NEC (see also Dermatitis, due
      to, sun) 692.82
varicose 454.1
   with ulcer 454.2
vegetans 686.8
verrucosa 117.2
xerotic 706.8
Dermatoarthritis, lipoid 272.8 [713.0]
Dermatochalasia, dermatochalasis 374.87
Dermatofibroma (lenticulare) (M8832/0) —
     see also Neoplasm, skin, benign
   protuberans (M8832/1) — see Neoplasm,
     skin, uncertain behavior
Dermatofibrosarcoma (protuberans)
     (M8832/3) — see Neoplasm, skin, malig-
     nant
Dermatographia 708.3
Dermatolysis (congenital) (exfoliativa) 757.39
   acquired 701.8
   eyelids 374.34
   palpebrarum 374.34
   senile 701.8
Dermatomegaly NEC 701.8

Dermatomucomyositis 710.3
Dermatomycosis 111.9
   furfuracea 111.0
   specified type NEC 111.8
Dermatomyositis (acute) (chronic) 710.3
Dermatoneuritis of children 985.0
Dermatophiliasis 134.1
Dermatophytide — see Dermatophytosis
Dermatophytosis (Epidermophyton) (infec-
     tion) (microsporum) (tinea) (Trichophy-
     ton) 110.9
   beard 110.0
   body 110.5
   deep seated 110.6
   fingernails 110.1
   foot 110.4
   groin 110.3
   hand 110.2
   nail 110.1
   perianal (area) 110.3
   scalp 110.0
   scrotal 110.8
   specified site NEC 110.8
   toenails 110.1
   vulva 110.8
Dermatopolyneuritis 985.0
Dermatorrhexis 756.83
   acquired 701.8
Dermatosclerosis — see also Scleroderma
     710.1
   localized 701.0
Dermatosis 709.9
   Andrews' 686.8
   atopic 691.8
   Bowen's (M8081/2) — see Neoplasm, skin,
     in situ
   bullous 694.9
      specified type NEC 694.8
   erythematosquamous 690.8
   exfoliativa 695.89
   factitial 698.4
   gonococcal 098.89
   herpetiformis 694.0
      juvenile 694.2
      senile 694.5
   hysterical 300.11
   linear IgA 694.8
   menstrual NEC 709.8
   neutrophilic, acute febrile 695.89
   occupational (see also Dermatitis) 692.9
   papulosa nigra 709.8
   pigmentary NEC 709.00
      progressive 709.09
      Schamberg's 709.09
      Siemens-Bloch 757.33
   progressive pigmentary 709.09
   psychogenic 316
   pustular subcorneal 694.1
   Schamberg's (progressive pigmentary)
     709.09
   senile NEC 709.3
   specified NEC 702.8
   Unna's (seborrheic dermatitis) 690.10
Dermographia 708.3
Dermographism 708.3
Dermoid (cyst) (M9084/0) — see also Neo-
     plasm, by site, benign
   with malignant transformation (M9084/3)
     183.0
Dermopathy
   infiltrative, with thyrotoxicosis 242.0 ☑
   nephrogenic fibrosing 701.8
   senile NEC 709.3
Dermophytosis — see Dermatophytosis
Descemet's membrane — see condition
Descemetocele 371.72
Descending — see condition
Descensus uteri (complete) (incomplete)
     (partial) (without vaginal wall prolapse)
     618.1
   with mention of vaginal wall prolapse —
     see Prolapse, uterovaginal
Desensitization to allergens V07.1
Desert
   rheumatism 114.0
   sore (see also Ulcer, skin) 707.9

☑ **Additional Digit Required — Refer to the Tabular List for Digit Selection**   ▽ **Subterms under main terms may continue to next column or page**

2014 ICD-9-CM   ▶◀ **Revised Text**   ● **New Line**   ▲ **Revised Code**   **Volume 2 — 77**

Dermatitis — Desert

Desertion (child) (newborn) 995.52
  adult 995.84
Desmoid (extra-abdominal) (tumor) (M8821/1) — *see also* Neoplasm, connective tissue, uncertain behavior
  abdominal (M8822/1) — *see* Neoplasm, connective tissue, uncertain behavior
Despondency 300.4
Desquamative dermatitis NEC 695.89
Destruction
  articular facet (*see also* Derangement, joint) 718.9 ☑
    vertebra 724.9
  bone 733.90
    syphilitic 095.5
  joint (*see also* Derangement, joint) 718.9 ☑
    sacroiliac 724.6
  kidney 593.89
  live fetus to facilitate birth NEC 763.89
  ossicles (ear) 385.24
  rectal sphincter 569.49
  septum (nasal) 478.19
  tuberculous NEC (*see also* Tuberculosis) 011.9 ☑
  tympanic membrane 384.82
  tympanum 385.89
  vertebral disc — *see* Degeneration, intervertebral disc
Destructiveness — *see also* Disturbance, conduct 312.9
  adjustment reaction 309.3
Detachment
  cartilage (*see also* Sprain, by site)
    knee — *see* Tear, meniscus
  cervix, annular 622.8
    complicating delivery 665.3 ☑
  choroid (old) (postinfectional) (simple) (spontaneous) 363.70
    hemorrhagic 363.72
    serous 363.71
  knee, medial meniscus (old) 717.3
    current injury 836.0
  ligament — *see* Sprain, by site
  placenta (premature) — *see* Placenta, separation
  retina (recent) 361.9
    with retinal defect (rhegmatogenous) 361.00
      giant tear 361.03
      multiple 361.02
      partial
        with
          giant tear 361.03
          multiple defects 361.02
          retinal dialysis (juvenile) 361.04
          single defect 361.01
      retinal dialysis (juvenile) 361.04
      single 361.01
      subtotal 361.05
      total 361.05
    delimited (old) (partial) 361.06
    old
      delimited 361.06
      partial 361.06
      total or subtotal 361.07
    pigment epithelium (RPE) (serous) 362.42
      exudative 362.42
      hemorrhagic 362.43
    rhegmatogenous (*see also* Detachment, retina, with retinal defect) 361.00
    serous (without retinal defect) 361.2
    specified type NEC 361.89
    traction with vitreoretinal organization) 361.81
  vitreous humor 379.21
Detergent asthma 507.8
Deterioration
  epileptic
    with behavioral disturbance 345.9 ☑ *[294.11]*
    without behavioral disturbance 345.9 ☑ *[294.10]*
  heart, cardiac (*see also* Degeneration, myocardial) 429.1

Deterioration — *continued*
  mental (*see also* Psychosis) 298.9
  myocardium, myocardial (*see also* Degeneration, myocardial) 429.1
  senile (simple) 797
  transplanted organ — *see* Complications, transplant, organ, by site
de Toni-Fanconi syndrome (cystinosis) 270.0
Deuteranomaly 368.52
Deuteranopia (anomalous trichromat) (complete) (incomplete) 368.52
Deutschländer's disease — *see* Fracture, foot
Development
  abnormal, bone 756.9
  arrested 783.40
    bone 733.91
    child 783.40
      due to malnutrition (protein-calorie) 263.2
    fetus or newborn 764.9 ☑
    tracheal rings (congenital) 748.3
  defective, congenital (*see also* Anomaly)
    cauda equina 742.59
    left ventricle 746.9
      with atresia or hypoplasia of aortic orifice or valve with hypoplasia of ascending aorta 746.7
      in hypoplastic left heart syndrome 746.7
  delayed (*see also* Delay, development) 783.40
    arithmetical skills 315.1
    language (skills) 315.31
      and speech due to hearing loss 315.34
      expressive 315.31
      mixed receptive-expressive 315.32
    learning skill, specified NEC 315.2
    mixed skills 315.5
    motor coordination 315.4
    reading 315.00
    specified
      learning skill NEC 315.2
      type NEC, except learning 315.8
    speech 315.39
      and language due to hearing loss 315.34
      associated with hyperkinesia 314.1
      phonological 315.39
    spelling 315.09
    written expression 315.2
  imperfect, congenital (*see also* Anomaly)
    heart 746.9
    lungs 748.60
  improper (fetus or newborn) 764.9 ☑
  incomplete (fetus or newborn) 764.9 ☑
    affecting management of pregnancy 656.5 ☑
    bronchial tree 748.3
    organ or site not listed — *see* Hypoplasia
    respiratory system 748.9
  sexual, precocious NEC 259.1
  tardy, mental (*see also* Disability, intellectual) 319
Developmental — *see* condition
Devergie's disease (pityriasis rubra pilaris) 696.4
Deviation
  conjugate (eye) 378.87
    palsy 378.81
    spasm, spastic 378.82
  esophagus 530.89
  eye, skew 378.87
  mandible, opening and closing 524.53
  midline (jaw) (teeth) 524.29
    specified site NEC — *see* Malposition
  occlusal plane 524.76
  organ or site, congenital NEC — *see* Malposition, congenital
  septum (acquired) (nasal) 470
    congenital 754.0
  sexual 302.9
    bestiality 302.1
    coprophilia 302.89
    ego-dystonic
      homosexuality 302.0

Deviation — *continued*
  sexual — *continued*
    ego-dystonic — *continued*
      lesbianism 302.0
    erotomania 302.89
      Clérambault's 297.8
    exhibitionism (sexual) 302.4
    fetishism 302.81
      transvestic 302.3
    frotteurism 302.89
    homosexuality, ego-dystonic 302.0
      pedophilic 302.2
    lesbianism, ego-dystonic 302.0
    masochism 302.83
    narcissism 302.89
    necrophilia 302.89
    nymphomania 302.89
    pederosis 302.2
    pedophilia 302.2
    sadism 302.84
    sadomasochism 302.84
    satyriasis 302.89
    specified type NEC 302.89
    transvestic fetishism 302.3
    transvestism 302.3
    voyeurism 302.82
    zoophilia (erotica) 302.1
  teeth, midline 524.29
  trachea 519.19
  ureter (congenital) 753.4
Devic's disease 341.0
Device
  cerebral ventricle (communicating) in situ V45.2
  contraceptive — *see* Contraceptive, device
  drainage, cerebrospinal fluid V45.2
Devil's
  grip 074.1
  pinches (purpura simplex) 287.2
Devitalized tooth 522.9
Devonshire colic 984.9
  specified type of lead — *see* Table of Drugs and Chemicals
Dextraposition, aorta 747.21
  with ventricular septal defect, pulmonary stenosis or atresia, and hypertrophy of right ventricle 745.2
  in tetralogy of Fallot 745.2
Dextratransposition, aorta 745.11
Dextrinosis, limit (debrancher enzyme deficiency) 271.0
Dextrocardia (corrected) (false) (isolated) (secondary) (true) 746.87
  with
    complete transposition of viscera 759.3
    situs inversus 759.3
Dextroversion, kidney (left) 753.3
Dhobie itch 110.3
DHTR (delayed hemolytic transfusion reaction) — *see* Complications, transfusion
Diabetes, diabetic (brittle) (congenital) (familial) (mellitus) (severe) (slight) (without complication) 250.0 ☑

Note — Use the following fifth-digit subclassification with category 250:

0 type II or unspecified type, not stated as uncontrolled

Fifth-digit 0 is for use for type II patients, even if the patient requires insulin

1 type I [juvenile type], not stated as uncontrolled

2 type II or unspecified type, uncontrolled

Fifth-digit 2 is for use for type II patients, even if the patient requires insulin

3 type I [juvenile type], uncontrolled

  with
    coma (with ketoacidosis) 250.3 ☑
      due to secondary diabetes 249.3 ☑
      hyperosmolar (nonketotic) 250.2 ☑
        due to secondary diabetes 249.2 ☑

Diabetes, diabetic — *continued*
  with — *continued*
    complication NEC 250.9 ☑
      due to secondary diabetes 249.9 ☑
      specified NEC 250.8 ☑
        due to secondary diabetes 249.8 ☑
    gangrene 250.7 ☑ *[785.4]*
      due to secondary diabetes 249.7 ☑ *[785.4]*
    hyperglycemia — *code to* Diabetes, by type, with 5th digit for not stated as uncontrolled
    hyperosmolarity 250.2 ☑
      due to secondary diabetes 249.2 ☑
    ketosis, ketoacidosis 250.1 ☑
      due to secondary diabetes 249.1 ☑
    loss of protective sensation (LOPS) — *see* Diabetes, neuropathy
    osteomyelitis 250.8 ☑ *[731.8]*
      due to secondary diabetes 249.8 ☑ *[731.8]*
    specified manisfestations NEC 250.8 ☑
      due to secondary diabetes 249.8 ☑
  acetonemia 250.1 ☑
    due to secondary diabetes 249.1 ☑
  acidosis 250.1 ☑
    due to secondary diabetes 249.1 ☑
  amyotrophy 250.6 ☑ *[353.5]*
    due to secondary diabetes 249.6 ☑ *[353.5]*
  angiopathy, peripheral 250.7 ☑ *[443.81]*
    due to secondary diabetes 249.7 ☑ *[443.81]*
  asymptomatic 790.29
  autonomic neuropathy (peripheral) 250.6 ☑ *[337.1]*
    due to secondary diabetes 249.6 ☑ *[337.1]*
  bone change 250.8 ☑ *[731.8]*
    due to secondary diabetes 249.8 ☑ *[731.8]*
  borderline 790.29
  bronze, bronzed 275.01
  cataract 250.5 ☑ *[366.41]*
    due to secondary diabetes 249.5 ☑ *[366.41]*
  chemical induced — *see* Diabetes, secondary
  complicating pregnancy, childbirth, or puerperium 648.0 ☑
  coma (with ketoacidosis) 250.3 ☑
    due to secondary diabetes 249.3 ☑
    hyperglycemic 250.3 ☑
      due to secondary diabetes 249.3 ☑
    hyperosmolar (nonketotic) 250.2 ☑
      due to secondary diabetes 249.2 ☑
    hypoglycemic 250.3 ☑
      due to secondary diabetes 249.3 ☑
    insulin 250.3 ☑
      due to secondary diabetes 249.3 ☑
  complicating pregnancy, childbirth, or puerperium (maternal) (conditions classifiable to 249 and 250) 648.0 ☑
    affecting fetus or newborn 775.0
  complication NEC 250.9 ☑
    due to secondary diabetes 249.9 ☑
    specified NEC 250.8 ☑
      due to secondary diabetes 249.8 ☑
  dorsal sclerosis 250.6 ☑ *[340]*
    due to secondary diabetes 249.6 ☑ *[340]*
  drug-induced — *see also* Diabetes, secondary
    overdose or wrong substance given or taken — *see* Table of Drugs and Chemicals
  due to
    cystic fibrosis — *see* Diabetes, secondary
    infection — *see* Diabetes, secondary
  dwarfism-obesity syndrome 258.1
  gangrene 250.7 ☑ *[785.4]*
    due to secondary diabetes 249.7 ☑ *[785.4]*

Diabetes, diabetic — *continued*
gastroparesis 250.6 ☑ *[536.3]*
  due to secondary diabetes
    249.6 ☑ *[536.3]*
gestational 648.8 ☑
  complicating pregnancy, childbirth, or
    puerperium 648.8 ☑
glaucoma 250.5 ☑ *[365.44]*
  due to secondary diabetes
    249.5 ☑ *[365.44]*
glomerulosclerosis (intercapillary)
  250.4 ☑ *[581.81]*
  due to secondary diabetes
    249.4 ☑ *[581.81]*
glycogenosis, secondary 250.8 *[259.8]*
  due to secondary diabetes
    249.8 ☑ *[259.8]*
hemochromatosis (*see also* Hemochromatosis) 275.03
hyperosmolar coma 250.2 ☑
  due to secondary diabetes 249.2 ☑
hyperosmolarity 250.2 ☑
  due to secondary diabetes 249.2 ☑
hypertension-nephrosis syndrome
  250.4 ☑ *[581.81]*
  due to secondary diabetes
    249.4 ☑ *[581.81]*
hypoglycemia 250.8 ☑
  due to secondary diabetes 249.8 ☑
hypoglycemic shock 250.8 ☑
  due to secondary diabetes 249.8 ☑
inadequately controlled — code to Diabetes, by type, with 5th digit for not stated as uncontrolled
insipidus 253.5
  nephrogenic 588.1
  pituitary 253.5
  vasopressin-resistant 588.1
intercapillary glomerulosclerosis
  250.4 ☑ *[581.81]*
  due to secondary diabetes
    249.4 ☑ *[581.81]*
iritis 250.5 ☑ *[364.42]*
  due to secondary diabetes
    249.5 ☑ *[364.42]*
ketosis, ketoacidosis 250.1 ☑
  due to secondary diabetes 249.1 ☑
Kimmelstiel (-Wilson) disease or syndrome (intercapillary glomerulosclerosis)
  250.4 ☑ *[581.81]*
  due to secondary diabetes
    249.4 ☑ *[581.81]*
Lancereaux's (diabetes mellitus with marked emaciation) 250.8 ☑ *[261]*
  due to secondary diabetes
    249.8 ☑ *[261]*
latent (chemical) — *see* Diabetes, secondary
complicating pregnancy, childbirth, or puerperium 648.0 ☑
lipoidosis 250.8 ☑ *[272.7]*
  due to secondary diabetes
    249.8 ☑ *[272.7]*
macular edema 250.5 ☑ *[362.07]*
  due to secondary diabetes
    249.5 ☑ *[362.07]*
maternal
  with manifest disease in the infant 775.1
  affecting fetus or newborn 775.0
microaneurysms, retinal 250.5 ☑ *[362.01]*
  due to secondary diabetes
    249.5 ☑ *[362.01]*
mononeuropathy 250.6 ☑ *[355.9]*
  due to secondary diabetes
    249.6 ☑ *[355.9]*
neonatal, transient 775.1
nephropathy 250.4 ☑ *[583.81]*
  due to secondary diabetes
    249.4 ☑ *[583.81]*
nephrosis (syndrome) 250.4 ☑ *[581.81]*
  due to secondary diabetes
    249.4 ☑ *[581.81]*
neuralgia 250.6 ☑ *[357.2]*
  due to secondary diabetes
    249.6 ☑ *[357.2]*

Diabetes, diabetic — *continued*
neuritis 250.6 ☑ *[357.2]*
  due to secondary diabetes
    249.6 ☑ *[357.2]*
neurogenic arthropathy 250.6 ☑ *[713.5]*
  due to secondary diabetes
    249.6 ☑ *[713.5]*
neuropathy 250.6 ☑ *[357.2]*
  autonomic (peripheral) 250.6 ☑ *[337.1]*
    due to secondary diabetes
      249.6 ☑ *[337.1]*
  due to secondary diabetes
    249.6 ☑ *[357.2]*
nonclinical 790.29
osteomyelitis 250.8 ☑ *[731.8]*
  due to secondary diabetes
    249.8 ☑ *[731.8]*
out of control — code to Diabetes, by type, with 5th digit for uncontrolled
peripheral autonomic neuropathy
  250.6 ☑ *[337.1]*
  due to secondary diabetes
    249.6 ☑ *[337.1]*
phosphate 275.3
polyneuropathy 250.6 ☑ *[357.2]*
  due to secondary diabetes
    249.6 ☑ *[357.2]*
poorly controlled — code to Diabetes, by type, with 5th digit for not stated as uncontrolled
renal (true) 271.4
retinal
  edema 250.5 ☑ *[362.07]*
    due to secondary diabetes
      249.5 ☑ *[362.07]*
  hemorrhage 250.5 ☑ *[362.01]*
    due to secondary diabetes
      249.5 ☑ *[362.01]*
  microaneurysms 250.5 ☑ *[362.01]*
    due to secondary diabetes
      249.5 ☑ *[362.01]*
retinitis 250.5 ☑ *[362.01]*
  due to secondary diabetes
    249.5 ☑ *[362.01]*
retinopathy 250.5 ☑ *[362.01]*
  background 250.5 ☑ *[362.01]*
    due to secondary diabetes
      249.5 ☑ *[362.01]*
  due to secondary diabetes
    249.5 ☑ *[362.01]*
  nonproliferative 250.5 ☑ *[362.03]*
    due to secondary diabetes
      249.5 ☑ *[362.03]*
    mild 250.5 ☑ *[362.04]*
      due to secondary diabetes
        249.5 ☑ *[362.04]*
    moderate 250.5 ☑ *[362.05]*
      due to secondary diabetes
        249.5 ☑ *[362.05]*
    severe 250.5 ☑ *[362.06]*
      due to secondary diabetes
        249.5 ☑ *[362.06]*
  proliferative 250.5 ☑ *[362.02]*
    due to secondary diabetes
      249.5 ☑ *[362.02]*
secondary (chemical-induced) (due to chronic condition) (due to infection) (drug-induced) 249.0 ☑
  with
    coma (with ketoacidosis) 249.3 ☑
      hyperosmolar (nonketotic)
        249.2 ☑
    complication NEC 249.9 ☑
      specified NEC 249.8 ☑
    gangrene 249.7 ☑ *[785.4]*
    hyperosmolarity 249.2 ☑
    ketosis, ketoacidosis 249.1 ☑
    osteomyelitis 249.8 ☑ *[731.8]*
    specified manifestations NEC
      249.8 ☑
  acetonemia 249.1 ☑
  acidosis 249.1 ☑
  amyotrophy 249.6 ☑ *[353.5]*
  angiopathy, peripheral 249.7 ☑ *[443.81]*

Diabetes, diabetic — *continued*
secondary — *continued*
  autonomic neuropathy (peripheral)
    249.6 ☑ *[337.1]*
  bone change 249.8 ☑ *[731.8]*
  cataract 249.5 ☑ *[366.41]*
  coma (with ketoacidosis) 249.3 ☑
    hyperglycemic 249.3 ☑
    hyperosmolar (nonketotic) 249.2 ☑
    hypoglycemic 249.3 ☑
    insulin 249.3 ☑
  complicating pregnancy, childbirth, or puerperium (maternal) 648.0 ☑
    affecting fetus or newborn 775.0
  complication NEC 249.9 ☑
    specified NEC 249.8 ☑
  dorsal sclerosis 249.6 ☑ *[340]*
  due to overdose or wrong substance given or taken — *see* Table of Drugs and Chemicals
  gangrene 249.7 ☑ *[785.4]*
  gastroparesis 249.6 ☑ *[536.3]*
  glaucoma 249.5 ☑ *[365.44]*
  glomerulosclerosis (intercapillary)
    249.4 ☑ *[581.81]*
  glycogenosis, secondary 249.8 ☑ *[259.8]*
  hyperosmolar coma 249.2 ☑
  hyperosmolarity 249.2 ☑
  hypertension-nephrosis syndrome
    249.4 ☑ *[581.81]*
  hypoglycemia 249.8 ☑
  hypoglycemic shock 249.8 ☑
  intercapillary glomerulosclerosis
    249.4 ☑ *[581.81]*
  iritis 249.5 ☑ *[364.42]*
  ketosis, ketoacidosis 249.1 ☑
  Kimmelstiel (-Wilson) disease or syndrome (intercapillary glomerulosclerosis) 249.4 ☑ *[581.81]*
  Lancereaux's (diabetes mellitus with marked emaciation)
    249.8 ☑ *[261]*
  lipoidosis 249.8 ☑ *[272.7]*
  macular edema 249.5 ☑ *[362.07]*
  maternal
    with manifest disease in the infant 775.1
    affecting fetus or newborn 775.0
  microaneurysms, retinal
    249.5 ☑ *[362.01]*
  mononeuropathy 249.6 ☑ *[355.9]*
  nephropathy 249.4 ☑ *[583.81]*
  nephrosis (syndrome) 249.4 ☑ *[581.81]*
  neuralgia 249.6 ☑ *[357.2]*
  neuritis 249.6 ☑ *[357.2]*
  neurogenic arthropathy 249.6 ☑ *[713.5]*
  neuropathy 249.6 ☑ *[357.2]*
    autonomic (peripheral)
      249.6 ☑ *[337.1]*
  osteomyelitis 249.8 ☑ *[731.8]*
  peripheral autonomic neuropathy
    249.6 ☑ *[337.1]*
  polyneuropathy 249.6 ☑ *[357.2]*
  retinal
    edema 249.5 ☑ *[362.07]*
    hemorrhage 249.5 ☑ *[362.01]*
    microaneurysms 249.5 ☑ *[362.01]*
  retinitis 249.5 ☑ *[362.01]*
  retinopathy 249.5 ☑ *[362.01]*
    background 249.5 ☑ *[362.01]*
    nonproliferative 249.5 ☑ *[362.03]*
      mild 249.5 ☑ *[362.04]*
      moderate 249.5 ☑ *[362.05]*
      severe 249.5 ☑ *[362.06]*
    proliferative 249.5 ☑ *[362.02]*
  ulcer (skin) 249.8 ☑ *[707.9]*
    lower extemity 249.8 ☑ *[707.10]*
      ankle 249.8 ☑ *[707.13]*
      calf 249.8 ☑ *[707.12]*
      foot 249.8 ☑ *[707.15]*
      heel 249.8 ☑ *[707.14]*
      knee 249.8 ☑ *[707.19]*
      specified site NEC
        249.8 ☑ *[707.19]*

Diabetes, diabetic — *continued*
secondary — *continued*
  ulcer — *continued*
    lower extemity — *continued*
      thigh 249.8 ☑ *[707.11]*
      toes 249.8 ☑ *[707.15]*
    specified site NEC 249.8 ☑ *[707.8]*
    xanthoma 249.8 ☑ *[272.2]*
  steroid induced — *see also* Diabetes, secondary
    overdose or wrong substance given or taken 962.0
  stress 790.29
  subclinical 790.29
  subliminal 790.29
  sugar 250.0 ☑
ulcer (skin) 250.8 ☑ *[707.9]*
  due to secondary diabetes
    249.8 ☑ *[707.9]*
  lower extremity 250.8 ☑ *[707.10]*
    ankle 250.8 ☑ *[707.13]*
      due to secondary diabetes
        249.8 ☑ *[707.13]*
    calf 250.8 ☑ *[707.12]*
      due to secondary diabetes
        249.8 ☑ *[707.12]*
      due to secondary diabetes
        249.8 ☑ *[707.10]*
    foot 250.8 ☑ *[707.15]*
      due to secondary diabetes
        249.8 ☑ *[707.15]*
    heel 250.8 ☑ *[707.14]*
      due to secondary diabetes
        249.8 ☑ *[707.14]*
    knee 250.8 ☑ *[707.19]*
      due to secondary diabetes
        249.8 ☑ *[707.19]*
    specified site NEC 250.8 ☑ *[707.19]*
      due to secondary diabetes
        249.8 ☑ *[707.19]*
    thigh 250.8 ☑ *[707.11]*
      due to secondary diabetes
        249.8 ☑ *[707.11]*
    toes 250.8 ☑ *[707.15]*
      due to secondary diabetes
        249.8 ☑ *[707.15]*
  specified site NEC 250.8 ☑ *[707.8]*
    due to secondary diabetes
      249.8 ☑ *[707.8]*
xanthoma 250.8 ☑ *[272.2]*
  due to secondary diabetes
    249.8 ☑ *[272.2]*
Diacyclothrombopathia 287.1
Diagnosis deferred 799.9
Dialysis (intermittent) (treatment)
  anterior retinal (juvenile) (with detachment) 361.04
  extracorporeal V56.0
  hemodialysis V56.0
    status only V45.11
  peritoneal V56.8
    status only V45.11
  renal V56.0
    status only V45.11
  specified type NEC V56.8
Diamond-Blackfan anemia or syndrome (congenital hypoplastic anemia) 284.01
Diamond-Gardener syndrome (autoerythrocyte sensitization) 287.2
Diaper rash 691.0
Diaphoresis (excessive) NEC — *see also* Hyperhidrosis) 780.8
Diaphragm — *see* condition
Diaphragmalgia 786.52
Diaphragmitis 519.4
Diaphyseal aclasis 756.4
Diaphysitis 733.99
Diarrhea, diarrheal (acute) (autumn) (bilious) (bloody) (catarrhal) (choleraic) (chronic) (gravis) (green) (infantile) (lienteric) (noninfectious) (presumed noninfectious) (putrefactive) (secondary) (sporadic) (summer) (symptomatic) (thermic) 787.91
  achlorhydric 536.0

☑ **Additional Digit Required** — Refer to the Tabular List for Digit Selection

▽ **Subterms under main terms may continue to next column or page**

2014 ICD-9-CM

▶◀ **Revised Text**

● **New Line**

▲ **Revised Code**

Volume 2 — 79

Diabetes, diabetic — Diarrhea, diarrheal

Diarrhea, diarrheal — *continued*
  allergic 558.3
  amebic (*see also* Amebiasis) 006.9
    with abscess — *see* Abscess, amebic
    acute 006.0
    chronic 006.1
    nondysenteric 006.2
  bacillary — *see* Dysentery, bacillary
  bacterial NEC 008.5
  balantidial 007.0
  bile salt-induced 579.8
  cachectic NEC 787.91
  chilomastix 007.8
  choleriformis 001.1
  coccidial 007.2
  Cochin-China 579.1
    anguilluliasis 127.2
    psilosis 579.1
  Dientamoeba 007.8
  dietetic 787.91
  due to
    achylia gastrica 536.8
    Aerobacter aerogenes 008.2
    Bacillus coli — *see* Enteritis, E. coli
    bacteria NEC 008.5
    bile salts 579.8
    Capillaria
      hepatica 128.8
      philippinensis 127.5
    Clostridium perfringens (C) (F) 008.46
    Enterobacter aerogenes 008.2
    enterococci 008.49
    Escherichia coli — *see* Enteritis, E. coli
    Giardia lamblia 007.1
    Heterophyes heterophyes 121.6
    irritating foods 787.91
    Metagonimus yokogawai 121.5
    Necator americanus 126.1
    Paracolobactrum arizonae 008.1
    Paracolon bacillus NEC 008.47
      Arizona 008.1
    Proteus (bacillus) (mirabilis) (Morganii) 008.3
    Pseudomonas aeruginosa 008.42
    S. japonicum 120.2
    specified organism NEC 008.8
      bacterial 008.49
      viral NEC 008.69
    Staphylococcus 008.41
    Streptococcus 008.49
      anaerobic 008.46
    Strongyloides stercoralis 127.2
    Trichuris trichiuria 127.3
    virus NEC (*see also* Enteritis, viral) 008.69
  dysenteric 009.2
    due to specified organism NEC 008.8
  dyspeptic 787.91
  endemic 009.3
    due to specified organism NEC 008.8
  epidemic 009.2
    due to specified organism NEC 008.8
  fermentative 787.91
  flagellate 007.9
  Flexner's (ulcerative) 004.1
  functional 564.5
    following gastrointestinal surgery 564.4
    psychogenic 306.4
  giardial 007.1
  Giardia lamblia 007.1
  hill 579.1
  hyperperistalsis (nervous) 306.4
  infectious 009.2
    due to specified organism NEC 008.8
    presumed 009.3
  inflammatory 787.91
    due to specified organism NEC 008.8
  malarial (*see also* Malaria) 084.6
  mite 133.8
  mycotic 117.9
  nervous 306.4
  neurogenic 564.5
  parenteral NEC 009.2
  postgastrectomy 564.4
  postvagotomy 564.4
  prostaglandin induced 579.8
  protozoal NEC 007.9

Diarrhea, diarrheal — *continued*
  psychogenic 306.4
  septic 009.2
    due to specified organism NEC 008.8
  specified organism NEC 008.8
    bacterial 008.49
    viral NEC 008.69
  Staphylococcus 008.41
  Streptococcus 008.49
    anaerobic 008.46
  toxic 558.2
  travelers' 009.2
    due to specified organism NEC 008.8
  trichomonal 007.3
  tropical 579.1
  tuberculous 014.8 ☑
  ulcerative (chronic) (*see also* Colitis, ulcerative) 556.9
  viral (*see also* Enteritis, viral) 008.8
  zymotic NEC 009.2
Diastasis
  cranial bones 733.99
    congenital 756.0
  joint (traumatic) — *see* Dislocation, by site
  muscle 728.84
    congenital 756.89
  recti (abdomen) 728.84
    complicating delivery 665.8 ☑
    congenital 756.79
Diastema, teeth, tooth 524.30
Diastematomyelia 742.51
Diataxia, cerebral, infantile 343.0
Diathesis
  allergic V15.09
  bleeding (familial) 287.9
  cystine (familial) 270.0
  gouty 274.9
  hemorrhagic (familial) 287.9
    newborn NEC 776.0
  oxalic 271.8
  scrofulous (*see also* Tuberculosis) 017.2 ☑
  spasmophilic (*see also* Tetany) 781.7
  ulcer 536.9
  uric acid 274.9
Diaz's disease or osteochondrosis 732.5
Dibothriocephaliasis 123.4
  larval 123.5
Dibothriocephalus (infection) (infestation) (latus) 123.4
  larval 123.5
Dicephalus 759.4
Dichotomy, teeth 520.2
Dichromat, dichromata (congenital) 368.59
Dichromatopsia (congenital) 368.59
Dichuchwa 104.0
Dicroceliasis 121.8
Didelphys, didelphic — *see also* Double uterus 752.2
Didymitis — *see also* Epididymitis 604.90
Died — *see also* Death
  without
    medical attention (cause unknown) 798.9
    sign of disease 798.2
Dientamoeba diarrhea 007.8
Dietary
  inadequacy or deficiency 269.9
  surveillance and counseling V65.3
Dietl's crisis 593.4
Dieulafoy lesion (hemorrhagic)
  of
    duodenum 537.84
    esophagus 530.82
    intestine 569.86
    stomach 537.84
Difficult
  birth, affecting fetus or newborn 763.9
  delivery NEC 669.9 ☑
Difficulty
  feeding 783.3
    adult 783.3
    breast 676.8 ☑
    child 783.3
    elderly 783.3
    infant 783.3
    newborn 779.31

Difficulty — *continued*
  feeding — *continued*
    nonorganic (infant) NEC 307.59
  mechanical, gastroduodenal stoma 537.89
  reading 315.00
  specific, spelling 315.09
  swallowing (*see also* Dysphagia) 787.20
  walking 719.7
Diffuse — *see* condition
Diffused ganglion 727.42
Di George's syndrome (thymic hypoplasia) 279.11
Digestive — *see* condition
Di Guglielmo's disease or syndrome (M9841/3) 207.0 ☑
Dihydropyrimidine dehydrogenase disease (DPD) 277.6
Diktyoma (M9051/3) — *see* Neoplasm, by site, malignant
Dilaceration, tooth 520.4
Dilatation
  anus 564.89
    venule — *see* Hemorrhoids
  aorta (focal) (general) (*see also* Ectasia, aortic) 447.70
    with aneurysm 441.9
    congenital 747.29
    infectional 093.0
    ruptured 441.5
    syphilitic 093.0
  appendix (cystic) 543.9
  artery 447.8
  bile duct (common) (congenital) 751.69
    acquired 576.8
  bladder (sphincter) 596.89
    congenital 753.8
    in pregnancy or childbirth 654.4 ☑
      causing obstructed labor 660.2 ☑
        affecting fetus or newborn 763.1
  blood vessel 459.89
  bronchus, bronchi 494.0
    with acute exacerbation 494.1
  calyx (due to obstruction) 593.89
  capillaries 448.9
  cardiac (acute) (chronic) (*see also* Hypertrophy, cardiac) 429.3
    congenital 746.89
      valve NEC 746.89
      pulmonary 746.09
    hypertensive (*see also* Hypertension, heart) 402.90
  cavum septi pellucidi 742.4
  cecum 564.89
    psychogenic 306.4
  cervix (uteri) (*see also* Incompetency, cervix)
    incomplete, poor, slow
      affecting fetus or newborn 763.7
    complicating delivery 661.0 ☑
      affecting fetus or newborn 763.7
  colon 564.7
    congenital 751.3
    due to mechanical obstruction 560.89
    psychogenic 306.4
  common bile duct (congenital) 751.69
    acquired 576.8
      with calculus, choledocholithiasis, or stones — *see* Choledocholithiasis
  cystic duct 751.69
    acquired (any bile duct) 575.8
  duct, mammary 610.4
  duodenum 564.89
  esophagus 530.89
    congenital 750.4
    due to
      achalasia 530.0
      cardiospasm 530.0
  Eustachian tube, congenital 744.24
  fontanel 756.0
  gallbladder 575.8
    congenital 751.69
  gastric 536.8
    acute 536.1
    psychogenic 306.4
  heart (acute) (chronic) (*see also* Hypertrophy, cardiac) 429.3

Dilatation — *continued*
  heart (*see also* Hypertrophy, cardiac) — *continued*
    congenital 746.89
    hypertensive (*see also* Hypertension, heart) 402.90
    valve (*see also* Endocarditis)
      congenital 746.89
  ileum 564.89
    psychogenic 306.4
  inguinal rings — *see* Hernia, inguinal
  jejunum 564.89
    psychogenic 306.4
  kidney (calyx) (collecting structures) (cystic) (parenchyma) (pelvis) 593.89
  lacrimal passages 375.69
  lymphatic vessel 457.1
  mammary duct 610.4
  Meckel's diverticulum (congenital) 751.0
  meningeal vessels, congenital 742.8
  myocardium (acute) (chronic) (*see also* Hypertrophy, cardiac) 429.3
  organ or site, congenital NEC — *see* Distortion
  pancreatic duct 577.8
  pelvis, kidney 593.89
  pericardium — *see* Pericarditis
  pharynx 478.29
  prostate 602.8
  pulmonary
    artery (idiopathic) 417.8
      congenital 747.39
    valve, congenital 746.09
  pupil 379.43
  rectum 564.89
  renal 593.89
  saccule vestibularis, congenital 744.05
  salivary gland (duct) 527.8
  sphincter ani 564.89
  stomach 536.8
    acute 536.1
    psychogenic 306.4
  submaxillary duct 527.8
  trachea, congenital 748.3
  ureter (idiopathic) 593.89
    congenital 753.20
    due to obstruction 593.5
  urethra (acquired) 599.84
  vasomotor 443.9
  vein 459.89
  ventricular, ventricle (acute) (chronic) (*see also* Hypertrophy, cardiac) 429.3
    cerebral, congenital 742.4
    hypertensive (*see also* Hypertension, heart) 402.90
  venule 459.89
    anus — *see* Hemorrhoids
  vesical orifice 596.89
Dilated, dilation — *see* Dilatation
Diminished
  hearing (acuity) (*see also* Deafness) 389.9
  pulse pressure 785.9
  vision NEC 369.9
  vital capacity 794.2
Diminuta taenia 123.6
Diminution, sense or sensation (cold) (heat) (tactile) (vibratory) — *see also* Disturbance, sensation 782.0
Dimitri-Sturge-Weber disease (encephalocutaneous angiomatosis) 759.6
Dimple
  parasacral 685.1
    with abscess 685.0
  pilonidal 685.1
    with abscess 685.0
  postanal 685.1
    with abscess 685.0
Dioctophyma renale (infection) (infestation) 128.8
Dipetalonemiasis 125.4
Diphallus 752.69
Diphtheria, diphtheritic (gangrenous) (hemorrhagic) 032.9
  carrier (suspected) of V02.4
  cutaneous 032.85
  cystitis 032.84

☑ **Additional Digit Required** — Refer to the Tabular List for Digit Selection   ▽ Subterms under main terms may continue to next column or page

80 — Volume 2   ▶◀ **Revised Text**   ● **New Line**   ▲ **Revised Code**   **2014 ICD-9-CM**

Diphtheria, diphtheritic — *continued*
  faucial 032.0
  infection of wound 032.85
  inoculation (anti) (not sick) V03.5
  laryngeal 032.3
  myocarditis 032.82
  nasal anterior 032.2
  nasopharyngeal 032.1
  neurological complication 032.89
  peritonitis 032.83
  specified site NEC 032.89
Diphyllobothriasis (intestine) 123.4
  larval 123.5
Diplacusis 388.41
Diplegia (upper limbs) 344.2
  brain or cerebral 437.8
  congenital 343.0
  facial 351.0
    congenital 352.6
  infantile or congenital (cerebral) (spastic) (spinal) 343.0
  lower limbs 344.1
  syphilitic, congenital 090.49
Diplococcus, diplococcal — *see* condition
Diplomyelia 742.59
Diplopia 368.2
  refractive 368.15
Dipsomania — *see also* Alcoholism 303.9 ☑
  with psychosis (*see also* Psychosis, alcoholic) 291.9
Dipylidiasis 123.8
  intestine 123.8
Direction, teeth, abnormal 524.30
Dirt-eating child 307.52
Disability, disabilities
  heart — *see* Disease, heart
  intellectual 319
    borderline V62.89
    mild, IQ 50-70 317
    moderate, IQ 35-49 318.0
    profound, IQ under 20 318.2
    severe, IQ 20-34 318.1
  learning NEC 315.2
  special spelling 315.09
Disarticulation — *see also* Derangement, joint 718.9 ☑
  meaning
    amputation
      status — *see* Absence, by site
      traumatic — *see* Amputation, traumatic
    dislocation, traumatic or congenital — *see* Dislocation
Disaster, cerebrovascular — *see also* Disease, cerebrovascular, acute 436
Discharge
  anal NEC 787.99
  breast (female) (male) 611.79
  conjunctiva 372.89
  continued locomotor idiopathic (*see also* Epilepsy) 345.5 ☑
  diencephalic autonomic idiopathic (*see also* Epilepsy) 345.5 ☑
  ear 388.60
    blood 388.69
    cerebrospinal fluid 388.61
  excessive urine 788.42
  eye 379.93
  nasal 478.19
  nipple 611.79
  patterned motor idiopathic (*see also* Epilepsy) 345.5 ☑
  penile 788.7
  postnasal — *see* Sinusitis
  sinus, from mediastinum 510.0
  umbilicus 789.9
  urethral 788.7
    bloody 599.84
  vaginal 623.5
Discitis 722.90
  cervical, cervicothoracic 722.91
  lumbar, lumbosacral 722.93
  thoracic, thoracolumbar 722.92
Discogenic syndrome — *see* Displacement, intervertebral disc

Discoid
  kidney 753.3
  meniscus, congenital 717.5
  semilunar cartilage 717.5
Discoloration
  mouth 528.9
  nails 703.8
  teeth 521.7
    due to
      drugs 521.7
      metals (copper) (silver) 521.7
      pulpal bleeding 521.7
    during formation 520.8
    extrinsic 523.6
    intrinsic posteruptive 521.7
Discomfort
  chest 786.59
  visual 368.13
Discomycosis — *see* Actinomycosis
Discontinuity, ossicles, ossicular chain 385.23
Discrepancy
  centric occlusion
    maximum intercuspation 524.55
    of teeth 524.55
  leg length (acquired) 736.81
    congenital 755.30
  uterine size-date 649.6 ☑
Discrimination
  political V62.4
  racial V62.4
  religious V62.4
  sex V62.4
Disease, diseased — *see also* Syndrome
  Abrami's (acquired hemolytic jaundice) 283.9
  absorbent system 459.89
  accumulation — *see* Thesaurismosis
  acid-peptic 536.8
  Acosta's 993.2
  Adams-Stokes (-Morgagni) (syncope with heart block) 426.9
  Addison-Gull — *see* Xanthoma
  Addison's (bronze) (primary adrenal insufficiency) 255.41
    anemia (pernicious) 281.0
    tuberculous (*see also* Tuberculosis) 017.6 ☑
  adenoids (and tonsils) (chronic) 474.9
  adrenal (gland) (capsule) (cortex) 255.9
    hyperfunction 255.3
    hypofunction 255.41
    specified type NEC 255.8
  ainhum (dactylolysis spontanea) 136.0
  akamushi (scrub typhus) 081.2
  Akureyri (epidemic neuromyasthenia) 049.8
  Albarrán's (colibacilluria) 791.9
  Albers-Schönberg's (marble bones) 756.52
  Albert's 726.71
  Albright (-Martin) (-Bantam) 275.49
  Alibert-Bazin (M9700/3) 202.1 ☑
  Alibert's (mycosis fungoides) (M9700/3) 202.1 ☑
  alimentary canal 569.9
  alligator skin (ichthyosis congenita) 757.1
    acquired 701.1
  Almeida's (Brazilian blastomycosis) 116.1
  Alpers' 330.8
  alpine 993.2
  altitude 993.2
  alveoli, teeth 525.9
  Alzheimer's — *see* Alzheimer's
  amyloid (any site) 277.30
  anarthritic rheumatoid 446.5
  Anders' (adiposis tuberosa simplex) 272.8
  Andersen's (glycogenosis IV) 271.0
  Anderson's (angiokeratoma corporis diffusum) 272.7
  Andes 993.2
  Andrews' (bacterid) 686.8
  angiospastic, angiospasmodic 443.9
    cerebral 435.9
      with transient neurologic deficit 435.9
    vein 459.89

Disease, diseased — *see also* Syndrome — *continued*
  anterior
    chamber 364.9
    horn cell 335.9
      specified type NEC 335.8
  antral (chronic) 473.0
    acute 461.0
  anus NEC 569.49
  aorta (nonsyphilitic) 447.9
    syphilitic NEC 093.89
  aortic (heart) (valve) (*see also* Endocarditis, aortic) 424.1
  apollo 077.4
  aponeurosis 726.90
  appendix 543.9
  aqueous (chamber) 364.9
  arc-welders' lung 503
  Armenian 277.31
  Arnold-Chiari (*see also* Spina bifida) 741.0 ☑
  arterial 447.9
    occlusive (*see also* Occlusion, by site) 444.22
      with embolus or thrombus — *see* Occlusion, by site
      due to stricture or stenosis 447.1
    specified type NEC 447.8
  arteriocardiorenal (*see also* Hypertension, cardiorenal) 404.90
  arteriolar (generalized) (obliterative) 447.9
    specified type NEC 447.8
  arteriorenal (*see also* Hypertension, kidney)
  arteriosclerotic (*see also* Arteriosclerosis)
    cardiovascular 429.2
    coronary — *see* Arteriosclerosis, coronary
    heart — *see* Arteriosclerosis, coronary
    vascular — *see* Arteriosclerosis
  artery 447.9
    cerebral 437.9
    coronary — *see* Arteriosclerosis, coronary
    specified type NEC 447.8
  arthropod-borne NEC 088.9
    specified type NEC 088.89
  Asboe-Hansen's (incontinentia pigmenti) 757.33
  atticoantral, chronic (with posterior or superior marginal perforation of ear drum) 382.2
  auditory canal, ear 380.9
  Aujeszky's 078.89
  auricle, ear NEC 380.30
  Australian X 062.4
  autoimmune NEC 279.49
    hemolytic (cold type) (warm type) 283.0
    parathyroid 252.1
    thyroid 245.2
  aviators' (*see also* Effect, adverse, high altitude) 993.2
  ax(e)-grinders' 502
  Ayala's 756.89
  Ayerza's (pulmonary artery sclerosis with pulmonary hypertension) 416.0
  Azorean (of the nervous system) 334.8
  Babington's (familial hemorrhagic telangiectasia) 448.0
  back bone NEC 733.90
  bacterial NEC 040.89
    zoonotic NEC 027.9
      specified type NEC 027.8
  Baehr-Schiffrin (thrombotic thrombocytopenic purpura) 446.6
  Baelz's (cheilitis glandularis apostematosa) 528.5
  Baerensprung's (eczema marginatum) 110.3
  Balfour's (chloroma) 205.3 ☑
  balloon (*see also* Effect, adverse, high altitude) 993.2
  Balò's 341.1
  Bamberger (-Marie) (hypertrophic pulmonary osteoarthropathy) 731.2
  Bang's (Brucella abortus) 023.1
  Bannister's 995.1
  Banti's (with cirrhosis) (with portal hypertension) — *see* Cirrhosis, liver

Disease, diseased — *see also* Syndrome — *continued*
  Barcoo (*see also* Ulcer, skin) 707.9
  barium lung 503
  Barlow (-Möller) (infantile scurvy) 267
  barometer makers' 985.0
  Barraquer (-Simons) (progressive lipodystrophy) 272.6
  basal ganglia 333.90
    degenerative NEC 333.0
    specified NEC 333.89
  Basedow's (exophthalmic goiter) 242.0 ☑
  basement membrane NEC 583.89
    with
      pulmonary hemorrhage (Goodpasture's syndrome) 446.21 [583.81]
  Bateman's 078.0
    purpura (senile) 287.2
  Batten-Mayou (retina) 330.1 [362.71]
  Batten-Steinert 359.21
  Batten's 330.1 [362.71]
  Battey 031.0
  Baumgarten-Cruveilhier (cirrhosis of liver) 571.5
  bauxite-workers' 503
  Bayle's (dementia paralytica) 094.1
  Bazin's (primary) (*see also* Tuberculosis) 017.1 ☑
  Beard's (neurasthenia) 300.5
  Beau's (*see also* Degeneration, myocardial) 429.1
  Bechterew's (ankylosing spondylitis) 720.0
  Becker's
    idiopathic mural endomyocardial disease 425.2
    myotonia congenita, recessive form 359.22
  Begbie's (exophthalmic goiter) 242.0 ☑
  Behr's 362.50
  Beigel's (white piedra) 111.2
  Bekhterev's (ankylosing spondylitis) 720.0
  Bell's (*see also* Psychosis, affective) 296.0 ☑
  Bennett's (leukemia) 208.9 ☑
  Benson's 379.22
  Bergeron's (hysteroepilepsy) 300.11
  Berlin's 921.3
  Bernard-Soulier (thrombopathy) 287.1
  Bernhardt (-Roth) 355.1
  beryllium 503
  Besnier-Boeck (-Schaumann) (sarcoidosis) 135
  Best's 362.76
  Beurmann's (sporotrichosis) 117.1
  Bielschowsky (-Jansky) 330.1
  Biermer's (pernicious anemia) 281.0
  Biett's (discoid lupus erythematosus) 695.4
  bile duct (*see also* Disease, biliary) 576.9
  biliary (duct) (tract) 576.9
    with calculus, choledocholithiasis, or stones — *see* Choledocholithiasis
  Billroth's (meningocele) (*see also* Spina bifida) 741.9 ☑
  Binswanger's 290.12
  Bird's (oxaluria) 271.8
  bird fanciers' 495.2
  black lung 500
  bladder 596.9
    specified NEC 596.89
  bleeder's 286.0
  Bloch-Sulzberger (incontinentia pigmenti) 757.33
  Blocq's (astasia-abasia) 307.9
  blood (-forming organs) 289.9
    specified NEC 289.89
    vessel 459.9
  Bloodgood's 610.1
  Blount's (tibia vara) 732.4
  blue 746.9
  Bodechtel-Guttmann (subacute sclerosing panencephalitis) 046.2
  Boeck's (sarcoidosis) 135
  bone 733.90
    fibrocystic NEC 733.29
      jaw 526.2
    marrow 289.9

☑ **Additional Digit Required** — Refer to the Tabular List for Digit Selection   ⏵ **Subterms under main terms may continue to next column or page**

2014 ICD-9-CM   ▶◀ Revised Text   ● New Line   ▲ Revised Code   Volume 2 — 81

Disease, diseased — *see also* Syndrome — *continued*
bone — *continued*
   Paget's (osteitis deformans) 731.0
   specified type NEC 733.99
   von Recklinghausen's (osteitis fibrosa cystica) 252.01
Bonfils' — *see* Disease, Hodgkin's
Borna 062.9
Bornholm (epidemic pleurodynia) 074.1
Bostock's (*see also* Fever, hay) 477.9
Bouchard's (myopathic dilatation of the stomach) 536.1
Bouillaud's (rheumatic heart disease) 391.9
Bourneville (-Brissaud) (tuberous sclerosis) 759.5
Bouveret (-Hoffmann) (paroxysmal tachycardia) 427.2
bowel 569.9
   functional 564.9
      psychogenic 306.4
Bowen's (M8081/2) — *see* Neoplasm, skin, in situ
Bozzolo's (multiple myeloma) (M9730/3) 203.0 ☑
Bradley's (epidemic vomiting) 078.82
Brailsford-Morquio (mucopolysaccharidosis IV) 277.5
Brailsford's 732.3
   radius, head 732.3
   tarsal, scaphoid 732.5
brain 348.9
   Alzheimer's 331.0
      with dementia — *see* Alzheimer's, dementia
   arterial, artery 437.9
   arteriosclerotic 437.0
   congenital 742.9
   degenerative — *see* Degeneration, brain
   inflammatory (*see also* Encephalitis)
      late effect — *see* category 326
   organic 348.9
      arteriosclerotic 437.0
   parasitic NEC 123.9
   Pick's 331.11
      with dementia
         with behavioral disturbance 331.11 *[294.11]*
         without behavioral disturbance 331.11 *[294.10]*
   senile 331.2
braziers' 985.8
breast 611.9
   cystic (chronic) 610.1
   fibrocystic 610.1
   inflammatory 611.0
   Paget's (M8540/3) 174.0
   puerperal, postpartum NEC 676.3 ☑
   specified NEC 611.89
Breda's (*see also* Yaws) 102.9
Breisky's (kraurosis vulvae) 624.09
Bretonneau's (diphtheritic malignant angina) 032.0
Bright's (*see also* Nephritis) 583.9
   arteriosclerotic (*see also* Hypertension, kidney) 403.90
Brill-Symmers (follicular lymphoma) (M9690/3) 202.0 ☑
Brill-Zinsser (recrudescent typhus) 081.1
Brill's (recrudescent typhus) 081.1
   flea-borne 081.0
   louse-borne 081.1
Brinton's (leather bottle stomach) (M8142/3) 151.9
Brion-Kayser (*see also* Fever, paratyphoid) 002.9
broad
   beta 272.2
   ligament, noninflammatory 620.9
      specified NEC 620.8
Brocq-Duhring (dermatitis herpetiformis) 694.0
Brocq's 691.8
   meaning
      atopic (diffuse) neurodermatitis 691.8

Disease, diseased — *see also* Syndrome — *continued*
Brocq's — *continued*
   meaning — *continued*
      dermatitis herpetiformis 694.0
      lichen simplex chronicus 698.3
      parapsoriasis 696.2
      prurigo 698.2
Brodie's (joint) (*see also* Osteomyelitis) 730.1 ☑
bronchi 519.19
bronchopulmonary 519.19
bronze (Addison's) 255.41
   tuberculous (*see also* Tuberculosis) 017.6 ☑
Brown-Séquard 344.89
Bruck-de Lange (Amsterdam dwarf, intellectual disabilities, and brachycephaly) 759.89
Bruck's 733.99
Bruhl's (splenic anemia with fever) 285.8
Bruton's (X-linked agammaglobulinemia) 279.04
buccal cavity 528.9
Buchanan's (juvenile osteochondrosis, iliac crest) 732.1
Buchman's (osteochondrosis juvenile) 732.1
Budgerigar-Fanciers' 495.2
Büdinger-Ludloff-Läwen 717.89
Buerger's (thromboangiitis obliterans) 443.1
Bürger-Grütz (essential familial hyperlipemia) 272.3
Burns' (lower ulna) 732.3
bursa 727.9
Bury's (erythema elevatum diutinum) 695.89
Buschke's 710.1
Busquet's (*see also* Osteomyelitis) 730.1 ☑
Busse-Buschke (cryptococcosis) 117.5
C₂ (*see also* Alcoholism) 303.9 ☑
Caffey's (infantile cortical hyperostosis) 756.59
caisson 993.3
calculus 592.9
California 114.0
Calvé (-Perthes) (osteochondrosis, femoral capital) 732.1
Camurati-Engelmann (diaphyseal sclerosis) 756.59
Canavan's 330.0
capillaries 448.9
Carapata 087.1
cardiac — *see* Disease, heart
cardiopulmonary, chronic 416.9
cardiorenal (arteriosclerotic) (hepatic) (hypertensive) (vascular) (*see also* Hypertension, cardiorenal) 404.90
cardiovascular (arteriosclerotic) 429.2
   congenital 746.9
   hypertensive (*see also* Hypertension, heart) 402.90
      benign 402.10
      malignant 402.00
   renal (*see also* Hypertension, cardiorenal) 404.90
   syphilitic (asymptomatic) 093.9
carotid gland 259.8
Carrión's (Bartonellosis) 088.0
cartilage NEC 733.90
   specified NEC 733.99
Castellani's 104.8
cat-scratch 078.3
Cavare's (familial periodic paralysis) 359.3
Cazenave's (pemphigus) 694.4
cecum 569.9
celiac (adult) 579.0
   infantile 579.0
cellular tissue NEC 709.9
central core 359.0
cerebellar, cerebellum — *see* Disease, brain
cerebral (*see also* Disease, brain) 348.9
   arterial, artery 437.9
   degenerative — *see* Degeneration, brain
cerebrospinal 349.9
cerebrovascular NEC 437.9
   acute 436
      embolic — *see* Embolism, brain

Disease, diseased — *see also* Syndrome — *continued*
cerebrovascular — *continued*
   acute — *continued*
      late effect — *see* Late effect(s) (of) cerebrovascular disease
      puerperal, postpartum, childbirth 674.0 ☑
      thrombotic — *see* Thrombosis, brain
   arteriosclerotic 437.0
   embolic — *see* Embolism, brain
   ischemic, generalized NEC 437.1
   late effect — *see* Late effect(s) (of) cerebrovascular disease
   occlusive 437.1
   puerperal, postpartum, childbirth 674.0 ☑
   specified type NEC 437.8
   thrombotic — *see* Thrombosis, brain
ceroid storage 272.7
cervix (uteri)
   inflammatory 616.0
   noninflammatory 622.9
      specified NEC 622.8
Chabert's 022.9
Chagas' (*see also* Trypanosomiasis, American) 086.2
Chandler's (osteochondritis dissecans, hip) 732.7
Charcôt-Marie-Tooth 356.1
Charcôt's (joint) 094.0 *[713.5]*
   spinal cord 094.0
Charlouis' (*see also* Yaws) 102.9
Cheadle (-Möller) (-Barlow) (infantile scurvy) 267
Chédiak-Steinbrinck (-Higashi) (congenital gigantism of peroxidase granules) 288.2
cheek, inner 528.9
chest 519.9
Chiari's (hepatic vein thrombosis) 453.0
Chicago (North American blastomycosis) 116.0
chignon (white piedra) 111.2
chigoe, chigo (jigger) 134.1
childhood granulomatous 288.1
Chinese liver fluke 121.1
chlamydial NEC 078.88
cholecystic (*see also* Disease, gallbladder) 575.9
choroid 363.9
   degenerative (*see also* Degeneration, choroid) 363.40
   hereditary (*see also* Dystrophy, choroid) 363.50
   specified type NEC 363.8
Christian-Weber (nodular nonsuppurative panniculitis) 729.30
Christian's (chronic histiocytosis X) 277.89
Christmas 286.1
ciliary body 364.9
   specified NEC 364.89
circulatory (system) NEC 459.9
   chronic, maternal, affecting fetus or newborn 760.3
   specified NEC 459.89
   syphilitic 093.9
      congenital 090.5
Civatte's (poikiloderma) 709.09
climacteric 627.2
   male 608.89
coagulation factor deficiency (congenital) (*see also* Defect, coagulation) 286.9
Coats' 362.12
coccidioidal pulmonary 114.5
   acute 114.0
   chronic 114.4
   primary 114.0
   residual 114.4
Cockayne's (microcephaly and dwarfism) 759.89
Cogan's 370.52
cold
   agglutinin 283.0
      or hemoglobinuria 283.0

Disease, diseased — *see also* Syndrome — *continued*
cold — *continued*
   agglutinin — *continued*
      or hemoglobinuria — *continued*
         paroxysmal (cold) (nocturnal) 283.2
   hemagglutinin (chronic) 283.0
collagen NEC 710.9
   nonvascular 710.9
   specified NEC 710.8
   vascular (allergic) (*see also* Angiitis, hypersensitivity) 446.20
colon 569.9
   functional 564.9
      congenital 751.3
   ischemic 557.0
combined system (of spinal cord) 266.2 *[336.2]*
   with anemia (pernicious) 281.0 *[336.2]*
compressed air 993.3
Concato's (pericardial polyserositis) 423.2
   peritoneal 568.82
   pleural — *see* Pleurisy
congenital NEC 799.89
conjunctiva 372.9
   chlamydial 077.98
      specified NEC 077.8
   specified type NEC 372.89
   viral 077.99
      specified NEC 077.8
connective tissue, diffuse (*see also* Disease, collagen) 710.9
Conor and Bruch's (boutonneuse fever) 082.1
Conradi (-Hünermann) 756.59
Cooley's (erythroblastic anemia) 282.44
Cooper's 610.1
Corbus' 607.1
cork-handlers' 495.3
cornea (*see also* Keratopathy) 371.9
coronary (*see also* Ischemia, heart) 414.9
   congenital 746.85
   ostial, syphilitic 093.20
      aortic 093.22
      mitral 093.21
      pulmonary 093.24
      tricuspid 093.23
Corrigan's — *see* Insufficiency, aortic
Cotugno's 724.3
Coxsackie (virus) NEC 074.8
cranial nerve NEC 352.9
Creutzfeldt-Jakob (CJD) 046.19
   with dementia
      with behavioral disturbance 046.19 *[294.11]*
      without behavioral disturbance 046.19 *[294.10]*
   familial 046.19
   iatrogenic 046.19
   specified NEC 046.19
   sporadic 046.19
   variant (vCJD) 046.11
      with dementia
         with behavioral disturbance 046.11 *[294.11]*
         without behavioral disturbance 046.11 *[294.10]*
Crigler-Najjar (congenital hyperbilirubinemia) 277.4
Crocq's (acrocyanosis) 443.89
Crohn's (intestine) (*see also* Enteritis, regional) 555.9
Crouzon's (craniofacial dysostosis) 756.0
Cruchet's (encephalitis lethargica) 049.8
Cruveilhier's 335.21
Cruz-Chagas (*see also* Trypanosomiasis, American) 086.2
crystal deposition (*see also* Arthritis, due to, crystals) 712.9 ☑
Csillag's (lichen sclerosus et atrophicus) 701.0
Curschmann's 359.21
Cushing's (pituitary basophilism) 255.0
cystic
   breast (chronic) 610.1

☑ **Additional Digit Required** — Refer to the Tabular List for Digit Selection   ▽ **Subterms under main terms may continue to next column or page**

82 — Volume 2   ▶◀ **Revised Text**   ● **New Line**   ▲ **Revised Code**   **2014 ICD-9-CM**

Disease, diseased — *see also* Syndrome — *continued*
  hair — *continued*
    specified type NEC 704.8
  Hallervorden-Spatz 333.0
  Hallopeau's (lichen sclerosus et atrophicus) 701.0
  Hamman's (spontaneous mediastinal emphysema) 518.1
  Hand-Schüller-Christian (chronic histiocytosis X) 277.89
  hand, foot, and mouth 074.3
  Hanot's — *see* Cirrhosis, biliary
  Hansen's (leprosy) 030.9
    benign form 030.1
    malignant form 030.0
  Harada's 363.22
  Harley's (intermittent hemoglobinuria) 283.2
  Hartnup (pellagra-cerebellar ataxia-renal aminoaciduria) 270.0
  Hart's (pellagra-cerebellar ataxia-renal aminoaciduria) 270.0
  Hashimoto's (struma lymphomatosa) 245.2
  Hb — *see* Disease, hemoglobin
  heart (organic) 429.9
    with
      acute pulmonary edema (*see also* Failure, ventricular, left) 428.1
      hypertensive 402.91
        with renal failure 404.93
        benign 402.11
          with renal failure 404.13
        malignant 402.01
          with renal failure 404.03
      kidney disease — *see* Hypertension, cardiorenal
      rheumatic fever (conditions classifiable to 390)
        active 391.9
          with chorea 392.0
        inactive or quiescent (with chorea) 398.90
    amyloid 277.39 *[425.7]*
    aortic (valve) (*see also* Endocarditis, aortic) 424.1
    arteriosclerotic or sclerotic (minimal) (senile) — *see* Arteriosclerosis, coronary
    artery, arterial — *see* Arteriosclerosis, coronary
    atherosclerotic — *see* Arteriosclerosis, coronary
    beer drinkers' 425.5
    beriberi 265.0 *[425.7]*
    black 416.0
    congenital NEC 746.9
      cyanotic 746.9
      maternal, affecting fetus or newborn 760.3
      specified type NEC 746.89
    congestive (*see also* Failure, heart) 428.0
    coronary 414.9
    cryptogenic 429.9
    due to
      amyloidosis 277.39 *[425.7]*
      beriberi 265.0 *[425.7]*
      cardiac glycogenosis 271.0 *[425.7]*
      Friedreich's ataxia 334.0 *[425.8]*
      gout 274.82
      mucopolysaccharidosis 277.5 *[425.7]*
      myotonia atrophica 359.21 *[425.8]*
      progressive muscular dystrophy 359.1 *[425.8]*
      sarcoidosis 135 *[425.8]*
    fetal 746.9
      inflammatory 746.89
    fibroid (*see also* Myocarditis) 429.0
    functional 427.9
      postoperative 997.1
      psychogenic 306.2
    glycogen storage 271.0 *[425.7]*
    gonococcal NEC 098.85
    gouty 274.82
    hypertensive (*see also* Hypertension, heart) 402.90

Disease, diseased — *see also* Syndrome — *continued*
  heart — *continued*
    hypertensive (*see also* Hypertension, heart) — *continued*
      benign 402.10
      malignant 402.00
    hyperthyroid (*see also* Hyperthyroidism) 242.9 ☑ *[425.7]*
    incompletely diagnosed — *see* Disease, heart
    ischemic (chronic) (*see also* Ischemia, heart) 414.9
      acute (*see also* Infarct, myocardium) 410.9 ☑
        without myocardial infarction 411.89
          with coronary (artery) occlusion 411.81
      asymptomatic 412
      diagnosed on ECG or other special investigation but currently presenting no symptoms 412
    kyphoscoliotic 416.1
    mitral (*see also* Endocarditis, mitral) 394.9
    muscular (*see also* Degeneration, myocardial) 429.1
    postpartum 674.8 ☑
    psychogenic (functional) 306.2
    pulmonary (chronic) 416.9
      acute 415.0
      specified NEC 416.8
    rheumatic (chronic) (inactive) (old) (quiescent) (with chorea) 398.90
      active or acute 391.9
        with chorea (active) (rheumatic) (Sydenham's) 392.0
        specified type NEC 391.8
      maternal, affecting fetus or newborn 760.3
    rheumatoid — *see* Arthritis, rheumatoid
    sclerotic — *see* Arteriosclerosis, coronary
    senile (*see also* Myocarditis) 429.0
    specified type NEC 429.89
    syphilitic 093.89
      aortic 093.1
        aneurysm 093.0
      asymptomatic 093.89
      congenital 090.5
    thyroid (gland) (*see also* Hyper-thyroidism) 242.9 ☑ *[425.7]*
    thyrotoxic (*see also* Thyrotoxicosis) 242.9 ☑ *[425.7]*
    tuberculous (*see also* Tuberculosis) 017.9 ☑ *[425.8]*
    valve, valvular (obstructive) (regurgitant) (*see also* Endocarditis)
      congenital NEC (*see also* Anomaly, heart, valve) 746.9
      pulmonary 746.00
        specified type NEC 746.89
    vascular — *see* Disease, cardiovascular
  heavy-chain (gamma G) 273.2
  Heberden's 715.04
  Hebra's
    dermatitis exfoliativa 695.89
    erythema multiforme exudativum 695.19
    pityriasis
      maculata et circinata 696.3
      rubra 695.89
        pilaris 696.4
    prurigo 698.2
  Heerfordt's (uveoparotitis) 135
  Heidenhain's 290.10
    with dementia 290.10
  Heilmeyer-Schöner (M9842/3) 207.1 ☑
  Heine-Medin (*see also* Poliomyelitis) 045.9 ☑
  Heller-Döhle (syphilitic aortitis) 093.1
  Heller's (*see also* Psychosis, childhood) 299.1 ☑
  hematopoietic organs 289.9
  hemoglobin (Hb) 282.7
    with thalassemia 282.49

Disease, diseased — *see also* Syndrome — *continued*
  hemoglobin — *continued*
    abnormal (mixed) NEC 282.7
      with thalassemia 282.49
    AS genotype 282.5
    Bart's 282.43
    C (Hb-C) 282.7
      with other abnormal hemoglobin NEC 282.7
      elliptocytosis 282.7
      Hb-S (without crisis) 282.63
        with
          crisis 282.64
            vaso-occlusive pain 282.64
      sickle-cell (without crisis) 282.63
        with
          crisis 282.64
            vaso-occlusive pain 282.64
      thalassemia 282.49
    constant spring 282.7
    D (Hb-D) 282.7
      with other abnormal hemoglobin NEC 282.7
      Hb-S (without crisis) 282.68
        with crisis 282.69
      sickle-cell (without crisis) 282.68
        with crisis 282.69
      thalassemia 282.49
    E (Hb-E) 282.7
      with other abnormal hemoglobin NEC 282.7
      Hb-S (without crisis) 282.68
        with crisis 282.69
      sickle-cell (without crisis) 282.68
        with crisis 282.69
      thalassemia 282.47
    elliptocytosis 282.7
    F (Hb-F) 282.7
    G (Hb-G) 282.7
    H (Hb-H) 282.43
    hereditary persistence, fetal (HPFH) ("Swiss variety") 282.7
    high fetal gene 282.7
    I thalassemia 282.49
    M 289.7
    S (*see also* Disease, sickle-cell, Hb-S)
      thalassemia (without crisis) 282.41
        with
          crisis 282.42
            vaso-occlusive pain 282.42
    spherocytosis 282.7
    unstable, hemolytic 282.7
    Zurich (Hb-Zurich) 282.7
  hemolytic (fetus) (newborn) 773.2
    autoimmune (cold type) (warm type) 283.0
    due to or with
      incompatibility
        ABO (blood group) 773.1
        blood (group) (Duffy) (Kell) (Kidd) (Lewis) (M) (S) NEC 773.2
        Rh (blood group) (factor) 773.0
        Rh negative mother 773.0
    unstable hemoglobin 282.7
  hemorrhagic 287.9
    newborn 776.0
  Henoch (-Schönlein) (purpura nervosa) 287.0
  hepatic — *see* Disease, liver
  hepatolenticular 275.1
  heredodegenerative NEC
    brain 331.89
    spinal cord 336.8
  Hers' (glycogenosis VI) 271.0
  Herter (-Gee) (-Heubner) (nontropical sprue) 579.0
  Herxheimer's (diffuse idiopathic cutaneous atrophy) 701.8
  Heubner-Herter (nontropical sprue) 579.0
  Heubner's 094.89
  high fetal gene or hemoglobin thalassemia (*see also* Thalassemia) 282.40
  Hildenbrand's (typhus) 081.9
  Hippel's (retinocerebral angiomatosis) 759.6
  hip (joint) NEC 719.95

Disease, diseased — *see also* Syndrome — *continued*
  hip — *continued*
    congenital 755.63
    suppurative 711.05
    tuberculous (*see also* Tuberculosis) 015.1 ☑ *[730.85]*
  Hirschfeld's (acute diabetes mellitus) (*see also* Diabetes) 250.0 ☑
    due to secondary diabetes 249.0 ☑
  Hirschsprung's (congenital megacolon) 751.3
  His (-Werner) (trench fever) 083.1
  HIV 042
  Hodgkin's (M9650/3) 201.9 ☑

> **Note** — Use the following fifth-digit subclassification with category 201:
>
> 0 unspecified site
>
> 1 lymph nodes of head, face, and neck
>
> 2 intrathoracic lymph nodes
>
> 3 intra-abdominal lymph nodes
>
> 4 lymph nodes of axilla and upper limb
>
> 5 lymph nodes of inguinal region and lower limb
>
> 6 intrapelvic lymph nodes
>
> 7 spleen
>
> 8 lymph nodes of multiple sites

    lymphocytic-histiocytic predominance (M9651/3) 201.4 ☑
    lymphocytic
      depletion (M9653/3) 201.7 ☑
        diffuse fibrosis (M9654/3) 201.7 ☑
        reticular type (M9655/3) 201.7 ☑
      predominance (M9651/3) 201.4 ☑
    mixed cellularity (M9652/3) 201.6 ☑
    nodular sclerosis (M9656/3) 201.5 ☑
      cellular phase (M9657/3) 201.5 ☑
  Hodgson's 441.9
    ruptured 441.5
  Hoffa (-Kastert) (liposynovitis prepatellaris) 272.8
  Holla (*see also* Spherocytosis) 282.0
  homozygous-Hb-S 282.61
  hoof and mouth 078.4
  hookworm (*see also* Ancylostomiasis) 126.9
  Horton's (temporal arteritis) 446.5
  host-versus-graft (immune or nonimmune cause) 279.50
  HPFH (hereditary persistence of fetal hemoglobin) ("Swiss variety") 282.7
  Huchard's disease (continued arterial hypertension) 401.9
  Huguier's (uterine fibroma) 218.9
  human immunodeficiency (virus) 042
  hunger 251.1
  Hunt's
    dyssynergia cerebellaris myoclonica 334.2
    herpetic geniculate ganglionitis 053.11
  Huntington's 333.4
  Huppert's (multiple myeloma) (M9730/3) 203.0 ☑
  Hurler's (mucopolysaccharidosis I) 277.5
  Hutchinson-Boeck (sarcoidosis) 135
  Hutchinson-Gilford (progeria) 259.8
  Hutchinson's, meaning
    angioma serpiginosum 709.1
    cheiropompholyx 705.81
    prurigo estivalis 692.72
  hyaline (diffuse) (generalized) 728.9
    membrane (lung) (newborn) 769
  hydatid (*see also* Echinococcus) 122.9
  Hyde's (prurigo nodularis) 698.3
  hyperkinetic (*see also* Hyperkinesia) 314.9
    heart 429.82
  hypertensive (*see also* Hypertension) 401.9
  hypophysis 253.9
    hyperfunction 253.1

☑ **Additional Digit Required** — Refer to the Tabular List for Digit Selection   ⁿᵉᶜ **Subterms under main terms may continue to next column or page**

Disease, diseased — *see also* Syndrome — *continued*

hypophysis — *continued*
  hypofunction 253.2
Iceland (epidemic neuromyasthenia) 049.8
I cell 272.7
ill-defined 799.89
immunologic NEC 279.9
immunoproliferative 203.8 ☑
inclusion 078.5
  salivary gland 078.5
infancy, early NEC 779.9
infective NEC 136.9
inguinal gland 289.9
internal semilunar cartilage, cystic 717.5
intervertebral disc 722.90
  with myelopathy 722.70
  cervical, cervicothoracic 722.91
    with myelopathy 722.71
  lumbar, lumbosacral 722.93
    with myelopathy 722.73
  thoracic, thoracolumbar 722.92
    with myelopathy 722.72
intestine 569.9
  functional 564.9
    congenital 751.3
    psychogenic 306.4
  lardaceous 277.39
  organic 569.9
  protozoal NEC 007.9
iris 364.9
  specified NEC 364.89
iron
  metabolism (*see also* Hemochromatosis) 275.09
  storage (*see also* Hemochromatosis) 275.03
Isambert's (*see also* Tuberculosis, larynx) 012.3 ☑
Iselin's (osteochondrosis, fifth metatarsal) 732.5
island (scrub typhus) 081.2
itai-itai 985.5
Jadassohn-Pellizari's (anetoderma) 701.3
Jadassohn's (maculopapular erythroderma) 696.2
Jakob-Creutzfeldt (CJD) 046.19
  with dementia
    with behavioral disturbance 046.19 [294.11]
    without behavioral disturbance 046.19 [294.10]
  familial 046.19
  iatrogenic 046.19
  specified NEC 046.19
  sporadic 046.19
  variant (vCJD) 046.11
    with dementia
      with behavioral disturbance 046.11 [294.11]
      without behavioral disturbance 046.11 [294.10]
Jaksch (-Luzet) (pseudoleukemia infantum) 285.8
Janet's 300.89
Jansky-Bielschowsky 330.1
jaw NEC 526.9
  fibrocystic 526.2
Jensen's 363.05
Jeune's (asphyxiating thoracic dystrophy) 756.4
jigger 134.1
Johnson-Stevens (erythema multiforme exudativum) 695.13
joint NEC 719.9 ☑
  ankle 719.97
  Charcôt 094.0 [713.5]
  degenerative (*see also* Osteoarthrosis) 715.9 ☑
    multiple 715.09
    spine (*see also* Spondylosis) 721.90
  elbow 719.92
  foot 719.97
  hand 719.94
  hip 719.95

Disease, diseased — *see also* Syndrome — *continued*

joint — *continued*
  hypertrophic (chronic) (degenerative) (*see also* Osteoarthrosis) 715.9 ☑
    spine (*see also* Spondylosis) 721.90
  knee 719.96
  Luschka 721.90
  multiple sites 719.99
  pelvic region 719.95
  sacroiliac 724.6
  shoulder (region) 719.91
  specified site NEC 719.98
  spine NEC 724.9
    pseudoarthrosis following fusion 733.82
    sacroiliac 724.6
  wrist 719.93
Jourdain's (acute gingivitis) 523.00
Jüngling's (sarcoidosis) 135
Kahler (-Bozzolo) (multiple myeloma) (M9730/3) 203.0 ☑
Kalischer's 759.6
Kaposi's 757.33
  lichen ruber 697.8
    acuminatus 696.4
    moniliformis 697.8
  xeroderma pigmentosum 757.33
Kaschin-Beck (endemic polyarthritis) 716.00
  ankle 716.07
  arm 716.02
    lower (and wrist) 716.03
    upper (and elbow) 716.02
  foot (and ankle) 716.07
  forearm (and wrist) 716.03
  hand 716.04
  leg 716.06
    lower 716.06
    upper 716.05
  multiple sites 716.09
  pelvic region (hip) (thigh) 716.05
  shoulder region 716.01
  specified site NEC 716.08
Katayama 120.2
Kawasaki 446.1
Kedani (scrub typhus) 081.2
kidney (functional) (pelvis) (*see also* Disease, renal) 593.9
  chronic 585.9
    requiring chronic dialysis 585.6
    stage
      I 585.1
      II (mild) 585.2
      III (moderate) 585.3
      IV (severe) 585.4
      V 585.5
  cystic (congenital) 753.10
    multiple 753.19
    single 753.11
    specified NEC 753.19
  fibrocystic (congenital) 753.19
  in gout 274.10
  polycystic (congenital) 753.12
    adult type (APKD) 753.13
    autosomal dominant 753.13
    autosomal recessive 753.14
    childhood type (CPKD) 753.14
    infantile type 753.14
Kienböck's (carpal lunate) (wrist) 732.3
Kimmelstiel (-Wilson) (intercapillary glomerulosclerosis) 250.4 ☑ [581.81]
  due to secondary diabetes 249.4 ☑ [581.81]
Kinnier Wilson's (hepatolenticular degeneration) 275.1
kissing 075
Kleb's (*see also* Nephritis) 583.9
Klinger's 446.4
Klippel-Feil (brevicollis) 756.16
Klippel's 723.8
knight's 911.1
Köbner's (epidermolysis bullosa) 757.39
Koenig-Wichmann (pemphigus) 694.4
Köhler-Freiberg (infraction, metatarsal head) 732.5

Disease, diseased — *see also* Syndrome — *continued*

Köhler-Mouchet (osteoarthrosis juvenilis) 732.5
Köhler-Pellegrini-Stieda (calcification, knee joint) 726.62
Köhler's
  first (osteoarthrosis juvenilis) 732.5
  second (Freiberg's infraction, metatarsal head) 732.5
  patellar 732.4
  tarsal navicular (bone) (osteoarthrosis juvenilis) 732.5
Kok 759.89
König's (osteochondritis dissecans) 732.7
Korsakoff's (nonalcoholic) 294.0
  alcoholic 291.1
Kostmann's (infantile genetic agranulocytosis) 288.01
Krabbe's 330.0
Kraepelin-Morel (*see also* Schizophrenia) 295.9 ☑
Kraft-Weber-Dimitri 759.6
Kufs' 330.1
Kugelberg-Welander 335.11
Kuhnt-Junius 362.52
Kümmell's (-Verneuil) (spondylitis) 721.7
Kundrat's (lymphosarcoma) 200.1 ☑
kuru 046.0
Kussmaul (-Meier) (polyarteritis nodosa) 446.0
Kyasanur Forest 065.2
Kyrle's (hyperkeratosis follicularis in cutem penetrans) 701.1
labia
  inflammatory 616.10
  noninflammatory 624.9
    specified NEC 624.8
labyrinth, ear 386.8
lacrimal system (apparatus) (passages) 375.9
  gland 375.00
  specified NEC 375.89
Lafora's 333.2
Lagleyze-von Hippel (retinocerebral angiomatosis) 759.6
Lancereaux-Mathieu (leptospiral jaundice) 100.0
Landry's 357.0
Lane's 569.89
lardaceous (any site) 277.39
Larrey-Weil (leptospiral jaundice) 100.0
Larsen (-Johansson) (juvenile osteopathia patellae) 732.4
larynx 478.70
Lasègue's (persecution mania) 297.9
Leber's 377.16
Lederer's (acquired infectious hemolytic anemia) 283.19
Legg-Calvé-Perthes (capital femoral osteochondrosis) 732.1
Legg-Calvé-Waldenström (femoral capital osteochondrosis) 732.1
Legg-Perthes (femoral capital osteochondosis) 732.1
Legg's (capital femoral osteochondrosis) 732.1
Legionnaires' 482.84
Leigh's 330.8
Leiner's (exfoliative dermatitis) 695.89
Leloir's (lupus erythematosus) 695.4
Lenegre's 426.0
lens (eye) 379.39
Leriche's (osteoporosis, posttraumatic) 733.7
Letterer-Siwe (acute histiocytosis X) (M9722/3) 202.5 ☑
Lev's (acquired complete heart block) 426.0
Lewandowski-Lutz (epidermodysplasia verruciformis) 078.19
Lewandowski's (*see also* Tuberculosis) 017.0 ☑
Lewy body 331.82
  with dementia
    with behavioral disturbance 331.82 [294.11]
    without behavioral disturbance 331.82 [294.10]

Disease, diseased — *see also* Syndrome — *continued*

Leyden's (periodic vomiting) 536.2
Libman-Sacks (verrucous endocarditis) 710.0 [424.91]
Lichtheim's (subacute combined sclerosis with pernicious anemia) 281.0 [336.2]
ligament 728.9
light chain 203.0 ☑
Lightwood's (renal tubular acidosis) 588.89
Lignac's (cystinosis) 270.0
Lindau-von Hippel (angiomatosis retinocerebellosa) 759.6
Lindau's (retinocerebral angiomatosis) 759.6
lipidosis 272.7
lipoid storage NEC 272.7
Lipschütz's 616.50
lip NEC 528.5
Little's — *see* Palsy, cerebral
liver 573.9
  alcoholic 571.3
    acute 571.1
    chronic 571.3
  chronic 571.9
    alcoholic 571.3
  cystic, congenital 751.62
  drug-induced 573.3
  due to
    chemicals 573.3
    fluorinated agents 573.3
    hypersensitivity drugs 573.3
    isoniazids 573.3
  end stage NEC 572.8
    due to hepatitis — *see* Hepatitis
  fibrocystic (congenital) 751.62
  glycogen storage 271.0
  organic 573.9
  polycystic (congenital) 751.62
Lobo's (keloid blastomycosis) 116.2
Lobstein's (brittle bones and blue sclera) 756.51
locomotor system 334.9
Lorain's (pituitary dwarfism) 253.3
Lou Gehrig's 335.20
Lucas-Championnière (fibrinous bronchitis) 466.0
Ludwig's (submaxillary cellulitis) 528.3
luetic — *see* Syphilis
lumbosacral region 724.6
lung NEC 518.89
  black 500
  congenital 748.60
  cystic 518.89
    congenital 748.4
  fibroid (chronic) (*see also* Fibrosis, lung) 515
  fluke 121.2
    oriental 121.2
  in
    amyloidosis 277.39 [517.8]
    polymyositis 710.4 [517.8]
    sarcoidosis 135 [517.8]
    Sjögren's syndrome 710.2 [517.8]
    syphilis 095.1
    systemic lupus erythematosus 710.0 [517.8]
    systemic sclerosis 710.1 [517.2]
  interstitial (chronic) 515
    acute 136.3
    respiratory bronchiolitis 516.34
  nonspecific, chronic 496
  obstructive (chronic) (COPD) 496
    with
      acute
        bronchitis 491.22
        exacerbation NEC 491.21
      alveolitis, allergic (*see also* Alveolitis, allergic) 495.9
      asthma (chronic) (obstructive) 493.2 ☑
  bronchiectasis 494.0
    with acute exacerbation 494.1
  bronchitis (chronic) 491.20
    with
      acute bronchitis 491.22

Disease, diseased — *see also* Syndrome — *continued*

lung — *continued*
  obstructive — *continued*
    with — *continued*
      bronchitis — *continued*
        with — *continued*
          exacerbation (acute) 491.21
        decompensated 491.21
          with exacerbation 491.21
      emphysema NEC 492.8
      diffuse (with fibrosis) 496
  of childhood, specific NEC 516.69
  polycystic 518.89
    asthma (chronic) (obstructive) 493.2 ☑
    congenital 748.4
  purulent (cavitary) 513.0
  restrictive 518.89
  rheumatoid 714.81
    diffuse interstitial 714.81
  specified NEC 518.89
Lutembacher's (atrial septal defect with mitral stenosis) 745.5
Lutz-Miescher (elastosis perforans serpiginosa) 701.1
Lutz-Splendore-de Almeida (Brazilian blastomycosis) 116.1
Lyell's (toxic epidermal necrolysis) 695.15
  due to drug
    correct substance properly administered 695.15
    overdose or wrong substance given or taken 977.9
      specific drug — *see* Table of Drugs and Chemicals
Lyme 088.81
lymphatic (gland) (system) 289.9
  channel (noninfective) 457.9
  vessel (noninfective) 457.9
    specified NEC 457.8
lymphoproliferative (chronic) (M9970/1) 238.79
  X linked 759.89
Machado-Joseph 334.8
Madelung's (lipomatosis) 272.8
Madura (actinomycotic) 039.9
  mycotic 117.4
Magitot's 526.4
Majocchi's (purpura annularis telangiectodes) 709.1
malarial (*see also* Malaria) 084.6
Malassez's (cystic) 608.89
Malibu 919.8
  infected 919.9
malignant (M8000/3) (*see also* Neoplasm, by site, malignant)
  previous, affecting management of pregnancy V23.89
Manson's 120.1
maple bark 495.6
maple syrup (urine) 270.3
Marburg (virus) 078.89
Marchiafava (-Bignami) 341.8
Marfan's 090.49
  congenital syphilis 090.49
  meaning Marfan's syndrome 759.82
Marie-Bamberger (hypertrophic pulmonary osteoarthropathy) (secondary) 731.2
  primary or idiopathic (acropachyderma) 757.39
  pulmonary (hypertrophic osteoarthropathy) 731.2
Marie-Strümpell (ankylosing spondylitis) 720.0
Marion's (bladder neck obstruction) 596.0
Marsh's (exophthalmic goiter) 242.0 ☑
Martin's 715.27
mast cell 757.33
  systemic (M9741/3) 202.6 ☑
mastoid (*see also* Mastoiditis) 383.9
  process 385.9
maternal, unrelated to pregnancy NEC, affecting fetus or newborn 760.9
Mathieu's (leptospiral jaundice) 100.0

Disease, diseased — *see also* Syndrome — *continued*

Mauclaire's 732.3
Mauriac's (erythema nodosum syphiliticum) 091.3
Maxcy's 081.0
McArdle (-Schmid-Pearson) (glycogenosis V) 271.0
mediastinum NEC 519.3
Medin's (*see also* Poliomyelitis) 045.9 ☑
Mediterranean 282.40
  with hemoglobinopathy 282.49
medullary center (idiopathic) (respiratory) 348.89
Meige's (chronic hereditary edema) 757.0
Meleda 757.39
Ménétrier's (hypertrophic gastritis) 535.2 ☑
Ménière's (active) 386.00
  cochlear 386.02
  cochleovestibular 386.01
  inactive 386.04
  in remission 386.04
  vestibular 386.03
meningeal — *see* Meningitis
mental (*see also* Psychosis) 298.9
Merzbacher-Pelizaeus 330.0
mesenchymal 710.9
mesenteric embolic 557.0
metabolic NEC 277.9
metal polishers' 502
metastatic — *see* Metastasis
Mibelli's 757.39
microdrepanocytic 282.41
microvascular — code to condition
microvillus
  atrophy 751.5
  inclusion (MVD) 751.5
Miescher's 709.3
Mikulicz's (dryness of mouth, absent or decreased lacrimation) 527.1
Milkman (-Looser) (osteomalacia with pseudofractures) 268.2
Miller's (osteomalacia) 268.2
Mills' 335.29
Milroy's (chronic hereditary edema) 757.0
Minamata 985.0
Minor's 336.1
Minot-von Willebrand-Jürgens (angiohemophilia) 286.4
Minot's (hemorrhagic disease, newborn) 776.0
Mitchell's (erythromelalgia) 443.82
mitral — *see* Endocarditis, mitral
Mljet (mal de Meleda) 757.39
Möbius', Moebius' 346.2 ☑
Moeller's 267
Möller (-Barlow) (infantile scurvy) 267
Mönckeberg's (*see also* Arteriosclerosis, extremities) 440.20
Mondor's (thrombophlebitis of breast) 451.89
Monge's 993.2
Morel-Kraepelin (*see also* Schizophrenia) 295.9 ☑
Morgagni-Adams-Stokes (syncope with heart block) 426.9
Morgagni's (syndrome) (hyperostosis frontalis interna) 733.3
Morquio (-Brailsford) (-Ullrich) (mucopolysaccharidosis IV) 277.5
Morton's (with metatarsalgia) 355.6
Morvan's 336.0
motor neuron (bulbar) (mixed type) 335.20
Mouchet's (juvenile osteochondrosis, foot) 732.5
mouth 528.9
Moyamoya 437.5
mu-chain 273.2
Mucha's (acute parapsoriasis varioliformis) 696.2
mucolipidosis (I) (II) (III) 272.7
Münchmeyer's (exostosis luxurians) 728.11
Murri's (intermittent hemoglobinuria) 283.2
muscle 359.9
  inflammatory 728.9
  ocular 378.9

Disease, diseased — *see also* Syndrome — *continued*

musculoskeletal system 729.90
mushroom workers' 495.5
Myà's (congenital dilation, colon) 751.3
mycotic 117.9
myeloproliferative (chronic) (M9960/1) 238.79
myocardium, myocardial (*see also* Degeneration, myocardial) 429.1
  hypertensive (*see also* Hypertension, heart 402.90
  primary (idiopathic) 425.4
myoneural 358.9
Naegeli's 287.1
nail 703.9
  specified type NEC 703.8
Nairobi sheep 066.1
nasal 478.19
  cavity NEC 478.19
  sinus (chronic) — *see* Sinusitis
navel (newborn) NEC 779.89
  delayed separation of umbilical cord 779.83
nemaline body 359.0
neoplastic, generalized (M8000/6) 199.0
nerve — *see* Disorder, nerve
nervous system (central) 349.9
  autonomic, peripheral (*see also* Neuropathy, peripheral, autonomic) 337.9
  congenital 742.9
  inflammatory — *see* Encephalitis
  parasympathetic (*see also* Neuropathy, peripheral, autonomic) 337.9
  peripheral NEC 355.9
  prion NEC 046.79
  specified NEC 349.89
  sympathetic (*see also* Neuropathy, peripheral, autonomic) 337.9
  vegetative (*see also* Neuropathy, peripheral, autonomic) 337.9
Nettleship's (urticaria pigmentosa) 757.33
Neumann's (pemphigus vegetans) 694.4
neurologic (central) NEC (*see also* Disease, nervous system) 349.9
  peripheral NEC 355.9
neuromuscular system NEC 358.9
Newcastle 077.8
Nicolas (-Durand) — Favre (climatic bubo) 099.1
Niemann-Pick (lipid histiocytosis) 272.7
nipple 611.9
  Paget's (M8540/3) 174.0
Nishimoto (-Takeuchi) 437.5
nonarthropod-borne NEC 078.89
  central nervous system NEC 049.9
  enterovirus NEC 078.89
nonautoimmune hemolytic NEC 283.10
Nonne-Milroy-Meige (chronic hereditary edema) 757.0
Norrie's (congenital progressive oculoacousticocerebral degeneration) 743.8
nose 478.19
nucleus pulposus — *see* Disease, intervertebral disc
nutritional 269.9
  maternal, affecting fetus or newborn 760.4
oasthouse, urine 270.2
obliterative vascular 447.1
Odelberg's (juvenile osteochondrosis) 732.1
Oguchi's (retina) 368.61
Ohara's (*see also* Tularemia) 021.9
Ollier's (chondrodysplasia) 756.4
Opitz's (congestive splenomegaly) 289.51
Oppenheim-Urbach (necrobiosis lipoidica diabeticorum) 250.8 ☑ [709.3]
  due to secondary diabetes 249.8 ☑ [709.3]
Oppenheim's 358.8
optic nerve NEC 377.49
orbit 376.9
  specified NEC 376.89
Oriental liver fluke 121.1
Oriental lung fluke 121.2
Ormond's 593.4

Disease, diseased — *see also* Syndrome — *continued*

Osgood-Schlatter 732.4
Osgood's tibia (tubercle) 732.4
Osler-Rendu (familial hemorrhagic telangiectasia) 448.0
Osler (-Vaquez) (polycythemia vera) (M9950/1) 238.4
osteofibrocystic 252.01
Otto's 715.35
outer ear 380.9
ovary (noninflammatory) NEC 620.9
  cystic 620.2
  polycystic 256.4
  specified NEC 620.8
Owren's (congenital) (*see also* Defect, coagulation) 286.3
Paas' 756.59
Paget's (osteitis deformans) 731.0
  with infiltrating duct carcinoma of the breast (M8541/3) — *see* Neoplasm, breast, malignant
  bone 731.0
    osteosarcoma in (M9184/3) — *see* Neoplasm, bone, malignant
  breast (M8540/3) 174.0
  extramammary (M8542/3) (*see also* Neoplasm, skin, malignant)
    anus 154.3
    skin 173.59
  malignant (M8540/3)
    breast 174.0
    specified site NEC (M8542/3) — *see* Neoplasm, skin, malignant
    unspecified site 174.0
  mammary (M8540/3) 174.0
  nipple (M8540/3) 174.0
palate (soft) 528.9
Paltauf-Sternberg 201.9 ☑
pancreas 577.9
  cystic 577.2
    congenital 751.7
  fibrocystic 277.00
Panner's 732.3
  capitellum humeri 732.3
  head of humerus 732.3
  tarsal navicular (bone) (osteochondrosis) 732.5
panvalvular — *see* Endocarditis, mitral
parametrium 629.9
parasitic NEC 136.9
  cerebral NEC 123.9
  intestinal NEC 129
  mouth 112.0
  skin NEC 134.9
  specified type — *see* Infestation
  tongue 112.0
parathyroid (gland) 252.9
  specified NEC 252.8
Parkinson's 332.0
parodontal 523.9
Parrot's (syphilitic osteochondritis) 090.0
Parry's (exophthalmic goiter) 242.0 ☑
Parson's (exophthalmic goiter) 242.0 ☑
Pavy's 593.6
Paxton's (white piedra) 111.2
Payr's (splenic flexure syndrome) 569.89
pearl-workers' (chronic osteomyelitis) (*see also* Osteomyelitis) 730.1 ☑
Pel-Ebstein — *see* Disease, Hodgkin's
Pelizaeus-Merzbacher 330.0
  with dementia
    with behavioral disturbance 330.0 [294.11]
    without behavioral disturbance 330.0 [294.10]
Pellegrini-Stieda (calcification, knee joint) 726.62
pelvis, pelvic
  female NEC 629.9
    specified NEC 629.89
  gonococcal (acute) 098.19
    chronic or duration of 2 months or over 098.39
  infection (*see also* Disease, pelvis, inflammatory) 614.9

☑ **Additional Digit Required** — Refer to the Tabular List for Digit Selection   ⓦ **Subterms under main terms may continue to next column or page**

86 — Volume 2   ▶◀ **Revised Text**   ● **New Line**   ▲ **Revised Code**   2014 ICD-9-CM

Disease, diseased — *see also* Syndrome — *continued*
pelvis, pelvic — *continued*
inflammatory (female) (PID) 614.9
with
abortion — *see* Abortion, by type, with sepsis
ectopic pregnancy (*see also* categories 633.0–633.9) 639.0
molar pregnancy (*see also* categories 630–632) 639.0
acute 614.3
chronic 614.4
complicating pregnancy 646.6 ☑
affecting fetus or newborn 760.8
following
abortion 639.0
ectopic or molar pregnancy 639.0
peritonitis (acute) 614.5
chronic NEC 614.7
puerperal, postpartum, childbirth 670.8 ☑
specified NEC 614.8
organ, female NEC 629.9
specified NEC 629.89
peritoneum, female NEC 629.9
specified NEC 629.89
penis 607.9
inflammatory 607.2
peptic NEC 536.9
acid 536.8
periapical tissues NEC 522.9
pericardium 423.9
specified type NEC 423.8
perineum
female
inflammatory 616.9
specified NEC 616.89
noninflammatory 624.9
specified NEC 624.8
male (inflammatory) 682.2
periodic (familial) (Reimann's) NEC 277.31
paralysis 359.3
periodontal NEC 523.9
specified NEC 523.8
periosteum 733.90
peripheral
arterial 443.9
autonomic nervous system (*see also* Neuropathy, autonomic) 337.9
nerve NEC (*see also* Neuropathy) 356.9
multiple — *see* Polyneuropathy
vascular 443.9
specified type NEC 443.89
peritoneum 568.9
pelvic, female 629.9
specified NEC 629.89
Perrin-Ferraton (snapping hip) 719.65
persistent mucosal (middle ear) (with posterior or superior marginal perforation of ear drum) 382.2
Perthes' (capital femoral osteochondrosis) 732.1
Petit's (*see also* Hernia, lumbar) 553.8
Peutz-Jeghers 759.6
Peyronie's 607.85
Pfeiffer's (infectious mononucleosis) 075
pharynx 478.20
Phocas' 610.1
photochromogenic (acid-fast bacilli) (pulmonary) 031.0
nonpulmonary 031.9
Pick's
brain 331.11
with dementia
with behavioral disturbance 331.11 [294.11]
without behavioral disturbance 331.11 [294.10]
cerebral atrophy 331.11
with dementia
with behavioral disturbance 331.11 [294.11]
without behavioral disturbance 331.11 [294.10]
lipid histiocytosis 272.7

Disease, diseased — *see also* Syndrome — *continued*
Pick's — *continued*
liver (pericardial pseudocirrhosis of liver) 423.2
pericardium (pericardial pseudocirrhosis of liver) 423.2
polyserositis (pericardial pseudocirrhosis of liver) 423.2
Pierson's (osteochondrosis) 732.1
pigeon fanciers' or breeders' 495.2
pineal gland 259.8
pink 985.0
Pinkus' (lichen nitidus) 697.1
pinworm 127.4
pituitary (gland) 253.9
hyperfunction 253.1
hypofunction 253.2
pituitary snuff-takers' 495.8
placenta
affecting fetus or newborn 762.2
complicating pregnancy or childbirth 656.7 ☑
pleura (cavity) (*see also* Pleurisy) 511.0
Plummer's (toxic nodular goiter) 242.3 ☑
pneumatic
drill 994.9
hammer 994.9
policeman's 729.2
Pollitzer's (hidradenitis suppurativa) 705.83
polycystic (congenital) 759.89
congenital 748.4
kidney or renal 753.12
adult type (APKD) 753.13
autosomal dominant 753.13
autosomal recessive 753.14
childhood type (CPKD) 753.14
infantile type 753.14
liver or hepatic 751.62
lung or pulmonary 518.89
ovary, ovaries 256.4
spleen 759.0
polyethylene 996.45
Pompe's (glycogenosis II) 271.0
Poncet's (tuberculous rheumatism) (*see also* Tuberculosis) 015.9 ☑
Posada-Wernicke 114.9
Potain's (pulmonary edema) 514
Pott's (*see also* Tuberculosis) 015.0 ☑ [730.88]
osteomyelitis 015.0 ☑ [730.88]
paraplegia 015.0 ☑ [730.88]
spinal curvature 015.0 ☑ [737.43]
spondylitis 015.0 ☑ [720.81]
Potter's 753.0
Poulet's 714.2
pregnancy NEC (*see also* Pregnancy) 646.9 ☑
Preiser's (osteoporosis) 733.09
Pringle's (tuberous sclerosis) 759.5
Profichet's 729.90
prostate 602.9
specified type NEC 602.8
protozoal NEC 136.8
intestine, intestinal NEC 007.9
pseudo-Hurler's (mucolipidosis III) 272.7
psychiatric (*see also* Psychosis) 298.9
psychotic (*see also* Psychosis) 298.9
Puente's (simple glandular cheilitis) 528.5
puerperal NEC (*see also* Puerperal) 674.9 ☑
pulmonary (*see also* Disease, lung)
amyloid 277.39 [517.8]
artery 417.9
circulation, circulatory 417.9
specified NEC 417.8
diffuse obstructive (chronic) 496
with
acute bronchitis 491.22
asthma (chronic) (obstructive) 493.2 ☑
exacerbation NEC (acute) 491.21
heart (chronic) 416.9
specified NEC 416.8
hypertensive (vascular) 416.0
cardiovascular 416.0
obstructive diffuse (chronic) 496

Disease, diseased — *see also* Syndrome — *continued*
pulmonary (*see also* Disease, lung) — *continued*
obstructive diffuse — *continued*
with
acute bronchitis 491.22
asthma (chronic) (obstructive) 493.2 ☑
bronchitis (chronic) 491.20
with
exacerbation (acute) 491.21
acute 491.22
exacerbation NEC (acute) 491.21
decompensated 491.21
with exacerbation 491.21
valve (*see also* Endocarditis, pulmonary) 424.3
pulp (dental) NEC 522.9
pulseless 446.7
Putnam's (subacute combined sclerosis with pernicious anemia) 281.0 [336.2]
Pyle (-Cohn) (craniometaphyseal dysplasia) 756.89
pyramidal tract 333.90
Quervain's
tendon sheath 727.04
thyroid (subacute granulomatous thyroiditis) 245.1
Quincke's — *see* Edema, angioneurotic
Quinquaud (acne decalvans) 704.09
rag sorters' 022.1
Raynaud's (paroxysmal digital cyanosis) 443.0
reactive airway — *see* Asthma
Recklinghausen-Applebaum (hemochromatosis) (*see also* Hemochromatosis) 275.03
Recklinghausen's (M9540/1) 237.71
bone (osteitis fibrosa cystica) 252.01
Reclus' (cystic) 610.1
rectum NEC 569.49
Refsum's (heredopathia atactica polyneuritiformis) 356.3
Reichmann's (gastrosuccorrhea) 536.8
Reimann's (periodic) 277.31
Reiter's 099.3
renal (functional) (pelvis) (*see also* Disease, kidney) 593.9
with
edema (*see also* Nephrosis) 581.9
exudative nephritis 583.89
lesion of interstitial nephritis 583.89
stated generalized cause — *see* Nephritis
acute 593.9
basement membrane NEC 583.89
with
pulmonary hemorrhage (Goodpasture's syndrome) 446.21 [583.81]
chronic (*see also* Disease, kidney, chronic) 585.9
complicating pregnancy or puerperium NEC 646.2 ☑
with hypertension — *see* Toxemia, of pregnancy
affecting fetus or newborn 760.1
cystic, congenital (*see also* Cystic, disease, kidney) 753.10
diabetic 250.4 ☑ [583.81]
due to secondary diabetes 249.4 ☑ [581.81]
due to
amyloidosis 277.39 [583.81]
diabetes mellitus 250.4 ☑ [583.81]
due to secondary diabetes 249.4 ☑ [581.81]
systemic lupus erythematosis 710.0 [583.81]
end-stage 585.6
exudative 583.89
fibrocystic (congenital) 753.19
gonococcal 098.19 [583.81]

Disease, diseased — *see also* Syndrome — *continued*
renal (*see also* Disease, kidney) — *continued*
gouty 274.10
hypertensive (*see also* Hypertension, kidney) 403.90
immune complex NEC 583.89
interstitial (diffuse) (focal) 583.89
lupus 710.0 [583.81]
maternal, affecting fetus or newborn 760.1
hypertensive 760.0
phosphate-losing (tubular) 588.0
polycystic (congenital) 753.12
adult type (APKD) 753.13
autosomal dominant 753.13
autosomal recessive 753.14
childhood type (CPKD) 753.14
infantile type 753.14
specified lesion or cause NEC (*see also* Glomerulonephritis) 583.89
subacute 581.9
syphilitic 095.4
tuberculous (*see also* Tuberculosis) 016.0 ☑ [583.81]
tubular (*see also* Nephrosis, tubular) 584.5
Rendu-Osler-Weber (familial hemorrhagic telangiectasia) 448.0
renovascular (arteriosclerotic) (*see also* Hypertension, kidney) 403.90
respiratory (tract) 519.9
acute or subacute (upper) NEC 465.9
due to fumes or vapors 506.3
multiple sites NEC 465.8
noninfectious 478.9
streptococcal 034.0
chronic 519.9
arising in the perinatal period 770.7
due to fumes or vapors 506.4
due to
aspiration of liquids or solids 508.9
external agents NEC 508.9
specified NEC 508.8
fumes or vapors 506.9
acute or subacute NEC 506.3
chronic 506.4
fetus or newborn NEC 770.9
obstructive 496
smoke inhalation 508.2
specified type NEC 519.8
upper (acute) (infectious) NEC 465.9
multiple sites NEC 465.8
noninfectious NEC 478.9
streptococcal 034.0
retina, retinal NEC 362.9
Batten's or Batten-Mayou 330.1 [362.71]
degeneration 362.89
vascular lesion 362.17
rheumatic (*see also* Arthritis) 716.8 ☑
heart — *see* Disease, heart, rheumatic
rheumatoid (heart) — *see* Arthritis, rheumatoid
rickettsial NEC 083.9
specified type NEC 083.8
Riedel's (ligneous thyroiditis) 245.3
Riga (-Fede) (cachectic aphthae) 529.0
Riggs' (compound periodontitis) 523.40
Ritter's 695.81
Rivalta's (cervicofacial actinomycosis) 039.3
Robles' (onchocerciasis) 125.3 [360.13]
Roger's (congenital interventricular septal defect) 745.4
Rokitansky's (*see also* Necrosis, liver) 570
Romberg's 349.89
Rosenthal's (factor XI deficiency) 286.2
Rossbach's (hyperchlorhydria) 536.8
psychogenic 306.4
Roth (-Bernhardt) 355.1
Runeberg's (progressive pernicious anemia) 281.0
Rust's (tuberculous spondylitis) (*see also* Tuberculosis) 015.0 ☑ [720.81]
Rustitskii's (multiple myeloma) (M9730/3) 203.0 ☑

Disease, diseased — *see also* Syndrome — *continued*

Ruysch's (Hirschsprung's disease) 751.3
Sachs (-Tay) 330.1
sacroiliac NEC 724.6
salivary gland or duct NEC 527.9
  inclusion 078.5
    streptococcal 034.0
  virus 078.5
Sander's (paranoia) 297.1
Sandhoff's 330.1
sandworm 126.9
Savill's (epidemic exfoliative dermatitis) 695.89
Schamberg's (progressive pigmentary dermatosis) 709.09
Schaumann's (sarcoidosis) 135
Schenck's (sporotrichosis) 117.1
Scheuermann's (osteochondrosis) 732.0
Schilder (-Flatau) 341.1
Schimmelbusch's 610.1
Schlatter-Osgood 732.4
Schlatter's tibia (tubercle) 732.4
Schmorl's 722.30
  cervical 722.39
  lumbosacral 722.32
  specified region NEC 722.39
  thoracic, thoracolumbar 722.31
Scholz's 330.0
Schönlein (-Henoch) (purpura rheumatica) 287.0
Schottmüller's (*see also* Fever, paratyphoid) 002.9
Schüller-Christian (chronic histiocytosis X) 277.89
Schultz's (agranulocytosis) 288.09
Schwalbe-Ziehen-Oppenheimer 333.6
Schwartz-Jampel 359.23
Schweninger-Buzzi (macular atrophy) 701.3
sclera 379.19
scrofulous (*see also* Tuberculosis) 017.2 ☑
scrotum 608.9
sebaceous glands NEC 706.9
Secretan's (posttraumatic edema) 782.3
semilunar cartilage, cystic 717.5
seminal vesicle 608.9
Senear-Usher (pemphigus erythematosus) 694.4
serum NEC 999.59
Sever's (osteochondrosis calcaneum) 732.5
sexually transmitted — *see* Disease, venereal
Sézary's (reticulosis) (M9701/3) 202.2 ☑
Shaver's (bauxite pneumoconiosis) 503
Sheehan's (postpartum pituitary necrosis) 253.2
shimamushi (scrub typhus) 081.2
shipyard 077.1
sickle cell 282.60
  with
    crisis 282.62
    Hb-S disease 282.61
    other abnormal hemoglobin (Hb-D) (Hb-E) (Hb-G) (Hb-J) (Hb-K) (Hb-O) (Hb-P) (high fetal gene) (without crisis) 282.68
      with crisis 282.69
  elliptocytosis 282.60
  Hb-C (without crisis) 282.63
    with
      crisis 282.64
      vaso-occlusive pain 282.64
  Hb-S 282.61
    with
      crisis 282.62
      Hb-C (without crisis) 282.63
        with
          crisis 282.64
          vaso-occlusive pain 282.64
      other abnormal hemoglobin (Hb-D) (Hb-E) (Hb-G) (Hb-J) (Hb-K) (Hb-O) (Hb-P) (high fetal gene) (without crisis) 282.68
        with crisis 282.69
  spherocytosis 282.60

Disease, diseased — *see also* Syndrome — *continued*

sickle cell — *continued*
  thalassemia (without crisis) 282.41
    with
      crisis 282.42
      vaso-occlusive pain 282.42
Siegal-Cattan-Mamou (periodic) 277.31
silo fillers' 506.9
Simian B 054.3
Simmonds' (pituitary cachexia) 253.2
Simons' (progressive lipodystrophy) 272.6
Sinding-Larsen (juvenile osteopathia patellae) 732.4
sinus (*see also* Sinusitis)
  brain 437.9
  specified NEC 478.19
Sirkari's 085.0
sixth (*see also* Exanthem subitum) 058.10
Sjögren (-Gougerot) 710.2
  with lung involvement 710.2 *[517.8]*
Skevas-Zerfus 989.5
skin NEC 709.9
  due to metabolic disorder 277.9
  specified type NEC 709.8
sleeping (*see also* Narcolepsy) 347.00
  meaning sleeping sickness (*see also* Trypanosomiasis) 086.5
small vessel 443.9
Smith-Strang (oasthouse urine) 270.2
Sneddon-Wilkinson (subcorneal pustular dermatosis) 694.1
South African creeping 133.8
Spencer's (epidemic vomiting) 078.82
Spielmeyer-Stock 330.1
Spielmeyer-Vogt 330.1
spine, spinal 733.90
  combined system (*see also* Degeneration, combined) 266.2 *[336.2]*
    with pernicious anemia 281.0 *[336.2]*
  cord NEC 336.9
    congenital 742.9
  demyelinating NEC 341.8
  joint (*see also* Disease, joint, spine) 724.9
  tuberculous 015.0 ☑ *[730.8]* ☑
spinocerebellar 334.9
  specified NEC 334.8
spleen (organic) (postinfectional) 289.50
  amyloid 277.39
  lardaceous 277.39
  polycystic 759.0
  specified NEC 289.59
sponge divers' 989.5
Stanton's (melioidosis) 025
Stargardt's 362.75
Startle 759.89
Steinert's 359.21
Sternberg's — *see* Disease, Hodgkin's
Stevens-Johnson (erythema multiforme exudativum) 695.13
Sticker's (erythema infectiosum) 057.0
Stieda's (calcification, knee joint) 726.62
Still's (juvenile rheumatoid arthritis) 714.30
  adult onset 714.2
Stiller's (asthenia) 780.79
Stokes-Adams (syncope with heart block) 426.9
Stokes' (exophthalmic goiter) 242.0 ☑
Stokvis (-Talma) (enterogenous cyanosis) 289.7
stomach NEC (organic) 537.9
  functional 536.9
    psychogenic 306.4
  lardaceous 277.39
stonemasons' 502
storage
  glycogen (*see also* Disease, glycogen storage) 271.0
  lipid 272.7
  mucopolysaccharide 277.5
striatopallidal system 333.90
  specified NEC 333.89
Strümpell-Marie (ankylosing spondylitis) 720.0

Disease, diseased — *see also* Syndrome — *continued*

Stuart-Prower (congenital factor X deficiency) (*see also* Defect, coagulation) 286.3
Stuart's (congenital factor X deficiency) (*see also* Defect, coagulation) 286.3
Sturge (-Weber) (-Dimitri) (encephalocutaneous angiomatosis) 759.6
Stuttgart 100.89
Sudeck's 733.7
supporting structures of teeth NEC 525.9
suprarenal (gland) (capsule) 255.9
  hyperfunction 255.3
  hypofunction 255.41
Sutton's 709.09
Sutton and Gull's — *see* Hypertension, kidney
sweat glands NEC 705.9
  specified type NEC 705.89
sweating 078.2
Sweeley-Klionsky 272.7
Swift (-Feer) 985.0
swimming pool (bacillus) 031.1
swineherd's 100.89
Sylvest's (epidemic pleurodynia) 074.1
Symmers (follicular lymphoma) (M9690/3) 202.0 ☑
sympathetic nervous system (*see also* Neuropathy, peripheral, autonomic) 337.9
synovium 727.9
syphilitic — *see* Syphilis
systemic tissue mast cell (M9741/3) 202.6 ☑
Taenzer's 757.4
Takayasu's (pulseless) 446.7
Talma's 728.85
Tangier (familial high-density lipoprotein deficiency) 272.5
Tarral-Besnier (pityriasis rubra pilaris) 696.4
Tay-Sachs 330.1
Taylor's 701.8
tear duct 375.69
teeth, tooth 525.9
  hard tissues 521.9
    specified NEC 521.89
  pulp NEC 522.9
tendon 727.9
  inflammatory NEC 727.9
terminal vessel 443.9
testis 608.9
Thaysen-Gee (nontropical sprue) 579.0
Thomsen's 359.22
Thomson's (congenital poikiloderma) 757.33
Thornwaldt's, Tornwaldt's (pharyngeal bursitis) 478.29
throat 478.20
  septic 034.0
thromboembolic (*see also* Embolism) 444.9
thymus (gland) 254.9
  specified NEC 254.8
thyroid (gland) NEC 246.9
  heart (*see also* Hyperthyroidism) 242.9 ☑ *[425.7]*
  lardaceous 277.39
  specified NEC 246.8
Tietze's 733.6
Tommaselli's
  correct substance properly administered 599.70
  overdose or wrong substance given or taken 961.4
tongue 529.9
tonsils, tonsillar (and adenoids) (chronic) 474.9
  specified NEC 474.8
tooth, teeth 525.9
  hard tissues 521.9
    specified NEC 521.89
  pulp NEC 522.9
Tornwaldt's (pharyngeal bursitis) 478.29
Tourette's 307.23
trachea 519.19
tricuspid — *see* Endocarditis, tricuspid
triglyceride-storage, type I, II, III 272.7

Disease, diseased — *see also* Syndrome — *continued*

triple vessel (coronary arteries) — *see* Arteriosclerosis, coronary
trisymptomatic, Gourgerot's 709.1
trophoblastic (*see also* Hydatidiform mole) 630
  previous, affecting management of pregnancy V23.1
tsutsugamushi (scrub typhus) 081.2
tube (fallopian), noninflammatory 620.9
  specified NEC 620.8
tuberculous NEC (*see also* Tuberculosis) 011.9 ☑
tubo-ovarian
  inflammatory (*see also* Salpingo-oophoritis) 614.2
  noninflammatory 620.9
  specified NEC 620.8
tubotympanic, chronic (with anterior perforation of ear drum) 382.1
tympanum 385.9
Uhl's 746.84
umbilicus (newborn) NEC 779.89
  delayed separation 779.83
Underwood's (sclerema neonatorum) 778.1
undiagnosed 799.9
Unna's (seborrheic dermatitis) 690.18
unstable hemoglobin hemolytic 282.7
Unverricht (-Lundborg) 345.1 ☑
Urbach-Oppenheim (necrobiosis lipoidica diabeticorum) 250.8 ☑ *[709.3]*
  due to secondary diabetes 249.8 ☑ *[709.3]*
Urbach-Wiethe (lipoid proteinosis) 272.8
ureter 593.9
urethra 599.9
  specified type NEC 599.84
urinary (tract) 599.9
  bladder 596.9
    specified NEC 596.89
  maternal, affecting fetus or newborn 760.1
Usher-Senear (pemphigus erythematosus) 694.4
uterus (organic) 621.9
  infective (*see also* Endometritis) 615.9
  inflammatory (*see also* Endometritis) 615.9
  noninflammatory 621.9
    specified type NEC 621.8
uveal tract
  anterior 364.9
  posterior 363.9
vagabonds' 132.1
vagina, vaginal
  inflammatory 616.10
  noninflammatory 623.9
    specified NEC 623.8
Valsuani's (progressive pernicious anemia, puerperal) 648.2 ☑
  complicating pregnancy or puerperium 648.2 ☑
valve, valvular — *see also* Endocarditis
  congenital NEC (*see also* Anomaly, heart, valve) 746.9
  pulmonary 746.00
    specified type NEC 746.89
van Bogaert-Nijssen (-Peiffer) 330.0
van Creveld-von Gierke (glycogenosis I) 271.0
van den Bergh's (enterogenous cyanosis) 289.7
van Neck's (juvenile osteochondrosis) 732.1
Vaquez (-Osler) (polycythemia vera) (M9950/1) 238.4
vascular 459.9
  arteriosclerotic — *see* Arteriosclerosis
  hypertensive — *see* Hypertension
  obliterative 447.1
    peripheral 443.9
  occlusive 459.9
  peripheral (occlusive) 443.9
    in (due to) (with) diabetes mellitus 250.7 ☑ *[443.81]*

Disease, diseased — *see also* Syndrome — *continued*

vascular — *continued*
  peripheral — *continued*
    in diabetes mellitus — *continued*
      in (due to) (with) secondary diabetes 249.7 ☑ [443.81]
      specified type NEC 443.89
vas deferens 608.9
vasomotor 443.9
vasospastic 443.9
vein 459.9
venereal 099.9
  chlamydial NEC 099.50
    anus 099.52
    bladder 099.53
    cervix 099.53
    epididymis 099.54
    genitourinary NEC 099.55
      lower 099.53
      specified NEC 099.54
    pelvic inflammatory disease 099.54
    perihepatic 099.56
    peritoneum 099.56
    pharynx 099.51
    rectum 099.52
    specified site NEC 099.59
    testis 099.54
    vagina 099.53
    vulva 099.53
  complicating pregnancy, childbirth, or puerperium 647.2 ☑
  fifth 099.1
  sixth 099.1
  specified nature or type NEC 099.8
    chlamydial — *see* Disease, venereal, chlamydial
Verneuil's (syphilitic bursitis) 095.7
Verse's (calcinosis intervertebralis) 275.49 [722.90]
vertebra, vertebral NEC 733.90
  disc — *see* Disease, Intervertebral disc
vibration NEC 994.9
Vidal's (lichen simplex chronicus) 698.3
Vincent's (trench mouth) 101
Virchow's 733.99
virus (filterable) NEC 078.89
  arbovirus NEC 066.9
  arthropod-borne NEC 066.9
  central nervous system NEC 049.9
    specified type NEC 049.8
  complicating pregnancy, childbirth, or puerperium 647.6 ☑
  contact (with) V01.79
    varicella V01.71
  exposure to V01.79
    varicella V01.71
  Marburg 078.89
  maternal
    with fetal damage affecting management of pregnancy 655.3 ☑
  nonarthropod-borne NEC 078.89
    central nervous system NEC 049.9
      specified NEC 049.8
  vaccination, prophylactic (against) V04.89
vitreous 379.29
vocal cords NEC 478.5
Vogt-Spielmeyer 330.1
Vogt's (Cecile) 333.71
Volhard-Fahr (malignant nephrosclerosis) 403.00
Volkmann's
  acquired 958.6
von Bechterew's (ankylosing spondylitis) 720.0
von Economo's (encephalitis lethargica) 049.8
von Eulenburg's (congenital paramyotonia) 359.29
von Gierke's (glycogenosis I) 271.0
von Graefe's 378.72
von Hippel-Lindau (angiomatosis retinocerebellosa) 759.6
von Hippel's (retinocerebral angiomatosis) 759.6

Disease, diseased — *see also* Syndrome — *continued*

von Jaksch's (pseudoleukemia infantum) 285.8
von Recklinghausen-Applebaum (hemochromatosis) (*see also* Hemochromatosis) 275.03
von Recklinghausen's (M9540/1) 237.71
  bone (osteitis fibrosa cystica) 252.01
von Willebrand (-Jürgens) (angiohemophilia) 286.4
von Zambusch's (lichen sclerosus et atrophicus) 701.0
Voorhoeve's (dyschondroplasia) 756.4
Vrolik's (osteogenesis imperfecta) 756.51
vulva
  inflammatory 616.10
  noninflammatory 624.9
    specified NEC 624.8
Wagner's (colloid milium) 709.3
Waldenström's (osteochondrosis capital femoral) 732.1
Wallgren's (obstruction of splenic vein with collateral circulation) 459.89
Wardrop's (with lymphangitis) 681.9
  finger 681.02
  toe 681.11
Wassilieff's (leptospiral jaundice) 100.0
wasting NEC 799.4
  due to malnutrition 261
  paralysis 335.21
Waterhouse-Friderichsen 036.3
waxy (any site) 277.39
Weber-Christian (nodular nonsuppurative panniculitis) 729.30
Wegner's (syphilitic osteochondritis) 090.0
Weil's (leptospiral jaundice) 100.0
  of lung 100.0
Weir Mitchell's (erythromelalgia) 443.82
Werdnig-Hoffmann 335.0
Werlhof's (*see also* Purpura, thrombocytopenic) 287.39
Wermer's 258.01
Werner-His (trench fever) 083.1
Werner-Schultz (agranulocytosis) 288.09
Werner's (progeria adultorum) 259.8
Wernicke-Posadas 114.9
Wernicke's (superior hemorrhagic polioencephalitis) 265.1
Whipple's (intestinal lipodystrophy) 040.2
whipworm 127.3
White's (congenital) (keratosis follicularis) 757.39
white
  blood cell 288.9
    specified NEC 288.8
  spot 701.0
Whitmore's (melioidosis) 025
Widal-Abrami (acquired hemolytic jaundice) 283.9
Wilkie's 557.1
Wilkinson-Sneddon (subcorneal pustular dermatosis) 694.1
Willis' (diabetes mellitus) (*see also* Diabetes) 250.0 ☑
  due to secondary diabetes 249.0 ☑
Wilson-Brocq (dermatitis exfoliativa) 695.89
Wilson's (hepatolenticular degeneration) 275.1
winter vomiting 078.82
Wise's 696.2
Wohlfart-Kugelberg-Welander 335.11
Woillez's (acute idiopathic pulmonary congestion) 518.52
Wolman's (primary familial xanthomatosis) 272.7
wool-sorters' 022.1
Zagari's (xerostomia) 527.7
Zahorsky's (exanthem subitum) 058.10
Ziehen-Oppenheim 333.6
zoonotic, bacterial NEC 027.9
  specified type NEC 027.8
Disfigurement (due to scar) 709.2
  head V48.6
  limb V49.4
  neck V48.7

Disfigurement — *continued*
  trunk V48.7
Disgerminoma — *see* Dysgerminoma
Disinsertion, retina 361.04
Disintegration, complete, of the body 799.89
  traumatic 869.1
Disk kidney 753.3
Dislocatable hip, congenital — *see also* Dislocation, hip, congenital 754.30
Dislocation (articulation) (closed) (displacement) (simple) (subluxation) 839.8

> Note — "Closed" includes simple, complete, partial, uncomplicated, and unspecified dislocation.
>
> "Open" includes dislocation specified as infected or compound and dislocation with foreign body.
>
> "Chronic," "habitual," "old," or "recurrent" dislocations should be coded as indicated under the entry "Dislocation, recurrent," and "pathological" as indicated under the entry "Dislocation, pathological."
>
> For late effect of dislocation see Late, effect, dislocation.

with fracture — *see* Fracture, by site
acromioclavicular (joint) (closed) 831.04
  open 831.14
anatomical site (closed)
  specified NEC 839.69
    open 839.79
  unspecified or ill-defined 839.8
    open 839.9
ankle (scaphoid bone) (closed) 837.0
  open 837.1
arm (closed) 839.8
  open 839.9
astragalus (closed) 837.0
  open 837.1
atlanto-axial (closed) 839.01
  open 839.11
atlas (closed) 839.01
  open 839.11
axis (closed) 839.02
  open 839.12
back (closed) 839.8
  open 839.9
Bell-Daly 723.8
breast bone (closed) 839.61
  open 839.71
capsule, joint — *see* Dislocation, by site
carpal (bone) — *see* Dislocation, wrist
carpometacarpal (joint) (closed) 833.04
  open 833.14
cartilage (joint) (*see also* Dislocation, by site)
  knee — *see* Tear, meniscus
cervical, cervicodorsal, or cervicothoracic (spine) (vertebra) — *see* Dislocation, vertebra, cervical
chiropractic (*see also* Lesion, nonallopathic) 739.9
chondrocostal — *see* Dislocation, costochondral
chronic — *see* Dislocation, recurrent
clavicle (closed) 831.04
  open 831.14
coccyx (closed) 839.41
  open 839.51
collar bone (closed) 831.04
  open 831.14
compound (open) NEC 839.9
congenital NEC 755.8
  hip (*see also* Dislocation, hip, congenital) 754.30
  lens 743.37
  rib 756.3
  sacroiliac 755.69
  spine NEC 756.19
  vertebra 756.19
coracoid (closed) 831.09
  open 831.19
costal cartilage (closed) 839.69
  open 839.79
costochondral (closed) 839.69

Dislocation — *continued*
costochondral — *continued*
  open 839.79
cricoarytenoid articulation (closed) 839.69
  open 839.79
cricothyroid (cartilage) articulation (closed) 839.69
  open 839.79
dorsal vertebrae (closed) 839.21
  open 839.31
ear ossicle 385.23
elbow (closed) 832.00
  anterior (closed) 832.01
    open 832.11
  congenital 754.89
  divergent (closed) 832.09
    open 832.19
  lateral (closed) 832.04
    open 832.14
  medial (closed) 832.03
    open 832.13
  open 832.10
  posterior (closed) 832.02
    open 832.12
  recurrent 718.32
  specified type NEC 832.09
    open 832.19
eye 360.81
  lateral 376.36
eyeball 360.81
  lateral 376.36
femur
  distal end (closed) 836.50
    anterior 836.52
      open 836.62
    lateral 836.54
      open 836.64
    medial 836.53
      open 836.63
    open 836.60
    posterior 836.51
      open 836.61
  proximal end (closed) 835.00
    anterior (pubic) 835.03
      open 835.13
    obturator 835.02
      open 835.12
    open 835.10
    posterior 835.01
      open 835.11
fibula
  distal end (closed) 837.0
    open 837.1
  proximal end (closed) 836.59
    open 836.69
finger(s) (phalanx) (thumb) (closed) 834.00
  interphalangeal (joint) 834.02
    open 834.12
  metacarpal (bone), distal end 834.01
    open 834.11
  metacarpophalangeal (joint) 834.01
    open 834.11
  open 834.10
  recurrent 718.34
foot (closed) 838.00
  open 838.10
  recurrent 718.37
forearm (closed) 839.8
  open 839.9
fracture — *see* Fracture, by site
glenoid (closed) 831.09
  open 831.19
habitual — *see* Dislocation, recurrent
hand (closed) 839.8
  open 839.9
hip (closed) 835.00
  anterior 835.03
    obturator 835.02
      open 835.12
    open 835.13
  congenital (unilateral) 754.30
    with subluxation of other hip 754.35
    bilateral 754.31
  developmental 718.75
  open 835.10
  posterior 835.01

☑ **Additional Digit Required — Refer to the Tabular List for Digit Selection**

△ **Subterms under main terms may continue to next column or page**

2014 ICD-9-CM

►◄ Revised Text   ● New Line   ▲ Revised Code

Volume 2 — 89

Disease, diseased — Dislocation

Dislocation — *continued*
hip — *continued*
posterior — *continued*
open 835.11
recurrent 718.35
humerus (closed) 831.00
distal end (*see also* Dislocation, elbow)
832.00
open 831.10
proximal end (closed) 831.00
anterior (subclavicular) (subcoracoid)
(subglenoid) (closed) 831.01
open 831.11
inferior (closed) 831.03
open 831.13
posterior (closed) 831.02
open 831.12
implant — *see* Complications, mechanical
incus 385.23
infracoracoid (closed) 831.01
open 831.11
innominate (pubic junction) (sacral junction)
(closed) 839.69
acetabulum (*see also* Dislocation, hip)
835.00
open 839.79
interphalangeal (joint)
finger or hand (closed) 834.02
open 834.12
foot or toe (closed) 838.06
open 838.16
jaw (cartilage) (meniscus) (closed) 830.0
open 830.1
recurrent 524.69
joint NEC (closed) 839.8
developmental 718.7 ☑
open 839.9
pathological — *see* Dislocation, pathological
recurrent — *see* Dislocation, recurrent
knee (closed) 836.50
anterior 836.51
open 836.61
congenital (with genu recurvatum)
754.41
habitual 718.36
lateral 836.54
open 836.64
medial 836.53
open 836.63
old 718.36
open 836.60
posterior 836.52
open 836.62
recurrent 718.36
rotatory 836.59
open 836.69
lacrimal gland 375.16
leg (closed) 839.8
open 839.9
lens (crystalline) (complete) (partial) 379.32
anterior 379.33
congenital 743.37
ocular implant 996.53
posterior 379.34
traumatic 921.3
ligament — *see* Dislocation, by site
lumbar (vertebrae) (closed) 839.20
open 839.30
lumbosacral (vertebrae) (closed) 839.20
congenital 756.19
open 839.30
mandible (closed) 830.0
open 830.1
maxilla (inferior) (closed) 830.0
open 830.1
meniscus (knee) (*see also* Tear, meniscus)
other sites — *see* Dislocation, by site
metacarpal (bone)
distal end (closed) 834.01
open 834.11
proximal end (closed) 833.05
open 833.15
metacarpophalangeal (joint) (closed) 834.01
open 834.11

Dislocation — *continued*
metatarsal (bone) (closed) 838.04
open 838.14
metatarsophalangeal (joint) (closed) 838.05
open 838.15
midcarpal (joint) (closed) 833.03
open 833.13
midtarsal (joint) (closed) 838.02
open 838.12
Monteggia's — *see* Dislocation, hip
multiple locations (except fingers only or
toes only) (closed) 839.8
open 839.9
navicular (bone) foot (closed) 837.0
open 837.1
neck (*see also* Dislocation, vertebra, cervical)
839.00
Nélaton's — *see* Dislocation, ankle
nontraumatic (joint) — *see* Dislocation,
pathological
nose (closed) 839.69
open 839.79
not recurrent, not current injury — *see* Dislocation, pathological
occiput from atlas (closed) 839.01
open 839.11
old — *see* Dislocation, recurrent
open (compound) NEC 839.9
ossicle, ear 385.23
paralytic (flaccid) (spastic) — *see* Dislocation, pathological
patella (closed) 836.3
congenital 755.64
open 836.4
pathological NEC 718.20
ankle 718.27
elbow 718.22
foot 718.27
hand 718.24
hip 718.25
knee 718.26
lumbosacral joint 724.6
multiple sites 718.29
pelvic region 718.25
sacroiliac 724.6
shoulder (region) 718.21
specified site NEC 718.28
spine 724.8
sacroiliac 724.6
wrist 718.23
pelvis (closed) 839.69
acetabulum (*see also* Dislocation, hip)
835.00
open 839.79
phalanx
foot or toe (closed) 838.09
open 838.19
hand or finger (*see also* Dislocation, finger) 834.00
postpoliomyelitic — *see* Dislocation,
pathological
prosthesis, internal — *see* Complications,
mechanical
radiocarpal (joint) (closed) 833.02
open 833.12
radioulnar (joint)
distal end (closed) 833.01
open 833.11
proximal end (*see also* Dislocation, elbow) 832.00
radius
distal end (closed) 833.00
open 833.10
proximal end (closed) 832.01
open 832.11
recurrent (*see also* Derangement, joint, recurrent) 718.3 ☑
elbow 718.32
hip 718.35
joint NEC 718.38
knee 718.36
lumbosacral (joint) 724.6
patella 718.36
sacroiliac 724.6
shoulder 718.31
temporomandibular 524.69

Dislocation — *continued*
rib (cartilage) (closed) 839.69
congenital 756.3
open 839.79
sacrococcygeal (closed) 839.42
open 839.52
sacroiliac (joint) (ligament) (closed) 839.42
congenital 755.69
open 839.52
recurrent 724.6
sacrum (closed) 839.42
open 839.52
scaphoid (bone)
ankle or foot (closed) 837.0
open 837.1
wrist (closed) (*see also* Dislocation, wrist)
833.00
open 833.10
scapula (closed) 831.09
open 831.19
semilunar cartilage, knee — *see* Tear,
meniscus
septal cartilage (nose) (closed) 839.69
open 839.79
septum (nasal) (old) 470
sesamoid bone — *see* Dislocation, by site
shoulder (blade) (ligament) (closed) 831.00
anterior (subclavicular) (subcoracoid)
(subglenoid) (closed) 831.01
open 831.11
chronic 718.31
inferior 831.03
open 831.13
open 831.10
posterior (closed) 831.02
open 831.12
recurrent 718.31
skull — *see* Injury, intracranial
Smith's — *see* Dislocation, foot
spine (articular process) (*see also* Dislocation, vertebra) (closed) 839.40
atlanto-axial (closed) 839.01
open 839.11
recurrent 723.8
cervical, cervicodorsal, cervicothoracic
(closed) (*see also* Dislocation,
vertebrae, cervical) 839.00
open 839.10
recurrent 723.8
coccyx 839.41
open 839.51
congenital 756.19
due to birth trauma 767.4
open 839.50
recurrent 724.9
sacroiliac 839.42
recurrent 724.6
sacrum (sacrococcygeal) (sacroiliac)
839.42
open 839.52
spontaneous — *see* Dislocation, pathological
sternoclavicular (joint) (closed) 839.61
open 839.71
sternum (closed) 839.61
open 839.71
subastragalar — *see* Dislocation, foot
subglenoid (closed) 831.01
open 831.11
symphysis
jaw (closed) 830.0
open 830.1
mandibular (closed) 830.0
open 830.1
pubis (closed) 839.69
open 839.79
tarsal (bone) (joint) 838.01
open 838.11
tarsometatarsal (joint) 838.03
open 838.13
temporomandibular (joint) (closed) 830.0
open 830.1
recurrent 524.69
thigh
distal end (*see also* Dislocation, femur,
distal end) 836.50

Dislocation — *continued*
thigh — *continued*
proximal end (*see also* Dislocation, hip)
835.00
thoracic (vertebrae) (closed) 839.21
open 839.31
thumb(s) (*see also* Dislocation, finger) 834.00
thyroid cartilage (closed) 839.69
open 839.79
tibia
distal end (closed) 837.0
open 837.1
proximal end (closed) 836.50
anterior 836.51
open 836.61
lateral 836.54
open 836.64
medial 836.53
open 836.63
posterior 836.52
open 836.62
rotatory 836.59
open 836.69
tibiofibular
distal (closed) 837.0
open 837.1
superior (closed) 836.59
open 836.69
toe(s) (closed) 838.09
open 838.19
trachea (closed) 839.69
open 839.79
ulna
distal end (closed) 833.09
open 833.19
proximal end — *see* Dislocation, elbow
vertebra (articular process) (body) (closed)
(traumatic) 839.40
cervical, cervicodorsal or cervicothoracic
(closed) 839.00
first (atlas) 839.01
open 839.11
second (axis) 839.02
open 839.12
third 839.03
open 839.13
fourth 839.04
open 839.14
fifth 839.05
open 839.15
sixth 839.06
open 839.16
seventh 839.07
open 839.17
congenital 756.19
multiple sites 839.08
open 839.18
open 839.10
congenital 756.19
dorsal 839.21
open 839.31
recurrent 724.9
lumbar, lumbosacral 839.20
open 839.30
non-traumatic — *see* Displacement, intervertebral disc
open NEC 839.50
recurrent 724.9
specified region NEC 839.49
open 839.59
thoracic 839.21
open 839.31
wrist (carpal bone) (scaphoid) (semilunar)
(closed) 833.00
carpometacarpal (joint) 833.04
open 833.14
metacarpal bone, proximal end 833.05
open 833.15
midcarpal (joint) 833.03
open 833.13
open 833.10
radiocarpal (joint) 833.02
open 833.12
radioulnar (joint) 833.01
open 833.11

☑ **Additional Digit Required — Refer to the Tabular List for Digit Selection**

▽ **Subterms under main terms may continue to next column or page**

Dislocation — continued
  wrist — continued
    recurrent 718.33
    specified site NEC 833.09
      open 833.19
  xiphoid cartilage (closed) 839.61
    open 839.71
Dislodgement
  artificial skin graft 996.55
  decellularized allodermis graft 996.55
Disobedience, hostile (covert) (overt) — see also Disturbance, conduct 312.0 ☑
Disorder — see also Disease
  academic underachievement, childhood and adolescence 313.83
  accommodation 367.51
    drug-induced 367.89
    toxic 367.89
  adjustment (see also Reaction, adjustment) 309.9
    with
      anxiety 309.24
      anxiety and depressed mood 309.28
      depressed mood 309.0
      disturbance of conduct 309.3
      disturbance of emotions and conduct 309.4
  adrenal (capsule) (cortex) (gland) 255.9
    specified type NEC 255.8
  adrenogenital 255.2
  affective (see also Psychosis, affective) 296.90
    atypical 296.81
  aggressive, unsocialized (see also Disturbance, conduct) 312.0 ☑
  alcohol, alcoholic (see also Alcohol) 291.9
    induced mood 291.89
  allergic — see Allergy
  amino acid (metabolic) (see also Disturbance, metabolism, amino acid) 270.9
    albinism 270.2
    alkaptonuria 270.2
    argininosuccinicaciduria 270.6
    beta-amino-isobutyricaciduria 277.2
    cystathioninuria 270.4
    cystinosis 270.0
    cystinuria 270.0
    glycinuria 270.0
    homocystinuria 270.4
    imidazole 270.5
    maple syrup (urine) disease 270.3
    neonatal, transitory 775.89
    oasthouse urine disease 270.2
    ochronosis 270.2
    phenylketonuria 270.1
    phenylpyruvic oligophrenia 270.1
    purine NEC 277.2
    pyrimidine NEC 277.2
    renal transport NEC 270.0
    specified type NEC 270.8
    transport NEC 270.0
      renal 270.0
    xanthinuria 277.2
  amnestic (see also Amnestic syndrome) 294.8
    alcohol-induced persisting 291.1
    drug-induced persisting 292.83
    in conditions classified elsewhere 294.0
  anaerobic glycolysis with anemia 282.3
  anxiety (see also Anxiety) 300.00
    due to or associated with physical condition 293.84
  arteriole 447.9
    specified type NEC 447.8
  artery 447.9
    specified type NEC 447.8
  articulation — see Disorder, joint
  Asperger's 299.8 ☑
  attachment of infancy or early childhood 313.89
  attention deficit 314.00
    with hyperactivity 314.01
    predominantly
      combined hyperactive/inattentive 314.01

Disorder — see also Disease — continued
  attention deficit — continued
    predominantly — continued
      hyperactive/impulsive 314.01
      inattentive 314.00
    residual type 314.8
  auditory processing disorder 388.45
    acquired 388.45
    developmental 315.32
  autistic 299.0 ☑
  autoimmune NEC 279.49
    hemolytic (cold type) (warm type) 283.0
    parathyroid 252.1
    thyroid 245.2
  avoidant, childhood or adolescence 313.21
  balance
    acid-base 276.9
      mixed (with hypercapnia) 276.4
    electrolyte 276.9
    fluid 276.9
  behavior NEC (see also Disturbance, conduct) 312.9
    disruptive 312.9
  bilirubin excretion 277.4
  bipolar (affective) (alternating) 296.80

> Note — Use the following fifth-digit subclassification with categories 296.0–296.6:
>
> 0   unspecifed
>
> 1   mild
>
> 2   moderate
>
> 3   severe, without mention of psychotic behavior
>
> 4   severe, specified as with psychotic behavior
>
> 5   in partial or unspecified remission
>
> 6   in full remission

    atypical 296.7
    currently
      depressed 296.5 ☑
      hypomanic 296.4 ☑
      manic 296.4 ☑
    mixed 296.6 ☑
    specified type NEC 296.89
    type I 296.7
      most recent episode (or current)
        depressed 296.5 ☑
        hypomanic 296.4 ☑
        manic 296.4 ☑
        mixed 296.6 ☑
        unspecified 296.7
      single manic episode 296.0 ☑
    type II (recurrent major depressive episodes with hypomania) 296.89
  bladder 596.9
    functional NEC 596.59
    specified NEC 596.89
  bleeding 286.9
  bone NEC 733.90
    specified NEC 733.99
  brachial plexus 353.0
  branched-chain amino-acid degradation 270.3
  breast 611.9
    puerperal, postpartum 676.3 ☑
    specified NEC 611.89
  Briquet's 300.81
  bursa 727.9
    shoulder region 726.10
  carbohydrate metabolism, congenital 271.9
  cardiac, functional 427.9
    postoperative 997.1
    psychogenic 306.2
  cardiovascular, psychogenic 306.2
  cartilage NEC 733.90
    articular 718.00
      ankle 718.07
      elbow 718.02
      foot 718.07
      hand 718.04
      hip 718.05
      knee 717.9

Disorder — see also Disease — continued
  cartilage — continued
    articular — continued
      multiple sites 718.09
      pelvic region 718.05
      shoulder region 718.01
      specified
        site NEC 718.08
        type NEC 733.99
      wrist 718.03
  catatonic — see Catatonia
  central auditory processing 315.32
    acquired 388.45
    developmental 315.32
  cervical region NEC 723.9
  cervical root (nerve) NEC 353.2
  character NEC (see also Disorder, personality) 301.9
  ciliary body 364.9
    specified NEC 364.89
  coagulation (factor) (see also Defect, coagulation) 286.9
    factor VIII (congenital) (functional) 286.0
    factor IX (congenital) (functional) 286.1
    neonatal, transitory 776.3
  coccyx 724.70
    specified NEC 724.79
  cognitive 294.9
  colon 569.9
    functional 564.9
      congenital 751.3
  communication 307.9
  conduct (see also Disturbance, conduct) 312.9
    adjustment reaction 309.3
    adolescent onset type 312.82
    childhood onset type 312.81
    compulsive 312.30
      specified type NEC 312.39
    hyperkinetic 314.2
    onset unspecified 312.89
    socialized (type) 312.20
      aggressive 312.23
      unaggressive 312.21
    specified NEC 312.89
  conduction, heart 426.9
    specified NEC 426.89
  conflict
    sexual orientation 302.0
  congenital
    glycosylation (CDG) 271.8
  convulsive (secondary) (see also Convulsions) 780.39
    due to injury at birth 767.0
    idiopathic 780.39
  coordination 781.3
  cornea NEC 371.89
    due to contact lens 371.82
  corticosteroid metabolism NEC 255.2
  cranial nerve — see Disorder, nerve, cranial
  cyclothymic 301.13
  degradation, branched-chain amino acid 270.3
  delusional 297.1
  dentition 520.6
  depersonalization 300.6
  depressive NEC 311
    atypical 296.82
    major (see also Psychosis, affective) 296.2 ☑
      recurrent episode 296.3 ☑
      single episode 296.2 ☑
  development, specific 315.9
    associated with hyperkinesia 314.1
    coordination 315.4
    language 315.31
      and speech due to hearing loss 315.34
    learning 315.2
      arithmetical 315.1
      reading 315.00
    mixed 315.5
    motor coordination 315.4
    specified type NEC 315.8
    speech 315.39

Disorder — see also Disease — continued
  development, specific — continued
    speech — continued
      and language due to hearing loss 315.34
  diaphragm 519.4
  digestive 536.9
    fetus or newborn 777.9
      specified NEC 777.8
    psychogenic 306.4
  disintegrative, childhood 299.1 ☑
  dissociative 300.15
    identity 300.14
    nocturnal 307.47
  drug-related 292.9
  dysmorphic body 300.7
  dysthymic 300.4
  ear 388.9
    degenerative NEC 388.00
    external 380.9
      specified 380.89
    pinna 380.30
    specified type NEC 388.8
    vascular NEC 388.00
  eating NEC 307.50
  electrolyte NEC 276.9
    with
      abortion — see Abortion, by type, with metabolic disorder
      ectopic pregnancy (see also categories 633.0–633.9) 639.4
      molar pregnancy (see also categories 630–632) 639.4
    acidosis 276.2
      metabolic 276.2
      respiratory 276.2
    alkalosis 276.3
      metabolic 276.3
      respiratory 276.3
    following
      abortion 639.4
      ectopic or molar pregnancy 639.4
    neonatal, transitory NEC 775.5
  emancipation as adjustment reaction 309.22
  emotional (see also Disorder, mental, nonpsychotic) V40.9
  endocrine 259.9
    specified type NEC 259.8
  esophagus 530.9
    functional 530.5
    psychogenic 306.4
  explosive
    intermittent 312.34
    isolated 312.35
  expressive language 315.31
  eye 379.90
    globe — see Disorder, globe
    ill-defined NEC 379.99
    limited duction NEC 378.63
    specified NEC 379.8
  eyelid 374.9
    degenerative 374.50
    sensory 374.44
    specified type NEC 374.89
    vascular 374.85
  factitious (with combined psychological and physical signs and symptoms) (with predominantly physical signs and symptoms) 300.19
    with predominantly psychological signs and symptoms 300.16
  factor, coagulation (see also Defect, coagulation) 286.9
    IX (congenital) (funcitonal) 286.1
    VIII (congenital) (functional) 286.0
  fascia 728.9
  fatty acid oxidation 277.85
  feeding — see Feeding
  female sexual arousal 302.72
  fluency 315.35
    adult onset 307.0
    childhood onset 315.35
    due to late effect of cerebrovascular accident 438.14
    in conditions classified elsewhere 784.52
  fluid NEC 276.9

☑ **Additional Digit Required** — Refer to the Tabular List for Digit Selection   ▽ **Subterms under main terms may continue to next column or page**

Disorder — *see also* Disease — *continued*
 gastric (functional) 536.9
  motility 536.8
  psychogenic 306.4
  secretion 536.8
 gastrointestinal (functional) NEC 536.9
  newborn (neonatal) 777.9
   specified NEC 777.8
  psychogenic 306.4
 gender (child) 302.6
  adult 302.85
 gender identity (childhood) 302.6
  adolescents 302.85
  adults (-life) 302.85
 genitourinary system, psychogenic 306.50
 globe 360.9
  degenerative 360.20
   specified NEC 360.29
  specified type NEC 360.89
 hearing (*see also* Deafness)
  conductive type (air) (*see also* Deafness, conductive) 389.00
  mixed conductive and sensorineural 389.20
   bilateral 389.22
   unilateral 389.21
  nerve
   bilateral 389.12
   unilateral 389.13
  perceptive (*see also* Deafness, perceptive) 389.10
  sensorineural type NEC (*see also* Deafness, sensorineural 389.10
 heart action 427.9
  postoperative 997.1
 hematological, transient neonatal 776.9
  specified type NEC 776.8
 hematopoietic organs 289.9
 hemorrhagic NEC 287.9
  due to intrinsic circulating anticoagulants, antibodies, or inhibitors 286.59
   with
    acquired hemophilia 286.52
    antiphospholipid antibody 286.53
  specified type NEC 287.8
 hemostasis (*see also* Defect, coagulation) 286.9
 homosexual conflict 302.0
 hypomanic (chronic) 301.11
 identity
  childhood and adolescence 313.82
   gender 302.6
 immune mechanism (immunity) 279.9
  single complement (C1-C9) 279.8
  specified type NEC 279.8
 impulse control (*see also* Disturbance, conduct, compulsive) 312.30
 infant sialic acid storage 271.8
 integument, fetus or newborn 778.9
  specified type NEC 778.8
 interactional psychotic (childhood) (*see also* Psychosis, childhood) 299.1 ☑
 intermittent explosive 312.34
 intervertebral disc 722.90
  cervical, cervicothoracic 722.91
  lumbar, lumbosacral 722.93
  thoracic, thoracolumbar 722.92
 intestinal 569.9
  functional NEC 564.9
   congenital 751.3
   postoperative 564.4
  psychogenic 306.4
 introverted, of childhood and adolescence 313.22
 involuntary emotional expression (IEED) 310.81
 iris 364.9
  specified NEC 364.89
 iron, metabolism 275.09
  specified type NEC 275.09
 isolated explosive 312.35
 joint NEC 719.90
  ankle 719.97
  elbow 719.92
  foot 719.97

Disorder — *see also* Disease — *continued*
 joint — *continued*
  hand 719.94
  hip 719.95
  knee 719.96
  multiple sites 719.99
  pelvic region 719.95
  psychogenic 306.0
  shoulder (region) 719.91
  specified site NEC 719.98
  temporomandibular 524.60
   sounds on opening or closing 524.64
   specified NEC 524.69
  wrist 719.93
 kidney 593.9
  functional 588.9
   specified NEC 588.89
 labyrinth, labyrinthine 386.9
  specified type NEC 386.8
 lactation 676.9 ☑
 language (developmental) (expressive) 315.31
  mixed receptive-expressive 315.32
 learning 315.9
 ligament 728.9
 ligamentous attachments, peripheral (*see also* Enthesopathy)
  spine 720.1
 limb NEC 729.90
  psychogenic 306.0
 lipid
  metabolism, congenital 272.9
  storage 272.7
 lipoprotein deficiency (familial) 272.5
 low back NEC 724.9
  psychogenic 306.0
 lumbosacral
  plexus 353.1
  root (nerve) NEC 353.4
 lymphoproliferative (chronic) NEC (M9970/1) 238.79
  post-transplant (PTLD) 238.77
 major depressive (*see also* Psychosis, affective) 296.2 ☑
  recurrent episode 296.3 ☑
  single episode 296.2 ☑
 male erectile 607.84
  nonorganic origin 302.72
 manic (*see also* Psychosis, affective) 296.0 ☑
  atypical 296.81
 mathematics 315.1
 meniscus NEC (*see also* Disorder, cartilage, articular) 718.0 ☑
 menopausal 627.9
  specified NEC 627.8
 menstrual 626.9
  psychogenic 306.52
  specified NEC 626.8
 mental (nonpsychotic) 300.9
  affecting management of pregnancy, childbirth, or puerperium 648.4 ☑
  drug-induced 292.9
   hallucinogen persisting perception 292.89
   specified type NEC 292.89
  due to or associated with
   alcoholism 291.9
   drug consumption NEC 292.9
    specified type NEC 292.89
   physical condition NEC 293.9
  induced by drug 292.9
   specified type NEC 292.89
  neurotic (*see also* Neurosis) 300.9
  of infancy, childhood or adolescence 313.9
  persistent
   other
    due to conditions classified elsewhere 294.8
   unspecified
    due to conditions classified elsewhere 294.9
  presenile 310.1
   psychotic NEC 290.10

Disorder — *see also* Disease — *continued*
 mental — *continued*
  previous, affecting management of pregnancy V23.89
  psychoneurotic (*see also* Neurosis) 300.9
  psychotic (*see also* Psychosis) 298.9
   brief 298.8
   senile 290.20
  specific, following organic brain damage 310.9
   cognitive or personality change of other type 310.1
   frontal lobe syndrome 310.0
   postconcussional syndrome 310.2
   specified type NEC 310.89
  transient
   in conditions classified elsewhere 293.9
 metabolism NEC 277.9
  with
   abortion — *see* Abortion, by type, with metabolic disorder
   ectopic pregnancy (*see also* categories 633.0–633.9) 639.4
   molar pregnancy (*see also* categories 630–632) 639.4
  alkaptonuria 270.2
  amino acid (*see also* Disorder, amino acid) 270.9
   specified type NEC 270.8
  ammonia 270.6
  arginine 270.6
  argininosuccinic acid 270.6
  basal 794.7
  bilirubin 277.4
  calcium 275.40
  carbohydrate 271.9
   specified type NEC 271.8
  cholesterol 272.9
  citrulline 270.6
  copper 275.1
  corticosteroid 255.2
  cystine storage 270.0
  cystinuria 270.0
  fat 272.9
  fatty acid oxidation 277.85
  following
   abortion 639.4
   ectopic or molar pregnancy 639.4
  fructosemia 271.2
  fructosuria 271.2
  fucosidosis 271.8
  galactose-1-phosphate uridyl transferase 271.1
  glutamine 270.7
  glycine 270.7
  glycogen storage NEC 271.0
   hepatorenal 271.0
  hemochromatosis (*see also* Hemochromatosis) 275.03
  in labor and delivery 669.0 ☑
  iron 275.09
  lactose 271.3
  lipid 272.9
   specified type NEC 272.8
   storage 272.7
  lipoprotein (*see also* Hyperlipemia deficiency (familial)) 272.5
  lysine 270.7
  magnesium 275.2
  mannosidosis 271.8
  mineral 275.9
   specified type NEC 275.8
  mitochondrial 277.87
  mucopolysaccharide 277.5
  nitrogen 270.9
  ornithine 270.6
  oxalosis 271.8
  pentosuria 271.8
  phenylketonuria 270.1
  phosphate 275.3
  phosphorous 275.3
  plasma protein 273.9
   specified type NEC 273.8
  porphyrin 277.1
  purine 277.2

Disorder — *see also* Disease — *continued*
 metabolism — *continued*
  pyrimidine 277.2
  serine 270.7
  sodium 276.9
  specified type NEC 277.89
  steroid 255.2
  threonine 270.7
  urea cycle 270.6
  xylose 271.8
 micturition NEC 788.69
  psychogenic 306.53
 misery and unhappiness, of childhood and adolescence 313.1
 mitochondrial metabolism 277.87
 mitral valve 424.0
 mood (*see also* Disorder, bipolar) 296.90
  alcohol-induced 291.89
  episodic 296.90
   specified NEC 296.99
  in conditions classified elsewhere 293.83
 motor tic 307.20
  chronic 307.22
  transient (childhood) 307.21
 movement NEC 333.90
  hysterical 300.11
  medication-induced 333.90
  periodic limb 327.51
  sleep related, unspecified 780.58
   other organic 327.59
  specified type NEC 333.99
  stereotypic 307.3
 mucopolysaccharide 277.5
 muscle 728.9
  psychogenic 306.0
  specified type NEC 728.3
 muscular attachments, peripheral (*see also* Enthesopathy)
  spine 720.1
 musculoskeletal system NEC 729.90
  psychogenic 306.0
 myeloproliferative (chronic) NEC (M9960/1) 238.79
 myoneural 358.9
  due to lead 358.2
  specified type NEC 358.8
  toxic 358.2
 myotonic 359.29
 neck region NEC 723.9
 nerve 349.9
  abducens NEC 378.54
  accessory 352.4
  acoustic 388.5
  auditory 388.5
  auriculotemporal 350.8
  axillary 353.0
  cerebral — *see* Disorder, nerve, cranial
  cranial 352.9
   first 352.0
   second 377.49
   third
    partial 378.51
    total 378.52
   fourth 378.53
   fifth 350.9
   sixth 378.54
   seventh NEC 351.9
   eighth 388.5
   ninth 352.2
   tenth 352.3
   eleventh 352.4
   twelfth 352.5
   multiple 352.6
  entrapment — *see* Neuropathy, entrapment
  facial 351.9
   specified NEC 351.8
  femoral 355.2
  glossopharyngeal NEC 352.2
  hypoglossal 352.5
  iliohypogastric 355.79
  ilioinguinal 355.79
  intercostal 353.8
  lateral
   cutaneous of thigh 355.1
   popliteal 355.3

☑ **Additional Digit Required — Refer to the Tabular List for Digit Selection**   ⩔ **Subterms under main terms may continue to next column or page**

92 — Volume 2   ▶◀ **Revised Text**   ● **New Line**   ▲ **Revised Code**   **2014 ICD-9-CM**

Disorder — *see also* Disease — *continued*

nerve — *continued*
　lower limb NEC 355.8
　medial, popliteal 355.4
　median NEC 354.1
　obturator 355.79
　oculomotor
　　partial 378.51
　　total 378.52
　olfactory 352.0
　optic 377.49
　　hypoplasia 377.43
　　ischemic 377.41
　　nutritional 377.33
　　toxic 377.34
　peroneal 355.3
　phrenic 354.8
　plantar 355.6
　pneumogastric 352.3
　posterior tibial 355.5
　radial 354.3
　recurrent laryngeal 352.3
　root 353.9
　　specified NEC 353.8
　saphenous 355.79
　sciatic NEC 355.0
　specified NEC 355.9
　　lower limb 355.79
　　upper limb 354.8
　spinal 355.9
　sympathetic NEC 337.9
　trigeminal 350.9
　　specified NEC 350.8
　trochlear 378.53
　ulnar 354.2
　upper limb NEC 354.9
　vagus 352.3
nervous system NEC 349.9
　autonomic (peripheral) (*see also* Neuropathy, peripheral, autonomic) 337.9
　cranial 352.9
　parasympathetic (*see also* Neuropathy, peripheral, autonomic) 337.9
　specified type NEC 349.89
　sympathetic (*see also* Neuropathy, peripheral, autonomic) 337.9
　vegetative (*see also* Neuropathy, peripheral, autonomic) 337.9
neurohypophysis NEC 253.6
neurological NEC 781.99
　peripheral NEC 355.9
neuromuscular NEC 358.9
　hereditary NEC 359.1
　specified NEC 358.8
　toxic 358.2
neurotic 300.9
　specified type NEC 300.89
neutrophil, polymorphonuclear (functional) 288.1
nightmare 307.47
night terror 307.46
obsessive-compulsive 300.3
oppositional defiant, childhood and adolescence 313.81
optic
　chiasm 377.54
　　associated with
　　　inflammatory disorders 377.54
　　　neoplasm NEC 377.52
　　　　pituitary 377.51
　　　pituitary disorders 377.51
　　　vascular disorders 377.53
　nerve 377.49
　radiations 377.63
　tracts 377.63
orbit 376.9
　specified NEC 376.89
orgasmic
　female 302.73
　male 302.74
overanxious, of childhood and adolescence 313.0
oxidation, fatty acid 277.85
pancreas, internal secretion (other than diabetes mellitus) 251.9
　specified type NEC 251.8

Disorder — *see also* Disease — *continued*

panic 300.01
　with agoraphobia 300.21
papillary muscle NEC 429.81
paranoid 297.9
　induced 297.3
　shared 297.3
parathyroid 252.9
　specified type NEC 252.8
paroxysmal, mixed 780.39
pentose phosphate pathway with anemia 282.2
periodic limb movement 327.51
peroxisomal 277.86
personality 301.9
　affective 301.10
　aggressive 301.3
　amoral 301.7
　anancastic, anankastic 301.4
　antisocial 301.7
　asocial 301.7
　asthenic 301.6
　avoidant 301.82
　borderline 301.83
　compulsive 301.4
　cyclothymic 301.13
　dependent-passive 301.6
　dyssocial 301.7
　emotional instability 301.59
　epileptoid 301.3
　explosive 301.3
　following organic brain damage 310.1
　histrionic 301.50
　hyperthymic 301.11
　hypomanic (chronic) 301.11
　hypothymic 301.12
　hysterical 301.50
　immature 301.89
　inadequate 301.6
　introverted 301.21
　labile 301.59
　moral deficiency 301.7
　narcissistic 301.81
　obsessional 301.4
　obsessive-compulsive 301.4
　overconscientious 301.4
　paranoid 301.0
　passive-aggressive 301.84
　passive (-dependent) 301.6
　pathological NEC 301.9
　pseudosocial 301.7
　psychopathic 301.9
　schizoid 301.20
　　introverted 301.21
　　schizotypal 301.22
　schizotypal 301.22
　seductive 301.59
　type A 301.4
　unstable 301.59
pervasive developmental 299.9 ☑
　childhood-onset 299.8 ☑
　specified NEC 299.8 ☑
phonological 315.39
pigmentation, choroid (congenital) 743.53
pinna 380.30
　specified type NEC 380.39
pituitary, thalamic 253.9
　anterior NEC 253.4
　iatrogenic 253.7
　postablative 253.7
　specified NEC 253.8
pityriasis-like NEC 696.8
platelets (blood) 287.1
polymorphonuclear neutrophils (functional) 288.1
porphyrin metabolism 277.1
post-transplant lymphoproliferative (PTLD) 238.77
post-traumatic stress (PTSD) 309.81
postmenopausal 627.9
　specified type NEC 627.8
posttraumatic stress 309.81
　acute 309.81
　brief 309.81
　chronic 309.81
premenstrual dysphoric (PMDD) 625.4

Disorder — *see also* Disease — *continued*

psoriatic-like NEC 696.8
psychic, with diseases classified elsewhere 316
psychogenic NEC (*see also* condition) 300.9
　allergic NEC
　　respiratory 306.1
　anxiety 300.00
　　atypical 300.00
　　generalized 300.02
　appetite 307.59
　articulation, joint 306.0
　asthenic 300.5
　blood 306.8
　cardiovascular (system) 306.2
　compulsive 300.3
　cutaneous 306.3
　depressive 306.3
　digestive (system) 306.4
　dysmenorrheic 306.52
　dyspneic 306.1
　eczematous 306.3
　endocrine (system) 306.6
　eye 306.7
　feeding 307.59
　functional NEC 306.9
　gastric 306.4
　gastrointestinal (system) 306.4
　genitourinary (system) 306.50
　heart (function) (rhythm) 306.2
　hemic 306.8
　hyperventilatory 306.1
　hypochondriacal 300.7
　hysterical 300.10
　intestinal 306.4
　joint 306.0
　learning 315.2
　limb 306.0
　lymphatic (system) 306.8
　menstrual 306.52
　micturition 306.53
　monoplegic NEC 306.0
　motor 307.9
　muscle 306.0
　musculoskeletal 306.0
　neurocirculatory 306.2
　obsessive 300.3
　occupational 300.89
　organ or part of body NEC 306.9
　organs of special sense 306.7
　paralytic NEC 306.0
　phobic 300.20
　physical NEC 306.9
　pruritic 306.3
　rectal 306.4
　respiratory (system) 306.1
　rheumatic 306.0
　sexual (function) 302.70
　　specified type NEC 302.79
　sexual orientation conflict 302.0
　skin (allergic) (eczematous) (pruritic) 306.3
　sleep 307.40
　　initiation or maintenance 307.41
　　　persistent 307.42
　　　transient 307.41
　　movement 780.58
　　sleep terror 307.46
　　specified type NEC 307.49
　specified part of body NEC 306.8
　stomach 306.4
psychomotor NEC 307.9
　hysterical 300.11
psychoneurotic (*see also* Neurosis) 300.9
　mixed NEC 300.89
psychophysiologic (*see also* Disorder, psychosomatic) 306.9
psychosexual identity (childhood) 302.6
　adult-life 302.85
psychosomatic NEC 306.9
　allergic NEC
　　respiratory 306.1
　articulation, joint 306.0
　cardiovascular (system) 306.2
　cutaneous 306.3
　digestive (system) 306.4

Disorder — *see also* Disease — *continued*

psychosomatic — *continued*
　dysmenorrheic 306.52
　dyspneic 306.1
　endocrine (system) 306.6
　eye 306.7
　gastric 306.4
　gastrointestinal (system) 306.4
　genitourinary (system) 306.50
　heart (functional) (rhythm) 306.2
　hyperventilatory 306.1
　intestinal 306.4
　joint 306.0
　limb 306.0
　lymphatic (system) 306.8
　menstrual 306.52
　micturition 306.53
　monoplegic NEC 306.0
　muscle 306.0
　musculoskeletal 306.0
　neurocirculatory 306.2
　organs of special sense 306.7
　paralytic NEC 306.0
　pruritic 306.3
　rectal 306.4
　respiratory (system) 306.1
　rheumatic 306.0
　sexual (function) 302.70
　skin 306.3
　specified part of body NEC 306.8
　specified type NEC 302.79
　stomach 306.4
psychotic (*see also* Psychosis) 298.9
　brief 298.8
purine metabolism NEC 277.2
pyrimidine metabolism NEC 277.2
reactive attachment of infancy or early childhood 313.89
reading, developmental 315.00
reflex 796.1
REM sleep behavior 327.42
renal function, impaired 588.9
　specified type NEC 588.89
renal transport NEC 588.89
respiration, respiratory NEC 519.9
　due to
　　aspiration of liquids or solids 508.9
　　inhalation of fumes or vapors 506.9
　　smoke inhalation 508.2
　psychogenic 306.1
retina 362.9
　specified type NEC 362.89
rumination 307.53
sacroiliac joint NEC 724.6
sacrum 724.6
schizo-affective (*see also* Schizophrenia) 295.7 ☑
schizoid, childhood or adolescence 313.22
schizophreniform 295.4 ☑
schizotypal personality 301.22
secretion, thyrocalcitonin 246.0
seizure 345.9 ☑
　recurrent 345.9 ☑
　　epileptic — *see* Epilepsy
semantic pragmatic 315.39
　with autism 299.0 ☑
sense of smell 781.1
　psychogenic 306.7
separation anxiety 309.21
sexual (*see also* Deviation, sexual) 302.9
　aversion 302.79
　desire, hypoactive 302.71
　function, psychogenic 302.70
shyness, of childhood and adolescence 313.21
single complement (C1-C9) 279.8
skin NEC 709.9
　fetus or newborn 778.9
　　specified type 778.8
　psychogenic (allergic) (eczematous) (pruritic) 306.3
　specified type NEC 709.8
　vascular 709.1
sleep 780.50
　with apnea — *see* Apnea, sleep
　alcohol induced 291.82

☑ **Additional Digit Required — Refer to the Tabular List for Digit Selection**　　　　　　　▽ **Subterms under main terms may continue to next column or page**

2014 ICD-9-CM　　　　▶◀ Revised Text　　　　● New Line　　　　▲ Revised Code　　　　**Volume 2 — 93**

Disorder — Disorder

Disorder — *see also* Disease — *continued*

sleep — *continued*

arousal 307.46

confusional 327.41

circadian rhythm 327.30

advanced sleep phase type 327.32

alcohol induced 291.82

delayed sleep phase type 327.31

drug induced 292.85

free running type 327.34

in conditions classified elsewhere 327.37

irregular sleep-wake type 327.33

jet lag type 327.35

other 327.39

shift work type 327.36

drug induced 292.85

initiation or maintenance (*see also* Insomnia) 780.52

nonorganic origin (transient) 307.41

persistent 307.42

nonorganic origin 307.40

specified type NEC 307.49

organic specified type NEC 327.8

periodic limb movement 327.51

specified NEC 780.59

wake

cycle — *see* Disorder, sleep, circadian rhythm

schedule — *see* Disorer, sleep, circadian rhythm

social, of childhood and adolescence 313.22

soft tissue 729.90

specified type NEC 729.99

somatization 300.81

somatoform (atypical) (undifferentiated) 300.82

severe 300.81

specified type NEC 300.89

speech NEC 784.59

nonorganic origin 307.9

spine NEC 724.9

ligamentous or muscular attachments, peripheral 720.1

steroid metabolism NEC 255.2

stomach (functional) (*see also* Disorder, gastric) 536.9

psychogenic 306.4

storage, iron 275.09

stress (*see also* Reaction, stress, acute) 308.3

posttraumatic

acute 309.81

brief 309.81

chronic 309.81

substitution 300.11

suspected — *see* Observation

synovium 727.9

temperature regulation, fetus or newborn 778.4

temporomandibular joint NEC 524.60

sounds on opening or closing 524.64

specified NEC 524.69

tendon 727.9

shoulder region 726.10

thoracic root (nerve) NEC 353.3

thyrocalcitonin secretion 246.0

thyroid (gland) NEC 246.9

specified type NEC 246.8

tic 307.20

chronic (motor or vocal) 307.22

motor-verbal 307.23

organic origin 333.1

transient (of childhood) 307.21

tooth NEC 525.9

development NEC 520.9

specified type NEC 520.8

eruption 520.6

specified type NEC 525.8

Tourette's 307.23

transport, carbohydrate 271.9

specified type NEC 271.8

tubular, phosphate-losing 588.0

tympanic membrane 384.9

unaggressive, unsocialized (*see also* Disturbance, conduct) 312.1 ☑

Disorder — *see also* Disease — *continued*

undersocialized, unsocialized (*see also* Disturbance, conduct)

aggressive (type) 312.0 ☑

unaggressive (type) 312.1 ☑

vision, visual NEC 368.9

binocular NEC 368.30

cortex 377.73

associated with

inflammatory disorders 377.73

neoplasms 377.71

vascular disorders 377.72

pathway NEC 377.63

associated with

inflammatory disorders 377.63

neoplasms 377.61

vascular disorders 377.62

vocal tic

chronic 307.22

wakefulness (*see also* Hypersomnia) 780.54

nonorganic origin (transient) 307.43

persistent 307.44

written expression 315.2

Disorganized globe 360.29

Displacement, displaced

> Note — For acquired displacement of bones, cartilage, joints, tendons, due to injury, see also Dislocation.
>
> Displacements at ages under one year should be considered congenital, provided there is no indication the condition was acquired after birth.

acquired traumatic of bone, cartilage, joint, tendon NEC (without fracture) (*see also* Dislocation) 839.8

with fracture — *see* Fracture, by site

adrenal gland (congenital) 759.1

alveolus and teeth, vertical 524.75

appendix, retrocecal (congenital) 751.5

auricle (congenital) 744.29

bladder (acquired) 596.89

congenital 753.8

brachial plexus (congenital) 742.8

brain stem, caudal 742.4

canaliculus lacrimalis 743.65

cardia, through esophageal hiatus 750.6

cerebellum, caudal 742.4

cervix — *see* Displacement, uterus

colon (congenital) 751.4

device, implant, or graft — *see* Complications, mechanical

epithelium

columnar of cervix 622.10

cuboidal, beyond limits of external os (uterus) 752.49

esophageal mucosa into cardia of stomach, congenital 750.4

esophagus (acquired) 530.89

congenital 750.4

eyeball (acquired) (old) 376.36

congenital 743.8

current injury 871.3

lateral 376.36

fallopian tube (acquired) 620.4

congenital 752.19

opening (congenital) 752.19

gallbladder (congenital) 751.69

gastric mucosa 750.7

into

duodenum 750.7

esophagus 750.7

Meckel's diverticulum, congenital 750.7

globe (acquired) (lateral) (old) 376.36

current injury 871.3

graft

artificial skin graft 996.55

decellularized allodermis graft 996.55

heart (congenital) 746.87

acquired 429.89

hymen (congenital) (upward) 752.49

internal prosthesis NEC — *see* Complications, mechanical

intervertebral disc (with neuritis, radiculitis, sciatica, or other pain) 722.2

Displacement, displaced — *continued*

intervertebral disc — *continued*

with myelopathy 722.70

cervical, cervicodorsal, cervicothoracic 722.0

with myelopathy 722.71

due to major trauma — *see* Dislocation, vertebra, cervical

due to trauma — *see* Dislocation, vertebra

lumbar, lumbosacral 722.10

with myelopathy 722.73

due to major trauma — *see* Dislocation, vertebra, lumbar

thoracic, thoracolumbar 722.11

with myelopathy 722.72

due to major trauma — *see* Dislocation, vertebra, thoracic

intrauterine device 996.32

kidney (acquired) 593.0

congenital 753.3

lacrimal apparatus or duct (congenital) 743.65

macula (congenital) 743.55

Meckel's diverticulum (congenital) 751.0

nail (congenital) 757.5

acquired 703.8

opening of Wharton's duct in mouth 750.26

organ or site, congenital NEC — *see* Malposition, congenital

ovary (acquired) 620.4

congenital 752.0

free in peritoneal cavity (congenital) 752.0

into hernial sac 620.4

oviduct (acquired) 620.4

congenital 752.19

parathyroid (gland) 252.8

parotid gland (congenital) 750.26

punctum lacrimale (congenital) 743.65

sacroiliac (congenital) (joint) 755.69

current injury — *see* Dislocation, sacroiliac

old 724.6

spine (congenital) 756.19

spleen, congenital 759.0

stomach (congenital) 750.7

acquired 537.89

subglenoid (closed) 831.01

sublingual duct (congenital) 750.26

teeth, tooth 524.30

horizontal 524.33

vertical 524.34

tongue (congenital) (downward) 750.19

trachea (congenital) 748.3

ureter or ureteric opening or orifice (congenital) 753.4

uterine opening of oviducts or fallopian tubes 752.19

uterus, uterine (*see also* Malposition, uterus) 621.6

congenital 752.39

ventricular septum 746.89

with rudimentary ventricle 746.89

xyphoid bone (process) 738.3

Disproportion 653.9 ☑

affecting fetus or newborn 763.1

breast, reconstructed 612.1

between native and reconstructed 612.1

caused by

conjoined twins 678.1 ☑

contraction, pelvis (general) 653.1 ☑

inlet 653.2 ☑

midpelvic 653.8 ☑

midplane 653.8 ☑

outlet 653.3 ☑

fetal

ascites 653.7 ☑

hydrocephalus 653.6 ☑

hydrops 653.7 ☑

meningomyelocele 653.7 ☑

sacral teratoma 653.7 ☑

tumor 653.7 ☑

hydrocephalic fetus 653.6 ☑

pelvis, pelvic, abnormality (bony) NEC 653.0 ☑

Disproportion — *continued*

caused by — *continued*

unusually large fetus 653.5 ☑

causing obstructed labor 660.1 ☑

cephalopelvic, normally formed fetus 653.4 ☑

causing obstructed labor 660.1 ☑

fetal NEC 653.5 ☑

causing obstructed labor 660.1 ☑

fetopelvic, normally formed fetus 653.4 ☑

causing obstructed labor 660.1 ☑

mixed maternal and fetal origin, normally formed fetus 653.4 ☑

pelvis, pelvic (bony) NEC 653.1 ☑

causing obstructed labor 660.1 ☑

specified type NEC 653.8 ☑

Disruption

cesarean wound 674.1 ☑

family V61.09

due to

child in

care of non-parental family member V61.06

foster care V61.06

welfare custody V61.05

death of family member V61.07

divorce V61.03

estrangement V61.09

parent-child V61.04

extended absence of family member NEC V61.08

family member

on military deployment V61.01

return from military deployment V61.02

legal separation V61.03

gastrointestinal anastomosis 997.49

ligament(s) (*see also* Sprain)

knee

current injury — *see* Dislocation, knee

old 717.89

capsular 717.85

collateral (medial) 717.82

lateral 717.81

cruciate (posterior) 717.84

anterior 717.83

specified site NEC 717.85

marital V61.10

involving

divorce V61.03

estrangement V61.09

operation wound (external) (*see also* Dehiscence) 998.32

internal 998.31

organ transplant, anastomosis site — *see* Complications, transplant, organ, by site

ossicles, ossicular chain 385.23

traumatic — *see* Fracture, skull, base

parenchyma

liver (hepatic) — *see* Laceration, liver, major

spleen — *see* Laceration, spleen, parenchyma, massive

phase-shift, of 24-hour sleep-wake cycle, unspecified 780.55

nonorganic origin 307.45

sleep-wake cycle (24-hour), unspecified 780.55

circadian rhythm 327.33

nonorganic origin 307.45

suture line (external) (*see also* Dehiscence) 998.32

internal 998.31

wound 998.30

cesarean operation 674.1 ☑

episiotomy 674.2 ☑

operation (surgical) 998.32

cesarean 674.1 ☑

internal 998.31

perineal (obstetric) 674.2 ☑

uterine 674.1 ☑

Disruptio uteri — *see also* Rupture, uterus

complicating delivery — *see* Delivery, complicated, rupture, uterus

Dissatisfaction with
- employment V62.29
- school environment V62.3

Dissecting — *see* condition

Dissection
- aorta 441.00
  - abdominal 441.02
  - thoracic 441.01
  - thoracoabdominal 441.03
- artery, arterial
  - carotid 443.21
  - coronary 414.12
  - iliac 443.22
  - renal 443.23
  - specified NEC 443.29
  - vertebral 443.24
- vascular 459.9
- wound — *see* Wound, open, by site

Disseminated — *see* condition

Dissociated personality NEC 300.15

Dissociation
- auriculoventricular or atrioventricular (any degree) (AV) 426.89
  - with heart block 426.0
- interference 426.89
- isorhythmic 426.89
- rhythm
  - atrioventricular (AV) 426.89
  - interference 426.89

Dissociative
- identity disorder 300.14
- reaction NEC 300.15

Dissolution, vertebra — *see also* Osteoporosis 733.00

Distention
- abdomen (gaseous) 787.3
- bladder 596.89
- cecum 569.89
- colon 569.89
- gallbladder 575.8
- gaseous (abdomen) 787.3
- intestine 569.89
- kidney 593.89
- liver 573.9
- seminal vesicle 608.89
- stomach 536.8
  - acute 536.1
  - psychogenic 306.4
- ureter 593.5
- uterus 621.8

Distichia, distichiasis (eyelid) 743.63

Disto-occlusion (division I) (division II) 524.22

Distoma hepaticum infestation 121.3

Distomiasis 121.9
- bile passages 121.3
  - due to Clonorchis sinensis 121.1
- hemic 120.9
- hepatic (liver) 121.3
  - due to Clonorchis sinensis (clonorchiasis) 121.1
- intestinal 121.4
- liver 121.3
  - due to Clonorchis sinensis 121.1
- lung 121.2
- pulmonary 121.2

Distomolar (fourth molar) 520.1
- causing crowding 524.31

Distortion (congenital)
- adrenal (gland) 759.1
- ankle (joint) 755.69
- anus 751.5
- aorta 747.29
- appendix 751.5
- arm 755.59
- artery (peripheral) NEC (*see also* Distortion, peripheral vascular system) 747.60
  - cerebral 747.81
  - coronary 746.85
  - pulmonary 747.39
  - retinal 743.58
  - umbilical 747.5
- auditory canal 744.29
  - causing impairment of hearing 744.02
- bile duct or passage 751.69
- bladder 753.8
- brain 742.4

Distortion — *continued*
- bronchus 748.3
- cecum 751.5
- cervix (uteri) 752.49
- chest (wall) 756.3
- clavicle 755.51
- clitoris 752.49
- coccyx 756.19
- colon 751.5
- common duct 751.69
- cornea 743.41
- cricoid cartilage 748.3
- cystic duct 751.69
- duodenum 751.5
- ear 744.3
  - auricle 744.29
    - causing impairment of hearing 744.02
  - causing impairment of hearing 744.09
  - external 744.29
    - causing impairment of hearing 744.02
  - inner 744.05
  - middle, except ossicles 744.03
    - ossicles 744.04
  - ossicles 744.04
- endocrine (gland) NEC 759.2
- epiglottis 748.3
- Eustachian tube 744.24
- eye 743.8
  - adnexa 743.69
- face bone(s) 756.0
- fallopian tube 752.19
- femur 755.69
- fibula 755.69
- finger(s) 755.59
- foot 755.67
- gallbladder 751.69
- genitalia, genital organ(s)
  - female 752.89
    - external 752.49
    - internal NEC 752.89
  - male 752.89
    - penis 752.69
- glottis 748.3
- gyri 742.4
- hand bone(s) 755.59
- heart (auricle) (ventricle) 746.89
  - valve (cusp) 746.89
- hepatic duct 751.69
- humerus 755.59
- hymen 752.49
- ileum 751.5
- intestine (large) (small) 751.5
  - with anomalous adhesions, fixation or malrotation 751.4
- jaw NEC 524.89
- jejunum 751.5
- kidney 753.3
- knee (joint) 755.64
- labium (majus) (minus) 752.49
- larynx 748.3
- leg 755.69
- lens 743.36
- liver 751.69
- lumbar spine 756.19
  - with disproportion (fetopelvic) 653.0 ☑
    - affecting fetus or newborn 763.1
    - causing obstructed labor 660.1 ☑
- lumbosacral (joint) (region) 756.19
- lung (fissures) (lobe) 748.69
- nerve 742.8
- nose 748.1
- organ
  - of Corti 744.05
  - of site not listed — *see* Anomaly, specified type NEC
- ossicles, ear 744.04
- ovary 752.0
- oviduct 752.19
- pancreas 751.7
- parathyroid (gland) 759.2
- patella 755.64
- peripheral vascular system NEC 747.60
  - gastrointestinal 747.61
  - lower limb 747.64

Distortion — *continued*
- peripheral vascular system — *continued*
  - renal 747.62
  - spinal 747.82
  - upper limb 747.63
- pituitary (gland) 759.2
- radius 755.59
- rectum 751.5
- rib 756.3
- sacroiliac joint 755.69
- sacrum 756.19
- scapula 755.59
- shoulder girdle 755.59
- site not listed — *see* Anomaly, specified type NEC
- skull bone(s) 756.0
  - with
    - anencephalus 740.0
    - encephalocele 742.0
    - hydrocephalus 742.3
      - with spina bifida (*see also* Spina bifida) 741.0 ☑
    - microcephalus 742.1
- spinal cord 742.59
- spine 756.19
- spleen 759.0
- sternum 756.3
- thorax (wall) 756.3
- thymus (gland) 759.2
- thyroid (gland) 759.2
  - cartilage 748.3
- tibia 755.69
- toe(s) 755.66
- tongue 750.19
- trachea (cartilage) 748.3
- ulna 755.59
- ureter 753.4
  - causing obstruction 753.20
- urethra 753.8
  - causing obstruction 753.6
- uterus 752.39
- vagina 752.49
- vein (peripheral) NEC (*see also* Distortion, peripheral vascular system) 747.60
  - great 747.49
  - portal 747.49
  - pulmonary 747.49
- vena cava (inferior) (superior) 747.49
- vertebra 756.19
- visual NEC 368.15
  - shape or size 368.14
- vulva 752.49
- wrist (bones) (joint) 755.59

Distress
- abdomen 789.0 ☑
- colon 564.9
- emotional V40.9
- epigastric 789.0 ☑
- fetal (syndrome) 768.4
  - affecting management of pregnancy or childbirth 656.8 ☑
  - liveborn infant 768.4
    - first noted
      - before onset of labor 768.2
      - during labor and delivery 768.3
  - stillborn infant (death before onset of labor) 768.0
  - death during labor 768.1
- gastrointestinal (functional) 536.9
  - psychogenic 306.4
- intestinal (functional) NEC 564.9
  - psychogenic 306.4
- intrauterine — *see* Distress, fetal
- leg 729.5
- maternal 669.0 ☑
- mental V40.9
- respiratory 786.09
  - acute (adult) 518.82
  - adult syndrome (following trauma and surgery) 518.52
    - specified NEC 518.82
  - fetus or newborn 770.89
  - syndrome (idiopathic) (newborn) 769
- stomach 536.9
  - psychogenic 306.4

Distribution vessel, atypical NEC 747.60

Distribution vessel, atypical — *continued*
- coronary artery 746.85
- spinal 747.82

Districhiasis 704.2

Disturbance — *see also* Disease
- absorption NEC 579.9
  - calcium 269.3
  - carbohydrate 579.8
  - fat 579.8
  - protein 579.8
  - specified type NEC 579.8
  - vitamin (*see also* Deficiency, vitamin) 269.2
- acid-base equilibrium 276.9
- activity and attention, simple, with hyperkinesis 314.01
- amino acid (metabolic) (*see also* Disorder, amino acid) 270.9
  - imidazole 270.5
  - maple syrup (urine) disease 270.3
  - transport 270.0
- assimilation, food 579.9
- attention, simple 314.00
  - with hyperactivity 314.01
- auditory, nerve, except deafness 388.5
- behavior (*see also* Disturbance, conduct) 312.9
- blood clotting (hypoproteinemia) (mechanism) (*see also* Defect, coagulation) 286.9
- central nervous system NEC 349.9
- cerebral nerve NEC 352.9
- circulatory 459.9
- conduct 312.9

> *Note* — *Use the following fifth-digit subclassification with categories 312.0–312.2:*
>
> 0   *unspecified*
>
> 1   *mild*
>
> 2   *moderate*
>
> 3   *severe*

- adjustment reaction 309.3
- adolescent onset type 312.82
- childhood onset type 312.81
- compulsive 312.30
  - intermittent explosive disorder 312.34
  - isolated explosive disorder 312.35
  - kleptomania 312.32
  - pathological gambling 312.31
  - pyromania 312.33
- hyperkinetic 314.2
- intermittent explosive 312.34
- isolated explosive 312.35
- mixed with emotions 312.4
- socialized (type) 312.20
  - aggressive 312.23
  - unaggressive 312.21
- specified type NEC 312.89
- undersocialized, unsocialized
  - aggressive (type) 312.0 ☑
  - unaggressive (type) 312.1 ☑
- coordination 781.3
- cranial nerve NEC 352.9
- deep sensibility — *see* Disturbance, sensation
- digestive 536.9
  - psychogenic 306.4
- electrolyte — *see* Imbalance, electrolyte
- emotions specific to childhood or adolescence 313.9
  - with
    - academic underachievement 313.83
    - anxiety and fearfulness 313.0
    - elective mutism 313.23
    - identity disorder 313.82
    - jealousy 313.3
    - misery and unhappiness 313.1
    - oppositional defiant disorder 313.81
    - overanxiousness 313.0
    - sensitivity 313.21
    - shyness 313.21
    - social withdrawal 313.22
    - withdrawal reaction 313.22

☑ Additional Digit Required — Refer to the Tabular List for Digit Selection   ▽ Subterms under main terms may continue to next column or page

2014 ICD-9-CM   ▶◀ Revised Text   ● New Line   ▲ Revised Code   Volume 2 — 95

Disturbance — *see also* Disease — *continued*
  emotions specific to childhood or adolescence — *continued*
    involving relationship problems 313.3
    mixed 313.89
    specified type NEC 313.89
  endocrine (gland) 259.9
    neonatal, transitory 775.9
      specified NEC 775.89
  equilibrium 780.4
  feeding (elderly) (infant) 783.3
    newborn 779.31
    nonorganic origin NEC 307.59
    psychogenic NEC 307.59
  fructose metabolism 271.2
  gait 781.2
    hysterical 300.11
  gastric (functional) 536.9
    motility 536.8
    psychogenic 306.4
    secretion 536.8
  gastrointestinal (functional) 536.9
    psychogenic 306.4
  habit, child 307.9
  hearing, except deafness 388.40
  heart, functional (conditions classifiable to 426, 427, 428)
    due to presence of (cardiac) prosthesis 429.4
    postoperative (immediate) 997.1
      long-term effect of cardiac surgery 429.4
    psychogenic 306.2
  hormone 259.9
  innervation uterus, sympathetic, parasympathetic 621.8
  keratinization NEC
    gingiva 523.10
    lip 528.5
    oral (mucosa) (soft tissue) 528.79
      residual ridge mucosa
        excessive 528.72
        minimal 528.71
    tongue 528.79
  labyrinth, labyrinthine (vestibule) 386.9
  learning, specific NEC 315.2
  memory (*see also* Amnesia) 780.93
    mild, following organic brain damage 310.89
  mental (*see also* Disorder, mental) 300.9
    associated with diseases classified elsewhere 316
  metabolism (acquired) (congenital) (*see also* Disorder, metabolism) 277.9
    with
      abortion — *see* Abortion, by type, with metabolic disorder
      ectopic pregnancy (*see also* categories 633.0–633.9) 639.4
      molar pregnancy (*see also* categories 630–632) 639.4
    amino acid (*see also* Disorder, amino acid) 270.9
      aromatic NEC 270.2
      branched-chain 270.3
      specified type NEC 270.8
      straight-chain NEC 270.7
      sulfur-bearing 270.4
      transport 270.0
    ammonia 270.6
    arginine 270.6
    argininosuccinic acid 270.6
    carbohydrate NEC 271.9
    cholesterol 272.9
    citrulline 270.6
    cystathionine 270.4
    fat 272.9
    following
      abortion 639.4
      ectopic or molar pregnancy 639.4
    general 277.9
      carbohydrate 271.9
      iron 275.09
      phosphate 275.3
      sodium 276.9

Disturbance — *see also* Disease — *continued*
  metabolism (*see also* Disorder, metabolism) — *continued*
    glutamine 270.7
    glycine 270.7
    histidine 270.5
    homocystine 270.4
    in labor or delivery 669.0 ☑
    iron 275.09
    isoleucine 270.3
    leucine 270.3
    lipoid 272.9
      specified type NEC 272.8
    lysine 270.7
    methionine 270.4
    neonatal, transitory 775.9
      specified type NEC 775.89
    nitrogen 788.99
    ornithine 270.6
    phosphate 275.3
    phosphatides 272.7
    serine 270.7
    sodium NEC 276.9
    threonine 270.7
    tryptophan 270.2
    tyrosine 270.2
    urea cycle 270.6
    valine 270.3
  motor 796.1
  nervous functional 799.21
  neuromuscular mechanism (eye) due to syphilis 094.84
  nutritional 269.9
    nail 703.8
  ocular motion 378.87
    psychogenic 306.7
  oculogyric 378.87
    psychogenic 306.7
  oculomotor NEC 378.87
    psychogenic 306.7
  olfactory nerve 781.1
  optic nerve NEC 377.49
  oral epithelium, including tongue 528.79
    residual ridge mucosa
      excessive 528.72
      minimal 528.71
  personality (pattern) (trait) (*see also* Disorder, personality) 301.9
    following organic brain damage 310.1
  polyglandular 258.9
  psychomotor 307.9
  pupillary 379.49
  reflex 796.1
  rhythm, heart 427.9
    postoperative (immediate) 997.1
      long-term effect of cardiac surgery 429.4
    psychogenic 306.2
  salivary secretion 527.7
  sensation (cold) (heat) (localization) (tactile discrimination localization) (texture) (vibratory) NEC 782.0
    hysterical 300.11
    skin 782.0
    smell 781.1
    taste 781.1
  sensory (*see also* Disturbance, sensation) 782.0
    innervation 782.0
  situational (transient) (*see also* Reaction, adjustment) 309.9
    acute 308.3
  sleep 780.50
    with apnea — *see* Apnea, sleep
    initiation or maintenance (*see also* Insomnia) 780.52
      nonorganic origin 307.41
    nonorganic origin 307.40
      specified type NEC 307.49
    specified NEC 780.59
      nonorganic origin 307.49
    wakefulness (*see also* Hypersomnia) 780.54
      nonorganic origin 307.43
  sociopathic 301.7

Disturbance — *see also* Disease — *continued*
  speech NEC 784.59
    developmental 315.39
      associated with hyperkinesis 314.1
    secondary to organic lesion 784.59
  stomach (functional) (*see also* Disturbance, gastric) 536.9
  sympathetic (nerve) (*see also* Neuropathy, peripheral, autonomic) 337.9
  temperature sense 782.0
    hysterical 300.11
  tooth
    eruption 520.6
    formation 520.4
    structure, hereditary NEC 520.5
  touch (*see also* Disturbance, sensation) 782.0
  vascular 459.9
    arteriosclerotic — *see* Arteriosclerosis
  vasomotor 443.9
  vasospastic 443.9
  vestibular labyrinth 386.9
  vision, visual NEC 368.9
    psychophysical 368.16
    specified NEC 368.8
    subjective 368.10
  voice and resonance 784.40
  wakefulness (initiation or maintenance) (*see also* Hypersomnia) 780.54
    nonorganic origin 307.43
Disulfiduria, beta-mercaptolactate-cysteine 270.0
Disuse atrophy, bone 733.7
Ditthomska syndrome 307.81
Diuresis 788.42
Divers'
  palsy or paralysis 993.3
  squeeze 993.3
Diverticula, diverticulosis, diverticulum (acute) (multiple) (perforated) (ruptured) 562.10
  with diverticulitis 562.11
  aorta (Kommerell's) 747.21
  appendix (noninflammatory) 543.9
  bladder (acquired) (sphincter) 596.3
    congenital 753.8
  broad ligament 620.8
  bronchus (congenital) 748.3
    acquired 494.0
      with acute exacerbation 494.1
  calyx, calyceal (kidney) 593.89
  cardia (stomach) 537.1
  cecum 562.10
    with
      diverticulitis 562.11
        with hemorrhage 562.13
      hemorrhage 562.12
    congenital 751.5
  colon (acquired) 562.10
    with
      diverticulitis 562.11
        with hemorrhage 562.13
      hemorrhage 562.12
    congenital 751.5
  duodenum 562.00
    with
      diverticulitis 562.01
        with hemorrhage 562.03
      hemorrhage 562.02
    congenital 751.5
  epiphrenic (esophagus) 530.6
  esophagus (congenital) 750.4
    acquired 530.6
    epiphrenic 530.6
    pulsion 530.6
    traction 530.6
    Zenker's 530.6
  Eustachian tube 381.89
  fallopian tube 620.8
  gallbladder (congenital) 751.69
  gastric 537.1
  heart (congenital) 746.89
  ileum 562.00
    with
      diverticulitis 562.01
        with hemorrhage 562.03

Diverticula, diverticulosis, diverticulum — *continued*
  ileum — *continued*
    with — *continued*
      hemorrhage 562.02
  intestine (large) 562.10
    with
      diverticulitis 562.11
        with hemorrhage 562.13
      hemorrhage 562.12
    congenital 751.5
    small 562.00
      with
        diverticulitis 562.01
          with hemorrhage 562.03
        hemorrhage 562.02
      congenital 751.5
  jejunum 562.00
    with
      diverticulitis 562.01
        with hemorrhage 562.03
      hemorrhage 562.02
  kidney (calyx) (pelvis) 593.89
    with calculus 592.0
  Kommerell's 747.21
  laryngeal ventricle (congenital) 748.3
  Meckel's (displaced) (hypertrophic) 751.0
  midthoracic 530.6
  organ or site, congenital NEC — *see* Distortion
  pericardium (conginital) (cyst) 746.89
    acquired (true) 423.8
  pharyngoesophageal (pulsion) 530.6
  pharynx (congenital) 750.27
  pulsion (esophagus) 530.6
  rectosigmoid 562.10
    with
      diverticulitis 562.11
        with hemorrhage 562.13
      hemorrhage 562.12
    congenital 751.5
  rectum 562.10
    with
      diverticulitis 562.11
        with hemorrhage 562.13
      hemorrhage 562.12
  renal (calyces) (pelvis) 593.89
    with calculus 592.0
  Rokitansky's 530.6
  seminal vesicle 608.0
  sigmoid 562.10
    with
      diverticulitis 562.11
        with hemorrhage 562.13
      hemorrhage 562.12
    congenital 751.5
  small intestine 562.00
    with
      diverticulitis 562.01
        with hemorrhage 562.03
      hemorrhage 562.02
  stomach (cardia) (juxtacardia) (juxtapyloric) (acquired) 537.1
    congenital 750.7
  subdiaphragmatic 530.6
  trachea (congenital) 748.3
    acquired 519.19
  traction (esophagus) 530.6
  ureter (acquired) 593.89
    congenital 753.4
  ureterovesical orifice 593.89
  urethra (acquired) 599.2
    congenital 753.8
  ventricle, left (congenital) 746.89
  vesical (urinary) 596.3
    congenital 753.8
  Zenker's (esophagus) 530.6
Diverticulitis (acute) — *see also* Diverticula 562.11
  with hemorrhage 562.13
  bladder (urinary) 596.3
  cecum (perforated) 562.11
    with hemorrhage 562.13
  colon (perforated) 562.11
    with hemorrhage 562.13
  duodenum 562.01

Diverticulitis — see also Diverticula — continued
  duodenum — continued
    with hemorrhage 562.03
  esophagus 530.6
  ileum (perforated) 562.01
    with hemorrhage 562.03
  intestine (large) (perforated) 562.11
    with hemorrhage 562.13
    small 562.01
      with hemorrhage 562.03
  jejunum (perforated) 562.01
    with hemorrhage 562.03
  Meckel's (perforated) 751.0
  pharyngoesophageal 530.6
  rectosigmoid (perforated) 562.11
    with hemorrhage 562.13
  rectum 562.11
    with hemorrhage 562.13
  sigmoid (old) (perforated) 562.11
    with hemorrhage 562.13
  small intestine (perforated) 562.01
    with hemorrhage 562.03
  vesical (urinary) 596.3
Diverticulosis — see Diverticula
Division
  cervix uteri 622.8
    external os into two openings by frenum 752.44
  external (cervical) into two openings by frenum 752.44
  glans penis 752.69
  hymen 752.49
  labia minora (congenital) 752.49
  ligament (partial or complete) (current) (see also Sprain, by site)
    with open wound — see Wound, open, by site
  muscle (partial or complete) (current) (see also Sprain, by site)
    with open wound — see Wound, open, by site
  nerve — see Injury, nerve, by site
  penis glans 752.69
  spinal cord — see Injury, spinal, by site
  vein 459.9
    traumatic — see Injury, vascular, by site
Divorce V61.03
Dix-Hallpike neurolabyrinthitis 386.12
Dizziness 780.4
  hysterical 300.11
  psychogenic 306.9
Doan-Wiseman syndrome (primary splenic neutropenia) 289.53
Dog bite — see Wound, open, by site
Döhle-Heller aortitis 093.1
Döhle body-panmyelopathic syndrome 288.2
Dolichocephaly, dolichocephalus 754.0
Dolichocolon 751.5
Dolichostenomelia 759.82
Donohue's syndrome (leprechaunism) 259.8
Donor
  blood V59.01
    other blood components V59.09
    stem cells V59.02
    whole blood V59.01
  bone V59.2
    marrow V59.3
  cornea V59.5
  egg (oocyte) (ovum) V59.70
    over age 35 V59.73
      anonymous recipient V59.73
      designated recipient V59.74
    under age 35 V59.71
      anonymous recipient V59.71
      designated recipient V59.72
  heart V59.8
  kidney V59.4
  liver V59.6
  lung V59.8
  lymphocyte V59.8
  organ V59.9
    specified NEC V59.8
  potential, examination of V70.8
  skin V59.1

Donor — continued
  specified organ or tissue NEC V59.8
  sperm V59.8
  stem cells V59.02
  tissue V59.9
    specified type NEC V59.8
Donovanosis (granuloma venereum) 099.2
DOPS (diffuse obstructive pulmonary syndrome) 496
Double
  albumin 273.8
  aortic arch 747.21
  auditory canal 744.29
  auricle (heart) 746.82
  bladder 753.8
  external (cervical) os 752.44
  kidney with double pelvis (renal) 753.3
  larynx 748.3
  meatus urinarius 753.8
  organ or site NEC — see Accessory
  orifice
    heart valve NEC 746.89
    pulmonary 746.09
  outlet, right ventricle 745.11
  pelvis (renal) with double ureter 753.4
  penis 752.69
  tongue 750.13
  ureter (one or both sides) 753.4
    with double pelvis (renal) 753.4
  urethra 753.8
  urinary meatus 753.8
  uterus (any degree) 752.2
    with doubling of cervix and vagina 752.2
    in pregnancy or childbirth 654.0 ☑
      affecting fetus or newborn 763.89
  vagina 752.47
    with doubling of cervix and uterus 752.2
  vision 368.2
  vocal cords 748.3
  vulva 752.49
  whammy (syndrome) 360.81
Douglas' pouch, cul-de-sac — see condition
Down-growth, epithelial (anterior chamber) 364.61
Down's disease or syndrome (mongolism) 758.0
DPD (dihydropyrimidine dehydrogenase deficiency) 277.6
Dracontiasis 125.7
Dracunculiasis 125.7
Dracunculosis 125.7
Drainage
  abscess (spontaneous) — see Abscess
  anomalous pulmonary veins to hepatic veins or right atrium 747.41
  stump (amputation) (surgical) 997.62
  suprapubic, bladder 596.89
Dream state, hysterical 300.13
Drepanocytic anemia — see also Disease, sickle cell 282.60
Dresbach's syndrome (elliptocytosis) 282.1
Dreschera (infection) 118
  hawaiiensis 117.8
Dressler's syndrome (postmyocardial infarction) 411.0
Dribbling (post-void) 788.35
Drift, ulnar 736.09
Drinking (alcohol) — see also Alcoholism
  excessive, to excess NEC (see also Abuse, drugs, nondependent) 305.0 ☑
    bouts, periodic 305.0 ☑
    continual 303.9 ☑
    episodic 305.0 ☑
    habitual 303.9 ☑
    periodic 305.0 ☑
Drip, postnasal (chronic) 784.91
  due to
    allergic rhinitis — see Rhinitis, allergic
    common cold 460
    gastroesophageal reflux — see Reflux, gastroesophageal
    nasopharyngitis — see Nasopharyngitis
    other known condition — code to condition
    sinusitis — see Sinusitis
Drivers' license examination V70.3

Droop
  Cooper's 611.81
  facial 781.94
Drop
  finger 736.29
  foot 736.79
  hematocrit (precipitous) 790.01
  hemoglobin 790.01
  toe 735.8
  wrist 736.05
Dropped
  dead 798.1
  heart beats 426.6
Dropsy, dropsical — see also Edema 782.3
  abdomen 789.59
  amnion (see also Hydramnios) 657.0 ☑
  brain — see Hydrocephalus
  cardiac (see also Failure, heart) 428.0
  cardiorenal (see also Hypertension, cardiorenal) 404.90
  chest 511.9
  fetus or newborn 778.0
    due to isoimmunization 773.3
  gangrenous (see also Gangrene) 785.4
  heart (see also Failure, heart) 428.0
  hepatic — see Cirrhosis, liver
  infantile — see Hydrops, fetalis
  kidney (see also Nephrosis) 581.9
  liver — see Cirrhosis, liver
  lung 514
  malarial (see also Malaria) 084.9
  neonatorum — see Hydrops, fetalis
  nephritic 581.9
  newborn — see Hydrops, fetalis
  nutritional 269.9
  ovary 620.8
  pericardium (see also Pericarditis) 423.9
  renal (see also Nephrosis) 581.9
  uremic — see Uremia
Drowned, drowning (near) 994.1
  lung 518.52
Drowsiness 780.09
Drug — see also condition
  addiction (see also listing under Dependence) 304.9 ☑
  adverse effect, correct substance properly administered 995.20
  allergy 995.27
  dependence (see also listing under Dependence) 304.9 ☑
  habit (see also listing under Dependence) 304.9 ☑
  hypersensitivity 995.27
  induced
    circadian rhythm sleep disorder 292.85
    hypersomnia 292.85
    insomnia 292.85
    mental disorder 292.9
      anxiety 292.89
      mood 292.84
      sexual 292.89
      sleep 292.85
      specified type 292.89
    parasomnia 292.85
    persisting
      amnestic disorder 292.83
      dementia 292.82
    psychotic disorder
      with
        delusions 292.11
        hallucinations 292.12
    sleep disorder 292.85
  intoxication 292.89
  overdose — see Table of Drugs and Chemicals
  poisoning — see Table of Drugs and Chemicals
  therapy (maintenance) status NEC
    chemotherapy, antineoplastic V58.11
    immunotherapy, antineoplastic V58.12
    long-term (current) (prophylactic) use V58.69
      anti-inflammatories, non-steroidal (NSAID) V58.64
      antibiotics V58.62
      anticoagulants V58.61

Drug — see also condition — continued
  therapy status — continued
    long-term use — continued
      antiplatelets V58.63
      antithrombotics V58.63
      aspirin V58.66
      bisphosphonates V58.68
      high-risk medications NEC V58.69
      insulin V58.67
      methadone for pain control V58.69
      opiate analgesic V58.69
      steroids V58.65
    methadone 304.00
  wrong substance given or taken in error — see Table of Drugs and Chemicals
Drunkenness — see also Abuse, drugs, nondependent 305.0 ☑
  acute in alcoholism (see also Alcoholism) 303.0 ☑
  chronic (see also Alcoholism) 303.9 ☑
  pathologic 291.4
  simple (acute) 305.0 ☑
    in alcoholism 303.0 ☑
  sleep 307.47
Drusen
  optic disc or papilla 377.21
  retina (colloid) (hyaloid degeneration) 362.57
    hereditary 362.77
Drusenfieber 075
Dry, dryness — see also condition
  eye 375.15
    syndrome 375.15
  larynx 478.79
  mouth 527.7
  nose 478.19
  skin syndrome 701.1
  socket (teeth) 526.5
  throat 478.29
DSAP (disseminated superficial actinic porokeratosis) 692.75
DSTR (delayed serologic transfusion reaction)
  due to or resulting from
    incompatibility
      ABO 999.69
      non-ABO antigen (minor) (Duffy) (Kell) (Kidd) (Lewis) (M) (N) (P) (S) 999.79
      Rh antigen (C) (c) (D) (E) (e) 999.74
Duane-Stilling-Türk syndrome (ocular retraction syndrome) 378.71
Duane's retraction syndrome 378.71
Dubin-Johnson disease or syndrome 277.4
Dubini's disease (electric chorea) 049.8
Dubois' abscess or disease 090.5
Duchenne-Aran myelopathic, muscular atrophy (nonprogressive) (progressive) 335.21
Duchenne-Griesinger disease 359.1
Duchenne's
  disease 094.0
    locomotor ataxia 094.0
    muscular dystrophy 359.1
    pseudohypertrophy, muscles 359.1
  paralysis 335.22
  syndrome 335.22
Ducrey's
  bacillus 099.0
  chancre 099.0
  disease (chancroid) 099.0
Duct, ductus — see condition
Duengero 061
Duhring's disease (dermatitis herpetiformis) 694.0
Dukes (-Filatov) disease 057.8
Dullness
  cardiac (decreased) (increased) 785.3
Dumb ague — see also Malaria 084.6
Dumbness — see also Aphasia 784.3
Dumdum fever 085.0
Dumping syndrome (postgastrectomy) 564.2
  nonsurgical 536.8
Duodenitis (nonspecific) (peptic) 535.60
  with hemorrhage 535.61
  due to
    Strongyloides stercoralis 127.2

☑ **Additional Digit Required** — Refer to the Tabular List for Digit Selection   ▽ **Subterms under main terms may continue to next column or page**

Duodenocholangitis 575.8
Duodenum, duodenal — *see* condition
Duplay's disease, periarthritis, or syndrome 726.2
Duplex — *see also* Accessory
    kidney 753.3
    placenta — *see* Placenta, abnormal
    uterus 752.2
Duplication — *see also* Accessory
    anus 751.5
    aortic arch 747.21
    appendix 751.5
    biliary duct (any) 751.69
    bladder 753.8
    cecum 751.5
        and appendix 751.5
    cervical, cervix 752.44
    clitoris 752.49
    cystic duct 751.69
    digestive organs 751.8
    duodenum 751.5
    esophagus 750.4
    fallopian tube 752.19
    frontonasal process 756.0
    gallbladder 751.69
    ileum 751.5
    intestine (large) (small) 751.5
    jejunum 751.5
    kidney 753.3
    liver 751.69
    nose 748.1
    pancreas 751.7
    penis 752.69
    respiratory organs NEC 748.9
    salivary duct 750.22
    spinal cord (incomplete) 742.51
    stomach 750.7
    ureter 753.4
    vagina 752.47
    vas deferens 752.89
    vocal cords 748.3
Dupré's disease or syndrome (meningism) 781.6
Dupuytren's
    contraction 728.6
    disease (muscle contracture) 728.6
    fracture (closed) 824.4
        ankle (closed) 824.4
            open 824.5
        fibula (closed) 824.4
            open 824.5
        open 824.5
        radius (closed) 813.42
            open 813.52
    muscle contracture 728.6
Durand-Nicolas-Favre disease (climatic bubo) 099.1
Durotomy, incidental (inadvertent) — *see also* Tear, dural 349.31
Duroziez's disease (congenital mitral stenosis) 746.5
Dust
    conjunctivitis 372.05
    reticulation (occupational) 504
Dutton's
    disease (trypanosomiasis) 086.9
    relapsing fever (West African) 087.1
Dwarf, dwarfism 259.4
    with infantilism (hypophyseal) 253.3
    achondroplastic 756.4
    Amsterdam 759.89
    bird-headed 759.89
    congenital 259.4
    constitutional 259.4
    hypophyseal 253.3
    infantile 259.4
    Levi type 253.3
    Lorain-Levi (pituitary) 253.3
    Lorain type (pituitary) 253.3
    metatropic 756.4
    nephrotic-glycosuric, with hypophos-phatemic rickets 270.0
    nutritional 263.2
    ovarian 758.6
    pancreatic 577.8
    pituitary 253.3

Dwarf, dwarfism — *continued*
    polydystrophic 277.5
    primordial 253.3
    psychosocial 259.4
    renal 588.0
        with hypertension — *see* Hypertension, kidney
    Russell's (uterine dwarfism and craniofacial dysostosis) 759.89
Dyke-Young anemia or syndrome (acquired macrocytic hemolytic anemia) (secondary) (symptomatic) 283.9
Dynia abnormality — *see also* Defect, coagulation 286.9
Dysacousis 388.40
Dysadrenocortism 255.9
    hyperfunction 255.3
    hypofunction 255.41
Dysarthria 784.51
    due to late effect of cerebrovascular disease (*see also* Late effect(s) (of) cerebrovascular disease) 438.13
Dysautonomia — *see also* Neuropathy, peripheral, autonomic 337.9
    familial 742.8
Dysbarism 993.3
Dysbasia 719.7
    angiosclerotica intermittens 443.9
        due to atherosclerosis 440.21
    hysterical 300.11
    lordotica (progressiva) 333.6
    nonorganic origin 307.9
    psychogenic 307.9
Dysbetalipoproteinemia (familial) 272.2
Dyscalculia 315.1
Dyschezia — *see also* Constipation 564.00
Dyschondroplasia (with hemangiomata) 756.4
    Voorhoeve's 756.4
Dyschondrosteosis 756.59
Dyschromia 709.00
Dyscollagenosis 710.9
Dyscoria 743.41
Dyscraniopyophalangy 759.89
Dyscrasia
    blood 289.9
        with antepartum hemorrhage 641.3 ☑
            hemorrhage, subungual 287.8
            puerperal, postpartum 666.3 ☑
    ovary 256.8
    plasma cell 273.9
    pluriglandular 258.9
    polyglandular 258.9
Dysdiadochokinesia 781.3
Dysectasia, vesical neck 596.89
Dysendocrinism 259.9
Dysentery, dysenteric (bilious) (catarrhal) (diarrhea) (epidemic) (gangrenous) (hemorrhagic) (infectious) (sporadic) (tropical) (ulcerative) 009.0
    abscess, liver (*see also* Abscess, amebic) 006.3
    amebic (*see also* Amebiasis) 006.9
        with abscess — *see* Abscess, amebic
        acute 006.0
        carrier (suspected) of V02.2
        chronic 006.1
        arthritis (*see also* Arthritis, due to, dysentery) 009.0 [711.3] ☑
        bacillary 004.9 [711.3] ☑
    asylum 004.9
    bacillary 004.9
        arthritis 004.9 [711.3] ☑
        Boyd 004.2
        Flexner 004.1
        Schmitz (-Stutzer) 004.0
        Shiga 004.0
        Shigella 004.9
            group A 004.0
            group B 004.1
            group C 004.2
            group D 004.3
            specified type NEC 004.8
        Sonne 004.3
        specified type NEC 004.8
    bacterium 004.9
    balantidial 007.0

Dysentery, dysenteric — *continued*
    Balantidium coli 007.0
    Boyd's 004.2
    Chilomastix 007.8
    Chinese 004.9
    choleriform 001.1
    coccidial 007.2
    Dientamoeba fragilis 007.8
    due to specified organism NEC — *see* Enteritis, due to, by organism
    Embadomonas 007.8
    Endolimax nana — *see* Dysentery, amebic
    Entamoba, entamebic — *see* Dysentery, amebic
    Flexner-Boyd 004.2
    Flexner's 004.1
    giardial 007.1
    Giardia lamblia 007.1
    Hiss-Russell 004.1
    lamblia 007.1
    leishmanial 085.0
    malarial (*see also* Malaria) 084.6
    metazoal 127.9
    Monilia 112.89
    protozoal NEC 007.9
    Russell's 004.8
    salmonella 003.0
    schistosomal 120.1
    Schmitz (-Stutzer) 004.0
    Shiga 004.0
    Shigella NEC (*see also* Dysentery, bacillary) 004.9
        boydii 004.2
        dysenteriae 004.0
            Schmitz 004.0
            Shiga 004.0
        flexneri 004.1
        group A 004.0
        group B 004.1
        group C 004.2
        group D 004.3
        Schmitz 004.0
        Shiga 004.0
        Sonnei 004.3
    Sonne 004.3
    strongyloidiasis 127.2
    trichomonal 007.3
    tuberculous (*see also* Tuberculosis) 014.8 ☑
    viral (*see also* Enteritis, viral) 008.8
Dysequilibrium 780.4
Dysesthesia 782.0
    hysterical 300.11
Dysfibrinogenemia (congenital) — *see also* Defect, coagulation 286.3
Dysfunction
    adrenal (cortical) 255.9
        hyperfunction 255.3
        hypofunction 255.41
    associated with sleep stages or arousal from sleep 780.56
        nonorganic origin 307.47
    bladder NEC 596.59
    bleeding, uterus 626.8
    brain, minimal (*see also* Hyperkinesia) 314.9
    cerebral 348.30
    colon 564.9
        psychogenic 306.4
    colostomy or enterostomy 569.62
    cystic duct 575.8
    diastolic 429.9
        with heart failure — *see* Failure, heart
        due to
            cardiomyopathy — *see* Cardiomyopathy
            hypertension — *see* Hypertension, heart
    endocrine NEC 259.9
    endometrium 621.8
    enteric stoma 569.62
    enterostomy 569.62
    erectile 607.84
        nonorganic origin 302.72
    esophagostomy 530.87
    Eustachian tube 381.81
    gallbladder 575.8
    gastrointestinal 536.9

Dysfunction — *continued*
    gland, glandular NEC 259.9
    heart 427.9
        postoperative (immediate) 997.1
            long-term effect of cardiac surgery 429.4
    hemoglobin 289.89
    hepatic 573.9
    hepatocellular NEC 573.9
    hypophysis 253.9
        hyperfunction 253.1
        hypofunction 253.2
        posterior lobe 253.6
            hypofunction 253.5
    kidney (*see also* Disease, renal) 593.9
    labyrinthine 386.50
        specified NEC 386.58
    liver 573.9
        constitutional 277.4
    minimal brain (child) (*see also* Hyperkinesia) 314.9
    ovary, ovarian 256.9
        hyperfunction 256.1
            estrogen 256.0
        hypofunction 256.39
            postablative 256.2
        postablative 256.2
        specified NEC 256.8
    papillary muscle 429.81
        with myocardial infarction 410.8 ☑
    parathyroid 252.8
        hyperfunction 252.00
        hypofunction 252.1
    pineal gland 259.8
    pituitary (gland) 253.9
        hyperfunction 253.1
        hypofunction 253.2
        posterior 253.6
            hypofunction 253.5
    placental — *see* Placenta, insufficiency
    platelets (blood) 287.1
    polyglandular 258.9
        specified NEC 258.8
    psychosexual 302.70
        with
            dyspareunia (functional) (psychogenic) 302.76
            frigidity 302.72
            impotence 302.72
            inhibition
                orgasm
                    female 302.73
                    male 302.74
                sexual
                    desire 302.71
                    excitement 302.72
            premature ejaculation 302.75
            sexual aversion 302.79
            specified disorder NEC 302.79
            vaginismus 306.51
    pylorus 537.9
    rectum 564.9
        psychogenic 306.4
    segmental (*see also* Dysfunction, somatic) 739.9
    senile 797
    sexual 302.70
    sinoatrial node 427.81
    somatic 739.9
        abdomen 739.9
        acromioclavicular 739.7
        cervical 739.1
        cervicothoracic 739.1
        costochondral 739.8
        costovertebral 739.8
        extremities
            lower 739.6
            upper 739.7
        head 739.0
        hip 739.5
        lumbar, lumbosacral 739.3
        occipitocervical 739.0
        pelvic 739.5
        pubic 739.5
        rib cage 739.8
        sacral 739.4

Dysfunction — *continued*
somatic — *continued*
  sacrococcygeal 739.4
  sacroiliac 739.4
  specified site NEC 739.9
  sternochondral 739.8
  sternoclavicular 739.7
  temporomandibular 739.0
  thoracic, thoracolumbar 739.2
 stomach 536.9
  psychogenic 306.4
 suprarenal 255.9
  hyperfunction 255.3
  hypofunction 255.41
 symbolic NEC 784.60
  specified type NEC 784.69
 systolic 429.9
  with heart failure — *see* Failure, heart
 temporomandibular (joint) (joint-pain-syndrome) NEC 524.60
  sounds on opening or closing 524.64
  specified NEC 524.69
 testicular 257.9
  hyperfunction 257.0
  hypofunction 257.2
  specified type NEC 257.8
 thymus 254.9
 thyroid 246.9
  complicating pregnancy, childbirth, or puerperium 648.1 ☑
  hyperfunction — *see* Hyperthyroidism
  hypofunction — *see* Hypothyroidism
 uterus, complicating delivery 661.9 ☑
  affecting fetus or newborn 763.7
  hypertonic 661.4 ☑
  hypotonic 661.2 ☑
   primary 661.0 ☑
   secondary 661.1 ☑
 velopharyngeal (acquired) 528.9
  congenital 750.29
 ventricular 429.9
  with congestive heart failure (*see also* Failure, heart) 428.0
  due to
   cardiomyopathy — *see* Cardiomyopathy
   hypertension — *see* Hypertension, heart
  left, reversible following sudden emotional stress 429.83
 vesicourethral NEC 596.59
 vestibular 386.50
  specified type NEC 386.58
Dysgammaglobulinemia 279.06
Dysgenesis
 gonadal (due to chromosomal anomaly) 758.6
  pure 752.7
 kidney(s) 753.0
 ovarian 758.6
 renal 753.0
 reticular 279.2
 seminiferous tubules 758.6
 tidal platelet 287.31
Dysgerminoma (M9060/3)
 specified site — *see* Neoplasm, by site, malignant
 unspecified site
  female 183.0
  male 186.9
Dysgeusia 781.1
Dysgraphia 781.3
Dyshidrosis 705.81
Dysidrosis 705.81
Dysinsulinism 251.8
Dyskaryotic cervical smear 795.09
Dyskeratosis — *see also* Keratosis 701.1
 bullosa hereditaria 757.39
 cervix 622.10
 congenital 757.39
 follicularis 757.39
  vitamin A deficiency 264.8
 gingiva 523.8
 oral soft tissue NEC 528.79
 tongue 528.79
 uterus NEC 621.8

Dyskinesia 781.3
 biliary 575.8
 esophagus 530.5
 hysterical 300.11
 intestinal 564.89
 neuroleptic-induced tardive 333.85
 nonorganic origin 307.9
 orofacial 333.82
  due to drugs 333.85
 psychogenic 307.9
 subacute, due to drugs 333.85
 tardive (oral) 333.85
Dyslalia 784.59
 developmental 315.39
Dyslexia 784.61
 developmental 315.02
 secondary to organic lesion 784.61
Dyslipidemia 272.4
Dysmaturity — *see also* Immaturity 765.1 ☑
 lung 770.4
 pulmonary 770.4
Dysmenorrhea (essential) (exfoliative) (functional) (intrinsic) (membranous) (primary) (secondary) 625.3
 psychogenic 306.52
Dysmetabolic syndrome X 277.7
Dysmetria 781.3
Dysmorodystrophia mesodermalis congenita 759.82
Dysnomia 784.3
Dysorexia 783.0
 hysterical 300.11
Dysostosis
 cleidocranial, cleidocranialis 755.59
 craniofacial 756.0
 Fairbank's (idiopathic familial generalized osteophytosis) 756.50
 mandibularis 756.0
 mandibulofacial, incomplete 756.0
 multiplex 277.5
 orodigitofacial 759.89
Dyspareunia (female) 625.0
 male 608.89
 psychogenic 302.76
Dyspepsia (allergic) (congenital) (fermentative) (flatulent) (functional) (gastric) (gastrointestinal) (neurogenic) (occupational) (reflex) 536.8
 acid 536.8
 atonic 536.3
  psychogenic 306.4
 diarrhea 787.91
  psychogenic 306.4
 intestinal 564.89
  psychogenic 306.4
 nervous 306.4
 neurotic 306.4
 psychogenic 306.4
Dysphagia 787.20
 cervical 787.29
 functional 300.11
 hysterical 300.11
 nervous 300.11
 neurogenic 787.29
 oral phase 787.21
 oropharyngeal phase 787.22
 pharyngeal phase 787.23
 pharyngoesophageal phase 787.24
 psychogenic 306.4
 sideropenic 280.8
 spastica 530.5
 specified NEC 787.29
Dysphagocytosis, congenital 288.1
Dysphasia 784.59
Dysphonia 784.42
 clericorum 784.49
 functional 300.11
 hysterical 300.11
 psychogenic 306.1
 spastica 478.79
Dyspigmentation — *see also* Pigmentation
 eyelid (acquired) 374.52
Dyspituitarism 253.9
 hyperfunction 253.1
 hypofunction 253.2
 posterior lobe 253.6

Dysplasia — *see also* Anomaly
 alveolar capillary, with vein misalignment 516.64
 anus 569.44
  intraepithelial neoplasia I (AIN I) (histologically confirmed) 569.44
  intraepithelial neoplasia II (AIN II) (histologically confirmed) 569.44
  intraepithelial neoplasia III (AIN III) 230.6
  anal canal 230.5
  mild (histologically confirmed) 569.44
  moderate (histologically confirmed) 569.44
  severe 230.6
   anal canal 230.5
 artery
  fibromuscular NEC 447.8
   carotid 447.8
   renal 447.3
 bladder 596.89
 bone (fibrous) NEC 733.29
  diaphyseal, progressive 756.59
  jaw 526.89
  monostotic 733.29
  polyostotic 756.54
  solitary 733.29
 brain 742.9
 bronchopulmonary, fetus or newborn 770.7
 cervix (uteri) 622.10
  cervical intraepithelial neoplasia I (CIN I) 622.11
  cervical intraepithelial neoplasia II (CIN II) 622.12
  cervical intraepithelial neoplasia III (CIN III) 233.1
  CIN I 622.11
  CIN II 622.12
  CIN III 233.1
  mild 622.11
  moderate 622.12
  severe 233.1
 chondroectodermal 756.55
 chondromatose 756.4
 colon 211.3
 craniocarpotarsal 759.89
 craniometaphyseal 756.89
 dentinal 520.5
 diaphyseal, progressive 756.59
 ectodermal (anhidrotic) (Bason) (Clouston's) (congenital) (Feinmesser) (hereditary) (hidrotic) (Marshall) (Robinson's) 757.31
 epiphysealis 756.9
  multiplex 756.56
  punctata 756.59
 epiphysis 756.9
  multiple 756.56
 epithelial
  epiglottis 478.79
  uterine cervix 622.10
 erythroid NEC 289.89
 eye (*see also* Microphthalmos) 743.10
 familial metaphyseal 756.89
 fibromuscular, artery NEC 447.8
  carotid 447.8
  renal 447.3
 fibrous
  bone NEC 733.29
  diaphyseal, progressive 756.59
  jaw 526.89
  monostotic 733.29
  polyostotic 756.54
  solitary 733.29
 high-grade, focal — *see* Neoplasm, by site, benign
 hip (congenital) 755.63
  with dislocation (*see also* Dislocation, hip, congenital) 754.30
 hypohidrotic ectodermal 757.31
 joint 755.8
 kidney 753.15
 leg 755.69
 linguofacialis 759.89
 lung 748.5
 macular 743.55
 mammary (benign) (gland) 610.9

Dysplasia — *see also* Anomaly — *continued*
 mammary — *continued*
  cystic 610.1
  specified type NEC 610.8
 metaphyseal 756.9
  familial 756.89
 monostotic fibrous 733.29
 muscle 756.89
 myeloid NEC 289.89
 nervous system (general) 742.9
 neuroectodermal 759.6
 oculoauriculovertebral 756.0
 oculodentodigital 759.89
 olfactogenital 253.4
 osteo-onycho-arthro (hereditary) 756.89
 periosteum 733.99
 polyostotic fibrous 756.54
 progressive diaphyseal 756.59
 prostate 602.3
  intraepithelial neoplasia I [PIN I] 602.3
  intraepithelial neoplasia II [PIN II] 602.3
  intraepithelial neoplasia III [PIN III] 233.4
 renal 753.15
 renofacialis 753.0
 retinal NEC 743.56
 retrolental (*see also* Retinopathy of prematurity) 362.21
 skin 709.8
 spinal cord 742.9
 thymic, with immunodeficiency 279.2
 vagina 623.0
  mild 623.0
  moderate 623.0
  severe 233.31
 vocal cord 478.5
 vulva 624.8
  intraepithelial neoplasia I (VIN I) 624.01
  intraepithelial neoplasia II (VIN II) 624.02
  intraepithelial neoplasia III (VIN III) 233.32
  mild 624.01
  moderate 624.02
  severe 233.32
  VIN I 624.01
  VIN II 624.02
  VIN III 233.32
Dyspnea (nocturnal) (paroxysmal) 786.09
 asthmatic (bronchial) (*see also* Asthma) 493.9 ☑
  with bronchitis (*see also* Asthma) 493.9 ☑
   chronic 493.2 ☑
 cardiac (*see also* Failure, ventricular, left) 428.1
 cardiac (*see also* Failure, ventricular, left) 428.1
 functional 300.11
 hyperventilation 786.01
 hysterical 300.11
 Monday morning 504
 newborn 770.89
 psychogenic 306.1
 uremic — *see* Uremia
Dyspraxia 781.3
 syndrome 315.4
Dysproteinemia 273.8
 transient with copper deficiency 281.4
Dysprothrombinemia (constitutional) — *see also* Defect, coagulation 286.3
Dysreflexia, autonomic 337.3
Dysrhythmia
 cardiac 427.9
  postoperative (immediate) 997.1
   long-term effect of cardiac surgery 429.4
  specified type NEC 427.89
 cerebral or cortical 348.30
Dyssecretosis, mucoserous 710.2
Dyssocial reaction, without manifest psychiatric disorder
 adolescent V71.02
 adult V71.01
 child V71.02
Dyssomnia NEC 780.56
 nonorganic origin 307.47

☑ **Additional Digit Required** — Refer to the Tabular List for Digit Selection   ⬆ **Subterms under main terms may continue to next column or page**

2014 ICD-9-CM   ▶◀ **Revised Text**   ● **New Line**   ▲ **Revised Code**   **Volume 2 — 99**

Dysfunction — Dyssomnia

Dysplenism 289.4
Dyssynergia
  biliary (see also Disease, biliary) 576.8
  cerebellaris myoclonica 334.2
  detrusor sphincter (bladder) 596.55
  ventricular 429.89
Dystasia, hereditary areflexic 334.3
Dysthymia 300.4
Dysthymic disorder 300.4
Dysthyroidism 246.9
Dystocia 660.9 ☑
  affecting fetus or newborn 763.1
  cervical 661.2 ☑
    affecting fetus or newborn 763.7
  contraction ring 661.4 ☑
    affecting fetus or newborn 763.7
  fetal 660.9 ☑
    abnormal size 653.5 ☑
    affecting fetus or newborn 763.1
    deformity 653.7 ☑
  maternal 660.9 ☑
    affecting fetus or newborn 763.1
  positional 660.0 ☑
    affecting fetus or newborn 763.1
  shoulder (girdle) 660.4 ☑
    affecting fetus or newborn 763.1
  uterine NEC 661.4 ☑
    affecting fetus or newborn 763.7
Dystonia
  acute
    due to drugs 333.72
      neuroleptic-induced acute 333.72
  deformans progressiva 333.6
  lenticularis 333.6
  musculorum deformans 333.6
  torsion (idiopathic) 333.6
    acquired 333.79
    fragments (of) 333.89
    genetic 333.6
    symptomatic 333.79
Dystonic
  movements 781.0
Dystopia kidney 753.3
Dystrophia myotonica 359.2 ☑
Dystrophy, dystrophia 783.9
  adiposogenital 253.8
  asphyxiating thoracic 756.4
  Becker's type 359.22
  brevicollis 756.16
  Bruch's membrane 362.77
  cervical (sympathetic) NEC 337.09
  chondro-osseous with punctate epiphyseal
    dysplasia 756.59
  choroid (hereditary) 363.50
    central (areolar) (partial) 363.53
      total (gyrate) 363.54
    circinate 363.53
    circumpapillary (partial) 363.51
      total 363.52
    diffuse
      partial 363.56
      total 363.57
    generalized
      partial 363.56
      total 363.57
    gyrate
      central 363.54
      generalized 363.57
    helicoid 363.52
    peripapillary — see Dystrophy, choroid,
      circumpapillary
    serpiginous 363.54
  cornea (hereditary) 371.50
    anterior NEC 371.52
    Cogan's 371.52
    combined 371.57
    crystalline 371.56
    endothelial (Fuchs') 371.57
    epithelial 371.50
      juvenile 371.51
      microscopic cystic 371.52
    granular 371.53
    lattice 371.54
    macular 371.55
    marginal (Terrien's) 371.48
    Meesman's 371.51

Dystrophy, dystrophia — continued
  cornea — continued
    microscopic cystic (epithelial) 371.52
    nodular, Salzmann's 371.46
    polymorphous 371.58
    posterior NEC 371.58
    ring-like 371.52
    Salzmann's nodular 371.46
    stromal NEC 371.56
  dermatochondrocorneal 371.50
  Duchenne's 359.1
  due to malnutrition 263.9
  Erb's 359.1
  familial
    hyperplastic periosteal 756.59
    osseous 277.5
  foveal 362.77
  Fuchs', cornea 371.57
  Gowers' muscular 359.1
  hair 704.2
  hereditary, progressive muscular 359.1
  hypogenital, with diabetic tendency 759.81
  Landouzy-Déjérine 359.1
  Leyden-Möbius 359.1
  mesodermalis congenita 759.82
  muscular 359.1
    congenital (hereditary) 359.0
      myotonic 359.22
    distal 359.1
    Duchenne's 359.1
    Erb's 359.1
    fascioscapulohumeral 359.1
    Gowers' 359.1
    hereditary (progressive) 359.1
    Landouzy-Déjérine 359.1
    limb-girdle 359.1
    myotonic 359.21
    progressive (hereditary) 359.1
      Charcôt-Marie-Tooth 356.1
    pseudohypertrophic (infantile) 359.1
  myocardium, myocardial (see also Degener-
    ation, myocardial) 429.1
  myotonic 359.21
  myotonica 359.21
  nail 703.8
    congenital 757.5
  neurovascular (traumatic) (see also Neuropa-
    thy, peripheral, autonomic) 337.9
  nutritional 263.9
  ocular 359.1
  oculocerebrorenal 270.8
  oculopharyngeal 359.1
  ovarian 620.8
  papillary (and pigmentary) 701.1
  pelvicrural atrophic 359.1
  pigmentary (see also Acanthosis) 701.2
  pituitary (gland) 253.8
  polyglandular 258.8
  posttraumatic sympathetic — see Dystro-
    phy, sympathetic
  progressive ophthalmoplegic 359.1
  reflex neuromuscular — see Dystrophy,
    sympathetic
  retina, retinal (hereditary) 362.70
    albipunctate 362.74
    Bruch's membrane 362.77
    cone, progressive 362.75
    hyaline 362.77
    in
      Bassen-Kornzweig syndrome
        272.5 [362.72]
      cerebroretinal lipidosis 330.1 [362.71]
      Refsum's disease 356.3 [362.72]
      systemic lipidosis 272.7 [362.71]
    juvenile (Stargardt's) 362.75
    pigmentary 362.74
    pigment epithelium 362.76
    progressive cone (-rod) 362.75
    pseudoinflammatory foveal 362.77
    rod, progressive 362.75
    sensory 362.75
    vitelliform 362.76
  Salzmann's nodular 371.46
  scapuloperoneal 359.1
  skin NEC 709.9
  sympathetic (posttraumatic) (reflex) 337.20

Dystrophy, dystrophia — continued
  sympathetic — continued
    lower limb 337.22
    specified site NEC 337.29
    upper limb 337.21
  tapetoretinal NEC 362.74
  thoracic asphyxiating 756.4
  unguium 703.8
    congenital 757.5
  vitreoretinal (primary) 362.73
    secondary 362.66
  vulva 624.09
Dysuria 788.1
  psychogenic 306.53

Eagle-Barrett syndrome 756.71
Eales' disease (syndrome) 362.18
Ear — see also condition
  ache 388.70
    otogenic 388.71
    referred 388.72
  lop 744.29
  piercing V50.3
  swimmers' acute 380.12
  tank 380.12
  tropical 111.8 [380.15]
  wax 380.4
Earache 388.70
  otogenic 388.71
  referred 388.72
Early satiety 780.94
Eaton-Lambert syndrome — see also Syndrome, Lambert-Eaton) 358.30
Eberth's disease (typhoid fever) 002.0
Ebstein's
  anomaly or syndrome (downward displace-
    ment, tricuspid valve into right ven-
    tricle) 746.2
  disease (diabetes) 250.4 ☑ [581.81]
    due to secondary diabetes
      249.4 ☑ [581.81]
Eccentro-osteochondrodysplasia 277.5
Ecchondroma (M9210/0) — see Neoplasm,
  bone, benign
Ecchondrosis (M9210/1) 238.0
Ecchordosis physaliphora 756.0
Ecchymosis (multiple) 459.89
  conjunctiva 372.72
  eye (traumatic) 921.0
  eyelids (traumatic) 921.1
  newborn 772.6
  spontaneous 782.7
  traumatic — see Contusion
ECD (Erdheim-Chester disease) 277.89
Echinococciasis — see Echinococcus
Echinococcosis — see Echinococcus
Echinococcus (infection) 122.9
  granulosus 122.4
    liver 122.0
    lung 122.1
    orbit 122.3 [376.13]
    specified site NEC 122.3
    thyroid 122.2
  liver NEC 122.8
    granulosus 122.0
    multilocularis 122.5
  lung NEC 122.9
    granulosus 122.1
    multilocularis 122.6
  multilocularis 122.7
    liver 122.5
    specified site NEC 122.6
  orbit 122.9 [376.13]
    granulosus 122.3 [376.13]
    multilocularis 122.6 [376.13]
  specified site NEC 122.9
    granulosus 122.3
    multilocularis 122.6 [376.13]
  thyroid NEC 122.9
    granulosus 122.2
    multilocularis 122.6
Echinorhynchiasis 127.7
Echinostomiasis 121.8
Echolalia 784.69
ECHO virus infection NEC 079.1

Eclampsia, eclamptic (coma) (convulsions)
  (delirium) 780.39
  female, child-bearing age NEC — see
    Eclampsia, pregnancy
  gravidarum — see Eclampsia, pregnancy
  male 780.39
  not associated with pregnancy or childbirth
    780.39
  pregnancy, childbirth, or puerperium
    642.6 ☑
    with pre-existing hypertension 642.7 ☑
    affecting fetus or newborn 760.0
  uremic 586
Eclipse blindness (total) 363.31
Economic circumstance affecting care V60.9
  specified type NEC V60.89
Economo's disease (encephalitis lethargica)
  049.8
Ectasia, ectasis
  annuloaortic 424.1
  aorta (see also Ectasia, aortic) 447.70
    with aneurysm 441.9
      ruptured 441.5
  aortic 447.70
    with aneurysm 441.9
      abdominal 447.72
      thoracic 447.71
      thoracoabdominal 447.73
  breast 610.4
  capillary 448.9
  cornea (marginal) (postinfectional) 371.71
  duct (mammary) 610.4
  gastric antral vascular (GAVE) 537.82
    with hemorrhage 537.83
    without hemorrhage 537.82
  kidney 593.89
  mammary duct (gland) 610.4
  papillary 448.9
  renal 593.89
  salivary gland (duct) 527.8
  scar, cornea 371.71
  sclera 379.11
Ecthyma 686.8
  contagiosum 051.2
  gangrenosum 686.09
  infectiosum 051.2
Ectocardia 746.87
Ectodermal dysplasia, congenital 757.31
Ectodermosis erosiva pluriorificialis 695.19
Ectopic, ectopia (congenital) 759.89
  abdominal viscera 751.8
    due to defect in anterior abdominal wall
      756.79
  ACTH syndrome 255.0
  adrenal gland 759.1
  anus 751.5
  auricular beats 427.61
  beats 427.60
  bladder 753.5
  bone and cartilage in lung 748.69
  brain 742.4
  breast tissue 757.6
  cardiac 746.87
  cerebral 742.4
  cordis 746.87
  endometrium 617.9
  gallbladder 751.69
  gastric mucosa 750.7
  gestation — see Pregnancy, ectopic
  heart 746.87
  hormone secretion NEC 259.3
  hyperparathyroidism 259.3
  kidney (crossed) (intrathoracic) (pelvis)
    753.3
    in pregnancy or childbirth 654.4 ☑
      causing obstructed labor 660.2 ☑
  lens 743.37
  lentis 743.37
  mole — see Pregnancy, ectopic
  organ or site NEC — see Malposition, con-
    genital
  ovary 752.0
  pancreas, pancreatic tissue 751.7
  pregnancy — see Pregnancy, ectopic
  pupil 364.75
  renal 753.3

☑ Additional Digit Required — Refer to the Tabular List for Digit Selection   ⛶ Subterms under main terms may continue to next column or page

100 — Volume 2   ▶◀ Revised Text   ● New Line   ▲ Revised Code   2014 ICD-9-CM

Ectopic, ectopia — *continued*
　sebaceous glands of mouth 750.26
　secretion
　　ACTH 255.0
　　adrenal hormone 259.3
　　adrenalin 259.3
　　adrenocorticotropin 255.0
　　antidiuretic hormone (ADH) 259.3
　　epinephrine 259.3
　　hormone NEC 259.3
　　norepinephrine 259.3
　　pituitary (posterior) 259.3
　spleen 759.0
　testis 752.51
　thyroid 759.2
　ureter 753.4
　ventricular beats 427.69
　vesicae 753.5
Ectrodactyly 755.4
　finger (*see also* Absence, finger, congenital)
　　755.29
　toe (*see also* Absence, toe, congenital)
　　755.39
Ectromelia 755.4
　lower limb 755.30
　upper limb 755.20
Ectropion 374.10
　anus 569.49
　cervix 622.0
　　with mention of cervicitis 616.0
　cicatricial 374.14
　congenital 743.62
　eyelid 374.10
　　cicatricial 374.14
　　congenital 743.62
　　mechanical 374.12
　　paralytic 374.12
　　senile 374.11
　　spastic 374.13
　iris (pigment epithelium) 364.54
　lip (congenital) 750.26
　　acquired 528.5
　mechanical 374.12
　paralytic 374.12
　rectum 569.49
　senile 374.11
　spastic 374.13
　urethra 599.84
　uvea 364.54
Eczema (acute) (allergic) (chronic) (erythematous) (fissum) (occupational) (rubrum) (squamous) 692.9
　asteatotic 706.8
　atopic 691.8
　contact NEC 692.9
　dermatitis NEC 692.9
　due to specified cause — *see* Dermatitis, due to
　dyshidrotic 705.81
　external ear 380.22
　flexural 691.8
　gouty 274.89
　herpeticum 054.0
　hypertrophicum 701.8
　hypostatic — *see* Varicose, vein
　impetiginous 684
　infantile (acute) (chronic) (due to any substance) (intertriginous) (seborrheic)
　　690.12
　intertriginous NEC 692.9
　　infantile 690.12
　intrinsic 691.8
　lichenified NEC 692.9
　marginatum 110.3
　nummular 692.9
　pustular 686.8
　seborrheic 690.18
　　infantile 690.12
　solare 692.72
　stasis (lower extremity) 454.1
　　ulcerated 454.2
　vaccination, vaccinatum 999.0
　varicose (lower extremity) — *see* Varicose, vein
　verrucosum callosum 698.3
Eczematoid, exudative 691.8

Eddowes' syndrome (brittle bones and blue sclera) 756.51
Edema, edematous 782.3
　with nephritis (*see also* Nephrosis) 581.9
　allergic 995.1
　angioneurotic (allergic) (any site) (with urticaria) 995.1
　　hereditary 277.6
　angiospastic 443.9
　Berlin's (traumatic) 921.3
　brain (cytotoxic) (vasogenic) 348.5
　　due to birth injury 767.8
　　fetus or newborn 767.8
　cardiac (*see also* Failure, heart) 428.0
　cardiovascular (*see also* Failure, heart) 428.0
　cerebral — *see* Edema, brain
　cerebrospinal vessel — *see* Edema, brain
　cervix (acute) (uteri) 622.8
　　puerperal, postpartum 674.8 ☑
　chronic hereditary 757.0
　circumscribed, acute 995.1
　　hereditary 277.6
　complicating pregnancy (gestational)
　　646.1 ☑
　　with hypertension — *see* Toxemia, of pregnancy
　conjunctiva 372.73
　connective tissue 782.3
　cornea 371.20
　　due to contact lenses 371.24
　　idiopathic 371.21
　　secondary 371.22
　cystoid macular 362.53
　due to
　　lymphatic obstruction — *see* Edema, lymphatic
　　salt retention 276.0
　epiglottis — *see* Edema, glottis
　essential, acute 995.1
　　hereditary 277.6
　extremities, lower — *see* Edema, legs
　eyelid NEC 374.82
　familial, hereditary (legs) 757.0
　famine 262
　fetus or newborn 778.5
　genital organs
　　female 629.89
　　male 608.86
　gestational 646.1 ☑
　　with hypertension — *see* Toxemia, of pregnancy
　glottis, glottic, glottides (obstructive) (passive) 478.6
　　allergic 995.1
　　hereditary 277.6
　　due to external agent — *see* Condition, respiratory, acute, due to specified agent
　heart (*see also* Failure, heart) 428.0
　　newborn 779.89
　heat 992.7
　hereditary (legs) 757.0
　inanition 262
　infectious 782.3
　intracranial 348.5
　　due to injury at birth 767.8
　iris 364.89
　joint (*see also* Effusion, joint) 719.0 ☑
　larynx (*see also* Edema, glottis) 478.6
　legs 782.3
　　due to venous obstruction 459.2
　　hereditary 757.0
　localized 782.3
　　due to venous obstruction 459.2
　　lower extremity 459.2
　lower extremities — *see* Edema, legs
　lung 514
　　acute 518.4
　　　with heart disease or failure (*see also* Failure, ventricular, left) 428.1
　　　congestive 428.0
　　　chemical (due to fumes or vapors) 506.1
　　　due to
　　　　external agent(s) NEC 508.9
　　　　specified NEC 508.8

Edema, edematous — *continued*
　lung — *continued*
　　acute — *continued*
　　　due to — *continued*
　　　　fumes and vapors (chemical) (inhalation) 506.1
　　　　radiation 508.0
　　　chemical (acute) 506.1
　　　　chronic 506.4
　　　chronic 514
　　　　chemical (due to fumes or vapors) 506.4
　　　　due to
　　　　　external agent(s) NEC 508.9
　　　　　　specified NEC 508.8
　　　　　fumes or vapors (chemical) (inhalation) 506.4
　　　　　radiation 508.1
　　　due to
　　　　external agent 508.9
　　　　　specified NEC 508.8
　　　　high altitude 993.2
　　　　near drowning 994.1
　　　postoperative 518.4
　　　terminal 514
　lymphatic 457.1
　　due to mastectomy operation 457.0
　macula 362.83
　　cystoid 362.53
　　diabetic 250.5 ☑ [362.07]
　　　due to secondary diabetes
　　　　249.5 ☑ [362.07]
　malignant (*see also* Gangrene, gas) 040.0
　Milroy's 757.0
　nasopharynx 478.25
　neonatorum 778.5
　nutritional (newborn) 262
　　with dyspigmentation, skin and hair 260
　optic disc or nerve — *see* Papilledema
　orbit 376.33
　　circulatory 459.89
　palate (soft) (hard) 528.9
　pancreas 577.8
　penis 607.83
　periodic 995.1
　　hereditary 277.6
　pharynx 478.25
　pitting 782.3
　pulmonary — *see* Edema, lung
　Quincke's 995.1
　　hereditary 277.6
　renal (*see also* Nephrosis) 581.9
　retina (localized) (macular) (peripheral)
　　362.83
　　cystoid 362.53
　　diabetic 250.5 ☑ [362.07]
　　　due to secondary diabetes
　　　　249.5 ☑ [362.07]
　salt 276.0
　scrotum 608.86
　seminal vesicle 608.86
　spermatic cord 608.86
　spinal cord 336.1
　starvation 262
　stasis (*see also* Hypertension, venous) 459.30
　subconjunctival 372.73
　subglottic (*see also* Edema, glottis) 478.6
　supraglottic (*see also* Edema, glottis) 478.6
　testis 608.86
　toxic NEC 782.3
　traumatic NEC 782.3
　tunica vaginalis 608.86
　vas deferens 608.86
　vocal cord — *see* Edema, glottis
　vulva (acute) 624.8
Edentia (complete) (partial) — *see also* Absence, tooth 520.0
　acquired (*see also* Edentulism) 525.40
　　due to
　　　caries 525.13
　　　extraction 525.10
　　　periodontal disease 525.12
　　　specified NEC 525.19
　　　trauma 525.11
　　causing malocclusion 524.30
　congenital (deficiency of tooth buds) 520.0

Edentulism 525.40
　complete 525.40
　　class I 525.41
　　class II 525.42
　　class III 525.43
　　class IV 525.44
　partial 525.50
　　class I 525.51
　　class II 525.52
　　class III 525.53
　　class IV 525.54
Edsall's disease 992.2
Educational handicap V62.3
Edwards' syndrome 758.2
Effect, adverse NEC
　abnormal gravitational (G) forces or states 994.9
　air pressure — *see* Effect, adverse, atmospheric pressure
　altitude (high) — *see* Effect, adverse, high altitude
　anesthetic
　　in labor and delivery NEC 668.9 ☑
　　affecting fetus or newborn 763.5
　antitoxin — *see* Complications, vaccination
　atmospheric pressure 993.9
　　due to explosion 993.4
　　high 993.3
　　low — *see* Effect, adverse, high altitude
　　specified effect NEC 993.8
　biological, correct substance properly administered (*see also* Effect, adverse, drug) 995.20
　blood (derivatives) (serum) (transfusion) — *see* Complications, transfusion
　chemical substance NEC 989.9
　　specified — *see* Table of Drugs and Chemicals
　cobalt, radioactive (*see also* Effect, adverse, radioactive substance) 990
　cold (temperature) (weather) 991.9
　　chilblains 991.5
　　frostbite — *see* Frostbite
　　specified effect NEC 991.8
　drugs and medicinals 995.20
　　correct substance properly administered 995.20
　　overdose or wrong substance given or taken 977.9
　　specified drug — *see* Table of Drugs and Chemicals
　electric current (shock) 994.8
　　burn — *see* Burn, by site
　electricity (electrocution) (shock) 994.8
　　burn — *see* Burn, by site
　exertion (excessive) 994.5
　exposure 994.9
　　exhaustion 994.4
　external cause NEC 994.9
　fallout (radioactive) NEC 990
　fluoroscopy NEC 990
　foodstuffs
　　anaphylactic reaction or shock due to food NEC — *see* Anaphylactic reaction or shock, due to food
　　noxious 988.9
　　　specified type NEC (*see also* Poisoning, by name of noxious foodstuff) 988.8
　gases, fumes, or vapors — *see* Table of Drugs and Chemicals
　glue (airplane) sniffing 304.6 ☑
　heat — *see* Heat
　high altitude NEC 993.2
　　anoxia 993.2
　　on
　　　ears 993.0
　　　sinuses 993.1
　　polycythemia 289.0
　hot weather — *see* Heat
　hunger 994.2
　immersion, foot 991.4
　immunization — *see* Complications, vaccination
　immunological agents — *see* Complications, vaccination

☑ **Additional Digit Required — Refer to the Tabular List for Digit Selection**　　　　　　　▽ **Subterms under main terms may continue to next column or page**

2014 ICD-9-CM　　　▶◀ Revised Text　　　● New Line　　　▲ Revised Code　　　　　　　　　　　Volume 2 — 101

Effect, adverse — *continued*
  implantation (removable) of isotope or radium NEC 990
  infrared (radiation) (rays) NEC 990
    burn — *see* Burn, by site
    dermatitis or eczema 692.82
  infusion — *see* Complications, infusion
  ingestion or injection of isotope (therapeutic) NEC 990
  irradiation NEC (*see also* Effect, adverse, radiation) 990
  isotope (radioactive) NEC 990
  lack of care (child) (infant) (newborn) 995.52
    adult 995.84
  lightning 994.0
    burn — *see* Burn, by site
  Lirugin — *see* Complications, vaccination
  medicinal substance, correct, properly administered (*see also* Effect, adverse, drugs) 995.20
  mesothorium NEC 990
  motion 994.6
  noise, inner ear 388.10
  other drug, medicinal and biological substance 995.29
  overheated places — *see* Heat
  polonium NEC 990
  psychosocial, of work environment V62.1
  radiation (diagnostic) (fallout) (infrared) (natural source) (therapeutic) (tracer) (ultraviolet) (x-ray) NEC 990
    with pulmonary manifestations
      acute 508.0
      chronic 508.1
    dermatitis or eczema 692.82
      due to sun NEC (*see also* Dermatitis, due to, sun) 692.70
    fibrosis of lungs 508.1
    maternal with suspected damage to fetus affecting management of pregnancy 655.6 ☑
    pneumonitis 508.0
  radioactive substance NEC 990
    dermatitis or eczema 692.82
  radioactivity NEC 990
  radiotherapy NEC 990
    dermatitis or eczema 692.82
  radium NEC 990
  reduced temperature 991.9
    frostbite — *see* Frostbite
    immersion, foot (hand) 991.4
    specified effect NEC 991.8
  roentgenography NEC 990
  roentgenoscopy NEC 990
  roentgen rays NEC 990
  serum (prophylactic) (therapeutic) NEC 999.59
  specified NEC 995.89
    external cause NEC 994.9
  strangulation 994.7
  submersion 994.1
  teletherapy NEC 990
  thirst 994.3
  transfusion — *see* Complications, transfusion
  ultraviolet (radiation) (rays) NEC 990
    burn (*see also* Burn, by site)
      from sun (*see also* Sunburn) 692.71
    dermatitis or eczema 692.82
      due to sun NEC (*see also* Dermatitis, due to, sun) 692.70
  uranium NEC 990
  vaccine (any) — *see* Complications, vaccination
  weightlessness 994.9
  whole blood (*see also* Complications, transfusion)
    overdose or wrong substance given (*see also* Table of Drugs and Chemicals) 964.7
  working environment V62.1
  x-rays NEC 990
    dermatitis or eczema 692.82
Effect, remote
  of cancer — *see* condition
Effects, late — *see* Late, effect (of)

Effluvium, telogen 704.02
Effort
  intolerance 306.2
  syndrome (aviators) (psychogenic) 306.2
Effusion
  amniotic fluid (*see also* Rupture, membranes, premature) 658.1 ☑
  brain (serous) 348.5
  bronchial (*see also* Bronchitis) 490
  cerebral 348.5
  cerebrospinal (*see also* Meningitis) 322.9
    vessel 348.5
  chest — *see* Effusion, pleura
  intracranial 348.5
  joint 719.00
    ankle 719.07
    elbow 719.02
    foot 719.07
    hand 719.04
    hip 719.05
    knee 719.06
    multiple sites 719.09
    pelvic region 719.05
    shoulder (region) 719.01
    specified site NEC 719.08
    wrist 719.03
  meninges (*see also* Meningitis) 322.9
  pericardium, pericardial (*see also* Pericarditis) 423.9
    acute 420.90
  peritoneal (chronic) 568.82
  pleura, pleurisy, pleuritic, pleuropericardial 511.9
    bacterial, nontuberculous 511.1
    fetus or newborn 511.9
    malignant 511.81
    nontuberculous 511.9
      bacterial 511.1
      pneumococcal 511.1
      staphylococcal 511.1
      streptococcal 511.1
    traumatic 862.29
      with open wound 862.39
    tuberculous (*see also* Tuberculosis, pleura) 012.0 ☑
      primary progressive 010.1 ☑
  pulmonary — *see* Effusion, pleura
  spinal (*see also* Meningitis) 322.9
  thorax, thoracic — *see* Effusion, pleura
Egg (oocyte) (ovum)
  donor V59.70
    over age 35 V59.73
      anonymous recipient V59.73
      designated recipient V59.74
    under age 35 V59.71
      anonymous recipient V59.71
      designated recipient V59.72
Eggshell nails 703.8
  congenital 757.5
Ego-dystonic
  homosexuality 302.0
  lesbianism 302.0
  sexual orientation 302.0
Egyptian splenomegaly 120.1
Ehlers-Danlos syndrome 756.83
Ehrlichiosis 082.40
  chaffeensis 082.41
  specified type NEC 082.49
Eichstedt's disease (pityriasis versicolor) 111.0
EIN (endometrial intraepithelial neoplasia) 621.35
Eisenmenger's complex or syndrome (ventricular septal defect) 745.4
Ejaculation, semen
  painful 608.89
    psychogenic 306.59
  premature 302.75
  retrograde 608.87
Ekbom syndrome (restless legs) 333.94
Ekman's syndrome (brittle bones and blue sclera) 756.51
Elastic skin 756.83
  acquired 701.8
Elastofibroma (M8820/0) — *see* Neoplasm, connective tissue, benign

Elastoidosis
  cutanea nodularis 701.8
  cutis cystica et comedonica 701.8
Elastoma 757.39
  juvenile 757.39
  Miescher's (elastosis perforans serpiginosa) 701.1
Elastomyofibrosis 425.3
Elastosis 701.8
  atrophicans 701.8
  perforans serpiginosa 701.1
  reactive perforating 701.1
  senilis 701.8
  solar (actinic) 692.74
Elbow — *see* condition
Electric
  current, electricity, effects (concussion) (fatal) (nonfatal) (shock) 994.8
    burn — *see* Burn, by site
  feet (foot) syndrome 266.2
  shock from electroshock gun (taser) 994.8
Electrocution 994.8
Electrolyte imbalance 276.9
  with
    abortion — *see* Abortion, by type, with metabolic disorder
    ectopic pregnancy (*see also* categories 633.0–633.9) 639.4
    hyperemesis gravidarum (before 22 completed weeks gestation) 643.1 ☑
    molar pregnancy (*see also* categories 630–632) 639.4
  following
    abortion 639.4
    ectopic or molar pregnancy 639.4
Elephantiasis (nonfilarial) 457.1
  arabicum (*see also* Infestation, filarial) 125.9
  congenita hereditaria 757.0
  congenital (any site) 757.0
  due to
    Brugia (malayi) 125.1
    mastectomy operation 457.0
    Wuchereria (bancrofti) 125.0
      malayi 125.1
  eyelid 374.83
  filarial (*see also* Infestation, filarial) 125.9
  filariensis (*see also* Infestation, filarial) 125.9
  gingival 523.8
  glandular 457.1
  graecorum 030.9
  lymphangiectatic 457.1
  lymphatic vessel 457.1
    due to mastectomy operation 457.0
  neuromatosa 237.71
  postmastectomy 457.0
  scrotum 457.1
  streptococcal 457.1
  surgical 997.99
    postmastectomy 457.0
  telangiectodes 457.1
  vulva (nonfilarial) 624.8
Elephant man syndrome 237.71
Elevated — *see* Elevation
  findings on laboratory examination — *see* Findings, abnormal, without diagnosis (examination) (laboratory test)
  GFR (glomerular filtration rate) — *see* Findings, abnormal, without diagnosis (examination) (laboratory test)
Elevation
  17-ketosteroids 791.9
  acid phosphatase 790.5
  alkaline phosphatase 790.5
  amylase 790.5
  antibody titers 795.79
  basal metabolic rate (BMR) 794.7
  blood pressure (*see also* Hypertension) 401.9
    reading (incidental) (isolated) (nonspecific), no diagnosis of hypertension 796.2
  blood sugar 790.29
  body temperature (of unknown origin) (*see also* Pyrexia) 780.60
  C-reactive protein (CRP) 790.95
  cancer antigen 125 [CA 125] 795.82

Elevation — *continued*
  carcinoembryonic antigen [CEA] 795.81
  cholesterol 272.0
    with high triglycerides 272.2
  conjugate, eye 378.81
  CRP (C-reactive protein) 790.95
  diaphragm, congenital 756.6
  GFR (glomerular filtration rate) — *see* Findings, abnormal, without diagnosis (examination) (laboratory test)
  glucose
    fasting 790.21
    tolerance test 790.22
  immunoglobulin level 795.79
  indolacetic acid 791.9
  lactic acid dehydrogenase (LDH) level 790.4
  leukocytes 288.60
  lipase 790.5
  lipoprotein a level 272.8
  liver function test (LFT) 790.6
    alkaline phosphatase 790.5
    aminotransferase 790.4
    bilirubin 782.4
    hepatic enzyme NEC 790.5
    lactate dehydrogenase 790.4
  lymphocytes 288.61
  prostate specific antigen (PSA) 790.93
  renin 790.99
    in hypertension (*see also* Hypertension, renovascular) 405.91
  Rh titer (*see also* Complications, transfusion) 999.70
  scapula, congenital 755.52
  sedimentation rate 790.1
  SGOT 790.4
  SGPT 790.4
  transaminase 790.4
  triglycerides 272.1
    with high cholesterol 272.2
  vanillylmandelic acid 791.9
  venous pressure 459.89
  VMA 791.9
  white blood cell count 288.60
    specified NEC 288.69
Elliptocytosis (congenital) (hereditary) 282.1
  Hb-C (disease) 282.7
  hemoglobin disease 282.7
  sickle-cell (disease) 282.60
    trait 282.5
Ellis-van Creveld disease or syndrome (chondroectodermal dysplasia) 756.55
Ellison-Zollinger syndrome (gastric hypersecretion with pancreatic islet cell tumor) 251.5
Elongation, elongated (congenital) — *see also* Distortion
  bone 756.9
  cervix (uteri) 752.49
    acquired 622.6
    hypertrophic 622.6
  colon 751.5
  common bile duct 751.69
  cystic duct 751.69
  frenulum, penis 752.69
  labia minora, acquired 624.8
  ligamentum patellae 756.89
  petiolus (epiglottidis) 748.3
  styloid bone (process) 733.99
  tooth, teeth 520.2
  uvula 750.26
    acquired 528.9
Elschnig bodies or pearls 366.51
El Tor cholera 001.1
Emaciation (due to malnutrition) 261
Emancipation disorder 309.22
Embadomoniasis 007.8
Embarrassment heart, cardiac — *see* Disease, heart
Embedded
  fragment (status) — *see* Foreign body, retained
  splinter (status) — *see* Foreign body, retained
  tooth, teeth 520.6
    root only 525.3
Embolic — *see* condition

☑ **Additional Digit Required** — Refer to the Tabular List for Digit Selection   ▽ **Subterms under main terms may continue to next column or page**

102 — Volume 2   ▶◀ **Revised Text**   ● **New Line**   ▲ **Revised Code**   **2014 ICD-9-CM**

Embolism 444.9
  with
    abortion — see Abortion, by type, with embolism
    ectopic pregnancy (see also categories 633.0–633.9) 639.6
    molar pregnancy (see also categories 630–632) 639.6
  air (any site) 958.0
    with
      abortion — see Abortion, by type, with embolism
      ectopic pregnancy (see also categories 633.0–633.9) 639.6
      molar pregnancy (see also categories 630–632) 639.6
    due to implanted device — see Complications, due to (presence of) any device, implant, or graft classified to 996.0–996.5 NEC
    following
      abortion 639.6
      ectopic or molar pregnancy 639.6
      infusion, perfusion, or transfusion 999.1
    in pregnancy, childbirth, or puerperium 673.0 ☑
    traumatic 958.0
  amniotic fluid (pulmonary) 673.1 ☑
    with
      abortion — see Abortion, by type, with embolism
      ectopic pregnancy (see also categories 633.0–633.9) 639.6
      molar pregnancy (see also categories 630–632) 639.6
    following
      abortion 639.6
      ectopic or molar pregnancy 639.6
  aorta, aortic 444.1
    abdominal 444.09
      saddle 444.01
    bifurcation 444.09
    saddle 444.01
    thoracic 444.1
  artery 444.9
    auditory, internal 433.8 ☑
    basilar (see also Occlusion, artery, basilar) 433.0 ☑
    bladder 444.89
    carotid (common) (internal) (see also Occlusion, artery, carotid) 433.1 ☑
    cerebellar (anterior inferior) (posterior inferior) (superior) 433.8 ☑
    cerebral (see also Embolism, brain) 434.1 ☑
    choroidal (anterior) 433.8 ☑
    communicating posterior 433.8 ☑
    coronary (see also Infarct, myocardium) 410.9 ☑
      without myocardial infarction 411.81
    extremity 444.22
      lower 444.22
      upper 444.21
    hypophyseal 433.8 ☑
    mesenteric (with gangrene) 557.0
    ophthalmic (see also Occlusion, retina) 362.30
    peripheral 444.22
    pontine 433.8 ☑
    precerebral NEC — see Occlusion, artery, precerebral
    pulmonary — see Embolism, pulmonary
    pyemic 449
      pulmonary 415.12
    renal 593.81
    retinal (see also Occlusion, retina) 362.30
    septic 449
      pulmonary 415.12
    specified site NEC 444.89
    vertebral (see also Occlusion, artery, vertebral) 433.2 ☑
  auditory, internal 433.8 ☑
  basilar (artery) (see also Occlusion, artery, basilar) 433.0 ☑

Embolism — continued
  birth, mother — see Embolism, obstetrical
  blood-clot
    with
      abortion — see Abortion, by type, with embolism
      ectopic pregnancy (see also categories 633.0–633.9) 639.6
      molar pregnancy (see also categories 630–632) 639.6
    following
      abortion 639.6
      ectopic or molar pregnancy 639.6
    in pregnancy, childbirth, or puerperium 673.2 ☑
  brain 434.1 ☑
    with
      abortion — see Abortion, by type, with embolism
      ectopic pregnancy (see also categories 633.0–633.9) 639.6
      molar pregnancy (see also categories 630–632) 639.6
    following
      abortion 639.6
      ectopic or molar pregnancy 639.6
    late effect — see Late effect(s) (of) cerebrovascular disease
    puerperal, postpartum, childbirth 674.0 ☑
  capillary 448.9
  cardiac (see also Infarct, myocardium) 410.9 ☑
  carotid (artery) (common) (internal) (see also Occlusion, artery, carotid) 433.1 ☑
  cavernous sinus (venous) — see Embolism, intracranial venous sinus
  cerebral (see also Embolism, brain) 434.1 ☑
  cholesterol — see Atheroembolism
  choroidal (anterior) (artery) 433.8 ☑
  coronary (artery or vein) (systemic) (see also Infarct, myocardium) 410.9 ☑
    without myocardial infarction 411.81
  due to (presence of) any device, implant, or graft classifiable to 996.0–996.5 — see Complications, due to (presence of) any device, implant, or graft classified to 996.0–996.5 NEC
  encephalomalacia (see also Embolism, brain) 434.1 ☑
  extremities 444.22
    lower 444.22
    upper 444.21
  eye 362.30
  fat (cerebral) (pulmonary) (systemic) 958.1
    with
      abortion — see Abortion, by type, with embolism
      ectopic pregnancy (see also categories 633.0–633.9) 639.6
      molar pregnancy (see also categories 630–632) 639.6
    complicating delivery or puerperium 673.8 ☑
    following
      abortion 639.6
      ectopic or molar pregnancy 639.6
    in pregnancy, childbirth, or the puerperium 673.8 ☑
  femoral (artery) 444.22
    vein 453.6
      deep 453.41
    following
      abortion 639.6
      ectopic or molar pregnancy 639.6
      infusion, perfusion, or transfusion
        air 999.1
        thrombus 999.2
  heart (fatty) (see also Infarct, myocardium) 410.9 ☑
  hepatic (vein) 453.0
  iliac (artery) 444.81
  iliofemoral 444.81
  in pregnancy, childbirth, or puerperium (pulmonary) — see Embolism, obstetrical

Embolism — continued
  intestine (artery) (vein) (with gangrene) 557.0
  intracranial (see also Embolism, brain) 434.1 ☑
    venous sinus (any) 325
      late effect — see category 326
      nonpyogenic 437.6
        in pregnancy or puerperium 671.5 ☑
  kidney (artery) 593.81
  lateral sinus (venous) — see Embolism, intracranial venous sinus
  longitudinal sinus (venous) — see Embolism, intracranial venous sinus
  lower extremity 444.22
  lung (massive) — see Embolism, pulmonary
  meninges (see also Embolism, brain) 434.1 ☑
  mesenteric (artery) (with gangrene) 557.0
  multiple NEC 444.9
  obstetrical (pulmonary) 673.2 ☑
    air 673.0 ☑
    amniotic fluid (pulmonary) 673.1 ☑
    blood-clot 673.2 ☑
    cardiac 674.8 ☑
    fat 673.8 ☑
    heart 674.8 ☑
    pyemic 673.3 ☑
    septic 673.3 ☑
    specified NEC 674.8 ☑
  ophthalmic (see also Occlusion, retina) 362.30
  paradoxical NEC 444.9
  penis 607.82
  peripheral arteries NEC 444.22
    lower 444.22
    upper 444.21
  pituitary 253.8
  popliteal (artery) 444.22
  portal (vein) 452
  postoperative NEC 997.2
    cerebral 997.02
    mesenteric artery 997.71
    other vessels 997.79
    peripheral vascular 997.2
    pulmonary 415.11
      septic 415.11
    renal artery 997.72
  precerebral artery (see also Occlusion, artery, precerebral) 433.9 ☑
  puerperal — see Embolism, obstetrical
  pulmonary (acute) (artery) (vein) 415.19
    with
      abortion — see Abortion, by type, with embolism
      ectopic pregnancy (see also categories 633.0–633.9) 639.6
      molar pregnancy (see also categories 630–632) 639.6
    chronic 416.2
    following
      abortion 639.6
      ectopic or molar pregnancy 639.6
    healed or old V12.55
    iatrogenic 415.11
    in pregnancy, childbirth, or puerperium — see Embolism, obstetrical
    personal history of V12.55
    postoperative 415.11
    septic 415.12
  pyemic (multiple) (see also Septicemia) 415.12
    with
      abortion — see Abortion, by type, with embolism
      ectopic pregnancy (see also categories 633.0–633.9) 639.6
      molar pregnancy (see also categories 630–632) 639.6
    Aerobacter aerogenes 415.12
    enteric gram-negative bacilli 415.12
    Enterobacter aerogenes 415.12
    Escherichia coli 415.12
    following
      abortion 639.6

Embolism — continued
  pyemic (see also Septicemia) — continued
    following — continued
      ectopic or molar pregnancy 639.6
    Hemophilus influenzae 415.12
    pneumococcal 415.12
    Proteus vulgaris 415.12
    Pseudomonas (aeruginosa) 415.12
    puerperal, postpartum, childbirth (any organism) 673.3 ☑
    Serratia 415.12
    specified organism NEC 415.12
    staphylococcal 415.12
      aureus 415.12
      specified organism NEC 415.12
    streptococcal 415.12
  renal (artery) 593.81
    vein 453.3
  retina, retinal (see also Occlusion, retina) 362.30
  saddle
    abdominal aorta 444.01
    pulmonary artery 415.13
  septic 415.12
    arterial 449
  septicemic — see Embolism, pyemic
  sinus — see Embolism, intracranial venous sinus
  soap
    with
      abortion — see Abortion, by type, with embolism
      ectopic pregnancy (see also categories 633.0–633.9) 639.6
      molar pregnancy (see also categories 630–632) 639.6
    following
      abortion 639.6
      ectopic or molar pregnancy 639.6
  spinal cord (nonpyogenic) 336.1
    in pregnancy or puerperium 671.5 ☑
    pyogenic origin 324.1
      late effect — see category 326
  spleen, splenic (artery) 444.89
  thrombus (thromboembolism) following infusion, perfusion, or transfusion 999.2
  upper extremity 444.21
  vein 453.9
    with inflammation or phlebitis — see Thrombophlebitis
    antecubital (acute) 453.81
      chronic 453.71
    axillary (acute) 453.84
      chronic 453.74
    basilic (acute) 453.81
      chronic 453.71
    brachial (acute) 453.82
      chronic 453.72
    brachiocephalic (acute) (innominate) 453.87
      chronic 453.77
    cephalic (acute) 453.81
      chronic 453.71
    cerebral (see also Embolism, brain) 434.1 ☑
    coronary (see also Infarct, myocardium) 410.9 ☑
      without myocardial infarction 411.81
    hepatic 453.0
    internal jugular (acute) 453.86
      chronic 453.76
    lower extremity (superficial) 453.6
      deep 453.40
        acute 453.40
          calf 453.42
          distal (lower leg) 453.42
          femoral 453.41
          iliac 453.41
          lower leg 453.42
          peroneal 453.42
          popliteal 453.41
          proximal (upper leg) 453.41
          thigh 453.41
          tibial 453.42

☑ Additional Digit Required — Refer to the Tabular List for Digit Selection   Subterms under main terms may continue to next column or page

2014 ICD-9-CM   ►◄ Revised Text   ● New Line   ▲ Revised Code   Volume 2 — 103

Index   Embolism — Embolism

Embolism — continued
- vein — continued
  - lower extremity — continued
    - deep — continued
      - chronic 453.50
        - calf 453.52
        - disal (lower leg) 453.52
        - femoral 453.51
        - iliac 453.51
        - lower leg 453.52
        - peroneal 453.52
        - popliteal 453.51
        - proximal (upper leg) 453.51
        - thigh 453.51
        - tibial 453.52
      - saphenous (greater) (lesser) 453.6
      - superficial 453.6
  - mesenteric (with gangrene) 557.0
  - portal 452
  - pulmonary — see Embolism, pulmonary
  - radial (acute) 453.82
    - chronic 453.72
  - renal 453.3
  - saphenous (greater) (lesser) 453.6
  - specified NEC (acute) 453.89
    - with inflammation or phlebitis — see Thrombophlebitis
    - chronic 453.79
  - subclavian (acute) 453.85
    - chronic 453.75
  - superior vena cava (acute) 453.87
    - chronic 453.77
  - thoracic (acute) 453.87
    - chronic 453.77
  - ulnar (acute) 453.82
    - chronic 453.72
  - upper extremity (acute) 453.83
    - chronic 453.73
      - deep 453.72
        - superficial 453.71
      - deep 453.82
      - superficial 453.81
  - vena cava
    - inferior 453.2
    - superior (acute) 453.87
      - chronic 453.77
  - vessels of brain (see also Embolism, brain) 434.1 ☑

Embolization — see Embolism

Embolus — see Embolism

Embryoma (M9080/1) — see also Neoplasm, by site, uncertain behavior
- benign (M9080/0) — see Neoplasm, by site, benign
- kidney (M8960/3) 189.0
- liver (M8970/3) 155.0
- malignant (M9080/3) (see also Neoplasm, by site, malignant)
  - kidney (M8960/3) 189.0
  - liver (M8970/3) 155.0
  - testis (M9070/3) 186.9
    - undescended 186.0
- testis (M9070/3) 186.9
  - undescended 186.0

Embryonic
- circulation 747.9
- heart 747.9
- vas deferens 752.89

Embryopathia NEC 759.9

Embryotomy, fetal 763.89

Embryotoxon 743.43
- interfering with vision 743.42

Emesis — see also Vomiting
- bilious 787.04
- gravidarum — see Hyperemesis, gravidarum

Emissions, nocturnal (semen) 608.89

Emotional
- crisis — see Crisis, emotional
- disorder (see also Disorder, mental) 300.9
- instability (excessive) 301.3
- lability 799.24
- overlay — see Reaction, adjustment
- upset 300.9

Emotionality, pathological 301.3

Emotogenic disease — see also Disorder, psychogenic 306.9

Emphysema (atrophic) (centriacinar) (centrilobular) (chronic) (diffuse) (essential) (hypertrophic) (interlobular) (lung) (obstructive) (panlobular) (paracatricial) (paracinar) (postural) (pulmonary) (senile) (subpleural) (traction) (unilateral) (unilobular) (vesicular) 492.8
- with bronchitis
  - chronic 491.20
    - with
      - acute bronchitis 491.22
      - exacerbation (acute) 491.21
- bullous (giant) 492.0
- cellular tissue 958.7
  - surgical 998.81
- compensatory 518.2
- congenital 770.2
- conjunctiva 372.89
- connective tissue 958.7
  - surgical 998.81
- due to fumes or vapors 506.4
- eye 376.89
- eyelid 374.85
  - surgical 998.81
  - traumatic 958.7
- fetus or newborn (interstitial) (mediastinal) (unilobular) 770.2
- heart 416.9
- interstitial 518.1
  - congenital 770.2
  - fetus or newborn 770.2
- laminated tissue 958.7
  - surgical 998.81
- mediastinal 518.1
  - fetus or newborn 770.2
- newborn (interstitial) (mediastinal) (unilobular) 770.2
- obstructive diffuse with fibrosis 492.8
- orbit 376.89
- subcutaneous 958.7
  - due to trauma 958.7
  - nontraumatic 518.1
  - surgical 998.81
- surgical 998.81
- thymus (gland) (congenital) 254.8
- traumatic 958.7
- tuberculous (see also Tuberculosis, pulmonary) 011.9 ☑

Employment examination (certification) V70.5

Empty sella (turcica) syndrome 253.8

Empyema (chest) (diaphragmatic) (double) (encapsulated) (general) (interlobar) (lung) (medial) (necessitatis) (perforating chest wall) (pleura) (pneumococcal) (residual) (sacculated) (streptococcal) (supradiaphragmatic) 510.9
- with fistula 510.0
- accessory sinus (chronic) (see also Sinusitis) 473.9
- acute 510.9
  - with fistula 510.0
- antrum (chronic) (see also Sinusitis, maxillary) 473.0
- brain (any part) (see also Abscess, brain) 324.0
- ethmoidal (sinus) (chronic) (see also Sinusitis, ethmoidal) 473.2
- extradural (see also Abscess, extradural) 324.9
- frontal (sinus) (chronic) (see also Sinusitis, frontal) 473.1
- gallbladder (see also Cholecystitis, acute) 575.0
- mastoid (process) (acute) (see also Mastoiditis, acute) 383.00
- maxilla, maxillary 526.4
  - sinus (chronic) (see also Sinusitis, maxillary) 473.0
- nasal sinus (chronic) (see also Sinusitis) 473.9
- sinus (accessory) (nasal) (see also Sinusitis) 473.9
- sphenoidal (chronic) (sinus) (see also Sinusitis, sphenoidal) 473.3
- subarachnoid (see also Abscess, extradural) 324.9
- subdural (see also Abscess, extradural) 324.9

Empyema — continued
- tuberculous (see also Tuberculosis, pleura) 012.0 ☑
- ureter (see also Ureteritis) 593.89
- ventricular (see also Abscess, brain) 324.0

Enameloma 520.2

Encephalitis (bacterial) (chronic) (hemorrhagic) (idiopathic) (nonepidemic) (spurious) (subacute) 323.9
- acute (see also Encephalitis, viral)
  - disseminated (postinfectious) NEC 136.9 [323.61]
    - postimmunization or postvaccination 323.51
  - inclusional 049.8
  - inclusion body 049.8
  - necrotizing 049.8
- arboviral, arbovirus NEC 064
- arthropod-borne (see also Encephalitis, viral, arthropod-borne) 064
- Australian X 062.4
- Bwamba fever 066.3
- California (virus) 062.5
- Central European 063.2
- Czechoslovakian 063.2
- Dawson's (inclusion body) 046.2
- diffuse sclerosing 046.2
- due to
  - actinomycosis 039.8 [323.41]
  - cat-scratch disease 078.3 [323.01]
  - human herpesvirus 6 058.21
  - human herpesvirus 7 058.29
  - human herpesvirus NEC 058.29
  - human immunodeficiency virus (HIV) disease 042 [323.01]
  - infectious mononucleosis 075 [323.01]
  - malaria (see also Malaria) 084.6 [323.2]
  - Negishi virus 064
  - ornithosis 073.7 [323.01]
  - other infection classified elsewhere 136.9 [323.41]
  - prophylactic inoculation against smallpox 323.51
  - rickettsiosis (see also Rickettsiosis) 083.9 [323.1]
  - rubella 056.01
  - toxoplasmosis (acquired) 130.0
    - congenital (active) 771.2 [323.41]
  - typhus (fever) (see also Typhus) 081.9 [323.1]
  - vaccination (smallpox) 323.51
- Eastern equine 062.2
- endemic 049.8
- epidemic 049.8
- equine (acute) (infectious) (viral) 062.9
  - Eastern 062.2
  - Venezuelan 066.2
  - Western 062.1
- Far Eastern 063.0
- following vaccination or other immunization procedure 323.51
- herpes 054.3
- human herpesvirus 6 058.21
- human herpesvirus 7 058.29
- human herpesvirus NEC 058.29
- Ilheus (virus) 062.8
- inclusion body 046.2
- infectious (acute) (virus) NEC 049.8
- influenzal (see also Influenza) 487.8 [323.41]
  - lethargic 049.8
- Japanese (B type) 062.0
- La Crosse 062.5
- Langat 063.8
- late effect — see Late, effect, encephalitis
- lead 984.9 [323.71]
- lethargic (acute) (infectious) (influenzal) 049.8
- lethargica 049.8
- louping ill 063.1
- lupus 710.0 [323.81]
- lymphatica 049.0
- Mengo 049.8
- meningococcal 036.1
- mumps 072.2
- Murray Valley 062.4
- myoclonic 049.8

Encephalitis — continued
- Negishi virus 064
- otitic NEC 382.4 [323.41]
- parasitic NEC 123.9 [323.41]
- periaxialis (concentrica) (diffusa) 341.1
- postchickenpox 052.0
- postexanthematous NEC 057.9 [323.62]
- postimmunization 323.51
- postinfectious NEC 136.9 [323.62]
- postmeasles 055.0
- posttraumatic 323.81
- postvaccinal (smallpox) 323.51
- postvaricella 052.0
- postviral NEC 079.99 [323.62]
  - postexanthematous 057.9 [323.62]
    - specified NEC 057.8 [323.62]
- Powassan 063.8
- progressive subcortical (Binswanger's) 290.12
- Rasmussen 323.81
- Rio Bravo 049.8
- rubella 056.01
- Russian
  - autumnal 062.0
  - spring-summer type (taiga) 063.0
- saturnine 984.9 [323.71]
- Semliki Forest 062.8
- serous 048
- slow-acting virus NEC 046.8
- specified cause NEC 323.81
- St. Louis type 062.3
- subacute sclerosing 046.2
- subcorticalis chronica 290.12
- summer 062.0
- suppurative 324.0
- syphilitic 094.81
  - congenital 090.41
- tick-borne 063.9
- torula, torular 117.5 [323.41]
- toxic NEC 989.9 [323.71]
- toxoplasmic (acquired) 130.0
  - congenital (active) 771.2 [323.41]
- trichinosis 124 [323.41]
- Trypanosomiasis (see also Trypanosomiasis) 086.9 [323.2]
- tuberculous (see also Tuberculosis) 013.6 ☑
- type B (Japanese) 062.0
- type C 062.3
- van Bogaert's 046.2
- Venezuelan 066.2
- Vienna type 049.8
- viral, virus 049.9
  - arthropod-borne NEC 064
  - mosquito-borne 062.9
    - Australian X disease 062.4
    - California virus 062.5
    - Eastern equine 062.2
    - Ilheus virus 062.8
    - Japanese (B type) 062.0
    - Murray Valley 062.4
    - specified type NEC 062.8
    - St. Louis 062.3
    - type B 062.0
    - type C 062.3
    - Western equine 062.1
  - tick-borne 063.9
    - biundulant 063.2
    - Central European 063.2
    - Czechoslovakian 063.2
    - diphasic meningoencephalitis 063.2
    - Far Eastern 063.0
    - Langat 063.8
    - louping ill 063.1
    - Powassan 063.8
    - Russian spring-summer (taiga) 063.0
    - specified type NEC 063.8
    - vector unknown 064
    - Western equine 062.1
  - slow acting NEC 046.8
  - specified type NEC 049.8
  - vaccination, prophylactic (against) V05.0
- von Economo's 049.8
- Western equine 062.1
- West Nile type 066.41

Encephalocele 742.0
  orbit 376.81
Encephalocystocele 742.0
Encephaloduroarteriomyosynangiosis (EDAMS) 437.5
Encephalomalacia (brain) (cerebellar) (cerebral) (cerebrospinal) — see also Softening, brain 348.89
  due to
    hemorrhage (see also Hemorrhage, brain) 431
    recurrent spasm of artery 435.9
  embolic (cerebral) (see also Embolism, brain) 434.1 ☑
  subcorticalis chronicus arteriosclerotica 290.12
  thrombotic (see also Thrombosis, brain) 434.0 ☑
Encephalomeningitis — see Meningoencephalitis
Encephalomeningocele 742.0
Encephalomeningomyelitis — see Meningoencephalitis
Encephalomeningopathy — see also Meningoencephalitis 349.9
Encephalomyelitis (chronic) (granulomatous) (myalgic, benign) — see also Encephalitis 323.9
  abortive disseminated 049.8
  acute disseminated (ADEM) (postinfectious) 136.9 [323.61]
    infectious 136.9 [323.61]
    noninfectious 323.81
    postimmunization 323.51
  due to
    cat-scratch disease 078.3 [323.01]
    infectious mononucleosis 075 [323.01]
    ornithosis 073.7 [323.01]
    vaccination (any) 323.51
  equine (acute) (infectious) 062.9
    Eastern 062.2
    Venezuelan 066.2
    Western 062.1
  funicularis infectiosa 049.8
  late effect — see Late, effect, encephalitis
  Munch-Peterson's 049.8
  postchickenpox 052.0
  postimmunization 323.51
  postmeasles 055.0
  postvaccinal (smallpox) 323.51
  rubella 056.01
  specified cause NEC 323.81
  syphilitic 094.81
  West Nile 066.41
Encephalomyelocele 742.0
Encephalomyelomeningitis — see Meningoencephalitis
Encephalomyeloneuropathy 349.9
Encephalomyelopathy 349.9
  subacute necrotizing (infantile) 330.8
Encephalomyeloradiculitis (acute) 357.0
Encephalomyeloradiculoneuritis (acute) 357.0
Encephalomyeloradiculopathy 349.9
Encephalomyocarditis 074.23
Encephalopathia hyperbilirubinemica, newborn 774.7
  due to isoimmunization (conditions classifiable to 773.0–773.2) 773.4
Encephalopathy (acute) 348.30
  alcoholic 291.2
  anoxic — see Damage, brain, anoxic
  arteriosclerotic 437.0
    late effect — see Late effect(s) (of) cerebrovascular disease
  bilirubin, newborn 774.7
    due to isoimmunization 773.4
  congenital 742.9
  demyelinating (callosal) 341.8
  due to
    birth injury (intracranial) 767.8
    dialysis 294.8
      transient 293.9
    drugs — (see also Table of Drugs and Chemicals) 349.82
    hyperinsulinism — see Hyperinsulinism

Encephalopathy — continued
  due to — continued
    influenza (virus) (see also Influenza) 487.8
      identified
        avian 488.09
        (novel) 2009 H1N1 488.19
    lack of vitamin (see also Deficiency, vitamin) 269.2
    nicotinic acid deficiency 291.2
    serum (nontherapeutic) (therapeutic) 999.59
    syphilis 094.81
    trauma (postconcussional) 310.2
      current (see also Concussion, brain) 850.9
        with skull fracture — see Fracture, skull, by site, with intracranial injury
    vaccination 323.51
  hepatic 572.2
  hyperbilirubinemic, newborn 774.7
    due to isoimmunization (conditions classifiable to 773.0–773.2) 773.4
  hypertensive 437.2
  hypoglycemic 251.2
  hypoxic (see also Damage, brain, anoxic)
    ischemic (HIE) 768.70
      mild 768.71
      moderate 768.72
      severe 768.73
  infantile cystic necrotizing (congenital) 341.8
  lead 984.9 [323.71]
  leukopolio 330.0
  metabolic (see also Delirium) 348.31
    drug induced 349.82
    toxic 349.82
  necrotizing
    hemorrhagic (acute) 323.61
    subacute 330.8
  other specified type NEC 348.39
  pellagrous 265.2
  portal-systemic 572.2
  postcontusional 310.2
  posttraumatic 310.2
  saturnine 984.9 [323.71]
  septic 348.31
  spongioform, subacute (viral) 046.19
  subacute
    necrotizing 330.8
    spongioform 046.19
    viral, spongioform 046.19
  subcortical progressive (Schilder) 341.1
    chronic (Binswanger's) 290.12
  toxic 349.82
    metabolic 349.82
  traumatic (postconcussional) 310.2
    current (see also Concussion, brain) 850.9
      with skull fracture — see Fracture, skull, by site, with intracranial injury
  vitamin B deficiency NEC 266.9
  Wernicke's (superior hemorrhagic polioencephalitis) 265.1
Encephalorrhagia — see also Hemorrhage, brain 432.9
  healed or old V12.54
  late effect — see Late effect(s) (of) cerebrovascular disease
Encephalosis, posttraumatic 310.2
Enchondroma (M9220/0) — see also Neoplasm, bone, benign
  multiple, congenital 756.4
Enchondromatosis (cartilaginous) (congenital) (multiple) 756.4
Enchondroses, multiple (cartilaginous) (congenital) 756.4
Encopresis — see also Incontinence, feces 787.60
  nonorganic origin 307.7
Encounter for — see also Admission for —
  administrative purpose only V68.9
    referral of patient without examination or treatment V68.81
    specified purpose NEC V68.89

Encounter for — see also Admission for — continued
  chemotherapy, (oral) (intravenous), antineoplastic V58.11
  determination of fetal viability of pregnancy V23.87
  dialysis
    extracorporeal (renal) V56.0
    peritoneal V56.8
  disability examination V68.01
  end-of-life care V66.7
  hospice care V66.7
  immunizations (childhood) appropriate for age V20.2
  immunotherapy, antineoplastic V58.12
  joint prosthesis insertion following prior explantation of joint prosthesis V54.82
  palliative care V66.7
  paternity testing V70.4
  radiotherapy V58.0
  respirator [ventilator] dependence
    during
      mechanical failure V46.14
      power failure V46.12
    for weaning V46.13
  routine infant and child vision and hearing testing V20.2
  school examination V70.3
    following surgery V67.09
  screening mammogram NEC V76.12
    for high-risk patient V76.11
  terminal care V66.7
  weaning from respirator [ventilator] V46.13
Encystment — see Cyst
End-of-life care V66.7
Endamebiasis — see Amebiasis
Endamoeba — see Amebiasis
Endarteritis (bacterial, subacute) (infective) (septic) 447.6
  brain, cerebral or cerebrospinal 437.4
    late effect — see Late effect(s) (of) cerebrovascular disease
  coronary (artery) — see Arteriosclerosis, coronary
  deformans — see Arteriosclerosis
  embolic (see also Embolism) 444.9
  obliterans (see also Arteriosclerosis)
    pulmonary 417.8
  pulmonary 417.8
  retina 362.18
  senile — see Arteriosclerosis
  syphilitic 093.89
    brain or cerebral 094.89
    congenital 090.5
    spinal 094.89
  tuberculous (see also Tuberculosis) 017.9 ☑
Endemic — see condition
Endocarditis (chronic) (indeterminate) (interstitial) (marantic) (nonbacterial thrombotic) (residual) (sclerotic) (sclerous) (senile) (valvular) 424.90
  with
    rheumatic fever (conditions classifiable to 390)
      active — see Endocarditis, acute, rheumatic
      inactive or quiescent (with chorea) 397.9
  acute or subacute 421.9
    rheumatic (aortic) (mitral) (pulmonary) (tricuspid) 391.1
      with chorea (acute) (rheumatic) (Sydenham's) 392.0
  aortic (heart) (nonrheumatic) (valve) 424.1
    with
      mitral (valve) disease 396.9
        active or acute 391.1
          with chorea (acute) (rheumatic) (Sydenham's) 392.0
        bacterial 421.0
      rheumatic fever (conditions classifiable to 390)
        active — see Endocarditis, acute, rheumatic

Endocarditis — continued
  aortic — continued
    with
      rheumatic fever — continued
        inactive or quiescent (with chorea) 395.9
          with mitral disease 396.9
    acute or subacute 421.9
    arteriosclerotic 424.1
    congenital 746.89
    hypertensive 424.1
    rheumatic (chronic) (inactive) 395.9
      with mitral (valve) disease 396.9
        active or acute 391.1
          with chorea (acute) (rheumatic) (Sydenham's) 392.0
      active or acute 391.1
        with chorea (acute) (rheumatic) (Sydenham's) 392.0
    specified cause, except rheumatic 424.1
    syphilitic 093.22
  arteriosclerotic or due to arteriosclerosis 424.99
  atypical verrucous (Libman-Sacks) 710.0 [424.91]
  bacterial (acute) (any valve) (chronic) (subacute) 421.0
  blastomycotic 116.0 [421.1]
  candidal 112.81
  congenital 425.3
  constrictive 421.0
  Coxsackie 074.22
  due to
    blastomycosis 116.0 [421.1]
    candidiasis 112.81
    Coxsackie (virus) 074.22
    disseminated lupus erythematosus 710.0 [424.91]
    histoplasmosis (see also Histoplasmosis) 115.94
    hypertension (benign) 424.99
    moniliasis 112.81
    prosthetic cardiac valve 996.61
    Q fever 083.0 [421.1]
    serratia marcescens 421.0
    typhoid (fever) 002.0 [421.1]
  fetal 425.3
  gonococcal 098.84
  hypertensive 424.99
  infectious or infective (acute) (any valve) (chronic) (subacute) 421.0
  lenta (acute) (any valve) (chronic) (subacute) 421.0
  Libman-Sacks 710.0 [424.91]
  Loeffler's (parietal fibroplastic) 421.0
  malignant (acute) (any valve) (chronic) (subacute) 421.0
  meningococcal 036.42
  mitral (chronic) (double) (fibroid) (heart) (inactive) (valve) (with chorea) 394.9
    with
      aortic (valve) disease 396.9
        active or acute 391.1
          with chorea (acute) (rheumatic) (Sydenham's) 392.0
      rheumatic fever (conditions classifiable to 390)
        active — see Endocarditis, acute, rheumatic
        inactive or quiescent (with chorea) 394.9
          with aortic valve disease 396.9
    active or acute 391.1
      with chorea (acute) (rheumatic) (Sydenham's) 392.0
    bacterial 421.0
    arteriosclerotic 424.0
    congenital 746.89
    hypertensive 424.0
    nonrheumatic 424.0
      acute or subacute 421.9
    syphilitic 093.21
  monilial 112.81

Endocarditis — *continued*
  mycotic (acute) (any valve) (chronic) (subacute) 421.0
  pneumococcic (acute) (any valve) (chronic) (subacute) 421.0
  pulmonary (chronic) (heart) (valve) 424.3
    with
      rheumatic fever (conditions classifiable to 390)
        active — *see* Endocarditis, acute, rheumatic
        inactive or quiescent (with chorea) 397.1
  acute or subacute 421.9
    rheumatic 391.1
      with chorea (acute) (rheumatic) (Sydenham's) 392.0
  arteriosclerotic or due to arteriosclerosis 424.3
  congenital 746.09
  hypertensive or due to hypertension (benign) 424.3
  rheumatic (chronic) (inactive) (with chorea) 397.1
    active or acute 391.1
      with chorea (acute) (rheumatic) (Sydenham's) 392.0
  syphilitic 093.24
  purulent (acute) (any valve) (chronic) (subacute) 421.0
  rheumatic (chronic) (inactive) (with chorea) 397.9
    active or acute (aortic) (mitral) (pulmonary) (tricuspid) 391.1
      with chorea (acute) (rheumatic) (Sydenham's) 392.0
  septic (acute) (any valve) (chronic) (subacute) 421.0
  specified cause, except rheumatic 424.99
  streptococcal (acute) (any valve) (chronic) (subacute) 421.0
  subacute — *see* Endocarditis, acute
  suppurative (any valve) (acute) (chronic) (subacute) 421.0
  syphilitic NEC 093.20
  toxic (*see also* Endocarditis, acute) 421.9
  tricuspid (chronic) (heart) (inactive) (rheumatic) (valve) (with chorea) 397.0
    with
      rheumatic fever (conditions classifiable to 390)
        active — *see* Endocarditis, acute, rheumatic
        inactive or quiescent (with chorea) 397.0
    active or acute 391.1
      with chorea (acute) (rheumatic) (Sydenham's) 392.0
    arteriosclerotic 424.2
    congenital 746.89
    hypertensive 424.2
    nonrheumatic 424.2
      acute or subacute 421.9
    specified cause, except rheumatic 424.2
    syphilitic 093.23
  tuberculous (*see also* Tuberculosis) 017.9 ☑ *[424.91]*
  typhoid 002.0 *[421.1]*
  ulcerative (acute) (any valve) (chronic) (subacute) 421.0
  vegetative (acute) (any valve) (chronic) (subacute) 421.0
  verrucous (acute) (any valve) (chronic) (subacute) NEC 710.0 *[424.91]*
    nonbacterial 710.0 *[424.91]*
    nonrheumatic 710.0 *[424.91]*
Endocardium, endocardial — *see also* condition
  cushion defect 745.60
    specified type NEC 745.69
Endocervicitis — *see also* Cervicitis 616.0
  due to
    intrauterine (contraceptive) device 996.65
  gonorrheal (acute) 098.15

Endocervicitis — *see also* Cervicitis — *continued*
  gonorrheal — *continued*
    chronic or duration of 2 months or over 098.35
  hyperplastic 616.0
  syphilitic 095.8
  trichomonal 131.09
  tuberculous (*see also* Tuberculosis) 016.7 ☑
Endocrine — *see* condition
Endocrinopathy, pluriglandular 258.9
Endodontitis 522.0
Endomastoiditis — *see also* Mastoiditis 383.9
Endometrioma 617.9
Endometriosis 617.9
  appendix 617.5
  bladder 617.8
  bowel 617.5
  broad ligament 617.3
  cervix 617.0
  colon 617.5
  cul-de-sac (Douglas') 617.3
  exocervix 617.0
  fallopian tube 617.2
  female genital organ NEC 617.8
  gallbladder 617.8
  in scar of skin 617.6
  internal 617.0
  intestine 617.5
  lung 617.8
  myometrium 617.0
  ovary 617.1
  parametrium 617.3
  pelvic peritoneum 617.3
  peritoneal (pelvic) 617.3
  rectovaginal septum 617.4
  rectum 617.5
  round ligament 617.3
  skin 617.6
  specified site NEC 617.8
  stromal (M8931/1) 236.0
  umbilicus 617.8
  uterus 617.0
    internal 617.0
  vagina 617.4
  vulva 617.8
Endometritis (nonspecific) (purulent) (septic) (suppurative) 615.9
  with
    abortion — *see* Abortion, by type, with sepsis
    ectopic pregnancy (*see also* categories 633.0–633.9) 639.0
    molar pregnancy (*see also* categories 630–632) 639.0
  acute 615.0
  blennorrhagic 098.16
    acute 098.16
    chronic or duration of 2 months or over 098.36
  cervix, cervical (*see also* Cervicitis) 616.0
    hyperplastic 616.0
  chronic 615.1
  complicating pregnancy 670.1 ☑
    affecting fetus or newborn 760.8
    septic 670.2 ☑
  decidual 615.9
  following
    abortion 639.0
    ectopic or molar pregnancy 639.0
  gonorrheal (acute) 098.16
    chronic or duration of 2 months or over 098.36
  hyperplastic (*see also* Hyperplasia, endometrium) 621.30
    cervix 616.0
  polypoid — *see* Endometritis, hyperplastic
  puerperal, postpartum, childbirth 670.1 ☑
    septic 670.2 ☑
  senile (atrophic) 615.9
  subacute 615.0
  tuberculous (*see also* Tuberculosis) 016.7 ☑
Endometrium — *see* condition
Endomyocardiopathy, South African 425.2
Endomyocarditis — *see* Endocarditis
Endomyofibrosis 425.0

Endomyometritis — *see also* Endometritis 615.9
Endopericarditis — *see* Endocarditis
Endoperineuritis — *see* Disorder, nerve
Endophlebitis — *see also* Phlebitis 451.9
  leg 451.2
    deep (vessels) 451.19
    superficial (vessels) 451.0
  portal (vein) 572.1
  retina 362.18
  specified site NEC 451.89
  syphilitic 093.89
Endophthalmia — *see also* Endophthalmitis 360.00
  gonorrheal 098.42
Endophthalmitis (globe) (infective) (metastatic) (purulent) (subacute) 360.00
  acute 360.01
  bleb associated 379.63
  chronic 360.03
  parasitic 360.13
  phacoanaphylactic 360.19
  specified type NEC 360.19
  sympathetic 360.11
Endosalpingioma (M9111/1) 236.2
Endosalpingiosis 629.89
Endosteitis — *see* Osteomyelitis
Endothelioma, bone (M9260/3) — *see* Neoplasm, bone, malignant
Endotheliosis 287.8
  hemorrhagic infectional 287.8
Endotoxemia — code to condition
Endotoxic shock 785.52
  postoperative 998.02
Endotrachelitis — *see also* Cervicitis 616.0
Enema rash 692.89
Engel-von Recklinghausen disease or syndrome (osteitis fibrosa cystica) 252.01
Engelmann's disease (diaphyseal sclerosis) 756.9
English disease — *see also* Rickets 268.0
Engman's disease (infectious eczematoid dermatitis) 690.8
Engorgement
  breast 611.79
    newborn 778.7
    puerperal, postpartum 676.2 ☑
  liver 573.9
  lung 514
  pulmonary 514
  retina, venous 362.37
  stomach 536.8
  venous, retina 362.37
Enlargement, enlarged — *see also* Hypertrophy
  abdomen 789.3 ☑
  adenoids 474.12
    and tonsils 474.10
  alveolar process or ridge 525.8
  apertures of diaphragm (congenital) 756.6
  blind spot, visual field 368.42
  gingival 523.8
  heart, cardiac (*see also* Hypertrophy, cardiac) 429.3
  lacrimal gland, chronic 375.03
  liver (*see also* Hypertrophy, liver) 789.1
  lymph gland or node 785.6
  orbit 376.46
  organ or site, congenital NEC — *see* Anomaly, specified type NEC
  parathyroid (gland) 252.01
  pituitary fossa 793.0
  prostate (simple) (soft) 600.00
    with
      other lower urinary tract symptoms (LUTS) 600.01
      urinary
        obstruction 600.01
        retention 600.01
  sella turcica 793.0
  spleen (*see also* Splenomegaly) 789.2
    congenital 759.0
  thymus (congenital) (gland) 254.0
  thyroid (gland) (*see also* Goiter) 240.9
  tongue 529.8
  tonsils 474.11

Enlargement, enlarged — *see also* Hypertrophy — *continued*
  tonsils — *continued*
    and adenoids 474.10
  uterus 621.2
Enophthalmos 376.50
  due to
    atrophy of orbital tissue 376.51
    surgery 376.52
    trauma 376.52
Enostosis 526.89
Entamebiasis — *see* Amebiasis
Entamebic — *see* Amebiasis
Entanglement, umbilical cord(s) 663.3 ☑
  with compression 663.2 ☑
  affecting fetus or newborn 762.5
  around neck with compression 663.1 ☑
  twins in monoamniotic sac 663.2 ☑
Enteralgia 789.0 ☑
Enteric — *see* condition
Enteritis (acute) (catarrhal) (choleraic) (chronic) (congestive) (diarrheal) (exudative) (follicular) (hemorrhagic) (infantile) (lienteric) (noninfectious) (perforative) (phlegmonous) (presumed noninfectious) (pseudomembranous) 558.9
  adaptive 564.9
  aertrycke infection 003.0
  allergic 558.3
  amebic (*see also* Amebiasis) 006.9
    with abscess — *see* Abscess, amebic
    acute 006.0
      with abscess — *see* Abscess, amebic
      nondysenteric 006.2
    chronic 006.1
      with abscess — *see* Abscess, amebic
      nondysenteric 006.2
    nondysenteric 006.2
  anaerobic (cocci) (gram-negative) (gram-positive) (mixed) NEC 008.46
  bacillary NEC 004.9
  bacterial NEC 008.5
    specified NEC 008.49
  Bacteroides (fragilis) (melaninogeniscus) (oralis) 008.46
  Butyrivibrio (fibriosolvens) 008.46
  Campylobacter 008.43
  Candida 112.85
  Chilomastix 007.8
  choleriformis 001.1
  chronic 558.9
    ulcerative (*see also* Colitis, ulcerative) 556.9
  cicatrizing (chronic) 555.0
  Clostridium
    botulinum 005.1
    difficile 008.45
    haemolyticum 008.46
    novyi 008.46
    perfringens (C) (F) 008.46
    specified type NEC 008.46
  coccidial 007.2
  dietetic 558.9
  due to
    achylia gastrica 536.8
    adenovirus 008.62
    Aerobacter aerogenes 008.2
    anaerobes (*see also* Enteritis, anaerobic) 008.46
    Arizona (bacillus) 008.1
    astrovirus 008.66
    Bacillus coli — *see* Enteritis, E. coli
    bacteria NEC 008.5
      specified NEC 008.49
    Bacteroides (*see also* Enteritis, Bacteroides) 008.46
    Butyrivibrio (fibriosolvens) 008.46
    calicivirus 008.65
    Camplyobacter 008.43
    Clostridium — *see* Enteritis, Clostridium
    Cockle agent 008.64
    Coxsackie (virus) 008.67
    Ditchling agent 008.64
    ECHO virus 008.67
    Enterobacter aerogenes 008.2
    enterococci 008.49

☑ **Additional Digit Required** — Refer to the Tabular List for Digit Selection   ﹂ **Subterms under main terms may continue to next column or page**

106 — Volume 2   ▶◀ **Revised Text**   ● **New Line**   ▲ **Revised Code**   **2014 ICD-9-CM**

Enteritis — continued

due to — continued
  enterovirus NEC 008.67
  Escherichia coli — see Enteritis, E. coli
  Eubacterium 008.46
  Fusobacterium (nucleatum) 008.46
  gram-negative bacteria NEC 008.47
    anaerobic NEC 008.46
  Hawaii agent 008.63
  irritating foods 558.9
  Klebsiella aerogenes 008.47
  Marin County agent 008.66
  Montgomery County agent 008.63
  norovirus 008.63
  Norwalk-like agent 008.63
  Norwalk virus 008.63
  Otofuke agent 008.63
  Paracolobactrum arizonae 008.1
  paracolon bacillus NEC 008.47
    Arizona 008.1
  Paramatta agent 008.64
  Peptococcus 008.46
  Peptostreptococcus 008.46
  Proprionibacterium 008.46
  Proteus (bacillus) (mirabilis) (morganii) 008.3
  Pseudomonas aeruginosa 008.42
  Rotavirus 008.61
  Sapporo agent 008.63
  small round virus (SRV) NEC 008.64
    featureless NEC 008.63
    structured NEC 008.63
  Snow Mountain (SM) agent 008.63
  specified
    bacteria NEC 008.49
    organism, nonbacterial NEC 008.8
    virus NEC 008.69
  Staphylococcus 008.41
  Streptococcus 008.49
    anaerobic 008.46
  Taunton agent 008.63
  Torovirus 008.69
  Treponema 008.46
  Veillonella 008.46
  virus 008.8
    specified type NEC 008.69
  Wollan (W) agent 008.64
  Yersinia enterocolitica 008.44
dysentery — see Dysentery
E. coli 008.00
  enterohemorrhagic 008.04
  enteroinvasive 008.03
  enteropathogenic 008.01
  enterotoxigenic 008.02
  specified type NEC 008.09
el tor 001.1
embadomonial 007.8
eosinophilic 558.41
epidemic 009.0
Eubacterium 008.46
fermentative 558.9
fulminant 557.0
Fusobacterium (nucleatum) 008.46
gangrenous (see also Enteritis, due to, by organism) 009.0
giardial 007.1
gram-negative bacteria NEC 008.47
  anaerobic NEC 008.46
infectious NEC (see also Enteritis, due to, by organism) 009.0
presumed 009.1
influenzal (see also Influenza) 487.8
ischemic 557.9
  acute 557.0
  chronic 557.1
  due to mesenteric artery insufficiency 557.1
membranous 564.9
mucous 564.9
myxomembranous 564.9
necrotic (see also Enteritis, due to, by organism) 009.0
necroticans 005.2
necrotizing of fetus or newborn (see also Enterocolitis, necrotizing, newborn) 777.50

Enteritis — continued

neurogenic 564.9
newborn 777.8
  necrotizing (see also Enterocolitis, necrotizing, newborn) 777.50
parasitic NEC 129
paratyphoid (fever) (see also Fever, paratyphoid) 002.9
Peptococcus 008.46
Peptostreptococcus 008.46
Proprionibacterium 008.46
protozoal NEC 007.9
radiation 558.1
regional (of) 555.9
  intestine
    large (bowel, colon, or rectum) 555.1
      with small intestine 555.2
    small (duodenum, ileum, or jejunum) 555.0
      with large intestine 555.2
Salmonella infection 003.0
salmonellosis 003.0
segmental (see also Enteritis, regional) 555.9
septic (see also Enteritis, due to, by organism) 009.0
Shigella 004.9
simple 558.9
spasmodic 564.9
spastic 564.9
staphylococcal 008.41
  due to food 005.0
streptococcal 008.49
  anaerobic 008.46
toxic 558.2
Treponema (denticola) (macrodentium) 008.46
trichomonal 007.3
tuberculous (see also Tuberculosis) 014.8 ☑
typhosa 002.0
ulcerative (chronic) (see also Colitis, ulcerative) 556.9
Veillonella 008.46
viral 008.8
  adenovirus 008.62
  enterovirus 008.67
  specified virus NEC 008.69
Yersinia enterocolitica 008.44
zymotic 009.0
Enteroarticular syndrome 099.3
Enterobiasis 127.4
Enterobius vermicularis 127.4
Enterocele — see also Hernia 553.9
  pelvis, pelvic (acquired) (congenital) 618.6
  vagina, vaginal (acquired) (congenital) 618.6
Enterocolitis — see also Enteritis
fetus or newborn (see also Enterocolitis, necrotizing, newborn) 777.8
  necrotizing 777.50
fulminant 557.0
granulomatous 555.2
hemorrhagic (acute) 557.0
  chronic 557.1
necrotizing (acute) (membranous) 557.0
  newborn 777.50
    with
      perforation 777.53
      pneumatosis and perforation 777.53
      pneumatosis without perforation 777.52
      without pneumatosis, without perforation 777.51
      stage I 777.51
      stage II 777.52
      stage III 777.53
primary necrotizing (see also Enterocolitis, necrotizing, newborn) 777.50
pseudomembranous 008.45
  newborn 008.45
radiation 558.1
  newborn (see also Enterocolitis, necrotizing, newborn) 777.50
ulcerative 556.0
Enterocystoma 751.5
Enterogastritis — see Enteritis
Enterogenous cyanosis 289.7

Enterolith, enterolithiasis (impaction) 560.39
with hernia (see also Hernia, by site, with obstruction)
gangrenous — see Hernia, by site, with gangrene
Enteropathy 569.9
exudative (of Gordon) 579.8
gluten 579.0
hemorrhagic, terminal 557.0
protein-losing 579.8
Enteroperitonitis — see also Peritonitis 567.9
Enteroptosis 569.89
Enterorrhagia 578.9
Enterospasm 564.9
psychogenic 306.4
Enterostenosis — see also Obstruction, intestine 560.9
Enterostomy status V44.4
with complication 569.60
Enthesopathy 726.90
ankle and tarsus 726.70
elbow region 726.30
  specified NEC 726.39
hip 726.5
knee 726.60
peripheral NEC 726.8
shoulder region 726.10
  adhesive 726.0
spinal 720.1
wrist and carpus 726.4
Entrance, air into vein — see Embolism, air
Entrapment, nerve — see Neuropathy, entrapment
Entropion (eyelid) 374.00
cicatricial 374.04
congenital 743.62
late effect of trachoma (healed) 139.1
mechanical 374.02
paralytic 374.02
senile 374.01
spastic 374.03
Enucleation of eye (current) (traumatic) 871.3
Enuresis 788.30
habit disturbance 307.6
nocturnal 788.36
  psychogenic 307.6
nonorganic origin 307.6
psychogenic 307.6
Enzymopathy 277.9
Eosinopenia 288.59
Eosinophilia 288.3
with
  angiolymphoid hyperplasia (ALHE) 228.01
allergic 288.3
hereditary 288.3
idiopathic 288.3
infiltrative 518.3
Loeffler's 518.3
myalgia syndrome 710.5
pulmonary (tropical) 518.3
secondary 288.3
tropical 518.3
Eosinophilic — see also condition
fasciitis 728.89
granuloma (bone) 277.89
infiltration lung 518.3
Ependymitis (acute) (cerebral) (chronic) (granular) — see also Meningitis 322.9
Ependymoblastoma (M9392/3)
specified site — see Neoplasm, by site, malignant
unspecified site 191.9
Ependymoma (epithelial) (malignant) (M9391/3)
anaplastic type (M9392/3)
  specified site — see Neoplasm, by site, malignant
  unspecified site 191.9
benign (M9391/0)
  specified site — see Neoplasm, by site, benign
  unspecified site 225.0
myxopapillary (M9394/1) 237.5
papillary (M9393/1) 237.5

Ependymoma — continued
specified site — see Neoplasm, by site, malignant
unspecified site 191.9
Ependymopathy 349.2
spinal cord 349.2
Ephelides, ephelis 709.09
Ephemeral fever — see also Pyrexia 780.60
Epiblepharon (congenital) 743.62
Epicanthus, epicanthic fold (congenital) (eyelid) 743.63
Epicondylitis (elbow) (lateral) 726.32
medial 726.31
Epicystitis — see also Cystitis 595.9
Epidemic — see condition
Epidermidalization, cervix — see condition
Epidermidization, cervix — see condition
Epidermis, epidermal — see condition
Epidermization, cervix — see condition
Epidermodysplasia verruciformis 078.19
Epidermoid
cholesteatoma — see Cholesteatoma
inclusion (see also Cyst, skin) 706.2
Epidermolysis
acuta (combustiformis) (toxica) 695.15
bullosa 757.39
necroticans combustiformis 695.15
  due to drug
    correct substance properly administered 695.15
    overdose or wrong substance given or taken 977.9
    specified drug — see Table of Drugs and Chemicals
Epidermophytid — see Dermatophytosis
Epidermophytosis (infected) — see Dermatophytosis
Epidermosis, ear (middle) — see also Cholesteatoma 385.30
Epididymis — see condition
Epididymitis (nonvenereal) 604.90
with abscess 604.0
acute 604.99
blennorrhagic (acute) 098.0
  chronic or duration of 2 months or over 098.2
caseous (see also Tuberculosis) 016.4 ☑
chlamydial 099.54
diphtheritic 032.89 [604.91]
filarial 125.9 [604.91]
gonococcal (acute) 098.0
  chronic or duration of 2 months or over 098.2
recurrent 604.99
residual 604.99
syphilitic 095.8 [604.91]
tuberculous (see also Tuberculosis) 016.4 ☑
Epididymo-orchitis — see also Epididymitis 604.90
with abscess 604.0
chlamydial 099.54
gonococcal (acute) 098.13
  chronic or duration of 2 months or over 098.33
Epidural — see condition
Epigastritis — see also Gastritis 535.5 ☑
Epigastrium, epigastric — see condition
Epigastrocele — see also Hernia, epigastric 553.29
Epiglottiditis (acute) 464.30
with obstruction 464.31
chronic 476.1
viral 464.30
  with obstruction 464.31
Epiglottis — see condition
Epiglottitis (acute) 464.30
with obstruction 464.31
chronic 476.1
viral 464.30
  with obstruction 464.31
Epignathus 759.4
Epilepsia
partialis continua (see also Epilepsy) 345.7 ☑
procursiva (see also Epilepsy) 345.8 ☑

☑ **Additional Digit Required — Refer to the Tabular List for Digit Selection**

▽ **Subterms under main terms may continue to next column or page**

2014 ICD-9-CM

▶◀ Revised Text   ● New Line   ▲ Revised Code

Volume 2 — 107

Enteritis — Epilepsia

Epilepsy, epileptic (idiopathic) 345.9 ☑

Note — use the following fifth-digit
subclassification with categories 345.0,
345.1, 345.4–345.9:

0   without mention of intractable
    epilepsy

1   with intractable epilepsy

     pharmacoresistant (pharmaco-
     logically resistant)

     poorly controlled

     refractory (medically)

     treatment resistant

abdominal 345.5 ☑
absence (attack) 345.0 ☑
akinetic 345.0 ☑
   psychomotor 345.4 ☑
automatism 345.4 ☑
autonomic diencephalic 345.5 ☑
brain 345.9 ☑
Bravais-Jacksonian 345.5 ☑
cerebral 345.9 ☑
climacteric 345.9 ☑
clonic 345.1 ☑
clouded state 345.9 ☑
coma 345.3
communicating 345.4 ☑
complicating pregnancy, childbirth, or the
   puerperium 649.4 ☑
congenital 345.9 ☑
convulsions 345.9 ☑
cortical (focal) (motor) 345.5 ☑
cursive (running) 345.8 ☑
cysticercosis 123.1
deterioration
   with behavioral disturbance
     345.9 ☑ [294.11]
   without behavioral disturbance
     345.9 ☑ [294.10]
due to syphilis 094.89
equivalent 345.5 ☑
fit 345.9 ☑
focal (motor) 345.5 ☑
gelastic 345.8 ☑
generalized 345.9 ☑
   convulsive 345.1 ☑
   flexion 345.1 ☑
   nonconvulsive 345.0 ☑
grand mal (idiopathic) 345.1 ☑
Jacksonian (motor) (sensory) 345.5 ☑
Kojevnikoff's, Kojevnikov's, Kojewnikoff's
   345.7 ☑
laryngeal 786.2
limbic system 345.4 ☑
localization related (focal) (partial) and
   epileptic syndromes
   with
     complex partial seizures 345.4 ☑
     simple partial seizures 345.5 ☑
major (motor) 345.1 ☑
minor 345.0 ☑
mixed (type) 345.9 ☑
motor partial 345.5 ☑
musicogenic 345.1 ☑
myoclonus, myoclonic 345.1 ☑
   progressive (familial) 345.1 ☑
nonconvulsive, generalized 345.0 ☑
parasitic NEC 123.9
partial (focalized) 345.5 ☑
   with
     impairment of consciousness
       345.4 ☑
     memory and ideational disturbances
       345.4 ☑
     without impairment of consciousness
       345.5 ☑
   abdominal type 345.5 ☑
   motor type 345.5 ☑
   psychomotor type 345.4 ☑
   psychosensory type 345.4 ☑
   secondarily generalized 345.4 ☑
   sensory type 345.5 ☑

Epilepsy, epileptic — continued
partial — continued
   somatomotor type 345.5 ☑
   somatosensory type 345.5 ☑
   temporal lobe type 345.4 ☑
   visceral type 345.5 ☑
   visual type 345.5 ☑
peripheral 345.9 ☑
petit mal 345.0 ☑
photokinetic 345.8 ☑
progressive myoclonic (familial) 345.1 ☑
psychic equivalent 345.5 ☑
psychomotor 345.4 ☑
psychosensory 345.4 ☑
reflex 345.1 ☑
seizure 345.9 ☑
senile 345.9 ☑
sensory-induced 345.5 ☑
sleep (see also Narcolepsy) 347.00
somatomotor type 345.5 ☑
somatosensory 345.5 ☑
specified type NEC 345.8 ☑
status (grand mal) 345.3
   focal motor 345.7 ☑
   petit mal 345.2
   psychomotor 345.7 ☑
   temporal lobe 345.7 ☑
symptomatic 345.9 ☑
temporal lobe 345.4 ☑
tonic (-clonic) 345.1 ☑
traumatic (injury unspecified) 907.0
   injury specified — see Late, effect (of)
     specified injury
twilight 293.0
uncinate (gyrus) 345.4 ☑
Unverricht (-Lundborg) (familial myoclonic)
   345.1 ☑
visceral 345.5 ☑
visual 345.5 ☑
Epileptiform
convulsions 780.39
seizure 780.39
Epiloia 759.5
Epimenorrhea 626.2
Epipharyngitis — see also Nasopharyngitis
   460
Epiphora 375.20
due to
   excess lacrimation 375.21
   insufficient drainage 375.22
Epiphyseal arrest 733.91
femoral head 732.2
Epiphyseolysis, epiphysiolysis — see also
   Osteochondrosis 732.9
Epiphysitis — see also Osteochondrosis 732.9
juvenile 732.6
marginal (Scheuermann's) 732.0
os calcis 732.5
syphilitic (congenital) 090.0
vertebral (Scheuermann's) 732.0
Epiplocele — see also Hernia 553.9
Epiploitis — see also Peritonitis 567.9
Epiplosarcomphalocele — see also Hernia,
   umbilicus 553.1
Episcleritis 379.00
gouty 274.89 [379.09]
nodular 379.02
periodica fugax 379.01
   angioneurotic — see Edema, angioneu-
     rotic
specified NEC 379.09
staphylococcal 379.00
suppurative 379.00
syphilitic 095.0
tuberculous (see also Tuberculosis)
   017.3 [379.09]
Episode
brain (see also Disease, cerebrovascular,
   acute) 436
cerebral (see also Disease, cerebrovascular,
   acute) 436
depersonalization (in neurotic state) 300.6
hyporesponsive 780.09
psychotic (see also Psychosis) 298.9
   organic, transient 293.9

Episode — continued
schizophrenic (acute) NEC (see also
   Schizophrenia) 295.4 ☑
Epispadias
female 753.8
male 752.62
Episplenitis 289.59
Epistaxis (multiple) 784.7
hereditary 448.0
vicarious menstruation 625.8
Epithelioma (malignant) (M8011/3) — see also
   Neoplasm, by site, malignant
adenoides cysticum (M8100/0) — see Neoplasm, skin, benign
basal cell (M8090/3) — see Neoplasm, skin,
   malignant
benign (M8011/0) — see Neoplasm, by site,
   benign
Bowen's (M8081/2) — see Neoplasm, skin,
   in situ
calcifying (benign) (Malherbe's) (M8110/0)
   — see Neoplasm, skin, benign
external site — see Neoplasm, skin, malignant
intraepidermal, Jadassohn (M8096/0) — see
   Neoplasm, skin, benign
squamous cell (M8070/3) — see Neoplasm,
   by site, malignant
Epitheliopathy
pigment, retina 363.15
posterior multifocal placoid (acute) 363.15
Epithelium, epithelial — see condition
Epituberculosis (allergic) (with atelectasis) —
   see also Tuberculosis 010.8 ☑
Eponychia 757.5
Epstein-Barr infection (viral) 075
chronic 780.79 [139.8]
Epstein's
nephrosis or syndrome (see also Nephrosis)
   581.9
pearl (mouth) 528.4
Epulis (giant cell) (gingiva) 523.8
Equinia 024
Equinovarus (congenital) 754.51
acquired 736.71
Equivalent
angina 413.9
convulsive (abdominal) (see also Epilepsy)
   345.5 ☑
epileptic (psychic) (see also Epilepsy)
   345.5 ☑
Erb-Goldflam disease or syndrome 358.00
Erb's
disease 359.1
palsy, paralysis (birth) (brachial) (newborn)
   767.6
spinal (spastic) syphilitic 094.89
pseudohypertrophic muscular dystrophy
   359.1
Erb (-Duchenne) paralysis (birth injury)
   (newborn) 767.6
Erdheim-Chester disease (ECD) 277.89
Erdheim's syndrome (acromegalic
   macrospondylitis) 253.0
Erection, painful (persistent) 607.3
Ergosterol deficiency (vitamin D) 268.9
with
   osteomalacia 268.2
   rickets (see also Rickets) 268.0
Ergotism (ergotized grain) 988.2
from ergot used as drug (migraine therapy)
   correct substance properly administered
     349.82
   overdose or wrong substance given or
     taken 975.0
Erichsen's disease (railway spine) 300.16
Erlacher-Blount syndrome (tibia vara) 732.4
Erosio interdigitalis blastomycetica 112.3
Erosion
arteriosclerotic plaque — see Arteriosclerosis, by site
artery NEC 447.2
   without rupture 447.8
bone 733.99
bronchus 519.19
cartilage (joint) 733.99

Erosion — continued
cervix (uteri) (acquired) (chronic) (congenital) 622.0
   with mention of cervicitis 616.0
cornea (recurrent) (see also Keratitis) 371.42
   traumatic 918.1
dental (idiopathic) (occupational) 521.30
   extending into
     dentine 521.32
     pulp 521.33
   generalized 521.35
   limited to enamel 521.31
   localized 521.34
duodenum, postpyloric — see Ulcer, duodenum
esophagus 530.89
gastric 535.4 ☑
implanted vaginal mesh
   in, into
     pelvic floor muscles 629.31
     surrounding organ(s) or tissue 629.31
intestine 569.89
lymphatic vessel 457.8
pylorus, pyloric (ulcer) 535.4 ☑
sclera 379.16
spine, aneurysmal 094.89
spleen 289.59
stomach 535.4 ☑
teeth (idiopathic) (occupational) (see also
   Erosion, dental) 521.30
   due to
     medicine 521.30
     persistent vomiting 521.30
urethra 599.84
uterus 621.8
vaginal prosthetic materials NEC
   in, into
     pelvic floor muscles 629.31
     surrounding organ(s) or tissue 629.31
vertebra 733.99
Erotomania 302.89
Clérambault's 297.8
Error
in diet 269.9
refractive 367.9
   astigmatism (see also Astigmatism)
     367.20
   drug-induced 367.89
   hypermetropia 367.0
   hyperopia 367.0
   myopia 367.1
   presbyopia 367.4
   toxic 367.89
Eructation 787.3
nervous 306.4
psychogenic 306.4
Eruption
creeping 126.9
drug — see Dermatitis, due to, drug
Hutchinson, summer 692.72
Kaposi's varicelliform 054.0
napkin (psoriasiform) 691.0
polymorphous
   light (sun) 692.72
     other source 692.82
psoriasiform, napkin 691.0
recalcitrant pustular 694.8
ringed 695.89
skin (see also Dermatitis) 782.1
   creeping (meaning hookworm) 126.9
   due to
     chemical(s) NEC 692.4
       internal use 693.8
     drug — see Dermatitis, due to, drug
     prophylactic inoculation or vaccina-
       tion against disease — see
       Dermatitis, due to, vaccine
     smallpox vaccination NEC — see
       Dermatitis, due to, vaccine
   erysipeloid 027.1
   feigned 698.4
   Hutchinson, summer 692.72
   Kaposi's, varicelliform 054.0
     vaccinia 999.0
   lichenoid, axilla 698.3
   polymorphous, due to light 692.72

☑ **Additional Digit Required** — Refer to the Tabular List for Digit Selection   ⩔ **Subterms under main terms may continue to next column or page**

108 — Volume 2   ▶◀ **Revised Text**   ● **New Line**   ▲ **Revised Code**   **2014 ICD-9-CM**

Eruption — *continued*
  skin (*see also* Dermatitis) — *continued*
    toxic NEC 695.0
    vesicular 709.8
  teeth, tooth
    accelerated 520.6
    delayed 520.6
    difficult 520.6
    disturbance of 520.6
    in abnormal sequence 520.6
    incomplete 520.6
    late 520.6
    natal 520.6
    neonatal 520.6
    obstructed 520.6
    partial 520.6
    persistent primary 520.6
    premature 520.6
    prenatal 520.6
  vesicular 709.8
Erysipelas (gangrenous) (infantile) (newborn)
  (phlegmonous) (suppurative) 035
  external ear 035 *[380.13]*
  puerperal, postpartum, childbirth 670.8 ☑
Erysipelatoid (Rosenbach's) 027.1
Erysipeloid (Rosenbach's) 027.1
Erythema, erythematous (generalized) 695.9
  ab igne — *see* Burn, by site, first degree
  annulare (centrifugum) (rheumaticum)
    695.0
  arthriticum epidemicum 026.1
  brucellum (*see also* Brucellosis) 023.9
  bullosum 695.19
  caloricum — *see* Burn, by site, first degree
  chronicum migrans 088.81
  circinatum 695.19
  diaper 691.0
  due to
    chemical (contact) NEC 692.4
      internal 693.8
    drug (internal use) 693.0
      contact 692.3
  elevatum diutinum 695.89
  endemic 265.2
  epidemic, arthritic 026.1
  figuratum perstans 695.0
  gluteal 691.0
  gyratum (perstans) (repens) 695.19
  heat — *see* Burn, by site, first degree
  ichthyosiforme congenitum 757.1
  induratum (primary) (scrofulosorum) (*see
    also* Tuberculosis) 017.1 ☑
    nontuberculous 695.2
  infantum febrile 057.8
  infectional NEC 695.9
  infectiosum 057.0
  inflammation NEC 695.9
  intertrigo 695.89
  iris 695.10
  lupus (discoid) (localized) (*see also* Lupus,
    erythematosus) 695.4
  marginatum 695.0
    rheumaticum — *see* Fever, rheumatic
  medicamentosum — *see* Dermatitis, due
    to, drug
  migrans 529.1
    chronicum 088.81
  multiforme 695.10
    bullosum 695.19
    conjunctiva 695.19
    exudativum (Hebra) 695.19
    major 695.12
    minor 695.11
    pemphigoides 694.5
  napkin 691.0
  neonatorum 778.8
  nodosum 695.2
    tuberculous (*see also* Tuberculosis)
      017.1 ☑
  nummular, nummulare 695.19
  palmar 695.0
  palmaris hereditarium 695.0
  pernio 991.5
  perstans solare 692.72
  rash, newborn 778.8
  scarlatiniform (exfoliative) (recurrent) 695.0

Erythema, erythematous — *continued*
  simplex marginatum 057.8
  solare (*see also* Sunburn) 692.71
  streptogenes 696.5
  toxic, toxicum NEC 695.0
    newborn 778.8
  tuberculous (primary) (*see also* Tuberculosis)
    017.0 ☑
  venenatum 695.0
Erythematosus — *see* condition
Erythematous — *see* condition
Erythermalgia (primary) 443.82
Erythralgia 443.82
Erythrasma 039.0
Erythredema 985.0
  polyneuritica 985.0
  polyneuropathy 985.0
Erythremia (acute) (M9841/3) 207.0 ☑
  chronic (M9842/3) 207.1 ☑
  secondary 289.0
Erythroblastopenia (acquired) 284.89
  congenital 284.01
Erythroblastophthisis 284.01
Erythroblastosis (fetalis) (newborn) 773.2
  due to
    ABO
      antibodies 773.1
      incompatibility, maternal/fetal 773.1
      isoimmunization 773.1
    Rh
      antibodies 773.0
      incompatibility, maternal/fetal 773.0
      isoimmunization 773.0
Erythrocyanosis (crurum) 443.89
Erythrocythemia — *see* Erythremia
Erythrocytopenia 285.9
Erythrocytosis (megalosplenic)
  familial 289.6
  oval, hereditary (*see also* Elliptocytosis)
    282.1
  secondary 289.0
  stress 289.0
Erythroderma — *see also* Erythema 695.9
  desquamativa (in infants) 695.89
  exfoliative 695.89
  ichthyosiform, congenital 757.1
  infantum 695.89
  maculopapular 696.2
  neonatorum 778.8
  psoriaticum 696.1
  secondary 695.9
Erythrodysesthesia, palmar plantar (PPE)
  693.0
Erythrogenesis imperfecta 284.09
Erythroleukemia (M9840/3) 207.0 ☑
Erythromelalgia 443.82
Erythromelia 701.8
Erythropenia 285.9
Erythrophagocytosis 289.9
Erythrophobia 300.23
Erythroplakia
  oral mucosa 528.79
  tongue 528.79
Erythroplasia (Queyrat) (M8080/2)
  specified site — *see* Neoplasm, skin, in situ
  unspecified site 233.5
Erythropoiesis, idiopathic ineffective 285.0
Escaped beats, heart 427.60
  postoperative 997.1
Escherichia coli (E. coli) — *see* Infection, Escherichia coli
Esoenteritis — *see* Enteritis
Esophagalgia 530.89
Esophagectasis 530.89
  due to cardiospasm 530.0
Esophagismus 530.5
Esophagitis (alkaline) (chemical) (chronic) (infectional) (necrotic) (peptic) (postoperative) (regurgitant) 530.10
  acute 530.12
  candidal 112.84
  eosinophilic 530.13
  reflux 530.11
  specified NEC 530.19
  tuberculous (*see also* Tuberculosis) 017.8 ☑
  ulcerative 530.19

Esophagocele 530.6
Esophagodynia 530.89
Esophagomalacia 530.89
Esophagoptosis 530.89
Esophagospasm 530.5
Esophagostenosis 530.3
Esophagostomiasis 127.7
Esophagostomy
  complication 530.87
    infection 530.86
    malfunctioning 530.87
    mechanical 530.87
Esophagotracheal — *see* condition
Esophagus — *see* condition
Esophoria 378.41
  convergence, excess 378.84
  divergence, insufficiency 378.85
Esotropia (nonaccommodative) 378.00
  accommodative 378.35
  alternating 378.05
    with
      A pattern 378.06
      specified noncomitancy NEC 378.08
      V pattern 378.07
      X pattern 378.08
      Y pattern 378.08
    intermittent 378.22
  intermittent 378.20
    alternating 378.22
    monocular 378.21
  monocular 378.01
    with
      A pattern 378.02
      specified noncomitancy NEC 378.04
      V pattern 378.03
      X pattern 378.04
      Y pattern 378.04
    intermittent 378.21
Espundia 085.5
Essential — *see* condition
Esterapenia 289.89
Esthesioneuroblastoma (M9522/3) 160.0
Esthesioneurocytoma (M9521/3) 160.0
Esthesioneuroepithelioma (M9523/3) 160.0
Esthiomene 099.1
Estivo-autumnal
  fever 084.0
  malaria 084.0
Estrangement V61.09
Estriasis 134.0
Ethanolaminuria 270.8
Ethanolism — *see also* Alcoholism 303.9 ☑
Ether dependence, dependency — *see also*
  Dependence 304.6 ☑
Etherism — *see also* Dependence 304.6 ☑
Ethmoid, ethmoidal — *see* condition
Ethmoiditis (chronic) (nonpurulent) (purulent)
  — *see also* Sinusitis, ethmoidal 473.2
  influenzal (*see also* Influenza) 487.1
  Woakes' 471.1
Ethylism — *see also* Alcoholism 303.9 ☑
Eulenburg's disease (congenital paramyoto-
  nia) 359.29
Eunuchism 257.2
Eunuchoidism 257.2
  hypogonadotropic 257.2
European blastomycosis 117.5
Eustachian — *see* condition
Euthyroidism 244.9
Euthyroid sick syndrome 790.94
Evaluation
  fetal lung maturity 659.8 ☑
  for suspected condition (*see also* Observa-
    tion) V71.9
    abuse V71.81
    exposure
      anthrax V71.82
      biologic agent NEC V71.83
      SARS V71.83
    neglect V71.81
    newborn — *see* Observation, suspected,
      condition, newborn
    specified condition NEC V71.89
  mental health V70.2
    requested by authority V70.1
  nursing care V63.8

Evaluation — *continued*
  social service V63.8
Evans' syndrome (thrombocytopenic purpura)
  287.32
Event, apparent life threatening in newborn
  and infant (ALTE) 799.82
Eventration
  colon into chest — *see* Hernia, diaphragm
  diaphragm (congenital) 756.6
Eversion
  bladder 596.89
  cervix (uteri) 622.0
    with mention of cervicitis 616.0
  foot NEC 736.79
    congenital 755.67
  lacrimal punctum 375.51
  punctum lacrimale (postinfectional) (senile)
    375.51
  ureter (meatus) 593.89
  urethra (meatus) 599.84
  uterus 618.1
    complicating delivery 665.2 ☑
      affecting fetus or newborn 763.89
    puerperal, postpartum 674.8 ☑
Evidence
  of malignancy
    cytologic
      without histologic confirmation
        anus 796.76
        cervix 795.06
        vagina 795.16
Evisceration
  birth injury 767.8
  bowel (congenital) — *see* Hernia, ventral
  congenital (*see also* Hernia, ventral) 553.29
  operative wound 998.32
  traumatic NEC 869.1
    eye 871.3
Evulsion — *see* Avulsion
Ewing's
  angioendothelioma (M9260/3) — *see* Neo-
    plasm, bone, malignant
  sarcoma (M9260/3) — *see* Neoplasm, bone,
    malignant
  tumor (M9260/3) — *see* Neoplasm, bone,
    malignant
Exaggerated lumbosacral angle (with imping-
  ing spine) 756.12
Examination (general) (routine) (of) (for) V70.9
  allergy V72.7
  annual V70.0
  cardiovascular preoperative V72.81
  cervical Papanicolaou smear V76.2
    as a part of routine gynecological exam-
      ination V72.31
    to confirm findings of recent normal
      smear following initial abnormal
      smear V72.32
  child care (routine) V20.2
  clinical research investigation (normal con-
    trol patient) (participant) V70.7
  dental V72.2
  developmental testing (child) (infant) V20.2
  donor (potential) V70.8
  ear V72.19
  eye V72.0
  follow-up (routine) (following) V67.9
    cancer chemotherapy V67.2
    chemotherapy V67.2
    disease NEC V67.59
    high-risk medication NEC V67.51
    injury NEC V67.59
    population survey V70.6
    postpartum V24.2
    psychiatric V67.3
    psychotherapy V67.3
    radiotherapy V67.1
    specified surgery NEC V67.09
    surgery V67.00
    vaginal pap smear V67.01
  following
    accident (motor vehicle) V71.4
    alleged rape or seduction (victim or cul-
      prit) V71.5
    inflicted injury (victim or culprit) NEC
      V71.6

☑ **Additional Digit Required — Refer to the Tabular List for Digit Selection**   ▽ **Subterms under main terms may continue to next column or page**

Examination — *continued*
following — *continued*
rape or seduction, alleged (victim or culprit) V71.5
treatment (for) V67.9
combined V67.6
fracture V67.4
involving high-risk medication NEC V67.51
mental disorder V67.3
specified condition NEC V67.59
gynecological V72.31
for contraceptive maintenance V25.40
intrauterine device V25.42
pill V25.41
specified method NEC V25.49
health (of)
armed forces personnel V70.5
checkup V70.0
child, routine V20.2
defined subpopulation NEC V70.5
inhabitants of institutions V70.5
occupational V70.5
pre-employment screening V70.5
preschool children V70.5
for admission to school V70.3
prisoners V70.5
for entrance into prison V70.3
prostitutes V70.5
refugees V70.5
school children V70.5
students V70.5
hearing V72.19
following failed hearing screening V72.11
infant
8 to 28 days old V20.32
over 28 days old, routine V20.2
under 8 days old V20.31
laboratory V72.60
ordered as part of a routine general medical examination V72.62
pre-operative V72.63
pre-procedural V72.63
specified NEC V72.69
lactating mother V24.1
medical (for) (of) V70.9
administrative purpose NEC V70.3
admission to
old age home V70.3
prison V70.3
school V70.3
adoption V70.3
armed forces personnel V70.5
at health care facility V70.0
camp V70.3
child, routine V20.2
clinical research (control) (normal comparison) (participant) V70.7
defined subpopulation NEC V70.5
donor (potential) V70.8
driving license V70.3
general V70.9
routine V70.0
specified reason NEC V70.8
immigration V70.3
inhabitants of institutions V70.5
insurance certification V70.3
marriage V70.3
medicolegal reasons V70.4
naturalization V70.3
occupational V70.5
population survey V70.6
pre-employment V70.5
preschool children V70.5
for admission to school V70.3
prison V70.3
prisoners V70.5
for entrance into prison V70.3
prostitutes V70.5
refugees V70.5
school children V70.5
specified reason NEC V70.8
sport competition V70.3
students V70.5
medicolegal reason V70.4

Examination — *continued*
pelvic (annual) (periodic) V72.31
periodic (annual) (routine) V70.0
postpartum
immediately after delivery V24.0
routine follow-up V24.2
pregnancy (unconfirmed) (possible) V72.40
negative result V72.41
positive result V72.42
prenatal V22.1
first pregnancy V22.0
high-risk pregnancy V23.9
specified problem NEC V23.89
to determine fetal viability V23.87
preoperative V72.84
cardiovascular V72.81
respiratory V72.82
specified NEC V72.83
preprocedural V72.84
cardiovascular V72.81
general physical V72.83
respiratory V72.82
specified NEC V72.83
prior to chemotherapy V72.83
psychiatric V70.2
follow-up not needing further care V67.3
requested by authority V70.1
radiological NEC V72.5
respiratory preoperative V72.82
screening — *see* Screening
sensitization V72.7
skin V72.7
hypersensitivity V72.7
special V72.9
specified type or reason NEC V72.85
preoperative V72.83
specified NEC V72.83
teeth V72.2
vaginal Papanicolaou smear V76.47
following hysterectomy for malignant condition V67.01
victim or culprit following
alleged rape or seduction V71.5
inflicted injury NEC V71.6
vision V72.0
well baby V20.2
Exanthem, exanthema — *see also* Rash 782.1
Boston 048
epidemic, with meningitis 048
lichenoid psoriasiform 696.2
subitum 058.10
due to
human herpesvirus 6 058.11
human herpesvirus 7 058.12
viral, virus NEC 057.9
specified type NEC 057.8
Excess, excessive, excessively
alcohol level in blood 790.3
carbohydrate tissue, localized 278.1
carotene (dietary) 278.3
cold 991.9
specified effect NEC 991.8
convergence 378.84
crying 780.95
of
adolescent 780.95
adult 780.95
baby 780.92
child 780.95
infant (baby) 780.92
newborn 780.92
development, breast 611.1
diaphoresis (*see also* Hyperhidrosis) 780.8
distance, interarch 524.28
divergence 378.85
drinking (alcohol) NEC (*see also* Abuse, drugs, nondependent) 305.0 ☑
continual (*see also* Alcoholism) 303.9 ☑
habitual (*see also* Alcoholism) 303.9 ☑
eating 783.6
eyelid fold (congenital) 743.62
fat 278.02
in heart (*see also* Degeneration, myocardial) 429.1
tissue, localized 278.1
foreskin 605

Excess, excessive, excessively — *continued*
gas 787.3
gastrin 251.5
glucagon 251.4
heat (*see also* Heat) 992.9
horizontal
overjet 524.26
overlap 524.26
interarch distance 524.28
intermaxillary vertical dimension 524.37
interocclusal distance of teeth 524.37
large
colon 564.7
congenital 751.3
fetus or infant 766.0
with obstructed labor 660.1 ☑
affecting management of pregnancy 656.6 ☑
causing disproportion 653.5 ☑
newborn (weight of 4500 grams or more) 766.0
organ or site, congenital NEC — *see* Anomaly, specified type NEC
lid fold (congenital) 743.62
long
colon 751.5
organ or site, congenital NEC — *see* Anomaly, specified type NEC
umbilical cord (entangled)
affecting fetus or newborn 762.5
in pregnancy or childbirth 663.3 ☑
with compression 663.2 ☑
menstruation 626.2
number of teeth 520.1
causing crowding 524.31
nutrients (dietary) NEC 783.6
potassium (K) 276.7
salivation (*see also* Ptyalism) 527.7
secretion (*see also* Hypersecretion)
milk 676.6 ☑
sputum 786.4
sweat (*see also* Hyperhidrosis) 780.8
short
organ or site, congenital NEC — *see* Anomaly, specified type NEC
umbilical cord
affecting fetus or newborn 762.6
in pregnancy or childbirth 663.4 ☑
skin NEC 701.9
eyelid 743.62
acquired 374.30
sodium (Na) 276.0
spacing of teeth 524.32
sputum 786.4
sweating (*see also* Hyperhidrosis) 780.8
tearing (ducts) (eye) (*see also* Epiphora) 375.20
thirst 783.5
due to deprivation of water 994.3
tissue in reconstructed breast 612.0
tuberosity 524.07
vitamin
A (dietary) 278.2
administered as drug (chronic) (prolonged excessive intake) 278.2
reaction to sudden overdose 963.5
D (dietary) 278.4
administered as drug (chronic) (prolonged excessive intake) 278.4
reaction to sudden overdose 963.5
weight 278.02
gain 783.1
of pregnancy 646.1 ☑
loss 783.21
Excitability, abnormal, under minor stress 309.29
Excitation
catatonic (*see also* Schizophrenia) 295.2 ☑
psychogenic 298.1
reactive (from emotional stress, psychological trauma) 298.1
Excitement
manic (*see also* Psychosis, affective) 296.0 ☑

Excitement — *continued*
manic (*see also* Psychosis, affective) — *continued*
recurrent episode 296.1 ☑
single episode 296.0 ☑
mental, reactive (from emotional stress, psychological trauma) 298.1
state, reactive (from emotional stress, psychological trauma) 298.1
Excluded pupils 364.76
Excoriation (traumatic) — *see also* Injury, superficial, by site 919.8
neurotic 698.4
Excyclophoria 378.44
Excyclotropia 378.33
Exencephalus, exencephaly 742.0
Exercise
breathing V57.0
remedial NEC V57.1
therapeutic NEC V57.1
Exfoliation
skin
due to erythematous condition 695.50
involving (percent of body surface)
less than 10 percent 695.50
10-19 percent 695.51
20-29 percent 695.52
30-39 percent 695.53
40-49 percent 695.54
50-59 percent 695.55
60-69 percent 695.56
70-79 percent 695.57
80-89 percent 695.58
90 percent or more 695.59
teeth
due to systemic causes 525.0
Exfoliative — *see also* condition
dermatitis 695.89
Exhaustion, exhaustive (physical NEC) 780.79
battle (*see also* Reaction, stress, acute) 308.9
cardiac (*see also* Failure, heart) 428.9
delirium (*see also* Reaction, stress, acute) 308.9
due to
cold 991.8
excessive exertion 994.5
exposure 994.4
overexertion 994.5
fetus or newborn 779.89
heart (*see also* Failure, heart) 428.9
heat 992.5
due to
salt depletion 992.4
water depletion 992.3
manic (*see also* Psychosis, affective) 296.0 ☑
recurrent episode 296.1 ☑
single episode 296.0 ☑
maternal, complicating delivery 669.8 ☑
affecting fetus or newborn 763.89
mental 300.5
myocardium, myocardial (*see also* Failure, heart) 428.9
nervous 300.5
old age 797
postinfectional NEC 780.79
psychogenic 300.5
psychosis (*see also* Reaction, stress, acute) 308.9
senile 797
dementia 290.0
Exhibitionism (sexual) 302.4
Exomphalos 756.72
Exophoria 378.42
convergence, insufficiency 378.83
divergence, excess 378.85
Exophthalmic
cachexia 242.0 ☑
goiter 242.0 ☑
ophthalmoplegia 242.0 ☑ *[376.22]*
Exophthalmos 376.30
congenital 743.66
constant 376.31
endocrine NEC 259.9 *[376.22]*
hyperthyroidism 242.0 ☑ *[376.21]*
intermittent NEC 376.34
malignant 242.0 ☑ *[376.21]*

☑ **Additional Digit Required — Refer to the Tabular List for Digit Selection**   ◥ **Subterms under main terms may continue to next column or page**

110 — Volume 2   ▶◀ Revised Text   ● New Line   ▲ Revised Code   2014 ICD-9-CM

Exophthalmos — *continued*
pulsating 376.35
endocrine NEC 259.9 *[376.22]*
thyrotoxic 242.0 ☑ *[376.21]*
Exostosis 726.91
cartilaginous (M9210/0) — *see* Neoplasm, bone, benign
congenital 756.4
ear canal, external 380.81
gonococcal 098.89
hip 726.5
intracranial 733.3
jaw (bone) 526.81
luxurians 728.11
multiple (cancellous) (congenital) (hereditary) 756.4
nasal bones 726.91
orbit, orbital 376.42
osteocartilaginous (M9210/0) — *see* Neoplasm, bone, benign
spine 721.8
with spondylosis — *see* Spondylosis
syphilitic 095.5
wrist 726.4
Exotropia 378.10
alternating 378.15
with
A pattern 378.16
specified noncomitancy NEC 378.18
V pattern 378.17
X pattern 378.18
Y pattern 378.18
intermittent 378.24
intermittent 378.20
alternating 378.24
monocular 378.23
monocular 378.11
with
A pattern 378.12
specified noncomitancy NEC 378.14
V pattern 378.13
X pattern 378.14
Y pattern 378.14
intermittent 378.23
Explanation of
investigation finding V65.4 ☑
medication V65.4 ☑
Exposure (suspected) 994.9
algae bloom V87.32
cold 991.9
specified effect NEC 991.8
effects of 994.9
exhaustion due to 994.4
implanted vaginal mesh
into vagina 629.32
through vaginal wall 629.32
to
AIDS virus V01.79
anthrax V01.81
aromatic
amines V87.11
dyes V87.19
arsenic V87.01
asbestos V15.84
benzene V87.12
body fluids (hazardous) V15.85
cholera V01.0
chromium compounds V87.09
communicable disease V01.9
specified type NEC V01.89
dyes V87.2
aromatic V87.19
Escherichia coli (E. coli) V01.83
German measles V01.4
gonorrhea V01.6
hazardous
aromatic compounds NEC V87.19
body fluids V15.85
chemicals NEC V87.2
metals V87.09
substances V87.39
HIV V01.79
human immunodeficiency virus V01.79
lead V15.86
meningococcus V01.84
mold V87.31

Exposure — *continued*
to — *continued*
nickel dust V87.09
parasitic disease V01.89
poliomyelitis V01.2
polycyclic aromatic hydrocarbons V87.19
potentially hazardous body fluids V15.85
rabies V01.5
rubella V01.4
SARS-associated coronavirus V01.82
smallpox V01.3
syphilis V01.6
tuberculosis V01.1
uranium V87.02
varicella V01.71
venereal disease V01.6
viral disease NEC V01.79
varicella V01.71
vaginal prosthetic materials NEC
into vagina 629.32
through vaginal wall 629.32
Exsanguination, fetal 772.0
Exstrophy
abdominal content 751.8
bladder (urinary) 753.5
Extensive — *see* condition
Extra — *see also* Accessory
rib 756.3
cervical 756.2
Extraction
with hook 763.89
breech NEC 669.6 ☑
affecting fetus or newborn 763.0
cataract postsurgical V45.61
manual NEC 669.8 ☑
affecting fetus or newborn 763.89
Extrasystole 427.60
atrial 427.61
postoperative 997.1
ventricular 427.69
Extrauterine gestation or pregnancy — *see* Pregnancy, ectopic
Extravasation
blood 459.0
lower extremity 459.0
chemotherapy, vesicant 999.81
chyle into mesentery 457.8
pelvicalyceal 593.4
pyelosinus 593.4
urine 788.8
from ureter 788.8
vesicant
agent NEC 999.82
chemotherapy 999.81
Extremity — *see* condition
Extrophy — *see* Exstrophy
Extroversion
bladder 753.5
uterus 618.1
complicating delivery 665.2 ☑
affecting fetus or newborn 763.89
postpartal (old) 618.1
Extruded tooth 524.34
Extrusion
alveolus and teeth 524.75
breast implant (prosthetic) 996.54
device, implant, or graft — *see* Complications, mechanical
eye implant (ball) (globe) 996.59
intervertebral disc — *see* Displacement, intervertebral disc
lacrimal gland 375.43
mesh (reinforcing) 996.59
ocular lens implant 996.53
prosthetic device NEC — *see* Complications, mechanical
vitreous 379.26
Exudate, pleura — *see* Effusion, pleura
Exudates, retina 362.82
Exudative — *see* condition
Eye, eyeball, eyelid — *see* condition
Eyestrain 368.13
Eyeworm disease of Africa 125.2

F

Faber's anemia or syndrome (achlorhydric anemia) 280.9
Fabry's disease (angiokeratoma corporis diffusum) 272.7
Face, facial — *see* condition
Facet of cornea 371.44
Faciocephalalgia, autonomic — *see also* Neuropathy, peripheral, autonomic 337.9
Facioscapulohumeral myopathy 359.1
Factitious disorder, illness — *see* Illness, factitious
Factor
deficiency — *see* Deficiency, factor
psychic, associated with diseases classified elsewhere 316
risk — *see* Problem
V Leiden mutation 289.81
Fahr-Volhard disease (malignant nephrosclerosis) 403.00
Failure, failed
adenohypophyseal 253.2
attempted abortion (legal) (*see also* Abortion, failed) 638.9
bone marrow (anemia) 284.9
acquired (secondary) 284.89
congenital 284.09
idiopathic 284.9
cardiac (*see also* Failure, heart) 428.9
newborn 779.89
cardiorenal (chronic) 428.9
hypertensive (*see also* Hypertension, cardiorenal) 404.93
cardiorespiratory 799.1
specified during or due to a procedure 997.1
long-term effect of cardiac surgery 429.4
cardiovascular (chronic) 428.9
cerebrovascular 437.8
cervical dilatation in labor 661.0 ☑
affecting fetus or newborn 763.7
circulation, circulatory 799.89
fetus or newborn 779.89
peripheral 785.50
postoperative 998.00
compensation — *see* Disease, heart
congestive (*see also* Failure, heart) 428.0
conscious sedation, during procedure 995.24
coronary (*see also* Insufficiency, coronary) 411.89
dental implant 525.79
due to
infection 525.71
lack of attached gingiva 525.72
occlusal trauma (caused by poor prosthetic design) 525.72
parafunctional habits 525.72
periodontal infection (peri-implantitis) 525.72
poor oral hygiene 525.72
unintentional loading 525.71
endosseous NEC 525.79
mechanical 525.73
osseointegration 525.71
due to
complications of systemic disease 525.71
poor bone quality 525.71
premature loading 525.71
iatrogenic 525.71
prior to intentional prosthetic loading 525.71
post-osseointegration
biological 525.72
iatrogenic 525.72
due to complications of systemic disease 525.72
mechanical 525.73
pre-integration 525.71
pre-osseointegration 525.71
dental prosthesis causing loss of dental implant 525.73

Failure, failed — *continued*
dental restoration
marginal integrity 525.61
periodontal anatomical integrity 525.65
descent of head (at term) 652.5 ☑
affecting fetus or newborn 763.1
in labor 660.0 ☑
affecting fetus or newborn 763.1
device, implant, or graft — *see* Complications, mechanical
engagement of head NEC 652.5 ☑
in labor 660.0 ☑
extrarenal 788.99
fetal head to enter pelvic brim 652.5 ☑
affecting fetus or newborn 763.1
in labor 660.0 ☑
affecting fetus or newborn 763.1
forceps NEC 660.7 ☑
affecting fetus or newborn 763.1
fusion (joint) (spinal) 996.49
growth in childhood 783.43
heart (acute) (sudden) 428.9
with
abortion — *see* Abortion, by type, with specified complication NEC
acute pulmonary edema (*see also* Failure, ventricular, left) 428.1
with congestion (*see also* Failure, heart) 428.0
decompensation (*see also* Failure, heart) 428.0
dilation — *see* Disease, heart
ectopic pregnancy (*see also* categories 633.0–633.9) 639.8
molar pregnancy (*see also* categories 630–632) 639.8
arteriosclerotic 440.9
combined left-right sided 428.0
combined systolic and diastolic 428.40
acute 428.41
acute on chronic 428.43
chronic 428.42
compensated (*see also* Failure, heart) 428.0
complicating
abortion — *see* Abortion, by type, with specified complication NEC
delivery (cesarean) (instrumental) 669.4 ☑
ectopic pregnancy (*see also* categories 633.0–633.9) 639.8
molar pregnancy (*see also* categories 630–632) 639.8
obstetric anesthesia or sedation 668.1 ☑
surgery 997.1
congestive (compensated) (decompensated) (*see also* Failure, heart) 428.0
with rheumatic fever (conditions classifiable to 390)
active 391.8
inactive or quiescent (with chorea) 398.91
fetus or newborn 779.89
hypertensive (*see also* Hypertension, heart) 402.91
with renal disease (*see also* Hypertension, cardiorenal) 404.91
with renal failure 404.93
benign 402.11
malignant 402.01
rheumatic (chronic) (inactive) (with chorea) 398.91
active or acute 391.8
with chorea (Sydenham's) 392.0
decompensated (*see also* Failure, heart) 428.0
degenerative (*see also* Degeneration, myocardial) 429.1
diastolic 428.30
acute 428.31

Failure, failed — Fatigue

Failure, failed — *continued*
heart — *continued*
diastolic — *continued*
acute on chronic 428.33
chronic 428.32
due to presence of (cardiac) prosthesis 429.4
fetus or newborn 779.89
following
abortion 639.8
cardiac surgery 429.4
ectopic or molar pregnancy 639.8
high output NEC 428.9
hypertensive (*see also* Hypertension, heart) 402.91
with renal disease (*see also* Hypertension, cardiorenal) 404.91
with renal failure 404.93
benign 402.11
malignant 402.01
left (ventricular) (*see also* Failure, ventricular, left) 428.1
with right-sided failure (see also Failure, heart) 428.0
low output (syndrome) NEC 428.9
organic — *see* Disease, heart
postoperative (immediate) 997.1
long term effect of cardiac surgery 429.4
rheumatic (chronic) (congestive) (inactive) 398.91
right (secondary to left heart failure, conditions classifiable to 428.1) (ventricular) (*see also* Failure, heart) 428.0
senile 797
specified during or due to a procedure 997.1
long-term effect of cardiac surgery 429.4
systolic 428.20
acute 428.21
acute on chronic 428.23
chronic 428.22
thyrotoxic (*see also* Thyrotoxicosis) 242.9 ☑ [425.7]
valvular — *see* Endocarditis
hepatic 572.8
acute 570
due to a procedure 997.49
hepatorenal 572.4
hypertensive heart (*see also* Hypertension, heart) 402.91
benign 402.11
malignant 402.01
induction (of labor) 659.1 ☑
abortion (legal) (*see also* Abortion, failed) 638.9
affecting fetus or newborn 763.89
by oxytocic drugs 659.1 ☑
instrumental 659.0 ☑
mechanical 659.0 ☑
medical 659.1 ☑
surgical 659.0 ☑
initial alveolar expansion, newborn 770.4
involution, thymus (gland) 254.8
kidney — *see* Failure, renal
lactation 676.4 ☑
Leydig's cell, adult 257.2
liver 572.8
acute 570
medullary 799.89
mitral — *see* Endocarditis, mitral
moderate sedation, during procedure 995.24
myocardium, myocardial (*see also* Failure, heart) 428.9
chronic (*see also* Failure, heart) 428.0
congestive (*see also* Failure, heart) 428.0
ovarian (primary) 256.39
iatrogenic 256.2
postablative 256.2
postirradiation 256.2
postsurgical 256.2
ovulation 628.0
prerenal 788.99

Failure, failed — *continued*
renal (kidney) 586
with
abortion — *see* Abortion, by type, with renal failure
ectopic pregnancy (*see also* categories 633.0–633.9) 639.3
edema (*see also* Nephrosis) 581.9
hypertension (*see also* Hypertension, kidney) 403.91
hypertensive heart disease (conditions classifiable to 402) 404.92
with heart failure 404.93
benign 404.12
with heart failure 404.13
malignant 404.02
with heart failure 404.03
molar pregnancy (*see also* categories 630–632) 639.3
tubular necrosis (acute) 584.5
acute 584.9
with lesion of
necrosis
cortical (renal) 584.6
medullary (renal) (papillary) 584.7
tubular 584.5
specified pathology NEC 584.8
chronic 585.9
hypertensive or with hypertension (*see also* Hypertension, kidney) 403.91
due to a procedure 997.5
following
abortion 639.3
crushing 958.5
ectopic or molar pregnancy 639.3
labor and delivery (acute) 669.3 ☑
hypertensive (*see also* Hypertension, kidney) 403.91
puerperal, postpartum 669.3 ☑
respiration, respiratory 518.81
acute 518.81
following trauma and surgery 518.51
acute and chronic 518.84
following trauma and surgery 518.53
center 348.89
newborn 770.84
chronic 518.83
following trauma and surgery or shock 518.51
newborn 770.84
rotation
cecum 751.4
colon 751.4
intestine 751.4
kidney 753.3
sedation, during procedure
conscious 995.24
moderate 995.24
segmentation (*see also* Fusion)
fingers (*see also* Syndactylism, fingers) 755.11
toes (*see also* Syndactylism, toes) 755.13
seminiferous tubule, adult 257.2
senile (general) 797
with psychosis 290.20
testis, primary (seminal) 257.2
to progress 661.2 ☑
to thrive
adult 783.7
child 783.41
newborn 779.34
transplant 996.80
bone marrow 996.85
organ (immune or nonimmune cause) 996.80
bone marrow 996.85
heart 996.83
intestines 996.87
kidney 996.81
liver 996.82
lung 996.84
pancreas 996.86
specified NEC 996.89

Failure, failed — *continued*
transplant — *continued*
skin 996.52
artificial 996.55
decellularized allodermis 996.55
temporary allograft or pigskin graft — omit code
stem cell(s) 996.88
from
peripheral blood 996.88
umbilical cord 996.88
trial of labor NEC 660.6 ☑
affecting fetus or newborn 763.1
tubal ligation 998.89
urinary 586
vacuum extraction
abortion — *see* Abortion, failed
delivery NEC 660.7 ☑
affecting fetus or newborn 763.1
vasectomy 998.89
ventouse NEC 660.7 ☑
affecting fetus or newborn 763.1
ventricular (*see also* Failure, heart) 428.9
left 428.1
with rheumatic fever (conditions classifiable to 390)
active 391.8
with chorea 392.0
inactive or quiescent (with chorea) 398.91
hypertensive (*see also* Hypertension, heart) 402.91
benign 402.11
malignant 402.01
rheumatic (chronic) (inactive) (with chorea) 398.91
active or acute 391.8
with chorea 392.0
right (*see also* Failure, heart) 428.0
vital centers, fetus or newborn 779.89
weight gain in childhood 783.41
Fainting (fit) (spell) 780.2
Falciform hymen 752.49
Fallen arches 734
Falling, any organ or part — *see* Prolapse
Fall, maternal, affecting fetus or newborn 760.5
Fallopian
insufflation
fertility testing V26.21
following sterilization reversal V26.22
tube — *see* condition
Fallot's
pentalogy 745.2
tetrad or tetralogy 745.2
triad or trilogy 746.09
Fallout, radioactive (adverse effect) NEC 990
False — *see also* condition
bundle branch block 426.50
bursa 727.89
croup 478.75
joint 733.82
labor (pains) 644.1 ☑
opening, urinary, male 752.69
passage, urethra (prostatic) 599.4
positive
serological test for syphilis 795.6
Wassermann reaction 795.6
pregnancy 300.11
Family, familial — *see also* condition
affected by
family member
currently on deployment (military) V61.01
returned from deployment (military) (current or past conflict) V61.02
disruption (*see also* Disruption, family) V61.09
estrangement V61.09
hemophagocytic
lymphohistiocytosis 288.4
reticulosis 288.4
Li-Fraumeni (syndrome) V84.01
planning advice V25.09

Family, familial — *see also* condition — *continued*
planning advice — *continued*
natural
procreative V26.41
to avoid pregnancy V25.04
problem V61.9
specified circumstance NEC V61.8
retinoblastoma (syndrome) 190.5
Famine 994.2
edema 262
Fanconi's anemia (congenital pancytopenia) 284.09
Fanconi (-de Toni) (-Debré) syndrome (cystinosis) 270.0
Farber (-Uzman) syndrome or disease (disseminated lipogranulomatosis) 272.8
Farcin 024
Farcy 024
Farmers'
lung 495.0
skin 692.74
Farsightedness 367.0
Fascia — *see* condition
Fasciculation 781.0
Fasciculitis optica 377.32
Fasciitis 729.4
eosinophilic 728.89
necrotizing 728.86
nodular 728.79
perirenal 593.4
plantar 728.71
pseudosarcomatous 728.79
traumatic (old) NEC 728.79
current — *see* Sprain, by site
Fasciola hepatica infestation 121.3
Fascioliasis 121.3
Fasciolopsiasis (small intestine) 121.4
Fasciolopsis (small intestine) 121.4
Fast pulse 785.0
Fat
embolism (cerebral) (pulmonary) (systemic) 958.1
with
abortion — *see* Abortion, by type, with embolism
ectopic pregnancy (*see also* categories 633.0–633.9) 639.6
molar pregnancy (*see also* categories 630–632) 639.6
complicating delivery or puerperium 673.8 ☑
following
abortion 639.6
ectopic or molar pregnancy 639.6
in pregnancy, childbirth, or the puerperium 673.8 ☑
excessive 278.02
in heart (*see also* Degeneration, myocardial) 429.1
general 278.02
hernia, herniation 729.30
eyelid 374.34
knee 729.31
orbit 374.34
retro-orbital 374.34
retropatellar 729.31
specified site NEC 729.39
indigestion 579.8
in stool 792.1
localized (pad) 278.1
heart (*see also* Degeneration, myocardial) 429.1
knee 729.31
retropatellar 729.31
necrosis (*see also* Fatty, degeneration)
breast (aseptic) (segmental) 611.3
mesentery 567.82
omentum 567.82
peritoneum 567.82
pad 278.1
Fatal familial insomnia (FFI) 046.72
Fatal syncope 798.1
Fatigue 780.79
auditory deafness (*see also* Deafness) 389.9
chronic, syndrome 780.71

Fatigue — *continued*
   combat (*see also* Reaction, stress, acute)
      308.9
   during pregnancy 646.8 ☑
   general 780.79
      psychogenic 300.5
   heat (transient) 992.6
   muscle 729.89
   myocardium (*see also* Failure, heart) 428.9
   nervous 300.5
   neurosis 300.5
   operational 300.89
   postural 729.89
   posture 729.89
   psychogenic (general) 300.5
   senile 797
   syndrome NEC 300.5
      chronic 780.71
   undue 780.79
   voice 784.49
Fatness 278.02
Fatty — *see also* condition
   apron 278.1
   degeneration (diffuse) (general) NEC 272.8
      localized — *see* Degeneration, by site,
         fatty
      placenta — *see* Placenta, abnormal
   heart (enlarged) (*see also* Degeneration,
      myocardial) 429.1
   infiltration (diffuse) (general) (*see also* De-
      generation, by site, fatty) 272.8
      heart (enlarged) (*see also* Degeneration,
         myocardial) 429.1
   liver 571.8
      alcoholic 571.0
   necrosis — *see* Degeneration, fatty
   phanerosis 272.8
Fauces — *see* condition
Fauchard's disease (periodontitis) 523.40
Faucitis 478.29
Faulty — *see also* condition
   position of teeth 524.30
Favism (anemia) 282.2
Favre-Racouchot disease (elastoidosis cutanea nodularis) 701.8
Favus 110.9
   beard 110.0
   capitis 110.0
   corporis 110.5
   eyelid 110.8
   foot 110.4
   hand 110.2
   scalp 110.0
   specified site NEC 110.8
Feared complaint unfounded V65.5
Fear, fearfulness (complex) (reaction) 300.20
   child 313.0
   of
      animals 300.29
      closed spaces 300.29
      crowds 300.29
      eating in public 300.23
      heights 300.29
      open spaces 300.22
         with panic attacks 300.21
      public speaking 300.23
      streets 300.22
         with panic attacks 300.21
      travel 300.22
         with panic attacks 300.21
      washing in public 300.23
   transient 308.0
Febricula (continued) (simple) — *see also*
   Pyrexia 780.60
Febrile — *see also* Pyrexia 780.60
   convulsion (simple) 780.31
      complex 780.32
   nonhemolytic transfusion reaction (FNHTR)
      780.66
   seizure (simple) 780.31
      atypical 780.32
      complex 780.32
      complicated 780.32
Febris — *see also* Fever 780.60
   aestiva (*see also* Fever, hay) 477.9
   flava (*see also* Fever, yellow) 060.9

Febris — *see also* Fever — *continued*
   melitensis 023.0
   pestis (*see also* Plague) 020.9
   puerperalis 672.0 ☑
   recurrens (*see also* Fever, relapsing) 087.9
      pediculo vestimenti 087.0
   rubra 034.1
   typhoidea 002.0
   typhosa 002.0
Fecal — *see* condition
Fecalith (impaction) 560.32
   with hernia (*see also* Hernia, by site, with
      obstruction)
      gangrenous — *see* Hernia, by site, with
         gangrene
   appendix 543.9
   congenital 777.1
Fede's disease 529.0
Feeble-minded 317
**Feeble rapid pulse due to shock following
   injury** 958.4
Feeding
   faulty (elderly) (infant) 783.3
      newborn 779.31
   formula check V20.2
   improper (elderly) (infant) 783.3
      newborn 779.31
   problem (elderly) (infant) 783.3
      newborn 779.31
      nonorganic origin 307.59
Feeling of foreign body in throat 784.99
Feer's disease 985.0
Feet — *see* condition
Feigned illness V65.2
Feil-Klippel syndrome (brevicollis) 756.16
Feinmesser's (hidrotic) **ectodermal dysplasia**
   757.31
Felix's disease (juvenile osteochondrosis, hip)
   732.1
Felon (any digit) (with lymphangitis) 681.01
   herpetic 054.6
Felty's syndrome (rheumatoid arthritis with
   splenomegaly and leukopenia) 714.1
Feminism in boys 302.6
Feminization, testicular 259.51
   with pseudohermaphroditism, male 259.51
Femoral hernia — *see* Hernia, femoral
Femora vara 736.32
Femur, femoral — *see* condition
Fenestrata placenta — *see* Placenta, abnormal
Fenestration, fenestrated — *see also* Imperfect, closure
   aorta-pulmonary 745.0
   aorticopulmonary 745.0
   aortopulmonary 745.0
   cusps, heart valve NEC 746.89
      pulmonary 746.09
   hymen 752.49
   pulmonic cusps 746.09
Fenwick's disease 537.89
Fermentation (gastric) (gastrointestinal)
   (stomach) 536.8
   intestine 564.89
      psychogenic 306.4
   psychogenic 306.4
Fernell's disease (aortic aneurysm) 441.9
Fertile eunuch syndrome 257.2
Fertility, meaning multiparity — *see* Multiparity
Fetal
   alcohol syndrome 760.71
   anemia 678.0 ☑
      thrombocytopenia 678.0 ☑
      twin to twin transfusion 678.0 ☑
Fetalis uterus 752.39
Fetid
   breath 784.99
   sweat 705.89
Fetishism 302.81
   transvestic 302.3
Fetomaternal hemorrhage
   affecting management of pregnancy
      656.0 ☑
      fetus or newborn 772.0
Fetus, fetal — *see also* condition
   papyraceous 779.89

Fetus, fetal — *see also* condition —
   continued
   type lung tissue 770.4
Fever 780.60
   with chills 780.60
      in malarial regions (*see also* Malaria)
         084.6
   abortus NEC 023.9
   aden 061
   African tick-borne 087.1
   American
      mountain tick 066.1
      spotted 082.0
   and ague (*see also* Malaria) 084.6
   aphthous 078.4
   arbovirus hemorrhagic 065.9
   Assam 085.0
   Australian A or Q 083.0
   Bangkok hemorrhagic 065.4
   biliary, Charcôt's intermittent — *see* Chole-
      docholithiasis
   bilious, hemoglobinuric 084.8
   blackwater 084.8
   blister 054.9
   Bonvale Dam 780.79
   boutonneuse 082.1
   brain 323.9
      late effect — *see* category 326
   breakbone 061
   Bullis 082.8
   Bunyamwera 066.3
   Burdwan 085.0
   Bwamba (encephalitis) 066.3
   Cameroon (*see also* Malaria) 084.6
   Canton 081.9
   cat-scratch 078.3
   catarrhal (acute) 460
      chronic 472.0
   cerebral 323.9
      late effect — *see* category 326
   cerebrospinal (meningococcal) (*see also*
      Meningitis, cerebrospinal) 036.0
   Chagres 084.0
   Chandipura 066.8
   changuinola 066.0
   Charcôt's (biliary) (hepatic) (intermittent)
      — *see* Choledocholithiasis
   Chikungunya (viral) 066.3
      hemorrhagic 065.4
   childbed 670.8 ☑
   Chitral 066.0
   Colombo (*see also* Fever, paratyphoid) 002.9
   Colorado tick (virus) 066.1
   congestive
      malarial (*see also* Malaria) 084.6
      remittent (*see also* Malaria) 084.6
   Congo virus 065.0
   continued 780.60
      malarial 084.0
   Corsican (*see also* Malaria) 084.6
   Crimean hemorrhagic 065.0
   Cyprus (*see also* Brucellosis) 023.9
   dandy 061
   deer fly (*see also* Tularemia) 021.9
   dehydration, newborn 778.4
   dengue (virus) 061
      hemorrhagic 065.4
   desert 114.0
   due to heat 992.0
   Dumdum 085.0
   enteric 002.0
   ephemeral (of unknown origin) (*see also*
      Pyrexia) 780.60
   epidemic, hemorrhagic of the Far East 065.0
   erysipelatous (*see also* Erysipelas) 035
   estivo-autumnal (malarial) 084.0
   etiocholanolone 277.31
   famine (*see also* Fever, relapsing)
      meaning typhus — *see* Typhus
   Far Eastern hemorrhagic 065.0
   five day 083.1
   Fort Bragg 100.89
   gastroenteric 002.0
   gastromalarial (*see also* Malaria) 084.6
   Gibraltar (*see also* Brucellosis) 023.9
   glandular 075

Fever — *continued*
   Guama (viral) 066.3
   Haverhill 026.1
   hay (allergic) (with rhinitis) 477.9
      with
         asthma (bronchial) (*see also* Asthma)
            493.0 ☑
      due to
         dander, animal (cat) (dog) 477.2
         dust 477.8
         fowl 477.8
         hair, animal (cat) (dog) 477.2
         pollen, any plant or tree 477.0
         specified allergen other than pollen
            477.8
   heat (effects) 992.0
   hematuric, bilious 084.8
   hemoglobinuric (malarial) 084.8
      bilious 084.8
   hemorrhagic (arthropod-borne) NEC 065.9
      with renal syndrome 078.6
      arenaviral 078.7
      Argentine 078.7
      Bangkok 065.4
      Bolivian 078.7
      Central Asian 065.0
      chikungunya 065.4
      Crimean 065.0
      dengue (virus) 065.4
      Ebola 065.8
      epidemic 078.6
         of Far East 065.0
      Far Eastern 065.0
      Junin virus 078.7
      Korean 078.6
      Kyasanur forest 065.2
      Machupo virus 078.7
      mite-borne NEC 065.8
      mosquito-borne 065.4
      Omsk 065.1
      Philippine 065.4
      Russian (Yaroslav) 078.6
      Singapore 065.4
      Southeast Asia 065.4
      Thailand 065.4
      tick-borne NEC 065.3
   hepatic (*see also* Cholecystitis) 575.8
      intermittent (Charcôt's) — *see* Choledo-
         cholithiasis
   herpetic (*see also* Herpes) 054.9
   Hyalomma tick 065.0
   icterohemorrhagic 100.0
   inanition 780.60
      newborn 778.4
   in conditions classified elsewhere 780.61
   infective NEC 136.9
   intermittent (bilious) (*see also* Malaria) 084.6
      hepatic (Charcôt) — *see* Choledocholithi-
         asis
      of unknown origin (*see also* Pyrexia)
         780.60
   pernicious 084.0
   iodide
      correct substance properly administered
         780.60
      overdose or wrong substance given or
         taken 975.5
   Japanese river 081.2
   jungle yellow 060.0
   Junin virus, hemorrhagic 078.7
   Katayama 120.2
   Kedani 081.2
   Kenya 082.1
   Korean hemorrhagic 078.6
   Lassa 078.89
   Lone Star 082.8
   lung — *see* Pneumonia
   Machupo virus, hemorrhagic 078.7
   malaria, malarial (*see also* Malaria) 084.6
   Malta (*see also* Brucellosis) 023.9
   Marseilles 082.1
   marsh (*see also* Malaria) 084.6
   Mayaro (viral) 066.3
   Mediterranean (*see also* Brucellosis) 023.9
      familial 277.31
      tick 082.1

☑ **Additional Digit Required — Refer to the Tabular List for Digit Selection**

▽ **Subterms under main terms may continue to next column or page**

2014 ICD-9-CM

▶◀ **Revised Text**   ● **New Line**   ▲ **Revised Code**

Volume 2 — 113

Fatigue — Fever

Fever — *continued*
- meningeal — *see* Meningitis
- metal fumes NEC 985.8
- Meuse 083.1
- Mexican — *see* Typhus, Mexican
- Mianeh 087.1
- miasmatic (*see also* Malaria) 084.6
- miliary 078.2
- milk, female 672.0 ☑
- mill 504
- mite-borne hemorrhagic 065.8
- Monday 504
- mosquito-borne NEC 066.3
  - hemorrhagic NEC 065.4
- mountain 066.1
  - meaning
    - Rocky Mountain spotted 082.0
    - undulant fever (*see also* Brucellosis) 023.9
  - tick (American) 066.1
- Mucambo (viral) 066.3
- mud 100.89
- Neapolitan (*see also* Brucellosis) 023.9
- neutropenic 288.00
- newborn (environmentally-induced) 778.4
- nine-mile 083.0
- nonexanthematous tick 066.1
- North Asian tick-borne typhus 082.2
- Omsk hemorrhagic 065.1
- O'nyong-nyong (viral) 066.3
- Oropouche (viral) 066.3
- Oroya 088.0
- paludal (*see also* Malaria) 084.6
- Panama 084.0
- pappataci 066.0
- paratyphoid 002.9
  - A 002.1
  - B (Schottmüller's) 002.2
  - C (Hirschfeld) 002.3
- parrot 073.9
- periodic 277.31
- pernicious, acute 084.0
- persistent (of unknown origin) (*see also* Pyrexia) 780.60
- petechial 036.0
- pharyngoconjunctival 077.2
  - adenoviral type 3 077.2
- Philippine hemorrhagic 065.4
- phlebotomus 066.0
- Piry 066.8
- Pixuna (viral) 066.3
- Plasmodium ovale 084.3
- pleural (*see also* Pleurisy) 511.0
- pneumonic — *see* Pneumonia
- polymer fume 987.8
- postimmunization 780.63
- postoperative 780.62
  - due to infection 998.59
- posttransfusion 780.66
- postvaccination 780.63
- pretibial 100.89
- puerperal, postpartum 672.0 ☑
- putrid — *see* Septicemia
- pyemic — *see* Septicemia
- Q 083.0
  - with pneumonia 083.0 [484.8]
- quadrilateral 083.0
- quartan (malaria) 084.2
- Queensland (coastal) 083.0
  - seven-day 100.89
- Quintan (A) 083.1
- quotidian 084.0
- rabbit (*see also* Tularemia) 021.9
- rat-bite 026.9
  - due to
    - Spirillum minor or minus 026.0
    - Spirochaeta morsus muris 026.0
    - Streptobacillus moniliformis 026.1
- recurrent — *see* Fever, relapsing
- relapsing 087.9
  - Carter's (Asiatic) 087.0
  - Dutton's (West African) 087.1
  - Koch's 087.9
  - louse-borne (epidemic) 087.0
  - Novy's (American) 087.1
  - Obermeyer's (European) 087.0

Fever — *continued*
- relapsing — *continued*
  - spirillum NEC 087.9
  - tick-borne (endemic) 087.1
- remittent (bilious) (congestive) (gastric) (*see also* Malaria) 084.6
- rheumatic (active) (acute) (chronic) (subacute) 390
  - with heart involvement 391.9
    - carditis 391.9
    - endocarditis (aortic) (mitral) (pulmonary) (tricuspid) 391.1
    - multiple sites 391.8
    - myocarditis 391.2
    - pancarditis, acute 391.8
    - pericarditis 391.0
    - specified type NEC 391.8
    - valvulitis 391.1
  - cardiac hypertrophy 398.99
  - inactive or quiescent
    - with cardiac hypertrophy 398.99
    - carditis 398.90
    - endocarditis 397.9
      - aortic (valve) 395.9
        - with mitral (valve) disease 396.9
      - mitral (valve) 394.9
        - with aortic (valve) disease 396.9
      - pulmonary (valve) 397.1
      - tricuspid (valve) 397.0
    - heart conditions (classifiable to 429.3, 429.6, 429.9) 398.99
      - failure (congestive) (conditions classifiable to 428.0, 428.9) 398.91
      - left ventricular failure (conditions classifiable to 428.1) 398.91
      - myocardial degeneration (conditions classifiable to 429.1) 398.0
    - myocarditis (conditions classifiable to 429.0) 398.0
    - pancarditis 398.99
    - pericarditis 393
- Rift Valley (viral) 066.3
- Rocky Mountain spotted 082.0
- rose 477.0
- Ross river (viral) 066.3
- Russian hemorrhagic 078.6
- sandfly 066.0
- San Joaquin (valley) 114.0
- São Paulo 082.0
- scarlet 034.1
- septic — *see* Septicemia
- seven-day 061
  - Japan 100.89
  - Queensland 100.89
- shin bone 083.1
- Singapore hemorrhagic 065.4
- solar 061
- sore 054.9
- South African tick-bite 087.1
- Southeast Asia hemorrhagic 065.4
- spinal — *see* Meningitis
- spirillary 026.0
- splenic (*see also* Anthrax) 022.9
- spotted (Rocky Mountain) 082.0
  - American 082.0
  - Brazilian 082.0
  - Colombian 082.0
  - meaning
    - cerebrospinal meningitis 036.0
    - typhus 082.9
- spring 309.23
- steroid
  - correct substance properly administered 780.60
  - overdose or wrong substance given or taken 962.0
- streptobacillary 026.1
- subtertian 084.0
- Sumatran mite 081.2
- sun 061
- swamp 100.89
- sweating 078.2
- swine 003.8

Fever — *continued*
- sylvatic yellow 060.0
- Tahyna 062.5
- tertian — *see* Malaria, tertian
- Thailand hemorrhagic 065.4
- thermic 992.0
- three day 066.0
  - with Coxsackie exanthem 074.8
- tick-bite NEC 066.1
- tick-borne NEC 066.1
  - hemorrhagic NEC 065.3
- tick
  - American mountain 066.1
  - Colorado 066.1
  - Kemerovo 066.1
  - Mediterranean 082.1
  - mountain 066.1
  - nonexanthematous 066.1
  - Quaranfil 066.1
- transitory of newborn 778.4
- trench 083.1
- tsutsugamushi 081.2
- typhogastric 002.0
- typhoid (abortive) (ambulant) (any site) (hemorrhagic) (infection) (intermittent) (malignant) (rheumatic) 002.0
- typhomalarial (*see also* Malaria) 084.6
- typhus — *see* Typhus
- undulant (*see also* Brucellosis) 023.9
- unknown origin (*see also* Pyrexia) 780.60
- uremic — *see* Uremia
- uveoparotid 135
- valley (Coccidioidomycosis) 114.0
- Venezuelan equine 066.2
- Volhynian 083.1
- Wesselsbron (viral) 066.3
- West
  - African 084.8
  - Nile (viral) 066.40
    - with
      - cranial nerve disorders 066.42
      - encephalitis 066.41
      - optic neuritis 066.42
      - other complications 066.49
      - other neurologic manifestations 066.42
      - polyradiculitis 066.42
- Whitmore's 025
- Wolhynian 083.1
- worm 128.9
- Yaroslav hemorrhagic 078.6
- yellow 060.9
  - jungle 060.0
  - sylvatic 060.0
  - urban 060.1
  - vaccination, prophylactic (against) V04.4
- Zika (viral) 066.3

Fibrillation
- atrial (established) (paroxysmal) 427.31
- auricular (atrial) (established) 427.31
- cardiac (ventricular) 427.41
- coronary (*see also* Infarct, myocardium) 410.9 ☑
- heart (ventricular) 427.41
- muscular 728.9
- postoperative 997.1
- ventricular 427.41

Fibrin
- ball or bodies, pleural (sac) 511.0
- chamber, anterior (eye) (gelatinous exudate) 364.04

Fibrinogenolysis (hemorrhagic) — *see* Fibrinolysis

Fibrinogenopenia (congenital) (hereditary) — *see also* Defect, coagulation 286.3
- acquired 286.6

Fibrinolysis (acquired) (hemorrhagic) (pathologic) 286.6
- with
  - abortion — *see* Abortion, by type, with hemorrhage, delayed or excessive
  - ectopic pregnancy (*see also* categories 633.0–633.9) 639.1
  - molar pregnancy (*see also* categories 630–632) 639.1
- antepartum or intrapartum 641.3 ☑

Fibrinolysis — *continued*
- antepartum or intrapartum — *continued*
  - affecting fetus or newborn 762.1
- following
  - abortion 639.1
  - ectopic or molar pregnancy 639.1
- newborn, transient 776.2
- postpartum 666.3 ☑

Fibrinopenia (hereditary) — *see also* Defect, coagulation 286.3
- acquired 286.6

Fibrinopurulent — *see* condition

Fibrinous — *see* condition

Fibro-odontoma, ameloblastic (M9290/0) 213.1
- upper jaw (bone) 213.0

Fibro-osteoma (M9262/0) — *see* Neoplasm, bone, benign

Fibroadenoma (M9010/0)
- cellular intracanalicular (M9020/0) 217
- giant (intracanalicular) (M9020/0) 217
- intracanalicular (M9011/0)
  - cellular (M9020/0) 217
  - giant (M9020/0) 217
  - specified site — *see* Neoplasm, by site, benign
  - unspecified site 217
- juvenile (M9030/0) 217
- pericanicular (M9012/0)
  - specified site — *see* Neoplasm, by site, benign
  - unspecified site 217
- phyllodes (M9020/0) 217
- prostate 600.20
  - with
    - other lower urinary tract symptoms (LUTS) 600.21
    - urinary
      - obstruction 600.21
      - retention 600.21
- specified site — *see* Neoplasm, by site, benign
- unspecified site 217

Fibroadenosis, breast (chronic) (cystic) (diffuse) (periodic) (segmental) 610.2

Fibroangioma (M9160/0) — *see also* Neoplasm, by site, benign
- juvenile (M9160/0)
  - specified site — *see* Neoplasm, by site, benign
  - unspecified site 210.7

Fibrocellulitis progressiva ossificans 728.11

Fibrochondrosarcoma (M9220/3) — *see* Neoplasm, cartilage, malignant

Fibrocystic
- disease 277.00
  - bone NEC 733.29
  - breast 610.1
  - jaw 526.2
  - kidney (congenital) 753.19
  - liver 751.62
  - lung 518.89
    - congenital 748.4
  - pancreas 277.00
- kidney (congenital) 753.19

Fibrodysplasia ossificans multiplex (progressiva) 728.11

Fibroelastosis (cordis) (endocardial) (endomyocardial) 425.3

Fibroid (tumor) (M8890/0) — *see also* Neoplasm, connective tissue, benign
- disease, lung (chronic) (*see also* Fibrosis, lung) 515
- heart (disease) (*see also* Myocarditis) 429.0
- induration, lung (chronic) (*see also* Fibrosis, lung) 515
- in pregnancy or childbirth 654.1 ☑
  - affecting fetus or newborn 763.89
  - causing obstructed labor 660.2 ☑
    - affecting fetus or newborn 763.1
- liver — *see* Cirrhosis, liver
- lung (*see also* Fibrosis, lung) 515
- pneumonia (chronic) (*see also* Fibrosis, lung) 515

☑ **Additional Digit Required — Refer to the Tabular List for Digit Selection**   ▽ **Subterms under main terms may continue to next column or page**

114 — Volume 2   ▶◀ Revised Text   ● New Line   ▲ Revised Code   2014 ICD-9-CM

Fibroid — *see also* Neoplasm, connective tissue, benign — *continued*
uterus (M8890/0) (*see also* Leiomyoma, uterus) 218.9
Fibrolipoma (M8851/0) — *see also* Lipoma, by site 214.9
Fibroliposarcoma (M8850/3) — *see* Neoplasm, connective tissue, malignant
Fibroma (M8810/0) — *see also* Neoplasm, connective tissue, benign
ameloblastic (M9330/0) 213.1
upper jaw (bone) 213.0
bone (nonossifying) 733.99
ossifying (M9262/0) — *see* Neoplasm, bone, benign
cementifying (M9274/0) — *see* Neoplasm, bone, benign
chondromyxoid (M9241/0) — *see* Neoplasm, bone, benign
desmoplastic (M8823/1) — *see* Neoplasm, connective tissue, uncertain behavior
facial (M8813/0) — *see* Neoplasm, connective tissue, benign
invasive (M8821/1) — *see* Neoplasm, connective tissue, uncertain behavior
molle (M8851/0) (*see also* Lipoma, by site) 214.9
myxoid (M8811/0) — *see* Neoplasm, connective tissue, benign
nasopharynx, nasopharyngeal (juvenile) (M9160/0) 210.7
nonosteogenic (nonossifying) — *see* Dysplasia, fibrous
odontogenic (M9321/0) 213.1
upper jaw (bone) 213.0
ossifying (M9262/0) — *see* Neoplasm, bone, benign
periosteal (M8812/0) — *see* Neoplasm, bone, benign
prostate 600.20
with
other lower urinary tract symptoms (LUTS) 600.21
urinary
obstruction 600.21
retention 600.21
soft (M8851/0) (*see also* Lipoma, by site) 214.9
Fibromatosis 728.79
abdominal (M8822/1) — *see* Neoplasm, connective tissue, uncertain behavior
aggressive (M8821/1) — *see* Neoplasm, connective tissue, uncertain behavior
congenital generalized (CGF) 759.89
Dupuytren's 728.6
gingival 523.8
plantar fascia 728.71
proliferative 728.79
pseudosarcomatous (proliferative) (subcutaneous) 728.79
subcutaneous pseudosarcomatous (proliferative) 728.79
Fibromyalgia 729.1
Fibromyoma (M8890/0) — *see also* Neoplasm, connective tissue, benign
uterus (corpus) (*see also* Leiomyoma, uterus) 218.9
in pregnancy or childbirth 654.1 ☑
affecting fetus or newborn 763.89
causing obstructed labor 660.2 ☑
affecting fetus or newborn 763.1
Fibromyositis — *see also* Myositis 729.1
scapulohumeral 726.2
Fibromyxolipoma (M8852/0) — *see also* Lipoma, by site 214.9
Fibromyxoma (M8811/0) — *see* Neoplasm, connective tissue, benign
Fibromyxosarcoma (M8811/3) — *see* Neoplasm, connective tissue, malignant
Fibroplasia, retrolental (*see also* Retinopathy of prematurity) 362.21
Fibropurulent — *see* condition
Fibrosarcoma (M8810/3) — *see also* Neoplasm, connective tissue, malignant
ameloblastic (M9330/3) 170.1
upper jaw (bone) 170.0

Fibrosarcoma — *see also* Neoplasm, connective tissue, malignant — *continued*
congenital (M8814/3) — *see* Neoplasm, connective tissue, malignant
fascial (M8813/3) — *see* Neoplasm, connective tissue, malignant
infantile (M8814/3) — *see* Neoplasm, connective tissue, malignant
odontogenic (M9330/3) 170.1
upper jaw (bone) 170.0
periosteal (M8812/3) — *see* Neoplasm, bone, malignant
Fibrosclerosis
breast 610.3
corpora cavernosa (penis) 607.89
familial multifocal NEC 710.8
multifocal (idiopathic) NEC 710.8
penis (corpora cavernosa) 607.89
Fibrosis, fibrotic
adrenal (gland) 255.8
alveolar (diffuse) 516.31
amnion 658.8 ☑
anal papillae 569.49
anus 569.49
appendix, appendiceal, noninflammatory 543.9
arteriocapillary — *see* Arteriosclerosis
bauxite (of lung) 503
biliary 576.8
due to Clonorchis sinensis 121.1
bladder 596.89
interstitial 595.1
localized submucosal 595.1
panmural 595.1
bone, diffuse 756.59
breast 610.3
capillary (*see also* Arteriosclerosis)
lung (chronic) (*see also* Fibrosis, lung) 515
cardiac (*see also* Myocarditis) 429.0
cervix 622.8
chorion 658.8 ☑
corpus cavernosum 607.89
cystic (of pancreas) 277.00
with
manifestations
gastrointestinal 277.03
pulmonary 277.02
specified NEC 277.09
meconium ileus 277.01
pulmonary exacerbation 277.02
due to (presence of) any device, implant, or graft — *see* Complications, due to (presence of) any device, implant, or graft classified to 996.0–996.5 NEC
ejaculatory duct 608.89
endocardium (*see also* Endocarditis) 424.90
endomyocardial (African) 425.0
epididymis 608.89
eye muscle 378.62
graphite (of lung) 503
heart (*see also* Myocarditis) 429.0
hepatic (*see also* Cirrhosis, liver)
due to Clonorchis sinensis 121.1
hepatolienal — *see* Cirrhosis, liver
hepatosplenic — *see* Cirrhosis, liver
infrapatellar fat pad 729.31
interstitial pulmonary, newborn 770.7
intrascrotal 608.89
kidney (*see also* Sclerosis, renal) 587
liver — *see* Cirrhosis, liver
lung (atrophic) (capillary) (chronic) (confluent) (massive) (perialveolar) (peribronchial) 515
with
anthracosilicosis (occupational) 500
anthracosis (occupational) 500
asbestosis (occupational) 501
bagassosis (occupational) 495.1
bauxite 503
berylliosis (occupational) 503
byssinosis (occupational) 504
calcicosis (occupational) 502
chalicosis (occupational) 502
dust reticulation (occupational) 504

Fibrosis, fibrotic — *continued*
lung — *continued*
with — *continued*
farmers' lung 495.0
gannister disease (occupational) 502
graphite 503
pneumoconiosis (occupational) 505
pneumosiderosis (occupational) 503
siderosis (occupational) 503
silicosis (occupational) 502
tuberculosis (*see also* Tuberculosis) 011.4 ☑
diffuse (idiopathic) (interstitial) 516.31
due to
bauxite 503
fumes or vapors (chemical) (inhalation) 506.4
graphite 503
following radiation 508.1
postinflammatory 515
silicotic (massive) (occupational) 502
tuberculous (*see also* Tuberculosis) 011.4 ☑
lymphatic gland 289.3
median bar 600.90
with
other lower urinary tract symptoms (LUTS) 600.91
urinary
obstruction 600.91
retention 600.91
mediastinum (idiopathic) 519.3
meninges 349.2
muscle NEC 728.2
iatrogenic (from injection) 999.9
myocardium, myocardial (*see also* Myocarditis) 429.0
oral submucous 528.8
ovary 620.8
oviduct 620.8
pancreas 577.8
cystic 277.00
with
manifestations
gastrointestinal 277.03
pulmonary 277.02
specified NEC 277.09
meconium ileus 277.01
pulmonary exacerbation 277.02
penis 607.89
periappendiceal 543.9
periarticular (*see also* Ankylosis) 718.5 ☑
pericardium 423.1
perineum, in pregnancy or childbirth 654.8 ☑
affecting fetus or newborn 763.89
causing obstructed labor 660.2 ☑
affecting fetus or newborn 763.1
perineural NEC 355.9
foot 355.6
periureteral 593.89
placenta — *see* Placenta, abnormal
pleura 511.0
popliteal fat pad 729.31
preretinal 362.56
prostate (chronic) 600.90
with
other lower urinary tract symptoms (LUTS) 600.91
urinary
obstruction 600.91
retention 600.91
pulmonary (chronic) (*see also* Fibrosis, lung) 515
alveolar capillary block 516.8
idiopathic 516.31
interstitial
diffuse (idiopathic) 516.31
newborn 770.7
radiation — *see* Effect, adverse, radiation
rectal sphincter 569.49
retroperitoneal, idiopathic 593.4
sclerosing mesenteric (idiopathic) 567.82
scrotum 608.89
seminal vesicle 608.89

Fibrosis, fibrotic — *continued*
senile 797
skin NEC 709.2
spermatic cord 608.89
spleen 289.59
bilharzial (*see also* Schistosomiasis) 120.9
subepidermal nodular (M8832/0) — *see* Neoplasm, skin, benign
submucous NEC 709.2
oral 528.8
tongue 528.8
syncytium — *see* Placenta, abnormal
testis 608.89
chronic, due to syphilis 095.8
thymus (gland) 254.8
tunica vaginalis 608.89
ureter 593.89
urethra 599.84
uterus (nonneoplastic) 621.8
bilharzial (*see also* Schistosomiasis) 120.9
neoplastic (*see also* Leiomyoma, uterus) 218.9
vagina 623.8
valve, heart (*see also* Endocarditis) 424.90
vas deferens 608.89
vein 459.89
lower extremities 459.89
vesical 595.1
Fibrositis (periarticular) (rheumatoid) 729.0
humeroscapular region 726.2
nodular, chronic
Jaccoud's 714.4
rheumatoid 714.4
ossificans 728.11
scapulohumeral 726.2
Fibrothorax 511.0
Fibrotic — *see* Fibrosis
Fibrous — *see* condition
Fibroxanthoma (M8831/0) — *see also* Neoplasm, connective tissue, benign
atypical (M8831/1) — *see* Neoplasm, connective tissue, uncertain behavior
malignant (M8831/3) — *see* Neoplasm, connective tissue, malignant
Fibroxanthosarcoma (M8831/3) — *see* Neoplasm, connective tissue, malignant
Fiedler's
disease (leptospiral jaundice) 100.0
myocarditis or syndrome (acute isolated myocarditis) 422.91
Fiessinger-Leroy (-Reiter) syndrome 099.3
Fiessinger-Rendu syndrome (erythema muliforme exudativum) 695.19
Fifth disease (eruptive) 057.0
venereal 099.1
Filaria, filarial — *see* Infestation, filarial
Filariasis — *see also* Infestation, filarial 125.9
bancroftian 125.0
Brug's 125.1
due to
bancrofti 125.0
Brugia (Wuchereria) (malayi) 125.1
Loa loa 125.2
malayi 125.1
organism NEC 125.6
Wuchereria (bancrofti) 125.0
malayi 125.1
Malayan 125.1
ozzardi 125.5
specified type NEC 125.6
Filatoff's, Filatov's, Filatow's disease (infectious mononucleosis) 075
File-cutters' disease 984.9
specified type of lead — *see* Table of Drugs and Chemicals
Filling defect
biliary tract 793.3
bladder 793.5
duodenum 793.4
gallbladder 793.3
gastrointestinal tract 793.4
intestine 793.4
kidney 793.5
stomach 793.4
ureter 793.5

☑ **Additional Digit Required** — Refer to the Tabular List for Digit Selection
⬇ **Subterms under main terms may continue to next column or page**
2014 ICD-9-CM
▶◀ **Revised Text** ● **New Line** ▲ **Revised Code**
Volume 2 — 115

Filtering bleb, eye (postglaucoma) (status)
 V45.69
 with complication or rupture 997.99
 postcataract extraction (complication)
  997.99
Fimbrial cyst (congenital) 752.11
Fimbriated hymen 752.49
Financial problem affecting care V60.2
Findings, (abnormal), without diagnosis
 (examination) (laboratory test) 796.4
 17-ketosteroids, elevated 791.9
 acetonuria 791.6
 acid phosphatase 790.5
 albumin-globulin ratio 790.99
 albuminuria 791.0
 alcohol in blood 790.3
 alkaline phosphatase 790.5
 amniotic fluid 792.3
 amylase 790.5
 anisocytosis 790.09
 antenatal screening 796.5
 anthrax, positive 795.31
 antibody titers, elevated 795.79
 anticardiolipin antibody 795.79
 antigen-antibody reaction 795.79
 antiphosphatidylglycerol antibody 795.79
 antiphosphatidylinositol antibody 795.79
 antiphosphatidylserine antibody 795.79
 antiphospholipid antibody 795.79
 bacteriuria 791.9
 ballistocardiogram 794.39
 bicarbonate 276.9
 bile in urine 791.4
 bilirubin 277.4
 bleeding time (prolonged) 790.92
 blood culture, positive 790.7
 blood gas level (arterial) 790.91
 blood sugar level 790.29
  high 790.29
   fasting glucose 790.21
    glucose tolerance test 790.22
  low 251.2
 C-reactive protein (CRP) 790.95
 calcium 275.40
 cancer antigen 125 [CA 125] 795.82
 carbonate 276.9
 carcinoembryonic antigen [CEA] 795.81
 casts, urine 791.7
 catecholamines 791.9
 cells, urine 791.7
 cerebrospinal fluid (color) (content) (pressure) 792.0
 cervical
  high risk human papillomavirus (HPV)
   DNA test positive 795.05
  low risk human papillomavirus (HPV)
   DNA test positive 795.09
  non-atypical endometrial cells 795.09
 chloride 276.9
 cholesterol 272.9
  high 272.0
   with high triglycerides 272.2
 chromosome analysis 795.2
 chyluria 791.1
 circulation time 794.39
 cloudy dialysis effluent 792.5
 cloudy urine 791.9
 coagulation study 790.92
 cobalt, blood 790.6
 color of urine (unusual) NEC 791.9
 copper, blood 790.6
 creatinine clearance 794.4
 crystals, urine 791.9
 culture, positive NEC 795.39
  blood 790.7
  HIV V08
  human immunodeficiency virus V08
  nose 795.39
   Staphylococcus — see Carrier (suspected) of, Staphylococcus
  skin lesion NEC 795.39
  spinal fluid 792.0
  sputum 795.39
  stool 792.1
  throat 795.39
  urine 791.9

Findings, (abnormal), without diagnosis —
 continued
 culture, positive — *continued*
  viral
   human immunodeficiency V08
  wound 795.39
 cytology specified site NEC 796.9
 echocardiogram 793.2
 echoencephalogram 794.01
 echogram NEC — *see* Findings, abnormal, structure
 electro-oculogram (EOG) 794.12
 electrocardiogram (ECG) (EKG) 794.31
 electroencephalogram (EEG) 794.02
 electrolyte level, urinary 791.9
 electromyogram (EMG) 794.17
  ocular 794.14
 electroretinogram (ERG) 794.11
 enzymes, serum NEC 790.5
 fibrinogen titer coagulation study 790.92
 filling defect — *see* Filling defect
 function study NEC 794.9
  auditory 794.15
  bladder 794.9
  brain 794.00
  cardiac 794.30
  endocrine NEC 794.6
   thyroid 794.5
  kidney 794.4
  liver 794.8
  nervous system
   central 794.00
   peripheral 794.19
  oculomotor 794.14
  pancreas 794.9
  placenta 794.9
  pulmonary 794.2
  retina 794.11
  special senses 794.19
  spleen 794.9
  vestibular 794.16
 gallbladder, nonvisualization 793.3
 glucose 790.29
  elevated
   fasting 790.21
   tolerance test 790.22
 glycosuria 791.5
 heart
  shadow 793.2
  sounds 785.3
 hematinuria 791.2
 hematocrit
  drop (precipitous) 790.01
  elevated 282.7
  low 285.9
 hematologic NEC 790.99
 hematuria 599.70
 hemoglobin
  drop 790.01
  elevated 282.7
  low 285.9
 hemoglobinuria 791.2
 histological NEC 795.4
 hormones 259.9
 immunoglobulins, elevated 795.79
 indolacetic acid, elevated 791.9
 iron 790.6
 karyotype 795.2
 ketonuria 791.6
 lactic acid dehydrogenase (LDH) 790.4
 lead 790.6
 lipase 790.5
 lipids NEC 272.9
 lithium, blood 790.6
 liver function test 790.6
 lung field (shadow) 793.19
  coin lesion 793.11
 magnesium, blood 790.6
 mammogram 793.80
  calcification 793.89
  calculus 793.89
  dense breasts 793.82
  inconclusive 793.82
   due to dense breasts 793.82
  microcalcification 793.81
 mediastinal shift 793.2

Findings, (abnormal), without diagnosis —
 continued
 melanin, urine 791.9
 microbiologic NEC 795.39
 mineral, blood NEC 790.6
 myoglobinuria 791.3
 nasal swab, anthrax 795.31
 neonatal screening 796.6
 nitrogen derivatives, blood 790.6
 nonvisualization of gallbladder 793.3
 nose culture, positive 795.39
 odor of urine (unusual) NEC 791.9
 oxygen saturation 790.91
 Papanicolaou (smear) 796.9
  anus 796.70
   with
    atypical squamous cells
     cannot exclude high grade
      squamous intraepithelial lesion (ASC-H)
      796.72
     of undetermined significance
      (ASC-US) 796.71
    cytologic evidence of malignancy
     796.76
    high grade squamous intraepithelial lesion (HGSIL) 796.74
    low grade squamous intraepithelial lesion (LGSIL) 796.73
  glandular 796.70
  specified finding NEC 796.79
  cervix 795.00
   with
    atypical squamous cells
     cannot exclude high grade
      squamous intraepithelial lesion (ASC-H)
      795.02
     of undetermined significance
      (ASC-US) 795.01
    cytologic evidence of malignancy
     795.06
    high grade squamous intraepithelial lesion (HGSIL) 795.04
    low grade squamous intraepithelial lesion (LGSIL) 795.03
    non-atypical endometrial cells
     795.09
   dyskaryotic 795.09
   non-atypical endometrial cells 795.09
   nonspecific finding NEC 795.09
  other site 796.9
  vagina 795.10
   with
    atypical squamous cells
     cannot exclude high grade
      squamous intraepithelial lesion (ASC-H)
      795.12
     of undetermined significance
      (ASC-US) 795.11
    cytologic evidence of malignancy
     795.16
    high grade squamous intraepithelial lesion (HGSIL) 795.14
    low grade squamous intraepithelial lesion (LGSIL) 795.13
   glandular 795.10
   specified NEC 795.19
 peritoneal fluid 792.9
 phonocardiogram 794.39
 phosphorus 275.3
 pleural fluid 792.9
 pneumoencephalogram 793.0
 PO_2-oxygen ratio 790.91
 poikilocytosis 790.09
 potassium
  deficiency 276.8
  excess 276.7
 PPD 795.51
 prostate specific antigen (PSA) 790.93
 protein, serum NEC 790.99
 proteinuria 791.0
 prothrombin time (partial) (prolonged) (PT)
  (PTT) 790.92
 pyuria 791.9

Findings, (abnormal), without diagnosis —
 continued
 radiologic (x-ray) 793.99
  abdomen 793.6
  biliary tract 793.3
  breast 793.89
   abnormal mammogram NOS 793.80
   mammographic
    calcification 793.89
    calculus 793.89
    microcalcification 793.81
  gastrointestinal tract 793.4
  genitourinary organs 793.5
  head 793.0
  image test inconclusive due to excess
   body fat 793.91
  intrathoracic organs NEC 793.2
  lung 793.19
  musculoskeletal 793.7
  placenta 793.99
  retroperitoneum 793.6
  skin 793.99
  skull 793.0
  subcutaneous tissue 793.99
 red blood cell 790.09
  count 790.09
  morphology 790.09
  sickling 790.09
  volume 790.09
 saliva 792.4
 scan NEC 794.9
  bladder 794.9
  bone 794.9
  brain 794.09
  kidney 794.4
  liver 794.8
  lung 794.2
  pancreas 794.9
  placental 794.9
  spleen 794.9
  thyroid 794.5
 sedimentation rate, elevated 790.1
 semen 792.2
 serological (for)
  human immunodeficiency virus (HIV)
   inconclusive 795.71
   positive V08
  syphilis — *see* Findings, serology for
   syphilis
 serology for syphilis
  false positive 795.6
  positive 097.1
   false 795.6
   follow-up of latent syphilis — *see*
    Syphilis, latent
   only finding — *see* Syphilis, latent
 serum 790.99
  blood NEC 790.99
  enzymes NEC 790.5
  proteins 790.99
 SGOT 790.4
 SGPT 790.4
 sickling of red blood cells 790.09
 skin test, positive 795.79
  tuberculin (without active tuberculosis)
   795.51
 sodium 790.6
  deficiency 276.1
  excess 276.0
 specified NEC 796.9
 spermatozoa 792.2
 spinal fluid 792.0
  culture, positive 792.0
 sputum culture, positive 795.39
  for acid-fast bacilli 795.39
 stool NEC 792.1
  bloody 578.1
   occult 792.1
  color 792.1
  culture, positive 792.1
  occult blood 792.1
 stress test 794.39
 structure, body (echogram) (thermogram)
  (ultrasound) (x-ray) NEC 793.99
  abdomen 793.6
  breast 793.89

☑ **Additional Digit Required** — Refer to the Tabular List for Digit Selection
▽ **Subterms under main terms may continue to next column or page**

116 — Volume 2
▶◀ **Revised Text**
● **New Line**
▲ **Revised Code**
2014 ICD-9-CM

Findings, (abnormal), without diagnosis — *continued*
  structure, body — *continued*
    breast — *continued*
      abnormal mammogram 793.80
      mammographic
        calcification 793.89
        calculus 793.89
        microcalcification 793.81
    gastrointestinal tract 793.4
    genitourinary organs 793.5
    head 793.0
      echogram (ultrasound) 794.01
    intrathoracic organs NEC 793.2
    lung 793.19
    musculoskeletal 793.7
    placenta 793.99
    retroperitoneum 793.6
    skin 793.99
    subcutaneous tissue NEC 793.99
  synovial fluid 792.9
  thermogram — *see* Findings, abnormal, structure
  throat culture, positive 795.39
  thyroid (function) 794.5
    metabolism (rate) 794.5
    scan 794.5
    uptake 794.5
  total proteins 790.99
  toxicology (drugs) (heavy metals) 796.0
  transaminase (level) 790.4
  triglycerides 272.9
    high 272.1
      with high cholesterol 272.2
  tuberculin skin test (without active tuberculosis) 795.51
  tumor markers NEC 795.89
  ultrasound (*see also* Findings, abnormal, structure)
    cardiogram 793.2
  uric acid, blood 790.6
  urine, urinary constituents 791.9
    acetone 791.6
    albumin 791.0
    bacteria 791.9
    bile 791.4
    blood 599.70
    casts or cells 791.7
    chyle 791.1
    culture, positive 791.9
    glucose 791.5
    hemoglobin 791.2
    ketone 791.6
    protein 791.0
    pus 791.9
    sugar 791.5
  vaginal
    fluid 792.9
    high risk human papillomavirus (HPV) DNA test positive 795.15
    low risk human papillomavirus (HPV) DNA test positive 795.19
  vanillylmandelic acid, elevated 791.9
  vectorcardiogram (VCG) 794.39
  ventriculogram (cerebral) 793.0
  VMA, elevated 791.9
  Wassermann reaction
    false positive 795.6
    positive 097.1
      follow-up of latent syphilis — *see* Syphilis, latent
      only finding — *see* Syphilis, latent
  white blood cell 288.9
    count 288.9
      elevated 288.60
      low 288.50
    differential 288.9
    morphology 288.9
  wound culture 795.39
  xerography 793.89
  zinc, blood 790.6
Finger — *see* condition
Finnish type nephrosis (congenital) 759.89
Fire, St. Anthony's — *see also* Erysipelas 035
Fish
  hook stomach 537.89

Fish — *continued*
  meal workers' lung 495.8
Fisher's syndrome 357.0
Fissure, fissured
  abdominal wall (congenital) 756.79
  anus, anal 565.0
    congenital 751.5
  buccal cavity 528.9
  clitoris (congenital) 752.49
  ear, lobule (congenital) 744.29
  epiglottis (congenital) 748.3
  larynx 478.79
    congenital 748.3
  lip 528.5
    congenital (*see also* Cleft, lip) 749.10
  nipple 611.2
    puerperal, postpartum 676.1 ☑
  palate (congenital) (*see also* Cleft, palate) 749.00
  postanal 565.0
  rectum 565.0
  skin 709.8
    streptococcal 686.9
  spine (congenital) (*see also* Spina bifida) 741.9 ☑
  sternum (congenital) 756.3
  tongue (acquired) 529.5
    congenital 750.13
Fistula (sinus) 686.9
  abdomen (wall) 569.81
    bladder 596.2
    intestine 569.81
    ureter 593.82
    uterus 619.2
  abdominorectal 569.81
  abdominosigmoidal 569.81
  abdominothoracic 510.0
  abdominouterine 619.2
    congenital 752.39
  abdominovesical 596.2
  accessory sinuses (*see also* Sinusitis) 473.9
  actinomycotic — *see* Actinomycosis
  alveolar
    antrum (*see also* Sinusitis, maxillary) 473.0
    process 522.7
  anorectal 565.1
  antrobuccal (*see also* Sinusitis, maxillary) 473.0
  antrum (*see also* Sinusitis, maxillary) 473.0
  anus, anal (infectional) (recurrent) 565.1
    congenital 751.5
    tuberculous (*see also* Tuberculosis) 014.8 ☑
  aortic sinus 747.29
  aortoduodenal 447.2
  appendix, appendicular 543.9
  arteriovenous (acquired) 447.0
    brain 437.3
      congenital 747.81
        ruptured (*see also* Hemorrhage, subarachnoid) 430
      ruptured (*see also* Hemorrhage, subarachnoid) 430
    cerebral 437.3
      congenital 747.81
    congenital (peripheral) 747.60
      brain — *see* Fistula, arteriovenous, brain, congenital
      coronary 746.85
      gastrointestinal 747.61
      lower limb 747.64
      pulmonary 747.39
      renal 747.62
      specified site NEC 747.69
      upper limb 747.63
    coronary 414.19
      congenital 746.85
    heart 414.19
    pulmonary (vessels) 417.0
      congenital 747.39
    surgically created (for dialysis) V45.11
      complication NEC 996.73
        atherosclerosis — *see* Arteriosclerosis, extremities
        embolism 996.74

Fistula — *continued*
  arteriovenous — *continued*
    surgically created — *continued*
      complication — *continued*
        infection or inflammation 996.62
        mechanical 996.1
        occlusion NEC 996.74
        thrombus 996.74
    traumatic — *see* Injury, blood vessel, by site
  artery 447.2
  aural 383.81
    congenital 744.49
  auricle 383.81
    congenital 744.49
  Bartholin's gland 619.8
  bile duct (*see also* Fistula, biliary) 576.4
  biliary (duct) (tract) 576.4
    congenital 751.69
  bladder (neck) (sphincter) 596.2
    into seminal vesicle 596.2
  bone 733.99
  brain 348.89
    arteriovenous — *see* Fistula, arteriovenous, brain
  branchial (cleft) 744.41
  branchiogenous 744.41
  breast 611.0
    puerperal, postpartum 675.1 ☑
  bronchial 510.0
  bronchocutaneous, bronchomediastinal, bronchopleural, bronchopleuromediastinal (infective) 510.0
    tuberculous (*see also* Tuberculosis) 011.3 ☑
  bronchoesophageal 530.89
    congenital 750.3
  buccal cavity (infective) 528.3
  canal, ear 380.89
  carotid-cavernous
    congenital 747.81
      with hemorrhage 430
    traumatic 900.82
      with hemorrhage (*see also* Hemorrhage, brain, traumatic) 853.0 ☑
        late effect 908.3
  cecosigmoidal 569.81
  cecum 569.81
  cerebrospinal (fluid) 349.81
  cervical, lateral (congenital) 744.41
  cervicoaural (congenital) 744.49
  cervicosigmoidal 619.1
  cervicovesical 619.0
  cervix 619.8
  chest (wall) 510.0
  cholecystocolic (*see also* Fistula, gallbladder) 575.5
  cholecystocolonic (*see also* Fistula, gallbladder) 575.5
  cholecystoduodenal (*see also* Fistula, gallbladder) 575.5
  cholecystoenteric (*see also* Fistula, gallbladder) 575.5
  cholecystogastric (*see also* Fistula, gallbladder) 575.5
  cholecystointestinal (*see also* Fistula, gallbladder) 575.5
  choledochoduodenal 576.4
  cholocolic (*see also* Fistula, gallbladder) 575.5
  coccyx 685.1
    with abscess 685.0
  colon 569.81
  colostomy 569.69
  colovaginal (acquired) 619.1
  common duct (bile duct) 576.4
  congenital, NEC — *see* Anomaly, specified type NEC
  cornea, causing hypotony 360.32
  coronary, arteriovenous 414.19
    congenital 746.85
  costal region 510.0
  cul-de-sac, Douglas' 619.8
  cutaneous 686.9

Fistula — *continued*
  cystic duct (*see also* Fistula, gallbladder) 575.5
    congenital 751.69
  cystostomy 596.83
  dental 522.7
  diaphragm 510.0
    bronchovisceral 510.0
    pleuroperitoneal 510.0
    pulmonoperitoneal 510.0
  duodenum 537.4
  ear (canal) (external) 380.89
  entero-uterine 619.1
    congenital 752.39
  enterocolic 569.81
  enterocutaneous 569.81
  enteroenteric 569.81
  enterovaginal 619.1
    congenital 752.49
  enterovesical 596.1
  epididymis 608.89
    tuberculous (*see also* Tuberculosis) 016.4 ☑
  esophagobronchial 530.89
    congenital 750.3
  esophagocutaneous 530.89
  esophagopleurocutaneous 530.89
  esophagotracheal 530.84
    congenital 750.3
  esophagus 530.89
    congenital 750.4
  ethmoid (*see also* Sinusitis, ethmoidal) 473.2
  eyeball (cornea) (sclera) 360.32
  eyelid 373.11
  fallopian tube (external) 619.2
  fecal 569.81
    congenital 751.5
  from periapical lesion 522.7
  frontal sinus (*see also* Sinusitis, frontal) 473.1
  gallbladder 575.5
    with calculus, cholelithiasis, stones (*see also* Cholelithiasis) 574.2 ☑
    congenital 751.69
  gastric 537.4
  gastrocolic 537.4
    congenital 750.7
    tuberculous (*see also* Tuberculosis) 014.8 ☑
  gastroenterocolic 537.4
  gastroesophageal 537.4
  gastrojejunal 537.4
  gastrojejunocolic 537.4
  genital
    organs
      female 619.9
        specified site NEC 619.8
      male 608.89
    tract-skin (female) 619.2
  hepatopleural 510.0
  hepatopulmonary 510.0
  horseshoe 565.1
  ileorectal 569.81
  ileosigmoidal 569.81
  ileostomy 569.69
  ileovesical 596.1
  ileum 569.81
  in ano 565.1
    tuberculous (*see also* Tuberculosis) 014.8 ☑
  inner ear (*see also* Fistula, labyrinth) 386.40
  intestine 569.81
  intestinocolonic (abdominal) 569.81
  intestinoureteral 593.82
  intestinouterine 619.1
  intestinovaginal 619.1
    congenital 752.49
  intestinovesical 596.1
  involving female genital tract 619.9
    digestive-genital 619.1
    genital tract-skin 619.2
    specified site NEC 619.8
    urinary-genital 619.0
  ischiorectal (fossa) 566
  jejunostomy 569.69
  jejunum 569.81
  joint 719.80

Fistula — Fitz-Hugh and Curtis syndrome

Fitz-Hugh and Curtis syndrome — *continued*
  due to — *continued*
    Neisseria gonorrhoeae (gonococcal peritonitis) 098.86
Fitz's syndrome (acute hemorrhagic pancreatitis) 577.0
Fixation
  joint — *see* Ankylosis
  larynx 478.79
  pupil 364.76
  stapes 385.22
    deafness (*see also* Deafness, conductive) 389.04
  uterus (acquired) — *see* Malposition, uterus
  vocal cord 478.5
Flaccid — *see also* condition
  foot 736.79
  forearm 736.09
  palate, congenital 750.26
Flail
  chest 807.4
    newborn 767.3
  joint (paralytic) 718.80
    ankle 718.87
    elbow 718.82
    foot 718.87
    hand 718.84
    hip 718.85
    knee 718.86
    multiple sites 718.89
    pelvic region 718.85
    shoulder (region) 718.81
    specified site NEC 718.88
    wrist 718.83
Flajani (-Basedow) syndrome or disease (exophthalmic goiter) 242.0 ☑
Flap, liver 572.8
Flare, anterior chamber (aqueous) (eye) 364.04
Flashback phenomena (drug) (hallucinogenic) 292.89
Flat
  chamber (anterior) (eye) 360.34
  chest, congenital 754.89
  electroencephalogram (EEG) 348.89
  foot (acquired) (fixed type) (painful) (postural) (spastic) 734
    congenital 754.61
      rocker bottom 754.61
      vertical talus 754.61
    rachitic 268.1
    rocker bottom (congenital) 754.61
    vertical talus, congenital 754.61
  organ or site, congenital NEC — *see* Anomaly, specified type NEC
  pelvis 738.6
    with disproportion (fetopelvic) 653.2 ☑
      affecting fetus or newborn 763.1
      causing obstructed labor 660.1 ☑
        affecting fetus or newborn 763.1
    congenital 755.69
Flatau-Schilder disease 341.1
Flattening
  head, femur 736.39
  hip 736.39
  lip (congenital) 744.89
  nose (congenital) 754.0
    acquired 738.0
Flatulence 787.3
Flatus 787.3
  vaginalis 629.89
Flax dressers' disease 504
Flea bite — *see* Injury, superficial, by site
Fleischer (-Kayser) ring (corneal pigmentation) 275.1 *[371.14]*
Fleischner's disease 732.3
Fleshy mole 631.8
Flexibilitas cerea — *see also* Catalepsy 300.11
Flexion
  cervix — *see* Flexion, uterus
  contracture, joint (*see also* Contraction, joint) 718.4 ☑
  deformity, joint (*see also* Contraction, joint) 736.9

Flexion — *continued*
  deformity, joint (*see also* Contraction, joint) — *continued*
    hip, congenital (*see also* Subluxation, congenital, hip) 754.32
    uterus (*see also* Malposition, uterus) 621.6
Flexner-Boyd dysentery 004.2
Flexner's
  bacillus 004.1
  diarrhea (ulcerative) 004.1
  dysentery 004.1
Flexure — *see* condition
Floater, vitreous 379.24
Floating
  cartilage (joint) (*see also* Disorder, cartilage, articular) 718.0 ☑
    knee 717.6
  gallbladder (congenital) 751.69
  kidney 593.0
    congenital 753.3
  liver (congenital) 751.69
  rib 756.3
  spleen 289.59
Flooding 626.2
Floor — *see* condition
Floppy
  infant NEC 781.99
  iris syndrome 364.81
  valve syndrome (mitral) 424.0
Flu — *see also* Influenza
  bird (*see also* Influenza, avian) 488.02
  gastric NEC 008.8
  swine — *see* Influenza (novel) 2009 H1N1
Fluctuating blood pressure 796.4
Fluid
  abdomen 789.59
  chest (*see also* Pleurisy, with effusion) 511.9
  heart (*see also* Failure, heart) 428.0
  joint (*see also* Effusion, joint) 719.0 ☑
  loss (acute) 276.50
    with
      hypernatremia 276.0
      hyponatremia 276.1
  lung (*see also* Edema, lung)
    encysted 511.89
  peritoneal cavity 789.59
    malignant 789.51
  pleural cavity (*see also* Pleurisy, with effusion) 511.9
  retention 276.69
Flukes NEC — *see also* Infestation, fluke 121.9
  blood NEC (*see also* Infestation, Schistosoma) 120.9
  liver 121.3
Fluor (albus) (vaginalis) 623.5
  trichomonal (Trichomonas vaginalis) 131.00
Fluorosis (dental) (chronic) 520.3
Flushing 782.62
  menopausal 627.2
Flush syndrome 259.2
Flutter
  atrial or auricular 427.32
  heart (ventricular) 427.42
    atrial 427.32
  impure 427.32
  postoperative 997.1
  ventricular 427.42
Flux (bloody) (serosanguineous) 009.0
FNHTR (febrile nonhemolytic transfusion reaction) 780.66
Focal — *see* condition
Fochier's abscess — *see* Abscess, by site
Focus, Assmann's — *see also* Tuberculosis 011.0 ☑
Fogo selvagem 694.4
Foix-Alajouanine syndrome 336.1
Folds, anomalous — *see also* Anomaly, specified type NEC
  Bowman's membrane 371.31
  Descemet's membrane 371.32
  epicanthic 743.63
  heart 746.89
  posterior segment of eye, congenital 743.54
Folie à deux 297.3
Follicle
  cervix (nabothian) (ruptured) 616.0

Follicle — *continued*
  graafian, ruptured, with hemorrhage 620.0
  nabothian 616.0
Folliclis (primary) — *see also* Tuberculosis 017.0 ☑
Follicular — *see also* condition
  cyst (atretic) 620.0
Folliculitis 704.8
  abscedens et suffodiens 704.8
  decalvans 704.09
  gonorrheal (acute) 098.0
    chronic or duration of 2 months or more 098.2
  keloid, keloidalis 706.1
  pustular 704.8
  ulerythematosa reticulata 701.8
Folliculosis, conjunctival 372.02
Følling's disease (phenylketonuria) 270.1
Follow-up (examination) (routine) (following) V67.9
  cancer chemotherapy V67.2
  chemotherapy V67.2
  fracture V67.4
  high-risk medication V67.51
  injury NEC V67.59
  postpartum
    immediately after delivery V24.0
    routine V24.2
  psychiatric V67.3
  psychotherapy V67.3
  radiotherapy V67.1
  specified condition NEC V67.59
  specified surgery NEC V67.09
  surgery V67.00
    vaginal pap smear V67.01
  treatment V67.9
    combined NEC V67.6
    fracture V67.4
    involving high-risk medication NEC V67.51
    mental disorder V67.3
    specified NEC V67.59
Fong's syndrome (hereditary osteoonychodysplasia) 756.89
Food
  allergy 693.1
  anaphylactic reaction or shock due to food
  asphyxia (from aspiration or inhalation) (*see also* Asphyxia, food) 933.1
  choked on (*see also* Asphyxia, food) 933.1
  deprivation 994.2
    specified kind of food NEC 269.8
  intoxication (*see also* Poisoning, food) 005.9
  lack of 994.2
  poisoning (*see also* Poisoning, food) 005.9
  refusal or rejection NEC 307.59
  strangulation or suffocation (*see also* Asphyxia, food) 933.1
  toxemia (*see also* Poisoning, food) 005.9
Foot — *see also* condition
  and mouth disease 078.4
  process disease 581.3
Foramen ovale (nonclosure) (patent) (persistent) 745.5
Forbes-Albright syndrome (nonpuerperal amenorrhea and lactation associated with pituitary tumor) 253.1
Forbes' (glycogen storage) disease 271.0
Forced birth or delivery NEC 669.8 ☑
  affecting fetus or newborn NEC 763.89
Forceps
  delivery NEC 669.5 ☑
    affecting fetus or newborn 763.2
Fordyce-Fox disease (apocrine miliaria) 705.82
Fordyce's disease (ectopic sebaceous glands) (mouth) 750.26
Forearm — *see* condition
Foreign body

> *Note* — For foreign body with open wound, or other injury, see Wound, open, or the type of injury specified.

  accidentally left during a procedure 998.4
  anterior chamber (eye) 871.6
    magnetic 871.5
      retained or old 360.51
    retained or old 360.61

Foreign body — *continued*
  ciliary body (eye) 871.6
    magnetic 871.5
      retained or old 360.52
    retained or old 360.62
  entering through orifice (current) (old)
    accessory sinus 932
    air passage (upper) 933.0
      lower 934.8
    alimentary canal 938
    alveolar process 935.0
    antrum (Highmore) 932
    anus 937
    appendix 936
    asphyxia due to (*see also* Asphyxia, food) 933.1
    auditory canal 931
    auricle 931
    bladder 939.0
    bronchioles 934.8
    bronchus (main) 934.1
    buccal cavity 935.0
    canthus (inner) 930.1
    cecum 936
    cervix (canal) uterine 939.1
    coil, ileocecal 936
    colon 936
    conjunctiva 930.1
    conjunctival sac 930.1
    cornea 930.0
    digestive organ or tract NEC 938
    duodenum 936
    ear (external) 931
    esophagus 935.1
    eye (external) 930.9
      combined sites 930.8
      intraocular — *see* Foreign body, by site
      specified site NEC 930.8
    eyeball 930.8
      intraocular — *see* Foreign body, intraocular
    eyelid 930.1
      retained or old 374.86
    frontal sinus 932
    gastrointestinal tract 938
    genitourinary tract 939.9
    globe 930.8
      penetrating 871.6
        magnetic 871.5
          retained or old 360.50
        retained or old 360.60
    gum 935.0
    Highmore's antrum 932
    hypopharynx 933.0
    ileocecal coil 936
    ileum 936
    inspiration (of) 933.1
    intestine (large) (small) 936
    lacrimal apparatus, duct, gland, or sac 930.2
    larynx 933.1
    lung 934.8
    maxillary sinus 932
    mouth 935.0
    nasal sinus 932
    nasopharynx 933.0
    nose (passage) 932
    nostril 932
    oral cavity 935.0
    palate 935.0
    penis 939.3
    pharynx 933.0
    pyriform sinus 933.0
    rectosigmoid 937
      junction 937
    rectum 937
    respiratory tract 934.9
      specified part NEC 934.8
    sclera 930.1
    sinus 932
      accessory 932
      frontal 932
      maxillary 932
      nasal 932
      pyriform 933.0

☑ **Additional Digit Required** — Refer to the Tabular List for Digit Selection   ▽ **Subterms under main terms may continue to next column or page**

2014 ICD-9-CM   ▶◀ **Revised Text**   ● **New Line**   ▲ **Revised Code**   **Volume 2 — 119**

Foreign body — *continued*
  entering through orifice — *continued*
    small intestine 936
    stomach (hairball) 935.2
    suffocation by (*see also* Asphyxia, food) 933.1
    swallowed 938
      tongue 933.0
    tear ducts or glands 930.2
    throat 933.0
    tongue 935.0
      swallowed 933.0
    tonsil, tonsillar 933.0
      fossa 933.0
    trachea 934.0
    ureter 939.0
    urethra 939.0
    uterus (any part) 939.1
    vagina 939.2
    vulva 939.2
    wind pipe 934.0
  feeling of, in throat 784.99
  granuloma (old) 728.82
    bone 733.99
    in operative wound (inadvertently left) 998.4
      due to surgical material intentionally left — *see* Complications, due to (presence of) any device, implant, or graft classified to 996.0–996.5 NEC
    muscle 728.82
    skin 709.4
    soft tissue 709.4
    subcutaneous tissue 709.4
  in
    bone (residual) 733.99
    open wound — *see* Wound, open, by site complicated
    soft tissue (residual) 729.6
  inadvertently left in operation wound (causing adhesions, obstruction, or perforation) 998.4
  ingestion, ingested NEC 938
  inhalation or inspiration (*see also* Asphyxia, food) 933.1
  internal organ, not entering through an orifice — *see* Injury, internal, by site, with open wound
  intraocular (nonmagnetic) 871.6
    combined sites 871.6
      magnetic 871.5
        retained or old 360.59
      retained or old 360.69
    magnetic 871.5
      retained or old 360.50
    retained or old 360.60
    specified site NEC 871.6
      magnetic 871.5
        retained or old 360.59
      retained or old 360.69
    iris (nonmagnetic) 871.6
      magnetic 871.5
        retained or old 360.52
      retained or old 360.62
    lens (nonmagnetic) 871.6
      magnetic 871.5
        retained or old 360.53
      retained or old 360.63
  lid, eye 930.1
  ocular muscle 870.4
    retained or old 376.6
  old or residual
    bone 733.99
    eyelid 374.86
    middle ear 385.83
    muscle 729.6
      ocular 376.6
    retrobulbar 376.6
    skin 729.6
      with granuloma 709.4
    soft tissue 729.6
      with granuloma 709.4
    subcutaneous tissue 729.6
      with granuloma 709.4
  operation wound, left accidentally 998.4

Foreign body — *continued*
  orbit 870.4
    retained or old 376.6
  posterior wall, eye 871.6
    magnetic 871.5
      retained or old 360.55
    retained or old 360.65
  respiratory tree 934.9
    specified site NEC 934.8
  retained (old) (nonmagnetic) (in) V90.9
    anterior chamber (eye) 360.61
      magnetic 360.51
    ciliary body 360.62
      magnetic 360.52
    eyelid 374.86
    fragment(s)
      acrylics V90.2
      animal quills V90.31
      animal spines V90.31
      cement V90.83
      concrete V90.83
      crystalline V90.83
      depleted
        isotope V90.09
        uranium V90.01
      diethylhexylphthalates V90.2
      glass V90.81
      isocyanate V90.2
      metal V90.10
        magnetic V90.11
        nonmagnetic V90.12
      organic NEC V90.39
      plastic V90.2
      radioactive
        nontherapeutic V90.09
        specified NEC V90.09
      stone V90.83
      tooth V90.32
      wood V90.33
    globe 360.60
      magnetic 360.50
    intraocular 360.60
      magnetic 360.50
      specified site NEC 360.69
        magnetic 360.59
    iris 360.62
      magnetic 360.52
    lens 360.63
      magnetic 360.53
    muscle 729.6
    orbit 376.6
    posterior wall of globe 360.65
      magnetic 360.55
    retina 360.65
      magnetic 360.55
    retrobulbar 376.6
    skin 729.6
      with granuloma 709.4
    soft tissue 729.6
      with granuloma 709.4
    specified NEC V90.89
    subcutaneous tissue 729.6
      with granuloma 709.4
    vitreous 360.64
      magnetic 360.54
  retina 871.6
    magnetic 871.5
      retained or old 360.55
    retained or old 360.65
  superficial, without major open wound (*see also* Injury, superficial, by site) 919.6
  swallowed NEC 938
  throat, feeling of 784.99
  vitreous (humor) 871.6
    magnetic 871.5
      retained or old 360.54
    retained or old 360.64
Forking, aqueduct of Sylvius 742.3
  with spina bifida (*see also* Spina bifida) 741.0 ☑
Formation
  bone in scar tissue (skin) 709.3
  connective tissue in vitreous 379.25
  Elschnig pearls (postcataract extraction) 366.51
  hyaline in cornea 371.49

Formation — *continued*
  sequestrum in bone (due to infection) (*see also* Osteomyelitis) 730.1 ☑
  valve
    colon, congenital 751.5
    ureter (congenital) 753.29
Formication 782.0
Fort Bragg fever 100.89
Fossa — *see also* condition
  pyriform — *see* condition
Foster-Kennedy syndrome 377.04
Foster care (status) V60.81
Fothergill's
  disease, meaning scarlatina anginosa 034.1
  neuralgia (*see also* Neuralgia, trigeminal) 350.1
Foul breath 784.99
Found dead (cause unknown) 798.9
Foundling V20.0
Fournier's disease (idiopathic gangrene) 608.83
  female 616.89
Fourth
  cranial nerve — *see* condition
  disease 057.8
  molar 520.1
Foville's syndrome 344.89
Fox-Fordyce disease (apocrine miliaria) 705.82
Fox's
  disease (apocrine miliaria) 705.82
  impetigo (contagiosa) 684
Fracture (abduction) (adduction) (avulsion) (compression) (crush) (dislocation) (oblique) (separation) (closed) 829.0

> *Note* — For fracture of any of the following sites with fracture of other bones — see Fracture, multiple.
>
> "Closed" includes the following descriptions of fractures, with or without delayed healing, unless they are specified as open or compound:
>
> | comminuted | linear |
> |---|---|
> | depressed | simple |
> | elevated | slipped epiphysis |
> | fissured | spiral |
> | greenstick | unspecified |
> | impacted | |
>
> "Open" includes the following descriptions of fractures, with or without delayed healing:
>
> | compound | puncture |
> |---|---|
> | infected | with foreign body |
> | missile | |
>
> For late effect of fracture, see Late, effect, fracture, by site.

  with
    internal injuries in same region (conditions classifiable to 860–869) (*see also* Injury, internal, by site)
    pelvic region — *see* Fracture, pelvis
  acetabulum (with visceral injury) (closed) 808.0
    open 808.1
  acromion (process) (closed) 811.01
    open 811.11
  alveolus (closed) 802.8
    open 802.9
  ankle (malleolus) (closed) 824.8
    bimalleolar (Dupuytren's) (Pott's) 824.4
      open 824.5
    bone 825.21
      open 825.31
    lateral malleolus only (fibular) 824.2
      open 824.3
    medial malleolus only (tibial) 824.0
      open 824.1
    open 824.9
    pathologic 733.16
    talus 825.21

Fracture — *continued*
  ankle — *continued*
    talus — *continued*
      open 825.31
    trimalleolar 824.6
      open 824.7
  antrum — *see* Fracture, skull, base
  arm (closed) 818.0
    and leg(s) (any bones) 828.0
      open 828.1
    both (any bones) (with rib(s)) (with sternum) 819.0
      open 819.1
    lower 813.80
      open 813.90
    open 818.1
    upper — *see* Fracture, humerus
  astragalus (closed) 825.21
    open 825.31
  atlas — *see* Fracture, vertebra, cervical, first
  axis — *see* Fracture, vertebra, cervical, second
  back — *see* Fracture, vertebra, by site
  Barton's — *see* Fracture, radius, lower end
  basal (skull) — *see* Fracture, skull, base
  Bennett's (closed) 815.01
    open 815.11
  bimalleolar (closed) 824.4
    open 824.5
  bone (closed) NEC 829.0
    birth injury NEC 767.3
    open 829.1
    pathologic NEC (*see also* Fracture, pathologic) 733.10
    stress NEC (*see also* Fracture, stress) 733.95
  boot top — *see* Fracture, fibula
  boxers' — *see* Fracture, metacarpal bone(s)
  breast bone — *see* Fracture, sternum
  bucket handle (semilunar cartilage) — *see* Tear, meniscus
  buckle — *see* Fracture, torus
  burst — *see* Fracture, traumatic, by site
  bursting — *see* Fracture, phalanx, hand, distal
  calcaneus (closed) 825.0
    open 825.1
  capitate (bone) (closed) 814.07
    open 814.17
  capitellum (humerus) (closed) 812.49
    open 812.59
  carpal bone(s) (wrist NEC) (closed) 814.00
    open 814.10
    specified site NEC 814.09
      open 814.19
  cartilage, knee (semilunar) — *see* Tear, meniscus
  cervical — *see* Fracture, vertebra, cervical
  chauffeur's — *see* Fracture, ulna, lower end
  chisel — *see* Fracture, radius, upper end
  chronic — *see* Fracture, pathologic
  clavicle (interligamentous part) (closed) 810.00
    acromial end 810.03
      open 810.13
    due to birth trauma 767.2
    open 810.10
    shaft (middle third) 810.02
      open 810.12
    sternal end 810.01
      open 810.11
  clayshovelers' — *see* Fracture, vertebra, cervical
  coccyx (*see also* Fracture, vertebra, coccyx)
    complicating delivery 665.6 ☑
  collar bone — *see* Fracture, clavicle
  Colles' (reversed) (closed) 813.41
    open 813.51
  comminuted — *see* Fracture, by site
  compression (*see also* Fracture, by site)
    nontraumatic — *see* Fracture, pathologic
  congenital 756.9
  coracoid process (closed) 811.02
    open 811.12
  coronoid process (ulna) (closed) 813.02
    mandible (closed) 802.23

☑ Additional Digit Required — Refer to the Tabular List for Digit Selection   ⟱ Subterms under main terms may continue to next column or page

120 — Volume 2   ▶◀ Revised Text   ● New Line   ▲ Revised Code   2014 ICD-9-CM

Fracture — *continued*
  coronoid process — *continued*
    mandible — *continued*
      open 802.33
    open 813.12
  corpus cavernosum penis 959.13
  costochondral junction — *see* Fracture, rib
  costosternal junction — *see* Fracture, rib
  cranium — *see* Fracture, skull, by site
  cricoid cartilage (closed) 807.5
    open 807.6
  cuboid (ankle) (closed) 825.23
    open 825.33
  cuneiform
    foot (closed) 825.24
      open 825.34
    wrist (closed) 814.03
      open 814.13
  dental implant 525.73
  dental restorative material
    with loss of material 525.64
    without loss of material 525.63
  due to
    birth injury — *see* Birth injury, fracture
    gunshot — *see* Fracture, by site, open
    neoplasm — *see* Fracture, pathologic
    osteoporosis — *see* Fracture, pathologic
  Dupuytren's (ankle) (fibula) (closed) 824.4
    open 824.5
    radius 813.42
      open 813.52
  Duverney's — *see* Fracture, ilium
  elbow (*see also* Fracture, humerus, lower
      end)
    olecranon (process) (closed) 813.01
      open 813.11
    supracondylar (closed) 812.41
      open 812.51
  ethmoid (bone) (sinus) — *see* Fracture, skull,
      base
  face bone(s) (closed) NEC 802.8
    with
      other bone(s) — *see* Fracture, multi-
          ple, skull
      skull (*see also* Fracture, skull)
        involving other bones — *see*
            Fracture, multiple, skull
    open 802.9
  fatigue — *see* Fracture, march
  femur, femoral (closed) 821.00
    cervicotrochanteric 820.03
      open 820.13
    condyles, epicondyles 821.21
      open 821.31
    distal end — *see* Fracture, femur, lower
        end
    epiphysis (separation)
      capital 820.01
        open 820.11
      head 820.01
        open 820.11
      lower 821.22
        open 821.32
      trochanteric 820.01
        open 820.11
      upper 820.01
        open 820.11
    head 820.09
      open 820.19
    lower end or extremity (distal end)
        (closed) 821.20
      condyles, epicondyles 821.21
        open 821.31
      epiphysis (separation) 821.22
        open 821.32
      multiple sites 821.29
        open 821.39
      open 821.30
      specified site NEC 821.29
        open 821.39
      supracondylar 821.23
        open 821.33
      T-shaped 821.21
        open 821.31
    neck (closed) 820.8
      base (cervicotrochanteric) 820.03

Fracture — *continued*
  femur, femoral — *continued*
    neck — *continued*
      base — *continued*
        open 820.13
      extracapsular 820.20
        open 820.30
      intertrochanteric (section) 820.21
        open 820.31
      intracapsular 820.00
        open 820.10
      intratrochanteric 820.21
        open 820.31
      midcervical 820.02
        open 820.12
      open 820.9
      pathologic 733.14
        specified part NEC 733.15
      specified site NEC 820.09
        open 820.19
      stress 733.96
      transcervical 820.02
        open 820.12
      transtrochanteric 820.20
        open 820.30
    open 821.10
    pathologic 733.14
      specified part NEC 733.15
    peritrochanteric (section) 820.20
      open 820.30
    shaft (lower third) (middle third) (upper
        third) 821.01
      open 821.11
      stress 733.97
    subcapital 820.09
      open 820.19
    subtrochanteric (region) (section) 820.22
      open 820.32
    supracondylar 821.23
      open 821.33
    T-shaped, into knee joint 821.21
      open 821.31
    transepiphyseal 820.01
      open 820.11
    trochanter (greater) (lesser) (*see also*
        Fracture, femur, neck, by site)
        820.20
      open 820.30
    upper end 820.8
      open 820.9
  fibula (closed) 823.81
    with tibia 823.82
      open 823.92
    distal end 824.8
      open 824.9
    epiphysis
      lower 824.8
        open 824.9
      upper — *see* Fracture, fibula, upper
          end
    head — *see* Fracture, fibula, upper end
    involving ankle 824.2
      open 824.3
    lower end or extremity 824.8
      open 824.9
    malleolus (external) (lateral) 824.2
      open 824.3
    open NEC 823.91
    pathologic 733.16
    proximal end — *see* Fracture, fibula,
        upper end
    shaft 823.21
      with tibia 823.22
        open 823.32
        open 823.31
      stress 733.93
    torus 823.41
      with tibia 823.42
    upper end or extremity (epiphysis)
        (head) (proximal end) (styloid)
        823.01
      with tibia 823.02
        open 823.12
      open 823.11
  finger(s), of one hand (closed) (*see also*
      Fracture, phalanx, hand) 816.00

Fracture — *continued*
  finger(s), of one hand (*see also* Fracture,
      phalanx, hand) — *continued*
    with
      metacarpal bone(s), of same hand
          817.0
        open 817.1
      thumb of same hand 816.03
        open 816.13
    open 816.10
  foot, except toe(s) alone (closed) 825.20
    open 825.30
  forearm (closed) NEC 813.80
    lower end (distal end) (lower epiphysis)
        813.40
      open 813.50
    open 813.90
    shaft 813.20
      open 813.30
    upper end (proximal end) (upper epiph-
        ysis) 813.00
      open 813.10
  fossa, anterior, middle, or posterior — *see*
      Fracture, skull, base
  Fracture (abduction) (adduction) (avulsion)
      (compression) (crush) (dislocation)
      (oblique) (separation) (closed) 829.0
  frontal (bone) (*see also* Fracture, skull, vault)
    sinus — *see* Fracture, skull, base
  Galeazzi's — *see* Fracture, radius, lower end
  glenoid (cavity) (fossa) (scapula) (closed)
      811.03
    open 811.13
  Gosselin's — *see* Fracture, ankle
  greenstick — *see* Fracture, by site
  grenade-throwers' — *see* Fracture, humerus,
      shaft
  gutter — *see* Fracture, skull, vault
  hamate (closed) 814.08
    open 814.18
  hand, one (closed) 815.00
    carpals 814.00
      open 814.10
      specified site NEC 814.09
        open 814.19
    metacarpals 815.00
      open 815.10
    multiple, bones of one hand 817.0
      open 817.1
    open 815.10
    phalanges (*see also* Fracture, phalanx,
        hand) 816.00
      open 816.10
  healing
    aftercare (*see also* Aftercare, fracture)
        V54.89
    change of cast V54.89
    complications — *see* condition
    convalescence V66.4
    removal of
      cast V54.89
      fixation device
        external V54.89
        internal V54.01
  heel bone (closed) 825.0
    open 825.1
  Hill-Sachs 812.09
  hip (closed) (*see also* Fracture, femur, neck)
      820.8
    open 820.9
    pathologic 733.14
  humerus (closed) 812.20
    anatomical neck 812.02
      open 812.12
    articular process (*see also* Fracture
        humerus, condyle(s)) 812.44
      open 812.54
    capitellum 812.49
      open 812.59
    condyle(s) 812.44
      lateral (external) 812.42
        open 812.52
      medial (internal epicondyle) 812.43
        open 812.53
      open 812.54

Fracture — *continued*
  humerus — *continued*
    distal end — *see* Fracture, humerus,
        lower end
    epiphysis
      lower (*see also* Fracture, humerus,
          condyle(s)) 812.44
        open 812.54
      upper 812.09
        open 812.19
    external condyle 812.42
      open 812.52
    great tuberosity 812.03
      open 812.13
    head 812.09
      open 812.19
    internal epicondyle 812.43
      open 812.53
    lesser tuberosity 812.09
      open 812.19
    lower end or extremity (distal end) (*see
        also* Fracture, humerus, by site)
        812.40
      multiple sites NEC 812.49
        open 812.59
      open 812.50
      specified site NEC 812.49
        open 812.59
    neck 812.01
      open 812.11
    open 812.30
    pathologic 733.11
    proximal end — *see* Fracture, humerus,
        upper end
    shaft 812.21
      open 812.31
    supracondylar 812.41
      open 812.51
    surgical neck 812.01
      open 812.11
    T-shaped 812.44
      open 812.54
    trochlea 812.49
      open 812.59
    tuberosity — *see* Fracture, humerus,
        upper end
    upper end or extremity (proximal end)
        (*see also* Fracture, humerus, by
        site) 812.00
      open 812.10
      specified site NEC 812.09
        open 812.19
  hyoid bone (closed) 807.5
    open 807.6
  hyperextension — *see* Fracture, radius,
      lower end
  ilium (with visceral injury) (closed) 808.41
    open 808.51
  impaction, impacted — *see* Fracture, by site
  incus — *see* Fracture, skull, base
  innominate bone (with visceral injury)
      (closed) 808.49
    open 808.59
  instep, of one foot (closed) 825.20
    with toe(s) of same foot 827.0
      open 827.1
    open 825.30
  insufficiency — *see* Fracture, pathologic, by
      site
  internal
    ear — *see* Fracture, skull, base
    semilunar cartilage, knee — *see* Tear,
        meniscus, medial
  intertrochanteric — *see* Fracture, femur,
      neck, intertrochanteric
  ischium (with visceral injury) (closed) 808.42
    open 808.52
  jaw (bone) (lower) (closed) (*see also* Frac-
      ture, mandible) 802.20
    angle 802.25
      open 802.35
    open 802.30
    upper — *see* Fracture, maxilla
  knee
    cap (closed) 822.0
      open 822.1

☑ **Additional Digit Required** — Refer to the Tabular List for Digit Selection

▽ **Subterms under main terms may continue to next column or page**

Fracture — *continued*
  knee — *continued*
    cartilage (semilunar) — *see* Tear,
      meniscus
    labyrinth (osseous) — *see* Fracture, skull,
      base
  larynx (closed) 807.5
    open 807.6
  late effect — *see* Late, effects (of), fracture
  Le Fort's — *see* Fracture, maxilla
  leg (closed) 827.0
    with rib(s) or sternum 828.0
      open 828.1
    both (any bones) 828.0
      open 828.1
    lower — *see* Fracture, tibia
      open 827.1
    upper — *see* Fracture, femur
  limb
    lower (multiple) (closed) NEC 827.0
      open 827.1
    upper (multiple) (closed) NEC 818.0
      open 818.1
  long bones, due to birth trauma — *see* Birth
    injury, fracture
  lower end or extremity (anterior lip) (poste-
    rior) 824.8
    open 824.9
  lumbar — *see* Fracture, vertebra, lumbar
  lunate bone (closed) 814.02
    open 814.12
  malar bone (closed) 802.4
    open 802.5
  Malgaigne's (closed) 808.43
    open 808.53
  malleolus (closed) 824.8
    bimalleolar 824.4
      open 824.5
    lateral 824.2
      and medial (*see also* Fracture, malle-
        olus, bimalleolar)
        with lip of tibia — *see* Fracture,
          malleolus, trimalleolar
      open 824.3
    medial (closed) 824.0
      and lateral (*see also* Fracture, malleo-
        lus, bimalleolar)
        with lip of tibia — *see* Fracture,
          malleolus, trimalleolar
      open 824.1
    open 824.9
    trimalleolar (closed) 824.6
      open 824.7
  malleus — *see* Fracture, skull, base
  malunion 733.81
  mandible (closed) 802.20
    angle 802.25
      open 802.35
    body 802.28
      alveolar border 802.27
        open 802.37
        open 802.38
      symphysis 802.26
        open 802.36
    condylar process 802.21
      open 802.31
    coronoid process 802.23
      open 802.33
    multiple sites 802.29
      open 802.39
    open 802.30
    ramus NEC 802.24
      open 802.34
    subcondylar 802.22
      open 802.32
  manubrium — *see* Fracture, sternum
  march 733.95
    femoral neck 733.96
    fibula 733.93
    metatarsals 733.94
    pelvis 733.98
    shaft of femur 733.97
    tibia 733.93
  maxilla, maxillary (superior) (upper jaw)
    (closed) 802.4
    inferior — *see* Fracture, mandible

Fracture — *continued*
  maxilla, maxillary — *continued*
    open 802.5
  meniscus, knee — *see* Tear, meniscus
  metacarpus, metacarpal (bone(s)), of one
    hand (closed) 815.00
    with phalanx, phalanges, hand (finger(s))
      (thumb) of same hand 817.0
      open 817.1
    base 815.02
      first metacarpal 815.01
        open 815.11
        open 815.12
      thumb 815.01
        open 815.11
    multiple sites 815.09
      open 815.19
    neck 815.04
      open 815.14
    open 815.10
    shaft 815.03
      open 815.13
  metatarsus, metatarsal (bone(s)), of one foot
    (closed) 825.25
    with tarsal bone(s) 825.29
      open 825.39
    open 825.35
  Monteggia's (closed) 813.03
    open 813.13
  Moore's — *see* Fracture, radius, lower end
  multangular bone (closed)
    larger 814.05
      open 814.15
    smaller 814.06
      open 814.16
  multiple (closed) 829.0

> *Note* — *Multiple fractures of sites clas-*
> *sifiable to the same three- or four-digit*
> *category are coded to that category,*
> *except for sites classifiable to 810–818*
> *or 820–827 in different limbs.*
>
> *Multiple fractures of sites classifiable to*
> *different fourth-digit subdivisions within*
> *the same three-digit category should*
> *be dealt with according to coding rules.*
>
> *Multiple fractures of sites classifiable to*
> *different three-digit categories (identifi-*
> *able from the listing under "Fracture"),*
> *and of sites classifiable to 810–818 or*
> *820–827 in different limbs should be*
> *coded according to the following list,*
> *which should be referred to in the fol-*
> *lowing priority order: skull or face*
> *bones, pelvis or vertebral column, legs,*
> *arms.*

    arm (multiple bones in same arm except
      in hand alone) (sites classifiable
      to 810–817 with sites classifiable
      to a different three-digit category
      in 810–817 in same arm) (closed)
      818.0
      open 818.1
    arms, both or arm(s) with rib(s) or ster-
      num (sites classifiable to 810–818
      with sites classifiable to same
      range of categories in other limb
      or to 807) (closed) 819.0
      open 819.1
    bones of trunk NEC (closed) 809.0
      open 809.1
    hand, metacarpal bone(s) with phalanx
      or phalanges of same hand (sites
      classifiable to 815 with sites clas-
      sifiable to 816 in same hand)
      (closed) 817.0
      open 817.1
    leg (multiple bones in same leg) (sites
      classifiable to 820–826 with sites
      classifiable to a different
      three-digit category in that range
      in same leg) (closed) 827.0
      open 827.1

Fracture — *continued*
  multiple — *continued*
    legs, both or leg(s) with arm(s), rib(s), or
      sternum (sites classifiable to
      820–827 with sites classifiable to
      same range of categories in other
      leg or to 807 or 810–819) (closed)
      828.0
      open 828.1
    open 829.1
    pelvis with other bones except skull or
      face bones (sites classifiable to
      808 with sites classifiable to
      805–807 or 810–829) (closed)
      809.0
      open 809.1
    skull, specified or unspecified bones, or
      face bone(s) with any other
      bone(s) (sites classifiable to
      800–803 with sites classifiable to
      805–829) (closed) 804.0 ☑

> *Note* — *Use the following fifth-digit*
> *subclassification with categories 800,*
> *801, 803, and 804:*
>
> *0   unspecified state of consciousness*
>
> *1   with no loss of consciousness*
>
> *2   with brief [less than one hour]*
>   *loss of consciousness*
>
> *3   with moderate [1–24 hours] loss*
>   *of consciousness*
>
> *4   with prolonged [more than 24*
>   *hours] loss of consciousness and*
>   *return to pre-existing conscious*
>   *level*
>
> *5   with prolonged [more than 24*
>   *hours] loss of consciousness,*
>   *without return to pre-existing*
>   *conscious level*
>
> *Use fifth-digit 5 to designate when a*
> *patient is unconscious and dies before*
> *regaining consciousness, regardless of*
> *the duration of the loss of consciousness*
>
> *6   with loss of consciousness of un-*
>   *specified duration*
>
> *9   with concussion, unspecified*

      with
        contusion, cerebral 804.1 ☑
        epidural hemorrhage 804.2 ☑
        extradural hemorrhage 804.2 ☑
        hemorrhage (intracranial) NEC
          804.3 ☑
        intracranial injury NEC 804.4 ☑
        laceration, cerebral 804.1 ☑
        subarachnoid hemorrhage
          804.2 ☑
        subdural hemorrhage 804.2 ☑
      open 804.5 ☑
        with
          contusion, cerebral 804.6 ☑
          epidural hemorrhage
            804.7 ☑
          extradural hemorrhage
            804.7 ☑
          hemorrhage (intracranial) NEC
            804.8 ☑
          intracranial injury NEC
            804.9 ☑
          laceration, cerebral 804.6 ☑
          subarachnoid hemorrhage
            804.7 ☑
          subdural hemorrhage
            804.7 ☑
    vertebral column with other bones, ex-
      cept skull or face bones (sites
      classifiable to 805 or 806 with
      sites classifiable to 807–808 or
      810–829) (closed) 809.0
      open 809.1
  nasal (bone(s)) (closed) 802.0
    open 802.1
  sinus — *see* Fracture, skull, base

Fracture — *continued*
  navicular
    carpal (wrist) (closed) 814.01
      open 814.11
    tarsal (ankle) (closed) 825.22
      open 825.32
  neck — *see* Fracture, vertebra, cervical
  neural arch — *see* Fracture, vertebra, by site
  nonunion 733.82
  nose, nasal, (bone) (septum) (closed) 802.0
    open 802.1
  occiput — *see* Fracture, skull, base
  odontoid process — *see* Fracture, vertebra,
    cervical
  olecranon (process) (ulna) (closed) 813.01
    open 813.11
  open 829.1
  orbit, orbital (bone) (region) (closed) 802.8
    floor (blow-out) 802.6
      open 802.7
    open 802.9
    roof — *see* Fracture, skull, base
    specified part NEC 802.8
      open 802.9
  os
    calcis (closed) 825.0
      open 825.1
    magnum (closed) 814.07
      open 814.17
    pubis (with visceral injury) (closed) 808.2
      open 808.3
    triquetrum (closed) 814.03
      open 814.13
  osseous
    auditory meatus — *see* Fracture, skull,
      base
    labyrinth — *see* Fracture, skull, base
  ossicles, auditory (incus) (malleus) (stapes)
    — *see* Fracture, skull, base
  osteoporotic — *see* Fracture, pathologic
  palate (closed) 802.8
    open 802.9
  paratrooper — *see* Fracture, tibia, lower end
  parietal bone — *see* Fracture, skull, vault
  parry — *see* Fracture, Monteggia's
  patella (closed) 822.0
    open 822.1
  pathologic (cause unknown) 733.10
    ankle 733.16
    femur (neck) 733.14
      specified NEC 733.15
    fibula 733.16
    hip 733.14
    humerus 733.11
    radius (distal) 733.12
    specified site NEC 733.19
    tibia 733.16
    ulna 733.12
    vertebrae (collapse) 733.13
    wrist 733.12
  pedicle (of vertebral arch) — *see* Fracture,
    vertebra, by site
  pelvis, pelvic (bone(s)) (with visceral injury)
    (closed) 808.8
    multiple
      with
        disruption of pelvic circle 808.43
          open 808.53
        disruption of pelvic ring 808.43
          open 808.53
      without
        disruption of pelvic circle 808.44
          open 808.54
        disruption of pelvic ring 808.44
          open 808.54
    open 808.9
    rim (closed) 808.49
      open 808.59
    stress 733.98
  peritrochanteric (closed) 820.20
    open 820.30
  phalanx, phalanges, of one
    foot (closed) 826.0
      with bone(s) of same lower limb
        827.0
        open 827.1

Fracture — *continued*
  phalanx, phalanges, of one — *continued*
    foot — *continued*
      open 826.1
    hand (closed) 816.00
      with metacarpal bone(s) of same
        hand 817.0
        open 817.1
      distal 816.02
        open 816.12
      middle 816.01
        open 816.11
      multiple sites NEC 816.03
        open 816.13
      open 816.10
      proximal 816.01
        open 816.11
  pisiform (closed) 814.04
    open 814.14
  pond — *see* Fracture, skull, vault
  Pott's (closed) 824.4
    open 824.5
  prosthetic device, internal — *see* Complications, mechanical
  pubis (with visceral injury) (closed) 808.2
    open 808.3
  Quervain's (closed) 814.01
    open 814.11
  radius (alone) (closed) 813.81
    with ulna NEC 813.83
      open 813.93
    distal end — *see* Fracture, radius, lower end
    epiphysis
      lower — *see* Fracture, radius, lower end
      upper — *see* Fracture, radius, upper end
    head — *see* Fracture, radius, upper end
    lower end or extremity (distal end) (lower epiphysis) 813.42
      with ulna (lower end) 813.44
        open 813.54
      open 813.52
      torus 813.45
        with ulna 813.47
    neck — *see* Fracture, radius, upper end
    open NEC 813.91
    pathologic 733.12
    proximal end — *see* Fracture, radius, upper end
    shaft (closed) 813.21
      with ulna (shaft) 813.23
        open 813.33
      open 813.31
    upper end 813.07
      with ulna (upper end) 813.08
        open 813.18
      epiphysis 813.05
        open 813.15
      head 813.05
        open 813.15
      multiple sites 813.07
        open 813.17
      neck 813.06
        open 813.16
      open 813.17
      specified site NEC 813.07
        open 813.17
  ramus
    inferior or superior (with visceral injury) (closed) 808.2
      open 808.3
    ischium — *see* Fracture, ischium
    mandible 802.24
      open 802.34

Fracture — *continued*
  rib(s) (closed) 807.0 ☑

> Note — Use the following fifth-digit subclassification with categories 807.0–807.1:
> 0 rib(s), unspecified
> 1 one rib
> 2 two ribs
> 3 three ribs
> 4 four ribs
> 5 five ribs
> 6 six ribs
> 7 seven ribs
> 8 eight or more ribs
> 9 multiple ribs, unspecified

    with flail chest (open) 807.4
    open 807.1 ☑
  root, tooth 873.63
    complicated 873.73
  sacrum — *see* Fracture, vertebra, sacrum
  scaphoid
    ankle (closed) 825.22
      open 825.32
    wrist (closed) 814.01
      open 814.11
  scapula (closed) 811.00
    acromial, acromion (process) 811.01
      open 811.11
    body 811.09
      open 811.19
    coracoid process 811.02
      open 811.12
    glenoid (cavity) (fossa) 811.03
      open 811.13
    neck 811.03
      open 811.13
    open 811.10
  semilunar
    bone, wrist (closed) 814.02
      open 814.12
    cartilage (interior) (knee) — *see* Tear, meniscus
  sesamoid bone — *see* Fracture, by site
  Shepherd's (closed) 825.21
    open 825.31
  shoulder (*see also* Fracture, humerus, upper end)
    blade — *see* Fracture, scapula
  silverfork — *see* Fracture, radius, lower end
  sinus (ethmoid) (frontal) (maxillary) (nasal) (sphenoidal) — *see* Fracture, skull, base
  Skillern's — *see* Fracture, radius, shaft

Fracture — *continued*
  skull (multiple NEC) (with face bones) (closed) 803.0 ☑

> Note — Use the following fifth-digit subclassification with categories 800, 801, 803, and 804:
> 0 unspecified state of consciousness
> 1 with no loss of consciousness
> 2 with brief [less than one hour] loss of consciousness
> 3 with moderate [1-24 hours] loss of consciousness
> 4 with prolonged [more than 24 hours] loss of consciousness and return to pre-existing conscious level
> 5 with prolonged [more than 24 hours] loss of consciousness, without return to pre-existing conscious level
>
> Use fifth-digit 5 to designate when a patient is unconscious and dies before regaining consciousness, regardless of the duration of the loss of consciousness
>
> 6 with loss of consciousness of unspecified duration
> 9 with concussion, unspecified

    with
      contusion, cerebral 803.1 ☑
      epidural hemorrhage 803.2 ☑
      extradural hemorrhage 803.2 ☑
      hemorrhage (intracranial) NEC 803.3 ☑
      intracranial injury NEC 803.4 ☑
      laceration, cerebral 803.1 ☑
      other bones — *see* Fracture, multiple, skull
      subarachnoid hemorrhage 803.2 ☑
      subdural hemorrhage 803.2 ☑
    base (antrum) (ethmoid bone) (fossa) (internal ear) (nasal sinus) (occiput) (sphenoid) (temporal bone) (closed) 801.0 ☑
      with
        contusion, cerebral 801.1 ☑
        epidural hemorrhage 801.2 ☑
        extradural hemorrhage 801.2 ☑
        hemorrhage (intracranial) NEC 801.3 ☑
        intracranial injury NEC 801.4 ☑
        laceration, cerebral 801.1 ☑
        subarachnoid hemorrhage 801.2 ☑
        subdural hemorrhage 801.2 ☑
      open 801.5 ☑
        with
          contusion, cerebral 801.6 ☑
          epidural hemorrhage 801.7 ☑
          extradural hemorrhage 801.7 ☑
          hemorrhage (intracranial) NEC 801.8 ☑
          intracranial injury NEC 801.9 ☑
          laceration, cerebral 801.6 ☑
          subarachnoid hemorrhage 801.7 ☑
          subdural hemorrhage 801.7 ☑
    birth injury 767.3
    face bones — *see* Fracture, face bones
    open 803.5 ☑

Fracture — *continued*
  skull — *continued*
    open — *continued*
      with
        contusion, cerebral 803.6 ☑
        epidural hemorrhage 803.7 ☑
        extradural hemorrhage 803.7 ☑
        hemorrhage (intracranial) NEC 803.8 ☑
        intracranial injury NEC 803.9 ☑
        laceration, cerebral 803.6 ☑
        subarachnoid hemorrhage 803.7 ☑
        subdural hemorrhage 803.7 ☑
    vault (frontal bone) (parietal bone) (vertex) (closed) 800.0 ☑
      with
        contusion, cerebral 800.1 ☑
        epidural hemorrhage 800.2 ☑
        extradural hemorrhage 800.2 ☑
        hemorrhage (intracranial) NEC 800.3 ☑
        intracranial injury NEC 800.4 ☑
        laceration, cerebral 800.1 ☑
        subarachnoid hemorrhage 800.2 ☑
        subdural hemorrhage 800.2 ☑
      open 800.5 ☑
        with
          contusion, cerebral 800.6 ☑
          epidural hemorrhage 800.7 ☑
          extradural hemorrhage 800.7 ☑
          hemorrhage (intracranial) NEC 800.8 ☑
          intracranial injury NEC 800.9 ☑
          laceration, cerebral 800.6 ☑
          subarachnoid hemorrhage 800.7 ☑
          subdural hemorrhage 800.7 ☑
  Smith's 813.41
    open 813.51
  sphenoid (bone) (sinus) — *see* Fracture, skull, base
  spine (*see also* Fracture, vertebra, by site due to birth trauma) 767.4
  spinous process — *see* Fracture, vertebra, by site
  spontaneous — *see* Fracture, pathologic
  sprinters' — *see* Fracture, ilium
  stapes — *see* Fracture, skull, base
  stave (*see also* Fracture, metacarpus, metacarpal bone(s))
    spine — *see* Fracture, tibia, upper end
  sternum (closed) 807.2
    with flail chest (open) 807.4
    open 807.3
  Stieda's — *see* Fracture, femur, lower end
  stress 733.95
    femoral neck 733.96
    fibula 733.93
    metatarsals 733.94
    pelvis 733.98
    shaft of femur 733.97
    specified site NEC 733.95
    tibia 733.93
  styloid process
    metacarpal (closed) 815.02
      open 815.12
    radius — *see* Fracture, radius, lower end
    temporal bone — *see* Fracture, skull, base

Fracture — *continued*
  styloid process — *continued*
    ulna — *see* Fracture, ulna, lower end
  supracondylar, elbow 812.41
    open 812.51
  symphysis pubis (with visceral injury)
      (closed) 808.2
    open 808.3
  talus (ankle bone) (closed) 825.21
    open 825.31
  tarsus, tarsal bone(s) (with metatarsus) of
      one foot (closed) NEC 825.29
    open 825.39
  temporal bone (styloid) — *see* Fracture,
      skull, base
  tendon — *see* Sprain, by site
  thigh — *see* Fracture, femur, shaft
  thumb (and finger(s)) of one hand (closed)
      (*see also* Fracture, phalanx, hand)
      816.00
    with metacarpal bone(s) of same hand
      817.0
      open 817.1
    metacarpal(s) — *see* Fracture, metacar-
      pus
    open 816.10
  thyroid cartilage (closed) 807.5
    open 807.6
  tibia (closed) 823.80
    with fibula 823.82
      open 823.92
    condyles — *see* Fracture, tibia, upper
      end
    distal end 824.8
      open 824.9
    epiphysis
      lower 824.8
        open 824.9
      upper — *see* Fracture, tibia, upper
        end
    head (involving knee joint) — *see* Frac-
      ture, tibia, upper end
    intercondyloid eminence — *see* Frac-
      ture, tibia, upper end
    involving ankle 824.0
      open 824.9
    lower end or extremity (anterior lip)
      (posterior lip) 824.8
      open 824.9
    malleolus (internal) (medial) 824.0
      open 824.1
    open NEC 823.90
    pathologic 733.16
    proximal end — *see* Fracture, tibia, up-
      per end
    shaft 823.20
      with fibula 823.22
        open 823.32
      open 823.30
    spine — *see* Fracture, tibia, upper end
    stress 733.93
    torus 823.40
      with fibula 823.42
    tuberosity — *see* Fracture, tibia, upper
      end
    upper end or extremity (condyle) (epiph-
      ysis) (head) (spine) (proximal end)
      (tuberosity) 823.00
      with fibula 823.02
        open 823.12
      open 823.10
  toe(s), of one foot (closed) 826.0
    with bone(s) of same lower limb 827.0
      open 827.1
    open 826.1
  tooth (root) 873.63
    complicated 873.73
  torus
    fibula 823.41
      with tibia 823.42
    humerus 812.49
    radius (alone) 813.45
      with ulna 813.47
    tibia 823.40
      with fibula 823.42
    ulna (alone) 813.46

Fracture — *continued*
  torus — *continued*
    ulna — *continued*
      with radius 813.47
  trachea (closed) 807.5
    open 807.6
  transverse process — *see* Fracture, vertebra,
      by site
  trapezium (closed) 814.05
    open 814.15
  trapezoid bone (closed) 814.06
    open 814.16
  trimalleolar (closed) 824.6
    open 824.7
  triquetral (bone) (closed) 814.03
    open 814.13
  trochanter (greater) (lesser) (closed) (*see also*
      Fracture, femur, neck, by site) 820.20
    open 820.30
  trunk (bones) (closed) 809.0
    open 809.1
  tuberosity (external) — *see* Fracture, by site
  ulna (alone) (closed) 813.82
    with radius NEC 813.83
      open 813.93
    coronoid process (closed) 813.02
      open 813.12
    distal end — *see* Fracture, ulna, lower
      end
    epiphysis
      lower — *see* Fracture, ulna, lower
        end
      upper — *see* Fracture, ulna, upper
        end
    head — *see* Fracture, ulna, lower end
    lower end (distal end) (head) (lower
      epiphysis) (styloid process)
      813.43
      with radius (lower end) 813.44
        open 813.54
      open 813.53
    olecranon process (closed) 813.01
      open 813.11
    open NEC 813.92
    pathologic 733.12
    proximal end — *see* Fracture, ulna, up-
      per end
    shaft 813.22
      with radius (shaft) 813.23
        open 813.33
      open 813.32
    styloid process — *see* Fracture, ulna,
      lower end
    torus 813.46
      with radius 813.47
    transverse — *see* Fracture, ulna, by site
    upper end (epiphysis) 813.04
      with radius (upper end) 813.08
        open 813.18
      multiple sites 813.04
        open 813.14
      open 813.14
      specified site NEC 813.04
        open 813.14
  unciform (closed) 814.08
    open 814.18
  vertebra, vertebral (back) (body) (column)
      (neural arch) (pedicle) (spine)
      (spinous process) (transverse pro-
      cess) (closed) 805.8
    with
      hematomyelia — *see* Fracture, verte-
        bra, by site, with spinal cord
        injury
      injury to
        cauda equina — *see* Fracture,
          vertebra, sacrum, with
          spinal cord injury
        nerve — *see* Fracture, vertebra,
          by site, with spinal cord
          injury
      paralysis — *see* Fracture, vertebra,
        by site, with spinal cord injury
      paraplegia — *see* Fracture, vertebra,
        by site, with spinal cord injury

Fracture — *continued*
  vertebra, vertebral — *continued*
    with — *continued*
      quadriplegia — *see* Fracture, verte-
        bra, by site, with spinal cord
        injury
      spinal concussion — *see* Fracture,
        vertebra, by site, with spinal
        cord injury
      spinal cord injury (closed) NEC 806.8

> *Note* — Use the following fifth-digit
> subclassification with categories
> 806.0–806.3:
>
> C_1–C_4 or unspecified level and D_1–D_6
> (T_1–T_6) or unspecified level with
>
> 0 unspecified spinal cord injury
>
> 1 complete lesion of cord
>
> 2 anterior cord syndrome
>
> 3 central cord syndrome
>
> 4 specified injury NEC
>
> C_5–C_7 level and D_7–D_{12} level with:
>
> 5 unspecified spinal cord injury
>
> 6 complete lesion of cord
>
> 7 anterior cord syndrome
>
> 8 central cord syndrome
>
> 9 specified injury NEC

        cervical 806.0 ☑
          open 806.1 ☑
        dorsal, dorsolumbar 806.2 ☑
          open 806.3 ☑
        open 806.9
        thoracic, thoracolumbar 806.2 ☑
          open 806.3 ☑
      atlanto-axial — *see* Fracture, vertebra,
        cervical
      cervical (hangman) (teardrop) (closed)
        805.00
        with spinal cord injury — *see* Frac-
          ture, vertebra, with spinal
          cord injury, cervical
        first (atlas) 805.01
          open 805.11
        second (axis) 805.02
          open 805.12
        third 805.03
          open 805.13
        fourth 805.04
          open 805.14
        fifth 805.05
          open 805.15
        sixth 805.06
          open 805.16
        seventh 805.07
          open 805.17
        multiple sites 805.08
          open 805.18
        open 805.10
      chronic 733.13
      coccyx (closed) 805.6
        with spinal cord injury (closed)
          806.60
          cauda equina injury 806.62
          complete lesion 806.61
            open 806.71
            open 806.72
          open 806.70
          specified type NEC 806.69
            open 806.79
        open 805.7
      collapsed 733.13
      compression, not due to trauma 733.13
      dorsal (closed) 805.2
        with spinal cord injury — *see* Frac-
          ture, vertebra, with spinal
          cord injury, dorsal
        open 805.3
      dorsolumbar (closed) 805.2

Fracture — *continued*
  vertebra, vertebral — *continued*
    dorsolumbar — *continued*
      with spinal cord injury — *see* Frac-
        ture, vertebra, with spinal
        cord injury, dorsal
      open 805.3
    due to osteoporosis 733.13
    fetus or newborn 767.4
    lumbar (closed) 805.4
      with spinal cord injury (closed) 806.4
        open 806.5
      open 805.5
    nontraumatic 733.13
    open NEC 805.9
    pathologic (any site) 733.13
    sacrum (closed) 805.6
      with spinal cord injury 806.60
        cauda equina injury 806.62
        complete lesion 806.61
          open 806.71
          open 806.72
        open 806.70
        specified type NEC 806.69
          open 806.79
      open 805.7
    site unspecified (closed) 805.8
      with spinal cord injury (closed) 806.8
        open 806.9
      open 805.9
    stress (any site) 733.95
    thoracic (closed) 805.2
      with spinal cord injury — *see* Frac-
        ture, vertebra, with spinal
        cord injury, thoracic
      open 805.3
    vertex — *see* Fracture, skull, vault
    vomer (bone) 802.0
      open 802.1
    Wagstaffe's — *see* Fracture, ankle
    wrist (closed) 814.00
      open 814.10
      pathologic 733.12
    xiphoid (process) — *see* Fracture, sternum
    zygoma (zygomatic arch) (closed) 802.4
      open 802.5
Fragile X syndrome 759.83
Fragilitas
  crinium 704.2
  hair 704.2
  ossium 756.51
    with blue sclera 756.51
  unguium 703.8
    congenital 757.5
Fragility
  bone 756.51
    with deafness and blue sclera 756.51
  capillary (hereditary) 287.8
  hair 704.2
  nails 703.8
Fragmentation — *see* Fracture, by site
Frailty 797
Frambesia, frambesial (tropica) — *see also*
    Yaws 102.9
  initial lesion or ulcer 102.0
  primary 102.0
Frambeside
  gummatous 102.4
  of early yaws 102.2
Frambesioma 102.1
Franceschetti's syndrome (mandibulofacial
    dysostosis) 756.0
Francis' disease — *see also* Tularemia 021.9
Franklin's disease (heavy chain) 273.2
Frank's essential thrombocytopenia — *see
    also* Purpura, thrombocytopenic 287.39
Fraser's syndrome 759.89
Freckle 709.09
  malignant melanoma in (M8742/3) — *see*
    Melanoma
  melanotic (of Hutchinson) (M8742/2) — *see*
    Neoplasm, skin, in situ
  retinal 239.81
Freeman-Sheldon syndrome 759.89
Freezing 991.9
  specified effect NEC 991.8

Freiberg's
  disease (osteochondrosis, second metatarsal) 732.5
  infraction of metatarsal head 732.5
  osteochondrosis 732.5
Frei's disease (climatic bubo) 099.1
Fremitus, friction, cardiac 785.3
Frenulum linguae 750.0
Frenum
  external os 752.44
  tongue 750.0
Frequency (urinary) NEC 788.41
  micturition 788.41
  nocturnal 788.43
  polyuria 788.42
  psychogenic 306.53
Frey's syndrome (auriculotemporal syndrome) 705.22
Friction
  burn (see also Injury, superficial, by site) 919.0
  fremitus, cardiac 785.3
  precordial 785.3
  sounds, chest 786.7
Friderichsen-Waterhouse syndrome or disease 036.3
Friedländer's
  B (bacillus) NEC (see also condition) 041.3
    sepsis or septicemia 038.49
  disease (endarteritis obliterans) — see Arteriosclerosis
Friedreich's
  ataxia 334.0
  combined systemic disease 334.0
  disease 333.2
    combined systemic 334.0
  myoclonia 333.2
  sclerosis (spinal cord) 334.0
Friedrich-Erb-Arnold syndrome (acropachyderma) 757.39
Frigidity 302.72
  psychic or psychogenic 302.72
Fröhlich's disease or syndrome (adiposogenital dystrophy) 253.8
Froin's syndrome 336.8
Frommel-Chiari syndrome 676.6 ☑
Frommel's disease 676.6 ☑
Frontal — see also condition
  lobe syndrome 310.0
Frostbite 991.3
  face 991.0
  foot 991.2
  hand 991.1
  specified site NEC 991.3
Frotteurism 302.89
Frozen 991.9
  pelvis 620.8
  shoulder 726.0
Fructosemia 271.2
Fructosuria (benign) (essential) 271.2
Fuchs'
  black spot (myopic) 360.21
  corneal dystrophy (endothelial) 371.57
  heterochromic cyclitis 364.21

Fucosidosis 271.8
Fugue 780.99
  dissociative 300.13
  hysterical (dissociative) 300.13
  reaction to exceptional stress (transient) 308.1
Fukuhara syndrome 277.87
Fuller Albright's syndrome (osteitis fibrosa disseminata) 756.59
Fuller's earth disease 502
Fulminant, fulminating — see condition
Functional — see condition
Functioning
  borderline intellectual V62.89
Fundus — see also condition
  flavimaculatus 362.76
Fungemia 117.9
Fungus, fungous
  cerebral 348.89
  disease NEC 117.9
  infection — see Infection, fungus
  testis (see also Tuberculosis) 016.5 ☑ [608.81]
Funiculitis (acute) 608.4
  chronic 608.4
  endemic 608.4
  gonococcal (acute) 098.14
    chronic or duration of 2 months or over 098.34
  tuberculous (see also Tuberculosis) 016.5 ☑
Funnel
  breast (acquired) 738.3
    congenital 754.81
    late effect of rickets 268.1
  chest (acquired) 738.3
    congenital 754.81
    late effect of rickets 268.1
  pelvis (acquired) 738.6
    with disproportion (fetopelvic) 653.3 ☑
      affecting fetus or newborn 763.1
      causing obstructed labor 660.1 ☑
        affecting fetus or newborn 763.1
    congenital 755.69
    tuberculous (see also Tuberculosis) 016.9 ☑
FUO — see also Pyrexia 780.60
Furfur 690.18
  microsporon 111.0
Furor, paroxysmal (idiopathic) — see also Epilepsy 345.8 ☑
Furriers' lung 495.8
Furrowed tongue 529.5
  congenital 750.13
Furrowing nail(s) (transverse) 703.8
  congenital 757.5
Furuncle 680.9
  abdominal wall 680.2
  ankle 680.6
  anus 680.5
  arm (any part, above wrist) 680.3
  auditory canal, external 680.0
  axilla 680.3
  back (any part) 680.2
  breast 680.2

Furuncle — continued
  buttock 680.5
  chest wall 680.2
  corpus cavernosum 607.2
  ear (any part) 680.0
  eyelid 373.13
  face (any part, except eye) 680.0
  finger (any) 680.4
  flank 680.2
  foot (any part) 680.7
  forearm 680.3
  gluteal (region) 680.5
  groin 680.2
  hand (any part) 680.4
  head (any part, except face) 680.8
  heel 680.7
  hip 680.6
  kidney (see also Abscess, kidney) 590.2
  knee 680.6
  labium (majus) (minus) 616.4
  lacrimal
    gland (see also Dacryoadenitis) 375.00
    passages (duct) (sac) (see also Dacryocystitis) 375.30
  leg, any part except foot 680.6
  malignant 022.0
  multiple sites 680.9
  neck 680.1
  nose (external) (septum) 680.0
  orbit 376.01
  partes posteriores 680.5
  pectoral region 680.2
  penis 607.2
  perineum 680.2
  pinna 680.0
  scalp (any part) 680.8
  scrotum 608.4
  seminal vesicle 608.0
  shoulder 680.3
  skin NEC 680.9
  specified site NEC 680.8
  spermatic cord 608.4
  temple (region) 680.0
  testis 604.90
  thigh 680.6
  thumb 680.4
  toe (any) 680.7
  trunk 680.2
  tunica vaginalis 608.4
  umbilicus 680.2
  upper arm 680.3
  vas deferens 608.4
  vulva 616.4
  wrist 680.4
Furunculosis — see also Furuncle 680.9
  external auditory meatus 680.0 [380.13]
Fusarium (infection) 118
Fusion, fused (congenital)
  anal (with urogenital canal) 751.5
  aorta and pulmonary artery 745.0
  astragaloscaphoid 755.67
  atria 745.5
  atrium and ventricle 745.69
  auditory canal 744.02

Fusion, fused — continued
  auricles, heart 745.5
  binocular, with defective stereopsis 368.33
  bone 756.9
  cervical spine — see Fusion, spine
  choanal 748.0
  commissure, mitral valve 746.5
  cranial sutures, premature 756.0
  cusps, heart valve NEC 746.89
    mitral 746.5
    tricuspid 746.89
  ear ossicles 744.04
  fingers (see also Syndactylism, fingers) 755.11
  hymen 752.42
  hymeno-urethral 599.89
    causing obstructed labor 660.1 ☑
      affecting fetus or newborn 763.1
  joint (acquired) (see also Ankylosis)
    congenital 755.8
  kidneys (incomplete) 753.3
  labium (majus) (minus) 752.49
  larynx and trachea 748.3
  limb 755.8
    lower 755.69
    upper 755.59
  lobe, lung 748.5
  lumbosacral (acquired) 724.6
    congenital 756.15
    surgical V45.4
  nares (anterior) (posterior) 748.0
  nose, nasal 748.0
  nostril(s) 748.0
  organ or site NEC — see Anomaly, specified type NEC
  ossicles 756.9
    auditory 744.04
  pulmonary valve segment 746.02
  pulmonic cusps 746.02
  ribs 756.3
  sacroiliac (acquired) (joint) 724.6
    congenital 755.69
    surgical V45.4
  skull, imperfect 756.0
  spine (acquired) 724.9
    arthrodesis status V45.4
    congenital (vertebra) 756.15
    postoperative status V45.4
  sublingual duct with submaxillary duct at opening in mouth 750.26
  talonavicular (bar) 755.67
  teeth, tooth 520.2
  testes 752.89
  toes (see also Syndactylism, toes) 755.13
  trachea and esophagus 750.3
  twins 759.4
  urethral-hymenal 599.89
  vagina 752.49
  valve cusps — see Fusion, cusps, heart valve
  ventricles, heart 745.4
  vertebra (arch) — see Fusion, spine
  vulva 752.49
Fusospirillosis (mouth) (tongue) (tonsil) 101
Fussy infant (baby) 780.91

☑ **Additional Digit Required — Refer to the Tabular List for Digit Selection**   ▽ **Subterms under main terms may continue to next column or page**

2014 ICD-9-CM   ▶◀ **Revised Text**   ● **New Line**   ▲ **Revised Code**   **Volume 2 — 125**

G

G-trisomy 758.0
Gafsa boil 085.1
Gain, weight (abnormal) (excessive) — see also Weight, gain 783.1
Gaisböck's disease or syndrome (polycythemia hypertonica) 289.0
Gait
  abnormality 781.2
    hysterical 300.11
  ataxic 781.2
    hysterical 300.11
  disturbance 781.2
    hysterical 300.11
  paralytic 781.2
  scissor 781.2
  spastic 781.2
  staggering 781.2
    hysterical 300.11
Galactocele (breast) (infected) 611.5
  puerperal, postpartum 676.8 ☑
Galactophoritis 611.0
  puerperal, postpartum 675.2 ☑
Galactorrhea 676.6 ☑
  not associated with childbirth 611.6
Galactosemia (classic) (congenital) 271.1
Galactosuria 271.1
Galacturia 791.1
  bilharziasis 120.0
Galen's vein — see condition
Gallbladder — see also condition
  acute (see also Disease, gallbladder) 575.0
Gall duct — see condition
Gallop rhythm 427.89
Gallstone (cholemic) (colic) (impacted) — see also Cholelithiasis
  causing intestinal obstruction 560.31
Gambling, pathological 312.31
Gammaloidosis 277.39
Gammopathy 273.9
  macroglobulinemia 273.3
  monoclonal (benign) (essential) (idiopathic) (with lymphoplasmacytic dyscrasia) 273.1
Gamna's disease (siderotic splenomegaly) 289.51
Gampsodactylia (congenital) 754.71
Gamstorp's disease (adynamia episodica hereditaria) 359.3
Gandy-Nanta disease (siderotic splenomegaly) 289.51
Gang activity, without manifest psychiatric disorder V71.09
  adolescent V71.02
  adult V71.01
  child V71.02
Gangliocytoma (M9490/0) — see Neoplasm, connective tissue, benign
Ganglioglioma (M9505/1) — see Neoplasm, by site, uncertain behavior
Ganglion 727.43
  Joint 727.41
  of yaws (early) (late) 102.6
  periosteal (see also Periostitis) 730.3 ☑
  tendon sheath (compound) (diffuse) 727.42
  tuberculous (see also Tuberculosis) 015.9 ☑
Ganglioneuroblastoma (M9490/3) — see Neoplasm, connective tissue, malignant
Ganglioneuroma (M9490/0) — see also Neoplasm, connective tissue, benign
  malignant (M9490/3) — see Neoplasm, connective tissue, malignant
Ganglioneuromatosis (M9491/0) — see Neoplasm, connective tissue, benign
Ganglionitis
  fifth nerve (see also Neuralgia, trigeminal) 350.1
  gasserian 350.1
  geniculate 351.1
    herpetic 053.11
    newborn 767.5
  herpes zoster 053.11
  herpetic geniculate (Hunt's syndrome) 053.11
Gangliosidosis 330.1

Gangosa 102.5
Gangrene, gangrenous (anemia) (artery) (cellulitis) (dermatitis) (dry) (infective) (moist) (pemphigus) (septic) (skin) (stasis) (ulcer) 785.4
  with
    arteriosclerosis (native artery) 440.24
      bypass graft 440.30
        autologous vein 440.31
        nonautologous biological 440.32
    diabetes (mellitus) 250.7 ☑ [785.4]
      due to secondary diabetes 249.7 ☑ [785.4]
  abdomen (wall) 785.4
  adenitis 683
  alveolar 526.5
  angina 462
    diphtheritic 032.0
  anus 569.49
  appendices epiploicae — see Gangrene, mesentery
  appendix — see Appendicitis, acute
  arteriosclerotic — see Arteriosclerosis, with, gangrene
  auricle 785.4
  Bacillus welchii (see also Gangrene, gas) 040.0
  bile duct (see also Cholangitis) 576.8
  bladder 595.89
  bowel — see Gangrene, intestine
  cecum — see Gangrene, intestine
  Clostridium perfringens or welchii (see also Gangrene, gas) 040.0
  colon — see Gangrene, intestine
  connective tissue 785.4
  cornea 371.40
  corpora cavernosa (infective) 607.2
    noninfective 607.89
  cutaneous, spreading 785.4
  decubital (see also Ulcer, pressure) 707.00 [785.4]
  diabetic (any site) 250.7 ☑ [785.4]
    due to secondary diabetes 249.7 ☑ [785.4]
  dropsical 785.4
  emphysematous (see also Gangrene, gas) 040.0
  epidemic (ergotized grain) 988.2
  epididymis (infectional) (see also Epididymitis) 604.99
  erysipelas (see also Erysipelas) 035
  extremity (lower) (upper) 785.4
  gallbladder or duct (see also Cholecystitis, acute) 575.0
  gas (bacillus) 040.0
    with
      abortion — see Abortion, by type, with sepsis
      ectopic pregnancy (see also categories 633.0–633.9) 639.0
      molar pregnancy (see also categories 630–632) 639.0
    following
      abortion 639.0
      ectopic or molar pregnancy 639.0
      puerperal, postpartum, childbirth 670.8 ☑
  glossitis 529.0
  gum 523.8
  hernia — see Hernia, by site, with gangrene
  hospital noma 528.1
  intestine, intestinal (acute) (hemorrhagic) (massive) 557.0
    with
      hernia — see Hernia, by site, with gangrene
      mesenteric embolism or infarction 557.0
      obstruction (see also Obstruction, intestine) 560.9
  laryngitis 464.00
    with obstruction 464.01
  liver 573.8
  lung 513.0
    spirochetal 104.8
  lymphangitis 457.2

Gangrene, gangrenous — continued
  Meleney's (cutaneous) 686.09
  mesentery 557.0
    with
      embolism or infarction 557.0
      intestinal obstruction (see also Obstruction, intestine) 560.9
  mouth 528.1
  noma 528.1
  orchitis 604.90
  ovary (see also Salpingo-oophoritis) 614.2
  pancreas 577.0
  penis (infectional) 607.2
    noninfective 607.89
  perineum 785.4
  pharynx 462
  pneumonia 513.0
  Pott's 440.24
  presenile 443.1
  pulmonary 513.0
  pulp, tooth 522.1
  quinsy 475
  Raynaud's (symmetric gangrene) 443.0 [785.4]
  rectum 569.49
  retropharyngeal 478.24
  rupture — see Hernia, by site, with gangrene
  scrotum 608.4
    noninfective 608.83
  senile 440.24
  septic 034.0
  septic 034.0
  sore throat 462
  spermatic cord 608.4
    noninfective 608.89
  spine 785.4
  spirochetal NEC 104.8
  spreading cutaneous 785.4
  stomach 537.89
  stomatitis 528.1
  symmetrical 443.0 [785.4]
  testis (infectional) (see also Orchitis) 604.99
    noninfective 608.89
  throat 462
    diphtheritic 032.0
  thyroid (gland) 246.8
  tonsillitis (acute) 463
  tooth (pulp) 522.1
  tuberculous NEC (see also Tuberculosis) 011.9 ☑
  tunica vaginalis 608.4
    noninfective 608.89
  umbilicus 785.4
  uterus (see also Endometritis) 615.9
  uvulitis 528.3
  vas deferens 608.4
    noninfective 608.89
  vulva (see also Vulvitis) 616.10
Gannister disease (occupational) 502
  with tuberculosis — see Tuberculosis, pulmonary
Ganser's syndrome, hysterical 300.16
Gardner-Diamond syndrome (autoerythrocyte sensitization) 287.2
Gargoylism 277.5
Garré's
  disease (see also Osteomyelitis) 730.1 ☑
  osteitis (sclerosing) (see also Osteomyelitis) 730.1 ☑
  osteomyelitis (see also Osteomyelitis) 730.1 ☑
Garrod's pads, knuckle 728.79
Gartner's duct
  cyst 752.41
  persistent 752.41
Gas 787.3
  asphyxia, asphyxiation, inhalation, poisoning, suffocation NEC 987.9
    specified gas — see Table of Drugs and Chemicals
  bacillus gangrene or infection — see Gas, gangrene
  cyst, mesentery 568.89
  excessive 787.3
  gangrene 040.0

Gas — continued
  gangrene — continued
    with
      abortion — see Abortion, by type, with sepsis
      ectopic pregnancy (see also categories 633.0–633.9) 639.0
      molar pregnancy (see also categories 630–632) 639.0
    following
      abortion 639.0
      ectopic or molar pregnancy 639.0
      puerperal, postpartum, childbirth 670.8 ☑
  on stomach 787.3
  pains 787.3
Gastradenitis 535.0 ☑
Gastralgia 536.8
  psychogenic 307.89
Gastrectasis, gastrectasia 536.1
  psychogenic 306.4
Gastric — see condition
Gastrinoma (M8153/1)
  malignant (M8153/3)
    pancreas 157.4
    specified site NEC — see Neoplasm, by site, malignant
    unspecified site 157.4
  specified site — see Neoplasm, by site, uncertain behavior
  unspecified site 235.5
Gastritis 535.5 ☑

Note — Use the following fifth-digit subclassification for category 535:

0   without mention of hemorrhage

1   with hemorrhage

  acute 535.0 ☑
  alcoholic 535.3 ☑
  allergic 535.4 ☑
  antral 535.4 ☑
  atrophic-hyperplastic 535.1 ☑
  atrophic 535.1 ☑
  bile-induced 535.4 ☑
  catarrhal 535.0 ☑
  chronic (atrophic) 535.1 ☑
  cirrhotic 535.4 ☑
  corrosive (acute) 535.4 ☑
  dietetic 535.4 ☑
  due to diet deficiency 269.9 [535.4] ☑
  eosinophilic 535.7 ☑
  erosive 535.4 ☑
  follicular 535.4 ☑
    chronic 535.1 ☑
  giant hypertrophic 535.2 ☑
  glandular 535.4 ☑
    chronic 535.1 ☑
  hypertrophic (mucosa) 535.2 ☑
    chronic giant 211.1
  irritant 535.4 ☑
  nervous 306.4
  phlegmonous 535.0 ☑
  psychogenic 306.4
  sclerotic 535.4 ☑
  spastic 536.8
  subacute 535.0 ☑
  superficial 535.4 ☑
  suppurative 535.0 ☑
  toxic 535.4 ☑
  tuberculous (see also Tuberculosis) 017.9 ☑
Gastrocarcinoma (M8010/3) 151.9
Gastrocolic — see condition
Gastrocolitis — see Enteritis
Gastrodisciasis 121.8
Gastroduodenitis — see also Gastritis 535.5 ☑
  catarrhal 535.0 ☑
  infectional 535.0 ☑
  virus, viral 008.8
    specified type NEC 008.69
Gastrodynia 536.8
Gastroenteritis (acute) (catarrhal) (congestive) (hemorrhagic) (noninfectious) — see also Enteritis 558.9
  aertrycke infection 003.0

☑ Additional Digit Required — Refer to the Tabular List for Digit Selection   Ⓦ Subterms under main terms may continue to next column or page

2014 ICD-9-CM   ▶◀ Revised Text   ● New Line   ▲ Revised Code   Volume 2 — 127

Gastroenteritis — *see also* Enteritis — *continued*
allergic 558.3
chronic 558.9
ulcerative (*see also* Colitis, ulcerative) 556.9
dietetic 558.9
due to
antineoplastic chemotherapy 558.9
food poisoning (*see also* Poisoning, food) 005.9
radiation 558.1
eosinophilic 558.41
epidemic 009.0
functional 558.9
infectious (*see also* Enteritis, due to, by organism) 009.0
presumed 009.1
salmonella 003.0
septic (*see also* Enteritis, due to, by organism) 009.0
toxic 558.2
tuberculous (*see also* Tuberculosis) 014.8 ☑
ulcerative (*see also* Colitis, ulcerative) 556.9
viral NEC 008.8
specified type NEC 008.69
zymotic 009.0
Gastroenterocolitis — *see* Enteritis
Gastroenteropathy, protein-losing 579.8
Gastroenteroptosis 569.89
Gastroesophageal laceration-hemorrhage syndrome 530.7
Gastroesophagitis 530.19
Gastrohepatitis — *see also* Gastritis 535.5 ☑
Gastrointestinal — *see* condition
Gastrojejunal — *see* condition
Gastrojejunitis — *see also* Gastritis 535.5 ☑
Gastrojejunocolic — *see* condition
Gastroliths 537.89
Gastromalacia 537.89
Gastroparalysis 536.3
diabetic 250.6 ☑ [536.3]
due to secondary diabetes 249.6 ☑ [536.3]
Gastroparesis 536.3
diabetic 250.6 ☑ [536.3]
due to secondary diabetes 249.6 ☑ [536.3]
Gastropathy 537.9
congestive portal 537.89
erythematous 535.5 ☑
exudative 579.8
portal hypertensive 537.89
Gastroptosis 537.5
Gastrorrhagia 578.0
Gastrorrhea 536.8
psychogenic 306.4
Gastroschisis (congenital) 756.73
acquired 569.89
Gastrospasm (neurogenic) (reflex) 536.8
neurotic 306.4
psychogenic 306.4
Gastrostaxis 578.0
Gastrostenosis 537.89
Gastrostomy
attention to V55.1
complication 536.40
specified type 536.49
infection 536.41
malfunctioning 536.42
status V44.1
Gastrosuccorrhea (continuous) (intermittent) 536.8
neurotic 306.4
psychogenic 306.4
Gaucher's
disease (adult) (cerebroside lipidosis) (infantile) 272.7
hepatomegaly 272.7
splenomegaly (cerebroside lipidosis) 272.7
GAVE (gastric antral vascular ectasia) 537.82
with hemorrhage 537.83
without hemorrhage 537.82
Gayet-Wernicke's syndrome (superior hemorrhagic polioencephalitis) 265.1

Gayet's disease (superior hemorrhagic polioencephalitis) 265.1
Gee (-Herter) (-Heubner) (-Thaysen) disease or syndrome (nontropical sprue) 579.0
Gélineau's syndrome — *see also* Narcolepsy 347.00
Gemination, teeth 520.2
Gemistocytoma (M9411/3)
specified site — *see* Neoplasm, by site, malignant
unspecified site 191.9
General, generalized — *see* condtion
Genetic
susceptibility to
MEN (multiple endocrine neoplasia) V84.81
neoplasia
multiple endocrine (MEN) V84.81
neoplasm
malignant, of
breast V84.01
endometrium V84.04
other V84.09
ovary V84.02
prostate V84.03
specified disease NEC V84.89
Genital — *see* condition
warts 078.11
Genito-anorectal syndrome 099.1
Genitourinary system — *see* condition
Genu
congenital 755.64
extrorsum (acquired) 736.42
congenital 755.64
late effects of rickets 268.1
introrsum (acquired) 736.41
congenital 755.64
late effects of rickets 268.1
rachitic (old) 268.1
recurvatum (acquired) 736.5
congenital 754.40
with dislocation of knee 754.41
late effects of rickets 268.1
valgum (acquired) (knock-knee) 736.41
congenital 755.64
late effects of rickets 268.1
varum (acquired) (bowleg) 736.42
congenital 755.64
late effect of rickets 268.1
Geographic tongue 529.1
Geophagia 307.52
Geotrichosis 117.9
intestine 117.9
lung 117.9
mouth 117.9
Gephyrophobia 300.29
Gerbode defect 745.4
GERD (gastroesophageal reflux disease) 530.81
Gerhardt's
disease (erythromelalgia) 443.82
syndrome (vocal cord paralysis) 478.30
Gerlier's disease (epidemic vertigo) 078.81
German measles 056.9
exposure to V01.4
Germinoblastoma (diffuse) (M9614/3) 202.8 ☑
follicular (M9692/3) 202.0 ☑
Germinoma (M9064/3) — *see* Neoplasm, by site, malignant
Gerontoxon 371.41
Gerstmann-Sträussler-Scheinker syndrome (GSS) 046.71
Gerstmann's syndrome (finger agnosia) 784.69
Gestation (period) — *see also* Pregnancy
ectopic NEC (*see also* Pregnancy, ectopic) 633.90
with intrauterine pregnancy 633.91
multiple
placenta status
quadruplet
two or more monoamniotic fetuses V91.22
two or more monochorionic fetuses V91.21

Gestation — *see also* Pregnancy — *continued*
multiple — *continued*
placenta status — *continued*
quadruplet — *continued*
unable to determine number of placenta and number of amniotic sacs V91.29
unspecified number of placenta and unspecified number of amniotic sacs V91.20
specified (greater than quadruplets) NEC
two or more monoamniotic fetuses V91.92
two or more monochorionic fetuses V91.91
unable to determine number of placenta and number of amniotic sacs V91.99
unspecified number of placenta and unspecified number of amniotic sacs V91.90
triplet
two or more monoamniotic fetuses V91.12
two or more monochorionic fetuses V91.11
unable to determine number of placenta and number of amniotic sacs V91.19
unspecified number of placenta, unspecified number of amniotic sacs V91.10
twin
dichorionic/diamniotic (two placentae, two amniotic sacs) V91.03
monochorionic/diamniotic (one placenta, two amniotic sacs) V91.02
monochorionic/monoamniotic (one placenta, one amniotic sac) V91.01
unable to determine number of placenta and number of amniotic sacs V91.09
unspecified number of placenta, unspecified number of amniotic sacs V91.00
Gestational proteinuria 646.2 ☑
with hypertension — *see* Toxemia, of pregnancy
Ghon tubercle primary infection — *see also* Tuberculosis 010.0 ☑
Ghost
teeth 520.4
vessels, cornea 370.64
Ghoul hand 102.3
Gianotti Crosti syndrome 057.8
due to known virus — *see* Infection, virus
due to unknown virus 057.8
Giant
cell
epulis 523.8
peripheral (gingiva) 523.8
tumor, tendon sheath 727.02
colon (congenital) 751.3
esophagus (congenital) 750.4
kidney 753.3
urticaria 995.1
hereditary 277.6
Giardia lamblia infestation 007.1
Giardiasis 007.1
Gibert's disease (pityriasis rosea) 696.3
Gibraltar fever — *see* Brucellosis
Giddiness 780.4
hysterical 300.11
psychogenic 306.9
Gierke's disease (glycogenosis I) 271.0
Gigantism (cerebral) (hypophyseal) (pituitary) 253.0
Gilbert's disease or cholemia (familial nonhemolytic jaundice) 277.4
Gilchrist's disease (North American blastomycosis) 116.0

Gilford (-Hutchinson) disease or syndrome (progeria) 259.8
Gilles de la Tourette's disease (motor-verbal tic) 307.23
Gillespie's syndrome (dysplasia oculodentodigitalis) 759.89
Gingivitis 523.10
acute 523.00
necrotizing 101
non-plaque induced 523.01
plaque induced 523.00
catarrhal 523.00
chronic 523.10
non-plaque induced 523.11
desquamative 523.10
expulsiva 523.40
hyperplastic 523.10
marginal, simple 523.10
necrotizing, acute 101
non-plaque induced 523.11
pellagrous 265.2
plaque induced 523.10
ulcerative 523.10
acute necrotizing 101
Vincent's 101
Gingivoglossitis 529.0
Gingivopericementitis 523.40
Gingivosis 523.10
Gingivostomatitis 523.10
herpetic 054.2
Giovannini's disease 117.9
GISA (glycopeptide intermediate staphylococcus aureus) V09.8 ☑
Glanders 024
Gland, glandular — *see* condition
Glanzmann (-Naegeli) disease or thrombasthenia 287.1
Glassblowers' disease 527.1
Glaucoma (capsular) (inflammatory) (noninflammatory) (primary) 365.9
with increased episcleral venous pressure 365.82
absolute 360.42
acute 365.22
narrow angle 365.22
secondary 365.60
angle closure 365.20
acute 365.22
attack 365.22
chronic 365.23
crisis 365.22
intermittent 365.21
interval 365.21
primary 365.20
chronic 365.23
residual stage 365.24
subacute 365.21
angle recession 365.65
borderline 365.00
chronic 365.11
noncongestive 365.11
open angle 365.11
simple 365.11
closed angle — *see* Glaucoma, angle closure
congenital 743.20
associated with other eye anomalies 743.22
simple 743.21
congestive — *see* Glaucoma, narrow angle
corticosteroid-induced (glaucomatous stage) 365.31
residual stage 365.32
exfoliation 365.52
hemorrhagic 365.60
hypersecretion 365.81
infantile 365.14
congenital 743.20
associated with other eye anomalies 743.22
simple 743.21
inflammatory 365.62
in or with
aniridia 365.42
Axenfeld's anomaly 365.41
congenital syndromes NEC 759.89 [365.44]

Glaucoma — *continued*
  in or with — *continued*
    disorder of lens NEC 365.59
    inflammation, ocular 365.62
    iris
      anomalies NEC 365.42
      atrophy, essential 365.42
      bombé 365.61
    microcornea 365.43
    neurofibromatosis 237.71 [365.44]
    ocular
      cysts NEC 365.64
      disorders NEC 365.60
      trauma 365.65
      tumors NEC 365.64
    pupillary block or seclusion 365.61
    Rieger's anomaly or syndrome 365.41
    seclusion of pupil 365.61
    Sturge-Weber (-Dimitri) syndrome
      759.6 [365.44]
    systemic syndrome NEC 365.44
    tumor of globe 365.64
    vascular disorders NEC 365.63
  juvenile 365.14
  low tension 365.12
  malignant 365.83
  narrow angle (primary) 365.20
    acute 365.22
    chronic 365.23
    intermittent 365.21
    interval 365.21
    residual stage 365.24
    subacute 365.21
  neovascular 365.63
  newborn 743.20
    associated with other eye anomalies
      743.22
    simple 743.21
  noncongestive (chronic) 365.11
  nonobstructive (chronic) 365.11
  normal tension 365.12
  obstructive 365.60
    due to lens changes 365.59
  open angle 365.10
    with
      abnormal optic disc appearance or
        asymmetry 365.01
      borderline findings
        high risk 365.05
        intraocular pressure 365.01
        low risk 365.01
      cupping of optic discs 365.01
      thin central corneal thickness
        (pachymetry) 365.01
    high risk 365.05
    low risk 365.01
    primary 365.11
    residual stage 365.15
  phacoanaphylactic 365.59
  phacolytic 365.51
  phacomorphic
    acute 365.22
    borderline 365.06
  pigmentary 365.13
  pigment dispersion 365.13
  postinfectious 365.60
  pseudoexfoliation 365.52
  secondary NEC 365.60
    due to
      steroids 365.31
      surgery 365.60
  simple (chronic) 365.11
  simplex 365.11
  stage
    advanced 365.73
    early 365.71
    end-stage 365.73
    indeterminate 365.74
    mild 365.71
    moderate 365.72
    severe 365.73
    unspecified 365.70
  steroid
    induced 365.31
    responders 365.03
  suspect 365.00

Glaucoma — *continued*
  suspect — *continued*
    primary angle closure 365.02
  syphilitic 095.8
  traumatic NEC 365.65
    newborn 767.8
  uveitic 365.62
  wide angle (*see also* Glaucoma, open angle)
    365.10
Glaucomatous flecks (subcapsular) 366.31
Glazed tongue 529.4
Gleet 098.2
Glénard's disease or syndrome (enteroptosis)
  569.89
Glinski-Simmonds syndrome (pituitary
  cachexia) 253.2
Glioblastoma (multiforme) (M9440/3)
  with sarcomatous component (M9442/3)
    specified site — *see* Neoplasm, by site,
      malignant
    unspecified site 191.9
  giant cell (M9441/3)
    specified site — *see* Neoplasm, by site,
      malignant
    unspecified site 191.9
  specified site — *see* Neoplasm, by site, ma-
    lignant
  unspecified site 191.9
Glioma (malignant) (M9380/3)
  astrocytic (M9400/3)
    specified site — *see* Neoplasm, by site,
      malignant
    unspecified site 191.9
  mixed (M9382/3)
    specified site — *see* Neoplasm, by site,
      malignant
    unspecified site 191.9
  nose 748.1
  specified site NEC — *see* Neoplasm, by site,
    malignant
  subependymal (M9383/1) 237.5
  unspecified site 191.9
Gliomatosis cerebri (M9381/3) 191.0
Glioneuroma (M9505/1) — *see* Neoplasm, by
  site, uncertain behavior
Gliosarcoma (M9380/3)
  specified site — *see* Neoplasm, by site, ma-
    lignant
  unspecified site 191.9
Gliosis (cerebral) 349.89
  spinal 336.0
Glisson's
  cirrhosis — *see* Cirrhosis, portal
  disease (*see also* Rickets) 268.0
Glissonitis 573.3
Globinuria 791.2
Globus 306.4
  hystericus 300.11
Glomangioma (M8712/0) — *see also* Heman-
  gioma 228.00
Glomangiosarcoma (M8710/3) — *see* Neoplasm, connective tissue, malignant
Glomerular nephritis — *see also* Nephritis
  583.9
Glomerulitis — *see also* Nephritis 583.9
Glomerulonephritis — *see also* Nephritis 583.9
  with
    edema (*see also* Nephrosis) 581.9
    lesion of
      exudative nephritis 583.89
      interstitial nephritis (diffuse) (focal)
        583.89
      necrotizing glomerulitis 583.4
        acute 580.4
        chronic 582.4
      renal necrosis 583.9
        cortical 583.6
        medullary 583.7
      specified pathology NEC 583.89
        acute 580.89
        chronic 582.89
    necrosis, renal 583.9
      cortical 583.6
      medullary (papillary) 583.7
    specified pathology or lesion NEC 583.89
  acute 580.9

Glomerulonephritis — *see also* Nephritis —
  continued
  acute — *continued*
    with
      exudative nephritis 580.89
      interstitial nephritis (diffuse) (focal)
        580.89
      necrotizing glomerulitis 580.4
      extracapillary with epithelial crescents
        580.4
      poststreptococcal 580.0
      proliferative (diffuse) 580.0
      rapidly progressive 580.4
      specified pathology NEC 580.89
  arteriolar (*see also* Hypertension, kidney)
    403.90
  arteriosclerotic (*see also* Hypertension, kid-
    ney) 403.90
  ascending (*see also* Pyelitis) 590.80
  basement membrane NEC 583.89
    with
      pulmonary hemorrhage (Goodpas-
        ture's syndrome)
        446.21 [583.81]
  chronic 582.9
    with
      exudative nephritis 582.89
      interstitial nephritis (diffuse) (focal)
        582.89
      necrotizing glomerulitis 582.4
      specified pathology or lesion NEC
        582.89
    endothelial 582.2
    extracapillary with epithelial crescents
      582.4
    hypocomplementemic persistent 582.2
    lobular 582.2
    membranoproliferative 582.2
    membranous 582.1
      and proliferative (mixed) 582.2
      sclerosing 582.1
    mesangiocapillary 582.2
    mixed membranous and proliferative
      582.2
    proliferative (diffuse) 582.0
    rapidly progressive 582.4
    sclerosing 582.1
  cirrhotic — *see* Sclerosis, renal
  desquamative — *see* Nephrosis
  due to or associated with
    amyloidosis 277.39 [583.81]
      with nephrotic syndrome
        277.39 [581.81]
      chronic 277.39 [582.81]
    diabetes mellitus 250.4 ☑ [583.81]
      with nephrotic syndrome
        250.4 ☑ [581.81]
      due to secondary diabetes
        249.4 ☑ [581.81]
      due to secondary diabetes
        249.4 ☑ [581.81]
    diphtheria 032.89 [580.81]
    gonococcal infection (acute)
      098.19 [583.81]
      chronic or duration of 2 months or
        over 098.39 [583.81]
    infectious hepatitis 070.9 [580.81]
    malaria (with nephrotic syndrome)
      084.9 [581.81]
    mumps 072.79 [580.81]
    polyarteritis (nodosa) (with nephrotic
      syndrome) 446.0 [581.81]
    specified pathology NEC 583.89
      acute 580.89
      chronic 582.89
    streptotrichosis 039.8 [583.81]
    subacute bacterial endocarditis
      421.0 [580.81]
    syphilis (late) 095.4
      congenital 090.5 [583.81]
      early 091.69 [583.81]
    systemic lupus erythematosus
      710.0 [583.81]
      with nephrotic syndrome
        710.0 [581.81]
      chronic 710.0 [582.81]

Glomerulonephritis — *see also* Nephritis —
  continued
  due to or associated with — *continued*
    tuberculosis (*see also* Tuberculosis)
      016.0 ☑ [583.81]
    typhoid fever 002.0 [580.81]
  extracapillary with epithelial crescents 583.4
    acute 580.4
    chronic 582.4
  exudative 583.89
    acute 580.89
    chronic 582.89
  focal (*see also* Nephritis) 583.9
    embolic 580.4
  granular 582.89
  granulomatous 582.89
  hydremic (*see also* Nephrosis) 581.9
  hypocomplementemic persistent 583.2
    with nephrotic syndrome 581.2
    chronic 582.2
  immune complex NEC 583.89
  infective (*see also* Pyelitis) 590.80
  interstitial (diffuse) (focal) 583.89
    with nephrotic syndrome 581.89
    acute 580.89
    chronic 582.89
  latent or quiescent 582.9
  lobular 583.2
    with nephrotic syndrome 581.2
    chronic 582.2
  membranoproliferative 583.2
    with nephrotic syndrome 581.2
    chronic 582.2
  membranous 583.1
    with nephrotic syndrome 581.1
    and proliferative (mixed) 583.2
      with nephrotic syndrome 581.2
      chronic 582.2
    chronic 582.1
    sclerosing 582.1
      with nephrotic syndrome 581.1
  mesangiocapillary 583.2
    with nephrotic syndrome 581.2
    chronic 582.2
  minimal change 581.3
  mixed membranous and proliferative 583.2
    with nephrotic syndrome 581.2
    chronic 582.2
  necrotizing 583.4
    acute 580.4
    chronic 582.4
  nephrotic (*see also* Nephrosis) 581.9
  old — *see* Glomerulonephritis, chronic
  parenchymatous 581.89
  poststreptococcal 580.0
  proliferative (diffuse) 583.0
    with nephrotic syndrome 581.0
    acute 580.0
    chronic 582.0
  purulent (*see also* Pyelitis) 590.80
  quiescent — *see* Nephritis, chronic
  rapidly progressive 583.4
    acute 580.4
    chronic 582.4
  sclerosing membranous (chronic) 582.1
    with nephrotic syndrome 581.1
  septic (*see also* Pyelitis) 590.80
  specified pathology or lesion NEC 583.89
    with nephrotic syndrome 581.89
    acute 580.89
    chronic 582.89
  suppurative (acute) (disseminated) (*see also*
    Pyelitis) 590.80
  toxic — *see* Nephritis, acute
  tubal, tubular — *see* Nephrosis, tubular
  type II (Ellis) — *see* Nephrosis
  vascular — *see* Hypertension, kidney
Glomerulosclerosis — *see also* Sclerosis, renal
  587
  focal 582.1
    with nephrotic syndrome 581.1
  intercapillary (nodular) (with diabetes)
    250.4 ☑ [581.81]
    due to secondary diabetes
      249.4 ☑ [581.81]
Glossagra 529.6

☑ Additional Digit Required — Refer to the Tabular List for Digit Selection   ▽ Subterms under main terms may continue to next column or page

2014 ICD-9-CM   ▶◀ Revised Text   ● New Line   ▲ Revised Code   Volume 2 — 129

Glossalgia 529.6
Glossitis 529.0
  areata exfoliativa 529.1
  atrophic 529.4
  benign migratory 529.1
  gangrenous 529.0
  Hunter's 529.4
  median rhomboid 529.2
  Moeller's 529.4
  pellagrous 265.2
Glossocele 529.8
Glossodynia 529.6
  exfoliativa 529.4
Glossoncus 529.8
Glossophytia 529.3
Glossoplegia 529.8
Glossoptosis 529.8
Glossopyrosis 529.6
Glossotrichia 529.3
Glossy skin 701.9
Glottis — see condition
Glottitis — see Glossitis
Glucagonoma (M8152/0)
  malignant (M8152/3)
    pancreas 157.4
    specified site NEC — see Neoplasm, by site, malignant
    unspecified site 157.4
  pancreas 211.7
  specified site NEC — see Neoplasm, by site, benign
  unspecified site 211.7
Glucoglycinuria 270.7
Glue ear syndrome 381.20
Glue sniffing (airplane glue) — see also Dependence 304.6 ☑
Glycinemia (with methylmalonic acidemia) 270.7
Glycinuria (renal) (with ketosis) 270.0
Glycogen
  infiltration (see also Disease, glycogen storage) 271.0
  storage disease (see also Disease, glycogen storage) 271.0
Glycogenosis — see also Disease, glycogen storage 271.0
  cardiac 271.0 [425.7]
  Cori, types I-VII 271.0
  diabetic, secondary 250.8 ☑ [259.8]
    due to secondary diabetes 249.8 ☑ [259.8]
  diffuse (with hepatic cirrhosis) 271.0
  generalized 271.0
  glucose-6-phosphatase deficiency 271.0
  hepatophosphorylase deficiency 271.0
  hepatorenal 271.0
  myophosphorylase deficiency 271.0
  pulmonary interstitial 516.62
Glycopenia 251.2
Glycopeptide
  intermediate staphylococcus aureus (GISA) V09.8 ☑
  resistant
    enterococcus V09.8 ☑
    staphylococcus aureus (GRSA) V09.8 ☑
Glycoprolinuria 270.8
Glycosuria 791.5
  renal 271.4
Gnathostoma (spinigerum) (infection) (infestation) 128.1
  wandering swellings from 128.1
Gnathostomiasis 128.1
Goiter (adolescent) (colloid) (diffuse) (dipping) (due to iodine deficiency) (endemic) (euthyroid) (heart) (hyperplastic) (internal) (intrathoracic) (juvenile) (mixed type) (nonendemic) (parenchymatous) (plunging) (sporadic) (subclavicular) (substernal) 240.9
  with
    hyperthyroidism (recurrent) (see also Goiter, toxic) 242.0 ☑
    thyrotoxicosis (see also Goiter, toxic) 242.0 ☑
  adenomatous (see also Goiter, nodular) 241.9

Goiter — continued
  cancerous (M8000/3) 193
  complicating pregnancy, childbirth, or puerperium 648.1 ☑
  congenital 246.1
  cystic (see also Goiter, nodular) 241.9
  due to enzyme defect in synthesis of thyroid hormone (butane-insoluble iodine) (coupling) (deiodinase) (iodide trapping or organification) (iodotyrosine dehalogenase) (peroxidase) 246.1
  dyshormonogenic 246.1
  exophthalmic (see also Goiter, toxic) 242.0 ☑
  familial (with deaf-mutism) 243
  fibrous 245.3
  lingual 759.2
  lymphadenoid 245.2
  malignant (M8000/3) 193
  multinodular (nontoxic) 241.1
    toxic or with hyperthyroidism (see also Goiter, toxic) 242.2 ☑
  nodular (nontoxic) 241.9
    with
      hyperthyroidism (see also Goiter, toxic) 242.3 ☑
      thyrotoxicosis (see also Goiter, toxic) 242.3 ☑
    endemic 241.9
    exophthalmic (diffuse) (see also Goiter, toxic) 242.0 ☑
    multinodular (nontoxic) 241.1
    sporadic 241.9
    toxic (see also Goiter, toxic) 242.3 ☑
    uninodular (nontoxic) 241.0
  nontoxic (nodular) 241.9
    multinodular 241.1
    uninodular 241.0
  pulsating (see also Goiter, toxic) 242.0 ☑
  simple 240.0
  toxic 242.0 ☑

> **Note** — Use the following fifth-digit subclassification with category 242:
>
> 0 without mention of thyrotoxic crisis or storm
>
> 1 with mention of thyrotoxic crisis or storm

    adenomatous 242.3 ☑
      multinodular 242.2 ☑
      uninodular 242.1 ☑
    multinodular 242.2 ☑
    nodular 242.3 ☑
      multinodular 242.2 ☑
      uninodular 242.1 ☑
    uninodular 242.1 ☑
  uninodular (nontoxic) 241.0
    toxic or with hyperthyroidism (see also Goiter, toxic) 242.1 ☑
Goldberg (-Maxwell) (-Morris) syndrome (testicular feminization) 259.51
Goldblatt's
  hypertension 440.1
  kidney 440.1
Goldenhar's syndrome (oculoauriculovertebral dysplasia) 756.0
Goldflam-Erb disease or syndrome 358.00
Goldscheider's disease (epidermolysis bullosa) 757.39
Goldstein's disease (familial hemorrhagic telangiectasia) 448.0
Golfer's elbow 726.32
Goltz-Gorlin syndrome (dermal hypoplasia) 757.39
Gonadoblastoma (M9073/1)
  specified site — see Neoplasm, by site uncertain behavior
  unspecified site
    female 236.2
    male 236.4
Gonecystitis — see also Vesiculitis 608.0
Gongylonemiasis 125.6
  mouth 125.6
Goniosynechiae 364.73
Gonococcemia 098.89

Gonococcus, gonococcal (disease) (infection) — see also condition 098.0
  anus 098.7
  bursa 098.52
  chronic NEC 098.2
  complicating pregnancy, childbirth, or puerperium 647.1 ☑
    affecting fetus or newborn 760.2
  conjunctiva, conjunctivitis (neonatorum) 098.40
  dermatosis 098.89
  endocardium 098.84
  epididymo-orchitis 098.13
    chronic or duration of 2 months or over 098.33
  eye (newborn) 098.40
  fallopian tube (chronic) 098.37
    acute 098.17
  genitourinary (acute) (organ) (system) (tract) (see also Gonorrhea) 098.0
    lower 098.0
      chronic 098.2
    upper 098.10
      chronic 098.30
  heart NEC 098.85
  joint 098.50
  keratoderma 098.81
  keratosis (blennorrhagica) 098.81
  lymphatic (gland) (node) 098.89
  meninges 098.82
  orchitis (acute) 098.13
    chronic or duration of 2 months or over 098.33
  pelvis (acute) 098.19
    chronic or duration of 2 months or over 098.39
  pericarditis 098.83
  peritonitis 098.86
  pharyngitis 098.6
  pharynx 098.6
  proctitis 098.7
  pyosalpinx (chronic) 098.37
    acute 098.17
  rectum 098.7
  septicemia 098.89
  skin 098.89
  specified site NEC 098.89
  synovitis 098.51
  tendon sheath 098.51
  throat 098.6
  urethra (acute) 098.0
    chronic or duration of 2 months or over 098.2
  vulva (acute) 098.0
    chronic or duration of 2 months or over 098.2
Gonocytoma (M9073/1)
  specified site — see Neoplasm, by site, uncertain behavior
  unspecified site
    female 236.2
    male 236.4
Gonorrhea 098.0
  acute 098.0
  Bartholin's gland (acute) 098.0
    chronic or duration of 2 months or over 098.2
  bladder (acute) 098.11
    chronic or duration of 2 months or over 098.31
  carrier (suspected of) V02.7
  cervix (acute) 098.15
    chronic or duration of 2 months or over 098.35
  chronic 098.2
  complicating pregnancy, childbirth, or puerperium 647.1 ☑
    affecting fetus or newborn 760.2
  conjunctiva, conjunctivitis (neonatorum) 098.40
  contact V01.6
  Cowper's gland (acute) 098.0
    chronic or duration of 2 months or over 098.2
  duration of two months or over 098.2
  exposure to V01.6

Gonorrhea — continued
  fallopian tube (chronic) 098.37
    acute 098.17
  genitourinary (acute) (organ) (system) (tract) 098.0
    chronic 098.2
    duration of two months or over 098.2
  kidney (acute) 098.19
    chronic or duration of 2 months or over 098.39
  ovary (acute) 098.19
    chronic or duration of 2 months or over 098.39
  pelvis (acute) 098.19
    chronic or duration of 2 months or over 098.39
  penis (acute) 098.0
    chronic or duration of 2 months or over 098.2
  prostate (acute) 098.12
    chronic or duration of 2 months or over 098.32
  seminal vesicle (acute) 098.14
    chronic or duration of 2 months or over 098.34
  specified site NEC — see Gonococcus
  spermatic cord (acute) 098.14
    chronic or duration of 2 months or over 098.34
  urethra (acute) 098.0
    chronic or duration of 2 months or over 098.2
  vagina (acute) 098.0
    chronic or duration of 2 months or over 098.2
  vas deferens (acute) 098.14
    chronic or duration of 2 months or over 098.34
  vulva (acute) 098.0
    chronic or duration of 2 months or over 098.2
Goodpasture's syndrome (pneumorenal) 446.21
Good's syndrome 279.06
Gopalan's syndrome (burning feet) 266.2
Gordon's disease (exudative enteropathy) 579.8
Gorlin-Chaudhry-Moss syndrome 759.89
Gougerot-Blum syndrome (pigmented purpuric lichenoid dermatitis) 709.1
Gougerot-Carteaud disease or syndrome (confluent reticulate papillomatosis) 701.8
Gougerot-Hailey-Hailey disease (benign familial chronic pemphigus) 757.39
Gougerot (-Houwer) -Sjögren syndrome (keratoconjunctivitis sicca) 710.2
Gougerot's syndrome (trisymptomatic) 709.1
Gouley's syndrome (constrictive pericarditis) 423.2
Goundou 102.6
Gout, gouty 274.9
  with
    specified manifestations NEC 274.89
    tophi (tophus) 274.03
  acute 274.01
  arthritis 274.00
    acute 274.01
  arthropathy 274.00
    acute 274.01
    chronic (without mention of tophus (tophi)) 274.02
      with tophus (tophi) 274.03
  attack 274.01
  chronic 274.02
    tophaceous 274.03
  degeneration, heart 274.82
  diathesis 274.9
  eczema 274.89
  episcleritis 274.89 [379.09]
  external ear (tophus) 274.81
  flare 274.01
  glomerulonephritis 274.10
  iritis 274.89 [364.11]
  joint 274.00
  kidney 274.10

Gout, gouty — *continued*
  lead 984.9
    specified type of lead — *see* Table of Drugs and Chemicals
  nephritis 274.10
  neuritis 274.89 *[357.4]*
  phlebitis 274.89 *[451.9]*
  rheumatic 714.0
  saturnine 984.9
    specified type of lead — *see* Table of Drugs and Chemicals
  spondylitis 274.00
  synovitis 274.00
  syphilitic 095.8
  tophi 274.03
    ear 274.81
    heart 274.82
    specified site NEC 274.82
Gowers-Paton-Kennedy syndrome 377.04
Gowers'
  muscular dystrophy 359.1
  syndrome (vasovagal attack) 780.2
Gradenigo's syndrome 383.02
Graft-versus-host disease 279.50
  due to organ transplant NEC — *see* Complications, transplant, organ
Graham Steell's murmur (pulmonic regurgitation) — *see also* Endocarditis, pulmonary 424.3
Grain-handlers' disease or lung 495.8
Grain mite (itch) 133.8
Grand
  mal (idiopathic) (*see also* Epilepsy) 345.1 ☑
    hysteria of Charcôt 300.11
    nonrecurrent or isolated 780.39
  multipara
    affecting management of labor and delivery 659.4 ☑
    status only (not pregnant) V61.5
Granite workers' lung 502
Granular — *see also* condition
  inflammation, pharynx 472.1
  kidney (contracting) (*see also* Sclerosis, renal) 587
  liver — *see* Cirrhosis, liver
  nephritis — *see* Nephritis
Granulation tissue, abnormal — *see also* Granuloma
  abnormal or excessive 701.5
  postmastoidectomy cavity 383.33
  postoperative 701.5
  skin 701.5
Granulocytopenia, granulocytopenic (primary) 288.00
  malignant 288.09
Granulomatosis NEC 686.1
  disciformis chronica et progressiva 709.3
  infantiseptica 771.2
  lipoid 277.89
  lipophagic, intestinal 040.2
  miliary 027.0
  necrotizing, respiratory 446.4
  progressive, septic 288.1
  Wegener's (necrotizing respiratory) 446.4
Granulomatous tissue — *see* Granuloma
Granuloma NEC 686.1
  abdomen (wall) 568.89
    skin (pyogenicum) 686.1
      from residual foreign body 709.4
  annulare 695.89
  anus 569.49
  apical 522.6
  appendix 543.9
  aural 380.23
  beryllium (skin) 709.4
    lung 503
  bone (*see also* Osteomyelitis) 730.1 ☑
    eosinophilic 277.89
    from residual foreign body 733.99
  canaliculus lacrimalis 375.81
  cerebral 348.89
  cholesterin, middle ear 385.82
  coccidioidal (progressive) 114.3
    lung 114.4
    meninges 114.2
    primary (lung) 114.0

Granuloma — *continued*
  colon 569.89
  conjunctiva 372.61
  dental 522.6
  ear, middle (cholesterin) 385.82
    with otitis media — *see* Otitis media
  eosinophilic 277.89
    bone 277.89
    lung 277.89
    oral mucosa 528.9
  exuberant 701.5
  eyelid 374.89
  facial
    lethal midline 446.3
    malignant 446.3
  faciale 701.8
  fissuratum (gum) 523.8
  foot NEC 686.1
  foreign body (in soft tissue) NEC 728.82
    bone 733.99
    in operative wound 998.4
    muscle 728.82
    skin 709.4
    subcutaneous tissue 709.4
  fungoides 202.1 ☑
  gangraenescens 446.3
  giant cell (central) (jaw) (reparative) 526.3
    gingiva 523.8
    peripheral (gingiva) 523.8
  gland (lymph) 289.3
  Hodgkin's (M9661/3) 201.1 ☑
  ileum 569.89
  infectious NEC 136.9
  inguinale (Donovan) 099.2
    venereal 099.2
  intestine 569.89
  iridocyclitis 364.10
  jaw (bone) 526.3
    reparative giant cell 526.3
  kidney (*see also* Infection, kidney) 590.9
  lacrimal sac 375.81
  larynx 478.79
  lethal midline 446.3
  lipid 277.89
  lipoid 277.89
  liver 572.8
  lung (infectious) (*see also* Fibrosis, lung) 515
    coccidioidal 114.4
    eosinophilic 277.89
  lymph gland 289.3
  Majocchi's 110.6
  malignant, face 446.3
  mandible 526.3
  mediastinum 519.3
  midline 446.3
  monilial 112.3
  muscle 728.82
    from residual foreign body 728.82
  nasal sinus (*see also* Sinusitis) 473.9
  operation wound 998.59
    foreign body 998.4
    stitch (external) 998.89
      internal wound 998.89
    talc 998.7
  oral mucosa, eosinophilic or pyogenic 528.9
  orbit, orbital 376.11
  paracoccidioidal 116.1
  penis, venereal 099.2
  periapical 522.6
  peritoneum 568.89
    due to ova of helminths NEC (*see also* Helminthiasis) 128.9
  postmastoidectomy cavity 383.33
  postoperative — *see* Granuloma, operation wound
  prostate 601.8
  pudendi (ulcerating) 099.2
  pudendorum (ulcerative) 099.2
  pulp, internal (tooth) 521.49
  pyogenic, pyogenicum (skin) 686.1
    maxillary alveolar ridge 522.6
    oral mucosa 528.9
  rectum 569.49
  reticulohistiocytic 277.89
  rubrum nasi 705.89
  sarcoid 135

Granuloma — *continued*
  Schistosoma 120.9
  septic (skin) 686.1
  silica (skin) 709.4
  sinus (accessory) (infectional) (nasal) (*see also* Sinusitis) 473.9
  skin (pyogenicum) 686.1
    from foreign body or material 709.4
  sperm 608.89
  spine
    syphilitic (epidural) 094.89
    tuberculous (*see also* Tuberculosis) 015.0 ☑ *[730.88]*
  stitch (postoperative) 998.89
    internal wound 998.89
  suppurative (skin) 686.1
  suture (postoperative) 998.89
    internal wound 998.89
  swimming pool 031.1
  talc 728.82
    in operation wound 998.7
  telangiectaticum (skin) 686.1
  tracheostomy 519.09
  trichophyticum 110.6
  tropicum 102.4
  umbilicus 686.1
    newborn 771.4
  urethra 599.84
  uveitis 364.10
  vagina 099.2
  venereum 099.2
  vocal cords 478.5
  Wegener's (necrotizing respiratory granulomatosis) 446.4
Granulosis rubra nasi 705.89
Graphite fibrosis (of lung) 503
Graphospasm 300.89
  organic 333.84
Grating scapula 733.99
Gravel (urinary) — *see also* Calculus 592.9
Graves' disease (exophthalmic goiter) — *see also* Goiter, toxic 242.0 ☑
Gravis — *see* condition
Grawitz's tumor (hypernephroma) (M8312/3) 189.0
Grayness, hair (premature) 704.3
  congenital 757.4
Gray or grey syndrome (chloramphenicol) (newborn) 779.4
Greenfield's disease 330.0
Green sickness 280.9
Greenstick fracture — *see* Fracture, by site
Greig's syndrome (hypertelorism) 756.0
Grief 309.0
Griesinger's disease — *see also* Ancylostomiasis 126.9
Grinders'
  asthma 502
  lung 502
  phthisis (*see also* Tuberculosis) 011.4 ☑
Grinding, teeth 306.8
Grip
  Dabney's 074.1
  devil's 074.1
Grippe, grippal — *see also* Influenza
  Balkan 083.0
  intestinal (*see also* Influenza) 487.8
  summer 074.8
Grippy cold — *see also* Influenza 487.1
Grisel's disease 723.5
Groin — *see* condition
Grooved
  nails (transverse) 703.8
  tongue 529.5
    congenital 750.13
Ground itch 126.9
Growing pains, children 781.99
Growth (fungoid) (neoplastic) (new) (M8000/1) — *see also* Neoplasm, by site, unspecified nature
  adenoid (vegetative) 474.12
  benign (M8000/0) — *see* Neoplasm, by site, benign
  fetal, poor 764.9 ☑
    affecting management of pregnancy 656.5 ☑

Growth — *see also* Neoplasm, by site, unspecified nature — *continued*
  malignant (M8000/3) — *see* Neoplasm, by site, malignant
  rapid, childhood V21.0
  secondary (M8000/6) — *see* Neoplasm, by site, malignant, secondary
GRSA (glycopeptide resistant staphylococcus aureus) V09.8 ☑
Gruber's hernia — *see* Hernia, Gruber's
Gruby's disease (tinea tonsurans) 110.0
GSS (Gerstmann-Sträussler-Scheinker syndrome) 046.71
Guama fever 066.3
Gubler (-Millard) paralysis or syndrome 344.89
Guérin-Stern syndrome (arthrogryposis multiplex congenita) 754.89
Guertin's disease (electric chorea) 049.8
Guillain-Barré disease or syndrome 357.0
Guinea worms (infection) (infestation) 125.7
Guinon's disease (motor-verbal tic) 307.23
Gull and Sutton's disease — *see* Hypertension, kidney
Gull's disease (thyroid atrophy with myxedema) 244.8
Gum — *see* condition
Gumboil 522.7
Gumma (syphilitic) 095.9
  artery 093.89
    cerebral or spinal 094.89
  bone 095.5
    of yaws (late) 102.6
  brain 094.89
  cauda equina 094.89
  central nervous system NEC 094.9
  ciliary body 095.8 *[364.11]*
  congenital 090.5
    testis 090.5
  eyelid 095.8 *[373.5]*
  heart 093.89
  intracranial 094.89
  iris 095.8 *[364.11]*
  kidney 095.4
  larynx 095.8
  leptomeninges 094.2
  liver 095.3
  meninges 094.2
  myocardium 093.82
  nasopharynx 095.8
  neurosyphilitic 094.9
  nose 095.8
  orbit 095.8
  palate (soft) 095.8
  penis 095.8
  pericardium 093.81
  pharynx 095.8
  pituitary 095.8
  scrofulous (see also Tuberculosis) 017.0 ☑
  skin 095.8
  specified site NEC 095.8
  spinal cord 094.89
  tongue 095.8
  tonsil 095.8
  trachea 095.8
  tuberculous (*see also* Tuberculosis) 017.0 ☑
  ulcerative due to yaws 102.4
  ureter 095.8
  yaws 102.4
    bone 102.6
Gunn's syndrome (jaw-winking syndrome) 742.8
Gunshot wound — *see also* Wound, open, by site
  fracture — *see* Fracture, by site, open
  internal organs (abdomen, chest, or pelvis) — *see* Injury, internal, by site, with open wound
  intracranial — *see* Laceration, brain, with open intracranial wound
Günther's disease or syndrome (congenital erythropoietic porphyria) 277.1
Gustatory hallucination 780.1
Gynandrism 752.7

☑ **Additional Digit Required — Refer to the Tabular List for Digit Selection**   ▽ **Subterms under main terms may continue to next column or page**

2014 ICD-9-CM   ▶◀ Revised Text   ● New Line   ▲ Revised Code   **Volume 2 — 131**

Gout, gouty — Gynandrism

Gynandroblastoma (M8632/1)
specified site — *see* Neoplasm, by site, uncertain behavior
unspecified site
female 236.2
male 236.4
Gynandromorphism 752.7
Gynatresia (congenital) 752.49
Gynecoid pelvis, male 738.6
Gynecological examination V72.31
for contraceptive maintenance V25.40
Gynecomastia 611.1
Gynephobia 300.29
Gyrate scalp 757.39

H

Haas' disease (osteochondrosis head of humerus) 732.3
Habermann's disease (acute parapsoriasis varioliformis) 696.2
Habit, habituation
chorea 307.22
disturbance, child 307.9
drug (*see also* Dependence) 304.9 ☑
laxative (*see also* Abuse, drugs, nondependent) 305.9 ☑
spasm 307.20
chronic 307.22
transient (of childhood) 307.21
tic 307.20
chronic 307.22
transient (of childhood) 307.21
use of
nonprescribed drugs (*see also* Abuse, drugs, nondependent) 305.9 ☑
patent medicines (*see also* Abuse, drugs, nondependent) 305.9 ☑
vomiting 536.2
Hadfield-Clarke syndrome (pancreatic infantilism) 577.8
Haff disease 985.1
Hageman factor defect, deficiency, or disease — *see also* Defect, coagulation 286.3
Haglund-Läwen-Fründ syndrome 717.89
Haglund's disease (osteochondrosis os tibiale externum) 732.5
Hagner's disease (hypertrophic pulmonary osteoarthropathy) 731.2
Hag teeth, tooth 524.39
Hailey-Hailey disease (benign familial chronic pemphigus) 757.39
Hair — *see also* condition
plucking 307.9
Hairball in stomach 935.2
Hairy black tongue 529.3
Half vertebra 756.14
Halitosis 784.99
Hallermann-Streiff syndrome 756.0
Hallervorden-Spatz disease or syndrome 333.0
Hallopeau's
acrodermatitis (continua) 696.1
disease (lichen sclerosis et atrophicus) 701.0
Hallucination (auditory) (gustatory) (olfactory) (tactile) 780.1
alcohol-induced 291.3
drug-induced 292.12
visual 368.16
Hallucinosis 298.9
alcohol-induced (acute) 291.3
drug-induced 292.12
Hallus — *see* Hallux
Hallux 735.9
limitus 735.8
malleus (acquired) 735.3
rigidus (acquired) 735.2
congenital 755.66
late effects of rickets 268.1
valgus (acquired) 735.0
congenital 755.66
varus (acquired) 735.1
congenital 755.66
Halo, visual 368.15
Hamartoblastoma 759.6
Hamartoma 759.6

Hamartoma — *continued*
epithelial (gingival), odontogenic, central, or peripheral (M9321/0) 213.1
upper jaw (bone) 213.0
vascular 757.32
Hamartosis, hamartoses NEC 759.6
Hamman-Rich syndrome (diffuse interstitial pulmonary fibrosis) 516.33
Hamman's disease or syndrome (spontaneous mediastinal emphysema) 518.1
Hammer toe (acquired) 735.4
congenital 755.66
late effects of rickets 268.1
Hand-foot syndrome 693.0
Hand-Schüller-Christian disease or syndrome (chronic histiocytosis x) 277.89
Hand — *see* condition
Hanging (asphyxia) (strangulation) (suffocation) 994.7
Hangnail (finger) (with lymphangitis) 681.02
Hangover (alcohol) — *see also* Abuse, drugs, nondependent 305.0 ☑
Hanot-Chauffard (-Troisier) syndrome (bronze diabetes) 275.01
Hanot's cirrhosis or disease — *see* Cirrhosis, biliary
Hansen's disease (leprosy) 030.9
benign form 030.1
malignant form 030.0
Harada's disease or syndrome 363.22
Hard chancre 091.0
Hardening
artery — *see* Arteriosclerosis
brain 348.89
liver 571.8
Hard firm prostate 600.10
with
urinary
obstruction 600.11
retention 600.11
Harelip — *see also* Cleft, lip 749.10
Hare's syndrome (M8010/3) (carcinoma, pulmonary apex) 162.3
Harkavy's syndrome 446.0
Harlequin (fetus) 757.1
color change syndrome 779.89
Harley's disease (intermittent hemoglobinuria) 283.2
Harris'
lines 733.91
syndrome (organic hyperinsulinism) 251.1
Hart's disease or syndrome (pellagra-cerebellar ataxia-renal aminoaciduria) 270.0
Hartmann's pouch (abnormal sacculation of gallbladder neck) 575.8
of intestine V44.3
attention to V55.3
Hartnup disease (pellagra-cerebellar ataxia-renal aminoaciduria) 270.0
Harvester lung 495.0
Hashimoto's disease or struma (struma lymphomatosa) 245.2
Hassall-Henle bodies (corneal warts) 371.41
Haut mal — *see also* Epilepsy 345.1 ☑
Haverhill fever 026.1
Hawaiian wood rose dependence 304.5 ☑
Hawkins' keloid 701.4
Hay
asthma (*see also* Asthma) 493.0 ☑
fever (allergic) (with rhinitis) 477.9
with asthma (bronchial) (*see also* Asthma) 493.0 ☑
allergic, due to grass, pollen, ragweed, or tree 477.0
conjunctivitis 372.05
due to
dander, animal (cat) (dog) 477.2
dust 477.8
fowl 477.8
hair, animal (cat) (dog) 477.2
pollen 477.0
specified allergen other than pollen 477.8
Hayem-Faber syndrome (achlorhydric anemia) 280.9

Hayem-Widal syndrome (acquired hemolytic jaundice) 283.9
Haygarth's nodosities 715.04
Hazard-Crile tumor (M8350/3) 193
Hb (abnormal)
disease — *see* Disease, hemoglobin
trait — *see* Trait
H disease 270.0
Head — *see also* condition
banging 307.3
Headache 784.0
allergic 339.00
associated with sexual activity 339.82
cluster 339.00
chronic 339.02
episodic 339.01
daily
chronic 784.0
new persistent (NPDH) 339.42
drug induced 339.3
due to
loss, spinal fluid 349.0
lumbar puncture 349.0
saddle block 349.0
emotional 307.81
histamine 339.00
hypnic 339.81
lumbar puncture 349.0
medication overuse 339.3
menopausal 627.2
menstrual 346.4 ☑
migraine 346.9 ☑
nasal septum 784.0
nonorganic origin 307.81
orgasmic 339.82
post-traumatic 339.20
acute 339.21
chronic 339.22
postspinal 349.0
premenstrual 346.4 ☑
preorgasmic 339.82
primary
cough 339.83
exertional 339.84
stabbing 339.85
thunderclap 339.43
psychogenic 307.81
psychophysiologic 307.81
rebound 339.3
short lasting unilateral neuralgiform with conjunctival injection and tearing (SUNCT) 339.05
sick 346.9 ☑
spinal 349.0
complicating labor and delivery 668.8 ☑
postpartum 668.8 ☑
spinal fluid loss 349.0
syndrome
cluster 339.00
complicated NEC 339.44
periodic in child or adolescent 346.2 ☑
specified NEC 339.89
tension 307.81
type 339.10
chronic 339.12
episodic 339.11
vascular 784.0
migraine type 346.9 ☑
vasomotor 346.9 ☑
Health
advice V65.4 ☑
audit V70.0
checkup V70.0
education V65.4 ☑
hazard (*see also* History of) V15.9
falling V15.88
specified cause NEC V15.89
instruction V65.4 ☑
services provided because (of)
boarding school residence V60.6
holiday relief for person providing home care V60.5
inadequate
housing V60.1
resources V60.2
lack of housing V60.0

Health — *continued*
services provided because — *continued*
no care available in home V60.4
person living alone V60.3
poverty V60.3
residence in institution V60.6
specified cause NEC V60.89
vacation relief for person providing home care V60.5
Healthy
donor (*see also* Donor) V59.9
infant or child
accompanying sick mother V65.0
receiving care V20.1
person
accompanying sick relative V65.0
admitted for sterilization V25.2
receiving prophylactic inoculation or vaccination (*see also* Vaccination, prophylactic) V05.9
Hearing
conservation and treatment V72.12
examination V72.19
following failed hearing screening V72.11
Heart — *see* condition
Heartburn 787.1
psychogenic 306.4
Heat (effects) 992.9
apoplexy 992.0
burn (*see also* Burn, by site)
from sun (*see also* Sunburn) 692.71
collapse 992.1
cramps 992.2
dermatitis or eczema 692.89
edema 992.7
erythema — *see* Burn, by site
excessive 992.9
specified effect NEC 992.8
exhaustion 992.5
anhydrotic 992.3
due to
salt (and water) depletion 992.4
water depletion 992.3
fatigue (transient) 992.6
fever 992.0
hyperpyrexia 992.0
prickly 705.1
prostration — *see* Heat, exhaustion
pyrexia 992.0
rash 705.1
specified effect NEC 992.8
stroke 992.0
sunburn (*see also* Sunburn) 692.71
syncope 992.1
Heavy-chain disease 273.2
Heavy-for-dates (fetus or infant) 766.1
4500 grams or more 766.0
exceptionally 766.0
Hebephrenia, hebephrenic (acute) — *see also* Schizophrenia 295.1 ☑
dementia (praecox) (*see also* Schizophrenia) 295.1 ☑
schizophrenia (*see also* Schizophrenia) 295.1 ☑
Heberden's
disease or nodes 715.04
syndrome (angina pectoris) 413.9
Hebra's disease
dermatitis exfoliativa 695.89
erythema multiforme exudativum 695.19
pityriasis 695.89
maculata et circinata 696.3
rubra 695.89
pilaris 696.4
prurigo 698.2
Hebra, nose 040.1
Hedinger's syndrome (malignant carcinoid) 259.2
Heel — *see* condition
Heerfordt's disease or syndrome (uveoparotitis) 135
Hegglin's anomaly or syndrome 288.2
Heidenhain's disease 290.10
with dementia 290.10

Heilmeyer-Schöner disease (M9842/3) 207.1 ☑

Heine-Medin disease — *see also* Poliomyelitis 045.9 ☑

Heinz-body anemia, congenital 282.7

Heller's disease or syndrome (infantile psychosis) — *see also* Psychosis, childhood 299.1 ☑

H.E.L.L.P 642.5 ☑

Helminthiasis — *see also* Infestation, by specific parasite 128.9
  Ancylostoma (*see also* Ancylostoma) 126.9
  intestinal 127.9
    mixed types (types classifiable to more than one of the categories 120.0–127.7) 127.8
    specified type 127.7
  mixed types (intestinal) (types classifiable to more than one of the categories 120.0–127.7) 127.8
  Necator americanus 126.1
  specified type NEC 128.8
  Trichinella 124

Heloma 700

Hemangioblastoma (M9161/1) — *see also* Neoplasm, connective tissue, uncertain behavior
  malignant (M9161/3) — *see* Neoplasm, connective tissue, malignant

Hemangioblastomatosis, cerebelloretinal 759.6

Hemangioendothelioma (M9130/1) — *see also* Neoplasm, by site, uncertain behavior
  benign (M9130/0) 228.00
  bone (diffuse) (M9130/3) — *see* Neoplasm, bone, malignant
  malignant (M9130/3) — *see* Neoplasm, connective tissue, malignant
  nervous system (M9130/0) 228.09

Hemangioendotheliosarcoma (M9130/3) — *see* Neoplasm, connective tissue, malignant

Hemangiofibroma (M9160/0) — *see* Neoplasm, by site, benign

Hemangiolipoma (M8861/0) — *see* Lipoma

Hemangioma (M9120/0) 228.00
  arteriovenous (M9123/0) — *see* Hemangioma, by site
  brain 228.02
  capillary (M9131/0) — *see* Hemangioma, by site
  cavernous (M9121/0) — *see* Hemangioma, by site
  central nervous system NEC 228.09
  choroid 228.09
  heart 228.09
  infantile (M9131/0) — *see* Hemangioma, by site
  intra-abdominal structures 228.04
  intracranial structures 228.02
  intramuscular (M9132/0) — *see* Hemangioma, by site
  iris 228.09
  juvenile (M9131/0) — *see* Hemangioma, by site
  malignant (M9120/3) — *see* Neoplasm, connective tissue, malignant
  meninges 228.09
    brain 228.02
    spinal cord 228.09
  peritoneum 228.04
  placenta — *see* Placenta, abnormal
  plexiform (M9131/0) — *see* Hemangioma, by site
  racemose (M9123/0) — *see* Hemangioma, by site
  retina 228.03
  retroperitoneal tissue 228.04
  sclerosing (M8832/0) — *see* Neoplasm, skin, benign
  simplex (M9131/0) — *see* Hemangioma, by site
  skin and subcutaneous tissue 228.01
  specified site NEC 228.09
  spinal cord 228.09

Hemangioma — *continued*
  venous (M9122/0) — *see* Hemangioma, by site
  verrucous keratotic (M9142/0) — *see* Hemangioma, by site

Hemangiomatosis (systemic) 757.32
  involving single site — *see* Hemangioma

Hemangiopericytoma (M9150/1) — *see also* Neoplasm, connective tissue, uncertain behavior
  benign (M9150/0) — *see* Neoplasm, connective tissue, benign
  malignant (M9150/3) — *see* Neoplasm, connective tissue, malignant

Hemangiosarcoma (M9120/3) — *see* Neoplasm, connective tissue, malignant

Hemarthrosis (nontraumatic) 719.10
  ankle 719.17
  elbow 719.12
  foot 719.17
  hand 719.14
  hip 719.15
  knee 719.16
  multiple sites 719.19
  pelvic region 719.15
  shoulder (region) 719.11
  specified site NEC 719.18
  traumatic — *see* Sprain, by site
  wrist 719.13

Hematemesis 578.0
  with ulcer — *see* Ulcer, by site, with hemorrhage
  due to S. japonicum 120.2
  Goldstein's (familial hemorrhagic telangiectasia) 448.0
  newborn 772.4
    due to swallowed maternal blood 777.3

Hematidrosis 705.89

Hematinuria — *see also* Hemoglobinuria 791.2
  malarial 084.8
  paroxysmal 283.2

Hematite miners' lung 503

Hematobilia 576.8

Hematocele (congenital) (diffuse) (idiopathic) 608.83
  broad ligament 620.7
  canal of Nuck 629.0
  cord, male 608.83
  fallopian tube 620.8
  female NEC 629.0
  ischiorectal 569.89
  male NEC 608.83
  ovary 629.0
  pelvis, pelvic
    female 629.0
      with ectopic pregnancy (*see also* Pregnancy, ectopic) 633.90
      with intrauterine pregnancy 633.91
    male 608.83
  periuterine 629.0
  retrouterine 629.0
  scrotum 608.83
  spermatic cord (diffuse) 608.83
  testis 608.84
  traumatic — *see* Injury, internal, pelvis
  tunica vaginalis 608.83
  uterine ligament 629.0
  uterus 621.4
  vagina 623.6
  vulva 624.5

Hematocephalus 742.4

Hematochezia — *see also* Melena 578.1

Hematochyluria — *see also* Infestation, filarial 125.9

Hematocolpos 626.8

Hematocornea 371.12

Hematogenous — *see* condition

Hematoma (skin surface intact) (traumatic) — *see also* Contusion

> *Note* — Hematomas are coded according to origin and the nature and site of the hematoma or the accompanying injury. Hematomas of unspecified origin are coded as injuries of the sites involved, except:
>
> (a) hematomas of genital organs which are coded as diseases of the organ involved unless they complicate pregnancy or delivery
>
> (b) hematomas of the eye which are coded as diseases of the eye.
>
> For late effect of hematoma classifiable to 920–924 see Late, effect, contusion

  with
    crush injury — *see* Crush
    fracture — *see* Fracture, by site
    injury of internal organs (*see also* Injury, internal, by site)
      kidney — *see* Hematoma, kidney, traumatic
      liver — *see* Hematoma, liver, traumatic
      spleen — *see* Hematoma, spleen
    nerve injury — *see* Injury, nerve
    open wound — *see* Wound, open, by site
    skin surface intact — *see* Contusion
  abdomen (wall) — *see* Contusion, abdomen
  amnion 658.8 ☑
  aorta, dissecting 441.00
    abdominal 441.02
    thoracic 441.01
    thoracoabdominal 441.03
  aortic intramural — *see* Dissection, aorta
  arterial (complicating trauma) 904.9
    specified site — *see* Injury, blood vessel, by site
  auricle (ear) 380.31
  birth injury 767.8
    skull 767.19
  brain (traumatic) 853.0 ☑

> *Note* — Use the following fifth-digit subclassification with categories 851–854:
>
> 0   unspecified state of consciousness
>
> 1   with no loss of consciousness
>
> 2   with brief [less than one hour] loss of consciousness
>
> 3   with moderate [1–24 hours] loss of consciousness
>
> 4   with prolonged [more than 24 hours] loss of consciousness and return to pre–existing conscious level
>
> 5   with prolonged [more than 24 hours] loss of consciousness, without return to pre–existing conscious level
>
> Use fifth-digit 5 to designate when a patient is unconscious and dies before regaining consciousness, regardless of the duration of the loss of consciousness
>
> 6   with loss of consciousness of unspecified duration
>
> 9   with concussion, unspecified

    with
      cerebral
        contusion — *see* Contusion, brain
        laceration — *see* Laceration, brain
      open intracranial wound 853.1 ☑
      skull fracture — *see* Fracture, skull, by site
    extradural or epidural 852.4 ☑
      with open intracranial wound 852.5 ☑
    fetus or newborn 767.0

Hematoma — *see also* Contusion — *continued*
  brain — *continued*
    extradural or epidural — *continued*
      nontraumatic 432.0
    fetus or newborn NEC 767.0
    nontraumatic (*see also* Hemorrhage, brain) 431
      epidural or extradural 432.0
      newborn NEC 772.8
      subarachnoid, arachnoid, or meningeal (*see also* Hemorrhage, subarachnoid) 430
      subdural (*see also* Hemorrhage, subdural) 432.1
    subarachnoid, arachnoid, or meningeal 852.0 ☑
      with open intracranial wound 852.1 ☑
      fetus or newborn 772.2
      nontraumatic (*see also* Hemorrhage, subarachnoid) 430
    subdural 852.2 ☑
      with open intracranial wound 852.3 ☑
      fetus or newborn (localized) 767.0
      nontraumatic (*see also* Hemorrhage, subdural) 432.1
  breast (nontraumatic) 611.89
  broad ligament (nontraumatic) 620.7
    complicating delivery 665.7 ☑
    traumatic — *see* Injury, internal, broad ligament
  calcified NEC 959.9
  capitis 920
    due to birth injury 767.19
    newborn 767.19
  cerebral — *see* Hematoma, brain
  cesarean section wound 674.3 ☑
  chorion — *see* Placenta, abnormal
  complicating delivery (perineum) (vulva) 664.5 ☑
    pelvic 665.7 ☑
    vagina 665.7 ☑
  corpus
    cavernosum (nontraumatic) 607.82
    luteum (nontraumatic) (ruptured) 620.1
  dura (mater) — *see* Hematoma, brain, subdural
  epididymis (nontraumatic) 608.83
  epidural (traumatic) (*see also* Hematoma, brain, extradural)
    spinal — *see* Injury, spinal, by site
  episiotomy 674.3 ☑
  external ear 380.31
  extradural (*see also* Hematoma, brain, extradural)
    fetus or newborn 767.0
    nontraumatic 432.0
      fetus or newborn 767.0
  fallopian tube 620.8
  genital organ (nontraumatic)
    female NEC 629.89
    male NEC 608.83
    traumatic (external site) 922.4
      internal — *see* Injury, internal, genital organ
  graafian follicle (ruptured) 620.0
  internal organs (abdomen, chest, or pelvis) (*see also* Injury, internal, by site)
    kidney — *see* Hematoma, kidney, traumatic
    liver — *see* Hematoma, liver, traumatic
    spleen — *see* Hematoma, spleen
  intracranial — *see* Hematoma, brain
  kidney, cystic 593.81
    traumatic 866.01
      with open wound into cavity 866.11
  labia (nontraumatic) 624.5
  lingual (and other parts of neck, scalp, or face, except eye) 920
  liver (subcapsular) 573.8
    birth injury 767.8
    fetus or newborn 767.8
    traumatic NEC 864.01

☑ **Additional Digit Required** — Refer to the Tabular List for Digit Selection   ▽ **Subterms under main terms may continue to next column or page**

Hematoma — *see also* Contusion — *continued*
liver — *continued*
  traumatic — *continued*
    with
      laceration — *see* Laceration, liver
      open wound into cavity 864.11
mediastinum — *see* Injury, internal, mediastinum
meninges, meningeal (brain) (*see also* Hematoma, brain, subarachnoid)
spinal — *see* Injury, spinal, by site
mesosalpinx (nontraumatic) 620.8
  traumatic — *see* Injury, internal, pelvis
muscle (traumatic) — *see* Contusion, by site
  nontraumatic 729.92
nasal (septum) (and other part(s) of neck, scalp, or face, except eye) 920
obstetrical surgical wound 674.3 ☑
orbit, orbital (nontraumatic) 376.32
  traumatic 921.2
ovary (corpus luteum) (nontraumatic) 620.1
  traumatic — *see* Injury, internal, ovary
pelvis (female) (nontraumatic) 629.89
  complicating delivery 665.7 ☑
  male 608.83
  traumatic (*see also* Injury, internal, pelvis)
    specified organ NEC (*see also* Injury, internal, pelvis) 867.6
penis (nontraumatic) 607.82
pericranial (and neck, or face any part, except eye) 920
  due to injury at birth 767.19
perineal wound (obstetrical) 674.3 ☑
  complicating delivery 664.5 ☑
perirenal, cystic 593.81
pinna 380.31
placenta — *see* Placenta, abnormal
postoperative 998.12
retroperitoneal (nontraumatic) 568.81
  traumatic — *see* Injury, internal, retroperitoneum
retropubic, male 568.81
scalp (and neck, or face any part, except eye) 920
  fetus or newborn 767.19
scrotum (nontraumatic) 608.83
  traumatic 922.4
seminal vesicle (nontraumatic) 608.83
  traumatic — *see* Injury, internal, seminal, vesicle
soft tissue 729.92
spermatic cord (*see also* Injury, internal, spermatic cord)
  nontraumatic 608.83
spinal (cord) (meninges) (*see also* Injury, spinal, by site)
  fetus or newborn 767.4
  nontraumatic 336.1
spleen 865.01
  with
    laceration — *see* Laceration, spleen
    open wound into cavity 865.11
sternocleidomastoid, birth injury 767.8
sternomastoid, birth injury 767.8
subarachnoid (*see also* Hematoma, brain, subarachnoid)
  fetus or newborn 772.2
  nontraumatic (*see also* Hemorrhage, subarachnoid) 430
    newborn 772.2
subdural (*see also* Hematoma, brain, subdural)
  fetus or newborn (localized) 767.0
  nontraumatic (*see also* Hemorrhage, subdural) 432.1
subperiosteal (syndrome) 267
  traumatic — *see* Hematoma, by site
superficial, fetus or newborn 772.6
syncytium — *see* Placenta, abnormal
testis (nontraumatic) 608.83
  birth injury 767.8
  traumatic 922.4
tunica vaginalis (nontraumatic) 608.83
umbilical cord 663.6 ☑
  affecting fetus or newborn 762.6

Hematoma — *see also* Contusion — *continued*
uterine ligament (nontraumatic) 620.7
  traumatic — *see* Injury, internal, pelvis
uterus 621.4
  traumatic — *see* Injury, internal, pelvis
vagina (nontraumatic) (ruptured) 623.6
  complicating delivery 665.7 ☑
  traumatic 922.4
vas deferens (nontraumatic) 608.83
  traumatic — *see* Injury, internal, vas deferens
vitreous 379.23
vocal cord 920
vulva (nontraumatic) 624.5
  complicating delivery 664.5 ☑
  fetus or newborn 767.8
  traumatic 922.4
Hematometra 621.4
Hematomyelia 336.1
  with fracture of vertebra (*see also* Fracture, vertebra, by site, with spinal cord injury) 806.8
  fetus or newborn 767.4
Hematomyelitis 323.9
  late effect — *see* category 326
Hematoperitoneum — *see also* Hemoperitoneum 568.81
Hematopneumothorax — *see also* Hemothorax 511.89
Hematopoiesis, cyclic 288.02
Hematoporphyria (acquired) (congenital) 277.1
Hematoporphyrinuria (acquired) (congenital) 277.1
Hematorachis, hematorrhachis 336.1
  fetus or newborn 767.4
Hematosalpinx 620.8
  with
    ectopic pregnancy (*see also* categories 633.0–633.9) 639.2
    infectional (*see also* Salpingo-oophoritis) 614.2
    molar pregnancy (*see also* categories 630–632) 639.2
Hematospermia 608.82
Hematothorax — *see also* Hemothorax 511.89
Hematotympanum 381.03
Hematuria (benign) (essential) (idiopathic) 599.70
  due to S. hematobium 120.0
  endemic 120.0
  gross 599.71
  intermittent 599.70
  malarial 084.8
  microscopic 599.72
  paroxysmal 599.70
  sulfonamide
    correct substance properly administered 599.70
    overdose or wrong substance given or taken 961.0
  tropical (bilharziasis) 120.0
  tuberculous (*see also* Tuberculosis) 016.9 ☑
Hematuric bilious fever 084.8
Hemeralopia 368.10
Hemi-akinesia 781.8
Hemi-inattention 781.8
Hemiabiotrophy 799.89
Hemianalgesia — *see also* Disturbance, sensation 782.0
Hemianencephaly 740.0
Hemianesthesia — *see also* Disturbance, sensation 782.0
Hemianopia, hemianopsia (altitudinal) (homonymous) 368.46
  binasal 368.47
  bitemporal 368.47
  heteronymous 368.47
  syphilitic 095.8
Hemiasomatognosia 307.9
Hemiathetosis 781.0
Hemiatrophy 799.89
  cerebellar 334.8
  face 349.89
    progressive 349.89

Hemiatrophy — *continued*
  fascia 728.9
  leg 728.2
  tongue 529.8
Hemiballism (us) 333.5
Hemiblock (cardiac) (heart) (left) 426.2
Hemicardia 746.89
Hemicephalus, hemicephaly 740.0
Hemichorea 333.5
Hemicrania 346.9 ☑
  congenital malformation 740.0
  continua 339.41
  paroxysmal 339.03
    chronic 339.04
    episodic 339.03
Hemidystrophy — *see* Hemiatrophy
Hemiectromelia 755.4
Hemihypalgesia — *see also* Disturbance, sensation 782.0
Hemihypertrophy (congenital) 759.89
  cranial 756.0
Hemihypesthesia — *see also* Disturbance, sensation 782.0
Hemimelia 755.4
  lower limb 755.30
    paraxial (complete) (incomplete) (intercalary) (terminal) 755.32
      fibula 755.37
      tibia 755.36
    transverse (complete) (partial) 755.31
  upper limb 755.20
    paraxial (complete) (incomplete) (intercalary) (terminal) 755.22
      radial 755.26
      ulnar 755.27
    transverse (complete) (partial) 755.21
Hemiparalysis — *see also* Hemiplegia 342.9 ☑
Hemiparesis — *see also* Hemiplegia 342.9 ☑
Hemiparesthesia — *see also* Disturbance, sensation 782.0
Hemiplegia 342.9 ☑
  acute (*see also* Disease, cerebrovascular, acute) 436
  alternans facialis 344.89
  apoplectic (*see also* Disease, cerebrovascular, acute) 436
    late effect or residual
      affecting
        dominant side 438.21
        nondominant side 438.22
        unspecified side 438.20
  arteriosclerotic 437.0
    late effect or residual
      affecting
        dominant side 438.21
        nondominant side 438.22
        unspecified side 438.20
  ascending (spinal) NEC 344.89
  attack (*see also* Disease, cerebrovascular, acute) 436
  brain, cerebral (current episode) 437.8
    congenital 343.1
  cerebral — *see* Hemiplegia, brain
  congenital (cerebral) (spastic) (spinal) 343.1
  conversion neurosis (hysterical) 300.11
  cortical — *see* Hemiplegia, brain
  due to
    arteriosclerosis 437.0
      late effect or residual
        affecting
          dominant side 438.21
          nondominant side 438.22
          unspecified side 438.20
    cerebrovascular lesion (*see also* Disease, cerebrovascular, acute) 436
      late effect
        affecting
          dominant side 438.21
          nondominant side 438.22
          unspecified side 438.20
  embolic (current) (*see also* Embolism, brain) 434.1 ☑
    late effect
      affecting
        dominant side 438.21
        nondominant side 438.22

Hemiplegia — *continued*
  embolic (*see also* Embolism, brain) — *continued*
    late effect — *continued*
      affecting — *continued*
        unspecified side 438.20
  flaccid 342.0 ☑
  hypertensive (current episode) 437.8
  infantile (postnatal) 343.4
  late effect
    birth injury, intracranial or spinal 343.4
    cerebrovascular lesion — *see* Late effect(s) (of) cerebrovascular disease
    viral encephalitis 139.0
  middle alternating NEC 344.89
  newborn NEC 767.0
  seizure (current episode) (*see also* Disease, cerebrovascular, acute) 436
  spastic 342.1 ☑
    congenital or infantile 343.1
  specified NEC 342.8 ☑
  thrombotic (current) (*see also* Thrombosis, brain) 434.0 ☑
    late effect — *see* Late effect(s) (of) cerebrovascular disease
Hemisection, spinal cord — *see* Fracture, vertebra, by site, with spinal cord injury
Hemispasm 781.0
  facial 781.0
Hemispatial neglect 781.8
Hemisporosis 117.9
Hemitremor 781.0
Hemivertebra 756.14
Hemobilia 576.8
Hemocholecyst 575.8
Hemochromatosis (acquired) (liver) (myocardium) (secondary) 275.03
  with refractory anemia 238.72
  diabetic 275.03
  due to repeated red blood cell transfusions 275.02
  hereditary 275.01
  primary idiopathic 275.01
  specified NEC 275.03
  transfusion associated (red blood cell) 275.02
Hemodialysis V56.0
Hemoglobin — *see also* condition
  abnormal (disease) — *see* Disease, hemoglobin
  AS genotype 282.5
  fetal, hereditary persistence 282.7
  H Constant Spring 282.43
  H disease 282.43
  high-oxygen-affinity 289.0
  low NEC 285.9
  S (Hb-S), heterozygous 282.5
Hemoglobinemia 283.2
  due to blood transfusion NEC 999.89
    bone marrow 996.85
  paroxysmal 283.2
Hemoglobinopathy (mixed) — *see also* Disease, hemoglobin 282.7
  with thalassemia 282.49
  sickle-cell 282.60
    with thalassemia (without crisis) 282.41
      with
        crisis 282.42
        vaso-occlusive pain 282.42
Hemoglobinuria, hemoglobinuric 791.2
  with anemia, hemolytic, acquired (chronic) NEC 283.2
  cold (agglutinin) (paroxysmal) (with Raynaud's syndrome) 283.2
  due to
    exertion 283.2
    hemolysis (from external causes) NEC 283.2
  exercise 283.2
  fever (malaria) 084.8
  infantile 791.2
  intermittent 283.2
  malarial 084.8
  march 283.2
  nocturnal (paroxysmal) 283.2

☑ Additional Digit Required — Refer to the Tabular List for Digit Selection
▽ Subterms under main terms may continue to next column or page
134 — Volume 2
▶◀ Revised Text
● New Line
▲ Revised Code
2014 ICD-9-CM

Hemoglobinuria, hemoglobinuric — *continued*
paroxysmal (cold) (nocturnal) 283.2
Hemolymphangioma (M9175/0) 228.1
Hemolysis
fetal — *see* Jaundice, fetus or newborn
intravascular (disseminated) NEC 286.6
with
abortion — *see* Abortion, by type, with hemorrhage, delayed or excessive
ectopic pregnancy (*see also* categories 633.0–633.9) 639.1
hemorrhage of pregnancy 641.3 ☑
affecting fetus or newborn 762.1
molar pregnancy (*see also* categories 630–632) 639.1
acute 283.2
following
abortion 639.1
ectopic or molar pregnancy 639.1
neonatal — *see* Jaundice, fetus or newborn
transfusion NEC 999.89
bone marrow 996.85
Hemolytic — *see also* condition
anemia — *see* Anemia, hemolytic
uremic syndrome 283.11
Hemometra 621.4
Hemopericardium (with effusion) 423.0
newborn 772.8
traumatic (*see also* Hemothorax, traumatic) 860.2
with open wound into thorax 860.3
Hemoperitoneum 568.81
infectional (*see also* Peritonitis) 567.29
traumatic — *see* Injury, internal, peritoneum
Hemophagocytic syndrome 288.4
infection-associated 288.4
Hemophilia (familial) (hereditary) 286.0
A 286.0
carrier (asymptomatic) V83.01
symptomatic V83.02
acquired 286.52
autoimmune 286.52
B (Leyden) 286.1
C 286.2
calcipriva (*see also* Fibrinolysis) 286.7
classical 286.0
nonfamilial 286.7
secondary 286.52
vascular 286.4
Hemophilus influenzae NEC 041.5
arachnoiditis (basic) (brain) (spinal) 320.0
late effect — *see* category 326
bronchopneumonia 482.2
cerebral ventriculitis 320.0
late effect — *see* category 326
cerebrospinal inflammation 320.0
late effect — *see* category 326
infection NEC 041.5
leptomeningitis 320.0
late effect — *see* category 326
meningitis (cerebral) (cerebrospinal) (spinal) 320.0
late effect — *see* category 326
meningomyelitis 320.0
late effect — *see* category 326
pachymeningitis (adhesive) (fibrous) (hemorrhagic) (hypertrophic) (spinal) 320.0
late effect — *see* category 326
pneumonia (broncho-) 482.2
Hemophthalmos 360.43
Hemopneumothorax — *see also* Hemothorax 511.89
traumatic 860.4
with open wound into thorax 860.5
Hemoptysis 786.30
due to Paragonimus (westermani) 121.2
newborn 770.3
specified NEC 786.39
tuberculous (*see also* Tuberculosis, pulmonary) 011.9 ☑
Hemorrhage, hemorrhagic (nontraumatic) 459.0
abdomen 459.0

Hemorrhage, hemorrhagic — *continued*
accidental (antepartum) 641.2 ☑
affecting fetus or newborn 762.1
adenoid 474.8
adrenal (capsule) (gland) (medulla) 255.41
newborn 772.5
after labor — *see* Hemorrhage, postpartum
alveolar
lung, newborn 770.3
process 525.8
alveolus 525.8
amputation stump (surgical) 998.11
secondary, delayed 997.69
anemia (chronic) 280.0
acute 285.1
antepartum — *see* Hemorrhage, pregnancy
anus (sphincter) 569.3
apoplexy (stroke) 432.9
arachnoid — *see* Hemorrhage, subarachnoid
artery NEC 459.0
brain (*see also* Hemorrhage, brain) 431
middle meningeal — *see* Hemorrhage, subarachnoid
basilar (ganglion) (*see also* Hemorrhage, brain) 431
bladder 596.89
blood dyscrasia 289.9
bowel 578.9
newborn 772.4
brain (miliary) (nontraumatic) 431
with
birth injury 767.0
arachnoid — *see* Hemorrhage, subarachnoid
due to
birth injury 767.0
rupture of aneurysm (congenital) (*see also* Hemorrhage, subarachnoid) 430
mycotic 431
syphilis 094.89
epidural or extradural — *see* Hemorrhage, extradural
fetus or newborn (anoxic) (hypoxic) (due to birth trauma) (nontraumatic) 767.0
intraventricular 772.10
grade I 772.11
grade II 772.12
grade III 772.13
grade IV 772.14
iatrogenic 997.02
postoperative 997.02
puerperal, postpartum, childbirth 674.0 ☑
stem 431
subarachnoid, arachnoid, or meningeal — *see* Hemorrhage, subarachnoid
subdural — *see* Hemorrhage, subdural

Hemorrhage, hemorrhagic — *continued*
brain — *continued*
traumatic NEC 853.0 ☑

Note — *Use the following fifth-digit subclassification with categories 851–854:*

0   *unspecified state of consciousness*

1   *with no loss of consciousness*

2   *with brief [less than one hour] loss of consciousness*

3   *with moderate [1–24 hours] loss of consciousness*

4   *with prolonged [more than 24 hours] loss of consciousness and return to pre–existing conscious level*

5   *with prolonged [more than 24 hours] loss of consciousness, without return to pre–existing conscious level*

Use fifth-digit 5 to designate when a patient is unconscious and dies before regaining consciousness, regardless of the duration of the loss of consciousness

6   *with loss of consciousness of unspecified duration*

9   *with concussion, unspecified*

with
cerebral
contusion — *see* Contusion, brain
laceration — *see* Laceration, brain
open intracranial wound 853.1 ☑
skull fracture — *see* Fracture, skull, by site
extradural or epidural 852.4 ☑
with open intracranial wound 852.5 ☑
subarachnoid 852.0 ☑
with open intracranial wound 852.1 ☑
subdural 852.2 ☑
with open intracranial wound 852.3 ☑
breast 611.79
bronchial tube — *see* Hemorrhage, lung
bronchopulmonary — *see* Hemorrhage, lung
bronchus (cause unknown) (*see also* Hemorrhage, lung) 786.30
bulbar (*see also* Hemorrhage, brain) 431
bursa 727.89
capillary 448.9
primary 287.8
capsular — *see* Hemorrhage, brain
cardiovascular 429.89
cecum 578.9
cephalic (*see also* Hemorrhage, brain) 431
cerebellar (*see also* Hemorrhage, brain) 431
cerebellum (*see also* Hemorrhage, brain) 431
cerebral (*see also* Hemorrhage, brain) 431
fetus or newborn (anoxic) (traumatic) 767.0
cerebromeningeal (*see also* Hemorrhage, brain) 431
cerebrospinal (*see also* Hemorrhage, brain) 431
cerebrovascular accident — *see* Hemorrhage, brain
cerebrum (*see also* Hemorrhage, brain) 431
cervix (stump) (uteri) 622.8
cesarean section wound 674.3 ☑
chamber, anterior (eye) 364.41
childbirth — *see* Hemorrhage, complicating, delivery
choroid 363.61
expulsive 363.62
ciliary body 364.41
cochlea 386.8
colon — *see* Hemorrhage, intestine

Hemorrhage, hemorrhagic — *continued*
complicating
delivery 641.9 ☑
affecting fetus or newborn 762.1
associated with
afibrinogenemia 641.3 ☑
affecting fetus or newborn 763.89
coagulation defect 641.3 ☑
affecting fetus or newborn 763.89
hyperfibrinolysis 641.3 ☑
affecting fetus or newborn 763.89
hypofibrinogenemia 641.3 ☑
affecting fetus or newborn 763.89
due to
low-lying placenta 641.1 ☑
affecting fetus or newborn 762.0
placenta previa 641.1 ☑
affecting fetus or newborn 762.0
premature separation of placenta 641.2 ☑
affecting fetus or newborn 762.1
retained
placenta 666.0 ☑
secundines 666.2 ☑
trauma 641.8 ☑
affecting fetus or newborn 763.89
uterine leiomyoma 641.8 ☑
affecting fetus or newborn 763.89
surgical procedure 998.11
complication(s)
of dental implant placement 525.71
concealed NEC 459.0
congenital 772.9
conjunctiva 372.72
newborn 772.8
cord, newborn 772.0
slipped ligature 772.3
stump 772.3
corpus luteum (ruptured) 620.1
cortical (*see also* Hemorrhage, brain) 431
cranial 432.9
cutaneous 782.7
newborn 772.6
cystitis — *see* Cystitis
cyst, pancreas 577.2
delayed
with
abortion — *see* Abortion, by type, with hemorrhage, delayed or excessive
ectopic pregnancy (*see also* categories 633.0–633.9) 639.1
molar pregnancy (*see also* categories 630–632) 639.1
following
abortion 639.1
ectopic or molar pregnancy 639.1
postpartum 666.2 ☑
diathesis (familial) 287.9
newborn 776.0
disease 287.9
newborn 776.0
specified type NEC 287.8
disorder 287.9
due to intrinsic circulating anticoagulants, antibodies, or inhibitors 286.59
with
acquired hemophilia 286.52
antiphospholipid antibody 286.53
specified type NEC 287.8
due to
any device, implant or graft (presence of) classifiable to 996.0–996.5 — *see* Complications, due to (presence of) any device, implant, or graft classified to 996.0–996.5NEC

Hemorrhage, hemorrhagic — *continued*
   due to — *continued*
      intrinsic circulating anticoagulant, anti-
         bodies, or inhibitors 286.59
         with
            acquired hemophilia 286.52
            antiphospholipid antibody 286.53
      duodenum, duodenal 537.89
         ulcer — *see* Ulcer, duodenum, with
            hemorrhage
      dura mater — *see* Hemorrhage, subdural
   endotracheal — *see* Hemorrhage, lung
   epicranial subaponeurotic (massive) 767.11
   epidural — *see* Hemorrhage, extradural
   episiotomy 674.3 ✔
   esophagus 530.82
      varix (*see also* Varix, esophagus, bleed-
         ing) 456.0
   excessive
      with
         abortion — *see* Abortion, by type,
            with hemorrhage, delayed or
            excessive
         ectopic pregnancy (*see also* cate-
            gories 633.0–633.9) 639.1
         molar pregnancy (*see also* categories
            630–632) 639.1
      following
         abortion 639.1
         ectopic or molar pregnancy 639.1
   external 459.0
   extradural (traumatic) (*see also* Hemorrhage,
      brain, traumatic, extradural)
      birth injury 767.0
      fetus or newborn (anoxic) (traumatic)
         767.0
      nontraumatic 432.0
   eye 360.43
      chamber (anterior) (aqueous) 364.41
      fundus 362.81
   eyelid 374.81
   fallopian tube 620.8
   fetomaternal 772.0
      affecting management of pregnancy or
         puerperium 656.0 ✔
   fetus, fetal, affecting newborn 772.0
      from
         cut end of co-twin's cord 772.0
         placenta 772.0
         ruptured cord 772.0
         vasa previa 772.0
      into
         co-twin 772.0
         mother's circulation 772.0
            affecting management of preg-
               nancy or puerperium
               656.0 ✔
   fever (*see also* Fever, hemorrhagic) 065.9
      with renal syndrome 078.6
      arthropod-borne NEC 065.9
      Bangkok 065.4
      Crimean 065.0
      dengue virus 065.4
      epidemic 078.6
      Junin virus 078.7
      Korean 078.6
      Machupo virus 078.7
      mite-borne 065.8
      mosquito-borne 065.4
      Philippine 065.4
      Russian (Yaroslav) 078.6
      Singapore 065.4
      southeast Asia 065.4
      Thailand 065.4
      tick-borne NEC 065.3
   fibrinogenolysis (*see also* Fibrinolysis) 286.6
   fibrinolytic (acquired) (*see also* Fibrinolysis)
      286.6
   fontanel 767.19
   from tracheostomy stoma 519.09
   fundus, eye 362.81
   funis
      affecting fetus or newborn 772.0
      complicating delivery 663.8 ✔
   gastric (*see also* Hemorrhage, stomach)
      578.9

Hemorrhage, hemorrhagic — *continued*
   gastroenteric 578.9
      newborn 772.4
   gastrointestinal (tract) 578.9
      newborn 772.4
   genitourinary (tract) NEC 599.89
   gingiva 523.8
   globe 360.43
   gravidarum — *see* Hemorrhage, pregnancy
   gum 523.8
   heart 429.89
   hypopharyngeal (throat) 784.8
   intermenstrual 626.6
      irregular 626.6
      regular 626.5
   internal (organs) 459.0
      capsule (*see also* Hemorrhage, brain) 431
      ear 386.8
      newborn 772.8
   intestine 578.9
      congenital 772.4
      newborn 772.4
   into
      bladder wall 596.7
      bursa 727.89
      corpus luysii (*see also* Hemorrhage,
         brain) 431
   intra-abdominal 459.0
      during or following surgery 998.11
   intra-alveolar, newborn (lung) 770.3
   intracerebral (*see also* Hemorrhage, brain)
      431
   intracranial NEC 432.9
      puerperal, postpartum, childbirth
         674.0 ✔
      traumatic — *see* Hemorrhage, brain,
         traumatic
   intramedullary NEC 336.1
   intraocular 360.43
   intraoperative 998.11
   intrapartum — *see* Hemorrhage, complicat-
      ing, delivery
   intrapelvic
      female 629.89
      male 459.0
   intraperitoneal 459.0
   intrapontine (*see also* Hemorrhage, brain)
      431
   intrauterine 621.4
      complicating delivery — *see* Hemor-
         rhage, complicating, delivery
      in pregnancy or childbirth — *see* Hemor-
         rhage, pregnancy
      postpartum (*see also* Hemorrhage,
         postpartum) 666.1 ✔
   intraventricular (*see also* Hemorrhage, brain)
      431
      fetus or newborn (anoxic) (traumatic)
         772.10
         grade I 772.11
         grade II 772.12
         grade III 772.13
         grade IV 772.14
   intravesical 596.7
   iris (postinfectional) (postinflammatory)
      (toxic) 364.41
   joint (nontraumatic) 719.10
      ankle 719.17
      elbow 719.12
      foot 719.17
      forearm 719.13
      hand 719.14
      hip 719.15
      knee 719.16
      lower leg 719.16
      multiple sites 719.19
      pelvic region 719.15
      shoulder (region) 719.11
      specified site NEC 719.18
      thigh 719.15
      upper arm 719.12
      wrist 719.13
   kidney 593.81
   knee (joint) 719.16
   labyrinth 386.8
   leg NEC 459.0

Hemorrhage, hemorrhagic — *continued*
   lenticular striate artery (*see also* Hemor-
      rhage, brain) 431
   ligature, vessel 998.11
   liver 573.8
   lower extremity NEC 459.0
   lung 786.30
      newborn 770.3
      tuberculous (*see also* Tuberculosis, pul-
         monary) 011.9 ✔
   malaria 084.8
   marginal sinus 641.2 ✔
   massive subaponeurotic, birth injury 767.11
   maternal, affecting fetus or newborn 762.1
   mediastinum 786.30
   medulla (*see also* Hemorrhage, brain) 431
   membrane (brain) (*see also* Hemorrhage,
      subarachnoid) 430
      spinal cord — *see* Hemorrhage, spinal
         cord
   meninges, meningeal (brain) (middle) (*see
      also* Hemorrhage, subarachnoid) 430
      spinal cord — *see* Hemorrhage, spinal
         cord
   mesentery 568.81
   metritis 626.8
   midbrain (*see also* Hemorrhage, brain) 431
   mole 631.8
   mouth 528.9
   mucous membrane NEC 459.0
      newborn 772.8
   muscle 728.89
   nail (subungual) 703.8
   nasal turbinate 784.7
      newborn 772.8
   nasopharynx 478.29
   navel, newborn 772.3
   newborn 772.9
      adrenal 772.5
      alveolar (lung) 770.3
      brain (anoxic) (hypoxic) (due to birth
         trauma) 767.0
      cerebral (anoxic) (hypoxic) (due to birth
         trauma) 767.0
      conjunctiva 772.8
      cutaneous 772.6
      diathesis 776.0
      due to vitamin K deficiency 776.0
      epicranial subaponeurotic (massive)
         767.11
      gastrointestinal 772.4
      internal (organs) 772.8
      intestines 772.4
      intra-alveolar (lung) 770.3
      intracranial (from any perinatal cause)
         767.0
      intraventricular (from any perinatal
         cause) 772.10
         grade I 772.11
         grade II 772.12
         grade III 772.13
         grade IV 772.14
      lung 770.3
      pulmonary (massive) 770.3
      spinal cord, traumatic 767.4
      stomach 772.4
      subaponeurotic (massive) 767.11
      subarachnoid (from any perinatal cause)
         772.2
      subconjunctival 772.8
      subgaleal 767.11
      umbilicus 772.0
         slipped ligature 772.3
         vasa previa 772.0
   nipple 611.79
   nose 784.7
      newborn 772.8
   obstetrical surgical wound 674.3 ✔
   omentum 568.89
      newborn 772.4
   optic nerve (sheath) 377.42
   orbit 376.32
   ovary 620.8
   oviduct 620.8
   pancreas 577.8
   parathyroid (gland) (spontaneous) 252.8

Hemorrhage, hemorrhagic — *continued*
   parturition — *see* Hemorrhage, complicat-
      ing, delivery
   penis 607.82
   pericardium, pericarditis 423.0
   perineal wound (obstetrical) 674.3 ✔
   peritoneum, peritoneal 459.0
   peritonsillar tissue 474.8
      after operation on tonsils 998.11
      due to infection 475
   petechial 782.7
   pituitary (gland) 253.8
   placenta NEC 641.9 ✔
      affecting fetus or newborn 762.1
      from surgical or instrumental damage
         641.8 ✔
         affecting fetus or newborn 762.1
      previa 641.1 ✔
         affecting fetus or newborn 762.0
   pleura — *see* Hemorrhage, lung
   polioencephalitis, superior 265.1
   polymyositis — *see* Polymyositis
   pons (*see also* Hemorrhage, brain) 431
   pontine (*see also* Hemorrhage, brain) 431
   popliteal 459.0
   postcoital 626.7
   postextraction (dental) 998.11
   postmenopausal 627.1
   postnasal 784.7
   postoperative 998.11
   postpartum (atonic) (following delivery of
      placenta) 666.1 ✔
      delayed or secondary (after 24 hours)
         666.2 ✔
      retained placenta 666.0 ✔
      third stage 666.0 ✔
   pregnancy (concealed) 641.9 ✔
      accidental 641.2 ✔
         affecting fetus or newborn 762.1
      affecting fetus or newborn 762.1
      before 22 completed weeks gestation
         640.9 ✔
         affecting fetus or newborn 762.1
      due to
         abruptio placenta 641.2 ✔
            affecting fetus or newborn 762.1
         afibrinogenemia or other coagula-
            tion defect (conditions classifi-
            able to 286.0–286.9) 641.3 ✔
            affecting fetus or newborn 762.1
         coagulation defect 641.3 ✔
            affecting fetus or newborn 762.1
         hyperfibrinolysis 641.3 ✔
            affecting fetus or newborn 762.1
         hypofibrinogenemia 641.3 ✔
            affecting fetus or newborn 762.1
         leiomyoma, uterus 641.8 ✔
            affecting fetus or newborn 762.1
         low-lying placenta 641.1 ✔
            affecting fetus or newborn 762.1
         marginal sinus (rupture) 641.2 ✔
            affecting fetus or newborn 762.1
         placenta previa 641.1 ✔
            affecting fetus or newborn 762.0
         premature separation of placenta
            (normally implanted) 641.2 ✔
            affecting fetus or newborn 762.1
         threatened abortion 640.0 ✔
            affecting fetus or newborn 762.1
         trauma 641.8 ✔
            affecting fetus or newborn 762.1
      early (before 22 completed weeks gesta-
         tion) 640.9 ✔
         affecting fetus or newborn 762.1
      previous, affecting management of
         pregnancy or childbirth V23.49
      unavoidable — *see* Hemorrhage, preg-
         nancy, due to placenta previa
   prepartum (mother) — *see* Hemorrhage,
      pregnancy
   preretinal, cause unspecified 362.81
   prostate 602.1
   puerperal (*see also* Hemorrhage, postpar-
      tum) 666.1 ✔

✔ **Additional Digit Required** — Refer to the Tabular List for Digit Selection   ⓦ **Subterms under main terms may continue to next column or page**

136 — Volume 2   ▶◀ **Revised Text**   ● **New Line**   ▲ **Revised Code**   2014 ICD-9-CM

Hemorrhage, hemorrhagic — *continued*
pulmonary (*see also* Hemorrhage, lung) 786.30
  acute idiopathic in infants (AIPHI) (over 28 days old) 786.31
  newborn (massive) 770.3
  renal syndrome 446.21
purpura (primary) (*see also* Purpura, thrombocytopenic) 287.39
rectum (sphincter) 569.3
recurring, following initial hemorrhage at time of injury 958.2
renal 593.81
  pulmonary syndrome 446.21
respiratory tract (*see also* Hemorrhage, lung) 786.30
retina, retinal (deep) (superficial) (vessels) 362.81
  diabetic 250.5 ☑ [362.01]
    due to secondary diabetes 249.5 ☑ [362.01]
  due to birth injury 772.8
retrobulbar 376.89
retroperitoneal 459.0
retroplacental (*see also* Placenta, separation) 641.2 ☑
scalp 459.0
  due to injury at birth 767.19
scrotum 608.83
secondary (nontraumatic) 459.0
  following initial hemorrhage at time of injury 958.2
seminal vesicle 608.83
skin 782.7
  newborn 772.6
spermatic cord 608.83
spinal (cord) 336.1
  aneurysm (ruptured) 336.1
    syphilitic 094.89
  due to birth injury 767.4
  fetus or newborn 767.4
spleen 289.59
spontaneous NEC 459.0
  petechial 782.7
stomach 578.9
  newborn 772.4
  ulcer — *see* Ulcer, stomach, with hemorrhage
subaponeurotic, newborn 767.11
  massive (birth injury) 767.11
subarachnoid (nontraumatic) 430
  fetus or newborn (anoxic) (traumatic) 772.2
  puerperal, postpartum, childbirth 674.0 ☑
  traumatic — *see* Hemorrhage, brain, traumatic, subarachnoid
subconjunctival 372.72
  due to birth injury 772.8
  newborn 772.8
subcortical (*see also* Hemorrhage, brain) 431
subcutaneous 782.7
subdiaphragmatic 459.0
subdural (nontraumatic) 432.1
  due to birth injury 767.0
  fetus or newborn (anoxic) (hypoxic) (due to birth trauma) 767.0
  puerperal, postpartum, childbirth 674.0 ☑
  spinal 336.1
  traumatic — *see* Hemorrhage, brain, traumatic, subdural
subgaleal 767.11
subhyaloid 362.81
subperiosteal 733.99
subretinal 362.81
subtentorial (*see also* Hemorrhage, subdural) 432.1
subungual 703.8
  due to blood dyscrasia 287.8
suprarenal (capsule) (gland) 255.41
  fetus or newborn 772.5
tentorium (traumatic) (*see also* Hemorrhage, brain, traumatic)
  fetus or newborn 767.0

Hemorrhage, hemorrhagic — *continued*
tentorium (*see also* Hemorrhage, brain, traumatic) — *continued*
  nontraumatic — *see* Hemorrhage, subdural
testis 608.83
thigh 459.0
third stage 666.0 ☑
thorax — *see* Hemorrhage, lung
throat 784.8
thrombocythemia 238.71
thymus (gland) 254.8
thyroid (gland) 246.3
  cyst 246.3
tongue 529.8
tonsil 474.8
  postoperative 998.11
tooth socket (postextraction) 998.11
trachea — *see* Hemorrhage, lung
traumatic (*see also* nature of injury)
  brain — *see* Hemorrhage, brain, traumatic
  recurring or secondary (following initial hemorrhage at time of injury) 958.2
tuberculous NEC (*see also* Tuberculosis, pulmonary) 011.9 ☑
tunica vaginalis 608.83
ulcer — *see* Ulcer, by site, with hemorrhage
umbilicus, umbilical cord 772.0
  after birth, newborn 772.3
  complicating delivery 663.8 ☑
    affecting fetus or newborn 772.0
  slipped ligature 772.3
  stump 772.3
unavoidable (due to placenta previa) 641.1 ☑
  affecting fetus or newborn 762.0
upper extremity 459.0
urethra (idiopathic) 599.84
uterus, uterine (abnormal) 626.9
  climacteric 627.0
  complicating delivery — *see* Hemorrhage, complicating, delivery
  due to
    intrauterine contraceptive device 996.76
      perforating uterus 996.32
  functional or dysfunctional 626.8
  in pregnancy — *see* Hemorrhage, pregnancy
  intermenstrual 626.6
    irregular 626.6
    regular 626.5
  postmenopausal 627.1
  postpartum (*see also* Hemorrhage, postpartum) 666.1 ☑
  prepubertal 626.8
  pubertal 626.3
  puerperal (immediate) 666.1 ☑
vagina 623.8
vasa previa 663.5 ☑
  affecting fetus or newborn 772.0
vas deferens 608.83
ventricular (*see also* Hemorrhage, brain) 431
vesical 596.89
viscera 459.0
  newborn 772.8
vitreous (humor) (intraocular) 379.23
vocal cord 478.5
vulva 624.8
Hemorrhoids (anus) (rectum) (without complication) 455.6
  bleeding, prolapsed, strangulated, or ulcerated NEC 455.8
    external 455.5
    internal 455.2
  complicated NEC 455.8
  complicating pregnancy and puerperium 671.8 ☑
  external 455.3
    with complication NEC 455.5
    bleeding, prolapsed, strangulated, or ulcerated 455.5
    thrombosed 455.4
  internal 455.0

Hemorrhoids — *continued*
internal — *continued*
  with complication NEC 455.2
    bleeding, prolapsed, strangulated, or ulcerated 455.2
    thrombosed 455.1
  residual skin tag 455.9
  sentinel pile 455.9
  thrombosed NEC 455.7
    external 455.4
    internal 455.1
Hemosalpinx 620.8
Hemosiderosis 275.09
  dietary 275.09
  pulmonary (idiopathic) 275.09 [516.1]
  transfusion NEC 275.02
    bone marrow 996.85
Hemospermia 608.82
Hemothorax 511.89
  bacterial, nontuberculous 511.1
  newborn 772.8
  nontuberculous 511.89
    bacterial 511.1
  pneumococcal 511.1
  postoperative 998.11
  staphylococcal 511.1
  streptococcal 511.1
  traumatic 860.2
    with
      open wound into thorax 860.3
      pneumothorax 860.4
        with open wound into thorax 860.5
  tuberculous (*see also* Tuberculosis, pleura) 012.0 ☑
Hemotympanum 385.89
Hench-Rosenberg syndrome (palindromic arthritis) — *see also* Rheumatism, palindromic 719.3 ☑
Henle's warts 371.41
Henoch (-Schönlein)
  disease or syndrome (allergic purpura) 287.0
  purpura (allergic) 287.0
Henpue, henpuye 102.6
Heparin-induced thrombocytopenia (HIT) 289.84
Heparitinuria 277.5
Hepar lobatum 095.3
Hepatalgia 573.8
Hepatic — *see also* condition
  flexure syndrome 569.89
Hepatitis 573.3
  acute (*see also* Necrosis, liver) 570
    alcoholic 571.1
    infective 070.1
      with hepatic coma 070.0
  alcoholic 571.1
  ambic — *see* Abscess, liver, amebic
  anicteric (acute) — *see* Hepatitis, viral
  antigen-associated (HAA) — *see* Hepatitis, viral, type B
  Australian antigen (positive) — *see* Hepatitis, viral, type B
  autoimmune 571.42
  catarrhal (acute) 070.1
    with hepatic coma 070.0
    chronic 571.40
    newborn 070.1
      with hepatic coma 070.0
  chemical 573.3
  cholangiolitic 573.8
  cholestatic 573.8
  chronic 571.40
    active 571.49
    viral — *see* Hepatitis, viral
    aggressive 571.49
    persistent 571.41
    viral — *see* Hepatitis, viral
  cytomegalic inclusion virus 078.5 [573.1]
  diffuse 573.3
  "dirty needle" — *see* Hepatitis, viral
  drug-induced 573.3
  due to
    Coxsackie 074.8 [573.1]
    cytomegalic inclusion virus 078.5 [573.1]
    infectious mononucleosis 075 [573.1]

Hepatitis — *continued*
due to — *continued*
  malaria 084.9 [573.2]
  mumps 072.71
  secondary syphilis 091.62
  toxoplasmosis (acquired) 130.5
    congenital (active) 771.2
epidemic — *see* Hepatitis, viral, type A
fetus or newborn 774.4
fibrous (chronic) 571.49
  acute 570
from injection, inoculation, or transfusion (blood) (other substance) (plasma) (serum) (onset within 8 months after administration) — *see* Hepatitis, viral
fulminant (viral) (*see also* Hepatitis, viral) 070.9
  with hepatic coma 070.6
  type A 070.1
    with hepatic coma 070.0
  type B — *see* Hepatitis, viral, type B
giant cell (neonatal) 774.4
hemorrhagic 573.8
history of
  B V12.09
  C V12.09
homologous serum — *see* Hepatitis, viral
hypertrophic (chronic) 571.49
  acute 570
infectious, infective (acute) (chronic) (subacute) 070.1
  with hepatic coma 070.0
inoculation — *see* Hepatitis, viral
interstitial (chronic) 571.49
  acute 570
lupoid 571.49
malarial 084.9 [573.2]
malignant (*see also* Necrosis, liver) 570
neonatal (toxic) 774.4
newborn 774.4
parenchymatous (acute) (*see also* Necrosis, liver) 570
peliosis 573.3
persistent, chronic 571.41
plasma cell 571.49
postimmunization — *see* Hepatitis, viral
postnecrotic 571.49
posttransfusion — *see* Hepatitis, viral
recurrent 571.49
septic 573.3
serum — *see* Hepatitis, viral
  carrier (suspected of) V02.61
subacute (*see also* Necrosis, liver) 570
suppurative (diffuse) 572.0
syphilitic (late) 095.3
  congenital (early) 090.0 [573.2]
    late 090.5 [573.2]
  secondary 091.62
toxic (noninfectious) 573.3
  fetus or newborn 774.4
tuberculous (*see also* Tuberculosis) 017.9 ☑
viral (acute) (anicteric) (cholangiolitic) (cholestatic) (chronic) (subacute) 070.9
  with hepatic coma 070.6
  AU-SH type virus — *see* Hepatitis, viral, type B
  Australian antigen — *see* Hepatitis, viral, type B
  B-antigen — *see* Hepatitis, viral, type B
  Coxsackie 074.8 [573.1]
  cytomegalic inclusion 078.5 [573.1]
  IH (virus) — *see* Hepatitis, viral, type A
  infectious hepatitis virus — *see* Hepatitis, viral, type A
  serum hepatitis virus — *see* Hepatitis, viral, type B
  SH — *see* Hepatitis, viral, type B
  specified type NEC 070.59
    with hepatic coma 070.49
  type A 070.1
    with hepatic coma 070.0
  type B (acute) 070.30
    with
      hepatic coma 070.20
        with hepatitis delta 070.21

☑ **Additional Digit Required — Refer to the Tabular List for Digit Selection**   ▽ **Subterms under main terms may continue to next column or page**

2014 ICD-9-CM   ▶◀ Revised Text   ● New Line   ▲ Revised Code   **Volume 2 — 137**

Hemorrhage, hemorrhagic — Hepatitis

Hepatitis — *continued*
  viral — *continued*
    type B — *continued*
      with — *continued*
        hepatitis delta 070.31
          with hepatic coma 070.21
        carrier status V02.61
        chronic 070.32
          with
            hepatic coma 070.22
              with hepatitis delta 070.23
            hepatitis delta 070.33
              with hepatic coma 070.23
    type C
      acute 070.51
        with hepatic coma 070.41
      carrier status V02.62
      chronic 070.54
        with hepatic coma 070.44
      in remission 070.54
      unspecified 070.70
        with hepatic coma 070.71
    type delta (with hepatitis B carrier state) 070.52
      with
        active hepatitis B disease — *see* Hepatitis, viral, type B
      hepatic coma 070.42
    type E 070.53
      with hepatic coma 070.43
    vaccination and inoculation (prophylactic) V05.3
  Waldenström's (lupoid hepatitis) 571.49
Hepatization, lung (acute) — *see also* Pneumonia, lobar
  chronic (*see also* Fibrosis, lung) 515
Hepatoblastoma (M8970/3) 155.0
Hepatocarcinoma (M8170/3) 155.0
Hepatocholangiocarcinoma (M8180/3) 155.0
Hepatocholangioma, benign (M8180/0) 211.5
Hepatocholangitis 573.8
Hepatocystitis — *see also* Cholecystitis 575.10
Hepatodystrophy 570
Hepatolenticular degeneration 275.1
Hepatolithiasis — *see* Choledocholithiasis
Hepatoma (malignant) (M8170/3) 155.0
  benign (M8170/0) 211.5
  congenital (M8970/3) 155.0
  embryonal (M8970/3) 155.0
Hepatomegalia glycogenica diffusa 271.0
Hepatomegaly — *see also* Hypertrophy, liver 789.1
  congenital 751.69
    syphilitic 090.0
  due to Clonorchis sinensis 121.1
  Gaucher's 272.7
  syphilitic (congenital) 090.0
Hepatoptosis 573.8
Hepatorrhexis 573.8
Hepatosis, toxic 573.8
Hepatosplenomegaly 571.8
  due to S. japonicum 120.2
  hyperlipemic (Bürger-Grutz type) 272.3
Herald patch 696.3
Hereditary — *see* condition
Heredodegeneration 330.9
  macular 362.70
Heredopathia atactica polyneuritiformis 356.3
Heredosyphilis — *see also* Syphilis, congenital 090.9
Hermaphroditism (true) 752.7
  with specified chromosomal anomaly — *see* Anomaly, chromosomes, sex
Hernia, hernial (acquired) (recurrent) 553.9
  with
    gangrene (obstructed) NEC 551.9
    obstruction NEC 552.9
      and gangrene 551.9
  abdomen (wall) — *see* Hernia, ventral
  abdominal, specified site NEC 553.8
    with
      gangrene (obstructed) 551.8
      obstruction 552.8
        and gangrene 551.8
  appendix 553.8

Hernia, hernial — *continued*
  appendix — *continued*
    with
      gangrene (obstructed) 551.8
      obstruction 552.8
        and gangrene 551.8
  bilateral (inguinal) — *see* Hernia, inguinal
  bladder (sphincter)
    congenital (female) (male) 756.71
    female (*see also* Cystocele, female) 618.01
    male 596.89
  brain 348.4
    congenital 742.0
  broad ligament 553.8
  cartilage, vertebral — *see* Displacement, intervertebral disc
  cerebral 348.4
    congenital 742.0
    endaural 742.0
  ciliary body 364.89
    traumatic 871.1
  colic 553.9
    with
      gangrene (obstructed) 551.9
      obstruction 552.9
        and gangrene 551.9
  colon 553.9
    with
      gangrene (obstructed) 551.9
      obstruction 552.9
        and gangrene 551.9
  colostomy (stoma) 569.69
  Cooper's (retroperitoneal) 553.8
    with
      gangrene (obstructed) 551.8
      obstruction 552.8
        and gangrene 551.8
  crural — *see* Hernia, femoral
  cystostomy 596.83
  diaphragm, diaphragmatic 553.3
    with
      gangrene (obstructed) 551.3
      obstruction 552.3
        and gangrene 551.3
    congenital 756.6
    due to gross defect of diaphragm 756.6
    traumatic 862.0
      with open wound into cavity 862.1
  direct (inguinal) — *see* Hernia, inguinal
  disc, intervertebral — *see* Displacement, intervertebral disc
  diverticulum, intestine 553.9
    with
      gangrene (obstructed) 551.9
      obstruction 552.9
        and gangrene 551.9
  double (inguinal) — *see* Hernia, inguinal
  due to adhesion with obstruction 552.9
  duodenojejunal 553.8
    with
      gangrene (obstructed) 551.8
      obstruction 552.8
        and gangrene 551.8
  en glissade — *see* Hernia, inguinal
  enterostomy (stoma) 569.69
  epigastric 553.29
    with
      gangrene (obstruction) 551.29
      obstruction 552.29
        and gangrene 551.29
    recurrent 553.21
      with
        gangrene (obstructed) 551.21
        obstruction 552.21
          and gangrene 551.21
  esophageal hiatus (sliding) 553.3
    with
      gangrene (obstructed) 551.3
      obstruction 552.3
        and gangrene 551.3
    congenital 750.6
  external (inguinal) — *see* Hernia, inguinal
  fallopian tube 620.4
  fascia 728.89
  fat 729.30

Hernia, hernial — *continued*
  fat — *continued*
    eyelid 374.34
    orbital 374.34
    pad 729.30
      eye, eyelid 374.34
      knee 729.31
      orbit 374.34
      popliteal (space) 729.31
      specified site NEC 729.39
  femoral (unilateral) 553.00
    with
      gangrene (obstructed) 551.00
      obstruction 552.00
        with gangrene 551.00
    bilateral 553.02
      gangrenous (obstructed) 551.02
      obstructed 552.02
        with gangrene 551.02
      recurrent 553.03
        gangrenous (obstructed) 551.03
        obstructed 552.03
          with gangrene 551.03
    recurrent (unilateral) 553.01
      bilateral 553.03
        gangrenous (obstructed) 551.03
        obstructed 552.03
          with gangrene 551.01
      gangrenous (obstructed) 551.01
      obstructed 552.01
        with gangrene 551.01
  foramen
    Bochdalek 553.3
      with
        gangrene (obstructed) 551.3
        obstruction 552.3
          and gangrene 551.3
      congenital 756.6
    magnum 348.4
    Morgagni, Morgagnian 553.3
      with
        gangrene 551.3
        obstruction 552.3
          and gangrene 551.3
      congenital 756.6
  funicular (umbilical) 553.1
    with
      gangrene (obstructed) 551.1
      obstruction 552.1
        and gangrene 551.1
    spermatic cord — *see* Hernia, inguinal
  gangrenous — *see* Hernia, by site, with gangrene
  gastrointestinal tract 553.9
    with
      gangrene (obstructed) 551.9
      obstruction 552.9
        and gangrene 551.9
  gluteal — *see* Hernia, femoral
  Gruber's (internal mesogastric) 553.8
    with
      gangrene (obstructed) 551.8
      obstruction 552.8
        and gangrene 551.8
  Hesselbach's 553.8
    with
      gangrene (obstructed) 551.8
      obstruction 552.8
        and gangrene 551.8
  hiatal (esophageal) (sliding) 553.3
    with
      gangrene (obstructed) 551.3
      obstruction 552.3
        and gangrene 551.3
    congenital 750.6
  incarcerated (*see also* Hernia, by site, with obstruction) 552.9
    gangrenous (*see also* Hernia, by site, with gangrene) 551.9
  incisional 553.21
    with
      gangrene (obstructed) 551.21
      obstruction 552.21
        and gangrene 551.21
    lumbar — *see* Hernia, lumbar
    recurrent 553.21

Hernia, hernial — *continued*
  incisional — *continued*
    recurrent — *continued*
      with
        gangrene (obstructed) 551.21
        obstruction 552.21
          and gangrene 551.21
  indirect (inguinal) — *see* Hernia, inguinal
  infantile — *see* Hernia, inguinal
  infrapatellar fat pad 729.31
  inguinal (direct) (double) (encysted) (external) (funicular) (indirect) (infantile) (internal) (interstitial) (oblique) (scrotal) (sliding) 550.9 ☑

Note — Use the following fifth-digit subclassification with category 550:

0	unilateral or unspecified (not specified as recurrent)
1	unilateral or unspecified, recurrent
2	bilateral (not specified as recurrent)
3	bilateral, recurrent

    with
      gangrene (obstructed) 550.0 ☑
      obstruction 550.1 ☑
        and gangrene 550.0 ☑
  internal 553.8
    with
      gangrene (obstructed) 551.8
      obstruction 552.8
        and gangrene 551.8
    inguinal — *see* Hernia, inguinal
  interstitial 553.9
    with
      gangrene (obstructed) 551.9
      obstruction 552.9
        and gangrene 551.9
    inguinal — *see* Hernia, inguinal
  intervertebral cartilage or disc — *see* Displacement, intervertebral disc
  intestine, intestinal 553.9
    with
      gangrene (obstructed) 551.9
      obstruction 552.9
        and gangrene 551.9
  intra-abdominal 553.9
    with
      gangrene (obstructed) 551.9
      obstruction 552.9
        and gangrene 551.9
  intraparietal 553.9
    with
      gangrene (obstructed) 551.9
      obstruction 552.9
        and gangrene 551.9
  iris 364.89
    traumatic 871.1
  irreducible (*see also* Hernia, by site, with obstruction) 552.9
    gangrenous (with obstruction) (*see also* Hernia, by site, with gangrene) 551.9
  ischiatic 553.8
    with
      gangrene (obstructed) 551.8
      obstruction 552.8
        and gangrene 551.8
  ischiorectal 553.8
    with
      gangrene (obstructed) 551.8
      obstruction 552.8
        and gangrene 551.8
  lens 379.32
    traumatic 871.1
  linea
    alba — *see* Hernia, epigastric
    semilunaris — *see* Hernia, spigelian
  Littre's (diverticular) 553.9
    with
      gangrene (obstructed) 551.9
      obstruction 552.9
        and gangrene 551.9
  lumbar 553.8

Hernia, hernial — *continued*
  lumbar — *continued*
    with
      gangrene (obstructed) 551.8
        obstruction 552.8
          and gangrene 551.8
      intervertebral disc 722.10
    lung (subcutaneous) 518.89
      congenital 748.69
    mediastinum 519.3
    mesenteric (internal) 553.8
      with
        gangrene (obstructed) 551.8
          obstruction 552.8
            and gangrene 551.8
    mesocolon 553.8
      with
        gangrene (obstructed) 551.8
          obstruction 552.8
            and gangrene 551.8
    muscle (sheath) 728.89
    nucleus pulposus — *see* Displacement, in-
        tervertebral disc
    oblique (inguinal) — *see* Hernia, inguinal
    obstructive (*see also* Hernia, by site, with
        obstruction) 552.9
      gangrenous (with obstruction) (*see also*
          Hernia, by site, with gangrene)
          551.9
    obturator 553.8
      with
        gangrene (obstructed) 551.8
          obstruction 552.8
            and gangrene 551.8
    omental 553.8
      with
        gangrene (obstructed) 551.8
          obstruction 552.8
            and gangrene 551.8
    orbital fat (pad) 374.34
    ovary 620.4
    oviduct 620.4
    paracolostomy (stoma) 569.69
    paraduodenal 553.8
      with
        gangrene (obstructed) 551.8
          obstruction 552.8
            and gangrene 551.8
    paraesophageal 553.3
      with
        gangrene (obstructed) 551.3
          obstruction 552.3
            and gangrene 551.3
      congenital 750.6
    parahiatal 553.3
      with
        gangrene (obstructed) 551.3
          obstruction 552.3
            and gangrene 551.3
    paraumbilical 553.1
      with
        gangrene (obstructed) 551.1
          obstruction 552.1
            and gangrene 551.1
    parietal 553.9
      with
        gangrene (obstructed) 551.9
          obstruction 552.9
            and gangrene 551.9
    perineal 553.8
      with
        gangrene (obstructed) 551.8
          obstruction 552.8
            and gangrene 551.8
    peritoneal sac, lesser 553.8
      with
        gangrene (obstructed) 551.8
          obstruction 552.8
            and gangrene 551.8
    popliteal fat pad 729.31
    postoperative 553.21
      with
        gangrene (obstructed) 551.21
          obstruction 552.21
            and gangrene 551.21
    pregnant uterus 654.4 ☑

Hernia, hernial — *continued*
    prevesical 596.89
    properitoneal 553.8
      with
        gangrene (obstructed) 551.8
          obstruction 552.8
            and gangrene 551.8
    pudendal 553.8
      with
        gangrene (obstructed) 551.8
          obstruction 552.8
            and gangrene 551.8
    rectovaginal 618.6
    retroperitoneal 553.8
      with
        gangrene (obstructed) 551.8
          obstruction 552.8
            and gangrene 551.8
    Richter's (parietal) 553.9
      with
        gangrene (obstructed) 551.9
          obstruction 552.9
            and gangrene 551.9
    Rieux's, Riex's (retrocecal) 553.8
      with
        gangrene (obstructed) 551.8
          obstruction 552.8
            and gangrene 551.8
    sciatic 553.8
      with
        gangrene (obstructed) 551.8
          obstruction 552.8
            and gangrene 551.8
    scrotum, scrotal — *see* Hernia, inguinal
    sliding (inguinal) (*see also* Hernia, inguinal)
      hiatus — *see* Hernia, hiatal
    spigelian 553.29
      with
        gangrene (obstructed) 551.29
          obstruction 552.29
            and gangrene 551.29
    spinal (*see also* Spina bifida) 741.9 ☑
      with hydrocephalus 741.0 ☑
    strangulated (*see also* Hernia, by site, with
        obstruction) 552.9
      gangrenous (with obstruction) (*see also*
          Hernia, by site, with gangrene)
          551.9
    supraumbilicus (linea alba) — *see* Hernia,
        epigastric
    tendon 727.9
    testis (nontraumatic) 550.9 ☑
      meaning
        scrotal hernia 550.9 ☑
        symptomatic late syphilis 095.8
    Treitz's (fossa) 553.8
      with
        gangrene (obstructed) 551.8
          obstruction 552.8
            and gangrene 551.8
    tunica
      albuginea 608.89
      vaginalis 752.89
    umbilicus, umbilical 553.1
      with
        gangrene (obstructed) 551.1
          obstruction 552.1
            and gangrene 551.1
    ureter 593.89
      with obstruction 593.4
    uterus 621.8
      pregnant 654.4 ☑
    vaginal (posterior) 618.6
    Velpeau's (femoral) (*see also* Hernia,
        femoral) 553.00
    ventral 553.20
      with
        gangrene (obstructed) 551.20
          obstruction 552.20
            and gangrene 551.20
      incisional 553.21
      recurrent 553.21
        with
          gangrene (obstructed) 551.21
            obstruction 552.21
              and gangrene 551.21

Hernia, hernial — *continued*
    vesical
      congenital (female) (male) 756.71
      female (*see also* Cystocele, female)
          618.01
      male 596.89
    vitreous (into anterior chamber) 379.21
      traumatic 871.1
Herniation — *see also* Hernia
  brain (stem) 348.4
  cerebral 348.4
  gastric mucosa (into duodenal bulb) 537.89
  mediastinum 519.3
  nucleus pulposus — *see* Displacement, in-
      tervertebral disc
Herpangina 074.0
Herpes, herpetic 054.9
  auricularis (zoster) 053.71
    simplex 054.73
  blepharitis (zoster) 053.20
    simplex 054.41
  circinate 110.5
  circinatus 110.5
    bullous 694.5
  conjunctiva (simplex) 054.43
    zoster 053.21
  cornea (simplex) 054.43
    disciform (simplex) 054.43
    zoster 053.21
  encephalitis 054.3
  eye (zoster) 053.29
    simplex 054.40
  eyelid (zoster) 053.20
    simplex 054.41
  febrilis 054.9
  fever 054.9
  geniculate ganglionitis 053.11
  genital, genitalis 054.10
    specified site NEC 054.19
  gestationis 646.8 ☑
  gingivostomatitis 054.2
  iridocyclitis (simplex) 054.44
    zoster 053.22
  iris (any site) 695.10
  iritis (simplex) 054.44
  keratitis (simplex) 054.43
    dendritic 054.42
    disciform 054.43
    interstitial 054.43
      zoster 053.21
  keratoconjunctivitis (simplex) 054.43
    zoster 053.21
  labialis 054.9
    meningococcal 036.89
  lip 054.9
  meningitis (simplex) 054.72
    zoster 053.0
  ophthalmicus (zoster) 053.20
    simplex 054.40
  otitis externa (zoster) 053.71
    simplex 054.73
  penis 054.13
  perianal 054.10
  pharyngitis 054.79
  progenitalis 054.10
  scrotum 054.19
  septicemia 054.5
  simplex 054.9
    complicated 054.8
      ophthalmic 054.40
        specified NEC 054.49
      specified NEC 054.79
    congenital 771.2
    external ear 054.73
    keratitis 054.43
      dendritic 054.42
    meningitis 054.72
    myelitis 054.74
    neuritis 054.79
    specified complication NEC 054.79
      ophthalmic 054.49
    visceral 054.71
  stomatitis 054.2
  tonsurans 110.0
    maculosus (of Hebra) 696.3
  visceral 054.71

Herpes, herpetic — *continued*
  vulva 054.12
  vulvovaginitis 054.11
  whitlow 054.6
  zoster 053.9
    auricularis 053.71
    complicated 053.8
      specified NEC 053.79
    conjunctiva 053.21
    cornea 053.21
    ear 053.71
    eye 053.29
    geniculate 053.11
    keratitis 053.21
      interstitial 053.21
    myelitis 053.14
    neuritis 053.10
    ophthalmicus(a) 053.20
    oticus 053.71
    otitis externa 053.71
    specified complication NEC 053.79
    specified site NEC 053.9
    zosteriform, intermediate type 053.9
Herrick's
  anemia (hemoglobin S disease) 282.61
  syndrome (hemoglobin S disease) 282.61
Hers' disease (glycogenosis VI) 271.0
Herter (-Gee) disease or syndrome (nontrop-
    ical sprue) 579.0
Herter's infantilism (nontropical sprue) 579.0
Herxheimer's disease (diffuse idiopathic cuta-
    neous atrophy) 701.8
Herxheimer's reaction 995.91
Hesitancy, urinary 788.64
Hesselbach's hernia — *see* Hernia, Hessel-
    bach's
Heterochromia (congenital) 743.46
  acquired 364.53
  cataract 366.33
  cyclitis 364.21
  hair 704.3
  iritis 364.21
  retained metallic foreign body 360.62
    magnetic 360.52
  uveitis 364.21
Heterophoria 378.40
  alternating 378.45
  vertical 378.43
Heterophyes, small intestine 121.6
Heterophyiasis 121.6
Heteropsia 368.8
Heterotopia, heterotopic — *see also* Malposi-
    tion, congenital
  cerebralis 742.4
  pancreas, pancreatic 751.7
  spinalis 742.59
Heterotropia 378.30
  intermittent 378.20
    vertical 378.31
  vertical (constant) (intermittent) 378.31
Heubner-Herter disease or syndrome (non-
    tropical sprue) 579.0
Heubner's disease 094.89
Hexadactylism 755.0 ☑
Heyd's syndrome (hepatorenal) 572.4
HGSIL (high grade squamous intraepithelial
    lesion) (cytologic finding) (Pap smear
    finding)
  anus 796.74
  cervix 795.04
    biopsy finding — code to CIN II or CIN
        III
  vagina 795.14
Hibernoma (M8880/0) — *see* Lipoma
Hiccough 786.8
  epidemic 078.89
  psychogenic 306.1
Hiccup — *see also* Hiccough 786.8
Hicks (-Braxton) contractures 644.1 ☑
Hidden penis 752.65
Hidradenitis (axillaris) (suppurative) 705.83
Hidradenoma (nodular) (M8400/0) — *see also*
    Neoplasm, skin, benign
  clear cell (M8402/0) — *see* Neoplasm, skin,
      benign

☑ **Additional Digit Required — Refer to the Tabular List for Digit Selection**   ▽ **Subterms under main terms may continue to next column or page**

2014 ICD-9-CM   ▶◀ **Revised Text**   ● **New Line**   ▲ **Revised Code**   **Volume 2 — 139**

Hidradenoma — see also Neoplasm, skin, benign — continued
  papillary (M8405/0) — see Neoplasm, skin, benign
Hidrocystoma (M8404/0) — see Neoplasm, skin, benign
HIE (hypoxic-ischemic encephalopathy) 768.70
  mild 768.71
  moderate 768.72
  severe 768.73
High
  A$_2$ anemia 282.46
  altitude effects 993.2
    anoxia 993.2
    on
      ears 993.0
      sinuses 993.1
    polycythemia 289.0
  arch
    foot 755.67
    palate 750.26
  artery (arterial) tension (see also Hypertension) 401.9
    without diagnosis of hypertension 796.2
  basal metabolic rate (BMR) 794.7
  blood pressure (see also Hypertension) 401.9
    borderline 796.2
    incidental reading (isolated) (nonspecific), no diagnosis of hypertension 796.2
  cholesterol 272.0
    with high triglycerides 272.2
  compliance bladder 596.4
  diaphragm (congenital) 756.6
  frequency deafness (congenital) (regional) 389.8
  head at term 652.5 ☑
    affecting fetus or newborn 763.1
  output failure (cardiac) (see also Failure, heart) 428.9
  oxygen-affinity hemoglobin 289.0
  palate 750.26
  risk
    behavior — see Problem
    family situation V61.9
      specified circumstance NEC V61.8
    human papillomavirus (HPV) DNA test positive
      anal 796.75
      cervical 795.05
      vaginal 795.15
    individual NEC V62.89
    infant NEC V20.1
    patient taking drugs (prescribed) V67.51
      nonprescribed (see also Abuse, drugs, nondependent) 305.9 ☑
    pregnancy V23.9
      inadequate prenatal care V23.7
      inconclusive fetal viability V23.87
      specified problem NEC V23.89
  temperature (of unknown origin) (see also Pyrexia) 780.60
  thoracic rib 756.3
  triglycerides 272.1
    with high cholesterol 272.2
Hildenbrand's disease (typhus) 081.9
Hilger's syndrome 337.09
Hill diarrhea 579.1
Hilliard's lupus — see also Tuberculosis 017.0 ☑
Hilum — see condition
Hip — see condition
Hippel's disease (retinocerebral angiomatosis) 759.6
Hippus 379.49
Hirschfeld's disease (acute diabetes mellitus) — see also Diabetes 250.0 ☑
  due to secondary diabetes 249.0 ☑
Hirschsprung's disease or megacolon (congenital) 751.3
Hirsuties — see also Hypertrichosis 704.1
Hirsutism — see also Hypertrichosis 704.1
Hirudiniasis (external) (internal) 134.2
His-Werner disease (trench fever) 083.1
Hiss-Russell dysentery 004.1
Histamine cephalgia 339.00

Histidinemia 270.5
Histidinuria 270.5
Histiocytic syndromes 288.4
Histiocytoma (M8832/0) — see also Neoplasm, skin, benign
  fibrous (M8830/0) (see also Neoplasm, skin, benign)
    atypical (M8830/1) — see Neoplasm, connective tissue, uncertain behavior
    malignant (M8830/3) — see Neoplasm, connective tissue, malignant
Histiocytosis (acute) (chronic) (subacute) 277.89
  acute differentiated progressive (M9722/3) 202.5 ☑
  adult pulmonary Langerhans cell (PLCH) 516.5
  cholesterol 277.89
  essential 277.89
  lipid, lipoid (essential) 272.7
  lipochrome (familial) 288.1
  malignant (M9720/3) 202.3 ☑
  non-Langerhans cell 277.89
  polyostotic sclerosing 277.89
  X (chronic) 277.89
    acute (progressive) (M9722/3) 202.5 ☑
Histoplasmosis 115.90
  with
    endocarditis 115.94
    meningitis 115.91
    pericarditis 115.93
    pneumonia 115.95
    retinitis 115.92
    specified manifestation NEC 115.99
  African (due to Histoplasma duboisii) 115.10
    with
      endocarditis 115.14
      meningitis 115.11
      pericarditis 115.13
      pneumonia 115.15
      retinitis 115.12
      specified manifestation NEC 115.19
  American (due to Histoplasma capsulatum) 115.00
    with
      endocarditis 115.04
      meningitis 115.01
      pericarditis 115.03
      pneumonia 115.05
      retinitis 115.02
      specified manifestation NEC 115.09
  Darling's — see Histoplasmosis, American
  large form (see also Histoplasmosis, African) 115.10
  lung 115.05
  small form (see also Histoplasmosis, American) 115.00
History (personal) of
  abuse
    emotional V15.42
    neglect V15.42
    physical V15.41
    sexual V15.41
  affective psychosis V11.1
  alcoholism V11.3
    specified as drinking problem (see also Abuse, drugs, nondependent) 305.0 ☑
  allergy to V15.09
    analgesic agent NEC V14.6
    anesthetic NEC V14.4
    anti-infective agent NEC V14.3
    antibiotic agent NEC V14.1
      penicillin V14.0
    arachnid bite V15.06
    diathesis V15.09
    drug V14.9
      specified type NEC V14.8
    eggs V15.03
    food additives V15.05
    insect bite V15.06
    latex V15.07
    medicinal agents V14.9
      specified type NEC V14.8
    milk products V15.02

History of — continued
  allergy to — continued
    narcotic agent NEC V14.5
    nuts V15.05
      peanuts V15.01
    penicillin V14.0
    radiographic dye V15.08
    seafood V15.04
    serum V14.7
    specified food NEC V15.05
    specified nonmedicinal agents NEC V15.09
    spider bite V15.06
    sulfa V14.2
    sulfonamides V14.2
    therapeutic agent NEC V15.09
    vaccine V14.7
  anaphylactic reaction or shock V13.81
  anaphylaxis V13.81
  anemia V12.3
  arrest, sudden cardiac V12.53
  arthritis V13.4
  attack, transient ischemic (TIA) V12.54
  benign neoplasm of brain V12.41
  blood disease V12.3
  calculi, urinary V13.01
  cardiovascular disease V12.50
    myocardial infarction 412
  chemotherapy, antineoplastic V87.41
  child abuse V15.41
  cigarette smoking V15.82
  circulatory system disease V12.50
    myocardial infarction 412
  cleft lip and palate, corrected V13.64
  combat and operational stress reaction V11.4
  congenital malformation (corrected)
    circulatory system V13.65
    digestive system V13.67
    ear V13.64
    eye V13.64
    face V13.64
    genitourinary system V13.62
    heart V13.65
    integument V13.68
    limbs V13.68
    musculoskeletal V13.68
    neck V13.64
    nervous system V13.63
    respiratory system V13.66
    specified type NEC V13.69
  contraception V15.7
  death, sudden, successfully resuscitated V12.53
  deficit
    prolonged reversible ischemic neurologic (PRIND) V12.54
    reversible ischemic neurologic (RIND) V12.54
  diathesis, allergic V15.09
  digestive system disease V12.70
    peptic ulcer V12.71
    polyps, colonic V12.72
    specified NEC V12.79
  disease (of) V13.9
    blood-forming organs V12.3
    blood V12.3
    cardiovascular system V12.50
    circulatory system V12.50
      specified NEC V12.59
    digestive system V12.70
      peptic ulcer V12.71
      polyps, colonic V12.72
      specified NEC V12.79
    infectious V12.00
      malaria V12.03
      methicillin resistant Staphylococcus aureus (MRSA) V12.04
      MRSA (methicillin resistant Staphylococcus aureus) V12.04
      poliomyelitis V12.02
      specified NEC V12.09
      tuberculosis V12.01
    parasitic V12.00
      specified NEC V12.09
    respiratory system V12.60

History of — continued
  disease — continued
    respiratory system — continued
      pneumonia V12.61
      specified NEC V12.69
    skin V13.3
    specified site NEC V13.89
    subcutaneous tissue V13.3
    trophoblastic V13.1
      affecting management of pregnancy V23.1
  disorder (of) V13.9
    endocrine V12.29
      gestational diabetes V12.21
    genital system V13.29
    hematological V12.3
    immunity V12.29
    mental V11.9
      affective type V11.1
      manic-depressive V11.1
      neurosis V11.2
      schizophrenia V11.0
      specified type NEC V11.8
    metabolic V12.29
    musculoskeletal NEC V13.59
    nervous system V12.40
      specified type NEC V12.49
    obstetric V13.29
      affecting management of current pregnancy V23.49
      ectopic pregnancy V23.42
      pre-term labor V23.41
    pre-term labor V13.21
    sense organs V12.40
      specified type NEC V12.49
    specified site NEC V13.89
    urinary system V13.00
      calculi V13.01
      infection V13.02
      nephrotic syndrome V13.03
      specified NEC V13.09
  drug use
    nonprescribed (see also Abuse, drugs, nondependent) 305.9 ☑
    patent (see also Abuse, drugs, non-dependent) 305.9 ☑
  dysplasia
    cervical (conditions classifiable to 622.10-622.12) V13.22
    vaginal (conditions classifiable to 623.0) V13.23
    vulvar (conditions classifiable to 624.01-624.02) V13.24
  effect NEC of external cause V15.89
  embolism V12.51
    pulmonary V12.55
  emotional abuse V15.42
  encephalitis V12.42
  endocrine disorder V12.29
    gestational diabetes V12.21
  estrogen therapy V87.43
  extracorporeal membrane oxygenation (ECMO) V15.87
  failed
    conscious sedation V15.80
    moderate sedation V15.80
  falling V15.88
  family
    allergy V19.6
    anemia V18.2
    arteriosclerosis V17.49
    arthritis V17.7
    asthma V17.5
    blindness V19.0
    blood disorder NEC V18.3
    cardiovascular disease V17.49
    carrier, genetic disease V18.9
    cerebrovascular disease V17.1
    chronic respiratory condition NEC V17.6
    colonic polyps V18.51
    congenital anomalies V19.5
    consanguinity V19.7
    coronary artery disease V17.3
    cystic fibrosis V18.19
    deafness V19.2
    diabetes mellitus V18.0

☑ **Additional Digit Required — Refer to the Tabular List for Digit Selection**   ▽ **Subterms under main terms may continue to next column or page**

History of — *continued*
  family — *continued*
    digestive disorders V18.59
    disabilities, intellectual V18.4
    disease or disorder (of)
      allergic V19.6
      blood NEC V18.3
      cardiovascular NEC V17.49
      cerebrovascular V17.1
      colonic polyps V18.51
      coronary artery V17.3
      death, sudden cardiac (SCD) V17.41
      digestive V18.59
      ear NEC V19.3
      endocrine V18.19
        multiple neoplasia (MEN) syndrome V18.11
      eye NEC V19.19
        glaucoma V19.11
      genitourinary NEC V18.7
      glaucoma V19.11
      hypertensive V17.49
      infectious V18.8
      ischemic heart V17.3
      kidney V18.69
        polycystic V18.61
      mental V17.0
      metabolic V18.19
      musculoskeletal NEC V17.89
        osteoporosis V17.81
      neurological NEC V17.2
      parasitic V18.8
      psychiatric condition V17.0
      skin condition V19.4
    ear disorder NEC V19.3
    endocrine disease V18.19
      multiple neoplasia (MEN) syndrome V18.11
    epilepsy V17.2
    eye disorder NEC V19.19
      glaucoma V19.11
    genetic disease carrier V18.9
    genitourinary disease NEC V18.7
    glaucoma V19.11
    glomerulonephritis V18.69
    gout V18.19
    hay fever V17.6
    hearing loss V19.2
    hematopoietic neoplasia V16.7
    Hodgkin's disease V16.7
    Huntington's chorea V17.2
    hydrocephalus V19.5
    hypertension V17.49
    infarction, myocardial V17.3
    infectious disease V18.8
    intellectual disabilities V18.4
    ischemic heart disease V17.3
    kidney disease V18.69
      polycystic V18.61
    leukemia V16.6
    lymphatic malignant neoplasia NEC V16.7
    malignant neoplasm (of) NEC V16.9
      anorectal V16.0
      anus V16.0
      appendix V16.0
      bladder V16.52
      bone V16.8
      brain V16.8
      breast V16.3
        male V16.8
      bronchus V16.1
      cecum V16.0
      cervix V16.49
      colon V16.0
      duodenum V16.0
      esophagus V16.0
      eye V16.8
      gallbladder V16.0
      gastrointestinal tract V16.0
      genital organs V16.40
      hemopoietic NEC V16.7
      ileum V16.0
      ilium V16.8
      intestine V16.0
      intrathoracic organs NEC V16.2

History of — *continued*
  family — *continued*
    malignant neoplasm — *continued*
      kidney V16.51
      larynx V16.2
      liver V16.0
      lung V16.1
      lymphatic NEC V16.7
      ovary V16.41
      oviduct V16.41
      pancreas V16.0
      penis V16.49
      prostate V16.42
      rectum V16.0
      respiratory organs NEC V16.2
      skin V16.8
      specified site NEC V16.8
      stomach V16.0
      testis V16.43
      trachea V16.1
      ureter V16.59
      urethra V16.59
      urinary organs V16.59
      uterus V16.49
      vagina V16.49
      vulva V16.49
    MEN (multiple endocrine neoplasia syndrome) V18.11
    mental retardation — *see* History, family, intellectual disabilities
    metabolic disease NEC V18.19
    mongolism V19.5
    multiple
      endocrine neoplasia (MEN) syndrome V18.11
      myeloma V16.7
    musculoskeletal disease NEC V17.89
      osteoporosis V17.81
    myocardial infarction V17.3
    nephritis V18.69
    nephrosis V18.69
    osteoporosis V17.81
    parasitic disease V18.8
    polycystic kidney disease V18.61
    psychiatric disorder V17.0
    psychosis V17.0
    retinitis pigmentosa V19.19
    schizophrenia V17.0
    skin conditions V19.4
    specified condition NEC V19.8
    stroke (cerebrovascular) V17.1
    sudden cardiac death (SCD) V17.41
    visual loss V19.0
  foreign body fully removed V15.53
  fracture, healed
    pathologic V13.51
    stress V13.52
    traumatic V15.51
  genital system disorder V13.29
    pre-term labor V13.21
  gestational diabetes V12.21
  health hazard V15.9
    falling V15.88
    specified cause NEC V15.89
  hepatitis
    B V12.09
    C V12.09
  Hodgkin's disease V10.72
  hypospadias (corrected) V13.61
  immunity disorder V12.29
  immunosuppression therapy V87.46
  infarction, cerebral, without residual deficits V12.54
  infection
    central nervous system V12.42
    urinary (tract) V13.02
  infectious disease V12.00
    malaria V12.03
    methicillin resistant Staphylococcus aureus (MRSA) V12.04
    MRSA (methicillin resistant Staphylococcus aureus) V12.04
    poliomyelitis V12.02
    specified NEC V12.09
    tuberculosis V12.01
  injury NEC V15.59

History of — *continued*
  injury — *continued*
    traumatic brain V15.52
  insufficient prenatal care V23.7
  in utero procedure
    during pregnancy V15.21
    while a fetus V15.22
  irradiation V15.3
  leukemia V10.60
    lymphoid V10.61
    monocytic V10.63
    myeloid V10.62
    specified type NEC V10.69
  little or no prenatal care V23.7
  low birth weight (*see also* Status, low birth weight) V21.30
  lymphosarcoma V10.71
  malaria V12.03
  malignant carcinoid tumor V10.91
  malignant neoplasm (of) V10.90
    accessory sinus V10.22
    adrenal V10.88
    anus V10.06
    bile duct V10.09
    bladder V10.51
    bone V10.81
    brain V10.85
    breast V10.3
    bronchus V10.11
    cervix uteri V10.41
    colon V10.05
    connective tissue NEC V10.89
    corpus uteri V10.42
    digestive system V10.00
      specified part NEC V10.09
    duodenum V10.09
    endocrine gland NEC V10.88
    epididymis V10.48
    esophagus V10.03
    eye V10.84
    fallopian tube V10.44
    female genital organ V10.40
      specified site NEC V10.44
    gallbladder V10.09
    gastrointestinal tract V10.00
    gum V10.02
    hematopoietic NEC V10.79
    hypopharynx V10.02
    ileum V10.09
    intrathoracic organs NEC V10.20
    jejunum V10.09
    kidney V10.52
    large intestine V10.05
    larynx V10.21
    lip V10.02
    liver V10.07
    lung V10.11
    lymphatic NEC V10.79
    lymph glands or nodes NEC V10.79
    male genital organ V10.45
      specified site NEC V10.49
    mediastinum V10.29
    melanoma (of skin) V10.82
    middle ear V10.22
    mouth V10.02
      specified part NEC V10.02
    nasal cavities V10.22
    nasopharynx V10.02
    nervous system NEC V10.86
    nose V10.22
    oropharynx V10.02
    ovary V10.43
    pancreas V10.09
    parathyroid V10.88
    penis V10.49
    pharynx V10.02
    pineal V10.88
    pituitary V10.88
    placenta V10.44
    pleura V10.29
    prostate V10.46
    rectosigmoid junction V10.06
    rectum V10.06
    renal pelvis V10.53
    respiratory organs NEC V10.20
    salivary gland V10.02

History of — *continued*
  malignant neoplasm — *continued*
    skin V10.83
      melanoma V10.82
    small intestine NEC V10.09
    soft tissue NEC V10.89
    specified site NEC V10.89
    stomach V10.04
    testis V10.47
    thymus V10.29
    thyroid V10.87
    tongue V10.01
    trachea V10.12
    ureter V10.59
    urethra V10.59
    urinary organ V10.50
    uterine adnexa V10.44
    uterus V10.42
    vagina V10.44
    vulva V10.44
  malignant neuroendocrine tumor V10.91
  manic-depressive psychosis V11.1
  meningitis V12.42
  mental disorder V11.9
    affective type V11.1
      manic-depressive V11.1
    neurosis V11.2
    schizophrenia V11.0
    specified type NEC V11.8
  Merkel cell carcinoma V10.91
  metabolic disorder V12.29
  methicillin resistant Staphylococcus aureus (MRSA) V12.04
  MRSA (methicillin resistant Staphylococcus aureus) V12.04
  musculoskeletal disorder NEC V13.59
  myocardial infarction 412
  neglect (emotional) V15.42
  nephrotic syndrome V13.03
  nervous system disorder V12.40
    specified type NEC V12.49
  neurosis V11.2
  noncompliance with medical treatment V15.81
  nutritional deficiency V12.1
  obstetric disorder V13.29
    affecting management of current pregnancy V23.49
      ectopic pregnancy V23.42
      pre-term labor V23.41
    pre-term labor V13.21
  parasitic disease V12.00
    specified NEC V12.09
  perinatal problems V13.7
    low birth weight (*see also* Status, low birth weight) V21.30
  physical abuse V15.41
  poisoning V15.6
  poliomyelitis V12.02
  polyps, colonic V12.72
  poor obstetric V13.29
    affecting management of current pregnancy V23.49
      ectopic pregnancy V23.42
      pre-term labor V23.41
    pre-term labor V13.21
  prolonged reversible ischemic neurologic deficit (PRIND) V12.54
  psychiatric disorder V11.9
    affective type V11.1
      manic-depressive V11.1
    neurosis V11.2
    schizophrenia V11.0
    specified type NEC V11.8
  psychological trauma V15.49
    emotional abuse V15.42
    neglect V15.42
    physical abuse V15.41
    rape V15.41
  psychoneurosis V11.2
  radiation therapy V15.3
  rape V15.41
  respiratory system disease V12.60
    pneumonia V12.61
    specified NEC V12.69
  reticulosarcoma V10.71

☑ **Additional Digit Required** — Refer to the Tabular List for Digit Selection   ▽ **Subterms under main terms may continue to next column or page**

2014 ICD-9-CM   ▶◀ Revised Text   ● New Line   ▲ Revised Code   Volume 2 — 141

History of — continued
  return from military deployment V62.22
  reversible ischemic neurologic deficit (RIND)
    V12.54
  schizophrenia V11.0
  skin disease V13.3
  smoking (tobacco) V15.82
  steroid therapy V87.45
    inhaled V87.44
    systemic V87.45
  stroke without residual deficits V12.54
  subcutaneous tissue disease V13.3
  sudden
    cardiac
      arrest V12.53
      death (successfully resuscitated)
        V12.53
  surgery to
    great vessels V15.1
    heart V15.1
    in utero
      during pregnancy V15.21
      while a fetus V15.22
    organs NEC V15.29
  syndrome, nephrotic V13.03
  therapy
    antineoplastic drug V87.41
    drug NEC V87.49
    estrogen V87.43
    immunosuppression V87.46
    monoclonal drug V87.42
    steroid V87.45
      inhaled V87.44
      systemic V87.45
  thrombophlebitis V12.52
  thrombosis V12.51
    pulmonary V12.55
  tobacco use V15.82
  trophoblastic disease V13.1
    affecting management of pregnancy
      V23.1
  tuberculosis V12.01
  ulcer, peptic V12.71
  urinary system disorder V13.00
    calculi V13.01
    infection V13.02
    nephrotic syndrome V13.03
    specified NEC V13.09
HIT (heparin-induced thrombocytopenia)
  289.84
Hives (bold) — *see also* Urticaria 708.9
HIV infection (disease) (illness) — *see* Human
  immunodeficiency virus (disease) (illness) (infection)
Hoarseness 784.42
Hobnail liver — *see* Cirrhosis, portal
Hobo, hoboism V60.0
Hodgkin's
  disease (M9650/3) 201.9 ☑
    lymphocytic-histiocytic predominance
      (M9651/3) 201.4 ☑
    lymphocytic
      depletion (M9653/3) 201.7 ☑
        diffuse fibrosis (M9654/3)
          201.7 ☑
        reticular type (M9655/3) 201.7 ☑
      predominance (M9651/3) 201.4 ☑
    mixed cellularity (M9652/3) 201.6 ☑
    nodular sclerosis (M9656/3) 201.5 ☑
      cellular phase (M9657/3) 201.5 ☑
  granuloma (M9661/3) 201.1 ☑
  lymphogranulomatosis (M9650/3) 201.9 ☑
  lymphoma (M9650/3) 201.9 ☑
  lymphosarcoma (M9650/3) 201.9 ☑
  paragranuloma (M9660/3) 201.0 ☑
  sarcoma (M9662/3) 201.9 ☑
Hodgson's disease (aneurysmal dilatation of
  aorta) 441.9
  ruptured 441.5
Hodi-potsy 111.0
Hoffa (-Kastert) disease or syndrome (lIposynovitis prepatellaris) 272.8
Hoffmann-Bouveret syndrome (paroxysmal
  tachycardia) 427.2
Hoffman's syndrome 244.9 *[359.5]*

Hole
  macula 362.54
  optic disc, crater-like 377.22
  retina (macula) 362.54
    round 361.31
      with detachment 361.01
Holla disease — *see also* Spherocytosis 282.0
Holländer-Simons syndrome (progressive
  lipodystrophy) 272.6
Hollow foot (congenital) 754.71
  acquired 736.73
Holmes' syndrome (visual disorientation)
  368.16
Holoprosencephaly 742.2
  due to
    trisomy 13 758.1
    trisomy 18 758.2
Holthouse's hernia — *see* Hernia, inguinal
Homesickness 309.89
Homicidal ideation V62.85
Homocystinemia 270.4
Homocystinuria 270.4
Homologous serum jaundice (prophylactic)
  (therapeutic) — *see* Hepatitis, viral
Homosexuality — omit code
  ego-dystonic 302.0
  pedophilic 302.2
  problems with 302.0
Homozygous Hb-S disease 282.61
Honeycomb lung 518.89
  congenital 748.4
Hong Kong ear 117.3
HOOD (hereditary osteo-onychodysplasia)
  756.89
Hooded
  clitoris 752.49
  penis 752.69
Hookworm (anemia) (disease) (infestation) —
  see Ancylostomiasis
Hoppe-Goldflam syndrome 358.00
Hordeolum (external) (eyelid) 373.11
  internal 373.12
Horn
  cutaneous 702.8
    cheek 702.8
    eyelid 702.8
    penis 702.8
  iliac 756.89
  nail 703.8
    congenital 757.5
  papillary 700
Horner's
  syndrome (*see also* Neuropathy, peripheral,
    autonomic) 337.9
    traumatic 954.0
  teeth 520.4
Horseshoe kidney (congenital) 753.3
Horton's
  disease (temporal arteritis) 446.5
  headache or neuralgia 339.00
Hospice care V66.7
Hospitalism (in children) NEC 309.83
Hourglass contraction, contracture
  bladder 596.89
  gallbladder 575.2
    congenital 751.69
  stomach 536.8
    congenital 750.7
    psychogenic 306.4
  uterus 661.4 ☑
    affecting fetus or newborn 763.7
Household circumstance affecting care V60.9
  specified type NEC V60.89
Housemaid's knee 727.2
Housing circumstance affecting care V60.9
  specified type NEC V60.89
HTLV-I infection 079.51
HTLV-II infection 079.52
HTLV-III/LAV (disease) (illness) (infection) —
  see Human immunodeficiency virus
  (disease) (illness) (infection)
HTLV-III (disease) (illness) (infection) — *see*
  Human immunodeficiency virus (dis-
  ease) (illness) (infection)

HTR (hemolytic transfusion reaction)
  due to or resulting from
    incompatibility
      ABO 999.61
        acute 999.62
        delayed 999.63
      non-ABO antigen (minor) (Duffy)
        (Kell) (Kidd) (Lewis) (M) (N) (P)
        (S) 999.76
        acute 999.77
        delayed 999.78
      Rh antigen (C) (c) (D) (E) (e) 999.71
        acute 999.72
        delayed 999.73
Huchard's disease (continued arterial hypertension) 401.9
Hudson-Ståhli lines 371.11
Huguier's disease (uterine fibroma) 218.9
Human bite (open wound) — *see also* Wound,
  open, by site
  intact skin surface — *see* Contusion
Human immunodeficiency virus-2 infection
  079.53
Human immunodeficiency virus (disease)
  (illness) 042
  infection V08
    with symptoms, symptomatic 042
Human immunovirus (disease) (illness) (infection) — *see* Human immunodeficiency
  virus (disease) (illness) (infection)
Human papillomavirus 079.4
  high risk, DNA test positive
    anal 796.75
    cervical 795.05
    vaginal 795.15
  low risk, DNA test positive
    anal 796.79
    cervical 795.09
    vaginal 795.19
Human parvovirus 079.83
Human T-cell lymphotrophic virus-I infec-
tion 079.51
Human T-cell lymphotrophic virus-II infec-
tion 079.52
Human T-cell lymphotrophic virus-III (disease) (illness) (infection) — *see* Human
  immunodeficiency virus (disease) (ill-
  ness) (infection)
Humpback (acquired) 737.9
  congenital 756.19
Hum, venous — omit code
Hunchback (acquired) 737.9
  congenital 756.19
Hunger 994.2
  air, psychogenic 306.1
  disease 251.1
Hungry bone syndrome 275.5
Hunner's ulcer — *see also* Cystitis 595.1
Hunt's
  neuralgia 053.11
  syndrome (herpetic geniculate ganglionitis)
    053.11
    dyssynergia cerebellaris myoclonica
      334.2
Hunter's glossitis 529.4
Hunterian chancre 091.0
Hunter (-Hurler) syndrome (mucopolysaccharidosis II) 277.5
Huntington's
  chorea 333.4
  disease 333.4
Huppert's disease (multiple myeloma)
  (M9730/3) 203.0 ☑
Hurler (-Hunter) disease or syndrome (mu-
  copolysaccharidosis II) 277.5
Hürthle cell
  adenocarcinoma (M8290/3) 193
  adenoma (M8290/0) 226
  carcinoma (M8290/3) 193
  tumor (M8290/0) 226
Hutchinson-Boeck disease or syndrome
  (sarcoidosis) 135
Hutchinson-Gilford disease or syndrome
  (progeria) 259.8

Hutchinson's
  disease meaning
    angioma serpiginosum 709.1
    cheiropompholyx 705.81
    prurigo estivalis 692.72
    summer eruption, or summer prurigo
      692.72
  incisors 090.5
  melanotic freckle (M8742/2) (*see also* Neo-
    plasm, skin, in situ)
    malignant melanoma in (M8742/3) —
      see Melanoma
  teeth or incisors (congenital syphilis) 090.5
Hyaline
  degeneration (diffuse) (generalized) 728.9
    localized — *see* Degeneration, by site
  membrane (disease) (lung) (newborn) 769
Hyalinosis cutis et mucosae 272.8
Hyalin plaque, sclera, senile 379.16
Hyalitis (asteroid) 379.22
  syphilitic 095.8
Hydatid
  cyst or tumor (*see also* Echinococcus)
    fallopian tube 752.11
  mole — *see* Hydatidiform mole
  Morgagni (congenital) 752.89
    fallopian tube 752.11
Hydatidiform mole (benign) (complicating
  pregnancy) (delivered) (undelivered) 630
  invasive (M9100/1) 236.1
  malignant (M9100/1) 236.1
  previous, affecting management of pregnan-
    cy V23.1
Hydatidosis — *see* Echinococcus
Hyde's disease (prurigo nodularis) 698.3
Hydradenitis 705.83
Hydradenoma (M8400/0) — *see* Hidradenoma
Hydralazine lupus or syndrome
  correct substance properly administered
    695.4
  overdose or wrong substance given or taken
    972.6
Hydramnios 657.0 ☑
  affecting fetus or newborn 761.3
Hydrancephaly 742.3
  with spina bifida (*see also* Spina bifida)
    741.0 ☑
Hydranencephaly 742.3
  with spina bifida (*see also* Spina bifida)
    741.0 ☑
Hydrargyrism NEC 985.0
Hydrarthrosis — *see also* Effusion, joint
  719.0 ☑
  gonococcal 098.50
  intermittent (*see also* Rheumatism, palin-
    dromic) 719.3 ☑
  of yaws (early) (late) 102.6
  syphilitic 095.8
    congenital 090.5
Hydremia 285.9
Hydrencephalocele (congenital) 742.0
Hydrencephalomeningocele (congenital)
  742.0
Hydroa 694.0
  aestivale 692.72
  gestationis 646.8 ☑
  herpetiformis 694.0
  pruriginosa 694.0
  vacciniforme 692.72
Hydroadenitis 705.83
Hydrocalycosis — *see also* Hydronephrosis 59
  congenital 753.29
Hydrocalyx — *see also* Hydronephrosis 591
Hydrocele (calcified) (chylous) (idiopathic)
  (infantile) (inguinal canal) (recurrent)
  (senile) (spermatic cord) (testis) (tunica
  vaginalis) 603.9
  canal of Nuck (female) 629.1
    male 603.9
  congenital 778.6
  encysted 603.0
    congenital 778.6
  female NEC 629.89
  infected 603.1
  round ligament 629.89
  specified type NEC 603.8

☑ Additional Digit Required — Refer to the Tabular List for Digit Selection   ⌐ Subterms under main terms may continue to next column or page

142 — Volume 2   ▶◀ Revised Text   ● New Line   ▲ Revised Code   2014 ICD-9-CM

Hydrocele — continued
  specified type — continued
    congenital 778.6
  spinalis (see also Spina bifida) 741.9 ☑
  vulva 624.8
Hydrocephalic fetus
  affecting management or pregnancy 655.0 ☑
  causing disproportion 653.6 ☑
    with obstructed labor 660.1 ☑
      affecting fetus or newborn 763.1
Hydrocephalus (acquired) (external) (internal) (malignant) (noncommunicating) (obstructive) (recurrent) 331.4
  aqueduct of Sylvius stricture 742.3
    with spina bifida (see also Spina bifida) 741.0 ☑
  chronic 742.3
    with spina bifida (see also Spina bifida) 741.0 ☑
  communicating 331.3
  congenital (external) (internal) 742.3
    with spina bifida (see also Spina bifida) 741.0 ☑
  due to
    stricture of aqueduct of Sylvius 742.3
      with spina bifida (see also Spina bifida) 741.0 ☑
    toxoplasmosis (congenital) 771.2
  fetal affecting management of pregnancy 655.0 ☑
  foramen Magendie block (acquired) 331.3
    congenital 742.3
      with spina bifida (see also Spina bifida) 741.0 ☑
  newborn 742.3
    with spina bifida (see also Spina bifida) 741.0 ☑
  normal pressure 331.5
    idiopathic (INPH) 331.5
    secondary 331.3
  otitic 348.2
  syphilitic, congenital 090.49
  tuberculous (see also Tuberculosis) 013.8 ☑
Hydrocolpos (congenital) 623.8
Hydrocystoma (M8404/0) — see Neoplasm, skin, benign
Hydroencephalocele (congenital) 742.0
Hydroencephalomeningocele (congenital) 742.0
Hydrohematopneumothorax — see also Hemothorax 511.89
Hydromeningitis — see Meningitis
Hydromeningocele (spinal) — see also Spina bifida 741.9 ☑
  cranial 742.0
Hydrometra 621.8
Hydrometrocolpos 623.8
Hydromicrocephaly 742.1
Hydromphalus (congenital) (since birth) 757.39
Hydromyelia 742.53
Hydromyelocele — see also Spina bifida 741.9 ☑
Hydronephrosis 591
  atrophic 591
  congenital 753.29
  due to S. hematobium 120.0
  early 591
  functionless (infected) 591
  infected 591
  intermittent 591
  primary 591
  secondary 591
  tuberculous (see also Tuberculosis) 016.0 ☑
Hydropericarditis — see also Pericarditis 423.9
Hydropericardium — see also Pericarditis 423.9
Hydroperitoneum 789.59
Hydrophobia 071
Hydrophthalmos — see also Buphthalmia 743.20
Hydropneumohemothorax — see also Hemothorax 511.89
Hydropneumopericarditis — see also Pericarditis 423.9

Hydropneumopericardium — see also Pericarditis 423.9
Hydropneumothorax 511.89
  nontuberculous 511.89
    bacterial 511.1
    pneumococcal 511.1
    staphylococcal 511.1
    streptococcal 511.1
  traumatic 860.0
    with open wound into thorax 860.1
  tuberculous (see also Tuberculosis, pleura) 012.0 ☑
Hydrops 782.3
  abdominis 789.59
  amnii (complicating pregnancy) (see also Hydramnios) 657.0 ☑
  articulorum intermittens (see also Rheumatism, palindromic) 719.3 ☑
  cardiac (see also Failure, heart) 428.0
  congenital — see Hydrops, fetalis
  endolymphatic (see also Disease, Ménière's) 386.00
  fetal, fetalis or newborn 778.0
    due to
      alpha thalassemia 282.43
      isoimmunization 773.3
    not due to isoimmunization 778.0
  gallbladder 575.3
  idiopathic (fetus or newborn) 778.0
  joint (see also Effusion, joint) 719.0 ☑
  labyrinth (see also Disease, Ménière's) 386.00
  meningeal NEC 331.4
  nutritional 262
  pericardium — see Pericarditis
  pleura (see also Hydrothorax) 511.89
  renal (see also Nephrosis) 581.9
  spermatic cord (see also Hydrocele) 603.9
Hydropyonephrosis — see also Pyelitis 590.80
  chronic 590.00
Hydrorachis 742.53
Hydrorrhea (nasal) 478.19
  gravidarum 658.1 ☑
  pregnancy 658.1 ☑
Hydrosadenitis 705.83
Hydrosalpinx (fallopian tube) (follicularis) 614.1
Hydrothorax (double) (pleural) 511.89
  chylous (nonfilarial) 457.8
    filaria (see also Infestation, filarial) 125.9
  nontuberculous 511.89
    bacterial 511.1
    pneumococcal 511.1
    staphylococcal 511.1
    streptococcal 511.1
  traumatic 862.29
    with open wound into thorax 862.39
  tuberculous (see also Tuberculosis, pleura) 012.0 ☑
Hydroureter 593.5
  congenital 753.22
Hydroureteronephrosis — see also Hydronephrosis 591
Hydrourethra 599.84
Hydroxykynureninuria 270.2
Hydroxyprolinemia 270.8
Hydroxyprolinuria 270.8
Hygroma (congenital) (cystic) (M9173/0) 228.1
  prepatellar 727.3
  subdural — see Hematoma, subdural
Hymen — see condition
Hymenolepiasis (diminuta) (infection) (infestation) (nana) 123.6
Hymenolepsis (diminuta) (infection) (infestation) (nana) 123.6
Hypalgesia — see also Disturbance, sensation 782.0
Hyper-TBG-nemia 246.8
Hyperabduction syndrome 447.8
Hyperacidity, gastric 536.8
  psychogenic 306.4
Hyperactive, hyperactivity 314.01
  basal cell, uterine cervix 622.10
  bladder 596.51
  bowel (syndrome) 564.9
    sounds 787.5
  cervix epithelial (basal) 622.10

Hyperactive, hyperactivity — continued
  child 314.01
  colon 564.9
  gastrointestinal 536.8
    psychogenic 306.4
  intestine 564.9
  labyrinth (unilateral) 386.51
    with loss of labyrinthine reactivity 386.58
    bilateral 386.52
  nasal mucous membrane 478.19
  stomach 536.8
  thyroid (gland) (see also Thyrotoxicosis) 242.9 ☑
Hyperacusis 388.42
Hyperadrenalism (cortical) 255.3
  medullary 255.6
Hyperadrenocorticism 255.3
  congenital 255.2
  iatrogenic
    correct substance properly administered 255.3
    overdose or wrong substance given or taken 962.0
Hyperaffectivity 301.11
Hyperaldosteronism (atypical) (hyperplastic) (normoaldosteronal) (normotensive) (primary) 255.10
  secondary 255.14
Hyperalgesia — see also Disturbance, sensation 782.0
Hyperalimentation 783.6
  carotene 278.3
  specified NEC 278.8
  vitamin A 278.2
  vitamin D 278.4
Hyperaminoaciduria 270.9
  arginine 270.6
  citrulline 270.6
  cystine 270.0
  glycine 270.0
  lysine 270.7
  ornithine 270.6
  renal (types I, II, III) 270.0
Hyperammonemia (congenital) 270.6
Hyperamnesia 780.99
Hyperamylasemia 790.5
Hyperaphia 782.0
Hyperazotemia 791.9
Hyperbetalipoproteinemia (acquired) (essential) (familial) (hereditary) (primary) (secondary) 272.0
  with prebetalipoproteinemia 272.2
Hyperbilirubinemia 782.4
  congenital 277.4
  constitutional 277.4
  neonatal (transient) (see also Jaundice, fetus or newborn) 774.6
  of prematurity 774.2
Hyperbilirubinemica encephalopathia, newborn 774.7
  due to isoimmunization 773.4
Hypercalcemia, hypercalcemic (idiopathic) 275.42
  nephropathy 588.89
Hypercalciuria 275.40
Hypercapnia 786.09
  with mixed acid-based disorder 276.4
  fetal, affecting newborn 770.89
Hypercarotinemia 278.3
Hypercementosis 521.5
Hyperchloremia 276.9
Hyperchlorhydria 536.8
  neurotic 306.4
  psychogenic 306.4
Hypercholesterinemia — see Hypercholesterolemia
Hypercholesterolemia 272.0
  with hyperglyceridemia, endogenous 272.2
  essential 272.0
  familial 272.0
  hereditary 272.0
  primary 272.0
  pure 272.0
Hypercholesterolosis 272.0
Hyperchylia gastrica 536.8
  psychogenic 306.4

Hyperchylomicronemia (familial) (with hyperbetalipoproteinemia) 272.3
Hypercoagulation syndrome (primary) 289.81
  secondary 289.82
Hypercorticosteronism
  correct substance properly administered 255.3
  overdose or wrong substance given or taken 962.0
Hypercortisonism
  correct substance properly administered 255.3
  overdose or wrong substance given or taken 962.0
Hyperdynamic beta-adrenergic state or syndrome (circulatory) 429.82
Hyperekplexia 759.89
Hyperelectrolytemia 276.9
Hyperemesis 536.2
  arising during pregnancy — see Hyperemesis, gravidarum
  gravidarum (mild) (before 22 completed weeks gestation) 643.0 ☑
    with
      carbohydrate depletion 643.1 ☑
      dehydration 643.1 ☑
      electrolyte imbalance 643.1 ☑
      metabolic disturbance 643.1 ☑
    affecting fetus or newborn 761.8
    severe (with metabolic disturbance) 643.1 ☑
  psychogenic 306.4
Hyperemia (acute) 780.99
  anal mucosa 569.49
  bladder 596.7
  cerebral 437.8
  conjunctiva 372.71
  ear, internal, acute 386.30
  enteric 564.89
  eye 372.71
  eyelid (active) (passive) 374.82
  intestine 564.89
  iris 364.41
  kidney 593.81
  labyrinth 386.30
  liver (active) (passive) 573.8
  lung 514
  ovary 620.8
  passive 780.99
  pulmonary 514
  renal 593.81
  retina 362.89
  spleen 289.59
  stomach 537.89
Hyperesthesia (body surface) — see also Disturbance, sensation 782.0
  larynx (reflex) 478.79
    hysterical 300.11
  pharynx (reflex) 478.29
Hyperestrinism 256.0
Hyperestrogenism 256.0
Hyperestrogenosis 256.0
Hyperexplexia 759.89
Hyperextension, joint 718.80
  ankle 718.87
  elbow 718.82
  foot 718.87
  hand 718.84
  hip 718.85
  knee 718.86
  multiple sites 718.89
  pelvic region 718.85
  shoulder (region) 718.81
  specified site NEC 718.88
  wrist 718.83
Hyperfibrinolysis — see Fibrinolysis
Hyperfolliculinism 256.0
Hyperfructosemia 271.2
Hyperfunction
  adrenal (cortex) 255.3
    androgenic, acquired benign 255.3
    medulla 255.6
    virilism 255.2
  corticoadrenal NEC 255.3
  labyrinth — see Hyperactive, labyrinth
  medulloadrenal 255.6

☑ Additional Digit Required — Refer to the Tabular List for Digit Selection   Subterms under main terms may continue to next column or page

2014 ICD-9-CM   ▶◀ Revised Text   ● New Line   ▲ Revised Code   Volume 2 — 143

Hyperfunction — *continued*
- ovary 256.1
  - estrogen 256.0
- pancreas 577.8
- parathyroid (gland) 252.00
- pituitary (anterior) (gland) (lobe) 253.1
- testicular 257.0

Hypergammaglobulinemia 289.89
- monoclonal, benign (BMH) 273.1
- polyclonal 273.0
- Waldenström's 273.0

Hyperglobulinemia 273.8

Hyperglycemia 790.29
- maternal
  - affecting fetus or newborn 775.0
  - manifest diabetes in infant 775.1
- postpancreatectomy (complete) (partial) 251.3

Hyperglyceridemia 272.1
- endogenous 272.1
- essential 272.1
- familial 272.1
- hereditary 272.1
- mixed 272.3
- pure 272.1

Hyperglycinemia 270.7

Hypergonadism
- ovarian 256.1
- testicular (infantile) (primary) 257.0

Hyperheparinemia — *see also* Circulating, intrinsic anticoagulants 287.5

Hyperhidrosis, hyperidrosis 705.21
- axilla 705.21
- face 705.21
- focal (localized) 705.21
  - primary 705.21
    - axilla 705.21
    - face 705.21
    - palms 705.21
    - soles 705.21
  - secondary 705.22
    - axilla 705.22
    - face 705.22
    - palms 705.22
    - soles 705.22
- generalized 780.8
- palms 705.21
- psychogenic 306.3
- secondary 780.8
- soles 705.21

Hyperhistidinemia 270.5

Hyperinsulinism (ectopic) (functional) (organic) NEC 251.1
- iatrogenic 251.0
- reactive 251.2
- spontaneous 251.2
- therapeutic misadventure (from administration of insulin) 962.3

Hyperiodemia 276.9

Hyperirritability (cerebral), in newborn 779.1

Hyperkalemia 276.7

Hyperkeratosis — *see also* Keratosis 701.1
- cervix 622.2
- congenital 757.39
- cornea 371.89
- due to yaws (early) (late) (palmar or plantar) 102.3
- eccentrica 757.39
- figurata centrifuga atrophica 757.39
- follicularis 757.39
  - in cutem penetrans 701.1
- limbic (cornea) 371.89
- palmoplantaris climacterica 701.1
- pinta (carate) 103.1
- senile (with pruritus) 702.0
- tongue 528.79
- universalis congenita 757.1
- vagina 623.1
- vocal cord 478.5
- vulva 624.09

Hyperkinesia, hyperkinetic (disease) (reaction) (syndrome) 314.9
- with
  - attention deficit — *see* Disorder, attention deficit
    - conduct disorder 314.2

Hyperkinesia, hyperkinetic — *continued*
- with — *continued*
  - developmental delay 314.1
  - simple disturbance of activity and attention 314.01
  - specified manifestation NEC 314.8
- heart (disease) 429.82
- of childhood or adolescence NEC 314.9

Hyperlacrimation — *see also* Epiphora 375.20

Hyperlipemia — *see also* Hyperlipidemia 272.4

Hyperlipidemia 272.4
- carbohydrate-induced 272.1
- combined 272.2
- endogenous 272.1
- exogenous 272.3
- fat-induced 272.3
- group
  - A 272.0
  - B 272.1
  - C 272.2
  - D 272.3
- mixed 272.2
- specified type NEC 272.4

Hyperlipidosis 272.7
- hereditary 272.7

Hyperlipoproteinemia (acquired) (essential) (familial) (hereditary) (primary) (secondary) 272.4
- Fredrickson type
  - I 272.3
  - IIa 272.0
  - IIb 272.2
  - III 272.2
  - IV 272.1
  - V 272.3
- low-density-lipoid-type (LDL) 272.0
- very-low-density-lipoid-type (VLDL) 272.1

Hyperlucent lung, unilateral 492.8

Hyperluteinization 256.1

Hyperlysinemia 270.7

Hypermagnesemia 275.2
- neonatal 775.5

Hypermaturity (fetus or newborn)
- post-term infant 766.21
- prolonged gestation infant 766.22

Hypermenorrhea 626.2

Hypermetabolism 794.7

Hypermethioninemia 270.4

Hypermetropia (congenital) 367.0

Hypermobility
- cecum 564.9
- coccyx 724.71
- colon 564.9
  - psychogenic 306.4
- ileum 564.89
- joint (acquired) 718.80
  - ankle 718.87
  - elbow 718.82
  - foot 718.87
  - hand 718.84
  - hip 718.85
  - knee 718.86
  - multiple sites 718.89
  - pelvic region 718.85
  - shoulder (region) 718.81
  - specified site NEC 718.88
  - wrist 718.83
- kidney, congenital 753.3
- meniscus (knee) 717.5
- scapula 718.81
- stomach 536.8
  - psychogenic 306.4
- syndrome 728.5
- testis, congenital 752.52
- urethral 599.81

Hypermotility
- gastrointestinal 536.8
- intestine 564.9
  - psychogenic 306.4
- stomach 536.8

Hypernasality 784.43

Hypernatremia 276.0
- with water depletion 276.0

Hypernephroma (M8312/3) 189.0

Hyperopia 367.0

Hyperorexia 783.6

Hyperornithinemia 270.6

Hyperosmia — *see also* Disturbance, sensation 781.1

Hyperosmolality 276.0

Hyperosteogenesis 733.99

Hyperostosis 733.99
- calvarial 733.3
- cortical 733.3
  - infantile 756.59
- frontal, internal of skull 733.3
- interna frontalis 733.3
- monomelic 733.99
- skull 733.3
  - congenital 756.0
- vertebral 733.99
  - with spondylosis — *see* Spondylosis
  - ankylosing 721.6

Hyperovarianism 256.1

Hyperovarism, hyperovaria 256.1

Hyperoxaluria (primary) 271.8

Hyperoxia 987.8

Hyperparathyroidism 252.00
- ectopic 259.3
- other 252.08
- primary 252.01
- secondary (of renal origin) 588.81
  - non-renal 252.02
- tertiary 252.08

Hyperpathia — *see also* Disturbance, sensation 782.0
- psychogenic 307.80

Hyperperistalsis 787.4
- psychogenic 306.4

Hyperpermeability, capillary 448.9

Hyperphagia 783.6

Hyperphenylalaninemia 270.1

Hyperphoria 378.40
- alternating 378.45

Hyperphosphatemia 275.3

Hyperpiesia — *see also* Hypertension 401.9

Hyperpiesis — *see also* Hypertension 401.9

Hyperpigmentation — *see* Pigmentation

Hyperpinealism 259.8

Hyperpipecolatemia 270.7

Hyperpituitarism 253.1

Hyperplasia, hyperplastic
- adenoids (lymphoid tissue) 474.12
  - and tonsils 474.10
- adrenal (capsule) (cortex) (gland) 255.8
  - with
    - sexual precocity (male) 255.2
    - virilism, adrenal 255.2
    - virilization (female) 255.2
  - congenital 255.2
  - due to excess ACTH (ectopic) (pituitary) 255.0
  - medulla 255.8
- alpha cells (pancreatic)
  - with
    - gastrin excess 251.5
    - glucagon excess 251.4
- angiolymphoid, with eosinophilia (ALHE) 228.01
- appendix (lymphoid) 543.0
- artery, fibromuscular NEC 447.8
  - carotid 447.8
  - renal 447.3
- bone 733.99
  - marrow 289.9
- breast (*see also* Hypertrophy, breast) 611.1
  - ductal 610.8
    - atypical 610.8
- carotid artery 447.8
- cementation, cementum (teeth) (tooth) 521.5
- cervical gland 785.6
- cervix (uteri) 622.10
  - basal cell 622.10
  - congenital 752.49
  - endometrium 622.10
  - polypoid 622.10
- chin 524.05
- clitoris, congenital 752.49
- dentin 521.5
- endocervicitis 616.0

Hyperplasia, hyperplastic — *continued*
- endometrium, endometrial (adenomatous) (atypical) (cystic) (glandular) (polypoid) (uterus) 621.30
  - with atypia 621.33
  - without atypia
    - complex 621.32
    - simple 621.31
  - benign 621.34
  - cervix 622.10
- epithelial 709.8
  - focal, oral, including tongue 528.79
  - mouth (focal) 528.79
  - nipple 611.89
  - skin 709.8
  - tongue (focal) 528.79
  - vaginal wall 623.0
- erythroid 289.9
- fascialis ossificans (progressiva) 728.11
- fibromuscular, artery NEC 447.8
  - carotid 447.8
  - renal 447.3
- genital
  - female 629.89
  - male 608.89
- gingiva 523.8
- glandularis
  - cystica uteri 621.30
  - endometrium (uterus) 621.30
  - interstitialis uteri 621.30
- granulocytic 288.69
- gum 523.8
- hymen, congenital 752.49
- islands of Langerhans 251.1
- islet cell (pancreatic) 251.9
  - alpha cells
    - with excess
      - gastrin 251.5
      - glucagon 251.4
    - beta cells 251.1
- juxtaglomerular (complex) (kidney) 593.89
- kidney (congenital) 753.3
- liver (congenital) 751.69
- lymph node (gland) 785.6
- lymphoid (diffuse) (nodular) 785.6
  - appendix 543.0
  - intestine 569.89
- mandibular 524.02
  - alveolar 524.72
  - unilateral condylar 526.89
- Marchand multiple nodular (liver) — *see* Cirrhosis, postnecrotic
- maxillary 524.01
  - alveolar 524.71
- medulla, adrenal 255.8
- myometrium, myometrial 621.2
- neuroendocrine cell, of infancy 516.61
- nose (lymphoid) (polypoid) 478.19
- oral soft tissue (inflammatory) (irritative) (mucosa) NEC 528.9
  - gingiva 523.8
  - tongue 529.8
- organ or site, congenital NEC — *see* Anomaly, specified type NEC
- ovary 620.8
- palate, papillary 528.9
- pancreatic islet cells 251.9
  - alpha
    - with excess
      - gastrin 251.5
      - glucagon 251.4
  - beta 251.1
- parathyroid (gland) 252.01
- persistent, vitreous (primary) 743.51
- pharynx (lymphoid) 478.29
- prostate 600.90
  - with
    - other lower urinary tract symptoms (LUTS) 600.91
    - urinary
      - obstruction 600.91
      - retention 600.91
  - adenofibromatous 600.20
    - with
      - other lower urinary tract symptoms (LUTS) 600.21

Index

Hyperfunction — Hyperplasia, hyperplastic

Hyperplasia, hyperplastic — *continued*
  prostate — *continued*
    adenofibromatous — *continued*
      with — *continued*
        urinary
          obstruction 600.21
          retention 600.21
      nodular 600.10
        with
          urinary
            obstruction 600.11
            retention 600.11
  renal artery (fibromuscular) 447.3
  reticuloendothelial (cell) 289.9
  salivary gland (any) 527.1
  Schimmelbusch's 610.1
  suprarenal (capsule) (gland) 255.8
  thymus (gland) (persistent) 254.0
  thyroid (*see also* Goiter) 240.9
    primary 242.0 ☑
    secondary 242.2 ☑
  tonsil (lymphoid tissue) 474.11
    and adenoids 474.10
  urethrovaginal 599.89
  uterus, uterine (myometrium) 621.2
    endometrium (*see also* Hyperplasia, en-
      dometrium) 621.30
  vitreous (humor), primary persistent 743.51
  vulva 624.3
  zygoma 738.11
Hyperpnea — *see also* Hyperventilation 786.01
Hyperpotassemia 276.7
Hyperprebetalipoproteinemia 272.1
  with chylomicronemia 272.3
  familial 272.1

Hyperprolactinemia 253.1
Hyperprolinemia 270.8
Hyperproteinemia 273.8
Hyperprothrombinemia 289.89
Hyperpselaphesia 782.0
Hyperpyrexia 780.60
  heat (effects of) 992.0
  malarial (*see also* Malaria) 084.6
  malignant, due to anesthetic 995.86
  rheumatic — *see* Fever, rheumatic
  unknown origin (*see also* Pyrexia) 780.60
Hyperreactor, vascular 780.2
Hyperreflexia 796.1
  bladder, autonomic 596.54
    with cauda equina 344.61
  detrusor 344.61
Hypersalivation — *see also* Ptyalism 527.7
Hypersarcosinemia 270.8
Hypersecretion
  ACTH 255.3
  androgens (ovarian) 256.1
  calcitonin 246.0
  corticoadrenal 255.3
  cortisol 255.0
  estrogen 256.0
  gastric 536.8
    psychogenic 306.4
  gastrin 251.5
  glucagon 251.4
  hormone
    ACTH 255.3
    anterior pituitary 253.1
    growth NEC 253.0
    ovarian androgen 256.1
    testicular 257.0

Hypersecretion — *continued*
  hormone — *continued*
    thyroid stimulating 242.8 ☑
  insulin — *see* Hyperinsulinism
  lacrimal glands (*see also* Epiphora) 375.20
  medulloadrenal 255.6
  milk 676.6 ☑
  ovarian androgens 256.1
  pituitary (anterior) 253.1
  salivary gland (any) 527.7
  testicular hormones 257.0
  thyrocalcitonin 246.0
  upper respiratory 478.9
Hypersegmentation, hereditary 288.2
  eosinophils 288.2
  neutrophil nuclei 288.2
Hypersensitive, hypersensitiveness, hyper-
  sensitivity — *see also* Allergy
  angiitis 446.20
    specified NEC 446.29
  carotid sinus 337.01
  colon 564.9
    psychogenic 306.4
  DNA (deoxyribonucleic acid) NEC 287.2
  drug (*see also* Allergy, drug) 995.27
  due to correct medical substance properly
    administered 995.27
  esophagus 530.89
  insect bites — *see* Injury, superficial, by site
  labyrinth 386.58
  pain (*see also* Disturbance, sensation) 782.0
  pneumonitis NEC 495.9
  reaction (*see also* Allergy) 995.3
    upper respiratory tract NEC 478.8
  stomach (allergic) (nonallergic) 536.8

Hypersensitive, hypersensitiveness,
  hypersensitivity — *see also* Allergy —
  continued
  stomach — *continued*
    psychogenic 306.4
Hypersomatotropism (classic) 253.0
Hypersomnia, unspecified 780.54
  with sleep apnea, unspecified 780.53
  alcohol induced 291.82
  drug induced 292.85
  due to
    medical condition classified elsewhere
      327.14
    mental disorder 327.15
  idiopathic
    with long sleep time 327.11
    without long sleep time 327.12
  menstrual related 327.13
  nonorganic origin 307.43
    persistent (primary) 307.44
    transient 307.43
  organic 327.10
    other 327.19
  primary 307.44
  recurrent 327.13
Hypersplenia 289.4
Hypersplenism 289.4
Hypersteatosis 706.3
Hyperstimulation, ovarian 256.1
Hypersuprarenalism 255.3
Hypersusceptibility — *see* Allergy
Hypertelorism 756.0
  orbit, orbital 376.41

☑ **Additional Digit Required** — **Refer to the Tabular List for Digit Selection**　　　　　　　　　　▽ **Subterms under main terms may continue to next column or page**

2014 ICD-9-CM　　　　　▶◀ **Revised Text**　　　●　**New Line**　　　▲　**Revised Code**　　　　**Volume 2 — 145**

	Malignant	Benign	Unspecified
Hypertension, hypertensive (arterial) (arteriolar) (crisis) (degeneration) (disease) (essential) (fluctuating) (idiopathic) (intermittent) (labile) (low renin) (orthostatic) (paroxysmal) (primary) (systemic) (uncontrolled) (vascular)	401.0	401.1	401.9
with			
chronic kidney disease			
stage I through stage IV, or unspecified	403.00	403.10	403.90
stage V or end stage renal disese	403.01	403.11	403.91
heart involvement (conditions classifiable to 429.0–429.3, 429.8, 429.9 due to hypertension) (see also Hypertension, heart)	402.00	402.10	402.90
with kidney involvement — see Hypertension, cardiorenal			
renal (kidney) involvement (only conditions classifiable to 585, 587) (excludes conditions classifiable to 584) (see also Hypertension, kidney)	403.00	403.10	403.90
with heart involvement — see Hypertension, cardiorenal			
failure (and sclerosis) (see also Hypertension, kidney)	403.01	403.11	403.91
sclerosis without failure (see also Hypertension, kidney)	403.00	403.10	403.90
accelerated (see also Hypertension, by type, malignant))	401.0	—	—
antepartum — see Hypertension, complicating pregnancy, childbirth, or the puerperium			
borderline	—	—	796.2
cardiorenal (disease)	404.00	404.10	404.90
with			
chronic kidney disease			
stage I through stage IV, or unspecified	404.00	404.10	404.90
and heart failure	404.01	404.11	404.91
stage V or end stage renal disease	404.02	404.12	404.92
and heart failure	404.03	404.13	404.93
heart failure	404.01	404.11	404.91
and chronic kidney disease	404.01	404.11	404.91
stage I through stage IV or unspecified	404.01	404.11	404.91
stave V or end stage renal disease	404.03	404.13	404.93
cardiovascular disease (arteriosclerotic) (sclerotic)	402.00	402.10	402.90
with			
heart failure	402.01	402.11	402.91
renal involvement (conditions classifiable to 403) (see also Hypertension, cardiorenal)	404.00	404.10	404.90
cardiovascular renal (disease) (sclerosis) (see also Hypertension, cardiorenal)	404.00	404.10	404.90
cerebrovascular disease NEC	437.2	—	—
complicating pregnancy, childbirth, or the puerperium	642.2	642.0	642.9
with			
albuminuria (and edema) (mild)	—	—	642.4
severe	—	—	642.5
chronic kidney disease	642.2	—	—
and heart disease	642.2	—	—
edema (mild)	—	—	642.4
severe	—	—	642.5
heart disease	642.2	—	—
and chronic kidney disease	642.2	—	—
renal disease	642.2	—	—
and heart disease	642.2	—	—
chronic	642.2	642.0	—
with pre-eclampsia or eclampsia	642.7	—	—
fetus or newborn	760.0	—	—
essential	—	642.0	—
with pre-eclampsia or eclampsia	—	642.7	—
fetus or newborn	760.0	—	—
fetus or newborn	760.0	—	—
gestational	—	—	642.3
pre-existing	642.2	642.0	—
with pre-eclampsia or eclampsia	642.7	—	—
fetus or newborn	760.0	—	—
secondary to renal disease	642.1	—	—
with pre-eclampsia or eclampsia	642.7	—	—
fetus or newborn	760.0	—	—
transient	—	—	642.3
due to			
aldosteronism, primary	405.09	405.19	405.99
brain tumor	405.09	405.19	405.99
bulbar poliomyelitis	405.09	405.19	405.99
calculus			
kidney	405.09	405.19	405.99

	Malignant	Benign	Unspecified
Hypertension, hypertensive — continued			
due to — continued			
calculus — continued			
ureter	405.09	405.19	405.99
coarctation, aorta	405.09	405.19	405.99
Cushing's disease	405.09	405.19	405.99
glomerulosclerosis (see also Hypertension, kidney)	403.00	403.10	403.90
periarteritis nodosa	405.09	405.19	405.99
pheochromocytoma	405.09	405.19	405.99
polycystic kidney(s)	405.09	405.19	405.99
polycythemia	405.09	405.19	405.99
porphyria	405.09	405.19	405.99
pyelonephritis	405.09	405.19	405.99
renal (artery)			
aneurysm	405.01	405.11	405.91
anomaly	405.01	405.11	405.91
embolism	405.01	405.11	405.91
fibromuscular hyperplasia	405.01	405.11	405.91
occlusion	405.01	405.11	405.91
stenosis	405.01	405.11	405.91
thrombosis	405.01	405.11	405.91
encephalopathy	437.2	—	—
gestational (transient) NEC	—	—	642.3
Goldblatt's	440.1	—	—
heart (disease) (conditions classifiable to 429.0–429.3, 429.8, 429.9 due to hypertension)	402.00	402.10	402.90
with heart failure	402.01	402.11	402.91
hypertensive kidney disease (conditions classifiable to 403) (see also Hypertension, cardiorenal)	404.00	404.10	404.90
renal sclerosis (see also Hypertension, cardiorenal)	404.00	404.10	404.90
intracranial, benign	—	348.2	—
intraocular	—	—	365.04
kidney	403.00	403.10	403.90
with			
chronic kidney disease			
stage I through stage IV, or unspecified	403.00	403.10	403.90
stage V or end stage renal disese	403.01	403.11	403.91
heart involvement (conditions classifiable to 429.0–429.3, 429.8, 429.9 due to hypertension) (see also Hypertension, cardiorenal)	404.00	404.10	404.90
hypertensive heart (disease) (conditions classifiable to 402) (see also Hypertension, cardiorenal)	404.00	404.10	404.90
lesser circulation	—	—	416.0
necrotizing	401.0	—	—
ocular	—	—	365.04
pancreatic duct — code to underlying condition			
with			
chronic pancreatitis	—	—	577.1
portal (due to chronic liver disease)	—	—	572.3
postoperative	—	—	997.91
psychogenic	—	—	306.2
puerperal, postpartum — see Hypertension, complicating pregnancy, childbirth, or the puerperium			
pulmonary (artery) (secondary)	—	—	416.8
with			
cor pulmonale (chronic)	—	—	416.8
acute	—	—	415.0
right heart ventricular strain/failure	—	—	416.8
acute	—	—	415.0
idiopathic	—	—	416.0
primary	—	—	416.0
of newborn	—	—	747.83
secondary	—	—	416.8
renal (disease) (see also Hypertension, kidney)	403.00	403.10	403.90
renovascular NEC	405.01	405.11	405.91
secondary NEC	405.09	405.19	405.99
due to			
aldosteronism, primary	405.09	405.19	405.99
brain tumor	405.09	405.19	405.99
bulbar poliomyelitis	405.09	405.19	405.99
calculus			
kidney	405.09	405.19	405.99
ureter	405.09	405.19	405.99
coarctation, aorta	405.09	405.19	405.99
Cushing's disease	405.09	405.19	405.99
glomerulosclerosis (see also Hypertension, kidney)	403.00	403.10	403.90

☑ **Additional Digit Required — Refer to the Tabular List for Digit Selection**   ▼ **Subterms under main terms may continue to next column or page**

	Malignant	Benign	Unspecified
Hypertension, hypertensive — *continued*			
secondary — *continued*			
due to — *continued*			
periarteritis nodosa	405.09	405.19	405.99
pheochromocytoma	405.09	405.19	405.99
polycystic kidney(s)	405.09	405.19	405.99
polycythemia	405.09	405.19	405.99
porphyria	405.09	405.19	405.99
pyelonephritis	405.09	405.19	405.99
renal (artery)			
aneurysm	405.01	405.11	405.91
anomaly	405.01	405.11	405.91
embolism	405.01	405.11	405.91
fibromuscular hyperplasia	405.01	405.11	405.91
occlusion	405.01	405.11	405.91
stenosis	405.01	405.11	405.91
thrombosis	405.01	405.11	405.91
transient	—	—	796.2
of pregnancy	—	—	642.3
vascular degeneration	401.0	401.1	401.9
venous, chronic (asymptomatic) (idiopathic)	—	—	459.30
with			
complication, NEC	—	—	459.39
inflammation	—	—	459.32
with ulcer	—	—	459.33
ulcer	—	—	459.31
with inflammation	—	—	459.33
due to			
deep vein thrombosis (*see also* Syndrome, postphlebetic)	—	—	459.10

☑ **Additional Digit Required — Refer to the Tabular List for Digit Selection**   ▽ **Subterms under main terms may continue to next column or page**

2014 ICD-9-CM   ▶◀ **Revised Text**   ● **New Line**   ▲ **Revised Code**   **Volume 2 — 147**

Hypertensive urgency — see Hypertension
Hyperthecosis, ovary 256.8
Hyperthermia (of unknown origin) — see also
    Pyrexia 780.60
    malignant (due to anesthesia) 995.86
    newborn 778.4
Hyperthymergasia — see also Psychosis, affec-
    tive 296.0 ☑
    reactive (from emotional stress, psycholog-
      ical trauma) 298.1
    recurrent episode 296.1 ☑
    single episode 296.0 ☑
Hyperthymism 254.8
Hyperthyroid (recurrent) — see Hyperthy-
    roidism
Hyperthyroidism (latent) (preadult) (recurrent)
    (without goiter) 242.9 ☑

> Note — Use the following fifth-digit
> subclassification with category 242:
>
> 0   without mention of thyrotoxic
>   crisis or storm
>
> 1   with mention of thyrotoxic crisis
>   or storm

    with
      goiter (diffuse) 242.0 ☑
        adenomatous 242.3 ☑
          multinodular 242.2 ☑
          uninodular 242.1 ☑
        nodular 242.3 ☑
          multinodular 242.2 ☑
          uninodular 242.1 ☑
      thyroid nodule 242.1 ☑
    complicating pregnancy, childbirth, or
      puerperium 648.1 ☑
    neonatal (transient) 775.3
Hypertonia — see Hypertonicity
Hypertonicity
    bladder 596.51
    fetus or newborn 779.89
    gastrointestinal (tract) 536.8
    infancy 779.89
      due to electrolyte imbalance 779.89
    muscle 728.85
    stomach 536.8
      psychogenic 306.4
    uterus, uterine (contractions) 661.4 ☑
      affecting fetus or newborn 763.7
Hypertony — see Hypertonicity
Hypertransaminemia 790.4
Hypertrichosis 704.1
    congenital 757.4
    eyelid 374.54
    lanuginosa 757.4
      acquired 704.1
Hypertriglyceridemia, essential 272.1
Hypertrophy, hypertrophic
    adenoids (infectional) 474.12
      and tonsils (faucial) (infective) (lingual)
        (lymphoid) 474.10
    adrenal 255.8
    alveolar process or ridge 525.8
    anal papillae 569.49
    apocrine gland 705.82
    artery NEC 447.8
      carotid 447.8
      congenital (peripheral) NEC 747.60
        gastrointestinal 747.61
        lower limb 747.64
        renal 747.62
        specified NEC 747.69
        spinal 747.82
        upper limb 747.63
      renal 447.3
    arthritis (chronic) (see also Osteoarthrosis)
      715.9 ☑
      spine (see also Spondylosis) 721.90
    arytenoid 478.79
    asymmetrical (heart) 429.9
    auricular — see Hypertrophy, cardiac
    Bartholin's gland 624.8
    bile duct 576.8
    bladder (sphincter) (trigone) 596.89
    blind spot, visual field 368.42
    bone 733.99

Hypertrophy, hypertrophic — continued
    brain 348.89
    breast 611.1
      cystic 610.1
      fetus or newborn 778.7
      fibrocystic 610.1
      massive pubertal 611.1
      puerperal, postpartum 676.3 ☑
      senile (parenchymatous) 611.1
    cardiac (chronic) (idiopathic) 429.3
      with
        rheumatic fever (conditions classifi-
          able to 390)
          active 391.8
            with chorea 392.0
          inactive or quiescent (with
            chorea) 398.99
      congenital NEC 746.89
      fatty (see also Degeneration, myocardial)
        429.1
      hypertensive (see also Hypertension,
        heart) 402.90
      rheumatic (with chorea) 398.99
        active or acute 391.8
          with chorea 392.0
      valve (see also Endocarditis) 424.90
        congenital NEC 746.89
    cartilage 733.99
    cecum 569.89
    cervix (uteri) 622.6
      congenital 752.49
      elongation 622.6
    clitoris (cirrhotic) 624.2
      congenital 752.49
    colon 569.89
      congenital 751.3
    conjunctiva, lymphoid 372.73
    cornea 371.89
    corpora cavernosa 607.89
    duodenum 537.89
    endometrium (uterus) (see also Hyperplasia,
      endometrium) 621.30
      cervix 622.6
    epididymis 608.89
    esophageal hiatus (congenital) 756.6
      with hernia — see Hernia, diaphragm
    eyelid 374.30
    falx, skull 733.99
    fat pad 729.30
      infrapatellar 729.31
      knee 729.31
      orbital 374.34
      popliteal 729.31
      prepatellar 729.31
      retropatellar 729.31
      specified site NEC 729.39
    foot (congenital) 755.67
    frenum, frenulum (tongue) 529.8
      linguae 529.8
      lip 528.5
    gallbladder or cystic duct 575.8
    gastric mucosa 535.2 ☑
    gingiva 523.8
    gland, glandular (general) NEC 785.6
    gum (mucous membrane) 523.8
    heart (idiopathic) (see also Hypertrophy,
      cardiac)
      valve (see also Endocarditis)
        congenital NEC 746.89
    hemifacial 754.0
    hepatic — see Hypertrophy, liver
    hiatus (esophageal) 756.6
    hilus gland 785.6
    hymen, congenital 752.49
    ileum 569.89
    infrapatellar fat pad 729.31
    intestine 569.89
    jejunum 569.89
    kidney (compensatory) 593.1
      congenital 753.3
    labial frenulum 528.5
    labium (majus) (minus) 624.3
    lacrimal gland, chronic 375.03
    ligament 728.9
      spinal 724.8
    linguae frenulum 529.8

Hypertrophy, hypertrophic — continued
    lingual tonsil (infectional) 474.11
    lip (frenum) 528.5
      congenital 744.81
    liver 789.1
      acute 573.8
      cirrhotic — see Cirrhosis, liver
      congenital 751.69
      fatty — see Fatty, liver
    lymph gland 785.6
      tuberculous — see Tuberculosis, lymph
        gland
    mammary gland — see Hypertrophy, breast
    maxillary frenulum 528.5
    Meckel's diverticulum (congenital) 751.0
    medial meniscus, acquired 717.3
    median bar 600.90
      with
        other lower urinary tract symptoms
          (LUTS) 600.91
        urinary
          obstruction 600.91
          retention 600.91
    mediastinum 519.3
    meibomian gland 373.2
    meniscus, knee, congenital 755.64
    metatarsal head 733.99
    metatarsus 733.99
    mouth 528.9
    mucous membrane
      alveolar process 523.8
      nose 478.19
      turbinate (nasal) 478.0
    muscle 728.9
    muscular coat, artery NEC 447.8
      carotid 447.8
      renal 447.3
    myocardium (see also Hypertrophy, cardiac)
      429.3
      idiopathic 425.18
    myometrium 621.2
    nail 703.8
      congenital 757.5
    nasal 478.19
      alae 478.19
      bone 738.0
      cartilage 478.19
      mucous membrane (septum) 478.19
      sinus (see also Sinusitis) 473.9
      turbinate 478.0
    nasopharynx, lymphoid (infectional) (tissue)
      (wall) 478.29
    neck, uterus 622.6
    nipple 611.1
    normal aperture diaphragm (congenital)
      756.6
    nose (see also Hypertrophy, nasal) 478.19
    orbit 376.46
    organ or site, congenital NEC — see
      Anomaly, specified type NEC
    osteoarthropathy (pulmonary) 731.2
    ovary 620.8
    palate (hard) 526.89
      soft 528.9
    pancreas (congenital) 751.7
    papillae
      anal 569.49
      tongue 529.3
    parathyroid (gland) 252.01
    parotid gland 527.1
    penis 607.89
    phallus 607.89
      female (clitoris) 624.2
    pharyngeal tonsil 474.12
    pharyngitis 472.1
    pharynx 478.29
      lymphoid (infectional) (tissue) (wall)
        478.29
    pituitary (fossa) (gland) 253.8
    popliteal fat pad 729.31
    preauricular (lymph) gland (Hampstead)
      785.6
    prepuce (congenital) 605
      female 624.2
    prostate (asymptomatic) (early) (recurrent)
      600.90

Hypertrophy, hypertrophic — continued
    prostate — continued
      with
        other lower urinary tract symptoms
          (LUTS) 600.91
        urinary
          obstruction 600.91
          retention 600.91
      adenofibromatous 600.20
        with
          other lower urinary tract symp-
            toms (LUTS) 600.21
          urinary
            obstruction 600.21
            retention 600.21
      benign 600.00
        with
          other lower urinary tract symp-
            toms (LUTS) 600.01
          urinary
            obstruction 600.01
            retention 600.01
      congenital 752.89
    pseudoedematous hypodermal 757.0
    pseudomuscular 359.1
    pylorus (muscle) (sphincter) 537.0
      congenital 750.5
      infantile 750.5
    rectal sphincter 569.49
    rectum 569.49
    renal 593.1
    rhinitis (turbinate) 472.0
    salivary duct or gland 527.1
      congenital 750.26
    scaphoid (tarsal) 733.99
    scar 701.4
    scrotum 608.89
    sella turcica 253.8
    seminal vesicle 608.89
    sigmoid 569.89
    skin condition NEC 701.9
    spermatic cord 608.89
    spinal ligament 724.8
    spleen — see Splenomegaly
    spondylitis (spine) (see also Spondylosis)
      721.90
    stomach 537.89
    subaortic stenosis (idiopathic) 425.11
    sublingual gland 527.1
      congenital 750.26
    submaxillary gland 527.1
    suprarenal (gland) 255.8
    tendon 727.9
    testis 608.89
      congenital 752.89
    thymic, thymus (congenital) (gland) 254.0
    thyroid (gland) (see also Goiter) 240.9
      primary 242.0 ☑
      secondary 242.2 ☑
    toe (congenital) 755.65
      acquired 735.8
    tongue 529.8
      congenital 750.15
      frenum 529.8
      papillae (foliate) 529.3
    tonsil (faucial) (infective) (lingual) (lym-
      phoid) 474.11
      with
        adenoiditis 474.01
        tonsillitis 474.00
          and adenoiditis 474.02
      and adenoids 474.10
    tunica vaginalis 608.89
    turbinate (mucous membrane) 478.0
    ureter 593.89
    urethra 599.84
    uterus 621.2
      puerperal, postpartum 674.8 ☑
    uvula 528.9
    vagina 623.8
    vas deferens 608.89
    vein 459.89
    ventricle, ventricular (heart) (left) (right) (see
      also Hypertrophy, cardiac)
      congenital 746.89

☑ **Additional Digit Required** — Refer to the Tabular List for Digit Selection   ᵂ **Subterms under main terms may continue to next column or page**

148 — Volume 2   ▶◀ **Revised Text**   ● **New Line**   ▲ **Revised Code**   **2014 ICD-9-CM**

Hypertrophy, hypertrophic — *continued*
  ventricle, ventricular (*see also* Hypertrophy, cardiac) — *continued*
    due to hypertension (left) (right) (*see also* Hypertension, heart) 402.90
      benign 402.10
      malignant 402.00
    right with ventricular septal defect, pulmonary stenosis or atresia, and dextraposition of aorta 745.2
  verumontanum 599.89
  vesical 596.89
  vocal cord 478.5
  vulva 624.3
    stasis (nonfilarial) 624.3
Hypertropia (intermittent) (periodic) 378.31
Hypertyrosinemia 270.2
Hyperuricemia 790.6
Hypervalinemia 270.3
Hyperventilation (tetany) 786.01
  hysterical 300.11
  psychogenic 306.1
  syndrome 306.1
Hyperviscidosis 277.00
Hyperviscosity (of serum) (syndrome) NEC 273.3
  polycythemic 289.0
  sclerocythemic 282.8
Hypervitaminosis (dietary) NEC 278.8
  A (dietary) 278.2
  D (dietary) 278.4
  from excessive administration or use of vitamin preparations (chronic) 278.8
    reaction to sudden overdose 963.5
    vitamin A 278.2
      reaction to sudden overdose 963.5
    vitamin D 278.4
      reaction to sudden overdose 963.5
    vitamin K
      correct substance properly administered 278.8
      overdose or wrong substance given or taken 964.3
Hypervolemia 276.69
Hypesthesia — *see also* Disturbance, sensation 782.0
  cornea 371.81
Hyphema (anterior chamber) (ciliary body) (iris) 364.41
  traumatic 921.3
Hyphemia — *see* Hyphema
Hypo-ovarianism 256.39
Hypo-ovarism 256.39
Hypo-TBG-nemia 246.8
Hypoacidity, gastric 536.8
  psychogenic 306.4
Hypoactive labyrinth (function) — *see* Hypofunction, labyrinth
Hypoadrenalism 255.41
  tuberculous (*see also* Tuberculosis) 017.6 ☑
Hypoadrenocorticism 255.41
  pituitary 253.4
Hypoalbuminemia 273.8
Hypoaldosteronism 255.42
Hypoalphalipoproteinemia 272.5
Hypobarism 993.2
Hypobaropathy 993.2
Hypobetalipoproteinemia (familial) 272.5
Hypocalcemia 275.41
  cow's milk 775.4
  dietary 269.3
  neonatal 775.4
  phosphate-loading 775.4
Hypocalcification, teeth 520.4
Hypochloremia 276.9
Hypochlorhydria 536.8
  neurotic 306.4
  psychogenic 306.4
Hypocholesteremia 272.5
Hypochondria (reaction) 300.7
Hypochondriac 300.7
Hypochondriasis 300.7
Hypochromasia blood cells 280.9
Hypochromic anemia 280.9
  due to blood loss (chronic) 280.0
    acute 285.1

Hypochromic anemia — *continued*
  microcytic 280.9
Hypocoagulability — *see also* Defect, coagulation 286.9
Hypocomplementemia 279.8
Hypocythemia (progressive) 284.9
Hypodontia — *see also* Anodontia 520.0
Hypoeosinophilia 288.59
Hypoesthesia — *see also* Disturbance, sensation 782.0
  cornea 371.81
  tactile 782.0
Hypoestrinism 256.39
Hypoestrogenism 256.39
Hypoferremia 280.9
  due to blood loss (chronic) 280.0
Hypofertility
  female 628.9
  male 606.1
Hypofibrinogenemia 286.3
  acquired 286.6
  congenital 286.3
Hypofunction
  adrenal (gland) 255.41
    cortex 255.41
    medulla 255.5
    specified NEC 255.5
  cerebral 331.9
  corticoadrenal NEC 255.41
  intestinal 564.89
  labyrinth (unilateral) 386.53
    with loss of labyrinthine reactivity 386.55
    bilateral 386.54
      with loss of labyrinthine reactivity 386.56
  Leydig cell 257.2
  ovary 256.39
    postablative 256.2
  pituitary (anterior) (gland) (lobe) 253.2
    posterior 253.5
  testicular 257.2
    iatrogenic 257.1
    postablative 257.1
    postirradiation 257.1
    postsurgical 257.1
Hypogammaglobulinemia 279.00
  acquired primary 279.06
  non-sex-linked, congenital 279.06
  sporadic 279.06
  transient of infancy 279.09
Hypogenitalism (congenital) (female) (male) 752.89
  penis 752.69
Hypoglycemia (spontaneous) 251.2
  coma 251.0
    diabetic 250.3 ☑
      due to secondary diabetes 249.3 ☑
  diabetic 250.8 ☑
    due to secondary diabetes 249.8 ☑
  due to insulin 251.0
    therapeutic misadventure 962.3
  familial (idiopathic) 251.2
  following gastrointestinal surgery 579.3
  infantile (idiopathic) 251.2
  in infant of diabetic mother 775.0
  leucine-induced 270.3
  neonatal 775.6
  reactive 251.2
  specified NEC 251.1
Hypoglycemic shock 251.0
  diabetic 250.8 ☑
    due to secondary diabetes 249.8 ☑
  due to insulin 251.0
  functional (syndrome) 251.1
Hypogonadism
  female 256.39
  gonadotrophic (isolated) 253.4
  hypogonadotropic (isolated) (with anosmia) 253.4
  isolated 253.4
  male 257.2
    hereditary familial (Reifenstein's syndrome) 259.52
  ovarian (primary) 256.39
  pituitary (secondary) 253.4
  testicular (primary) (secondary) 257.2

Hypohidrosis 705.0
Hypohidrotic ectodermal dysplasia 757.31
Hypoidrosis 705.0
Hypoinsulinemia, postsurgical 251.3
  postpancreatectomy (complete) (partial) 251.3
Hypokalemia 276.8
Hypokinesia 780.99
Hypoleukia splenica 289.4
Hypoleukocytosis 288.50
Hypolipidemia 272.5
Hypolipoproteinemia 272.5
Hypomagnesemia 275.2
  neonatal 775.4
Hypomania, hypomanic reaction — *see also* Psychosis, affective 296.0 ☑
  recurrent episode 296.1 ☑
  single episode 296.0 ☑
Hypomastia (congenital) 611.82
Hypomenorrhea 626.1
Hypometabolism 783.9
Hypomotility
  gastrointestinal tract 536.8
    psychogenic 306.4
  intestine 564.89
    psychogenic 306.4
  stomach 536.8
    psychogenic 306.4
Hyponasality 784.44
Hyponatremia 276.1
Hypoparathyroidism (idiopathic) (surgically induced) 252.1
  neonatal 775.4
Hypoperfusion (in)
  newborn 779.89
Hypopharyngitis 462
Hypophoria 378.40
Hypophosphatasia 275.3
Hypophosphatemia (acquired) (congenital) (familial) 275.3
  renal 275.3
Hypophyseal, hypophysis — *see also* condition
  dwarfism 253.3
  gigantism 253.0
  syndrome 253.8
Hypophyseothalamic syndrome 253.8
Hypopiesis — *see* Hypotension
Hypopigmentation 709.00
  eyelid 374.53
Hypopinealism 259.8
Hypopituitarism (juvenile) (syndrome) 253.2
  due to
    hormone therapy 253.7
    hypophysectomy 253.7
    radiotherapy 253.7
  postablative 253.7
  postpartum hemorrhage 253.2
Hypoplasia, hypoplasis 759.89
  adrenal (gland) 759.1
  alimentary tract 751.8
    lower 751.2
    upper 750.8
  angiolymphoid, with eosinophilia (ALHE) 228.01
  anus, anal (canal) 751.2
  aorta 747.22
  aortic
    arch (tubular) 747.10
    orifice or valve with hypoplasia of ascending aorta and defective development of left ventricle (with mitral valve atresia) 746.7
  appendix 751.2
  areola 757.6
  arm (*see also* Absence, arm, congenital) 755.20
  artery (congenital) (peripheral) 747.60
    brain 747.81
    cerebral 747.81
    coronary 746.85
    gastrointestinal 747.61
    lower limb 747.64
    pulmonary 747.31
    renal 747.62
    retinal 743.58

Hypoplasia, hypoplasis — *continued*
  artery — *continued*
    specified NEC 747.69
    spinal 747.82
    umbilical 747.5
    upper limb 747.63
  auditory canal 744.29
    causing impairment of hearing 744.02
  biliary duct (common) or passage 751.61
  bladder 753.8
  bone NEC 756.9
    face 756.0
    malar 756.0
    mandible 524.04
      alveolar 524.74
    marrow 284.9
      acquired (secondary) 284.89
      congenital 284.09
      idiopathic 284.9
    maxilla 524.03
      alveolar 524.73
    skull (*see also* Hypoplasia, skull) 756.0
  brain 742.1
    gyri 742.2
    specified part 742.2
  breast (areola) 611.82
  bronchus (tree) 748.3
  cardiac 746.89
    valve — *see* Hypoplasia, heart, valve
    vein 746.89
  carpus (*see also* Absence, carpal, congenital) 755.28
  cartilaginous 756.9
  cecum 751.2
  cementum 520.4
    hereditary 520.5
  cephalic 742.1
  cerebellum 742.2
  cervix (uteri) 752.43
  chin 524.06
  clavicle 755.51
  coccyx 756.19
  colon 751.2
  corpus callosum 742.2
  cricoid cartilage 748.3
  dermal, focal (Goltz) 757.39
  digestive organ(s) or tract NEC 751.8
    lower 751.2
    upper 750.8
  ear 744.29
    auricle 744.23
    lobe 744.29
    middle, except ossicles 744.03
      ossicles 744.04
    ossicles 744.04
  enamel of teeth (neonatal) (postnatal) (prenatal) 520.4
    hereditary 520.5
  endocrine (gland) NEC 759.2
  endometrium 621.8
  epididymis 752.89
  epiglottis 748.3
  erythroid, congenital 284.01
  erythropoietic, chronic acquired 284.81
  esophagus 750.3
  Eustachian tube 744.24
  eye (*see also* Microphthalmos) 743.10
    lid 743.62
  face 744.89
    bone(s) 756.0
  fallopian tube 752.19
  femur (*see also* Absence, femur, congenital) 755.34
  fibula (*see also* Absence, fibula, congenital) 755.37
  finger (*see also* Absence, finger, congenital) 755.29
  focal dermal 757.39
  foot 755.31
  gallbladder 751.69
  genitalia, genital organ(s)
    female 752.89
      external 752.49
      internal NEC 752.89
      in adiposogenital dystrophy 253.8
    male 752.89

Hypoplasia, hypoplasis — *continued*
  genitalia, genital organ(s) — *continued*
    male — *continued*
      penis 752.69
  glottis 748.3
  hair 757.4
  hand 755.21
  heart 746.89
    left (complex) (syndrome) 746.7
    valve NEC 746.89
      pulmonary 746.01
  humerus (*see also* Absence, humerus, congenital) 755.24
  hymen 752.49
  intestine (small) 751.1
    large 751.2
  iris 743.46
  jaw 524.09
  kidney(s) 753.0
  labium (majus) (minus) 752.49
  labyrinth, membranous 744.05
  lacrimal duct (apparatus) 743.65
  larynx 748.3
  leg (*see also* Absence, limb, congenital, lower) 755.30
  limb 755.4
    lower (*see also* Absence, limb, congenital, lower) 755.30
    upper (*see also* Absence, limb, congenital, upper) 755.20
  liver 751.69
  lung (lobe) 748.5
  mammary (areolar) 611.82
  mandibular 524.04
    alveolar 524.74
    unilateral condylar 526.89
  maxillary 524.03
    alveolar 524.73
  medullary 284.9
  megakaryocytic 287.30
  metacarpus (*see also* Absence, metacarpal, congenital) 755.28
  metatarsus (*see also* Absence, metatarsal, congenital) 755.38
  muscle 756.89
    eye 743.69
  myocardium (congenital) (Uhl's anomaly) 746.84
  nail(s) 757.5
  nasolacrimal duct 743.65
  nervous system NEC 742.8
  neural 742.8
  nose, nasal 748.1
  ophthalmic (*see also* Microphthalmos) 743.10
  optic nerve 377.43
  organ
    of Corti 744.05
    or site NEC — *see* Anomaly, by site
  osseous meatus (ear) 744.03
  ovary 752.0
  oviduct 752.19
  pancreas 751.7
  parathyroid (gland) 759.2
  parotid gland 750.26
  patella 755.64
  pelvis, pelvic girdle 755.69
  penis 752.69
  peripheral vascular system (congenital) NEC 747.60
    gastrointestinal 747.61
    lower limb 747.64
    renal 747.62
    specified NEC 747.69
    spinal 747.82
    upper limb 747.63
  pituitary (gland) 759.2
  pulmonary 748.5

Hypoplasia, hypoplasis — *continued*
  pulmonary — *continued*
    arteriovenous 747.32
    artery 747.31
    valve 746.01
  punctum lacrimale 743.65
  radioulnar (*see also* Absence, radius, congenital, with ulna) 755.25
  radius (*see also* Absence, radius, congenital) 755.26
  rectum 751.2
  respiratory system NEC 748.9
  rib 756.3
  sacrum 756.19
  scapula 755.59
  shoulder girdle 755.59
  skin 757.39
  skull (bone) 756.0
    with
      anencephalus 740.0
      encephalocele 742.0
      hydrocephalus 742.3
        with spina bifida (*see also* Spina bifida) 741.0 ☑
      microcephalus 742.1
  spinal (cord) (ventral horn cell) 742.59
    vessel 747.82
  spine 756.19
  spleen 759.0
  sternum 756.3
  tarsus (*see also* Absence, tarsal, congenital) 755.38
  testis, testicle 752.89
  thymus (gland) 279.11
  thyroid (gland) 243
    cartilage 748.3
  tibiofibular (*see also* Absence, tibia, congenital, with fibula) 755.35
  toe (*see also* Absence, toe, congenital) 755.39
  tongue 750.16
  trachea (cartilage) (rings) 748.3
  Turner's (tooth) 520.4
  ulna (*see also* Absence, ulna, congenital) 755.27
  umbilical artery 747.5
  ureter 753.29
  uterus 752.32
  vagina 752.45
  vascular (peripheral) NEC (*see also* Hypoplasia, peripheral vascular system) 747.60
    brain 747.81
  vein(s) (peripheral) NEC (*see also* Hypoplasia, peripheral vascular system) 747.60
    brain 747.81
    cardiac 746.89
    great 747.49
    portal 747.49
    pulmonary 747.49
  vena cava (inferior) (superior) 747.49
  vertebra 756.19
  vulva 752.49
  zonule (ciliary) 743.39
  zygoma 738.12
Hypopotassemia 276.8
Hypoproaccelerinemia — *see also* Defect, coagulation 286.3
Hypoproconvertinemia (congenital) — *see also* Defect, coagulation 286.3
Hypoproteinemia (essential) (hypermetabolic) (idiopathic) 273.8
Hypoproteinosis 260
Hypoprothrombinemia (congenital) (hereditary) (idiopathic) — *see also* Defect, coagulation 286.3
  acquired 286.7
  newborn 776.3

Hypopselaphesia 782.0
Hypopyon (anterior chamber) (eye) 364.05
  iritis 364.05
  ulcer (cornea) 370.04
Hypopyrexia 780.99
Hyporeflex 796.1
Hyporeninemia, extreme 790.99
  in primary aldosteronism 255.10
Hyporesponsive episode 780.09
Hyposecretion
  ACTH 253.4
  ovary 256.39
    postablative 256.2
  salivary gland (any) 527.7
Hyposegmentation of neutrophils, hereditary 288.2
Hyposiderinemia 280.9
Hyposmolality 276.1
  syndrome 276.1
Hyposomatotropism 253.3
Hyposomnia, unspecified — *see also* Insomnia 780.52
  with sleep apnea, unspecified 780.51
Hypospadias (male) 752.61
  female 753.8
Hypospermatogenesis 606.1
Hyposphagma 372.72
Hyposplenism 289.59
Hypostasis, pulmonary 514
Hypostatic — *see* condition
Hyposthenuria 593.89
Hyposuprarenalism 255.41
Hypotension (arterial) (constitutional) 458.9
  chronic 458.1
  iatrogenic 458.29
  maternal, syndrome (following labor and delivery) 669.2 ☑
  of hemodialysis 458.21
  orthostatic (chronic) 458.0
    dysautonomic-dyskinetic syndrome 333.0
  permanent idiopathic 458.1
  postoperative 458.29
  postural 458.0
  specified type NEC 458.8
  transient 796.3
Hypothermia (accidental) 991.6
  anesthetic 995.89
  associated with low environmental temperature 991.6
  newborn NEC 778.3
  not associated with low environmental temperature 780.65
Hypothymergasia — *see also* Psychosis, affective 296.2 ☑
  recurrent episode 296.3 ☑
  single episode 296.2 ☑
Hypothyroidism (acquired) 244.9
  complicating pregnancy, childbirth, or puerperium 648.1 ☑
  congenital 243
  due to
    ablation 244.1
      radioactive iodine 244.1
      surgical 244.0
    iodine (administration) (ingestion) 244.2
      radioactive 244.1
    irradiation therapy 244.1
    p-aminosalicylic acid (PAS) 244.3
    phenylbutazone 244.3
    resorcinol 244.3
    specified cause NEC 244.8
    surgery 244.0
  goitrous (sporadic) 246.1
  iatrogenic NEC 244.3
  iodine 244.2
  pituitary 244.8
  postablative NEC 244.1

Hypothyroidism — *continued*
  postsurgical 244.0
  primary 244.9
  secondary NEC 244.8
  specified cause NEC 244.8
  sporadic goitrous 246.1
Hypotonia, hypotonicity, hypotony 781.3
  benign congenital 358.8
  bladder 596.4
  congenital 779.89
    benign 358.8
  eye 360.30
    due to
      fistula 360.32
      ocular disorder NEC 360.33
    following loss of aqueous or vitreous 360.33
    primary 360.31
  infantile muscular (benign) 359.0
  muscle 728.9
  uterus, uterine (contractions) — *see* Inertia, uterus
Hypotrichosis 704.09
  congenital 757.4
  lid (congenital) 757.4
    acquired 374.55
  postinfectional NEC 704.09
Hypotropia 378.32
Hypoventilation 786.09
  congenital central alveolar syndrome 327.25
  idiopathic sleep related nonobstructive alveolar 327.24
  obesity 278.03
  sleep related, in conditions classifiable elsewhere 327.26
Hypovitaminosis — *see also* Deficiency, vitamin 269.2
Hypovolemia 276.52
  surgical shock 998.09
  traumatic (shock) 958.4
Hypoxemia — *see also* Anoxia 799.02
  sleep related, in conditions classifiable elsewhere 327.26
Hypoxia — *see also* Anoxia 799.02
  cerebral 348.1
    during or resulting from a procedure 997.01
    newborn 770.88
      mild or moderate 768.6
      severe 768.5
  fetal, affecting newborn 770.88
  intrauterine — *see* Distress, fetal
  myocardial (*see also* Insufficiency, coronary) 411.89
    arteriosclerotic — *see* Arteriosclerosis, coronary
  newborn 770.88
  sleep related 327.24
Hypoxic-ischemic encephalopathy (HIE) 768.70
  mild 768.71
  moderate 768.72
  severe 768.73
Hypsarrhythmia — *see also* Epilepsy 345.6 ☑
Hysteralgia, pregnant uterus 646.8 ☑
Hysteria, hysterical 300.10
  anxiety 300.20
  Charcôt's gland 300.11
  conversion (any manifestation) 300.11
  dissociative type NEC 300.15
  psychosis, acute 298.1
Hysteroepilepsy 300.11
Hysterotomy, affecting fetus or newborn 763.89

☑ Additional Digit Required — Refer to the Tabular List for Digit Selection   ▽ Subterms under main terms may continue to next column or page

150 — Volume 2   ▶◀ Revised Text   ● New Line   ▲ Revised Code   2014 ICD-9-CM

I

Iatrogenic syndrome of excess cortisol 255.0
IBM (inclusion body myositis) 359.71
Iceland disease (epidemic neuromyasthenia) 049.8
Ichthyosis (congenita) 757.1
  acquired 701.1
  fetalis gravior 757.1
  follicularis 757.1
  hystrix 757.39
  lamellar 757.1
  lingual 528.6
  palmaris and plantaris 757.39
  simplex 757.1
  vera 757.1
  vulgaris 757.1
Ichthyotoxism 988.0
  bacterial (see also Poisoning, food) 005.9
Icteroanemia, hemolytic (acquired) 283.9
  congenital (see also Spherocytosis) 282.0
Icterus — see also Jaundice 782.4
  catarrhal — see Icterus, infectious
  conjunctiva 782.4
    newborn 774.6
  epidemic — see Icterus, infectious
  febrilis — see Icterus, infectious
  fetus or newborn — see Jaundice, fetus or newborn
  gravis (see also Necrosis, liver) 570
    complicating pregnancy 646.7 ☑
      affecting fetus or newborn 760.8
    fetus or newborn NEC 773.0
    obstetrical 646.7 ☑
      affecting fetus or newborn 760.8
  hematogenous (acquired) 283.9
  hemolytic (acquired) 283.9
    congenital (see also Spherocytosis) 282.0
  hemorrhagic (acute) 100.0
    leptospiral 100.0
    newborn 776.0
    spirochetal 100.0
  infectious 070.1
    with hepatic coma 070.0
    leptospiral 100.0
    spirochetal 100.0
  intermittens juvenilis 277.4
  malignant (see also Necrosis, liver) 570
  neonatorum (see also Jaundice, fetus or newborn) 774.6
  pernicious (see also Necrosis, liver) 570
  spirochetal 100.0
Ictus solaris, solis 992.0
Ideation
  homicidal V62.85
  suicidal V62.84
Identity disorder 313.82
  dissociative 300.14
  gender role (child) 302.6
    adult 302.85
  psychosexual (child) 302.6
    adult 302.85
Idioglossia 307.9
Idiopathic — see condition
Idiosyncrasy — see also Allergy 995.3
  drug, medicinal substance, and biological — see Allergy, drug
Idiot, idiocy (congenital) 318.2
  amaurotic (Bielschowsky) (-Jansky) (family) (infantile) (late) (juvenile) (late) (Vogt-Spielmeyer) 330.1
  microcephalic 742.1
  Mongolian 758.0
  oxycephalic 756.0
Id reaction (due to bacteria) 692.89
IEED (involuntary emotional expression disorder) 310.81
IFIS (intraoperative floppy iris syndrome) 364.81
IgE asthma 493.0 ☑
Ileitis (chronic) — see also Enteritis 558.9
  infectious 009.0
  noninfectious 558.9
  regional (ulcerative) 555.0
    with large intestine 555.2
  segmental 555.0

Ileitis — see also Enteritis — continued
  segmental — continued
    with large intestine 555.2
  terminal (ulcerative) 555.0
    with large intestine 555.2
Ileocolitis — see also Enteritis 558.9
  infectious 009.0
  regional 555.2
  ulcerative 556.1
Ileostomy status V44.2
  with complication 569.60
Ileotyphus 002.0
Ileum — see condition
Ileus (adynamic) (bowel) (colon) (inhibitory) (intestine) (neurogenic) (paralytic) 560.1
  arteriomesenteric duodenal 537.2
  due to gallstone (in intestine) 560.31
  duodenal, chronic 537.2
  following gastrointestinal surgery 997.49
  gallstone 560.31
  mechanical (see also Obstruction, intestine) 560.9
  meconium 777.1
    due to cystic fibrosis 277.01
  myxedema 564.89
  postoperative 997.49
  transitory, newborn 777.4
Iliac — see condition
Iliotibial band friction syndrome 728.89
Illegitimacy V61.6
Ill, louping 063.1
Illness — see also Disease
  factitious 300.19
    with
      combined psychological and physical signs and symptoms 300.19
      predominantly
        physical signs and symptoms 300.19
        psychological symptoms 300.16
    chronic (with physical symptoms) 301.51
  heart — see Disease, heart
  manic-depressive (see also Psychosis, affective) 296.80
  mental (see also Disorder, mental) 300.9
Imbalance 781.2
  autonomic (see also Neuropathy, peripheral, autonomic) 337.9
  electrolyte 276.9
    with
      abortion — see Abortion, by type, with metabolic disorder
      ectopic pregnancy (see also categories 633.0–633.9) 639.4
      hyperemesis gravidarum (before 22 completed weeks gestation) 643.1 ☑
      molar pregnancy (see also categories 630–632) 639.4
    following
      abortion 639.4
      ectopic or molar pregnancy 639.4
    neonatal, transitory NEC 775.5
  endocrine 259.9
  eye muscle NEC 378.9
    heterophoria — see Heterophoria
  glomerulotubular NEC 593.89
  hormone 259.9
  hysterical (see also Hysteria) 300.10
  labyrinth NEC 386.50
  posture 729.90
  sympathetic (see also Neuropathy, peripheral, autonomic) 337.9
Imbecile, imbecility 318.0
  moral 301.7
  old age 290.9
  senile 290.9
  specified IQ — see IQ
  unspecified IQ 318.0
Imbedding, intrauterine device 996.32
Imbibition, cholesterol (gallbladder) 575.6
Imerslund (-Gräsbeck) syndrome (anemia due to familial selective vitamin B₁₂ malabsorption) 281.1
Iminoacidopathy 270.8
Iminoglycinuria, familial 270.8

Immature — see also Immaturity
  personality 301.89
Immaturity 765.1 ☑
  extreme 765.0 ☑
  fetus or infant light-for-dates — see Light-for-dates
  lung, fetus or newborn 770.4
  organ or site NEC — see Hypoplasia
  pulmonary, fetus or newborn 770.4
  reaction 301.89
  sexual (female) (male) 259.0
Immersion 994.1
  foot 991.4
  hand 991.4
Immobile, immobility
  complete
    due to severe physical disability or frailty 780.72
  intestine 564.89
  joint — see Ankylosis
  syndrome (paraplegic) 728.3
Immunization
  ABO
    affecting management of pregnancy 656.2 ☑
    fetus or newborn 773.1
  complication — see Complications, vaccination
  Rh factor
    affecting management of pregnancy 656.1 ☑
    fetus or newborn 773.0
    from transfusion (see also Complications, transfusion) 999.70
Immunodeficiency 279.3
  with
    adenosine-deaminase deficiency 279.2
    defect, predominant
      B-cell 279.00
      T-cell 279.10
    hyperimmunoglobulinemia 279.2
    lymphopenia, hereditary 279.2
    thrombocytopenia and eczema 279.12
    thymic
      aplasia 279.2
      dysplasia 279.2
  autosomal recessive, Swiss-type 279.2
  common variable 279.06
  severe combined (SCID) 279.2
  to Rh factor
    affecting management of pregnancy 656.1 ☑
    fetus or newborn 773.0
  X-linked, with increased IgM 279.05
Immunotherapy, prophylactic V07.2
  antineoplastic V58.12
Impaction, impacted
  bowel, colon, rectum 560.30
    with hernia (see also Hernia, by site, with obstruction)
      gangrenous — see Hernia, by site, with gangrene
    by
      calculus 560.32
      gallstone 560.31
      fecal 560.32
      specified type NEC 560.32
  calculus — see Calculus
  cerumen (ear) (external) 380.4
  cuspid 520.6
  dental 520.6
  fecal, feces 560.32
    with hernia (see also Hernia, by site, with obstruction)
      gangrenous — see Hernia, by site, with gangrene
  fracture — see Fracture, by site
  gallbladder — see Cholelithiasis
  gallstone(s) — see Cholelithiasis
    in intestine (any part) 560.31
  intestine(s) 560.30
    with hernia (see also Hernia, by site, with obstruction)
      gangrenous — see Hernia, by site, with gangrene

Impaction, impacted — continued
  intestine(s) — continued
    by
      calculus 560.32
      gallstone 560.31
      fecal 560.32
      specified type NEC 560.32
  intrauterine device (IUD) 996.32
  molar 520.6
  shoulder 660.4 ☑
    affecting fetus or newborn 763.1
  tooth, teeth 520.6
  turbinate 733.99
Impaired, impairment (function)
  arm V49.1
    movement, involving
      musculoskeletal system V49.1
      nervous system V49.2
  auditory discrimination 388.43
  back V48.3
  body (entire) V49.89
  cognitive, mild, so stated 331.83
  combined visual hearing V49.85
  dual sensory V49.85
  glucose
    fasting 790.21
    tolerance test (oral) 790.22
  hearing (see also Deafness) 389.9
    combined with visual impairment V49.85
  heart — see Disease, heart
  kidney (see also Disease, renal) 593.9
    disorder resulting from 588.9
      specified NEC 588.89
  leg V49.1
    movement, involving
      musculoskeletal system V49.1
      nervous system V49.2
  limb V49.1
    movement, involving
      musculoskeletal system V49.1
      nervous system V49.2
  liver 573.8
  mastication 524.9
  mild cognitive, so stated 331.83
  mobility
    ear ossicles NEC 385.22
    incostapedial joint 385.22
    malleus 385.21
  myocardium, myocardial (see also Insufficiency, myocardial) 428.0
  neuromusculoskeletal NEC V49.89
    back V48.3
    head V48.2
    limb V49.2
    neck V48.3
    spine V48.3
    trunk V48.3
  rectal sphincter 787.99
  renal (see also Disease, renal) 593.9
    disorder resulting from 588.9
      specified NEC 588.89
  spine V48.3
  vision NEC 369.9
    both eyes NEC 369.3
      combined with hearing impairment V49.85
      moderate 369.74
        both eyes 369.25
          with impairment of lesser eye (specified as)
            blind, not further specified 369.15
            low vision, not further specified 369.23
            near-total 369.17
            profound 369.18
            severe 369.24
            total 369.16
        one eye 369.74
          with vision of other eye (specified as)
            near-normal 369.75
            normal 369.76
      near-total 369.64
        both eyes 369.04

☑ Additional Digit Required — Refer to the Tabular List for Digit Selection
▼ Subterms under main terms may continue to next column or page
2014 ICD-9-CM
▶◀ Revised Text
● New Line
▲ Revised Code
Volume 2 — 151

Impaired, impairment — continued
vision — continued
near-total — continued
both eyes — continued
with impairment of lesser eye
(specified as)
blind, not further specified
369.02
total 369.03
one eye 369.64
with vision of other eye (specified
as)
near normal 369.65
normal 369.66
one eye 369.60
with low vision of other eye 369.10
profound 369.67
both eyes 369.08
with impairment of lesser eye
(specified as)
blind, not further specified
369.05
near-total 369.07
total 369.06
one eye 369.67
with vision of other eye (specified
as)
near-normal 369.68
normal 369.69
severe 369.71
both eyes 369.22
with impairment of lesser eye
(specified as)
blind, not further specified
369.11
low vision, not further specified 369.21
near-total 369.13
profound 369.14
total 369.12
one eye 369.71
with vision of other eye (specified
as)
near-normal 369.72
normal 369.73
total
both eyes 369.01
one eye 369.61
with vision of other eye (specified
as)
near-normal 369.62
normal 369.63
Impaludism — see Malaria
Impediment, speech NEC 784.59
psychogenic 307.9
secondary to organic lesion 784.59
Impending
cerebrovascular accident or attack 435.9
coronary syndrome 411.1
delirium tremens 291.0
myocardial infarction 411.1
Imperception, auditory (acquired) (congenital) 389.9
Imperfect
aeration, lung (newborn) 770.5
closure (congenital)
alimentary tract NEC 751.8
lower 751.5
upper 750.8
atrioventricular ostium 745.69
atrium (secundum) 745.5
primum 745.61
branchial cleft or sinus 744.41
choroid 743.59
cricoid cartilage 748.3
cusps, heart valve NEC 746.89
pulmonary 746.09
ductus
arteriosus 747.0
Botalli 747.0
ear drum 744.29
causing impairment of hearing
744.03
endocardial cushion 745.60
epiglottis 748.3

Imperfect — continued
closure — continued
esophagus with communication to
bronchus or trachea 750.3
Eustachian valve 746.89
eyelid 743.62
face, facial (see also Cleft, lip) 749.10
foramen
Botalli 745.5
ovale 745.5
genitalia, genital organ(s) or system
female 752.89
external 752.49
internal NEC 752.89
uterus 752.39
male 752.89
penis 752.69
glottis 748.3
heart valve (cusps) NEC 746.89
interatrial ostium or septum 745.5
interauricular ostium or septum 745.5
interventricular ostium or septum 745.4
iris 743.46
kidney 753.3
larynx 748.3
lens 743.36
lip (see also Cleft, lip) 749.10
nasal septum or sinus 748.1
nose 748.1
omphalomesenteric duct 751.0
optic nerve entry 743.57
organ or site NEC — see Anomaly, specified type, by site
ostium
interatrial 745.5
interauricular 745.5
interventricular 745.4
palate (see also Cleft, palate) 749.00
preauricular sinus 744.46
retina 743.56
roof of orbit 742.0
sclera 743.47
septum
aortic 745.0
aorticopulmonary 745.0
atrial (secundum) 745.5
primum 745.61
between aorta and pulmonary artery
745.0
heart 745.9
interatrial (secundum) 745.5
primum 745.61
interauricular (secundum) 745.5
primum 745.61
interventricular 745.4
with pulmonary stenosis or atresia, dextraposition of aorta, and hypertrophy of
right ventricle 745.2
in tetralogy of Fallot 745.2
nasal 748.1
ventricular 745.4
with pulmonary stenosis or atresia, dextraposition of aorta, and hypertrophy of
right ventricle 745.2
in tetralogy of Fallot 745.2
skull 756.0
with
anencephalus 740.0
encephalocele 742.0
hydrocephalus 742.3
with spina bifida (see also
Spina bifida) 741.0 ☑
microcephalus 742.1
spine (with meningocele) (see also Spina
bifida) 741.90
thyroid cartilage 748.3
trachea 748.3
tympanic membrane 744.29
causing impairment of hearing
744.03
uterus (with communication to bladder,
intestine, or rectum) 752.39
uvula 749.02

Imperfect — continued
closure — continued
uvula — continued
with cleft lip (see also Cleft, palate,
with cleft lip) 749.20
vitelline duct 751.0
development — see Anomaly, by site
erection 607.84
fusion — see Imperfect, closure
inflation lung (newborn) 770.5
intestinal canal 751.5
poise 729.90
rotation — see Malrotation
septum, ventricular 745.4
Imperfectly descended testis 752.51
Imperforate (congenital) — see also Atresia
anus 751.2
bile duct 751.61
cervix (uteri) 752.49
esophagus 750.3
hymen 752.42
intestine (small) 751.1
large 751.2
jejunum 751.1
pharynx 750.29
rectum 751.2
salivary duct 750.23
urethra 753.6
urinary meatus 753.6
vagina 752.49
Impervious (congenital) — see also Atresia
anus 751.2
bile duct 751.61
esophagus 750.3
intestine (small) 751.1
large 751.5
rectum 751.2
urethra 753.6
Impetiginization of other dermatoses 684
Impetigo (any organism) (any site) (bullous)
(circinate) (contagiosa) (neonatorum)
(simplex) 684
Bockhart's (superficial folliculitis) 704.8
external ear 684 [380.13]
eyelid 684 [373.5]
Fox's (contagiosa) 684
furfuracea 696.5
herpetiformis 694.3
nonobstetrical 694.3
staphylococcal infection 684
ulcerative 686.8
vulgaris 684
Impingement, soft tissue between teeth
524.89
anterior 524.81
posterior 524.82
Implantation
anomalous (see also Anomaly, specified
type, by site)
ureter 753.4
cyst
external area or site (skin) NEC 709.8
iris 364.61
vagina 623.8
vulva 624.8
dermoid (cyst)
external area or site (skin) NEC 709.8
iris 364.61
vagina 623.8
vulva 624.8
placenta, low or marginal — see Placenta
previa
Implant, endometrial 617.9
Impotence (sexual) 607.84
organic origin NEC 607.84
psychogenic 302.72
Impoverished blood 285.9
Impression, basilar 756.0
Imprisonment V62.5
Improper
development, infant 764.9 ☑
Improperly tied umbilical cord (causing
hemorrhage) 772.3
Impulses, obsessional 300.3
Impulsive 799.23
neurosis 300.3

Impulsiveness 799.23
Inaction, kidney — see also Disease, renal
593.9
Inactive — see condition
Inadequate, inadequacy
aesthetics of dental restoration 525.67
biologic 301.6
cardiac and renal — see Hypertension, cardiorenal
constitutional 301.6
development
child 783.40
fetus 764.9 ☑
affecting management of pregnancy
656.5 ☑
genitalia
after puberty NEC 259.0
congenital — see Hypoplasia, genitalia
lungs 748.5
organ or site NEC — see Hypoplasia, by
site
dietary 269.9
distance, interarch 524.28
education V62.3
environment
economic problem V60.2
household condition NEC V60.1
poverty V60.2
unemployment V62.0
functional 301.6
household care, due to
family member
handicapped or ill V60.4
temporarily away from home V60.4
on vacation V60.5
technical defects in home V60.1
temporary absence from home of person
rendering care V60.4
housing (heating) (space) V60.1
interarch distance 524.28
material resources V60.2
mental (see also Disability, intellectual) 319
nervous system 799.29
personality 301.6
prenatal care in current pregnancy V23.7
pulmonary
function 786.09
newborn 770.89
ventilation, newborn 770.89
respiration 786.09
newborn 770.89
sample
cytology
anal 796.78
cervical 795.08
vaginal 795.18
social 301.6
Inanition 263.9
with edema 262
due to
deprivation of food 994.2
malnutrition 263.9
fever 780.60
Inappropriate
change in quantitative human chorionic
gonadotropin (hCG) in early pregnancy 631.0
level of quantitative human chorionic gonadotropin (hCG) for gestational age
in early pregnancy 631.0
secretion
ACTH 255.0
antidiuretic hormone (ADH) (excessive)
253.6
deficiency 253.5
ectopic hormone NEC 259.3
pituitary (posterior) 253.6
Inattention after or at birth 995.52
Inborn errors of metabolism — see Disorder,
metabolism
Incarceration, incarcerated
bubonocele (see also Hernia, inguinal, with
obstruction)
gangrenous — see Hernia, inguinal, with
gangrene

Incarceration, incarcerated — *continued*
  colon (by hernia) (*see also* Hernia, by site with obstruction)
    gangrenous — *see* Hernia, by site, with gangrene
  enterocele 552.9
    gangrenous 551.9
  epigastrocele 552.29
    gangrenous 551.29
  epiplocele 552.9
    gangrenous 551.9
  exomphalos 552.1
    gangrenous 551.1
  fallopian tube 620.8
  hernia (*see also* Hernia, by site, with obstruction)
    gangrenous — *see* Hernia, by site, with gangrene
  iris, in wound 871.1
  lens, in wound 871.1
  merocele (*see also* Hernia, femoral, with obstruction) 552.00
  omentum (by hernia) (*see also* Hernia, by site, with obstruction)
    gangrenous — *see* Hernia, by site, with gangrene
  omphalocele 756.72
  rupture (meaning hernia) (*see also* Hernia, by site, with obstruction) 552.9
    gangrenous (*see also* Hernia, by site, with gangrene) 551.9
  sarcoepiplocele 552.9
    gangrenous 551.9
  sarcoepiplomphalocele 552.1
    with gangrene 551.1
  uterus 621.8
    gravid 654.3 ☑
      causing obstructed labor 660.2 ☑
        affecting fetus or newborn 763.1
Incident, cerebrovascular — *see also* Disease, cerebrovascular, acute 436
Incineration (entire body) (from fire, conflagration, electricity, or lightning) — *see* Burn, multiple, specified sites
Incised wound
  external — *see* Wound, open, by site
  internal organs (abdomen, chest, or pelvis) — *see* Injury, internal, by site, with open wound
Incision, incisional
  hernia — *see* Hernia, incisional
  surgical, complication — *see* Complications, surgical procedures
  traumatic
    external — *see* Wound, open, by site
    internal organs (abdomen, chest, or pelvis) — *see* Injury, internal, by site, with open wound
Inclusion
  azurophilic leukocytic 288.2
  blennorrhea (neonatal) (newborn) 771.6
  cyst — *see* Cyst, skin
  gallbladder in liver (congenital) 751.69
Incompatibility
  ABO
    affecting management of pregnancy 656.2 ☑
    fetus or newborn 773.1
    infusion or transfusion reaction (*see also* Complications, transfusion) 999.60
  blood (group) (Duffy) (E) (K(ell)) (Kidd) (Lewis) (M) (N) (P) (S) NEC
    affecting management of pregnancy 656.2 ☑
    fetus or newborn 773.2
    infusion or transfusion reaction (*see also* Complications, transfusion) 999.75
  contour of existing restoration of tooth with oral health 525.65
  marital V61.10
    involving
      divorce V61.03
      estrangement V61.09

Incompatibility — *continued*
  non-ABO (*see also* Complications, transfusion) 999.75
  Rh (antigen) (C) (c) (D) (E) (e) (blood group) (factor)
    affecting management of pregnancy 656.1 ☑
    fetus or newborn 773.0
    infusion or transfusion reaction (*see also* Complications, transfusion) 999.70
  Rhesus — *see* Incompatibility, Rh
Incompetency, incompetence, incompetent
  annular
    aortic (valve) (*see also* Insufficiency, aortic) 424.1
    mitral (valve) (*see also* Insufficiency, mitral) 424.0
    pulmonary valve (heart) (*see also* Endocarditis, pulmonary) 424.3
  aortic (valve) (*see also* Insufficiency, aortic) 424.1
    syphilitic 093.22
  cardiac (orifice) 530.0
    valve — *see* Endocarditis
  cervix, cervical (os) 622.5
    in pregnancy 654.5 ☑
      affecting fetus or newborn 761.0
  chronotropic 426.89
    with
      autonomic dysfunction 337.9
      ischemic heart disease 414.9
      left ventricular dysfunction 429.89
      sinus node dysfunction 427.81
  esophagogastric (junction) (sphincter) 530.0
  heart valve, congenital 746.89
  mitral (valve) — *see* Insufficiency, mitral
  papillary muscle (heart) 429.81
  pelvic fundus
    pubocervical tissue 618.81
    rectovaginal tissue 618.82
  pulmonary valve (heart) (*see also* Endocarditis, pulmonary) 424.3
    congenital 746.09
  tricuspid (annular) (rheumatic) (valve) (*see also* Endocarditis, tricuspid) 397.0
  valvular — *see* Endocarditis
  vein, venous (saphenous) (varicose) (*see also* Varicose, vein) 454.9
  velopharyngeal (closure)
    acquired 528.9
    congenital 750.29
Incomplete — *see also* condition
  bladder emptying 788.21
  defecation 787.61
  expansion lungs (newborn) 770.5
  gestation (liveborn) — *see* Immaturity
  rotation — *see* Malrotation
Inconclusive
  image test due to excess body fat 793.91
  mammogram, mammography 793.82
    due to dense breasts 793.82
Incontinence 788.30
  without sensory awareness 788.34
  anal sphincter 787.60
  continuous leakage 788.37
  feces, fecal 787.60
    due to hysteria 300.11
    nonorganic origin 307.7
  hysterical 300.11
  mixed (male) (female) (urge and stress) 788.33
  overflow 788.38
  paradoxical 788.39
  rectal 787.60
  specified NEC 788.39
  stress (female) 625.6
    male NEC 788.32
  urethral sphincter 599.84
  urge 788.31
    and stress (male) (female) 788.33
  urine 788.30
    active 788.30
    due to
      cognitive impairment 788.91
      immobility 788.91

Incontinence — *continued*
  urine — *continued*
    due to — *continued*
      severe physical disability 788.91
    functional 788.91
    male 788.30
      stress 788.32
        and urge 788.33
    neurogenic 788.39
    nonorganic origin 307.6
    stress (female) 625.6
      male NEC 788.32
    urge 788.31
      and stress 788.33
Incontinentia pigmenti 757.33
Incoordinate
  uterus (action) (contractions) 661.4 ☑
    affecting fetus or newborn 763.7
Incoordination
  esophageal-pharyngeal (newborn) 787.24
  muscular 781.3
  papillary muscle 429.81
Increase, increased
  abnormal, in development 783.9
  androgens (ovarian) 256.1
  anticoagulants (antithrombin) (anti-II) (anti-VIIIa) (anti-IXa) (anti-XIa) (prothrombin) (*see also* Anticoagulants 286.59
    anti-IIa 287.8
    anti-Xa 287.8
    extrinsic 287.8
    postpartum 666.3 ☑
  cold sense (*see also* Disturbance, sensation) 782.0
  estrogen 256.0
  function
    adrenal (cortex) 255.3
      medulla 255.6
    pituitary (anterior) (gland) (lobe) 253.1
      posterior 253.6
  heat sense (*see also* Disturbance, sensation) 782.0
  intracranial pressure 781.99
    injury at birth 767.8
  light reflex of retina 362.13
  permeability, capillary 448.9
  pressure
    intracranial 781.99
      injury at birth 767.8
    intraocular 365.00
  pulsations 785.9
  pulse pressure 785.9
  sphericity, lens 743.36
  splenic activity 289.4
  venous pressure 459.89
    portal 572.3
Incrustation, cornea, lead or zinc 930.0
Incyclophoria 378.44
Incyclotropia 378.33
Indeterminate sex 752.7
India rubber skin 756.83
Indicanuria 270.2
Indigestion (bilious) (functional) 536.8
  acid 536.8
  catarrhal 536.8
  due to decomposed food NEC 005.9
  fat 579.8
  nervous 306.4
  psychogenic 306.4
Indirect — *see* condition
Indolent bubo NEC 099.8
Induced
  abortion — *see* Abortion, induced
  birth, affecting fetus or newborn 763.89
  delivery — *see* Delivery
  labor — *see* Delivery
Induration, indurated
  brain 348.89
  breast (fibrous) 611.79
    puerperal, postpartum 676.3 ☑
  broad ligament 620.8
  chancre 091.0
    anus 091.1
    congenital 090.0
    extragenital NEC 091.2
  corpora cavernosa (penis) (plastic) 607.89

Induration, indurated — *continued*
  liver (chronic) 573.8
    acute 573.8
  lung (black) (brown) (chronic) (fibroid) (*see also* Fibrosis, lung) 515
    essential brown 275.09 [516.1]
  penile 607.89
  phlebitic — *see* Phlebitis
  skin 782.8
  stomach 537.89
Induratio penis plastica 607.89
Industrial — *see* condition
Inebriety — *see also* Abuse, drugs, nondependent 305.0 ☑
Inefficiency
  kidney (*see also* Disease, renal) 593.9
  thyroid (acquired) (gland) 244.9
Inelasticity, skin 782.8
Inequality, leg (acquired) (length) 736.81
  congenital 755.30
Inertia
  bladder 596.4
    neurogenic 596.54
      with cauda equina syndrome 344.61
    stomach 536.8
      psychogenic 306.4
    uterus, uterine 661.2 ☑
      affecting fetus or newborn 763.7
      primary 661.0 ☑
      secondary 661.1 ☑
    vesical 596.4
      neurogenic 596.54
        with cauda equina syndrome 344.61
Infant — *see also* condition
  excessive crying of 780.92
  fussy (baby) 780.91
  held for adoption V68.89
  newborn — *see* Newborn
  post-term (gestation period over 40 completed weeks to 42 completed weeks) 766.21
  prolonged gestation of (period over 42 completed weeks) 766.22
  syndrome of diabetic mother 775.0
"Infant Hercules" syndrome 255.2
Infantile — *see also* condition
  genitalia, genitals 259.0
    in pregnancy or childbirth NEC 654.4 ☑
      affecting fetus or newborn 763.89
      causing obstructed labor 660.2 ☑
        affecting fetus or newborn 763.1
  heart 746.9
  kidney 753.3
  lack of care 995.52
  macula degeneration 362.75
  melanodontia 521.05
  os, uterus (*see also* Infantile, genitalia) 259.0
  pelvis 738.6
    with disproportion (fetopelvic) 653.1 ☑
      affecting fetus or newborn 763.1
      causing obstructed labor 660.1 ☑
        affecting fetus or newborn 763.1
  penis 259.0
  testis 257.2
  uterus (*see also* Infantile, genitalia) 259.0
  vulva 752.49
Infantilism 259.9
  with dwarfism (hypophyseal) 253.3
  Brissaud's (infantile myxedema) 244.9
  celiac 579.0
  Herter's (nontropical sprue) 579.0
  hypophyseal 253.3
  hypothalamic (with obesity) 253.8
  idiopathic 259.9
  intestinal 579.0
  pancreatic 577.8
  pituitary 253.3
  renal 588.0
  sexual (with obesity) 259.0
Infants, healthy liveborn — *see* Newborn
Infarct, infarction
  adrenal (capsule) (gland) 255.41
  amnion 658.8 ☑
  anterior (with contiguous portion of intraventricular septum) NEC (*see also* Infarct, myocardium) 410.1 ☑

☑ Additional Digit Required — Refer to the Tabular List for Digit Selection   ▽ Subterms under main terms may continue to next column or page

2014 ICD-9-CM   ▶◀ Revised Text   ● New Line   ▲ Revised Code   Volume 2 — 153

Index

Infarct, infarction — Infection, infected, infective

Infarct, infarction — *continued*
appendices epiploicae 557.0
bowel 557.0
brain (stem) 434.91
  embolic (*see also* Embolism, brain) 434.11
  healed or old without residuals V12.54
  iatrogenic 997.02
  lacunar 434.91
  late effect — *see* Late effect(s) (of) cerebrovascular disease
  postoperative 997.02
  puerperal, postpartum, childbirth 674.0 ☑
  thrombotic (*see also* Thrombosis, brain) 434.01
breast 611.89
Brewer's (kidney) 593.81
cardiac (*see also* Infarct, myocardium) 410.9 ☑
cerebellar (*see also* Infarct, brain) 434.91
  embolic (*see also* Embolism, brain) 434.11
cerebral (*see also* Infarct, brain) 434.91
  aborted 434.91
  embolic (*see also* Embolism, brain) 434.11
  thrombotic (*see also* Infarct, brain) 434.01
chorion 658.8 ☑
colon (acute) (agnogenic) (embolic) (hemorrhagic) (nonocclusive) (nonthrombotic) (occlusive) (segmental) (thrombotic) (with gangrene) 557.0
coronary artery (*see also* Infarct, myocardium) 410.9 ☑
cortical 434.91
embolic (*see also* Embolism) 444.9
fallopian tube 620.8
gallbladder 575.8
heart (*see also* Infarct, myocardium) 410.9 ☑
hepatic 573.4
hypophysis (anterior lobe) 253.8
impending (myocardium) 411.1
intestine (acute) (agnogenic) (embolic) (hemorrhagic) (nonocclusive) (nonthrombotic) (occlusive) (thrombotic) (with gangrene) 557.0
kidney 593.81
lacunar 434.91
liver 573.4
lung (embolic) (thrombotic) 415.19
  with
    abortion — *see* Abortion, by type, with, embolism
    ectopic pregnancy (*see also* categories 633.0–633.9) 639.6
    molar pregnancy (*see also* categories 630–632) 639.6
  following
    abortion 639.6
    ectopic or molar pregnancy 639.6
  iatrogenic 415.11
  in pregnancy, childbirth, or puerperium — *see* Embolism, obstetrical
  postoperative 415.11
  septic 415.12
lymph node or vessel 457.8
medullary (brain) — *see* Infarct, brain
meibomian gland (eyelid) 374.85
mesentery, mesenteric (embolic) (thrombotic) (with gangrene) 557.0
midbrain — *see* Infarct, brain
myocardium, myocardial (acute or with a stated duration of 8 weeks or less) (with hypertension) 410.9 ☑

Note — *Use the following fifth-digit subclassification with category 410:*

0 *episode unspecified*

1 *initial episode*

2 *subsequent episode without recurrence*

Infarct, infarction — *continued*
myocardium, myocardial — *continued*
  with symptoms after 8 weeks from date of infarction 414.8
  anterior (wall) (with contiguous portion of intraventricular septum) NEC 410.1 ☑
  anteroapical (with contiguous portion of intraventricular septum) 410.1 ☑
  anterolateral (wall) 410.0 ☑
  anteroseptal (with contiguous portion of intraventricular septum) 410.1 ☑
  apical-lateral 410.5 ☑
  atrial 410.8 ☑
  basal-lateral 410.5 ☑
  chronic (with symptoms after 8 weeks from date of infarction) 414.8
  diagnosed on ECG, but presenting no symptoms 412
  diaphragmatic wall (with contiguous portion of intraventricular septum) 410.4 ☑
  healed or old, currently presenting no symptoms 412
  high lateral 410.5 ☑
  impending 411.1
  inferior (wall) (with contiguous portion of intraventricular septum) 410.4 ☑
  inferolateral (wall) 410.2 ☑
  inferoposterior wall 410.3 ☑
  intraoperative 997.1
  lateral wall 410.5 ☑
  non-Q wave 410.7 ☑
  non-ST elevation (NSTEMI) 410.7 ☑
  nontransmural 410.7 ☑
  papillary muscle 410.8 ☑
  past (diagnosed on ECG or other special investigation, but currently presenting no symptoms) 412
    with symptoms NEC 414.8
  posterior (strictly) (true) (wall) 410.6 ☑
  posterobasal 410.6 ☑
  posteroinferior 410.3 ☑
  posterolateral 410.5 ☑
  postprocedural 997.1
  previous, currently presenting no symptoms 412
  Q wave (*see also* Infarct, myo-cardium, by site) 410.9 ☑
  septal 410.8 ☑
  specified site NEC 410.8 ☑
  ST elevation (STEMI) 410.9 ☑
    anterior (wall) 410.1 ☑
    anterolateral (wall) 410.0 ☑
    inferior (wall) 410.4 ☑
    inferolateral (wall) 410.2 ☑
    inferoposterior wall 410.3 ☑
    lateral wall 410.5 ☑
    posterior (strictly) (true) (wall) 410.6 ☑
    specified site NEC 410.8 ☑
  subendocardial 410.7 ☑
  syphilitic 093.82
  non-ST elevation myocardial infarction (NSTEMI) 410.7 ☑
  nontransmural 410.7 ☑
omentum 557.0
ovary 620.8
pancreas 577.8
papillary muscle (*see also* Infarct, myocardium) 410.8 ☑
parathyroid gland 252.8
pituitary (gland) 253.8
placenta (complicating pregnancy) 656.7 ☑
  affecting fetus or newborn 762.2
pontine — *see* Infarct, brain
posterior NEC (*see also* Infarct, myocardium) 410.6 ☑
prostate 602.8
pulmonary (artery) (hemorrhagic) (vein) 415.19

Infarct, infarction — *continued*
pulmonary — *continued*
  with
    abortion — *see* Abortion, by type, with embolism
    ectopic pregnancy (*see also* categories 633.0–633.9) 639.6
    molar pregnancy (*see also* categories 630–632) 639.6
  following
    abortion 639.6
    ectopic or molar pregnancy 639.6
  iatrogenic 415.11
  in pregnancy, childbirth, or puerperium — *see* Embolism, obstetrical
  postoperative 415.11
  septic 415.12
renal 593.81
  embolic or thrombotic 593.81
retina, retinal 362.84
  with occlusion — *see* Occlusion, retina
spinal (acute) (cord) (embolic) (nonembolic) 336.1
spleen 289.59
  embolic or thrombotic 444.89
subchorionic — *see* Infarct, placenta
subendocardial (*see also* Infarct, myocardium) 410.7 ☑
suprarenal (capsule) (gland) 255.41
syncytium — *see* Infarct, placenta
testis 608.83
thrombotic (*see also* Thrombosis) 453.9
  artery, arterial — *see* Embolism
thyroid (gland) 246.3
ventricle (heart) (*see also* Infarct, myocardium) 410.9 ☑

Infecting — *see* condition
Infection, infected, infective (opportunistic) 136.9
  with
    influenza viruses occurring in pigs or other animals — *see* Influenza, due to identified, novel influenza A virus
    lymphangitis — *see* Lymphangitis
  abortion — *see* Abortion, by type, with, sepsis
  abscess (skin) — *see* Abscess, by site
  Absidia 117.7
  acanthamoeba 136.21
  Acanthocheilonema (perstans) 125.4
    streptocerca 125.6
  accessory sinus (chronic) (*see also* Sinusitis) 473.9
  Achorion — *see* Dermatophytosis
  Acremonium falciforme 117.4
  acromioclavicular (joint) 711.91
  actinobacillus
    lignieresii 027.8
    mallei 024
    muris 026.1
  actinomadura — *see* Actinomycosis
  Actinomyces (israelii) (*see also* Actinomycosis)
    muris-ratti 026.1
  Actinomycetales (actinomadura) (Actinomyces) (Nocardia) (Streptomyces) — *see* Actinomycosis
  actinomycotic NEC (*see also* Actinomycosis) 039.9
  adenoid (chronic) 474.01
    acute 463
    and tonsil (chronic) 474.02
      acute or subacute 463
  adenovirus NEC 079.0
    in diseases classified elsewhere — *see* category 079 ☑
    unspecified nature or site 079.0
  Aerobacter aerogenes NEC 041.85
    enteritis 008.2
  aerogenes capsulatus (*see also* Gangrene, gas) 040.0
  aertrycke (*see also* Infection, Salmonella) 003.9
  ajellomyces dermatitidis 116.0

Infection, infected, infective — *continued*
alimentary canal NEC (*see also* Enteritis, due to, by organism) 009.0
Allescheria boydii 117.6
Alternaria 118
alveolus, alveolar (process) (pulpal origin) 522.4
ameba, amebic (histolytica) (*see also* Amebiasis) 006.9
  acute 006.0
  chronic 006.1
  free-living 136.29
  hartmanni 007.8
  specified
    site NEC 006.8
    type NEC 007.8
amniotic fluid or cavity 658.4 ☑
  affecting fetus or newborn 762.7
anaerobes (cocci) (gram-negative) (gram-positive) (mixed) NEC 041.84
anal canal 569.49
Ancylostoma braziliense 126.2
Angiostrongylus cantonensis 128.8
anisakiasis 127.1
Anisakis larva 127.1
anthrax (*see also* Anthrax) 022.9
antrum (chronic) (*see also* Sinusitis, maxillary) 473.0
anus (papillae) (sphincter) 569.49
arbor virus NEC 066.9
arbovirus NEC 066.9
argentophil-rod 027.0
Ascaris lumbricoides 127.0
ascomycetes 117.4
Aspergillus (flavus) (fumigatus) (terreus) 117.3
atypical
  acid-fast (bacilli) (*see also* Mycobacterium, atypical) 031.9
  mycobacteria (*see also* Mycobacterium, atypical) 031.9
auditory meatus (circumscribed) (diffuse) (external) (*see also* Otitis, externa) 380.10
auricle (ear) (*see also* Otitis, externa) 380.10
axillary gland 683
Babesiasis 088.82
Babesiosis 088.82
Bacillus NEC 041.89
  abortus 023.1
  anthracis (*see also* Anthrax) 022.9
  cereus (food poisoning) 005.89
  coli — *see* Infection, Escherichia coli
  coliform NEC 041.85
  Ducrey's (any location) 099.0
  Flexner's 004.1
  Friedländer's NEC 041.3
  fusiformis 101
  gas (gangrene) (*see also* Gangrene, gas) 040.0
  mallei 024
  melitensis 023.0
  paratyphoid, paratyphosus 002.9
    A 002.1
    B 002.2
    C 002.3
  Schmorl's 040.3
  Shiga 004.0
  suipestifer (*see also* Infection, Salmonella) 003.9
  swimming pool 031.1
  typhosa 002.0
  welchii (*see also* Gangrene, gas) 040.0
  Whitmore's 025
bacterial NEC 041.9
  specified NEC 041.89
    anaerobic NEC 041.84
    gram-negative NEC 041.85
      anaerobic NEC 041.84
Bacterium
  paratyphosum 002.9
    A 002.1
    B 002.2
    C 002.3
  typhosum 002.0

Infection, infected, infective — *continued*
  Bacteroides (fragilis) (melaninogenicus)
    (oralis) NEC 041.82
  balantidium coli 007.0
  Bartholin's gland 616.89
  Basidiobolus 117.7
  Bedsonia 079.98
    specified NEC 079.88
  bile duct 576.1
  bladder (*see also* Cystitis) 595.9
  Blastomyces, blastomycotic 116.0
    brasiliensis 116.1
    dermatitidis 116.0
    European 117.5
    loboi 116.2
    North American 116.0
    South American 116.1
  bleb
    postprocedural 379.60
      stage 1 379.61
      stage 2 379.62
      stage 3 379.63
  blood stream (*see also* Septicemia)
    catheter-related (CRBSI) 999.31
    central line-associated (CLABSI) 999.32
    due to central venous catheter 999.32
  bone 730.9 ☑
    specified — *see* Osteomyelitis
  Bordetella 033.9
    bronchiseptica 033.8
    parapertussis 033.1
    pertussis 033.0
  Borrelia
    bergdorfi 088.81
    vincentii (mouth) (pharynx) (tonsil) 101
  bovine stomatitis 059.11
  brain (*see also* Encephalitis) 323.9
    late effect — *see* category 326
    membranes (*see also* Meningitis) 322.9
    septic 324.0
      late effect — *see* category 326
      meninges (*see also* Meningitis) 320.9
  branchial cyst 744.42
  breast 611.0
    puerperal, postpartum 675.2 ☑
      with nipple 675.9 ☑
        specified type NEC 675.8 ☑
      nonpurulent 675.2 ☑
      purulent 675.1 ☑
  bronchus (*see also* Bronchitis) 490
    fungus NEC 117.9
  Brucella 023.9
    abortus 023.1
    canis 023.3
    melitensis 023.0
    mixed 023.8
    suis 023.2
  Brugia (Wuchereria) malayi 125.1
  bursa — *see* Bursitis
  buttocks (skin) 686.9
  Candida (albicans) (tropicalis) (*see also*
    Candidiasis) 112.9
    congenital 771.7
  Candiru 136.8
  Capillaria
    hepatica 128.8
    philippinensis 127.5
  cartilage 733.99
  catheter-related bloodstream (CRBSI) 999.31
  cat liver fluke 121.0
  cellulitis — *see* Cellulitis, by site
  central line-associated 999.31
    bloodstream 999.32
  Cephalosporum falciforme 117.4
  Cercomonas hominis (intestinal) 007.3
  cerebrospinal (*see also* Meningitis) 322.9
    late effect — *see* category 326
  cervical gland 683
  cervix (*see also* Cervicitis) 616.0
  cesarean section wound 674.3 ☑
  Chilomastix (intestinal) 007.8
  Chlamydia 079.98
    specified NEC 079.88
  cholera (*see also* Cholera) 001.9
  chorionic plate 658.8 ☑

Infection, infected, infective — *continued*
  Cladosporium
    bantianum 117.8
    carrionii 117.2
    mansoni 111.1
    trichoides 117.8
    wernecki 111.1
  Clonorchis (sinensis) (liver) 121.1
  Clostridium (haemolyticum) (novyi) NEC
    041.84
    botulinum 005.1
    histolyticum (*see also* Gangrene, gas)
      040.0
    oedematiens (*see also* Gangrene, gas)
      040.0
    perfringens 041.83
      due to food 005.2
    septicum (*see also* Gangrene, gas) 040.0
    sordellii (*see also* Gangrene, gas) 040.0
    welchii (*see also* Gangrene, gas) 040.0
      due to food 005.2
  Coccidioides (immitis) (*see also* Coccid-
    ioidomycosis) 114.9
  coccus NEC 041.89
  colon (*see also* Enteritis, due to, by organ-
    ism) 009.0
    bacillus — *see* Infection, Escherichia coli
  colostomy or enterostomy 569.61
  common duct 576.1
  complicating pregnancy, childbirth, or
    puerperium NEC 647.9 ☑
    affecting fetus or newborn 760.2
  Condiobolus 117.7
  congenital NEC 771.89
    Candida albicans 771.7
    chronic 771.2
    cytomegalovirus 771.1
    hepatitis, viral 771.2
    herpes simplex 771.2
    listeriosis 771.2
    malaria 771.2
    poliomyelitis 771.2
    rubella 771.0
    toxoplasmosis 771.2
    tuberculosis 771.2
    urinary (tract) 771.82
    vaccinia 771.2
  coronavirus 079.89
    SARS-associated 079.82
  corpus luteum (*see also* Salpingo-oophoritis)
    614.2
  Corynebacterium diphtheriae — *see* Diph-
    theria
  cotia virus 059.8
  Coxsackie (*see also* Coxsackie) 079.2
    endocardium 074.22
    heart NEC 074.20
    in diseases classified elsewhere — *see*
      category 079 ☑
    meninges 047.0
    myocardium 074.23
    pericardium 074.21
    pharynx 074.0
    specified disease NEC 074.8
    unspecified nature or site 079.2
  Cryptococcus neoformans 117.5
  Cryptosporidia 007.4
  Cunninghamella 117.7
  cyst — *see* Cyst
  Cysticercus cellulosae 123.1
  cystostomy 596.83
  cytomegalovirus 078.5
    congenital 771.1
  dental (pulpal origin) 522.4
  deuteromycetes 117.4
  Dicrocoelium dendriticum 121.8
  Dipetalonema (perstans) 125.4
    streptocerca 125.6
  diphtherial — *see* Diphtheria
  Diphyllobothrium (adult) (latum) (pacifi-
    cum) 123.4
    larval 123.5
  Diplogonoporus (grandis) 123.8
  Dipylidium (caninum) 123.8
  Dirofilaria 125.6
  dog tapeworm 123.8

Infection, infected, infective — *continued*
  Dracunculus medinensis 125.7
  Dreschlera 118
    hawaiiensis 117.8
  Ducrey's bacillus (any site) 099.0
  due to or resulting from
    central venous catheter (*see also* Compli-
      cations, due to, catheter, central
      venous) 999.31
      bloodstream 999.32
      localized 999.33
    device, implant, or graft (any) (presence
      of) — *see* Complications, infec-
      tion and inflammation, due to
      (presence of) any device, implant,
      or graft classified to 996.0–996.5
      NEC
    injection, inoculation, infusion, transfu-
      sion, or vaccination (prophylactic)
      (therapeutic) 999.39
      blood and blood products
        acute 999.34
    injury NEC — *see* Wound, open, by site,
      complicated
    surgery 998.59
  duodenum 535.6 ☑
  ear (*see also* Otitis)
    external (*see also* Otitis, externa) 380.10
    inner (*see also* Labyrinthitis) 386.30
    middle — *see* Otitis, media
  Eaton's agent NEC 041.81
  Eberthella typhosa 002.0
  Ebola 078.89
  ECHO virus 079.1
    in diseases classified elsewhere — *see*
      category 079 ☑
    unspecified nature or site 079.1
  echinococcosis 122.9
  Echinococcus (*see also* Echinococcus) 122.9
  Echinostoma 121.8
  Ehrlichiosis 082.40
    chaffeensis 082.41
    specified type NEC 082.49
  Endamoeba — *see* Infection, ameba
  endocardium (*see also* Endocarditis) 421.0
  endocervix (*see also* Cervicitis) 616.0
  Entamoeba — *see* Infection, ameba
  enteric (*see also* Enteritis, due to, by organ-
    ism) 009.0
  Enterobacter aerogenes NEC 041.85
  Enterobacter sakazakii 041.85
  Enterobius vermicularis 127.4
  enterococcus NEC 041.04
  enterovirus NEC 079.89
    central nervous system NEC 048
    enteritis 008.67
    meningitis 047.9
  Entomophthora 117.7
  Epidermophyton — *see* Dermatophytosis
  epidermophytosis — *see* Dermatophytosis
  episiotomy 674.3 ☑
  Epstein-Barr virus 075
    chronic 780.79 [139.8]
  erysipeloid 027.1
  Erysipelothrix (insidiosa) (rhusiopathiae)
    027.1
  erythema infectiosum 057.0
  Escherichia coli (E. coli) 041.49
    enteritis — *see* Enteritis, E. coli
    generalized 038.42
    intestinal — *see* Enteritis, E. coli
    non-Shiga toxin-producing 041.49
    Shiga toxin-producing (STEC) 041.43
      with
        unspecified O group 041.43
        non-O157 (with known O group)
          041.43
        O157 (with confirmation of Shiga
          toxin when H antigen is un-
          known, or is not H7) 041.41
        O157:H7 with or without confirma-
          tion of Shiga toxin-production
          041.41
        O157H:- (nonmotile) with confirma-
          tion of Shiga toxin 041.41
    specified NEC 041.42

Infection, infected, infective — *continued*
  esophagostomy 530.86
  ethmoidal (chronic) (sinus) (*see also* Sinusi-
    tis, ethmoidal) 473.2
  Eubacterium 041.84
  Eustachian tube (ear) 381.50
    acute 381.51
    chronic 381.52
  exanthema subitum (*see also* Exanthem
    subitum) 058.10
  exit site 999.33
  external auditory canal (meatus) (*see also*
    Otitis, externa) 380.10
  eyelid 373.9
    specified NEC 373.8
  eye NEC 360.00
  fallopian tube (*see also* Salpingo-oophoritis)
    614.2
  fascia 728.89
  Fasciola
    gigantica 121.3
    hepatica 121.3
  Fasciolopsis (buski) 121.4
  fetus (intra-amniotic) — *see* Infection, con-
    genital
  filarial — *see* Infestation, filarial
  finger (skin) 686.9
    abscess (with lymphangitis) 681.00
      pulp 681.01
    cellulitis (with lymphangitis) 681.00
    distal closed space (with lymphangitis)
      681.00
    nail 681.02
      fungus 110.1
  fish tapeworm 123.4
    larval 123.5
  flagellate, intestinal 007.9
  fluke — *see* Infestation, fluke
  focal
    teeth (pulpal origin) 522.4
    tonsils 474.00
      and adenoids 474.02
  Fonsecaea
    compactum 117.2
    pedrosoi 117.2
  food (*see also* Poisoning, food) 005.9
  foot (skin) 686.9
    fungus 110.4
  Francisella tularensis (*see also* Tularemia)
    021.9
  frontal sinus (chronic) (*see also* Sinusitis,
    frontal) 473.1
  fungus NEC 117.9
    beard 110.0
    body 110.5
    dermatiacious NEC 117.8
    foot 110.4
    groin 110.3
    hand 110.2
    nail 110.1
    pathogenic to compromised host only
      118
    perianal (area) 110.3
    scalp 110.0
    scrotum 110.8
    skin 111.9
      foot 110.4
      hand 110.2
    toenails 110.1
    trachea 117.9
  Fusarium 118
  Fusobacterium 041.84
  gallbladder (*see also* Cholecystitis, acute)
    575.0
  Gardnerella vaginalis 041.89
  gas bacillus (*see also* Gas, gangrene) 040.0
  gastric (*see also* Gastritis) 535.5 ☑
  Gastrodiscoides hominis 121.8
  gastroenteric (*see also* Enteritis, due to, by
    organism) 009.0
  gastrointestinal (*see also* Enteritis, due to,
    by organism) 009.0
  gastrostomy 536.41
  generalized NEC (*see also* Septicemia) 038.9
  genital organ or tract NEC
    female 614.9

Infection, infected, infective — Infection, infected, infective — Infection, infected, infective

Infection, infected, infective — *continued*
genital organ or tract — *continued*
female — *continued*
with
abortion — *see* Abortion, by type,
with sepsis
ectopic pregnancy (*see also* categories 633.0–633.9) 639.0
molar pregnancy (*see also* categories 630–632) 639.0
complicating pregnancy 646.6 ☑
affecting fetus or newborn 760.8
following
abortion 639.0
ectopic or molar pregnancy 639.0
puerperal, postpartum, childbirth
670.8 ☑
minor or localized 646.6 ☑
affecting fetus or newborn
760.8
male 608.4
genitourinary tract NEC 599.0
Ghon tubercle, primary (*see also* Tuberculosis) 010.0 ☑
Giardia lamblia 007.1
gingival (chronic) 523.10
acute 523.00
Vincent's 101
glanders 024
Glenosporopsis amazonica 116.2
Gnathostoma spinigerum 128.1
Gongylonema 125.6
gonococcal NEC (*see also* Gonococcus) 098.0
gram-negative bacilli NEC 041.85
anaerobic 041.84
guinea worm 125.7
gum (*see also* Infection, gingival) 523.10
Hantavirus 079.81
heart 429.89
Helicobacter pylori [H. pylori] 041.86
helminths NEC 128.9
intestinal 127.9
mixed (types classifiable to more
than one category in
120.0–127.7) 127.8
specified type NEC 127.7
specified type NEC 128.8
Hemophilus influenzae NEC 041.5
generalized 038.41
herpes (simplex) (*see also* Herpes, simplex)
054.9
congenital 771.2
zoster (*see also* Herpes, zoster) 053.9
eye NEC 053.29
Heterophyes heterophyes 121.6
Histoplasma (*see also* Histoplasmosis) 115.90
capsulatum (*see also* Histoplasmosis,
American) 115.00
duboisii (*see also* Histoplasmosis, African)
115.10
HIV V08
with symptoms, symptomatic 042
hookworm (*see also* Ancylostomiasis) 126.9
human herpesvirus 6 058.81
human herpesvirus 7 058.82
human herpesvirus 8 058.89
human herpesvirus NEC 058.89
human immunodeficiency virus V08
with symptoms, symptomatic 042
human papillomavirus 079.4
hydrocele 603.1
hydronephrosis 591
Hymenolepis 123.6
hypopharynx 478.29
inguinal glands 683
due to soft chancre 099.0
insertion site 999.33
intestine, intestinal (*see also* Enteritis, due
to, by organism) 009.0
intrauterine (*see also* Endometritis) 615.9
complicating delivery 646.6 ☑
isospora belli or hominis 007.2
Japanese B encephalitis 062.0
jaw (bone) (acute) (chronic) (lower) (subacute) (upper) 526.4
joint — *see* Arthritis, infectious or infective

Infection, infected, infective — *continued*
Kaposi's sarcoma-associated herpesvirus
058.89
kidney (cortex) (hematogenous) 590.9
with
abortion — *see* Abortion, by type,
with urinary tract infection
calculus 592.0
ectopic pregnancy (*see also* categories 633.0–633.9) 639.8
molar pregnancy (*see also* categories
630–632) 639.8
complicating pregnancy or puerperium
646.6 ☑
affecting fetus or newborn 760.1
following
abortion 639.8
ectopic or molar pregnancy 639.8
pelvis and ureter 590.3
Klebsiella pneumoniae NEC 041.3
knee (skin) NEC 686.9
joint — *see* Arthritis, infectious
Koch's (*see also* Tuberculosis, pulmonary)
011.9 ☑
labia (majora) (minora) (*see also* Vulvitis)
616.10
lacrimal
gland (*see also* Dacryoadenitis) 375.00
passages (duct) (sac) (*see also* Dacryocystitis) 375.30
larynx NEC 478.79
leg (skin) NEC 686.9
Leishmania (*see also* Leishmaniasis) 085.9
braziliensis 085.5
donovani 085.0
ethiopica 085.3
furunculosa 085.1
infantum 085.0
mexicana 085.4
tropica (minor) 085.1
major 085.2
Leptosphaeria senegalensis 117.4
leptospira (*see also* Leptospirosis) 100.9
Australis 100.89
Bataviae 100.89
pyrogenes 100.89
specified type NEC 100.89
leptospirochetal NEC (*see also* Leptospirosis)
100.9
Leptothrix — *see* Actinomycosis
Listeria monocytogenes (listeriosis) 027.0
congenital 771.2
liver fluke — *see* Infestation, fluke, liver
Loa loa 125.2
eyelid 125.2 [373.6]
Loboa loboi 116.2
local, skin (staphylococcal) (streptococcal)
NEC 686.9
abscess — *see* Abscess, by site
cellulitis — *see* Cellulitis, by site
ulcer (*see also* Ulcer, skin) 707.9
Loefflerella
mallei 024
whitmori 025
lung 518.89
atypical Mycobacterium 031.0
tuberculous (*see also* Tuberculosis,
pulmonary) 011.9 ☑
basilar 518.89
chronic 518.89
fungus NEC 117.9
spirochetal 104.8
virus — *see* Pneumonia, virus
lymph gland (axillary) (cervical) (inguinal)
683
mesenteric 289.2
lymphoid tissue, base of tongue or posterior
pharynx, NEC 474.00
madurella
grisea 117.4
mycetomii 117.4
major
with
abortion — *see* Abortion, by type,
with sepsis

Infection, infected, infective — *continued*
major — *continued*
with — *continued*
ectopic pregnancy (*see also* categories 633.0–633.9) 639.0
molar pregnancy (*see also* categories
630–632) 639.0
following
abortion 639.0
ectopic or molar pregnancy 639.0
puerperal, postpartum, childbirth
670.0 ☑
Malassezia furfur 111.0
Malleomyces
mallei 024
pseudomallei 025
mammary gland 611.0
puerperal, postpartum 675.2 ☑
Mansonella (ozzardi) 125.5
mastoid (suppurative) — *see* Mastoiditis
maxilla, maxillary 526.4
sinus (chronic) (*see also* Sinusitis, maxillary) 473.0
mediastinum 519.2
medina 125.7
meibomian
cyst 373.12
gland 373.12
melioidosis 025
meninges (*see also* Meningitis) 320.9
meningococcal (*see also* condition) 036.9
brain 036.1
cerebrospinal 036.0
endocardium 036.42
generalized 036.2
meninges 036.0
meningococcemia 036.2
specified site NEC 036.89
mesenteric lymph nodes or glands NEC
289.2
Metagonimus 121.5
metatarsophalangeal 711.97
methicillin
resistant Staphylococcus aureus (MRSA)
041.12
susceptible Staphylococcus aureus
(MSSA) 041.11
microorganism resistant to drugs — *see*
Resistance (to), drugs by microorganisms
Microsporidia 136.8
microsporum, microsporic — *see* Dermatophytosis
Mima polymorpha NEC 041.85
mixed flora NEC 041.89
Monilia (*see also* Candidiasis) 112.9
neonatal 771.7
monkeypox 059.01
Monosporium apiospermum 117.6
mouth (focus) NEC 528.9
parasitic 136.9
MRSA (methicillin resistant Staphylococcus
aureus) 041.12
MSSA (methicillin susceptible Staphylococcus aureus) 041.11
Mucor 117.7
muscle NEC 728.89
mycelium NEC 117.9
mycetoma
actinomycotic NEC (*see also* Actinomycosis) 039.9
mycotic NEC 117.4
Mycobacterium, mycobacterial (*see also*
Mycobacterium) 031.9
Mycoplasma NEC 041.81
mycotic NEC 117.9
pathogenic to compromised host only
118
skin NEC 111.9
systemic 117.9
myocardium NEC 422.90
nail (chronic) (with lymphangitis) 681.9
finger 681.02
fungus 110.1
ingrowing 703.0
toe 681.11

Infection, infected, infective — *continued*
nail — *continued*
toe — *continued*
fungus 110.1
nasal sinus (chronic) (*see also* Sinusitis) 473.9
nasopharynx (chronic) 478.29
acute 460
navel 686.9
newborn 771.4
Neisserian — *see* Gonococcus
Neotestudina rosatii 117.4
newborn, generalized 771.89
nipple 611.0
puerperal, postpartum 675.0 ☑
with breast 675.9 ☑
specified type NEC 675.8 ☑
Nocardia — *see* Actinomycosis
nose 478.19
nostril 478.19
obstetrical surgical wound 674.3 ☑
Oesophagostomum (apiostomum) 127.7
Oestrus ovis 134.0
Oidium albicans (*see also* Candidiasis) 112.9
Onchocerca (volvulus) 125.3
eye 125.3 [360.13]
eyelid 125.3 [373.6]
operation wound 998.59
Opisthorchis (felineus) (tenuicollis) (viverri-
ni) 121.0
orbit 376.00
chronic 376.10
orthopoxvirus 059.00
specified NEC 059.09
ovary (*see also* Salpingo-oophoritis) 614.2
Oxyuris vermicularis 127.4
pancreas 577.0
Paracoccidioides brasiliensis 116.1
Paragonimus (westermani) 121.2
parainfluenza virus 079.89
parameningococcus NEC 036.9
with meningitis 036.0
parapoxvirus 059.10
specified NEC 059.19
parasitic NEC 136.9
paratyphoid 002.9
type A 002.1
type B 002.2
type C 002.3
paraurethral ducts 597.89
parotid gland 527.2
Pasteurella NEC 027.2
multocida (cat-bite) (dog-bite) 027.2
pestis (*see also* Plague) 020.9
pseudotuberculosis 027.2
septica (cat-bite) (dog-bite) 027.2
tularensis (*see also* Tularemia) 021.9
pelvic, female (*see also* Disease, pelvis, inflammatory) 614.9
penis (glans) (retention) NEC 607.2
herpetic 054.13
Peptococcus 041.84
Peptostreptococcus 041.84
periapical (pulpal origin) 522.4
peridental 523.30
peridental 523.31
perineal wound (obstetrical) 674.3 ☑
periodontal 523.31
periorbital 376.00
chronic 376.10
perirectal 569.49
perirenal (*see also* Infection, kidney) 590.9
peritoneal (*see also* Peritonitis) 567.9
periureteral 593.89
periurethral 597.89
Petriellidium boydii 117.6
pharynx 478.29
Coxsackie virus 074.0
phlegmonous 462
posterior, lymphoid 474.00
Phialophora
gougerotii 117.8
jeanselmei 117.8
verrucosa 117.2
Piedraia hortai 111.3
pinna, acute 380.11
pinta 103.9
intermediate 103.1

☑ Additional Digit Required — Refer to the Tabular List for Digit Selection   ▽ Subterms under main terms may continue to next column or page

Infection, infected, infective — *continued*

pinta — *continued*
    late 103.2
    mixed 103.3
    primary 103.0
pinworm 127.4
pityrosporum furfur 111.0
pleuropneumonia-like organisms NEC (PP-LO) 041.81
pneumococcal NEC 041.2
    generalized (purulent) 038.2
Pneumococcus NEC 041.2
port 999.33
postoperative wound 998.59
posttraumatic NEC 958.3
postvaccinal 999.39
poxvirus 059.9
    specified NEC 059.8
prepuce NEC 607.1
Proprionibacterium 041.84
prostate (capsule) (*see also* Prostatitis) 601.9
Proteus (mirabilis) (morganii) (vulgaris) NEC 041.6
    enteritis 008.3
protozoal NEC 136.8
    intestinal NEC 007.9
Pseudomonas NEC 041.7
    mallei 024
    pneumonia 482.1
    pseudomallei 025
psittacosis 073.9
puerperal, postpartum (major) 670.0 ☑
    minor 646.6 ☑
pulmonary — *see* Infection, lung
purulent — *see* Abscess
putrid, generalized — *see* Septicemia
pyemic — *see* Septicemia
Pyrenochaeta romeroi 117.4
Q fever 083.0
rabies 071
rectum (sphincter) 569.49
renal (*see also* Infection, kidney) 590.9
    pelvis and ureter 590.3
reservoir 999.33
resistant to drugs — *see* Resistance (to), drugs by microorganisms
respiratory 519.8
    chronic 519.8
    influenzal (acute) (upper) (*see also* Influenza) 487.1
    lung 518.89
    rhinovirus 460
    syncytial virus 079.6
    upper (acute) (infectious) NEC 465.9
        with flu, grippe, or influenza (*see also* Influenza) 487.1
        influenzal (*see also* Influenza) 487.1
        multiple sites NEC 465.8
        streptococcal 034.0
        viral NEC 465.9
respiratory syncytial virus (RSV) 079.6
resulting from presence of shunt or other internal prosthetic device — *see* Complications, infection and inflammation, due to (presence of) any device, implant, or graft classified to 996.0–996.5 NEC
retroperitoneal 567.39
retrovirus 079.50
    human immunodeficiency virus type 2 (HIV2) 079.53
    human T-cell lymphotrophic virus type I (HTLV-I) 079.51
    human T-cell lymphotrophic virus type II (HTLV-II) 079.52
    specified NEC 079.59
Rhinocladium 117.1
Rhinosporidium — *see beri* 117.0
rhinovirus
    in diseases classified elsewhere — *see* category 079 ☑
    unspecified nature or site 079.3
Rhizopus 117.7
rickettsial 083.9
rickettsialpox 083.2
rubella (*see also* Rubella) 056.9

Infection, infected, infective — *continued*

rubella (*see also* Rubella) — *continued*
    congenital 771.0
Saccharomyces (*see also* Candidiasis) 112.9
Saksenaea 117.7
salivary duct or gland (any) 527.2
Salmonella (aertrycke) (callinarum) (choleraesuis) (enteritidis) (suipestifer) (typhimurium) 003.9
    with
        arthritis 003.23
        gastroenteritis 003.0
        localized infection 003.20
            specified type NEC 003.29
        meningitis 003.21
        osteomyelitis 003.24
        pneumonia 003.22
        septicemia 003.1
        specified manifestation NEC 003.8
    due to food (poisoning) (any serotype) (*see also* Poisoning, food, due to, Salmonella)
    hirschfeldii 002.3
    localized 003.20
        specified type NEC 003.29
    paratyphi 002.9
        A 002.1
        B 002.2
        C 002.3
    schottmuelleri 002.2
    specified type NEC 003.8
    typhi 002.0
    typhosa 002.0
saprophytic 136.8
Sarcocystis, lindemanni 136.5
SARS-associated coronavirus 079.82
scabies 133.0
Schistosoma — *see* Infestation, Schistosoma
Schmorl's bacillus 040.3
scratch or other superficial injury — *see* Injury, superficial, by site
scrotum (acute) NEC 608.4
sealpox 059.12
secondary, burn or open wound (dislocation) (fracture) 958.3
seminal vesicle (*see also* Vesiculitis) 608.0
septic
    generalized — *see* Septicemia
    localized, skin (*see also* Abscess) 682.9
septicemic — *see* Septicemia
seroma 998.51
Serratia (marcescens) 041.85
    generalized 038.44
sheep liver fluke 121.3
Shigella 004.9
    boydii 004.2
    dysenteriae 004.0
    flexneri 004.1
    group
        A 004.0
        B 004.1
        C 004.2
        D 004.3
    Schmitz (-Stutzer) 004.0
    schmitzii 004.0
    Shiga 004.0
    sonnei 004.3
    specified type NEC 004.8
Sin Nombre virus 079.81
sinus (*see also* Sinusitis) 473.9
    pilonidal 685.1
        with abscess 685.0
    skin NEC 686.9
Skene's duct or gland (*see also* Urethritis) 597.89
skin (local) (staphylococcal) (streptococcal) NEC 686.9
    abscess — *see* Abscess, by site
    cellulitis — *see* Cellulitis, by site
    due to fungus 111.9
        specified type NEC 111.8
    mycotic 111.9
        specified type NEC 111.8
    ulcer (*see also* Ulcer, skin) 707.9
slow virus 046.9
    specified condition NEC 046.8

Infection, infected, infective — *continued*

Sparganum (mansoni) (proliferum) 123.5
spermatic cord NEC 608.4
sphenoidal (chronic) (sinus) (*see also* Sinusitis, sphenoidal) 473.3
Spherophorus necrophorus 040.3
spinal cord NEC (*see also* Encephalitis) 323.9
    abscess 324.1
        late effect — *see* category 326
    late effect — *see* category 326
    meninges — *see* Meningitis
    streptococcal 320.2
Spirillum
    minus or minor 026.0
    morsus muris 026.0
    obermeieri 087.0
spirochetal NEC 104.9
    lung 104.8
    specified nature or site NEC 104.8
spleen 289.59
Sporothrix schenckii 117.1
Sporotrichum (schenckii) 117.1
Sporozoa 136.8
staphylococcal NEC 041.10
    aureus 041.11
        methicillin
            resistant (MRSA) 041.12
            susceptible (MSSA) 041.11
    food poisoning 005.0
    generalized (purulent) 038.10
        aureus 038.11
            methicillin
                resistant 038.12
                susceptible 038.11
        specified organism NEC 038.19
    pneumonia 482.40
        aureus 482.41
            methicillin
                resistant (MRSA) 482.42
                susceptible (MSSA) 482.41
        MRSA (methicillin resistant Staphylococcus aureus) 482.42
        MSSA (methicillin susceptible Staphylococcus aureus) 482.41
        specified type NEC 482.49
    septicemia 038.10
        aureus 038.11
            methicillin
                resistant (MRSA) 038.12
                susceptible (MSSA) 038.11
        MRSA (methicillin resistant Staphylococcus aureus) 038.12
        MSSA (methicillin susceptible Staphylococcus aureus) 038.11
        specified organism NEC 038.19
    specified NEC 041.19
steatoma 706.2
Stellantchasmus falcatus 121.6
Streptobacillus moniliformis 026.1
streptococcal NEC 041.00
    generalized (purulent) 038.0
    Group
        A 041.01
        B 041.02
        C 041.03
        D [enterococcus] 041.04
        G 041.05
    pneumonia — *see* Pneumonia, streptococcal
    septicemia 038.0
    sore throat 034.0
    specified NEC 041.09
Streptomyces — *see* Actinomycosis
streptotrichosis — *see* Actinomycosis
Strongyloides (stercoralis) 127.2
stump (amputation) (posttraumatic) (surgical) 997.62
    traumatic — *see* Amputation, traumatic, by site, complicated
subcutaneous tissue, local NEC 686.9
submaxillary region 528.9
suipestifer (*see also* Infection, Salmonella) 003.9
swimming pool bacillus 031.1

Infection, infected, infective — *continued*

syphilitic — *see* Syphilis
systemic — *see* Septicemia
Taenia — *see* Infestation, Taenia
Taeniarhynchus saginatus 123.2
tanapox 059.21
tapeworm — *see* Infestation, tapeworm
tendon (sheath) 727.89
Ternidens diminutus 127.7
testis (*see also* Orchitis) 604.90
thigh (skin) 686.9
threadworm 127.4
throat 478.29
    pneumococcal 462
    staphylococcal 462
    streptococcal 034.0
    viral NEC (*see also* Pharyngitis) 462
thumb (skin) 686.9
    abscess (with lymphangitis) 681.00
        pulp 681.01
    cellulitis (with lymphangitis) 681.00
    nail 681.02
thyroglossal duct 529.8
toe (skin) 686.9
    abscess (with lymphangitis) 681.10
    cellulitis (with lymphangitis) 681.10
    nail 681.11
        fungus 110.1
tongue NEC 529.0
    parasitic 112.0
tonsil (faucial) (lingual) (pharyngeal) 474.00
    acute or subacute 463
    and adenoid 474.02
    tag 474.00
tooth, teeth 522.4
    periapical (pulpal origin) 522.4
    peridental 523.30
    periodontal 523.31
    pulp 522.0
    socket 526.5
TORCH — *see* Infection, congenital NEC
    without active infection 760.2
Torula histolytica 117.5
Toxocara (cani) (cati) (felis) 128.0
Toxoplasma gondii (*see also* Toxoplasmosis) 130.9
trachea, chronic 491.8
    fungus 117.9
traumatic NEC 958.3
trematode NEC 121.9
trench fever 083.1
Treponema
    denticola 041.84
    macrodenticum 041.84
    pallidum (*see also* Syphilis) 097.9
Trichinella (spiralis) 124
Trichomonas 131.9
    bladder 131.09
    cervix 131.09
    hominis 007.3
    intestine 007.3
    prostate 131.03
    specified site NEC 131.8
    urethra 131.02
    urogenitalis 131.00
    vagina 131.01
    vulva 131.01
Trichophyton, trichophytid — *see* Dermatophytosis
Trichosporon (beigelii) cutaneum 111.2
Trichostrongylus 127.6
Trichuris (trichiuria) 127.3
Trombicula (irritans) 133.8
Trypanosoma (*see also* Trypanosomiasis) 086.9
    cruzi 086.2
tubal (*see also* Salpingo-oophoritis) 614.2
tuberculous NEC (*see also* Tuberculosis) 011.9 ☑
tubo-ovarian (*see also* Salpingo-oophoritis) 614.2
tunica vaginalis 608.4
tunnel 999.33
tympanic membrane — *see* Myringitis
typhoid (abortive) (ambulant) (bacillus) 002.0

Index

Infection, infected, infective — Infestation

Infection, infected, infective — *continued*
  typhus 081.9
    flea-borne (endemic) 081.0
    louse-borne (epidemic) 080
    mite-borne 081.2
    recrudescent 081.1
    tick-borne 082.9
      African 082.1
      North Asian 082.2
  umbilicus (septic) 686.9
    newborn NEC 771.4
  ureter 593.89
  urethra (*see also* Urethritis) 597.80
  urinary (tract) NEC 599.0
    with
      abortion — *see* Abortion, by type,
        with urinary tract infection
      ectopic pregnancy (*see also* cate-
        gories 633.0–633.9) 639.8
      molar pregnancy (*see also* categories
        630–632) 639.8
  candidal 112.2
  complicating pregnancy, childbirth, or
    puerperium 646.6 ☑
      affecting fetus or newborn 760.1
      asymptomatic 646.5 ☑
        affecting fetus or newborn 760.1
  diplococcal (acute) 098.0
    chronic 098.2
  due to Trichomonas (vaginalis) 131.00
    following
      abortion 639.8
      ectopic or molar pregnancy 639.8
    gonococcal (acute) 098.0
      chronic or duration of 2 months
        or over 098.2
  newborn 771.82
  trichomonal 131.00
  tuberculous (*see also* Tuberculosis)
    016.3 ☑
  uterus, uterine (*see also* Endometritis)
    615.9
  utriculus masculinus NEC 597.89
  vaccination 999.39
  vagina (granulation tissue) (wall) (*see
    also* Vaginitis) 616.10
  varicella 052.9
  varicose veins — *see* Varicose, veins
  variola 050.9
    major 050.0
    minor 050.1
  vas deferens NEC 608.4
  Veillonella 041.84
  verumontanum 597.89
  vesical (*see also* Cystitis) 595.9
  Vibrio
    cholerae 001.0
      El Tor 001.1
    parahaemolyticus (food poisoning)
      005.4
    vulnificus 041.85
  Vincent's (gums) (mouth) (tonsil) 101
  vaccination 999.39
  virus, viral 079.99
    adenovirus
      in diseases classified elsewhere —
        see category 079 ☑
      unspecified nature or site 079.0
    central nervous system NEC 049.9
      enterovirus 048
        meningitis 047.9
          specified type NEC 047.8
      slow virus 046.9
      specified condition NEC 046.8
    chest 519.8
    conjunctivitis 077.99
      specified type NEC 077.8
    coronavirus 079.89
      SARS-associated 079.82
    Coxsackie (*see also* Infection, Coxsackie)
      079.2
    Ebola 065.8
    ECHO
      in diseases classified elsewhere —
        see category 079 ☑
      unspecified nature or site 079.1

Infection, infected, infective — *continued*
  virus, viral — *continued*
    encephalitis 049.9
      arthropod-borne NEC 064
      tick-borne 063.9
        specified type NEC 063.8
    enteritis NEC (*see also* Enteritis, viral)
      008.8
    exanthem NEC 057.9
    Hantavirus 079.81
    human papilloma 079.4
    in diseases classified elsewhere — *see*
      category 079 ☑
    intestine (*see also* Enteritis, viral) 008.8
    lung — *see* Pneumonia, viral
    respiratory syncytial (RSV) 079.6
    retrovirus 079.50
    rhinovirus
      in diseases classified elsewhere —
        see category 079 ☑
      unspecified nature or site 079.3
    salivary gland disease 078.5
    slow 046.9
      specified condition NEC 046.8
    specified type NEC 079.89
      in diseases classified elsewhere —
        see category 079 ☑
    unspecified nature or site 079.99
    warts 078.10
      specified NEC 078.19
    yaba monkey tumor 059.22
  vulva (*see also* Vulvitis) 616.10
  whipworm 127.3
  Whitmore's bacillus 025
  wound (local) (posttraumatic) NEC 958.3
    with
      dislocation — *see* Dislocation, by site,
        open
      fracture — *see* Fracture, by site, open
      open wound — *see* Wound, open,
        by site, complicated
    postoperative 998.59
    surgical 998.59
  Wuchereria 125.0
    bancrofti 125.0
    malayi 125.1
  yaba monkey tumor virus 059.22
  yatapoxvirus 059.20
  yaws — *see* Yaws
  yeast (*see also* Candidiasis) 112.9
  yellow fever (*see also* Fever, yellow) 060.9
  Yersinia pestis (*see also* Plague) 020.9
  Zeis' gland 373.12
  zoonotic bacterial NEC 027.9
  Zopfia senegalensis 117.4
Infective, infectious — *see* condition
Inferiority complex 301.9
  constitutional psychopathic 301.9
Infertility
  female 628.9
    age related 628.8
    associated with
      adhesions, peritubal 614.6 *[628.2]*
      anomaly
        cervical mucus 628.4
        congenital
          cervix 628.4
          fallopian tube 628.2
          uterus 628.3
          vagina 628.4
      anovulation 628.0
      dysmucorrhea 628.4
      endometritis, tuberculous (*see also*
        Tuberculosis) 016.7 ☑ *[628.3]*
      Stein-Leventhal syndrome
        256.4 *[628.0]*
    due to
      adiposogenital dystrophy
        253.8 *[628.1]*
      anterior pituitary disorder NEC
        253.4 *[628.1]*
        hyperfunction 253.1 *[628.1]*
      cervical anomaly 628.4
      fallopian tube anomaly 628.2
      ovarian failure 256.39 *[628.0]*

Infertility — *continued*
  female — *continued*
    due to — *continued*
      Stein-Leventhal syndrome
        256.4 *[628.0]*
      uterine anomaly 628.3
      vaginal anomaly 628.4
    nonimplantation 628.3
    origin
      cervical 628.4
      pituitary-hypothalamus NEC
        253.8 *[628.1]*
        anterior pituitary NEC
          253.4 *[628.1]*
          hyperfunction NEC
            253.1 *[628.1]*
          dwarfism 253.3 *[628.1]*
          panhypopituitarism 253.2 *[628.1]*
      specified NEC 628.8
    tubal (block) (occlusion) (stenosis)
      628.2
      adhesions 614.6 *[628.2]*
    uterine 628.3
    vaginal 628.4
    previous, requiring supervision of preg-
      nancy V23.0
  male 606.9
    absolute 606.0
    due to
      azoospermia 606.0
      drug therapy 606.8
      extratesticular cause NEC 606.8
      germinal cell
        aplasia 606.0
        desquamation 606.1
      hypospermatogenesis 606.1
      infection 606.8
      obstruction, afferent ducts 606.8
      oligospermia 606.1
      radiation 606.8
      spermatogenic arrest (complete)
        606.0
        incomplete 606.1
      systemic disease 606.8
Infestation 134.9
  Acanthocheilonema (perstans) 125.4
    streptocerca 125.6
  Acariasis 133.9
    demodex folliculorum 133.8
    Sarcoptes scabiei 133.0
    trombiculae 133.8
  Agamofilaria streptocerca 125.6
  Ancylostoma, Ankylostoma 126.9
    americanum 126.1
    braziliense 126.2
    canium 126.8
    ceylanicum 126.3
    duodenale 126.0
    new world 126.1
    old world 126.0
  Angiostrongylus cantonensis 128.8
  anisakiasis 127.1
  Anisakis larva 127.1
  arthropod NEC 134.1
  Ascaris lumbricoides 127.0
  Bacillus fusiformis 101
  Balantidium coli 007.0
  beef tapeworm 123.2
  Bothriocephalus (latus) 123.4
    larval 123.5
  broad tapeworm 123.4
    larval 123.5
  Brugia malayi 125.1
  Candiru 136.8
  Capillaria
    hepatica 128.8
    philippinensis 127.5
  cat liver fluke 121.0
  Cercomonas hominis (intestinal) 007.3
  cestodes 123.9
    specified type NEC 123.8
  chigger 133.8
  chigoe 134.1
  Chilomastix 007.8
  Clonorchis (sinensis) (liver) 121.1
  coccidia 007.2

Infestation — *continued*
  complicating pregnancy, childbirth, or
    puerperium 647.9 ☑
      affecting fetus or newborn 760.8
  Cysticercus cellulosae 123.1
  Demodex folliculorum 133.8
  Dermatobia (hominis) 134.0
  Dibothriocephalus (latus) 123.4
    larval 123.5
  Dicrocoelium dendriticum 121.8
  Diphyllobothrium (adult) (intestinal) (latum)
    (pacificum) 123.4
    larval 123.5
  Diplogonoporus (grandis) 123.8
  Dipylidium (caninum) 123.8
  Distoma hepaticum 121.3
  dog tapeworm 123.8
  Dracunculus medinensis 125.7
  dragon worm 125.7
  dwarf tapeworm 123.6
  Echinococcus (*see also* Echinococcus) 122.9
  Echinostoma ilocanum 121.8
  Embadomonas 007.8
  Endamoeba (histolytica) — *see* Infection,
    ameba
  Entamoeba (histolytica) — *see* Infection,
    ameba
  Enterobius vermicularis 127.4
  Epidermophyton — *see* Dermatophytosis
  eyeworm 125.2
  Fasciola
    gigantica 121.3
    hepatica 121.3
  Fasciolopsis (buski) (small intestine) 121.4
    blood NEC (*see also* Schistosomiasis)
      120.9
    cat liver 121.0
    filarial 125.9
    due to
      Acanthocheilonema (perstans)
        125.4
        streptocerca 125.6
      Brugia (Wuchereria) malayi 125.1
      Dracunculus medinensis 125.7
      guinea worms 125.7
      Mansonella (ozzardi) 125.5
      Onchocerca volvulus 125.3
        eye 125.3 *[360.13]*
        eyelid 125.3 *[373.6]*
      Wuchereria (bancrofti) 125.0
        malayi 125.1
    specified type NEC 125.6
  fish tapeworm 123.4
    larval 123.5
  fluke 121.9
    intestinal (giant) 121.4
    liver (sheep) 121.3
      cat 121.0
      Chinese 121.1
      clonorchiasis 121.1
      fascioliasis 121.3
      Oriental 121.1
    lung (oriental) 121.2
    sheep liver 121.3
  fly larva 134.0
  Gasterophilus (intestinalis) 134.0
  Gastrodiscoides hominis 121.8
  Giardia lamblia 007.1
  Gnathostoma (spinigerum) 128.1
  Gongylonema 125.6
  guinea worm 125.7
  helminth NEC 128.9
    intestinal 127.9
      mixed (types classifiable to more
        than one category in
        120.0–127.7) 127.8
      specified type NEC 127.7
    specified type NEC 128.8
  Heterophyes heterophyes (small intestine)
    121.6
  hookworm (*see also* Infestation, ancy-
    lostoma) 126.9
  Hymenolepis (diminuta) (nana) 123.6
  intestinal NEC 129
  leeches (aquatic) (land) 134.2
  Leishmania — *see* Leishmaniasis

Infestation — *continued*
  lice (*see also* Infestation, pediculus) 132.9
  Linguatulidae, linguatula (pentastoma)
    (serrata) 134.1
  Loa loa 125.2
    eyelid 125.2 *[373.6]*
  louse (*see also* Infestation, pediculus) 132.9
    body 132.1
    head 132.0
    pubic 132.2
  maggots 134.0
  Mansonella (ozzardi) 125.5
  medina 125.7
  Metagonimus yokogawai (small intestine)
    121.5
  Microfilaria streptocerca 125.3
    eye 125.3 *[360.13]*
    eyelid 125.3 *[373.6]*
  Microsporon furfur 111.0
  microsporum — *see* Dermatophytosis
  mites 133.9
    scabic 133.0
    specified type NEC 133.8
  monilia (albicans) (*see also* Candidiasis)
    112.9
    vagina 112.1
    vulva 112.1
  mouth 112.0
  Necator americanus 126.1
  nematode (intestinal) 127.9
    Ancylostoma (*see also* Ancylostoma)
      126.9
    Ascaris lumbricoides 127.0
    conjunctiva NEC 128.9
    Dioctophyma 128.8
    Enterobius vermicularis 127.4
    Gnathostoma spinigerum 128.1
    Oesophagostomum (apiostomum) 127.7
    Physaloptera 127.4
    specified type NEC 127.7
    Strongyloides stercoralis 127.2
    Ternidens diminutus 127.7
    Trichinella spiralis 124
    Trichostrongylus 127.6
    Trichuris (trichiuria) 127.3
  Oesophagostomum (apiostomum) 127.7
  Oestrus ovis 134.0
  Onchocerca (volvulus) 125.3
    eye 125.3 *[360.13]*
    eyelid 125.3 *[373.6]*
  Opisthorchis (felineus) (tenuicollis) (viverri-
    ni) 121.0
  Oxyuris vermicularis 127.4
  Paragonimus (westermani) 121.2
  parasite, parasitic NEC 136.9
    eyelid 134.9 *[373.6]*
    intestinal 129
    mouth 112.0
    orbit 376.13
    skin 134.9
    tongue 112.0
  pediculus 132.9
    capitis (humanus) (any site) 132.0
    corporis (humanus) (any site) 132.1
    eyelid 132.0 *[373.6]*
    mixed (classifiable to more than one
      category in 132.0–132.2) 132.3
    pubis (any site) 132.2
  phthirus (pubis) (any site) 132.2
    with any infestation classifiable to 132.0,
      132.1 and 132.3
  pinworm 127.4
  pork tapeworm (adult) 123.0
  protozoal NEC 136.8
  pubic louse 132.2
  rat tapeworm 123.6
  red bug 133.8
  roundworm (large) NEC 127.0
  sand flea 134.1
  saprophytic NEC 136.8
  Sarcoptes scabiei 133.0
  scabies 133.0
  Schistosoma 120.9
    bovis 120.8
    cercariae 120.3
    hematobium 120.0

Infestation — *continued*
  Schistosoma — *continued*
    intercalatum 120.8
    japonicum 120.2
    mansoni 120.1
    mattheii 120.8
    specified
      site — *see* Schistosomiasis
      type NEC 120.8
    spindale 120.8
  screw worms 134.0
  skin NEC 134.9
  Sparganum (mansoni) (proliferum) 123.5
    larval 123.5
  specified type NEC 134.8
  Spirometra larvae 123.5
  Sporozoa NEC 136.8
  Stellantchasmus falcatus 121.6
  Strongyloides 127.2
  Strongylus (gibsoni) 127.7
  Taenia 123.3
    diminuta 123.6
    Echinococcus (*see also* Echinococcus)
      122.9
    mediocanellata 123.2
    nana 123.6
    saginata (mediocanellata) 123.2
    solium (intestinal form) 123.0
      larval form 123.1
  Taeniarhynchus saginatus 123.2
  tapeworm 123.9
    beef 123.2
    broad 123.4
      larval 123.5
    dog 123.8
    dwarf 123.6
    fish 123.4
      larval 123.5
    pork 123.0
    rat 123.6
  Ternidens diminutus 127.7
  Tetranychus molestissimus 133.8
  threadworm 127.4
  tongue 112.0
  Toxocara (cani) (cati) (felis) 128.0
  trematode(s) NEC 121.9
  Trichina spiralis 124
  Trichinella spiralis 124
  Trichocephalus 127.3
  Trichomonas 131.9
    bladder 131.09
    cervix 131.09
    intestine 007.3
    prostate 131.03
    specified site NEC 131.8
    urethra (female) (male) 131.02
    urogenital 131.00
    vagina 131.01
    vulva 131.01
  Trichophyton — *see* Dermatophytosis
  Trichostrongylus instabilis 127.6
  Trichuris (trichiuria) 127.3
  Trombicula (irritans) 133.8
  Trypanosoma — *see* Trypanosomiasis
  Tunga penetrans 134.1
  Uncinaria americana 126.1
  whipworm 127.3
  worms NEC 128.9
    intestinal 127.9
  Wuchereria 125.0
    bancrofti 125.0
    malayi 125.1

Infiltrate, infiltration
  with an iron compound 275.09
  amyloid (any site) (generalized) 277.39
  calcareous (muscle) NEC 275.49
    localized — *see* Degeneration, by site
  calcium salt (muscle) 275.49
  chemotherapy, vesicant 999.81
  corneal (*see also* Edema, cornea) 371.20
    eyelid 373.9
  fatty (diffuse) (generalized) 272.8
    localized — *see* Degeneration, by site,
      fatty
  glycogen, glycogenic (*see also* Disease,
    glycogen storage) 271.0

Infiltrate, infiltration — *continued*
  heart, cardiac
    fatty (*see also* Degeneration, myocardial)
      429.1
    glycogenic 271.0 *[425.7]*
  inflammatory in vitreous 379.29
  kidney (*see also* Disease, renal) 593.9
  leukemic (M9800/3) — *see* Leukemia
  liver 573.8
    fatty — *see* Fatty, liver
    glycogen (*see also* Disease, glycogen
      storage) 271.0
  lung (*see also* Infiltrate, pulmonary) 793.19
    eosinophilic 518.3
    x-ray finding only 793.19
  lymphatic (*see also* Leukemia, lymphatic)
    204.9 ☑
    gland, pigmentary 289.3
  muscle, fatty 728.9
  myelogenous (*see also* Leukemia, myeloid)
    205.9 ☑
  myocardium, myocardial
    fatty (*see also* Degeneration, myocardial)
      429.1
    glycogenic 271.0 *[425.7]*
  pulmonary 793.19
    with
      eosinophilia 518.3
      pneumonia — *see* Pneumonia, by
        type
    x-ray finding only 793.19
    Ranke's primary (*see also* Tuberculosis)
      010.0 ☑
  skin, lymphocytic (benign) 709.8
  thymus (gland) (fatty) 254.8
  urine 788.8
  vesicant
    agent NEC 999.82
    chemotherapy 999.81
  vitreous humor 379.29

Infirmity 799.89
  senile 797

Inflammation, inflamed, inflammatory (with
  exudation)
  abducens (nerve) 378.54
  accessory sinus (chronic) (*see also* Sinusitis)
    473.9
  adrenal (gland) 255.8
  alimentary canal — *see* Enteritis
  alveoli (teeth) 526.5
    scorbutic 267
  amnion — *see* Amnionitis
  anal canal 569.49
  antrum (chronic) (*see also* Sinusitis, maxil-
    lary) 473.0
  anus 569.49
  appendix (*see also* Appendicitis) 541
  arachnoid — *see* Meningitis
  areola 611.0
    puerperal, postpartum 675.0 ☑
  areolar tissue NEC 686.9
  artery — *see* Arteritis
  auditory meatus (external) (*see also* Otitis,
    externa) 380.10
  Bartholin's gland 616.89
  bile duct or passage 576.1
  bladder (*see also* Cystitis) 595.9
  bleb
    postprocedural 379.60
      stage 1 379.61
      stage 2 379.62
      stage 3 379.63
  bone — *see* Osteomyelitis
  bowel (*see also* Enteritis) 558.9
  brain (*see also* Encephalitis) 323.9
    late effect — *see* category 326
    membrane — *see* Meningitis
  breast 611.0
    puerperal, postpartum 675.2 ☑
  broad ligament (*see also* Disease, pelvis, in-
    flammatory) 614.4
    acute 614.3
  bronchus — *see* Bronchitis
  bursa — *see* Bursitis
  capsule
    liver 573.3

Inflammation, inflamed, inflammatory —
  continued
  capsule — *continued*
    spleen 289.59
  catarrhal (*see also* Catarrh) 460
    vagina 616.10
  cecum (*see also* Appendicitis) 541
  cerebral (*see also* Encephalitis) 323.9
    late effect — *see* category 326
    membrane — *see* Meningitis
  cerebrospinal (*see also* Meningitis) 322.9
    late effect — *see* category 326
    meningococcal 036.0
    tuberculous (*see also* Tuberculosis)
      013.6 ☑
  cervix (uteri) (*see also* Cervicitis) 616.0
  chest 519.9
  choroid NEC (*see also* Choroiditis) 363.20
  cicatrix (tissue) — *see* Cicatrix
  colon (*see also* Enteritis) 558.9
    granulomatous 555.1
    newborn 558.9
  connective tissue (diffuse) NEC 728.9
  cornea (*see also* Keratitis) 370.9
    with ulcer (*see also* Ulcer, cornea) 370.00
  corpora cavernosa (penis) 607.2
  cranial nerve — *see* Disorder, nerve, cranial
  diarrhea — *see* Diarrhea
  disc (intervertebral) (space) 722.90
    cervical, cervicothoracic 722.91
    lumbar, lumbosacral 722.93
    thoracic, thoracolumbar 722.92
  Douglas' cul-de-sac or pouch (chronic) (*see
    also* Disease, pelvis, inflammatory)
    614.4
    acute 614.3
  due to (presence of) any device, implant, or
    graft classifiable to 996.0–996.5 —
    see Complications, infection and in-
    flammation, due to (presence of) any
    device, implant, or graft classified to
    996.0–996.5 NEC
  duodenum 535.6 ☑
  dura mater — *see* Meningitis
  ear (*see also* Otitis)
    external (*see also* Otitis, externa) 380.10
    inner (*see also* Labyrinthitis) 386.30
    middle — *see* Otitis media
  esophagus 530.10
  ethmoidal (chronic) (sinus) (*see also* Sinusi-
    tis, ethmoidal) 473.2
  Eustachian tube (catarrhal) 381.50
    acute 381.51
    chronic 381.52
  extrarectal 569.49
  eye 379.99
  eyelid 373.9
    specified NEC 373.8
  fallopian tube (*see also* Salpingo-oophoritis)
    614.2
  fascia 728.9
  fetal membranes (acute) 658.4 ☑
    affecting fetus or newborn 762.7
  follicular, pharynx 472.1
  frontal (chronic) (sinus) (*see also* Sinusitis,
    frontal) 473.1
  gallbladder (*see also* Cholecystitis, acute)
    575.0
  gall duct (*see also* Cholecystitis) 575.10
  gastrointestinal (*see also* Enteritis) 558.9
  genital organ (diffuse) (internal)
    female 614.9
      with
        abortion — *see* Abortion, by type,
          with sepsis
        ectopic pregnancy (*see also* cate-
          gories 633.0–633.9) 639.0
        molar pregnancy (*see also* cate-
          gories 630–632) 639.0
      complicating pregnancy, childbirth,
        or puerperium 646.6 ☑
      affecting fetus or newborn 760.8
      following
        abortion 639.0
        ectopic or molar pregnancy 639.0
    male 608.4

☑ **Additional Digit Required** — Refer to the Tabular List for Digit Selection   ▽ **Subterms under main terms may continue to next column or page**

2014 ICD-9-CM   ▶◀ **Revised Text**   ● **New Line**   ▲ **Revised Code**   **Volume 2 — 159**

Inflammation, inflamed, inflammatory —
　　continued
　　gland (lymph) (*see also* Lymphadenitis)
　　　　289.3
　　glottis (*see also* Laryngitis) 464.00
　　　　with obstruction 464.01
　　granular, pharynx 472.1
　　gum 523.10
　　heart (*see also* Carditis) 429.89
　　hepatic duct 576.8
　　hernial sac — *see* Hernia, by site
　　ileum (*see also* Enteritis) 558.9
　　　　terminal or regional 555.0
　　　　　　with large intestine 555.2
　　intervertebral disc 722.90
　　　　cervical, cervicothoracic 722.91
　　　　lumbar, lumbosacral 722.93
　　　　thoracic, thoracolumbar 722.92
　　intestine (*see also* Enteritis) 558.9
　　jaw (acute) (bone) (chronic) (lower) (suppu-
　　　　rative) (upper) 526.4
　　jejunum — *see* Enteritis
　　joint NEC (*see also* Arthritis) 716.9 ☑
　　　　sacroiliac 720.2
　　kidney (*see also* Nephritis) 583.9
　　knee (joint) 716.66
　　　　tuberculous (active) (*see also* Tuberculo-
　　　　　　sis) 015.2 ☑
　　labium (majus) (minus) (*see also* Vulvitis)
　　　　616.10
　　lacrimal
　　　　gland (*see also* Dacryoadenitis) 375.00
　　　　passages (duct) (sac) (*see also* Dacryocys-
　　　　　　titis) 375.30
　　larynx (*see also* Laryngitis) 464.00
　　　　with obstruction 464.01
　　　　diphtheritic 032.3
　　leg NEC 686.9
　　lip 528.5
　　liver (capsule) (*see also* Hepatitis) 573.3
　　　　acute 570
　　　　chronic 571.40
　　　　suppurative 572.0
　　lung (acute) (*see also* Pneumonia) 486
　　　　chronic (interstitial) 518.89
　　lymphatic vessel (*see also* Lymphangitis)
　　　　457.2
　　lymph node or gland (*see also* Lymphadeni-
　　　　tis) 289.3
　　mammary gland 611.0
　　　　puerperal, postpartum 675.2 ☑
　　maxilla, maxillary 526.4
　　　　sinus (chronic) (*see also* Sinusitis, maxil-
　　　　　　lary) 473.0
　　membranes of brain or spinal cord — *see*
　　　　Meningitis
　　meninges — *see* Meningitis
　　mouth 528.00
　　muscle 728.9
　　myocardium (*see also* Myocarditis) 429.0
　　nasal sinus (chronic) (*see also* Sinusitis) 473.9
　　nasopharynx — *see* Nasopharyngitis
　　navel 686.9
　　　　newborn NEC 771.4
　　nerve NEC 729.2
　　nipple 611.0
　　　　puerperal, postpartum 675.0 ☑
　　nose 478.19
　　　　suppurative 472.0
　　oculomotor nerve 378.51
　　optic nerve 377.30
　　orbit (chronic) 376.10
　　　　acute 376.00
　　　　chronic 376.10
　　ovary (*see also* Salpingo-oophoritis) 614.2
　　oviduct (*see also* Salpingo-oophoritis) 614.2
　　pancreas — *see* Pancreatitis
　　parametrium (chronic) (*see also* Disease,
　　　　pelvis, inflammatory) 614.4
　　　　acute 614.3
　　parotid region 686.9
　　　　gland 527.2
　　pelvis, female (*see also* Disease, pelvis, in-
　　　　flammatory) 614.9
　　penis (corpora cavernosa) 607.2
　　perianal 569.49

Inflammation, inflamed, inflammatory —
　　continued
　　pericardium (*see also* Pericarditis) 423.9
　　perineum (female) (male) 686.9
　　perirectal 569.49
　　peritoneum (*see also* Peritonitis) 567.9
　　periuterine (*see also* Disease, pelvis, inflam-
　　　　matory) 614.9
　　perivesical (*see also* Cystitis) 595.9
　　petrous bone (*see also* Petrositis) 383.20
　　pharynx (*see also* Pharyngitis) 462
　　　　follicular 472.1
　　　　granular 472.1
　　pia mater — *see* Meningitis
　　pleura — *see* Pleurisy
　　postmastoidectomy cavity 383.30
　　　　chronic 383.33
　　pouch, internal ileoanal 569.71
　　prostate (*see also* Prostatitis) 601.9
　　rectosigmoid — *see* Rectosigmoiditis
　　rectum (*see also* Proctitis) 569.49
　　respiratory, upper (*see also* Infection, respi-
　　　　ratory, upper) 465.9
　　　　chronic, due to external agent — *see*
　　　　　　Condition, respiratory, chronic,
　　　　　　due to, external agent
　　　　due to
　　　　　　fumes or vapors (chemical) (inhala-
　　　　　　　　tion) 506.2
　　　　　　radiation 508.1
　　retina (*see also* Retinitis) 363.20
　　retrocecal (*see also* Appendicitis) 541
　　retroperitoneal (*see also* Peritonitis) 567.9
　　salivary duct or gland (any) (suppurative)
　　　　527.2
　　scorbutic, alveoli, teeth 267
　　scrotum 608.4
　　sigmoid — *see* Enteritis
　　sinus (*see also* Sinusitis) 473.9
　　Skene's duct or gland (*see also* Urethritis)
　　　　597.89
　　skin 686.9
　　spermatic cord 608.4
　　sphenoidal (sinus) (*see also* Sinusitis, sphe-
　　　　noidal) 473.3
　　spinal
　　　　cord (*see also* Encephalitis) 323.9
　　　　　　late effect — *see* category 326
　　　　membrane — *see* Meningitis
　　　　nerve — *see* Disorder, nerve
　　spine (*see also* Spondylitis) 720.9
　　spleen (capsule) 289.59
　　stomach — *see* Gastritis
　　stricture, rectum 569.49
　　subcutaneous tissue NEC 686.9
　　suprarenal (gland) 255.8
　　synovial (fringe) (membrane) — *see* Bursitis
　　tendon (sheath) NEC 726.90
　　testis (*see also* Orchitis) 604.90
　　thigh 686.9
　　throat (*see also* Sore throat) 462
　　thymus (gland) 254.8
　　thyroid (gland) (*see also* Thyroiditis) 245.9
　　tongue 529.0
　　tonsil — *see* Tonsillitis
　　trachea — *see* Tracheitis
　　trochlear nerve 378.53
　　tubal (*see also* Salpingo-oophoritis) 614.2
　　tuberculous NEC (*see also* Tuberculosis)
　　　　011.9 ☑
　　tubo-ovarian (*see also* Salpingo-oophoritis)
　　　　614.2
　　tunica vaginalis 608.4
　　tympanic membrane — *see* Myringitis
　　umbilicus, umbilical 686.9
　　　　newborn NEC 771.4
　　uterine ligament (*see also* Disease, pelvis,
　　　　inflammatory) 614.4
　　　　acute 614.3
　　uterus (catarrhal) (*see also* Endometritis)
　　　　615.9
　　uveal tract (anterior) (*see also* Iridocyclitis)
　　　　364.3
　　　　posterior — *see* Chorioretinitis
　　　　sympathetic 360.11
　　vagina (*see also* Vaginitis) 616.10

Inflammation, inflamed, inflammatory —
　　continued
　　vas deferens 608.4
　　vein (*see also* Phlebitis) 451.9
　　　　thrombotic 451.9
　　　　　　cerebral (*see also* Thrombosis, brain)
　　　　　　　　434.0 ☑
　　　　　　leg 451.2
　　　　　　　　deep (vessels) NEC 451.19
　　　　　　　　superficial (vessels) 451.0
　　　　　　lower extremity 451.2
　　　　　　　　deep (vessels) NEC 451.19
　　　　　　　　superficial (vessels) 451.0
　　vocal cord 478.5
　　vulva (*see also* Vulvitis) 616.10
Inflation, lung imperfect (newborn) 770.5
Influenza-like disease — *see also* Influenza
　　487.1
Influenza, influenzal 487.1
　　with
　　　　bronchitis 487.1
　　　　bronchopneumonia 487.0
　　　　cold (any type) 487.1
　　　　digestive manifestations 487.8
　　　　hemoptysis 487.1
　　　　involvement of
　　　　　　gastrointestinal tract 487.8
　　　　　　nervous system 487.8
　　　　laryngitis 487.1
　　　　manifestations NEC 487.8
　　　　　　respiratory 487.1
　　　　　　　　pneumonia 487.0
　　　　pharyngitis 487.1
　　　　pneumonia (any form classifiable to
　　　　　　480–483, 485–486) 487.0
　　　　respiratory manifestations NEC 487.1
　　　　sinusitis 487.1
　　　　sore throat 487.1
　　　　tonsillitis 487.1
　　　　tracheitis 487.1
　　　　upper respiratory infection (acute) 487.1
　　abdominal 487.8
　　A/H5N1 (*see also* Influenza, avian) 488.02
　　Asian 487.1
　　avian 488.02
　　　　with involvement of gastrointestinal
　　　　　　tract 488.09
　　　　bronchopneumonia 488.01
　　　　laryngitis 488.02
　　　　manifestations NEC 488.09
　　　　　　respiratory 488.02
　　　　pharyngitis 488.02
　　　　pneumonia (any form classifiable to 480-
　　　　　　483, 485-486) 488.01
　　　　respiratory infection (acute) (upper)
　　　　　　488.02
　　bronchial 487.1
　　bronchopneumonia 487.0
　　catarrhal 487.1
　　due to identified
　　　　animal origin influenza virus — *see* In-
　　　　　　fluenza, due to identified, novel
　　　　　　influenza A virus
　　　　avian influenza virus 488.02
　　　　　　with
　　　　　　　　manifestations NEC 488.09
　　　　　　　　　　respiratory 488.02
　　　　　　　　pneumonia (any form classifiable
　　　　　　　　　　to 480-483, 485-486)
　　　　　　　　　　488.01
　　　　(novel 2009) H1N1 influenza virus 488.12
　　　　　　with
　　　　　　　　manifestations NEC 488.19
　　　　　　　　　　respiratory 488.12
　　　　　　　　pneumonia 488.11
　　　　novel influenza A virus 488.82
　　　　　　with
　　　　　　　　encephalopathy 488.89
　　　　　　　　involvement of gastrointestinal
　　　　　　　　　　tract 488.89
　　　　　　　　laryngitis 488.82
　　　　　　　　manifestations NEC 488.89
　　　　　　　　　　respiratory (acute) (upper)
　　　　　　　　　　　　488.82
　　　　　　　　pharyngitis 488.82
　　　　　　　　pneumonia 488.81

Influenza, influenzal — *continued*
　　epidemic 487.1
　　gastric 487.8
　　intestinal 487.8
　　laryngitis 487.1
　　maternal affecting fetus or newborn 760.2
　　　　manifest influenza in infant 771.2
　　(novel) 2009 H1N1 488.12
　　　　with involvement of gastrointestinal
　　　　　　tract 488.19
　　　　bronchopneumonia 488.11
　　　　laryngitis 488.12
　　　　manifestations NEC 488.19
　　　　　　respiratory 488.12
　　　　pharyngitis 488.12
　　　　pneumonia (any form classifiable to 480-
　　　　　　483, 485-486) 488.11
　　　　respiratory infection (acute) (upper)
　　　　　　488.12
　　novel A/H1N1 (*see also* Influenza, (novel)
　　　　2009 H1N1) 488.12
　　novel influenza A viruses not previously
　　　　found in humans — *see* Influenza,
　　　　due to identified, novel influenza A
　　　　virus
　　pharyngitis 487.1
　　pneumonia (any form) 487.0
　　respiratory (upper) 487.1
　　specified NEC 487.1
　　stomach 487.8
　　vaccination, prophylactic (against) V04.81
Infraction, Freiberg's (metatarsal head) 732.5
Infraeruption, teeth 524.34
Infusion complication, misadventure, or
　　reaction — *see* Complication, infusion
Ingestion
　　chemical — *see* Table of Drugs and Chemi-
　　　　cals
　　drug or medicinal substance
　　　　overdose or wrong substance given or
　　　　　　taken 977.9
　　　　　　specified drug — *see* Table of Drugs
　　　　　　　　and Chemicals
　　foreign body NEC (*see also* Foreign body)
　　　　938
Ingrowing
　　hair 704.8
　　nail (finger) (toe) (infected) 703.0
Inguinal — *see also* condition
　　testis 752.51
Inhalation
　　carbon monoxide 986
　　flame
　　　　lung 947.1
　　　　mouth 947.0
　　food or foreign body (*see also* Asphyxia,
　　　　food or foreign body) 933.1
　　gas, fumes, or vapor (noxious) 987.9
　　　　specified agent — *see* Table of Drugs
　　　　　　and Chemicals
　　liquid or vomitus (*see also* Asphyxia, food
　　　　or foreign body) 933.1
　　lower respiratory tract NEC 934.9
　　meconium (fetus or newborn) 770.11
　　　　with respiratory symptoms 770.12
　　mucus (*see also* Asphyxia, mucus) 933.1
　　oil (causing suffocation) (*see also* Asphyxia,
　　　　food or foreign body) 933.1
　　pneumonia — *see* Pneumonia, aspiration
　　smoke 508.2
　　steam 987.9
　　stomach contents or secretions (*see also*
　　　　Asphyxia, food or foreign body) 933.1
　　　　in labor and delivery 668.0 ☑
Inhibition, inhibited
　　academic as adjustment reaction 309.23
　　orgasm
　　　　female 302.73
　　　　male 302.74
　　sexual
　　　　desire 302.71
　　　　excitement 302.72
　　work as adjustment reaction 309.23
Inhibitor
　　autoimmune, to clotting factors 286.52

☑ **Additional Digit Required** — Refer to the Tabular List for Digit Selection　　　　　　　　　　▽ **Subterms under main terms may continue to next column or page**

160 — Volume 2　　　　　　▶◀ **Revised Text**　　　　● **New Line**　　▲ **Revised Code**　　　　　　**2014 ICD-9-CM**

Inhibitor — *continued*
  systemic lupus erythematosus (presence of) 795.79
    with
      hemorrhagic disorder 286.53
      hypercoagulable state 289.81
Iniencephalus, iniencephaly 740.2
Injected eye 372.74
Injury 959.9

> *Note* — For abrasion, insect bite (non-venomous), blister, or scratch, see Injury, superficial.
>
> For laceration, traumatic rupture, tear, or penetrating wound of internal organs, such as heart, lung, liver, kidney, pelvic organs, whether or not accompanied by open wound in the same region, see Injury, internal.
>
> For nerve injury, see Injury, nerve.
>
> For late effect of injuries classifiable to 850–854, 860–869, 900–919, 950–959, see Late, effect, injury, by type.

  abdomen, abdominal (viscera) (*see also* Injury, internal, abdomen)
    muscle or wall 959.12
  acoustic, resulting in deafness 951.5
  adenoid 959.09
  adrenal (gland) — *see* Injury, internal, adrenal
  alveolar (process) 959.09
  ankle (and foot) (and knee) (and leg, except thigh) 959.7
  anterior chamber, eye 921.3
  anus 959.19
  aorta (thoracic) 901.0
    abdominal 902.0
  appendix — *see* Injury, internal, appendix
  arm, upper (and shoulder) 959.2
  artery (complicating trauma) (*see also* Injury, blood vessel, by site) 904.9
    cerebral or meningeal (*see also* Hemorrhage, brain, traumatic, subarachnoid) 852.0 ☑
  auditory canal (external) (meatus) 959.09
  auricle, auris, ear 959.09
  axilla 959.2
  back 959.19
  bile duct — *see* Injury, internal, bile duct
  birth (*see also* Birth, injury)
    canal NEC, complicating delivery 665.9 ☑
  bladder (sphincter) — *see* Injury, internal, bladder
  blast (air) (hydraulic) (immersion) (underwater) NEC 869.0
    with open wound into cavity NEC 869.1
    abdomen or thorax — *see* Injury, internal, by site
    brain — *see* Concussion, brain
    ear (acoustic nerve trauma) 951.5
      with perforation of tympanic membrane — *see* Wound, open, ear, drum
  blood vessel NEC 904.9
    abdomen 902.9
      multiple 902.87
      specified NEC 902.89
    aorta (thoracic) 901.0
      abdominal 902.0
    arm NEC 903.9
    axillary 903.00
      artery 903.01
      vein 903.02
    azygos vein 901.89
    basilic vein 903.1
    brachial (artery) (vein) 903.1
    bronchial 901.89
    carotid artery 900.00
      common 900.01
      external 900.02
      internal 900.03
    celiac artery 902.20
      specified branch NEC 902.24
    cephalic vein (arm) 903.1

Injury — *continued*
  blood vessel — *continued*
    colica dextra 902.26
    cystic
      artery 902.24
      vein 902.39
    deep plantar 904.6
    digital (artery) (vein) 903.5
      due to accidental puncture or laceration during procedure 998.2
    extremity
      lower 904.8
        multiple 904.7
        specified NEC 904.7
      upper 903.9
        multiple 903.8
        specified NEC 903.8
    femoral
      artery (superficial) 904.1
        above profunda origin 904.0
        common 904.0
      vein 904.2
    gastric
      artery 902.21
      vein 902.39
    head 900.9
      intracranial — *see* Injury, intracranial
      multiple 900.82
      specified NEC 900.89
    hemiazygos vein 901.89
    hepatic
      artery 902.22
      vein 902.11
    hypogastric 902.59
      artery 902.51
      vein 902.52
    ileocolic
      artery 902.26
      vein 902.31
    iliac 902.50
      artery 902.53
      specified branch NEC 902.59
      vein 902.54
    innominate
      artery 901.1
      vein 901.3
    intercostal (artery) (vein) 901.81
    jugular vein (external) 900.81
      internal 900.1
    leg NEC 904.8
    mammary (artery) (vein) 901.82
    mesenteric
      artery 902.20
        inferior 902.27
        specified branch NEC 902.29
        superior (trunk) 902.25
          branches, primary 902.26
      vein 902.39
        inferior 902.32
        superior (and primary subdivisions) 902.31
    neck 900.9
      multiple 900.82
      specified NEC 900.89
    ovarian 902.89
      artery 902.81
      vein 902.82
    palmar artery 903.4
    pelvis 902.9
      multiple 902.87
      specified NEC 902.89
    plantar (deep) (artery) (vein) 904.6
    popliteal 904.40
      artery 904.41
      vein 904.42
    portal 902.33
    pulmonary 901.40
      artery 901.41
      vein 901.42
    radial (artery) (vein) 903.2
    renal 902.40
      artery 902.41
      specified NEC 902.49
      vein 902.42
    saphenous
      artery 904.7

Injury — *continued*
  blood vessel — *continued*
    saphenous — *continued*
      vein (greater) (lesser) 904.3
    splenic
      artery 902.23
      vein 902.34
    subclavian
      artery 901.1
      vein 901.3
    suprarenal 902.49
    thoracic 901.9
      multiple 901.83
      specified NEC 901.89
    tibial 904.50
      artery 904.50
        anterior 904.51
        posterior 904.53
      vein 904.50
        anterior 904.52
        posterior 904.54
    ulnar (artery) (vein) 903.3
    uterine 902.59
      artery 902.55
      vein 902.56
    vena cava
      inferior 902.10
        specified branches NEC 902.19
      superior 901.2
  brachial plexus 953.4
    newborn 767.6
  brain (traumatic) NEC (*see also* Injury, intracranial) 854.0 ☑
    due to fracture of skull — *see* Fracture, skull, by site
  breast 959.19
  broad ligament — *see* Injury, internal, broad ligament
  bronchus, bronchi — *see* Injury, internal, bronchus
  brow 959.09
  buttock 959.19
  canthus, eye 921.1
  cathode ray 990
  cauda equina 952.4
    with fracture, vertebra — *see* Fracture, vertebra, sacrum
  cavernous sinus (*see also* Injury, intracranial) 854.0 ☑
  cecum — *see* Injury, internal, cecum
  celiac ganglion or plexus 954.1
  cerebellum (*see also* Injury, intracranial) 854.0 ☑
  cervix (uteri) — *see* Injury, internal, cervix
  cheek 959.09
  chest (*see also* Injury, internal, chest)
    wall 959.11
  childbirth (*see also* Birth, injury)
    maternal NEC 665.9 ☑
  chin 959.09
  choroid (eye) 921.3
  clitoris 959.14
  coccyx 959.19
    complicating delivery 665.6 ☑
  colon — *see* Injury, internal, colon
  common duct — *see* Injury, internal, common duct
  conjunctiva 921.1
    superficial 918.2
  cord
    spermatic — *see* Injury, internal, spermatic cord
    spinal — *see* Injury, spinal, by site
  cornea 921.3
    abrasion 918.1
      due to contact lens 371.82
    penetrating — *see* Injury, eyeball, penetrating
    superficial 918.1
      due to contact lens 371.82
    cortex (cerebral) (*see also* Injury, intracranial) 854.0 ☑
      visual 950.3
  costal region 959.11
  costochondral 959.11

Injury — *continued*
  cranial
    bones — *see* Fracture, skull, by site
    cavity (*see also* Injury, intracranial) 854.0 ☑
    nerve — *see* Injury, nerve, cranial
  crushing — *see* Crush
  cutaneous sensory nerve
    lower limb 956.4
    upper limb 955.5
  deep tissue — *see* Contusion, by site
    meaning pressure ulcer 707.25
  delivery (*see also* Birth, injury)
    maternal NEC 665.9 ☑
  Descemet's membrane — *see* Injury, eyeball, penetrating
  diaphragm — *see* Injury, internal, diaphragm
  diffuse axonal — *see* Injury, intracranial
  duodenum — *see* Injury, internal, duodenum
  ear (auricle) (canal) (drum) (external) 959.09
  elbow (and forearm) (and wrist) 959.3
  epididymis 959.14
  epigastric region 959.12
  epiglottis 959.09
  epiphyseal, current — *see* Fracture, by site
  esophagus — *see* Injury, internal, esophagus
  Eustachian tube 959.09
  extremity (lower) (upper) NEC 959.8
  eye 921.9
    penetrating eyeball — *see* Injury, eyeball, penetrating
    superficial 918.9
  eyeball 921.3
    penetrating 871.7
      with
        partial loss (of intraocular tissue) 871.2
        prolapse or exposure (of intraocular tissue) 871.1
        without prolapse 871.0
        foreign body (nonmagnetic) 871.6
          magnetic 871.5
    superficial 918.9
  eyebrow 959.09
  eyelid(s) 921.1
    laceration — *see* Laceration, eyelid
    superficial 918.0
  face (and neck) 959.09
  fallopian tube — *see* Injury, internal, fallopian tube
  finger(s) (nail) 959.5
  flank 959.19
  foot (and ankle) (and knee) (and leg, except thigh) 959.7
  forceps NEC 767.9
    scalp 767.19
  forearm (and elbow) (and wrist) 959.3
  forehead 959.09
  gallbladder — *see* Injury, internal, gallbladder
  gasserian ganglion 951.2
  gastrointestinal tract — *see* Injury, internal, gastrointestinal tract
  genital organ(s)
    with
      abortion — *see* Abortion, by type, with, damage to pelvic organs
      ectopic pregnancy (*see also* categories 633.0–633.9) 639.2
      molar pregnancy (*see also* categories 630–632) 639.2
    external 959.14
      fracture of corpus cavernosum penis 959.13
    following
      abortion 639.2
      ectopic or molar pregnancy 639.2
    internal — *see* Injury, internal, genital organs
    obstetrical trauma NEC 665.9 ☑
      affecting fetus or newborn 763.89
  gland
    lacrimal 921.1

☑ **Additional Digit Required** — Refer to the Tabular List for Digit Selection

☝ **Subterms under main terms may continue to next column or page**

2014 ICD-9-CM

▶◀ Revised Text   ● New Line   ▲ Revised Code

Volume 2 — 161

Inhibitor — Injury

Injury — *continued*
  gland — *continued*
    lacrimal — *continued*
      laceration 870.8
    parathyroid 959.09
    salivary 959.09
    thyroid 959.09
  globe (eye) (*see also* Injury, eyeball) 921.3
  grease gun — *see* Wound, open, by site, complicated
  groin 959.19
  gum 959.09
  hand(s) (except fingers) 959.4
  head NEC 959.01
    with
      loss of consciousness 850.5
      skull fracture — *see* Fracture, skull, by site
  heart — *see* Injury, internal, heart
  heel 959.7
  hip (and thigh) 959.6
  hymen 959.14
  hyperextension (cervical) (vertebra) 847.0
  ileum — *see* Injury, internal, ileum
  iliac region 959.19
  infrared rays NEC 990
  instrumental (during surgery) 998.2
    birth injury — *see* Birth, injury
    nonsurgical (*see also* Injury, by site) 959.9
  obstetrical 665.9 ☑
    affecting fetus or newborn 763.89
    bladder 665.5 ☑
    cervix 665.3 ☑
    high vaginal 665.4 ☑
    perineal NEC 664.9 ☑
    urethra 665.5 ☑
    uterus 665.5 ☑
  internal 869.0

> Note — For injury of internal organ(s) by foreign body entering through a natural orifice (e.g., inhaled, ingested, or swallowed) — see Foreign body, entering through orifice.
>
> For internal injury of any of the following sites with internal injury of any other of the sites — see Injury, internal, multiple.

    with
      fracture
        pelvis — *see* Fracture, pelvis
        specified site, except pelvis — *see* Injury, internal, by site
      open wound into cavity 869.1
    abdomen, abdominal (viscera) NEC 868.00
      with
        fracture, pelvis — *see* Fracture, pelvis
        open wound into cavity 868.10
      specified site NEC 868.09
        with open wound into cavity 868.19
    adrenal (gland) 868.01
      with open wound into cavity 868.11
    aorta (thoracic) 901.0
      abdominal 902.0
    appendix 863.85
      with open wound into cavity 863.95
    bile duct 868.02
      with open wound into cavity 868.12
    bladder (sphincter) 867.0
      with
        abortion — *see* Abortion, by type, with damage to pelvic organs
        ectopic pregnancy (*see also* categories 633.0–633.9) 639.2
        molar pregnancy (*see also* categories 630–632) 639.2
        open wound into cavity 867.1
      following
        abortion 639.2
        ectopic or molar pregnancy 639.2
      obstetrical trauma 665.5 ☑

  internal — *continued*
    bladder — *continued*
      obstetrical trauma — *continued*
        affecting fetus or newborn 763.89
    blood vessel — *see* Injury, blood vessel, by site
    broad ligament 867.6
      with open wound into cavity 867.7
    bronchus, bronchi 862.21
      with open wound into cavity 862.31
    cecum 863.89
      with open wound into cavity 863.99
    cervix (uteri) 867.4
      with
        abortion — *see* Abortion, by type, with damage to pelvic organs
        ectopic pregnancy (*see also* categories 633.0–633.9) 639.2
        molar pregnancy (*see also* categories 630–632) 639.2
        open wound into cavity 867.5
      following
        abortion 639.2
        ectopic or molar pregnancy 639.2
      obstetrical trauma 665.3 ☑
        affecting fetus or newborn 763.89
    chest (*see also* Injury, internal, intrathoracic organs) 862.8
      with open wound into cavity 862.9
    colon 863.40
      with
        open wound into cavity 863.50
        rectum 863.46
          with open wound into cavity 863.56
      ascending (right) 863.41
        with open wound into cavity 863.51
      descending (left) 863.43
        with open wound into cavity 863.53
      multiple sites 863.46
        with open wound into cavity 863.56
      sigmoid 863.44
        with open wound into cavity 863.54
      specified site NEC 863.49
        with open wound into cavity 863.59
      transverse 863.42
        with open wound into cavity 863.52
    common duct 868.02
      with open wound into cavity 868.12
    complicating delivery 665.9 ☑
      affecting fetus or newborn 763.89
    diaphragm 862.0
      with open wound into cavity 862.1
    duodenum 863.21
      with open wound into cavity 863.31
    esophagus (intrathoracic) 862.22
      with open wound into cavity 862.32
      cervical region 874.4
        complicated 874.5
    fallopian tube 867.6
      with open wound into cavity 867.7
    gallbladder 868.02
      with open wound into cavity 868.12
    gastrointestinal tract NEC 863.80
      with open wound into cavity 863.90
    genital organ NEC 867.6
      with open wound into cavity 867.7
    heart 861.00
      with open wound into thorax 861.10
    ileum 863.29
      with open wound into cavity 863.39
    intestine NEC 863.89
      with open wound into cavity 863.99
      large NEC 863.40
        with open wound into cavity 863.90
      small NEC 863.20

  internal — *continued*
    intestine — *continued*
      small — *continued*
        with open wound into cavity 863.30
    intra-abdominal (organ) 868.00
      with open wound into cavity 868.10
      multiple sites 868.09
        with open wound into cavity 868.19
      specified site NEC 868.09
        with open wound into cavity 868.19
    intrathoracic organs (multiple) 862.8
      with open wound into cavity 862.9
      diaphragm (only) — *see* Injury, internal, diaphragm
      heart (only) — *see* Injury, internal, heart
      lung (only) — *see* Injury, internal, lung
      specified site NEC 862.29
        with open wound into cavity 862.39
    intrauterine (*see also* Injury, internal, uterus) 867.4
      with open wound into cavity 867.5
    jejunum 863.29
      with open wound into cavity 863.39
    kidney (subcapsular) 866.00
      with
        disruption of parenchyma (complete) 866.03
          with open wound into cavity 866.13
        hematoma (without rupture of capsule) 866.01
          with open wound into cavity 866.11
        laceration 866.02
          with open wound into cavity 866.12
        open wound into cavity 866.10
    liver 864.00
      with
        contusion 864.01
          with open wound into cavity 864.11
        hematoma 864.01
          with open wound into cavity 864.11
        laceration 864.05
          with open wound into cavity 864.15
          major (disruption of hepatic parenchyma) 864.04
            with open wound into cavity 864.14
          minor (capsule only) 864.02
            with open wound into cavity 864.12
          moderate (involving parenchyma) 864.03
            with open wound into cavity 864.13
          multiple 864.04
        stellate 864.04
          with open wound into cavity 864.14
        open wound into cavity 864.10
    lung 861.20
      with open wound into thorax 861.30
      aspiration 507.0
      hemopneumothorax — *see* Hemopneumothorax, traumatic
      hemothorax — *see* Hemothorax, traumatic
      pneumohemothorax — *see* Pneumohemothorax, traumatic
      pneumothorax — *see* Pneumothorax, traumatic
      transfusion related, acute (TRALI) 518.7
    mediastinum 862.29
      with open wound into cavity 862.39

  internal — *continued*
    mesentery 863.89
      with open wound into cavity 863.99
    mesosalpinx 867.6
      with open wound into cavity 867.7
    multiple 869.0

> Note — Multiple internal injuries of sites classifiable to the same three- or four-digit category should be classified to that category.
>
> Multiple injuries classifiable to different fourth-digit subdivisions of 861 (heart and lung injuries) should be dealt with according to coding rules.

      internal
        with open wound into cavity 869.1
      intra-abdominal organ (sites classifiable to 863–868)
        with
          intrathoracic organ(s) (sites classifiable to 861–862) 869.0
            with open wound into cavity 869.1
          other intra-abdominal organ(s) (sites classifiable to 863–868, except where classifiable to the same three-digit category) 868.09
            with open wound into cavity 868.19
      intrathoracic organ (sites classifiable to 861–862)
        with
          intra-abdominal organ(s) (sites classifiable to 863–868) 869.0
            with open wound into cavity 869.1
          other intrathoracic organ(s) (sites classifiable to 861–862, except where classifiable to the same three-digit category) 862.8
            with open wound into cavity 862.9
    myocardium — *see* Injury, internal, heart
    ovary 867.6
      with open wound into cavity 867.7
    pancreas (multiple sites) 863.84
      with open wound into cavity 863.94
      body 863.82
        with open wound into cavity 863.92
      head 863.81
        with open wound into cavity 863.91
      tail 863.83
        with open wound into cavity 863.93
    pelvis, pelvic (organs) (viscera) 867.8
      with
        fracture, pelvis — *see* Fracture, pelvis
        open wound into cavity 867.9
      specified site NEC 867.6
        with open wound into cavity 867.7
    peritoneum 868.03
      with open wound into cavity 868.13
    pleura 862.29
      with open wound into cavity 862.39
    prostate 867.6
      with open wound into cavity 867.7
    rectum 863.45
      with
        colon 863.46
          with open wound into cavity 863.56
        open wound into cavity 863.55
    retroperitoneum 868.04

Injury — continued
  internal — continued
    retroperitoneum — continued
      with open wound into cavity 868.14
    round ligament 867.6
      with open wound into cavity 867.7
    seminal vesicle 867.6
      with open wound into cavity 867.7
    spermatic cord 867.6
      with open wound into cavity 867.7
      scrotal — see Wound, open, spermatic cord
    spleen 865.00
      with
        disruption of parenchyma (massive) 865.04
          with open wound into cavity 865.14
        hematoma (without rupture of capsule) 865.01
          with open wound into cavity 865.11
        open wound into cavity 865.10
        tear, capsular 865.02
          with open wound into cavity 865.12
          extending into parenchyma 865.03
            with open wound into cavity 865.13
    stomach 863.0
      with open wound into cavity 863.1
    suprarenal gland (multiple) 868.01
      with open wound into cavity 868.11
    thorax, thoracic (cavity) (organs) (multiple) (see also Injury, internal, intrathoracic organs) 862.8
      with open wound into cavity 862.9
    thymus (gland) 862.29
      with open wound into cavity 862.39
    trachea (intrathoracic) 862.29
      with open wound into cavity 862.39
      cervical region (see also Wound, open, trachea) 874.02
    ureter 867.2
      with open wound into cavity 867.3
    urethra (sphincter) 867.0
      with
        abortion — see Abortion, by type, with damage to pelvic organs
        ectopic pregnancy (see also categories 633.0–633.9) 639.2
        molar pregnancy (see also categories 630–632) 639.2
        open wound into cavity 867.1
      following
        abortion 639.2
        ectopic or molar pregnancy 639.2
      obstetrical trauma 665.5 ☑
        affecting fetus or newborn 763.89
    uterus 867.4
      with
        abortion — see Abortion, by type, with damage to pelvic organs
        ectopic pregnancy (see also categories 633.0–633.9) 639.2
        molar pregnancy (see also categories 630–632) 639.2
        open wound into cavity 867.5
      following
        abortion 639.2
        ectopic or molar pregnancy 639.2
      obstetrical trauma NEC 665.5 ☑
        affecting fetus or newborn 763.89
    vas deferens 867.6
      with open wound into cavity 867.7
    vesical (sphincter) 867.0
      with open wound into cavity 867.1
    viscera (abdominal) (see also Injury, internal, multiple) 868.00
      with
        fracture, pelvis — see Fracture, pelvis
        open wound into cavity 868.10

Injury — continued
  internal — continued
    viscera (see also Injury, internal, multiple) — continued
      thoracic NEC (see also Injury, internal, intrathoracic organs) 862.8
        with open wound into cavity 862.9
    interscapular region 959.19
    intervertebral disc 959.19
    intestine — see Injury, internal, intestine
    intra-abdominal (organs) NEC — see Injury, internal, intra-abdominal
    intracranial (traumatic) 854.0 ☑

> Note — Use the following fifth-digit subclassification with categories 851–854:
>
> 0 unspecified state of consciousness
>
> 1 with no loss of consciousness
>
> 2 with brief [less than one hour] loss of consciousness
>
> 3 with moderate [1–24 hours] loss of consciousness
>
> 4 with prolonged [more than 24 hours] loss of consciousness and return to pre–existing conscious level
>
> 5 with prolonged [more than 24 hours] loss of consciousness, without return to pre–existing conscious level
>
> Use fifth-digit 5 to designate when a patient is unconscious and dies before regaining consciousness, regardless of the duration of the loss of consciousness
>
> 6 with loss of consciousness of unspecified duration
>
> 9 with concussion, unspecified

      with
        open intracranial wound 854.1 ☑
        skull fracture — see Fracture, skull, by site
      contusion 851.8 ☑
        with open intracranial wound 851.9 ☑
        brain stem 851.4 ☑
          with open intracranial wound 851.5 ☑
        cerebellum 851.4 ☑
          with open intracranial wound 851.5 ☑
        cortex (cerebral) 851.0 ☑
          with open intracranial wound 851.2 ☑
      hematoma — see Injury, intracranial, hemorrhage
      hemorrhage 853.0 ☑
        with
          laceration — see Injury, intracranial, laceration
          open intracranial wound 853.1 ☑
        extradural 852.4 ☑
          with open intracranial wound 852.5 ☑
        subarachnoid 852.0 ☑
          with open intracranial wound 852.1 ☑
        subdural 852.2 ☑
          with open intracranial wound 852.3 ☑
      laceration 851.8 ☑
        with open intracranial wound 851.9 ☑
        brain stem 851.6 ☑
          with open intracranial wound 851.7 ☑
        cerebellum 851.6 ☑
          with open intracranial wound 851.7 ☑
        cortex (cerebral) 851.2 ☑

Injury — continued
  intracranial — continued
    laceration — continued
      cortex — continued
        with open intracranial wound 851.3 ☑
    intraocular — see Injury, eyeball, penetrating
    intrathoracic organs (multiple) — see Injury, internal, intrathoracic organs
    intrauterine — see Injury, internal, intrauterine
    iris 921.3
      penetrating — see Injury, eyeball, penetrating
    jaw 959.09
    jejunum — see Injury, internal, jejunum
    joint NEC 959.9
      old or residual 718.80
        ankle 718.87
        elbow 718.82
        foot 718.87
        hand 718.84
        hip 718.85
        knee 718.86
        multiple sites 718.89
        pelvic region 718.85
        shoulder (region) 718.81
        specified site NEC 718.88
        wrist 718.83
    kidney — see Injury, internal, kidney
      acute (nontraumatic) 584.9
    knee (and ankle) (and foot) (and leg, except thigh) 959.7
    labium (majus) (minus) 959.14
    labyrinth, ear 959.09
    lacrimal apparatus, gland, or sac 921.1
      laceration 870.8
    larynx 959.09
    late effect — see Late, effects (of), injury
    leg, except thigh (and ankle) (and foot) (and knee) 959.7
      upper or thigh 959.6
    lens, eye 921.3
      penetrating — see Injury, eyeball, penetrating
    lid, eye — see Injury, eyelid
    lip 959.09
    liver — see Injury, internal, liver
    lobe, parietal — see Injury, intracranial
    lumbar (region) 959.19
      plexus 953.5
    lumbosacral (region) 959.19
      plexus 953.5
    lung — see Injury, internal, lung
    malar region 959.09
    mastoid region 959.09
    maternal, during pregnancy, affecting fetus or newborn 760.5
    maxilla 959.09
    mediastinum — see Injury, internal, mediastinum
    membrane
      brain (see also Injury, intracranial) 854.0 ☑
      tympanic 959.09
    meningeal artery — see Hemorrhage, brain, traumatic, subarachnoid
    meninges (cerebral) — see Injury, intracranial
    mesenteric
      artery — see Injury, blood vessel, mesenteric, artery
      plexus, inferior 954.1
      vein — see Injury, blood vessel, mesenteric, vein
    mesentery — see Injury, internal, mesentery
    mesosalpinx — see Injury, internal, mesosalpinx
    middle ear 959.09
    midthoracic region 959.11
    mouth 959.09
    multiple (sites not classifiable to the same four–digit category in 959.0–959.7) 959.8
      internal 869.0

Injury — continued
  multiple — continued
    internal — continued
      with open wound into cavity 869.1
  musculocutaneous nerve 955.4
  nail
    finger 959.5
    toe 959.7
  nasal (septum) (sinus) 959.09
  nasopharynx 959.09
  neck (and face) 959.09
  nerve 957.9
    abducens 951.3
    abducent 951.3
    accessory 951.6
    acoustic 951.5
    ankle and foot 956.9
    anterior crural, femoral 956.1
    arm (see also Injury, nerve, upper limb) 955.9
    auditory 951.5
    axillary 955.0
    brachial plexus 953.4
    cervical sympathetic 954.0
    cranial 951.9
      first or olfactory 951.8
      second or optic 950.0
      third or oculomotor 951.0
      fourth or trochlear 951.1
      fifth or trigeminal 951.2
      sixth or abducens 951.3
      seventh or facial 951.4
      eighth, acoustic, or auditory 951.5
      ninth or glossopharyngeal 951.8
      tenth, pneumogastric, or vagus 951.8
      eleventh or accessory 951.6
      twelfth or hypoglossal 951.7
      newborn 767.7
    cutaneous sensory
      lower limb 956.4
      upper limb 955.5
    digital (finger) 955.6
      toe 956.5
    facial 951.4
      newborn 767.5
    femoral 956.1
    finger 955.9
    foot and ankle 956.9
    forearm 955.9
    glossopharyngeal 951.8
    hand and wrist 955.9
    head and neck, superficial 957.0
    hypoglossal 951.7
    involving several parts of body 957.8
    leg (see also Injury, nerve, lower limb) 956.9
    lower limb 956.9
      multiple 956.8
      specified site NEC 956.5
    lumbar plexus 953.5
    lumbosacral plexus 953.5
    median 955.1
      forearm 955.1
      wrist and hand 955.1
    multiple (in several parts of body) (sites not classifiable to the same three-digit category) 957.8
    musculocutaneous 955.4
    musculospiral 955.3
      upper arm 955.3
    oculomotor 951.0
    olfactory 951.8
    optic 950.0
    pelvic girdle 956.9
      multiple sites 956.8
      specified site NEC 956.5
    peripheral 957.9
      multiple (in several regions) (sites not classifiable to the same three-digit category) 957.8
      specified site NEC 957.1
    peroneal 956.3
      ankle and foot 956.3
      lower leg 956.3
    plantar 956.5
    plexus 957.9

Injury — continued
nerve — continued
plexus — continued
celiac 954.1
mesenteric, inferior 954.1
spinal 953.9
brachial 953.4
lumbosacral 953.5
multiple sites 953.8
sympathetic NEC 954.1
pneumogastric 951.8
radial 955.3
wrist and hand 955.3
sacral plexus 953.5
sciatic 956.0
thigh 956.0
shoulder girdle 955.9
multiple 955.8
specified site NEC 955.7
specified site NEC 957.1
spinal 953.9
plexus — see Injury, nerve, plexus, spinal
root 953.9
cervical 953.0
dorsal 953.1
lumbar 953.2
multiple sites 953.8
sacral 953.3
splanchnic 954.1
sympathetic NEC 954.1
cervical 954.0
thigh 956.9
tibial 956.5
ankle and foot 956.2
lower leg 956.5
posterior 956.2
toe 956.9
trigeminal 951.2
trochlear 951.1
trunk, excluding shoulder and pelvic girdles 954.9
specified site NEC 954.8
sympathetic NEC 954.1
ulnar 955.2
forearm 955.2
wrist (and hand) 955.2
upper limb 955.9
multiple 955.8
specified site NEC 955.7
vagus 951.8
wrist and hand 955.9
nervous system, diffuse 957.8
nose (septum) 959.09
obstetrical NEC 665.9 ☑
affecting fetus or newborn 763.89
occipital (region) (scalp) 959.09
lobe (see also Injury, intracranial) 854.0 ☑
optic 950.9
chiasm 950.1
cortex 950.3
nerve 950.0
pathways 950.2
orbit, orbital (region) 921.2
penetrating 870.3
with foreign body 870.4
ovary — see Injury, internal, ovary
paint-gun — see Wound, open, by site, complicated
palate (soft) 959.09
pancreas — see Injury, internal, pancreas
parathyroid (gland) 959.09
parietal (region) (scalp) 959.09
lobe — see Injury, intracranial
pelvic
floor 959.19
complicating delivery 664.1 ☑
affecting fetus or newborn 763.89
joint or ligament, complicating delivery 665.6 ☑
affecting fetus or newborn 763.89
organs (see also Injury, internal, pelvis)

Injury — continued
pelvic — continued
organs (see also Injury, internal, pelvis) — continued
with
abortion — see Abortion, by type, with damage to pelvic organs
ectopic pregnancy (see also categories 633.0–633.9) 639.2
molar pregnancy (see also categories 633.0–633.9) 639.2
following
abortion 639.2
ectopic or molar pregnancy 639.2
obstetrical trauma 665.5 ☑
affecting fetus or newborn 763.89
pelvis 959.19
penis 959.14
fracture of corpus cavernosum 959.13
perineum 959.14
peritoneum — see Injury, internal, peritoneum
periurethral tissue
with
abortion — see Abortion, by type, with damage to pelvic organs
ectopic pregnancy (see also categories 633.0–633.9) 639.2
molar pregnancy (see also categories 630–632) 639.2
complicating delivery 664.8 ☑
affecting fetus or newborn 763.89
following
abortion 639.2
ectopic or molar pregnancy 639.2
phalanges
foot 959.7
hand 959.5
pharynx 959.09
pleura — see Injury, internal, pleura
popliteal space 959.7
post-cardiac surgery (syndrome) 429.4
prepuce 959.14
prostate — see Injury, internal, prostate
pubic region 959.19
pudenda 959.14
radiation NEC 990
radioactive substance or radium NEC 990
rectovaginal septum 959.14
rectum — see Injury, internal, rectum
retina 921.3
penetrating — see Injury, eyeball, penetrating
retroperitoneal — see Injury, internal, retroperitoneum
roentgen rays NEC 990
round ligament — see Injury, internal, round ligament
sacral (region) 959.19
plexus 953.5
sacroiliac ligament NEC 959.19
sacrum 959.19
salivary ducts or glands 959.09
scalp 959.09
due to birth trauma 767.19
fetus or newborn 767.19
scapular region 959.2
sclera 921.3
penetrating — see Injury, eyeball, penetrating
superficial 918.2
scrotum 959.14
seminal vesicle — see Injury, internal, seminal vesicle
shoulder (and upper arm) 959.2
sinus
cavernous (see also Injury, intracranial) 854.0 ☑
nasal 959.09
skeleton NEC, birth injury 767.3
skin NEC 959.9
skull — see Fracture, skull, by site
soft tissue (of external sites) (severe) — see Wound, open, by site
specified site NEC 959.8

Injury — continued
spermatic cord — see Injury, internal, spermatic cord
spinal (cord) 952.9
with fracture, vertebra — see Fracture, vertebra, by site, with spinal cord injury
cervical (C$_1$-C$_4$) 952.00
with
anterior cord syndrome 952.02
central cord syndrome 952.03
complete lesion of cord 952.01
incomplete lesion NEC 952.04
posterior cord syndrome 952.04
C$_5$-C$_7$ level 952.05
with
anterior cord syndrome 952.07
central cord syndrome 952.08
complete lesion of cord 952.06
incomplete lesion NEC 952.09
posterior cord syndrome 952.09
specified type NEC 952.09
specified type NEC 952.04
dorsal (D$_1$-D$_6$) (T$_1$-T$_6$) (thoracic) 952.10
with
anterior cord syndrome 952.12
central cord syndrome 952.13
complete lesion of cord 952.11
incomplete lesion NEC 952.14
posterior cord syndrome 952.14
D$_7$-D$_{12}$ level (T$_7$-T$_{12}$) 952.15
with
anterior cord syndrome 952.17
central cord syndrome 952.18
complete lesion of cord 952.16
incomplete lesion NEC 952.19
posterior cord syndrome 952.19
specified type NEC 952.19
specified type NEC 952.14
lumbar 952.2
multiple sites 952.8
nerve (root) NEC — see Injury, nerve, spinal, root
plexus 953.9
brachial 953.4
lumbosacral 953.5
multiple sites 953.8
sacral 952.3
thoracic (see also Injury, spinal, dorsal) 952.10
spleen — see Injury, internal, spleen
stellate ganglion 954.1
sternal region 959.11
stomach — see Injury, internal, stomach
subconjunctival 921.1
subcutaneous 959.9
subdural — see Injury, intracranial
submaxillary region 959.09
submental region 959.09
subungual
fingers 959.5
toes 959.7

Injury — continued
superficial 919 ☑

Note — Use the following fourth-digit subdivisions with categories 910–919:

0 Abrasion or friction burn without mention of infection

1 Abrasion or friction burn, infected

2 Blister without mention of infection

3 Blister, infected

4 Insect bite, nonvenomous, without mention of infection

5 Insect bite, nonvenomous, infected

6 Superficial foreign body (splinter) without major open wound and without mention of infection

7 Superficial foreign body (splinter) without major open wound, infected

8 Other and unspecified superficial injury without mention of infection

9 Other and unspecified superficial injury, infected

For late effects of superficial injury, see category 906.2.

abdomen, abdominal (muscle) (wall) (and other part(s) of trunk) 911 ☑
ankle (and hip, knee, leg, or thigh) 916 ☑
anus (and other part(s) of trunk) 911 ☑
arm 913 ☑
upper (and shoulder) 912 ☑
auditory canal (external) (meatus) (and other part(s) of face, neck, or scalp, except eye) 910 ☑
axilla (and upper arm) 912 ☑
back (and other part(s) of trunk) 911 ☑
breast (and other part(s) of trunk) 911 ☑
brow (and other part(s) of face, neck, or scalp, except eye) 910 ☑
buttock (and other part(s) of trunk) 911 ☑
canthus, eye 918.0
cheek(s) (and other part(s) of face, neck, or scalp, except eye) 910 ☑
chest wall (and other part(s) of trunk) 911 ☑
chin (and other part(s) of face, neck, or scalp, except eye) 910 ☑
clitoris (and other part(s) of trunk) 911 ☑
conjunctiva 918.2
cornea 918.1
due to contact lens 371.82
costal region (and other part(s) of trunk) 911 ☑
ear(s) (auricle) (canal) (drum) (external) (and other part(s) of face, neck, or scalp, except eye) 910 ☑
elbow (and forearm) (and wrist) 913 ☑
epididymis (and other part(s) of trunk) 911 ☑
epigastric region (and other part(s) of trunk) 911 ☑
epiglottis (and other part(s) of face, neck, or scalp, except eye) 910 ☑
eyelid(s) (and periocular area) 918.0
eye(s) (and adnexa) NEC 918.9
face (any part(s), except eye) (and neck or scalp) 910 ☑
finger(s) (nail) (any) 915 ☑
flank (and other part(s) of trunk) 911 ☑
foot (phalanges) (and toe(s)) 917 ☑
forearm (and elbow) (and wrist) 913 ☑
forehead (and other part(s) of face, neck, or scalp, except eye) 910 ☑
globe (eye) 918.9

☑ Additional Digit Required — Refer to the Tabular List for Digit Selection

▽ Subterms under main terms may continue to next column or page

►◄ Revised Text   ● New Line   ▲ Revised Code

Injury — *continued*
　superficial — *continued*
　　groin (and other part(s) of trunk) 911 ☑
　　gum(s) (and other part(s) of face, neck, or scalp, except eye) 910 ☑
　　hand(s) (except fingers alone) 914 ☑
　　head (and other part(s) of face, neck, or scalp, except eye) 910 ☑
　　heel (and foot or toe) 917 ☑
　　hip (and ankle, knee, leg, or thigh) 916 ☑
　　iliac region (and other part(s) of trunk) 911 ☑
　　interscapular region (and other part(s) of trunk) 911 ☑
　　iris 918.9
　　knee (and ankle, hip, leg, or thigh) 916 ☑
　　labium (majus) (minus) (and other part(s) of trunk) 911 ☑
　　lacrimal (apparatus) (gland) (sac) 918.0
　　leg (lower) (upper) (and ankle, hip, knee, or thigh) 916 ☑
　　lip(s) (and other part(s) of face, neck, or scalp, except eye) 910 ☑
　　lower extremity (except foot) 916 ☑
　　lumbar region (and other part(s) of trunk) 911 ☑
　　malar region (and other part(s) of face, neck, or scalp, except eye) 910 ☑
　　mastoid region (and other part(s) of face, neck, or scalp, except eye) 910 ☑
　　midthoracic region (and other part(s) of trunk) 911 ☑
　　mouth (and other part(s) of face, neck, or scalp, except eye) 910 ☑
　　multiple sites (not classifiable to the same three-digit category) 919 ☑
　　nasal (septum) (and other part(s) of face, neck, or scalp, except eye) 910 ☑
　　neck (and face or scalp, any part(s), except eye) 910 ☑
　　nose (septum) (and other part(s) of face, neck, or scalp, except eye) 910 ☑
　　occipital region (and other part(s) of face, neck, or scalp, except eye) 910 ☑
　　orbital region 918.0
　　palate (soft) (and other part(s) of face, neck, or scalp, except eye) 910 ☑
　　parietal region (and other part(s) of face, neck, or scalp, except eye) 910 ☑
　　penis (and other part(s) of trunk) 911 ☑
　　perineum (and other part(s) of trunk) 911 ☑
　　periocular area 918.0
　　pharynx (and other part(s) of face, neck, or scalp, except eye) 910 ☑
　　popliteal space (and ankle, hip, leg, or thigh) 916 ☑
　　prepuce (and other part(s) of trunk) 911 ☑
　　pubic region (and other part(s) of trunk) 911 ☑
　　pudenda (and other part(s) of trunk) 911 ☑
　　sacral region (and other part(s) of trunk) 911 ☑
　　salivary (ducts) (glands) (and other part(s) of face, neck, or scalp, except eye) 910 ☑
　　scalp (and other part(s) of face or neck, except eye) 910 ☑
　　scapular region (and upper arm) 912 ☑
　　sclera 918.2
　　scrotum (and other part(s) of trunk) 911 ☑
　　shoulder (and upper arm) 912 ☑
　　skin NEC 919 ☑
　　specified site(s) NEC 919 ☑
　　sternal region (and other part(s) of trunk) 911 ☑
　　subconjunctival 918.2
　　subcutaneous NEC 919 ☑

Injury — *continued*
　superficial — *continued*
　　submaxillary region (and other part(s) of face, neck, or scalp, except eye) 910 ☑
　　submental region (and other part(s) of face, neck, or scalp, except eye) 910 ☑
　　supraclavicular fossa (and other part(s) of face, neck, or scalp, except eye) 910 ☑
　　supraorbital 918.0
　　temple (and other part(s) of face, neck, or scalp, except eye) 910 ☑
　　temporal region (and other part(s) of face, neck, or scalp, except eye) 910 ☑
　　testis (and other part(s) of trunk) 911 ☑
　　thigh (and ankle, hip, knee, or leg) 916 ☑
　　thorax, thoracic (external) (and other part(s) of trunk) 911 ☑
　　throat (and other part(s) of face, neck, or scalp, except eye) 910 ☑
　　thumb(s) (nail) 915 ☑
　　toe(s) (nail) (subungual) (and foot) 917 ☑
　　tongue (and other part(s) of face, neck, or scalp, except eye) 910 ☑
　　tooth, teeth (*see also* Abrasion, dental) 521.20
　　trunk (any part(s)) 911 ☑
　　tunica vaginalis 959.14
　　tympanum, tympanic membrane (and other part(s) of face, neck, or scalp, except eye) 910 ☑
　　upper extremity NEC 913 ☑
　　uvula (and other part(s) of face, neck, or scalp, except eye) 910 ☑
　　vagina (and other part(s) of trunk) 911 ☑
　　vulva (and other part(s) of trunk) 911 ☑
　　wrist (and elbow) (and forearm) 913 ☑
　supraclavicular fossa 959.19
　supraorbital 959.09
　surgical complication (external or internal site) 998.2
　symphysis pubis 959.19
　　complicating delivery 665.6 ☑
　　　affecting fetus or newborn 763.89
　temple 959.09
　temporal region 959.09
　testis 959.14
　thigh (and hip) 959.6
　thorax, thoracic (external) 959.11
　　cavity — *see* Injury, internal, thorax
　　internal — *see* Injury, internal, intrathoracic organs
　throat 959.09
　thumb(s) (nail) 959.5
　thymus — *see* Injury, internal, thymus
　thyroid (gland) 959.09
　toe (nail) (any) 959.7
　tongue 959.09
　tonsil 959.09
　tooth NEC 873.63
　　complicated 873.73
　trachea — *see* Injury, internal, trachea
　trunk 959.19
　tunica vaginalis 959.14
　tympanum, tympanic membrane 959.09
　ultraviolet rays NEC 990
　ureter — *see* Injury, internal, ureter
　urethra (sphincter) — *see* Injury, internal, urethra
　uterus — *see* Injury, internal, uterus
　uvula 959.09
　vagina 959.14
　vascular — *see* Injury, blood vessel
　vas deferens — *see* Injury, internal, vas deferens
　vein (*see also* Injury, blood vessel, by site) 904.9
　vena cava
　　inferior 902.10
　　superior 901.2

Injury — *continued*
　vesical (sphincter) — *see* Injury, internal, vesical
　viscera (abdominal) — *see* Injury, internal, viscera
　　with fracture, pelvis — *see* Fracture, pelvis
　visual 950.9
　　cortex 950.3
　vitreous (humor) 871.2
　vulva 959.14
　whiplash (cervical spine) 847.0
　wringer — *see* Crush, by site
　wrist (and elbow) (and forearm) 959.3
　x-ray NEC 990
Inoculation — *see also* Vaccination
　complication or reaction — *see* Complication, vaccination
INPH (idiopathic normal pressure hydrocephalus) 331.5
Insanity, insane — *see also* Psychosis 298.9
　adolescent (*see also* Schizophrenia) 295.9 ☑
　alternating (*see also* Psychosis, affective, circular) 296.7
　confusional 298.9
　　acute 293.0
　　subacute 293.1
　delusional 298.9
　paralysis, general 094.1
　　progressive 094.1
　paresis, general 094.1
　senile 290.20
Insect
　bite — *see* Injury, superficial, by site
　venomous, poisoning by 989.5
Insemination, artificial V26.1
Insensitivity
　adrenocorticotropin hormone (ACTH) 255.41
　androgen 259.50
　　complete 259.51
　　partial 259.52
Insertion
　cord (umbilical) lateral or velamentous 663.8 ☑
　　affecting fetus or newborn 762.6
　intrauterine contraceptive device V25.11
　placenta, vicious — *see* Placenta, previa
　subdermal implantable contraceptive V25.5
　velamentous, umbilical cord 663.8 ☑
　　affecting fetus or newborn 762.6
Insolation 992.0
　meaning sunstroke 992.0
Insomnia, unspecified 780.52
　with sleep apnea, unspecified 780.51
　adjustment 307.41
　alcohol induced 291.82
　behavioral, of childhood V69.5
　drug induced 292.85
　due to
　　medical condition classified elsewhere 327.01
　　mental disorder 327.02
　fatal familial (FFI) 046.72
　idiopathic 307.42
　nonorganic origin 307.41
　　persistent (primary) 307.42
　　transient 307.41
　organic 327.00
　　other 327.09
　paradoxical 307.42
　primary 307.42
　psychophysiological 307.42
　subjective complaint 307.49
Inspiration
　food or foreign body (*see also* Asphyxia, food or foreign body) 933.1
　mucus (*see also* Asphyxia, mucus) 933.1
Inspissated bile syndrome, newborn 774.4
Instability
　detrusor 596.59
　emotional (excessive) 301.3
　joint (posttraumatic) 718.80
　　ankle 718.87
　　elbow 718.82
　　foot 718.87

Instability — *continued*
　joint — *continued*
　　hand 718.84
　　hip 718.85
　　knee 718.86
　　lumbosacral 724.6
　　multiple sites 718.89
　　pelvic region 718.85
　　sacroiliac 724.6
　　shoulder (region) 718.81
　　specified site NEC 718.88
　　wrist 718.83
　lumbosacral 724.6
　nervous 301.89
　personality (emotional) 301.59
　thyroid, paroxysmal 242.9 ☑
　urethral 599.83
　vasomotor 780.2
Insufficiency, insufficient
　accommodation 367.4
　adrenal (gland) (acute) (chronic) 255.41
　　medulla 255.5
　　primary 255.41
　　specified site NEC 255.5
　adrenocortical 255.41
　anterior (occlusal) guidance 524.54
　anus 569.49
　aortic (valve) 424.1
　　with
　　　mitral (valve) disease 396.1
　　　　insufficiency, incompetence, or regurgitation 396.3
　　　　stenosis or obstruction 396.1
　　　stenosis or obstruction 424.1
　　　　with mitral (valve) disease 396.8
　　congenital 746.4
　　rheumatic 395.1
　　　with
　　　　mitral (valve) disease 396.1
　　　　　insufficiency, incompetence, or regurgitation 396.3
　　　　　stenosis or obstruction 396.1
　　　　stenosis or obstruction 395.2
　　　　　with mitral (valve) disease 396.8
　　specified cause NEC 424.1
　　syphilitic 093.22
　arterial 447.1
　　basilar artery 435.0
　　carotid artery 435.8
　　cerebral 437.1
　　coronary (acute or subacute) 411.89
　　mesenteric 557.1
　　peripheral 443.9
　　precerebral 435.9
　　vertebral artery 435.1
　　vertebrobasilar 435.3
　arteriovenous 459.9
　basilar artery 435.0
　biliary 575.8
　cardiac (*see also* Insufficiency, myocardial) 428.0
　　complicating surgery 997.1
　　due to presence of (cardiac) prosthesis 429.4
　　postoperative 997.1
　　　long-term effect of cardiac surgery 429.4
　　specified during or due to a procedure 997.1
　　　long-term effect of cardiac surgery 429.4
　cardiorenal (*see also* Hypertension, cardiorenal) 404.90
　cardiovascular (*see also* Disease, cardiovascular) 429.2
　　renal (*see also* Hypertension, cardiorenal) 404.90
　carotid artery 435.8
　cerebral (vascular) 437.9
　cerebrovascular 437.9
　　with transient focal neurological signs and symptoms 435.9
　　acute 437.1
　　　with transient focal neurological signs and symptoms 435.9

☑ **Additional Digit Required — Refer to the Tabular List for Digit Selection**　　　　　　▽ **Subterms under main terms may continue to next column or page**

2014 ICD-9-CM　　　　▶◀ **Revised Text**　　　● **New Line**　　　▲ **Revised Code**　　　**Volume 2 — 165**

Insufficiency, insufficient — continued
circulatory NEC 459.9
  fetus or newborn 779.89
convergence 378.83
coronary (acute or subacute) 411.89
  chronic or with a stated duration of over 8 weeks 414.8
corticoadrenal 255.41
dietary 269.9
divergence 378.85
food 994.2
gastroesophageal 530.89
gonadal
  ovary 256.39
  testis 257.2
gonadotropic hormone secretion 253.4
heart (see also Insufficiency, myocardial)
  fetus or newborn 779.89
  valve (see also Endocarditis) 424.90
    congenital NEC 746.89
hepatic 573.8
idiopathic autonomic 333.0
interocclusal distance of teeth (ridge) 524.36
kidney
  acute 593.9
  chronic 585.9
labyrinth, labyrinthine (function) 386.53
  bilateral 386.54
  unilateral 386.53
lacrimal 375.15
liver 573.8
lung (acute) (see also Insufficiency, pulmonary) 518.82
  following trauma and surgery 518.52
  newborn 770.89
mental (congenital) (see also Disability, intellectual) 319
mesenteric 557.1
mitral (valve) 424.0
  with
    aortic (valve) disease 396.3
      insufficiency, incompetence, or regurgitation 396.3
      stenosis or obstruction 396.2
    obstruction or stenosis 394.2
      with aortic valve disease 396.8
  congenital 746.6
  rheumatic 394.1
    with
      aortic (valve) disease 396.3
        insufficiency, incompetence, or regurgitation 396.3
        stenosis or obstruction 396.2
      obstruction or stenosis 394.2
        with aortic valve disease 396.8
    active or acute 391.1
      with chorea, rheumatic (Sydenham's) 392.0
  specified cause, except rheumatic 424.0
muscle
  heart — see Insufficiency, myocardial
  ocular (see also Strabismus) 378.9
myocardial, myocardium (with arteriosclerosis) 428.0
  with rheumatic fever (conditions classifiable to 390)
    active, acute, or subacute 391.2
      with chorea 392.0
    inactive or quiescent (with chorea) 398.0
  congenital 746.89
  due to presence of (cardiac) prosthesis 429.4
  fetus or newborn 779.89
  following cardiac surgery 429.4
  hypertensive (see also Hypertension, heart) 402.91
    benign 402.11
    malignant 402.01
  postoperative 997.1
    long-term effect of cardiac surgery 429.4
  rheumatic 398.0
    active, acute, or subacute 391.2
      with chorea (Sydenham's) 392.0
syphilitic 093.82

Insufficiency, insufficient — continued
nourishment 994.2
organic 799.89
ovary 256.39
  postablative 256.2
pancreatic 577.8
parathyroid (gland) 252.1
peripheral vascular (arterial) 443.9
pituitary (anterior) 253.2
  posterior 253.5
placental — see Placenta, insufficiency
platelets 287.5
prenatal care in current pregnancy V23.7
progressive pluriglandular 258.9
pseudocholinesterase 289.89
pulmonary (acute) 518.82
  following
    shock 518.52
    surgery 518.52
    trauma 518.52
  newborn 770.89
  valve (see also Endocarditis, pulmonary) 424.3
    congenital 746.09
pyloric 537.0
renal 593.9
  acute 593.9
  chronic 585.9
  due to a procedure 997.5
respiratory 786.09
  acute 518.82
    following trauma and surgery 518.52
  newborn 770.89
rotation — see Malrotation
suprarenal 255.41
  medulla 255.5
tarso-orbital fascia, congenital 743.66
tear film 375.15
testis 257.2
thyroid (gland) (acquired) (see also Hypothyroidism)
  congenital 243
tricuspid (see also Endocarditis, tricuspid) 397.0
  congenital 746.89
  syphilitic 093.23
urethral sphincter 599.84
valve, valvular (heart) (see also Endocarditis) 424.90
vascular 459.9
  intestine NEC 557.9
  mesenteric 557.1
  peripheral 443.9
  renal (see also Hypertension, kidney) 403.90
velopharyngeal
  acquired 528.9
  congenital 750.29
venous (peripheral) 459.81
ventricular — see Insufficiency, myocardial
vertebral artery 435.1
vertebrobasilar artery 435.3
weight gain during pregnancy 646.8 ☑
zinc 269.3
Insufflation
fallopian
  fertility testing V26.21
  following sterilization reversal V26.22
meconium 770.11
  with respiratory symptoms 770.12
Insular — see condition
Insulinoma (M8151/0)
malignant (M8151/3)
  pancreas 157.4
  specified site — see Neoplasm, by site, malignant
  unspecified site 157.4
pancreas 211.7
specified site — see Neoplasm, by site, benign
unspecified site 211.7
Insuloma — see Insulinoma
Insult
brain 437.9
  acute 436
cerebral 437.9

Insult — continued
cerebral — continued
  acute 436
  cerebrovascular 437.9
  acute 436
  vascular NEC 437.9
  acute 436
Insurance examination (certification) V70.3
Intemperance — see also Alcoholism 303.9 ☑
Interception of pregnancy (menstrual extraction) V25.3
Interference
balancing side 524.56
non-working side 524.56
Intermenstrual
bleeding 626.6
  irregular 626.6
  regular 626.5
hemorrhage 626.6
  irregular 626.6
  regular 626.5
pain(s) 625.2
Intermittent — see condition
Internal — see condition
Interproximal wear 521.10
Interrogation
cardiac defibrillator (automatic) (implantable) V53.32
cardiac pacemaker V53.31
cardiac (event) (loop) recorder V53.39
infusion pump (implanted) (intrathecal) V53.09
neurostimulator V53.02
Interruption
aortic arch 747.11
bundle of His 426.50
fallopian tube (for sterilization) V25.2
phase-shift, sleep cycle 307.45
repeated REM-sleep 307.48
sleep
  due to perceived environmental disturbances 307.48
  phase-shift, of 24-hour sleep-wake cycle 307.45
  repeated REM-sleep type 307.48
vas deferens (for sterilization) V25.2
Intersexuality 752.7
Interstitial — see condition
Intertrigo 695.89
  labialis 528.5
Intervertebral disc — see condition
Intestine, intestinal — see also condition
flu 487.8
Intolerance
carbohydrate NEC 579.8
cardiovascular exercise, with pain (at rest) (with less than ordinary activity) (with ordinary activity) V47.2
cold 780.99
dissacharide (hereditary) 271.3
drug
  correct substance properly administered 995.27
  wrong substance given or taken in error 977.9
  specified drug — see Table of Drugs and Chemicals
effort 306.2
fat NEC 579.8
foods NEC 579.8
fructose (hereditary) 271.2
glucose (-galactose) (congenital) 271.3
gluten 579.0
lactose (hereditary) (infantile) 271.3
lysine (congenital) 270.7
milk NEC 579.8
protein (familial) 270.7
starch NEC 579.8
sucrose (-isomaltose) (congenital) 271.3
Intoxicated NEC — see also Alcoholism 305.0 ☑
Intoxication
acid 276.2
acute
  alcoholic 305.0 ☑
    with alcoholism 303.0 ☑

Intoxication — continued
acute — continued
  alcoholic — continued
    hangover effects 305.0 ☑
  caffeine 305.9 ☑
  hallucinogenic (see also Abuse, drugs, nondependent) 305.3 ☑
alcohol (acute) 305.0 ☑
  with alcoholism 303.0 ☑
  hangover effects 305.0 ☑
  idiosyncratic 291.4
  pathological 291.4
alimentary canal 558.2
ammonia (hepatic) 572.2
caffeine 305.9 ☑
chemical (see also Table of Drugs and Chemicals)
  via placenta or breast milk 760.70
    alcohol 760.71
    anti-infective agents 760.74
    anticonvulsants
    antifungals
    antimetabolics
    cocaine 760.75
    "crack" 760.75
    hallucinogenic agents NEC 760.73
    medicinal agents NEC 760.79
    narcotics 760.72
    obstetric anesthetic or analgesic drug 763.5
    specified agent NEC 760.79
    suspected, affecting management of pregnancy 655.5 ☑
cocaine, through placenta or breast milk 760.75
delirium
  alcohol 291.0
  drug 292.81
drug 292.89
  with delirium 292.81
  correct substance properly administered (see also Allergy, drug) 995.27
  newborn 779.4
  obstetric anesthetic or sedation 668.9 ☑
    affecting fetus or newborn 763.5
  overdose or wrong substance given or taken — see Table of Drugs and Chemicals
  pathologic 292.2
  specific to newborn 779.4
  via placenta or breast milk 760.70
    alcohol 760.71
    anti-infective agents 760.74
    anticonvulsants 760.77
    antifungals 760.74
    antimetabolics 760.78
    cocaine 760.75
    "crack" 760.75
    hallucinogenic agents 760.73
    medicinal agents NEC 760.79
    narcotics 760.72
    obstetric anesthetic or analgesic drug 763.5
    specified agent NEC 760.79
    suspected, affecting management of pregnancy 655.5 ☑
enteric — see Intoxication, intestinal
fetus or newborn, via placenta or breast milk 760.70
  alcohol 760.71
  anti-infective agents 760.74
  anticonvulsants 760.77
  antifungals 760.74
  antimetabolics 760.78
  cocaine 760.75
  "crack" 760.75
  hallucinogenic agents 760.73
  medicinal agents NEC 760.79
  narcotics 760.72
  obstetric anesthetic or analgesic drug 763.5
  specified agent NEC 760.79
  suspected, affecting management of pregnancy 655.5 ☑
food — see Poisoning, food
gastrointestinal 558.2

☑ **Additional Digit Required** — Refer to the Tabular List for Digit Selection   ▽ **Subterms under main terms may continue to next column or page**

Intoxication — *continued*
　hallucinogenic (acute) 305.3 ☑
　hepatocerebral 572.2
　idiosyncratic alcohol 291.4
　intestinal 569.89
　　due to putrefaction of food 005.9
　methyl alcohol (*see also* Alcoholism)
　　305.0 ☑
　　with alcoholism 303.0 ☑
　non-foodborne due to toxins of Clostridium
　　botulinum [C. botulinum] — *see* Botulism
　pathologic 291.4
　　drug 292.2
　potassium (K) 276.7
　septic
　　with
　　　abortion — *see* Abortion, by type,
　　　　with sepsis
　　　ectopic pregnancy (*see also* categories 633.0–633.9) 639.0
　　　molar pregnancy (*see also* categories 630–632) 639.0
　　during labor 659.3 ☑
　　following
　　　abortion 639.0
　　　ectopic or molar pregnancy 639.0
　　generalized — *see* Septicemia
　　puerperal, postpartum, childbirth 670.2 ☑
　serum (prophylactic) (therapeutic) 999.59
　uremic — *see* Uremia
　water 276.69
Intracranial — *see* condition
Intrahepatic gallbladder 751.69
Intraligamentous — *see also* condition
　pregnancy — *see* Pregnancy, cornual
Intraocular — *see also* condition
　sepsis 360.00
Intrathoracic — *see also* condition
　kidney 753.3
　stomach — *see* Hernia, diaphragm
Intrauterine contraceptive device
　checking V25.42
　insertion V25.11
　in situ V45.51
　management V25.42
　prescription V25.02
　　repeat V25.42
　reinsertion V25.13
　removal V25.12
　　and reinsertion V25.13
　replacement V25.13
Intraventricular — *see* condition
Intrinsic deformity — *see* Deformity
Intruded tooth 524.34
Intrusion, repetitive, of sleep (due to environmental disturbances) (with atypical polysomnographic features) 307.48
Intumescent, lens (eye) NEC 366.9
　senile 366.12
Intussusception (colon) (enteric) (intestine) (rectum) 560.0
　appendix 543.9
　congenital 751.5
　fallopian tube 620.8
　ileocecal 560.0
　ileocolic 560.0
　ureter (with obstruction) 593.4
Invagination
　basilar 756.0
　colon or intestine 560.0
Invalid (since birth) 799.89
Invalidism (chronic) 799.89
Inversion
　albumin-globulin (A-G) ratio 273.8
　bladder 596.89
　cecum (*see also* Intussusception) 560.0
　cervix 622.8
　nipple 611.79
　　congenital 757.6
　　puerperal, postpartum 676.3 ☑
　optic papilla 743.57
　organ or site, congenital NEC — *see* Anomaly, specified type NEC
　sleep rhythm 327.39

Inversion — *continued*
　sleep rhythm — *continued*
　　nonorganic origin 307.45
　testis (congenital) 752.51
　uterus (postinfectional) (postpartal, old) 621.7
　　chronic 621.7
　　complicating delivery 665.2 ☑
　　　affecting fetus or newborn 763.89
　vagina — *see* Prolapse, vagina
Investigation
　allergens V72.7
　clinical research (control) (normal comparison) (participant) V70.7
Inviability — *see* Immaturity
Involuntary movement, abnormal 781.0
Involution, involutional — *see also* condition
　breast, cystic or fibrocystic 610.1
　depression (*see also* Psychosis, affective) 296.2 ☑
　　recurrent episode 296.3 ☑
　　single episode 296.2 ☑
　melancholia (*see also* Psychosis, affective) 296.2 ☑
　　recurrent episode 296.3 ☑
　　single episode 296.2 ☑
　ovary, senile 620.3
　paranoid state (reaction) 297.2
　paraphrenia (climacteric) (menopause) 297.2
　psychosis 298.8
　thymus failure 254.8
IQ
　under 20 318.2
　20-34 318.1
　35-49 318.0
　50-70 317
IRDS 769
Irideremia 743.45
Iridis rubeosis 364.42
　diabetic 250.5 ☑ [364.42]
　　due to secondary diabetes 249.5 ☑ [364.42]
Iridochoroiditis (panuveitis) 360.12
Iridocyclitis NEC 364.3
　acute 364.00
　　primary 364.01
　　recurrent 364.02
　chronic 364.10
　　in
　　　lepromatous leprosy 030.0 [364.11]
　　　sarcoidosis 135 [364.11]
　　　tuberculosis (*see also* Tuberculosis) 017.3 ☑ [364.11]
　due to allergy 364.04
　endogenous 364.01
　gonococcal 098.41
　granulomatous 364.10
　herpetic (simplex) 054.44
　　zoster 053.22
　hypopyon 364.05
　lens induced 364.23
　nongranulomatous 364.00
　primary 364.01
　recurrent 364.02
　rheumatic 364.10
　secondary 364.04
　　infectious 364.03
　　noninfectious 364.04
　subacute 364.00
　　primary 364.01
　　recurrent 364.02
　sympathetic 360.11
　syphilitic (secondary) 091.52
　tuberculous (chronic) (*see also* Tuberculosis) 017.3 ☑ [364.11]
Iridocyclochoroiditis (panuveitis) 360.12
Iridodialysis 364.76
Iridodonesis 364.89
Iridoplegia (complete) (partial) (reflex) 379.49
Iridoschisis 364.52
IRIS (Immune Reconstitution Inflammatory Syndrome) 995.90
Iris — *see* condition
Iritis 364.3
　acute 364.00

Iritis — *continued*
　acute — *continued*
　　primary 364.01
　　recurrent 364.02
　chronic 364.10
　　in
　　　sarcoidosis 135 [364.11]
　　　tuberculosis (*see also* Tuberculosis) 017.3 ☑ [364.11]
　diabetic 250.5 ☑ [364.42]
　　due to secondary diabetes 249.5 ☑ [364.42]
　due to
　　allergy 364.04
　　herpes simplex 054.44
　　leprosy 030.0 [364.11]
　endogenous 364.01
　gonococcal 098.41
　gouty 274.89 [364.11]
　granulomatous 364.10
　hypopyon 364.05
　lens induced 364.23
　nongranulomatous 364.00
　papulosa 095.8 [364.11]
　primary 364.01
　recurrent 364.02
　rheumatic 364.10
　secondary 364.04
　　infectious 364.03
　　noninfectious 364.04
　subacute 364.00
　　primary 364.01
　　recurrent 364.02
　sympathetic 360.11
　syphilitic (secondary) 091.52
　　congenital 090.0 [364.11]
　　late 095.8 [364.11]
　tuberculous (*see also* Tuberculosis) 017.3 ☑ [364.11]
　uratic 274.89 [364.11]
Iron-miners' lung 503
Iron
　deficiency anemia 280.9
　metabolism disease 275.09
　storage disease 275.09
Irradiated enamel (tooth, teeth) 521.89
Irradiation
　burn — *see* Burn, by site
　effects, adverse 990
Irreducible, irreducibility — *see* condition
Irregular, irregularity
　action, heart 427.9
　alveolar process 525.8
　bleeding NEC 626.4
　breathing 786.09
　colon 569.89
　contour
　　acquired 371.70
　　of cornea 743.41
　　　acquired 371.70
　　reconstructed breast 612.0
　dentin in pulp 522.3
　eye movements NEC 379.59
　menstruation (cause unknown) 626.4
　periods 626.4
　prostate 602.9
　pupil 364.75
　respiratory 786.09
　septum (nasal) 470
　shape, organ or site, congenital NEC — *see* Distortion
　sleep-wake rhythm (non-24-hour) 327.39
　　nonorganic origin 307.45
　vertebra 733.99
Irritability 799.22
　bladder 596.89
　　neurogenic 596.54
　　　with cauda equina syndrome 344.61
　bowel (syndrome) 564.1
　bronchial (*see also* Bronchitis) 490
　cerebral, newborn 779.1
　colon 564.1
　　psychogenic 306.4
　duodenum 564.89
　heart (psychogenic) 306.2
　ileum 564.89

Irritability — *continued*
　jejunum 564.89
　myocardium 306.2
　nervousness 799.21
　rectum 564.89
　stomach 536.9
　　psychogenic 306.4
　sympathetic (nervous system) (*see also* Neuropathy, peripheral, autonomic) 337.9
　urethra 599.84
　ventricular (heart) (psychogenic) 306.2
Irritable — *see also* Irritability 799.22
Irritation
　anus 569.49
　axillary nerve 353.0
　bladder 596.89
　brachial plexus 353.0
　brain (traumatic) (*see also* Injury, intracranial) 854.0 ☑
　　nontraumatic — *see* Encephalitis
　bronchial (*see also* Bronchitis) 490
　cerebral (traumatic) (*see also* Injury, intracranial) 854.0 ☑
　　nontraumatic — *see* Encephalitis
　cervical plexus 353.2
　cervix (*see also* Cervicitis) 616.0
　choroid, sympathetic 360.11
　cranial nerve — *see* Disorder, nerve, cranial
　digestive tract 536.9
　　psychogenic 306.4
　gastric 536.9
　　psychogenic 306.4
　gastrointestinal (tract) 536.9
　　functional 536.9
　　psychogenic 306.4
　globe, sympathetic 360.11
　intestinal (bowel) 564.9
　labyrinth 386.50
　lumbosacral plexus 353.1
　meninges (traumatic) (*see also* Injury, intracranial) 854.0 ☑
　　nontraumatic — *see* Meningitis
　myocardium 306.2
　nerve — *see* Disorder, nerve
　nervous 799.21
　nose 478.19
　penis 607.89
　perineum 709.9
　peripheral
　　autonomic nervous system (*see also* Neuropathy, peripheral, autonomic) 337.9
　　nerve — *see* Disorder, nerve
　peritoneum (*see also* Peritonitis) 567.9
　pharynx 478.29
　plantar nerve 355.6
　spinal (cord) (traumatic) (*see also* Injury, spinal, by site)
　　nerve (*see also* Disorder, nerve)
　　　root NEC 724.9
　　traumatic — *see* Injury, nerve, spinal
　　nontraumatic — *see* Myelitis
　stomach 536.9
　　psychogenic 306.4
　sympathetic nerve NEC (*see also* Neuropathy, peripheral, autonomic) 337.9
　ulnar nerve 354.2
　vagina 623.9
Isambert's disease 012.3 ☑
Ischemia, ischemic 459.9
　basilar artery (with transient neurologic deficit) 435.0
　bone NEC 733.40
　bowel (transient) 557.9
　　acute 557.0
　　chronic 557.1
　　due to mesenteric artery insufficiency 557.1
　brain (*see also* Ischemia, cerebral)
　　recurrent focal 435.9
　cardiac (*see also* Ischemia, heart) 414.9
　cardiomyopathy 414.8
　carotid artery (with transient neurologic deficit) 435.8
　cerebral (chronic) (generalized) 437.1

Ischemia, ischemic — *continued*
  cerebral — *continued*
    arteriosclerotic 437.0
    intermittent (with transient neurologic deficit) 435.9
    newborn 779.2
    puerperal, postpartum, childbirth 674.0 ☑
    recurrent focal (with transient neurologic deficit) 435.9
    transient (with transient neurologic deficit) 435.9
  colon 557.9
    acute 557.0
    chronic 557.1
    due to mesenteric artery insufficiency 557.1
  coronary (chronic) (*see also* Ischemia, heart) 414.9
  demand 411.89
  heart (chronic or with a stated duration of over 8 weeks) 414.9
    acute or with a stated duration of 8 weeks or less (*see also* Infarct, myocardium) 410.9 ☑
      without myocardial infarction 411.89
        with coronary (artery) occlusion 411.81
    subacute 411.89
  intestine (transient) 557.9
    acute 557.0
    chronic 557.1
    due to mesenteric artery insufficiency 557.1
  kidney 593.81
  labyrinth 386.50

Ischemia, ischemic — *continued*
  muscles, leg 728.89
  myocardium, myocardial (chronic or with a stated duration of over 8 weeks) 414.8
    acute (*see also* Infarct, myocardium) 410.9 ☑
      without myocardial infarction 411.89
        with coronary (artery) occlusion 411.81
  renal 593.81
  retina, retinal 362.84
  small bowel 557.9
    acute 557.0
    chronic 557.1
    due to mesenteric artery insufficiency 557.1
  spinal cord 336.1
  subendocardial (*see also* Insufficiency, coronary) 411.89
  supply (*see also* Angina) 414.9
  vertebral artery (with transient neurologic deficit) 435.1
Ischialgia — *see also* Sciatica 724.3
Ischiopagus 759.4
Ischium, ischial — *see* condition
Ischomenia 626.8
Ischuria 788.5
Iselin's disease or osteochondrosis 732.5
Islands of
  parotid tissue in
    lymph nodes 750.26
    neck structures 750.26
  submaxillary glands in
    fascia 750.26
    lymph nodes 750.26

Islands of — *continued*
  submaxillary glands in — *continued*
    neck muscles 750.26
Islet cell tumor, pancreas (M8150/0) 211.7
Isoimmunization NEC — *see also* Incompatibility 656.2 ☑
  anti-E 656.2 ☑
  fetus or newborn 773.2
    ABO blood groups 773.1
    Rhesus (Rh) factor 773.0
Isolation V07.0
  social V62.4
Isosporosis 007.2
Issue
  medical certificate NEC V68.09
    cause of death V68.09
    disability examination V68.01
    fitness V68.09
    incapacity V68.09
  repeat prescription NEC V68.1
    appliance V68.1
    contraceptive V25.40
      device NEC V25.49
        intrauterine V25.42
        specified type NEC V25.49
      pill V25.41
    glasses V68.1
    medicinal substance V68.1
Itch — *see also* Pruritus 698.9
  bakers' 692.89
  barbers' 110.0
  bricklayers' 692.89
  cheese 133.8
  clam diggers' 120.3
  coolie 126.9
  copra 133.8

Itch — *see also* Pruritus — *continued*
  Cuban 050.1
  dew 126.9
  dhobie 110.3
  eye 379.99
  filarial (*see also* Infestation, filarial) 125.9
  grain 133.8
  grocers' 133.8
  ground 126.9
  harvest 133.8
  jock 110.3
  Malabar 110.9
    beard 110.0
    foot 110.4
    scalp 110.0
  meaning scabies 133.0
  Norwegian 133.0
  perianal 698.0
  poultrymen's 133.8
  sarcoptic 133.0
  scrub 134.1
  seven year V61.10
    meaning scabies 133.0
  straw 133.8
  swimmers' 120.3
  washerwoman's 692.4
  water 120.3
  winter 698.8
Itsenko-Cushing syndrome (pituitary basophilism) 255.0
Ivemark's syndrome (asplenia with congenital heart disease) 759.0
Ivory bones 756.52
Ixodes 134.8
Ixodiasis 134.8

J

Jaccoud's nodular fibrositis, chronic (Jaccoud's syndrome) 714.4
Jackson's
  membrane 751.4
  paralysis or syndrome 344.89
  veil 751.4
Jacksonian
  epilepsy (see also Epilepsy) 345.5 ☑
  seizures (focal) (see also Epilepsy) 345.5 ☑
Jacob's ulcer (M8090/3) — see Neoplasm, skin, malignant, by site
Jacquet's dermatitis (diaper dermatitis) 691.0
Jadassohn-Lewandowski syndrome (pachyonychia congenita) 757.5
Jadassohn-Pellizari's disease (anetoderma) 701.3
Jadassohn-Tièche nevus (M8780/0) — see Neoplasm, skin, benign
Jadassohn's
  blue nevus (M8780/0) — see Neoplasm, skin, benign
  disease (maculopapular erythroderma) 696.2
  intraepidermal epithelioma (M8096/0) — see Neoplasm, skin, benign
Jaffe-Lichtenstein (-Uehlinger) syndrome 252.01
Jahnke's syndrome (encephalocutaneous angiomatosis) 759.6
Jakob-Creutzfeldt disease (CJD) (syndrome) 046.19
  with dementia
    with behavioral disturbance 046.19 [294.11]
    without behavioral disturbance 046.19 [294.10]
  familial 046.19
  iatrogenic 046.19
  specified NEC 046.19
  sporadic 046.19
  variant (vCJD) 046.11
    with dementia
      with behavioral disturbance 046.11 [294.11]
      without behavioral disturbance 046.11 [294.10]
Jaksch (-Luzet) disease or syndrome (pseudoleukemia infantum) 285.8
Jamaican
  neuropathy 349.82
  paraplegic tropical ataxic-spastic syndrome 349.82
Janet's disease (psychasthenia) 300.89
Janiceps 759.4
Jansky-Bielschowsky amaurotic familial idiocy 330.1
Japanese
  B type encephalitis 062.0
  river fever 081.2
  seven-day fever 100.89
Jaundice (yellow) 782.4
  acholuric (familial) (splenomegalic) (see also Spherocytosis) 282.0
    acquired 283.9
  breast milk 774.39
  catarrhal (acute) 070.1
    with hepatic coma 070.0
    chronic 571.9
    epidemic — see Jaundice, epidemic
  cholestatic (benign) 782.4
  chronic idiopathic 277.4
  epidemic (catarrhal) 070.1
    with hepatic coma 070.0
    leptospiral 100.0
    spirochetal 100.0
  febrile (acute) 070.1
    with hepatic coma 070.0
    leptospiral 100.0
    spirochetal 100.0
  fetus or newborn 774.6
    due to or associated with
      ABO
        absence or deficiency of enzyme system for bilirubin conjugation (congenital) 774.39

Jaundice — continued
  fetus or newborn — continued
    due to or associated with — continued
      antibodies 773.1
      blood group incompatibility NEC 773.2
      breast milk inhibitors to conjugation 774.39
        associated with preterm delivery 774.2
      bruising 774.1
      Crigler-Najjar syndrome 277.4 [774.31]
      delayed conjugation 774.30
        associated with preterm delivery 774.2
      development 774.39
      drugs or toxins transmitted from mother 774.1
      G-6-PD deficiency 282.2 [774.0]
      galactosemia 271.1 [774.5]
      Gilbert's syndrome 277.4 [774.31]
      hepatocellular damage 774.4
      hereditary hemolytic anemia (see also Anemia, hemolytic) 282.9 [774.0]
      hypothyroidism, congenital 243 [774.31]
      incompatibility, maternal/fetal 773.1
      incompatibility, maternal/fetal NEC 773.2
      infection 774.1
      inspissated bile syndrome 774.4
      isoimmunization 773.1
      isoimmunization NEC 773.2
      mucoviscidosis 277.01 [774.5]
      obliteration of bile duct, congenital 751.61 [774.5]
      polycythemia 774.1
      preterm delivery 774.2
      red cell defect 282.9 [774.0]
      Rh
        antibodies 773.0
        incompatibility, maternal/fetal 773.0
        isoimmunization 773.0
      spherocytosis (congenital) 282.0 [774.0]
      swallowed maternal blood 774.1
    physiological NEC 774.6
  from injection, inoculation, infusion, or transfusion (blood) (plasma) (serum) (other substance) (onset within 8 months after administration) — see Hepatitis, viral
  Gilbert's (familial nonhemolytic) 277.4
  hematogenous 283.9
  hemolytic (acquired) 283.9
    congenital (see also Spherocytosis) 282.0
  hemorrhagic (acute) 100.0
    leptospiral 100.0
    newborn 776.0
    spirochetal 100.0
  hepatocellular 573.8
  homologous (serum) — see Hepatitis, viral
  idiopathic, chronic 277.4
  infectious (acute) (subacute) 070.1
    with hepatic coma 070.0
    leptospiral 100.0
    spirochetal 100.0
  leptospiral 100.0
  malignant (see also Necrosis, liver) 570
  newborn (physiological) (see also Jaundice, fetus or newborn) 774.6
  nonhemolytic, congenital familial (Gilbert's) 277.4
  nuclear, newborn (see also Kernicterus of newborn) 774.7
  obstructive NEC (see also Obstruction, biliary) 576.8
  postimmunization — see Hepatitis, viral
  posttransfusion — see Hepatitis, viral
  regurgitation (see also Obstruction, biliary) 576.8

Jaundice — continued
  serum (homologous) (prophylactic) (therapeutic) — see Hepatitis, viral
  spirochetal (hemorrhagic) 100.0
  symptomatic 782.4
    newborn 774.6
Jaw-blinking 374.43
  congenital 742.8
Jaw-winking phenomenon or syndrome 742.8
Jaw — see condition
Jealousy
  alcoholic 291.5
  childhood 313.3
  sibling 313.3
Jejunitis — see also Enteritis 558.9
Jejunostomy status V44.4
Jejunum, jejunal — see condition
Jensen's disease 363.05
Jericho boil 085.1
Jerks, myoclonic 333.2
Jervell-Lange-Nielsen syndrome 426.82
Jeune's disease or syndrome (asphyxiating thoracic dystrophy) 756.4
Jigger disease 134.1
Job's syndrome (chronic granulomatous disease) 288.1
Jod-Basedow phenomenon 242.8 ☑
Johnson-Stevens disease (erythema multiforme exudativum) 695.13
Joint — see also condition
  Charcôt's 094.0 [713.5]
  false 733.82
  flail — see Flail, joint
  mice — see Loose, body, joint, by site
  sinus to bone 730.9 ☑
  von Gies' 095.8
Jordan's anomaly or syndrome 288.2
Josephs-Diamond-Blackfan anemia (congenital hypoplastic) 284.01
Joubert syndrome 759.89
Jumpers' knee 727.2
Jungle yellow fever 060.0
Jüngling's disease (sarcoidosis) 135
Junin virus hemorrhagic fever 078.7
Juvenile — see also condition
  delinquent 312.9
    group (see also Disturbance, conduct) 312.2 ☑
    neurotic 312.4

K

Kabuki syndrome 759.89
Kahler (-Bozzolo) disease (multiple myeloma) (M9730/3) 203.0 ☑
Kakergasia 300.9
Kakke 265.0
Kala-azar (Indian) (infantile) (Mediterranean) (Sudanese) 085.0
Kalischer's syndrome (encephalocutaneous angiomatosis) 759.6
Kallmann's syndrome (hypogonadotropic hypogonadism with anosmia) 253.4
Kanner's syndrome (autism) — see also Psychosis, childhood 299.0 ☑
Kaolinosis 502
Kaposi's
  disease 757.33
    lichen ruber 696.4
      acuminatus 696.4
      moniliformis 697.8
    xeroderma pigmentosum 757.33
  sarcoma (M9140/3) 176.9
    adipose tissue 176.1
    aponeurosis 176.1
    artery 176.1
    associated herpesvirus infection 058.89
    blood vessel 176.1
    bursa 176.1
    connective tissue 176.1
    external genitalia 176.8
    fascia 176.1
    fatty tissue 176.1
    fibrous tissue 176.1
    gastrointestinal tract NEC 176.3
    ligament 176.1

Kaposi's — continued
  sarcoma — continued
    lung 176.4
    lymph
      gland(s) 176.5
      node(s) 176.5
    lymphatic(s) NEC 176.1
    muscle (skeletal) 176.1
    oral cavity NEC 176.8
    palate 176.2
    scrotum 176.8
    skin 176.0
    soft tissue 176.1
    specified site NEC 176.8
    subcutaneous tissue 176.1
    synovia 176.1
    tendon (sheath) 176.1
    vein 176.1
    vessel 176.1
    viscera NEC 176.9
    vulva 176.8
  varicelliform eruption 054.0
  vaccinia 999.0
Kartagener's syndrome or triad (sinusitis, bronchiectasis, situs inversus) 759.3
Kasabach-Merritt syndrome (capillary hemangioma associated with thrombocytopenic purpura) 287.39
Kaschin-Beck disease (endemic polyarthritis) — see Disease, Kaschin-Beck
Kast's syndrome (dyschondroplasia with hemangiomas) 756.4
Katatonia — see Catatonia
Katayama disease or fever 120.2
Kathisophobia 781.0
Kawasaki disease 446.1
Kayser-Fleischer ring (cornea) (pseudosclerosis) 275.1 [371.14]
Kaznelson's syndrome (congenital hypoplastic anemia) 284.01
Kearns-Sayre syndrome 277.87
Kedani fever 081.2
Kelis 701.4
Kelly (-Patterson) syndrome (sideropenic dysphagia) 280.8
Keloid, cheloid 701.4
  Addison's (morphea) 701.0
  cornea 371.00
  Hawkins' 701.4
  scar 701.4
Keloma 701.4
Kenya fever 082.1
Keratectasia 371.71
  congenital 743.41
Keratinization NEC
  alveolar ridge mucosa
    excessive 528.72
    minimal 528.71
Keratitis (nodular) (nonulcerative) (simple) (zonular) NEC 370.9
  with ulceration (see also Ulcer, cornea) 370.00
  actinic 370.24
  arborescens 054.42
  areolar 370.22
  bullosa 370.8
  deep — see Keratitis, interstitial
  dendritic(a) 054.42
  desiccation 370.34
  diffuse interstitial 370.52
  disciform(is) 054.43
    varicella 052.7 [370.44]
  epithelialis vernalis 372.13 [370.32]
  exposure 370.34
  filamentary 370.23
  gonococcal (congenital) (prenatal) 098.43
  herpes, herpetic (simplex) NEC 054.43
    zoster 053.21
  hypopyon 370.04
  in
    chickenpox 052.7 [370.44]
    exanthema (see also Exanthem) 057.9 [370.44]
    paravaccinia (see also Paravaccinia) 051.9 [370.44]

Keratitis — *continued*
  in — *continued*
    smallpox (*see also* Smallpox)
      050.9 *[370.44]*
    vernal conjunctivitis 372.13 *[370.32]*
  interstitial (nonsyphilitic) 370.50
    with ulcer (*see also* Ulcer, cornea) 370.00
    diffuse 370.52
    herpes, herpetic (simplex) 054.43
      zoster 053.21
    syphilitic (congenital) (hereditary) 090.3
    tuberculous (*see also* Tuberculosis)
      017.3 ☑ *[370.59]*
  lagophthalmic 370.34
  macular 370.22
  neuroparalytic 370.35
  neurotrophic 370.35
  nummular 370.22
  oyster-shuckers' 370.8
  parenchymatous — *see* Keratitis, interstitial
  petrificans 370.8
  phlyctenular 370.31
  postmeasles 055.71
  punctata, punctate 370.21
    leprosa 030.0 *[370.21]*
    profunda 090.3
    superficial (Thygeson's) 370.21
  purulent 370.8
  pustuliformis profunda 090.3
  rosacea 695.3 *[370.49]*
  sclerosing 370.54
  specified type NEC 370.8
  stellate 370.22
  striate 370.22
  superficial 370.20
    with conjunctivitis (*see also* Keratoconjunctivitis) 370.40
    punctate (Thygeson's) 370.21
  suppurative 370.8
  syphilitic (congenital) (prenatal) 090.3
  trachomatous 076.1
    late effect 139.1
  tuberculous (phlyctenular) (see also Tuberculosis) 017.3 ☑ *[370.31]*
  ulcerated (*see also* Ulcer, cornea) 370.00
  vesicular 370.8
  welders' 370.24
  xerotic (*see also* Keratomalacia) 371.45
    vitamin A deficiency 264.4
Kerato-uveitis — *see also* Iridocyclitis 364.3
Keratoacanthoma 238.2
Keratocele 371.72
Keratoconjunctivitis — *see also* Keratitis
  370.40
  adenovirus type 8 077.1
  epidemic 077.1
  exposure 370.34
  gonococcal 098.43
  herpetic (simplex) 054.43
    zoster 053.21
  in
    chickenpox 052.7 *[370.44]*
    exanthema (*see also* Exanthem)
      057.9 *[370.44]*
    paravaccinia (*see also* Paravaccinia)
      051.9 *[370.44]*
    smallpox (*see also* Smallpox)
      050.9 *[370.44]*
  infectious 077.1
  neurotrophic 370.35
  phlyctenular 370.31
  postmeasles 055.71
  shipyard 077.1
  sicca (Sjögren's syndrome) 710.2
    not in Sjögren's syndrome 370.33
  specified type NEC 370.49
  tuberculous (phlyctenular) (*see also* Tuberculosis) 017.3 ☑ *[370.31]*
Keratoconus 371.60
  acute hydrops 371.62
  congenital 743.41
  stable 371.61
Keratocyst (dental) 526.0
Keratoderma, keratodermia (congenital)
  (palmaris et plantaris) (symmetrical)
  757.39

Keratoderma, keratodermia — *continued*
  acquired 701.1
  blennorrhagica 701.1
    gonococcal 098.81
  climacterium 701.1
  eccentrica 757.39
  gonorrheal 098.81
  punctata 701.1
  tylodes, progressive 701.1
Keratodermatocele 371.72
Keratoglobus 371.70
  congenital 743.41
    associated with buphthalmos 743.22
Keratohemia 371.12
Keratoiritis — *see also* Iridocyclitis 364.3
  syphilitic 090.3
  tuberculous (*see also* Tuberculosis)
    017.3 ☑ *[364.11]*
Keratolysis exfoliativa (congenital) 757.39
  acquired 695.89
  neonatorum 757.39
Keratoma 701.1
  congenital 757.39
  malignum congenitale 757.1
  palmaris et plantaris hereditarium 757.39
  senile 702.0
Keratomalacia 371.45
  vitamin A deficiency 264.4
Keratomegaly 743.41
Keratomycosis 111.1
  nigricans (palmaris) 111.1
Keratopathy 371.40
  band (*see also* Keratitis) 371.43
  bullous (*see also* Keratitis) 371.23
  degenerative (*see also* Degeneration,
    cornea) 371.40
  hereditary (*see also* Dystrophy, cornea)
    371.50
  discrete colliquative 371.49
Keratoscleritis, tuberculous — *see also* Tuberculosis 017.3 ☑ *[370.31]*
Keratosis 701.1
  actinic 702.0
  arsenical 692.4
  blennorrhagica 701.1
    gonococcal 098.81
  congenital (any type) 757.39
  ear (middle) (*see also* Cholesteatoma) 385.30
  female genital (external) 629.89
  follicularis 757.39
    acquired 701.1
    congenital (acneiformis) (Siemens')
      757.39
    spinulosa (decalvans) 757.39
    vitamin A deficiency 264.8
  follicular, vitamin A deficiency 264.8
  gonococcal 098.81
  larynx, laryngeal 478.79
  male genital (external) 608.89
  middle ear (*see also* Cholesteatoma) 385.30
  nigricans 701.2
    congenital 757.39
  obturans 380.21
  oral epithelium
    residual ridge mucosa
      excessive 528.72
      minimal 528.71
  palmaris et plantaris (symmetrical) 757.39
  penile 607.89
  pharyngeus 478.29
  pilaris 757.39
    acquired 701.1
  punctata (palmaris et plantaris) 701.1
  scrotal 608.89
  seborrheic 702.19
    inflamed 702.11
  senilis 702.0
  solar 702.0
  suprafollicularis 757.39
  tonsillaris 478.29
  vagina 623.1
  vegetans 757.39
  vitamin A deficiency 264.8
Keraunoparalysis 994.0
Kerion (celsi) 110.0

Kernicterus of newborn (not due to isoimmunization) 774.7
  due to isoimmunization (conditions classifiable to 773.0–773.2) 773.4
Ketoacidosis 276.2
  diabetic 250.1 ☑
    due to secondary diabetes 249.1 ☑
Ketonuria 791.6
  branched-chain, intermittent 270.3
Ketosis 276.2
  diabetic 250.1 ☑
    due to secondary diabetes 249.1 ☑
Kidney — *see* condition
Kienböck's
  disease 732.3
    adult 732.8
  osteochondrosis 732.3
Kimmelstiel (-Wilson) disease or syndrome
  (intercapillary glomerulosclerosis)
  250.4 ☑ *[581.81]*
  due to secondary diabetes 249.4 ☑ *[581.81]*
Kink, kinking
  appendix 543.9
  artery 447.1
  cystic duct, congenital 751.61
  hair (acquired) 704.2
  ileum or intestine (*see also* Obstruction, intestine) 560.9
  Lane's (*see also* Obstruction, intestine) 560.9
  organ or site, congenital NEC — *see*
    Anomaly, specified type NEC, by site
  ureter (pelvic junction) 593.3
    congenital 753.20
  vein(s) 459.2
    caval 459.2
    peripheral 459.2
Kinnier Wilson's disease (hepatolenticular
  degeneration) 275.1
Kissing
  osteophytes 721.5
  spine 721.5
  vertebra 721.5
Klauder's syndrome (erythema multiforme,
  exudativum) 695.19
Klebs' disease — *see also* Nephritis 583.9
Klein-Waardenburg syndrome (ptosisepicanthus) 270.2
Kleine-Levin syndrome 327.13
Kleptomania 312.32
Klinefelter's syndrome 758.7
Klinger's disease 446.4
Klippel-Feil disease or syndrome (brevicollis)
  756.16
Klippel-Trenaunay syndrome 759.89
Klippel's disease 723.8
Klumpke (-Déjérine) palsy, paralysis (birth)
  (newborn) 767.6
Klüver-Bucy (-Terzian) syndrome 310.0
Knee — *see* condition
Knifegrinders' rot — *see also* Tuberculosis
  011.4 ☑
Knock-knee (acquired) 736.41
  congenital 755.64
Knot
  intestinal, syndrome (volvulus) 560.2
  umbilical cord (true) 663.2 ☑
    affecting fetus or newborn 762.5
Knots, surfer 919.8
  infected 919.9
Knotting (of)
  hair 704.2
  intestine 560.2
Knuckle pads (Garrod's) 728.79
Köbner's disease (epidermolysis bullosa)
  757.39
Koch-Weeks conjunctivitis 372.03
Koch's
  infection (*see also* Tuberculosis, pulmonary)
    011.9 ☑
  relapsing fever 087.9
Koenig-Wichman disease (pemphigus) 694.4
Köhler-Mouchet disease (osteoarthrosis juvenilis) 732.5
Köhler-Pellegrini-Stieda disease or syndrome (calcification, knee joint) 726.62
Köhler's disease (osteochondrosis) 732.5

Köhler's disease — *continued*
  first (osteochondrosis juvenilis) 732.5
  second (Freiburg's infarction, metatarsal
    head) 732.5
  patellar 732.4
  tarsal navicular (bone) (osteoarthrosis juvenilis) 732.5
Koilonychia 703.8
  congenital 757.5
Kojevnikov's, Kojewnikoff's epilepsy — *see*
  also Epilepsy 345.7 ☑
König's
  disease (osteochondritis dissecans) 732.7
  syndrome 564.89
Koniophthisis — *see also* Tuberculosis
  011.4 ☑
Koplik's spots 055.9
Kopp's asthma 254.8
Korean hemorrhagic fever 078.6
Korsakoff (-Wernicke) disease, psychosis,
  or syndrome (nonalcoholic) 294.0
  alcoholic 291.1
Korsakov's disease — *see* Korsakoff's disease
Korsakow's disease — *see* Korsakoff's disease
Kostmann's disease or syndrome (infantile
  genetic agranulocytosis) 288.01
Krabbe's
  disease (leukodystrophy) 330.0
  syndrome
    congenital muscle hypoplasia 756.89
    cutaneocerebral angioma 759.6
Kraepelin-Morel disease — *see also*
  Schizophrenia 295.9 ☑
Kraft-Weber-Dimitri disease 759.6
Kraurosis
  ani 569.49
  penis 607.0
  vagina 623.8
  vulva 624.09
Kreotoxism 005.9
Krukenberg's
  spindle 371.13
  tumor (M8490/6) 198.6
Kufs' disease 330.1
Kugelberg-Welander disease 335.11
Kuhnt-Junius degeneration or disease
  362.52
Kulchitsky's cell carcinoma (carcinoid tumor
  of intestine) 259.2
Kümmell's disease or spondylitis 721.7
Kundrat's disease (lymphosarcoma) 200.1 ☑
Kunekune — *see* Dermatophytosis
Kunkel syndrome (lupoid hepatitis) 571.49
Kupffer cell sarcoma (M9124/3) 155.0
Kuru 046.0
Kussmaul's
  coma (diabetic) 250.3 ☑
    due to secondary diabetes 249.3 ☑
  disease (polyarteritis nodosa) 446.0
  respiration (air hunger) 786.09
Kwashiorkor (marasmus type) 260
Kyasanur Forest disease 065.2
Kyphoscoliosis, kyphoscoliotic (acquired) —
  see also Scoliosis 737.30
  congenital 756.19
  due to radiation 737.33
  heart (disease) 416.1
  idiopathic 737.30
  infantile
    progressive 737.32
    resolving 737.31
  late effect of rickets 268.1 *[737.43]*
  specified NEC 737.39
  thoracogenic 737.34
  tuberculous (*see also* Tuberculosis)
    015.0 ☑ *[737.43]*
Kyphosis, kyphotic (acquired) (postural)
  737.10
  adolescent postural 737.0
  congenital 756.19
  dorsalis juvenilis 732.0
  due to or associated with
    Charcôt-Marie-Tooth disease
      356.1 *[737.41]*
    mucopolysaccharidosis 277.5 *[737.41]*
    neurofibromatosis 237.71 *[737.41]*

☑ **Additional Digit Required** — Refer to the Tabular List for Digit Selection

▽ **Subterms under main terms may continue to next column or page**

170 — Volume 2

▶◀ Revised Text

● New Line   ▲ Revised Code

2014 ICD-9-CM

Kyphosis, kyphotic — *continued*
due to or associated with — *continued*
osteitis
deformans 731.0 *[737.41]*
fibrosa cystica 252.01 *[737.41]*
osteoporosis (*see also* Osteoporosis)
733.0 ☑ *[737.41]*
poliomyelitis (*see also* Poliomyelitis)
138 *[737.41]*
radiation 737.11
tuberculosis (*see also* Tuberculosis)
015.0 ☑ *[737.41]*
Kümmell's 721.7
late effect of rickets 268.1 *[737.41]*
Morquio-Brailsford type (spinal)
277.5 *[737.41]*
pelvis 738.6
postlaminectomy 737.12
specified cause NEC 737.19
syphilitic, congenital 090.5 *[737.41]*
tuberculous (*see also* Tuberculosis)
015.0 ☑ *[737.41]*
Kyrle's disease (hyperkeratosis follicularis in
cutem penetrans) 701.1

L

L-shaped kidney 753.3
L-xyloketosuria 271.8
Labia, labium — *see* condition
Labiated hymen 752.49
Labile
blood pressure 796.2
emotions, emotionality 301.3
vasomotor system 443.9
Lability, emotional 799.24
Labioglossal paralysis 335.22
Labium leporinum — *see also* Cleft, lip 749.10
Labor — *see also* Delivery
with complications — *see* Delivery, complicated
abnormal NEC 661.9 ☑
affecting fetus or newborn 763.7
arrested active phase 661.1 ☑
affecting fetus or newborn 763.7
desultory 661.2 ☑
affecting fetus or newborn 763.7
dyscoordinate 661.4 ☑
affecting fetus or newborn 763.7
early onset (22-36 weeks gestation)
644.2 ☑
failed
induction 659.1 ☑
mechanical 659.0 ☑
medical 659.1 ☑
surgical 659.0 ☑
trial (vaginal delivery) 660.6 ☑
false 644.1 ☑
forced or induced, affecting fetus or newborn 763.89
hypertonic 661.4 ☑
affecting fetus or newborn 763.7
hypotonic 661.2 ☑
affecting fetus or newborn 763.7
primary 661.0 ☑
affecting fetus or newborn 763.7
secondary 661.1 ☑
affecting fetus or newborn 763.7
incoordinate 661.4 ☑
affecting fetus or newborn 763.7
irregular 661.2 ☑
affecting fetus or newborn 763.7
long — *see* Labor, prolonged
missed (at or near term) 656.4 ☑
obstructed NEC 660.9 ☑
affecting fetus or newborn 763.1
due to female genital mutilation
660.8 ☑
specified cause NEC 660.8 ☑
affecting fetus or newborn 763.1
pains, spurious 644.1 ☑
precipitate 661.3 ☑
affecting fetus or newborn 763.6
premature 644.2 ☑
threatened 644.0 ☑
prolonged or protracted 662.1 ☑

Labor — *see also* Delivery — *continued*
prolonged or protracted — *continued*
first stage 662.0 ☑
affecting fetus or newborn 763.89
second stage 662.2 ☑
affecting fetus or newborn 763.89
affecting fetus or newborn 763.89
threatened NEC 644.1 ☑
undelivered 644.1 ☑
Labored breathing — *see also* Hyperventilation 786.09
Labyrinthitis (inner ear) (destructive) (latent)
386.30
circumscribed 386.32
diffuse 386.31
focal 386.32
purulent 386.33
serous 386.31
suppurative 386.33
syphilitic 095.8
toxic 386.34
viral 386.35
Laceration — *see also* Wound, open, by site
accidental, complicating surgery 998.2
Achilles tendon 845.09
with open wound 892.2
anus (sphincter) 879.6
with
abortion — *see* Abortion, by type,
with damage to pelvic organs
ectopic pregnancy (*see also* categories 633.0–633.9) 639.2
molar pregnancy (*see also* categories
630–632) 639.2
complicated 879.7
complicating delivery (healed) (old)
654.8 ☑
with laceration of anal or rectal mucosa 664.3 ☑
not associated with third-degree
perineal laceration 664.6 ☑
following
abortion 639.2
ectopic or molar pregnancy 639.2
nontraumatic, nonpuerperal (healed)
(old) 569.43
bladder (urinary)
with
abortion — *see* Abortion, by type,
with damage to pelvic organs
ectopic pregnancy (*see also* categories 633.0–633.9) 639.2
molar pregnancy (*see also* categories
630–632) 639.2
following
abortion 639.2
ectopic or molar pregnancy 639.2
obstetrical trauma 665.5 ☑
blood vessel — *see* Injury, blood vessel, by
site
bowel
with
abortion — *see* Abortion, by type,
with damage to pelvic organs
ectopic pregnancy (*see also* categories 633.0–633.9) 639.2
molar pregnancy (*see also* categories
630–632) 639.2
following
abortion 639.2
ectopic or molar pregnancy 639.2
obstetrical trauma 665.5 ☑

Laceration — *see also* Wound, open, by site —
continued
brain (cerebral) (membrane) (with hemorrhage) 851.8 ☑

> *Note* — Use the following fifth-digit
> *subclassification with categories*
> *851–854:*
>
> 0 unspecified state of consciousness
>
> 1 with no loss of consciousness
>
> 2 with brief [less than one hour]
>   loss of consciousness
>
> 3 with moderate [1–24 hours] loss
>   of consciousness
>
> 4 with prolonged [more than 24
>   hours] loss of consciousness and
>   return to pre–existing conscious
>   level
>
> 5 with prolonged [more than 24
>   hours] loss of consciousness,
>   without return to pre–existing
>   conscious level
>
> Use fifth-digit 5 to designate when a
> patient is unconscious and dies before
> regaining consciousness, regardless of
> the duration of the loss of consciousness
>
> 6 with loss of consciousness of un-
>   specified duration
>
> 9 with concussion, unspecified

with
open intracranial wound 851.9 ☑
skull fracture — *see* Fracture, skull,
by site
cerebellum 851.6 ☑
with open intracranial wound
851.7 ☑
cortex 851.2 ☑
with open intracranial wound
851.3 ☑
during birth 767.0
stem 851.6 ☑
with open intracranial wound
851.7 ☑
broad ligament
with
abortion — *see* Abortion, by type,
with damage to pelvic organs
ectopic pregnancy (*see also* categories 633.0–633.9) 639.2
molar pregnancy (*see also* categories
630–632) 639.2
following
abortion 639.2
ectopic or molar pregnancy 639.2
nontraumatic 620.6
obstetrical trauma 665.6 ☑
syndrome (nontraumatic) 620.6
capsule, joint — *see* Sprain, by site
cardiac — *see* Laceration, heart
causing eversion of cervix uteri (old) 622.0
central, complicating delivery 664.4 ☑
cerebellum — *see* Laceration, brain, cerebellum
cerebral (*see also* Laceration, brain)
during birth 767.0
cervix (uteri)
with
abortion — *see* Abortion, by type,
with damage to pelvic organs
ectopic pregnancy (*see also* categories 633.0–633.9) 639.2
molar pregnancy (*see also* categories
630–632) 639.2
following
abortion 639.2
ectopic or molar pregnancy 639.2
nonpuerperal, nontraumatic 622.3
obstetrical trauma (current) 665.3 ☑
old (postpartal) 622.3
traumatic — *see* Injury, internal, cervix
chordae heart 429.5
complicated 879.9

Laceration — *see also* Wound, open, by site —
continued
cornea — *see* Laceration, eyeball
superficial 918.1
cortex (cerebral) — *see* Laceration, brain,
cortex
esophagus 530.89
eye(s) — *see* Laceration, ocular
eyeball NEC 871.4
with prolapse or exposure of intraocular
tissue 871.1
penetrating — *see* Penetrating wound,
eyeball
specified as without prolapse of intraocular tissue 871.0
eyelid NEC 870.8
full thickness 870.1
involving lacrimal passages 870.2
skin (and periocular area) 870.0
penetrating — *see* Penetrating
wound, orbit
fourchette
with
abortion — *see* Abortion, by type,
with damage to pelvic organs
ectopic pregnancy (*see also* categories 633.0–633.9) 639.2
molar pregnancy (*see also* categories
630–632) 639.2
complicating delivery 664.0 ☑
following
abortion 639.2
ectopic or molar pregnancy 639.2
heart (without penetration of heart chambers) 861.02
with
open wound into thorax 861.12
penetration of heart chambers
861.03
with open wound into thorax
861.13
hernial sac — *see* Hernia, by site
internal organ (abdomen) (chest) (pelvis)
NEC — *see* Injury, internal, by site
NEC — *see* Injury, internal, by site
kidney (parenchyma) 866.02
with
complete disruption of parenchyma
(rupture) 866.03
with open wound into cavity
866.13
open wound into cavity 866.12
labia
complicating delivery 664.0 ☑
ligament (*see also* Sprain, by site)
with open wound — *see* Wound, open,
by site
liver 864.05
with open wound into cavity 864.15
major (disruption of hepatic parenchyma) 864.04
with open wound into cavity 864.14
minor (capsule only) 864.02
with open wound into cavity 864.12
moderate (involving parenchyma without major disruption) 864.03
with open wound into cavity 864.13
multiple 864.04
with open wound into cavity
864.14
stellate 864.04
with open wound into cavity 864.14
lung 861.22
with open wound into thorax 861.32
meninges — *see* Laceration, brain
meniscus (knee) (*see also* Tear, meniscus)
836.2
old 717.5
site other than knee (*see also* Sprain, by
site)
old NEC (*see also* Disorder, cartilage,
articular) 718.0 ☑
muscle (*see also* Sprain, by site)
with open wound — *see* Wound, open,
by site
myocardium — *see* Laceration, heart

Laceration — *see also* Wound, open, by site — *continued*
nerve — *see* Injury, nerve, by site
ocular NEC (*see also* Laceration, eyeball) 871.4
  adnexa NEC 870.8
    penetrating 870.3
      with foreign body 870.4
  orbit (eye) 870.8
    penetrating 870.3
      with foreign body 870.4
pelvic
  floor (muscles)
    with
      abortion — *see* Abortion, by type, with damage to pelvic organs
      ectopic pregnancy (*see also* categories 633.0–633.9) 639.2
      molar pregnancy (*see also* categories 630–632) 639.2
    complicating delivery 664.1 ☑
    following
      abortion 639.2
      ectopic or molar pregnancy 639.2
    nonpuerperal 618.7
    old (postpartal) 618.7
  organ NEC
    with
      abortion — *see* Abortion, by type, with damage to pelvic organs
      ectopic pregnancy (*see also* categories 633.0–633.9) 639.2
      molar pregnancy (*see also* categories 630–632) 639.2
    complicating delivery 665.5 ☑
      affecting fetus or newborn 763.89
    following
      abortion 639.2
      ectopic or molar pregnancy 639.2
    obstetrical trauma 665.5 ☑
perineum, perineal (old) (postpartal) 618.7
  with
    abortion — *see* Abortion, by type, with damage to pelvic floor
    ectopic pregnancy (*see also* categories 633.0–633.9) 639.2
    molar pregnancy (*see also* categories 630–632) 639.2
  complicating delivery 664.4 ☑
    first degree 664.0 ☑
    second degree 664.1 ☑
    third degree 664.2 ☑
    fourth degree 664.3 ☑
    anal sphincter (healed) (old) 654.8 ☑
      not associated with third-degree perineal laceration 664.6 ☑
    sphincter (anal) (healed) (old) 654.8 ☑
      not associated with third-degree perineal laceration 664.6 ☑
    central 664.4 ☑
    involving
      anal sphincter 664.2 ☑
      fourchette 664.0 ☑
      hymen 664.0 ☑
      labia 664.0 ☑
      pelvic floor 664.1 ☑
      perineal muscles 664.1 ☑
      rectovaginal septum 664.2 ☑
        with anal mucosa 664.3 ☑
      skin 664.0 ☑
      sphincter (anal) 664.2 ☑
        with anal mucosa 664.3 ☑
      vagina 664.0 ☑
      vaginal muscles 664.1 ☑
      vulva 664.0 ☑
    secondary 674.2 ☑
  following
    abortion 639.2
    ectopic or molar pregnancy 639.2
  male 879.6

Laceration — *see also* Wound, open, by site — *continued*
perineum, perineal — *continued*
  male — *continued*
    complicated 879.7
  muscles, complicating delivery 664.1 ☑
  nonpuerperal, current injury 879.6
    complicated 879.7
  secondary (postpartal) 674.2 ☑
peritoneum
  with
    abortion — *see* Abortion, by type, with damage to pelvic organs
    ectopic pregnancy (*see also* categories 633.0–633.9) 639.2
    molar pregnancy (*see also* categories 630–632) 639.2
  following
    abortion 639.2
    ectopic or molar pregnancy 639.2
  obstetrical trauma 665.5 ☑
periurethral tissue
  with
    abortion — *see* Abortion, by type, with damage to pelvic organs
    ectopic pregnancy (*see also* categories 633.0–633.9) 639.2
    molar pregnancy (*see also* categories 630–632) 639.2
  following
    abortion 639.2
    ectopic or molar pregnancy 639.2
  obstetrical trauma 664.8 ☑
rectovaginal (septum)
  with
    abortion — *see* Abortion, by type, with damage to pelvic organs
    ectopic pregnancy (*see also* categories 633.0–633.9) 639.2
    molar pregnancy (*see also* categories 630–632) 639.2
  complicating delivery 665.4 ☑
    with perineum 664.2 ☑
      involving anal or rectal mucosa 664.3 ☑
  following
    abortion 639.2
    ectopic or molar pregnancy 639.2
  nonpuerperal 623.4
  old (postpartal) 623.4
spinal cord (meninges) (*see also* Injury, spinal, by site)
  due to injury at birth 767.4
  fetus or newborn 767.4
spleen 865.09
  with
    disruption of parenchyma (massive) 865.04
      with open wound into cavity 865.14
    open wound into cavity 865.19
  capsule (without disruption of parenchyma) 865.02
    with open wound into cavity 865.12
  parenchyma 865.03
    with open wound into cavity 865.13
    massive disruption (rupture) 865.04
      with open wound into cavity 865.14
tendon 848.9
  with open wound — *see* Wound, open, by site
  Achilles 845.09
    with open wound 892.2
  lower limb NEC 844.9
    with open wound NEC 894.2
  upper limb NEC 840.9
    with open wound NEC 884.2
tentorium cerebelli — *see* Laceration, brain, cerebellum
tongue 873.64
  complicated 873.74
urethra
  with
    abortion — *see* Abortion, by type, with damage to pelvic organs

Laceration — *see also* Wound, open, by site — *continued*
urethra — *continued*
  with — *continued*
    ectopic pregnancy (*see also* categories 633.0–633.9) 639.2
    molar pregnancy (*see also* categories 630–632) 639.2
  following
    abortion 639.2
    ectopic or molar pregnancy 639.2
  nonpuerperal, nontraumatic 599.84
  obstetrical trauma 665.5 ☑
uterus
  with
    abortion — *see* Abortion, by type, with damage to pelvic organs
    ectopic pregnancy (*see also* categories 633.0–633.9) 639.2
    molar pregnancy (*see also* categories 630–632) 639.2
  following
    abortion 639.2
    ectopic or molar pregnancy 639.2
  nonpuerperal, nontraumatic 621.8
  obstetrical trauma NEC 665.5 ☑
  old (postpartal) 621.8
vagina
  with
    abortion — *see* Abortion, by type, with damage to pelvic organs
    ectopic pregnancy (*see also* categories 633.0–633.9) 639.2
    molar pregnancy (*see also* categories 630–632) 639.2
    perineal involvement, complicating delivery 664.0 ☑
  complicating delivery 665.4 ☑
    first degree 664.0 ☑
    second degree 664.1 ☑
    third degree 664.2 ☑
    fourth degree 664.3 ☑
    high 665.4 ☑
    muscles 664.1 ☑
    sulcus 665.4 ☑
    wall 665.4 ☑
  following
    abortion 639.2
    ectopic or molar pregnancy 639.2
  nonpuerperal, nontraumatic 623.4
  old (postpartal) 623.4
valve, heart — *see* Endocarditis
vulva
  with
    abortion — *see* Abortion, by type, with damage to pelvic organs
    ectopic pregnancy (*see also* categories 633.0–633.9) 639.2
    molar pregnancy (*see also* categories 630–632) 639.2
  complicating delivery 664.0 ☑
  following
    abortion 639.2
    ectopic or molar pregnancy 639.2
  nonpuerperal, nontraumatic 624.4
  old (postpartal) 624.4
Lachrymal — *see* condition
Lachrymonasal duct — *see* condition
Lack of
  adequate intermaxillary vertical dimension 524.36
  appetite (*see also* Anorexia) 783.0
  care
    in home V60.4
    of adult 995.84
    of infant (at or after birth) 995.52
  coordination 781.3
  development (*see also* Hypoplasia)
    physiological in childhood 783.40
  education V62.3
  energy 780.79
  financial resources V60.2
  food 994.2
    in environment V60.89
  growth in childhood 783.43
  heating V60.1

Lack of — *continued*
  housing (permanent) (temporary) V60.0
    adequate V60.1
  material resources V60.2
  medical attention 799.89
  memory (*see also* Amnesia) 780.93
    mild, following organic brain damage 310.89
  ovulation 628.0
  person able to render necessary care V60.4
  physical exercise V69.0
  physiologic development in childhood 783.40
  posterior occlusal support 524.57
  prenatal care in current pregnancy V23.7
  shelter V60.0
  sleep V69.4
  water 994.3
Lacrimal — *see* condition
Lacrimation, abnormal — *see also* Epiphora 375.20
Lacrimonasal duct — *see* condition
Lactation, lactating (breast) (puerperal) (postpartum)
  defective 676.4 ☑
  disorder 676.9 ☑
    specified type NEC 676.8 ☑
  excessive 676.6 ☑
  failed 676.4 ☑
  mastitis NEC 675.2 ☑
  mother (care and/or examination) V24.1
  nonpuerperal 611.6
  suppressed 676.5 ☑
Lacticemia 271.3
  excessive 276.2
Lactosuria 271.3
Lacunar skull 756.0
Laennec's cirrhosis (alcoholic) 571.2
  nonalcoholic 571.5
Lafora's disease 333.2
Lagleyze-von Hippel disease (retinocerebral angiomatosis) 759.6
Lag, lid (nervous) 374.41
Lagophthalmos (eyelid) (nervous) 374.20
  cicatricial 374.23
  keratitis (*see also* Keratitis) 370.34
  mechanical 374.22
  paralytic 374.21
La grippe — *see* Influenza
Lahore sore 085.1
Lakes, venous (cerebral) 437.8
Laki-Lorand factor deficiency — *see also* Defect, coagulation 286.3
Lalling 307.9
Lambliasis 007.1
Lame back 724.5
Lancereaux's diabetes (diabetes mellitus with marked emaciation) 250.8 ☑ *[261]*
  due to secondary diabetes 249.8 ☑ *[261]*
Landau-Kleffner syndrome 345.8 ☑
Landouzy-Déjérine dystrophy (fascioscapulohumeral atrophy) 359.1
Landry-Guillain-Barré syndrome 357.0
Landry's disease or paralysis 357.0
Lane's
  band 751.4
  disease 569.89
  kink (*see also* Obstruction, intestine) 560.9
Langdon Down's syndrome (mongolism) 758.0
Language abolition 784.69
Lanugo (persistent) 757.4
Laparoscopic surgical procedure converted to open procedure V64.41
Lardaceous
  degeneration (any site) 277.39
  disease 277.39
  kidney 277.39 *[583.81]*
  liver 277.39
Large
  baby (regardless of gestational age) 766.1
    exceptionally (weight of 4500 grams or more) 766.0
    of diabetic mother 775.0
  ear 744.22
  fetus (*see also* Oversize, fetus)

☑ **Additional Digit Required** — Refer to the Tabular List for Digit Selection
▼ **Subterms under main terms may continue to next column or page**
172 — Volume 2   ▶◀ Revised Text   ● New Line   ▲ Revised Code   2014 ICD-9-CM

Large — *continued*
  fetus (*see also* Oversize, fetus) — *continued*
    causing disproportion 653.5 ☑
      with obstructed labor 660.1 ☑
    for dates
      fetus or newborn (regardless of gestational age) 766.1
      affecting management of pregnancy 656.6 ☑
    exceptionally (weight of 4500 grams or more) 766.0
  physiological cup 743.57
  stature 783.9
  waxy liver 277.39
  white kidney — *see* Nephrosis
Larsen-Johansson disease (juvenile osteopathia patellae) 732.4
Larsen's syndrome (flattened facies and multiple congenital dislocations) 755.8
Larva migrans
  cutaneous NEC 126.9
    ancylostoma 126.9
  of Diptera in vitreous 128.0
  visceral NEC 128.0
Laryngeal — *see also* condition 786.2
  syncope 786.2
Laryngismus (acute) (infectious) (stridulous) 478.75
  congenital 748.3
  diphtheritic 032.3
Laryngitis (acute) (edematous) (fibrinous) (gangrenous) (infective) (infiltrative) (malignant) (membranous) (phlegmonous) (pneumococcal) (pseudomembranous) (septic) (subglottic) (suppurative) (ulcerative) (viral) 464.00
  with
    influenza, flu, or grippe (*see also* Influenza) 487.1
    obstruction 464.01
    tracheitis (*see also* Laryngotracheitis) 464.20
      with obstruction 464.21
      acute 464.20
        with obstruction 464.21
      chronic 476.1
  atrophic 476.0
  Borrelia vincentii 101
  catarrhal 476.0
  chronic 476.0
    with tracheitis (chronic) 476.1
    due to external agent — *see* Condition, respiratory, chronic, due to
  diphtheritic (membranous) 032.3
  due to external agent — *see* Inflammation, respiratory, upper, due to
  Hemophilus influenzae 464.00
    with obstruction 464.01
  H. influenzae 464.00
    with obstruction 464.01
  hypertrophic 476.0
  influenzal (*see also* Influenza) 487.1
  pachydermic 478.79
  sicca 476.0
  spasmodic 478.75
    acute 464.00
      with obstruction 464.01
  streptococcal 034.0
  stridulous 478.75
  syphilitic 095.8
    congenital 090.5
  tuberculous (*see also* Tuberculosis, larynx) 012.3 ☑
  Vincent's 101
Laryngocele (congenital) (ventricular) 748.3
Laryngofissure 478.79
  congenital 748.3
Laryngomalacia (congenital) 748.3
Laryngopharyngitis (acute) 465.0
  chronic 478.9
    due to external agent — *see* Condition, respiratory, chronic, due to
  due to external agent — *see* Inflammation, respiratory, upper, due to
  septic 034.0

Laryngoplegia — *see also* Paralysis, vocal cord 478.30
Laryngoptosis 478.79
Laryngospasm 478.75
  due to external agent — *see* Condition, respiratory, acute, due to
Laryngostenosis 478.74
  congenital 748.3
Laryngotracheitis (acute) (infectional) (viral) — *see also* Laryngitis 464.20
  with obstruction 464.21
  atrophic 476.1
  Borrelia vincenti 101
  catarrhal 476.1
  chronic 476.1
    due to external agent — *see* Condition, respiratory, chronic, due to
  diphtheritic (membranous) 032.3
  due to external agent — *see* Inflammation, respiratory, upper, due to
  H. influenzae 464.20
    with obstruction 464.21
  hypertrophic 476.1
  influenzal (*see also* Influenza) 487.1
  pachydermic 478.75
  sicca 476.1
  spasmodic 478.75
    acute 464.20
      with obstruction 464.21
  streptococcal 034.0
  stridulous 478.75
  syphilitic 095.5
    congenital 090.5
  tuberculous (*see also* Tuberculosis, larynx) 012.3 ☑
  Vincent's 101
Laryngotracheobronchitis — *see also* Bronchitis 490
  acute 466.0
  chronic 491.8
  viral 466.0
Laryngotracheobronchopneumonitis — *see* Pneumonia, broncho-
Larynx, laryngeal — *see* condition
Lasègue's disease (persecution mania) 297.9
Lassa fever 078.89
Lassitude — *see also* Weakness 780.79
Late — *see also* condition
  effect(s) (of) (*see also* condition)
    abscess
      intracranial or intraspinal (conditions classifiable to 324) — *see* category 326
    adverse effect of drug, medicinal or biological substance 909.5
    allergic reaction 909.9
    amputation
      postoperative (late) 997.60
      traumatic (injury classifiable to 885–887 and 895–897) 905.9
    burn (injury classifiable to 948–949) 906.9
      extremities NEC (injury classifiable to 943 or 945) 906.7
      hand or wrist (injury classifiable to 944) 906.6
      eye (injury classifiable to 940) 906.5
      face, head, and neck (injury classifiable to 941) 906.5
      specified site NEC (injury classifiable to 942 and 946–947) 906.8
    cerebrovascular disease (conditions classifiable to 430–437) 438.9
      with
        alterations of sensations 438.6
        aphasia 438.11
        apraxia 438.81
        ataxia 438.84
        cognitive deficits 438.0
        disturbances of vision 438.7
        dysarthria 438.13
        dysphagia 438.82
        dysphasia 438.12
        facial droop 438.83
        facial weakness 438.83
        fluency disorder 438.14

Late — *see also* condition — *continued*
  effect(s) (*see also* condition) — *continued*
    cerebrovascular disease — *continued*
      with — *continued*
        hemiplegia/hemiparesis
          affecting
            dominant side 438.21
            nondominant side 438.22
            unspecified side 438.20
        monoplegia of lower limb
          affecting
            dominant side 438.41
            nondominant side 438.42
            unspecified side 438.40
        monoplegia of upper limb
          affecting
            dominant side 438.31
            nondominant side 438.32
            unspecified side 438.30
        paralytic syndrome NEC
          affecting
            bilateral 438.53
            dominant side 438.51
            nondominant side 438.52
            unspecified side 438.50
        speech and language deficit 438.10
          specified type NEC 438.19
        stuttering 438.14
        vertigo 438.85
        specified type NEC 438.89
    childbirth complication(s) 677
    complication(s) of
      childbirth 677
      delivery 677
      pregnancy 677
      puerperium 677
      surgical and medical care (conditions classifiable to 996–999) 909.3
      trauma (conditions classifiable to 958) 908.6
    contusion (injury classifiable to 920–924) 906.3
    crushing (injury classifiable to 925–929) 906.4
    delivery complication(s) 677
    dislocation (injury classifiable to 830–839) 905.6
    encephalitis or encephalomyelitis (conditions classifiable to 323) — *see* category 326
      in infectious diseases 139.8
      viral (conditions classifiable to 049.8, 049.9, 062–064) 139.0
    external cause NEC (conditions classifiable to 995) 909.9
      certain conditions classifiable to categories 991-994 909.4
    foreign body in orifice (injury classifiable to 930–939) 908.5
    fracture (multiple) (injury classifiable to 828–829) 905.5
      extremity
        lower (injury classifiable to 821–827) 905.4
          neck of femur (injury classifiable to 820) 905.3
        upper (injury classifiable to 810–819) 905.2
      face and skull (injury classifiable to 800–804) 905.0
      skull and face (injury classifiable to 800–804) 905.0
      spine and trunk (injury classifiable to 805 and 807–809) 905.1
        with spinal cord lesion (injury classifiable to 806) 907.2
    infection
      pyogenic, intracranial — *see* category 326
    infectious diseases (conditions classifiable to 001–136) NEC 139.8
    injury (injury classifiable to 959) 908.9

Late — *see also* condition — *continued*
  effect(s) (*see also* condition) — *continued*
    injury — *continued*
      blood vessel 908.3
        abdomen and pelvis (injury classifiable to 902) 908.4
        extremity (injury classifiable to 903–904) 908.3
        head and neck (injury classifiable to 900) 908.3
        intracranial (injury classifiable to 850–854) 907.0
          with skull fracture 905.0
        thorax (injury classifiable to 901) 908.4
      internal organ NEC (injury classifiable to 867 and 869) 908.2
        abdomen (injury classifiable to 863–866 and 868) 908.1
        thorax (injury classifiable to 860–862) 908.0
      intracranial (injury classifiable to 850–854) 907.0
        with skull fracture (injury classifiable to 800–801 and 803–804) 905.0
      nerve NEC (injury classifiable to 957) 907.9
        cranial (injury classifiable to 950–951) 907.1
        peripheral NEC (injury classifiable to 957) 907.9
        lower limb and pelvic girdle (injury classifiable to 956) 907.5
        upper limb and shoulder girdle (injury classifiable to 955) 907.4
        roots and plexus(es), spinal (injury classifiable to 953) 907.3
        trunk (injury classifiable to 954) 907.3
      spinal
        cord (injury classifiable to 806 and 952) 907.2
        nerve root(s) and plexus(es) (injury classifiable to 953) 907.3
      superficial (injury classifiable to 910–919) 906.2
      tendon (tendon injury classifiable to 840–848, 880–884 with .2, and 890–894 with .2) 905.8
    meningitis
      bacterial (conditions classifiable to 320) — *see* category 326
      unspecified cause (conditions classifiable to 322) — *see* category 326
    myelitis (*see also* Late, effect(s) (of), encephalitis) — *see* category 326
    parasitic diseases (conditions classifiable to 001–136 NEC) 139.8
    phlebitis or thrombophlebitis of intracranial venous sinuses (conditions classifiable to 325) — *see* category 326
    poisoning due to drug, medicinal or biological substance (conditions classifiable to 960–979) 909.0
    poliomyelitis, acute (conditions classifiable to 045) 138
    pregnancy complication(s) 677
    puerperal complication(s) 677
    radiation (conditions classifiable to 990) 909.2
    rickets 268.1
    sprain and strain without mention of tendon injury (injury classifiable to 840–848, except tendon injury) 905.7
      tendon involvement 905.8

☑ **Additional Digit Required** — Refer to the Tabular List for Digit Selection   ▽ **Subterms under main terms may continue to next column or page**

2014 ICD-9-CM   ▶◀ Revised Text   ● New Line   ▲ Revised Code   **Volume 2 — 173**

Large — Late

Late — *see also* condition — *continued*
effect(s) (*see also* condition) — *continued*
  toxic effect of
    drug, medicinal or biological substance (conditions classifiable to 960–979) 909.0
    nonmedical substance (conditions classifiable to 980–989) 909.1
    trachoma (conditions classifiable to 076) 139.1
    tuberculosis 137.0
      bones and joints (conditions classifiable to 015) 137.3
      central nervous system (conditions classifiable to 013) 137.1
      genitourinary (conditions classifiable to 016) 137.2
      pulmonary (conditions classifiable to 010–012) 137.0
      specified organs NEC (conditions classifiable to 014, 017–018) 137.4
      viral encephalitis (conditions classifiable to 049.8, 049.9, 062–064) 139.0
    wound, open
      extremity (injury classifiable to 880–884 and 890–894, except .2) 906.1
      tendon (injury classifiable to 880–884 with .2 and 890–894 with .2) 905.8
      head, neck, and trunk (injury classifiable to 870–879) 906.0
  infant
    post-term (gestation period over 40 completed weeks to 42 completed weeks) 766.21
    prolonged gestation (period over 42 completed weeks) 766.22
Latent — *see* condition
Lateral — *see* condition
Laterocession — *see* Lateroversion
Lateroflexion — *see* Lateroversion
Lateroversion
  cervix — *see* Lateroversion, uterus
  uterus, uterine (cervix) (postinfectional) (postpartal, old) 621.6
    congenital 752.39
    in pregnancy or childbirth 654.4 ☑
      affecting fetus or newborn 763.89
Lathyrism 988.2
Launois-Bensaude's lipomatosis 272.8
Launois-Cléret syndrome (adiposogenital dystrophy) 253.8
Launois' syndrome (pituitary gigantism) 253.0
Laurence-Moon-Biedl syndrome (obesity, polydactyly, and intellectual disabilities) 759.89
LAV (disease) (illness) (infection) — *see* Human immunodeficiency virus (disease) (illness) (infection)
LAV/HTLV-III (disease) (illness) (infection) — *see* Human immunodeficiency virus (disease) (illness) (infection)
Lawford's syndrome (encephalocutaneous angiomatosis) 759.6
Laxative habit — *see also* Abuse, drugs, nondependent 305.9 ☑
Lax, laxity — *see also* Relaxation
  ligament 728.4
  skin (acquired) 701.8
    congenital 756.83
Lazy leukocyte syndrome 288.09
LCAD (long chain/very long chain acyl CoA dehydrogenase deficiency, VLCAD) 277.85
LCHAD (long chain 3-hydroxyacyl CoA dehydrogenase deficiency) 277.85
Lead — *see also* condition
  exposure (suspected) to V15.86
  incrustation of cornea 371.15
  poisoning 984.9
    specified type of lead — *see* Table of Drugs and Chemicals
Lead miners' lung 503

Leakage
amniotic fluid 658.1 ☑
  with delayed delivery 658.2 ☑
  affecting fetus or newborn 761.1
bile from drainage tube (T tube) 997.49
blood (microscopic), fetal, into maternal circulation 656.0 ☑
  affecting management of pregnancy or puerperium 656.0 ☑
device, implant, or graft — *see* Complications, mechanical
spinal fluid at lumbar puncture site 997.09
urine, continuous 788.37
Leaky heart — *see* Endocarditis
Learning defect, specific NEC (strephosymbolia) 315.2
Leather bottle stomach (M8142/3) 151.9
Leber's
  congenital amaurosis 362.76
  optic atrophy (hereditary) 377.16
Lederer-Brill syndrome (acquired infectious hemolytic anemia) 283.19
Lederer's anemia or disease (acquired infectious hemolytic anemia) 283.19
Leeches (aquatic) (land) 134.2
Left-sided neglect 781.8
Leg — *see* condition
Legal investigation V62.5
Legg (-Calvé) -Perthes disease or syndrome (osteochondrosis, femoral capital) 732.1
Legionnaires' disease 482.84
Leigh's disease 330.8
Leiner's disease (exfoliative dermatitis) 695.89
Leiofibromyoma (M8890/0) — *see also* Leiomyoma
  uterus (cervix) (corpus) (*see also* Leiomyoma, uterus) 218.9
Leiomyoblastoma (M8891/1) — *see* Neoplasm, connective tissue, uncertain behavior
Leiomyofibroma (M8890/0) — *see also* Neoplasm, connective tissue, benign
  uterus (cervix) (corpus) (*see also* Leiomyoma, uterus) 218.9
Leiomyoma (M8890/0) — *see also* Neoplasm, connective tissue, benign
  bizarre (M8893/0) — *see* Neoplasm, connective tissue, benign
  cellular (M8892/1) — *see* Neoplasm, connective tissue, uncertain behavior
  epithelioid (M8891/1) — *see* Neoplasm, connective tissue, uncertain behavior
  prostate (polypoid) 600.20
    with
      other lower urinary tract symptoms (LUTS) 600.21
      urinary
        obstruction 600.21
        retention 600.21
  uterus (cervix) (corpus) 218.9
    interstitial 218.1
    intramural 218.1
    submucous 218.0
    subperitoneal 218.2
    subserous 218.2
  vascular (M8894/0) — *see* Neoplasm, connective tissue, benign
Leiomyomatosis (intravascular) (M8890/1) — *see* Neoplasm, connective tissue, uncertain behavior
Leiomyosarcoma (M8890/3) — *see also* Neoplasm, connective tissue, malignant
  epithelioid (M8891/3) — *see* Neoplasm, connective tissue, malignant
Leishmaniasis 085.9
  American 085.1
    cutaneous 085.4
    mucocutaneous 085.5
  Asian desert 085.2
  Brazilian 085.5
  cutaneous 085.9
    acute necrotizing 085.2
    American 085.4
    Asian desert 085.2
    diffuse 085.3
    dry form 085.1

Leishmaniasis — *continued*
  cutaneous — *continued*
    Ethiopian 085.3
    eyelid 085.5 [373.6]
    late 085.1
    lepromatous 085.3
    recurrent 085.1
    rural 085.2
    ulcerating 085.1
    urban 085.1
    wet form 085.2
    zoonotic form 085.2
  dermal (*see also* Leishmaniasis, cutaneous)
    post kala-azar 085.0
  eyelid 085.5 [373.6]
  infantile 085.0
  Mediterranean 085.0
  mucocutaneous (American) 085.5
  naso-oral 085.5
  nasopharyngeal 085.5
  Old World 085.1
  tegumentaria diffusa 085.4
  vaccination, prophylactic (against) V05.2
  visceral (Indian) 085.0
Leishmanoid, dermal — *see also* Leishmaniasis, cutaneous
  post kala-azar 085.0
Leloir's disease 695.4
Lemiere syndrome 451.89
Lenegre's disease 426.0
Lengthening, leg 736.81
Lennox-Gastaut syndrome 345.0 ☑
  with tonic seizures 345.1 ☑
Lennox's syndrome — *see also* Epilepsy 345.0 ☑
Lens — *see* condition
Lenticonus (anterior) (posterior) (congenital) 743.36
Lenticular degeneration, progressive 275.1
Lentiglobus (posterior) (congenital) 743.36
Lentigo (congenital) 709.09
  juvenile 709.09
  Maligna (M8742/2) (*see also* Neoplasm, skin, in situ)
    melanoma (M8742/3) — *see* Melanoma
  senile 709.09
Leonine leprosy 030.0
Leontiasis
  ossium 733.3
  syphilitic 095.8
    congenital 090.5
Léopold-Lévi's syndrome (paroxysmal thyroid instability) 242.9 ☑
Lepore hemoglobin syndrome 282.45
Lepothrix 039.0
Lepra 030.9
  Willan's 696.1
Leprechaunism 259.8
Lepromatous leprosy 030.0
Leprosy 030.9
  anesthetic 030.1
  beriberi 030.1
  borderline (group B) (infiltrated) (neuritic) 030.3
  cornea (*see also* Leprosy, by type) 030.9 [371.89]
  dimorphous (group B) (infiltrated) (lepromatous) (neuritic) (tuberculoid) 030.3
  eyelid 030.0 [373.4]
  indeterminate (group I) (macular) (neuritic) (uncharacteristic) 030.2
  leonine 030.0
  lepromatous (diffuse) (infiltrated) (macular) (neuritic) (nodular) (type L) 030.0
  macular (early) (neuritic) (simple) 030.2
  maculoanesthetic 030.1
  mixed 030.0
  neuro 030.1
  nodular 030.0
  primary neuritic 030.3
  specified type or group NEC 030.8
  tubercular 030.1
  tuberculoid (macular) (maculoanesthetic) (major) (minor) (neuritic) (type T) 030.1
Leptocytosis, hereditary 282.40

Leptomeningitis (chronic) (circumscribed) (hemorrhagic) (nonsuppurative) — *see also* Meningitis 322.9
aseptic 047.9
  adenovirus 049.1
  Coxsackie virus 047.0
  ECHO virus 047.1
  enterovirus 047.9
  lymphocytic choriomeningitis 049.0
epidemic 036.0
late effect — *see* category 326
meningococcal 036.0
pneumococcal 320.1
syphilitic 094.2
tuberculous (*see also* Tuberculosis, meninges) 013.0 ☑
Leptomeningopathy — *see also* Meningitis 322.9
Leptospiral — *see* condition
Leptospirochetal — *see* condition
Leptospirosis 100.9
  autumnalis 100.89
  canicula 100.89
  grippotyphosa 100.89
  hebdomidis 100.89
  icterohemorrhagica 100.0
  nanukayami 100.89
  pomona 100.89
  Weil's disease 100.0
Leptothricosis — *see* Actinomycosis
Leptothrix infestation — *see* Actinomycosis
Leptotricosis — *see* Actinomycosis
Leptus dermatitis 133.8
Léri-Weill syndrome 756.59
Leriche's syndrome (aortic bifurcation occlusion) 444.09
Léris pleonosteosis 756.89
Lermoyez's syndrome — *see also* Disease, Ménière's 386.00
Lesbianism — *omit code*
  ego-dystonic 302.0
  problems with 302.0
Lesch-Nyhan syndrome (hypoxanthineguanine-phosphoribosyltransferase deficiency) 277.2
Lesion(s)
  abducens nerve 378.54
  alveolar process 525.8
  anorectal 569.49
  aortic (valve) — *see* Endocarditis, aortic
  auditory nerve 388.5
  basal ganglion 333.90
  bile duct (*see also* Disease, biliary) 576.8
  bladder 596.9
  bone 733.90
  brachial plexus 353.0
  brain 348.89
    congenital 742.9
    vascular (*see also* Lesion, cerebrovascular) 437.9
      degenerative 437.1
      healed or old without residuals V12.54
      hypertensive 437.2
      late effect — *see* Late effect(s) (of) cerebrovascular disease
  buccal 528.9
  calcified — *see* Calcification
  canthus 373.9
  carate — *see* Pinta, lesions
  cardia 537.89
  cardiac — *see also* Disease, heart
    congenital 746.9
    valvular — *see* Endocarditis
  cauda equina 344.60
    with neurogenic bladder 344.61
  cecum 569.89
  cerebral — *see* Lesion, brain
  cerebrovascular (*see also* Disease, cerebrovascular NEC) 437.9
    degenerative 437.1
      healed or old without residuals V12.54
    hypertensive 437.2
    specified type NEC 437.8
  cervical root (nerve) NEC 353.2

☑ **Additional Digit Required** — Refer to the Tabular List for Digit Selection   ▽ **Subterms under main terms may continue to next column or page**

174 — Volume 2   ▶◀ Revised Text   ● New Line   ▲ Revised Code   2014 ICD-9-CM

Lesion(s) — *continued*
chiasmal 377.54
  associated with
    inflammatory disorders 377.54
    neoplasm NEC 377.52
      pituitary 377.51
    pituitary disorders 377.51
    vascular disorders 377.53
chorda tympani 351.8
coin, lung 793.11
colon 569.89
congenital — *see* Anomaly
conjunctiva 372.9
coronary artery (*see also* Ischemia, heart) 414.9
cranial nerve 352.9
  first 352.0
  second 377.49
  third
    partial 378.51
    total 378.52
  fourth 378.53
  fifth 350.9
  sixth 378.54
  seventh 351.9
  eighth 388.5
  ninth 352.2
  tenth 352.3
  eleventh 352.4
  twelfth 352.5
cystic — *see* Cyst
degenerative — *see* Degeneration
dermal (skin) 709.9
Dieulafoy (hemorrhagic)
  of
    duodenum 537.84
    intestine 569.86
    stomach 537.84
duodenum 537.89
  with obstruction 537.3
eyelid 373.9
gasserian ganglion 350.8
gastric 537.89
gastroduodenal 537.89
gastrointestinal 569.89
glossopharyngeal nerve 352.2
heart (organic) (*see also* Disease, heart)
  vascular — *see* Disease, cardiovascular
helix (ear) 709.9
high grade myelodysplastic syndrome 238.73
hyperchromic, due to pinta (carate) 103.1
hyperkeratotic (*see also* Hyperkeratosis) 701.1
hypoglossal nerve 352.5
hypopharynx 478.29
hypothalamic 253.9
ileocecal coil 569.89
ileum 569.89
iliohypogastric nerve 355.79
ilioinguinal nerve 355.79
in continuity — *see* Injury, nerve, by site
inflammatory — *see* Inflammation
intestine 569.89
intracerebral — *see* Lesion, brain
intrachiasmal (optic) (*see also* Lesion, chiasmal) 377.54
intracranial, space-occupying NEC 784.2
joint 719.90
  ankle 719.97
  elbow 719.92
  foot 719.97
  hand 719.94
  hip 719.95
  knee 719.96
  multiple sites 719.99
  pelvic region 719.95
  sacroiliac (old) 724.6
  shoulder (region) 719.91
  specified site NEC 719.98
  wrist 719.93
keratotic (*see also* Keratosis) 701.1
kidney (*see also* Disease, renal) 593.9
laryngeal nerve (recurrent) 352.3
leonine 030.0
lip 528.5

Lesion(s) — *continued*
liver 573.8
low grade myelodysplastic syndrome 238.72
lumbosacral
  plexus 353.1
  root (nerve) NEC 353.4
lung 518.89
  coin 793.11
maxillary sinus 473.0
mitral — *see* Endocarditis, mitral
Morel Lavallée — *see* Hematoma, by site
motor cortex 348.89
nerve (*see also* Disorder, nerve) 355.9
nervous system 349.9
  congenital 742.9
nonallopathic NEC 739.9
  in region (of)
    abdomen 739.9
    acromioclavicular 739.7
    cervical, cervicothoracic 739.1
    costochondral 739.8
    costovertebral 739.8
    extremity
      lower 739.6
      upper 739.7
    head 739.0
    hip 739.5
    lower extremity 739.6
    lumbar, lumbosacral 739.3
    occipitocervical 739.0
    pelvic 739.5
    pubic 739.5
    rib cage 739.8
    sacral, sacrococcygeal, sacroiliac 739.4
    sternochondral 739.8
    sternoclavicular 739.7
    thoracic, thoracolumbar 739.2
    upper extremity 739.7
nose (internal) 478.19
obstructive — *see* Obstruction
obturator nerve 355.79
occlusive
  artery — *see* Embolism, artery
organ or site NEC — *see* Disease, by site
osteolytic 733.90
paramacular, of retina 363.32
peptic 537.89
periodontal, due to traumatic occlusion 523.8
perirectal 569.49
peritoneum (granulomatous) 568.89
pigmented (skin) 709.00
pinta — *see* Pinta, lesions
polypoid — *see* Polyp
prechiasmal (optic) (*see also* Lesion, chiasmal) 377.54
primary (*see also* Syphilis, primary)
  carate 103.0
  pinta 103.0
  yaws 102.0
pulmonary 518.89
  valve (*see also* Endocarditis, pulmonary) 424.3
pylorus 537.89
radiation NEC 990
radium NEC 990
rectosigmoid 569.89
retina, retinal (*see also* Retinopathy)
  vascular 362.17
retroperitoneal 568.89
romanus 720.1
sacroiliac (joint) 724.6
salivary gland 527.8
  benign lymphoepithelial 527.8
saphenous nerve 355.79
secondary — *see* Syphilis, secondary
sigmoid 569.89
sinus (accessory) (nasal) (*see also* Sinusitis) 473.9
skin 709.9
  suppurative 686.00
SLAP (superior glenoid labrum) 840.7
space-occupying, intracranial NEC 784.2
spinal cord 336.9
  congenital 742.9

Lesion(s) — *continued*
spinal cord — *continued*
  traumatic (complete) (incomplete) (transverse) (*see also* Injury, spinal, by site)
    with
      broken
        back — *see* Fracture, vertebra, by site, with spinal cord injury
        neck — *see* Fracture, vertebra, cervical, with spinal cord injury
      fracture, vertebra — *see* Fracture, vertebra, by site, with spinal cord injury
spleen 289.50
stomach 537.89
superior glenoid labrum (SLAP) 840.7
syphilitic — *see* Syphilis
tertiary — *see* Syphilis, tertiary
thoracic root (nerve) 353.3
tonsillar fossa 474.9
tooth, teeth 525.8
  white spot 521.01
traumatic NEC (*see also* nature and site of injury) 959.9
tricuspid (valve) — *see* Endocarditis, tricuspid
trigeminal nerve 350.9
ulcerated or ulcerative — *see* Ulcer
uterus NEC 621.9
vagina 623.8
vagus nerve 352.3
valvular — *see* Endocarditis
vascular 459.9
  affecting central nervous system (*see also* Lesion, cerebrovascular) 437.9
  following trauma (*see also* Injury, blood vessel, by site) 904.9
  retina 362.17
  traumatic — *see* Injury, blood vessel, by site
  umbilical cord 663.6 ☑
    affecting fetus or newborn 762.6
visual
  cortex NEC (*see also* Disorder, visual, cortex) 377.73
  pathway NEC (*see also* Disorder, visual, pathway) 377.63
warty — *see* Verruca
white spot, on teeth 521.01
x-ray NEC 990
Lethargic — *see* condition
Lethargy 780.79
Letterer-Siwe disease (acute histiocytosis X) (M9722/3) 202.5 ☑
Leucinosis 270.3
Leucocoria 360.44
Leucosarcoma (M9850/3) 207.8 ☑
Leukasmus 270.2
Leukemia, leukemic (congenital) (M9800/3) 208.9 ☑

> *Note – Use the following fifth-digit subclassification for categories 203–208:*
> 0 *without mention of having achieved remission*
>   *failed remission*
> 1 *with remission*
> 2 *in relapse*

acute NEC (M9801/3) 208.0 ☑
aleukemic NEC (M9804/3) 208.8 ☑
  granulocytic (M9864/3) 205.8 ☑
basophilic (M9870/3) 205.1 ☑
blast (cell) (M9801/3) 208.0 ☑
blastic (M9801/3) 208.0 ☑
  granulocytic (M9861/3) 205.0 ☑
chronic NEC (M9803/3) 208.1 ☑
compound (M9810/3) 207.8 ☑
eosinophilic (M9880/3) 205.1 ☑
giant cell (M9910/3) 207.2 ☑
granulocytic (M9860/3) 205.9 ☑
  acute (M9861/3) 205.0 ☑

Leukemia, leukemic — *continued*
granulocytic — *continued*
  aleukemic (M9864/3) 205.8 ☑
  blastic (M9861/3) 205.0 ☑
  chronic (M9863/3) 205.1 ☑
  subacute (M9862/3) 205.2 ☑
  subleukemic (M9864/3) 205.8 ☑
hairy cell (M9940/3) 202.4 ☑
hemoblastic (M9801/3) 208.0 ☑
histiocytic (M9890/3) 206.9 ☑
lymphatic (M9820/3) 204.9 ☑
  acute (M9821/3) 204.0 ☑
  aleukemic (M9824/3) 204.8 ☑
  chronic (M9823/3) 204.1 ☑
  subacute (M9822/3) 204.2 ☑
  subleukemic (M9824/3) 204.8 ☑
lymphoblastic (M9821/3) 204.0 ☑
lymphocytic (M9820/3) 204.9 ☑
  acute (M9821/3) 204.0 ☑
  aleukemic (M9824/3) 204.8 ☑
  chronic (M9823/3) 204.1 ☑
  granular
    large T-cell 204.8 ☑
  subacute (M9822/3) 204.2 ☑
  subleukemic (M9824/3) 204.8 ☑
lymphogenous (M9820/3) — *see* Leukemia, lymphoid
lymphoid (M9820/3) 204.9 ☑
  acute (M9821/3) 204.0 ☑
  aleukemic (M9824/3) 204.8 ☑
  blastic (M9821/3) 204.0 ☑
  chronic (M9823/3) 204.1 ☑
  subacute (M9822/3) 204.2 ☑
  subleukemic (M9824/3) 204.8 ☑
lymphosarcoma cell (M9850/3) 207.8 ☑
mast cell (M9900/3) 207.8 ☑
megakaryocytic (M9910/3) 207.2 ☑
megakaryocytoid (M9910/3) 207.2 ☑
mixed (cell) (M9810/3) 207.8 ☑
monoblastic (M9891/3) 206.0 ☑
monocytic (Schilling-type) (M9890/3) 206.9 ☑
  acute (M9891/3) 206.0 ☑
  aleukemic (M9894/3) 206.8 ☑
  chronic (M9893/3) 206.1 ☑
  Naegeli-type (M9863/3) 205.1 ☑
  subacute (M9892/3) 206.2 ☑
  subleukemic (M9894/3) 206.8 ☑
monocytoid (M9890/3) 206.9 ☑
  acute (M9891/3) 206.0 ☑
  aleukemic (M9894/3) 206.8 ☑
  chronic (M9893/3) 206.1 ☑
  myelogenous (M9863/3) 205.1 ☑
  subacute (M9892/3) 206.2 ☑
  subleukemic (M9894/3) 206.8 ☑
monomyelocytic (M9860/3) — *see* Leukemia, myelomonocytic
myeloblastic (M9861/3) 205.0 ☑
myelocytic (M9863/3) 205.1 ☑
  acute (M9861/3) 205.0 ☑
myelogenous (M9860/3) 205.9 ☑
  acute (M9861/3) 205.0 ☑
  aleukemic (M9864/3) 205.8 ☑
  chronic (M9863/3) 205.1 ☑
  monocytoid (M9863/3) 205.1 ☑
  subacute (M9862/3) 205.2 ☑
  subleukemic (M9864) 205.8 ☑
myeloid (M9860/3) 205.9 ☑
  acute (M9861/3) 205.0 ☑
  aleukemic (M9864/3) 205.8 ☑
  chronic (M9863/3) 205.1 ☑
  subacute (M9862/3) 205.2 ☑
  subleukemic (M9864/3) 205.8 ☑
myelomonocytic (M9860/3) 205.9 ☑
  acute (M9861/3) 205.0 ☑
  chronic (M9863/3) 205.1 ☑
Naegeli-type monocytic (M9863/3) 205.1 ☑
neutrophilic (M9865/3) 205.1 ☑
plasma cell (M9830/3) 203.1 ☑
plasmacytic (M9830/3) 203.1 ☑
prolymphocytic (M9825/3) — *see* Leukemia, lymphoid
promyelocytic, acute (M9866/3) 205.0 ☑

☑ **Additional Digit Required** — Refer to the Tabular List for Digit Selection   ▽ **Subterms under main terms may continue to next column or page**

2014 ICD-9-CM   ▶◀ **Revised Text**   ● **New Line**   ▲ **Revised Code**   **Volume 2 — 175**

Lesion(s) — Leukemia, leukemic

Leukemia, leukemic — *continued*
  Schilling-type monocytic (M9890/3) — *see* Leukemia, monocytic
  stem cell (M9801/3) 208.0 ☑
  subacute NEC (M9802/3) 208.2 ☑
  subleukemic NEC (M9804/3) 208.8 ☑
  thrombocytic (M9910/3) 207.2 ☑
  undifferentiated (M9801/3) 208.0 ☑
Leukemoid reaction (basophilic) (lymphocytic) (monocytic) (myelocytic) (neutrophilic) 288.62
Leukoaraiosis (hypertensive) 437.1
Leukoariosis — *see* Leukoaraiosis
Leukoclastic vasculitis 446.29
Leukocoria 360.44
Leukocythemia — *see* Leukemia
Leukocytopenia 288.50
Leukocytosis 288.60
  basophilic 288.8
  eosinophilic 288.3
  lymphocytic 288.8
  monocytic 288.8
  neutrophilic 288.8
Leukoderma 709.09
  syphilitic 091.3
    late 095.8
Leukodermia — *see also* Leukoderma 709.09
Leukodystrophy (cerebral) (globoid cell) (metachromatic) (progressive) (sudanophilic) 330.0
Leukoedema, mouth or tongue 528.79
Leukoencephalitis
  acute hemorrhagic (postinfectious) NEC 136.9 [323.61]
    postimmunization or postvaccinal 323.51
  subacute sclerosing 046.2
    van Bogaert's 046.2
  van Bogaert's (sclerosing) 046.2
Leukoencephalopathy — *see also* Encephalitis 323.9
  acute necrotizing hemorrhagic (postinfectious) 136.9 [323.61]
    postimmunization or postvaccinal 323.51
  arteriosclerotic 437.0
  Binswanger's 290.12
  metachromatic 330.0
  multifocal (progressive) 046.3
  progressive multifocal 046.3
  reversible, posterior 348.5
Leukoerythroblastosis 289.9
Leukoerythrosis 289.0
Leukokeratosis — *see also* Leukoplakia 702.8
  mouth 528.6
  nicotina palati 528.79
  tongue 528.6
Leukokoria 360.44
Leukokraurosis vulva, vulvae 624.09
Leukolymphosarcoma (M9850/3) 207.8 ☑
Leukoma (cornea) (interfering with central vision) 371.03
  adherent 371.04
Leukomalacia, periventricular 779.7
Leukomelanopathy, hereditary 288.2
Leukonychia (punctata) (striata) 703.8
  congenital 757.5
Leukopathia
  unguium 703.8
    congenital 757.5
Leukopenia 288.50
  basophilic 288.59
  cyclic 288.02
  eosinophilic 288.59
  familial 288.59
  malignant (*see also* Agranulocytosis) 288.09
  periodic 288.02
  transitory neonatal 776.7
Leukopenic — *see* condition
Leukoplakia 702.8
  anus 569.49
  bladder (postinfectional) 596.89
  buccal 528.6
  cervix (uteri) 622.2
  esophagus 530.83
  gingiva 528.6

Leukoplakia — *continued*
  kidney (pelvis) 593.89
  larynx 478.79
  lip 528.6
  mouth 528.6
  oral soft tissue (including tongue) (mucosa) 528.6
  palate 528.6
  pelvis (kidney) 593.89
  penis (infectional) 607.0
  rectum 569.49
  syphilitic 095.8
  tongue 528.6
  tonsil 478.29
  ureter (postinfectional) 593.89
  urethra (postinfectional) 599.84
  uterus 621.8
  vagina 623.1
  vesical 596.89
  vocal cords 478.5
  vulva 624.09
Leukopolioencephalopathy 330.0
Leukorrhea (vagina) 623.5
  due to trichomonas (vaginalis) 131.00
  trichomonal (Trichomonas vaginalis) 131.00
Leukosarcoma (M9850/3) 207.8 ☑
Leukosis (M9800/3) — *see* Leukemia
Lev's disease or syndrome (acquired complete heart block) 426.0
Levi's syndrome (pituitary dwarfism) 253.3
Levocardia (isolated) 746.87
  with situs inversus 759.3
Levulosuria 271.2
Lewandowski-Lutz disease (epidermodysplasia verruciformis) 078.19
Lewandowski's disease (primary) — *see also* Tuberculosis 017.0 ☑
Lewy body dementia 331.82
Lewy body disease 331.82
Leyden-Möbius dystrophy 359.1
Leyden's disease (periodic vomiting) 536.2
Leydig-Sertoli cell tumor (M8631/0)
  specified site — *see* Neoplasm, by site, benign
  unspecified site
    female 220
    male 222.0
Leydig cell
  carcinoma (M8650/3)
    specified site — *see* Neoplasm, by site, malignant
    unspecified site
      female 183.0
      male 186.9
  tumor (M8650/1)
    benign (M8650/0)
      specified site — *see* Neoplasm, by site, benign
      unspecified site
        female 220
        male 222.0
    malignant (M8650/3)
      specified site — *see* Neoplasm, by site, malignant
      unspecified site
        female 183.0
        male 186.9
    specified site — *see* Neoplasm, by site, uncertain behavior
    unspecified site
      female 236.2
      male 236.4
LGSIL (low grade squamous intraepithelial lesion)
  anus 796.73
  cervix 795.03
  vagina 795.13
Li-Fraumeni cancer syndrome V84.01
Liar, pathologic 301.7
Libman-Sacks disease or syndrome 710.0 [424.91]
Lice (infestation) 132.9
  body (pediculus corporis) 132.1
  crab 132.2
  head (pediculus capitis) 132.0

Lice — *continued*
  mixed (classifiable to more than one of the categories 132.0–132.2) 132.3
  pubic (pediculus pubis) 132.2
Lichen 697.9
  albus 701.0
  annularis 695.89
  atrophicus 701.0
  corneus obtusus 698.3
  myxedematous 701.8
  nitidus 697.1
  pilaris 757.39
    acquired 701.1
  planopilaris 697.0
  planus (acute) (chronicus) (hypertrophic) (verrucous) 697.0
    morphoeicus 701.0
    sclerosus (et atrophicus) 701.0
  ruber 696.4
    acuminatus 696.4
    moniliformis 697.8
    obtusus corneus 698.3
    of Wilson 697.0
    planus 697.0
  sclerosus (et atrophicus) 701.0
  scrofulosus (primary) (*see also* Tuberculosis) 017.0 ☑
  simplex (Vidal's) 698.3
    chronicus 698.3
    circumscriptus 698.3
  spinulosus 757.39
    mycotic 117.9
  striata 697.8
  urticatus 698.2
Lichenification 698.3
  nodular 698.3
Lichenoides tuberculosis (primary) — *see also* Tuberculosis 017.0 ☑
Lichtheim's disease or syndrome (subacute combined sclerosis with pernicious anemia) 281.0 [336.2]
Lien migrans 289.59
Lientery — *see also* Diarrhea 787.91
  infectious 009.2
Life circumstance problem NEC V62.89
Ligament — *see* condition
Light-for-dates (infant) 764.0 ☑
  with signs of fetal malnutrition 764.1 ☑
  affecting management of pregnancy 656.5 ☑
Light-headedness 780.4
Lightning (effects) (shock) (stroke) (struck by) 994.0
  burn — *see* Burn, by site
  foot 266.2
Lightwood's disease or syndrome (renal tubular acidosis) 588.89
Lignac's disease (cystinosis) 270.0
Lignac (-de Toni) (-Fanconi) (-Debré) syndrome (cystinosis) 270.0
Lignac (-Fanconi) syndrome (cystinosis) 270.0
Ligneous thyroiditis 245.3
Likoff's syndrome (angina in menopausal women) 413.9
Limb — *see* condition
Limitation of joint motion — *see also* Stiffness, joint 719.5 ☑
  sacroiliac 724.6
Limit dextrinosis 271.0
Limited
  cardiac reserve — *see* Disease, heart
  duction, eye NEC 378.63
  mandibular range of motion 524.52
Lindau's disease (retinocerebral angiomatosis) 759.6
Lindau (-von Hippel) disease (angiomatosis retinocerebellosa) 759.6
Linea corneae senilis 371.41
Lines
  Beau's (transverse furrows on fingernails) 703.8
  Harris' 733.91
  Hudson-Stähli 371.11
  Stähli's 371.11
Lingua
  geographical 529.1

Lingua — *continued*
  nigra (villosa) 529.3
  plicata 529.5
    congenital 750.13
  tylosis 528.6
Lingual (tongue) — *see also* condition
  thyroid 759.2
Linitis (gastric) 535.4 ☑
  plastica (M8142/3) 151.9
Lioderma essentialis (cum melanosis et telangiectasia) 757.33
Lip — *see also* condition
  biting 528.9
Lipalgia 272.8
Lipedema — *see* Edema
Lipemia — *see also* Hyperlipidemia 272.4
  retina, retinalis 272.3
Lipidosis 272.7
  cephalin 272.7
  cerebral (infantile) (juvenile) (late) 330.1
  cerebroretinal 330.1 [362.71]
  cerebroside 272.7
  cerebrospinal 272.7
  chemically-induced 272.7
  cholesterol 272.7
  diabetic 250.8 ☑ [272.7]
    due to secondary diabetes 249.8 ☑ [272.7]
  dystopic (hereditary) 272.7
  glycolipid 272.7
  hepatosplenomegalic 272.3
  hereditary, dystopic 272.7
  sulfatide 330.0
Lipoadenoma (M8324/0) — *see* Neoplasm, by site, benign
Lipoblastoma (M8881/0) — *see* Lipoma, by site
Lipoblastomatosis (M8881/0) — *see* Lipoma, by site
Lipochondrodystrophy 277.5
Lipochrome histiocytosis (familial) 288.1
Lipodermatosclerosis 729.39
Lipodystrophia progressiva 272.6
Lipodystrophy (progressive) 272.6
  insulin 272.6
  intestinal 040.2
  mesenteric 567.82
Lipofibroma (M8851/0) — *see* Lipoma, by site
Lipoglycoproteinosis 272.8
Lipogranuloma, sclerosing 709.8
Lipogranulomatosis (disseminated) 272.8
  kidney 272.8
Lipoid — *see also* condition
  histiocytosis 272.7
    essential 272.7
  nephrosis (*see also* Nephrosis) 581.3
  proteinosis of Urbach 272.8
Lipoidemia — *see also* Hyperlipidemia 272.4
Lipoidosis — *see also* Lipidosis 272.7
Lipoma (M8850/0) 214.9
  breast (skin) 214.1
  face 214.0
  fetal (M8881/0) (*see also* Lipoma, by site)
    fat cell (M8880/0) — *see* Lipoma, by site
  infiltrating (M8856/0) — *see* Lipoma, by site
  intra-abdominal 214.3
  intramuscular (M8856/0) — *see* Lipoma, by site
  intrathoracic 214.2
  kidney 214.3
  mediastinum 214.2
  muscle 214.8
  peritoneum 214.3
  retroperitoneum 214.3
  skin 214.1
    face 214.0
  spermatic cord 214.4
  spindle cell (M8857/0) — *see* Lipoma, by site
  stomach 214.3
  subcutaneous tissue 214.1
    face 214.0
  thymus 214.2
  thyroid gland 214.2
Lipomatosis (dolorosa) 272.8
  epidural 214.8

☑ **Additional Digit Required** — Refer to the Tabular List for Digit Selection   ▽ **Subterms under main terms may continue to next column or page**

Lipomatosis — *continued*
  fetal (M8881/0) — *see* Lipoma, by site
  Launois-Bensaude's 272.8
Lipomyohemangioma (M8860/0)
  specified site — *see* Neoplasm, connective tissue, benign
  unspecified site 223.0
Lipomyoma (M8860/0)
  specified site — *see* Neoplasm, connective tissue, benign
  unspecified site 223.0
Lipomyxoma (M8852/0) — *see* Lipoma, by site
Lipomyxosarcoma (M8852/3) — *see* Neoplasm, connective tissue, malignant
Lipophagocytosis 289.89
Lipoproteinemia (alpha) 272.4
  broad-beta 272.2
  floating-beta 272.2
  hyper-pre-beta 272.1
Lipoproteinosis (Rössle-Urbach-Wiethe) 272.8
Liposarcoma (M8850/3) — *see also* Neoplasm, connective tissue, malignant
  differentiated type (M8851/3) — *see* Neoplasm, connective tissue, malignant
  embryonal (M8852/3) — *see* Neoplasm, connective tissue, malignant
  mixed type (M8855/3) — *see* Neoplasm, connective tissue, malignant
  myxoid (M8852/3) — *see* Neoplasm, connective tissue, malignant
  pleomorphic (M8854/3) — *see* Neoplasm, connective tissue, malignant
  round cell (M8853/3) — *see* Neoplasm, connective tissue, malignant
  well differentiated type (M8851/3) — *see* Neoplasm, connective tissue, malignant
Liposynovitis prepatellaris 272.8
Lipping
  cervix 622.0
  spine (*see also* Spondylosis) 721.90
  vertebra (*see also* Spondylosis) 721.90
Lip pits (mucus), congenital 750.25
Lipschütz disease or ulcer 616.50
Lipuria 791.1
  bilharziasis 120.0
Liquefaction, vitreous humor 379.21
Lisping 307.9
Lissauer's paralysis 094.1
Lissencephalia, lissencephaly 742.2
Listerellose 027.0
Listeriose 027.0
Listeriosis 027.0
  congenital 771.2
  fetal 771.2
  suspected fetal damage affecting management of pregnancy 655.4 ☑
Listlessness 780.79
Lithemia 790.6
Lithiasis — *see also* Calculus
  hepatic (duct) — *see* Choledocholithiasis
  urinary 592.9
Lithopedion 779.9
  affecting management of pregnancy 656.8 ☑
Lithosis (occupational) 502
  with tuberculosis — *see* Tuberculosis, pulmonary
Lithuria 791.9
Litigation V62.5
Little
  league elbow 718.82
  stroke syndrome 435.9
Little's disease — *see* Palsy, cerebral
Littre's
  gland — *see* condition
  hernia — *see* Hernia, Littre's
Littritis — *see also* Urethritis 597.89
Livedo 782.61
  annularis 782.61
  racemose 782.61
  reticularis 782.61
Live flesh 781.0
Liver — *see also* condition
  donor V59.6

Livida, asphyxia
  newborn 768.6
Living
  alone V60.3
    with handicapped person V60.4
Lloyd's syndrome 258.1
Loa loa 125.2
Loasis 125.2
Lobe, lobar — *see* condition
Lobo's disease or blastomycosis 116.2
Lobomycosis 116.2
Lobotomy syndrome 310.0
Lobstein's disease (brittle bones and blue sclera) 756.51
Lobster-claw hand 755.58
Lobulation (congenital) — *see also* Anomaly, specified type NEC, by site
  kidney, fetal 753.3
  liver, abnormal 751.69
  spleen 759.0
Lobule, lobular — *see* condition
Local, localized — *see* condition
Locked-in state 344.81
Locked bowel or intestine — *see also* Obstruction, intestine 560.9
Locked twins 660.5 ☑
  affecting fetus or newborn 763.1
Locking
  joint (*see also* Derangement, joint) 718.90
  knee 717.9
Lockjaw — *see also* Tetanus 037
Locomotor ataxia (progressive) 094.0
Löffler's
  endocarditis 421.0
  eosinophilia or syndrome 518.3
  pneumonia 518.3
  syndrome (eosinophilic pneumonitis) 518.3
Löfgren's syndrome (sarcoidosis) 135
Loiasis 125.2
  eyelid 125.2 [373.6]
Loneliness V62.89
Lone star fever 082.8
Long-term (current) (prophylactic) **drug use** V58.69
  anti-inflammatories, non-steroidal (NSAID) V58.64
  antibiotics V58.62
  anticoagulants V58.61
  antiplatelets/antithrombotics V58.63
  aspirin V58.66
  bisphosphonates V58.68
  high-risk medications NEC V58.69
  insulin V58.67
  methadone for pain control V58.69
  opiate analgesic V58.69
  pain killers V58.69
    anti-inflammatories, non-steroidal (NSAID) V58.64
    aspirin V58.66
  steroids V58.65
  tamoxifen V07.51
Longitudinal stripes or grooves, nails 703.8
  congenital 757.5
Long labor 662.1 ☑
  affecting fetus or newborn 763.89
  first stage 662.0 ☑
  second stage 662.2 ☑
Loop
  intestine (*see also* Volvulus) 560.2
  intrascleral nerve 379.29
  vascular on papilla (optic) 743.57
Loose — *see also* condition
  body
    in tendon sheath 727.82
    joint 718.10
      ankle 718.17
      elbow 718.12
      foot 718.17
      hand 718.14
      hip 718.15
      knee 717.6
      multiple sites 718.19
      pelvic region 718.15
      prosthetic implant — *see* Complications, mechanical
      shoulder (region) 718.11

Loose — *see also* condition — *continued*
  body — *continued*
    joint — *continued*
      specified site NEC 718.18
      wrist 718.13
    cartilage (joint) (*see also* Loose, body, joint) 718.1 ☑
      knee 717.6
    facet (vertebral) 724.9
    prosthetic implant — *see* Complications, mechanical
    sesamoid, joint (*see also* Loose, body, joint) 718.1 ☑
    tooth, teeth 525.8
Loosening epiphysis 732.9
Looser (-Debray)-Milkman syndrome (osteomalacia with pseudofractures) 268.2
Lop ear (deformity) 744.29
Lorain-Levi syndrome (pituitary dwarfism) 253.3
Lorain's disease or syndrome (pituitary dwarfism) 253.3
Lordosis (acquired) (postural) 737.20
  congenital 754.2
  due to or associated with
    Charcôt-Marie-Tooth disease 356.1 [737.42]
    mucopolysaccharidosis 277.5 [737.42]
    neurofibromatosis 237.71 [737.42]
    osteitis
      deformans 731.0 [737.42]
      fibrosa cystica 252.01 [737.42]
    osteoporosis (*see also* Osteoporosis) 733.00 [737.42]
    poliomyelitis (*see also* Poliomyelitis) 138 [737.42]
    tuberculosis (*see also* Tuberculosis) 015.0 ☑ [737.42]
  late effect of rickets 268.1 [737.42]
  postlaminectomy 737.21
  postsurgical NEC 737.22
  rachitic 268.1 [737.42]
  specified NEC 737.29
  tuberculous (*see also* Tuberculosis) 015.0 ☑ [737.42]
Loss
  appetite 783.0
    hysterical 300.11
    nonorganic origin 307.59
    psychogenic 307.59
  blood — *see* Hemorrhage
  central vision 368.41
  consciousness 780.09
    transient 780.2
  control, sphincter, rectum 787.60
    nonorganic origin 307.7
  ear ossicle, partial 385.24
  elasticity, skin 782.8
  extremity or member, traumatic, current — *see* Amputation, traumatic
  fluid (acute) 276.50
    with
      hypernatremia 276.0
      hyponatremia 276.1
    fetus or newborn 775.5
  hair 704.00
  hearing (*see also* Deafness)
    central 389.14
    conductive (air) 389.00
      with sensorineural hearing loss 389.20
        bilateral 389.22
        unilateral 389.21
      bilateral 389.06
      combined types 389.08
      external ear 389.01
      inner ear 389.04
      middle ear 389.03
      multiple types 389.08
      tympanic membrane 389.02
      unilateral 389.05
    mixed conductive and sensorineural 389.20
      bilateral 389.22
      unilateral 389.21
    mixed type 389.20

Loss — *continued*
  hearing (*see also* Deafness) — *continued*
    mixed type — *continued*
      bilateral 389.22
      unilateral 389.21
    nerve
      bilateral 389.12
      unilateral 389.13
    neural
      bilateral 389.12
      unilateral 389.13
    noise-induced 388.12
    perceptive NEC (*see also* Loss, hearing, sensorineural) 389.10
    sensorineural 389.10
      with conductive hearing loss 389.20
        bilateral 389.22
        unilateral 389.21
      asymmetrical 389.16
      bilateral 389.18
      central 389.14
      neural 389.12
        bilateral 389.12
        unilateral 389.13
      sensory
        bilateral 389.11
        unilateral 389.17
      unilateral 389.15
    sensory
      bilateral 389.11
      unilateral 389.17
    specified type NEC 389.8
    sudden NEC 388.2
  height 781.91
  labyrinthine reactivity (unilateral) 386.55
    bilateral 386.56
  memory (*see also* Amnesia) 780.93
    mild, following organic brain damage 310.89
  mind (*see also* Psychosis) 298.9
  occlusal vertical dimension 524.37
  organ or part — *see* Absence, by site, acquired
  recurrent pregnancy — *see* Pregnancy, management affected by, abortion, habitual
  sensation 782.0
  sense of
    smell (*see also* Disturbance, sensation) 781.1
    taste (*see also* Disturbance, sensation) 781.1
    touch (*see also* Disturbance, sensation) 781.1
  sight (acquired) (complete) (congenital) — *see* Blindness
  spinal fluid
    headache 349.0
  substance of
    bone (*see also* Osteoporosis) 733.00
    cartilage 733.99
      ear 380.32
      vitreous (humor) 379.26
  tooth, teeth
    acquired 525.10
      due to
        caries 525.13
        extraction 525.10
        periodontal disease 525.12
        specified NEC 525.19
        trauma 525.11
  vision, visual (*see also* Blindness) 369.9
    both eyes (*see also* Blindness, both eyes) 369.3
    complete (*see also* Blindness, both eyes) 369.00
    one eye 369.8
    sudden 368.11
    transient 368.12
  vitreous 379.26
  voice (*see also* Aphonia) 784.41
  weight (cause unknown) 783.21
Lou Gehrig's disease 335.20
Louis-Bar syndrome (ataxia-telangiectasia) 334.8
Louping ill 063.1

☑ **Additional Digit Required** — Refer to the Tabular List for Digit Selection   ⓣ **Subterms under main terms may continue to next column or page**

2014 ICD-9-CM   ▶◀ Revised Text   ● New Line   ▲ Revised Code   Volume 2 — 177

Lipomatosis — Louping ill

Lousiness — *see* Lice
Low
  back syndrome 724.2
  basal metabolic rate (BMR) 794.7
  birthweight 765.1 ☑
    extreme (less than 1000 grams) 765.0 ☑
    for gestational age 764.0 ☑
    status (*see also* Status, low birth weight)
      V21.30
  bladder compliance 596.52
  blood pressure (*see also* Hypotension) 458.9
    reading (incidental) (isolated) (nonspecific) 796.3
  cardiac reserve — *see* Disease, heart
  compliance bladder 596.52
  frequency deafness — *see* Disorder, hearing
  function (*see also* Hypofunction)
    kidney (*see also* Disease, renal) 593.9
    liver 573.9
  hemoglobin 285.9
  implantation, placenta — *see* Placenta, previa
  insertion, placenta — *see* Placenta, previa
  lying
    kidney 593.0
    organ or site, congenital — *see* Malposition, congenital
    placenta — *see* Placenta, previa
  output syndrome (cardiac) (*see also* Failure, heart) 428.9
  platelets (blood) (*see also* Thrombocytopenia) 287.5
  reserve, kidney (*see also* Disease, renal) 593.9
  risk
    human papillomavirus (HPA) DNA test positive
      anal 796.79
      cervical 795.09
      vaginal 795.19
  salt syndrome 593.9
  tension glaucoma 365.12
  vision 369.9
    both eyes 369.20
    one eye 369.70
Lower extremity — *see* condition
Lowe (-Terrey-MacLachlan) syndrome (oculocerebrorenal dystrophy) 270.8
Lown (-Ganong) -Levine syndrome (short P-R interval, normal QRS complex, and paroxysmal supraventricular tachycardia) 426.81
LSD reaction — *see also* Abuse, drugs, nondependent 305.3 ☑
Lucas-Championnière disease (fibrinous bronchitis) 466.0
Lucey-Driscoll syndrome (jaundice due to delayed conjugation) 774.30
Ludwig's
  angina 528.3
  disease (submaxillary cellulitis) 528.3
Lues (venerea), **luetic** — *see* Syphilis
Luetscher's syndrome (dehydration) 276.51
Lumbago 724.2
  due to displacement, intervertebral disc 722.10
Lumbalgia 724.2
  due to displacement, intervertebral disc 722.10
Lumbar — *see* condition
Lumbarization, vertebra 756.15
Lumbermen's itch 133.8
Lump — *see also* Mass
  abdominal 789.3 ☑
  breast 611.72
  chest 786.6
  epigastric 789.3 ☑
  head 784.2
  kidney 753.3
  liver 789.1
  lung 786.6
  mediastinal 786.6
  neck 784.2
  nose or sinus 784.2
  pelvic 789.3 ☑
  skin 782.2

Lump — *see also* Mass — *continued*
  substernal 786.6
  throat 784.2
  umbilicus 789.3 ☑
Lunacy — *see also* Psychosis 298.9
Lunatomalacia 732.3
Lung — *see also* condition
  donor V59.8
  drug addict's 417.8
  mainliners' 417.8
  vanishing 492.0
Lupoid (miliary) **of Boeck** 135
Lupus 710.0
  anticoagulant 795.79
    with
      hemorrhagic disorder 286.53
      hypercoagulable state 289.81
  Cazenave's (erythematosus) 695.4
  discoid (local) 695.4
  disseminated 710.0
  erythematodes (discoid) (local) 695.4
  erythematosus (discoid) (local) 695.4
    disseminated 710.0
    eyelid 373.34
    systemic 710.0
      with
        encephalitis 710.0 *[323.81]*
        lung involvement 710.0 *[517.8]*
      inhibitor (presence of) 795.79
        with hypercoagulable state 289.81
  exedens 017.0 ☑
  eyelid (*see also* Tuberculosis)
    017.0 *[373.4]*
  Hilliard's 017.0 ☑
  hydralazine
    correct substance properly administered 695.4
    overdose or wrong substance given or taken 972.6
  miliaris disseminatus faciei 017.0 ☑
  nephritis 710.0 *[583.81]*
    acute 710.0 *[580.81]*
    chronic 710.0 *[582.81]*
  nontuberculous, not disseminated 695.4
  pernio (Besnier) 135
  tuberculous (*see also* Tuberculosis) 017.0 ☑
    eyelid (*see also* Tuberculosis)
      017.0 *[373.4]*
  vulgaris 017.0 ☑
Luschka's joint disease 721.90
Luteinoma (M8610/0) 220
Lutembacher's disease or syndrome (atrial septal defect with mitral stenosis) 745.5
Luteoma (M8610/0) 220
Lutz-Miescher disease (elastosis perforans serpiginosa) 701.1
Lutz-Splendore-de Almeida disease (Brazilian blastomycosis) 116.1
Luxatio
  bulbi due to birth injury 767.8
  coxae congenita (*see also* Dislocation, hip, congenital) 754.30
  erecta — *see* Dislocation, shoulder
  imperfecta — *see* Sprain, by site
  perinealis — *see* Dislocation, hip
Luxation — *see also* Dislocation, by site
  eyeball 360.81
    due to birth injury 767.8
    lateral 376.36
  genital organs (external) NEC — *see* Wound, open, genital organs
  globe (eye) 360.81
    lateral 376.36
  lacrimal gland (postinfectional) 375.16
  lens (old) (partial) 379.32
    congenital 743.37
      syphilitic 090.49 *[379.32]*
    Marfan's disease 090.49
    spontaneous 379.32
  penis — *see* Wound, open, penis
  scrotum — *see* Wound, open, scrotum
  testis — *see* Wound, open, testis
Lycanthropy — *see also* Psychosis 298.9
Lyell's disease or syndrome (toxic epidermal necrolysis) 695.15

Lyell's disease or syndrome — *continued*
  due to drug
    correct substance properly administered 695.15
    overdose or wrong substance given or taken 977.9
    specified drug — *see* Table of Drugs and Chemicals
Lyme disease 088.81
Lymph-hemangioma (M9120/0) — *see* Hemangioma, by site
Lymph
  gland or node — *see* condition
  scrotum (*see also* Infestation, filarial) 125.9
Lymphadenitis 289.3
  with
    abortion — *see* Abortion, by type, with sepsis
    ectopic pregnancy (*see also* categories 633.0–633.9) 639.0
    molar pregnancy (*see also* categories 630–632) 639.0
  acute 683
    mesenteric 289.2
  any site, except mesenteric 289.3
    acute 683
    chronic 289.1
    mesenteric (acute) (chronic) (nonspecific) (subacute) 289.2
    subacute 289.1
      mesenteric 289.2
  breast, puerperal, postpartum 675.2 ☑
  chancroidal (congenital) 099.0
  chronic 289.1
    mesenteric 289.2
  dermatopathic 695.89
  due to
    anthracosis (occupational) 500
    Brugia (Wuchereria) malayi 125.1
    diphtheria (toxin) 032.89
    lymphogranuloma venereum 099.1
    Wuchereria bancrofti 125.0
  following
    abortion 639.0
    ectopic or molar pregnancy 639.0
  generalized 289.3
  gonorrheal 098.89
  granulomatous 289.1
  infectional 683
  mesenteric (acute) (chronic) (nonspecific) (subacute) 289.2
    due to Bacillus typhi 002.0
    tuberculous (*see also* Tuberculosis) 014.8 ☑
  mycobacterial 031.8
  purulent 683
  pyogenic 683
  regional 078.3
  septic 683
  streptococcal 683
  subacute, unspecified site 289.1
  suppurative 683
  syphilitic (early) (secondary) 091.4
    late 095.8
  tuberculous — *see* Tuberculosis, lymph gland
  venereal 099.1
Lymphadenoid goiter 245.2
Lymphadenopathy-associated virus (disease) (illness) (infection) — *see* Human immunodeficiency virus (disease) (illness) (infection)
Lymphadenopathy (general) 785.6
  due to toxoplasmosis (acquired) 130.7
    congenital (active) 771.2
Lymphadenosis 785.6
  acute 075
Lymphangiectasis 457.1
  conjunctiva 372.89
  postinfectional 457.1
  scrotum 457.1
Lymphangiectatic elephantiasis, nonfilarial 457.1
Lymphangioendothelioma (M9170/0) 228.1
  malignant (M9170/3) — *see* Neoplasm, connective tissue, malignant

Lymphangioleiomyomatosis 516.4
Lymphangioma (M9170/0) 228.1
  capillary (M9171/0) 228.1
  cavernous (M9172/0) 228.1
  cystic (M9173/0) 228.1
  malignant (M9170/3) — *see* Neoplasm, connective tissue, malignant
Lymphangiomyoma (M9174/0) 228.1
Lymphangiomyomatosis 516.4
Lymphangiosarcoma (M9170/3) — *see* Neoplasm, connective tissue, malignant
Lymphangitis 457.2
  with
    abortion — *see* Abortion, by type, with sepsis
    abscess — *see* Abscess, by site
    cellulitis — *see* Abscess, by site
    ectopic pregnancy (*see also* categories 633.0–633.9) 639.0
    molar pregnancy (*see also* categories 630–632) 639.0
  acute (with abscess or cellulitis) 682.9
    specified site — *see* Abscess, by site
  breast, puerperal, postpartum 675.2 ☑
  chancroidal 099.0
  chronic (any site) 457.2
  due to
    Brugia (Wuchereria) malayi 125.1
    Wuchereria bancrofti 125.0
  following
    abortion 639.0
    ectopic or molar pregnancy 639.0
  gangrenous 457.2
  penis
    acute 607.2
    gonococcal (acute) 098.0
      chronic or duration of 2 months or more 098.2
  puerperal, postpartum, childbirth 670.8 ☑
  strumous, tuberculous (*see also* Tuberculosis) 017.2 ☑
  subacute (any site) 457.2
  tuberculous — *see* Tuberculosis, lymph gland
Lymphatic (vessel) — *see* condition
Lymphatism 254.8
  scrofulous (*see also* Tuberculosis) 017.2 ☑
Lymphectasia 457.1
Lymphedema — *see also* Elephantiasis 457.1
  acquired (chronic) 457.1
  chronic hereditary 757.0
  congenital 757.0
  idiopathic hereditary 757.0
  praecox 457.1
  secondary 457.1
  surgical NEC 997.99
    postmastectomy (syndrome) 457.0
Lymphoblastic — *see* condition
Lymphoblastoma (diffuse) (M9630/3) 200.1 ☑
  giant follicular (M9690/3) 202.0 ☑
  macrofollicular (M9690/3) 202.0 ☑
Lymphoblastosis, acute benign 075
Lymphocele 457.8
Lymphocythemia 288.51
Lymphocytic — *see also* condition
  chorioencephalitis (acute) (serous) 049.0
  choriomeningitis (acute) (serous) 049.0
Lymphocytoma (diffuse) (malignant) (M9620/3) 200.1 ☑
Lymphocytomatosis (M9620/3) 200.1 ☑
Lymphocytopenia 288.51
Lymphocytosis (symptomatic) 288.61
  infectious (acute) 078.89
Lymphoepithelioma (M8082/3) — *see* Neoplasm, by site, malignant
Lymphogranuloma (malignant) (M9650/3) 201.9 ☑
  inguinale 099.1
  venereal (any site) 099.1
    with stricture of rectum 099.1
  venereum 099.1
Lymphogranulomatosis (malignant) (M9650/3) 201.9 ☑
  benign (Boeck's sarcoid) (Schaumann's) 135
  Hodgkin's (M9650/3) 201.9 ☑

☑ **Additional Digit Required — Refer to the Tabular List for Digit Selection**

▽ **Subterms under main terms may continue to next column or page**

Lymphohistiocytosis, familial hemophagocytic 288.4
Lymphoid — *see* condition
Lympholeukoblastoma (M9850/3) 207.8 ☑
Lympholeukosarcoma (M9850/3) 207.8 ☑
Lymphoma (malignant) (M9590/3) 202.8 ☑

> *Note — Use the following fifth-digit subclassification with categories 200–202:*
>
> 0   *unspecified site, extranodal and solid organ sites*
>
> 1   *lymph nodes of head, face, and neck*
>
> 2   *intrathoracic lymph nodes*
>
> 3   *intra–abdominal lymph nodes*
>
> 4   *lymph nodes of axilla and upper limb*
>
> 5   *lymph nodes of inguinal region and lower limb*
>
> 6   *intrapelvic lymph nodes*
>
> 7   *spleen*
>
> 8   *lymph nodes of multiple sites*

  benign (M9590/0) — *see* Neoplasm, by site, benign
  Burkitt's type (lymphoblastic) (undifferentiated) (M9750/3) 200.2 ☑
  Castleman's (mediastinal lymph node hyperplasia) 785.6
  centroblastic-centrocytic
    diffuse (M9614/3) 202.8 ☑
    follicular (M9692/3) 202.0 ☑
  centroblastic type (diffuse) (M9632/3) 202.8 ☑
    follicular (M9697/3) 202.0 ☑
  centrocytic (M9622/3) 202.8 ☑
  compound (M9613/3) 200.8 ☑
  convoluted cell type (lymphoblastic) (M9602/3) 202.8 ☑
  diffuse NEC (M9590/3) 202.8 ☑
  large B cell 202.8 ☑
  follicular (giant) (M9690/3) 202.0 ☑
    center cell (diffuse) (M9615/3) 202.8 ☑
    cleaved (diffuse) (M9623/3) 202.8 ☑
      follicular (M9695/3) 202.0 ☑
      non-cleaved (diffuse) (M9633/3) 202.8 ☑
        follicular (M9698/3) 202.0 ☑
    centroblastic-centrocytic (M9692/3) 202.0 ☑
    centroblastic type (M9697/3) 202.0 ☑
    large cell (M9698/3) 202.0 ☑
    lymphocytic
      intermediate differentiation (M9694/3) 202.0 ☑
      poorly differentiated (M9696/3) 202.0 ☑
    mixed (cell type) (lymphocytic-histiocytic) (small cell and large cell) (M9691/3) 202.0 ☑
  germinocytic (M9622/3) 202.8 ☑
  giant, follicular or follicle (M9690/3) 202.0 ☑
  histiocytic (diffuse) (M9640/3) 200.0 ☑
    nodular (M9642/3) 200.0 ☑
    pleomorphic cell type (M9641/3) 200.0 ☑
  Hodgkin's (M9650/3) (*see also* Disease, Hodgkin's) 201.9 ☑
  immunoblastic (type) (M9612/3) 200.8 ☑
  large cell (M9640/3) 200.7 ☑
    anaplastic 200.6 ☑
    nodular (M9642/3) 202.0 ☑
    pleomorphic cell type (M9641/3) 200.0 ☑
  lymphoblastic (diffuse) (M9630/3) 200.1 ☑
    Burkitt's type (M9750/3) 200.2 ☑
    convoluted cell type (M9602/3) 202.8 ☑
  lymphocytic-histiocytic, mixed (diffuse) (M9613/3) 200.8 ☑
    follicular (M9691/3) 202.0 ☑

Lymphoma — *continued*
  lymphocytic-histiocytic, mixed — *continued*
    nodular (M9691/3) 202.0 ☑
  lymphocytic (cell type) (diffuse) (M9620/3) 200.1 ☑
    with plasmacytoid differentiation, diffuse (M9611/3) 200.8 ☑
    intermediate differentiation (diffuse) (M9621/3) 200.1 ☑
      follicular (M9694/3) 202.0 ☑
      nodular (M9694/3) 202.0 ☑
    nodular (M9690/3) 202.0 ☑
    poorly differentiated (diffuse) (M9630/3) 200.1 ☑
      follicular (M9696/3) 202.0 ☑
      nodular (M9696/3) 202.0 ☑
    well differentiated (diffuse) (M9620/3) 200.1 ☑
      follicular (M9693/3) 202.0 ☑
      nodular (M9693/3) 202.0 ☑
  lymphoplasmacytoid type (M9611/3) 200.8 ☑
  lymphosarcoma type (M9610/3) 200.1 ☑
  macrofollicular (M9690/3) 202.0 ☑
  mantle cell 200.4 ☑
  marginal zone 200.3 ☑
    extranodal B-cell 200.3 ☑
    nodal B-cell 200.3 ☑
    splenic B-cell 200.3 ☑
  mixed cell type (diffuse) (M9613/3) 200.8 ☑
    follicular (M9691/3) 202.0 ☑
    nodular (M9691/3) 202.0 ☑
  nodular (M9690/3) 202.0 ☑
    histiocytic (M9642/3) 200.0 ☑
    lymphocytic (M9690/3) 202.0 ☑
      intermediate differentiation (M9694/3) 202.0 ☑
      poorly differentiated (M9696/3) 202.0 ☑
    mixed (cell type) (lymphocytic-histiocytic) (small cell and large cell) (M9691/3) 202.0 ☑
  non-Hodgkin's type NEC (M9591/3) 202.8 ☑
  peripheral T-cell 202.7 ☑
  primary central nervous system 200.5 ☑
  reticulum cell (type) (M9640/3) 200.0 ☑
  small cell and large cell, mixed (diffuse) (M9613/3) 200.8 ☑
    follicular (M9691/3) 202.0 ☑
    nodular (M9691/3) 202.0 ☑
  stem cell (type) (M9601/3) 202.8 ☑
  T-cell 202.1 ☑
    peripheral 202.7 ☑
  undifferentiated (cell type) (non-Burkitt's) (M9600/3) 202.8 ☑
    Burkitt's type (M9750/3) 200.2 ☑
Lymphomatosis (M9590/3) — *see also* Lymphoma
  granulomatous 099.1
Lymphopathia
  venereum 099.1
  veneris 099.1
Lymphopenia 288.51
  familial 279.2
Lymphoreticulosis, benign (of inoculation) 078.3
Lymphorrhea 457.8
Lymphosarcoma (M9610/3) 200.1 ☑
  diffuse (M9610/3) 200.1 ☑
    with plasmacytoid differentiation (M9611/3) 200.8 ☑
    lymphoplasmacytic (M9611/3) 200.8 ☑
  follicular (giant) (M9690/3) 202.0 ☑
    lymphoblastic (M9696/3) 202.0 ☑
    lymphocytic, intermediate differentiation (M9694/3) 202.0 ☑
    mixed cell type (M9691/3) 202.0 ☑
  giant follicular (M9690/3) 202.0 ☑
  Hodgkin's (M9650/3) 201.9 ☑
  immunoblastic (M9612/3) 200.8 ☑
  lymphoblastic (diffuse) (M9630/3) 200.1 ☑
    follicular (M9696/3) 202.0 ☑
    nodular (M9696/3) 202.0 ☑

Lymphosarcoma — *continued*
  lymphocytic (diffuse) (M9620/3) 200.1 ☑
    intermediate differentiation (diffuse) (M9621/3) 200.1 ☑
      follicular (M9694/3) 202.0 ☑
      nodular (M9694/3) 202.0 ☑
  mixed cell type (diffuse) (M9613/3) 200.8 ☑
    follicular (M9691/3) 202.0 ☑
    nodular (M9691/3) 202.0 ☑
  nodular (M9690/3) 202.0 ☑
    lymphoblastic (M9696/3) 202.0 ☑
    lymphocytic, intermediate differentiation (M9694/3) 202.0 ☑
    mixed cell type (M9691/3) 202.0 ☑
  prolymphocytic (M9631/3) 200.1 ☑
  reticulum cell (M9640/3) 200.0 ☑
Lymphostasis 457.8
Lypemania — *see also* Melancholia 296.2 ☑
Lyssa 071

M

Macacus ear 744.29
Maceration
  fetus (cause not stated) 779.9
  wet feet, tropical (syndrome) 991.4
Machado-Joseph disease 334.8
Machupo virus hemorrhagic fever 078.7
Macleod's syndrome (abnormal transradiancy, one lung) 492.8
Macrocephalia, macrocephaly 756.0
Macrocheilia (congenital) 744.81
Macrochilia (congenital) 744.81
Macrocolon (congenital) 751.3
Macrocornea 743.41
  associated with buphthalmos 743.22
Macrocyte — *see* condition
Macrocytosis 289.89
Macrodactylia, macrodactylism (fingers) (thumbs) 755.57
  toes 755.65
Macrodontia 520.2
Macroencephaly 742.4
Macrogenia 524.05
Macrogenitosomia (female) (male) (praecox) 255.2
Macrogingivae 523.8
Macroglobulinemia (essential) (idiopathic) (monoclonal) (primary) (syndrome) (Waldenström's) 273.3
Macroglossia (congenital) 750.15
  acquired 529.8
Macrognathia, macrognathism (congenital) 524.00
  mandibular 524.02
    alveolar 524.72
  maxillary 524.01
    alveolar 524.71
Macrogyria (congenital) 742.4
Macrohydrocephalus — *see also* Hydrocephalus 331.4
Macromastia — *see also* Hypertrophy, breast 611.1
Macrophage activation syndrome 288.4
Macropsia 368.14
Macrosigmoid 564.7
  congenital 751.3
Macrospondylitis, acromegalic 253.0
Macrostomia (congenital) 744.83
Macrotia (external ear) (congenital) 744.22
Macula
  cornea, corneal
    congenital 743.43
      interfering with vision 743.42
    interfering with central vision 371.03
    not interfering with central vision 371.02
  degeneration (*see also* Degeneration, macula) 362.50
    hereditary (*see also* Dystrophy, retina) 362.70
  edema, cystoid 362.53
Maculae ceruleae 132.1
Macules and papules 709.8
Maculopathy, toxic 362.55
Madarosis 374.55

Madelung's
  deformity (radius) 755.54
  disease (lipomatosis) 272.8
  lipomatosis 272.8
Madness — *see also* Psychosis 298.9
  myxedema (acute) 293.0
    subacute 293.1
Madura
  disease (actinomycotic) 039.9
    mycotic 117.4
  foot (actinomycotic) 039.4
    mycotic 117.4
Maduromycosis (actinomycotic) 039.9
  mycotic 117.4
Maffucci's syndrome (dyschondroplasia with hemangiomas) 756.4
Magenblase syndrome 306.4
Main en griffe (acquired) 736.06
  congenital 755.59
Maintenance
  chemotherapy regimen or treatment V58.11
  dialysis regimen or treatment
    extracorporeal (renal) V56.0
    peritoneal V56.8
    renal V56.0
  drug therapy or regimen
    chemotherapy, antineoplastic V58.11
    immunotherapy, antineoplastic V58.12
  external fixation NEC V54.89
  methadone 304.00
  radiotherapy V58.0
  traction NEC V54.89
Majocchi's
  disease (purpura annularis telangiectodes) 709.1
  granuloma 110.6
Major — *see* condition
Mal
  cerebral (idiopathic) (*see also* Epilepsy) 345.9 ☑
  comital (*see also* Epilepsy) 345.9 ☑
  de los pintos (*see also* Pinta) 103.9
  de Meleda 757.39
  de mer 994.6
  lie — *see* Presentation, fetal
  perforant (*see also* Ulcer, lower extremity) 707.15
Malabar itch 110.9
  beard 110.0
  foot 110.4
  scalp 110.0
Malabsorption 579.9
  calcium 579.8
  carbohydrate 579.8
  disaccharide 271.3
  drug-induced 579.8
  due to bacterial overgrowth 579.8
  fat 579.8
  folate, congenital 281.2
  galactose 271.1
  glucose-galactose (congenital) 271.3
  intestinal 579.9
  isomaltose 271.3
  lactose (hereditary) 271.3
  methionine 270.4
  monosaccharide 271.8
  postgastrectomy 579.3
  postsurgical 579.3
  protein 579.8
  sucrose (-isomaltose) (congenital) 271.3
  syndrome 579.9
    postgastrectomy 579.3
    postsurgical 579.3
Malacia, bone 268.2
  juvenile (*see also* Rickets) 268.0
  Kienböck's (juvenile) (lunate) (wrist) 732.3
  adult 732.8
Malacoplakia
  bladder 596.89
  colon 569.89
  pelvis (kidney) 593.89
  ureter 593.89
  urethra 599.84
Malacosteon 268.2
  juvenile (*see also* Rickets) 268.0
Maladaptation — *see* Maladjustment

☑ Additional Digit Required — Refer to the Tabular List for Digit Selection   ▽ Subterms under main terms may continue to next column or page

2014 ICD-9-CM   ►◄ Revised Text   ● New Line   ▲ Revised Code   Volume 2 — 179

Maladie de Roger 745.4
Maladjustment
conjugal V61.10
  involving
    divorce V61.03
    estrangement V61.09
educational V62.3
family V61.9
  specified circumstance NEC V61.8
marital V61.10
  involving
    divorce V61.03
    estrangement V61.09
occupational V62.29
  current military deployment status V62.21
simple, adult (*see also* Reaction, adjustment) 309.9
situational acute (*see also* Reaction, adjustment) 309.9
social V62.4
Malaise 780.79
Malakoplakia — *see* Malacoplakia
Malaria, malarial (fever) 084.6
algid 084.9
any type, with
  algid malaria 084.9
  blackwater fever 084.8
  fever
    blackwater 084.8
    hemoglobinuric (bilious) 084.8
  hemoglobinuria, malarial 084.8
  hepatitis 084.9 *[573.2]*
  nephrosis 084.9 *[581.81]*
  pernicious complication NEC 084.9
    cardiac 084.9
    cerebral 084.9
cardiac 084.9
carrier (suspected) of V02.9
cerebral 084.9
complicating pregnancy, childbirth, or puerperium 647.4 ☑
congenital 771.2
congestion, congestive 084.6
  brain 084.9
continued 084.0
estivo-autumnal 084.0
falciparum (malignant tertian) 084.0
hematinuria 084.8
hematuria 084.8
hemoglobinuria 084.8
hemorrhagic 084.6
induced (therapeutically) 084.7
  accidental — *see* Malaria, by type
liver 084.9 *[573.2]*
malariae (quartan) 084.2
malignant (tertian) 084.0
mixed infections 084.5
monkey 084.4
ovale 084.3
pernicious, acute 084.0
Plasmodium, P.
  falciparum 084.0
  malariae 084.2
  ovale 084.3
  vivax 084.1
quartan 084.2
quotidian 084.0
recurrent 084.6
  induced (therapeutically) 084.7
    accidental — *see* Malaria, by type
remittent 084.6
specified types NEC 084.4
spleen 084.6
subtertian 084.0
tertian (benign) 084.1
  malignant 084.0
tropical 084.0
typhoid 084.6
vivax (benign tertian) 084.1
Malassez's disease (testicular cyst) 608.89
Malassimilation 579.9
Maldescent, testis 752.51
Maldevelopment — *see also* Anomaly, by site
brain 742.9
colon 751.5

Maldevelopment — *see also* Anomaly, by site — *continued*
hip (joint) 755.63
  congenital dislocation (*see also* Dislocation, hip, congenital) 754.30
mastoid process 756.0
middle ear, except ossicles 744.03
  ossicles 744.04
newborn (not malformation) 764.9 ☑
ossicles, ear 744.04
spine 756.10
toe 755.66
Male type pelvis 755.69
with disproportion (fetopelvic) 653.2 ☑
  affecting fetus or newborn 763.1
  causing obstructed labor 660.1 ☑
    affecting fetus or newborn 763.1
Malformation (congenital) — *see also* Anomaly
arteriovenous
  pulmonary 747.32
bone 756.9
bursa 756.9
Chiari
  type I 348.4
  type II (*see also* Spina bifida) 741.0 ☑
  type III 742.0
  type IV 742.2
circulatory system NEC 747.9
  specified type NEC 747.89
cochlea 744.05
digestive system NEC 751.9
  lower 751.5
  specified type NEC 751.8
  upper 750.9
eye 743.9
gum 750.9
heart NEC 746.9
  specified type NEC 746.89
  valve 746.9
internal ear 744.05
joint NEC 755.9
  specified type NEC 755.8
Mondini's (congenital) (malformation, cochlea) 744.05
muscle 756.9
nervous system (central) 742.9
pelvic organs or tissues
  in pregnancy or childbirth 654.9 ☑
    affecting fetus or newborn 763.89
    causing obstructed labor 660.2 ☑
      affecting fetus or newborn 763.1
placenta (*see also* Placenta, abnormal) 656.7 ☑
respiratory organs 748.9
  specified type NEC 748.8
Rieger's 743.44
sense organs NEC 742.9
  specified type NEC 742.8
skin 757.9
  specified type NEC 757.8
spinal cord 742.9
teeth, tooth NEC 520.9
tendon 756.9
throat 750.9
umbilical cord (complicating delivery) 663.9 ☑
  affecting fetus or newborn 762.6
umbilicus 759.9
urinary system NEC 753.9
  specified type NEC 753.8
venous — *see* Anomaly, vein
Malfunction — *see also* Dysfunction
arterial graft 996.1
cardiac pacemaker 996.01
catheter device — *see* Complications, mechanical, catheter
colostomy 569.62
  valve 569.62
cystostomy 596.82
  infection 596.81
  mechanical 596.82
  specified complication NEC 596.83
device, implant, or graft NEC — *see* Complications, mechanical
enteric stoma 569.62

Malfunction — *see also* Dysfunction — *continued*
enterostomy 569.62
esophagostomy 530.87
gastroenteric 536.8
gastrostomy 536.42
ileostomy
  valve 569.62
nephrostomy 997.5
pacemaker — *see* Complications, mechanical, pacemaker
prosthetic device, internal — *see* Complications, mechanical
tracheostomy 519.02
valve
  colostomy 569.62
  ileostomy 569.62
vascular graft or shunt 996.1
Malgaigne's fracture (closed) 808.43
open 808.53
Malherbe's
calcifying epithelioma (M8110/0) — *see* Neoplasm, skin, benign
tumor (M8110/0) — *see* Neoplasm, skin, benign
Malibu disease 919.8
infected 919.9
Malignancy (M8000/3) — *see* Neoplasm, by site, malignant
Malignant — *see* condition
Malingerer, malingering V65.2
Mallet, finger (acquired) 736.1
congenital 755.59
late effect of rickets 268.1
Malleus 024
Mallory-Weiss syndrome 530.7
Mallory's bodies 034.1
Malnutrition (calorie) 263.9
complicating pregnancy 648.9 ☑
degree
  first 263.1
  second 263.0
  third 262
  mild (protein) 263.1
  moderate (protein) 263.0
  severe 261
    protein-calorie 262
fetus 764.2 ☑
  "light-for-dates" 764.1 ☑
following gastrointestinal surgery 579.3
intrauterine or fetal 764.2 ☑
  fetus or infant "light-for-dates" 764.1 ☑
lack of care, or neglect (child) (infant) 995.52
  adult 995.84
malignant 260
mild (protein) 263.1
moderate (protein) 263.0
protein-calorie 263.9
  mild 263.1
  moderate 263.0
  severe 262
  specified type NEC 263.8
protein 260
severe 261
  protein-calorie NEC 262
Malocclusion (teeth) 524.4
angle's class I 524.21
angle's class II 524.22
angle's class III 524.23
due to
  abnormal swallowing 524.59
  accessory teeth (causing crowding) 524.31
  dentofacial abnormality NEC 524.89
  impacted teeth (causing crowding) 520.6
  missing teeth 524.30
  mouth breathing 524.59
  sleep postures 524.59
  supernumerary teeth (causing crowding) 524.31
  thumb sucking 524.59
  tongue, lip, or finger habits 524.59
  temporomandibular (joint) 524.69
Malposition
cardiac apex (congenital) 746.87
cervix — *see* Malposition, uterus

Malposition — *continued*
congenital
  adrenal (gland) 759.1
  alimentary tract 751.8
    lower 751.5
    upper 750.8
  aorta 747.21
  appendix 751.5
  arterial trunk 747.29
  artery (peripheral) NEC (*see also* Malposition, congenital, peripheral vascular system) 747.60
    coronary 746.85
    pulmonary 747.39
  auditory canal 744.29
    causing impairment of hearing 744.02
  auricle (ear) 744.29
    causing impairment of hearing 744.02
  cervical 744.43
  biliary duct or passage 751.69
  bladder (mucosa) 753.8
    exteriorized or extroverted 753.5
  brachial plexus 742.8
  brain tissue 742.4
  breast 757.6
  bronchus 748.3
  cardiac apex 746.87
  cecum 751.5
  clavicle 755.51
  colon 751.5
  digestive organ or tract NEC 751.8
    lower 751.5
    upper 750.8
  ear (auricle) (external) 744.29
    ossicles 744.04
  endocrine (gland) NEC 759.2
  epiglottis 748.3
  Eustachian tube 744.24
  eye 743.8
  facial features 744.89
  fallopian tube 752.19
  finger(s) 755.59
    supernumerary 755.01
  foot 755.67
  gallbladder 751.69
  gastrointestinal tract 751.8
  genitalia, genital organ(s) or tract
    female 752.89
      external 752.49
      internal NEC 752.89
    male 752.89
      penis 752.69
      scrotal transposition 752.81
  glottis 748.3
  hand 755.59
  heart 746.87
    dextrocardia 746.87
      with complete transposition of viscera 759.3
  hepatic duct 751.69
  hip (joint) (*see also* Dislocation, hip, congenital) 754.30
  intestine (large) (small) 751.5
    with anomalous adhesions, fixation, or malrotation 751.4
  joint NEC 755.8
  kidney 753.3
  larynx 748.3
  limb 755.8
    lower 755.69
    upper 755.59
  liver 751.69
  lung (lobe) 748.69
  nail(s) 757.5
  nerve 742.8
  nervous system NEC 742.8
  nose, nasal (septum) 748.1
  organ or site NEC — *see* Anomaly, specified type NEC, by site
  ovary 752.0
  pancreas 751.7
  parathyroid (gland) 759.2
  patella 755.64
  peripheral vascular system 747.60

☑ **Additional Digit Required** — Refer to the Tabular List for Digit Selection   ⬝ **Subterms under main terms may continue to next column or page**

180 — Volume 2   ▶◀ **Revised Text**   ● **New Line**   ▲ **Revised Code**   **2014 ICD-9-CM**

Malposition — *continued*
congenital — *continued*
peripheral vascular system — *continued*
gastrointestinal 747.61
lower limb 747.64
renal 747.62
specified NEC 747.69
spinal 747.82
upper limb 747.63
pituitary (gland) 759.2
respiratory organ or system NEC 748.9
rib (cage) 756.3
supernumerary in cervical region 756.2
scapula 755.59
shoulder 755.59
spinal cord 742.59
spine 756.19
spleen 759.0
sternum 756.3
stomach 750.7
symphysis pubis 755.69
testis (undescended) 752.51
thymus (gland) 759.2
thyroid (gland) (tissue) 759.2
cartilage 748.3
toe(s) 755.66
supernumerary 755.02
tongue 750.19
trachea 748.3
uterus 752.39
vein(s) (peripheral) NEC (*see also* Malposition, congenital, peripheral vascular system) 747.60
great 747.49
portal 747.49
pulmonary 747.49
vena cava (inferior) (superior) 747.49
device, implant, or graft — *see* Complications, mechanical
fetus NEC (*see also* Presentation, fetal) 652.9 ☑
with successful version 652.1 ☑
affecting fetus or newborn 763.1
before labor, affecting fetus or newborn 761.7
causing obstructed labor 660.0 ☑
in multiple gestation (one fetus or more) 652.6 ☑
with locking 660.5 ☑
causing obstructed labor 660.0 ☑
gallbladder (*see also* Disease, gallbladder) 575.8
gastrointestinal tract 569.89
congenital 751.8
heart (*see also* Malposition, congenital, heart) 746.87
intestine 569.89
congenital 751.5
pelvic organs or tissues
in pregnancy or childbirth 654.4 ☑
affecting fetus or newborn 763.89
causing obstructed labor 660.2 ☑
affecting fetus or newborn 763.1
placenta — *see* Placenta, previa
stomach 537.89
congenital 750.7
tooth, teeth 524.30
with impaction 520.6
uterus (acquired) (acute) (adherent) (any degree) (asymptomatic) (postinfectional) (postpartal, old) 621.6
anteflexion or anteversion (*see also* Anteversion, uterus) 621.6
congenital 752.39
flexion 621.6
lateral (*see also* Lateroversion, uterus) 621.6
in pregnancy or childbirth 654.4 ☑
affecting fetus or newborn 763.89
causing obstructed labor 660.2 ☑
affecting fetus or newborn 763.1
inversion 621.6
lateral (flexion) (version) (*see also* Lateroversion, uterus) 621.6

Malposition — *continued*
uterus — *continued*
lateroflexion (*see also* Lateroversion, uterus) 621.6
lateroversion (*see also* Lateroversion, uterus) 621.6
retroflexion or retroversion (*see also* Retroversion, uterus) 621.6
Malposture 729.90
Malpresentation, fetus — *see also* Presentation, fetal 652.9 ☑
Malrotation
cecum 751.4
colon 751.4
intestine 751.4
kidney 753.3
MALT (mucosa associated lymphoid tissue) 200.3 ☑
Malta fever — *see also* Brucellosis 023.9
Maltosuria 271.3
Maltreatment (of)
adult 995.80
emotional 995.82
multiple forms 995.85
neglect (nutritional) 995.84
physical 995.81
psychological 995.82
sexual 995.83
child 995.50
emotional 995.51
multiple forms 995.59
neglect (nutritional) 995.52
physical 995.54
shaken infant syndrome 995.55
psychological 995.51
sexual 995.53
spouse (*see also* Maltreatment, adult) 995.80
Malt workers' lung 495.4
Malum coxae senilis 715.25
Malunion, fracture 733.81
Mammillitis — *see also* Mastitis 611.0
puerperal, postpartum 675.2 ☑
Mammitis — *see also* Mastitis 611.0
puerperal, postpartum 675.2 ☑
Mammographic
calcification 793.89
calculus 793.89
microcalcification 793.81
Mammoplasia 611.1
Management
contraceptive V25.9
specified type NEC V25.8
procreative V26.9
specified type NEC V26.89
Mangled NEC — *see also* nature and site of injury 959.9
Mania (monopolar) — *see also* Psychosis, affective 296.0 ☑
alcoholic (acute) (chronic) 291.9
Bell's — *see* Mania, chronic
chronic 296.0 ☑
recurrent episode 296.1 ☑
single episode 296.0 ☑
compulsive 300.3
delirious (acute) 296.0 ☑
recurrent episode 296.1 ☑
single episode 296.0 ☑
epileptic (*see also* Epilepsy) 345.4 ☑
hysterical 300.10
inhibited 296.89
puerperal (after delivery) 296.0 ☑
recurrent episode 296.1 ☑
single episode 296.0 ☑
recurrent episode 296.1 ☑
senile 290.8
single episode 296.0 ☑
stupor 296.89
stuporous 296.89
unproductive 296.89
Manic-depressive insanity, psychosis, reaction, or syndrome — *see also* Psychosis, affective 296.80
circular (alternating) 296.7
currently
depressed 296.5 ☑
episode unspecified 296.7

Manic-depressive insanity, psychosis, reaction, or syndrome — *see also* Psychosis, affective — *continued*
circular — *continued*
currently — *continued*
hypomanic, previously depressed 296.4 ☑
manic 296.4 ☑
mixed 296.6 ☑
depressed (type), depressive 296.2 ☑
atypical 296.82
recurrent episode 296.3 ☑
single episode 296.2 ☑
hypomanic 296.0 ☑
recurrent episode 296.1 ☑
single episode 296.0 ☑
manic 296.0 ☑
atypical 296.81
recurrent episode 296.1 ☑
single episode 296.0 ☑
mixed NEC 296.89
perplexed 296.89
stuporous 296.89
Manifestations, rheumatoid
lungs 714.81
pannus — *see* Arthritis, rheumatoid
subcutaneous nodules — *see* Arthritis, rheumatoid
Mankowsky's syndrome (familial dysplastic osteopathy) 731.2
Mannoheptulosuria 271.8
Mannosidosis 271.8
Manson's
disease (schistosomiasis) 120.1
pyosis (pemphigus contagiosus) 684
schistosomiasis 120.1
Mansonellosis 125.5
Manual — *see* condition
Maple bark-strippers' lung 495.6
Maple bark disease 495.6
Maple syrup (urine) disease or syndrome 270.3
Marable's syndrome (celiac artery compression) 447.4
Marasmus 261
brain 331.9
due to malnutrition 261
intestinal 569.89
nutritional 261
senile 797
tuberculous NEC (*see also* Tuberculosis) 011.9 ☑
Marble
bones 756.52
skin 782.61
Marburg disease (virus) 078.89
March
foot 733.94
hemoglobinuria 283.2
Marchand multiple nodular hyperplasia (liver) 571.5
Marchesani (-Weill) syndrome (brachymorphism and ectopia lentis) 759.89
Marchiafava-Micheli syndrome (paroxysmal nocturnal hemoglobinuria) 283.2
Marchiafava (-Bignami) disease or syndrome 341.8
Marcus Gunn's syndrome (jaw-winking syndrome) 742.8
Marfan's
congenital syphilis 090.49
disease 090.49
syndrome (arachnodactyly) 759.82
meaning congenital syphilis 090.49
with luxation of lens 090.49 [379.32]
Marginal
implantation, placenta — *see* Placenta, previa
placenta — *see* Placenta, previa
sinus (hemorrhage) (rupture) 641.2 ☑
affecting fetus or newborn 762.1
Marie-Bamberger disease or syndrome (hypertrophic) (pulmonary) (secondary) 731.2
idiopathic (acropachyderma) 757.39
primary (acropachyderma) 757.39

Marie-Charcôt-Tooth neuropathic atrophy, muscle 356.1
Marie-Strümpell arthritis or disease (ankylosing spondylitis) 720.0
Marie's
cerebellar ataxia 334.2
syndrome (acromegaly) 253.0
Marihuana, marijuana
abuse (*see also* Abuse, drugs, nondependent) 305.2 ☑
dependence (*see also* Dependence) 304.3 ☑
Marion's disease (bladder neck obstruction) 596.0
Marital conflict V61.10
Mark
port wine 757.32
raspberry 757.32
strawberry 757.32
stretch 701.3
tattoo 709.09
Maroteaux-Lamy syndrome (mucopolysaccharidosis VI) 277.5
Marriage license examination V70.3
Marrow (bone)
arrest 284.9
megakaryocytic 287.30
poor function 289.9
Marseilles fever 082.1
Marshall's (hidrotic) **ectodermal dysplasia** 757.31
Marsh's disease (exophthalmic goiter) 242.0 ☑
Marsh fever — *see also* Malaria 084.6
Martin-Albright syndrome (pseudohypoparathyroidism) 275.49
Martin's disease 715.27
Martorell-Fabre syndrome (pulseless disease) 446.7
Masculinization, female, with adrenal hyperplasia 255.2
Masculinovoblastoma (M8670/0) 220
Masochism 302.83
Masons' lung 502
Mass
abdominal 789.3 ☑
anus 787.99
bone 733.90
breast 611.72
cheek 784.2
chest 786.6
cystic — *see* Cyst
ear 388.8
epigastric 789.3 ☑
eye 379.92
female genital organ 625.8
gum 784.2
head 784.2
intracranial 784.2
joint 719.60
ankle 719.67
elbow 719.62
foot 719.67
hand 719.64
hip 719.65
knee 719.66
multiple sites 719.69
pelvic region 719.65
shoulder (region) 719.61
specified site NEC 719.68
wrist 719.63
kidney (*see also* Disease, kidney) 593.9
lung 786.6
lymph node 785.6
malignant (M8000/3) — *see* Neoplasm, by site, malignant
mediastinal 786.6
mouth 784.2
muscle (limb) 729.89
neck 784.2
nose or sinus 784.2
palate 784.2
pelvis, pelvic 789.3 ☑
penis 607.89
perineum 625.8
rectum 787.99
scrotum 608.89

☑ **Additional Digit Required** — Refer to the Tabular List for Digit Selection   ⌄ **Subterms under main terms may continue to next column or page**

Mass — *continued*
  skin 782.2
  specified organ NEC — *see* Disease of specified organ or site
  splenic 789.2
  substernal 786.6
    thyroid (*see also* Goiter) 240.9
  superficial (localized) 782.2
  testes 608.89
  throat 784.2
  tongue 784.2
  umbilicus 789.3 ☑
  uterus 625.8
  vagina 625.8
  vulva 625.8
Massive — *see* condition
Mastalgia 611.71
  psychogenic 307.89
Mast cell
  disease 757.33
    systemic (M9741/3) 202.6 ☑
  leukemia (M9900/3) 207.8 ☑
  sarcoma (M9740/3 202.6 ☑
  tumor (M9740/1) 238.5
    malignant (M9740/3) 202.6 ☑
Masters-Allen syndrome 620.6
Mastitis (acute) (adolescent) (diffuse) (interstitial) (lobular) (nonpuerperal) (nonsuppurative) (parenchymatous) (phlegmonous) (simple) (subacute) (suppurative) 611.0
  chronic (cystic) (fibrocystic) 610.1
  cystic 610.1
    Schimmelbusch's type 610.1
  fibrocystic 610.1
  infective 611.0
  lactational 675.2 ☑
  lymphangitis 611.0
  neonatal (noninfective) 778.7
    infective 771.5
  periductal 610.4
  plasma cell 610.4
  puerperalis 675.2 ☑
  puerperal, postpartum, (interstitial) (nonpurulent) (parenchymatous) 675.2 ☑
    purulent 675.1 ☑
    stagnation 676.2 ☑
  retromammary 611.0
    puerperal, postpartum 675.1 ☑
  submammary 611.0
    puerperal, postpartum 675.1 ☑
Mastocytoma (M9740/1) 238.5
  malignant (M9740/3) 202.6 ☑
Mastocytosis 757.33
  malignant (M9741/3) 202.6 ☑
  systemic (M9741/3) 202.6 ☑
Mastodynia 611.71
  psychogenic 307.89
Mastoid — *see* condition
Mastoidalgia — *see also* Otalgia 388.70
Mastoiditis (coalescent) (hemorrhagic) (pneumococcal) (streptococcal) (suppurative) 383.9
  acute or subacute 383.00
    with
      Gradenigo's syndrome 383.02
      petrositis 383.02
      specified complication NEC 383.02
      subperiosteal abscess 383.01
  chronic (necrotic) (recurrent) 383.1
  tuberculous (*see also* Tuberculosis) 015.6 ☑
Mastopathy, mastopathia 611.9
  chronica cystica 610.1
  diffuse cystic 610.1
  estrogenic 611.89
  ovarian origin 611.89
Mastoplasia 611.1
Masturbation 307.9
Maternal condition, affecting fetus or newborn
  acute yellow atrophy of liver 760.8
  albuminuria 760.1
  anesthesia or analgesia 763.5
  blood loss 762.1
  chorioamnionitis 762.7

Maternal condition, affecting fetus or newborn — *continued*
  circulatory disease, chronic (conditions classifiable to 390–459, 745–747) 760.3
  congenital heart disease (conditions classifiable to 745–746) 760.3
  cortical necrosis of kidney 760.1
  death 761.6
  diabetes mellitus 775.0
    manifest diabetes in the infant 775.1
  disease NEC 760.9
    circulatory system, chronic (conditions classifiable to 390–459, 745–747) 760.3
    genitourinary system (conditions classifiable to 580–599) 760.1
    respiratory (conditions classifiable to 490–519, 748) 760.3
  eclampsia 760.0
  hemorrhage NEC 762.1
  hepatitis acute, malignant, or subacute 760.8
  hyperemesis (gravidarum) 761.8
  hypertension (arising during pregnancy) (conditions classifiable to 642) 760.0
  infection
    disease classifiable to 001-136 ☑, 760.2
    genital tract NEC 760.8
    urinary tract 760.1
  influenza 760.2
    manifest influenza in the infant 771.2
  injury (conditions classifiable to 800–996) 760.5
  malaria 760.2
    manifest malaria in infant or fetus 771.2
  malnutrition 760.4
  necrosis of liver 760.8
  nephritis (conditions classifiable to 580–583) 760.1
  nephrosis (conditions classifiable to 581) 760.1
  noxious substance transmitted via breast milk or placenta 760.70
    alcohol 760.71
    anti-infective agents 760.74
    anticonvulsants 760.77
    antifungals 760.74
    antimetabolics 760.78
    cocaine 760.75
    "crack" 760.75
    diethylstilbestrol [DES] 760.76
    hallucinogenic agents 760.73
    medicinal agents NEC 760.79
    narcotics 760.72
    obstetric anesthetic or analgesic drug 760.72
    specified agent NEC 760.79
  nutritional disorder (conditions classifiable to 260–269) 760.4
  operation unrelated to current delivery (*see also* Newborn, affected by) 760.64
  pre-eclampsia 760.0
  pyelitis or pyelonephritis, arising during pregnancy (conditions classifiable to 590) 760.1
  renal disease or failure 760.1
  respiratory disease, chronic (conditions classifiable to 490–519, 748) 760.3
  rheumatic heart disease (chronic) (conditions classifiable to 393–398) 760.3
  rubella (conditions classifiable to 056) 760.2
    manifest rubella in the infant or fetus 771.0
  surgery unrelated to current delivery (*see also* Newborn, affected by) 760.64
    to uterus or pelvic organs 760.64
  syphilis (conditions classifiable to 090–097) 760.2
    manifest syphilis in the infant or fetus 090.0
  thrombophlebitis 760.3
  toxemia (of pregnancy) 760.0
    pre-eclamptic 760.0
  toxoplasmosis (conditions classifiable to 130) 760.2

Maternal condition, affecting fetus or newborn — *continued*
  toxoplasmosis — *continued*
    manifest toxoplasmosis in the infant or fetus 771.2
  transmission of chemical substance through the placenta 760.70
    alcohol 760.71
    anti-infective 760.74
    anticonvulsants 760.77
    antifungals 760.74
    antimetabolics 760.78
    cocaine 760.75
    "crack" 760.75
    diethylstilbestrol [DES] 760.76
    hallucinogenic agents 760.73
    narcotics 760.72
    specified substance NEC 760.79
  uremia 760.1
  urinary tract conditions (conditions classifiable to 580–599) 760.1
  vomiting (pernicious) (persistent) (vicious) 761.8
Maternity — *see* Delivery
Matheiu's disease (leptospiral jaundice) 100.0
Mauclaire's disease or osteochondrosis 732.3
Maxcy's disease 081.0
Maxilla, maxillary — *see* condition
May (-Hegglin) anomaly or syndrome 288.2
Mayaro fever 066.3
Mazoplasia 610.8
MBD (minimal brain dysfunction), child — *see also* Hyperkinesia 314.9
MCAD (medium chain acyl CoA dehydrogenase deficiency) 277.85
McArdle (-Schmid-Pearson) disease or syndrome (glycogenosis V) 271.0
McCune-Albright syndrome (osteitis fibrosa disseminata) 756.59
MCLS (mucocutaneous lymph node syndrome) 446.1
McQuarrie's syndrome (idiopathic familial hypoglycemia) 251.2
Measles (black) (hemorrhagic) (suppressed) 055.9
  with
    encephalitis 055.0
    keratitis 055.71
    keratoconjunctivitis 055.71
    otitis media 055.2
    pneumonia 055.1
  complication 055.8
    specified type NEC 055.79
  encephalitis 055.0
  French 056.9
  German 056.9
  keratitis 055.71
  keratoconjunctivitis 055.71
  liberty 056.9
  otitis media 055.2
  pneumonia 055.1
  specified complications NEC 055.79
  vaccination, prophylactic (against) V04.2
Meat-wrappers' asthma 506.9
Meatitis, urethral — *see also* Urethritis 597.89
Meat poisoning — *see* Poisoning, food
Meatus, meatal — *see* condition
Meckel's
  diverticulitis 751.0
  diverticulum (displaced) (hypertrophic) 751.0
Meconium
  aspiration 770.11
    with
      pneumonia 770.12
      pneumonitis 770.12
      respiratory symptoms 770.12
    below vocal cords 770.11
      with respiratory symptoms 770.12
    syndrome 770.12
  delayed passage in newborn 777.1
  ileus 777.1
    due to cystic fibrosis 277.01
  in liquor 792.3
    noted during delivery 656.8 ☑
  insufflation 770.11

Meconium — *continued*
  insufflation — *continued*
    with respiratory symptoms 770.12
  obstruction
    fetus or newborn 777.1
      in mucoviscidosis 277.01
  passage of 792.3
    noted during delivery 763.84
  peritonitis 777.6
  plug syndrome (newborn) NEC 777.1
  staining 779.84
Median — *see also* condition
  arcuate ligament syndrome 447.4
  bar (prostate) 600.90
    with
      other lower urinary tract symptoms (LUTS) 600.91
      urinary
        obstruction 600.91
        retention 600.91
  rhomboid glossitis 529.2
  vesical orifice 600.90
    with
      other lower urinary tract symptoms (LUTS) 600.91
      urinary
        obstruction 600.91
        retention 600.91
Mediastinal shift 793.2
Mediastinitis (acute) (chronic) 519.2
  actinomycotic 039.8
  syphilitic 095.8
  tuberculous (*see also* Tuberculosis) 012.8 ☑
Mediastinopericarditis — *see also* Pericarditis 423.9
  acute 420.90
  chronic 423.8
    rheumatic 393
  rheumatic, chronic 393
Mediastinum, mediastinal — *see* condition
Medical services provided for — *see* Health services provided because (of)
Medicine poisoning (by overdose) (wrong substance given or taken in error) 977.9
  specified drug or substance — *see* Table of Drugs and Chemicals
Medin's disease (poliomyelitis) 045.9 ☑
Mediterranean
  anemia 282.40
    with other hemoglobinopathy 282.49
  disease or syndrome (hemopathic) 282.40
    with other hemoglobinopathy 282.49
  fever (*see also* Brucellosis) 023.9
    familial 277.31
  kala-azar 085.0
  leishmaniasis 085.0
  tick fever 082.1
Medulla — *see* condition
Medullary
  cystic kidney 753.16
  sponge kidney 753.17
Medullated fibers
  optic (nerve) 743.57
  retina 362.85
Medulloblastoma (M9470/3)
  desmoplastic (M9471/3) 191.6
  specified site — *see* Neoplasm, by site, malignant
  unspecified site 191.6
Medulloepithelioma (M9501/3) — *see also* Neoplasm, by site, malignant
  teratoid (M9502/3) — *see* Neoplasm, by site, malignant
Medullomyoblastoma (M9472/3)
  specified site — *see* Neoplasm, by site, malignant
  unspecified site 191.6
Meekeren-Ehlers-Danlos syndrome 756.83
Megacaryocytic — *see* condition
Megacolon (acquired) (functional) (not Hirschsprung's disease) 564.7
  aganglionic 751.3
  congenital, congenitum 751.3
  Hirschsprung's (disease) 751.3
  psychogenic 306.4
  toxic (*see also* Colitis, ulcerative) 556.9

☑ Additional Digit Required — Refer to the Tabular List for Digit Selection   🔻 Subterms under main terms may continue to next column or page

182 — Volume 2   ►◄ Revised Text   ● New Line   ▲ Revised Code   2014 ICD-9-CM

☑ Additional Digit Required — Refer to the Tabular List for Digit Selection
▽ Subterms under main terms may continue to next column or page
2014 ICD-9-CM
▶◀ Revised Text
● New Line
▲ Revised Code
Volume 2 — 183

Meningioma — see also Neoplasm, meninges, benign — continued
 hemangiopericytic (M9536/0) — see Neoplasm, meninges, benign
 malignant (M9530/3) — see Neoplasm, meninges, malignant
 meningiothelial (M9531/0) — see Neoplasm, meninges, benign
 meningotheliomatous (M9531/0) — see Neoplasm, meninges, benign
 mixed (M9537/0) — see Neoplasm, meninges, benign
 multiple (M9530/1) 237.6
 papillary (M9538/1) 237.6
 psammomatous (M9533/0) — see Neoplasm, meninges, benign
 syncytial (M9531/0) — see Neoplasm, meninges, benign
 transitional (M9537/0) — see Neoplasm, meninges, benign
Meningiomatosis (diffuse) (M9530/1) 237.6
Meningism — see also Meningismus 781.6
Meningismus (infectional) (pneumococcal) 781.6
 due to serum or vaccine 997.09 [321.8]
 influenzal NEC (see also Influenza) 487.8
Meningitis (basal) (basic) (basilar) (brain) (cerebral) (cervical) (congestive) (diffuse) (hemorrhagic) (infantile) (membranous) (metastatic) (nonspecific) (pontine) (progressive) (simple) (spinal) (subacute) (sympathetica) (toxic) 322.9
 abacterial NEC (see also Meningitis, aseptic) 047.9
 actinomycotic 039.8 [320.7]
 adenoviral 049.1
 Aerobacter aerogenes 320.82
 anaerobes (cocci) (gram-negative) (gram-positive) (mixed) (NEC) 320.81
 arbovirus NEC 066.9 [321.2]
  specified type NEC 066.8 [321.2]
 aseptic (acute) NEC 047.9
  adenovirus 049.1
  Coxsackie virus 047.0
  due to
   adenovirus 049.1
   Coxsackie virus 047.0
   ECHO virus 047.1
   enterovirus 047.9
   mumps 072.1
   poliovirus (see also Poliomyelitis) 045.2 ☑ [321.2]
  ECHO virus 047.1
  herpes (simplex) virus 054.72
   zoster 053.0
  leptospiral 100.81
  lymphocytic choriomeningitis 049.0
  noninfective 322.0
 Bacillus pyocyaneus 320.89
 bacterial NEC 320.9
  anaerobic 320.81
  gram-negative 320.82
   anaerobic 320.81
 Bacteroides (fragilis) (oralis) (melaninogenicus) 320.81
 cancerous (M8000/6) 198.4
 candidal 112.83
 carcinomatous (M8010/6) 198.4
 caseous (see also Tuberculosis, meninges) 013.0 ☑
 cerebrospinal (acute) (chronic) (diplococcal) (endemic) (epidemic) (fulminant) (infectious) (malignant) (meningococcal) (sporadic) 036.0
  carrier (suspected) of V02.59
 chronic NEC 322.2
 clear cerebrospinal fluid NEC 322.0
 Clostridium (haemolyticum) (novyi) NEC 320.81
 coccidioidomycosis 114.2
 Coxsackie virus 047.0
 cryptococcal 117.5 [321.0]
 diplococcal 036.0
  gram-negative 036.0
  gram-positive 320.1

Meningitis — continued
 Diplococcus pneumoniae 320.1
 due to
  actinomycosis 039.8 [320.7]
  adenovirus 049.1
  coccidiomycosis 114.2
  enterovirus 047.9
   specified NEC 047.8
  histoplasmosis (see also Histoplasmosis) 115.91
  Listerosis 027.0 [320.7]
  Lyme disease 088.81 [320.7]
  moniliasis 112.83
  mumps 072.1
  neurosyphilis 094.2
  nonbacterial organisms NEC 321.8
  oidiomycosis 112.83
  poliovirus (see also Poliomyelitis) 045.2 ☑ [321.2]
  preventive immunization, inoculation, or vaccination 997.09 [321.8]
  sarcoidosis 135 [321.4]
  sporotrichosis 117.1 [321.1]
  syphilis 094.2
   acute 091.81
   congenital 090.42
   secondary 091.81
  trypanosomiasis (see also Trypanosomiasis) 086.9 [321.3]
  whooping cough 033.9 [320.7]
 ECHO virus 047.1
 E. coli 320.82
 endothelial-leukocytic, benign, recurrent 047.9
 Enterobacter aerogenes 320.82
 enteroviral 047.9
  specified type NEC 047.8
 enterovirus 047.9
  specified NEC 047.8
 eosinophilic 322.1
 epidemic NEC 036.0
 Escherichia coli (E. coli) 320.82
 Eubacterium 320.81
 fibrinopurulent NEC 320.9
  specified type NEC 320.89
 Friedländer (bacillus) 320.82
 fungal NEC 117.9 [321.1]
 Fusobacterium 320.81
 gonococcal 098.82
 gram-negative bacteria NEC 320.82
  anaerobic 320.81
  cocci 036.0
   specified NEC 320.82
 gram-negative cocci NEC 036.0
  specified NEC 320.82
 gram-positive cocci NEC 320.9
 herpes (simplex) virus 054.72
  zoster 053.0
 H. influenzae 320.0
 infectious NEC 320.9
 influenzal 320.0
 Klebsiella pneumoniae 320.82
 late effect — see Late, effect, meningitis
 leptospiral (aseptic) 100.81
 Listerella (monocytogenes) 027.0 [320.7]
 Listeria monocytogenes 027.0 [320.7]
 lymphocytic (acute) (benign) (serous) 049.0
  choriomeningitis virus 049.0
 meningococcal (chronic) 036.0
 Mima polymorpha 320.82
 Mollaret's 047.9
 monilial 112.83
 mumps (virus) 072.1
 mycotic NEC 117.9 [321.1]
 Neisseria 036.0
 neurosyphilis 094.2
 nonbacterial NEC (see also Meningitis, aseptic) 047.9
 nonpyogenic NEC 322.0
 oidiomycosis 112.83
 ossificans 349.2
 Peptococcus 320.81
 Peptostreptococcus 320.81
 pneumococcal 320.1
 poliovirus (see also Poliomyelitis) 045.2 ☑ [321.2]

Meningitis — continued
 Proprionibacterium 320.81
 Proteus morganii 320.82
 Pseudomonas (aeruginosa) (pyocyaneus) 320.82
 purulent NEC 320.9
  specified organism NEC 320.89
 pyogenic NEC 320.9
  specified organism NEC 320.89
 Salmonella 003.21
 septic NEC 320.9
  specified organism NEC 320.89
 serosa circumscripta NEC 322.0
 serous NEC (see also Meningitis, aseptic) 047.9
  lymphocytic 049.0
  syndrome 348.2
 Serratia (marcescens) 320.82
 specified organism NEC 320.89
 sporadic cerebrospinal 036.0
 sporotrichosis 117.1 [321.1]
 staphylococcal 320.3
 sterile 997.09
 streptococcal (acute) 320.2
 suppurative 320.9
  specified organism NEC 320.89
 syphilitic 094.2
  acute 091.81
  congenital 090.42
  secondary 091.81
 torula 117.5 [321.0]
 traumatic (complication of injury) 958.8
 Treponema (denticola) (macrodenticum) 320.81
 trypanosomiasis 086.1 [321.3]
 tuberculous (see also Tuberculosis, meninges) 013.0 ☑
 typhoid 002.0 [320.7]
 Veillonella 320.81
 Vibrio vulnificus 320.82
 viral, virus NEC (see also Meningitis, aseptic) 047.9
 Wallgren's (see also Meningitis, aseptic) 047.9
Meningocele (congenital) (spinal) — see also Spina bifida 741.9 ☑
 acquired (traumatic) 349.2
 cerebral 742.0
 cranial 742.0
Meningocerebritis — see Meningoencephalitis
Meningococcemia (acute) (chronic) 036.2
Meningococcus, meningococcal — see also condition 036.9
 adrenalitis, hemorrhagic 036.3
 carditis 036.40
 carrier (suspected) of V02.59
 cerebrospinal fever 036.0
 encephalitis 036.1
 endocarditis 036.42
 exposure to V01.84
 infection NEC 036.9
 meningitis (cerebrospinal) 036.0
 myocarditis 036.43
 optic neuritis 036.81
 pericarditis 036.41
 septicemia (chronic) 036.2
Meningoencephalitis — see also Encephalitis 323.9
 acute NEC 048
 bacterial, purulent, pyogenic, or septic — see Meningitis
 chronic NEC 094.1
 diffuse NEC 094.1
 diphasic 063.2
 due to
  actinomycosis 039.8 [320.7]
  blastomycosis NEC (see also Blastomycosis) 116.0 [323.41]
  free-living amebae 136.29
  Listeria monocytogenes 027.0 [320.7]
  Lyme disease 088.81 [320.7]
  mumps 072.2
  Naegleria (amebae) (gruberi) (organisms) 136.29
  rubella 056.01

Meningoencephalitis — see also Encephalitis — continued
 due to — continued
  sporotrichosis 117.1 [321.1]
  toxoplasmosis (acquired) 130.0
   congenital (active) 771.2 [323.41]
  Trypanosoma 086.1 [323.2]
 epidemic 036.0
 herpes 054.3
 herpetic 054.3
 H. influenzae 320.0
 infectious (acute) 048
 influenzal 320.0
 late effect — see category 326
 Listeria monocytogenes 027.0 [320.7]
 lymphocytic (serous) 049.0
 mumps 072.2
 parasitic NEC 123.9 [323.41]
 pneumococcal 320.1
 primary amebic 136.29
 rubella 056.01
 serous 048
  lymphocytic 049.0
 specific 094.2
 staphylococcal 320.3
 streptococcal 320.2
 syphilitic 094.2
 toxic NEC 989.9 [323.71]
  due to
   carbon tetrachloride (vapor) 987.8 [323.71]
   hydroxyquinoline derivatives poisoning 961.3 [323.71]
   lead 984.9 [323.71]
   mercury 985.0 [323.71]
   thallium 985.8 [323.71]
 toxoplasmosis (acquired) 130.0
 trypanosomic 086.1 [323.2]
 tuberculous (see also Tuberculosis, meninges) 013.0 ☑
 virus NEC 048
Meningoencephalocele 742.0
 syphilitic 094.89
 congenital 090.49
Meningoencephalomyelitis — see also Meningoencephalitis 323.9
 acute NEC 048
  disseminated (postinfectious) 136.9 [323.61]
   postimmunization or postvaccination 323.51
 due to
  actinomycosis 039.8 [320.7]
  torula 117.5 [323.41]
  toxoplasma or toxoplasmosis (acquired) 130.0
   congenital (active) 771.2 [323.41]
 late effect — see category 326
Meningoencephalomyelopathy — see also Meningoencephalomyelitis 349.9
Meningoencephalopathy — see also Meningoencephalitis 348.39
Meningoencephalopoliomyelitis — see also Poliomyelitis, bulbar 045.0 ☑
 late effect 138
Meningomyelitis — see also Meningoencephalitis 323.9
 blastomycotic NEC (see also Blastomycosis) 116.0 [323.41]
 due to
  actinomycosis 039.8 [320.7]
  blastomycosis (see also Blastomycosis) 116.0 [323.41]
  Meningococcus 036.0
  sporotrichosis 117.1 [323.41]
  torula 117.5 [323.41]
 late effect — see category 326
 lethargic 049.8
 meningococcal 036.0
 syphilitic 094.2
 tuberculous (see also Tuberculosis, meninges) 013.0 ☑
Meningomyelocele — see also Spina bifida 741.9 ☑
 syphilitic 094.89

☑ Additional Digit Required — Refer to the Tabular List for Digit Selection   ▽ Subterms under main terms may continue to next column or page

184 — Volume 2   ▶◀ Revised Text   ● New Line   ▲ Revised Code   2014 ICD-9-CM

Meningomyeloneuritis — *see* Meningoencephalitis
Meningoradiculitis — *see* Meningitis
Meningovascular — *see* condition
Meniscocytosis 282.60
Menkes' syndrome — *see* Syndrome, Menkes'
Menolipsis 626.0
Menometrorrhagia 626.2
Menopause, menopausal (symptoms) (syndrome) 627.2
  arthritis (any site) NEC 716.3 ☑
  artificial 627.4
  bleeding 627.0
  crisis 627.2
  depression (*see also* Psychosis, affective) 296.2 ☑
    agitated 296.2 ☑
      recurrent episode 296.3 ☑
      single episode 296.2 ☑
    psychotic 296.2 ☑
      recurrent episode 296.3 ☑
      single episode 296.2 ☑
    recurrent episode 296.3 ☑
    single episode 296.2 ☑
    melancholia (*see also* Psychosis, affective) 296.2 ☑
      recurrent episode 296.3 ☑
      single episode 296.2 ☑
  paranoid state 297.2
  paraphrenia 297.2
  postsurgical 627.4
  premature 256.31
    postirradiation 256.2
    postsurgical 256.2
  psychoneurosis 627.2
  psychosis NEC 298.8
  surgical 627.4
  toxic polyarthritis NEC 716.39
Menorrhagia (primary) 626.2
  climacteric 627.0
  menopausal 627.0
  postclimacteric 627.1
  postmenopausal 627.1
  preclimacteric 627.0
  premenopausal 627.0
  puberty (menses retained) 626.3
Menorrhalgia 625.3
Menoschesis 626.8
Menostaxis 626.2
Menses, retention 626.8
Menstrual — *see also* Menstruation
  cycle, irregular 626.4
  disorders NEC 626.9
  extraction V25.3
  fluid, retained 626.8
  molimen 625.4
  period, normal V65.5
  regulation V25.3
Menstruation
  absent 626.0
  anovulatory 628.0
  delayed 626.8
  difficult 625.3
  disorder 626.9
    psychogenic 306.52
    specified NEC 626.8
  during pregnancy 640.8 ☑
  excessive 626.2
  frequent 626.2
  infrequent 626.1
  irregular 626.4
  latent 626.8
  membranous 626.8
  painful (primary) (secondary) 625.3
    psychogenic 306.52
  passage of clots 626.2
  precocious 259.1
  protracted 626.8
  retained 626.8
  retrograde 626.8
  scanty 626.1
  suppression 626.8
  vicarious (nasal) 625.8
Mentagra — *see also* Sycosis 704.8
Mental — *see also* condition

Mental — *see also* condition — *continued*
  deficiency (*see also* Disability, intellectual) 319
  deterioration (*see also* Psychosis) 298.9
  disorder (*see also* Disorder, mental) 300.9
  exhaustion 300.5
  insufficiency (congenital) (*see also* Disability, intellectual) 319
  observation without need for further medical care NEC V71.09
  retardation —*see* Disability, intellectual
  subnormality (*see also* Disability, intellectual) 319
    mild 317
    moderate 318.0
    profound 318.2
    severe 318.1
  upset (*see also* Disorder, mental) 300.9
Meralgia paresthetica 355.1
Mercurial — *see* condition
Mercurialism NEC 985.0
Merergasia 300.9
Merkel cell tumor — *see* Carcinoma, Merkel cell
Merocele — *see also* Hernia, femoral 553.00
Meromelia 755.4
  lower limb 755.30
    intercalary 755.32
      femur 755.34
        tibiofibular (complete) (incomplete) 755.33
      fibula 755.37
      metatarsal(s) 755.38
      tarsal(s) 755.38
      tibia 755.36
      tibiofibular 755.35
    terminal (complete) (partial) (transverse) 755.31
    longitudinal 755.32
      metatarsal(s) 755.38
      phalange(s) 755.39
      tarsal(s) 755.38
    transverse 755.31
  upper limb 755.20
    intercalary 755.22
      carpal(s) 755.28
      humeral 755.24
        radioulnar (complete) (incomplete) 755.23
      metacarpal(s) 755.28
      phalange(s) 755.29
      radial 755.26
      radioulnar 755.25
      ulnar 755.27
    terminal (complete) (partial) (transverse) 755.21
    longitudinal 755.22
      carpal(s) 755.28
      metacarpal(s) 755.28
      phalange(s) 755.29
    transverse 755.21
Merosmia 781.1
MERRF syndrome (myoclonus with epilepsy and with ragged red fibers) 277.87
Merycism — *see also* Vomiting
  psychogenic 307.53
Merzbacher-Pelizaeus disease 330.0
Mesaortitis — *see* Aortitis
Mesarteritis — *see* Arteritis
Mesencephalitis — *see also* Encephalitis 323.9
  late effect — *see* category 326
Mesenchymoma (M8990/1) — *see also* Neoplasm, connective tissue, uncertain behavior
  benign (M8990/0) — *see* Neoplasm, connective tissue, benign
  malignant (M8990/3) — *see* Neoplasm, connective tissue, malignant
Mesenteritis
  retractile 567.82
  sclerosing 567.82
Mesentery, mesenteric — *see* condition
Mesio-occlusion 524.23
Mesiodens, mesiodentes 520.1
  causing crowding 524.31
Mesocardia (with asplenia) 746.87

Mesocolon — *see* condition
Mesonephroma (malignant) (M9110/3) — *see also* Neoplasm, by site, malignant
  benign (M9110/0) — *see* Neoplasm, by site, benign
Mesophlebitis — *see* Phlebitis
Mesostromal dysgenesis 743.51
Mesothelioma (malignant) (M9050/3) — *see also* Neoplasm, by site, malignant
  benign (M9050/0) — *see* Neoplasm, by site, benign
  biphasic type (M9053/3) (*see also* Neoplasm, by site, malignant)
    benign (M9053/0) — *see* Neoplasm, by site, benign
  epithelioid (M9052/3) (*see also* Neoplasm, by site, malignant)
    benign (M9052/0) — *see* Neoplasm, by site, benign
  fibrous (M9051/3) (*see also* Neoplasm, by site, malignant)
    benign (M9051/0) — *see* Neoplasm, by site, benign
Metabolic syndrome 277.7
Metabolism disorder 277.9
  specified type NEC 277.89
Metagonimiasis 121.5
Metagonimus infestation (small intestine) 121.5
Metal
  pigmentation (skin) 709.00
  polishers' disease 502
Metalliferous miners' lung 503
Metamorphopsia 368.14
Metaplasia
  bone, in skin 709.3
  breast 611.89
  cervix — *omit code*
  endometrium (squamous) 621.8
  esophagus 530.85
  intestinal, of gastric mucosa 537.89
  kidney (pelvis) (squamous) (*see also* Disease, renal) 593.89
  myelogenous 289.89
  myeloid 289.89
    agnogenic 238.76
    megakaryocytic 238.76
  spleen 289.59
  squamous cell
    amnion 658.8 ☑
    bladder 596.89
    cervix — *see* condition
    trachea 519.19
    tracheobronchial tree 519.19
    uterus 621.8
      cervix — *see* condition
Metastasis, metastatic
  abscess — *see* Abscess
  calcification 275.40
  cancer, neoplasm, or disease
    from specified site (M8000/3) — *see* Neoplasm, by site, malignant
    to specified site (M8000/6) — *see* Neoplasm, by site, secondary
  deposits (in) (M8000/6) — *see* Neoplasm, by site, secondary
  mesentery, of neuroendocrine tumor 209.74
  pneumonia 038.8 [484.8]
  spread (to) (M8000/6) — *see* Neoplasm, by site, secondary
Metatarsalgia 726.70
  anterior 355.6
  due to Freiberg's disease 732.5
  Morton's 355.6
Metatarsus, metatarsal — *see also* condition
  abductus valgus (congenital) 754.60
  adductus varus (congenital) 754.53
  primus varus 754.52
  valgus (adductus) (congenital) 754.60
  varus (abductus) (congenital) 754.53
    primus 754.52
Methadone use 304.00
Methemoglobinemia 289.7
  acquired (with sulfhemoglobinemia) 289.7
  congenital 289.7
  enzymatic 289.7

Methemoglobinemia — *continued*
  Hb-M disease 289.7
  hereditary 289.7
  toxic 289.7
Methemoglobinuria — *see also* Hemoglobinuria 791.2
Methicillin
  resistant staphyloccocus aureus (MRSA) 041.12
    colonization V02.54
    personal history of V12.04
  susceptible staphylococcus aureus (MSSA) 041.11
    colonization V02.53
Methioninemia 270.4
Metritis (catarrhal) (septic) (suppurative) — *see also* Endometritis 615.9
  blennorrhagic 098.16
    chronic or duration of 2 months or over 098.36
  cervical (*see also* Cervicitis) 616.0
  gonococcal 098.16
    chronic or duration of 2 months or over 098.36
  hemorrhagic 626.8
  puerperal, postpartum, childbirth 670.1 ☑
  septic 670.2 ☑
  tuberculous (*see also* Tuberculosis) 016.7 ☑
Metropathia hemorrhagica 626.8
Metroperitonitis — *see also* Peritonitis, pelvic, female 614.5
Metrorrhagia 626.6
  arising during pregnancy — *see* Hemorrhage, pregnancy
  postpartum NEC 666.2 ☑
  primary 626.6
  psychogenic 306.59
  puerperal 666.2 ☑
Metrorrhexis — *see* Rupture, uterus
Metrosalpingitis — *see also* Salpingo-oophoritis 614.2
Metrostaxis 626.6
Metrovaginitis — *see also* Endometritis 615.9
  gonococcal (acute) 098.16
    chronic or duration of 2 months or over 098.36
Mexican fever — *see* Typhus, Mexican
Meyenburg-Altherr-Uehlinger syndrome 733.99
Meyer-Schwickerath and Weyers syndrome (dysplasia oculodentodigitalis) 759.89
Meynert's amentia (nonalcoholic) 294.0
  alcoholic 291.1
Mibelli's disease 757.39
Mice, joint — *see also* Loose, body, joint 718.1 ☑
  knee 717.6
Micheli-Rietti syndrome (thalassemia minor) 282.46
Michotte's syndrome 721.5
Micrencephalon, micrencephaly 742.1
Microalbuminuria 791.0
Microaneurysm, retina 362.14
  diabetic 250.5 ☑ *[362.01]*
    due to secondary diabetes 249.5 ☑ *[362.01]*
Microangiopathy 443.9
  diabetic (peripheral) 250.7 ☑ *[443.81]*
    due to secondary diabetes 249.7 ☑ *[443.81]*
    retinal 250.5 ☑ *[362.01]*
      due to secondary diabetes 249.5 ☑ *[362.01]*
  peripheral 443.9
    diabetic 250.7 ☑ *[443.81]*
      due to secondary diabetes 249.7 ☑ *[443.81]*
  retinal 362.18
    diabetic 250.5 ☑ *[362.01]*
      due to secondary diabetes 249.5 ☑ *[362.01]*
  thrombotic 446.6
    Moschcowitz's (thrombotic thrombocytopenic purpura) 446.6
Microcalcification, mammographic 793.81

☑ Additional Digit Required — Refer to the Tabular List for Digit Selection   ▽ Subterms under main terms may continue to next column or page

2014 ICD-9-CM   ▶◀ Revised Text   ● New Line   ▲ Revised Code   Volume 2 — 185

Microcephalus, microcephalic, microcephaly 742.1
  due to toxoplasmosis (congenital) 771.2
Microcheilia 744.82
Microcolon (congenital) 751.5
Microcornea (congenital) 743.41
Microcytic — *see condition*
Microdeletions NEC 758.33
Microdontia 520.2
Microdrepanocytosis (thalassemia-Hb-S disease) 282.41
  with sickle cell crisis 282.42
Microembolism
  atherothrombotic — *see* Atheroembolism
  retina 362.33
Microencephalon 742.1
Microfilaria streptocerca infestation 125.3
Microgastria (congenital) 750.7
Microgenia 524.06
Microgenitalia (congenital) 752.89
  penis 752.64
Microglioma (M9710/3)
  specified site — *see* Neoplasm, by site, malignant
  unspecified site 191.9
Microglossia (congenital) 750.16
Micrognathia, micrognathism (congenital) 524.00
  mandibular 524.04
    alveolar 524.74
  maxillary 524.03
    alveolar 524.73
Microgyria (congenital) 742.2
Microinfarct, heart — *see also* Insufficiency, coronary 411.89
Microlithiasis, alveolar, pulmonary 516.2
Micromastia 611.82
Micromyelia (congenital) 742.59
Micropenis 752.64
Microphakia (congenital) 743.36
Microphthalmia (congenital) — *see also* Microphthalmos 743.10
Microphthalmos (congenital) 743.10
  associated with eye and adnexal anomalies NEC 743.12
  due to toxoplasmosis (congenital) 771.2
  isolated 743.11
  simple 743.11
  syndrome 759.89
Micropsia 368.14
Microsporidiosis 136.8
Microsporon furfur infestation 111.0
Microsporosis — *see also* Dermatophytosis 110.9
  nigra 111.1
Microstomia (congenital) 744.84
Microthelia 757.6
Microthromboembolism — *see* Embolism
Microtia (congenital) (external ear) 744.23
Microtropia 378.34
Microvillus inclusion disease (MVD) 751.5
Micturition
  disorder NEC 788.69
    psychogenic 306.53
  frequency 788.41
    psychogenic 306.53
  nocturnal 788.43
  painful 788.1
    psychogenic 306.53
Middle
  ear — *see* condition
  lobe (right) syndrome 518.0
Midplane — *see* condition
Miescher-Leder syndrome or granulomatosis 709.3
Miescher's disease 709.3
  cheilitis 351.8
  granulomatosis disciformis 709.3
Mieten's syndrome 759.89

Migraine (idiopathic) 346.9 ☑
Note — The following fifth digit subclassification is for use with category 346:

0   *without mention of intractable migraine without mention of status migrainosus*
    without mention of refractory migraine without mention of status migrainosus
1   *with intractable migraine, so stated, without mention of status migrainosus*
    with refractory migraine, so stated, without mention of status migrainosus
2   *without mention of intractable migraine with status migrainosus*
    without mention of refractory migraine with status migrainosus
3   *with intractable migraine, so stated, with status migrainosus*
    with refractory migraine, so stated, with status migrainosus

  with aura (acute-onset) (without headache) (prolonged) (typical) 346.0 ☑
  without aura 346.1 ☑
    chronic 346.7 ☑
    transformed 346.7 ☑
  abdominal (syndrome) 346.2 ☑
  allergic (histamine) 346.2 ☑
  atypical 346.8 ☑
  basilar 346.0 ☑
  chronic without aura 346.7 ☑
  classic(al) 346.0 ☑
  common 346.1 ☑
  complicated 346.0 ☑
  hemiplegic 346.3 ☑
    familial 346.3 ☑
    sporadic 346.3 ☑
  lower-half 339.00
  menstrual 346.4 ☑
  menstrually related 346.4 ☑
  ophthalmic 346.8 ☑
  ophthalmoplegic 346.2 ☑
  premenstrual 346.4 ☑
  pure menstrual 346.4 ☑
  retinal 346.0 ☑
  specified form NEC 346.8 ☑
  transformed without aura 346.7 ☑
  variant 346.2 ☑
Migrant, social V60.0
Migratory, migrating — *see also* condition
  person V60.0
  testis, congenital 752.52
Mikulicz's disease or syndrome (dryness of mouth, absent or decreased lacrimation) 527.1
Milian atrophia blanche 701.3
Miliaria (crystallina) (rubra) (tropicalis) 705.1
  apocrine 705.82
Miliary — *see* condition
Milium — *see also* Cyst, sebaceous 706.2
  colloid 709.3
  eyelid 374.84
Milk-leg (deep vessels) 671.4 ☑
  complicating pregnancy 671.3 ☑
  nonpuerperal 451.19
  puerperal, postpartum, childbirth 671.4 ☑
Milk
  crust 690.11
  excess secretion 676.6 ☑
  fever, female 672.0 ☑
  poisoning 988.8
  retention 676.2 ☑
  sickness 988.8
  spots 423.1
Milkers' nodes 051.1
Milkman (-Looser) disease or syndrome (osteomalacia with pseudofractures) 268.2

Milky urine — *see also* Chyluria 791.1
Millar's asthma (laryngismus stridulus) 478.75
Millard-Gubler-Foville paralysis 344.89
Millard-Gubler paralysis or syndrome 344.89
Miller-Dieker syndrome 758.33
Miller's disease (osteomalacia) 268.2
Miller Fisher's syndrome 357.0
Milles' syndrome (encephalocutaneous angiomatosis) 759.6
Mills' disease 335.29
Millstone makers' asthma or lung 502
Milroy's disease (chronic hereditary edema) 757.0
Miners' — *see also* condition
  asthma 500
  elbow 727.2
  knee 727.2
  lung 500
  nystagmus 300.89
  phthisis (*see also* Tuberculosis) 011.4 ☑
  tuberculosis (*see also* Tuberculosis) 011.4 ☑
Minkowski-Chauffard syndrome — *see also* Spherocytosis 282.0
Minor — *see* condition
Minor's disease 336.1
Minot-von Willebrand (-Jürgens) disease or syndrome (angiohemophilia) 286.4
Minot's disease (hemorrhagic disease, newborn) 776.0
Minus (and plus) hand (intrinsic) 736.09
Miosis (persistent) (pupil) 379.42
Mirizzi's syndrome (hepatic duct stenosis) — *see also* Obstruction, biliary 576.2
  with calculus, cholelithiasis, or stones — *see* Choledocholithiasis
Mirror writing 315.09
  secondary to organic lesion 784.69
Misadventure (prophylactic) (therapeutic) — *see also* Complications 999.9
  administration of insulin 962.3
  infusion — *see* Complications, infusion
  local applications (of fomentations, plasters, etc.) 999.9
    burn or scald — *see* Burn, by site
  medical care (early) (late) NEC 999.9
    adverse effect of drugs or chemicals — *see* Table of Drugs and Chemicals
    burn or scald — *see* Burn, by site
  radiation NEC 990
  radiotherapy NEC 990
  surgical procedure (early) (late) — *see* Complications, surgical procedure
  transfusion — *see* Complications, transfusion
  vaccination or other immunological procedure — *see* Complications, vaccination
Misanthropy 301.7
Miscarriage — *see* Abortion, spontaneous
Mischief, malicious, child — *see also* Disturbance, conduct 312.0 ☑
Misdirection
  aqueous 365.83
Mismanagement, feeding 783.3
Misplaced, misplacement
  kidney (*see also* Disease, renal) 593.0
    congenital 753.3
  organ or site, congenital NEC — *see* Malposition, congenital
Missed
  abortion 632
  delivery (at or near term) 656.4 ☑
  labor (at or near term) 656.4 ☑
Misshapen reconstructed breast 612.0
Missing — *see also* Absence
  teeth (acquired) 525.10
    congenital (*see also* Anodontia) 520.0
    due to
      caries 525.13
      extraction 525.10
      periodontal disease 525.12
      specified NEC 525.19
      trauma 525.11
    vertebrae (congenital) 756.13
Misuse of drugs NEC — *see also* Abuse, drug, nondependent 305.9 ☑

Mitchell's disease (erythromelalgia) 443.82
Mite(s)
  diarrhea 133.8
  grain (itch) 133.8
  hair follicle (itch) 133.8
  in sputum 133.8
Mitochondrial encephalopathy, lactic acidosis and stroke-like episodes (MELAS syndrome) 277.87
Mitochondrial neurogastrointestinal encephalopathy syndrome (MNGIE) 277.87
Mitral — *see* condition
Mittelschmerz 625.2
Mixed — *see* condition
Mljet disease (mal de Meleda) 757.39
Mobile, mobility
  cecum 751.4
  coccyx 733.99
  excessive — *see* Hypermobility
  gallbladder 751.69
  kidney 593.0
    congenital 753.3
  organ or site, congenital NEC — *see* Malposition, congenital
  spleen 289.59
Mobitz heart block (atrioventricular) 426.10
  type I (Wenckebach's) 426.13
  type II 426.12
Möbius'
  disease 346.2 ☑
  syndrome
    congenital oculofacial paralysis 352.6
    ophthalmoplegic migraine 346.2 ☑
Moeller (-Barlow) disease (infantile scurvy) 267
  glossitis 529.4
Mohr's syndrome (types I and II) 759.89
Mola destruens (M9100/1) 236.1
Molarization, premolars 520.2
Molar pregnancy 631.8
  hydatidiform (delivered) (undelivered) 630
Molding, head (during birth) — *omit code*
Mold(s) in vitreous 117.9
Mole (pigmented) (M8720/0) — *see also* Neoplasm, skin, benign
  blood 631.8
  Breus' 631.8
  cancerous (M8720/3) — *see* Melanoma
  carneous 631.8
  destructive (M9100/1) 236.1
  ectopic — *see* Pregnancy, ectopic
  fleshy 631.8
  hemorrhagic 631.8
  hydatid, hydatidiform (benign) (complicating pregnancy) (delivered) (undelivered) (*see also* Hydatidiform mole) 630
    invasive (M9100/1) 236.1
    malignant (M9100/1) 236.1
    previous, affecting management of pregnancy V23.1
  invasive (hydatidiform) (M9100/1) 236.1
  malignant
    meaning
      malignant hydatidiform mole (M9100/1) 236.1
      melanoma (M8720/3) — *see* Melanoma
  nonpigmented (M8730/0) — *see* Neoplasm, skin, benign
  pregnancy NEC 631.8
  skin (M8720/0) — *see* Neoplasm, skin, benign
  stone 631.8
  tubal — *see* Pregnancy, tubal
  vesicular (*see also* Hydatidiform mole) 630
Molimen, molimina (menstrual) 625.4
Mollaret's meningitis 047.9
Mollities (cerebellar) (cerebral) 437.8
  ossium 268.2
Molluscum
  contagiosum 078.0
  epitheliale 078.0
  fibrosum (M8851/0) — *see* Lipoma, by site
  pendulum (M8851/0) — *see* Lipoma, by site

☑ **Additional Digit Required** — Refer to the Tabular List for Digit Selection   ⬔ **Subterms under main terms may continue to next column or page**

186 — Volume 2   ▶◀ **Revised Text**   ● **New Line**   ▲ **Revised Code**   **2014 ICD-9-CM**

Mönckeberg's arteriosclerosis, degeneration, disease, or sclerosis — *see also* Arteriosclerosis, extremities 440.20
Monday fever 504
Monday morning dyspnea or asthma 504
Mondini's malformation (cochlea) 744.05
Mondor's disease (thrombophlebitis of breast) 451.89
Mongolian, mongolianism, mongolism, mongoloid 758.0
   spot 757.33
Monilethrix (congenital) 757.4
Monilia infestation — *see* Candidiasis
Moniliasis — *see also* Candidiasis
   neonatal 771.7
   vulvovaginitis 112.1
Monkeypox 059.01
Monoarthritis 716.60
   ankle 716.67
   arm 716.62
      lower (and wrist) 716.63
      upper (and elbow) 716.62
   foot (and ankle) 716.67
   forearm (and wrist) 716.63
   hand 716.64
   leg 716.66
      lower 716.66
      upper 716.65
   pelvic region (hip) (thigh) 716.65
   shoulder (region) 716.61
   specified site NEC 716.68
Monoblastic — *see* condition
Monochromatism (cone) (rod) 368.54
Monocytic — *see* condition
Monocytopenia 288.59
Monocytosis (symptomatic) 288.63
Monofixation syndrome 378.34
Monomania — *see also* Psychosis 298.9
Mononeuritis 355.9
   cranial nerve — *see* Disorder, nerve, cranial
   femoral nerve 355.2
   lateral
      cutaneous nerve of thigh 355.1
      popliteal nerve 355.3
   lower limb 355.8
      specified nerve NEC 355.79
   medial popliteal nerve 355.4
   median nerve 354.1
   multiplex 354.5
   plantar nerve 355.6
   posterior tibial nerve 355.5
   radial nerve 354.3
   sciatic nerve 355.0
   ulnar nerve 354.2
   upper limb 354.9
      specified nerve NEC 354.8
   vestibular 388.5
Mononeuropathy — *see also* Mononeuritis 355.9
   diabetic NEC 250.6 ☑ *[355.9]*
      due to secondary diabetes 249.6 ☑ *[355.9]*
      lower limb 250.6 ☑ *[355.8]*
         due to secondary diabetes 249.6 ☑ *[355.8]*
      upper limb 250.6 ☑ *[354.9]*
         due to secondary diabetes 249.6 ☑ *[354.9]*
   iliohypogastric nerve 355.79
   ilioinguinal nerve 355.79
   obturator nerve 355.79
   saphenous nerve 355.79
Mononucleosis, infectious 075
   with hepatitis 075 *[573.1]*
Monoplegia 344.5
   brain (current episode) (*see also* Paralysis, brain) 437.8
      fetus or newborn 767.8
   cerebral (current episode) (*see also* Paralysis, brain) 437.8
   congenital or infantile (cerebral) (spastic) (spinal) 343.3
   embolic (current) (*see also* Embolism, brain) 434.1 ☑
      late effect — *see* Late effect(s) (of) cerebrovascular disease

Monoplegia — *continued*
   infantile (cerebral) (spastic) (spinal) 343.3
   lower limb 344.30
      affecting
         dominant side 344.31
         nondominant side 344.32
      due to late effect of cerebrovascular accident — *see* Late effect(s) (of) cerebrovascular accident
   newborn 767.8
   psychogenic 306.0
      specified as conversion reaction 300.11
   thrombotic (current) (*see also* Thrombosis, brain) 434.0 ☑
      late effect — *see* Late effect(s) (of) cerebrovascular disease
   transient 781.4
   upper limb 344.40
      affecting
         dominant side 344.41
         nondominant side 344.42
      due to late effect of cerebrovascular accident — *see* Late effect(s) (of) cerebrovascular accident
Monorchism, monorchidism 752.89
Monteggia's fracture (closed) 813.03
   open 813.13
Mood swings
   brief compensatory 296.99
   rebound 296.99
Mooren's ulcer (cornea) 370.07
Moore's syndrome — *see also* Epilepsy 345.5 ☑
Mooser-Neill reaction 081.0
Mooser bodies 081.0
Moral
   deficiency 301.7
   imbecility 301.7
Morax-Axenfeld conjunctivitis 372.03
Morbilli — *see also* Measles 055.9
Morbus
   anglicus, anglorum 268.0
   Beigel 111.2
   caducus (*see also* Epilepsy) 345.9 ☑
   caeruleus 746.89
   celiacus 579.0
   comitialis (see also Epilepsy) 345.9 ☑
   cordis (*see also* Disease, heart)
      valvulorum — *see* Endocarditis
   coxae 719.95
      tuberculous (*see also* Tuberculosis) 015.1 ☑
   hemorrhagicus neonatorum 776.0
   maculosus neonatorum 772.6
   renum 593.0
   senilis (*see also* Osteoarthrosis) 715.9 ☑
Morel-Kraepelin disease — *see also* Schizophrenia 295.9 ☑
Morel-Moore syndrome (hyperostosis frontalis interna) 733.3
Morel-Morgagni syndrome (hyperostosis frontalis interna) 733.3
Morgagni-Adams-Stokes syndrome (syncope with heart block) 426.9
Morgagni-Stewart-Morel syndrome (hyperostosis frontalis interna) 733.3
Morgagni
   cyst, organ, hydatid, or appendage 752.89
      fallopian tube 752.11
   disease or syndrome (hyperostosis frontalis interna) 733.3
Moria — *see also* Psychosis 298.9
Morning sickness 643.0 ☑
Moron 317
Morphea (guttate) (linear) 701.0
Morphine dependence — *see also* Dependence 304.0 ☑
Morphinism — *see also* Dependence 304.0 ☑
Morphinomania — *see also* Dependence 304.0 ☑
Morphoea 701.0
Morquio (-Brailsford) (-Ullrich) disease or syndrome (mucopolysaccharidosis IV) 277.5
   kyphosis 277.5

Morris syndrome (testicular feminization) 259.51
Morsus humanus (open wound) — *see also* Wound, open, by site
   skin surface intact — *see* Contusion
Mortification (dry) (moist) — *see also* Gangrene 785.4
Morton's
   disease 355.6
   foot 355.6
   metatarsalgia (syndrome) 355.6
   neuralgia 355.6
   neuroma 355.6
   syndrome (metatarsalgia) (neuralgia) 355.6
   toe 355.6
Morvan's disease 336.0
Mosaicism, mosaic (chromosomal) 758.9
   autosomal 758.5
   sex 758.81
Moschcowitz's syndrome (thrombotic thrombocytopenic purpura) 446.6
Mother yaw 102.0
Motion sickness (from travel, any vehicle) (from roundabouts or swings) 994.6
Mottled teeth (enamel) (endemic) (nonendemic) 520.3
Mottling enamel (endemic) (nonendemic) (teeth) 520.3
Mouchet's disease 732.5
Mould(s) (in vitreous) 117.9
Moulders'
   bronchitis 502
   tuberculosis (*see also* Tuberculosis) 011.4 ☑
Mounier-Kuhn syndrome 748.3
   with
      acute exacerbation 494.1
      bronchiectasis 494.0
         with (acute) exacerbation 494.1
   acquired 519.19
      with bronchiectasis 494.0
         with (acute) exacerbation 494.1
Mountain
   fever — *see* Fever, mountain
   sickness 993.2
      with polycythemia, acquired 289.0
      acute 289.0
   tick fever 066.1
Mouse, joint — *see also* Loose, body, joint 718.1 ☑
   knee 717.6
Mouth — *see* condition
Movable
   coccyx 724.71
   kidney (*see also* Disease, renal) 593.0
      congenital 753.3
   organ or site, congenital NEC — *see* Malposition, congenital
   spleen 289.59
Movement
   abnormal (dystonic) (involuntary) 781.0
   decreased fetal 655.7 ☑
   paradoxical facial 374.43
Moya Moya disease 437.5
Mozart's ear 744.29
MRSA (methicillin-resistant staphylococcus aureus) 041.12
   colonization V02.54
   personal history of V12.04
MSSA (methicillin susceptible staphylococcus aureus) 041.11
   colonization V02.53
Mu-chain disease 273.2
Mucha-Haberman syndrome (acute parapsoriasis varioliformis) 696.2
Mucha's disease (acute parapsoriasis varioliformis) 696.2
Mucinosis (cutaneous) (papular) 701.8
Mucocele
   appendix 543.9
   buccal cavity 528.9
   gallbladder (*see also* Disease, gallbladder) 575.3
   lacrimal sac 375.43
   orbit (eye) 376.81
   salivary gland (any) 527.6
   sinus (accessory) (nasal) 478.19

Mucocele — *continued*
   turbinate (bone) (middle) (nasal) 478.19
   uterus 621.8
Mucocutaneous lymph node syndrome (acute) (febrile) (infantile) 446.1
Mucoenteritis 564.9
Mucolipidosis I, II, III 272.7
Mucopolysaccharidosis (types 1-6) 277.5
   cardiopathy 277.5 *[425.7]*
Mucormycosis (lung) 117.7
Mucosa associated lymphoid tissue (MALT) 200.3 ☑
Mucositis — *see also* Inflammation, by site 528.00
   cervix (ulcerative) 616.81
   due to
      antineoplastic therapy (ulcerative) 528.01
      other drugs (ulcerative) 528.02
      specified NEC 528.09
   gastrointestinal (ulcerative) 538
   nasal (ulcerative) 478.11
   necroticans agranulocytica (*see also* Agranulocytosis) 288.09
   ulcerative 528.00
   vagina (ulcerative) 616.81
   vulva (ulcerative) 616.81
Mucous — *see also* condition
   patches (syphilitic) 091.3
      congenital 090.0
Mucoviscidosis 277.00
   with meconium obstruction 277.01
Mucus
   asphyxia or suffocation (*see also* Asphyxia, mucus) 933.1
      newborn 770.18
   in stool 792.1
   plug (*see also* Asphyxia, mucus) 933.1
      aspiration, of newborn 770.17
      tracheobronchial 519.19
         newborn 770.18
Muguet 112.0
Mulberry molars 090.5
Müllerian mixed tumor (M8950/3) — *see* Neoplasm, by site, malignant
Multicystic kidney 753.19
Multilobed placenta — *see* Placenta, abnormal
Multinodular prostate 600.10
   with
      urinary
         obstruction 600.11
         retention 600.11
Multiparity V61.5
   affecting
      fetus or newborn 763.89
      management of
         labor and delivery 659.4 ☑
         pregnancy V23.3
   requiring contraceptive management (*see also* Contraception) V25.9
Multipartita placenta — *see* Placenta, abnormal
Multiple, multiplex — *see also* condition
   birth
      affecting fetus or newborn 761.5
      healthy liveborn — *see* Newborn, multiple
   digits (congenital) 755.00
      fingers 755.01
      toes 755.02
   organ or site NEC — *see* Accessory
   personality 300.14
   renal arteries 747.62
Mumps 072.9
   with complication 072.8
      specified type NEC 072.79
   encephalitis 072.2
   hepatitis 072.71
   meningitis (aseptic) 072.1
   meningoencephalitis 072.2
   oophoritis 072.79
   orchitis 072.0
   pancreatitis 072.3
   polyneuropathy 072.72
   vaccination, prophylactic (against) V04.6

☑ **Additional Digit Required** — Refer to the Tabular List for Digit Selection   ▽ **Subterms under main terms may continue to next column or page**

Mumu — see also Infestation, filarial 125.9
Münchausen syndrome 301.51
Münchmeyer's disease or syndrome (exostosis luxurians) 728.11
Mural — see condition
Murmur (cardiac) (heart) (nonorganic) (organic) 785.2
  abdominal 787.5
  aortic (valve) (see also Endocarditis, aortic) 424.1
  benign — omit code
  cardiorespiratory 785.2
  diastolic — see condition
  Flint (see also Endocarditis, aortic) 424.1
  functional — omit code
  Graham Steell (pulmonic regurgitation) (see also Endocarditis, pulmonary) 424.3
  innocent — omit code
  insignificant — omit code
  midsystolic 785.2
  mitral (valve) — see Stenosis, mitral
  physiologic — see condition
  presystolic, mitral — see Insufficiency, mitral
  pulmonic (valve) (see also Endocarditis, pulmonary) 424.3
  Still's (vibratory) — omit code
  systolic (valvular) — see condition
  tricuspid (valve) — see Endocarditis, tricuspid
  undiagnosed 785.2
  valvular — see condition
  vibratory — omit code
Murri's disease (intermittent hemoglobinuria) 283.2
Muscae volitantes 379.24
Muscle, muscular — see condition
Musculoneuralgia 729.1
Mushrooming hip 718.95
Mushroom workers' (pickers') lung 495.5
Mutation(s)
  factor V Leiden 289.81
  prothrombin gene 289.81
  surfactant, of lung 516.63
Mutism — see also Aphasia 784.3
  akinetic 784.3
  deaf (acquired) (congenital) 389.7
  hysterical 300.11
  selective (elective) 313.23
    adjustment reaction 309.83
MVD (microvillus inclusion disease) 751.5
MVID (microvillus inclusion disease) 751.5
Myà's disease (congenital dilation, colon) 751.3
Myalgia (intercostal) 729.1
  eosinophilia syndrome 710.5
  epidemic 074.1
    cervical 078.89
  psychogenic 307.89
  traumatic NEC 959.9
Myasthenia 358.00
  cordis — see Failure, heart
  gravis 358.00
    with exacerbation (acute) 358.01
    in crisis 358.01
    neonatal 775.2
    pseudoparalytica 358.00
  stomach 536.8
    psychogenic 306.4
  syndrome
    in
      botulism 005.1 [358.1]
      diabetes mellitus 250.6 ☑ [358.1]
        due to secondary diabetes 249.6 ☑ [358.1]
      hypothyroidism (see also Hypothyroidism) 244.9 [358.1]
      malignant neoplasm NEC 199.1 [358.1]
      pernicious anemia 281.0 [358.1]
      thyrotoxicosis (see also Thyrotoxicosis) 242.9 ☑ [358.1]
Myasthenic 728.87
Mycelium infection NEC 117.9
Mycetismus 988.1
Mycetoma (actinomycotic) 039.9
  bone 039.8

Mycetoma — continued
  bone — continued
    mycotic 117.4
  foot 039.4
    mycotic 117.4
  madurae 039.9
    mycotic 117.4
  maduromycotic 039.9
    mycotic 117.4
  mycotic 117.4
  nocardial 039.9
Mycobacteriosis — see Mycobacterium
Mycobacterium, mycobacterial (infection) 031.9
  acid-fast (bacilli) 031.9
  anonymous (see also Mycobacterium, atypical) 031.9
  atypical (acid-fast bacilli) 031.9
    cutaneous 031.1
    pulmonary 031.0
      tuberculous (see also Tuberculosis, pulmonary) 011.9 ☑
    specified site NEC 031.8
  avium 031.0
    intracellulare complex bacteremia (MAC) 031.2
  balnei 031.1
  Battey 031.1
  cutaneous 031.1
  disseminated 031.2
    avium-intracellulare complex (DMAC) 031.2
  fortuitum 031.0
  intracellulare (battey bacillus) 031.0
  kakerifu 031.8
  kansasii 031.0
  kasongo 031.8
  leprae — see Leprosy
  luciflavum 031.0
  marinum 031.1
  pulmonary 031.0
    tuberculous (see also Tuberculosis, pulmonary) 011.9 ☑
  scrofulaceum 031.1
  tuberculosis (human, bovine) (see also Tuberculosis)
    avian type 031.0
  ulcerans 031.1
  xenopi 031.0
Mycosis, mycotic 117.9
  cutaneous NEC 111.9
  ear 111.8 [380.15]
  fungoides (M9700/3) 202.1 ☑
  mouth 112.0
  pharynx 117.9
  skin NEC 111.9
  stomatitis 112.0
  systemic NEC 117.9
  tonsil 117.9
  vagina, vaginitis 112.1
Mydriasis (persistent) (pupil) 379.43
Myelatelia 742.59
Myelinoclasis, perivascular, acute (postinfectious) NEC 136.9 [323.61]
  postimmunization or postvaccinal 323.51
Myelinosis, central pontine 341.8
Myelitis (ascending) (cerebellar) (childhood) (chronic) (descending) (diffuse) (disseminated) (pressure) (progressive) (spinal cord) (subacute) — see also Encephalitis 323.9
  acute (transverse) 341.20
    idiopathic 341.22
    in conditions classified elsewhere 341.21
  due to
    other infection classified elsewhere 136.9 [323.42]
    specified cause NEC 323.82
    vaccination (any) 323.52
    viral diseases classified elsewhere 323.02
  herpes simplex 054.74
  herpes zoster 053.14
  late effect — see category 326
  optic neuritis in 341.0
  postchickenpox 052.2
  postimmunization 323.52

Myelitis — see also Encephalitis — continued
  postinfectious 136.9 [323.63]
  postvaccinal 323.52
  postvaricella 052.2
  syphilitic (transverse) 094.89
  toxic 989.9 [323.72]
  transverse 323.82
    acute 341.20
      idiopathic 341.22
    in conditions classified elsewhere 341.21
    idiopathic 341.22
  tuberculous (see also Tuberculosis) 013.6 ☑
  virus 049.9
Myelo-osteo-musculodysplasia hereditaria 756.89
Myeloblastic — see condition
Myelocele — see also Spina bifida 741.9 ☑
  with hydrocephalus 741.0 ☑
Myelocystocele — see also Spina bifida 741.9 ☑
Myelocytic — see condition
Myelocytoma 205.1 ☑
Myelodysplasia (spinal cord) 742.59
  meaning myelodysplastic syndrome — see Syndrome, myelodysplastic
Myeloencephalitis — see Encephalitis
Myelofibrosis 289.83
  with myeloid metaplasia 238.76
  idiopathic (chronic) 238.76
  megakaryocytic 238.79
  primary 238.76
  secondary 289.83
Myelogenous — see condition
Myeloid — see condition
Myelokathexis 288.09
Myeloleukodystrophy 330.0
Myelolipoma (M8870/0) — see Neoplasm, by site, benign
Myeloma (multiple) (plasma cell) (plasmacytic) (M9730/3) 203.0 ☑
  monostotic (M9731/1) 238.6
  solitary (M9731/1) 238.6
Myelomalacia 336.8
Myelomata, multiple (M9730/3) 203.0 ☑
Myelomatosis (M9730/3) 203.0 ☑
Myelomeningitis — see Meningoencephalitis
Myelomeningocele (spinal cord) — see also Spina bifida 741.9 ☑
  fetal, causing fetopelvic disproportion 653.7 ☑
Myelopathic — see condition
Myelopathy (spinal cord) 336.9
  cervical 721.1
  diabetic 250.6 ☑ [336.3]
    due to secondary diabetes 249.6 ☑ [336.3]
  drug-induced 336.8
  due to or with
    carbon tetrachloride 987.8 [323.72]
    degeneration or displacement, intervertebral disc 722.70
      cervical, cervicothoracic 722.71
      lumbar, lumbosacral 722.73
      thoracic, thoracolumbar 722.72
    hydroxyquinoline derivatives 961.3 [323.72]
    infection — see Encephalitis
    intervertebral disc disorder 722.70
      cervical, cervicothoracic 722.71
      lumbar, lumbosacral 722.73
      thoracic, thoracolumbar 722.72
    lead 984.9 [323.72]
    mercury 985.0 [323.72]
    neoplastic disease (see also Neoplasm, by site) 239.9 [336.3]
    pernicious anemia 281.0 [336.3]
    spondylosis 721.91
      cervical 721.1
      lumbar, lumbosacral 721.42
      thoracic 721.41
    thallium 985.8 [323.72]
  lumbar, lumbosacral 721.42
  necrotic (subacute) 336.1
  radiation-induced 336.8

Myelopathy — continued
  spondylogenic NEC 721.91
    cervical 721.1
    lumbar, lumbosacral 721.42
    thoracic 721.41
  thoracic 721.41
  toxic NEC 989.9 [323.72]
  transverse (see also Myelitis) 323.82
  vascular 336.1
Myelophthisis 284.2
Myeloproliferative disease (M9960/1) 238.79
Myeloradiculitis — see also Polyneuropathy 357.0
Myeloradiculodysplasia (spinal) 742.59
Myelosarcoma (M9930/3) 205.3 ☑
Myelosclerosis 289.89
  with myeloid metaplasia (M9961/1) 238.76
  disseminated, of nervous system 340
  megakaryocytic (M9961/1) 238.79
Myelosis (M9860/3) — see also Leukemia, myeloid 205.9 ☑
  acute (M9861/3) 205.0 ☑
  aleukemic (M9864/3) 205.8 ☑
  chronic (M9863/3) 205.1 ☑
  erythremic (M9840/3) 207.0 ☑
    acute (M9841/3) 207.0 ☑
  megakaryocytic (M9920/3) 207.2 ☑
  nonleukemic (chronic) 288.8
  subacute (M9862/3) 205.2 ☑
Myesthenia — see Myasthenia
Myiasis (cavernous) 134.0
  orbit 134.0 [376.13]
Myoadenoma, prostate 600.20
  with
    other lower urinary tract symptoms (LUTS) 600.21
    urinary
      obstruction 600.21
      retention 600.21
Myoblastoma
  granular cell (M9580/0) (see also Neoplasm, connective tissue, benign)
    malignant (M9580/3) — see Neoplasm, connective tissue, malignant
  tongue (M9580/0) 210.1
Myocardial — see condition
Myocardiopathy (congestive) (constrictive) (familial) (idiopathic) (infiltrative) (obstructive) (primary) (restrictive) (sporadic) 425.4
  alcoholic 425.5
  amyloid 277.39 [425.7]
  beriberi 265.0 [425.7]
  cobalt-beer 425.5
  due to
    amyloidosis 277.39 [425.7]
    beriberi 265.0 [425.7]
    cardiac glycogenosis 271.0 [425.7]
    Chagas' disease 086.0
    Friedreich's ataxia 334.0 [425.8]
    influenza (see also Influenza) 487.8 [425.8]
    mucopolysaccharidosis 277.5 [425.7]
    myotonia atrophica 359.21 [425.8]
    progressive muscular dystrophy 359.1 [425.8]
    sarcoidosis 135 [425.8]
  glycogen storage 271.0 [425.7]
  hypertrophic 425.18
    nonobstructive 425.18
    obstructive 425.11
  metabolic NEC 277.9 [425.7]
  nutritional 269.9 [425.7]
  obscure (African) 425.2
  peripartum 674.5 ☑
  postpartum 674.5 ☑
  secondary 425.9
  thyrotoxic (see also Thyrotoxicosis) 242.9 ☑ [425.7]
  toxic NEC 425.9
Myocarditis (fibroid) (interstitial) (old) (progressive) (senile) (with arteriosclerosis) 429.0
  with
    rheumatic fever (conditions classifiable to 390) 398.0

☑ **Additional Digit Required** — Refer to the Tabular List for Digit Selection   ▽ **Subterms under main terms may continue to next column or page**

188 — Volume 2   ▶◀ Revised Text   ● New Line   ▲ Revised Code   **2014 ICD-9-CM**

Myocarditis — *continued*
  with — *continued*
    rheumatic fever — *continued*
      active (*see also* Myocarditis, acute, rheumatic) 391.2
      inactive or quiescent (with chorea) 398.0
  active (nonrheumatic) 422.90
    rheumatic 391.2
      with chorea (acute) (rheumatic) (Sydenham's) 392.0
  acute or subacute (interstitial) 422.90
    due to Streptococcus (beta-hemolytic) 391.2
    idiopathic 422.91
    rheumatic 391.2
      with chorea (acute) (rheumatic) (Sydenham's) 392.0
    specified type NEC 422.99
  aseptic of newborn 074.23
  bacterial (acute) 422.92
  chagasic 086.0
  chronic (interstitial) 429.0
  congenital 746.89
  constrictive 425.4
  Coxsackie (virus) 074.23
  diphtheritic 032.82
  due to or in
    Coxsackie (virus) 074.23
    diphtheria 032.82
    epidemic louse-borne typhus 080 *[422.0]*
    influenza (*see also* Influenza) 487.8 *[422.0]*
    Lyme disease 088.81 *[422.0]*
    scarlet fever 034.1 *[422.0]*
    toxoplasmosis (acquired) 130.3
    tuberculosis (*see also* Tuberculosis) 017.9 ☑ *[422.0]*
    typhoid 002.0 *[422.0]*
    typhus NEC 081.9 *[422.0]*
  eosinophilic 422.91
  epidemic of newborn 074.23
  Fiedler's (acute) (isolated) (subacute) 422.91
  giant cell (acute) (subacute) 422.91
  gonococcal 098.85
  granulomatous (idiopathic) (isolated) (nonspecific) 422.91
  hypertensive (*see also* Hypertension, heart) 402.90
  idiopathic 422.91
    granulomatous 422.91
  infective 422.92
  influenzal (*see also* Influenza) 487.8 *[422.0]*
  isolated (diffuse) (granulomatous) 422.91
  malignant 422.99
  meningococcal 036.43
  nonrheumatic, active 422.90
  parenchymatous 422.90
  pneumococcal (acute) (subacute) 422.92
  rheumatic (chronic) (inactive) (with chorea) 398.0
    active or acute 391.2
      with chorea (acute) (rheumatic) (Sydenham's) 392.0
  septic 422.92
  specific (giant cell) (productive) 422.91
  staphylococcal (acute) (subacute) 422.92
  suppurative 422.92
  syphilitic (chronic) 093.82
  toxic 422.93
    rheumatic (*see also* Myocarditis, acute rheumatic) 391.2
  tuberculous (*see also* Tuberculosis) 017.9 ☑ *[422.0]*
  typhoid 002.0 *[422.0]*
  valvular — *see* Endocarditis
  viral, except Coxsackie 422.91
    Coxsackie 074.23
    of newborn (Coxsackie) 074.23
Myocardium, myocardial — *see* condition
Myocardosis — *see also* Cardiomyopathy 425.4
Myoclonia (essential) 333.2
  epileptica 345.1 ☑
  Friedrich's 333.2
  massive 333.2

Myoclonic
  epilepsy, familial (progressive) 345.1 ☑
  jerks 333.2
Myoclonus (familial essential) (multifocal) (simplex) 333.2
  with epilepsy and with ragged red fibers (MERRF syndrome) 277.87
  facial 351.8
  massive (infantile) 333.2
  palatal 333.2
  pharyngeal 333.2
Myocytolysis 429.1
Myodiastasis 728.84
Myoendocarditis — *see also* Endocarditis
  acute or subacute 421.9
Myoepithelioma (M8982/0) — *see* Neoplasm, by site, benign
Myofascitis (acute) 729.1
  low back 724.2
Myofibroma (M8890/0) — *see also* Neoplasm, connective tissue, benign
  uterus (cervix) (corpus) (*see also* Leiomyoma) 218.9
Myofibromatosis
  infantile 759.89
Myofibrosis 728.2
  heart (*see also* Myocarditis) 429.0
  humeroscapular region 726.2
  scapulohumeral 726.2
Myofibrositis — *see also* Myositis 729.1
  scapulohumeral 726.2
Myogelosis (occupational) 728.89
Myoglobinuria 791.3
Myoglobulinuria, primary 791.3
Myokymia — *see also* Myoclonus
  facial 351.8
Myolipoma (M8860/0)
  specified site — *see* Neoplasm, connective tissue, benign
  unspecified site 223.0
Myoma (M8895/0) — *see also* Neoplasm, connective tissue, benign
  cervix (stump) (uterus) (*see also* Leiomyoma) 218.9
  malignant (M8895/3) — *see* Neoplasm, connective tissue, malignant
  prostate 600.20
    with
      other lower urinary tract symptoms (LUTS) 600.21
      urinary
        obstruction 600.21
        retention 600.21
  uterus (cervix) (corpus) (*see also* Leiomyoma) 218.9
    in pregnancy or childbirth 654.1 ☑
      affecting fetus or newborn 763.89
      causing obstructed labor 660.2 ☑
        affecting fetus or newborn 763.1
Myomalacia 728.9
  cordis, heart (*see also* Degeneration, myocardial) 429.1
Myometritis — *see also* Endometritis 615.9
Myometrium — *see* condition
Myonecrosis, clostridial 040.0
Myopathy 359.9
  alcoholic 359.4
  amyloid 277.39 *[359.6]*
  benign, congenital 359.0
  central core 359.0
  centronuclear 359.0
  congenital (benign) 359.0
  critical illness 359.81
  distal 359.1
  due to drugs 359.4
  endocrine 259.9 *[359.5]*
    specified type NEC 259.8 *[359.5]*
  extraocular muscles 376.82
  facioscapulohumeral 359.1
  in
    Addison's disease 255.41 *[359.5]*
    amyloidosis 277.39 *[359.6]*
    cretinism 243 *[359.5]*
    Cushing's syndrome 255.0 *[359.5]*
    disseminated lupus erythematosus 710.0 *[359.6]*

Myopathy — *continued*
  in — *continued*
    giant cell arteritis 446.5 *[359.6]*
    hyperadrenocorticism NEC 255.3 *[359.5]*
    hyperparathyroidism 252.01 *[359.5]*
    hypopituitarism 253.2 *[359.5]*
    hypothyroidism (*see also* Hypothyroidism) 244.9 *[359.5]*
    malignant neoplasm NEC (M8000/3) 199.1 *[359.6]*
    myxedema (*see also* Myxedema) 244.9 *[359.5]*
    polyarteritis nodosa 446.0 *[359.6]*
    rheumatoid arthritis 714.0 *[359.6]*
    sarcoidosis 135 *[359.6]*
    scleroderma 710.1 *[359.6]*
    Sjögren's disease 710.2 *[359.6]*
    thyrotoxicosis (*see also* Thyrotoxicosis) 242.9 ☑ *[359.5]*
  inflammatory 359.79
    immune NEC 359.79
    specified NEC 359.79
  intensive care (ICU) 359.81
  limb-girdle 359.1
  myotubular 359.0
  necrotizing, acute 359.81
  nemaline 359.0
  ocular 359.1
  oculopharyngeal 359.1
  of critical illness 359.81
  primary 359.89
  progressive NEC 359.89
  proximal myotonic (PROMM) 359.21
  quadriplegic, acute 359.81
  rod body 359.0
  scapulohumeral 359.1
  specified type NEC 359.89
  toxic 359.4
Myopericarditis — *see also* Pericarditis 423.9
Myopia (axial) (congenital) (increased curvature or refraction, nucleus of lens) 367.1
  degenerative, malignant 360.21
  malignant 360.21
  progressive high (degenerative) 360.21
Myosarcoma (M8895/3) — *see* Neoplasm, connective tissue, malignant
Myosis (persistent) 379.42
  stromal (endolymphatic) (M8931/1) 236.0
Myositis 729.1
  clostridial 040.0
  due to posture 729.1
  epidemic 074.1
  fibrosa or fibrous (chronic) 728.2
    Volkmann's (complicating trauma) 958.6
  inclusion body (IBM) 359.71
  infective 728.0
  interstitial 728.81
  multiple — *see* Polymyositis
  occupational 729.1
  orbital, chronic 376.12
  ossificans 728.12
    circumscribed 728.12
    progressive 728.11
    traumatic 728.12
  progressive fibrosing 728.11
  purulent 728.0
  rheumatic 729.1
  rheumatoid 729.1
  suppurative 728.0
  syphilitic 095.6
  traumatic (old) 729.1
Myospasia impulsiva 307.23
Myotonia (acquisita) (intermittens) 728.85
  atrophica 359.21
  congenita 359.22
    acetazolamide responsive 359.22
    dominant form 359.22
    recessive form 359.22
  drug-induced 359.24
  dystrophica 359.21
  fluctuans 359.29
  levior 359.22
  permanens 359.29
Myotonic pupil 379.46
Myriapodiasis 134.1

Myringitis
  with otitis media — *see* Otitis media
  acute 384.00
    specified type NEC 384.09
  bullosa hemorrhagica 384.01
  bullous 384.01
  chronic 384.1
Mysophobia 300.29
Mytilotoxism 988.0
Myxadenitis labialis 528.5
Myxedema (adult) (idiocy) (infantile) (juvenile) (thyroid gland) — *see also* Hypothyroidism 244.9
  circumscribed 242.9 ☑
  congenital 243
  cutis 701.8
  localized (pretibial) 242.9 ☑
  madness (acute) 293.0
    subacute 293.1
  papular 701.8
  pituitary 244.8
  postpartum 674.8 ☑
  pretibial 242.9 ☑
  primary 244.9
Myxochondrosarcoma (M9220/3) — *see* Neoplasm, cartilage, malignant
Myxofibroma (M8811/0) — *see also* Neoplasm, connective tissue, benign
  odontogenic (M9320/0) 213.1
  upper jaw (bone) 213.0
Myxofibrosarcoma (M8811/3) — *see* Neoplasm, connective tissue, malignant
Myxolipoma (M8852/0) — *see also* Lipoma, by site 214.9
Myxoliposarcoma (M8852/3) — *see* Neoplasm, connective tissue, malignant
Myxoma (M8840/0) — *see also* Neoplasm, connective tissue, benign
  odontogenic (M9320/0) 213.1
  upper jaw (bone) 213.0
Myxosarcoma (M8840/3) — *see* Neoplasm, connective tissue, malignant

N

Naegeli's
  disease (hereditary hemorrhagic thrombasthenia) 287.1
  leukemia, monocytic (M9863/3) 205.1 ☑
  syndrome (incontinentia pigmenti) 757.33
Naffziger's syndrome 353.0
Naga sore — *see also* Ulcer, skin 707.9
Nägele's pelvis 738.6
  with disproportion (fetopelvic) 653.0 ☑
    affecting fetus or newborn 763.1
    causing obstructed labor 660.1 ☑
      affecting fetus or newborn 763.1
Nager-de Reynier syndrome (dysostosis mandibularis) 756.0
Nail — *see also* condition
  biting 307.9
  patella syndrome (hereditary osteoonychodysplasia) 756.89
Nanism, nanosomia — *see also* Dwarfism 259.4
  hypophyseal 253.3
  pituitary 253.3
  renis, renalis 588.0
Nanukayami 100.89
Napkin rash 691.0
Narcissism 301.81
Narcolepsy 347.00
  with cataplexy 347.01
  in conditions classified elsewhere 347.10
    with cataplexy 347.11
Narcosis
  carbon dioxide (respiratory) 786.09
  due to drug
    correct substance properly administered 780.09
    overdose or wrong substance given or taken 977.9
      specified drug — *see* Table of Drugs and Chemicals
Narcotism (chronic) — *see also* Dependence 304.9 ☑

☑ **Additional Digit Required** — Refer to the Tabular List for Digit Selection   ▽ **Subterms under main terms may continue to next column or page**

2014 ICD-9-CM   ▶◀ **Revised Text**   ● **New Line**   ▲ **Revised Code**   **Volume 2 — 189**

Narcotism (chronic) — see also Dependence
— continued
  acute
    correct substance properly administered 349.82
    overdose or wrong substance given or taken 967.8
      specified drug — see Table of Drugs and Chemicals
NARP (ataxia and retinitis pigmentosa) 277.87
Narrow
  anterior chamber angle 365.02
  pelvis (inlet) (outlet) — see Contraction, pelvis
Narrowing
  artery NEC 447.1
    auditory, internal 433.8 ☑
    basilar 433.0 ☑
      with other precerebral artery 433.3 ☑
        bilateral 433.3 ☑
    carotid 433.1 ☑
      with other precerebral artery 433.3 ☑
        bilateral 433.3 ☑
    cerebellar 433.8 ☑
    choroidal 433.8 ☑
    communicating posterior 433.8 ☑
    coronary (see also Arteriosclerosis, coronary)
      congenital 746.85
      due to syphilis 090.5
    hypophyseal 433.8 ☑
    pontine 433.8 ☑
    precerebral NEC 433.9 ☑
      multiple or bilateral 433.3 ☑
      specified NEC 433.8 ☑
    vertebral 433.2 ☑
      with other precerebral artery 433.3 ☑
        bilateral 433.3 ☑
  auditory canal (external) (see also Stricture, ear canal, acquired) 380.50
  cerebral arteries 437.0
  cicatricial — see Cicatrix
  congenital — see Anomaly, congenital
  coronary artery — see Narrowing, artery, coronary
  ear, middle 385.22
  Eustachian tube (see also Obstruction, Eustachian tube) 381.60
  eyelid 374.46
    congenital 743.62
  intervertebral disc or space NEC — see Degeneration, intervertebral disc
  joint space, hip 719.85
  larynx 478.74
  lids 374.46
    congenital 743.62
  mesenteric artery (with gangrene) 557.0
  palate 524.89
  palpebral fissure 374.46
  retinal artery 362.13
  ureter 593.3
  urethra (see also Stricture, urethra) 598.9
Narrowness, abnormal, eyelid 743.62
Nasal — see condition
Nasolacrimal — see condition
Nasopharyngeal — see also condition
  bursa 478.29
  pituitary gland 759.2
  torticollis 723.5
Nasopharyngitis (acute) (infective) (subacute) 460
  chronic 472.2
    due to external agent — see Condition, respiratory, chronic, due to
  due to external agent — see Condition, respiratory, due to
  septic 034.0
  streptococcal 034.0
  suppurative (chronic) 472.2
  ulcerative (chronic) 472.2
Nasopharynx, nasopharyngeal — see condition
Natal tooth, teeth 520.6

Nausea — see also Vomiting 787.02
  with vomiting 787.01
  epidemic 078.82
  gravidarum — see Hyperemesis, gravidarum
  marina 994.6
Navel — see condition
Neapolitan fever — see also Brucellosis 023.9
Near-syncope 780.2
Near drowning 994.1
Nearsightedness 367.1
Nebécourt's syndrome 253.3
Nebula, cornea (eye) 371.01
  congenital 743.43
    interfering with vision 743.42
Necator americanus infestation 126.1
Necatoriasis 126.1
Neck — see condition
Necrencephalus — see also Softening, brain 437.8
Necrobacillosis 040.3
Necrobiosis 799.89
  brain or cerebral (see also Softening, brain) 437.8
  lipoidica 709.3
    diabeticorum 250.8 ☑ [709.3]
      due to secondary diabetes 249.8 ☑ [709.3]
Necrodermolysis 695.15
Necrolysis, toxic epidermal 695.15
  due to drug
    correct substance properly administered 695.15
    overdose or wrong substance given or taken 977.9
      specified drug — see Table of Drugs and Chemicals
  Stevens-Johnson syndrome overlap (SJS-TEN overlap syndrome) 695.14
Necrophilia 302.89
Necrosis, necrotic
  adrenal (capsule) (gland) 255.8
  antrum, nasal sinus 478.19
  aorta (hyaline) (see also Aneurysm, aorta) 441.9
    cystic medial 441.00
      abdominal 441.02
      thoracic 441.01
      thoracoabdominal 441.03
    ruptured 441.5
  arteritis 446.0
  artery 447.5
  aseptic, bone 733.40
    femur (head) (neck) 733.42
      medial condyle 733.43
    humoral head 733.41
    jaw 733.45
    medial femoral condyle 733.43
    specific site NEC 733.49
    talus 733.44
  avascular, bone NEC (see also Necrosis, aseptic, bone) 733.40
  bladder (aseptic) (sphincter) 596.89
  bone (see also Osteomyelitis) 730.1 ☑
    acute 730.0 ☑
    aseptic or avascular 733.40
      femur (head) (neck) 733.42
        medial condyle 733.43
      humoral head 733.41
      jaw 733.45
      medial femoral condyle 733.43
      specified site NEC 733.49
      talus 733.44
    ethmoid 478.19
    ischemic 733.40
    jaw 526.4
      aseptic 733.45
    marrow 289.89
    Paget's (osteitis deformans) 731.0
    tuberculous — see Tuberculosis, bone
  brain (softening) (see also Softening, brain) 437.8
  breast (aseptic) (fat) (segmental) 611.3
  bronchus, bronchi 519.19
  central nervous system NEC (see also Softening, brain) 437.8
  cerebellar (see also Softening, brain) 437.8

Necrosis, necrotic — continued
  cerebral (softening) (see also Softening, brain) 437.8
  cerebrospinal (softening) (see also Softening, brain) 437.8
  colon 557.0
  cornea (see also Keratitis) 371.40
  cortical, kidney 583.6
  cystic medial (aorta) 441.00
    abdominal 441.02
    thoracic 441.01
    thoracoabdominal 441.03
  dental 521.09
    pulp 522.1
  due to swallowing corrosive substance — see Burn, by site
  ear (ossicle) 385.24
  esophagus 530.89
  ethmoid (bone) 478.19
  eyelid 374.50
  fat, fatty (generalized) (see also Degeneration, fatty) 272.8
    abdominal wall 567.82
    breast (aseptic) (segmental) 611.3
    intestine 569.89
    localized — see Degeneration, by site, fatty
    mesentery 567.82
    omentum 567.82
    pancreas 577.8
    peritoneum 567.82
    skin (subcutaneous) 709.3
      newborn 778.1
  femur (aseptic) (avascular) 733.42
    head 733.42
    medial condyle 733.43
    neck 733.42
  gallbladder (see also Cholecystitis, acute) 575.0
  gangrenous 785.4
  gastric 537.89
  glottis 478.79
  heart (myocardium) — see Infarct, myocardium
  hepatic (see also Necrosis, liver) 570
  hip (aseptic) (avascular) 733.42
  intestine (acute) (hemorrhagic) (massive) 557.0
  ischemic 785.4
  jaw 526.4
    aseptic 733.45
  kidney (bilateral) 583.9
    acute 584.9
    cortical 583.6
      acute 584.6
        with
          abortion — see Abortion, by type, with renal failure
          ectopic pregnancy (see also categories 633.0–633.9) 639.3
          molar pregnancy (see also categories 630–632) 639.3
        complicating pregnancy 646.2 ☑
          affecting fetus or newborn 760.1
        following labor and delivery 669.3 ☑
    medullary (papillary) (see also Pyelitis) 590.80
      in
        acute renal failure 584.7
        nephritis, nephropathy 583.7
    papillary (see also Pyelitis) 590.80
      in
        acute renal failure 584.7
        nephritis, nephropathy 583.7
    tubular 584.5
      with
        abortion — see Abortion, by type, with renal failure
        ectopic pregnancy (see also categories 633.0–633.9) 639.3
        molar pregnancy (see also categories 630–632) 639.3

Necrosis, necrotic — continued
  kidney — continued
    tubular — continued
      complicating
        abortion 639.3
        ectopic or molar pregnancy 639.3
        pregnancy 646.2 ☑
          affecting fetus or newborn 760.1
      following labor and delivery 669.3 ☑
      traumatic 958.5
  larynx 478.79
  liver (acute) (congenital) (diffuse) (massive) (subacute) 570
    with
      abortion — see Abortion, by type, with specified complication NEC
      ectopic pregnancy (see also categories 633.0–633.9) 639.8
      molar pregnancy (see also categories 630–632) 639.8
    complicating pregnancy 646.7 ☑
      affecting fetus or newborn 760.8
    following
      abortion 639.8
      ectopic or molar pregnancy 639.8
    obstetrical 646.7 ☑
    postabortal 639.8
    puerperal, postpartum 674.8 ☑
    toxic 573.3
  lung 513.0
  lymphatic gland 683
  mammary gland 611.3
  mastoid (chronic) 383.1
  mesentery 557.0
    fat 567.82
  mitral valve — see Insufficiency, mitral
  myocardium, myocardial — see Infarct, myocardium
  nose (septum) 478.19
  omentum 557.0
    with mesenteric infarction 557.0
    fat 567.82
  orbit, orbital 376.10
  ossicles, ear (aseptic) 385.24
  ovary (see also Salpingo-oophoritis) 614.2
  pancreas (aseptic) (duct) (fat) 577.8
    acute 577.0
    infective 577.0
  papillary, kidney (see also Pyelitis) 590.80
  perineum 624.8
  peritoneum 557.0
    with mesenteric infarction 557.0
    fat 567.82
  pharynx 462
    in granulocytopenia 288.09
  phosphorus 983.9
  pituitary (gland) (postpartum) (Sheehan) 253.2
  placenta (see also Placenta, abnormal) 656.7 ☑
  pneumonia 513.0
  pulmonary 513.0
  pulp (dental) 522.1
  pylorus 537.89
  radiation — see Necrosis, by site
  radium — see Necrosis, by site
  renal — see Necrosis, kidney
  sclera 379.19
  scrotum 608.89
  skin or subcutaneous tissue 709.8
    due to burn — see Burn, by site
    gangrenous 785.4
  spine, spinal (column) 730.18
    acute 730.18
    cord 336.1
  spleen 289.59
  stomach 537.89
  stomatitis 528.1
  subcutaneous fat 709.3
    fetus or newborn 778.1
  subendocardial — see Infarct, myocardium
  suprarenal (capsule) (gland) 255.8
  teeth, tooth 521.09
  testis 608.89

☑ **Additional Digit Required** — Refer to the Tabular List for Digit Selection   ⩗ **Subterms under main terms may continue to next column or page**

Character Analysis Comp II 9-4-13

Consider: (to support)

- name
- Appearance
- Actions
- speech
- Thoughts + feelings
- Past/bio

Character traits

- manipulative
- selfish
- cold-hearted
- deceiving
- obnoxious
- promiscous
- world-wise
- stubborn

Essay   Thesis - last
                     sentence

I. Introduction (1 paragraph)
    A. Lead (hook)
        1. Background info (general truth)
        2. Appropriate passage from text
        3. Definition
        4. Question *
        5. Quotation from secondary source
        6. Startling statement

Potential techniques }

long ones ↓
↓ ←
(Italics or) B. "Title" + Author - (use ~~one~~ entire name) use last
  quotes   name
↓
short
stories   C. Brief summary - plot (overview) (2-4 lines)
           D. Thesis statement - only (1)
               1. 3 traits ☆
               2. 3 methods

II. Body (3 paragraphs)
        A. Topic sentence   1.) one trait
        B. Introduce quote
        C. Quotation
(3-5)   D. Analyze quotation (most important) your explanation
        E. Transition ~~quote~~
        F. Introduce quote
        G. Quotation
        H. Analyze

III Conclusion (1) (summary)
  A. restate thesis
  B. review key points
  C. Clincher - ~~leave readers with~~

3 good clinchers
  - what can we learn from this character
  - circle back to the lead
  - bring in title, + play with the words,
    how it describes the story.

Necrosis, necrotic — *continued*
    thymus (gland) 254.8
    tonsil 474.8
    trachea 519.19
    tuberculous NEC — *see* Tuberculosis
    tubular (acute) (anoxic) (toxic) 584.5
        due to a procedure 997.5
    umbilical cord, affecting fetus or newborn
        762.6
    vagina 623.8
    vertebra (lumbar) 730.18
        acute 730.18
        tuberculous (*see also* Tuberculosis)
            015.0 ☑ *[730.8]* ☑
    vesical (aseptic) (bladder) 596.89
    vulva 624.8

Necrosis, necrotic — *continued*
    x-ray — *see* Necrosis, by site
Necrospermia 606.0
Necrotizing angiitis 446.0
Negativism 301.7
Neglect (child) (newborn) NEC 995.52
    adult 995.84
    after or at birth 995.52
    hemispatial 781.8
    left-sided 781.8
    sensory 781.8
    visuospatial 781.8
Negri bodies 071
Neill-Dingwall syndrome (microcephaly and
    dwarfism) 759.89
Neisserian infection NEC — *see* Gonococcus

Nematodiasis NEC — *see also* Infestation, Ne-
    matode 127.9
    ancylostoma (*see also* Ancylostomiasis)
        126.9
Neoformans cryptococcus infection 117.5
Neonatal — *see also* condition
    abstinence syndrome 779.5
    adrenoleukodystrophy 277.86
    teeth, tooth 520.6
Neonatorum — *see* condition
Neoplasia
    anal intraepithelial I (AIN I) (histologically
        confirmed) 569.44
    anal intraepithelial II (AIN II) (histologically
        confirmed) 569.44
    anal intraepithelial III (AIN III) 230.6

Neoplasia — *continued*
    anal intraepithelial III — *continued*
        anal canal 230.5
    endometrial intraepithelial (EIN) 621.35
    multiple endocrine (MEN)
        type I 258.01
        type IIA 258.02
        type IIB 258.03
    vaginal intraepithelial I (VAIN I) 623.0
    vaginal intraepithelial II (VAIN II) 623.0
    vaginal intraepithelial III (VAIN III) 233.31
    vulvular intraepithelial I (VIN I) 624.01
    vulvular intraepithelial II (VIN II) 624.02
    vulvular intraepithelial III (VIN III) 233.32

☑ **Additional Digit Required** — Refer to the Tabular List for Digit Selection   ▽ **Subterms under main terms may continue to next column or page**

2014 ICD-9-CM   ▶◀ **Revised Text**   ● **New Line**   ▲ **Revised Code**   **Volume 2 — 191**

	Malignant — Primary	Malignant — Secondary	Malignant — Ca in situ	Benign	Uncertain Behavior	Unspecified
Neoplasm, neoplastic	199.1	—	234.9	229.9	238.9	239.9

> Notes — 1. The list below gives the code numbers for neoplasms by anatomical site. For each site there are six possible code numbers according to whether the neoplasm in question is malignant, benign, in situ, of uncertain behavior, or of unspecified nature. The description of the neoplasm will often indicate which of the six columns is appropriate; e.g., malignant melanoma of skin, benign fibroadenoma of breast, carcinoma in situ of cervix uteri.
>
> Where such descriptors are not present, the remainder of the Index should be consulted where guidance is given to the appropriate column for each morphological (histological) variety listed; e.g., Mesonephroma — see Neoplasm, malignant; Embryoma — see also Neoplasm, uncertain behavior; Disease, Bowen's — see Neoplasm, skin, in situ. However, the guidance in the Index can be overridden if one of the descriptors mentioned above is present; e.g., malignant adenoma of colon is coded to 153.9 and not to 211.3 as the adjective "malignant" overrides the Index entry "Adenoma — see also Neoplasm, benign."
>
> 2. Sites marked with the sign * (e.g., face NEC*) should be classified to malignant neoplasm of skin of these sites if the variety of neoplasm is a squamous cell carcinoma or an epidermoid carcinoma, and to benign neoplasm of skin of these sites if the variety of neoplasm is a papilloma (any type).

	Malignant — Primary	Malignant — Secondary	Malignant — Ca in situ	Benign	Uncertain Behavior	Unspecified
abdomen, abdominal	195.2	198.89	234.8	229.8	238.8	239.89
cavity	195.2	198.89	234.8	229.8	238.8	239.89
organ	195.2	198.89	234.8	229.8	238.8	239.89
viscera	195.2	198.89	234.8	229.8	238.8	239.89
wall	173.50	198.2	232.5	216.5	238.2	239.2
basal cell carcinoma	173.51	—	—	—	—	—
connective tissue	171.5	198.89	—	215.5	238.1	239.2
specified type NEC	173.59	—	—	—	—	—
squamous cell carcinoma	173.52	—	—	—	—	—
abdominopelvic	195.8	198.89	234.8	229.8	238.8	239.89
accessory sinus — see Neoplasm, sinus						
acoustic nerve	192.0	198.4	—	225.1	237.9	239.7
acromion (process)	170.4	198.5	—	213.4	238.0	239.2
adenoid (pharynx) (tissue)	147.1	198.89	230.0	210.7	235.1	239.0
adipose tissue (see also Neoplasm, connective tissue)	171.9	198.89	—	215.9	238.1	239.2
adnexa (uterine)	183.9	198.82	233.39	221.8	236.3	239.5
adrenal (cortex) (gland) (medulla)	194.0	198.7	234.8	227.0	237.2	239.7
ala nasi (external)	173.30	198.2	232.3	216.3	238.2	239.2
alimentary canal or tract NEC	159.9	197.8	230.9	211.9	235.5	239.0
alveolar	143.9	198.89	230.0	210.4	235.1	239.0
mucosa	143.9	198.89	230.0	210.4	235.1	239.0
lower	143.1	198.89	230.0	210.4	235.1	239.0
upper	143.0	198.89	230.0	210.4	235.1	239.0
ridge or process	170.1	198.5	—	213.1	238.0	239.2
carcinoma	143.9	—	—	—	—	—
lower	143.1	—	—	—	—	—
upper	143.0	—	—	—	—	—
lower	170.1	198.5	—	213.1	238.0	239.2
mucosa	143.9	198.89	230.0	210.4	235.1	239.0
lower	143.1	198.89	230.0	210.4	235.1	239.0
upper	143.0	198.89	230.0	210.4	235.1	239.0
upper	170.0	198.5	—	213.0	238.0	239.2
sulcus	145.1	198.89	230.0	210.4	235.1	239.0
alveolus	143.9	198.89	230.0	210.4	235.1	239.0
lower	143.1	198.89	230.0	210.4	235.1	239.0
upper	143.0	198.89	230.0	210.4	235.1	239.0
ampulla of Vater	156.2	197.8	230.8	211.5	235.3	239.0
ankle NEC*	195.5	198.89	232.7	229.8	238.8	239.89
anorectum, anorectal (junction)	154.8	197.5	230.7	211.4	235.2	239.0
antecubital fossa or space*	195.4	198.89	232.6	229.8	238.8	239.89
Neoplasm, neoplastic — continued						
antrum (Highmore) (maxillary)	160.2	197.3	231.8	212.0	235.9	239.1
pyloric	151.2	197.8	230.2	211.1	235.2	239.0
tympanicum	160.1	197.3	231.8	212.0	235.9	239.1
anus, anal	154.3	197.5	230.6	211.4	235.5	239.0
canal	154.2	197.5	230.5	211.4	235.5	239.0
contiguous sites with rectosigmoid junction or rectum	154.8	—	—	—	—	—
margin (see also Neoplasm, anus, skin)	173.50	198.2	232.5	216.6	238.2	239.2
skin	173.50	198.2	232.5	216.5	238.2	239.2
basal cell carcinoma	173.51	—	—	—	—	—
specified type NEC	173.59	—	—	—	—	—
squamous cell carcinoma	173.52	—	—	—	—	—
sphincter	154.2	197.5	230.5	211.4	235.5	239.0
aorta (thoracic)	171.4	198.89	—	215.4	238.1	239.2
abdominal	171.5	198.89	—	215.5	238.1	239.2
aortic body	194.6	198.89	—	227.6	237.3	239.7
aponeurosis	171.9	198.89	—	215.9	238.1	239.2
palmar	171.2	198.89	—	215.2	238.1	239.2
plantar	171.3	198.89	—	215.3	238.1	239.2
appendix	153.5	197.5	230.3	211.3	235.2	239.0
arachnoid (cerebral)	192.1	198.4	—	225.2	237.6	239.7
spinal	192.3	198.4	—	225.4	237.6	239.7
areola (female)	174.0	198.81	233.0	217	238.3	239.3
male	175.0	198.81	233.0	217	238.3	239.3
arm NEC*	195.4	198.89	232.6	229.8	238.8	239.89
artery — see Neoplasm, connective tissue						
aryepiglottic fold	148.2	198.89	230.0	210.8	235.1	239.0
hypopharyngeal aspect	148.2	198.89	230.0	210.8	235.1	239.0
laryngeal aspect	161.1	197.3	231.0	212.1	235.6	239.1
marginal zone	148.2	198.89	230.0	210.8	235.1	239.0
arytenoid (cartilage)	161.3	197.3	231.0	212.1	235.6	239.1
fold — see Neoplasm, aryepiglottic						
associated with transplanted organ	199.2	—	—	—	—	—
atlas	170.2	198.5	—	213.2	238.0	239.2
atrium, cardiac	164.1	198.89	—	212.7	238.8	239.89
auditory						
canal (external) (skin) (see also Neoplasm, skin, ear)	173.20	198.2	232.2	216.2	238.2	239.2
internal	160.1	197.3	231.8	212.0	235.9	239.1
nerve	192.0	198.4	—	225.1	237.9	239.7
tube	160.1	197.3	231.8	212.0	235.9	239.1
Eustachian	160.1	197.3	231.8	212.0	235.9	239.1
opening	147.2	198.89	230.0	210.7	235.1	239.0
auricle, ear see also Neoplasm, skin, ear	173.20	198.2	232.2	216.2	238.2	239.2
cartilage	171.0	198.89	—	215.0	238.1	239.2
auricular canal (external) (see also Neoplasm, skin, ear)	173.20	198.2	232.2	216.2	238.2	239.2
internal	160.1	197.3	231.8	212.0	235.9	239.1
autonomic nerve or nervous system NEC	171.9	198.89	—	215.9	238.1	239.2
axilla, axillary	195.1	198.89	234.8	229.8	238.8	239.89
fold (see also Neoplasm, skin, trunk)	173.50	198.2	232.5	216.5	238.2	239.2

☑ Additional Digit Required — Refer to the Tabular List for Digit Selection ▽ Subterms under main terms may continue to next column or page

	Malignant					
	Primary	Secondary	Ca in situ	Benign	Uncertain Behavior	Unspecified
Neoplasm, neoplastic— *continued*						
back NEC*	195.8	198.89	232.5	229.8	238.8	239.89
Bartholin's gland	184.1	198.82	233.32	221.2	236.3	239.5
basal ganglia	191.0	198.3	—	225.0	237.5	239.6
basis pedunculi	191.7	198.3	—	225.0	237.5	239.6
bile or biliary (tract)	156.9	197.8	230.8	211.5	235.3	239.0
canaliculi (biliferi) (intrahepatic)	155.1	197.8	230.8	211.5	235.3	239.0
canals, interlobular	155.1	197.8	230.8	211.5	235.3	239.0
contiguous sites	156.8	—	—	—	—	—
duct or passage (common) (cystic) (extrahepatic)	156.1	197.8	230.8	211.5	235.3	239.0
contiguous sites with gallbladder	156.8	—	—	—	—	—
interlobular	155.1	197.8	230.8	211.5	235.3	239.0
intrahepatic	155.1	197.8	230.8	211.5	235.3	239.0
and extrahepatic	156.9	197.8	230.8	211.5	235.3	239.0
bladder (urinary)	188.9	198.1	233.7	223.3	236.7	239.4
contiguous sites	188.8	—	—	—	—	—
dome	188.1	198.1	233.7	223.3	236.7	239.4
neck	188.5	198.1	233.7	223.3	236.7	239.4
orifice	188.9	198.1	233.7	223.3	236.7	239.4
ureteric	188.6	198.1	233.7	223.3	236.7	239.4
urethral	188.5	198.1	233.7	223.3	236.7	239.4
sphincter	188.8	198.1	233.7	223.3	236.7	239.4
trigone	188.0	198.1	233.7	223.3	236.7	239.4
urachus	188.7	—	233.7	223.3	236.7	239.4
wall	188.9	198.1	233.7	223.3	236.7	239.4
anterior	188.3	198.1	233.7	223.3	236.7	239.4
lateral	188.2	198.1	233.7	223.3	236.7	239.4
posterior	188.4	198.1	233.7	223.3	236.7	239.4
blood vessel — *see* Neoplasm, connective tissue						
bone (periosteum)	170.9	198.5	—	213.9	238.0	239.2

Note — Carcinomas and adenocarcinomas, of any type other than intraosseous or odontogenic, of the sites listed under "Neoplasm, bone" should be considered as constituting metastatic spread from an unspecified primary site and coded to 198.5 for morbidity coding.

	Malignant					
	Primary	Secondary	Ca in situ	Benign	Uncertain Behavior	Unspecified
acetabulum	170.6	198.5	—	213.6	238.0	239.2
acromion (process)	170.4	198.5	—	213.4	238.0	239.2
ankle	170.8	198.5	—	213.8	238.0	239.2
arm NEC	170.4	198.5	—	213.4	238.0	239.2
astragalus	170.8	198.5	—	213.8	238.0	239.2
atlas	170.2	198.5	—	213.2	238.0	239.2
axis	170.2	198.5	—	213.2	238.0	239.2
back NEC	170.2	198.5	—	213.2	238.0	239.2
calcaneus	170.8	198.5	—	213.8	238.0	239.2
calvarium	170.0	198.5	—	213.0	238.0	239.2
carpus (any)	170.5	198.5	—	213.5	238.0	239.2
cartilage NEC	170.9	198.5	—	213.9	238.0	239.2
clavicle	170.3	198.5	—	213.3	238.0	239.2
clivus	170.0	198.5	—	213.0	238.0	239.2
coccygeal vertebra	170.6	198.5	—	213.6	238.0	239.2
coccyx	170.6	198.5	—	213.6	238.0	239.2
costal cartilage	170.3	198.5	—	213.3	238.0	239.2
costovertebral joint	170.3	198.5	—	213.3	238.0	239.2
cranial	170.0	198.5	—	213.0	238.0	239.2
cuboid	170.8	198.5	—	213.8	238.0	239.2
cuneiform	170.9	198.5	—	213.9	238.0	239.2
ankle	170.8	198.5	—	213.8	238.0	239.2
wrist	170.5	198.5	—	213.5	238.0	239.2
digital	170.9	198.5	—	213.9	238.0	239.2
finger	170.5	198.5	—	213.5	238.0	239.2
toe	170.8	198.5	—	213.8	238.0	239.2

	Malignant					
	Primary	Secondary	Ca in situ	Benign	Uncertain Behavior	Unspecified
Neoplasm, neoplastic— *continued* bone — *continued*						
elbow	170.4	198.5	—	213.4	238.0	239.2
ethmoid (labyrinth)	170.0	198.5	—	213.0	238.0	239.2
face	170.0	198.5	—	213.0	238.0	239.2
lower jaw	170.1	198.5	—	213.1	238.0	239.2
femur (any part)	170.7	198.5	—	213.7	238.0	239.2
fibula (any part)	170.7	198.5	—	213.7	238.0	239.2
finger (any)	170.5	198.5	—	213.5	238.0	239.2
foot	170.8	198.5	—	213.8	238.0	239.2
forearm	170.4	198.5	—	213.4	238.0	239.2
frontal	170.0	198.5	—	213.0	238.0	239.2
hand	170.5	198.5	—	213.5	238.0	239.2
heel	170.8	198.5	—	213.8	238.0	239.2
hip	170.6	198.5	—	213.6	238.0	239.2
humerus (any part)	170.4	198.5	—	213.4	238.0	239.2
hyoid	170.0	198.5	—	213.0	238.0	239.2
ilium	170.6	198.5	—	213.6	238.0	239.2
innominate	170.6	198.5	—	213.6	238.0	239.2
intervertebral cartilage or disc	170.2	198.5	—	213.2	238.0	239.2
ischium	170.6	198.5	—	213.6	238.0	239.2
jaw (lower)	170.1	198.5	—	213.1	238.0	239.2
upper	170.0	198.5	—	213.0	238.0	239.2
knee	170.7	198.5	—	213.7	238.0	239.2
leg NEC	170.7	198.5	—	213.7	238.0	239.2
limb NEC	170.9	198.5	—	213.9	238.0	239.2
lower (long bones)	170.7	198.5	—	213.7	238.0	239.2
short bones	170.8	198.5	—	213.8	238.0	239.2
upper (long bones)	170.4	198.5	—	213.4	238.0	239.2
short bones	170.5	198.5	—	213.5	238.0	239.2
long	170.9	198.5	—	213.9	238.0	239.2
lower limbs NEC	170.7	198.5	—	213.7	238.0	239.2
upper limbs NEC	170.4	198.5	—	213.4	238.0	239.2
malar	170.0	198.5	—	213.0	238.0	239.2
mandible	170.1	198.5	—	213.1	238.0	239.2
marrow NEC	202.9	198.5	—	—	—	238.79
mastoid	170.0	198.5	—	213.0	238.0	239.2
maxilla, maxillary (superior)	170.0	198.5	—	213.0	238.0	239.2
inferior	170.1	198.5	—	213.1	238.0	239.2
metacarpus (any)	170.5	198.5	—	213.5	238.0	239.2
metatarsus (any)	170.8	198.5	—	213.8	238.0	239.2
navicular (ankle)	170.8	198.5	—	213.8	238.0	239.2
hand	170.5	198.5	—	213.5	238.0	239.2
nose, nasal	170.0	198.5	—	213.0	238.0	239.2
occipital	170.0	198.5	—	213.0	238.0	239.2
orbit	170.0	198.5	—	213.0	238.0	239.2
parietal	170.0	198.5	—	213.0	238.0	239.2
patella	170.8	198.5	—	213.8	238.0	239.2
pelvic	170.6	198.5	—	213.6	238.0	239.2
phalanges	170.9	198.5	—	213.9	238.0	239.2
foot	170.8	198.5	—	213.8	238.0	239.2
hand	170.5	198.5	—	213.5	238.0	239.2
pubic	170.6	198.5	—	213.6	238.0	239.2
radius (any part)	170.4	198.5	—	213.4	238.0	239.2
rib	170.3	198.5	—	213.3	238.0	239.2
sacral vertebra	170.6	198.5	—	213.6	238.0	239.2
sacrum	170.6	198.5	—	213.6	238.0	239.2
scaphoid (of hand)	170.5	198.5	—	213.5	238.0	239.2
of ankle	170.8	198.5	—	213.8	238.0	239.2
scapula (any part)	170.4	198.5	—	213.4	238.0	239.2
sella turcica	170.0	198.5	—	213.0	238.0	239.2
short	170.9	198.5	—	213.9	238.0	239.2
lower limb	170.8	198.5	—	213.8	238.0	239.2

☑ Additional Digit Required — Refer to the Tabular List for Digit Selection   ▽ Subterms under main terms may continue to next column or page

194 — Volume 2   ▶◀ Revised Text   ● New Line   ▲ Revised Code   2014 ICD-9-CM

Neoplasm, neoplastic—	Malignant					
	Primary	Secondary	Ca in situ	Benign	Uncertain Behavior	Unspecified
continued						
bone — *continued*						
short — *continued*						
upper limb	170.5	198.5	—	213.5	238.0	239.2
shoulder	170.4	198.5	—	213.4	238.0	239.2
skeleton, skeletal NEC	170.9	198.5	—	213.9	238.0	239.2
skull	170.0	198.5	—	213.0	238.0	239.2
sphenoid	170.0	198.5	—	213.0	238.0	239.2
spine, spinal (column)	170.2	198.5	—	213.2	238.0	239.2
coccyx	170.6	198.5	—	213.6	238.0	239.2
sacrum	170.6	198.5	—	213.6	238.0	239.2
sternum	170.3	198.5	—	213.3	238.0	239.2
tarsus (any)	170.8	198.5	—	213.8	238.0	239.2
temporal	170.0	198.5	—	213.0	238.0	239.2
thumb	170.5	198.5	—	213.5	238.0	239.2
tibia (any part)	170.7	198.5	—	213.7	238.0	239.2
toe (any)	170.8	198.5	—	213.8	238.0	239.2
trapezium	170.5	198.5	—	213.5	238.0	239.2
trapezoid	170.5	198.5	—	213.5	238.0	239.2
turbinate	170.0	198.5	—	213.0	238.0	239.2
ulna (any part)	170.4	198.5	—	213.4	238.0	239.2
unciform	170.5	198.5	—	213.5	238.0	239.2
vertebra (column)	170.2	198.5	—	213.2	238.0	239.2
coccyx	170.6	198.5	—	213.6	238.0	239.2
sacrum	170.6	198.5	—	213.6	238.0	239.2
vomer	170.0	198.5	—	213.0	238.0	239.2
wrist	170.5	198.5	—	213.5	238.0	239.2
xiphoid process	170.3	198.5	—	213.3	238.0	239.2
zygomatic	170.0	198.5	—	213.0	238.0	239.2
book-leaf (mouth)	145.8	198.89	230.0	210.4	235.1	239.0
bowel — *see* Neoplasm, intestine						
brachial plexus	171.2	198.89	—	215.2	238.1	239.2
brain NEC	191.9	198.3	—	225.0	237.5	239.6
basal ganglia	191.0	198.3	—	225.0	237.5	239.6
cerebellopontine angle	191.6	198.3	—	225.0	237.5	239.6
cerebellum NOS	191.6	198.3	—	225.0	237.5	239.6
cerebrum	191.0	198.3	—	225.0	237.5	239.6
choroid plexus	191.5	198.3	—	225.0	237.5	239.6
contiguous sites	191.8	—	—	—	—	—
corpus callosum	191.8	198.3	—	225.0	237.5	239.6
corpus striatum	191.0	198.3	—	225.0	237.5	239.6
cortex (cerebral)	191.0	198.3	—	225.0	237.5	239.6
frontal lobe	191.1	198.3	—	225.0	237.5	239.6
globus pallidus	191.0	198.3	—	225.0	237.5	239.6
hippocampus	191.2	198.3	—	225.0	237.5	239.6
hypothalamus	191.0	198.3	—	225.0	237.5	239.6
internal capsule	191.0	198.3	—	225.0	237.5	239.6
medulla oblongata	191.7	198.3	—	225.0	237.5	239.6
meninges	192.1	198.4	—	225.2	237.6	239.7
midbrain	191.7	198.3	—	225.0	237.5	239.6
occipital lobe	191.4	198.3	—	225.0	237.5	239.6
parietal lobe	191.3	198.3	—	225.0	237.5	239.6
peduncle	191.7	198.3	—	225.0	237.5	239.6
pons	191.7	198.3	—	225.0	237.5	239.6
stem	191.7	198.3	—	225.0	237.5	239.6
tapetum	191.8	198.3	—	225.0	237.5	239.6
temporal lobe	191.2	198.3	—	225.0	237.5	239.6
thalamus	191.0	198.3	—	225.0	237.5	239.6
uncus	191.2	198.3	—	225.0	237.5	239.6
ventricle (floor)	191.5	198.3	—	225.0	237.5	239.6
branchial (cleft) (vestiges)	146.8	198.89	230.0	210.6	235.1	239.0
breast (connective tissue) (female) (glandular tissue) (soft parts)	174.9	198.81	233.0	217	238.3	239.3
areola	174.0	198.81	233.0	217	238.3	239.3
male	175.0	198.81	233.0	217	238.3	239.3
axillary tail	174.6	198.81	233.0	217	238.3	239.3

Neoplasm, neoplastic—	Malignant					
	Primary	Secondary	Ca in situ	Benign	Uncertain Behavior	Unspecified
continued						
breast — *continued*						
central portion	174.1	198.81	233.0	217	238.3	239.3
contiguous sites	174.8	—	—	—	—	—
ectopic sites	174.8	198.81	233.0	217	238.3	239.3
inner	174.8	198.81	233.0	217	238.3	239.3
lower-inner quadrant	174.3	198.81	233.0	217	238.3	239.3
lower-outer quadrant	174.5	198.81	233.0	217	238.3	239.3
lower	174.8	198.81	233.0	217	238.3	239.3
male	175.9	198.81	233.0	217	238.3	239.3
areola	175.0	198.81	233.0	217	238.3	239.3
ectopic tissue	175.9	198.81	233.0	217	238.3	239.3
nipple	175.0	198.81	233.0	217	238.3	239.3
mastectomy site (skin) (*see also* Neoplasm, mastectomy site)	173.50	198.2	—	—	—	—
specified as breast tissue	174.8	198.81	—	—	—	—
midline	174.8	198.81	233.0	217	238.3	239.3
nipple	174.0	198.81	233.0	217	238.3	239.3
male	175.0	198.81	233.0	217	238.3	239.3
outer	174.8	198.81	233.0	217	238.3	239.3
skin (*see also* Neoplasm, mastectomy site)	173.50	198.2	232.5	216.5	238.2	239.2
tail (axillary)	174.6	198.81	233.0	217	238.3	239.3
upper-inner quadrant	174.2	198.81	233.0	217	238.3	239.3
upper-outer quadrant	174.4	198.81	233.0	217	238.3	239.3
upper	174.8	198.81	233.0	217	238.3	239.3
broad ligament	183.3	198.82	233.39	221.0	236.3	239.5
bronchiogenic, bronchogenic (lung)	162.9	197.0	231.2	212.3	235.7	239.1
bronchiole	162.9	197.0	231.2	212.3	235.7	239.1
bronchus	162.9	197.0	231.2	212.3	235.7	239.1
carina	162.2	197.0	231.2	212.3	235.7	239.1
contiguous sites with lung or trachea	162.8	—	—	—	—	—
lower lobe of lung	162.5	197.0	231.2	212.3	235.7	239.1
main	162.2	197.0	231.2	212.3	235.7	239.1
middle lobe of lung	162.4	197.0	231.2	212.3	235.7	239.1
upper lobe of lung	162.3	197.0	231.2	212.3	235.7	239.1
brow	173.30	198.2	232.3	216.3	238.2	239.2
basal cell carcinoma	173.31	—	—	—	—	—
specified type NEC	173.39	—	—	—	—	—
squamous cell carcinoma	173.32	—	—	—	—	—
buccal (cavity)	145.9	198.89	230.0	210.4	235.1	239.0
commissure	145.0	198.89	230.0	210.4	235.1	239.0
groove (lower) (upper)	145.1	198.89	230.0	210.4	235.1	239.0
mucosa	145.0	198.89	230.0	210.4	235.1	239.0
sulcus (lower) (upper)	145.1	198.89	230.0	210.4	235.1	239.0
bulbourethral gland	189.3	198.1	233.9	223.81	236.99	239.5
bursa — *see* Neoplasm, connective tissue						
buttock NEC*	195.3	198.89	232.5	229.8	238.8	239.89
calf*	195.5	198.89	232.7	229.8	238.8	239.89
calvarium	170.0	198.5	—	213.0	238.0	239.2
calyx, renal	189.1	198.0	233.9	223.1	236.91	239.5
canal						
anal	154.2	197.5	230.5	211.4	235.5	239.0

☑ **Additional Digit Required** — Refer to the Tabular List for Digit Selection   ▽ **Subterms under main terms may continue to next column or page**

2014 ICD-9-CM   ▶◀ Revised Text   ● New Line   ▲ Revised Code   **Volume 2 — 195**

Neoplasm, canal — Neoplasm, common duct

	Malignant			Benign	Uncertain Behavior	Unspecified
	Primary	Secondary	Ca in situ			
Neoplasm, neoplastic — *continued*						
canal — *continued*						
auditory (external) (*see also* Neoplasm, skin, ear)	173.20	198.2	232.2	216.2	238.2	239.2
auricular (external) (*see also* Neoplasm, skin, ear)	173.20	198.2	232.2	216.2	238.2	239.2
canaliculi, biliary (biliferi) (intrahepatic)	155.1	197.8	230.8	211.5	235.3	239.0
canthus (eye) (inner) (outer)	173.10	198.2	232.1	216.1	238.2	239.2
basal cell carcinoma	173.11	—	—	—	—	—
specified type NEC	173.19	—	—	—	—	—
squamous cell carcinoma	173.12	—	—	—	—	—
capillary — *see* Neoplasm, connective tissue						
caput coli	153.4	197.5	230.3	211.3	235.2	239.0
cardia (gastric)	151.0	197.8	230.2	211.1	235.2	239.0
cardiac orifice (stomach)	151.0	197.8	230.2	211.1	235.2	239.0
cardio-esophageal junction	151.0	197.8	230.2	211.1	235.2	239.0
cardio-esophagus	151.0	197.8	230.2	211.1	235.2	239.0
carina (bronchus)	162.2	197.0	231.2	212.3	235.7	239.1
carotid (artery)	171.0	198.89	—	215.0	238.1	239.2
body	194.5	198.89	—	227.5	237.3	239.7
carpus (any bone)	170.5	198.5	—	213.5	238.0	239.2
cartilage (articular) (joint) NEC (*see also* Neoplasm, bone)	170.9	198.5	—	213.9	238.0	239.2
arytenoid	161.3	197.3	231.0	212.1	235.6	239.1
auricular	171.0	198.89	—	215.0	238.1	239.2
bronchi	162.2	197.3	—	212.3	235.7	239.1
connective tissue — *see* Neoplasm, connective tissue						
costal	170.3	198.5	—	213.3	238.0	239.2
cricoid	161.3	197.3	231.0	212.1	235.6	239.1
cuneiform	161.3	197.3	231.0	212.1	235.6	239.1
ear (external)	171.0	198.89	—	215.0	238.1	239.2
ensiform	170.3	198.5	—	213.3	238.0	239.2
epiglottis	161.1	197.3	231.0	212.1	235.6	239.1
anterior surface	146.4	198.89	230.0	210.6	235.1	239.0
eyelid	171.0	198.89	—	215.0	238.1	239.2
intervertebral	170.2	198.5	—	213.2	238.0	239.2
larynx, laryngeal	161.3	197.3	231.0	212.1	235.6	239.1
nose, nasal	160.0	197.3	231.8	212.0	235.9	239.1
pinna	171.0	198.89	—	215.0	238.1	239.2
rib	170.3	198.5	—	213.3	238.0	239.2
semilunar (knee)	170.7	198.5	—	213.7	238.0	239.2
thyroid	161.3	197.3	231.0	212.1	235.6	239.1
trachea	162.0	197.3	231.1	212.2	235.7	239.1
cauda equina	192.2	198.3	—	225.3	237.5	239.7
cavity						
buccal	145.9	198.89	230.0	210.4	235.1	239.0
nasal	160.0	197.3	231.8	212.0	235.9	239.1
oral	145.9	198.89	230.0	210.4	235.1	239.0
peritoneal	158.9	197.6	—	211.8	235.4	239.0
tympanic	160.1	197.3	231.8	212.0	235.9	239.1
cecum	153.4	197.5	230.3	211.3	235.2	239.0
central						
nervous system — *see* Neoplasm, nervous system						
white matter	191.0	198.3	—	225.0	237.5	239.6
Neoplasm, neoplastic — *continued*						
cerebellopontine (angle)	191.6	198.3	—	225.0	237.5	239.6
cerebellum, cerebellar	191.6	198.3	—	225.0	237.5	239.6
cerebrum, cerebral (cortex) (hemisphere) (white matter)	191.0	198.3	—	225.0	237.5	239.6
meninges	192.1	198.4	—	225.2	237.6	239.7
peduncle	191.7	198.3	—	225.0	237.5	239.6
ventricle (any)	191.5	198.3	—	225.0	237.5	239.6
cervical region	195.0	198.89	234.8	229.8	238.8	239.89
cervix (cervical) (uteri) (uterus)	180.9	198.82	233.1	219.0	236.0	239.5
canal	180.0	198.82	233.1	219.0	236.0	239.5
contiguous sites	180.8	—	—	—	—	—
endocervix (canal) (gland)	180.0	198.82	233.1	219.0	236.0	239.5
exocervix	180.1	198.82	233.1	219.0	236.0	239.5
external os	180.1	198.82	233.1	219.0	236.0	239.5
internal os	180.0	198.82	233.1	219.0	236.0	239.5
nabothian gland	180.0	198.82	233.1	219.0	236.0	239.5
squamocolumnar junction	180.8	198.82	233.1	219.0	236.0	239.5
stump	180.8	198.82	233.1	219.0	236.0	239.5
cheek	195.0	198.89	234.8	229.8	238.8	239.89
external	173.30	198.2	232.3	216.3	238.2	239.2
basal cell carcinoma	173.31	—	—	—	—	—
specified type NEC	173.39	—	—	—	—	—
squamous cell carcinoma	173.32	—	—	—	—	—
inner aspect	145.0	198.89	230.0	210.4	235.1	239.0
internal	145.0	198.89	230.0	210.4	235.1	239.0
mucosa	145.0	198.89	230.0	210.4	235.1	239.0
chest (wall) NEC	195.1	198.89	234.8	229.8	238.8	239.89
chiasma opticum	192.0	198.4	—	225.1	237.9	239.7
chin	173.30	198.2	232.3	216.3	238.2	239.2
basal cell carcinoma	173.31	—	—	—	—	—
specified type NEC	173.39	—	—	—	—	—
squamous cell carcinoma	173.32	—	—	—	—	—
choana	147.3	198.89	230.0	210.7	235.1	239.0
cholangiole	155.1	197.8	230.8	211.5	235.3	239.0
choledochal duct	156.1	197.8	230.8	211.5	235.3	239.0
choroid	190.6	198.4	234.0	224.6	238.8	239.81
plexus	191.5	198.3	—	225.0	237.5	239.6
ciliary body	190.0	198.4	234.0	224.0	238.8	239.89
clavicle	170.3	198.5	—	213.3	238.0	239.2
clitoris	184.3	198.82	233.32	221.2	236.3	239.5
clivus	170.0	198.5	—	213.0	238.0	239.2
cloacogenic zone	154.8	197.5	230.7	211.4	235.5	239.0
coccygeal						
body or glomus	194.6	198.89	—	227.6	237.3	239.7
vertebra	170.6	198.5	—	213.6	238.0	239.2
coccyx	170.6	198.5	—	213.6	238.0	239.2
colon — *see also* Neoplasm, intestine, large	153.9	197.5	230.3	211.3	235.2	239.0
with rectum	154.0	197.5	230.4	211.4	235.2	239.0
columnella (*see also* Neoplasm, skin, face)	173.30	198.2	232.3	216.3	238.2	239.2
column, spinal — *see* Neoplasm, spine						
commissure						
labial, lip	140.6	198.89	230.0	210.4	235.1	239.0
laryngeal	161.0	197.3	231.0	212.1	235.6	239.1
common (bile) duct	156.1	197.8	230.8	211.5	235.3	239.0

☑ **Additional Digit Required** — Refer to the Tabular List for Digit Selection

▽ Subterms under main terms may continue to next column or page

	Malignant					
	Primary	Secondary	Ca in situ	Benign	Uncertain Behavior	Unspecified
Neoplasm, neoplastic — *continued*						
concha (*see also* Neoplasm, skin, ear)	173.20	198.2	232.2	216.2	238.2	239.2
nose	160.0	197.3	231.8	212.0	235.9	239.1
conjunctiva	190.3	198.4	234.0	224.3	238.8	239.89
connective tissue NEC	171.9	198.89	—	215.9	238.1	239.2

Note — For neoplasms of connective tissue (blood vessel, bursa, fascia, ligament, muscle, peripheral nerves, sympathetic and parasympathetic nerves and ganglia, synovia, tendon, etc.) or of morphological types that indicate connective tissue, code according to the list under "Neoplasm, connective tissue"; for sites that do not appear in this list, code to neoplasm of that site; e.g.,

liposarcoma, shoulder 171.2

leiomyosarcoma, stomach 151.9

neurofibroma, chest wall 215.4

Morphological types that indicate connective tissue appear in the proper place in the alphabetic index with the instruction "see Neoplasm, connective tissue..."

	Primary	Secondary	Ca in situ	Benign	Uncertain Behavior	Unspecified
abdomen	171.5	198.89	—	215.5	238.1	239.2
abdominal wall	171.5	198.89	—	215.5	238.1	239.2
ankle	171.3	198.89	—	215.3	238.1	239.2
antecubital fossa or space	171.2	198.89	—	215.2	238.1	239.2
arm	171.2	198.89	—	215.2	238.1	239.2
auricle (ear)	171.0	198.89	—	215.0	238.1	239.2
axilla	171.4	198.89	—	215.4	238.1	239.2
back	171.7	198.89	—	215.7	238.1	239.2
breast (female) (*see also* Neoplasm, breast)	174.9	198.81	233.0	217	238.3	239.3
male	175.9	198.81	233.0	217	238.3	239.3
buttock	171.6	198.89	—	215.6	238.1	239.2
calf	171.3	198.89	—	215.3	238.1	239.2
cervical region	171.0	198.89	—	215.0	238.1	239.2
cheek	171.0	198.89	—	215.0	238.1	239.2
chest (wall)	171.4	198.89	—	215.4	238.1	239.2
chin	171.0	198.89	—	215.0	238.1	239.2
contiguous sites	171.8	—	—	—	—	—
diaphragm	171.4	198.89	—	215.4	238.1	239.2
ear (external)	171.0	198.89	—	215.0	238.1	239.2
elbow	171.2	198.89	—	215.2	238.1	239.2
extrarectal	171.6	198.89	—	215.6	238.1	239.2
extremity	171.8	198.89	—	215.8	238.1	239.2
lower	171.3	198.89	—	215.3	238.1	239.2
upper	171.2	198.89	—	215.2	238.1	239.2
eyelid	171.0	198.89	—	215.0	238.1	239.2
face	171.0	198.89	—	215.0	238.1	239.2
finger	171.2	198.89	—	215.2	238.1	239.2
flank	171.7	198.89	—	215.7	238.1	239.2
foot	171.3	198.89	—	215.3	238.1	239.2
forearm	171.2	198.89	—	215.2	238.1	239.2
forehead	171.0	198.89	—	215.0	238.1	239.2
gastric	171.5	198.89	—	215.5	238.1	—
gastrointestinal	171.5	198.89	—	215.5	238.1	—
gluteal region	171.6	198.89	—	215.6	238.1	239.2
great vessels NEC	171.4	198.89	—	215.4	238.1	239.2
groin	171.6	198.89	—	215.6	238.1	239.2
hand	171.2	198.89	—	215.2	238.1	239.2
head	171.0	198.89	—	215.0	238.1	239.2
heel	171.3	198.89	—	215.3	238.1	239.2
hip	171.3	198.89	—	215.3	238.1	239.2
hypochondrium	171.5	198.89	—	215.5	238.1	239.2
iliopsoas muscle	171.6	198.89	—	215.5	238.1	239.2
infraclavicular region	171.4	198.89	—	215.4	238.1	239.2
inguinal (canal) (region)	171.6	198.89	—	215.6	238.1	239.2
intestine	171.5	198.89	—	215.5	238.1	—
intrathoracic	171.4	198.89	—	215.4	238.1	239.2
ischiorectal fossa	171.6	198.89	—	215.6	238.1	239.2
jaw	143.9	198.89	230.0	210.4	235.1	239.0

	Malignant					
	Primary	Secondary	Ca in situ	Benign	Uncertain Behavior	Unspecified
Neoplasm, neoplastic — *continued* connective tissue — *continued*						
knee	171.3	198.89	—	215.3	238.1	239.2
leg	171.3	198.89	—	215.3	238.1	239.2
limb NEC	171.9	198.89	—	215.8	238.1	239.2
lower	171.3	198.89	—	215.3	238.1	239.2
upper	171.2	198.89	—	215.2	238.1	239.2
nates	171.6	198.89	—	215.6	238.1	239.2
neck	171.0	198.89	—	215.0	238.1	239.2
orbit	190.1	198.4	234.0	224.1	238.8	239.89
para-urethral	171.6	198.89	—	215.6	238.1	239.2
pararectal	171.6	198.89	—	215.6	238.1	239.2
paravaginal	171.6	198.89	—	215.6	238.1	239.2
pelvis (floor)	171.6	198.89	—	215.6	238.1	239.2
pelvo-abdominal	171.8	198.89	—	215.8	238.1	239.2
perineum	171.6	198.89	—	215.6	238.1	239.2
perirectal (tissue)	171.6	198.89	—	215.6	238.1	239.2
periurethral (tissue)	171.6	198.89	—	215.6	238.1	239.2
popliteal fossa or space	171.3	198.89	—	215.3	238.1	239.2
presacral	171.6	198.89	—	215.6	238.1	239.2
psoas muscle	171.5	198.89	—	215.5	238.1	239.2
pterygoid fossa	171.0	198.89	—	215.0	238.1	239.2
rectovaginal septum or wall	171.6	198.89	—	215.6	238.1	239.2
rectovesical	171.6	198.89	—	215.6	238.1	239.2
retroperitoneum	158.0	197.6	—	211.8	235.4	239.0
sacrococcygeal region	171.6	198.89	—	215.6	238.1	239.2
scalp	171.0	198.89	—	215.0	238.1	239.2
scapular region	171.4	198.89	—	215.4	238.1	239.2
shoulder	171.2	198.89	—	215.2	238.1	239.2
skin (dermis) NEC	173.90	198.2	232.9	216.9	238.2	239.2
stomach	171.5	198.89	—	215.5	238.1	—
submental	171.0	198.89	—	215.0	238.1	239.2
supraclavicular region	171.0	198.89	—	215.0	238.1	239.2
temple	171.0	198.89	—	215.0	238.1	239.2
temporal region	171.0	198.89	—	215.0	238.1	239.2
thigh	171.3	198.89	—	215.3	238.1	239.2
thoracic (duct) (wall)	171.4	198.89	—	215.4	238.1	239.2
thorax	171.4	198.89	—	215.4	238.1	239.2
thumb	171.2	198.89	—	215.2	238.1	239.2
toe	171.3	198.89	—	215.3	238.1	239.2
trunk	171.7	198.89	—	215.7	238.1	239.2
umbilicus	171.5	198.89	—	215.5	238.1	239.2
vesicorectal	171.6	198.89	—	215.6	238.1	239.2
wrist	171.2	198.89	—	215.2	238.1	239.2
conus medullaris	192.2	198.3		225.3	237.5	239.7
cord (true) (vocal)	161.0	197.3	231.0	212.1	235.6	239.1
false	161.1	197.3	231.0	212.1	235.6	239.1
spermatic	187.6	198.82	233.6	222.8	236.6	239.5
spinal (cervical) (lumbar) (thoracic)	192.2	198.3	—	225.3	237.5	239.7
cornea (limbus)	190.4	198.4	234.0	224.4	238.8	239.89
corpus						
albicans	183.0	198.6	233.39	220	236.2	239.5
callosum, brain	191.8	198.3	—	225.0	237.5	239.6
cavernosum	187.3	198.82	233.5	222.1	236.6	239.5
gastric	151.4	197.8	230.2	211.1	235.2	239.0
penis	187.3	198.82	233.5	222.1	236.6	239.5
striatum, cerebrum	191.0	198.3		225.0	237.5	239.6
uteri	182.0	198.82	233.2	219.1	236.0	239.5
isthmus	182.1	198.82	233.2	219.1	236.0	239.5
cortex						
adrenal	194.0	198.7	234.8	227.0	237.2	239.7
cerebral	191.0	198.3	—	225.0	237.5	239.6
costal cartilage	170.3	198.5	—	213.3	238.0	239.2

	Malignant			Benign	Uncertain Behavior	Unspecified
	Primary	Secondary	Ca in situ			

Neoplasm, neoplastic — *continued*

	Primary	Secondary	Ca in situ	Benign	Uncertain Behavior	Unspecified
costovertebral joint	170.3	198.5	—	213.3	238.0	239.2
Cowper's gland	189.3	198.1	233.9	223.81	236.99	239.5
cranial (fossa, any)	191.9	198.3	—	225.0	237.5	239.6
meninges	192.1	198.4	—	225.2	237.6	239.7
nerve (any)	192.0	198.4	—	225.1	237.9	239.7
craniobuccal pouch	194.3	198.89	234.8	227.3	237.0	239.7
craniopharyngeal (duct) (pouch)	194.3	198.89	234.8	227.3	237.0	239.7
cricoid	148.0	198.89	230.0	210.8	235.1	239.0
cartilage	161.3	197.3	231.0	212.1	235.6	239.1
cricopharynx	148.0	198.89	230.0	210.8	235.1	239.0
crypt of Morgagni	154.8	197.5	230.7	211.4	235.2	239.0
crystalline lens	190.0	198.4	234.0	224.0	238.8	239.89
cul-de-sac (Douglas')	158.8	197.6	—	211.8	235.4	239.0
cuneiform cartilage	161.3	197.3	231.0	212.1	235.6	239.1
cutaneous — *see* Neoplasm, skin						
cutis — *see* Neoplasm, skin						
cystic (bile) duct (common)	156.1	197.8	230.8	211.5	235.3	239.0
dermis — *see* Neoplasm, skin						
diaphragm	171.4	198.89	—	215.4	238.1	239.2
digestive organs, system, tube, or tract NEC	159.9	197.8	230.9	211.9	235.5	239.0
contiguous sites with peritoneum	159.8	—	—	—	—	—
disc, intervertebral	170.2	198.5	—	213.2	238.0	239.2
disease, generalized	199.0	—	234.9	229.9	238.9	—
disseminated	199.0	—	234.9	229.9	238.9	—
Douglas' cul-de-sac or pouch	158.8	197.6	—	211.8	235.4	239.0
duodenojejunal junction	152.8	197.4	230.7	211.2	235.2	239.0
duodenum	152.0	197.4	230.7	211.2	235.2	239.0
dura (cranial) (mater)	192.1	198.4	—	225.2	237.6	239.7
cerebral	192.1	198.4	—	225.2	237.6	239.7
spinal	192.3	198.4	—	225.4	237.6	239.7
ear (external) (*see also* Neoplasm, ear, skin)	173.20	198.2	232.2	216.2	238.2	239.2
auricle or auris (*see also* Neoplasm, ear, skin)	173.20	198.2	232.2	216.2	238.2	239.2
canal, external (*see also* Neoplasm, ear, skin)	173.20	198.2	232.2	216.2	238.2	239.2
cartilage	171.0	198.89	—	215.0	238.1	239.2
external meatus (*see also* Neoplasm, ear, skin)	173.20	198.2	232.2	216.2	238.2	239.2
inner	160.1	197.3	231.8	212.0	235.9	239.89
lobule (*see also* Neoplasm, ear, skin)	173.20	198.2	232.2	216.2	238.2	239.2
middle	160.1	197.3	231.8	212.0	235.9	239.89
contiguous sites with accessory sinuses or nasal cavities	160.8	—	—	—	—	—
skin	173.20	198.2	232.2	216.2	238.2	239.2
basal cell carcinoma	173.21	—	—	—	—	—
specified type NEC	173.29	—	—	—	—	—
squamous cell carcinoma	173.22	—	—	—	—	—
earlobe	173.20	198.2	232.2	216.2	238.2	239.2

Neoplasm, neoplastic — *continued*

	Primary	Secondary	Ca in situ	Benign	Uncertain Behavior	Unspecified
earlobe — *continued*						
basal cell carcinoma	173.21	—	—	—	—	—
specified type NEC	173.29	—	—	—	—	—
squamous cell carcinoma	173.22	—	—	—	—	—
ejaculatory duct	187.8	198.82	233.6	222.8	236.6	239.5
elbow NEC*	195.4	198.89	232.6	229.8	238.8	239.89
endocardium	164.1	198.89	—	212.7	238.8	239.89
endocervix (canal) (gland)	180.0	198.82	233.1	219.0	236.0	239.5
endocrine gland NEC	194.9	198.89	—	227.9	237.4	239.7
pluriglandular NEC	194.8	198.89	234.8	227.8	237.4	239.7
endometrium (gland) (stroma)	182.0	198.82	233.2	219.1	236.0	239.5
ensiform cartilage	170.3	198.5	—	213.3	238.0	239.2
enteric — *see* Neoplasm, intestine						
ependyma (brain)	191.5	198.3	—	225.0	237.5	239.6
epicardium	164.1	198.89	—	212.7	238.8	239.89
epididymis	187.5	198.82	233.6	222.3	236.6	239.5
epidural	192.9	198.4	—	225.9	237.9	239.7
epiglottis	161.1	197.3	231.0	212.1	235.6	239.1
anterior aspect or surface	146.4	198.89	230.0	210.6	235.1	239.0
cartilage	161.3	197.3	231.0	212.1	235.6	239.1
free border (margin)	146.4	198.89	230.0	210.6	235.1	239.0
junctional region	146.5	198.89	230.0	210.6	235.1	239.0
posterior (laryngeal) surface	161.1	197.3	231.0	212.1	235.6	239.1
suprahyoid portion	161.1	197.3	231.0	212.1	235.6	239.1
esophagogastric junction	151.0	197.8	230.2	211.1	235.2	239.0
esophagus	150.9	197.8	230.1	211.0	235.5	239.0
abdominal	150.2	197.8	230.1	211.0	235.5	239.0
cervical	150.0	197.8	230.1	211.0	235.5	239.0
contiguous sites	150.8	—	—	—	—	—
distal (third)	150.5	197.8	230.1	211.0	235.5	239.0
lower (third)	150.5	197.8	230.1	211.0	235.5	239.0
middle (third)	150.4	197.8	230.1	211.0	235.5	239.0
proximal (third)	150.3	197.8	230.1	211.0	235.5	239.0
specified part NEC	150.8	197.8	230.1	211.0	235.5	239.0
thoracic	150.1	197.8	230.1	211.0	235.5	239.0
upper (third)	150.3	197.8	230.1	211.0	235.5	239.0
ethmoid (sinus)	160.3	197.3	231.8	212.0	235.9	239.1
bone or labyrinth	170.0	198.5	—	213.0	238.0	239.2
Eustachian tube	160.1	197.3	231.8	212.0	235.9	239.1
exocervix	180.1	198.82	233.1	219.0	236.0	239.5
external meatus (ear) (*see also* Neoplasm, skin, ear)	173.20	198.2	232.2	216.2	238.2	239.2
os, cervix uteri	180.1	198.82	233.1	219.0	236.0	239.5
extradural	192.9	198.4	—	225.9	237.9	239.7
extrahepatic (bile) duct	156.1	197.8	230.8	211.5	235.3	239.0
contiguous sites with gallbladder	156.8	—	—	—	—	—
extraocular muscle	190.1	198.4	234.0	224.1	238.8	239.89
extrarectal	195.3	198.89	234.8	229.8	238.8	239.89
extremity*	195.8	198.89	232.8	229.8	238.8	239.89
lower*	195.5	198.89	232.7	229.8	238.8	239.89
upper*	195.4	198.89	232.6	229.8	238.8	239.89
eyeball	190.0	198.4	234.0	224.0	238.8	239.89
eyebrow	173.30	198.2	232.3	216.3	238.2	239.2

	Malignant					
	Primary	Secondary	Ca in situ	Benign	Uncertain Behavior	Unspecified
Neoplasm, neoplastic — *continued*						
eyebrow — *continued*						
basal cell						
carcinoma	173.31	—	—	—	—	—
specified type						
NEC	173.39	—	—	—	—	—
squamous cell						
carcinoma	173.32	—	—	—	—	—
eyelid (lower) (skin)						
(upper)	173.10	198.2	232.1	216.1	238.2	239.2
basal cell						
carcinoma	173.11	—	—	—	—	—
cartilage	171.0	198.89	—	215.0	238.1	239.2
specified type						
NEC	173.19	—	—	—	—	—
squamous cell						
carcinoma	173.12	—	—	—	—	—
eye NEC	190.9	198.4	234.0	224.9	238.8	239.89
contiguous sites	190.8	—	—	—	—	—
specified sites						
NEC	190.8	198.4	234.0	224.8	238.8	239.89
face NEC*	195.0	198.89	232.3	229.8	238.8	239.89
fallopian tube						
(accessory)	183.2	198.82	233.39	221.0	236.3	239.5
falx (cerebelli)						
(cerebri)	192.1	198.4		225.2	237.6	239.7
fascia (*see also* Neoplasm, connective tissue)						
palmar	171.2	198.89	—	215.2	238.1	239.2
plantar	171.3	198.89	—	215.3	238.1	239.2
fatty tissue — *see* Neoplasm, connective tissue						
fauces, faucial NEC	146.9	198.89	230.0	210.6	235.1	239.0
pillars	146.2	198.89	230.0	210.6	235.1	239.0
tonsil	146.0	198.89	230.0	210.5	235.1	239.0
femur (any part)	170.7	198.5	—	213.7	238.0	239.2
fetal membrane	181	198.82	233.2	219.8	236.1	239.5
fibrous tissue — *see* Neoplasm, connective tissue						
fibula (any part)	170.7	198.5	—	213.7	238.0	239.2
filum terminale	192.2	198.3		225.3	237.5	239.7
finger NEC*	195.4	198.89	232.6	229.8	238.8	239.89
flank NEC*	195.8	198.89	232.5	229.8	238.8	239.89
follicle, nabothian	180.0	198.82	233.1	219.0	236.0	239.5
foot NEC*	195.5	198.89	232.7	229.8	238.8	239.89
forearm NEC*	195.4	198.89	232.6	229.8	238.8	239.89
forehead (skin)	173.30	198.2	232.3	216.3	238.2	239.2
basal cell						
carcinoma	173.31	—	—	—	—	—
specified type						
NEC	173.39	—	—	—	—	—
squamous cell						
carcinoma	173.32	—	—	—	—	—
foreskin	187.1	198.82	233.5	222.1	236.6	239.5
fornix						
pharyngeal	147.3	198.89	230.0	210.7	235.1	239.0
vagina	184.0	198.82	233.31	221.1	236.3	239.5
fossa (of)						
anterior (cranial)	191.9	198.3	—	225.0	237.5	239.6
cranial	191.9	198.3	—	225.0	237.5	239.6
ischiorectal	195.3	198.89	234.8	229.8	238.8	239.89
middle (cranial)	191.9	198.3	—	225.0	237.5	239.6
pituitary	194.3	198.89	234.8	227.3	237.0	239.7
posterior (cranial)	191.9	198.3	—	225.0	237.5	239.6
pterygoid	171.0	198.89	—	215.0	238.1	239.2
pyriform	148.1	198.89	230.0	210.8	235.1	239.0
Rosenmüller	147.2	198.89	230.0	210.7	235.1	239.0
tonsillar	146.1	198.89	230.0	210.6	235.1	239.0
fourchette	184.4	198.82	233.32	221.2	236.3	239.5
frenulum						
labii — *see* Neoplasm, lip, internal						

	Malignant					
	Primary	Secondary	Ca in situ	Benign	Uncertain Behavior	Unspecified
Neoplasm, neoplastic — *continued*						
frenulum — *continued*						
linguae	141.3	198.89	230.0	210.1	235.1	239.0
frontal						
bone	170.0	198.5	—	213.0	238.0	239.2
lobe, brain	191.1	198.3	—	225.0	237.5	239.6
meninges	192.1	198.4	—	225.2	237.6	239.7
pole	191.1	198.3	—	225.0	237.5	239.6
sinus	160.4	197.3	231.8	212.0	235.9	239.1
fundus						
stomach	151.3	197.8	230.2	211.1	235.2	239.0
uterus	182.0	198.82	233.2	219.1	236.0	239.5
gallbladder	156.0	197.8	230.8	211.5	235.3	239.0
contiguous sites with extrahepatic bile ducts	156.8	—	—	—	—	—
gall duct (extrahepatic)	156.1	197.8	230.8	211.5	235.3	239.0
intrahepatic	155.1	197.8	230.8	211.5	235.3	239.0
ganglia (*see also* Neoplasm, connective tissue)	171.9	198.89	—	215.9	238.1	239.2
basal	191.0	198.3	—	225.0	237.5	239.6
ganglion (*see also* Neoplasm, connective tissue)	171.9	198.89	—	215.9	238.1	239.2
cranial nerve	192.0	198.4	—	225.1	237.9	239.7
Gartner's duct	184.0	198.82	233.31	221.1	236.3	239.5
gastric — *see* Neoplasm, stomach						
gastrocolic	159.8	197.8	230.9	211.9	235.5	239.0
gastroesophageal junction	151.0	197.8	230.2	211.1	235.2	239.0
gastrointestinal (tract) NEC	159.9	197.8	230.9	211.9	235.5	239.0
generalized	199.0	—	234.9	229.9	238.9	—
genital organ or tract						
female NEC	184.9	198.82	233.39	221.9	236.3	239.5
contiguous sites	184.8	—	—	—	—	—
specified site NEC	184.8	198.82	233.39	221.8	236.3	239.5
male NEC	187.9	198.82	233.6	222.9	236.6	239.5
contiguous sites	187.8	—	—	—	—	—
specified site NEC	187.8	198.82	233.6	222.8	236.6	239.5
genitourinary tract						
female	184.9	198.82	233.39	221.9	236.3	239.5
male	187.9	198.82	233.6	222.9	236.6	239.5
gingiva (alveolar) (marginal)	143.9	198.89	230.0	210.4	235.1	239.0
lower	143.1	198.89	230.0	210.4	235.1	239.0
mandibular	143.1	198.89	230.0	210.4	235.1	239.0
maxillary	143.0	198.89	230.0	210.4	235.1	239.0
upper	143.0	198.89	230.0	210.4	235.1	239.0
gland, glandular (lymphatic) (system) (*see also* Neoplasm, lymph gland)						
endocrine NEC	194.9	198.89		227.9	237.4	239.7
salivary — *see* Neoplasm, salivary, gland						
glans penis	187.2	198.82	233.5	222.1	236.6	239.5
globus pallidus	191.0	198.3		225.0	237.5	239.6
glomus						
coccygeal	194.6	198.89	—	227.6	237.3	239.7
jugularis	194.6	198.89	—	227.6	237.3	239.7
glosso-epiglottic fold(s)	146.4	198.89	230.0	210.6	235.1	239.0
glossopalatine fold	146.2	198.89	230.0	210.6	235.1	239.0
glossopharyngeal sulcus	146.1	198.89	230.0	210.6	235.1	239.0

☑ **Additional Digit Required** — Refer to the Tabular List for Digit Selection

📖 **Subterms under main terms may continue to next column or page**

Neoplasm, neoplastic— *continued*

| | Malignant | | | | | |
	Primary	Secondary	Ca in situ	Benign	Uncertain Behavior	Unspecified
glottis	161.0	197.3	231.0	212.1	235.6	239.1
gluteal region*	195.3	198.89	232.5	229.8	238.8	239.89
great vessels NEC	171.4	198.89	—	215.4	238.1	239.2
groin NEC	195.3	198.89	232.5	229.8	238.8	239.89
gum	143.9	198.89	230.0	210.4	235.1	239.0
contiguous sites	143.8	—	—	—	—	—
lower	143.1	198.89	230.0	210.4	235.1	239.0
upper	143.0	198.89	230.0	210.4	235.1	239.0
hand NEC*	195.4	198.89	232.6	229.8	238.8	239.89
head NEC*	195.0	198.89	232.4	229.8	238.8	239.89
heart	164.1	198.89	—	212.7	238.8	239.89
contiguous sites with mediastinum or thymus	164.8	—	—	—	—	—
heel NEC*	195.5	198.89	232.7	229.8	238.8	239.89
helix (*see also* Neoplasm, skin, ear)	173.20	198.2	232.2	216.2	238.2	239.2
hematopoietic, hemopoietic tissue NEC	202.8	198.89	—	—	—	238.79
hemisphere, cerebral	191.0	198.3	—	225.0	237.5	239.6
hemorrhoidal zone	154.2	197.5	230.5	211.4	235.5	239.0
hepatic	155.2	197.7	230.8	211.5	235.3	239.0
duct (bile)	156.1	197.8	230.8	211.5	235.3	239.0
flexure (colon)	153.0	197.5	230.3	211.3	235.2	239.0
primary	155.0	—	—	—	—	—
hilus of lung	162.2	197.0	231.2	212.3	235.7	239.1
hippocampus, brain	191.2	198.3	—	225.0	237.5	239.6
hip NEC*	195.5	198.89	232.7	229.8	238.8	239.89
humerus (any part)	170.4	198.5	—	213.4	238.0	239.2
hymen	184.0	198.82	233.31	221.1	236.3	239.5
hypopharynx, hypopharyngeal NEC	148.9	198.89	230.0	210.8	235.1	239.0
contiguous sites	148.8	—	—	—	—	—
postcricoid region	148.0	198.89	230.0	210.8	235.1	239.0
posterior wall	148.3	198.89	230.0	210.8	235.1	239.0
pyriform fossa (sinus)	148.1	198.89	230.0	210.8	235.1	239.0
specified site NEC	148.8	198.89	230.0	210.8	235.1	239.0
wall	148.9	198.89	230.0	210.8	235.1	239.0
posterior	148.3	198.89	230.0	210.8	235.1	239.0
hypophysis	194.3	198.89	234.8	227.3	237.0	239.7
hypothalamus	191.0	198.3	—	225.0	237.5	239.6
ileocecum, ileocecal (coil) (junction) (valve)	153.4	197.5	230.3	211.3	235.2	239.0
ileum	152.2	197.4	230.7	211.2	235.2	239.0
ilium	170.6	198.5	—	213.6	238.0	239.2
immunoproliferative NEC	203.8	—	—	—	—	—
infraclavicular (region)*	195.1	198.89	232.5	229.8	238.8	239.89
inguinal (region)*	195.3	198.89	232.5	229.8	238.8	239.89
insula	191.0	198.3	—	225.0	237.5	239.6
insular tissue (pancreas)	157.4	197.8	230.9	211.7	235.5	239.0
brain	191.0	198.3	—	225.0	237.5	239.6
interarytenoid fold	148.2	198.89	230.0	210.8	235.1	239.0
hypopharyngeal aspect	148.2	198.89	230.0	210.8	235.1	239.0
laryngeal aspect	161.1	197.3	231.0	212.1	235.6	239.1
marginal zone	148.2	198.89	230.0	210.8	235.1	239.0
interdental papillae	143.9	198.89	230.0	210.4	235.1	239.0
lower	143.1	198.89	230.0	210.4	235.1	239.0
upper	143.0	198.89	230.0	210.4	235.1	239.0
internal						
capsule	191.0	198.3	—	225.0	237.5	239.6
os (cervix)	180.0	198.82	233.1	219.0	236.0	239.5

Neoplasm, neoplastic— *continued*

| | Malignant | | | | | |
	Primary	Secondary	Ca in situ	Benign	Uncertain Behavior	Unspecified
intervertebral cartilage or disc	170.2	198.5	—	213.2	238.0	239.2
intestine, intestinal	159.0	197.8	230.7	211.9	235.2	239.0
large	153.9	197.5	230.3	211.3	235.2	239.0
appendix	153.5	197.5	230.3	211.3	235.2	239.0
caput coli	153.4	197.5	230.3	211.3	235.2	239.0
cecum	153.4	197.5	230.3	211.3	235.2	239.0
colon	153.9	197.5	230.3	211.3	235.2	239.0
and rectum	154.0	197.5	230.4	211.4	235.2	239.0
ascending*	153.6	197.5	230.3	211.3	235.2	239.0
caput	153.4	197.5	230.3	211.3	235.2	239.0
contiguous sites	153.8	—	—	—	—	—
descending	153.2	197.5	230.3	211.3	235.2	239.0
distal	153.2	197.5	230.3	211.3	235.2	239.0
left	153.2	197.5	230.3	211.3	235.2	239.0
pelvic	153.3	197.5	230.3	211.3	235.2	239.0
right	153.6	197.5	230.3	211.3	235.2	239.0
sigmoid (flexure)	153.3	197.5	230.3	211.3	235.2	239.0
transverse	153.1	197.5	230.3	211.3	235.2	239.0
contiguous sites	153.8	—	—	—	—	—
hepatic flexure	153.0	197.5	230.3	211.3	235.2	239.0
ileocecum, ileocecal (coil) (valve)	153.4	197.5	230.3	211.3	235.2	239.0
sigmoid flexure (lower) (upper)	153.3	197.5	230.3	211.3	235.2	239.0
splenic flexure	153.7	197.5	230.3	211.3	235.2	239.0
small	152.9	197.4	230.7	211.2	235.2	239.0
contiguous sites	152.8	—	—	—	—	—
duodenum	152.0	197.4	230.7	211.2	235.2	239.0
ileum	152.2	197.4	230.7	211.2	235.2	239.0
jejunum	152.1	197.4	230.7	211.2	235.2	239.0
tract NEC	159.0	197.8	230.7	211.9	235.2	239.0
intra-abdominal	195.2	198.89	234.8	229.8	238.8	239.89
intracranial NEC	191.9	198.3	—	225.0	237.5	239.6
intrahepatic (bile) duct	155.1	197.8	230.8	211.5	235.3	239.0
intraocular	190.0	198.4	234.0	224.0	238.8	239.89
intraorbital	190.1	198.4	234.0	224.1	238.8	239.89
intrasellar	194.3	198.89	234.8	227.3	237.0	239.7
intrathoracic (cavity) (organs NEC)	195.1	198.89	234.8	229.8	238.8	239.89
contiguous sites with respiratory organs	165.8	—	—	—	—	—
iris	190.0	198.4	234.0	224.0	238.8	239.89
ischiorectal (fossa)	195.3	198.89	234.8	229.8	238.8	239.89
ischium	170.6	198.5	—	213.6	238.0	239.2
island of Reil	191.0	198.3	—	225.0	237.5	239.6
islands or islets of Langerhans	157.4	197.8	230.9	211.7	235.5	239.0
isthmus uteri	182.1	198.82	233.2	219.1	236.0	239.5
jaw	195.0	198.89	234.8	229.8	238.8	239.89
bone	170.1	198.5	—	213.1	238.0	239.2
carcinoma	143.9	—	—	—	—	—
lower	143.1	—	—	—	—	—
upper	143.0	—	—	—	—	—
lower	170.1	198.5	—	213.1	238.0	239.2
upper	170.0	198.5	—	213.0	238.0	239.2
carcinoma (any type) (lower) (upper)	195.0	—	—	—	—	—
skin (*see also* Neoplasm, skin, face)	173.30	198.2	232.3	216.3	238.2	239.2
soft tissues	143.9	198.89	230.0	210.4	235.1	239.0
lower	143.1	198.89	230.0	210.4	235.1	239.0
upper	143.0	198.89	230.0	210.4	235.1	239.0
jejunum	152.1	197.4	230.7	211.2	235.2	239.0

☑ **Additional Digit Required** — Refer to the Tabular List for Digit Selection   ▽ **Subterms under main terms may continue to next column or page**

Neoplasm, neoplastic—continued	Malignant — Primary	Malignant — Secondary	Malignant — Ca in situ	Benign	Uncertain Behavior	Unspecified
joint NEC (see also Neoplasm, bone)	170.9	198.5	—	213.9	238.0	239.2
acromioclavicular	170.4	198.5	—	213.4	238.0	239.2
bursa or synovial membrane — see Neoplasm, connective tissue						
costovertebral	170.3	198.5	—	213.3	238.0	239.2
sternocostal	170.3	198.5	—	213.3	238.0	239.2
temporomandibular	170.1	198.5	—	213.1	238.0	239.2
junction						
anorectal	154.8	197.5	230.7	211.4	235.5	239.0
cardioesophageal	151.0	197.8	230.2	211.1	235.2	239.0
esophagogastric	151.0	197.8	230.2	211.1	235.2	239.0
gastroesophageal	151.0	197.8	230.2	211.1	235.2	239.0
hard and soft palate	145.5	198.89	230.0	210.4	235.1	239.0
ileocecal	153.4	197.5	230.3	211.3	235.2	239.0
pelvirectal	154.0	197.5	230.4	211.4	235.2	239.0
pelviureteric	189.1	198.0	233.9	223.1	236.91	239.5
rectosigmoid	154.0	197.5	230.4	211.4	235.2	239.0
squamocolumnar, of cervix	180.8	198.82	233.1	219.0	236.0	239.5
kidney (parenchyma)	189.0	198.0	233.9	223.0	236.91	239.5
calyx	189.1	198.0	233.9	223.1	236.91	239.5
hilus	189.1	198.0	233.9	223.1	236.91	239.5
pelvis	189.1	198.0	233.9	223.1	236.91	239.5
knee NEC*	195.5	198.89	232.7	229.8	238.8	239.89
labia (skin)	184.4	198.82	233.32	221.2	236.3	239.5
majora	184.1	198.82	233.32	221.2	236.3	239.5
minora	184.2	198.82	233.32	221.2	236.3	239.5
labial (see also Neoplasm, lip) sulcus (lower) (upper)	145.1	198.89	230.0	210.4	235.1	239.0
labium (skin)	184.4	198.82	233.32	221.2	236.3	239.5
majus	184.1	198.82	233.32	221.2	236.3	239.5
minus	184.2	198.82	233.32	221.2	236.3	239.5
lacrimal						
canaliculi	190.7	198.4	234.0	224.7	238.8	239.89
duct (nasal)	190.7	198.4	234.0	224.7	238.8	239.89
gland	190.2	198.4	234.0	224.2	238.8	239.89
punctum	190.7	198.4	234.0	224.7	238.8	239.89
sac	190.7	198.4	234.0	224.7	238.8	239.89
Langerhans, islands or islets	157.4	197.8	230.9	211.7	235.5	239.0
laryngopharynx	148.9	198.89	230.0	210.8	235.1	239.0
larynx, laryngeal NEC	161.9	197.3	231.0	212.1	235.6	239.1
aryepiglottic fold	161.1	197.3	231.0	212.1	235.6	239.1
cartilage (arytenoid) (cricoid) (cuneiform) (thyroid)	161.3	197.3	231.0	212.1	235.6	239.1
commissure (anterior) (posterior)	161.0	197.3	231.0	212.1	235.6	239.1
contiguous sites	161.8	—	—	—	—	—
extrinsic NEC	161.1	197.3	231.0	212.1	235.6	239.1
meaning hypopharynx	148.9	198.89	230.0	210.8	235.1	239.0
interarytenoid fold	161.1	197.3	231.0	212.1	235.6	239.1
intrinsic	161.0	197.3	231.0	212.1	235.6	239.1
ventricular band	161.1	197.3	231.0	212.1	235.6	239.1
leg NEC*	195.5	198.89	232.7	229.8	238.8	239.89
lens, crystalline	190.0	198.4	234.0	224.0	238.8	239.89
lid (lower) (upper)	173.10	198.2	232.1	216.1	238.2	239.2
basal cell carcinoma	173.11	—	—	—	—	—
specified type NEC	173.19	—	—	—	—	—
squamous cell carcinoma	173.12	—	—	—	—	—

Neoplasm, neoplastic—continued	Malignant — Primary	Malignant — Secondary	Malignant — Ca in situ	Benign	Uncertain Behavior	Unspecified
ligament (see also Neoplasm, connective tissue)						
broad	183.3	198.82	233.39	221.0	236.3	239.5
Mackenrodt's	183.8	198.82	233.39	221.8	236.3	239.5
non-uterine — see Neoplasm, connective tissue						
round	183.5	198.82	—	221.0	236.3	239.5
sacro-uterine	183.4	198.82	—	221.0	236.3	239.5
uterine	183.4	198.82	—	221.0	236.3	239.5
utero-ovarian	183.8	198.82	233.39	221.8	236.3	239.5
uterosacral	183.4	198.82	—	221.0	236.3	239.5
limb*	195.8	198.89	232.8	229.8	238.8	239.89
lower*	195.5	198.89	232.7	229.8	238.8	239.89
upper*	195.4	198.89	232.6	229.8	238.8	239.89
limbus of cornea	190.4	198.4	234.0	224.4	238.8	239.89
lingual NEC (see also Neoplasm, tongue)	141.9	198.89	230.0	210.1	235.1	239.0
lingula, lung	162.3	197.0	231.2	212.3	235.7	239.1
lip (external) (lipstick area) (vermillion border)	140.9	198.89	230.0	210.0	235.1	239.0
buccal aspect — see Neoplasm, lip, internal						
commissure	140.6	198.89	230.0	210.4	235.1	239.0
contiguous sites	140.8	—	—	—	—	—
with oral cavity or pharynx	149.8	—	—	—	—	—
frenulum — see Neoplasm, lip, internal						
inner aspect — see Neoplasm, lip, internal						
internal (buccal) (frenulum) (mucosa) (oral)	140.5	198.89	230.0	210.0	235.1	239.0
lower	140.4	198.89	230.0	210.0	235.1	239.0
upper	140.3	198.89	230.0	210.0	235.1	239.0
lower	140.1	198.89	230.0	210.0	235.1	239.0
internal (buccal) (frenulum) (mucosa) (oral)	140.4	198.89	230.0	210.0	235.1	239.0
mucosa — see Neoplasm, lip, internal						
oral aspect — see Neoplasm, lip, internal						
skin (commissure) (lower) (upper)	173.00	198.2	232.0	216.0	238.2	239.2
basal cell carcinoma	173.01	—	—	—	—	—
specified type NEC	173.09	—	—	—	—	—
squamous cell carcinoma	173.02	—	—	—	—	—
upper	140.0	198.89	230.0	210.0	235.1	239.0
internal (buccal) (frenulum) (mucosa) (oral)	140.3	198.89	230.0	210.0	235.1	239.0
liver	155.2	197.7	230.8	211.5	235.3	239.0
primary	155.0	—	—	—	—	—
lobe						
azygos	162.3	197.0	231.2	212.3	235.7	239.1
frontal	191.1	198.3	—	225.0	237.5	239.6
lower	162.5	197.0	231.2	212.3	235.7	239.1
middle	162.4	197.0	231.2	212.3	235.7	239.1
occipital	191.4	198.3	—	225.0	237.5	239.6

☑ **Additional Digit Required** — Refer to the Tabular List for Digit Selection

▽ **Subterms under main terms may continue to next column or page**

Neoplasm, neoplastic — *continued*

	Malignant			Benign	Uncertain Behavior	Unspecified
	Primary	Secondary	Ca in situ			
lobe — *continued*						
parietal	191.3	198.3	—	225.0	237.5	239.6
temporal	191.2	198.3	—	225.0	237.5	239.6
upper	162.3	197.0	231.2	212.3	235.7	239.1
lumbosacral plexus	171.6	198.4	—	215.6	238.1	239.2
lung	162.9	197.0	231.2	212.3	235.7	239.1
azygos lobe	162.3	197.0	231.2	212.3	235.7	239.1
carina	162.2	197.0	231.2	212.3	235.7	239.1
contiguous sites with bronchus or trachea	162.8	—	—	—	—	—
hilus	162.2	197.0	231.2	212.3	235.7	239.1
lingula	162.3	197.0	231.2	212.3	235.7	239.1
lobe NEC	162.9	197.0	231.2	212.3	235.7	239.1
lower lobe	162.5	197.0	231.2	212.3	235.7	239.1
main bronchus	162.2	197.0	231.2	212.3	235.7	239.1
middle lobe	162.4	197.0	231.2	212.3	235.7	239.1
upper lobe	162.3	197.0	231.2	212.3	235.7	239.1
lymph, lymphatic channel NEC (*see also* Neoplasm, connective tissue)	171.9	198.89	—	215.9	238.1	239.2
gland						
(secondary)	—	196.9	—	229.0	238.8	239.89
abdominal	—	196.2	—	229.0	238.8	239.89
aortic	—	196.2	—	229.0	238.8	239.89
arm	—	196.3	—	229.0	238.8	239.89
auricular (anterior) (posterior)	—	196.0	—	229.0	238.8	239.89
axilla, axillary	—	196.3	—	229.0	238.8	239.89
brachial	—	196.3	—	229.0	238.8	239.89
bronchial	—	196.1	—	229.0	238.8	239.89
bronchopulmonary	—	196.1	—	229.0	238.8	239.89
celiac	—	196.2	—	229.0	238.8	239.89
cervical	—	196.0	—	229.0	238.8	239.89
cervicofacial	—	196.0	—	229.0	238.8	239.89
Cloquet	—	196.5	—	229.0	238.8	239.89
colic	—	196.2	—	229.0	238.8	239.89
common duct	—	196.2	—	229.0	238.8	239.89
cubital	—	196.3	—	229.0	238.8	239.89
diaphragmatic	—	196.1	—	229.0	238.8	239.89
epigastric, inferior	—	196.6	—	229.0	238.8	239.89
epitrochlear	—	196.3	—	229.0	238.8	239.89
esophageal	—	196.1	—	229.0	238.8	239.89
face	—	196.0	—	229.0	238.8	239.89
femoral	—	196.5	—	229.0	238.8	239.89
gastric	—	196.2	—	229.0	238.8	239.89
groin	—	196.5	—	229.0	238.8	239.89
head	—	196.0	—	229.0	238.8	239.89
hepatic	—	196.2	—	229.0	238.8	239.89
hilar (pulmonary)	—	196.1	—	229.0	238.8	239.89
splenic	—	196.2	—	229.0	238.8	239.89
hypogastric	—	196.6	—	229.0	238.8	239.89
ileocolic	—	196.2	—	229.0	238.8	239.89
iliac	—	196.6	—	229.0	238.8	239.89
infraclavicular	—	196.3	—	229.0	238.8	239.89
inguina, inguinal	—	196.5	—	229.0	238.8	239.89
innominate	—	196.1	—	229.0	238.8	239.89
intercostal	—	196.1	—	229.0	238.8	239.89
intestinal	—	196.2	—	229.0	238.8	239.89
intra-abdominal	—	196.2	—	229.0	238.8	239.89
intrapelvic	—	196.6	—	229.0	238.8	239.89
intrathoracic	—	196.1	—	229.0	238.8	239.9
jugular	—	196.0	—	229.0	238.8	239.89
leg	—	196.5	—	229.0	238.8	239.89
limb						
lower	—	196.5	—	229.0	238.8	239.9
upper	—	196.3	—	229.0	238.8	239.89
lower limb	—	196.5	—	229.0	238.8	239.9
lumbar	—	196.2	—	229.0	238.8	239.89

Neoplasm, neoplastic — *continued*

	Malignant			Benign	Uncertain Behavior	Unspecified
	Primary	Secondary	Ca in situ			
lymph, lymphatic — *continued*						
gland — *continued*						
mandibular	—	196.0	—	229.0	238.8	239.89
mediastinal	—	196.1	—	229.0	238.8	239.89
mesenteric (inferior) (superior)	—	196.2	—	229.0	238.8	239.89
midcolic	—	196.2	—	229.0	238.8	239.89
multiple sites in categories 196.0–196.6	—	196.8	—	229.0	238.8	239.89
neck	—	196.0	—	229.0	238.8	239.89
obturator	—	196.6	—	229.0	238.8	239.89
occipital	—	196.0	—	229.0	238.8	239.89
pancreatic	—	196.2	—	229.0	238.8	239.89
para-aortic	—	196.2	—	229.0	238.8	239.89
paracervical	—	196.6	—	229.0	238.8	239.89
parametrial	—	196.6	—	229.0	238.8	239.89
parasternal	—	196.1	—	229.0	238.8	239.89
parotid	—	196.0	—	229.0	238.8	239.89
pectoral	—	196.3	—	229.0	238.8	239.89
pelvic	—	196.6	—	229.0	238.8	239.89
peri-aortic	—	196.2	—	229.0	238.8	239.89
peripancreatic	—	196.2	—	229.0	238.8	239.89
popliteal	—	196.5	—	229.0	238.8	239.89
porta hepatis	—	196.2	—	229.0	238.8	239.89
portal	—	196.2	—	229.0	238.8	239.89
preauricular	—	196.0	—	229.0	238.8	239.89
prelaryngeal	—	196.0	—	229.0	238.8	239.89
presymphysial	—	196.6	—	229.0	238.8	239.89
pretracheal	—	196.0	—	229.0	238.8	239.89
primary (any site) NEC	202.9	—	—	—	—	—
pulmonary (hiler)	—	196.1	—	229.0	238.8	239.89
pyloric	—	196.2	—	229.0	238.8	239.89
retroperitoneal	—	196.2	—	229.0	238.8	239.89
retropharyngeal	—	196.0	—	229.0	238.8	239.89
Rosenmüller's	—	196.5	—	229.0	238.8	239.89
sacral	—	196.6	—	229.0	238.8	239.89
scalene	—	196.0	—	229.0	238.8	239.89
site NEC	—	196.9	—	229.0	238.8	239.89
splenic (hilar)	—	196.2	—	229.0	238.8	239.89
subclavicular	—	196.3	—	229.0	238.8	239.89
subinguinal	—	196.5	—	229.0	238.8	239.89
sublingual	—	196.0	—	229.0	238.8	239.89
submandibular	—	196.0	—	229.0	238.8	239.89
submaxillary	—	196.0	—	229.0	238.8	239.89
submental	—	196.0	—	229.0	238.8	239.89
subscapular	—	196.3	—	229.0	238.8	239.89
supraclavicular	—	196.0	—	229.0	238.8	239.89
thoracic	—	196.1	—	229.0	238.8	239.89
tibial	—	196.5	—	229.0	238.8	239.89
tracheal	—	196.1	—	229.0	238.8	239.89
tracheobronchial	—	196.1	—	229.0	238.8	239.89
upper limb	—	196.3	—	229.0	238.8	239.89
Virchow's	—	196.0	—	229.0	238.8	239.89
node (*see also* Neoplasm, lymph gland)						
primary NEC	202.9	—	—	—	—	—
vessel (*see also* Neoplasm, connective tissue)	171.9	198.89	—	215.9	238.1	239.2
Mackenrodt's ligament	183.8	198.82	233.39	221.8	236.3	239.5
malar	170.0	198.5	—	213.0	238.0	239.2
region — *see* Neoplasm, cheek						
mammary gland — *see* Neoplasm, breast						
mandible	170.1	198.5	—	213.1	238.0	239.2
alveolar						

☑ **Additional Digit Required** — Refer to the Tabular List for Digit Selection   Subterms under main terms may continue to next column or page

202 — Volume 2   ►◄ Revised Text   ● New Line   ▲ Revised Code   2014 ICD-9-CM

Neoplasm, neoplastic — continued	Malignant			Benign	Uncertain Behavior	Unspecified
	Primary	Secondary	Ca in situ			
mandible — continued						
alveolar — continued						
mucosa	143.1	198.89	230.0	210.4	235.1	239.0
mucose	143.1	198.89	230.0	210.4	235.1	239.0
ridge or process	170.1	198.5	—	213.1	238.0	239.2
carcinoma	143.1	—	—	—	—	—
carcinoma	143.1	—	—	—	—	—
marrow (bone) NEC	202.9	198.5	—	—	—	238.79
mastectomy site (skin)	173.50	198.2				
basal cell carcinoma	173.51	—	—	—	—	—
specified as breast tissue	174.8	198.81				
specified type NEC	173.59	—	—	—	—	—
squamous cell carcinoma	173.52	—	—	—	—	—
mastoid (air cells) (antrum) (cavity)	160.1	197.3	231.8	212.0	235.9	239.1
bone or process	170.0	198.5	—	213.0	238.0	239.2
maxilla, maxillary (superior)	170.0	198.5	—	213.0	238.0	239.2
alveolar						
mucosa	143.0	198.89	230.0	210.4	235.1	239.0
ridge or process	170.0	198.5	—	213.0	238.0	239.2
carcinoma	143.0	—	—	—	—	—
antrum	160.2	197.3	231.8	212.0	235.9	239.1
carcinoma	143.0	—	—	—	—	—
inferior — see Neoplasm, mandible						
sinus	160.2	197.3	231.8	212.0	235.9	239.1
meatus						
external (ear) (see also Neoplasm, skin, ear)	173.20	198.2	232.2	216.2	238.2	239.2
Meckel's diverticulum	152.3	197.4	230.7	211.2	235.2	239.0
mediastinum, mediastinal	164.9	197.1	—	212.5	235.8	239.89
anterior	164.2	197.1	—	212.5	235.8	239.89
contiguous sites with heart and thymus	164.8	—	—	—	—	—
posterior	164.3	197.1	—	212.5	235.8	239.89
medulla						
adrenal	194.0	198.7	234.8	227.0	237.2	239.7
oblongata	191.7	198.3	—	225.0	237.5	239.6
meibomian gland	173.10	198.2	232.1	216.1	238.2	239.2
basal cell carcinoma	173.11	—	—	—	—	—
specified type NEC	173.19	—	—	—	—	—
squamous cell carcinoma	173.12	—	—	—	—	—
meninges (brain) (cerebral) (cranial) (intracranial)	192.1	198.4	—	225.2	237.6	239.7
spinal (cord)	192.3	198.4	—	225.4	237.6	239.7
meniscus, knee joint (lateral) (medial)	170.7	198.5	—	213.7	238.0	239.2
mesentery, mesenteric	158.8	197.6	—	211.8	235.4	239.0
mesoappendix	158.8	197.6	—	211.8	235.4	239.0
mesocolon	158.8	197.6	—	211.8	235.4	239.0
mesopharynx — see Neoplasm, oropharynx						
mesosalpinx	183.3	198.82	233.39	221.0	236.3	239.5
mesovarium	183.3	198.82	233.39	221.0	236.3	239.5

Neoplasm, neoplastic — continued	Malignant			Benign	Uncertain Behavior	Unspecified
	Primary	Secondary	Ca in situ			
metacarpus (any bone)	170.5	198.5	—	213.5	238.0	239.2
metastatic NEC (see also Neoplasm, by site, secondary)	—	199.1	—	—	—	—
metatarsus (any bone)	170.8	198.5	—	213.8	238.0	239.2
midbrain	191.7	198.3	—	225.0	237.5	239.6
milk duct — see Neoplasm, breast						
mons						
pubis	184.4	198.82	233.32	221.2	236.3	239.5
veneris	184.4	198.82	233.32	221.2	236.3	239.5
motor tract	192.9	198.4	—	225.9	237.9	239.7
brain	191.9	198.3	—	225.0	237.5	239.6
spinal	192.2	198.3	—	225.3	237.5	239.7
mouth	145.9	198.89	230.0	210.4	235.1	239.0
contiguous sites	145.8	—	—	—	—	—
floor	144.9	198.89	230.0	210.3	235.1	239.0
anterior portion	144.0	198.89	230.0	210.3	235.1	239.0
contiguous sites	144.8	—	—	—	—	—
lateral portion	144.1	198.89	230.0	210.3	235.1	239.0
roof	145.5	198.89	230.0	210.4	235.1	239.0
specified part NEC	145.8	198.89	230.0	210.4	235.1	239.0
vestibule	145.1	198.89	230.0	210.4	235.1	239.0
mucosa						
alveolar (ridge or process)	143.9	198.89	230.0	210.4	235.1	239.0
lower	143.1	198.89	230.0	210.4	235.1	239.0
upper	143.0	198.89	230.0	210.4	235.1	239.0
buccal	145.0	198.89	230.0	210.4	235.1	239.0
cheek	145.0	198.89	230.0	210.4	235.1	239.0
lip — see Neoplasm, lip, internal						
nasal	160.0	197.3	231.8	212.0	235.9	239.1
oral	145.0	198.89	230.0	210.4	235.1	239.0
Müllerian duct						
female	184.8	198.82	233.39	221.8	236.3	239.5
male	187.8	198.82	233.6	222.8	236.6	239.5
multiple sites NEC	199.0	—	234.9	229.9	238.9	—
muscle (see also Neoplasm, connective tissue)						
extraocular	190.1	198.4	234.0	224.1	238.8	239.89
myocardium	164.1	198.89	—	212.7	238.8	239.89
myometrium	182.0	198.82	233.2	219.1	236.0	239.5
myopericardium	164.1	198.89	—	212.7	238.8	239.89
nabothian gland (follicle)	180.0	198.82	233.1	219.0	236.0	239.5
nail	173.90	198.2	232.9	216.9	238.2	239.2
finger (see also Neoplasm, skin, limb, upper)	173.60	198.2	232.6	216.6	238.2	239.2
toe (see also Neoplasm, skin, limb, lower)	173.70	198.2	232.7	216.7	238.2	239.2
nares, naris (anterior) (posterior)	160.0	197.3	231.8	212.0	235.9	239.1
nasal — see Neoplasm, nose						
nasolabial groove (see also Neoplasm, skin, face)	173.30	198.2	232.3	216.3	238.2	239.2
nasolacrimal duct	190.7	198.4	234.0	224.7	238.8	239.89
nasopharynx, nasopharyngeal	147.9	198.89	230.0	210.7	235.1	239.0
contiguous sites	147.8	—	—	—	—	—
floor	147.3	198.89	230.0	210.7	235.1	239.0
roof	147.0	198.89	230.0	210.7	235.1	239.0
specified site NEC	147.8	198.89	230.0	210.7	235.1	239.0
wall	147.9	198.89	230.0	210.7	235.1	239.0

	Malignant			Benign	Uncertain Behavior	Unspecified
	Primary	Secondary	Ca in situ			
Neoplasm, neoplastic — *continued*						
nasopharynx, nasopharyngeal — *continued*						
wall — *continued*						
anterior	147.3	198.89	230.0	210.7	235.1	239.0
lateral	147.2	198.89	230.0	210.7	235.1	239.0
posterior	147.1	198.89	230.0	210.7	235.1	239.0
superior	147.0	198.89	230.0	210.7	235.1	239.0
nates (*see also* Neoplasm, skin, trunk)	173.50	198.2	232.5	216.5	238.2	239.2
neck NEC*	195.0	198.89	234.8	229.8	238.8	239.89
skin	173.40	198.2	232.4	216.4	238.2	239.2
basal cell carcinoma	173.41	—	—	—	—	—
specified type NEC	173.49	—	—	—	—	—
squamous cell carcinoma	173.42	—	—	—	—	—
nerve (autonomic) (ganglion) (parasympathetic) (peripheral) (sympathetic) (*see also* Neoplasm, connective tissue)						
abducens	192.0	198.4	—	225.1	237.9	239.7
accessory (spinal)	192.0	198.4	—	225.1	237.9	239.7
acoustic	192.0	198.4	—	225.1	237.9	239.7
auditory	192.0	198.4	—	225.1	237.9	239.7
brachial	171.2	198.89	—	215.2	238.1	239.2
cranial (any)	192.0	198.4	—	225.1	237.9	239.7
facial	192.0	198.4	—	225.1	237.9	239.7
femoral	171.3	198.89	—	215.3	238.1	239.2
glossopharyngeal	192.0	198.4	—	225.1	237.9	239.7
hypoglossal	192.0	198.4	—	225.1	237.9	239.7
intercostal	171.4	198.89	—	215.4	238.1	239.2
lumbar	171.7	198.89	—	215.7	238.1	239.2
median	171.2	198.89	—	215.2	238.1	239.2
obturator	171.3	198.89	—	215.3	238.1	239.2
oculomotor	192.0	198.4	—	225.1	237.9	239.7
olfactory	192.0	198.4	—	225.1	237.9	239.7
optic	192.0	198.4	—	225.1	237.9	239.7
peripheral NEC	171.9	198.89	—	215.9	238.1	239.2
radial	171.2	198.89	—	215.2	238.1	239.2
sacral	171.6	198.89	—	215.6	238.1	239.2
sciatic	171.3	198.89	—	215.3	238.1	239.2
spinal NEC	171.9	198.89	—	215.9	238.1	239.2
trigeminal	192.0	198.4	—	225.1	237.9	239.7
trochlear	192.0	198.4	—	225.1	237.9	239.7
ulnar	171.2	198.89	—	215.2	238.1	239.2
vagus	192.0	198.4	—	225.1	237.9	239.7
nervous system (central) NEC	192.9	198.4	—	225.9	237.9	239.7
autonomic NEC	171.9	198.89	—	215.9	238.1	239.2
brain (*see also* Neoplasm, brain) membrane or meninges	192.1	198.4	—	225.2	237.6	239.7
contiguous sites	192.8	—	—	—	—	—
parasympathetic NEC*	171.9	198.89	—	215.9	238.1	239.2
sympathetic NEC*	171.9	198.89	—	215.9	238.1	239.2
nipple (female)	174.0	198.81	233.0	217	238.3	239.3
male	175.0	198.81	233.0	217	238.3	239.3
nose, nasal	195.0	198.89	234.8	229.8	238.8	239.89
ala (external) (*see also* Neoplasm, nose, skin)	173.30	198.2	232.3	216.3	238.2	239.2
bone	170.0	198.5	—	213.0	238.0	239.2
cartilage	160.0	197.3	231.8	212.0	235.9	239.1
Neoplasm, neoplastic — *continued*						
nose, nasal — *continued*						
cavity	160.0	197.3	231.8	212.0	235.9	239.1
contiguous sites with accessory sinuses or middle ear	160.8	—	—	—	—	—
choana	147.3	198.89	230.0	210.7	235.1	239.0
external (skin) (*see also* Neoplasm, nose, skin)	173.30	198.2	232.3	216.3	238.2	239.2
fossa	160.0	197.3	231.8	212.0	235.9	239.1
internal	160.0	197.3	231.8	212.0	235.9	239.1
mucosa	160.0	197.3	231.8	212.0	235.9	239.1
septum	160.0	197.3	231.8	212.0	235.9	239.1
posterior margin	147.3	198.89	230.0	210.7	235.1	239.0
sinus — *see* Neoplasm, sinus						
skin	173.30	198.2	232.3	216.3	238.2	239.2
basal cell carcinoma	173.31	—	—	—	—	—
specified type NEC	173.39	—	—	—	—	—
squamous cell carcinoma	173.32	—	—	—	—	—
turbinate (mucosa)	160.0	197.3	231.8	212.0	235.9	239.1
bone	170.0	198.5	—	213.0	238.0	239.2
vestibule	160.0	197.3	231.8	212.0	235.9	239.1
nostril	160.0	197.3	231.8	212.0	235.9	239.1
nucleus pulposus	170.2	198.5	—	213.2	238.0	239.2
occipital bone	170.0	198.5	—	213.0	238.0	239.2
lobe or pole, brain	191.4	198.3	—	225.0	237.5	239.6
odontogenic — *see* Neoplasm, jaw bone						
oesophagus — *see* Neoplasm, esophagus						
olfactory nerve or bulb	192.0	198.4	—	225.1	237.9	239.7
olive (brain)	191.7	198.3	—	225.0	237.5	239.6
omentum	158.8	197.6	—	211.8	235.4	239.0
operculum (brain)	191.0	198.3	—	225.0	237.5	239.6
optic nerve, chiasm, or tract	192.0	198.4	—	225.1	237.9	239.7
oral (cavity)	145.9	198.89	230.0	210.4	235.1	239.0
contiguous sites with lip or pharynx	149.8	—	—	—	—	—
ill-defined	149.9	198.89	230.0	210.4	235.1	239.0
mucosa	145.9	198.89	230.0	210.4	235.1	239.0
orbit	190.1	198.4	234.0	224.1	238.8	239.89
bone	170.0	198.5	—	213.0	238.0	239.2
eye	190.1	198.4	234.0	224.1	238.8	239.89
soft parts	190.1	198.4	234.0	224.1	238.8	239.89
organ of Zuckerkandl	194.6	198.89	—	227.6	237.3	239.7
oropharynx	146.9	198.89	230.0	210.6	235.1	239.0
branchial cleft (vestige)	146.8	198.89	230.0	210.6	235.1	239.0
contiguous sites	146.8	—	—	—	—	—
junctional region	146.5	198.89	230.0	210.6	235.1	239.0
lateral wall	146.6	198.89	230.0	210.6	235.1	239.0
pillars of fauces	146.2	198.89	230.0	210.6	235.1	239.0
posterior wall	146.7	198.89	230.0	210.6	235.1	239.0
specified part NEC	146.8	198.89	230.0	210.6	235.1	239.0
vallecula	146.3	198.89	230.0	210.6	235.1	239.0
os						
external	180.1	198.82	233.1	219.0	236.0	239.5

Neoplasm, neoplastic—continued

	Malignant					
	Primary	Secondary	Ca in situ	Benign	Uncertain Behavior	Unspecified
os — continued						
internal	180.0	198.82	233.1	219.0	236.0	239.5
ovary	183.0	198.6	233.39	220	236.2	239.5
oviduct	183.2	198.82	233.39	221.0	236.3	239.5
palate	145.5	198.89	230.0	210.4	235.1	239.0
hard	145.2	198.89	230.0	210.4	235.1	239.0
junction of hard and soft palate	145.5	198.89	230.0	210.4	235.1	239.0
soft	145.3	198.89	230.0	210.4	235.1	239.0
nasopharyngeal surface	147.3	198.89	230.0	210.7	235.1	239.0
posterior surface	147.3	198.89	230.0	210.7	235.1	239.0
superior surface	147.3	198.89	230.0	210.7	235.1	239.0
palatoglossal arch	146.2	198.89	230.0	210.6	235.1	239.0
palatopharyngeal arch	146.2	198.89	230.0	210.6	235.1	239.0
pallium	191.0	198.3	—	225.0	237.5	239.6
palpebra	173.10	198.2	232.1	216.1	238.2	239.2
basal cell carcinoma	173.11	—	—	—	—	—
specified type NEC	173.19	—	—	—	—	—
squamous cell carcinoma	173.12	—	—	—	—	—
pancreas	157.9	197.8	230.9	211.6	235.5	239.0
body	157.1	197.8	230.9	211.6	235.5	239.0
contiguous sites	157.8	—	—	—	—	—
duct (of Santorini) (of Wirsung)	157.3	197.8	230.9	211.6	235.5	239.0
ectopic tissue	157.8	197.8	230.9	211.6	235.5	239.0
head	157.0	197.8	230.9	211.6	235.5	239.0
islet cells	157.4	197.8	230.9	211.7	235.5	239.0
neck	157.8	197.8	230.9	211.6	235.5	239.0
tail	157.2	197.8	230.9	211.6	235.5	239.0
para-aortic body	194.6	198.89	—	227.6	237.3	239.7
paraganglion NEC	194.6	198.89	—	227.6	237.3	239.7
parametrium	183.4	198.82	—	221.0	236.3	239.5
paranephric	158.0	197.6	—	211.8	235.4	239.0
pararectal	195.3	198.89	—	229.8	238.8	239.89
parasagittal (region)	195.0	198.89	234.8	229.8	238.8	239.89
parasellar	192.9	198.4	—	225.9	237.9	239.7
parathyroid (gland)	194.1	198.89	234.8	227.1	237.4	239.7
paraurethral	195.3	198.89	—	229.8	238.8	239.89
gland	189.4	198.1	233.9	223.89	236.99	239.5
paravaginal	195.3	198.89	—	229.8	238.8	239.89
parenchyma, kidney	189.0	198.0	233.9	223.0	236.91	239.5
parietal						
bone	170.0	198.5	—	213.0	238.0	239.2
lobe, brain	191.3	198.3	—	225.0	237.5	239.6
paroophoron	183.3	198.82	233.39	221.0	236.3	239.5
parotid (duct) (gland)	142.0	198.89	230.0	210.2	235.0	239.0
parovarium	183.3	198.82	233.39	221.0	236.3	239.5
patella	170.8	198.5	—	213.8	238.0	239.2
peduncle, cerebral	191.7	198.3	—	225.0	237.5	239.6
pelvirectal junction	154.0	197.5	230.4	211.4	235.2	239.0
pelvis, pelvic	195.3	198.89	234.8	229.8	238.8	239.89
bone	170.6	198.5	—	213.6	238.0	239.2
floor	195.3	198.89	234.8	229.8	238.8	239.89
renal	189.1	198.0	233.9	223.1	236.91	239.5
viscera	195.3	198.89	234.8	229.8	238.8	239.89
wall	195.3	198.89	234.8	229.8	238.8	239.89
pelvo-abdominal	195.8	198.89	234.8	229.8	238.8	239.89
penis	187.4	198.82	233.5	222.1	236.6	239.5
body	187.3	198.82	233.5	222.1	236.6	239.5
corpus (cavernosum)	187.3	198.82	233.5	222.1	236.6	239.5
glans	187.2	198.82	233.5	222.1	236.6	239.5
skin NEC	187.4	198.82	233.5	222.1	236.6	239.5
periadrenal (tissue)	158.0	197.6	—	211.8	235.4	239.0

Neoplasm, neoplastic—continued

	Malignant					
	Primary	Secondary	Ca in situ	Benign	Uncertain Behavior	Unspecified
perianal (skin) (see also Neoplasm, skin, anus)	173.50	198.2	232.5	216.5	238.2	239.2
pericardium	164.1	198.89	—	212.7	238.8	239.89
perinephric	158.0	197.6	—	211.8	235.4	239.0
perineum	195.3	198.89	234.8	229.8	238.8	239.89
periodontal tissue NEC	143.9	198.89	230.0	210.4	235.1	239.0
periosteum — see Neoplasm, bone						
peripancreatic	158.0	197.6	—	211.8	235.4	239.0
peripheral nerve NEC	171.9	198.89	—	215.9	238.1	239.2
perirectal (tissue)	195.3	198.89	—	229.8	238.8	239.89
perirenal (tissue)	158.0	197.6	—	211.8	235.4	239.0
peritoneum, peritoneal (cavity)	158.9	197.6	—	211.8	235.4	239.0
contiguous sites	158.8	—	—	—	—	—
with digestive organs	159.8	—	—	—	—	—
parietal	158.8	197.6	—	211.8	235.4	239.0
pelvic	158.8	197.6	—	211.8	235.4	239.0
specified part NEC	158.8	197.6	—	211.8	235.4	239.0
peritonsillar (tissue)	195.0	198.89	234.8	229.8	238.8	239.89
periurethral tissue	195.3	198.89	—	229.8	238.8	239.89
phalanges	170.9	198.5	—	213.9	238.0	239.2
foot	170.8	198.5	—	213.8	238.0	239.2
hand	170.5	198.5	—	213.5	238.0	239.2
pharynx, pharyngeal	149.0	198.89	230.0	210.9	235.1	239.0
bursa	147.1	198.89	230.0	210.7	235.1	239.0
fornix	147.3	198.89	230.0	210.7	235.1	239.0
recess	147.2	198.89	230.0	210.7	235.1	239.0
region	149.0	198.89	230.0	210.9	235.1	239.0
tonsil	147.1	198.89	230.0	210.7	235.1	239.0
wall (lateral) (posterior)	149.0	198.89	230.0	210.9	235.1	239.0
pia mater (cerebral) (cranial)	192.1	198.4	—	225.2	237.6	239.7
spinal	192.3	198.4	—	225.4	237.6	239.7
pillars of fauces	146.2	198.89	230.0	210.6	235.1	239.0
pineal (body) (gland)	194.4	198.89	234.8	227.4	237.1	239.7
pinna (ear) NEC (see also Neoplasm, skin, ear)	173.20	198.2	232.2	216.2	238.2	239.2
cartilage	171.0	198.89	—	215.0	238.1	239.2
piriform fossa or sinus	148.1	198.89	230.0	210.8	235.1	239.0
pituitary (body) (fossa) (gland) (lobe)	194.3	198.89	234.8	227.3	237.0	239.7
placenta	181	198.82	233.2	219.8	236.1	239.5
pleura, pleural (cavity)	163.9	197.2	—	212.4	235.8	239.1
contiguous sites	163.8	—	—	—	—	—
parietal	163.0	197.2	—	212.4	235.8	239.1
visceral	163.1	197.2	—	212.4	235.8	239.1
plexus						
brachial	171.2	198.89	—	215.2	238.1	239.2
cervical	171.0	198.89	—	215.0	238.1	239.2
choroid	191.5	198.3	—	225.0	237.5	239.6
lumbosacral	171.6	198.89	—	215.6	238.1	239.2
sacral	171.6	198.89	—	215.6	238.1	239.2
pluri-endocrine	194.8	198.89	234.8	227.8	237.4	239.7
pole						
frontal	191.1	198.3	—	225.0	237.5	239.6
occipital	191.4	198.3	—	225.0	237.5	239.6
pons (varolii)	191.7	198.3	—	225.0	237.5	239.6
popliteal fossa or space*	195.5	198.89	234.8	229.8	238.8	239.89
postcricoid (region)	148.0	198.89	230.0	210.8	235.1	239.0

Neoplasm, os — Neoplasm, postcricoid

	Malignant					
	Primary	Secondary	Ca in situ	Benign	Uncertain Behavior	Unspecified
Neoplasm, neoplastic— *continued*						
posterior fossa (cranial)	191.9	198.3	—	225.0	237.5	239.6
postnasal space	147.9	198.89	230.0	210.7	235.1	239.0
prepuce	187.1	198.82	233.5	222.1	236.6	239.5
prepylorus	151.1	197.8	230.2	211.1	235.2	239.0
presacral (region)	195.3	198.89	—	229.8	238.8	239.89
prostate (gland)	185	198.82	233.4	222.2	236.5	239.5
utricle	189.3	198.1	233.9	223.81	236.99	239.5
pterygoid fossa	171.0	198.89	—	215.0	238.1	239.2
pubic bone	170.6	198.5	—	213.6	238.0	239.2
pudenda, pudendum (female)	184.4	198.82	233.32	221.2	236.3	239.5
pulmonary	162.9	197.0	231.2	212.3	235.7	239.1
putamen	191.0	198.3	—	225.0	237.5	239.6
pyloric						
antrum	151.2	197.8	230.2	211.1	235.2	239.0
canal	151.1	197.8	230.2	211.1	235.2	239.0
pylorus	151.1	197.8	230.2	211.1	235.2	239.0
pyramid (brain)	191.7	198.3	—	225.0	237.5	239.6
pyriform fossa or sinus	148.1	198.89	230.0	210.8	235.1	239.0
radius (any part)	170.4	198.5	—	213.4	238.0	239.2
Rathke's pouch	194.3	198.89	234.8	227.3	237.0	239.7
rectosigmoid (colon) (junction)	154.0	197.5	230.4	211.4	235.2	239.0
contiguous sites with anus or rectum	154.8	—	—	—	—	—
rectouterine pouch	158.8	197.6	—	211.8	235.4	239.0
rectovaginal septum or wall	195.3	198.89	234.8	229.8	238.8	239.89
rectovesical septum	195.3	198.89	234.8	229.8	238.8	239.89
rectum (ampulla)	154.1	197.5	230.4	211.4	235.2	239.0
and colon	154.0	197.5	230.4	211.4	235.2	239.0
contiguous sites with anus or rectosigmoid junction	154.8	—	—	—	—	—
renal	189.0	198.0	233.9	223.0	236.91	239.5
calyx	189.1	198.0	233.9	223.1	236.91	239.5
hilus	189.1	198.0	233.9	223.1	236.91	239.5
parenchyma	189.0	198.0	233.9	223.0	236.91	239.5
pelvis	189.1	198.0	233.9	223.1	236.91	239.5
respiratory organs or system NEC	165.9	197.3	231.9	212.9	235.9	239.1
contiguous sites with intrathoracic organs	165.8	—	—	—	—	—
specified sites NEC	165.8	197.3	231.8	212.8	235.9	239.1
tract NEC	165.9	197.3	231.9	212.9	235.9	239.1
upper	165.0	197.3	231.9	212.9	235.9	239.1
retina	190.5	198.4	234.0	224.5	238.8	239.81
retro-orbital	195.0	198.89	234.8	229.8	238.8	239.89
retrobulbar	190.1	198.4	—	224.1	238.8	239.89
retrocecal	158.0	197.6	—	211.8	235.4	239.0
retromolar (area) (triangle) (trigone)	145.6	198.89	230.0	210.4	235.1	239.0
retroperitoneal (space) (tissue)	158.0	197.6	—	211.8	235.4	239.0
contiguous sites	158.8	—	—	—	—	—
retroperitoneum	158.0	197.6	—	211.8	235.4	239.0
contiguous sites	158.8	—	—	—	—	—
retropharyngeal	149.0	198.89	230.0	210.9	235.1	239.0
retrovesical (septum)	195.3	198.89	234.8	229.8	238.8	239.89
rhinencephalon	191.0	198.3	—	225.0	237.5	239.6
rib	170.3	198.5	—	213.3	238.0	239.2
Rosenmüller's fossa	147.2	198.89	230.0	210.7	235.1	239.0
round ligament	183.5	198.82	—	221.0	236.3	239.5

	Malignant					
	Primary	Secondary	Ca in situ	Benign	Uncertain Behavior	Unspecified
Neoplasm, neoplastic— *continued*						
sacrococcyx, sacrococcygeal	170.6	198.5	—	213.6	238.0	239.2
region	195.3	198.89	234.8	229.8	238.8	239.89
sacrouterine ligament	183.4	198.82	—	221.0	236.3	239.5
sacrum, sacral (vertebra)	170.6	198.5	—	213.6	238.0	239.2
salivary gland or duct (major)	142.9	198.89	230.0	210.2	235.0	239.0
contiguous sites	142.8	—	—	—	—	—
minor NEC	145.9	198.89	230.0	210.4	235.1	239.0
parotid	142.0	198.89	230.0	210.2	235.0	239.0
pluriglandular	142.8	198.89	—	210.2	235.0	239.0
sublingual	142.2	198.89	230.0	210.2	235.0	239.0
submandibular	142.1	198.89	230.0	210.2	235.0	239.0
submaxillary	142.1	198.89	230.0	210.2	235.0	239.0
salpinx (uterine)	183.2	198.82	233.39	221.0	236.3	239.5
Santorini's duct	157.3	197.8	230.9	211.6	235.5	239.0
scalp	173.40	198.2	232.4	216.4	238.2	239.2
basal cell carcinoma	173.41	—	—	—	—	—
specified type NEC	173.49	—	—	—	—	—
squamous cell carcinoma	173.42	—	—	—	—	—
scapula (any part)	170.4	198.5	—	213.4	238.0	239.2
scapular region	195.1	198.89	234.8	229.8	238.8	239.89
scar NEC (*see also* Neoplasm, skin)	173.90	198.2	232.9	216.9	238.2	239.2
sciatic nerve	171.3	198.89	—	215.3	238.1	239.2
sclera	190.0	198.4	234.0	224.0	238.8	239.89
scrotum (skin)	187.7	198.82	—	222.4	236.6	239.5
sebaceous gland — *see* Neoplasm, skin						
sella turcica	194.3	198.89	234.8	227.3	237.0	239.7
bone	170.0	198.5	—	213.0	238.0	239.2
semilunar cartilage (knee)	170.7	198.5	—	213.7	238.0	239.2
seminal vesicle	187.8	198.82	233.6	222.8	236.6	239.5
septum						
nasal	160.0	197.3	231.8	212.0	235.9	239.1
posterior margin	147.3	198.89	230.0	210.7	235.1	239.0
rectovaginal	195.3	198.89	234.8	229.8	238.8	239.89
rectovesical	195.3	198.89	234.8	229.8	238.8	239.89
urethrovaginal	184.9	198.82	233.39	221.9	236.3	239.5
vesicovaginal	184.9	198.82	233.39	221.9	236.3	239.5
shoulder NEC*	195.4	198.89	232.6	229.8	238.8	239.89
sigmoid flexure (lower) (upper)	153.3	197.5	230.3	211.3	235.2	239.0
sinus (accessory)	160.9	197.3	231.8	212.0	235.9	239.1
bone (any)	170.0	198.5	—	213.0	238.0	239.2
contiguous sites with middle ear or nasal cavities	160.8	—	—	—	—	—
ethmoidal	160.3	197.3	231.8	212.0	235.9	239.1
frontal	160.4	197.3	231.8	212.0	235.9	239.1
maxillary	160.2	197.3	231.8	212.0	235.9	239.1
nasal, paranasal NEC	160.9	197.3	231.8	212.0	235.9	239.1
pyriform	148.1	198.89	230.0	210.8	235.1	239.0
sphenoidal	160.5	197.3	231.8	212.0	235.9	239.1
skeleton, skeletal NEC	170.9	198.5	—	213.9	238.0	239.2
Skene's gland	189.4	198.1	233.9	223.89	236.99	239.5
skin NOS	173.90	198.2	232.9	216.9	238.2	239.2
abdominal wall	173.50	198.2	232.5	216.5	238.2	239.2
basal cell carcinoma	173.51	—	—	—	—	—
specified type NEC	173.59	—	—	—	—	—
squamous cell carcinoma	173.52	—	—	—	—	—

☑ Additional Digit Required — Refer to the Tabular List for Digit Selection   ▽ Subterms under main terms may continue to next column or page

206 — Volume 2   ▶◀ Revised Text   ● New Line   ▲ Revised Code   2014 ICD-9-CM

	Malignant Primary	Malignant Secondary	Malignant Ca in situ	Benign	Uncertain Behavior	Unspecified
Neoplasm, neoplastic— *continued*						
skin — *continued*						
ala nasi (*see also* Neoplasm, skin, face)	173.30	198.2	232.3	216.3	238.2	239.2
ankle (*see also* Neoplasm, skin, limb, lower)	173.70	198.2	232.7	216.7	238.2	239.2
antecubital space (*see also* Neoplasm, skin, limb, upper)	173.60	198.2	232.6	216.6	238.2	239.2
anus	173.50	198.2	232.5	216.5	238.2	239.2
basal cell carcinoma	173.51	—	—	—	—	—
specified type NEC	173.59	—	—	—	—	—
squamous cell carcinoma	173.52	—	—	—	—	—
arm (*see also* Neoplasm, skin, limb, upper)	173.60	198.2	232.6	216.6	238.2	239.2
auditory canal (external) (*see also* Neoplasm, skin, ear)	173.20	198.2	232.2	216.2	238.2	239.2
auricle (ear) (*see also* Neoplasm, skin, ear)	173.20	198.2	232.2	216.2	238.2	239.2
auricular canal (external) (*see also* Neoplasm, skin, ear)	173.20	198.2	232.2	216.2	238.2	239.2
axilla, axillary fold (*see also* Neoplasm, skin, trunk)	173.50	198.2	232.5	216.5	238.2	239.2
back	173.50	198.2	232.5	216.5	238.2	239.2
basal cell carcinoma	173.51	—	—	—	—	—
specified type NEC	173.59	—	—	—	—	—
squamous cell carcinoma	173.52	—	—	—	—	—
basal cell carcinoma, unspecified site	173.91	—	—	—	—	—
breast (*see also* Neoplasm, skin, trunk)	173.50	198.2	232.5	216.5	238.2	239.2
brow (*see also* Neoplasm, skin, face)	173.30	198.2	232.3	216.3	238.2	239.2
buttock (*see also* Neoplasm, skin, trunk)	173.50	198.2	232.5	216.5	238.2	239.2
calf (*see also* Neoplasm, skin, limb, lower)	173.70	198.2	232.7	216.7	238.2	239.2
canthus (eye) (inner) (outer)	173.10	198.2	232.1	216.1	238.2	239.2
basal cell carcinoma	173.11	—	—	—	—	—
specified type NEC	173.19	—	—	—	—	—
squamous cell carcinoma	173.12	—	—	—	—	—
cervical region (*see also* Neoplasm, skin, neck)	173.40	198.2	232.4	216.4	238.2	239.2
cheek (external) (*see also* Neoplasm, skin, face)	173.30	198.2	232.3	216.3	238.2	239.2
chest (wall) (*see also* Neoplasm, skin, trunk)	173.50	198.2	232.5	216.5	238.2	239.2
chin (*see also* Neoplasm, skin, face)	173.30	198.2	232.3	216.3	238.2	239.2
Neoplasm, neoplastic— *continued*						
skin — *continued*						
clavicular area (*see also* Neoplasm, skin, trunk)	173.50	198.2	232.5	216.5	238.2	239.2
clitoris	—	198.82	233.32	221.2	236.3	239.5
columnella (*see also* Neoplasm, skin, face)	173.30	198.2	232.3	216.3	238.2	239.2
concha (*see also* Neoplasm, skin, ear)	173.20	198.2	232.2	216.2	238.2	239.2
contiguous sites	173.80	—	—			
basal cell carcinoma	173.81	—	—	—	—	—
specified type NEC	173.89	—	—	—	—	—
squamous cell carcinoma	173.82	—	—	—	—	—
ear (external)	173.20	198.2	232.2	216.2	238.2	239.2
basal cell carcinoma	173.21	—	—	—	—	—
specified type NEC	173.29	—	—	—	—	—
squamous cell carcinoma	173.22	—	—	—	—	—
elbow (*see also* Neoplasm, skin, limb, upper)	173.60	198.2	232.6	216.6	238.2	239.2
eyebrow (*see also* Neoplasm, skin, face)	173.30	198.2	232.3	216.3	238.2	239.2
eyelid	173.10	198.2	232.1	—	238.2	239.2
basal cell carcinoma	173.11	—	—	—	—	—
specified type NEC	173.19	—	—	—	—	—
squamous cell carcinoma	173.12	—	—	—	—	—
face NEC	173.30	198.2	232.3	216.3	238.2	239.2
basal cell carcinoma	173.31	—	—	—	—	—
specified type NEC	173.39	—	—	—	—	—
squamous cell carcinoma	173.32	—	—	—	—	—
female genital organs (external)	184.4	198.82	233.30	221.2	236.3	239.5
clitoris	184.3	198.82	233.32	221.2	236.3	239.5
labium NEC	184.4	198.82	233.32	221.2	236.3	239.5
majus	184.1	198.82	233.32	221.2	236.3	239.5
minus	184.2	198.82	233.32	221.2	236.3	239.5
pudendum	184.4	198.82	233.32	221.2	236.3	239.5
vulva	184.4	198.82	233.32	221.2	236.3	239.5
finger (*see also* Neoplasm, skin, limb, upper)	173.60	198.2	232.6	216.6	238.2	239.2
flank (*see also* Neoplasm, skin, trunk)	173.50	198.2	232.5	216.5	238.2	239.2
foot (*see also* Neoplasm, skin, limb, lower)	173.70	198.2	232.7	216.7	238.2	239.2
forearm (*see also* Neoplasm, skin, limb, upper)	173.60	198.2	232.6	216.6	238.2	239.2
forehead (*see also* Neoplasm, skin, face)	173.30	198.2	232.3	216.3	238.2	239.2
glabella (*see also* Neoplasm, skin, face)	173.30	198.2	232.3	216.3	238.2	239.2
gluteal region (*see also* Neoplasm, skin, trunk)	173.50	198.2	232.5	216.5	238.2	239.2
groin (*see also* Neoplasm, skin, trunk)	173.50	198.2	232.5	216.5	238.2	239.2

☑ Additional Digit Required — Refer to the Tabular List for Digit Selection

▽ Subterms under main terms may continue to next column or page

	Malignant			Benign	Uncertain Behavior	Unspecified
	Primary	Secondary	Ca in situ			
Neoplasm, neoplastic — *continued*						
skin — *continued*						
hand (*see also* Neoplasm, skin, limb, upper)	173.60	198.2	232.6	216.6	238.2	239.2
head NEC (*see also* Neoplasm, skin, scalp)	173.40	198.2	232.4	216.4	238.2	239.2
heel (*see also* Neoplasm, skin, limb, lower)	173.70	198.2	232.7	216.7	238.2	239.2
helix (*see also* Neoplasm, skin, ear)	173.20	198.2	—	216.2	238.2	239.2
hip	173.70	198.2	232.7	216.7	238.2	239.2
basal cell carcinoma	173.71	—	—	—	—	—
specified type NEC	173.79	—	—	—	—	—
squamous cell carcinoma	173.72	—	—	—	—	—
infraclavicular region (*see also* Neoplasm, skin, trunk)	173.50	198.2	232.5	216.5	238.2	239.2
inguinal region (*see also* Neoplasm, skin, trunk)	173.50	198.2	232.5	216.5	238.2	239.2
jaw (*see also* Neoplasm, skin, face)	173.30	198.2	232.3	216.3	238.2	239.2
knee (*see also* Neoplasm, skin, limb, lower)	173.70	198.2	232.7	216.7	238.2	239.2
labia						
majora	184.1	198.82	233.32	221.2	236.3	239.5
minora	184.2	198.82	233.32	221.2	236.3	239.5
leg (*see also* Neoplasm, skin, limb, lower)	173.70	198.2	232.7	216.7	238.2	239.2
lid (lower) (upper)	173.10	198.2	232.1	216.1	238.2	239.2
basal cell carcinoma	173.11	—	—	—	—	—
specified type NEC	173.19	—	—	—	—	—
squamous cell carcinoma	173.12	—	—	—	—	—
limb NEC	173.90	198.2	232.9	216.9	238.2	239.5
lower	173.70	198.2	232.7	216.7	238.2	239.2
basal cell carcinoma	173.71	—	—	—	—	—
specified type NEC	173.79	—	—	—	—	—
squamous cell carcinoma	173.72	—	—	—	—	—
upper	173.60	198.2	232.6	216.6	238.2	239.2
basal cell carcinoma	173.61	—	—	—	—	—
specified type NEC	173.69	—	—	—	—	—
squamous cell carcinoma	173.62	—	—	—	—	—
lip (lower) (upper)	173.00	198.2	232.0	216.0	238.2	239.2
basal cell carcinoma	173.01	—	—	—	—	—
specified type NEC	173.09	—	—	—	—	—
squamous cell carcinoma	173.02	—	—	—	—	—
male genital organs	187.9	198.82	233.6	222.9	236.6	239.5
penis	187.4	198.82	233.5	222.1	236.6	239.5
prepuce	187.1	198.82	233.5	222.1	236.6	239.5
scrotum	187.7	198.82	233.6	222.4	236.6	239.5
Neoplasm, neoplastic — *continued*						
skin — *continued*						
mastectomy site (*see also* Neoplasm, skin, trunk)	173.50	198.2	—	—	—	—
specified as breast tissue	174.8	198.81	—	—	—	—
meatus, acoustic (external) (*see also* Neoplasm, skin, ear)	173.20	198.2	232.2	216.2	238.2	239.2
nates (*see also* Neoplasm, skin, trunk)	173.50	198.2	232.5	216.5	238.2	239.0
neck	173.40	198.2	232.4	216.4	238.2	239.2
basal cell carcinoma	173.41	—	—	—	—	—
specified type NEC	173.49	—	—	—	—	—
squamous cell carcinoma	173.42	—	—	—	—	—
nose (external) (*see also* Neoplasm, skin, face)	173.30	198.2	232.3	216.3	238.2	239.2
palm (*see also* Neoplasm, skin, limb, upper)	173.60	198.2	232.6	216.6	238.2	239.2
palpebra	173.10	198.2	232.1	216.1	238.2	239.2
basal cell carcinoma	173.11	—	—	—	—	—
specified type NEC	173.19	—	—	—	—	—
squamous cell carcinoma	173.12	—	—	—	—	—
penis NEC	187.4	198.82	233.5	222.1	236.6	239.5
perianal (*see also* Neoplasm, skin, anus)	173.50	198.2	232.5	216.5	238.2	239.2
perineum (*see also* Neoplasm, skin, anus)	173.50	198.2	232.5	216.5	238.2	239.2
pinna (*see also* Neoplasm, skin, ear)	173.20	198.2	232.2	216.2	238.2	239.2
plantar (*see also* Neoplasm, skin, limb, lower)	173.70	198.2	232.7	216.7	238.2	239.2
popliteal fossa or space (*see also* Neoplasm, skin, limb, lower)	173.70	198.2	232.7	216.7	238.2	239.2
prepuce	187.1	198.82	233.5	222.1	236.6	239.5
pubes (*see also* Neoplasm, skin, trunk)	173.50	198.2	232.5	216.5	238.2	239.2
sacrococcygeal region (*see also* Neoplasm, skin, trunk)	173.50	198.2	232.5	216.5	238.2	239.2
scalp	173.40	198.2	232.4	216.4	238.2	239.2
basal cell carcinoma	173.41	—	—	—	—	—
specified type NEC	173.49	—	—	—	—	—
squamous cell carcinoma	173.42	—	—	—	—	—
scapular region (*see also* Neoplasm, skin, trunk)	173.50	198.2	232.5	216.5	238.2	239.2
scrotum	187.7	198.82	233.6	222.4	236.6	239.5
shoulder	173.60	198.2	232.6	216.6	238.2	239.2
basal cell carcinoma	173.61	—	—	—	—	—
specified type NEC	173.69	—	—	—	—	—
squamous cell carcinoma	173.62	—	—	—	—	—

	Malignant					
	Primary	Secondary	Ca in situ	Benign	Uncertain Behavior	Unspecified
Neoplasm, neoplastic — continued						
skin — continued						
sole (foot) (see also Neoplasm, skin, limb, lower)	173.70	198.2	232.7	216.7	238.2	239.2
specified sites NEC	173.80	198.2	232.8	216.8	—	239.2
basal cell carcinoma	173.81	—	—	—	—	—
specified type NEC	173.89	—	—	—	—	—
squamous cell carcinoma	173.82	—	—	—	—	—
specified type NEC, unspecified site	173.99	—	—	—	—	—
squamous cell carcinoma, unspecified site	173.92	—	—	—	—	—
submammary fold (see also Neoplasm, skin, trunk)	173.50	198.2	232.5	216.5	238.2	239.2
supraclavicular region (see also Neoplasm, skin, neck)	173.40	198.2	232.4	216.4	238.2	239.2
temple (see also Neoplasm, skin, face)	173.30	198.2	232.3	216.3	238.2	239.2
thigh (see also Neoplasm, skin, limb, lower)	173.70	198.2	232.7	216.7	238.2	239.2
thoracic wall (see also Neoplasm, skin, trunk)	173.50	198.2	232.5	216.5	238.2	239.2
thumb (see also Neoplasm, skin, limb, upper)	173.60	198.2	232.6	216.6	238.2	239.2
toe (see also Neoplasm, skin, limb, lower)	173.70	198.2	232.7	216.7	238.2	239.2
tragus (see also Neoplasm, skin, ear)	173.20	198.2	232.2	216.2	238.2	239.2
trunk	173.50	198.2	232.5	216.5	238.2	239.2
basal cell carcinoma	173.51	—	—	—	—	—
specified type NEC	173.59	—	—	—	—	—
squamous cell carcinoma	173.52	—	—	—	—	—
umbilicus (see also Neoplasm, skin, trunk)	173.50	198.2	232.5	216.5	238.2	239.2
vulva	184.4	198.82	233.32	221.2	236.3	239.5
wrist (see also Neoplasm, skin, limb, upper)	173.60	198.2	232.6	216.6	238.2	239.2
skull	170.0	198.5	—	213.0	238.0	239.2
soft parts or tissues — see Neoplasm, connective tissue						
specified site — see Neoplasm, skin						
specified site NEC	195.8	198.89	234.8	229.8	238.8	239.89
spermatic cord	187.6	198.82	233.6	222.8	236.6	239.5
sphenoid	160.5	197.3	231.8	212.0	235.9	239.1
bone	170.0	198.5	—	213.0	238.0	239.2
sinus	160.5	197.3	231.8	212.0	235.9	239.1
sphincter						
anal	154.2	197.5	230.5	211.4	235.5	239.0
of Oddi	156.1	197.8	230.8	211.5	235.3	239.0
spine, spinal (column)	170.2	198.5	—	213.2	238.0	239.2
bulb	191.7	198.3	—	225.0	237.5	239.6
coccyx	170.6	198.5	—	213.6	238.0	239.2
cord (cervical) (lumbar) (sacral) (thoracic)	192.2	198.3	—	225.3	237.5	239.7
dura mater	192.3	198.4	—	225.4	237.6	239.7
lumbosacral	170.2	198.5	—	213.2	238.0	239.2
membrane	192.3	198.4	—	225.4	237.6	239.7
meninges	192.3	198.4	—	225.4	237.6	239.7
nerve (root)	171.9	198.89	—	215.9	238.1	239.2
pia mater	192.3	198.4	—	225.4	237.6	239.7
root	171.9	198.89	—	215.9	238.1	239.2
sacrum	170.6	198.5	—	213.6	238.0	239.2
spleen, splenic NEC	159.1	197.8	230.9	211.9	235.5	239.0
flexure (colon)	153.7	197.5	230.3	211.3	235.2	239.0
stem, brain	191.7	198.3	—	225.0	237.5	239.6
Stensen's duct	142.0	198.89	230.0	210.2	235.0	239.0
sternum	170.3	198.5	—	213.3	238.0	239.2
stomach	151.9	197.8	230.2	211.1	235.2	239.0
antrum (pyloric)	151.2	197.8	230.2	211.1	235.2	239.0
body	151.4	197.8	230.2	211.1	235.2	239.0
cardia	151.0	197.8	230.2	211.1	235.2	239.0
cardiac orifice	151.0	197.8	230.2	211.1	235.2	239.0
contiguous sites	151.8	—	—	—	—	—
corpus	151.4	197.8	230.2	211.1	235.2	239.0
fundus	151.3	197.8	230.2	211.1	235.2	239.0
greater curvature NEC	151.6	197.8	230.2	211.1	235.2	239.0
lesser curvature NEC	151.5	197.8	230.2	211.1	235.2	239.0
prepylorus	151.1	197.8	230.2	211.1	235.2	239.0
pylorus	151.1	197.8	230.2	211.1	235.2	239.0
wall NEC	151.9	197.8	230.2	211.1	235.2	239.0
anterior NEC	151.8	197.8	230.2	211.1	235.2	239.0
posterior NEC	151.8	197.8	230.2	211.1	235.2	239.0
stroma, endometrial	182.0	198.82	233.2	219.1	236.0	239.5
stump, cervical	180.8	198.82	233.1	219.0	236.0	239.5
subcutaneous (nodule) (tissue) NEC — see Neoplasm, connective tissue						
subdural	192.1	198.4	—	225.2	237.6	239.7
subglottis, subglottic	161.2	197.3	231.0	212.1	235.6	239.1
sublingual	144.9	198.89	230.0	210.3	235.1	239.0
gland or duct	142.2	198.89	230.0	210.2	235.0	239.0
submandibular gland	142.1	198.89	230.0	210.2	235.0	239.0
submaxillary gland or duct	142.1	198.89	230.0	210.2	235.0	239.0
submental	195.0	198.89	234.8	229.8	238.8	239.89
subpleural	162.9	197.0	—	212.3	235.7	239.1
substernal	164.2	197.1	—	212.5	235.8	239.89
sudoriferous, sudoriparous gland, site unspecified	173.90	198.2	232.9	216.9	238.2	239.2
specified site — see Neoplasm, skin						
supraclavicular region	195.0	198.89	234.8	229.8	238.8	239.89
supraglottis	161.1	197.3	231.0	212.1	235.6	239.1
suprarenal (capsule) (cortex) (gland) (medulla)	194.0	198.7	234.8	227.0	237.2	239.7
suprasellar (region)	191.9	198.3	—	225.0	237.5	239.6
sweat gland (apocrine) (eccrine), site unspecified	173.90	198.2	232.9	216.9	238.2	239.2
sympathetic nerve or nervous system NEC	171.9	198.89	—	215.9	238.1	239.2

Neoplasm, neoplastic— *continued*

	Malignant			Benign	Uncertain Behavior	Unspecified
	Primary	Secondary	Ca in situ			
symphysis pubis	170.6	198.5	—	213.6	238.0	239.2
synovial membrane — *see* Neoplasm, connective tissue						
tapetum, brain	191.8	198.3	—	225.0	237.5	239.6
tarsus (any bone)	170.8	198.5	—	213.8	238.0	239.2
temple (skin) (*see also* Neoplasm, skin, face)	173.30	198.2	232.3	216.3	238.2	239.2
temporal						
bone	170.0	198.5	—	213.0	238.0	239.2
lobe or pole	191.2	198.3	—	225.0	237.5	239.6
region	195.0	198.89	234.8	229.8	238.8	239.89
skin (*see also* Neoplasm, skin, face)	173.30	198.2	232.3	216.3	238.2	239.2
tendon (sheath) — *see* Neoplasm, connective tissue						
tentorium (cerebelli)	192.1	198.4	—	225.2	237.6	239.7
testis, testes (descended) (scrotal)	186.9	198.82	233.6	222.0	236.4	239.5
ectopic	186.0	198.82	233.6	222.0	236.4	239.5
retained	186.0	198.82	233.6	222.0	236.4	239.5
undescended	186.0	198.82	233.6	222.0	236.4	239.5
thalamus	191.0	198.3	—	225.0	237.5	239.6
thigh NEC*	195.5	198.89	234.8	229.8	238.8	239.89
thorax, thoracic (cavity) (organs NEC)	195.1	198.89	234.8	229.8	238.8	239.89
duct	171.4	198.89	—	215.4	238.1	239.2
wall NEC	195.1	198.89	234.8	229.8	238.8	239.89
throat	149.0	198.89	230.0	210.9	235.1	239.0
thumb NEC*	195.4	198.89	232.6	229.8	238.8	239.89
thymus (gland)	164.0	198.89	—	212.6	235.8	239.89
contiguous sites with heart and mediastinum	164.8	—	—	—	—	—
thyroglossal duct	193	198.89	234.8	226	237.4	239.7
thyroid (gland)	193	198.89	234.8	226	237.4	239.7
cartilage	161.3	197.3	231.0	212.1	235.6	239.1
tibia (any part)	170.7	198.5	—	213.7	238.0	239.2
toe NEC*	195.5	198.89	232.7	229.8	238.8	239.89
tongue	141.9	198.89	230.0	210.1	235.1	239.0
anterior (two-thirds) NEC	141.4	198.89	230.0	210.1	235.1	239.0
dorsal surface	141.1	198.89	230.0	210.1	235.1	239.0
ventral surface	141.3	198.89	230.0	210.1	235.1	239.0
base (dorsal surface)	141.0	198.89	230.0	210.1	235.1	239.0
border (lateral)	141.2	198.89	230.0	210.1	235.1	239.0
contiguous sites	141.8	—	—	—	—	—
dorsal surface NEC	141.1	198.89	230.0	210.1	235.1	239.0
fixed part NEC	141.0	198.89	230.0	210.1	235.1	239.0
foreamen cecum	141.1	198.89	230.0	210.1	235.1	239.0
frenulum linguae	141.3	198.89	230.0	210.1	235.1	239.0
junctional zone	141.5	198.89	230.0	210.1	235.1	239.0
margin (lateral)	141.2	198.89	230.0	210.1	235.1	239.0
midline NEC	141.1	198.89	230.0	210.1	235.1	239.0
mobile part NEC	141.4	198.89	230.0	210.1	235.1	239.0
posterior (third)	141.0	198.89	230.0	210.1	235.1	239.0
root	141.0	198.89	230.0	210.1	235.1	239.0
surface (dorsal)	141.1	198.89	230.0	210.1	235.1	239.0
base	141.0	198.89	230.0	210.1	235.1	239.0
ventral	141.3	198.89	230.0	210.1	235.1	239.0
tip	141.2	198.89	230.0	210.1	235.1	239.0
tonsil	141.6	198.89	230.0	210.1	235.1	239.0
tonsil	146.0	198.89	230.0	210.5	235.1	239.0
fauces, faucial	146.0	198.89	230.0	210.5	235.1	239.0
lingual	141.6	198.89	230.0	210.1	235.1	239.0
palatine	146.0	198.89	230.0	210.5	235.1	239.0
pharyngeal	147.1	198.89	230.0	210.7	235.1	239.0

Neoplasm, neoplastic— *continued*

	Malignant			Benign	Uncertain Behavior	Unspecified
	Primary	Secondary	Ca in situ			
tonsil — *continued*						
pillar (anterior) (posterior)	146.2	198.89	230.0	210.6	235.1	239.0
tonsillar fossa	146.1	198.89	230.0	210.6	235.1	239.0
tooth socket NEC	143.9	198.89	230.0	210.4	235.1	239.0
trachea (cartilage) (mucosa)	162.0	197.3	231.1	212.2	235.7	239.1
contiguous sites with bronchus or lung	162.8	—	—	—	—	—
tracheobronchial	162.8	197.3	231.1	212.2	235.7	239.1
contiguous sites with lung	162.8	—	—	—	—	—
tragus (*see also* Neoplasm, skin, ear)	173.20	198.2	232.2	216.2	238.2	239.2
trunk NEC*	195.8	198.89	232.5	229.8	238.8	239.89
tubo-ovarian	183.8	198.82	233.39	221.8	236.3	239.5
tunica vaginalis	187.8	198.82	233.6	222.8	236.6	239.5
turbinate (bone)	170.0	198.5	—	213.0	238.0	239.2
nasal	160.0	197.3	231.8	212.0	235.9	239.1
tympanic cavity	160.1	197.3	231.8	212.0	235.9	239.1
ulna (any part)	170.4	198.5	—	213.4	238.0	239.2
umbilicus, umbilical (*see also* Neoplasm, skin, trunk)	173.50	198.2	232.5	216.5	238.2	239.2
uncus, brain	191.2	198.3	—	225.0	237.5	239.6
unknown site or unspecified	199.1	199.1	234.9	229.9	238.9	239.9
urachus	188.7	198.1	233.7	223.3	236.7	239.4
ureter-bladder junction)	188.6	198.1	233.7	223.3	236.7	239.4
ureter, ureteral	189.2	198.1	233.9	223.2	236.91	239.5
orifice (bladder)	188.6	198.1	233.7	223.3	236.7	239.4
urethra, urethral (gland)	189.3	198.1	233.9	223.81	236.99	239.5
orifice, internal	188.5	198.1	233.7	223.3	236.7	239.4
urethrovaginal (septum)	184.9	198.82	233.39	221.9	236.3	239.5
urinary organ or system NEC	189.9	198.1	233.9	223.9	236.99	239.5
bladder — *see* Neoplasm, bladder						
contiguous sites	189.8	—	—	—	—	—
specified sites NEC	189.8	198.1	233.9	223.89	236.99	239.5
utero-ovarian	183.8	198.82	233.39	221.8	236.3	239.5
ligament	183.3	198.82	—	221.0	236.3	239.5
uterosacral ligament	183.4	198.82	—	221.0	236.3	239.5
uterus, uteri, uterine	179	198.82	233.2	219.9	236.0	239.5
adnexa NEC	183.9	198.82	233.39	221.8	236.3	239.5
contiguous sites	183.8	—	—	—	—	—
body	182.0	198.82	233.2	219.1	236.0	239.5
contiguous sites	182.8	—	—	—	—	—
cervix	180.9	198.82	233.1	219.0	236.0	239.5
cornu	182.0	198.82	233.2	219.1	236.0	239.5
corpus	182.0	198.82	233.2	219.1	236.0	239.5
endocervix (canal) (gland)	180.0	198.82	233.1	219.0	236.0	239.5
endometrium	182.0	198.82	233.2	219.1	236.0	239.5
exocervix	180.1	198.82	233.1	219.0	236.0	239.5
external os	180.1	198.82	233.1	219.0	236.0	239.5
fundus	182.0	198.82	233.2	219.1	236.0	239.5
internal os	180.0	198.82	233.1	219.0	236.0	239.5
isthmus	182.1	198.82	233.2	219.1	236.0	239.5
ligament	183.4	198.82	—	221.0	236.3	239.5
broad	183.3	198.82	233.39	221.0	236.3	239.5
round	183.5	198.82	—	221.0	236.3	239.5
lower segment	182.1	198.82	233.2	219.1	236.0	239.5
myometrium	182.0	198.82	233.2	219.1	236.0	239.5

	Malignant					
	Primary	Secondary	Ca in situ	Benign	Uncertain Behavior	Unspecified
Neoplasm, neoplastic — continued						
uterus, uteri, uterine — continued						
squamocolumnar junction	180.8	198.82	233.1	219.0	236.0	239.5
tube	183.2	198.82	233.39	221.0	236.3	239.5
utricle, prostatic	189.3	198.1	233.9	223.81	236.99	239.5
uveal tract	190.0	198.4	234.0	224.0	238.8	239.89
uvula	145.4	198.89	230.0	210.4	235.1	239.0
vagina, vaginal (fornix) (vault) (wall)	184.0	198.82	233.31	221.1	236.3	239.5
vaginovesical	184.9	198.82	233.39	221.9	236.3	239.5
septum	184.9	198.82	233.39	221.9	236.3	239.5
vallecula (epiglottis)	146.3	198.89	230.0	210.6	235.1	239.0
vascular — see Neoplasm, connective tissue						
vas deferens	187.6	198.82	233.6	222.8	236.6	239.5
Vater's ampulla	156.2	197.8	230.8	211.5	235.3	239.0
vein, venous — see Neoplasm, connective tissue						
vena cava (abdominal) (inferior)	171.5	198.89	—	215.5	238.1	239.2
superior	171.4	198.89	—	215.4	238.1	239.2
ventricle (cerebral) (floor) (fourth) (lateral) (third)	191.5	198.3	—	225.0	237.5	239.6
cardiac (left) (right)	164.1	198.89		212.7	238.8	239.89
ventricular band of larynx	161.1	197.3	231.0	212.1	235.6	239.1
ventriculus — see Neoplasm, stomach						
vermillion border — see Neoplasm, lip						
vermis, cerebellum	191.6	198.3	—	225.0	237.5	239.6
vertebra (column)	170.2	198.5	—	213.2	238.0	239.2
coccyx	170.6	198.5	—	213.6	238.0	239.2
sacrum	170.6	198.5	—	213.6	238.0	239.2
vesical — see Neoplasm, bladder						
vesicle, seminal	187.8	198.82	233.6	222.8	236.6	239.5
vesicocervical tissue	184.9	198.82	233.39	221.9	236.3	239.5
vesicorectal	195.3	198.89	234.8	229.8	238.8	239.89
vesicovaginal	184.9	198.82	233.39	221.9	236.3	239.5
septum	184.9	198.82	233.39	221.9	236.3	239.5
vessel (blood) — see Neoplasm, connective tissue						
vestibular gland, greater	184.1	198.82	233.32	221.2	236.3	239.5
vestibule						
mouth	145.1	198.89	230.0	210.4	235.1	239.0
nose	160.0	197.3	231.8	212.0	235.9	239.1
Virchow's gland	—	196.0	—	229.0	238.8	239.89
viscera NEC	195.8	198.89	234.8	229.8	238.8	239.89
vocal cords (true)	161.0	197.3	231.0	212.1	235.6	239.1
false	161.1	197.3	231.0	212.1	235.6	239.1
vomer	170.0	198.5	—	213.0	238.0	239.2
vulva	184.4	198.82	233.32	221.2	236.3	239.5
vulvovaginal gland	184.4	198.82	233.32	221.2	236.3	239.5
Waldeyer's ring	149.1	198.89	230.0	210.9	235.1	239.0
Wharton's duct	142.1	198.89	230.0	210.2	235.0	239.0
white matter (central) (cerebral)	191.0	198.3	—	225.0	237.5	239.6
windpipe	162.0	197.3	231.1	212.2	235.7	239.1
Wirsung's duct	157.3	197.8	230.9	211.6	235.5	239.0
wolffian (body) (duct)						
female	184.8	198.82	233.39	221.8	236.3	239.5
male	187.8	198.82	233.6	222.8	236.6	239.5
womb — see Neoplasm, uterus						

	Malignant					
	Primary	Secondary	Ca in situ	Benign	Uncertain Behavior	Unspecified
Neoplasm, neoplastic — continued						
wrist NEC*	195.4	198.89	232.6	229.8	238.8	239.89
xiphoid process	170.3	198.5	—	213.3	238.0	239.2
Zuckerkandl's organ	194.6	198.89	—	227.6	237.3	239.7

☑ Additional Digit Required — Refer to the Tabular List for Digit Selection   Subterms under main terms may continue to next column or page

2014 ICD-9-CM   ▶◀ Revised Text   ● New Line   ▲ Revised Code   Volume 2 — 211

Index

Neovascularization — Nephrosis, nephrotic

Neovascularization
- choroid 362.16
- ciliary body 364.42
- cornea 370.60
  - deep 370.63
  - localized 370.61
- iris 364.42
- retina 362.16
- subretinal 362.16

Nephralgia 788.0

Nephritis, nephritic (albuminuric) (azotemic) (congenital) (degenerative) (diffuse) (disseminated) (epithelial) (familial) (focal) (granulomatous) (hemorrhagic) (infantile) (nonsuppurative, excretory) (uremic) 583.9
- with
  - edema — *see* Nephrosis
  - lesion of
    - glomerulonephritis
      - hypocomplementemic persistent 583.2
        - with nephrotic syndrome 581.2
        - chronic 582.2
      - lobular 583.2
        - with nephrotic syndrome 581.2
        - chronic 582.2
      - membranoproliferative 583.2
        - with nephrotic syndrome 581.2
        - chronic 582.2
      - membranous 583.1
        - with nephrotic syndrome 581.1
        - chronic 582.1
      - mesangiocapillary 583.2
        - with nephrotic syndrome 581.2
        - chronic 582.2
      - mixed membranous and proliferative 583.2
        - with nephrotic syndrome 581.2
        - chronic 582.2
      - proliferative (diffuse) 583.0
        - with nephrotic syndrome 581.0
        - acute 580.0
        - chronic 582.0
      - rapidly progressive 583.4
        - acute 580.4
        - chronic 582.4
    - interstitial nephritis (diffuse) (focal) 583.89
      - with nephrotic syndrome 581.89
      - acute 580.89
      - chronic 582.89
    - necrotizing glomerulitis 583.4
      - acute 580.4
      - chronic 582.4
    - renal necrosis 583.9
      - cortical 583.6
      - medullary 583.7
    - specified pathology NEC 583.89
      - with nephrotic syndrome 581.89
      - acute 580.89
      - chronic 582.89
- necrosis, renal 583.9
  - cortical 583.6
  - medullary (papillary) 583.7
- nephrotic syndrome (*see also* Nephrosis) 581.9
- papillary necrosis 583.7
- specified pathology NEC 583.89
- acute 580.9
  - extracapillary with epithelial crescents 580.4
  - hypertensive (*see also* Hypertension, kidney) 403.90
  - necrotizing 580.4
  - poststreptococcal 580.0
  - proliferative (diffuse) 580.0
  - rapidly progressive 580.4
  - specified pathology NEC 580.89

Nephritis, nephritic — *continued*
- amyloid 277.39 *[583.81]*
  - chronic 277.39 *[582.81]*
- arteriolar (*see also* Hypertension, kidney) 403.90
- arteriosclerotic (*see also* Hypertension, kidney) 403.90
- ascending (*see also* Pyelitis) 590.80
- atrophic 582.9
- basement membrane NEC 583.89
  - with
    - pulmonary hemorrhage (Goodpasture's syndrome) 446.21 *[583.81]*
- calculous, calculus 592.0
- cardiac (*see also* Hypertension, kidney) 403.90
- cardiovascular (*see also* Hypertension, kidney) 403.90
- chronic 582.9
  - arteriosclerotic (*see also* Hypertension, kidney) 403.90
  - hypertensive (*see also* Hypertension, kidney) 403.90
- cirrhotic (*see also* Sclerosis, renal) 587
- complicating pregnancy, childbirth, or puerperium 646.2 ☑
  - with hypertension 642.1 ☑
  - affecting fetus or newborn 760.0
  - affecting fetus or newborn 760.1
- croupous 580.9
- desquamative — *see* Nephrosis
- due to
  - amyloidosis 277.39 *[583.81]*
    - chronic 277.39 *[582.81]*
  - arteriosclerosis (*see also* Hypertension, kidney) 403.90
  - diabetes mellitus 250.4 ☑ *[583.81]*
    - with nephrotic syndrome 250.4 ☑ *[581.81]*
      - due to secondary diabetes 249.4 ☑ *[583.81]*
    - due to secondary diabetes 249.4 ☑ *[583.81]*
  - diphtheria 032.89 *[580.81]*
  - gonococcal infection (acute) 098.19 *[583.81]*
    - chronic or duration of 2 months or over 098.39 *[583.81]*
  - gout 274.10
  - infectious hepatitis 070.9 *[580.81]*
  - mumps 072.79 *[580.81]*
  - specified kidney pathology NEC 583.89
    - acute 580.89
    - chronic 582.89
  - streptotrichosis 039.8 *[583.81]*
  - subacute bacterial endocarditis 421.0 *[580.81]*
  - systemic lupus erythematosus 710.0 *[583.81]*
    - chronic 710.0 *[582.81]*
  - typhoid fever 002.0 *[580.81]*
- endothelial 582.2
- end stage (chronic) (terminal) NEC 585.6
- epimembranous 581.1
- exudative 583.89
  - with nephrotic syndrome 581.89
  - acute 580.89
  - chronic 582.89
- gonococcal (acute) 098.19 *[583.81]*
  - chronic or duration of 2 months or over 098.39 *[583.81]*
- gouty 274.10
- hereditary (Alport's syndrome) 759.89
- hydremic — *see* Nephrosis
- hypertensive (*see also* Hypertension, kidney) 403.90
- hypocomplementemic persistent 583.2
  - with nephrotic syndrome 581.2
  - chronic 582.2
- immune complex NEC 583.89
- infective (*see also* Pyelitis) 590.80
- interstitial (diffuse) (focal) 583.89
  - with nephrotic syndrome 581.89
  - acute 580.89
  - chronic 582.89

Nephritis, nephritic — *continued*
- latent or quiescent — *see* Nephritis, chronic
- lead 984.9
  - specified type of lead — *see* Table of Drugs and Chemicals
- lobular 583.2
  - with nephrotic syndrome 581.2
  - chronic 582.2
- lupus 710.0 *[583.81]*
  - acute 710.0 *[580.81]*
  - chronic 710.0 *[582.81]*
- membranoproliferative 583.2
  - with nephrotic syndrome 581.2
  - chronic 582.2
- membranous 583.1
  - with nephrotic syndrome 581.1
  - chronic 582.1
- mesangiocapillary 583.2
  - with nephrotic syndrome 581.2
  - chronic 582.2
- minimal change 581.3
- mixed membranous and proliferative 583.2
  - with nephrotic syndrome 581.2
  - chronic 582.2
- necrotic, necrotizing 583.4
  - acute 580.4
  - chronic 582.4
- nephrotic — *see* Nephrosis
- old — *see* Nephritis, chronic
- parenchymatous 581.89
- polycystic 753.12
  - adult type (APKD) 753.13
  - autosomal dominant 753.13
  - autosomal recessive 753.14
  - childhood type (CPKD) 753.14
  - infantile type 753.14
- poststreptococcal 580.0
- pregnancy — *see* Nephritis, complicating pregnancy
- proliferative 583.0
  - with nephrotic syndrome 581.0
  - acute 580.0
  - chronic 582.0
- purulent (*see also* Pyelitis) 590.80
- rapidly progressive 583.4
  - acute 580.4
  - chronic 582.4
- salt-losing or salt-wasting (*see also* Disease, renal) 593.9
- saturnine 584.9
  - specified type of lead — *see* Table of Drugs and Chemicals
- septic (*see also* Pyelitis) 590.80
- specified pathology NEC 583.89
  - acute 580.89
  - chronic 582.89
- staphylococcal (*see also* Pyelitis) 590.80
- streptotrichosis 039.8 *[583.81]*
- subacute (*see also* Nephrosis) 581.9
- suppurative (*see also* Pyelitis) 590.80
- syphilitic (late) 095.4
  - congenital 090.5 *[583.81]*
  - early 091.69 *[583.81]*
- terminal (chronic) (end-stage) NEC 585.6
- toxic — *see* Nephritis, acute
- tubal, tubular — *see* Nephrosis, tubular
- tuberculous (*see also* Tuberculosis) 016.0 ☑ *[583.81]*
- type II (Ellis) — *see* Nephrosis
- vascular — *see* Hypertension, kidney
- war 580.9

Nephroblastoma (M8960/3) 189.0
- epithelial (M8961/3) 189.0
- mesenchymal (M8962/3) 189.0

Nephrocalcinosis 275.49

Nephrocystitis, pustular — *see also* Pyelitis 590.80

Nephrolithiasis (congenital) (pelvis) (recurrent) 592.0
- uric acid 274.11

Nephroma (M8960/3) 189.0
- mesoblastic (M8960/1) 236.9 ☑

Nephronephritis — *see also* Nephrosis 581.9

Nephronophthisis 753.16

Nephropathy — *see also* Nephritis 583.9

Nephropathy — *see also* Nephritis — *continued*
- with
  - exudative nephritis 583.89
  - interstitial nephritis (diffuse) (focal) 583.89
  - medullary necrosis 583.7
  - necrosis 583.9
    - cortical 583.6
    - medullary or papillary 583.7
  - papillary necrosis 583.7
  - specified lesion or cause NEC 583.89
- analgesic 583.89
  - with medullary necrosis, acute 584.7
- arteriolar (*see also* Hypertension, kidney) 403.90
- arteriosclerotic (*see also* Hypertension, kidney) 403.90
- complicating pregnancy 646.2 ☑
- diabetic 250.4 ☑ *[583.81]*
  - due to secondary diabetes 249.4 ☑ *[583.81]*
- gouty 274.10
  - specified type NEC 274.19
- hereditary amyloid 277.31
- hypercalcemic 588.89
- hypertensive (*see also* Hypertension, kidney) 403.90
- hypokalemic (vacuolar) 588.89
- IgA 583.9
- obstructive 593.89
  - congenital 753.20
- phenacetin 584.7
- phosphate-losing 588.0
- potassium depletion 588.89
- proliferative (*see also* Nephritis, proliferative) 583.0
- protein-losing 588.89
- salt-losing or salt-wasting (*see also* Disease, renal) 593.9
- sickle-cell (*see also* Disease, sickle-cell) 282.60 *[583.81]*
- toxic 584.5
- vasomotor 584.5
- water-losing 588.89

Nephroptosis — *see also* Disease, renal 593.0
- congenital (displaced) 753.3

Nephropyosis — *see also* Abscess, kidney 590.2

Nephrorrhagia 593.81

Nephrosclerosis (arteriolar) (arteriosclerotic) (chronic) (hyaline) — *see also* Hypertension, kidney 403.90
- gouty 274.10
- hyperplastic (arteriolar) (*see also* Hypertension, kidney) 403.90
- senile (*see also* Sclerosis, renal) 587

Nephrosis, nephrotic (Epstein's) (syndrome) 581.9
- with
  - lesion of
    - focal glomerulosclerosis 581.1
    - glomerulonephritis
      - endothelial 581.2
      - hypocomplementemic persistent 581.2
      - lobular 581.2
      - membranoproliferative 581.2
      - membranous 581.1
      - mesangiocapillary 581.2
      - minimal change 581.3
      - mixed membranous and proliferative 581.2
      - proliferative 581.0
      - segmental hyalinosis 581.1
      - specified pathology NEC 581.89
- acute — *see* Nephrosis, tubular
- anoxic — *see* Nephrosis, tubular
- arteriosclerotic (*see also* Hypertension, kidney) 403.90
- chemical — *see* Nephrosis, tubular
- cholemic 572.4
- complicating pregnancy, childbirth, or puerperium — *see* Nephritis, complicating pregnancy
- diabetic 250.4 ☑ *[581.81]*

Nephrosis, nephrotic — *continued*
 diabetic — *continued*
  due to secondary diabetes
   249.4 ☑ *[581.81]*
  Finnish type (congenital) 759.89
  hemoglobinuric — *see* Nephrosis, tubular
  in
   amyloidosis 277.39 *[581.81]*
   diabetes mellitus 250.4 ☑ *[581.81]*
    due to secondary diabetes
     249.4 ☑ *[581.81]*
   epidemic hemorrhagic fever 078.6
   malaria 084.9 *[581.81]*
   polyarteritis 446.0 *[581.81]*
   systemic lupus erythematosus
    710.0 *[581.81]*
 ischemic — *see* Nephrosis, tubular
 lipoid 581.3
 lower nephron — *see* Nephrosis, tubular
 lupoid 710.0 *[581.81]*
 lupus 710.0 *[581.81]*
 malarial 084.9 *[581.81]*
 minimal change 581.3
 necrotizing — *see* Nephrosis, tubular
 osmotic (sucrose) 588.89
 polyarteritic 446.0 *[581.81]*
 radiation 581.9
 specified lesion or cause NEC 581.89
 syphilitic 095.4
 toxic — *see* Nephrosis, tubular
 tubular (acute) 584.5
  due to a procedure 997.5
  radiation 581.9
Nephrosonephritis hemorrhagic (endemic)
  078.6
Nephrostomy status V44.6
 with complication 997.5
Nerve — *see* condition
Nerves 799.21
Nervous — *see also* condition 799.21
 breakdown 300.9
 heart 306.2
 stomach 306.4
 tension 799.21
Nervousness 799.21
Nesidioblastoma (M8150/0)
 pancreas 211.7
 specified site NEC — *see* Neoplasm, by site,
  benign
 unspecified site 211.7
Netherton's syndrome (ichthyosiform erythroderma) 757.1
Nettle rash 708.8
Nettleship's disease (urticaria pigmentosa)
  757.33
Neumann's disease (pemphigus vegetans)
  694.4
Neuralgia, neuralgic (acute) — *see also* Neuritis 729.2
 accessory (nerve) 352.4
 acoustic (nerve) 388.5
 ankle 355.8
 anterior crural 355.8
 anus 787.99
 arm 723.4
 auditory (nerve) 388.5
 axilla 353.0
 bladder 788.1
 brachial 723.4
 brain — *see* Disorder, nerve, cranial
 broad ligament 625.9
 cerebral — *see* Disorder, nerve, cranial
 ciliary 339.00
 cranial nerve (*see also* Disorder, nerve, cranial)
   fifth or trigeminal (*see also* Neuralgia,
    trigeminal) 350.1
 ear 388.71
  middle 352.1
 facial 351.8
 finger 354.9
 flank 355.8
 foot 355.8
 forearm 354.9
 Fothergill's (*see also* Neuralgia, trigeminal)
  350.1

Neuralgia, neuralgic — *see also* Neuritis —
  continued
 Fothergill's (*see also* Neuralgia, trigeminal)
  — *continued*
   postherpetic 053.12
 glossopharyngeal (nerve) 352.1
 groin 355.8
 hand 354.9
 heel 355.8
 Horton's 339.00
 Hunt's 053.11
 hypoglossal (nerve) 352.5
 iliac region 355.8
 infraorbital (*see also* Neuralgia, trigeminal)
  350.1
 inguinal 355.8
 intercostal (nerve) 353.8
  postherpetic 053.19
 jaw 352.1
 kidney 788.0
 knee 355.8
 loin 355.8
 malarial (*see also* Malaria) 084.6
 mastoid 385.89
 maxilla 352.1
 median thenar 354.1
 metatarsal 355.6
 middle ear 352.1
 migrainous 339.00
 Morton's 355.6
 nerve, cranial — *see* Disorder, nerve, cranial
 nose 352.0
 occipital 723.8
 olfactory (nerve) 352.0
 ophthalmic 377.30
  postherpetic 053.19
 optic (nerve) 377.30
 penis 607.9
 perineum 355.8
 pleura 511.0
 postherpetic NEC 053.19
  geniculate ganglion 053.11
  ophthalmic 053.19
  trifacial 053.12
  trigeminal 053.12
 pubic region 355.8
 radial (nerve) 723.4
 rectum 787.99
 sacroiliac joint 724.3
 sciatic (nerve) 724.3
 scrotum 608.9
 seminal vesicle 608.9
 shoulder 354.9
 Sluder's 337.09
 specified nerve NEC — *see* Disorder, nerve
 spermatic cord 608.9
 sphenopalatine (ganglion) 337.09
 subscapular (nerve) 723.4
 suprascapular (nerve) 723.4
 testis 608.89
 thenar (median) 354.1
 thigh 355.8
 tongue 352.5
 trifacial (nerve) (*see also* Neuralgia, trigeminal) 350.1
 trigeminal (nerve) 350.1
  postherpetic 053.12
 tympanic plexus 388.71
 ulnar (nerve) 723.4
 vagus (nerve) 352.3
 wrist 354.9
 writers' 300.89
  organic 333.84
Neurapraxia — *see* Injury, nerve, by site
Neurasthenia 300.5
 cardiac 306.2
 gastric 306.4
 heart 306.2
 postfebrile 780.79
 postviral 780.79
Neurilemmoma (M9560/0) — *see also* Neoplasm, connective tissue, benign
 acoustic (nerve) 225.1
 malignant (M9560/3) (*see also* Neoplasm,
  connective tissue, malignant)
   acoustic (nerve) 192.0

Neurilemmosarcoma (M9560/3) — *see* Neoplasm, connective tissue, malignant
Neurilemoma — *see* Neurilemmoma
Neurinoma (M9560/0) — *see* Neurilemmoma
Neurinomatosis (M9560/1) — *see also* Neoplasm, connective tissue, uncertain behavior
 centralis 759.5
Neuritis — *see also* Neuralgia 729.2
 abducens (nerve) 378.54
 accessory (nerve) 352.4
 acoustic (nerve) 388.5
  syphilitic 094.86
 alcoholic 357.5
  with psychosis 291.1
 amyloid, any site 277.39 *[357.4]*
 anterior crural 355.8
 arising during pregnancy 646.4 ☑
 arm 723.4
 ascending 355.2
 auditory (nerve) 388.5
 brachial (nerve) NEC 723.4
  due to displacement, intervertebral disc
   722.0
 cervical 723.4
 chest (wall) 353.8
 costal region 353.8
 cranial nerve (*see also* Disorder, nerve, cranial)
   first or olfactory 352.0
   second or optic 377.30
   third or oculomotor 378.52
   fourth or trochlear 378.53
   fifth or trigeminal (*see also* Neuralgia,
    trigeminal) 350.1
   sixth or abducens 378.54
   seventh or facial 351.8
    newborn 767.5
   eighth or acoustic 388.5
   ninth or glossopharyngeal 352.1
   tenth or vagus 352.3
   eleventh or accessory 352.4
   twelfth or hypoglossal 352.5
 Déjérine-Sottas 356.0
 diabetic 250.6 ☑ *[357.2]*
  due to secondary diabetes
   249.6 ☑ *[357.2]*
 diphtheritic 032.89 *[357.4]*
 due to
  beriberi 265.0 *[357.4]*
  displacement, prolapse, protrusion, or
   rupture of intervertebral disc
   722.2
    cervical 722.0
    lumbar, lumbosacral 722.10
    thoracic, thoracolumbar 722.11
  herniation, nucleus pulposus 722.2
    cervical 722.0
    lumbar, lumbosacral 722.10
    thoracic, thoracolumbar 722.11
 endemic 265.0 *[357.4]*
 facial (nerve) 351.8
  newborn 767.5
 general — *see* Polyneuropathy
 geniculate ganglion 351.1
  due to herpes 053.11
 glossopharyngeal (nerve) 352.1
 gouty 274.89 *[357.4]*
 hypoglossal (nerve) 352.5
 ilioinguinal (nerve) 355.8
 in diseases classified elsewhere — *see*
  Polyneuropathy, in
 infectious (multiple) 357.0
 intercostal (nerve) 353.8
 interstitial hypertrophic progressive NEC
  356.9
 leg 355.8
 lumbosacral NEC 724.4
 median (nerve) 354.1
  thenar 354.1
 multiple (acute) (infective) 356.9
  endemic 265.0 *[357.4]*
 multiplex endemica 265.0 *[357.4]*
 nerve root (*see also* Radiculitis) 729.2
 oculomotor (nerve) 378.52
 olfactory (nerve) 352.0

Neuritis — *see also* Neuralgia — *continued*
 optic (nerve) 377.30
  in myelitis 341.0
  meningococcal 036.81
 pelvic 355.5
 peripheral (nerve) (*see also* Neuropathy,
  peripheral)
   complicating pregnancy or puerperium
    646.4 ☑
   specified nerve NEC — *see* Mononeuritis
 pneumogastric (nerve) 352.3
 postchickenpox 052.7
 postherpetic 053.19
 progressive hypertrophic interstitial NEC
  356.9
 puerperal, postpartum 646.4 ☑
 radial (nerve) 723.4
 retrobulbar 377.32
  syphilitic 094.85
 rheumatic (chronic) 729.2
 sacral region 355.8
 sciatic (nerve) 724.3
  due to displacement of intervertebral
   disc 722.10
 serum 999.59
 specified nerve NEC — *see* Disorder, nerve
 spinal (nerve) 355.9
  root (*see also* Radiculitis) 729.2
 subscapular (nerve) 723.4
 suprascapular (nerve) 723.4
 syphilitic 095.8
 thenar (median) 354.1
 thoracic NEC 724.4
 toxic NEC 357.7
 trochlear (nerve) 378.53
 ulnar (nerve) 723.4
 vagus (nerve) 352.3
Neuro-avitaminosis 269.2
Neuroangiomatosis, encephalofacial 759.6
Neuroastrocytoma (M9505/1) — *see* Neoplasm, by site, uncertain behavior
Neuroblastoma (M9500/3)
 olfactory (M9522/3) 160.0
 specified site — *see* Neoplasm, by site, malignant
 unspecified site 194.0
Neurochorioretinitis — *see also* Chorioretinitis
  363.20
Neurocirculatory asthenia 306.2
Neurocytoma (M9506/0) — *see* Neoplasm, by
  site, benign
Neurodermatitis (circumscribed) (circumscripta) (local) 698.3
 atopic 691.8
 diffuse (Brocq) 691.8
 disseminated 691.8
 nodulosa 698.3
Neuroencephalomyelopathy, optic 341.0
Neuroendocrine tumor — *see* Tumor, neuroendocrine
Neuroepithelioma (M9503/3) — *see also*
  Neoplasm, by site, malignant
 olfactory (M9521/3) 160.0
Neurofibroma (M9540/0) — *see also* Neoplasm, connective tissue, benign
 melanotic (M9541/0) — *see* Neoplasm,
  connective tissue, benign
 multiple (M9540/1) 237.70
  type 1 237.71
  type 2 237.72
 plexiform (M9550/0) — *see* Neoplasm,
  connective tissue, benign
Neurofibromatosis (multiple) (M9540/1)
  237.70
 acoustic 237.72
 malignant (M9540/3) — *see* Neoplasm,
  connective tissue, malignant
 Schwannomatosis 237.73
 specified type NEC 237.79
 type 1 237.71
 type 2 237.72
 von Recklinghausen's 237.71
Neurofibrosarcoma (M9540/3) — *see* Neoplasm, connective tissue, malignant
Neurogenic — *see also* condition

☑ Additional Digit Required — Refer to the Tabular List for Digit Selection
▶◀ Revised Text ● New Line ▲ Revised Code
▽ Subterms under main terms may continue to next column or page
2014 ICD-9-CM
Volume 2 — 213

Neurogenic — see also condition —
  continued
  bladder (atonic) (automatic) (autonomic)
    (flaccid) (hypertonic) (hypotonic)
    (inertia) (infranuclear) (irritable)
    (motor) (nonreflex) (nuclear) (paraly-
    sis) (reflex) (sensory) (spastic)
    (supranuclear) (uninhibited) 596.54
    with cauda equina syndrome 344.61
  bowel 564.81
  heart 306.2
Neuroglioma (M9505/1) — see Neoplasm,
  by site, uncertain behavior
Neurolabyrinthitis (of Dix and Hallpike) 386.12
Neurolathyrism 988.2
Neuroleprosy 030.1
Neuroleptic malignant syndrome 333.92
Neurolipomatosis 272.8
Neuroma (M9570/0) — see also Neoplasm,
  connective tissue, benign
  acoustic (nerve) (M9560/0) 225.1
  amputation (traumatic) (see also Injury,
    nerve, by site)
    surgical complication (late) 997.61
  appendix 211.3
  auditory nerve 225.1
  digital 355.6
    toe 355.6
  interdigital (toe) 355.6
  intermetatarsal 355.6
  Morton's 355.6
  multiple 237.70
    type 1 237.71
    type 2 237.72
  nonneoplastic 355.9
    arm NEC 354.9
    leg NEC 355.8
    lower extremity NEC 355.8
    specified site NEC — see Mononeuritis,
      by site
    upper extremity NEC 354.9
  optic (nerve) 225.1
  plantar 355.6
  plexiform (M9550/0) — see Neoplasm,
    connective tissue, benign
  surgical (nonneoplastic) 355.9
    arm NEC 354.9
    leg NEC 355.8
    lower extremity NEC 355.8
    upper extremity NEC 354.9
  traumatic (see also Injury, nerve, by site)
    old — see Neuroma, nonneoplastic
Neuromyalgia 729.1
Neuromyasthenia (epidemic) 049.8
Neuromyelitis 341.8
  ascending 357.0
  optica 341.0
Neuromyopathy NEC 358.9
Neuromyositis 729.1
Neuronevus (M8725/0) — see Neoplasm, skin,
  benign
Neuronitis 357.0
  ascending (acute) 355.2
  vestibular 386.12
Neuroparalytic — see condition
Neuropathy, neuropathic — see also Disorder,
  nerve 355.9
  acute motor 357.82
  alcoholic 357.5
    with psychosis 291.1
  arm NEC 354.9
  ataxia and retinitis pigmentosa (NARP syn-
    drome) 277.87
  autonomic (peripheral) — see Neuropathy,
    peripheral, autonomic
  axillary nerve 353.0
  brachial plexus 353.0
  cervical plexus 353.2
  chronic
    progressive segmentally demyelinating
      357.89
    relapsing demyelinating 357.89
  congenital sensory 356.2
  Déjérine-Sottas 356.0
  diabetic 250.6 ☑ [357.2]
    autonomic (peripheral) 250.6 ☑ [337.1]

Neuropathy, neuropathic — see also Disorder,
  nerve — continued
  diabetic — continued
    due to secondary diabetes
      249.6 ☑ [357.2]
    autonomic (peripheral)
      249.6 ☑ [337.1]
  entrapment 355.9
    iliohypogastric nerve 355.79
    ilioinguinal nerve 355.79
    lateral cutaneous nerve of thigh 355.1
    median nerve 354.0
    obturator nerve 355.79
    peroneal nerve 355.3
    posterior tibial nerve 355.5
    saphenous nerve 355.79
    ulnar nerve 354.2
  facial nerve 351.9
  hereditary 356.9
    peripheral 356.0
    sensory (radicular) 356.2
  hypertrophic
    Charcôt-Marie-Tooth 356.1
    Déjérine-Sottas 356.0
    interstitial 356.9
    Refsum 356.3
  intercostal nerve 354.8
  ischemic — see Disorder, nerve
  Jamaican (ginger) 357.7
  leg NEC 355.8
  lower extremity NEC 355.8
  lumbar plexus 353.1
  median nerve 354.1
  motor
    acute 357.82
    multiple (acute) (chronic) (see also
      Polyneuropathy) 356.9
  optic 377.39
    ischemic 377.41
    nutritional 377.33
    toxic 377.34
  peripheral (nerve) (see also Polyneuropathy)
    356.9
    arm NEC 354.9
    autonomic 337.9
      amyloid 277.39 [337.1]
      idiopathic 337.00
      in
        amyloidosis 277.39 [337.1]
        diabetes (mellitus)
          250.6 ☑ [337.1]
          due to secondary diabetes
            249.6 ☑ [337.1]
        diseases classified elsewhere
          337.1
        gout 274.89 [337.1]
        hyperthyroidism 242.9 ☑ [337.1]
      due to
        antitetanus serum 357.6
        arsenic 357.7
        drugs 357.6
        lead 357.7
        organophosphate compounds 357.7
        toxic agent NEC 357.7
    hereditary 356.0
    idiopathic 356.9
      progressive 356.4
      specified type NEC 356.8
    in diseases classified elsewhere — see
      Polyneuropathy, in
    leg NEC 355.8
    lower extremity NEC 355.8
    upper extremity NEC 354.9
  plantar nerves 355.6
  progressive
    hypertrophic interstitial 356.9
    inflammatory 357.89
  radicular NEC 729.2
    brachial 723.4
    cervical NEC 723.4
    hereditary sensory 356.2
    lumbar 724.4
    lumbosacral 724.4
    thoracic NEC 724.4
  sacral plexus 353.1
  sciatic 355.0

Neuropathy, neuropathic — see also Disorder,
  nerve — continued
  spinal nerve NEC 355.9
    root (see also Radiculitis) 729.2
  toxic 357.7
  trigeminal sensory 350.8
  ulnar nerve 354.2
  upper extremity NEC 354.9
  uremic 585.9 [357.4]
  vitamin B$_{12}$ 266.2 [357.4]
    with anemia (pernicious) 281.0 [357.4]
    due to dietary deficiency
      281.1 [357.4]
Neurophthisis — see also Disorder, nerve
  diabetic 250.6 ☑ [357.2]
    due to secondary diabetes
      249.6 ☑ [357.2]
  peripheral 356.9
Neuropraxia — see Injury, nerve
Neuroretinitis 363.05
  syphilitic 094.85
Neurosarcoma (M9540/3) — see Neoplasm,
  connective tissue, malignant
Neurosclerosis — see Disorder, nerve
Neurosis, neurotic 300.9
  accident 300.16
  anancastic, anankastic 300.3
  anxiety (state) 300.00
    generalized 300.02
    panic type 300.01
  asthenic 300.5
  bladder 306.53
  cardiac (reflex) 306.2
  cardiovascular 306.2
  climacteric, unspecified type 627.2
  colon 306.4
  compensation 300.16
  compulsive, compulsion 300.3
  conversion 300.11
  craft 300.89
  cutaneous 306.3
  depersonalization 300.6
  depressive (reaction) (type) 300.4
  endocrine 306.6
  environmental 300.89
  fatigue 300.5
  functional (see also Disorder, psychosomat-
    ic) 306.9
  gastric 306.4
  gastrointestinal 306.4
  genitourinary 306.50
  heart 306.2
  hypochondriacal 300.7
  hysterical 300.10
    conversion type 300.11
    dissociative type 300.15
  impulsive 300.3
  incoordination 306.0
    larynx 306.1
    vocal cord 306.1
  intestine 306.4
  larynx 306.1
    hysterical 300.11
    sensory 306.1
  menopause, unspecified type 627.2
  mixed NEC 300.89
  musculoskeletal 306.0
  obsessional 300.3
    phobia 300.3
  obsessive-compulsive 300.3
  occupational 300.89
  ocular 306.7
  oral (see also Disorder, fluency) 315.35
  organ (see also Disorder, psychosomatic)
    306.9
  pharynx 306.1
  phobic 300.20
  posttraumatic (acute) (situational) 309.81
    chronic 309.81
  psychasthenic (type) 300.89
  railroad 300.16
  rectum 306.4
  respiratory 306.1
  rumination 306.4
  senile 300.89
  sexual 302.70

Neurosis, neurotic — continued
  situational 300.89
  specified type NEC 300.89
  state 300.9
    with depersonalization episode 300.6
  stomach 306.4
  vasomotor 306.2
  visceral 306.4
  war 300.16
Neurospongioblastosis diffusa 759.5
Neurosyphilis (arrested) (early) (inactive) (late)
  (latent) (recurrent) 094.9
  with ataxia (cerebellar) (locomotor) (spastic)
    (spinal) 094.0
  acute meningitis 094.2
  aneurysm 094.89
  arachnoid (adhesive) 094.2
  arteritis (any artery) 094.89
  asymptomatic 094.3
  congenital 090.40
  dura (mater) 094.89
  general paresis 094.1
  gumma 094.9
  hemorrhagic 094.9
  juvenile (asymptomatic) (meningeal) 090.40
  leptomeninges (aseptic) 094.2
  meningeal 094.2
  meninges (adhesive) 094.2
  meningovascular (diffuse) 094.2
  optic atrophy 094.84
  parenchymatous (degenerative) 094.1
  paresis (see also Paresis, general) 094.1
  paretic (see also Paresis, general) 094.1
  relapse 094.9
  remission in (sustained) 094.9
  serological 094.3
  specified nature or site NEC 094.89
  tabes (dorsalis) 094.0
    juvenile 090.40
  tabetic 094.0
    juvenile 090.40
  taboparesis 094.1
    juvenile 090.40
  thrombosis 094.89
  vascular 094.89
Neurotic — see also Neurosis 300.9
  excoriation 698.4
    psychogenic 306.3
Neurotmesis — see Injury, nerve, by site
Neurotoxemia — see Toxemia
Neutro-occlusion 524.21
Neutropenia, neutropenic (idiopathic) (pernicious) (primary) 288.00
  chronic 288.09
    hypoplastic 288.09
  congenital (nontransient) 288.01
  cyclic 288.02
  drug induced 288.03
  due to infection 288.04
  fever 288.00
  genetic 288.01
  immune 288.09
  infantile 288.01
  malignant 288.09
  neonatal, transitory (isoimmune) (maternal
    transfer) 776.7
  periodic 288.02
  splenic 289.53
  splenomegaly 289.53
  toxic 288.09
Neutrophilia, hereditary giant 288.2
Nevocarcinoma (M8720/3) — see Melanoma
Nevus (M8720/0) — see also Neoplasm, skin,
  benign

Note — Except where otherwise indicated, varieties of nevus in the list below
that are followed by a morphology code
number (M----/0) should be coded by
site as for "Neoplasm, skin, benign."

  acanthotic 702.8
  achromic (M8730/0)
  amelanotic (M8730/0)
  anemic, anemicus 709.09
  angiomatous (M9120/0) (see also Heman-
    gioma) 228.00
  araneus 448.1

Nevus — *see also* Neoplasm, skin, benign — *continued*
avasculosus 709.09
balloon cell (M8722/0)
bathing trunk (M8761/1) 238.2
blue (M8780/0)
  cellular (M8790/0)
  giant (M8790/0)
  Jadassohn's (M8780/0)
  malignant (M8780/3) — *see* Melanoma
capillary (M9131/0) (*see also* Hemangioma) 228.00
cavernous (M9121/0) (*see also* Hemangioma) 228.00
cellular (M8720/0)
  blue (M8790/0)
comedonicus 757.33
compound (M8760/0)
conjunctiva (M8720/0) 224.3
dermal (M8750/0)
  and epidermal (M8760/0)
epithelioid cell (and spindle cell) (M8770/0)
flammeus 757.32
  osteohypertrophic 759.89
hairy (M8720/0)
halo (M8723/0)
hemangiomatous (M9120/0) (*see also* Hemangioma) 228.00
intradermal (M8750/0)
intraepidermal (M8740/0)
involuting (M8724/0)
Jadassohn's (blue) (M8780/0)
junction, junctional (M8740/0)
  malignant melanoma in (M8740/3) — *see* Melanoma
juvenile (M8770/0)
lymphatic (M9170/0) 228.1
magnocellular (M8726/0)
  specified site — *see* Neoplasm, by site, benign
  unspecified site 224.0
malignant (M8720/3) — *see* Melanoma
meaning hemangioma (M9120/0) (*see also* Hemangioma) 228.00
melanotic (pigmented) (M8720/0)
multiplex 759.5
nonneoplastic 448.1
nonpigmented (M8730/0)
nonvascular (M8720/0)
oral mucosa, white sponge 750.26
osteohypertrophic, flammeus 759.89
papillaris (M8720/0)
papillomatosus (M8720/0)
pigmented (M8720/0)
  giant (M8761/1) (*see also* Neoplasm, skin, uncertain behavior)
    malignant melanoma in (M8761/3) — *see* Melanoma
  systematicus 757.33
pilosus (M8720/0)
port wine 757.32
sanguineous 757.32
sebaceous (senile) 702.8
senile 448.1
spider 448.1
spindle cell (and epithelioid cell) (M8770/0)
stellar 448.1
strawberry 757.32
syringocystadenomatous papilliferous (M8406/0)
unius lateris 757.33
Unna's 757.32
vascular 757.32
verrucous 757.33
white sponge (oral mucosa) 750.26
Newborn (infant) (liveborn)
abstinence syndrome 779.5
affected by
  amniocentesis 760.61
  maternal abuse of drugs (gestational) (via placenta) (via breast milk) (*see also* Noxious, substances transmitted through placenta or breast milk (affecting fetus or newborn)) 760.70
  methamphetamine(s) 760.72

Newborn — *continued*
affected by — *continued*
  procedure
    amniocentesis 760.61
    in utero NEC 760.62
    surgical on mother
      during pregnancy NEC 760.63
      previous not associated with pregnancy 760.64
apnea 770.81
  obstructive 770.82
  specified NEC 770.82
breast buds 779.89
cardiomyopathy 425.4
  congenital 425.3
convulsion 779.0
electrolyte imbalance NEC (transitory) 775.5
fever (environmentally-induced) 778.4
gestation
  24 completed weeks 765.22
  25-26 completed weeks 765.23
  27-28 completed weeks 765.24
  29-30 completed weeks 765.25
  31-32 completed weeks 765.26
  33-34 completed weeks 765.27
  35-36 completed weeks 765.28
  37 or more completed weeks 765.29
  less than 24 completed weeks 765.21
  unspecified completed weeks 765.20
infection 771.89
  candida 771.7
  mastitis 771.5
  specified NEC 771.89
  urinary tract 771.82
mastitis 771.5
multiple NEC
  born in hospital (without mention of cesarean delivery or section) V37.00
    with cesarean delivery or section V37.01
  born outside hospital
    hospitalized V37.1
    not hospitalized V37.2
  mates all liveborn
    born in hospital (without mention of cesarean delivery or section) V34.00
      with cesarean delivery or section V34.01
    born outside hospital
      hospitalized V34.1
      not hospitalized V34.2
  mates all stillborn
    born in hospital (without mention of cesarean delivery or section) V35.00
      with cesarean delivery or section V35.01
    born outside hospital
      hospitalized V35.1
      not hospitalized V35.2
  mates liveborn and stillborn
    born in hospital (without mention of cesarean delivery or section) V36.00
      with cesarean delivery or section V36.01
    born outside hospital
      hospitalized V36.1
      not hospitalized V36.2
omphalitis 771.4
seizure 779.0
sepsis 771.81
single
  born in hospital (without mention of cesarean delivery or section) V30.00
    with cesarean delivery or section V30.01
  born outside hospital
    hospitalized V30.1
    not hospitalized V30.2
specified condition NEC 779.89

Newborn — *continued*
twin NEC
  born in hospital (without mention of cesarean delivery or section) V33.00
    with cesarean delivery or section V33.01
  born outside hospital
    hospitalized V33.1
    not hospitalized V33.2
  mate liveborn
    born in hospital V31.0 ☑
    born outside hospital
      hospitalized V31.1
      not hospitalized V31.2
  mate stillborn
    born in hospital V32.0 ☑
    born outside hospital
      hospitalized V32.1
      not hospitalized V32.2
unspecified as to single or multiple birth
  born in hospital (without mention of cesarean delivery or section) V39.00
    with cesarean delivery or section V39.01
  born outside hospital
    hospitalized V39.1
    not hospitalized V39.2
weight check V20.32
Newcastle's conjunctivitis or disease 077.8
Nezelof's syndrome (pure alymphocytosis) 279.13
Niacin (amide) **deficiency** 265.2
Nicolas-Durand-Favre disease (climatic bubo) 099.1
Nicolas-Favre disease (climatic bubo) 099.1
Nicotinic acid (amide) **deficiency** 265.2
Niemann-Pick disease (lipid histiocytosis) (splenomegaly) 272.7
Night
blindness (*see also* Blindness, night) 368.60
  congenital 368.61
  vitamin A deficiency 264.5
cramps 729.82
sweats 780.8
terrors, child 307.46
Nightmare 307.47
REM-sleep type 307.47
Nipple — *see* condition
Nisbet's chancre 099.0
Nishimoto (-Takeuchi) disease 437.5
Nitritoid crisis or reaction — *see* Crisis, nitritoid
Nitrogen retention, extrarenal 788.99
Nitrosohemoglobinemia 289.89
Njovera 104.0
No
diagnosis 799.9
disease (found) V71.9
room at the inn V65.0
Nocardiasis — *see* Nocardiosis
Nocardiosis 039.9
with pneumonia 039.1
lung 039.1
specified type NEC 039.8
Nocturia 788.43
psychogenic 306.53
Nocturnal — *see also* condition
dyspnea (paroxysmal) 786.09
emissions 608.89
enuresis 788.36
  psychogenic 307.6
frequency (micturition) 788.43
  psychogenic 306.53
Nodal rhythm disorder 427.89
Nodding of head 781.0
Node(s) — *see also* Nodule(s)
Heberden's 715.04
larynx 478.79
lymph — *see* condition
milkers' 051.1
Osler's 421.0
rheumatic 729.89
Schmorl's 722.30
  lumbar, lumbosacral 722.32

Node(s) — *see also* Nodule(s) — *continued*
Schmorl's — *continued*
  specified region NEC 722.39
  thoracic, thoracolumbar 722.31
singers' 478.5
skin NEC 782.2
tuberculous — *see* Tuberculosis, lymph gland
vocal cords 478.5
Nodosities, Haygarth's 715.04
Nodule(s), nodular
actinomycotic (*see also* Actinomycosis) 039.9
arthritic — *see* Arthritis, nodosa
breast 793.89
cutaneous 782.2
Haygarth's 715.04
inflammatory — *see* Inflammation
juxta-articular 102.7
  syphilitic 095.7
  yaws 102.7
larynx 478.79
lung
  emphysematous 492.8
  solitary 793.11
milkers' 051.1
prostate 600.10
  with
    urinary
      obstruction 600.11
      retention 600.11
pulmonary, solitary (subsegmental branch of the bronchial tree) 793.11
  multiple 793.19
retrocardiac 785.9
rheumatic 729.89
rheumatoid — *see* Arthritis, rheumatoid
scrotum (inflammatory) 608.4
singers' 478.5
skin NEC 782.2
solitary, lung 793.11
  emphysematous 492.8
subcutaneous 782.2
thyroid (gland) (nontoxic) (uninodular) 241.0
  with
    hyperthyroidism 242.1 ☑
    thyrotoxicosis 242.1 ☑
  toxic or with hyperthyroidism 242.1 ☑
vocal cords 478.5
Noma (gangrenous) (hospital) (infective) 528.1
auricle (*see also* Gangrene) 785.4
mouth 528.1
pudendi (*see also* Vulvitis) 616.10
vulvae (*see also* Vulvitis) 616.10
Nomadism V60.0
Non-adherence
artificial skin graft 996.55
decellularized allodermis graft 996.55
Non-autoimmune hemolytic anemia NEC 283.10
Non-working side interference 524.56
Nonclosure — *see also* Imperfect, closure
ductus
  arteriosus 747.0
  Botalli 747.0
Eustachian valve 746.89
foramen
  Botalli 745.5
  ovale 745.5
Noncompliance with medical treatment V15.81
renal dialysis V45.12
Nondescent (congenital) — *see also* Malposition, congenital
cecum 751.4
colon 751.4
testis 752.51
Nondevelopment
brain 742.1
  specified part 742.2
heart 746.89
organ or site, congenital NEC — *see* Hypoplasia
Nonengagement
head NEC 652.5 ☑
  in labor 660.1 ☑

Nonengagement — *continued*
  head — *continued*
    in labor — *continued*
      affecting fetus or newborn 763.1
Nonexanthematous tick fever 066.1
Nonexpansion, lung (newborn) NEC 770.4
Nonfunctioning
  cystic duct (*see also* Disease, gallbladder)
    575.8
  gallbladder (*see also* Disease, gallbladder)
    575.8
  kidney (*see also* Disease, renal) 593.9
  labyrinth 386.58
Nonhealing
  stump (surgical) 997.69
  wound, surgical 998.83
Nonimplantation of ovum, causing infertility 628.3
Noninsufflation, fallopian tube 628.2
Nonne-Milroy-Meige syndrome (chronic hereditary edema) 757.0
Nonovulation 628.0
Nonpatent fallopian tube 628.2
Nonpneumatization, lung NEC 770.4
Nonreflex bladder 596.54
  with cauda equina 344.61
Nonretention of food — *see* Vomiting
Nonrotation — *see* Malrotation
Nonsecretion, urine — *see also* Anuria 788.5
  newborn 753.3
Nonunion
  fracture 733.82
  organ or site, congenital NEC — *see* Imperfect, closure
  symphysis pubis, congenital 755.69
  top sacrum, congenital 756.19
Nonviability 765.0 ☑
Nonvisualization, gallbladder 793.3
Nonvitalized tooth 522.9
Normal
  delivery — *see* category 650
  menses V65.5

Normal — *continued*
  state (feared complaint unfounded) V65.5
Normoblastosis 289.89
Normocytic anemia (infectional) 285.9
  due to blood loss (chronic) 280.0
    acute 285.1
Norrie's disease (congenital) (progressive oculoacousticocerebral degeneration) 743.8
North American blastomycosis 116.0
Norwegian itch 133.0
Nosebleed 784.7
Nose, nasal — *see* condition
Nosomania 298.9
Nosophobia 300.29
Nostalgia 309.89
Notched lip, congenital — *see also* Cleft, lip 749.10
Notching nose, congenital (tip) 748.1
Notch of iris 743.46
Nothnagel's
  syndrome 378.52
  vasomotor acroparesthesia 443.89
Novy's relapsing fever (American) 087.1
Noxious
  foodstuffs, poisoning by
    fish 988.0
    fungi 988.1
    mushrooms 988.1
    plants (food) 988.2
    shellfish 988.0
    specified type NEC 988.8
    toadstool 988.1
  substances transmitted through placenta or breast milk (affecting fetus or newborn) 760.70
    acetretin 760.78
    alcohol 760.71
    aminopterin 760.78
    anti-infective agents 760.74
    antiandrogens 760.79
    anticonvulsant 760.77

Noxious — *continued*
  substances transmitted through placenta or breast milk — *continued*
    antifungal 760.74
    antimetabolic 760.78
    atorvastatin 760.78
    carbamazepine 760.77
    cocaine 760.75
    "crack" 760.75
    diethylstilbestrol (DES) 760.76
    divalproex sodium 760.77
    endocrine disrupting chemicals 760.79
    estrogens 760.79
    etretinate 760.78
    fluconazole 760.74
    fluvastatin 760.78
    hallucinogenic agents NEC 760.73
    hormones 760.79
    lithium 760.79
    lovastatin 760.78
    medicinal agents NEC 760.79
    methotrexate 760.78
    misoprostil 760.79
    narcotics 760.72
    obstetric anesthetic or analgesic 763.5
    phenobarbital 760.77
    phenytoin 760.77
    pravastatin 760.78
    progestins 760.79
    retinoic acid 760.78
    simvastatin 760.78
    solvents 760.79
    specified agent NEC 760.79
    statins 760.78
    suspected, affecting management of pregnancy 655.5 ☑
    tetracycline 760.74
    thalidomide 760.79
    trimethadione 760.77
    valproate 760.77
    valproic acid 760.77
    vitamin A 760.78

NPDH (new persistent daily headache) 339.42
Nuchal hitch (arm) 652.8 ☑
Nucleus pulposus — *see* condition
Numbness 782.0
Nuns' knee 727.2
Nursemaid's
  elbow 832.2
  shoulder 831.0 ☑
Nutmeg liver 573.8
Nutrition, deficient or insufficient (particular kind of food) 269.9
  due to
    insufficient food 994.2
    lack of
      care (child) (infant) 995.52
        adult 995.84
      food 994.2
Nyctalopia — *see also* Blindness, night 368.60
  vitamin A deficiency 264.5
Nycturia 788.43
  psychogenic 306.53
Nymphomania 302.89
Nystagmus 379.50
  associated with vestibular system disorders 379.54
  benign paroxysmal positional 386.11
  central positional 386.2
  congenital 379.51
  deprivation 379.53
  dissociated 379.55
  latent 379.52
  miners' 300.89
  positional
    benign paroxysmal 386.11
    central 386.2
  specified NEC 379.56
  vestibular 379.54
  visual deprivation 379.53

☑ **Additional Digit Required** — **Refer to the Tabular List for Digit Selection**

▽ **Subterms under main terms may continue to next column or page**

216 — Volume 2

▶◀ **Revised Text**

● **New Line**　▲ **Revised Code**

2014 ICD-9-CM

O

Oasthouse urine disease 270.2
Obermeyer's relapsing fever (European) 087.0
Obesity (constitutional) (exogenous) (familial) (nutritional) (simple) 278.00
  adrenal 255.8
  complicating pregnancy, childbirth, or puerperium 649.1 ☑
  due to hyperalimentation 278.00
  endocrine NEC 259.9
  endogenous 259.9
  Fröhlich's (adiposogenital dystrophy) 253.8
  glandular NEC 259.9
  hypothyroid (see also Hypothyroidism) 244.9
  hypoventilation syndrome 278.03
  morbid 278.01
  of pregnancy 649.1 ☑
  pituitary 253.8
  severe 278.01
  thyroid (see also Hypothyroidism) 244.9
Oblique — see also condition
  lie before labor, affecting fetus or newborn 761.7
Obliquity, pelvis 738.6
Obliteration
  abdominal aorta 446.7
  appendix (lumen) 543.9
  artery 447.1
  ascending aorta 446.7
  bile ducts 576.8
    with calculus, choledocholithiasis, or stones — see Choledocholithiasis
    congenital 751.61
      jaundice from 751.61 [774.5]
  common duct 576.8
    with calculus, choledocholithiasis, or stones — see Choledocholithiasis
    congenital 751.61
  cystic duct 575.8
    with calculus, choledocholithiasis, or stones — see Choledocholithiasis
  disease, arteriolar 447.1
  endometrium 621.8
  eye, anterior chamber 360.34
  fallopian tube 628.2
  lymphatic vessel 457.1
    postmastectomy 457.0
  organ or site, congenital NEC — see Atresia
  placental blood vessels — see Placenta, abnormal
  supra-aortic branches 446.7
  ureter 593.89
  urethra 599.84
  vein 459.9
  vestibule (oral) 525.8
Observation (for) V71.9
  without need for further medical care V71.9
  accident NEC V71.4
    at work V71.3
  criminal assault V71.6
  deleterious agent ingestion V71.89
  disease V71.9
    cardiovascular V71.7
    heart V71.7
    mental V71.09
    specified condition NEC V71.89
  foreign body ingestion V71.89
  growth and development variations V21.8
  injuries (accidental) V71.4
    inflicted NEC V71.6
      during alleged rape or seduction V71.5
  malignant neoplasm, suspected V71.1
  postpartum
    immediately after delivery V24.0
    routine follow-up V24.2
  pregnancy
    high-risk V23.9
      inconclusive fetal viability V23.87
      specified problem NEC V23.89
    normal (without complication) V22.1
      with nonobstetric complication V22.2
      first V22.0
  rape or seduction, alleged V71.5
    injury during V71.5

Observation — continued
  suicide attempt, alleged V71.89
  suspected (undiagnosed) (unproven)
    abuse V71.81
    cardiovascular disease V71.7
    child or wife battering victim V71.6
    concussion (cerebral) V71.6
    condition NEC V71.89
      infant — see Observation, suspected, condition, newborn
      maternal and fetal
        amniotic cavity and membrane problem V89.01
        cervical shortening V89.05
        fetal anomaly V89.03
        fetal growth problem V89.04
        oligohydramnios V89.01
        other specified problem NEC V89.09
        placental problem V89.02
        polyhydramnios V89.01
      newborn V29.9
        cardiovascular disease V29.8
        congenital anomaly V29.8
        genetic V29.3
        infectious V29.0
        ingestion foreign object V29.8
        injury V29.8
        metabolic V29.3
        neoplasm V29.8
        neurological V29.1
        poison, poisoning V29.8
        respiratory V29.2
        specified NEC V29.8
    exposure
      anthrax V71.82
      biologic agent NEC V71.83
      SARS V71.83
    infectious disease not requiring isolation V71.89
    malignant neoplasm V71.1
    mental disorder V71.09
    neglect V71.81
    neoplasm
      benign V71.89
      malignant V71.1
    specified condition NEC V71.89
    tuberculosis V71.2
  tuberculosis, suspected V71.2
Obsession, obsessional 300.3
  ideas and mental images 300.3
  impulses 300.3
  neurosis 300.3
  phobia 300.3
  psychasthenia 300.3
  ruminations 300.3
  state 300.3
  syndrome 300.3
Obsessive-compulsive 300.3
  neurosis 300.3
  personality 301.4
  reaction 300.3
Obstetrical trauma NEC (complicating delivery) 665.9 ☑
  with
    abortion — see Abortion, by type, with damage to pelvic organs
    ectopic pregnancy (see also categories 633.0–633.9) 639.2
    molar pregnancy (see also categories 630–632) 639.2
  affecting fetus or newborn 763.89
  following
    abortion 639.2
    ectopic or molar pregnancy 639.2
Obstipation (see also Constipation 564.00
  psychogenic 306.4
Obstruction, obstructed, obstructive
  airway NEC 519.8
    with
      allergic alveolitis NEC 495.9
      asthma NEC (see also Asthma) 493.9 ☑
      bronchiectasis 494.0
        with acute exacerbation 494.1

Obstruction, obstructed, obstructive — continued
  airway — continued
    with
      bronchitis (chronic) (see also Bronchitis, with, obstruction) 491.20
      emphysema NEC 492.8
      chronic 496
        with
          allergic alveolitis NEC 495.5
          asthma NEC (see also Asthma) 493.2 ☑
          bronchiectasis 494.0
            with acute exacerbation 494.1
          bronchitis (chronic) (see also Bronchitis, with, obstruction) 491.20
          emphysema NEC 492.8
    due to
      bronchospasm 519.11
      foreign body 934.9
      inhalation of fumes or vapors 506.9
      laryngospasm 478.75
  alimentary canal (see also Obstruction, intestine) 560.9
  ampulla of Vater 576.2
    with calculus, cholelithiasis, or stones — see Choledocholithiasis
  aortic (heart) (valve) (see also Stenosis, aortic) 424.1
    rheumatic (see also Stenosis, aortic, rheumatic) 395.0
  aortoiliac 444.09
  aqueduct of Sylvius 331.4
    congenital 742.3
      with spina bifida (see also Spina bifida) 741.0 ☑
  Arnold-Chiari (see also Spina bifida) 741.0 ☑
  artery (see also Embolism, artery) 444.9
    basilar (complete) (partial) (see also Occlusion, artery, basilar) 433.0 ☑
    carotid (complete) (partial) (see also Occlusion, artery, carotid) 433.1 ☑
    precerebral — see Occlusion, artery, precerebral NEC
    retinal (central) (see also Occlusion, retina) 362.30
    vertebral (complete) (partial) (see also Occlusion, artery, vertebral) 433.2 ☑
  asthma (chronic) (with obstructive pulmonary disease) 493.2 ☑
  band (intestinal) 560.81
  bile duct or passage (see also Obstruction, biliary) 576.2
    congenital 751.61
      jaundice from 751.61 [774.5]
  biliary (duct) (tract) 576.2
    with calculus 574.51
      with cholecystitis (chronic) 574.41
        acute 574.31
    congenital 751.61
      jaundice from 751.61 [774.5]
    gallbladder 575.2
      with calculus 574.21
        with cholecystitis (chronic) 574.11
          acute 574.01
  bladder neck (acquired) 596.0
    congenital 753.6
  bowel (see also Obstruction, intestine) 560.9
  bronchus 519.19
  canal, ear (see also Stricture, ear canal, acquired) 380.50
  cardia 537.89
  caval veins (inferior) (superior) 459.2
  cecum (see also Obstruction, intestine) 560.9
  circulatory 459.9
  colon (see also Obstruction, intestine) 560.9
    sympathicotonic 560.89
  common duct (see also Obstruction, biliary) 576.2
    congenital 751.61
  coronary (artery) (heart) (see also Arteriosclerosis, coronary)
    acute (see also Infarct, myocardium) 410.9 ☑

Obstruction, obstructed, obstructive — continued
  coronary (see also Arteriosclerosis, coronary) — continued
    acute (see also Infarct, myocardium) — continued
      without myocardial infarction 411.81
  cystic duct (see also Obstruction, gallbladder) 575.2
    congenital 751.61
  device, implant, or graft — see Complications, due to (presence of) any device, implant, or graft classified to 996.0–996.5 NEC
  due to foreign body accidentally left in operation wound 998.4
  duodenum 537.3
    congenital 751.1
    due to
      compression NEC 537.3
      cyst 537.3
      intrinsic lesion or disease NEC 537.3
      scarring 537.3
      torsion 537.3
      ulcer 532.91
      volvulus 537.3
  ejaculatory duct 608.89
  endocardium 424.90
    arteriosclerotic 424.99
    specified cause, except rheumatic 424.99
  esophagus 530.3
  eustachian tube (complete) (partial) 381.60
    cartilaginous
      extrinsic 381.63
      intrinsic 381.62
    due to
      cholesteatoma 381.61
      osseous lesion NEC 381.61
      polyp 381.61
      osseous 381.61
  fallopian tube (bilateral) 628.2
  fecal 560.32
    with hernia (see also Hernia, by site, with obstruction)
      gangrenous — see Hernia, by site, with gangrene
  foramen of Monro (congenital) 742.3
    with spina bifida (see also Spina bifida) 741.0 ☑
  foreign body — see Foreign body
  gallbladder 575.2
    with calculus, cholelithiasis, or stones 574.21
      with cholecystitis (chronic) 574.11
        acute 574.01
    congenital 751.69
      jaundice from 751.69 [774.5]
  gastric outlet 537.0
  gastrointestinal (see also Obstruction, intestine) 560.9
  glottis 478.79
  hepatic 573.8
    duct (see also Obstruction, biliary) 576.2
      congenital 751.61
  icterus (see also Obstruction, biliary) 576.8
    congenital 751.61
  ileocecal coil (see also Obstruction, intestine) 560.9
  ileum (see also Obstruction, intestine) 560.9
  iliofemoral (artery) 444.81
  internal anastomosis — see Complications, mechanical, graft
  intestine (mechanical) (neurogenic) (paroxysmal) (postinfectional) (reflex) 560.9
    with
      adhesions (intestinal) (peritoneal) 560.81
      hernia (see also Hernia, by site, with obstruction)
        gangrenous — see Hernia, by site, with gangrene
    adynamic (see also Ileus) 560.1
    by gallstone 560.31
    congenital or infantile (small) 751.1
      large 751.2

Obstruction, obstructed, obstructive —
continued
  intestine — *continued*
    due to
      Ascaris lumbricoides 127.0
      mural thickening 560.89
      procedure 997.49
        involving urinary tract 997.5
    impaction 560.32
    infantile — *see* Obstruction, intestine,
      congenital
    newborn
      due to
        fecaliths 777.1
        inspissated milk 777.2
        meconium (plug) 777.1
          in mucoviscidosis 277.01
        transitory 777.4
      specified cause NEC 560.89
      transitory, newborn 777.4
      volvulus 560.2
    intracardiac ball valve prosthesis 996.02
    jaundice (*see also* Obstruction, biliary) 576.8
      congenital 751.61
    jejunum (*see also* Obstruction, intestine)
      560.9
    kidney 593.89
    labor 660.9 ☑
      affecting fetus or newborn 763.1
      by
        bony pelvis (conditions classifiable
          to 653.0–653.9) 660.1 ☑
        deep transverse arrest 660.3 ☑
        impacted shoulder 660.4 ☑
        locked twins 660.5 ☑
        malposition (fetus) (conditions classi-
          fiable to 652.0–652.9)
          660.0 ☑
        head during labor 660.3 ☑
        persistent occipitoposterior position
          660.3 ☑
        soft tissue, pelvic (conditions classifi-
          able to 654.0–654.9) 660.2 ☑
    lacrimal
      canaliculi 375.53
        congenital 743.65
        punctum 375.52
        sac 375.54
      lacrimonasal duct 375.56
        congenital 743.65
        neonatal 375.55
    lacteal, with steatorrhea 579.2
    laryngitis (*see also* Laryngitis) 464.01
    larynx 478.79
      congenital 748.3
    liver 573.8
      cirrhotic (*see also* Cirrhosis, liver) 571.5
    lung 518.89
      with
        asthma — *see* Asthma
        bronchitis (chronic) 491.20
        emphysema NEC 492.8
      airway, chronic 496
      chronic NEC 496
        with
          asthma (chronic) (obstructive)
            493.2 ☑
      disease, chronic 496
        with
          asthma (chronic) (obstructive)
            493.2 ☑
      emphysematous 492.8
    lymphatic 457.1
    meconium
      fetus or newborn 777.1
        in mucoviscidosis 277.01
      newborn due to fecaliths 777.1
    mediastinum 519.3
    mitral (rheumatic) — *see* Stenosis, mitral
    nasal 478.19
      duct 375.56
        neonatal 375.55
      sinus — *see* Sinusitis
    nasolacrimal duct 375.56
      congenital 743.65
      neonatal 375.55

Obstruction, obstructed, obstructive —
continued
  nasopharynx 478.29
  nose 478.19
  organ or site, congenital NEC — *see* Atresia
  pancreatic duct 577.8
  parotid gland 527.8
  pelviureteral junction (*see also* Obstruction,
    ureter) 593.4
  pharynx 478.29
  portal (circulation) (vein) 452
  prostate 600.90
    with
      other lower urinary tract symptoms
        (LUTS) 600.91
      urinary
        obstruction 600.91
        retention 600.91
    valve (urinary) 596.0
  pulmonary
    valve (heart) (*see also* Endocarditis, pul-
      monary) 424.3
    vein, isolated 747.49
  pyemic — *see* Septicemia
  pylorus (acquired) 537.0
    congenital 750.5
    infantile 750.5
  rectosigmoid (*see also* Obstruction, intes-
    tine) 560.9
  rectum 569.49
  renal 593.89
  respiratory 519.8
    chronic 496
  retinal (artery) (vein) (central) (*see also* Oc-
    clusion, retina) 362.30
  salivary duct (any) 527.8
    with calculus 527.5
  sigmoid (*see also* Obstruction, intestine)
    560.9
  sinus (accessory) (nasal) (*see also* Sinusitis)
    473.9
  Stensen's duct 527.8
  stomach 537.89
    acute 536.1
    congenital 750.7
  submaxillary gland 527.8
    with calculus 527.5
  thoracic duct 457.1
  thrombotic — *see* Thrombosis
  tooth eruption 520.6
  trachea 519.19
  tracheostomy airway 519.09
  tricuspid — *see* Endocarditis, tricuspid
  upper respiratory, congenital 748.8
  ureter (functional) 593.4
    congenital 753.20
    due to calculus 592.1
  ureteropelvic junction, congenital 753.21
  ureterovesical junction, congenital 753.22
  urethra 599.60
    congenital 753.6
  urinary (moderate) 599.60
    organ or tract (lower) 599.60
      due to
        benign prostatic hypertrophy
          (BPH) - see category 600
      specified NEC 599.69
        due to
          benign prostatic hypertrophy
            (BPH) — see category
            600
    prostatic valve 596.0
  uropathy 599.60
  uterus 621.8
  vagina 623.2
  valvular — *see* Endocarditis
  vascular graft or shunt 996.1
    atherosclerosis — *see* Arteriosclerosis,
      coronary
    embolism 996.74
    occlusion NEC 996.74
    thrombus 996.74
  vein, venous 459.2
    caval (inferior) (superior) 459.2
    thrombotic — *see* Thrombosis
  vena cava (inferior) (superior) 459.2

Obstruction, obstructed, obstructive —
continued
  ventricular shunt 996.2
  vesical 596.0
  vesicourethral orifice 596.0
  vessel NEC 459.9
Obturator — *see* condition
Occlusal
  plane deviation 524.76
  wear, teeth 521.10
Occlusion
  anus 569.49
    congenital 751.2
    infantile 751.2
  aortoiliac (chronic) 444.09
  aqueduct of Sylvius 331.4
    congenital 742.3
      with spina bifida (*see also* Spina bifi-
        da) 741.0 ☑
  arteries of extremities, lower 444.22
    without thrombus or embolus (*see also*
      Arteriosclerosis, extremities)
      440.20
    due to stricture or stenosis 447.1
    upper 444.21
      without thrombus or embolus (*see
        also* Arteriosclerosis, extremi-
        ties) 440.20
      due to stricture or stenosis 447.1
  artery NEC (*see also* Embolism, artery) 444.9
    auditory, internal 433.8 ☑
    basilar 433.0 ☑
      with other precerebral artery
        433.3 ☑
      bilateral 433.3 ☑
    brain or cerebral (*see also* Infarct, brain)
      434.9 ☑
    carotid 433.1 ☑
      with other precerebral artery
        433.3 ☑
      bilateral 433.3 ☑
    cerebellar (anterior inferior) (posterior
      inferior) (superior) 433.8 ☑
    cerebral (*see also* Infarct, brain) 434.9 ☑
    choroidal (anterior) 433.8 ☑
    chronic total
      coronary 414.2
      extremity(ies) 440.4
    communicating posterior 433.8 ☑
    complete
      coronary 414.2
      extremity(ies) 440.4
    coronary (thrombotic) (*see also* Infarct,
      myocardium) 410.9 ☑
      acute 410.9 ☑
        without myocardial infarction
          411.81
      chronic total 414.2
      complete 414.2
      healed or old 412
      total 414.2
    extremity(ies)
      chronic total 440.4
      complete 440.4
      total 440.4
    hypophyseal 433.8 ☑
    iliac (artery) 444.81
    mesenteric (embolic) (thrombotic) (with
      gangrene) 557.0
    pontine 433.8 ☑
    precerebral NEC 433.9 ☑
      late effect — *see* Late effect(s) (of)
        cerebrovascular disease
      multiple or bilateral 433.3 ☑
      puerperal, postpartum, childbirth
        674.0 ☑
      specified NEC 433.8 ☑
    renal 593.81
    retinal — *see* Occlusion, retina, artery
    spinal 433.8 ☑
    vertebral 433.2 ☑
      with other precerebral artery
        433.3 ☑
      bilateral 433.3 ☑

Occlusion — *continued*
  basilar (artery) — *see* Occlusion, artery,
    basilar
  bile duct (any) (*see also* Obstruction, biliary)
    576.2
  bowel (*see also* Obstruction, intestine) 560.9
  brain (artery) (vascular) (*see also* Infarct,
    brain) 434.9 ☑
  breast (duct) 611.89
  carotid (artery) (common) (internal) — *see*
    Occlusion, artery, carotid
  cerebellar (anterior inferior) (artery) (poste-
    rior inferior) (superior) 433.8 ☑
  cerebral (artery) (*see also* Infarct, brain)
    434.9 ☑
  cerebrovascular (*see also* Infarct, brain)
    434.9 ☑
    diffuse 437.0
  cervical canal (*see also* Stricture, cervix)
    622.4
    by falciparum malaria 084.0
  cervix (uteri) (*see also* Stricture, cervix) 622.4
  choanal 748.0
  choroidal (artery) 433.8 ☑
  colon (*see also* Obstruction, intestine) 560.9
  communicating posterior artery 433.8 ☑
  coronary (artery) (thrombotic) (*see also* In-
    farct, myocardium) 410.9 ☑
    without myocardial infarction 411.81
    acute 410.9 ☑
      without myocardial infarction 411.81
    healed or old 412
  cystic duct (*see also* Obstruction, gallblad-
    der) 575.2
    congenital 751.69
  disto
    division I 524.22
    division II 524.22
  embolic — *see* Embolism
  fallopian tube 628.2
    congenital 752.19
  gallbladder (*see also* Obstruction, gallblad-
    der) 575.2
    congenital 751.69
      jaundice from 751.69 [774.5]
  gingiva, traumatic 523.8
  hymen 623.3
    congenital 752.42
  hypophyseal (artery) 433.8 ☑
  iliac artery 444.81
  intestine (*see also* Obstruction, intestine)
    560.9
  kidney 593.89
  lacrimal apparatus — *see* Stenosis, lacrimal
  lung 518.89
  lymph or lymphatic channel 457.1
  mammary duct 611.89
  mesenteric artery (embolic) (thrombotic)
    (with gangrene) 557.0
  nose 478.1 ☑
    congenital 748.0
  organ or site, congenital NEC — *see* Atresia
  oviduct 628.2
    congenital 752.19
  periodontal, traumatic 523.8
  peripheral arteries (lower extremity) 444.22
    without thrombus or embolus (*see also*
      Arteriosclerosis, extremities)
      440.20
    due to stricture or stenosis 447.1
    upper extremity 444.21
      without thrombus or embolus (*see
        also* Arteriosclerosis, extremi-
        ties) 440.20
      due to stricture or stenosis 447.1
  pontine (artery) 433.8 ☑
  posterior lingual, of mandibular teeth
    524.29
  precerebral artery — *see* Occlusion, artery,
    precerebral NEC
  puncta lacrimalia 375.52
  pupil 364.74
  pylorus (*see also* Stricture, pylorus) 537.0
  renal artery 593.81
  retina, retinal (vascular) 362.30
    artery, arterial 362.30

Orchitis — *continued*
  gangrenous 604.99
  gonococcal (acute) 098.13
    chronic or duration of 2 months or over 098.33
  mumps 072.0
  parotidea 072.0
  suppurative 604.99
  syphilitic 095.8 *[604.91]*
  tuberculous (*see also* Tuberculosis) 016.5 ☑ *[608.81]*
Orf 051.2
Organic — *see also* condition
  heart — *see* Disease, heart
  insufficiency 799.89
Oriental
  bilharziasis 120.2
  schistosomiasis 120.2
  sore 085.1
Orientation
  ego-dystonic sexual 302.0
Orifice — *see* condition
Origin, both great vessels from right ventricle 745.11
Ormond's disease or syndrome 593.4
Ornithosis 073.9
  with
    complication 073.8
      specified NEC 073.7
    pneumonia 073.0
    pneumonitis (lobular) 073.0
Orodigitofacial dysostosis 759.89
Oropouche fever 066.3
Orotaciduria, oroticaciduria (congenital) (hereditary) (pyrimidine deficiency) 281.4
Oroya fever 088.0
Orthodontics V58.5
  adjustment V53.4
  aftercare V58.5
  fitting V53.4
Orthopnea 786.02
Orthoptic training V57.4
Osgood-Schlatter
  disease 732.4
  osteochondrosis 732.4
Osler-Rendu disease (familial hemorrhagic telangiectasia) 448.0
Osler-Vaquez disease (M9950/1) (polycythemia vera) 238.4
Osler-Weber-Rendu syndrome (familial hemorrhagic telangiectasia) 448.0
Osler's
  disease (M9950/1) (polycythemia vera) 238.4
  nodes 421.0
Osmidrosis 705.89
Osseous — *see* condition
Ossification
  artery — *see* Arteriosclerosis
  auricle (ear) 380.39
  bronchus 519.19
  cardiac (*see also* Degeneration, myocardial) 429.1
  cartilage (senile) 733.99
  coronary (artery) — *see* Arteriosclerosis, coronary
  diaphragm 728.10
  ear 380.39
    middle (*see also* Otosclerosis) 387.9
  falx cerebri 349.2
  fascia 728.10
  fontanel
    defective or delayed 756.0
    premature 756.0
  heart (*see also* Degeneration, myocardial) 429.1
    valve — *see* Endocarditis
  larynx 478.79
  ligament
    posterior longitudinal 724.8
      cervical 723.7
  meninges (cerebral) 349.2
    spinal 336.8
  multiple, eccentric centers 733.99
  muscle 728.10

Ossification — *continued*
  muscle — *continued*
    heterotopic, postoperative 728.13
  myocardium, myocardial (*see also* Degeneration, myocardial) 429.1
  penis 607.81
  periarticular 728.89
  sclera 379.16
  tendon 727.82
  trachea 519.19
  tympanic membrane (*see also* Tympanosclerosis) 385.00
  vitreous (humor) 360.44
Osteitis — *see also* Osteomyelitis 730.2 ☑
  acute 730.0 ☑
  alveolar 526.5
  chronic 730.1 ☑
  condensans (ilii) 733.5
  deformans (Paget's) 731.0
    due to or associated with malignant neoplasm (*see also* Neoplasm, bone, malignant) 170.9 *[731.1]*
  due to yaws 102.6
  fibrosa NEC 733.29
    cystica (generalisata) 252.01
    disseminata 756.59
    osteoplastica 252.01
  fragilitans 756.51
  Garré's (sclerosing) 730.1 ☑
  infectious (acute) (subacute) 730.0 ☑
    chronic or old 730.1 ☑
  jaw (acute) (chronic) (lower) (neonatal) (suppurative) (upper) 526.4
  parathyroid 252.01
  petrous bone (*see also* Petrositis) 383.20
  pubis 733.5
  sclerotic, nonsuppurative 730.1 ☑
  syphilitic 095.5
  tuberculosa
    cystica (of Jüngling) 135
    multiplex cystoides 135
Osteo-onycho-arthro dysplasia 756.89
Osteo-onychodysplasia, hereditary 756.89
Osteoarthritica spondylitis (spine) — *see also* Spondylosis 721.90
Osteoarthritis — *see also* Osteoarthrosis 715.9 ☑
  distal interphalangeal 715.9 ☑
  hyperplastic 731.2
  interspinalis (*see also* Spondylosis) 721.90
  spine, spinal NEC (*see also* Spondylosis) 721.90
Osteoarthropathy — *see also* Osteoarthrosis 715.9 ☑
  chronic idiopathic hypertrophic 757.39
  familial idiopathic 757.39
  hypertrophic pulmonary 731.2
    secondary 731.2
  idiopathic hypertrophic 757.39
  primary hypertrophic 731.2
  pulmonary hypertrophic 731.2
  secondary hypertrophic 731.2
Osteoarthrosis (degenerative) (hypertrophic) (rheumatoid) 715.9 ☑

Note — Use the following fifth-digit subclassification with category 715:

0   site unspecified

1   shoulder region

2   upper arm

3   forearm

4   hand

5   pelvic region and thigh

6   lower leg

7   ankle and foot

8   other specified sites except spine

9   multiple sites

  Deformans alkaptonurica 270.2
  generalized 715.09
  juvenilis (Köhler's) 732.5
  localized 715.3 ☑
    idiopathic 715.1 ☑

Osteoarthrosis — *continued*
  localized — *continued*
    primary 715.1 ☑
    secondary 715.2 ☑
  multiple sites, not specified as generalized 715.89
  polyarticular 715.09
  spine (*see also* Spondylosis) 721.90
  temporomandibular joint 524.69
Osteoblastoma (M9200/0) — *see* Neoplasm, bone, benign
Osteochondritis — *see also* Osteochondrosis 732.9
  dissecans 732.7
    hip 732.7
  ischiopubica 732.1
  multiple 756.59
  syphilitic (congenital) 090.0
Osteochondrodermodysplasia 756.59
Osteochondrodystrophy 277.5
  deformans 277.5
  familial 277.5
  fetalis 756.4
Osteochondrolysis 732.7
Osteochondroma (M9210/0) — *see also* Neoplasm, bone, benign
  multiple, congenital 756.4
Osteochondromatosis (M9210/1) 238.0
  synovial 727.82
Osteochondromyxosarcoma (M9180/3) — *see* Neoplasm, bone, malignant
Osteochondropathy NEC 732.9
Osteochondrosarcoma (M9180/3) — *see* Neoplasm, bone, malignant
Osteochondrosis 732.9
  acetabulum 732.1
  adult spine 732.8
  astragalus 732.5
  Blount's 732.4
  Buchanan's (juvenile osteochondrosis of iliac crest) 732.1
  Buchman's (juvenile osteochondrosis) 732.1
  Burns' 732.3
  calcaneus 732.5
  capitular epiphysis (femur) 732.1
  carpal
    lunate (wrist) 732.3
    scaphoid 732.3
  coxae juvenilis 732.1
  deformans juvenilis (coxae) (hip) 732.1
    Scheuermann's 732.0
    spine 732.0
    tibia 732.4
    vertebra 732.0
  Diaz's (astragalus) 732.5
  dissecans (knee) (shoulder) 732.7
  femoral capital epiphysis 732.1
  femur (head) (juvenile) 732.1
  foot (juvenile) 732.5
  Freiberg's (disease) (second metatarsal) 732.5
  Haas' 732.3
  Haglund's (os tibiale externum) 732.5
  hand (juvenile) 732.3
  head of
    femur 732.1
    humerus (juvenile) 732.3
  hip (juvenile) 732.1
  humerus (juvenile) 732.3
  iliac crest (juvenile) 732.1
  ilium (juvenile) 732.1
  ischiopubic synchondrosis 732.1
  Iselin's (osteochondrosis fifth metatarsal) 732.5
  juvenile, juvenilis 732.6
    arm 732.3
    capital femoral epiphysis 732.1
    capitellum humeri 732.3
    capitular epiphysis 732.1
    carpal scaphoid 732.3
    clavicle, sternal epiphysis 732.6
    coxae 732.1
    deformans 732.1
    foot 732.5
    hand 732.3
    hip and pelvis 732.1

Osteochondrosis — *continued*
  juvenile, juvenilis — *continued*
    lower extremity, except foot 732.4
    lunate, wrist 732.3
    medial cuneiform bone 732.5
    metatarsal (head) 732.5
    metatarsophalangeal 732.5
    navicular, ankle 732.5
    patella 732.4
    primary patellar center (of Köhler) 732.4
    specified site NEC 732.6
    spine 732.0
    tarsal scaphoid 732.5
    tibia (epiphysis) (tuberosity) 732.4
    upper extremity 732.3
    vertebra (body) (Calvé) 732.0
      epiphyseal plates (of Scheuermann) 732.0
  Kienböck's (disease) 732.3
  Köhler's (disease) (navicular, ankle) 732.5
    patellar 732.4
    tarsal navicular 732.5
  Legg-Calvé-Perthes (disease) 732.1
  lower extremity (juvenile) 732.4
  lunate bone 732.3
  Mauclaire's 732.3
  metacarpal heads (of Mauclaire) 732.3
  metatarsal (fifth) (head) (second) 732.5
  navicular, ankle 732.5
  os calcis 732.5
  Osgood-Schlatter 732.4
  os tibiale externum 732.5
  Panner's 732.3
  patella (juvenile) 732.4
  patellar center
    primary (of Köhler) 732.4
    secondary (of Sinding-Larsen) 732.4
  pelvis (juvenile) 732.1
  Pierson's 732.1
  radial head (juvenile) 732.3
  Scheuermann's 732.0
  Sever's (calcaneum) 732.5
  Sinding-Larsen (secondary patellar center) 732.4
  spine (juvenile) 732.0
    adult 732.8
  symphysis pubis (of Pierson) (juvenile) 732.1
  syphilitic (congenital) 090.0
  tarsal (navicular) (scaphoid) 732.5
  tibia (proximal) (tubercle) 732.4
  tuberculous — *see* Tuberculosis, bone
  ulna 732.3
  upper extremity (juvenile) 732.3
  van Neck's (juvenile osteochondrosis) 732.1
  vertebral (juvenile) 732.0
    adult 732.8
Osteoclastoma (M9250/1) 238.0
  malignant (M9250/3) — *see* Neoplasm, bone, malignant
Osteocopic pain 733.90
Osteodynia 733.90
Osteodystrophy
  azotemic 588.0
  chronica deformans hypertrophica 731.0
  congenital 756.50
    specified type NEC 756.59
  deformans 731.0
  fibrosa localisata 731.0
  parathyroid 252.01
  renal 588.0
Osteofibroma (M9262/0) — *see* Neoplasm, bone, benign
Osteofibrosarcoma (M9182/3) — *see* Neoplasm, bone, malignant
Osteogenesis imperfecta 756.51
Osteogenic — *see* condition
Osteoma (M9180/0) — *see also* Neoplasm, bone, benign
  osteoid (M9191/0) (*see also* Neoplasm, bone, benign)
    giant (M9200/0) — *see* Neoplasm, bone, benign
Osteomalacia 268.2
  chronica deformans hypertrophica 731.0
  due to vitamin D deficiency 268.2
  infantile (*see also* Rickets) 268.0

☑ **Additional Digit Required** — Refer to the Tabular List for Digit Selection

220 — Volume 2

►◄ **Revised Text**

● **New Line**   ▲ **Revised Code**

Subterms under main terms may continue to next column or page

2014 ICD-9-CM

Osteomalacia — continued
   juvenile (see also Rickets) 268.0
   oncogenic 275.8
   pelvis 268.2
   vitamin D-resistant 275.3
Osteomalacic bone 268.2
Osteomalacosis 268.2
Osteomyelitis (general) (infective) (localized)
   (neonatal) (purulent) (pyogenic) (septic)
   (staphylococcal) (streptococcal) (suppurative) (with periostitis) 730.2 ☑

> Note — Use the following fifth-digit
> subclassification with category 730:
> 0   site unspecified
> 1   shoulder region
> 2   upper arm
> 3   forearm
> 4   hand
> 5   pelvic region and thigh
> 6   lower leg
> 7   ankle and foot
> 8   other specified sites
> 9   multiple sites

   acute or subacute 730.0 ☑
   chronic or old 730.1 ☑
   due to or associated with
      diabetes mellitus 250.8 ☑ [731.8]
         due to secondary diabetes
            249.8 ☑ [731.8]
      tuberculosis (see also Tuberculosis, bone)
         015.9 ☑ [730.8] ☑
         limb bones 015.5 ☑ [730.8] ☑
         specified bones NEC
            015.7 ☑ [730.8] ☑
         spine 015.0 ☑ [730.8] ☑
      typhoid 002.0 [730.8] ☑
   Garré's 730.1 ☑
   jaw (acute) (chronic) (lower) (neonatal)
      (suppurative) (upper) 526.4
   nonsuppurating 730.1 ☑
   orbital 376.03
   petrous bone (see also Petrositis) 383.20
   Salmonella 003.24
   sclerosing, nonsuppurative 730.1 ☑
   sicca 730.1 ☑
   syphilitic 095.5
      congenital 090.0 [730.8] ☑
   tuberculous — see Tuberculosis, bone
   typhoid 002.0 [730.8] ☑
Osteomyelofibrosis 289.89
Osteomyelosclerosis 289.89
Osteonecrosis 733.40
   meaning osteomyelitis 730.1 ☑
Osteopathia
   condensans disseminata 756.53
   hyperostotica multiplex infantilis 756.59
   hypertrophica toxica 731.2
   striata 756.4
Osteopathy resulting from poliomyelitis —
   see also Poliomyelitis 045.9 ☑ [730.7] ☑
   familial dysplastic 731.2
Osteopecilia 756.53
Osteopenia 733.90
   borderline 733.90
Osteoperiostitis — see also Osteomyelitis
   730.2 ☑
   ossificans toxica 731.2
   toxica ossificans 731.2
Osteopetrosis (familial) 756.52
Osteophyte — see Exostosis
Osteophytosis — see Exostosis
Osteopoikilosis 756.53
Osteoporosis-osteomalacia syndrome 268.2
Osteoporosis (generalized) 733.00
   circumscripta 731.0
   disuse 733.03
   drug-induced 733.09
   idiopathic 733.02
   postmenopausal 733.01
   posttraumatic 733.7

Osteoporosis — continued
   screening V82.81
   senile 733.01
   specified type NEC 733.09
Osteopsathyrosis 756.51
Osteoradionecrosis, jaw 526.89
Osteosarcoma (M9180/3) — see also Neoplasm, bone, malignant
   chondroblastic (M9181/3) — see Neoplasm,
      bone, malignant
   fibroblastic (M9182/3) — see Neoplasm,
      bone, malignant
   in Paget's disease of bone (M9184/3) — see
      Neoplasm, bone, malignant
   juxtacortical (M9190/3) — see Neoplasm,
      bone, malignant
   parosteal (M9190/3) — see Neoplasm, bone,
      malignant
   telangiectatic (M9183/3) — see Neoplasm,
      bone, malignant
Osteosclerosis 756.52
   fragilis (generalisata) 756.52
Osteosclerotic anemia 289.89
Osteosis
   acromegaloid 757.39
   cutis 709.3
   parathyroid 252.01
   renal fibrocystic 588.0
Österreicher-Turner syndrome 756.89
Ostium
   atrioventriculare commune 745.69
   primum (arteriosum) (defect) (persistent)
      745.61
   secundum (arteriosum) (defect) (patent)
      (persistent) 745.5
Ostrum-Furst syndrome 756.59
Os, uterus — see condition
Otalgia 388.70
   otogenic 388.71
   referred 388.72
Othematoma 380.31
Otitic hydrocephalus 348.2
Otitis 382.9
   with effusion 381.4
      purulent 382.4
      secretory 381.4
      serous 381.4
      suppurative 382.4
   acute 382.9
   adhesive (see also Adhesions, middle ear)
      385.10
   chronic 382.9
      with effusion 381.3
      mucoid, mucous (simple) 381.20
      purulent 382.3
      secretory 381.3
      serous 381.10
      suppurative 382.3
   diffuse parasitic 136.8
   externa (acute) (diffuse) (hemorrhagica)
      380.10
      actinic 380.22
      candidal 112.82
      chemical 380.22
      chronic 380.23
         mycotic — see Otitis, externa, my-
            cotic
         specified type NEC 380.23
      circumscribed 380.10
      contact 380.22
      due to
         erysipelas 035 [380.13]
         impetigo 684 [380.13]
         seborrheic dermatitis 690.10 [380.13]
      eczematoid 380.22
      furuncular 680.0 [380.13]
      infective 380.10
         chronic 380.16
      malignant 380.14
      mycotic (chronic) 380.15
         due to
            aspergillosis 117.3 [380.15]
            moniliasis 112.82
            otomycosis 111.8 [380.15]
      reactive 380.22
      specified type NEC 380.22

Otitis — continued
   externa — continued
      tropical 111.8 [380.15]
   insidiosa (see also Otosclerosis) 387.9
   interna (see also Labyrinthitis) 386.30
   media (hemorrhagic) (staphylococcal)
      (streptococcal) 382.9
      acute 382.9
         with effusion 381.00
         allergic 381.04
            mucoid 381.05
            sanguineous 381.06
            serous 381.04
         catarrhal 381.00
         exudative 381.00
         mucoid 381.02
            allergic 381.05
         necrotizing 382.00
            with spontaneous rupture of ear
               drum 382.01
         in
            influenza (see also Influenza)
               487.8 [382.02]
            measles 055.2
            scarlet fever 034.1 [382.02]
         nonsuppurative 381.00
         purulent 382.00
            with spontaneous rupture of ear
               drum 382.01
         sanguineous 381.03
            allergic 381.06
         secretory 381.01
         seromucinous 381.02
         serous 381.01
            allergic 381.04
         suppurative 382.00
            with spontaneous rupture of ear
               drum 382.01
           due to
            influenza (see also Influenza)
               487.8 [382.02]
            scarlet fever 034.1 [382.02]
         transudative 381.00
      adhesive (see also Adhesions, middle ear)
         385.10
      allergic 381.4
         acute 381.04
            mucoid 381.05
            sanguineous 381.06
            serous 381.04
         chronic 381.3
      catarrhal 381.4
         acute 381.00
         chronic (simple) 381.10
      chronic 382.9
         with effusion 381.3
         adhesive (see also Adhesions, middle
            ear) 385.10
         allergic 381.3
         atticoantral, suppurative (with poste-
            rior or superior marginal per-
            foration of ear drum) 382.2
         benign suppurative (with anterior
            perforation of ear drum) 382.1
         catarrhal 381.10
         exudative 381.3
         mucinous 381.20
         mucoid, mucous (simple) 381.20
         mucosanguineous 381.29
         nonsuppurative 381.3
         purulent 382.3
         secretory 381.3
         seromucinous 381.3
         serosanguineous 381.19
         serous (simple) 381.10
         suppurative 382.3
           atticoantral (with posterior or su-
            perior marginal perfora-
            tion of ear drum) 382.2
           benign (with anterior perforation
            of ear drum) 382.1
           tuberculous (see also Tuberculo-
            sis) 017.4 ☑
         tubotympanic 382.1
         transudative 381.3
      exudative 381.4

Otitis — continued
   media — continued
      exudative — continued
         acute 381.00
         chronic 381.3
      fibrotic (see also Adhesions, middle ear)
         385.10
      mucoid, mucous 381.4
         acute 381.02
         chronic (simple) 381.20
      mucosanguineous, chronic 381.29
      nonsuppurative 381.4
         acute 381.00
         chronic 381.3
      postmeasles 055.2
      purulent 382.4
         acute 382.00
           with spontaneous rupture of ear
             drum 382.01
         chronic 382.3
      sanguineous, acute 381.03
         allergic 381.06
      secretory 381.4
         acute or subacute 381.01
         chronic 381.3
      seromucinous 381.4
         acute or subacute 381.02
         chronic 381.3
      serosanguineous, chronic 381.19
      serous 381.4
         acute or subacute 381.01
         chronic (simple) 381.10
      subacute — see Otitis, media, acute
      suppurative 382.4
         acute 382.00
           with spontaneous rupture of ear
             drum 382.01
         chronic 382.3
           atticoantral 382.2
           benign 382.1
           tuberculous (see also Tuberculo-
            sis) 017.4 ☑
           tubotympanic 382.1
      transudative 381.4
         acute 381.00
         chronic 381.3
      tuberculous (see also Tuberculosis)
         017.4 ☑
      postmeasles 055.2
Otoconia 386.8
Otolith syndrome 386.19
Otomycosis 111.8 [380.15]
   in
      aspergillosis 117.3 [380.15]
      moniliasis 112.82
Otopathy 388.9
Otoporosis — see also Otosclerosis 387.9
Otorrhagia 388.69
   traumatic — see nature of injury
Otorrhea 388.60
   blood 388.69
   cerebrospinal (fluid) 388.61
Otosclerosis (general) 387.9
   cochlear (endosteal) 387.2
   involving
      otic capsule 387.2
      oval window
         nonobliterative 387.0
         obliterative 387.1
      round window 387.2
   nonobliterative 387.0
   obliterative 387.1
   specified type NEC 387.8
Otospongiosis — see also Otosclerosis 387.9
Otto's disease or pelvis 715.35
Outburst, aggressive — see also Disturbance,
   conduct 312.0 ☑
   in children or adolescents 313.9
Outcome of delivery
   multiple birth NEC V27.9
      all liveborn V27.5
      all stillborn V27.7
      some liveborn V27.6
      unspecified V27.9
   single V27.9
      liveborn V27.0

☑ **Additional Digit Required** — Refer to the Tabular List for Digit Selection   ▽ **Subterms under main terms may continue to next column or page**

2014 ICD-9-CM   ►◄ Revised Text   ● New Line   ▲ Revised Code   **Volume 2 — 221**

Outcome of delivery — continued
single — continued
stillborn V27.1
twins V27.9
both liveborn V27.2
both stillborn V27.4
one liveborn, one stillborn V27.3
Outlet — see also condition
syndrome (thoracic) 353.0
Outstanding ears (bilateral) 744.29
Ovalocytosis (congenital) (hereditary) — see also Elliptocytosis 282.1
Ovarian — see also condition
pregnancy — see Pregnancy, ovarian
remnant syndrome 620.8
vein syndrome 593.4
Ovaritis (cystic) — see also Salpingo-oophoritis 614.2
Ovary, ovarian — see condition
Overactive — see also Hyperfunction
bladder 596.51
eye muscle (see also Strabismus) 378.9
hypothalamus 253.8
thyroid (see also Thyrotoxicosis) 242.9 ☑
Overactivity, child 314.01
Overbite (deep) (excessive) (horizontal) (vertical) 524.29
Overbreathing — see also Hyperventilation 786.01
Overconscientious personality 301.4
Overdevelopment — see also Hypertrophy
breast (female) (male) 611.1
nasal bones 738.0
prostate, congenital 752.89
Overdistention — see Distention
Overdose overdosage (drug) 977.9
specified drug or substance — see Table of Drugs and Chemicals
Overeating 783.6
nonorganic origin 307.51
Overexertion (effects) (exhaustion) 994.5
Overexposure (effects) 994.9
exhaustion 994.4
Overfeeding — see also Overeating 783.6
Overfill, endodontic 526.62
Overgrowth, bone NEC 733.99
Overhanging
tooth restoration 525.62
unrepairable, dental restorative materials 525.62
Overheated (effects) (places) — see Heat
Overinhibited child 313.0
Overjet 524.29
excessive horizontal 524.26
Overlaid, overlying (suffocation) 994.7
Overlap
excessive horizontal 524.26
Overlapping toe (acquired) 735.8
congenital (fifth toe) 755.66
Overload
fluid 276.69
due to transfusion (blood) (blood components) 276.61
iron, due to repeated red blood cell transfusions 275.02
potassium (K) 276.7
sodium (Na) 276.0
transfusion associated circulatory (TACO) 276.61
Overnutrition — see also Hyperalimentation 783.6
Overproduction — see also Hypersecretion
ACTH 255.3
cortisol 255.0
growth hormone 253.0
thyroid-stimulating hormone (TSH) 242.8 ☑
Overriding
aorta 747.21
finger (acquired) 736.29
congenital 755.59
toe (acquired) 735.8
congenital 755.66
Oversize
fetus (weight of 4500 grams or more) 766.0
affecting management of pregnancy 656.6 ☑

Oversize — continued
fetus — continued
causing disproportion 653.5 ☑
with obstructed labor 660.1 ☑
affecting fetus or newborn 763.1
Overstimulation, ovarian 256.1
Overstrained 780.79
heart — see Hypertrophy, cardiac
Overweight — see also Obesity 278.02
Overwork 780.79
Oviduct — see condition
Ovotestis 752.7
Ovulation (cycle)
failure or lack of 628.0
pain 625.2
Ovum
blighted 631.8
donor V59.70
over age 35 V59.73
anonymous recipient V59.73
designated recipient V59.74
under age 35 V59.71
anonymous recipient V59.71
designated recipient V59.72
dropsical 631.8
pathologic 631.8
Owren's disease or syndrome (parahemophilia) — see also Defect, coagulation 286.3
Oxalosis 271.8
Oxaluria 271.8
Ox heart — see Hypertrophy, cardiac
OX syndrome 758.6
Oxycephaly, oxycephalic 756.0
syphilitic, congenital 090.0
Oxyuriasis 127.4
Oxyuris vermicularis (infestation) 127.4
Ozena 472.0

P

Pacemaker syndrome 429.4
Pachyderma, pachydermia 701.8
laryngis 478.5
laryngitis 478.79
larynx (verrucosa) 478.79
Pachydermatitis 701.8
Pachydermatocele (congenital) 757.39
acquired 701.8
Pachydermatosis 701.8
Pachydermoperiostitis
secondary 731.2
Pachydermoperiostosis
primary idiopathic 757.39
secondary 731.2
Pachymeningitis (adhesive) (basal) (brain) (cerebral) (cervical) (chronic) (circumscribed) (external) (fibrous) (hemorrhagic) (hypertrophic) (internal) (purulent) (spinal) (suppurative) — see also Meningitis 322.9
gonococcal 098.82
Pachyonychia (congenital) 757.5
acquired 703.8
Pachyperiosteodermia
primary or idiopathic 757.39
secondary 731.2
Pachyperiostosis
primary or idiopathic 757.39
secondary 731.2
Pacinian tumor (M9507/0) — see Neoplasm, skin, benign
Pads, knuckle or Garrod's 728.79
Paget-Schroetter syndrome (intermittent venous claudication) 453.89
Paget's disease (osteitis deformans) 731.0
with infiltrating duct carcinoma of the breast (M8541/3) — see Neoplasm, breast, malignant
bone 731.0
osteosarcoma in (M9184/3) — see Neoplasm, bone, malignant
breast (M8540/3) 174.0
extramammary (M8542/3) (see also Neoplasm, skin, malignant)
anus 154.3
skin 173.59

Paget's disease — continued
malignant (M8540/3)
breast 174.0
specified site NEC (M8542/3) — see Neoplasm, skin, malignant
unspecified site 174.0
mammary (M8540/3) 174.0
necrosis of bone 731.0
nipple (M8540/3) 174.0
osteitis deformans 731.0
Pain(s) (see also Painful) 780.96
abdominal 789.0 ☑
acute 338.19
due to trauma 338.11
postoperative 338.18
post-thoracotomy 338.12
adnexa (uteri) 625.9
alimentary, due to vascular insufficiency 557.9
anginoid (see also Pain, precordial) 786.51
anus 569.42
arch 729.5
arm 729.5
axillary 729.5
back (postural) 724.5
low 724.2
psychogenic 307.89
bile duct 576.9
bladder 788.99
bone 733.90
breast 611.71
psychogenic 307.89
broad ligament 625.9
cancer associated 338.3
cartilage NEC 733.90
cecum 789.0 ☑
cervicobrachial 723.3
chest (central) 786.50
atypical 786.59
midsternal 786.51
musculoskeletal 786.59
noncardiac 786.59
substernal 786.51
wall (anterior) 786.52
chronic 338.29
associated with significant psychosocial dysfunction 338.4
due to trauma 338.21
postoperative 338.28
post-thoracotomy 338.22
syndrome 338.4
coccyx 724.79
colon 789.0 ☑
common duct 576.9
coronary — see Angina
costochondral 786.52
diaphragm 786.52
due to (presence of) any device, implant, or graft classifiable to 996.0–996.5 — see Complications, due to (presence of) any device, implant, or graft classified to 996.0–996.5 NEC
malignancy (primary) (secondary) 338.3
ear (see also Otalgia) 388.70
epigastric, epigastrium 789.06
extremity (lower) (upper) 729.5
eye 379.91
face, facial 784.0
atypical 350.2
nerve 351.8
false (labor) 644.1 ☑
female genital organ NEC 625.9
psychogenic 307.89
finger 729.5
flank 789.0 ☑
foot 729.5
gallbladder 575.9
gas (intestinal) 787.3
gastric 536.8
generalized 780.96
genital organ
female 625.9
male 608.9
psychogenic 307.89
groin 789.0 ☑
growing 781.99

Pain(s) (see also Painful) — continued
hand 729.5
head (see also Headache) 784.0
heart (see also Pain, precordial) 786.51
infraorbital (see also Neuralgia, trigeminal) 350.1
intermenstrual 625.2
jaw 784.92
joint 719.40
ankle 719.47
elbow 719.42
foot 719.47
hand 719.44
hip 719.45
knee 719.46
multiple sites 719.49
pelvic region 719.45
psychogenic 307.89
shoulder (region) 719.41
specified site NEC 719.48
wrist 719.43
kidney 788.0
labor, false or spurious 644.1 ☑
laryngeal 784.1
leg 729.5
limb 729.5
low back 724.2
lumbar region 724.2
mandible, mandibular 784.92
mastoid (see also Otalgia) 388.70
maxilla 784.92
menstrual 625.3
metacarpophalangeal (joint) 719.44
metatarsophalangeal (joint) 719.47
mouth 528.9
muscle 729.1
intercostal 786.59
musculoskeletal (see also Pain, by site) 729.1
nasal 478.19
nasopharynx 478.29
neck NEC 723.1
psychogenic 307.89
neoplasm related (acute) (chronic) 338.3
nerve NEC 729.2
neuromuscular 729.1
nose 478.19
ocular 379.91
ophthalmic 379.91
orbital region 379.91
osteocopic 733.90
ovary 625.9
psychogenic 307.89
over heart (see also Pain, precordial) 786.51
ovulation 625.2
pelvic (female) 625.9
male NEC 789.0 ☑
psychogenic 307.89
psychogenic 307.89
penis 607.9
psychogenic 307.89
pericardial (see also Pain, precordial) 786.51
perineum
female 625.9
male 608.9
pharynx 478.29
pleura, pleural, pleuritic 786.52
post-thoracotomy 338.12
acute 338.12
chronic 338.22
postoperative 338.18
acute 338.18
chronic 338.28
preauricular 388.70
precordial (region) 786.51
psychogenic 307.89
premenstrual 625.4
psychogenic 307.80
cardiovascular system 307.89
gastrointestinal system 307.89
genitourinary system 307.89
heart 307.89
musculoskeletal system 307.89
respiratory system 307.89
skin 306.3
radicular (spinal) (see also Radiculitis) 729.2
rectum 569.42

☑ Additional Digit Required — Refer to the Tabular List for Digit Selection

🔲 Subterms under main terms may continue to next column or page

222 — Volume 2

►◄ Revised Text

● New Line

▲ Revised Code

2014 ICD-9-CM

Pain(s) (*see also* Painful) — *continued*
- respiration 786.52
- retrosternal 786.51
- rheumatic NEC 729.0
  - muscular 729.1
- rib 786.50
- root (spinal) (*see also* Radiculitis) 729.2
- round ligament (stretch) 625.9
- sacroiliac 724.6
- sciatic 724.3
- scrotum 608.9
  - psychogenic 307.89
- seminal vesicle 608.9
- sinus 478.19
- skin 782.0
- spermatic cord 608.9
- spinal root (*see also* Radiculitis) 729.2
- stomach 536.8
  - psychogenic 307.89
- substernal 786.51
- testis 608.9
  - psychogenic 307.89
- thoracic spine 724.1
  - with radicular and visceral pain 724.4
- throat 784.1
- tibia 733.90
- toe 729.5
- tongue 529.6
- tooth 525.9
- total hip replacement 996.77
- total knee replacement 996.77
- trigeminal (*see also* Neuralgia, trigeminal) 350.1
- tumor associated 338.3
- umbilicus 789.05
- ureter 788.0
- urinary (organ) (system) 788.0
- uterus 625.9
  - psychogenic 307.89
- vagina 625.9
- vertebrogenic (syndrome) 724.5
- vesical 788.99
- vulva 625.9
- xiphoid 733.90

Painful — *see also* Pain
- arc syndrome 726.19
- coitus
  - female 625.0
  - male 608.89
  - psychogenic 302.76
- ejaculation (semen) 608.89
  - psychogenic 302.79
- erection 607.3
- feet syndrome 266.2
- menstruation 625.3
  - psychogenic 306.52
- micturition 788.1
- ophthalmoplegia 378.55
- respiration 786.52
- scar NEC 709.2
- urination 788.1
- wire sutures 998.89

Painters' colic 984.9
- specified type of lead — *see* Table of Drugs and Chemicals

Palate — *see* condition

Palatoplegia 528.9

Palatoschisis — *see also* Cleft, palate 749.00

Palilalia 784.69

Palindromic arthritis — *see also* Rheumatism, palindromic 719.3 ☑

Palliative care V66.7

Pallor 782.61
- temporal, optic disc 377.15

Palmar — *see also* condition
- fascia — *see* condition

Palpable
- cecum 569.89
- kidney 593.89
- liver 573.9
- lymph nodes 785.6
- ovary 620.8
- prostate 602.9
- spleen (*see also* Splenomegaly) 789.2
- uterus 625.8

Palpitation (heart) 785.1

Palpitation — *continued*
- psychogenic 306.2

Palsy — *see also* Paralysis 344.9
- atrophic diffuse 335.20
- Bell's 351.0
  - newborn 767.5
- birth 767.7
- brachial plexus 353.0
  - fetus or newborn 767.6
- brain (*see also* Palsy, cerebral)
  - noncongenital or noninfantile 344.89
    - late effect — *see* Late effect(s) (of) cerebrovascular disease
  - syphilitic 094.89
    - congenital 090.49
- bulbar (chronic) (progressive) 335.22
  - pseudo NEC 335.23
  - supranuclear NEC 344.8 ☑
- cerebral (congenital) (infantile) (spastic) 343.9
  - athetoid 333.71
  - diplegic 343.0
    - late effect — *see* Late effect(s) (of) cerebrovascular disease
  - hemiplegic 343.1
  - monoplegic 343.3
  - noncongenital or noninfantile 437.8
    - late effect — *see* Late effect(s) (of) cerebrovascular disease
  - paraplegic 343.0
  - quadriplegic 343.2
  - spastic, not congenital or infantile 344.89
  - syphilitic 094.89
    - congenital 090.49
  - tetraplegic 343.2
- cranial nerve (*see also* Disorder, nerve, cranial)
  - multiple 352.6
- creeping 335.21
- divers' 993.3
- Erb's (birth injury) 767.6
- facial 351.0
  - newborn 767.5
- glossopharyngeal 352.2
- Klumpke (-Déjérine) 767.6
- lead 984.9
  - specified type of lead — *see* Table of Drugs and Chemicals
- median (tardy) 354.0
- peroneal nerve (acute) (tardy) 355.3
- progressive supranuclear 333.0
- pseudobulbar NEC 335.23
- radial nerve (acute) 354.3
- seventh nerve 351.0
  - newborn 767.5
- shaking (*see also* Parkinsonism) 332.0
- spastic (cerebral) (spinal) 343.9
  - hemiplegic 343.1
- specified nerve NEC — *see* Disorder, nerve
- supranuclear NEC 356.8
  - progressive 333.0
- ulnar nerve (tardy) 354.2
- wasting 335.21

Paltauf-Sternberg disease 201.9 ☑

Paludism — *see* Malaria

Panama fever 084.0

Panaris (with lymphangitis) 681.9
- finger 681.02
- toe 681.11

Panaritium (with lymphangitis) 681.9
- finger 681.02
- toe 681.11

Panarteritis (nodosa) 446.0
- brain or cerebral 437.4

Pancake heart 793.2
- with cor pulmonale (chronic) 416.9

Pancarditis (acute) (chronic) 429.89
- with
  - rheumatic
    - fever (active) (acute) (chronic) (subacute) 391.8
      - inactive or quiescent 398.99
- rheumatic, acute 391.8
  - chronic or inactive 398.99

Pancoast-Tobias syndrome (M8010/3) (carcinoma, pulmonary apex) 162.3

Pancoast's syndrome or tumor (carcinoma, pulmonary apex) (M8010/3) 162.3

Pancolitis 556.6

Pancreas, pancreatic — *see* condition

Pancreatitis 577.0
- acute (edematous) (hemorrhagic) (recurrent) 577.0
- annular 577.0
- apoplectic 577.0
- calcerceous 577.0
- chronic (infectious) 577.1
  - recurrent 577.1
- cystic 577.2
- fibrous 577.8
- gangrenous 577.0
- hemorrhagic (acute) 577.0
- interstitial (chronic) 577.1
  - acute 577.0
- malignant 577.0
- mumps 072.3
- painless 577.1
- recurrent 577.1
- relapsing 577.1
- subacute 577.0
- suppurative 577.0
- syphilitic 095.8

Pancreatolithiasis 577.8

Pancytolysis 289.9

Pancytopenia (acquired) 284.19
- with
  - malformations 284.09
  - myelodysplastic syndrome — *see* Syndrome, myelodysplastic
- congenital 284.09
- due to
  - antineoplastic chemotherapy 284.11
  - drug, specified NEC 284.12
- specified NEC 284.19

Panencephalitis — *see also* Encephalitis
- subacute, sclerosing 046.2

Panhematopenia 284.81
- congenital 284.09
- constitutional 284.09
- splenic, primary 289.4

Panhemocytopenia 284.81
- congenital 284.09
- constitutional 284.09

Panhypogonadism 257.2

Panhypopituitarism 253.2
- prepubertal 253.3

Panic (attack) (state) 300.01
- reaction to exceptional stress (transient) 308.0

Panmyelopathy, familial constitutional 284.09

Panmyelophthisis 284.2
- acquired (secondary) 284.81
- congenital 284.2
- idiopathic 284.9

Panmyelosis (acute) (M9951/1) 238.79

Panner's disease 732.3
- capitellum humeri 732.3
- head of humerus 732.3
- tarsal navicular (bone) (osteochondrosis) 732.5

Panneuritis endemica 265.0 *[357.4]*

Panniculitis 729.30
- back 724.8
- knee 729.31
- mesenteric 567.82
- neck 723.6
- nodular, nonsuppurative 729.30
- sacral 724.8
- specified site NEC 729.39

Panniculus adiposus (abdominal) 278.1

Pannus (corneal) 370.62
- abdominal (symptomatic) 278.1
- allergic eczematous 370.62
- degenerativus 370.62
- keratic 370.62
- rheumatoid — *see* Arthritis, rheumatoid
- trachomatosus, trachomatous (active) 076.1 *[370.62]*
  - late effect 139.1

Panophthalmitis 360.02

Panotitis — *see* Otitis media

Pansinusitis (chronic) (hyperplastic) (nonpurulent) (purulent) 473.8
- acute 461.8
- due to fungus NEC 117.9
- tuberculous (*see also* Tuberculosis) 012.8 ☑

Panuveitis 360.12
- sympathetic 360.11

Panvalvular disease — *see* Endocarditis, mitral

Papageienkrankheit 073.9

Papanicolaou smear
- anus 796.70
  - with
    - atypical squamous cells
      - cannot exclude high grade squamous intraepithelial lesion (ASC-H) 796.72
      - of undetermined significance (ASC-US) 796.71
    - cytologic evidence of malignancy 796.76
    - high grade squamous intraepithelial lesion (HGSIL) 796.74
    - low grade squamous intraepithelial lesion (LGSIL) 796.73
  - glandular 796.70
  - specified finding NEC 796.79
  - unsatisfactory cytology 796.78
- cervix (screening test) V76.2
  - as part of gynecological examination V72.31
  - for suspected malignant neoplasm V76.2
    - no disease found V71.1
  - inadequate cytology sample 795.08
  - nonspecific abnormal finding 795.00
    - with
      - atypical squamous cells
        - cannot exclude high grade squamous intraepithelial lesion (ASC-H) 795.02
        - of undetermined significance (ASC-US) 795.01
      - cytologic evidence of malignancy 795.06
      - high grade squamous intraepithelial lesion (HGSIL) 795.04
      - low grade squamous intraepithelial lesion (LGSIL) 795.03
    - nonspecific finding NEC 795.09
  - to confirm findings of recent normal smear following initial abnormal smear V72.32
  - satisfactory smear but lacking transformation zone 795.07
  - unsatisfactory cervical cytology 795.08
- other specified site (*see also* Screening, malignant neoplasm)
  - for suspected malignant neoplasm (*see also* Screening, malignant neoplasm)
    - no disease found V71.1
  - nonspecific abnormal finding 796.9
- vagina V76.47
  - with
    - atypical squamous cells
      - cannot exclude high grade squamous intraepithelial lesion (ASC-H) 795.12
      - of undetermined significance (ASC-US) 795.11
    - cytologic evidence of malignancy 795.16
    - high grade squamous intraepithelial lesion (HGSIL) 795.14
    - low grade squamous intraepithelial lesion (LGSIL) 795.13
  - abnormal NEC 795.19
  - following hysterectomy for malignant condition V67.01
  - inadequate cytology sample 795.18
  - unsatisfactory cytology 795.18

Papilledema 377.00
- associated with
  - decreased ocular pressure 377.02

☑ **Additional Digit Required** — Refer to the Tabular List for Digit Selection   ▽ **Subterms under main terms may continue to next column or page**

2014 ICD-9-CM   ►◄ **Revised Text**   ● **New Line**   ▲ **Revised Code**   **Volume 2 — 223**

Pain(s) — Papilledema

Papilledema — continued
  associated with — continued
    increased intracranial pressure 377.01
    retinal disorder 377.03
  choked disc 377.00
  infectional 377.00
Papillitis 377.31
  anus 569.49
  chronic lingual 529.4
  necrotizing, kidney 584.7
  optic 377.31
  rectum 569.49
  renal, necrotizing 584.7
  tongue 529.0
Papilloma (M8050/0) — see also Neoplasm,
  by site, benign

> Note — Except where otherwise indicated, the morphological varieties of papilloma in the list below should be coded by site as for "Neoplasm, benign."

  acuminatum (female) (male) 078.11
  bladder (urinary) (transitional cell)
    (M8120/1) 236.7
    benign (M8120/0) 223.3
  choroid plexus (M9390/0) 225.0
    anaplastic type (M9390/3) 191.5
    malignant (M9390/3) 191.5
  ductal (M8503/0)
  dyskeratotic (M8052/0)
  epidermoid (M8052/0)
  hyperkeratotic (M8052/0)
  intracystic (M8504/0)
  intraductal (M8503/0)
  inverted (M8053/0)
  keratotic (M8052/0)
  parakeratotic (M8052/0)
  pinta (primary) 103.0
  renal pelvis (transitional cell) (M8120/1)
    236.99
    benign (M8120/0) 223.1
  Schneiderian (M8121/0)
    specified site — see Neoplasm, by site,
      benign
    unspecified site 212.0
  serous surface (M8461/0)
    borderline malignancy (M8461/1)
      specified site — see Neoplasm, by
        site, uncertain behavior
      unspecified site 236.2
    specified site — see Neoplasm, by site,
      benign
    unspecified site 220
  squamous (cell) (M8052/0)
  transitional (cell) (M8120/0)
    bladder (urinary) (M8120/1) 236.7
    inverted type (M8121/1) — see Neoplasm, by site, uncertain behavior
    renal pelvis (M8120/1) 236.91
    ureter (M8120/1) 236.91
    ureter (transitional cell) (M8120/1) 236.91
      benign (M8120/0) 223.2
    urothelial (M8120/1) — see Neoplasm, by site, uncertain behavior
  verrucous (M8051/0)
  villous (M8261/1) — see Neoplasm, by site, uncertain behavior
  yaws, plantar or palmar 102.1
Papillomata, multiple, of yaws 102.1
Papillomatosis (M8060/0) — see also Neoplasm, by site, benign
  confluent and reticulate 701.8
  cutaneous 701.8
  ductal, breast 610.1
  Gougerot-Carteaud (confluent reticulate) 701.8
  intraductal (diffuse) (M8505/0) — see Neoplasm, by site, benign
  subareolar duct (M8506/0) 217
Papillon-Léage and Psaume syndrome
  (orodigitofacial dysostosis) 759.89
Papule 709.8
  carate (primary) 103.0
  fibrous, of nose (M8724/0) 216.3
  pinta (primary) 103.0
Papulosis
  lymphomatoid 709.8

Papulosis — continued
  malignant 447.8
Papyraceous fetus 779.89
  complicating pregnancy 646.0 ☑
Para-urethritis 597.89
  gonococcal (acute) 098.0
    chronic or duration of 2 months or over 098.2
Paracephalus 759.7
Parachute mitral valve 746.5
Paracoccidioidomycosis 116.1
  mucocutaneous-lymphangitic 116.1
  pulmonary 116.1
  visceral 116.1
Paracoccidioidomycosis — see Paracoccidioidomycosis
Paracusis 388.40
Paradentosis 523.5
Paradoxical facial movements 374.43
Paraffinoma 999.9
Paraganglioma (M8680/1)
  adrenal (M8700/0) 227.0
    malignant (M8700/3) 194.0
  aortic body (M8691/1) 237.3
    malignant (M8691/3) 194.6
  carotid body (M8692/1) 237.3
    malignant (M8692/3) 194.5
  chromaffin (M8700/0) (see also Neoplasm, by site, benign)
    malignant (M8700/3) — see Neoplasm, by site, malignant
  extra-adrenal (M8693/1)
    malignant (M8693/3)
      specified site — see Neoplasm, by site, malignant
      unspecified site 194.6
    specified site — see Neoplasm, by site, uncertain behavior
    unspecified site 237.3
  glomus jugulare (M8690/1) 237.3
    malignant (M8690/3) 194.6
  jugular (M8690/1) 237.3
    malignant (M8690/3) 194.6
  nonchromaffin (M8693/1)
    malignant (M8693/3)
      specified site — see Neoplasm, by site, malignant
      unspecified site 194.6
    specified site — see Neoplasm, by site, uncertain behavior
    unspecified site 237.3
  parasympathetic (M8682/1)
    specified site — see Neoplasm, by site, uncertain behavior
    unspecified site 237.3
  specified site — see Neoplasm, by site, uncertain behavior
  sympathetic (M8681/1)
    specified site — see Neoplasm, by site, uncertain behavior
    unspecified site 237.3
  unspecified site 237.3
Parageusia 781.1
  psychogenic 306.7
Paragonimiasis 121.2
Paragranuloma, Hodgkin's (M9660/3)
  201.0 ☑
Parahemophilia — see also Defect, coagulation 286.3
Parakeratosis 690.8
  psoriasiformis 696.2
  variegata 696.2
Paralysis, paralytic (complete) (incomplete) 344.9
  with
    broken
      back — see Fracture, vertebra, by site, with spinal cord injury
      neck — see Fracture, vertebra, cervical, with spinal cord injury
    fracture, vertebra — see Fracture, vertebra, by site, with spinal cord injury

Paralysis, paralytic — continued
  with — continued
    syphilis 094.89
  abdomen and back muscles 355.9
  abdominal muscles 355.9
  abducens (nerve) 378.54
  abductor 355.9
    lower extremity 355.8
    upper extremity 354.9
  accessory nerve 352.4
  accommodation 367.51
    hysterical 300.11
  acoustic nerve 388.5
  agitans 332.0
    arteriosclerotic 332.0
  alternating 344.89
    oculomotor 344.89
  amyotrophic 335.20
  ankle 355.8
  anterior serratus 355.9
  anus (sphincter) 569.49
  apoplectic (current episode) (see also Disease, cerebrovascular, acute) 436
    late effect — see Late effect(s) (of) cerebrovascular disease
  arm 344.40
    affecting
      dominant side 344.41
      nondominant side 344.42
    both 344.2
    hysterical 300.11
    late effect — see Late effect(s) (of) cerebrovascular disease
    psychogenic 306.0
    transient 781.4
    traumatic NEC (see also Injury, nerve, upper limb) 955.9
  arteriosclerotic (current episode) 437.0
    late effect — see Late effect(s) (of) cerebrovascular disease
  ascending (spinal), acute 357.0
  associated, nuclear 344.89
  asthenic bulbar 358.00
  ataxic NEC 334.9
    general 094.1
  athetoid 333.71
  atrophic 356.9
    infantile, acute (see also Poliomyelitis, with paralysis) 045.1 ☑
    muscle NEC 355.9
    progressive 335.21
    spinal (acute) (see also Poliomyelitis, with paralysis) 045.1 ☑
  attack (see also Disease, cerebrovascular, acute) 436
  axillary 353.0
  Babinski-Nageotte's 344.89
  Bell's 351.0
    newborn 767.5
  Benedikt's 344.89
  birth (injury) 767.7
    brain 767.0
    intracranial 767.0
    spinal cord 767.4
  bladder (sphincter) 596.53
    neurogenic 596.54
      with cauda equina syndrome 344.61
    puerperal, postpartum, childbirth 665.5 ☑
    sensory 596.54
      with cauda equina 344.61
    spastic 596.54
      with cauda equina 344.61
  bowel, colon, or intestine (see also Ileus) 560.1
  brachial plexus 353.0
    due to birth injury 767.6
    newborn 767.6
  brain
    congenital — see Palsy, cerebral
    current episode 437.8
    diplegia 344.2
    hemiplegia 342.9 ☑
      late effect — see Late effect(s) (of) cerebrovascular disease
    infantile — see Palsy, cerebral

Paralysis, paralytic — continued
  brain — continued
    late effect — see Late effect(s) (of) cerebrovascular disease
    monoplegia (see also Monoplegia)
      late effect — see Late effect(s) (of) cerebrovascular disease
    paraplegia 344.1
    quadriplegia — see Quadriplegia
    syphilitic, congenital 090.49
    triplegia 344.89
  bronchi 519.19
  Brown-Séquard's 344.89
  bulbar (chronic) (progressive) 335.22
    infantile (see also Poliomyelitis, bulbar) 045.0 ☑
    poliomyelitic (see also Poliomyelitis, bulbar) 045.0 ☑
    pseudo 335.23
    supranuclear 344.89
  bulbospinal 358.00
  cardiac (see also Failure, heart) 428.9
  cerebral
    current episode 437.8
    spastic, infantile — see Palsy, cerebral
  cerebrocerebellar 437.8
    diplegic infantile 343.0
  cervical
    plexus 353.2
    sympathetic NEC 337.09
  Céstan-Chenais 344.89
  Charcôt-Marie-Tooth type 356.1
  childhood — see Palsy, cerebral
  Clark's 343.9
  colon (see also Ileus) 560.1
  compressed air 993.3
  compression
    arm NEC 354.9
    cerebral — see Paralysis, brain
    leg NEC 355.8
    lower extremity NEC 355.8
    upper extremity NEC 354.9
  congenital (cerebral) (spastic) (spinal) — see Palsy, cerebral
  conjugate movement (of eye) 378.81
    cortical (nuclear) (supranuclear) 378.81
  convergence 378.83
  cordis (see also Failure, heart) 428.9
  cortical (see also Paralysis, brain) 437.8
  cranial or cerebral nerve (see also Disorder, nerve, cranial) 352.9
  creeping 335.21
  crossed leg 344.89
  crutch 953.4
  deglutition 784.99
    hysterical 300.11
  dementia 094.1
  descending (spinal) NEC 335.9
  diaphragm (flaccid) 519.4
    due to accidental section of phrenic nerve during procedure 998.2
  digestive organs NEC 564.89
  diplegic — see Diplegia
  divergence (nuclear) 378.85
  divers' 993.3
  Duchenne's 335.22
  due to intracranial or spinal birth injury — see Palsy, cerebral
  embolic (current episode) (see also Embolism, brain) 434.1 ☑
    late effect — see Late effect(s) (of) cerebrovascular disease
  enteric (see also Ileus) 560.1
    with hernia — see Hernia, by site, with obstruction
  Erb (-Duchenne) (birth) (newborn) 767.6
  Erb's syphilitic spastic spinal 094.89
  esophagus 530.89
  essential, infancy (see also Poliomyelitis) 045.9 ☑
  extremity
    lower — see Paralysis, leg
    spastic (hereditary) 343.3
      noncongenital or noninfantile 344.1
    transient (cause unknown) 781.4
    upper — see Paralysis, arm

☑ **Additional Digit Required** — Refer to the Tabular List for Digit Selection
🔄 **Subterms under main terms may continue to next column or page**

224 — Volume 2
▶◀ Revised Text
● New Line
▲ Revised Code
2014 ICD-9-CM

Paralysis, paralytic — *continued*
  eye muscle (extrinsic) 378.55
    intrinsic 367.51
  facial (nerve) 351.0
    birth injury 767.5
    congenital 767.5
    following operation NEC 998.2
    newborn 767.5
  familial 359.3
    periodic 359.3
    spastic 334.1
  fauces 478.29
  finger NEC 354.9
  foot NEC 355.8
  gait 781.2
  gastric nerve 352.3
  gaze 378.81
  general 094.1
    ataxic 094.1
    insane 094.1
    juvenile 090.40
    progressive 094.1
    tabetic 094.1
  glossopharyngeal (nerve) 352.2
  glottis (*see also* Paralysis, vocal cord) 478.30
  gluteal 353.4
  Gubler (-Millard) 344.89
  hand 354.9
    hysterical 300.11
    psychogenic 306.0
  heart (*see also* Failure, heart) 428.9
  hemifacial, progressive 349.89
  hemiplegic — *see* Hemiplegia
  hyperkalemic periodic (familial) 359.3
  hypertensive (current episode) 437.8
  hypoglossal (nerve) 352.5
  hypokalemic periodic 359.3
  Hyrtl's sphincter (rectum) 569.49
  hysterical 300.11
  ileus (*see also* Ileus) 560.1
  infantile (*see also* Poliomyelitis) 045.9 ☑
    atrophic acute 045.1 ☑
    bulbar 045.0 ☑
    cerebral — *see* Palsy, cerebral
    paralytic 045.1 ☑
    progressive acute 045.9 ☑
    spastic — *see* Palsy, cerebral
    spinal 045.9 ☑
  infective (*see also* Poliomyelitis) 045.9 ☑
  inferior nuclear 344.9
  insane, general or progressive 094.1
  internuclear 378.86
  interosseous 355.9
  intestine (*see also* Ileus) 560.1
  intracranial (current episode) (*see also*
      Paralysis, brain) 437.8
    due to birth injury 767.0
  iris 379.49
    due to diphtheria (toxin) 032.81 [379.49]
  ischemic, Volkmann's (complicating trauma)
      958.6
  isolated sleep, recurrent
  Jackson's 344.89
  jake 357.7
  Jamaica ginger (jake) 357.7
  Landry's 357.0
  laryngeal nerve (recurrent) (superior) (*see
      also* Paralysis, vocal cord) 478.30
  larynx (*see also* Paralysis, vocal cord) 478.30
    due to diphtheria (toxin) 032.3
  late effect
    due to
      birth injury, brain or spinal (cord) —
          see Palsy, cerebral
      edema, brain or cerebral — *see*
          Paralysis, brain
      lesion
        late effect — *see* Late effect(s) (of)
            cerebrovascular disease
        spinal (cord) — *see* Paralysis,
            spinal
  lateral 335.24
  lead 984.9

Paralysis, paralytic — *continued*
  lead — *continued*
    specified type of lead — *see* Table of
        Drugs and Chemicals
  left side — *see* Hemiplegia
  leg 344.30
    affecting
      dominant side 344.31
      nondominant side 344.32
    both (*see also* Paraplegia) 344.1
    crossed 344.89
    hysterical 300.11
    psychogenic 306.0
    transient or transitory 781.4
      traumatic NEC (*see also* Injury, nerve,
          lower limb) 956.9
  levator palpebrae superioris 374.31
  limb NEC 344.5
    all four — *see* Quadriplegia
    quadriplegia — *see* Quadriplegia
  lip 528.5
  Lissauer's 094.1
  local 355.9
  lower limb (*see also* Paralysis, leg)
    both (*see also* Paraplegia) 344.1
  lung 518.89
    newborn 770.89
  median nerve 354.1
  medullary (tegmental) 344.89
  mesencephalic NEC 344.89
    tegmental 344.89
  middle alternating 344.89
  Millard-Gubler-Foville 344.89
  monoplegic — *see* Monoplegia
  motor NEC 344.9
    cerebral — *see* Paralysis, brain
    spinal — *see* Paralysis, spinal
  multiple
    cerebral — *see* Paralysis, brain
    spinal — *see* Paralysis, spinal
  muscle (flaccid) 359.9
    due to nerve lesion NEC 355.9
    eye (extrinsic) 378.55
      intrinsic 367.51
      oblique 378.51
    iris sphincter 364.89
    ischemic (complicating trauma) (Volk-
        mann's) 958.6
    pseudohypertrophic 359.1
  muscular (atrophic) 359.9
    progressive 335.21
  musculocutaneous nerve 354.9
  musculospiral 354.9
  nerve (*see also* Disorder, nerve)
    third or oculomotor (partial) 378.51
      total 378.52
    fourth or trochlear 378.53
    sixth or abducens 378.54
    seventh or facial 351.0
      birth injury 767.5
      due to
        injection NEC 999.9
        operation NEC 997.09
      newborn 767.5
    accessory 352.4
    auditory 388.5
    birth injury 767.7
    cranial or cerebral (*see also* Disorder,
        nerve, cranial) 352.9
    facial 351.0
      birth injury 767.5
      newborn 767.5
    laryngeal (*see also* Paralysis, vocal cord)
        478.30
    newborn 767.7
    phrenic 354.8
      newborn 767.7
    radial 354.3
      birth injury 767.6
      newborn 767.6
    syphilitic 094.89
    traumatic NEC (*see also* Injury, nerve, by
        site) 957.9
    trigeminal 350.9
    ulnar 354.2
  newborn NEC 767.0

Paralysis, paralytic — *continued*
  normokalemic periodic 359.3
  obstetrical, newborn 767.7
  ocular 378.9
  oculofacial, congenital 352.6
  oculomotor (nerve) (partial) 378.51
    alternating 344.89
    external bilateral 378.55
    total 378.52
  olfactory nerve 352.0
  palate 528.9
  palatopharyngolaryngeal 352.6
  paratrigeminal 350.9
  periodic (familial) (hyperkalemic) (hy-
      pokalemic) (normokalemic) (potassi-
      um sensitive) (secondary) 359.3
  peripheral
    autonomic nervous system — *see* Neu-
        ropathy, peripheral, autonomic
    nerve NEC 355.9
  peroneal (nerve) 355.3
  pharynx 478.29
  phrenic nerve 354.8
  plantar nerves 355.6
  pneumogastric nerve 352.3
  poliomyelitis (current) (*see also* Poliomyeli-
      tis, with paralysis) 045.1 ☑
    bulbar 045.0 ☑
  popliteal nerve 355.3
  pressure (*see also* Neuropathy, entrapment)
      355.9
  progressive 335.21
    atrophic 335.21
    bulbar 335.22
    general 094.1
    hemifacial 349.89
    infantile, acute (*see also* Poliomyelitis)
        045.9 ☑
    multiple 335.20
  pseudobulbar 335.23
  pseudohypertrophic 359.1
    muscle 359.1
  psychogenic 306.0
  pupil, pupillary 379.49
  quadriceps 355.8
  quadriplegic (*see also* Quadriplegia)
      344.0 ☑
  radial nerve 354.3
    birth injury 767.6
  rectum (sphincter) 569.49
  rectus muscle (eye) 378.55
  recurrent
    isolated sleep 327.43
    laryngeal nerve (*see also* Paralysis, vocal
        cord) 478.30
  respiratory (muscle) (system) (tract) 786.09
    center NEC 344.89
      fetus or newborn 770.87
    congenital 768.9
    newborn 768.9
  right side — *see* Hemiplegia
  Saturday night 354.3
  saturnine 984.9
    specified type of lead — *see* Table of
        Drugs and Chemicals
  sciatic nerve 355.0
  secondary — *see* Paralysis, late effect
  seizure (cerebral) (current episode) (*see also*
      Disease, cerebrovascular, acute) 436
    late effect — *see* Late effect(s) (of) cere-
        brovascular disease
  senile NEC 344.9
  serratus magnus 355.9
  shaking (*see also* Parkinsonism) 332.0
  shock (*see also* Disease, cerebrovascular,
      acute) 436
    late effect — *see* Late effect(s) (of) cere-
        brovascular disease
  shoulder 354.9
  soft palate 528.9
  spasmodic — *see* Paralysis, spastic
  spastic 344.9
    cerebral infantile — *see* Palsy, cerebral
    congenital (cerebral) — *see* Palsy, cere-
        bral
    familial 334.1

Paralysis, paralytic — *continued*
  spastic — *continued*
    hereditary 334.1
    infantile 343.9
    noncongenital or noninfantile, cerebral
        344.9
    syphilitic 094.0
      spinal 094.89
  sphincter, bladder (*see also* Paralysis, blad-
      der) 596.53
  spinal (cord) NEC 344.1
    accessory nerve 352.4
    acute (*see also* Poliomyelitis) 045.9 ☑
    ascending acute 357.0
    atrophic (acute) (*see also* Poliomyelitis,
        with paralysis) 045.1 ☑
      spastic, syphilitic 094.89
    congenital NEC 343.9
    hemiplegic — *see* Hemiplegia
    hereditary 336.8
    infantile (*see also* Poliomyelitis) 045.9 ☑
    late effect NEC 344.89
    monoplegic — *see* Monoplegia
    nerve 355.9
    progressive 335.10
    quadriplegic — *see* Quadriplegia
    spastic NEC 343.9
    traumatic — *see* Injury, spinal, by site
  sternomastoid 352.4
  stomach 536.3
    diabetic 250.6 ☑ [536.3]
      due to secondary diabetes
          249.6 ☑ [536.3]
    nerve (nondiabetic) 352.3
  stroke (current episode) — *see* Infarct, brain
    late effect — *see* Late effect(s) (of) cere-
        brovascular disease
  subscapularis 354.8
  superior nuclear NEC 334.9
  supranuclear 356.8
  sympathetic
    cervical NEC 337.09
    nerve NEC (*see also* Neuropathy, periph-
        eral, autonomic) 337.9
    nervous system — *see* Neuropathy, pe-
        ripheral, autonomic
  syndrome 344.9
    specified NEC 344.89
  syphilitic spastic spinal (Erb's) 094.89
  tabetic general 094.1
  thigh 355.8
  throat 478.29
    diphtheritic 032.0
    muscle 478.29
  thrombotic (current episode) (*see also*
      Thrombosis, brain) 434.0 ☑
    late effect — *see* Late effect(s) (of) cere-
        brovascular disease
  thumb NEC 354.9
  tick (-bite) 989.5
  Todd's (postepileptic transitory paralysis)
      344.89
  toe 355.6
  tongue 529.8
  transient
    arm or leg NEC 781.4
    traumatic NEC (*see also* Injury, nerve, by
        site) 957.9
  trapezius 352.4
  traumatic, transient NEC (*see also* Injury,
      nerve, by site) 957.9
  trembling (*see also* Parkinsonism) 332.0
  triceps brachii 354.9
  trigeminal nerve 350.9
  trochlear nerve 378.53
  ulnar nerve 354.2
  upper limb (*see also* Paralysis, arm)
    both (*see also* Diplegia) 344.2
  uremic — *see* Uremia
  uveoparotitic 135
  uvula 528.9
    hysterical 300.11
    postdiphtheritic 032.0
  vagus nerve 352.3
  vasomotor NEC 337.9
  velum palati 528.9

☑ **Additional Digit Required — Refer to the Tabular List for Digit Selection**   ▽ **Subterms under main terms may continue to next column or page**

Paralysis, paralytic — *continued*
vesical (*see also* Paralysis, bladder) 596.53
vestibular nerve 388.5
visual field, psychic 368.16
vocal cord 478.30
bilateral (partial) 478.33
complete 478.34
complete (bilateral) 478.34
unilateral (partial) 478.31
complete 478.32
Volkmann's (complicating trauma) 958.6
wasting 335.21
Weber's 344.89
wrist NEC 354.9
Paramedial orifice, urethrovesical 753.8
Paramenia 626.9
Parametritis (chronic) — *see also* Disease, pelvis, inflammatory 614.4
acute 614.3
puerperal, postpartum, childbirth 670.8 ☑
Parametrium, parametric — *see* condition
Paramnesia — *see also* Amnesia 780.93
Paramolar 520.1
causing crowding 524.31
Paramyloidosis 277.30
Paramyoclonus multiplex 333.2
Paramyotonia 359.29
congenita (of von Eulenburg) 359.29
Paraneoplastic syndrome — *see* condition
Parangi — *see also* Yaws 102.9
Paranoia 297.1
alcoholic 291.5
querulans 297.8
senile 290.20
Paranoid
dementia (*see also* Schizophrenia) 295.3 ☑
praecox (acute) 295.3 ☑
senile 290.20
personality 301.0
psychosis 297.9
alcoholic 291.5
climacteric 297.2
drug-induced 292.11
involutional 297.2
menopausal 297.2
protracted reactive 298.4
psychogenic 298.4
acute 298.3
senile 290.20
reaction (chronic) 297.9
acute 298.3
schizophrenia (acute) (*see also* Schizophrenia) 295.3 ☑
state 297.9
alcohol-induced 291.5
climacteric 297.2
drug-induced 292.11
due to or associated with
arteriosclerosis (cerebrovascular) 290.42
presenile brain disease 290.12
senile brain disease 290.20
involutional 297.2
menopausal 297.2
senile 290.20
simple 297.0
specified type NEC 297.8
tendencies 301.0
traits 301.0
trends 301.0
type, psychopathic personality 301.0
Paraparesis — *see also* Paraplegia 344.1
Paraphasia 784.3
Paraphilia — *see also* Deviation, sexual 302.9
Paraphimosis (congenital) 605
chancroidal 099.0
Paraphrenia, paraphrenic (late) 297.2
climacteric 297.2
dementia (*see also* Schizophrenia) 295.3 ☑
involutional 297.2
menopausal 297.2
schizophrenia (acute) (*see also* Schizophrenia) 295.3 ☑
Paraplegia 344.1

Paraplegia — *continued*
with
broken back — *see* Fracture, vertebra, by site, with spinal cord injury
fracture, vertebra — *see* Fracture, vertebra, by site, with spinal cord injury
ataxic — *see* Degeneration, combined, spinal cord
brain (current episode) (*see also* Paralysis, brain) 437.8
cerebral (current episode) (*see also* Paralysis, brain) 437.8
congenital or infantile (cerebral) (spastic) (spinal) 343.0
cortical — *see* Paralysis, brain
familial spastic 334.1
functional (hysterical) 300.11
hysterical 300.11
infantile 343.0
late effect 344.1
Pott's (*see also* Tuberculosis) 015.0 ☑ [730.88]
psychogenic 306.0
spastic
Erb's spinal 094.89
hereditary 334.1
not infantile or congenital 344.1
spinal (cord)
traumatic NEC — *see* Injury, spinal, by site
syphilitic (spastic) 094.89
traumatic NEC — *see* Injury, spinal, by site
Paraproteinemia 273.2
benign (familial) 273.1
monoclonal 273.1
secondary to malignant or inflammatory disease 273.1
Parapsoriasis 696.2
en plaques 696.2
guttata 696.2
lichenoides chronica 696.2
retiformis 696.2
varioliformis (acuta) 696.2
Parascarlatina 057.8
Parasitic — *see also* condition
disease NEC (*see also* Infestation, parasitic) 136.9
contact V01.89
exposure to V01.89
intestinal NEC 129
skin NEC 134.9
stomatitis 112.0
sycosis 110.0
beard 110.0
scalp 110.0
twin 759.4
Parasitism NEC 136.9
intestinal NEC 129
skin NEC 134.9
specified — *see* Infestation
Parasitophobia 300.29
Parasomnia 307.47
alcohol induced 291.82
drug induced 292.85
nonorganic origin 307.47
organic 327.40
in conditions classified elsewhere 327.44
other 327.49
Paraspadias 752.69
Paraspasm facialis 351.8
Parathyroid gland — *see* condition
Parathyroiditis (autoimmune) 252.1
Parathyroprival tetany 252.1
Paratrachoma 077.0
Paratyphilitis — *see also* Appendicitis 541
Paratyphoid (fever) — *see* Fever, paratyphoid
Paratyphus — *see* Fever, paratyphoid
Paraurethral duct 753.8
Paravaccinia NEC 051.9
milkers' node 051.1
Paravaginitis — *see also* Vaginitis 616.10
Parencephalitis — *see also* Encephalitis 323.9
late effect — *see* category 326
Parergasia 298.9
Paresis — *see also* Paralysis 344.9

Paresis — *see also* Paralysis — *continued*
accommodation 367.51
bladder (spastic) (sphincter) (*see also* Paralysis, bladder) 596.53
tabetic 094.0
bowel, colon, or intestine (*see also* Ileus) 560.1
brain or cerebral — *see* Paralysis, brain
extrinsic muscle, eye 378.55
general 094.1
arrested 094.1
brain 094.1
cerebral 094.1
insane 094.1
juvenile 090.40
remission 090.49
progressive 094.1
remission (sustained) 094.1
tabetic 094.1
heart (*see also* Failure, heart) 428.9
infantile (*see also* Poliomyelitis) 045.9 ☑
insane 094.1
juvenile 090.40
late effect — *see* Paralysis, late effect
luetic (general) 094.1
peripheral progressive 356.9
pseudohypertrophic 359.1
senile NEC 344.9
stomach 536.3
diabetic 250.6 ☑ [536.3]
due to secondary diabetes 249.6 ☑ [536.3]
syphilitic (general) 094.1
congenital 090.40
transient, limb 781.4
vesical (sphincter) NEC 596.53
Paresthesia — *see also* Disturbance, sensation 782.0
Berger's (paresthesia of lower limb) 782.0
Bernhardt 355.1
Magnan's 782.0
Paretic — *see* condition
Parinaud's
conjunctivitis 372.02
oculoglandular syndrome 372.02
ophthalmoplegia 378.81
syndrome (paralysis of conjugate upward gaze) 378.81
Parkes Weber and Dimitri syndrome (encephalocutaneous angiomatosis) 759.6
Parkinson's disease, syndrome, or tremor — *see* Parkinsonism
Parkinsonism (arteriosclerotic) (idiopathic) (primary) 332.0
associated with orthostatic hypotension (idiopathic) (symptomatic) 333.0
due to drugs 332.1
neuroleptic-induced 332.1
secondary 332.1
syphilitic 094.82
Parodontitis 523.40
Parodontosis 523.5
Paronychia (with lymphangitis) 681.9
candidal (chronic) 112.3
chronic 681.9
candidal 112.3
finger 681.02
toe 681.11
finger 681.02
toe 681.11
tuberculous (primary) (*see also* Tuberculosis) 017.0 ☑
Parorexia NEC 307.52
hysterical 300.11
Parosmia 781.1
psychogenic 306.7
Parotid gland — *see* condition
Parotiditis — *see also* Parotitis 527.2
epidemic 072.9
infectious 072.9
Parotitis 527.2
allergic 527.2
chronic 527.2
epidemic (*see also* Mumps) 072.9
infectious (*see also* Mumps) 072.9
noninfectious 527.2

Parotitis — *continued*
nonspecific toxic 527.2
not mumps 527.2
postoperative 527.2
purulent 527.2
septic 527.2
suppurative (acute) 527.2
surgical 527.2
toxic 527.2
Paroxysmal — *see also* condition
dyspnea (nocturnal) 786.09
Parrot's disease (syphilitic osteochondritis) 090.0
Parrot fever 073.9
Parry-Romberg syndrome 349.89
Parry's disease or syndrome (exophthalmic goiter) 242.0 ☑
Parsonage-Aldren-Turner syndrome 353.5
Parsonage-Turner syndrome 353.5
Parson's disease (exophthalmic goiter) 242.0 ☑
Pars planitis 363.21
Particolored infant 757.39
Parturition — *see* Delivery
Parvovirus 079.83
B19 079.83
human 079.83
Passage
false, urethra 599.4
meconium noted during delivery 763.84
of sounds or bougies (*see also* Attention to artificial opening) V55.9
Passive — *see* condition
Pasteurella septica 027.2
Pasteurellosis — *see also* Infection, Pasteurella 027.2
PAT (paroxysmal atrial tachycardia) 427.0
Patau's syndrome (trisomy D1) 758.1
Patch
herald 696.3
Patches
mucous (syphilitic) 091.3
congenital 090.0
smokers' (mouth) 528.6
Patellar — *see* condition
Patellofemoral syndrome 719.46
Patent — *see also* Imperfect closure
atrioventricular ostium 745.69
canal of Nuck 752.41
cervix 622.5
complicating pregnancy 654.5 ☑
affecting fetus or newborn 761.0
ductus arteriosus or Botalli 747.0
Eustachian
tube 381.7
valve 746.89
foramen
Botalli 745.5
ovale 745.5
interauricular septum 745.5
interventricular septum 745.4
omphalomesenteric duct 751.0
os (uteri) — *see* Patent, cervix
ostium secundum 745.5
urachus 753.7
vitelline duct 751.0
Paternity testing V70.4
Paterson-Kelly syndrome or web (sideropenic dysphagia) 280.8
Paterson (-Brown) (-Kelly) syndrome (sideropenic dysphagia) 280.8
Paterson's syndrome (sideropenic dysphagia) 280.8
Pathologic, pathological — *see also* condition
asphyxia 799.01
drunkenness 291.4
emotionality 301.3
fracture — *see* Fracture, pathologic
liar 301.7
personality 301.9
resorption, tooth 521.40
external 521.42
internal 521.41
specified NEC 521.49
sexuality (*see also* Deviation, sexual) 302.9
Pathology (of) — *see also* Disease

Pathology — *see also* Disease — *continued*
  periradicular, associated with previous endodontic treatment 526.69
Patterned motor discharge, idiopathic —
  see also Epilepsy 345.5 ☑
Patulous — *see also* Patent
  anus 569.49
  Eustachian tube 381.7
Pause, sinoatrial 427.81
Pavor nocturnus 307.46
Pavy's disease 593.6
Paxton's disease (white piedra) 111.2
Payr's disease or syndrome (splenic flexure syndrome) 569.89
PBA (pseudobulbar affect) 310.81
Pearl-workers' disease (chronic osteomyelitis) — *see also* Osteomyelitis 730.1 ☑
Pearls
  Elschnig 366.51
  enamel 520.2
Pectenitis 569.49
Pectenosis 569.49
Pectoral — *see* condition
Pectus
  carinatum (congenital) 754.82
    acquired 738.3
      rachitic (*see also* Rickets) 268.0
  excavatum (congenital) 754.81
    acquired 738.3
      rachitic (*see also* Rickets) 268.0
  recurvatum (congenital) 754.81
    acquired 738.3
Pedatrophia 261
Pederosis 302.2
Pediculosis (infestation) 132.9
  capitis (head louse) (any site) 132.0
  corporis (body louse) (any site) 132.1
  eyelid 132.0 [373.6]
  mixed (classifiable to more than one category in 132.0–132.2) 132.3
  pubis (pubic louse) (any site) 132.2
  vestimenti 132.1
  vulvae 132.2
Pediculus (infestation) — *see* Pediculosis
Pedophilia 302.2
Peg-shaped teeth 520.2
Pel-Ebstein disease — *see* Disease, Hodgkin's
Pelade 704.01
Pel's crisis 094.0
Pelger-Huët anomaly or syndrome (hereditary hyposegmentation) 288.2
Peliosis (rheumatica) 287.0
Pelizaeus-Merzbacher
  disease 330.0
  sclerosis, diffuse cerebral 330.0
Pellagra-cerebellar-ataxia-renal aminoaciduria syndrome 270.0
Pellagra (alcoholic or with alcoholism) 265.2
  with polyneuropathy 265.2 [357.4]
Pellegrini's disease (calcification, knee joint) 726.62
Pellegrini (-Stieda) disease or syndrome (calcification, knee joint) 726.62
Pellizzi's syndrome (pineal) 259.8
Pelvic — *see also* condition
  congestion-fibrosis syndrome 625.5
  kidney 753.3
Pelvioectasis 591
Pelviolithiasis 592.0
Pelviperitonitis
  female (*see also* Peritonitis, pelvic, female) 614.5
  male (*see also* Peritonitis) 567.21
Pelvis, pelvic — *see also* condition or type
  infantile 738.6
  Nägele's 738.6
  obliquity 738.6
  Robert's 755.69
Pemphigoid 694.5
  benign, mucous membrane 694.60
    with ocular involvement 694.61
  bullous 694.5
  cicatricial 694.60
    with ocular involvement 694.61
  juvenile 694.2
Pemphigus 694.4

Pemphigus — *continued*
  benign 694.5
    chronic familial 757.39
  Brazilian 694.4
  circinatus 694.0
  congenital, traumatic 757.39
  conjunctiva 694.61
  contagiosus 684
  erythematodes 694.4
  erythematosus 694.4
  foliaceus 694.4
  frambesiodes 694.4
  gangrenous (*see also* Gangrene) 785.4
  malignant 694.4
  neonatorum, newborn 684
  ocular 694.61
  papillaris 694.4
  seborrheic 694.4
  South American 694.4
  syphilitic (congenital) 090.0
  vegetans 694.4
  vulgaris 694.4
  wildfire 694.4
Pendred's syndrome (familial goiter with deaf-mutism) 243
Pendulous
  abdomen 701.9
    in pregnancy or childbirth 654.4 ☑
      affecting fetus or newborn 763.89
  breast 611.89
Penetrating wound — *see also* Wound, open, by site
  with internal injury — *see* Injury, internal, by site, with open wound
  eyeball 871.7
    with foreign body (nonmagnetic) 871.6
      magnetic 871.5
  ocular (*see also* Penetrating wound, eyeball) 871.7
    adnexa 870.3
      with foreign body 870.4
  orbit 870.3
    with foreign body 870.4
Penetration, pregnant uterus by instrument
  with
    abortion — *see* Abortion, by type, with damage to pelvic organs
    ectopic pregnancy (*see also* categories 633.0–633.9) 639.2
    molar pregnancy (*see also* categories 630–632) 639.2
  complication of delivery 665.1 ☑
    affecting fetus or newborn 763.89
  following
    abortion 639.2
    ectopic or molar pregnancy 639.2
Penfield's syndrome — *see also* Epilepsy 345.5 ☑
Penicilliosis of lung 117.3
Penis — *see* condition
Penitis 607.2
Pentalogy (of Fallot) 745.2
Penta X syndrome 758.81
Pentosuria (benign) (essential) 271.8
Peptic acid disease 536.8
Peregrinating patient V65.2
Perforated — *see* Perforation
Perforation, perforative (nontraumatic)
  antrum (*see also* Sinusitis, maxillary) 473.0
  appendix 540.0
    with peritoneal abscess 540.1
  atrial septum, multiple 745.5
  attic, ear 384.22
    healed 384.81
  bile duct, except cystic (*see also* Disease, biliary) 576.3
    cystic 575.4
  bladder (urinary) 596.6
    with
      abortion — *see* Abortion, by type, with damage to pelvic organs
      ectopic pregnancy (*see also* categories 633.0–633.9) 639.2
      molar pregnancy (*see also* categories 630–632) 639.2

Perforation, perforative — *continued*
  bladder — *continued*
    following
      abortion 639.2
      ectopic or molar pregnancy 639.2
    obstetrical trauma 665.5 ☑
  bowel 569.83
    with
      abortion — *see* Abortion, by type, with damage to pelvic organs
      ectopic pregnancy (*see also* categories 633.0–633.9) 639.2
      molar pregnancy (*see also* categories 630–632) 639.2
    fetus or newborn 777.6
    following
      abortion 639.2
      ectopic or molar pregnancy 639.2
    obstetrical trauma 665.5 ☑
  broad ligament
    with
      abortion — *see* Abortion, by type, with damage to pelvic organs
      ectopic pregnancy (*see also* categories 633.0–633.9) 639.2
      molar pregnancy (*see also* categories 630–632) 639.2
    following
      abortion 639.2
      ectopic or molar pregnancy 639.2
    obstetrical trauma 665.6 ☑
  by
    device, implant, or graft — *see* Complications, mechanical
    foreign body left accidentally in operation wound 998.4
    instrument (any) during a procedure, accidental 998.2
  cecum 540.0
    with peritoneal abscess 540.1
  cervix (uteri) (*see also* Injury, internal, cervix)
    with
      abortion — *see* Abortion, by type, with damage to pelvic organs
      ectopic pregnancy (*see also* categories 633.0–633.9) 639.2
      molar pregnancy (*see also* categories 630–632) 639.2
    following
      abortion 639.2
      ectopic or molar pregnancy 639.2
    obstetrical trauma 665.3 ☑
  colon 569.83
  common duct (bile) 576.3
  cornea (*see also* Ulcer, cornea) 370.00
    due to ulceration 370.06
  cystic duct 575.4
  diverticulum (*see also* Diverticula) 562.10
    small intestine 562.00
  duodenum, duodenal (ulcer) — *see* Ulcer, duodenum, with perforation
  ear drum — *see* Perforation, tympanum
  enteritis — *see* Enteritis
  esophagus 530.4
  ethmoidal sinus (*see also* Sinusitis, ethmoidal) 473.2
  foreign body (external site) (*see also* Wound, open, by site, complicated)
    internal site, by ingested object — *see* Foreign body
  frontal sinus (*see also* Sinusitis, frontal) 473.1
  gallbladder or duct (*see also* Disease, gallbladder) 575.4
  gastric (ulcer) — *see* Ulcer, stomach, with perforation
  heart valve — *see* Endocarditis
  ileum (*see also* Perforation, intestine) 569.83
  instrumental
    external — *see* Wound, open, by site
    pregnant uterus, complicating delivery 665.9 ☑
    surgical (accidental) (blood vessel) (nerve) (organ) 998.2
  intestine 569.83

Perforation, perforative — *continued*
  intestine — *continued*
    with
      abortion — *see* Abortion, by type, with damage to pelvic organs
      ectopic pregnancy (*see also* categories 633.0–633.9) 639.2
      molar pregnancy (*see also* categories 630–632) 639.2
    fetus or newborn 777.6
    obstetrical trauma 665.5 ☑
    ulcerative NEC 569.83
  jejunum, jejunal 569.83
    ulcer — *see* Ulcer, gastrojejunal, with perforation
  mastoid (antrum) (cell) 383.89
  maxillary sinus (*see also* Sinusitis, maxillary) 473.0
  membrana tympani — *see* Perforation, tympanum
  nasal
    septum 478.19
      congenital 748.1
      syphilitic 095.8
    sinus (*see also* Sinusitis) 473.9
      congenital 748.1
  palate (hard) 526.89
    soft 528.9
      syphilitic 095.8
        syphilitic 095.8
  palatine vault 526.89
    syphilitic 095.8
      congenital 090.5
  pelvic
    floor
      with
        abortion — *see* Abortion, by type, with damage to pelvic organs
        ectopic pregnancy (*see also* categories 633.0–633.9) 639.2
        molar pregnancy (*see also* categories 630–632) 639.2
      obstetrical trauma 664.1 ☑
    organ
      with
        abortion — *see* Abortion, by type, with damage to pelvic organs
        ectopic pregnancy (*see also* categories 633.0–633.9) 639.2
        molar pregnancy (*see also* categories 630–632) 639.2
      following
        abortion 639.2
        ectopic or molar pregnancy 639.2
      obstetrical trauma 665.5 ☑
  perineum — *see* Laceration, perineum
  periurethral tissue
    with
      abortion — *see* Abortion, by type, with damage to pelvic organs
      ectopic pregnancy (*see also* categories 633.0–633.9) 639.2
      molar pregnancy (*see also* categories 630–632) 639.2
  pharynx 478.29
  pylorus, pyloric (ulcer) — *see* Ulcer, stomach, with perforation
  rectum 569.49
  root canal space 526.61
  sigmoid 569.83
  sinus (accessory) (chronic) (nasal) (*see also* Sinusitis) 473.9
  sphenoidal sinus (*see also* Sinusitis, sphenoidal) 473.3
  stomach (due to ulcer) — *see* Ulcer, stomach, with perforation
  surgical (accidental) (by instrument) (blood vessel) (nerve) (organ) 998.2
  traumatic
    external — *see* Wound, open, by site
    eye (*see also* Penetrating wound, ocular) 871.7
    internal organ — *see* Injury, internal, by site

☑ **Additional Digit Required** — Refer to the Tabular List for Digit Selection   ▽ **Subterms under main terms may continue to next column or page**

2014 ICD-9-CM   ▶◀ **Revised Text**   ● **New Line**   ▲ **Revised Code**   **Volume 2 — 227**

Perforation, perforative — *continued*
tympanum (membrane) (persistent posttraumatic) (postinflammatory) 384.20
with
otitis media — *see* Otitis media
attic 384.22
central 384.21
healed 384.81
marginal NEC 384.23
multiple 384.24
pars flaccida 384.22
total 384.25
traumatic — *see* Wound, open, ear,
drum
typhoid, gastrointestinal 002.0
ulcer — *see* Ulcer, by site, with perforation
ureter 593.89
urethra
with
abortion — *see* Abortion, by type,
with damage to pelvic organs
ectopic pregnancy (*see also* categories 633.0–633.9) 639.2
molar pregnancy (*see also* categories
630–632) 639.2
following
abortion 639.2
ectopic or molar pregnancy 639.2
obstetrical trauma 665.5 ☑
uterus (*see also* Injury, internal, uterus)
with
abortion — *see* Abortion, by type,
with damage to pelvic organs
ectopic pregnancy (*see also* categories 633.0–633.9) 639.2
molar pregnancy (*see also* categories
630–632) 639.2
by intrauterine contraceptive device
996.32
following
abortion 639.2
ectopic or molar pregnancy 639.2
obstetrical trauma — *see* Injury, internal,
uterus, obstetrical trauma
uvula 528.9
syphilitic 095.8
vagina — *see* Laceration, vagina
viscus NEC 799.89
traumatic 868.00
with open wound into cavity 868.10
Peri-ileitis (subacute) 569.89
Periadenitis mucosa necrotica recurrens
528.2
Periangiitis 446.0
Periantritis 535.4 ☑
Periappendicitis (acute) — *see also* Appendicitis 541
Periarteritis (disseminated) (infectious)
(necrotizing) (nodosa) 446.0
Periarthritis (joint) 726.90
Duplay's 726.2
gonococcal 098.50
humeroscapularis 726.2
scapulohumeral 726.2
shoulder 726.2
wrist 726.4
Periarthrosis (angioneural) — *see* Periarthritis
Peribronchitis 491.9
tuberculous (*see also* Tuberculosis) 011.3 ☑
Pericapsulitis, adhesive (shoulder) 726.0
Pericarditis (granular) (with decompensation)
(with effusion) 423.9
with
rheumatic fever (conditions classifiable
to 390)
active (*see also* Pericarditis,
rheumatic) 391.0
inactive or quiescent 393
actinomycotic 039.8 *[420.0]*
acute (nonrheumatic) 420.90
with chorea (acute) (rheumatic) (Sydenham's) 392.0
bacterial 420.99
benign 420.91
hemorrhagic 420.90
idiopathic 420.91

Pericarditis — *continued*
acute — *continued*
infective 420.90
nonspecific 420.91
rheumatic 391.0
with chorea (acute) (rheumatic)
(Sydenham's) 392.0
sicca 420.90
viral 420.91
adhesive or adherent (external) (internal)
423.1
acute — *see* Pericarditis, acute
rheumatic (external) (internal) 393
amebic 006.8 *[420.0]*
bacterial (acute) (subacute) (with serous or
seropurulent effusion) 420.99
calcareous 423.2
cholesterol (chronic) 423.8
acute 420.90
chronic (nonrheumatic) 423.8
rheumatic 393
constrictive 423.2
Coxsackie 074.21
due to
actinomycosis 039.8 *[420.0]*
amebiasis 006.8 *[420.0]*
Coxsackie (virus) 074.21
histoplasmosis (*see also* Histoplasmosis)
115.93
nocardiosis 039.8 *[420.0]*
tuberculosis (*see also* Tuberculosis)
017.9 ☑ *[420.0]*
fibrinocaseous (*see also* Tuberculosis)
017.9 ☑ *[420.0]*
fibrinopurulent 420.99
fibrinous — *see* Pericarditis, rheumatic
fibropurulent 420.99
fibrous 423.1
gonococcal 098.83
hemorrhagic 423.0
idiopathic (acute) 420.91
infective (acute) 420.90
meningococcal 036.41
neoplastic (chronic) 423.8
acute 420.90
nonspecific 420.91
obliterans, obliterating 423.1
plastic 423.1
pneumococcal (acute) 420.99
postinfarction 411.0
purulent (acute) 420.99
rheumatic (active) (acute) (with effusion)
(with pneumonia) 391.0
with chorea (acute) (rheumatic) (Sydenham's) 392.0
chronic or inactive (with chorea) 393
septic (acute) 420.99
serofibrinous — *see* Pericarditis, rheumatic
staphylococcal (acute) 420.99
streptococcal (acute) 420.99
suppurative (acute) 420.99
syphilitic 093.81
tuberculous (acute) (chronic) (*see also* Tuberculosis) 017.9 ☑ *[420.0]*
uremic 585.9 *[420.0]*
viral (acute) 420.91
Pericardium, pericardial — *see* condition
Pericellulitis — *see also* Cellulitis 682.9
Pericementitis 523.40
acute 523.30
chronic (suppurative) 523.40
Pericholecystitis — *see also* Cholecystitis
575.10
Perichondritis
auricle 380.00
acute 380.01
chronic 380.02
bronchus 491.9
ear (external) 380.00
acute 380.01
chronic 380.02
larynx 478.71
syphilitic 095.8
typhoid 002.0 *[478.71]*
nose 478.19
pinna 380.00

Perichondritis — *continued*
pinna — *continued*
acute 380.01
chronic 380.02
trachea 478.9
Periclasia 523.5
Pericolitis 569.89
Pericoronitis (chronic) 523.40
acute 523.33
Pericystitis — *see also* Cystitis 595.9
Pericytoma (M9150/1) — *see also* Neoplasm,
connective tissue, uncertain behavior
benign (M9150/0) — *see* Neoplasm, connective tissue, benign
malignant (M9150/3) — *see* Neoplasm,
connective tissue, malignant
Peridacryocystitis, acute 375.32
Peridiverticulitis — *see also* Diverticulitis
562.11
Periduodenitis 535.6 ☑
Periendocarditis — *see also* Endocarditis
424.90
acute or subacute 421.9
Periepididymitis — *see also* Epididymitis
604.90
Perifolliculitis (abscedens) 704.8
capitis, abscedens et suffodiens 704.8
dissecting, scalp 704.8
scalp 704.8
superficial pustular 704.8
Perigastritis (acute) 535.0 ☑
Perigastrojejunitis (acute) 535.0 ☑
Perihepatitis (acute) 573.3
chlamydial 099.56
gonococcal 098.86
Perilabyrinthitis (acute) — *see* Labyrinthitis
Perimeningitis — *see* Meningitis
Perimetritis — *see also* Endometritis 615.9
Perimetrosalpingitis — *see also* Salpingo-
oophoritis 614.2
Perineocele 618.05
Perinephric — *see* condition
Perinephritic — *see* condition
Perinephritis — *see also* Infection, kidney
590.9
purulent (*see also* Abscess, kidney) 590.2
Perineum, perineal — *see* condition
Perineuritis NEC 729.2
Periodic — *see also* condition
disease (familial) 277.31
edema 995.1
hereditary 277.6
fever 277.31
headache syndromes in child or adolescent
346.2 ☑
limb movement disorder 327.51
paralysis (familial) 359.3
peritonitis 277.31
polyserositis 277.31
somnolence (*see also* Narcolepsy) 347.00
Periodontal
cyst 522.8
pocket 523.8
Periodontitis (chronic) (complex) (compound)
(simplex) 523.40
acute 523.33
aggressive 523.30
generalized 523.32
localized 523.31
apical 522.6
acute (pulpal origin) 522.4
generalized 523.42
localized 523.41
Periodontoclasia 523.5
Periodontosis 523.5
Periods — *see also* Menstruation
heavy 626.2
irregular 626.4
Perionychia (with lymphangitis) 681.9
finger 681.02
toe 681.11
Perioophoritis — *see also* Salpingo-oophoritis
614.2
Periorchitis — *see also* Orchitis 604.90
Periosteum, periosteal — *see* condition

Periostitis (circumscribed) (diffuse) (infective)
730.3 ☑

Note — *Use the following fifth-digit
subclassification with category 730:*

0	site unspecified
1	shoulder region
2	upper arm
3	forearm
4	hand
5	pelvic region and thigh
6	lower leg
7	ankle and foot
8	other specified sites
9	multiple sites

with osteomyelitis (*see also* Osteomyelitis)
730.2 ☑
acute or subacute 730.0 ☑
chronic or old 730.1 ☑
albuminosa, albuminosus 730.3 ☑
alveolar 526.5
alveolodental 526.5
dental 526.5
gonorrheal 098.89
hyperplastica, generalized 731.2
jaw (lower) (upper) 526.4
monomelic 733.99
orbital 376.02
syphilitic 095.5
congenital 090.0 *[730.8]* ☑
secondary 091.61
tuberculous (*see also* Tuberculosis, bone)
015.9 ☑ *[730.8]* ☑
yaws (early) (hypertrophic) (late) 102.6
Periostosis — *see also* Periostitis 730.3 ☑
with osteomyelitis (*see also* Osteomyelitis)
730.2 ☑
acute or subacute 730.0 ☑
chronic or old 730.1 ☑
hyperplastic 756.59
Peripartum cardiomyopathy 674.5 ☑
Periphlebitis — *see also* Phlebitis 451.9
lower extremity 451.2
deep (vessels) 451.19
superficial (vessels) 451.0
portal 572.1
retina 362.18
superficial (vessels) 451.0
tuberculous (*see also* Tuberculosis) 017.9 ☑
retina 017.3 ☑ *[362.18]*
Peripneumonia — *see* Pneumonia
Periproctitis 569.49
Periprostatitis — *see also* Prostatitis 601.9
Perirectal — *see* condition
Perirenal — *see* condition
Perisalpingitis — *see also* Salpingo-oophoritis
614.2
Perisigmoiditis 569.89
Perisplenitis (infectional) 289.59
Perispondylitis — *see* Spondylitis
Peristalsis reversed or visible 787.4
Peritendinitis — *see also* Tenosynovitis 726.90
adhesive (shoulder) 726.0
Perithelioma (M9150/1) — *see* Pericytoma
Peritoneum, peritoneal — *see also* condition
equilibration test V56.32
Peritonitis (acute) (adhesive) (fibrinous)
(hemorrhagic) (idiopathic) (localized)
(perforative) (primary) (with adhesions)
(with effusion) 567.9
with or following
abortion — *see* Abortion, by type, with
sepsis
abscess 567.21
appendicitis 540.0
with peritoneal abscess 540.1
ectopic pregnancy (*see also* categories
633.0–633.9) 639.0
molar pregnancy (*see also* categories
630–632) 639.0
aseptic 998.7

☑ **Additional Digit Required** — Refer to the Tabular List for Digit Selection   ▽ **Subterms under main terms may continue to next column or page**

228 — Volume 2   ▶◀ **Revised Text**   ● **New Line**   ▲ **Revised Code**   **2014 ICD-9-CM**

Peritonitis — *continued*
bacterial 567.29
spontaneous 567.23
bile, biliary 567.81
chemical 998.7
chlamydial 099.56
chronic proliferative 567.89
congenital NEC 777.6
diaphragmatic 567.22
diffuse NEC 567.29
diphtheritic 032.83
disseminated NEC 567.29
due to
bile 567.81
foreign
body or object accidentally left during a procedure (instrument) (sponge) (swab) 998.4
substance accidentally left during a procedure (chemical) (powder) (talc) 998.7
talc 998.7
urine 567.89
fibrinopurulent 567.29
fibrinous 567.29
fibrocaseous (*see also* Tuberculosis) 014.0 ☑
fibropurulent 567.29
general, generalized (acute) 567.21
gonococcal 098.86
in infective disease NEC 136.9 *[567.0]*
meconium (newborn) 777.6
pancreatic 577.8
paroxysmal, benign 277.31
pelvic
female (acute) 614.5
chronic NEC 614.7
with adhesions 614.6
puerperal, postpartum, childbirth 670.8 ☑
male (acute) 567.21
periodic (familial) 277.31
phlegmonous 567.29
pneumococcal 567.1
postabortal 639.0
proliferative, chronic 567.89
puerperal, postpartum, childbirth 670.8 ☑
purulent 567.29
septic 567.29
spontaneous bacterial 567.23
staphylococcal 567.29
streptococcal 567.29
subdiaphragmatic 567.29
subphrenic 567.29
suppurative 567.29
syphilitic 095.2
congenital 090.0 *[567.0]*
talc 998.7
tuberculous (*see also* Tuberculosis) 014.0 ☑
urine 567.89
Peritonsillar — *see* condition
Peritonsillitis 475
Perityphlitis — *see also* Appendicitis 541
Periureteritis 593.89
Periurethral — *see* condition
Periurethritis (gangrenous) 597.89
Periuterine — *see* condition
Perivaginitis — *see also* Vaginitis 616.10
Perivasculitis, retinal 362.18
Perivasitis (chronic) 608.4
Periventricular leukomalacia 779.7
Perivesiculitis (seminal) — *see also* Vesiculitis 608.0
Perlèche 686.8
due to
moniliasis 112.0
riboflavin deficiency 266.0
Pernicious — *see* condition
Pernio, perniosis 991.5
Persecution
delusion 297.9
social V62.4
Perseveration (tonic) 784.69
Persistence, persistent (congenital) 759.89
anal membrane 751.2
arteria stapedia 744.04
atrioventricular canal 745.69

Persistence, persistent — *continued*
bloody ejaculate 792.2
branchial cleft 744.41
bulbus cordis in left ventricle 745.8
canal of Cloquet 743.51
capsule (opaque) 743.51
cilioretinal artery or vein 743.51
cloaca 751.5
communication — *see* Fistula, congenital
convolutions
aortic arch 747.21
fallopian tube 752.19
oviduct 752.19
uterine tube 752.19
double aortic arch 747.21
ductus
arteriosus 747.0
Botalli 747.0
fetal
circulation 747.83
form of cervix (uteri) 752.49
hemoglobin (hereditary) ("Swiss variety") 282.7
pulmonary hypertension 747.83
foramen
Botalli 745.5
ovale 745.5
Gartner's duct 752.41
hemoglobin, fetal (hereditary) (HPFH) 282.7
hyaloid
artery (generally incomplete) 743.51
system 743.51
hymen (tag)
in pregnancy or childbirth 654.8 ☑
causing obstructed labor 660.2 ☑
lanugo 757.4
left
posterior cardinal vein 747.49
root with right arch of aorta 747.21
superior vena cava 747.49
Meckel's diverticulum 751.0
mesonephric duct 752.89
fallopian tube 752.11
mucosal disease (middle ear) (with posterior or superior marginal perforation of ear drum) 382.2
nail(s), anomalous 757.5
occiput, anterior or posterior 660.3 ☑
fetus or newborn 763.1
omphalomesenteric duct 751.0
organ or site NEC — *see* Anomaly, specified type NEC
ostium
atrioventriculare commune 745.69
primum 745.61
secundum 745.5
ovarian rests in fallopian tube 752.19
pancreatic tissue in intestinal tract 751.5
primary (deciduous)
teeth 520.6
vitreous hyperplasia 743.51
pulmonary hypertension 747.83
pupillary membrane 743.46
iris 743.46
Rhesus (Rh) titer (*see also* Complications, transfusion) 999.70
right aortic arch 747.21
sinus
urogenitalis 752.89
venosus with imperfect incorporation in right auricle 747.49
thymus (gland) 254.8
hyperplasia 254.0
thyroglossal duct 759.2
thyrolingual duct 759.2
truncus arteriosus or communis 745.0
tunica vasculosa lentis 743.39
umbilical sinus 753.7
urachus 753.7
vegetative state 780.03
vitelline duct 751.0
wolffian duct 752.89
Person (with)
admitted for clinical research, as participant or control subject V70.7

Person — *continued*
affected by
family member
currently on deployment (military) V61.01
returned from deployment (military) (current or past conflict) V61.02
awaiting admission to adequate facility elsewhere V63.2
undergoing social agency investigation V63.8
concern (normal) about sick person in family V61.49
consulting on behalf of another V65.19
pediatric
pre-adoption visit for adoptive parents V65.11
pre-birth visit for expectant parents V65.11
currently deployed in theater or in support of military war, peacekeeping and humanitarian operations V62.21
feared
complaint in whom no diagnosis was made V65.5
condition not demonstrated V65.5
feigning illness V65.2
healthy, accompanying sick person V65.0
history of military war, peacekeeping and humanitarian deployment (current or past conflict) V62.22
living (in)
without
adequate
financial resources V60.2
housing (heating) (space) V60.1
housing (permanent) (temporary) V60.0
material resources V60.2
person able to render necessary care V60.2
shelter V60.0
alone V60.3
boarding school V60.6
residence remote from hospital or medical care facility V63.0
residential institution V60.6
medical services in home not available V63.1
on waiting list V63.2
undergoing social agency investigation V63.8
sick or handicapped in family V61.49
"worried well" V65.5
Personality
affective 301.10
aggressive 301.3
amoral 301.7
anancastic, anankastic 301.4
antisocial 301.7
asocial 301.7
asthenic 301.6
avoidant 301.82
borderline 301.83
change 310.1
compulsive 301.4
cycloid 301.13
cyclothymic 301.13
dependent 301.6
depressive (chronic) 301.12
disorder, disturbance NEC 301.9
with
antisocial disturbance 301.7
pattern disturbance NEC 301.9
sociopathic disturbance 301.7
trait disturbance 301.9
dual 300.14
dyssocial 301.7
eccentric 301.89
"haltlose" type 301.89
emotionally unstable 301.59
epileptoid 301.3
explosive 301.3
fanatic 301.0
histrionic 301.50
hyperthymic 301.11

Personality — *continued*
hypomanic 301.11
hypothymic 301.12
hysterical 301.50
immature 301.89
inadequate 301.6
labile 301.59
masochistic 301.89
morally defective 301.7
multiple 300.14
narcissistic 301.81
obsessional 301.4
obsessive-compulsive 301.4
overconscientious 301.4
paranoid 301.0
passive-aggressive 301.84
passive (-dependent) 301.6
pathologic NEC 301.9
pattern defect or disturbance 301.9
pseudosocial 301.7
psychoinfantile 301.59
psychoneurotic NEC 301.89
psychopathic 301.9
with
amoral trend 301.7
antisocial trend 301.7
asocial trend 301.7
pathologic sexuality (*see also* Deviation, sexual) 302.9
mixed types 301.9
schizoid 301.20
type A 301.4
unstable (emotional) 301.59
Perthes' disease (capital femoral osteochondrosis) 732.1
Pertussis — *see also* Whooping cough 033.9
vaccination, prophylactic (against) V03.6
Peruvian wart 088.0
Perversion, perverted
appetite 307.52
hysterical 300.11
function
pineal gland 259.8
pituitary gland 253.9
anterior lobe
deficient 253.2
excessive 253.1
posterior lobe 253.6
placenta — *see* Placenta, abnormal
sense of smell or taste 781.1
psychogenic 306.7
sexual (*see also* Deviation, sexual) 302.9
Pervious, congenital — *see also* Imperfect, closure
ductus arteriosus 747.0
Pes (congenital) — *see also* Talipes 754.70
abductus (congenital) 754.60
acquired 736.79
acquired NEC 736.79
planus 734
adductus (congenital) 754.79
acquired 736.79
cavus 754.71
acquired 736.73
planovalgus (congenital) 754.69
acquired 736.79
planus (acquired) (any degree) 734
congenital 754.61
rachitic 268.1
valgus (congenital) 754.61
acquired 736.79
varus (congenital) 754.50
acquired 736.79
Pest — *see also* Plague 020.9
Pestis — *see also* Plague 020.9
bubonica 020.0
fulminans 020.0
minor 020.8
pneumonica — *see* Plague, pneumonic
Petechial
fever 036.0
typhus 081.9
Petechia, petechiae 782.7
fetus or newborn 772.6
Petges-Cléjat or Petges-Clégat syndrome (poikilodermatomyositis) 710.3

Pick-Niemann disease (lipid histiocytosis) 272.7

Pick's
cerebral atrophy 331.11
with dementia
with behavioral disturbance 331.11 [294.11]
without behavioral disturbance 331.11 [294.10]
disease
brain 331.11
dementia in
with behavioral disturbance 331.11 [294.11]
without behavioral disturbance 331.11 [294.10]
lipid histiocytosis 272.7
liver (pericardial pseudocirrhosis of liver) 423.2
pericardium (pericardial pseudocirrhosis of liver) 423.2
polyserositis (pericardial pseudocirrhosis of liver) 423.2
syndrome
heart (pericardial pseudocirrhosis of liver) 423.2
liver (pericardial pseudocirrhosis of liver) 423.2
tubular adenoma (M8640/0)
specified site — see Neoplasm, by site, benign
unspecified site
female 220
male 222.0

Pickwickian syndrome (cardiopulmonary obesity) 278.03

Piebaldism, classic 709.09

Piedra 111.2
beard 111.2
black 111.3
white 111.2
black 111.3
scalp 111.3
black 111.3
white 111.2
white 111.2

Pierre Marie-Bamberger syndrome (hypertrophic pulmonary osteoarthropathy) 731.2

Pierre Marie's syndrome (pulmonary hypertrophic osteoarthropathy) 731.2

Pierre Mauriac's syndrome (diabetes-dwarfism-obesity) 258.1

Pierre Robin deformity or syndrome (congenital) 756.0

Pierson's disease or osteochondrosis 732.1

Pigeon
breast or chest (acquired) 738.3
congenital 754.82
rachitic (see also Rickets) 268.0
breeders' disease or lung 495.2
fanciers' disease or lung 495.2
toe 735.8

Pigmentation (abnormal) 709.00
anomaly 709.00
congenital 757.33
specified NEC 709.09
conjunctiva 372.55
cornea 371.10
anterior 371.11
posterior 371.13
stromal 371.12
lids (congenital) 757.33
acquired 374.52
limbus corneae 371.10
metals 709.00
optic papilla, congenital 743.57
retina (congenital) (grouped) (nevoid) 743.53
acquired 362.74
scrotum, congenital 757.33

Piles — see Hemorrhoids

Pili
annulati or torti (congenital) 757.4
incarnati 704.8

Pill roller hand (intrinsic) 736.09

Pilomatrixoma (M8110/0) — see Neoplasm, skin, benign

Pilonidal — see condition

Pimple 709.8

PIN I (prostatic intraepithelial neoplasia I) 602.3

PIN II (prostatic intraepithelial neoplasia II) 602.3

PIN III (prostatic intraepithelial neoplasia III) 233.4

Pinched nerve — see Neuropathy, entrapment

Pineal body or gland — see condition

Pinealoblastoma (M9362/3) 194.4

Pinealoma (M9360/1) 237.1
malignant (M9360/3) 194.4

Pineoblastoma (M9362/3) 194.4

Pineocytoma (M9361/1) 237.1

Pinguecula 372.51

Pingueculitis 372.34

Pinhole meatus — see also Stricture, urethra 598.9

Pink
disease 985.0
eye 372.03
puffer 492.8

Pinkus' disease (lichen nitidus) 697.1

Pinpoint
meatus (see also Stricture, urethra) 598.9
os uteri (see also Stricture, cervix) 622.4

Pinselhaare (congenital) 757.4

Pinta 103.9
cardiovascular lesions 103.2
chancre (primary) 103.0
erythematous plaques 103.1
hyperchromic lesions 103.1
hyperkeratosis 103.1
lesions 103.9
cardiovascular 103.2
hyperchromic 103.1
intermediate 103.1
late 103.2
mixed 103.3
primary 103.0
skin (achromic) (cicatricial) (dyschromic) 103.2
hyperchromic 103.1
mixed (achromic and hyperchromic) 103.3
papule (primary) 103.0
skin lesions (achromic) (cicatricial) (dyschromic) 103.2
hyperchromic 103.1
mixed (achromic and hyperchromic) 103.3
vitiligo 103.2

Pintid 103.0

Pinworms (disease) (infection) (infestation) 127.4

Piry fever 066.8

Pistol wound — see Gunshot wound

Pitchers' elbow 718.82

Pithecoid pelvis 755.69
with disproportion (fetopelvic) 653.2 ☑
affecting fetus or newborn 763.1
causing obstructed labor 660.1 ☑

Pithiatism 300.11

Pit, lip (mucus), **congenital** 750.25

Pitted — see also Pitting
teeth 520.4

Pitting (edema) — see also Edema 782.3
lip 782.3
nail 703.8
congenital 757.5

Pituitary gland — see condition

Pituitary snuff-takers' disease 495.8

Pityriasis 696.5
alba 696.5
capitis 690.11
circinata (et maculata) 696.3
Hebra's (exfoliative dermatitis) 695.89
lichenoides et varioliformis 696.2
maculata (et circinata) 696.3
nigra 111.1
pilaris 757.39
acquired 701.1
Hebra's 696.4
rosea 696.3

Pityriasis — continued
rotunda 696.3
rubra (Hebra) 695.89
pilaris 696.4
sicca 690.18
simplex 690.18
specified type NEC 696.5
streptogenes 696.5
versicolor 111.0
scrotal 111.0

Placenta, placental
ablatio 641.2 ☑
affecting fetus or newborn 762.1
abnormal, abnormality 656.7 ☑
with hemorrhage 641.8 ☑
affecting fetus or newborn 762.1
affecting fetus or newborn 762.2
abruptio 641.2 ☑
affecting fetus or newborn 762.1
accessory lobe — see Placenta, abnormal
accreta (without hemorrhage) 667.0 ☑
with hemorrhage 666.0 ☑
adherent (without hemorrhage) 667.0 ☑
with hemorrhage 666.0 ☑
apoplexy — see Placenta, separation
battledore — see Placenta, abnormal
bilobate — see Placenta, abnormal
bipartita — see Placenta, abnormal
carneous mole 631.8
centralis — see Placenta, previa
circumvallata — see Placenta, abnormal
cyst (amniotic) — see Placenta, abnormal
deficiency — see Placenta, insufficiency
degeneration — see Placenta, insufficiency
detachment (partial) (premature) (with hemorrhage) 641.2 ☑
affecting fetus or newborn 762.1
dimidiata — see Placenta, abnormal
disease 656.7 ☑
affecting fetus or newborn 762.2
duplex — see Placenta, abnormal
dysfunction — see Placenta, insufficiency
fenestrata — see Placenta, abnormal
fibrosis — see Placenta, abnormal
fleshy mole 631.8
hematoma — see Placenta, abnormal
hemorrhage NEC — see Placenta, separation
hormone disturbance or malfunction — see Placenta, abnormal
hyperplasia — see Placenta, abnormal
increta (without hemorrhage) 667.0 ☑
with hemorrhage 666.0 ☑
infarction 656.7 ☑
affecting fetus or newborn 762.2
insertion, vicious — see Placenta, previa
insufficiency
affecting
fetus or newborn 762.2
management of pregnancy 656.5 ☑
lateral — see Placenta, previa
low-lying — see Placenta, previa
low implantation or insertion — see Placenta, previa
malformation — see Placenta, abnormal
malposition — see Placenta, previa
marginalis, marginata — see Placenta, previa
marginal sinus (hemorrhage) (rupture) 641.2 ☑
affecting fetus or newborn 762.1
membranacea — see Placenta, abnormal
multilobed — see Placenta, abnormal
multipartita — see Placenta, abnormal
necrosis — see Placenta, abnormal
percreta (without hemorrhage) 667.0 ☑
with hemorrhage 666.0 ☑
polyp 674.4 ☑
previa (central) (centralis) (complete) (lateral) (marginal) (marginalis) (partial) (partialis) (total) (with hemorrhage) 641.1 ☑
without hemorrhage (before labor and delivery) (during pregnancy) 641.0 ☑
affecting fetus or newborn 762.0

Placenta, placental — continued
previa — continued
noted
before labor, without hemorrhage (with cesarean delivery) 641.0 ☑
during pregnancy (without hemorrhage) 641.0 ☑
retention (with hemorrhage) 666.0 ☑
without hemorrhage 667.0 ☑
fragments, complicating puerperium (delayed hemorrhage) 666.2 ☑
without hemorrhage 667.1 ☑
postpartum, puerperal 666.2 ☑
separation (normally implanted) (partial) (premature) (with hemorrhage) 641.2 ☑
affecting fetus or newborn 762.1
septuplex — see Placenta, abnormal
small — see Placenta, insufficiency
softening (premature) — see Placenta, abnormal
spuria — see Placenta, abnormal
succenturiata — see Placenta, abnormal
syphilitic 095.8
transfusion syndromes 762.3
transmission of chemical substance — see Absorption, chemical, through placenta
trapped (with hemorrhage) 666.0 ☑
without hemorrhage 667.0 ☑
trilobate — see Placenta, abnormal
tripartita — see Placenta, abnormal
triplex — see Placenta, abnormal
varicose vessel — see Placenta, abnormal
vicious insertion — see Placenta, previa

Placentitis
affecting fetus or newborn 762.7
complicating pregnancy 658.4 ☑

Plagiocephaly (skull) 754.0

Plague 020.9
abortive 020.8
ambulatory 020.8
bubonic 020.0
cellulocutaneous 020.1
lymphatic gland 020.0
pneumonic 020.5
primary 020.3
secondary 020.4
pulmonary — see Plague, pneumonic
pulmonic — see Plague, pneumonic
septicemic 020.2
tonsillar 020.9
septicemic 020.2
vaccination, prophylactic (against) V03.3

Planning, family V25.09
contraception V25.9
natural
procreative V26.41
to avoid pregnancy V25.04
procreation V26.49
natural V26.41

Plaque
artery, arterial — see Arteriosclerosis
calcareous — see Calcification
Hollenhorst's (retinal) 362.33
tongue 528.6

Plasma cell myeloma 203.0 ☑

Plasmacytoma, plasmocytoma (solitary) (M9731/1) 238.6
benign (M9731/0) — see Neoplasm, by site, benign
malignant (M9731/3) 203.8 ☑

Plasmacytopenia 288.59

Plasmacytosis 288.64

Plaster ulcer — see also Ulcer, pressure 707.00

Plateau iris syndrome (without glaucoma) 364.82
with glaucoma 365.23

Platybasia 756.0

Platyonychia (congenital) 757.5
acquired 703.8

Platypelloid pelvis 738.6
with disproportion (fetopelvic) 653.2 ☑
affecting fetus or newborn 763.1
causing obstructed labor 660.1 ☑

☑ Additional Digit Required — Refer to the Tabular List for Digit Selection   ▽ Subterms under main terms may continue to next column or page

2014 ICD-9-CM   ▶◀ Revised Text   ● New Line   ▲ Revised Code   Volume 2 — 231

Platypelloid pelvis — *continued*
  with disproportion — *continued*
    causing obstructed labor — *contin-ued*
      affecting fetus or newborn 763.1
  congenital 755.69
Platyspondylia 756.19
Plethora 782.62
  newborn 776.4
Pleuralgia 786.52
Pleura, pleural — *see* condition
Pleurisy (acute) (adhesive) (chronic) (costal) (diaphragmatic) (double) (dry) (fetid) (fibrinous) (fibrous) (interlobar) (latent) (lung) (old) (plastic) (primary) (residual) (sicca) (sterile) (subacute) (unresolved) (with adherent pleura) 511.0
  with
    effusion (without mention of cause) 511.9
      bacterial, nontuberculous 511.1
        nontuberculous NEC 511.9
          bacterial 511.1
      pneumococcal 511.1
      specified type NEC 511.89
      staphylococcal 511.1
      streptococcal 511.1
      tuberculous (*see also* Tuberculosis, pleura) 012.0 ☑
        primary, progressive 010.1 ☑
    influenza, flu, or grippe (*see also* Influenza) 487.1
    tuberculosis — *see* Pleurisy, tuberculous
  encysted 511.89
  exudative (*see also* Pleurisy, with effusion) 511.9
    bacterial, nontuberculous 511.1
  fibrinopurulent 510.9
    with fistula 510.0
  fibropurulent 510.9
    with fistula 510.0
  hemorrhagic 511.89
  influenzal (*see also* Influenza) 487.1
  pneumococcal 511.0
    with effusion 511.1
  purulent 510.9
    with fistula 510.0
  septic 510.9
    with fistula 510.0
  serofibrinous (*see also* Pleurisy, with effusion) 511.9
    bacterial, nontuberculous 511.1
  seropurulent 510.9
    with fistula 510.0
  serous (*see also* Pleurisy, with effusion) 511.9
    bacterial, nontuberculous 511.1
  staphylococcal 511.0
    with effusion 511.1
  streptococcal 511.0
    with effusion 511.1
  suppurative 510.9
    with fistula 510.0
  traumatic (post) (current) 862.29
    with open wound into cavity 862.39
  tuberculous (with effusion) (*see also* Tuberculosis, pleura) 012.0 ☑
    primary, progressive 010.1 ☑
Pleuritis sicca — *see* Pleurisy
Pleurobronchopneumonia — *see also* Pneumonia, broncho- 485
Pleurodynia 786.52
  epidemic 074.1
  viral 074.1
Pleurohepatitis 573.8
Pleuropericarditis — *see also* Pericarditis 423.9
  acute 420.90
Pleuropneumonia (acute) (bilateral) (double) (septic) — *see also* Pneumonia 486
  chronic (*see also* Fibrosis, lung) 515
Pleurorrhea — *see also* Hydrothorax 511.89
Plexitis, brachial 353.0
Plica
  knee 727.83
  polonica 132.0
  syndrome 727.83
  tonsil 474.8

Plicae dysphonia ventricularis 784.49
Plicated tongue 529.5
  congenital 750.13
Plug
  bronchus NEC 519.19
  meconium (newborn) NEC 777.1
  mucus — *see* Mucus, plug
Plumbism 984.9
  specified type of lead — *see* Table of Drugs and Chemicals
Plummer-Vinson syndrome (sideropenic dysphagia) 280.8
Plummer's disease (toxic nodular goiter) 242.3 ☑
Pluricarential syndrome of infancy 260
Plurideficiency syndrome of infancy 260
Plus (and minus) hand (intrinsic) 736.09
PMDD (premenstrual dysphoric disorder) 625.4
PMS 625.4
Pneumathemia — *see* Air, embolism, by type
Pneumatic drill or hammer disease 994.9
Pneumatocele (lung) 518.89
  intracranial 348.89
  tension 492.0
Pneumatosis
  cystoides intestinalis 569.89
  peritonei 568.89
  pulmonum 492.8
Pneumaturia 599.84
Pneumoblastoma (M8981/3) — *see* Neoplasm, lung, malignant
Pneumocephalus 348.89
Pneumococcemia 038.2
Pneumococcus, pneumococcal — *see* condition
Pneumoconiosis (due to) (inhalation of) 505
  aluminum 503
  asbestos 501
  bagasse 495.1
  bauxite 503
  beryllium 503
  carbon electrode makers' 503
  coal
    miners' (simple) 500
    workers' (simple) 500
  cotton dust 504
  diatomite fibrosis 502
  dust NEC 504
    inorganic 503
    lime 502
    marble 502
    organic NEC 504
  fumes or vapors (from silo) 506.9
  graphite 503
  hard metal 503
  mica 502
  moldy hay 495.0
  rheumatoid 714.81
  silicate NEC 502
  silica NEC 502
    and carbon 500
  talc 502
Pneumocystis carinii pneumonia 136.3
Pneumocystis jiroveci pneumonia 136.3
Pneumocystosis 136.3
  with pneumonia 136.3
Pneumoenteritis 025
Pneumohemopericardium — *see also* Pericarditis 423.9
Pneumohemothorax — *see also* Hemothorax 511.89
  traumatic 860.4
    with open wound into thorax 860.5
Pneumohydropericardium — *see also* Pericarditis 423.9
Pneumohydrothorax — *see also* Hydrothorax 511.89
Pneumomediastinum 518.1
  congenital 770.2
  fetus or newborn 770.2
Pneumomycosis 117.9

Pneumonia (acute) (Alpenstich) (benign) (bilateral) (brain) (cerebral) (circumscribed) (congestive) (creeping) (delayed resolution) (double) (epidemic) (fever) (flash) (fulminant) (fungoid) (granulomatous) (hemorrhagic) (incipient) (infantile) (infectious) (infiltration) (insular) (intermittent) (latent) (lobe) (migratory) (newborn) (organized) (overwhelming) (primary) (progressive) (pseudolobar) (purulent) (resolved) (secondary) (senile) (septic) (suppurative) (terminal) (true) (unresolved) (vesicular) 486
  with influenza, flu, or grippe 487.0
    due to
      identified (virus)
        avian 488.01
        (novel) 2009 H1N1 488.11
        novel influenza A 488.81
  adenoviral 480.0
  adynamic 514
  alba 090.0
  allergic 518.3
  alveolar — *see* Pneumonia, lobar
  anaerobes 482.81
  anthrax 022.1 [484.5]
  apex, apical — *see* Pneumonia, lobar
  ascaris 127.0 [484.8]
  aspiration 507.0
    due to
      aspiration of microorganisms
        bacterial 482.9
          specified type NEC 482.89
        specified organism NEC 483.8
          bacterial NEC 482.89
        viral 480.9
          specified type NEC 480.8
      food (regurgitated) 507.0
      gastric secretions 507.0
      milk 507.0
      oils, essences 507.1
      solids, liquids NEC 507.8
      vomitus 507.0
    fetal 770.18
      due to
        blood 770.16
        clear amniotic fluid 770.14
        meconium 770.12
        postnatal stomach contents 770.86
    newborn 770.18
      due to
        blood 770.16
        clear amniotic fluid 770.14
        meconium 770.12
        postnatal stomach contents 770.86
  asthenic 514
  atypical (disseminated) (focal) (primary) 486
    with influenza (*see also* Influenza) 487.0
  bacillus 482.9
    specified type NEC 482.89
  bacterial 482.9
    specified type NEC 482.89
  Bacteroides (fragilis) (oralis) (melaninogenicus) 482.81
  basal, basic, basilar — *see* Pneumonia, by type
  bronchiolitis obliterans organized (BOOP) 516.8
  broncho-, bronchial (confluent) (croupous) (diffuse) (disseminated) (hemorrhagic) (involving lobes) (lobar) (terminal) 485
    with influenza 487.0
      due to
        identified (virus)
          avian 488.01
          (novel) 2009 H1N1 488.11
          novel influenza A 488.81
    allergic 518.3
    aspiration (*see also* Pneumonia, aspiration) 507.0
    bacterial 482.9
      specified type NEC 482.89
    capillary 466.19

Pneumonia — *continued*
  broncho-, bronchial — *continued*
    capillary — *continued*
      with bronchospasm or obstruction 466.19
    chronic (*see also* Fibrosis, lung) 515
    congenital (infective) 770.0
    diplococcal 481
    Eaton's agent 483.0
    Escherichia coli (E. coli) 482.82
    Friedländer's bacillus 482.0
    Hemophilus influenzae 482.2
    hiberno-vernal 083.0 [484.8]
    hypostatic 514
    influenzal (*see also* Influenza) 487.0
    inhalation (*see also* Pneumonia, aspiration) 507.0
      due to fumes or vapors (chemical) 506.0
    Klebsiella 482.0
    lipid 507.1
      endogenous 516.8
    Mycoplasma (pneumoniae) 483.0
    ornithosis 073.0
    pleuropneumonia-like organisms (PPLO) 483.0
    pneumococcal 481
    Proteus 482.83
    Pseudomonas 482.1
    specified organism NEC 483.8
      bacterial NEC 482.89
    staphylococcal 482.40
      aureus 482.41
      methicillin
        resistant (MRSA) 482.42
        susceptible (MSSA) 482.41
      specified type NEC 482.49
    streptococcal — *see* Pneumonia, streptococcal
    typhoid 002.0 [484.8]
    viral, virus (*see also* Pneumonia, viral) 480.9
  Butyrivibrio (fibriosolvens) 482.81
  Candida 112.4
  capillary 466.19
    with bronchospasm or obstruction 466.19
  caseous (*see also* Tuberculosis) 011.6 ☑
  catarrhal — *see* Pneumonia, broncho-
  central — *see* Pneumonia, lobar
  Chlamydia, chlamydial 483.1
    pneumoniae 483.1
    psittaci 073.0
    specified type NEC 483.1
    trachomatis 483.1
  cholesterol 516.8
  chronic (*see also* Fibrosis, lung) 515
  cirrhotic (chronic) (*see also* Fibrosis, lung) 515
  Clostridium (haemolyticum) (novyi) NEC 482.81
  confluent — *see* Pneumonia, broncho-
  congenital (infective) 770.0
    aspiration 770.18
  croupous — *see* Pneumonia, lobar
  cryptogenic organizing 516.36
  cytomegalic inclusion 078.5 [484.1]
  deglutition (*see also* Pneumonia, aspiration) 507.0
  desquamative interstitial 516.37
  diffuse — *see* Pneumonia, broncho-
  diplococcal, diplococcus (broncho-) (lobar) 481
  disseminated (focal) — *see* Pneumonia, broncho-
  due to
    adenovirus 480.0
    anaerobes 482.81
    Bacterium anitratum 482.83
    Chlamydia, chlamydial 483.1
      pneumoniae 483.1
      psittaci 073.0
      specified type NEC 483.1
      trachomatis 483.1
    coccidioidomycosis 114.0
    Diplococcus (pneumoniae) 481

Pneumonia — *continued*
  due to — *continued*
    Eaton's agent 483.0
    Escherichia coli (E. coli) 482.82
    Friedländer's bacillus 482.0
    fumes or vapors (chemical) (inhalation)
      506.0
    fungus NEC 117.9 *[484.7]*
      coccidioidomycosis 114.0
    Hemophilus influenzae (H. influenzae)
      482.2
    Herellea 482.83
    influenza (*see also* Influenza) 487.0
    Klebsiella pneumoniae 482.0
    Mycoplasma (pneumoniae) 483.0
    parainfluenza virus 480.2
    pleuropneumonia-like organism (PPLO)
      483.0
    Pneumococcus 481
    Pneumocystis carinii 136.3
    Pneumocystis jiroveci 136.3
    Proteus 482.83
    Pseudomonas 482.1
    respiratory syncytial virus 480.1
    rickettsia 083.9 *[484.8]*
    SARS-associated coronavirus 480.3
    specified
      bacteria NEC 482.89
      organism NEC 483.8
      virus NEC 480.8
    Staphylococcus 482.40
      aureus 482.41
        methicillin
          resistant (MRSA) 482.42
          susceptible (MSSA) 482.41
      specified type NEC 482.49
    Streptococcus (*see also* Pneumonia,
      streptococcal)
      pneumoniae 481
    virus (*see also* Pneumonia, viral) 480.9
    SARS-associated coronavirus 480.3
  Eaton's agent 483.0
  embolic, embolism — (*see* Embolism, pul-
    monary
  eosinophilic 518.3
  Escherichia coli (E. coli) 482.82
  Eubacterium 482.81
  fibrinous — *see* Pneumonia, lobar
  fibroid (chronic) (*see also* Fibrosis, lung) 515
  fibrous (*see also* Fibrosis, lung) 515
  Friedländer's bacillus 482.0
  Fusobacterium (nucleatum) 482.81
  gangrenous 513.0
  giant cell (*see also* Pneumonia, viral) 480.9
  gram-negative bacteria NEC 482.83
    anaerobic 482.81
  grippal (*see also* Influenza) 487.0
  Hemophilus influenzae (bronchial) (lobar)
    482.2
  hypostatic (broncho-) (lobar) 514
  in
    actinomycosis 039.1
    anthrax 022.1 *[484.5]*
    aspergillosis 117.3 *[484.6]*
    candidiasis 112.4
    coccidioidomycosis 114.0
    cytomegalic inclusion disease
      078.5 *[484.1]*
    histoplasmosis (*see also* Histoplasmosis)
      115.95
    infectious disease NEC 136.9 *[484.8]*
    measles 055.1
    mycosis, systemic NEC 117.9 *[484.7]*
    nocardiasis, nocardiosis 039.1
    ornithosis 073.0
    pneumocystosis 136.3
    psittacosis 073.0
    Q fever 083.0 *[484.8]*
    salmonellosis 003.22
    toxoplasmosis 130.4
    tularemia 021.2
    typhoid (fever) 002.0 *[484.8]*
    varicella 052.1
    whooping cough (*see also* Whooping
      cough) 033.9 *[484.3]*
  infective, acquired prenatally 770.0

Pneumonia — *continued*
  influenzal (broncho) (lobar) (virus) (*see also*
    Influenza) 487.0
  inhalation (*see also* Pneumonia, aspiration)
    507.0
    fumes or vapors (chemical) 506.0
  interstitial 516.8
    with influenzal (*see also* Influenza) 487.0
    acute
      due to Pneumocystis (carinii) (jirove-
        ci) 136.3
      meaning:
        acute interstitial pneumonitis
          516.33
        atypical pneumonia — *see*
          Pneumonia, atypical
        bacterial pneumonia — *see*
          Pneumonia, bacterial
    chronic (*see also* Fibrosis, lung) 515
    desquamative 516.37
    hypostatic 514
    idiopathic 516.30
      lymphoid 516.35
    lipoid 507.1
    lymphoid (due to known underlying
      cause) 516.8
    non-specific (due to known underlying
      cause) 516.8
    organizing (due to known underlying
      cause) 516.8
    plasma cell 136.3
    Pseudomonas 482.1
  intrauterine (infective) 770.0
    aspiration 770.18
      blood 770.16
      clear amniotic fluid 770.14
      meconium 770.12
      postnatal stomach contents 770.86
  Klebsiella pneumoniae 482.0
  Legionnaires' 482.84
  lipid, lipoid (exogenous) (interstitial) 507.1
    endogenous 516.8
  lobar (diplococcal) (disseminated) (double)
    (interstitial) (pneumococcal, any
    type) 481
    with influenza (*see also* Influenza) 487.0
    bacterial 482.9
      specified type NEC 482.89
    chronic (*see also* Fibrosis, lung) 515
    Escherichia coli (E. coli) 482.82
    Friedländer's bacillus 482.0
    Hemophilus influenzae (H. influenzae)
      482.2
    hypostatic 514
    influenzal (*see also* Influenza) 487.0
    Klebsiella 482.0
    ornithosis 073.0
    Proteus 482.83
    Pseudomonas 482.1
    psittacosis 073.0
    specified organism NEC 483.8
      bacterial NEC 482.89
    staphylococcal 482.40
      aureus 482.41
        methicillin
          resistant (MRSA) 482.42
          susceptible (MSSA) 482.41
      specified type NEC 482.49
    streptococcal — *see* Pneumonia, strep-
      tococcal
    viral, virus (*see also* Pneumonia, viral)
      480.9
  lobular (confluent) — *see* Pneumonia,
    broncho-
  Löffler's 518.3
  massive — *see* Pneumonia, lobar
  meconium aspiration 770.12
  metastatic NEC 038.8 *[484.8]*
  methicillin resistant Staphylococcus aureus
    (MRSA) 482.42
  methicillin susceptible Staphylococcus au-
    reus (MSSA) 482.41
  MRSA (methicillin resistant Staphylococcus
    aureus) 482.42
  MSSA (methicillin susceptible Staphylococ-
    cus aureus) 482.41

Pneumonia — *continued*
  multilobar — *see* Pneumonia, by type
  Mycoplasma (pneumoniae) 483.0
  necrotic 513.0
  nitrogen dioxide 506.9
  orthostatic 514
  parainfluenza virus 480.2
  parenchymatous (*see also* Fibrosis, lung) 515
  passive 514
  patchy — *see* Pneumonia, broncho-
  Peptococcus 482.81
  Peptostreptococcus 482.81
  plasma cell 136.3
  pleurolobar — *see* Pneumonia, lobar
  pleuropneumonia-like organism (PPLO)
    483.0
  pneumococcal (broncho) (lobar) 481
  Pneumocystis (carinii) (jiroveci) 136.3
  postinfectional NEC 136.9 *[484.8]*
  postmeasles 055.1
  postoperative 997.39
    aspiration 997.32
  primary atypical 486
  Proprionibacterium 482.81
  Proteus 482.83
  Pseudomonas 482.1
  psittacosis 073.0
  radiation 508.0
  respiratory syncytial virus 480.1
  resulting from a procedure 997.39
    aspiration 997.32
  rheumatic 390 *[517.1]*
  Salmonella 003.22
  SARS-associated coronavirus 480.3
  segmented, segmental — *see* Pneumonia,
    broncho-
  Serratia (marcescens) 482.83
  specified
    bacteria NEC 482.89
    organism NEC 483.8
    virus NEC 480.8
  spirochetal 104.8 *[484.8]*
  staphylococcal (broncho) (lobar) 482.40
    aureus 482.41
      methicillin
        resistant 482.42
        susceptible (MSSA) 482.41
    specified type NEC 482.49
  static, stasis 514
  streptococcal (broncho) (lobar) NEC 482.30
    Group
      A 482.31
      B 482.32
      specified NEC 482.39
    pneumoniae 481
    specified type NEC 482.39
  Streptococcus pneumoniae 481
  traumatic (complication) (early) (secondary)
    958.8
  tuberculous (any) (*see also* Tuberculosis)
    011.6 ☑
  tularemic 021.2
  TWAR agent 483.1
  varicella 052.1
  Veillonella 482.81
  ventilator associated 997.31
  viral, virus (broncho) (interstitial) (lobar)
    480.9
    with influenza, flu, or grippe (*see also*
      Influenza) 487.0
    adenoviral 480.0
    parainfluenza 480.2
    respiratory syncytial 480.1
    SARS-associated coronavirus 480.3
    specified type NEC 480.8
  white (congenital) 090.0
Pneumonic — *see* condition
Pneumonitis (acute) (primary) — *see also*
  Pneumonia 486
  allergic 495.9
    specified type NEC 495.8
  aspiration 507.0
    due to fumes or gases 506.0
    fetal 770.18
      due to
        blood 770.16

Pneumonitis — *see also* Pneumonia —
  continued
  aspiration — *continued*
    fetal — *continued*
      due to — *continued*
        clear amniotic fluid 770.14
        meconium 770.12
        postnatal stomach contents
          770.86
    newborn 770.18
      due to
        blood 770.16
        clear amniotic fluid 770.14
        meconium 770.12
        postnatal stomach contents
          770.86
    obstetric 668.0 ☑
  chemical 506.0
    due to fumes or gases 506.0
    resulting from a procedure 997.32
  cholesterol 516.8
  chronic (*see also* Fibrosis, lung) 515
  congenital rubella 771.0
  crack 506.0
  due to
    crack (cocaine) 506.0
    fumes or vapors 506.0
    inhalation
      food (regurgitated), milk, vomitus
        507.0
      oils, essences 507.1
      saliva 507.0
      solids, liquids NEC 507.8
    toxoplasmosis (acquired) 130.4
      congenital (active) 771.2 *[484.8]*
  eosinophilic 518.3
  fetal aspiration 770.18
    due to
      blood 770.16
      clear amniotic fluid 770.14
      meconium 770.12
      postnatal stomach contents 770.86
  hypersensitivity 495.9
  interstitial (chronic) (*see also* Fibrosis, lung)
    515
    acute 516.33
    idiopathic
      lymphocytic 516.35
      non-specific 516.32
    lymphoid 516.8
  lymphoid, interstitial 516.8
  meconium aspiration 770.12
  postanesthetic
    correct substance properly administered
      507.0
    obstetric 668.0 ☑
    overdose or wrong substance given
      968.4
      specified anesthetic — *see* Table of
        Drugs and Chemicals
  postoperative 997.3 ☑
    aspiration 997.32
    obstetric 668.0 ☑
  radiation 508.0
  rubella, congenital 771.0
  "ventilation" 495.7
  ventilator associated 997.31
  wood-dust 495.8
Pneumonoconiosis — *see* Pneumoconiosis
Pneumoparotid 527.8
Pneumopathy NEC 518.89
  alveolar 516.9
    specified NEC 516.8
  due to dust NEC 504
  parietoalveolar 516.9
    specified condition NEC 516.8
Pneumopericarditis — *see also* Pericarditis
  423.9
  acute 420.90
Pneumopericardium — *see also* Pericarditis
  congenital 770.2
  fetus or newborn 770.2
  traumatic (post) (*see also* Pneumothorax,
    traumatic) 860.0
    with open wound into thorax 860.1
Pneumoperitoneum 568.89

☑ **Additional Digit Required** — Refer to the Tabular List for Digit Selection   ⩩ **Subterms under main terms may continue to next column or page**

Polyneuropathy (peripheral) 356.9
  alcoholic 357.5
  amyloid 277.39 *[357.4]*
  arsenical 357.7
  critical illness 357.82
  demyelinating, chronic inflammatory (CIDP) 357.81
  diabetic 250.6 ☑ *[357.2]*
    due to secondary diabetes 249.6 ☑ *[357.2]*
  due to
    antitetanus serum 357.6
    arsenic 357.7
    drug or medicinal substance 357.6
      correct substance properly administered 357.6
      overdose or wrong substance given or taken 977.9
      specified drug — *see* Table of Drugs and Chemicals
    lack of vitamin NEC 269.2 *[357.4]*
    lead 357.7
    organophosphate compounds 357.7
    pellagra 265.2 *[357.4]*
    porphyria 277.1 *[357.4]*
    serum 357.6
    toxic agent NEC 357.7
  hereditary 356.0
  idiopathic 356.9
    progressive 356.4
  in
    amyloidosis 277.39 *[357.4]*
    avitaminosis 269.2 *[357.4]*
      specified NEC 269.1 *[357.4]*
    beriberi 265.0 *[357.4]*
    collagen vascular disease NEC 710.9 *[357.1]*
    deficiency
      B-complex NEC 266.2 *[357.4]*
      vitamin B 266.1 *[357.4]*
      vitamin B6 266.9 *[357.4]*
    diabetes 250.6 ☑ *[357.2]*
      due to secondary diabetes 249.6 ☑ *[357.2]*
    diphtheria (*see also* Diphtheria) 032.89 *[357.4]*
    disseminated lupus erythematosus 710.0 *[357.1]*
    herpes zoster 053.13
    hypoglycemia 251.2 *[357.4]*
    malignant neoplasm (M8000/3) NEC 199.1 *[357.3]*
    mumps 072.72
    pellagra 265.2 *[357.4]*
    polyarteritis nodosa 446.0 *[357.1]*
    porphyria 277.1 *[357.4]*
    rheumatoid arthritis 714.0 *[357.1]*
    sarcoidosis 135 *[357.4]*
    uremia 585.9 *[357.4]*
  lead 357.7
  nutritional 269.9 *[357.4]*
    specified NEC 269.8 *[357.4]*
  postherpetic 053.13
  progressive 356.4
  sensory (hereditary) 356.2
  specified NEC 356.8
Polyonychia 757.5
Polyopia 368.2
  refractive 368.15
Polyorchism, polyorchidism (three testes) 752.89
Polyorrhymenitis (peritoneal) — *see also* Polyserositis 568.82
  pericardial 423.2
Polyostotic fibrous dysplasia 756.54
Polyotia 744.1
Polyphagia 783.6
Polypoid — *see* condition
Polyposis — *see also* Polyp
  coli (adenomatous) (M8220/0) 211.3
    adenocarcinoma in (M8220/3) 153.9
    carcinoma in (M8220/3) 153.9
  familial (M8220/0) 211.3
  intestinal (adenomatous) (M8220/0) 211.3
  multiple (M8221/0) — *see* Neoplasm, by site, benign

Polyp, polypus

| *Note* — Polyps of organs or sites that do not appear in the list below should be coded to the residual category for diseases of the organ or site concerned. |

  accessory sinus 471.8
  adenoid tissue 471.0
  adenomatous (M8210/0) (*see also* Neoplasm, by site, benign)
    adenocarcinoma in (M8210/3) — *see* Neoplasm, by site, malignant
    carcinoma in (M8210/3) — *see* Neoplasm, by site, malignant
    multiple (M8221/0) — *see* Neoplasm, by site, benign
  antrum 471.8
  anus, anal (canal) (nonadenomatous) 569.0
    adenomatous 211.4
  Bartholin's gland 624.6
  bladder (M8120/1) 236.7
  broad ligament 620.8
  cervix (uteri) 622.7
    adenomatous 219.0
    in pregnancy or childbirth 654.6 ☑
      affecting fetus or newborn 763.89
      causing obstructed labor 660.2 ☑
    mucous 622.7
    nonneoplastic 622.7
  choanal 471.0
  cholesterol 575.6
  clitoris 624.6
  colon (M8210/0) (*see also* Polyp, adenomatous) 211.3
  corpus uteri 621.0
  dental 522.0
  ear (middle) 385.30
  endometrium 621.0
  ethmoidal (sinus) 471.8
  fallopian tube 620.8
  female genital organs NEC 624.8
  frontal (sinus) 471.8
  gallbladder 575.6
  gingiva 523.8
  gum 523.8
  labia 624.6
  larynx (mucous) 478.4
  malignant (M8000/3) — *see* Neoplasm, by site, malignant
  maxillary (sinus) 471.8
  middle ear 385.30
  myometrium 621.0
  nares
    anterior 471.9
    posterior 471.0
  nasal (mucous) 471.9
    cavity 471.0
    septum 471.9
  nasopharyngeal 471.0
  neoplastic (M8210/0) — *see* Neoplasm, by site, benign
  nose (mucous) 471.9
  oviduct 620.8
  paratubal 620.8
  pharynx 478.29
    congenital 750.29
  placenta, placental 674.4 ☑
  prostate 600.20
    with
      other lower urinary tract symptoms (LUTS) 600.21
      urinary
        obstruction 600.21
        retention 600.21
  pudenda 624.6
  pulp (dental) 522.0
  rectosigmoid 211.4
  rectum (nonadenomatous) 569.0´
    adenomatous 211.4
  septum (nasal) 471.9
  sinus (accessory) (ethmoidal) (frontal) (maxillary) (sphenoidal) 471.8
  sphenoidal (sinus) 471.8
  stomach (M8210/0) 211.1
  tube, fallopian 620.8
  turbinate, mucous membrane 471.8
  ureter 593.89

Polyp, polypus — *continued*
  urethra 599.3
  uterine
    ligament 620.8
    tube 620.8
  uterus (body) (corpus) (mucous) 621.0
    in pregnancy or childbirth 654.1 ☑
      affecting fetus or newborn 763.89
      causing obstructed labor 660.2 ☑
  vagina 623.7
  vocal cord (mucous) 478.4
  vulva 624.6
Polyradiculitis (acute) 357.0
Polyradiculoneuropathy (acute) (segmentally demyelinating) 357.0
Polysarcia 278.00
Polyserositis (peritoneal) 568.82
  due to pericarditis 423.2
  paroxysmal (familial) 277.31
  pericardial 423.2
  periodic (familial) 277.31
  pleural — *see* Pleurisy
  recurrent 277.31
  tuberculous (*see also* Tuberculosis, polyserositis) 018.9 ☑
Polysialia 527.7
Polysplenia syndrome 759.0
Polythelia 757.6
Polytrichia — *see also* Hypertrichosis 704.1
Polyunguia (congenital) 757.5
  acquired 703.8
Polyuria 788.42
Pompe's disease (glycogenosis II) 271.0
Pompholyx 705.81
Poncet's disease (tuberculous rheumatism) — *see also* Tuberculosis 015.9 ☑
Pond fracture — *see* Fracture, skull, vault
Ponos 085.0
Pons, pontine — *see* condition
Poor
  aesthetics of existing restoration of tooth 525.67
  contractions, labor 661.2 ☑
    affecting fetus or newborn 763.7
  fetal growth NEC 764.9 ☑
    affecting management of pregnancy 656.5 ☑
  incorporation
    artificial skin graft 996.55
    decellularized allodermis graft 996.55
  obstetrical history V13.29
    affecting management of current pregnancy V23.49
      ectopic pregnancy V23.42
      pre-term labor V23.41
    pre-term labor V13.21
  sucking reflex (newborn) 796.1
  vision NEC 369.9
Poradenitis, nostras 099.1
Porencephaly (congenital) (developmental) (true) 742.4
  acquired 348.0
  nondevelopmental 348.0
  traumatic (post) 310.2
Porocephaliasis 134.1
Porokeratosis 757.39
  disseminated superficial actinic (DSAP) 692.75
Poroma, eccrine (M8402/0) — *see* Neoplasm, skin, benign
Porphyria (acute) (congenital) (constitutional) (erythropoietic) (familial) (hepatica) (idiopathic) (idiosyncratic) (intermittent) (latent) (mixed hepatic) (photosensitive) (South African genetic) (Swedish) 277.1
  acquired 277.1
  cutaneatarda
    hereditaria 277.1
    symptomatica 277.1
  due to drugs
    correct substance properly administered 277.1
    overdose or wrong substance given or taken 977.9
    specified drug — *see* Table of Drugs and Chemicals

Porphyria — *continued*
  secondary 277.1
  toxic NEC 277.1
  variegata 277.1
Porphyrinuria (acquired) (congenital) (secondary) 277.1
Porphyruria (acquired) (congenital) 277.1
Portal — *see* condition
Port wine nevus or mark 757.32
Posadas-Wernicke disease 114.9
Position
  fetus, abnormal (*see also* Presentation, fetal) 652.9 ☑
  teeth, faulty (*see also* Anomaly, position tooth) 524.30
Positive
  culture (nonspecific) 795.39
    AIDS virus V08
    blood 790.7
    HIV V08
    human immunodeficiency virus V08
    nose 795.39
      Staphylococcus — *see* Carrier (suspected) of, Staphylococcus
    skin lesion NEC 795.39
    spinal fluid 792.0
    sputum 795.39
    stool 792.1
    throat 795.39
    urine 791.9
    wound 795.39
  findings, anthrax 795.31
  HIV V08
  human immunodeficiency virus (HIV) V08
  PPD 795.51
  serology
    AIDS virus V08
      inconclusive 795.71
    HIV V08
      inconclusive 795.71
    human immunodeficiency virus (HIV) V08
      inconclusive 795.71
    syphilis 097.1
      with signs or symptoms — *see* Syphilis, by site and stage
      false 795.6
  skin test 795.7 ☑
    tuberculin (without active tuberculosis) 795.51
  VDRL 097.1
    with signs or symptoms — *see* Syphilis, by site and stage
    false 795.6
  Wassermann reaction 097.1
    false 795.6
Post-dates (pregnancy) — *see* Pregnancy
Post-term (pregnancy) 645.1 ☑
  infant (gestation period over 40 completed weeks to 42 completed weeks) 766.21
Post-transplant lymphoproliferative disorder (PTLD) 238.77
Post-traumatic stress disorder (PTSD) 309.81
Post-typhoid abscess 002.0
Postcardiotomy syndrome 429.4
Postcaval ureter 753.4
Postcholecystectomy syndrome 576.0
Postclimacteric bleeding 627.1
Postcommissurotomy syndrome 429.4
Postconcussional syndrome 310.2
Postcontusional syndrome 310.2
Postcricoid region — *see* condition
Postencephalitic — *see also* condition
  syndrome 310.89
Posterior — *see* condition
Posterolateral sclerosis (spinal cord) — *see* Degeneration, combined
Postexanthematous — *see* condition
Postfebrile — *see* condition
Postgastrectomy dumping syndrome 564.2
Posthemiplegic chorea 344.89
Posthemorrhagic anemia (chronic) 280.0
  acute 285.1
  newborn 776.5
Posthepatitis syndrome 780.79

☑ **Additional Digit Required** — Refer to the Tabular List for Digit Selection   ᵂ **Subterms under main terms may continue to next column or page**

2014 ICD-9-CM   ▶◀ **Revised Text**   ● **New Line**   ▲ **Revised Code**   **Volume 2 — 235**

Postherpetic neuralgia (intercostal) (syndrome) (zoster) 053.19
  geniculate ganglion 053.11
  ophthalmica 053.19
  trigeminal 053.12
Posthitis 607.1
Postimmunization complication or reaction — see Complications, vaccination
Postinfectious — see condition
Postinfluenzal syndrome 780.79
Postlaminectomy syndrome 722.80
  cervical, cervicothoracic 722.81
  kyphosis 737.12
  lumbar, lumbosacral 722.83
  thoracic, thoracolumbar 722.82
Postleukotomy syndrome 310.0
Postlobectomy syndrome 310.0
Postmastectomy lymphedema (syndrome) 457.0
Postmaturity, postmature (fetus or newborn) (gestation period over 42 completed weeks) 766.22
  affecting management of pregnancy
    post-term pregnancy 645.1 ☑
    prolonged pregnancy 645.2 ☑
  syndrome 766.22
Postmeasles — see also condition
  complication 055.8
    specified NEC 055.79
Postmenopausal
  endometrium (atrophic) 627.8
    suppurative (see also Endometritis) 615.9
  hormone replacement therapy V07.4
  status (age related) (natural) V49.81
Postnasal drip 784.91
Postnatal — see condition
Postoperative — see also condition
  confusion state 293.9
  psychosis 293.9
  status NEC (see also Status (post)) V45.89
Postpancreatectomy hyperglycemia 251.3
Postpartum — see also condition
  anemia 648.2 ☑
  cardiomyopathy 674.5 ☑
  observation
    immediately after delivery V24.0
    routine follow-up V24.2
Postperfusion syndrome NEC 999.89
  bone marrow 996.85
Postpoliomyelitic — see condition
Postsurgery status NEC — see also Status (post V45.89
Posttraumatic — see condition
Posttraumatic brain syndrome, nonpsychotic 310.2
Postures, hysterical 300.11
Postvaccinal reaction or complication — see Complications, vaccination
Postvagotomy syndrome 564.2
Postvalvulotomy syndrome 429.4
Postvasectomy sperm count V25.8
Potain's disease (pulmonary edema) 514
Potain's syndrome (gastrectasis with dyspepsia) 536.1
Pott's
  curvature (spinal) (see also Tuberculosis) 015.0 ☑ [737.43]
  disease or paraplegia (see also Tuberculosis) 015.0 ☑ [730.88]
  fracture (closed) 824.4
    open 824.5
  gangrene 440.24
  osteomyelitis (see also Tuberculosis) 015.0 ☑ [730.88]
  spinal curvature (see also Tuberculosis) 015.0 ☑ [737.43]
  tumor, puffy (see also Osteomyelitis) 730.2 ☑
Potter's
  asthma 502
  disease 753.0
  facies 754.0
  lung 502
  syndrome (with renal agenesis) 753.0

Pouch
  bronchus 748.3
  Douglas' — see condition
  esophagus, esophageal (congenital) 750.4
    acquired 530.6
  gastric 537.1
  Hartmann's (abnormal sacculation of gallbladder neck) 575.8
  of intestine V44.3
    attention to V55.3
  pharynx, pharyngeal (congenital) 750.27
Pouchitis 569.71
Poulet's disease 714.2
Poultrymen's itch 133.8
Poverty V60.2
PPE (palmar plantar erythrodysesthesia) 693.0
Prader-Labhart-Willi-Fanconi syndrome (hypogenital dystrophy with diabetic tendency) 759.81
Prader-Willi syndrome (hypogenital dystrophy with diabetic tendency) 759.81
Pre-AIDS — see Human immunodeficiency virus (disease) (illness) (infection)
Pre-syncope 780.2
Preachers' voice 784.49
Preauricular appendage 744.1
Prebetalipoproteinemia (acquired) (essential) (familial) (hereditary) (primary) (secondary) 272.1
  with chylomicronemia 272.3
Precipitate labor 661.3 ☑
  affecting fetus or newborn 763.6
Preclimacteric bleeding 627.0
  menorrhagia 627.0
Precocious
  adrenarche 259.1
  menarche 259.1
  menstruation 259.1
  pubarche 259.1
  puberty NEC 259.1
  sexual development NEC 259.1
  thelarche 259.1
Precocity, sexual (constitutional) (cryptogenic) (female) (idiopathic) (male) NEC 259.1
  with adrenal hyperplasia 255.2
Precordial pain 786.51
  psychogenic 307.89
Predeciduous teeth 520.2
Prediabetes, prediabetic 790.29
  complicating pregnancy, childbirth, or puerperium 648.8 ☑
  fetus or newborn 775.89
Predislocation status of hip, at birth — see also Subluxation, congenital, hip 754.32
Preeclampsia (mild) 642.4 ☑
  with pre-existing hypertension 642.7 ☑
  affecting fetus or newborn 760.0
  severe 642.5 ☑
  superimposed on pre-existing hypertensive disease 642.7 ☑
Preeruptive color change, teeth, tooth 520.8
Preexcitation 426.7
  atrioventricular conduction 426.7
  ventricular 426.7
Preglaucoma 365.00
Pregnancy (single) (uterine) (without sickness) V22.2

Note — Use the following fifth-digit subclassification with categories 640–649, 651–679:

0 unspecified as to episode of care

1 delivered, with or without mention of antepartum condition

2 delivered, with mention of postpartum complication

3 antepartum condition or complication

4 postpartum condition or complication

  abdominal (ectopic) 633.00
    with intrauterine pregnancy 633.01
    affecting fetus or newborn 761.4
  abnormal NEC 646.9 ☑

Pregnancy — continued
  ampullar — see Pregnancy, tubal
  biochemical 631.0
  broad ligament — see Pregnancy, cornual
  cervical — see Pregnancy, cornual
  chemical 631.0
  combined (extrauterine and intrauterine) — see Pregnancy, cornual
  complicated (by) 646.9 ☑
    abnormal, abnormality NEC 646.9 ☑
      cervix 654.6 ☑
      cord (umbilical) 663.9 ☑
      glucose tolerance (conditions classifiable to 790.21–790.29) 648.8 ☑
      pelvic organs or tissues NEC 654.9 ☑
      pelvis (bony) 653.0 ☑
      perineum or vulva 654.8 ☑
      placenta, placental (vessel) 656.7 ☑
      position
        cervix 654.4 ☑
        placenta 641.1 ☑
          without hemorrhage 641.0 ☑
        uterus 654.4 ☑
      size, fetus 653.5 ☑
      uterus (congenital) 654.0 ☑
    abscess or cellulitis
      bladder 646.6 ☑
      genitourinary tract (conditions classifiable to 590, 595, 597, 599.0, 614.0–614.5, 614.7–614.9, 615) 646.6 ☑
      kidney 646.6 ☑
      urinary tract NEC 646.6 ☑
    adhesion, pelvic peritoneal 648.9 ☑
    air embolism 673.0 ☑
    albuminuria 646.2 ☑
      with hypertension — see Toxemia, of pregnancy
    amnionitis 658.4 ☑
    amniotic fluid embolism 673.1 ☑
    anemia (conditions classifiable to 280–285) 648.2 ☑
    appendicitis 648.9 ☑
    atrophy, yellow (acute) (liver) (subacute) 646.7 ☑
    bacilluria, asymptomatic 646.5 ☑
    bacteriuria, asymptomatic 646.5 ☑
    bariatric surgery status 649.2 ☑
    bicornis or bicornuate uterus 654.0 ☑
    biliary problems 646.8 ☑
    bone and joint disorders (conditions classifiable to 720–724 or conditions affecting lower limbs classifiable to 711–719, 725–738) 648.7 ☑
    breech presentation (buttocks) (complete) (frank) 652.2 ☑
      with successful version 652.1 ☑
    cardiovascular disease (conditions classifiable to 390–398, 410–429) 648.6 ☑
      congenital (conditions classifiable to 745–747) 648.5 ☑
    cerebrovascular disorders (conditions classifiable to 430–434, 436–437) 674.0 ☑
    cervicitis (conditions classifiable to 616.0) 646.6 ☑
    chloasma (gravidarum) 646.8 ☑
    cholelithiasis 646.8 ☑
    cholestasis 646.7 ☑
    chorea (gravidarum) — see Eclampsia, pregnancy
    coagulation defect 649.3 ☑
    conjoined twins 678.1 ☑
    contraction, pelvis (general) 653.1 ☑
      inlet 653.2 ☑
      outlet 653.3 ☑
    convulsions (eclamptic) (uremic) 642.6 ☑
      with pre-existing hypertension 642.7 ☑

Pregnancy — continued
  complicated — continued
    current disease or condition (nonobstetric)
      abnormal glucose tolerance 648.8 ☑
      anemia 648.2 ☑
      biliary tract 646.7 ☑
      bone and joint (lower limb) 648.7 ☑
      cardiovascular 648.6 ☑
        congenital 648.5 ☑
      cerebrovascular 674.0 ☑
      diabetes (conditions classifiable to 249 and 250) 648.0 ☑
      drug dependence 648.3 ☑
      female genital mutilation 648.9 ☑
      genital organ or tract 646.6 ☑
      gonorrheal 647.1 ☑
      hypertensive 642.2 ☑
        chronic kidney 642.2 ☑
        renal 642.1 ☑
      infectious 647.9 ☑
        specified type NEC 647.8 ☑
      liver 646.7 ☑
      malarial 647.4 ☑
      nutritional deficiency 648.9 ☑
      parasitic NEC 647.8 ☑
      periodontal disease 648.9 ☑
      renal 646.2 ☑
        hypertensive 642.1 ☑
      rubella 647.5 ☑
      specified condition NEC 648.9 ☑
      syphilitic 647.0 ☑
      thyroid 648.1 ☑
      tuberculous 647.3 ☑
      urinary 646.6 ☑
      venereal 647.2 ☑
      viral NEC 647.6 ☑
    cystitis 646.6 ☑
    cystocele 654.4 ☑
    death of fetus (near term) 656.4 ☑
      early pregnancy (before 22 completed weeks gestation) 632
    deciduitis 646.6 ☑
    decreased fetal movements 655.7 ☑
    diabetes (mellitus) (conditions classifiable to 249 and 250) 648.0 ☑
    disorders of liver and biliary tract 646.7 ☑
    displacement, uterus NEC 654.4 ☑
    disproportion — see Disproportion
    double uterus 654.0 ☑
    drug dependence (conditions classifiable to 304) 648.3 ☑
    dysplasia, cervix 654.6 ☑
    early onset of delivery (spontaneous) 644.2 ☑
    eclampsia, eclamptic (coma) (convulsions) (delirium) (nephritis) (uremia) 642.6 ☑
      with pre-existing hypertension 642.7 ☑
    edema 646.1 ☑
      with hypertension — see Toxemia, of pregnancy
    effusion, amniotic fluid 658.1 ☑
      delayed delivery following 658.2 ☑
    embolism
      air 673.0 ☑
      amniotic fluid 673.1 ☑
      blood-clot 673.2 ☑
      cerebral 674.0 ☑
      pulmonary NEC 673.2 ☑
      pyemic 673.3 ☑
      septic 673.3 ☑
    emesis (gravidarum) — see Pregnancy, complicated, vomiting
    endometritis (conditions classifiable to 615.0–615.9) 670.1 ☑
      decidual 646.6 ☑
    epilepsy 649.4 ☑
    excessive weight gain NEC 646.1 ☑
    face presentation 652.4 ☑
    failure, fetal head to enter pelvic brim 652.5 ☑

☑ Additional Digit Required — Refer to the Tabular List for Digit Selection   ▽ Subterms under main terms may continue to next column or page

236 — Volume 2   ▶◀ Revised Text   ● New Line   ▲ Revised Code   2014 ICD-9-CM

Pregnancy — *continued*
  complicated — *continued*
    false labor (pains) 644.1 ☑
    fatigue 646.8 ☑
    fatty metamorphosis of liver 646.7 ☑
    female genital mutilation 648.9 ☑
    fetal
      anemia 678.0 ☑
      complications from in utero proce-
        dure 679.1 ☑
      conjoined twins 678.1 ☑
      death (near term) 656.4 ☑
        early (before 22 completed weeks
          gestation) 632
      deformity 653.7 ☑
      distress 656.8 ☑
      hematologic conditions 678.0 ☑
      reduction of multiple fetuses reduced
        to single fetus 651.7 ☑
      thrombocytopenia 678.0 ☑
      twin to twin transfusion 678.0 ☑
    fibroid (tumor) (uterus) 654.1 ☑
    footling presentation 652.8 ☑
      with successful version 652.1 ☑
    gallbladder disease 646.8 ☑
    gastric banding status 649.2 ☑
    gastric bypass status for obesity
    genital herpes (asymptomatic) (history
      of) (inactive) 647.6 ☑
    goiter 648.1 ☑
    gonococcal infection (conditions classifi-
      able to 098) 647.1 ☑
    gonorrhea (conditions classifiable to
      098) 647.1 ☑
    hemorrhage 641.9 ☑
      accidental 641.2 ☑
      before 22 completed weeks gesta-
        tion NEC 640.9 ☑
      cerebrovascular 674.0 ☑
      due to
        afibrinogenemia or other coagu-
          lation defect (conditions
          classifiable to 286.0–286.9)
          641.3 ☑
        leiomyoma, uterine 641.8 ☑
        marginal sinus (rupture) 641.2 ☑
        premature separation, placenta
          641.2 ☑
        trauma 641.8 ☑
      early (before 22 completed weeks
        gestation) 640.9 ☑
      threatened abortion 640.0 ☑
      unavoidable 641.1 ☑
    hepatitis (acute) (malignant) (subacute)
      646.7 ☑
      viral 647.6 ☑
    herniation of uterus 654.4 ☑
    high head at term 652.5 ☑
    hydatidiform mole (delivered) (undeliv-
      ered) 630
    hydramnios 657.0 ☑
    hydrocephalic fetus 653.6 ☑
    hydrops amnii 657.0 ☑
    hydrorrhea 658.1 ☑
    hyperemesis (gravidarum) — *see* Hyper-
      emesis, gravidarum
    hypertension — *see* Hypertension,
      complicating pregnancy
    hypertensive
      chronic kidney disease 642.2 ☑
      heart and chronic kidney disease
        642.2 ☑
      heart and renal disease 642.2 ☑
      heart disease 642.2 ☑
      renal disease 642.2 ☑
    hypertensive heart and chronic kidney
      disease 642.2 ☑
    hyperthyroidism 648.1 ☑
    hypothyroidism 648.1 ☑
    hysteralgia 646.8 ☑
    icterus gravis 646.7 ☑
    incarceration, uterus 654.3 ☑
    incompetent cervix (os) 654.5 ☑
    infection 647.9 ☑

Pregnancy — *continued*
  complicated — *continued*
    infection — *continued*
      amniotic fluid 658.4 ☑
      bladder 646.6 ☑
      genital organ (conditions classifiable
        to 614.0–614.5, 614.7–614.9,
        615) 646.6 ☑
      kidney (conditions classifiable to
        590.0–590.9) 646.6 ☑
      urinary (tract) 646.6 ☑
        asymptomatic 646.5 ☑
    infective and parasitic diseases NEC
      647.8 ☑
    inflammation
      bladder 646.6 ☑
      genital organ (conditions classifiable
        to 614.0–614.5, 614.7–614.9,
        615) 646.6 ☑
      urinary tract NEC 646.6 ☑
    insufficient weight gain 646.8 ☑
    insulin resistance 648.8 ☑
    intrauterine fetal death (near term) NEC
      656.4 ☑
      early (before 22 completed weeks'
        gestation) 632
    malaria (conditions classifiable to 084)
      647.4 ☑
    malformation, uterus (congenital)
      654.0 ☑
    malnutrition (conditions classifiable to
      260–269) 648.9 ☑
    malposition
      fetus — *see* Pregnancy, complicated,
        malpresentation
      uterus or cervix 654.4 ☑
    malpresentation 652.9 ☑
      with successful version 652.1 ☑
      in multiple gestation 652.6 ☑
      specified type NEC 652.8 ☑
    marginal sinus hemorrhage or rupture
      641.2 ☑
    maternal complications from in utero
      procedure 679.0 ☑
    maternal drug abuse 648.4 ☑
    maternal obesity syndrome 646.1 ☑
    menstruation 640.8 ☑
    mental disorders (conditions classifiable
      to 290–303, 305.0, 305.2-305.9,
      306–316, 317–319) 648.4 ☑
    mentum presentation 652.4 ☑
    missed
      abortion 632
      delivery (at or near term) 656.4 ☑
      labor (at or near term) 656.4 ☑
    necrosis
      genital organ or tract (conditions
        classifiable to 614.0–614.5,
        614.7–614.9, 615) 646.6 ☑
      liver (conditions classifiable to 570)
        646.7 ☑
      renal, cortical 646.2 ☑
    nephritis or nephrosis (conditions classi-
      fiable to 580–589) 646.2 ☑
      with hypertension 642.1 ☑
    nephropathy NEC 646.2 ☑
    neuritis (peripheral) 646.4 ☑
    nutritional deficiency (conditions classi-
      fiable to 260–269) 648.9 ☑
    obesity 649.1 ☑
      surgery status 649.2 ☑
    oblique lie or presentation 652.3 ☑
      with successful version 652.1 ☑
    obstetrical trauma NEC 665.9 ☑
    oligohydramnios NEC 658.0 ☑
    onset of contractions before 37 weeks
      644.0 ☑
    oversize fetus 653.5 ☑
    papyraceous fetus 646.0 ☑
    patent cervix 654.5 ☑
    pelvic inflammatory disease (conditions
      classifiable to 614.0–614.5,
      614.7–614.9, 615) 646.6 ☑
    pelvic peritoneal adhesion 648.9 ☑

Pregnancy — *continued*
  complicated — *continued*
    placenta, placental
      abnormality 656.7 ☑
      abruptio or ablatio 641.2 ☑
      detachment 641.2 ☑
      disease 656.7 ☑
      infarct 656.7 ☑
      low implantation 641.1 ☑
        without hemorrhage 641.0 ☑
      malformation 656.7 ☑
      malposition 641.1 ☑
        without hemorrhage 641.0 ☑
      marginal sinus hemorrhage 641.2 ☑
      previa 641.1 ☑
        without hemorrhage 641.0 ☑
      separation (premature) (undelivered)
        641.2 ☑
    placentitis 658.4 ☑
    pneumonia 648.9 ☑
    polyhydramnios 657.0 ☑
    postmaturity
      post-term 645.1 ☑
      prolonged 645.2 ☑
    pre-eclampsia (mild) 642.4 ☑
      severe 642.5 ☑
      superimposed on pre-existing hyper-
        tensive disease 642.7 ☑
    prediabetes 648.8 ☑
    premature rupture of membranes
      658.1 ☑
      with delayed delivery 658.2 ☑
    previous
      ectopic pregnancy V23.42
      infertility V23.0
      in utero procedure during previous
        pregnancy V23.86
      nonobstetric condition V23.89
      poor obstetrical history V23.49
      premature delivery V23.41
      trophoblastic disease (conditions
        classifiable to 630) V23.1
    prolapse, uterus 654.4 ☑
    proteinuria (gestational) 646.2 ☑
      with hypertension — *see* Toxemia,
        of pregnancy
    pruritus (neurogenic) 646.8 ☑
    psychosis or psychoneurosis 648.4 ☑
    ptyalism 646.8 ☑
    pyelitis (conditions classifiable to
      590.0–590.9) 646.6 ☑
    renal disease or failure NEC 646.2 ☑
      with secondary hypertension
        642.1 ☑
        hypertensive 642.2 ☑
    retention, retained dead ovum 631.8
    retroversion, uterus 654.3 ☑
    Rh immunization, incompatibility, or
      sensitization 656.1 ☑
    rubella (conditions classifiable to 056)
      647.5 ☑
    rupture
      amnion (premature) 658.1 ☑
        with delayed delivery 658.2 ☑
      marginal sinus (hemorrhage)
        641.2 ☑
      membranes (premature) 658.1 ☑
        with delayed delivery 658.2 ☑
      uterus (before onset of labor)
        665.0 ☑
    salivation (excessive) 646.8 ☑
    salpingo–oophoritis (conditions classifi-
      able to 614.0–614.2) 646.6 ☑
    septicemia (conditions classifiable to
      038.0–038.9) 647.8 ☑
      postpartum 670.2 ☑
      puerperal 670.2 ☑
    smoking 649.0 ☑
    spasms, uterus (abnormal) 646.8 ☑
    specified condition NEC 646.8 ☑
    spotting 649.5 ☑
    spurious labor pains 644.1 ☑
    status post
      bariatric surgery 649.2 ☑

Pregnancy — *continued*
  complicated — *continued*
    status post — *continued*
      gastric banding 649.2 ☑
      gastric bypass for obesity 649.2 ☑
      obesity surgery 649.2 ☑
    superfecundation 651.9 ☑
    superfetation 651.9 ☑
    syphilis (conditions classifiable to
      090–097) 647.0 ☑
    threatened
      abortion 640.0 ☑
      premature delivery 644.2 ☑
      premature labor 644.0 ☑
    thrombophlebitis (superficial) 671.2 ☑
      deep 671.3 ☑
      septic 670.3 ☑
    thrombosis 671.2 ☑
      venous (superficial) 671.2 ☑
      deep 671.3 ☑
    thyroid dysfunction (conditions classifi-
      able to 240–246) 648.1 ☑
    thyroiditis 648.1 ☑
    thyrotoxicosis 648.1 ☑
    tobacco use disorder 649.0 ☑
    torsion of uterus 654.4 ☑
    toxemia — *see* Toxemia, of pregnancy
    transverse lie or presentation 652.3 ☑
      with successful version 652.1 ☑
    trauma 648.9 ☑
      obstetrical 665.9 ☑
    tuberculosis (conditions classifiable to
      010–018) 647.3 ☑
    tumor
      cervix 654.6 ☑
      ovary 654.4 ☑
      pelvic organs or tissue NEC 654.4 ☑
      uterus (body) 654.1 ☑
        cervix 654.6 ☑
      vagina 654.7 ☑
      vulva 654.8 ☑
    unstable lie 652.0 ☑
    uremia — *see* Pregnancy, complicated,
      renal disease
    urethritis 646.6 ☑
    vaginitis or vulvitis (conditions classifi-
      able to 616.1) 646.6 ☑
    varicose
      placental vessels 656.7 ☑
      veins (legs) 671.0 ☑
        perineum 671.1 ☑
        vulva 671.1 ☑
    varicosity, labia or vulva 671.1 ☑
    venereal disease NEC (conditions classi-
      fiable to 099) 647.2 ☑
    venous complication 671.9 ☑
    viral disease NEC (conditions classifiable
      to 042, 050–055, 057–079,
      795.05, 795.15, 796.75) 647.6 ☑
    vomiting (incoercible) (pernicious) (per-
      sistent) (uncontrollable) (vicious)
      643.9 ☑
      due to organic disease or other cause
        643.8 ☑
      early — *see* Hyperemesis, gravi-
        darum
      late (after 22 completed weeks gesta-
        tion) 643.2 ☑
    young maternal age 659.8 ☑
  complications NEC 646.9 ☑
  cornual 633.80
    with intrauterine pregnancy 633.81
    affecting fetus or newborn 761.4
  death, maternal NEC 646.9 ☑
  delivered — *see* Delivery
  ectopic (ruptured) NEC 633.90
    with intrauterine pregnancy 633.91
    abdominal — *see* Pregnancy, abdominal
    affecting fetus or newborn 761.4
    combined (extrauterine and intrauter-
      ine) — *see* Pregnancy, cornual
    ovarian — *see* Pregnancy, ovarian
    specified type NEC 633.80
      with intrauterine pregnancy 633.81

☑ **Additional Digit Required** — Refer to the Tabular List for Digit Selection   ▽ **Subterms under main terms may continue to next column or page**

2014 ICD-9-CM   ▶◀ **Revised Text**   ● **New Line**   ▲ **Revised Code**   **Volume 2 — 237**

Premyeloma 273.1
Prenatal
  care, normal pregnancy V22.1
    first V22.0
  death, cause unknown — *see* Death, fetus
  screening — *see* Antenatal, screening
  teeth 520.6
Prepartum — *see* condition
Preponderance, left or right ventricular
  429.3
Prepuce — *see* condition
PRES (posterior reversible encephalopathy
  syndrome) 348.39
Presbycardia 797
  hypertensive (*see also* Hypertension, heart)
  402.90
Presbycusis 388.01
Presbyesophagus 530.89
Presbyophrenia 310.1
Presbyopia 367.4
Prescription of contraceptives NEC V25.02
  diaphragm V25.02
  oral (pill) V25.01
    emergency V25.03
    postcoital V25.03
    repeat V25.41
  repeat V25.40
    oral (pill) V25.41
Presenile — *see also* condition
  aging 259.8
  dementia (*see also* Dementia, presenile)
  290.10
Presenility 259.8
Presentation, fetal
  abnormal 652.9 ☑
    with successful version 652.1 ☑
    before labor, affecting fetus or newborn
    761.7
    causing obstructed labor 660.0 ☑
      affecting fetus or newborn, any, ex-
      cept breech 763.1
    in multiple gestation (one or more)
    652.6 ☑
    specified NEC 652.8 ☑
  arm 652.7 ☑
    causing obstructed labor 660.0 ☑
  breech (buttocks) (complete) (frank)
  652.2 ☑
    with successful version 652.1 ☑
    before labor, affecting fetus or new-
    born 761.7
    before labor, affecting fetus or newborn
    761.7
  brow 652.4 ☑
    causing obstructed labor 660.0 ☑
  buttocks 652.2 ☑
  chin 652.4 ☑
  complete 652.2 ☑
  compound 652.8 ☑
  cord 663.0 ☑
  extended head 652.4 ☑
  face 652.4 ☑
    to pubes 652.8 ☑
  footling 652.8 ☑
  frank 652.2 ☑
  hand, leg, or foot NEC 652.8 ☑
  incomplete 652.8 ☑
  mentum 652.4 ☑
  multiple gestation (one fetus or more)
  652.6 ☑
  oblique 652.3 ☑
    with successful version 652.1 ☑
  shoulder 652.8 ☑
    affecting fetus or newborn 763.1
  transverse 652.3 ☑
    with successful version 652.1 ☑
  umbilical cord 663.0 ☑
  unstable 652.0 ☑
Prespondylolisthesis (congenital) (lumbosacral) 756.11
Pressure
  area, skin ulcer (*see also* Ulcer, pressure)
  707.00
  atrophy, spine 733.99
  birth, fetus or newborn NEC 767.9

Pressure — *continued*
  brachial plexus 353.0
  brain 348.4
    injury at birth 767.0
  cerebral — *see* Pressure, brain
  chest 786.59
  cone, tentorial 348.4
    injury at birth 767.0
  funis — *see* Compression, umbilical cord
  hyposystolic (*see also* Hypotension) 458.9
  increased
    intracranial 781.99
      due to
        benign intracranial hypertension
        348.2
        hydrocephalus — *see* hydro-
        cephalus
      injury at birth 767.8
    intraocular 365.00
  lumbosacral plexus 353.1
  mediastinum 519.3
  necrosis (chronic) (skin) (*see also* Decubitus)
  707.00
  nerve — *see* Compression, nerve
  paralysis (*see also* Neuropathy, entrapment)
  355.9
  pre-ulcer skin changes limited to persistent
    focal erythema (*see also* Ulcer, pres-
    sure) 707.21
  sore (chronic) (*see also* Ulcer, pressure)
  707.00
  spinal cord 336.9
  ulcer (chronic) (*see also* Ulcer, pressure)
  707.00
  umbilical cord — *see* Compression, umbilical cord
  venous, increased 459.89
Preterm infant NEC 765.1 ☑
  extreme 765.0 ☑
Priapism (penis) 607.3
Prickling sensation — *see also* Disturbance,
  sensation 782.0
Prickly heat 705.1
Primary — *see also* condition
  angle closure suspect 365.02
Primigravida, elderly
  affecting
    fetus or newborn 763.89
    management of pregnancy, labor, and
    delivery 659.5 ☑
Primipara, old
  affecting
    fetus or newborn 763.89
    management of pregnancy, labor, and
    delivery 659.5 ☑
Primula dermatitis 692.6
Primus varus (bilateral) (metatarsus) 754.52
PRIND (prolonged reversible ischemic neurologic deficit) 434.91
  history of (personal) V12.54
Pringle's disease (tuberous sclerosis) 759.5
Prinzmetal-Massumi syndrome (anterior
  chest wall) 786.52
Prinzmetal's angina 413.1
Prizefighter ear 738.7
Problem (with) V49.9
  academic V62.3
  acculturation V62.4
  adopted child V61.24
  aged
    in-law V61.3
    parent V61.3
    person NEC V61.8
  alcoholism in family V61.41
  anger reaction (*see also* Disturbance, conduct) 312.0 ☑
  behavioral V40.9
    specified NEC V40.39
  behavior, child 312.9
  betting V69.3
  biological child V61.23
  cardiorespiratory NEC V47.2
  career choice V62.29
  care of sick or handicapped person in family
  or household V61.49
  communication V40.1

Problem — *continued*
  conscience regarding medical care V62.6
  delinquency (juvenile) 312.9
  diet, inappropriate V69.1
  digestive NEC V47.3
  ear NEC V41.3
  eating habits, inappropriate V69.1
  economic V60.2
    affecting care V60.9
      specified circumstance NEC V60.89
  educational V62.3
  enuresis, child 307.6
  exercise, lack of V69.0
  eye NEC V41.1
  family V61.9
    specified circumstance NEC V61.8
  fear reaction, child 313.0
  feeding (elderly) (infant) 783.3
    newborn 779.31
    nonorganic 307.59
  fetal, affecting management of pregnancy
  656.9 ☑
    specified type NEC 656.8 ☑
  financial V60.2
  foster child V61.25
  functional V41.9
    specified type NEC V41.8
  gambling V69.3
  genital NEC V47.5
  head V48.9
    deficiency V48.0
    disfigurement V48.6
    mechanical V48.2
    motor V48.2
    movement of V48.2
    sensory V48.4
    specified condition NEC V48.8
  hearing V41.2
  high-risk sexual behavior V69.2
  identity 313.82
  influencing health status NEC V49.89
  internal organ NEC V47.9
    deficiency V47.0
    mechanical or motor V47.1
  interpersonal NEC V62.81
  jealousy, child 313.3
  learning V40.0
  legal V62.5
  life circumstance NEC V62.89
  lifestyle V69.9
    specified NEC V69.8
  limb V49.9
    deficiency V49.0
    disfigurement V49.4
    mechanical V49.1
    motor V49.2
    movement, involving
      musculoskeletal system V49.1
      nervous system V49.2
    sensory V49.3
    specified condition NEC V49.5
  litigation V62.5
  living alone V60.3
  loneliness NEC V62.89
  marital V61.10
    involving
      divorce V61.03
      estrangement V61.09
      psychosexual disorder 302.9
      sexual function V41.7
    relationship V61.10
  mastication V41.6
  medical care, within family V61.49
  mental V40.9
    specified NEC V40.2
  mental hygiene, adult V40.9
  multiparity V61.5
  nail biting, child 307.9
  neck V48.9
    deficiency V48.1
    disfigurement V48.7
    mechanical V48.3
    motor V48.3
    movement V48.3
    sensory V48.5
    specified condition NEC V48.8

Problem — *continued*
  neurological NEC 781.99
  none (feared complaint unfounded) V65.5
  occupational V62.29
  parent-child V61.20
    adopted child V61.24
    biological child V61.23
    foster child V61.25
    relationship V61.20
  partner V61.10
    relationship V61.10
  personality (*see also* Disorder, personality)
  301.9
  personal NEC V62.89
    interpersonal conflict NEC V62.81
  phase of life V62.89
  placenta, affecting management of pregnancy 656.9 ☑
    specified type NEC 656.8 ☑
  poverty V60.2
  presence of sick or handicapped person in
    family or household V61.49
  psychiatric 300.9
  psychosocial V62.9
    specified type NEC V62.89
  relational NEC V62.81
  relationship, childhood 313.3
  religious or spiritual belief
    other than medical care V62.89
    regarding medical care V62.6
  self-damaging behavior V69.8
  sexual
    behavior, high-risk V69.2
    function NEC V41.7
  sibling
    relational V61.8
    relationship V61.8
  sight V41.0
  sleep disorder, child 307.40
  sleep, lack of V69.4
  smell V41.5
  speech V40.1
  spite reaction, child (*see also* Disturbance,
    conduct) 312.0 ☑
  spoiled child reaction (*see also* Disturbance,
    conduct) 312.1 ☑
  substance abuse in family V61.42
  swallowing V41.6
  tantrum, child (*see also* Disturbance, con-
    duct) 312.1 ☑
  taste V41.5
  thumb sucking, child 307.9
  tic (child) 307.21
  trunk V48.9
    deficiency V48.1
    disfigurement V48.7
    mechanical V48.3
    motor V48.3
    movement V48.3
    sensory V48.5
    specified condition NEC V48.8
  unemployment V62.0
  urinary NEC V47.4
  voice production V41.4
Procedure (surgical) **not done** NEC V64.3
  because of
    contraindication V64.1
    patient's decision V64.2
      for reasons of conscience or religion
      V62.6
    specified reason NEC V64.3
Procidentia
  anus (sphincter) 569.1
  rectum (sphincter) 569.1
  stomach 537.89
  uteri 618.1
Proctalgia 569.42
  fugax 564.6
  spasmodic 564.6
    psychogenic 307.89
Proctitis 569.49
  amebic 006.8
  chlamydial 099.52
  gonococcal 098.7
  granulomatous 555.1
  idiopathic 556.2

☑ Additional Digit Required — Refer to the Tabular List for Digit Selection   ▽ Subterms under main terms may continue to next column or page

Proctitis — continued
　idiopathic — continued
　　with ulcerative sigmoiditis 556.3
　tuberculous (see also Tuberculosis) 014.8 ☑
　ulcerative (chronic) (nonspecific) 556.2
　　with ulcerative sigmoiditis 556.3
Proctocele
　female (without uterine prolapse) 618.04
　　with uterine prolapse 618.4
　　　complete 618.3
　　　incomplete 618.2
　male 569.49
Proctocolitis, idiopathic 556.2
　with ulcerative sigmoiditis 556.3
Proctoptosis 569.1
Proctosigmoiditis 569.89
　ulcerative (chronic) 556.3
Proctospasm 564.6
　psychogenic 306.4
Prodromal-AIDS — see Human immunodeficiency virus (disease) (illness) (infection)
Profichet's disease or syndrome 729.90
Progeria (adultorum) (syndrome) 259.8
Prognathism (mandibular) (maxillary) 524.10
Progonoma (melanotic) (M9363/0) — see Neoplasm, by site, benign
Progressive — see condition
Prolapse, prolapsed
　anus, anal (canal) (sphincter) 569.1
　arm or hand, complicating delivery 652.7 ☑
　　causing obstructed labor 660.0 ☑
　　　affecting fetus or newborn 763.1
　　fetus or newborn 763.1
　bladder (acquired) (mucosa) (sphincter)
　　congenital (female) (male) 756.71
　　female (see also Cystocele, female) 618.01
　　male 596.89
　breast implant (prosthetic) 996.54
　cecostomy 569.69
　cecum 569.89
　cervix, cervical (hypertrophied) 618.1
　　anterior lip, obstructing labor 660.2 ☑
　　　affecting fetus or newborn 763.1
　　congenital 752.49
　　postpartal (old) 618.1
　　stump 618.84
　ciliary body 871.1
　colon (pedunculated) 569.89
　colostomy 569.69
　conjunctiva 372.73
　cord — see Prolapse, umbilical cord
　cystostomy 596.83
　disc (intervertebral) — see Displacement, intervertebral disc
　duodenum 537.89
　eye implant (orbital) 996.59
　　lens (ocular) 996.53
　fallopian tube 620.4
　fetal extremity, complicating delivery 652.8 ☑
　　causing obstructed labor 660.0 ☑
　　　fetus or newborn 763.1
　funis — see Prolapse, umbilical cord
　gastric (mucosa) 537.89
　genital, female 618.9
　　specified NEC 618.89
　globe 360.81
　ileostomy bud 569.69
　intervertebral disc — see Displacement, intervertebral disc
　intestine (small) 569.89
　iris 364.89
　　traumatic 871.1
　kidney (see also Disease, renal) 593.0
　　congenital 753.3
　laryngeal muscles or ventricle 478.79
　leg, complicating delivery 652.8 ☑
　　causing obstructed labor 660.0 ☑
　　　fetus or newborn 763.1
　liver 573.8
　meatus urinarius 599.5
　mitral valve 424.0
　ocular lens implant 996.53
　organ or site, congenital NEC — see Malposition, congenital

Prolapse, prolapsed — continued
　ovary 620.4
　pelvic (floor), female 618.89
　perineum, female 618.89
　pregnant uterus 654.4 ☑
　rectum (mucosa) (sphincter) 569.1
　　due to Trichuris trichiuria 127.3
　spleen 289.59
　stomach 537.89
　umbilical cord
　　affecting fetus or newborn 762.4
　　complicating delivery 663.0 ☑
　ureter 593.89
　　with obstruction 593.4
　ureterovesical orifice 593.89
　urethra (acquired) (infected) (mucosa) 599.5
　　congenital 753.8
　uterovaginal 618.4
　　complete 618.3
　　incomplete 618.2
　　specified NEC 618.89
　uterus (first degree) (second degree) (third degree) (complete) (without vaginal wall prolapse) 618.1
　　with mention of vaginal wall prolapse — see Prolapse, uterovaginal
　　congenital 752.39
　　in pregnancy or childbirth 654.4 ☑
　　　affecting fetus or newborn 763.1
　　　causing obstructed labor 660.2 ☑
　　　　affecting fetus or newborn 763.1
　　postpartal (old) 618.1
　uveal 871.1
　vagina (anterior) (posterior) (vault) (wall) (without uterine prolapse) 618.00
　　with uterine prolapse 618.4
　　　complete 618.3
　　　incomplete 618.2
　　paravaginal 618.02
　　posthysterectomy 618.5
　　specified NEC 618.09
　vitreous (humor) 379.26
　　traumatic 871.1
　womb — see Prolapse, uterus
Prolapsus, female 618.9
Proliferative — see condition
Prolinemia 270.8
Prolinuria 270.8
Prolonged, prolongation
　bleeding time (see also Defect, coagulation) 790.92
　　"idiopathic" (in von Willebrand's disease) 286.4
　coagulation time (see also Defect, coagulation) 790.92
　gestation syndrome 766.22
　labor 662.1 ☑
　　affecting fetus or newborn 763.89
　　first stage 662.0 ☑
　　second stage 662.2 ☑
　pregnancy 645.2 ☑
　PR interval 426.11
　prothrombin time (see also Defect, coagulation) 790.92
　QT interval 794.31
　　syndrome 426.82
　rupture of membranes (24 hours or more prior to onset of labor) 658.2 ☑
　uterine contractions in labor 661.4 ☑
　　affecting fetus or newborn 763.7
Prominauris 744.29
Prominence
　auricle (ear) (congenital) 744.29
　　acquired 380.32
　ischial spine or sacral promontory
　　with disproportion (fetopelvic) 653.3 ☑
　　　affecting fetus or newborn 763.1
　　　causing obstructed labor 660.1 ☑
　　　　affecting fetus or newborn 763.1
　nose (congenital) 748.1
　　acquired 738.0
PROMM (proximal myotonic myotonia) 359.21
Pronation
　ankle 736.79
　foot 736.79
　　congenital 755.67

Prophylactic
　administration of
　　antibiotics, long-term V58.62
　　　short-term — omit code
　　antitoxin, any V07.2
　　antivenin V07.2
　　chemotherapeutic agent NEC V07.39
　　　fluoride V07.31
　　diphtheria antitoxin V07.2
　　drug V07.39
　　exemestar (Aromasin) V07.52
　　gamma globulin V07.2
　　immune sera (gamma globulin) V07.2
　　RhoGAM V07.2
　　tetanus antitoxin V07.2
　chemotherapy NEC V07.39
　　fluoride V07.31
　hormone replacement (postmenopausal) V07.4
　immunotherapy V07.2
　measure V07.9
　　specified type NEC V07.8
　medication V07.39
　postmenopausal hormone replacement V07.4
　sterilization V25.2
Proptosis (ocular) — see also Exophthalmos 376.30
　thyroid 242.0 ☑
Propulsion
　eyeball 360.81
Prosecution, anxiety concerning V62.5
Prosopagnosia 368.16
Prostate, prostatic — see condition
Prostatism 600.90
　with
　　other lower urinary tract symptoms (LUTS) 600.91
　　urinary
　　　obstruction 600.91
　　　retention 600.91
Prostatitis (congestive) (suppurative) 601.9
　acute 601.0
　cavitary 601.8
　chlamydial 099.54
　chronic 601.1
　diverticular 601.8
　due to Trichomonas (vaginalis) 131.03
　fibrous 600.90
　　with
　　　other lower urinary tract symptoms (LUTS) 600.91
　　　urinary
　　　　obstruction 600.91
　　　　retention 600.91
　gonococcal (acute) 098.12
　　chronic or duration of 2 months or over 098.32
　granulomatous 601.8
　hypertrophic 600.00
　　with
　　　other lower urinary tract symptoms (LUTS) 600.01
　　　urinary
　　　　obstruction 600.01
　　　　retention 600.01
　specified type NEC 601.8
　subacute 601.1
　trichomonal 131.03
　tuberculous (see also Tuberculosis) 016.5 ☑ [601.4]
Prostatocystitis 601.3
Prostatorrhea 602.8
Prostatoseminovesiculitis, trichomonal 131.03
Prostration 780.79
　heat 992.5
　　anhydrotic 992.3
　　due to
　　　salt (and water) depletion 992.4
　　　water depletion 992.3
　nervous 300.5
　newborn 779.89
　senile 797
Protanomaly 368.51

Protanopia (anomalous trichromat) (complete) (incomplete) 368.51
Protection (against) (from) — see Prophylactic
Protein
　deficiency 260
　malnutrition 260
　sickness (prophylactic) (therapeutic) 999.59
Proteinemia 790.99
Proteinosis
　alveolar, lung or pulmonary 516.0
　lipid 272.8
　lipoid (of Urbach) 272.8
Proteinuria — see also Albuminuria 791.0
　Bence-Jones NEC 791.0
　gestational 646.2 ☑
　　with hypertension — see Toxemia, of pregnancy
　orthostatic 593.6
　postural 593.6
Proteolysis, pathologic 286.6
Protocoproporphyria 277.1
Protoporphyria (erythrohepatic) (erythropoietic) 277.1
Protrusio acetabuli 718.65
Protrusion
　acetabulum (into pelvis) 718.65
　device, implant, or graft — see Complications, mechanical
　ear, congenital 744.29
　intervertebral disc — see Displacement, intervertebral disc
　nucleus pulposus — see Displacement, intervertebral disc
Proud flesh 701.5
Prune belly (syndrome) 756.71
Prurigo (ferox) (gravis) (Hebra's) (hebrae) (mitis) (simplex) 698.2
　agria 698.3
　asthma syndrome 691.8
　Besnier's (atopic dermatitis) (infantile eczema) 691.8
　eczematodes allergicum 691.8
　estivalis (Hutchinson's) 692.72
　Hutchinson's 692.72
　nodularis 698.3
　psychogenic 306.3
Pruritus, pruritic 698.9
　ani 698.0
　　psychogenic 306.3
　conditions NEC 698.9
　　psychogenic 306.3
　due to Onchocerca volvulus 125.3
　ear 698.9
　essential 698.9
　genital organ(s) 698.1
　　psychogenic 306.3
　gravidarum 646.8 ☑
　hiemalis 698.8
　neurogenic (any site) 306.3
　perianal 698.0
　psychogenic (any site) 306.3
　scrotum 698.1
　　psychogenic 306.3
　senile, senilis 698.8
　Trichomonas 131.9
　vulva, vulvae 698.1
　　psychogenic 306.3
Psammocarcinoma (M8140/3) — see Neoplasm, by site, malignant
Pseudarthrosis, pseudoarthrosis (bone) 733.82
　joint following fusion V45.4
Pseudo-Argyll-Robertson pupil 379.45
Pseudo-Hurler's disease (mucolipidosis III) 272.7
Pseudo-obstruction
　intestine (chronic) (idiopathic) (intermittent secondary) (primary) 564.89
　　acute 560.89
Pseudo-Turner's syndrome 759.89
Pseudoacanthosis
　nigricans 701.8
Pseudoaneurysm — see Aneurysm
Pseudoangina (pectoris) — see Angina
Pseudoangioma 452
Pseudoarteriosus 747.89

☑ **Additional Digit Required — Refer to the Tabular List for Digit Selection**　　　　　　　▽ **Subterms under main terms may continue to next column or page**

240 — Volume 2　　　　　　　▶◀ **Revised Text**　　　● **New Line**　　　▲ **Revised Code**　　　　　　　**2014 ICD-9-CM**

Pseudoarthrosis — see Pseudarthrosis
Pseudoataxia 799.89
Pseudobulbar affect (PBA) 310.81
Pseudobursa 727.89
Pseudocholera 025
Pseudochromidrosis 705.89
Pseudocirrhosis, liver, pericardial 423.2
Pseudocoarctation 747.21
Pseudocowpox 051.1
Pseudocoxalgia 732.1
Pseudocroup 478.75
Pseudocyesis 300.11
Pseudocyst
  lung 518.89
  pancreas 577.2
  retina 361.19
Pseudodementia 300.16
Pseudoelephantiasis neuroarthritica 757.0
Pseudoemphysema 518.89
Pseudoencephalitis
  superior (acute) hemorrhagic 265.1
Pseudoerosion cervix, congenital 752.49
Pseudoexfoliation, lens capsule 366.11
Pseudofracture (idiopathic) (multiple) (spontaneous) (symmetrical) 268.2
Pseudoglanders 025
Pseudoglioma 360.44
Pseudogout — see Chondrocalcinosis
Pseudohallucination 780.1
Pseudohemianesthesia 782.0
Pseudohemophilia (Bernuth's) (hereditary) (typeB) 286.4
  type A 287.8
  vascular 287.8
Pseudohermaphroditism 752.7
  with chromosomal anomaly — see Anomaly, chromosomal
  adrenal 255.2
  female (without adrenocortical disorder) 752.7
    with adrenocortical disorder 255.2
    adrenal 255.2
  male (without gonadal disorder) 752.7
    with
      adrenocortical disorder 255.2
      cleft scrotum 752.7
      feminizing testis 259.51
      gonadal disorder 257.9
      adrenal 255.2
Pseudohole, macula 362.54
Pseudohydrocephalus 348.2
Pseudohypertrophic muscular dystrophy (Erb's) 359.1
Pseudohypertrophy, muscle 359.1
Pseudohypoparathyroidism 275.49
Pseudoinfluenza — see also Influenza 487.1
Pseudoinsomnia 307.49
Pseudoleukemia 288.8
  infantile 285.8
Pseudomembranous — see condition
Pseudomeningocele (cerebral) (infective) 349.2
  postprocedural 997.01
  spinal 349.2
Pseudomenstruation 626.8
Pseudomucinous
  cyst (ovary) (M8470/0) 220
  peritoneum 568.89
Pseudomyeloma 273.1
Pseudomyxoma peritonei (M8480/6) 197.6
Pseudoneuritis optic (nerve) 377.24
  papilla 377.24
    congenital 743.57
Pseudoneuroma — see Injury, nerve, by site
Pseudopapilledema 377.24
Pseudoparalysis
  arm or leg 781.4
  atonic, congenital 358.8
Pseudopelade 704.09
Pseudophakia V43.1
Pseudopolycythemia 289.0
Pseudopolyposis, colon 556.4
Pseudoporencephaly 348.0
Pseudopseudohypoparathyroidism 275.49
Pseudopsychosis 300.16
Pseudopterygium 372.52

Pseudoptosis (eyelid) 374.34
Pseudorabies 078.89
Pseudoretinitis, pigmentosa 362.65
Pseudorickets 588.0
  senile (Pozzi's) 731.0
Pseudorubella 057.8
Pseudoscarlatina 057.8
Pseudosclerema 778.1
Pseudosclerosis (brain)
  Jakob's 046.19
  of Westphal (-Strümpell) (hepatolenticular degeneration) 275.1
  spastic 046.19
    with dementia
      with behavioral disturbance 046.19 *[294.11]*
      without behavioral disturbance 046.19 *[294.10]*
Pseudoseizure 780.39
  non-psychiatric 780.39
  psychiatric 300.11
Pseudotabes 799.89
  diabetic 250.6 ☑ *[337.1]*
    due to secondary diabetes 249.6 ☑ *[337.1]*
Pseudotetanus — see also Convulsions 780.39
Pseudotetany 781.7
  hysterical 300.11
Pseudothalassemia 285.0
Pseudotrichinosis 710.3
Pseudotruncus arteriosus 747.29
Pseudotuberculosis, pasteurella (infection) 027.2
Pseudotumor
  cerebri 348.2
  orbit (inflammatory) 376.11
Pseudoxanthoma elasticum 757.39
Psilosis (sprue) (tropical) 579.1
  Monilia 112.89
  nontropical 579.0
  not sprue 704.00
Psittacosis 073.9
Psoitis 728.89
Psora NEC 696.1
Psoriasis 696.1
  any type, except arthropathic 696.1
  arthritic, arthropathic 696.0
  buccal 528.6
  flexural 696.1
  follicularis 696.1
  guttate 696.1
  inverse 696.1
  mouth 528.6
  nummularis 696.1
  psychogenic 316 *[696.1]*
  punctata 696.1
  pustular 696.1
  rupioides 696.1
  vulgaris 696.1
Psorospermiasis 136.4
Psorospermosis 136.4
  follicularis (vegetans) 757.39
Psychalgia 307.80
Psychasthenia 300.89
  compulsive 300.3
  mixed compulsive states 300.3
  obsession 300.3
Psychiatric disorder or problem NEC 300.9
Psychogenic — see also condition
  factors associated with physical conditions 316
Psychoneurosis, psychoneurotic — see also
  Neurosis 300.9
  anxiety (state) 300.00
  climacteric 627.2
  compensation 300.16
  compulsion 300.3
  conversion hysteria 300.11
  depersonalization 300.6
  depressive type 300.4
  dissociative hysteria 300.15
  hypochondriacal 300.7
  hysteria 300.10
    conversion type 300.11
    dissociative type 300.15
  mixed NEC 300.89

Psychoneurosis, psychoneurotic — see also
  Neurosis — continued
  neurasthenic 300.5
  obsessional 300.3
  obsessive-compulsive 300.3
  occupational 300.89
  personality NEC 301.89
  phobia 300.20
  senile NEC 300.89
Psychopathic — see also condition
  constitution, posttraumatic 310.2
    with psychosis 293.9
  personality 301.9
    amoral trends 301.7
    antisocial trends 301.7
    asocial trends 301.7
    mixed types 301.7
  state 301.9
Psychopathy, sexual — see also Deviation, sexual 302.9
Psychophysiologic, psychophysiological condition — see Reaction, psychophysiologic
Psychose passionelle 297.8
Psychosexual identity disorder 302.6
  adult-life 302.85
  childhood 302.6
Psychosis 298.9
  acute hysterical 298.1
  affecting management of pregnancy, childbirth, or puerperium 648.4 ☑
  affective (see also Disorder, mood) 296.90

> Note — Use the following fifth-digit subclassification with categories 296.0–296.6:
>
> 0   unspecified
>
> 1   mild
>
> 2   moderate
>
> 3   severe, without mention of psychotic behavior
>
> 4   severe, specified as with psychotic behavior
>
> 5   in partial or unspecified remission
>
> 6   in full remission

    drug-induced 292.84
    due to or associated with physical condition 293.83
    involutional 293.83
      recurrent episode 296.3 ☑
      single episode 296.2 ☑
    manic-depressive 296.80
      circular (alternating) 296.7
        currently depressed 296.5 ☑
        currently manic 296.4 ☑
      depressed type 296.2 ☑
        atypical 296.82
        recurrent episode 296.3 ☑
        single episode 296.2 ☑
      manic 296.0 ☑
        atypical 296.81
        recurrent episode 296.1 ☑
        single episode 296.0 ☑
      mixed type NEC 296.89
      specified type NEC 296.89
    senile 290.21
    specified type NEC 296.99
  alcoholic 291.9
    with
      anxiety 291.89
      delirium tremens 291.0
      delusions 291.5
      dementia 291.2
      hallucinosis 291.3
      jealousy 291.5
      mood disturbance 291.89
      paranoia 291.5
      persisting amnesia 291.1
      sexual dysfunction 291.89
      sleep disturbance 291.89
    amnestic confabulatory 291.1
    delirium tremens 291.0
    hallucinosis 291.3

Psychosis — continued
  alcoholic — continued
    Korsakoff's, Korsakov's, Korsakow's 291.1
    paranoid type 291.5
    pathological intoxication 291.4
    polyneuritic 291.1
    specified type NEC 291.89
  alternating (see also Psychosis, manic-depressive, circular) 296.7
  anergastic (see also Psychosis, organic) 294.9
  arteriosclerotic 290.40
    with
      acute confusional state 290.41
      delirium 290.41
      delusions 290.42
      depressed mood 290.43
    depressed type 290.43
    paranoid type 290.42
    simple type 290.40
    uncomplicated 290.40
  atypical 298.9
    depressive 296.82
    manic 296.81
  borderline (schizophrenia) (see also Schizophrenia) 295.5 ☑
    of childhood (see also Psychosis, childhood) 299.8 ☑
    prepubertal 299.8 ☑
  brief reactive 298.8
  childhood, with origin specific to 299.9 ☑

> Note — Use the following fifth-digit subclassification with category 299:
>
> 0   current or active state
>
> 1   residual state

    atypical 299.8 ☑
    specified type NEC 299.8 ☑
  circular (see also Psychosis, manic-depressive, circular) 296.7
  climacteric (see also Psychosis, involutional) 298.8
  confusional 298.9
    acute 293.0
    reactive 298.2
    subacute 293.1
  depressive (see also Psychosis, affective) 296.2 ☑
    atypical 296.82
    involutional 296.2 ☑
      with hypomania (bipolar II) 296.89
      recurrent episode 296.3 ☑
      single episode 296.2 ☑
    psychogenic 298.0
    reactive (emotional stress) (psychological trauma) 298.0
    recurrent episode 296.3 ☑
      with hypomania (bipolar II) 296.89
    single episode 296.2 ☑
  disintegrative, childhood (see also Psychosis, childhood) 299.1 ☑
  drug 292.9
    with
      affective syndrome 292.84
      amnestic syndrome 292.83
      anxiety 292.89
      delirium 292.81
        withdrawal 292.0
      delusions 292.11
      dementia 292.82
      depressive state 292.84
      hallucinations 292.12
      hallucinosis 292.12
      mood disorder 292.84
      mood disturbance 292.84
      organic personality syndrome NEC 292.89
      sexual dysfunction 292.89
      sleep disturbance 292.89
      withdrawal syndrome (and delirium) 292.0
    affective syndrome 292.84
    delusions 292.11
    hallucinatory state 292.12
    hallucinosis 292.12
    paranoid state 292.11

☑ Additional Digit Required — Refer to the Tabular List for Digit Selection   ▽ Subterms under main terms may continue to next column or page

2014 ICD-9-CM   ▶◀ Revised Text   ● New Line   ▲ Revised Code   **Volume 2 — 241**

Index

Pseudoarthrosis — Psychosis

Psychosis — *continued*
  drug — *continued*
    specified type NEC 292.89
    withdrawal syndrome (and delirium) 292.0
  due to or associated with physical condition (*see also* Psychosis, organic) 293.9
  epileptic NEC 293.9
  excitation (psychogenic) (reactive) 298.1
  exhaustive (*see also* Reaction, stress, acute) 308.9
  hypomanic (*see also* Psychosis, affective) 296.0 ☑
    recurrent episode 296.1 ☑
    single episode 296.0 ☑
  hysterical 298.8
    acute 298.1
  in
    conditions classified elsewhere
      with
        delusions 293.81
        hallucinations 293.82
    pregnancy, childbirth, or puerperium 648.4 ☑
  incipient 298.8
    schizophrenic (*see also* Schizophrenia) 295.5 ☑
  induced 297.3
  infantile (*see also* Psychosis, childhood) 299.0 ☑
  infective 293.9
    acute 293.0
    subacute 293.1
  interactional (childhood) (*see also* Psychosis, childhood) 299.1 ☑
  involutional 298.8
    depressive (*see also* Psychosis, affective) 296.2 ☑
      recurrent episode 296.3 ☑
      single episode 296.2 ☑
    melancholic 296.2 ☑
      recurrent episode 296.3 ☑
      single episode 296.2 ☑
    paranoid state 297.2
    paraphrenia 297.2
  Korsakoff's, Korakov's, Korsakow's (nonalcoholic) 294.0
    alcoholic 291.1
  mania (phase) (*see also* Psychosis, affective) 296.0 ☑
    recurrent episode 296.1 ☑
    single episode 296.0 ☑
  manic-depressive 296.80
    circular 296.7
      currently
        depressed 296.5 ☑
        manic 296.4 ☑
      mixed 296.6 ☑
    depressive 296.2 ☑
      recurrent episode 296.3 ☑
        with hypomania (bipolar II) 296.89
      single episode 296.2 ☑
    hypomanic 296.0 ☑
      recurrent episode 296.1 ☑
      single episode 296.0 ☑
    manic 296.0 ☑
      atypical 296.81
      recurrent episode 296.1 ☑
      single episode 296.0 ☑
    mixed NEC 296.89
    perplexed 296.89
    stuporous 296.89
  manic (*see also* Psychosis, affective) 296.0 ☑
    atypical 296.81
    recurrent episode 296.1 ☑
    single episode 296.0 ☑
  menopausal (*see also* Psychosis, involutional) 298.8
  mixed schizophrenic and affective (*see also* Schizophrenia) 295.7 ☑
  multi-infarct (cerebrovascular) (*see also* Psychosis, arteriosclerotic) 290.40
  organic NEC 294.9

Psychosis — *continued*
  organic — *continued*
    due to or associated with
      addiction
        alcohol (*see also* Psychosis, alcoholic) 291.9
        drug (*see also* Psychosis, drug) 292.9
      alcohol intoxication, acute (*see also* Psychosis, alcoholic) 291.9
      alcoholism (*see also* Psychosis, alcoholic) 291.9
      arteriosclerosis (cerebral) (*see also* Psychosis, arteriosclerotic) 290.40
      cerebrovascular disease
        acute (psychosis) 293.0
        arteriosclerotic (*see also* Psychosis, arteriosclerotic) 290.40
      childbirth — *see* Psychosis, puerperal
      dependence
        alcohol (*see also* Psychosis, alcoholic) 291.9
        drug 292.9
      disease
        alcoholic liver (*see also* Psychosis, alcoholic) 291.9
        brain
          arteriosclerotic (*see also* Psychosis, arteriosclerotic) 290.40
          cerebrovascular
            acute (psychosis) 293.0
            arteriosclerotic (*see also* Psychosis, arteriosclerotic) 290.40
        endocrine or metabolic 293.9
          acute (psychosis) 293.0
          subacute (psychosis) 293.1
        Jakob-Creutzfeldt 046.19
          with behavioral disturbance 046.19 *[294.11]*
          without behavioral disturbance 046.19 *[294.10]*
          familial 046.19
          iatrogenic 046.19
          specified NEC 046.19
          sporadic 046.19
          variant 046.11
            with dementia
              with behavioral disturbance 046.11 *[294.11]*
              without behavioral disturbance 046.11 *[294.10]*
        liver, alcoholic (*see also* Psychosis, alcoholic) 291.9
      disorder
        cerebrovascular
          acute (psychosis) 293.0
        endocrine or metabolic 293.9
          acute (psychosis) 293.0
          subacute (psychosis) 293.1
      epilepsy
        with behavioral disturbance 345.9 *[294.11]*
        without behavioral disturbance 345.9 *[294.10]*
        transient (acute) 293.0
      Huntington's chorea
        with behavioral disturbance 333.4 *[294.11]*
        without behavioral disturbance 333.4 *[294.10]*
      infection
        brain 293.9
          acute (psychosis) 293.0
          chronic 294.8
          subacute (psychosis) 293.1
        intracranial NEC 293.9
          acute (psychosis) 293.0
          chronic 294.8
          subacute (psychosis) 293.1

Psychosis — *continued*
  organic — *continued*
    due to or associated with — *continued*
      intoxication
        alcoholic (acute) (*see also* Psychosis, alcoholic) 291.9
        pathological 291.4
        drug (*see also* Psychosis, drug) 292.9
      ischemia
        cerebrovascular (generalized) (*see also* Psychosis, arteriosclerotic) 290.40
      Jakob-Creutzfeldt disease (syndrome) 046.19
        with behavioral disturbance 046.19 *[294.11]*
        without behavioral disturbance 046.19 *[294.10]*
        variant 046.11
          with dementia
            with behavioral disturbance 046.11 *[294.11]*
            without behavioral disturbance 046.11 *[294.10]*
      multiple sclerosis
        with behavioral disturbance 340 *[294.11]*
        without behavioral disturbance 340 *[294.10]*
      physical condition NEC 293.9
        with
          delusions 293.81
          hallucinations 293.82
      presenility 290.10
      puerperium — *see* Psychosis, puerperal
      sclerosis, multiple
        with behavioral disturbance 340 *[294.11]*
        without behavioral disturbance 340 *[294.10]*
      senility 290.20
      status epilepticus
        with behavioral disturbance 345.3 *[294.11]*
        without behavioral disturbance 345.3 *[294.10]*
      trauma
        brain (birth) (from electrical current) (surgical) 293.9
        acute (psychosis) 293.0
        chronic 294.8
        subacute (psychosis) 293.1
        unspecified physical condition 293.9
          with
            delusion 293.81
            hallucinations 293.82
    infective 293.9
      acute (psychosis) 293.0
      subacute 293.1
    posttraumatic 293.9
      acute 293.0
      subacute 293.1
    specified type NEC 294.8
    transient 293.9
      with
        anxiety 293.84
        delusions 293.81
        depression 293.83
        hallucinations 293.82
      depressive type 293.83
      hallucinatory type 293.82
      paranoid type 293.81
      specified type NEC 293.89
  paranoic 297.1
  paranoid (chronic) 297.9
    alcoholic 291.5
    chronic 297.1
    climacteric 297.2
    involutional 297.2
    menopausal 297.2

Psychosis — *continued*
  paranoid — *continued*
    protracted reactive 298.4
    psychogenic 298.4
      acute 298.3
    schizophrenic (*see also* Schizophrenia) 295.3 ☑
    senile 290.20
  paroxysmal 298.9
    senile 290.20
  polyneuritic, alcoholic 291.1
  postoperative 293.9
  postpartum — *see* Psychosis, puerperal
  prepsychotic (*see also* Schizophrenia) 295.5 ☑
  presbyophrenic (type) 290.8
  presenile (*see also* Dementia, presenile) 290.10
  prison 300.16
  psychogenic 298.8
    depressive 298.0
    paranoid 298.4
      acute 298.3
  puerperal
    specified type — *see* categories 295-298 ☑
    unspecified type 293.89
      acute 293.0
      chronic 293.89
      subacute 293.1
  reactive (emotional stress) (psychological trauma) 298.8
    brief 298.8
    confusion 298.2
    depressive 298.0
    excitation 298.1
  schizo-affective (depressed) (excited) (*see also* Schizophrenia) 295.7 ☑
  schizophrenia, schizophrenic (*see also* Schizophrenia) 295.9 ☑
    borderline type 295.5 ☑
      of childhood (*see also* Psychosis, childhood) 299.8 ☑
    catatonic (excited) (withdrawn) 295.2 ☑
    childhood type (*see also* Psychosis, childhood) 299.9 ☑
    hebephrenic 295.1 ☑
    incipient 295.5 ☑
    latent 295.5 ☑
    paranoid 295.3 ☑
    prepsychotic 295.5 ☑
    prodromal 295.5 ☑
    pseudoneurotic 295.5 ☑
    pseudopsychopathic 295.5 ☑
    schizophreniform 295.4 ☑
    simple 295.0 ☑
    undifferentiated type 295.9 ☑
  schizophreniform 295.4 ☑
  senile NEC 290.20
    with
      delusional features 290.20
      depressive features 290.21
    depressed type 290.21
    paranoid type 290.20
    simple deterioration 290.20
    specified type — *see* categories 295-298 ☑
  shared 297.3
  situational (reactive) 298.8
  symbiotic (childhood) (*see also* Psychosis, childhood) 299.1 ☑
  toxic (acute) 293.9
Psychotic — *see also* condition 298.9
  episode 298.9
    due to or associated with physical conditions (*see also* Psychosis, organic) 293.9
Pterygium (eye) 372.40
  central 372.43
  colli 744.5
  double 372.44
  peripheral (stationary) 372.41
    progressive 372.42
  recurrent 372.45
Ptilosis 374.55

☑ **Additional Digit Required** — Refer to the Tabular List for Digit Selection   ▽ **Subterms under main terms may continue to next column or page**

Psychosis — Ptilosis

242 — Volume 2   ▶◀ Revised Text   ● New Line   ▲ Revised Code   **2014 ICD-9-CM**

PTLD (post-transplant lymphoproliferative disorder) 238.77
Ptomaine (poisoning) — *see also* Poisoning, food 005.9
Ptosis (adiposa) 374.30
  breast 611.81
  cecum 569.89
  colon 569.89
  congenital (eyelid) 743.61
    specified site NEC — *see* Anomaly, specified type NEC
  epicanthus syndrome 270.2
  eyelid 374.30
    congenital 743.61
    mechanical 374.33
    myogenic 374.32
    paralytic 374.31
  gastric 537.5
  intestine 569.89
  kidney (*see also* Disease, renal) 593.0
    congenital 753.3
  liver 573.8
  renal (*see also* Disease, renal) 593.0
    congenital 753.3
  splanchnic 569.89
  spleen 289.59
  stomach 537.5
  viscera 569.89
PTP (posttransfusion purpura) 287.41
PTSD (Post-traumatic stress disorder) 309.81
Ptyalism 527.7
  hysterical 300.11
  periodic 527.2
  pregnancy 646.8 ☑
  psychogenic 306.4
Ptyalolithiasis 527.5
Pubalgia 848.8
Pubarche, precocious 259.1
Pubertas praecox 259.1
Puberty V21.1
  abnormal 259.9
  bleeding 626.3
  delayed 259.0
  precocious (constitutional) (cryptogenic) (idiopathic) NEC 259.1
    due to
      adrenal
        cortical hyperfunction 255.2
        hyperplasia 255.2
      cortical hyperfunction 255.2
      ovarian hyperfunction 256.1
        estrogen 256.0
      pineal tumor 259.8
      testicular hyperfunction 257.0
  premature 259.1
    due to
      adrenal cortical hyperfunction 255.2
      pineal tumor 259.8
      pituitary (anterior) hyperfunction 253.1
Puckering, macula 362.56
Pudenda, pudendum — *see* condition
Puente's disease (simple glandular cheilitis) 528.5
Puerperal
  abscess
    areola 675.1 ☑
    Bartholin's gland 646.6 ☑
    breast 675.1 ☑
    cervix (uteri) 670.8 ☑
    fallopian tube 670.8 ☑
    genital organ 670.8 ☑
    kidney 646.6 ☑
    mammary 675.1 ☑
    mesosalpinx 670.8 ☑
    nabothian 646.6 ☑
    nipple 675.0 ☑
    ovary, ovarian 670.8 ☑
    oviduct 670.8 ☑
    para-uterine 670.8 ☑
    parametric 670.8 ☑
    pelvic 670.8 ☑
    perimetric 670.8 ☑
    periuterine 670.8 ☑
    retro-uterine 670.8 ☑
    subareolar 675.1 ☑

Puerperal — *continued*
  abscess — *continued*
    suprapelvic 670.8 ☑
    tubal (ruptured) 670.8 ☑
    tubo-ovarian 670.8 ☑
    urinary tract NEC 646.6 ☑
    uterine, uterus 670.8 ☑
    vagina (wall) 646.6 ☑
    vaginorectal 646.6 ☑
    vulvovaginal gland 646.6 ☑
  accident 674.9 ☑
  adnexitis 670.8 ☑
  afibrinogenemia, or other coagulation defect 666.3 ☑
  albuminuria (acute) (subacute) 646.2 ☑
    pre-eclamptic 642.4 ☑
  anemia (conditions classifiable to 280–285) 648.2 ☑
  anuria 669.3 ☑
  apoplexy 674.0 ☑
  asymptomatic bacteriuria 646.5 ☑
  atrophy, breast 676.3 ☑
  blood dyscrasia 666.3 ☑
  caked breast 676.2 ☑
  cardiomyopathy 674.5 ☑
  cellulitis — *see* Puerperal, abscess
  cerebrovascular disorder (conditions classifiable to 430–434, 436–437) 674.0 ☑
  cervicitis (conditions classifiable to 616.0) 646.6 ☑
  coagulopathy (any) 666.3 ☑
  complications 674.9 ☑
    specified type NEC 674.8 ☑
  convulsions (eclamptic) (uremic) 642.6 ☑
    with pre-existing hypertension 642.7 ☑
  cracked nipple 676.1 ☑
  cystitis 646.6 ☑
  cystopyelitis 646.6 ☑
  deciduitis (acute) 670.8 ☑
  delirium NEC 293.9
  diabetes (mellitus) (conditions classifiable to 249 and 250) 648.0 ☑
  disease 674.9 ☑
    breast NEC 676.3 ☑
    cerebrovascular (acute) 674.0 ☑
    nonobstetric NEC (*see also* Pregnancy, complicated, current disease or condition) 648.9 ☑
    pelvis inflammatory 670.8 ☑
    renal NEC 646.2 ☑
    tubo-ovarian 670.8 ☑
    Valsuani's (progressive pernicious anemia) 648.2 ☑
  disorder
    lactation 676.9 ☑
      specified type NEC 676.8 ☑
    nonobstetric NEC (*see also* Pregnancy, complicated, current disease or condition) 648.9 ☑
  disruption
    cesarean wound 674.1 ☑
    episiotomy wound 674.2 ☑
    perineal laceration wound 674.2 ☑
  drug dependence (conditions classifiable to 304) 648.3 ☑
  eclampsia 642.6 ☑
    with pre-existing hypertension 642.7 ☑
  embolism (pulmonary) 673.2 ☑
    air 673.0 ☑
    amniotic fluid 673.1 ☑
    blood-clot 673.2 ☑
    brain or cerebral 674.0 ☑
    cardiac 674.8 ☑
    fat 673.8 ☑
    intracranial sinus (venous) 671.5 ☑
    pyemic 673.3 ☑
    septic 673.3 ☑
    spinal cord 671.5 ☑
  endometritis (conditions classifiable to 615.0–615.9) 670.1 ☑
  endophlebitis — *see* Puerperal, phlebitis
  endotrachelitis 646.6 ☑
  engorgement, breasts 676.2 ☑
  erysipelas 670.8 ☑

Puerperal — *continued*
  failure
    lactation 676.4 ☑
    renal, acute 669.3 ☑
  fever 672 ☑
    meaning pyrexia (of unknown origin) 672.0 ☑
    meaning sepsis 670.2 ☑
  fissure, nipple 676.1 ☑
  fistula
    breast 675.1 ☑
    mammary gland 675.1 ☑
    nipple 675.0 ☑
  galactophoritis 675.2 ☑
  galactorrhea 676.6 ☑
  gangrene
    gas 670.8 ☑
      with sepsis 670.2 ☑
    uterus 670.8 ☑
  gonorrhea (conditions classifiable to 098) 647.1 ☑
  hematoma, subdural 674.0 ☑
  hematosalpinx, infectional 670.8 ☑
  hemiplegia, cerebral 674.0 ☑
  hemorrhage 666.1 ☑
    brain 674.0 ☑
    bulbar 674.0 ☑
    cerebellar 674.0 ☑
    cerebral 674.0 ☑
    cortical 674.0 ☑
    delayed (after 24 hours) (uterine) 666.2 ☑
    extradural 674.0 ☑
    internal capsule 674.0 ☑
    intracranial 674.0 ☑
    intrapontine 674.0 ☑
    meningeal 674.0 ☑
    pontine 674.0 ☑
    subarachnoid 674.0 ☑
    subcortical 674.0 ☑
    subdural 674.0 ☑
    uterine, delayed 666.2 ☑
    ventricular 674.0 ☑
  hemorrhoids 671.8 ☑
  hepatorenal syndrome 674.8 ☑
  hypertrophy
    breast 676.3 ☑
    mammary gland 676.3 ☑
  induration breast (fibrous) 676.3 ☑
  infarction
    lung — *see* Puerperal, embolism
    pulmonary — *see* Puerperal, embolism
  infection
    Bartholin's gland 646.6 ☑
    breast 675.2 ☑
      with nipple 675.9 ☑
        specified type NEC 675.8 ☑
    cervix 646.6 ☑
    endocervix 646.6 ☑
    fallopian tube 670.8 ☑
    generalized 670.0 ☑
    genital tract (major) 670.0 ☑
      minor or localized 646.6 ☑
    kidney (bacillus coli) 646.6 ☑
    mammary gland 675.2 ☑
      with nipple 675.9 ☑
        specified type NEC 675.8 ☑
    nipple 675.0 ☑
      with breast 675.9 ☑
        specified type NEC 675.8 ☑
    ovary 670.8 ☑
    pelvic 670.8 ☑
    peritoneum 670.8 ☑
    renal 646.6 ☑
    tubo-ovarian 670.8 ☑
    urinary (tract) NEC 646.6 ☑
      asymptomatic 646.5 ☑
    uterus, uterine 670.8 ☑
    vagina 646.6 ☑
  inflammation (*see also* Puerperal, infection)
    areola 675.1 ☑
    Bartholin's gland 646.6 ☑
    breast 675.2 ☑

Puerperal — *continued*
  inflammation (*see also* Puerperal, infection) — *continued*
    broad ligament 670.8 ☑
    cervix (uteri) 646.6 ☑
    fallopian tube 670.8 ☑
    genital organs 670.8 ☑
      localized 646.6 ☑
    mammary gland 675.2 ☑
    nipple 675.0 ☑
    ovary 670.8 ☑
    oviduct 670.8 ☑
    pelvis 670.8 ☑
    periuterine 670.8 ☑
    tubal 670.8 ☑
    vagina 646.6 ☑
    vein — *see* Puerperal, phlebitis
  inversion, nipple 676.3 ☑
  ischemia, cerebral 674.0 ☑
  lymphangitis 670.8 ☑
    breast 675.2 ☑
  malaria (conditions classifiable to 084) 647.4 ☑
  malnutrition 648.9 ☑
  mammillitis 675.0 ☑
  mammitis 675.2 ☑
  mania 296.0
    recurrent episode 296.1
    single episode 296.0
  mastitis 675.2 ☑
    purulent 675.1 ☑
    retromammary 675.1 ☑
    submammary 675.1 ☑
  melancholia 296.2 ☑
    recurrent episode 296.3 ☑
    single episode 296.2 ☑
  mental disorder (conditions classifiable to 290–303, 305.0, 305.2–305.9, 306–316, 317–319) 648.4 ☑
  metritis (suppurative) 670.1 ☑
    septic 670.2 ☑
  metroperitonitis 670.8 ☑
  metrorrhagia 666.2 ☑
  metrosalpingitis 670.8 ☑
  metrovaginitis 670.8 ☑
  milk leg 671.4 ☑
  monoplegia, cerebral 674.0 ☑
  necrosis
    kidney, tubular 669.3 ☑
    liver (acute) (subacute) (conditions classifiable to 570) 674.8 ☑
    ovary 670.8 ☑
    renal cortex 669.3 ☑
  nephritis or nephrosis (conditions classifiable to 580–589) 646.2 ☑
    with hypertension 642.1 ☑
  nutritional deficiency (conditions classifiable to 260–269) 648.9 ☑
  occlusion, precerebral artery 674.0 ☑
  oliguria 669.3 ☑
  oophoritis 670.8 ☑
  ovaritis 670.8 ☑
  paralysis
    bladder (sphincter) 665.5 ☑
    cerebral 674.0 ☑
  paralytic stroke 674.0 ☑
  parametritis 670.8 ☑
  paravaginitis 646.6 ☑
  pelviperitonitis 670.8 ☑
  perimetritis 670.8 ☑
  perimetrosalpingitis 670.8 ☑
  perinephritis 646.6 ☑
  perioophoritis 670.8 ☑
  periphlebitis — *see* Puerperal, phlebitis
  perisalpingitis 670.8 ☑
  peritoneal infection 670.8 ☑
  peritonitis (pelvic) 670.8 ☑
  perivaginitis 646.6 ☑
  phlebitis 671.2 ☑
    deep 671.4 ☑
    intracranial sinus (venous) 671.5 ☑
    pelvic 671.4 ☑
    specified site NEC 671.5 ☑

☑ **Additional Digit Required** — Refer to the Tabular List for Digit Selection   ▽ **Subterms under main terms may continue to next column or page**

2014 ICD-9-CM   ▶◀ **Revised Text**   ● **New Line**   ▲ **Revised Code**   **Volume 2 — 243**

Puerperal — *continued*
phlebitis — *continued*
superficial 671.2 ✓
phlegmasia alba dolens 671.4 ✓
placental polyp 674.4 ✓
pneumonia, embolic — *see* Puerperal, embolism
pre-eclampsia (mild) 642.4 ✓
with pre-existing hypertension 642.7 ✓
severe 642.5 ✓
prediabetes 648.8 ✓
psychosis, unspecified (*see also* Psychosis, puerperal) 293.89
pyelitis 646.6 ✓
pyelocystitis 646.6 ✓
pyelohydronephrosis 646.6 ✓
pyelonephritis 646.6 ✓
pyelonephrosis 646.6 ✓
pyemia 670.2 ✓
pyo-oophoritis 670.8 ✓
pyocystitis 646.6 ✓
pyohemia 670.2 ✓
pyometra 670.8 ✓
pyonephritis 646.6 ✓
pyonephrosis 646.6 ✓
pyosalpingitis 670.8 ✓
pyosalpinx 670.8 ✓
pyrexia (of unknown origin) 672.0 ✓
renal
disease NEC 646.2 ✓
failure, acute 669.3 ✓
retention
decidua (fragments) (with delayed hemorrhage) 666.2 ✓
without hemorrhage 667.1 ✓
placenta (fragments) (with delayed hemorrhage) 666.2 ✓
without hemorrhage 667.1 ✓
secundines (fragments) (with delayed hemorrhage) 666.2 ✓
without hemorrhage 667.1 ✓
retracted nipple 676.0 ✓
rubella (conditions classifiable to 056) 647.5 ✓
salpingitis 670.8 ✓
salpingo-oophoritis 670.8 ✓
salpingo-ovaritis 670.8 ✓
salpingoperitonitis 670.8 ✓
sapremia 670.2 ✓
secondary perineal tear 674.2 ✓
sepsis (pelvic) 670.2 ✓
septicemia 670.2 ✓
subinvolution (uterus) 674.8 ✓
sudden death (cause unknown) 674.9 ✓
suppuration — *see* Puerperal, abscess
syphilis (conditions classifiable to 090–097) 647.0 ✓
tetanus 670.8 ✓
thelitis 675.0 ✓
thrombocytopenia 666.3 ✓
thrombophlebitis (superficial) 671.2 ✓
deep 671.4 ✓
pelvic 671.4 ✓
septic 670.3 ✓
specified site NEC 671.5 ✓
thrombosis (venous) — *see* Thrombosis, puerperal
thyroid dysfunction (conditions classifiable to 240–246) 648.1 ✓
toxemia (*see also* Toxemia, of pregnancy) 642.4 ✓
eclamptic 642.6 ✓
with pre-existing hypertension 642.7 ✓
pre-eclamptic (mild) 642.4 ✓
with
convulsions 642.6 ✓
pre-existing hypertension 642.7 ✓
severe 642.5 ✓
tuberculosis (conditions classifiable to 010–018) 647.3 ✓
uremia 669.3 ✓

Puerperal — *continued*
vaginitis (conditions classifiable to 616.1) 646.6 ✓
varicose veins (legs) 671.0 ✓
vulva or perineum 671.1 ✓
venous complication 671.9 ✓
vulvitis (conditions classifiable to 616.1) 646.6 ✓
vulvovaginitis (conditions classifiable to 616.1) 646.6 ✓
white leg 671.4 ✓
Pulled muscle — *see* Sprain, by site
Pulmolithiasis 518.89
Pulmonary — *see* condition
Pulmonitis (unknown etiology) 486
Pulpitis (acute) (anachoretic) (chronic) (hyperplastic) (putrescent) (suppurative) (ulcerative) 522.0
Pulpless tooth 522.9
Pulse
alternating 427.89
psychogenic 306.2
bigeminal 427.89
fast 785.0
feeble, rapid, due to shock following injury 958.4
rapid 785.0
slow 427.89
strong 785.9
trigeminal 427.89
water-hammer (*see also* Insufficiency, aortic) 424.1
weak 785.9
Pulseless disease 446.7
Pulsus
alternans or trigeminy 427.89
psychogenic 306.2
Punch drunk 310.2
Puncta lacrimalia occlusion 375.52
Punctiform hymen 752.49
Puncture (traumatic) — *see also* Wound, open, by site
accidental, complicating surgery 998.2
bladder, nontraumatic 596.6
by
device, implant, or graft — *see* Complications, mechanical
foreign body
internal organs (*see also* Injury, internal, by site)
by ingested object — *see* Foreign body
left accidentally in operation wound 998.4
instrument (any) during a procedure, accidental 998.2
internal organs, abdomen, chest, or pelvis — *see* Injury, internal, by site
kidney, nontraumatic 593.89
Pupil — *see* condition
Pupillary membrane 364.74
persistent 743.46
Pupillotonia 379.46
pseudotabetic 379.46
Purpura 287.2
abdominal 287.0
allergic 287.0
anaphylactoid 287.0
annularis telangiectodes 709.1
arthritic 287.0
autoerythrocyte sensitization 287.2
autoimmune 287.0
bacterial 287.0
Bateman's (senile) 287.2
capillary fragility (hereditary) (idiopathic) 287.8
cryoglobulinemic 273.2
devil's pinches 287.2
fibrinolytic (*see also* Fibrinolysis) 286.6
fulminans, fulminous 286.6
gangrenous 287.0
hemorrhagic (*see also* Purpura, thrombocytopenic) 287.39
nodular 272.7
nonthrombocytopenic 287.0
thrombocytopenic 287.39

Purpura — *continued*
Henoch-Schönlein (allergic) 287.0
Henoch's (purpura nervosa) 287.0
hypergammaglobulinemic (benign primary) (Waldenström's) 273.0
idiopathic 287.31
nonthrombocytopenic 287.0
thrombocytopenic 287.31
immune thrombocytopenic 287.31
infectious 287.0
malignant 287.0
neonatorum 772.6
nervosa 287.0
newborn NEC 772.6
nonthrombocytopenic 287.2
hemorrhagic 287.0
idiopathic 287.0
nonthrombopenic 287.2
peliosis rheumatica 287.0
pigmentaria, progressiva 709.09
posttransfusion (PTP) 287.41
from whole blood (fresh) or blood products 287.41
primary 287.0
primitive 287.0
red cell membrane sensitivity 287.2
rheumatica 287.0
Schönlein (-Henoch) (allergic) 287.0
scorbutic 267
senile 287.2
simplex 287.2
symptomatica 287.0
telangiectasia annularis 709.1
thrombocytopenic (*see also* Thrombocytopenia) 287.30
congenital 287.33
essential 287.30
hereditary 287.31
idiopathic 287.31
immune 287.31
neonatal, transitory (*see also* Thrombocytopenia, neonatal transitory) 776.1
primary 287.30
puerperal, postpartum 666.3 ✓
thrombotic 446.6
thrombohemolytic (*see also* Fibrinolysis) 286.6
thrombopenic (*see also* Thrombocytopenia) 287.30
congenital 287.33
essential 287.30
thrombotic 446.6
thrombocytic 446.6
thrombocytopenic 446.6
toxic 287.0
variolosa 050.0
vascular 287.0
visceral symptoms 287.0
Werlhof's (*see also* Purpura, thrombocytopenic) 287.39
Purpuric spots 782.7
Purulent — *see* condition
Pus
absorption, general — *see* Septicemia
in
stool 792.1
urine 791.9
tube (rupture) (*see also* Salpingo-oophoritis) 614.2
Pustular rash 782.1
Pustule 686.9
malignant 022.0
nonmalignant 686.9
Putnam-Dana syndrome (subacute combined sclerosis with pernicious anemia) 281.0 *[336.2]*
Putnam's disease (subacute combined sclerosis with pernicious anemia) 281.0 *[336.2]*
Putrefaction, intestinal 569.89
Putrescent pulp (dental) 522.1
Pyarthritis — *see* Pyarthrosis
Pyarthrosis — *see also* Arthritis, pyogenic 711.0 ✓
tuberculous — *see* Tuberculosis, joint

Pycnoepilepsy, pycnolepsy (idiopathic) — *see also* Epilepsy 345.0 ✓
Pyelectasia 593.89
Pyelectasis 593.89
Pyelitis (congenital) (uremic) 590.80
with
abortion — *see* Abortion, by type, with specified complication NEC
contracted kidney 590.00
ectopic pregnancy (*see also* categories 633.0–633.9) 639.8
molar pregnancy (*see also* categories 630–632) 639.8
acute 590.10
with renal medullary necrosis 590.11
chronic 590.00
with
renal medullary necrosis 590.01
complicating pregnancy, childbirth, or puerperium 646.6 ✓
affecting fetus or newborn 760.1
cystica 590.3
following
abortion 639.8
ectopic or molar pregnancy 639.8
gonococcal 098.19
chronic or duration of 2 months or over 098.39
tuberculous (*see also* Tuberculosis) 016.0 ✓ *[590.81]*
Pyelo-ureteritis cystica 590.3
Pyelocaliectasis 593.89
Pyelocystitis — *see also* Pyelitis 590.80
Pyelohydronephrosis 591
Pyelonephritis — *see also* Pyelitis 590.80
acute 590.10
with renal medullary necrosis 590.11
chronic 590.00
syphilitic (late) 095.4
tuberculous (*see also* Tuberculosis) 016.0 ✓ *[590.81]*
Pyelonephrosis — *see also* Pyelitis 590.80
chronic 590.00
Pyelophlebitis 451.89
Pyemia, pyemic (purulent) — *see also* Septicemia 038.9
abscess — *see* Abscess
arthritis (*see also* Arthritis, pyogenic) 711.0 ✓
Bacillus coli 038.42
embolism (*see also* Septicemia) 415.12
fever 038.9
infection 038.9
joint (*see also* Arthritis, pyogenic) 711.0 ✓
liver 572.1
meningococcal 036.2
newborn 771.81
phlebitis — *see* Phlebitis
pneumococcal 038.2
portal 572.1
postvaccinal 999.39
puerperal 670.2 ✓
specified organism NEC 038.8
staphylococcal 038.10
aureus 038.11
methicillin
resistant 038.12
susceptible 038.11
specified organism NEC 038.19
streptococcal 038.0
tuberculous — *see* Tuberculosis, miliary
Pygopagus 759.4
Pykno-epilepsy, pyknolepsy (idiopathic) — *see also* Epilepsy 345.0 ✓
Pyle (-Cohn) disease (craniometaphyseal dysplasia) 756.89
Pylephlebitis (suppurative) 572.1
Pylethrombophlebitis 572.1
Pylethrombosis 572.1
Pyloritis — *see also* Gastritis 535.5 ✓
Pylorospasm (reflex) 537.81
congenital or infantile 750.5
neurotic 306.4
newborn 750.5
psychogenic 306.4
Pylorus, pyloric — *see* condition

✓ **Additional Digit Required — Refer to the Tabular List for Digit Selection**   ⬛ **Subterms under main terms may continue to next column or page**

Pyo-oophoritis — see also Salpingo-oophoritis 614.2
Pyo-ovarium — see also Salpingo-oophoritis 614.2
Pyoarthrosis — see Pyarthrosis
Pyocele
  mastoid 383.00
  sinus (accessory) (nasal) (see also Sinusitis) 473.9
  turbinate (bone) 473.9
  urethra (see also Urethritis) 597.0
Pyococcal dermatitis 686.00
Pyococcide, skin 686.00
Pyocolpos — see also Vaginitis 616.10
Pyocyaneus dermatitis 686.09
Pyocystitis — see Cystitis 595.9
Pyoderma, pyodermia 686.00
  gangrenosum 686.01
  specified type NEC 686.09
  vegetans 686.8
Pyodermatitis 686.00
  vegetans 686.8
Pyogenic — see condition
Pyohemia — see Septicemia
Pyohydronephrosis — see also Pyelitis 590.80
Pyometra 615.9
Pyometritis — see also Endometritis 615.9
Pyometrium — see also Endometritis 615.9
Pyomyositis 728.0
  ossificans 728.19
  tropical (bungpagga) 040.81
Pyonephritis — see also Pyelitis 590.80
  chronic 590.80
Pyonephrosis (congenital) — see also Pyelitis 590.80
  acute 590.10
Pyopericarditis 420.99
Pyopericardium 420.99
Pyophlebitis — see Phlebitis
Pyopneumopericardium 420.99
Pyopneumothorax (infectional) 510.9
  with fistula 510.0
  subdiaphragmatic (see also Peritonitis) 567.29
  subphrenic (see also Peritonitis) 567.29
  tuberculous (see also Tuberculosis, pleura) 012.0 ☑
Pyorrhea (alveolar) (alveolaris) 523.40
  degenerative 523.5
Pyosalpingitis — see also Salpingo-oophoritis 614.2
Pyosalpinx — see also Salpingo-oophoritis 614.2
Pyosepticemia — see Septicemia
Pyosis
  Corlett's (impetigo) 684
  Manson's (pemphigus contagiosus) 684
Pyothorax 510.9
  with fistula 510.0
  tuberculous (see also Tuberculosis, pleura) 012.0 ☑
Pyoureter 593.89
  tuberculous (see also Tuberculosis) 016.2 ☑
Pyramidopallidonigral syndrome 332.0
Pyrexia (of unknown origin) (P.U.O.) 780.60
  atmospheric 992.0
  during labor 659.2 ☑
  environmentally-induced newborn 778.4
  heat 992.0
  newborn, environmentally-induced 778.4
  puerperal 672.0 ☑
Pyroglobulinemia 273.8
Pyromania 312.33
Pyrosis 787.1
Pyrroloporphyria 277.1
Pyuria (bacterial) 791.9

Q

Q fever 083.0
  with pneumonia 083.0 [484.8]
Quadricuspid aortic valve 746.89
Quadrilateral fever 083.0
Quadriparesis — see Quadriplegia
  meaning muscle weakness 728.87
Quadriplegia 344.00

Quadriplegia — continued
  with fracture, vertebra (process) — see Fracture, vertebra, cervical, with spinal cord injury
  brain (current episode) 437.8
  C1-C4
    complete 344.01
    incomplete 344.02
  C5-C7
    complete 344.03
    incomplete 344.04
  cerebral (current episode) 437.8
  congenital or infantile (cerebral) (spastic) (spinal) 343.2
  cortical 437.8
  embolic (current episode) (see also Embolism, brain) 434.1 ☑
  functional 780.72
  infantile (cerebral) (spastic) (spinal) 343.2
  newborn NEC 767.0
  specified NEC 344.09
  thrombotic (current episode) (see also Thrombosis, brain) 434.0 ☑
  traumatic — see Injury, spinal, cervical
Quadruplet
  affected by maternal complications of pregnancy 761.5
  healthy liveborn — see Newborn, multiple
  pregnancy (complicating delivery) NEC 651.8 ☑
    with fetal loss and retention of one or more fetus(es) 651.5 ☑
    following (elective) fetal reduction 651.7 ☑
Quarrelsomeness 301.3
Quartan
  fever 084.2
  malaria (fever) 084.2
Queensland fever 083.0
  coastal 083.0
  seven-day 100.89
Quervain's disease 727.04
  thyroid (subacute granulomatous thyroiditis) 245.1
Queyrat's erythroplasia (M8080/2)
  specified site — see Neoplasm, skin, in situ
  unspecified site 233.5
Quincke's disease or edema — see Edema, angioneurotic
Quinquaud's disease (acne decalvans) 704.09
Quinsy (gangrenous) 475
Quintan fever 083.1
Quintuplet
  affected by maternal complications of pregnancy 761.5
  healthy liveborn — see Newborn, multiple
  pregnancy (complicating delivery) NEC 651.2 ☑
    with fetal loss and retention of one or more fetus(es) 651.6 ☑
    following (elective) fetal reduction 651.7 ☑
Quotidian
  fever 084.0
  malaria (fever) 084.0

R

Rabbia 071
Rabbit fever — see also Tularemia 021.9
Rabies 071
  contact V01.5
  exposure to V01.5
  inoculation V04.5
    reaction — see Complications, vaccination
  vaccination, prophylactic (against) V04.5
Rachischisis — see also Spina bifida 741.9 ☑
Rachitic — see also condition
  deformities of spine 268.1
  pelvis 268.1
    with disproportion (fetopelvic) 653.2 ☑
      affecting fetus or newborn 763.1
      causing obstructed labor 660.1 ☑
        affecting fetus or newborn 763.1
Rachitis, rachitism — see also Rickets

Rachitis, rachitism — see also Rickets — continued
  acute 268.0
  fetalis 756.4
  renalis 588.0
  tarda 268.0
Racket nail 757.5
Radial nerve — see condition
Radiation effects or sickness — see also Effect, adverse, radiation
  cataract 366.46
  dermatitis 692.82
    sunburn (see also Sunburn) 692.71
Radiculitis (pressure) (vertebrogenic) 729.2
  accessory nerve 723.4
  anterior crural 724.4
  arm 723.4
  brachial 723.4
  cervical NEC 723.4
  due to displacement of intervertebral disc — see Neuritis, due to, displacement intervertebral disc
  leg 724.4
  lumbar 724.4
  lumbosacral 724.4
  rheumatic 729.2
  syphilitic 094.89
  thoracic (with visceral pain) 724.4
Radiculomyelitis 357.0
  toxic, due to
    Clostridium tetani 037
    Corynebacterium diphtheriae 032.89
Radiculopathy — see also Radiculitis 729.2
Radioactive substances, adverse effect — see Effect, adverse, radioactive substance
Radiodermal burns (acute) (chronic) (occupational) — see Burn, by site
Radiodermatitis 692.82
Radionecrosis — see Effect, adverse, radiation
Radiotherapy session V58.0
Radium, adverse effect — see Effect, adverse, radioactive substance
Raeder-Harbitz syndrome (pulseless disease) 446.7
Rage — see also Disturbance, conduct 312.0 ☑
  meaning rabies 071
Rag sorters' disease 022.1
Raillietiniasis 123.8
Railroad neurosis 300.16
Railway spine 300.16
Raised — see Elevation
Raiva 071
Rake teeth, tooth 524.39
Rales 786.7
Ramifying renal pelvis 753.3
Ramsay Hunt syndrome (herpetic geniculate ganglionitis) 053.11
  meaning dyssynergia cerebellaris myoclonica 334.2
Ranke's primary infiltration — see also Tuberculosis 010.0 ☑
Ranula 527.6
  congenital 750.26
Rape
  adult 995.83
  alleged, observation or examination V71.5
  child 995.53
Rapid
  feeble pulse, due to shock, following injury 958.4
  heart (beat) 785.0
    psychogenic 306.2
  respiration 786.06
    psychogenic 306.1
  second stage (delivery) 661.3 ☑
    affecting fetus or newborn 763.6
  time-zone change syndrome 327.35
Rarefaction, bone 733.99
Rash 782.1
  canker 034.1
  diaper 691.0
  drug (internal use) 693.0
    contact 692.3
  ECHO 9 virus 078.89
  enema 692.89
  food (see also Allergy, food) 693.1

Rash — continued
  heat 705.1
  napkin 691.0
  nettle 708.8
  pustular 782.1
  rose 782.1
    epidemic 056.9
    of infants 057.8
  scarlet 034.1
  serum (prophylactic) (therapeutic) 999.59
  toxic 782.1
  wandering tongue 529.1
Rasmussen's aneurysm — see also Tuberculosis 011.2 ☑
Rat-bite fever 026.9
  due to Streptobacillus moniliformis 026.1
  spirochetal (morsus muris) 026.0
Rathke's pouch tumor (M9350/1) 237.0
Raymond (-Céstan) syndrome 433.8 ☑
Raynaud's
  disease or syndrome (paroxysmal digital cyanosis) 443.0
  gangrene (symmetric) 443.0 [785.4]
  phenomenon (paroxysmal digital cyanosis) (secondary) 443.0
RDS 769
Reaction
  acute situational maladjustment (see also Reaction, adjustment) 309.9
  adaptation (see also Reaction, adjustment) 309.9
  adjustment 309.9
    with
      anxious mood 309.24
        with depressed mood 309.28
      conduct disturbance 309.3
        combined with disturbance of emotions 309.4
      depressed mood 309.0
        brief 309.0
          with anxious mood 309.28
        prolonged 309.1
      elective mutism 309.83
      mixed emotions and conduct 309.4
      mutism, elective 309.83
      physical symptoms 309.82
      predominant disturbance (of)
        conduct 309.3
        emotions NEC 309.29
          mixed 309.28
        mixed, emotions and conduct 309.4
        specified type NEC 309.89
      specific academic or work inhibition 309.23
      withdrawal 309.83
    depressive 309.0
      with conduct disturbance 309.4
      brief 309.0
      prolonged 309.1
    specified type NEC 309.89
  adverse food NEC 995.7
  affective (see also Psychosis, affective) 296.90
    specified type NEC 296.99
  aggressive 301.3
    unsocialized (see also Disturbance, conduct) 312.0 ☑
  allergic (see also Allergy) 995.3
    drug, medicinal substance, and biological — see Allergy, drug
    due to correct medical substance properly administered 995.27
    food — see Allergy, food
    serum 999.59
  anaphylactic — see Anaphylactic reaction
  anesthesia — see Anesthesia, complication
  anger 312.0 ☑
  antisocial 301.7
  antitoxin (prophylactic) (therapeutic) — see Complications, vaccination
  anxiety 300.00
  Arthus 995.21
  asthenic 300.5
  compulsive 300.3

Reaction — *continued*
  conversion (anesthetic) (autonomic) (hyperkinetic) (mixed paralytic) (paresthetic) 300.11
  deoxyribonuclease (DNA) (DNase) hypersensitivity NEC 287.2
  depressive 300.4
    acute 309.0
    affective (*see also* Psychosis, affective) 296.2 ☑
      recurrent episode 296.3 ☑
      single episode 296.2 ☑
    brief 309.0
    manic (*see also* Psychosis, affective) 296.80
    neurotic 300.4
    psychoneurotic 300.4
    psychotic 298.0
  dissociative 300.15
  drug NEC (*see also* Table of Drugs and Chemicals) 995.20
    allergic (*see also* Allergy, drug) 995.27
    correct substance properly administered 995.20
    obstetric anesthetic or analgesic NEC 668.9 ☑
      affecting fetus or newborn 763.5
      specified drug — *see* Table of Drugs and Chemicals
    overdose or poisoning 977.9
      specified drug — *see* Table of Drugs and Chemicals
    specific to newborn 779.4
    transmitted via placenta or breast milk — *see* Absorption, drug, through placenta
    withdrawal NEC 292.0
      infant of dependent mother 779.5
    wrong substance given or taken in error 977.9
      specified drug — *see* Table of Drugs and Chemicals
  dyssocial 301.7
  dystonic, acute, due to drugs 333.72
  erysipeloid 027.1
  fear 300.20
    child 313.0
  fluid loss, cerebrospinal 349.0
  food (*see also* Allergy, food)
    adverse NEC 995.7
    anaphylactic shock — *see* Anaphylactic reaction or shock, due to, food
  foreign
    body NEC 728.82
      in operative wound (inadvertently left) 998.4
        due to surgical material intentionally left — *see* Complications, due to (presence of) any device, implant, or graft classified to 996.0–996.5 NEC
      substance accidentally left during a procedure (chemical) (powder) (talc) 998.7
      body or object (instrument) (sponge) (swab) 998.4
  graft-versus-host (GVH) 279.50
  grief (acute) (brief) 309.0
    prolonged 309.1
  gross stress (*see also* Reaction, stress, acute) 308.9
  group delinquent (*see also* Disturbance, conduct) 312.2 ☑
  Herxheimer's 995.91
  hyperkinetic (*see also* Hyperkinesia) 314.9
  hypochondriacal 300.7
  hypoglycemic, due to insulin 251.0
    therapeutic misadventure 962.3
  hypomanic (*see also* Psychosis, affective) 296.0 ☑
    recurrent episode 296.1 ☑
    single episode 296.0 ☑
  hysterical 300.10
    conversion type 300.11
    dissociative 300.15

Reaction — *continued*
  id (bacterial cause) 692.89
  immaturity NEC 301.89
    aggressive 301.3
    emotional instability 301.59
  immunization — *see* Complications, vaccination
  incompatibility
    blood group (*see also* Complications, transfusion) 999.80
      ABO (due to transfusion of blood or blood products) (*see also* Complications, transfusion) 999.60
      minor blood group 999.89
      non-ABO — *see also* Complications, transfusion 999.75
      Rh antigen (C) (c) (D) (E) (e) (factor) (infusion) (transfusion) (*see also* Complications, transfusion) 999.70
  inflammatory — *see* Infection
  infusion — *see* Complications, infusion
  inoculation (immune serum) — *see* Complications, vaccination
  insulin 995.23
  involutional
    paranoid 297.2
    psychotic (*see also* Psychosis, affective, depressive) 296.2 ☑
  leukemoid (basophilic) (lymphocytic) (monocytic) (myelocytic) (neutrophilic) 288.62
  LSD (*see also* Abuse, drugs, nondependent) 305.3 ☑
  lumbar puncture 349.0
  manic-depressive (*see also* Psychosis, affective) 296.80
    depressed 296.2 ☑
      recurrent episode 296.3 ☑
      single episode 296.2 ☑
    hypomanic 296.0 ☑
  neurasthenic 300.5
  neurogenic (*see also* Neurosis) 300.9
  neurotic-depressive 300.4
  neurotic NEC 300.9
  nitritoid — *see* Crisis, nitritoid
  nonspecific
    to
      cell mediated immunity measurement of gamma interferon antigen response without active tuberculosis 795.52
      QuantiFERON-TB test (QFT) without active tuberculosis 795.52
      tuberculin test (*see also* Reaction, tuberculin skin test) 795.51
  obsessive compulsive 300.3
  organic 293.9
    acute 293.0
    subacute 293.1
  overanxious, child or adolescent 313.0
  paranoid (chronic) 297.9
    acute 298.3
    climacteric 297.2
    involutional 297.2
    menopausal 297.2
    senile 290.20
    simple 297.0
  passive
    aggressive 301.84
    dependency 301.6
  personality (*see also* Disorder, personality) 301.9
  phobic 300.20
  postradiation — *see* Effect, adverse, radiation
  psychogenic NEC 300.9
  psychoneurotic (*see also* Neurosis) 300.9
    anxiety 300.00
    compulsive 300.3
    conversion 300.11
    depersonalization 300.6
    depressive 300.4
    dissociative 300.15
    hypochondriacal 300.7
    hysterical 300.10

Reaction — *continued*
  psychoneurotic (*see also* Neurosis) — *continued*
    hysterical — *continued*
      conversion type 300.11
      dissociative type 300.15
    neurasthenic 300.5
    obsessive-compulsive 300.3
    obsessive 300.3
    phobic 300.20
    tension state 300.9
  psychophysiologic NEC (*see also* Disorder, psychosomatic) 306.9
    cardiovascular 306.2
    digestive 306.4
    endocrine 306.6
    gastrointestinal 306.4
    genitourinary 306.50
    heart 306.2
    hemic 306.8
    intestinal (large) (small) 306.4
    laryngeal 306.1
    lymphatic 306.8
    musculoskeletal 306.0
    pharyngeal 306.1
    respiratory 306.1
    skin 306.3
    special sense organs 306.7
  psychosomatic (*see also* Disorder, psychosomatic) 306.9
  psychotic (*see also* Psychosis) 298.9
    depressive 298.0
    due to or associated with physical condition (*see also* Psychosis, organic) 293.9
    involutional (*see also* Psychosis, affective) 296.2 ☑
      recurrent episode 296.3 ☑
      single episode 296.2 ☑
  pupillary (myotonic) (tonic) 379.46
  radiation — *see* Effect, adverse, radiation
  runaway (*see also* Disturbance, conduct)
    socialized 312.2 ☑
    undersocialized, unsocialized 312.1 ☑
  scarlet fever toxin — *see* Complications, vaccination
  schizophrenic (*see also* Schizophrenia) 295.9 ☑
    latent 295.5 ☑
  serological for syphilis — *see* Serology for syphilis
  serum (prophylactic) (therapeutic) 999.59
    anaphylactic 999.49
    due to
      administration of blood and blood products 999.51
        anaphylactic 999.41
      vaccination 999.52
        anaphylactic 999.41
    immediate 999.49
  situational (*see also* Reaction, adjustment) 309.9
    acute, to stress 308.3
    adjustment (*see also* Reaction, adjustment) 309.9
  somatization (*see also* Disorder, psychosomatic) 306.9
  spinal puncture 349.0
  spite, child (*see also* Disturbance, conduct) 312.0 ☑
  stress, acute 308.9
    with predominant disturbance (of)
      consciousness 308.1
      emotions 308.0
      mixed 308.4
      psychomotor 308.2
      specified type NEC 308.3
    bone or cartilage — *see* Fracture, stress
  surgical procedure — *see* Complications, surgical procedure
  tetanus antitoxin — *see* Complications, vaccination
  toxin-antitoxin — *see* Complications, vaccination

Reaction — *continued*
  transfusion (blood) (bone marrow) (lymphocytes) (allergic) (*see also* Complications, transfusion) 999.80
  tuberculin skin test, nonspecific (without active tuberculosis) 795.51
    positive (without active tuberculosis) 795.51
  ultraviolet — *see* Effect, adverse, ultraviolet
  undersocialized, unsocialized (*see also* Disturbance, conduct)
    aggressive (type) 312.0 ☑
    unaggressive (type) 312.1 ☑
  vaccination (any) — *see* Complications, vaccination
  white graft (skin) 996.52
  withdrawing, child or adolescent 313.22
  x-ray — *see* Effect, adverse, x-rays
Reactive depression — *see also* Reaction, depressive 300.4
  neurotic 300.4
  psychoneurotic 300.4
  psychotic 298.0
Rebound tenderness 789.6 ☑
Recalcitrant patient V15.81
Recanalization, thrombus — *see* Thrombosis
Recession, receding
  chamber angle (eye) 364.77
  chin 524.06
  gingival (postinfective) (postoperative) 523.20
    generalized 523.25
    localized 523.24
    minimal 523.21
    moderate 523.22
    severe 523.23
Recklinghausen-Applebaum disease (hemochromatosis) 275.03
Recklinghausen's disease (M9540/1) 237.71
  bones (osteitis fibrosa cystica) 252.01
Reclus' disease (cystic) 610.1
Recrudescent typhus (fever) 081.1
Recruitment, auditory 388.44
Rectalgia 569.42
Rectitis 569.49
Rectocele
  female (without uterine prolapse) 618.04
    with uterine prolapse 618.4
      complete 618.3
      incomplete 618.2
    in pregnancy or childbirth 654.4 ☑
      causing obstructed labor 660.2 ☑
        affecting fetus or newborn 763.1
  male 569.49
  vagina, vaginal (outlet) 618.04
Rectosigmoiditis 569.89
  ulcerative (chronic) 556.3
Rectosigmoid junction — *see* condition
Rectourethral — *see* condition
Rectovaginal — *see* condition
Rectovesical — *see* condition
Rectum, rectal — *see* condition
Recurrent — *see* condition
  pregnancy loss — *see* Pregnancy, management affected by, abortion, habitual
Red bugs 133.8
Red cedar asthma 495.8
Redness
  conjunctiva 379.93
  eye 379.93
  nose 478.19
Reduced ventilatory or vital capacity 794.2
Reduction
  function
    kidney (*see also* Disease, renal) 593.9
    liver 573.8
  ventilatory capacity 794.2
  vital capacity 794.2
Redundant, redundancy
  abdomen 701.9
  anus 751.5
  cardia 537.89
  clitoris 624.2
  colon (congenital) 751.5
  foreskin (congenital) 605
  intestine 751.5

☑ **Additional Digit Required — Refer to the Tabular List for Digit Selection**   ▽ **Subterms under main terms may continue to next column or page**

246 — Volume 2   ▶◀ Revised Text   ● New Line   ▲ Revised Code   2014 ICD-9-CM

Redundant, redundancy — *continued*
  labia 624.3
  organ or site, congenital NEC — *see* Accessory
  panniculus (abdominal) 278.1
  prepuce (congenital) 605
  pylorus 537.89
  rectum 751.5
  scrotum 608.89
  sigmoid 751.5
  skin (of face) 701.9
    eyelids 374.30
  stomach 537.89
  uvula 528.9
  vagina 623.8
Reduplication — *see* Duplication
Referral
  adoption (agency) V68.89
  nursing care V63.8
  patient without examination or treatment V68.81
  social services V63.8
Reflex — *see also* condition
  blink, deficient 374.45
  hyperactive gag 478.29
  neurogenic bladder NEC 596.54
    atonic 596.54
      with cauda equina syndrome 344.61
  vasoconstriction 443.9
  vasovagal 780.2
Reflux 530.81
  acid 530.81
  esophageal 530.81
    with esophagitis 530.11
  esophagitis 530.11
  gastroesophageal 530.81
  mitral — *see* Insufficiency, mitral
  ureteral — *see* Reflux, vesicoureteral
  vesicoureteral 593.70
    with
      reflux nephropathy 593.73
        bilateral 593.72
        unilateral 593.71
Reformed gallbladder 576.0
Reforming, artificial openings — *see also* Attention to, artificial, opening V55.9
Refractive error — *see also* Error, refractive 367.9
Refsum's disease or syndrome (heredopathia atactica polyneuritiformis) 356.3
Refusal of
  food 307.59
    hysterical 300.11
  treatment because of, due to
    patient's decision NEC V64.2
    reason of conscience or religion V62.6
Regaud
  tumor (M8082/3) — *see* Neoplasm, nasopharynx, malignant
  type carcinoma (M8082/3) — *see* Neoplasm, nasopharynx, malignant
Regional — *see* condition
Regulation feeding (elderly) (infant) 783.3
  newborn 779.31
Regurgitated
  food, choked on 933.1
  stomach contents, choked on 933.1
Regurgitation 787.03
  aortic (valve) (*see also* Insufficiency, aortic) 424.1
    congenital 746.4
    syphilitic 093.22
  food (*see also* Vomiting)
    with reswallowing — *see* Rumination
    newborn 779.33
  gastric contents — *see* Vomiting
  heart — *see* Endocarditis
  mitral (valve) (*see also* Insufficiency, mitral)
    congenital 746.6
  myocardial — *see* Endocarditis
  pulmonary (heart) (valve) (*see also* Endocarditis, pulmonary) 424.3
  stomach — *see* Vomiting
  tricuspid — *see* Endocarditis, tricuspid
  valve, valvular — *see* Endocarditis
  vesicoureteral — *see* Reflux, vesicoureteral

Rehabilitation V57.9
  multiple types V57.89
  occupational V57.21
  specified type NEC V57.89
  speech (-language) V57.3
  vocational V57.22
Reichmann's disease or syndrome (gastrosuccorrhea) 536.8
Reifenstein's syndrome (hereditary familial hypogonadism, male) 259.52
Reilly's syndrome or phenomenon — *see also* Neuropathy, peripheral, autonomic 337.9
Reimann's periodic disease 277.31
Reinsertion, contraceptive device V25.42
  intrauterine V25.13
Reiter's disease, syndrome, or urethritis 099.3 *[711.1]* ☑
Rejection
  food, hysterical 300.11
  transplant 996.80
    bone marrow 996.85
    corneal 996.51
    organ (immune or nonimmune cause) 996.80
      bone marrow 996.85
      heart 996.83
      intestines 996.87
      kidney 996.81
      liver 996.82
      lung 996.84
      pancreas 996.86
      specified NEC 996.89
    skin 996.52
      artificial 996.55
      decellularized allodermis 996.55
    stem cells(s) 996.88
      from
        peripheral blood 996.88
        umbilical cord 996.88
Relapsing fever 087.9
  Carter's (Asiatic) 087.0
  Dutton's (West African) 087.1
  Koch's 087.9
  louse-borne (epidemic) 087.0
  Novy's (American) 087.1
  Obermeyer's (European) 087.0
  Spirillum 087.9
  tick-borne (endemic) 087.1
Relaxation
  anus (sphincter) 569.49
    due to hysteria 300.11
  arch (foot) 734
    congenital 754.61
  back ligaments 728.4
  bladder (sphincter) 596.59
  cardio-esophageal 530.89
  cervix (*see also* Incompetency, cervix) 622.5
  diaphragm 519.4
  inguinal rings — *see* Hernia, inguinal
  joint (capsule) (ligament) (paralytic) (*see also* Derangement, joint) 718.90
    congenital 755.8
  lumbosacral joint 724.6
  pelvic floor 618.89
  pelvis 618.89
  perineum 618.89
  posture 729.90
  rectum (sphincter) 569.49
  sacroiliac (joint) 724.6
  scrotum 608.89
  urethra (sphincter) 599.84
  uterus (outlet) 618.89
  vagina (outlet) 618.89
  vesical 596.59
Remains
  canal of Cloquet 743.51
  capsule (opaque) 743.51
Remittent fever (malarial) 084.6
Remnant
  canal of Cloquet 743.51
  capsule (opaque) 743.51
  cervix, cervical stump (acquired) (postoperative) 622.8
  cystic duct, postcholecystectomy 576.0
  fingernail 703.8

Remnant — *continued*
  fingernail — *continued*
    congenital 757.5
  meniscus, knee 717.5
  thyroglossal duct 759.2
  tonsil 474.8
    infected 474.00
  urachus 753.7
Remote effect of cancer — *see* condition
Removal (of)
  catheter (urinary) (indwelling) V53.6
    from artificial opening — *see* Attention to, artificial, opening
    non-vascular V58.82
    vascular V58.81
  cerebral ventricle (communicating) shunt V53.01
  device (*see also* Fitting (of))
    contraceptive V25.12
      with reinsertion V25.13
    fixation
      external V54.89
      internal V54.01
      traction V54.89
  drains V58.49
  dressing
    wound V58.30
      nonsurgical V58.30
      surgical V58.31
  ileostomy V55.2
  Kirschner wire V54.89
  nonvascular catheter V58.82
  pin V54.01
  plaster cast V54.89
  plate (fracture) V54.01
  rod V54.01
  screw V54.01
  splint, external V54.89
  staples V58.32
  subdermal implantable contraceptive V25.43
  sutures V58.32
  traction device, external V54.89
  vascular catheter V58.81
  wound packing V58.30
    nonsurgical V58.30
    surgical V58.31
Ren
  arcuatus 753.3
  mobile, mobilis (*see also* Disease, renal) 593.0
    congenital 753.3
  unguliformis 753.3
Renal — *see also* condition
  glomerulohyalinosis-diabetic syndrome 250.4 ☑ *[581.81]*
    due to secondary diabetes 249.4 ☑ *[581.81]*
Rendu-Osler-Weber disease or syndrome (familial hemorrhagic telangiectasia) 448.0
Reninoma (M8361/1) 236.91
Rénon-Delille syndrome 253.8
Repair
  pelvic floor, previous, in pregnancy or childbirth 654.4 ☑
    affecting fetus or newborn 763.89
  scarred tissue V51.8
Replacement by artificial or mechanical device or prosthesis of — *see also* Fitting (of
  artificial skin V43.83
  bladder V43.5
  blood vessel V43.4
  breast V43.82
  eye globe V43.0
  heart
    with
      assist device V43.21
      fully implantable artificial heart V43.22
    valve V43.3
  intestine V43.89
  joint V43.60
    ankle V43.66
    elbow V43.62

Replacement by artificial or mechanical device or prosthesis of — *see also* Fitting (of — *continued*
  joint — *continued*
    finger V43.69
    hip (partial) (total) V43.64
    knee V43.65
    shoulder V43.61
    specified NEC V43.69
    wrist V43.63
  kidney V43.89
  larynx V43.81
  lens V43.1
  limb(s) V43.7
  liver V43.89
  lung V43.89
  organ NEC V43.89
  pancreas V43.89
  skin (artificial) V43.83
  tissue NEC V43.89
Reprogramming
  cardiac pacemaker V53.31
Request for expert evidence V68.2
Reserve, decreased or low
  cardiac — *see* Disease, heart
  kidney (*see also* Disease, renal) 593.9
Residual — *see also* condition
  bladder 596.89
  foreign body — *see* Retention, foreign body
  state, schizophrenic (*see also* Schizophrenia) 295.6 ☑
  urine 788.69
Resistance, resistant (to)
  activated protein C 289.81

Note — *use the following subclassification for categories V09.5, V09.7, V09.8, V09.9:*

0   without mention of resistance to multiple drugs

1   with resistance to multiple drugs

      V09.5 quinolones and fluoroquinolones

      V09.7 antimycobacterial agents

      V09.8 specified drugs NEC

      V09.9 unspecified drugs
---

  drugs by microorganisms V09.9 ☑
    Amikacin V09.4
    aminoglycosides V09.4
    Amodiaquine V09.5 ☑
    Amoxicillin V09.0
    Ampicillin V09.0
    antimycobacterial agents V09.7 ☑
    Azithromycin V09.2
    Azlocillin V09.0
    Aztreonam V09.1
    B-lactam antibiotics V09.1
    Bacampicillin V09.0
    Bacitracin V09.8 ☑
    Benznidazole V09.8 ☑
    Capreomycin V09.7 ☑
    Carbenicillin V09.0
    Cefaclor V09.1
    Cefadroxil V09.1
    Cefamandole V09.1
    Cefatetan V09.1
    Cefazolin V09.1
    Cefixime V09.1
    Cefonicid V09.1
    Cefoperazone V09.1
    Ceforanide V09.1
    Cefotaxime V09.1
    Cefoxitin V09.1
    Ceftazidime V09.1
    Ceftizoxime V09.1
    Ceftriaxone V09.1
    Cefuroxime V09.1
    Cephalexin V09.1
    Cephaloglycin V09.1
    Cephaloridine V09.1
    Cephalosporins V09.1
    Cephalothin V09.1
    Cephapirin V09.1

☑ **Additional Digit Required** — Refer to the Tabular List for Digit Selection   ▼ **Subterms under main terms may continue to next column or page**

2014 ICD-9-CM   ▶◀ **Revised Text**   ● **New Line**   ▲ **Revised Code**   **Volume 2 — 247**

Resistance, resistant — *continued*
  drugs by microorganisms — *continued*
    Cephradine V09.1
    Chloramphenicol V09.8 ☑
    Chloroquine V09.5 ☑
    Chlorguanide V09.8 ☑
    Chlorproguanil V09.8 ☑
    Chlortetracycline V09.3
    Cinoxacin V09.5 ☑
    Ciprofloxacin V09.5 ☑
    Clarithromycin V09.2
    Clindamycin V09.8 ☑
    Clioquinol V09.5 ☑
    Clofazimine V09.7 ☑
    Cloxacillin V09.0
    Cyclacillin V09.0
    Cycloserine V09.7 ☑
    Dapsone [DZ] V09.7 ☑
    Demeclocycline V09.3
    Dicloxacillin V09.0
    Doxycycline V09.3
    Enoxacin V09.5 ☑
    Erythromycin V09.2
    Ethambutol [EMB] V09.7 ☑
    Ethionamide [ETA] V09.7 ☑
    fluoroquinolones V09.5 ☑
    Gentamicin V09.4
    Halofantrine V09.8 ☑
    Imipenem V09.1
    Iodoquinol V09.5 ☑
    Isoniazid [INH] V09.7 ☑
    Kanamycin V09.4
    macrolides V09.2
    Mafenide V09.6
    MDRO (multiple drug resistant organisms) NOS V09.91
    Mefloquine V09.8 ☑
    Melasoprol V09.8 ☑
    Methacycline V09.3
    Methenamine V09.8 ☑
    Methicillin — *see* Infection, Methicillin V09.0
    Metronidazole V09.8 ☑
    Mezlocillin V09.0
    Minocycline V09.3
    multiple drug resistant organisms NOS V09.91
    Nafcillin V09.0
    Nalidixic acid V09.5 ☑
    Natamycin V09.2
    Neomycin V09.4
    Netilmicin V09.4
    Nimorazole V09.8 ☑
    Nitrofurantoin V09.8 ☑
    Nitrofurtimox V09.8 ☑
    Norfloxacin V09.5 ☑
    Nystatin V09.2
    Ofloxacin V09.5 ☑
    Oleandomycin V09.2
    Oxacillin V09.0
    Oxytetracycline V09.3
    Para-amino salicylic acid [PAS] V09.7 ☑
    Paromomycin V09.4
    Penicillin (G) (V) (VK) V09.0
    penicillins V09.0
    Pentamidine V09.8 ☑
    Piperacillin V09.0
    Primaquine V09.5 ☑
    Proguanil V09.8 ☑
    Pyrazinamide [PZA] V09.7 ☑
    Pyrimethamine/Sulfalene V09.8 ☑
    Pyrimethamine/Sulfodoxine V09.8 ☑
    Quinacrine V09.5 ☑
    Quinidine V09.8 ☑
    Quinine V09.8 ☑
    quinolones V09.5 ☑
    Rifabutin V09.7 ☑
    Rifampin [RIF] V09.7 ☑
    Rifamycin V09.7 ☑
    Rolitetracycline V09.3
    specified drugs NEC V09.8 ☑
    Spectinomycin V09.8 ☑
    Spiramycin V09.2
    Streptomycin [SM] V09.4
    Sulfacetamide V09.6
    Sulfacytine V09.6
    Sulfadiazine V09.6
    Sulfadoxine V09.6
    Sulfamethoxazole V09.6
    Sulfapyridine V09.6
    Sulfasalizine V09.6
    Sulfasoxazole V09.6
    sulfonamides V09.6
    Sulfoxone V09.7 ☑
    tetracycline V09.3
    tetracyclines V09.3
    Thiamphenicol V09.8 ☑
    Ticarcillin V09.0
    Tinidazole V09.8 ☑
    Tobramycin V09.4
    Triamphenicol V09.8 ☑
    Trimethoprim V09.8 ☑
    Vancomycin V09.8 ☑
  insulin 277.7
    complicating pregnancy 648.8 ☑
  thyroid hormone 246.8

Resorption
  biliary 576.8
    purulent or putrid (*see also* Cholecystitis) 576.8
  dental (roots) 521.40
    alveoli 525.8
    pathological
      external 521.42
      internal 521.41
      specified NEC 521.49
  septic — *see* Septicemia
  teeth (roots) 521.40
    pathological
      external 521.42
      internal 521.41
      specified NEC 521.49

Respiration
  asymmetrical 786.09
  bronchial 786.09
  Cheyne-Stokes (periodic respiration) 786.04
  decreased, due to shock following injury 958.4
  disorder of 786.00
    psychogenic 306.1
    specified NEC 786.09
  failure 518.81
    acute 518.81
      following trauma and surgery 518.51
    acute and chronic 518.84
      following trauma and surgery 518.53
    chronic 518.83
    following trauma and surgery 518.51
    newborn 770.84
  insufficiency 786.09
    acute 518.82
    newborn NEC 770.89
  Kussmaul (air hunger) 786.09
  painful 786.52
  periodic 786.09
    high altitude 327.22
  poor 786.09
    newborn NEC 770.89
  sighing 786.7
    psychogenic 306.1
  wheezing 786.07

Respiratory — *see also* condition
  distress 786.09
    acute 518.82
    fetus or newborn NEC 770.89
    syndrome (newborn) 769
      adult (following trauma and surgery) 518.52
      specified NEC 518.82
  failure 518.81
    acute 518.81
      following trauma and surgery 518.51
    acute and chronic 518.84
      following trauma and surgery 518.53
    chronic 518.83
    following trauma and surgery 518.51

Respiratory syncytial virus (RSV) 079.6
  bronchiolitis 466.11
  pneumonia 480.1

Respiratory syncytial virus (RSV) — *continued*
  vaccination, prophylactic (against) V04.82

Response
  photoallergic 692.72
  phototoxic 692.72

Restless legs syndrome (RLS) 333.94

Restlessness 799.29

Restoration of organ continuity from previous sterilization (tuboplasty) (vasoplasty) V26.0

Rest, rests
  mesonephric duct 752.89
    fallopian tube 752.11
  ovarian, in fallopian tubes 752.19
  wolffian duct 752.89

Restriction of housing space V60.1

Restzustand, schizophrenic — *see also* Schizophrenia 295.6 ☑

Retained — *see* Retention

Retardation
  development, developmental, specific (*see also* Disorder, development, specific) 315.9
    learning, specific 315.2
      arithmetical 315.1
      language (skills) 315.31
        expressive 315.31
        mixed receptive-expressive 315.32
      mathematics 315.1
      reading 315.00
        phonological 315.39
      written expression 315.2
    motor 315.4
  endochondral bone growth 733.91
  growth (physical) in childhood 783.43
    due to malnutrition 263.2
    fetal (intrauterine) 764.9 ☑
      affecting management of pregnancy 656.5 ☑
  intrauterine growth 764.9 ☑
    affecting management of pregnancy 656.5 ☑
  mental — *see* Disability, intellectual
  motor, specific 315.4
  physical 783.43
    child 783.43
      due to malnutrition 263.2
    fetus (intrauterine) 764.9 ☑
      affecting management of pregnancy 656.5 ☑
  psychomotor NEC 307.9
  reading 315.00

Retching — *see* Vomiting

Retention, retained
  bladder (*see also* Retention, urine) 788.20
    psychogenic 306.53
  carbon dioxide 276.2
  cholelithiasis, following cholecystectomy 997.41
  cyst — *see* Cyst
  dead
    fetus (after 22 completed weeks gestation) 656.4 ☑
      early fetal death (before 22 completed weeks gestation) 632
    ovum 631.8
  decidua (following delivery) (fragments) (with hemorrhage) 666.2 ☑
    without hemorrhage 667.1 ☑
  deciduous tooth 520.6
  dental root 525.3
  fecal (*see also* Constipation) 564.00
  fluid 276.69
  foreign body (*see also* Foreign body, retained)
    bone 733.99
    current trauma — *see* Foreign body, by site or type
    middle ear 385.83
    muscle 729.6
    soft tissue NEC 729.6
  gallstones, following cholecystectomy 997.41
  gastric 536.8

Retention, retained — *continued*
  membranes (following delivery) (with hemorrhage) 666.2 ☑
    with abortion — *see* Abortion, by type
    without hemorrhage 667.1 ☑
  menses 626.8
  milk (puerperal) 676.2 ☑
  nitrogen, extrarenal 788.99
  placenta (total) (with hemorrhage) 666.0 ☑
    with abortion — *see* Abortion, by type
    without hemorrhage 667.0 ☑
    portions or fragments 666.2 ☑
      without hemorrhage 667.1 ☑
  products of conception
    early pregnancy (fetal death before 22 completed weeks gestation) 632
    following
      abortion — *see* Abortion, by type
      delivery 666.2 ☑
        with hemorrhage 666.2 ☑
        without hemorrhage 667.1 ☑
  secundines (following delivery) (with hemorrhage) 666.2 ☑
    with abortion — *see* Abortion, by type
    without hemorrhage 667.1 ☑
    complicating puerperium (delayed hemorrhage) 666.2 ☑
  smegma, clitoris 624.8
  urine NEC 788.20
    bladder, incomplete emptying 788.21
    due to
      benign prostatic hypertrophy (BPH) — *see* category 600
    due to
      benign prostatic hypertrophy (BPH) — *see* category 600
    psychogenic 306.53
    specified NEC 788.29
  water (in tissue) (*see also* Edema) 782.3

Reticulation, dust (occupational) 504

Reticulocytosis NEC 790.99

Reticuloendotheliosis
  acute infantile (M9722/3) 202.5 ☑
  leukemic (M9940/3) 202.4
  malignant (M9720/3) 202.3 ☑
  nonlipid (M9722/3) 202.5 ☑

Reticulohistiocytoma (giant cell) 277.89

Reticulohistiocytosis, multicentric 272.8

Reticulolymphosarcoma (diffuse) (M9613/3) 200.8 ☑
  follicular (M9691/3) 202.0 ☑
  nodular (M9691/3) 202.0 ☑

Reticulosarcoma (M9640/3) 200.0 ☑
  nodular (M9642/3) 200.0 ☑
  pleomorphic cell type (M9641/3) 200.0 ☑

Reticulosis (skin)
  acute of infancy (M9722/3) 202.5 ☑
  familial hemophagocytic 288.4
  histiocytic medullary (M9721/3) 202.3 ☑
  lipomelanotic 695.89
  malignant (M9720/3) 202.3 ☑
  Sézary's (M9701/3) 202.2 ☑

Retina, retinal — *see* condition

Retinitis — *see also* Chorioretinitis 363.20
  albuminurica 585.9 *[363.10]*
  arteriosclerotic 440.8 *[362.13]*
  central angiospastic 362.41
  Coat's 362.12
  diabetic 250.5 ☑ *[362.01]*
    due to secondary diabetes 249.5 ☑ *[362.01]*
  disciformis 362.52
  disseminated 363.10
    metastatic 363.14
    neurosyphilitic 094.83
    pigment epitheliopathy 363.15
  exudative 362.12
  focal 363.00
    in histoplasmosis 115.92
      capsulatum 115.02
      duboisii 115.12
    juxtapapillary 363.05
    macular 363.06
    paramacular 363.06
    peripheral 363.08

☑ Additional Digit Required — Refer to the Tabular List for Digit Selection   ▽ Subterms under main terms may continue to next column or page

Retinitis — *see also* Chorioretinitis — *continued*
  focal — *continued*
    posterior pole NEC 363.07
  gravidarum 646.8 ☑
  hemorrhagica externa 362.12
  juxtapapillary (Jensen's) 363.05
  luetic — *see* Retinitis, syphilitic
  metastatic 363.14
  pigmentosa 362.74
  proliferans 362.29
  proliferating 362.29
  punctata albescens 362.76
  renal 585.9 [363.13]
  syphilitic (secondary) 091.51
    congenital 090.0 [363.13]
    early 091.51
    late 095.8 [363.13]
  syphilitica, central, recurrent 095.8 [363.13]
  tuberculous (*see also* Tuberculous)
    017.3 ☑ [363.13]
Retinoblastoma (M9510/3) 190.5
  differentiated type (M9511/3) 190.5
  undifferentiated type (M9512/3) 190.5
Retinochoroiditis — *see also* Chorioretinitis
  363.20
  central angiospastic 362.41
  disseminated 363.10
    metastatic 363.14
    neurosyphilitic 094.83
    pigment epitheliopathy 363.15
    syphilitic 094.83
  due to toxoplasmosis (acquired) (focal)
    130.2
  focal 363.00
    in histoplasmosis 115.92
      capsulatum 115.02
      duboisii 115.12
    juxtapapillary (Jensen's) 363.05
    macular 363.06
    paramacular 363.06
    peripheral 363.08
    posterior pole NEC 363.07
  juxtapapillaris 363.05
  syphilitic (disseminated) 094.83
Retinopathy (background) 362.10
  arteriosclerotic 440.8 [362.13]
  atherosclerotic 440.8 [362.13]
  central serous 362.41
  circinate 362.10
  Coat's 362.12
  diabetic 250.5 ☑ [362.01]
    due to secondary diabetes
      249.5 ☑ [362.01]
    nonproliferative 250.5 ☑ [362.03]
      due to secondary diabetes
        249.5 ☑ [362.03]
      mild 250.5 ☑ [362.04]
        due to secondary diabetes
          249.5 ☑ [362.04]
      moderate 250.5 ☑ [362.05]
        due to secondary diabetes
          249.5 ☑ [362.05]
      severe 250.5 ☑ [362.06]
        due to secondary diabetes
          249.5 ☑ [362.06]
    proliferative 250.5 ☑ [362.02]
      due to secondary diabetes
        249.5 ☑ [362.02]
  exudative 362.12
  hypertensive 362.11
  nonproliferative
    diabetic 250.5 ☑ [362.03]
      due to secondary diabetes
        249.5 ☑ [362.03]
      mild 250.5 ☑ [362.04]
        due to secondary diabetes
          249.5 ☑ [362.04]
      moderate 250.5 ☑ [362.05]
        due to secondary diabetes
          249.5 ☑ [362.05]
      severe 250.5 ☑ [362.06]
        due to secondary diabetes
          249.5 ☑ [362.06]
  of prematurity 362.20
    cicatricial 362.21

Retinopathy — *continued*
  of prematurity — *continued*
    stage
      0 362.22
      1 362.23
      2 362.24
      3 362.25
      4 362.26
      5 362.27
  pigmentary, congenital 362.74
  proliferative 362.29
    diabetic 250.5 ☑ [362.02]
      due to secondary diabetes
        249.5 ☑ [362.02]
    sickle-cell 282.60 [362.29]
  solar 363.31
Retinoschisis 361.10
  bullous 361.12
  congenital 743.56
  flat 361.11
  juvenile 362.73
Retractile testis 752.52
Retraction
  cervix — *see* Retraction, uterus
  drum (membrane) 384.82
  eyelid 374.41
  finger 736.29
  head 781.0
  lid 374.41
  lung 518.89
  mediastinum 519.3
  nipple 611.79
    congenital 757.6
    puerperal, postpartum 676.0 ☑
  palmar fascia 728.6
  pleura (*see also* Pleurisy) 511.0
  ring, uterus (Bandl's) (pathological) 661.4 ☑
    affecting fetus or newborn 763.7
  sternum (congenital) 756.3
    acquired 738.3
    during respiration 786.9
  substernal 738.3
  supraclavicular 738.8
  syndrome (Duane's) 378.71
  uterus 621.6
  valve (heart) — *see* Endocarditis
Retrobulbar — *see* condition
Retrocaval ureter 753.4
Retrocecal — *see also* condition
  appendix (congenital) 751.5
Retrocession — *see* Retroversion
Retrodisplacement — *see* Retroversion
Retroflection, retroflexion — *see* Retroversion
Retrognathia, retrognathism (mandibular) (maxillary) 524.10
Retrograde
  ejaculation 608.87
  menstruation 626.8
Retroiliac ureter 753.4
Retroperineal — *see* condition
Retroperitoneal — *see* condition
Retroperitonitis 567.39
Retropharyngeal — *see* condition
Retroplacental — *see* condition
Retroposition — *see* Retroversion
Retroprosthetic membrane 996.51
Retrosternal thyroid (congenital) 759.2
Retroversion, retroverted
  cervix — *see* Retroversion, uterus
  female NEC (*see also* Retroversion, uterus)
    621.6
  iris 364.70
  testis (congenital) 752.51
  uterus, uterine (acquired) (acute) (adherent) (any degree) (asymptomatic) (cervix) (postinfectional) (postpartal, old)
    621.6
    congenital 752.39
    in pregnancy or childbirth 654.3 ☑
      affecting fetus or newborn 763.89
      causing obstructed labor 660.2 ☑
        affecting fetus or newborn 763.1
Retrusion, premaxilla (developmental) 524.04
Rett's syndrome 330.8

Reverse, reversed
  peristalsis 787.4
Reye-Sheehan syndrome (postpartum pituitary necrosis) 253.2
Reye's syndrome 331.81
Rhabdomyolysis (idiopathic) 728.88
Rhabdomyoma (M8900/0) — *see also* Neoplasm, connective tissue, benign
  adult (M8904/0) — *see* Neoplasm, connective tissue, benign
  fetal (M8903/0) — *see* Neoplasm, connective tissue, benign
  glycogenic (M8904/0) — *see* Neoplasm, connective tissue, benign
Rhabdomyosarcoma (M8900/3) — *see also* Neoplasm, connective tissue, malignant
  alveolar (M8920/3) — *see* Neoplasm, connective tissue, malignant
  embryonal (M8910/3) — *see* Neoplasm, connective tissue, malignant
  mixed type (M8902/3) — *see* Neoplasm, connective tissue, malignant
  pleomorphic (M8901/3) — *see* Neoplasm, connective tissue, malignant
Rhabdosarcoma (M8900/3) — *see* Rhabdomyosarcoma
Rh antigen (C) (c) (D) (E) (e) (factor)
  hemolytic disease 773.0
  incompatibility, immunization, or sensitization
    affecting management of pregnancy
      656.1 ☑
    fetus or newborn 773.0
    transfusion reaction (*see also* Complications, transfusion) 999.70
  negative mother, affecting fetus or newborn
    773.0
  titer elevated (*see also* Complications, transfusion) 999.70
  transfusion reaction (*see also* Complications, transfusion) 999.70
Rhesus (factor) (Rh) incompatibility — *see* Rh, incompatibility
Rheumaticosis — *see* Rheumatism
Rheumatism, rheumatic (acute NEC) 729.0
  adherent pericardium 393
  arthritis
    acute or subacute — *see* Fever, rheumatic
    chronic 714.0
      spine 720.0
    articular (chronic) NEC (*see also* Arthritis)
      716.9 ☑
    acute or subacute — *see* Fever, rheumatic
  back 724.9
  blennorrhagic 098.59
  carditis — *see* Disease, heart, rheumatic
  cerebral — *see* Fever, rheumatic
  chorea (acute) — *see* Chorea, rheumatic
  chronic NEC 729.0
  coronary arteritis 391.9
    chronic 398.99
  degeneration, myocardium (*see also* Degeneration, myocardium, with rheumatic fever) 398.0
  desert 114.0
  febrile — *see* Fever, rheumatic
  fever — *see* Fever, rheumatic
  gonococcal 098.59
  gout 714.0
  heart
    disease (*see also* Disease, heart, rheumatic) 398.90
    failure (chronic) (congestive) (inactive) 398.91
    hemopericardium — *see* Rheumatic, pericarditis
    hydropericardium — *see* Rheumatic, pericarditis
  inflammatory (acute) (chronic) (subacute) — *see* Fever, rheumatic
  intercostal 729.0
    meaning Tietze's disease 733.6
  joint (chronic) NEC (*see also* Arthritis)
    716.9 ☑

Rheumatism, rheumatic — *continued*
  joint (*see also* Arthritis) — *continued*
    acute — *see* Fever, rheumatic
  mediastinopericarditis — *see* Rheumatic, pericarditis
  muscular 729.0
  myocardial degeneration (*see also* Degeneration, myocardium, with rheumatic fever) 398.0
  myocarditis (chronic) (inactive) (with chorea) 398.0
    active or acute 391.2
      with chorea (acute) (rheumatic) (Sydenham's) 392.0
  myositis 729.1
  neck 724.9
  neuralgic 729.0
  neuritis (acute) (chronic) 729.2
  neuromuscular 729.0
  nodose — *see* Arthritis, nodosa
  nonarticular 729.0
  palindromic 719.30
    ankle 719.37
    elbow 719.32
    foot 719.37
    hand 719.34
    hip 719.35
    knee 719.36
    multiple sites 719.39
    pelvic region 719.35
    shoulder (region) 719.31
    specified site NEC 719.38
    wrist 719.33
  pancarditis, acute 391.8
    with chorea (acute) (rheumatic) (Sydenham's) 392.0
    chronic or inactive 398.99
  pericarditis (active) (acute) (with effusion) (with pneumonia) 391.0
    with chorea (acute) (rheumatic) (Sydenham's) 392.0
    chronic or inactive 393
  pericardium — *see* Rheumatic, pericarditis
  pleuropericarditis — *see* Rheumatic, pericarditis
  pneumonia 390 [517.1]
  pneumonitis 390 [517.1]
  pneumopericarditis — *see* Rheumatic, pericarditis
  polyarthritis
    acute or subacute — *see* Fever, rheumatic
    chronic 714.0
  polyarticular NEC (*see also* Arthritis) 716.9 ☑
  psychogenic 306.0
  radiculitis 729.2
  sciatic 724.3
  septic — *see* Fever, rheumatic
  spine 724.9
  subacute NEC 729.0
  torticollis 723.5
  tuberculous NEC (*see also* Tuberculosis)
    015.9 ☑
  typhoid fever 002.0
Rheumatoid — *see also* condition
  lungs 714.81
Rhinitis (atrophic) (catarrhal) (chronic) (croupous) (fibrinous) (hyperplastic) (hypertrophic) (membranous) (purulent) (suppurative) (ulcerative) 472.0
  with
    hay fever (*see also* Fever, hay) 477.9
      with asthma (bronchial) 493.0 ☑
    sore throat — *see* Nasopharyngitis
  acute 460
  allergic (nonseasonal) (seasonal) (*see also* Fever, hay) 477.9
    with asthma (*see also* Asthma) 493.0 ☑
    due to food 477.1
  granulomatous 472.0
  infective 460
  obstructive 472.0
  pneumococcal 460
  syphilitic 095.8
    congenital 090.0
  tuberculous (*see also* Tuberculosis) 012.8 ☑

☑ **Additional Digit Required** — Refer to the Tabular List for Digit Selection   ▽ **Subterms under main terms may continue to next column or page**

2014 ICD-9-CM   ▶◀ Revised Text   ● New Line   ▲ Revised Code   **Volume 2 — 249**

Rhinitis — *continued*
  vasomotor (*see also* Fever, hay) 477.9
Rhinoantritis (chronic) 473.0
  acute 461.0
Rhinodacryolith 375.57
Rhinolalia (aperta) (clausa) (open) 784.43
Rhinolith 478.19
  nasal sinus (*see also* Sinusitis) 473.9
Rhinomegaly 478.19
Rhinopharyngitis (acute) (subacute) — *see also* Nasopharyngitis 460
  chronic 472.2
  destructive ulcerating 102.5
  mutilans 102.5
Rhinophyma 695.3
Rhinorrhea 478.19
  cerebrospinal (fluid) 349.81
  paroxysmal (*see also* Fever, hay) 477.9
  spasmodic (*see also* Fever, hay) 477.9
Rhinosalpingitis 381.50
  acute 381.51
  chronic 381.52
Rhinoscleroma 040.1
Rhinosporidiosis 117.0
Rhinovirus infection 079.3
Rhizomelic chrondrodysplasia punctata 277.86
Rhizomelique, pseudopolyarthritic 446.5
Rhoads and Bomford anemia (refractory) 238.72
Rhus
  diversiloba dermatitis 692.6
  radicans dermatitis 692.6
  toxicodendron dermatitis 692.6
  venenata dermatitis 692.6
  verniciflua dermatitis 692.6
Rhythm
  atrioventricular nodal 427.89
  disorder 427.9
    coronary sinus 427.89
    ectopic 427.89
    nodal 427.89
  escape 427.89
  heart, abnormal 427.9
    fetus or newborn — *see* Abnormal, heart rate
  idioventricular 426.89
    accelerated 427.89
  nodal 427.89
  sleep, inversion 327.39
    nonorganic origin 307.45
Rhytidosis facialis 701.8
Rib — *see also* condition
  cervical 756.2
Riboflavin deficiency 266.0
Rice bodies — *see also* Loose, body, joint 718.1 ☑
  knee 717.6
Richter's hernia — *see* Hernia, Richter's
Ricinism 988.2
Rickets (active) (acute) (adolescent) (adult) (chest wall) (congenital) (current) (infantile) (intestinal) 268.0
  celiac 579.0
  fetal 756.4
  hemorrhagic 267
  hypophosphatemic with nephrotic-glycosuric dwarfism 270.0
  kidney 588.0
  late effect 268.1
  renal 588.0
  scurvy 267
  vitamin D-resistant 275.3
Rickettsial disease 083.9
  specified type NEC 083.8
Rickettsialpox 083.2
Rickettsiosis NEC 083.9
  specified type NEC 083.8
  tick-borne 082.9
    specified type NEC 082.8
  vesicular 083.2
Ricord's chancre 091.0
Riddoch's syndrome (visual disorientation) 368.16
Rider's
  bone 733.99

Rider's — *continued*
  chancre 091.0
Ridge, alveolus — *see also* condition
  edentulous
    atrophy 525.20
      mandible 525.20
        minimal 525.21
        moderate 525.22
        severe 525.23
      maxilla 525.20
        minimal 525.24
        moderate 525.25
        severe 525.26
    flabby 525.20
Ridged ear 744.29
Riedel's
  disease (ligneous thyroiditis) 245.3
  lobe, liver 751.69
  struma (ligneous thyroiditis) 245.3
  thyroiditis (ligneous) 245.3
Rieger's anomaly or syndrome (mesodermal dysgenesis, anterior ocular segment) 743.44
Riehl's melanosis 709.09
Rietti-Greppi-Micheli anemia or syndrome 282.46
Rieux's hernia — *see* Hernia, Rieux's
Rift Valley fever 066.3
Riga-Fede disease (cachectic aphthae) 529.0
Riga's disease (cachectic aphthae) 529.0
Riggs' disease (compound periodontitis) 523.40
Right middle lobe syndrome 518.0
Rigid, rigidity — *see also* condition
  abdominal 789.4 ☑
  articular, multiple congenital 754.89
  back 724.8
  cervix uteri
    in pregnancy or childbirth 654.6 ☑
      affecting fetus or newborn 763.89
      causing obstructed labor 660.2 ☑
        affecting fetus or newborn 763.1
  hymen (acquired) (congenital) 623.3
  nuchal 781.6
  pelvic floor
    in pregnancy or childbirth 654.4 ☑
      affecting fetus or newborn 763.89
      causing obstructed labor 660.2 ☑
        affecting fetus or newborn 763.1
  perineum or vulva
    in pregnancy or childbirth 654.8 ☑
      affecting fetus or newborn 763.89
      causing obstructed labor 660.2 ☑
        affecting fetus or newborn 763.1
  spine 724.8
  vagina
    in pregnancy or childbirth 654.7 ☑
      affecting fetus or newborn 763.89
      causing obstructed labor 660.2 ☑
        affecting fetus or newborn 763.1
Rigors 780.99
Riley-Day syndrome (familial dysautonomia) 742.8
RIND (reversible ischemic neurological deficit) 434.91
  history of (personal) V12.54
Ring(s)
  aorta 747.21
  Bandl's, complicating delivery 661.4 ☑
    affecting fetus or newborn 763.7
  contraction, complicating delivery 661.4 ☑
    affecting fetus or newborn 763.7
  esophageal (congenital) 750.3
  Fleischer (-Kayser) (cornea) 275.1 *[371.14]*
  hymenal, tight (acquired) (congenital) 623.3
  Kayser-Fleischer (cornea) 275.1 *[371.14]*
  retraction, uterus, pathological 661.4 ☑
    affecting fetus or newborn 763.7
  Schatzki's (esophagus) (congenital) (lower) 750.3
    acquired 530.3
  Soemmering's 366.51
  trachea, abnormal 748.3
  vascular (congenital) 747.21
  Vossius' 921.3
    late effect 366.21

Ringed hair (congenital) 757.4
Ringing in the ear — *see also* Tinnitus 388.30
Ringworm 110.9
  beard 110.0
  body 110.5
  Burmese 110.9
  corporeal 110.5
  foot 110.4
  groin 110.3
  hand 110.2
  honeycomb 110.0
  nails 110.1
  perianal (area) 110.3
  scalp 110.0
  specified site NEC 110.8
  Tokelau 110.5
Rise, venous pressure 459.89
Risk
  factor — *see* Problem
  falling V15.88
  suicidal 300.9
Ritter's disease (dermatitis exfoliativa neonatorum) 695.81
Rivalry, sibling 313.3
Rivalta's disease (cervicofacial actinomycosis) 039.3
River blindness 125.3 *[360.13]*
Robert's pelvis 755.69
  with disproportion (fetopelvic) 653.0 ☑
    affecting fetus or newborn 763.1
    causing obstructed labor 660.1 ☑
      affecting fetus or newborn 763.1
Robinson's (hidrotic) **ectodermal dysplasia** 757.31
Robin's syndrome 756.0
Robles' disease (onchocerciasis) 125.3 *[360.13]*
Rochalimea — *see* Rickettsial disease
Rocky Mountain fever (spotted) 082.0
Rodent ulcer (M8090/3) — *see also* Neoplasm, skin, malignant
  cornea 370.07
Roentgen ray, adverse effect — *see* Effect, adverse, x-ray
Roetheln 056.9
Roger's disease (congenital interventricular septal defect) 745.4
Rokitansky-Aschoff sinuses (mucosal outpouching of gallbladder) — *see also* Disease, gallbladder 575.8
Rokitansky-Kuster-Hauser syndrome (congenital absence vagina) 752.45
Rokitansky's
  disease (*see also* Necrosis, liver) 570
  tumor 620.2
Rollet's chancre (syphilitic) 091.0
Rolling of head 781.0
Romano-Ward syndrome (prolonged QT interval syndrome) 426.82
Romanus lesion 720.1
Romberg's disease or syndrome 349.89
Roof, mouth — *see* condition
Rosacea 695.3
  acne 695.3
  keratitis 695.3 *[370.49]*
Rosary, rachitic 268.0
Rose
  cold 477.0
  fever 477.0
  rash 782.1
    epidemic 056.9
    of infants 057.8
Rosen-Castleman-Liebow syndrome (pulmonary proteinosis) 516.0
Rosenbach's erysipelatoid or erysipeloid 027.1
Rosenthal's disease (factor XI deficiency) 286.2
Roseola 057.8
  infantum, infantilis (*see also* Exanthem subitum) 058.10
Rossbach's disease (hyperchlorhydria) 536.8
  psychogenic 306.4
Rössle-Urbach-Wiethe lipoproteinosis 272.8
Ross river fever 066.3
Rostan's asthma (cardiac) — *see* Failure, ventricular, left 428.1
Rot-Bernhardt disease 355.1

Rot
  Barcoo (*see also* Ulcer, skin) 707.9
  knife-grinders' (*see also* Tuberculosis) 011.4 ☑
Rotation
  anomalous, incomplete or insufficient — *see* Malrotation
  cecum (congenital) 751.4
  colon (congenital) 751.4
  manual, affecting fetus or newborn 763.89
  spine, incomplete or insufficient 737.8
  tooth, teeth 524.35
  vertebra, incomplete or insufficient 737.8
Röteln 056.9
Roth-Bernhardt disease or syndrome 355.1
Roth's disease or meralgia 355.1
Rothmund (-Thomson) syndrome 757.33
Rotor's disease or syndrome (idiopathic hyperbilirubinemia) 277.4
Rotundum ulcus — *see* Ulcer, stomach
Round
  back (with wedging of vertebrae) 737.10
    late effect of rickets 268.1
  hole, retina 361.31
    with detachment 361.01
  ulcer (stomach) — *see* Ulcer, stomach
  worms (infestation) (large) NEC 127.0
Roussy-Lévy syndrome 334.3
Routine postpartum follow-up V24.2
Roy (-Jutras) syndrome (acropachyderma) 757.39
Rubella (German measles) 056.9
  complicating pregnancy, childbirth, or puerperium 647.5 ☑
  complication 056.8
    neurological 056.00
      encephalomyelitis 056.01
      specified type NEC 056.09
    specified type NEC 056.79
  congenital 771.0
  contact V01.4
  exposure to V01.4
  maternal
    with suspected fetal damage affecting management of pregnancy 655.3 ☑
    affecting fetus or newborn 760.2
      manifest rubella in infant 771.0
  specified complications NEC 056.79
  vaccination, prophylactic (against) V04.3
Rubeola (measles) — *see also* Measles 055.9
  complicated 055.8
  meaning rubella (*see also* Rubella) 056.9
  scarlatinosis 057.8
Rubeosis iridis 364.42
  diabetica 250.5 ☑ *[364.42]*
    due to secondary diabetes 249.5 ☑ *[364.42]*
Rubinstein-Taybi's syndrome (brachydactylia, short stature and intellectual disabilities) 759.89
Rudimentary (congenital) — *see also* Agenesis
  arm 755.22
  bone 756.9
  cervix uteri 752.43
  eye (*see also* Microphthalmos) 743.10
  fallopian tube 752.19
  leg 755.32
  lobule of ear 744.21
  patella 755.64
  respiratory organs in thoracopagus 759.4
  tracheal bronchus 748.3
  uterine horn 752.39
  uterus 752.39
    in male 752.7
    solid or with cavity 752.39
  vagina 752.45
Rud's syndrome (mental deficiency, epilepsy, and infantilism) 759.89
Ruiter-Pompen (-Wyers) syndrome (angiokeratoma corporis diffusum) 272.7
Ruled out condition — *see also* Observation, suspected V71.9
Rumination — *see also* Vomiting
  disorder 307.53
  neurotic 300.3

☑ Additional Digit Required — Refer to the Tabular List for Digit Selection ⬙ Subterms under main terms may continue to next column or page

250 — Volume 2 ▶◀ Revised Text ● New Line ▲ Revised Code 2014 ICD-9-CM

Rumination — *see also* Vomiting — *continued*
- obsessional 300.3
- psychogenic 307.53

Runaway reaction — *see also* Disturbance, conduct
- socialized 312.2 ☑
- undersocialized, unsocialized 312.1 ☑

Runeberg's disease (progressive pernicious anemia) 281.0

Runge's syndrome (postmaturity) 766.22

Runny nose 784.99

Rupia 091.3
- congenital 090.0
- tertiary 095.9

Rupture, ruptured 553.9
- abdominal viscera NEC 799.89
  - obstetrical trauma 665.5 ☑
- abscess (spontaneous) — *see* Abscess, by site
- amnion — *see* Rupture, membranes
- aneurysm — *see* Aneurysm
- anus (sphincter) — *see* Laceration, anus
- aorta, aortic 441.5
  - abdominal 441.3
  - arch 441.1
  - ascending 441.1
  - descending 441.5
    - abdominal 441.3
    - thoracic 441.1
  - syphilitic 093.0
  - thoracoabdominal 441.6
  - thorax, thoracic 441.1
  - transverse 441.1
  - traumatic (thoracic) 901.0
    - abdominal 902.0
  - valve or cusp (*see also* Endocarditis, aortic) 424.1
- appendix (with peritonitis) 540.0
  - with peritoneal abscess 540.1
  - traumatic — *see* Injury, internal, gastrointestinal tract
- arteriovenous fistula, brain (congenital) 430
- artery 447.2
  - brain (*see also* Hemorrhage, brain) 431
  - coronary (*see also* Infarct, myocardium) 410.9 ☑
  - heart (*see also* Infarct, myocardium) 410.9 ☑
  - pulmonary 417.8
  - traumatic (complication) (*see also* Injury, blood vessel, by site) 904.9
- bile duct, except cystic (*see also* Disease, biliary) 576.3
  - cystic 575.4
  - traumatic — *see* Injury, internal, intraabdominal
- bladder (sphincter) 596.6
  - with
    - abortion — *see* Abortion, by type, with damage to pelvic organs
    - ectopic pregnancy (*see also* categories 633.0–633.9) 639.2
    - molar pregnancy (*see also* categories 630–632) 639.2
  - following
    - abortion 639.2
    - ectopic or molar pregnancy 639.2
  - nontraumatic 596.6
  - obstetrical trauma 665.5 ☑
  - spontaneous 596.6
  - traumatic — *see* Injury, internal, bladder
- blood vessel (*see also* Hemorrhage) 459.0
  - brain (*see also* Hemorrhage, brain) 431
  - heart (*see also* Infarct, myocardium) 410.9 ☑
  - traumatic (complication) (*see also* Injury, blood vessel, by site) 904.9
- bone — *see* Fracture, by site
- bowel 569.89
  - traumatic — *see* Injury, internal, intestine
- Bowman's membrane 371.31
- brain
  - aneurysm (congenital) (*see also* Hemorrhage, subarachnoid) 430

Rupture, ruptured — *continued*
- brain — *continued*
  - aneurysm (*see also* Hemorrhage, subarachnoid) — *continued*
    - late effect — *see* Late effect(s) (of) cerebrovascular disease
    - syphilitic 094.87
  - hemorrhagic (*see also* Hemorrhage, brain) 431
  - injury at birth 767.0
  - syphilitic 094.89
- capillaries 448.9
- cardiac (*see also* Infarct, myocardium) 410.9 ☑
- cartilage (articular) (current) (*see also* Sprain, by site)
  - knee — *see* Tear, meniscus
  - semilunar — *see* Tear, meniscus
- cecum (with peritonitis) 540.0
  - with peritoneal abscess 540.1
  - traumatic 863.89
    - with open wound into cavity 863.99
- cerebral aneurysm (congenital) (*see also* Hemorrhage, subarachnoid) 430
  - late effect — *see* Late effect(s) (of) cerebrovascular disease
- cervix (uteri)
  - with
    - abortion — *see* Abortion, by type, with damage to pelvic organs
    - ectopic pregnancy (*see also* categories 633.0–633.9) 639.2
    - molar pregnancy (*see also* categories 630–632) 639.2
  - following
    - abortion 639.2
    - ectopic or molar pregnancy 639.2
  - obstetrical trauma 665.3 ☑
  - traumatic — *see* Injury, internal, cervix
- chordae tendineae 429.5
- choroid (direct) (indirect) (traumatic) 363.63
- circle of Willis (*see also* Hemorrhage, subarachnoid) 430
  - late effect — *see* Late effect(s) (of) cerebrovascular disease
- colon 569.89
  - traumatic — *see* Injury, internal, colon
- cornea (traumatic) (*see also* Rupture, eye)
  - due to ulcer 370.00
- coronary (artery) (thrombotic) (*see also* Infarct, myocardium) 410.9 ☑
- corpus luteum (infected) (ovary) 620.1
- cyst — *see* Cyst
- cystic duct (*see also* Disease, gallbladder) 575.4
- Descemet's membrane 371.33
  - traumatic — *see* Rupture, eye
- diaphragm (*see also* Hernia, diaphragm)
  - traumatic — *see* Injury, internal, diaphragm
- diverticulum
  - bladder 596.3
  - intestine (large) (*see also* Diverticula) 562.10
    - small 562.00
- duodenal stump 537.89
- duodenum (ulcer) — *see* Ulcer, duodenum, with perforation
- ear drum (*see also* Perforation, tympanum) 384.20
  - with otitis media — *see* Otitis media
  - traumatic — *see* Wound, open, ear
- esophagus 530.4
  - traumatic 862.22
    - with open wound into cavity 862.32
    - cervical region — *see* Wound, open, esophagus
- eye (without prolapse of intraocular tissue) 871.0
  - with
    - exposure of intraocular tissue 871.1
    - partial loss of intraocular tissue 871.2
    - prolapse of intraocular tissue 871.1
  - due to burn 940.5
- fallopian tube 620.8

Rupture, ruptured — *continued*
- fallopian tube — *continued*
  - due to pregnancy — *see* Pregnancy, tubal
  - traumatic — *see* Injury, internal, fallopian tube
- fontanel 767.3
- free wall (ventricle) (*see also* Infarct, myocardium) 410.9 ☑
- gallbladder or duct (*see also* Disease, gallbladder) 575.4
  - traumatic — *see* Injury, internal, gallbladder
- gastric (*see also* Rupture, stomach) 537.89
  - vessel 459.0
- globe (eye) (traumatic) — *see* Rupture, eye
- graafian follicle (hematoma) 620.0
- heart (auricle) (ventricle) (*see also* Infarct, myocardium) 410.9 ☑
  - infectional 422.90
  - traumatic — *see* Rupture, myocardium, traumatic
- hymen 623.8
- internal
  - organ, traumatic (*see also* Injury, internal, by site)
    - heart — *see* Rupture, myocardium, traumatic
    - kidney — *see* Rupture, kidney
    - liver — *see* Rupture, liver
    - spleen — *see* Rupture, spleen, traumatic
  - semilunar cartilage — *see* Tear, meniscus
- intervertebral disc — *see* Displacement, intervertebral disc
  - traumatic (current) — *see* Dislocation, vertebra
- intestine 569.89
  - traumatic — *see* Injury, internal, intestine
- intracranial, birth injury 767.0
- iris 364.76
  - traumatic — *see* Rupture, eye
- joint capsule — *see* Sprain, by site
- kidney (traumatic) 866.03
  - with open wound into cavity 866.13
  - due to birth injury 767.8
  - nontraumatic 593.89
- lacrimal apparatus (traumatic) 870.2
- lens (traumatic) 366.20
- ligament (*see also* Sprain, by site)
  - with open wound — *see* Wound, open, by site
  - old (*see also* Disorder, cartilage, articular) 718.0 ☑
- liver (traumatic) 864.04
  - with open wound into cavity 864.14
  - due to birth injury 767.8
  - nontraumatic 573.8
- lymphatic (node) (vessel) 457.8
- marginal sinus (placental) (with hemorrhage) 641.2 ☑
  - affecting fetus or newborn 762.1
- meaning hernia — *see* Hernia
- membrana tympani (*see also* Perforation, tympanum) 384.20
  - with otitis media — *see* Otitis media
  - traumatic — *see* Wound, open, ear
- membranes (spontaneous)
  - artificial
    - delayed delivery following 658.3 ☑
      - affecting fetus or newborn 761.1
    - fetus or newborn 761.1
  - delayed delivery following 658.2 ☑
    - affecting fetus or newborn 761.1
  - premature (less than 24 hours prior to onset of labor) 658.1 ☑
    - affecting fetus or newborn 761.1
    - delayed delivery following 658.2 ☑
      - affecting fetus or newborn 761.1
- meningeal artery (*see also* Hemorrhage, subarachnoid) 430
  - late effect — *see* Late effect(s) (of) cerebrovascular disease
- meniscus (knee) (*see also* Tear, meniscus)

Rupture, ruptured — *continued*
- meniscus (*see also* Tear, meniscus) — *continued*
  - old (*see also* Derangement, meniscus) 717.5
    - site other than knee — *see* Disorder, cartilage, articular
  - site other than knee — *see* Sprain, by site
- mesentery 568.89
  - traumatic — *see* Injury, internal, mesentery
- mitral — *see* Insufficiency, mitral
- muscle (traumatic) NEC (*see also* Sprain, by site)
  - with open wound — *see* Wound, open, by site
  - nontraumatic 728.83
- musculotendinous cuff (nontraumatic) (shoulder) 840.4
- mycotic aneurysm, causing cerebral hemorrhage (*see also* Hemorrhage, subarachnoid) 430
  - late effect — *see* Late effect(s) (of) cerebrovascular disease
- myocardium, myocardial (*see also* Infarct, myocardium) 410.9 ☑
  - traumatic 861.03
    - with open wound into thorax 861.13
- nontraumatic (meaning hernia) (*see also* Hernia, by site) 553.9
  - obstructed (*see also* Hernia, by site, with obstruction) 552.9
  - gangrenous (*see also* Hernia, by site, with gangrene) 551.9
- operation wound (*see also* Dehiscence) 998.32
  - internal 998.31
- ovary, ovarian 620.8
  - corpus luteum 620.1
  - follicle (graafian) 620.0
- oviduct 620.8
  - due to pregnancy — *see* Pregnancy, tubal
- pancreas 577.8
  - traumatic — *see* Injury, internal, pancreas
- papillary muscle (ventricular) 429.6
- pelvic
  - floor, complicating delivery 664.1 ☑
  - organ NEC — *see* Injury, pelvic, organs
- penis (traumatic) — *see* Wound, open, penis
- perineum 624.8
  - during delivery (*see also* Laceration, perineum, complicating delivery) 664.4 ☑
- pharynx (nontraumatic) (spontaneous) 478.29
- pregnant uterus (before onset of labor) 665.0 ☑
- prostate (traumatic) — *see* Injury, internal, prostate
- pulmonary
  - artery 417.8
  - valve (heart) (*see also* Endocarditis, pulmonary) 424.3
  - vein 417.8
  - vessel 417.8
- pupil, sphincter 364.75
- pus tube (*see also* Salpingo-oophoritis) 614.2
- pyosalpinx (*see also* Salpingo-oophoritis) 614.2
- rectum 569.49
  - traumatic — *see* Injury, internal, rectum
- retina, retinal (traumatic) (without detachment) 361.30
  - with detachment (*see also* Detachment, retina, with retinal defect) 361.00
- rotator cuff (capsule) (traumatic) 840.4
  - nontraumatic (complete) 727.61
    - partial 726.13
- sclera 871.0
- semilunar cartilage, knee (*see also* Tear, meniscus) 836.2

☑ Additional Digit Required — Refer to the Tabular List for Digit Selection　　　　　　　　　▽ Subterms under main terms may continue to next column or page

2014 ICD-9-CM　　　▶◀ Revised Text　　　● New Line　　　▲ Revised Code　　　　　　　　Volume 2 — 251

Rupture, ruptured — *continued*
 semilunar cartilage, knee (*see also* Tear, meniscus) — *continued*
  old (*see also* Derangement, meniscus) 717.5
 septum (cardiac) 410.8 ☑
 sigmoid 569.89
  traumatic — *see* Injury, internal, colon, sigmoid
 sinus of Valsalva 747.29
 spinal cord (*see also* Injury, spinal, by site)
  due to injury at birth 767.4
  fetus or newborn 767.4
  syphilitic 094.89
  traumatic (*see also* Injury, spinal, by site)
   with fracture — *see* Fracture, vertebra, by site, with spinal cord injury
 spleen 289.59
  congenital 767.8
  due to injury at birth 767.8
  malarial 084.9
  nontraumatic 289.59
  spontaneous 289.59
  traumatic 865.04
   with open wound into cavity 865.14
 splenic vein 459.0
 stomach 537.89
  due to injury at birth 767.8
  traumatic — *see* Injury, internal, stomach
  ulcer — *see* Ulcer, stomach, with perforation
 synovium 727.50
  specified site NEC 727.59
 tendon (traumatic) (*see also* Sprain, by site)
  with open wound — *see* Wound, open, by site
  Achilles 845.09
   nontraumatic 727.67
  ankle 845.09
   nontraumatic 727.68
  biceps (long bead) 840.8
   nontraumatic 727.62
  foot 845.10
   interphalangeal (joint) 845.13

Rupture, ruptured — *continued*
 tendon (*see also* Sprain, by site) — *continued*
  foot — *continued*
   metatarsophalangeal (joint) 845.12
   nontraumatic 727.68
   specified site NEC 845.19
   tarsometatarsal (joint) 845.11
  hand 842.10
   carpometacarpal (joint) 842.11
   interphalangeal (joint) 842.13
   metacarpophalangeal (joint) 842.12
   nontraumatic 727.63
    extensors 727.63
    flexors 727.64
   specified site NEC 842.19
  nontraumatic 727.60
   specified site NEC 727.69
  patellar 844.8
   nontraumatic 727.66
  quadriceps 844.8
   nontraumatic 727.65
  rotator cuff (capsule) 840.4
   nontraumatic (complete) 727.61
    partial 726.13
  wrist 842.00
   carpal (joint) 842.01
   nontraumatic 727.63
    extensors 727.63
    flexors 727.64
   radiocarpal (joint) (ligament) 842.02
   radioulnar (joint), distal 842.09
   specified site NEC 842.09
 testis (traumatic) 878.2
  complicated 878.3
  due to syphilis 095.8
 thoracic duct 457.8
 tonsil 474.8
 traumatic
  with open wound — *see* Wound, open, by site
  aorta — *see* Rupture, aorta, traumatic
  ear drum — *see* Wound, open, ear, drum
  external site — *see* Wound, open, by site
  eye 871.2
  globe (eye) — *see* Wound, open, eyeball

Rupture, ruptured — *continued*
 traumatic — *continued*
  internal organ (abdomen, chest, or pelvis) (*see also* Injury, internal, by site)
   heart — *see* Rupture, myocardium, traumatic
   kidney — *see* Rupture, kidney
   liver — *see* Rupture, liver
   spleen — *see* Rupture, spleen, traumatic
  ligament, muscle, or tendon (*see also* Sprain, by site)
   with open wound — *see* Wound, open, by site
  meaning hernia — *see* Hernia
 tricuspid (heart) (valve) — *see* Endocarditis, tricuspid
 tube, tubal 620.8
  abscess (*see also* Salpingo-oophoritis) 614.2
  due to pregnancy — *see* Pregnancy, tubal
 tympanum, tympanic (membrane) (*see also* Perforation, tympanum) 384.20
  with otitis media — *see* Otitis media
  traumatic — *see* Wound, open, ear, drum
 umbilical cord 663.8 ☑
  fetus or newborn 772.0
 ureter (traumatic) (*see also* Injury, internal, ureter) 867.2
  nontraumatic 593.89
 urethra 599.84
  with
   abortion — *see* Abortion, by type, with damage to pelvic organs
   ectopic pregnancy (*see also* categories 633.0–633.9) 639.2
   molar pregnancy (*see also* categories 630–632) 639.2
  following
   abortion 639.2
   ectopic or molar pregnancy 639.2
  obstetrical trauma 665.5 ☑
  traumatic — *see* Injury, internal urethra

Rupture, ruptured — *continued*
 uterosacral ligament 620.8
 uterus (traumatic) (*see also* Injury, internal uterus)
  affecting fetus or newborn 763.89
  during labor 665.1 ☑
  nonpuerperal, nontraumatic 621.8
  nontraumatic 621.8
  pregnant (during labor) 665.1 ☑
   before labor 665.0 ☑
 vagina 878.6
  complicated 878.7
  complicating delivery — *see* Laceration, vagina, complicating delivery
 valve, valvular (heart) — *see* Endocarditis
 varicose vein — *see* Varicose, vein
 varix — *see* Varix
 vena cava 459.0
 ventricle (free wall) (left) (*see also* Infarct, myocardium) 410.9 ☑
 vesical (urinary) 596.6
  traumatic — *see* Injury, internal, bladder
 vessel (blood) 459.0
  pulmonary 417.8
 viscus 799.89
 vulva 878.4
  complicated 878.5
  complicating delivery 664.0 ☑
Russell's dwarf (uterine dwarfism and craniofacial dysostosis) 759.89
Russell's dysentery 004.8
Russell (-Silver) syndrome (congenital hemihypertrophy and short stature) 759.89
Russian spring-summer type encephalitis 063.0
Rust's disease (tuberculous spondylitis) 015.0 ☑ *[720.81]*
Rustitskii's disease (multiple myeloma) (M9730/3) 203.0 ☑
Ruysch's disease (Hirschsprung's disease) 751.3
Rytand-Lipsitch syndrome (complete atrioventricular block) 426.0

☑ Additional Digit Required — Refer to the Tabular List for Digit Selection ▽ Subterms under main terms may continue to next column or page

252 — Volume 2 ▶◀ Revised Text ● New Line ▲ Revised Code 2014 ICD-9-CM

S

Saber
  shin 090.5
  tibia 090.5
Saccharomyces infection — *see also* Candidiasis 112.9
Saccharopinuria 270.7
Saccular — *see* condition
Sacculation
  aorta (nonsyphilitic) (*see also* Aneurysm, aorta) 441.9
    ruptured 441.5
    syphilitic 093.0
  bladder 596.3
  colon 569.89
  intralaryngeal (congenital) (ventricular) 748.3
  larynx (congenital) (ventricular) 748.3
  organ or site, congenital — *see* Distortion
  pregnant uterus, complicating delivery 654.4 ☑
    affecting fetus or newborn 763.1
    causing obstructed labor 660.2 ☑
      affecting fetus or newborn 763.1
  rectosigmoid 569.89
  sigmoid 569.89
  ureter 593.89
  urethra 599.2
  vesical 596.3
Sachs (-Tay) disease (amaurotic familial idiocy) 330.1
Sacks-Libman disease 710.0 [424.91]
Sac, lacrimal — *see* condition
Sacralgia 724.6
Sacralization
  fifth lumbar vertebra 756.15
  incomplete (vertebra) 756.15
Sacrodynia 724.6
Sacroiliac joint — *see* condition
Sacroiliitis NEC 720.2
Sacrum — *see* condition
Saddle
  back 737.8
  embolus
    abdominal aorta 444.01
    pulmonary artery 415.13
  injury — code to condition
  nose 738.0
    congenital 754.0
    due to syphilis 090.5
Sadism (sexual) 302.84
Saemisch's ulcer 370.04
Saenger's syndrome 379.46
Sago spleen 277.39
Sailors' skin 692.74
Saint
  Anthony's fire (*see also* Erysipelas) 035
  Guy's dance — *see* Chorea
  Louis-type encephalitis 062.3
  triad (*see also* Hernia, diaphragm) 553.3
  Vitus' dance — *see* Chorea
Salicylism
  correct substance properly administered 535.4 ☑
  overdose or wrong substance given or taken 965.1
Salivary duct or gland — *see also* condition
  virus disease 078.5
Salivation (excessive) — *see also* Ptyalism 527.7
Salmonella (aertrycke) (choleraesuis) (enteritidis) (gallinarum) (suipestifer) (typhimurium) — *see also* Infection, Salmonella 003.9
  arthritis 003.23
  carrier (suspected) of V02.3
  meningitis 003.21
  osteomyelitis 003.24
  pneumonia 003.22
  septicemia 003.1
  typhosa 002.0
    carrier (suspected) of V02.1
Salmonellosis 003.0
  with pneumonia 003.22

Salpingitis (catarrhal) (fallopian tube) (nodular) (pseudofollicular) (purulent) (septic) — *see also* Salpingo-oophoritis 614.2
  ear 381.50
    acute 381.51
    chronic 381.52
  Eustachian (tube) 381.50
    acute 381.51
    chronic 381.52
  follicularis 614.1
  gonococcal (chronic) 098.37
    acute 098.17
  interstitial, chronic 614.1
  isthmica nodosa 614.1
  old — *see* Salpingo-oophoritis, chronic
  puerperal, postpartum, childbirth 670.8 ☑
  specific (chronic) 098.37
    acute 098.17
  tuberculous (acute) (chronic) (*see also* Tuberculosis) 016.6 ☑
  venereal (chronic) 098.37
    acute 098.17
Salpingo-oophoritis (catarrhal) (purulent) (ruptured) (septic) (suppurative) 614.2
  acute 614.0
    with
      abortion — *see* Abortion, by type, with sepsis
      ectopic pregnancy (*see also* categories 633.0–633.9) 639.0
      molar pregnancy (*see also* categories 630–632) 639.0
    following
      abortion 639.0
      ectopic or molar pregnancy 639.0
    gonococcal 098.17
    puerperal, postpartum, childbirth 670.8 ☑
    tuberculous (*see also* Tuberculosis) 016.6 ☑
  chronic 614.1
    gonococcal 098.37
    tuberculous (see also Tuberculosis) 016.6 ☑
  complicating pregnancy 646.6 ☑
    affecting fetus or newborn 760.8
  gonococcal (chronic) 098.37
    acute 098.17
  old — *see* Salpingo-oophoritis, chronic
  puerperal 670.8 ☑
  specific — *see* Salpingo-oophoritis, gonococcal
  subacute (*see also* Salpingo-oophoritis, acute) 614.0
  tuberculous (acute) (chronic) (*see also* Tuberculosis) 016.6 ☑
  venereal — *see* Salpingo-oophoritis, gonococcal
Salpingo-ovaritis — *see also* Salpingo-oophoritis 614.2
Salpingocele 620.4
Salpingoperitonitis — *see also* Salpingo-oophoritis 614.2
Salt-losing
  nephritis (*see also* Disease, renal) 593.9
  syndrome (*see also* Disease, renal) 593.9
Salt-rheum — *see also* Eczema 692.9
Salzmann's nodular dystrophy 371.46
Sampling
  chorionic villus V28.89
Sampson's cyst or tumor 617.1
Sandblasters'
  asthma 502
  lung 502
Sander's disease (paranoia) 297.1
Sandfly fever 066.0
Sandhoff's disease 330.1
Sanfilippo's syndrome (mucopolysaccharidosis III) 277.5
Sanger-Brown's ataxia 334.2
San Joaquin Valley fever 114.0
Sao Paulo fever or typhus 082.0
Saponification, mesenteric 567.89
Sapremia — *see* Septicemia
Sarcocele (benign)
  syphilitic 095.8

Sarcocele — *continued*
  syphilitic — *continued*
    congenital 090.5
Sarcoepiplocele — *see also* Hernia 553.9
Sarcoepiplomphalocele — *see also* Hernia, umbilicus 553.1
Sarcoid (any site) 135
  with lung involvement 135 [517.8]
  Boeck's 135
  Darier-Roussy 135
  Spiegler-Fendt 686.8
Sarcoidosis 135
  cardiac 135 [425.8]
  lung 135 [517.8]
Sarcoma (M8800/3) — *see also* Neoplasm, connective tissue, malignant
  alveolar soft part (M9581/3) — *see* Neoplasm, connective tissue, malignant
  ameloblastic (M9330/3) 170.1
    upper jaw (bone) 170.0
  botryoid (M8910/3) — *see* Neoplasm, connective tissue, malignant
  botryoides (M8910/3) — *see* Neoplasm, connective tissue, malignant
  cerebellar (M9480/3) 191.6
    circumscribed (arachnoidal) (M9471/3) 191.6
  circumscribed (arachnoidal) cerebellar (M9471/3) 191.6
  clear cell, of tendons and aponeuroses (M9044/3) — *see* Neoplasm, connective tissue, malignant
  embryonal (M8991/3) — *see* Neoplasm, connective tissue, malignant
  endometrial (stromal) (M8930/3) 182.0
    isthmus 182.1
  endothelial (M9130/3) (*see also* Neoplasm, connective tissue, malignant)
    bone (M9260/3) — *see* Neoplasm, bone, malignant
  epithelioid cell (M8804/3) — *see* Neoplasm, connective tissue, malignant
  Ewing's (M9260/3) — *see* Neoplasm, bone, malignant
  follicular dendritic cell 202.9 ☑
  germinoblastic (diffuse) (M9632/3) 202.8 ☑
    follicular (M9697/3) 202.0
  giant cell (M8802/3) (*see also* Neoplasm, connective tissue, malignant)
    bone (M9250/3) — *see* Neoplasm, bone, malignant
  glomoid (M8710/3) — *see* Neoplasm, connective tissue, malignant
  granulocytic (M9930/3) 205.3 ☑
  hemangioendothelial (M9130/3) — *see* Neoplasm, connective tissue, malignant
  hemorrhagic, multiple (M9140/3) — *see* Kaposi's, sarcoma
  Hodgkin's (M9662/3) 201.2 ☑
  immunoblastic (M9612/3) 200.8 ☑
  interdigitating dendritic cell 202.9 ☑
  Kaposi's (M9140/3) — *see* Kaposi's, sarcoma
  Kupffer cell (M9124/3) 155.0
  Langerhans cell 202.9 ☑
  leptomeningeal (M9530/3) — *see* Neoplasm, meninges, malignant
  lymphangioendothelial (M9170/3) — *see* Neoplasm, connective tissue, malignant
  lymphoblastic (M9630/3) 200.1 ☑
  lymphocytic (M9620/3) 200.1 ☑
  mast cell (M9740/3) 202.6 ☑
  melanotic (M8720/3) — *see* Melanoma
  meningeal (M9530/3) — *see* Neoplasm, meninges, malignant
  meningothelial (M9530/3) — *see* Neoplasm, meninges, malignant
  mesenchymal (M8800/3) (*see also* Neoplasm, connective tissue, malignant)
    mixed (M8990/3) — *see* Neoplasm, connective tissue, malignant
  mesothelial (M9050/3) — *see* Neoplasm, by site, malignant

Sarcoma — *see also* Neoplasm, connective tissue, malignant — *continued*
  monstrocellular (M9481/3)
    specified site — *see* Neoplasm, by site, malignant
    unspecified site 191.9
  myeloid (M9930/3) 205.3 ☑
  neurogenic (M9540/3) — *see* Neoplasm, connective tissue, malignant
  odontogenic (M9270/3) 170.1
    upper jaw (bone) 170.0
  osteoblastic (M9180/3) — *see* Neoplasm, bone, malignant
  osteogenic (M9180/3) (*see also* Neoplasm, bone, malignant)
    juxtacortical (M9190/3) — *see* Neoplasm, bone, malignant
    periosteal (M9190/3) — *see* Neoplasm, bone, malignant
  periosteal (M8812/3) (*see also* Neoplasm, bone, malignant)
    osteogenic (M9190/3) — *see* Neoplasm, bone, malignant
  plasma cell (M9731/3) 203.8 ☑
  pleomorphic cell (M8802/3) — *see* Neoplasm, connective tissue, malignant
  reticuloendothelial (M9720/3) 202.3 ☑
  reticulum cell (M9640/3) 200.0 ☑
    nodular (M9642/3) 200.0 ☑
    pleomorphic cell type (M9641/3) 200.0 ☑
  round cell (M8803/3) — *see* Neoplasm, connective tissue, malignant
  small cell (M8803/3) — *see* Neoplasm, connective tissue, malignant
  spindle cell (M8801/3) — *see* Neoplasm, connective tissue, malignant
  stromal (endometrial) (M8930/3) 182.0
    isthmus 182.1
  synovial (M9040/3) (*see also* Neoplasm, connective tissue, malignant)
    biphasic type (M9043/3) — *see* Neoplasm, connective tissue, malignant
    epithelioid cell type (M9042/3) — *see* Neoplasm, connective tissue, malignant
    spindle cell type (M9041/3) — *see* Neoplasm, connective tissue, malignant
Sarcomatosis
  meningeal (M9539/3) — *see* Neoplasm, meninges, malignant
  specified site NEC (M8800/3) — *see* Neoplasm, connective tissue, malignant
  unspecified site (M8800/6) 171.9
Sarcosinemia 270.8
Sarcosporidiosis 136.5
Satiety, early 780.94
Satisfactory smear but lacking transformation zone
  anal 796.77
  cervical 795.07
Saturnine — *see* condition
Saturnism 984.9
  specified type of lead — *see* Table of Drugs and Chemicals
Satyriasis 302.89
Sauriasis — *see* Ichthyosis
Sauriderma 757.39
Sauriosis — *see* Ichthyosis
Savill's disease (epidemic exfoliative dermatitis) 695.89
SBE (subacute bacterial endocarditis) 421.0
Scabies (any site) 133.0
Scabs 782.8
Scaglietti-Dagnini syndrome (acromegalic macrospondylitis) 253.0
Scald, scalded — *see also* Burn, by site
  skin syndrome 695.81
Scalenus anticus (anterior) syndrome 353.0
Scales 782.8
Scalp — *see* condition
Scaphocephaly 756.0
Scaphoiditis, tarsal 732.5
Scapulalgia 733.90

☑ **Additional Digit Required** — Refer to the Tabular List for Digit Selection

2014 ICD-9-CM

▶◀ **Revised Text**   ● **New Line**   ▲ **Revised Code**

🔻 **Subterms under main terms may continue to next column or page**

Volume 2 — 253

Saber — Scapulalgia

Scapulohumeral myopathy 359.1
Scarabiasis 134.1
Scarlatina 034.1
   anginosa 034.1
   maligna 034.1
   myocarditis, acute 034.1 *[422.0]*
      old (*see also* Myocarditis) 429.0
   otitis media 034.1 *[382.02]*
   ulcerosa 034.1
Scarlatinella 057.8
Scarlet fever (albuminuria) (angina) (convulsions) (lesions of lid) (rash) 034.1
Scar, scarring — *see also* Cicatrix 709.2
   adherent 709.2
   atrophic 709.2
   cervix
      in pregnancy or childbirth 654.6 ☑
         affecting fetus or newborn 763.89
         causing obstructed labor 660.2 ☑
            affecting fetus or newborn 763.1
   cheloid 701.4
   chorioretinal 363.30
      disseminated 363.35
      macular 363.32
      peripheral 363.34
      posterior pole NEC 363.33
   choroid (*see also* Scar, chorioretinal) 363.30
   compression, pericardial 423.9
   congenital 757.39
   conjunctiva 372.64
   cornea 371.00
      xerophthalmic 264.6
   due to previous cesarean delivery, compli-
      cating pregnancy or childbirth
      654.2 ☑
         affecting fetus or newborn 763.89
   duodenal (bulb) (cap) 537.3
   hypertrophic 701.4
   keloid 701.4
   labia 624.4
   lung (base) 518.89
   macula 363.32
      disseminated 363.35
      peripheral 363.34
   muscle 728.89
   myocardium, myocardial 412
   painful 709.2
   papillary muscle 429.81
   posterior pole NEC 363.33
      macular — *see* Scar, macula
   postnecrotic (hepatic) (liver) 571.9
   psychic V15.49
   retina (*see also* Scar, chorioretinal) 363.30
   trachea 478.9
   uterus 621.8
      in pregnancy or childbirth NEC 654.9 ☑
         affecting fetus or newborn 763.89
         due to previous cesarean delivery
         654.2 ☑
   vulva 624.4
Schamberg's disease, dermatitis, or der-
   matosis (progressive pigmentary dermatosis) 709.09
Schatzki's ring (esophagus) (lower) (congenital) 750.3
   acquired 530.3
Schaufenster krankheit 413.9
Schaumann's
   benign lymphogranulomatosis 135
   disease (sarcoidosis) 135
   syndrome (sarcoidosis) 135
Scheie's syndrome (mucopolysaccharidosis
   IS) 277.5
Schenck's disease (sporotrichosis) 117.1
Scheuermann's disease or osteochondrosis
   732.0
Scheuthauer-Marie-Sainton syndrome
   (cleidocranialis dysostosis) 755.59
Schilder (-Flatau) disease 341.1
Schilling-type monocytic leukemia
   (M9890/3) 206.9 ☑
Schimmelbusch's disease, cystic mastitis,
   or hyperplasia 610.1
Schirmer's syndrome (encephalocutaneous
   angiomatosis) 759.6
Schistocelia 756.79

Schistoglossia 750.13
Schistosoma infestation — *see* Infestation,
   Schistosoma
Schistosomiasis 120.9
   Asiatic 120.2
   bladder 120.0
   chestermani 120.8
   colon 120.1
   cutaneous 120.3
   due to
      S. hematobium 120.0
      S. japonicum 120.2
      S. mansoni 120.1
      S. mattheii 120.8
   eastern 120.2
   genitourinary tract 120.0
   intestinal 120.1
   lung 120.2
   Manson's (intestinal) 120.1
   Oriental 120.2
   pulmonary 120.2
   specified type NEC 120.8
   vesical 120.0
Schizencephaly 742.4
Schizo-affective psychosis — *see also*
   Schizophrenia 295.7 ☑
Schizodontia 520.2
Schizoid personality 301.20
   introverted 301.21
   schizotypal 301.22
Schizophrenia, schizophrenic (reaction)
   295.9 ☑

Note — Use the following fifth-digit
subclassification with category 295:

0   unspecified

1   subchronic

2   chronic

3   subchronic with acute exacerba-
    tion

4   chronic with acute exacerbation

5   in remission

   acute (attack) NEC 295.8 ☑
      episode 295.4 ☑
   atypical form 295.8 ☑
   borderline 295.5 ☑
   catalepsy 295.2 ☑
   catatonic (type) (acute) (excited) (with-
      drawn) 295.2 ☑
   childhood (type) (*see also* Psychosis, child-
      hood) 299.9 ☑
   chronic NEC 295.6 ☑
   coenesthesiopathic 295.8 ☑
   cyclic (type) 295.7 ☑
   disorganized (type) 295.1 ☑
   flexibilitas cerea 295.2 ☑
   hebephrenic (type) (acute) 295.1 ☑
   incipient 295.5 ☑
   latent 295.5 ☑
   paranoid (type) (acute) 295.3 ☑
   paraphrenic (acute) 295.3 ☑
   prepsychotic 295.5 ☑
   primary (acute) 295.0 ☑
   prodromal 295.5 ☑
   pseudoneurotic 295.5 ☑
   pseudopsychopathic 295.5 ☑
   reaction 295.9 ☑
   residual type (state) 295.6 ☑
   restzustand 295.6 ☑
   schizo-affective (type) (depressed) (excited)
      295.7 ☑
   schizophreniform type 295.4 ☑
   simple (type) (acute) 295.0 ☑
   simplex (acute) 295.0 ☑
   specified type NEC 295.8 ☑
   syndrome of childhood NEC (*see also* Psy-
      chosis, childhood) 299.9 ☑
   undifferentiated type 295.9 ☑
      acute 295.8 ☑
      chronic 295.6 ☑
Schizothymia 301.20
   introverted 301.21

Schizothymia — *continued*
   schizotypal 301.22
Schlafkrankheit 086.5
Schlatter-Osgood disease (osteochondrosis,
   tibial tubercle) 732.4
Schlatter's tibia (osteochondrosis) 732.4
Schloffer's tumor — *see also* Peritonitis 567.29
Schmidt's syndrome
   sphallo-pharyngo-laryngeal hemiplegia
      352.6
   thyroid-adrenocortical insufficiency 258.1
   vagoaccessory 352.6
Schmincke
   carcinoma (M8082/3) — *see* Neoplasm, na-
      sopharynx, malignant
   tumor (M8082/3) — *see* Neoplasm, na-
      sopharynx, malignant
Schmitz (-Stutzer) dysentery 004.0
Schmorl's disease or nodes 722.30
   lumbar, lumbosacral 722.32
   specified region NEC 722.39
   thoracic, thoracolumbar 722.31
Schneiderian
   carcinoma (M8121/3)
      specified site — *see* Neoplasm, by site,
         malignant
      unspecified site 160.0
   papilloma (M8121/0)
      specified site — *see* Neoplasm, by site,
         benign
      unspecified site 212.0
Schneider's syndrome 047.9
Schnitzler syndrome 273.1
Schoffer's tumor — *see also* Peritonitis 567.29
Scholte's syndrome (malignant carcinoid)
   259.2
Scholz's disease 330.0
Scholz (-Bielschowsky-Henneberg) syn-
   drome 330.0
Schönlein (-Henoch) disease (primary) (pur-
   pura) (rheumatic) 287.0
School examination V70.3
   following surgery V67.09
Schottmüller's disease — *see also* Fever,
   paratyphoid 002.9
Schroeder's syndrome (endocrine-hyperten-
   sive) 255.3
Schüller-Christian disease or syndrome
   (chronic histiocytosis X) 277.89
Schultz's disease or syndrome (agranulocyto-
   sis) 288.09
Schultze's acroparesthesia, simple 443.89
Schwalbe-Ziehen-Oppenheimer disease
   333.6
Schwannoma (M9560/0) — *see also* Neoplasm,
   connective tissue, benign
   malignant (M9560/3) — *see* Neoplasm,
      connective tissue, malignant
Schwannomatosis 237.73
Schwartz-Bartter syndrome (inappropriate
   secretion of antidiuretic hormone) 253.6
Schwartz (-Jampel) syndrome 359.23
Schweninger-Buzzi disease (macular atrophy)
   701.3
Sciatic — *see* condition
Sciatica (infectional) 724.3
   due to
      displacement of intervertebral disc
         722.10
      herniation, nucleus pulposus 722.10
   wallet 724.3
Scimitar syndrome (anomalous venous
   drainage, right lung to inferior vena cava) 747.49
Sclera — *see* condition
Sclerectasia 379.11
Scleredema
   adultorum 710.1
   Buschke's 710.1
   newborn 778.1
Sclerema
   adiposum (newborn) 778.1
   adultorum 710.1
   edematosum (newborn) 778.1
   neonatorum 778.1
   newborn 778.1

Scleriasis — *see* Scleroderma
Scleritis 379.00
   with corneal involvement 379.05
   anterior (annular) (localized) 379.03
   brawny 379.06
   granulomatous 379.09
   posterior 379.07
   specified NEC 379.09
   suppurative 379.09
   syphilitic 095.0
   tuberculous (nodular) (*see also* Tuberculosis)
      017.3 ☑ *[379.09]*
Sclerochoroiditis — *see also* Scleritis 379.00
Scleroconjunctivitis — *see also* Scleritis 379.00
Sclerocystic ovary (syndrome) 256.4
Sclerodactylia 701.0
Scleroderma, sclerodermia (acrosclerotic)
   (diffuse) (generalized) (progressive)
   (pulmonary) 710.1
   circumscribed 701.0
   linear 701.0
   localized (linear) 701.0
   newborn 778.1
Sclerokeratitis 379.05
   meaning sclerosing keratitis 370.54
   tuberculous (*see also* Tuberculosis)
      017.3 ☑ *[379.09]*
Scleromalacia
   multiple 731.0
   perforans 379.04
Scleroma, trachea 040.1
Scleromyxedema 701.8
Scleroperikeratitis 379.05
Sclerose en plaques 340
Sclerosis, sclerotic
   adrenal (gland) 255.8
   Alzheimer's 331.0
      with dementia — *see* Alzheimer's, de-
         mentia
   amyotrophic (lateral) 335.20
   annularis fibrosi
      aortic 424.1
      mitral 424.0
   aorta, aortic 440.0
      valve (*see also* Endocarditis, aortic) 424.1
   artery, arterial, arteriolar, arteriovascular —
      see Arteriosclerosis
   ascending multiple 340
   Balo's (concentric) 341.1
   basilar — *see* Sclerosis, brain
   bone (localized) NEC 733.99
   brain (general) (lobular) 348.89
      Alzheimer's — *see* Alzheimer's, demen-
         tia
      artery, arterial 437.0
      atrophic lobar 331.0
         with dementia
            with behavioral disturbance
               331.0 *[294.11]*
            without behavioral disturbance
               331.0 *[294.10]*
      diffuse 341.1
         familial (chronic) (infantile) 330.0
         infantile (chronic) (familial) 330.0
         Pelizaeus-Merzbacher type 330.0
      disseminated 340
      hereditary 334.2
      hippocampal 348.81
      infantile (degenerative) (diffuse) 330.0
      insular 340
      Krabbe's 330.0
      mesial temporal 348.81
      miliary 340
      multiple 340
      Pelizaeus-Merzbacher 330.0
      progressive familial 330.0
      senile 437.0
      temporal 348.81
         mesial 348.81
      tuberous 759.5
   bulbar, progressive 340
   bundle of His 426.50
      left 426.3
      right 426.4
   cardiac — *see* Arteriosclerosis, coronary

☑ **Additional Digit Required** — Refer to the Tabular List for Digit Selection
▼ **Subterms under main terms may continue to next column or page**

254 — Volume 2   ▶◀ Revised Text   ● New Line   ▲ Revised Code   **2014 ICD-9-CM**

Sclerosis, sclerotic — *continued*
  cardiorenal (*see also* Hypertension, cardiorenal) 404.90
  cardiovascular (*see also* Disease, cardiovascular) 429.2
    renal (*see also* Hypertension, cardiorenal) 404.90
  centrolobar, familial 330.0
  cerebellar — *see* Sclerosis, brain
  cerebral — *see* Sclerosis, brain
  cerebrospinal 340
    disseminated 340
    multiple 340
  cerebrovascular 437.0
  choroid 363.40
    diffuse 363.56
  combined (spinal cord) (*see also* Degeneration, combined)
    multiple 340
  concentric, Baló's 341.1
  cornea 370.54
  coronary (artery) — *see* Arteriosclerosis, coronary
  corpus cavernosum
    female 624.8
    male 607.89
  Dewitzky's
    aortic 424.1
    mitral 424.0
  diffuse NEC 341.1
  disease, heart — *see* Arteriosclerosis, coronary
  disseminated 340
  dorsal 340
  dorsolateral (spinal cord) — *see* Degeneration, combined
  endometrium 621.8
  extrapyramidal 333.90
  eye, nuclear (senile) 366.16
  Friedreich's (spinal cord) 334.0
  funicular (spermatic cord) 608.89
  gastritis 535.4 ☑
  general (vascular) — *see* Arteriosclerosis
  gland (lymphatic) 457.8
  hepatic 571.9
  hereditary
    cerebellar 334.2
    spinal 334.0
  hippocampal 348.81
  idiopathic cortical (Garré's) (*see also* Osteomyelitis) 730.1 ☑
  ilium, piriform 733.5
  insular 340
    pancreas 251.8
  Islands of Langerhans 251.8
  kidney — *see* Sclerosis, renal
  larynx 478.79
  lateral 335.24
    amyotrophic 335.20
    descending 335.24
    primary 335.24
    spinal 335.24
  liver 571.9
  lobar, atrophic (of brain) 331.0
    with dementia
      with behavioral disturbance 331.0 [294.11]
      without behavioral disturbance 331.0 [294.10]
  lung (*see also* Fibrosis, lung) 515
  mastoid 383.1
  mesial temporal 348.81
  mitral — *see* Endocarditis, mitral
  Mönckeberg's (medial) (*see also* Arteriosclerosis, extremities) 440.20
  multiple (brain stem) (cerebral) (generalized) (spinal cord) 340
  myocardium, myocardial — *see* Arteriosclerosis, coronary
  nuclear (senile), eye 366.16
  ovary 620.8
  pancreas 577.8
  penis 607.89
  peripheral arteries (*see also* Arteriosclerosis, extremities) 440.20
  plaques 340

Sclerosis, sclerotic — *continued*
  pluriglandular 258.8
  polyglandular 258.8
  posterior (spinal cord) (syphilitic) 094.0
  posterolateral (spinal cord) — *see* Degeneration, combined
  prepuce 607.89
  primary lateral 335.24
  progressive systemic 710.1
  pulmonary (*see also* Fibrosis, lung) 515
    artery 416.0
    valve (heart) (*see also* Endocarditis, pulmonary) 424.3
  renal 587
    with
      cystine storage disease 270.0
      hypertension (*see also* Hypertension, kidney) 403.90
      hypertensive heart disease (conditions classifiable to 402) (*see also* Hypertension, cardiorenal) 404.90
      arteriolar (hyaline) (*see also* Hypertension, kidney) 403.90
      hyperplastic (*see also* Hypertension, kidney) 403.90
  retina (senile) (vascular) 362.17
  rheumatic
    aortic valve 395.9
    mitral valve 394.9
  Schilder's 341.1
  senile — *see* Arteriosclerosis
  spinal (cord) (general) (progressive) (transverse) 336.8
    ascending 357.0
    combined (*see also* Degeneration, combined)
      multiple 340
      syphilitic 094.89
    disseminated 340
    dorsolateral — *see* Degeneration, combined
    hereditary (Friedreich's) (mixed form) 334.0
    lateral (amyotrophic) 335.24
    multiple 340
    posterior (syphilitic) 094.0
  stomach 537.89
  subendocardial, congenital 425.3
  systemic (progressive) 710.1
    with lung involvement 710.1 [517.2]
  temporal 348.81
    mesial 348.81
  tricuspid (heart) (valve) — *see* Endocarditis, tricuspid
  tuberous (brain) 759.5
  tympanic membrane (*see also* Tympanosclerosis) 385.00
  valve, valvular (heart) — *see* Endocarditis
  vascular — *see* Arteriosclerosis
  vein 459.89
Sclerotenonitis 379.07
Sclerotitis — *see also* Scleritis 379.00
  syphilitic 095.0
  tuberculous (*see also* Tuberculosis) 017.3 ☑ [379.09]
Scoliosis (acquired) (postural) 737.30
  congenital 754.2
  due to or associated with
    Charcôt-Marie-Tooth disease 356.1 [737.43]
    mucopolysaccharidosis 277.5 [737.43]
    neurofibromatosis 237.71 [737.43]
    osteitis
      deformans 731.0 [737.43]
      fibrosa cystica 252.01 [737.43]
    osteoporosis (*see also* Osteoporosis) 733.00 [737.43]
    poliomyelitis 138 [737.43]
    radiation 737.33
    tuberculosis (*see also* Tuberculosis) 015.0 ☑ [737.43]
  idiopathic 737.30
    infantile
      progressive 737.32
      resolving 737.31

Scoliosis — *continued*
  paralytic 737.39
  rachitic 268.1
  sciatic 724.3
  specified NEC 737.39
  thoracogenic 737.34
  tuberculous (*see also* Tuberculosis) 015.0 ☑ [737.43]
Scoliotic pelvis 738.6
  with disproportion (fetopelvic) 653.0 ☑
    affecting fetus or newborn 763.1
    causing obstructed labor 660.1 ☑
      affecting fetus or newborn 763.1
Scorbutus, scorbutic 267
  anemia 281.8
Scotoma (ring) 368.44
  arcuate 368.43
  Bjerrum 368.43
  blind spot area 368.42
  central 368.41
  centrocecal 368.41
  paracecal 368.42
  paracentral 368.41
  scintillating 368.12
  Seidel 368.43
Scratch — *see* Injury, superficial, by site
Scratchy throat 784.99
Screening (for) V82.9
  alcoholism V79.1
  anemia, deficiency NEC V78.1
    iron V78.0
  anomaly, congenital V82.89
  antenatal, of mother V28.9
    alphafetoprotein levels, raised V28.1
    based on amniocentesis V28.2
      chromosomal anomalies V28.0
      raised alphafetoprotein levels V28.1
    fetal growth retardation using ultrasonics V28.4
      ultrasonics V28.4
    genomic V28.89
    isoimmunization V28.5
    malformations using ultrasonics V28.3
    proteomic V28.89
    raised alphafetoprotein levels V28.1
    risk
      pre-term labor V28.82
    specified condition NEC V28.89
    Streptococcus B V28.6
  arterial hypertension V81.1
  arthropod-borne viral disease NEC V73.5
  asymptomatic bacteriuria V81.5
  bacterial
    and spirochetal sexually transmitted diseases V74.5
    conjunctivitis V74.4
    disease V74.9
      sexually transmitted V74.5
      specified condition NEC V74.8
  bacteriuria, asymptomatic V81.5
  blood disorder NEC V78.9
    specified type NEC V78.8
  bronchitis, chronic V81.3
  brucellosis V74.8
  cancer — *see* Screening, malignant neoplasm
  cardiovascular disease NEC V81.2
  cataract V80.2
  Chagas' disease V75.3
  chemical poisoning V82.5
  cholera V74.0
  cholesterol level V77.91
  chromosomal
    anomalies
      by amniocentesis, antenatal V28.0
      maternal postnatal V82.4
    athletes V70.3
  colonoscopy V76.51
  condition
    cardiovascular NEC V81.2
    eye NEC V80.2
    genitourinary NEC V81.6
    neurological NEC V80.09
    respiratory NEC V81.4
    skin V82.0
    specified NEC V82.89

Screening — *continued*
  congenital
    anomaly V82.89
      eye V80.2
    dislocation of hip V82.3
    eye condition or disease V80.2
  conjunctivitis, bacterial V74.4
  contamination NEC (*see also* Poisoning) V82.5
  coronary artery disease V81.0
  cystic fibrosis V77.6
  deficiency anemia NEC V78.1
    iron V78.0
  dengue fever V73.5
  depression V79.0
  developmental handicap V79.9
    in early childhood V79.3
    specified type NEC V79.8
  diabetes mellitus V77.1
  diphtheria V74.3
  disease or disorder V82.9
    bacterial V74.9
      specified NEC V74.8
    blood-forming organ V78.9
      specified type NEC V78.8
    blood V78.9
      specified type NEC V78.8
    cardiovascular NEC V81.2
      hypertensive V81.1
      ischemic V81.0
    Chagas' V75.3
    chlamydial V73.98
      specified NEC V73.88
    ear NEC V80.3
    endocrine NEC V77.99
    eye NEC V80.2
    genitourinary NEC V81.6
    heart NEC V81.2
      hypertensive V81.1
      ischemic V81.0
    HPV (human papillomavirus) V73.81
    human papillomavirus V73.81
    immunity NEC V77.99
    infectious NEC V75.9
    lipoid NEC V77.91
    mental V79.9
      specified type NEC V79.8
    metabolic NEC V77.99
      inborn NEC V77.7
    neurological NEC V80.09
    nutritional NEC V77.99
    rheumatic NEC V82.2
    rickettsial V75.0
    sexually transmitted V74.5
      bacterial V74.5
      spirochetal V74.5
    sickle-cell V78.2
      trait V78.2
    specified type NEC V82.89
    thyroid V77.0
    vascular NEC V81.2
      ischemic V81.0
    venereal V74.5
    viral V73.99
      arthropod-borne NEC V73.5
      specified type NEC V73.89
  dislocation of hip, congenital V82.3
  drugs in athletes V70.3
  elevated titer V82.9
  emphysema (chronic) V81.3
  encephalitis, viral (mosquito or tick borne) V73.5
  endocrine disorder NEC V77.99
  eye disorder NEC V80.2
    congenital V80.2
  fever
    dengue V73.5
    hemorrhagic V73.5
    yellow V73.4
  filariasis V75.6
  galactosemia V77.4
  genetic V82.79
    disease carrier status V82.71
  genitourinary condition NEC V81.6
  glaucoma V80.1
  gonorrhea V74.5

☑ **Additional Digit Required** — Refer to the Tabular List for Digit Selection   ▽ **Subterms under main terms may continue to next column or page**

2014 ICD-9-CM   ▶◀ **Revised Text**   ● **New Line**   ▲ **Revised Code**   **Volume 2 — 255**

Screening — continued
  gout V77.5
  Hansen's disease V74.2
  heart disease NEC V81.2
    hypertensive V81.1
    ischemic V81.0
  heavy metal poisoning V82.5
  helminthiasis, intestinal V75.7
  hematopoietic malignancy V76.89
  hemoglobinopathies NEC V78.3
  hemorrhagic fever V73.5
  Hodgkin's disease V76.89
  hormones in athletes V70.3
  HPV (human papillomavirus) V73.81
  human papillomavirus (HPV) V73.81
  hypercholesterolemia V77.91
  hyperlipidemia V77.91
  hypertension V81.1
  immunity disorder NEC V77.99
  inborn errors of metabolism NEC V77.7
  infection
    bacterial V74.9
      specified type NEC V74.8
    mycotic V75.4
    parasitic NEC V75.8
  infectious disease V75.9
    specified type NEC V75.8
  ingestion of radioactive substance V82.5
  intellectual disabilities V79.2
  intestinal helminthiasis V75.7
  iron deficiency anemia V78.0
  ischemic heart disease V81.0
  lead poisoning V82.5
  leishmaniasis V75.2
  leprosy V74.2
  leptospirosis V74.8
  leukemia V76.89
  lipoid disorder NEC V77.91
  lymphoma V76.89
  malaria V75.1
  malignant neoplasm (of) V76.9
    bladder V76.3
    blood V76.89
    breast V76.10
      mammogram NEC V76.12
        for high-risk patient V76.11
      specified type NEC V76.19
    cervix V76.2
    colon V76.51
    colorectal V76.51
    hematopoietic system V76.89
    intestine V76.50
      colon V76.51
      small V76.52
    lung V76.0
    lymph (glands) V76.89
    nervous system V76.81
    oral cavity V76.42
    other specified neoplasm NEC V76.89
    ovary V76.46
    prostate V76.44
    rectum V76.41
    respiratory organs V76.0
    skin V76.43
    specified sites NEC V76.49
    testis V76.45
    vagina V76.47
      following hysterectomy for malig-
        nant condition V67.01
  malnutrition V77.2
  mammogram NEC V76.12
    for high-risk patient V76.11
  maternal postnatal chromosomal anomalies
    V82.4
  measles V73.2
  mental
    disorder V79.9
      specified type NEC V79.8
    retardation — see Screening, intellectual
      disabilities
  metabolic disorder NEC V77.99
  metabolic errors, inborn V77.7
  mucoviscidosis V77.6
  multiphasic V82.6
  mycosis V75.4
  mycotic infection V75.4

Screening — continued
  nephropathy V81.5
  neurological condition NEC V80.09
  nutritional disorder V77.99
  obesity V77.8
  osteoporosis V82.81
  parasitic infection NEC V75.8
  phenylketonuria V77.3
  plague V74.8
  poisoning
    chemical NEC V82.5
      contaminated water supply V82.5
        heavy metal V82.5
  poliomyelitis V73.0
  postnatal chromosomal anomalies, mater-
    nal V82.4
  prenatal — see Screening, antenatal
  pulmonary tuberculosis V74.1
  radiation exposure V82.5
  renal disease V81.5
  respiratory condition NEC V81.4
  rheumatic disorder NEC V82.2
  rheumatoid arthritis V82.1
  rickettsial disease V75.0
  rubella V73.3
  schistosomiasis V75.5
  senile macular lesions of eye V80.2
  sexually transmitted diseases V74.5
    bacterial V74.5
    spirochetal V74.5
  sickle-cell anemia, disease, or trait V78.2
  skin condition V82.0
  sleeping sickness V75.3
  smallpox V73.1
  special V82.9
    specified condition NEC V82.89
  specified type NEC V82.89
  spirochetal disease V74.9
    sexually transmitted V74.5
    specified type NEC V74.8
  stimulants in athletes V70.3
  syphilis V74.5
  tetanus V74.8
  thyroid disorder V77.0
  trachoma V73.6
  traumatic brain injury V80.01
  trypanosomiasis V75.3
  tuberculosis, pulmonary V74.1
  venereal disease V74.5
  viral encephalitis
    mosquito-borne V73.5
    tick-borne V73.5
  whooping cough V74.8
  worms, intestinal V75.7
  yaws V74.6
  yellow fever V73.4
Scrofula — see also Tuberculosis 017.2 ☑
Scrofulide (primary) — see also Tuberculosis
    017.0 ☑
Scrofuloderma, scrofulodermia (any site)
    (primary) — see also Tuberculosis
    017.0 ☑
Scrofulosis (universal) — see also Tuberculosis
    017.2 ☑
Scrofulosis lichen (primary) — see also Tuber-
    culosis 017.0 ☑
Scrofulous — see condition
Scrotal tongue 529.5
  congenital 750.13
Scrotum — see condition
Scurvy (gum) (infantile) (rickets) (scorbutic) 267
Sea-blue histiocyte syndrome 272.7
Seabright-Bantam syndrome (pseudohy-
    poparathyroidism) 275.49
Sealpox 059.12
Seasickness 994.6
Seatworm 127.4
Sebaceous
  cyst (see also Cyst, sebaceous) 706.2
  gland disease NEC 706.9
Sebocystomatosis 706.2
Seborrhea, seborrheic 706.3
  adiposa 706.3
  capitis 690.11
  congestiva 695.4
  corporis 706.3

Seborrhea, seborrheic — continued
  dermatitis 690.10
    infantile 690.12
  diathesis in infants 695.89
  eczema 690.18
    infantile 690.12
  keratosis 702.19
    inflamed 702.11
  nigricans 705.89
  sicca 690.18
  wart 702.19
    inflamed 702.11
Seckel's syndrome 759.89
Seclusion pupil 364.74
Seclusiveness, child 313.22
Secondary — see also condition
  neoplasm — see Neoplasm, by site, malig-
    nant, secondary
Secretan's disease or syndrome (posttraumat-
    ic edema) 782.3
Secretion
  antidiuretic hormone, inappropriate (syn-
    drome) 253.6
  catecholamine, by pheochromocytoma
    255.6
  hormone
    antidiuretic, inappropriate (syndrome)
      253.6
    by
      carcinoid tumor 259.2
      pheochromocytoma 255.6
    ectopic NEC 259.3
  urinary
    excessive 788.42
    suppression 788.5
Section
  cesarean
    affecting fetus or newborn 763.4
    post mortem, affecting fetus or newborn
      761.6
    previous, in pregnancy or childbirth
      654.2 ☑
      affecting fetus or newborn 763.89
  nerve, traumatic — see Injury, nerve, by site
Seeligmann's syndrome (ichthyosis congeni-
    ta) 757.1
Segmentation, incomplete (congenital) —
    see also Fusion
  bone NEC 756.9
  lumbosacral (joint) 756.15
  vertebra 756.15
    lumbosacral 756.15
Seizure(s) 780.39
  akinetic (idiopathic) (see also Epilepsy)
    345.0 ☑
    psychomotor 345.4 ☑
  apoplexy, apoplectic (see also Disease,
    cerebrovascular, acute) 436
  atonic (see also Epilepsy) 345.0 ☑
  autonomic 300.11
  brain or cerebral (see also Disease, cere-
    brovascular, acute) 436
  convulsive (see also Convulsions) 780.39
  cortical (focal) (motor) (see also Epilepsy)
    345.5 ☑
  disorder (see also Epilepsy) 345.9 ☑
    due to stroke 438.89
  epilepsy, epileptic (cryptogenic) (see also
    Epilepsy) 345.9 ☑
  epileptiform, epileptoid 780.39
    focal (see also Epilepsy) 345.5 ☑
  febrile (simple) 780.31
    with status epilepticus 345.3
    atypical 780.32
    complex 780.32
    complicated 780.32
  heart — see Disease, heart
  hysterical 300.11
  Jacksonian (focal) (see also Epilepsy)
    345.5 ☑
    motor type 345.5 ☑
    sensory type 345.5 ☑
  migraine triggered 346.0 ☑
  newborn 779.0
  paralysis (see also Disease, cerebrovascular,
    acute) 436

Seizure(s) — continued
  posttraumatic 780.33
  recurrent 345.8 ☑
    epileptic — see Epilepsy
  repetitive 780.39
    epileptic — see Epilepsy
  salaam (see also Epilepsy) 345.6 ☑
  uncinate (see also Epilepsy) 345.4 ☑
Self-mutilation 300.9
Semicoma 780.09
Semiconsciousness 780.09
Seminal
  vesicle — see condition
  vesiculitis (see also Vesiculitis) 608.0
Seminoma (M9061/3)
  anaplastic type (M9062/3)
    specified site — see Neoplasm, by site,
      malignant
    unspecified site 186.9
  specified site — see Neoplasm, by site, ma-
    lignant
  spermatocytic (M9063/3)
    specified site — see Neoplasm, by site,
      malignant
    unspecified site 186.9
  unspecified site 186.9
Semliki Forest encephalitis 062.8
Senear-Usher disease or syndrome (pemphi-
    gus erythematosus) 694.4
Senecio jacobae dermatitis 692.6
Senectus 797
Senescence 797
Senile — see also condition 797
  cervix (atrophic) 622.8
  degenerative atrophy, skin 701.3
  endometrium (atrophic) 621.8
  fallopian tube (atrophic) 620.3
  heart (failure) 797
  lung 492.8
  ovary (atrophic) 620.3
  syndrome 259.8
  vagina, vaginitis (atrophic) 627.3
  wart 702.0
Senility 797
  with
    acute confusional state 290.3
    delirium 290.3
    mental changes 290.9
    psychosis NEC (see also Psychosis, senile)
      290.20
  premature (syndrome) 259.8
Sensation
  burning (see also Disturbance, sensation)
    782.0
    tongue 529.6
  choking 784.99
  loss of (see also Disturbance, sensation)
    782.0
  prickling (see also Disturbance, sensation)
    782.0
  tingling (see also Disturbance, sensation)
    782.0
Sense loss (touch) — see also Disturbance,
    sensation 782.0
  smell 781.1
  taste 781.1
Sensibility disturbance NEC (cortical) (deep)
    (vibratory) — see also Disturbance, sen-
    sation 782.0
Sensitive dentine 521.89
Sensitiver Beziehungswahn 297.8
Sensitivity, sensitization — see also Allergy
  autoerythrocyte 287.2
  carotid sinus 337.01
  child (excessive) 313.21
  cold, autoimmune 283.0
  methemoglobin 289.7
  suxamethonium 289.89
  tuberculin, without clinical or radiological
    symptoms 795.51
Sensory
  extinction 781.8
  neglect 781.8
Separation
  acromioclavicular — see Dislocation,
    acromioclavicular

☑ **Additional Digit Required** — Refer to the Tabular List for Digit Selection   ▽ **Subterms under main terms may continue to next column or page**

256 — Volume 2   ▶◀ **Revised Text**   ● **New Line**   ▲ **Revised Code**   **2014 ICD-9-CM**

Separation — *continued*
anxiety, abnormal 309.21
apophysis, traumatic — *see* Fracture, by site
choroid 363.70
hemorrhagic 363.72
serous 363.71
costochondral (simple) (traumatic) — *see* Dislocation, costochondral
delayed
umbilical cord 779.83
epiphysis, epiphyseal
nontraumatic 732.9
upper femoral 732.2
traumatic — *see* Fracture, by site
fracture — *see* Fracture, by site
infundibulum cardiac from right ventricle by a partition 746.83
joint (current) (traumatic) — *see* Dislocation, by site
placenta (normally implanted) — *see* Placenta, separation
pubic bone, obstetrical trauma 665.6 ☑
retina, retinal (*see also* Detachment, retina) 361.9
layers 362.40
sensory (*see also* Retinoschisis) 361.10
pigment epithelium (exudative) 362.42
hemorrhagic 362.43
sternoclavicular (traumatic) — *see* Dislocation, sternoclavicular
symphysis pubis, obstetrical trauma 665.6 ☑
tracheal ring, incomplete (congenital) 748.3

Sepsis (generalized) 995.91
with
abortion — *see* Abortion, by type, with sepsis
acute organ dysfunction 995.92
ectopic pregnancy (*see also* categories 633.0–633.9) 639.0
molar pregnancy (*see also* categories 630–632) 639.0
multiple organ dysfunction (MOD) 995.92
buccal 528.3
complicating labor 659.3 ☑
dental (pulpal origin) 522.4
female genital organ NEC 614.9
fetus (intrauterine) 771.81
following
abortion 639.0
ectopic or molar pregnancy 639.0
infusion, perfusion, or transfusion 999.39
Friedländer's 038.49
intra-abdominal 567.22
intraocular 360.00
localized — code to specific localized infection
in operation wound 998.59
skin (*see also* Abscess) 682.9
malleus 024
nadir 038.9
newborn (organism unspecified) NEC 771.81
oral 528.3
puerperal, postpartum, childbirth (pelvic) 670.2 ☑
resulting from infusion, injection, transfusion, or vaccination 999.39
severe 995.92
skin, localized (*see also* Abscess) 682.9
umbilical (newborn) (organism unspecified) 771.89
tetanus 771.3
urinary 599.0
meaning sepsis 995.91
meaning urinary tract infection 599.0
Septate — *see also* Septum
Septic — *see also* condition
adenoids 474.01
and tonsils 474.02
arm (with lymphangitis) 682.3
embolus — *see* Embolism
finger (with lymphangitis) 681.00
foot (with lymphangitis) 682.7
gallbladder (*see also* Cholecystitis) 575.8

Septic — *see also* condition — *continued*
hand (with lymphangitis) 682.4
joint (*see also* Arthritis, septic) 711.0 ☑
kidney (*see also* Infection, kidney) 590.9
leg (with lymphangitis) 682.6
mouth 528.3
nail 681.9
finger 681.02
toe 681.11
shock (endotoxic) 785.52
postoperative 998.02
sore (*see also* Abscess) 682.9
throat 034.0
milk-borne 034.0
streptococcal 034.0
spleen (acute) 289.59
teeth (pulpal origin) 522.4
throat 034.0
thrombus — *see* Thrombosis
toe (with lymphangitis) 681.10
tonsils 474.00
and adenoids 474.02
umbilical cord (newborn) (organism unspecified) 771.89
uterus (*see also* Endometritis) 615.9
Septicemia, septicemic (generalized) (suppurative) 038.9
with
abortion — *see* Abortion, by type, with sepsis
ectopic pregnancy (*see also* categories 633.0–633.9) 639.0
molar pregnancy (*see also* categories 630–632) 639.0
Aerobacter aerogenes 038.49
anaerobic 038.3
anthrax 022.3
Bacillus coli 038.42
Bacteroides 038.3
Clostridium 038.3
complicating labor 659.3 ☑
cryptogenic 038.9
enteric gram-negative bacilli 038.40
Enterobacter aerogenes 038.49
Erysipelothrix (insidiosa) (rhusiopathiae) 027.1
Escherichia coli 038.42
following
abortion 639.0
ectopic or molar pregnancy 639.0
infusion, injection, transfusion, or vaccination 999.39
Friedländer's (bacillus) 038.49
gangrenous 038.9
gonococcal 098.89
gram-negative (organism) 038.40
anaerobic 038.3
Hemophilus influenzae 038.41
herpes (simplex) 054.5
herpetic 054.5
Listeria monocytogenes 027.0
meningeal — *see* Meningitis
meningococcal (chronic) (fulminating) 036.2
methicillin
resistant Staphylococcus aureus (MRSA) 038.12
susceptible Staphylococcus aureus (MSSA) 038.11
MRSA (methicillin resistant Staphylococcus aureus) 038.12
MSSA (methicillin susceptible Staphylococcus aureus) 038.11
navel, newborn (organism unspecified) 771.89
newborn (organism unspecified) 771.81
plague 020.2
pneumococcal 038.2
postabortal 639.0
postoperative 998.59
Proteus vulgaris 038.49
Pseudomonas (aeruginosa) 038.43
puerperal, postpartum 670.2 ☑
Salmonella (aertrycke) (callinarum) (choleraesuis) (enteritidis) (suipestifer) 003.1
Serratia 038.44
Shigella (*see also* Dysentery, bacillary) 004.9

Septicemia, septicemic — *continued*
specified organism NEC 038.8
staphylococcal 038.10
aureus 038.11
methicillin
resistant (MRSA) 038.12
susceptible (MSSA) 038.11
specified organism NEC 038.19
streptococcal (anaerobic) 038.0
Streptococcus pneumoniae 038.2
suipestifer 003.1
umbilicus, newborn (organism unspecified) 771.89
viral 079.99
Yersinia enterocolitica 038.49
Septum, septate (congenital) — *see also* Anomaly, specified type NEC
anal 751.2
aqueduct of Sylvius 742.3
with spina bifida (*see also* Spina bifida) 741.0 ☑
hymen 752.49
uterus (complete) (partial) 752.35
vagina
in pregnancy or childbirth 654.7 ☑
affecting fetus or newborn 763.89
causing obstructed labor 660.2 ☑
affecting fetus or newborn 763.1
longitudinal (with or without obstruction) 752.47
transverse 752.46
Sequestration
lung (congenital) (extralobar) (intralobar) 748.5
orbit 376.10
pulmonary artery (congenital) 747.39
splenic 289.52
Sequestrum
bone (*see also* Osteomyelitis) 730.1 ☑
jaw 526.4
dental 525.8
jaw bone 526.4
sinus (accessory) (nasal) (*see also* Sinusitis) 473.9
maxillary 473.0
Sequoiosis asthma 495.8
Serology for syphilis
doubtful
with signs or symptoms — *see* Syphilis, by site and stage
follow-up of latent syphilis — *see* Syphilis, latent
false positive 795.6
negative, with signs or symptoms — *see* Syphilis, by site and stage
positive 097.1
with signs or symptoms — *see* Syphilis, by site and stage
false 795.6
follow-up of latent syphilis — *see* Syphilis, latent
only finding — *see* Syphilis, latent
reactivated 097.1
Seroma (postoperative) (non-infected) 998.13
infected 998.51
post-traumatic 729.91
Seropurulent — *see* condition
Serositis, multiple 569.89
pericardial 423.2
peritoneal 568.82
pleural — *see* Pleurisy
Serotonin syndrome 333.99
Serous — *see* condition
Sertoli-Leydig cell tumor (M8631/0)
specified site — *see* Neoplasm, by site, benign
unspecified site
female 220
male 222.0
Sertoli cell
adenoma (M8640/0)
specified site — *see* Neoplasm, by site, benign
unspecified site
female 220
male 222.0

Sertoli cell — *continued*
carcinoma (M8640/3)
specified site — *see* Neoplasm, by site, malignant
unspecified site 186.9
syndrome (germinal aplasia) 606.0
tumor (M8640/0)
with lipid storage (M8641/0)
specified site — *see* Neoplasm, by site, benign
unspecified site
female 220
male 222.0
specified site — *see* Neoplasm, by site, benign
unspecified site
female 220
male 222.0
Serum
allergy, allergic reaction 999.59
shock 999.49
arthritis 999.59 [713.6]
complication or reaction NEC 999.59
disease NEC 999.59
hepatitis 070.3 ☑
intoxication 999.59
jaundice (homologous) — *see* Hepatitis, viral, type B
neuritis 999.59
poisoning NEC 999.59
rash NEC 999.59
reaction NEC 999.59
sickness NEC 999.59
Sesamoiditis 733.99
Seven-day fever 061
of
Japan 100.89
Queensland 100.89
Sever's disease or osteochondrosis (calcaneum) 732.5
Sex chromosome mosaics 758.81
Sex reassignment surgery status (*see also* Trans-sexualism) 302.50
Sextuplet
affected by maternal complications of pregnancy 761.5
healthy liveborn — *see* Newborn, multiple
pregnancy (complicating delivery) NEC 651.8 ☑
with fetal loss and retention of one or more fetus(es) 651.6 ☑
following (elective) fetal reduction 651.7 ☑
Sexual
anesthesia 302.72
deviation (*see also* Deviation, sexual) 302.9
disorder (*see also* Deviation, sexual) 302.9
frigidity (female) 302.72
function, disorder of (psychogenic) 302.70
specified type NEC 302.79
immaturity (female) (male) 259.0
impotence 607.84
organic origin NEC 607.84
psychogenic 302.72
precocity (constitutional) (cryptogenic) (female) (idiopathic) (male) NEC 259.1
with adrenal hyperplasia 255.2
sadism 302.84
Sexuality, pathological — *see also* Deviation, sexual 302.9
Sézary's disease, reticulosis, or syndrome (M9701/3) 202.2 ☑
Shadow, lung 793.19
Shaken infant syndrome 995.55
Shaking
head (tremor) 781.0
palsy or paralysis (*see also* Parkinsonism) 332.0
Shallowness, acetabulum 736.39
Shaver's disease or syndrome (bauxite pneumoconiosis) 503
Shearing
artificial skin graft 996.55
decellularized allodermis graft 996.55
Sheath (tendon) — *see* condition

☑ **Additional Digit Required** — Refer to the Tabular List for Digit Selection   ▽ **Subterms under main terms may continue to next column or page**

2014 ICD-9-CM   ▶◀ Revised Text   ● New Line   ▲ Revised Code   **Volume 2 — 257**

Shedding
- nail 703.8
- teeth, premature, primary (deciduous) 520.6

Sheehan's disease or syndrome (postpartum pituitary necrosis) 253.2

Shelf, rectal 569.49

Shell
- shock (current) (see also Reaction, stress, acute) 308.9
  - lasting state 300.16
- teeth 520.5

Shield kidney 753.3

Shifting
- pacemaker 427.89
- sleep-work schedule (affecting sleep) 327.36

Shift, mediastinal 793.2

Shiga's
- bacillus 004.0
- dysentery 004.0

Shigella (dysentery) — see also Dysentery, bacillary 004.9
- carrier (suspected) of V02.3

Shigellosis — see also Dysentery, bacillary 004.9

Shingles — see also Herpes, zoster 053.9
- eye NEC 053.29

Shin splints 844.9

Shipyard eye or disease 077.1

Shirodkar suture, in pregnancy 654.5 ☑

Shock 785.50
- with
  - abortion — see Abortion, by type, with shock
  - ectopic pregnancy (see also categories 633.0–633.9) 639.5
  - molar pregnancy (see also categories 630–632) 639.5
- allergic — see Anaphylactic reaction or shock
- anaclitic 309.21
- anaphylactic — see also Anaphylactic reaction or shock
  - due to administration of blood and blood products 999.41
- anaphylactoid — see Anaphylactic reaction or shock
- anesthetic
  - correct substance properly administered 995.4
  - overdose or wrong substance given 968.4
    - specified anesthetic — see Table of Drugs and Chemicals
- birth, fetus or newborn NEC 779.89
- cardiogenic 785.51
- chemical substance — see Table of Drugs and Chemicals
- circulatory 785.59
- complicating
  - abortion — see Abortion, by type, with shock
  - ectopic pregnancy (see also categories 633.0–633.9) 639.5
  - labor and delivery 669.1 ☑
  - molar pregnancy (see also categories 630–632) 639.5
- culture 309.29
- due to
  - drug 995.0
    - correct substance properly administered 995.0
    - overdose or wrong substance given or taken 977.9
    - specified drug — see Table of Drugs and Chemicals
  - food — see Anaphylactic shock, due to, food
- during labor and delivery 669.1 ☑
- electric 994.8
  - from electroshock gun (taser) 994.8
- endotoxic 785.52
  - due to surgical procedure 998.02
  - postoperative 998.02
- following
  - abortion 639.5
  - ectopic or molar pregnancy 639.5

Shock — continued
- following — continued
  - injury (immediate) (delayed) 958.4
  - labor and delivery 669.1 ☑
- gram-negative 785.52
  - postoperative 998.02
- hematogenic 785.59
- hemorrhagic
  - due to
    - disease 785.59
    - surgery (intraoperative) (postoperative) 998.09
    - trauma 958.4
- hypovolemic NEC 785.59
  - surgical 998.09
  - traumatic 958.4
- insulin 251.0
  - therapeutic misadventure 962.3
- kidney 584.5
  - traumatic (following crushing) 958.5
- lightning 994.0
- lung 518.82
  - related to trauma and surgery 518.52
- nervous (see also Reaction, stress, acute) 308.9
- obstetric 669.1 ☑
  - with
    - abortion — see Abortion, by type, with shock
    - ectopic pregnancy (see also categories 633.0–633.9) 639.5
    - molar pregnancy (see also categories 630–632) 639.5
  - following
    - abortion 639.5
    - ectopic or molar pregnancy 639.5
- paralysis, paralytic (see also Disease, cerebrovascular, acute) 436
  - late effect — see Late effect(s) (of) cerebrovascular disease
- pleural (surgical) 998.09
  - due to trauma 958.4
- postoperative 998.00
  - with
    - abortion — see Abortion, by type, with shock
    - ectopic pregnancy (see also categories 633.0–633.9) 639.5
    - molar pregnancy (see also categories 630–632) 639.5
  - cardiogenic 998.01
  - following
    - abortion 639.5
    - ectopic or molar pregnancy 639.5
  - hypovolemic 998.09
  - septic (endotoxic) (gram-negative) 998.02
  - specified NEC 998.09
- psychic (see also Reaction, stress, acute) 308.9
  - past history (of) V15.49
- psychogenic (see also Reaction, stress, acute) 308.9
- septic 785.52
  - with
    - abortion — see Abortion, by type, with shock
    - ectopic pregnancy (see also categories 633.0–633.9) 639.5
    - molar pregnancy (see also categories 630–632) 639.5
  - due to
    - surgical procedure 998.02
    - transfusion NEC 999.89
      - bone marrow 996.85
  - following
    - abortion 639.5
    - ectopic or molar pregnancy 639.5
    - surgical procedure 998.02
    - transfusion NEC 999.89
      - bone marrow 996.85
  - postoperative 998.02
- spinal (see also Injury, spinal, by site)
  - with spinal bone injury — see Fracture, vertebra, by site, with spinal cord injury

Shock — continued
- surgical 998.00
- therapeutic misadventure NEC (see also Complications) 998.89
- thyroxin 962.7
- toxic 040.82
- transfusion — see Complications, transfusion
- traumatic (immediate) (delayed) 958.4

Shoemakers' chest 738.3

Short, shortening, shortness
- Achilles tendon (acquired) 727.81
- arm 736.89
  - congenital 755.20
- back 737.9
- bowel syndrome 579.3
- breath 786.05
- cervical, cervix 649.7 ☑
  - gravid uterus 649.7 ☑
  - non-gravid uterus 622.5
    - acquired 622.5
    - congenital 752.49
- chain acyl CoA dehydrogenase deficiency (SCAD) 277.85
- common bile duct, congenital 751.69
- cord (umbilical) 663.4 ☑
  - affecting fetus or newborn 762.6
- cystic duct, congenital 751.69
- esophagus (congenital) 750.4
- femur (acquired) 736.81
  - congenital 755.34
- frenulum linguae 750.0
- frenum, lingual 750.0
- hamstrings 727.81
- hip (acquired) 736.39
  - congenital 755.63
- leg (acquired) 736.81
  - congenital 755.30
- metatarsus (congenital) 754.79
  - acquired 736.79
- organ or site, congenital NEC — see Distortion
- P-R interval syndrome 426.81
- palate (congenital) 750.26
- radius (acquired) 736.09
  - congenital 755.26
- round ligament 629.89
- sleeper 307.49
- stature, constitutional (hereditary) (idiopathic) 783.43
- tendon 727.81
  - Achilles (acquired) 727.81
    - congenital 754.79
  - congenital 756.89
- thigh (acquired) 736.81
  - congenital 755.34
- tibialis anticus 727.81
- umbilical cord 663.4 ☑
  - affecting fetus or newborn 762.6
- urethra 599.84
- uvula (congenital) 750.26
- vagina 623.8

Shortsightedness 367.1

Shoshin (acute fulminating beriberi) 265.0

Shoulder — see condition

Shovel-shaped incisors 520.2

Shower, thromboembolic — see Embolism

Shunt (status)
- aortocoronary bypass V45.81
- arterial-venous (dialysis) V45.11
- arteriovenous, pulmonary (acquired) 417.0
  - congenital 747.39
  - traumatic (complication) 901.40
- cerebral ventricle (communicating) in situ V45.2
- coronary artery bypass V45.81
- surgical, prosthetic, with complications — see Complications, shunt
- vascular NEC V45.89

Shutdown
- renal 586
  - with
    - abortion — see Abortion, by type, with renal failure
    - ectopic pregnancy (see also categories 633.0–633.9) 639.3

Shutdown — continued
- renal — continued
  - with — continued
    - molar pregnancy (see also categories 630–632) 639.3
  - complicating
    - abortion 639.3
    - ectopic or molar pregnancy 639.3
  - following labor and delivery 669.3 ☑

Shwachman's syndrome 288.02

Shy-Drager syndrome (orthostatic hypotension with multisystem degeneration) 333.0

Sialadenitis (any gland) (chronic) (suppurative) 527.2
- epidemic — see Mumps

Sialadenosis, periodic 527.2

Sialaporia 527.7

Sialectasia 527.8

Sialitis 527.2

Sialoadenitis — see also Sialadenitis 527.2

Sialoangitis 527.2

Sialodochitis (fibrinosa) 527.2

Sialodocholithiasis 527.5

Sialolithiasis 527.5

Sialorrhea — see also Ptyalism 527.7
- periodic 527.2

Sialosis 527.8
- rheumatic 710.2

Siamese twin 759.4
- complicating pregnancy 678.1 ☑

Sicard's syndrome 352.6

Sicca syndrome (keratoconjunctivitis) 710.2

Sick 799.9
- cilia syndrome 759.89
- or handicapped person in family V61.49

Sickle-cell
- anemia (see also Disease, sickle-cell) 282.60
- disease (see also Disease, sickle-cell) 282.60
- hemoglobin
  - C disease (without crisis) 282.63
    - with
      - crisis 282.64
      - vaso-occlusive pain 282.64
  - D disease (without crisis) 282.68
    - with crisis 282.69
  - E disease (without crisis) 282.68
    - with crisis 282.69
  - thalassemia (without crisis) 282.41
    - with
      - crisis 282.42
      - vaso-occlusive pain 282.42
  - trait 282.5

Sicklemia — see also Disease, sickle-cell 282.60
- trait 282.5

Sickness
- air (travel) 994.6
- airplane 994.6
- alpine 993.2
- altitude 993.2
- Andes 993.2
- aviators' 993.2
- balloon 993.2
- car 994.6
- compressed air 993.3
- decompression 993.3
- green 280.9
- harvest 100.89
- milk 988.8
- morning 643.0 ☑
- motion 994.6
- mountain 993.2
  - acute 289.0
- protein (see also Complications, vaccination) 999.59
- radiation NEC 990
- roundabout (motion) 994.6
- sea 994.6
- serum NEC 999.59
- sleeping (African) 086.5
  - by Trypanosoma 086.5
    - gambiense 086.3
    - rhodesiense 086.4
  - Gambian 086.3
  - late effect 139.8
  - Rhodesian 086.4

☑ Additional Digit Required — Refer to the Tabular List for Digit Selection   ▽ Subterms under main terms may continue to next column or page

258 — Volume 2   ▶◀ Revised Text   ● New Line   ▲ Revised Code   2014 ICD-9-CM

Sickness — *continued*
sweating 078.2
swing (motion) 994.6
train (railway) (travel) 994.6
travel (any vehicle) 994.6
Sick sinus syndrome 427.81
Sideropenia — *see also* Anemia, iron deficiency 280.9
Siderosis (lung) (occupational) 503
central nervous system (CNS) 437.8
cornea 371.15
eye (bulbi) (vitreous) 360.23
lens 360.23
Siegal-Cattan-Mamou disease (periodic) 277.31
Siemens' syndrome
ectodermal dysplasia 757.31
keratosis follicularis spinulosa (decalvans) 757.39
Sighing respiration 786.7
Sigmoid
flexure — *see* condition
kidney 753.3
Sigmoiditis — *see* Enteritis
Silfverskiöld's syndrome 756.50
Silicosis, silicotic (complicated) (occupational) (simple) 502
fibrosis, lung (confluent) (massive) (occupational) 502
non-nodular 503
pulmonum 502
Silicotuberculosis — *see also* Tuberculosis 011.4 ☑
Silo fillers' disease 506.9
Silver's syndrome (congenital hemihypertrophy and short stature) 759.89
Silver wire arteries, retina 362.13
Silvestroni-Bianco syndrome (thalassemia minima) 282.49
Simian crease 757.2
Simmonds' cachexia or disease (pituitary cachexia) 253.2
Simons' disease or syndrome (progressive lipodystrophy) 272.6
Simple, simplex — *see* condition
Sinding-Larsen disease (juvenile osteopathia patellae) 732.4
Singapore hemorrhagic fever 065.4
Singers' node or nodule 478.5
Single
atrium 745.69
coronary artery 746.85
umbilical artery 747.5
ventricle 745.3
Singultus 786.8
epidemicus 078.89
Sinus — *see also* Fistula
abdominal 569.81
arrest 426.6
arrhythmia 427.89
bradycardia 427.89
chronic 427.81
branchial cleft (external) (internal) 744.41
coccygeal (infected) 685.1
with abscess 685.0
dental 522.7
dermal (congenital) 685.1
with abscess 685.0
draining — *see* Fistula
infected, skin NEC 686.9
marginal, ruptured or bleeding 641.2 ☑
affecting fetus or newborn 762.1
pause 426.6
pericranii 742.0
pilonidal (infected) (rectum) 685.1
with abscess 685.0
preauricular 744.46
rectovaginal 619.1
sacrococcygeal (dermoid) (infected) 685.1
with abscess 685.0
skin
infected NEC 686.9
noninfected — *see* Ulcer, skin
tachycardia 427.89
tarsi syndrome 726.79
testis 608.89

Sinus — *see also* Fistula — *continued*
tract (postinfectional) — *see* Fistula
urachus 753.7
Sinuses, Rokitansky-Aschoff — *see also* Disease, gallbladder 575.8
Sinusitis-bronchiectasis-situs inversus (syndrome) (triad) 759.3
Sinusitis (accessory) (nasal) (hyperplastic) (nonpurulent) (purulent) (chronic) 473.9
with influenza, flu, or grippe (*see also* Influenza) 487.1
acute 461.9
ethmoidal 461.2
frontal 461.1
maxillary 461.0
specified type NEC 461.8
sphenoidal 461.3
allergic (*see also* Fever, hay) 477.9
antrum — *see* Sinusitis, maxillary
due to
fungus, any sinus 117.9
high altitude 993.1
ethmoidal 473.2
acute 461.2
frontal 473.1
acute 461.1
influenzal (*see also* Influenza) 487.1
maxillary 473.0
acute 461.0
specified site NEC 473.8
sphenoidal 473.3
acute 461.3
syphilitic, any sinus 095.8
tuberculous, any sinus (*see also* Tuberculosis) 012.8 ☑
Sioloangitis 527.2
Sipple's syndrome (medullary thyroid carcinoma-pheochromocytoma) 258.02
Sirenomelia 759.89
Siriasis 992.0
Sirkari's disease 085.0
SIRS (systemic inflammatory response syndrome) 995.90
due to
infectious process 995.91
with acute organ dysfunction 995.92
non-infectious process 995.93
with acute organ dysfunction 995.94
Siti 104.0
Sitophobia 300.29
Situational
disturbance (transient) (*see also* Reaction, adjustment) 309.9
acute 308.3
maladjustment, acute (*see also* Reaction, adjustment) 309.9
reaction (*see also* Reaction, adjustment) 309.9
acute 308.3
Situation, psychiatric 300.9
Situs inversus or transversus 759.3
abdominalis 759.3
thoracis 759.3
Sixth disease
due to
human herpesvirus 6 058.11
human herpesvirus 7 058.12
Sjögren-Larsson syndrome (ichthyosis congenita) 757.1
Sjögren (-Gougerot) syndrome or disease (keratoconjunctivitis sicca) 710.2
with lung involvement 710.2 [517.8]
SJS-TEN (Stevens-Johnson syndrome - toxic epidermal necrolysis overlap syndrome) 695.14
Skeletal — *see* condition
Skene's gland — *see* condition
Skenitis — *see also* Urethritis 597.89
gonorrheal (acute) 098.0
chronic or duration of 2 months or over 098.2
Skerljevo 104.0
Skevas-Zerfus disease 989.5
Skin — *see also* condition
donor V59.1
hidebound 710.9

SLAP lesion (superior glenoid labrum) 840.7
Slate-dressers' lung 502
Slate-miners' lung 502
Sleep
deprivation V69.4
disorder 780.50
with apnea — *see* Apnea, sleep
child 307.40
movement, unspecified 780.58
nonorganic origin 307.40
specified type NEC 307.49
disturbance 780.50
with apnea — *see* Apnea, sleep
nonorganic origin 307.40
specified type NEC 307.49
drunkenness 307.47
movement disorder, unspecified 780.58
paroxysmal (*see also* Narcolepsy) 347.00
related movement disorder, unspecified 780.58
rhythm inversion 327.39
nonorganic origin 307.45
walking 307.46
hysterical 300.13
Sleeping sickness 086.5
late effect 139.8
Sleeplessness — *see also* Insomnia 780.52
menopausal 627.2
nonorganic origin 307.41
Slipped, slipping
epiphysis (postinfectional) 732.9
traumatic (old) 732.9
current — *see* Fracture, by site
upper femoral (nontraumatic) 732.2
intervertebral disc — *see* Displacement, intervertebral disc
ligature, umbilical 772.3
patella 717.89
rib 733.99
sacroiliac joint 724.6
tendon 727.9
ulnar nerve, nontraumatic 354.2
vertebra NEC (*see also* Spondylolisthesis) 756.12
Slocumb's syndrome 255.3
Sloughing (multiple) (skin) 686.9
abscess — *see* Abscess, by site
appendix 543.9
bladder 596.89
fascia 728.9
graft — *see* Complications, graft
phagedena (*see also* Gangrene) 785.4
reattached extremity (*see also* Complications, reattached extremity) 996.90
rectum 569.49
scrotum 608.89
tendon 727.9
transplanted organ (*see also* Rejection, transplant, organ, by site) 996.80
ulcer (*see also* Ulcer, skin) 707.9
Slow
feeding newborn 779.31
fetal, growth NEC 764.9 ☑
affecting management of pregnancy 656.5 ☑
Slowing
heart 427.89
urinary stream 788.62
Sluder's neuralgia or syndrome 337.09
Slurred, slurring, speech 784.59
Small-for-dates — *see also* Light-for-dates 764.0 ☑
affecting management of pregnancy 656.5 ☑
Smallpox 050.9
contact V01.3
exposure to V01.3
hemorrhagic (pustular) 050.0
malignant 050.0
modified 050.2
vaccination
complications — *see* Complications, vaccination
prophylactic (against) V04.1
Small, smallness
cardiac reserve — *see* Disease, heart

Small, smallness — *continued*
for dates
fetus or newborn 764.0 ☑
with malnutrition 764.1 ☑
affecting management of pregnancy 656.5 ☑
infant, term 764.0 ☑
with malnutrition 764.1 ☑
affecting management of pregnancy 656.5 ☑
introitus, vagina 623.3
kidney, unknown cause 589.9
bilateral 589.1
unilateral 589.0
ovary 620.8
pelvis
with disproportion (fetopelvic) 653.1 ☑
affecting fetus or newborn 763.1
causing obstructed labor 660.1 ☑
affecting fetus or newborn 763.1
placenta — *see* Placenta, insufficiency
uterus 621.8
white kidney 582.9
Smearing, fecal 787.62
Smith-Lemli Opitz syndrome (cerebrohepatorenal syndrome) 759.89
Smith-Magenis syndrome 758.33
Smith-Strang disease (oasthouse urine) 270.2
Smith's fracture (separation) (closed) 813.41
open 813.51
Smokers'
bronchitis 491.0
cough 491.0
syndrome (*see also* Abuse, drugs, nondependent) 305.1
throat 472.1
tongue 528.6
Smoking complicating pregnancy, childbirth, or the puerperium 649.0 ☑
Smothering spells 786.09
Snaggle teeth, tooth 524.39
Snapping
finger 727.05
hip 719.65
jaw 524.69
temporomandibular joint sounds on opening or closing 524.64
knee 717.9
thumb 727.05
Sneddon-Wilkinson disease or syndrome (subcorneal pustular dermatosis) 694.1
Sneezing 784.99
intractable 478.19
Sniffing
cocaine (*see also* Dependence) 304.2 ☑
ether (*see also* Dependence) 304.6 ☑
glue (airplane) (*see also* Dependence) 304.6 ☑
Snoring 786.09
Snow blindness 370.24
Snuffles (nonsyphilitic) 460
syphilitic (infant) 090.0
Social migrant V60.0
Sodoku 026.0
Soemmering's ring 366.51
Soft — *see also* condition
enlarged prostate 600.00
with
other lower urinary tract symptoms (LUTS) 600.01
urinary
obstruction 600.01
retention 600.01
nails 703.8
Softening
bone 268.2
brain (necrotic) (progressive) 348.89
arteriosclerotic 437.0
congenital 742.4
due to cerebrovascular accident 438.89
embolic (*see also* Embolism, brain) 434.1 ☑
hemorrhagic (*see also* Hemorrhage, brain) 431
occlusive 434.9 ☑

☑ **Additional Digit Required — Refer to the Tabular List for Digit Selection**   ▽ **Subterms under main terms may continue to next column or page**

2014 ICD-9-CM   ▶◀ Revised Text   ● New Line   ▲ Revised Code   **Volume 2 — 259**

Softening — *continued*
  brain — *continued*
    thrombotic (*see also* Thrombosis, brain) 434.0 ☑
  cartilage 733.92
  cerebellar — *see* Softening, brain
  cerebral — *see* Softening, brain
  cerebrospinal — *see* Softening, brain
  myocardial, heart (*see also* Degeneration, myocardial) 429.1
  nails 703.8
  spinal cord 336.8
  stomach 537.89
Soiling, fecal 787.62
Solar fever 061
Soldier's
  heart 306.2
  patches 423.1
Solitary
  cyst
    bone 733.21
    kidney 593.2
  kidney (congenital) 753.0
  tubercle, brain (*see also* Tuberculosis, brain) 013.2 ☑
  ulcer, bladder 596.89
Somatization reaction, somatic reaction — *see also* Disorder, psychosomatic 306.9
  disorder 300.81
Somatoform disorder 300.82
  atypical 300.82
  severe 300.81
  undifferentiated 300.82
Somnambulism 307.46
  hysterical 300.13
Somnolence 780.09
  nonorganic origin 307.43
  periodic 349.89
Sonne dysentery 004.3
Soor 112.0
Sore
  Delhi 085.1
  desert (*see also* Ulcer, skin) 707.9
  eye 379.99
  Lahore 085.1
  mouth 528.9
    canker 528.2
    due to dentures 528.9
  muscle 729.1
  Naga (*see also* Ulcer, skin) 707.9
  oriental 085.1
  pressure (*see also* Ulcer, pressure) 707.00
    with gangrene (*see also* Ulcer, pressure) 707.00 [785.4]
  skin NEC 709.9
  soft 099.0
  throat 462
    with influenza, flu, or grippe (*see also* Influenza) 487.1
    acute 462
    chronic 472.1
    clergyman's 784.49
    coxsackie (virus) 074.0
    diphtheritic 032.0
    epidemic 034.0
    gangrenous 462
    herpetic 054.79
    influenzal (*see also* Influenza) 487.1
    malignant 462
    purulent 462
    putrid 462
    septic 034.0
    streptococcal (ulcerative) 034.0
    ulcerated 462
    viral NEC 462
      Coxsackie 074.0
    tropical (*see also* Ulcer, skin) 707.9
    veldt (*see also* Ulcer, skin) 707.9
Sotos' syndrome (cerebral gigantism) 253.0
Sounds
  friction, pleural 786.7
  succussion, chest 786.7
  temporomandibular joint
    on opening or closing 524.64
South African cardiomyopathy syndrome 425.2

South American
  blastomycosis 116.1
  trypanosomiasis — *see* Trypanosomiasis
Southeast Asian hemorrhagic fever 065.4
Spacing, teeth, abnormal 524.30
  excessive 524.32
Spade-like hand (congenital) 754.89
Spading nail 703.8
  congenital 757.5
Spanemia 285.9
Spanish collar 605
Sparganosis 123.5
Spasmodic — *see* condition
Spasmophilia — *see also* Tetany 781.7
Spasm, spastic, spasticity — *see also* condition 781.0
  accommodation 367.53
  ampulla of Vater (*see also* Disease, gallbladder) 576.8
  anus, ani (sphincter) (reflex) 564.6
    psychogenic 306.4
  artery NEC 443.9
    basilar 435.0
    carotid 435.8
    cerebral 435.9
      specified artery NEC 435.8
    retinal (*see also* Occlusion, retinal, artery) 362.30
    vertebral 435.1
    vertebrobasilar 435.3
  Bell's 351.0
  bladder (sphincter, external or internal) 596.89
  bowel 564.9
    psychogenic 306.4
  bronchus, bronchiole 519.11
  cardia 530.0
  cardiac — *see* Angina
  carpopedal (*see also* Tetany) 781.7
  cecum 564.9
    psychogenic 306.4
  cerebral (arteries) (vascular) 435.9
    specified artery NEC 435.8
  cerebrovascular 435.9
  cervix, complicating delivery 661.4 ☑
    affecting fetus or newborn 763.7
  ciliary body (of accommodation) 367.53
  colon 564.1
    psychogenic 306.4
  common duct (*see also* Disease, biliary) 576.8
  compulsive 307.22
  conjugate 378.82
  convergence 378.84
  coronary (artery) — *see* Angina
  diaphragm (reflex) 786.8
    psychogenic 306.1
  duodenum, duodenal (bulb) 564.89
  esophagus (diffuse) 530.5
    psychogenic 306.4
  facial 351.8
  fallopian tube 620.8
  gait 781.2
  gastrointestinal (tract) 536.8
    psychogenic 306.4
  glottis 478.75
    hysterical 300.11
    psychogenic 306.1
      specified as conversion reaction 300.11
    reflex through recurrent laryngeal nerve 478.75
  habit 307.20
    chronic 307.22
    transient (of childhood) 307.21
  heart — *see* Angina
  hourglass — *see* Contraction, hourglass
  hysterical 300.11
  infantile (*see also* Epilepsy) 345.6 ☑
  internal oblique, eye 378.51
  intestinal 564.9
    psychogenic 306.4
  larynx, laryngeal 478.75
    hysterical 300.11
    psychogenic 306.1

Spasm, spastic, spasticity — *see also* condition — *continued*
  larynx, laryngeal — *continued*
    psychogenic — *continued*
      specified as conversion reaction 300.11
    levator palpebrae superioris 333.81
  lightning (*see also* Epilepsy) 345.6 ☑
  mobile 781.0
  muscle 728.85
    back 724.8
    psychogenic 306.0
  nerve, trigeminal 350.1
  nervous 306.0
  nodding 307.3
    infantile (*see also* Epilepsy) 345.6 ☑
  occupational 300.89
  oculogyric 378.87
  ophthalmic artery 362.30
  orbicularis 781.0
  perineal 625.8
  peroneo-extensor (*see also* Flat, foot) 734
  pharynx (reflex) 478.29
    hysterical 300.11
    psychogenic 306.1
      specified as conversion reaction 300.11
  pregnant uterus, complicating delivery 661.4 ☑
  psychogenic 306.0
  pylorus 537.81
    adult hypertrophic 537.0
    congenital or infantile 750.5
    psychogenic 306.4
  rectum (sphincter) 564.6
    psychogenic 306.4
  retinal artery NEC (*see also* Occlusion, retina, artery) 362.30
  sacroiliac 724.6
  salaam (infantile) (*see also* Epilepsy) 345.6 ☑
  saltatory 781.0
  sigmoid 564.9
    psychogenic 306.4
  sphincter of Oddi (*see also* Disease, gallbladder) 576.5
  stomach 536.8
    neurotic 306.4
  throat 478.29
    hysterical 300.11
    psychogenic 306.1
      specified as conversion reaction 300.11
  tic 307.20
    chronic 307.22
    transient (of childhood) 307.21
  tongue 529.8
  torsion 333.6
  trigeminal nerve 350.1
    postherpetic 053.12
  ureter 593.89
  urethra (sphincter) 599.84
  uterus 625.8
    complicating labor 661.4 ☑
      affecting fetus or newborn 763.7
  vagina 625.1
    psychogenic 306.51
  vascular NEC 443.9
  vasomotor NEC 443.9
  vein NEC 459.89
  vesical (sphincter, external or internal) 596.89
  viscera 789.0 ☑
Spasmus nutans 307.3
Spastic — *see also* Spasm
  child 343.9
Spasticity — *see also* Spasm
  cerebral, child 343.9
Speakers' throat 784.49
Specific, specified — *see* condition
Speech
  defect, disorder, disturbance, impediment NEC 784.59
    psychogenic 307.9
  (language) therapy V57.3
Spells 780.39

Spells — *continued*
  breath-holding 786.9
Spencer's disease (epidemic vomiting) 078.82
Spens' syndrome (syncope with heart block) 426.9
Spermatic cord — *see* condition
Spermatocele 608.1
  congenital 752.89
Spermatocystitis 608.4
Spermatocytoma (M9063/3)
  specified site — *see* Neoplasm, by site, malignant
  unspecified site 186.9
Spermatorrhea 608.89
Sperm counts
  fertility testing V26.21
  following sterilization reversal V26.22
  postvasectomy V25.8
Sphacelus — *see also* Gangrene 785.4
Sphenoidal — *see* condition
Sphenoiditis (chronic) — *see also* Sinusitis, sphenoidal 473.3
Sphenopalatine ganglion neuralgia 337.09
Sphericity, increased, lens 743.36
Spherocytosis (congenital) (familial) (hereditary) 282.0
  hemoglobin disease 282.7
  sickle-cell (disease) 282.60
Spherophakia 743.36
Sphincter — *see* condition
Sphincteritis, sphincter of Oddi — *see also* Cholecystitis 576.8
Sphingolipidosis 272.7
Sphingolipodystrophy 272.7
Sphingomyelinosis 272.7
Spicule tooth 520.2
Spider
  finger 755.59
  nevus 448.1
  vascular 448.1
Spiegler-Fendt sarcoid 686.8
Spielmeyer-Stock disease 330.1
Spielmeyer-Vogt disease 330.1
Spina bifida (aperta) 741.9 ☑

> Note — Use the following fifth-digit subclassification with category 741:
>
> 0   unspecified region
> 1   cervical region
> 2   dorsal [thoracic] region
> 3   lumbar region

  with hydrocephalus 741.0 ☑
    fetal (suspected), affecting management of pregnancy 655.0 ☑
  occulta 756.17
Spindle, Krukenberg's 371.13
Spine, spinal — *see* condition
Spiradenoma (eccrine) (M8403/0) — *see* Neoplasm, skin, benign
Spirillosis NEC — *see also* Fever, relapsing 087.9
Spirillum minus 026.0
Spirillum obermeieri infection 087.0
Spirochetal — *see* condition
Spirochetosis 104.9
  arthritic, arthritica 104.9 [711.8] ☑
  bronchopulmonary 104.8
  icterohemorrhagica 100.0
  lung 104.8
Spitting blood — *see also* Hemoptysis 786.30
Splanchnomegaly 569.89
Splanchnoptosis 569.89
Spleen, splenic — *see also* condition
  agenesis 759.0
  flexure syndrome 569.89
  neutropenia syndrome 289.53
  sequestration syndrome 289.52
Splenectasis — *see also* Splenomegaly 789.2
Splenitis (interstitial) (malignant) (nonspecific) 289.59
  malarial (*see also* Malaria) 084.6
  tuberculous (*see also* Tuberculosis) 017.7 ☑
Splenocele 289.59
Splenomegalia — *see* Splenomegaly
Splenomegalic — *see* condition

☑ **Additional Digit Required** — Refer to the Tabular List for Digit Selection   ⬇ **Subterms under main terms may continue to next column or page**

260 — Volume 2   ▶◀ **Revised Text**   ● **New Line**   ▲ **Revised Code**   **2014 ICD-9-CM**

Splenomegaly 789.2
Bengal 789.2
cirrhotic 289.51
congenital 759.0
congestive, chronic 289.51
cryptogenic 789.2
Egyptian 120.1
Gaucher's (cerebroside lipidosis) 272.7
idiopathic 789.2
malarial (see also Malaria) 084.6
neutropenic 289.53
Niemann-Pick (lipid histiocytosis) 272.7
siderotic 289.51
syphilitic 095.8
congenital 090.0
tropical (Bengal) (idiopathic) 789.2
Splenopathy 289.50
Splenopneumonia — see Pneumonia
Splenoptosis 289.59
Splinter — see Injury, superficial, by site
Split, splitting
heart sounds 427.89
lip, congenital (see also Cleft, lip) 749.10
nails 703.8
urinary stream 788.61
Spoiled child reaction — see also Disturbance, conduct 312.1 ☑
Spondylarthritis — see also Spondylosis 721.90
Spondylarthrosis — see also Spondylosis 721.90
Spondylitis 720.9
ankylopoietica 720.0
ankylosing (chronic) 720.0
atrophic 720.9
ligamentous 720.9
chronic (traumatic) (see also Spondylosis) 721.90
deformans (chronic) (see also Spondylosis) 721.90
gonococcal 098.53
gouty 274.00
hypertrophic (see also Spondylosis) 721.90
infectious NEC 720.9
juvenile (adolescent) 720.0
Kümmell's 721.7
Marie-Strümpell (ankylosing) 720.0
muscularis 720.9
ossificans ligamentosa 721.6
osteoarthritica (see also Spondylosis) 721.90
posttraumatic 721.7
proliferative 720.0
rheumatoid 720.0
rhizomelica 720.0
sacroiliac NEC 720.2
senescent (see also Spondylosis) 721.90
senile (see also Spondylosis) 721.90
static (see also Spondylosis) 721.90
traumatic (chronic) (see also Spondylosis) 721.90
tuberculous (see also Tuberculosis) 015.0 ☑ [720.81]
typhosa 002.0 [720.81]
Spondyloarthrosis — see also Spondylosis 721.90
Spondylolisthesis (congenital) (lumbosacral) 756.12
with disproportion (fetopelvic) 653.3 ☑
affecting fetus or newborn 763.1
causing obstructed labor 660.1 ☑
affecting fetus or newborn 763.1
acquired 738.4
degenerative 738.4
traumatic 738.4
acute (lumbar) — see Fracture, vertebra, lumbar
site other than lumbosacral — see Fracture, vertebra, by site
Spondylolysis (congenital) 756.11
acquired 738.4
cervical 756.19
lumbosacral region 756.11
with disproportion (fetopelvic) 653.3 ☑
affecting fetus or newborn 763.1
causing obstructed labor 660.1 ☑
affecting fetus or newborn 763.1

Spondylopathy
inflammatory 720.9
specified type NEC 720.89
traumatic 721.7
Spondylose rhizomelique 720.0
Spondylosis 721.90
with
disproportion 653.3 ☑
affecting fetus or newborn 763.1
causing obstructed labor 660.1 ☑
affecting fetus or newborn 763.1
myelopathy NEC 721.91
cervical, cervicodorsal 721.0
with myelopathy 721.1
inflammatory 720.9
lumbar, lumbosacral 721.3
with myelopathy 721.42
sacral 721.3
with myelopathy 721.42
thoracic 721.2
with myelopathy 721.41
traumatic 721.7
Sponge
divers' disease 989.5
inadvertently left in operation wound 998.4
kidney (medullary) 753.17
Spongioblastoma (M9422/3)
multiforme (M9440/3)
specified site — see Neoplasm, by site, malignant
unspecified site 191.9
polare (M9423/3)
specified site — see Neoplasm, by site, malignant
unspecified site 191.9
primitive polar (M9443/3)
specified site — see Neoplasm, by site, malignant
unspecified site 191.9
specified site — see Neoplasm, by site, malignant
unspecified site 191.9
Spongiocytoma (M9400/3)
specified site — see Neoplasm, by site, malignant
unspecified site 191.9
Spongioneuroblastoma (M9504/3) — see Neoplasm, by site, malignant
Spontaneous — see also condition
fracture — see Fracture, pathologic
Spoon nail 703.8
congenital 757.5
Sporadic — see condition
Sporotrichosis (bones) (cutaneous) (disseminated) (epidermal) (lymphatic) (lymphocutaneous) (mucous membranes) (pulmonary) (skeletal) (visceral) 117.1
Sporotrichum schenckii infection 117.1
Spots, spotting
atrophic (skin) 701.3
Bitôt's (in the young child) 264.1
café au lait 709.09
cayenne pepper 448.1
complicating pregnancy 649.5 ☑
cotton wool (retina) 362.83
de Morgan's (senile angiomas) 448.1
Fúchs' black (myopic) 360.21
intermenstrual
irregular 626.6
regular 626.5
interpalpebral 372.53
Koplik's 055.9
liver 709.09
Mongolian (pigmented) 757.33
of pregnancy 649.5 ☑
purpuric 782.7
ruby 448.1
Spotted fever — see Fever, spotted
Sprain, strain (joint) (ligament) (muscle) (tendon) 848.9
abdominal wall (muscle) 848.8
Achilles tendon 845.09
acromioclavicular 840.0
ankle 845.00
and foot 845.00
anterior longitudinal, cervical 847.0

Sprain, strain — continued
arm 840.9
upper 840.9
and shoulder 840.9
astragalus 845.00
atlanto-axial 847.0
atlanto-occipital 847.0
atlas 847.0
axis 847.0
back (see also Sprain, spine) 847.9
breast bone 848.40
broad ligament — see Injury, internal, broad ligament
calcaneofibular 845.02
carpal 842.01
carpometacarpal 842.11
cartilage
costal, without mention of injury to sternum 848.3
involving sternum 848.42
ear 848.8
knee 844.9
with current tear (see also Tear, meniscus) 836.2
semilunar (knee) 844.8
with current tear (see also Tear, meniscus) 836.2
septal, nose 848.0
thyroid region 848.2
xiphoid 848.49
cervical, cervicodorsal, cervicothoracic 847.0
chondrocostal, without mention of injury to sternum 848.3
involving sternum 848.42
chondrosternal 848.42
chronic (joint) — see Derangement, joint
clavicle 840.9
coccyx 847.4
collar bone 840.9
collateral, knee (medial) (tibial) 844.1
lateral (fibular) 844.0
recurrent or old 717.89
lateral 717.81
medial 717.82
coracoacromial 840.8
coracoclavicular 840.1
coracohumeral 840.2
coracoid (process) 840.9
coronary, knee 844.8
costal cartilage, without mention of injury to sternum 848.3
involving sternum 848.42
cricoarytenoid articulation 848.2
cricothyroid articulation 848.2
cruciate
knee 844.2
old 717.89
anterior 717.83
posterior 717.84
deltoid
ankle 845.01
shoulder 840.8
dorsal (spine) 847.1
ear cartilage 848.8
elbow 841.9
and forearm 841.9
specified site NEC 841.8
femur (proximal end) 843.9
distal end 844.9
fibula (proximal end) 844.9
distal end 845.00
fibulocalcaneal 845.02
finger(s) 842.10
foot 845.10
and ankle 845.00
forearm 841.9
and elbow 841.9
specified site NEC 841.8
glenoid (shoulder) (see also SLAP lesion) 840.8
hand 842.10
hip 843.9
and thigh 843.9
humerus (proximal end) 840.9
distal end 841.9
iliofemoral 843.0

Sprain, strain — continued
infraspinatus 840.3
innominate
acetabulum 843.9
pubic junction 848.5
sacral junction 846.1
internal
collateral, ankle 845.01
semilunar cartilage 844.8
with current tear (see also Tear, meniscus) 836.2
old 717.5
interphalangeal
finger 842.13
toe 845.13
ischiocapsular 843.1
jaw (cartilage) (meniscus) 848.1
old 524.69
knee 844.9
and leg 844.9
old 717.5
collateral
lateral 717.81
medial 717.82
cruciate
anterior 717.83
posterior 717.84
late effect — see Late, effects (of), sprain
lateral collateral, knee 844.0
old 717.81
leg 844.9
and knee 844.9
ligamentum teres femoris 843.8
low back 846.9
lumbar (spine) 847.2
lumbosacral 846.0
chronic or old 724.6
mandible 848.1
old 524.69
maxilla 848.1
medial collateral, knee 844.1
old 717.82
meniscus
jaw 848.1
old 524.69
knee 844.8
with current tear (see also Tear, meniscus) 836.2
old 717.5
mandible 848.1
old 524.69
specified site NEC 848.8
metacarpal 842.10
distal 842.12
proximal 842.11
metacarpophalangeal 842.12
metatarsal 845.10
metatarsophalangeal 845.12
midcarpal 842.19
midtarsal 845.19
multiple sites, except fingers alone or toes alone 848.8
neck 847.0
nose (septal cartilage) 848.0
occiput from atlas 847.0
old — see Derangement, joint
orbicular, hip 843.8
patella(r) 844.8
old 717.89
pelvis 848.5
phalanx
finger 842.10
toe 845.10
radiocarpal 842.02
radiohumeral 841.2
radioulnar 841.9
distal 842.09
radius, radial (proximal end) 841.9
and ulna 841.9
distal 842.09
collateral 841.0
distal end 842.00
recurrent — see Sprain, by site
rib (cage), without mention of injury to sternum 848.3
involving sternum 848.42

Index

Sprain, strain — Status

Sprain, strain — *continued*
- rotator cuff (capsule) 840.4
- round ligament (*see also* Injury, internal, round ligament)
  - femur 843.8
- sacral (spine) 847.3
- sacrococcygeal 847.3
- sacroiliac (region) 846.9
  - chronic or old 724.6
  - ligament 846.1
  - specified site NEC 846.8
- sacrospinatus 846.2
- sacrospinous 846.2
- sacrotuberous 846.3
- scaphoid bone, ankle 845.00
- scapula(r) 840.9
- semilunar cartilage (knee) 844.8
  - with current tear (*see also* Tear, meniscus) 836.2
  - old 717.5
- septal cartilage (nose) 848.0
- shoulder 840.9
  - and arm, upper 840.9
  - blade 840.9
- specified site NEC 848.8
- spine 847.9
  - cervical 847.0
  - coccyx 847.4
  - dorsal 847.1
  - lumbar 847.2
  - lumbosacral 846.0
    - chronic or old 724.6
  - sacral 847.3
  - sacroiliac (*see also* Sprain, sacroiliac) 846.9
    - chronic or old 724.6
  - thoracic 847.1
- sternoclavicular 848.41
- sternum 848.40
- subglenoid (*see also* SLAP lesion) 840.8
- subscapularis 840.5
- supraspinatus 840.6
- symphysis
  - jaw 848.1
    - old 524.69
  - mandibular 848.1
    - old 524.69
  - pubis 848.5
- talofibular 845.09
- tarsal 845.10
- tarsometatarsal 845.11
- temporomandibular 848.1
  - old 524.69
- teres
  - ligamentum femoris 843.8
  - major or minor 840.8
- thigh (proximal end) 843.9
  - and hip 843.9
  - distal end 844.9
- thoracic (spine) 847.1
- thorax 848.8
- thumb 842.10
- thyroid cartilage or region 848.2
- tibia (proximal end) 844.9
  - distal end 845.00
- tibiofibular
  - distal 845.03
  - superior 844.3
- toe(s) 845.10
- trachea 848.8
- trapezoid 840.8
- ulna, ulnar (proximal end) 841.9
  - collateral 841.1
  - distal end 842.00
- ulnohumeral 841.3
- vertebrae (*see also* Sprain, spine) 847.9
  - cervical, cervicodorsal, cervicothoracic 847.0
- wrist (cuneiform) (scaphoid) (semilunar) 842.00
- xiphoid cartilage 848.49
Sprengel's deformity (congenital) 755.52
Spring fever 309.23
Sprue 579.1
- celiac 579.0
- idiopathic 579.0

Sprue — *continued*
- meaning thrush 112.0
- nontropical 579.0
- tropical 579.1
Spur — *see also* Exostosis
- bone 726.91
  - calcaneal 726.73
- calcaneal 726.73
- iliac crest 726.5
- nose (septum) 478.19
  - bone 726.91
- septal 478.19
Spuria placenta — *see* Placenta, abnormal
Spurway's syndrome (brittle bones and blue sclera) 756.51
Sputum, abnormal (amount) (color) (excessive) (odor) (purulent) 786.4
- bloody 786.30
Squamous — *see also* condition
- cell metaplasia
  - bladder 596.89
  - cervix — *see* condition
- epithelium in
  - cervical canal (congenital) 752.49
  - uterine mucosa (congenital) 752.39
- metaplasia
  - bladder 596.89
  - cervix — *see* condition
Squashed nose 738.0
- congenital 754.0
Squeeze, divers' 993.3
Squint — *see also* Strabismus 378.9
- accommodative (*see also* Esotropia) 378.00
- concomitant (*see also* Heterotropia) 378.30
Stab — *see also* Wound, open, by site
- internal organs — *see* Injury, internal, by site, with open wound
Staggering gait 781.2
- hysterical 300.11
Staghorn calculus 592.0
Stain, staining
- meconium 779.84
- port wine 757.32
- tooth, teeth (hard tissues) 521.7
  - due to
    - accretions 523.6
    - deposits (betel) (black) (green) (materia alba) (orange) (tobacco) 523.6
    - metals (copper) (silver) 521.7
    - nicotine 523.6
    - pulpal bleeding 521.7
    - tobacco 523.6
Stälh's
- ear 744.29
- pigment line (cornea) 371.11
Stälhi's pigment lines (cornea) 371.11
Stammering — *see also* Disorder, fluency 315.35
Standstill
- atrial 426.6
- auricular 426.6
- cardiac (*see also* Arrest, cardiac) 427.5
- sinoatrial 426.6
- sinus 426.6
- ventricular (*see also* Arrest, cardiac) 427.5
Stannosis 503
Stanton's disease (melioidosis) 025
Staphylitis (acute) (catarrhal) (chronic) (gangrenous) (membranous) (suppurative) (ulcerative) 528.3
Staphylococcemia 038.10
- aureus 038.11
- specified organism NEC 038.19
Staphylococcus, staphylococcal — *see* condition
Staphyloderma (skin) 686.00
Staphyloma 379.11
- anterior, localized 379.14
- ciliary 379.11
- cornea 371.73
- equatorial 379.13
- posterior 379.12
- posticum 379.12
- ring 379.15
- sclera NEC 379.11

Starch eating 307.52
Stargardt's disease 362.75
Starvation (inanition) (due to lack of food) 994.2
- edema 262
- voluntary NEC 307.1
Stasis
- bile (duct) (*see also* Disease, biliary) 576.8
- bronchus (*see also* Bronchitis) 490
- cardiac (*see also* Failure, heart) 428.0
- cecum 564.89
- colon 564.89
- dermatitis (*see also* Varix, with stasis dermatitis) 454.1
- duodenal 536.8
- eczema (*see also* Varix, with stasis dermatitis) 454.1
- edema (*see also* Hypertension, venous) 459.30
- foot 991.4
- gastric 536.3
- ileocecal coil 564.89
- ileum 564.89
- intestinal 564.89
- jejunum 564.89
- kidney 586
- liver 571.9
  - cirrhotic — *see* Cirrhosis, liver
- lymphatic 457.8
- pneumonia 514
- portal 571.9
- pulmonary 514
- rectal 564.89
- renal 586
  - tubular 584.5
- stomach 536.3
- ulcer
  - with varicose veins 454.0
  - without varicose veins 459.81
- urine NEC (*see also* Retention, urine) 788.20
- venous 459.81
State
- affective and paranoid, mixed, organic psychotic 294.8
- agitated 307.9
  - acute reaction to stress 308.2
- anxiety (neurotic) (*see also* Anxiety) 300.00
  - specified type NEC 300.09
- apprehension (*see also* Anxiety) 300.00
  - specified type NEC 300.09
- climacteric, female 627.2
  - following induced menopause 627.4
- clouded
  - epileptic (*see also* Epilepsy) 345.9 ☑
  - paroxysmal (idiopathic) (*see also* Epilepsy) 345.9 ☑
- compulsive (mixed) (with obsession) 300.3
- confusional 298.9
  - acute 293.0
    - with
      - arteriosclerotic dementia 290.41
      - presenile brain disease 290.11
      - senility 290.3
    - alcoholic 291.0
    - drug-induced 292.81
  - epileptic 293.0
  - postoperative 293.9
  - reactive (emotional stress) (psychological trauma) 298.2
  - subacute 293.1
- constitutional psychopathic 301.9
- convulsive (*see also* Convulsions) 780.39
- depressive NEC 311
  - induced by drug 292.84
  - neurotic 300.4
- dissociative 300.15
- hallucinatory 780.1
  - induced by drug 292.12
- hypercoagulable (primary) 289.81
  - secondary 289.82
- hyperdynamic beta-adrenergic circulatory 429.82
- locked-in 344.81
- menopausal 627.2
  - artificial 627.4
  - following induced menopause 627.4

State — *continued*
- neurotic NEC 300.9
  - with depersonalization episode 300.6
- obsessional 300.3
- oneiroid (*see also* Schizophrenia) 295.4 ☑
- panic 300.01
- paranoid 297.9
  - alcohol-induced 291.5
  - arteriosclerotic 290.42
  - climacteric 297.2
  - drug-induced 292.11
  - in
    - presenile brain disease 290.12
    - senile brain disease 290.20
  - involutional 297.2
  - menopausal 297.2
  - senile 290.20
  - simple 297.0
- postleukotomy 310.0
- pregnant (*see also* Pregnancy) V22.2
- psychogenic, twilight 298.2
- psychotic, organic (*see also* Psychosis, organic) 294.9
  - mixed paranoid and affective 294.8
  - senile or presenile NEC 290.9
  - transient NEC 293.9
    - with
      - anxiety 293.84
      - delusions 293.81
      - depression 293.83
      - hallucinations 293.82
- residual schizophrenic (*see also* Schizophrenia) 295.6 ☑
- tension (*see also* Anxiety) 300.9
- transient organic psychotic 293.9
  - anxiety type 293.84
  - depressive type 293.83
  - hallucinatory type 293.83
  - paranoid type 293.81
  - specified type NEC 293.89
- twilight
  - epileptic 293.0
  - psychogenic 298.2
- vegetative (persistent) 780.03
Status (post)
- absence
  - epileptic (*see also* Epilepsy) 345.2
  - of organ, acquired (postsurgical) — *see* Absence, by site, acquired
- administration of tPA(rtPA) in a different institution within the last 24 hours prior to admission to facility V45.88
- anastomosis of intestine (for bypass) V45.3
- anginosus 413.9
- angioplasty, percutaneous transluminal coronary V45.82
- ankle prosthesis V43.66
- aortocoronary bypass or shunt V45.81
- arthrodesis V45.4
- artificially induced condition NEC V45.89
- artificial opening (of) V44.9
  - gastrointestinal tract NEC V44.4
  - specified site NEC V44.8
  - urinary tract NEC V44.6
  - vagina V44.7
- aspirator V46.0
- asthmaticus (*see also* Asthma) 493.9 ☑
- awaiting organ transplant V49.83
- bariatric surgery V45.86
  - complicating pregnancy, childbirth, or the puerperium 649.2 ☑
- bed confinement V49.84
- breast
  - correction V43.82
  - implant removal V45.83
  - reconstruction V43.82
- cardiac
  - device (in situ) V45.00
    - carotid sinus V45.09
      - fitting or adjustment V53.39
    - defibrillator, automatic implantable (with synchronous cardiac pacemaker) V45.02
    - pacemaker V45.01
      - fitting or adjustment V53.31
  - carotid sinus stimulator V45.09

☑ **Additional Digit Required** — Refer to the Tabular List for Digit Selection   ▽ **Subterms under main terms may continue to next column or page**

262 — Volume 2   ►◄ Revised Text   ● New Line   ▲ Revised Code   2014 ICD-9-CM

Status — *continued*
  cataract extraction V45.61
  chemotherapy V66.2
    current V58.69
  circumcision, female 629.20
  clitorectomy (female genital mutilation type I) 629.21
    with excision of labia minora (female genital mutilation type II) 629.22
  colonization — *see* Carrier (suspected) of
  colostomy V44.3
  contraceptive device V45.59
    intrauterine V45.51
    subdermal V45.52
  convulsivus idiopathicus (*see also* Epilepsy) 345.3
  coronary artery bypass or shunt V45.81
  cutting
    female genital 629.20
      specified NEC 629.29
      type I 629.21
      type II 629.22
      type III 629.23
      type IV 629.29
  cystostomy V44.50
    appendico-vesicostomy V44.52
    cutaneous-vesicostomy V44.51
    specified type NEC V44.59
  defibrillator, automatic implantable cardiac (with synchronous cardiac pacemaker) V45.02
  delinquent immunization V15.83
  dental crowns V45.84
  dental fillings V45.84
  dental restoration V45.84
  dental sealant V49.82
  dialysis (hemo) (peritoneal) V45.11
  donor V59.9
  do not resuscitate V49.86
  drug therapy or regimen V67.59
    high-risk medication NEC V67.51
  elbow prosthesis V43.62
  embedded
    fragment — *see* Foreign body, retained
    splinter — *see* Foreign body, retained
  enterostomy V44.4
  epileptic, epilepticus (absence) (grand mal) (*see also* Epilepsy) 345.3
    focal motor 345.7 ☑
    partial 345.7 ☑
    petit mal 345.2
    psychomotor 345.7 ☑
    temporal lobe 345.7 ☑
  estrogen receptor
    negative [ER-] V86.1
    positive [ER+] V86.0
  explantation of joint prosthesis NEC V88.29
    hip V88.21
    knee V88.22
  eye (adnexa) surgery V45.69
  female genital
    cutting 629.20
      specified NEC 629.29
      type I 629.21
      type II 629.22
      type III 629.23
      type IV 629.29
    mutilation 629.20
      type I 629.21
      type II 629.22
      type III 629.23
      type IV 629.29
  filtering bleb (eye) (postglaucoma) V45.69
    with rupture or complication 997.99
    postcataract extraction (complication) 997.99
  finger joint prosthesis V43.69
  foster care V60.81
  gastric
    banding V45.86
      complicating pregnancy, childbirth, or the puerperium 649.2 ☑
    bypass for obesity V45.86
      complicating pregnancy, childbirth, or the puerperium 649.2 ☑
  gastrostomy V44.1

Status — *continued*
  grand mal 345.3
  heart valve prosthesis V43.3
  hemodialysis V45.11
  hip prosthesis (joint) (partial) (total) V43.64
    explantation V88.21
  hysterectomy V88.01
    partial with remaining cervical stump V88.02
    total V88.01
  ileostomy V44.2
  infibulation (female genital mutilation type III) 629.23
  insulin pump V45.85
  intestinal bypass V45.3
  intrauterine contraceptive device V45.51
  jejunostomy V44.4
  joint prosthesis NEC V43.69
    explantation V88.29
  knee joint prosthesis V43.65
    explantation V88.22
  lacunaris 437.8
  lacunosis 437.8
  lapsed immunization schedule V15.83
  low birth weight V21.30
    less than 500 grams V21.31
    1000–1499 grams V21.33
    1500–1999 grams V21.34
    2000–2500 grams V21.35
    500–999 grams V21.32
  lymphaticus 254.8
  malignant neoplasm, ablated or excised — *see* History, malignant neoplasm
  marmoratus 333.79
  military deployment V62.22
  mutilation, female 629.20
    type I 629.21
    type II 629.22
    type III 629.23
    type IV 629.29
  nephrostomy V44.6
  neuropacemaker NEC V45.89
    brain V45.89
    carotid sinus V45.09
    neurologic NEC V45.89
  obesity surgery V45.86
    complicating pregnancy, childbirth, or the puerperium 649.2 ☑
  organ replacement
    by artificial or mechanical device or prosthesis of
      artery V43.4
      artificial skin V43.83
      bladder V43.5
      blood vessel V43.4
      breast V43.82
      eye globe V43.0
      heart
        assist device V43.21
        fully implantable artificial heart V43.22
        valve V43.3
      intestine V43.89
      joint V43.60
        ankle V43.66
        elbow V43.62
        finger V43.69
        hip (partial) (total) V43.64
        knee V43.65
        shoulder V43.61
        specified NEC V43.69
        wrist V43.63
      kidney V43.89
      larynx V43.81
      lens V43.1
      limb(s) V43.7
      liver V43.89
      lung V43.89
      organ NEC V43.89
      pancreas V43.89
      skin (artificial) V43.83
      tissue NEC V43.89
      vein V43.4
    by organ transplant (heterologous) (homologous) — *see* Status, transplant

Status — *continued*
  pacemaker
    brain V45.89
    cardiac V45.01
    carotid sinus V45.09
    neurologic NEC V45.89
    specified site NEC V45.89
  percutaneous transluminal coronary angioplasty V45.82
  peritoneal dialysis V45.11
  petit mal 345.2
  physical restraints V49.87
  postcommotio cerebri 310.2
  postmenopausal (age related) (natural) V49.81
  postoperative NEC V45.89
  postpartum NEC V24.2
    care immediately following delivery V24.0
    routine follow-up V24.2
  postsurgical NEC V45.89
  renal dialysis V45.11
    noncompliance V45.12
  respirator [ventilator] V46.11
    encounter
      during
        mechanical failure V46.14
        power failure V46.12
      for weaning V46.13
  retained foreign body — *see* Foreign body, retained
  reversed jejunal transposition (for bypass) V45.3
  sex reassignment surgery (*see also* Transsexualism) 302.50
  shoulder prosthesis V43.61
  shunt
    aortocoronary bypass V45.81
    arteriovenous (for dialysis) V45.11
    cerebrospinal fluid V45.2
    vascular NEC V45.89
      aortocoronary (bypass) V45.81
    ventricular (communicating) (for drainage) V45.2
  sterilization
    tubal ligation V26.51
    vasectomy V26.52
  subdermal contraceptive device V45.52
  thymicolymphaticus 254.8
  thymicus 254.8
  thymolymphaticus 254.8
  tooth extraction 525.10
  tracheostomy V44.0
  transplant
    blood vessel V42.89
    bone V42.4
      marrow V42.81
    cornea V42.5
    heart V42.1
      valve V42.2
    intestine V42.84
    kidney V42.0
    liver V42.7
    lung V42.6
    organ V42.9
      removal (due to complication, failure, rejection or infection) V45.87
      specified site NEC V42.89
    pancreas V42.83
    peripheral stem cells V42.82
    skin V42.3
    stem cells, peripheral V42.82
    tissue V42.9
      specified type NEC V42.89
    vessel, blood V42.89
  tubal ligation V26.51
  underimmunization V15.83
  ureterostomy V44.6
  urethrostomy V44.6
  vagina, artificial V44.7
  vascular shunt NEC V45.89
    aortocoronary (bypass) V45.81
  vasectomy V26.52
  ventilator [respirator] V46.11

Status — *continued*
  ventilator [respirator] — *continued*
    encounter
      during
        mechanical failure V46.14
        power failure V46.12
      for weaning V46.13
  wheelchair confinement V46.3
  wrist prosthesis V43.63
Stave fracture — *see* Fracture, metacarpus, metacarpal bone(s)
Steal
  subclavian artery 435.2
  vertebral artery 435.1
Stealing, solitary, child problem — *see also* Disturbance, conduct 312.1 ☑
Steam burn — *see* Burn, by site
Steatocystoma multiplex 706.2
Steatoma (infected) 706.2
  eyelid (cystic) 374.84
    infected 373.13
Steatorrhea (chronic) 579.8
  with lacteal obstruction 579.2
  idiopathic 579.0
    adult 579.0
    infantile 579.0
  pancreatic 579.4
  primary 579.0
  secondary 579.8
  specified cause NEC 579.8
  tropical 579.1
Steatosis 272.8
  heart (*see also* Degeneration, myocardial) 429.1
  kidney 593.89
  liver 571.8
Steele-Richardson (-Olszewski) Syndrome 333.0
Stein-Leventhal syndrome (polycystic ovary) 256.4
Steinbrocker's syndrome — *see also* Neuropathy, peripheral, autonomic 337.9
Steinert's disease 359.21
Stein's syndrome (polycystic ovary) 256.4
STEMI (ST elevation myocardial infarction — *see also* — Infarct, myocardium, ST elevation 410.9 ☑
Stenocardia — *see also* Angina 413.9
Stenocephaly 756.0
Stenosis (cicatricial) — *see also* Stricture
  ampulla of Vater 576.2
    with calculus, cholelithiasis, or stones — *see* Choledocholithiasis
  anus, anal (canal) (sphincter) 569.2
    congenital 751.2
  aorta (ascending) 747.22
    arch 747.10
    arteriosclerotic 440.0
    calcified 440.0
  aortic (valve) 424.1
    with
      mitral (valve)
        insufficiency or incompetence 396.2
        stenosis or obstruction 396.0
    atypical 396.0
    congenital 746.3
    rheumatic 395.0
      with
        insufficiency, incompetency or regurgitation 395.2
          with mitral (valve) disease 396.8
        mitral (valve)
          disease (stenosis) 396.0
          insufficiency or incompetence 396.2
          stenosis or obstruction 396.0
    specified cause, except rheumatic 424.1
    syphilitic 093.22
  aqueduct of Sylvius (congenital) 742.3
    with spina bifida (*see also* Spina bifida) 741.0 ☑
    acquired 331.4
  artery NEC (*see also* Arteriosclerosis) 447.1
    basilar — *see* Narrowing, artery, basilar

☑ **Additional Digit Required** — Refer to the Tabular List for Digit Selection   ▽ **Subterms under main terms may continue to next column or page**

2014 ICD-9-CM   ▶◀ **Revised Text**   ● **New Line**   ▲ **Revised Code**   **Volume 2 — 263**

Stenosis — see also Stricture — continued
artery (see also Arteriosclerosis) — continued
carotid (common) (internal) — see Narrowing, artery, carotid
celiac 447.4
cerebral 437.0
due to
embolism (see also Embolism, brain) 434.1 ☑
thrombus (see also Thrombosis, brain) 434.0 ☑
extremities 440.20
precerebral — see Narrowing, artery, precerebral
pulmonary (congenital) 747.31
acquired 417.8
renal 440.1
vertebral — see Narrowing, artery, vertebral
bile duct or biliary passage (see also Obstruction, biliary) 576.2
congenital 751.61
bladder neck (acquired) 596.0
congenital 753.6
brain 348.89
bronchus 519.19
syphilitic 095.8
cardia (stomach) 537.89
congenital 750.7
cardiovascular (see also Disease, cardiovascular) 429.2
carotid artery — see Narrowing, artery, carotid
cervix, cervical (canal) 622.4
congenital 752.49
in pregnancy or childbirth 654.6 ☑
affecting fetus or newborn 763.89
causing obstructed labor 660.2 ☑
affecting fetus or newborn 763.1
colon (see also Obstruction, intestine) 560.9
congenital 751.2
colostomy 569.62
common bile duct (see also Obstruction, biliary) 576.2
congenital 751.61
coronary (artery) — see Arteriosclerosis, coronary
cystic duct (see also Obstruction, gallbladder) 575.2
congenital 751.61
due to (presence of) any device, implant, or graft classifiable to 996.0–996.5 — see Complications, due to (presence of) any device, implant, or graft classified to 996.0–996.5 NEC
duodenum 537.3
congenital 751.1
ejaculatory duct NEC 608.89
endocervical os — see Stenosis, cervix
enterostomy 569.62
esophagostomy 530.87
esophagus 530.3
congenital 750.3
syphilitic 095.8
congenital 090.5
external ear canal 380.50
secondary to
inflammation 380.53
surgery 380.52
trauma 380.51
gallbladder (see also Obstruction, gallbladder) 575.2
glottis 478.74
heart valve (acquired) (see also Endocarditis)
congenital NEC 746.89
aortic 746.3
mitral 746.5
pulmonary 746.02
tricuspid 746.1
hepatic duct (see also Obstruction, biliary) 576.2
hymen 623.3
hypertrophic subaortic (idiopathic) 425.11
infundibulum cardiac 746.83

Stenosis — see also Stricture — continued
intestine (see also Obstruction, intestine) 560.9
congenital (small) 751.1
large 751.2
lacrimal
canaliculi 375.53
duct 375.56
congenital 743.65
punctum 375.52
congenital 743.65
sac 375.54
congenital 743.65
lacrimonasal duct 375.56
congenital 743.65
neonatal 375.55
larynx 478.74
congenital 748.3
syphilitic 095.8
congenital 090.5
mitral (valve) (chronic) (inactive) 394.0
with
aortic (valve)
disease (insufficiency) 396.1
insufficiency or incompetence 396.1
stenosis or obstruction 396.0
incompetency, insufficiency or regurgitation 394.2
with aortic valve disease 396.8
active or acute 391.1
with chorea (acute) (rheumatic) (Sydenham's) 392.0
congenital 746.5
specified cause, except rheumatic 424.0
syphilitic 093.21
myocardium, myocardial (see also Degeneration, myocardial) 429.1
hypertrophic subaortic (idiopathic) 425.11
nares (anterior) (posterior) 478.19
congenital 748.0
nasal duct 375.56
congenital 743.65
nasolacrimal duct 375.56
congenital 743.65
neonatal 375.55
organ or site, congenital NEC — see Atresia
papilla of Vater 576.2
with calculus, cholelithiasis, or stones — see Choledocholithiasis
pulmonary (artery) (congenital) 747.31
with ventricular septal defect, dextraposition of aorta and hypertrophy of right ventricle 745.2
acquired 417.8
infundibular 746.83
in tetralogy of Fallot 745.2
subvalvular 746.83
valve (see also Endocarditis, pulmonary) 424.3
congenital 746.02
vein 747.49
acquired 417.8
vessel NEC 417.8
pulmonic (congenital) 746.02
infundibular 746.83
subvalvular 746.83
pylorus (hypertrophic) 537.0
adult 537.0
congenital 750.5
infantile 750.5
rectum (sphincter) (see also Stricture, rectum) 569.2
renal artery 440.1
salivary duct (any) 527.8
sphincter of Oddi (see also Obstruction, biliary) 576.2
spinal 724.00
cervical 723.0
lumbar, lumbosacral (without neurogenic claudication) 724.02
with neurogenic claudication 724.03
nerve (root) NEC 724.9
specified region NEC 724.09
thoracic, thoracolumbar 724.01

Stenosis — see also Stricture — continued
stomach, hourglass 537.6
subaortic 746.81
hypertrophic (idiopathic) 425.11
supra (valvular)-aortic 747.22
trachea 519.19
congenital 748.3
syphilitic 095.8
tuberculous (see also Tuberculosis) 012.8 ☑
tracheostomy 519.02
tricuspid (valve) (see also Endocarditis, tricuspid) 397.0
congenital 746.1
nonrheumatic 424.2
tubal 628.2
ureter (see also Stricture, ureter) 593.3
congenital 753.29
urethra (see also Stricture, urethra) 598.9
vagina 623.2
congenital 752.49
in pregnancy or childbirth 654.7 ☑
affecting fetus or newborn 763.89
causing obstructed labor 660.2 ☑
affecting fetus or newborn 763.1
valve (cardiac) (heart) (see also Endocarditis) 424.90
congenital NEC 746.89
aortic 746.3
mitral 746.5
pulmonary 746.02
tricuspid 746.1
urethra 753.6
valvular (see also Endocarditis) 424.90
congenital NEC 746.89
urethra 753.6
vascular graft or shunt 996.1
atherosclerosis — see Arteriosclerosis, extremities
embolism 996.74
occlusion NEC 996.74
thrombus 996.74
vena cava (inferior) (superior) 459.2
congenital 747.49
ventricular shunt 996.2
vulva 624.8
Stent jail 996.72
Stercolith — see also Fecalith 560.32
appendix 543.9
Stercoraceous, stercoral ulcer 569.82
anus or rectum 569.41
Stereopsis, defective
with fusion 368.33
without fusion 368.32
Stereotypes NEC 307.3
Sterility
female — see Infertility, female
male (see also Infertility, male) 606.9
Sterilization, admission for V25.2
status
tubal ligation V26.51
vasectomy V26.52
Sternalgia — see also Angina 413.9
Sternopagus 759.4
Sternum bifidum 756.3
Sternutation 784.99
Steroid
effects (adverse) (iatrogenic)
cushingoid
correct substance properly administered 255.0
overdose or wrong substance given or taken 962.0
diabetes — see Diabetes, secondary
correct substance properly administered 251.8
overdose or wrong substance given or taken 962.0
due to
correct substance properly administered 255.8
overdose or wrong substance given or taken 962.0
fever
correct substance properly administered 780.60

Steroid — continued
effects — continued
fever — continued
overdose or wrong substance given or taken 962.0
withdrawal
correct substance properly administered 255.41
overdose or wrong substance given or taken 962.0
responder 365.03
Stevens-Johnson disease or syndrome (erythema multiforme exudativum) 695.13
toxic epidermal necrolysis overlap (SJS-TEN overlap syndrome) 695.14
Stewart-Morel syndrome (hyperostosis frontalis interna) 733.3
Sticker's disease (erythema infectiosum) 057.0
Stickler syndrome 759.89
Sticky eye 372.03
Stieda's disease (calcification, knee joint) 726.62
Stiff-baby 759.89
Stiff-man syndrome 333.91
Stiff
back 724.8
neck (see also Torticollis) 723.5
Stiffness, joint NEC 719.50
ankle 719.57
back 724.8
elbow 719.52
finger 719.54
hip 719.55
knee 719.56
multiple sites 719.59
sacroiliac 724.6
shoulder 719.51
specified site NEC 719.58
spine 724.9
surgical fusion V45.4
wrist 719.53
Stigmata, congenital syphilis 090.5
Still-Felty syndrome (rheumatoid arthritis with splenomegaly and leukopenia) 714.1
Stillbirth, stillborn NEC 779.9
Still's disease or syndrome 714.30
adult onset 714.2
Stiller's disease (asthenia) 780.79
Stilling-Türk-Duane syndrome (ocular retraction syndrome) 378.71
Stimulation, ovary 256.1
Sting (animal) (bee) (fish) (insect) (jellyfish) (Portuguese man-o-war) (wasp) (venomous) 989.5
anaphylactic shock or reaction 989.5
plant 692.6
Stippled epiphyses 756.59
Stitch
abscess 998.59
burst (in external operation wound) (see also Dehiscence) 998.32
internal 998.31
in back 724.5
Stojano's (subcostal) **syndrome** 098.86
Stokes-Adams syndrome (syncope with heart block) 426.9
Stokes' disease (exophthalmic goiter) 242.0 ☑
Stokvis' (-Talma) disease (enterogenous cyanosis) 289.7
Stomach — see condition
Stoma malfunction
colostomy 569.62
cystostomy 596.82
infection 596.81
mechanical 596.82
specified complication NEC 596.83
enterostomy 569.62
esophagostomy 530.87
gastrostomy 536.42
ileostomy 569.62
nephrostomy 997.5
tracheostomy 519.02
ureterostomy 997.5
Stomatitis 528.00
angular 528.5

Stomatitis — continued
  angular — continued
    due to dietary or vitamin deficiency 266.0
  aphthous 528.2
  bovine 059.11
  candidal 112.0
  catarrhal 528.00
  denture 528.9
  diphtheritic (membranous) 032.0
  due to
    dietary deficiency 266.0
    thrush 112.0
    vitamin deficiency 266.0
  epidemic 078.4
  epizootic 078.4
  follicular 528.00
  gangrenous 528.1
  herpetic 054.2
  herpetiformis 528.2
  malignant 528.00
  membranous acute 528.00
  monilial 112.0
  mycotic 112.0
  necrotic 528.1
    ulcerative 101
  necrotizing ulcerative 101
  parasitic 112.0
  septic 528.00
  specified NEC 528.09
  spirochetal 101
  suppurative (acute) 528.00
  ulcerative 528.00
    necrotizing 101
  ulceromembranous 101
  vesicular 528.00
    with exanthem 074.3
  Vincent's 101
Stomatocytosis 282.8
Stomatomycosis 112.0
Stomatorrhagia 528.9
Stone(s) — see also Calculus
  bladder 594.1
    diverticulum 594.0
  cystine 270.0
  heart syndrome (see also Failure, ventricular, left) 428.1
  kidney 592.0
  prostate 602.0
  pulp (dental) 522.2
  renal 592.0
  salivary duct or gland (any) 527.5
  ureter 592.1
  urethra (impacted) 594.2
  urinary (duct) (impacted) (passage) 592.9
    bladder 594.1
      diverticulum 594.0
    lower tract NEC 594.9
    specified site 594.8
  xanthine 277.2
Stonecutters' lung 502
  tuberculous (see also Tuberculosis) 011.4 ☑
Stonemasons'
  asthma, disease, or lung 502
    tuberculous (see also Tuberculosis) 011.4 ☑
  phthisis (see also Tuberculosis) 011.4 ☑
Stoppage
  bowel (see also Obstruction, intestine) 560.9
  heart (see also Arrest, cardiac) 427.5
  intestine (see also Obstruction, intestine) 560.9
  urine NEC (see also Retention, urine) 788.20
Storm, thyroid (apathetic) — see also Thyrotoxicosis 242.9 ☑
Strabismus (alternating) (congenital) (nonparalytic) 378.9
  concomitant (see also Heterotropia) 378.30
    convergent (see also Esotropia) 378.00
    divergent (see also Exotropia) 378.10
  convergent (see also Esotropia) 378.00
  divergent (see also Exotropia) 378.10
  due to adhesions, scars — see Strabismus, mechanical
  in neuromuscular disorder NEC 378.73
    intermittent 378.20

Strabismus — continued
  in neuromuscular disorder — continued
    intermittent — continued
      vertical 378.31
  latent 378.40
    convergent (esophoria) 378.41
    divergent (exophoria) 378.42
    vertical 378.43
  mechanical 378.60
    due to
      Brown's tendon sheath syndrome 378.61
      specified musculofascial disorder NEC 378.62
  paralytic 378.50
    third or oculomotor nerve (partial) 378.51
      total 378.52
    fourth or trochlear nerve 378.53
    sixth or abducens nerve 378.54
  specified type NEC 378.73
  vertical (hypertropia) 378.31
Strain — see also Sprain, by site
  eye NEC 368.13
  heart — see Disease, heart
  meaning gonorrhea — see Gonorrhea
  on urination 788.65
  physical NEC V62.89
  postural 729.90
  psychological NEC V62.89
Strands
  conjunctiva 372.62
  vitreous humor 379.25
Strangulation, strangulated 994.7
  appendix 543.9
  asphyxiation or suffocation by 994.7
  bladder neck 596.0
  bowel — see Strangulation, intestine
  colon — see Strangulation, intestine
  cord (umbilical) — see Compression, umbilical cord
  due to birth injury 767.8
  food or foreign body (see also Asphyxia, food) 933.1
  hemorrhoids 455.8
    external 455.5
    internal 455.2
  hernia (see also Hernia, by site, with obstruction)
    gangrenous — see Hernia, by site, with gangrene
  intestine (large) (small) 560.2
    with hernia (see also Hernia, by site, with obstruction)
      gangrenous — see Hernia, by site, with gangrene
    congenital (small) 751.1
      large 751.2
  mesentery 560.2
  mucus (see also Asphyxia, mucus) 933.1
    newborn 770.18
  omentum 560.2
  organ or site, congenital NEC — see Atresia
  ovary 620.8
    due to hernia 620.4
  penis 607.89
    foreign body 939.3
  rupture (see also Hernia, by site, with obstruction) 552.9
    gangrenous (see also Hernia, by site, with gangrene) 551.9
  stomach, due to hernia (see also Hernia, by site, with obstruction) 552.9
    with gangrene (see also Hernia, by site, with gangrene) 551.9
  umbilical cord — see Compression, umbilical cord
  vesicourethral orifice 596.0
Strangury 788.1
Strawberry
  gallbladder (see also Disease, gallbladder) 575.6
  mark 757.32
  tongue (red) (white) 529.3
Straw itch 133.8
Streak, ovarian 752.0

Strephosymbolia 315.01
  secondary to organic lesion 784.69
Streptobacillary fever 026.1
Streptobacillus moniliformis 026.1
Streptococcemia 038.0
Streptococcicosis — see Infection, streptococcal
Streptococcus, streptococcal — see condition
Streptoderma 686.00
Streptomycosis — see Actinomycosis
Streptothricosis — see Actinomycosis
Streptothrix — see Actinomycosis
Streptotrichosis — see Actinomycosis
Stress 308.9
  fracture — see Fracture, stress
  polycythemia 289.0
  reaction (gross) (see also Reaction, stress, acute) 308.9
Stretching, nerve — see Injury, nerve, by site
Striae (albicantes) (atrophicae) (cutis distensae) (distensae) 701.3
Striations of nails 703.8
Stricture — see also Stenosis 799.89
  ampulla of Vater 576.2
    with calculus, cholelithiasis, or stones — see Choledocholithiasis
  anus (sphincter) 569.2
    congenital 751.2
    infantile 751.2
  aorta (ascending) 747.22
    arch 747.10
    arteriosclerotic 440.0
    calcified 440.0
  aortic (valve) (see also Stenosis, aortic) 424.1
    congenital 746.3
  aqueduct of Sylvius (congenital) 742.3
    with spina bifida (see also Spina bifida) 741.0 ☑
    acquired 331.4
  artery 447.1
    basilar — see Narrowing, artery, basilar
    carotid (common) (internal) — see Narrowing, artery, carotid
    celiac 447.4
    cerebral 437.0
      congenital 747.81
      due to
        embolism (see also Embolism, brain) 434.1 ☑
        thrombus (see also Thrombosis, brain) 434.0 ☑
    congenital (peripheral) 747.60
      cerebral 747.81
      coronary 746.85
      gastrointestinal 747.61
      lower limb 747.64
      renal 747.62
      retinal 743.58
      specified NEC 747.69
      spinal 747.82
      umbilical 747.5
      upper limb 747.63
    coronary — see Arteriosclerosis, coronary
      congenital 746.85
    precerebral — see Narrowing, artery, precerebral NEC
    pulmonary (congenital) 747.31
      acquired 417.8
    renal 440.1
    vertebral — see Narrowing, artery, vertebral
  auditory canal (congenital) (external) 744.02
    acquired (see also Stricture, ear canal, acquired) 380.50
  bile duct or passage (any) (postoperative) (see also Obstruction, biliary) 576.2
    congenital 751.61
  bladder 596.89
    congenital 753.6
    neck 596.0
      congenital 753.6
  bowel (see also Obstruction, intestine) 560.9
  brain 348.89
  bronchus 519.19
    syphilitic 095.8

Stricture — see also Stenosis — continued
  cardia (stomach) 537.89
    congenital 750.7
  cardiac (see also Disease, heart)
    orifice (stomach) 537.89
  cardiovascular (see also Disease, cardiovascular) 429.2
  carotid artery — see Narrowing, artery, carotid
  cecum (see also Obstruction, intestine) 560.9
  cervix, cervical (canal) 622.4
    congenital 752.49
    in pregnancy or childbirth 654.6 ☑
      affecting fetus or newborn 763.89
      causing obstructed labor 660.2 ☑
        affecting fetus or newborn 763.1
  colon (see also Obstruction, intestine) 560.9
    congenital 751.2
  colostomy 569.62
  common bile duct (see also Obstruction, biliary) 576.2
    congenital 751.61
  coronary (artery) — see Arteriosclerosis, coronary
    congenital 746.85
  cystic duct (see also Obstruction, gallbladder) 575.2
    congenital 751.61
  cystostomy 596.83
  digestive organs NEC, congenital 751.8
  duodenum 537.3
    congenital 751.1
  ear canal (external) (congenital) 744.02
    acquired 380.50
      secondary to
        inflammation 380.53
        surgery 380.52
        trauma 380.51
  ejaculatory duct 608.85
  enterostomy 569.62
  esophagostomy 530.87
  esophagus (corrosive) (peptic) 530.3
    congenital 750.3
    syphilitic 095.8
      congenital 090.5
  eustachian tube (see also Obstruction, Eustachian tube) 381.60
    congenital 744.24
  fallopian tube 628.2
    gonococcal (chronic) 098.37
      acute 098.17
    tuberculous (see also Tuberculosis) 016.6 ☑
  gallbladder (see also Obstruction, gallbladder) 575.2
    congenital 751.69
  glottis 478.74
  heart (see also Disease, heart)
    congenital NEC 746.89
    valve (see also Endocarditis)
      congenital NEC 746.89
        aortic 746.3
        mitral 746.5
        pulmonary 746.02
        tricuspid 746.1
  hepatic duct (see also Obstruction, biliary) 576.2
  hourglass, of stomach 537.6
  hymen 623.3
  hypopharynx 478.29
  intestine (see also Obstruction, intestine) 560.9
    congenital (small) 751.1
      large 751.2
    ischemic 557.1
  lacrimal
    canaliculi 375.53
      congenital 743.65
    punctum 375.52
      congenital 743.65
    sac 375.54
      congenital 743.65
  lacrimonasal duct 375.56
    congenital 743.65
    neonatal 375.55
  larynx 478.79

☑ **Additional Digit Required** — Refer to the Tabular List for Digit Selection   ▽ **Subterms under main terms may continue to next column or page**

2014 ICD-9-CM   ▶◀ **Revised Text**   ● **New Line**   ▲ **Revised Code**   **Volume 2 — 265**

Stricture — see also Stenosis — continued
  larynx — continued
    congenital 748.3
    syphilitic 095.8
      congenital 090.5
  lung 518.89
  meatus
    ear (congenital) 744.02
      acquired (see also Stricture, ear canal, acquired) 380.50
    osseous (congenital) (ear) 744.03
      acquired (see also Stricture, ear canal, acquired) 380.50
    urinarius (see also Stricture, urethra) 598.9
      congenital 753.6
  mitral (valve) (see also Stenosis, mitral) 394.0
    congenital 746.5
    specified cause, except rheumatic 424.0
  myocardium, myocardial (see also Degeneration, myocardial) 429.1
    hypertrophic subaortic (idiopathic) 425.11
  nares (anterior) (posterior) 478.19
    congenital 748.0
  nasal duct 375.56
    congenital 743.65
    neonatal 375.55
  nasolacrimal duct 375.56
    congenital 743.65
    neonatal 375.55
  nasopharynx 478.29
    syphilitic 095.8
  nephrostomy 997.5
  nose 478.19
    congenital 748.0
  nostril (anterior) (posterior) 478.19
    congenital 748.0
  organ or site, congenital NEC — see Atresia
  osseous meatus (congenital) (ear) 744.03
    acquired (see also Stricture, ear canal, acquired) 380.50
  os uteri (see also Stricture, cervix) 622.4
  oviduct — see Stricture, fallopian tube
  pelviureteric junction 593.3
  pharynx (dilation) 478.29
  prostate 602.8
  pulmonary, pulmonic
    artery (congenital) 747.31
      acquired 417.8
      noncongenital 417.8
    infundibulum (congenital) 746.83
    valve (see also Endocarditis, pulmonary) 424.3
      congenital 746.02
    vein (congenital) 747.49
      acquired 417.8
    vessel NEC 417.8
  punctum lacrimale 375.52
    congenital 743.65
  pylorus (hypertrophic) 537.0
    adult 537.0
    congenital 750.5
    infantile 750.5
  rectosigmoid 569.89
  rectum (sphincter) 569.2
    congenital 751.2
    due to
      chemical burn 947.3
      irradiation 569.2
      lymphogranuloma venereum 099.1
    gonococcal 098.7
    inflammatory 099.1
    syphilitic 095.8
    tuberculous (see also Tuberculosis) 014.8 ☑
  renal artery 440.1
  salivary duct or gland (any) 527.8
  sigmoid (flexure) (see also Obstruction, intestine) 560.9
  spermatic cord 608.85
  stoma (following) (of)
    colostomy 569.62
    cystostomy 596.83
    enterostomy 569.62
    esophagostomy 530.87

Stricture — see also Stenosis — continued
  stoma — continued
    gastrostomy 536.42
    ileostomy 569.62
    nephrostomy 997.5
    tracheostomy 519.02
    ureterostomy 997.5
  stomach 537.89
    congenital 750.7
    hourglass 537.6
  subaortic 746.81
    hypertrophic (acquired) (idiopathic) 425.11
  subglottic 478.74
  syphilitic NEC 095.8
  tendon (sheath) 727.81
  trachea 519.19
    congenital 748.3
    syphilitic 095.8
    tuberculous (see also Tuberculosis) 012.8 ☑
  tracheostomy 519.02
  tricuspid (valve) (see also Endocarditis, tricuspid) 397.0
    congenital 746.1
    nonrheumatic 424.2
  tunica vaginalis 608.85
  ureter (postoperative) 593.3
    congenital 753.29
    tuberculous (see also Tuberculosis) 016.2 ☑
  ureteropelvic junction 593.3
    congenital 753.21
  ureterovesical orifice 593.3
    congenital 753.22
  urethra (anterior) (meatal) (organic) (posterior) (spasmodic) 598.9
    associated with schistosomiasis (see also Schistosomiasis) 120.9 [598.01]
    congenital (valvular) 753.6
    due to
      infection 598.00
        syphilis 095.8 [598.01]
      trauma 598.1
    gonococcal 098.2 [598.01]
    gonorrheal 098.2 [598.01]
    infective 598.00
    late effect of injury 598.1
    postcatheterization 598.2
    postobstetric 598.1
    postoperative 598.2
    specified cause NEC 598.8
    syphilitic 095.8 [598.01]
    traumatic 598.1
    valvular, congenital 753.6
  urinary meatus (see also Stricture, urethra) 598.9
    congenital 753.6
  uterus, uterine 621.5
    os (external) (internal) — see Stricture, cervix
  vagina (outlet) 623.2
    congenital 752.49
  valve (cardiac) (heart) (see also Endocarditis) 424.90
    congenital (cardiac) (heart) NEC 746.89
      aortic 746.3
      mitral 746.5
      pulmonary 746.02
      tricuspid 746.1
      urethra 753.6
    valvular (see also Endocarditis) 424.90
  vascular graft or shunt 996.1
    atherosclerosis — see Arteriosclerosis, extremities
    embolism 996.74
    occlusion NEC 996.74
    thrombus 996.74
  vas deferens 608.85
    congenital 752.89
  vein 459.2
  vena cava (inferior) (superior) NEC 459.2
    congenital 747.49
  ventricular shunt 996.2
  vesicourethral orifice 596.0
    congenital 753.6

Stricture — see also Stenosis — continued
  vulva (acquired) 624.8
Stridor 786.1
  congenital (larynx) 748.3
Stridulous — see condition
Strippling of nails 703.8
Stroke 434.91
  apoplectic (see also Disease, cerebrovascular, acute) 436
  brain — see Infarct, brain
  embolic 434.11
  epileptic — see Epilepsy
  healed or old V12.54
  heart — see Disease, heart
  heat 992.0
  hemorrhagic — see Hemorrhage, brain
  iatrogenic 997.02
  in evolution 434.91
  ischemic 434.91
  late effect — see Late effect(s) (of) cerebrovascular disease
  lightning 994.0
  paralytic — see Infarct, brain
  postoperative 997.02
  progressive 435.9
  thrombotic 434.01
Stromatosis, endometrial (M8931/1) 236.0
Strong pulse 785.9
Strongyloides stercoralis infestation 127.2
Strongyloidiasis 127.2
Strongyloidosis 127.2
Strongylus (gibsoni) infestation 127.7
Strophulus (newborn) 779.89
  pruriginosus 698.2
Struck by lightning 994.0
Struma — see also Goiter 240.9
  fibrosa 245.3
  Hashimoto (struma lymphomatosa) 245.2
  lymphomatosa 245.2
  nodosa (simplex) 241.9
    endemic 241.9
    multinodular 241.1
    sporadic 241.9
    toxic or with hyperthyroidism 242.3 ☑
      multinodular 242.2 ☑
      uninodular 242.1 ☑
    toxicosa 242.3 ☑
      multinodular 242.2 ☑
      uninodular 242.1 ☑
    uninodular 241.0
  ovarii (M9090/0) 220
    and carcinoid (M9091/1) 236.2
    malignant (M9090/3) 183.0
  Riedel's (ligneous thyroiditis) 245.3
  scrofulous (see also Tuberculosis) 017.2 ☑
  tuberculous (see also Tuberculosis) 017.2 ☑
    abscess 017.2 ☑
    adenitis 017.2 ☑
    lymphangitis 017.2 ☑
    ulcer 017.2 ☑
Strumipriva cachexia — see also Hypothyroidism 244.9
Strümpell-Marie disease or spine (ankylosing spondylitis) 720.0
Strümpell-Westphal pseudosclerosis (hepatolenticular degeneration) 275.1
Stuart-Prower factor deficiency (congenital factor X deficiency) — see also Defect, coagulation 286.3
Stuart's disease (congenital factor X deficiency) — see also Defect, coagulation 286.3
Students' elbow 727.2
Stuffy nose 478.19
Stump — see also Amputation
  cervix, cervical (healed) 622.8
Stupor 780.09
  catatonic (see also Schizophrenia) 295.2 ☑
  circular (see also Psychosis, manic-depressive, circular) 296.7
  manic-depressive (see also Psychosis, affective) 296.89
  manic 296.89
  mental (anergic) (delusional) 298.9
  psychogenic 298.8
  reaction to exceptional stress (transient) 308.2

Stupor — continued
  traumatic NEC (see also Injury, intracranial) with spinal (cord)
    lesion — see Injury, spinal, by site
    shock — see Injury, spinal, by site
Sturge-Kalischer-Weber syndrome (encephalocutaneous angiomatosis) 759.6
Sturge (-Weber) (-Dimitri) disease or syndrome (encephalocutaneous angiomatosis) 759.6
Stuttering 315.35
  adult onset 307.0
  childhood onset 315.35
  due to late effect of cerebrovascular disease (see also Late effect(s) (of) cerebrovascular disease) 438.14
  in conditions classified elsewhere 784.52
Sty, stye 373.11
  external 373.11
  internal 373.12
  meibomian 373.12
Subacidity, gastric 536.8
  psychogenic 306.4
Subacute — see condition
Subarachnoid — see condition
Subclavian steal syndrome 435.2
Subcortical — see condition
Subcostal syndrome 098.86
  nerve compression 354.8
Subcutaneous, subcuticular — see condition
Subdelirium 293.1
Subdural — see condition
Subendocardium — see condition
Subependymoma (M9383/1) 237.5
Suberosis 495.3
Subglossitis — see Glossitis
Subhemophilia 286.0
Subinvolution (uterus) 621.1
  breast (postlactational) (postpartum) 611.89
  chronic 621.1
  puerperal, postpartum 674.8 ☑
Sublingual — see condition
Sublinguitis 527.2
Subluxation — see also Dislocation, by site
  congenital NEC (see also Malposition, congenital)
    hip (unilateral) 754.32
      with dislocation of other hip 754.35
      bilateral 754.33
    joint
      lower limb 755.69
      shoulder 755.59
      upper limb 755.59
    lower limb (joint) 755.69
    shoulder (joint) 755.59
    upper limb (joint) 755.59
  lens 379.32
    anterior 379.33
    posterior 379.34
  radial head 832.2
  rotary, cervical region of spine — see Fracture, vertebra, cervical
Submaxillary — see condition
Submersion (fatal) (nonfatal) 994.1
Submissiveness (undue), in child 313.0
Submucous — see condition
Subnormal, subnormality
  accommodation (see also Disorder, accommodation) 367.9
  mental (see also Disability, intellectual) 319
    mild 317
    moderate 318.0
    profound 318.2
    severe 318.1
  temperature (accidental) 991.6
    not associated with low environmental temperature 780.99
Subphrenic — see condition
Subscapular nerve — see condition
Subseptus uterus 752.35
Subsiding appendicitis 542
Substance abuse in family V61.42
Substernal thyroid — see also Goiter 240.9
  congenital 759.2
Substitution disorder 300.11
Subtentorial — see condition

☑ Additional Digit Required — Refer to the Tabular List for Digit Selection
▽ Subterms under main terms may continue to next column or page
266 — Volume 2
▶◀ Revised Text   ● New Line   ▲ Revised Code
2014 ICD-9-CM

Subtertian
 fever 084.0
 malaria (fever) 084.0
Subthyroidism (acquired) — *see also* Hypothyroidism 244.9
 congenital 243
Succenturiata placenta — *see* Placenta, abnormal
Succussion sounds, chest 786.7
Sucking thumb, child 307.9
Sudamen 705.1
Sudamina 705.1
Sudanese kala-azar 085.0
Sudden
 death, cause unknown (less than 24 hours)
   798.1
  cardiac (SCD)
   family history of V17.41
   personal history of, successfully resus-
    citated V12.53
  during childbirth 669.9 ☑
  infant 798.0
  puerperal, postpartum 674.9 ☑
 hearing loss NEC 388.2
 heart failure (*see also* Failure, heart) 428.9
 infant death syndrome 798.0
Sudeck's atrophy, disease, or syndrome
  733.7
SUDS (sudden unexplained death) 798.2
Suffocation — *see also* Asphyxia 799.01
 by
  bed clothes 994.7
  bunny bag 994.7
  cave-in 994.7
  constriction 994.7
  drowning 994.1
  inhalation
   food or foreign body (*see also* Asphyx-
     ia, food or foreign body) 933.1
   oil or gasoline (*see also* Asphyxia,
     food or foreign body) 933.1
  overlying 994.7
  plastic bag 994.7
  pressure 994.7
  strangulation 994.7
 during birth 768.1
 mechanical 994.7
Sugar
 blood
  high 790.29
  low 251.2
 in urine 791.5
Suicide, suicidal (attempted)
 by poisoning — *see* Table of Drugs and
   Chemicals
 ideation V62.84
 risk 300.9
 tendencies 300.9
 trauma NEC (*see also* nature and site of injury) 959.9
Suipestifer infection — *see also* Infection,
  Salmonella 003.9
Sulfatidosis 330.0
Sulfhemoglobinemia, sulphemoglobinemia
  (acquired) (congenital) 289.7
Sumatran mite fever 081.2
Summer — *see* condition
Sunburn 692.71
 first degree 692.71
 second degree 692.76
 third degree 692.77
 dermatitis 692.71
 due to
  other ultraviolet radiation 692.82
  tanning bed 692.82
SUNCT (short lasting unilateral neuralgiform
  headache with conjunctival injection
  and tearing) 339.05
Sunken
 acetabulum 718.85
 fontanels 756.0
Sunstroke 992.0
Superfecundation 651.9 ☑
 with fetal loss and retention of one or more
   fetus(es) 651.6 ☑
 following (elective) fetal reduction 651.7 ☑

Superfetation 651.9 ☑
 with fetal loss and retention of one or more
   fetus(es) 651.6 ☑
 following (elective) fetal reduction 651.7 ☑
Superinvolution uterus 621.8
Supernumerary (congenital)
 aortic cusps 746.89
 auditory ossicles 744.04
 bone 756.9
 breast 757.6
 carpal bones 755.56
 cusps, heart valve NEC 746.89
  mitral 746.5
  pulmonary 746.09
 digit(s) 755.00
  finger 755.01
  toe 755.02
 ear (lobule) 744.1
 fallopian tube 752.19
 finger 755.01
 hymen 752.49
 kidney 753.3
 lacrimal glands 743.64
 lacrimonasal duct 743.65
 lobule (ear) 744.1
 mitral cusps 746.5
 muscle 756.82
 nipples 757.6
 organ or site NEC — *see* Accessory
 ossicles, auditory 744.04
 ovary 752.0
 oviduct 752.19
 pulmonic cusps 746.09
 rib 756.3
  cervical or first 756.2
   syndrome 756.2
 roots (of teeth) 520.2
 spinal vertebra 756.19
 spleen 759.0
 tarsal bones 755.67
 teeth 520.1
  causing crowding 524.31
 testis 752.89
 thumb 755.01
 toe 755.02
 uterus 752.2
 vagina 752.49
 vertebra 756.19
Supervision (of)
 contraceptive method previously prescribed
   V25.40
  intrauterine device V25.42
  oral contraceptive (pill) V25.41
  specified type NEC V25.49
  subdermal implantable contraceptive
    V25.43
 dietary (for) V65.3
  allergy (food) V65.3
  colitis V65.3
  diabetes mellitus V65.3
  food allergy intolerance V65.3
  gastritis V65.3
  hypercholesterolemia V65.3
  hypoglycemia V65.3
  intolerance (food) V65.3
  obesity V65.3
  specified NEC V65.3
 lactation V24.1
 newborn health
  8 to 28 days old V20.32
  under 8 days old V20.31
 pregnancy — *see* Pregnancy, supervision
   of
Supplemental teeth 520.1
 causing crowding 524.31
Suppression
 binocular vision 368.31
 lactation 676.5 ☑
 menstruation 626.8
 ovarian secretion 256.39
 renal 586
 urinary secretion 788.5
 urine 788.5
Suppuration, suppurative — *see also* condition

Suppuration, suppurative — *see also*
  condition — *continued*
 accessory sinus (chronic) (*see also* Sinusitis)
   473.9
 adrenal gland 255.8
 antrum (chronic) (*see also* Sinusitis, maxillary) 473.0
 bladder (*see also* Cystitis) 595.89
 bowel 569.89
 brain 324.0
  late effect 326
 breast 611.0
  puerperal, postpartum 675.1 ☑
 dental periosteum 526.5
 diffuse (skin) 686.00
 ear (middle) (*see also* Otitis media) 382.4
  external (*see also* Otitis, externa) 380.10
  internal 386.33
 ethmoidal (sinus) (chronic) (*see also* Sinusitis, ethmoidal) 473.2
 fallopian tube (*see also* Salpingo-oophoritis)
   614.2
 frontal (sinus) (chronic) (*see also* Sinusitis,
   frontal) 473.1
 gallbladder (*see also* Cholecystitis, acute)
   575.0
 gum 523.30
 hernial sac — *see* Hernia, by site
 intestine 569.89
 joint (*see also* Arthritis, suppurative)
   711.0 ☑
 labyrinthine 386.33
 lung 513.0
 mammary gland 611.0
  puerperal, postpartum 675.1 ☑
 maxilla, maxillary 526.4
  sinus (chronic) (*see also* Sinusitis, maxil-
    lary) 473.0
 muscle 728.0
 nasal sinus (chronic) (*see also* Sinusitis) 473.9
 pancreas 577.0
 parotid gland 527.2
 pelvis, pelvic
  female (*see also* Disease, pelvis, inflam-
    matory) 614.4
   acute 614.3
  male (*see also* Peritonitis) 567.21
 pericranial (*see also* Osteomyelitis) 730.2 ☑
 salivary duct or gland (any) 527.2
 sinus (nasal) (*see also* Sinusitis) 473.9
 sphenoidal (sinus) (chronic) (*see also* Sinusitis, sphenoidal) 473.3
 thymus (gland) 254.1
 thyroid (gland) 245.0
 tonsil 474.8
 uterus (*see also* Endometritis) 615.9
 vagina 616.10
 wound (*see also* Wound, open, by site,
   complicated)
  dislocation — *see* Dislocation, by site,
    compound
  fracture — *see* Fracture, by site, open
  scratch or other superficial injury — *see*
    Injury, superficial, by site
Supraeruption, teeth 524.34
Supraglottitis 464.50
 with obstruction 464.51
Suprapubic drainage 596.89
Suprarenal (gland) — *see* condition
Suprascapular nerve — *see* condition
Suprasellar — *see* condition
Supraspinatus syndrome 726.10
Surfer knots 919.8
 infected 919.9
Surgery
 cosmetic NEC V50.1
  breast reconstruction following mastec-
    tomy V51.0
  following healed injury or operation
    V51.8
  hair transplant V50.0
 elective V50.9
  breast
   augmentation or reduction V50.1
   reconstruction following mastectomy
     V51.0

Surgery — *continued*
 elective — *continued*
  circumcision, ritual or routine (in ab-
    sence of medical indication)
    V50.2
  cosmetic NEC V50.1
  ear piercing V50.3
  face-lift V50.1
  following healed injury or operation
    V51.8
  hair transplant V50.0
 not done because of
  contraindication V64.1
  patient's decision V64.2
  specified reason NEC V64.3
 plastic
  breast
   augmentation or reduction V50.1
   reconstruction following mastectomy
     V51.0
  cosmetic V50.1
  face-lift V50.1
  following healed injury or operation
    V51.8
  repair of scarred tissue (following healed
    injury or operation) V51.8
  specified type NEC V50.8
 previous, in pregnancy or childbirth
  cervix 654.6 ☑
   affecting fetus or newborn (*see also*
     Newborn, affected by) 760.63
   causing obstructed labor 660.2 ☑
    affecting fetus or newborn 763.1
  pelvic soft tissues NEC 654.9 ☑
   affecting fetus or newborn (*see also*
     Newborn, affected by) 760.63
   causing obstructed labor 660.2 ☑
    affecting fetus or newborn 763.1
  perineum or vulva 654.8 ☑
  uterus NEC 654.9 ☑
   affecting fetus or newborn (*see also*
     Newborn, affected by) 760.63
   causing obstructed labor 660.2 ☑
    affecting fetus or newborn 763.1
   due to previous cesarean delivery
     654.2 ☑
  vagina 654.7 ☑
Surgical
 abortion — *see* Abortion, legal
 emphysema 998.81
 kidney (*see also* Pyelitis) 590.80
 operation NEC 799.9
 procedures, complication or misadventure
   — *see* Complications, surgical procedure
 shock 998.00
Survey
 fetal anatomic V28.81
Susceptibility
 genetic
  to
   MEN (multiple endocrine neoplasia)
     V84.81
   neoplasia
    multiple endocrine (MEN) V84.81
   neoplasm
    malignant, of
     breast V84.01
     endometrium V84.04
     other V84.09
     ovary V84.02
     prostate V84.03
    specified disease V84.89
Suspected condition, ruled out — *see also*
  Observation, suspected V71.9
 specified condition NEC V71.89
Suspended uterus, in pregnancy or child-
  birth 654.4 ☑
 affecting fetus or newborn 763.89
 causing obstructed labor 660.2 ☑
  affecting fetus or newborn 763.1
Sutton and Gull's disease (arteriolar
  nephrosclerosis) — *see also* Hypertension, kidney 403.90
Sutton's disease 709.09

Subtertian — Sutton's disease

☑ Additional Digit Required — Refer to the Tabular List for Digit Selection   ▽ Subterms under main terms may continue to next column or page

2014 ICD-9-CM   ▶◀ Revised Text   ● New Line   ▲ Revised Code   Volume 2 — 267

Suture
  burst (in external operation wound) (see also Dehiscence) 998.32
    internal 998.31
  inadvertently left in operation wound 998.4
  removal V58.32
  Shirodkar, in pregnancy (with or without cervical incompetence) 654.5 ☑
Swab inadvertently left in operation wound 998.4
Swallowed, swallowing
  difficulty (see also Dysphagia) 787.20
  foreign body NEC (see also Foreign body) 938
Swamp fever 100.89
Swan neck hand (intrinsic) 736.09
Sweat(s), sweating
  disease or sickness 078.2
  excessive (see also Hyperhidrosis) 780.8
  fetid 705.89
  fever 078.2
  gland disease 705.9
    specified type NEC 705.89
  miliary 078.2
  night 780.8
Sweeley-Klionsky disease (angiokeratoma corporis diffusum) 272.7
Sweet's syndrome (acute febrile neutrophilic dermatosis) 695.89
Swelling 782.3
  abdominal (not referable to specific organ) 789.3 ☑
  adrenal gland, cloudy 255.8
  ankle 719.07
  anus 787.99
  arm 729.81
  breast 611.72
  Calabar 125.2
  cervical gland 785.6
  cheek 784.2
  chest 786.6
  ear 388.8
  epigastric 789.3 ☑
  extremity (lower) (upper) 729.81
  eye 379.92
  female genital organ 625.8
  finger 729.81
  foot 729.81
  glands 785.6
  gum 784.2
  hand 729.81
  head 784.2
  inflammatory — see Inflammation
  joint (see also Effusion, joint) 719.0 ☑
    tuberculous — see Tuberculosis, joint
  kidney, cloudy 593.89
  leg 729.81
  limb 729.81
  liver 573.8
  lung 786.6
  lymph nodes 785.6
  mediastinal 786.6
  mouth 784.2
  muscle (limb) 729.81
  neck 784.2
  nose or sinus 784.2
  palate 784.2
  pelvis 789.3 ☑
  penis 607.83
  perineum 625.8
  rectum 787.99
  scrotum 608.86
  skin 782.2
  splenic (see also Splenomegaly) 789.2
  substernal 786.6
  superficial, localized (skin) 782.2
  testicle 608.86
  throat 784.2
  toe 729.81
  tongue 784.2
  tubular (see also Disease, renal) 593.9
  umbilicus 789.3 ☑
  uterus 625.8
  vagina 625.8
  vulva 625.8

Swelling — continued
  wandering, due to Gnathostoma (spinigerum) 128.1
  white — see Tuberculosis, arthritis
Swift's disease 985.0
Swimmers'
  ear (acute) 380.12
  itch 120.3
Swimming in the head 780.4
Swollen — see also Swelling
  glands 785.6
Swyer-James syndrome (unilateral hyperlucent lung) 492.8
Swyer's syndrome (XY pure gonadal dysgenesis) 752.7
Sycosis 704.8
  barbae (not parasitic) 704.8
  contagiosa 110.0
  lupoid 704.8
  mycotic 110.0
  parasitic 110.0
  vulgaris 704.8
Sydenham's chorea — see Chorea, Sydenham's
Sylvatic yellow fever 060.0
Sylvest's disease (epidemic pleurodynia) 074.1
Symblepharon 372.63
  congenital 743.62
Symonds' syndrome 348.2
Sympathetic — see condition
Sympatheticotonia — see also Neuropathy, peripheral, autonomic 337.9
Sympathicoblastoma (M9500/3)
  specified site — see Neoplasm, by site, malignant
  unspecified site 194.0
Sympathicogonioma (M9500/3) — see Sympathicoblastoma
Sympathoblastoma (M9500/3) — see Sympathicoblastoma
Sympathogonioma (M9500/3) — see Sympathicoblastoma
Symphalangy — see also Syndactylism 755.10
Symptoms, specified (general) NEC 780.99
  abdomen NEC 789.9
  bone NEC 733.90
  breast NEC 611.79
  cardiac NEC 785.9
  cardiovascular NEC 785.9
  chest NEC 786.9
  cognition 799.59
  development NEC 783.9
  digestive system NEC 787.99
  emotional state NEC 799.29
  eye NEC 379.99
  gastrointestinal tract NEC 787.99
  genital organs NEC
    female 625.9
    male 608.9
  head and neck NEC 784.99
  heart NEC 785.9
  jaw 784.92
  joint NEC 719.60
    ankle 719.67
    elbow 719.62
    foot 719.67
    hand 719.64
    hip 719.65
    knee 719.66
    multiple sites 719.69
    pelvic region 719.65
    shoulder (region) 719.61
    specified site NEC 719.68
    temporomandibular 524.69
    wrist 719.63
  larynx NEC 784.99
  limbs NEC 729.89
  lymphatic system NEC 785.9
  maxilla 784.92
  menopausal 627.2
  metabolism NEC 783.9
  mouth NEC 528.9
  muscle NEC 728.9
  musculoskeletal NEC 781.99
    limbs NEC 729.89
  nervous system NEC 781.99

Symptoms, specified — continued
  neurotic NEC 300.9
  nutrition, metabolism, and development NEC 783.9
  pelvis NEC 789.9
    female 625.9
  peritoneum NEC 789.9
  respiratory system NEC 786.9
  skin and integument NEC 782.9
  subcutaneous tissue NEC 782.9
  throat NEC 784.99
  tonsil NEC 784.99
  urinary system NEC 788.99
  vascular NEC 785.9
Sympus 759.89
Synarthrosis 719.80
  ankle 719.87
  elbow 719.82
  foot 719.87
  hand 719.84
  hip 719.85
  knee 719.86
  multiple sites 719.89
  pelvic region 719.85
  shoulder (region) 719.81
  specified site NEC 719.88
  wrist 719.83
Syncephalus 759.4
Synchondrosis 756.9
  abnormal (congenital) 756.9
  ischiopubic (van Neck's) 732.1
Synchysis (senile) (vitreous humor) 379.21
  scintillans 379.22
Syncope (near) (pre-) 780.2
  anginosa 413.9
  bradycardia 427.89
  cardiac 780.2
  carotid sinus 337.01
  complicating delivery 669.2 ☑
  due to lumbar puncture 349.0
  fatal 798.1
  heart 780.2
  heat 992.1
  laryngeal 786.2
  tussive 786.2
  vasoconstriction 780.2
  vasodepressor 780.2
  vasomotor 780.2
  vasovagal 780.2
Syncytial infarct — see Placenta, abnormal
Syndactylism, syndactyly (multiple sites) 755.10
  fingers (without fusion of bone) 755.11
    with fusion of bone 755.12
  toes (without fusion of bone) 755.13
    with fusion of bone 755.14
Syndrome — see also Disease
  with 5q deletion 238.74
  5q minus 238.74
  abdominal
    acute 789.0 ☑
    migraine 346.2 ☑
    muscle deficiency 756.79
  Abercrombie's (amyloid degeneration) 277.39
  abnormal innervation 374.43
  abstinence
    alcohol 291.81
    drug 292.0
    neonatal 779.5
  Abt-Letterer-Siwe (acute histiocytosis X) (M9722/3) 202.5 ☑
  Achard-Thiers (adrenogenital) 255.2
  acid pulmonary aspiration 997.39
    obstetric (Mendelson's) 668.0 ☑
  acquired immune deficiency 042
  acquired immunodeficiency 042
  acrocephalosyndactylism 755.55
  acute abdominal 789.0 ☑
  acute chest 517.3
  acute coronary 411.1
  Adair-Dighton (brittle bones and blue sclera, deafness) 756.51
  Adams-Stokes (-Morgagni) (syncope with heart block) 426.9
  Addisonian 255.41

Syndrome — see also Disease — continued
  Adie (-Holmes) (pupil) 379.46
  adiposogenital 253.8
  adrenal
    hemorrhage 036.3
    meningococcic 036.3
  adrenocortical 255.3
  adrenogenital (acquired) (congenital) 255.2
    feminizing 255.2
    iatrogenic 760.79
    virilism (acquired) (congenital) 255.2
  affective organic NEC 293.89
    drug-induced 292.84
  afferent loop NEC 537.89
  African macroglobulinemia 273.3
  Ahumada-Del Castillo (nonpuerperal galactorrhea and amenorrhea) 253.1
  air blast concussion — see Injury, internal, by site
  Alagille 759.89
  Albright-McCune-Sternberg (osteitis fibrosa disseminata) 756.59
  Albright (-Martin) (pseudohypoparathyroidism) 275.49
  alcohol withdrawal 291.81
  Alder's (leukocyte granulation anomaly) 288.2
  Aldrich (-Wiskott) (eczema-thrombocytopenia) 279.12
  Alibert-Bazin (mycosis fungoides) (M9700/3) 202.1 ☑
  Alice in Wonderland 293.89
  alien hand 781.8
  Allen-Masters 620.6
  Alligator baby (ichthyosis congenita) 757.1
  Alport's (hereditary hematuria-nephropathy-deafness) 759.89
  Alvarez (transient cerebral ischemia) 435.9
  alveolar capillary block 516.8
  Alzheimer's 331.0
    with dementia — see Alzheimer's, dementia
  amnestic (confabulatory) 294.0
    alcohol-induced persisting 291.1
    drug-induced 292.83
    posttraumatic 294.0
  amotivational 292.89
  amyostatic 275.1
  amyotrophic lateral sclerosis 335.20
  androgen insensitivity 259.51
    partial 259.52
  Angelman 759.89
  angina (see also Angina) 413.9
  ankyloglossia superior 750.0
  anterior
    chest wall 786.52
    compartment (tibial) 958.8
    spinal artery 433.8 ☑
      compression 721.1
    tibial (compartment) 958.8
  antibody deficiency 279.00
    agammaglobulinemic 279.00
    congenital 279.04
    hypogammaglobulinemic 279.00
  anticardiolipin antibody 289.81
  antimongolism 758.39
  antiphospholipid antibody 289.81
  Anton (-Babinski) (hemiasomatognosia) 307.9
  anxiety (see also Anxiety) 300.00
    organic 293.84
  aortic
    arch 446.7
    bifurcation (occlusion) 444.09
    ring 747.21
  Apert-Gallais (adrenogenital) 255.2
  Apert's (acrocephalosyndactyly) 755.55
  aphasia-apraxia-alexia 784.69
  apical ballooning 429.83
  "approximate answers" 300.16
  arcuate ligament (-celiac axis) 447.4
  arcus aortae 446.7
  arc welders' 370.24
  argentaffin, argintaffinoma 259.2
  Argonz-Del Castillo (nonpuerperal galactorrhea and amenorrhea) 253.1

☑ Additional Digit Required — Refer to the Tabular List for Digit Selection   ▽ Subterms under main terms may continue to next column or page

268 — Volume 2   ▶◀ Revised Text   ● New Line   ▲ Revised Code   2014 ICD-9-CM

Syndrome — *see also* Disease — *continued*

Argyll Robertson's (syphilitic) 094.89
  nonsyphilitic 379.45
arm-shoulder (*see also* Neuropathy, peripheral, autonomic) 337.9
Armenian 277.31
Arnold-Chiari (*see also* Spina bifida) 741.0 ☑
  type I 348.4
  type II 741.0 ☑
  type III 742.0
  type IV 742.2
Arrillaga-Ayerza (pulmonary artery sclerosis with pulmonary hypertension) 416.0
arteriomesenteric duodenum occlusion 537.89
arteriovenous steal 996.73
arteritis, young female (obliterative brachiocephalic) 446.7
aseptic meningitis — *see* Meningitis, aseptic
Asherman's 621.5
Asperger's 299.8 ☑
asphyctic (*see also* Anxiety) 300.00
aspiration, of newborn (massive) 770.18
  meconium 770.12
ataxia-telangiectasia 334.8
Audry's (acropachyderma) 757.39
auriculotemporal 350.8
autoimmune lymphoproliferative (ALPS) 279.41
autosomal (*see also* Abnormal, autosomes NEC)
  deletion 758.39
    5p 758.31
    22q11.2 758.32
Avellis' 344.89
Axenfeld's 743.44
Ayerza (-Arrillaga) (pulmonary artery sclerosis with pulmonary hypertension) 416.0
Baader's (erythema multiforme exudativum) 695.19
Baastrup's 721.5
Babinski-Fröhlich (adiposogenital dystrophy) 253.8
Babinski-Nageotte 344.89
Babinski (-Vaquez) (cardiovascular syphilis) 093.89
Bagratuni's (temporal arteritis) 446.5
Bakwin-Krida (craniometaphyseal dysplasia) 756.89
Balint's (psychic paralysis of visual disorientation) 368.16
Ballantyne (-Runge) (postmaturity) 766.22
ballooning posterior leaflet 424.0
Banti's — *see* Cirrhosis, liver
Bard-Pic's (carcinoma, head of pancreas) 157.0
Bardet-Biedl (obesity, polydactyly, and intellectual disabilities) 759.89
Barlow's (mitral valve prolapse) 424.0
Barlow (-Möller) (infantile scurvy) 267
Baron Munchausen's 301.51
Barré-Guillain 357.0
Barré-Liéou (posterior cervical sympathetic) 723.2
Barrett's (chronic peptic ulcer of esophagus) 530.85
Bársony-Polgár (corkscrew esophagus) 530.5
Bársony-Teschendorf (corkscrew esophagus) 530.5
Barth 759.89
Bartter's (secondary hyperaldosteronism with juxtaglomerular hyperplasia) 255.13
basal cell nevus 759.89
Basedow's (exophthalmic goiter) 242.0 ☑
basilar artery 435.0
basofrontal 377.04
Bassen-Kornzweig (abetalipoproteinemia) 272.5
Batten-Steinert 359.21
battered
  adult 995.81
  baby or child 995.54
  spouse 995.81

Syndrome — *see also* Disease — *continued*

Baumgarten-Cruveilhier (cirrhosis of liver) 571.5
Beals 759.82
Bearn-Kunkel (-Slater) (lupoid hepatitis) 571.49
Beau's (*see also* Degeneration, myocardial) 429.1
Bechterew-Strümpell-Marie (ankylosing spondylitis) 720.0
Beck's (anterior spinal artery occlusion) 433.8 ☑
Beckwith (-Wiedemann) 759.89
Behçet's 136.1
Bekhterev-Strümpell-Marie (ankylosing spondylitis) 720.0
Benedikt's 344.89
Béquez César (-Steinbrinck-Chédiak-Higashi) (congenital gigantism of peroxidase granules) 288.2
Bernard-Horner (*see also* Neuropathy, peripheral, autonomic) 337.9
Bernard-Sergent (acute adrenocortical insufficiency) 255.41
Bernhardt-Roth 355.1
Bernheim's (*see also* Failure, heart) 428.0
Bertolotti's (sacralization of fifth lumbar vertebra) 756.15
Besnier-Boeck-Schaumann (sarcoidosis) 135
Bianchi's (aphasia-apraxia-alexia syndrome) 784.69
Biedl-Bardet (obesity, polydactyly, and intellectual disabilities) 759.89
Biemond's (obesity, polydactyly, and intellectual disabilities) 759.89
big spleen 289.4
bilateral polycystic ovarian 256.4
Bing-Horton's 339.00
Biörck (-Thorson) (malignant carcinoid) 259.2
Birt-Hogg-Dube 759.89
Blackfan-Diamond (congenital hypoplastic anemia) 284.01
black lung 500
black widow spider bite 989.5
bladder neck (*see also* Incontinence, urine) 788.30
blast (concussion) — *see* Blast, injury
blind loop (postoperative) 579.2
Bloch-Siemens (incontinentia pigmenti) 757.33
Bloch-Sulzberger (incontinentia pigmenti) 757.33
Bloom (-Machacek) (-Torre) 757.39
Blount-Barber (tibia vara) 732.4
blue
  bloater 491.20
    with
      acute bronchitis 491.22
      exacerbation (acute) 491.21
  diaper 270.0
  drum 381.02
  sclera 756.51
  toe 445.02
Boder-Sedgwick (ataxia-telangiectasia) 334.8
Boerhaave's (spontaneous esophageal rupture) 530.4
Bonnevie-Ullrich 758.6
Bonnier's 386.19
Borjeson-Forssman-Lehmann 759.89
Bouillaud's (rheumatic heart disease) 391.9
Bourneville (-Pringle) (tuberous sclerosis) 759.5
Bouveret (-Hoffmann) (paroxysmal tachycardia) 427.2
brachial plexus 353.0
Brachman-de Lange (Amsterdam dwarf, intellectual disabilities, and brachycephaly) 759.89
bradycardia-tachycardia 427.81
Brailsford-Morquio (dystrophy) (mucopolysaccharidosis IV) 277.5
brain (acute) (chronic) (nonpsychotic) (organic) (with behavioral reaction) (with neurotic reaction) 310.9

Syndrome — *see also* Disease — *continued*

brain — *continued*
  with
    presenile brain disease (*see also* Dementia, presenile) 290.10
    psychosis, psychotic reaction (*see also* Psychosis, organic) 294.9
  chronic alcoholic 291.2
  congenital (*see also* Disability, intellectual) 319
  postcontusional 310.2
  posttraumatic
    nonpsychotic 310.2
    psychotic 293.9
      acute 293.0
      chronic (*see also* Psychosis, organic) 294.8
      subacute 293.1
    psycho-organic (*see also* Syndrome, psycho-organic) 310.9
    psychotic (*see also* Psychosis, organic) 294.9
  senile (*see also* Dementia, senile) 290.0
branchial arch 744.41
Brandt's (acrodermatitis enteropathica) 686.8
Brennemann's 289.2
Briquet's 300.81
Brissaud-Meige (infantile myxedema) 244.9
broad ligament laceration 620.6
Brock's (atelectasis due to enlarged lymph nodes) 518.0
broken heart 429.83
Brown-Séquard 344.89
brown spot 756.59
Brown's tendon sheath 378.61
Brugada 746.89
Brugsch's (acropachyderma) 757.39
bubbly lung 770.7
Buchem's (hyperostosis corticalis) 733.3
Budd-Chiari (hepatic vein thrombosis) 453.0
Büdinger-Ludloff-Läwen 717.89
bulbar 335.22
  lateral (*see also* Disease, cerebrovascular, acute) 436
Bullis fever 082.8
bundle of Kent (anomalous atrioventricular excitation) 426.7
Bürger-Grütz (essential familial hyperlipemia) 272.3
Burke's (pancreatic insufficiency and chronic neutropenia) 577.8
Burnett's (milk-alkali) 275.42
Burnier's (hypophyseal dwarfism) 253.3
burning feet 266.2
Bywaters' 958.5
Caffey's (infantile cortical hyperostosis) 756.59
Calvé-Legg-Perthes (osteochondrosis, femoral capital) 732.1
Caplan (-Colinet) syndrome 714.81
capsular thrombosis (*see also* Thrombosis, brain) 434.0 ☑
carbohydrate-deficient glycoprotein (CDGS) 271.8
carcinogenic thrombophlebitis 453.1
carcinoid 259.2
cardiac asthma (*see also* Failure, ventricular, left) 428.1
cardiacos negros 416.0
cardiofaciocutaneous 759.89
cardiopulmonary obesity 278.03
cardiorenal (*see also* Hypertension, cardiorenal) 404.90
cardiorespiratory distress (idiopathic), newborn 769
cardiovascular renal (*see also* Hypertension, cardiorenal) 404.90
cardiovasorenal 272.7
Carini's (ichthyosis congenita) 757.1
carotid
  artery (internal) 435.8
  body or sinus 337.01
carpal tunnel 354.0
Carpenter's 759.89

Syndrome — *see also* Disease — *continued*

Cassidy (-Scholte) (malignant carcinoid) 259.2
cat-cry 758.31
cauda equina 344.60
causalgia 355.9
  lower limb 355.71
  upper limb 354.4
cavernous sinus 437.6
celiac 579.0
  artery compression 447.4
  axis 447.4
central pain 338.0
cerebellomedullary malformation (*see also* Spina bifida) 741.0 ☑
cerebral gigantism 253.0
cerebrohepatorenal 759.89
cervical (root) (spine) NEC 723.8
  disc 722.71
  posterior, sympathetic 723.2
  rib 353.0
  sympathetic paralysis 337.09
  traumatic (acute) NEC 847.0
cervicobrachial (diffuse) 723.3
cervicocranial 723.2
cervicodorsal outlet 353.2
Céstan-Chenais 344.89
Céstan's 344.89
Céstan (-Raymond) 433.8 ☑
chancriform 114.1
Charcôt-Marie-Tooth 356.1
Charcôt-Weiss-Baker 337.01
Charcôt's (intermittent claudication) 443.9
  angina cruris 443.9
  due to atherosclerosis 440.21
CHARGE association 759.89
Cheadle (-Möller) (-Barlow) (infantile scurvy) 267
Chédiak-Higashi (-Steinbrinck) (congenital gigantism of peroxidase granules) 288.2
chest wall 786.52
Chiari-Frommel 676.6 ☑
Chiari's (hepatic vein thrombosis) 453.0
chiasmatic 368.41
Chilaiditi's (subphrenic displacement, colon) 751.4
chondroectodermal dysplasia 756.55
chorea-athetosis-agitans 275.1
Christian's (chronic histiocytosis X) 277.89
chromosome 4 short arm deletion 758.39
chronic pain 338.4
Churg-Strauss 446.4
Clarke-Hadfield (pancreatic infantilism) 577.8
Claude's 352.6
Claude Bernard-Horner (*see also* Neuropathy, peripheral, autonomic) 337.9
Clérambault's
  automatism 348.89
  erotomania 297.8
Clifford's (postmaturity) 766.22
climacteric 627.2
Clouston's (hidrotic ectodermal dysplasia) 757.31
clumsiness 315.4
Cockayne-Weber (epidermolysis bullosa) 757.39
Cockayne's (microencephaly and dwarfism) 759.89
Coffin-Lowry 759.89
Cogan's (nonsyphilitic interstitial keratitis) 370.52
cold injury (newborn) 778.2
Collet (-Sicard) 352.6
combined immunity deficiency 279.2
compartment(al) (anterior) (deep) (posterior) 958.8
  nontraumatic
    abdomen 729.73
    arm 729.71
    buttock 729.72
    fingers 729.71
    foot 729.72
    forearm 729.71
    hand 729.71

☑ **Additional Digit Required** — Refer to the Tabular List for Digit Selection   ▽ **Subterms under main terms may continue to next column or page**

2014 ICD-9-CM   ▶◄ **Revised Text**   ● **New Line**   ▲ **Revised Code**   **Volume 2 — 269**

Syndrome — *see also* Disease — *continued*
compartment — *continued*
 nontraumatic — *continued*
  hip 729.72
  leg 729.72
  lower extremity 729.72
  shoulder 729.71
  specified site NEC 729.79
  thigh 729.72
  toes 729.72
  upper extremity 729.71
  wrist 729.71
 post-surgical (*see also* Syndrome, compartment, non-traumatic) 998.89
 traumatic 958.90
  adomen 958.93
  arm 958.91
  buttock 958.92
  fingers 958.91
  foot 958.92
  forearm 958.91
  hand 958.91
  hip 958.92
  leg 958.92
  lower extremity 958.92
  shoulder 958.91
  specified site NEC 958.99
  thigh 958.92
  tibial 958.92
  toes 958.92
  upper extremity 958.91
  wrist 958.91
 complex regional pain — *see also* Dystrophy, sympathetic
  type I — *see* Dystrophy, sympathetic (posttraumatic) (reflex)
  type II — *see* Causalgia
 compression 958.5
  cauda equina 344.60
   with neurogenic bladder 344.61
 concussion 310.2
 congenital
  affecting more than one system 759.7
   specified type NEC 759.89
  congenital central alveolar hypoventilation 327.25
  facial diplegia 352.6
  muscular hypertrophy-cerebral 759.89
 congestion-fibrosis (pelvic) 625.5
 conjunctivourethrosynovial 099.3
 Conn (-Louis) (primary aldosteronism) 255.12
 Conradi (-Hünermann) (chondrodysplasia calcificans congenita) 756.59
 conus medullaris 336.8
 Cooke-Apert-Gallais (adrenogenital) 255.2
 Cornelia de Lange's (Amsterdam dwarf, intellectual disabilities, and brachycephaly) 759.8
 coronary insufficiency or intermediate 411.1
 cor pulmonale 416.9
 corticosexual 255.2
 Costen's (complex) 524.60
 costochondral junction 733.6
 costoclavicular 353.0
 costovertebral 253.0
 Cotard's (paranoia) 297.1
 Cowden 759.6
 craniovertebral 723.2
 Creutzfeldt-Jakob 046.19
  with dementia
   with behavioral disturbance 046.19 [294.11]
   without behavioral disturbance 046.19 [294.10]
  variant 046.11
   with dementia
    with behavioral disturbance 046.11 [294.11]
    without behavioral disturbance 046.11 [294.10]
 cri-du-chat 758.31
 crib death 798.0
 cricopharyngeal 787.20
 Crigler-Najjar (congenital hyperbilirubinemia) 277.4

Syndrome — *see also* Disease — *continued*
crocodile tears 351.8
Cronkhite-Canada 211.3
croup 464.4
CRST (cutaneous systemic sclerosis) 710.1
crush 958.5
crushed lung (*see also* Injury, internal, lung) 861.20
Cruveilhier-Baumgarten (cirrhosis of liver) 571.5
cubital tunnel 354.2
Cuiffini-Pancoast (M8010/3) (carcinoma, pulmonary apex) 162.3
Curschmann (-Batten) (-Steinert) 359.21
Cushing's (iatrogenic) (idiopathic) (pituitary basophilism) (pituitary-dependent) 255.0
 overdose or wrong substance given or taken 962.0
Cyriax's (slipping rib) 733.99
cystic duct stump 576.0
Da Costa's (neurocirculatory asthenia) 306.2
Dameshek's (erythroblastic anemia) 282.49
Dana-Putnam (subacute combined sclerosis with pernicious anemia) 281.0 [336.2]
Danbolt (-Closs) (acrodermatitis enteropathica) 686.8
Dandy-Walker (atresia, foramen of Magendie) 742.3
 with spina bifida (*see also* Spina bifida) 741.0 ☑
Danlos' 756.83
Davies-Colley (slipping rib) 733.99
dead fetus 641.3 ☑
defeminization 255.2
defibrination (*see also* Fibrinolysis) 286.6
Degos' 447.8
Deiters' nucleus 386.19
Déjérine-Roussy 338.0
Déjérine-Thomas 333.0
de Lange's (Amsterdam dwarf, intellectual disabilities, and brachycephaly) (Cornelia) 759.89
Del Castillo's (germinal aplasia) 606.0
deletion chromosomes 758.39
delusional
 induced by drug 292.11
dementia-aphonia, of childhood (*see also* Psychosis, childhood) 299.1 ☑
demyelinating NEC 341.9
denial visual hallucination 307.9
depersonalization 300.6
de Quervain's 259.51
Dercum's (adiposis dolorosa) 272.8
de Toni-Fanconi (-Debré) (cystinosis) 270.0
diabetes-dwarfism-obesity (juvenile) 258.1
diabetes-nephrosis 250.4 ☑ [581.81]
 due to secondary diabetes 249.4 ☑ [581.81]
diabetes mellitus-hypertension-nephrosis 250.4 ☑ [581.81]
 due to secondary diabetes 249.4 ☑ [581.81]
diabetes mellitus in newborn infant 775.1
diabetic amyotrophy 250.6 ☑ [353.5]
 due to secondary diabetes 249.6 ☑ [353.5]
Diamond-Blackfan (congenital hypoplastic anemia) 284.01
Diamond-Gardener (autoerythrocyte sensitization) 287.2
DIC (diffuse or disseminated intravascular coagulopathy) (*see also* Fibrinolysis) 286.6
diencephalohypophyseal NEC 253.8
diffuse cervicobrachial 723.3
diffuse obstructive pulmonary 496
DiGeorge's (thymic hypoplasia) 279.11
Dighton's 756.51
Di Guglielmo's (erythremic myelosis) (M9841/3) 207.0 ☑
disequilibrium 276.9
disseminated platelet thrombosis 446.6
Ditthomska 307.81
Doan-Wiseman (primary splenic neutropenia) 289.53

Syndrome — *see also* Disease — *continued*
Döhle body-panmyelopathic 288.2
Donohue's (leprechaunism) 259.8
dorsolateral medullary (*see also* Disease, cerebrovascular, acute) 436
double athetosis 333.71
double whammy 360.81
Down's (mongolism) 758.0
Dresbach's (elliptocytosis) 282.1
Dressler's (postmyocardial infarction) 411.0
 hemoglobinuria 283.2
 postcardiotomy 429.4
drug withdrawal, infant, of dependent mother 779.5
dry skin 701.1
 eye 375.15
DSAP (disseminated superficial actinic porokeratosis) 692.75
Duane-Stilling-Türk (ocular retraction syndrome) 378.71
Duane's (retraction) 378.71
Dubin-Johnson (constitutional hyperbilirubinemia) 277.4
Dubin-Sprinz (constitutional hyperbilirubinemia) 277.4
Duchenne's 335.22
due to abnormality
 autosomal NEC (*see also* Abnormal, autosomes NEC) 758.5
  13 758.1
  18 758.2
  21 or 22 758.0
  D1 758.1
  E3 758.2
  G 758.0
 chromosomal 758.89
 sex 758.81
dumping 564.2
 nonsurgical 536.8
Duplay's 726.2
Dupré's (meningism) 781.6
Dyke-Young (acquired macrocytic hemolytic anemia) 283.9
dyspraxia 315.4
dystocia, dystrophia 654.9 ☑
Eagle-Barret 756.71
Eales' 362.18
Eaton-Lambert (*see also* Syndrome, Lambert-Eaton) 358.30
Ebstein's (downward displacement, tricuspid valve into right ventricle) 746.2
ectopic ACTH secretion 255.0
eczema-thrombocytopenia 279.12
Eddowes' (brittle bones and blue sclera) 756.51
Edwards' 758.2
efferent loop 537.89
effort (aviators') (psychogenic) 306.2
Ehlers-Danlos 756.83
Eisenmenger's (ventricular septal defect) 745.4
Ekbom's (restless legs) 333.94
Ekman's (brittle bones and blue sclera) 756.51
electric feet 266.2
Elephant man 237.71
Ellis-van Creveld (chondroectodermal dysplasia) 756.55
Ellison-Zollinger (gastric hypersecretion with pancreatic islet cell tumor) 251.5
embryonic fixation 270.2
empty sella (turcica) 253.8
endocrine-hypertensive 255.3
Engel-von Recklinghausen (osteitis fibrosa cystica) 252.01
enteroarticular 099.3
entrapment — *see* Neuropathy, entrapment
eosinophilia myalgia 710.5
epidemic vomiting 078.82
Epstein's — *see* Nephrosis
Erb (-Oppenheim)-Goldflam 358.00
Erdheim-Chester 277.89
Erdheim's (acromegalic macrospondylitis) 253.0
Erlacher-Blount (tibia vara) 732.4
erythrocyte fragmentation 283.19

Syndrome — *see also* Disease — *continued*
euthyroid sick 790.94
Evans' (thrombocytopenic purpura) 287.32
excess cortisol, iatrogenic 255.0
exhaustion 300.5
extrapyramidal 333.90
eyelid-malar-mandible 756.0
eye retraction 378.71
Faber's (achlorhydric anemia) 280.9
Fabry (-Anderson) (angiokeratoma corporis diffusum) 272.7
facet 724.8
Fallot's 745.2
falx (*see also* Hemorrhage, brain) 431
familial eczema-thrombocytopenia 279.12
Fanconi (-de Toni) (-Debré) (cystinosis) 270.0
Fanconi's (anemia) (congenital pancytopenia) 284.09
Farber (-Uzman) (disseminated lipogranulomatosis) 272.8
fatigue NEC 300.5
 chronic 780.71
faulty bowel habit (idiopathic megacolon) 564.7
FDH (focal dermal hypoplasia) 757.39
fecal reservoir 560.39
Feil-Klippel (brevicollis) 756.16
Felty's (rheumatoid arthritis with splenomegaly and leukopenia) 714.1
fertile eunuch 257.2
fetal alcohol 760.71
 late effect 760.71
fibrillation-flutter 427.32
fibrositis (periarticular) 729.0
Fiedler's (acute isolated myocarditis) 422.91
Fiessinger-Leroy (-Reiter) 099.3
Fiessinger-Rendu (erythema multiforme exudativum) 695.19
first arch 756.0
Fisher's 357.0
fish odor 270.8
Fitz-Hugh and Curtis 098.86
 due to
  Chlamydia trachomatis 099.56
  Neisseria gonorrhoeae (gonococcal peritonitis) 098.86
Fitz's (acute hemorrhagic pancreatitis) 577.0
Flajani (-Basedow) (exophthalmic goiter) 242.0 ☑
flat back
 acquired 737.29
 postprocedural 738.5
floppy
 infant 781.99
 iris 364.81
 valve (mitral) 424.0
flush 259.2
Foix-Alajouanine 336.1
Fong's (hereditary osteo-onychodysplasia) 756.89
foramen magnum 348.4
Forbes-Albright (nonpuerperal amenorrhea and lactation associated with pituitary tumor) 253.1
Foster-Kennedy 377.04
Foville's (peduncular) 344.89
fragile X 759.83
Franceschetti's (mandibulofacial dysostosis) 756.0
Fraser's 759.89
Freeman-Sheldon 759.89
Frey's (auriculotemporal) 705.22
Friderichsen-Waterhouse 036.3
Friedrich-Erb-Arnold (acropachyderma) 757.39
Fröhlich's (adiposogenital dystrophy) 253.8
Froin's 336.8
Frommel-Chiari 676.6 ☑
frontal lobe 310.0
Fukuhara 277.87
Fuller Albright's (osteitis fibrosa disseminata) 756.59
functional
 bowel 564.9
 prepubertal castrate 752.89

Syndrome — *see also* Disease — *continued*

Gaisböck's (polycythemia hypertonica) 289.0

ganglion (basal, brain) 333.90

geniculi 351.1

Ganser's, hysterical 300.16

Gardner-Diamond (autoerythrocyte sensitization) 287.2

gastroesophageal junction 530.0

gastroesophageal laceration-hemorrhage 530.7

gastrojejunal loop obstruction 537.89

Gayet-Wernicke's (superior hemorrhagic polioencephalitis) 265.1

Gee-Herter-Heubner (nontropical sprue) 579.0

Gélineau's (*see also* Narcolepsy) 347.00

genito-anorectal 099.1

Gerhardt's (vocal cord paralysis) 478.30

Gerstmann-Sträussler-Scheinker (GSS) 046.71

Gerstmann's (finger agnosia) 784.69

Gianotti Crosti 057.8

due to known virus — *see* Infection, virus

due to unknown virus 057.8

Gilbert's 277.4

Gilford (-Hutchinson) (progeria) 259.8

Gilles de la Tourette's 307.23

Gillespie's (dysplasia oculodentodigitalis) 759.89

Glénard's (enteroptosis) 569.89

Glinski-Simmonds (pituitary cachexia) 253.2

glucuronyl transferase 277.4

glue ear 381.20

Goldberg (-Maxwell) (-Morris) (testicular feminization) 259.51

Goldenhar's (oculoauriculovertebral dysplasia) 756.0

Goldflam-Erb 358.00

Goltz-Gorlin (dermal hypoplasia) 757.39

Good's 279.06

Goodpasture's (pneumorenal) 446.21

Gopalan's (burning feet) 266.2

Gorlin-Chaudhry-Moss 759.89

Gorlin's 759.89

Gougerot-Blum (pigmented purpuric lichenoid dermatitis) 709.1

Gougerot-Carteaud (confluent reticulate papillomatosis) 701.8

Gougerot (-Houwer)-Sjögren (keratoconjunctivitis sicca) 710.2

Gouley's (constrictive pericarditis) 423.2

Gowers-Paton-Kennedy 377.04

Gowers' (vasovagal attack) 780.2

Gradenigo's 383.02

gray or grey (chloramphenicol) (newborn) 779.4

Greig's (hypertelorism) 756.0

GSS (Gerstmann-Sträussler-Scheinker) 046.71

Gubler-Millard 344.89

Guérin-Stern (arthrogryposis multiplex congenita) 754.89

Guillain-Barré (-Strohl) 357.0

Gunn's (jaw-winking syndrome) 742.8

Günther's (congenital erythropoietic porphyria) 277.1

gustatory sweating 350.8

H₃O 759.81

Hadfield-Clarke (pancreatic infantilism) 577.8

Haglund-Läwen-Fründ 717.89

hairless women 257.8

hair tourniquet (*see also* Injury, superficial, by site)

finger 915.8

infected 915.9

penis 911.8

infected 911.9

toe 917.8

infected 917.9

Hallermann-Streiff 756.0

Hallervorden-Spatz 333.0

Hamman-Rich (diffuse interstitial pulmonary fibrosis) 516.33

Syndrome — *see also* Disease — *continued*

Hamman's (spontaneous mediastinal emphysema) 518.1

hand-foot 693.0

Hand-Schüller-Christian (chronic histiocytosis X) 277.89

Hanot-Chauffard (-Troisier) (bronze diabetes) 275.01

Harada's 363.22

Hare's (M8010/3) (carcinoma, pulmonary apex) 162.3

Harkavy's 446.0

harlequin color change 779.89

Harris' (organic hyperinsulinism) 251.1

Hart's (pellagra-cerebellar ataxia-renal aminoaciduria) 270.0

Hayem-Faber (achlorhydric anemia) 280.9

Hayem-Widal (acquired hemolytic jaundice) 283.9

headache — *see* Headache, syndrome

Heberden's (angina pectoris) 413.9

Hedinger's (malignant carcinoid) 259.2

Hegglin's 288.2

Heller's (infantile psychosis) (*see also* Psychosis, childhood) 299.1 ☑

H.E.L.L.P 642.5 ☑

hemolytic-uremic (adult) (child) 283.11

hemophagocytic 288.4

infection-associated 288.4

Henoch-Schönlein (allergic purpura) 287.0

hepatic flexure 569.89

hepatopulmonary 573.5

hepatorenal 572.4

due to a procedure 997.49

following delivery 674.8 ☑

hepatourologic 572.4

Herrick's (hemoglobin S disease) 282.61

Herter (-Gee) (nontropical sprue) 579.0

Heubner-Herter (nontropical sprue) 579.0

Heyd's (hepatorenal) 572.4

HHHO 759.81

high grade myelodysplastic 238.73

with 5q deletion 238.73

Hilger's 337.09

histiocytic 288.4

Hoffa (-Kastert) (liposynovitis prepatellaris) 272.8

Hoffmann-Bouveret (paroxysmal tachycardia) 427.2

Hoffmann-Werdnig 335.0

Hoffmann's 244.9 [359.5]

Holländer-Simons (progressive lipodystrophy) 272.6

Holmes-Adie 379.46

Holmes' (visual disorientation) 368.16

Hoppe-Goldflam 358.00

Horner's (*see also* Neuropathy, peripheral, autonomic) 337.9

traumatic — *see* Injury, nerve, cervical sympathetic

hospital addiction 301.51

hungry bone 275.5

Hunt's (herpetic geniculate ganglionitis) 053.11

dyssynergia cerebellaris myoclonica 334.2

Hunter (-Hurler) (mucopolysaccharidosis II) 277.5

hunterian glossitis 529.4

Hurler (-Hunter) (mucopolysaccharidosis II) 277.5

Hutchinson-Boeck (sarcoidosis) 135

Hutchinson-Gilford (progeria) 259.8

Hutchinson's incisors or teeth 090.5

hydralazine

correct substance properly administered 695.4

overdose or wrong substance given or taken 972.6

hydraulic concussion (abdomen) (*see also* Injury, internal, abdomen) 868.00

hyperabduction 447.8

hyperactive bowel 564.9

Syndrome — *see also* Disease — *continued*

hyperaldosteronism with hypokalemic alkalosis (Bartter's) 255.13

hypercalcemic 275.42

hypercoagulation NEC 289.89

hypereosinophilic (idiopathic) 288.3

hyperkalemic 276.7

hyperkinetic (*see also* Hyperkinesia)

heart 429.82

hyperlipemia-hemolytic anemia-icterus 571.1

hypermobility 728.5

hypernatremia 276.0

hyperosmolarity 276.0

hyperperfusion 997.01

hypersomnia-bulimia 349.89

hypersplenic 289.4

hypersympathetic (*see also* Neuropathy, peripheral, autonomic) 337.9

hypertransfusion, newborn 776.4

hyperventilation, psychogenic 306.1

hyperviscosity (of serum) NEC 273.3

polycythemic 289.0

sclerothymic 282.8

hypoglycemic (familial) (neonatal) 251.2

functional 251.1

hypokalemic 276.8

hypophyseal 253.8

hypophyseothalamic 253.8

hypopituitarism 253.2

hypoplastic left heart 746.7

hypopotassemia 276.8

hyposmolality 276.1

hypotension, maternal 669.2 ☑

hypothenar hammer 443.89

hypotonia-hypomentia-hypogonadism-obesity 759.81

ICF (intravascular coagulation-fibrinolysis) (*see also* Fibrinolysis) 286.6

idiopathic cardiorespiratory distress, newborn 769

idiopathic nephrotic (infantile) 581.9

iliotibial band 728.89

Imerslund (-Gräsbeck) (anemia due to familial selective vitamin B₁₂ malabsorption) 281.1

immobility (paraplegic) 728.3

immune reconstitution inflammatory (IRIS) 995.90

immunity deficiency, combined 279.2

impending coronary 411.1

impingement

shoulder 726.2

vertebral bodies 724.4

inappropriate secretion of antidiuretic hormone (ADH) 253.6

incomplete

mandibulofacial 756.0

infant

death, sudden (SIDS) 798.0

Hercules 255.2

of diabetic mother 775.0

shaken 995.55

infantilism 253.3

inferior vena cava 459.2

influenza-like (*see also* Influenza) 487.1

inspissated bile, newborn 774.4

insufficient sleep 307.44

intermediate coronary (artery) 411.1

internal carotid artery (*see also* Occlusion, artery, carotid) 433.1 ☑

interspinous ligament 724.8

intestinal

carcinoid 259.2

gas 787.3

knot 560.2

intraoperative floppy iris (IFIS) 364.81

intravascular

coagulation-fibrinolysis (ICF) (*see also* Fibrinolysis) 286.6

coagulopathy (*see also* Fibrinolysis) 286.6

inverted Marfan's 759.89

IRDS (idiopathic respiratory distress, newborn) 769

irritable

bowel 564.1

Syndrome — *see also* Disease — *continued*

irritable — *continued*

heart 306.2

weakness 300.5

ischemic bowel (transient) 557.9

chronic 557.1

due to mesenteric artery insufficiency 557.1

Itsenko-Cushing (pituitary basophilism) 255.0

IVC (intravascular coagulopathy) (*see also* Fibrinolysis) 286.6

Ivemark's (asplenia with congenital heart disease) 759.0

Jaccoud's 714.4

Jackson's 344.89

Jadassohn-Lewandowski (pachyonychia congenita) 757.5

Jaffe-Lichtenstein (-Uehlinger) 252.01

Jahnke's (encephalocutaneous angiomatosis) 759.6

Jakob-Creutzfeldt 046.19

with dementia

with behavioral disturbance 046.19 [294.11]

without behavioral disturbance 046.19 [294.10]

variant 046.11

with dementia

with behavioral disturbance 046.11 [294.11]

without behavioral disturbance 046.11 [294.10]

Jaksch-Hayem (-Luzet) (pseudoleukemia infantum) 285.8

Jaksch's (pseudoleukemia infantum) 285.8

jaw-winking 742.8

jejunal 564.2

Jervell-Lange-Nielsen 426.82

jet lag 327.35

Jeune's (asphyxiating thoracic dystrophy of newborn) 756.4

Job's (chronic granulomatous disease) 288.1

Jordan's 288.2

Joseph-Diamond-Blackfan (congenital hypoplastic anemia) 284.01

Joubert 759.89

jugular foramen 352.6

Kabuki 759.89

Kahler's (multiple myeloma) (M9730/3) 203.0 ☑

Kalischer's (encephalocutaneous angiomatosis) 759.6

Kallmann's (hypogonadotropic hypogonadism with anosmia) 253.4

Kanner's (autism) (*see also* Psychosis, childhood) 299.0 ☑

Kartagener's (sinusitis, bronchiectasis, situs inversus) 759.3

Kasabach-Merritt (capillary hemangioma associated with thrombocytopenic purpura) 287.39

Kast's (dyschondroplasia with hemangiomas) 756.4

Kaznelson's (congenital hypoplastic anemia) 284.01

Kearns-Sayre 277.87

Kelly's (sideropenic dysphagia) 280.8

Kimmelstiel-Wilson (intercapillary glomerulosclerosis) 250.4 ☑ [581.81]

due to secondary diabetes 249.4 ☑ [581.81]

Klauder's (erythema multiforme exudativum) 695.19

Klein-Waardenburg (ptosis-epicanthus) 270.2

Kleine-Levin 327.13

Klinefelter's 758.7

Klippel-Feil (brevicollis) 756.16

Klippel-Trenaunay 759.89

Klumpke (-Déjérine) (injury to brachial plexus at birth) 767.6

Klüver-Bucy (-Terzian) 310.0

Köhler-Pellegrini-Stieda (calcification, knee joint) 726.62

König's 564.89

☑ **Additional Digit Required** — Refer to the Tabular List for Digit Selection ▽ **Subterms under main terms may continue to next column or page**

2014 ICD-9-CM ▶◀ **Revised Text** ● **New Line** ▲ **Revised Code** **Volume 2 — 271**

Syndrome — Syndrome

Syndrome — see also Disease — continued

Korsakoff's (nonalcoholic) 294.0
Korsakoff (-Wernicke) (nonalcoholic) 294.0
  alcoholic 291.1
  alcoholic 291.1
Kostmann's (infantile genetic agranulocytosis) 288.01
Krabbe's
  congenital muscle hypoplasia 756.89
  cutaneocerebral angioma 759.6
Kunkel (lupoid hepatitis) 571.49
labyrinthine 386.50
laceration, broad ligament 620.6
Lambert-Eaton 358.30
  in
    diseases classified elsewhere 358.39
    neoplastic disease 358.31
Landau-Kieffner 345.8 ☑
Langdon Down (mongolism) 758.0
Larsen's (flattened facies and multiple congenital dislocations) 755.8
lateral
  cutaneous nerve of thigh 355.1
  medullary (see also Disease, cerebrovascular acute) 436
Launois-Cléret (adiposogenital dystrophy) 253.8
Launois' (pituitary gigantism) 253.0
Laurence-Moon (-Bardet)-Biedl (obesity, polydactyly, and intellectual disabilities) 759.89
Lawford's (encephalocutaneous angiomatosis) 759.6
lazy
  leukocyte 288.09
  posture 728.3
Lederer-Brill (acquired infectious hemolytic anemia) 283.19
Legg-Calvé-Perthes (osteochondrosis capital femoral) 732.1
Lemiere 451.89
Lennox-Gastaut syndrome 345.0 ☑
  with tonic seizures 345.1 ☑
Lennox's (see also Epilepsy) 345.0 ☑
lenticular 275.1
Léopold-Lévi's (paroxysmal thyroid instability) 242.9 ☑
Lepore hemoglobin 282.45
Léri-Weill 756.59
Leriche's (aortic bifurcation occlusion) 444.09
Lermoyez's (see also Disease, Ménière's) 386.00
Lesch-Nyhan (hypoxanthine-guanine-phosphoribosyltransferase deficiency) 277.2
leukoencephalopathy, reversible, posterior 348.5
Lev's (acquired complete heart block) 426.0
Levi's (pituitary dwarfism) 253.3
Lévy-Roussy 334.3
Li-Fraumeni V84.01
Lichtheim's (subacute combined sclerosis with pernicious anemia) 281.0 [336.2]
Lightwood's (renal tubular acidosis) 588.89
Lignac (-de Toni) (-Fanconi) (-Debré) (cystinosis) 270.0
Likoff's (angina in menopausal women) 413.9
liver-kidney 572.4
Lloyd's 258.1
lobotomy 310.0
Löffler's (eosinophilic pneumonitis) 518.3
Löfgren's (sarcoidosis) 135
long arm 18 or 21 deletion 758.39
Looser (-Debray)-Milkman (osteomalacia with pseudofractures) 268.2
Lorain-Levi (pituitary dwarfism) 253.3
Louis-Bar (ataxia-telangiectasia) 334.8
low
  atmospheric pressure 993.2
  back 724.2
    psychogenic 306.0
  output (cardiac) (see also Failure, heart) 428.9

Syndrome — see also Disease — continued

Lowe-Terrey-MacLachlan (oculocerebrorenal dystrophy) 270.8
Lowe's (oculocerebrorenal dystrophy) 270.8
lower radicular, newborn 767.4
Lown (-Ganong)-Levine (short P-R interval, normal QRS complex, and supraventricular tachycardia) 426.81
Lucey-Driscoll (jaundice due to delayed conjugation) 774.30
Luetscher's (dehydration) 276.51
lumbar vertebral 724.4
Lutembacher's (atrial septal defect with mitral stenosis) 745.5
Lyell's (toxic epidermal necrolysis) 695.15
  due to drug
    correct substance properly administered 695.15
    overdose or wrong substance given or taken 977.9
    specified drug — see Table of Drugs and Chemicals
MacLeod's 492.8
macrogenitosomia praecox 259.8
macroglobulinemia 273.3
macrophage activation 288.4
Maffucci's (dyschondroplasia with hemangiomas) 756.4
Magenblase 306.4
magnesium-deficiency 781.7
malabsorption 579.9
  postsurgical 579.3
  spinal fluid 331.3
Mal de Debarquement 780.4
malignant carcinoid 259.2
Mallory-Weiss 530.7
mandibulofacial dysostosis 756.0
manic-depressive (see also Psychosis, affective) 296.80
Mankowsky's (familial dysplastic osteopathy) 731.2
maple syrup (urine) 270.3
Marable's (celiac artery compression) 447.4
Marchesani (-Weill) (brachymorphism and ectopia lentis) 759.89
Marchiafava-Bignami 341.8
Marchiafava-Micheli (paroxysmal nocturnal hemoglobinuria) 283.2
Marcus Gunn's (jaw-winking syndrome) 742.8
Marfan's (arachnodactyly) 759.82
  meaning congenital syphilis 090.49
    with luxation of lens 090.49 [379.32]
Marie's (acromegaly) 253.0
  primary or idiopathic (acropachyderma) 757.39
  secondary (hypertrophic pulmonary osteoarthropathy) 731.2
Markus-Adie 379.46
Maroteaux-Lamy (mucopolysaccharidosis VI) 277.5
Martin-Albright (pseudohypoparathyroidism) 275.49
Martin's 715.27
Martorell-Fabré (pulseless disease) 446.7
massive aspiration of newborn 770.18
Masters-Allen 620.6
mastocytosis 757.33
maternal hypotension 669.2 ☑
maternal obesity 646.1 ☑
May (-Hegglin) 288.2
McArdle (-Schmid) (-Pearson) (glycogenosis V) 271.0
McCune-Albright (osteitis fibrosa disseminata) 756.59
McQuarrie's (idiopathic familial hypoglycemia) 251.2
meconium
  aspiration 770.12
  plug (newborn) NEC 777.1
median arcuate ligament 447.4
mediastinal fibrosis 519.3
Meekeren-Ehlers-Danlos 756.83
Meige (blepharospasm-oromandibular dystonia) 333.82
  -Milroy (chronic hereditary edema) 757.0

Syndrome — see also Disease — continued

MELAS (mitochondrial encephalopathy, lactic acidosis and stroke-like episodes) 277.87
Melkersson (-Rosenthal) 351.8
MEN (multiple endocrine neoplasia)
  type I 258.01
  type IIA 258.02
  type IIB 258.03
Mende's (ptosis-epicanthus) 270.2
Mendelson's (resulting from a procedure) 997.32
  during labor 668.0 ☑
  obstetric 668.0 ☑
Ménétrier's (hypertrophic gastritis) 535.2 ☑
Ménière's (see also Disease, Ménière's) 386.00
meningo-eruptive 047.1
Menkes' 759.89
  glutamic acid 759.89
  maple syrup (urine) disease 270.3
menopause 627.2
  postartificial 627.4
menstruation 625.4
MERRF (myoclonus with epilepsy and with ragged red fibers) 277.87
mesenteric
  artery, superior 557.1
  vascular insufficiency (with gangrene) 557.1
metabolic 277.7
metastatic carcinoid 259.2
Meyenburg-Altherr-Uehlinger 733.99
Meyer-Schwickerath and Weyers (dysplasia oculodentodigitalis) 759.89
Micheli-Rietti (thalassemia minor) 282.46
Michotte's 721.5
micrognathia-glossoptosis 756.0
microphthalmos (congenital) 759.89
midbrain 348.89
middle
  lobe (lung) (right) 518.0
  radicular 353.0
Miescher's
  familial acanthosis nigricans 701.2
  granulomatosis disciformis 709.3
Mieten's 759.89
migraine 346.0 ☑
Mikity-Wilson (pulmonary dysmaturity) 770.7
Mikulicz's (dryness of mouth, absent or decreased lacrimation) 527.1
milk alkali (milk drinkers') 275.42
Milkman (-Looser) (osteomalacia with pseudofractures) 268.2
Millard-Gubler 344.89
Miller-Dieker 758.33
Miller Fisher's 357.0
Milles' (encephalocutaneous angiomatosis) 759.6
Minkowski-Chauffard (see also Spherocytosis) 282.0
Mirizzi's (hepatic duct stenosis) 576.2
  with calculus, cholelithiasis, or stones — see Choledocholithiasis
mitochondrial neurogastrointestinal encephalopathy (MNGIE) 277.87
mitral
  click (-murmur) 785.2
  valve prolapse 424.0
MNGIE (mitochondrial neurogastrointestinal encephalopathy) 277.87
Möbius'
  congenital oculofacial paralysis 352.6
  ophthalmoplegic migraine 346.2 ☑
Mohr's (types I and II) 759.89
monofixation 378.34
Moore's (see also Epilepsy) 345.5 ☑
Morel-Moore (hyperostosis frontalis interna) 733.3
Morel-Morgani (hyperostosis frontalis interna) 733.3
Morgagni-Adams-Stokes (syncope with heart block) 426.9
Morgagni (-Stewart-Morel) (hyperostosis frontalis interna) 733.3

Syndrome — see also Disease — continued

Morquio (-Brailsford) (-Ullrich) (mucopolysaccharidosis IV) 277.5
Morris (testicular feminization) 259.51
Morton's (foot) (metatarsalgia) (metatarsal neuralgia) (neuralgia) (neuroma) (toe) 355.6
Moschcowitz (-Singer-Symmers) (thrombotic thrombocytopenic purpura) 446.6
Mounier-Kuhn 748.3
  with
    acute exacerbation 494.1
    bronchiectasis 494.0
      with (acute) exacerbation 494.1
  acquired 519.19
    with bronchiectasis 494.0
      with (acute) exacerbation 494.1
Mucha-Haberman (acute parapsoriasis varioliformis) 696.2
mucocutaneous lymph node (acute) (febrile) (infantile) (MCLS) 446.1
multiple
  deficiency 260
  endocrine neoplasia (MEN)
    type I 258.01
    type IIA 258.02
    type IIB 258.03
  operations 301.51
Munchausen's 301.51
Münchmeyer's (exostosis luxurians) 728.11
Murchison-Sanderson — see Disease, Hodgkin's
myasthenic — see Myasthenia, syndrome
myelodysplastic 238.75
  with 5q deletion 238.74
  high grade with 5q deletion 238.73
  lesions, low grade 238.72
  therapy-related 289.83
myeloproliferative (chronic) (M9960/1) 238.79
myofascial pain NEC 729.1
Naffziger's 353.0
Nager-de Reynier (dysostosis mandibularis) 756.0
nail-patella (hereditary osteo-onychodysplasia) 756.89
NARP (neuropathy, ataxia and retinitis pigmentosa) 277.87
Nebécourt's 253.3
Neill-Dingwall (microencephaly and dwarfism) 759.89
nephrotic (see also Nephrosis) 581.9
  diabetic 250.4 ☑ [581.81]
    due to secondary diabetes 249.4 ☑ [581.81]
Netherton's (ichthyosiform erythroderma) 757.1
neurocutaneous 759.6
neuroleptic malignant 333.92
Nezelof's (pure alymphocytosis) 279.13
Niemann-Pick (lipid histiocytosis) 272.7
Nonne-Milroy-Meige (chronic hereditary edema) 757.0
nonsense 300.16
Noonan's 759.89
Nothnagel's
  ophthalmoplegia-cerebellar ataxia 378.52
  vasomotor acroparesthesia 443.89
nucleus ambiguous-hypoglossal 352.6
OAV (oculoauriculovertebral dysplasia) 756.0
obesity hypoventilation 278.03
obsessional 300.3
oculocutaneous 364.24
oculomotor 378.81
oculourethroarticular 099.3
Ogilvie's (sympathicotonic colon obstruction) 560.89
ophthalmoplegia-cerebellar ataxia 378.52
Oppenheim-Urbach (necrobiosis lipoidica diabeticorum) 250.8 ☑ [709.3]
  due to secondary diabetes 249.8 ☑ [709.3]
oral-facial-digital 759.89

Syndrome — *see also* Disease — *continued*
- organic
  - affective NEC 293.83
    - drug-induced 292.84
  - anxiety 293.84
  - delusional 293.81
    - alcohol-induced 291.5
    - drug-induced 292.11
    - due to or associated with
      - arteriosclerosis 290.42
        - presenile brain disease 290.12
        - senility 290.20
  - depressive 293.83
    - drug-induced 292.84
    - due to or associated with
      - arteriosclerosis 290.43
        - presenile brain disease 290.13
        - senile brain disease 290.21
  - hallucinosis 293.82
    - drug-induced 292.84
- organic affective 293.83
  - induced by drug 292.84
- organic personality 310.1
  - induced by drug 292.89
- Ormond's 593.4
- orodigitofacial 759.89
- orthostatic hypotensive-dysautonomic dyskinetic 333.0
- Osler-Weber-Rendu (familial hemorrhagic telangiectasia) 448.0
- osteodermopathic hyperostosis 757.39
- osteoporosis-osteomalacia 268.2
- Österreicher-Turner (hereditary osteo-ony-chodysplasia) 756.89
- os trigonum 755.69
- Ostrum-Furst 756.59
- otolith 386.19
- otopalatodigital 759.89
- outlet (thoracic) 353.0
- ovarian remnant 620.8
- Owren's (*see also* Defect, coagulation) 286.3
- OX 758.6
- pacemaker 429.4
- Paget-Schroetter (intermittent venous claudication) 453.89
- pain (*see also* Pain)
  - central 338.0
  - chronic 338.4
  - complex regional 355.9
    - type I 337.20
      - lower limb 337.22
      - specified site NEC 337.29
      - upper limb 337.21
    - type II
      - lower limb 355.71
      - upper limb 354.4
  - myelopathic 338.0
  - thalamic (hyperesthetic) 338.0
- painful
  - apicocostal vertebral (M8010/3) 162.3
  - arc 726.19
  - bruising 287.2
  - feet 266.2
- Pancoast's (carcinoma, pulmonary apex) (M8010/3) 162.3
- panhypopituitary (postpartum) 253.2
- papillary muscle 429.81
  - with myocardial infarction 410.8 ☑
- Papillon-Léage and Psaume (orodigitofacial dysostosis) 759.89
- parabiotic (transfusion)
  - donor (twin) 772.0
  - recipient (twin) 776.4
- paralysis agitans 332.0
- paralytic 344.9
  - specified type NEC 344.89
- paraneoplastic — *see* condition
- Parinaud's (paralysis of conjugate upward gaze) 378.81
  - oculoglandular 372.02
- Parkes Weber and Dimitri (encephalocutaneous angiomatosis) 759.6
- Parkinson's (*see also* Parkinsonism) 332.0
- parkinsonian (*see also* Parkinsonism) 332.0
- Parry-Romberg 349.89
- Parry's (exophthalmic goiter) 242.0 ☑

Syndrome — *see also* Disease — *continued*
- Parsonage-Aldren-Turner 353.5
- Parsonage-Turner 353.5
- Patau's (trisomy D1) 758.1
- patella clunk 719.66
- patellofemoral 719.46
- Paterson (-Brown) (-Kelly) (sideropenic dysphagia) 280.8
- Payr's (splenic flexure syndrome) 569.89
- pectoral girdle 447.8
- pectoralis minor 447.8
- Pelger-Huët (hereditary hyposegmentation) 288.2
- pellagra-cerebellar ataxia-renal aminoaciduria 270.0
- pellagroid 265.2
- Pellegrini-Stieda 726.62
- Pellizzi's (pineal) 259.8
- Pendred's (familial goiter with deaf-mutism) 243
- Penfield's (*see also* Epilepsy) 345.5 ☑
- Penta X 758.81
- peptic ulcer — *see* Ulcer, peptic 533.9 ☑
- perabduction 447.8
- periodic 277.31
- periurethral fibrosis 593.4
- persistent fetal circulation 747.83
- Petges-Cléjat (poikilodermatomyositis) 710.3
- Peutz-Jeghers 759.6
- Pfeiffer (acrocephalosyndactyly) 755.55
- phantom limb 353.6
- pharyngeal pouch 279.11
- Pick-Herxheimer (diffuse idiopathic cutaneous atrophy) 701.8
- Pick's (pericardial pseudocirrhosis of liver) 423.2
  - heart 423.2
  - liver 423.2
- Pickwickian (cardiopulmonary obesity) 278.03
- PIE (pulmonary infiltration with eosinophilia) 518.3
- Pierre Marie-Bamberger (hypertrophic pulmonary osteoarthropathy) 731.2
- Pierre Mauriac's (diabetes-dwarfism-obesity) 258.1
- Pierre Robin 756.0
- pigment dispersion, iris 364.53
- pineal 259.8
- pink puffer 492.8
- pituitary 253.0
- placental
  - dysfunction 762.2
  - insufficiency 762.2
  - transfusion 762.3
- plantar fascia 728.71
- plateau iris (without glaucoma) 364.82
  - with glaucoma 365.23
- plica knee 727.83
- Plummer-Vinson (sideropenic dysphagia) 280.8
- pluricarential of infancy 260
- plurideficiency of infancy 260
- pluriglandular (compensatory) 258.8
- Poland 756.81
- polycarential of infancy 260
- polyglandular 258.8
- polysplenia 759.0
- pontine 433.8 ☑
- popliteal
  - artery entrapment 447.8
  - web 756.89
- post-gastric surgery 564.2
- postartificial menopause 627.4
- postcardiac injury
  - postcardiotomy 429.4
  - postmyocardial infarction 411.0
- postcardiotomy 429.4
- post chemoembolization — code to associated conditions
- postcholecystectomy 576.0
- postcommissurotomy 429.4
- postconcussional 310.2
- postcontusional 310.2

Syndrome — *see also* Disease — *continued*
- postencephalitic 310.89
- posterior
  - cervical sympathetic 723.2
  - fossa compression 348.4
  - inferior cerebellar artery (*see also* Disease, cerebrovascular, acute) 436
  - reversible encephalopathy (PRES) 348.39
- postgastrectomy (dumping) 564.2
- posthepatitis 780.79
- postherpetic (neuralgia) (zoster) 053.19
  - geniculate ganglion 053.11
  - ophthalmica 053.19
- postimmunization — *see* Complications, vaccination
- postinfarction 411.0
- postinfluenza (asthenia) 780.79
- postirradiation 990
- postlaminectomy 722.80
  - cervical, cervicothoracic 722.81
  - lumbar, lumbosacral 722.83
  - thoracic, thoracolumbar 722.82
- postleukotomy 310.0
- postlobotomy 310.0
- postmastectomy lymphedema 457.0
- postmature (of newborn) 766.22
- postmyocardial infarction 411.0
- postoperative NEC 998.9
  - blind loop 579.2
- postpartum panhypopituitary 253.2
- postperfusion NEC 999.89
  - bone marrow 996.85
- postpericardiotomy 429.4
- postphlebitic (asymptomatic) 459.10
  - with
    - complications NEC 459.19
    - inflammation 459.12
      - and ulcer 459.13
    - stasis dermatitis 459.12
      - with ulcer 459.13
    - ulcer 459.11
      - with inflammation 459.13
- postpolio (myelitis) 138
- postvagotomy 564.2
- postvalvulotomy 429.4
- postviral (asthenia) NEC 780.79
- Potain's (gastrectasis with dyspepsia) 536.1
- potassium intoxication 276.7
- Potter's 753.0
- Prader (-Labhart) -Willi (-Fanconi) 759.81
- preinfarction 411.1
- preleukemic 238.75
- premature senility 259.8
- premenstrual 625.4
- premenstrual tension 625.4
- pre ulcer 536.9
- Prinzmetal-Massumi (anterior chest wall syndrome) 786.52
- Profichet's 729.90
- progeria 259.8
- progressive pallidal degeneration 333.0
- prolonged gestation 766.22
- Proteus (dermal hypoplasia) 757.39
- prune belly 756.71
- prurigo-asthma 691.8
- pseudo-Turner's 759.89
- pseudocarpal tunnel (sublimis) 354.0
- pseudohermaphroditism-virilism-hirsutism 255.2
- pseudoparalytica 358.00
- psycho-organic 293.9
  - acute 293.0
  - anxiety type 293.84
  - depressive type 293.83
  - hallucinatory type 293.82
  - nonpsychotic severity 310.1
    - specified focal (partial) NEC 310.89
  - paranoid type 293.81
  - specified type NEC 293.89
  - subacute 293.1
- pterygolymphangiectasia 758.6
- ptosis-epicanthus 270.2
- pulmonary
  - arteriosclerosis 416.0
  - hypoperfusion (idiopathic) 769
  - renal (hemorrhagic) 446.21

Syndrome — *see also* Disease — *continued*
- pulseless 446.7
- Putnam-Dana (subacute combined sclerosis with pernicious anemia) 281.0 *[336.2]*
- pyloroduodenal 537.89
- pyramidopallidonigral 332.0
- pyriformis 355.0
- QT interval prolongation 426.82
- radicular NEC 729.2
  - lower limbs 724.4
  - upper limbs 723.4
    - newborn 767.4
- Raeder-Harbitz (pulseless disease) 446.7
- Ramsay Hunt's
  - dyssynergia cerebellaris myoclonica 334.2
  - herpetic geniculate ganglionitis 053.11
- rapid time-zone change 327.35
- Raymond (-Céstan) 433.8 ☑
- Raynaud's (paroxysmal digital cyanosis) 443.0
- RDS (respiratory distress syndrome, newborn) 769
- Refsum's (heredopathia atactica polyneuritiformis) 356.3
- Reichmann's (gastrosuccorrhea) 536.8
- Reifenstein's (hereditary familial hypogonadism, male) 259.52
- Reilly's (*see also* Neuropathy, peripheral, autonomic) 337.9
- Reiter's 099.3
- renal glomerulohyalinosis-diabetic 250.4 ☑ *[581.81]*
  - due to secondary diabetes 249.4 ☑ *[581.81]*
- Rendu-Osler-Weber (familial hemorrhagic telangiectasia) 448.0
- renofacial (congenital biliary fibroangiomatosis) 753.0
- Rénon-Delille 253.8
- respiratory distress (idiopathic) (newborn) 769
  - adult (following trauma and surgery) 518.82
  - specified NEC 518.82
  - type II 770.6
- restless legs (RLS) 333.94
- retinoblastoma (familial) 190.5
- retraction (Duane's) 378.71
- retroperitoneal fibrosis 593.4
- retroviral seroconversion (acute) V08
- Rett's 330.8
- Reye-Sheehan (postpartum pituitary necrosis) 253.2
- Reye's 331.81
- Riddoch's (visual disorientation) 368.16
- Ridley's (*see also* Failure, ventricular, left) 428.1
- Rieger's (mesodermal dysgenesis, anterior ocular segment) 743.44
- Rietti-Greppi-Micheli (thalassemia minor) 282.46
- right ventricular obstruction — *see* Failure, heart
- Riley-Day (familial dysautonomia) 742.8
- Robin's 756.0
- Rokitansky-Kuster-Hauser (congenital absence, vagina) 752.45
- Romano-Ward (prolonged QT interval syndrome) 426.82
- Romberg's 349.89
- Rosen-Castleman-Liebow (pulmonary proteinosis) 516.0
- rotator cuff, shoulder 726.10
- Roth's 355.1
- Rothmund's (congenital poikiloderma) 757.33
- Rotor's (idiopathic hyperbilirubinemia) 277.4
- Roussy-Lévy 334.3
- Roy (-Jutras) (acropachyderma) 757.39
- rubella (congenital) 771.0
- Rubinstein-Taybi's (brachydactylia, short stature, and intellectual disabilities) 759.89

☑ **Additional Digit Required** — Refer to the Tabular List for Digit Selection   ▽ **Subterms under main terms may continue to next column or page**

Syndrome — *see also* Disease — *continued*
- Rud's (mental deficiency, epilepsy, and infantilism) 759.89
- Ruiter-Pompen (-Wyers) (angiokeratoma corporis diffusum) 272.7
- Runge's (postmaturity) 766.22
- Russell (-Silver) (congenital hemihypertrophy and short stature) 759.89
- Rytand-Lipsitch (complete atrioventricular block) 426.0
- sacralization-scoliosis-sciatica 756.15
- sacroiliac 724.6
- Saenger's 379.46
- salt-losing (*see also* Disease, renal) 593.9
- salt
  - depletion (*see also* Disease, renal) 593.9
    - due to heat NEC 992.8
      - causing heat exhaustion or prostration 992.4
  - low (*see also* Disease, renal) 593.9
- Sanfilippo's (mucopolysaccharidosis III) 277.5
- Scaglietti-Dagnini (acromegalic macrospondylitis) 253.0
- scalded skin 695.81
- scalenus anticus (anterior) 353.0
- scapulocostal 354.8
- scapuloperoneal 359.1
- scapulovertebral 723.4
- Schaumann's (sarcoidosis) 135
- Scheie's (mucopolysaccharidosis IS) 277.5
- Scheuthauer-Marie-Sainton (cleidocranialis dysostosis) 755.59
- Schirmer's (encephalocutaneous angiomatosis) 759.6
- schizophrenic, of childhood NEC (*see also* Psychosis, childhood) 299.9 ☑
- Schmidt's
  - sphallo-pharyngo-laryngeal hemiplegia 352.6
  - thyroid-adrenocortical insufficiency 258.1
  - vagoaccessory 352.6
- Schneider's 047.9
- Schnitzler 273.1
- Scholte's (malignant carcinoid) 259.2
- Scholz (-Bielschowsky-Henneberg) 330.0
- Schroeder's (endocrine-hypertensive) 255.3
- Schüller-Christian (chronic histiocytosis X) 277.89
- Schultz's (agranulocytosis) 288.09
- Schwartz-Bartter (inappropriate secretion of antidiuretic hormone) 253.6
- Schwartz (-Jampel) 359.23
- Scimitar (anomalous venous drainage, right lung to inferior vena cava) 747.49
- sclerocystic ovary 256.4
- sea-blue histiocyte 272.7
- Seabright-Bantam (pseudohypoparathyroidism) 275.49
- Seckel's 759.89
- Secretan's (posttraumatic edema) 782.3
- secretoinhibitor (keratoconjunctivitis sicca) 710.2
- Seeligmann's (ichthyosis congenita) 757.1
- Senear-Usher (pemphigus erythematosus) 694.4
- senilism 259.8
- seroconversion, retroviral (acute) V08
- serotonin 333.99
- serous meningitis 348.2
- Sertoli cell (germinal aplasia) 606.0
- sex chromosome mosaic 758.81
- Sézary's (reticulosis) (M9701/3) 202.2 ☑
- shaken infant 995.55
- Shaver's (bauxite pneumoconiosis) 503
- Sheehan's (postpartum pituitary necrosis) 253.2
- shock (traumatic) 958.4
  - kidney 584.5
    - following crush injury 958.5
  - lung 518.82
    - related to trauma and surgery 518.52
  - neurogenic 308.9
  - psychic 308.9
- Shone's 746.84

Syndrome — *see also* Disease — *continued*
- short
  - bowel 579.3
  - P-R interval 426.81
- shoulder-arm (*see also* Neuropathy, peripheral, autonomic) 337.9
- shoulder-girdle 723.4
- shoulder-hand (*see also* Neuropathy, peripheral, autonomic) 337.9
- Shwachman's 288.02
- Shy-Drager (orthostatic hypotension with multisystem degeneration) 333.0
- Sicard's 352.6
- sicca (keratoconjunctivitis) 710.2
- sick
  - cell 276.1
  - cilia 759.89
  - sinus 427.81
- sideropenic 280.8
- Siemens'
  - ectodermal dysplasia 757.31
  - keratosis follicularis spinulosa (decalvans) 757.39
- Silfverskiöld's (osteochondrodystrophy, extremities) 756.50
- Silver's (congenital hemihypertrophy and short stature) 759.89
- Silvestroni-Bianco (thalassemia minima) 282.46
- Simons' (progressive lipodystrophy) 272.6
- sinusitis-bronchiectasis-situs inversus 759.3
- sinus tarsi 726.79
- Sipple's (medullary thyroid carcinoma-pheochromocytoma) 258.02
- Sjögren-Larsson (ichthyosis congenita) 757.1
- Sjögren (-Gougerot) (keratoconjunctivitis sicca) 710.2
  - with lung involvement 710.2 *[517.8]*
- SJS-TEN (Stevens-Johnson syndrome - toxic epidermal necrolysis overlap) 695.14
- Slocumb's 255.3
- Sluder's 337.09
- Smith-Lemli-Opitz (cerebrohepatorenal syndrome) 759.89
- Smith-Magenis 758.33
- smokers' 305.1
- Sneddon-Wilkinson (subcorneal pustular dermatosis) 694.1
- Sotos' (cerebral gigantism) 253.0
- South African cardiomyopathy 425.2
- spasmodic
  - upward movement, eye(s) 378.82
  - winking 307.20
- Spens' (syncope with heart block) 426.9
- spherophakia-brachymorphia 759.89
- spinal cord injury (*see also* Injury, spinal, by site)
  - with fracture, vertebra — *see* Fracture, vertebra, by site, with spinal cord injury
  - cervical — *see* Injury, spinal, cervical
  - fluid malabsorption (acquired) 331.3
- splenic
  - agenesis 759.0
  - flexure 569.89
  - neutropenia 289.53
  - sequestration 289.52
- Spurway's (brittle bones and blue sclera) 756.51
- staphylococcal scalded skin 695.81
- Stein-Leventhal (polycystic ovary) 256.4
- Stein's (polycystic ovary) 256.4
- Steinbrocker's (*see also* Neuropathy, peripheral, autonomic) 337.9
- Stevens-Johnson (erythema multiforme exudativum) 695.13
  - toxic epidermal necrolysis overlap (SJS-TEN overlap syndrome) 695.14
- Stewart-Morel (hyperostosis frontalis interna) 733.3
- Stickler 759.89
- stiff-baby 759.89
- stiff-man 333.91
- Still-Felty (rheumatoid arthritis with splenomegaly and leukopenia) 714.1

Syndrome — *see also* Disease — *continued*
- Still's (juvenile rheumatoid arthritis) 714.30
- Stilling-Türk-Duane (ocular retraction syndrome) 378.71
- Stojano's (subcostal) 098.86
- Stokes (-Adams) (syncope with heart block) 426.9
- Stokvis-Talma (enterogenous cyanosis) 289.7
- stone heart (*see also* Failure, ventricular, left) 428.1
- straight-back 756.19
- stroke (*see also* Disease, cerebrovascular, acute) 436
  - little 435.9
- Sturge-Kalischer-Weber (encephalotrigeminal angiomatosis) 759.6
- Sturge-Weber (-Dimitri) (encephalocutaneous angiomatosis) 759.6
- subclavian-carotid obstruction (chronic) 446.7
- subclavian steal 435.2
- subcoracoid-pectoralis minor 447.8
- subcostal 098.86
  - nerve compression 354.8
- subperiosteal hematoma 267
- subphrenic interposition 751.4
- sudden infant death (SIDS) 798.0
- Sudeck-Leriche 733.7
- Sudeck's 733.7
- superior
  - cerebellar artery (*see also* Disease, cerebrovascular, acute) 436
  - mesenteric artery 557.1
  - pulmonary sulcus (tumor) (M8010/3) 162.3
  - semi-circular canal dehiscence 386.8
  - vena cava 459.2
- suprarenal cortical 255.3
- supraspinatus 726.10
- Susac 348.39
- swallowed blood 777.3
- sweat retention 705.1
- Sweet's (acute febrile neutrophilic dermatosis) 695.89
- Swyer-James (unilateral hyperlucent lung) 492.8
- Swyer's (XY pure gonadal dysgenesis) 752.7
- Symonds' 348.2
- sympathetic
  - cervical paralysis 337.09
  - pelvic 625.5
- syndactylic oxycephaly 755.55
- syphilitic-cardiovascular 093.89
- systemic
  - fibrosclerosing 710.8
  - inflammatory response (SIRS) 995.90
    - due to
      - infectious process 995.91
        - with acute organ dysfunction 995.92
      - non-infectious process 995.93
        - with acute organ dysfunction 995.94
- systolic click (-murmur) 785.2
- Tabagism 305.1
- tachycardia-bradycardia 427.81
- Takayasu (-Onishi) (pulseless disease) 446.7
- Takotsubo 429.83
- Tapia's 352.6
- tarsal tunnel 355.5
- Taussig-Bing (transposition, aorta and overriding pulmonary artery) 745.11
- Taybi's (otopalatodigital) 759.89
- Taylor's 625.5
- teething 520.7
- tegmental 344.89
- telangiectasis-pigmentation-cataract 757.33
- temporal 383.02
  - lobectomy behavior 310.0
- temporomandibular joint-pain-dysfunction [TMJ] NEC 524.60
  - specified NEC 524.69
- Terry's (*see also* Retinopathy of prematurity) 362.21
- testicular feminization 259.51

Syndrome — *see also* Disease — *continued*
- testis, nonvirilizing 257.8
- tethered (spinal) cord 742.59
- thalamic 338.0
- Thibierge-Weissenbach (cutaneous systemic sclerosis) 710.1
- Thiele 724.6
- thoracic outlet (compression) 353.0
- thoracogenous rheumatic (hypertrophic pulmonary osteoarthropathy) 731.2
- Thorn's (*see also* Disease, renal) 593.9
- Thorson-Biörck (malignant carcinoid) 259.2
- thrombopenia-hemangioma 287.39
- thyroid-adrenocortical insufficiency 258.1
- Tietze's 733.6
- time-zone (rapid) 327.35
- Tobias' (carcinoma, pulmonary apex) (M8010/3) 162.3
- toilet seat 926.0
- Tolosa-Hunt 378.55
- Toni-Fanconi (cystinosis) 270.0
- Touraine-Solente-Golé (acropachyderma) 757.39
- Touraine's (hereditary osteo-onychodysplasia) 756.89
- toxic
  - oil 710.5
  - shock 040.82
- transfusion
  - fetal-maternal 772.0
  - twin
    - donor (infant) 772.0
    - recipient (infant) 776.4
- transient left ventricular apical ballooning 429.83
- Treacher Collins' (incomplete mandibulofacial dysostosis) 756.0
- trigeminal plate 259.8
- triple X female 758.81
- trisomy NEC 758.5
  - 13 or D₁ 758.1
  - 16-18 or E 758.2
  - 18 or E₃ 758.2
  - 20 758.5
  - 21 or G (mongolism) 758.0
  - 22 or G (mongolism) 758.0
  - G 758.0
- Troisier-Hanot-Chauffard (bronze diabetes) 275.01
- tropical wet feet 991.4
- Trousseau's (thrombophlebitis migrans visceral cancer) 453.1
- tumor lysis (following antineoplastic drug therapy) (spontaneous) 277.88
- Türk's (ocular retraction syndrome) 378.71
- Turner-Varny 758.6
- Turner's 758.6
- Twiddler's (due to)
  - automatic implantable defibrillator 996.04
  - pacemaker 996.01
- twin-to-twin transfusion 762.3
  - recipient twin 776.4
- Uehlinger's (acropachyderma) 757.39
- Ullrich-Feichtiger 759.89
- Ullrich (-Bonnevie) (-Turner) 758.6
- underwater blast injury (abdominal) (*see also* Injury, internal, abdomen) 868.00
- universal joint, cervix 620.6
- Unverricht-Wagner (dermatomyositis) 710.3
- Unverricht (-Lundborg) 345.1 ☑
- upward gaze 378.81
- Urbach-Oppenheim (necrobiosis lipoidica diabeticorum) 250.8 ☑ *[709.3]*
  - due to secondary diabetes 249.8 ☑ *[709.3]*
- Urbach-Wiethe (lipoid proteinosis) 272.8
- uremia, chronic 585.9
- urethral 597.81
- urethro-oculoarticular 099.3
- urethro-oculosynovial 099.3
- urohepatic 572.4
- uveocutaneous 364.24
- uveomeningeal, uveomeningitis 363.22
- vagohypoglossal 352.6

☑ **Additional Digit Required** — Refer to the Tabular List for Digit Selection ▽ **Subterms under main terms may continue to next column or page**

274 — Volume 2   ▶◀ **Revised Text**   ● **New Line**   ▲ **Revised Code**   **2014 ICD-9-CM**

Syndrome — see also Disease — continued
vagovagal 780.2
van Buchem's (hyperostosis corticalis) 733.3
van der Hoeve-Halbertsma-Waardenburg (ptosis-epicanthus) 270.2
van der Hoeve-Waardenburg-Gualdi (ptosis-epicanthus) 270.2
van der Hoeve's (brittle bones and blue sclera, deafness) 756.51
vanishing twin 651.33
van Neck-Odelberg (juvenile osteochondrosis) 732.1
vascular splanchnic 557.0
vasomotor 443.9
vasovagal 780.2
VATER 759.89
Velo-cardio-facial 758.32
vena cava (inferior) (superior) (obstruction) 459.2
Verbiest's (claudicatio intermittens spinalis) 435.1
Vernet's 352.6
vertebral
    artery 435.1
        compression 721.1
    lumbar 724.4
    steal 435.1
vertebrogenic (pain) 724.5
vertiginous NEC 386.9
video display tube 723.8
Villaret's 352.6
Vinson-Plummer (sideropenic dysphagia) 280.8
virilizing adrenocortical hyperplasia, congenital 255.2
virus, viral 079.99
visceral larval migrans 128.0
visual disorientation 368.16
vitamin B$_6$ deficiency 266.1
vitreous touch 997.99
Vogt-Koyanagi 364.24
Vogt's (corpus striatum) 333.71
Volkmann's 958.6
von Bechterew-Strümpell (ankylosing spondylitis) 720.0
von Graefe's 378.72
von Hippel-Lindau (angiomatosis retinocerebellosa) 759.6
von Schroetter's (intermittent venous claudication) 453.89
von Willebrand (-Jürgens) (angiohemophilia) 286.4
Waardenburg-Klein (ptosis epicanthus) 270.2
Wagner (-Unverricht) (dermatomyositis) 710.3
Waldenström-Kjellberg (sideropenic dysphagia) 280.8
Waldenström's (macroglobulinemia) 273.3
Wallenberg's (posterior inferior cerebellar artery) (see also Disease, cerebrovascular, acute) 436
Waterhouse (-Friderichsen) 036.3
water retention 276.69
Weber-Christian (nodular nonsuppurative panniculitis) 729.30
Weber-Cockayne (epidermolysis bullosa) 757.39
Weber-Dimitri (encephalocutaneous angiomatosis) 759.6
Weber-Gubler 344.89
Weber-Leyden 344.89
Weber-Osler (familial hemorrhagic telangiectasia) 448.0
Weber's 344.89
Wegener's (necrotizing respiratory granulomatosis) 446.4
Weill-Marchesani (brachymorphism and ectopia lentis) 759.89
Weingarten's (tropical eosinophilia) 518.3
Weiss-Baker (carotid sinus syncope) 337.01
Weissenbach-Thibierge (cutaneous systemic sclerosis) 710.1
Werdnig-Hoffmann 335.0
Werlhof-Wichmann (see also Purpura, thrombocytopenic) 287.39

Syndrome — see also Disease — continued
Wermer's (polyendocrine adenomatosis) 258.01
Werner's (progeria adultorum) 259.8
Wernicke-Korsakoff (nonalcoholic) 294.0
    alcoholic 291.1
Wernicke's (nonalcoholic) (superior hemorrhagic polioencephalitis) 265.1
Westphal-Strümpell (hepatolenticular degeneration) 275.1
wet
    brain (alcoholic) 303.9 ☑
    feet (maceration) (tropical) 991.4
    lung
        adult 518.52
        newborn 770.6
whiplash 847.0
Whipple's (intestinal lipodystrophy) 040.2
"whistling face" (craniocarpotarsal dystrophy) 759.89
Widal (-Abrami) (acquired hemolytic jaundice) 283.9
Wilkie's 557.1
Wilkinson-Sneddon (subcorneal pustular dermatosis) 694.1
Willan-Plumbe (psoriasis) 696.1
Willebrand (-Jürgens) (angiohemophilia) 286.4
Willi-Prader (hypogenital dystrophy with diabetic tendency) 759.81
Wilson-Mikity 770.7
Wilson's (hepatolenticular degeneration) 275.1
Wiskott-Aldrich (eczema-thrombocytopenia) 279.12
withdrawal
    alcohol 291.81
    drug 292.0
        infant of dependent mother 779.5
Woakes' (ethmoiditis) 471.1
Wolff-Parkinson-White (anomalous atrioventricular excitation) 426.7
Wright's (hyperabduction) 447.8
X
    cardiac 413.9
    dysmetabolic 277.7
xiphoidalgia 733.99
XO 758.6
XXX 758.81
XXXXY 758.81
XXY 758.7
yellow vernix (placental dysfunction) 762.2
Zahorsky's 074.0
Zellweger 277.86
Zieve's (jaundice, hyperlipemia and hemolytic anemia) 571.1
Zollinger-Ellison (gastric hypersecretion with pancreatic islet cell tumor) 251.5
Zuelzer-Ogden (nutritional megaloblastic anemia) 281.2
Synechia (iris) (pupil) 364.70
    anterior 364.72
        peripheral 364.73
    intrauterine (traumatic) 621.5
    posterior 364.71
    vulvae, congenital 752.49
Synesthesia — see also Disturbance, sensation 782.0
Synodontia 520.2
Synophthalmus 759.89
Synorchidism 752.89
Synorchism 752.89
Synostosis (congenital) 756.59
    astragaloscaphoid 755.67
    radioulnar 755.53
    talonavicular (bar) 755.67
    tarsal 755.67
Synovial — see condition
Synovioma (M9040/3) — see also Neoplasm, connective tissue, malignant
    benign (M9040/0) — see Neoplasm, connective tissue, benign
Synoviosarcoma (M9040/3) — see Neoplasm, connective tissue, malignant
Synovitis (see also Tenosynovitis) 727.00
    chronic crepitant, wrist 727.2

Synovitis (see also Tenosynovitis) — continued
    due to crystals — see Arthritis, due to crystals
    gonococcal 098.51
    gouty 274.00
    specified NEC 727.09
    syphilitic 095.7
        congenital 090.0
    traumatic, current — see Sprain, by site
    tuberculous — see Tuberculosis, synovitis
    villonodular 719.20
        ankle 719.27
        elbow 719.22
        foot 719.27
        hand 719.24
        hip 719.25
        knee 719.26
        multiple sites 719.29
        pelvic region 719.25
        shoulder (region) 719.21
        specified site NEC 719.28
        wrist 719.23
Syphilide 091.3
    congenital 090.0
    newborn 090.0
    tubercular 095.8
        congenital 090.0
Syphilis, syphilitic (acquired) 097.9
    with lung involvement 095.1
    abdomen (late) 095.2
    acoustic nerve 094.86
    adenopathy (secondary) 091.4
    adrenal (gland) 095.8
        with cortical hypofunction 095.8
    age under 2 years NEC (see also Syphilis, congenital) 090.9
        acquired 097.9
    alopecia (secondary) 091.82
    anemia 095.8
    aneurysm (artery) (ruptured) 093.89
        aorta 093.0
        central nervous system 094.89
        congenital 090.5
    anus 095.8
        primary 091.1
        secondary 091.3
    aorta, aortic (arch) (abdominal) (insufficiency) (pulmonary) (regurgitation) (stenosis) (thoracic) 093.89
        aneurysm 093.0
    arachnoid (adhesive) 094.2
    artery 093.89
        cerebral 094.89
        spinal 094.89
    arthropathy (neurogenic) (tabetic) 094.0 [713.5]
    asymptomatic — see Syphilis, latent
    ataxia, locomotor (progressive) 094.0
    atrophoderma maculatum 091.3
    auricular fibrillation 093.89
    Bell's palsy 094.89
    bladder 095.8
    bone 095.5
        secondary 091.61
    brain 094.89
    breast 095.8
    bronchus 095.8
    bubo 091.0
    bulbar palsy 094.89
    bursa (late) 095.7
    cardiac decompensation 093.89
    cardiovascular (early) (late) (primary) (secondary) (tertiary) 093.9
        specified type and site NEC 093.89
    causing death under 2 years of age (see also Syphilis, congenital) 090.9
        stated to be acquired NEC 097.9
    central nervous system (any site) (early) (late) (latent) (primary) (recurrent) (relapse) (secondary) (tertiary) 094.9
        with
            ataxia 094.0
            paralysis, general 094.1
                juvenile 090.40
            paresis (general) 094.1

Syphilis, syphilitic — continued
    central nervous system — continued
        with — continued
            paresis — continued
                juvenile 090.40
                tabes (dorsalis) 094.0
                    juvenile 090.40
                taboparesis 094.1
                    juvenile 090.40
            aneurysm (ruptured) 094.87
            congenital 090.40
            juvenile 090.40
            remission in (sustained) 094.9
            serology doubtful, negative, or positive 094.9
            specified nature or site NEC 094.89
            vascular 094.89
        cerebral 094.89
            meningovascular 094.2
            nerves 094.89
            sclerosis 094.89
            thrombosis 094.89
        cerebrospinal 094.89
            tabetic 094.0
        cerebrovascular 094.89
    cervix 095.8
    chancre (multiple) 091.0
        extragenital 091.2
        Rollet's 091.2
    Charcôt's joint 094.0 [713.5]
    choked disc 094.89 [377.00]
    chorioretinitis 091.51
        congenital 090.0 [363.13]
        late 094.83
    choroiditis 091.51
        congenital 090.0 [363.13]
        late 094.83
        prenatal 090.0 [363.13]
    choroidoretinitis (secondary) 091.51
        congenital 090.0 [363.13]
        late 094.83
    ciliary body (secondary) 091.52
        late 095.8 [364.11]
    colon (late) 095.8
    combined sclerosis 094.89
    complicating pregnancy, childbirth or puerperium 647.0 ☑
        affecting fetus or newborn 760.2
    condyloma (latum) 091.3
    congenital 090.9
        with
            encephalitis 090.41
            paresis (general) 090.40
            tabes (dorsalis) 090.40
            taboparesis 090.40
        chorioretinitis, choroiditis 090.0 [363.13]
        early or less than 2 years after birth NEC 090.2
            with manifestations 090.0
            latent (without manifestations) 090.1
                negative spinal fluid test 090.1
                serology, positive 090.1
            symptomatic 090.0
        interstitial keratitis 090.3
        juvenile neurosyphilis 090.40
        late or 2 years or more after birth NEC 090.7
            chorioretinitis, choroiditis 090.5 [363.13]
            interstitial keratitis 090.3
            juvenile neurosyphilis NEC 090.40
            latent (without manifestations) 090.6
                negative spinal fluid test 090.6
                serology, positive 090.6
            symptomatic or with manifestations NEC 090.5
            interstitial keratitis 090.3
    conjugal 097.9
        tabes 094.0
    conjunctiva 095.8 [372.10]
    contact V01.6
    cord, bladder 094.0
    cornea, late 095.8 [370.59]
    coronary (artery) 093.89
        sclerosis 093.89
    coryza 095.8

☑ Additional Digit Required — Refer to the Tabular List for Digit Selection
▽ Subterms under main terms may continue to next column or page
2014 ICD-9-CM   ▶◀ Revised Text   ● New Line   ▲ Revised Code
Volume 2 — 275

Syphilis, syphilitic — *continued*
 coryza — *continued*
  congenital 090.0
 cranial nerve 094.89
 cutaneous — *see* Syphilis, skin
 dacryocystitis 095.8
 degeneration, spinal cord 094.89
 d'emblée 095.8
 dementia 094.1
  paralytica 094.1
   juvenilis 090.40
 destruction of bone 095.5
 dilatation, aorta 093.0
 due to blood transfusion 097.9
 dura mater 094.89
 ear 095.8
  inner 095.8
   nerve (eighth) 094.86
   neurorecurrence 094.86
 early NEC 091.0
  cardiovascular 093.9
  central nervous system 094.9
   paresis 094.1
   tabes 094.0
  latent (without manifestations) (less
    than 2 years after infection) 092.9
  negative spinal fluid test 092.9
  serological relapse following treat-
    ment 092.0
  serology positive 092.9
  paresis 094.1
  relapse (treated, untreated) 091.7
  skin 091.3
  symptomatic NEC 091.89
   extragenital chancre 091.2
   primary, except extragenital chancre
     091.0
   secondary (*see also* Syphilis, sec-
     ondary) 091.3
    relapse (treated, untreated) 091.7
  tabes 094.0
  ulcer 091.3
 eighth nerve 094.86
 endemic, nonvenereal 104.0
 endocarditis 093.20
  aortic 093.22
  mitral 093.21
  pulmonary 093.24
  tricuspid 093.23
 epididymis (late) 095.8
 epiglottis 095.8
 epiphysitis (congenital) 090.0
 esophagus 095.8
 Eustachian tube 095.8
 exposure to V01.6
 eye 095.8 *[363.13]*
  neuromuscular mechanism 094.85
 eyelid 095.8 *[373.5]*
  with gumma 095.8 *[373.5]*
  ptosis 094.89
 fallopian tube 095.8
 fracture 095.5
 gallbladder (late) 095.8
 gastric 095.8
  crisis 094.0
  polyposis 095.8
 general 097.9
  paralysis 094.1
   juvenile 090.40
 genital (primary) 091.0
 glaucoma 095.8
 gumma (late) NEC 095.9
  cardiovascular system 093.9
  central nervous system 094.9
  congenital 090.5
  heart or artery 093.89
 heart 093.89
  block 093.89
  decompensation 093.89
  disease 093.89
  failure 093.89
  valve (*see also* Syphilis, endocarditis)
    093.20
 hemianesthesia 094.89
 hemianopsia 095.8
 hemiparesis 094.89

Syphilis, syphilitic — *continued*
 hemiplegia 094.89
 hepatic artery 093.89
 hepatitis 095.3
 hepatomegaly 095.3
  congenital 090.0
 hereditaria tarda (*see also* Syphilis, congenital, late) 090.7
 hereditary (*see also* Syphilis, congenital)
   090.9
  interstitial keratitis 090.3
 Hutchinson's teeth 090.5
 hyalitis 095.8
 inactive — *see* Syphilis, latent
 infantum NEC (*see also* Syphilis, congenital)
   090.9
 inherited — *see* Syphilis, congenital
 internal ear 095.8
 intestine (late) 095.8
 iris, iritis (secondary) 091.52
  late 095.8 *[364.11]*
 joint (late) 095.8
 keratitis (congenital) (early) (interstitial)
   (late) (parenchymatous) (punctata
   profunda) 090.3
 kidney 095.4
 lacrimal apparatus 095.8
 laryngeal paralysis 095.8
 larynx 095.8
 late 097.0
  cardiovascular 093.9
  central nervous system 094.9
  latent or 2 years or more after infection
    (without manifestations) 096
   negative spinal fluid test 096
   serology positive 096
  paresis 094.1
  specified site NEC 095.8
  symptomatic or with symptoms 095.9
  tabes 094.0
 latent 097.1
  central nervous system 094.9
  date of infection unspecified 097.1
  early or less than 2 years after infection
    092.9
  late or 2 years or more after infection 096
  serology
   doubtful
    follow-up of latent syphilis 097.1
     central nervous system 094.9
     date of infection unspecified
       097.1
     early or less than 2 years after
       infection 092.9
     late or 2 years or more after
       infection 096
   positive, only finding 097.1
    date of infection unspecified
      097.1
    early or less than 2 years after in-
      fection 097.1
    late or 2 years or more after infec-
      tion 097.1
 lens 095.8
 leukoderma 091.3
  late 095.8
 lienis 095.8
 lip 091.3
  chancre 091.2
  late 095.8
  primary 091.2
 Lissauer's paralysis 094.1
 liver 095.3
  secondary 091.62
 locomotor ataxia 094.0
 lung 095.1
 lymphadenitis (secondary) 091.4
 lymph gland (early) (secondary) 091.4
  late 095.8
 macular atrophy of skin 091.3
  striated 095.8
 maternal, affecting fetus or newborn 760.2
  manifest syphilis in newborn — *see*
    Syphilis, congenital
 mediastinum (late) 095.8

Syphilis, syphilitic — *continued*
 meninges (adhesive) (basilar) (brain) (spinal
   cord) 094.2
 meningitis 094.2
  acute 091.81
  congenital 090.42
 meningoencephalitis 094.2
 meningovascular 094.2
  congenital 090.49
 mesarteritis 093.89
  brain 094.89
  spine 094.89
 middle ear 095.8
 mitral stenosis 093.21
 monoplegia 094.89
 mouth (secondary) 091.3
  late 095.8
 mucocutaneous 091.3
  late 095.8
 mucous
  membrane 091.3
   late 095.8
  patches 091.3
   congenital 090.0
 mulberry molars 090.5
 muscle 095.6
 myocardium 093.82
 myositis 095.6
 nasal sinus 095.8
 neonatorum NEC (*see also* Syphilis, congenital) 090.9
 nerve palsy (any cranial nerve) 094.89
 nervous system, central 094.9
 neuritis 095.8
  acoustic nerve 094.86
 neurorecidive of retina 094.83
 neuroretinitis 094.85
 newborn (*see also* Syphilis, congenital) 090.9
 nodular superficial 095.8
 nonvenereal, endemic 104.0
 nose 095.8
  saddle back deformity 090.5
  septum 095.8
   perforated 095.8
 occlusive arterial disease 093.89
 ophthalmic 095.8 *[363.13]*
 ophthalmoplegia 094.89
 optic nerve (atrophy) (neuritis) (papilla)
   094.84
 orbit (late) 095.8
 orchitis 095.8
 organic 097.9
 osseous (late) 095.5
 osteochondritis (congenital) 090.0
 osteoporosis 095.5
 ovary 095.8
 oviduct 095.8
 palate 095.8
  gumma 095.8
  perforated 090.5
 pancreas (late) 095.8
 pancreatitis 095.8
 paralysis 094.89
  general 094.1
  juvenile 090.40
 paraplegia 094.89
 paresis (general) 094.1
  juvenile 090.40
 paresthesia 094.89
 Parkinson's disease or syndrome 094.82
 paroxysmal tachycardia 093.89
 pemphigus (congenital) 090.0
 penis 091.0
  chancre 091.0
  late 095.8
 pericardium 093.81
 perichondritis, larynx 095.8
 periosteum 095.5
  congenital 090.0
  early 091.61
  secondary 091.61
 peripheral nerve 095.8
 petrous bone (late) 095.5
 pharynx 095.8
  secondary 091.3
 pituitary (gland) 095.8

Syphilis, syphilitic — *continued*
 placenta 095.8
 pleura (late) 095.8
 pneumonia, white 090.0
 pontine (lesion) 094.89
 portal vein 093.89
 primary NEC 091.2
  anal 091.1
  and secondary (*see also* Syphilis, sec-
    ondary) 091.9
  cardiovascular 093.9
  central nervous system 094.9
  extragenital chancre NEC 091.2
  fingers 091.2
  genital 091.0
  lip 091.2
  specified site NEC 091.2
  tonsils 091.2
 prostate 095.8
 psychosis (intracranial gumma) 094.89
 ptosis (eyelid) 094.89
 pulmonary (late) 095.1
  artery 093.89
 pulmonum 095.1
 pyelonephritis 095.4
 recently acquired, symptomatic NEC 091.89
 rectum 095.8
 respiratory tract 095.8
 retina
  late 094.83
  neurorecidive 094.83
 retrobulbar neuritis 094.85
 salpingitis 095.8
 sclera (late) 095.0
 sclerosis
  cerebral 094.89
  coronary 093.89
  multiple 094.89
  subacute 094.89
 scotoma (central) 095.8
 scrotum 095.8
 secondary (and primary) 091.9
  adenopathy 091.4
  anus 091.3
  bone 091.61
  cardiovascular 093.9
  central nervous system 094.9
  chorioretinitis, choroiditis 091.51
  hepatitis 091.62
  liver 091.62
  lymphadenitis 091.4
  meningitis, acute 091.81
  mouth 091.3
  mucous membranes 091.3
  periosteum 091.61
  periostitis 091.61
  pharynx 091.3
  relapse (treated) (untreated) 091.7
  skin 091.3
  specified form NEC 091.89
  tonsil 091.3
  ulcer 091.3
  viscera 091.69
  vulva 091.3
 seminal vesicle (late) 095.8
 seronegative
  with signs or symptoms — *see* Syphilis,
    by site or stage
 seropositive
  with signs or symptoms — *see* Syphilis,
    by site and stage
  follow-up of latent syphilis — *see*
    Syphilis, latent
  only finding — *see* Syphilis, latent
 seventh nerve (paralysis) 094.89
 sinus 095.8
 sinusitis 095.8
 skeletal system 095.5
 skin (early) (secondary) (with ulceration)
   091.3
  late or tertiary 095.8
 small intestine 095.8
 spastic spinal paralysis 094.0
 spermatic cord (late) 095.8
 spinal (cord) 094.89

☑ Additional Digit Required — Refer to the Tabular List for Digit Selection
Ⓦ Subterms under main terms may continue to next column or page

276 — Volume 2
▶◀ Revised Text
● New Line
▲ Revised Code
2014 ICD-9-CM

Syphilis, syphilitic — continued
  spinal — continued
    with
      paresis 094.1
      tabes 094.0
  spleen 095.8
  splenomegaly 095.8
  spondylitis 095.5
  staphyloma 095.8
  stigmata (congenital) 090.5
  stomach 095.8
  synovium (late) 095.7
  tabes dorsalis (early) (late) 094.0
    juvenile 090.40
  tabetic type 094.0
    juvenile 090.40
  taboparesis 094.1
    juvenile 090.40
  tachycardia 093.89
  tendon (late) 095.7
  tertiary 097.0
    with symptoms 095.8
    cardiovascular 093.9
    central nervous system 094.9
    multiple NEC 095.8
    specified site NEC 095.8
  testis 095.8
  thorax 095.8
  throat 095.8
  thymus (gland) 095.8
  thyroid (late) 095.8
  tongue 095.8
  tonsil (lingual) 095.8
    primary 091.2
    secondary 091.3
  trachea 095.8
  tricuspid valve 093.23
  tumor, brain 094.89
  tunica vaginalis (late) 095.8
  ulcer (any site) (early) (secondary) 091.3
    late 095.9
    perforating 095.9
      foot 094.0
  urethra (stricture) 095.8
  urogenital 095.8
  uterus 095.8
  uveal tract (secondary) 091.50
    late 095.8 [363.13]
  uveitis (secondary) 091.50
    late 095.8 [363.13]
  uvula (late) 095.8
    perforated 095.8
  vagina 091.0
    late 095.8
  valvulitis NEC 093.20
  vascular 093.89
    brain or cerebral 094.89
  vein 093.89
    cerebral 094.89
  ventriculi 095.8
  vesicae urinariae 095.8
  viscera (abdominal) 095.2
    secondary 091.69
  vitreous (hemorrhage) (opacities) 095.8
  vulva 091.0
    late 095.8
    secondary 091.3
Syphiloma 095.9
  cardiovascular system 093.9
  central nervous system 094.9
  circulatory system 093.9
  congenital 090.5
Syphilophobia 300.29
Syringadenoma (M8400/0) — see also Neoplasm, skin, benign
  papillary (M8406/0) — see Neoplasm, skin, benign
Syringobulbia 336.0
Syringocarcinoma (M8400/3) — see Neoplasm, skin, malignant
Syringocystadenoma (M8400/0) — see also Neoplasm, skin, benign
  papillary (M8406/0) — see Neoplasm, skin, benign
Syringocystoma (M8407/0) — see Neoplasm, skin, benign

Syringoma (M8407/0) — see also Neoplasm, skin, benign
  chondroid (M8940/0) — see Neoplasm, by site, benign
Syringomyelia 336.0
Syringomyelitis 323.9
  late effect — see category 326
Syringomyelocele — see also Spina bifida 741.9 ☑
Syringopontia 336.0
System, systemic — see also condition
  disease, combined — see Degeneration, combined
  fibrosclerosing syndrome 710.8
  inflammatory response syndrome (SIRS) 995.90
    due to
      infectious process 995.91
        with acute organ dysfunction 995.92
      non-infectious process 995.93
        with acute organ dysfunction 995.94
  lupus erythematosus 710.0
    inhibitor 795.79

T

T-shaped incisors 520.2
Tab — see Tag
Tabacism 989.84
Tabacosis 989.84
Tabardillo 080
  flea-borne 081.0
  louse-borne 080
Tabes, tabetic
  with
    central nervous system syphilis 094.0
    Charcôt's joint 094.0 [713.5]
    cord bladder 094.0
    crisis, viscera (any) 094.0
    paralysis, general 094.1
    paresis (general) 094.1
    perforating ulcer 094.0
  arthropathy 094.0 [713.5]
  bladder 094.0
  bone 094.0
  cerebrospinal 094.0
  congenital 090.40
  conjugal 094.0
  dorsalis 094.0
    neurosyphilis 094.0
  early 094.0
  juvenile 090.40
  latent 094.0
  mesenterica (see also Tuberculosis) 014.8 ☑
  paralysis insane, general 094.1
  peripheral (nonsyphilitic) 799.89
  spasmodic 094.0
    not dorsal or dorsalis 343.9
  syphilis (cerebrospinal) 094.0
Taboparalysis 094.1
Taboparesis (remission) 094.1
  with
    Charcôt's joint 094.1 [713.5]
    cord bladder 094.1
    perforating ulcer 094.1
  juvenile 090.40
Tache noir 923.20
Tachyalimentation 579.3
Tachyarrhythmia, tachyrhythmia — see also Tachycardia
  paroxysmal with sinus bradycardia 427.81
Tachycardia 785.0
  atrial 427.89
  auricular 427.89
  AV nodal re-entry (re-entrant) 427.89
  junctional ectopic 427.0
  newborn 779.82
  nodal 427.89
    nonparoxysmal atrioventricular 426.89
  nonparoxysmal atrioventricular (nodal) 426.89
  nonsustained 427.2
  paroxysmal 427.2
    with sinus bradycardia 427.81
    atrial (PAT) 427.0

Tachycardia — continued
  paroxysmal — continued
    atrial — continued
      psychogenic 316 [427.0]
      atrioventricular (AV) 427.0
        psychogenic 316 [427.0]
      essential 427.2
      junctional 427.0
      nodal 427.0
      psychogenic 316 [427.2]
        atrial 316 [427.0]
        supraventricular 316 [427.0]
        ventricular 316 [427.1]
      supraventricular 427.0
        psychogenic 316 [427.0]
      ventricular 427.1
        psychogenic 316 [427.1]
  postoperative 997.1
  psychogenic 306.2
  sick sinus 427.81
  sinoauricular 427.89
  sinus 427.89
  supraventricular 427.89
  sustained 427.2
    supraventricular 427.0
    ventricular 427.1
  ventricular (paroxysmal) 427.1
    psychogenic 316 [427.1]
Tachygastria 536.8
Tachypnea 786.06
  hysterical 300.11
  newborn (idiopathic) (transitory) 770.6
  psychogenic 306.1
  transitory, of newborn 770.6
TACO (transfusion associated circulatory overload) 276.61
Taenia (infection) (infestation) — see also Infestation, taenia 123.3
  diminuta 123.6
  echinococcal infestation (see also Echinococcus) 122.9
  nana 123.6
  saginata infestation 123.2
  solium (intestinal form) 123.0
    larval form 123.1
Taeniasis (intestine) — see also Infestation, taenia 123.3
  saginata 123.2
  solium 123.0
Taenzer's disease 757.4
Tag (hypertrophied skin) (infected) 701.9
  adenoid 474.8
  anus 455.9
  endocardial (see also Endocarditis) 424.90
  hemorrhoidal 455.9
  hymen 623.8
  perineal 624.8
  preauricular 744.1
  rectum 455.9
  sentinel 455.9
  skin 701.9
    accessory 757.39
    anus 455.9
    congenital 757.39
    preauricular 744.1
    rectum 455.9
  tonsil 474.8
  urethra, urethral 599.84
  vulva 624.8
Tahyna fever 062.5
Takayasu (-Onishi) disease or syndrome (pulseless disease) 446.7
Takotsubo syndrome 429.83
Talc granuloma 728.82
  in operation wound 998.7
Talcosis 502
Talipes (congenital) 754.70
  acquired NEC 736.79
    planus 734
  asymmetric 754.79
    acquired 736.79
  calcaneovalgus 754.62
    acquired 736.76
  calcaneovarus 754.59
    acquired 736.76
  calcaneus 754.79

Talipes — continued
  calcaneus — continued
    acquired 736.76
  cavovarus 754.59
    acquired 736.75
  cavus 754.71
    acquired 736.73
  equinovalgus 754.69
    acquired 736.72
  equinovarus 754.51
    acquired 736.71
  equinus 754.79
    acquired, NEC 736.72
  percavus 754.71
    acquired 736.73
  planovalgus 754.69
    acquired 736.79
  planus (acquired) (any degree) 734
    congenital 754.61
    due to rickets 268.1
  valgus 754.60
    acquired 736.79
  varus 754.50
    acquired 736.79
Talma's disease 728.85
Talon noir 924.20
  hand 923.20
  heel 924.20
  toe 924.3
Tamponade heart (Rose's) — see also Pericarditis 423.3
Tanapox 059.21
Tangier disease (familial high-density lipoprotein deficiency) 272.5
Tank ear 380.12
Tantrum (childhood) — see also Disturbance, conduct 312.1 ☑
Tapeworm (infection) (infestation) — see also Infestation, tapeworm 123.9
Tapia's syndrome 352.6
Tarantism 297.8
Target-oval cell anemia 285.8
  with thalassemia — see Thalassemia
Tarlov's cyst 355.9
Tarral-Besnier disease (pityriasis rubra pilaris) 696.4
Tarsalgia 729.2
Tarsal tunnel syndrome 355.5
Tarsitis (eyelid) 373.00
  syphilitic 095.8 [373.00]
  tuberculous (see also Tuberculosis) 017.0 ☑ [373.4]
Tartar (teeth) 523.6
Tattoo (mark) 709.09
Taurodontism 520.2
Taussig-Bing defect, heart, or syndrome (transposition, aorta and overriding pulmonary artery) 745.11
Tay-Sachs
  amaurotic familial idiocy 330.1
  disease 330.1
Taybi's syndrome (otopalatodigital) 759.89
Tay's choroiditis 363.41
Taylor's
  disease (diffuse idiopathic cutaneous atrophy) 701.8
  syndrome 625.5
TBI (traumatic brain injury) — see also Injury, intracranial 854.0 ☑
  with skull fracture — see Fracture, skull, by site
Tear stone 375.57
Tear, torn (traumatic) — see also Wound, open, by site
  annular fibrosis 722.51
  anus, anal (sphincter) 863.89
    with open wound in cavity 863.99
    complicating delivery (healed) (old) 654.8 ☑
      with mucosa 664.3 ☑
      not associated with third-degree perineal laceration 664.6 ☑
    nontraumatic, nonpuerperal (healed) (old) 569.43
  articular cartilage, old (see also Disorder, cartilage, articular) 718.0 ☑

☑ Additional Digit Required — Refer to the Tabular List for Digit Selection

▽ Subterms under main terms may continue to next column or page

2014 ICD-9-CM

▶◀ Revised Text   ● New Line   ▲ Revised Code

Volume 2 — 277

Syphilis, syphilitic — Tear, torn

Tear, torn — *see also* Wound, open, by site — *continued*
  bladder
    with
      abortion — *see* Abortion, by type, with damage to pelvic organs
      ectopic pregnancy (*see also* categories 633.0–633.9) 639.2
      molar pregnancy (*see also* categories 630–632) 639.2
    following
      abortion 639.2
      ectopic or molar pregnancy 639.2
    obstetrical trauma 665.5 ☑
  bowel
    with
      abortion — *see* Abortion, by type, with damage to pelvic organs
      ectopic pregnancy (*see also* categories 633.0–633.9) 639.2
      molar pregnancy (*see also* categories 630–632) 639.2
    following
      abortion 639.2
      ectopic or molar pregnancy 639.2
    obstetrical trauma 665.5 ☑
  broad ligament
    with
      abortion — *see* Abortion, by type, with damage to pelvic organs
      ectopic pregnancy (*see also* categories 633.0–633.9) 639.2
      molar pregnancy (*see also* categories 630–632) 639.2
    following
      abortion 639.2
      ectopic or molar pregnancy 639.2
    obstetrical trauma 665.6 ☑
  bucket handle (knee) (meniscus) — *see* Tear, meniscus
  capsule
    joint — *see* Sprain, by site
    spleen — *see* Laceration, spleen, capsule
  cartilage (*see also* Sprain, by site)
    articular, old (*see also* Disorder, cartilage, articular) 718.0 ☑
    knee — *see* Tear, meniscus
    semilunar (knee) (current injury) — *see* Tear, meniscus
  cervix
    with
      abortion — *see* Abortion, by type, with damage to pelvic organs
      ectopic pregnancy (*see also* categories 633.0–633.9) 639.2
      molar pregnancy (*see also* categories 630–632) 639.2
    following
      abortion 639.2
      ectopic or molar pregnancy 639.2
    obstetrical trauma (current) 665.3 ☑
    old 622.3
  dural 349.31
    accidental puncture or laceration during a procedure 349.31
    incidental (inadvertent) 349.31
    nontraumatic NEC 349.39
  internal organ (abdomen, chest, or pelvis) — *see* Injury, internal, by site
  ligament (*see also* Sprain, by site)
    with open wound — *see* Wound, open, by site
  meniscus (knee) (current injury) 836.2
    bucket handle 836.0
      old 717.0
    lateral 836.1
      anterior horn 836.1
        old 717.42
      bucket handle 836.1
        old 717.41
      old 717.40
      posterior horn 836.1
        old 717.43
      specified site NEC 836.1
        old 717.49
    medial 836.0

Tear, torn — *see also* Wound, open, by site — *continued*
  meniscus — *continued*
    medial — *continued*
      anterior horn 836.0
        old 717.1
      bucket handle 836.0
        old 717.0
      posterior horn 836.0
        old 717.2
    old NEC 717.5
    site other than knee — *see* Sprain, by site
  muscle (*see also* Sprain, by site)
    with open wound — *see* Wound, open by site
  pelvic
    floor, complicating delivery 664.1 ☑
    organ NEC
      with
        abortion — *see* Abortion, by type, with damage to pelvic organs
        ectopic pregnancy (*see also* categories 633.0–633.9) 639.2
        molar pregnancy (*see also* categories 630–632) 639.2
      following
        abortion 639.2
        ectopic or molar pregnancy 639.2
      obstetrical trauma 665.5 ☑
  perineum (*see also* Laceration, perineum)
    obstetrical trauma 665.5 ☑
  periurethral tissue
    with
      abortion — *see* Abortion, by type, with damage to pelvic organs
      ectopic pregnancy (*see also* categories 633.0–633.9) 639.2
      molar pregnancy (*see also* categories 630–632) 639.2
    following
      abortion 639.2
      ectopic or molar pregnancy 639.2
    obstetrical trauma 664.8 ☑
  rectovaginal septum — *see* Laceration, rectovaginal septum
  retina, retinal (recent) (with detachment) 361.00
    without detachment 361.30
    dialysis (juvenile) (with detachment) 361.04
    giant (with detachment) 361.03
    horseshoe (without detachment) 361.32
    multiple (with detachment) 361.02
      without detachment 361.33
    old
      delimited (partial) 361.06
      partial 361.06
      total or subtotal 361.07
    partial (without detachment)
      giant 361.03
      multiple defects 361.02
      old (delimited) 361.06
      single defect 361.01
    round hole (without detachment) 361.31
    single defect (with detachment) 361.01
    total or subtotal (recent) 361.05
      old 361.07
  rotator cuff (traumatic) 840.4
    current injury 840.4
    degenerative 726.10
    nontraumatic (complete) 727.61
      partial 726.13
  semilunar cartilage, knee (*see also* Tear, meniscus) 836.2
    old 717.5
  tendon (*see also* Sprain, by site)
    with open wound — *see* Wound, open by site
  tentorial, at birth 767.0
  umbilical cord
    affecting fetus or newborn 772.0
    complicating delivery 663.8 ☑

Tear, torn — *see also* Wound, open, by site — *continued*
  urethra
    with
      abortion — *see* Abortion, by type, with damage to pelvic organs
      ectopic pregnancy (*see also* categories 633.0–633.9) 639.2
      molar pregnancy (*see also* categories 630–632) 639.2
    following
      abortion 639.2
      ectopic or molar pregnancy 639.2
    obstetrical trauma 665.5 ☑
  uterus — *see* Injury, internal, uterus
  vagina — *see* Laceration, vagina
  vessel, from catheter 998.2
  vulva, complicating delivery 664.0 ☑
Teething 520.7
  syndrome 520.7
Teeth, tooth — *see also* condition
  grinding 306.8
  prenatal 520.6
Tegmental syndrome 344.89
Telangiectasia, telangiectasis (verrucous) 448.9
  ataxic (cerebellar) 334.8
  familial 448.0
  hemorrhagic, hereditary (congenital) (senile) 448.0
  hereditary hemorrhagic 448.0
  retina 362.15
  spider 448.1
Telecanthus (congenital) 743.63
Telescoped bowel or intestine — *see also* Intussusception 560.0
Teletherapy, adverse effect NEC 990
Telogen effluvium 704.02
Temperature
  body, high (of unknown origin) (*see also* Pyrexia) 780.60
  cold, trauma from 991.9
    newborn 778.2
    specified effect NEC 991.8
  high
    body (of unknown origin) (*see also* Pyrexia) 780.60
    trauma from — *see* Heat
Temper tantrum (childhood) — *see also* Disturbance, conduct 312.1 ☑
Temple — *see* condition
Temporal — *see also* condition
  lobe syndrome 310.0
Temporomandibular joint-pain-dysfunction syndrome 524.60
Temporosphenoidal — *see* condition
Tendency
  bleeding (*see also* Defect, coagulation) 286.9
  homosexual, ego-dystonic 302.0
  paranoid 301.0
  suicide 300.9
Tenderness
  abdominal (generalized) (localized) 789.6 ☑
  rebound 789.6 ☑
  skin 782.0
Tendinitis, tendonitis — *see also* Tenosynovitis 726.90
  Achilles 726.71
  adhesive 726.90
    shoulder 726.0
  calcific 727.82
    shoulder 726.11
  gluteal 726.5
  patellar 726.64
  peroneal 726.79
  pes anserinus 726.61
  psoas 726.5
  tibialis (anterior) (posterior) 726.72
  trochanteric 726.5
Tendon — *see* condition
Tendosynovitis — *see* Tenosynovitis
Tendovaginitis — *see* Tenosynovitis
Tenesmus 787.99
  rectal 787.99
  vesical 788.99
Tenia — *see* Taenia

Teniasis — *see* Taeniasis
Tennis elbow 726.32
Tenonitis — *see also* Tenosynovitis
  eye (capsule) 376.04
Tenontosynovitis — *see* Tenosynovitis
Tenontothecitis — *see* Tenosynovitis
Tenophyte 727.9
Tenosynovitis (*see also* Synovitis) 727.00
  adhesive 726.90
    shoulder 726.0
  ankle 727.06
  bicipital (calcifying) 726.12
  buttock 727.09
  due to crystals — *see* Arthritis, due to crystals
  elbow 727.09
  finger 727.05
  foot 727.06
  gonococcal 098.51
  hand 727.05
  hip 727.09
  knee 727.09
  radial styloid 727.04
  shoulder 726.10
    adhesive 726.0
  specified NEC 727.09
  spine 720.1
  supraspinatus 726.10
  toe 727.06
  tuberculous — *see* Tuberculosis, tenosynovitis
  wrist 727.05
Tenovaginitis — *see* Tenosynovitis
Tension
  arterial, high (*see also* Hypertension) 401.9
    without diagnosis of hypertension 796.2
  headache 307.81
  intraocular (elevated) 365.00
  nervous 799.21
  ocular (elevated) 365.00
  pneumothorax 512.0
    iatrogenic 512.1
    postoperative 512.1
    spontaneous 512.0
  premenstrual 625.4
  state 300.9
Tentorium — *see* condition
Teratencephalus 759.89
Teratism 759.7
Teratoblastoma (malignant) (M9080/3) — *see* Neoplasm, by site, malignant
Teratocarcinoma (M9081/3) — *see also* Neoplasm, by site, malignant
  liver 155.0
Teratoma (solid) (M9080/1) — *see also* Neoplasm, by site, uncertain behavior
  adult (cystic) (M9080/0) — *see* Neoplasm, by site, benign
  and embryonal carcinoma, mixed (M9081/3) — *see* Neoplasm, by site, malignant
  benign (M9080/0) — *see* Neoplasm, by site, benign
  combined with choriocarcinoma (M9101/3) — *see* Neoplasm, by site, malignant
  cystic (adult) (M9080/0) — *see* Neoplasm, by site, benign
  differentiated type (M9080/0) — *see* Neoplasm, by site, benign
  embryonal (M9080/3) (*see also* Neoplasm, by site, malignant)
    liver 155.0
  fetal
    sacral, causing fetopelvic disproportion 653.7 ☑
  immature (M9080/3) — *see* Neoplasm, by site, malignant
  liver (M9080/3) 155.0
    adult, benign, cystic, differentiated type or mature (M9080/0) 211.5
  malignant (M9080/3) (*see also* Neoplasm, by site, malignant)
    anaplastic type (M9082/3) — *see* Neoplasm, by site, malignant
    intermediate type (M9083/3) — *see* Neoplasm, by site, malignant
    liver (M9080/3) 155.0

Teratoma — *see also* Neoplasm, by site, uncertain behavior — *continued*
  malignant (*see also* Neoplasm, by site, malignant) — *continued*
    trophoblastic (M9102/3)
      specified site — *see* Neoplasm, by site, malignant
      unspecified site 186.9
    undifferentiated type (M9082/3) — *see* Neoplasm, by site, malignant
  mature (M9080/0) — *see* Neoplasm, by site, benign
  malignant (M9080/3) — *see* Neoplasm, by site, malignant
  ovary (M9080/0) 220
    embryonal, immature, or malignant (M9080/3) 183.0
  suprasellar (M9080/3) — *see* Neoplasm, by site, malignant
  testis (M9080/3) 186.9
    adult, benign, cystic, differentiated type or mature (M9080/0) 222.0
    undescended 186.0
Terminal care V66.7
Termination
  anomalous (*see also* Malposition, congenital)
    portal vein 747.49
    right pulmonary vein 747.42
  pregnancy (legal) (therapeutic) — *see* Abortion, legal 635.9 ☑
    fetus NEC 779.6
    illegal (*see also* Abortion, illegal) 636.9 ☑
Ternidens diminutus infestation 127.7
Terrors, night (child) 307.46
Terry's syndrome (*see also* Retinopathy of prematurity) 362.21
Tertiary — *see* condition
Tessellated fundus, retina (tigroid) 362.89
Test(s)
  adequacy
    hemodialysis V56.31
    peritoneal dialysis V56.32
  AIDS virus V72.69
  allergen V72.7
  bacterial disease NEC (*see also* Screening, by name of disease) V74.9
  basal metabolic rate V72.69
  blood
    alcohol V70.4
    drug V70.4
      for therapeutic drug monitoring V58.83
      for routine general physical examination V72.62
    prior to treatment or procedure V72.63
    typing V72.86
      Rh typing V72.86
  developmental, infant or child V20.2
  Dick V74.8
  fertility V26.21
  genetic
    female V26.32
    for genetic disease carrier status
      female V26.31
      male V26.34
    male V26.39
  hearing V72.19
    following failed hearing screening V72.11
    routine, for infant and child V20.2
  HIV V72.69
  human immunodeficiency virus V72.69
  immunity status V72.61
  Kveim V82.89
  laboratory V72.60
    for medicolegal reason V70.4
    ordered as part of a routine general medical examination V72.62
    pre-operative V72.63
    pre-procedural V72.63
    specified NEC V72.69
  male partner of female with recurrent pregnancy loss V26.35
  Mantoux (for tuberculosis) V74.1

Test(s) — *continued*
  mycotic organism V75.4
  nuchal translucency V28.89
  parasitic agent NEC V75.8
  paternity V70.4
  peritoneal equilibration V56.32
  pregnancy
    negative result V72.41
    positive result V72.42
      first pregnancy V72.42
    unconfirmed V72.40
  preoperative V72.84
    cardiovascular V72.81
    respiratory V72.82
    specified NEC V72.83
  procreative management NEC V26.29
    genetic disease carrier status
      female V26.31
      male V26.34
  Rh typing V72.86
  sarcoidosis V82.89
  Schick V74.3
  Schultz-Charlton V74.8
  skin, diagnostic
    allergy V72.7
    bacterial agent NEC (*see also* Screening, by name of disease) V74.9
    Dick V74.8
    hypersensitivity V72.7
    Kveim V82.89
    Mantoux V74.1
    mycotic organism V75.4
    parasitic agent NEC V75.8
    sarcoidosis V82.89
    Schick V74.3
    Schultz-Charlton V74.8
    tuberculin V74.1
    specified type NEC V72.85
  tuberculin V74.1
  vision V72.0
    routine, for infant and child V20.2
  Wassermann
    positive (*see also* Serology for syphilis, positive) 097.1
    false 795.6
Testicle, testicular, testis — *see also* condition
  feminization (syndrome) 259.51
Tetanus, tetanic (cephalic) (convulsions) 037
  with
    abortion — *see* Abortion, by type, with sepsis
    ectopic pregnancy (*see also* categories 633.0–633.9) 639.0
    molar pregnancy — *see* categories 630–632 639.0
  following
    abortion 639.0
    ectopic or molar pregnancy 639.0
  inoculation V03.7
    reaction (due to serum) — *see* Complications, vaccination
  neonatorum 771.3
  puerperal, postpartum, childbirth 670.8 ☑
Tetany, tetanic 781.7
  alkalosis 276.3
  associated with rickets 268.0
  convulsions 781.7
    hysterical 300.11
  functional (hysterical) 300.11
  hyperkinetic 781.7
    hysterical 300.11
  hyperpnea 786.01
    hysterical 300.11
    psychogenic 306.1
  hyperventilation 786.01
    hysterical 300.11
    psychogenic 306.1
  hypocalcemic, neonatal 775.4
  hysterical 300.11
  neonatal 775.4
  parathyroid (gland) 252.1
  parathyroprival 252.1
  postoperative 252.1
  postthyroidectomy 252.1
  pseudotetany 781.7
    hysterical 300.11

Tetany, tetanic — *continued*
  psychogenic 306.1
    specified as conversion reaction 300.11
Tetralogy of Fallot 745.2
Tetraplegia — *see* Quadriplegia
Thailand hemorrhagic fever 065.4
Thalassanemia 282.40
Thalassemia (disease) 282.40
  with other hemoglobinopathy 282.49
  alpha (major) (severe) (triple gene defect) 282.43
    silent carrier 282.46
  beta (homozygous) (major) (severe) 282.44
  delta-beta (homozygous) 282.45
  dominant 282.49
  Hb-S (without crisis) 282.41
    with
      crisis 282.42
      vaso-occlusive pain 282.42
  hemoglobin
    C (Hb-C) 282.49
    D (Hb-D) 282.49
    E-beta 282.47
    E (Hb-E) 282.49
    H (Hb-H) 282.49
    I (Hb-I) 282.49
  high fetal gene (*see also* Thalassemia) 282.40
  high fetal hemoglobin (*see also* Thalassemia) 282.40
  intermedia 282.44
  major 282.44
  minor (alpha) (beta) 282.46
  mixed 282.49
  sickle-cell (without crisis) 282.41
    with
      crisis 282.42
      vaso-occlusive pain 282.42
  specified NEC 282.49
  trait (alpha) (beta) (delta-beta) 282.46
Thalassemic variants 282.49
Thaysen-Gee disease (nontropical sprue) 579.0
Thecoma (M8600/0) 220
  malignant (M8600/3) 183.0
Thelarche, precocious 259.1
Thelitis 611.0
  puerperal, postpartum 675.0 ☑
Therapeutic — *see* condition
Therapy V57.9
  blood transfusion, without reported diagnosis V58.2
  breathing V57.0
  chemotherapy, antineoplastic V58.11
    fluoride V07.31
    prophylactic NEC V07.39
  dialysis (intermittent) (treatment)
    extracorporeal V56.0
    peritoneal V56.8
    renal V56.0
    specified type NEC V56.8
  exercise NEC V57.1
    breathing V57.0
  extracorporeal dialysis (renal) V56.0
  fluoride prophylaxis V07.31
  hemodialysis V56.0
  hormone replacement (postmenopausal) V07.4
  immunotherapy antineoplastic V58.12
  long term oxygen therapy V46.2
  occupational V57.21
  orthoptic V57.4
  orthotic V57.81
  peritoneal dialysis V56.8
  physical NEC V57.1
  postmenopausal hormone replacement V07.4
  radiation V58.0
  speech (-language) V57.3
  vocational V57.22
Thermalgesia 782.0
Thermalgia 782.0
Thermanalgesia 782.0
Thermanesthesia 782.0
Thermic — *see* condition
Thermography (abnormal) 793.99
  breast 793.89

Thermoplegia 992.0
Thesaurismosis
  amyloid 277.39
  bilirubin 277.4
  calcium 275.40
  cystine 270.0
  glycogen (*see also* Disease, glycogen storage) 271.0
  kerasin 272.7
  lipoid 272.7
  melanin 255.41
  phosphatide 272.7
  urate 274.9
Thiaminic deficiency 265.1
  with beriberi 265.0
Thibierge-Weissenbach syndrome (cutaneous systemic sclerosis) 710.1
Thickened endometrium 793.5
Thickening
  bone 733.99
    extremity 733.99
  breast 611.79
  hymen 623.3
  larynx 478.79
  nail 703.8
    congenital 757.5
  periosteal 733.99
  pleura (*see also* Pleurisy) 511.0
  skin 782.8
  subepiglottic 478.79
  tongue 529.8
  valve, heart — *see* Endocarditis
Thiele syndrome 724.6
Thigh — *see* condition
Thinning vertebra — *see also* Osteoporosis 733.00
Thirst, excessive 783.5
  due to deprivation of water 994.3
Thomsen's disease 359.22
Thomson's disease (congenital poikiloderma) 757.33
Thoracic — *see also* condition
  kidney 753.3
  outlet syndrome 353.0
  stomach — *see* Hernia, diaphragm
Thoracogastroschisis (congenital) 759.89
Thoracopagus 759.4
Thoracoschisis 756.3
Thoracoscopic surgical procedure converted to open procedure V64.42
Thorax — *see* condition
Thorn's syndrome — *see also* Disease, renal 593.9
Thornwaldt's, Tornwaldt's
  bursitis (pharyngeal) 478.29
  cyst 478.26
  disease (pharyngeal bursitis) 478.29
Thorson-Biörck syndrome (malignant carcinoid) 259.2
Threadworm (infection) (infestation) 127.4
Threatened
  abortion or miscarriage 640.0 ☑
    with subsequent abortion (*see also* Abortion, spontaneous) 634.9 ☑
    affecting fetus 762.1
  labor 644.1 ☑
    affecting fetus or newborn 761.8
    premature 644.0 ☑
  miscarriage 640.0 ☑
    affecting fetus 762.1
  premature
    delivery 644.2 ☑
      affecting fetus or newborn 761.8
    labor 644.0 ☑
      before 22 completed weeks gestation 640.0 ☑
Three-day fever 066.0
Threshers' lung 495.0
Thrix annulata (congenital) 757.4
Throat — *see* condition
Thrombasthenia (Glanzmann's) (hemorrhagic) (hereditary) 287.1
Thromboangiitis 443.1
  obliterans (general) 443.1
    cerebral 437.1

☑ Additional Digit Required — Refer to the Tabular List for Digit Selection   ▽ Subterms under main terms may continue to next column or page

2014 ICD-9-CM   ►◄ Revised Text   ● New Line   ▲ Revised Code   Volume 2 — 279

Teratoma — Thromboangiitis

Index

Thromboangiitis — Thrombosis, thrombotic

Thrombosis, thrombotic — *continued*
  lower extremity — *continued*
    deep vessels — *continued*
      acute — *continued*
        femoral 453.41
        iliac 453.41
        lower leg 453.42
        peroneal 453.42
        popliteal 453.41
        proximal (upper leg) 453.41
        thigh 453.41
        tibial 453.42
      chronic 453.50
        calf 453.52
        distal (lower leg) 453.52
        femoral 453.51
        iliac 453.51
        lower leg 453.52
        peroneal 453.52
        popliteal 453.51
        proximal (upper leg) 453.51
        thigh 453.51
        tibial 453.52
    personal history of V12.51
    saphenous (greater) (lesser) 453.6
    superficial 453.6
  lung 415.19
    iatrogenic 415.11
    personal history of V12.55
    postoperative 415.11
    septic 415.12
  marantic, dural sinus 437.6
  meninges (brain) (*see also* Thrombosis, brain) 434.0 ☑
  mesenteric (artery) (with gangrene) 557.0
    vein (inferior) (superior) 557.0
  mitral — *see* Insufficiency, mitral
  mural (heart chamber) (*see also* Infarct, myocardium) 410.9 ☑
    without
      cardiac condition 429.89
      coronary artery disease 429.89
      myocardial infarction 429.89
    due to syphilis 093.89
    following myocardial infarction 429.79
    healed or specified as old 412
  omentum (with gangrene) 557.0
  ophthalmic (artery) (*see also* Occlusion, retina) 362.30
  pampiniform plexus (male) 608.83
    female 620.8
  parietal (*see also* Infarct, myocardium) 410.9 ☑
  penis, penile 607.82
  peripheral arteries 444.22
    lower 444.22
    upper 444.21
  platelet 446.6
  portal 452
    due to syphilis 093.89
    infectional or septic 572.1
  precerebral artery (*see also* Occlusion, artery, precerebral NEC)
  pregnancy 671.2 ☑
    deep (vein) 671.3 ☑
    superficial (vein) 671.2 ☑
  puerperal, postpartum, childbirth 671.2 ☑
    brain (artery) 674.0 ☑
      venous 671.5 ☑
    cardiac 674.8 ☑
    cerebral (artery) 674.0 ☑
      venous 671.5 ☑
    deep (vein) 671.4 ☑
    intracranial sinus (nonpyogenic) (venous) 671.5 ☑
    pelvic 671.4 ☑
    pulmonary (artery) 673.2 ☑
    specified site NEC 671.5 ☑
    superficial 671.2 ☑
  pulmonary (artery) (vein) 415.19
    iatrogenic 415.11
    personal history of V12.55
    postoperative 415.11
    septic 415.12
  renal (artery) 593.81
    vein 453.3

Thrombosis, thrombotic — *continued*
  resulting from presence of shunt or other internal prosthetic device — *see* Complications, due to (presence of) any device, implant, or graft classified to 996.0–996.5 NEC
  retina, retinal (artery) 362.30
    arterial branch 362.32
    central 362.31
    partial 362.33
    vein
      central 362.35
      tributary (branch) 362.36
  saphenous vein (greater) (lesser) 453.6
  scrotum 608.83
  seminal vesicle 608.83
  sigmoid (venous) sinus — *see* Thrombosis, intracranial venous sinus 325
  silent NEC 453.9
  sinus, intracranial (venous) (any) (*see also* Thrombosis, intracranial venous sinus) 325
  softening, brain (*see also* Thrombosis, brain) 434.0 ☑
  specified site NEC (acute) 453.89
    chronic 453.79
  spermatic cord 608.83
  spinal cord 336.1
    due to syphilis 094.89
    in pregnancy or puerperium 671.5 ☑
    pyogenic origin 324.1
    late effect — *see* category 326
  spleen, splenic 289.59
    artery 444.89
  testis 608.83
  traumatic (complication) (early) (*see also* Injury, blood vessel, by site) 904.9
  tricuspid — *see* Endocarditis, tricuspid
  tumor — *see* Neoplasm, by site
  tunica vaginalis 608.83
  umbilical cord (vessels) 663.6 ☑
    affecting fetus or newborn 762.6
  upper extremity (acute) 453.83
    chronic 453.73
    deep 453.72
    superficial 453.71
    deep 453.82
    superficial 453.81
  vas deferens 608.83
  vein
    antecubital (acute) 453.81
      chronic 453.71
    axillary (acute) 453.84
      chronic 453.74
    basilic (acute) 453.81
      chronic 453.71
    brachial (acute) 453.82
      chronic 453.72
    brachiocephalic (innominate) (acute) 453.87
      chronic 453.77
    cephalic (acute) 453.81
      chronic 453.71
    deep 453.40
      personal history of V12.51
    internal jugular (acute) 453.86
      chronic 453.76
    lower extremity — *see* Thrombosis, lower extremity
    personal history of V12.51
    radial (acute) 453.82
      chronic 453.72
    saphenous (greater) (lesser) 453.6
    specified site NEC (acute) 453.89
      chronic 453.79
    subclavian (acute) 453.85
      chronic 453.75
    superior vena cava (acute) 453.87
      chronic 453.77
    thoracic (acute) 453.87
      chronic 453.77
    ulnar (acute) 453.82
      chronic 453.72
    upper extremity — *see* Thrombosis, upper extremity

Thrombosis, thrombotic — *continued*
  vena cava
    inferior 453.2
      personal history of V12.51
    superior (acute) 453.87
      chronic 453.77
Thrombus — *see* Thrombosis
Thrush 112.0
  newborn 771.7
Thumb — *see also* condition
  gamekeeper's 842.12
  sucking (child problem) 307.9
Thygeson's superficial punctate keratitis 370.21
Thymergasia — *see also* Psychosis, affective 296.80
Thymitis 254.8
Thymoma (benign) (M8580/0) 212.6
  malignant (M8580/3) 164.0
Thymus, thymic (gland) — *see* condition
Thyrocele — *see also* Goiter 240.9
Thyroglossal — *see also* condition
  cyst 759.2
  duct, persistent 759.2
Thyroid (body) (gland) — *see also* condition
  hormone resistance 246.8
  lingual 759.2
Thyroiditis 245.9
  acute (pyogenic) (suppurative) 245.0
    nonsuppurative 245.0
  autoimmune 245.2
  chronic (nonspecific) (sclerosing) 245.8
    fibrous 245.3
    lymphadenoid 245.2
    lymphocytic 245.2
    lymphoid 245.2
  complicating pregnancy, childbirth, or puerperium 648.1 ☑
  de Quervain's (subacute granulomatous) 245.1
  fibrous (chronic) 245.3
  giant (cell) (follicular) 245.1
  granulomatous (de Quervain's) (subacute) 245.1
  Hashimoto's (struma lymphomatosa) 245.2
  iatrogenic 245.4
  invasive (fibrous) 245.3
  ligneous 245.3
  lymphocytic (chronic) 245.2
  lymphoid 245.2
  lymphomatous 245.2
  pseudotuberculous 245.1
  pyogenic 245.0
  radiation 245.4
  Riedel's (ligneous) 245.3
  subacute 245.1
  suppurative 245.0
  tuberculous (*see also* Tuberculosis) 017.5 ☑
  viral 245.1
  woody 245.3
Thyrolingual duct, persistent 759.2
Thyromegaly 240.9
Thyrotoxic
  crisis or storm (*see also* Thyrotoxicosis) 242.9 ☑
  heart failure (*see also* Thyrotoxicosis) 242.9 ☑ *[425.7]*
Thyrotoxicosis 242.9 ☑

> *Note* — Use the following fifth-digit subclassification with category 242:
>
> 0   without mention of thyrotoxic crisis or storm
>
> 1   with mention of thyrotoxic crisis or storm

  with
    goiter (diffuse) 242.0 ☑
      adenomatous 242.3 ☑
        multinodular 242.2 ☑
        uninodular 242.1 ☑
      nodular 242.3 ☑
        multinodular 242.2 ☑
        uninodular 242.1 ☑
    infiltrative
      dermopathy 242.0 ☑

Thyrotoxicosis — *continued*
  with — *continued*
    infiltrative — *continued*
      ophthalmopathy 242.0 ☑
      thyroid acropachy 242.0 ☑
  complicating pregnancy, childbirth, or puerperium 648.1 ☑
  due to
    ectopic thyroid nodule 242.4 ☑
    ingestion of (excessive) thyroid material 242.8 ☑
    specified cause NEC 242.8 ☑
  factitia 242.8 ☑
  heart 242.9 ☑ *[425.7]*
  neonatal (transient) 775.3
TIA (transient ischemic attack) 435.9
  with transient neurologic deficit 435.9
  late effect — *see* Late effect(s) (of) cerebrovascular disease
Tibia vara 732.4
Tic 307.20
  breathing 307.20
  child problem 307.21
  compulsive 307.22
  convulsive 307.20
  degenerative (generalized) (localized) 333.3
    facial 351.8
  douloureux (*see also* Neuralgia, trigeminal) 350.1
    atypical 350.2
  habit 307.20
    chronic (motor or vocal) 307.22
    transient (of childhood) 307.21
  lid 307.20
    transient (of childhood) 307.21
  motor-verbal 307.23
  occupational 300.89
  orbicularis 307.20
    transient (of childhood) 307.21
  organic origin 333.3
  postchoreic — *see* Chorea
  psychogenic 307.20
    compulsive 307.22
  salaam 781.0
  spasm 307.20
    chronic (motor or vocal) 307.22
    transient (of childhood) 307.21
Tick-bite fever NEC 066.1
  African 087.1
  Colorado (virus) 066.1
  Rocky Mountain 082.0
Tick (-borne) fever NEC 066.1
  American mountain 066.1
  Colorado 066.1
  hemorrhagic NEC 065.3
    Crimean 065.0
    Kyasanur Forest 065.2
    Omsk 065.1
  mountain 066.1
  nonexanthematous 066.1
Tick paralysis 989.5
Tics and spasms, compulsive 307.22
Tietze's disease or syndrome 733.6
Tight, tightness
  anus 564.89
  chest 786.59
  fascia (lata) 728.9
  foreskin (congenital) 605
  hymen 623.3
  introitus (acquired) (congenital) 623.3
  rectal sphincter 564.89
  tendon 727.81
    Achilles (heel) 727.81
  urethral sphincter 598.9
Tilting vertebra 737.9
Timidity, child 313.21
Tin-miners' lung 503
Tinea (intersecta) (tarsi) 110.9
  amiantacea 110.0
  asbestina 110.0
  barbae 110.0
  beard 110.0
  black dot 110.0
  blanca 111.2
  capitis 110.0
  corporis 110.5

☑ Additional Digit Required — Refer to the Tabular List for Digit Selection   ▽ Subterms under main terms may continue to next column or page

2014 ICD-9-CM   ▶◀ Revised Text   ● New Line   ▲ Revised Code   Volume 2 — 281

Tinea — *continued*
  cruris 110.3
  decalvans 704.09
  flava 111.0
  foot 110.4
  furfuracea 111.0
  imbricata (Tokelau) 110.5
  lepothrix 039.0
  manuum 110.2
  microsporic (*see also* Dermatophytosis) 110.9
  nigra 111.1
  nodosa 111.2
  pedis 110.4
  scalp 110.0
  specified site NEC 110.8
  sycosis 110.0
  tonsurans 110.0
  trichophytic (*see also* Dermatophytosis) 110.9
  unguium 110.1
  versicolor 111.0
Tingling sensation — *see also* Disturbance, sensation 782.0
Tinnitus (aurium) 388.30
  audible 388.32
  objective 388.32
  subjective 388.31
Tipped, teeth 524.33
Tipping
  pelvis 738.6
    with disproportion (fetopelvic) 653.0 ☑
      affecting fetus or newborn 763.1
      causing obstructed labor 660.1 ☑
        affecting fetus or newborn 763.1
  teeth 524.33
Tiredness 780.79
Tissue — *see* condition
Tobacco
  abuse (affecting health) NEC (*see also* Abuse, drugs, nondependent) 305.1
  heart 989.84
  use disorder complicating pregnancy, childbirth, or the puerperium 649.0 ☑
Tobias' syndrome (carcinoma, pulmonary apex) (M8010/3) 162.3
Tocopherol deficiency 269.1
Todd's
  cirrhosis — *see* Cirrhosis, biliary
  paralysis (postepileptic transitory paralysis) 344.89
Toe — *see* condition
Toilet, artificial opening — *see also* Attention to, artificial, opening V55.9
Tokelau ringworm 110.5
Tollwut 071
Tolosa-Hunt syndrome 378.55
Tommaselli's disease
  correct substance properly administered 599.70
  overdose or wrong substance given or taken 961.4
Tongue — *see also* condition
  worms 134.1
Tongue tie 750.0
Toni-Fanconi syndrome (cystinosis) 270.0
Tonic pupil 379.46
Tonsil — *see* condition
Tonsillitis (acute) (catarrhal) (croupous) (follicular) (gangrenous) (infective) (lacunar) (lingual) (malignant) (membranous) (phlegmonous) (pneumococcal) (pseudomembranous) (purulent) (septic) (staphylococcal) (subacute) (suppurative) (toxic) (ulcerative) (vesicular) (viral) 463
  with influenza, flu, or grippe (*see also* Influenza) 487.1
  chronic 474.00
  diphtheritic (membranous) 032.0
  hypertrophic 474.00
  influenzal (*see also* Influenza) 487.1
  parenchymatous 475
  streptococcal 034.0
  tuberculous (*see also* Tuberculosis) 012.8 ☑

Tonsillitis — *continued*
  Vincent's 101
Tonsillopharyngitis 465.8
Toothache 525.9
Tooth, teeth — *see* condition
Topagnosis 782.0
Tophi (gouty) 274.03
  ear 274.81
  heart 274.82
  specified site NEC 274.82
TORCH infection — *see also* Infection, congenital 760.2
Torn — *see* Tear, torn
Tornwaldt's bursitis (disease) (pharyngeal bursitis) 478.29
  cyst 478.26
Torpid liver 573.9
Torsion
  accessory tube 620.5
  adnexa (female) 620.5
  aorta (congenital) 747.29
    acquired 447.1
  appendix
    epididymis 608.24
    testis 608.23
  bile duct 576.8
    with calculus, choledocholithiasis or stones — *see* Choledocholithiasis
    congenital 751.69
  bowel, colon, or intestine 560.2
  cervix — *see* Malposition, uterus
  duodenum 537.3
  dystonia — *see* Dystonia, torsion
  epididymis 608.24
    appendix 608.24
  fallopian tube 620.5
  gallbladder (*see also* Disease, gallbladder) 575.8
    congenital 751.69
  gastric 537.89
  hydatid of Morgagni (female) 620.5
  kidney (pedicle) 593.89
  Meckel's diverticulum (congenital) 751.0
  mesentery 560.2
  omentum 560.2
  organ or site, congenital NEC — *see* Anomaly, specified type NEC
  ovary (pedicle) 620.5
    congenital 752.0
  oviduct 620.5
  penis 607.89
    congenital 752.69
  renal 593.89
  spasm — *see* Dystonia, torsion
  spermatic cord 608.22
    extravaginal 608.21
    intravaginal 608.22
  spleen 289.59
  testicle, testis 608.20
    appendix 608.23
  tibia 736.89
  umbilical cord — *see* Compression, umbilical cord
  uterus (*see also* Malposition, uterus) 621.6
Torticollis (intermittent) (spastic) 723.5
  congenital 754.1
    sternomastoid 754.1
    due to birth injury 767.8
  hysterical 300.11
  ocular 781.93
  psychogenic 306.0
    specified as conversion reaction 300.11
  rheumatic 723.5
  rheumatoid 714.0
  spasmodic 333.83
  traumatic, current NEC 847.0
Tortuous
  artery 447.1
  fallopian tube 752.19
  organ or site, congenital NEC — *see* Distortion
  renal vessel (congenital) 747.62
  retina vessel (congenital) 743.58
    acquired 362.17
  ureter 593.4
  urethra 599.84

Tortuous — *continued*
  vein — *see* Varicose, vein
Torula, torular (infection) 117.5
  histolytica 117.5
  lung 117.5
Torulosis 117.5
Torus
  fracture
    fibula 823.41
      with tibia 823.42
    humerus 812.49
    radius (alone) 813.45
      with ulna 813.47
    tibia 823.40
      with fibula 823.42
    ulna (alone) 813.46
      with radius 813.47
  mandibularis 526.81
  palatinus 526.81
Touch, vitreous 997.99
Touraine-Solente-Golé syndrome (acropachyderma) 757.39
Touraine's syndrome (hereditary osteo-onychodysplasia) 756.89
Tourette's disease (motor-verbal tic) 307.23
Tower skull 756.0
  with exophthalmos 756.0
Toxemia 799.89
  with
    abortion — *see* Abortion, by type, with toxemia
    bacterial — *see* Septicemia
  biliary (*see also* Disease, biliary) 576.8
  burn — *see* Burn, by site
  congenital NEC 779.89
  eclamptic 642.6 ☑
    with pre-existing hypertension 642.7 ☑
  erysipelatous (*see also* Erysipelas) 035
  fatigue 799.89
  fetus or newborn NEC 779.89
  food (*see also* Poisoning, food) 005.9
  gastric 537.89
  gastrointestinal 558.2
  intestinal 558.2
  kidney (*see also* Disease, renal) 593.9
  lung 518.89
  malarial NEC (*see also* Malaria) 084.6
  maternal (of pregnancy), affecting fetus or newborn 760.0
  myocardial — *see* Myocarditis, toxic
  of pregnancy (mild) (pre-eclamptic) 642.4 ☑
    with
      convulsions 642.6 ☑
      pre-existing hypertension 642.7 ☑
    affecting fetus or newborn 760.0
    severe 642.5 ☑
  pre-eclamptic — *see* Toxemia, of pregnancy
  puerperal, postpartum — *see* Toxemia, of pregnancy
  pulmonary 518.89
  renal (*see also* Disease, renal) 593.9
  septic (*see also* Septicemia) 038.9
  small intestine 558.2
  staphylococcal 038.10
    aureus 038.11
    due to food 005.0
    specified organism NEC 038.19
  stasis 799.89
  stomach 537.89
  uremic (*see also* Uremia) 586
  urinary 586
Toxemica cerebropathia psychica (nonalcoholic) 294.0
  alcoholic 291.1
Toxic (poisoning) — *see also* condition
  from drug or poison — *see* Table of Drugs and Chemicals
  oil syndrome 710.5
  shock syndrome 040.82
  thyroid (gland) (*see also* Thyrotoxicosis) 242.9 ☑
Toxicemia — *see* Toxemia
Toxicity
  dilantin
    asymptomatic 796.0

Toxicity — *continued*
  dilantin — *continued*
    symptomatic — *see* Table of Drugs and Chemicals
  drug
    asymptomatic 796.0
    symptomatic — *see* Table of Drugs and Chemicals
  fava bean 282.2
  from drug or poison
    asymptomatic 796.0
    symptomatic — *see* Table of Drugs and Chemicals
Toxicosis — *see also* Toxemia 799.89
  capillary, hemorrhagic 287.0
Toxinfection 799.89
  gastrointestinal 558.2
Toxocariasis 128.0
Toxoplasma infection, generalized 130.9
Toxoplasmosis (acquired) 130.9
  with pneumonia 130.4
  congenital, active 771.2
  disseminated (multisystemic) 130.8
  maternal
    with suspected damage to fetus affecting management of pregnancy 655.4 ☑
    affecting fetus or newborn 760.2
    manifest toxoplasmosis in fetus or newborn 771.2
  multiple sites 130.8
  multisystemic disseminated 130.8
  specified site NEC 130.7
Trabeculation, bladder 596.89
Trachea — *see* condition
Tracheitis (acute) (catarrhal) (infantile) (membranous) (plastic) (pneumococcal) (septic) (suppurative) (viral) 464.10
  with
    bronchitis 490
      acute or subacute 466.0
      chronic 491.8
      tuberculosis — *see* Tuberculosis, pulmonary
    laryngitis (acute) 464.20
      with obstruction 464.21
      chronic 476.1
      tuberculous (*see also* Tuberculosis, larynx) 012.3 ☑
    obstruction 464.11
  chronic 491.8
    with
      bronchitis (chronic) 491.8
      laryngitis (chronic) 476.1
    due to external agent — *see* Condition, respiratory, chronic, due to
  diphtheritic (membranous) 032.3
  due to external agent — *see* Inflammation, respiratory, upper, due to
  edematous 464.11
  influenzal (*see also* Influenza) 487.1
  streptococcal 034.0
  syphilitic 095.8
  tuberculous (*see also* Tuberculosis) 012.8 ☑
Trachelitis (nonvenereal) — *see also* Cervicitis 616.0
  trichomonal 131.09
Tracheobronchial — *see* condition
Tracheobronchitis — *see also* Bronchitis 490
  acute or subacute 466.0
    with bronchospasm or obstruction 466.0
  chronic 491.8
  influenzal (*see also* Influenza) 487.1
  senile 491.8
Tracheobronchomegaly (congenital) 748.3
  with bronchiectasis 494.0
    with (acute) exacerbation 494.1
  acquired 519.19
    with bronchiectasis 494.0
      with (acute) exacerbation 494.1
Tracheobronchopneumonitis — *see* Pneumonia, broncho
Tracheocele (external) (internal) 519.19
  congenital 748.3
Tracheomalacia 519.19
  congenital 748.3

Tracheopharyngitis (acute) 465.8
  chronic 478.9
    due to external agent — *see* Condition, respiratory, chronic, due to
    due to external agent — *see* Inflammation, respiratory, upper, due to
Tracheostenosis 519.19
  congenital 748.3
Tracheostomy
  attention to V55.0
  complication 519.00
  granuloma 519.09
  hemorrhage 519.09
  infection 519.01
  malfunctioning 519.02
  obstruction 519.09
  sepsis 519.01
  status V44.0
  stenosis 519.02
Trachoma, trachomatous 076.9
  active (stage) 076.1
  contraction of conjunctiva 076.1
  dubium 076.0
  healed or late effect 139.1
  initial (stage) 076.0
  Türck's (chronic catarrhal laryngitis) 476.0
Trachyphonia 784.49
Traction, vitreomacular 379.27
Training
  insulin pump V65.46
  orthoptic V57.4
  orthotic V57.81
Train sickness 994.6
Trait
  hemoglobin
    abnormal NEC 282.7
      with thalassemia 282.46
    C (*see also* Disease, hemoglobin, C) 282.7
      with elliptocytosis 282.7
    S (Hb-S) 282.5
    Lepore 282.49
      with other abnormal hemoglobin NEC 282.49
  paranoid 301.0
  sickle-cell 282.5
    with
      elliptocytosis 282.5
      spherocytosis 282.5
    thalassemia (alpha) (beta) (delta-beta) 282.46
Traits, paranoid 301.0
Tramp V60.0
Trance 780.09
  hysterical 300.13
Trans-sexualism 302.50
  with
    asexual history 302.51
    heterosexual history 302.53
    homosexual history 302.52
Transaminasemia 790.4
Transfusion, blood
  without reported diagnosis V58.2
  donor V59.01
    stem cells V59.02
  fetal twin to twin 678.0 ☑
  incompatible (*see also* Complications, transfusion) 999.80
    ABO (*see also* Complications, transfusion) 999.60
    minor blood group 999.89
    non-ABO (*see also* Complications, transfusion) 999.75
    Rh (antigen) (C) (c) (D) (E) (e) (*see also* Complications, transfusion) 999.70
  reaction or complication — *see* Complications, transfusion
  related acute lung injury (TRALI) 518.7
  syndrome
    fetomaternal 772.0
    twin-to-twin
      blood loss (donor twin) 772.0
      recipient twin 776.4
  twin to twin fetal 678.0 ☑
Transient — *see also* condition
  alteration of awareness 780.02

Transient — *see also* condition — continued
  blindness 368.12
  deafness (ischemic) 388.02
  global amnesia 437.7
  hyperglycemia (post-procedural) 790.29
  hypoglycemia (post-procedural) 251.2
  person (homeless) NEC V60.0
Transitional, lumbosacral joint of vertebra 756.19
Translocation
  autosomes NEC 758.5
    13-15 758.1
    16-18 758.2
    21 or 22 758.0
    balanced in normal individual 758.4
    D₁ 758.1
    E₃ 758.2
    G 758.0
  balanced autosomal in normal individual 758.4
  chromosomes NEC 758.89
  Down's syndrome 758.0
Translucency, iris 364.53
Transmission of chemical substances through the placenta (affecting fetus or newborn) 760.70
  alcohol 760.71
  anti-infective agents 760.74
  anticonvulsants 760.77
  antifungals 760.74
  antimetabolics 760.78
  cocaine 760.75
  "crack" 760.75
  diethylstilbestrol [DES] 760.76
  hallucinogenic agents 760.73
  medicinal agents NEC 760.79
  narcotics 760.72
  obstetric anesthetic or analgesic drug 763.5
  specified agent NEC 760.79
  suspected, affecting management of pregnancy 655.5 ☑
Transplant(ed)
  bone V42.4
    marrow V42.81
  complication (*see also* Complications, due to (presence of) any device, implant, or graft classified to 996.0–996.5 NEC)
    bone marrow 996.85
    corneal graft NEC 996.79
      infection or inflammation 996.69
      reaction 996.51
      rejection 996.51
    organ (failure) (immune or nonimmune cause) (infection) (rejection) 996.80
      bone marrow 996.85
      heart 996.83
      intestines 996.87
      kidney 996.81
      liver 996.82
      lung 996.84
      pancreas 996.86
      specified NEC 996.89
    previously removed due to complication, failure, rejection or infection V45.87
    removal status V45.87
    skin NEC 996.79
      infection or inflammation 996.69
      rejection 996.52
        artificial 996.55
        decellularized allodermis 996.55
    stem cell(s) 996.88
      from
        peripheral blood 996.88
        umbilical cord 996.88
  cornea V42.5
  hair V50.0
  heart V42.1
    valve V42.2
  intestine V42.84
  kidney V42.0
  liver V42.7
  lung V42.6

Transplant(ed) — continued
  organ V42.9
    specified NEC V42.89
  pancreas V42.83
  peripheral stem cells V42.82
  skin V42.3
  stem cells, peripheral V42.82
  tissue V42.9
    specified NEC V42.89
Transplants, ovarian, endometrial 617.1
Transposed — *see* Transposition
Transposition (congenital) — *see also* Malposition, congenital
  abdominal viscera 759.3
  aorta (dextra) 745.11
  appendix 751.5
  arterial trunk 745.10
  colon 751.5
  great vessels (complete) 745.10
    both originating from right ventricle 745.11
    corrected 745.12
    double outlet right ventricle 745.11
    incomplete 745.11
    partial 745.11
    specified type NEC 745.19
  heart 746.87
    with complete transposition of viscera 759.3
  intestine (large) (small) 751.5
  pulmonary veins 747.49
  reversed jejunal (for bypass) (status) V45.3
  scrotal 752.81
  stomach 750.7
    with general transposition of viscera 759.3
  teeth, tooth 524.30
  vessels (complete) 745.10
    partial 745.11
  viscera (abdominal) (thoracic) 759.3
Transverse — *see also* condition
  arrest (deep), in labor 660.3 ☑
    affecting fetus or newborn 763.1
  lie 652.3 ☑
    before labor, affecting fetus or newborn 761.7
    causing obstructed labor 660.0 ☑
      affecting fetus or newborn 763.1
    during labor, affecting fetus or newborn 763.1
Transvestism, transvestitism (transvestic fetishism) 302.3
Trapped placenta (with hemorrhage) 666.0 ☑
  without hemorrhage 667.0 ☑
Traumatic — *see also* condition
  brain injury (TBI) (*see also* Injury, intracranial) 854.0 ☑
    with skull fracture — *see* Fracture, skull, by site
Trauma, traumatism — *see also* Injury, by site 959.9
  birth — *see* Birth, injury NEC
  causing hemorrhage of pregnancy or delivery 641.8 ☑
  complicating
    abortion — *see* Abortion, by type, with damage to pelvic organs
    ectopic pregnancy (*see also* categories 633.0–633.9) 639.2
    molar pregnancy (*see also* categories 630–632) 639.2
  during delivery NEC 665.9 ☑
  following
    abortion 639.2
    ectopic or molar pregnancy 639.2
  maternal, during pregnancy, affecting fetus or newborn 760.5
  neuroma — *see* Injury, nerve, by site
  previous major, affecting management of pregnancy, childbirth, or puerperium V23.89
  psychic (current) (*see also* Reaction, adjustment)
    previous (history) V15.49
  psychologic, previous (affecting health) V15.49

Trauma, traumatism — *see also* Injury, by site — continued
  transient paralysis — *see* Injury, nerve, by site
Treacher Collins' syndrome (incomplete facial dysostosis) 756.0
Treitz's hernia — *see* Hernia, Treitz's
Trematode infestation NEC 121.9
Trematodiasis NEC 121.9
Trembles 988.8
Trembling paralysis — *see also* Parkinsonism 332.0
Tremor 781.0
  essential (benign) 333.1
  familial 333.1
  flapping (liver) 572.8
  hereditary 333.1
  hysterical 300.11
  intention 333.1
  medication-induced postural 333.1
  mercurial 985.0
  muscle 728.85
  Parkinson's (*see also* Parkinsonism) 332.0
  psychogenic 306.0
    specified as conversion reaction 300.11
  senilis 797
  specified type NEC 333.1
Trench
  fever 083.1
  foot 991.4
  mouth 101
  nephritis — *see* Nephritis, acute
Treponema pallidum infection — *see also* Syphilis 097.9
Treponematosis 102.9
  due to
    T. pallidum — *see* Syphilis
    T. pertenue (yaws) (*see also* Yaws) 102.9
Triad
  Kartagener's 759.3
  Reiter's (complete) (incomplete) 099.3
  Saint's (*see also* Hernia, diaphragm) 553.3
Trichiasis 704.2
  cicatricial 704.2
  eyelid 374.05
    with entropion (*see also* Entropion) 374.00
Trichinella spiralis (infection) (infestation) 124
Trichinelliasis 124
Trichinellosis 124
Trichiniasis 124
Trichinosis 124
Trichobezoar 938
  intestine 936
  stomach 935.2
Trichocephaliasis 127.3
Trichocephalosis 127.3
Trichocephalus infestation 127.3
Trichoclasis 704.2
Trichoepithelioma (M8100/0) — *see also* Neoplasm, skin, benign
  breast 217
  genital organ NEC — *see* Neoplasm, by site, benign
  malignant (M8100/3) — *see* Neoplasm, skin, malignant
Trichofolliculoma (M8101/0) — *see* Neoplasm, skin, benign
Tricholemmoma (M8102/0) — *see* Neoplasm, skin, benign
Trichomatosis 704.2
Trichomoniasis 131.9
  bladder 131.09
  cervix 131.09
  intestinal 007.3
  prostate 131.03
  seminal vesicle 131.09
  specified site NEC 131.8
  urethra 131.02
  urogenitalis 131.00
  vagina 131.01
  vulva 131.01
  vulvovaginal 131.01
Trichomycosis 039.0
  axillaris 039.0
  nodosa 111.2

☑ **Additional Digit Required — Refer to the Tabular List for Digit Selection**   ▽ **Subterms under main terms may continue to next column or page**

2014 ICD-9-CM   ▶◀ **Revised Text**   ● **New Line**   ▲ **Revised Code**   **Volume 2 — 283**

Trichomycosis — *continued*
  nodularis 111.2
  rubra 039.0
Trichonocardiosis (axillaris) (palmellina) 039.0
Trichonodosis 704.2
Trichophytide — *see* Dermatophytosis
Trichophytid, trichophyton infection — *see also* Dermatophytosis 110.9
Trichophytobezoar 938
  intestine 936
  stomach 935.2
Trichophytosis — *see* Dermatophytosis
Trichoptilosis 704.2
Trichorrhexis (nodosa) 704.2
Trichosporosis nodosa 111.2
Trichostasis spinulosa (congenital) 757.4
Trichostrongyliasis (small intestine) 127.6
Trichostrongylosis 127.6
Trichostrongylus (instabilis) infection 127.6
Trichotillomania 312.39
Trichromat, anomalous (congenital) 368.59
Trichromatopsia, anomalous (congenital) 368.59
Trichuriasis 127.3
Trichuris trichiuria (any site) (infection) (infestation) 127.3
Tricuspid (valve) — *see* condition
Trifid — *see also* Accessory
  kidney (pelvis) 753.3
  tongue 750.13
Trigeminal neuralgia — *see also* Neuralgia, trigeminal 350.1
Trigeminoencephaloangiomatosis 759.6
Trigeminy 427.89
  postoperative 997.1
Trigger finger (acquired) 727.03
  congenital 756.89
Trigonitis (bladder) (chronic) (pseudomembranous) 595.3
  tuberculous (*see also* Tuberculosis) 016.1 ☑
Trigonocephaly 756.0
Trihexosidosis 272.7
Trilobate placenta — *see* Placenta, abnormal
Trilocular heart 745.8
Trimethylaminuria 270.8
Tripartita placenta — *see* Placenta, abnormal
Triple — *see also* Accessory
  kidneys 753.3
  uteri 752.2
  X female 758.81
Triplegia 344.89
  congenital or infantile 343.8
Triplet
  affected by maternal complications of pregnancy 761.5
  healthy liveborn — *see* Newborn, multiple
  pregnancy (complicating delivery) NEC 651.1 ☑
    with fetal loss and retention of one or more fetus(es) 651.4 ☑
    following (elective) fetal reduction 651.7 ☑
Triplex placenta — *see* Placenta, abnormal
Triplication — *see* Accessory
Trismus 781.0
  neonatorum 771.3
  newborn 771.3
Trisomy (syndrome) NEC 758.5
  13 (partial) 758.1
  16-18 758.2
  18 (partial) 758.2
  21 (partial) 758.0
  22 758.0
  autosomes NEC 758.5
  D_1 758.1
  E_3 758.2
  G (group) 758.0
  group D_1 758.1
  group E 758.2
  group G 758.0
Tritanomaly 368.53
Tritanopia 368.53
Troisier-Hanot-Chauffard syndrome (bronze diabetes) 275.01
Trombidiosis 133.8
Trophedema (hereditary) 757.0

Trophedema — *continued*
  congenital 757.0
Trophoblastic disease — *see also* Hydatidiform mole 630
  previous, affecting management of pregnancy V23.1
Tropholymphedema 757.0
Trophoneurosis NEC 356.9
  arm NEC 354.9
  disseminated 710.1
  facial 349.89
  leg NEC 355.8
  lower extremity NEC 355.8
  upper extremity NEC 354.9
Tropical — *see also* condition
  maceration feet (syndrome) 991.4
  wet foot (syndrome) 991.4
Trouble — *see also* Disease
  bowel 569.9
  heart — *see* Disease, heart
  intestine 569.9
  kidney (*see also* Disease, renal) 593.9
  nervous 799.21
  sinus (*see also* Sinusitis) 473.9
Trousseau's syndrome (thrombophlebitis migrans) 453.1
Truancy, childhood — *see also* Disturbance, conduct
  socialized 312.2 ☑
  undersocialized, unsocialized 312.1 ☑
Truncus
  arteriosus (persistent) 745.0
  common 745.0
  communis 745.0
Trunk — *see* condition
Trychophytide — *see* Dermatophytosis
Trypanosoma infestation — *see* Trypanosomiasis
Trypanosomiasis 086.9
  with meningoencephalitis 086.9 [323.2]
  African 086.5
    due to Trypanosoma 086.5
      gambiense 086.3
      rhodesiense 086.4
  American 086.2
    with
      heart involvement 086.0
      other organ involvement 086.1
    without mention of organ involvement 086.2
  Brazilian — *see* Trypanosomiasis, American
  Chagas' — *see* Trypanosomiasis, American
  due to Trypanosoma
    cruzi — *see* Trypanosomiasis, American
    gambiense 086.3
    rhodesiense 086.4
  gambiensis, Gambian 086.3
  North American — *see* Trypanosomiasis, American
  rhodesiensis, Rhodesian 086.4
  South American — *see* Trypanosomiasis, American
Tsutsugamushi fever 081.2
Tubercle — *see also* Tuberculosis
  brain, solitary 013.2 ☑
  Darwin's 744.29
  epithelioid noncaseating 135
  Ghon, primary infection 010.0 ☑
Tuberculid, tuberculide (indurating) (lichenoid) (miliary) (papulonecrotic) (primary) (skin) (subcutaneous) — *see also* Tuberculosis 017.0 ☑
Tuberculoma — *see also* Tuberculosis
  brain (any part) 013.2 ☑
  meninges (cerebral) (spinal) 013.1 ☑
  spinal cord 013.4 ☑

Tuberculosis, tubercular, tuberculous (calcification) (calcified) (caseous) (chromogenic acid-fast bacilli) (congenital) (degeneration) (disease) (fibrocaseous) (fistula) (gangrene) (interstitial) (isolated circumscribed lesions) (necrosis) (parenchymatous) (ulcerative) 011.9 ☑

> *Note* — Use the following fifth-digit subclassification with categories 010–018:
>
> 0   unspecified
>
> 1   bacteriological or histological examination not done
>
> 2   bacteriological or histological examination unknown (at present)
>
> 3   tubercle bacilli found (in sputum) by microscopy
>
> 4   tubercle bacilli not found (in sputum) by microscopy, but found by bacterial culture
>
> 5   tubercle bacilli not found by bacteriological examination, but tuberculosis confirmed histologically
>
> 6   tubercle bacilli not found by bacteriological or histological examination, but tuberculosis confirmed by other methods [inoculation of animals]
>
> For tuberculous conditions specified as late effects or sequelae, see category 137.

  abdomen 014.8 ☑
    lymph gland 014.8 ☑
  abscess 011.9 ☑
    arm 017.9 ☑
    bone (*see also* Osteomyelitis, due to, tuberculosis) 015.9 ☑ [730.8]
      hip 015.1 ☑ [730.85]
      knee 015.2 ☑ [730.86]
      sacrum 015.0 ☑ [730.88]
      specified site NEC 015.7 ☑ [730.88]
      spinal 015.0 ☑ [730.88]
      vertebra 015.0 ☑ [730.88]
    brain 013.3 ☑
    breast 017.9 ☑
    Cowper's gland 016.5 ☑
    dura (mater) 013.8 ☑
      brain 013.3 ☑
      spinal cord 013.5 ☑
    epidural 013.8 ☑
      brain 013.3 ☑
      spinal cord 013.5 ☑
    frontal sinus — *see* Tuberculosis, sinus
    genital organs NEC 016.9 ☑
      female 016.7 ☑
      male 016.5 ☑
    genitourinary NEC 016.9 ☑
    gland (lymphatic) — *see* Tuberculosis, lymph gland
    hip 015.1 ☑
    iliopsoas 015.0 ☑ [730.88]
    intestine 014.8 ☑
    ischiorectal 014.8 ☑
    joint 015.9 ☑
      hip 015.1 ☑
      knee 015.2 ☑
      specified joint NEC 015.8 ☑
      vertebral 015.0 ☑ [730.88]
    kidney 016.0 ☑ [590.81]
    knee 015.2 ☑
    lumbar 015.0 ☑ [730.88]
    lung 011.2 ☑
      primary, progressive 010.8 ☑
    meninges (cerebral) (spinal) 013.0 ☑
    pelvic 016.9 ☑
      female 016.7 ☑
      male 016.5 ☑
    perianal 014.8 ☑
      fistula 014.8 ☑
    perinephritic 016.0 ☑ [590.81]

Tuberculosis, tubercular, tuberculous — *continued*
  abscess — *continued*
    perineum 017.9 ☑
    perirectal 014.8 ☑
    psoas 015.0 ☑ [730.88]
    rectum 014.8 ☑
    retropharyngeal 012.8 ☑
    sacrum 015.0 ☑ [730.88]
    scrofulous 017.2 ☑
    scrotum 016.5 ☑
    skin 017.0 ☑
      primary 017.0 ☑
    spinal cord 013.5 ☑
    spine or vertebra (column) 015.0 ☑ [730.88]
    strumous 017.2 ☑
    subdiaphragmatic 014.8 ☑
    testis 016.5 ☑
    thigh 017.9 ☑
    urinary 016.3 ☑
      kidney 016.0 ☑ [590.81]
    uterus 016.7 ☑
  accessory sinus — *see* Tuberculosis, sinus
  Addison's disease 017.6 ☑
  adenitis (*see also* Tuberculosis, lymph gland) 017.2 ☑
  adenoids 012.8 ☑
  adenopathy (*see also* Tuberculosis, lymph gland) 017.2 ☑
    tracheobronchial 012.1 ☑
      primary progressive 010.8 ☑
  adherent pericardium 017.9 ☑ [420.0]
  adnexa (uteri) 016.7 ☑
  adrenal (capsule) (gland) 017.6 ☑
  air passage NEC 012.8 ☑
  alimentary canal 014.8 ☑
  anemia 017.9 ☑
  ankle (joint) 015.8 ☑
    bone 015.5 ☑ [730.87]
  anus 014.8 ☑
  apex (*see also* Tuberculosis, pulmonary) 011.9 ☑
  apical (*see also* Tuberculosis, pulmonary) 011.9 ☑
  appendicitis 014.8 ☑
  appendix 014.8 ☑
  arachnoid 013.0 ☑
  artery 017.9 ☑
  arthritis (chronic) (synovial) 015.9 ☑ [711.40]
    ankle 015.8 ☑ [730.87]
    hip 015.1 ☑ [711.45]
    knee 015.2 ☑ [711.46]
    specified site NEC 015.8 ☑ [711.48]
    spine or vertebra (column) 015.0 ☑ [720.81]
    wrist 015.8 ☑ [730.83]
  articular — *see* Tuberculosis, joint
  ascites 014.0 ☑
  asthma (*see also* Tuberculosis, pulmonary) 011.9 ☑
  axilla, axillary 017.2 ☑
    gland 017.2 ☑
  bilateral (*see also* Tuberculosis, pulmonary) 011.9 ☑
  bladder 016.1 ☑
  bone (*see also* Osteomyelitis, due to, tuberculosis) 015.9 ☑ [730.8]
    hip 015.1 ☑ [730.85]
    knee 015.2 ☑ [730.86]
    limb NEC 015.5 ☑ [730.88]
    sacrum 015.0 ☑ [730.88]
    specified site NEC 015.7 ☑ [730.88]
    spinal or vertebral column 015.0 ☑ [730.88]
  bowel 014.8 ☑
    miliary 018.9 ☑
  brain 013.2 ☑
  breast 017.9 ☑
  broad ligament 016.7 ☑
  bronchi, bronchial, bronchus 011.3 ☑
    ectasia, ectasis 011.5 ☑
    fistula 011.3 ☑

Tuberculosis, tubercular, tuberculous — *continued*
  bronchi, bronchial, bronchus — *continued*
    fistula — *continued*
      primary, progressive 010.8 ☑
    gland 012.1 ☑
      primary, progressive 010.8 ☑
      isolated 012.2 ☑
      lymph gland or node 012.1 ☑
        primary, progressive 010.8 ☑
  bronchiectasis 011.5 ☑
  bronchitis 011.3 ☑
  bronchopleural 012.0 ☑
  bronchopneumonia, bronchopneumonic 011.6 ☑
  bronchorrhagia 011.3 ☑
  bronchotracheal 011.3 ☑
    isolated 012.2 ☑
  bronchus — *see* Tuberculosis, bronchi
  bronze disease (Addison's) 017.6 ☑
  buccal cavity 017.9 ☑
  bulbourethral gland 016.5 ☑
  bursa (*see also* Tuberculosis, joint) 015.9 ☑
  cachexia NEC (*see also* Tuberculosis, pulmonary) 011.9 ☑
  cardiomyopathy 017.9 ☑ *[425.8]*
  caries (*see also* Tuberculosis, bone) 015.9 ☑ *[730.8]*
  cartilage (*see also* Tuberculosis, bone) 015.9 ☑ *[730.8]*
    intervertebral 015.0 ☑ *[730.88]*
  catarrhal (*see also* Tuberculosis, pulmonary) 011.9 ☑
  cecum 014.8 ☑
  cellular tissue (primary) 017.0 ☑
  cellulitis (primary) 017.0 ☑
  central nervous system 013.9 ☑
    specified site NEC 013.8 ☑
  cerebellum (current) 013.2 ☑
  cerebral (current) 013.2 ☑
    meninges 013.0 ☑
  cerebrospinal 013.6 ☑
    meninges 013.0 ☑
  cerebrum (current) 013.2 ☑
  cervical 017.2 ☑
    gland 017.2 ☑
    lymph nodes 017.2 ☑
  cervicitis (uteri) 016.7 ☑
  cervix 016.7 ☑
  chest (*see also* Tuberculosis, pulmonary) 011.9 ☑
  childhood type or first infection 010.0 ☑
  choroid 017.3 ☑ *[363.13]*
  choroiditis 017.3 ☑ *[363.13]*
  ciliary body 017.3 ☑ *[364.11]*
  colitis 014.8 ☑
  colliers' 011.4 ☑
  colliquativa (primary) 017.0 ☑
  colon 014.8 ☑
    ulceration 014.8 ☑
  complex, primary 010.0 ☑
  complicating pregnancy, childbirth, or puerperium 647.3 ☑
    affecting fetus or newborn 760.2
  congenital 771.2
  conjunctiva 017.3 ☑ *[370.31]*
  connective tissue 017.9 ☑
    bone — *see* Tuberculosis, bone
  contact V01.1
  converter (tuberculin skin test) (without disease) 795.51
  cornea (ulcer) 017.3 ☑ *[370.31]*
  Cowper's gland 016.5 ☑
  coxae 015.1 ☑ *[730.85]*
  coxalgia 015.1 ☑ *[730.85]*
  cul-de-sac of Douglas 014.8 ☑
  curvature, spine 015.0 ☑ *[737.40]*
  cutis (colliquativa) (primary) 017.0 ☑
  cystitis 016.1 ☑
  cyst, ovary 016.6 ☑
  dacryocystitis 017.3 ☑ *[375.32]*
  dactylitis 015.5 ☑
  diarrhea 014.8 ☑

Tuberculosis, tubercular, tuberculous — *continued*
  diffuse (*see also* Tuberculosis, miliary) 018.9 ☑
    lung — *see* Tuberculosis, pulmonary
    meninges 013.0 ☑
  digestive tract 014.8 ☑
  disseminated (*see also* Tuberculosis, miliary) 018.9 ☑
    meninges 013.0 ☑
  duodenum 014.8 ☑
  dura (mater) 013.9 ☑
    abscess 013.8 ☑
      cerebral 013.3 ☑
      spinal 013.5 ☑
  dysentery 014.8 ☑
  ear (inner) (middle) 017.4 ☑
    bone 015.6 ☑
    external (primary) 017.0 ☑
    skin (primary) 017.0 ☑
  elbow 015.8 ☑
  emphysema — *see* Tuberculosis, pulmonary
  empyema 012.0 ☑
  encephalitis 013.6 ☑
  endarteritis 017.9 ☑
  endocarditis (any valve) 017.9 ☑ *[424.91]*
  endocardium (any valve) 017.9 ☑ *[424.91]*
  endocrine glands NEC 017.9 ☑
  endometrium 016.7 ☑
  enteric, enterica 014.8 ☑
  enteritis 014.8 ☑
  enterocolitis 014.8 ☑
  epididymis 016.4 ☑
  epididymitis 016.4 ☑
  epidural abscess 013.8 ☑
    brain 013.3 ☑
    spinal cord 013.5 ☑
  epiglottis 012.3 ☑
  episcleritis 017.3 ☑ *[379.00]*
  erythema (induratum) (nodosum) (primary) 017.1 ☑
  esophagus 017.8 ☑
  Eustachian tube 017.4 ☑
  exposure to V01.1
  exudative 012.0 ☑
    primary, progressive 010.1 ☑
  eye 017.3 ☑
  eyelid (primary) 017.0 ☑
    lupus 017.0 ☑ *[373.4]*
  fallopian tube 016.6 ☑
  fascia 017.9 ☑
  fauces 012.8 ☑
  finger 017.9 ☑
  first infection 010.0 ☑
  fistula, perirectal 014.8 ☑
  Florida 011.6 ☑
  foot 017.9 ☑
  funnel pelvis 137.3
  gallbladder 017.9 ☑
  galloping (*see also* Tuberculosis, pulmonary) 011.9 ☑
  ganglionic 015.9 ☑
  gastritis 017.9 ☑
  gastrocolic fistula 014.8 ☑
  gastroenteritis 014.8 ☑
  gastrointestinal tract 014.8 ☑
  general, generalized 018.9 ☑
    acute 018.0 ☑
    chronic 018.8 ☑
  genital organs NEC 016.9 ☑
    female 016.7 ☑
    male 016.5 ☑
  genitourinary NEC 016.9 ☑
  genu 015.2 ☑
  glandulae suprarenalis 017.6 ☑
  glandular, general 017.2 ☑
  glottis 012.3 ☑
  grinders' 011.4 ☑
  groin 017.2 ☑
  gum 017.9 ☑
  hand 017.9 ☑
  heart 017.9 ☑ *[425.8]*
  hematogenous — *see* Tuberculosis, miliary

Tuberculosis, tubercular, tuberculous — *continued*
  hemoptysis (*see also* Tuberculosis, pulmonary) 011.9 ☑
  hemorrhage NEC (*see also* Tuberculosis, pulmonary) 011.9 ☑
  hemothorax 012.0 ☑
  hepatitis 017.9 ☑
  hilar lymph nodes 012.1 ☑
    primary, progressive 010.8 ☑
  hip (disease) (joint) 015.1 ☑
    bone 015.1 ☑ *[730.85]*
  hydrocephalus 013.8 ☑
  hydropneumothorax 012.0 ☑
  hydrothorax 012.0 ☑
  hypoadrenalism 017.6 ☑
  hypopharynx 012.8 ☑
  ileocecal (hyperplastic) 014.8 ☑
  ileocolitis 014.8 ☑
  ileum 014.8 ☑
  iliac spine (superior) 015.0 ☑ *[730.88]*
  incipient NEC (*see also* Tuberculosis, pulmonary) 011.9 ☑
  indurativa (primary) 017.1 ☑
  infantile 010.0 ☑
  infection NEC 011.9 ☑
    without clinical manifestation 010.0 ☑
  infraclavicular gland 017.2 ☑
  inguinal gland 017.2 ☑
  inguinalis 017.2 ☑
  intestine (any part) 014.8 ☑
  iris 017.3 ☑ *[364.11]*
  iritis 017.3 ☑ *[364.11]*
  ischiorectal 014.8 ☑
  jaw 015.7 ☑ *[730.88]*
  jejunum 014.8 ☑
  joint 015.9 ☑
    hip 015.1 ☑
    knee 015.2 ☑
    specified site NEC 015.8 ☑
    vertebral 015.0 ☑ *[730.88]*
  keratitis 017.3 ☑ *[370.31]*
    interstitial 017.3 ☑ *[370.59]*
  keratoconjunctivitis 017.3 ☑ *[370.31]*
  kidney 016.0 ☑
  knee (joint) 015.2 ☑
  kyphoscoliosis 015.0 ☑ *[737.43]*
  kyphosis 015.0 ☑ *[737.41]*
  lacrimal apparatus, gland 017.3 ☑
  laryngitis 012.3 ☑
  larynx 012.3 ☑
  latent 795.51
  leptomeninges, leptomeningitis (cerebral) (spinal) 013.0 ☑
  lichenoides (primary) 017.0 ☑
  linguae 017.9 ☑
  lip 017.9 ☑
  liver 017.9 ☑
  lordosis 015.0 ☑ *[737.42]*
  lung — *see* Tuberculosis, pulmonary
  luposa 017.0 ☑
    eyelid 017.0 ☑ *[373.4]*
  lymphadenitis — *see* Tuberculosis, lymph gland
  lymphangitis — *see* Tuberculosis, lymph gland
  lymphatic (gland) (vessel) — *see* Tuberculosis, lymph gland
  lymph gland or node (peripheral) 017.2 ☑
    abdomen 014.8 ☑
    bronchial 012.1 ☑
      primary, progressive 010.8 ☑
    cervical 017.2 ☑
    hilar 012.1 ☑
      primary, progressive 010.8 ☑
    intrathoracic 012.1 ☑
      primary, progressive 010.8 ☑
    mediastinal 012.1 ☑
      primary, progressive 010.8 ☑
    mesenteric 014.8 ☑
    peripheral 017.2 ☑
    retroperitoneal 014.8 ☑
    tracheobronchial 012.1 ☑

Tuberculosis, tubercular, tuberculous — *continued*
  lymph gland or node — *continued*
    tracheobronchial — *continued*
      primary, progressive 010.8 ☑
  malignant NEC (*see also* Tuberculosis, pulmonary) 011.9 ☑
  mammary gland 017.9 ☑
  marasmus NEC (*see also* Tuberculosis, pulmonary) 011.9 ☑
  mastoiditis 015.6 ☑
  maternal, affecting fetus or newborn 760.2
  mediastinal (lymph) gland or node 012.1 ☑
    primary, progressive 010.8 ☑
  mediastinitis 012.8 ☑
    primary, progressive 010.8 ☑
  mediastinopericarditis 017.9 ☑ *[420.0]*
  mediastinum 012.8 ☑
    primary, progressive 010.8 ☑
  medulla 013.9 ☑
    brain 013.2 ☑
    spinal cord 013.4 ☑
  melanosis, Addisonian 017.6 ☑
  membrane, brain 013.0 ☑
  meninges (cerebral) (spinal) 013.0 ☑
  meningitis (basilar) (brain) (cerebral) (cerebrospinal) (spinal) 013.0 ☑
  meningoencephalitis 013.0 ☑
  mesentery, mesenteric 014.8 ☑
    lymph gland or node 014.8 ☑
  miliary (any site) 018.9 ☑
    acute 018.0 ☑
    chronic 018.8 ☑
    specified type NEC 018.8 ☑
  millstone makers' 011.4 ☑
  miners' 011.4 ☑
  moulders' 011.4 ☑
  mouth 017.9 ☑
  multiple 018.9 ☑
    acute 018.0 ☑
    chronic 018.8 ☑
  muscle 017.9 ☑
  myelitis 013.6 ☑
  myocarditis 017.9 ☑ *[422.0]*
  myocardium 017.9 ☑ *[422.0]*
  nasal (passage) (sinus) 012.8 ☑
  nasopharynx 012.8 ☑
  neck gland 017.2 ☑
  nephritis 016.0 ☑ *[583.81]*
  nerve 017.9 ☑
  nose (septum) 012.8 ☑
  ocular 017.3 ☑
  old NEC 137.0
    without residuals V12.01
  omentum 014.8 ☑
  oophoritis (acute) (chronic) 016.6 ☑
  optic 017.3 ☑ *[377.39]*
    nerve trunk 017.3 ☑ *[377.39]*
    papilla, papillae 017.3 ☑ *[377.39]*
  orbit 017.3 ☑
  orchitis 016.5 ☑ *[608.81]*
  organ, specified NEC 017.9 ☑
  orificialis (primary) 017.0 ☑
  osseous (*see also* Tuberculosis, bone) 015.9 ☑ *[730.8]* ☑
  osteitis (*see also* Tuberculosis, bone) 015.9 ☑ *[730.8]* ☑
  osteomyelitis (*see also* Tuberculosis, bone) 015.9 ☑ *[730.8]* ☑
  otitis (media) 017.4 ☑
  ovaritis (acute) (chronic) 016.6 ☑
  ovary (acute) (chronic) 016.6 ☑
  oviducts (acute) (chronic) 016.6 ☑
  pachymeningitis 013.0 ☑
  palate (soft) 017.9 ☑
  pancreas 017.9 ☑
  papulonecrotic (primary) 017.0 ☑
  parathyroid glands 017.9 ☑
  paronychia (primary) 017.0 ☑
  parotid gland or region 017.9 ☑
  pelvic organ NEC 016.9 ☑
    female 016.7 ☑
    male 016.5 ☑

☑ **Additional Digit Required** — Refer to the Tabular List for Digit Selection   ▽ **Subterms under main terms may continue to next column or page**

2014 ICD-9-CM   ▶◀ **Revised Text**   ● **New Line**   ▲ **Revised Code**   **Volume 2 — 285**

Tuberculosis, tubercular, tuberculous — *continued*
- pelvis (bony) 015.7 ☑ *[730.85]*
- penis 016.5 ☑
- peribronchitis 011.3 ☑
- pericarditis 017.9 ☑ *[420.0]*
- pericardium 017.9 ☑ *[420.0]*
- perichondritis, larynx 012.3 ☑
- perineum 017.9 ☑
- periostitis (*see also* Tuberculosis, bone) 015.9 ☑ *[730.8]* ☑
- periphlebitis 017.9 ☑
  - eye vessel 017.3 ☑ *[362.18]*
  - retina 017.3 ☑ *[362.18]*
- perirectal fistula 014.8 ☑
- peritoneal gland 014.8 ☑
- peritoneum 014.0 ☑
- peritonitis 014.0 ☑
- pernicious NEC (*see also* Tuberculosis, pulmonary) 011.9 ☑
- pharyngitis 012.8 ☑
- pharynx 012.8 ☑
- phlyctenulosis (conjunctiva) 017.3 ☑ *[370.31]*
- phthisis NEC (*see also* Tuberculosis, pulmonary) 011.9 ☑
- pituitary gland 017.9 ☑
- placenta 016.7 ☑
- pleura, pleural, pleurisy, pleuritis (fibrinous) (obliterative) (purulent) (simple plastic) (with effusion) 012.0 ☑
  - primary, progressive 010.1 ☑
- pneumonia, pneumonic 011.6 ☑
- pneumothorax 011.7 ☑
- polyserositis 018.9 ☑
  - acute 018.0 ☑
  - chronic 018.8 ☑
- potters' 011.4 ☑
- prepuce 016.5 ☑
- primary 010.9 ☑
  - complex 010.0 ☑
  - complicated 010.8 ☑
    - with pleurisy or effusion 010.1 ☑
  - progressive 010.8 ☑
    - with pleurisy or effusion 010.1 ☑
  - skin 017.0 ☑
- proctitis 014.8 ☑
- prostate 016.5 ☑ *[601.4]*
- prostatitis 016.5 ☑ *[601.4]*
- pulmonaris (*see also* Tuberculosis, pulmonary) 011.9 ☑
- pulmonary (artery) (incipient) (malignant) (multiple round foci) (pernicious) (reinfection stage) 011.9 ☑
  - cavitated or with cavitation 011.2 ☑
    - primary, progressive 010.8 ☑
  - childhood type or first infection 010.0 ☑
  - chromogenic acid-fast bacilli 795.39
  - fibrosis or fibrotic 011.4 ☑
  - infiltrative 011.0 ☑
    - primary, progressive 010.9 ☑
  - nodular 011.1 ☑
  - specified NEC 011.8 ☑
  - sputum positive only 795.39
  - status following surgical collapse of lung NEC 011.9 ☑
- pyelitis 016.0 ☑ *[590.81]*
- pyelonephritis 016.0 ☑ *[590.81]*
- pyemia — *see* Tuberculosis, miliary
- pyonephrosis 016.0 ☑
- pyopneumothorax 012.0 ☑
- pyothorax 012.0 ☑
- rectum (with abscess) 014.8 ☑
  - fistula 014.8 ☑
- reinfection stage (*see also* Tuberculosis, pulmonary) 011.9 ☑
- renal 016.0 ☑
- renis 016.0 ☑
- reproductive organ 016.7 ☑
- respiratory NEC (*see also* Tuberculosis, pulmonary) 011.9 ☑
  - specified site NEC 012.8 ☑
- retina 017.3 ☑ *[363.13]*

Tuberculosis, tubercular, tuberculous — *continued*
- retroperitoneal (lymph gland or node) 014.8 ☑
  - gland 014.8 ☑
- retropharyngeal abscess 012.8 ☑
- rheumatism 015.9 ☑
- rhinitis 012.8 ☑
- sacroiliac (joint) 015.8 ☑
- sacrum 015.0 ☑ *[730.88]*
- salivary gland 017.9 ☑
- salpingitis (acute) (chronic) 016.6 ☑
- sandblasters' 011.4 ☑
- sclera 017.3 ☑ *[379.09]*
- scoliosis 015.0 ☑ *[737.43]*
- scrofulous 017.2 ☑
- scrotum 016.5 ☑
- seminal tract or vesicle 016.5 ☑ *[608.81]*
- senile NEC (*see also* Tuberculosis, pulmonary) 011.9 ☑
- septic NEC (*see also* Tuberculosis, miliary) 018.9 ☑
- shoulder 015.8 ☑
  - blade 015.7 ☑ *[730.8]* ☑
- sigmoid 014.8 ☑
- sinus (accessory) (nasal) 012.8 ☑
  - bone 015.7 ☑ *[730.88]*
  - epididymis 016.4 ☑
- skeletal NEC (*see also* Osteomyelitis, due to tuberculosis) 015.9 ☑ *[730.8]* ☑
- skin (any site) (primary) 017.0 ☑
- small intestine 014.8 ☑
- soft palate 017.9 ☑
- spermatic cord 016.5 ☑
- spinal
  - column 015.0 ☑ *[730.88]*
  - cord 013.4 ☑
  - disease 015.0 ☑ *[730.88]*
  - medulla 013.4 ☑
  - membrane 013.0 ☑
  - meninges 013.0 ☑
- spine 015.0 ☑ *[730.88]*
- spleen 017.7 ☑
- splenitis 017.7 ☑
- spondylitis 015.0 ☑ *[720.81]*
- spontaneous pneumothorax — *see* Tuberculosis, pulmonary
- sternoclavicular joint 015.8 ☑
- stomach 017.9 ☑
- stonemasons' 011.4 ☑
- struma 017.2 ☑
- subcutaneous tissue (cellular) (primary) 017.0 ☑
- subcutis (primary) 017.0 ☑
- subdeltoid bursa 017.9 ☑
- submaxillary 017.9 ☑
  - region 017.9 ☑
- supraclavicular gland 017.2 ☑
- suprarenal (capsule) (gland) 017.6 ☑
- swelling, joint (*see also* Tuberculosis, joint) 015.9 ☑
- symphysis pubis 015.7 ☑ *[730.88]*
- synovitis 015.9 ☑ *[727.01]*
  - hip 015.1 ☑ *[727.01]*
  - knee 015.2 ☑ *[727.01]*
  - specified site NEC 015.8 ☑ *[727.01]*
  - spine or vertebra 015.0 ☑ *[727.01]*
- systemic — *see* Tuberculosis, miliary
- tarsitis (eyelid) 017.0 ☑ *[373.4]*
  - ankle (bone) 015.5 ☑ *[730.87]*
- tendon (sheath) — *see* Tuberculosis, tenosynovitis
- tenosynovitis 015.9 ☑ *[727.01]*
  - hip 015.1 ☑ *[727.01]*
  - knee 015.2 ☑ *[727.01]*
  - specified site NEC 015.8 ☑ *[727.01]*
  - spine or vertebra 015.0 ☑ *[727.01]*
- testis 016.5 ☑ *[608.81]*
- throat 012.8 ☑
- thymus gland 017.9 ☑
- thyroid gland 017.5 ☑
- toe 017.9 ☑
- tongue 017.9 ☑

Tuberculosis, tubercular, tuberculous — *continued*
- tonsil (lingual) 012.8 ☑
- tonsillitis 012.8 ☑
- trachea, tracheal 012.8 ☑
  - gland 012.1 ☑
    - primary, progressive 010.8 ☑
    - isolated 012.2 ☑
- tracheobronchial 011.3 ☑
  - glandular 012.1 ☑
    - primary, progressive 010.8 ☑
    - isolated 012.2 ☑
  - lymph gland or node 012.1 ☑
    - primary, progressive 010.8 ☑
- tubal 016.6 ☑
- tunica vaginalis 016.5 ☑
- typhlitis 014.8 ☑
- ulcer (primary) (skin) 017.0 ☑
  - bowel or intestine 014.8 ☑
  - specified site NEC — *see* Tuberculosis, by site
- unspecified site — *see* Tuberculosis, pulmonary
- ureter 016.2 ☑
- urethra, urethral 016.3 ☑
- urinary organ or tract 016.3 ☑
  - kidney 016.0 ☑
- uterus 016.7 ☑
- uveal tract 017.3 ☑ *[363.13]*
- uvula 017.9 ☑
- vaccination, prophylactic (against) V03.2
- vagina 016.7 ☑
- vas deferens 016.5 ☑
- vein 017.9 ☑
- verruca (primary) 017.0 ☑
- verrucosa (cutis) (primary) 017.0 ☑
- vertebra (column) 015.0 ☑ *[730.88]*
- vesiculitis 016.5 ☑ *[608.81]*
- viscera NEC 014.8 ☑
- vulva 016.7 ☑ *[616.51]*
- wrist (joint) 015.8 ☑
  - bone 015.5 ☑ *[730.83]*

Tuberculum
- auriculae 744.29
- occlusal 520.2
- paramolare 520.2

Tuberosity
- jaw, excessive 524.07
- maxillary, entire 524.07

Tuberous sclerosis (brain) 759.5

Tube, tubal, tubular — *see also* condition
- ligation, admission for V25.2

Tubo-ovarian — *see* condition

Tuboplasty, after previous sterilization V26.0

Tubotympanitis 381.10

Tularemia 021.9
- with
  - conjunctivitis 021.3
  - pneumonia 021.2
- bronchopneumonic 021.2
- conjunctivitis 021.3
- cryptogenic 021.1
- disseminated 021.8
- enteric 021.1
- generalized 021.8
- glandular 021.8
- intestinal 021.1
- oculoglandular 021.3
- ophthalmic 021.3
- pneumonia 021.2
- pulmonary 021.2
- specified NEC 021.8
- typhoidal 021.1
- ulceroglandular 021.0
- vaccination, prophylactic (against) V03.4

Tularensis conjunctivitis 021.3

Tumefaction — *see also* Swelling
- liver (*see also* Hypertrophy, liver) 789.1

Tumor (M8000/1) — *see also* Neoplasm, by site, unspecified nature
- Abrikossov's (M9580/0) (*see also* Neoplasm, connective tissue, benign)
  - malignant (M9580/3) — *see* Neoplasm, connective tissue, malignant

Tumor — *see also* Neoplasm, by site, unspecified nature — *continued*
- acinar cell (M8550/1) — *see* Neoplasm, by site, uncertain behavior
- acinic cell (M8550/1) — *see* Neoplasm, by site, uncertain behavior
- adenomatoid (M9054/0) (*see also* Neoplasm, by site, benign)
  - odontogenic (M9300/0) 213.1
    - upper jaw (bone) 213.0
- adnexal (skin) (M8390/0) — *see* Neoplasm, skin, benign
- adrenal
  - cortical (benign) (M8370/0) 227.0
    - malignant (M8370/3) 194.0
  - rest (M8671/0) — *see* Neoplasm, by site, benign
- alpha cell (M8152/0)
  - malignant (M8152/3)
    - pancreas 157.4
    - specified site NEC — *see* Neoplasm, by site, malignant
    - unspecified site 157.4
  - pancreas 211.7
  - specified site NEC — *see* Neoplasm, by site, benign
  - unspecified site 211.7
- aneurysmal (*see also* Aneurysm) 442.9
- aortic body (M8691/1) 237.3
  - malignant (M8691/3) 194.6
- argentaffin (M8241/1) — *see* Neoplasm, by site, uncertain behavior
- basal cell (M8090/1) (*see also* Neoplasm, skin, uncertain behavior)
- benign (M8000/0) — *see* Neoplasm, by site, benign
- beta cell (M8151/0)
  - malignant (M8151/3)
    - pancreas 157.4
    - specified site — *see* Neoplasm, by site, malignant
    - unspecified site 157.4
  - pancreas 211.7
  - specified site NEC — *see* Neoplasm, by site, benign
  - unspecified site 211.7
- blood — *see* Hematoma
- Brenner (M9000/0) 220
  - borderline malignancy (M9000/1) 236.2
  - malignant (M9000/3) 183.0
  - proliferating (M9000/1) 236.2
- Brooke's (M8100/0) — *see* Neoplasm, skin, benign
- brown fat (M8880/0) — *see* Lipoma, by site
- Burkitt's (M9750/3) 200.2 ☑
- calcifying epithelial odontogenic (M9340/0) 213.1
  - upper jaw (bone) 213.0
- carcinoid (M8240/1) 209.60
  - benign 209.60
    - appendix 209.51
    - ascending colon 209.53
    - bronchus 209.61
    - cecum 209.52
    - colon 209.50
    - descending colon 209.55
    - duodenum 209.41
    - foregut 209.65
    - hindgut 209.67
    - ileum 209.43
    - jejunum 209.42
    - kidney 209.64
    - large intestine 209.50
    - lung 209.61
    - midgut 209.66
    - rectum 209.57
    - sigmoid colon 209.56
    - small intestine 209.40
    - specified NEC 209.69
    - stomach 209.63
    - thymus 209.62
    - transverse colon 209.54
  - malignant (of) 209.20
    - appendix 209.11
    - ascending colon 209.13
    - bronchus 209.21

Tumor — see also Neoplasm, by site, unspecified nature — continued
carcinoid — continued
  malignant — continued
    cecum 209.12
    colon 209.10
    descending colon 209.15
    duodenum 209.01
    foregut 209.25
    hindgut 209.27
    ileum 209.03
    jejunum 209.02
    kidney 209.24
    large intestine 209.10
    lung 209.21
    midgut 209.26
    rectum 209.17
    sigmoid colon 209.16
    small intestine 209.00
    specified NEC 209.29
    stomach 209.23
    thymus 209.22
    transverse colon 209.14
  secondary — see Tumor, neuroendocrine, secondary
carotid body (M8692/1) 237.3
  malignant (M8692/3) 194.5
Castleman's (mediastinal lymph node hyperplasia) 785.6
cells (M8001/1) (see also Neoplasm, by site, unspecified nature)
  benign (M8001/0) — see Neoplasm, by site, benign
  malignant (M8001/3) — see Neoplasm, by site, malignant
  uncertain whether benign or malignant (M8001/1) — see Neoplasm, by site, uncertain nature
cervix
  in pregnancy or childbirth 654.6 ☑
    affecting fetus or newborn 763.89
    causing obstructed labor 660.2 ☑
      affecting fetus or newborn 763.1
chondromatous giant cell (M9230/0) — see Neoplasm, bone, benign
chromaffin (M8700/0) (see also Neoplasm, by site, benign)
  malignant (M8700/3) — see Neoplasm, by site, malignant
Cock's peculiar 706.2
Codman's (benign chondroblastoma) (M9230/0) — see Neoplasm, bone, benign
dentigerous, mixed (M9282/0) 213.1
  upper jaw (bone) 213.0
dermoid (M9084/0) — see Neoplasm, by site, benign
  with malignant transformation (M9084/3) 183.0
desmoid (extra-abdominal) (M8821/1) (see also Neoplasm, connective tissue, uncertain behavior)
  abdominal (M8822/1) — see Neoplasm, connective tissue, uncertain behavior
embryonal (mixed) (M9080/1) (see also Neoplasm, by site, uncertain behavior)
  liver (M9080/3) 155.0
endodermal sinus (M9071/3)
  specified site — see Neoplasm, by site, malignant
  unspecified site
    female 183.0
    male 186.9
epithelial
  benign (M8010/0) — see Neoplasm, by site, benign
  malignant (M8010/3) — see Neoplasm, by site, malignant
Ewing's (M9260/3) — see Neoplasm, bone, malignant
fatty — see Lipoma
fetal, causing disproportion 653.7 ☑
  causing obstructed labor 660.1 ☑
fibroid (M8890/0) — see Leiomyoma

Tumor — see also Neoplasm, by site, unspecified nature — continued
G cell (M8153/1)
  malignant (M8153/3)
    pancreas 157.4
    specified site NEC — see Neoplasm, by site, malignant
    unspecified site 157.4
  specified site — see Neoplasm, by site, uncertain behavior
  unspecified site 235.5
giant cell (type) (M8003/1) (see also Neoplasm, by site, unspecified nature)
  bone (M9250/1) 238.0
    malignant (M9250/3) — see Neoplasm, bone, malignant
  chondromatous (M9230/0) — see Neoplasm, bone, benign
  malignant (M8003/3) — see Neoplasm, by site, malignant
  peripheral (gingiva) 523.8
  soft parts (M9251/1) (see also Neoplasm, connective tissue, uncertain behavior)
    malignant (M9251/3) — see Neoplasm, connective tissue, malignant
  tendon sheath 727.02
glomus (M8711/0) (see also Hemangioma, by site)
  jugulare (M8690/1) 237.3
    malignant (M8690/3) 194.6
gonadal stromal (M8590/1) — see Neoplasm, by site, uncertain behavior
granular cell (M9580/0) (see also Neoplasm, connective tissue, benign)
  malignant (M9580/3) — see Neoplasm, connective tissue, malignant
granulosa cell-theca cell (M8621/1) 236.2
  malignant (M8621/3) 183.0
granulosa cell (M8620/1) 236.2
  malignant (M8620/3) 183.0
Grawitz's (hypernephroma) (M8312/3) 189.0
hazard-crile (M8350/3) 193
hemorrhoidal — see Hemorrhoids
hilar cell (M8660/0) 220
Hürthle cell (benign) (M8290/0) 226
  malignant (M8290/3) 193
hydatid (see also Echinococcus) 122.9
hypernephroid (M8311/1) (see also Neoplasm, by site, uncertain behavior)
interstitial cell (M8650/1) (see also Neoplasm, by site, uncertain behavior)
  benign (M8650/0) — see Neoplasm, by site, benign
  malignant (M8650/3) — see Neoplasm, by site, malignant
islet cell (M8150/0)
  malignant (M8150/3)
    pancreas 157.4
    specified site — see Neoplasm, by site, malignant
    unspecified site 157.4
  pancreas 211.7
  specified site NEC — see Neoplasm, by site, benign
  unspecified site 211.7
juxtaglomerular (M8361/1) 236.91
Krukenberg's (M8490/6) 198.6
Leydig cell (M8650/1)
  benign (M8650/0)
    specified site — see Neoplasm, by site, benign
    unspecified site
      female 220
      male 222.0
  malignant (M8650/3)
    specified site — see Neoplasm, by site, malignant
    unspecified site
      female 183.0
      male 186.9
  specified site — see Neoplasm, by site, uncertain behavior
  unspecified site
    female 236.2

Tumor — see also Neoplasm, by site, unspecified nature — continued
Leydig cell — continued
  unspecified site — continued
    male 236.4
lipid cell, ovary (M8670/0) 220
lipoid cell, ovary (M8670/0) 220
lymphomatous, benign (M9590/0) (see also Neoplasm, by site, benign)
lysis syndrome (following antineoplastic drug therapy) (spontaneous) 277.88
Malherbe's (M8110/0) — see Neoplasm, skin, benign
malignant (M8000/3) (see also Neoplasm, by site, malignant)
  fusiform (type) (M8004/3) — see Neoplasm, by site, malignant
  giant cell (type) (M8003/3) — see Neoplasm, by site, malignant
  mixed NEC (M8940/3) — see Neoplasm, by site, malignant
  small cell (type) (M8002/3) — see Neoplasm, by site, malignant
  spindle cell (type) (M8004/3) — see Neoplasm, by site, malignant
mast cell (M9740/1) 238.5
  malignant (M9740/3) 202.6 ☑
melanotic, neuroectodermal (M9363/0) — see Neoplasm, by site, benign
Merkel cell — see Carcinoma, Merkel cell
mesenchymal
  malignant (M8800/3) — see Neoplasm, connective tissue, malignant
  mixed (M8990/1) — see Neoplasm, connective tissue, uncertain behavior
mesodermal, mixed (M8951/3) (see also Neoplasm, by site, malignant)
  liver 155.0
mesonephric (M9110/1) (see also Neoplasm, by site, uncertain behavior)
  malignant (M9110/3) — see Neoplasm, by site, malignant
metastatic
  from specified site (M8000/3) — see Neoplasm, by site, malignant
  to specified site (M8000/6) — see Neoplasm, by site, malignant, secondary
mixed NEC (M8940/0) (see also Neoplasm, by site, benign)
  malignant (M8940/3) — see Neoplasm, by site, malignant
mucocarcinoid, malignant (M8243/3) — see Neoplasm, by site, malignant
mucoepidermoid (M8430/1) — see Neoplasm, by site, uncertain behavior
Müllerian, mixed (M8950/3) — see Neoplasm, by site, malignant
myoepithelial (M8982/0) — see Neoplasm, by site, benign
neuroendocrine 209.60
  malignant poorly differentiated 209.30
  secondary 209.70
    bone 209.73
    distant lymph nodes 209.71
    liver 209.72
    peritoneum 209.74
    site specified NEC 209.79
neurogenic olfactory (M9520/3) 160.0
nonencapsulated sclerosing (M8350/3) 193
odontogenic (M9270/1) 238.0
  adenomatoid (M9300/0) 213.1
    upper jaw (bone) 213.0
  benign (M9270/0) 213.1
    upper jaw (bone) 213.0
  calcifying epithelial (M9340/0) 213.1
    upper jaw (bone) 213.0
  malignant (M9270/3) 170.1
    upper jaw (bone) 170.0
  squamous (M9312/0) 213.1
    upper jaw (bone) 213.0
ovarian stromal (M8590/1) 236.2
ovary
  in pregnancy or childbirth 654.4 ☑
    affecting fetus or newborn 763.89

Tumor — see also Neoplasm, by site, unspecified nature — continued
ovary — continued
  in pregnancy or childbirth — continued
    causing obstructed labor 660.2 ☑
      affecting fetus or newborn 763.1
pacinian (M9507/0) — see Neoplasm, skin, benign
Pancoast's (M8010/3) 162.3
papillary — see Papilloma
pelvic, in pregnancy or childbirth 654.9 ☑
  affecting fetus or newborn 763.89
  causing obstructed labor 660.2 ☑
    affecting fetus or newborn 763.1
phantom 300.11
plasma cell (M9731/1) 238.6
  benign (M9731/0) — see Neoplasm, by site, benign
  malignant (M9731/3) 203.8 ☑
polyvesicular vitelline (M9071/3)
  specified site — see Neoplasm, by site, malignant
  unspecified site
    female 183.0
    male 186.9
Pott's puffy (see also Osteomyelitis) 730.2 ☑
Rathke's pouch (M9350/1) 237.0
regaud's (M8082/3) — see Neoplasm, nasopharynx, malignant
rete cell (M8140/0) 222.0
retinal anlage (M9363/0) — see Neoplasm, by site, benign
Rokitansky's 620.2
salivary gland type, mixed (M8940/0) (see also Neoplasm, by site, benign)
  malignant (M8940/3) — see Neoplasm, by site, malignant
Sampson's 617.1
Schloffer's (see also Peritonitis) 567.29
Schmincke (M8082/3) — see Neoplasm, nasopharynx, malignant
sebaceous (see also Cyst, sebaceous) 706.2
secondary (M8000/6) — see Neoplasm, by site, secondary
  carcinoid — see Tumor, neuroendocrine, secondary
  neuroendocrine — see Tumor, neuroendocrine, secondary
Sertoli-Leydig cell (M8631/0)
  specified site — see Neoplasm, by site, benign
  unspecified site
    female 220
    male 222.0
Sertoli cell (M8640/0)
  with lipid storage (M8641/0)
    specified site — see Neoplasm, by site, benign
    unspecified site
      female 220
      male 222.0
  specified site — see Neoplasm, by site, benign
  unspecified site
    female 220
    male 222.0
sex cord (-stromal) (M8590/1) — see Neoplasm, by site, uncertain behavior
skin appendage (M8390/0) — see Neoplasm, skin, benign
soft tissue
  benign (M8800/0) — see Neoplasm, connective tissue, benign
  malignant (M8800/3) — see Neoplasm, connective tissue, malignant
sternomastoid 754.1
stromal
  abdomen
    benign 215.5
    malignant NEC 171.5
    uncertain behavior 238.1
  digestive system 238.1
    benign 215.5
    malignant NEC 171.5
    uncertain behavior 238.1

☑ Additional Digit Required — Refer to the Tabular List for Digit Selection   ▽ Subterms under main terms may continue to next column or page

2014 ICD-9-CM   ▶◀ Revised Text   ● New Line   ▲ Revised Code   Volume 2 — 287

Tumor — *see also* Neoplasm, by site, unspecified nature — *continued*
  stromal — *continued*
    endometrium (endometrial) 236.0
    gastric 238.1
      benign 215.5
      malignant 151.9
      uncertain behavior 238.1
    gastrointestinal 238.1
      benign 215.5
      malignant NEC 171.9
      uncertain behavior 238.1
    intestine (small) 238.1
      benign 215.5
      malignant 152.9
      uncertain behavior 238.1
    stomach 238.1
      benign 215.5
      malignant 151.9
      uncertain behavior 238.1
  superior sulcus (lung) (pulmonary) (syndrome) (M8010/3) 162.3
  suprasulcus (M8010/3) 162.3
  sweat gland (M8400/1) (*see also* Neoplasm, skin, uncertain behavior)
    benign (M8400/0) — *see* Neoplasm, skin, benign
    malignant (M8400/3) — *see* Neoplasm, skin, malignant
  syphilitic brain 094.89
    congenital 090.49
  testicular stromal (M8590/1) 236.4
  theca-lutein (M8610/0) 220
  theca cell-granulosa cell (M8621/1) 236.2
  theca cell (M8600/0) 220
  turban (M8200/0) 216.4
  uterus
    in pregnancy or childbirth 654.1 ☑
      affecting fetus or newborn 763.89
      causing obstructed labor 660.2 ☑
        affecting fetus or newborn 763.1
  vagina
    in pregnancy or childbirth 654.7 ☑
      affecting fetus or newborn 763.89
      causing obstructed labor 660.2 ☑
        affecting fetus or newborn 763.1
  varicose (*see also* Varicose, vein) 454.9
  von Recklinghausen's (M9540/1) 237.71
  vulva
    in pregnancy or childbirth 654.8 ☑
      affecting fetus or newborn 763.89
      causing obstructed labor 660.2 ☑
        affecting fetus or newborn 763.1
  Warthin's (salivary gland) (M8561/0) 210.2
  White-Darier 757.39
  white (*see also* Tuberculosis, arthritis)
  Wilms' (nephroblastoma) (M8960/3) 189.0
  yolk sac (M9071/3)
    specified site — *see* Neoplasm, by site, malignant
    unspecified site
      female 183.0
      male 186.9
Tumorlet (M8040/1) — *see* Neoplasm, by site, uncertain behavior
Tungiasis 134.1
Tunica vasculosa lentis 743.39
Tunnel vision 368.45
Turban tumor (M8200/0) 216.4
Türck's trachoma (chronic catarrhal laryngitis) 476.0
Türk's syndrome (ocular retraction syndrome) 378.71
Turner-Kieser syndrome (hereditary osteo-onychodysplasia) 756.89
Turner-Varny syndrome 758.6
Turner's
  hypoplasia (tooth) 520.4
  syndrome 758.6
  tooth 520.4
Turricephaly 756.0
Tussis convulsiva — *see also* Whooping cough 033.9
Twiddler's syndrome (due to)
  automatic implantable defibrillator 996.04
  pacemaker 996.01

Twin
  affected by maternal complications of pregnancy 761.5
  conjoined 759.4
    fetal 678.1 ☑
  healthy liveborn — *see* Newborn, twin
  pregnancy (complicating delivery) NEC 651.0 ☑
    with fetal loss and retention of one fetus 651.3 ☑
    conjoined 678.1 ☑
    following (elective) fetal reduction 651.7 ☑
Twinning, teeth 520.2
Twist, twisted
  bowel, colon, or intestine 560.2
  hair (congenital) 757.4
  mesentery 560.2
  omentum 560.2
  organ or site, congenital NEC — *see* Anomaly, specified type NEC
  ovarian pedicle 620.5
    congenital 752.0
  umbilical cord — *see* Compression, umbilical cord
Twitch 781.0
Tylosis 700
  buccalis 528.6
  gingiva 523.8
  linguae 528.6
  palmaris et plantaris 757.39
Tympanism 787.3
Tympanites (abdominal) (intestine) 787.3
Tympanitis — *see* Myringitis
Tympanosclerosis 385.00
  involving
    combined sites NEC 385.09
      with tympanic membrane 385.03
    tympanic membrane 385.01
      with ossicles 385.02
        and middle ear 385.03
Tympanum — *see* condition
Tympany
  abdomen 787.3
  chest 786.7
Typhlitis — *see also* Appendicitis 541
Typhoenteritis 002.0
Typhogastric fever 002.0
Typhoid (abortive) (ambulant) (any site) (fever) (hemorrhagic) (infection) (intermittent) (malignant) (rheumatic) 002.0
  with pneumonia 002.0 [484.8]
  abdominal 002.0
  carrier (suspected) of V02.1
  cholecystitis (current) 002.0
  clinical (Widal and blood test negative) 002.0
  endocarditis 002.0 [421.1]
  inoculation reaction — *see* Complications, vaccination
  meningitis 002.0 [320.7]
  mesenteric lymph nodes 002.0
  myocarditis 002.0 [422.0]
  osteomyelitis (*see also* Osteomyelitis, due to, typhoid) 002.0 [730.8] ☑
  perichondritis, larynx 002.0 [478.71]
  pneumonia 002.0 [484.8]
  spine 002.0 [720.81]
  ulcer (perforating) 002.0
  vaccination, prophylactic (against) V03.1
  Widal negative 002.0
Typhomalaria (fever) — *see also* Malaria 084.6
Typhomania 002.0
Typhoperitonitis 002.0
Typhus (fever) 081.9
  abdominal, abdominalis 002.0
  African tick 082.1
  amarillic (*see also* Fever, Yellow) 060.9
  brain 081.9
  cerebral 081.9
  classical 080
  endemic (flea-borne) 081.0
  epidemic (louse-borne) 080
  exanthematic SAI 080
    brilli SAI 081.1
    Mexicanus SAI 081.0

Typhus — *continued*
  exanthematicus SAI — *continued*
    pediculo vestimenti causa 080
    typhus murinus 081.0
  exanthematic NEC 080
  flea-borne 081.0
  Indian tick 082.1
  Kenya tick 082.1
  louse-borne 080
  Mexican 081.0
    flea-borne 081.0
    louse-borne 080
    tabardillo 080
  mite-borne 081.2
  murine 081.0
  North Asian tick-borne 082.2
  petechial 081.9
  Queensland tick 082.3
  rat 081.0
  recrudescent 081.1
  recurrent (*see also* Fever, relapsing) 087.9
  São Paulo 082.0
  scrub (China) (India) (Malaya) (New Guinea) 081.2
  shop (of Malaya) 081.0
  Siberian tick 082.2
  tick-borne NEC 082.9
  tropical 081.2
  vaccination, prophylactic (against) V05.8
Tyrosinemia 270.2
  neonatal 775.89
Tyrosinosis (Medes) (Sakai) 270.2
Tyrosinuria 270.2
Tyrosyluria 270.2

U

Uehlinger's syndrome (acropachyderma) 757.39
Uhl's anomaly or disease (hypoplasia of myocardium, right ventricle) 746.84
Ulcerosa scarlatina 034.1
Ulcer, ulcerated, ulcerating, ulceration, ulcerative 707.9
  with gangrene 707.9 [785.4]
  abdomen (wall) (*see also* Ulcer, skin) 707.8
  ala, nose 478.19
  alveolar process 526.5
  amebic (intestine) 006.9
    skin 006.6
  anastomotic — *see* Ulcer, gastrojejunal
  anorectal 569.41
  antral — *see* Ulcer, stomach
  anus (sphincter) (solitary) 569.41
    varicose — *see* Varicose, ulcer, anus
  aorta — *see* Aneuysm
  aphthous (oral) (recurrent) 528.2
    genital organ(s)
      female 616.50
      male 608.89
    mouth 528.2
  arm (*see also* Ulcer, skin) 707.8
  arteriosclerotic plaque — *see* Arteriosclerosis, by site
  artery NEC 447.2
    without rupture 447.8
  atrophic NEC — *see* Ulcer, skin
  Barrett's (chronic peptic ulcer of esophagus) 530.85
  bile duct 576.8
  bladder (solitary) (sphincter) 596.89
    bilharzial (*see also* Schistosomiasis) 120.9 [595.4]
    submucosal (*see also* Cystitis) 595.1
    tuberculous (*see also* Tuberculosis) 016.1 ☑
  bleeding NEC — *see* Ulcer, peptic, with hemorrhage
  bone 730.9 ☑
  bowel (*see also* Ulcer, intestine) 569.82
  breast 611.0
  bronchitis 491.8
  bronchus 519.19
  buccal (cavity) (traumatic) 528.9
  burn (acute) — *see* Ulcer, duodenum
  Buruli 031.1
  buttock (*see also* Ulcer, skin) 707.8

Ulcer, ulcerated, ulcerating, ulceration, ulcerative — *continued*
  buttock (*see also* Ulcer, skin) — *continued*
    decubitus (*see also* Ulcer, pressure) 707.00
  cancerous (M8000/3) — *see* Neoplasm, by site, malignant
  cardia — *see* Ulcer, stomach
  cardio-esophageal (peptic) 530.20
    with bleeding 530.21
  cecum (*see also* Ulcer, intestine) 569.82
  cervix (uteri) (trophic) 622.0
    with mention of cervicitis 616.0
  chancroidal 099.0
  chest (wall) (*see also* Ulcer, skin) 707.8
  Chiclero 085.4
  chin (pyogenic) (*see also* Ulcer, skin) 707.8
  chronic (cause unknown) (*see also* Ulcer, skin)
    penis 607.89
  Cochin-China 085.1
  colitis — *see* Colitis, ulcerative
  colon (*see also* Ulcer, intestine) 569.82
  conjunctiva (acute) (postinfectional) 372.00
  cornea (infectional) 370.00
    with perforation 370.06
    annular 370.02
    catarrhal 370.01
    central 370.03
    dendritic 054.42
    marginal 370.01
    mycotic 370.05
    phlyctenular, tuberculous (*see also* Tuberculosis) 017.3 ☑ [370.31]
    ring 370.02
    rodent 370.07
    serpent, serpiginous 370.04
    superficial marginal 370.01
    tuberculous (*see also* Tuberculosis) 017.3 ☑ [370.31]
  corpus cavernosum (chronic) 607.89
  crural — *see* Ulcer, lower extremity
  Curling's — *see* Ulcer, duodenum
  Cushing's — *see* Ulcer, peptic
  cystitis (interstitial) 595.1
  decubitus (unspecified site) (*see also* Ulcer, pressure) 707.00
    with gangrene 707.00 [785.4]
    ankle 707.06
    back
      lower 707.03
      upper 707.02
    buttock 707.05
    coccyx 707.03
    elbow 707.01
    head 707.09
    heel 707.07
    hip 707.04
    other site 707.09
    sacrum 707.03
    shoulder blades 707.02
  dendritic 054.42
  diabetes, diabetic (mellitus) 250.8 ☑ [707.9]
    due to secondary diabetes 249.8 ☑ [707.9]
    lower limb 250.8 ☑ [707.10]
      ankle 250.8 ☑ [707.13]
        due to secondary diabetes 249.8 ☑ [707.13]
      calf 250.8 ☑ [707.12]
        due to secondary diabetes 249.8 ☑ [707.12]
        due to secondary diabetes 249.8 ☑ [707.10]
      foot 250.8 ☑ [707.15]
        due to secondary diabetes 249.8 ☑ [707.15]
      heel 250.8 ☑ [707.14]
        due to secondary diabetes 249.8 ☑ [707.14]
      knee 250.8 ☑ [707.19]
        due to secondary diabetes 249.8 ☑ [707.19]
      specified site NEC 250.8 ☑ [707.19]

Ulcer, ulcerated, ulcerating, ulceration, ulcerative — *continued*
diabetes, diabetic — *continued*
  lower limb — *continued*
    specified site — *continued*
      due to secondary diabetes
        249.8 ☑ *[707.19]*
      thigh 250.8 ☑ *[707.11]*
        due to secondary diabetes
          249.8 ☑ *[707.11]*
      toes 250.8 ☑ *[707.15]*
        due to secondary diabetes
          249.8 ☑ *[707.15]*
    specified site NEC 250.8 ☑ *[707.8]*
      due to secondary diabetes
        249.8 ☑ *[707.8]*
Dieulafoy — *see* Lesion, Dieulafoy
due to
  infection NEC — *see* Ulcer, skin
  radiation, radium — *see* Ulcer, by site
  trophic disturbance (any region) — *see* Ulcer, skin
  x-ray — *see* Ulcer, by site
duodenum, duodenal (eroded) (peptic) 532.9 ☑

Note — *Use the following fifth-digit subclassification with categories 531–534:*
0   *without mention of obstruction*
1   *with obstruction*

  with
    hemorrhage (chronic) 532.4 ☑
      and perforation 532.6 ☑
    perforation (chronic) 532.5 ☑
      and hemorrhage 532.6 ☑
  acute 532.3 ☑
    with
      hemorrhage 532.0 ☑
        and perforation 532.2 ☑
      perforation 532.1 ☑
        and hemorrhage 532.2 ☑
  bleeding (recurrent) — *see* Ulcer, duodenum, with hemorrhage
  chronic 532.7 ☑
    with
      hemorrhage 532.4 ☑
        and perforation 532.6 ☑
      perforation 532.5 ☑
        and hemorrhage 532.6 ☑
  penetrating — *see* Ulcer, duodenum, with perforation
  perforating — *see* Ulcer, duodenum, with perforation
dysenteric NEC 009.0
elusive 595.1
endocarditis (any valve) (acute) (chronic) (subacute) 421.0
enteritis — *see* Colitis, ulcerative
enterocolitis 556.0
epiglottis 478.79
esophagus (peptic) 530.20
  with bleeding 530.21
  due to ingestion
    aspirin 530.20
    chemicals 530.20
    medicinal agents 530.20
  fungal 530.20
  infectional 530.20
  varicose (*see also* Varix, esophagus) 456.1
    bleeding (*see also* Varix, esophagus, bleeding) 456.0
eyelid (region) 373.01
eye NEC 360.00
  dendritic 054.42
face (*see also* Ulcer, skin) 707.8
fauces 478.29
Fenwick (-Hunner) (solitary) (*see also* Cystitis) 595.1
fistulous NEC — *see* Ulcer, skin
foot (indolent) (*see also* Ulcer, lower extremity) 707.15
  perforating 707.15
    leprous 030.1
    syphilitic 094.0

Ulcer, ulcerated, ulcerating, ulceration, ulcerative — *continued*
foot (*see also* Ulcer, lower extremity) — *continued*
  trophic 707.15
  varicose 454.0
    inflamed or infected 454.2
frambesial, initial or primary 102.0
gallbladder or duct 575.8
gall duct 576.8
gangrenous (*see also* Gangrene) 785.4
gastric — *see* Ulcer, stomach
gastrocolic — *see* Ulcer, gastrojejunal
gastroduodenal — *see* Ulcer, peptic
gastroesophageal — *see* Ulcer, stomach
gastrohepatic — *see* Ulcer, stomach
gastrointestinal — *see* Ulcer, gastrojejunal
gastrojejunal (eroded) (peptic) 534.9 ☑

Note — *Use the following fifth-digit subclassification with categories 531–534:*
0   *without mention of obstruction*
1   *with obstruction*

  with
    hemorrhage (chronic) 534.4 ☑
      and perforation 534.6 ☑
    perforation 534.5 ☑
      and hemorrhage 534.6 ☑
  acute 534.3 ☑
    with
      hemorrhage 534.0 ☑
        and perforation 534.2 ☑
      perforation 534.1 ☑
        and hemorrhage 534.2 ☑
  bleeding (recurrent) — *see* Ulcer, gastrojejunal, with hemorrhage
  chronic 534.7 ☑
    with
      hemorrhage 534.4 ☑
        and perforation 534.6 ☑
      perforation 534.5 ☑
        and hemorrhage 534.6 ☑
  penetrating — *see* Ulcer, gastrojejunal, with perforation
  perforating — *see* Ulcer, gastrojejunal, with perforation
gastrojejunocolic — *see* Ulcer, gastrojejunal
genital organ
  female 629.89
  male 608.89
gingiva 523.8
gingivitis 523.10
glottis 478.79
granuloma of pudenda 099.2
groin (*see also* Ulcer, skin) 707.8
gum 523.8
gumma, due to yaws 102.4
hand (*see also* Ulcer, skin) 707.8
hard palate 528.9
heel (*see also* Ulcer, lower extremity) 707.14
  decubitus (*see also* Ulcer, pressure) 707.07
hemorrhoids 455.8
  external 455.5
  internal 455.2
hip (*see also* Ulcer, skin) 707.8
  decubitus (*see also* Ulcer, pressure) 707.04
Hunner's 595.1
hypopharynx 478.29
hypopyon (chronic) (subacute) 370.04
hypostaticum — *see* Ulcer, varicose
ileocolitis 556.1
ileum (*see also* Ulcer, intestine) 569.82
intestine, intestinal 569.82
  with perforation 569.83
  amebic 006.9
  duodenal — *see* Ulcer, duodenum
  granulocytopenic (with hemorrhage) 288.09
  marginal 569.82
  perforating 569.83
  small, primary 569.82
  stercoraceous 569.82

Ulcer, ulcerated, ulcerating, ulceration, ulcerative — *continued*
intestine, intestinal — *continued*
  stercoral 569.82
  tuberculous (*see also* Tuberculosis) 014.8 ☑
  typhoid (fever) 002.0
  varicose 456.8
ischemic 707.9
  lower extremity (*see also* Ulcer, lower extremity) 707.10
    ankle 707.13
    calf 707.12
    foot 707.15
    heel 707.14
    knee 707.19
    specified site NEC 707.19
    thigh 707.11
    toes 707.15
jejunum, jejunal — *see* Ulcer, gastrojejunal
keratitis (*see also* Ulcer, cornea) 370.00
knee — *see* Ulcer, lower extremity
labium (majus) (minus) 616.50
laryngitis (*see also* Laryngitis) 464.00
  with obstruction 464.01
larynx (aphthous) (contact) 478.79
  diphtheritic 032.3
leg — *see* Ulcer, lower extremity
lip 528.5
Lipschütz's 616.50
lower extremity (atrophic) (chronic) (neurogenic) (perforating) (pyogenic) (trophic) (tropical) 707.10
  with gangrene (*see also* Ulcer, lower extremity) 707.10 *[785.4]*
    arteriosclerotic 440.24
  ankle 707.13
    arteriosclerotic 440.23
      with gangrene 440.24
  calf 707.12
  decubitus (*see also* Ulcer, pressure) 707.00
    with gangrene 707.00 *[785.4]*
    ankle 707.06
    buttock 707.05
    heel 707.07
    hip 707.04
  foot 707.15
  heel 707.14
  knee 707.19
  specified site NEC 707.19
  thigh 707.11
  toes 707.15
  varicose 454.0
    inflamed or infected 454.2
luetic — *see* Ulcer, syphilitic
lung 518.89
  tuberculous (*see also* Tuberculosis) 011.2 ☑
malignant (M8000/3) — *see* Neoplasm, by site, malignant
marginal NEC — *see* Ulcer, gastrojejunal
meatus (urinarius) 597.89
Meckel's diverticulum 751.0
Meleney's (chronic undermining) 686.09
Mooren's (cornea) 370.07
mouth (traumatic) 528.9
mycobacterial (skin) 031.1
nasopharynx 478.29
navel cord (newborn) 771.4
neck (*see also* Ulcer, skin) 707.8
  uterus 622.0
neurogenic NEC — *see* Ulcer, skin
nose, nasal (infectional) (passage) 478.19
  septum 478.19
    varicose 456.8
skin — *see* Ulcer, skin
spirochetal NEC 104.8
oral mucosa (traumatic) 528.9
palate (soft) 528.9
penetrating NEC — *see* Ulcer, peptic, with perforation
penis (chronic) 607.89

Ulcer, ulcerated, ulcerating, ulceration, ulcerative — *continued*
peptic (site unspecified) 533.9 ☑

Note — *Use the following fifth-digit subclassification with categories 531–534:*
0   *without mention of obstruction*
1   *with obstruction*

  with
    hemorrhage 533.4 ☑
      and perforation 533.6 ☑
    perforation (chronic) 533.5 ☑
      and hemorrhage 533.6 ☑
  acute 533.3 ☑
    with
      hemorrhage 533.0 ☑
        and perforation 533.2 ☑
      perforation 533.1 ☑
        and hemorrhage 533.2 ☑
  bleeding (recurrent) — *see* Ulcer, peptic, with hemorrhage
  chronic 533.7 ☑
    with
      hemorrhage 533.4 ☑
        and perforation 533.6 ☑
      perforation 533.5 ☑
        and hemorrhage 533.6 ☑
  penetrating — *see* Ulcer, peptic, with perforation
  perforating NEC (*see also* Ulcer, peptic, with perforation) 533.5 ☑
skin 707.9
perineum (*see also* Ulcer, skin) 707.8
peritonsillar 474.8
phagedenic (tropical) NEC — *see* Ulcer, skin
pharynx 478.29
phlebitis — *see* Phlebitis
plaster (*see also* Ulcer, pressure) 707.00
popliteal space — *see* Ulcer, lower extremity
postpyloric — *see* Ulcer, duodenum
prepuce 607.89
prepyloric — *see* Ulcer, stomach
pressure 707.00
  with
    abrasion, blister, partial thickness skin loss involving epidermis and/or dermis 707.22
    full thickness skin loss involving damage or necrosis of subcutaneous tissue 707.23
    gangrene 707.00 *[785.4]*
    necrosis of soft tissue through to underlying muscle, tendon, or bone 707.24
  ankle 707.06
  back
    lower 707.03
    upper 707.02
  buttock 707.05
  coccyx 707.03
  elbow 707.01
  head 707.09
  healed — omit code
  healing — code to Ulcer, pressure, by stage
  heel 707.07
  hip 707.04
  other site 707.09
  sacrum 707.03
  shoulder blades 707.02
  stage
    I (healing) 707.21
    II (healing) 707.22
    III (healing) 707.23
    IV (healing) 707.24
    unspecified (healing) 707.20
  unstageable 707.25
primary of intestine 569.82
  with perforation 569.83
proctitis 556.2
  with ulcerative sigmoiditis 556.3
prostate 601.8
pseudopeptic — *see* Ulcer, peptic
pyloric — *see* Ulcer, stomach

☑ **Additional Digit Required** — Refer to the Tabular List for Digit Selection   ▽ **Subterms under main terms may continue to next column or page**

Ulcer, ulcerated, ulcerating, ulceration, ulcerative — *continued*
  rectosigmoid 569.82
    with perforation 569.83
  rectum (sphincter) (solitary) 569.41
    stercoraceous, stercoral 569.41
    varicose — *see* Varicose, ulcer, anus
  retina (*see also* Chorioretinitis) 363.20
  rodent (M8090/3) (*see also* Neoplasm, skin, malignant)
    cornea 370.07
  round — *see* Ulcer, stomach
  sacrum (region) (*see also* Ulcer, skin) 707.8
  Saemisch's 370.04
  scalp (*see also* Ulcer, skin) 707.8
  sclera 379.09
  scrofulous (*see also* Tuberculosis) 017.2 ☑
  scrotum 608.89
    tuberculous (*see also* Tuberculosis) 016.5 ☑
    varicose 456.4
  seminal vesicle 608.89
  sigmoid 569.82
    with perforation 569.83
  skin (atrophic) (chronic) (neurogenic) (non-healing) (perforating) (pyogenic) (trophic) 707.9
    with gangrene 707.9 *[785.4]*
    amebic 006.6
    decubitus (*see also* Ulcer, pressure) 707.00
      with gangrene 707.00 *[785.4]*
      in granulocytopenia 288.09
    lower extremity (*see also* Ulcer, lower extremity) 707.10
      with gangrene 707.10 *[785.4]*
        arteriosclerotic 440.24
      ankle 707.13
      arteriosclerotic 440.23
        with gangrene 440.24
      calf 707.12
      foot 707.15
      heel 707.14
      knee 707.19
      specified site NEC 707.19
      thigh 707.11
      toes 707.15
    mycobacterial 031.1
    syphilitic (early) (secondary) 091.3
    tuberculous (primary) (*see also* Tuberculosis) 017.0 ☑
    varicose — *see* Ulcer, varicose
  sloughing NEC — *see* Ulcer, skin
  soft palate 528.9
  solitary, anus or rectum (sphincter) 569.41
  sore throat 462
    streptococcal 034.0
  spermatic cord 608.89
  spine (tuberculous) 015.0 ☑ *[730.88]*
  stasis (leg) (venous) 454.0
    with varicose veins 454.0
    without varicose veins 459.81
    inflamed or infected 454.2
  stercoral, stercoraceous 569.82
    with perforation 569.83
    anus or rectum 569.41
  stoma, stomal — *see* Ulcer, gastrojejunal
  stomach (eroded) (peptic) (round) 531.9 ☑

> *Note* — Use the following fifth-digit subclassification with categories 531–534:
>
> 0   *without mention of obstruction*
>
> 1   *with obstruction*

    with
      hemorrhage 531.4 ☑
        and perforation 531.6 ☑
      perforation (chronic) 531.5 ☑
        and hemorrhage 531.6 ☑
      acute 531.3 ☑
        with
          hemorrhage 531.0 ☑
            and perforation 531.2 ☑
          perforation 531.1 ☑
            and hemorrhage 531.2 ☑

Ulcer, ulcerated, ulcerating, ulceration, ulcerative — *continued*
  stomach — *continued*
    bleeding (recurrent) — *see* Ulcer, stomach, with hemorrhage
    chronic 531.7 ☑
      with
        hemorrhage 531.4 ☑
          and perforation 531.6 ☑
        perforation 531.5 ☑
          and hemorrhage 531.6 ☑
    penetrating — *see* Ulcer, stomach, with perforation
    perforating — *see* Ulcer, stomach, with perforation
  stomatitis 528.00
  stress — *see* Ulcer, peptic
  strumous (tuberculous) (*see also* Tuberculosis) 017.2 ☑
  submental (*see also* Ulcer, skin) 707.8
  submucosal, bladder 595.1
  syphilitic (any site) (early) (secondary) 091.3
    late 095.9
    perforating 095.9
      foot 094.0
  testis 608.89
  thigh — *see* Ulcer, lower extremity
  throat 478.29
    diphtheritic 032.0
  toe — *see* Ulcer, lower extremity
  tongue (traumatic) 529.0
  tonsil 474.8
    diphtheritic 032.0
  trachea 519.19
  trophic — *see* Ulcer, skin
  tropical NEC (*see also* Ulcer, skin) 707.9
  tuberculous — *see* Tuberculosis, ulcer
  tunica vaginalis 608.89
  turbinate 730.9 ☑
  typhoid (fever) 002.0
    perforating 002.0
  umbilicus (newborn) 771.4
  unspecified site NEC — *see* Ulcer, skin
  urethra (meatus) (*see also* Urethritis) 597.89
  uterus 621.8
    cervix 622.0
      with mention of cervicitis 616.0
    neck 622.0
      with mention of cervicitis 616.0
  vagina 616.89
  valve, heart 421.0
  varicose (lower extremity, any part) 454.0
    anus — *see* Varicose, ulcer, anus
    broad ligament 456.5
    esophagus (*see also* Varix, esophagus) 456.1
      bleeding (*see also* Varix, esophagus, bleeding) 456.0
    inflamed or infected 454.2
    nasal septum 456.8
    perineum 456.6
    rectum — *see* Varicose, ulcer, anus
    scrotum 456.4
    specified site NEC 456.8
    sublingual 456.3
    vulva 456.6
  vas deferens 608.89
  vesical (*see also* Ulcer, bladder) 596.89
  vulva (acute) (infectional) 616.50
    Behçet's syndrome 136.1 *[616.51]*
    herpetic 054.12
    tuberculous 016.7 ☑ *[616.51]*
  vulvobuccal, recurring 616.50
  x-ray — *see* Ulcer, by site
  yaws 102.4
Ulcus — *see also* Ulcer
  cutis tuberculosum (*see also* Tuberculosis) 017.0 ☑
  duodeni — *see* Ulcer, duodenum
  durum 091.0
    extragenital 091.2
  gastrojejunale — *see* Ulcer, gastrojejunal
  hypostaticum — *see* Ulcer, varicose
  molle (cutis) (skin) 099.0
  serpens corneae (pneumococcal) 370.04
  ventriculi — *see* Ulcer, stomach

Ulegyria 742.4
Ulerythema
  acneiforma 701.8
  centrifugum 695.4
  ophryogenes 757.4
Ullrich-Feichtiger syndrome 759.89
Ullrich (-Bonnevie) (-Turner) syndrome 758.6
Ulnar — *see* condition
Ulorrhagia 523.8
Ulorrhea 523.8
Umbilicus, umbilical — *see also* condition
  cord necrosis, affecting fetus or newborn 762.6
Unacceptable
  existing dental restoration
    contours 525.65
    morphology 525.65
Unavailability of medical facilities (at) V63.9
  due to
    investigation by social service agency V63.8
    lack of services at home V63.1
    remoteness from facility V63.0
    waiting list V63.2
    home V63.1
    outpatient clinic V63.0
    specified reason NEC V63.8
Uncinaria americana infestation 126.1
Uncinariasis — *see also* Ancylostomiasis 126.9
Unconscious, unconsciousness 780.09
Underdevelopment — *see also* Undeveloped
  sexual 259.0
Underfill, endodontic 526.63
Undernourishment 269.9
Undernutrition 269.9
Under observation — *see* Observation
Underweight 783.22
  for gestational age — *see* Light-for-dates
Underwood's disease (sclerema neonatorum) 778.1
Undescended — *see also* Malposition, congenital
  cecum 751.4
  colon 751.4
  testis 752.51
Undetermined diagnosis or cause 799.9
Undeveloped, undevelopment — *see also* Hypoplasia
  brain (congenital) 742.1
  cerebral (congenital) 742.1
  fetus or newborn 764.9 ☑
  heart 746.89
  lung 748.5
  testis 257.2
  uterus 259.0
Undiagnosed (disease) 799.9
Undulant fever — *see also* Brucellosis 023.9
Unemployment, anxiety concerning V62.0
Unequal leg (acquired) (length) 736.81
  congenital 755.30
Unerupted teeth, tooth 520.6
Unextracted dental root 525.3
Unguis incarnatus 703.0
Unicornis uterus 752.33
Unicornuate uterus (with or without a separate uterine horn) 752.33
Unicorporeus uterus 752.39
Uniformis uterus 752.39
Unilateral — *see also* condition
  development, breast 611.89
  organ or site, congenital NEC — *see* Agenesis
  vagina 752.49
Unilateralis uterus 752.39
Unilocular heart 745.8
Uninhibited bladder 596.54
  with cauda equina syndrome 344.61
  neurogenic — *see also* Neurogenic, bladder 596.54
Union, abnormal — *see also* Fusion
  divided tendon 727.89
  larynx and trachea 748.3
Universal
  joint, cervix 620.6
  mesentery 751.4

Unknown
  cause of death 799.9
  diagnosis 799.9
Unna's disease (seborrheic dermatitis) 690.10
Unresponsiveness, adrenocorticotropin (ACTH) 255.41
Unsatisfactory
  cytology smear
    anal 796.78
    cervical 795.08
    vaginal 795.18
  restoration, tooth (existing) 525.60
    specified NEC 525.69
Unsoundness of mind — *see also* Psychosis 298.9
Unspecified cause of death 799.9
Unstable
  back NEC 724.9
  colon 569.89
  joint — *see* Instability, joint
  lie 652.0 ☑
    affecting fetus or newborn (before labor) 761.7
    causing obstructed labor 660.0 ☑
      affecting fetus or newborn 763.1
  lumbosacral joint (congenital) 756.19
    acquired 724.6
  sacroiliac 724.6
  spine NEC 724.9
Untruthfulness, child problem — *see also* Disturbance, conduct 312.0 ☑
Unverricht-Wagner syndrome (dermatomyositis) 710.3
Unverricht (-Lundborg) disease, syndrome, or epilepsy 345.1 ☑
Upper respiratory — *see* condition
Upset
  gastric 536.8
    psychogenic 306.4
  gastrointestinal 536.8
    psychogenic 306.4
    virus (*see also* Enteritis, viral) 008.8
  intestinal (large) (small) 564.9
    psychogenic 306.4
  menstruation 626.9
  mental 300.9
  stomach 536.8
    psychogenic 306.4
Urachus — *see also* condition
  patent 753.7
  persistent 753.7
Uratic arthritis 274.00
Urbach-Oppenheim disease or syndrome (necrobiosis lipoidica diabeticorum) 250.8 ☑ *[709.3]*
  due to secondary diabetes 249.8 ☑ *[709.3]*
Urbach-Wiethe disease or syndrome (lipoid proteinosis) 272.8
Urbach's lipoid proteinosis 272.8
Urban yellow fever 060.1
Urea, blood, high — *see* Uremia
Uremia, uremic (absorption) (amaurosis) (amblyopia) (aphasia) (apoplexy) (coma) (delirium) (dementia) (dropsy) (dyspnea) (fever) (intoxication) (mania) (paralysis) (poisoning) (toxemia) (vomiting) 586
  with
    abortion — *see* Abortion, by type, with renal failure
    ectopic pregnancy (*see also* categories 633.0–633.9) 639.3
    hypertension (*see also* Hypertension, kidney) 403.91
    molar pregnancy (*see also* categories 630–632) 639.3
  chronic 585.9
  complicating
    abortion 639.3
    ectopic or molar pregnancy 639.3
    hypertension (*see also* Hypertension, kidney) 403.91
    labor and delivery 669.3 ☑
  congenital 779.89
  extrarenal 788.99
  hypertensive (chronic) (*see also* Hypertension, kidney) 403.91

☑ **Additional Digit Required** — Refer to the Tabular List for Digit Selection   ▽ **Subterms under main terms may continue to next column or page**

290 — Volume 2   ►◄ Revised Text   ● New Line   ▲ Revised Code   2014 ICD-9-CM

Uremia, uremic — *continued*
   maternal NEC, affecting fetus or newborn
      760.1
   neuropathy 585.9 *[357.4]*
   pericarditis 585.9 *[420.0]*
   prerenal 788.99
   pyelitic (*see also* Pyelitis) 590.80
Ureteralgia 788.0
Ureterectasis 593.89
Ureteritis 593.89
   cystica 590.3
   due to calculus 592.1
   gonococcal (acute) 098.19
      chronic or duration of 2 months or over
         098.39
   nonspecific 593.89
Ureterocele (acquired) 593.89
   congenital 753.23
Ureterolith 592.1
Ureterolithiasis 592.1
Ureterostomy status V44.6
   with complication 997.5
Ureter, ureteral — *see* condition
Urethralgia 788.99
Urethra, urethral — *see* condition
Urethritis (abacterial) (acute) (allergic) (anteri-
   or) (chronic) (nonvenereal) (posterior)
   (recurrent) (simple) (subacute) (ulcerative) (undifferentiated) 597.80
   diplococcal (acute) 098.0
      chronic or duration of 2 months or over
         098.2
   due to Trichomonas (vaginalis) 131.02
   gonococcal (acute) 098.0
      chronic or duration of 2 months or over
         098.2
   nongonococcal (sexually transmitted)
      099.40
      Chlamydia trachomatis 099.41
      Reiter's 099.3
      specified organism NEC 099.49
   nonspecific (sexually transmitted) (*see also*
      Urethritis, nongonococcal) 099.40
   not sexually transmitted 597.80
   Reiter's 099.3
   trichomonal or due to Trichomonas (vagi-
      nalis) 131.02
   tuberculous (*see also* Tuberculosis) 016.3 ☑
   venereal NEC (*see also* Urethritis, nongono-
      coccal) 099.40
Urethro-oculoarticular syndrome 099.3
Urethro-oculosynovial syndrome 099.3
Urethrocele
   female 618.03
      with uterine prolapse 618.4
         complete 618.3
         incomplete 618.2
   male 599.5
Urethrolithiasis 594.2
Urethrorectal — *see* condition
Urethrorrhagia 599.84
Urethrorrhea 788.7
Urethrostomy status V44.6
   with complication 997.5

Urethrotrigonitis 595.3
Urethrovaginal — *see* condition
Urgency
   fecal 787.63
   hypertensive — *see* Hypertension
Urhidrosis, uridrosis 705.89
Uric acid
   diathesis 274.9
   in blood 790.6
Uricacidemia 790.6
Uricemia 790.6
Uricosuria 791.9
Urination
   frequent 788.41
   painful 788.1
   urgency 788.63
Urinemia — *see* Uremia
Urine, urinary — *see also* condition
   abnormality NEC 788.69
   blood in (*see also* Hematuria) 599.70
   discharge, excessive 788.42
   enuresis 788.30
      nonorganic origin 307.6
   extravasation 788.8
   frequency 788.41
   hesitancy 788.64
   incontinence 788.30
      active 788.30
      female 788.30
         stress 625.6
            and urge 788.33
      male 788.30
         stress 788.32
            and urge 788.33
      mixed (stress and urge) 788.33
      neurogenic 788.39
      nonorganic origin 307.6
      overflow 788.38
      stress (female) 625.6
         male NEC 788.32
   intermittent stream 788.61
   pus in 791.9
   retention or stasis NEC 788.20
      bladder, incomplete emptying 788.21
      psychogenic 306.53
      specified NEC 788.29
   secretion
      deficient 788.5
      excessive 788.42
      frequency 788.41
   strain 788.65
   stream
      intermittent 788.61
      slowing 788.62
      splitting 788.61
      weak 788.62
   urgency 788.63
Urinoma NEC 599.9
   bladder 596.89
   kidney 593.89
   renal 593.89
   ureter 593.89
   urethra 599.84
Uroarthritis, infectious 099.3

Urodialysis 788.5
Urolithiasis 592.9
Uronephrosis 593.89
Uropathy 599.9
   obstructive 599.60
Urosepsis 599.0
   meaning sepsis 995.91
   meaning urinary tract infection 599.0
Urticaria 708.9
   with angioneurotic edema 995.1
      hereditary 277.6
   allergic 708.0
   cholinergic 708.5
   chronic 708.8
   cold, familial 708.2
   dermatographic 708.3
   due to
      cold or heat 708.2
      drugs 708.0
      food 708.0
      inhalants 708.0
      plants 708.8
      serum 999.59
   factitial 708.3
   giant 995.1
      hereditary 277.6
   gigantea 995.1
      hereditary 277.6
   idiopathic 708.1
   larynx 995.1
      hereditary 277.6
   neonatorum 778.8
   nonallergic 708.1
   papulosa (Hebra) 698.2
   perstans hemorrhagica 757.39
   pigmentosa 757.33
   recurrent periodic 708.8
   serum 999.59
   solare 692.72
   specified type NEC 708.8
   thermal (cold) (heat) 708.2
   vibratory 708.4
Urticarioides acarodermatitis 133.9
Use of
   agents affecting estrogen receptors and
      estrogen levels NEC V07.59
   anastrozole (Arimidex) V07.52
   aromatase inhibitors V07.52
   estrogen receptor downregulators V07.59
   exemestane (Aromasin) V07.52
   fulvestrant (Faslodex) V07.59
   gonadotropin-releasing hormone (GnRH)
      agonist V07.59
   goserelin acetate (Zoladex) V07.59
   letrozole (Femara) V07.52
   leuprolide acetate (leuprorelin) (Lupron)
      V07.59
   megestrol acetate (Megace) V07.59
   methadone 304.00
   nonprescribed drugs (*see also* Abuse, drugs,
      nondependent) 305.9 ☑
   patent medicines (*see also* Abuse, drugs,
      nondependent) 305.9 ☑
   raloxifene (Evista) V07.51

Use of — *continued*
   selective estrogen receptor modulators
      (SERMs) V07.51
   tamoxifen (Nolvadex) V07.51
   toremifene (Fareston) V07.51
Usher-Senear disease (pemphigus erythemato-
   sus) 694.4
Uta 085.5
Uterine size-date discrepancy 649.6 ☑
Uteromegaly 621.2
Uterovaginal — *see* condition
Uterovesical — *see* condition
Uterus — *see also* condition
   with only one functioning horn 752.33
Utriculitis (utriculus prostaticus) 597.89
Uveal — *see* condition
Uveitis (anterior) — *see also* Iridocyclitis 364.3
   acute or subacute 364.00
      due to or associated with
         gonococcal infection 098.41
         herpes (simplex) 054.44
            zoster 053.22
      primary 364.01
      recurrent 364.02
      secondary (noninfectious) 364.04
         infectious 364.03
   allergic 360.11
   chronic 364.10
      due to or associated with
         sarcoidosis 135 *[364.11]*
         tuberculosis (*see also* Tuberculosis)
            017.3 ☑ *[364.11]*
   due to
      operation 360.11
      toxoplasmosis (acquired) 130.2
         congenital (active) 771.2
   granulomatous 364.10
   heterochromic 364.21
   lens-induced 364.23
   nongranulomatous 364.00
   posterior 363.20
      disseminated — *see* Chorioretinitis, dis-
         seminated
      focal — *see* Chorioretinitis, focal
   recurrent 364.02
   sympathetic 360.11
   syphilitic (secondary) 091.50
      congenital 090.0 *[363.13]*
      late 095.8 *[363.13]*
   tuberculous (*see also* Tuberculosis)
      017.3 ☑ *[364.11]*
Uveoencephalitis 363.22
Uveokeratitis — *see also* Iridocyclitis 364.3
Uveoparotid fever 135
Uveoparotitis 135
Uvula — *see* condition
Uvulitis (acute) (catarrhal) (chronic) (gangrenous) (membranous) (suppurative)
   (ulcerative) 528.3

☑ Additional Digit Required — Refer to the Tabular List for Digit Selection   Subterms under main terms may continue to next column or page

2014 ICD-9-CM   ▶◀ Revised Text   ● New Line   ▲ Revised Code   Volume 2 — 291

V

Vaccination
complication or reaction — *see* Complications, vaccination
delayed V64.00
not carried out V64.00
because of
acute illness V64.01
allergy to vaccine or component V64.04
caregiver refusal V64.05
chronic illness V64.02
guardian refusal V64.05
immune compromised state V64.03
parent refusal V64.05
patient had disease being vaccinated against V64.08
patient refusal V64.06
reason NEC V64.09
religious reasons V64.07
prophylactic (against) V05.9
arthropod-borne viral
disease NEC V05.1
encephalitis V05.0
chickenpox V05.4
cholera (alone) V03.0
with typhoid-paratyphoid (cholera + TAB) V06.0
common cold V04.7
diphtheria (alone) V03.5
with
poliomyelitis (DTP+ polio) V06.3
tetanus V06.5
pertussis combined (DTP) (DTaP) V06.1
typhoid-paratyphoid (DTP + TAB) V06.2
disease (single) NEC V05.9
bacterial NEC V03.9
specified type NEC V03.89
combination NEC V06.9
specified type NEC V06.8
specified type NEC V05.8
encephalitis, viral, arthropod-borne V05.0
Hemophilus influenzae, type B [Hib] V03.81
hepatitis, viral V05.3
influenza V04.81
with
Streptococcus pneumoniae [pneumococcus] V06.6
leishmaniasis V05.2
measles (alone) V04.2
with mumps-rubella (MMR) V06.4
mumps (alone) V04.6
with measles and rubella (MMR) V06.4
pertussis alone V03.6
plague V03.3
poliomyelitis V04.0
with diphtheria-tetanus-pertussis (DTP + polio) V06.3
rabies V04.5
respiratory syncytial virus (RSV) V04.82
rubella (alone) V04.3
with measles and mumps (MMR) V06.4
smallpox V04.1
Streptococcus pneumoniae [pneumococcus] V03.82
with
influenza V06.6
tetanus toxoid (alone) V03.7
with diphtheria [Td] [DT] V06.5
with
pertussis (DTP) (DTaP) V06.1
with poliomyelitis (DTP+polio) V06.3
tuberculosis (BCG) V03.2
tularemia V03.4
typhoid-paratyphoid (TAB) (alone) V03.1
with diphtheria-tetanus-pertussis (TAB + DTP) V06.2
varicella V05.4

Vaccination — *continued*
prophylactic — *continued*
viral
disease NEC V04.89
encephalitis, arthropod-borne V05.0
hepatitis V05.3
yellow fever V04.4
Vaccinia (generalized) 999.0
without vaccination 051.02
congenital 771.2
conjunctiva 999.39
eyelids 999.0 *[373.5]*
localized 999.39
nose 999.39
not from vaccination 051.02
eyelid 051.02 *[373.5]*
sine vaccinatione 051.02
Vacuum
extraction of fetus or newborn 763.3
in sinus (accessory) (nasal) (*see also* Sinusitis) 473.9
Vagabond V60.0
Vagabondage V60.0
Vagabonds' disease 132.1
Vaginalitis (tunica) 608.4
Vagina, vaginal — *see also* condition
high risk human papillomavirus (HPV) DNA test positive 795.15
low risk human papillomavirus (HPV) DNA test positive 795.19
Vaginismus (reflex) 625.1
functional 306.51
hysterical 300.11
psychogenic 306.51
Vaginitis (acute) (chronic) (circumscribed) (diffuse) (emphysematous) (Hemophilus vaginalis) (nonspecific) (nonvenereal) (ulcerative) 616.10
with
abortion — *see* Abortion, by type, with sepsis
ectopic pregnancy (*see also* categories 633.0–633.9) 639.0
molar pregnancy (*see also* categories 630–632) 639.0
adhesive, congenital 752.49
atrophic, postmenopausal 627.3
bacterial 616.10
blennorrhagic (acute) 098.0
chronic or duration of 2 months or over 098.2
candidal 112.1
chlamydial 099.53
complicating pregnancy or puerperium 646.6 ☑
affecting fetus or newborn 760.8
congenital (adhesive) 752.49
due to
C. albicans 112.1
Trichomonas (vaginalis) 131.01
following
abortion 639.0
ectopic or molar pregnancy 639.0
gonococcal (acute) 098.0
chronic or duration of 2 months or over 098.2
granuloma 099.2
Monilia 112.1
mycotic 112.1
pinworm 127.4 *[616.11]*
postirradiation 616.10
postmenopausal atrophic 627.3
senile (atrophic) 627.3
syphilitic (early) 091.0
late 095.8
trichomonal 131.01
tuberculous (*see also* Tuberculosis) 016.7 ☑
venereal NEC 099.8
Vaginosis — *see* Vaginitis
Vagotonia 352.3
Vagrancy V60.0
VAIN I (vaginal intraepithelial neoplasia I) 623.0
VAIN II (vaginal intraepithelial neoplasia II) 623.0
VAIN III (vaginal intraepithelial neoplasia III) 233.31

Vallecula — *see* condition
Valley fever 114.0
Valsuani's disease (progressive pernicious anemia, puerperal) 648.2 ☑
Valve, valvular (formation) — *see also* condition
cerebral ventricle (communicating) in situ V45.2
cervix, internal os 752.49
colon 751.5
congenital NEC — *see* Atresia
formation, congenital NEC — *see* Atresia
heart defect — *see* Anomaly, heart, valve
ureter 753.29
pelvic junction 753.21
vesical orifice 753.22
urethra 753.6
Valvulitis (chronic) — *see also* Endocarditis 424.90
rheumatic (chronic) (inactive) (with chorea) 397.9
active or acute (aortic) (mitral) (pulmonary) (tricuspid) 391.1
syphilitic NEC 093.20
aortic 093.22
mitral 093.21
pulmonary 093.24
tricuspid 093.23
Valvulopathy — *see* Endocarditis
van Bogaert-Nijssen (-Peiffer) disease 330.0
van Bogaert's leukoencephalitis (sclerosing) (subacute) 046.2
van Buchem's syndrome (hyperostosis corticalis) 733.3
Vancomycin (glycopeptide)
intermediate staphylococcus aureus (VISA/GISA) V09.8 ☑
resistant
enterococcus (VRE) V09.8 ☑
staphylococcus aureus (VRSA/GRSA) V09.8 ☑
van Creveld-von Gierke disease (glycogenosis I) 271.0
van den Bergh's disease (enterogenous cyanosis) 289.7
van der Hoeve-Halbertsma-Waardenburg syndrome (ptosis-epicanthus) 270.2
van der Hoeve-Waardenburg-Gualdi syndrome (ptosis epicanthus) 270.2
van der Hoeve's syndrome (brittle bones and blue sclera, deafness) 756.51
Vanillism 692.89
Vanishing lung 492.0
Vanishing twin 651.33
van Neck (-Odelberg) disease or syndrome (juvenile osteochondrosis) 732.1
Vapor asphyxia or suffocation NEC 987.9
specified agent — *see* Table of Drugs and Chemicals
Vaquez-Osler disease (polycythemia vera) (M9950/1) 238.4
Vaquez's disease (M9950/1) 238.4
Variance, lethal ball, prosthetic heart valve 996.02
Variants, thalassemic 282.49
Variations in hair color 704.3
Varicella 052.9
with
complication 052.8
specified NEC 052.7
pneumonia 052.1
vaccination and inoculation (prophylactic) V05.4
exposure to V01.71
vaccination and inoculation (against) (prophylactic) V05.4
Varices — *see* Varix
Varicocele (scrotum) (thrombosed) 456.4
ovary 456.5
perineum 456.6
spermatic cord (ulcerated) 456.4
Varicose
aneurysm (ruptured) (*see also* Aneurysm) 442.9
dermatitis (lower extremity) — *see* Varicose, vein, inflamed or infected

Varicose — *continued*
eczema — *see* Varicose, vein
phlebitis — *see* Varicose, vein, inflamed or infected
placental vessel — *see* Placenta, abnormal
tumor — *see* Varicose, vein
ulcer (lower extremity, any part) 454.0
anus 455.8
external 455.5
internal 455.2
esophagus (*see also* Varix, esophagus) 456.1
bleeding (*see also* Varix, esophagus, bleeding) 456.0
inflamed or infected 454.2
nasal septum 456.8
perineum 456.6
rectum — *see* Varicose, ulcer, anus
scrotum 456.4
specified site NEC 456.8
vein (lower extremity) (ruptured) (*see also* Varix) 454.9
with
complications NEC 454.8
edema 454.8
inflammation or infection 454.1
ulcerated 454.2
pain 454.8
stasis dermatitis 454.1
with ulcer 454.2
swelling 454.8
ulcer 454.0
inflamed or infected 454.2
anus — *see* Hemorrhoids
broad ligament 456.5
congenital (peripheral) 747.60
gastrointestinal 747.61
lower limb 747.64
renal 747.62
specified NEC 747.69
upper limb 747.63
esophagus (ulcerated) (*see also* Varix, esophagus) 456.1
bleeding (*see also* Varix, esophagus, bleeding) 456.0
inflamed or infected 454.1
with ulcer 454.2
in pregnancy or puerperium 671.0 ☑
vulva or perineum 671.1 ☑
nasal septum (with ulcer) 456.8
pelvis 456.5
perineum 456.6
in pregnancy, childbirth, or puerperium 671.1 ☑
rectum — *see* Hemorrhoids
scrotum (ulcerated) 456.4
specified site NEC 456.8
sublingual 456.3
ulcerated 454.0
inflamed or infected 454.2
umbilical cord, affecting fetus or newborn 762.6
urethra 456.8
vulva 456.6
in pregnancy, childbirth, or puerperium 671.1 ☑
vessel (*see also* Varix)
placenta — *see* Placenta, abnormal
Varicosis, varicosities, varicosity — *see also* Varix 454.9
Variola 050.9
hemorrhagic (pustular) 050.0
major 050.0
minor 050.1
modified 050.2
Varioloid 050.2
Variolosa, purpura 050.0
Varix (lower extremity) (ruptured) 454.9
with
complications NEC 454.8
edema 454.8
inflammation or infection 454.1
with ulcer 454.2
pain 454.0
stasis dermatitis 454.1
with ulcer 454.2

Vaccination — Varix

☑ **Additional Digit Required** — Refer to the Tabular List for Digit Selection　　　　　　🔄 **Subterms under main terms may continue to next column or page**

2014 ICD-9-CM　　　　▶◀ **Revised Text**　　　● **New Line**　　　▲ **Revised Code**　　　　**Volume 2 — 293**

Varix — continued
  with — continued
    swelling 454.8
    ulcer 454.0
      with inflammation or infection 454.2
  aneurysmal (see also Aneurysm) 442.9
  anus — see Hemorrhoids
  arteriovenous (congenital) (peripheral) NEC
    747.60
    gastrointestinal 747.61
    lower limb 747.64
    renal 747.62
    specified NEC 747.69
    spinal 747.82
    upper limb 747.63
  bladder 456.5
  broad ligament 456.5
  congenital (peripheral) 747.60
  esophagus (ulcerated) 456.1
    bleeding 456.0
      in
        cirrhosis of liver 571.5 [456.20]
        portal hypertension
          572.3 [456.20]
    congenital 747.69
      in
        cirrhosis of liver 571.5 [456.21]
          with bleeding 571.5 [456.20]
        portal hypertension
          572.3 [456.21]
          with bleeding 572.3 [456.20]
  gastric 456.8
  inflamed or infected 454.1
    ulcerated 454.2
  in pregnancy or puerperium 671.0 ☑
    perineum 671.1 ☑
    vulva 671.1 ☑
  labia (majora) 456.6
  orbit 456.8
    congenital 747.69
  ovary 456.5
  papillary 448.1
  pelvis 456.5
  perineum 456.6
    in pregnancy or puerperium 671.1 ☑
  pharynx 456.8
  placenta — see Placenta, abnormal
  prostate 456.8
  rectum — see Hemorrhoids
  renal papilla 456.8
  retina 362.17
  scrotum (ulcerated) 456.4
  sigmoid colon 456.8
  specified site NEC 456.8
  spinal (cord) (vessels) 456.8
  spleen, splenic (vein) (with phlebolith) 456.8
  sublingual 456.3
  ulcerated 454.0
    inflamed or infected 454.2
  umbilical cord, affecting fetus or newborn
    762.6
  uterine ligament 456.5
  vocal cord 456.8
  vulva 456.6
    in pregnancy, childbirth, or puerperium
      671.1 ☑
Vasa previa 663.5 ☑
  affecting fetus or newborn 762.6
  hemorrhage from, affecting fetus or new-
    born 772.0
Vascular — see also condition
  loop on papilla (optic) 743.57
  sheathing, retina 362.13
  spasm 443.9
  spider 448.1
Vascularity, pulmonary, congenital 747.39
Vascularization
  choroid 362.16
  cornea 370.60
    deep 370.63
    localized 370.61
  retina 362.16
  subretinal 362.16
Vasculitis 447.6
  allergic 287.0
  cryoglobulinemic 273.2

Vasculitis — continued
  disseminated 447.6
  kidney 447.8
  leukocytoclastic 446.29
  nodular 695.2
  retinal 362.18
  rheumatic — see Fever, rheumatic
Vasculopathy
  cardiac allograft 996.83
Vas deferens — see condition
Vas deferentitis 608.4
Vasectomy, admission for V25.2
Vasitis 608.4
  nodosa 608.4
  scrotum 608.4
  spermatic cord 608.4
  testis 608.4
  tuberculous (see also Tuberculosis) 016.5 ☑
  tunica vaginalis 608.4
  vas deferens 608.4
Vasodilation 443.9
Vasomotor — see condition
Vasoplasty, after previous sterilization V26.0
Vasoplegia, splanchnic — see also Neuropathy, peripheral, autonomic 337.9
Vasospasm 443.9
  cerebral (artery) 435.9
    with transient neurologic deficit 435.9
  coronary 413.1
  nerve
    arm NEC 354.9
    autonomic 337.9
    brachial plexus 353.0
    cervical plexus 353.2
    leg NEC 355.8
    lower extremity NEC 355.8
    peripheral NEC 355.9
    spinal NEC 355.9
    sympathetic 337.9
    upper extremity NEC 354.9
  peripheral NEC 443.9
  retina (artery) (see also Occlusion, retinal,
    artery) 362.30
Vasospastic — see condition
Vasovagal attack (paroxysmal) 780.2
  psychogenic 306.2
Vater's ampulla — see condition
VATER syndrome 759.89
vCJD (variant Creutzfeldt-Jakob disease) 046.11
Vegetation, vegetative
  adenoid (nasal fossa) 474.2
  consciousness (persistent) 780.03
  endocarditis (acute) (any valve) (chronic)
    (subacute) 421.0
  heart (mycotic) (valve) 421.0
  state (persistent) 780.03
Veil
  Jackson's 751.4
  over face (causing asphyxia) 768.9
Vein, venous — see condition
Veldt sore — see also Ulcer, skin 707.9
Velo-cardio-facial syndrome 758.32
Velpeau's hernia — see Hernia, femoral
Venereal
  balanitis NEC 099.8
  bubo 099.1
  disease 099.9
    specified nature or type NEC 099.8
  granuloma inguinale 099.2
  lymphogranuloma (Durand-Nicolas-Favre),
    any site 099.1
  salpingitis 098.37
  urethritis (see also Urethritis, nongonococ-
    cal) 099.40
  vaginitis NEC 099.8
  warts 078.11
Vengefulness, in child — see also Disturbance,
    conduct 312.0 ☑
Venofibrosis 459.89
Venom, venomous
  bite or sting (animal or insect) 989.5
  poisoning 989.5
Venous — see condition
Ventouse delivery NEC 669.5 ☑
  affecting fetus or newborn 763.3
Ventral — see condition

Ventricle, ventricular — see also condition
  escape 427.69
  standstill (see also Arrest, cardiac) 427.5
Ventriculitis, cerebral — see also Meningitis
  322.9
Ventriculostomy status V45.2
Verbiest's syndrome (claudicatio intermittens
  spinalis) 435.1
Vernet's syndrome 352.6
Verneuil's disease (syphilitic bursitis) 095.7
Verruca (filiformis) 078.10
  acuminata (any site) 078.11
  necrogenica (primary) (see also Tuberculosis)
    017.0 ☑
  peruana 088.0
  peruviana 088.0
  plana (juvenilis) 078.19
  plantaris 078.12
  seborrheica 702.19
    inflamed 702.11
  senilis 702.0
  tuberculosa (primary) (see also Tuberculosis)
    017.0 ☑
  venereal 078.11
  viral 078.10
    specified NEC 078.19
  vulgaris 078.10
Verrucosities — see also Verruca 078.10
Verrucous endocarditis (acute) (any valve)
  (chronic) (subacute) 710.0 [424.91]
  nonbacterial 710.0 [424.91]
Verruga
  peruana 088.0
  peruviana 088.0
Verse's disease (calcinosis intervertebralis)
  275.49 [722.90]
Version
  before labor, affecting fetus or newborn
    761.7
  cephalic (correcting previous malposition)
    652.1 ☑
    affecting fetus or newborn 763.1
  cervix — see Version, uterus
  uterus (postinfectional) (postpartal, old) (see
    also Malposition, uterus) 621.6
    forward — see Anteversion, uterus
    lateral — see Lateroversion, uterus
Vertebra, vertebral — see condition
Vertigo 780.4
  auditory 386.19
  aural 386.19
  benign paroxysmal positional 386.11
  central origin 386.2
  cerebral 386.2
  Dix and Hallpike (epidemic) 386.12
  endemic paralytic 078.81
  epidemic 078.81
    Dix and Hallpike 386.12
    Gerlier's 078.81
    Pedersen's 386.12
    vestibular neuronitis 386.12
  epileptic — see Epilepsy
  Gerlier's (epidemic) 078.81
  hysterical 300.11
  labyrinthine 386.10
  laryngeal 786.2
  malignant positional 386.2
  Ménière's (see also Disease, Ménière's)
    386.00
  menopausal 627.2
  otogenic 386.19
  paralytic 078.81
  paroxysmal positional, benign 386.11
  Pedersen's (epidemic) 386.12
  peripheral 386.10
    specified type NEC 386.19
  positional
    benign paroxysmal 386.11
    malignant 386.2
Verumontanitis (chronic) — see also Urethritis
  597.89
Vesania — see also Psychosis 298.9
Vesical — see condition
Vesicle
  cutaneous 709.8
  seminal — see condition

Vesicle — continued
  skin 709.8
Vesicocolic — see condition
Vesicoperineal — see condition
Vesicorectal — see condition
Vesicourethrorectal — see condition
Vesicovaginal — see condition
Vesicular — see condition
Vesiculitis (seminal) 608.0
  amebic 006.8
  gonorrheal (acute) 098.14
    chronic or duration of 2 months or over
      098.34
  trichomonal 131.09
  tuberculous (see also Tuberculosis)
    016.5 ☑ [608.81]
Vestibulitis (ear) — see also Labyrinthitis
  386.30
  nose (external) 478.19
  vulvar 625.71
Vestibulopathy, acute peripheral (recurrent)
  386.12
Vestige, vestigial — see also Persistence
  branchial 744.41
  structures in vitreous 743.51
Vibriosis NEC 027.9
Vidal's disease (lichen simplex chronicus)
  698.3
Video display tube syndrome 723.8
Vienna-type encephalitis 049.8
Villaret's syndrome 352.6
Villous — see condition
VIN I (vulvar intraepithelial neoplasia I) 624.01
VIN II (vulvar intraepithelial neoplasia II) 624.02
VIN III (vulvar intraepithelial neoplasia III)
  233.32
Vincent's
  angina 101
  bronchitis 101
  disease 101
  gingivitis 101
  infection (any site) 101
  laryngitis 101
  stomatitis 101
  tonsillitis 101
Vinson-Plummer syndrome (sideropenic
  dysphagia) 280.8
Viosterol deficiency — see also Deficiency,
  calciferol 268.9
Virchow's disease 733.99
Viremia 790.8
Virilism (adrenal) (female) NEC 255.2
  with
    3-beta-hydroxysteroid dehydrogenase
      defect 255.2
    11-hydroxylase defect 255.2
    21-hydroxylase defect 255.2
    adrenal
      hyperplasia 255.2
      insufficiency (congenital) 255.2
    cortical hyperfunction 255.2
Virilization (female) (suprarenal) — see also
  Virilism 255.2
  isosexual 256.4
Virulent bubo 099.0
Virus, viral — see also condition
  infection NEC (see also Infection, viral)
    079.99
  septicemia 079.99
  yaba monkey tumor 059.22
VISA (vancomycin intermediate staphylococcus
  aureus) V09.8 ☑
Viscera, visceral — see condition
Visceroptosis 569.89
Visible peristalsis 787.4
Vision, visual
  binocular, suppression 368.31
  blurred, blurring 368.8
    hysterical 300.11
  defect, defective (see also Impaired, vision)
    369.9
  disorientation (syndrome) 368.16
  disturbance NEC (see also Disturbance, vi-
    sion) 368.9
    hysterical 300.11
  examination V72.0

☑ Additional Digit Required — Refer to the Tabular List for Digit Selection   ▽ Subterms under main terms may continue to next column or page

Vision, visual — *continued*
  field, limitation 368.40
  fusion, with defective steropsis 368.33
  hallucinations 368.16
  halos 368.16
  loss 369.9
    both eyes (*see also* Blindness, both eyes)
      369.3
    complete (*see also* Blindness, both eyes)
      369.00
    one eye 369.8
    sudden 368.16
    low (both eyes) 369.20
      one eye (other eye normal) (*see also* Impaired, vision) 369.70
      blindness, other eye 369.10
    perception, simultaneous without fusion
      368.32
    tunnel 368.45
Vitality, lack or want of 780.79
  newborn 779.89
Vitamin deficiency NEC — *see also* Deficiency, vitamin 269.2
Vitelline duct, persistent 751.0
Vitiligo 709.01
  due to pinta (carate) 103.2
  eyelid 374.53
  vulva 624.8
Vitium cordis — *see* Disease, heart
Vitreous — *see also* condition
  touch syndrome 997.99
VLCAD (long chain/very long chain acyl CoA dehydrogenase deficiency, LCAD) 277.85
Vocal cord — *see* condition
Vocational rehabilitation V57.22
Vogt-Koyanagi syndrome 364.24
Vogt-Spielmeyer disease (amaurotic familial idiocy) 330.1
Vogt's (Cecile) disease or syndrome 333.7 ☑
Voice
  change (*see also* Dysphonia) 784.49
  loss (*see also* Aphonia) 784.41
Volhard-Fahr disease (malignant nephrosclerosis) 403.00
Volhynian fever 083.1
Volkmann's ischemic contracture or paralysis (complicating trauma) 958.6
Voluntary starvation 307.1
Volvulus (bowel) (colon) (intestine) 560.2
  with
    hernia (*see also* Hernia, by site, with obstruction)
      gangrenous — *see* Hernia, by site, with gangrene
      perforation 560.2
  congenital 751.5
  duodenum 537.3
  fallopian tube 620.5
  oviduct 620.5
  stomach (due to absence of gastrocolic ligament) 537.89
Vomiting 787.03
  with nausea 787.01
  allergic 535.4 ☑
  asphyxia 933.1
  bilious (cause unknown) 787.04
    following gastrointestinal surgery 564.3
    newborn 779.32
  blood (*see also* Hematemesis) 578.0
  causing asphyxia, choking, or suffocation (*see also* Asphyxia, food) 933.1
  cyclical 536.2
    associated with migraine 346.2 ☑
    psychogenic 306.4
  epidemic 078.82
  fecal matter 569.87
  following gastrointestinal surgery 564.3
  functional 536.8
    psychogenic 306.4
  habit 536.2
  hysterical 300.11
  nervous 306.4
  neurotic 306.4
  newborn 779.33
    bilious 779.32
  of or complicating pregnancy 643.9 ☑

Vomiting — *continued*
  of or complicating pregnancy — *continued*
    due to
      organic disease 643.8 ☑
      specific cause NEC 643.8 ☑
    early — *see* Hyperemesis, gravidarum
    late (after 22 completed weeks of gestation) 643.2 ☑
  pernicious or persistent 536.2
    complicating pregnancy — *see* Hyperemesis, gravidarum
  psychogenic 306.4
  physiological 787.03
    bilious 787.04
  psychic 306.4
  psychogenic 307.54
  stercoral 569.89
  uncontrollable 536.2
    psychogenic 306.4
  uremic — *see* Uremia
  winter 078.82
von Bechterew (-Strumpell) disease or syndrome (ankylosing spondylitis) 720.0
von Bezold's abscess 383.01
von Economo's disease (encephalitis lethargica) 049.8
von Eulenburg's disease (congenital paramyotonia) 359.29
von Gierke's disease (glycogenosis I) 271.0
von Gies' joint 095.8
von Graefe's disease or syndrome 378.72
von Hippel (-Lindau) disease or syndrome (retinocerebral angiomatosis) 759.6
von Jaksch's anemia or disease (pseudoleukemia infantum) 285.8
von Recklinghausen-Applebaum disease (hemochromatosis) — *see also* Hemochromatosis 275.03
von Recklinghausen's
  disease or syndrome (nerves) (skin) (M9540/1) 237.71
  bones (osteitis fibrosa cystica) 252.01
  tumor (M9540/1) 237.71
von Schroetter's syndrome (intermittent venous claudication) 453.89
von Willebrand (-Jürgens) (-Minot) disease or syndrome (angiohemophilia) 286.4
von Zambusch's disease (lichen sclerosus et atrophicus) 701.0
Voorhoeve's disease or dyschondroplasia 756.4
Vossius' ring 921.3
  late effect 366.21
Voyeurism 302.82
VRE (vancomycin resistant enterococcus) V09.8 ☑
Vrolik's disease (osteogenesis imperfecta) 756.51
VRSA (vancomycin resistant staphylococcus aureus) V09.8 ☑
Vulva — *see* condition
Vulvismus 625.1
Vulvitis (acute) (allergic) (chronic) (gangrenous) (hypertrophic) (intertriginous) 616.10
  with
    abortion — *see* Abortion, by type, with sepsis
    ectopic pregnancy (*see also* categories 633.0–633.9) 639.0
    molar pregnancy (*see also* categories 630–632) 639.0
  adhesive, congenital 752.49
  blennorrhagic (acute) 098.0
    chronic or duration of 2 months or over 098.2
  chlamydial 099.53
  complicating pregnancy or puerperium 646.6 ☑
  due to Ducrey's bacillus 099.0
  following
    abortion 639.0
    ectopic or molar pregnancy 639.0
  gonococcal (acute) 098.0

Vulvitis — *continued*
  gonococcal — *continued*
    chronic or duration of 2 months or over 098.2
  herpetic 054.11
  leukoplakic 624.09
  monilial 112.1
  puerperal, postpartum, childbirth 646.6 ☑
  syphilitic (early) 091.0
    late 095.8
  trichomonal 131.01
Vulvodynia 625.70
  specified NEC 625.79
Vulvorectal — *see* condition
Vulvovaginitis — *see also* Vulvitis 616.10
  amebic 006.8
  chlamydial 099.53
  gonococcal (acute) 098.0
    chronic or duration of 2 months or over 098.2
  herpetic 054.11
  monilial 112.1
  trichomonal (Trichomonas vaginalis) 131.01

W

Waardenburg-Klein syndrome (ptosis-epicanthus) 270.2
Waardenburg's syndrome 756.89
  meaning ptosis-epicanthus 270.2
Wagner's disease (colloid milium) 709.3
Wagner (-Unverricht) syndrome (dermatomyositis) 710.3
Waiting list, person on V63.2
  undergoing social agency investigation V63.8
Wakefulness disorder — *see also* Hypersomnia 780.54
  nonorganic origin 307.43
Waldenström-Kjellberg syndrome (sideropenic dysphagia) 280.8
Waldenström's
  disease (osteochondrosis, capital femoral) 732.1
  hepatitis (lupoid hepatitis) 571.49
  hypergammaglobulinemia 273.0
  macroglobulinemia 273.3
  purpura, hypergammaglobulinemic 273.0
  syndrome (macroglobulinemia) 273.3
Walking
  difficulty 719.7
    psychogenic 307.9
  sleep 307.46
    hysterical 300.13
Wall, abdominal — *see* condition
Wallenberg's syndrome (posterior inferior cerebellar artery) — *see also* Disease, cerebrovascular, acute 436
Wallgren's
  disease (obstruction of splenic vein with collateral circulation) 459.89
  meningitis (*see also* Meningitis, aseptic) 047.9
Wandering
  acetabulum 736.39
  gallbladder 751.69
  in diseases classified elsewhere V40.31
  kidney, congenital 753.3
  organ or site, congenital NEC — *see* Malposition, congenital
  pacemaker (atrial) (heart) 427.89
  spleen 289.59
Wardrop's disease (with lymphangitis) 681.9
  finger 681.02
  toe 681.11
War neurosis 300.16
Wart (digitate) (filiform) (infectious) (viral) 078.10
  common 078.19
  external genital organs (venereal) 078.11
  fig 078.19
  flat 078.19
  genital 078.11
  Hassall-Henle's (of cornea) 371.41
  Henle's (of cornea) 371.41
  juvenile 078.19
  moist 078.10

Wart — *continued*
  Peruvian 088.0
  plantar 078.12
  prosector (*see also* Tuberculosis) 017.0 ☑
  seborrheic 702.19
    inflamed 702.11
  senile 702.0
  specified NEC 078.19
  syphilitic 091.3
  tuberculous (*see also* Tuberculosis) 017.0 ☑
  venereal (female) (male) 078.11
Warthin's tumor (salivary gland) (M8561/0) 210.2
Washerwoman's itch 692.4
Wassilieff's disease (leptospiral jaundice) 100.0
Wasting
  disease 799.4
    due to malnutrition 261
    extreme (due to malnutrition) 261
  muscular NEC 728.2
  palsy, paralysis 335.21
  pelvic muscle 618.83
Water-hammer pulse — *see also* Insufficiency, aortic 424.1
Water-losing nephritis 588.89
Water
  clefts 366.12
  deprivation of 994.3
  in joint (*see also* Effusion, joint) 719.0 ☑
  intoxication 276.69
  itch 120.3
  lack of 994.3
  loading 276.69
  on
    brain — *see* Hydrocephalus
    chest 511.89
  poisoning 276.69
Waterbrash 787.1
Waterhouse (-Friderichsen) disease or syndrome 036.3
Watermelon stomach 537.82
  with hemorrhage 537.83
  without hemorrhage 537.82
Wax in ear 380.4
Waxy
  degeneration, any site 277.39
  disease 277.39
  kidney 277.39 [583.81]
  liver (large) 277.39
  spleen 277.39
Weak, weakness (generalized) 780.79
  arches (acquired) 734
    congenital 754.61
  bladder sphincter 596.59
  congenital 779.89
  eye muscle — *see* Strabismus
  facial 781.94
  foot (double) — *see* Weak, arches
  heart, cardiac (*see also* Failure, heart) 428.9
    congenital 746.9
  mind 317
  muscle (generalized) 728.87
  myocardium (*see also* Failure, heart) 428.9
  newborn 779.89
  pelvic fundus
    pubocervical tissue 618.81
    rectovaginal tissue 618.82
  pulse 785.9
  senile 797
  urinary stream 788.62
  valvular — *see* Endocarditis
Wear, worn, tooth, teeth (approximal) (hard tissues) (interproximal) (occlusal) — *see also* Attrition, teeth 521.10
Weather, weathered
  effects of
    cold NEC 991.9
      specified effect NEC 991.8
    hot (*see also* Heat) 992.9
  skin 692.74
Weber-Christian disease or syndrome (nodular nonsuppurative panniculitis) 729.30
Weber-Cockayne syndrome (epidermolysis bullosa) 757.39

Weber-Dimitri syndrome 759.6
Weber-Gubler syndrome 344.89
Weber-Leyden syndrome 344.89
Weber-Osler syndrome (familial hemorrhagic telangiectasia) 448.0
Weber's paralysis or syndrome 344.89
Web, webbed (congenital) — see also Anomaly, specified type NEC
   canthus 743.63
   digits (see also Syndactylism) 755.10
   duodenal 751.5
   esophagus 750.3
   fingers (see also Syndactylism, fingers) 755.11
   larynx (glottic) (subglottic) 748.2
   neck (pterygium colli) 744.5
   Paterson-Kelly (sideropenic dysphagia) 280.8
   popliteal syndrome 756.89
   toes (see also Syndactylism, toes) 755.13
Wedge-shaped or wedging vertebra — see also Osteoporosis 733.00
Wegener's granulomatosis or syndrome 446.4
Wegner's disease (syphilitic osteochondritis) 090.0
Weight
   gain (abnormal) (excessive) 783.1
      during pregnancy 646.1 ☑
         insufficient 646.8 ☑
   less than 1000 grams at birth 765.0 ☑
   loss (cause unknown) 783.21
Weightlessness 994.9
Weil's disease (leptospiral jaundice) 100.0
Weill-Marchesani syndrome (brachymorphism and ectopia lentis) 759.89
Weingarten's syndrome (tropical eosinophilia) 518.3
Weir Mitchell's disease (erythromelalgia) 443.82
Weiss-Baker syndrome (carotid sinus syncope) 337.01
Weissenbach-Thibierge syndrome (cutaneous systemic sclerosis) 710.1
Wen — see also Cyst, sebaceous 706.2
Wenckebach's phenomenon, heart block (second degree) 426.13
Werdnig-Hoffmann syndrome (muscular atrophy) 335.0
Werlhof-Wichmann syndrome — see also Purpura, thrombocytopenic 287.39
Werlhof's disease — see also Purpura, thrombocytopenic 287.39
Wermer's syndrome or disease (polyendocrine adenomatosis) 258.01
Werner-His disease (trench fever) 083.1
Werner-Schultz disease (agranulocytosis) 288.09
Werner's disease or syndrome (progeria adultorum) 259.8
Wernicke-Korsakoff syndrome or psychosis (nonalcoholic) 294.0
   alcoholic 291.1
Wernicke-Posadas disease — see also Coccidioidomycosis 114.9
Wernicke's encephalopathy, disease, or syndrome (superior hemorrhagic polioencephalitis) 265.1
Wesselsbron fever 066.3
West African fever 084.8
West Nile
   encephalitis 066.41
   encephalomyelitis 066.41
   fever 066.40
      with
         cranial nerve disorders 066.42
         encephalitis 066.41
         optic neuritis 066.42
         other complications 066.49
         other neurologic manifestations 066.42
         polyradiculitis 066.42
   virus 066.40
Westphal-Strümpell syndrome (hepatolenticular degeneration) 275.1

Wet
   brain (alcoholic) (see also Alcoholism) 303.9 ☑
   feet, tropical (syndrome) (maceration) 991.4
   lung (syndrome)
      adult 518.52
      newborn 770.6
Wharton's duct — see condition
Wheal 709.8
Wheelchair confinement status V46.3
Wheezing 786.07
Whiplash injury or syndrome 847.0
Whipple's disease or syndrome (intestinal lipodystrophy) 040.2
Whipworm 127.3
"Whistling face" syndrome (craniocarpotarsal dystrophy) 759.89
White — see also condition
   kidney
      large — see Nephrosis
      small 582.9
   leg, puerperal, postpartum, childbirth 671.4 ☑
      nonpuerperal 451.19
   mouth 112.0
   patches of mouth 528.6
   sponge nevus of oral mucosa 750.26
   spot lesions, teeth 521.01
White's disease (congenital) (keratosis follicularis) 757.39
Whitehead 706.2
Whitlow (with lymphangitis) 681.01
   herpetic 054.6
Whitmore's disease or fever (melioidosis) 025
Whooping cough 033.9
   with pneumonia 033.9 [484.3]
   due to
      Bordetella
         bronchoseptica 033.8
            with pneumonia 033.8 [484.3]
         parapertussis 033.1
            with pneumonia 033.1 [484.3]
         pertussis 033.0
            with pneumonia 033.0 [484.3]
      specified organism NEC 033.8
         with pneumonia 033.8 [484.3]
   vaccination, prophylactic (against) V03.6
Wichmann's asthma (laryngismus stridulus) 478.75
Widal (-Abrami) syndrome (acquired hemolytic jaundice) 283.9
Widening aorta — see also Ectasia, aortic 447.70
   with aneurysm 441.9
   ruptured 441.5
Wilkie's disease or syndrome 557.1
Wilkinson-Sneddon disease or syndrome (subcorneal pustular dermatosis) 694.1
Willan-Plumbe syndrome (psoriasis) 696.1
Willan's lepra 696.1
Willebrand (-Jürgens) syndrome or thrombopathy (angiohemophilia) 286.4
Willi-Prader syndrome (hypogenital dystrophy with diabetic tendency) 759.81
Willis' disease (diabetes mellitus) — see also Diabetes 250.0 ☑
   due to secondary diabetes 249.0 ☑
Wilms' tumor or neoplasm (nephroblastoma) (M8960/3) 189.0
Wilson-Brocq disease (dermatitis exfoliativa) 695.89
Wilson-Mikity syndrome 770.7
Wilson's
   disease or syndrome (hepatolenticular degeneration) 275.1
   hepatolenticular degeneration 275.1
   lichen ruber 697.0
Window — see also Imperfect, closure aorticopulmonary 745.0
Winged scapula 736.89
Winter — see also condition
   vomiting disease 078.82
Wise's disease 696.2
Wiskott-Aldrich syndrome (eczema-thrombocytopenia) 279.12

Withdrawal symptoms, syndrome
   alcohol 291.81
      delirium (acute) 291.0
         chronic 291.1
      newborn 760.71
   drug or narcotic 292.0
      newborn, infant of dependent mother 779.5
   steroid NEC
      correct substance properly administered 255.41
      overdose or wrong substance given or taken 962.0
Withdrawing reaction, child or adolescent 313.22
Witts' anemia (achlorhydric anemia) 280.9
Witzelsucht 301.9
Woakes' syndrome (ethmoiditis) 471.1
Wohlfart-Kugelberg-Welander disease 335.11
Woillez's disease (acute idiopathic pulmonary congestion) 518.52
Wolff-Parkinson-White syndrome (anomalous atrioventricular excitation) 426.7
Wolhynian fever 083.1
Wolman's disease (primary familial xanthomatosis) 272.7
Wood asthma 495.8
Wool-sorters' disease 022.1
Woolly, wooly hair (congenital) (nevus) 757.4
Word
   blindness (congenital) (developmental) 315.01
      secondary to organic lesion 784.61
   deafness (secondary to organic lesion) 784.69
      developmental 315.31
Worm-eaten soles 102.3
Worm(s) (colic) (fever) (infection) (infestation) — see also Infestation 128.9
   guinea 125.7
   in intestine NEC 127.9
Worn out — see also Exhaustion 780.79
   artificial heart valve 996.02
   cardiac defibrillator (with synchronous cardiac pacemaker) V53.32
   cardiac pacemaker lead or battery V53.31
   joint prosthesis (see also Complications, mechanical, device NEC, prosthetic NEC, joint) 996.46
"Worried well" V65.5
Wound, open (by cutting or piercing instrument) (by firearms) (cut) (dissection) (incised) (laceration) (perforating) (puncture) (with initial hemorrhage, not internal) 879.8

> Note — For fracture with open wound, see Fracture.
>
> For laceration, traumatic rupture, tear or penetrating wound of internal organs, such as heart, lung, liver, kidney, pelvic organs, etc., whether or not accompanied by open wound or fracture in the same region, see Injury, internal.
>
> For contused wound, see Contusion. For crush injury, see Crush. For abrasion, insect bite (nonvenomous), blister, or scratch, see Injury, superficial.
>
> Complicated includes wounds with:
>   delayed healing
>   delayed treatment
>   foreign body
>   primary infection
>
> For late effect of open wound, see Late, effect, wound, open, by site.

   abdomen, abdominal (external) (muscle) 879.2
      complicated 879.3
      wall (anterior) 879.2
         complicated 879.3
         lateral 879.4
            complicated 879.5
   alveolar (process) 873.62

Wound, open — continued
   alveolar — continued
      complicated 873.72
   ankle 891.0
      with tendon involvement 891.2
      complicated 891.1
   anterior chamber, eye (see also Wound, open, intraocular) 871.9
   anus 863.89
   arm 884.0
      with tendon involvement 884.2
      complicated 884.1
      forearm 881.00
         with tendon involvement 881.20
         complicated 881.10
      multiple sites — see Wound, open, multiple, upper limb
      upper 880.03
         with tendon involvement 880.23
         complicated 880.13
         multiple sites (with axillary or shoulder regions) 880.09
            with tendon involvement 880.29
            complicated 880.19
   artery — see Injury, blood vessel, by site
   auditory
      canal (external) (meatus) 872.02
         complicated 872.12
      ossicles (incus) (malleus) (stapes) 872.62
         complicated 872.72
   auricle, ear 872.01
      complicated 872.11
   axilla 880.02
      with tendon involvement 880.22
      complicated 880.12
         with tendon involvement 880.29
      involving other sites of upper arm 880.09
         complicated 880.19
   back 876.0
      complicated 876.1
   bladder — see Injury, internal, bladder
   blood vessel — see Injury, blood vessel, by site
   brain — see Injury, intracranial, with open intracranial wound
   breast 879.0
      complicated 879.1
   brow 873.42
      complicated 873.52
   buccal mucosa 873.61
      complicated 873.71
   buttock 877.0
      complicated 877.1
   calf 891.0
      with tendon involvement 891.2
      complicated 891.1
   canaliculus lacrimalis 870.8
      with laceration of eyelid 870.2
   canthus, eye 870.8
      laceration — see Laceration, eyelid
   cavernous sinus — see Injury, intracranial
   cerebellum — see Injury, intracranial
   cervical esophagus 874.4
      complicated 874.5
   cervix — see Injury, internal, cervix
   cheek(s) (external) 873.41
      complicated 873.51
      internal 873.61
         complicated 873.71
   chest (wall) (external) 875.0
      complicated 875.1
   chin 873.44
      complicated 873.54
   choroid 363.63
   ciliary body (eye) (see also Wound, open, intraocular) 871.9
   clitoris 878.8
      complicated 878.9
   cochlea 872.64
      complicated 872.74
   complicated 879.9
   conjunctiva — see Wound, open, intraocular
   cornea (nonpenetrating) (see also Wound, open, intraocular) 871.9
   costal region 875.0
      complicated 875.1

☑ Additional Digit Required — Refer to the Tabular List for Digit Selection   ▽ Subterms under main terms may continue to next column or page

296 — Volume 2   ▶◀ Revised Text   ● New Line   ▲ Revised Code   2014 ICD-9-CM

Wound, open — *continued*
  Descemet's membrane (*see also* Wound, open, intraocular) 871.9
  digit(s)
    foot 893.0
      with tendon involvement 893.2
      complicated 893.1
    hand 883.0
      with tendon involvement 883.2
      complicated 883.1
  drumhead, ear 872.61
    complicated 872.71
  ear 872.8
    canal 872.02
      complicated 872.12
    complicated 872.9
    drum 872.61
      complicated 872.71
    external 872.00
      complicated 872.10
    multiple sites 872.69
      complicated 872.79
    ossicles (incus) (malleus) (stapes) 872.62
      complicated 872.72
    specified part NEC 872.69
      complicated 872.79
  elbow 881.01
    with tendon involvement 881.21
    complicated 881.11
  epididymis 878.2
    complicated 878.3
  epigastric region 879.2
    complicated 879.3
  epiglottis 874.01
    complicated 874.11
  esophagus (cervical) 874.4
    complicated 874.5
    thoracic — *see* Injury, internal, esophagus
  Eustachian tube 872.63
    complicated 872.73
  extremity
    lower (multiple) NEC 894.0
      with tendon involvement 894.2
      complicated 894.1
    upper (multiple) NEC 884.0
      with tendon involvement 884.2
      complicated 884.1
  eye(s) (globe) — *see* Wound, open, intraocular
  eyeball NEC 871.9
    laceration (*see also* Laceration, eyeball) 871.4
    penetrating (*see also* Penetrating wound, eyeball) 871.7
  eyebrow 873.42
    complicated 873.52
  eyelid NEC 870.8
    laceration — *see* Laceration, eyelid
  face 873.40
    complicated 873.50
    multiple sites 873.49
      complicated 873.59
    specified part NEC 873.49
      complicated 873.59
  fallopian tube — *see* Injury, internal, fallopian tube
  finger(s) (nail) (subungual) 883.0
    with tendon involvement 883.2
    complicated 883.1
  flank 879.4
    complicated 879.5
  foot (any part except toe(s) alone) 892.0
    with tendon involvement 892.2
    complicated 892.1
  forearm 881.00
    with tendon involvement 881.20
    complicated 881.10
  forehead 873.42
    complicated 873.52
  genital organs (external) NEC 878.8
    complicated 878.9
    internal — *see* Injury, internal, by site
  globe (eye) (*see also* Wound, open, eyeball) 871.9
  groin 879.4

Wound, open — *continued*
  groin — *continued*
    complicated 879.5
  gum(s) 873.62
    complicated 873.72
  hand (except finger(s) alone) 882.0
    with tendon involvement 882.2
    complicated 882.1
  head NEC 873.8
    with intracranial injury — *see* Injury, intracranial
      due to or associated with skull fracture — *see* Fracture, skull
    complicated 873.9
    scalp — *see* Wound, open, scalp
  heel 892.0
    with tendon involvement 892.2
    complicated 892.1
  high-velocity (grease gun) — *see* Wound, open, complicated, by site
  hip 890.0
    with tendon involvement 890.2
    complicated 890.1
  hymen 878.6
    complicated 878.7
  hypochondrium 879.4
    complicated 879.5
  hypogastric region 879.2
    complicated 879.3
  iliac (region) 879.4
    complicated 879.5
  incidental to
    dislocation — *see* Dislocation, open, by site
    fracture — *see* Fracture, open, by site
    intracranial injury — *see* Injury, intracranial, with open intracranial wound
    nerve injury — *see* Injury, nerve, by site
  inguinal region 879.4
    complicated 879.5
  instep 892.0
    with tendon involvement 892.2
    complicated 892.1
  interscapular region 876.0
    complicated 876.1
  intracranial — *see* Injury, intracranial, with open intracranial wound
  intraocular 871.9
    with
      partial loss (of intraocular tissue) 871.2
      prolapse or exposure (of intraocular tissue) 871.1
      without prolapse (of intraocular tissue) 871.0
    laceration (*see also* Laceration, eyeball) 871.4
    penetrating 871.7
      with foreign body (nonmagnetic) 871.6
      magnetic 871.5
  iris (*see also* Wound, open, eyeball) 871.9
  jaw (fracture not involved) 873.44
    with fracture — *see* Fracture, jaw
    complicated 873.54
  knee 891.0
    with tendon involvement 891.2
    complicated 891.1
  labium (majus) (minus) 878.4
    complicated 878.5
  lacrimal apparatus, gland, or sac 870.8
    with laceration of eyelid 870.2
  larynx 874.01
    with trachea 874.00
      complicated 874.10
    complicated 874.11
  leg (multiple) 891.0
    with tendon involvement 891.2
    complicated 891.1
    lower 891.0
      with tendon involvement 891.2
      complicated 891.1
    thigh 890.0
      with tendon involvement 890.2
      complicated 890.1

Wound, open — *continued*
  leg — *continued*
    upper 890.0
      with tendon involvement 890.2
      complicated 890.1
  lens (eye) (alone) (*see also* Cataract, traumatic) 366.20
    with involvement of other eye structures — *see* Wound, open, eyeball
  limb
    lower (multiple) NEC 894.0
      with tendon involvement 894.2
      complicated 894.1
    upper (multiple) NEC 884.0
      with tendon involvement 884.2
      complicated 884.1
  lip 873.43
    complicated 873.53
  loin 876.0
    complicated 876.1
  lumbar region 876.0
    complicated 876.1
  malar region 873.41
    complicated 873.51
  mastoid region 873.49
    complicated 873.59
  mediastinum — *see* Injury, internal, mediastinum
  midthoracic region 875.0
    complicated 875.1
  mouth 873.60
    complicated 873.70
    floor 873.64
      complicated 873.74
    multiple sites 873.69
      complicated 873.79
    specified site NEC 873.69
      complicated 873.79
  multiple, unspecified site(s) 879.8

> **Note** — Multiple open wounds of sites classifiable to the same four-digit category should be classified to that category unless they are in different limbs.
>
> Multiple open wounds of sites classifiable to different four-digit categories, or to different limbs, should be coded separately.

    complicated 879.9
    lower limb(s) (one or both) (sites classifiable to more than one three-digit category in 890 to 893) 894.0
      with tendon involvement 894.2
      complicated 894.1
    upper limb(s) (one or both) (sites classifiable to more than one three-digit category in 880 to 883) 884.0
      with tendon involvement 884.2
      complicated 884.1
  muscle — *see* Sprain, by site
  nail
    finger(s) 883.0
      complicated 883.1
    thumb 883.0
      complicated 883.1
    toe(s) 893.0
      complicated 893.1
  nape (neck) 874.8
    complicated 874.9
    specified part NEC 874.8
      complicated 874.9
  nasal (*see also* Wound, open, nose)
    cavity 873.22
      complicated 873.32
    septum 873.21
      complicated 873.31
    sinuses 873.23
      complicated 873.33
  nasopharynx 873.22
    complicated 873.32
  neck 874.8
    complicated 874.9
    nape 874.8
      complicated 874.9
    specified part NEC 874.8

Wound, open — *continued*
  neck — *continued*
    specified part — *continued*
      complicated 874.9
  nerve — *see* Injury, nerve, by site
  non-healing surgical 998.83
  nose 873.20
    complicated 873.30
    multiple sites 873.29
      complicated 873.39
    septum 873.21
      complicated 873.31
    sinuses 873.23
      complicated 873.33
  occipital region — *see* Wound, open, scalp
  ocular NEC 871.9
    adnexa 870.9
      specified region NEC 870.8
    laceration (*see also* Laceration, ocular) 871.4
    muscle (extraocular) 870.3
      with foreign body 870.4
      eyelid 870.1
      intraocular — *see* Wound, open, eyeball
    penetrating (*see also* Penetrating wound, ocular) 871.7
  orbit 870.8
    penetrating 870.3
      with foreign body 870.4
  orbital region 870.9
  ovary — *see* Injury, internal, pelvic organs
  palate 873.65
    complicated 873.75
  palm 882.0
    with tendon involvement 882.2
    complicated 882.1
  parathyroid (gland) 874.2
    complicated 874.3
  parietal region — *see* Wound, open, scalp
  pelvic floor or region 879.6
    complicated 879.7
  penis 878.0
    complicated 878.1
  perineum 879.6
    complicated 879.7
  periocular area 870.8
    laceration of skin 870.0
  pharynx 874.4
    complicated 874.5
  pinna 872.01
    complicated 872.11
  popliteal space 891.0
    with tendon involvement 891.2
    complicated 891.1
  prepuce 878.0
    complicated 878.1
  pubic region 879.2
    complicated 879.3
  pudenda 878.8
    complicated 878.9
  rectovaginal septum 878.8
    complicated 878.9
  sacral region 877.0
    complicated 877.1
  sacroiliac region 877.0
    complicated 877.1
  salivary (ducts) (glands) 873.69
    complicated 873.79
  scalp 873.0
    complicated 873.1
  scalpel, fetus or newborn 767.8
  scapular region 880.01
    with tendon involvement 880.21
    complicated 880.11
    involving other sites of upper arm 880.09
      with tendon involvement 880.29
      complicated 880.19
  sclera (*see also* Wound, open, intraocular) 871.9
  scrotum 878.2
    complicated 878.3
  seminal vesicle — *see* Injury, internal, pelvic organs
  shin 891.0
    with tendon involvement 891.2

☑ **Additional Digit Required** — Refer to the Tabular List for Digit Selection   ꟽ **Subterms under main terms may continue to next column or page**

2014 ICD-9-CM   ▶◀ Revised Text   ● New Line   ▲ Revised Code   Volume 2 — 297

Wound, open — *continued*
  shin — *continued*
    complicated 891.1
  shoulder 880.00
    with tendon involvement 880.20
    complicated 880.10
    involving other sites of upper arm 880.09
      with tendon involvement 880.29
      complicated 880.19
  skin NEC 879.8
    complicated 879.9
  skull (*see also* Injury, intracranial, with open intracranial wound)
    with skull fracture — *see* Fracture, skull
  spermatic cord (scrotal) 878.2
    complicated 878.3
    pelvic region — *see* Injury, internal, spermatic cord
  spinal cord — *see* Injury, spinal
  sternal region 875.0
    complicated 875.1
  subconjunctival — *see* Wound, open, intraocular
  subcutaneous NEC 879.8
    complicated 879.9
  submaxillary region 873.44
    complicated 873.54
  submental region 873.44
    complicated 873.54
  subungual
    finger(s) (thumb) — *see* Wound, open, finger
    toe(s) — *see* Wound, open, toe
  supraclavicular region 874.8
    complicated 874.9
  supraorbital 873.42
    complicated 873.52
  surgical, non-healing 998.83
  temple 873.49
    complicated 873.59
  temporal region 873.49
    complicated 873.59
  testis 878.2
    complicated 878.3
  thigh 890.0
    with tendon involvement 890.2
    complicated 890.1
  thorax, thoracic (external) 875.0
    complicated 875.1
  throat 874.8
    complicated 874.9
  thumb (nail) (subungual) 883.0
    with tendon involvement 883.2
    complicated 883.1
  thyroid (gland) 874.2
    complicated 874.3
  toe(s) (nail) (subungual) 893.0
    with tendon involvement 893.2
    complicated 893.1
  tongue 873.64
    complicated 873.74
  tonsil — *see* Wound, open, neck
  trachea (cervical region) 874.02
    with larynx 874.00
      complicated 874.10
    complicated 874.12
    intrathoracic — *see* Injury, internal, trachea
  trunk (multiple) NEC 879.6
    complicated 879.7
    specified site NEC 879.6
      complicated 879.7

Wound, open — *continued*
  tunica vaginalis 878.2
    complicated 878.3
  tympanic membrane 872.61
    complicated 872.71
  tympanum 872.61
    complicated 872.71
  umbilical region 879.2
    complicated 879.3
  ureter — *see* Injury, internal, ureter
  urethra — *see* Injury, internal, urethra
  uterus — *see* Injury, internal, uterus
  uvula 873.69
    complicated 873.79
  vagina 878.6
    complicated 878.7
  vas deferens — *see* Injury, internal, vas deferens
  vitreous (humor) 871.2
  vulva 878.4
    complicated 878.5
  wrist 881.02
    with tendon involvement 881.22
    complicated 881.12
Wright's syndrome (hyperabduction) 447.8
  pneumonia 390 [517.1]
Wringer injury — *see* Crush injury, by site
Wrinkling of skin 701.8
Wrist — *see also* condition
  drop (acquired) 736.05
Wrong drug (given in error) NEC 977.9
  specified drug or substance — *see* Table of Drugs and Chemicals
Wry neck — *see also* Torticollis
  congenital 754.1
Wuchereria infestation 125.0
  bancrofti 125.0
  Brugia malayi 125.1
  malayi 125.1
Wuchereriasis 125.0
Wuchereriosis 125.0
Wuchernde struma langhans (M8332/3) 193

X

X-ray
  effects, adverse, NEC 990
  of chest
    for suspected tuberculosis V71.2
    routine V72.5
Xanthelasma 272.2
  eyelid 272.2 [374.51]
  palpebrarum 272.2 [374.51]
Xanthelasmatosis (essential) 272.2
Xanthelasmoidea 757.33
Xanthine stones 277.2
Xanthinuria 277.2
Xanthofibroma (M8831/0) — *see* Neoplasm, connective tissue, benign
Xanthoma(s), xanthomatosis 272.2
  with
    hyperlipoproteinemia
      type I 272.3
      type III 272.2
      type IV 272.1
      type V 272.3
  bone 272.7
  craniohypophyseal 277.89
  cutaneotendinous 272.7
  diabeticorum 250.8 ☑ [272.2]
    due to secondary diabetes 249.8 ☑ [272.2]

Xanthoma(s), xanthomatosis — *continued*
  disseminatum 272.7
  eruptive 272.2
  eyelid 272.2 [374.51]
  familial 272.7
  hereditary 272.7
  hypercholesterinemic 272.0
  hypercholesterolemic 272.0
  hyperlipemic 272.4
  hyperlipidemic 272.4
  infantile 272.7
  joint 272.7
  juvenile 272.7
  multiple 272.7
  multiplex 272.7
  primary familial 272.7
  tendon (sheath) 272.7
  tuberosum 272.2
  tuberous 272.2
  tubo-eruptive 272.2
Xanthosis 709.09
  surgical 998.81
Xenophobia 300.29
Xeroderma (congenital) 757.39
  acquired 701.1
    eyelid 373.33
  eyelid 373.33
  pigmentosum 757.33
  vitamin A deficiency 264.8
Xerophthalmia 372.53
  vitamin A deficiency 264.7
Xerosis
  conjunctiva 372.53
    with Bitôt's spot 372.53
      vitamin A deficiency 264.1
      vitamin A deficiency 264.0
  cornea 371.40
    with corneal ulceration 370.00
      vitamin A deficiency 264.3
    vitamin A deficiency 264.2
  cutis 706.8
  skin 706.8
Xerostomia 527.7
Xiphodynia 733.90
Xiphoidalgia 733.90
Xiphoiditis 733.99
Xiphopagus 759.4
XO syndrome 758.6
XXX syndrome 758.81
XXXXY syndrome 758.81
XXY syndrome 758.7
Xyloketosuria 271.8
Xylosuria 271.8
Xylulosuria 271.8
XYY syndrome 758.81

Y

Yaba monkey tumor virus 059.22
Yawning 786.09
  psychogenic 306.1
Yaws 102.9
  bone or joint lesions 102.6
  butter 102.1
  chancre 102.0
  cutaneous, less than five years after infection 102.2
  early (cutaneous) (macular) (maculopapular) (micropapular) (papular) 102.2
    frambeside 102.2
    skin lesions NEC 102.2

Yaws — *continued*
  eyelid 102.9 [373.4]
  ganglion 102.6
  gangosis, gangosa 102.5
  gumma, gummata 102.4
    bone 102.6
  gummatous
    frambeside 102.4
    osteitis 102.6
    periostitis 102.6
  hydrarthrosis 102.6
  hyperkeratosis (early) (late) (palmar) (plantar) 102.3
  initial lesions 102.0
  joint lesions 102.6
  juxta-articular nodules 102.7
  late nodular (ulcerated) 102.4
  latent (without clinical manifestations) (with positive serology) 102.8
  mother 102.0
  mucosal 102.7
  multiple papillomata 102.1
  nodular, late (ulcerated) 102.4
  osteitis 102.6
  papilloma, papillomata (palmar) (plantar) 102.1
  periostitis (hypertrophic) 102.6
  ulcers 102.4
  wet crab 102.1
Yeast infection — *see also* Candidiasis 112.9
Yellow
  atrophy (liver) 570
    chronic 571.8
    resulting from administration of blood, plasma, serum, or other biological substance (within 8 months of administration) — *see* Hepatitis, viral
  fever — *see* Fever, yellow
  jack (*see also* Fever, yellow) 060.9
  jaundice (*see also* Jaundice) 782.4
  vernix syndrome 762.2
Yersinia septica 027.8

Z

Zagari's disease (xerostomia) 527.7
Zahorsky's disease (exanthema subitum) (*see also* Exanthem subitum) 058.10
  syndrome (herpangina) 074.0
Zellweger syndrome 277.86
Zenker's diverticulum (esophagus) 530.6
Ziehen-Oppenheim disease 333.6
Zieve's syndrome (jaundice, hyperlipemia, and hemolytic anemia) 571.1
Zika fever 066.3
Zollinger-Ellison syndrome (gastric hypersecretion with pancreatic islet cell tumor) 251.5
Zona — *see also* Herpes, zoster 053.9
Zoophilia (erotica) 302.1
Zoophobia 300.29
Zoster (herpes) — *see also* Herpes, zoster 053.9
Zuelzer (-Ogden) anemia or syndrome (nutritional megaloblastic anemia) 281.2
Zygodactyly — *see also* Syndactylism 755.10
Zygomycosis 117.7
Zymotic — *see* condition

☑ **Additional Digit Required** — Refer to the Tabular List for Digit Selection   Subterms under main terms may continue to next column or page

SECTION 2

Alphabetic Index to Poisoning and External Causes of Adverse Effects of Drugs and Other Chemical Substances

TABLE OF DRUGS AND CHEMICALS

This table contains a classification of drugs and other chemical substances to identify poisoning states and external causes of adverse effects.

Each of the listed substances in the table is assigned a code according to the poisoning classification (960-989). These codes are used when there is a statement of poisoning, overdose, wrong substance given or taken, or intoxication.

The table also contains a listing of external causes of adverse effects. An adverse effect is a pathologic manifestation due to ingestion or exposure to drugs or other chemical substances (e.g., dermatitis, hypersensitivity reaction, aspirin gastritis). The adverse effect is to be identified by the appropriate code found in Section 1, Index to Diseases and Injuries. An external cause code can then be used to identify the circumstances involved. The table headings pertaining to external causes are defined below:

Accidental poisoning (E850-E869) — accidental overdose of drug, wrong substance given or taken, drug taken inadvertently, accidents in the usage of drugs and biologicals in medical and surgical procedures, and to show external causes of poisonings classifiable to 980-989.

Therapeutic use (E930-E949) — a correct substance properly administered in therapeutic or prophylactic dosage as the external cause of adverse effects.

Suicide attempt (E950-E952) — instances in which self-inflicted injuries or poisonings are involved.

Assault (E961-E962) — injury or poisoning inflicted by another person with the intent to injure or kill.

Undetermined (E980-E982) — to be used when the intent of the poisoning or injury cannot be determined whether it was intentional or accidental.

The American Hospital Formulary Service list numbers are included in the table to help classify new drugs not identified in the table by name. The AHFS list numbers are keyed to the continually revised American Hospital Formulary Service (AHFS).* These listings are found in the table under the main term **Drug**.

Excluded from the table are radium and other radioactive substances. The classification of adverse effects and complications pertaining to these substances will be found in Section 1, Index to Diseases and Injuries, and Section 3, Index to External Causes of Injuries.

Although certain substances are indexed with one or more subentries, the majority are listed according to one use or state. It is recognized that many substances may be used in various ways, in medicine and in industry, and may cause adverse effects whatever the state of the agent (solid, liquid, or fumes arising from a liquid). In cases in which the reported data indicates a use or state not in the table, or which is clearly different from the one listed, an attempt should be made to classify the substance in the form which most nearly expresses the reported facts.

*American Hospital Formulary Service, 2 vol. (Washington, D.C.: American Society of Hospital Pharmacists, 1959-)

☑ Additional Digit Required — Refer to the Tabular List for Digit Selection   ▽ Subterms under main terms may continue to next column or page

2014 ICD-9-CM   ▶◀ Revised Text   ● New Line   ▲ Revised Code   Volume 2 — 299

Substance	Poisoning	Accident	Therapeutic Use	Suicide Attempt	Assault	Undetermined
1-propanol	980.3	E860.4	—	E950.9	E962.1	E980.9
2-propanol	980.2	E860.3	—	E950.9	E962.1	E980.9
2, 4-D (dichlorophenoxyacetic acid)	989.4	E863.5	—	E950.6	E962.1	E980.7
2, 4-toluene diisocyanate	983.0	E864.0	—	E950.7	E962.1	E980.6
2, 4, 5-T (trichlorophenoxyacetic acid)	989.2	E863.5	—	E950.6	E962.1	E980.7
14-hydroxydihydromorphinone	965.09	E850.2	E935.2	E950.0	E962.0	E980.0
ABOB	961.7	E857	E931.7	E950.4	E962.0	E980.4
Abrus (seed)	988.2	E865.3	—	E950.9	E962.1	E980.9
Absinthe	980.0	E860.1	—	E950.9	E962.1	E980.9
beverage	980.0	E860.0	—	E950.9	E962.1	E980.9
Acenocoumarin, acenocoumarol	964.2	E858.2	E934.2	E950.4	E962.0	E980.4
Acepromazine	969.1	E853.0	E939.1	E950.3	E962.0	E980.3
Acetal	982.8	E862.4	—	E950.9	E962.1	E980.9
Acetaldehyde (vapor)	987.8	E869.8	—	E952.8	E962.2	E982.8
liquid	989.89	E866.8	—	E950.9	E962.1	E980.9
Acetaminophen	965.4	E850.4	E935.4	E950.0	E962.0	E980.0
Acetaminosalol	965.1	E850.3	E935.3	E950.0	E962.0	E980.0
Acetanilid(e)	965.4	E850.4	E935.4	E950.0	E962.0	E980.0
Acetarsol, acetarsone	961.1	E857	E931.1	E950.4	E962.0	E980.4
Acetazolamide	974.2	E858.5	E944.2	E950.4	E962.0	E980.4
Acetic						
acid	983.1	E864.1	—	E950.7	E962.1	E980.6
with sodium acetate (ointment)	976.3	E858.7	E946.3	E950.4	E962.0	E980.4
irrigating solution	974.5	E858.5	E944.5	E950.4	E962.0	E980.4
lotion	976.2	E858.7	E946.2	E950.4	E962.0	E980.4
anhydride	983.1	E864.1	—	E950.7	E962.1	E980.6
ether (vapor)	982.8	E862.4	—	E950.9	E962.1	E980.9
Acetohexamide	962.3	E858.0	E932.3	E950.4	E962.0	E980.4
Acetomenaphthone	964.3	E858.2	E934.3	E950.4	E962.0	E980.4
Acetomorphine	965.01	E850.0	E935.0	E950.0	E962.0	E980.0
Acetone (oils) (vapor)	982.8	E862.4	—	E950.9	E962.1	E980.9
Acetophenazine (maleate)	969.1	E853.0	E939.1	E950.3	E962.0	E980.3
Acetophenetidin	965.4	E850.4	E935.4	E950.0	E962.0	E980.0
Acetophenone	982.0	E862.4	—	E950.9	E962.1	E980.9
Acetorphine	965.09	E850.2	E935.2	E950.0	E962.0	E980.0
Acetosulfone (sodium)	961.8	E857	E931.8	E950.4	E962.0	E980.4
Acetrizoate (sodium)	977.8	E858.8	E947.8	E950.4	E962.0	E980.4
Acetylcarbromal	967.3	E852.2	E937.3	E950.2	E962.0	E980.2
Acetylcholine (chloride)	971.0	E855.3	E941.0	E950.4	E962.0	E980.4
Acetylcysteine	975.5	E858.6	E945.5	E950.4	E962.0	E980.4
Acetyldigitoxin	972.1	E858.3	E942.1	E950.4	E962.0	E980.4
Acetyldihydrocodeine	965.09	E850.2	E935.2	E950.0	E962.0	E980.0
Acetyldihydrocodeinone	965.09	E850.2	E935.2	E950.0	E962.0	E980.0
Acetylene (gas) (industrial)	987.1	E868.1	—	E951.8	E962.2	E981.8
incomplete combustion of — see Carbon monoxide, fuel, utility						
tetrachloride (vapor)	982.3	E862.4	—	E950.9	E962.1	E980.9
Acetyliodosalicylic acid	965.1	E850.3	E935.3	E950.0	E962.0	E980.0
Acetylphenylhydrazine	965.8	E850.8	E935.8	E950.0	E962.0	E980.0
Acetylsalicylic acid	965.1	E850.3	E935.3	E950.0	E962.0	E980.0
Achromycin	960.4	E856	E930.4	E950.4	E962.0	E980.4
ophthalmic preparation	976.5	E858.7	E946.5	E950.4	E962.0	E980.4
topical NEC	976.0	E858.7	E946.0	E950.4	E962.0	E980.4
Acidifying agents	963.2	E858.1	E933.2	E950.4	E962.0	E980.4
Acids (corrosive) NEC	983.1	E864.1	—	E950.7	E962.1	E980.6
Aconite (wild)	988.2	E865.4	—	E950.9	E962.1	E980.9
Aconitine (liniment)	976.8	E858.7	E946.8	E950.4	E962.0	E980.4
Aconitum ferox	988.2	E865.4	—	E950.9	E962.1	E980.9
Acridine	983.0	E864.0	—	E950.7	E962.1	E980.6
vapor	987.8	E869.8	—	E952.8	E962.2	E982.8
Acriflavine	961.9	E857	E931.9	E950.4	E962.0	E980.4
Acrisorcin	976.0	E858.7	E946.0	E950.4	E962.0	E980.4
Acrolein (gas)	987.8	E869.8	—	E952.8	E962.2	E982.8
liquid	989.89	E866.8	—	E950.9	E962.1	E980.9
Actaea spicata	988.2	E865.4	—	E950.9	E962.1	E980.9
Acterol	961.5	E857	E931.5	E950.4	E962.0	E980.4
ACTH	962.4	E858.0	E932.4	E950.4	E962.0	E980.4
Acthar	962.4	E858.0	E932.4	E950.4	E962.0	E980.4
Actinomycin (C) (D)	960.7	E856	E930.7	E950.4	E962.0	E980.4
Adalin (acetyl)	967.3	E852.2	E937.3	E950.2	E962.0	E980.2
Adenosine (phosphate)	977.8	E858.8	E947.8	E950.4	E962.0	E980.4
ADH	962.5	E858.0	E932.5	E950.4	E962.0	E980.4
Adhesives	989.89	E866.6	—	E950.9	E962.1	E980.9
Adicillin	960.0	E856	E930.0	E950.4	E962.0	E980.4
Adiphenine	975.1	E855.6	E945.1	E950.4	E962.0	E980.4
Adjunct, pharmaceutical	977.4	E858.8	E947.4	E950.4	E962.0	E980.4
Adrenal (extract, cortex or medulla) (glucocorticoids) (hormones) (mineralocorticoids)	962.0	E858.0	E932.0	E950.4	E962.0	E980.4
ENT agent	976.6	E858.7	E946.6	E950.4	E962.0	E980.4
ophthalmic preparation	976.5	E858.7	E946.5	E950.4	E962.0	E980.4
topical NEC	976.0	E858.7	E946.0	E950.4	E962.0	E980.4
Adrenalin	971.2	E855.5	E941.2	E950.4	E962.0	E980.4
Adrenergic blocking agents	971.3	E855.6	E941.3	E950.4	E962.0	E980.4
Adrenergics	971.2	E855.5	E941.2	E950.4	E962.0	E980.4
Adrenochrome (derivatives)	972.8	E858.3	E942.8	E950.4	E962.0	E980.4
Adrenocorticotropic hormone	962.4	E858.0	E932.4	E950.4	E962.0	E980.4
Adrenocorticotropin	962.4	E858.0	E932.4	E950.4	E962.0	E980.4
Adriamycin	960.7	E856	E930.7	E950.4	E962.0	E980.4
Aerosol spray — see Sprays						
Aerosporin	960.8	E856	E930.8	E950.4	E962.0	E980.4
ENT agent	976.6	E858.7	E946.6	E950.4	E962.0	E980.4
ophthalmic preparation	976.5	E858.7	E946.5	E950.4	E962.0	E980.4
topical NEC	976.0	E858.7	E946.0	E950.4	E962.0	E980.4
Aethusa cynapium	988.2	E865.4	—	E950.9	E962.1	E980.9
Afghanistan black	969.6	E854.1	E939.6	E950.3	E962.0	E980.3
Aflatoxin	989.7	E865.9	—	E950.9	E962.1	E980.9
African boxwood	988.2	E865.4	—	E950.9	E962.1	E980.9
Agar (-agar)	973.3	E858.4	E943.3	E950.4	E962.0	E980.4
Agricultural agent NEC	989.89	E863.9	—	E950.6	E962.1	E980.7
Agrypnal	967.0	E851	E937.0	E950.1	E962.0	E980.1
Air contaminant(s), source or type not specified	987.9	E869.9	—	E952.9	E962.2	E982.9
specified type — see specific substance						
Akee	988.2	E865.4	—	E950.9	E962.1	E980.9
Akrinol	976.0	E858.7	E946.0	E950.4	E962.0	E980.4
Alantolactone	961.6	E857	E931.6	E950.4	E962.0	E980.4
Albamycin	960.8	E856	E930.8	E950.4	E962.0	E980.4
Albumin (normal human serum)	964.7	E858.2	E934.7	E950.4	E962.0	E980.4
Albuterol	975.7	E858.6	E945.7	E950.4	E962.0	E980.4
Alcohol	980.9	E860.9	—	E950.9	E962.1	E980.9
absolute	980.0	E860.1	—	E950.9	E962.1	E980.9
beverage	980.0	E860.0	E947.8	E950.9	E962.1	E980.9
amyl	980.3	E860.4	—	E950.9	E962.1	E980.9
antifreeze	980.1	E860.2	—	E950.9	E962.1	E980.9
butyl	980.3	E860.4	—	E950.9	E962.1	E980.9
dehydrated	980.0	E860.1	—	E950.9	E962.1	E980.9
beverage	980.0	E860.0	E947.8	E950.9	E962.1	E980.9
denatured	980.0	E860.1	—	E950.9	E962.1	E980.9
deterrents	977.3	E858.8	E947.3	E950.4	E962.0	E980.4
diagnostic (gastric function)	977.8	E858.8	E947.8	E950.4	E962.0	E980.4
ethyl	980.0	E860.1	—	E950.9	E962.1	E980.9
beverage	980.0	E860.0	E947.8	E950.9	E962.1	E980.9
grain	980.0	E860.1	—	E950.9	E962.1	E980.9
beverage	980.0	E860.0	E947.8	E950.9	E962.1	E980.9
industrial	980.9	E860.9	—	E950.9	E962.1	E980.9
isopropyl	980.2	E860.3	—	E950.9	E962.1	E980.9
methyl	980.1	E860.2	—	E950.9	E962.1	E980.9
preparation for consumption	980.0	E860.0	E947.8	E950.9	E962.1	E980.9
propyl	980.3	E860.4	—	E950.9	E962.1	E980.9
secondary	980.2	E860.3	—	E950.9	E962.1	E980.9
radiator	980.1	E860.2	—	E950.9	E962.1	E980.9
rubbing	980.2	E860.3	—	E950.9	E962.1	E980.9
specified type NEC	980.8	E860.8	—	E950.9	E962.1	E980.9
surgical	980.9	E860.9	—	E950.9	E962.1	E980.9
vapor (from any type of alcohol)	987.8	E869.8	—	E952.8	E962.2	E982.8
wood	980.1	E860.2	—	E950.9	E962.1	E980.9
Alcuronium chloride	975.2	E858.6	E945.2	E950.4	E962.0	E980.4
Aldactone	974.4	E858.5	E944.4	E950.4	E962.0	E980.4
Aldicarb	989.3	E863.2	—	E950.6	E962.1	E980.7
Aldomet	972.6	E858.3	E942.6	E950.4	E962.0	E980.4
Aldosterone	962.0	E858.0	E932.0	E950.4	E962.0	E980.4
Aldrin (dust)	989.2	E863.0	—	E950.6	E962.1	E980.7
Algeldrate	973.0	E858.4	E943.0	E950.4	E962.0	E980.4
Alidase	963.4	E858.1	E933.4	E950.4	E962.0	E980.4
Aliphatic thiocyanates	989.0	E866.8	—	E950.9	E962.1	E980.9

Nontherapeutic use substance

◀ Revised Text   ● New Line   ▲ Revised Code   ▽ Subterms under main terms may continue to next column or page

	Poisoning	Accident	Therapeutic Use	Suicide Attempt	Assault	Undetermined
Alka-seltzer	965.1	E850.3	E935.3	E950.0	E962.0	E980.0
Alkaline antiseptic solution (aromatic)	976.6	E858.7	E946.6	E950.4	E962.0	E980.4
Alkalinizing agents (medicinal)	963.3	E858.1	E933.3	E950.4	E962.0	E980.4
Alkalis, caustic	983.2	E864.2	—	E950.7	E962.1	E980.6
Alkalizing agents (medicinal)	963.3	E858.1	E933.3	E950.4	E962.0	E980.4
Alkavervir	972.6	E858.3	E942.6	E950.4	E962.0	E980.4
Allegron	969.05	E854.0	E939.0	E950.3	E962.0	E980.3
Alleve — Naproxen						
Allobarbital, allobarbitone	967.0	E851	E937.0	E950.1	E962.0	E980.1
Allopurinol	974.7	E858.5	E944.7	E950.4	E962.0	E980.4
Allylestrenol	962.2	E858.0	E932.2	E950.4	E962.0	E980.4
Allylisopropylacetylurea	967.8	E852.8	E937.8	E950.2	E962.0	E980.2
Allylisopropylmalonylurea	967.0	E851	E937.0	E950.1	E962.0	E980.1
Allyltribromide	967.3	E852.2	E937.3	E950.2	E962.0	E980.2
Aloe, aloes, aloin	973.1	E858.4	E943.1	E950.4	E962.0	E980.4
Alosetron	973.8	E858.4	E943.8	E950.4	E962.0	E980.4
Aloxidone	966.0	E855.0	E936.0	E950.4	E962.0	E980.4
Aloxiprin	965.1	E850.3	E935.3	E950.0	E962.0	E980.0
Alpha-1 blockers	971.3	E855.6	E941.3	E950.4	E962.0	E980.4
Alpha amylase	963.4	E858.1	E933.4	E950.4	E962.0	E980.4
Alphaprodine (hydrochloride)	965.09	E850.2	E935.2	E950.0	E962.0	E980.0
Alpha tocopherol	963.5	E858.1	E933.5	E950.4	E962.0	E980.4
Alseroxylon	972.6	E858.3	E942.6	E950.4	E962.0	E980.4
Alum (ammonium) (potassium)	983.2	E864.2	—	E950.7	E962.1	E980.6
medicinal (astringent) NEC	976.2	E858.7	E946.2	E950.4	E962.0	E980.4
Aluminium, aluminum (gel) (hydroxide)	973.0	E858.4	E943.0	E950.4	E962.0	E980.4
acetate solution	976.2	E858.7	E946.2	E950.4	E962.0	E980.4
aspirin	965.1	E850.3	E935.3	E950.0	E962.0	E980.0
carbonate	973.0	E858.4	E943.0	E950.4	E962.0	E980.4
glycinate	973.0	E858.4	E943.0	E950.4	E962.0	E980.4
nicotinate	972.2	E858.3	E942.2	E950.4	E962.0	E980.4
ointment (surgical) (topical)	976.3	E858.7	E946.3	E950.4	E962.0	E980.4
phosphate	973.0	E858.4	E943.0	E950.4	E962.0	E980.4
subacetate	976.2	E858.7	E946.2	E950.4	E962.0	E980.4
topical NEC	976.3	E858.7	E946.3	E950.4	E962.0	E980.4
Alurate	967.0	E851	E937.0	E950.1	E962.0	E980.1
Alverine (citrate)	975.1	E858.6	E945.1	E950.4	E962.0	E980.4
Alvodine	965.09	E850.2	E935.2	E950.0	E962.0	E980.0
Amanita phalloides	988.1	E865.5	—	E950.9	E962.1	E980.9
Amantadine (hydrochloride)	966.4	E855.0	E936.4	E950.4	E962.0	E980.4
Ambazone	961.9	E857	E931.9	E950.4	E962.0	E980.4
Ambenonium	971.0	E855.3	E941.0	E950.4	E962.0	E980.4
Ambutonium bromide	971.1	E855.4	E941.1	E950.4	E962.0	E980.4
Ametazole	977.8	E858.8	E947.8	E950.4	E962.0	E980.4
Amethocaine (infiltration) (topical)	968.5	E855.2	E938.5	E950.4	E962.0	E980.4
nerve block (peripheral) (plexus)	968.6	E855.2	E938.6	E950.4	E962.0	E980.4
spinal	968.7	E855.2	E938.7	E950.4	E962.0	E980.4
Amethopterin	963.1	E858.1	E933.1	E950.4	E962.0	E980.4
Amfepramone	977.0	E858.8	E947.0	E950.4	E962.0	E980.4
Amidon	965.02	E850.1	E935.1	E950.0	E962.0	E980.0
Amidopyrine	965.5	E850.5	E935.5	E950.0	E962.0	E980.0
Aminacrine	976.0	E858.7	E946.0	E950.4	E962.0	E980.4
Aminitrozole	961.5	E857	E931.5	E950.4	E962.0	E980.4
Aminoacetic acid	974.5	E858.5	E944.5	E950.4	E962.0	E980.4
Amino acids	974.5	E858.5	E944.5	E950.4	E962.0	E980.4
Aminocaproic acid	964.4	E858.2	E934.4	E950.4	E962.0	E980.4
Aminoethylisothiourium	963.8	E858.1	E933.8	E950.4	E962.0	E980.4
Aminoglutethimide	966.3	E855.0	E936.3	E950.4	E962.0	E980.4
Aminometradine	974.3	E858.5	E944.3	E950.4	E962.0	E980.4
Aminopentamide	971.1	E855.4	E941.1	E950.4	E962.0	E980.4
Aminophenazone	965.5	E850.5	E935.5	E950.0	E962.0	E980.0
Aminophenol	983.0	E864.0	—	E950.7	E962.1	E980.6
Aminophenylpyridone	969.5	E853.8	E939.5	E950.3	E962.0	E980.3
Aminophylline	975.7	E858.6	E945.7	E950.4	E962.0	E980.4
Aminopterin	963.1	E858.1	E933.1	E950.4	E962.0	E980.4
Aminopyrine	965.5	E850.5	E935.5	E950.0	E962.0	E980.0
Aminosalicylic acid	961.8	E857	E931.8	E950.4	E962.0	E980.4
Amiphenazole	970.1	E854.3	E940.1	E950.4	E962.0	E980.4
Amiquinsin	972.6	E858.3	E942.6	E950.4	E962.0	E980.4

	Poisoning	Accident	Therapeutic Use	Suicide Attempt	Assault	Undetermined
Amisometradine	974.3	E858.5	E944.3	E950.4	E962.0	E980.4
Amitriptyline	969.05	E854.0	E939.0	E950.3	E962.0	E980.3
Ammonia (fumes) (gas) (vapor)	987.8	E869.8	—	E952.8	E962.2	E982.8
liquid (household) NEC	983.2	E861.4	—	E950.7	E962.1	E980.6
spirit, aromatic	970.89	E854.3	E940.8	E950.4	E962.0	E980.4
Ammoniated mercury	976.0	E858.7	E946.0	E950.4	E962.0	E980.4
Ammonium						
carbonate	983.2	E864.2	—	E950.7	E962.1	E980.6
chloride (acidifying agent)	963.2	E858.1	E933.2	E950.4	E962.0	E980.4
expectorant	975.5	E858.6	E945.5	E950.4	E962.0	E980.4
compounds (household) NEC	983.2	E861.4	—	E950.7	E962.1	E980.6
fumes (any usage)	987.8	E869.8	—	E952.8	E962.2	E982.8
industrial	983.2	E864.2	—	E950.7	E962.1	E980.6
ichthyosulfonate	976.4	E858.7	E946.4	E950.4	E962.0	E980.4
mandelate	961.9	E857	E931.9	E950.4	E962.0	E980.4
Amobarbital	967.0	E851	E937.0	E950.1	E962.0	E980.1
Amodiaquin(e)	961.4	E857	E931.4	E950.4	E962.0	E980.4
Amopyroquin(e)	961.4	E857	E931.4	E950.4	E962.0	E980.4
Amphenidone	969.5	E853.8	E939.5	E950.3	E962.0	E980.3
Amphetamine	969.72	E854.2	E939.7	E950.3	E962.0	E980.3
Amphomycin	960.8	E856	E930.8	E950.4	E962.0	E980.4
Amphotericin B	960.1	E856	E930.1	E950.4	E962.0	E980.4
topical	976.0	E858.7	E946.0	E950.4	E962.0	E980.4
Ampicillin	960.0	E856	E930.0	E950.4	E962.0	E980.4
Amprotropine	971.1	E855.4	E941.1	E950.4	E962.0	E980.4
Amygdalin	977.8	E858.8	E947.8	E950.4	E962.0	E980.4
Amyl						
acetate (vapor)	982.8	E862.4	—	E950.9	E962.1	E980.9
alcohol	980.3	E860.4	—	E950.9	E962.1	E980.9
nitrite (medicinal)	972.4	E858.3	E942.4	E950.4	E962.0	E980.4
Amylase (alpha)	963.4	E858.1	E933.4	E950.4	E962.0	E980.4
Amylene hydrate	980.8	E860.8	—	E950.9	E962.1	E980.9
Amylobarbitone	967.0	E851	E937.0	E950.1	E962.0	E980.1
Amylocaine	968.9	E855.2	E938.9	E950.4	E962.0	E980.4
infiltration (subcutaneous)	968.5	E855.2	E938.5	E950.4	E962.0	E980.4
nerve block (peripheral) (plexus)	968.6	E855.2	E938.6	E950.4	E962.0	E980.4
spinal	968.7	E855.2	E938.7	E950.4	E962.0	E980.4
topical (surface)	968.5	E855.2	E938.5	E950.4	E962.0	E980.4
Amytal (sodium)	967.0	E851	E937.0	E950.1	E962.0	E980.1
Analeptics	970.0	E854.3	E940.0	E950.4	E962.0	E980.4
Analgesics	965.9	E850.9	E935.9	E950.0	E962.0	E980.0
aromatic NEC	965.4	E850.4	E935.4	E950.0	E962.0	E980.0
non-narcotic NEC	965.7	E850.7	E935.7	E950.0	E962.0	E980.0
specified NEC	965.8	E850.8	E935.8	E950.0	E962.0	E980.0
Anamirta cocculus	988.2	E865.3	—	E950.9	E962.1	E980.9
Ancillin	960.0	E856	E930.0	E950.4	E962.0	E980.4
Androgens (anabolic congeners)	962.1	E858.0	E932.1	E950.4	E962.0	E980.4
Androstalone	962.1	E858.0	E932.1	E950.4	E962.0	E980.4
Androsterone	962.1	E858.0	E932.1	E950.4	E962.0	E980.4
Anemone pulsatilla	988.2	E865.4	—	E950.9	E962.1	E980.9
Anesthesia, anesthetic (general) NEC	968.4	E855.1	E938.4	E950.4	E962.0	E980.4
block (nerve) (plexus)	968.6	E855.2	E938.6	E950.4	E962.0	E980.4
gaseous NEC	968.2	E855.1	E938.2	E950.4	E962.0	E980.4
halogenated hydrocarbon derivatives NEC	968.2	E855.1	E938.2	E950.4	E962.0	E980.4
infiltration (intradermal) (subcutaneous) (submucosal)	968.5	E855.2	E938.5	E950.4	E962.0	E980.4
intravenous	968.3	E855.1	E938.3	E950.4	E962.0	E980.4
local NEC	968.9	E855.2	E938.9	E950.4	E962.0	E980.4
nerve blocking (peripheral) (plexus)	968.6	E855.2	E938.6	E950.4	E962.0	E980.4
rectal NEC	968.3	E855.1	E938.3	E950.4	E962.0	E980.4
spinal	968.7	E855.2	E938.7	E950.4	E962.0	E980.4
surface	968.5	E855.2	E938.5	E950.4	E962.0	E980.4
topical	968.5	E855.2	E938.5	E950.4	E962.0	E980.4
Aneurine	963.5	E858.1	E933.5	E950.4	E962.0	E980.4
Anginine — see Glyceryl trinitrate						
Angio-Conray	977.8	E858.8	E947.8	E950.4	E962.0	E980.4
Angiotensin	971.2	E855.5	E941.2	E950.4	E962.0	E980.4
Anhydrohydroxyprogesterone	962.2	E858.0	E932.2	E950.4	E962.0	E980.4
Anhydron	974.3	E858.5	E944.3	E950.4	E962.0	E980.4
Anileridine	965.09	E850.2	E935.2	E950.0	E962.0	E980.0

Substance	Poisoning	Accident	Therapeutic Use	Suicide Attempt	Assault	Undetermined
Aniline (dye) (liquid)	983.0	E864.0	—	E950.7	E962.1	E980.6
analgesic	965.4	E850.4	E935.4	E950.0	E962.0	E980.0
derivatives, therapeutic NEC	965.4	E850.4	E935.4	E950.0	E962.0	E980.0
vapor	987.8	E869.8	—	E952.8	E962.2	E982.8
Aniscoropine	971.1	E855.4	E941.1	E950.4	E962.0	E980.4
Anisindione	964.2	E858.2	E934.2	E950.4	E962.0	E980.4
Anorexic agents	977.0	E858.8	E947.0	E950.4	E962.0	E980.4
Ant (bite) (sting)	—	E905.5	—	E950.9	E962.1	E980.9
Antabuse	977.3	E858.8	E947.3	E950.4	E962.0	E980.4
Antacids	973.0	E858.4	E943.0	E950.4	E962.0	E980.4
Antazoline	963.0	E858.1	E933.0	E950.4	E962.0	E980.4
Anthralin	976.4	E858.7	E946.4	E950.4	E962.0	E980.4
Anthramycin	960.7	E856	E930.7	E950.4	E962.0	E980.4
Anti-common cold agents NEC	975.6	E858.6	E945.6	E950.4	E962.0	E980.4
Anti-infectives NEC	961.9	E857	E931.9	E950.4	E962.0	E980.4
antibiotics	960.9	E856	E930.9	E950.4	E962.0	E980.4
specified NEC	960.8	E856	E930.8	E950.4	E962.0	E980.4
antihelmintic	961.6	E857	E931.6	E950.4	E962.0	E980.4
antimalarial	961.4	E857	E931.4	E950.4	E962.0	E980.4
antimycobacterial NEC	961.8	E857	E931.8	E950.4	E962.0	E980.4
antibiotics	960.6	E856	E930.6	E950.4	E962.0	E980.4
antiprotozoal NEC	961.5	E857	E931.5	E950.4	E962.0	—
blood	961.4	E857	E931.4	E950.4	E962.0	E980.4
antiviral	961.7	E857	E931.7	E950.4	E962.0	E980.4
arsenical	961.1	E857	E931.1	E950.4	E962.0	E980.4
ENT agents	976.6	E858.7	E946.6	E950.4	E962.0	E980.4
heavy metals NEC	961.2	E857	E931.2	E950.4	E962.0	E980.4
local	976.0	E858.7	E946.0	E950.4	E962.0	E980.4
ophthalmic preparation	976.5	E858.7	E946.5	E950.4	E962.0	E980.4
topical NEC	976.0	E858.7	E946.0	E950.4	E962.0	E980.4
Anti-inflammatory agents (topical)	976.0	E858.7	E946.0	E950.4	E962.0	E980.4
Anti-Parkinsonism agents	966.4	E855.0	E936.4	E950.4	E962.0	E980.4
Antiadrenergics	971.3	E855.6	E941.3	E950.4	E962.0	E980.4
Antiallergic agents	963.0	E858.1	E933.0	E950.4	E962.0	E980.4
Antianemic agents NEC	964.1	E858.2	E934.1	E950.4	E962.0	E980.4
Antiaris toxicaria	988.2	E865.4	—	E950.9	E962.1	E980.9
Antiarteriosclerotic agents	972.2	E858.3	E942.2	E950.4	E962.0	E980.4
Antiasthmatics	975.7	E858.6	E945.7	E950.4	E962.0	E980.4
Antibiotics	960.9	E856	E930.9	E950.4	E962.0	E980.4
antifungal	960.1	E856	E930.1	E950.4	E962.0	E980.4
antimycobacterial	960.6	E856	E930.6	E950.4	E962.0	E980.4
antineoplastic	960.7	E856	E930.7	E950.4	E962.0	E980.4
cephalosporin (group)	960.5	E856	E930.5	E950.4	E962.0	E980.4
chloramphenicol (group)	960.2	E856	E930.2	E950.4	E962.0	E980.4
macrolides	960.3	E856	E930.3	E950.4	E962.0	E980.4
specified NEC	960.8	E856	E930.8	E950.4	E962.0	E980.4
tetracycline (group)	960.4	E856	E930.4	E950.4	E962.0	E980.4
Anticancer agents NEC	963.1	E858.1	E933.1	E950.4	E962.0	E980.4
antibiotics	960.7	E856	E930.7	E950.4	E962.0	E980.4
Anticholinergics	971.1	E855.4	E941.1	E950.4	E962.0	E980.4
Anticholinesterase (organophosphorus) (reversible)	971.0	E855.3	E941.0	E950.4	E962.0	E980.4
Anticoagulants	964.2	E858.2	E934.2	E950.4	E962.0	E980.4
antagonists	964.5	E858.2	E934.5	E950.4	E962.0	E980.4
Anticonvulsants NEC	966.3	E855.0	E936.3	E950.4	E962.0	E980.4
Antidepressants	969.00	E854.0	E939.0	E950.3	E962.0	E980.3
monoamine oxidase inhibitors (MAOI)	969.01	E854.0	E939.0	E950.3	E962.0	E980.3
specified type NEC	969.09	E854.0	E939.0	E950.3	E962.0	E980.3
SSNRI (selective serotonin and norepinephrine reuptake inhibitors)	969.02	E854.0	E939.0	E950.3	E962.0	E980.3
SSRI (selective serotonin reuptake inhibitors)	969.03	E854.0	E939.0	E950.3	E962.0	E980.3
tetracyclic	969.04	E854.0	E939.0	E950.3	E962.0	E980.3
tricyclic	969.05	E854.0	E939.0	E950.3	E962.0	E980.3
Antidiabetic agents	962.3	E858.0	E932.3	E950.4	E962.0	E980.4
Antidiarrheal agents	973.5	E858.4	E943.5	E950.4	E962.0	E980.4
Antidiuretic hormone	962.5	E858.0	E932.5	E950.4	E962.0	E980.4
Antidotes NEC	977.2	E858.8	E947.2	E950.4	E962.0	E980.4
Antiemetic agents	963.0	E858.1	E933.0	E950.4	E962.0	E980.4
Antiepilepsy agent NEC	966.3	E855.0	E936.3	E950.4	E962.0	E980.4
Antifertility pills	962.2	E858.0	E932.2	E950.4	E962.0	E980.4
Antiflatulents	973.8	E858.4	E943.8	E950.4	E962.0	E980.4
Antifreeze	989.89	E866.8	—	E950.9	E962.1	E980.9
alcohol	980.1	E860.2	—	E950.9	E962.1	E980.9

Substance	Poisoning	Accident	Therapeutic Use	Suicide Attempt	Assault	Undetermined
Antifreeze — *continued*						
ethylene glycol	982.8	E862.4	—	E950.9	E962.1	E980.9
Antifungals (nonmedicinal) (sprays)	989.4	E863.6	—	E950.6	E962.1	E980.7
medicinal NEC	961.9	E857	E931.9	E950.4	E962.0	E980.4
antibiotic	960.1	E856	E930.1	E950.4	E962.0	E980.4
topical	976.0	E858.7	E946.0	E950.4	E962.0	E980.4
Antigastric secretion agents	973.0	E858.4	E943.0	E950.4	E962.0	E980.4
Antihelmintics	961.6	E857	E931.6	E950.4	E962.0	E980.4
Antihemophilic factor (human)	964.7	E858.2	E934.7	E950.4	E962.0	E980.4
Antihistamine	963.0	E858.1	E933.0	E950.4	E962.0	E980.4
Antihypertensive agents NEC	972.6	E858.3	E942.6	E950.4	E962.0	E980.4
Antiknock (tetraethyl lead)	984.1	E862.1	—	E950.9	—	E980.9
Antilipemics	972.2	E858.3	E942.2	E950.4	E962.0	E980.4
Antimalarials	961.4	E857	E931.4	E950.4	E962.0	E980.4
Antimony (compounds) (vapor) NEC	985.4	E866.2	—	E950.9	E962.1	E980.9
anti-infectives	961.2	E857	E931.2	E950.4	E962.0	E980.4
pesticides (vapor)	985.4	E863.4	—	E950.6	E962.2	E980.7
potassium tartrate	961.2	E857	E931.2	E950.4	E962.0	E980.4
tartrated	961.2	E857	E931.2	E950.4	E962.0	E980.4
Antimuscarinic agents	971.1	E855.4	E941.1	E950.4	E962.0	E980.4
Antimycobacterials NEC	961.8	E857	E931.8	E950.4	E962.0	E980.4
antibiotics	960.6	E856	E930.6	E950.4	E962.0	E980.4
Antineoplastic agents	963.1	E858.1	E933.1	E950.4	E962.0	E980.4
antibiotics	960.7	E856	E930.7	E950.4	E962.0	E980.4
Antiphlogistics	965.69	E850.6	E935.6	E950.0	E962.0	E980.0
Antiprotozoals NEC	961.5	E857	E931.5	E950.4	E962.0	E980.4
blood	961.4	E857	E931.4	E950.4	E962.0	E980.4
Antipruritics (local)	976.1	E858.7	E946.1	E950.4	E962.0	E980.4
Antipsychotic agents NEC	969.3	E853.8	E939.3	E950.3	E962.0	E980.3
Antipyretics	965.9	E850.9	E935.9	E950.0	E962.0	E980.0
specified NEC	965.8	E850.8	E935.8	E950.0	E962.0	E980.0
Antipyrine	965.5	E850.5	E935.5	E950.0	E962.0	E980.0
Antirabies serum (equine)	979.9	E858.8	E949.9	E950.4	E962.0	E980.4
Antirheumatics	965.69	E850.6	E935.6	E950.0	E962.0	E980.0
Antiseborrheics	976.4	E858.7	E946.4	E950.4	E962.0	E980.4
Antiseptics (external) (medicinal)	976.0	E858.7	E946.0	E950.4	E962.0	E980.4
Antistine	963.0	E858.1	E933.0	E950.4	E962.0	E980.4
Antithyroid agents	962.8	E858.0	E932.8	E950.4	E962.0	E980.4
Antitoxin, any	979.9	E858.8	E949.9	E950.4	E962.0	E980.4
Antituberculars	961.8	E857	E931.8	E950.4	E962.0	E980.4
antibiotics	960.6	E856	E930.6	E950.4	E962.0	E980.4
Antitussives	975.4	E858.6	E945.4	E950.4	E962.0	E980.4
Antivaricose agents (sclerosing)	972.7	E858.3	E942.7	E950.4	E962.0	E980.4
Antivenin (crotaline) (spider-bite)	979.9	E858.8	E949.9	E950.4	E962.0	E980.4
Antivert	963.0	E858.1	E933.0	E950.4	E962.0	E980.4
Antivirals NEC	961.7	E857	E931.7	E950.4	E962.0	E980.4
Ant poisons — *see* Pesticides						
Antrol	989.4	E863.4	—	E950.6	E962.1	E980.7
fungicide	989.4	E863.6	—	E950.6	E962.1	E980.7
Apomorphine hydrochloride (emetic)	973.6	E858.4	E943.6	E950.4	E962.0	E980.4
Appetite depressants, central	977.0	E858.8	E947.0	E950.4	E962.0	E980.4
Apresoline	972.6	E858.3	E942.6	E950.4	E962.0	E980.4
Aprobarbital, aprobarbitone	967.0	E851	E937.0	E950.1	E962.0	E980.1
Apronalide	967.8	E852.8	E937.8	E950.2	E962.0	E980.2
Aqua fortis	983.1	E864.1	—	E950.7	E962.1	E980.6
Arachis oil (topical)	976.3	E858.7	E946.3	E950.4	E962.0	E980.4
cathartic	973.2	E858.4	E943.2	E950.4	E962.0	E980.4
Aralen	961.4	E857	E931.4	E950.4	E962.0	E980.4
Arginine salts	974.5	E858.5	E944.5	E950.4	E962.0	E980.4
Argyrol	976.0	E858.7	E946.0	E950.4	E962.0	E980.4
ENT agent	976.6	E858.7	E946.6	E950.4	E962.0	E980.4
ophthalmic preparation	976.5	E858.7	E946.5	E950.4	E962.0	E980.4
Aristocort	962.0	E858.0	E932.0	E950.4	E962.0	E980.4
ENT agent	976.6	E858.7	E946.6	E950.4	E962.0	E980.4
ophthalmic preparation	976.5	E858.7	E946.5	E950.4	E962.0	E980.4
topical NEC	976.0	E858.7	E946.0	E950.4	E962.0	E980.4
Aromatics, corrosive	983.0	E864.0	—	E950.7	E962.1	E980.6
disinfectants	983.0	E861.4	—	E950.7	E962.1	E980.6

Nontherapeutic use substance

Subterms under main terms may continue to next column or page

	Poisoning	Accident	Therapeutic Use	Suicide Attempt	Assault	Undetermined
Arsenate of lead (insecticide)	985.1	E863.4	—	E950.8	E962.1	E980.8
herbicide	985.1	E863.5	—	E950.8	E962.1	E980.8
Arsenic, arsenicals (compounds) (dust) (fumes) (vapor) NEC	985.1	E866.3	—	E950.8	E962.1	E980.8
anti-infectives	961.1	E857	E931.1	E950.4	E962.0	E980.4
pesticide (dust) (fumes)	985.1	E863.4	—	E950.8	E962.1	E980.8
Arsine (gas)	985.1	E866.3	—	E950.8	E962.1	E980.8
Arsphenamine (silver)	961.1	E857	E931.1	E950.4	E962.0	E980.4
Arsthinol	961.1	E857	E931.1	E950.4	E962.0	E980.4
Artane	971.1	E855.4	E941.1	E950.4	E962.0	E980.4
Arthropod (venomous) NEC	989.5	E905.5	—	E950.9	E962.1	E980.9
Asbestos	989.81	E866.8	—	E950.9	E962.1	E980.9
Ascaridole	961.6	E857	E931.6	E950.4	E962.0	E980.4
Ascorbic acid	963.5	E858.1	E933.5	E950.4	E962.0	E980.4
Asiaticoside	976.0	E858.7	E946.0	E950.4	E962.0	E980.4
Aspidium (oleoresin)	961.6	E857	E931.6	E950.4	E962.0	E980.4
Aspirin	965.1	E850.3	E935.3	E950.0	E962.0	E980.0
Astringents (local)	976.2	E858.7	E946.2	E950.4	E962.0	E980.4
Atabrine	961.3	E857	E931.3	E950.4	E962.0	E980.4
Ataractics	969.5	E853.8	E939.5	E950.3	E962.0	E980.3
Atonia drug, intestinal	973.3	E858.4	E943.3	E950.4	E962.0	E980.4
Atophan	974.7	E858.5	E944.7	E950.4	E962.0	E980.4
Atropine	971.1	E855.4	E941.1	E950.4	E962.0	E980.4
Attapulgite	973.5	E858.4	E943.5	E950.4	E962.0	E980.4
Attenuvax	979.4	E858.8	E949.4	E950.4	E962.0	E980.4
Aureomycin	960.4	E856	E930.4	E950.4	E962.0	E980.4
ophthalmic preparation	976.5	E858.7	E946.5	E950.4	E962.0	E980.4
topical NEC	976.0	E858.7	E946.0	E950.4	E962.0	E980.4
Aurothioglucose	965.69	E850.6	E935.6	E950.0	E962.0	E980.0
Aurothioglycanide	965.69	E850.6	E935.6	E950.0	E962.0	E980.0
Aurothiomalate	965.69	E850.6	E935.6	E950.0	E962.0	E980.0
Automobile fuel	981	E862.1	—	E950.9	E962.1	E980.9
Autonomic nervous system agents NEC	971.9	E855.9	E941.9	E950.4	E962.0	E980.4
Avlosulfon	961.8	E857	E931.8	E950.4	E962.0	E980.4
Avomine	967.8	E852.8	E937.8	E950.2	E962.0	E980.2
Azacyclonol	969.5	E853.8	E939.5	E950.3	E962.0	E980.3
Azapetine	971.3	E855.6	E941.3	E950.4	E962.0	E980.4
Azaribine	963.1	E858.1	E933.1	E950.4	E962.0	E980.4
Azaserine	960.7	E856	E930.7	E950.4	E962.0	E980.4
Azathioprine	963.1	E858.1	E933.1	E950.4	E962.0	E980.4
Azosulfamide	961.0	E857	E931.0	E950.4	E962.0	E980.4
Azulfidine	961.0	E857	E931.0	E950.4	E962.0	E980.4
Azuresin	977.8	E858.8	E947.8	E950.4	E962.0	E980.4
Bacimycin	976.0	E858.7	E946.0	E950.4	E962.0	E980.4
ophthalmic preparation	976.5	E858.7	E946.5	E950.4	E962.0	E980.4
Bacitracin	960.8	E856	E930.8	E950.4	E962.0	E980.4
ENT agent	976.6	E858.7	E946.6	E950.4	E962.0	E980.4
ophthalmic preparation	976.5	E858.7	E946.5	E950.4	E962.0	E980.4
topical NEC	976.0	E858.7	E946.0	E950.4	E962.0	E980.4
Baking soda	963.3	E858.1	E933.3	E950.4	E962.0	E980.4
BAL	963.8	E858.1	E933.8	E950.4	E962.0	E980.4
Bamethan (sulfate)	972.5	E858.3	E942.5	E950.4	E962.0	E980.4
Bamipine	963.0	E858.1	E933.0	E950.4	E962.0	E980.4
Baneberry	988.2	E865.4	—	E950.9	E962.1	E980.9
Banewort	988.2	E865.4	—	E950.9	E962.1	E980.9
Barbenyl	967.0	E851	E937.0	E950.1	E962.0	E980.1
Barbital, barbitone	967.0	E851	E937.0	E950.1	E962.0	E980.1
Barbiturates, barbituric acid	967.0	E851	E937.0	E950.1	E962.0	E980.1
anesthetic (intravenous)	968.3	E855.1	E938.3	E950.4	E962.0	E980.4
Barium (carbonate) (chloride) (sulfate)	985.8	E866.4	—	E950.9	E962.1	E980.9
diagnostic agent	977.8	E858.8	E947.8	E950.4	E962.0	E980.4
pesticide	985.8	E863.4	—	E950.6	E962.1	E980.7
rodenticide	985.8	E863.7	—	E950.6	E962.1	E980.7
Barrier cream	976.3	E858.7	E946.3	E950.4	E962.0	E980.4
Battery acid or fluid	983.1	E864.1	—	E950.7	E962.1	E980.6
Bay rum	980.8	E860.8	—	E950.9	E962.1	E980.9
BCG vaccine	978.0	E858.8	E948.0	E950.4	E962.0	E980.4
Bearsfoot	988.2	E865.4	—	E950.9	E962.1	E980.9
Beclamide	966.3	E855.0	E936.3	E950.4	E962.0	E980.4
Bee (sting) (venom)	989.5	E905.3	—	E950.9	E962.1	E980.9
Belladonna (alkaloids)	971.1	E855.4	E941.1	E950.4	E962.0	E980.4
Bemegride	970.0	E854.3	E940.0	E950.4	E962.0	E980.4
Benactyzine	969.8	E855.8	E939.8	E950.3	E962.0	E980.3
Benadryl	963.0	E858.1	E933.0	E950.4	E962.0	E980.4
Bendrofluazide	974.3	E858.5	E944.3	E950.4	E962.0	E980.4
Bendroflumethiazide	974.3	E858.5	E944.3	E950.4	E962.0	E980.4
Benemid	974.7	E858.5	E944.7	E950.4	E962.0	E980.4
Benethamine penicillin G	960.0	E856	E930.0	E950.4	E962.0	E980.4
Benisone	976.0	E858.7	E946.0	E950.4	E962.0	E980.4
Benoquin	976.8	E858.7	E946.8	E950.4	E962.0	E980.4
Benoxinate	968.5	E855.2	E938.5	E950.4	E962.0	E980.4
Bentonite	976.3	E858.7	E946.3	E950.4	E962.0	E980.4
Benzalkonium (chloride)	976.0	E858.7	E946.0	E950.4	E962.0	E980.4
ophthalmic preparation	976.5	E858.7	E946.5	E950.4	E962.0	E980.4
Benzamidosalicylate (calcium)	961.8	E857	E931.8	E950.4	E962.0	E980.4
Benzathine penicillin	960.0	E856	E930.0	E950.4	E962.0	E980.4
Benzcarbimine	963.1	E858.1	E933.1	E950.4	E962.0	E980.4
Benzedrex	971.2	E855.5	E941.2	E950.4	E962.0	E980.4
Benzedrine (amphetamine)	969.72	E854.2	E939.7	E950.3	E962.0	E980.3
Benzene (acetyl) (dimethyl) (methyl) (solvent) (vapor)	982.0	E862.4	—	E950.9	E962.1	E980.9
hexachloride (gamma) (insecticide) (vapor)	989.2	E863.0	—	E950.6	E962.1	E980.7
Benzethonium	976.0	E858.7	E946.0	E950.4	E962.0	E980.4
Benzhexol (chloride)	966.4	E855.0	E936.4	E950.4	E962.0	E980.4
Benzilonium	971.1	E855.4	E941.1	E950.4	E962.0	E980.4
Benzin(e) — see Ligroin						
Benziodarone	972.4	E858.3	E942.4	E950.4	E962.0	E980.4
Benzocaine	968.5	E855.2	E938.5	E950.4	E962.0	E980.4
Benzodiapin	969.4	E853.2	E939.4	E950.3	E962.0	E980.4
Benzodiazepines (tranquilizers) NEC	969.4	E853.2	E939.4	E950.3	E962.0	E980.3
Benzoic acid (with salicylic acid) (anti-infective)	976.0	E858.7	E946.0	E950.4	E962.0	E980.4
Benzoin	976.3	E858.7	E946.3	E950.4	E962.0	E980.4
Benzol (vapor)	982.0	E862.4	—	E950.9	E962.1	E980.9
Benzomorphan	965.09	E850.2	E935.2	E950.0	E962.0	E980.0
Benzonatate	975.4	E858.6	E945.4	E950.4	E962.0	E980.4
Benzothiadiazides	974.3	E858.5	E944.3	E950.4	E962.0	E980.4
Benzoylpas	961.8	E857	E931.8	E950.4	E962.0	E980.4
Benzperidol	969.5	E853.8	E939.5	E950.3	E962.0	E980.3
Benzphetamine	977.0	E858.8	E947.0	E950.4	E962.0	E980.4
Benzpyrinium	971.0	E855.3	E941.0	E950.4	E962.0	E980.4
Benzquinamide	963.0	E858.1	E933.0	E950.4	E962.0	E980.4
Benzthiazide	974.3	E858.5	E944.3	E950.4	E962.0	E980.4
Benztropine	971.1	E855.4	E941.1	E950.4	E962.0	E980.4
Benzyl						
acetate	982.8	E862.4	—	E950.9	E962.1	E980.9
benzoate (anti-infective)	976.0	E858.7	E946.0	E950.4	E962.0	E980.4
morphine	965.09	E850.2	E935.2	E950.0	E962.0	E980.0
penicillin	960.0	E856	E930.0	E950.4	E962.0	E980.4
Bephenium hydroxynapthoate	961.6	E857	E931.6	E950.4	E962.0	E980.4
Bergamot oil	989.89	E866.8	—	E950.9	E962.1	E980.9
Berries, poisonous	988.2	E865.3	—	E950.9	E962.1	E980.9
Beryllium (compounds) (fumes)	985.3	E866.4	—	E950.9	E962.1	E980.9
Beta-carotene	976.3	E858.7	E946.3	E950.4	E962.0	E980.4
Beta-Chlor	967.1	E852.0	E937.1	E950.2	E962.0	E980.2
Betamethasone	962.0	E858.0	E932.0	E950.4	E962.0	E980.4
topical	976.0	E858.7	E946.0	E950.4	E962.0	E980.4
Betazole	977.8	E858.8	E947.8	E950.4	E962.0	E980.4
Bethanechol	971.0	E855.3	E941.0	E950.4	E962.0	E980.4
Bethanidine	972.6	E858.3	E942.6	E950.4	E962.0	E980.4
Betula oil	976.3	E858.7	E946.3	E950.4	E962.0	E980.4
Bhang	969.6	E854.1	E939.6	E950.3	E962.0	E980.3
Bialamicol	961.5	E857	E931.5	E950.4	E962.0	E980.4
Bichloride of mercury — see Mercury, chloride						
Bichromates (calcium) (crystals) (potassium) (sodium)	983.9	E864.3	—	E950.7	E962.1	E980.6
fumes	987.8	E869.8	—	E952.8	E962.2	E982.8
Biguanide derivatives, oral	962.3	E858.0	E932.3	E950.4	E962.0	E980.4
Biligrafin	977.8	E858.8	E947.8	E950.4	E962.0	E980.4
Bilopaque	977.8	E858.8	E947.8	E950.4	E962.0	E980.4
Bioflavonoids	972.8	E858.3	E942.8	E950.4	E962.0	E980.4
Biological substance NEC	979.9	E858.8	E949.9	E950.4	E962.0	E980.4
Biperiden	966.4	E855.0	E936.4	E950.4	E962.0	E980.4
Bisacodyl	973.1	E858.4	E943.1	E950.4	E962.0	E980.4
Bishydroxycoumarin	964.2	E858.2	E934.2	E950.4	E962.0	E980.4
Bismarsen	961.1	E857	E931.1	E950.4	E962.0	E980.4

	Poisoning	Accident	Therapeutic Use	Suicide Attempt	Assault	Undetermined
Bismuth (compounds)						
NEC	985.8	E866.4	—	E950.9	E962.1	E980.9
anti-infectives	961.2	E857	E931.2	E950.4	E962.0	E980.4
subcarbonate	973.5	E858.4	E943.5	E950.4	E962.0	E980.4
sulfarsphenamine	961.1	E857	E931.1	E950.4	E962.0	E980.4
Bisphosphonates						
intravenous	963.1	E858.1	E933.7	E950.4	E962.0	E980.4
oral	963.1	E858.1	E933.6	E950.4	E962.0	E980.4
Bithionol	961.6	E857	E931.6	E950.4	E962.0	E980.4
Bitter almond oil	989.0	E866.8	—	E950.9	E962.1	E980.9
Bittersweet	988.2	E865.4	—	E950.9	E962.1	E980.9
Black						
flag	989.4	E863.4	—	E950.6	E962.1	E980.7
henbane	988.2	E865.4	—	E950.9	E962.1	E980.9
leaf (40)	989.4	E863.4	—	E950.6	E962.1	E980.7
widow spider (bite)	989.5	E905.1	—	E950.9	E962.1	E980.9
antivenin	979.9	E858.8	E949.9	E950.4	E962.0	E980.4
Blast furnace gas (carbon monoxide from)	986	E868.8	—	E952.1	E962.2	E982.1
Bleaching solutions	983.9	E864.3	—	E950.7	E962.1	E980.6
Bleach NEC	983.9	E864.3	—	E950.7	E962.1	E980.6
Bleomycin (sulfate)	960.7	E856	E930.7	E950.4	E962.0	E980.4
Blockain	968.9	E855.2	E938.9	E950.4	E962.0	E980.4
infiltration (subcutaneous)	968.5	E855.2	E938.5	E950.4	E962.0	E980.4
nerve block (peripheral) (plexus)	968.6	E855.2	E938.6	E950.4	E962.0	E980.4
topical (surface)	968.5	E855.2	E938.5	E950.4	E962.0	E980.4
Blood (derivatives) (natural) (plasma) (whole)	964.7	E858.2	E934.7	E950.4	E962.0	E980.4
affecting agent	964.9	E858.2	E934.9	E950.4	E962.0	E980.4
specified NEC	964.8	E858.2	E934.8	E950.4	E962.0	E980.4
substitute (macromolecular)	964.8	E858.2	E934.8	E950.4	E962.0	E980.4
Blue velvet	965.09	E850.2	E935.2	E950.0	E962.0	E980.0
Bone meal	989.89	E866.5	—	E950.9	E962.1	E980.9
Bonine	963.0	E858.1	E933.0	E950.4	E962.0	E980.4
Boracic acid	976.0	E858.7	E946.0	E950.4	E962.0	E980.4
ENT agent	976.6	E858.7	E946.6	E950.4	E962.0	E980.4
ophthalmic preparation	976.5	E858.7	E946.5	E950.4	E962.0	E980.4
Borate (cleanser) (sodium)	989.6	E861.3	—	E950.9	E962.1	E980.9
Borax (cleanser)	989.6	E861.3	—	E950.9	E962.1	E980.9
Boric acid	976.0	E858.7	E946.0	E950.4	E962.0	E980.4
ENT agent	976.6	E858.7	E946.6	E950.4	E962.0	E980.4
ophthalmic preparation	976.5	E858.7	E946.5	E950.4	E962.0	E980.4
Boron hydride NEC	989.89	E866.8	—	E950.9	E962.1	E980.9
fumes or gas	987.8	E869.8	—	E952.8	E962.2	E982.8
Botox	975.3	E858.6	E945.3	E950.4	E962.0	E980.4
Brake fluid vapor	987.8	E869.8	—	E952.8	E962.2	E982.8
Brass (compounds) (fumes)	985.8	E866.4	—	E950.9	E962.1	E980.9
Brasso	981	E861.3	—	E950.9	E962.1	E980.9
Bretylium (tosylate)	972.6	E858.3	E942.6	E950.4	E962.0	E980.4
Brevital (sodium)	968.3	E855.1	E938.3	E950.4	E962.0	E980.4
British antilewisite	963.8	E858.1	E933.8	E950.4	E962.0	E980.4
Bromal (hydrate)	967.3	E852.2	E937.3	E950.2	E962.0	E980.2
Bromelains	963.4	E858.1	E933.4	E950.4	E962.0	E980.4
Bromides NEC	967.3	E852.2	E937.3	E950.2	E962.0	E980.2
Bromine (vapor)	987.8	E869.8	—	E952.8	E962.2	E982.8
compounds (medicinal)	967.3	E852.2	E937.3	E950.2	E962.0	E980.2
Bromisovalum	967.3	E852.2	E937.3	E950.2	E962.0	E980.2
Bromo-seltzer	965.4	E850.4	E935.4	E950.0	E962.0	E980.0
Bromobenzyl cyanide	987.5	E869.3	—	E952.8	E962.2	E982.8
Bromodiphenhydramine	963.0	E858.1	E933.0	E950.4	E962.0	E980.4
Bromoform	967.3	E852.2	E937.3	E950.2	E962.0	E980.2
Bromophenol blue reagent	977.8	E858.8	E947.8	E950.4	E962.0	E980.4
Bromosalicylhydroxamic acid	961.8	E857	E931.8	E950.4	E962.0	E980.4
Brompheniramine	963.0	E858.1	E933.0	E950.4	E962.0	E980.4
Bromural	967.3	E852.2	E937.3	E950.2	E962.0	E980.2
Brown spider (bite) (venom)	989.5	E905.1	—	E950.9	E962.1	E980.9
Brucia	988.2	E865.3	—	E950.9	E962.1	E980.9
Brucine	989.1	E863.7	—	E950.6	E962.1	E980.7
Brunswick green — see Copper						
Bruten — see Ibuprofen						
Bryonia (alba) (dioica)	988.2	E865.4	—	E950.9	E962.1	E980.9
Buclizine	969.5	E853.8	E939.5	E950.3	E962.0	E980.3
Bufferin	965.1	E850.3	E935.3	E950.0	E962.0	E980.0
Bufotenine	969.6	E854.1	E939.6	E950.3	E962.0	E980.3
Buphenine	971.2	E855.5	E941.2	E950.4	E962.0	E980.4
Bupivacaine	968.9	E855.2	E938.9	E950.4	E962.0	E980.4
infiltration (subcutaneous)	968.5	E855.2	E938.5	E950.4	E962.0	E980.4
nerve block (peripheral) (plexus)	968.6	E855.2	E938.6	E950.4	E962.0	E980.4
Busulfan	963.1	E858.1	E933.1	E950.4	E962.0	E980.4
Butabarbital (sodium)	967.0	E851	E937.0	E950.1	E962.0	E980.1
Butabarbitone	967.0	E851	E937.0	E950.1	E962.0	E980.1
Butabarpal	967.0	E851	E937.0	E950.1	E962.0	E980.1
Butacaine	968.5	E855.2	E938.5	E950.4	E962.0	E980.4
Butallylonal	967.0	E851	E937.0	E950.1	E962.0	E980.1
Butane (distributed in mobile container)	987.0	E868.0	—	E951.1	E962.2	E981.1
distributed through pipes	987.0	E867	—	E951.0	E962.2	E981.0
incomplete combustion of — see Carbon monoxide, butane						
Butanol	980.3	E860.4	—	E950.9	E962.1	E980.9
Butanone	982.8	E862.4	—	E950.9	E962.1	E980.9
Butaperazine	969.1	E853.0	E939.1	E950.3	E962.0	E980.3
Butazolidin	965.5	E850.5	E935.5	E950.0	E962.0	E980.0
Butethal	967.0	E851	E937.0	E950.1	E962.0	E980.1
Butethamate	971.1	E855.4	E941.1	E950.4	E962.0	E980.4
Buthalitone (sodium)	968.3	E855.1	E938.3	E950.4	E962.0	E980.4
Butisol (sodium)	967.0	E851	E937.0	E950.1	E962.0	E980.1
Butobarbital, butobarbitone	967.0	E851	E937.0	E950.1	E962.0	E980.1
Butriptyline	969.05	E854.0	E939.0	E950.3	E962.0	E980.3
Buttercups	988.2	E865.4	—	E950.9	E962.1	E980.9
Butter of antimony — see Antimony						
Butyl						
acetate (secondary)	982.8	E862.4	—	E950.9	E962.1	E980.9
alcohol	980.3	E860.4	—	E950.9	E962.1	E980.9
carbinol	980.8	E860.8	—	E950.9	E962.1	E980.9
carbitol	982.8	E862.4	—	E950.9	E962.1	E980.9
cellosolve	982.8	E862.4	—	E950.9	E962.1	E980.9
chloral (hydrate)	967.1	E852.0	E937.1	E950.2	E962.0	E980.2
formate	982.8	E862.4	—	E950.9	E962.1	E980.9
scopolammonium bromide	971.1	E855.4	E941.1	E950.4	E962.0	E980.4
Butyn	968.5	E855.2	E938.5	E950.4	E962.0	E980.4
Butyrophenone (-based tranquilizers)	969.2	E853.1	E939.2	E950.3	E962.0	E980.3
Cacodyl, cacodylic acid — see Arsenic						
Cactinomycin	960.7	E856	E930.7	E950.4	E962.0	E980.4
Cade oil	976.4	E858.7	E946.4	E950.4	E962.0	E980.4
Cadmium (chloride) (compounds) (dust) (fumes) (oxide)	985.5	E866.4	—	E950.9	E962.1	E980.9
sulfide (medicinal) NEC	976.4	E858.7	E946.4	E950.4	E962.0	E980.4
Caffeine	969.71	E854.2	E939.7	E950.3	E962.0	E980.3
Calabar bean	988.2	E865.4	—	E950.9	E962.1	E980.9
Caladium seguinium	988.2	E865.4	—	E950.9	E962.1	E980.9
Calamine (liniment) (lotion)	976.3	E858.7	E946.3	E950.4	E962.0	E980.4
Calciferol	963.5	E858.1	E933.5	E950.4	E962.0	E980.4
Calcium (salts) NEC	974.5	E858.5	E944.5	E950.4	E962.0	E980.4
acetylsalicylate	965.1	E850.3	E935.3	E950.0	E962.0	E980.0
benzamidosalicylate	961.8	E857	E931.8	E950.4	E962.0	E980.4
carbaspirin	965.1	E850.3	E935.3	E950.0	E962.0	E980.0
carbimide (citrated)	977.3	E858.8	E947.3	E950.4	E962.0	E980.4
carbonate (antacid)	973.0	E858.4	E943.0	E950.4	E962.0	E980.4
cyanide (citrated)	977.3	E858.8	E947.3	E950.4	E962.0	E980.4
dioctyl sulfosuccinate	973.2	E858.4	E943.2	E950.4	E962.0	E980.4
disodium edathamil	963.8	E858.1	E933.8	E950.4	E962.0	E980.4
disodium edetate	963.8	E858.1	E933.8	E950.4	E962.0	E980.4
EDTA	963.8	E858.1	E933.8	E950.4	E962.0	E980.4
hydrate, hydroxide	983.2	E864.2	—	E950.7	E962.1	E980.6
mandelate	961.9	E857	E931.9	E950.4	E962.0	E980.4
oxide	983.2	E864.2	—	E950.7	E962.1	E980.6
Calomel — see Mercury, chloride						
Caloric agents NEC	974.5	E858.5	E944.5	E950.4	E962.0	E980.4
Calusterone	963.1	E858.1	E933.1	E950.4	E962.0	E980.4
Camoquin	961.4	E857	E931.4	E950.4	E962.0	E980.4
Camphor (oil)	976.1	E858.7	E946.1	E950.4	E962.0	E980.4
Candeptin	976.0	E858.7	E946.0	E950.4	E962.0	E980.4

Nontherapeutic use substance

Subterms under main terms may continue to next column or page

	Poisoning	Accident	Therapeutic Use	Suicide Attempt	Assault	Undetermined
			External Cause (E-Code)			
Candicidin	976.0	E858.7	E946.0	E950.4	E962.0	E980.4
Cannabinols	969.6	E854.1	E939.6	E950.3	E962.0	E980.3
Cannabis (derivatives) (indica) (sativa)	969.6	E854.1	E939.6	E950.3	E962.0	E980.3
Canned heat	980.1	E860.2	—	E950.9	E962.1	E980.9
Cantharides, cantharidin, cantharis	976.8	E858.7	E946.8	E950.4	E962.0	E980.4
Capillary agents	972.8	E858.3	E942.8	E950.4	E962.0	E980.4
Capreomycin	960.6	E856	E930.6	E950.4	E962.0	E980.4
Captodiame, captodiamine	969.5	E853.8	E939.5	E950.3	E962.0	E980.3
Caramiphen (hydrochloride)	971.1	E855.4	E941.1	E950.4	E962.0	E980.4
Carbachol	971.0	E855.3	E941.0	E950.4	E962.0	E980.4
Carbacrylamine resins	974.5	E858.5	E944.5	E950.4	E962.0	E980.4
Carbamate (sedative)	967.8	E852.8	E937.8	E950.2	E962.0	E980.2
herbicide	989.3	E863.5		E950.6	E962.1	E980.7
insecticide	989.3	E863.2	—	E950.6	E962.1	E980.7
Carbamazepine	966.3	E855.0	E936.3	E950.4	E962.0	E980.4
Carbamic esters	967.8	E852.8	E937.8	E950.2	E962.0	E980.2
Carbamide	974.4	E858.5	E944.4	E950.4	E962.0	E980.4
topical	976.8	E858.7	E946.8	E950.4	E962.0	E980.4
Carbamylcholine chloride	971.0	E855.3	E941.0	E950.4	E962.0	E980.4
Carbarsone	961.1	E857	E931.1	E950.4	E962.0	E980.4
Carbaryl	989.3	E863.2		E950.6	E962.1	E980.7
Carbaspirin	965.1	E850.3	E935.3	E950.0	E962.0	E980.0
Carbazochrome	972.8	E858.3	E942.8	E950.4	E962.0	E980.4
Carbenicillin	960.0	E856	E930.0	E950.4	E962.0	E980.4
Carbenoxolone	973.8	E858.4	E943.8	E950.4	E962.0	E980.4
Carbetapentane	975.4	E858.6	E945.4	E950.4	E962.0	E980.4
Carbimazole	962.8	E858.0	E932.8	E950.4	E962.0	E980.4
Carbinol	980.1	E860.2	—	E950.9	E962.1	E980.9
Carbinoxamine	963.0	E858.1	E933.0	E950.4	E962.0	E980.4
Carbitol	982.8	E862.4	—	E950.9	E962.1	E980.9
Carbocaine	968.9	E855.2	E938.9	E950.4	E962.0	E980.4
infiltration (subcutaneous)	968.5	E855.2	E938.5	E950.4	E962.0	E980.4
nerve block (peripheral) (plexus)	968.6	E855.2	E938.6	E950.4	E962.0	E980.4
topical (surface)	968.5	E855.2	E938.5	E950.4	E962.0	E980.4
Carbol-fuchsin solution	976.0	E858.7	E946.0	E950.4	E962.0	E980.4
Carbolic acid — see also Phenol)	983.0	E864.0	—	E950.7	E962.1	E980.6
Carbomycin	960.8	E856	E930.8	E950.4	E962.0	E980.4
Carbon						
bisulfide (liquid) (vapor)	982.2	E862.4		E950.9	E962.1	E980.9
dioxide (gas)	987.8	E869.8	—	E952.8	E962.2	E982.8
disulfide (liquid) (vapor)	982.2	E862.4		E950.9	E962.1	E980.9
monoxide (from incomplete combustion of) (in) NEC	986	E868.9	—	E952.1	E962.2	E982.1
blast furnace gas	986	E868.8	—	E952.1	E962.2	E982.1
butane (distributed in mobile container)	986	E868.0	—	E951.1	E962.2	E981.1
distributed through pipes	986	E867		E951.0	E962.2	E981.0
charcoal fumes	986	E868.3	—	E952.1	E962.2	E982.1
coal						
gas (piped)	986	E867		E951.0	E962.2	E981.0
solid (in domestic stoves, fireplaces)	986	E868.3		E952.1	E962.2	E982.1
coke (in domestic stoves, fireplaces)	986	E868.3		E952.1	E962.2	E982.1
exhaust gas (motor) not in transit	986	E868.2	—	E952.0	E962.2	E982.0
combustion engine, any not in watercraft	986	E868.2		E952.0	E962.2	E982.0
farm tractor, not in transit	986	E868.2	—	E952.0	E962.2	E982.0
gas engine	986	E868.2		E952.0	E962.2	E982.0
motor pump	986	E868.2		E952.0	E962.2	E982.0
motor vehicle, not in transit	986	E868.2	—	E952.0	E962.2	E982.0
fuel (in domestic use)	986	E868.3	—	E952.1	E962.2	E982.1
gas (piped)	986	E867		E951.0	E962.2	E981.0
in mobile container	986	E868.0	—	E951.1	E962.2	E981.1
utility	986	E868.1	—	E951.8	E962.2	E981.1
in mobile container	986	E868.0	—	E951.1	E962.2	E981.1
piped (natural)	986	E867		E951.0	E962.2	E981.0
illuminating gas	986	E868.1	—	E951.8	E962.2	E981.8

	Poisoning	Accident	Therapeutic Use	Suicide Attempt	Assault	Undetermined
			External Cause (E-Code)			
Carbon — continued						
monoxide — continued						
industrial fuels or gases, any	986	E868.8	—	E952.1	E962.2	E982.1
kerosene (in domestic stoves, fireplaces)	986	E868.3	—	E952.1	E962.2	E982.1
kiln gas or vapor	986	E868.8	—	E952.1	E962.2	E982.1
motor exhaust gas, not in transit	986	E868.2	—	E952.0	E962.2	E982.0
piped gas (manufactured) (natural)	986	E867	—	E951.0	E962.2	E981.0
producer gas	986	E868.8	—	E952.1	E962.2	E982.1
propane (distributed in mobile container)	986	E868.0	—	E951.1	E962.2	E981.1
distributed through pipes	986	E867	—	E951.0	E962.2	E981.0
specified source NEC	986	E868.8	—	E952.1	E962.2	E982.1
stove gas	986	E868.1	—	E951.8	E962.2	E981.8
piped	986	E867	—	E951.0	E962.2	E981.0
utility gas	986	E868.1	—	E951.8	E962.2	E981.8
piped	986	E867	—	E951.0	E962.2	E981.0
water gas	986	E868.1	—	E951.8	E962.2	E981.8
wood (in domestic stoves, fireplaces)	986	E868.3	—	E952.1	E962.2	E982.1
tetrachloride (vapor) NEC	987.8	E869.8	—	E952.8	E962.2	E982.8
liquid (cleansing agent) NEC	982.1	E861.3	—	E950.9	E962.1	E980.9
solvent	982.1	E862.4	—	E950.9	E962.1	E980.9
Carbonic acid (gas)	987.8	E869.8	—	E952.8	E962.2	E982.8
anhydrase inhibitors	974.2	E858.5	E944.2	E950.4	E962.0	E980.4
Carbowax	976.3	E858.7	E946.3	E950.4	E962.0	E980.4
Carbrital	967.0	E851	E937.0	E950.1	E962.0	E980.1
Carbromal (derivatives)	967.3	E852.2	E937.3	E950.2	E962.0	E980.2
Cardiac						
depressants	972.0	E858.3	E942.0	E950.4	E962.0	E980.4
rhythm regulators	972.0	E858.3	E942.0	E950.4	E962.0	E980.4
Cardio-green	977.8	E858.8	E947.8	E950.4	E962.0	E980.4
Cardiografin	977.8	E858.8	E947.8	E950.4	E962.0	E980.4
Cardiotonic glycosides	972.1	E858.3	E942.1	E950.4	E962.0	E980.4
Cardiovascular agents NEC	972.9	E858.3	E942.9	E950.4	E962.0	E980.4
Cardrase	974.2	E858.5	E944.2	E950.4	E962.0	E980.4
Carfusin	976.0	E858.7	E946.0	E950.4	E962.0	E980.4
Carisoprodol	968.0	E855.1	E938.0	E950.4	E962.0	E980.4
Carmustine	963.1	E858.1	E933.1	E950.4	E962.0	E980.4
Carotene	963.5	E858.1	E933.5	E950.4	E962.0	E980.4
Carphenazine (maleate)	969.1	E853.0	E939.1	E950.3	E962.0	E980.3
Carter's Little Pills	973.1	E858.4	E943.1	E950.4	E962.0	E980.4
Cascara (sagrada)	973.1	E858.4	E943.1	E950.4	E962.0	E980.4
Cassava	988.2	E865.4	—	E950.9	E962.1	E980.9
Castellani's paint	976.0	E858.7	E946.0	E950.4	E962.0	E980.4
Castor						
bean	988.2	E865.3	—	E950.9	E962.1	E980.9
oil	973.1	E858.4	E943.1	E950.4	E962.0	E980.4
Caterpillar (sting)	989.5	E905.5	—	E950.9	E962.1	E980.9
Catha (edulis)	970.89	E854.3	E940.8	E950.4	E962.0	E980.4
Cathartics NEC	973.3	E858.4	E943.3	E950.4	E962.0	E980.4
contact	973.1	E858.4	E943.1	E950.4	E962.0	E980.4
emollient	973.2	E858.4	E943.2	E950.4	E962.0	E980.4
intestinal irritants	973.1	E858.4	E943.1	E950.4	E962.0	E980.4
saline	973.3	E858.4	E943.3	E950.4	E962.0	E980.4
Cathomycin	960.8	E856	E930.8	E950.4	E962.0	E980.4
Caustic(s)	983.9	E864.4	—	E950.7	E962.1	E980.6
alkali	983.2	E864.2	—	E950.7	E962.1	E980.6
hydroxide	983.2	E864.2	—	E950.7	E962.1	E980.6
potash	983.2	E864.2	—	E950.7	E962.1	E980.6
soda	983.2	E864.2	—	E950.7	E962.1	E980.6
specified NEC	983.9	E864.3	—	E950.7	E962.1	E980.6
Ceepryn	976.0	E858.7	E946.0	E950.4	E962.0	E980.4
ENT agent	976.6	E858.7	E946.6	E950.4	E962.0	E980.4
lozenges	976.6	E858.7	E946.6	E950.4	E962.0	E980.4
Celestone	962.0	E858.0	E932.0	E950.4	E962.0	E980.4
topical	976.0	E858.7	E946.0	E950.4	E962.0	E980.4
Cellosolve	982.8	E862.4	—	E950.9	E962.1	E980.9
Cell stimulants and proliferants	976.8	E858.7	E946.8	E950.4	E962.0	E980.4
Cellulose derivatives, cathartic	973.3	E858.4	E943.3	E950.4	E962.0	E980.4
nitrates (topical)	976.3	E858.7	E946.3	E950.4	E962.0	E980.4
Centipede (bite)	989.5	E905.4	—	E950.9	E962.1	E980.9
Central nervous system						
depressants	968.4	E855.1	E938.4	E950.4	E962.0	E980.4

	External Cause (E-Code)					
	Poisoning	Accident	Therapeutic Use	Suicide Attempt	Assault	Undetermined
Central nervous system —						
continued						
depressants — *continued*						
anesthetic (general)						
NEC	968.4	E855.1	E938.4	E950.4	E962.0	E980.4
gases NEC	968.2	E855.1	E938.2	E950.4	E962.0	E980.4
intravenous	968.3	E855.1	E938.3	E950.4	E962.0	E980.4
barbiturates	967.0	E851	E937.0	E950.1	E962.0	E980.1
bromides	967.3	E852.2	E937.3	E950.2	E962.0	E980.2
cannabis sativa	969.6	E854.1	E939.6	E950.3	E962.0	E980.3
chloral hydrate	967.1	E852.0	E937.1	E950.2	E962.0	E980.2
hallucinogenics	969.6	E854.1	E939.6	E950.3	E962.0	E980.3
hypnotics	967.9	E852.9	E937.9	E950.2	E962.0	E980.2
specified NEC	967.8	E852.8	E937.8	E950.2	E962.0	E980.2
muscle relaxants	968.0	E855.1	E938.0	E950.4	E962.0	E980.4
paraldehyde	967.2	E852.1	E937.2	E950.2	E962.0	E980.2
sedatives	967.9	E852.9	E937.9	E950.2	E962.0	E980.2
mixed NEC	967.6	E852.5	E937.6	E950.2	E962.0	E980.2
specified NEC	967.8	E852.8	E937.8	E950.2	E962.0	E980.2
muscle-tone depressants	968.0	E855.1	E938.0	E950.4	E962.0	E980.4
stimulants	970.9	E854.3	E940.9	E950.4	E962.0	E980.4
amphetamines	969.72	E854.2	E939.7	E950.3	E962.0	E980.3
analeptics	970.0	E854.3	E940.0	E950.4	E962.0	E980.4
antidepressants	969.00	E854.0	E939.0	E950.3	E962.0	E980.3
opiate antagonists	970.1	E854.3	E940.0	E950.4	E962.0	E980.4
specified NEC	970.89	E854.3	E940.8	E950.4	E962.0	E980.4
Cephalexin	960.5	E856	E930.5	E950.4	E962.0	E980.4
Cephaloglycin	960.5	E856	E930.5	E950.4	E962.0	E980.4
Cephaloridine	960.5	E856	E930.5	E950.4	E962.0	E980.4
Cephalosporins NEC	960.5	E856	E930.5	E950.4	E962.0	E980.4
N (adicillin)	960.0	E856	E930.0	E950.4	E962.0	E980.4
Cephalothin (sodium)	960.5	E856	E930.5	E950.4	E962.0	E980.4
Cerbera (odallam)	988.2	E865.4	—	E950.9	E962.1	E980.9
Cerberin	972.1	E858.3	E942.1	E950.4	E962.0	E980.4
Cerebral stimulants	970.9	E854.3	E940.9	E950.4	E962.0	E980.4
psychotherapeutic	969.79	E854.2	E939.7	E950.3	E962.0	E980.3
specified NEC	970.89	E854.3	E940.8	E950.4	E962.0	E980.4
Cetalkonium (chloride)	976.0	E858.7	E946.0	E950.4	E962.0	E980.4
Cetoxime	963.0	E858.1	E933.0	E950.4	E962.0	E980.4
Cetrimide	976.2	E858.7	E946.2	E950.4	E962.0	E980.4
Cetylpyridinium	976.0	E858.7	E946.0	E950.4	E962.0	E980.4
ENT agent	976.6	E858.7	E946.6	E950.4	E962.0	E980.4
lozenges	976.6	E858.7	E946.6	E950.4	E962.0	E980.4
Cevadilla — see Sabadilla						
Cevitamic acid	963.5	E858.1	E933.5	E950.4	E962.0	E980.4
Chalk, precipitated	973.0	E858.4	E943.0	E950.4	E962.0	E980.4
Charcoal						
fumes (carbon monoxide)	986	E868.3	—	E952.1	E962.2	E982.1
industrial	986	E868.8	—	E952.1	E962.2	E982.1
medicinal (activated)	973.0	E858.4	E943.0	E950.4	E962.0	E980.4
Chelating agents NEC	977.2	E858.8	E947.2	E950.4	E962.0	E980.4
Chelidonium majus	988.2	E865.4	—	E950.9	E962.1	E980.9
Chemical substance	989.9	E866.9	—	E950.9	E962.1	E980.9
specified NEC	989.89	E866.8	—	E950.9	E962.1	E980.9
Chemotherapy, antineoplastic	963.1	E858.1	E933.1	E950.4	E962.0	E980.4
Chenopodium (oil)	961.6	E857	E931.6	E950.4	E962.0	E980.4
Cherry laurel	988.2	E865.4	—	E950.9	E962.1	E980.9
Chiniofon	961.3	E857	E931.3	E950.4	E962.0	E980.4
Chlophedianol	975.4	E858.6	E945.4	E950.4	E962.0	E980.4
Chlor-Trimeton	963.0	E858.1	E933.0	E950.4	E962.0	E980.4
Chloral (betaine) (formamide) (hydrate)	967.1	E852.0	E937.1	E950.2	E962.0	E980.2
Chloralamide	967.1	E852.0	E937.1	E950.2	E962.0	E980.2
Chlorambucil	963.1	E858.1	E933.1	E950.4	E962.0	E980.4
Chloramphenicol	960.2	E856	E930.2	E950.4	E962.0	E980.4
ENT agent	976.6	E858.7	E946.6	E950.4	E962.0	E980.4
ophthalmic preparation	976.5	E858.7	E946.5	E950.4	E962.0	E980.4
topical NEC	976.0	E858.7	E946.0	E950.4	E962.0	E980.4
Chlorate(s) (potassium) (sodium) NEC	983.9	E864.3	—	E950.7	E962.1	E980.6
herbicides	989.4	E863.5	—	E950.6	E962.1	E980.7
Chlorcyclizine	963.0	E858.1	E933.0	E950.4	E962.0	E980.4
Chlordan(e) (dust)	989.2	E863.0	—	E950.6	E962.1	E980.7
Chlordantoin	976.0	E858.7	E946.0	E950.4	E962.0	E980.4
Chlordiazepoxide	969.4	E853.2	E939.4	E950.3	E962.0	E980.3
Chloresium	976.8	E858.7	E946.8	E950.4	E962.0	E980.4
Chlorethiazol	967.1	E852.0	E937.1	E950.2	E962.0	E980.2
Chlorethyl — *see* Ethyl, chloride						
Chloretone	967.1	E852.0	E937.1	E950.2	E962.0	E980.2

	External Cause (E-Code)					
	Poisoning	Accident	Therapeutic Use	Suicide Attempt	Assault	Undetermined
Chlorex	982.3	E862.4	—	E950.9	E962.1	E980.9
Chlorhexadol	967.1	E852.0	E937.1	E950.2	E962.0	E980.2
Chlorhexidine (hydrochloride)	976.0	E858.7	E946.0	E950.4	E962.0	E980.4
Chlorhydroxyquinolin	976.0	E858.7	E946.0	E950.4	E962.0	E980.4
Chloride of lime (bleach)	983.9	E864.3	—	E950.7	E962.1	E980.6
Chlorinated						
camphene	989.2	E863.0	—	E950.6	E962.1	E980.7
diphenyl	989.89	E866.8	—	E950.9	E962.1	E980.9
hydrocarbons NEC	989.2	E863.0	—	E950.6	E962.1	E980.7
solvent	982.3	E862.4	—	E950.9	E962.1	E980.9
lime (bleach)	983.9	E864.3	—	E950.7	E962.1	E980.6
naphthalene — see Naphthalene						
pesticides NEC	989.2	E863.0	—	E950.6	E962.1	E980.7
soda — see Sodium, hypochlorite						
Chlorine (fumes) (gas)	987.6	E869.8	—	E952.8	E962.2	E982.8
bleach	983.9	E864.3	—	E950.7	E962.1	E980.6
compounds NEC	983.9	E864.3	—	E950.7	E962.1	E980.6
disinfectant	983.9	E861.4	—	E950.7	E962.1	E980.6
releasing agents NEC	983.9	E864.3	—	E950.7	E962.1	E980.6
Chlorisondamine	972.3	E858.3	E942.3	E950.4	E962.0	E980.4
Chlormadinone	962.2	E858.0	E932.2	E950.4	E962.0	E980.4
Chlormerodrin	974.0	E858.5	E944.0	E950.4	E962.0	E980.4
Chlormethiazole	967.1	E852.0	E937.1	E950.2	E962.0	E980.2
Chlormethylenecycline	960.4	E856	E930.4	E950.4	E962.0	E980.4
Chlormezanone	969.5	E853.8	E939.5	E950.3	E962.0	E980.3
Chloroacetophenone	987.5	E869.3	—	E952.8	E962.2	E982.8
Chloroaniline	983.0	E864.0	—	E950.7	E962.1	E980.6
Chlorobenzene, chlorobenzol	982.0	E862.4	—	E950.9	E962.1	E980.9
Chlorobutanol	967.1	E852.0	E937.1	E950.2	E962.0	E980.2
Chlorodinitrobenzene	983.0	E864.0	—	E950.7	E962.1	E980.6
dust or vapor	987.8	E869.8	—	E952.8	E962.2	E982.8
Chloroethane — *see* Ethyl, chloride						
Chloroform (fumes) (vapor)	987.8	E869.8	—	E952.8	E962.2	E982.8
anesthetic (gas)	968.2	E855.1	E938.2	E950.4	E962.0	E980.4
liquid NEC	968.4	E855.1	E938.4	E950.4	E962.0	E980.4
solvent	982.3	E862.4	—	E950.9	E962.1	E980.9
Chloroguanide	961.4	E857	E931.4	E950.4	E962.0	E980.4
Chloromycetin	960.2	E856	E930.2	E950.4	E962.0	E980.4
ENT agent	976.6	E858.7	E946.6	E950.4	E962.0	E980.4
ophthalmic preparation	976.5	E858.7	E946.5	E950.4	E962.0	E980.4
otic solution	976.6	E858.7	E946.6	E950.4	E962.0	E980.4
topical NEC	976.0	E858.7	E946.0	E950.4	E962.0	E980.4
Chloronitrobenzene	983.0	E864.0	—	E950.7	E962.1	E980.6
dust or vapor	987.8	E869.8	—	E952.8	E962.2	E982.8
Chlorophenol	983.0	E864.0	—	E950.7	E962.1	E980.6
Chlorophenothane	989.2	E863.0	—	E950.6	E962.1	E980.7
Chlorophyll (derivatives)	976.8	E858.7	E946.8	E950.4	E962.0	E980.4
Chloropicrin (fumes)	987.8	E869.8	—	E952.8	E962.2	E982.8
fumigant	989.4	E863.8	—	E950.6	E962.1	E980.7
fungicide	989.4	E863.6	—	E950.6	E962.1	E980.7
pesticide (fumes)	989.4	E863.4	—	E950.6	E962.1	E980.7
Chloroprocaine	968.9	E855.2	E938.9	E950.4	E962.0	E980.4
infiltration (subcutaneous)	968.5	E855.2	E938.5	E950.4	E962.0	E980.4
nerve block (peripheral) (plexus)	968.6	E855.2	E938.6	E950.4	E962.0	E980.4
Chloroptic	976.5	E858.7	E946.5	E950.4	E962.0	E980.4
Chloropurine	963.1	E858.1	E933.1	E950.4	E962.0	E980.4
Chloroquine (hydrochloride) (phosphate)	961.4	E857	E931.4	E950.4	E962.0	E980.4
Chlorothen	963.0	E858.1	E933.0	E950.4	E962.0	E980.4
Chlorothiazide	974.3	E858.5	E944.3	E950.4	E962.0	E980.4
Chlorotrianisene	962.2	E858.0	E932.2	E950.4	E962.0	E980.4
Chlorovinyldichloroarsine	985.1	E866.3	—	E950.8	E962.1	E980.8
Chloroxylenol	976.0	E858.7	E946.0	E950.4	E962.0	E980.4
Chlorphenesin (carbamate)	968.0	E855.1	E938.0	E950.4	E962.0	E980.4
topical (antifungal)	976.0	E858.7	E946.0	E950.4	E962.0	E980.4
Chlorpheniramine	963.0	E858.1	E933.0	E950.4	E962.0	E980.4
Chlorphenoxamine	966.4	E855.0	E936.4	E950.4	E962.0	E980.4
Chlorphentermine	977.0	E858.8	E947.0	E950.4	E962.0	E980.4
Chlorproguanil	961.4	E857	E931.4	E950.4	E962.0	E980.4
Chlorpromazine	969.1	E853.0	E939.1	E950.3	E962.0	E980.3
Chlorpropamide	962.3	E858.0	E932.3	E950.4	E962.0	E980.4
Chlorprothixene	969.3	E853.8	E939.3	E950.3	E962.0	E980.3

Nontherapeutic use substance   ▽ Subterms under main terms may continue to next column or page

	Poisoning	Accident	Therapeutic Use	Suicide Attempt	Assault	Undetermined
External Cause (E-Code)						
Chlorquinaldol	976.0	E858.7	E946.0	E950.4	E962.0	E980.4
Chlortetracycline	960.4	E856	E930.4	E950.4	E962.0	E980.4
Chlorthalidone	974.4	E858.5	E944.4	E950.4	E962.0	E980.4
Chlortrianisene	962.2	E858.0	E932.2	E950.4	E962.0	E980.4
Chlorzoxazone	968.0	E855.1	E938.0	E950.4	E962.0	E980.4
Choke damp	987.8	E869.8	—	E952.8	E962.2	E982.8
Cholebrine	977.8	E858.8	E947.8	E950.4	E962.0	E980.4
Cholera vaccine	978.2	E858.8	E948.2	E950.4	E962.0	E980.4
Cholesterol-lowering agents	972.2	E858.3	E942.2	E950.4	E962.0	E980.4
Cholestyramine (resin)	972.2	E858.3	E942.2	E950.4	E962.0	E980.4
Cholic acid	973.4	E858.4	E943.4	E950.4	E962.0	E980.4
Choline						
dihydrogen citrate	977.1	E858.8	E947.1	E950.4	E962.0	E980.4
salicylate	965.1	E850.3	E935.3	E950.0	E962.0	E980.0
theophyllinate	974.1	E858.5	E944.1	E950.4	E962.0	E980.4
Cholinergics	971.0	E855.3	E941.0	E950.4	E962.0	E980.4
Cholografin	977.8	E858.8	E947.8	E950.4	E962.0	E980.4
Chorionic gonadotropin	962.4	E858.0	E932.4	E950.4	E962.0	E980.4
Chromates	983.9	E864.3	—	E950.7	E962.1	E980.6
dust or mist	987.8	E869.8		E952.8	E962.2	E982.8
lead	984.0	E866.0	—	E950.9	E962.1	E980.9
paint	984.0	E861.5		E950.9	E962.1	E980.9
Chromic acid	983.9	E864.3	—	E950.7	E962.1	E980.6
dust or mist	987.8	E869.8		E952.8	E962.2	E982.8
Chromium	985.6	E866.4	—	E950.9	E962.1	E980.9
compounds — see Chromates						
Chromonar	972.4	E858.3	E942.4	E950.4	E962.0	E980.4
Chromyl chloride	983.9	E864.3		E950.7	E962.1	E980.6
Chrysarobin (ointment)	976.4	E858.7	E946.4	E950.4	E962.0	E980.4
Chrysazin	973.1	E858.4	E943.1	E950.4	E962.0	E980.4
Chymar	963.4	E858.1	E933.4	E950.4	E962.0	E980.4
ophthalmic preparation	976.5	E858.7	E946.5	E950.4	E962.0	E980.4
Chymotrypsin	963.4	E858.1	E933.4	E950.4	E962.0	E980.4
ophthalmic preparation	976.5	E858.7	E946.5	E950.4	E962.0	E980.4
Cicuta maculata or virosa	988.2	E865.4	—	E950.9	E962.1	E980.9
Cigarette lighter fluid	981	E862.1		E950.9	E962.1	E980.9
Cinchocaine (spinal)	968.7	E855.2	E938.7	E950.4	E962.0	E980.4
topical (surface)	968.5	E855.2	E938.5	E950.4	E962.0	E980.4
Cinchona	961.4	E857	E931.4	E950.4	E962.0	E980.4
Cinchonine alkaloids	961.4	E857	E931.4	E950.4	E962.0	E980.4
Cinchophen	974.7	E858.5	E944.7	E950.4	E962.0	E980.4
Cinnarizine	963.0	E858.1	E933.0	E950.4	E962.0	E980.4
Citanest	968.9	E855.2	E938.9	E950.4	E962.0	E980.4
infiltration (subcutaneous)	968.5	E855.2	E938.5	E950.4	E962.0	E980.4
nerve block (peripheral) (plexus)	968.6	E855.2	E938.6	E950.4	E962.0	E980.4
Citric acid	989.89	E866.8		E950.9	E962.1	E980.9
Citrovorum factor	964.1	E858.2	E934.1	E950.4	E962.0	E980.4
Claviceps purpurea	988.2	E865.4		E950.9	E962.1	E980.9
Cleaner, cleansing agent, type not specified	989.89	E861.9	—	E950.9	E962.1	E980.9
of paint or varnish	982.8	E862.9		E950.9	E962.1	E980.9
specified type NEC	989.89	E861.3	—	E950.9	E962.1	E980.9
Clematis vitalba	988.2	E865.4		E950.9	E962.1	E980.9
Clemizole	963.0	E858.1	E933.0	E950.4	E962.0	E980.4
penicillin	960.0	E856	E930.0	E950.4	E962.0	E980.4
Clidinium	971.1	E855.4	E941.1	E950.4	E962.0	E980.4
Clindamycin	960.8	E856	E930.8	E950.4	E962.0	E980.4
Cliradon	965.09	E850.2	E935.2	E950.0	E962.0	E980.0
Clocortolone	962.0	E858.0	E932.0	E950.4	E962.0	E980.4
Clofedanol	975.4	E858.6	E945.4	E950.4	E962.0	E980.4
Clofibrate	972.2	E858.3	E942.2	E950.4	E962.0	E980.4
Clomethiazole	967.1	E852.0	E937.1	E950.2	E962.0	E980.2
Clomiphene	977.8	E858.8	E947.8	E950.4	E962.0	E980.4
Clonazepam	969.4	E853.2	E939.4	E950.3	E962.0	E980.3
Clonidine	972.6	E858.3	E942.6	E950.4	E962.0	E980.4
Clopamide	974.3	E858.5	E944.3	E950.4	E962.0	E980.4
Clorazepate	969.4	E853.2	E939.4	E950.3	E962.0	E980.3
Clorexolone	974.4	E858.5	E944.4	E950.4	E962.0	E980.4
Clorox (bleach)	983.9	E864.3		E950.7	E962.1	E980.6
Clortermine	977.0	E858.8	E947.0	E950.4	E962.0	E980.4
Clotrimazole	976.0	E858.7	E946.0	E950.4	E962.0	E980.4
Cloxacillin	960.0	E856	E930.0	E950.4	E962.0	E980.4
Coagulants NEC	964.5	E858.2	E934.5	E950.4	E962.0	E980.4
Coal (carbon monoxide from) — see also Carbon, monoxide, coal						
oil — see Kerosene						
External Cause (E-Code)						
Coal — see also Carbon, monoxide, coal — continued						
tar NEC	983.0	E864.0	—	E950.7	E962.1	E980.6
fumes	987.8	E869.8	—	E952.8	E962.2	E982.8
medicinal (ointment)	976.4	E855.2	E946.4	E950.4	E962.0	E980.4
analgesics NEC	965.5	E850.5	E935.5	E950.0	E962.0	E980.0
naphtha (solvent)	981	E862.0		E950.9	E962.1	E980.9
Cobalt (fumes) (industrial)	985.8	E866.4	—	E950.9	E962.1	E980.9
Cobra (venom)	989.5	E905.0	—	E950.9	E962.1	E980.9
Coca (leaf)	970.81	E854.3	E940.8	E950.4	E962.0	E980.4
Cocaine (hydrochloride) (salt)	970.81	E854.3	E940.8	E950.4	E962.0	E980.4
topical anesthetic	968.5	E855.2	E938.5	E950.4	E962.0	E980.4
Coccidioidin	977.8	E858.8	E947.8	E950.4	E962.0	E980.4
Cocculus indicus	988.2	E865.3	—	E950.9	E962.1	E980.9
Cochineal	989.89	E866.8	—	E950.9	E962.1	E980.9
medicinal products	977.4	E858.8	E947.4	E950.4	E962.0	E980.4
Codeine	965.09	E850.2	E935.2	E950.0	E962.0	E980.0
Coffee	989.89	E866.8	—	E950.9	E962.1	E980.9
Cogentin	971.1	E855.4	E941.1	E950.4	E962.0	E980.4
Coke fumes or gas (carbon monoxide)	986	E868.3	—	E952.1	E962.2	E982.1
industrial use	986	E868.8	—	E952.1	E962.2	E982.1
Colace	973.2	E858.4	E943.2	E950.4	E962.0	E980.4
Colchicine	974.7	E858.5	E944.7	E950.4	E962.0	E980.4
Colchicum	988.2	E865.3	—	E950.9	E962.1	E980.9
Cold cream	976.3	E858.7	E946.3	E950.4	E962.0	E980.4
Colestipol	972.2	E858.3	E942.2	E950.4	E962.0	E980.4
Colistimethate	960.8	E856	E930.8	E950.4	E962.0	E980.4
Colistin	960.8	E856	E930.8	E950.4	E962.0	E980.4
Collagen	977.8	E866.8	E947.8	E950.9	E962.1	E980.9
Collagenase	976.8	E858.7	E946.8	E950.4	E962.0	E980.4
Collodion (flexible)	976.3	E858.7	E946.3	E950.4	E962.0	E980.4
Colocynth	973.1	E858.4	E943.1	E950.4	E962.0	E980.4
Coloring matter — see Dye(s)						
Combustion gas — see Carbon, monoxide						
Compazine	969.1	E853.0	E939.1	E950.3	E962.0	E980.3
Compound						
42 (warfarin)	989.4	E863.7	—	E950.6	E962.1	E980.7
269 (endrin)	989.2	E863.0	—	E950.6	E962.1	E980.7
497 (dieldrin)	989.2	E863.0	—	E950.6	E962.1	E980.7
1080 (sodium fluoroacetate)	989.4	E863.7	—	E950.6	E962.1	E980.7
3422 (parathion)	989.3	E863.1	—	E950.6	E962.1	E980.7
3911 (phorate)	989.3	E863.1	—	E950.6	E962.1	E980.7
3956 (toxaphene)	989.2	E863.0	—	E950.6	E962.1	E980.7
4049 (malathion)	989.3	E863.1	—	E950.6	E962.1	E980.7
4124 (dicapthon)	989.4	E863.4	—	E950.6	E962.1	E980.7
E (cortisone)	962.0	E858.0	E932.0	E950.4	E962.0	E980.4
F (hydrocortisone)	962.0	E858.0	E932.0	E950.4	E962.0	E980.4
Congo red	977.8	E858.8	E947.8	E950.4	E962.0	E980.4
Coniine, conine	965.7	E850.7	E935.7	E950.0	E962.0	E980.0
Conium (maculatum)	988.2	E865.4	—	E950.9	E962.1	E980.9
Conjugated estrogens (equine)	962.2	E858.0	E932.2	E950.4	E962.0	E980.4
Contac	975.6	E858.6	E945.6	E950.4	E962.0	E980.4
Contact lens solution	976.5	E858.7	E946.5	E950.4	E962.0	E980.4
Contraceptives (oral)	962.2	E858.0	E932.2	E950.4	E962.0	E980.4
vaginal	976.8	E858.7	E946.8	E950.4	E962.0	E980.4
Contrast media (roentgenographic)	977.8	E858.8	E947.8	E950.4	E962.0	E980.4
Convallaria majalis	988.2	E865.4	—	E950.9	E962.1	E980.9
Copperhead snake (bite) (venom)	989.5	E905.0	—	E950.9	E962.1	E980.9
Copper (dust) (fumes) (salts) NEC	985.8	E866.4	—	E950.9	E962.1	E980.9
arsenate, arsenite	985.1	E866.3	—	E950.8	E962.1	E980.8
insecticide	985.1	E863.4	—	E950.6	E962.1	E980.8
emetic	973.6	E858.4	E943.6	E950.4	E962.0	E980.4
fungicide	985.8	E863.6	—	E950.6	E962.1	E980.7
insecticide	985.8	E863.4	—	E950.6	E962.1	E980.7
oleate	976.0	E858.7	E946.0	E950.4	E962.0	E980.4
sulfate	983.9	E864.3	—	E950.7	E962.1	E980.6
cupric	973.6	E858.4	E943.6	E950.4	E962.0	E980.4
cuprous	983.9	E864.3	—	E950.7	E962.1	E980.6
fungicide	983.9	E863.6	—	E950.7	E962.1	E980.6
Coral (sting)	989.5	E905.6	—	E950.9	E962.1	E980.9
snake (bite) (venom)	989.5	E905.0	—	E950.9	E962.1	E980.9
Cordran	976.0	E858.7	E946.0	E950.4	E962.0	E980.4
Corn cures	976.4	E858.7	E946.4	E950.4	E962.0	E980.4
Cornhusker's lotion	976.3	E858.7	E946.3	E950.4	E962.0	E980.4

Index

Corn starch — Decamethonium

	Poisoning	Accident	Therapeutic Use	Suicide Attempt	Assault	Undetermined
Corn starch	976.3	E858.7	E946.3	E950.4	E962.0	E980.4
Corrosive	983.9	E864.4	—	E950.7	E962.1	E980.6
acids NEC	983.1	E864.1	—	E950.7	E962.1	E980.6
aromatics	983.0	E864.0	—	E950.7	E962.1	E980.6
disinfectant	983.0	E861.4	—	E950.7	E962.1	E980.6
fumes NEC	987.9	E869.9	—	E952.9	E962.2	E982.9
specified NEC	983.9	E864.3	—	E950.7	E962.1	E980.6
sublimate — see Mercury, chloride						
Cort-Dome	962.0	E858.0	E932.0	E950.4	E962.0	E980.4
ENT agent	976.6	E858.7	E946.6	E950.4	E962.0	E980.4
ophthalmic preparation	976.5	E858.7	E946.5	E950.4	E962.0	E980.4
topical NEC	976.0	E858.7	E946.0	E950.4	E962.0	E980.4
Cortate	962.0	E858.0	E932.0	E950.4	E962.0	E980.4
Cortef	962.0	E858.0	E932.0	E950.4	E962.0	E980.4
ENT agent	976.6	E858.7	E946.6	E950.4	E962.0	E980.4
ophthalmic preparation	976.5	E858.7	E946.5	E950.4	E962.0	E980.4
topical NEC	976.0	E858.7	E946.0	E950.4	E962.0	E980.4
Corticosteroids (fluorinated)	962.0	E858.0	E932.0	E950.4	E962.0	E980.4
ENT agent	976.6	E858.7	E946.6	E950.4	E962.0	E980.4
ophthalmic preparation	976.5	E858.7	E946.5	E950.4	E962.0	E980.4
topical NEC	976.0	E858.7	E946.0	E950.4	E962.0	E980.4
Corticotropin	962.4	E858.0	E932.4	E950.4	E962.0	E980.4
Cortisol	962.0	E858.0	E932.0	E950.4	E962.0	E980.4
ENT agent	976.6	E858.7	E946.6	E950.4	E962.0	E980.4
ophthalmic preparation	976.5	E858.7	E946.5	E950.4	E962.0	E980.4
topical NEC	976.0	E858.7	E946.0	E950.4	E962.0	E980.4
Cortisone derivatives (acetate)	962.0	E858.0	E932.0	E950.4	E962.0	E980.4
ENT agent	976.6	E858.7	E946.6	E950.4	E962.0	E980.4
ophthalmic preparation	976.5	E858.7	E946.5	E950.4	E962.0	E980.4
topical NEC	976.0	E858.7	E946.0	E950.4	E962.0	E980.4
Cortogen	962.0	E858.0	E932.0	E950.4	E962.0	E980.4
ENT agent	976.6	E858.7	E946.6	E950.4	E962.0	E980.4
ophthalmic preparation	976.5	E858.7	E946.5	E950.4	E962.0	E980.4
Cortone	962.0	E858.0	E932.0	E950.4	E962.0	E980.4
ENT agent	976.6	E858.7	E946.6	E950.4	E962.0	E980.4
ophthalmic preparation	976.5	E858.7	E946.5	E950.4	E962.0	E980.4
Cortril	962.0	E858.0	E932.0	E950.4	E962.0	E980.4
ENT agent	976.6	E858.7	E946.6	E950.4	E962.0	E980.4
ophthalmic preparation	976.5	E858.7	E946.5	E950.4	E962.0	E980.4
topical NEC	976.0	E858.7	E946.0	E950.4	E962.0	E980.4
Cosmetics	989.89	E866.7	—	E950.9	E962.1	E980.9
Cosyntropin	977.8	E858.8	E947.8	E950.4	E962.0	E980.4
Cotarnine	964.5	E858.2	E934.5	E950.4	E962.0	E980.4
Cottonseed oil	976.3	E858.7	E946.3	E950.4	E962.0	E980.4
Cough mixtures (antitussives)	975.4	E858.6	E945.4	E950.4	E962.0	E980.4
containing opiates	965.09	E850.2	E935.2	E950.0	E962.0	E980.0
expectorants	975.5	E858.6	E945.5	E950.4	E962.0	E980.4
Coumadin	964.2	E858.2	E934.2	E950.4	E962.0	E980.4
rodenticide	989.4	E863.7	—	E950.6	E962.1	E980.7
Coumarin	964.2	E858.2	E934.2	E950.4	E962.0	E980.4
Coumetarol	964.2	E858.2	E934.2	E950.4	E962.0	E980.4
Cowbane	988.2	E865.4	—	E950.9	E962.1	E980.9
Cozyme	963.5	E858.1	E933.5	E950.4	E962.0	E980.4
Crack	970.81	E854.3	E940.8	E950.4	E962.0	E980.4
Creolin	983.0	E864.0	—	E950.7	E962.1	E980.6
disinfectant	983.0	E861.4	—	E950.7	E962.1	E980.6
Creosol (compound)	983.0	E864.0	—	E950.7	E962.1	E980.6
Creosote (beechwood) (coal tar)	983.0	E864.0	—	E950.7	E962.1	E980.6
medicinal (expectorant)	975.5	E858.6	E945.5	E950.4	E962.0	E980.4
syrup	975.5	E858.6	E945.5	E950.4	E962.0	E980.4
Cresol	983.0	E864.0	—	E950.7	E962.1	E980.6
disinfectant	983.0	E861.4	—	E950.7	E962.1	E980.6
Cresylic acid	983.0	E864.0	—	E950.7	E962.1	E980.6
Cropropamide	965.7	E850.7	E935.7	E950.0	E962.0	E980.0
with crotethamide	970.0	E854.3	E940.0	E950.4	E962.0	E980.4
Crotamiton	976.0	E858.7	E946.0	E950.4	E962.0	E980.4
Crotethamide	965.7	E850.7	E935.7	E950.0	E962.0	E980.0
with cropropamide	970.0	E854.3	E940.0	E950.4	E962.0	E980.4
Croton (oil)	973.1	E858.4	E943.1	E950.4	E962.0	E980.4
chloral	967.1	E852.0	E937.1	E950.2	E962.0	E980.2
Crude oil	981	E862.1	—	E950.9	E962.1	E980.9
Cryogenine	965.8	E850.8	E935.8	E950.0	E962.0	E980.0
Cryolite (pesticide)	989.4	E863.4	—	E950.6	E962.1	E980.7
Cryptenamine	972.6	E858.3	E942.6	E950.4	E962.0	E980.4
Crystal violet	976.0	E858.7	E946.0	E950.4	E962.0	E980.4
Cuckoopint	988.2	E865.4	—	E950.9	E962.1	E980.9
Cumetharol	964.2	E858.2	E934.2	E950.4	E962.0	E980.4

	Poisoning	Accident	Therapeutic Use	Suicide Attempt	Assault	Undetermined
Cupric sulfate	973.6	E858.4	E943.6	E950.4	E962.0	E980.4
Cuprous sulfate	983.9	E864.3	—	E950.7	E962.1	E980.6
Curare, curarine	975.2	E858.6	E945.2	E950.4	E962.0	E980.4
Cyanic acid — see Cyanide(s)						
Cyanide(s) (compounds) (hydrogen) (potassium) (sodium) NEC	989.0	E866.8	—	E950.9	E962.1	E980.9
dust or gas (inhalation) NEC	987.7	E869.8	—	E952.8	E962.2	E982.8
fumigant	989.0	E863.8	—	E950.6	E962.1	E980.7
mercuric — see Mercury						
pesticide (dust) (fumes)	989.0	E863.4	—	E950.6	E962.1	E980.7
Cyanocobalamin	964.1	E858.2	E934.1	E950.4	E962.0	E980.4
Cyanogen (chloride) (gas) NEC	987.8	E869.8	—	E952.8	E962.2	E982.8
Cyclaine	968.5	E855.2	E938.5	E950.4	E962.0	E980.4
Cyclamen europaeum	988.2	E865.4	—	E950.9	E962.1	E980.9
Cyclandelate	972.5	E858.3	E942.5	E950.4	E962.0	E980.4
Cyclazocine	965.09	E850.2	E935.2	E950.0	E962.0	E980.0
Cyclizine	963.0	E858.1	E933.0	E950.4	E962.0	E980.4
Cyclobarbital, cyclobarbitone	967.0	E851	E937.0	E950.1	E962.0	E980.1
Cycloguanil	961.4	E857	E931.4	E950.4	E962.0	E980.4
Cyclohexane	982.0	E862.4	—	E950.9	E962.1	E980.9
Cyclohexanol	980.8	E860.8	—	E950.9	E962.1	E980.9
Cyclohexanone	982.8	E862.4	—	E950.9	E962.1	E980.9
Cyclomethycaine	968.5	E855.2	E938.5	E950.4	E962.0	E980.4
Cyclopentamine	971.2	E855.5	E941.2	E950.4	E962.0	E980.4
Cyclopenthiazide	974.3	E858.5	E944.3	E950.4	E962.0	E980.4
Cyclopentolate	971.1	E855.4	E941.1	E950.4	E962.0	E980.4
Cyclophosphamide	963.1	E858.1	E933.1	E950.4	E962.0	E980.4
Cyclopropane	968.2	E855.1	E938.2	E950.4	E962.0	E980.4
Cycloserine	960.6	E856	E930.6	E950.4	E962.0	E980.4
Cyclothiazide	974.3	E858.5	E944.3	E950.4	E962.0	E980.4
Cycrimine	966.4	E855.0	E936.4	E950.4	E962.0	E980.4
Cymarin	972.1	E858.3	E942.1	E950.4	E962.0	E980.4
Cyproheptadine	963.0	E858.1	E933.0	E950.4	E962.0	E980.4
Cyprolidol	969.09	E854.0	E939.0	E950.3	E962.0	E980.3
Cytarabine	963.1	E858.1	E933.1	E950.4	E962.0	E980.4
Cytisus						
laburnum	988.2	E865.4	—	E950.9	E962.1	E980.9
scoparius	988.2	E865.4	—	E950.9	E962.1	E980.9
Cytomel	962.7	E858.0	E932.7	E950.4	E962.0	E980.4
Cytosine (antineoplastic)	963.1	E858.1	E933.1	E950.4	E962.0	E980.4
Cytoxan	963.1	E858.1	E933.1	E950.4	E962.0	E980.4
D-Con (rodenticide)	989.4	E863.7	—	E950.6	E962.1	E980.7
D-lysergic acid diethylamide	969.6	E854.1	E939.6	E950.3	E962.0	E980.3
Dacarbazine	963.1	E858.1	E933.1	E950.4	E962.0	E980.4
Dactinomycin	960.7	E856	E930.7	E950.4	E962.0	E980.4
DADPS	961.8	E857	E931.8	E950.4	E962.0	E980.4
Dakin's solution (external)	976.0	E858.7	E946.0	E950.4	E962.0	E980.4
Dalmane	969.4	E853.2	E939.4	E950.3	E962.0	E980.3
DAM	977.2	E858.8	E947.2	E950.4	E962.0	E980.4
Danilone	964.2	E858.2	E934.2	E950.4	E962.0	E980.4
Danthron	973.1	E858.4	E943.1	E950.4	E962.0	E980.4
Dantrolene	975.2	E858.6	E945.2	E950.4	E962.0	E980.4
Daphne (gnidium) (mezereum)	988.2	E865.4	—	E950.9	E962.1	E980.9
berry	988.2	E865.3	—	E950.9	E962.1	E980.9
Dapsone	961.8	E857	E931.8	E950.4	E962.0	E980.4
Daraprim	961.4	E857	E931.4	E950.4	E962.0	E980.4
Darnel	988.2	E865.3	—	E950.9	E962.1	E980.9
Darvon	965.8	E850.8	E935.8	E950.0	E962.0	E980.0
Daunorubicin	960.7	E856	E930.7	E950.4	E962.0	E980.4
DBI	962.3	E858.0	E932.3	E950.4	E962.0	E980.4
DDS	961.8	E857	E931.8	E950.4	E962.0	E980.4
DDT	989.2	E863.0	—	E950.6	E962.1	E980.7
Deadly nightshade	988.2	E865.4	—	E950.9	E962.1	E980.9
berry	988.2	E865.3	—	E950.9	E962.1	E980.9
Deanol	969.79	E854.2	E939.7	E950.3	E962.0	E980.3
Debrisoquine	972.6	E858.3	E942.6	E950.4	E962.0	E980.4
Decaborane	989.89	E866.8	—	E950.9	E962.1	E980.9
fumes	987.8	E869.8	—	E952.8	E962.2	E982.8
Decadron	962.0	E858.0	E932.0	E950.4	E962.0	E980.4
ENT agent	976.6	E858.7	E946.6	E950.4	E962.0	E980.4
ophthalmic preparation	976.5	E858.7	E946.5	E950.4	E962.0	E980.4
topical NEC	976.0	E858.7	E946.0	E950.4	E962.0	E980.4
Decahydronaphthalene	982.0	E862.4	—	E950.9	E962.1	E980.9
Decalin	982.0	E862.4	—	E950.9	E962.1	E980.9
Decamethonium	975.2	E858.6	E945.2	E950.4	E962.0	E980.4

	Poisoning	Accident	Therapeutic Use	Suicide Attempt	Assault	Undetermined
External Cause (E-Code)						
Decholin	973.4	E858.4	E943.4	E950.4	E962.0	E980.4
sodium (diagnostic)	977.8	E858.8	E947.8	E950.4	E962.0	E980.4
Declomycin	960.4	E856	E930.4	E950.4	E962.0	E980.4
Deferoxamine	963.8	E858.1	E933.8	E950.4	E962.0	E980.4
Dehydrocholic acid	973.4	E858.4	E943.4	E950.4	E962.0	E980.4
Dekalin	982.0	E862.4	—	E950.9	E962.1	E980.9
Delalutin	962.2	E858.0	E932.2	E950.4	E962.0	E980.4
Delphinium	988.2	E865.3	—	E950.9	E962.1	E980.9
Deltasone	962.0	E858.0	E932.0	E950.4	E962.0	E980.4
Deltra	962.0	E858.0	E932.0	E950.4	E962.0	E980.4
Delvinal	967.0	E851	E937.0	E950.1	E962.0	E980.1
Demecarium (bromide)	971.0	E855.3	E941.0	E950.4	E962.0	E980.4
Demeclocycline	960.4	E856	E930.4	E950.4	E962.0	E980.4
Demecolcine	963.1	E858.1	E933.1	E950.4	E962.0	E980.4
Demelanizing agents	976.8	E858.7	E946.8	E950.4	E962.0	E980.4
Demerol	965.09	E850.2	E935.2	E950.0	E962.0	E980.0
Demethylchlortetracy-						
cline	960.4	E856	E930.4	E950.4	E962.0	E980.4
Demethyltetracycline	960.4	E856	E930.4	E950.4	E962.0	E980.4
Demeton	989.3	E863.1	—	E950.6	E962.1	E980.7
Demulcents	976.3	E858.7	E946.3	E950.4	E962.0	E980.4
Demulen	962.2	E858.0	E932.2	E950.4	E962.0	E980.4
Denatured alcohol	980.0	E860.1	—	E950.9	E962.1	E980.9
Dendrid	976.5	E858.7	E946.5	E950.4	E962.0	E980.4
Dental agents, topical	976.7	E858.7	E946.7	E950.4	E962.0	E980.4
Deodorant spray (feminine						
hygiene)	976.8	E858.7	E946.8	E950.4	E962.0	E980.4
Deoxyribonuclease	963.4	E858.1	E933.4	E950.4	E962.0	E980.4
Depressants						
appetite, central	977.0	E858.8	E947.0	E950.4	E962.0	E980.4
cardiac	972.0	E858.3	E942.0	E950.4	E962.0	E980.4
central nervous system (anes-						
thetic)	968.4	E855.1	E938.4	E950.4	E962.0	E980.4
psychotherapeutic	969.5	E853.9	E939.5	E950.3	E962.0	E980.3
Dequalinium	976.0	E858.7	E946.0	E950.4	E962.0	E980.4
Dermolate	976.2	E858.7	E946.2	E950.4	E962.0	E980.4
DES	962.2	E858.0	E932.2	E950.4	E962.0	E980.4
Desenex	976.0	E858.7	E946.0	E950.4	E962.0	E980.4
Deserpidine	972.6	E858.3	E942.6	E950.4	E962.0	E980.4
Desipramine	969.05	E854.0	E939.0	E950.3	E962.0	E980.3
Deslanoside	972.1	E858.3	E942.1	E950.4	E962.0	E980.4
Desocodeine	965.09	E850.2	E935.2	E950.0	E962.0	E980.0
Desomorphine	965.09	E850.2	E935.2	E950.0	E962.0	E980.0
Desonide	976.0	E858.7	E946.0	E950.4	E962.0	E980.4
Desoxycorticosterone						
derivatives	962.0	E858.0	E932.0	E950.4	E962.0	E980.4
Desoxyephedrine	969.72	E854.2	E939.7	E950.3	E962.0	E980.3
DET	969.6	E854.1	E939.6	E950.3	E962.0	E980.3
Detergents (ingested) (synthet-						
ic)	989.6	E861.0	—	E950.9	E962.1	E980.9
ENT agent	976.6	E858.7	E946.6	E950.4	E962.0	E980.4
external medication	976.2	E858.7	E946.2	E950.4	E962.0	E980.4
ophthalmic preparation	976.5	E858.7	E946.5	E950.4	E962.0	E980.4
topical NEC	976.0	E858.7	E946.0	E950.4	E962.0	E980.4
Deterrent, alcohol	977.3	E858.8	E947.3	E950.4	E962.0	E980.4
Detrothyronine	962.7	E858.0	E932.7	E950.4	E962.0	E980.4
Dettol (external medica-						
tion)	976.0	E858.7	E946.0	E950.4	E962.0	E980.4
Dexamethasone	962.0	E858.0	E932.0	E950.4	E962.0	E980.4
Dexamphetamine	969.72	E854.2	E939.7	E950.3	E962.0	E980.3
Dexedrine	969.72	E854.2	E939.7	E950.3	E962.0	E980.3
Dexpanthenol	963.5	E858.1	E933.5	E950.4	E962.0	E980.4
Dextran	964.8	E858.2	E934.8	E950.4	E962.0	E980.4
Dextriferron	964.0	E858.2	E934.0	E950.4	E962.0	E980.4
Dextroamphetamine	969.72	E854.2	E939.7	E950.3	E962.0	E980.3
Dextro calcium pantothen-						
ate	963.5	E858.1	E933.5	E950.4	E962.0	E980.4
Dextromethorphan	975.4	E858.6	E945.4	E950.4	E962.0	E980.4
Dextromoramide	965.09	E850.2	E935.2	E950.0	E962.0	E980.0
Dextro pantothenyl alco-						
hol	963.5	E858.1	E933.5	E950.4	E962.0	E980.4
topical	976.8	E858.7	E946.8	E950.4	E962.0	E980.4
Dextropropoxyphene (hy-						
drochloride)	965.8	E850.8	E935.8	E950.0	E962.0	E980.0
Dextrorphan	965.09	E850.2	E935.2	E950.0	E962.0	E980.0
Dextrose NEC	974.5	E858.5	E944.5	E950.4	E962.0	E980.4
Dextrothyroxin	962.7	E858.0	E932.7	E950.4	E962.0	E980.4
DFP	971.0	E855.3	E941.0	E950.4	E962.0	E980.4
DHE-45	972.9	E858.3	E942.9	E950.4	E962.0	E980.4
Diabinese	962.3	E858.0	E932.3	E950.4	E962.0	E980.4
Diacetyl monoxime	977.2	E858.8	E947.2	E950.4	E962.0	E980.4
Diacetylmorphine	965.01	E850.0	E935.0	E950.0	E962.0	E980.0

	Poisoning	Accident	Therapeutic Use	Suicide Attempt	Assault	Undetermined
External Cause (E-Code)						
Diagnostic agents	977.8	E858.8	E947.8	E950.4	E962.0	E980.4
Dial (soap)	976.2	E858.7	E946.2	E950.4	E962.0	E980.4
sedative	967.0	E851	E937.0	E950.1	E962.0	E980.1
Diallylbarbituric acid	967.0	E851	E937.0	E950.1	E962.0	E980.1
Diaminodiphenylsulfone	961.8	E857	E931.8	E950.4	E962.0	E980.4
Diamorphine	965.01	E850.0	E935.0	E950.0	E962.0	E980.0
Diamox	974.2	E858.5	E944.2	E950.4	E962.0	E980.4
Diamthazole	976.0	E858.7	E946.0	E950.4	E962.0	E980.4
Diaphenylsulfone	961.8	E857	E931.8	E950.4	E962.0	E980.4
Diasone (sodium)	961.8	E857	E931.8	E950.4	E962.0	E980.4
Diazepam	969.4	E853.2	E939.4	E950.3	E962.0	E980.3
Diazinon	989.3	E863.1	—	E950.6	E962.1	E980.7
Diazomethane (gas)	987.8	E869.8	—	E952.8	E962.2	E982.8
Diazoxide	972.5	E858.3	E942.5	E950.4	E962.0	E980.4
Dibenamine	971.3	E855.6	E941.3	E950.4	E962.0	E980.4
Dibenzheptropine	963.0	E858.1	E933.0	E950.4	E962.0	E980.4
Dibenzyline	971.3	E855.6	E941.3	E950.4	E962.0	E980.4
Diborane (gas)	987.8	E869.8	—	E952.8	E962.2	E982.8
Dibromomannitol	963.1	E858.1	E933.1	E950.4	E962.0	E980.4
Dibucaine (spinal)	968.7	E855.2	E938.7	E950.4	E962.0	E980.4
topical (surface)	968.5	E855.2	E938.5	E950.4	E962.0	E980.4
Dibunate sodium	975.4	E858.6	E945.4	E950.4	E962.0	E980.4
Dibutoline	971.1	E855.4	E941.1	E950.4	E962.0	E980.4
Dicapthon	989.4	E863.4	—	E950.6	E962.1	E980.7
Dichloralphenazone	967.1	E852.0	E937.1	E950.2	E962.0	E980.2
Dichlorodifluo-						
romethane	987.4	E869.2	—	E952.8	E962.2	E982.8
Dichloroethane	982.3	E862.4	—	E950.9	E962.1	E980.9
Dichloroethylene	982.3	E862.4	—	E950.9	E962.1	E980.9
Dichloroethyl sulfide	987.8	E869.8	—	E952.8	E962.2	E982.8
Dichlorohydrin	982.3	E862.4	—	E950.9	E962.1	E980.9
Dichloromethane (solvent)						
(vapor)	982.3	E862.4	—	E950.9	E962.1	E980.9
Dichlorophen(e)	961.6	E857	E931.6	E950.4	E962.0	E980.4
Dichlorphenamide	974.2	E858.5	E944.2	E950.4	E962.0	E980.4
Dichlorvos	989.3	E863.1	—	E950.6	E962.1	E980.7
Diclofenac sodium	965.69	E850.6	E935.6	E950.0	E962.0	E980.0
Dicoumarin, dicumarol	964.2	E858.2	E934.2	E950.4	E962.0	E980.4
Dicyanogen (gas)	987.8	E869.8	—	E952.8	E962.2	E982.8
Dicyclomine	971.1	E855.4	E941.1	E950.4	E962.0	E980.4
Dieldrin (vapor)	989.2	E863.0	—	E950.6	E962.1	E980.7
Dienestrol	962.2	E858.0	E932.2	E950.4	E962.0	E980.4
Dietetics	977.0	E858.8	E947.0	E950.4	E962.0	E980.4
Diethazine	966.4	E855.0	E936.4	E950.4	E962.0	E980.4
Diethyl						
barbituric acid	967.0	E851	E937.0	E950.1	E962.0	E980.1
carbamazine	961.6	E857	E931.6	E950.4	E962.0	E980.4
carbinol	980.8	E860.8	—	E950.9	E962.1	E980.9
carbonate	982.8	E862.4	—	E950.9	E962.1	E980.9
dioxide	982.8	E862.4	—	E950.9	E962.1	E980.9
ether (vapor) — see Ether(s)						
glycol (monoacetate) (mo-						
noethyl ether)	982.8	E862.4	—	E950.9	E962.1	E980.9
propion	977.0	E858.8	E947.0	E950.4	E962.0	E980.4
stilbestrol	962.2	E858.0	E932.2	E950.4	E962.0	E980.4
Diethylene						
dioxide	982.8	E862.4	—	E950.9	E962.1	E980.9
glycol (monoacetate) (mo-						
noethyl ether)	982.8	E862.4	—	E950.9	E962.1	E980.9
Diethylsulfone-diethyl-						
methane	967.8	E852.8	E937.8	E950.2	E962.0	E980.2
Difencloxazine	965.09	E850.2	E935.2	E950.0	E962.0	E980.0
Diffusin	963.4	E858.1	E933.4	E950.4	E962.0	E980.4
Diflos	971.0	E855.3	E941.0	E950.4	E962.0	E980.4
Digestants	973.4	E858.4	E943.4	E950.4	E962.0	E980.4
Digitalin(e)	972.1	E858.3	E942.1	E950.4	E962.0	E980.4
Digitalis glycosides	972.1	E858.3	E942.1	E950.4	E962.0	E980.4
Digitoxin	972.1	E858.3	E942.1	E950.4	E962.0	E980.4
Digoxin	972.1	E858.3	E942.1	E950.4	E962.0	E980.4
Dihydrocodeine	965.09	E850.2	E935.2	E950.0	E962.0	E980.0
Dihydrocodeinone	965.09	E850.2	E935.2	E950.0	E962.0	E980.0
Dihydroergocristine	972.9	E858.3	E942.9	E950.4	E962.0	E980.4
Dihydroergotamine	972.9	E858.3	E942.9	E950.4	E962.0	E980.4
Dihydroergotoxine	972.9	E858.3	E942.9	E950.4	E962.0	E980.4
Dihydrohydroxy-						
codeinone	965.09	E850.2	E935.2	E950.0	E962.0	E980.0
Dihydrohydroxymorphi-						
none	965.09	E850.2	E935.2	E950.0	E962.0	E980.0
Dihydroisocodeine	965.09	E850.2	E935.2	E950.0	E962.0	E980.0
Dihydromorphine	965.09	E850.2	E935.2	E950.0	E962.0	E980.0
Dihydromorphinone	965.09	E850.2	E935.2	E950.0	E962.0	E980.0
Dihydrostreptomycin	960.6	E856	E930.6	E950.4	E962.0	E980.4

Nontherapeutic use substance

▽ Subterms under main terms may continue to next column or page

▶◀ Revised Text   ● New Line   ▲ Revised Code

	External Cause (E-Code)				
	Poisoning	Accident	Therapeutic Use	Suicide Attempt	Assault	Undetermined
Dihydrotachysterol	962.6	E858.0	E932.6	E950.4	E962.0	E980.4
Dihydroxyan-thraquinone	973.1	E858.4	E943.1	E950.4	E962.0	E980.4
Dihydroxycodeinone	965.09	E850.2	E935.2	E950.0	E962.0	E980.0
Diiodohydroxyquin	961.3	E857	E931.3	E950.4	E962.0	E980.4
topical	976.0	E858.7	E946.0	E950.4	E962.0	E980.4
Diiodohydroxyquinoline	961.3	E857	E931.3	E950.4	E962.0	E980.4
Dilantin	966.1	E855.0	E936.1	E950.4	E962.0	E980.4
Dilaudid	965.09	E850.2	E935.2	E950.0	E962.0	E980.0
Diloxanide	961.5	E857	E931.5	E950.4	E962.0	E980.4
Dimefline	970.0	E854.3	E940.0	E950.4	E962.0	E980.4
Dimenhydrinate	963.0	E858.1	E933.0	E950.4	E962.0	E980.4
Dimercaprol	963.8	E858.1	E933.8	E950.4	E962.0	E980.4
Dimercaptopropanol	963.8	E858.1	E933.8	E950.4	E962.0	E980.4
Dimetane	963.0	E858.1	E933.0	E950.4	E962.0	E980.4
Dimethicone	976.3	E858.7	E946.3	E950.4	E962.0	E980.4
Dimethindene	963.0	E858.1	E933.0	E950.4	E962.0	E980.4
Dimethisoquin	968.5	E855.2	E938.5	E950.4	E962.0	E980.4
Dimethisterone	962.2	E858.0	E932.2	E950.4	E962.0	E980.4
Dimethoxanate	975.4	E858.6	E945.4	E950.4	E962.0	E980.4
Dimethyl						
arsine, arsinic acid — see Arsenic						
carbinol	980.2	E860.3	—	E950.9	E962.1	E980.9
diguanide	962.3	E858.0	E932.3	E950.4	E962.0	E980.4
ketone	982.8	E862.4	—	E950.9	E962.1	E980.9
vapor	987.8	E869.8	—	E952.8	E962.2	E982.8
meperidine	965.09	E850.2	E935.2	E950.0	E962.0	E980.0
parathion	989.3	E863.1	—	E950.6	E962.1	E980.7
polysiloxane	973.8	E858.4	E943.8	E950.4	E962.0	E980.4
sulfate (fumes)	987.8	E869.8	—	E952.8	E962.2	E982.8
liquid	983.9	E864.3	—	E950.7	E962.1	E980.6
sulfoxide NEC	982.8	E862.4	—	E950.9	E962.1	E980.9
medicinal	976.4	E858.7	E946.4	E950.4	E962.0	E980.4
triptamine	969.6	E854.1	E939.6	E950.3	E962.0	E980.3
tubocurarine	975.2	E858.6	E945.2	E950.4	E962.0	E980.4
Dindevan	964.2	E858.2	E934.2	E950.4	E962.0	E980.4
Dinitro-orthocresol (herbicide)	989.4	E863.5	—	E950.6	E962.1	E980.7
insecticide	989.4	E863.4	—	E950.6	E962.1	E980.7
Dinitrobenzene	983.0	E864.0	—	E950.7	E962.1	E980.6
vapor	987.8	E869.8	—	E952.8	E962.2	E982.8
Dinitro (-ortho-) cresol (herbicide) (spray)	989.4	E863.5	—	E950.6	E962.1	E980.7
insecticide	989.4	E863.4	—	E950.6	E962.1	E980.7
Dinitrophenol (herbicide) (spray)	989.4	E863.5	—	E950.6	E962.1	E980.7
insecticide	989.4	E863.4	—	E950.6	E962.1	E980.7
Dinoprost	975.0	E858.6	E945.0	E950.4	E962.0	E980.4
Dioctyl sulfosuccinate (calcium) (sodium)	973.2	E858.4	E943.2	E950.4	E962.0	E980.4
Diodoquin	961.3	E857	E931.3	E950.4	E962.0	E980.4
Dione derivatives NEC	966.3	E855.0	E936.3	E950.4	E962.0	E980.4
Dionin	965.09	E850.2	E935.2	E950.0	E962.0	E980.0
Dioxane	982.8	E862.4	—	E950.9	E962.1	E980.9
Dioxin — see Herbicide						
Dioxyline	972.5	E858.3	E942.5	E950.4	E962.0	E980.4
Dipentene	982.8	E862.4	—	E950.9	E962.1	E980.9
Diphemanil	971.1	E855.4	E941.1	E950.4	E962.0	E980.4
Diphenadione	964.2	E858.2	E934.2	E950.4	E962.0	E980.4
Diphenhydramine	963.0	E858.1	E933.0	E950.4	E962.0	E980.4
Diphenidol	963.0	E858.1	E933.0	E950.4	E962.0	E980.4
Diphenoxylate	973.5	E858.4	E943.5	E950.4	E962.0	E980.4
Diphenylchloroarsine	985.1	E866.3	—	E950.8	E962.1	E980.8
Diphenylhydantoin (sodium)	966.1	E855.0	E936.1	E950.4	E962.0	E980.4
Diphenylpyraline	963.0	E858.1	E933.0	E950.4	E962.0	E980.4
Diphtheria						
antitoxin	979.9	E858.8	E949.9	E950.4	E962.0	E980.4
toxoid	978.5	E858.8	E948.5	E950.4	E962.0	E980.4
with tetanus toxoid	978.9	E858.8	E948.9	E950.4	E962.0	E980.4
with pertussis component	978.6	E858.8	E948.6	E950.4	E962.0	E980.4
vaccine	978.5	E858.8	E948.5	E950.4	E962.0	E980.4
Dipipanone	965.09	E850.2	E935.2	E950.0	E962.0	E980.0
Diplovax	979.5	E858.8	E949.5	E950.4	E962.0	E980.4
Diprophylline	975.1	E858.6	E945.1	E950.4	E962.0	E980.4
Dipyridamole	972.4	E858.3	E942.4	E950.4	E962.0	E980.4
Dipyrone	965.5	E850.5	E935.5	E950.0	E962.0	E980.0
Diquat	989.4	E863.5	—	E950.6	E962.1	E980.7
Disinfectant NEC	983.9	E861.4	—	E950.7	E962.1	E980.6
alkaline	983.2	E861.4	—	E950.7	E962.1	E980.6
Disinfectant — continued						
aromatic	983.0	E861.4	—	E950.7	E962.1	E980.6
Disipal	966.4	E855.0	E936.4	E950.4	E962.0	E980.4
Disodium edetate	963.8	E858.1	E933.8	E950.4	E962.0	E980.4
Disulfamide	974.4	E858.5	E944.4	E950.4	E962.0	E980.4
Disulfanilamide	961.0	E857	E931.0	E950.4	E962.0	E980.4
Disulfiram	977.3	E858.8	E947.3	E950.4	E962.0	E980.4
Dithiazanine	961.6	E857	E931.6	E950.4	E962.0	E980.4
Dithioglycerol	963.8	E858.1	E933.8	E950.4	E962.0	E980.4
Dithranol	976.4	E858.7	E946.4	E950.4	E962.0	E980.4
Diucardin	974.3	E858.5	E944.3	E950.4	E962.0	E980.4
Diupres	974.3	E858.5	E944.3	E950.4	E962.0	E980.4
Diuretics NEC	974.4	E858.5	E944.4	E950.4	E962.0	E980.4
carbonic acid anhydrase inhibitors	974.2	E858.5	E944.2	E950.4	E962.0	E980.4
mercurial	974.0	E858.5	E944.0	E950.4	E962.0	E980.4
osmotic	974.4	E858.5	E944.4	E950.4	E962.0	E980.4
purine derivatives	974.1	E858.5	E944.1	E950.4	E962.0	E980.4
saluretic	974.3	E858.5	E944.3	E950.4	E962.0	E980.4
Diuril	974.3	E858.5	E944.3	E950.4	E962.0	E980.4
Divinyl ether	968.2	E855.1	E938.2	E950.4	E962.0	E980.4
DMCT	960.4	E856	E930.4	E950.4	E962.0	E980.4
DMSO	982.8	E862.4	—	E950.9	E962.1	E980.9
DMT	969.6	E854.1	E939.6	E950.3	E962.0	E980.3
DNOC	989.4	E863.5	—	E950.6	E962.1	E980.7
DOCA	962.0	E858.0	E932.0	E950.4	E962.0	E980.4
Dolophine	965.02	E850.1	E935.1	E950.0	E962.0	E980.0
Doloxene	965.8	E850.8	E935.8	E950.0	E962.0	E980.0
DOM	969.6	E854.1	E939.6	E950.3	E962.0	E980.3
Domestic gas — see Gas, utility						
Domiphen (bromide) (lozenges)	976.6	E858.7	E946.6	E950.4	E962.0	E980.4
Dopa (levo)	966.4	E855.0	E936.4	E950.4	E962.0	E980.4
Dopamine	971.2	E855.5	E941.2	E950.4	E962.0	E980.4
Doriden	967.5	E852.4	E937.5	E950.2	E962.0	E980.2
Dormiral	967.0	E851	E937.0	E950.1	E962.0	E980.1
Dormison	967.8	E852.8	E937.8	E950.2	E962.0	E980.2
Dornase	963.4	E858.1	E933.4	E950.4	E962.0	E980.4
Dorsacaine	968.5	E855.2	E938.5	E950.4	E962.0	E980.4
Dothiepin hydrochloride	969.05	E854.0	E939.0	E950.3	E962.0	E980.3
Doxapram	970.0	E854.3	E940.0	E950.4	E962.0	E980.4
Doxepin	969.05	E854.0	E939.0	E950.3	E962.0	E980.3
Doxorubicin	960.7	E856	E930.7	E950.4	E962.0	E980.4
Doxycycline	960.4	E856	E930.4	E950.4	E962.0	E980.4
Doxylamine	963.0	E858.1	E933.0	E950.4	E962.0	E980.4
Dramamine	963.0	E858.1	E933.0	E950.4	E962.0	E980.4
Drano (drain cleaner)	983.2	E864.2	—	E950.7	E962.1	E980.6
Dromoran	965.09	E850.2	E935.2	E950.0	E962.0	E980.0
Dromostanolone	962.1	E858.0	E932.1	E950.4	E962.0	E980.4
Droperidol	969.2	E853.1	E939.2	E950.3	E962.0	E980.3
Drotrecogin alfa	964.2	E858.2	E934.2	E950.4	E962.0	E980.4
Drug	977.9	E858.9	E947.9	E950.5	E962.0	E980.5
AHFS List						
4:00 antihistamine drugs	963.0	E858.1	E933.0	E950.4	E962.0	E980.4
8:04 amebacides	961.5	E857	E931.5	E950.4	E962.0	E980.4
arsenical anti-infectives	961.1	E857	E931.1	E950.4	E962.0	E980.4
quinoline derivatives	961.3	E857	E931.3	E950.4	E962.0	E980.4
8:08 anthelmintics	961.6	E857	E931.6	E950.4	E962.0	E980.4
quinoline derivatives	961.3	E857	E931.3	E950.4	E962.0	E980.4
8:12.04 antifungal antibiotics	960.1	E856	E930.1	E950.4	E962.0	E980.4
8:12.06 cephalosporins	960.5	E856	E930.5	E950.4	E962.0	E980.4
8:12.08 chloramphenicol	960.2	E856	E930.2	E950.4	E962.0	E980.4
8:12.12 erythromycins	960.3	E856	E930.3	E950.4	E962.0	E980.4
8:12.16 penicillins	960.0	E856	E930.0	E950.4	E962.0	E980.4
8:12.20 streptomycins	960.6	E856	E930.6	E950.4	E962.0	E980.4
8:12.24 tetracyclines	960.4	E856	E930.4	E950.4	E962.0	E980.4
8:12.28 other antibiotics	960.8	E856	E930.8	E950.4	E962.0	E980.4
antimycobacterial	960.6	E856	E930.6	E950.4	E962.0	E980.4
macrolides	960.3	E856	E930.3	E950.4	E962.0	E980.4
8:16 antituberculars	961.8	E857	E931.8	E950.4	E962.0	E980.4
antibiotics	960.6	E856	E930.6	E950.4	E962.0	E980.4
8:18 antivirals	961.7	E857	E931.7	E950.4	E962.0	E980.4
8:20 plasmodicides (antimalarials)	961.4	E857	E931.4	E950.4	E962.0	E980.4
8:24 sulfonamides	961.0	E857	E931.0	E950.4	E962.0	E980.4
8:26 sulfones	961.8	E857	E931.8	E950.4	E962.0	E980.4
8:28 treponemicides	961.2	E857	E931.2	E950.4	E962.0	E980.4
8:32 trichomonacides	961.5	E857	E931.5	E950.4	E962.0	E980.4
nitrofuran derivatives	961.9	E857	E931.9	E950.4	E962.0	E980.4
quinoline derivatives	961.3	E857	E931.3	E950.4	E962.0	E980.4

Nontherapeutic use substance

Subterms under main terms may continue to next column or page

		External Cause (E-Code)							External Cause (E-Code)				
	Poisoning	Accident	Therapeutic Use	Suicide Attempt	Assault	Undeter-mined		Poisoning	Accident	Therapeutic Use	Suicide Attempt	Assault	Undeter-mined
Drug — *continued*							**Drug** — *continued*						
8:36 urinary germicides	961.9	E857	E931.9	E950.4	E962.0	E980.4	28:16.04 antidepressants	969.00	E854.0	E939.0	E950.3	E962.0	E980.3
quinoline derivatives	961.3	E857	E931.3	E950.4	E962.0	E980.4	28:16.08 tranquilizers	969.5	E853.9	E939.5	E950.3	E962.0	E980.3
8:40 other anti-infectives	961.9	E857	E931.9	E950.4	E962.0	E980.4	benzodiazepine-based	969.4	E853.2	E939.4	E950.3	E962.0	E980.3
10:00 antineoplastic							butyrophenone-based	969.2	E853.1	E939.2	E950.3	E962.0	E980.3
agents	963.1	E858.1	E933.1	E950.4	E962.0	E980.4	major NEC	969.3	E853.8	E939.3	E950.3	E962.0	E980.3
antibiotics	960.7	E856	E930.7	E950.4	E962.0	E980.4	phenothiazine-based	969.1	E853.0	E939.1	E950.3	E962.0	E980.3
progestogens	962.2	E858.0	E932.2	E950.4	E962.0	E980.4	28:16.12 other psychothera-						
12:04 parasympathomimetic							peutic agents	969.8	E855.8	E939.8	E950.3	E962.0	E980.3
(cholinergic) agents	971.0	E855.3	E941.0	E950.4	E962.0	E980.4	28:20 respiratory and cerebral						
12:08 parasympatholytic							stimulants	970.9	E854.3	E940.9	E950.4	E962.0	E980.4
(cholinergic-blocking)							analeptics	970.0	E854.3	E940.0	E950.4	E962.0	E980.4
agents	971.1	E855.4	E941.1	E950.4	E962.0	E980.4	anorexigenic agents	977.0	E858.8	E947.0	E950.4	E962.0	E980.4
12:12 Sympathomimetic							psychostimulants	969.70	E854.2	E939.7	E950.3	E962.0	E980.3
(adrenergic) agents	971.2	E855.5	E941.2	E950.4	E962.0	E980.4	specified NEC	970.89	E854.3	E940.8	E950.4	E962.0	E980.4
12:16 sympatholytic (adrener-							28:24 sedatives and hyp-						
gic-blocking) agents	971.3	E855.6	E941.3	E950.4	E962.0	E980.4	notics	967.9	E852.9	E937.9	E950.2	E962.0	E980.2
12:20 skeletal muscle relax-							barbiturates	967.0	E851	E937.0	E950.1	E962.0	E980.1
ants							benzodiazepine-based tran-						
central nervous system							quilizers	969.4	E853.2	E939.4	E950.3	E962.0	E980.3
muscle-tone depres-							chloral hydrate (group)	967.1	E852.0	E937.1	E950.2	E962.0	E980.2
sants	968.0	E855.1	E938.0	E950.4	E962.0	E980.4	glutethamide group	967.5	E852.4	E937.5	E950.2	E962.0	E980.2
myoneural blocking							intravenous anesthetics	968.3	E855.1	E938.3	E950.4	E962.0	E980.4
agents	975.2	E858.6	E945.2	E950.4	E962.0	E980.4	methaqualone (com-						
16:00 blood derivatives	964.7	E858.2	E934.7	E950.4	E962.0	E980.4	pounds)	967.4	E852.3	E937.4	E950.2	E962.0	E980.2
20:04.04 iron prepara-							paraldehyde	967.2	E852.1	E937.2	E950.2	E962.0	E980.2
tions	964.0	E858.2	E934.0	E950.4	E962.0	E980.4	phenothiazine-based tran-						
20:04.08 liver and stomach							quilizers	969.1	E853.0	E939.1	E950.3	E962.0	E980.3
preparations	964.1	E858.2	E934.1	E950.4	E962.0	E980.4	specified NEC	967.8	E852.8	E937.8	E950.2	E962.0	E980.2
20:04 antianemia drugs	964.1	E858.2	E934.1	E950.4	E962.0	E980.4	thiobarbiturates	968.3	E855.1	E938.3	E950.4	E962.0	E980.4
20:12.04 anticoagulants	964.2	E858.2	E934.2	E950.4	E962.0	E980.4	tranquilizer NEC	969.5	E853.9	E939.5	E950.3	E962.0	E980.3
20:12.08 antiheparin							36:04 to 36:88 diagnostic						
agents	964.5	E858.2	E934.5	E950.4	E962.0	E980.4	agents	977.8	E858.8	E947.8	E950.4	E962.0	E980.4
20:12.12 coagulants	964.5	E858.2	E934.5	E950.4	E962.0	E980.4	40:00 electrolyte, caloric, and						
20:12.16 hemostatics							water balance agents						
NEC	964.5	E858.2	E934.5	E950.4	E962.0	E980.4	NEC	974.5	E858.5	E944.5	E950.4	E962.0	E980.4
capillary active drugs	972.8	E858.3	E942.8	E950.4	E962.0	E980.4	40:04 acidifying agents	963.2	E858.1	E933.2	E950.4	E962.0	E980.4
24:04 cardiac drugs	972.9	E858.3	E942.9	E950.4	E962.0	E980.4	40:08 alkalinizing agents	963.3	E858.1	E933.3	E950.4	E962.0	E980.4
cardiotonic agents	972.1	E858.3	E942.1	E950.4	E962.0	E980.4	40:10 ammonia detoxi-						
rhythm regulators	972.0	E858.3	E942.0	E950.4	E962.0	E980.4	cants	974.5	E858.5	E944.5	E950.4	E962.0	E980.4
24:06 antilipemic agents	972.2	E858.3	E942.2	E950.4	E962.0	E980.4	40:12 replacement solu-						
thyroid derivatives	962.7	E858.0	E932.7	E950.4	E962.0	E980.4	tions	974.5	E858.5	E944.5	E950.4	E962.0	E980.4
24:08 hypotensive							plasma expanders	964.8	E858.2	E934.8	E950.4	E962.0	E980.4
agents	972.6	E858.3	E942.6	E950.4	E962.0	E980.4	40:16 sodium-removing						
adrenergic blocking							resins	974.5	E858.5	E944.5	E950.4	E962.0	E980.4
agents	971.3	E855.6	E941.3	E950.4	E962.0	E980.4	40:18 potassium-removing						
ganglion blocking							resins	974.5	E858.5	E944.5	E950.4	E962.0	E980.4
agents	972.3	E858.3	E942.3	E950.4	E962.0	E980.4	40:20 caloric agents	974.5	E858.5	E944.5	E950.4	E962.0	E980.4
vasodilators	972.5	E858.3	E942.5	E950.4	E962.0	E980.4	40:24 salt and sugar substi-						
24:12 vasodilating agents							tutes	974.5	E858.5	E944.5	E950.4	E962.0	E980.4
NEC	972.5	E858.3	E942.5	E950.4	E962.0	E980.4	40:28 diuretics NEC	974.4	E858.5	E944.4	E950.4	E962.0	E980.4
coronary	972.4	E858.3	E942.4	E950.4	E962.0	E980.4	carbonic acid anhydrase in-						
nicotinic acid deriva-							hibitors	974.2	E858.5	E944.2	E950.4	E962.0	E980.4
tives	972.2	E858.3	E942.2	E950.4	E962.0	E980.4	mercurials	974.0	E858.5	E944.0	E950.4	E962.0	E980.4
24:16 sclerosing agents	972.7	E858.3	E942.7	E950.4	E962.0	E980.4	purine derivatives	974.1	E858.5	E944.1	E950.4	E962.0	E980.4
28:04 general anesthetics	968.4	E855.1	E938.4	E950.4	E962.0	E980.4	saluretics	974.3	E858.5	E944.3	E950.4	E962.0	E980.4
gaseous anesthetics	968.2	E855.1	E938.2	E950.4	E962.0	E980.4	thiazides	974.3	E858.5	E944.3	E950.4	E962.0	E980.4
halothane	968.1	E855.1	E938.1	E950.4	E962.0	E980.4	40:36 irrigating solutions	974.5	E858.5	E944.5	E950.4	E962.0	E980.4
intravenous anesthetics	968.3	E855.1	E938.3	E950.4	E962.0	E980.4	40:40 uricosuric agents	974.7	E858.5	E944.7	E950.4	E962.0	E980.4
28:08 analgesics and antipyret-							44:00 enzymes	963.4	E858.1	E933.4	E950.4	E962.0	E980.4
ics	965.9	E850.9	E935.9	E950.0	E962.0	E980.0	fibrinolysis-affecting						
antirheumatics	965.69	E850.6	E935.6	E950.0	E962.0	E980.0	agents	964.4	E858.2	E934.4	E950.4	E962.0	E980.4
aromatic analgesics	965.4	E850.4	E935.4	E950.0	E962.0	E980.0	gastric agents	973.4	E858.4	E943.4	E950.4	E962.0	E980.4
non-narcotic NEC	965.7	E850.7	E935.7	E950.0	E962.0	E980.0	48:00 expectorants and cough						
opium alkaloids	965.00	E850.2	E935.2	E950.0	E962.0	E980.0	preparations						
heroin	965.01	E850.0	E935.0	E950.0	E962.0	E980.0	antihistamine agents	963.0	E858.1	E933.0	E950.4	E962.0	E980.4
methadone	965.02	E850.1	E935.1	E950.0	E962.0	E980.0	antitussives	975.4	E858.6	E945.4	E950.4	E962.0	E980.4
specified type NEC	965.09	E850.2	E935.2	E950.0	E962.0	E980.0	codeine derivatives	965.09	E850.2	E935.2	E950.0	E962.0	E980.0
pyrazole derivatives	965.5	E850.5	E935.5	E950.0	E962.0	E980.0	expectorants	975.5	E858.6	E945.5	E950.4	E962.0	E980.4
salicylates	965.1	E850.3	E935.3	E950.0	E962.0	E980.0	narcotic agents NEC	965.09	E850.2	E935.2	E950.0	E962.0	E980.0
specified NEC	965.8	E850.8	E935.8	E950.0	E962.0	E980.0	52:04.04 antibiotics (EENT)						
28:10 narcotic antago-							ENT agent	976.6	E858.7	E946.6	E950.4	E962.0	E980.4
nists	970.1	E854.3	E940.1	E950.4	E962.0	E980.4	ophthalmic preparation	976.5	E858.7	E946.5	E950.4	E962.0	E980.4
28:12 anticonvulsants	966.3	E855.0	E936.3	E950.4	E962.0	E980.4	52:04.06 antivirals (EENT)						
barbiturates	967.0	E851	E937.0	E950.1	E962.0	E980.1	ENT agent	976.6	E858.7	E946.6	E950.4	E962.0	E980.4
benzodiazepine-based tran-							ophthalmic preparation	976.5	E858.7	E946.5	E950.4	E962.0	E980.4
quilizers	969.4	E853.2	E939.4	E950.3	E962.0	E980.3	52:04.08 sulfonamides (EENT)						
bromides	967.3	E852.2	E937.3	E950.2	E962.0	E980.2	ENT agent	976.6	E858.7	E946.6	E950.4	E962.0	E980.4
hydantoin derivatives	966.1	E855.0	E936.1	E950.4	E962.0	E980.4	ophthalmic preparation	976.5	E858.7	E946.5	E950.4	E962.0	E980.4
oxazolidine (deriva-							52:04.12 miscellaneous anti-						
tives)	966.0	E855.0	E936.0	E950.4	E962.0	E980.4	infectives (EENT)						
succinimides	966.2	E855.0	E936.2	E950.4	E962.0	E980.4	ENT agent	976.6	E858.7	E946.6	E950.4	E962.0	E980.4

Nontherapeutic use substance

☞ Subterms under main terms may continue to next column or page

Index

Drug — Drug

Drug — continued	Poisoning	Accident	Therapeutic Use	Suicide Attempt	Assault	Undetermined
52:04.12 miscellaneous anti-infectives — *continued*						
ophthalmic preparation	976.5	E858.7	E946.5	E950.4	E962.0	E980.4
52:04 anti-infectives (EENT)						
ENT agent	976.6	E858.7	E946.6	E950.4	E962.0	E980.4
ophthalmic preparation	976.5	E858.7	E946.5	E950.4	E962.0	E980.4
52:08 anti-inflammatory agents (EENT)						
ENT agent	976.6	E858.7	E946.6	E950.4	E962.0	E980.4
ophthalmic preparation	976.5	E858.7	E946.5	E950.4	E962.0	E980.4
52:10 carbonic anhydrase inhibitors	974.2	E858.5	E944.2	E950.4	E962.0	E980.4
52:12 contact lens solutions	976.5	E858.7	E946.5	E950.4	E962.0	E980.4
52:16 local anesthetics (EENT)	968.5	E855.2	E938.5	E950.4	E962.0	E980.4
52:20 miotics	971.0	E855.3	E941.0	E950.4	E962.0	E980.4
52:24 mydriatics						
adrenergics	971.2	E855.5	E941.2	E950.4	E962.0	E980.4
anticholinergics	971.1	E855.4	E941.1	E950.4	E962.0	E980.4
antimuscarinics	971.1	E855.4	E941.1	E950.4	E962.0	E980.4
parasympatholytics	971.1	E855.4	E941.1	E950.4	E962.0	E980.4
spasmolytics	971.1	E855.4	E941.1	E950.4	E962.0	E980.4
sympathomimetics	971.2	E855.5	E941.2	E950.4	E962.0	E980.4
52:28 mouth washes and gargles	976.6	E858.7	E946.6	E950.4	E962.0	E980.4
52:32 vasoconstrictors (EENT)	971.2	E855.5	E941.2	E950.4	E962.0	E980.4
52:36 unclassified agents (EENT)						
ENT agent	976.6	E858.7	E946.6	E950.4	E962.0	E980.4
ophthalmic preparation	976.5	E858.7	E946.5	E950.4	E962.0	E980.4
56:04 antacids and adsorbents	973.0	E858.4	E943.0	E950.4	E962.0	E980.4
56:08 antidiarrhea agents	973.5	E858.4	E943.5	E950.4	E962.0	E980.4
56:10 antiflatulents	973.8	E858.4	E943.8	E950.4	E962.0	E980.4
56:12 cathartics NEC	973.3	E858.4	E943.3	E950.4	E962.0	E980.4
emollients	973.2	E858.4	E943.2	E950.4	E962.0	E980.4
irritants	973.1	E858.4	E943.1	E950.4	E962.0	E980.4
56:16 digestants	973.4	E858.4	E943.4	E950.4	E962.0	E980.4
56:20 emetics and antiemetics						
antiemetics	963.0	E858.1	E933.0	E950.4	E962.0	E980.4
emetics	973.6	E858.4	E943.6	E950.4	E962.0	E980.4
56:24 lipotropic agents	977.1	E858.8	E947.1	E950.4	E962.0	E980.4
56:40 miscellaneous G.I. drugs	973.8	E858.4	E943.8	E950.4	E962.0	E980.4
60:00 gold compounds	965.69	E850.6	E935.6	E950.0	E962.0	E980.0
64:00 heavy metal antagonists	963.8	E858.1	E933.8	E950.4	E962.0	E980.4
68:04 adrenals	962.0	E858.0	E932.0	E950.4	E962.0	E980.4
68:08 androgens	962.1	E858.0	E932.1	E950.4	E962.0	E980.4
68:12 contraceptives, oral	962.2	E858.0	E932.2	E950.4	E962.0	E980.4
68:16 estrogens	962.2	E858.0	E932.2	E950.4	E962.0	E980.4
68:18 gonadotropins	962.4	E858.0	E932.4	E950.4	E962.0	E980.4
68:20.08 insulins	962.3	E858.0	E932.3	E950.4	E962.0	E980.4
68:20 insulins and antidiabetic agents	962.3	E858.0	E932.3	E950.4	E962.0	E980.4
68:24 parathyroid	962.6	E858.0	E932.6	E950.4	E962.0	E980.4
68:28 pituitary (posterior)	962.5	E858.0	E932.5	E950.4	E962.0	E980.4
anterior	962.4	E858.0	E932.4	E950.4	E962.0	E980.4
68:32 progestogens	962.2	E858.0	E932.2	E950.4	E962.0	E980.4
68:34 other corpus luteum hormones NEC	962.2	E858.0	E932.2	E950.4	E962.0	E980.4
68:36 thyroid and antithyroid						
antithyroid	962.8	E858.0	E932.8	E950.4	E962.0	E980.4
thyroid (derivatives)	962.7	E858.0	E932.7	E950.4	E962.0	E980.4
72:00 local anesthetics						
NEC	968.9	E855.2	E938.9	E950.4	E962.0	E980.4
infiltration (intradermal) (subcutaneous) (submucosal)	968.5	E855.2	E938.5	E950.4	E962.0	E980.4
nerve blocking (peripheral) (plexus) (regional)	968.6	E855.2	E938.6	E950.4	E962.0	E980.4
spinal	968.7	E855.2	E938.7	E950.4	E962.0	E980.4
topical (surface)	968.5	E855.2	E938.5	E950.4	E962.0	E980.4
76:00 oxytocics	975.0	E858.6	E945.0	E950.4	E962.0	E980.4
78:00 radioactive agents	990	—	—	—	—	—
80:04 serums NEC	979.9	E858.8	E949.9	E950.4	E962.0	E980.4

Drug — continued	Poisoning	Accident	Therapeutic Use	Suicide Attempt	Assault	Undetermined
80:04 serums — *continued*						
immune gamma globulin (human)	964.6	E858.2	E934.6	E950.4	E962.0	E980.4
80:08 toxoids NEC	978.8	E858.8	E948.8	E950.4	E962.0	E980.4
diphtheria	978.5	E858.8	E948.5	E950.4	E962.0	E980.4
and diphtheria	978.9	E858.8	E948.9	E950.4	E962.0	E980.4
with pertussis component	978.6	E858.8	E948.6	E950.4	E962.0	E980.4
and tetanus	978.9	E858.8	E948.9	E950.4	E962.0	E980.4
with pertussis component	978.6	E858.8	E948.6	E950.4	E962.0	E980.4
tetanus	978.4	E858.8	E948.4	E950.4	E962.0	E980.4
80:12 vaccines	979.9	E858.8	E949.9	E950.4	E962.0	E980.4
bacterial NEC	978.8	E858.8	E948.8	E950.4	E962.0	E980.4
with						
other bacterial components	978.9	E858.8	E948.9	E950.4	E962.0	E980.4
pertussis component	978.6	E858.8	E948.6	E950.4	E962.0	E980.4
viral and rickettsial components	979.7	E858.8	E949.7	E950.4	E962.0	E980.4
rickettsial NEC	979.6	E858.8	E949.6	E950.4	E962.0	E980.4
with						
bacterial component	979.7	E858.8	E949.7	E950.4	E962.0	E980.4
pertussis component	978.6	E858.8	E948.6	E950.4	E962.0	E980.4
viral component	979.7	E858.8	E949.7	E950.4	E962.0	E980.4
viral NEC	979.6	E858.8	E949.6	E950.4	E962.0	E980.4
with						
bacterial component	979.7	E858.8	E949.7	E950.4	E962.0	E980.4
pertussis component	978.6	E858.8	E948.6	E950.4	E962.0	E980.4
rickettsial component	979.7	E858.8	E949.7	E950.4	E962.0	E980.4
84:04.04 antibiotics (skin and mucous membrane)	976.0	E858.7	E946.0	E950.4	E962.0	E980.4
84:04.08 fungicides (skin and mucous membrane)	976.0	E858.7	E946.0	E950.4	E962.0	E980.4
84:04.12 scabicides and pediculicides (skin and mucous membrane)	976.0	E858.7	E946.0	E950.4	E962.0	E980.4
84:04.16 miscellaneous local anti-infectives (skin and mucous membrane)	976.0	E858.7	E946.0	E950.4	E962.0	E980.4
84:06 anti-inflammatory agents (skin and mucous membrane)	976.0	E858.7	E946.0	E950.4	E962.0	E980.4
84:08 antipruritics and local anesthetics						
antipruritics	976.1	E858.7	E946.1	E950.4	E962.0	E980.4
local anesthetics	968.5	E855.2	E938.5	E950.4	E962.0	E980.4
84:12 astringents	976.2	E858.7	E946.2	E950.4	E962.0	E980.4
84:16 cell stimulants and proliferants	976.8	E858.7	E946.8	E950.4	E962.0	E980.4
84:20 detergents	976.2	E858.7	E946.2	E950.4	E962.0	E980.4
84:24 emollients, demulcents, and protectants	976.3	E858.7	E946.3	E950.4	E962.0	E980.4
84:28 keratolytic agents	976.4	E858.7	E946.4	E950.4	E962.0	E980.4
84:32 keratoplastic agents	976.4	E858.7	E946.4	E950.4	E962.0	E980.4
84:36 miscellaneous agents (skin and mucous membrane)	976.8	E858.7	E946.8	E950.4	E962.0	E980.4
86:00 spasmolytic agents	975.1	E858.6	E945.1	E950.4	E962.0	E980.4
antiasthmatics	975.7	E858.6	E945.7	E950.4	E962.0	E980.4
papaverine	972.5	E858.3	E942.5	E950.4	E962.0	E980.4
theophylline	974.1	E858.5	E944.1	E950.4	E962.0	E980.4
88:04 vitamin A	963.5	E858.1	E933.5	E950.4	E962.0	E980.4
88:08 vitamin B complex	963.5	E858.1	E933.5	E950.4	E962.0	E980.4
hematopoietic vitamin	964.1	E858.2	E934.1	E950.4	E962.0	E980.4
nicotinic acid derivatives	972.2	E858.3	E942.2	E950.4	E962.0	E980.4
88:12 vitamin C	963.5	E858.1	E933.5	E950.4	E962.0	E980.4
88:16 vitamin D	963.5	E858.1	E933.5	E950.4	E962.0	E980.4
88:20 vitamin E	963.5	E858.1	E933.5	E950.4	E962.0	E980.4
88:24 vitamin K activity	964.3	E858.2	E934.3	E950.4	E962.0	E980.4
88:28 multivitamin preparations	963.5	E858.1	E933.5	E950.4	E962.0	E980.4

Nontherapeutic use substance

⚕ Subterms under main terms may continue to next column or page

►◄ Revised Text   ● New Line   ▲ Revised Code

Drug	Poisoning	Accident	Therapeutic Use	Suicide Attempt	Assault	Undetermined
Drug — *continued*						
92:00 unclassified therapeutic agents	977.8	E858.8	E947.8	E950.4	E962.0	E980.4
specified NEC	977.8	E858.8	E947.8	E950.4	E962.0	E980.4
Duboisine	971.1	E855.4	E941.1	E950.4	E962.0	E980.4
Dulcolax	973.1	E858.4	E943.1	E950.4	E962.0	E980.4
Duponol (C) (EP)	976.2	E858.7	E946.2	E950.4	E962.0	E980.4
Durabolin	962.1	E858.0	E932.1	E950.4	E962.0	E980.4
Dyclone	968.5	E855.2	E938.5	E950.4	E962.0	E980.4
Dyclonine	968.5	E855.2	E938.5	E950.4	E962.0	E980.4
Dydrogesterone	962.2	E858.0	E932.2	E950.4	E962.0	E980.4
Dyes NEC	989.89	E866.8	—	E950.9	E962.1	E980.9
diagnostic agents	977.8	E858.8	E947.8	E950.4	E962.0	E980.4
pharmaceutical NEC	977.4	E858.8	E947.4	E950.4	E962.0	E980.4
Dyfols	971.0	E855.3	E941.0	E950.4	E962.0	E980.4
Dymelor	962.3	E858.0	E932.3	E950.4	E962.0	E980.4
Dynamite	989.89	E866.8	—	E950.9	E962.1	E980.9
fumes	987.8	E869.8	—	E952.8	E962.2	E982.8
Dyphylline	975.1	E858.6	E945.1	E950.4	E962.0	E980.4
Ear preparations	976.6	E858.7	E946.6	E950.4	E962.0	E980.4
Echothiopate, ecoth-iopate	971.0	E855.3	E941.0	E950.4	E962.0	E980.4
Ecstasy	969.72	E854.2	E939.7	E950.3	E962.0	E980.3
Ectylurea	967.8	E852.8	E937.8	E950.2	E962.0	E980.2
Edathamil disodium	963.8	E858.1	E933.8	E950.4	E962.0	E980.4
Edecrin	974.4	E858.5	E944.4	E950.4	E962.0	E980.4
Edetate, disodium (calcium)	963.8	E858.1	E933.8	E950.4	E962.0	E980.4
Edrophonium	971.0	E855.3	E941.0	E950.4	E962.0	E980.4
Elase	976.8	E858.7	E946.8	E950.4	E962.0	E980.4
Elaterium	973.1	E858.4	E943.1	E950.4	E962.0	E980.4
Elder	988.2	E865.4	—	E950.9	E962.1	E980.9
berry (unripe)	988.2	E865.3	—	E950.9	E962.1	E980.9
Electrolytes NEC	974.5	E858.5	E944.5	E950.4	E962.0	E980.4
Electrolytic agent NEC	974.5	E858.5	E944.5	E950.4	E962.0	E980.4
Embramine	963.0	E858.1	E933.0	E950.4	E962.0	E980.4
Emetics	973.6	E858.4	E943.6	E950.4	E962.0	E980.4
Emetine (hydrochloride)	961.5	E857	E931.5	E950.4	E962.0	E980.4
Emollients	976.3	E858.7	E946.3	E950.4	E962.0	E980.4
Emylcamate	969.5	E853.8	E939.5	E950.3	E962.0	E980.3
Encyprate	969.09	E854.0	E939.0	E950.3	E962.0	E980.3
Endocaine	968.5	E855.2	E938.5	E950.4	E962.0	E980.4
Endrin	989.2	E863.0	—	E950.6	E962.1	E980.7
Enflurane	968.2	E855.1	E938.2	E950.4	E962.0	E980.4
Enovid	962.2	E858.0	E932.2	E950.4	E962.0	E980.4
ENT preparations (anti-infectives)	976.6	E858.7	E946.6	E950.4	E962.0	E980.4
Enzodase	963.4	E858.1	E933.4	E950.4	E962.0	E980.4
Enzymes NEC	963.4	E858.1	E933.4	E950.4	E962.0	E980.4
Epanutin	966.1	E855.0	E936.1	E950.4	E962.0	E980.4
Ephedra (tincture)	971.2	E855.5	E941.2	E950.4	E962.0	E980.4
Ephedrine	971.2	E855.5	E941.2	E950.4	E962.0	E980.4
Epiestriol	962.2	E858.0	E932.2	E950.4	E962.0	E980.4
Epilim — see Sodium valproate						
Epinephrine	971.2	E855.5	E941.2	E950.4	E962.0	E980.4
Epsom salt	973.3	E858.4	E943.3	E950.4	E962.0	E980.4
Equanil	969.5	E853.8	E939.5	E950.3	E962.0	E980.3
Equisetum (diuretic)	974.4	E858.5	E944.4	E950.4	E962.0	E980.4
Ergometrine	975.0	E858.6	E945.0	E950.4	E962.0	E980.4
Ergonovine	975.0	E858.6	E945.0	E950.4	E962.0	E980.4
Ergotamine (tartrate) (for migraine) NEC	972.9	E858.3	E942.9	E950.4	E962.0	E980.4
Ergotrate	975.0	E858.6	E945.0	E950.4	E962.0	E980.4
Ergot NEC	988.2	E865.4	—	E950.9	E962.1	E980.9
medicinal (alkaloids)	975.0	E858.6	E945.0	E950.4	E962.0	E980.4
Erythrityl tetranitrate	972.4	E858.3	E942.4	E950.4	E962.0	E980.4
Erythrol tetranitrate	972.4	E858.3	E942.4	E950.4	E962.0	E980.4
Erythromycin	960.3	E856	E930.3	E950.4	E962.0	E980.4
ophthalmic preparation	976.5	E858.7	E946.5	E950.4	E962.0	E980.4
topical NEC	976.0	E858.7	E946.0	E950.4	E962.0	E980.4
Eserine	971.0	E855.3	E941.0	E950.4	E962.0	E980.4
Eskabarb	967.0	E851	E937.0	E950.1	E962.0	E980.1
Eskalith	969.8	E855.8	E939.8	E950.3	E962.0	E980.3
Estradiol (cypionate) (dipropionate) (valerate)	962.2	E858.0	E932.2	E950.4	E962.0	E980.4
Estriol	962.2	E858.0	E932.2	E950.4	E962.0	E980.4
Estrogens (with progestogens)	962.2	E858.0	E932.2	E950.4	E962.0	E980.4
Estrone	962.2	E858.0	E932.2	E950.4	E962.0	E980.4
Etafedrine	971.2	E855.5	E941.2	E950.4	E962.0	E980.4
Ethacrynate sodium	974.4	E858.5	E944.4	E950.4	E962.0	E980.4
Ethacrynic acid	974.4	E858.5	E944.4	E950.4	E962.0	E980.4
Ethambutol	961.8	E857	E931.8	E950.4	E962.0	E980.4
Ethamide	974.2	E858.5	E944.2	E950.4	E962.0	E980.4
Ethamivan	970.0	E854.3	E940.0	E950.4	E962.0	E980.4
Ethamsylate	964.5	E858.2	E934.5	E950.4	E962.0	E980.4
Ethanol	980.0	E860.1	—	E950.9	E962.1	E980.9
beverage	980.0	E860.0	—	E950.9	E962.1	E980.9
Ethchlorvynol	967.8	E852.8	E937.8	E950.2	E962.0	E980.2
Ethebenecid	974.7	E858.5	E944.7	E950.4	E962.0	E980.4
Ether(s) (diethyl) (ethyl) (vapor)	987.8	E869.8	—	E952.8	E962.2	E982.8
anesthetic	968.2	E855.1	E938.2	E950.4	E962.0	E980.4
petroleum — see Ligroin						
solvent	982.8	E862.4	—	E950.9	E962.1	E980.9
Ethidine chloride (vapor)	987.8	E869.8	—	E952.8	E962.2	E982.8
liquid (solvent)	982.3	E862.4	—	E950.9	E962.1	E980.9
Ethinamate	967.8	E852.8	E937.8	E950.2	E962.0	E980.2
Ethinylestradiol	962.2	E858.0	E932.2	E950.4	E962.0	E980.4
Ethionamide	961.8	E857	E931.8	E950.4	E962.0	E980.4
Ethisterone	962.2	E858.0	E932.2	E950.4	E962.0	E980.4
Ethobral	967.0	E851	E937.0	E950.1	E962.0	E980.1
Ethocaine (infiltration) (topical)	968.5	E855.2	E938.5	E950.4	E962.0	E980.4
nerve block (peripheral) (plexus)	968.6	E855.2	E938.6	E950.4	E962.0	E980.4
spinal	968.7	E855.2	E938.7	E950.4	E962.0	E980.4
Ethoheptazine (citrate)	965.7	E850.7	E935.7	E950.0	E962.0	E980.0
Ethopropazine	966.4	E855.0	E936.4	E950.4	E962.0	E980.4
Ethosuximide	966.2	E855.0	E936.2	E950.4	E962.0	E980.4
Ethotoin	966.1	E855.0	E936.1	E950.4	E962.0	E980.4
Ethoxazene	961.9	E857	E931.9	E950.4	E962.0	E980.4
Ethoxzolamide	974.2	E858.5	E944.2	E950.4	E962.0	E980.4
Ethyl						
acetate (vapor)	982.8	E862.4	—	E950.9	E962.1	E980.9
alcohol	980.0	E860.1	—	E950.9	E962.1	E980.9
beverage	980.0	E860.0	—	E950.9	E962.1	E980.9
aldehyde (vapor)	987.8	E869.8	—	E952.8	E962.2	E982.8
liquid	989.89	E866.8	—	E950.9	E962.1	E980.9
aminobenzoate	968.5	E855.2	E938.5	E950.4	E962.0	E980.4
biscoumacetate	964.2	E858.2	E934.2	E950.4	E962.0	E980.4
bromide (anesthetic)	968.2	E855.1	E938.2	E950.4	E962.0	E980.4
carbamate (antineoplastic)	963.1	E858.1	E933.1	E950.4	E962.0	E980.4
carbinol	980.3	E860.4	—	E950.9	E962.1	E980.9
chaulmoograte	961.8	E857	E931.8	E950.4	E962.0	E980.4
chloride (vapor)	987.8	E869.8	—	E952.8	E962.2	E982.8
anesthetic (local)	968.5	E855.2	E938.5	E950.4	E962.0	E980.4
inhaled	968.2	E855.1	E938.2	E950.4	E962.0	E980.4
solvent	982.3	E862.4	—	E950.9	E962.1	E980.9
estranol	962.1	E858.0	E932.1	E950.4	E962.0	E980.4
ether — see Ether(s)						
formate (solvent) NEC	982.8	E862.4	—	E950.9	E962.1	E980.9
iodoacetate	987.5	E869.3	—	E952.8	E962.2	E982.8
lactate (solvent) NEC	982.8	E862.4	—	E950.9	E962.1	E980.9
methylcarbinol	980.8	E860.8	—	E950.9	E962.1	E980.9
morphine	965.09	E850.2	E935.2	E950.0	E962.0	E980.0
Ethylene (gas)	987.1	E869.8	—	E952.8	E962.2	E982.8
anesthetic (general)	968.2	E855.1	E938.2	E950.4	E962.0	E980.4
chlorohydrin (vapor)	982.3	E862.4	—	E950.9	E962.1	E980.9
dichloride (vapor)	982.3	E862.4	—	E950.9	E962.1	E980.9
glycol(s) (any) (vapor)	982.8	E862.4	—	E950.9	E962.1	E980.9
Ethylidene						
chloride NEC	982.3	E862.4	—	E950.9	E962.1	E980.9
diethyl ether	982.8	E862.4	—	E950.9	E962.1	E980.9
Ethynodiol	962.2	E858.0	E932.2	E950.4	E962.0	E980.4
Etidocaine	968.9	E855.2	E938.9	E950.4	E962.0	E980.4
infiltration (subcutaneous)	968.5	E855.2	E938.5	E950.4	E962.0	E980.4
nerve (peripheral) (plexus)	968.6	E855.2	E938.6	E950.4	E962.0	E980.4
Etilfen	967.0	E851	E937.0	E950.1	E962.0	E980.1
Etomide	965.7	E850.7	E935.7	E950.0	E962.0	E980.0
Etorphine	965.09	E850.2	E935.2	E950.0	E962.0	E980.0
Etoval	967.0	E851	E937.0	E950.1	E962.0	E980.1
Etryptamine	969.01	E854.0	E939.0	E950.3	E962.0	E980.3
Eucaine	968.5	E855.2	E938.5	E950.4	E962.0	E980.4
Eucalyptus (oil) NEC	975.5	E858.6	E945.5	E950.4	E962.0	E980.4
Eucatropine	971.1	E855.4	E941.1	E950.4	E962.0	E980.4
Eucodal	965.09	E850.2	E935.2	E950.0	E962.0	E980.0
Euneryl	967.0	E851	E937.0	E950.1	E962.0	E980.1
Euphthalmine	971.1	E855.4	E941.1	E950.4	E962.0	E980.4
Eurax	976.0	E858.7	E946.0	E950.4	E962.0	E980.4

Nontherapeutic use substance

Subterms under main terms may continue to next column or page

	Poisoning	Accident	Therapeutic Use	Suicide Attempt	Assault	Undetermined
External Cause (E-Code)						
Euresol	976.4	E858.7	E946.4	E950.4	E962.0	E980.4
Euthroid	962.7	E858.0	E932.7	E950.4	E962.0	E980.4
Evans blue	977.8	E858.8	E947.8	E950.4	E962.0	E980.4
Evipal	967.0	E851	E937.0	E950.1	E962.0	E980.1
sodium	968.3	E855.1	E938.3	E950.4	E962.0	E980.4
Evipan	967.0	E851	E937.0	E950.1	E962.0	E980.1
sodium	968.3	E855.1	E938.3	E950.4	E962.0	E980.4
Ex-Lax (phenolphthalein)	973.1	E858.4	E943.1	E950.4	E962.0	E980.4
Exalgin	965.4	E850.4	E935.4	E950.0	E962.0	E980.0
Excipients, pharmaceutical	977.4	E858.8	E947.4	E950.4	E962.0	E980.4
Exhaust gas — see Carbon, monoxide						
Expectorants	975.5	E858.6	E945.5	E950.4	E962.0	E980.4
External medications (skin)						
(mucous membrane)	976.9	E858.7	E946.9	E950.4	E962.0	E980.4
dental agent	976.7	E858.7	E946.7	E950.4	E962.0	E980.4
ENT agent	976.6	E858.7	E946.6	E950.4	E962.0	E980.4
ophthalmic preparation	976.5	E858.7	E946.5	E950.4	E962.0	E980.4
specified NEC	976.8	E858.7	E946.8	E950.4	E962.0	E980.4
Eye agents (anti-infective)	976.5	E858.7	E946.5	E950.4	E962.0	E980.4
Factor IX complex (human)	964.5	E858.2	E934.5	E950.4	E962.0	E980.4
Fecal softeners	973.2	E858.4	E943.2	E950.4	E962.0	E980.4
Fenbutrazate	977.0	E858.8	E947.0	E950.4	E962.0	E980.4
Fencamfamin	970.89	E854.3	E940.8	E950.4	E962.0	E980.4
Fenfluramine	977.0	E858.8	E947.0	E950.4	E962.0	E980.4
Fenoprofen	965.61	E850.6	E935.6	E950.0	E962.0	E980.0
Fentanyl	965.09	E850.2	E935.2	E950.0	E962.0	E980.0
Fentazin	969.1	E853.0	E939.1	E950.3	E962.0	E980.3
Fenticlor, fentichlor	976.0	E858.7	E946.0	E950.4	E962.0	E980.4
Fer de lance (bite) (venom)	989.5	E905.0	—	E950.9	E962.1	E980.9
Ferric — see Iron						
Ferrocholinate	964.0	E858.2	E934.0	E950.4	E962.0	E980.4
Ferrous fumerate, gluconate, lactate, salt NEC, sulfate (medicinal)	964.0	E858.2	E934.0	E950.4	E962.0	E980.4
Ferrum — see Iron						
Fertilizers NEC	989.89	E866.5	—	E950.9	E962.1	E980.4
with herbicide mixture	989.4	E863.5	—	E950.6	E962.1	E980.7
Fibrinogen (human)	964.7	E858.2	E934.7	E950.4	E962.0	E980.4
Fibrinolysin	964.4	E858.2	E934.4	E950.4	E962.0	E980.4
Fibrinolysis-affecting agents	964.4	E858.2	E934.4	E950.4	E962.0	E980.4
Filix mas	961.6	E857	E931.6	E950.4	E962.0	E980.4
Fiorinal	965.1	E850.3	E935.3	E950.0	E962.0	E980.0
Fire damp	987.1	E869.8	—	E952.8	E962.2	E982.8
Fish, nonbacterial or noxious	988.0	E865.2	—	E950.9	E962.1	E980.9
shell	988.0	E865.1	—	E950.9	E962.1	E980.9
Flagyl	961.5	E857	E931.5	E950.4	E962.0	E980.4
Flavoxate	975.1	E858.6	E945.1	E950.4	E962.0	E980.4
Flaxedil	975.2	E858.6	E945.2	E950.4	E962.0	E980.4
Flaxseed (medicinal)	976.3	E858.7	E946.3	E950.4	E962.0	E980.4
Flomax	971.3	E855.6	E941.3	E950.4	E962.0	E980.4
Florantyrone	973.4	E858.4	E943.4	E950.4	E962.0	E980.4
Floraquin	961.3	E857	E931.3	E950.4	E962.0	E980.4
Florinef	962.0	E858.0	E932.0	E950.4	E962.0	E980.4
ENT agent	976.6	E858.7	E946.6	E950.4	E962.0	E980.4
ophthalmic preparation	976.5	E858.7	E946.5	E950.4	E962.0	E980.4
topical NEC	976.0	E858.7	E946.0	E950.4	E962.0	E980.4
Flowers of sulfur	976.4	E858.7	E946.4	E950.4	E962.0	E980.4
Floxuridine	963.1	E858.1	E933.1	E950.4	E962.0	E980.4
Flucytosine	961.9	E857	E931.9	E950.4	E962.0	E980.4
Fludrocortisone	962.0	E858.0	E932.0	E950.4	E962.0	E980.4
ENT agent	976.6	E858.7	E946.6	E950.4	E962.0	E980.4
ophthalmic preparation	976.5	E858.7	E946.5	E950.4	E962.0	E980.4
topical NEC	976.0	E858.7	E946.0	E950.4	E962.0	E980.4
Flumethasone	976.0	E858.7	E946.0	E950.4	E962.0	E980.4
Flumethiazide	974.3	E858.5	E944.3	E950.4	E962.0	E980.4
Flumidin	961.7	E857	E931.7	E950.4	E962.0	E980.4
Flunitrazepam	969.4	E853.2	E939.4	E950.3	E962.0	E980.3
Fluocinolone	976.0	E858.7	E946.0	E950.4	E962.0	E980.4
Fluocortolone	962.0	E858.0	E932.0	E950.4	E962.0	E980.4
Fluohydrocortisone	962.0	E858.0	E932.0	E950.4	E962.0	E980.4
ENT agent	976.6	E858.7	E946.6	E950.4	E962.0	E980.4
ophthalmic preparation	976.5	E858.7	E946.5	E950.4	E962.0	E980.4
topical NEC	976.0	E858.7	E946.0	E950.4	E962.0	E980.4
Fluonid	976.0	E858.7	E946.0	E950.4	E962.0	E980.4
Fluopromazine	969.1	E853.0	E939.1	E950.3	E962.0	E980.3

	Poisoning	Accident	Therapeutic Use	Suicide Attempt	Assault	Undetermined
External Cause (E-Code)						
Fluoracetate	989.4	E863.7	—	E950.6	E962.1	E980.7
Fluorescein (sodium)	977.8	E858.8	E947.8	E950.4	E962.0	E980.4
Fluoride(s) (pesticides) (sodium) NEC	989.4	E863.4	—	E950.6	E962.1	E980.7
hydrogen — see Hydrofluoric acid						
medicinal	976.7	E858.7	E946.7	E950.4	E962.0	E980.4
not pesticide NEC	983.9	E864.4	—	E950.7	E962.1	E980.6
stannous	976.7	E858.7	E946.7	E950.4	E962.0	E980.4
Fluorinated corticosteroids	962.0	E858.0	E932.0	E950.4	E962.0	E980.4
Fluorine (compounds) (gas)	987.8	E869.8	—	E952.8	E962.2	E982.8
salt — see Fluoride(s)						
Fluoristan	976.7	E858.7	E946.7	E950.4	E962.0	E980.4
Fluoroacetate	989.4	E863.7	—	E950.6	E962.1	E980.7
Fluorodeoxyuridine	963.1	E858.1	E933.1	E950.4	E962.0	E980.4
Fluorometholone (topical) NEC	976.0	E858.7	E946.0	E950.4	E962.0	E980.4
ophthalmic preparation	976.5	E858.7	E946.5	E950.4	E962.0	E980.4
Fluorouracil	963.1	E858.1	E933.1	E950.4	E962.0	E980.4
Fluothane	968.1	E855.1	E938.1	E950.4	E962.0	E980.4
Fluoxetine hydrochloride	969.03	E854.0	E939.0	E950.3	E962.0	E980.3
Fluoxymesterone	962.1	E858.0	E932.1	E950.4	E962.0	E980.4
Fluphenazine	969.1	E853.0	E939.1	E950.3	E962.0	E980.3
Fluprednisolone	962.0	E858.0	E932.0	E950.4	E962.0	E980.4
Flurandrenolide	976.0	E858.7	E946.0	E950.4	E962.0	E980.4
Flurazepam (hydrochloride)	969.4	E853.2	E939.4	E950.3	E962.0	E980.3
Flurbiprofen	965.61	E850.6	E935.6	E950.0	E962.0	E980.0
Flurobate	976.0	E858.7	E946.0	E950.4	E962.0	E980.4
Flurothyl	969.8	E855.8	E939.8	E950.3	E962.0	E980.3
Fluroxene	968.2	E855.1	E938.2	E950.4	E962.0	E980.4
Folacin	964.1	E858.2	E934.1	E950.4	E962.0	E980.4
Folic acid	964.1	E858.2	E934.1	E950.4	E962.0	E980.4
Follicle stimulating hormone	962.4	E858.0	E932.4	E950.4	E962.0	E980.4
Food, foodstuffs, nonbacterial or noxious	988.9	E865.9	—	E950.9	E962.1	E980.9
berries, seeds	988.2	E865.3	—	E950.9	E962.1	E980.9
fish	988.0	E865.2	—	E950.9	E962.1	E980.9
mushrooms	988.1	E865.5	—	E950.9	E962.1	E980.9
plants	988.2	E865.9	—	E950.9	E962.1	E980.9
specified type NEC	988.2	E865.4	—	E950.9	E962.1	E980.9
shellfish	988.0	E865.1	—	E950.9	E962.1	E980.9
specified NEC	988.8	E865.8	—	E950.9	E962.1	E980.9
Fool's parsley	988.2	E865.4	—	E950.9	E962.1	E980.9
Formaldehyde (solution)	989.89	E861.4	—	E950.9	E962.1	E980.9
fungicide	989.4	E863.6	—	E950.6	E962.1	E980.7
gas or vapor	987.8	E869.8	—	E952.8	E962.2	E982.8
Formalin	989.89	E861.4	—	E950.9	E962.1	E980.9
fungicide	989.4	E863.6	—	E950.6	E962.1	E980.7
vapor	987.8	E869.8	—	E952.8	E962.2	E982.8
Formic acid	983.1	E864.1	—	E950.7	E962.1	E980.6
automobile	981	E862.1		E950.9	E962.1	E980.9
exhaust gas, not in transit	986	E868.2	—	E952.0	E962.2	E982.0
vapor NEC	987.1	E869.8	—	E952.8	E962.2	E982.8
gas (domestic use) (see also Carbon, monoxide, fuel)						
utility	987.1	E868.1	—	E951.8	E962.2	E981.8
incomplete combustion of — see Carbon, monoxide, fuel, utility						
in mobile container	987.0	E868.0	—	E951.1	E962.2	E981.1
piped (natural)	987.1	E867	—	E951.0	E962.2	E981.0
industrial, incomplete combustion	986	E868.3	—	E952.1	E962.2	E982.1
vapor	987.8	E869.8	—	E952.8	E962.2	E982.8
Fowler's solution	985.1	E866.3	—	E950.8	E962.1	E980.8
Foxglove	988.2	E865.4	—	E950.9	E962.1	E980.9
Fox green	977.8	E858.8	E947.8	E950.4	E962.0	E980.4
Framycetin	960.8	E856	E930.8	E950.4	E962.0	E980.4
Frangula (extract)	973.1	E858.4	E943.1	E950.4	E962.0	E980.4
Frei antigen	977.8	E858.8	E947.8	E950.4	E962.0	E980.4
Freons	987.4	E869.2	—	E952.8	E962.2	E982.8
Fructose	974.5	E858.5	E944.5	E950.4	E962.0	E980.4
Frusemide	974.4	E858.5	E944.4	E950.4	E962.0	E980.4
FSH	962.4	E858.0	E932.4	E950.4	E962.0	E980.4
Fuel						
Fugillin	960.8	E856	E930.8	E950.4	E962.0	E980.4

Nontherapeutic use substance

Subterms under main terms may continue to next column or page

	Poisoning	Accident	Therapeutic Use	Suicide Attempt	Assault	Undetermined
Fulminate of mercury	985.0	E866.1	—	E950.9	E962.1	E980.9
Fulvicin	960.1	E856	E930.1	E950.4	E962.0	E980.4
Fumadil	960.8	E856	E930.8	E950.4	E962.0	E980.4
Fumagillin	960.8	E856	E930.8	E950.4	E962.0	E980.4
Fumes (from)	987.9	E869.9	—	E952.9	E962.2	E982.9
carbon monoxide — see Carbon, monoxide						
charcoal (domestic use)	986	E868.3	—	E952.1	E962.2	E982.1
chloroform — see Chloroform						
coke (in domestic stoves, fireplaces)	986	E868.3	—	E952.1	E962.2	E982.1
corrosive NEC	987.8	E869.8	—	E952.8	E962.2	E982.8
ether — see Ether(s)						
freons	987.4	E869.2	—	E952.8	E962.2	E982.8
hydrocarbons	987.1	E869.8	—	E952.8	E962.2	E982.8
petroleum (liquefied)	987.0	E868.0	—	E951.1	E962.2	E981.1
distributed through pipes (pure or mixed with air)	987.0	E867	—	E951.0	E962.2	E981.0
lead — see Lead						
metals — see specified metal						
nitrogen dioxide	987.2	E869.0	—	E952.8	E962.2	E982.8
pesticides — see Pesticides						
petroleum (liquefied)	987.0	E868.0	—	E951.1	E962.2	E981.1
distributed through pipes (pure or mixed with air)	987.0	E867	—	E951.0	E962.2	E981.0
polyester	987.8	E869.8	—	E952.8	E962.2	E982.8
specified, source other (see also substance specified)	987.8	E869.8	—	E952.8	E962.2	E982.8
sulfur dioxide	987.3	E869.1	—	E952.8	E962.2	E982.8
Fumigants	989.4	E863.8	—	E950.6	E962.1	E980.7
Fungicides — see also Antifungals	989.4	E863.6	—	E950.6	E962.1	E980.7
Fungi, noxious, used as food	988.1	E865.5	—	E950.9	E962.1	E980.9
Fungizone	960.1	E856	E930.1	E950.4	E962.0	E980.4
topical	976.0	E858.7	E946.0	E950.4	E962.0	E980.4
Furacin	976.0	E858.7	E946.0	E950.4	E962.0	E980.4
Furadantin	961.9	E857	E931.9	E950.4	E962.0	E980.4
Furazolidone	961.9	E857	E931.9	E950.4	E962.0	E980.4
Furnace (coal burning) (domestic), gas from	986	E868.3	—	E952.1	E962.2	E982.1
industrial	986	E868.8	—	E952.1	E962.2	E982.1
Furniture polish	989.89	E861.2	—	E950.9	E962.1	E980.9
Furosemide	974.4	E858.5	E944.4	E950.4	E962.0	E980.4
Furoxone	961.9	E857	E931.9	E950.4	E962.0	E980.4
Fusel oil (amyl) (butyl) (propyl)	980.3	E860.4	—	E950.9	E962.1	E980.9
Fusidic acid	960.8	E856	E930.8	E950.4	E962.0	E980.4
Gallamine	975.2	E858.6	E945.2	E950.4	E962.0	E980.4
Gallotannic acid	976.2	E858.7	E946.2	E950.4	E962.0	E980.4
Gamboge	973.1	E858.4	E943.1	E950.4	E962.0	E980.4
Gamimune	964.6	E858.2	E934.6	E950.4	E962.0	E980.4
Gamma-benzene hexachloride (vapor)	989.2	E863.0	—	E950.6	E962.1	E980.7
Gamma globulin	964.6	E858.2	E934.6	E950.4	E962.0	E980.4
Gamma hydroxy butyrate (GHB)	968.4	E855.1	E938.4	E950.4	E962.0	E980.4
Gamulin	964.6	E858.2	E934.6	E950.4	E962.0	E980.4
Ganglionic blocking agents	972.3	E858.3	E942.3	E950.4	E962.0	E980.4
Ganja	969.6	E854.1	E939.6	E950.3	E962.0	E980.3
Garamycin	960.8	E856	E930.8	E950.4	E962.0	E980.4
ophthalmic preparation	976.5	E858.7	E946.5	E950.4	E962.0	E980.4
topical NEC	976.0	E858.7	E946.0	E950.4	E962.0	E980.4
Gardenal	967.0	E851	E937.0	E950.1	E962.0	E980.1
Gardepanyl	967.0	E851	E937.0	E950.1	E962.0	E980.1
Gas	987.9	E869.9	—	E952.9	E962.2	E982.9
acetylene	987.1	E868.1	—	E951.8	E962.2	E981.8
incomplete combustion of — see Carbon, monoxide, fuel, utility						
air contaminants, source or type not specified	987.9	E869.9	—	E952.9	E962.2	E982.9
anesthetic (general) NEC	968.2	E855.1	E938.2	E950.4	E962.0	E980.4
blast furnace	986	E868.8	—	E952.1	E962.2	E982.1
butane — see Butane						
carbon monoxide — see Carbon, monoxide						

	Poisoning	Accident	Therapeutic Use	Suicide Attempt	Assault	Undetermined
Gas — continued						
chlorine	987.6	E869.8	—	E952.8	E962.2	E982.8
coal — see Carbon, monoxide, coal						
cyanide	987.7	E869.8	—	E952.8	E962.2	E982.8
dicyanogen	987.8	E869.8	—	E952.8	E962.2	E982.8
domestic — see Gas, utility						
exhaust — see Carbon, monoxide, exhaust gas						
from wood- or coal-burning stove or fireplace	986	E868.3	—	E952.1	E962.2	E982.1
fuel (domestic use) (see also Carbon, monoxide, fuel)						
industrial use	986	E868.8	—	E952.1	E962.2	E982.1
utility	987.1	E868.1	—	E951.8	E962.2	E981.8
incomplete combustion of — see Carbon, monoxide, fuel, utility						
in mobile container	987.0	E868.0	—	E951.1	E962.2	E981.1
piped (natural)	987.1	E867	—	E951.0	E962.2	E981.0
garage	986	E868.2	—	E952.0	E962.2	E982.0
hydrocarbon NEC	987.1	E869.8	—	E952.8	E962.2	E982.8
incomplete combustion of — see Carbon, monoxide, fuel, utility						
liquefied (mobile container)	987.0	E868.0	—	E951.1	E962.2	E981.1
piped	987.0	E867	—	E951.0	E962.2	E981.0
hydrocyanic acid	987.7	E869.8	—	E952.8	E962.2	E982.8
illuminating — see Gas, utility						
incomplete combustion, any — see Carbon, monoxide						
kiln	986	E868.8	—	E952.1	E962.2	E982.1
lacrimogenic	987.5	E869.3	—	E952.8	E962.2	E982.8
marsh	987.1	E869.8	—	E952.8	E962.2	E982.8
motor exhaust, not in transit	986	E868.8	—	E952.1	E962.2	E982.1
mustard — see Mustard, gas						
natural	987.1	E867	—	E951.0	E962.2	E981.0
nerve (war)	987.9	E869.9	—	E952.9	E962.2	E982.9
oils	981	E862.1	—	E950.9	E962.1	E980.9
petroleum (liquefied) (distributed in mobile containers)	987.0	E868.0	—	E951.1	E962.2	E981.1
piped (pure or mixed with air)	987.0	E867	—	E951.1	E962.2	E981.1
piped (manufactured) (natural) NEC	987.1	E867	—	E951.0	E962.2	E981.0
producer	986	E868.8	—	E952.1	E962.2	E982.1
propane — see Propane						
refrigerant (freon)	987.4	E869.2	—	E952.8	E962.2	E982.8
not freon	987.9	E869.9	—	E952.9	E962.2	E982.9
sewer	987.8	E869.8	—	E952.8	E962.2	E982.8
specified source NEC (see also substance specified)	987.8	E869.8	—	E952.8	E962.2	E982.8
stove — see Gas, utility						
tear	987.5	E869.3	—	E952.8	E962.2	E982.8
utility (for cooking, heating, or lighting) (piped) NEC	987.1	E868.1	—	E951.8	E962.2	E981.8
incomplete combustion of — see Carbon, monoxide, fuel, utility						
in mobile container	987.0	E868.0	—	E951.1	E962.2	E981.1
piped (natural)	987.1	E867	—	E951.0	E962.2	E981.0
water	987.1	E868.1	—	E951.8	E962.2	E981.8
incomplete combustion of — see Carbon, monoxide, fuel, utility						
Gaseous substance — see Gas						
Gasoline, gasolene	981	E862.1	—	E950.9	E962.1	E980.9
vapor	987.1	E869.8	—	E952.8	E962.2	E982.8
Gastric enzymes	973.4	E858.4	E943.4	E950.4	E962.0	E980.4
Gastrografin	977.8	E858.8	E947.8	E950.4	E962.0	E980.4
Gastrointestinal agents	973.9	E858.4	E943.9	E950.4	E962.0	E980.4
specified NEC	973.8	E858.4	E943.8	E950.4	E962.0	E980.4
Gaultheria procumbens	988.2	E865.4	—	E950.9	E962.1	E980.9
Gelatin (intravenous)	964.8	E858.2	E934.8	E950.4	E962.0	E980.4
absorbable (sponge)	964.5	E858.2	E934.5	E950.4	E962.0	E980.4
Gelfilm	976.8	E858.7	E946.8	E950.4	E962.0	E980.4
Gelfoam	964.5	E858.2	E934.5	E950.4	E962.0	E980.4

Fulminate of mercury — Gelfoam

Substance	Poisoning	External Cause (E-Code)				
		Accident	Therapeutic Use	Suicide Attempt	Assault	Undetermined
Gelsemine	970.89	E854.3	E940.8	E950.4	E962.0	E980.4
Gelsemium (semper-virens)	988.2	E865.4	—	E950.9	E962.1	E980.9
Gemonil	967.0	E851	E937.0	E950.1	E962.0	E980.1
Gentamicin	960.8	E856	E930.8	E950.4	E962.0	E980.4
ophthalmic preparation	976.5	E858.7	E946.5	E950.4	E962.0	E980.4
topical NEC	976.0	E858.7	E946.0	E950.4	E962.0	E980.4
Gentian violet	976.0	E858.7	E946.0	E950.4	E962.0	E980.4
Gexane	976.0	E858.7	E946.0	E950.4	E962.0	E980.4
Gila monster (venom)	989.5	E905.0	—	E950.9	E962.1	E980.9
Ginger, Jamaica	989.89	E866.8	—	E950.9	E962.1	E980.9
Gitalin	972.1	E858.3	E942.1	E950.4	E962.0	E980.4
Gitoxin	972.1	E858.3	E942.1	E950.4	E962.0	E980.4
Glandular extract (medicinal) NEC	977.9	E858.9	E947.9	E950.5	E962.0	E980.5
Glaucarubin	961.5	E857	E931.5	E950.4	E962.0	E980.4
Globin zinc insulin	962.3	E858.0	E932.3	E950.4	E962.0	E980.4
Glucagon	962.3	E858.0	E932.3	E950.4	E962.0	E980.4
Glucochloral	967.1	E852.0	E937.1	E950.2	E962.0	E980.2
Glucocorticoids	962.0	E858.0	E932.0	E950.4	E962.0	E980.4
Glucose	974.5	E858.5	E944.5	E950.4	E962.0	E980.4
oxidase reagent	977.8	E858.8	E947.8	E950.4	E962.0	E980.4
Glucosulfone sodium	961.8	E857	E931.8	E950.4	E962.0	E980.4
Glue(s)	989.89	E866.6	—	E950.9	E962.1	E980.9
Glutamic acid (hydrochlo-ride)	973.4	E858.4	E943.4	E950.4	E962.0	E980.4
Glutaraldehyde	989.89	E861.4	—	E950.9	E962.1	E980.9
Glutathione	963.8	E858.1	E933.8	E950.4	E962.0	E980.4
Glutethimide (group)	967.5	E852.4	E937.5	E950.2	E962.0	E980.2
Glycerin (lotion)	976.3	E858.7	E946.3	E950.4	E962.0	E980.4
Glycerol (topical)	976.3	E858.7	E946.3	E950.4	E962.0	E980.4
Glyceryl						
guaiacolate	975.5	E858.6	E945.5	E950.4	E962.0	E980.4
triacetate (topical)	976.0	E858.7	E946.0	E950.4	E962.0	E980.4
trinitrate	972.4	E858.3	E942.4	E950.4	E962.0	E980.4
Glycine	974.5	E858.5	E944.5	E950.4	E962.0	E980.4
Glycobiarsol	961.1	E857	E931.1	E950.4	E962.0	E980.4
Glycols (ether)	982.8	E862.4	—	E950.9	E962.1	E980.9
Glycopyrrolate	971.1	E855.4	E941.1	E950.4	E962.0	E980.4
Glymidine	962.3	E858.0	E932.3	E950.4	E962.0	E980.4
Gold (compounds) (salts)	965.69	E850.6	E935.6	E950.0	E962.0	E980.0
Golden sulfide of antimo-ny	985.4	E866.2	—	E950.9	E962.1	E980.9
Goldylocks	988.2	E865.4	—	E950.9	E962.1	E980.9
Gonadal tissue extract	962.9	E858.0	E932.9	E950.4	E962.0	E980.4
female	962.2	E858.0	E932.2	E950.4	E962.0	E980.4
male	962.1	E858.0	E932.1	E950.4	E962.0	E980.4
Gonadotropin	962.4	E858.0	E932.4	E950.4	E962.0	E980.4
Gramicidin	960.8	E856	E930.8	E950.4	E962.0	E980.4
Gratiola officinalis	988.2	E865.4	—	E950.9	E962.1	E980.9
Grease	989.89	E866.8	—	E950.9	E962.1	E980.9
Green hellebore	988.2	E865.4	—	E950.9	E962.1	E980.9
Green soap	976.2	E858.7	E946.2	E950.4	E962.0	E980.4
Grifulvin	960.1	E856	E930.1	E950.4	E962.0	E980.4
Griseofulvin	960.1	E856	E930.1	E950.4	E962.0	E980.4
Growth hormone	962.4	E858.0	E932.4	E950.4	E962.0	E980.4
Guaiacol	975.5	E858.6	E945.5	E950.4	E962.0	E980.4
Guaiac reagent	977.8	E858.8	E947.8	E950.4	E962.0	E980.4
Guaifenesin	975.5	E858.6	E945.5	E950.4	E962.0	E980.4
Guaiphenesin	975.5	E858.6	E945.5	E950.4	E962.0	E980.4
Guanatol	961.4	E857	E931.4	E950.4	E962.0	E980.4
Guanethidine	972.6	E858.3	E942.6	E950.4	E962.0	E980.4
Guano	989.89	E866.5	—	E950.9	E962.1	E980.9
Guanochlor	972.6	E858.3	E942.6	E950.4	E962.0	E980.4
Guanoctine	972.6	E858.3	E942.6	E950.4	E962.0	E980.4
Guanoxan	972.6	E858.3	E942.6	E950.4	E962.0	E980.4
Hair treatment agent NEC	976.4	E858.7	E946.4	E950.4	E962.0	E980.4
Halcinonide	976.0	E858.7	E946.0	E950.4	E962.0	E980.4
Halethazole	976.0	E858.7	E946.0	E950.4	E962.0	E980.4
Hallucinogens	969.6	E854.1	E939.6	E950.3	E962.0	E980.3
Haloperidol	969.2	E853.1	E939.2	E950.3	E962.0	E980.3
Haloprogin	976.0	E858.7	E946.0	E950.4	E962.0	E980.4
Halotex	976.0	E858.7	E946.0	E950.4	E962.0	E980.4
Halothane	968.1	E855.1	E938.1	E950.4	E962.0	E980.4
Halquinols	976.0	E858.7	E946.0	E950.4	E962.0	E980.4
Hand sanitizer	976.0	E858.7	E946.0	E950.4	E962.0	E980.4
Harmonyl	972.6	E858.3	E942.6	E950.4	E962.0	E980.4
Hartmann's solution	974.5	E858.5	E944.5	E950.4	E962.0	E980.4
Hashish	969.6	E854.1	E939.6	E950.3	E962.0	E980.3

Substance	Poisoning	External Cause (E-Code)				
		Accident	Therapeutic Use	Suicide Attempt	Assault	Undetermined
Hawaiian wood rose seeds	969.6	E854.1	E939.6	E950.3	E962.0	E980.3
Headache cures, drugs, pow-ders NEC	977.9	E858.9	E947.9	E950.5	E962.0	E980.9
Heavenly Blue (morning glo-ry)	969.6	E854.1	E939.6	E950.3	E962.0	E980.3
Heavy metal antagonists	963.8	E858.1	E933.8	E950.4	E962.0	E980.4
anti-infectives	961.2	E857	E931.2	E950.4	E962.0	E980.4
Hedaquinium	976.0	E858.7	E946.0	E950.4	E962.0	E980.4
Hedge hyssop	988.2	E865.4	—	E950.9	E962.1	E980.9
Heet	976.8	E858.7	E946.8	E950.4	E962.0	E980.4
Helenin	961.6	E857	E931.6	E950.4	E962.0	E980.4
Hellebore (black) (green) (white)	988.2	E865.4	—	E950.9	E962.1	E980.9
Hemlock	988.2	E865.4	—	E950.9	E962.1	E980.9
Hemostatics	964.5	E858.2	E934.5	E950.4	E962.0	E980.4
capillary active drugs	972.8	E858.3	E942.8	E950.4	E962.0	E980.4
Henbane	988.2	E865.4	—	E950.9	E962.1	E980.9
Heparin (sodium)	964.2	E858.2	E934.2	E950.4	E962.0	E980.4
Heptabarbital, heptabarbi-tone	967.0	E851	E937.0	E950.1	E962.0	E980.1
Heptachlor	989.2	E863.0	—	E950.6	E962.1	E980.7
Heptalgin	965.09	E850.2	E935.2	E950.0	E962.0	E980.0
Herbicides	989.4	E863.5	—	E950.6	E962.1	E980.7
Heroin	965.01	E850.0	E935.0	E950.0	E962.0	E980.0
Herplex	976.5	E858.7	E946.5	E950.4	E962.0	E980.4
HES	964.8	E858.2	E934.8	E950.4	E962.0	E980.4
Hetastarch	964.8	E858.2	E934.8	E950.4	E962.0	E980.4
Hexa-germ	976.2	E858.7	E946.2	E950.4	E962.0	E980.4
Hexachlorocyclohexane	989.2	E863.0	—	E950.6	E962.1	E980.7
Hexachlorophene	976.2	E858.7	E946.2	E950.4	E962.0	E980.4
Hexadimethrine (bro-mide)	964.5	E858.2	E934.5	E950.4	E962.0	E980.4
Hexafluorenium	975.2	E858.6	E945.2	E950.4	E962.0	E980.4
Hexahydrophenol	980.8	E860.8	—	E950.9	E962.1	E980.9
Hexalin	980.8	E860.8	—	E950.9	E962.1	E980.9
Hexamethonium	972.3	E858.3	E942.3	E950.4	E962.0	E980.4
Hexamethyleneamine	961.9	E857	E931.9	E950.4	E962.0	E980.4
Hexamine	961.9	E857	E931.9	E950.4	E962.0	E980.4
Hexanone	982.8	E862.4	—	E950.9	E962.1	E980.9
Hexapropymate	967.8	E852.8	E937.8	E950.2	E962.0	E980.2
Hexestrol	962.2	E858.0	E932.2	E950.4	E962.0	E980.4
Hexethal (sodium)	967.0	E851	E937.0	E950.1	E962.0	E980.1
Hexetidine	976.0	E858.7	E946.0	E950.4	E962.0	E980.4
Hexobarbital, hexobarbi-tone	967.0	E851	E937.0	E950.1	E962.0	E980.1
sodium (anesthetic)	968.3	E855.1	E938.3	E950.4	E962.0	E980.4
soluble	968.3	E855.1	E938.3	E950.4	E962.0	E980.4
Hexocyclium	971.1	E855.4	E941.1	E950.4	E962.0	E980.4
Hexoestrol	962.2	E858.0	E932.2	E950.4	E962.0	E980.4
Hexone	982.8	E862.4	—	E950.9	E962.1	E980.9
Hexylcaine	968.5	E855.2	E938.5	E950.4	E962.0	E980.4
Hexylresorcinol	961.6	E857	E931.6	E950.4	E962.0	E980.4
Hinkle's pills	973.1	E858.4	E943.1	E950.4	E962.0	E980.4
Histalog	977.8	E858.8	E947.8	E950.4	E962.0	E980.4
Histamine (phosphate)	972.5	E858.3	E942.5	E950.4	E962.0	E980.4
Histoplasmin	977.8	E858.8	E947.8	E950.4	E962.0	E980.4
Holly berries	988.2	E865.3	—	E950.9	E962.1	E980.9
Homatropine	971.1	E855.4	E941.1	E950.4	E962.0	E980.4
Homo-tet	964.6	E858.2	E934.6	E950.4	E962.0	E980.4
Hormones (synthetic substi-tute) NEC	962.9	E858.0	E932.9	E950.4	E962.0	E980.4
adrenal cortical steroids	962.0	E858.0	E932.0	E950.4	E962.0	E980.4
antidiabetic agents	962.3	E858.0	E932.3	E950.4	E962.0	E980.4
follicle stimulating	962.4	E858.0	E932.4	E950.4	E962.0	E980.4
gonadotropic	962.4	E858.0	E932.4	E950.4	E962.0	E980.4
growth	962.4	E858.0	E932.4	E950.4	E962.0	E980.4
ovarian (substitutes)	962.2	E858.0	E932.2	E950.4	E962.0	E980.4
parathyroid (derivatives)	962.6	E858.0	E932.6	E950.4	E962.0	E980.4
pituitary (posterior)	962.5	E858.0	E932.5	E950.4	E962.0	E980.4
anterior	962.4	E858.0	E932.4	E950.4	E962.0	E980.4
thyroid (derivative)	962.7	E858.0	E932.7	E950.4	E962.0	E980.4
Hornet (sting)	989.5	E905.3	—	E950.9	E962.1	E980.9
Horticulture agent NEC	989.4	E863.9	—	E950.6	E962.1	E980.7
Hyaluronidase	963.4	E858.1	E933.4	E950.4	E962.0	E980.4
Hyazyme	963.4	E858.1	E933.4	E950.4	E962.0	E980.4
Hycodan	965.09	E850.2	E935.2	E950.0	E962.0	E980.0
Hydantoin derivatives	966.1	E855.0	E936.1	E950.4	E962.0	E980.4
Hydeltra	962.0	E858.0	E932.0	E950.4	E962.0	E980.4
Hydergine	971.3	E855.6	E941.3	E950.4	E962.0	E980.4
Hydrabamine penicillin	960.0	E856	E930.0	E950.4	E962.0	E980.4

Nontherapeutic use substance

Subterms under main terms may continue to next column or page

	Poisoning	Accident	Therapeutic Use	Suicide Attempt	Assault	Undetermined
Hydralazine, hydrallazine	972.6	E858.3	E942.6	E950.4	E962.0	E980.4
Hydrargaphen	976.0	E858.7	E946.0	E950.4	E962.0	E980.4
Hydrazine	983.9	E864.3	—	E950.7	E962.1	E980.6
Hydriodic acid	975.5	E858.6	E945.5	E950.4	E962.0	E980.4
Hydrocarbon gas	987.1	E869.8	—	E952.8	E962.2	E982.8
incomplete combustion of — see Carbon, monoxide, fuel, utility						
liquefied (mobile container)	987.0	E868.0	—	E951.1	E962.2	E981.1
piped (natural)	987.0	E867	—	E951.0	E962.2	E981.0
Hydrochloric acid (liquid)	983.1	E864.1	—	E950.7	E962.1	E980.6
medicinal	973.4	E858.4	E943.4	E950.4	E962.0	E980.4
vapor	987.8	E869.8	—	E952.8	E962.2	E982.8
Hydrochlorothiazide	974.3	E858.5	E944.3	E950.4	E962.0	E980.4
Hydrocodone	965.09	E850.2	E935.2	E950.0	E962.0	E980.0
Hydrocortisone	962.0	E858.0	E932.0	E950.4	E962.0	E980.4
ENT agent	976.6	E858.7	E946.6	E950.4	E962.0	E980.4
ophthalmic preparation	976.5	E858.7	E946.5	E950.4	E962.0	E980.4
topical NEC	976.0	E858.7	E946.0	E950.4	E962.0	E980.4
Hydrocortone	962.0	E858.0	E932.0	E950.4	E962.0	E980.4
ENT agent	976.6	E858.7	E946.6	E950.4	E962.0	E980.4
ophthalmic preparation	976.5	E858.7	E946.5	E950.4	E962.0	E980.4
topical NEC	976.0	E858.7	E946.0	E950.4	E962.0	E980.4
Hydrocyanic acid — see Cyanide(s)						
Hydroflumethiazide	974.3	E858.5	E944.3	E950.4	E962.0	E980.4
Hydrofluoric acid (liquid)	983.1	E864.1	—	E950.7	E962.1	E980.6
vapor	987.8	E869.8	—	E952.8	E962.2	E982.8
Hydrogen	987.8	E869.8	—	E952.8	E962.2	E982.8
arsenide	985.1	E866.3	—	E950.8	E962.1	E980.8
arseniureted	985.1	E866.3	—	E950.8	E962.1	E980.8
cyanide (salts)	989.0	E866.8	—	E950.9	E962.1	E980.9
gas	987.7	E869.8	—	E952.8	E962.2	E982.8
fluoride (liquid)	983.1	E864.1	—	E950.7	E962.1	E980.6
vapor	987.8	E869.8	—	E952.8	E962.2	E982.8
peroxide (solution)	976.6	E858.7	E946.6	E950.4	E962.0	E980.4
phosphureted	987.8	E869.8	—	E952.8	E962.2	E982.8
sulfide (gas)	987.8	E869.8	—	E952.8	E962.2	E982.8
arseniureted	985.1	E866.3	—	E950.8	E962.1	E980.8
sulfureted	987.8	E869.8	—	E952.8	E962.2	E982.8
Hydromorphinol	965.09	E850.2	E935.2	E950.0	E962.0	E980.0
Hydromorphinone	965.09	E850.2	E935.2	E950.0	E962.0	E980.0
Hydromorphone	965.09	E850.2	E935.2	E950.0	E962.0	E980.0
Hydromox	974.3	E858.5	E944.3	E950.4	E962.0	E980.4
Hydrophilic lotion	976.3	E858.7	E946.3	E950.4	E962.0	E980.4
Hydroquinone	983.0	E864.0	—	E950.7	E962.1	E980.6
vapor	987.8	E869.8	—	E952.8	E962.2	E982.8
Hydrosulfuric acid (gas)	987.8	E869.8	—	E952.8	E962.2	E982.8
Hydrous wool fat (lotion)	976.3	E858.7	E946.3	E950.4	E962.0	E980.4
Hydroxide, caustic	983.2	E864.2	—	E950.7	E962.1	E980.6
Hydroxocobalamin	964.1	E858.2	E934.1	E950.4	E962.0	E980.4
Hydroxyamphetamine	971.2	E855.5	E941.2	E950.4	E962.0	E980.4
Hydroxychloroquine	961.4	E857	E931.4	E950.4	E962.0	E980.4
Hydroxydihydrocodeinone	965.09	E850.2	E935.2	E950.0	E962.0	E980.0
Hydroxyethyl starch	964.8	E858.2	E934.8	E950.4	E962.0	E980.4
Hydroxyphenamate	969.5	E853.8	E939.5	E950.3	E962.0	E980.3
Hydroxyphenylbutazone	965.5	E850.5	E935.5	E950.0	E962.0	E980.0
Hydroxyprogesterone	962.2	E858.0	E932.2	E950.4	E962.0	E980.4
Hydroxyquinoline derivatives	961.3	E857	E931.3	E950.4	E962.0	E980.4
Hydroxystilbamidine	961.5	E857	E931.5	E950.4	E962.0	E980.4
Hydroxyurea	963.1	E858.1	E933.1	E950.4	E962.0	E980.4
Hydroxyzine	969.5	E853.8	E939.5	E950.3	E962.0	E980.3
Hyoscine (hydrobromide)	971.1	E855.4	E941.1	E950.4	E962.0	E980.4
Hyoscyamine	971.1	E855.4	E941.1	E950.4	E962.0	E980.4
Hyoscyamus (albus) (niger)	988.2	E865.4	—	E950.9	E962.1	E980.9
Hypaque	977.8	E858.8	E947.8	E950.4	E962.0	E980.4
Hypertussis	964.6	E858.2	E934.6	E950.4	E962.0	E980.4
Hypnotics NEC	967.9	E852.9	E937.9	E950.2	E962.0	E980.2
Hypochlorites — see Sodium, hypochlorite						
Hypotensive agents NEC	972.6	E858.3	E942.6	E950.4	E962.0	E980.4
I-thyroxine sodium	962.7	E858.0	E932.7	E950.4	E962.0	E980.4
Ibufenac	965.69	E850.6	E935.6	E950.0	E962.0	E980.0
Ibuprofen	965.61	E850.6	E935.6	E950.0	E962.0	E980.0
ICG	977.8	E858.8	E947.8	E950.4	E962.0	E980.4
Ichthammol	976.4	E858.7	E946.4	E950.4	E962.0	E980.4
Ichthyol	976.4	E858.7	E946.4	E950.4	E962.0	E980.4
Idoxuridine	976.5	E858.7	E946.5	E950.4	E962.0	E980.4
IDU	976.5	E858.7	E946.5	E950.4	E962.0	E980.4
Iletin	962.3	E858.0	E932.3	E950.4	E962.0	E980.4
Ilex	988.2	E865.4	—	E950.9	E962.1	E980.9
Illuminating gas — see Gas, utility						
Ilopan	963.5	E858.1	E933.5	E950.4	E962.0	E980.4
Ilotycin	960.3	E856	E930.3	E950.4	E962.0	E980.4
ophthalmic preparation	976.5	E858.7	E946.5	E950.4	E962.0	E980.4
topical NEC	976.0	E858.7	E946.0	E950.4	E962.0	E980.4
Imipramine	969.05	E854.0	E939.0	E950.3	E962.0	E980.3
Immu-G	964.6	E858.2	E934.6	E950.4	E962.0	E980.4
Immu-tetanus	964.6	E858.2	E934.6	E950.4	E962.0	E980.4
Immuglobin	964.6	E858.2	E934.6	E950.4	E962.0	E980.4
Immune serum globulin	964.6	E858.2	E934.6	E950.4	E962.0	E980.4
Immunosuppressive agents	963.1	E858.1	E933.1	E950.4	E962.0	E980.4
Indandione (derivatives)	964.2	E858.2	E934.2	E950.4	E962.0	E980.4
Inderal	972.0	E858.3	E942.0	E950.4	E962.0	E980.4
Indian hemp	969.6	E854.1	E939.6	E950.3	E962.0	E980.3
tobacco	988.2	E865.4	—	E950.9	E962.1	E980.9
Indigo carmine	977.8	E858.8	E947.8	E950.4	E962.0	E980.4
Indocin	965.69	E850.6	E935.6	E950.0	E962.0	E980.0
Indocyanine green	977.8	E858.8	E947.8	E950.4	E962.0	E980.4
Indomethacin	965.69	E850.6	E935.6	E950.0	E962.0	E980.0
Industrial alcohol	980.9	E860.9	—	E950.9	E962.1	E980.9
fumes	987.8	E869.8	—	E952.8	E962.2	E982.8
solvents (fumes) (vapors)	982.8	E862.9	—	E950.9	E962.1	E980.9
Influenza vaccine	979.6	E858.8	E949.6	E950.4	E962.0	E982.8
Ingested substances NEC	989.9	E866.9	—	E950.9	E962.1	E980.9
INH (isoniazid)	961.8	E857	E931.8	E950.4	E962.0	E980.4
Inhalation, gas (noxious) — see Gas						
Ink	989.89	E866.8	—	E950.9	E962.1	E980.9
Innovar	967.6	E852.5	E937.6	E950.2	E962.0	E980.2
Inositol niacinate	972.2	E858.3	E942.2	E950.4	E962.0	E980.4
Inproquone	963.1	E858.1	E933.1	E950.4	E962.0	E980.4
Insecticides — see also Pesticides	989.4	E863.4	—	E950.6	E962.1	E980.7
chlorinated	989.2	E863.0	—	E950.6	E962.1	E980.7
mixtures	989.4	E863.3	—	E950.6	E962.1	E980.7
organochlorine (compounds)	989.2	E863.0	—	E950.6	E962.1	E980.7
organophosphorus (compounds)	989.3	E863.1	—	E950.6	E962.1	E980.7
Insect (sting), venomous	989.5	E905.5	—	E950.9	E962.1	E980.9
Insular tissue extract	962.3	E858.0	E932.3	E950.4	E962.0	E980.4
Insulin (amorphous) (globin) (isophane) (Lente) (NPH) (protamine) (Semilente) (Ultralente) (zinc)	962.3	E858.0	E932.3	E950.4	E962.0	E980.4
Intranarcon	968.3	E855.1	E938.3	E950.4	E962.0	E980.4
Inulin	977.8	E858.8	E947.8	E950.4	E962.0	E980.4
Invert sugar	974.5	E858.5	E944.5	E950.4	E962.0	E980.4
Inza — see Naproxen						
Iodide NEC — see also Iodine	976.0	E858.7	E946.0	E950.4	E962.0	E980.4
mercury (ointment)	976.0	E858.7	E946.0	E950.4	E962.0	E980.4
methylate	976.0	E858.7	E946.0	E950.4	E962.0	E980.4
potassium (expectorant) NEC	975.5	E858.6	E945.5	E950.4	E962.0	E980.4
Iodinated glycerol	975.5	E858.6	E945.5	E950.4	E962.0	E980.4
Iodine (antiseptic, external) (tincture) NEC	976.0	E858.7	E946.0	E950.4	E962.0	E980.4
diagnostic	977.8	E858.8	E947.8	E950.4	E962.0	E980.4
for thyroid conditions (antithyroid)	962.8	E858.0	E932.8	E950.4	E962.0	E980.4
vapor	987.8	E869.8	—	E952.8	E962.2	E982.8
Iodized oil	977.8	E858.8	E947.8	E950.4	E962.0	E980.4
Iodobismitol	961.2	E857	E931.2	E950.4	E962.0	E980.4
Iodochlorhydroxyquin	961.3	E857	E931.3	E950.4	E962.0	E980.4
topical	976.0	E858.7	E946.0	E950.4	E962.0	E980.4
Iodoform	976.0	E858.7	E946.0	E950.4	E962.0	E980.4
Iodopanoic acid	977.8	E858.8	E947.8	E950.4	E962.0	E980.4
Iodophthalein	977.8	E858.8	E947.8	E950.4	E962.0	E980.4
Ion exchange resins	974.5	E858.5	E944.5	E950.4	E962.0	E980.4
Iopanoic acid	977.8	E858.8	E947.8	E950.4	E962.0	E980.4
Iophendylate	977.8	E858.8	E947.8	E950.4	E962.0	E980.4
Iothiouracil	962.8	E858.0	E932.8	E950.4	E962.0	E980.4
Ipecac	973.6	E858.4	E943.6	E950.4	E962.0	E980.4

	Poisoning	External Cause (E-Code)				
		Accident	Therapeutic Use	Suicide Attempt	Assault	Undetermined
Ipecacuanha	973.6	E858.4	E943.6	E950.4	E962.0	E980.4
Ipodate	977.8	E858.8	E947.8	E950.4	E962.0	E980.4
Ipral	967.0	E851	E937.0	E950.1	E962.0	E980.1
Ipratropium	975.1	E858.6	E945.1	E950.4	E962.0	E980.4
Iproniazid	969.01	E854.0	E939.0	E950.3	E962.0	E980.3
Iron (compounds) (medicinal) (preparations)	964.0	E858.2	E934.0	E950.4	E962.0	E980.4
dextran	964.0	E858.2	E934.0	E950.4	E962.0	E980.4
nonmedicinal (dust) (fumes) NEC	985.8	E866.4	—	E950.9	E962.1	E980.9
Irritant drug	977.9	E858.9	E947.9	E950.5	E962.0	E980.5
Ismelin	972.6	E858.3	E942.6	E950.4	E962.0	E980.4
Isoamyl nitrite	972.4	E858.3	E942.4	E950.4	E962.0	E980.4
Isobutyl acetate	982.8	E862.4	—	E950.9	E962.1	E980.9
Isocarboxazid	969.01	E854.0	E939.0	E950.3	E962.0	E980.3
Isoephedrine	971.2	E855.5	E941.2	E950.4	E962.0	E980.4
Isoetharine	971.2	E855.5	E941.2	E950.4	E962.0	E980.4
Isofluorophate	971.0	E855.3	E941.0	E950.4	E962.0	E980.4
Isoniazid (INH)	961.8	E857	E931.8	E950.4	E962.0	E980.4
Isopentaquine	961.4	E857	E931.4	E950.4	E962.0	E980.4
Isophane insulin	962.3	E858.0	E932.3	E950.4	E962.0	E980.4
Isopregnenone	962.2	E858.0	E932.2	E950.4	E962.0	E980.4
Isoprenaline	971.2	E855.5	E941.2	E950.4	E962.0	E980.4
Isopropamide	971.1	E855.4	E941.1	E950.4	E962.0	E980.4
Isopropanol	980.2	E860.3	—	E950.9	E962.1	E980.9
topical (germicide)	976.0	E858.7	E946.0	E950.4	E962.0	E980.4
Isopropyl						
acetate	982.8	E862.4	—	E950.9	E962.1	E980.9
alcohol	980.2	E860.3	—	E950.9	E962.1	E980.9
topical (germicide)	976.0	E858.7	E946.0	E950.4	E962.0	E980.4
ether	982.8	E862.4	—	E950.9	E962.1	E980.9
Isoproterenol	971.2	E855.5	E941.2	E950.4	E962.0	E980.4
Isosorbide dinitrate	972.4	E858.3	E942.4	E950.4	E962.0	E980.4
Isothipendyl	963.0	E858.1	E933.0	E950.4	E962.0	E980.4
Isoxazolyl penicillin	960.0	E856	E930.0	E950.4	E962.0	E980.4
Isoxsuprine hydrochloride	972.5	E858.3	E942.5	E950.4	E962.0	E980.4
Jaborandi (pilocarpus) (extract)	971.0	E855.3	E941.0	E950.4	E962.0	E980.4
Jalap	973.1	E858.4	E943.1	E950.4	E962.0	E980.4
Jamaica						
dogwood (bark)	965.7	E850.7	E935.7	E950.0	E962.0	E980.0
ginger	989.89	E866.8	—	E950.9	E962.1	E980.9
Jatropha	988.2	E865.4	—	E950.9	E962.1	E980.9
curcas	988.2	E865.3	—	E950.9	E962.1	E980.9
Jectofer	964.0	E858.2	E934.0	E950.4	E962.0	E980.4
Jellyfish (sting)	989.5	E905.6	—	E950.9	E962.1	E980.9
Jequirity (bean)	988.2	E865.3	—	E950.9	E962.1	E980.9
Jimson weed	988.2	E865.4	—	E950.9	E962.1	E980.9
seeds	988.2	E865.3	—	E950.9	E962.1	E980.9
Juniper tar (oil) (ointment)	976.4	E858.7	E946.4	E950.4	E962.0	E980.4
Kallikrein	972.5	E858.3	E942.5	E950.4	E962.0	E980.4
Kanamycin	960.6	E856	E930.6	E950.4	E962.0	E980.4
Kantrex	960.6	E856	E930.6	E950.4	E962.0	E980.4
Kaolin	973.5	E858.4	E943.5	E950.4	E962.0	E980.4
Karaya (gum)	973.3	E858.4	E943.3	E950.4	E962.0	E980.4
Kemithal	968.3	E855.1	E938.3	E950.4	E962.0	E980.4
Kenacort	962.0	E858.0	E932.0	E950.4	E962.0	E980.4
Keratolytics	976.4	E858.7	E946.4	E950.4	E962.0	E980.4
Keratoplastics	976.4	E858.7	E946.4	E950.4	E962.0	E980.4
Kerosene, kerosine (fuel) (solvent) NEC	981	E862.1	—	E950.9	E962.1	E980.9
insecticide	981	E863.4	—	E950.6	E962.1	E980.7
vapor	987.1	E869.8	—	E952.8	E962.2	E982.8
Ketamine	968.3	E855.1	E938.3	E950.4	E962.0	E980.4
Ketobemidone	965.09	E850.2	E935.2	E950.0	E962.0	E980.0
Ketols	982.8	E862.4	—	E950.9	E962.1	E980.9
Ketone oils	982.8	E862.4	—	E950.9	E962.1	E980.9
Ketoprofen	965.61	E850.6	E935.6	E950.0	E962.0	E980.0
Kiln gas or vapor (carbon monoxide)	986	E868.8	—	E952.1	E962.2	E982.1
Konsyl	973.3	E858.4	E943.3	E950.4	E962.0	E980.4
Kosam seed	988.2	E865.3	—	E950.9	E962.1	E980.9
Krait (venom)	989.5	E905.0	—	E950.9	E962.1	E980.9
Kwell (insecticide)	989.2	E863.0	—	E950.6	E962.1	E980.7
anti-infective (topical)	976.0	E858.7	E946.0	E950.4	E962.0	E980.4
L-dopa	966.4	E855.0	E936.4	E950.4	E962.0	E980.4
L-Tryptophan — *see* amino acid						
Laburnum (flowers) (seeds)	988.2	E865.3	—	E950.9	E962.1	E980.9

	Poisoning	External Cause (E-Code)				
		Accident	Therapeutic Use	Suicide Attempt	Assault	Undetermined
Laburnum — *continued*						
leaves	988.2	E865.4	—	E950.9	E962.1	E980.9
Lacquers	989.89	E861.6	—	E950.9	E962.1	E980.9
Lacrimogenic gas	987.5	E869.3	—	E952.8	E962.2	E982.8
Lactic acid	983.1	E864.1	—	E950.7	E962.1	E980.6
Lactobacillus acidophilus	973.5	E858.4	E943.5	E950.4	E962.0	E980.4
Lactoflavin	963.5	E858.1	E933.5	E950.4	E962.0	E980.4
Lactuca (virosa) (extract)	967.8	E852.8	E937.8	E950.2	E962.0	E980.2
Lactucarium	967.8	E852.8	E937.8	E950.2	E962.0	E980.2
Laevulose	974.5	E858.5	E944.5	E950.4	E962.0	E980.4
Lanatoside (C)	972.1	E858.3	E942.1	E950.4	E962.0	E980.4
Lanolin (lotion)	976.3	E858.7	E946.3	E950.4	E962.0	E980.4
Largactil	969.1	E853.0	E939.1	E950.3	E962.0	E980.3
Larkspur	988.2	E865.3	—	E950.9	E962.1	E980.9
Laroxyl	969.05	E854.0	E939.0	E950.3	E962.0	E980.3
Lasix	974.4	E858.5	E944.4	E950.4	E962.0	E980.4
Latex	989.82	E866.8	—	E950.9	E962.1	E980.9
Lathyrus (seed)	988.2	E865.3	—	E950.9	E962.1	E980.9
Laudanum	965.09	E850.2	E935.2	E950.0	E962.0	E980.0
Laudexium	975.2	E858.6	E945.2	E950.4	E962.0	E980.4
Laurel, black or cherry	988.2	E865.4	—	E950.9	E962.1	E980.9
Laurolinium	976.0	E858.7	E946.0	E950.4	E962.0	E980.4
Lauryl sulfoacetate	976.2	E858.7	E946.2	E950.4	E962.0	E980.4
Laxatives NEC	973.3	E858.4	E943.3	E950.4	E962.0	E980.4
emollient	973.2	E858.4	E943.2	E950.4	E962.0	E980.4
Lead (dust) (fumes) (vapor) NEC	984.9	E866.0	—	E950.9	E962.1	E980.9
acetate (dust)	984.1	E866.0	—	E950.9	E962.1	E980.9
anti-infectives	961.2	E857	E931.2	E950.4	E962.0	E980.4
antiknock compound (tetraethyl)	984.1	E862.1	—	E950.9	E962.1	E980.9
arsenate, arsenite (dust) (insecticide) (vapor)	985.1	E863.4	—	E950.8	E962.1	E980.8
herbicide	985.1	E863.5	—	E950.8	E962.1	E980.8
carbonate	984.0	E866.0	—	E950.9	E962.1	E980.9
paint	984.0	E861.5	—	E950.9	E962.1	E980.9
chromate	984.0	E866.0	—	E950.9	E962.1	E980.9
paint	984.0	E861.5	—	E950.9	E962.1	E980.9
dioxide	984.0	E866.0	—	E950.9	E962.1	E980.9
inorganic (compound)	984.0	E866.0	—	E950.9	E962.1	E980.9
paint	984.0	E861.5	—	E950.9	E962.1	E980.9
iodide	984.0	E866.0	—	E950.9	E962.1	E980.9
pigment (paint)	984.0	E861.5	—	E950.9	E962.1	E980.9
monoxide (dust)	984.0	E866.0	—	E950.9	E962.1	E980.9
paint	984.0	E861.5	—	E950.9	E962.1	E980.9
organic	984.1	E866.0	—	E950.9	E962.1	E980.9
oxide	984.0	E866.0	—	E950.9	E962.1	E980.9
paint	984.0	E861.5	—	E950.9	E962.1	E980.9
paint	984.0	E861.5	—	E950.9	E962.1	E980.9
salts	984.0	E866.0	—	E950.9	E962.1	E980.9
specified compound NEC	984.8	E866.0	—	E950.9	E962.1	E980.9
tetra-ethyl	984.1	E862.1	—	E950.9	E962.1	E980.9
Lebanese red	969.6	E854.1	E939.6	E950.3	E962.0	E980.3
Lente Iletin (insulin)	962.3	E858.0	E932.3	E950.4	E962.0	E980.4
Leptazol	970.0	E854.3	E940.0	E950.4	E962.0	E980.4
Leritine	965.09	E850.2	E935.2	E950.0	E962.0	E980.0
Letter	962.7	E858.0	E932.7	E950.4	E962.0	E980.4
Lettuce opium	967.8	E852.8	E937.8	E950.2	E962.0	E980.2
Leucovorin (factor)	964.1	E858.2	E934.1	E950.4	E962.0	E980.4
Leukeran	963.1	E858.1	E933.1	E950.4	E962.0	E980.4
Levalbuterol	975.7	E858.6	E945.7	E950.4	E962.0	E980.4
Levallorphan	970.1	E854.3	E940.1	E950.4	E962.0	E980.4
Levanil	967.8	E852.8	E937.8	E950.2	E962.0	E980.2
Levarterenol	971.2	E855.5	E941.2	E950.4	E962.0	E980.4
Levo-dromoran	965.09	E850.2	E935.2	E950.0	E962.0	E980.0
Levo-iso-methadone	965.02	E850.1	E935.1	E950.0	E962.0	E980.0
Levodopa	966.4	E855.0	E936.4	E950.4	E962.0	E980.4
Levoid	962.7	E858.0	E932.7	E950.4	E962.0	E980.4
Levomepromazine	967.8	E852.8	E937.8	E950.2	E962.0	E980.2
Levoprome	967.8	E852.8	E937.8	E950.2	E962.0	E980.2
Levopropoxyphene	975.4	E858.6	E945.4	E950.4	E962.0	E980.4
Levorphan, levophanol	965.09	E850.2	E935.2	E950.0	E962.0	E980.0
Levothyroxine (sodium)	962.7	E858.0	E932.7	E950.4	E962.0	E980.4
Levsin	971.1	E855.4	E941.1	E950.4	E962.0	E980.4
Levulose	974.5	E858.5	E944.5	E950.4	E962.0	E980.4
Lewisite (gas)	985.1	E866.3	—	E950.8	E962.1	E980.8
Librium	969.4	E853.2	E939.4	E950.3	E962.0	E980.3
Lidex	976.0	E858.7	E946.0	E950.4	E962.0	E980.4
Lidocaine (infiltration) (topical)	968.5	E855.2	E938.5	E950.4	E962.0	E980.4

		External Cause (E-Code)				
	Poisoning	Accident	Therapeutic Use	Suicide Attempt	Assault	Undetermined
Lidocaine — *continued*						
nerve block (peripheral) (plexus)	968.6	E855.2	E938.6	E950.4	E962.0	E980.4
spinal	968.7	E855.2	E938.7	E950.4	E962.0	E980.4
Lighter fluid	981	E862.1	—	E950.9	E962.1	E980.9
Lignocaine (infiltration) (topical)	968.5	E855.2	E938.5	E950.4	E962.0	E980.4
nerve block (peripheral) (plexus)	968.6	E855.2	E938.6	E950.4	E962.0	E980.4
spinal	968.7	E855.2	E938.7	E950.4	E962.0	E980.4
Ligroin(e) (solvent)	981	E862.0	—	E950.9	E962.1	E980.9
vapor	987.1	E869.8	—	E952.8	E962.2	E982.8
Ligustrum vulgare	988.2	E865.3	—	E950.9	E962.1	E980.9
Lily of the valley	988.2	E865.4	—	E950.9	E962.1	E980.9
Lime (chloride)	983.2	E864.2	—	E950.7	E962.1	E980.6
solution, sulferated	976.4	E858.7	E946.4	E950.4	E962.0	E980.4
Limonene	982.8	E862.4	—	E950.9	E962.1	E980.9
Lincomycin	960.8	E856	E930.8	E950.4	E962.0	E980.4
Lindane (insecticide) (vapor)	989.2	E863.0	—	E950.6	E962.1	E980.7
anti-infective (topical)	976.0	E858.7	E946.0	E950.4	E962.0	E980.4
Liniments NEC	976.9	E858.7	E946.9	E950.4	E962.0	E980.4
Linoleic acid	972.2	E858.3	E942.2	E950.4	E962.0	E980.4
Liothyronine	962.7	E858.0	E932.7	E950.4	E962.0	E980.4
Liotrix	962.7	E858.0	E932.7	E950.4	E962.0	E980.4
Lipancreatin	973.4	E858.4	E943.4	E950.4	E962.0	E980.4
Lipo-Lutin	962.2	E858.0	E932.2	E950.4	E962.0	E980.4
Lipotropic agents	977.1	E858.8	E947.1	E950.4	E962.0	E980.4
Liquefied petroleum gases	987.0	E868.0	—	E951.1	E962.2	E981.1
piped (pure or mixed with air)	987.0	E867	—	E951.0	E962.2	E981.0
Liquid petrolatum	973.2	E858.4	E943.2	E950.4	E962.0	E980.4
substance	989.9	E866.9	—	E950.9	E962.1	E980.9
specified NEC	989.89	E866.8	—	E950.9	E962.1	E980.9
Lirugen	979.4	E858.8	E949.4	E950.4	E962.0	E980.4
Lithane	969.8	E855.8	E939.8	E950.3	E962.0	E980.3
Lithium	985.8	E866.4	—	E950.9	E962.1	E980.9
carbonate	969.8	E855.8	E939.8	E950.3	E962.0	E980.3
Lithonate	969.8	E855.8	E939.8	E950.3	E962.0	E980.3
Liver (extract) (injection) (preparations)	964.1	E858.2	E934.1	E950.4	E962.0	E980.4
Lizard (bite) (venom)	989.5	E905.0	—	E950.9	E962.1	E980.9
LMD	964.8	E858.2	E934.8	E950.4	E962.0	E980.4
Lobelia	988.2	E865.4	—	E950.9	E962.1	E980.9
Lobeline	970.0	E854.3	E940.0	E950.4	E962.0	E980.4
Locorten	976.0	E858.7	E946.0	E950.4	E962.0	E980.4
Lolium temulentum	988.2	E865.3	—	E950.9	E962.1	E980.9
Lomotil	973.5	E858.4	E943.5	E950.4	E962.0	E980.4
Lomustine	963.1	E858.1	E933.1	E950.4	E962.0	E980.4
Lophophora williamsii	969.6	E854.1	E939.6	E950.3	E962.0	E980.3
Lorazepam	969.4	E853.2	E939.4	E950.3	E962.0	E980.3
Lotions NEC	976.9	E858.7	E946.9	E950.4	E962.0	E980.4
Lotronex	973.8	E858.4	E943.8	E950.4	E962.0	E980.4
Lotusate	967.0	E851	E937.0	E950.1	E962.0	E980.1
Lowila	976.2	E858.7	E946.2	E950.4	E962.0	E980.4
Loxapine	969.3	E853.8	E939.3	E950.3	E962.0	E980.3
Lozenges (throat)	976.6	E858.7	E946.6	E950.4	E962.0	E980.4
LSD (25)	969.6	E854.1	E939.6	E950.3	E962.0	E980.3
Lubricating oil NEC	981	E862.2	—	E950.9	E962.1	E980.9
Lucanthone	961.6	E857	E931.6	E950.4	E962.0	E980.4
Luminal	967.0	E851	E937.0	E950.1	E962.0	E980.1
Lung irritant (gas) NEC	987.9	E869.9	—	E952.9	E962.2	E982.9
Lutocylol	962.2	E858.0	E932.2	E950.4	E962.0	E980.4
Lutromone	962.2	E858.0	E932.2	E950.4	E962.0	E980.4
Lututrin	975.0	E858.6	E945.0	E950.4	E962.0	E980.4
Lye (concentrated)	983.2	E864.2	—	E950.7	E962.1	E980.6
Lygranum (skin test)	977.8	E858.8	E947.8	E950.4	E962.0	E980.4
Lymecycline	960.4	E856	E930.4	E950.4	E962.0	E980.4
Lymphogranuloma venereum antigen	977.8	E858.8	E947.8	E950.4	E962.0	E980.4
Lynestrenol	962.2	E858.0	E932.2	E950.4	E962.0	E980.4
Lyovac Sodium Edecrin	974.4	E858.5	E944.4	E950.4	E962.0	E980.4
Lypressin	962.5	E858.0	E932.5	E950.4	E962.0	E980.4
Lysergic acid (amide) (diethylamide)	969.6	E854.1	E939.6	E950.3	E962.0	E980.3
Lysergide	969.6	E854.1	E939.6	E950.3	E962.0	E980.3
Lysine vasopressin	962.5	E858.0	E932.5	E950.4	E962.0	E980.4
Lysol	983.0	E864.0	—	E950.7	E962.1	E980.6
Lytta (vitatta)	976.8	E858.7	E946.8	E950.4	E962.0	E980.4
M-vac	979.4	E858.8	E949.4	E950.4	E962.0	E980.4
Mace	987.5	E869.3	—	E952.8	E962.2	E982.8

		External Cause (E-Code)				
	Poisoning	Accident	Therapeutic Use	Suicide Attempt	Assault	Undetermined
Macrolides (antibiotics)	960.3	E856	E930.3	E950.4	E962.0	E980.4
Mafenide	976.0	E858.7	E946.0	E950.4	E962.0	E980.4
Magaldrate	973.0	E858.4	E943.0	E950.4	E962.0	E980.4
Magic mushroom	969.6	E854.1	E939.6	E950.3	E962.0	E980.3
Magnamycin	960.8	E856	E930.8	E950.4	E962.0	E980.4
Magnesia magma	973.0	E858.4	E943.0	E950.4	E962.0	E980.4
Magnesium (compounds) (fumes) NEC	985.8	E866.4	—	E950.9	E962.1	E980.9
antacid	973.0	E858.4	E943.0	E950.4	E962.0	E980.4
carbonate	973.0	E858.4	E943.0	E950.4	E962.0	E980.4
cathartic	973.3	E858.4	E943.3	E950.4	E962.0	E980.4
citrate	973.3	E858.4	E943.3	E950.4	E962.0	E980.4
hydroxide	973.0	E858.4	E943.0	E950.4	E962.0	E980.4
oxide	973.0	E858.4	E943.0	E950.4	E962.0	E980.4
sulfate (oral)	973.3	E858.4	E943.3	E950.4	E962.0	E980.4
intravenous	966.3	E855.0	E936.3	E950.4	E962.0	E980.4
trisilicate	973.0	E858.4	E943.0	E950.4	E962.0	E980.4
Malathion (insecticide)	989.3	E863.1	—	E950.6	E962.1	E980.7
Male fern (oleoresin)	961.6	E857	E931.6	E950.4	E962.0	E980.4
Mandelic acid	961.9	E857	E931.9	E950.4	E962.0	E980.4
Manganese compounds (fumes) NEC	985.2	E866.4	—	E950.9	E962.1	E980.9
Mannitol (diuretic) (medicinal) NEC	974.4	E858.5	E944.4	E950.4	E962.0	E980.4
hexanitrate	972.4	E858.3	E942.4	E950.4	E962.0	E980.4
mustard	963.1	E858.1	E933.1	E950.4	E962.0	E980.4
Mannomustine	963.1	E858.1	E933.1	E950.4	E962.0	E980.4
MAO inhibitors	969.01	E854.0	E939.0	E950.3	E962.0	E980.3
Mapharsen	961.1	E857	E931.1	E950.4	E962.0	E980.4
Marcaine	968.9	E855.2	E938.9	E950.4	E962.0	E980.4
infiltration (subcutaneous)	968.5	E855.2	E938.5	E950.4	E962.0	E980.4
nerve block (peripheral) (plexus)	968.6	E855.2	E938.6	E950.4	E962.0	E980.4
Marezine	963.0	E858.1	E933.0	E950.4	E962.0	E980.4
Marihuana, marijuana (derivatives)	969.6	E854.1	E939.6	E950.3	E962.0	E980.3
Marine animals or plants (sting)	989.5	E905.6	—	E950.9	E962.1	E980.9
Marplan	969.01	E854.0	E939.0	E950.3	E962.0	E980.3
Marsh gas	987.1	E869.8	—	E952.8	E962.2	E982.8
Marsilid	969.01	E854.0	E939.0	E950.3	E962.0	E980.3
Matulane	963.1	E858.1	E933.1	E950.4	E962.0	E980.4
Mazindol	977.0	E858.8	E947.0	E950.4	E962.0	E980.4
MDMA	969.72	E854.2	E939.7	E950.3	E962.0	E980.3
Meadow saffron	988.2	E865.3	—	E950.9	E962.1	E980.9
Measles vaccine	979.4	E858.8	E949.4	E950.4	E962.0	E980.4
Meat, noxious or nonbacterial	988.8	E865.0	—	E950.9	E962.1	E980.9
Mebanazine	969.01	E854.0	E939.0	E950.3	E962.0	E980.3
Mebaral	967.0	E851	E937.0	E950.1	E962.0	E980.1
Mebendazole	961.6	E857	E931.6	E950.4	E962.0	E980.4
Mebeverine	975.1	E858.6	E945.1	E950.4	E962.0	E980.4
Mebhydroline	963.0	E858.1	E933.0	E950.4	E962.0	E980.4
Mebrophenhydramine	963.0	E858.1	E933.0	E950.4	E962.0	E980.4
Mebutamate	969.5	E853.8	E939.5	E950.3	E962.0	E980.3
Mecamylamine (chloride)	972.3	E858.3	E942.3	E950.4	E962.0	E980.4
Mechlorethamine hydrochloride	963.1	E858.1	E933.1	E950.4	E962.0	E980.4
Meclizine (hydrochloride)	963.0	E858.1	E933.0	E950.4	E962.0	E980.4
Meclofenoxate	970.0	E854.3	E940.0	E950.4	E962.0	E980.4
Meclozine (hydrochloride)	963.0	E858.1	E933.0	E950.4	E962.0	E980.4
Medazepam	969.4	E853.2	E939.4	E950.3	E962.0	E980.3
Medicine, medicinal substance	977.9	E858.9	E947.9	E950.5	E962.0	E980.5
specified NEC	977.8	E858.8	E947.8	E950.4	E962.0	E980.4
Medinal	967.0	E851	E937.0	E950.1	E962.0	E980.1
Medomin	967.0	E851	E937.0	E950.1	E962.0	E980.1
Medroxyprogesterone	962.2	E858.0	E932.2	E950.4	E962.0	E980.4
Medrysone	976.5	E858.7	E946.5	E950.4	E962.0	E980.4
Mefenamic acid	965.7	E850.7	E935.7	E950.0	E962.0	E980.0
Megahallucinogen	969.6	E854.1	E939.6	E950.3	E962.0	E980.3
Megestrol	962.2	E858.0	E932.2	E950.4	E962.0	E980.4
Meglumine	977.8	E858.8	E947.8	E950.4	E962.0	E980.4
Meladinin	976.3	E858.7	E946.3	E950.4	E962.0	E980.4
Melanizing agents	976.3	E858.7	E946.3	E950.4	E962.0	E980.4
Melarsoprol	961.1	E857	E931.1	E950.4	E962.0	E980.4
Melia azedarach	988.2	E865.3	—	E950.9	E962.1	E980.9
Mellaril	969.1	E853.0	E939.1	E950.3	E962.0	E980.3
Meloxine	976.3	E858.7	E946.3	E950.4	E962.0	E980.4
Melphalan	963.1	E858.1	E933.1	E950.4	E962.0	E980.4

Nontherapeutic use substance

▷◁ Revised Text   ● New Line   ▲ Revised Code

Subterms under main terms may continue to next column or page

	Poisoning	Accident	Therapeutic Use	Suicide Attempt	Assault	Undeter-mined
Menadiol sodium diphos-phate	964.3	E858.2	E934.3	E950.4	E962.0	E980.4
Menadione (sodium bisul-fite)	964.3	E858.2	E934.3	E950.4	E962.0	E980.4
Menaphthone	964.3	E858.2	E934.3	E950.4	E962.0	E980.4
Meningococcal vaccine	978.8	E858.8	E948.8	E950.4	E962.0	E980.4
Menningovax-C	978.8	E858.8	E948.8	E950.4	E962.0	E980.4
Menotropins	962.4	E858.0	E932.4	E950.4	E962.0	E980.4
Menthol NEC	976.1	E858.7	E946.1	E950.4	E962.0	E980.4
Mepacrine	961.3	E857	E931.3	E950.4	E962.0	E980.4
Meparfynol	967.8	E852.8	E937.8	E950.2	E962.0	E980.2
Mepazine	969.1	E853.0	E939.1	E950.3	E962.0	E980.3
Mepenzolate	971.1	E855.4	E941.1	E950.4	E962.0	E980.4
Meperidine	965.09	E850.2	E935.2	E950.0	E962.0	E980.0
Mephenamin(e)	966.4	E855.0	E936.4	E950.4	E962.0	E980.4
Mephenesin (carbamate)	968.0	E855.1	E938.0	E950.4	E962.0	E980.4
Mephenoxalone	969.5	E853.8	E939.5	E950.3	E962.0	E980.3
Mephentermine	971.2	E855.5	E941.2	E950.4	E962.0	E980.4
Mephenytoin	966.1	E855.0	E936.1	E950.4	E962.0	E980.4
Mephobarbital	967.0	E851	E937.0	E950.1	E962.0	E980.1
Mepiperphenidol	971.1	E855.4	E941.1	E950.4	E962.0	E980.4
Mepivacaine	968.9	E855.2	E938.9	E950.4	E962.0	E980.4
infiltration (subcuta-neous)	968.5	E855.2	E938.5	E950.4	E962.0	E980.4
nerve block (peripheral) (plexus)	968.6	E855.2	E938.6	E950.4	E962.0	E980.4
topical (surface)	968.5	E855.2	E938.5	E950.4	E962.0	E980.4
Meprednisone	962.0	E858.0	E932.0	E950.4	E962.0	E980.4
Meprobam	969.5	E853.8	E939.5	E950.3	E962.0	E980.3
Meprobamate	969.5	E853.8	E939.5	E950.3	E962.0	E980.3
Mepyramine (maleate)	963.0	E858.1	E933.0	E950.4	E962.0	E980.4
Meralluride	974.0	E858.5	E944.0	E950.4	E962.0	E980.4
Merbaphen	974.0	E858.5	E944.0	E950.4	E962.0	E980.4
Merbromin	976.0	E858.7	E946.0	E950.4	E962.0	E980.4
Mercaptomerin	974.0	E858.5	E944.0	E950.4	E962.0	E980.4
Mercaptopurine	963.1	E858.1	E933.1	E950.4	E962.0	E980.4
Mercumatilin	974.0	E858.5	E944.0	E950.4	E962.0	E980.4
Mercuramide	974.0	E858.5	E944.0	E950.4	E962.0	E980.4
Mercuranin	976.0	E858.7	E946.0	E950.4	E962.0	E980.4
Mercurochrome	976.0	E858.7	E946.0	E950.4	E962.0	E980.4
Mercury, mercuric, mer-curous (compounds) (cyanide) (fumes) (nonmedic-inal) (vapor) NEC	985.0	E866.1	—	E950.9	E962.1	E980.9
ammoniated	976.0	E858.7	E946.0	E950.4	E962.0	E980.4
anti-infective	961.2	E857	E931.2	E950.4	E962.0	E980.4
topical	976.0	E858.7	E946.0	E950.4	E962.0	E980.4
chloride (antiseptic) NEC	976.0	E858.7	E946.0	E950.4	E962.0	E980.4
fungicide	985.0	E863.6	—	E950.6	E962.1	E980.7
diuretic compounds	974.0	E858.5	E944.0	E950.4	E962.0	E980.4
fungicide	985.0	E863.6	—	E950.6	E962.1	E980.7
organic (fungicide)	985.0	E863.6	—	E950.6	E962.1	E980.7
Merethoxylline	974.0	E858.5	E944.0	E950.4	E962.0	E980.4
Mersalyl	974.0	E858.5	E944.0	E950.4	E962.0	E980.4
Merthiolate (topical)	976.0	E858.7	E946.0	E950.4	E962.0	E980.4
ophthalmic preparation	976.5	E858.7	E946.5	E950.4	E962.0	E980.4
Meruvax	979.4	E858.8	E949.4	E950.4	E962.0	E980.4
Mescal buttons	969.6	E854.1	E939.6	E950.3	E962.0	E980.3
Mescaline (salts)	969.6	E854.1	E939.6	E950.3	E962.0	E980.3
Mesoridazine besylate	969.1	E853.0	E939.1	E950.3	E962.0	E980.3
Mestanolone	962.1	E858.0	E932.1	E950.4	E962.0	E980.4
Mestranol	962.2	E858.0	E932.2	E950.4	E962.0	E980.4
Metacresylacetate	976.0	E858.7	E946.0	E950.4	E962.0	E980.4
Metaldehyde (snail killer) NEC	989.4	E863.4	—	E950.6	E962.1	E980.7
Metals (heavy) (nonmedici-nal) NEC	985.9	E866.4	—	E950.9	E962.1	E980.9
dust, fumes, or vapor NEC	985.9	E866.4	—	E950.9	E962.1	E980.9
light NEC	985.9	E866.4	—	E950.9	E962.1	E980.9
dust, fumes, or vapor NEC	985.9	E866.4	—	E950.9	E962.1	E980.9
pesticides (dust) (vapor)	985.9	E863.4	—	E950.6	E962.1	E980.7
Metamucil	973.3	E858.4	E943.3	E950.4	E962.0	E980.4
Metaphen	976.0	E858.7	E946.0	E950.4	E962.0	E980.4
Metaproterenol	975.1	E858.6	E945.1	E950.4	E962.0	E980.4
Metaraminol	972.8	E858.3	E942.8	E950.4	E962.0	E980.4
Metaxalone	968.0	E855.1	E938.0	E950.4	E962.0	E980.4
Metformin	962.3	E858.0	E932.3	E950.4	E962.0	E980.4
Methacycline	960.4	E856	E930.4	E950.4	E962.0	E980.4
Methadone	965.02	E850.1	E935.1	E950.0	E962.0	E980.0
Methallenestril	962.2	E858.0	E932.2	E950.4	E962.0	E980.4

	Poisoning	Accident	Therapeutic Use	Suicide Attempt	Assault	Undeter-mined
Methamphetamine	969.72	E854.2	E939.7	E950.3	E962.0	E980.3
Methandienone	962.1	E858.0	E932.1	E950.4	E962.0	E980.4
Methandriol	962.1	E858.0	E932.1	E950.4	E962.0	E980.4
Methandrostenolone	962.1	E858.0	E932.1	E950.4	E962.0	E980.4
Methane gas	987.1	E869.8	—	E952.8	E962.2	E982.8
Methanol	980.1	E860.2	—	E950.9	E962.1	E980.9
vapor	987.8	E869.8	—	E952.8	E962.2	E982.8
Methantheline	971.1	E855.4	E941.1	E950.4	E962.0	E980.4
Methaphenilene	963.0	E858.1	E933.0	E950.4	E962.0	E980.4
Methapyrilene	963.0	E858.1	E933.0	E950.4	E962.0	E980.4
Methaqualone (com-pounds)	967.4	E852.3	E937.4	E950.2	E962.0	E980.2
Metharbital, methar-bitone	967.0	E851	E937.0	E950.1	E962.0	E980.1
Methazolamide	974.2	E858.5	E944.2	E950.4	E962.0	E980.4
Methdilazine	963.0	E858.1	E933.0	E950.4	E962.0	E980.4
Methedrine	969.72	E854.2	E939.7	E950.3	E962.0	E980.3
Methenamine (mande-late)	961.9	E857	E931.9	E950.4	E962.0	E980.4
Methenolone	962.1	E858.0	E932.1	E950.4	E962.0	E980.4
Methergine	975.0	E858.6	E945.0	E950.4	E962.0	E980.4
Methiacil	962.8	E858.0	E932.8	E950.4	E962.0	E980.4
Methicillin (sodium)	960.0	E856	E930.0	E950.4	E962.0	E980.4
Methimazole	962.8	E858.0	E932.8	E950.4	E962.0	E980.4
Methionine	977.1	E858.8	E947.1	E950.4	E962.0	E980.4
Methisazone	961.7	E857	E931.7	E950.4	E962.0	E980.4
Methitural	967.0	E851	E937.0	E950.1	E962.0	E980.1
Methixene	971.1	E855.4	E941.1	E950.4	E962.0	E980.4
Methobarbital, methobarbi-tone	967.0	E851	E937.0	E950.1	E962.0	E980.1
Methocarbamol	968.0	E855.1	E938.0	E950.4	E962.0	E980.4
Methohexital, methohexi-tone (sodium)	968.3	E855.1	E938.3	E950.4	E962.0	E980.4
Methoin	966.1	E855.0	E936.1	E950.4	E962.0	E980.4
Methopholine	965.7	E850.7	E935.7	E950.0	E962.0	E980.0
Methorate	975.4	E858.6	E945.4	E950.4	E962.0	E980.4
Methoserpidine	972.6	E858.3	E942.6	E950.4	E962.0	E980.4
Methotrexate	963.1	E858.1	E933.1	E950.4	E962.0	E980.4
Methotrimeprazine	967.8	E852.8	E937.8	E950.2	E962.0	E980.2
Methoxa-Dome	976.3	E858.7	E946.3	E950.4	E962.0	E980.4
Methoxamine	971.2	E855.5	E941.2	E950.4	E962.0	E980.4
Methoxsalen	976.3	E858.7	E946.3	E950.4	E962.0	E980.4
Methoxybenzyl peni-cillin	960.0	E856	E930.0	E950.4	E962.0	E980.4
Methoxychlor	989.2	E863.0	—	E950.6	E962.1	E980.7
Methoxyflurane	968.2	E855.1	E938.2	E950.4	E962.0	E980.4
Methoxyphenamine	971.2	E855.5	E941.2	E950.4	E962.0	E980.4
Methoxypromazine	969.1	E853.0	E939.1	E950.3	E962.0	E980.3
Methoxypsoralen	976.3	E858.7	E946.3	E950.4	E962.0	E980.4
Methscopolamine (bro-mide)	971.1	E855.4	E941.1	E950.4	E962.0	E980.4
Methsuximide	966.2	E855.0	E936.2	E950.4	E962.0	E980.4
Methyclothiazide	974.3	E858.5	E944.3	E950.4	E962.0	E980.4
Methyl						
acetate	982.8	E862.4	—	E950.9	E962.1	E980.9
acetone	982.8	E862.4	—	E950.9	E962.1	E980.9
alcohol	980.1	E860.2	—	E950.9	E962.1	E980.9
amphetamine	969.72	E854.2	E939.7	E950.3	E962.0	E980.3
androstanolone	962.1	E858.0	E932.1	E950.4	E962.0	E980.4
atropine	971.1	E855.4	E941.1	E950.4	E962.0	E980.4
benzene	982.0	E862.4	—	E950.9	E962.1	E980.9
bromide (gas)	987.8	E869.8	—	E952.8	E962.2	E982.8
fumigant	987.8	E863.8	—	E950.6	E962.2	E980.7
butanol	980.8	E860.8	—	E950.9	E962.1	E980.9
carbinol	980.1	E860.2	—	E950.9	E962.1	E980.9
cellosolve	982.8	E862.4	—	E950.9	E962.1	E980.9
cellulose	973.3	E858.4	E943.3	E950.4	E962.0	E980.4
chloride (gas)	987.8	E869.8	—	E952.8	E962.2	E982.8
cyclohexane	982.8	E862.4	—	E950.9	E962.1	E980.9
cyclohexanone	982.8	E862.4	—	E950.9	E962.1	E980.9
dihydromorphinone	965.09	E850.2	E935.2	E950.0	E962.0	E980.0
ergometrine	975.0	E858.6	E945.0	E950.4	E962.0	E980.4
ergonovine	975.0	E858.6	E945.0	E950.4	E962.0	E980.4
ethyl ketone	982.8	E862.4	—	E950.9	E962.1	E980.9
hydrazine	983.9	E864.3	—	E950.7	E962.1	E980.6
isobutyl ketone	982.8	E862.4	—	E950.9	E962.1	E980.9
morphine NEC	965.09	E850.2	E935.2	E950.0	E962.0	E980.0
parafynol	967.8	E852.8	E937.8	E950.2	E962.0	E980.2
parathion	989.3	E863.1	—	E950.6	E962.1	E980.7
pentynol NEC	967.8	E852.8	E937.8	E950.2	E962.0	E980.2
peridol	969.2	E853.1	E939.2	E950.3	E962.0	E980.3
phenidate	969.73	E854.2	E939.7	E950.3	E962.0	E980.3

	Poisoning	Accident	Therapeutic Use	Suicide Attempt	Assault	Undetermined
Methyl — *continued*						
prednisolone	962.0	E858.0	E932.0	E950.4	E962.0	E980.4
ENT agent	976.6	E858.7	E946.6	E950.4	E962.0	E980.4
ophthalmic preparation	976.5	E858.7	E946.5	E950.4	E962.0	E980.4
topical NEC	976.0	E858.7	E946.0	E950.4	E962.0	E980.4
propylcarbinol	980.8	E860.8	—	E950.9	E962.1	E980.9
rosaniline NEC	976.0	E858.7	E946.0	E950.4	E962.0	E980.4
salicylate NEC	976.3	E858.7	E946.3	E950.4	E962.0	E980.4
sulfate (fumes)	987.8	E869.8	—	E952.8	E962.2	E982.8
liquid	983.9	E864.3	—	E950.7	E962.1	E980.6
sulfonal	967.8	E852.8	E937.8	E950.2	E962.0	E980.2
testosterone	962.1	E858.0	E932.1	E950.4	E962.0	E980.4
thiouracil	962.8	E858.0	E932.8	E950.4	E962.0	E980.4
Methylated spirit	980.0	E860.1		E950.9	E962.1	E980.9
Methyldopa	972.6	E858.3	E942.6	E950.4	E962.0	E980.4
Methylene						
blue	961.9	E857	E931.9	E950.4	E962.0	E980.4
chloride or dichloride (solvent) NEC	982.3	E862.4	—	E950.9	E962.1	E980.9
Methylhexabital	967.0	E851	E937.0	E950.1	E962.0	E980.1
Methylparaben (ophthalmic)	976.5	E858.7	E946.5	E950.4	E962.0	E980.4
Methyprylon	967.5	E852.4	E937.5	E950.2	E962.0	E980.2
Methysergide	971.3	E855.6	E941.3	E950.4	E962.0	E980.4
Metoclopramide	963.0	E858.1	E933.0	E950.4	E962.0	E980.4
Metofoline	965.7	E850.7	E935.7	E950.0	E962.0	E980.0
Metopon	965.09	E850.2	E935.2	E950.0	E962.0	E980.0
Metronidazole	961.5	E857	E931.5	E950.4	E962.0	E980.4
Metycaine	968.9	E855.2	E938.9	E950.4	E962.0	E980.4
infiltration (subcutaneous)	968.5	E855.2	E938.5	E950.4	E962.0	E980.4
nerve block (peripheral) (plexus)	968.6	E855.2	E938.6	E950.4	E962.0	E980.4
topical (surface)	968.5	E855.2	E938.5	E950.4	E962.0	E980.4
Metyrapone	977.8	E858.8	E947.8	E950.4	E962.0	E980.4
Mevinphos	989.3	E863.1	—	E950.6	E962.1	E980.7
Mezereon (berries)	988.2	E865.3	—	E950.9	E962.1	E980.9
Micatin	976.0	E858.7	E946.0	E950.4	E962.0	E980.4
Miconazole	976.0	E858.7	E946.0	E950.4	E962.0	E980.4
Midol	965.1	E850.3	E935.3	E950.0	E962.0	E980.0
Mifepristone	962.9	E858.0	E932.9	E950.4	E962.0	E980.4
Milk of magnesia	973.0	E858.4	E943.0	E950.4	E962.0	E980.4
Millipede (tropical) (venomous)	989.5	E905.4	—	E950.9	E962.1	E980.9
Miltown	969.5	E853.8	E939.5	E950.3	E962.0	E980.3
Mineral						
oil (medicinal)	973.2	E858.4	E943.2	E950.4	E962.0	E980.4
nonmedicinal	981	E862.1	—	E950.9	E962.1	E980.9
topical	976.3	E858.7	E946.3	E950.4	E962.0	E980.4
salts NEC	974.6	E858.5	E944.6	E950.4	E962.0	E980.4
spirits	981	E862.0	—	E950.9	E962.1	E980.9
Minocycline	960.4	E856	E930.4	E950.4	E962.0	E980.4
Mithramycin (antineoplastic)	960.7	E856	E930.7	E950.4	E962.0	E980.4
Mitobronitol	963.1	E858.1	E933.1	E950.4	E962.0	E980.4
Mitomycin (antineoplastic)	960.7	E856	E930.7	E950.4	E962.0	E980.4
Mitotane	963.1	E858.1	E933.1	E950.4	E962.0	E980.4
Moderil	972.6	E858.3	E942.6	E950.4	E962.0	E980.4
Mogadon — *see* Nitrazepam						
Molindone	969.3	E853.8	E939.3	E950.3	E962.0	E980.3
Monistat	976.0	E858.7	E946.0	E950.4	E962.0	E980.4
Monkshood	988.2	E865.4	—	E950.9	E962.1	E980.9
Monoamine oxidase inhibitors	969.01	E854.0	E939.0	E950.3	E962.0	E980.3
Monochlorobenzene	982.0	E862.4	—	E950.9	E962.1	E980.9
Monosodium glutamate	989.89	E866.8	—	E950.9	E962.1	E980.9
Monoxide, carbon — *see* Carbon, monoxide						
Moperone	969.2	E853.1	E939.2	E950.3	E962.0	E980.3
Morning glory seeds	969.6	E854.1	E939.6	E950.3	E962.0	E980.3
Moroxydine (hydrochloride)	961.7	E857	E931.7	E950.4	E962.0	E980.4
Morphazinamide	961.8	E857	E931.8	E950.4	E962.0	E980.4
Morphinans	965.09	E850.2	E935.2	E950.0	E962.0	E980.0
Morphine NEC	965.09	E850.2	E935.2	E950.0	E962.0	E980.0
antagonists	970.1	E854.3	E940.1	E950.4	E962.0	E980.4
Morpholinylethylmorphine	965.09	E850.2	E935.2	E950.0	E962.0	E980.0
Morrhuate sodium	972.7	E858.3	E942.7	E950.4	E962.0	E980.4
Moth balls — *see also* Pesticides	989.4	E863.4	—	E950.6	E962.1	E980.7
Moth balls — *see also* Pesticides — *continued*						
naphthalene	983.0	E863.4	—	E950.7	E962.1	E980.6
Motor exhaust gas — *see* Carbon, monoxide, exhaust gas						
Mouth wash	976.6	E858.7	E946.6	E950.4	E962.0	E980.4
Mucolytic agent	975.5	E858.6	E945.5	E950.4	E962.0	E980.4
Mucomyst	975.5	E858.6	E945.5	E950.4	E962.0	E980.4
Mucous membrane agents (external)	976.9	E858.7	E946.9	E950.4	E962.0	E980.4
specified NEC	976.8	E858.7	E946.8	E950.4	E962.0	E980.4
Mumps						
immune globulin (human)	964.6	E858.2	E934.6	E950.4	E962.0	E980.4
skin test antigen	977.8	E858.8	E947.8	E950.4	E962.0	E980.4
vaccine	979.6	E858.8	E949.6	E950.4	E962.0	E980.4
Mumpsvax	979.6	E858.8	E949.6	E950.4	E962.0	E980.4
Muriatic acid — *see* Hydrochloric acid						
Muscarine	971.0	E855.3	E941.0	E950.4	E962.0	E980.4
Muscle affecting agents						
NEC	975.3	E858.6	E945.3	E950.4	E962.0	E980.4
oxytocic	975.0	E858.6	E945.0	E950.4	E962.0	E980.4
relaxants	975.3	E858.6	E945.3	E950.4	E962.0	E980.4
central nervous system	968.0	E855.1	E938.0	E950.4	E962.0	E980.4
skeletal	975.2	E858.6	E945.2	E950.4	E962.0	E980.4
smooth	975.1	E858.6	E945.1	E950.4	E962.0	E980.4
Mushrooms, noxious	988.1	E865.5	—	E950.9	E962.1	E980.9
Mussel, noxious	988.0	E865.1	—	E950.9	E962.1	E980.9
Mustard (emetic)	973.6	E858.4	E943.6	E950.4	E962.0	E980.4
gas	987.8	E869.8	—	E952.8	E962.2	E982.8
nitrogen	963.1	E858.1	E933.1	E950.4	E962.0	E980.4
Mustine	963.1	E858.1	E933.1	E950.4	E962.0	E980.4
Mycifradin	960.8	E856	E930.8	E950.4	E962.0	E980.4
topical	976.0	E858.7	E946.0	E950.4	E962.0	E980.4
Mycitracin	960.8	E856	E930.8	E950.4	E962.0	E980.4
ophthalmic preparation	976.5	E858.7	E946.5	E950.4	E962.0	E980.4
Mycostatin	960.1	E856	E930.1	E950.4	E962.0	E980.4
topical	976.0	E858.7	E946.0	E950.4	E962.0	E980.4
Mydriacyl	971.1	E855.4	E941.1	E950.4	E962.0	E980.4
Myelobromal	963.1	E858.1	E933.1	E950.4	E962.0	E980.4
Myleran	963.1	E858.1	E933.1	E950.4	E962.0	E980.4
Myochrysin(e)	965.69	E850.6	E935.6	E950.0	E962.0	E980.0
Myoneural blocking agents	975.2	E858.6	E945.2	E950.4	E962.0	E980.4
Myristica fragrans	988.2	E865.3	—	E950.9	E962.1	E980.9
Myristicin	988.2	E865.3	—	E950.9	E962.1	E980.9
Mysoline	966.3	E855.0	E936.3	E950.4	E962.0	E980.4
Nafcillin (sodium)	960.0	E856	E930.0	E950.4	E962.0	E980.4
Nail polish remover	982.8	E862.4	—	E950.9	E962.1	E908.9
Nalidixic acid	961.9	E857	E931.9	E950.4	E962.0	E980.4
Nalorphine	970.1	E854.3	E940.1	E950.4	E962.0	E980.4
Naloxone	970.1	E854.3	E940.1	E950.4	E962.0	E980.4
Nandrolone (decanoate) (phenproprioate)	962.1	E858.0	E932.1	E950.4	E962.0	E980.4
Naphazoline	971.2	E855.5	E941.2	E950.4	E962.0	E980.4
Naphtha (painter's) (petroleum)	981	E862.0	—	E950.9	E962.1	E980.9
solvent	981	E862.0	—	E950.9	E962.1	E980.9
vapor	987.1	E869.8	—	E952.8	E962.2	E982.8
Naphthalene (chlorinated)	983.0	E864.0	—	E950.7	E962.1	E980.6
insecticide or moth repellent	983.0	E863.4	—	E950.7	E962.1	E980.6
vapor	987.8	E869.8	—	E952.8	E962.2	E982.8
Naphthol	983.0	E864.0	—	E950.7	E962.1	E980.6
Naphthylamine	983.0	E864.0	—	E950.7	E962.1	E980.6
Naprosyn — *see* Naproxen						
Naproxen	965.61	E850.6	E935.6	E950.0	E962.0	E980.0
Narcotic (drug)	967.9	E852.9	E937.9	E950.2	E962.0	E980.2
analgesic NEC	965.8	E850.8	E935.8	E950.0	E962.0	E980.0
antagonist	970.1	E854.3	E940.1	E950.4	E962.0	E980.4
specified NEC	967.8	E852.8	E937.8	E950.2	E962.0	E980.2
Narcotine	975.4	E858.6	E945.4	E950.4	E962.0	E980.4
Nardil	969.01	E854.0	E939.0	E950.3	E962.0	E980.3
Natrium cyanide — *see* Cyanide(s)						
Natural						
blood (product)	964.7	E858.2	E934.7	E950.4	E962.0	E980.4
gas (piped)	987.1	E867	—	E951.0	E962.2	E981.0
incomplete combustion	986	E867	—	E951.0	E962.2	E981.0

		External Cause (E-Code)				
	Poisoning	Accident	Therapeutic Use	Suicide Attempt	Assault	Undetermined
Nealbarbital, nealbarbitone	967.0	E851	E937.0	E950.1	E962.0	E980.1
Nectadon	975.4	E858.6	E945.4	E950.4	E962.0	E980.4
Nematocyst (sting)	989.5	E905.6	—	E950.9	E962.1	E980.9
Nembutal	967.0	E851	E937.0	E950.1	E962.0	E980.1
Neoarsphenamine	961.1	E857	E931.1	E950.4	E962.0	E980.4
Neocinchophen	974.7	E858.5	E944.7	E950.4	E962.0	E980.4
Neomycin	960.8	E856	E930.8	E950.4	E962.0	E980.4
ENT agent	976.6	E858.7	E946.6	E950.4	E962.0	E980.4
ophthalmic preparation	976.5	E858.7	E946.5	E950.4	E962.0	E980.4
topical NEC	976.0	E858.7	E946.0	E950.4	E962.0	E980.4
Neonal	967.0	E851	E937.0	E950.1	E962.0	E980.1
Neoprontosil	961.0	E857	E931.0	E950.4	E962.0	E980.4
Neosalvarsan	961.1	E857	E931.1	E950.4	E962.0	E980.4
Neosilversalvarsan	961.1	E857	E931.1	E950.4	E962.0	E980.4
Neosporin	960.8	E856	E930.8	E950.4	E962.0	E980.4
ENT agent	976.6	E858.7	E946.6	E950.4	E962.0	E980.4
opthalmic preparation	976.5	E858.7	E946.5	E950.4	E962.0	E980.4
topical NEC	976.0	E858.7	E946.0	E950.4	E962.0	E980.4
Neostigmine	971.0	E855.3	E941.0	E950.4	E962.0	E980.4
Neraval	967.0	E851	E937.0	E950.1	E962.0	E980.1
Neravan	967.0	E851	E937.0	E950.1	E962.0	E980.1
Nerium oleander	988.2	E865.4	—	E950.9	E962.1	E980.9
Nerve gases (war)	987.9	E869.9	—	E952.9	E962.2	E982.9
Nesacaine	968.9	E855.2	E938.9	E950.4	E962.0	E980.4
infiltration (subcutaneous)	968.5	E855.2	E938.5	E950.4	E962.0	E980.4
nerve block (peripheral) (plexus)	968.6	E855.2	E938.6	E950.4	E962.0	E980.4
Neurobarb	967.0	E851	E937.0	E950.1	E962.0	E980.1
Neuroleptics NEC	969.3	E853.8	E939.3	E950.3	E962.0	E980.3
Neuroprotective agent	977.8	E858.8	E947.8	E950.4	E962.0	E980.4
Neutral spirits	980.0	E860.1	—	E950.9	E962.1	E980.9
beverage	980.0	E860.0	—	E950.9	E962.1	E980.9
Niacin, niacinamide	972.2	E858.3	E942.2	E950.4	E962.0	E980.4
Nialamide	969.01	E854.0	E939.0	E950.3	E962.0	E980.3
Nickle (carbonyl) (compounds) (fumes) (tetracarbonyl) (vapor)	985.8	E866.4	—	E950.9	E962.1	E980.9
Niclosamide	961.6	E857	E931.6	E950.4	E962.0	E980.4
Nicomorphine	965.09	E850.2	E935.2	E950.0	E962.0	E980.0
Nicotinamide	972.2	E858.3	E942.2	E950.4	E962.0	E980.4
Nicotine (insecticide) (spray) (sulfate) NEC	989.4	E863.4	—	E950.6	E962.1	E980.7
not insecticide	989.89	E866.8	—	E950.9	E962.1	E980.9
Nicotinic acid (derivatives)	972.2	E858.3	E942.2	E950.4	E962.0	E980.4
Nicotinyl alcohol	972.2	E858.3	E942.2	E950.4	E962.0	E980.4
Nicoumalone	964.2	E858.2	E934.2	E950.4	E962.0	E980.4
Nifenazone	965.5	E850.5	E935.5	E950.0	E962.0	E980.0
Nifuraldezone	961.9	E857	E931.9	E950.4	E962.0	E980.4
Nightshade (deadly)	988.2	E865.4	—	E950.9	E962.1	E980.9
Nikethamide	970.0	E854.3	E940.0	E950.4	E962.0	E980.4
Nilstat	960.1	E856	E930.1	E950.4	E962.0	E980.4
topical	976.0	E858.7	E946.0	E950.4	E962.0	E980.4
Nimodipine	977.8	E858.8	E947.8	E950.4	E962.0	E980.4
Niridazole	961.6	E857	E931.6	E950.4	E962.0	E980.4
Nisentil	965.09	E850.2	E935.2	E950.0	E962.0	E980.0
Nitrates	972.4	E858.3	E942.4	E950.4	E962.0	E980.4
Nitrazepam	969.4	E853.2	E939.4	E950.3	E962.0	E980.3
Nitric						
acid (liquid)	983.1	E864.1	—	E950.7	E962.1	E980.6
vapor	987.8	E869.8	—	E952.8	E962.2	E982.8
oxide (gas)	987.2	E869.0	—	E952.8	E962.2	E982.8
Nitrite, amyl (medicinal) (vapor)	972.4	E858.3	E942.4	E950.4	E962.0	E980.4
Nitroaniline	983.0	E864.0	—	E950.7	E962.1	E980.6
vapor	987.8	E869.8	—	E952.8	E962.2	E982.8
Nitrobenzene, nitrobenzol	983.0	E864.0	—	E950.7	E962.1	E980.6
vapor	987.8	E869.8	—	E952.8	E962.2	E982.8
Nitrocellulose	976.3	E858.7	E946.3	E950.4	E962.0	E980.4
Nitrofuran derivatives	961.9	E857	E931.9	E950.4	E962.0	E980.4
Nitrofurantoin	961.9	E857	E931.9	E950.4	E962.0	E980.4
Nitrofurazone	976.0	E858.7	E946.0	E950.4	E962.0	E980.4
Nitrogen (dioxide) (gas) (oxide)	987.2	E869.0	—	E952.8	E962.2	E982.8
mustard (antineoplastic)	963.1	E858.1	E933.1	E950.4	E962.0	E980.4
nonmedicinal	989.89	E866.8	—	E950.9	E962.1	E980.9
fumes	987.8	E869.8	—	E952.8	E962.2	E982.8
Nitroglycerin, nitroglycerol (medicinal)	972.4	E858.3	E942.4	E950.4	E962.0	E980.4
Nitrohydrochloric acid	983.1	E864.1	—	E950.7	E962.1	E980.6
Nitromersol	976.0	E858.7	E946.0	E950.4	E962.0	E980.4
Nitronaphthalene	983.0	E864.0	—	E950.7	E962.2	E980.6
Nitrophenol	983.0	E864.0	—	E950.7	E962.2	E980.6
Nitrothiazol	961.6	E857	E931.6	E950.4	E962.0	E980.4
Nitrotoluene, nitrotoluol	983.0	E864.0	—	E950.7	E962.1	E980.6
vapor	987.8	E869.8	—	E952.8	E962.2	E982.8
Nitrous	968.2	E855.1	E938.2	E950.4	E962.0	E980.4
acid (liquid)	983.1	E864.1	—	E950.7	E962.1	E980.6
fumes	987.2	E869.0	—	E952.8	E962.2	E982.8
oxide (anesthetic) NEC	968.2	E855.1	E938.2	E950.4	E962.0	E980.4
Nitrozone	976.0	E858.7	E946.0	E950.4	E962.0	E980.4
Noctec	967.1	E852.0	E937.1	E950.2	E962.0	E980.2
Noludar	967.5	E852.4	E937.5	E950.2	E962.0	E980.2
Noptil	967.0	E851	E937.0	E950.1	E962.0	E980.1
Noradrenalin	971.2	E855.5	E941.2	E950.4	E962.0	E980.4
Noramidopyrine	965.5	E850.5	E935.5	E950.0	E962.0	E980.0
Norepinephrine	971.2	E855.5	E941.2	E950.4	E962.0	E980.4
Norethandrolone	962.1	E858.0	E932.1	E950.4	E962.0	E980.4
Norethindrone	962.2	E858.0	E932.2	E950.4	E962.0	E980.4
Norethisterone	962.2	E858.0	E932.2	E950.4	E962.0	E980.4
Norethynodrel	962.2	E858.0	E932.2	E950.4	E962.0	E980.4
Norlestrin	962.2	E858.0	E932.2	E950.4	E962.0	E980.4
Norlutin	962.2	E858.0	E932.2	E950.4	E962.0	E980.4
Normison — see Benzodiazepines						
Normorphine	965.09	E850.2	E935.2	E950.0	E962.0	E980.0
Nortriptyline	969.05	E854.0	E939.0	E950.3	E962.0	E980.3
Noscapine	975.4	E858.6	E945.4	E950.4	E962.0	E980.4
Nose preparations	976.6	E858.7	E946.6	E950.4	E962.0	E980.4
Novobiocin	960.8	E856	E930.8	E950.4	E962.0	E980.4
Novocain (infiltration) (topical)	968.5	E855.2	E938.5	E950.4	E962.0	E980.4
nerve block (peripheral) (plexus)	968.6	E855.2	E938.6	E950.4	E962.0	E980.4
spinal	968.7	E855.2	E938.7	E950.4	E962.0	E980.4
Noxythiolin	961.9	E857	E931.9	E950.4	E962.0	E980.4
NPH Iletin (insulin)	962.3	E858.0	E932.3	E950.4	E962.0	E980.4
Numorphan	965.09	E850.2	E935.2	E950.0	E962.0	E980.0
Nunol	967.0	E851	E937.0	E950.1	E962.0	E980.1
Nupercaine (spinal anesthetic)	968.7	E855.2	E938.7	E950.4	E962.0	E980.4
topical (surface)	968.5	E855.2	E938.5	E950.4	E962.0	E980.4
Nutmeg oil (liniment)	976.3	E858.7	E946.3	E950.4	E962.0	E980.4
Nux vomica	989.1	E863.7	—	E950.6	E962.1	E980.7
Nydrazid	961.8	E857	E931.8	E950.4	E962.0	E980.4
Nylidrin	971.2	E855.5	E941.2	E950.4	E962.0	E980.4
Nystatin	960.1	E856	E930.1	E950.4	E962.0	E980.4
topical	976.0	E858.7	E946.0	E950.4	E962.0	E980.4
Nytol	963.0	E858.1	E933.0	E950.4	E962.0	E980.4
Oblivion	967.8	E852.8	E937.8	E950.2	E962.0	E980.2
Octyl nitrite	972.4	E858.3	E942.4	E950.4	E962.0	E980.4
Oestradiol (cypionate) (dipropionate) (valerate)	962.2	E858.0	E932.2	E950.4	E962.0	E980.4
Oestriol	962.2	E858.0	E932.2	E950.4	E962.0	E980.4
Oestrone	962.2	E858.0	E932.2	E950.4	E962.0	E980.4
Oil (of) NEC	989.89	E866.8	—	E950.9	E962.1	E980.9
bitter almond	989.0	E866.8	—	E950.9	E962.1	E980.9
camphor	976.1	E858.7	E946.1	E950.4	E962.0	E980.4
colors	989.89	E861.6	—	E950.9	E962.1	E980.9
fumes	987.8	E869.8	—	E952.8	E962.2	E982.8
lubricating	981	E862.2	—	E950.9	E962.1	E980.9
specified source, other — see substance specified						
vitriol (liquid)	983.1	E864.1	—	E950.7	E962.1	E980.6
fumes	987.8	E869.8	—	E952.8	E962.2	E982.8
wintergreen (bitter) NEC	976.3	E858.7	E946.3	E950.4	E962.0	E980.4
Ointments NEC	976.9	E858.7	E946.9	E950.4	E962.0	E980.4
Oleander	988.2	E865.4	—	E950.9	E962.1	E980.9
Oleandomycin	960.3	E856	E930.3	E950.4	E962.0	E980.4
Oleovitamin A	963.5	E858.1	E933.5	E950.4	E962.0	E980.4
Oleum ricini	973.1	E858.4	E943.1	E950.4	E962.0	E980.4
Olive oil (medicinal) NEC	973.2	E858.4	E943.2	E950.4	E962.0	E980.4
OMPA	989.3	E863.1	—	E950.6	E962.1	E980.7
Oncovin	963.1	E858.1	E933.1	E950.4	E962.0	E980.4
Ophthaine	968.5	E855.2	E938.5	E950.4	E962.0	E980.4
Ophthetic	968.5	E855.2	E938.5	E950.4	E962.0	E980.4
Opiates, opioids, opium NEC	965.00	E850.2	E935.2	E950.0	E962.0	E980.0
antagonists	970.1	E854.3	E940.1	E950.4	E962.0	E980.4
Oracon	962.2	E858.0	E932.2	E950.4	E962.0	E980.4
Oragrafin	977.8	E858.8	E947.8	E950.4	E962.0	E980.4

Nontherapeutic use substance

▽ Subterms under main terms may continue to next column or page

	Poisoning	External Cause (E-Code)				
		Accident	Therapeutic Use	Suicide Attempt	Assault	Undetermined
Oral contraceptives	962.2	E858.0	E932.2	E950.4	E962.0	E980.4
Orciprenaline	975.1	E858.6	E945.1	E950.4	E962.0	E980.4
Organidin	975.5	E858.6	E945.5	E950.4	E962.0	E980.4
Organophosphates	989.3	E863.1	—	E950.6	E962.1	E980.7
Orimune	979.5	E858.8	E949.5	E950.4	E962.0	E980.4
Orinase	962.3	E858.0	E932.3	E950.4	E962.0	E980.4
Orphenadrine	966.4	E855.0	E936.4	E950.4	E962.0	E980.4
Ortal (sodium)	967.0	E851	E937.0	E950.1	E962.0	E980.1
Ortho-Novum	962.2	E858.0	E932.2	E950.4	E962.0	E980.4
Orthoboric acid	976.0	E858.7	E946.0	E950.4	E962.0	E980.4
ENT agent	976.6	E858.7	E946.6	E950.4	E962.0	E980.4
ophthalmic preparation	976.5	E858.7	E946.5	E950.4	E962.0	E980.4
Orthocaine	968.5	E855.2	E938.5	E950.4	E962.0	E980.4
Orthotolidine (reagent)	977.8	E858.8	E947.8	E950.4	E962.0	E980.4
Osmic acid (liquid)	983.1	E864.1	—	E950.7	E962.1	E980.6
fumes	987.8	E869.8	—	E952.8	E962.2	E982.8
Osmotic diuretics	974.4	E858.5	E944.4	E950.4	E962.0	E980.4
Ouabain	972.1	E858.3	E942.1	E950.4	E962.0	E980.4
Ovarian hormones (synthetic substitutes)	962.2	E858.0	E932.2	E950.4	E962.0	E980.4
Ovral	962.2	E858.0	E932.2	E950.4	E962.0	E980.4
Ovulation suppressants	962.2	E858.0	E932.2	E950.4	E962.0	E980.4
Ovulen	962.2	E858.0	E932.2	E950.4	E962.0	E980.4
Oxacillin (sodium)	960.0	E856	E930.0	E950.4	E962.0	E980.4
Oxalic acid	983.1	E864.1	—	E950.7	E962.1	E980.6
Oxanamide	969.5	E853.8	E939.5	E950.3	E962.0	E980.3
Oxandrolone	962.1	E858.0	E932.1	E950.4	E962.0	E980.4
Oxaprozin	965.61	E850.6	E935.6	E950.0	E962.0	E980.0
Oxazepam	969.4	E853.2	E939.4	E950.3	E962.0	E980.3
Oxazolidine derivatives	966.0	E855.0	E936.0	E950.4	E962.0	E980.4
Ox bile extract	973.4	E858.4	E943.4	E950.4	E962.0	E980.4
Oxedrine	971.2	E855.5	E941.2	E950.4	E962.0	E980.4
Oxeladin	975.4	E858.6	E945.4	E950.4	E962.0	E980.4
Oxethazaine NEC	968.5	E855.2	E938.5	E950.4	E962.0	E980.4
Oxidizing agents NEC	983.9	E864.3	—	E950.7	E962.1	E980.6
Oxolinic acid	961.3	E857	E931.3	E950.4	E962.0	E980.4
Oxophenarsine	961.1	E857	E931.1	E950.4	E962.0	E980.4
Oxsoralen	976.3	E858.7	E946.3	E950.4	E962.0	E980.4
Oxtriphylline	975.7	E858.6	E945.7	E950.4	E962.0	E980.4
Oxybuprocaine	968.5	E855.2	E938.5	E950.4	E962.0	E980.4
Oxybutynin	975.1	E858.6	E945.1	E950.4	E962.0	E980.4
Oxycodone	965.09	E850.2	E935.2	E950.0	E962.0	E980.0
Oxygen	987.8	E869.8	—	E952.8	E962.2	E982.8
Oxylone	976.0	E858.7	E946.0	E950.4	E962.0	E980.4
ophthalmic preparation	976.5	E858.7	E946.5	E950.4	E962.0	E980.4
Oxymesterone	962.1	E858.0	E932.1	E950.4	E962.0	E980.4
Oxymetazoline	971.2	E855.5	E941.2	E950.4	E962.0	E980.4
Oxymetholone	962.1	E858.0	E932.1	E950.4	E962.0	E980.4
Oxymorphone	965.09	E850.2	E935.2	E950.0	E962.0	E980.0
Oxypertine	969.09	E854.0	E939.0	E950.3	E962.0	E980.3
Oxyphenbutazone	965.5	E850.5	E935.5	E950.0	E962.0	E980.0
Oxyphencyclimine	971.1	E855.4	E941.1	E950.4	E962.0	E980.4
Oxyphenisatin	973.1	E858.4	E943.1	E950.4	E962.0	E980.4
Oxyphenonium	971.1	E855.4	E941.1	E950.4	E962.0	E980.4
Oxyquinoline	961.3	E857	E931.3	E950.4	E962.0	E980.4
Oxytetracycline	960.4	E856	E930.4	E950.4	E962.0	E980.4
Oxytocics	975.0	E858.6	E945.0	E950.4	E962.0	E980.4
Oxytocin	975.0	E858.6	E945.0	E950.4	E962.0	E980.4
Ozone	987.8	E869.8	—	E952.8	E962.2	E982.8
PABA	976.3	E858.7	E946.3	E950.4	E962.0	E980.4
Packed red cells	964.7	E858.2	E934.7	E950.4	E962.0	E980.4
Paint NEC	989.89	E861.6	—	E950.9	E962.1	E980.9
cleaner	982.8	E862.9	—	E950.9	E962.1	E980.9
fumes NEC	987.8	E869.8	—	E952.8	E962.1	E982.8
lead (fumes)	984.0	E861.5	—	E950.9	E962.1	E980.9
solvent NEC	982.8	E862.9	—	E950.9	E962.1	E980.9
stripper	982.8	E862.9	—	E950.9	E962.1	E980.9
Palfium	965.09	E850.2	E935.2	E950.0	E962.0	E980.0
Palivizumab	979.9	E858.8	E949.6	E950.4	E962.0	E980.4
Paludrine	961.4	E857	E931.4	E950.4	E962.0	E980.4
PAM	977.2	E855.8	E947.2	E950.4	E962.0	E980.4
Pamaquine (naphthoate)	961.4	E857	E931.4	E950.4	E962.0	E980.4
Pamprin	965.1	E850.3	E935.3	E950.0	E962.0	E980.0
Panadol	965.4	E850.4	E935.4	E950.0	E962.0	E980.0
Pancreatic dornase (mucolytic)	963.4	E858.1	E933.4	E950.4	E962.0	E980.4
Pancreatin	973.4	E858.4	E943.4	E950.4	E962.0	E980.4
Pancrelipase	973.4	E858.4	E943.4	E950.4	E962.0	E980.4
Pangamic acid	963.5	E858.1	E933.5	E950.4	E962.0	E980.4
Panthenol	963.5	E858.1	E933.5	E950.4	E962.0	E980.4
topical	976.8	E858.7	E946.8	E950.4	E962.0	E980.4
Pantopaque	977.8	E858.8	E947.8	E950.4	E962.0	E980.4
Pantopon	965.00	E850.2	E935.2	E950.0	E962.0	E980.4
Pantothenic acid	963.5	E858.1	E933.5	E950.4	E962.0	E980.4
Panwarfin	964.2	E858.2	E934.2	E950.4	E962.0	E980.4
Papain	973.4	E858.4	E943.4	E950.4	E962.0	E980.4
Papaverine	972.5	E858.3	E942.5	E950.4	E962.0	E980.4
Para-aminobenzoic acid	976.3	E858.7	E946.3	E950.4	E962.0	E980.4
Para-aminophenol derivatives	965.4	E850.4	E935.4	E950.0	E962.0	E980.0
Para-aminosalicylic acid (derivatives)	961.8	E857	E931.8	E950.4	E962.0	E980.4
Paracetaldehyde (medicinal)	967.2	E852.1	E937.2	E950.2	E962.0	E980.2
Paracetamol	965.4	E850.4	E935.4	E950.0	E962.0	E980.0
Paracodin	965.09	E850.2	E935.2	E950.0	E962.0	E980.0
Paradione	966.0	E855.0	E936.0	E950.4	E962.0	E980.4
Paraffin(s) (wax)	981	E862.3	—	E950.9	E962.1	E980.9
liquid (medicinal)	973.2	E858.4	E943.2	E950.4	E962.0	E980.4
nonmedicinal (oil)	981	E962.1	—	E950.9	—	E980.9
Paraldehyde (medicinal)	967.2	E852.1	E937.2	E950.2	E962.0	E980.2
Paramethadione	966.0	E855.0	E936.0	E950.4	E962.0	E980.4
Paramethasone	962.0	E858.0	E932.0	E950.4	E962.0	E980.4
Paraquat	989.4	E863.5	—	E950.6	E962.1	E980.7
Parasympatholytics	971.1	E855.4	E941.1	E950.4	E962.0	E980.4
Parasympathomimetics	971.0	E855.3	E941.0	E950.4	E962.0	E980.4
Parathion	989.3	E863.1	—	E950.6	E962.1	E980.7
Parathormone	962.6	E858.0	E932.6	E950.4	E962.0	E980.4
Parathyroid (derivatives)	962.6	E858.0	E932.6	E950.4	E962.0	E980.4
Paratyphoid vaccine	978.1	E858.8	E948.1	E950.4	E962.0	E980.4
Paredrine	971.2	E855.5	E941.2	E950.4	E962.0	E980.4
Paregoric	965.00	E850.2	E935.2	E950.0	E962.0	E980.0
Pargyline	972.3	E858.3	E942.3	E950.4	E962.0	E980.4
Paris green	985.1	E866.3	—	E950.8	E962.1	E980.8
insecticide	985.1	E863.4	—	E950.8	E962.1	E980.8
Parnate	969.01	E854.0	E939.0	E950.3	E962.0	E980.3
Paromomycin	960.8	E856	E930.8	E950.4	E962.0	E980.4
Paroxypropione	963.1	E858.1	E933.1	E950.4	E962.0	E980.4
Parzone	965.09	E850.2	E935.2	E950.0	E962.0	E980.0
PAS	961.8	E857	E931.8	E950.4	E962.0	E980.4
PCBs	981	E862.3	—	E950.9	E962.1	E980.9
PCP (pentachlorophenol)	989.4	E863.6	—	E950.6	E962.1	E980.7
herbicide	989.4	E863.5	—	E950.6	E962.1	E980.7
insecticide	989.4	E863.4	—	E950.6	E962.1	E980.7
phencyclidine	968.3	E855.1	E938.3	E950.4	E962.0	E980.4
Peach kernel oil (emulsion)	973.2	E858.4	E943.2	E950.4	E962.0	E980.4
Peanut oil (emulsion) NEC	973.2	E858.4	E943.2	E950.4	E962.0	E980.4
topical	976.3	E858.7	E946.3	E950.4	E962.0	E980.4
Pearly Gates (morning glory seeds)	969.6	E854.1	E939.6	E950.3	E962.0	E980.3
Pecazine	969.1	E853.0	E939.1	E950.3	E962.0	E980.3
Pecilocin	960.1	E856	E930.1	E950.4	E962.0	E980.4
Pectin (with kaolin) NEC	973.5	E858.4	E943.5	E950.4	E962.0	E980.4
Pelletierine tannate	961.6	E857	E931.6	E950.4	E962.0	E980.4
Pemoline	969.79	E854.2	E939.7	E950.3	E962.0	E980.3
Pempidine	972.3	E858.3	E942.3	E950.4	E962.0	E980.4
Penamecillin	960.0	E856	E930.0	E950.4	E962.0	E980.4
Penethamate hydriodide	960.0	E856	E930.0	E950.4	E962.0	E980.4
Penicillamine	963.8	E858.1	E933.8	E950.4	E962.0	E980.4
Penicillin (any type)	960.0	E856	E930.0	E950.4	E962.0	E980.4
Penicillinase	963.4	E858.1	E933.4	E950.4	E962.0	E980.4
Pentachlorophenol (fungicide)	989.4	E863.6	—	E950.6	E962.1	E980.7
herbicide	989.4	E863.5	—	E950.6	E962.1	E980.7
insecticide	989.4	E863.4	—	E950.6	E962.1	E980.7
Pentaerythritol	972.4	E858.3	E942.4	E950.4	E962.0	E980.4
chloral	967.1	E852.0	E937.1	E950.2	E962.0	E980.2
tetranitrate NEC	972.4	E858.3	E942.4	E950.4	E962.0	E980.4
Pentagastrin	977.8	E858.8	E947.8	E950.4	E962.0	E980.4
Pentalin	982.3	E862.4	—	E950.9	E962.1	E980.9
Pentamethonium (bromide)	972.3	E858.3	E942.3	E950.4	E962.0	E980.4
Pentamidine	961.5	E857	E931.5	E950.4	E962.0	E980.4
Pentanol	980.8	E860.8	—	E950.9	E962.1	E980.9
Pentaquine	961.4	E857	E931.4	E950.4	E962.0	E980.4
Pentazocine	965.8	E850.8	E935.8	E950.0	E962.0	E980.0
Penthienate	971.1	E855.4	E941.1	E950.4	E962.0	E980.4
Pentobarbital, pentobarbitone (sodium)	967.0	E851	E937.0	E950.1	E962.0	E980.1
Pentolinium (tartrate)	972.3	E858.3	E942.3	E950.4	E962.0	E980.4
Penthotal	968.3	E855.1	E938.3	E950.4	E962.0	E980.4
Pentylenetetrazol	970.0	E854.3	E940.0	E950.4	E962.0	E980.4

	External Cause (E-Code)					
	Poisoning	Accident	Therapeutic Use	Suicide Attempt	Assault	Undetermined
Pentylsalicylamide	961.8	E857	E931.8	E950.4	E962.0	E980.4
Pepsin	973.4	E858.4	E943.4	E950.4	E962.0	E980.4
Peptavlon	977.8	E858.8	E947.8	E950.4	E962.0	E980.4
Percaine (spinal)	968.7	E855.2	E938.7	E950.4	E962.0	E980.4
topical (surface)	968.5	E855.2	E938.5	E950.4	E962.0	E980.4
Perchloroethylene (vapor)	982.3	E862.4	—	E950.9	E962.1	E980.9
medicinal	961.6	E857	E931.6	E950.4	E962.0	E980.4
Percodan	965.09	E850.2	E935.2	E950.0	E962.0	E980.0
Percogesic	965.09	E850.2	E935.2	E950.0	E962.0	E980.0
Percorten	962.0	E858.0	E932.0	E950.4	E962.0	E980.4
Pergonal	962.4	E858.0	E932.4	E950.4	E962.0	E980.4
Perhexiline	972.4	E858.3	E942.4	E950.4	E962.0	E980.4
Periactin	963.0	E858.1	E933.0	E950.4	E962.0	E980.4
Periclor	967.1	E852.0	E937.1	E950.2	E962.0	E980.2
Pericyazine	969.1	E853.0	E939.1	E950.3	E962.0	E980.3
Peritrate	972.4	E858.3	E942.4	E950.4	E962.0	E980.4
Permanganates NEC	983.9	E864.3	—	E950.7	E962.1	E980.6
potassium (topical)	976.0	E858.7	E946.0	E950.4	E962.0	E980.4
Pernocton	967.0	E851	E937.0	E950.1	E962.0	E980.1
Pernoston	967.0	E851	E937.0	E950.1	E962.0	E980.1
Peronin(e)	965.09	E850.2	E935.2	E950.0	E962.0	E980.0
Perphenazine	969.1	E853.0	E939.1	E950.3	E962.0	E980.3
Pertofrane	969.05	E854.0	E939.0	E950.3	E962.0	E980.3
Pertussis						
immune serum (human)	964.6	E858.2	E934.6	E950.4	E962.0	E980.4
vaccine (with diphtheria toxoid) (with tetanus toxoid)	978.6	E858.8	E948.6	E950.4	E962.0	E980.4
Peruvian balsam	976.8	E858.7	E946.8	E950.4	E962.0	E980.4
Pesticides (dust) (fumes) (vapor)	989.4	E863.4	—	E950.6	E962.1	E980.7
arsenic	985.1	E863.4	—	E950.8	E962.1	E980.8
chlorinated	989.2	E863.0	—	E950.6	E962.1	E980.7
cyanide	989.0	E863.4	—	E950.6	E962.1	E980.7
kerosene	981	E863.4	—	E950.6	E962.1	E980.7
mixture (of compounds)	989.4	E863.3	—	E950.6	E962.1	E980.7
naphthalene	983.0	E863.4	—	E950.7	E962.1	E980.6
organochlorine (compounds)	989.2	E863.0	—	E950.6	E962.1	E980.7
petroleum (distillate) (products) NEC	981	E863.4	—	E950.6	E962.1	E980.7
specified ingredient NEC	989.4	E863.4	—	E950.6	E962.1	E980.7
strychnine	989.1	E863.4	—	E950.6	E962.1	E980.7
thallium	985.8	E863.7	—	E950.6	E962.1	E980.7
Pethidine (hydrochloride)	965.09	E850.2	E935.2	E950.0	E962.0	E980.0
Petrichloral	967.1	E852.0	E937.1	E950.2	E962.0	E980.2
Petrol	981	E862.1	—	E950.9	E962.1	E980.9
vapor	987.1	E869.8	—	E952.8	E962.2	E982.8
Petrolatum (jelly) (ointment)	976.3	E858.7	E946.3	E950.4	E962.0	E980.4
hydrophilic	976.3	E858.7	E946.3	E950.4	E962.0	E980.4
liquid	973.2	E858.4	E943.2	E950.4	E962.0	E980.4
topical	976.3	E858.7	E946.3	E950.4	E962.0	E980.4
nonmedicinal	981	E862.1	—	E950.9	E962.1	E980.9
Petroleum (cleaners) (fuels) (products) NEC	981	E862.1	—	E950.9	E962.1	E980.9
benzin(e) — see Ligroin						
ether — see Ligroin						
jelly — see Petrolatum						
naphtha — see Ligroin						
pesticide	981	E863.4	—	E950.6	E962.1	E980.7
solids	981	E862.3	—	E950.9	E962.1	E980.9
solvents	981	E862.0	—	E950.9	E962.1	E980.9
vapor	987.1	E869.8	—	E952.8	E962.2	E982.8
Peyote	969.6	E854.1	E939.6	E950.3	E962.0	E980.3
Phanodorm, phanodorn	967.0	E851	E937.0	E950.1	E962.0	E980.1
Phanquinone, phanquone	961.5	E857	E931.5	E950.4	E962.0	E980.4
Pharmaceutical excipient or adjunct	977.4	E858.8	E947.4	E950.4	E962.0	E980.4
Phenacemide	966.3	E855.0	E936.3	E950.4	E962.0	E980.4
Phenacetin	965.4	E850.4	E935.4	E950.0	E962.0	E980.0
Phenadoxone	965.09	E850.2	E935.2	E950.0	E962.0	E980.0
Phenaglycodol	969.5	E853.8	E939.5	E950.3	E962.0	E980.3
Phenantoin	966.1	E855.0	E936.1	E950.4	E962.0	E980.4
Phenaphthazine reagent	977.8	E858.8	E947.8	E950.4	E962.0	E980.4
Phenazocine	965.09	E850.2	E935.2	E950.0	E962.0	E980.0
Phenazone	965.5	E850.5	E935.5	E950.0	E962.0	E980.0
Phenazopyridine	976.1	E858.7	E946.1	E950.4	E962.0	E980.4
Phenbenicillin	960.0	E856	E930.0	E950.4	E962.0	E980.4
Phenbutrazate	977.0	E858.8	E947.0	E950.4	E962.0	E980.4
Phencyclidine	968.3	E855.1	E938.3	E950.4	E962.0	E980.4
Phendimetrazine	977.0	E858.8	E947.0	E950.4	E962.0	E980.4
Phenelzine	969.01	E854.0	E939.0	E950.3	E962.0	E980.3
Phenergan	967.8	E852.8	E937.8	E950.2	E962.0	E980.2
Phenethicillin (potassium)	960.0	E856	E930.0	E950.4	E962.0	E980.4
Phenetsal	965.1	E850.3	E935.3	E950.0	E962.0	E980.0
Pheneturide	966.3	E855.0	E936.3	E950.4	E962.0	E980.4
Phenformin	962.3	E858.0	E932.3	E950.4	E962.0	E980.4
Phenglutarimide	971.1	E855.4	E941.1	E950.4	E962.0	E980.4
Phenicarbazide	965.8	E850.8	E935.8	E950.0	E962.0	E980.0
Phenindamine (tartrate)	963.0	E858.1	E933.0	E950.4	E962.0	E980.4
Phenindione	964.2	E858.2	E934.2	E950.4	E962.0	E980.4
Pheniprazine	969.01	E854.0	E939.0	E950.3	E962.0	E980.3
Pheniramine (maleate)	963.0	E858.1	E933.0	E950.4	E962.0	E980.4
Phenmetrazine	977.0	E858.8	E947.0	E950.4	E962.0	E980.4
Phenobal	967.0	E851	E937.0	E950.1	E962.0	E980.1
Phenobarbital	967.0	E851	E937.0	E950.1	E962.0	E980.1
Phenobarbitone	967.0	E851	E937.0	E950.1	E962.0	E980.1
Phenoctide	976.0	E858.7	E946.0	E950.4	E962.0	E980.4
Phenolphthalein	973.1	E858.4	E943.1	E950.4	E962.0	E980.4
Phenolsulfonphthalein	977.8	E858.8	E947.8	E950.4	E962.0	E980.4
Phenol (derivatives) NEC	983.0	E864.0	—	E950.7	E962.1	E980.6
disinfectant	983.0	E864.0	—	E950.7	E962.1	E980.6
pesticide	989.4	E863.4	—	E950.6	E962.1	E980.7
red	977.8	E858.8	E947.8	E950.4	E962.0	E980.4
Phenomorphan	965.09	E850.2	E935.2	E950.0	E962.0	E980.0
Phenonyl	967.0	E851	E937.0	E950.1	E962.0	E980.1
Phenoperidine	965.09	E850.2	E935.2	E950.0	E962.0	E980.0
Phenoquin	974.7	E858.5	E944.7	E950.4	E962.0	E980.4
Phenothiazines (tranquilizers) NEC	969.1	E853.0	E939.1	E950.3	E962.0	E980.3
insecticide	989.3	E863.4	—	E950.6	E962.1	E980.7
Phenoxybenzamine	971.3	E855.6	E941.3	E950.4	E962.0	E980.4
Phenoxymethyl penicillin	960.0	E856	E930.0	E950.4	E962.0	E980.4
Phenprocoumon	964.2	E858.2	E934.2	E950.4	E962.0	E980.4
Phensuximide	966.2	E855.0	E936.2	E950.4	E962.0	E980.4
Phentermine	977.0	E858.8	E947.0	E950.4	E962.0	E980.4
Phentolamine	971.3	E855.6	E941.3	E950.4	E962.0	E980.4
Phenyl						
butazone	965.5	E850.5	E935.5	E950.0	E962.0	E980.0
enediamine	983.0	E864.0	—	E950.7	E962.1	E980.6
hydrazine	983.0	E864.0	—	E950.7	E962.1	E980.6
antineoplastic	963.1	E858.1	E933.1	E950.4	E962.0	E980.4
mercuric compounds — see Mercury						
salicylate	976.3	E858.7	E946.3	E950.4	E962.0	E980.4
Phenylephrine	971.2	E855.5	E941.2	E950.4	E962.0	E980.4
Phenylethylbiguanide	962.3	E858.0	E932.3	E950.4	E962.0	E980.4
Phenylpropanolamine	971.2	E855.5	E941.2	E950.4	E962.0	E980.4
Phenylsulfthion	989.3	E863.1	—	E950.6	E962.1	E980.7
Phenyramidol, phenyramidon	965.7	E850.7	E935.7	E950.0	E962.0	E980.0
Phenytoin	966.1	E855.0	E936.1	E950.4	E962.0	E980.4
pHisoHex	976.2	E858.7	E946.2	E950.4	E962.0	E980.4
Pholcodine	965.09	E850.2	E935.2	E950.0	E962.0	E980.0
Phorate	989.3	E863.1	—	E950.6	E962.1	E980.7
Phosdrin	989.3	E863.1	—	E950.6	E962.1	E980.7
Phosgene (gas)	987.8	E869.8	—	E952.8	E962.2	E982.8
Phosphate (tricresyl)	989.89	E866.8	—	E950.9	E962.1	E980.9
organic	989.3	E863.1	—	E950.6	E962.1	E980.7
solvent	982.8	E862.4	—	E950.9	E926.1	E980.9
Phosphine	987.8	E869.8	—	E952.8	E962.2	E982.8
fumigant	987.8	E863.8	—	E950.6	E962.1	E980.7
Phospholine	971.0	E855.3	E941.0	E950.4	E962.0	E980.4
Phosphoric acid	983.1	E864.1	—	E950.7	E962.1	E980.6
Phosphorus (compounds) NEC	983.9	E864.3	—	E950.7	E962.1	E980.6
rodenticide	983.9	E863.7	—	E950.7	E962.1	E980.6
Phthalimidoglutarimide	967.8	E852.8	E937.8	E950.2	E962.0	E980.2
Phthalylsulfathiazole	961.0	E857	E931.0	E950.4	E962.0	E980.4
Phylloquinone	964.3	E858.2	E934.3	E950.4	E962.0	E980.4
Physeptone	965.02	E850.1	E935.1	E950.0	E962.0	E980.0
Physostigma venenosum	988.2	E865.4	—	E950.9	E962.1	E980.9
Physostigmine	971.0	E855.3	E941.0	E950.4	E962.0	E980.4
Phytolacca decandra	988.2	E865.4	—	E950.9	E962.1	E980.9
Phytomenadione	964.3	E858.2	E934.3	E950.4	E962.0	E980.4
Phytonadione	964.3	E858.2	E934.3	E950.4	E962.0	E980.4
Picric (acid)	983.0	E864.0	—	E950.7	E962.1	E980.6
Picrotoxin	970.0	E854.3	E940.0	E950.4	E962.0	E980.4

Nontherapeutic use substance

▽ Subterms under main terms may continue to next column or page

	Poisoning	Accident	Therapeutic Use	Suicide Attempt	Assault	Undeter-mined
Pilocarpine	971.0	E855.3	E941.0	E950.4	E962.0	E980.4
Pilocarpus (jaborandi) extract	971.0	E855.3	E941.0	E950.4	E962.0	E980.4
Pimaricin	960.1	E856	E930.1	E950.4	E962.0	E980.4
Piminodine	965.09	E850.2	E935.2	E950.0	E962.0	E980.0
Pine oil, pinesol (disinfectant)	983.9	E861.4	—	E950.7	E962.1	E980.6
Pinkroot	961.6	E857	E931.6	E950.4	E962.0	E980.4
Pipadone	965.09	E850.2	E935.2	E950.0	E962.0	E980.0
Pipamazine	963.0	E858.1	E933.0	E950.4	E962.0	E980.4
Pipazethate	975.4	E858.6	E945.4	E950.4	E962.0	E980.4
Pipenzolate	971.1	E855.4	E941.1	E950.4	E962.0	E980.4
Piperacetazine	969.1	E853.0	E939.1	E950.3	E962.0	E980.3
Piperazine NEC	961.6	E857	E931.6	E950.4	E962.0	E980.4
estrone sulfate	962.2	E858.0	E932.2	E950.4	E962.0	E980.4
Piper cubeba	988.2	E865.4	—	E950.9	E962.1	E980.9
Piperidione	975.4	E858.6	E945.4	E950.4	E962.0	E980.4
Piperidolate	971.1	E855.4	E941.1	E950.4	E962.0	E980.4
Piperocaine	968.9	E855.2	E938.9	E950.4	E962.0	E980.4
infiltration (subcutaneous)	968.5	E855.2	E938.5	E950.4	E962.0	E980.4
nerve block (peripheral) (plexus)	968.6	E855.2	E938.6	E950.4	E962.0	E980.4
topical (surface)	968.5	E855.2	E938.5	E950.4	E962.0	E980.4
Pipobroman	963.1	E858.1	E933.1	E950.4	E962.0	E980.4
Pipradrol	970.89	E854.3	E940.8	E950.4	E962.0	E980.4
Piscidia (bark) (erythrina)	965.7	E850.7	E935.7	E950.0	E962.0	E980.0
Pitch	983.0	E864.0	—	E950.7	E962.1	E980.6
Pitkin's solution	968.7	E855.2	E938.7	E950.4	E962.0	E980.4
Pitocin	975.0	E858.6	E945.0	E950.4	E962.0	E980.4
Pitressin (tannate)	962.5	E858.0	E932.5	E950.4	E962.0	E980.4
Pituitary extracts (posterior)	962.5	E858.0	E932.5	E950.4	E962.0	E980.4
anterior	962.4	E858.0	E932.4	E950.4	E962.0	E980.4
Pituitrin	962.5	E858.0	E932.5	E950.4	E962.0	E980.4
Placental extract	962.9	E858.0	E932.9	E950.4	E962.0	E980.4
Placidyl	967.8	E852.8	E937.8	E950.2	E962.0	E980.2
Plague vaccine	978.3	E858.8	E948.3	E950.4	E962.0	E980.4
Plant foods or fertilizers NEC	989.89	E866.5	—	E950.9	E962.1	E980.9
mixed with herbicides	989.4	E863.5	—	E950.6	E962.1	E980.7
Plants, noxious, used as food	988.2	E865.9	—	E950.9	E962.1	E980.9
berries and seeds	988.2	E865.3	—	E950.9	E962.1	E980.9
specified type NEC	988.2	E865.4	—	E950.9	E962.1	E980.9
Plasma (blood)	964.7	E858.2	E934.7	E950.4	E962.0	E980.4
expanders	964.8	E858.2	E934.8	E950.4	E962.0	E980.4
Plasmanate	964.7	E858.2	E934.7	E950.4	E962.0	E980.4
Plegicil	969.1	E853.0	E939.1	E950.3	E962.0	E980.3
Podophyllin	976.4	E858.7	E946.4	E950.4	E962.0	E980.4
Podophyllum resin	976.4	E858.7	E946.4	E950.4	E962.0	E980.4
Poisonous berries	988.2	E865.3	—	E950.9	E962.1	E980.9
Poison NEC	989.9	E866.9	—	E950.9	E962.1	E980.9
Pokeweed (any part)	988.2	E865.4	—	E950.9	E962.1	E980.9
Poldine	971.1	E855.4	E941.1	E950.4	E962.0	E980.4
Poliomyelitis vaccine	979.5	E858.8	E949.5	E950.4	E962.0	E980.4
Poliovirus vaccine	979.5	E858.8	E949.5	E950.4	E962.0	E980.4
Polish (car) (floor) (furniture) (metal) (silver)	989.89	E861.2	—	E950.9	E962.1	E980.9
abrasive	989.89	E861.3	—	E950.9	E962.1	E980.9
porcelain	989.89	E861.3	—	E950.9	E962.1	E980.9
Poloxalkol	973.2	E858.4	E943.2	E950.4	E962.0	E980.4
Polyaminostyrene resins	974.5	E858.5	E944.5	E950.4	E962.0	E980.4
Polychlorinated biphenyl — see PCBs						
Polycycline	960.4	E856	E930.4	E950.4	E962.0	E980.4
Polyester resin hardener	982.8	E862.4	—	E950.9	E962.1	E980.9
fumes	987.8	E869.8	—	E952.8	E962.2	E982.8
Polyestradiol (phosphate)	962.2	E858.0	E932.2	E950.4	E962.0	E980.4
Polyethanolamine alkyl sulfate	976.2	E858.7	E946.2	E950.4	E962.0	E980.4
Polyethylene glycol	976.3	E858.7	E946.3	E950.4	E962.0	E980.4
Polyferose	964.0	E858.2	E934.0	E950.4	E962.0	E980.4
Polymyxin B	960.8	E856	E930.8	E950.4	E962.0	E980.4
ENT agent	976.6	E858.7	E946.6	E950.4	E962.0	E980.4
ophthalmic preparation	976.5	E858.7	E946.5	E950.4	E962.0	E980.4
topical NEC	976.0	E858.7	E946.0	E950.4	E962.0	E980.4
Polynoxylin(e)	976.0	E858.7	E946.0	E950.4	E962.0	E980.4
Polyoxymethyleneurea	976.0	E858.7	E946.0	E950.4	E962.0	E980.4
Polytetrafluoroethylene (inhaled)	987.8	E869.8	—	E952.8	E962.2	E982.8

	Poisoning	Accident	Therapeutic Use	Suicide Attempt	Assault	Undeter-mined
Polythiazide	974.3	E858.5	E944.3	E950.4	E962.0	E980.4
Polyvinylpyrrolidone	964.8	E858.2	E934.8	E950.4	E962.0	E980.4
Pontocaine (hydrochloride) (infiltration) (topical)	968.5	E855.2	E938.5	E950.4	E962.0	E980.4
nerve block (peripheral) (plexus)	968.6	E855.2	E938.6	E950.4	E962.0	E980.4
spinal	968.7	E855.2	E938.7	E950.4	E962.0	E980.4
Pot	969.6	E854.1	E939.6	E950.3	E962.0	E980.3
Potash (caustic)	983.2	E864.2	—	E950.7	E962.1	E980.6
Potassic saline injection (lactated)	974.5	E858.5	E944.5	E950.4	E962.0	E980.4
Potassium (salts) NEC	974.5	E858.5	E944.5	E950.4	E962.0	E980.4
aminosalicylate	961.8	E857	E931.8	E950.4	E962.0	E980.4
arsenite (solution)	985.1	E866.3	—	E950.8	E962.1	E980.8
bichromate	983.9	E864.3	—	E950.7	E962.1	E980.6
bisulfate	983.9	E864.3	—	E950.7	E962.1	E980.6
bromide (medicinal) NEC	967.3	E852.2	E937.3	E950.2	E962.0	E980.2
carbonate	983.2	E864.2	—	E950.7	E962.1	E980.6
chlorate NEC	983.9	E864.3	—	E950.7	E962.1	E980.6
cyanide — see Cyanide						
hydroxide	983.2	E864.2	—	E950.7	E962.1	E980.6
iodide (expectorant) NEC	975.5	E858.6	E945.5	E950.4	E962.0	E980.4
nitrate	989.89	E866.8	—	E950.9	E962.1	E980.9
oxalate	983.9	E864.3	—	E950.7	E962.1	E980.6
perchlorate NEC	977.8	E858.8	E947.8	E950.4	E962.0	E980.4
antithyroid	962.8	E858.0	E932.8	E950.4	E962.0	E980.4
permanganate	976.0	E858.7	E946.0	E950.4	E962.0	E980.4
nonmedicinal	983.9	E864.3	—	E950.7	E962.1	E980.6
Povidone-iodine (anti-infective) NEC	976.0	E858.7	E946.0	E950.4	E962.0	E980.4
Practolol	972.0	E858.3	E942.0	E950.4	E962.0	E980.4
Pralidoxime (chloride)	977.2	E858.8	E947.2	E950.4	E962.0	E980.4
Pramoxine	968.5	E855.2	E938.5	E950.4	E962.0	E980.4
Prazosin	972.6	E858.3	E942.6	E950.4	E962.0	E980.4
Prednisolone	962.0	E858.0	E932.0	E950.4	E962.0	E980.4
ENT agent	976.6	E858.7	E946.6	E950.4	E962.0	E980.4
ophthalmic preparation	976.5	E858.7	E946.5	E950.4	E962.0	E980.4
topical NEC	976.0	E858.7	E946.0	E950.4	E962.0	E980.4
Prednisone	962.0	E858.0	E932.0	E950.4	E962.0	E980.4
Pregnanediol	962.2	E858.0	E932.2	E950.4	E962.0	E980.4
Pregneninolone	962.2	E858.0	E932.2	E950.4	E962.0	E980.4
Preludin	977.0	E858.8	E947.0	E950.4	E962.0	E980.4
Premarin	962.2	E858.0	E932.2	E950.4	E962.0	E980.4
Prenylamine	972.4	E858.3	E942.4	E950.4	E962.0	E980.4
Preparation H	976.8	E858.7	E946.8	E950.4	E962.0	E980.4
Preservatives	989.89	E866.8	—	E950.9	E962.1	E980.9
Pride of China	988.2	E865.3	—	E950.9	E962.1	E980.9
Prilocaine	968.9	E855.2	E938.9	E950.4	E962.0	E980.4
infiltration (subcutaneous)	968.5	E855.2	E938.5	E950.4	E962.0	E980.4
nerve block (peripheral) (plexus)	968.6	E855.2	E938.6	E950.4	E962.0	E980.4
Primaquine	961.4	E857	E931.4	E950.4	E962.0	E980.4
Primidone	966.3	E855.0	E936.3	E950.4	E962.0	E980.4
Primula (veris)	988.2	E865.4	—	E950.9	E962.1	E980.9
Prinadol	965.09	E850.2	E935.2	E950.0	E962.0	E980.0
Priscol, Priscoline	971.3	E855.6	E941.3	E950.4	E962.0	E980.4
Privet	988.2	E865.4	—	E950.9	E962.1	E980.9
Privine	971.2	E855.5	E941.2	E950.4	E962.0	E980.4
Pro-Banthine	971.1	E855.4	E941.1	E950.4	E962.0	E980.4
Probarbital	967.0	E851	E937.0	E950.1	E962.0	E980.1
Probenecid	974.7	E858.5	E944.7	E950.4	E962.0	E980.4
Procainamide (hydrochloride)	972.0	E858.3	E942.0	E950.4	E962.0	E980.4
Procaine (hydrochloride) (infiltration) (topical)	968.5	E855.2	E938.5	E950.4	E962.0	E980.4
nerve block (peripheral) (plexus)	968.6	E855.2	E938.6	E950.4	E962.0	E980.4
penicillin G	960.0	E856	E930.0	E950.4	E962.0	E980.4
spinal	968.7	E855.2	E938.7	E950.4	E962.0	E980.4
Procalmidol	969.5	E853.8	E939.5	E950.3	E962.0	E980.3
Procarbazine	963.1	E858.1	E933.1	E950.4	E962.0	E980.4
Prochlorperazine	969.1	E853.0	E939.1	E950.3	E962.0	E980.3
Procyclidine	966.4	E855.0	E936.4	E950.4	E962.0	E980.4
Producer gas	986	E868.8	—	E952.1	E962.2	E982.1
Profenamine	966.4	E855.0	E936.4	E950.4	E962.0	E980.4
Profenil	975.1	E858.6	E945.1	E950.4	E962.0	E980.4
Progesterones	962.2	E858.0	E932.2	E950.4	E962.0	E980.4
Progestin	962.2	E858.0	E932.2	E950.4	E962.0	E980.4
Progestogens (with estrogens)	962.2	E858.0	E932.2	E950.4	E962.0	E980.4
Progesterone	962.2	E858.0	E932.2	E950.4	E962.0	E980.4

▽ **Subterms under main terms may continue to next column or page**

	Poisoning	Accident	Therapeutic Use	Suicide Attempt	Assault	Undeter-mined
Proguanil	961.4	E857	E931.4	E950.4	E962.0	E980.4
Prolactin	962.4	E858.0	E932.4	E950.4	E962.0	E980.4
Proloid	962.7	E858.0	E932.7	E950.4	E962.0	E980.4
Proluton	962.2	E858.0	E932.2	E950.4	E962.0	E980.4
Promacetin	961.8	E857	E931.8	E950.4	E962.0	E980.4
Promazine	969.1	E853.0	E939.1	E950.3	E962.0	E980.3
Promedol	965.09	E850.2	E935.2	E950.0	E962.0	E980.0
Promethazine	967.8	E852.8	E937.8	E950.2	E962.0	E980.2
Promin	961.8	E857	E931.8	E950.4	E962.0	E980.4
Pronestyl (hydrochloride)	972.0	E858.3	E942.0	E950.4	E962.0	E980.4
Pronetalol, pronethalol	972.0	E858.3	E942.0	E950.4	E962.0	E980.4
Prontosil	961.0	E857	E931.0	E950.4	E962.0	E980.4
Propamidine isethionate	961.5	E857	E931.5	E950.4	E962.0	E980.4
Propanal (medicinal)	967.8	E852.8	E937.8	E950.2	E962.0	E980.2
Propane (gas) (distributed in mobile container)	987.0	E868.0	—	E951.1	E962.2	E981.1
distributed through pipes	987.0	E867	—	E951.0	E962.2	E981.0
incomplete combustion of — see Carbon monoxide, Propane						
Propanidid	968.3	E855.1	E938.3	E950.4	E962.0	E980.4
Propanol	980.3	E860.4	—	E950.9	E962.1	E980.9
Propantheline	971.1	E855.4	E941.1	E950.4	E962.0	E980.4
Proparacaine	968.5	E855.2	E938.5	E950.4	E962.0	E980.4
Propatyl nitrate	972.4	E858.3	E942.4	E950.4	E962.0	E980.4
Propicillin	960.0	E856	E930.0	E950.4	E962.0	E980.4
Propiolactone (vapor)	987.8	E869.8	—	E952.8	E962.2	E982.8
Propiomazine	967.8	E852.8	E937.8	E950.2	E962.0	E980.2
Propionaldehyde (medicinal)	967.8	E852.8	E937.8	E950.2	E962.0	E980.2
Propionate compound	976.0	E858.7	E946.0	E950.4	E962.0	E980.4
Propion gel	976.0	E858.7	E946.0	E950.4	E962.0	E980.4
Propitocaine	968.9	E855.2	E938.9	E950.4	E962.0	E980.4
infiltration (subcutaneous)	968.5	E855.2	E938.5	E950.4	E962.0	E980.4
nerve block (peripheral) (plexus)	968.6	E855.2	E938.6	E950.4	E962.0	E980.4
Propoxur	989.3	E863.2	—	E950.6	E962.1	E980.7
Propoxycaine	968.9	E855.2	E938.9	E950.4	E962.0	E980.4
infiltration (subcutaneous)	968.5	E855.2	E938.5	E950.4	E962.0	E980.4
nerve block (peripheral) (plexus)	968.6	E855.2	E938.6	E950.4	E962.0	E980.4
topical (surface)	968.5	E855.2	E938.5	E950.4	E962.0	E980.4
Propoxyphene (hydrochloride)	965.8	E850.8	E935.8	E950.0	E962.0	E980.0
Propranolol	972.0	E858.3	E942.0	E950.4	E962.0	E980.4
Propyl						
alcohol	980.3	E860.4	—	E950.9	E962.1	E980.9
carbinol	980.3	E860.4	—	E950.9	E962.1	E980.9
hexadrine	971.2	E855.5	E941.2	E950.4	E962.0	E980.4
iodone	977.8	E858.8	E947.8	E950.4	E962.0	E980.4
thiouracil	962.8	E858.0	E932.8	E950.4	E962.0	E980.4
Propylene	987.1	E869.8	—	E952.8	E962.2	E982.8
Propylparaben (ophthalmic)	976.5	E858.7	E946.5	E950.4	E962.0	E980.4
Proscillaridin	972.1	E858.3	E942.1	E950.4	E962.0	E980.4
Prostaglandins	975.0	E858.6	E945.0	E950.4	E962.0	E980.4
Prostigmin	971.0	E855.3	E941.0	E950.4	E962.0	E980.4
Protamine (sulfate)	964.5	E858.2	E934.5	E950.4	E962.0	E980.4
zinc insulin	962.3	E858.0	E932.3	E950.4	E962.0	E980.4
Protectants (topical)	976.3	E858.7	E946.3	E950.4	E962.0	E980.4
Protein hydrolysate	974.5	E858.5	E944.5	E950.4	E962.0	E980.4
Prothiaden — *see* Dothiepin hydrochloride						
Prothionamide	961.8	E857	E931.8	E950.4	E962.0	E980.4
Prothipendyl	969.5	E853.8	E939.5	E950.3	E962.0	E980.3
Protokylol	971.2	E855.5	E941.2	E950.4	E962.0	E980.4
Protopam	977.2	E858.8	E947.2	E950.4	E962.0	E980.4
Protoveratrine(s) (A) (B)	972.6	E858.3	E942.6	E950.4	E962.0	E980.4
Protriptyline	969.05	E854.0	E939.0	E950.3	E962.0	E980.3
Provera	962.2	E858.0	E932.2	E950.4	E962.0	E980.4
Provitamin A	963.5	E858.1	E933.5	E950.4	E962.0	E980.4
Proxymetacaine	968.5	E855.2	E938.5	E950.4	E962.0	E980.4
Proxyphylline	975.1	E858.6	E945.1	E950.4	E962.0	E980.4
Prozac — *see* Fluoxetine hydrochloride						
Prunus						
laurocerasus	988.2	E865.4	—	E950.9	E962.1	E980.9
virginiana	988.2	E865.4	—	E950.9	E962.1	E980.9
Prussic acid	989.0	E866.8	—	E950.9	E962.1	E980.9

	Poisoning	Accident	Therapeutic Use	Suicide Attempt	Assault	Undeter-mined
Prussic acid — *continued*						
vapor	987.7	E869.8	—	E952.8	E962.2	E982.8
Pseudoephedrine	971.2	E855.5	E941.2	E950.4	E962.0	E980.4
Psilocin	969.6	E854.1	E939.6	E950.3	E962.0	E980.3
Psilocybin	969.6	E854.1	E939.6	E950.3	E962.0	E980.3
PSP	977.8	E858.8	E947.8	E950.4	E962.0	E980.4
Psychedelic agents	969.6	E854.1	E939.6	E950.3	E962.0	E980.3
Psychodysleptics	969.6	E854.1	E939.6	E950.3	E962.0	E980.3
Psychostimulants	969.70	E854.2	E939.7	E950.3	E962.0	E980.3
Psychotherapeutic agents	969.9	E855.9	E939.9	E950.3	E962.0	E980.3
antidepressants	969.00	E854.0	E939.0	E950.3	E962.0	E980.3
specified NEC	969.8	E855.8	E939.8	E950.3	E962.0	E980.3
tranquilizers NEC	969.5	E853.9	E939.5	E950.3	E962.0	E980.3
Psychotomimetic agents	969.6	E854.1	E939.6	E950.3	E962.0	E980.3
Psychotropic agents	969.9	E854.8	E939.9	E950.3	E962.0	E980.3
specified NEC	969.8	E854.8	E939.8	E950.3	E962.0	E980.3
Psyllium	973.3	E858.4	E943.3	E950.4	E962.0	E980.4
Pteroylglutamic acid	964.1	E858.2	E934.1	E950.4	E962.0	E980.4
Pteroyltriglutamate	963.1	E858.1	E933.1	E950.4	E962.0	E980.4
PTFE	987.8	E869.8	—	E952.8	E962.2	E982.8
Pulsatilla	988.2	E865.4	—	E950.9	E962.1	E980.9
Purex (bleach)	983.9	E864.3	—	E950.7	E962.1	E980.6
Purine diuretics	974.1	E858.5	E944.1	E950.4	E962.0	E980.4
Purinethol	963.1	E858.1	E933.1	E950.4	E962.0	E980.4
PVP	964.8	E858.2	E934.8	E950.4	E962.0	E980.4
Pyrabital	965.7	E850.7	E935.7	E950.0	E962.0	E980.0
Pyramidon	965.5	E850.5	E935.5	E950.0	E962.0	E980.0
Pyrantel (pamoate)	961.6	E857	E931.6	E950.4	E962.0	E980.4
Pyrathiazine	963.0	E858.1	E933.0	E950.4	E962.0	E980.4
Pyrazinamide	961.8	E857	E931.8	E950.4	E962.0	E980.4
Pyrazinoic acid (amide)	961.8	E857	E931.8	E950.4	E962.0	E980.4
Pyrazole (derivatives)	965.5	E850.5	E935.5	E950.0	E962.0	E980.0
Pyrazolone (analgesics)	965.5	E850.5	E935.5	E950.0	E962.0	E980.0
Pyrethrins, pyrethrum	989.4	E863.4	—	E950.6	E962.1	E980.7
Pyribenzamine	963.0	E858.1	E933.0	E950.4	E962.0	E980.4
Pyridine (liquid) (vapor)	982.0	E862.4	—	E950.9	E962.1	E980.9
aldoxime chloride	977.2	E858.8	E947.2	E950.4	E962.0	E980.4
Pyridium	976.1	E858.7	E946.1	E950.4	E962.0	E980.4
Pyridostigmine	971.0	E855.3	E941.0	E950.4	E962.0	E980.4
Pyridoxine	963.5	E858.1	E933.5	E950.4	E962.0	E980.4
Pyrilamine	963.0	E858.1	E933.0	E950.4	E962.0	E980.4
Pyrimethamine	961.4	E857	E931.4	E950.4	E962.0	E980.4
Pyrogallic acid	983.0	E864.0	—	E950.7	E962.1	E980.6
Pyroxylin	976.3	E858.7	E946.3	E950.4	E962.0	E980.4
Pyrrobutamine	963.0	E858.1	E933.0	E950.4	E962.0	E980.4
Pyrrocitine	968.5	E855.2	E938.5	E950.4	E962.0	E980.4
Pyrvinium (pamoate)	961.6	E857	E931.6	E950.4	E962.0	E980.4
PZI	962.3	E858.0	E932.3	E950.4	E962.0	E980.4
Quaalude	967.4	E852.3	E937.4	E950.2	E962.0	E980.2
Quaternary ammonium derivatives	971.1	E855.4	E941.1	E950.4	E962.0	E980.4
Quicklime	983.2	E864.2	—	E950.7	E962.1	E980.6
Quinacrine	961.3	E857	E931.3	E950.4	E962.0	E980.4
Quinaglute	972.0	E858.3	E942.0	E950.4	E962.0	E980.4
Quinalbarbitone	967.0	E851	E937.0	E950.1	E962.0	E980.1
Quinestradiol	962.2	E858.0	E932.2	E950.4	E962.0	E980.4
Quinethazone	974.3	E858.5	E944.3	E950.4	E962.0	E980.4
Quinidine (gluconate) (polygalacturonate) (salts) (sulfate)	972.0	E858.3	E942.0	E950.4	E962.0	E980.4
Quinine	961.4	E857	E931.4	E950.4	E962.0	E980.4
Quiniobine	961.3	E857	E931.3	E950.4	E962.0	E980.4
Quinolines	961.3	E857	E931.3	E950.4	E962.0	E980.4
Quotane	968.5	E855.2	E938.5	E950.4	E962.0	E980.4
Rabies						
immune globulin (human)	964.6	E858.2	E934.6	E950.4	E962.0	E980.4
vaccine	979.1	E858.8	E949.1	E950.4	E962.0	E980.4
Racemoramide	965.09	E850.2	E935.2	E950.0	E962.0	E980.0
Racemorphan	965.09	E850.2	E935.2	E950.0	E962.0	E980.0
Radiator alcohol	980.1	E860.2	—	E950.9	E962.1	E980.9
Radio-opaque (drugs) (materials)	977.8	E858.8	E947.8	E950.4	E962.0	E980.4
Ranunculus	988.2	E865.4	—	E950.9	E962.1	E980.9
Rat poison	989.4	E863.7	—	E950.6	E962.1	E980.7
Rattlesnake (venom)	989.5	E905.0	—	E950.9	E962.1	E980.9
Raudixin	972.6	E858.3	E942.6	E950.4	E962.0	E980.4
Rautensin	972.6	E858.3	E942.6	E950.4	E962.0	E980.4
Rautina	972.6	E858.3	E942.6	E950.4	E962.0	E980.4
Rautotal	972.6	E858.3	E942.6	E950.4	E962.0	E980.4
Rauwiloid	972.6	E858.3	E942.6	E950.4	E962.0	E980.4

Nontherapeutic use substance

▽ Subterms under main terms may continue to next column or page

	Poisoning	Accident	Therapeutic Use	Suicide Attempt	Assault	Undetermined
			External Cause (E-Code)			
Rauwoldin	972.6	E858.3	E942.6	E950.4	E962.0	E980.4
Rauwolfia (alkaloids)	972.6	E858.3	E942.6	E950.4	E962.0	E980.4
Realgar	985.1	E866.3	—	E950.8	E962.1	E980.8
Red cells, packed	964.7	E858.2	E934.7	E950.4	E962.0	E980.4
Reducing agents, industrial NEC	983.9	E864.3	—	E950.7	E962.1	E980.6
Refrigerant gas (freon)	987.4	E869.2	—	E952.8	E962.2	E982.8
central nervous system	968.0	E855.1	E938.0	E950.4	E962.0	E980.4
not freon	987.9	E869.9	—	E952.9	E962.2	E982.9
Regroton	974.4	E858.5	E944.4	E950.4	E962.0	E980.4
Rela	968.0	E855.1	E938.0	E950.4	E962.0	E980.4
Relaxants, skeletal muscle (autonomic)	975.2	E858.6	E945.2	E950.4	E962.0	E980.4
Renese	974.3	E858.5	E944.3	E950.4	E962.0	E980.4
Renografin	977.8	E858.8	E947.8	E950.4	E962.0	E980.4
Replacement solutions	974.5	E858.5	E944.5	E950.4	E962.0	E980.4
Rescinnamine	972.6	E858.3	E942.6	E950.4	E962.0	E980.4
Reserpine	972.6	E858.3	E942.6	E950.4	E962.0	E980.4
Resorcin, resorcinol	976.4	E858.7	E946.4	E950.4	E962.0	E980.4
Respaire	975.5	E858.6	E945.5	E950.4	E962.0	E980.4
Respiratory agents NEC	975.8	E858.6	E945.8	E950.4	E962.0	E980.4
Retinoic acid	976.8	E858.7	E946.8	E950.4	E962.0	E980.4
Retinol	963.5	E858.1	E933.5	E950.4	E962.0	E980.4
Rh (D) immune globulin (human)	964.6	E858.2	E934.6	E950.4	E962.0	E980.4
Rhodine	965.1	E850.3	E935.3	E950.0	E962.0	E980.0
RhoGAM	964.6	E858.2	E934.6	E950.4	E962.0	E980.4
Riboflavin	963.5	E858.1	E933.5	E950.4	E962.0	E980.4
Ricin	989.89	E866.8	—	E950.9	E962.1	E980.9
Ricinus communis	988.2	E865.3	—	E950.9	E962.1	E980.9
Rickettsial vaccine NEC	979.6	E858.8	E949.6	E950.4	E962.0	E980.4
with viral and bacterial vaccine	979.7	E858.8	E949.7	E950.4	E962.0	E980.4
Rifampin	960.6	E856	E930.6	E950.4	E962.0	E980.4
Rimifon	961.8	E857	E931.8	E950.4	E962.0	E980.4
Ringer's injection (lactated)	974.5	E858.5	E944.5	E950.4	E962.0	E980.4
Ristocetin	960.8	E856	E930.8	E950.4	E962.0	E980.4
Ritalin	969.73	E854.2	E939.7	E950.3	E962.0	E980.3
Roach killers — see Pesticides						
Rocky Mountain spotted fever vaccine	979.6	E858.8	E949.6	E950.4	E962.0	E980.4
Rodenticides	989.4	E863.7	—	E950.6	E962.1	E980.7
Rohypnol	969.4	E853.2	E939.4	E950.3	E962.0	E980.3
Rolaids	973.0	E858.4	E943.0	E950.4	E962.0	E980.4
Rolitetracycline	960.4	E856	E930.4	E950.4	E962.0	E980.4
Romilar	975.4	E858.6	E945.4	E950.4	E962.0	E980.4
Rose water ointment	976.3	E858.7	E946.3	E950.4	E962.0	E980.4
Rosuvastatin calcium	972.1	E858.3	E942.2	E950.4	E962.0	E980.4
Rotenone	989.4	E863.7	—	E950.6	E962.1	E980.7
Rotoxamine	963.0	E858.1	E933.0	E950.4	E962.0	E980.4
Rough-on-rats	989.4	E863.7	—	E950.6	E962.1	E980.7
RU486	962.9	E858.0	E932.9	E950.4	E962.0	E980.4
Rubbing alcohol	980.2	E860.3	—	E950.9	E962.1	E980.9
Rubella virus vaccine	979.4	E858.8	E949.4	E950.4	E962.0	E980.4
Rubelogen	979.4	E858.8	E949.4	E950.4	E962.0	E980.4
Rubeovax	979.4	E858.8	E949.4	E950.4	E962.0	E980.4
Rubidomycin	960.7	E856	E930.7	E950.4	E962.0	E980.4
Rue	988.2	E865.4	—	E950.9	E962.1	E980.9
Ruta	988.2	E865.4	—	E950.9	E962.1	E980.9
Sabadilla (medicinal)	976.0	E858.7	E946.0	E950.4	E962.0	E980.4
pesticide	989.4	E863.4	—	E950.6	E962.1	E980.7
Sabin oral vaccine	979.5	E858.8	E949.5	E950.4	E962.0	E980.4
Saccharated iron oxide	964.0	E858.2	E934.0	E950.4	E962.0	E980.4
Saccharin	974.5	E858.5	E944.5	E950.4	E962.0	E980.4
Safflower oil	972.2	E858.3	E942.2	E950.4	E962.0	E980.4
Salbutamol sulfate	975.7	E858.6	E945.7	E950.4	E962.0	E980.4
Salicylamide	965.1	E850.3	E935.3	E950.0	E962.0	E980.0
Salicylate(s)	965.1	E850.3	E935.3	E950.0	E962.0	E980.0
methyl	976.3	E858.7	E946.3	E950.4	E962.0	E980.4
theobromine calcium	974.1	E858.5	E944.1	E950.4	E962.0	E980.4
Salicylazosulfapyridine	961.0	E857	E931.0	E950.4	E962.0	E980.4
Salicylhydroxamic acid	976.0	E858.7	E946.0	E950.4	E962.0	E980.4
Salicylic acid (keratolytic) NEC	976.4	E858.7	E946.4	E950.4	E962.0	E980.4
congeners	965.1	E850.3	E935.3	E950.0	E962.0	E980.0
salts	965.1	E850.3	E935.3	E950.0	E962.0	E980.0
Saliniazid	961.8	E857	E931.8	E950.4	E962.0	E980.4
Salol	976.3	E858.7	E946.3	E950.4	E962.0	E980.4
Salt (substitute) NEC	974.5	E858.5	E944.5	E950.4	E962.0	E980.4
Saluretics	974.3	E858.5	E944.3	E950.4	E962.0	E980.4
Saluron	974.3	E858.5	E944.3	E950.4	E962.0	E980.4
Salvarsan 606 (neosilver) (silver)	961.1	E857	E931.1	E950.4	E962.0	E980.4
Sambucus canadensis	988.2	E865.4	—	E950.9	E962.1	E980.9
berry	988.2	E865.3	—	E950.9	E962.1	E980.9
Sandril	972.6	E858.3	E942.6	E950.4	E962.0	E980.4
Sanguinaria canadensis	988.2	E865.4	—	E950.9	E962.1	E980.9
Saniflush (cleaner)	983.9	E861.3	—	E950.7	E962.1	E980.6
Santonin	961.6	E857	E931.6	E950.4	E962.0	E980.4
Santyl	976.8	E858.7	E946.8	E950.4	E962.0	E980.4
Sarkomycin	960.7	E856	E930.7	E950.4	E962.0	E980.4
Saroten	969.05	E854.0	E939.0	E950.3	E962.0	E980.3
Saturnine — see Lead						
Savin (oil)	976.4	E858.7	E946.4	E950.4	E962.0	E980.4
Scammony	973.1	E858.4	E943.1	E950.4	E962.0	E980.4
Scarlet red	976.8	E858.7	E946.8	E950.4	E962.0	E980.4
Scheele's green	985.1	E866.3	—	E950.8	E962.1	E980.8
insecticide	985.1	E863.4	—	E950.8	E962.1	E980.8
Schradan	989.3	E863.1	—	E950.6	E962.1	E980.7
Schweinfurt(h) green	985.1	E866.3	—	E950.8	E962.1	E980.8
insecticide	985.1	E863.4	—	E950.8	E962.1	E980.8
Scilla — see Squill						
Sclerosing agents	972.7	E858.3	E942.7	E950.4	E962.0	E980.4
Scopolamine	971.1	E855.4	E941.1	E950.4	E962.0	E980.4
Scouring powder	989.89	E861.3	—	E950.9	E962.1	E980.9
Sea						
anemone (sting)	989.5	E905.6	—	E950.9	E962.1	E980.9
cucumber (sting)	989.5	E905.6	—	E950.9	E962.1	E980.9
snake (bite) (venom)	989.5	E905.0	—	E950.9	E962.1	E980.9
urchin spine (puncture)	989.5	E905.6	—	E950.9	E962.1	E980.9
Secbutabarbital	967.0	E851	E937.0	E950.1	E962.0	E980.1
Secbutabarbitone	967.0	E851	E937.0	E950.1	E962.0	E980.1
Secobarbital	967.0	E851	E937.0	E950.1	E962.0	E980.1
Seconal	967.0	E851	E937.0	E950.1	E962.0	E980.1
Secretin	977.8	E858.8	E947.8	E950.4	E962.0	E980.4
Sedatives, nonbarbiturate	967.9	E852.9	E937.9	E950.2	E962.0	E980.2
specified NEC	967.8	E852.8	E937.8	E950.2	E962.0	E980.2
Sedormid	967.8	E852.8	E937.8	E950.2	E962.0	E980.2
Seed (plant)	988.2	E865.3	—	E950.9	E962.1	E980.9
disinfectant or dressing	989.89	E866.5	—	E950.9	E962.1	E980.9
Selective serotonin and norepinephrine reuptake inhibitors (SSNRI)	969.02	E854.0	E939.0	E950.3	E962.0	E980.3
Selective serotonin reuptake inhibitors (SSRI)	969.03	E854.0	E939.0	E950.3	E962.0	E980.3
Selenium (fumes) NEC	985.8	E866.4	—	E950.9	E962.1	E980.9
disulfide or sulfide	976.4	E858.7	E946.4	E950.4	E962.0	E980.4
Selsun	976.4	E858.7	E946.4	E950.4	E962.0	E980.4
Senna	973.1	E858.4	E943.1	E950.4	E962.0	E980.4
Septisol	976.2	E858.7	E946.2	E950.4	E962.0	E980.4
Serax	969.4	E853.2	E939.4	E950.3	E962.0	E980.3
Serenesil	967.8	E852.8	E937.8	E950.2	E962.0	E980.2
Serenium (hydrochloride)	961.9	E857	E931.9	E950.4	E962.0	E980.4
Serepax — see Oxazepam						
Sernyl	968.3	E855.1	E938.3	E950.4	E962.0	E980.4
Serotonin	977.8	E858.8	E947.8	E950.4	E962.0	E980.4
Serpasil	972.6	E858.3	E942.6	E950.4	E962.0	E980.4
Sewer gas	987.8	E869.8	—	E952.8	E962.2	E982.8
Shampoo	989.6	E861.0	—	E950.9	E962.1	E980.9
Shellfish, nonbacterial or noxious	988.0	E865.1	—	E950.9	E962.1	E980.9
Silicones NEC	989.83	E866.8	E947.8	E950.9	E962.1	E980.9
Silvadene	976.0	E858.7	E946.0	E950.4	E962.0	E980.4
Silver (compound) (medicinal) NEC	976.0	E858.7	E946.0	E950.4	E962.0	E980.4
anti-infectives	976.0	E858.7	E946.0	E950.4	E962.0	E980.4
arsphenamine	961.1	E857	E931.1	E950.4	E962.0	E980.4
nitrate	976.0	E858.7	E946.0	E950.4	E962.0	E980.4
ophthalmic preparation	976.5	E858.7	E946.5	E950.4	E962.0	E980.4
toughened (keratolytic)	976.4	E858.7	E946.4	E950.4	E962.0	E980.4
nonmedicinal (dust)	985.8	E866.4	—	E950.9	E962.1	E980.9
protein (mild) (strong)	976.0	E858.7	E946.0	E950.4	E962.0	E980.4
salvarsan	961.1	E857	E931.1	E950.4	E962.0	E980.4
Simethicone	973.8	E858.4	E943.8	E950.4	E962.0	E980.4
Sinequan	969.05	E854.0	E939.0	E950.3	E962.0	E980.3
Singoserp	972.6	E858.3	E942.6	E950.4	E962.0	E980.4
Sintrom	964.2	E858.2	E934.2	E950.4	E962.0	E980.4
Sitosterols	972.2	E858.3	E942.2	E950.4	E962.0	E980.4
Skeletal muscle relaxants	975.2	E858.6	E945.2	E950.4	E962.0	E980.4
Skin						
agents (external)	976.9	E858.7	E946.9	E950.4	E962.0	E980.4

Index

Skin — Squirting cucumber

		External Cause (E-Code)			
	Poisoning	Accident	Therapeutic Use	Suicide Attempt	Assault	Undetermined

	Poisoning	Accident	Therapeutic Use	Suicide Attempt	Assault	Undetermined
Skin — *continued*						
agents — *continued*						
specified NEC	976.8	E858.7	E946.8	E950.4	E962.0	E980.4
test antigen	977.8	E858.8	E947.8	E950.4	E962.0	E980.4
Sleep-eze	963.0	E858.1	E933.0	E950.4	E962.0	E980.4
Sleeping draught (drug) (pill) (tablet)	967.9	E852.9	E937.9	E950.2	E962.0	E980.2
Smallpox vaccine	979.0	E858.8	E949.0	E950.4	E962.0	E980.4
Smelter fumes NEC	985.9	E866.4	—	E950.9	E962.1	E980.9
Smog	987.3	E869.1	—	E952.8	E962.2	E982.8
Smoke NEC	987.9	E869.9	—	E952.9	E962.2	E982.9
Smooth muscle relaxant	975.1	E858.6	E945.1	E950.4	E962.0	E980.4
Snail killer	989.4	E863.4	—	E950.6	E962.1	E980.7
Snake (bite) (venom)	989.5	E905.0	—	E950.9	E962.1	E980.9
Snuff	989.89	E866.8	—	E950.9	E962.1	E980.9
Soap (powder) (product)	989.6	E861.1	—	E950.9	E962.1	E980.9
bicarb	963.3	E858.1	E933.3	E950.4	E962.0	E980.4
chlorinated — see Sodium, hypochlorite						
medicinal, soft	976.2	E858.7	E946.2	E950.4	E962.0	E980.4
Soda (caustic)	983.2	E864.2	—	E950.7	E962.1	E980.6
Sodium						
acetosulfone	961.8	E857	E931.8	E950.4	E962.0	E980.4
acetrizoate	977.8	E858.8	E947.8	E950.4	E962.0	E980.4
amytal	967.0	E851	E937.0	E950.1	E962.0	E980.1
arsenate — see Arsenic						
bicarbonate	963.3	E858.1	E933.3	E950.4	E962.0	E980.4
bichromate	983.9	E864.3	—	E950.7	E962.1	E980.6
biphosphate	963.2	E858.1	E933.2	E950.4	E962.0	E980.4
bisulfate	983.9	E864.3	—	E950.7	E962.1	E980.6
borate (cleanser)	989.6	E861.3	—	E950.9	E962.1	E980.9
bromide NEC	967.3	E852.2	E937.3	E950.2	E962.0	E980.2
cacodylate (nonmedicinal)						
NEC	978.8	E858.8	E948.8	E950.4	E962.0	E980.4
anti-infective	961.1	E857	E931.1	E950.4	E962.0	E980.4
herbicide	989.4	E863.5	—	E950.6	E962.1	E980.7
calcium edetate	963.8	E858.1	E933.8	E950.4	E962.0	E980.4
carbonate	983.2	E864.2	—	E950.7	E962.1	E980.6
chlorate NEC	983.9	E864.3	—	E950.7	E962.1	E980.6
herbicide	983.9	E863.5	—	E950.7	E962.1	E980.6
chloride NEC	974.5	E858.5	E944.5	E950.4	E962.0	E980.4
chromate	983.9	E864.3	—	E950.7	E962.1	E980.6
citrate	963.3	E858.1	E933.3	E950.4	E962.0	E980.4
cyanide — see Cyanide(s)						
cyclamate	974.5	E858.5	E944.5	E950.4	E962.0	E980.4
diatrizoate	977.8	E858.8	E947.8	E950.4	E962.0	E980.4
dibunate	975.4	E858.6	E945.4	E950.4	E962.0	E980.4
dioctyl sulfosuccinate	973.2	E858.4	E943.2	E950.4	E962.0	E980.4
edetate	963.8	E858.1	E933.8	E950.4	E962.0	E980.4
ethacrynate	974.4	E858.5	E944.4	E950.4	E962.0	E980.4
fluoracetate (dust) (rodenticide)	989.4	E863.7	—	E950.6	E962.1	E980.7
fluoride — see Fluoride(s)						
free salt	974.5	E858.5	E944.5	E950.4	E962.0	E980.4
glucosulfone	961.8	E857	E931.8	E950.4	E962.0	E980.4
hydroxide	983.2	E864.2	—	E950.7	E962.1	E980.6
hypochlorite (bleach)						
NEC	983.9	E864.3	—	E950.7	E962.1	E980.6
disinfectant	983.9	E861.4	—	E950.7	E962.1	E980.6
medicinal (anti-infective) (external)	976.0	E858.7	E946.0	E950.4	E962.0	E980.4
vapor	987.8	E869.8	—	E952.8	E962.2	E982.8
hyposulfite	976.0	E858.7	E946.0	E950.4	E962.0	E980.4
indigotindisulfonate	977.8	E858.8	E947.8	E950.4	E962.0	E980.4
iodide	977.8	E858.8	E947.8	E950.4	E962.0	E980.4
iothalamate	977.8	E858.8	E947.8	E950.4	E962.0	E980.4
iron edetate	964.0	E858.2	E934.0	E950.4	E962.0	E980.4
L-triiodothyronine	962.7	E858.0	E932.7	E950.4	E962.0	E980.4
lactate	963.3	E858.1	E933.3	E950.4	E962.0	E980.4
lauryl sulfate	976.2	E858.7	E946.2	E950.4	E962.0	E980.4
metrizoate	977.8	E858.8	E947.8	E950.4	E962.0	E980.4
monofluoracetate (dust) (rodenticide)	989.4	E863.7	—	E950.6	E962.1	E980.7
morrhuate	972.7	E858.3	E942.7	E950.4	E962.0	E980.4
nafcillin	960.0	E856	E930.0	E950.4	E962.0	E980.4
nitrate (oxidizing agent)	983.9	E864.3	—	E950.7	E962.1	E980.6
nitrite (medicinal)	972.4	E858.3	E942.4	E950.4	E962.0	E980.4
nitroferricyanide	972.6	E858.3	E942.6	E950.4	E962.0	E980.4
nitroprusside	972.6	E858.3	E942.6	E950.4	E962.0	E980.4
para-aminohippurate	977.8	E858.8	E947.8	E950.4	E962.0	E980.4
perborate (nonmedicinal) NEC	989.89	E866.8	—	E950.9	E962.1	E980.9

		External Cause (E-Code)			
	Poisoning	Accident	Therapeutic Use	Suicide Attempt	Assault	Undetermined

	Poisoning	Accident	Therapeutic Use	Suicide Attempt	Assault	Undetermined
Sodium — *continued*						
perborate — *continued*						
medicinal	976.6	E858.7	E946.6	E950.4	E962.0	E980.4
soap	989.6	E861.1	—	E950.9	E962.1	E980.9
percarbonate — see Sodium, perborate						
phosphate	973.3	E858.4	E943.3	E950.4	E962.0	E980.4
polystyrene sulfonate	974.5	E858.5	E944.5	E950.4	E962.0	E980.4
propionate	976.0	E858.7	E946.0	E950.4	E962.0	E980.4
psylliate	972.7	E858.3	E942.7	E950.4	E962.0	E980.4
removing resins	974.5	E858.5	E944.5	E950.4	E962.0	E980.4
salicylate	965.1	E850.3	E935.3	E950.0	E962.0	E980.0
sulfate	973.3	E858.4	E943.3	E950.4	E962.0	E980.4
sulfoxone	961.8	E857	E931.8	E950.4	E962.0	E980.4
tetradecyl sulfate	972.7	E858.3	E942.7	E950.4	E962.0	E980.4
thiopental	968.3	E855.1	E938.3	E950.4	E962.0	E980.4
thiosalicylate	965.1	E850.3	E935.3	E950.0	E962.0	E980.0
thiosulfate	976.0	E858.7	E946.0	E950.4	E962.0	E980.4
tolbutamide	977.8	E858.8	E947.8	E950.4	E962.0	E980.4
tyropanoate	977.8	E858.8	E947.8	E950.4	E962.0	E980.4
valproate	966.3	E855.0	E936.3	E950.4	E962.0	E980.4
Solanine	977.8	E858.8	E947.8	E950.4	E962.0	E980.4
Solanum dulcamara	988.2	E865.4	—	E950.9	E962.1	E980.9
Solapsone	961.8	E857	E931.8	E950.4	E962.0	E980.4
Solasulfone	961.8	E857	E931.8	E950.4	E962.0	E980.4
Soldering fluid	983.1	E864.1	—	E950.7	E962.1	E980.6
Solid substance	989.9	E866.9	—	E950.9	E962.1	E980.9
specified NEC	989.9	E866.8	—	E950.9	E962.1	E980.9
Solvents, industrial	982.8	E862.9	—	E950.9	E962.1	E980.9
naphtha	981	E862.0	—	E950.9	E962.1	E980.9
petroleum	981	E862.0	—	E950.9	E962.1	E980.9
specified NEC	982.8	E862.4	—	E950.9	E962.1	E980.9
Soma	968.0	E855.1	E938.0	E950.4	E962.0	E980.4
Somatotropin	962.4	E858.0	E932.4	E950.4	E962.0	E980.4
Sominex	963.0	E858.1	E933.0	E950.4	E962.0	E980.4
Somnos	967.1	E852.0	E937.1	E950.2	E962.0	E980.2
Somonal	967.0	E851	E937.0	E950.1	E962.0	E980.1
Soneryl	967.0	E851	E937.0	E950.1	E962.0	E980.1
Soothing syrup	977.9	E858.9	E947.9	E950.5	E962.0	E980.5
Sopor	967.4	E852.3	E937.4	E950.2	E962.0	E980.2
Soporific drug	967.9	E852.9	E937.9	E950.2	E962.0	E980.2
specified type NEC	967.8	E852.8	E937.8	E950.2	E962.0	E980.2
Sorbitol NEC	977.4	E858.8	E947.4	E950.4	E962.0	E980.4
Sotradecol	972.7	E858.3	E942.7	E950.4	E962.0	E980.4
Spacoline	975.1	E858.6	E945.1	E950.4	E962.0	E980.4
Spanish fly	976.8	E858.7	E946.8	E950.4	E962.0	E980.4
Sparine	969.1	E853.0	E939.1	E950.3	E962.0	E980.3
Sparteine	975.0	E858.6	E945.0	E950.4	E962.0	E980.4
Spasmolytics	975.1	E858.6	E945.1	E950.4	E962.0	E980.4
anticholinergics	971.1	E855.4	E941.1	E950.4	E962.0	E980.4
Spectinomycin	960.8	E856	E930.8	E950.4	E962.0	E980.4
Speed	969.72	E854.2	E939.7	E950.3	E962.0	E980.3
Spermicides	976.8	E858.7	E946.8	E950.4	E962.0	E980.4
Spider (bite) (venom)	989.5	E905.1	—	E950.9	E962.1	E980.9
antivenin	979.9	E858.8	E949.9	E950.4	E962.0	E980.4
Spigelia (root)	961.6	E857	E931.6	E950.4	E962.0	E980.4
Spiperone	969.2	E853.1	E939.2	E950.3	E962.0	E980.3
Spiramycin	960.3	E856	E930.3	E950.4	E962.0	E980.4
Spirilene	969.5	E853.8	E939.5	E950.3	E962.0	E980.3
Spirit(s) (neutral) NEC	980.0	E860.1	—	E950.9	E962.1	E980.9
beverage	980.0	E860.0	—	E950.9	E962.1	E980.9
industrial	980.9	E860.9	—	E950.9	E962.1	E980.9
mineral	981	E862.0	—	E950.9	E962.1	E980.9
of salt — see Hydrochloric acid						
surgical	980.9	E860.9	—	E950.9	E962.1	E980.9
Spironolactone	974.4	E858.5	E944.4	E950.4	E962.0	E980.4
Sponge, absorbable (gelatin)	964.5	E858.2	E934.5	E950.4	E962.0	E980.4
Sporostacin	976.0	E858.7	E946.0	E950.4	E962.0	E980.4
Sprays (aerosol)	989.89	E866.8	—	E950.9	E962.1	E980.9
cosmetic	989.89	E866.7	—	E950.9	E962.1	E980.9
medicinal NEC	977.9	E858.9	E947.9	E950.5	E962.0	E980.5
pesticides — see Pesticides						
specified content — see substance specified						
Spurge flax	988.2	E865.4	—	E950.9	E962.1	E980.9
Spurges	988.2	E865.4	—	E950.9	E962.1	E980.9
Squill (expectorant) NEC	975.5	E858.6	E945.5	E950.4	E962.0	E980.4
rat poison	989.4	E863.7	—	E950.6	E962.1	E980.7
Squirting cucumber (cathartic)	973.1	E858.4	E943.1	E950.4	E962.0	E980.4

Nontherapeutic use substance

328 — Volume 2   ▶◀ Revised Text   ● New Line   ▲ Revised Code   ▽ Subterms under main terms may continue to next column or page   2014 ICD-9-CM

Substance	Poisoning	Accident	Therapeutic Use	Suicide Attempt	Assault	Undetermined
SSNRI (selective serotonin and norepinephrine reuptake inhibitors)	969.02	E854.0	E939.0	E950.3	E962.0	E980.3
SSRI (selective serotonin reuptake inhibitors)	969.03	E854.0	E939.0	E950.3	E962.0	E980.3
Stains	989.89	E866.8	—	E950.9	E962.1	E980.9
Stannous — see also Tin fluoride	976.7	E858.7	E946.7	E950.4	E962.0	E980.4
Stanolone	962.1	E858.0	E932.1	E950.4	E962.0	E980.4
Stanozolol	962.1	E858.0	E932.1	E950.4	E962.0	E980.4
Staphisagria or stavesacre (pediculicide)	976.0	E858.7	E946.0	E950.4	E962.0	E980.4
Stelazine	969.1	E853.0	E939.1	E950.3	E962.0	E980.3
Stemetil	969.1	E853.0	E939.1	E950.3	E962.0	E980.3
Sterculia (cathartic) (gum)	973.3	E858.4	E943.3	E950.4	E962.0	E980.4
Sternutator gas	987.8	E869.8	—	E952.8	E962.2	E982.8
Steroids NEC	962.0	E858.0	E932.0	E950.4	E962.0	E980.4
ENT agent	976.6	E858.7	E946.6	E950.4	E962.0	E980.4
ophthalmic preparation	976.5	E858.7	E946.5	E950.4	E962.0	E980.4
topical NEC	976.0	E858.7	E946.0	E950.4	E962.0	E980.4
Stibine	985.8	E866.4	—	E950.9	E962.1	E980.9
Stibophen	961.2	E857	E931.2	E950.4	E962.0	E980.4
Stilbamide, stilbamidine	961.5	E857	E931.5	E950.4	E962.0	E980.4
Stilbestrol	962.2	E858.0	E932.2	E950.4	E962.0	E980.4
Stimulants (central nervous system)	970.9	E854.3	E940.9	E950.4	E962.0	E980.4
analeptics	970.0	E854.3	E940.0	E950.4	E962.0	E980.4
opiate antagonist	970.1	E854.3	E940.1	E950.4	E962.0	E980.4
psychotherapeutic NEC	969.09	E854.0	E939.0	E950.3	E962.0	E980.3
specified NEC	970.89	E854.3	E940.8	E950.4	E962.0	E980.4
Storage batteries (acid) (cells)	983.1	E864.1	—	E950.7	E962.1	E980.6
Stovaine	968.9	E855.2	E938.9	E950.4	E962.0	E980.4
infiltration (subcutaneous)	968.5	E855.2	E938.5	E950.4	E962.0	E980.4
nerve block (peripheral) (plexus)	968.6	E855.2	E938.6	E950.4	E962.0	E980.4
spinal	968.7	E855.2	E938.7	E950.4	E962.0	E980.4
topical (surface)	968.5	E855.2	E938.5	E950.4	E962.0	E980.4
Stovarsal	961.1	E857	E931.1	E950.4	E962.0	E980.4
Stove gas — see Gas, utility						
Stoxil	976.5	E858.7	E946.5	E950.4	E962.0	E980.4
STP	969.6	E854.1	E939.6	E950.3	E962.0	E980.3
Stramonium (medicinal) NEC	971.1	E855.4	E941.1	E950.4	E962.0	E980.4
natural state	988.2	E865.4	—	E950.9	E962.1	E980.9
Streptodornase	964.4	E858.2	E934.4	E950.4	E962.0	E980.4
Streptoduocin	960.6	E856	E930.6	E950.4	E962.0	E980.4
Streptokinase	964.4	E858.2	E934.4	E950.4	E962.0	E980.4
Streptomycin	960.6	E856	E930.6	E950.4	E962.0	E980.4
Streptozocin	960.7	E856	E930.7	E950.4	E962.0	E980.4
Stripper (paint) (solvent)	982.8	E862.9	—	E950.9	E962.1	E980.9
Strobane	989.2	E863.0	—	E950.6	E962.1	E980.7
Strophanthin	972.1	E858.3	E942.1	E950.4	E962.0	E980.4
Strophanthus hispidus or kombe	988.2	E865.4		E950.9	E962.1	E980.9
Strychnine (rodenticide) (salts)	989.1	E863.7	—	E950.6	E962.1	E980.7
medicinal NEC	970.89	E854.3	E940.8	E950.4	E962.0	E980.4
Strychnos (ignatii) — see Strychnine						
Styramate	968.0	E855.1	E938.0	E950.4	E962.0	E980.4
Styrene	983.0	E864.0	—	E950.7	E962.1	E980.6
Succinimide (anticonvulsant)	966.2	E855.0	E936.2	E950.4	E962.0	E980.4
mercuric — see Mercury						
Succinylcholine	975.2	E858.6	E945.2	E950.4	E962.0	E980.4
Succinylsulfathiazole	961.0	E857	E931.0	E950.4	E962.0	E980.4
Sucrose	974.5	E858.5	E944.5	E950.4	E962.0	E980.4
Sulfacetamide	961.0	E857	E931.0	E950.4	E962.0	E980.4
ophthalmic preparation	976.5	E858.7	E946.5	E950.4	E962.0	E980.4
Sulfachlorpyridazine	961.0	E857	E931.0	E950.4	E962.0	E980.4
Sulfacytine	961.0	E857	E931.0	E950.4	E962.0	E980.4
Sulfadiazine	961.0	E857	E931.0	E950.4	E962.0	E980.4
silver (topical)	976.0	E858.7	E946.0	E950.4	E962.0	E980.4
Sulfadimethoxine	961.0	E857	E931.0	E950.4	E962.0	E980.4
Sulfadimidine	961.0	E857	E931.0	E950.4	E962.0	E980.4
Sulfaethidole	961.0	E857	E931.0	E950.4	E962.0	E980.4
Sulfafurazole	961.0	E857	E931.0	E950.4	E962.0	E980.4
Sulfaguanidine	961.0	E857	E931.0	E950.4	E962.0	E980.4
Sulfamerazine	961.0	E857	E931.0	E950.4	E962.0	E980.4
Sulfameter	961.0	E857	E931.0	E950.4	E962.0	E980.4

Substance	Poisoning	Accident	Therapeutic Use	Suicide Attempt	Assault	Undetermined
Sulfamethizole	961.0	E857	E931.0	E950.4	E962.0	E980.4
Sulfamethoxazole	961.0	E857	E931.0	E950.4	E962.0	E980.4
Sulfamethoxydiazine	961.0	E857	E931.0	E950.4	E962.0	E980.4
Sulfamethoxypyridazine	961.0	E857	E931.0	E950.4	E962.0	E980.4
Sulfamethylthiazole	961.0	E857	E931.0	E950.4	E962.0	E980.4
Sulfamylon	976.0	E858.7	E946.0	E950.4	E962.0	E980.4
Sulfan blue (diagnostic dye)	977.8	E858.8	E947.8	E950.4	E962.0	E980.4
Sulfanilamide	961.0	E857	E931.0	E950.4	E962.0	E980.4
Sulfanilylguanidine	961.0	E857	E931.0	E950.4	E962.0	E980.4
Sulfaphenazole	961.0	E857	E931.0	E950.4	E962.0	E980.4
Sulfaphenylthiazole	961.0	E857	E931.0	E950.4	E962.0	E980.4
Sulfaproxyline	961.0	E857	E931.0	E950.4	E962.0	E980.4
Sulfapyridine	961.0	E857	E931.0	E950.4	E962.0	E980.4
Sulfapyrimidine	961.0	E857	E931.0	E950.4	E962.0	E980.4
Sulfarsphenamine	961.1	E857	E931.1	E950.4	E962.0	E980.4
Sulfasalazine	961.0	E857	E931.0	E950.4	E962.0	E980.4
Sulfasomizole	961.0	E857	E931.0	E950.4	E962.0	E980.4
Sulfasuxidine	961.0	E857	E931.0	E950.4	E962.0	E980.4
Sulfinpyrazone	974.7	E858.5	E944.7	E950.4	E962.0	E980.4
Sulfisoxazole	961.0	E857	E931.0	E950.4	E962.0	E980.4
ophthalmic preparation	976.5	E858.7	E946.5	E950.4	E962.0	E980.4
Sulfomyxin	960.8	E856	E930.8	E950.4	E962.0	E980.4
Sulfonal	967.8	E852.8	E937.8	E950.2	E962.0	E980.2
Sulfonamides (mixtures)	961.0	E857	E931.0	E950.4	E962.0	E980.4
Sulfones	961.8	E857	E931.8	E950.4	E962.0	E980.4
Sulfonethylmethane	967.8	E852.8	E937.8	E950.2	E962.0	E980.2
Sulfonmethane	967.8	E852.8	E937.8	E950.2	E962.0	E980.2
Sulfonphthal, sulfonphthol	977.8	E858.8	E947.8	E950.4	E962.0	E980.4
Sulfonylurea derivatives, oral	962.3	E858.0	E932.3	E950.4	E962.0	E980.4
Sulfoxone	961.8	E857	E931.8	E950.4	E962.0	E980.4
Sulfur, sulfureted, sulfuric, sulfurous, sulfuryl (compounds) NEC	989.89	E866.8	—	E950.9	E962.1	E980.9
acid	983.1	E864.1	—	E950.7	E962.1	E980.6
dioxide	987.3	E869.1	—	E952.8	E962.2	E982.8
ether — see Ether(s)						
hydrogen	987.8	E869.8	—	E952.8	E962.2	E982.8
medicinal (keratolytic) (ointment) NEC	976.4	E858.7	E946.4	E950.4	E962.0	E980.4
pesticide (vapor)	989.4	E863.4	—	E950.6	E962.1	E980.7
vapor NEC	987.8	E869.8	—	E952.8	E962.2	E982.8
Sulkowitch's reagent	977.8	E858.8	E947.8	E950.4	E962.0	E980.4
Sulphadione	961.8	E857	E931.8	E950.4	E962.0	E980.4
Sulph — see also Sulf-						
Sulthiame, sultiame	966.3	E855.0	E936.3	E950.4	E962.0	E980.4
Superinone	975.5	E858.6	E945.5	E950.4	E962.0	E980.4
Suramin	961.5	E857	E931.5	E950.4	E962.0	E980.4
Surfacaine	968.5	E855.2	E938.5	E950.4	E962.0	E980.4
Surital	968.3	E855.1	E938.3	E950.4	E962.0	E980.4
Sutilains	976.8	E858.7	E946.8	E950.4	E962.0	E980.4
Suxamethonium (bromide) (chloride) (iodide)	975.2	E858.6	E945.2	E950.4	E962.0	E980.4
Suxethonium (bromide)	975.2	E858.6	E945.2	E950.4	E962.0	E980.4
Sweet oil (birch)	976.3	E858.7	E946.3	E950.4	E962.0	E980.4
Sym-dichloroethyl ether	982.3	E862.4	—	E950.9	E962.1	E980.9
Sympatholytics	971.3	E855.6	E941.3	E950.4	E962.0	E980.4
Sympathomimetics	971.2	E855.5	E941.2	E950.4	E962.0	E980.4
Synagis	979.6	E858.8	E949.6	E950.4	E962.0	E980.4
Synalar	976.0	E858.7	E946.0	E950.4	E962.0	E980.4
Synthroid	962.7	E858.0	E932.7	E950.4	E962.0	E980.4
Syntocinon	975.0	E858.6	E945.0	E950.4	E962.0	—
Syrosingopine	972.6	E858.3	E942.6	E950.4	E962.0	E980.4
Systemic agents (primarily)	963.9	E858.1	E933.9	E950.4	E962.0	E980.4
specified NEC	963.8	E858.1	E933.8	E950.4	E962.0	E980.4
Tablets — see also specified substance	977.9	E858.9	E947.9	E950.5	E962.0	E980.5
Tace	962.2	E858.0	E932.2	E950.4	E962.0	E980.4
Tacrine	971.0	E855.3	E941.0	E950.4	E962.0	E980.4
Talbutal	967.0	E851	E937.0	E950.1	E962.0	E980.1
Talc	976.3	E858.7	E946.3	E950.4	E962.0	E980.4
Talcum	976.3	E858.7	E946.3	E950.4	E962.0	E980.4
Tamsulosin	971.3	E855.6	E941.3	E950.4	E962.0	E980.4
Tandearil, tanderil	965.5	E850.5	E935.5	E950.0	E962.0	E980.0
Tannic acid	983.1	E864.1	—	E950.7	E962.1	E980.6
medicinal (astringent)	976.2	E858.7	E946.2	E950.4	E962.0	E980.4
Tannin — see Tannic acid						
Tansy	988.2	E865.4	—	E950.9	E962.1	E980.9
TAO	960.3	E856	E930.3	E950.4	E962.0	E980.4

Nontherapeutic use substance

▼ Subterms under main terms may continue to next column or page

SSNRI — TAO

	Poisoning	Accident	Therapeutic Use	Suicide Attempt	Assault	Undetermined
Tapazole	962.8	E858.0	E932.8	E962.0	E962.0	E980.4
Taractan	969.3	E853.8	E939.3	E950.3	E962.0	E980.3
Tarantula (venomous)	989.5	E905.1	—	E950.9	E962.1	E980.9
Tartar emetic (anti-infective)	961.2	E857	E931.2	E950.4	E962.0	E980.4
Tartaric acid	983.1	E864.1	—	E950.7	E962.1	E980.6
Tartrated antimony (anti-infective)	961.2	E857	E931.2	E950.4	E962.0	E980.4
Tar NEC	983.0	E864.0	—	E950.7	E962.1	E980.6
camphor — see Naphthalene						
fumes	987.8	E869.8	—	E952.8	E962.2	E982.8
TCA — see Trichloroacetic acid						
TDI	983.0	E864.0	—	E950.7	E962.1	E980.6
vapor	987.8	E869.8	—	E952.8	E962.2	E982.8
Tear gas	987.5	E869.3	—	E952.8	E962.2	E982.8
Teclothiazide	974.3	E858.5	E944.3	E950.4	E962.0	E980.4
Tegretol	966.3	E855.0	E936.3	E950.4	E962.0	E980.4
Telepaque	977.8	E858.8	E947.8	E950.4	E962.0	E980.4
Tellurium	985.8	E866.4	—	E950.9	E962.1	E980.9
fumes	985.8	E866.4	—	E950.9	E962.1	E980.9
TEM	963.1	E858.1	E933.1	E950.4	E962.0	E980.4
Temazepan — see Benzodiazepines						
TEPA	963.1	E858.1	E933.1	E950.4	E962.0	E980.4
TEPP	989.3	E863.1	—	E950.6	E962.1	E980.7
Terbutaline	971.2	E855.5	E941.2	E950.4	E962.0	E980.4
Teroxalene	961.6	E857	E931.6	E950.4	E962.0	E980.4
Terpin hydrate	975.5	E858.6	E945.5	E950.4	E962.0	E980.4
Terramycin	960.4	E856	E930.4	E950.4	E962.0	E980.4
Tessalon	975.4	E858.6	E945.4	E950.4	E962.0	E980.4
Testosterone	962.1	E858.0	E932.1	E950.4	E962.0	E980.4
Tetanus (vaccine)	978.4	E858.8	E948.4	E950.4	E962.0	E980.4
antitoxin	979.9	E858.8	E949.9	E950.4	E962.0	E980.4
immune globulin (human)	964.6	E858.2	E934.6	E950.4	E962.0	E980.4
toxoid	978.4	E858.8	E948.4	E950.4	E962.0	E980.4
with diphtheria toxoid	978.9	E858.8	E948.9	E950.4	E962.0	E980.4
with pertussis	978.6	E858.8	E948.6	E950.4	E962.0	E980.4
Tetrabenazine	969.5	E853.8	E939.5	E950.3	E962.0	E980.3
Tetracaine (infiltration) (topical)	968.5	E855.2	E938.5	E950.4	E962.0	E980.4
nerve block (peripheral) (plexus)	968.6	E855.2	E938.6	E950.4	E962.0	E980.4
spinal	968.7	E855.2	E938.7	E950.4	E962.0	E980.4
Tetrachlorethylene — see Tetrachloroethylene						
Tetrachlormethiazide	974.3	E858.5	E944.3	E950.4	E962.0	E980.4
Tetrachloroethane (liquid) (vapor)	982.3	E862.4	—	E950.9	E962.1	E980.9
paint or varnish	982.3	E861.6	—	E950.9	E962.1	E980.9
Tetrachloroethylene (liquid) (vapor)	982.3	E862.4	—	E950.9	E962.1	E980.9
medicinal	961.6	E857	E931.6	E950.4	E962.0	E980.4
Tetrachloromethane — see Carbon, tetrachloride						
Tetracycline	960.4	E856	E930.4	E950.4	E962.0	E980.4
ophthalmic preparation	976.5	E858.7	E946.5	E950.4	E962.0	E980.4
topical NEC	976.0	E858.7	E946.0	E950.4	E962.0	E980.4
Tetraethylammonium chloride	972.3	E858.3	E942.3	E950.4	E962.0	E980.4
Tetraethyl lead (antiknock compound)	984.1	E862.1	—	E950.9	E962.1	E980.9
Tetraethyl pyrophosphate	989.3	E863.1	—	E950.6	E962.1	E980.7
Tetraethylthiuram disulfide	977.3	E858.8	E947.3	E950.4	E962.0	E980.4
Tetrahydroaminoacridine	971.0	E855.3	E941.0	E950.4	E962.0	E980.4
Tetrahydrocannabinol	969.6	E854.1	E939.6	E950.3	E962.0	E980.3
Tetrahydronaphthalene	982.0	E862.4	—	E950.9	E962.1	E980.9
Tetrahydrozoline	971.2	E855.5	E941.2	E950.4	E962.0	E980.4
Tetralin	982.0	E862.4	—	E950.9	E962.1	E980.9
Tetramethylthiuram (disulfide) NEC	989.4	E863.6	—	E950.6	E962.1	E980.7
medicinal	976.2	E858.7	E946.2	E950.4	E962.0	E980.4
Tetronal	967.8	E852.8	E937.8	E950.2	E962.0	E980.2
Tetryl	983.0	E864.0	—	E950.7	E962.1	E980.6
Thalidomide	967.8	E852.8	E937.8	E950.2	E962.0	E980.2
Thallium (compounds) (dust) NEC	985.8	E866.4	—	E950.9	E962.1	E980.9
pesticide (rodenticide)	985.8	E863.7	—	E950.6	E962.1	E980.7
THC	969.6	E854.1	E939.6	E950.3	E962.0	E980.3

	Poisoning	Accident	Therapeutic Use	Suicide Attempt	Assault	Undetermined
Thebacon	965.09	E850.2	E935.2	E950.0	E962.0	E980.0
Thebaine	965.09	E850.2	E935.2	E950.0	E962.0	E980.0
Theobromine (calcium salicylate)	974.1	E858.5	E944.1	E950.4	E962.0	E980.4
Theophylline (diuretic)	974.1	E858.5	E944.1	E950.4	E962.0	E980.4
ethylenediamine	975.7	E858.6	E945.7	E950.4	E962.0	E980.4
Thiabendazole	961.6	E857	E931.6	E950.4	E962.0	E980.4
Thialbarbital, thialbarbitone	968.3	E855.1	E938.3	E950.4	E962.0	E980.4
Thiamine	963.5	E858.1	E933.5	E950.4	E962.0	E980.4
Thiamylal (sodium)	968.3	E855.1	E938.3	E950.4	E962.0	E980.4
Thiazesim	969.09	E854.0	E939.0	E950.3	E962.0	E980.3
Thiazides (diuretics)	974.3	E858.5	E944.3	E950.4	E962.0	E980.4
Thiethylperazine	963.0	E858.1	E933.0	E950.4	E962.0	E980.4
Thimerosal (topical)	976.0	E858.7	E946.0	E950.4	E962.0	E980.4
ophthalmic preparation	976.5	E858.7	E946.5	E950.4	E962.0	E980.4
Thio-TEPA, thiotepa	963.1	E858.1	E933.1	E950.4	E962.0	E980.4
Thioacetazone	961.8	E857	E931.8	E950.4	E962.0	E980.4
Thiobarbiturates	968.3	E855.1	E938.3	E950.4	E962.0	E980.4
Thiobismol	961.2	E857	E931.2	E950.4	E962.0	E980.4
Thiocarbamide	962.8	E858.0	E932.8	E950.4	E962.0	E980.4
Thiocarbarsone	961.1	E857	E931.1	E950.4	E962.0	E980.4
Thiocarlide	961.8	E857	E931.8	E950.4	E962.0	E980.4
Thioguanine	963.1	E858.1	E933.1	E950.4	E962.0	E980.4
Thiomercaptomerin	974.0	E858.5	E944.0	E950.4	E962.0	E980.4
Thiomerin	974.0	E858.5	E944.0	E950.4	E962.0	E980.4
Thiopental, thiopentone (sodium)	968.3	E855.1	E938.3	E950.4	E962.0	E980.4
Thiopropazate	969.1	E853.0	E939.1	E950.3	E962.0	E980.3
Thioproperazine	969.1	E853.0	E939.1	E950.3	E962.0	E980.3
Thioridazine	969.1	E853.0	E939.1	E950.3	E962.0	E980.3
Thiothixene	969.3	E853.8	E939.3	E950.3	E962.0	E980.3
Thiouracil	962.8	E858.0	E932.8	E950.4	E962.0	E980.4
Thiourea	962.8	E858.0	E932.8	E950.4	E962.0	E980.4
Thiphenamil	971.1	E855.4	E941.1	E950.4	E962.0	E980.4
Thiram NEC	989.4	E863.6	—	E950.6	E962.1	E980.7
medicinal	976.2	E858.7	E946.2	E950.4	E962.0	E980.4
Thonzylamine	963.0	E858.1	E933.0	E950.4	E962.0	E980.4
Thorazine	969.1	E853.0	E939.1	E950.3	E962.0	E980.3
Thornapple	988.2	E865.4	—	E950.9	E962.1	E980.9
Throat preparation (lozenges) NEC	976.6	E858.7	E946.6	E950.4	E962.0	E980.4
Thrombin	964.5	E858.2	E934.5	E950.4	E962.0	E980.4
Thrombolysin	964.4	E858.2	E934.4	E950.4	E962.0	E980.4
Thymol	983.0	E864.0	—	E950.7	E962.1	E980.6
Thymus extract	962.9	E858.0	E932.9	E950.4	E962.0	E980.4
Thyroglobulin	962.7	E858.0	E932.7	E950.4	E962.0	E980.4
Thyroid (derivatives) (extract)	962.7	E858.0	E932.7	E950.4	E962.0	E980.4
Thyrolar	962.7	E858.0	E932.7	E950.4	E962.0	E980.4
Thyrothrophin, thyrotropin	977.8	E858.8	E947.8	E950.4	E962.0	E980.4
Thyroxin(e)	962.7	E858.0	E932.7	E950.4	E962.0	E980.4
Tigan	963.0	E858.1	E933.0	E950.4	E962.0	E980.4
Tigloidine	968.0	E855.1	E938.0	E950.4	E962.0	E980.4
Tinactin	976.0	E858.7	E946.0	E950.4	E962.0	E980.4
Tincture, iodine — see Iodine						
Tindal	969.1	E853.0	E939.1	E950.3	E962.0	E980.3
Tin (chloride) (dust) (oxide) NEC	985.8	E866.4	—	E950.9	E962.1	E980.9
anti-infectives	961.2	E857	E931.2	E950.4	E962.0	E980.4
Titanium (compounds) (vapor)	985.8	E866.4	—	E950.9	E962.1	E980.9
ointment	976.3	E858.7	E946.3	E950.4	E962.0	E980.4
Titroid	962.7	E858.0	E932.7	E950.4	E962.0	E980.4
TMTD — see Tetramethylthiuram disulfide						
TNT	989.89	E866.8	—	E950.9	E962.1	E980.9
fumes	987.8	E869.8	—	E952.8	E962.2	E982.8
Toadstool	988.1	E865.5	—	E950.9	E962.1	E980.9
Tobacco NEC	989.84	E866.8	—	E950.9	E962.1	E980.9
Indian	988.2	E865.4	—	E950.9	E962.1	E980.9
smoke, second-hand	987.8	E869.4	—	—	—	—
Tocopherol	963.5	E858.1	E933.5	E950.4	E962.0	E980.4
Tocosamine	975.0	E858.6	E945.0	E950.4	E962.0	E980.4
Tofranil	969.05	E854.0	E939.0	E950.3	E962.0	E980.3
Toilet deodorizer	989.89	E866.8	—	E950.9	E962.1	E980.9
Tolazamide	962.3	E858.0	E932.3	E950.4	E962.0	E980.4
Tolazoline	971.3	E855.6	E941.3	E950.4	E962.0	E980.4
Tolbutamide	962.3	E858.0	E932.3	E950.4	E962.0	E980.4
sodium	977.8	E858.8	E947.8	E950.4	E962.0	E980.4
Tolmetin	965.69	E850.6	E935.6	E950.0	E962.0	E980.0

	Poisoning	Accident	Therapeutic Use	Suicide Attempt	Assault	Undetermined
Tolnaftate	976.0	E858.7	E946.0	E950.4	E962.0	E980.4
Tolpropamine	976.1	E858.7	E946.1	E950.4	E962.0	E980.4
Tolserol	968.0	E855.1	E938.0	E950.4	E962.0	E980.4
Toluene (liquid) (vapor)	982.0	E862.4	—	E950.9	E962.1	E980.9
diisocyanate	983.0	E864.0	—	E950.7	E962.1	E980.6
Toluidine	983.0	E864.0	—	E950.7	E962.1	E980.6
vapor	987.8	E869.8	—	E952.8	E962.2	E982.8
Toluol (liquid) (vapor)	982.0	E862.4	—	E950.9	E962.1	E980.9
Tolylene-2, 4-diiso-cyanate	983.0	E864.0	—	E950.7	E962.1	E980.6
Tonics, cardiac	972.1	E858.3	E942.1	E950.4	E962.0	E980.4
Toxaphene (dust) (spray)	989.2	E863.0	—	E950.6	E962.1	E980.7
Toxoids NEC	978.8	E858.8	E948.8	E950.4	E962.0	E980.4
Tractor fuel NEC	981	E862.1	—	E950.9	E962.1	E980.9
Tragacanth	973.3	E858.4	E943.3	E950.4	E962.0	E980.4
Tramazoline	971.2	E855.5	E941.2	E950.4	E962.0	E980.4
Tranquilizers	969.5	E853.9	E939.5	E950.3	E962.0	E980.3
benzodiazepine-based	969.4	E853.2	E939.4	E950.3	E962.0	E980.3
butyrophenone-based	969.2	E853.1	E939.2	E950.3	E962.0	E980.3
major NEC	969.3	E853.8	E939.3	E950.3	E962.0	E980.3
phenothiazine-based	969.1	E853.0	E939.1	E950.3	E962.0	E980.3
specified NEC	969.5	E853.8	E939.5	E950.3	E962.0	E980.3
Trantoin	961.9	E857	E931.9	E950.4	E962.0	E980.4
Tranxene	969.4	E853.2	E939.4	E950.3	E962.0	E980.3
Tranylcypromine (sulfate)	969.01	E854.0	E939.0	E950.3	E962.0	E980.3
Trasentine	975.1	E858.6	E945.1	E950.4	E962.0	E980.4
Travert	974.5	E858.5	E944.5	E950.4	E962.0	E980.4
Trecator	961.8	E857	E931.8	E950.4	E962.0	E980.4
Tretinoin	976.8	E858.7	E946.8	E950.4	E962.0	E980.4
Triacetin	976.0	E858.7	E946.0	E950.4	E962.0	E980.4
Triacetyloleandomycin	960.3	E856	E930.3	E950.4	E962.0	E980.4
Triamcinolone	962.0	E858.0	E932.0	E950.4	E962.0	E980.4
ENT agent	976.6	E858.7	E946.6	E950.4	E962.0	E980.4
medicinal (keratolytic)	976.4	E858.7	E946.4	E950.4	E962.0	E980.4
ophthalmic preparation	976.5	E858.7	E946.5	E950.4	E962.0	E980.4
topical NEC	976.0	E858.7	E946.0	E950.4	E962.0	E980.4
Triamterene	974.4	E858.5	E944.4	E950.4	E962.0	E980.4
Triaziquone	963.1	E858.1	E933.1	E950.4	E962.0	E980.4
Tribromacetaldehyde	967.3	E852.2	E937.3	E950.2	E962.0	E980.2
Tribromoethanol	968.2	E855.1	E938.2	E950.4	E962.0	E980.4
Tribromomethane	967.3	E852.2	E937.3	E950.2	E962.0	E980.2
Trichlorethane	982.3	E862.4	—	E950.9	E962.1	E980.9
Trichlormethiazide	974.3	E858.5	E944.3	E950.4	E962.0	E980.4
Trichloroacetic acid	983.1	E864.1	—	E950.7	E962.1	E980.6
Trichloroethanol	967.1	E852.0	E937.1	E950.2	E962.0	E980.2
Trichloroethylene (liquid) (vapor)	982.3	E862.4	—	E950.9	E962.1	E980.9
anesthetic (gas)	968.2	E855.1	E938.2	E950.4	E962.0	E980.4
Trichloroethyl phosphate	967.1	E852.0	E937.1	E950.2	E962.0	E980.2
Trichlorofluoromethane NEC	987.4	E869.2	—	E952.8	E962.2	E982.8
Trichlorotriethylamine	963.1	E858.1	E933.1	E950.4	E962.0	E980.4
Trichomonacides NEC	961.5	E857	E931.5	E950.4	E962.0	E980.4
Trichomycin	960.1	E856	E930.1	E950.4	E962.0	E980.4
Triclofos	967.1	E852.0	E937.1	E950.2	E962.0	E980.2
Tricresyl phosphate	989.89	E866.8	—	E950.9	E962.1	E980.9
solvent	982.8	E862.4	—	E950.9	E962.1	E980.9
Tricyclamol	966.4	E855.0	E936.4	E950.4	E962.0	E980.4
Tridesilon	976.0	E858.7	E946.0	E950.4	E962.0	E980.4
Tridihexethyl	971.1	E855.4	E941.1	E950.4	E962.0	E980.4
Tridione	966.0	E855.0	E936.0	E950.4	E962.0	E980.4
Triethanolamine NEC	983.2	E864.2	—	E950.7	E962.1	E980.6
detergent	983.2	E861.0	—	E950.7	E962.1	E980.6
trinitrate	972.4	E858.3	E942.4	E950.4	E962.0	E980.4
Triethanomelamine	963.1	E858.1	E933.1	E950.4	E962.0	E980.4
Triethylene melamine	963.1	E858.1	E933.1	E950.4	E962.0	E980.4
Triethylenephosphoramide	963.1	E858.1	E933.1	E950.4	E962.0	E980.4
Triethylenethiophosphoramide	963.1	E858.1	E933.1	E950.4	E962.0	E980.4
Trifluoperazine	969.1	E853.0	E939.1	E950.3	E962.0	E980.3
Trifluperidol	969.2	E853.1	E939.2	E950.3	E962.0	E980.3
Triflupromazine	969.1	E853.0	E939.1	E950.3	E962.0	E980.3
Trihexyphenidyl	971.1	E855.4	E941.1	E950.4	E962.0	E980.4
Triiodothyronine	962.7	E858.0	E932.7	E950.4	E962.0	E980.4
Trilene	968.2	E855.1	E938.2	E950.4	E962.0	E980.4
Trimeprazine	963.0	E858.1	E933.0	E950.4	E962.0	E980.4
Trimetazidine	972.4	E858.3	E942.4	E950.4	E962.0	E980.4
Trimethadione	966.0	E855.0	E936.0	E950.4	E962.0	E980.4
Trimethaphan	972.3	E858.3	E942.3	E950.4	E962.0	E980.4
Trimethidinium	972.3	E858.3	E942.3	E950.4	E962.0	E980.4
Trimethobenzamide	963.0	E858.1	E933.0	E950.4	E962.0	E980.4
Trimethylcarbinol	980.8	E860.8	—	E950.9	E962.1	E980.9
Trimethylpsoralen	976.3	E858.7	E946.3	E950.4	E962.0	E980.4
Trimeton	963.0	E858.1	E933.0	E950.4	E962.0	E980.4
Trimipramine	969.05	E854.0	E939.0	E950.3	E962.0	E980.3
Trimustine	963.1	E858.1	E933.1	E950.4	E962.0	E980.4
Trinitrin	972.4	E858.3	E942.4	E950.4	E962.0	E980.4
Trinitrophenol	983.0	E864.0	—	E950.7	E962.1	E980.6
Trinitrotoluene	989.89	E866.8	—	E950.9	E962.1	E980.9
fumes	987.8	E869.8	—	E952.8	E962.2	E982.8
Trional	967.8	E852.8	E937.8	E950.2	E962.0	E980.2
Trioxide of arsenic — see Arsenic						
Trioxsalen	976.3	E858.7	E946.3	E950.4	E962.0	E980.4
Tripelennamine	963.0	E858.1	E933.0	E950.4	E962.0	E980.4
Triperidol	969.2	E853.1	E939.2	E950.3	E962.0	E980.3
Triprolidine	963.0	E858.1	E933.0	E950.4	E962.0	E980.4
Trisoralen	976.3	E858.7	E946.3	E950.4	E962.0	E980.4
Troleandomycin	960.3	E856	E930.3	E950.4	E962.0	E980.4
Trolnitrate (phosphate)	972.4	E858.3	E942.4	E950.4	E962.0	E980.4
Trometamol	963.3	E858.1	E933.3	E950.4	E962.0	E980.4
Tromethamine	963.3	E858.1	E933.3	E950.4	E962.0	E980.4
Tronothane	968.5	E855.2	E938.5	E950.4	E962.0	E980.4
Tropicamide	971.1	E855.4	E941.1	E950.4	E962.0	E980.4
Troxidone	966.0	E855.0	E936.0	E950.4	E962.0	E980.4
Tryparsamide	961.1	E857	E931.1	E950.4	E962.0	E980.4
Trypsin	963.4	E858.1	E933.4	E950.4	E962.0	E980.4
Tryptizol	969.05	E854.0	E939.0	E950.3	E962.0	E980.3
Tuaminoheptane	971.2	E855.5	E941.2	E950.4	E962.0	E980.4
Tuberculin (old)	977.8	E858.8	E947.8	E950.4	E962.0	E980.4
Tubocurare	975.2	E858.6	E945.2	E950.4	E962.0	E980.4
Tubocurarine	975.2	E858.6	E945.2	E950.4	E962.0	E980.4
Turkish green	969.6	E854.1	E939.6	E950.3	E962.0	E980.3
Turpentine (spirits of) (liquid) (vapor)	982.8	E862.4	—	E950.9	E962.1	E980.9
Tybamate	969.5	E853.8	E939.5	E950.3	E962.0	E980.3
Tyloxapol	975.5	E858.6	E945.5	E950.4	E962.0	E980.4
Tymazoline	971.2	E855.5	E941.2	E950.4	E962.0	E980.4
Typhoid vaccine	978.1	E858.8	E948.1	E950.4	E962.0	E980.4
Typhus vaccine	979.2	E858.8	E949.2	E950.4	E962.0	E980.4
Tyrothricin	976.0	E858.7	E946.0	E950.4	E962.0	E980.4
ENT agent	976.6	E858.7	E946.6	E950.4	E962.0	E980.4
ophthalmic preparation	976.5	E858.7	E946.5	E950.4	E962.0	E980.4
Undecenoic acid	976.0	E858.7	E946.0	E950.4	E962.0	E980.4
Undecylenic acid	976.0	E858.7	E946.0	E950.4	E962.0	E980.4
Unna's boot	976.3	E858.7	E946.3	E950.4	E962.0	E980.4
Uracil mustard	963.1	E858.1	E933.1	E950.4	E962.0	E980.4
Uramustine	963.1	E858.1	E933.1	E950.4	E962.0	E980.4
Urari	975.2	E858.6	E945.2	E950.4	E962.0	E980.4
Urea	974.4	E858.5	E944.4	E950.4	E962.0	E980.4
topical	976.8	E858.7	E946.8	E950.4	E962.0	E980.4
Urethan(e) (antineoplastic)	963.1	E858.1	E933.1	E950.4	E962.0	E980.4
Urginea (maritima) (scilla) — see Squill						
Uric acid metabolism agents NEC	974.7	E858.5	E944.7	E950.4	E962.0	E980.4
Urokinase	964.4	E858.2	E934.4	E950.4	E962.0	E980.4
Urokon	977.8	E858.8	E947.8	E950.4	E962.0	E980.4
Urotropin	961.9	E857	E931.9	E950.4	E962.0	E980.4
Urtica	988.2	E865.4	—	E950.9	E962.1	E980.9
Utility gas — see Gas, utility						
Vaccine NEC	979.9	E858.8	E949.9	E950.4	E962.0	E980.4
bacterial NEC	978.8	E858.8	E948.8	E950.4	E962.0	E980.4
with						
other bacterial component	978.9	E858.8	E948.9	E950.4	E962.0	E980.4
pertussis component	978.6	E858.8	E948.6	E950.4	E962.0	E980.4
viral-rickettsial component	979.7	E858.8	E949.7	E950.4	E962.0	E980.4
mixed NEC	978.9	E858.8	E948.9	E950.4	E962.0	E980.4
BCG	978.0	E858.8	E948.0	E950.4	E962.0	E980.4
cholera	978.2	E858.8	E948.2	E950.4	E962.0	E980.4
diphtheria	978.5	E858.8	E948.5	E950.4	E962.0	E980.4
influenza	979.6	E858.8	E949.6	E950.4	E962.0	E980.4
measles	979.4	E858.8	E949.4	E950.4	E962.0	E980.4
meningococcal	978.8	E858.8	E948.8	E950.4	E962.0	E980.4
mumps	979.6	E858.8	E949.6	E950.4	E962.0	E980.4
paratyphoid	978.1	E858.8	E948.1	E950.4	E962.0	E980.4

	Poisoning	Accident	Therapeutic Use	Suicide Attempt	Assault	Undetermined
Vaccine — *continued*						
pertussis (with diphtheria toxoid) (with tetanus toxoid)	978.6	E858.8	E948.6	E950.4	E962.0	E980.4
plague	978.3	E858.8	E948.3	E950.4	E962.0	E980.4
poliomyelitis	979.5	E858.8	E949.5	E950.4	E962.0	E980.4
poliovirus	979.5	E858.8	E949.5	E950.4	E962.0	E980.4
rabies	979.1	E858.8	E949.1	E950.4	E962.0	E980.4
respiratory syncytial virus	979.6	E858.8	E949.6	E950.4	E962.0	E980.4
rickettsial NEC	979.6	E858.8	E949.6	E950.4	E962.0	E980.4
with						
bacterial component	979.7	E858.8	E949.7	E950.4	E962.0	E980.4
pertussis component	978.6	E858.8	E948.6	E950.4	E962.0	E980.4
viral component	979.7	E858.8	E949.7	E950.4	E962.0	E980.4
Rocky mountain spotted fever	979.6	E858.8	E949.6	E950.4	E962.0	E980.4
rotavirus	979.6	E858.8	E949.6	E950.4	E962.0	E980.4
rubella virus	979.4	E858.8	E949.4	E950.4	E962.0	E980.4
sabin oral	979.5	E858.8	E949.5	E950.4	E962.0	E980.4
smallpox	979.0	E858.8	E949.0	E950.4	E962.0	E980.4
tetanus	978.4	E858.8	E948.4	E950.4	E962.0	E980.4
typhoid	978.1	E858.8	E948.1	E950.4	E962.0	E980.4
typhus	979.2	E858.8	E949.2	E950.4	E962.0	E980.4
viral NEC	979.6	E858.8	E949.6	E950.4	E962.0	E980.4
with						
bacterial component	979.7	E858.8	E949.7	E950.4	E962.0	E980.4
pertussis component	978.6	E858.8	E948.6	E950.4	E962.0	E980.4
rickettsial component	979.7	E858.8	E949.7	E950.4	E962.0	E980.4
yellow fever	979.3	E858.8	E949.3	E950.4	E962.0	E980.4
Vaccinia immune globulin (human)	964.6	E858.2	E934.6	E950.4	E962.0	E980.4
Vaginal contraceptives	976.8	E858.7	E946.8	E950.4	E962.0	E980.4
Valethamate	971.1	E855.4	E941.1	E950.4	E962.0	E980.4
Valisone	976.0	E858.7	E946.0	E950.4	E962.0	E980.4
Valium	969.4	E853.2	E939.4	E950.3	E962.0	E980.3
Valmid	967.8	E852.8	E937.8	E950.2	E962.0	E980.2
Vanadium	985.8	E866.4	—	E950.9	E962.1	E980.9
Vancomycin	960.8	E856	E930.8	E950.4	E962.0	E980.4
Vapor — *see also* Gas	987.9	E869.9	—	E952.9	E962.2	E982.9
kiln (carbon monoxide)	986	E868.8	—	E952.1	E962.2	E982.1
lead — *see* Lead						
specified source NEC (*see also* specific substance)	987.8	E869.8	—	E952.8	E962.2	E982.8
Varidase	964.4	E858.2	E934.4	E950.4	E962.0	E980.4
Varnish	989.89	E861.6	—	E950.9	E962.1	E980.9
cleaner	982.8	E862.9	—	E950.9	E962.1	E980.9
Vaseline	976.3	E858.7	E946.3	E950.4	E962.0	E980.4
Vasodilan	972.5	E858.3	E942.5	E950.4	E962.0	E980.4
Vasodilators NEC	972.5	E858.3	E942.5	E950.4	E962.0	E980.4
coronary	972.4	E858.3	E942.4	E950.4	E962.0	E980.4
Vasopressin	962.5	E858.0	E932.5	E950.4	E962.0	E980.4
Vasopressor drugs	962.5	E858.0	E932.5	E950.4	E962.0	E980.4
Venom, venomous (bite) (sting)	989.5	E905.9	—	E950.9	E962.1	E980.9
arthropod NEC	989.5	E905.5	—	E950.9	E962.1	E980.9
bee	989.5	E905.3	—	E950.9	E962.1	E980.9
centipede	989.5	E905.4	—	E950.9	E962.1	E980.9
hornet	989.5	E905.3	—	E950.9	E962.1	E980.9
lizard	989.5	E905.0	—	E950.9	E962.1	E980.9
marine animals or plants	989.5	E905.6	—	E950.9	E962.1	E980.9
millipede (tropical)	989.5	E905.4	—	E950.9	E962.1	E980.9
plant NEC	989.5	E905.7	—	E950.9	E962.1	E980.9
marine	989.5	E905.6	—	E950.9	E962.1	E980.9
scorpion	989.5	E905.2	—	E950.9	E962.1	E980.9
snake	989.5	E905.0	—	E950.9	E962.1	E980.9
specified NEC	989.5	E905.8	—	E950.9	E962.1	E980.9
spider	989.5	E905.1	—	E950.9	E962.1	E980.9
wasp	989.5	E905.3	—	E950.9	E962.1	E980.9
Ventolin — *see* Salbutamol sulfate						
Veramon	967.0	E851	E937.0	E950.1	E962.0	E980.1
Veratrum						
album	988.2	E865.4	—	E950.9	E962.1	E980.9
alkaloids	972.6	E858.3	E942.6	E950.4	E962.0	E980.4
viride	988.2	E865.4	—	E950.9	E962.1	E980.9
Verdigris — *see also* Copper	985.8	E866.4	—	E950.9	E962.1	E980.9
Veronal	967.0	E851	E937.0	E950.1	E962.0	E980.1
Veroxil	961.6	E857	E931.6	E950.4	E962.0	E980.4
Versidyne	965.7	E850.7	E935.7	E950.0	E962.0	E980.0
Viagra	972.5	E858.3	E942.5	E950.4	E962.0	E980.4
Vienna						

	Poisoning	Accident	Therapeutic Use	Suicide Attempt	Assault	Undetermined
Vienna — *continued*						
green	985.1	E866.3	—	E950.8	E962.1	E980.8
insecticide	985.1	E863.4	—	E950.6	E962.1	E980.7
red	989.89	E866.8	—	E950.9	E962.1	E980.9
pharmaceutical dye	977.4	E858.8	E947.4	E950.4	E962.0	E980.4
Vinbarbital, vinbarbitone	967.0	E851	E937.0	E950.1	E962.0	E980.1
Vinblastine	963.1	E858.1	E933.1	E950.4	E962.0	E980.4
Vincristine	963.1	E858.1	E933.1	E950.4	E962.0	E980.4
Vinesthene, vinethene	968.2	E855.1	E938.2	E950.4	E962.0	E980.4
Vinyl						
bital	967.0	E851	E937.0	E950.1	E962.0	E980.1
ether	968.2	E855.1	E938.2	E950.4	E962.0	E980.4
Vioform	961.3	E857	E931.3	E950.4	E962.0	E980.4
topical	976.0	E858.7	E946.0	E930.4	E962.0	E980.4
Viomycin	960.6	E856	E930.6	E950.4	E962.0	E980.4
Viosterol	963.5	E858.1	E933.5	E950.4	E962.0	E980.4
Viper (venom)	989.5	E905.0	—	E950.9	E962.1	E980.9
Viprynium (embonate)	961.6	E857	E931.6	E950.4	E962.0	E980.4
Virugon	961.7	E857	E931.7	E950.4	E962.0	E980.4
Visine	976.5	E858.7	E946.5	E950.4	E962.0	E980.4
Vitamins NEC	963.5	E858.1	E933.5	E950.4	E962.0	E980.4
B$_{12}$	964.1	E858.2	E934.1	E950.4	E962.0	E980.4
hematopoietic	964.1	E858.2	E934.1	E950.4	E962.0	E980.4
K	964.3	E858.2	E934.3	E950.4	E962.0	E980.4
Vleminckx's solution	976.4	E858.7	E946.4	E950.4	E962.0	E980.4
Voltaren — *see* Diclofenac sodium						
Warfarin (potassium) (sodium)	964.2	E858.2	E934.2	E950.4	E962.0	E980.4
rodenticide	989.4	E863.7	—	E950.6	E962.1	E980.7
Wasp (sting)	989.5	E905.3	—	E950.9	E962.1	E980.9
Water						
balance agents NEC	974.5	E858.5	E944.5	E950.4	E962.0	E980.4
gas	987.1	E868.1	—	E951.8	E962.2	E981.8
incomplete combustion of — *see* Carbon, monoxide, fuel, utility						
hemlock	988.2	E865.4	—	E950.9	E962.1	E980.9
moccasin (venom)	989.5	E905.0	—	E950.9	E962.1	E980.9
Wax (paraffin) (petroleum)	981	E862.3	—	E950.9	E962.1	E980.9
automobile	989.89	E861.2	—	E950.9	E962.1	E980.9
floor	981	E862.0	—	E950.9	E962.1	E980.9
Weed killers NEC	989.4	E863.5	—	E950.6	E962.1	E980.7
Welldorm	967.1	E852.0	E937.1	E950.2	E962.0	E980.2
White						
arsenic — *see* Arsenic						
hellebore	988.2	E865.4	—	E950.9	E962.1	E980.9
lotion (keratolytic)	976.4	E858.7	E946.4	E950.4	E962.0	E980.4
spirit	981	E862.0	—	E950.9	E962.1	E980.9
Whitewashes	989.89	E861.6	—	E950.9	E962.1	E980.9
Whole blood	964.7	E858.2	E934.7	E950.4	E962.0	E980.4
Wild						
black cherry	988.2	E865.4	—	E950.9	E962.1	E980.9
poisonous plants NEC	988.2	E865.4	—	E950.9	E962.1	E980.9
Window cleaning fluid	989.89	E861.3	—	E950.9	E962.1	E980.9
Wintergreen (oil)	976.3	E858.7	E946.3	E950.4	E962.0	E980.4
Witch hazel	976.2	E858.7	E946.2	E950.4	E962.0	E980.4
Wood						
alcohol	980.1	E860.2	—	E950.9	E962.1	E980.9
spirit	980.1	E860.2	—	E950.9	E962.1	E980.9
Woorali	975.2	E858.6	E945.2	E950.4	E962.0	E980.4
Wormseed, American	961.6	E857	E931.6	E950.4	E962.0	E980.4
Xanthine diuretics	974.1	E858.5	E944.1	E950.4	E962.0	E980.4
Xanthocillin	960.0	E856	E930.0	E950.4	E962.0	E980.4
Xanthotoxin	976.3	E858.7	E946.3	E950.4	E962.0	E980.4
Xigris	964.2	E858.2	E934.2	E950.4	E962.0	E980.4
Xylene (liquid) (vapor)	982.0	E862.4	—	E950.9	E962.1	E980.9
Xylocaine (infiltration) (topical)	968.5	E855.2	E938.5	E950.4	E962.0	E980.4
nerve block (peripheral) (plexus)	968.6	E855.2	E938.6	E950.4	E962.0	E980.4
spinal	968.7	E855.2	E938.7	E950.4	E962.0	E980.4
Xylol (liquid) (vapor)	982.0	E862.4	—	E950.9	E962.1	E980.9
Xylometazoline	971.2	E855.5	E941.2	E950.4	E962.0	E980.4
Yellow						
fever vaccine	979.3	E858.8	E949.3	E950.4	E962.0	E980.4
jasmine	988.2	E865.4	—	E950.9	E962.1	E980.9
Yew	988.2	E865.4	—	E950.9	E962.1	E980.9
Zactane	965.7	E850.7	E935.7	E950.0	E962.0	E980.0
Zaroxolyn	974.3	E858.5	E944.3	E950.4	E962.0	E980.4
Zephiran (topical)	976.0	E858.7	E946.0			

Index — Vaccine NEC — Zephiran

	Poisoning	External Cause (E-Code)				
		Accident	Therapeutic Use	Suicide Attempt	Assault	Undeter-mined
Zephiran — *continued*						
ophthalmic preparation	976.5	E858.7	E946.5	E950.4	E962.0	E980.4
Zerone	980.1	E860.2	—	E950.9	E962.1	E980.9
Zinc (compounds) (fumes)						
(salts) (vapor) NEC	985.8	E866.4	—	E950.9	E962.1	E980.9
anti-infectives	976.0	E858.7	E946.0	E950.4	E962.0	E980.4
antivaricose	972.7	E858.3	E942.7	E950.4	E962.0	E980.4
bacitracin	976.0	E858.7	E946.0	E950.4	E962.0	E980.4
chloride	976.2	E858.7	E946.2	E950.4	E962.0	E980.4
gelatin	976.3	E858.7	E946.3	E950.4	E962.0	E980.4
oxide	976.3	E858.7	E946.3	E950.4	E962.0	E980.4
peroxide	976.0	E858.7	E946.0	E950.4	E962.0	E980.4
pesticides	985.8	E863.4	—	E950.6	E962.1	E980.7
phosphide (rodenticide)	985.8	E863.7	—	E950.6	E962.1	E980.7
stearate	976.3	E858.7	E946.3	E950.4	E962.0	E980.4
sulfate (antivaricose)	972.7	E858.3	E942.7	E950.4	E962.0	E980.4
ENT agent	976.6	E858.7	E946.6	E950.4	E962.0	E980.4
ophthalmic solution	976.5	E858.7	E946.5	E950.4	E962.0	E980.4
topical NEC	976.0	E858.7	E946.0	E950.4	E962.0	E980.4
undecylenate	976.0	E858.7	E946.0	E950.4	E962.0	E980.4
Zovant	964.2	E858.2	E934.2	E950.4	E962.0	E980.4
Zoxazolamine	968.0	E855.1	E938.0	E950.4	E962.0	E980.4
Zygadenus (venenosus)	988.2	E865.4	—	E950.9	E962.1	E980.9
Zyprexa	969.3	E853.8	E939.3	E950.3	E962.0	E980.3

SECTION 3

Alphabetic Index to External Causes of Injury and Poisoning (E Code)

This section contains the index to the codes which classify environmental events, circumstances, and other conditions as the cause of injury and other adverse effects. Where a code from the section Supplementary Classification of External Causes of Injury and Poisoning (E800-E999) is applicable, it is intended that the E code shall be used in addition to a code from the main body of the classification, Chapters 1 to 17.

The alphabetic index to the E codes is organized by main terms which describe the accident, circumstance, event, or specific agent which caused the injury or other adverse effect.

Note — Transport accidents (E800-E848) include accidents involving:

- *aircraft and spacecraft (E840-E845)*
- *watercraft (E830-E838)*
- *motor vehicle (E810-E825)*
- *railway (E800-E807)*
- *other road vehicles (E826-E829)*

For definitions and examples related to transport accidents — see Volume 1 code categories E800-E848.

The fourth-digit subdivisions for use with categories E800-E848 to identify the injured person are found at the end of this section.

For identifying the place in which an accident or poisoning occurred (circumstances classifiable to categories E850-E869 and E880-E928) — see the listing in this section under "Accident, occurring."

See the Table of Drugs and Chemicals (Section 2 of this volume) for identifying the specific agent involved in drug overdose or a wrong substance given or taken in error, and for intoxication or poisoning by a drug or other chemical substance.

The specific adverse effect, reaction, or localized toxic effect to a correct drug or substance properly administered in therapeutic or prophylactic dosage should be classified according to the nature of the adverse effect (e.g., allergy, dermatitis, tachycardia) listed in Section 1 of this volume.

☑ Additional Digit Required — Refer to the Tabular List for Digit Selection   ▽ Subterms under main terms may continue to next column or page

334 — Volume 2   ►◄ Revised Text   ● New Line   ▲ Revised Code   2014 ICD-9-CM

A

Abandonment
causing exposure to weather conditions —
see Exposure
child, with intent to injure or kill E968.4
helpless person, infant, newborn E904.0
with intent to injure or kill E968.4
Abortion, criminal, injury to child E968.8
Abuse (alleged) (suspected)
adult
by
child E967.4
ex-partner E967.3
ex-spouse E967.3
father E967.0
grandchild E967.7
grandparent E967.6
mother E967.2
non-related caregiver E967.8
other relative E967.7
other specified person E967.1
partner E967.3
sibling E967.5
spouse E967.3
stepfather E967.0
stepmother E967.2
unspecified person E967.9
child
by
boyfriend of parent or guardian
E967.0
child E967.4
father E967.0
female partner of parent or guardian
E967.2
girlfriend of parent or guardian
E967.2
grandchild E967.7
grandparent E967.6
male partner of parent or guardian
E967.0
mother E967.2
non-related caregiver E967.8
other relative E967.7
other specified person(s) E967.1
sibling E967.5
stepfather E967.0
stepmother E967.2
unspecified person E967.9
Accident (to) E928.9
aircraft (in transit) (powered) E841 ☑
at landing, take-off E840 ☑
due to, caused by cataclysm — *see* categories E908 ☑, E909 ☑
late effect of E929.1
unpowered (*see also* Collision, aircraft,
unpowered) E842 ☑
while alighting, boarding E843 ☑
amphibious vehicle
on
land — *see* Accident, motor vehicle
water — *see* Accident, watercraft
animal-drawn vehicle NEC E827 ☑
animal, ridden NEC E828 ☑
balloon (*see also* Collision, aircraft, unpowered) E842 ☑
caused by, due to
abrasive wheel (metalworking) E919.3
animal NEC E906.9
being ridden (in sport or transport)
E828 ☑
avalanche NEC E909.2
band saw E919.4
bench saw E919.4
bore, earth-drilling or mining (land)
(seabed) E919.1
bulldozer E919.7
cataclysmic
earth surface movement or eruption
E909.9
storm E908.9
chain
hoist E919.2
agricultural operations E919.0
mining operations E919.1

Accident (to) — *continued*
caused by, due to — *continued*
chain — *continued*
saw E920.1
circular saw E919.4
cold (excessive) (*see also* Cold, exposure
to) E901.9
combine E919.0
conflagration — *see* Conflagration
corrosive liquid, substance NEC E924.1
cotton gin E919.8
crane E919.2
agricultural operations E919.0
mining operations E919.1
cutting or piercing instrument (*see also*
Cut) E920.9
dairy equipment E919.8
derrick E919.2
agricultural operations E919.0
mining operations E919.1
drill E920.1
earth (land) (seabed) E919.1
hand (powered) E920.1
not powered E920.4
metalworking E919.3
woodworking E919.4
earth(-)
drilling machine E919.1
moving machine E919.7
scraping machine E919.7
electric
current (*see also* Electric shock)
E925.9
motor (*see also* Accident, machine,
by type of machine)
current (of) — *see* Electric shock
elevator (building) (grain) E919.2
agricultural operations E919.0
mining operations E919.1
environmental factors NEC E928.9
excavating machine E919.7
explosive material (*see also* Explosion)
E923.9
farm machine E919.0
firearm missile — *see* Shooting
fire, flames (*see also* Fire)
conflagration — *see* Conflagration
forging (metalworking) machine E919.3
forklift (truck) E919.2
agricultural operations E919.0
mining operations E919.1
gas turbine E919.5
harvester E919.0
hay derrick, mower, or rake E919.0
heat (excessive) (*see also* Heat) E900.9
hoist (*see also* Accident, caused by, due
to, lift) E919.2
chain — *see* Accident, caused by, due
to, chain
shaft E919.1
hot
liquid E924.0
caustic or corrosive E924.1
object (not producing fire or flames)
E924.8
substance E924.9
caustic or corrosive E924.1
liquid (metal) NEC E924.0
specified type NEC E924.8
human bite E928.3
ignition — *see* Ignition
internal combustion engine E919.5
landslide NEC E909.2
lathe (metalworking) E919.3
turnings E920.8
woodworking E919.4
lift, lifting (appliances) E919.2
agricultural operations E919.0
mining operations E919.1
shaft E919.1
lightning NEC E907
machine, machinery (*see also* Accident,
machine)
drilling, metal E919.3
manufacturing, for manufacture of
beverages E919.8

Accident (to) — *continued*
caused by, due to — *continued*
machine, machinery (*see also* Accident,
machine) — *continued*
manufacturing, for manufacture of
— *continued*
clothing E919.8
foodstuffs E919.8
paper E919.8
textiles E919.8
milling, metal E919.3
moulding E919.4
power press, metal E919.3
printing E919.8
rolling mill, metal E919.3
sawing E919.8
specified type NEC E919.8
spinning E919.8
weaving E919.8
natural factor NEC E928.9
overhead plane E919.4
plane E920.4
overhead E919.4
powered
hand tool NEC E920.1
saw E919.4
hand E920.1
printing machine E919.8
pulley (block) E919.2
agricultural operations E919.0
mining operations E919.1
transmission E919.6
radial saw E919.4
radiation — *see* Radiation
reaper E919.0
road scraper E919.7
when in transport under its own
power — *see* categories
E810-E825 ☑
roller coaster E919.8
sander E919.4
saw E920.4
band E919.4
bench E919.4
chain E920.1
circular E919.4
hand E920.4
powered E920.1
powered, except hand E919.4
radial E919.4
sawing machine, metal E919.3
shaft
hoist E919.1
lift E919.1
transmission E919.6
shears E920.4
hand E920.4
powered E920.1
mechanical E919.3
shovel E920.4
steam E919.7
spinning machine E919.8
steam (*see also* Burning, steam)
engine E919.5
shovel E919.7
thresher E919.0
thunderbolt NEC E907
tractor E919.0
when in transport under its own
power — *see* categories
E810-E825 ☑
transmission belt, cable, chain, gear,
pinion, pulley, shaft E919.6
turbine (gas) (water driven) E919.5
under-cutter E919.1
weaving machine E919.8
winch E919.2
agricultural operations E919.0
mining operations E919.1
diving E883.0
with insufficient air supply E913.2
glider (hang) (*see also* Collision, aircraft, unpowered) E842 ☑
hovercraft
on
land — *see* Accident, motor vehicle

Accident (to) — *continued*
hovercraft — *continued*
on — *continued*
water — *see* Accident, watercraft
ice yacht (*see also* Accident, vehicle NEC)
E848
in
medical, surgical procedure
as, or due to misadventure — *see*
Misadventure
causing an abnormal reaction or later
complication without men-
tion of misadventure — *see*
Reaction, abnormal
kite carrying a person (*see also* Collision, involving aircraft, unpowered) E842 ☑
land yacht (*see also* Accident, vehicle NEC)
E848
late effect of — *see* Late effect
launching pad E845 ☑
machine, machinery (*see also* Accident,
caused by, due to, by specific type of
machine) E919.9
agricultural including animal-powered
E919.0
earth-drilling E919.1
earth moving or scraping E919.7
excavating E919.7
involving transport under own power
on highway or transport vehicle
— *see* categories
E810-E825 ☑, E840-E845 ☑
lifting (appliances) E919.2
metalworking E919.3
mining E919.1
prime movers, except electric motors
E919.5
electric motors — *see* Accident, machine, by specific type of machine
recreational E919.8
specified type NEC E919.8
transmission E919.6
watercraft (deck) (engine room) (galley)
(laundry) (loading) E836 ☑
woodworking or forming E919.4
motor vehicle (on public highway) (traffic)
E819 ☑
due to cataclysm — *see* categories
E908 ☑, E909 ☑
involving
collision (*see also* Collision, motor
vehicle) E812 ☑
nontraffic, not on public highway — *see*
categories E820-E825 ☑
not involving collision — *see* categories
E816-E819 ☑
nonmotor vehicle NEC E829 ☑
nonroad — *see* Accident, vehicle NEC
road, except pedal cycle, animal-drawn
vehicle, or animal being ridden
E829 ☑
nonroad vehicle NEC — *see* Accident, vehicle NEC
not elsewhere classifiable involving
cable car (not on rails) E847
on rails E829 ☑
coal car in mine E846
hand truck — *see* Accident, vehicle NEC
logging car E846
sled(ge), meaning snow or ice vehicle
E848
tram, mine or quarry E846
truck
mine or quarry E846
self-propelled, industrial E846
station baggage E846
tub, mine or quarry E846
vehicle NEC E848
snow and ice E848
used only on industrial premises
E846
wheelbarrow E848
occurring (at) (in)
apartment E849.0
baseball field, diamond E849.4

☑ **Additional Digit Required** — Refer to the Tabular List for Digit Selection

Subterms under main terms may continue to next column or page

2014 ICD-9-CM

▶◄ **Revised Text**

● **New Line**

▲ **Revised Code**

Volume 2 — 335

Accident (to) — *continued*
occurring — *continued*
  construction site, any E849.3
  dock E849.8
    yard E849.3
  dormitory E849.7
  factory (building) (premises) E849.3
  farm E849.1
    buildings E849.1
    house E849.0
  football field E849.4
  forest E849.8
  garage (place of work) E849.3
    private (home) E849.0
  gravel pit E849.2
  gymnasium E849.4
  highway E849.5
  home (private) (residential) E849.0
    institutional E849.7
  hospital E849.7
  hotel E849.6
  house (private) (residential) E849.0
    movie E849.6
    public E849.6
  institution, residential E849.7
  jail E849.7
  mine E849.2
  motel E849.6
  movie house E849.6
  office (building) E849.6
  orphanage E849.7
  park (public) E849.4
    mobile home E849.8
    trailer E849.8
  parking lot or place E849.8
  place
    industrial NEC E849.3
    parking E849.8
    public E849.8
      specified place NEC E849.5
    recreational NEC E849.4
    sport NEC E849.4
  playground (park) (school) E849.4
  prison E849.6
  public building NEC E849.6
  quarry E849.2
  railway
    line NEC E849.8
    yard E849.3
  residence
    home (private) E849.0
  resort (beach) (lake) (mountain)
      (seashore) (vacation) E849.4
  restaurant E849.6
  sand pit E849.2
  school (building) (private) (public) (state)
      E849.6
    reform E849.7
    riding E849.4
  seashore E849.8
    resort E849.4
  shop (place of work) E849.3
    commercial E849.6
  skating rink E849.4
  sports palace E849.4
  stadium E849.4
  store E849.6
  street E849.5
  swimming pool (public) E849.4
    private home or garden E849.0
  tennis court, public E849.4
  theatre, theater E849.6
  trailer court E849.8
  tunnel E849.8
    under construction E849.2
  warehouse E849.3
  yard
    dock E849.3
    industrial E849.3
    private (home) E849.0
    railway E849.3
off-road type motor vehicle (not on public
    highway) NEC E821 ☑
  on public highway — *see* categories
    E810–E819 ☑
pedal cycle E826 ☑

Accident (to) — *continued*
railway E807 ☑
  due to cataclysm — *see* categories
      E908 ☑, E909 ☑
  involving
    avalanche E909.2
    burning by engine, locomotive, train
        (*see also* Explosion, railway
        engine) E803 ☑
    collision (*see also* Collision, railway)
        E800 ☑
    derailment (*see also* Derailment, rail-
        way) E802 ☑
    explosion (*see also* Explosion, railway
        engine) E803 ☑
    fall (*see also* Fall, from, railway rolling
        stock) E804 ☑
    fire (*see also* Explosion, railway en-
        gine) E803 ☑
    hitting by, being struck by
        object falling in, on, from, rolling
            stock, train, vehicle
            E806 ☑
        rolling stock, train, vehicle
            E805 ☑
    overturning, railway rolling stock,
        train, vehicle (*see also* Derail-
        ment, railway) E802 ☑
    running off rails, railway (*see also*
        Derailment, railway) E802 ☑
    specified circumstances NEC E806 ☑
    train or vehicle hit by
        avalanche E909.2
        falling object (earth, rock, tree)
            E806 ☑
            due to cataclysm — *see* cate-
                gories
                E908 ☑, E909 ☑
        landslide E909.2
roller skate E885.1
scooter (nonmotorized) E885.0
skateboard E885.2
ski(ing) E885.3
    jump E884.9
    lift or tow (with chair or gondola) E847
snowboard E885.4
snow vehicle, motor driven (not on public
    highway) E820 ☑
  on public highway — *see* categories
    E810–E819 ☑
spacecraft E845 ☑
specified cause NEC E928.8
street car E829 ☑
traffic NEC E819 ☑
vehicle NEC (with pedestrian) E848
  battery powered
    airport passenger vehicle E846
    truck (baggage) (mail) E846
  powered commercial or industrial (with
      other vehicle or object within
      commercial or industrial premis-
      es) E846
watercraft E838 ☑
  with
    drowning or submersion resulting
        from
        accident other than to watercraft
            E832 ☑
        accident to watercraft E830 ☑
    injury, except drowning or submer-
        sion, resulting from
        accident other than to watercraft
            — *see* categories
            E833–E838 ☑
        accident to watercraft E831 ☑
  due to, caused by cataclysm — *see* cate-
      gories E908 ☑, E909 ☑
  machinery E836 ☑
Acid throwing E961
Acosta syndrome E902.0
Activity (involving) E030
  aerobic and step exercise (class) E009.2
  alpine skiing E003.2
  animal care NEC E019.9
  arts and handcrafts NEC E012.9

Activity — *continued*
athletics NEC E008.9
  played
    as a team or group NEC E007.9
    individually NEC E006.9
baking E015.2
ballet E005.0
barbells E010.2
baseball E007.3
BASE (Building, Antenna, Span, Earth)
    jumping E004.2
basketball E007.6
bathing (personal) E013.0
beach volleyball E007.7
bike riding E006.4
boogie boarding E002.7
bowling E006.3
boxing E008.0
brass instrument playing E018.3
building and construction E016.2
bungee jumping E004.3
calisthenics E009.1
canoeing (in calm and turbulent water)
    E002.5
capture the flag E007.8
cardiorespiratory exercise NEC E009.9
caregiving (providing) NEC E014.9
  bathing E014.0
  lifting E014.1
cellular
  communication device E011.1
  telephone E011.1
challenge course E009.4
cheerleading E005.4
circuit training E009.3
cleaning
  floor E013.4
climbing NEC E004.9
  mountain E004.0
  rock E004.0
  wall climbing E004.0
combatives E008.4
computer
  keyboarding E011.0
  technology NEC E011.9
confidence course E009.4
construction (building) E016.2
cooking and baking E015.2
cooking and grilling NEC E015.9
cool down exercises E009.1
cricket E007.9
crocheting E012.0
cross country skiing E003.3
dancing (all types) E005.0
digging
  dirt E016.0
dirt digging E016.0
dishwashing E015.0
diving (platform) (springboard) E002.1
  underwater E002.4
dodge ball E007.8
downhill skiing E003.2
drum playing E018.1
dumbbells E010.2
electronic
  devices NEC E011.9
    hand held interactive E011.1
  game playing (using) (with)
    interactive device E011.1
    keyboard or other stationary device
        E011.0
elliptical machine E009.0
exercise(s)
  machines (primarily for)
    cardiorespiratory conditioning
        E009.0
    muscle strengthening E010.0
  muscle strengthening (non-machine)
      NEC E010.9
external motion NEC E017.9
  roller coaster E017.0
field hockey E007.4
figure skating (pairs) (singles) E003.0
flag football E007.1
floor mopping and cleaning E013.4
food preparation and clean up E015.0

Activity — *continued*
football (American) NOS E007.0
  flag E007.1
  tackle E007.0
  touch E007.1
four square E007.8
free weights E010.2
frisbee (ultimate) E008.3
furniture
  building E012.2
  finishing E012.2
  repair E012.2
game playing (electronic)
  using
    interactive device E011.1
    keyboard or other stationary device
        E011.0
gardening E016.1
golf E006.2
grass drills E009.5
grilling and smoking food E015.1
grooming and shearing an animal E019.2
guerilla drills E009.5
gymnastics (rhythmic) E005.2
handball E008.2
handcrafts NEC E012.9
hand held interactive electronic device
    E011.1
hang gliding E004.4
hiking (on level or elevated terrain) E001.0
hockey (ice) E003.1
  field E007.4
horseback riding E006.1
household maintenance NEC E013.9
ice NEC E003.9
  dancing E003.0
  hockey E003.1
  skating E003.0
inline roller skating E006.0
ironing E013.3
judo E008.4
jumping jacks E009.1
jumping rope E006.5
jumping (off) NEC E004.9
  BASE (Building, Antenna, Span, Earth)
      E004.2
  bungee E004.3
  jacks E009.1
  rope E006.5
karate E008.4
kayaking (in calm and turbulent water)
    E002.5
keyboarding (computer) E011.0
kickball E007.8
knitting E012.0
lacrosse E007.4
land maintenance NEC E016.9
landscaping E016.1
laundry E013.1
machines (exercise) primarily for cardiores-
    piratory conditioning E009.0
maintenance
  building E016.9
  household NEC E013.9
  land E016.9
  property E016.9
marching (on level or elevated terrain)
    E001.0
martial arts E008.4
microwave oven E015.2
milking an animal E019.1
mopping (floor) E013.4
mountain climbing E004.0
muscle strengthening
  exercises (non-machine) NEC E010.9
  machines E010.0
musical keyboard (electronic) playing E018.0
nordic skiing E003.3
obstacle course E009.4
oven (microwave) E015.2
packing up and unpacking in moving to a
    new residence E013.5
parasailing E002.9
percussion instrument playing NEC E018.1
personal
  bathing and showering E013.0

Activity — *continued*
personal — *continued*
hygiene NEC E013.8
showering E013.0
physical
games generally associated with school recess, summer camp and children E007.8
training NEC E009.9
piano playing E018.0
pilates E010.3
platform diving E002.1
playing musical instrument
brass instrument E018.3
drum E018.1
musical keyboard (electronic) E018.0
percussion instrument NEC E018.1
piano E018.0
string instrument E018.2
wind instrument E018.3
property maintenance NEC E016.9
pruning (garden and lawn) E016.1
pull-ups E010.1
push-ups E010.1
racquetball E008.2
rafting (in calm and turbulent water) E002.5
raking (leaves) E016.0
rappelling E004.1
refereeing a sports activity E029.0
residential relocation E013.5
rhythmic
gymnastics E005.2
movement NEC E005.9
riding
horseback E006.1
roller coaster E017.0
rock climbing E004.0
roller coaster riding E017.0
roller skating (inline) E006.0
rough housing and horseplay E029.2
rowing (in calm and turbulent water) E002.5
rugby E007.2
running E001.1
SCUBA diving E002.4
sewing E012.1
shoveling E016.0
dirt E016.0
snow E016.0
showering (personal) E013.0
sit-ups E010.1
skateboarding E006.0
skating (ice) E003.0
roller E006.0
skiing (alpine) (downhill) E003.2
cross country E003.3
nordic E003.3
sledding (snow) E003.2
smoking and grilling food E015.1
snorkeling E002.4
snow NEC E003.9
boarding E003.2
shoveling E016.0
sledding E003.2
tubing E003.2
soccer E007.5
softball E007.3
specified NEC E029.9
spectator at an event E029.1
sports played as a team or group NEC E007.9
sports played individually NEC E006.9
sports NEC E008.9
springboard diving E002.1
squash E008.2
stationary bike E009.0
step (stepping) exercise (class) E009.2
stepper machine E009.0
stove E015.2
string instrument playing E018.2
surfing E002.7
swimming E002.0
tackle football E007.0
tap dancing E005.0
tennis E008.2
tobogganing E003.2
touch football E007.1
track and field events (non-running) E006.6

Activity — *continued*
track and field events — *continued*
running E001.1
trampoline E005.3
treadmill E009.0
trimming shrubs E016.1
tubing (in calm and turbulent water) E002.5
snow E003.2
ultimate frisbee E008.3
underwater diving E002.4
unpacking in moving to a new residence E013.5
use of stove, oven and microwave oven E015.2
vacuuming E013.2
volleyball (beach) (court) E007.7
wake boarding E002.6
walking (on level or elevated terrain) E001.0
an animal E019.0
walking an animal E019.0
wall climbing E004.0
warm up and cool down exercises E009.1
water NEC E002.9
aerobics E002.3
craft NEC E002.9
exercise E002.3
polo E002.2
skiing E002.6
sliding E002.8
survival training and testing E002.9
weeding (garden and lawn) E016.1
wind instrument playing E018.3
windsurfing E002.7
wrestling E008.1
yoga E005.1
Activity status E000.9
child assisting in compensated work of other family member E000.8
civilian
done for
financial or other compensation E000.0
pay or income E000.0
family member assisting in compensated work of other family member E000.8
for income E000.0
hobby or leisure E000.8
military E000.1
off duty E000.8
off duty military E000.8
recreation E000.8
specified NEC E000.8
sport not for income E000.8
student E000.8
volunteer E000.2
Aero-otitis media — *see* Effects of, air pressure
Aeroneurosis E902.1
Aerosinusitis — *see* Effects of, air pressure
After-effect, late — *see* Late effect
Air
blast
in
terrorism E979.2
war operations E993.9
embolism (traumatic) NEC E928.9
in
infusion or transfusion E874.1
perfusion E874.2
sickness E903
Alpine sickness E902.0
Altitude sickness — *see* Effects of, air pressure
Anaphylactic shock, anaphylaxis — *see also* Table of Drugs and Chemicals E947.9
due to bite or sting (venomous) — *see* Bite, venomous
Andes disease E902.0
Apoplexy
heat — *see* Heat
Arachnidism E905.1
Arson E968.0
Asphyxia, asphyxiation
by
chemical
in
terrorism E979.7

Asphyxia, asphyxiation — *continued*
by — *continued*
chemical — *continued*
in — *continued*
war operations E997.2
explosion — *see* Explosion
food (bone) (regurgitated food) (seed) E911
foreign object, except food E912
fumes
in
terrorism (chemical weapons) E979.7
war operations E997.2
gas (*see also* Table of Drugs and Chemicals)
in
terrorism E979.7
war operations E997.2
legal
execution E978
intervention (tear) E972
tear E972
mechanical means (*see also* Suffocation) E913.9
from
conflagration — *see* Conflagration
fire (*see also* Fire) E899
in
terrorism E979.3
war operations E990.9
ignition — *see* Ignition
Aspiration
foreign body — *see* Foreign body, aspiration
mucus, not of newborn (with asphyxia, obstruction respiratory passage, suffocation) E912
phlegm (with asphyxia, obstruction respiratory passage, suffocation) E912
vomitus (with asphyxia, obstruction respiratory passage, suffocation) (*see also* Foreign body, aspiration, food) E911
Assassination (attempt) — *see also* Assault E968.9
Assault (homicidal) (by) (in) E968.9
acid E961
swallowed E962.1
air gun E968.6
BB gun E968.6
bite NEC E968.8
of human being E968.7
bomb ((placed in) car or house) E965.8
antipersonnel E965.5
letter E965.7
petrol E965.6
brawl (hand) (fists) (foot) E960.0
burning, burns (by fire) E968.0
acid E961
swallowed E962.1
caustic, corrosive substance E961
swallowed E962.1
chemical from swallowing caustic, corrosive substance NEC E962.1
hot liquid E968.3
scalding E968.3
vitriol E961
swallowed E962.1
caustic, corrosive substance E961
swallowed E962.1
cut, any part of body E966
dagger E966
drowning E964
explosive(s) E965.9
bomb (*see also* Assault, bomb) E965.8
dynamite E965.8
fight (hand) (fists) (foot) E960.0
with weapon E968.9
blunt or thrown E968.2
cutting or piercing E966
firearm — *see* Shooting, homicide
fire E968.0
firearm(s) — *see* Shooting, homicide
garrotting E963
gunshot (wound) — *see* Shooting, homicide
hanging E963
injury NEC E968.9

Assault — *continued*
knife E966
late effect of E969
ligature E963
poisoning E962.9
drugs or medicinals E962.0
gas(es) or vapors, except drugs and medicinals E962.2
solid or liquid substances, except drugs and medicinals E962.1
puncture, any part of body E966
pushing
before moving object, train, vehicle E968.5
from high place E968.1
rape E960.1
scalding E968.3
shooting — *see* Shooting, homicide
sodomy E960.1
stab, any part of body E966
strangulation E963
submersion E964
suffocation E963
transport vehicle E968.5
violence NEC E968.9
vitriol E961
swallowed E962.1
weapon E968.9
blunt or thrown E968.2
cutting or piercing E966
firearm — *see* Shooting, homicide
wound E968.9
cutting E966
gunshot — *see* Shooting, homicide
knife E966
piercing E966
puncture E966
stab E966
Attack by animal NEC E906.9
Avalanche E909.2
falling on or hitting
motor vehicle (in motion) (on public highway) E909.2
railway train E909.2
Aviators' disease E902.1

B

Barotitis, barodontalgia, barosinusitis, barotrauma (otitic) (sinus) — *see* Effects of, air pressure
Battered
baby or child (syndrome) — *see* Abuse, child; category E967 ☑
person other than baby or child — *see* Assault
Bayonet wound — *see also* Cut, by bayonet E920.3
in
legal intervention E974
terrorism E979.8
war operations E995.2
Bean in nose E912
Bed set on fire NEC E898.0
Beheading (by guillotine)
homicide E966
legal execution E978
Bending, injury
due to
repetitive movement E927.3
sudden strenuous movement E927.0
Bends E902.0
Bite
animal NEC E906.5
other specified (except arthropod) E906.3
venomous NEC E905.9
arthropod (nonvenomous) NEC E906.4
venomous — *see* Sting
black widow spider E905.1
cat E906.3
centipede E905.4
cobra E905.0
copperhead snake E905.0
coral snake E905.0
dog E906.0
fer de lance E905.0

☑ **Additional Digit Required** — Refer to the Tabular List for Digit Selection   ▽ **Subterms under main terms may continue to next column or page**

2014 ICD-9-CM   ▶◀ **Revised Text**   ● **New Line**   ▲ **Revised Code**   **Volume 2 — 337**

Bite — *continued*
  gila monster E905.0
  human being
    accidental E928.3
    assault E968.7
  insect (nonvenomous) E906.4
    venomous — *see* Sting
  krait E905.0
  late effect of — *see* Late effect
  lizard E906.2
    venomous E905.0
  mamba E905.0
  marine animal
    nonvenomous E906.3
      snake E906.2
    venomous E905.6
      snake E905.0
  millipede E906.4
    venomous E905.4
  moray eel E906.3
  rat E906.1
  rattlesnake E905.0
  rodent, except rat E906.3
  serpent — *see* Bite, snake
  shark E906.3
  snake (venomous) E905.0
    nonvenomous E906.2
    sea E905.0
  spider E905.1
    nonvenomous E906.4
  tarantula (venomous) E905.1
  venomous NEC E905.9
    by specific animal — *see category*
      E905 ☑
  viper E905.0
  water moccasin E905.0
Blast (air)
  from nuclear explosion E996 ☑
  in
    terrorism E979.2
      from nuclear explosion E979.5
      underwater E979.0
    war operations E993.9
      from nuclear explosion — *see* War
        operations, injury due to, nu-
        clear weapons
      underwater E992.9
Blizzard E908.3
Blow E928.9
  by law-enforcing agent, police (on duty)
    E975
    with blunt object (baton) (nightstick)
      (stave) (truncheon) E973
Blowing up — *see also* Explosion E923.9
Brawl (hand) (fists) (foot) E960.0
Breakage (accidental)
  cable of cable car not on rails E847
  ladder (causing fall) E881.0
  part (any) of
    animal-drawn vehicle E827 ☑
    ladder (causing fall) E881.0
    motor vehicle
      in motion (on public highway)
        E818 ☑
        not on public highway E825 ☑
    nonmotor road vehicle, except animal-
      drawn vehicle or pedal cycle
      E829 ☑
    off-road type motor vehicle (not on
      public highway) NEC E821 ☑
      on public highway E818 ☑
    pedal cycle E826 ☑
    scaffolding (causing fall) E881.1
    snow vehicle, motor-driven (not on
      public highway) E820 ☑
      on public highway E818 ☑
    vehicle NEC — *see* Accident, vehicle
Broken
  glass
    fall on E888.0
    injury by E920.8
  power line (causing electric shock) E925.1
Bumping against, into (accidentally)
  object (moving) E917.9
    caused by crowd E917.1
      with subsequent fall E917.6

Bumping against, into — *continued*
  object — *continued*
    furniture E917.3
      with subsequent fall E917.7
    in
      running water E917.2
      sports E917.0
        with subsequent fall E917.5
    stationary E917.4
      with subsequent fall E917.8
  person(s) E917.9
    with fall E886.0
      in sports E886.0
    as, or caused by, a crowd E917.1
      with subsequent fall E917.6
    in sports E917.0
      with fall E886.0
Burning, burns (accidental) (by) (from) (on)
  E899
  acid (any kind) E924.1
    swallowed — *see* Table of Drugs and
      Chemicals
  airgun E928.7
  bedclothes (*see also* Fire, specified NEC)
    E898.0
  blowlamp (*see also* Fire, specified NEC)
    E898.1
  blowtorch (*see also* Fire, specified NEC)
    E898.1
  boat, ship, watercraft — *see* categories
    E830 ☑, E831 ☑, E837 ☑
  bonfire (controlled) E897
    uncontrolled E892
  candle (*see also* Fire, specified NEC) E898.1
  caustic liquid, substance E924.1
    swallowed — *see* Table of Drugs and
      Chemicals
  chemical E924.1
    from swallowing caustic, corrosive sub-
      stance — *see* Table of Drugs and
      Chemicals
    in
      terrorism E979.7
      war operations E997.2
  cigar(s) or cigarette(s) (*see also* Fire, speci-
    fied NEC) E898.1
  clothes, clothing, nightdress — *see* Ignition,
    clothes
    with conflagration — *see* Conflagration
  conflagration — *see* Conflagration
  corrosive liquid, substance E924.1
    swallowed — *see* Table of Drugs and
      Chemicals
  electric current (*see also* Electric shock)
    E925.9
  firearm E928.7
  fire, flames (*see also* Fire) E899
  flare, Verey pistol E922.8
  heat
    from appliance (electrical) E924.8
    in local application, or packing during
      medical or surgical procedure
      E873.5
  homicide (attempt) (*see also* Assault, burn-
    ing) E968.0
  hot
    liquid E924.0
      caustic or corrosive E924.1
    object (not producing fire or flames)
      E924.8
    substance E924.9
      caustic or corrosive E924.1
      liquid (metal) NEC E924.0
      specified type NEC E924.8
    tap water E924.2
  ignition (*see also* Ignition)
    clothes, clothing, nightdress (*see also*
      Ignition, clothes)
      with conflagration — *see* Conflagra-
        tion
    highly inflammable material (benzine)
      (fat) (gasoline) (kerosene) (paraf-
      fin) (petrol) E894
    in
      terrorism E979.3
      from nuclear explosion E979.5

Burning, burns — *continued*
  in — *continued*
    terrorism — *continued*
      petrol bomb E979.3
    war operations (from fire-producing de-
      vice or conventional weapon)
      E990.9
      from nuclear explosion (*see also* War
        operations, injury due to, nu-
        clear weapons) E996.2
      incendiary bomb E990.0
      petrol bomb E990.0
  inflicted by other person
    stated as
      homicidal, intentional (*see also* As-
        sault, burning) E968.0
      undetermined whether accidental or
        intentional (*see also* Burn,
        stated as undetermined
        whether accidental or inten-
        tional) E988.1
  internal, from swallowed caustic, corrosive
    liquid, substance — *see* Table of
    Drugs and Chemicals
  lamp (*see also* Fire, specified NEC) E898.1
  late effect of NEC E929.4
  lighter (cigar) (cigarette) (*see also* Fire,
    specified NEC) E898.1
  lightning E907
  liquid (boiling) (hot) (molten) E924.0
    caustic, corrosive (external) E924.1
      swallowed — *see* Table of Drugs and
        Chemicals
  local application of externally applied sub-
    stance in medical or surgical care
    E873.5
  machinery — *see* Accident, machine
  matches (*see also* Fire, specified NEC) E898.1
  medicament, externally applied E873.5
  metal, molten E924.0
  object (hot) E924.8
    producing fire or flames — *see* Fire
  oven (electric) (gas) E924.8
  pipe (smoking) (*see also* Fire, specified NEC)
    E898.1
  radiation — *see* Radiation
  railway engine, locomotive, train (*see also*
    Explosion, railway engine) E803 ☑
  self-inflicted (unspecified whether acciden-
    tal or intentional) E988.1
    caustic or corrosive substance NEC
      E988.7
    stated as intentional, purposeful E958.1
      caustic or corrosive substance NEC
        E958.7
    stated as undetermined whether accidental
      or intentional E988.1
      caustic or corrosive substance NEC
        E988.7
  steam E924.0
    pipe E924.8
  substance (hot) E924.9
    boiling or molten E924.0
    caustic, corrosive (external) E924.1
      swallowed — *see* Table of Drugs and
        Chemicals
  suicidal (attempt) NEC E958.1
    caustic substance E958.7
    late effect of E959
  tanning bed E926.2
  therapeutic misadventure
    overdose of radiation E873.2
  torch, welding (*see also* Fire, specified NEC)
    E898.1
  trash fire (*see also* Burning, bonfire) E897
  vapor E924.0
  vitriol E924.1
  x-rays E926.3
    in medical, surgical procedure — *see*
      Misadventure, failure, in dosage,
      radiation
Butted by animal E906.8

C

Cachexia, lead or saturnine E866.0

Cachexia, lead or saturnine — *continued*
  from pesticide NEC (*see also* Table of Drugs
    and Chemicals) E863.4
Caisson disease E902.2
Capital punishment (any means) E978
Car sickness E903
Casualty (not due to war) NEC E928.9
  terrorism E979.8
  war (*see also* War operations) E995.9
Cat
  bite E906.3
  scratch E906.8
Cataclysmic (any injury)
  earth surface movement or eruption E909.9
    specified type NEC E909.8
  storm or flood resulting from storm E908.9
    specified type NEC E909.8
Catching fire — *see* Ignition
Caught
  between
    objects (moving) (stationary and mov-
      ing) E918
      and machinery — *see* Accident, ma-
        chine
  by cable car, not on rails E847
  in
    machinery (moving parts of) — *see*, Ac-
      cident, machine
    object E918
Cave-in (causing asphyxia, suffocation (by
  pressure)) — *see also* Suffocation, due
  to, cave-in E913.3
  with injury other than asphyxia or suffoca-
    tion E916
    with asphyxia or suffocation (*see also*
      Suffocation, due to, cave-in)
      E913.3
  struck or crushed by E916
    with asphyxia or suffocation (*see also*
      Suffocation, due to, cave-in)
      E913.3
Change(s) in air pressure — *see also* Effects
  of, air pressure
  sudden, in aircraft (ascent) (descent) (caus-
    ing aeroneurosis or aviators' disease)
    E902.1
Chilblains E901.0
  due to manmade conditions E901.1
Choking (on) (any object except food or vomitus) E912
  apple E911
  bone E911
  food, any type (regurgitated) E911
  mucus or phlegm E912
  seed E911
Civil insurrection — *see* War operations
Cloudburst E908.8
Cold, exposure to (accidental) (excessive)
  (extreme) (place) E901.9
  causing chilblains or immersion foot E901.0
  due to
    manmade conditions E901.1
    specified cause NEC E901.8
    weather (conditions) E901.0
  late effect of NEC E929.5
  self-inflicted (undetermined whether acci-
    dental or intentional) E988.3
    suicidal E958.3
  suicide E958.3
Colic, lead, painter's, or saturnine — *see*
  category E866 ☑
Collapse
  building E916
    burning (uncontrolled fire) E891.8
      in terrorism E979.3
      private E890.8
  dam E909.3
  due to heat — *see* Heat
  machinery — *see* Accident, machine or ve-
    hicle
  man-made structure E909.3
  postoperative NEC E878.9
  structure
    burning (uncontrolled fire) NEC E891.8
      in terrorism E979.3

☑ **Additional Digit Required** — Refer to the Tabular List for Digit Selection

▼ **Subterms under main terms may continue to next column or page**

Collision (accidental)

Note — In the case of collisions between different types of vehicles, persons and objects, priority in classification is in the following order:

    Aircraft

    Watercraft

    Motor vehicle

    Railway vehicle

    Pedal cycle

    Animal-drawn vehicle

    Animal being ridden

    Streetcar or other nonmotor road vehicle

    Other vehicle

    Pedestrian or person using pedestrian conveyance

    Object (except where falling from or set in motion by vehicle etc. listed above)

In the listing below, the combinations are listed only under the vehicle etc. having priority. For definitions, see Supplementary Classification of External Causes of Injury and Poisoning (E800-E999).

aircraft (with object or vehicle) (fixed) (movable) (moving) E841 ☑
  with
    person (while landing, taking off) (without accident to aircraft) E844 ☑
  powered (in transit) (with unpowered aircraft) E841 ☑
    while landing, taking off E840 ☑
  unpowered E842 ☑
  while landing, taking off E840 ☑
animal-drawn vehicle E827 ☑
  and
    animal (being ridden) (herded) (unattended) E827 ☑
    nonmotor road vehicle, except pedal cycle E827 ☑
    object (fallen) (fixed) (movable) (moving) not falling from or set in motion by vehicle of higher priority E827 ☑
    pedestrian (conveyance or vehicle) E827 ☑
    streetcar E827 ☑
animal being ridden (in sport or transport) E828 ☑
  and
    animal (being ridden) (herded) (unattended) E828 ☑
    nonmotor road vehicle, except pedal cycle or animal-drawn vehicle E828 ☑
    object (fallen) (fixed) (movable) (moving) not falling from or set in motion by vehicle of higher priority E828 ☑
    pedestrian (conveyance or vehicle) E828 ☑
motor vehicle (on public highway) (traffic accident) E812 ☑
  after leaving, running off, public highway (without antecedent collision) (without re-entry) E816 ☑
  with antecedent collision on public highway — see categories E810-E815 ☑
  with re-entrance collision with another motor vehicle E811 ☑
  and
    abutment (bridge) (overpass) E815 ☑
    animal-drawn vehicle E813 ☑

Collision — continued

motor vehicle — continued
  and — continued
    animal (herded) (unattended) E815 ☑
    carrying person, property E813 ☑
    another motor vehicle (abandoned) (disabled) (parked) (stalled) (stopped) E812 ☑
      with, involving re-entrance (on same roadway) (across median strip) E811 ☑
    any object, person, or vehicle off the public highway resulting from a noncollision motor vehicle nontraffic accident E816 ☑
    avalanche, fallen or not moving E815 ☑
      falling E909.2
    boundary fence E815 ☑
    culvert E815 ☑
    fallen
      stone E815 ☑
      tree E815 ☑
    guard post or guard rail E815 ☑
    inter-highway divider E815 ☑
    landslide, fallen or not moving E815 ☑
      moving E909 ☑
    machinery (road) E815 ☑
    nonmotor road vehicle NEC E813 ☑
    object (any object, person, or vehicle off the public highway resulting from a noncollision motor vehicle nontraffic accident) E815 ☑
      off, normally not on, public highway resulting from a noncollision motor vehicle traffic accident E816 ☑
    pedal cycle E813 ☑
    pedestrian (conveyance) E814 ☑
    person (using pedestrian conveyance) E814 ☑
    post or pole (lamp) (light) (signal) (telephone) (utility) E815 ☑
    railway rolling stock, train, vehicle E810 ☑
    safety island E815 ☑
    street car E813 ☑
    traffic signal, sign, or marker (temporary) E815 ☑
    tree E815 ☑
    tricycle E813 ☑
    wall of cut made for road E815 ☑
  due to cataclysm — see categories E908 ☑, E909 ☑
  not on public highway, nontraffic accident E822 ☑
  and
    animal-drawn vehicle E822 ☑
    animal (carrying person, property) (herded) (unattended) E822 ☑
    another motor vehicle (moving), except off-road motor vehicle E822 ☑
      stationary E823 ☑
    avalanche, fallen, not moving E823 ☑
      moving E909.2
    landslide, fallen, not moving E823 ☑
      moving E909.2
    nonmotor vehicle (moving) E822 ☑
      stationary E823 ☑
    object (fallen) (normally) (fixed) (movable but not in motion) (stationary) E823 ☑
      moving, except when falling from, set in motion by, aircraft or cataclysm E822 ☑
    pedal cycle (moving) E822 ☑

Collision — continued

motor vehicle — continued
  not on public highway, nontraffic accident — continued
    and — continued
      pedal cycle — continued
        stationary E823 ☑
      pedestrian (conveyance) E822 ☑
      person (using pedestrian conveyance) E822 ☑
      railway rolling stock, train, vehicle (moving) E822 ☑
        stationary E823 ☑
      road vehicle (any) (moving) E822 ☑
        stationary E823 ☑
      tricycle (moving) E822 ☑
        stationary E823 ☑
    off-road type motor vehicle (not on public highway) E821 ☑
    and
      animal (being ridden) (-drawn vehicle) E821 ☑
      another off-road motor vehicle, except snow vehicle E821 ☑
      other motor vehicle, not on public highway E821 ☑
      other object or vehicle NEC, fixed or movable, not set in motion by aircraft, motor vehicle on highway, or snow vehicle, motor driven E821 ☑
      pedal cycle E821 ☑
      pedestrian (conveyance) E821 ☑
      railway train E821 ☑
    on public highway — see Collision, motor vehicle
pedal cycle E826 ☑
  and
    animal-drawn vehicle E826 ☑
    animal (carrying person, property) (herded) (unherded) E826 ☑
    another pedal cycle E826 ☑
    nonmotor road vehicle E826 ☑
    object (fallen) (fixed) (movable) (moving) not falling from or set in motion by aircraft, motor vehicle, or railway train NEC E826 ☑
    pedestrian (conveyance) E826 ☑
    person (using pedestrian conveyance) E826 ☑
    street car E826 ☑
pedestrian(s) (conveyance) E917.9
  with fall E886.9
    in sports E886.0
  and
    crowd, human stampede E917.1
      with subsequent fall E917.6
    furniture E917.3
      with subsequent fall E917.7
    machinery — see Accident, machine
    object (fallen) (moving) not falling from NEC, fixed or set in motion by any vehicle classifiable to E800-E848 ☑, E917.9
      with subsequent fall E917.6
      caused by a crowd E917.1
        with subsequent fall E917.6
      furniture E917.3
        with subsequent fall E917.7
      in
        running water E917.2
          with drowning or submersion — see Submersion
        sports E917.0
          with subsequent fall E917.5
        stationary E917.4
          with subsequent fall E917.8
    vehicle, nonmotor, nonroad E848
    in
      running water E917.2

Collision — continued

pedestrian(s) — continued
  in — continued
    running water — continued
      with drowning or submersion — see Submersion
    sports E917.0
      with fall E886.0
  person(s) (using pedestrian conveyance) (see also Collision, pedestrian) E917.9
railway (rolling stock) (train) (vehicle) (with (subsequent) derailment, explosion, fall or fire) E800
  with antecedent derailment E802 ☑
  and
    animal (carrying person) (herded) (unattended) E801 ☑
    another railway train or vehicle E800 ☑
    buffers E801 ☑
    fallen tree on railway E801 ☑
    farm machinery, nonmotor (in transport) (stationary) E801 ☑
    gates E801 ☑
    nonmotor vehicle E801 ☑
    object (fallen) (fixed) (movable) (moving) not falling from, set in motion by, aircraft or motor vehicle NEC E801 ☑
    pedal cycle E801 ☑
    pedestrian (conveyance) E805 ☑
    person (using pedestrian conveyance) E805 ☑
    platform E801 ☑
    rock on railway E801 ☑
    street car E801 ☑
snow vehicle, motor-driven (not on public highway) E820 ☑
  and
    animal (being ridden) (-drawn vehicle) E820 ☑
    another off-road motor vehicle E820 ☑
    other motor vehicle, not on public highway E820 ☑
    other object or vehicle NEC, fixed or movable, not set in motion by aircraft or motor vehicle on highway E820 ☑
    pedal cycle E820 ☑
    pedestrian (conveyance) E820 ☑
    railway train E820 ☑
  on public highway — see Collision, motor vehicle
street car(s) E829 ☑
  and
    animal, herded, not being ridden, unattended E829 ☑
    nonmotor road vehicle NEC E829 ☑
    object (fallen) (fixed) (movable) (moving) not falling from or set in motion by aircraft, animal-drawn vehicle, animal being ridden, motor vehicle, pedal cycle, or railway train E829 ☑
    pedestrian (conveyance) E829 ☑
    person (using pedestrian conveyance) E829 ☑
vehicle
  animal-drawn — see Collision, animal-drawn vehicle
  motor — see Collision, motor vehicle
  nonmotor
    nonroad E848
    and
      another nonmotor, nonroad vehicle E848

☑ Additional Digit Required — Refer to the Tabular List for Digit Selection   ▽ Subterms under main terms may continue to next column or page

2014 ICD-9-CM   ▶◀ Revised Text   ● New Line   ▲ Revised Code   Volume 2 — 339

Collision — *continued*
  vehicle — *continued*
    nonmotor — *continued*
      nonroad — *continued*
        and — *continued*
          object (fallen) (fixed) (movable) (moving) not falling from or set in motion by aircraft, animal-drawn vehicle, animal being ridden, motor vehicle, nonmotor road vehicle, pedal cycle, railway train, or streetcar E848
       road, except animal being ridden, animal-drawn vehicle, or pedal cycle E829 ☑
       and
        animal, herded, not being ridden, unattended E829 ☑
        another nonmotor road vehicle, except animal being ridden, animal-drawn vehicle, or pedal cycle E829 ☑
        object (fallen) (fixed) (movable) (moving) not falling from or set in motion by, aircraft, animal-drawn vehicle, animal being ridden, motor vehicle, pedal cycle, or railway train E829 ☑
        pedestrian (conveyance) E829 ☑
        person (using pedestrian conveyance) E829 ☑
        vehicle, nonmotor, nonroad E829 ☑
  watercraft E838 ☑
    and
      person swimming or water skiing E838 ☑
    causing
      drowning, submersion E830 ☑
      injury except drowning, submersion E831 ☑
Combustion, spontaneous — *see* Ignition
Complication of medical or surgical procedure or treatment
  as an abnormal reaction — *see* Reaction, abnormal
  delayed, without mention of misadventure — *see* Reaction, abnormal
  due to misadventure — *see* Misadventure
Compression
  divers' squeeze E902.2
  trachea by
    food E911
    foreign body, except food E912
Conflagration
  building or structure, except private dwelling (barn) (church) (convalescent or residential home) (factory) (farm outbuilding) (hospital) (hotel) (institution) (educational) (domitory) (residential) (school) (shop) (store) (theater) E891.9
    with or causing (injury due to)
      accident or injury NEC E891.9
        specified circumstance NEC E891.8
      burns, burning E891.3
      carbon monoxide E891.2
      fumes E891.2
        polyvinylchloride (PVC) or similar material E891.1
      smoke E891.2
      causing explosion E891.0
    in terrorism E979.3
  not in building or structure E892

Conflagration — *continued*
  private dwelling (apartment) (boarding house) (camping place) (caravan) (farmhouse) (home (private)) (house) (lodging house) (private garage) (rooming house) (tenement) E890.9
    with or causing (injury due to)
      accident or injury NEC E890.9
        specified circumstance NEC E890.8
      burns, burning E890.3
      carbon monoxide E890.2
      fumes E890.2
        polyvinylchloride (PVC) or similar material E890.1
      smoke E890.2
      causing explosion E890.0
Constriction, external
  caused by
    hair E928.4
    other object E928.5
Contact with
  dry ice E901.1
  liquid air, hydrogen, nitrogen E901.1
Cramp(s)
  Heat — *see* Heat
  swimmers (*see also* category E910) E910.2
    not in recreation or sport E910.3
Cranking (car) (truck) (bus) (engine), injury by E917.9
Crash
  aircraft (in transit) (powered) E841 ☑
    at landing, take-off E840 ☑
    in
      terrorism E979.1
      war operations E994.9
    on runway NEC E840 ☑
    stated as
      homicidal E968.8
      suicidal E958.6
      undetermined whether accidental or intentional E988.6
    unpowered E842 ☑
  glider E842 ☑
  motor vehicle (*see also* Accident, motor vehicle)
    homicidal E968.5
    suicidal E958.5
    undetermined whether accidental or intentional E988.5
Crushed (accidentally) E928.9
  between
    boat(s), ship(s), watercraft (and dock or pier) (without accident to watercraft) E838 ☑
      after accident to, or collision, watercraft E831 ☑
    objects (moving) (stationary and moving) E918
  by
    avalanche NEC E909.2
    boat, ship, watercraft after accident to, collision, watercraft E831 ☑
    cave-in E916
      with asphyxiation or suffocation (*see also* Suffocation, due to, cave-in) E913.3
    crowd, human stampede E917.1
    falling
      aircraft (*see also* Accident, aircraft) E841 ☑
        in
          terrorism E979.1
          war operations E994.8
      earth, material E916
        with asphyxiation or suffocation (*see also* Suffocation, due to, cave-in) E913.3
      object E916
        on ship, watercraft E838 ☑
        while loading, unloading watercraft E838 ☑
    firearm E928.7
    landslide NEC E909.2
    lifeboat after abandoning ship E831 ☑
    machinery — *see* Accident, machine

Crushed — *continued*
  by — *continued*
    railway rolling stock, train, vehicle (part of) E805 ☑
    slide trigger mechanism, scope or other part of gun E928.7
    street car E829 ☑
    vehicle NEC — *see* Accident, vehicle NEC
  in
    machinery — *see* Accident, machine
    object E918
    transport accident — *see* categories E800-E848 ☑
  late effect of NEC E929.9
Cut, cutting (any part of body) (accidental) E920.9
  by
    arrow E920.8
    axe E920.4
    bayonet (*see also* Bayonet wound) E920.3
      in war operations E995.2
    blender E920.2
    broken glass E920.8
      following fall E888.0
    can opener E920.4
      powered E920.2
    chisel E920.4
    circular saw E919.4
    cutting or piercing instrument (*see also* category) E920 ☑
      following fall E888.0
      late effect of E929.8
    dagger E920.3
    dart E920.8
    drill — *see* Accident, caused by drill
    edge of stiff paper E920.8
    electric
      beater E920.2
      fan E920.2
      knife E920.2
      mixer E920.2
    firearm component E928.7
    fork E920.4
    garden fork E920.4
    hand saw or tool (not powered) E920.4
      powered E920.1
    hedge clipper E920.4
      powered E920.1
    hoe E920.4
    ice pick E920.4
    knife E920.3
      electric E920.2
      in war operations E995.2
    lathe turnings E920.8
    lawn mower E920.4
      powered E920.0
      riding E919.8
    machine — *see* Accident, machine
    meat
      grinder E919.8
      slicer E919.8
    nails E920.8
    needle E920.4
      hypodermic E920.5
    object, edged, pointed, sharp — *see* category E920 ☑
      following fall E888.0
    paper cutter E920.4
    piercing instrument (*see also* category) E920 ☑
      late effect of E929.8
    pitchfork E920.4
    powered
      can opener E920.2
      garden cultivator E920.1
        riding E919.8
      hand saw E920.1
      hand tool NEC E920.1
      hedge clipper E920.1
      household appliance or implement E920.2
      lawn mower (hand) E920.0
        riding E919.8
      rivet gun E920.1
      staple gun E920.1

Cut, cutting — *continued*
  by — *continued*
    rake E920.4
    saw
      circular E919.4
      hand E920.4
    scissors E920.4
    screwdriver E920.4
    sewing machine (electric) (powered) E920.2
      not powered E920.4
    shears E920.4
    shovel E920.4
    slide trigger mechanism, scope or other part of gun E928.7
    spade E920.4
    splinters E920.8
    sword E920.3
      in war operations E995.2
    tin can lid E920.8
    wood slivers E920.8
  homicide (attempt) E966
  inflicted by other person
    stated as
      intentional, homicidal E966
      undetermined whether accidental or intentional E986
  late effect of NEC E929.8
  legal
    execution E978
    intervention E974
  self-inflicted (unspecified whether accidental or intentional) E986
    stated as intentional, purposeful E956
  stated as undetermined whether accidental or intentional E986
  suicidal (attempt) E956
  terrorism E979.8
  war operations E995.2
Cyclone E908.1

D

Death due to injury occurring one year or more previous — *see* Late effect
Decapitation (accidental circumstances) NEC E928.9
  homicidal E966
  legal execution (by guillotine) E978
Deprivation — *see also* Privation
  homicidal intent E968.4
Derailment (accidental)
  railway (rolling stock) (train) (vehicle) (with subsequent collision) E802 ☑
    with
      collision (antecedent) (*see also* Collision, railway) E800 ☑
      explosion (subsequent) (without antecedent collision) E802 ☑
        antecedent collision E803 ☑
      fall (without collision (antecedent)) E802 ☑
      fire (without collision (antecedent)) E802 ☑
  street car E829 ☑
Descent
  parachute (voluntary) (without accident to aircraft) E844 ☑
    due to accident to aircraft — *see* categories E840-E842 ☑
Desertion
  child, with intent to injure or kill E968.4
  helpless person, infant, newborn E904.0
    with intent to injure or kill E968.4
Destitution — *see* Privation
Dirty bomb (*see also* War operations, injury due to, nuclear weapons) E996.9
Disability, late effect or sequela of injury — *see* Late effect
Disease
  Andes E902.0
  aviators' E902.1
  caisson E902.2
  range E902.0
Divers' disease, palsy, paralysis, squeeze E902.0

Dog bite E906.0
Dragged by
    cable car (not on rails) E847
        on rails E829 ☑
    motor vehicle (on highway) E814 ☑
        not on highway, nontraffic accident
           E825 ☑
    street car E829 ☑
Drinking poison (accidental) — *see* Table of
    Drugs and Chemicals
Drowning — *see* Submersion
Dust in eye E914

E

Earth falling (on) (with asphyxia or suffocation
    (by pressure)) — *see also* Suffocation,
    due to, cave-in E913.3
    as, or due to, a cataclysm (involving any
        transport vehicle) — *see* categories
        E908 ☑, E909 ☑
    not due to cataclysmic action E913.3
        motor vehicle (in motion) (on public
           highway) E813 ☑
           not on public highway E825 ☑
        nonmotor road vehicle NEC E829 ☑
        pedal cycle E826 ☑
        railway rolling stock, train, vehicle
           E806 ☑
        street car E829 ☑
        struck or crushed by E916
           with asphyxiation or suffocation
               E913.3
           with injury other than asphyxia, suf-
               focation E916
Earthquake (any injury) E909.0
Effect(s) (adverse) of
    air pressure E902.9
        at high altitude E902.9
           in aircraft E902.1
           residence or prolonged visit (causing
               conditions classifiable to
               E902.0) E902.0
        due to
           diving E902.2
           specified cause NEC E902.8
        in aircraft E902.1
    cold, excessive (exposure to) (*see also* Cold,
        exposure to) E901.9
    heat (excessive) (*see also* Heat) E900.9
    hot
        place — *see* Heat
        weather E900.0
    insulation — *see* Heat
    late — *see* Late effect of
    motion E903
    nuclear explosion or weapon
        in
           terrorism E979.5
           war operations (*see also* War opera-
               tions, injury due to, nuclear
               weapons) E996.9
    radiation — *see* Radiation
    terrorism, secondary E979.9
    travel E903
Electric shock, electrocution (accidental)
    (from exposed wire, faulty appliance,
    high voltage cable, live rail, open socket)
    (by) (in) E925.9
    appliance or wiring
        domestic E925.0
        factory E925.2
        farm (building) E925.8
           house E925.0
        home E925.0
        industrial (conductor) (control appara-
           tus) (transformer) E925.2
        outdoors E925.8
        public building E925.8
        residential institution E925.8
        school E925.8
        specified place NEC E925.8
    caused by other person
        stated as
           intentional, homicidal E968.8

Electric shock, electrocution — *continued*
    caused by other person — *continued*
        stated as — *continued*
           undetermined whether accidental or
               intentional E988.4
    electric power generating plant, distribution
        station E925.1
    electroshock gun (taser) (stun gun) E925.8
        caused by other person E968.8
        legal intervention E975
        stated as accidental E925.8
        stated as intentional E968.8
        due to legal intervention E975
        stated as intentional self-harm (suicidal
           attempt) E958.4
        stated as undetermined whether acciden-
           tal or intentional E988.4
        suicide (attempt) E958.4
    homicidal (attempt) E968.8
    legal execution E978
    lightning E907
    machinery E925.9
        domestic E925.0
        factory E925.2
        farm E925.8
        home E925.0
    misadventure in medical or surgical proce-
        dure
        in electroshock therapy E873.4
    self-inflicted (undetermined whether acci-
        dental or intentional) E988.4
        stated as intentional E958.4
        stated as undetermined whether accidental
           or intentional E988.4
    suicidal (attempt) E958.4
    transmission line E925.1
Electrocution — *see* Electric shock
Embolism
    air (traumatic) NEC — *see* Air, embolism
Encephalitis
    lead or saturnine E866.0
        from pesticide NEC E863.4
Entanglement
    in
        bedclothes, causing suffocation E913.0
        wheel of pedal cycle E826 ☑
Entry of foreign body, material, any — *see*
    Foreign body
Execution, legal (any method) E978
**Exertion, excessive physical, from pro-
    longed activity** E927.2
Exhaustion
    cold — *see* Cold, exposure to
    due to excessive exertion E927.2
    heat — *see* Heat
Explosion (accidental) (in) (of) (on) E923.9
    acetylene E923.2
    aerosol can E921.8
    aircraft (in transit) (powered) E841 ☑
        at landing, take-off E840 ☑
        in
           terrorism E979.1
           war operations
               from
                   enemy fire or explosive(s)
                      (device placed on air-
                      craft) E994.0
                  own onboard explosives
                      E994.1
        unpowered E842 ☑
    air tank (compressed) (in machinery) E921.1
    anesthetic gas in operating theatre E923.2
    automobile tire NEC E921.8
        causing transport accident — *see* cate-
           gories E810-E825 ☑
    blasting (cap) (materials) E923.1
    boiler (machinery), not on transport vehicle
        E921.0
        steamship — *see* Explosion, watercraft
    bomb E923.8
        in
           terrorism E979.2
           war operations E993.8
               after cessation of hostilities
                  E998.1

Explosion — *continued*
    bomb — *continued*
        in — *continued*
           war operations — *continued*
               atom, hydrogen or nuclear (*see
                  also* War operations, injury
                  due to, nuclear weapons)
                  E996.9
               injury by fragments from E991.9
                 antipersonnel bomb E991.3
    butane E923.2
    caused by
        other person
           stated as
               intentional, homicidal — *see* As-
                  sault, explosive
               undetermined whether acciden-
                  tal or homicidal E985.5
    coal gas E923.2
    detonator E923.1
    dynamite E923.1
    explosive (material) NEC E923.9
        gas(es) E923.2
        missile E923.8
           in
               terrorism E979.2
               war operations E993.1
                  injury by fragments from
                    E991.9
                    antipersonnel bomb
                      E991.3
        used in blasting operations E923.1
    fire-damp E923.2
    fireworks E923.0
    gas E923.2
        cylinder (in machinery) E921.1
        pressure tank (in machinery) E921.1
    gasoline (fumes) (tank) not in moving motor
        vehicle E923.2
    grain store (military) (munitions) E923.8
    grenade E923.8
        in
           terrorism E979.2
           war operations E993.8
               injury by fragments from E991.4
    homicide (attempt) — *see* Assault, explosive
    hot water heater, tank (in machinery) E921.0
    in mine (of explosive gases) NEC E923.2
    late effect of NEC E929.8
    machinery (*see also* Accident, machine)
        pressure vessel — *see* Explosion, pres-
           sure vessel
    methane E923.2
    missile E923.8
        in
           terrorism E979.2
           war operations E993.1
               injury by fragments from E991.4
    motor vehicle (part of)
        in motion (on public highway) E818 ☑
           not on public highway E825 ☑
    munitions (dump) (factory) E923.8
        in
           terrorism E979.2
           war operations E993.9
    of mine E923.8
        in
           terrorism
               at sea or in harbor E979.0
               land E979.2
               marine E979.0
           war operations
               after cessation of hostilities
                 E998.0
               at sea or in harbor E992.2
               land E993.8
                 after cessation of hostilities
                   E998.0
                 injury by fragments from
                    E991.4
               marine E992.2
    own weapons
        in
           terrorism (*see also* Suicide) E979.2
           war operations E993.7
               injury by fragments from E991.9

Explosion — *continued*
    own weapons — *continued*
        in — *continued*
           war operations — *continued*
               injury by fragments from — *con-
                 tinued*
                 antipersonnel bomb E991.3
    pressure
        cooker E921.8
        gas tank (in machinery) E921.1
        vessel (in machinery) E921.9
           on transport vehicle — *see* cate-
               gories E800-E848 ☑
           specified type NEC E921.8
    propane E923.2
    railway engine, locomotive, train (boiler)
        (with subsequent collision, derail-
        ment, fall) E803 ☑
        with
           collision (antecedent) (*see also* Colli-
               sion, railway) E800 ☑
           derailment (antecedent) E802 ☑
           fire (without antecedent collision or
               derailment) E803 ☑
    secondary fire resulting from — *see* Fire
    self-inflicted (unspecified whether acciden-
        tal or intentional) E985.5
        stated as intentional, purposeful E955.5
    shell (artillery) E923.8
        in
           terrorism E979.2
           war operations E993.2
               injury by fragments from E991.4
    stated as undetermined whether caused
        accidentally or purposely inflicted
        E985.5
    steam or water lines (in machinery) E921.0
    suicide (attempted) E955.5
    terrorism — *see* Terrorism, explosion
    torpedo E923.8
        in
           terrorism E979.0
           war operations E992.0
    transport accident — *see* categories
        E800-E848 ☑
    war operations — *see* War operations, ex-
        plosion
    watercraft (boiler) E837 ☑
        causing drowning, submersion (after
           jumping from watercraft) E830 ☑
Exposure (weather) (conditions) (rain) (wind)
    E904.3
    with homicidal intent E968.4
    environmental
        to
           algae bloom E928.6
           blue-green algae bloom E928.6
           brown tide E928.6
           cyanobacteria bloom E928.6
           Florida red tide E928.6
           harmful alage
               and toxins E928.6
               bloom E928.6
           pfiesteria piscicida E928.6
           red tide E928.6
    excessive E904.3
        cold (*see also* Cold, exposure to) E901.9
           self-inflicted — *see* Cold, exposure
               to, self-inflicted
        heat (*see also* Heat) E900.9
    helpless person, infant, newborn due to
        abandonment or neglect E904.0
    noise E928.1
    prolonged in deep-freeze unit or refrigerator
        E901.1
    radiation — *see* Radiation
    resulting from transport accident — *see*
        categories E800-E848 ☑
    smoke from, due to
        fire — *see* Fire
        tobacco, second-hand E869.4
    vibration E928.2
External cause status E000.9
    child assisting in compensated work of
        other family member E000.8

External cause status — *continued*
  civilian
    done for
      financial or other compensation
        E000.0
      pay or income E000.0
    family member assisting in compensated
      work of other family member E000.8
    for income E000.0
    hobby or leisure E000.8
    military E000.1
      off duty E000.8
    off duty military E000.8
    recreation E000.8
    specified NEC E000.8
    sport not for income E000.8
    student E000.8
    volunteer E000.2

F

Fallen on by
  animal (horse) (not being ridden) E906.8
    being ridden (in sport or transport)
      E828 ☑

Fall, falling (accidental) E888.9
  building E916
    burning E891.8
      private E890.8
  down
    escalator E880.0
    ladder E881.0
      in boat, ship, watercraft E833 ☑
    staircase E880.9
    stairs, steps — *see* Fall, from, stairs
  earth (with asphyxia or suffocation (by
    pressure)) (*see also* Earth, falling)
    E913.3
  from, off
    aircraft (at landing, take-off) (in-transit)
      (while alighting, boarding)
      E843 ☑
      resulting from accident to aircraft —
        see categories E840-E842 ☑
    animal-drawn vehicle E827 ☑
    animal (in sport or transport) E828 ☑
    balcony E882
    bed E884.4
    bicycle E826 ☑
    boat, ship, watercraft (into water)
      E832 ☑
      after accident to, collision, fire on
        E830 ☑
        and subsequently struck by (part
          of) boat E831 ☑
        and subsequently struck by (part of)
          while alighting, boat E831 ☑
      burning, crushed, sinking E830 ☑
        and subsequently struck by (part
          of) boat E831 ☑
    bridge E882
    building E882
      burning (uncontrolled fire) E891.8
        in terrorism E979.3
      private E890.8
    bunk in boat, ship, watercraft E834 ☑
      due to accident to watercraft
        E831 ☑
    cable car (not on rails) E847
      on rails E829 ☑
    car — *see* Fall from motor vehicle
    chair E884.2
    cliff E884.1
    commode E884.6
    curb (sidewalk) E880.1
    elevation aboard ship E834 ☑
      due to accident to ship E831 ☑
    embankment E884.9
    escalator E880.0
    fire escape E882
    flagpole E882
    furniture NEC E884.5
    gangplank (into water) (*see also* Fall,
      from, boat) E832 ☑
      to deck, dock E834 ☑
    hammock on ship E834 ☑

Fall, falling — *continued*
  from, off — *continued*
    hammock on ship — *continued*
      due to accident to watercraft
        E831 ☑
    haystack E884.9
    heelies E885.1
    high place E884.9
      stated as undetermined whether ac-
        cidental or intentional — *see*
        Jumping, from, high place
    horse (in sport or transport) E828 ☑
    in-line skates E885.1
    ladder E881.0
      in boat, ship, watercraft E833 ☑
        due to accident to watercraft
          E831 ☑
    machinery (*see also* Accident, machine)
      not in operation E884.9
    motorized
      mobility scooter E884.3
      wheelchair E884.3
    motor vehicle (in motion) (on public
      highway) E818 ☑
      not on public highway E825 ☑
        stationary, except while alighting,
          boarding, entering, leav-
          ing E884.9
        while alighting, boarding, enter-
          ing, leaving E824 ☑
      stationary, except while alighting,
        boarding, entering, leaving
        E884.9
      while alighting, boarding, entering,
        leaving, except off-road type
        motor vehicle E817 ☑
      off-road type — *see* Fall, from,
        off-road type motor vehi-
        cle
    nonmotor road vehicle (while alighting,
      boarding) NEC E829 ☑
      stationary, except while alighting,
        boarding, entering, leaving
        E884.9
    off road type motor vehicle (not on
      public highway) NEC E821 ☑
    on public highway E818 ☑
      while alighting, boarding, enter-
        ing, leaving E817 ☑
    snow vehicle — *see* Fall from snow
      vehicle, motor-driven
  one
    deck to another on ship E834 ☑
      due to accident to ship E831 ☑
    level to another NEC E884.9
      boat, ship, or watercraft E834 ☑
        due to accident to watercraft
          E831 ☑
    pedal cycle E826 ☑
    playground equipment E884.0
    railway rolling stock, train, vehicle (while
      alighting, boarding) E804 ☑
      with
        collision (*see also* Collision, rail-
          way) E800 ☑
        derailment (*see also* Derailment,
          railway) E802 ☑
        explosion (*see also* Explosion,
          railway engine) E803 ☑
    rigging (aboard ship) E834 ☑
      due to accident to watercraft
        E831 ☑
    roller skates E885.1
    scaffolding E881.1
    scooter (nonmotorized) E885.0
      motorized mobility E884.3
    sidewalk (curb) E880.1
      moving E885.9
    skateboard E885.2
    skis E885.3
    snowboard E885.4
    snow vehicle, motor-driven (not on
      public highway) E820 ☑
      on public highway E818 ☑

Fall, falling — *continued*
  from, off — *continued*
    snow vehicle, motor-driven — *contin-
      ued*
      on public highway — *continued*
        while alighting, boarding, enter-
          ing, leaving E817 ☑
    stairs, steps E880.9
      boat, ship, watercraft E833 ☑
        due to accident to watercraft
          E831 ☑
      motor bus, motor vehicle — *see* Fall,
        from, motor vehicle, while
        alighting, boarding
      street car E829 ☑
    stationary vehicle NEC E884.9
    stepladder E881.0
    street car (while boarding, alighting)
      E829 ☑
      stationary, except while boarding or
        alighting E884.9
    structure NEC E882
      burning (uncontrolled fire) E891.8
        in terrorism E979.3
    table E884.9
    toilet E884.6
    tower E882
    tree E884.9
    turret E882
    vehicle NEC (*see also* Accident, vehicle
      NEC)
      stationary E884.9
    viaduct E882
    wall E882
    wheelchair (electric) (motorized) E884.3
    wheelies E885.1
    window E882
  in, on
    aircraft (at landing, take-off) (in-transit)
      E843 ☑
      resulting from accident to aircraft —
        see categories E840-E842 ☑
    boat, ship, watercraft E835 ☑
      due to accident to watercraft
        E831 ☑
      one level to another NEC E834 ☑
      on ladder, stairs E833 ☑
    cutting or piercing instrument or ma-
      chine E888.0
    deck (of boat, ship, watercraft) E835 ☑
      due to accident to watercraft
        E831 ☑
    escalator E880.0
    gangplank E835 ☑
    glass, broken E888.0
    knife E888.0
    ladder E881.0
      in boat, ship, watercraft E833 ☑
        due to accident to watercraft
          E831 ☑
    object
      edged, pointed or sharp E888.0
      other E888.1
    pitchfork E888.0
    railway rolling stock, train, vehicle (while
      alighting, boarding) E804 ☑
      with
        collision (*see also* Collision, rail-
          way) E800 ☑
        derailment (*see also* Derailment,
          railway) E802 ☑
        explosion (see also Explosion,
          railway engine) E803 ☑
    scaffolding E881.1
    scissors E888.0
    staircase, stairs, steps (*see also* Fall, from,
      stairs) E880.9
    street car E829 ☑
    water transport (*see also* Fall, in, boat)
      E835 ☑
  into
    cavity E883.9
    dock E883.9
      from boat, ship, watercraft (*see also*
        Fall, from, boat) E832 ☑

Fall, falling — *continued*
  into — *continued*
    hold (of ship) E834 ☑
      due to accident to watercraft
        E831 ☑
    hole E883.9
    manhole E883.2
    moving part of machinery — *see* Acci-
      dent, machine
    opening in surface NEC E883.9
    pit E883.9
    quarry E883.9
    shaft E883.9
    storm drain E883.2
    tank E883.9
    water (with drowning or submersion)
      E910.9
    well E883.1
  late effect of NEC E929.3
  object (*see also* Hit by, object, falling) E916
  other E888.8
  over
    animal E885.9
    cliff E884.1
    embankment E884.9
    small object E885.9
  overboard (*see also* Fall, from, boat) E832 ☑
  resulting in striking against object E888.1
    sharp E888.0
  rock E916
  same level NEC E888.9
    aircraft (any kind) E843 ☑
      resulting from accident to aircraft —
        see categories E840-E842 ☑
    boat, ship, watercraft E835 ☑
      due to accident to, collision, water-
        craft E831 ☑
    from
      collision, pushing, shoving, by or
        with other person(s) E886.9
        as, or caused by, a crowd E917.6
        in sports E886.0
      in-line skates E885.1
      roller skates E885.1
      scooter (nonmotorized) E885.0
      skateboard E885.2
      slipping stumbling, tripping E885 ☑
      snowboard E885.4
  snowslide E916
    as avalanche E909.2
  stone E916
  through
    hatch (on ship) E834 ☑
      due to accident to watercraft
        E831 ☑
    roof E882
    window E882
  timber E916
  while alighting from, boarding, entering,
    leaving
    aircraft (any kind) E843 ☑
    motor bus, motor vehicle — *see* Fall,
      from, motor vehicle, while
      alighting, boarding
    nonmotor road vehicle NEC E829 ☑
    railway train E804 ☑
    street car E829 ☑
Fell or jumped from high place, so stated —
  see Jumping, from, high place
Felo-de-se — *see also* Suicide E958.9
Fever
  heat — *see* Heat
  thermic — *see* Heat
Fight (hand) (fist) (foot) — *see also* Assault,
  fight E960.0
Fire (accidental) (caused by great heat from
  appliance (electrical), hot object or hot
  substance) (secondary, resulting from
  explosion) E899
  conflagration — *see* Conflagration
  controlled, normal (in brazier, fireplace,
    furnace, or stove) (charcoal) (coal)
    (coke) (electric) (gas) (wood)
    bonfire E897
    brazier, not in building or structure E89?

☑ **Additional Digit Required** — Refer to the Tabular List for Digit Selection   🔺 **Subterms under main terms may continue to next column or page**

342 — Volume 2   ▶◀ **Revised Text**   ● **New Line**   ▲ **Revised Code**   **2014 ICD-9-CM**

Fire, hot object or hot substance — *continued*
  controlled, normal — *continued*
    in building or structure, except private dwelling (barn) (church) (convalescent or residential home) (factory) (farm outbuilding) (hospital) (hotel) (institution (educational) (dormitory) (residential) (private garage) (school) (shop) (store) (theatre) E896
    in private dwelling (apartment) (boarding house) (camping place) (caravan) (farmhouse) (home (private)) (house) (lodging house) (rooming house) (tenement) E895
    not in building or structure E897
    trash E897
  forest (uncontrolled) E892
  grass (uncontrolled) E892
  hay (uncontrolled) E892
  homicide (attempt) E968.0
    late effect of E969
  in, on, starting in E892
    aircraft (in transit) (powered) E841 ☑
      at landing, take-off E840 ☑
      stationary E892
      unpowered (balloon) (glider) E842 ☑
    balloon E842 ☑
    boat, ship, watercraft — *see* categories E830 ☑, E831 ☑, E837 ☑
    building or structure, except private dwelling (barn) (church) (convalescent or residential home) (factory) (farm outbuilding) (hospital) (hotel) (institution (educational) (dormitory) (residential) (private garage) (school) (shop) (store) (theatre) (*see also* Conflagration, building or structure, except private dwelling) E891.9
    forest (uncontrolled) E892
    glider E842 ☑
    grass (uncontrolled) E892
    hay (uncontrolled) E892
    lumber (uncontrolled) E892
    machinery — *see* Accident, machine
    mine (uncontrolled) E892
    motor vehicle (in motion) (on public highway) E818 ☑
      not on public highway E825 ☑
      stationary E892
    prairie (uncontrolled) E892
    private dwelling (apartment) (boarding house) (camping place) (caravan) (farmhouse) (home (private)) (house) (lodging house) (private garage) (rooming house) (tenement) (*see also* Conflagration, private dwelling) E890.9
    railway rolling stock, train, vehicle (*see also* Explosion, railway engine) E803 ☑
      stationary E892
    room NEC E898.1
    street car (in motion) E829 ☑
      stationary E892
    terrorism (by fire-producing device) E979.3
      fittings or furniture (burning building) (uncontrolled fire) E979.3
      from nuclear explosion E979.5
    transport vehicle, stationary NEC E892
    tunnel (uncontrolled) E892
    war operations (by fire-producing device or conventional weapon) E990.9
      from nuclear explosion (*see also* War operations, injury due to, nuclear weapons) E996.2
      incendiary bomb E990.0
      petrol bomb E990.0
  late effect of NEC E929.4
  lumber (uncontrolled) E892
  mine (uncontrolled) E892
  prairie (uncontrolled) E892

Fire, hot object or hot substance — *continued*
  self-inflicted (unspecified whether accidental or intentional) E988.1
    stated as Intentional, purposeful E958.1
  specified NEC E898.1
    with
      conflagration — *see* Conflagration
      ignition (of)
        clothing — *see* Ignition, clothes
        highly inflammable material (benzine) (fat) (gasoline) (kerosene) (paraffin) (petrol) E894
  started by other person
    stated as
      with intent to injure or kill E968.0
      undetermined whether or not with intent to injure or kill E988.1
  suicide (attempted) E958.1
    late effect of E959
  tunnel (uncontrolled) E892
Fireball effects from nuclear explosion
  in
    terrorism E979.5
    war operations (*see also* War operations, injury due to, nuclear weapons) E996.2
Fireworks (explosion) E923.0
Flash burns from explosion — *see also* Explosion E923.9
Flood (any injury) (resulting from storm) E908.2
  caused by collapse of dam or manmade structure E909.3
Forced landing (aircraft) E840 ☑
Foreign body, object or material (entrance into) (accidental)
  air passage (causing injury) E915
    with asphyxia, obstruction, suffocation E912
      food or vomitus E911
    nose (with asphyxia, obstruction, suffocation) E912
      causing injury without asphyxia, obstruction, suffocation E915
  alimentary canal (causing injury) (with obstruction) E915
    with asphyxia, obstruction respiratory passage, suffocation E912
      food E911
    mouth E915
      with asphyxia, obstruction, suffocation E912
        food E911
    pharynx E915
      with asphyxia, obstruction, suffocation E912
        food E911
  aspiration (with asphyxia, obstruction respiratory passage, suffocation) E912
    causing injury without asphyxia, obstruction respiratory passage, suffocation E915
    food (regurgitated) (vomited) E911
      causing injury without asphyxia, obstruction respiratory passage, suffocation E915
    mucus (not of newborn) E912
    phlegm E912
  bladder (causing injury or obstruction) E915
  bronchus, bronchi — *see* Foreign body, air passages
  conjunctival sac E914
  digestive system — *see* Foreign body, alimentary canal
  ear (causing injury or obstruction) E915
  esophagus (causing injury or obstruction) (*see also* Foreign body, alimentary canal) E915
  eye (any part) E914
  eyelid E914
  hairball (stomach) (with obstruction) E915
  ingestion — *see* Foreign body, alimentary canal
  inhalation — *see* Foreign body, aspiration

Foreign body, object or material — *continued*
  intestine (causing injury or obstruction) E915
  iris E914
  lacrimal apparatus E914
  larynx — *see* Foreign body, air passage
  late effect of NEC E929.8
  lung — *see* Foreign body, air passage
  mouth — *see* Foreign body, alimentary canal, mouth
  nasal passage — *see* Foreign body, air passage, nose
  nose — *see* Foreign body, air passage, nose
  ocular muscle E914
  operation wound (left in) — *see* Misadventure, foreign object
  orbit E914
  pharynx — *see* Foreign body, alimentary canal, pharynx
  rectum (causing injury or obstruction) E915
  stomach (hairball) (causing injury or obstruction) E915
  tear ducts or glands E914
  trachea — *see* Foreign body, air passage
  urethra (causing injury or obstruction) E915
  vagina (causing injury or obstruction) E915
Found dead, injured
  from exposure (to) — *see* Exposure
  on
    public highway E819 ☑
    railway right of way E807 ☑
Fracture (circumstances unknown or unspecified) E887
  due to specified external means — *see* manner of accident
  late effect of NEC E929.3
  occurring in water transport NEC E835 ☑
Freezing — *see* Cold, exposure to
Frostbite E901.0
  due to manmade conditions E901.1
Frozen — *see* Cold, exposure to

G

Garrotting, homicidal (attempted) E963
Gored E906.8
Gunshot wound — *see also* Shooting E922.9

H

Hailstones, injury by E904.3
Hairball (stomach) (with obstruction) E915
Hanged himself — *see also* Hanging, self-inflicted E983.0
Hang gliding E842 ☑
Hanging (accidental) E913.8
  caused by other person
    in accidental circumstances E913.8
    stated as
      intentional, homicidal E963
      undetermined whether accidental or intentional E983.0
  homicide (attempt) E963
  in bed or cradle E913.0
  legal execution E978
  self-inflicted (unspecified whether accidental or intentional) E983.0
    in accidental circumstances E913.8
    stated as intentional, purposeful E953.0
    stated as undetermined whether accidental or intentional E983.0
  suicidal (attempt) E953.0
Heat (apoplexy) (collapse) (cramps) (effects of) (excessive) (exhaustion) (fever) (prostration) (stroke) E900.9
  due to
    manmade conditions (as listed in E900.1, except boat, ship, watercraft) E900.1
    weather (conditions) E900.0
  from
    electric heating appartus causing burning E924.8
    nuclear explosion
      in
        terrorism E979.5

Heat — *continued*
  from — *continued*
    nuclear explosion — *continued*
      in — *continued*
        war operations (*see also* War operations, injury due to, nuclear weapons) E996.2
    generated in, boiler, engine, evaporator, fire room of boat, ship, watercraft E838 ☑
    inappropriate in local application or packing in medical or surgical procedure E873.5
  late effect of NEC E989
Hemorrhage
  delayed following medical or surgical treatment without mention of misadventure — *see* Reaction, abnormal
  during medical or surgical treatment as misadventure — *see* Misadventure, cut
High
  altitude, effects E902.9
  level of radioactivity, effects — *see* Radiation
  pressure effects (*see also* Effects of, air pressure)
    from rapid descent in water (causing caisson or divers' disease, palsy, or paralysis) E902.2
  temperature, effects — *see* Heat
Hit, hitting (accidental) by
  aircraft (propeller) (without accident to aircraft) E844 ☑
    unpowered E842 ☑
  avalanche E909.2
  being thrown against object in or part of motor vehicle (in motion) (on public highway) E818 ☑
    not on public highway E825 ☑
    nonmotor road vehicle NEC E829 ☑
    street car E829 ☑
  boat, ship, watercraft
    after fall from watercraft E838 ☑
      damaged, involved in accident E831 ☑
    while swimming, water skiing E838 ☑
  bullet (*see also* Shooting) E922.9
    from air gun E922.4
    in
      terrorism E979.4
      war operations E991.2
        rubber E991.0
  flare, Verey pistol (*see also* Shooting) E922.8
  hailstones E904.3
  landslide E909.2
  law-enforcing agent (on duty) E975
    with blunt object (baton) (night stick) (stave) (truncheon) E973
  machine — *see* Accident, machine
  missile
    firearm (*see also* Shooting) E922.9
    in
      terrorism — *see* Terrorism, missile
      war operations — *see* War operations, missile
  motor vehicle (on public highway) (traffic accident) E814 ☑
    not on public highway, nontraffic accident E822 ☑
  nonmotor road vehicle NEC E829 ☑
  object
    falling E916
      from, in, on
        aircraft E844 ☑
          due to accident to aircraft — *see* categories E840-E842 ☑
          unpowered E842 ☑
        boat, ship, watercraft E838 ☑
          due to accident to watercraft E831 ☑
        building E916
          burning (uncontrolled fire) E891.8
          in terrorism E979.3

☑ Additional Digit Required — Refer to the Tabular List for Digit Selection
Ⓦ Subterms under main terms may continue to next column or page

Hit, hitting by — *continued*
  object — *continued*
    falling — *continued*
      from, in, on — *continued*
        building — *continued*
          burning — *continued*
            private E890.8
      cataclysmic
        earth surface movement or
          eruption E909.9
        storm E908.9
      cave-in E916
        with asphyxiation or suffoca-
          tion (*see also* Suffoca-
          tion, due to, cave-in)
          E913.3
      earthquake E909.0
      motor vehicle (in motion) (on
        public highway) E818 ☑
        not on public highway
          E825 ☑
        stationary E916
      nonmotor road vehicle NEC
        E829 ☑
      pedal cycle E826 ☑
      railway rolling stock, train, vehicle
        E806 ☑
      street car E829 ☑
      structure, burning NEC E891.8
      vehicle, stationary E916
    moving NEC — *see* Striking against, ob-
      ject
    projected NEC — *see* Striking against,
      object
    set in motion by
      compressed air or gas, spring, strik-
        ing, throwing — *see* Striking
        against, object
      explosion — *see* Explosion
    thrown into, on, or towards
      motor vehicle (in motion) (on public
        highway) E818 ☑
        not on public highway E825 ☑
      nonmotor road vehicle NEC E829 ☑
      pedal cycle E826 ☑
      street car E829 ☑
  off-road type motor vehicle (not on public
    highway) E821 ☑
    on public highway E814 ☑
  other person(s) E917.9
    with blunt or thrown object E917.9
      in sports E917.0
        with subsequent fall E917.5
      intentionally, homicidal E968.2
    as, or caused by, a crowd E917.1
      with subsequent fall E917.6
    in sports E917.0
  pedal cycle E826 ☑
  police (on duty) E975
    with blunt object (baton) (nightstick)
      (stave) (truncheon) E973
  railway, rolling stock, train, vehicle (part of)
    E805 ☑
  shot — *see* Shooting
  snow vehicle, motor-driven (not on public
    highway) E820 ☑
    on public highway E814 ☑
  street car E829 ☑
  vehicle NEC — *see* Accident, vehicle NEC
Homicide, homicidal (attempt) (justifiable) —
  see also Assault E968.9
Hot
  liquid, object, substance, accident caused
    by (*see also* Accident, caused by, hot,
    by type of substance)
    late effect of E929.8
  place, effects — *see* Heat
  weather, effects E900.0
Humidity, causing problem E904.3
Hunger E904.1
  resulting from
    abandonment or neglect E904.0
    transport accident — *see* categories
      E800–E848 ☑
Hurricane (any injury) E908.0

Hypobarism, hypobaropathy — *see* Effects
  of, air pressure
Hypothermia — *see* Cold, exposure to

I

Ictus
  caloris — *see* Heat
  solaris E900.0
Ignition (accidental)
  anesthetic gas in operating theatre E923.2
  bedclothes
    with
      conflagration — *see* Conflagration
      ignition (of)
        clothing — *see* Ignition, clothes
        highly inflammable material
          (benzine) (fat) (gasoline)
          (kerosene) (paraffin)
          (petrol) E894
  benzine E894
  clothes, clothing (from controlled fire) (in
    building) E893.9
    with conflagration — *see* Conflagration
    from
      bonfire E893.2
      highly inflammable material E894
      sources or material as listed in E893.8
      trash fire E893.2
      uncontrolled fire — *see* Conflagra-
        tion
    in
      private dwelling E893.0
      specified building or structure, ex-
        cept private dwelling E893.1
      not in building or structure E893.2
  explosive material — *see* Explosion
  fat E894
  gasoline E894
  kerosene E894
  material
    explosive — *see* Explosion
    highly inflammable E894
      with conflagration — *see* Conflagra-
        tion
      with explosion E923.2
    nightdress — *see* Ignition, clothes
  paraffin E894
  petrol E894
Immersion — *see* Submersion
Implantation of quills of porcupine E906.8
Inanition (from) E904.9
  hunger — *see* Lack of, food
    resulting from homicidal intent E968.4
  thirst — *see* Lack of, water
Inattention after, at birth E904.0
  homicidal, infanticidal intent E968.4
Infanticide — *see also* Assault
Ingestion
  foreign body (causing injury) (with obstruc-
    tion) — *see* Foreign body, alimentary
    canal
  poisonous substance NEC — *see* Table of
    Drugs and Chemicals
Inhalation
  excessively cold substance, manmade
    E901.1
  foreign body — *see* Foreign body, aspiration
  liquid air, hydrogen, nitrogen E901.1
  mucus, not of newborn (with asphyxia, ob-
    struction respiratory passage, suffo-
    cation) E912
  phlegm (with asphyxia, obstruction respira-
    tory passage, suffocation) E912
  poisonous gas — *see* Table of Drugs and
    Chemicals
  smoke from, due to
    fire — *see* Fire
    tobacco, second-hand E869.4
  vomitus (with asphyxia, obstruction respira-
    tory passage, suffocation) E911
Injury, injured (accidental(ly)) NEC E928.9
  by, caused by, from
    air rifle (BB gun) E922.4
    animal (not being ridden) NEC E906.9
      being ridden (in sport or transport)
        E828 ☑

Injury, injured — *continued*
  by, caused by, from — *continued*
    assault (*see also* Assault) E968.9
    avalanche E909.2
    bayonet (*see also* Bayonet wound)
      E920.3
    being thrown against some part of, or
      object in
      motor vehicle (in motion) (on public
        highway) E818 ☑
        not on public highway E825 ☑
      nonmotor road vehicle NEC E829 ☑
      off-road motor vehicle NEC E821 ☑
      railway train E806 ☑
      snow vehicle, motor-driven E820 ☑
      street car E829 ☑
    bending
      due to
        repetitive movement E927.3
        sudden strenuous movement
          E927.0
    bite, human E928.3
    broken glass E920.8
    bullet — *see* Shooting
    cave-in (*see also* Suffocation, due to,
      cave-in) E913.3
      without asphyxiation or suffocation
        E916
      earth surface movement or eruption
        E909.9
      storm E908.9
    cloudburst E908.8
    component of firearm or air gun E928.7
    cutting or piercing instrument (*see also*
      Cut) E920.9
    cyclone E908.1
    earthquake E909.0
    earth surface movement or eruption
      E909.9
    electric current (*see also* Electric shock)
      E925.9
    explosion (*see also* Explosion) E923.9
      of gun part E928.7
    fire — *see* Fire
    flare, Verey pistol E922.8
    flood E908.2
    foreign body — *see* Foreign body
    gun recoil E928.7
    hailstones E904.3
    hurricane E908.0
    landslide E909.2
    law-enforcing agent, police, in course of
      legal intervention — *see* Legal
      intervention
    lightning E907
    live rail or live wire — *see* Electric shock
    machinery (*see also* Accident, machine)
      aircraft, without accident to aircraft
        E844 ☑
      boat, ship, watercraft (deck) (engine
        room) (galley) (laundry)
        (loading) E836 ☑
    mechanism of firearm or air gun E928.7
    missile
      explosive E923.8
      firearm — *see* Shooting
      in
        terrorism — *see* Terrorism, mis-
          sile
        war operations — *see* War opera-
          tions, missile
    moving part of motor vehicle (in motion)
      (on public highway) E818 ☑
      not on public highway, nontraffic
        accident E825 ☑
      while alighting, boarding, entering,
        leaving — *see* Fall, from, mo-
        tor vehicle, while alighting,
        boarding
    nail E920.8
    needle (sewing) E920.4
      hypodermic E920.5
    noise E928.1

Injury, injured — *continued*
  by, caused by, from — *continued*
    object
      fallen on
        motor vehicle (in motion) (on
          public highway) E818 ☑
          not on public highway
            E825 ☑
      falling — *see* Hit by, object, falling
      paintball gun E922.5
      radiation — *see* Radiation
      railway rolling stock, train, vehicle (part
        of) E805 ☑
        door or window E806 ☑
      recoil of firearm E928.7
      rotating propeller, aircraft E844 ☑
      rough landing of off-road type motor
        vehicle (after leaving ground or
        rough terrain) E821 ☑
      snow vehicle E820 ☑
      saber (*see also* Wound, saber) E920.3
      shot — *see* Shooting
      sound waves E928.1
      splinter or sliver, wood E920.8
      straining
        due to
          repetitive movement E927.3
          sudden strenuous movement
            E927.0
      street car (door) E829 ☑
      suicide (attempt) E958.9
      sword E920.3
      terrorism — *see* Terrorism
      third rail — *see* Electric shock
      thunderbolt E907
      tidal wave E909.4
        caused by storm E908.0
      tornado E908.1
      torrential rain E908.2
      twisting
        due to
          repetitive movement E927.3
          sudden strenuous movement
            E927.0
      vehicle NEC — *see* Accident, vehicle NEC
      vibration E928.2
      volcanic eruption E909.1
      weapon burst, in war operations E993.9
      weightlessness (in spacecraft, real or
        simulated) E928.0
      wood splinter or sliver E920.8
    due to
      civil insurrection — *see* War operations
        occurring after cessation of hostilities
          E998.9
      terrorism — *see* Terrorism
      war operations — *see* War operations
        occurring after cessation of hostilities
          E998.9
      weapon of mass destruction [WMD]
        E997.3
    homicidal (*see also* Assault) E968.9
    inflicted (by)
      in course of arrest (attempted), suppres-
        sion of disturbance, maintenance
        of order, by law enforcing agents
        — *see* Legal intervention
      law-enforcing agent (on duty) — *see*
        Legal intervention
      other person
        stated as
          accidental E928.9
          homicidal, intentional — *see* As-
            sault
          undetermined whether acciden-
            tal or intentional — *see*
            Injury, stated as undeter-
            mined
      police (on duty) — *see* Legal interven-
        tion
    in, on
      civil insurrection — *see* War operations
      fight E960.0
      parachute descent (voluntary) (without
        accident to aircraft) E844 ☑

☑ **Additional Digit Required** — Refer to the Tabular List for Digit Selection   ▽ **Subterms under main terms may continue to next column or page**

Injury, injured — *continued*
  in, on — *continued*
    parachute descent — *continued*
      with accident to aircraft — *see* categories E840-E842 ☑
    public highway E819 ☑
    railway right of way E807 ☑
    terrorism — *see* Terrorism
    war operations — *see* War operations
  late effect of E929.9
  purposely (inflicted) by other person(s) — *see* Assault
  self-inflicted (unspecified whether accidental or intentional) E988.9
    stated as
      accidental E928.9
      intentionally, purposely E958.9
  specified cause NEC E928.8
  stated as
    hanging E983.0
    knife E986
    late effect of E989
    puncture (any part of body) E986
    shooting — *see* Shooting, stated as undetermined whether accidental or intentional
    specified means NEC E988.8
    stab (any part of body) E986
    strangulation — *see* Suffocation, stated as undetermined whether accidental or intentional
    submersion E984
    suffocation — *see* Suffocation, stated as undetermined whether accidental or intentional
  undetermined whether accidentally or purposely inflicted (by) E988.9
    cut (any part of body) E986
    cutting or piercing instrument (classifiable to E920) E986
    drowning E984
    explosive(s) (missile) E985.5
    falling from high place E987.9
      manmade structure, except residential E987.1
      natural site E987.2
      residential premises E987.0
  to child due to criminal abortion E968.8

Insufficient nourishment — *see also* Lack of, food
  homicidal intent E968.4
Insulation, effects — *see* Heat
Interruption of respiration by
  food lodged in esophagus E911
  foreign body, except food, in esophagus E912
Intervention, legal — *see* Legal intervention
Intoxication, drug or poison — *see* Table of Drugs and Chemicals
Irradiation — *see* Radiation

Jammed (accidentally)
  between objects (moving) (stationary and moving) E918
  in object E918
Jumped or fell from high place, so stated — *see* Jumping, from, high place, stated as in undetermined circumstances
Jumping
  before train, vehicle or other moving object (unspecified whether accidental or intentional) E988.0
    stated as
      intentional, purposeful E958.0
      suicidal (attempt) E958.0
  from
    aircraft
      by parachute (voluntarily) (without accident to aircraft) E844 ☑
      due to accident to aircraft — *see* categories E840-E842 ☑
    boat, ship, watercraft (into water)
      after accident to, fire on, watercraft E830 ☑

Jumping — *continued*
  from — *continued*
    boat, ship, watercraft — *continued*
      after accident to, fire on, watercraft — *continued*
        and subsequently struck by (part of) boat E831 ☑
      burning, crushed, sinking E830 ☑
        and subsequently struck by (part of) boat E831 ☑
      voluntarily, without accident (to boat) with injury other than drowning or submersion E883.0
    building (*see also* Jumping, from, high place)
      burning (uncontrolled fire) E891.8
        in terrorism E979.3
        private E890.8
    cable car (not on rails) E847
      on rails E829 ☑
    high place
      in accidental circumstances or in sport — *see* categories E880-E884 ☑
      stated as
        with intent to injure self E957.9
          man-made structures NEC E957.1
          natural sites E957.2
          residential premises E957.0
        in undetermined circumstances E987.9
          man-made structures NEC E987.1
          natural sites E987.2
          residential premises E987.0
        suicidal (attempt) E957.9
          man-made structures NEC E957.1
          natural sites E957.1
          residential premises E957.0
    motor vehicle (in motion) (on public highway) — *see* Fall, from, motor vehicle
    nonmotor road vehicle NEC E829 ☑
    street car E829 ☑
    structure (*see also* Jumping, from, high place)
      burning NEC (uncontrolled fire) E891.8
        in terrorism E979.3
  into water
    with injury other than drowning or submersion E883.0
    drowning or submersion — *see* Submersion
  from, off, watercraft — *see* Jumping, from, boat
Justifiable homicide — *see* Assault

Kicked by
  animal E906.8
  person(s) (accidentally) E917.9
    with intent to injure or kill E960.0
    as, or caused by a crowd E917.1
      with subsequent fall E917.6
    in fight E960.0
    in sports E917.0
      with subsequent fall E917.5
Kicking against
  object (moving) E917.9
    in sports E917.0
      with subsequent fall E917.5
    stationary E917.4
      with subsequent fall E917.8
  person — *see* Striking against, person
Killed, killing (accidentally) NEC — *see also* Injury E928.9
  in
    action — *see* War operations
    brawl, fight (hand) (fists) (foot) E960.0
    by weapon (*see also* Assault)
      cutting, piercing E966
      firearm — *see* Shooting, homicide

Killed, killing — *see also* Injury — *continued*
  self
    stated as
      accident E928.9
      suicide — *see* Suicide
    unspecified whether accidental or suicidal E988.9
Knocked down (accidentally) (by) NEC E928.9
  animal (not being ridden) E906.8
    being ridden (in sport or transport) E828 ☑
  blast from explosion (*see also* Explosion) E923.9
  crowd, human stampede E917.6
  late effect of — *see* Late effect
  person (accidentally) E917.9
    in brawl, fight E960.0
    in sports E917.5
  transport vehicle — *see* vehicle involved under Hit by
  while boxing E917.5

Laceration NEC E928.9
Lack of
  air (refrigerator or closed place), suffocation by E913.2
  care (helpless person) (infant) (newborn) E904.0
    homicidal intent E968.4
  food except as result of transport accident E904.1
    helpless person, infant, newborn due to abandonment or neglect E904.0
  water except as result of transport accident E904.2
    helpless person, infant, newborn due to abandonment or neglect E904.0
Landslide E909.2
  falling on, hitting
    motor vehicle (any) (in motion) (on or off public highway) E909.2
    railway rolling stock, train, vehicle E909.2
Late effect of
  accident NEC (accident classifiable to E928.9) E929.9
    specified NEC (accident classifiable to E9I0–E928.8) E929.8
  assault E969
  fall, accidental (accident classifiable to E880–E888) E929.3
  fire, accident caused by (accident classifiable to E890–E899) E929.4
  homicide, attempt (any means) E969
  injury due to terrorism E999.1
  injury undetermined whether accidentally or purposely inflicted (injury classifiable to E980–E988) E989
  legal intervention (injury classifiable to E970–E976) E977
  medical or surgical procedure, test or therapy
    as, or resulting in, or from
      abnormal or delayed reaction or complication — *see* Reaction, abnormal
      misadventure — *see* Misadventure
  motor vehicle accident (accident classifiable to E810–E825) E929.0
  natural or environmental factor, accident due to (accident classifiable to E900–E909) E929.5
  poisoning, accidental (accident classifiable to E850–E858, E860–E869) E929.2
  suicide, attempt (any means) E959
  transport accident NEC (accident classifiable to E800–E807, E826–E838, E840–E848) E929.1
  war operations, injury due to (injury classifiable to E990–E998) E999.0
Launching pad accident E845 ☑
Legal
  execution, any method E978
  intervention (by) (injury from) E976
    baton E973

Legal — *continued*
  intervention — *continued*
    bayonet E974
    blow E975
    blunt object (baton) (nightstick) (stave) (truncheon) E973
    cutting or piercing instrument E974
    dynamite E971
    execution, any method E973
    explosive(s) (shell) E971
    firearm(s) E970
    gas (asphyxiation) (poisoning) (tear) E972
    grenade E971
    late effect of E977
    machine gun E970
    manhandling E975
    mortar bomb E971
    nightstick E973
    revolver E970
    rifle E970
    specified means NEC E975
    stabbing E974
    stave E973
    truncheon E973
Lifting, injury
  due to
    repetitive movement E927.3
    sudden strenuous movement E927.0
Lightning (shock) (stroke) (struck by) E907
Liquid (noncorrosive) in eye E914
  corrosive E924.1
Loss of control
  motor vehicle (on public highway) (without antecedent collision) E816 ☑
    with
      antecedent collision on public highway — *see* Collision, motor vehicle
      involving any object, person or vehicle not on public highway E816 ☑
    not on public highway, nontraffic accident E825 ☑
      with antecedent collision — *see* Collision, motor vehicle, not on public highway
    on public highway — *see* Collision, motor vehicle
    off-road type motor vehicle (not on public highway) E821 ☑
      on public highway — *see* Loss of control, motor vehicle
    snow vehicle, motor-driven (not on public highway) E820 ☑
      on public highway — *see* Loss of control, motor vehicle
Lost at sea E832 ☑
  with accident to watercraft E830 ☑
  in war operations E995.8
Low
  pressure, effects — *see* Effects of, air pressure
  temperature, effects — *see* Cold, exposure to
Lying before train, vehicle or other moving object (unspecified whether accidental or intentional) E988.0
  stated as intentional, purposeful, suicidal (attempt) E958.0
Lynching — *see also* Assault E968.9

Malfunction, atomic power plant in water transport E838 ☑
Mangled (accidentally) NEC E928.9
Manhandling (in brawl, fight) E960.0
  legal intervention E975
Manslaughter (nonaccidental) — *see* Assault
Marble in nose E912
Mauled by animal E906.8
Medical procedure, complication of
  delayed or as an abnormal reaction without mention of misadventure — *see* Reaction, abnormal

Medical procedure, complication of — *continued*
  due to or as a result of misadventure — *see* Misadventure
Melting of fittings and furniture in burning
  in terrorism E979.3
Minamata disease E865.2
Misadventure(s) to patient(s) during surgical or medical care E876.9
  contaminated blood, fluid, drug or biological substance (presence of agents and toxins as listed in E875) E875.9
    administered (by) NEC E875.9
      infusion E875.0
      injection E875.1
      specified means NEC E875.2
      transfusion E875.0
      vaccination E875.1
  cut, cutting, puncture, perforation or hemorrhage (accidental) (inadvertent) (inappropriate) (during) E870.9
    aspiration of fluid or tissue (by puncture or catheterization, except heart) E870.5
    biopsy E870.8
      needle (aspirating) E870.5
    blood sampling E870.5
    catheterization E870.5
      heart E870.6
    dialysis (kidney) E870.2
    endoscopic examination E870.4
    enema E870.7
    infusion E870.1
    injection E870.3
    lumbar puncture E870.5
    needle biopsy E870.5
    paracentesis, abdominal E870.5
    perfusion E870.2
    specified procedure NEC E870.8
    surgical operation E870.0
    thoracentesis E870.5
    transfusion E870.1
    vaccination E870.3
  excessive amount of blood or other fluid during transfusion or infusion E873.0
  failure
    in dosage E873.9
      electroshock therapy E873.4
      inappropriate temperature (too hot or too cold) in local application and packing E873.5
      infusion
        excessive amount of fluid E873.0
        incorrect dilution of fluid E873.1
      insulin-shock therapy E873.4
      nonadministration of necessary drug or medicinal E873.6
      overdose (*see also* Overdose)
        radiation, in therapy E873.2
      radiation
        inadvertent exposure of patient (receiving radiation for test or therapy) E873.3
        not receiving radiation for test or therapy — *see* Radiation
        overdose E873.2
      specified procedure NEC E873.8
      transfusion
        excessive amount of blood E873.0
    mechanical, of instrument or apparatus (during procedure) E874.9
      aspiration of fluid or tissue (by puncture or catheterization, except of heart) E874.4
      biopsy E874.8
        needle (aspirating) E874.4
      blood sampling E874.4
      catheterization E874.4
        heart E874.5
      dialysis (kidney) E874.2
      endoscopic examination E874.3
      enema E874.8
      infusion E874.1
      injection E874.8
      lumbar puncture E874.4

Misadventure(s) to patient(s) during surgical or medical care — *continued*
  failure — *continued*
    mechanical, of instrument or apparatus — *continued*
      needle biopsy E874.4
      paracentesis, abdominal E874.4
      perfusion E874.2
      specified procedure NEC E874.8
      surgical operation E874.0
      thoracentesis E874.4
      transfusion E874.1
      vaccination E874.8
    sterile precautions (during procedure) E872.9
      aspiration of fluid or tissue (by puncture or catheterization, except heart) E872.5
      biopsy E872.8
        needle (aspirating) E872.5
      blood sampling E872.5
      catheterization E872.5
        heart E872.6
      dialysis (kidney) E872.2
      endoscopic examination E872.4
      enema E872.8
      infusion E872.1
      injection E872.3
      lumbar puncture E872.5
      needle biopsy E872.5
      paracentesis, abdominal E872.5
      perfusion E872.2
      removal of catheter or packing E872.5
      specified procedure NEC E872.8
      surgical operation E872.0
      thoracentesis E872.5
      transfusion E872.1
      vaccination E872.3
    suture or ligature during surgical procedure E876.2
    to introduce or to remove tube or instrument E876.4
    foreign object left in body — *see* Misadventure, foreign object
  foreign object left in body (during procedure) E871.9
    aspiration of fluid or tissue (by puncture or catheterization, except heart) E871.5
    biopsy E871.8
      needle (aspirating) E871.5
    blood sampling E871.5
    catheterization E871.5
      heart E871.6
    dialysis (kidney) E871.2
    endoscopic examination E871.4
    enema E871.8
    infusion E871.1
    injection E871.3
    lumbar puncture E871.5
    needle biopsy E871.5
    paracentesis, abdominal E871.5
    perfusion E871.2
    removal of catheter or packing E871.7
    specified procedure NEC E871.8
    surgical operation E871.0
    thoracentesis E871.5
    transfusion E871.1
    vaccination E871.3
  hemorrhage — *see* Misadventure, cut
  inadvertent exposure of patient to radiation (being received for test or therapy) E873.3
  inappropriate
    temperature (too hot or too cold) in local application or packing E873.5
    infusion (*see also* Misadventure, by specific type, infusion)
      excessive amount of fluid E873.0
      incorrect dilution of fluid E873.1
      wrong fluid E876.1
    mismatched blood in transfusion E876.0
    nonadministration of necessary drug or medicinal E873.6
  overdose (*see also* Overdose)

Misadventure(s) to patient(s) during surgical or medical care — *continued*
  overdose (*see also* Overdose) — *continued*
    radiation, in therapy E873.2
  perforation — *see* Misadventure, cut
  performance of correct operation (procedure) on wrong
    body part E876.7
    side E876.7
    site E876.7
  performance of operation (procedure)
    intended for another patient E876.6
    on patient not scheduled for surgery E876.6
    on wrong patient E876.6
  performance of wrong operation on correct patient E876.5
  puncture — *see* Misadventure, cut
  specified type NEC E876.8
    failure
      suture or ligature during surgical operation E876.2
      to introduce or to remove tube or instrument E876.4
      foreign object left in body E871.9
    infusion of wrong fluid E876.1
    performance of inappropriate operation E876.5
    transfusion of mismatched blood E876.0
    wrong
      fluid in infusion E876.1
      placement of endotracheal tube during anesthetic procedure E876.3
  transfusion (*see also* Misadventure, by specific type, transfusion)
    excessive amount of blood E873.0
    mismatched blood E876.0
  wrong
    device implanted into correct surgical site E876.5
    drug given in error — *see* Table of Drugs and Chemicals
    fluid in infusion E876.1
    placement of endotracheal tube during anesthetic procedure E876.3
    procedure (operation) performed on the correct patient E876.5
Motion (effects) E903
  sickness E903
Mountain sickness E902.0
Mucus aspiration or inhalation, not of newborn (with asphyxia, obstruction respiratory passage, suffocation) E912
Mudslide of cataclysmic nature E909.2
Murder (attempt) — *see also* Assault E968.9

N

Nail, injury by E920.8
Needlestick (sewing needle) E920.4
  hypodermic E920.5
Neglect — *see also* Privation
  criminal E968.4
  homicidal intent E968.4
Noise (causing injury) (pollution) E928.1
Nuclear weapon — *see also* War operations, injury due to, nuclear weapons E996.9

O

Object
  falling
    from, in, on, hitting
      aircraft E844 ☑
        due to accident to aircraft — *see* categories E840-E842 ☑
      machinery (*see also* Accident, machine)
        not in operation E916
      motor vehicle (in motion) (on public highway) E818 ☑
        not on public highway E825 ☑
        stationary E916
      nonmotor road vehicle NEC E829 ☑

Object — *continued*
  falling — *continued*
    from, in, on, hitting — *continued*
      motor vehicle — *continued*
        pedal cycle E826 ☑
        person E916
        railway rolling stock, train, vehicle E806 ☑
        street car E829 ☑
        watercraft E838 ☑
          due to accident to watercraft E831 ☑
    set in motion by
      accidental explosion of pressure vessel — *see* category E921 ☑
      firearm — *see* category E922 ☑
      machine(ry) — *see* Accident, machine
      transport vehicle — *see* categories E800-E848 ☑
    thrown from, in, on, towards
      aircraft E844 ☑
      cable car (not on rails) E847
        on rails E829 ☑
      motor vehicle (in motion) (on public highway) E818 ☑
        not on public highway E825 ☑
      nonmotor road vehicle NEC E829 ☑
      pedal cycle E826 ☑
      street car E829 ☑
      vehicle NEC — *see* Accident, vehicle NEC
Obstruction
  air passages, larynx, respiratory passages
    by
      external means NEC — *see* Suffocation
      food, any type (regurgitated) (vomited) E911
      material or object, except food E912
      mucus E912
      phlegm E912
      vomitus E911
  digestive tract, except mouth or pharynx
    by
      food, any type E915
      foreign body (any) E915
  esophagus
    without asphyxia or obstruction of respiratory passage E915
      food E911
      foreign body, except food E912
  mouth or pharynx
    by
      food, any type E911
      material or object, except food E912
  respiration — *see* Obstruction, air passages
Oil in eye E914
Overdose
  anesthetic (drug) — *see* Table of Drugs and Chemicals
  drug — *see* Table of Drugs and Chemicals
Overexertion E927.9
  from
    lifting
      repetitive movement E927.3
      sudden strenuous movement E927.0
    maintaining prolonged positions E927.1
      holding E927.1
      sitting E927.1
      standing E927.1
    prolonged static position E927.1
    pulling
      repetitive movement E927.3
      sudden strenuous movement E927.0
    pushing
      repetitive movement E927.3
      sudden strenuous movement E927.0
  specified NEC E927.8
  sudden strenuous movement E927.0
Overexposure (accidental) (to)
  cold (*see also* Cold, exposure to) E901.9
    due to manmade conditions E901.1
  heat (*see also* Heat) E900.9
  radiation — *see* Radiation
  radioactivity — *see* Radiation
  sun, except sunburn E900.0
  weather — *see* Exposure

☑ **Additional Digit Required** — Refer to the Tabular List for Digit Selection   ▽ **Subterms under main terms may continue to next column or page**

Overexposure — *continued*
  wind — *see* Exposure
Overheated — *see also* Heat E900.9
Overlaid E913.0
Overturning (accidental)
  animal-drawn vehicle E827 ☑
  boat, ship, watercraft
    causing
      drowning, submersion E830 ☑
      injury except drowning, submersion E831 ☑
  machinery — *see* Accident, machine
  motor vehicle (*see also* Loss of control, motor vehicle) E816 ☑
    with antecedent collision on public highway — *see* Collision, motor vehicle
    not on public highway, nontraffic accident E825 ☑
      with antecedent collision — *see* Collision, motor vehicle, not on public highway
  nonmotor road vehicle NEC E829 ☑
  off-road type motor vehicle — *see* Loss of control, off-road type motor vehicle
  pedal cycle E826 ☑
  railway rolling stock, train, vehicle (*see also* Derailment, railway) E802 ☑
  street car E829 ☑
  vehicle NEC — *see* Accident, vehicle NEC

P

Palsy, divers' E902.2
Parachuting (voluntary) (without accident to aircraft) E844 ☑
  due to accident to aircraft — *see* categories E840-E842 ☑
Paralysis
  divers' E902.2
  lead or saturnine E866.0
    from pesticide NEC E863.4
Pecked by bird E906.8
Performance of correct operation (procedure) **on wrong**
  body part E876.7
  side E876.7
  site E876.7
Performance of operation (procedure)
  intended for another patient E876.6
  on patient not scheduled for surgery E876.6
  on wrong patient E876.6
Performance of wrong operation on correct patient E876.5
Phlegm aspiration or inhalation (with asphyxia, obstruction respiratory passage, suffocation) E912
Piercing — *see also* Cut E920.9
  by slide trigger mechanism, scope or other part of gun E928.7
Pinched
  between objects (moving) (stationary and moving) E918
  by slide trigger mechanism, scope or other part of gun E928.7
  in object E918
Pinned under
  machine(ry) — *see* Accident, machine
Place of occurrence of accident — *see* Accident (to), occurring (at) (in)
Plumbism E866.0
  from insecticide NEC E863.4
Poisoning (accidental) (by) — *see also* Table of Drugs and Chemicals
  carbon monoxide
    generated by
      aircraft in transit E844 ☑
      motor vehicle
        in motion (on public highway) E818 ☑
        not on public highway E825 ☑
      watercraft (in transit) (not in transit) E838 ☑

Poisoning — *see also* Table of Drugs and Chemicals — *continued*
  caused by injection of poisons or toxins into or through skin by plant thorns, spines, or other mechanism E905.7
    marine or sea plants E905.6
  fumes or smoke due to
    conflagration — *see* Conflagration
    explosion or fire — *see* Fire
    ignition — *see* Ignition
  gas
    in legal intervention E972
    legal execution, by E978
    on watercraft E838 ☑
    used as anesthetic — *see* Table of Drugs and Chemicals
    in
      terrorism (chemical weapons) E979.7
      war operations E997.2
        execution E978
        intervention
          by gas E972
  late effect of — *see* Late effect
  legal
Pressure, external, causing asphyxia, suffocation — *see also* Suffocation E913.9
Privation E904.9
  food (*see also* Lack of, food) E904.1
  helpless person, infant, newborn due to abandonment or neglect E904.0
  late effect of NEC E929.5
  resulting from transport accident — *see* categories E800-E848 ☑
  water (*see also* Lack of, water) E904.2
Projected objects, striking against or struck by — *see* Striking against, object
Prolonged stay in
  high altitude (causing conditions as listed in E902.0) E902.0
  weightless environment E928.0
Prostration
  heat — *see* Heat
Pulling, injury
  due to
    repetitive movement E927.3
    sudden strenuous movement E927.0
Puncture, puncturing — *see also* Cut E920.9
  by
    plant thorns or spines E920.8
      toxic reaction E905.7
        marine or sea plants E905.6
    sea-urchin spine E905.6
Pushing (injury in) (overexertion)
  by other person(s) (accidental) E917.9
    with fall E886.9
      in sports E886.0
    as, or caused by, a crowd, human stampede E917.1
      with subsequent fall E917.6
    before moving vehicle or object
      stated as
        intentional, homicidal E968.5
        undetemined whether accidental or intentional E988.8
    from
      high place
        in accidental circum-stances — *see* categories E880-E884 ☑
        stated as
          intentional, homicidal E968.1
          undetermined whether accidental or intentional E987.9
          man-made structure, except residential E987.1
          natural site E987.2
          residential E987.0
      motor vehicle (*see also* Fall, from, motor vehicle) E818 ☑
        stated as
          intentional, homicidal E968.5
          undetermined whether accidental or intentional E988.8

Pushing — *continued*
  by other person(s) — *continued*
    in sports E917.0
      with fall E886.0
  due to
    repetitive movement E927.3
    sudden strenuous movement E927.0

R

Radiation (exposure to) E926.9
  abnormal reaction to medical test or therapy E879.2
  arc lamps E926.2
  atomic power plant (malfunction) NEC E926.9
    in water transport E838 ☑
  electromagnetic, ionizing E926.3
  gamma rays E926.3
    in
      terrorism (from or following nuclear explosion) (direct) (secondary) E979.5
      laser E979.8
      war operations (*see also* War operations, injury due to, nuclear weapons) E996.3
        laser(s) E997.0
      water transport E838 ☑
  inadvertent exposure of patient (receiving test or therapy) E873.3
  infrared (heaters and lamps) E926.1
    excessive heat E900.1
  ionized, ionizing (particles, artificially accelerated) E926.8
    electromagnetic E926.3
  isotopes, radioactive — *see* Radiation, radioactive isotopes
  laser(s) E926.4
    in
      terrorism E979.8
      war operations E997.0
    misadventure in medical care — *see* Misadventure, failure, in dosage, radiation
  late effect of NEC E929.8
    excessive heat from — *see* Heat
  light sources (visible) (ultraviolet) E926.2
  misadventure in medical or surgical procedure — *see* Misadventure, failure, in dosage, radiation
  overdose (in medical or surgical procedure) E873.2
  radar E926.0
  radioactive isotopes E926.5
    atomic power plant malfunction E926.5
      in water transport E838 ☑
    misadventure in medical or surgical treatment — *see* Misadventure, failure, in dosage, radiation
  radiobiologicals — *see* Radiation, radioactive isotopes
  radiofrequency E926.0
  radiopharmaceuticals — *see* Radiation, radioactive isotopes
  radium NEC E926.9
  sun E926.2
    excessive heat from E900.0
  tanning bed E926.2
  welding arc or torch E926.2
    excessive heat from E900.1
  x-rays (hard) (soft) E926.3
    misadventure in medical or surgical treatment — *see* Misadventure, failure, in dosage, radiation
Rape E960.1
Reaction, abnormal to or following (medical or surgical procedure) E879.9
  amputation (of limbs) E878.5
  anastomosis (arteriovenous) (blood vessel) (gastrojejunal) (skin) (tendon) (natural, artificial material, tissue) E878.2
    external stoma, creation of E878.3
  aspiration (of fluid) E879.4
    tissue E879.8
  biopsy E879.8

Reaction, abnormal to or following — *continued*
  blood
    sampling E879.7
    transfusion
      procedure E879.8
  bypass — *see* Reaction, abnormal, anastomosis
  catheterization
    cardiac E879.0
    urinary E879.6
  colostomy E878.3
  cystostomy E878.3
  dialysis (kidney) E879.1
  drugs or biologicals — *see* Table of Drugs and Chemicals
  duodenostomy E878.3
  electroshock therapy E879.3
  formation of external stoma E878.3
  gastrostomy E878.3
  graft — *see* Reaction, abnormal, anastomosis
  hypothermia E879.8
  implant, implantation (of)
    artificial
      internal device (cardiac pacemaker) (electrodes in brain) (heart valve prosthesis) (orthopedic) E878.1
      material or tissue (for anastomosis or bypass) E878.2
        with creation of external stoma E878.3
    natural tissues (for anastomosis or bypass) E878.2
      with creation of external stoma E878.3
    as transplantion — *see* Reaction, abnormal, transplant
  infusion
    procedure E879.8
  injection
    procedure E879.8
      specific type of procedure) E879.9
  insertion of gastric or duodenal sound E879.5
  insulin-shock therapy E879.3
  lumbar puncture E879.4
  perfusion E879.1
  procedures other than surgical operation (*see also* Reaction, abnormal, by specified procedure NEC E879.8
  radiological procedure or therapy E879.2
  removal of organ (partial) (total) NEC E878.6
    with
      anastomosis, bypass or graft E878.2
      formation of external stoma E878.3
      implant of artificial internal device E878.1
      transplant(ation)
        partial organ E878.4
        whole organ E878.0
  sampling
    blood E879.7
    fluid NEC E879.4
    tissue E879.8
  shock therapy E879.3
  surgical operation (*see also* Reaction, abnormal, by specified type of operation) E878.9
    restorative NEC E878.4
      with
        anastomosis, bypass or graft E878.2
        fomation of external stoma E878.3
        implant(ation) — *see* Reaction, abnormal, implant
        transplant(ation) — *see* Reaction, abnormal, transplant
    specified operation NEC E878.8
  thoracentesis E879.4
  transfusion
    procedure E879.8
  transplant, transplantation (heart) (kidney) (liver) E878.0

Overexposure — Reaction, abnormal to or following

☑ **Additional Digit Required — Refer to the Tabular List for Digit Selection**　　　　　　　▽ **Subterms under main terms may continue to next column or page**

2014 ICD-9-CM　　　▶◀ Revised Text　　　● New Line　　　▲ Revised Code　　　**Volume 2 — 347**

Reaction, abnormal to or following — *continued*
  transplant, transplantation — *continued*
    partial organ E878.4
    ureterostomy E878.3
    vaccination E879.8
Reduction in
  atmospheric pressure (*see also* Effects of, air pressure)
    while surfacing from
      deep water diving causing caisson or divers' disease, palsy or paralysis E902.2
      underground E902.8
Repetitive movements NEC E927.8
Residual (effect) — *see* Late effect
Rock falling on or hitting (accidentally)
  motor vehicle (in motion) (on public highway) E818 ☑
    not on public highway E825 ☑
  nonmotor road vehicle NEC E829 ☑
  pedal cycle E826 ☑
  person E916
  railway rolling stock, train, vehicle E806 ☑
Running off, away
  animal-drawn vehicle E827 ☑
  animal (being ridden) (in sport or transport) E828 ☑
    not being ridden E906.8
  rails, railway (*see also* Derailment) E802 ☑
  roadway
    motor vehicle (without antecedent collision) E816 ☑
      with
        antecedent collision — *see* Collision motor vehicle
        subsequent collision
          involving any object, person or vehicle not on public highway E816 ☑
          on public highway E811 ☑
    nontraffic accident E825 ☑
      with antecedent collision — *see* Collision, motor vehicle, not on public highway
    nonmotor road vehicle NEC E829 ☑
    pedal cycle E826 ☑
Run over (accidentally) (by)
  animal-drawn vehicle E827 ☑
  animal (not being ridden) E906.8
    being ridden (in sport or transport) E828 ☑
  machinery — *see* Accident, machine
  motor vehicle (on public highway) — *see* Hit by, motor vehicle
  nonmotor road vehicle NEC E829 ☑
  railway train E805 ☑
  street car E829 ☑
  vehicle NEC E848

S

Saturnism E866.0
  from insecticide NEC E863.4
Scald, scalding (accidental) (by) (from) (in) E924.0
  acid — *see* Scald, caustic
  boiling tap water E924.2
  caustic or corrosive liquid, substance E924.1
    swallowed — *see* Table of Drugs and Chemicals
  homicide (attempt) — *see* Assault, burning
  inflicted by other person
    stated as
      intentional or homicidal E968.3
      undetermined whether accidental or intentional E988.2
  late effect of NEC E929.8
  liquid (boiling) (hot) E924.0
  local application of externally applied substance in medical or surgical care E873.5
  molten metal E924.0
  self-inflicted (unspecified whether accidental or intentional) E988.2
    stated as intentional, purposeful E958.2

Scald, scalding — *continued*
  stated as undetermined whether accidental or intentional E988.2
  steam E924.0
  tap water (boiling) E924.2
  transport accident — *see* categories E800-E848 ☑
  vapor E924.0
Scratch, cat E906.8
Sea
  sickness E903
Self-mutilation — *see* Suicide
Sequelae (of)
  in
    terrorism E999.1
    war operations E999.0
Shock
  anaphylactic (*see also* Table of Drugs and Chemicals) E947.9
    due to
      bite (venomous) — *see* Bite, venomous NEC
      sting — *see* Sting
  electric (*see also* Electric shock) E925.9
  from electric appliance or current (*see also* Electric shock) E925.9
Shooting, shot (accidental(ly)) E922.9
  air gun E922.4
  BB gun E922.4
  hand gun (pistol) (revolver) E922.0
  himself (*see also* Shooting, self-inflicted) E985.4
    hand gun (pistol) (revolver) E985.0
    military firearm, except hand gun E985.3
      hand gun (pistol) (revolver) E985.0
    rifle (hunting) E985.2
      military E985.3
    shotgun (automatic) E985.1
    specified firearm NEC E985.4
    Verey pistol E985.4
  homicide (attempt) E965.4
    air gun E968.6
    BB gun E968.6
    hand gun (pistol) (revolver) E965.0
    military firearm, except hand gun E965.3
      hand gun (pistol) (revolver) E965.0
    paintball gun E965.4
    rifle (hunting) E965.2
      military E965.3
    shotgun (automatic) E965.1
    specified firearm NEC E965.4
    Verey pistol E965.4
  in
    terrorism — *see* Terrorism, shooting
    war operations — *see* War operations, shooting
  inflicted by other person
    in accidental circumstances E922.9
      hand gun (pistol) (revolver) E922.0
      military firearm, except hand gun E922.3
        hand gun (pistol) (revolver) E922.0
      rifle (hunting) E922.2
        military E922.3
      shotgun (automatic) E922.1
      specified firearm NEC E922.8
      Verey pistol E922.8
    stated as
      intentional, homicidal E965.4
        hand gun (pistol) (revolver) E965.0
        military firearm, except hand gun E965.3
          hand gun (pistol) (revolver) E965.0
        paintball gun E965.4
        rifle (hunting) E965.2
          military E965.3
        shotgun (automatic) E965.1
        specified firearm E965.4
        Verey pistol E965.4
      undetermined whether accidental or intentional E985.4
        air gun E985.6
        BB gun E985.6

Shooting, shot — *continued*
  inflicted by other person — *continued*
    stated as — *continued*
      undetermined whether accidental or intentional — *continued*
        hand gun (pistol) (revolver) E985.0
        military firearm, except hand gun E985.3
          hand gun (pistol) (revolver) E985.0
        paintball gun E985.7
        rifle (hunting) E985.2
        shotgun (automatic) E985.1
        specified firearm NEC E985.4
        Verey pistol E985.4
  legal
    execution E978
    intervention E970
  military firearm, except hand gun E922.3
    hand gun (pistol) (revolver) E922.0
  paintball gun E922.5
  rifle (hunting) E922.2
    military E922.3
  self-inflicted (unspecified whether accidental or intentional) E985.4
    air gun E985.6
    BB gun E985.6
    hand gun (pistol) (revolver) E985.0
    military firearm, except hand gun E985.3
      hand gun (pistol) (revolver) E985.0
    paintball gun E985.7
    rifle (hunting) E985.2
      military E985.3
    shotgun (automatic) E985.1
    specified firearm NEC E985.4
    stated as
      accidental E922.9
        hand gun (pistol) (revolver) E922.0
        military firearm, except hand gun E922.3
          hand gun (pistol) (revolver) E922.0
        paintball gun E922.5
        rifle (hunting) E922.2
          military E922.3
        shotgun (automatic) E922.1
        specified firearm NEC E922.8
        Verey pistol E922.8
      intentional, purposeful E955.4
        hand gun (pistol) (revolver) E955.0
        military firearm, except hand gun E955.3
          hand gun (pistol) (revolver) E955.0
        paintball gun E955.7
        rifle (hunting) E955.2
          military E955.3
        shotgun (automatic) E955.1
        specified firearm NEC E955.4
        Verey pistol E955.4
    shotgun (automatic) E922.1
    specified firearm NEC E922.8
    stated as undetermined whether accidental or intentional E985.4
      hand gun (pistol) (revolver) E985.0
      military firearm, except hand gun E985.3
        hand gun (pistol) (revolver) E985.0
      paintball gun E985.7
      rifle (hunting) E985.2
        military E985.3
      shotgun (automatic) E985.1
      specified firearm NEC E985.4
      Verey pistol E985.4
    suicidal (attempt) E955.4
      air gun E955.6
      BB gun E955.6
      hand gun (pistol) (revolver) E955.0
      military firearm, except hand gun E955.3
        hand gun (pistol) (revolver) E955.0
      paintball gun E955.7
      rifle (hunting) E955.2
        military E955.3
      shotgun (automatic) E955.1

Shooting, shot — *continued*
  suicidal — *continued*
    specified firearm NEC E955.4
    Verey pistol E955.4
  Verey pistol E922.8
Shoving (accidentally) by other person — *see also* Pushing by other person E917.9
Sickness
  air E903
  alpine E902.0
  car E903
  motion E903
  mountain E902.0
  sea E903
  travel E903
Sinking (accidental)
  boat, ship, watercraft (causing drowning, submersion) E830 ☑
    causing injury except drowning, submersion E831 ☑
Siriasis E900.0
Skydiving E844 ☑
Slashed wrists — *see also* Cut, self-inflicted E986
Slipping (accidental)
  on
    deck (of boat, ship, watercraft) (icy) (oily) (wet) E835 ☑
    ice E885.9
    ladder of ship E833 ☑
      due to accident to watercraft E831 ☑
    mud E885.9
    oil E885.9
    snow E885.9
    stairs of ship E833 ☑
      due to accident to watercraft E831 ☑
    surface
      slippery E885 ☑
      wet E885 ☑
Sliver, wood, injury by E920.8
Smothering, smothered — *see also* Suffocation E913.9
Smouldering building or structure in terrorism E979.3
Sodomy (assault) E960.1
Solid substance in eye (any part) or adnexa E914
Sound waves (causing injury) E928.1
Splinter, injury by E920.8
Stab, stabbing E966
  accidental — *see* Cut
Starvation E904.1
  helpless person, infant, newborn — *see* Lack of food
  homicidal intent E968.4
  late effect of NEC E929.5
  resulting from accident connected with transport — *see* categories E800-E848 ☑
Stepped on
  by
    animal (not being ridden) E906.8
      being ridden (in sport or transport) E828 ☑
    crowd E917.1
    person E917.9
      in sports E917.0
  in sports E917.0
Stepping on
  object (moving) E917.9
    in sports E917.0
      with subsequent fall E917.5
    stationary E917.4
      with subsequent fall E917.8
  person E917.9
    as, or caused by a crowd E917.1
      with subsequent fall E917.6
    in sports E917.0
Sting E905.9
  ant E905.5
  bee E905.3
  caterpillar E905.5
  coral E905.6
  hornet E905.3

☑ **Additional Digit Required** — Refer to the Tabular List for Digit Selection   ▽ **Subterms under main terms may continue to next column or page**

348 — Volume 2   ▶◀ **Revised Text**   ● **New Line**   ▲ **Revised Code**   **2014 ICD-9-CM**

Sting — *continued*
  insect NEC E905.5
  jellyfish E905.6
  marine animal or plant E905.6
  nematocysts E905.6
  scorpion E905.2
  sea anemone E905.6
  sea cucumber E905.6
  wasp E905.3
  yellow jacket E905.3
Storm E908.9
  specified type NEC E908.8
Straining, injury
  due to
    repetitive movement E927.3
    sudden strenuous movement E927.0
Strangling — *see* Suffocation
Strangulation — *see* Suffocation
Strenuous movements (in recreational or other activities) NEC E927.8
Striking against
  bottom (when jumping or diving into water) E883.0
  object (moving) E917.9
    caused by crowd E917.1
      with subsequent fall E917.6
    furniture E917.3
      with subsequent fall E917.7
    in
      running water E917.2
        with drowning or submersion — *see* Submersion
      sports E917.0
        with subsequent fall E917.5
    stationary E917.4
      with subsequent fall E917.8
  person(s) E917.9
    with fall E886.9
      in sports E886.0
    as, or caused by, a crowd E917.1
      with subsequent fall E917.6
        in sports E917.0
          with fall E886.0
Stroke
  heat — *see* Heat
  lightning E907
Struck by — *see also* Hit by
  bullet
    in
      terrorism E979.4
      war operations E991.2
        rubber E991.0
  lightning E907
  missile
    in terrorism — *see* Terrorism, missile
  object
    falling
      from, in, on
        building
          burning (uncontrolled fire)
            in terrorism E979.3
  thunderbolt E907
Stumbling over animal, carpet, curb, rug or (small) object (with fall) E885.9
  without fall — *see* Striking against, object
Submersion (accidental) E910.8
  boat, ship, watercraft (causing drowning, submersion) E830 ☑
    causing injury except drowning, submersion E831 ☑
  by other person
    in accidental circumstances — *see* category E910 ☑
    intentional, homicidal E964
    stated as undetermined whether accidental or intentional E984
  due to
    accident
      machinery — *see* Accident, machine
      to boat, ship, watercraft E830 ☑
      transport — *see* categories E800-E848 ☑
    avalanche E909.2
    cataclysmic
      earth surface movement or eruption E909.9

Submersion (accidental) — *continued*
  due to — *continued*
    cataclysmic — *continued*
      storm E908.9
      cloudburst E908.8
      cyclone E908.1
    fall
      from
        boat, ship, watercraft (not involved in accident) E832 ☑
          burning, crushed E830 ☑
            involved in accident, collision E830 ☑
        gangplank (into water) E832 ☑
      overboard NEC E832 ☑
    flood E908.2
    hurricane E908.0
    jumping into water E910.8
      from boat, ship, watercraft
        burning, crushed, sinking E830 ☑
          involved in accident, collision E830 ☑
        not involved in accident, for swim E910.2
        in recreational activity (without diving equipment) E910.2
          with or using diving equipment E910.1
        to rescue another person E910.3
  homicide (attempt) E964
  in
    bathtub E910.4
    specified activity, not sport, transport or recreational E910.3
    sport or recreational activity (without diving equipment) E910.2
      with or using diving equipment E910.1
    water skiing E910.0
    swimming pool NEC E910.8
    terrorism E979.8
    war operations E995.4
      intentional E995.3
    water transport E832 ☑
      due to accident to boat, ship, watercraft E830 ☑
  landslide E909.2
  overturning boat, ship, watercraft E909.2
  sinking boat, ship, watercraft E909.2
  submersion boat, ship, watercraft E909.2
  tidal wave E909.4
    caused by storm E908.0
  torrential rain E908.2
  late effect of NEC E929.8
  quenching tank E910.8
  self-inflicted (unspecified whether accidental or intentional) E984
    in accidental circumstances — *see* category E910 ☑
    stated as intentional, purposeful E954
    stated as undetermined whether accidental or intentional E984
  suicidal (attempted) E954
  while
    attempting rescue of another person E910.3
    engaged in
      marine salvage E910.3
      underwater construction or repairs E910.3
    fishing, not from boat E910.2
    hunting, not from boat E910.2
    ice skating E910.2
    pearl diving E910.3
    placing fishing nets E910.3
    playing in water E910.2
    scuba diving E910.1
      nonrecreational E910.3
    skin diving E910.1
    snorkel diving E910.2
    spear fishing underwater E910.1
    surfboarding E910.2
    swimming (swimming pool) E910.2
    wading (in water) E910.2
    water skiing E910.0

Sucked
  into
    jet (aircraft) E844 ☑
Suffocation (accidental) (by external means) (by pressure) (mechanical) E913.9
  caused by other person
    in accidental circumstances — *see* category E913 ☑
    stated as
      intentional, homicidal E963
      undetermined whether accidental or intentional E983.9
        by, in
          hanging E983.0
          plastic bag E983.1
          specified means NEC E983.8
  due to, by
    avalanche E909.2
    bedclothes E913.0
    bib E913.0
    blanket E913.0
    cave-in E913.3
      caused by cataclysmic earth surface movement or eruption E909.9
    conflagration — *see* Conflagration
    explosion — *see* Explosion
    falling earth, other substance E913.3
    fire — *see* Fire
    food, any type (ingestion) (inhalation) (regurgitated) (vomited) E911
    foreign body, except food (ingestion) (inhalation) E912
    ignition — *see* Ignition
    landslide E909.2
    machine(ry) — *see* Accident, machine
    material, object except food entering by nose or mouth, ingested, inhaled E912
    mucus (aspiration) (inhalation), not of newborn E912
    phlegm (aspiration) (inhalation) E912
    pillow E913.0
    plastic bag — *see* Suffocation, in, plastic bag
    sheet (plastic) E913.0
    specified means NEC E913.8
    vomitus (aspiration) (inhalation) E911
  homicidal (attempt) E963
    in war operations E995.3
  in
    airtight enclosed place E913.2
    baby carriage E913.0
    bed E913.0
    closed place E913.2
    cot, cradle E913.0
    perambulator E913.0
    plastic bag (in accidental circumstances) E913.1
      homicidal, purposely inflicted by other person E963
      self-inflicted (unspecified whether accidental or intentional) E983.1
        in accidental circumstances E913.1
        intentional, suicidal E953.1
        stated as undetermined whether accidentally or purposely inflicted E983.1
      suicidal, purposely self-inflicted E953.1
    refrigerator E913.2
    war operations E995.3
  self-inflicted (*see also* Suffocation, stated as undetermined whether accidental or intentional) E953.9
    in accidental circumstances — *see* category E913 ☑
    stated as intentional, purposeful — *see* Suicide, suffocation
    stated as undetermined whether accidental or intentional E983.9
      by, in
        hanging E983.0
        plastic bag E983.1
        specified means NEC E983.8

Suffocation — *continued*
  suicidal — *see* Suicide, suffocation
Suicide, suicidal (attempted) (by) E958.9
  burning, burns E958.1
  caustic substance E958.7
    poisoning E950.7
    swallowed E950.7
  cold, extreme E958.3
  cut (any part of body) E956
  cutting or piercing instrument (classifiable to E920) E956
  drowning E954
  electrocution E958.4
  explosive(s) (classifiable to E923) E955.5
  fire E958.1
  firearm (classifiable to E922) — *see* Shooting, suicidal
  hanging E953.0
  jumping
    before moving object, train, vehicle E958.0
    from high place — *see* Jumping, from, high place, stated as, suicidal
  knife E956
  late effect of E959
  motor vehicle, crashing of E958.5
  poisoning — *see* Table of Drugs and Chemicals
  puncture (any part of body) E956
  scald E958.2
  shooting — *see* Shooting, suicidal
  specified means NEC E958.8
  stab (any part of body) E956
  strangulation — *see* Suicide, suffocation
  submersion E954
  suffocation E953.9
    by, in
      hanging E953.0
      plastic bag E953.1
      specified means NEC E953.8
  wound NEC E958.9
Sunburn E926.2
Sunstroke E900.0
Supersonic waves (causing injury) E928.1
Surgical procedure, complication of
  delayed or as an abnormal reaction without mention of misadventure — *see* Reaction, abnormal
  due to or as a result of misadventure — *see* Misadventure
Swallowed, swallowing
  foreign body — *see* Foreign body, alimentary canal
  poison — *see* Table of Drugs and Chemicals
  substance
    caustic — *see* Table of Drugs and Chemicals
    corrosive — *see* Table of Drugs and Chemicals
    poisonous — *see* Table of Drugs and Chemicals
Swimmers cramp — *see also* category E910 E910.2
  not in recreation or sport E910.3
Syndrome, battered
  baby or child — *see* Abuse, child
  wife — *see* Assault

T

Tackle in sport E886.0
Terrorism (injury) (by) (in) E979.8
  air blast E979.2
  aircraft burned, destroyed, exploded, shot down E979.1
    used as a weapon E979.1
  anthrax E979.6
  asphyxia from
    chemical (weapons) E979.7
    fire, conflagration (caused by fire-producing device) E979.3
      from nuclear explosion E979.5
    gas or fumes E979.7
  bayonet E979.8
  biological agents E979.6
  blast (air) (effects) E979.2
    from nuclear explosion E979.5

☑ Additional Digit Required — Refer to the Tabular List for Digit Selection   ▽ Subterms under main terms may continue to next column or page

2014 ICD-9-CM   ▶◀ Revised Text   ● New Line   ▲ Revised Code   Volume 2 — 349

Terrorism — *continued*
blast — *continued*
  underwater E979.0
  bomb (antipersonnel) (mortar) (explosion) (fragments) E979.2
  bullet(s) (from carbine, machine gun, pistol, rifle, shotgun) E979.4
  burn from
    chemical E979.7
    fire, conflagration (caused by fire-producing device) E979.3
      from nuclear explosion E979.5
    gas E979.7
  burning aircraft E979.1
  chemical E979.7
  cholera E979.6
  conflagration E979.3
  crushed by falling aircraft E979.1
  depth-charge E979.0
  destruction of aircraft E979.1
  disability, as sequelae one year or more after injury E999.1
  drowning E979.8
  effect
    of nuclear weapon (direct) (secondary) E979.5
    secondary NEC E979.9
    sequelae E999.1
  explosion (artillery shell) (breech-block) (cannon block) E979.2
    aircraft E979.1
    bomb (antipersonnel) (mortar) E979.2
      nuclear (atom) (hydrogen) E979.5
    depth-charge E979.0
    grenade E979.2
    injury by fragments from E979.2
    land-mine E979.2
    marine weapon E979.0
    mine (land) E979.2
      at sea or in harbor E979.0
      marine E979.0
    missile (explosive) NEC E979.2
    munitions (dump) (factory) E979.2
    nuclear (weapon) E979.5
      other direct and secondary effects of E979.5
    sea-based artillery shell E979.0
    torpedo E979.0
  exposure to ionizing radiation from nuclear explosion E979.5
  falling aircraft E979.1
  firearms E979.4
  fireball effects from nuclear explosion E979.5
  fire or fire-producing device E979.3
  fragments from artillery shell, bomb NEC, grenade, guided missile, land-mine, rocket, shell, shrapnel E979.2
  gas or fumes E979.7
  grenade (explosion) (fragments) E979.2
  guided missile (explosion) (fragments) E979.2
    nuclear E979.5
  heat from nuclear explosion E979.5
  hot substances E979.3
  hydrogen cyanide E979.7
  land-mine (explosion) (fragments) E979.2
  laser(s) E979.8
  late effect of E999.1
  lewisite E979.7
  lung irritant (chemical) (fumes) (gas) E979.7
  marine mine E979.0
  mine E979.2
    at sea E979.0
    in harbor E979.0
    land (explosion) (fragments) E979.2
    marine E979.0
  missile (explosion) (fragments) (guided) E979.2
    marine E979.0
    nuclear weapons E979.5
  mortar bomb (explosion) (fragments) E979.2
  mustard gas E979.7
  nerve gas E979.7
  nuclear weapons E979.5
  pellets (shotgun) E979.4

Terrorism — *continued*
  petrol bomb E979.3
  phosgene E979.7
  piercing object E979.8
  poisoning (chemical) (fumes) (gas) E979.7
  radiation, ionizing from nuclear explosion E979.5
  rocket (explosion) (fragments) E979.2
  saber, sabre E979.8
  sarin E979.7
  screening smoke E979.7
  sequelae effect (of) E999.1
  shell (aircraft) (artillery) (cannon) (land-based) (explosion) (fragments) E979.2
    sea-based E979.0
  shooting E979.4
    bullet(s) E979.4
    pellet(s) (rifle) (shotgun) E979.4
  shrapnel E979.2
  smallpox E979.7
  stabbing object(s) E979.8
  submersion E979.8
  torpedo E979.0
  underwater blast E979.0
  vesicant (chemical) (fumes) (gas) E979.7
  weapon burst E979.2
Thermic fever E900.0
Thermoplegia E900.9
Thirst — *see also* Lack of water
  resulting from accident connected with transport — *see* categories E800-E848 ☑
Thrown (accidently)
  against object in or part of vehicle
    by motion of vehicle
      aircraft E844 ☑
      boat, ship, watercraft E838 ☑
      motor vehicle (on public highway) E818 ☑
        not on public highway E825 ☑
      off-road type (not on public highway) E821 ☑
        on public highway E818 ☑
      snow vehicle E820 ☑
        on public highway E818 ☑
      nonmotor road vehicle NEC E829 ☑
      railway rolling stock, train, vehicle E806 ☑
      street car E829 ☑
  from
    animal (being ridden) (in sport or transport) E828 ☑
    high place, homicide (attempt) E968.1
    machinery — *see* Accident, machine
    vehicle NEC — *see* Accident, vehicle NEC
  off — *see* Thrown, from
  overboard (by motion of boat, ship, watercraft) E832 ☑
    by accident to boat, ship, watercraft E830 ☑
Thunderbolt NEC E907
Tidal wave (any injury) E909.4
  caused by storm E908.0
Took
  overdose of drug — *see* Table of Drugs and Chemicals
  poison — *see* Table of Drugs and Chemicals
Tornado (any injury) E908.1
Torrential rain (any injury) E908.2
Traffic accident NEC E819 ☑
Trampled by animal E906.8
  being ridden (in sport or transport) E828 ☑
Trapped (accidently)
  between
    objects (moving) (stationary and moving) E918
  by
    door of
      elevator E918
      motor vehicle (on public highway) (while alighting, boarding) — *see* Fall, from, motor vehicle, while alighting
      railway train (underground) E806 ☑

Trapped — *continued*
  by — *continued*
    door of — *continued*
      street car E829 ☑
      subway train E806 ☑
  in object E918
Trauma
  cumulative
    from
      repetitive
        impact E927.4
        motion or movements E927.3
    sudden from strenuous movement E927.0
Travel (effects) E903
  sickness E903
Tree
  falling on or hitting E916
    motor vehicle (in motion) (on public highway) E818 ☑
      not on public highway E825 ☑
    nonmotor road vehicle NEC E829 ☑
    pedal cycle E826 ☑
    person E916
    railway rolling stock, train, vehicle E806 ☑
    street car E829 ☑
Trench foot E901.0
Tripping over animal, carpet, curb, rug, or small object (with fall) E885 ☑
  without fall — *see* Striking against, object
Tsunami E909.4
Twisting, injury
  due to
    repetitive movement E927.3
    sudden strenuous movement E927.0

V

Violence, nonaccidental — *see also* Assault E968.9
Volcanic eruption (any injury) E909.1
Vomitus in air passages (with asphyxia, obstruction or suffocation) E911

W

War operations (during hostilities) (injury) (by) (in) E995.9
  after cessation of hostilities, injury due to E998.9
  air blast E993.9
  aircraft burned, destroyed, exploded, shot down E994 ☑
  asphyxia from
    chemical E997.2
    fire, conflagration (caused by fire producing device or conventional weapon) E990.9
      from nuclear explosion (*see also* War operations, injury due to, nuclear weapons) E996.8
      incendiary bomb E990.0
      petrol bomb E990.0
    fumes E997.2
    gas E997.2
  baton (nightstick) E995.1
  battle wound NEC E995.8
  bayonet E995.2
  biological warfare agents E997.1
  blast (air) (effects) E993.9
    from nuclear explosion — *see* War operations, injury due to, nuclear weapons
    underwater E992.9
  bomb (mortar) (explosion) E993.2
    after cessation of hostilities E998.1
    fragments, injury by E991.4
      antipersonnel E991.3
  bullet(s) (from carbine, machine gun, pistol, rifle, shotgun) E991.2
    rubber E991.0
  burn from
    chemical E997.2
    fire, conflagration (caused by fire-producing device or conventional weapon) E990.9

War operations — *continued*
  burn from — *continued*
    fire, conflagration — *continued*
      from
        conventional weapon E990.3
        flamethrower E990.1
        incendiary bomb E990.0
        incendiary bullet E990.2
        nuclear explosion E996.2
        petrol bomb E990.0
    gas E997.2
  burning aircraft E994.3
  chemical E997.2
  chlorine E997.2
  conventional warfare, specified form NEC E995.8
  crushing by falling aircraft E994.8
  depth charge E992.1
  destruction of aircraft E994.9
  detonation of own munitions (ammunition) (artillery) (mortars), unintentional E993.6
  disability as sequela one year or more after injury E999.0
  discharge of own munitions launch device (autocannons) (automatic grenade launchers) (missile launchers) (small arms), unintentional E993.7
  drowning E995.4
  effect nuclear weapon (*see also* War operations, injury due to, nuclear weapons) E996.9
  explosion (breech block) (cannon shell) E993.9
    after cessation of hostilities
      bomb placed in war E998.1
      mine placed in war E998.0
    aircraft E994.1
      due to
        enemy fire or explosives E994.0
        own onboard explosives E994.1
    artillery shell E993.2
    bomb (mortar) E993.2
      aerial E993.0
      atom (*see also* War operations, injury due to, nuclear weapons) E996.9
      hydrogen (*see also* War operations, injury due to, nuclear weapons) E996.9
      injury by fragments from E991.4
        antipersonnel E991.3
      nuclear (*see also* War operations, injury due to, nuclear weapons) E996.9
    depth charge E992.1
    injury by fragments from E991.4
      antipersonnel E991.3
    marine weapon NEC E992.8
    mine
      at sea or in harbor E992.2
      land E993.8
        injury by fragments from E991.4
      marine E992.2
    missile, guided E993.1
    mortar E993.2
    munitions (accidental) (being used in war) (dump) (factory) E993.9
      own E993.7
        ammunition (artillery) (mortars) E993.6
        launch device (autocannons) (automatic grenade launchers) (missile launchers) (small arms) E993.7
    nuclear (weapon) (*see also* War operations, injury due to, nuclear weapons) E996.9
    own weapons (accidental) E993.7
      injury by fragments from E991.9
        antipersonnel E991.3
    sea-based artillery shell E992.3
    specified NEC E993.8
    torpedo E992.0

War operations — *continued*

 exposure to ionizing radiation from nuclear explosion (*see also* War operations, injury due to, nuclear weapons) E996.3

falling aircraft E994.8

fireball effects from nuclear explosion E996.2

fire or fire-producing device E990.9
 flamethrower E990.1
 incendiary bomb E990.0
 incendiary bullet E990.2
 indirectly caused from conventional weapon E990.3
 petrol bomb E990.0

fragments from
 antipersonnel bomb E991.3
 artillery shell E991.4
 bomb NEC E991.4
 grenade E991.4
 guided missile E991.4
 land mine E991.4
 rocket E991.4
 shell E991.4
 shrapnel E991.9

fumes E997.2

gas E997.2

grenade (explosion) E993.8
 fragments, injury by E991.4

guided missile (explosion) E993.1
 fragments, injury by E991.4
 nuclear (*see also* War operations, injury due to, nuclear weapons) E996.9

heat from nuclear explosion E996.2

injury due to
 aerial bomb E993.0
 air blast E993.9
 aircraft shot down E994.0
 artillery shell E993.2
 blast E993.9
  wave E993.9
  wind E993.9
 bomb E993.8
 but occurring after cessation of hostilities
  explosion of bombs E998.1
  explosion of mines E998.0
  specified NEC E998.8
 conventional warfare E995.9
  specified form NEC E995.8
 depth charge E992.1
 destruction of aircraft E994.9
  due to
   air to air missile E994.0
   collision with other aircraft E994.2
   enemy fire or explosives E994.0
   on board explosion (explosives) E994.1
   on board fire E994.3
   rocket propelled grenade [RPG] E994.0
   small arms fire E994.0
   surface to air missile E994.0
   specified NEC E994.8
 dirty bomb (*see also* War operations, injury due to, nuclear weapons) E996.9
 drowning E995.4
 explosion (direct pressure) (indirect pressure) (due to) E993.9
  depth charge E992.1

War operations — *continued*

injury due to — *continued*
 explosion — *continued*
  improvised explosive device [IED]
   person borne E993.3
   roadside E993.5
   specified NEC E993.5
   transport vehicle (air) (land) (water) E993.4
   vehicle (air) (land) (water) borne E993.4
  marine mines (in harbor) (at sea) E992.2
  marine weapons E992.9
   specified NEC E992.8
  sea based artillery shell E992.3
  specified NEC E993.8
  torpedo E992.0
  unintentional (of own)
   autocannons E993.7
   automatic grenade launchers E993.7
   launch device discharge E993.7
   missile launchers E993.7
   munitions detonation (ammunition) (artillery) (mortars) E993.6
   small arms E993.7

fragments (from) E991.9
 artillery E991.8
 artillery shells E991.4
 autocannons E991.8
 automatic grenade launchers [AGL] E991.8
 bombs E991.4
  antipersonnel E991.3
 detonation of unexploded ordnance [UXO] E991.4
 grenade E991.4
 guided missile E991.4
 improvised explosive device [IED]
  person borne E991.5
  roadside E991.7
  specified NEC E991.7
  transport vehicle (air) (land) (water) borne E991.6
  vehicle (air) (land) (water) borne E991.6
 land mine E991.4
 missile launchers E991.8
 mortars E991.8
 munitions (artillery shells) (bombs) (grenades) (rockets) (shells) E991.4
 rockets E991.4
 shells E991.4
 small arms E991.8
 specified NEC E991.9
 weapons (artillery) (autocannons) (mortars) (small arms) E991.8

grenade E993.8

guided missile E993.1

hand to hand combat, unarmed E995.0

improvised explosive device [IED]
 person borne E993.3
 roadside E993.5
 specified NEC E993.5
 transport vehicle (air) (land) (water) borne E993.4
 vehicle (air) (land) (water) borne E993.4

inability to surface or obtain air E995.4

War operations — *continued*

injury due to — *continued*
 land mine E993.8
 marine mines (in harbor) (at sea) E992.2
 marine weapons E992.9
  specified NEC E992.8
 mortar E993.2
 nuclear weapons E996.9
  beta burns E996.3
  blast debris E996.1
  blast pressure E996.0
  burns due to thermal radiation E996.2
  direct blast effect E996.0
  fallout exposure E996.3
  fireball effect E996.2
  flash burns E996.2
  heat effect E996.2
  indirect blast effect E996.1
  nuclear radiation effects E996.3
  radiation exposure (acute) E996.3
  radiation sickness E996.3
  secondary effects E996.3
  specified effects NEC E996.8
  thermal radiation effect E996.2
 piercing object E995.2
 restriction of airway, intentional E995.3
 sea based artillery shell E992.3
 shrapnel E991.9
 stave E995.1
 strangulation E995.3
 strike by blunt object (baton) (nightstick) (stave) E995.1
 submersion (accidental) (unintentional) E995.4
  intentional E995.3
 suffocation E995.3
  accidental E995.4
 torpedo E992.0
 underwater blast E992.9
 weapon of mass destruction [WMD] E997.3

knife E995.2

lacrimator (gas) (chemical) E997.2

land mine (explosion) E993.8
 after cessation of hostilities E998.0
 fragments, injury by E991.4

laser(s) E997.0

late effect of E999.0

lewisite E997.2

lung irritant (chemical) (fumes) (gas) E997.2

marine mine E992.2

mine
 after cessation of hostilities E998.0
 at sea E992.2
 in harbor E992.2
 land (explosion) E993.8
  fragments, injury by E991.4
 marine E992.2

missile (guided) (explosion) E993.1
 fragments, injury by E991.4
 marine E992.8
 nuclear (*see also* War operations, injury due to, nuclear weapons) E996.9

mortar bomb (explosion) E993.2
 fragments, injury by E991.4

mustard gas E997.2

nerve gas E997.2

phosgene E997.2

piercing object E995.2

poisoning (chemical) (fumes) (gas) E997.2

War operations — *continued*

 radiation, ionizing from nuclear explosion (*see also* War operations, injury due to, nuclear weapons) E996.3

rocket (explosion) E993.8
 fragments, injury by E991.4

saber, sabre E995.2

screening smoke E997.8

shell (aircraft) (artillery) (cannon) (land based) (explosion) E993.2
 fragments, injury by E991.4
 sea-based E992.3

shooting E991.2
 after cessation of hostilities E998.8
 bullet(s) E991.2
  rubber E991.0
 pellet(s) (rifle) E991.1
 shrapnel E991.9
 submersion E995 ☑
 torpedo E992 ☑

stave E995.2

strike by blunt object (baton) (nightstick) (stave) E995.1

submersion E995.4
 intentional E995.3

sword E995.2

torpedo E992.0

unconventional warfare, except by nuclear weapon E997.9
 biological (warfare) E997.1
 gas, fumes, chemicals E997.2
 laser(s) E997.0
 specified type NEC E997.8

underwater blast E992.9

vesicant (chemical) (fumes) (gas) E997.2

weapon burst E993.9

Washed
 away by flood — *see* Flood
 away by tidal wave — *see* Tidal wave
 off road by storm (transport vehicle) E908.9
 overboard E832 ☑

Weapon of mass destruction [WMD] E997.3

Weather exposure — *see also* Exposure
 cold E901.0
 hot E900.0

Weightlessness (causing injury) (effects of) (in spacecraft, real or simulated) E928.0

Wound (accidental) NEC — *see also* Injury E928.9
 battle (*see also* War operations) E995.9
 bayonet E920.3
  in
   legal intervention E974
   war operations E995.2
 gunshot — *see* Shooting
 incised — *see* Cut
 saber, sabre E920.3
  in war operations E995.2

Wrong
 body part, performance of correct operation (procedure) on E876.7
 device implanted into correct surgical site E876.5
 patient, performance of operation (procedure) on E876.6
 procedure (operation) performed on correct patient E876.5
 side, performance of correct operation (procedure) on E876.7
 site, performance of correct operation (procedure) on E876.7

☑ Additional Digit Required — Refer to the Tabular List for Digit Selection   ▽ Subterms under main terms may continue to next column or page

2014 ICD-9-CM   ▶◀ Revised Text   ● New Line   ▲ Revised Code   Volume 2 — 351

Railway Accidents (E800-E807)

The following fourth-digit subdivisions are for use with categories E800-E807 to identify the injured person:

.0 Railway employee
Any person who by virtue of his employment in connection with a railway, whether by the railway company or not, is at increased risk of involvement in a railway accident, such as:
  catering staff on train
  postal staff on train
  driver
  railway fireman
  guard
  shunter
  porter
  sleeping car attendant

.1 Passenger on railway
Any authorized person traveling on a train, except a railway employee
  EXCLUDES   intending passenger waiting at station (.8)
              unauthorized rider on railway vehicle (.8)

.2 Pedestrian See definition (r), E-Codes-2

.3 Pedal cyclist See definition (p), E-Codes-2

.8 Other specified person Intending passenger waiting at station
Unauthorized rider on railway vehicle

.9 Unspecified person

Motor Vehicle Traffic and Nontraffic Accidents (E810-E825)

The following fourth-digit subdivisions are for use with categories E810-E819 and E820-E825 to identify the injured person:

.0 Driver of motor vehicle other than motorcycle See definition (1), E-Codes-2

.1 Passenger in motor vehicle other than motorcycle See definition (1), E-Codes-2

.2 Motorcyclist See definition (1), E-Codes-2

.3 Passenger on motorcycle See definition (1), E-Codes-2

.4 Occupant of streetcar

.5 Rider of animal; occupant of animal-drawn vehicle

.6 Pedal cyclist See definition (p), E-Codes-2

.7 Pedestrian See definition (r), E-Codes-2

.8 Other specified person
Occupant of vehicle other than above
Person in railway train involved in accident
Unauthorized rider of motor vehicle

.9 Unspecified person

Other Road Vehicle Accidents (E826-E829)

(animal-drawn vehicle, streetcar, pedal cycle, and other nonmotor road vehicle accidents)

The following fourth-digit subdivisions are for use with categories E826-E829 to identify the injured person:

.0 Pedestrian See definition (r), E-Codes-2

.1 Pedal cyclist (does not apply to codes E827, E828, E829) See definition (p), E-Codes-2

.2 Rider of animal (does not apply to code E829)

.3 Occupant of animal-drawn vehicle (does not apply to codes E828, E829)

.4 Occupant of streetcar

.8 Other specified person

.9 Unspecified person

Water Transport Accidents (E830-E838)

The following fourth-digit subdivisions are for use with categories E830-E838 to identify the injured person:

.0 Occupant of small boat, unpowered

.1 Occupant of small boat, powered See definition (t), E-Codes-2
  EXCLUDES   water skier (.4)

.2 Occupant of other watercraft — crew
Persons:
  engaged in operation of watercraft
    providing passenger services [cabin attendants, ship's physician, catering personnel]
    working on ship during voyage in other capacity [musician in band, operators of shops and beauty parlors]

.3 Occupant of other watercraft — other than crew
Passenger
Occupant of lifeboat, other than crew, after abandoning ship

.4 Water skier

.5 Swimmer

.6 Dockers, stevedores
Longshoreman employed on the dock in loading and unloading ships

.8 Other specified person
Immigration and custom officials on board ship
Persons:
  accompanying passenger or member of crew visiting boat
Pilot (guiding ship into port)

.9 Unspecified person

Air and Space Transport Accidents (E840-E845)

The following fourth-digit subdivisions are for use with categories E840-E845 to identify the injured person:

.0 Occupant of spacecraft
  Crew
  Passenger (civilian)   in military aircraft [air force]
  (military)   [army] [national guard] [navy]
  Troops

.1 Occupant of military aircraft, any
  EXCLUDES   occupants of aircraft operated under jurisdiction of police
              departments (.5) parachutist (.7)

.2 Crew of commercial aircraft (powered) in surface to surface transport

.3 Other occupant of commercial aircraft (powered) in surface to surface transport
Flight personnel:
  not part of crew
  on familiarization flight Passenger on aircraft

.4 Occupant of commercial aircraft (powered) in surface to air transport
Occupant [crew] [passenger] of aircraft (powered) engaged in activities, such as:
  air drops of emergency supplies
    air drops of parachutists, except from military craft
    crop dusting
    lowering of construction material [bridge or telephone pole]
    sky writing

.5 Occupant of other powered aircraft
Occupant [crew] [passenger] of aircraft (powered) engaged in activities, such as:
  aerial spraying (crops)(fire retardants)
  aerobatic flying
  aircraft racing
  rescue operation
  storm surveillance
  traffic surveillance
Occupant of private plane NOS

.6 Occupant of unpowered aircraft, except parachutist
Occupant of aircraft classifiable to E842

.7 Parachutist (military)(other)
Person making voluntary descent
  EXCLUDES   person making descent after accident to aircraft (.1-.6)

.8 Ground crew, airline employee
Persons employed at airfields (civil)(military) or launching pads, not occupants of aircraft

.9 Other person

☑ **Additional Digit Required — Refer to the Tabular List for Digit Selection**   ▽ **Subterms under main terms may continue to next column or page**

1. Infectious and Parasitic Diseases (001-139)

NOTE Categories for "late effects" of infectious and parasitic diseases are to be found at 137-139.

INCLUDES diseases generally recognized as communicable or transmissible as well as a few diseases of unknown but possibly infectious origin

EXCLUDES acute respiratory infections (460-466)
carrier or suspected carrier of infectious organism (V02.0-V02.9)
certain localized infections
influenza (487.0-487.8, 488.01-488.19)

Intestinal Infectious Diseases (001-009)

EXCLUDES helminthiases (120.0-129)

√4ᵗʰ **001 Cholera**
DEF: An acute infectious enteritis caused by a potent enterotoxin produced by *Vibrio cholerae*; changes the permeability of the mucosa of the intestines and leads to diarrhea and dehydration.

001.0 Due to Vibrio cholerae   `CC`
CC Exd: 001.0-001.9

001.1 Due to Vibrio cholerae el tor   `CC`
CC Exd: See code: 001.0

001.9 Cholera, unspecified   `CC`
CC Exd: See code: 001.0

√4ᵗʰ **002 Typhoid and paratyphoid fevers**
DEF: Typhoid fever: an acute generalized illness caused by *Salmonella typhi*; clinical features are fever, headache, abdominal pain, cough, toxemia, leukopenia, abnormal pulse, rose spots on the skin, bacteremia, hyperplasia of intestinal lymph nodes, mesenteric lymphadenopathy, and Peyer's patches in the intestines.
DEF: Paratyphoid fever: a prolonged febrile illness, caused by salmonella serotypes other than *S. typhi*, especially *S. enteritidis* serotypes paratyphi A and B and *S. choleraesuis*.

002.0 Typhoid fever   `CC`
Typhoid (fever) (infection) [any site]
CC Exd: 002.0-002.9

002.1 Paratyphoid fever A   `CC`
CC Exd: See code: 002.0

002.2 Paratyphoid fever B   `CC`
CC Exd: See code: 002.0

002.3 Paratyphoid fever C   `CC`
CC Exd: See code: 002.0

002.9 Paratyphoid fever, unspecified   `CC`
CC Exd: See code: 002.0

√4ᵗʰ **003 Other salmonella infections**
INCLUDES infection or food poisoning by Salmonella [any serotype]
DEF: Infections caused by a genus of gram-negative, anaerobic bacteria of the family *Enterobacteriaceae*; major symptoms are enteric fevers, acute gastroenteritis and septicemia.

003.0 Salmonella gastroenteritis   `CC`
Salmonellosis
CC Exd: 002.0, 002.9-003.0, 004.9-005.2, 007.5, 008.00-009.0, 040.41-040.42, 536.8, 558.2-558.9, 564.1, 567.21, 567.23, 567.31-567.39, 567.89, 777.50-777.53, 777.8

003.1 Salmonella septicemia   `MCC` `HIV`
CC Exd: 03.1, 020.2, 022.3, 036.2, 038.0-038.9, 040.89-041.3, 041.41-041.85, 041.89-041.9, 054.5, 139.8, 771.81, 771.83-771.89, 995.90-995.94, V09.0-V09.91

√5ᵗʰ **003.2 Localized salmonella infections**

003.20 Localized salmonella infection, unspecified   `HIV`

003.21 Salmonella meningitis   `MCC` `HIV`
CC Exd: 003.21, 013.00-013.16, 036.0, 047.0-047.9, 049.0-049.1, 072.1, 078.88-078.89, 079.81, 079.88-079.99, 090.42, 091.81, 094.2, 098.89, 100.81, 112.83, 114.2, 115.01, 115.11, 115.91, 130.0, 139.8, 320.0-322.9, 349.89-349.9

003.22 Salmonella pneumonia   `MCC` `HIV`
CC Exd: 003.22, 011.00-012.16, 012.80-012.86, 017.90-017.96, 020.3-020.5, 021.3, 022.1, 031.0, 039.1, 073.0, 115.05, 115.15, 115.95, 122.1, 130.4, 136.3, 480.0-480.2, 480.8-487.1, 488.0-488.1, 495.0-495.7, 500, 502-508.9, 517.1, 517.8, 518.89, 519.8-519.9

003.23 Salmonella arthritis   `CC` `HIV`
CC Exd: 003.23, 015.80-015.96, 036.82, 056.71, 098.50-098.51, 098.59, 098.89, 711.00-714.0, 715.00, 715.09-715.10, 715.18-716.99, 718.00-718.08, 719.00-719.10, 719.18-719.69, 719.80-719.99

003.24 Salmonella osteomyelitis   `CC` `HIV`
CC Exd: 003.24, 015.50-015.56, 015.70-015.76, 015.90-015.96, 730.00-730.39, 730.80-730.99

003.29 Other   `CC` `HIV`
CC Exd: 003.29

003.8 Other specified salmonella infections   `CC` `HIV`
CC Exd: 003.8

003.9 Salmonella infection, unspecified   `CC` `HIV`
CC Exd: 003.9

√4ᵗʰ **004 Shigellosis**
INCLUDES bacillary dysentery
DEF: Acute infectious dysentery caused by the genus *Shigella*, of the family *Enterobacteriaceae*; affecting the colon causing blood-stained stools, tenesmus, abdominal cramps and fever.

004.0 Shigella dysenteriae   `CC`
Infection by group A Shigella (Schmitz) (Shiga)
CC Exd: 001.1, 002.0, 002.9-003.0, 004.0, 004.9-005.2, 006.0-006.2, 006.9, 007.1-007.9, 008.1-008.3, 008.5, 008.8-009.0, 014.80-014.86, 040.41-040.42, 112.85, 129, 487.8, 488.09, 488.19, 536.3, 536.8, 555.0-557.9, 558.2-558.9, 564.1, 775.0-775.7, 775.9, 777.50-777.53, 777.8

004.1 Shigella flexneri
Infection by group B Shigella

004.2 Shigella boydii
Infection by group C Shigella

004.3 Shigella sonnei
Infection by group D Shigella

004.8 Other specified Shigella infections

004.9 Shigellosis, unspecified

√4ᵗʰ **005 Other food poisoning (bacterial)**
EXCLUDES salmonella infections (003.0-003.9)
toxic effect of:
food contaminants (989.7)
noxious foodstuffs (988.0-988.9)
DEF: Enteritis caused by ingesting contaminated foods and characterized by diarrhea, abdominal pain, vomiting; symptoms may be mild or life threatening.

005.0 Staphylococcal food poisoning   `CC`
Staphylococcal toxemia specified as due to food
CC Exd: 001.0-009.3, 040.41-040.42

005.1 Botulism food poisoning   `CC`
Botulism NOS
Food poisoning due to Clostridium botulinum
EXCLUDES infant botulism (040.41)
wound botulism (040.42)
CC Exd: 005.0-005.2, 008.45-008.46, 040.41-040.42

005.2 Food poisoning due to Clostridium perfringens [C. welchii]   `CC`
Enteritis necroticans
CC Exd: 003.0, 004.9-005.2, 007.5, 008.00-009.0, 040.41-040.42, 487.8, 488.09, 488.19, 536.3, 536.8, 558.2-558.9, 564.1, 567.21, 567.23, 567.31-567.39, 567.89, 777.50-777.53, 777.8

005.3 Food poisoning due to other Clostridia   `CC`
CC Exd: See code: 005.0

005.4 Food poisoning due to Vibrio parahaemolyticus   `CC`
CC Exd: See code: 005.0

√5ᵗʰ **005.8 Other bacterial food poisoning**
EXCLUDES salmonella food poisoning (003.0-003.9)

005.81 Food poisoning due to Vibrio vulnificus   `CC`
CC Exd: See code: 005.0

005.89 Other bacterial food poisoning   `CC`
Food poisoning due to Bacillus cereus
CC Exd: See code: 005.0

005.9 Food poisoning, unspecified

Additional Digit Required   Unacceptable PDx   Manifestation Code   Hospital Acquired Condition   ▶◀ Revised Text   ● New Code   ▲ Revised Code Title

√4th 006 Amebiasis

INCLUDES infection due to Entamoeba histolytica

EXCLUDES *amebiasis due to organisms other than Entamoeba histolytica (007.8)*

DEF: Infection of the large intestine caused by *Entamoeba histolytica;* usually asymptomatic but symptoms may range from mild diarrhea to profound life-threatening dysentery. Extraintestinal complications include hepatic abscess, which may rupture, causing life-threatening infections.

006.0 Acute amebic dysentery without mention of abscess `CC`
Acute amebiasis
DEF: Sudden, severe *Entamoeba histolytica* infection causing bloody stools.
CC Exd: 006.0-006.1, 007.5

006.1 Chronic intestinal amebiasis without mention of abscess `CC`
Chronic:
   amebiasis
   amebic dysentery
CC Exd: See code: 006.0

006.2 Amebic nondysenteric colitis `CC`
DEF: *Entamoeba histolytica* infection with inflamed colon but no dysentery.
CC Exd: 003.0, 004.9-005.0, 005.2, 006.0-006.2, 006.9, 007.1-009.0, 129, 487.8, 488.09, 488.19, 536.3, 536.8, 555.0-557.9, 558.2-558.9, 564.1, 777.50-777.53, 777.8

006.3 Amebic liver abscess `MCC`
Hepatic amebiasis
CC Exd: 006.3, 572.0

006.4 Amebic lung abscess `MCC`
Amebic abscess of lung (and liver)
CC Exd: 006.4, 513.0

006.5 Amebic brain abscess `MCC`
Amebic abscess of brain (and liver) (and lung)
CC Exd: 006.5, 324.0

006.6 Amebic skin ulceration
Cutaneous amebiasis

006.8 Amebic infection of other sites `CC`
Amebic: Ameboma
   appendicitis
   balanitis
EXCLUDES *specific infections by free-living amebae (136.21-136.29)*
CC Exd: 006.0-006.5, 006.8

006.9 Amebiasis, unspecified
Amebiasis NOS

√4th 007 Other protozoal intestinal diseases

INCLUDES protozoal:
   colitis
   diarrhea
   dysentery

007.0 Balantidiasis
Infection by Balantidium coli

007.1 Giardiasis `CC`
Infection by Giardia lamblia
Lambliasis
CC Exd: 003.0, 004.9-005.0, 005.2, 006.0-006.2, 006.9, 007.1-009.0, 129, 487.8, 488.09, 488.19, 536.3, 536.8, 558.2-558.9, 564.1

007.2 Coccidiosis `CC` `HIV`
Infection by Isospora belli and Isospora hominis Isosporiasis
CC Exd: See code: 007.1

007.3 Intestinal trichomoniasis
DEF: Colitis, diarrhea, or dysentery caused by the protozoa *Trichomonas.*

007.4 Cryptosporidiosis `CC`
DEF: An intestinal infection by protozoan parasites causing intractable diarrhea in patients with AIDS and other immunosuppressed individuals.
CC Exd: See code: 007.1
AHA: 4Q, '97, 30

007.5 Cyclosporiasis `CC`
DEF: An infection of the small intestine by the protozoal organism, *Cyclospora cayetenanesis,* spread to humans through ingestion of contaminated water or food. Symptoms include watery diarrhea, loss of appetite, increased gas, stomach cramps, nausea, vomiting, muscle aches, low grade fever, and fatigue.
CC Exd: 003.0, 004.9-005.0, 005.2, 006.0-006.2, 006.9, 007.1-009.0, 129, 487.8, 488.09, 488.19, 536.3, 536.8, 558.2-558.9, 564.1, 567.21, 567.23, 567.31-567.39, 567.89
AHA: 4Q, '00, 38

007.8 Other specified protozoal intestinal diseases `CC`
Amebiasis due to organisms other than Entamoeba histolytica
CC Exd: See code: 007.1

007.9 Unspecified protozoal intestinal disease `CC`
Flagellate diarrhea
Protozoal dysentery NOS
CC Exd: See code: 007.1

√4th 008 Intestinal infections due to other organisms

INCLUDES any condition classifiable to 009.0-009.3 with mention of the responsible organisms

EXCLUDES *food poisoning by these organisms (005.0-005.9)*

√5th 008.0 Escherichia coli [E. coli]
AHA: 4Q, '92, 17

008.00 E. coli, unspecified `CC`
E. coli enteritis NOS
CC Exd: 003.0, 004.9-005.0, 005.2, 007.5, 008.00-009.0, 487.8, 488.09, 488.19, 536.3, 536.8, 558.2-558.9, 564.1, 567.21, 567.23, 567.31-567.39, 567.89, 777.50-777.53, 777.8

008.01 Enteropathogenic E. coli `CC`
DEF: *E. coli* causing inflammation of intestines.
CC Exd: See code: 008.00

008.02 Enterotoxigenic E. coli `CC`
DEF: A toxic reaction to *E. coli* of the intestinal mucosa, causing voluminous watery secretions.
CC Exd: See code: 008.00

008.03 Enteroinvasive E. coli `CC`
DEF: *E. coli* infection penetrating intestinal mucosa.
CC Exd: See code: 008.00

008.04 Enterohemorrhagic E. coli `CC`
DEF: *E. coli* infection penetrating the intestinal mucosa, producing microscopic ulceration and bleeding.
CC Exd: See code: 008.00
AHA: 4Q, '11, 83

008.09 Other intestinal E. coli infections `CC`
CC Exd: See code: 008.00

008.1 Arizona group of paracolon bacilli `CC`
CC Exd: See code: 008.00

008.2 Aerobacter aerogenes `CC`
Enterobacter aeogenes
CC Exd: See code: 008.00

008.3 Proteus (mirabilis) (morganii) `CC`
CC Exd: See code: 008.00

√5th 008.4 Other specified bacteria
AHA: 4Q, '92, 18

008.41 Staphylococcus `CC`
Staphylococcal enterocolitis
CC Exd: 001.1, 002.0, 002.9-003.0, 004.9-005.2, 006.0-006.2, 006.9, 007.1-009.0, 014.80-014.86, 040.41-040.42, 112.85, 129, 487.8, 488.09, 488.19, 536.3, 536.8, 555.0-557.9, 558.2-558.9, 564.1, 775.0-775.7, 775.9, 777.50-777.53, 777.8

008.42 Pseudomonas `CC`
CC Exd: See code: 008.41
AHA: 2Q, '89, 10

008.43 Campylobacter `CC`
CC Exd: See code 008.41

008.44 Yersinia enterocolitica `CC`
CC Exd: See code 008.41

N Newborn Age: 0   P Pediatric Age: 0-17   M Maternity Age: 12-55   A Adult Age: 15-124   `MCC` Major CC Condition   `CC` CC Condition   `HIV` HIV Related D

2 – Volume 1   2014 ICD-9-C

008.45 Clostridium difficile `CC`
Pseudomembranous colitis

DEF: An overgrowth of a species of bacterium that is a part of the normal colon flora in human infants and sometimes in adults; produces a toxin that causes pseudomembranous enterocolitis typically is seen in patients undergoing antibiotic therapy.
CC Excl: See code 008.41
A04.7 Enterocolitis due to clostridium difficile `I-10`

008.46 Other anaerobes `CC`
Anaerobic enteritis NOS
Bacteroides (fragilis)
Gram-negative anaerobes
CC Excl: See code 008.41

008.47 Other gram-negative bacteria `CC`
Gram-negative enteritis NOS
EXCLUDES gram-negative anaerobes (008.46)
CC Excl: See code 008.41

008.49 Other `CC`
CC Excl: See code 008.41
AHA: 2Q, '89, 10; 1Q, '88, 6

008.5 Bacterial enteritis, unspecified `CC`
CC Excl: 001.1, 002.0, 002.9-003.0, 004.9-005.0, 005.2, 006.0-006.2, 006.9, 007.1-009.0, 014.80-014.86, 112.85, 129, 487.8, 488.09, 488.19, 536.3, 536.8, 558.2-558.9, 564.1, 567.21, 567.23, 567.31-567.39, 567.89, 777.50-777.53, 777.8

√5th **008.6 Enteritis due to specified virus**
AHA: 4Q, '92, 18

008.61 Rotavirus `CC`
CC Excl: 003.0, 004.9-005.0, 005.2, 006.0-006.2, 006.9, 007.1-009.0, 014.80-014.86, 112.85, 129, 487.8, 488.09, 488.19, 536.3, 536.8, 558.2-558.9, 564.1, 567.21, 567.23, 567.31-567.39, 567.89, 777.50-777.53, 777.8

008.62 Adenovirus `CC`
CC Excl: See code: 008.61

008.63 Norwalk virus `CC`
Norovirus
Norwalk-like agent
CC Excl: See code: 008.61

008.64 Other small round viruses [SRVs] `CC`
Small round virus NOS
CC Excl: See code: 008.61

008.65 Calicivirus `CC`
DEF: Enteritis due to a subgroup of *Picornaviruses*.
CC Excl: See code: 008.61

008.66 Astrovirus `CC`
CC Excl: See code: 008.61

008.67 Enterovirus NEC `CC`
Coxsackie virus
Echovirus
EXCLUDES poliovirus (045.0-045.9)
CC Excl: See code: 008.61

008.69 Other viral enteritis `CC`
Torovirus
CC Excl: See code: 008.61
AHA: 1Q, '03, 10

008.8 Other organism, not elsewhere classified
Viral:
enteritis NOS
gastroenteritis
EXCLUDES influenza with involvement of gastrointestinal tract (487.8, 488.09, 488.19)
A08.4 Viral intestinal infection unspecified `I-10`

√4th **009 Ill-defined intestinal infections**
EXCLUDES diarrheal disease or intestinal infection due to specified organism (001.0-008.8)
diarrhea following gastrointestinal surgery (564.4)
intestinal malabsorption (579.0-579.9)
ischemic enteritis (557.0-557.9)
other noninfectious gastroenteritis and colitis (558.1-558.9)
regional enteritis (555.0-555.9)
ulcerative colitis (556)

009.0 Infectious colitis, enteritis, and gastroenteritis `CC`
Colitis
Enteritis   } septic
Gastroenteritis

Dysentery: Dysentery:
NOS   hemorrhagic
catarrhal

DEF: Colitis: An inflammation of mucous membranes of the colon.
DEF: Enteritis: An inflammation of mucous membranes of the small intestine.
DEF: Gastroenteritis: An inflammation of mucous membranes of stomach and intestines.
CC Excl: 001.0-009.3, 040.41-040.42
AHA: 3Q, '99, 4
A09 Infectious gastroenteritis and colitis unspec `I-10`

009.1 Colitis, enteritis, and gastroenteritis of presumed infectious origin `CC`
EXCLUDES colitis NOS (558.9)
enteritis NOS (558.9)
gastroenteritis NOS (558.9)
CC Excl: 009.1
AHA: 3Q, '99, 6

009.2 Infectious diarrhea `CC`
Diarrhea: Infectious diarrheal disease NOS
dysenteric
epidemic
CC Excl: See code: 009.0

009.3 Diarrhea of presumed infectious origin `CC`
EXCLUDES diarrhea NOS (787.91)
CC Excl: 009.3
AHA: N-D, '87, 7

Tuberculosis (010-018)

INCLUDES infection by Mycobacterium tuberculosis (human) (bovine)
EXCLUDES congenital tuberculosis (771.2)
late effects of tuberculosis (137.0-137.4)

The following fifth-digit subclassification is for use with categories 010-018:
0 unspecified
1 bacteriological or histological examination not done
2 bacteriological or histological examination unknown (at present)
3 tubercle bacilli found (in sputum) by microscopy
4 tubercle bacilli not found (in sputum) by microscopy, but found by bacterial culture
5 tubercle bacilli not found by bacteriological examination, but tuberculosis confirmed histologically
6 tubercle bacilli not found by bacteriological or histological examination but tuberculosis confirmed by other methods [inoculation of animals]

DEF: An infection by *Mycobacterium tuberculosis* causing the formation of small, rounded nodules, called tubercles, that can disseminate throughout the body via lymph and blood vessels. Localized tuberculosis is most often seen in the lungs.b

010 Primary tuberculous infection
DEF: Tuberculosis of the lungs occurring when the patient is first infected.

§ √5th **010.0 Primary tuberculous infection** `CC` `HIV`
[0-6] *EXCLUDES* nonspecific reaction to test for tuberculosis without active tuberculosis (795.51-795.52)
positive PPD (795.51)
positive tuberculin skin test without active tuberculosis (795.51)
CC Excl: 010.00-018.96
DEF: Hilar or paratracheal lymph node enlargement in pulmonary tuberculosis.

---

§ Requires fifth digit. Valid digits are in [brackets] under each code. See beginning of section 010-018 for codes and definitions.

Additional Digit Required   Unacceptable PDx   Manifestation Code   Hospital Acquired Condition   ►◄ Revised Text   ● New Code   ▲ Revised Code Title

14 ICD-9-CM   **Volume 1 – 3**

Infectious and Parasitic Diseases

010.1–014.8

§ ✓5ᵗʰ **010.1 Tuberculous pleurisy in primary progressive**   CC HIV
[0-6]   **tuberculosis**
     CC Exd: See code: 010.0
     DEF: Inflammation and exudation in the lining of the tubercular lung.

§ ✓5ᵗʰ **010.8 Other primary progressive tuberculosis**   CC HIV
[0-6]   EXCLUDES *tuberculous erythema nodosum (017.1)*
     CC Exd: See code: 010.0

§ ✓5ᵗʰ **010.9 Primary tuberculous infection, unspecified**   CC HIV
[0-6]   CC Exd: See code: 010.0

✓4ᵗʰ **011 Pulmonary tuberculosis**
     Use additional code to identify any associated silicosis (502)

§ ✓5ᵗʰ **011.0 Tuberculosis of lung, infiltrative**   CC HIV
[0-6]   CC Exd: For code 011.00: 011.00-012.86, 017.90-018.96, 031.0,
     031.2-031.9, 041.81-041.9, 137.0, 139.8, 480.0-480.2, 480.8-487.1,
     488.01-488.02, 488.11-488.12, 494.0-508.9, 517.1, 518.89

§ ✓5ᵗʰ **011.1 Tuberculosis of lung, nodular**   CC HIV
[0-6]   CC Exd: See code: 011.0

§ ✓5ᵗʰ **011.2 Tuberculosis of lung with cavitation**   CC HIV
[0-6]   CC Exd: See code: 011.0

§ ✓5ᵗʰ **011.3 Tuberculosis of bronchus**   CC HIV
[0-6]   EXCLUDES *isolated bronchial tuberculosis (012.2)*
     CC Exd: See code: 011.0

§ ✓5ᵗʰ **011.4 Tuberculous fibrosis of lung**   CC HIV
[0-6]   CC Exd: See code: 011.0

§ ✓5ᵗʰ **011.5 Tuberculous bronchiectasis**   CC HIV
[0-6]   CC Exd: See code: 011.0

§ ✓5ᵗʰ **011.6 Tuberculous pneumonia [any form]**   MCC HIV
[0-6]   DEF: Inflammatory pulmonary reaction to tuberculous cells.
     CC Exd: For codes 011.60-011.65: See code 011.0; For code 011.66: 011.66,
     139.8, 480.0-480.2, 480.8-487.1, 488.01-488.02, 488.11-488.12,
     494.0-508.9, 517.1, 518.89

§ ✓5ᵗʰ **011.7 Tuberculous pneumothorax**   CC HIV
[0-6]   DEF: Spontaneous rupture of damaged tuberculous pulmonary
     tissue.
     CC Exd: See code: 011.0

§ ✓5ᵗʰ **011.8 Other specified pulmonary tuberculosis**   CC HIV
[0-6]   CC Exd: See code: 011.0

§ ✓5ᵗʰ **011.9 Pulmonary tuberculosis, unspecified**   CC HIV
[0-6]   Respiratory tuberculosis NOS
     Tuberculosis of lung NOS
     CC Exd: See code: 011.0

✓4ᵗʰ **012 Other respiratory tuberculosis**
     EXCLUDES *respiratory tuberculosis, unspecified (011.9)*

§ ✓5ᵗʰ **012.0 Tuberculous pleurisy**   CC HIV
[0-6]   Tuberculosis of pleura
     Tuberculous empyema
     Tuberculous hydrothorax
     EXCLUDES *pleurisy with effusion without mention of cause*
         (511.9)
         tuberculous pleurisy in primary progressive
         tuberculosis (010.1)
     DEF: Inflammation and exudation in the lining of the tubercular lung.
     CC Exd: 011.00-012.86, 017.90-018.96, 031.0, 031.2-031.9,
     041.81-041.9, 137.0, 139.8, 480.0-480.2, 480.8-487.1, 488,
     494.0-508.9, 517.1, 518.89

§ ✓5ᵗʰ **012.1 Tuberculosis of intrathoracic lymph nodes**   CC HIV
[0-6]   Tuberculosis of lymph nodes:
     hilar
     mediastinal
     tracheobronchial
     Tuberculous tracheobronchial adenopathy
     EXCLUDES *that specified as primary (010.0-010.9)*
     CC Exd: See code: 012.0

§ ✓5ᵗʰ **012.2 Isolated tracheal or bronchial tuberculosis**   CC
[0-6]   CC Exd: 010.00-014.86, 018.00-018.96

§ ✓5ᵗʰ **012.3 Tuberculous laryngitis**   CC
[0-6]   Tuberculosis of glottis
     CC Exd: See code: 012.2

§ ✓5ᵗʰ **012.8 Other specified respiratory tuberculosis**   CC H
[0-6]   Tuberculosis of: Tuberculosis of:
     mediastinum   nose (septum)
     nasopharynx   sinus [any nasal]
     CC Exd: See code: 012.2

✓4ᵗʰ **013 Tuberculosis of meninges and central nervous system**

§ ✓5ᵗʰ **013.0 Tuberculous meningitis**   MCC
[0-6]   Tuberculosis of meninges (cerebral) (spinal)
     Tuberculous:
     leptomeningitis
     meningoencephalitis
     EXCLUDES *tuberculoma of meninges (013.1)*
     CC Exd: 003.21, 013.00-013.16, 013.40-013.56, 013.80-013.96,
     017.90-017.96, 031.2-031.9, 036.0, 041.81-041.9, 047.0-047.9,
     049.0-049.1, 053.0, 054.72, 072.1, 090.42, 091.81, 094.2, 098.89,
     100.81, 112.83, 114.2, 115.01, 115.11, 115.91, 130.0, 137.1, 139.8,
     320.0-322.9, 349.89-349.9, 357.0

§ ✓5ᵗʰ **013.1 Tuberculoma of meninges**   MCC H
[0-6]   CC Exd: See code: 013.0

§ ✓5ᵗʰ **013.2 Tuberculoma of brain**   MCC H
[0-6]   Tuberculosis of brain (current disease)
     CC Exd: 013.20-013.36, 013.60-013.96, 017.90-017.96, 031.2-031.9,
     041.81-041.9, 137.1, 139.8

§ ✓5ᵗʰ **013.3 Tuberculous abscess of brain**   MCC H
[0-6]   CC Exd: See code: 013.2

§ ✓5ᵗʰ **013.4 Tuberculoma of spinal cord**   MCC H
[0-6]   CC Exd: 013.00-013.16, 013.40-013.56, 013.80-013.96, 017.90-017.96,
     031.2-031.9, 041.81-041.9, 137.1, 139.8

§ ✓5ᵗʰ **013.5 Tuberculous abscess of spinal cord**   MCC H
[0-6]   CC Exd: See code: 013.4

§ ✓5ᵗʰ **013.6 Tuberculous encephalitis or myelitis**   MCC H
[0-6]   CC Exd: See code: 013.2

§ ✓5ᵗʰ **013.8 Other specified tuberculosis of central**   MCC H
[0-6]   **nervous system**
     CC Exd: 013.80-013.96, 017.90-017.96, 031.2-031.9, 041.81-041.9,
     137.1, 139.8

§ ✓5ᵗʰ **013.9 Unspecified tuberculosis of central nervous**   MCC H
[0-6]   **system**
     Tuberculosis of central nervous system NOS
     CC Exd: See code: 013.8

✓4ᵗʰ **014 Tuberculosis of intestines, peritoneum, and mesenteric glands**

§ ✓5ᵗʰ **014.0 Tuberculous peritonitis**   MCC H
[0-6]   Tuberculous ascites
     DEF: Tuberculous inflammation of the membrane lining the
     abdomen.
     CC Exd: 014.00-014.86, 017.90-017.96, 031.2-031.9, 041.81-041.9,
     139.8

§ ✓5ᵗʰ **014.8 Other**   CC H
[0-6]   Tuberculosis (of):
     anus
     intestine (large) (small)
     mesenteric glands
     rectum
     retroperitoneal (lymph nodes)
     Tuberculous enteritis
     CC Exd: For codes 014.80, 014.82-014.86: 014.00-014.86, 017.90-017.96
     031.2-031.9, 041.81-041.9, 139.8; For code 014.81: 014.81, 139.8

---

§   Requires fifth digit. Valid digits are in [brackets] under each code. See beginning of section 010-018 for codes and definitions.

N Newborn Age: 0   P Pediatric Age: 0-17   M Maternity Age: 12-55   A Adult Age: 15-124   MCC Major CC Condition   CC CC Condition   HIV HIV Related D

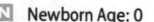

4 – Volume 1   2014 ICD-9-C

Infectious and Parasitic Diseases

015–017.8

✓4th **015 Tuberculosis of bones and joints**

Use additional code to identify manifestation, as:
  tuberculous:
    arthropathy (711.4)
    necrosis of bone (730.8)
    osteitis (730.8)
    osteomyelitis (730.8)
    synovitis (727.01)
    tenosynovitis (727.01)

§ ✓5th **015.0 Vertebral column**   CC HIV
[0-6]   Pott's disease

Use additional code to identify manifestation, as:
    curvature of spine [Pott's] (737.4)
    kyphosis (737.4)
    spondylitis (720.81)
CC Excl: 015.00-015.06

§ ✓5th **015.1 Hip**   CC HIV
[0-6]   CC Excl: 015.10-015.16

§ ✓5th **015.2 Knee**   CC HIV
[0-6]   CC Excl: 015.20-015.26

§ ✓5th **015.5 Limb bones**   CC HIV
[0-6]   Tuberculous dactylitis
     CC Excl: 015.10-015.56

§ ✓5th **015.6 Mastoid**   CC HIV
[0-6]   Tuberculous mastoiditis
     CC Excl: 015.60-015.66

§ ✓5th **015.7 Other specified bone**   CC HIV
[0-6]   CC Excl: For code 015.70: 015.00-015.70; For code 015.71: 015.00-015.66, 015.71; For code 015.72: 015.00-015.66, 015.72; For code 015.73: 015.00-015.66, 015.73; For code 015.74: 015.00-015.66, 015.74; For code 015.75: 015.00-015.66, 015.75; For code 015.76: 015.00-015.66, 015.76

§ ✓5th **015.8 Other specified joint**   CC HIV
[0-6]   CC Excl: 015.80-015.86

§ ✓5th **015.9 Tuberculosis of unspecified bones and joints**   CC HIV
[0-6]   CC Excl: For codes 015.90, 015.92-015.96: 015.00-015.66, 015.80-015.96; For codes 015.91: 015.00-015.66, 015.80-015.93, 015.95-015.96

✓4th **016 Tuberculosis of genitourinary system**

§ ✓5th **016.0 Kidney**   CC HIV
[0-6]   Renal tuberculosis

Use additional code to identify manifestation, as:
    tuberculous:
      nephropathy (583.81)
      pyelitis (590.81)
      pyelonephritis (590.81)
CC Excl: 016.00-016.36, 016.90-016.96, 017.90-017.96, 031.2-031.9, 041.81-041.9, 137.2, 139.8

§ ✓5th **016.1 Bladder**   CC HIV
[0-6]   CC Excl: See code: 016.0

§ ✓5th **016.2 Ureter**   CC HIV
[0-6]   CC Excl: See code: 016.0

§ ✓5th **016.3 Other urinary organs**   CC HIV
[0-6]   CC Excl: See code: 016.0

§ ✓5th **016.4 Epididymis**   CC HIV ♂
[0-6]   CC Excl: 016.40-016.56, 016.90-016.96, 017.90-017.96, 031.2-031.9, 041.81-041.9, 137.2, 139.8

§ ✓5th **016.5 Other male genital organs**   CC HIV ♂
[0-6]   Use additional code to identify manifestation, as:
    tuberculosis of:
      prostate (601.4)
      seminal vesicle (608.81)
      testis (608.81)
CC Excl: See code: 016.4

§ ✓5th **016.6 Tuberculous oophoritis and salpingitis**   CC HIV ♀
[0-6]   CC Excl: 016.60-016.96, 017.90-017.96, 031.2-031.9, 041.81-041.9, 137.2, 139.8

§ ✓5th **016.7 Other female genital organs**   CC HIV ♀
[0-6]   Tuberculous:
    cervicitis
    endometritis
     CC Excl: See code: 016.6

§ ✓5th **016.9 Genitourinary tuberculosis, unspecified**   CC HIV
[0-6]   CC Excl: 016.90-016.96, 017.90-017.96, 031.2-031.9, 041.81-041.9, 137.2, 139.8

✓4th **017 Tuberculosis of other organs**

§ ✓5th **017.0 Skin and subcutaneous cellular tissue**   CC HIV
[0-6]

Lupus:	Tuberculosis:
exedens	colliquativa
vulgaris	cutis
Scrofuloderma	lichenoides
	papulonecrotica
	verrucosa cutis

EXCLUDES   lupus erythematosus (695.4)
         disseminated (710.0)
       lupus NOS (710.0)
       nonspecific reaction to test for tuberculosis without
         active tuberculosis (795.51-795.52)
       positive PPD (795.51)
       positive tuberculin skin test without active
         tuberculosis (795.51)
CC Excl: 010.00-018.96

§ ✓5th **017.1 Erythema nodosum with hypersensitivity**   HIV
[0-6] **reaction in tuberculosis**
Bazin's disease
Erythema:
  induratum
  nodosum, tuberculous
Tuberculosis indurativa
EXCLUDES   erythema nodosum NOS (695.2)
DEF: Tender, inflammatory, bilateral nodules appearing on the shins and thought to be an allergic reaction to tuberculotoxin.

§ ✓5th **017.2 Peripheral lymph nodes**   CC HIV
[0-6]   Scrofula
Scrofulous abscess
Tuberculous adenitis
EXCLUDES   tuberculosis of lymph nodes:
       bronchial and mediastinal (012.1)
       mesenteric and retroperitoneal (014.8)
       tuberculous tracheobronchial adenopathy (012.1)
DEF: Scrofula: Old name for tuberculous cervical lymphadenitis.
CC Excl: 017.20-017.26, 017.90-017.96, 031.2-031.9, 041.81-041.9, 139.8

§ ✓5th **017.3 Eye**   CC HIV
[0-6]   Use additional code to identify manifestation, as:
    tuberculous:
      chorioretinitis, disseminated (363.13)
      episcleritis (379.09)
      interstitial keratitis (370.59)
      iridocyclitis, chronic (364.11)
      keratoconjunctivitis (phlyctenular) (370.31)
CC Excl: 017.30-017.36, 017.90-017.96, 031.2-031.9, 041.81-041.9, 139.8

§ ✓5th **017.4 Ear**   CC HIV
[0-6]   Tuberculosis of ear
Tuberculous otitis media
EXCLUDES   tuberculous mastoiditis (015.6)
CC Excl: 017.40-017.46, 017.90-017.96, 031.2-031.9, 041.81-041.9, 139.8

§ ✓5th **017.5 Thyroid gland**   CC HIV
[0-6]   CC Excl: 017.50-017.56, 017.90-017.96, 031.2-031.9, 041.81-041.9, 139.8

§ ✓5th **017.6 Adrenal glands**   CC HIV
[0-6]   Addison's disease, tuberculous
CC Excl: 017.60-017.66, 017.90-017.96, 031.2-031.9, 041.81-041.9, 139.8

§ ✓5th **017.7 Spleen**   CC HIV
[0-6]   CC Excl: 017.70-017.76, 017.90-017.96, 031.2-031.9, 041.81-041.9, 139.8

§ ✓5th **017.8 Esophagus**   CC HIV
[0-6]   CC Excl: 017.80-017.96, 031.2-031.9, 041.81-041.9, 139.8

Requires fifth digit. Valid digits are in [brackets] under each code. See beginning of section 010-018 for codes and definitions.

Additional Digit Required   Unacceptable PDx   Manifestation Code   Hospital Acquired Condition   ▶◀ Revised Text   ● New Code   ▲ Revised Code Title

2014 ICD-9-CM   Volume 1 – 5

Infectious and Parasitic Diseases

017.9–023.9

§ ✓5ᵗʰ **017.9 Other specified organs**   `CC` `HIV`
[0-6]   Use additional code to identify manifestation, as:
     tuberculosis of:
       endocardium [any valve] (424.91)
       myocardium (422.0)
       pericardium (420.0)
     CC Exd: 017.90-017.96, 031.2-031.9, 041.81-041.9, 139.8

✓4ᵗʰ **018 Miliary tuberculosis**
   INCLUDES tuberculosis:
     disseminated
     generalized
     miliary, whether of a single specified site, multiple sites,
       or unspecified site
     polyserositis
   DEF: A form of tuberculosis caused by caseous material carried through the bloodstream planting seedlike tubercles in various body organs.

§ ✓5ᵗʰ **018.0 Acute miliary tuberculosis**   `MCC` `HIV`
[0-6]   **CC Exd:** 017.90-018.96, 031.2-031.9, 041.81-041.9, 139.8

§ ✓5ᵗʰ **018.8 Other specified miliary tuberculosis**   `MCC` `HIV`
[0-6]   **CC Exd:** See code: 018.0

§ ✓5ᵗʰ **018.9 Miliary tuberculosis, unspecified**   `MCC` `HIV`
[0-6]   **CC Exd:** See code: 018.0

Zoonotic Bacterial Diseases (020-027)

✓4ᵗʰ **020 Plague**
   INCLUDES infection by Yersinia [Pasteurella] pestis

020.0 Bubonic   `MCC`
   DEF: Most common acute and severe form of plague characterized by lymphadenopathy (buboes), chills, fever and headache.
   CC Exd: 020.0-020.9

020.1 Cellulocutaneous   `MCC`
   DEF: Plague characterized by inflammation and necrosis of skin.
   CC Exd: See code: 020.0

020.2 Septicemic   `MCC`
   DEF: Plague characterized by massive infection in the bloodstream.
   CC Exd: 020.0-020.9, 771.81, 771.83-771.89, 995.90-995.94

020.3 Primary pneumonic   `MCC`
   DEF: Plague characterized by massive pulmonary infection.
   CC Exd: 011.00-012.16, 012.80-012.86, 017.90-017.96, 020.0-020.9, 021.3, 022.1, 031.0, 039.1, 073.0, 115.05, 115.15, 115.95, 122.1, 130.4, 136.3, 480.0-487.1, 488.01-488.02, 488.11-488.12, 495.0-495.9, 500-502

020.4 Secondary pneumonic   `MCC`
   DEF: Lung infection as a secondary complication of plague.
   CC Exd: 011.73-011.93, 480.3

020.5 Pneumonic, unspecified   `MCC`
   CC Exd: 020.5, 480.3

020.8 Other specified types of plague   `MCC`
   Abortive plague   Pestis minor
   Ambulatory plague
   CC Exd: 020.8

020.9 Plague, unspecified   `MCC`
   CC Exd: 020.9

✓4ᵗʰ **021 Tularemia**
   INCLUDES deerfly fever
     infection by Francisella [Pasteurella] tularensis
     rabbit fever
   DEF: A febrile disease transmitted by the bites of deer flies, fleas and ticks, by inhalations of aerosolized *F. tularensis* or by ingestion of contaminated food or water; patients quickly develop fever, chills, weakness, headache, backache and malaise.

021.0 Ulceroglandular tularemia   `CC`
   DEF: Lesions occur at the site *Francisella tularensis* organism enters body, usually the fingers or hands.
   CC Exd: 021.0

021.1 Enteric tularemia   `CC`
   Tularemia:
     cryptogenic
     intestinal
     typhoidal
   CC Exd: 021.1

021.2 Pulmonary tularemia   `CC`
   Bronchopneumonic tularemia
   CC Exd: 482.49-487.1, 488.01-488.02, 488.11-488.12, 495.0-495.9, 500-508.9, 517.1, 517.8, 518.89, 519.8-519.9

021.3 Oculoglandular tularemia   `CC`
   DEF: Painful conjunctival infection by *Francisella tularensis* organism with possible corneal, preauricular lymph, or lacrimal involvement.
   CC Exd: 021.3, 480.3

021.8 Other specified tularemia   `CC`
   Tularemia:
     generalized or disseminated
     glandular
   CC Exd: 021.0-021.9

021.9 Unspecified tularemia   `CC`
   CC Exd: See code: 021.8

✓4ᵗʰ **022 Anthrax**
   DEF: A bacterial disease usually transmitted by contact with infected animals or their discharges; primary routes of inoculation are cutaneous, gastrointestinal and inhalation.
   AHA: 4Q '02, 70

022.0 Cutaneous anthrax   `CC`
   Malignant pustule
   CC Exd: 022.0

022.1 Pulmonary anthrax   `MCC`
   Respiratory anthrax
   Wool-sorters' disease
   CC Exd: 011.00-012.16, 012.80-012.86, 017.90-017.96, 020.3-020.5, 021.3, 022.1, 031.0, 039.1, 073.0, 115.05, 115.15, 115.95, 122.1, 130.4, 136.3, 480.0-487.1, 488.01-488.02, 488.11-488.12, 494.0-495.9, 500-508.9, 517.1, 517.8, 518.89, 519.8-519.9

022.2 Gastrointestinal anthrax   `CC`
   CC Exd: 022.2

022.3 Anthrax septicemia   `MCC`
   CC Exd: 003.1, 020.2, 022.3, 036.2, 038.0-038.9, 040.89-041.3, 041.41-041.9, 054.5, 139.8, 771.81, 771.83-771.89, 995.90-995.94, V09.0-V09.91

022.8 Other specified manifestations of anthrax   `CC`
   CC Exd: 022.8

022.9 Anthrax, unspecified   `CC`
   CC Exd: 022.0-022.9

✓4ᵗʰ **023 Brucellosis**
   INCLUDES fever:
     Malta
     Mediterranean
     undulant
   DEF: An infectious disease caused by gram-negative, aerobic coccobacilli organisms transmitted to humans through contact with infected tissue or dairy products; fever, sweating, weakness and aching are symptoms.

023.0 Brucella melitensis
   DEF: Infection from direct or indirect contact with infected sheep or goats.

023.1 Brucella abortus
   DEF: Infection from direct or indirect contact with infected cattle.

023.2 Brucella suis
   DEF: Infection from direct or indirect contact with infected swine.

023.3 Brucella canis
   DEF: Infection from direct or indirect contact with infected dogs.

023.8 Other brucellosis   `CC`
   Infection by more than one organism
   CC Exd: 023.0-023.9

023.9 Brucellosis, unspecified   `CC`
   CC Exd: See code: 023.8

---

§   Requires fifth digit. Valid digits are in [brackets] under each code. See beginning of section 010-018 for codes and definitions.

N Newborn Age: 0   P Pediatric Age: 0-17   M Maternity Age: 12-55   A Adult Age: 15-124   `MCC` Major CC Condition   `CC` CC Condition   `HIV` HIV Related D

6 – Volume 1   2014 ICD-9-C

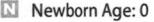

024　Glanders　　`CC`
　　Infection by:
　　　actinobacillus mallei
　　　malleomyces mallei
　　　pseudomonas mallei
　　Farcy
　　Malleus
　　DEF: Equine infection causing mucosal inflammation and skin ulcers in humans.
　　CC Exd: 024

025　Melioidosis　　`CC`
　　Infection by:
　　　malleomyces pseudomallei
　　　pseudomonas pseudomallei
　　　whitmore's bacillus
　　Pseudoglanders
　　DEF: Rare infection caused by *Pseudomonas pseudomallei;* clinical symptoms range from localized infection to fatal septicemia.
　　CC Exd: 025

✓4ᵗʰ **026　Rat-bite fever**

026.0　Spirillary fever　　`CC`
　　Rat-bite fever due to Spirillum minor [S. minus]
　　Sodoku
　　CC Exd: 026.0-026.9

026.1　Streptobacillary fever　　`CC`
　　Epidemic arthritic erythema
　　Haverhill fever
　　Rat-bite fever due to Streptobacillus moniliformis
　　CC Exd: See code: 026.0

026.9　Unspecified rat-bite fever　　`CC`
　　CC Exd: See code: 026.0

✓4ᵗʰ **027　Other zoonotic bacterial diseases**

027.0　Listeriosis　　`CC`
　　Infection ⎫
　　Septicemia ⎬ by Listeria monocytogenes
　　Use additional code to identify manifestation, as meningitis (320.7)
　　EXCLUDES congenital listeriosis (771.2)
　　CC Exd: 027.0-027.9

027.1　Erysipelothrix infection
　　Erysipeloid (of Rosenbach)
　　Infection ⎫ by Erysipelothrix insidiosa [E.
　　Septicemia ⎬ rhusiopathiae]
　　DEF: Usually associated with handling of fish, meat, or poultry; symptoms range from localized inflammation to septicemia.

027.2　Pasteurellosis　　`CC`
　　Pasteurella pseudotuberculosis infection
　　Mesenteric adenitis ⎫ by Pasteurella multocida
　　Septic infection (cat ⎬ [P. septica]
　　　bite) (dog bite) ⎭
　　EXCLUDES infection by:
　　　　Francisella [Pasteurella] tularensis (021.0-021.9)
　　　　Yersinia [Pasteurella] pestis (020.0-020.9)
　　DEF: Swelling, abscesses, or septicemia from *Pasteurella multocida,* commonly transmitted to humans by a dog or cat scratch.
　　CC Exd: See code: 027.0
　　AHA: ▶3Q, '12, 13◀

027.8　Other specified zoonotic bacterial diseases　　`CC`
　　CC Exd: See code: 027.0

027.9　Unspecified zoonotic bacterial disease　　`CC`
　　CC Exd: See code: 027.0

Other Bacterial Diseases (030-041)

　　EXCLUDES bacterial venereal diseases (098.0-099.9)
　　　　bartonellosis (088.0)

✓4ᵗʰ **030　Leprosy**
　　INCLUDES Hansen's disease
　　　　infection by Mycobacterium leprae

030.0　Lepromatous [type L]　　`CC`
　　Lepromatous leprosy (macular) (diffuse) (infiltrated) (nodular) (neuritic)
　　DEF: Infectious, disseminated leprosy bacilli with lesions and deformities.
　　CC Exd: 030.0

030.1　Tuberculoid [type T]　　`CC`
　　Tuberculoid leprosy (macular) (maculoanesthetic) (major) (minor) (neuritic)
　　DEF: Relatively benign, self-limiting leprosy with neuralgia and scales.
　　CC Exd: 030.1

030.2　Indeterminate [group I]　　`CC`
　　Indeterminate [uncharacteristic] leprosy (macular) (neuritic)
　　DEF: Uncharacteristic leprosy, frequently an early manifestation.
　　CC Exd: 030.2

030.3　Borderline [group B]　　`CC`
　　Borderline or dimorphous leprosy (infiltrated) (neuritic)
　　DEF: Transitional form of leprosy, neither lepromatous nor tuberculoid.
　　CC Exd: 030.3

030.8　Other specified leprosy　　`CC`
　　CC Exd: 030.8

030.9　Leprosy, unspecified　　`CC`
　　CC Exd: 030.9

✓4ᵗʰ **031　Diseases due to other mycobacteria**

031.0　Pulmonary　　`CC`
　　Battey disease
　　Infection by Mycobacterium:
　　　avium
　　　intracellulare [Battey bacillus]
　　　kansasii
　　CC Exd: 011.00-012.86, 017.90-017.96, 031.0, 031.2-031.9, 041.81-041.9, 137.0, 139.8, 480.0-480.2, 480.8-487.1, 488.01-488.02, 488.11-488.12, 494.0-508.9, 517.1, 518.89

031.1　Cutaneous　　`CC`
　　Buruli ulcer
　　Infection by Mycobacterium:
　　　marinum [M. balnei]
　　　ulcerans
　　CC Exd: 031.0-031.9

031.2　Disseminated　　`CC` `HIV`
　　Disseminated mycobacterium avium-intracellulare complex (DMAC)
　　Mycobacterium avium-intracellulare complex (MAC) bacteremia
　　DEF: Disseminated mycobacterium avium-intracellulare complex (DMAC): A serious systemic form of MAC commonly observed in patients in the late course of AIDS.
　　DEF: Mycobacterium avium-intracellulare complex (MAC) bacterium: Human pulmonary disease, lymphadenitis in children and systemic disease in immunocompromised individuals caused by a slow growing, gram-positive, aerobic organism.
　　CC Exd: See code: 031.1
　　AHA: 4Q, '97, 31

031.8　Other specified mycobacterial diseases　　`CC` `HIV`
　　CC Exd: See code: 031.1

031.9　Unspecified diseases due to mycobacteria　　`CC` `HIV`
　　Atypical mycobacterium infection NOS
　　CC Exd: See code: 031.1

✓4ᵗʰ **032　Diphtheria**
　　INCLUDES infection by Corynebacterium diphtheriae

032.0　Faucial diphtheria　　`CC`
　　Membranous angina, diphtheritic
　　DEF: Diphtheria of the throat.
　　CC Exd: 032.0-032.9

032.1　Nasopharyngeal diphtheria　　`CC`
　　CC Exd: See code: 032.0

032.2　Anterior nasal diphtheria　　`CC`
　　CC Exd: See code: 032.0

032.3　Laryngeal diphtheria　　`CC`
　　Laryngotracheitis, diphtheritic
　　CC Exd: See code: 032.0

✓5ᵗʰ **032.8　Other specified diphtheria**

032.81　Conjunctival diphtheria　　`CC`
　　Pseudomembranous diphtheritic conjunctivitis
　　CC Exd: See code: 032.0

Infectious and Parasitic Diseases

032.82–038.12

032.82 Diphtheritic myocarditis `CC`
CC Excl: 032.82, 074.20, 074.22-074.23, 093.82, 390, 391.2-391.9, 398.0-398.90, 398.99, 422.0-422.99, 429.0, 429.71-429.79, 459.89-459.9

032.83 Diphtheritic peritonitis `CC`
CC Excl: 014.00-014.06, 032.83, 090.0, 095.2, 098.86, 099.56, 540.0-540.1, 567.0-567.1, 567.22, 567.29, 567.81, 567.9, 569.87-569.9, 577.8, 614.5-614.7, 639.0, 670.00-670.84, 777.6, 998.7

032.84 Diphtheritic cystitis `CC`
CC Excl: See code: 032.0

032.85 Cutaneous diphtheria `CC`
CC Excl: See code: 032.0

032.89 Other `CC`
CC Excl: See code: 032.0

032.9 Diphtheria, unspecified `CC`
CC Excl: See code: 032.0

√4ᵗʰ **033 Whooping cough**
INCLUDES pertussis
Use additional code to identify any associated pneumonia (484.3)
DEF: An acute, highly contagious respiratory tract infection caused by *Bordetella pertussis* and *B. bronchiseptica;* characteristic paroxysmal cough.

033.0 Bordetella pertussis [B. pertussis] `CC`
CC Excl: 033.0-033.9

033.1 Bordetella parapertussis [B. parapertussis] `CC`
CC Excl: See code: 033.0

033.8 Whooping cough due to other specified organism `CC`
Bordetella bronchiseptica [B. bronchiseptica]
CC Excl: See code: 033.0

033.9 Whooping cough, unspecified organism `CC`
CC Excl: See code: 033.0

√4ᵗʰ **034 Streptococcal sore throat and scarlet fever**

034.0 Streptococcal sore throat
Septic:
  angina
  sore throat
Streptococcal:
  angina
  laryngitis
  pharyngitis
  tonsillitis

J02.0 Streptococcal pharyngitis `I-10`

034.1 Scarlet fever `CC`
Scarlatina
EXCLUDES parascarlatina (057.8)
DEF: Streptococcal infection and fever with red rash spreading from trunk.
CC Excl: 034.0-035

035 Erysipelas
EXCLUDES postpartum or puerperal erysipelas (670.8)
DEF: An acute superficial cellulitis involving the dermal lymphatics; it is often caused by group A streptococci.

√4ᵗʰ **036 Meningococcal infection**

036.0 Meningococcal meningitis `MCC`
Cerebrospinal fever (meningococcal)
Meningitis:
  cerebrospinal
  epidemic
CC Excl: 003.21, 013.00-013.16, 036.0, 036.89-036.9, 041.81-041.9, 047.0-047.9, 049.0-049.1, 053.0, 054.72, 072.1, 090.42, 091.81, 094.2, 098.89, 100.81, 112.83, 114.2, 115.01, 115.11, 115.91, 130.0, 139.8, 320.0-322.9, 349.89-349.9, 357.0

036.1 Meningococcal encephalitis `MCC`
CC Excl: 036.1, 036.89-036.9, 041.81-041.9, 139.8

036.2 Meningococcemia `MCC`
Meningococcal septicemia
CC Excl: 003.1, 020.2, 036.2, 036.89-036.9, 038.0-038.9, 041.81-041.9, 054.5, 139.8, 995.90-995.94

036.3 Waterhouse-Friderichsen syndrome, meningococcal `MCC`
Meningococcal hemorrhagic adrenalitis
Meningococcic adrenal syndrome
Waterhouse-Friderichsen syndrome NOS
CC Excl: 036.3, 036.89-036.9, 041.81-041.9, 139.8

√5ᵗʰ **036.4 Meningococcal carditis**

036.40 Meningococcal carditis, unspecified `MCC`
CC Excl: 036.40, 036.89-036.9, 041.81-041.9, 139.8

036.41 Meningococcal pericarditis `MCC`
DEF: Meningococcal infection of the outer membrane of the heart.
CC Excl: 036.41, 036.89-036.9, 041.81-041.9, 139.8

036.42 Meningococcal endocarditis `MCC`
DEF: Meningococcal infection of the membranes lining the cavities of the heart.
CC Excl: 036.42, 036.89-036.9, 041.81-041.9, 139.8

036.43 Meningococcal myocarditis `MCC`
DEF: Meningococcal infection of the muscle of the heart.
CC Excl: 036.43, 041.81-041.9, 139.8

√5ᵗʰ **036.8 Other specified meningococcal infections**

036.81 Meningococcal optic neuritis `CC`
CC Excl: 036.81, 036.89-036.9, 041.81-041.9, 139.8

036.82 Meningococcal arthropathy `CC`
CC Excl: 036.82-036.9, 041.81-041.9, 139.8

036.89 Other `CC`
CC Excl: 036.89-036.9, 041.81-041.9, 139.8

036.9 Meningococcal infection, unspecified `CC`
Meningococcal infection NOS
CC Excl: See code: 036.89

037 Tetanus `MCC`
EXCLUDES tetanus:
  complicating:
    abortion (634-638 with .0, 639.0)
    ectopic or molar pregnancy (639.0)
  neonatorum (771.3)
  puerperal (670.8)
DEF: An acute, often fatal, infectious disease caused by the anaerobic, spore-forming bacillus *Clostridium tetani;* the bacillus enters the body through a contaminated wound, burns, surgical wounds, or cutaneous ulcers. Symptoms: lockjaw, spasms, seizures, and paralysis.
CC Excl: 037, 139.8

√4ᵗʰ **038 Septicemia**
Use additional code for systemic inflammatory response syndrome (SIRS) (995.91-995.92)
EXCLUDES bacteremia (790.7)
  during labor (659.3)
  following ectopic or molar pregnancy (639.0)
  following infusion, injection, transfusion, or vaccination (999.3)
  postpartum, puerperal (670)
  septicemia (sepsis) of newborn (771.81)
  that complicating abortion (634-638 with .0, 639.0)
DEF: A systemic disease associated with the presence and persistence of pathogenic microorganisms or their toxins in the blood.
AHA: ▶3Q, '12, 11-12;◀1Q, '12, 19; 2Q, '10, 4; 2Q, '04, 16; 4Q, '88, 10; 3Q, '88, 12
TIP: When septicemia is due to a complication of care, sequence the complication code first (e.g., due to device or injury).

038.0 Streptococcal septicemia `MCC` `HIV`
CC Excl: 003.1, 020.2, 036.2, 038.0-038.9, 040.82-041.3, 041.41-041.9, 054.5, 139.8, 995.90-995.94, V09.0-V09.91
AHA: 4Q, '03, 79; 2Q, '96, 5

√5ᵗʰ **038.1 Staphylococcal septicemia**
AHA: 4Q, '97, 32

038.10 Staphylococcal septicemia, unspecified `MCC` `HIV`
CC Excl: See code: 038.0

038.11 Methicillin susceptible Staphylococcus aureus septicemia `MCC` `HIV`
MSSA septicemia
Staphylococcus aureus septicemia NOS
CC Excl: See code: 038.0
AHA: 4Q, '08, 69-70;1Q, '05, 7; 2Q, '00, 5; 4Q, '98, 42
A41.01 Sepsis d/t Methicillin susceptible Staphylococcus aureus `I-10`

038.12 Methicillin resistant Staphylococcus aureus septicemia `MCC` `HIV`
CC Excl: See code: 038.0
AHA: 4Q, '11, 153; 3Q, '11, 15; 4Q, '08, 69-73

N Newborn Age: 0   P Pediatric Age: 0-17   M Maternity Age: 12-55   A Adult Age: 15-124   MCC Major CC Condition   CC CC Condition   HIV HIV Related Dx

8 – Volume 1 · February 2013   2014 ICD-9-CM

038.19 Other staphylococcal septicemia `MCC` `HIV`
    CC Exd: See code: 038.0
    AHA: 2Q, '00, 5
    A41.1 Sepsis due to other specified `I-10`

038.2 Pneumococcal septicemia `MCC` `HIV`
    [Streptococcus pneumoniae septicemia]
    CC Exd: See code 038.0
    AHA: 2Q, '96, 5; 1Q, '91, 13

038.3 Septicemia due to anaerobes `MCC` `HIV`
    Septicemia due to bacteroides
    EXCLUDES   gas gangrene (040.0)
                that due to anaerobic streptococci (038.0)
    DEF: Infection of blood by microorganisms that thrive without oxygen.
    CC Exd: See code 038.0

√5ᵗʰ **038.4 Septicemia due to other gram-negative organisms**
    DEF: Infection of blood by microorganisms categorized as gram-negative by Gram's method of staining for identification of bacteria.

    038.40 Gram-negative organism, unspecified `MCC` `HIV`
        Gram-negative septicemia NOS
        CC Exd: See code 038.0

    038.41 Hemophilus influenzae [H. influenzae] `MCC` `HIV`
        CC Exd: See code 038.0

    038.42 Escherichia coli [E. coli] `MCC` `HIV`
        CC Exd: See code 038.0
        AHA: 4Q, '03, 73
        A41.51 Sepsis due to Escherichia coli [E coli] `I-10`

    038.43 Pseudomonas `MCC` `HIV`
        CC Exd: See code 038.0

    038.44 Serratia `MCC` `HIV`
        CC Exd: See code 038.0

    038.49 Other `MCC` `HIV`
        CC Exd: See code 038.0
        AHA: ▶3Q, '12, 13◀
        A41.59 Other Gram-negative sepsis `I-10`

038.8 Other specified septicemias `MCC` `HIV`
    EXCLUDES   septicemia (due to):
                 anthrax (022.3)
                 gonococcal (098.89)
                 herpetic (054.5)
                 meningococcal (036.2)
                 septicemic plague (020.2)
    CC Exd: See code 038.0

038.9 Unspecified septicemia `MCC` `HIV`
    Septicemia NOS
    EXCLUDES   bacteremia NOS (790.7)
    CC Exd: See code 038.0
    AHA: 4Q, '07, 97; 2Q, '05, 18-19; 2Q, '04, 16; 4Q, '03, 79; 2Q, '00, 3; 3Q, '99, 5, 9; 1Q, '98, 5; 3Q, '96, 16; 2Q, '96, 6
    TIP: Ensure that documentation includes clinical evidence of systemic infection; do not code if documentation indicates "urosepsis" only.
    A41.9 Sepsis unspecified `I-10`

√4ᵗʰ **039 Actinomycotic infections**
    INCLUDES   actinomycotic mycetoma
                 infection by Actinomycetales, such as species of Actinomyces, Actinomadura, Nocardia, Streptomyces
                 maduromycosis (actinomycotic)
                 schizomycetoma (actinomycotic)
    DEF: Inflammatory lesions and abscesses at site of infection by Actinomyces israelii.

039.0 Cutaneous `CC` `HIV`
    Erythrasma
    Trichomycosis axillaris
    CC Exd: 039.0, 039.8-039.9

039.1 Pulmonary `CC` `HIV`
    Thoracic actinomycosis
    CC Exd: 039.1, 039.8-039.9, 480.3

039.2 Abdominal `CC` `HIV`
    CC Exd: 039.2, 039.8-039.9

039.3 Cervicofacial `CC` `HIV`
    CC Exd: 039.3, 039.8-039.9

039.4 Madura foot `CC` `HIV`
    EXCLUDES   madura foot due to mycotic infection (117.4)
    CC Exd: 039.4-039.9

039.8 Of other specified sites `CC` `HIV`
    CC Exd: 039.0-039.9

039.9 Of unspecified site `CC` `HIV`
    Actinomycosis NOS
    Maduromycosis NOS
    Nocardiosis NOS
    CC Exd: See code: 039.8

√4ᵗʰ **040 Other bacterial diseases**
    EXCLUDES   bacteremia NOS (790.7)
                 bacterial infection NOS (041.9)

040.0 Gas gangrene `MCC`
    Gas bacillus infection or gangrene
    Infection by Clostridium:
        histolyticum
        oedematiens
        perfringens [welchii]
        septicum
        sordellii
    Malignant edema
    Myonecrosis, clostridial
    Myositis, clostridial
    CC Exd: 040.0, 139.8
    AHA: 1Q, '95, 11

040.1 Rhinoscleroma
    DEF: Growths on the nose and nasopharynx caused by Klebsiella rhinoscleromatis.

040.2 Whipple's disease `CC`
    Intestinal lipodystrophy
    CC Exd: 040.2

040.3 Necrobacillosis `CC`
    DEF: Infection with Fusobacterium necrophorum causing abscess or necrosis.
    CC Exd: 040.3
    AHA: 4Q, '07, 85

√5ᵗʰ **040.4 Other specified botulism**
    Non-foodborne intoxication due to toxins of Clostridium botulinum [C. botulinum]
    EXCLUDES   botulism NOS (005.1)
                 food poisoning due to toxins of Clostridium botulinum (005.1)

    040.41 Infant botulism `P` `CC`
        DEF: Colonization of Clostridium botulinum spores in the large intestine; release of neurotoxins results in constipation; may progress to neuromuscular paralysis; affects infants of less than six months.
        CC Exd: 005.0-005.2, 008.45-008.46, 040.41-040.42
        AHA: 4Q, '07, 60

    040.42 Wound botulism `CC`
        Non-foodborne botulism NOS
        Use additional code to identify complicated open wound
        CC Exd: See code 040.41
        AHA: 4Q, '07, 60

√5ᵗʰ **040.8 Other specified bacterial diseases**

    040.81 Tropical pyomyositis `CC`
        CC Exd: 040.81, 040.89

    040.82 Toxic shock syndrome `MCC`
        Use additional code to identify the organism
        DEF: Syndrome caused by staphylococcal exotoxin that may rapidly progress to severe and intractable shock; symptoms include sunburn-like rash with peeling of skin on palms and soles, sudden onset high fever, vomiting, diarrhea, myalgia, and hypotension.
        CC Exd: 040.82, 338.0-338.4, 780.64-780.65, 780.91-780.99, 785.50-785.59, 785.9, 799.81-799.89
        AHA: 4Q, '02, 44

    040.89 Other
        AHA: N-D, '86, 7

Infectious and Parasitic Diseases

041–042

√4ᵗʰ **041 Bacterial infection in conditions classified elsewhere and of unspecified site**

> **NOTE** This category is provided to be used as an additional code to identify the bacterial agent in diseases classified elsewhere. This category will also be used to classify bacterial infections of unspecified nature or site.
>
> **EXCLUDES** *septicemia (038.0-038.9)*
>
> AHA: 2Q, '01, 12; J-A, '84, 19

√5ᵗʰ **041.0 Streptococcus**

  041.00 Streptococcus, unspecified

  041.01 Group A
    AHA: 1Q, '02, 3

  041.02 Group B
    B95.1 Streptococcus group B cause of dz   I-10

  041.03 Group C

  041.04 Group D [Enterococcus]
    B95.2 Enterococcus as the cause of dz class   I-10

  041.05 Group G

  041.09 Other Streptococcus
    B95.4 Oth streptococcus cause of dz class elsewhere   I-10

√5ᵗʰ **041.1 Staphylococcus**

  041.10 Staphylococcus, unspecified
    AHA: 2Q, '06, 15

  041.11 Methicillin susceptible Staphylococcus aureus
    MSSA
    Staphylococcus aureus NOS
    AHA: 4Q, '08, 69-70; 2Q, '06, 16; 4Q, '03, 104, 106; 2Q, '01, 11; 4Q, '98, 42, 54; 4Q, '97, 32
    A49.01 Methicillin suscep staph infection, unsp site   I-10

  041.12 Methicillin resistant Staphylococcus aureus
    Methicillin-resistant staphylococcus aureus (MRSA)
    AHA: 4Q, '09, 98; 4Q, '08, 69-70, 73
    TIP: Do not assign if combination code (with localized infection) available, or if only colonization or carrier status documented.

  041.19 Other Staphylococcus
    AHA: 2Q, '11, 7; 2Q, '08, 3
    B95.7 Other staphylococcus cause of dz class   I-10

041.2 Pneumococcus

041.3 Klebsiella pneumoniae
  AHA: 4Q, '08, 149

√5ᵗʰ **041.4 Escherichia coli [E. coli]**
  AHA: 4Q, '11, 81-83

  041.41 Shiga toxin-producing Escherichia coli [E. coli] (STEC) O157
    E. coli O157:H- (nonmotile) with confirmation of Shiga toxin
    E. coli O157 with confirmation of Shiga toxin when H antigen is unknown, or is not H7
    O157:H7 Escherichia coli [E.coli] with or without confirmation of Shiga toxin-production
    Shiga toxin-producing Escherichia coli [E.coli] O157:H7 with or without confirmation of Shiga toxin-production
    STEC O157:H7 with or without confirmation of Shiga toxin-production
    AHA: 4Q, '11, 83

  041.42 Other specified Shiga toxin-producing Escherichia coli [E. coli] (STEC)
    Non-O157 Shiga toxin-producing Escherichia coli [E.coli]
    Non-O157 Shiga toxin-producing Escherichia coli [E.coli] with known O group

  041.43 Shiga toxin-producing Escherichia coli [E. coli] (STEC), unspecified
    Shiga toxin-producing Escherichia coli [E. coli] with unspecified O group
    STEC NOS

  041.49 Other and unspecified Escherichia coli [E. coli]
    Escherichia coli [E. coli] NOS
    Non-Shiga toxin-producing E. Coli
    AHA: 4Q, '11, 155
    B96.20 Unsp Escherichia coli as cause of diseases classd elswhr   I-10

041.5 Hemophilus influenzae [H. influenzae]

041.6 Proteus (mirabilis) (morganii)

041.7 Pseudomonas
  AHA: 1Q, '10, 9; 4Q, '02, 45
  B96.5 Pseudomonas as the cause of dz class elsewhere   I-1

√5ᵗʰ **041.8 Other specified bacterial infections**

  041.81 Mycoplasma
    Eaton's agent
    Pleuropneumonia-like organisms [PPLO]

  041.82 Bacteroides fragilis
    DEF: Anaerobic gram-negative bacilli of the gastrointestinal tract; frequently implicated in intra-abdominal infection; commonly resistant to antibiotics.

  041.83 Clostridium perfringens

  041.84 Other anaerobes
    Gram-negative anaerobes
    EXCLUDES *Helicobacter pylori (041.86)*

  041.85 Other gram-negative organisms
    Aerobacter aerogenes
    Gram-negative bacteria NOS
    Mima polymorpha
    Serratia
    EXCLUDES *gram-negative anaerobes (041.84)*
    AHA: 1Q, '95, 18

  041.86 Helicobacter pylori [H. pylori]
    AHA: 4Q, '95, 60
    B96.81 Helicobacter pylori cause of dz class elsewhere   I-

  041.89 Other specified bacteria
    AHA: 2Q, '06, 7; 2Q, '03, 7
    A49.8 Other bacterial infections of unspecified site   I-

041.9 Bacterial infection, unspecified
  AHA: 2Q, '91, 9

Human Immunodeficiency Virus (HIV) Infection (042)

042 Human immunodeficiency virus [HIV] disease   MC
  Acquired immune deficiency syndrome
  Acquired immunodeficiency syndrome
  AIDS
  AIDS-like syndrome
  AIDS-related complex
  ARC
  HIV infection, symptomatic
  Use additional code(s) to identify all manifestations of HIV
  Use additional code to identify HIV-2 infection (079.53)
  EXCLUDES *asymptomatic HIV infection status (V08)*
      exposure to HIV virus (V01.79)
      nonspecific serologic evidence of HIV (795.71)
  CC Excl: 042, 139.8
  AHA: 3Q, '10, 13; 4Q, '07, 63; 3Q, '06, 15; 1Q, '05, 7; 2Q, '04, 11; 1Q, '04, 5; 1Q, '03, 15; 1Q, '99, 14; 4Q, '97, 30, 31; 1Q, '93, 21; 2Q, '92, 11; 3Q, '90, 17; J-A, '88
  TIP: Code only confirmed cases of HIV infection/illness; may be coded from provider's diagnostic statement.
  B20 Human immunodeficiency virus [HIV] disease   I-

N Newborn Age: 0   P Pediatric Age: 0-17   M Maternity Age: 12-55   A Adult Age: 15-124   MCC Major CC Condition   CC CC Condition   HIV HIV Related

10 – Volume 1   2014 ICD-9-
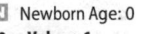

Poliomyelitis and Other Non-Arthropod-borne Viral Diseases and Prion Diseases of Central Nervous System (045-049)

☑4ᵗʰ 045 Acute poliomyelitis

EXCLUDES *late effects of acute poliomyelitis (138)*

The following fifth-digit subclassification is for use with category 045:
- 0 poliovirus, unspecified type
- 1 poliovirus type I
- 2 poliovirus type II
- 3 poliovirus type III

§ ☑5ᵗʰ 045.0 Acute paralytic poliomyelitis specified as bulbar   MCC
[0-3]

Infantile paralysis (acute)
Poliomyelitis (acute) (anterior) } specified as bulbar

Polioencephalitis (acute) (bulbar)
Polioencephalomyelitis (acute) (anterior) (bulbar)

DEF: Acute paralytic infection occurring where the brain merges with the spinal cord; affecting breathing, swallowing, and heart rate.
CC Exd: 045.00-045.13

§ ☑5ᵗʰ 045.1 Acute poliomyelitis with other paralysis   MCC
[0-3]

Paralysis:
  acute atrophic, spinal
  infantile, paralytic
Poliomyelitis (acute)
  anterior } with paralysis except bulbar
  epidemic

DEF: Paralytic infection affecting peripheral or spinal nerves.
CC Exd: See code: 045.0

§ ☑5ᵗʰ 045.2 Acute nonparalytic poliomyelitis
[0-3]

Poliomyelitis (acute)
  anterior } specified as nonparalytic
  epidemic

DEF: Nonparalytic infection causing pain, stiffness, and paresthesias.

§ ☑5ᵗʰ 045.9 Acute poliomyelitis, unspecified
[0-3]

Infantile paralysis
Poliomyelitis (acute) } unspecified whether paralytic or
  anterior   nonparalytic
  epidemic

☑4ᵗʰ 046 Slow virus infections and prion diseases of central nervous system

046.0 Kuru   CC

DEF: A chronic, progressive, fatal nervous system disorder; clinical symptoms include cerebellar ataxia, trembling, spasticity and progressive dementia.
CC Exd: 046.0-046.9

☑5ᵗʰ 046.1 Jakob-Creutzfeldt disease

Use additional code to identify dementia:
  with behavioral disturbance (294.11)
  without behavioral disturbance (294.10)

046.11 Variant Creutzfeldt-Jakob disease   CC
vCJD

AHA: 4Q, '08, 73-75
CC Exd: 013.60-013.66, 046.0-046.9, 048-049.0, 049.8, 052.0, 052.2, 054.3, 054.74, 056.01, 057.8-058.29, 059.00-059.9, 062.0-064, 066.2-066.3, 072.2, 073.7, 079.99, 081.9, 083.9, 090.41, 094.81, 117.5, 124, 130.0, 290.12, 323.01-323.9, 341.1, 487.8, 488.09, 488.19, 771.2, 984.9

046.19 Other and unspecified Creutzfeldt-Jakob disease   CC
CJD
Familial Creutzfeldt-Jakob disease
Iatrogenic Creutzfeldt-Jakob disease
Jakob-Creutzfeldt disease, unspecified
Sporadic Creutzfeldt-Jakob disease
Subacute spongiform encephalopathy

EXCLUDES *variant Creutzfeldt-Jakob disease (vCJD) (046.11)*

DEF: Communicable, progressive spongiform encephalopathy thought to be caused by an infectious particle known as a "prion" (proteinaceous infection particle); a progressive, fatal disease manifested principally by mental deterioration.
CC Exd: See code: 046.11
AHA: 4Q, '08, 73-75

046.2 Subacute sclerosing panencephalitis   CC
Dawson's inclusion body encephalitis
Van Bogaert's sclerosing leukoencephalitis
CC Exd: 046.2, 139.8
DEF: Progressive viral infection causing cerebral dysfunction, blindness, dementia, and death (SSPE).

046.3 Progressive multifocal leukoencephalopathy   CC HIV
Multifocal leukoencephalopathy NOS
DEF: Infection affecting cerebral cortex in patients with weakened immune systems.
CC Exd: 013.60-013.66, 046.0-046.9, 048-049.0, 049.8, 052.0, 052.2, 054.3, 054.74, 056.01, 057.8-058.29, 059.00-059.9, 062.0-064, 066.2-066.3, 072.2, 073.7, 075, 081.9, 083.9, 090.41, 094.81, 117.5, 124, 130.0, 290.12, 323.01-323.9, 341.1, 487.8, 488.09, 488.19, 771.2, 984.9

☑5ᵗʰ 046.7 Other specified prion diseases of central nervous system

EXCLUDES *Creutzfeldt-Jakob disease (046.11-046.19)*
Jakob-Creutzfeldt disease (046.11-046.19)
kuru (046.0)
variant Creutzfeldt-Jakob disease (vCJD) (046.11)

046.71 Gerstmann-Sträussler-Scheinker syndrome   CC HIV
GSS syndrome
AHA: 4Q, '08, 73-75
CC Exd: 046.0-046.9, 066.40-066.49, 079.82

046.72 Fatal familial insomnia   CC HIV
FFI
AHA: 4Q, '08, 73-75
CC Exd: See code: 046.71

046.79 Other and unspecified prion disease of central nervous system   CC HIV
CC Exd: See code: 046.71

046.8 Other specified slow virus infection of central nervous system   CC HIV
CC Exd: 046.0-046.9, 066.40-066.49, 079.82

046.9 Unspecified slow virus infection of central nervous system   CC HIV
CC Exd: 046.0-046.9

☑4ᵗʰ 047 Meningitis due to enterovirus

INCLUDES meningitis:
  abacterial
  aseptic
  viral

EXCLUDES *meningitis due to:*
adenovirus (049.1)
arthropod-borne virus (060.0-066.9)
leptospira (100.81)
virus of:
  herpes simplex (054.72)
  herpes zoster (053.0)
  lymphocytic choriomeningitis (049.0)
  mumps (072.1)
  poliomyelitis (045.0-045.9)
any other infection specifically classified elsewhere

AHA: J-F, '87, 6

047.0 Coxsackie virus   CC
CC Exd: 003.21, 013.00-013.16, 036.0, 047.0-047.9, 049.0-049.1, 072.1, 078.88-078.89, 079.81, 079.88-079.99, 090.42, 091.81, 094.2, 098.89, 100.81, 112.83, 114.2, 115.01, 115.11, 115.91, 130.0, 139.8, 320.0-322.9, 349.89-349.9, 357.0

047.1 ECHO virus   CC
Meningo-eruptive syndrome
CC Exd: See code: 047.0

047.8 Other specified viral meningitis   CC
CC Exd: See code: 047.0

047.9 Unspecified viral meningitis   CC
Viral meningitis NOS
CC Exd: See code: 047.0
A87.9 Viral meningitis unspecified   I-10

Requires fifth digit. Valid digits are in [brackets] under each code. See category 045 for codes and definitions.

4ᵗʰ 5ᵗʰ   Additional Digit Required   Unacceptable PDx   Manifestation Code   Hospital Acquired Condition   ▶◀ Revised Text   ● New Code   ▲ Revised Code Title

2014 ICD-9-CM   Volume 1 – 11

048 Other enterovirus diseases of central nervous system `CC`
Boston exanthem
CC Excl: 013.60-013.66, 046.2, 046.71-046.8, 048-049.0, 049.8, 052.0, 052.2, 054.3, 054.74, 056.01, 057.8-058.29, 059.00-059.9, 062.0-064, 066.2-066.49, 072.2, 073.7, 075, 079.82, 079.99, 081.9, 083.9, 090.41, 094.81, 117.5, 124, 130.0, 290.12, 323.01-323.9, 341.1, 487.8, 488.00, 488.19, 771.2, 984.9

√4th 049 Other non-arthropod-borne viral diseases of central nervous system
EXCLUDES *late effects of viral encephalitis (139.0)*

049.0 Lymphocytic choriomeningitis `CC`
Lymphocytic:
    meningitis (serous) (benign)
    meningoencephalitis (serous) (benign)
CC Excl: 003.21, 013.00-013.16, 036.0, 047.0-047.9, 049.0-049.1, 066.40-066.49, 072.1, 078.88-078.89, 079.81-079.82, 079.88-079.99, 090.42, 091.81, 094.2, 098.89, 100.81, 112.83, 114.2, 115.01, 115.11, 115.91, 130.0, 139.8, 320.0-322.9, 349.89-349.9, 357.0

049.1 Meningitis due to adenovirus `CC`
DEF: Inflammation of lining of brain caused by Arenaviruses and usually occurring in adults in fall and winter months.
CC Excl: 003.21, 013.00-013.16, 036.0, 047.0-047.9, 049.0-049.1, 072.1, 078.88-078.89, 079.81, 079.88-079.99, 090.42, 091.81, 094.2, 098.89, 100.81, 112.83, 114.2, 115.01, 115.11, 115.91, 130.0, 139.8, 320.0-322.9, 349.89-349.9, 357.0

049.8 Other specified non-arthropod-borne viral diseases of central nervous system `CC` `HIV`
Encephalitis: Encephalitis:
  acute: lethargica
    inclusion body   Rio Bravo
    necrotizing   von Economo's disease
    epidemic
EXCLUDES *human herpesvirus 6 encephalitis (058.21)*
               other human herpesvirus encephalitis (058.29)
CC Excl: 013.60-013.66, 046.2, 046.71-046.8, 048-049.0, 049.8, 052.0, 052.2, 054.3, 054.74, 056.01, 057.8-058.29, 059.00-059.9, 062.0-064, 066.2-066.49, 072.2, 073.7, 075, 079.82, 079.99, 081.9, 083.9, 090.41, 094.81, 117.5, 124, 130.0, 290.12, 323.01-323.9, 341.1, 382.4, 487.8, 488.09, 488.19, 710.0, 771.2, 984.9

049.9 Unspecified non-arthropod-borne viral diseases of central nervous system `CC` `HIV`
Viral encephalitis NOS
CC Excl: 013.60-013.66, 046.2, 046.71-046.8, 048-049.0, 049.8-049.9, 052.0, 052.2, 054.3, 054.74, 056.01, 057.8-058.29, 059.00-059.9, 062.0-064, 066.2-066.3, 072.2, 073.7, 075, 079.99, 081.9, 083.9, 090.41, 094.81, 117.5, 124, 130.0, 290.12, 323.01-323.9, 341.1, 382.4, 487.8, 488.09, 488.19, 710.0, 771.2, 984.9

Viral Diseases Generally Accompanied by Exanthem (050-059)
EXCLUDES *arthropod-borne viral diseases (060.0-066.9)*
             Boston exanthem (048)

√4th 050 Smallpox

050.0 Variola major `CC`
Hemorrhagic (pustular)   Malignant smallpox
  smallpox   Purpura variolosa
DEF: Form of smallpox known for its high mortality; exists only in laboratories.
CC Excl: 050.0-052.9

050.1 Alastrim `CC`
Variola minor
DEF: Mild form of smallpox known for its low mortality rate.
CC Excl: See code: 050.0

050.2 Modified smallpox `CC`
Varioloid
DEF: Mild form occurring in patients with history of infection or vaccination.
CC Excl: See code: 050.0

050.9 Smallpox, unspecified `CC`
CC Excl: See code: 050.0

√4th 051 Cowpox and paravaccinia

√5th 051.0 Cowpox and vaccinia not from vaccination

051.01 Cowpox
DEF: A disease contracted by milking infected cows; vesicles usually appear on the fingers, hands and adjacent areas and usually disappear without scarring; other symptoms: local edema, lymphangitis and regional lymphadenitis with or without fever.
AHA: 4Q, '08, 76-77

051.02 Vaccinia not from vaccination
EXCLUDES *vaccinia (generalized) (from vaccination) (999.0)*
AHA: 4Q, '08, 76-77

051.1 Pseudocowpox
Milkers' node
DEF: Hand lesions and mild fever in dairy workers caused by exposure to paravaccinia.

051.2 Contagious pustular dermatitis
Ecthyma contagiosum   Orf
DEF: Skin eruptions caused by exposure to poxvirus-infected sheep or goats.

051.9 Paravaccinia, unspecified

√4th 052 Chickenpox
DEF: Contagious infection by *Varicella-zoster* virus causing rash with pustules and fever.

052.0 Postvaricella encephalitis `MCC`
Postchickenpox encephalitis
CC Excl: 051.9-052.0, 052.2-052.9, 078.88-078.89, 079.81, 079.88-079.99, 139.8

052.1 Varicella (hemorrhagic) pneumonitis `MCC`
CC Excl: 051.9, 052.1-052.9, 078.88-078.89, 079.81, 079.88-079.99, 139.8

052.2 Postvaricella myelitis `MCC`
Postchickenpox myelitis
CC Excl: 051.9, 052.2-052.9, 053.14, 054.74, 078.88-078.89, 079.81, 079.88-079.99, 139.8, 323.01-323.02, 323.41-323.82, 341.20-341.22
AHA: 4Q, '06, 58-63

052.7 With other specified complications `CC`
CC Excl: 051.9, 052.2-052.9, 078.88-078.89, 079.81, 079.88-079.99, 139.8
AHA: 1Q, '02, 3

052.8 With unspecified complication `CC`
CC Excl: See code: 052.7

052.9 Varicella without mention of complication `CC`
Chickenpox NOS   Varicella NOS
CC Excl: See code: 052.7

√4th 053 Herpes zoster
INCLUDES shingles
          zona
DEF: Self-limiting infection by *Varicella-zoster* virus causing unilateral eruptions and neuralgia along affected nerves.

053.0 With meningitis `MCC` `HIV`
DEF: *Varicella-zoster* virus infection causing inflammation of the lining of the brain and/or spinal cord.
CC Excl: 003.21, 013.00-013.16, 036.0, 047.0-047.9, 049.0-049.1, 053.0-053.19, 053.79-053.9, 054.72, 054.74-054.9, 058.81-058.89, 072.1, 078.88-078.89, 079.81, 079.88-079.99, 090.42, 091.81, 094.2, 098.89, 100.81, 112.83, 114.2, 115.01, 115.11, 115.91, 130.0, 139.8, 320.0-322.9, 349.89-349.9, 357.0

√5th 053.1 With other nervous system complications

053.10 With unspecified nervous system complication `CC` `HIV`
CC Excl: 053.0-053.19, 053.79-053.9, 054.72, 054.74-054.9, 058.81-058.89, 078.88-078.89, 079.81, 079.88-079.99, 139.

053.11 Geniculate herpes zoster `CC` `HIV`
Herpetic geniculate ganglionitis
DEF: Unilateral eruptions and neuralgia along the facial nerve geniculum affecting face and outer and middle ear.
CC Excl: See code: 053.10

053.12 Postherpetic trigeminal neuralgia `CC` `HIV`
DEF: Severe oral or nasal pain following a herpes zoster infection.
CC Excl: See code: 053.10

`N` Newborn Age: 0   `P` Pediatric Age: 0-17   `M` Maternity Age: 12-55   `A` Adult Age: 15-124   `MCC` Major CC Condition   `CC` CC Condition   `HIV` HIV Related D

12 – Volume 1   2014 ICD-9-CM

053.13 Postherpetic polyneuropathy   `CC` `HIV`
> **DEF:** Multiple areas of pain following a herpes zoster infection.
> **CC Excl:** See code: 053.10

053.14 Herpes zoster myelitis   `MCC`
> **CC Excl:** 052.2, 053.0-053.19, 053.79-053.9, 054.72, 054.74-054.9, 058.81-058.89, 078.88-078.89, 079.81, 079.88-079.99, 139.8, 323.01-323.02, 323.41-323.82, 341.20-341.22
> **AHA:** 4Q, '06, 58-63

053.19 Other   `CC` `HIV`
> **CC Excl:** See code: 053.10

✓5ᵗʰ **053.2 With ophthalmic complications**

053.20 Herpes zoster dermatitis of eyelid   `CC` `HIV`
> Herpes zoster ophthalmicus
> **CC Excl:** 053.20-053.29

053.21 Herpes zoster keratoconjunctivitis   `CC` `HIV`
> **CC Excl:** See code: 053.20

053.22 Herpes zoster iridocyclitis   `CC` `HIV`
> **CC Excl:** See code: 053.20

053.29 Other   `CC` `HIV`
> **CC Excl:** See code: 053.20

✓5ᵗʰ **053.7 With other specified complications**

053.71 Otitis externa due to herpes zoster   `CC` `HIV`
> **CC Excl:** 053.71

053.79 Other   `CC` `HIV`
> **CC Excl:** 053.0-054.71, 054.73-054.9, 058.21-058.89, 078.88-078.89, 079.81, 079.88-079.99, 139.8

053.8 With unspecified complication   `CC` `HIV`
> **CC Excl:** See code: 053.79

053.9 Herpes zoster without mention of complication   `HIV`
> Herpes zoster NOS
> B02.9 Zoster without complications   `I-10`

✓4ᵗʰ **054 Herpes simplex**
> `EXCLUDES` *congenital herpes simplex (771.2)*

054.0 Eczema herpeticum   `HIV`
> Kaposi's varicelliform eruption
> **DEF:** Herpes simplex virus invading site of preexisting skin inflammation.

✓5ᵗʰ **054.1 Genital herpes**
> **AHA:** J-F, '87, 15, 16

054.10 Genital herpes, unspecified   `HIV`
> Herpes progenitalis
> **AHA:** 2Q, '10, 10
> A60.00 Herpesviral infection urogenital system unspec   `I-10`

054.11 Herpetic vulvovaginitis   `HIV` ♀

054.12 Herpetic ulceration of vulva   `HIV` ♀

054.13 Herpetic infection of penis   `HIV` ♂

054.19 Other   `HIV`

054.2 Herpetic gingivostomatitis   `CC` `HIV`
> **CC Excl:** 054.2

054.3 Herpetic meningoencephalitis   `MCC` `HIV`
> Herpes encephalitis
> Simian B disease
> `EXCLUDES` *human herpesvirus 6 encephalitis (058.21)*
> *other human herpesvirus encephalitis (058.29)*
> **DEF:** Inflammation of the brain and its lining, caused by infection of herpes simplex 1 in adults and simplex 2 in newborns.
> **CC Excl:** 054.3, 054.74-054.9, 058.21-058.89, 139.8

✓5ᵗʰ **054.4 With ophthalmic complications**

054.40 With unspecified ophthalmic complication   `CC` `HIV`
> **CC Excl:** 054.40-054.49, 054.79-054.9, 058.81-058.89

054.41 Herpes simplex dermatitis of eyelid   `CC` `HIV`
> **CC Excl:** See code: 054.40

054.42 Dendritic keratitis   `CC` `HIV`
> **CC Excl:** See code: 054.40

054.43 Herpes simplex disciform keratitis   `CC` `HIV`
> **CC Excl:** See code: 054.40

054.44 Herpes simplex iridocyclitis   `CC` `HIV`
> **CC Excl:** See code: 054.40

054.49 Other   `CC` `HIV`
> **CC Excl:** See code: 054.40

054.5 Herpetic septicemia   `MCC` `HIV`
> **CC Excl:** 003.1, 020.2, 036.2, 038.0-038.9, 054.5, 054.74-054.9, 058.81-058.89, 139.8, 995.90-995.94
> **AHA:** 2Q, '00, 5

054.6 Herpetic whitlow   `HIV`
> Herpetic felon
> **DEF:** A primary infection of the terminal segment of a finger by herpes simplex; intense itching and pain start the disease, vesicles form, and tissue ultimately is destroyed.

✓5ᵗʰ **054.7 With other specified complications**

054.71 Visceral herpes simplex   `CC` `HIV`
> **CC Excl:** 054.71-054.72, 054.74-054.9, 058.81-058.89, 139.8

054.72 Herpes simplex meningitis   `MCC` `HIV`
> **CC Excl:** 003.21, 013.00-013.16, 036.0, 047.0-047.9, 049.0-049.1, 053.0, 054.72, 054.74-054.9, 058.81-058.89, 072.1, 090.42, 091.81, 094.2, 098.89, 100.81, 112.83, 114.2, 115.01, 115.11, 115.91, 130.0, 139.8, 320.0-322.9, 349.89-349.9, 357.0

054.73 Herpes simplex otitis externa   `HIV`

054.74 Herpes simplex myelitis   `MCC`
> **CC Excl:** 052.2, 053.14, 054.74-054.9, 058.81-058.89, 078.88-078.89, 079.81, 079.88-079.99, 139.8, 323.01-323.02, 323.41-323.82, 341.20-341.22
> **AHA:** 4Q, '06, 58-63

054.79 Other   `CC` `HIV`
> **CC Excl:** 054.74-054.9, 058.81-058.89, 078.88-078.89, 079.81, 079.88-079.99, 139.8

054.8 With unspecified complication   `HIV`

054.9 Herpes simplex without mention of complication   `HIV`
> B00.9 Herpesviral infection unspecified   `I-10`

✓4ᵗʰ **055 Measles**
> `INCLUDES` morbilli
> rubeola

055.0 Postmeasles encephalitis   `MCC`
> **CC Excl:** 055.0, 055.79-055.9, 078.88-078.89, 079.81, 079.88-079.99, 139.8

055.1 Postmeasles pneumonia   `MCC`
> **CC Excl:** 055.1, 055.79-055.9, 078.88-078.89, 079.81, 079.88-079.99, 139.8

055.2 Postmeasles otitis media

✓5ᵗʰ **055.7 With other specified complications**

055.71 Measles keratoconjunctivitis   `CC`
> Measles keratitis
> **CC Excl:** 055.71-055.9, 078.88-078.89, 079.81, 079.88-079.99, 139.8

055.79 Other   `CC`
> **CC Excl:** 055.79-055.9, 078.88-078.89, 079.81, 079.88-079.99, 139.8

055.8 With unspecified complication

055.9 Measles without mention of complication

✓4ᵗʰ **056 Rubella**
> `INCLUDES` German measles
> `EXCLUDES` *congenital rubella (771.0)*
> **DEF:** Acute but usually benign togavirus infection causing fever, sore throat, and rash; associated with complications to fetus as a result of maternal infection.

✓5ᵗʰ **056.0 With neurological complications**

056.00 With unspecified neurological complication   `CC`
> **CC Excl:** 056.00-056.09, 056.79-056.9, 078.88-078.89, 079.81, 079.88-079.99, 139.8

056.01 Encephalomyelitis due to rubella   `MCC`
> Encephalitis } due to rubella
> Meningoencephalitis
> **CC Excl:** See code: 056.00

4ᵗʰ 5ᵗʰ Additional Digit Required   `Unacceptable PDx`   `Manifestation Code`   Hospital Acquired Condition   ▶◀ Revised Text   ● New Code   ▲ Revised Code Title

2014 ICD-9-CM   Volume 1 – 13

Infectious and Parasitic Diseases

056.09–062.1

056.09 Other   `CC`
     CC Exd: See code: 056.00

√5ᵗʰ **056.7 With other specified complications**

   056.71 Arthritis due to rubella   `CC`
     CC Exd: 056.71-056.9, 078.88-078.89, 079.81, 079.88-079.99, 139.8

   056.79 Other   `CC`
     CC Exd: 056.00-056.09, 056.79-056.9, 078.88-078.89, 079.81, 079.88-079.99, 139.8

056.8 With unspecified complications

056.9 Rubella without mention of complication

√4ᵗʰ **057 Other viral exanthemata**
     DEF: Skin eruptions or rashes and fever caused by viruses, including poxviruses.

   057.0 Erythema infectiosum [fifth disease]   `CC`
     DEF: A moderately contagious, benign, epidemic disease, usually seen in children, of probable viral etiology; a red macular rash appears on face and may spread to the limbs and trunk.
     CC Exd: 057.0, 079.83

   057.8 Other specified viral exanthemata
     Dukes (-Filatow) disease   Parascarlatina
     Fourth disease   Pseudoscarlatina
     EXCLUDES   exanthema subitum [sixth disease] (058.10-058.12)
        roseola infantum (058.10-058.12)

   057.9 Viral exanthem, unspecified

√4ᵗʰ **058 Other human herpesvirus**
     EXCLUDES   congenital herpes (771.2)
        cytomegalovirus (078.5)
        Epstein-Barr virus (075)
        herpes NOS (054.0-054.9)
        herpes simplex (054.0-054.9)
        herpes zoster (053.0-053.9)
        human herpesvirus NOS (054.0-054.9)
        human herpesvirus 1 (054.0-054.9)
        human herpesvirus 2 (054.0-054.9)
        human herpesvirus 3 (052.0-053.9)
        human herpesvirus 4 (075)
        human herpesvirus 5 (078.5)
        varicella (052.0-052.9)
        varicella-zoster virus (052.0-053.9)
     AHA: 4Q, '07, 61

√5ᵗʰ **058.1 Roseola infantum**
     Exanthema subitum [sixth disease]

   058.10 Roseola infantum, unspecified   `P`
     Exanthema subitum [sixth disease], unspecified
     AHA: 4Q, '07, 63

   058.11 Roseola infantum due to human herpesvirus 6   `P`
     Exanthema subitum [sixth disease] due to human herpesvirus 6

   058.12 Roseola infantum due to human herpesvirus 7   `P`
     Exanthema subitum [sixth disease] due to human herpesvirus 7

√5ᵗʰ **058.2 Other human herpesvirus encephalitis**
     EXCLUDES   herpes encephalitis NOS (054.3)
        herpes simplex encephalitis (054.3)
        human herpesvirus encephalitis NOS (054.3)
        simian B herpesvirus encephalitis (054.3)

   058.21 Human herpesvirus 6 encephalitis   `MCC` `HIV`
     CC Exd: 054.3, 054.74-054.9, 058.21-058.89, 139.8

   058.29 Other human herpesvirus encephalitis   `MCC` `HIV`
     Human herpesvirus 7 encephalitis
     CC Exd: See code: 058.21

√5ᵗʰ **058.8 Other human herpesvirus infections**

   058.81 Human herpesvirus 6 infection

   058.82 Human herpesvirus 7 infection

   058.89 Other human herpesvirus infection
     Human herpesvirus 8 infection
     Kaposi's sarcoma-associated herpesvirus infection
     AHA: 4Q, '07, 63

√4ᵗʰ **059 Other poxvirus infections**
     EXCLUDES   contagious pustular dermatitis (051.2)
        cowpox (051.01)
        ecthyma contagiosum (051.2)
        milker's nodule (051.1)
        orf (051.2)
        paravaccinia NOS (051.9)
        pseudocowpox (051.1)
        smallpox (050.0-050.9)
        vaccinia (generalized) (from vaccination) (999.0)
        vaccinia not from vaccination (051.02)
     AHA: 4Q, '08, 76-78

√5ᵗʰ **059.0 Other orthopoxvirus infections**

   059.00 Orthopoxvirus infection, unspecified

   059.01 Monkeypox   `CC`
     CC Exd: 051.01-051.02, 057.0-057.9, 059.00-059.9

   059.09 Other orthopoxvirus infection

√5ᵗʰ **059.1 Other parapoxvirus infections**

   059.10 Parapoxvirus infection, unspecified

   059.11 Bovine stomatitis

   059.12 Sealpox

   059.19 Other parapoxvirus infections

√5ᵗʰ **059.2 Yatapoxvirus infections**

   059.20 Yatapoxvirus infection, unspecified

   059.21 Tanapox   `CC`
     CC Exd: See code: 059.01

   059.22 Yaba monkey tumor virus

059.8 Other poxvirus infections

059.9 Poxvirus infections, unspecified

Arthropod-borne Viral Diseases (060-066)
     Use additional code to identify any associated meningitis (321.2)
     EXCLUDES   late effects of viral encephalitis (139.0)

√4ᵗʰ **060 Yellow fever**
     DEF: Fever and jaundice from infection by mosquito-borne virus of genus *Flavivirus*.

   060.0 Sylvatic   `CC`
     Yellow fever: Yellow fever:
      jungle   sylvan
     DEF: Yellow fever transmitted from animal to man, via mosquito.
     CC Exd: 060.0-060.9

   060.1 Urban   `CC`
     DEF: Yellow fever transmitted from man to man, via mosquito.
     CC Exd: See code: 060.0

   060.9 Yellow fever, unspecified   `CC`
     CC Exd: See code: 060.0

061 Dengue   `CC`
     Breakbone fever
     EXCLUDES   hemorrhagic fever caused by dengue virus (065.4)
     DEF: Acute, self-limiting infection by mosquito-borne virus characterized by fever and generalized aches.
     CC Exd: 061

√4ᵗʰ **062 Mosquito-borne viral encephalitis**

   062.0 Japanese encephalitis   `MCC`
     Japanese B encephalitis
     DEF: *Flavivirus* causing inflammation of the brain, with a wide range of clinical manifestations.
     CC Exd: 013.60-013.66, 046.2, 046.71-046.8, 048-049.0, 049.8, 052.0, 052.2, 054.3, 054.74, 056.01, 057.8-058.29, 059.00-059.9, 062.0-064, 066.2-066.49, 072.2, 073.7, 075, 079.82, 079.99, 081.9, 083.9, 090.41, 094.81, 117.5, 124, 130.0, 290.12, 323.01-323.9, 341.1, 487.8, 771.2, 984.9

   062.1 Western equine encephalitis   `MCC`
     DEF: Alphavirus WEE infection causing inflammation of the brain, found in areas west of the Mississippi; transmitted horse to mosquito to man.
     CC Exd: See code: 062.0

`N` Newborn Age: 0   `P` Pediatric Age: 0-17   `M` Maternity Age: 12-55   `A` Adult Age: 15-124   `MCC` Major CC Condition   `CC` CC Condition   `HIV` HIV Related Dx

14 – Volume 1   2014 ICD-9-CM

062.2 Eastern equine encephalitis `MCC`

EXCLUDES *Venezuelan equine encephalitis (066.2)*

DEF: Alphavirus EEE causing inflammation of the brain and spinal cord, found from Canada to South America and Mexico; transmitted horse to mosquito to man.

CC Exd: See code: 062.0

062.3 St. Louis encephalitis `MCC`

DEF: Epidemic form caused by *Flavivirus* and transmitted by mosquito, and characterized by fever, difficulty in speech, and headache.

CC Exd: See code: 062.0

062.4 Australian encephalitis `MCC`

Australian arboencephalitis
Australian X disease
Murray Valley encephalitis

DEF: *Flavivirus* causing inflammation of the brain, occurring in Australia and New Guinea.

CC Exd: See code: 062.0

062.5 California virus encephalitis `MCC`

Encephalitis: Tahyna fever
   California
   La Crosse

DEF: Bunyamwere virus causing inflammation of the brain.

CC Exd: See code: 062.0

062.8 Other specified mosquito-borne viral encephalitis `MCC`

Encephalitis by Ilheus virus

EXCLUDES *West Nile virus (066.40-066.49)*

CC Exd: See code: 062.0

062.9 Mosquito-borne viral encephalitis, unspecified `MCC`

CC Exd: See code: 062.0

✓4ᵗʰ 063 Tick-borne viral encephalitis

INCLUDES diphasic meningoencephalitis

063.0 Russian spring-summer [taiga] encephalitis `MCC`

CC Exd: See code: 062.0

063.1 Louping ill `MCC`

DEF: Inflammation of brain caused by virus transmitted sheep to tick to man; incidence usually limited to British Isles.

CC Exd: See code: 062.0

063.2 Central European encephalitis `MCC`

DEF: Inflammation of brain caused by virus transmitted by tick; limited to central Europe and presenting with two distinct phases.

CC Exd: See code: 062.0

063.8 Other specified tick-borne viral encephalitis `MCC`

Langat encephalitisPowassan encephalitis

CC Exd: See code: 062.0

063.9 Tick-borne viral encephalitis, unspecified `MCC`

CC Exd: See code: 062.0

064 Viral encephalitis transmitted by other and unspecified arthropods `MCC`

Arthropod-borne viral encephalitis, vector unknown
Negishi virus encephalitis

EXCLUDES *viral encephalitis NOS (049.9)*

CC Exd: See code: 062.0

✓4ᵗʰ 065 Arthropod-borne hemorrhagic fever

065.0 Crimean hemorrhagic fever [CHF Congo virus] `CC`

Central Asian hemorrhagic fever

CC Exd: 065.0-066.9

065.1 Omsk hemorrhagic fever `CC`

CC Exd: See code: 065.0

065.2 Kyasanur Forest disease `CC`

CC Exd: See code: 065.0

065.3 Other tick-borne hemorrhagic fever `CC`

CC Exd: See code: 065.0

065.4 Mosquito-borne hemorrhagic fever `CC`

Chikungunya hemorrhagic fever
Dengue hemorrhagic fever

EXCLUDES *Chikungunya fever (066.3)*
dengue (061)
yellow fever (060.0-060.9)

CC Exd: See code: 065.0

065.8 Other specified arthropod-borne hemorrhagic fever `CC`

Mite-borne hemorrhagic fever

CC Exd: See code: 065.0

065.9 Arthropod-borne hemorrhagic fever, unspecified `CC`

Arbovirus hemorrhagic fever NOS

CC Exd: See code: 065.0

✓4ᵗʰ 066 Other arthropod-borne viral diseases

066.0 Phlebotomus fever `CC`

Changuinola fever
Sandfly fever

DEF: Sandfly-borne viral infection occurring in Asia, Mideast and South America.

CC Exd: See code: 065.0

066.1 Tick-borne fever `CC`

Nairobi sheep disease   Tick fever:
Tick fever: Kemerovo
   American mountain   Quaranfil
   Colorado

CC Exd: See code: 065.0

066.2 Venezuelan equine fever `CC`

Venezuelan equine encephalitis

DEF: Alphavirus VEE infection causing inflammation of the brain, usually limited to South America, Mexico, and Florida; transmitted horse to mosquito to man.

CC Exd: 013.60-013.66, 046.2, 046.71-046.8, 048-049.0, 049.8, 052.0, 052.2, 054.3, 054.74, 056.01, 057.8-058.29, 059.00-059.9, 062.0-066.9, 072.2, 073.7, 075, 079.82, 079.99, 081.9, 083.9, 090.41, 094.81, 117.5, 124, 130.0, 290.12, 323.01-323.9, 341.1, 487.8, 488.09, 488.19, 771.2, 984.9

066.3 Other mosquito-borne fever `CC`

Fever (viral):   Fever (viral):
   Bunyamwera   Oropouche
   Bwamba   Pixuna
   Chikungunya   Rift valley
   Guama   Ross river
   Mayaro   Wesselsbron
   Mucambo   Zika
   O'Nyong-Nyong

EXCLUDES *dengue (061)*
yellow fever (060.0-060.9)

CC Exd: See code: 066.2

✓5ᵗʰ 066.4 West Nile fever

DEF: Mosquito-borne fever causing fatal inflammation of the brain, the lining of the brain, or of the lining of the brain and spinal cord.

AHA: 4Q, '02, 44

066.40 West Nile fever, unspecified `MCC`

West Nile fever NOS
West Nile fever without complications
West Nile virus NOS

CC Exd: 013.60-013.66, 046.2, 046.71-046.8, 048-049.0, 049.8, 052.0, 052.2, 054.3, 054.74, 056.01, 057.8-058.29, 059.00-059.9, 062.0-066.3, 066.8-066.9, 072.2, 073.7, 075, 079.99, 081.9, 083.9, 090.41, 094.81, 117.5, 124, 130.0, 323.01-323.9, 341.1, 487.8, 488.09, 488.19, 771.2

066.41 West Nile fever with encephalitis `MCC`

West Nile encephalitis
West Nile encephalomyelitis

CC Exd: See code: 066.40

AHA: 4Q, '04, 51

066.42 West Nile fever with other neurologic manifestation `MCC`

Use additional code to specify the neurologic manifestation

CC Exd: See code: 066.40

AHA: 4Q, '04, 51

066.49 West Nile fever with other complications `MCC`

Use additional code to specify the other conditions

CC Exd: See code: 066.40

066.8 Other specified arthropod-borne viral diseases `CC`

Chandipura fever
Piry fever

CC Exd: 065.0-066.9

066.9 Arthropod-borne viral disease, unspecified `CC`

Arbovirus infection NOS

CC Exd: 065.0-066.9

⁴ᵗʰ⁄₅ᵗʰ Additional Digit Required   Unacceptable PDx   Manifestation Code   Hospital Acquired Condition   ▶◀ Revised Text   ● New Code   ▲ Revised Code Title

014 ICD-9-CM   **Volume 1 – 15**

Infectious and Parasitic Diseases

070–073.0

Other Diseases Due to Viruses and Chlamydiae (070-079)

✓4ᵗʰ **070 Viral hepatitis**

INCLUDES viral hepatitis (acute) (chronic)

EXCLUDES *cytomegalic inclusion virus hepatitis (078.5)*

The following fifth-digit subclassification is for use with categories 070.2 and 070.3:

0 acute or unspecified, without mention of hepatitis delta
1 acute or unspecified, with hepatitis delta
2 chronic, without mention of hepatitis delta
3 chronic, with hepatitis delta

DEF: Hepatitis A: HAV infection is self-limiting with flulike symptoms; transmission, fecal-oral.
DEF: Hepatitis B: HBV infection can be chronic and systemic; transmission, bodily fluids.
DEF: Hepatitis C: HCV infection can be chronic and systemic; transmission, blood transfusion and unidentified agents.
DEF: Hepatitis D (delta): HDV occurs only in the presence of hepatitis B virus.
DEF: Hepatitis E: HEV is epidemic form; transmission and nature under investigation.
AHA: 2Q, '07, 5

070.0 Viral hepatitis A with hepatic coma   MCC
     CC Exd: 070.0-070.9, 078.88-078.89, 079.81, 079.88-079.99, 139.8

070.1 Viral hepatitis A without mention of hepatic coma   CC
     Infectious hepatitis
     CC Exd: See code: 070.0

§ ✓5ᵗʰ **070.2 Viral hepatitis B with hepatic coma**   MCC
     [0-3]   **CC Exd:** See code: 070.0
     AHA: 4Q, '91, 28; **For code 070.20:** 2Q, '07, 6

§ ✓5ᵗʰ **070.3 Viral hepatitis B without mention of hepatic coma**   CC
     [0-3]   Serum hepatitis
     CC Exd: See code: 070.0
     AHA: 1Q, '93, 28; 4Q, '91, 28
     B16.9 Acute hep B w/o delta-agent & w/o hepatic coma   I-10

✓5ᵗʰ **070.4 Other specified viral hepatitis with hepatic coma**
     AHA: 4Q, '91, 28

     070.41 Acute hepatitis C with hepatic coma   MCC
         CC Exd: See code: 070.0

     070.42 Hepatitis delta without mention of active hepatitis B disease with hepatic coma   MCC
         Hepatitis delta with hepatitis B carrier state
         CC Exd: See code: 070.0

     070.43 Hepatitis E with hepatic coma   MCC
         CC Exd: See code: 070.0

     070.44 Chronic hepatitis C with hepatic coma   MCC
         CC Exd: See code: 070.0
         AHA: 2Q, '07, 5

     070.49 Other specified viral hepatitis with hepatic coma   MCC
         CC Exd: See code: 070.0

✓5ᵗʰ **070.5 Other specified viral hepatitis without mention of hepatic coma**
     AHA: 4Q, '91, 28

     070.51 Acute hepatitis C without mention of hepatic coma   CC
         CC Exd: See code: 070.0

     070.52 Hepatitis delta without mention of active hepatititis B disease or hepatic coma   CC
         CC Exd: See code: 070.0

     070.53 Hepatitis E without mention of hepatic coma   CC
         CC Exd: See code: 070.0

     070.54 Chronic hepatitis C without mention of hepatic coma
         AHA: 1Q, '11, 23; 4Q, '08, 120; 3Q, '07, 7; 2Q, '06, 13
         B18.2 Chronic viral hepatitis C   I-10

     070.59 Other specified viral hepatitis without mention of hepatic coma   CC
         CC Exd: See code: 070.0

070.6 Unspecified viral hepatitis with hepatic coma   MCC
     EXCLUDES *unspecified viral hepatitis C with hepatic coma (070.71)*
     CC Exd: See code: 070.0

✓5ᵗʰ **070.7 Unspecified viral hepatitis C**

     070.70 Unspecified viral hepatitis C without hepatic coma
         Unspecified viral hepatitis C NOS
         AHA: 4Q, '04, 52
         B19.20 Unspecified viral hepatits C w/o hepatic coma   I-10

     070.71 Unspecified viral hepatitis C with hepatic coma   MCC
         CC Exd: See code: 070.0
         AHA: 4Q, '04, 52

070.9 Unspecified viral hepatitis without mention of hepatic coma   CC
     Viral hepatitis NOS
     EXCLUDES *unspecified viral hepatitis C without hepatic coma (070.70)*
     CC Exd: See code: 070.0

071 Rabies   CC
     Hydrophobia
     Lyssa
     DEF: Acute infectious disease of the CNS caused by a rhabdovirus; usually spread by bites by infected animals; progresses from fever, restlessness, and extreme excitability, to hydrophobia, seizures, confusion and death.
     CC Exd: 071

✓4ᵗʰ **072 Mumps**
     DEF: Acute infectious disease caused by paramyxovirus; usually seen in children less than 15 years of age; salivary glands are typically enlarged, involves other organs, such as testes, pancreas and meninges.

     072.0 Mumps orchitis   CC ♂
         CC Exd: 072.0, 072.79-072.9, 078.88-078.89, 079.81, 079.88-079.99, 139.8

     072.1 Mumps meningitis   MCC
         CC Exd: 003.21, 013.00-013.16, 036.0, 047.0-047.9, 049.0-049.1, 053.0, 054.72, 072.1, 072.79-072.9, 078.88-078.89, 079.81, 079.88-079.99, 090.42, 091.81, 094.2, 098.89, 100.81, 112.83, 114.2, 115.01, 115.11, 115.91, 130.0, 139.8, 320.0-322.9, 349.89-349.9, 357.0

     072.2 Mumps encephalitis   MCC
         Mumps meningoencephalitis
         CC Exd: 072.2, 072.79-072.9, 078.88-078.89, 079.81, 079.88-079.99, 139.8

     072.3 Mumps pancreatitis   CC
         CC Exd: 072.3, 072.79-072.9, 078.88-078.89, 079.81, 079.88-079.99, 139.8

✓5ᵗʰ **072.7 Mumps with other specified complications**

     072.71 Mumps hepatitis   CC
         CC Exd: 072.71, 072.79-072.9, 078.88-078.89, 079.81, 079.88-079.99, 139.8

     072.72 Mumps polyneuropathy   CC
         CC Exd: 072.72-072.9, 078.88-078.89, 079.81, 079.88-079.99, 139.8

     072.79 Other   CC
         CC Exd: 072.79-072.9, 078.88-078.89, 079.81, 079.88-079.99, 139.8

     072.8 Mumps with unspecified complication   CC
         CC Exd: 072.79-072.9, 078.88-078.89, 079.81, 079.88-079.99

     072.9 Mumps without mention of complication
         Epidemic parotitis
         Infectious parotitis

✓4ᵗʰ **073 Ornithosis**
     INCLUDES parrot fever
              psittacosis
     DEF: *Chlamydia psittaci* infection often transmitted from birds to humans.

     073.0 With pneumonia   MCC
         Lobular pneumonitis due to ornithosis
         CC Exd: 011.00-012.16, 012.80-012.86, 017.90-017.96, 020.3-020.5, 021.3, 022.1, 031.0, 039.1, 073.0, 073.8-073.9, 115.05, 115.15, 115.95, 122.1, 130.4, 136.3, 480.0-487.1, 488.01-488.02, 488.11-488.12, 495.0-495.9, 500-508.9, 517.1, 517.8, 518.89, 519.8-519.9

---

§   Requires fifth digit. Valid digits are in [brackets] under each code. See category 070 for codes and definitions.

N Newborn Age: 0   P Pediatric Age: 0-17   M Maternity Age: 12-55   A Adult Age: 15-124   MCC Major CC Condition   CC CC Condition   HIV HIV Related Dx

16 – Volume 1   **2014 ICD-9-CM**

073.7 With other specified complications `CC`
CC Excl: 013.60-013.66, 046.2, 046.71-046.8, 048-049.0, 049.8, 052.0, 052.2, 054.3, 054.74, 056.01, 057.8-058.29, 059.00-059.9, 062.0-064, 066.2-066.49, 072.2, 073.0-073.9, 079.82, 079.99, 081.9, 083.9, 090.41, 094.81, 117.5, 124, 130.0, 290.12, 323.01-323.9, 341.1, 487.8, 488.09, 488.19, 771.2, 984.9

073.8 With unspecified complication `CC`
CC Excl: 073.0, 073.8-073.9

073.9 Ornithosis, unspecified `CC`
CC Excl: See code: 073.8

✓4ᵗʰ **074 Specific diseases due to Coxsackie virus**
EXCLUDES Coxsackie virus:
  infection NOS (079.2)
  meningitis (047.0)

074.0 Herpangina
Vesicular pharyngitis
DEF: Acute infectious coxsackie virus infection causing throat lesions, fever, and vomiting; generally affects children in summer.

074.1 Epidemic pleurodynia
Bornholm disease   Epidemic:
Devil's grip   myalgia
                            myositis
DEF: Paroxysmal pain in chest, accompanied by fever and usually limited to children and young adults; caused by coxsackie virus.

✓5ᵗʰ **074.2 Coxsackie carditis**

074.20 Coxsackie carditis, unspecified `CC`
CC Excl: 074.20, 074.22-074.23, 093.82, 390, 391.2-391.9, 398.0-398.90, 398.99, 422.0-422.99, 429.0, 429.71-429.79, 459.89-459.9

074.21 Coxsackie pericarditis `CC`
DEF: Coxsackie infection of the outer lining of the heart.
CC Excl: 074.21, 093.81, 391.0, 393, 420.0-420.99, 423.3-423.9, 459.89-459.9

074.22 Coxsackie endocarditis `CC`
DEF: Coxsackie infection within the heart's cavities.
CC Excl: 002.0, 036.42, 074.22, 083.0, 093.20-093.24, 098.84, 112.81, 115.94, 116.0, 390, 391.1, 391.8-392.0, 394.0-395.9, 396.9-397.9, 398.90, 398.99, 421.0-421.9, 424.0-424.99, 425.3, 459.89-459.9, 746.09, 746.89, 996.61

074.23 Coxsackie myocarditis `CC`
Aseptic myocarditis of newborn
DEF: Coxsackie infection of the muscle of the heart.
CC Excl: See code: 074.20

074.3 Hand, foot, and mouth disease
Vesicular stomatitis and exanthem
DEF: Mild coxsackie infection causing lesions on hands, feet and oral mucosa, most commonly seen in preschool children.

074.8 Other specified diseases due to Coxsackie virus
Acute lymphonodular pharyngitis

075 Infectious mononucleosis
Glandular fever   Pfeiffer's disease
Monocytic angina
DEF: Acute infection by Epstein-Barr virus causing fever, sore throat, enlarged lymph glands and spleen, and fatigue; usually seen in teens and young adults.
AHA: 3Q, '01, 13; M-A, '87, 8

✓4ᵗʰ **076 Trachoma**
EXCLUDES late effect of trachoma (139.1)
DEF: A chronic infectious disease of the cornea and conjunctiva caused by a strain of the bacteria Chlamydia trachomatis; the infection can cause photophobia, pain, excessive tearing and sometimes blindness.

076.0 Initial stage
Trachoma dubium

076.1 Active stage
Granular conjunctivitis (trachomatous)
Trachomatous:
  follicular conjunctivitis
  pannus

076.9 Trachoma, unspecified
Trachoma NOS

✓4ᵗʰ **077 Other diseases of conjunctiva due to viruses and Chlamydiae**
EXCLUDES ophthalmic complications of viral diseases classified elsewhere

077.0 Inclusion conjunctivitis
Paratrachoma   Swimming pool conjunctivitis
EXCLUDES inclusion blennorrhea (neonatal) (771.6)
DEF: Pus in conjunctiva caused by Chlamydiae trachomatis.

077.1 Epidemic keratoconjunctivitis
Shipyard eye
DEF: Highly contagious corneal or conjunctival infection caused by adenovirus type 8; symptoms include inflammation and corneal infiltrates.

077.2 Pharyngoconjunctival fever
Viral pharyngoconjunctivitis

077.3 Other adenoviral conjunctivitis
Acute adenoviral follicular conjunctivitis

077.4 Epidemic hemorrhagic conjunctivitis
Apollo:
  conjunctivitis
  disease
Conjunctivitis due to enterovirus type 70
Hemorrhagic conjunctivitis (acute) (epidemic)

077.8 Other viral conjunctivitis
Newcastle conjunctivitis

✓5ᵗʰ **077.9 Unspecified diseases of conjunctiva due to viruses and Chlamydiae**

077.98 Due to Chlamydiae

077.99 Due to viruses
Viral conjunctivitis NOS
B30.9 Viral conjunctivitis, unspecified `I-10`

✓4ᵗʰ **078 Other diseases due to viruses and Chlamydiae**
EXCLUDES viral infection NOS (079.0-079.9)
viremia NOS (790.8)

078.0 Molluscum contagiosum
DEF: Benign poxvirus infection causing small bumps on the skin or conjunctiva; transmitted by close contact.

✓5ᵗʰ **078.1 Viral warts**
Viral warts due to human papilloma virus
DEF: A keratotic papilloma of the epidermis caused by the human papilloma virus; the superficial vegetative lesions last for varying durations and eventually regress spontaneously.
AHA: 2Q, '97, 9; 4Q, '93, 22

078.10 Viral warts, unspecified
Verruca:
  NOS
  Vulgaris
Warts (infectious)

078.11 Condyloma acuminatum
Condyloma NOS   Genital warts NOS
DEF: Clusters of mucosa or epidermal lesions on external genitalia; viral infection is sexually transmitted.

078.12 Plantar wart
Verruca plantaris
AHA: 4Q, '08, 78-79

078.19 Other specified viral warts
Common wart
Flat wart
Veruca planna

078.2 Sweating fever
Miliary fever   Sweating disease
DEF: A viral infection characterized by profuse sweating; various papular, vesicular and other eruptions cause the blockage of sweat glands.

078.3 Cat-scratch disease `CC`
Benign lymphoreticulosis (of inoculation)
Cat-scratch fever
CC Excl: 078.3, 079.82

Infectious and Parasitic Diseases

078.4–079.99

078.4 Foot and mouth disease
Aphthous fever   Epizootic:
Epizootic: stomatitis
  aphthae
DEF: Ulcers on oral mucosa, legs, and feet after exposure to infected animal.

078.5 Cytomegaloviral disease   `CC` `HIV`
Cytomegalic inclusion disease
Salivary gland virus disease
Use additional code to identify manifestation, as:
  cytomegalic inclusion virus:
    hepatitis (573.1)
    pneumonia (484.1)
  EXCLUDES congenital cytomegalovirus infection (771.1)
DEF: A herpesvirus associated with serious disease morbidity including fever, leukopenia, pneumonia, retinitis, hepatitis and organ transplant; often leads to hepatomegaly, splenomegaly and thrombocytopenia; a common post-transplant complication.
CC Excl: 078.5-078.7, 078.89-079.50, 079.59, 079.81-079.82, 079.89, 079.99
AHA: 3Q, '11, 5; 1Q, '03, 10; 3Q, '98, 4; 2Q, '93, 11; 1Q, '89, 9

078.6 Hemorrhagic nephrosonephritis   `CC`
Hemorrhagic fever: Hemorrhagic fever:
  epidemic   Russian
  Korean   with renal syndrome
DEF: Viral infection causing kidney dysfunction and bleeding disorders.
CC Excl: 016.00-016.06, 016.30-016.36, 016.90-016.96, 017.90-017.96, 078.6, 079.82, 098.10, 098.19, 098.30-098.31, 098.89, 112.2, 131.00, 131.8-131.9, 249.40-249.41, 249.80-249.91, 250.40-250.43, 250.80-250.93, 274.10, 274.19, 580.0-584.9, 586-591, 593.0-593.2, 593.89-593.9, 599.70-599.9

078.7 Arenaviral hemorrhagic fever   `CC`
Hemorrhagic fever: Hemorrhagic fever:
  Argentine   Junin virus
  Bolivian   Machupo virus
CC Excl: 078.5-079.82, 079.88-079.99

`√5ᵗʰ` **078.8 Other specified diseases due to viruses and Chlamydiae**
  EXCLUDES epidemic diarrhea (009.2)
                   lymphogranuloma venereum (099.1)

  078.81 Epidemic vertigo

  078.82 Epidemic vomiting syndrome
    Winter vomiting disease

  078.88 Other specified diseases due to Chlamydiae
    AHA: 4Q, '96, 22

  078.89 Other specified diseases due to viruses
    Epidemic cervical myalgia
    Marburg disease

`√4ᵗʰ` **079 Viral and chlamydial infection in conditions classified elsewhere and of unspecified site**
  NOTE This category is provided to be used as an additional code to identify the viral agent in diseases classifiable elsewhere. This category will also be used to classify virus infection of unspecified nature or site.

  079.0 Adenovirus

  079.1 ECHO virus
    DEF: An "orphan" enteric RNA virus, certain serotypes of which are associated with human disease, especially aseptic meningitis.

  079.2 Coxsackie virus
    DEF: A heterogenous group of viruses associated with aseptic meningitis, myocarditis, pericarditis, and acute onset juvenile diabetes.

  079.3 Rhinovirus
    DEF: Rhinoviruses affect primarily the upper respiratory tract. Over 100 distinct types infect humans.

  079.4 Human papillomavirus
    DEF: Viral infection caused by the genus *Papillomavirus* causing cutaneous and genital warts, including verruca vulgaris and condyloma acuminatum; certain types are associated with cervical dysplasia, cancer and other genital malignancies.
    AHA: 2Q, '97, 9; 4Q, '93, 22
    TIP: Do not assign for viral warts; see instead subcategory 078.1.

`√5ᵗʰ` **079.5 Retrovirus**
  EXCLUDES human immunodeficiency virus, type 1 [HIV-1] (042)
                   human T-cell lymphotrophic virus, type III [HTLV-III] (042)
                   lymphadenopathy-associated virus [LAV] (042)
  DEF: A large group of RNA viruses that carry reverse transcriptase and include the leukoviruses and lentiviruses.
  AHA: 4Q, '93, 22, 23

  079.50 Retrovirus, unspecified

  079.51 Human T-cell lymphotrophic virus, type I [HTLV-I]   `CC`
    CC Excl: 079.51-079.59, 079.81-079.82, 079.88-079.99

  079.52 Human T-cell lymphotrophic virus, type II [HTLV-II]   `CC`
    CC Excl: 079.50-079.59, 079.81-079.82, 079.88-079.99

  079.53 Human immunodeficiency virus, type 2 [HIV-2]   `CC`
    CC Excl: 042, 079.50-079.59, 079.81-079.82, 079.88-079.99

  079.59 Other specified retrovirus

  079.6 Respiratory syncytial virus [RSV]
    DEF: The major respiratory pathogen of young children, causing severe bronchitis and bronchopneumonia, and minor infection in adults.
    AHA: 4Q, '96, 27, 28

`√5ᵗʰ` **079.8 Other specified viral and chlamydial infections**
    AHA: 1Q, '88, 12

  079.81 Hantavirus   `CC`
    DEF: An infection caused by the Muerto Canyon virus whose primary rodent reservoir is the deer mouse Peromyscus maniculatus; commonly characterized by fever, myalgias, headache, cough.
    CC Excl: 070.70-070.71, 078.5-079.82, 079.88-079.99
    AHA: 4Q, '95, 60

  079.82 SARS-associated coronavirus   `CC`
    DEF: A life-threatening respiratory disease, severe acute respiratory syndrome (SARS); etiology coronavirus; presenting symptoms may range from mild to severe forms of flu-like conditions; fever, chills, cough, headache, myalgia; diagnosis of SARS is based upon clinical, laboratory, and epidemiological criteria.
    CC Excl: 011.00-012.16, 012.80-012.86, 017.90-017.96, 021.2, 031.0, 039.1, 079.82, 079.89, 115.05, 115.15, 115.95, 122.1, 130.4, 136.3, 480.0-480.2, 480.8-487.1, 488.01-488.02, 488.11-488.12, 494.0-508.9, 517.1, 517.8, 518.89, 519.8-519.9, 748.61
    AHA: 4Q, '03, 46

  079.83 Parvovirus B19   `CC`
    Human parvovirus
    Parvovirus NOS
    EXCLUDES erythema infectiosum [fifth disease] (057.0)
    DEF: The only known parvovirus to cause disease in humans; manifestation is erythema infectiosum; also associated with polyarthropathy, chronic anemia, red cell aplasia, and fetal hydrops.
    CC Excl: 057.0, 079.83
    AHA: 4Q, '07, 64

  079.88 Other specified chlamydial infection

  079.89 Other specified viral infection

`√5ᵗʰ` **079.9 Unspecified viral and chlamydial infections**
  EXCLUDES viremia NOS (790.8)
  AHA: 2Q, '91, 8

  079.98 Unspecified chlamydial infection
    Chlamydial infections NOS

  079.99 Unspecified viral infection
    Viral infections NOS
    B97.89 Other viral agents cause of dz class elsewhere   `I-10`

`N` Newborn Age: 0   `P` Pediatric Age: 0-17   `M` Maternity Age: 12-55   `A` Adult Age: 15-124   `MCC` Major CC Condition   `CC` CC Condition   `HIV` HIV Related Dx

18 – Volume 1

2014 ICD-9-CM

Rickettsioses and Other Arthropod-Borne Diseases (080-088)

EXCLUDES arthropod-borne viral diseases (060.0-066.9)

080 Louse-borne [epidemic] typhus   CC

Typhus (fever):   Typhus (fever):
    classical   exanthematic NOS
    epidemic   louse-borne

DEF: *Rickettsia prowazekii;* causes severe headache, rash, high fever.
CC Exd: 080-083.9, 085.0-088.9

✓4ᵗʰ 081 Other typhus

081.0 Murine [endemic] typhus   CC
Typhus (fever):   Typhus (fever):
    endemic   flea-borne
DEF: Milder typhus caused by *Rickettsia typhi (mooseri);* transmitted by rat flea.
CC Exd: See code: 080

081.1 Brill's disease   CC
Brill-Zinsser diseaseRecrudescent typhus (fever)
CC Exd: See code: 080

081.2 Scrub typhus   CC
Japanese river fever   Mite-borne typhus
Kedani fever   Tsutsugamushi
DEF: Typhus caused by *Rickettsia tsutsugamushi* transmitted by chigger.
CC Exd: See code: 080

081.9 Typhus, unspecified   CC
Typhus (fever) NOS
CC Exd: 013.60-013.66, 046.2, 046.71-046.8, 048-049.0, 049.8, 052.0, 052.2, 054.3, 054.74, 056.01, 057.8-058.29, 059.00-059.9, 062.0-064, 066.2-066.49, 072.2, 073.7, 079.82, 079.99-084.0, 085.0-088.9, 090.41, 094.81, 117.5, 124, 130.0, 290.12, 323.01-323.9, 341.1, 487.8, 488.09, 488.19, 771.2, 984.9

✓4ᵗʰ 082 Tick-borne rickettsioses

082.0 Spotted fevers   CC
Rocky mountain spotted fever
Sao Paulo fever
CC Exd: See code: 080

082.1 Boutonneuse fever   CC
African tick typhus   Marseilles fever
India tick typhus   Mediterranean tick fever
Kenya tick typhus
CC Exd: See code: 080

082.2 North Asian tick fever   CC
Siberian tick typhus
CC Exd: See code: 080

082.3 Queensland tick typhus   CC
CC Exd: See code: 080

✓5ᵗʰ 082.4 Ehrlichiosis
AHA: 3Q, '06, 11; 4Q, '00, 38

082.40 Ehrlichiosis, unspecified   CC
CC Exd: See code: 080

082.41 Ehrlichiosis chaffeensis [E. chaffeensis]   CC
DEF: A febrile illness caused by bacterial infection, also called human monocytic ehrlichiosis (HME). Causal organism is *Ehrlichia chaffeensis,* transmitted by the Lone Star tick. Symptoms include fever, chills, myalgia, nausea, vomiting, diarrhea, confusion, and severe headache occurring one week after a tick bite. Clinical findings are lymphadenopathy, rash, thrombocytopenia, leukopenia, and abnormal liver function tests.
CC Exd: See code: 080

082.49 Other ehrlichiosis   CC
CC Exd: See code: 080

082.8 Other specified tick-borne rickettsioses   CC
Lone star fever
CC Exd: See code: 080
AHA: 4Q, '99, 19

082.9 Tick-borne rickettsiosis, unspecified   CC
Tick-borne typhus NOS
CC Exd: See code: 080

✓4ᵗʰ 083 Other rickettsioses

083.0 Q fever   CC
DEF: Infection of *Coxiella burnettii* usually acquired through airborne organisms.
CC Exd: See code: 080

083.1 Trench fever   CC
Quintan fever
Wolhynian fever
CC Exd: See code: 080

083.2 Rickettsialpox   CC
Vesicular rickettsiosis
DEF: Infection of *Rickettsia akari* usually acquired through a mite bite.
CC Exd: 082.0-083.9

083.8 Other specified rickettsioses   CC
CC Exd: See code: 083.2

083.9 Rickettsiosis, unspecified   CC
CC Exd: See code: 083.2

✓4ᵗʰ 084 Malaria

NOTE Subcategories 084.0-084.6 exclude the listed conditions with mention of pernicious complications (084.8-084.9).

EXCLUDES congenital malaria (771.2)

DEF: Mosquito-borne disease causing high fever and prostration and cataloged by species of *Plasmodium: P. falciparum, P. malariae, P. ovale,* and *P. vivax.*

084.0 Falciparum malaria [malignant tertian]   MCC
Malaria (fever):
    by Plasmodium falciparum
    subtertian
CC Exd: 084.0-086.9

084.1 Vivax malaria [benign tertian]   CC
Malaria (fever) by Plasmodium vivax
CC Exd: 084.0-088.9

084.2 Quartan malaria   CC
Malaria (fever) by Plasmodium malariae
Malariae malaria
CC Exd: See code: 084.0

084.3 Ovale malaria   CC
Malaria (fever) by Plasmodium ovale
CC Exd: See code: 084.0

084.4 Other malaria   CC
Monkey malaria
CC Exd: See code: 084.0

084.5 Mixed malaria   CC
Malaria (fever) by more than one parasite
CC Exd: See code: 084.0

084.6 Malaria, unspecified   CC
Malaria (fever) NOS
CC Exd: 079.82, 084.0-086.9

084.7 Induced malaria   CC
Therapeutically induced malaria
EXCLUDES accidental infection from syringe, blood transfusion, etc. (084.0-084.6, above, according to parasite species)
    transmission from mother to child during delivery (771.2)
CC Exd: 084.1-086.9

084.8 Blackwater fever   CC
Hemoglobinuric:
    fever (bilious)
    malaria
Malarial hemoglobinuria
DEF: Severe hemic and renal complication of *Plasmodium falciparum* infection.
CC Exd: See code: 084.0

084.9 Other pernicious complications of malaria   CC
Algid malaria
Cerebral malaria
Use additional code to identify complication, as:
    malarial:
       hepatitis (573.2)
       nephrosis (581.81)
CC Exd: See code: 084.0

✓4ᵗʰ / ✓5ᵗʰ Additional Digit Required   Unacceptable PDx   Manifestation Code   Hospital Acquired Condition   ▶◀ Revised Text   ● New Code   ▲ Revised Code Title

2014 ICD-9-CM   **Volume 1 – 19**

080–084.9

Infectious and Parasitic Diseases

085–090.1

☑4ᵗʰ 085 Leishmaniasis

085.0 Visceral [kala-azar]   CC
Dumdum fever
Infection by Leishmania:
    donovani
    infantum
Leishmaniasis:
    dermal, post-kala-azar
    Mediterranean
    visceral (Indian)
CC Excl: 080–088.9

085.1 Cutaneous, urban   CC
Aleppo boil
Baghdad boil
Delhi boil
Infection by Leishmania tropica (minor)
Leishmaniasis, cutaneous:
    dry form
    late
    recurrent
    ulcerating
Oriental sore
CC Excl: See code: 085.0

085.2 Cutaneous, Asian desert   CC
Infection by Leishmania tropica major
Leishmaniasis, cutaneous:
    acute necrotizing
    rural
    wet form
    zoonotic form
CC Excl: See code: 085.0

085.3 Cutaneous, Ethiopian   CC
Infection by Leishmania ethiopica
Leishmaniasis, cutaneous:
    diffuse
    lepromatous
CC Excl: See code: 085.0

085.4 Cutaneous, American   CC
Chiclero ulcer
Infection by Leishmania mexicana
Leishmaniasis tegumentaria diffusa
CC Excl: See code: 085.0

085.5 Mucocutaneous (American)   CC
Espundia
Infection by Leishmania braziliensis
Uta
CC Excl: See code: 085.0

085.9 Leishmaniasis, unspecified   CC
CC Excl: See code: 085.0

☑4ᵗʰ 086 Trypanosomiasis
Use additional code to identify manifestations, as:
    trypanosomiasis:
      encephalitis (323.2)
      meningitis (321.3)

086.0 Chagas' disease with heart involvement   CC
American trypanosomiasis ⎫ with heart
Infection by Trypanosoma cruzi ⎭ involvement
   Any condition classifiable to 086.2 with heart involvement
CC Excl: 086.0, 139.8

086.1 Chagas' disease with other organ involvement   CC
American trypanosomiasis ⎫ with involvement of organ
Infection by Trypanosoma cruzi ⎭ other than heart
   Any condition classifiable to 086.2 with involvement of organ other than heart
CC Excl: 080–088.9

086.2 Chagas' disease without mention of organ involvement   CC
American trypanosomiasis
Infection by Trypanosoma cruzi
CC Excl: See code: 086.1

086.3 Gambian trypanosomiasis   CC
Gambian sleeping sickness
Infection by Trypanosoma gambiense
CC Excl: See code: 086.1

086.4 Rhodesian trypanosomiasis   CC
Infection by Trypanosoma rhodesiense
Rhodesian sleeping sickness
CC Excl: See code: 086.1

086.5 African trypanosomiasis, unspecified
Sleeping sickness NOS
CC Excl: See code: 086.1

086.9 Trypanosomiasis, unspecified   CC
CC Excl: 013.60–013.66, 046.2, 046.71–046.8, 048–049.0, 049.8, 052.0, 052.2, 054.3, 054.74, 056.01, 057.8–058.29, 059.00–059.9, 062.0–064, 066.2–066.3, 072.2, 073.7, 075, 078.3, 079.99–088.9, 090.41, 094.81, 117.5, 124, 130.0, 290.12, 323.01–323.9, 341.1, 382.4, 487.8, 488.09, 488.19, 771.2, 984.9

☑4ᵗʰ 087 Relapsing fever
INCLUDES recurrent fever
DEF: Infection of *Borrelia;* symptoms are episodic and include fever and arthralgia.

087.0 Louse-borne   CC
CC Excl: 080–083.9, 085.0–088.9

087.1 Tick-borne   CC
CC Excl: See code: 087.0

087.9 Relapsing fever, unspecified   CC
CC Excl: See code: 087.0

☑4ᵗʰ 088 Other arthropod-borne diseases

088.0 Bartonellosis   CC
Carrión's disease   Verruga peruana
Oroya fever
CC Excl: See code: 087.0

☑5ᵗʰ 088.8 Other specified arthropod-borne diseases

088.81 Lyme disease   CC
Erythema chronicum migrans
DEF: A recurrent multisystem disorder caused by the spirochete *Borrelia burgdorferi* with the carrier being the tick; begins with lesions of erythema chronicum migrans; followed by arthritis of the large joints, myalgia, malaise, and neurological and cardiac manifestations.
CC Excl: See code: 087.0
AHA: 4Q, '91, 15; 3Q, '90, 14; 2Q, '89, 10
TIP: Do not assign if patient has been cured of Lyme disease but has residual chronic condition; refer instead to late-effect code 139.8.

088.82 Babesiosis   CC
Babesiasis
DEF: A tick-borne disease caused by infection of *Babesia,* characterized by fever, malaise, listlessness, severe anemia and hemoglobinuria.
CC Excl: 080–088.9
AHA: 4Q, '93, 23

088.89 Other

088.9 Arthropod-borne disease, unspecified

Syphilis and other Venereal Diseases (090-099)

EXCLUDES nonvenereal endemic syphilis (104.0)
urogenital trichomoniasis (131.0)

☑4ᵗʰ 090 Congenital syphilis
DEF: Infection by spirochete *Treponema pallidum* acquired in utero from the infected mother.

090.0 Early congenital syphilis, symptomatic   CC
Congenital syphilitic: Congenital syphilitic:
    choroiditis   splenomegaly
    coryza (chronic)   Syphilitic (congenital):
    hepatomegaly   epiphysitis
    mucous patches   osteochondritis
    periostitis   pemphigus
   Any congenital syphilitic condition specified as early or manifest less than two years after birth
CC Excl: 090.0–097.9

090.1 Early congenital syphilis, latent
Congenital syphilis without clinical manifestations, with positive serological reaction and negative spinal fluid test, less than two years after birth

---

N Newborn Age: 0   P Pediatric Age: 0-17   M Maternity Age: 12-55   A Adult Age: 15-124   MCC Major CC Condition   CC CC Condition   HIV HIV Related Dx

20 – Volume 1   2014 ICD-9-CM

090.2 Early congenital syphilis, unspecified `CC`
Congenital syphilis NOS, less than two years after birth
CC Excl: 090.0-099.9, 139.8

090.3 Syphilitic interstitial keratitis `CC`
Syphilitic keratitis:
    parenchymatous
    punctata profunda
    EXCLUDES *interstitial keratitis NOS (370.50)*
CC Excl: See code: 090.0

√5ᵗʰ **090.4 Juvenile neurosyphilis**
Use additional code to identify any associated mental
    disorder
DEF: *Treponema pallidum* infection involving the nervous system.

  090.40 Juvenile neurosyphilis, unspecified `CC`
    Congenital neurosyphilis
    Dementia paralytica juvenilis
    Juvenile:
      general paresis
      tabes
      taboparesis
    CC Excl: 090.0-097.9, 099.40-099.9, 139.8

  090.41 Congenital syphilitic encephalitis `MCC`
    DEF: Congenital *Treponema pallidum* infection involving the brain.
    CC Excl: See code: 090.40

  090.42 Congenital syphilitic meningitis `MCC`
    DEF: Congenital *Treponema pallidum* infection involving the lining of the brain and/or spinal cord.
    CC Excl: 003.21, 013.00-013.16, 036.0, 047.0-047.9, 049.0-049.1, 053.0, 054.72, 072.1, 090.0-097.9, 098.89, 099.40-099.9, 100.81, 112.83, 114.2, 115.01, 115.11, 115.91, 130.0, 139.8, 320.0-322.9, 349.89-349.9, 357.0

  090.49 Other `CC`
    CC Excl: See code: 090.40

090.5 Other late congenital syphilis, symptomatic `CC`
    Gumma due to congenital syphilis
    Hutchinson's teeth
    Syphilitic saddle nose
    Any congenital syphilitic condition specified as late or
      manifest two years or more after birth
    CC Excl: 090.0-097.9

090.6 Late congenital syphilis, latent
Congenital syphilis without clinical manifestations, with
    positive serological reaction and negative spinal fluid
    test, two years or more after birth

090.7 Late congenital syphilis, unspecified
Congenital syphilis NOS, two years or more after birth

090.9 Congenital syphilis, unspecified

√4ᵗʰ **091 Early syphilis, symptomatic**
    EXCLUDES *early cardiovascular syphilis (093.0-093.9)*
                early neurosyphilis (094.0-094.9)

091.0 Genital syphilis (primary)
    Genital chancre
    DEF: Genital lesion at the site of initial infection by *Treponema pallidum.*

091.1 Primary anal syphilis
    DEF: Anal lesion at the site of initial infection by *Treponema pallidum.*

091.2 Other primary syphilis
    Primary syphilis of:
      breast
      fingers
      lip
      tonsils
    DEF: Lesion at the site of initial infection by *Treponema pallidum.*

091.3 Secondary syphilis of skin or mucous membranes `CC`
    Condyloma latum
    Secondary syphilis of:
      anus
      mouth
      pharynx
      skin
      tonsils
      vulva
    DEF: Transitory or chronic lesions following initial syphilis infection.
    CC Excl: 090.0-097.9

091.4 Adenopathy due to secondary syphilis `CC`
    Syphilitic adenopathy (secondary)
    Syphilitic lymphadenitis (secondary)
    CC Excl: 090.0-097.9

√5ᵗʰ **091.5 Uveitis due to secondary syphilis**

  091.50 Syphilitic uveitis, unspecified `CC`
    CC Excl: 090.0-097.9

  091.51 Syphilitic chorioretinitis (secondary) `CC`
    DEF: Inflammation of choroid and retina as a secondary infection.
    CC Excl: 090.0-097.9

  091.52 Syphilitic iridocyclitis (secondary) `CC`
    DEF: Inflammation of iris and ciliary body as a secondary infection.
    CC Excl: 090.0-097.9

√5ᵗʰ **091.6 Secondary syphilis of viscera and bone**

  091.61 Secondary syphilitic periostitis `CC`
    DEF: Inflammation of outer layers of bone as a secondary infection.
    CC Excl: 015.90-015.96, 090.0-099.9, 102.6, 730.10-730.19, 730.30-730.39, 733.99

  091.62 Secondary syphilitic hepatitis `CC`
    Secondary syphilis of liver
    CC Excl: 090.0-099.9, 571.42-571.9, 573.1-573.3, 573.8-573.9

  091.69 Other viscera `CC`
    CC Excl: 090.0-099.9, 139.8

091.7 Secondary syphilis, relapse `CC`
    Secondary syphilis, relapse (treated) (untreated)
    DEF: Return of symptoms of syphilis following asymptomatic period.
    CC Excl: 090.0-099.9, 139.8

√5ᵗʰ **091.8 Other forms of secondary syphilis**

  091.81 Acute syphilitic meningitis (secondary) `MCC`
    DEF: Sudden, severe inflammation of the lining of the brain and/or spinal cord as a secondary infection.
    CC Excl: 003.21, 013.00-013.16, 036.0, 047.0-047.9, 049.0-049.1, 072.1, 078.88-078.89, 079.81, 079.88-079.99, 090.0-099.9, 100.81, 112.83, 114.2, 115.01, 115.11, 115.91, 130.0, 139.8, 320.0-322.9, 349.89-349.9, 357.0

  091.82 Syphilitic alopecia `CC`
    DEF: Hair loss following initial syphilis infection.
    CC Excl: 090.0-099.9

  091.89 Other `CC`
    CC Excl: 090.0-099.9, 139.8

091.9 Unspecified secondary syphilis `CC`
    CC Excl: 090.0-099.9, 139.8

√4ᵗʰ **092 Early syphilis, latent**
    INCLUDES syphilis (acquired) without clinical manifestations, with positive serological reaction and negative spinal fluid test, less than two years after infection

092.0 Early syphilis, latent, serological relapse after treatment

092.9 Early syphilis, latent, unspecified

√4ᵗʰ **093 Cardiovascular syphilis**

093.0 Aneurysm of aorta, specified as syphilitic `CC`
    Dilatation of aorta, specified as syphilitic
    CC Excl: 090.0-097.9, 099.40-099.9, 139.8

093.1 Syphilitic aortitis `CC`
    DEF: Inflammation of the aorta — the main artery leading from the heart.
    CC Excl: See code: 093.0

Infectious and Parasitic Diseases

093.2–097.9

√5ᵗʰ **093.2 Syphilitic endocarditis**
     DEF: Inflammation of the tissues lining the cavities of the heart.

     093.20 Valve, unspecified   `CC`
        Syphilitic ostial coronary disease
        CC Exd: See code: 093.0

     093.21 Mitral valve   `CC`
        CC Exd: See code: 093.0

     093.22 Aortic valve   `CC`
        Syphilitic aortic incompetence or stenosis
        CC Exd: See code: 093.0

     093.23 Tricuspid valve   `CC`
        CC Exd: See code: 093.0

     093.24 Pulmonary valve   `CC`
        CC Exd: See code: 093.0

√5ᵗʰ **093.8 Other specified cardiovascular syphilis**

     093.81 Syphilitic pericarditis   `CC`
        DEF: Inflammation of the outer lining of the heart.
        CC Exd: See code: 093.0

     093.82 Syphilitic myocarditis   `CC`
        DEF: Inflammation of the muscle of the heart.
        CC Exd: See code: 093.0

     093.89 Other   `CC`
        CC Exd: See code: 093.0

093.9 Cardiovascular syphilis, unspecified   `CC`
     CC Exd: See code: 093.0

√4ᵗʰ **094 Neurosyphilis**
     Use additional code to identify any associated mental disorder

     094.0 Tabes dorsalis   `CC`
        Locomotor ataxia (progressive)
        Posterior spinal sclerosis (syphilitic)
        Tabetic neurosyphilis
        Use additional code to identify manifestation, as:
           neurogenic arthropathy [Charcot's joint disease] (713.5)
        DEF: Progressive degeneration of nerves associated with long-term syphilis; causing pain, wasting away, incontinence, and ataxia.
        CC Exd: 090.0-097.9, 099.40-099.9, 139.8
        AHA: ▶3Q, '12, 4◀

     094.1 General paresis   `CC`
        Dementia paralytica
        General paralysis (of the insane) (progressive)
        Paretic neurosyphilis
        Taboparesis
        DEF: Degeneration of brain associated with long-term syphilis, causing loss of brain function, progressive dementia, and paralysis.
        CC Exd: 090.0-097.9, 099.40-099.9, 139.8

     094.2 Syphilitic meningitis   `MCC`
        Meningovascular syphilis
        EXCLUDES   acute syphilitic meningitis (secondary) (091.81)
        DEF: Inflammation of the lining of the brain and/or spinal cord.
        CC Exd: 003.21, 013.00-013.16, 036.0, 047.0-047.9, 049.0-049.1, 053.0, 054.72, 072.1, 090.0-097.9, 098.89, 099.40-099.9, 100.81, 112.83, 114.2, 115.01, 115.11, 115.91, 130.0, 139.8, 320.0-322.9, 349.89-349.9, 357.0

     094.3 Asymptomatic neurosyphilis   `CC`
        CC Exd: 090.0-097.9, 099.40-099.9, 139.8

√5ᵗʰ **094.8 Other specified neurosyphilis**

     094.81 Syphilitic encephalitis   `MCC`
        CC Exd: 090.0-097.9, 099.40-099.9, 139.8

     094.82 Syphilitic Parkinsonism   `CC`
        DEF: Decreased motor function, tremors, and muscular rigidity.
        CC Exd: 090.0-099.9, 332.0-333.0

     094.83 Syphilitic disseminated retinochoroiditis   `CC`
        DEF: Inflammation of retina and choroid due to neurosyphilis.
        CC Exd: 017.30-017.36, 090.0-099.9, 115.02, 115.12, 362.01, 362.12-362.13, 362.29, 362.41, 362.52, 362.76, 363.00, 363.05-363.10, 363.13-363.15, 646.80-646.84, 679.12, 679.14

     094.84 Syphilitic optic atrophy   `CC`
        DEF: Degeneration of the eye and its nerves due to neurosyphilis.
        CC Exd: 003.21, 013.00-013.16, 036.0, 047.0-047.9, 049.0-049.1, 072.1, 078.88-078.89, 079.81, 079.88-079.99, 090.0-099.9, 100.81, 112.83, 114.2, 115.01, 115.11, 115.91, 130.0, 139.8, 320.0-322.9, 349.89-349.9, 357.0

     094.85 Syphilitic retrobulbar neuritis   `CC`
        DEF: Inflammation of the posterior optic nerve due to neurosyphilis.
        CC Exd: 090.0-099.9, 377.32

     094.86 Syphilitic acoustic neuritis   `CC`
        DEF: Inflammation of acoustic nerve due to neurosyphilis.
        CC Exd: 090.0-099.9, 388.5

     094.87 Syphilitic ruptured cerebral aneurysm   `MCC`
        CC Exd: 090.0-097.9, 099.40-099.9, 139.8

     094.89 Other   `CC`
        CC Exd: 090.0-097.9, 099.40-099.9, 139.8

     094.9 Neurosyphilis, unspecified   `CC`
        Gumma (syphilitic) ⎫
        Syphilis (early) (late) ⎬ of central nervous system
        Syphiloma ⎭ NOS
        CC Exd: 090.0-097.9, 099.40-099.9, 139.8

√4ᵗʰ **095 Other forms of late syphilis, with symptoms**
     INCLUDES   gumma (syphilitic)
             syphilis, late, tertiary, or unspecified stage

     095.0 Syphilitic episcleritis   `CC`
        CC Exd: 017.30-017.36, 090.0-099.9, 379.00-379.02, 379.09

     095.1 Syphilis of lung   `CC`
        CC Exd: 090.0-099.9

     095.2 Syphilitic peritonitis   `CC`
        CC Exd: 014.00-014.06, 032.83, 090.0-099.9, 540.0-540.1, 567.0-567.1, 567.22, 567.29, 567.81, 567.9, 569.87-569.9, 577.8, 614.5-614.7, 639.0, 670.00-670.84, 777.6, 998.7

     095.3 Syphilis of liver   `CC`
        CC Exd: 090.0-099.9

     095.4 Syphilis of kidney   `CC`
        CC Exd: 090.0-099.9

     095.5 Syphilis of bone   `CC`
        CC Exd: 090.0-099.9

     095.6 Syphilis of muscle   `CC`
        Syphilitic myositis
        CC Exd: 090.0-099.9

     095.7 Syphilis of synovium, tendon, and bursa   `CC`
        Syphilitic:
          bursitis
          synovitis
        CC Exd: 090.0-099.9

     095.8 Other specified forms of late symptomatic syphilis   `CC`
        EXCLUDES   cardiovascular syphilis (093.0-093.9)
               neurosyphilis (094.0-094.9)
        CC Exd: 090.0-099.9

     095.9 Late symptomatic syphilis, unspecified   `CC`
        CC Exd: 090.0-099.9

096 Late syphilis, latent
     Syphilis (acquired) without clinical manifestations, with positive serological reaction and negative spinal fluid test, two years or more after infection

√4ᵗʰ **097 Other and unspecified syphilis**

     097.0 Late syphilis, unspecified

     097.1 Latent syphilis, unspecified
        Positive serological reaction for syphilis

     097.9 Syphilis, unspecified
        Syphilis (acquired) NOS
        EXCLUDES   syphilis NOS causing death under two years of age (090.9)

`N` Newborn Age: 0   `P` Pediatric Age: 0-17   `M` Maternity Age: 12-55   `A` Adult Age: 15-124   `MCC` Major CC Condition   `CC` CC Condition   `HIV` HIV Related Dx

22 – Volume 1 · February 2013   2014 ICD-9-CM

√4ᵗʰ **098 Gonococcal infections**
DEF: *Neisseria gonorrhoeae* infection generally acquired in utero or in sexual congress.

098.0 Acute, of lower genitourinary tract   CC
Gonococcal: Gonorrhea (acute):
  Bartholinitis (acute)   NOS
  urethritis (acute)   genitourinary (tract) NOS
  vulvovaginitis (acute)
CC Excl: 098.0-098.39, 098.89, 099.40-099.9, 139.8

√5ᵗʰ **098.1 Acute, of upper genitourinary tract**

098.10 Gonococcal infection (acute) of upper genitourinary tract, site unspecified   CC
CC Excl: See code: 098.0

098.11 Gonococcal cystitis (acute) upper   CC
Gonorrhea (acute) of bladder
CC Excl: See code: 098.0

098.12 Gonococcal prostatitis (acute)   CC ♂
CC Excl: See code: 098.0

098.13 Gonococcal epididymo-orchitis (acute)   CC ♂
Gonococcal orchitis (acute)
DEF: Acute inflammation of the testes.
CC Excl: See code: 098.0

098.14 Gonococcal seminal vesiculitis (acute)   CC ♂
Gonorrhea (acute) of seminal vesicle
CC Excl: See code: 098.0

098.15 Gonococcal cervicitis (acute)   CC ♀
Gonorrhea (acute) of cervix
CC Excl: See code: 098.0

098.16 Gonococcal endometritis (acute)   CC ♀
Gonorrhea (acute) of uterus
CC Excl: See code: 098.0

098.17 Gonococcal salpingitis, specified as acute   CC ♀
DEF: Acute inflammation of the fallopian tubes.
CC Excl: See code: 098.0

098.19 Other   CC
CC Excl: See code: 098.0

098.2 Chronic, of lower genitourinary tract
Gonoccocal:
  Bartholinitis
  urethritis   } specified as chronic or
  vulvovaginitis   with duration of two
Gonorrhea: months or more
  NOS
  genitourinary (tract)
Any condition classifiable to 098.0 specified as chronic or with duration of two months or more

√5ᵗʰ **098.3 Chronic, of upper genitourinary tract**
INCLUDES   any condition classifiable to 098.1 stated as chronic or with a duration of two months or more

098.30 Chronic gonococcal infection of upper genitourinary tract, site unspecified

098.31 Gonococcal cystitis, chronic
Gonorrhea of bladder, chronic
Any condition classifiable to 098.11, specified as chronic

098.32 Gonococcal prostatitis, chronic   ♂
Any condition classifiable to 098.12, specified as chronic

098.33 Gonococcal epididymo-orchitis, chronic   ♂
Chronic gonococcal orchitis
Any condition classifiable to 098.13, specified as chronic
DEF: Chronic inflammation of the testes.

098.34 Gonococcal seminal vesiculitis, chronic   ♂
Gonorrhea of seminal vesicle, chronic
Any condition classifiable to 098.14, specified as chronic

098.35 Gonococcal cervicitis, chronic   ♀
Gonorrhea of cervix, chronic
Any condition classifiable to 098.15, specified as chronic

098.36 Gonococcal endometritis, chronic   ♀
Any condition classifiable to 098.16, specified as chronic
DEF: Chronic inflammation of the uterus.

098.37 Gonococcal salpingitis (chronic)   ♀
DEF: Chronic inflammation of the fallopian tubes.

098.39 Other

√5ᵗʰ **098.4 Gonococcal infection of eye**

098.40 Gonococcal conjunctivitis (neonatorum)   CC
Gonococcal ophthalmia (neonatorum)
DEF: Infection of conjunctiva present at birth.
CC Excl: 090.0-099.9

098.41 Gonococcal iridocyclitis   CC
DEF: Inflammation and infection of iris and ciliary body.
CC Excl: 090.0-099.9

098.42 Gonococcal endophthalmia   CC
DEF: Inflammation and infection of contents of eyeball.
CC Excl: 090.0-099.9

098.43 Gonococcal keratitis   CC
DEF: Inflammation and infection of the cornea.
CC Excl: 090.0-099.9

098.49 Other   CC
CC Excl: 090.0-099.9

√5ᵗʰ **098.5 Gonococcal infection of joint**

098.50 Gonococcal arthritis   CC
Gonococcal infection of joint NOS
CC Excl: 003.23, 015.80-015.96, 017.90-017.96, 036.82, 056.71, 090.0-099.9, 711.00-714.0, 715.00, 715.09-715.10, 715.18-716.99, 718.00-718.08, 719.00-719.10, 719.18-719.69, 719.80-719.99

098.51 Gonococcal synovitis and tenosynovitis   CC
CC Excl: See code: 098.50

098.52 Gonococcal bursitis   CC
DEF: Inflammation of the sac-like cavities in a joint.
CC Excl: See code: 098.50

098.53 Gonococcal spondylitis   CC
CC Excl: See code: 098.50

098.59 Other   CC
Gonococcal rheumatism
CC Excl: See code: 098.50

098.6 Gonococcal infection of pharynx

098.7 Gonococcal infection of anus and rectum
Gonococcal proctitis

√5ᵗʰ **098.8 Gonococcal infection of other specified sites**

098.81 Gonococcal keratosis (blennorrhagica)   CC
DEF: Pustular skin lesions caused by *Neisseria gonorrhoeae*.
CC Excl: 098.40-098.49, 098.81

098.82 Gonococcal meningitis   MCC
DEF: Inflammation of lining of brain and/or spinal cord.
CC Excl: 003.21, 013.00-013.16, 036.0, 047.0-047.9, 049.0-049.1, 072.1, 078.88-078.89, 079.81, 079.88-079.99, 090.0-099.9, 100.81, 112.83, 114.2, 115.01, 115.11, 115.91, 130.0, 139.8, 320.0-322.9, 349.89-349.9, 357.0

098.83 Gonococcal pericarditis   MCC
DEF: Inflammation of the outer lining of the heart.
CC Excl: 074.21, 090.0-099.9, 391.0, 393, 420.0-420.99, 423.3-423.9, 459.89-459.9

098.84 Gonococcal endocarditis   MCC
DEF: Inflammation of tissues lining the cavities of heart.
CC Excl: 002.0, 036.42, 074.22, 083.0, 090.0-099.9, 112.81, 115.94, 116.0, 390, 391.1, 391.8-392.0, 394.0-395.9, 396.9-397.9, 398.90, 398.99, 421.0-421.9, 424.0-424.99, 425.3, 459.89-459.9, 711.00, 711.08-711.09, 746.09, 746.89, 996.61

Infectious and Parasitic Diseases

098.85–102.2

098.85 Other gonococcal heart disease `CC`
CC Excl: 002.0, 036.42, 074.20, 074.22-074.23, 083.0, 090.0-099.9, 112.81, 115.94, 116.0, 390, 391.1-392.0, 394.0-395.9, 396.9-398.90, 398.99, 421.0-422.99, 424.0-424.99, 425.3, 429.0, 429.71-429.79, 459.89-459.9, 711.00, 711.08-711.09, 746.09, 746.89, 996.61

098.86 Gonococcal peritonitis `CC`
DEF: Inflammation of the membrane lining the abdomen.
CC Excl: 014.00-014.06, 032.83, 090.0-099.9, 540.0-540.1, 567.0-567.1, 567.22, 567.29, 567.81, 567.9, 569.89-569.9, 577.8, 614.5-614.7, 639.0, 670.00-670.04, 777.6, 998.7

098.89 Other `CC`
Gonococcemia
CC Excl: 090.0-099.9, 588.81-588.89

✔4ᵗʰ 099 Other venereal diseases

099.0 Chancroid
Bubo (inguinal):
  chancroidal
  due to Hemophilus ducreyi
Chancre:
  Ducrey's
  simple
  soft
Ulcus molle (cutis)(skin)
DEF: A sexually transmitted disease caused by *Haemophilus ducreyi;* identified by a painful primary ulcer at the site of inoculation (usually external genitalia) with related lymphadenitis.

099.1 Lymphogranuloma venereum
Climatic or tropical bubo
(Durand-) Nicolas-Favre disease
Esthiomene
Lymphogranuloma inguinale
DEF: Sexually transmitted infection of *Chlamydia trachomatis* causing skin lesions.

099.2 Granuloma inguinale
Donovanosis
Granuloma pudendi (ulcerating)
Granuloma venereum
Pudendal ulcer
DEF: Chronic, sexually transmitted infection of *Calymmatobacterium granulomatis* causing progressive, anogenital skin ulcers.

099.3 Reiter's disease
Reactive arthritis
Reiter's syndrome
Use additional code for associated:
  arthropathy (711.1)
  conjunctivitis (372.33)
DEF: A symptom complex of unknown etiology consisting of urethritis, conjunctivitis, arthritis and myocutaneous lesions; occurs most commonly in young men and patients with HIV. Also a form of reactive arthritis.

✔5ᵗʰ 099.4 Other nongonococcal urethritis [NGU]

099.40 Unspecified
Nonspecific urethritis

099.41 Chlamydia trachomatis

099.49 Other specified organism

✔5ᵗʰ 099.5 Other venereal diseases due to Chlamydia trachomatis
EXCLUDES   Chlamydia trachomatis infection of conjunctiva (076.0-076.9, 077.0, 077.9)
           Lymphogranuloma venereum (099.1)
DEF: Venereal diseases caused by *Chlamydia trachomatis* at other sites besides the urethra (e.g., pharynx, anus and rectum, conjunctiva and peritoneum).

099.50 Unspecified site

099.51 Pharynx

099.52 Anus and rectum

099.53 Lower genitourinary sites
Use additional code to specify site of infection, such as:
  bladder (595.4)
  cervix (616.0)
  vagina and vulva (616.11)
    EXCLUDES   urethra (099.41)

099.54 Other genitourinary sites
Use additional code to specify site of infection, such as:
  pelvic inflammatory disease NOS (614.9)
  testis and epididymis (604.91)

099.55 Unspecified genitourinary site

099.56 Peritoneum `CC`
Perihepatitis
CC Excl: 014.00-014.06, 032.83, 090.0-099.9, 540.0-540.1, 567.0-567.1, 567.22, 567.29, 567.81, 567.9, 569.89-569.9, 577.8, 614.5-614.7, 639.0, 670.00-670.04, 777.6, 998.7

099.59 Other specified site

099.8 Other specified venereal diseases

099.9 Venereal disease, unspecified

Other Spirochetal Diseases (100-104)

✔4ᵗʰ 100 Leptospirosis
DEF: A blood infection of any spirochete of the genus *Leptospire*; transmitted to humans by exposure to contaminated animal tissues or water. Patients present with flulike symptoms, characteristic muscle aches involving the thighs and low back.

100.0 Leptospirosis icterohemorrhagica `CC`
Leptospiral or spirochetal jaundice (hemorrhagic)
Weil's disease
CC Excl: 100.0-100.9

✔5ᵗʰ 100.8 Other specified leptospiral infections

100.81 Leptospiral meningitis (aseptic) `MCC`
CC Excl: 003.21, 013.00-013.16, 036.0, 047.0-047.9, 049.0-049.1, 072.1, 078.88-078.89, 079.81, 079.88-079.99, 090.42, 091.81, 094.2, 098.89, 100.0-100.9, 112.83, 114.2, 115.01, 115.11, 115.91, 130.0, 139.8, 320.0-322.9, 349.89-349.9, 357.0

100.89 Other `CC`
Fever: Infection by Leptospira:
  Fort Bragg   australis
  pretibial   bataviae
  swamp   pyrogenes
CC Excl: See code: 100.0

100.9 Leptospirosis, unspecified `CC`
CC Excl: See code: 100.0

101 Vincent's angina `CC`
Acute necrotizing ulcerative:
  gingivitis
  stomatitis
Fusospirochetal pharyngitis
Spirochetal stomatitis
Trench mouth
Vincent's:
  gingivitis
  infection [any site]
DEF: Painful ulceration with edema and hypermic patches of the oropharyngeal and throat membranes; it is caused by spreading of acute ulcerative gingivitis.
CC Excl: 101

✔4ᵗʰ 102 Yaws
INCLUDES   frambesia
           pian
DEF: An infectious, endemic, tropical disease caused by *Treponema pertenue* usually affects persons 15 years old or younger; a primary cutaneous lesion develops, then a granulomatous skin eruption, and occasionally lesions that destroy skin and bone.

102.0 Initial lesions
Chancre of yaws   Initial frambesial ulcer
Frambesia, initial or primary   Mother yaw

102.1 Multiple papillomata and wet crab yaws
Butter yaws
Frambesioma
Pianoma
Plantar or palmar papilloma of yaws

102.2 Other early skin lesions
Cutaneous yaws, less than five years after infection
Early yaws (cutaneous) (macular) (papular) (maculopapular) (micropapular)
Frambeside of early yaws

N Newborn Age: 0   P Pediatric Age: 0-17   M Maternity Age: 12-55   A Adult Age: 15-124   MCC Major CC Condition   CC CC Condition   HIV HIV Related D

24 – Volume 1   2014 ICD-9-C

102.3 Hyperkeratosis
Ghoul hand
Hyperkeratosis, palmar or plantar (early) (late) due to yaws
Worm-eaten soles
DEF: Overgrowth of skin of palm or bottoms of feet, due to yaws.

102.4 Gummata and ulcers
Gummatous frambeside
Nodular late yaws (ulcerated)
DEF: Rubbery lesions and areas of dead skin caused by yaws.

102.5 Gangosa
Rhinopharyngitis mutilans
DEF: Massive, mutilating lesions of the nose and oral cavity caused by yaws.

102.6 Bone and joint lesions
Goundou
Gumma, bone   } of yaws (late)
Gummatous osteitis or periostitis

Hydrarthrosis
Osteitis   } of yaws (early) (late)
Periostitis (hypertrophic)

102.7 Other manifestations
Juxta-articular nodules of yaws
Mucosal yaws

102.8 Latent yaws
Yaws without clinical manifestations, with positive serology

102.9 Yaws, unspecified

√4ᵗʰ **103 Pinta**
DEF: A chronic form of treponematosis, endemic in areas of tropical America; it is identified by the presence of red, violet, blue, coffee-colored or white spots on the skin.

103.0 Primary lesions
Chancre (primary)
Papule (primary)   } of pinta [carate]
Pintid

103.1 Intermediate lesions
Erythematous plaques
Hyperchronic lesions } of pinta [carate]
Hyperkeratosis

103.2 Late lesions
Cardiovascular lesions
Skin lesions:
   achromic
   cicatricial   } of pinta [carate]
   dyschromic
Vitiligo

103.3 Mixed lesions
Achromic and hyperchromic skin lesions of pinta [carate]

103.9 Pinta, unspecified

√4ᵗʰ **104 Other spirochetal infection**

104.0 Nonvenereal endemic syphilis
Bejel
Njovera
DEF: *Treponema pallidum, T. pertenue,* or *T. caroteum* infection transmitted non-sexually, causing lesions on mucosa and skin.

104.8 Other specified spirochetal infections
EXCLUDES *relapsing fever (087.0-087.9)*
syphilis (090.0-097.9)

104.9 Spirochetal infection, unspecified

Mycoses (110-118)

Use additional code to identify manifestation as:
arthropathy (711.6)
meningitis (321.0-321.1)
otitis externa (380.15)
EXCLUDES *infection by Actinomycetales, such as species of Actinomyces, Actinomadura, Nocardia, Streptomyces (039.0-039.9)*

√4ᵗʰ **110 Dermatophytosis**
INCLUDES infection by species of Epidermophyton, Microsporum, and Trichophyton
tinea, any type except those in 111
DEF: Superficial infection of the skin caused by a parasitic fungus.

110.0 Of scalp and beard
Kerion
Sycosis, mycotic
Trichophytic tinea [black dot tinea], scalp

110.1 Of nail
Dermatophytic onychia
Onychomycosis
Tinea unguium
B35.1 Tinea unguium   I-10

110.2 Of hand
Tinea manuum

110.3 Of groin and perianal area
Dhobie itch
Eczema marginatum
Tinea cruris

110.4 Of foot
Athlete's foot
Tinea pedis

110.5 Of the body
Herpes circinatus
Tinea imbricata [Tokelau]

110.6 Deep seated dermatophytosis
Granuloma trichophyticum
Majocchi's granuloma

110.8 Of other specified sites

110.9 Of unspecified site
Favus NOS
Microsporic tinea NOS
Ringworm NOS

√4ᵗʰ **111 Dermatomycosis, other and unspecified**

111.0 Pityriasis versicolor
Infection by Malassezia [Pityrosporum] furfur
Tinea flava
Tinea versicolor

111.1 Tinea nigra
Infection by Cladosporium species
Keratomycosis nigricans
Microsporosis nigra
Pityriasis nigra
Tinea palmaris nigra

111.2 Tinea blanca
Infection by Trichosporon (beigelii) cutaneum
White piedra

111.3 Black piedra
Infection by Piedraia hortai

111.8 Other specified dermatomycoses

111.9 Dermatomycosis, unspecified

√4ᵗʰ **112 Candidiasis**
INCLUDES infection by Candida species
moniliasis
EXCLUDES *neonatal monilial infection (771.7)*
DEF: Fungal infection caused by *Candida*; usually seen in mucous membranes or skin.

112.0 Of mouth   CC HIV
Thrush (oral)
CC Exd: 112.0-112.9, 117.9, 139.8
B37.0 Candidal stomatitis   I-10

√4ᵗʰ/5ᵗʰ Additional Digit Required   Unacceptable PDx   Manifestation Code   Hospital Acquired Condition   ▶◀ Revised Text   ● New Code   ▲ Revised Code Title

2014 ICD-9-CM   **Volume 1 – 25**

Infectious and Parasitic Diseases

112.1–116.0

112.1 Of vulva and vagina   ♀
Candidal vulvovaginitis
Monilial vulvovaginitis
B37.3 Candidiasis of vulva and vagina   `I-10`

[8] **112.2 Of other urogenital sites**   `CC`
Candidal balanitis
CC Excl: 112.2, 112.4-112.9, 588.81-588.89
AHA: ▶3Q, '12, 11-12;◀ 4Q, '03, 105; 4Q, '96, 33

112.3 Of skin and nails   `HIV`
Candidal intertrigo
Candidal onychia
Candidal perionyxis [paronychia]
B37.2 Candidiasis of skin and nail   `I-10`

112.4 Of lung   `MCC` `HIV`
Candidal pneumonia
CC Excl: See code: 112.0
AHA: 2Q, '98, 7

112.5 Disseminated   `MCC` `HIV`
Systemic candidiasis
CC Excl: See code: 112.0
AHA: ▶3Q, '12, 11-12;◀2Q, '00, 5; 2Q, '89, 10
TIP: ▶Report for candidal sepsis, followed by the appropriate subcategory 995.9 code. If due to underlying candidal UTI, code also 112.2.◀

√5ᵗʰ **112.8 Of other specified sites**

112.81 Candidal endocarditis   `MCC` `HIV`
CC Excl: See code: 112.0

112.82 Candidal otitis externa   `CC` `HIV`
Otomycosis in moniliasis
CC Excl: See code: 112.0

112.83 Candidal meningitis   `MCC` `HIV`
CC Excl: 003.21, 013.00-013.16, 036.0, 047.0-047.9, 049.0-049.1, 053.0, 054.72, 072.1, 090.42, 091.81, 094.2, 098.89, 100.81, 112.0-112.9, 114.2, 115.01, 115.11, 115.91, 117.9, 130.0, 139.8, 320.0-322.9, 349.89-349.9, 357.0

112.84 Candidal esophagitis   `CC` `HIV`
CC Excl: See code: 112.0
AHA: 4Q, '92, 19
B37.81 Candidal esophagitis   `I-10`

112.85 Candidal enteritis   `CC` `HIV`
CC Excl: See code: 112.0
AHA: 4Q, '92, 19

112.89 Other   `CC` `HIV`
CC Excl: 112.4-112.9
AHA: 1Q, '92, 17; 3Q, '91, 20

112.9 Of unspecified site   `HIV`

√4ᵗʰ **114 Coccidioidomycosis**
INCLUDES infection by Coccidioides (immitis)
Posada-Wernicke disease
DEF: A fungal disease caused by inhalation of dust particles containing arthrospores of *Coccidioides immitis;* a self-limited respiratory infection; the primary form is known as San Joaquin fever, desert fever or valley fever.
AHA: 4Q, '93, 23

114.0 Primary coccidioidomycosis (pulmonary)   `CC` `HIV`
Acute pulmonary coccidioidomycosis
Coccidioidomycotic pneumonitis
Desert rheumatism
Pulmonary coccidioidomycosis
San Joaquin Valley fever
DEF: Acute, self-limiting *Coccidioides immitis* infection of the lung.
CC Excl: 114.0, 114.3-114.9, 117.9, 139.8
B38.0 Acute pulmonary coccidioidomycosis   `I-10`

114.1 Primary extrapulmonary coccidioidomycosis   `CC` `HIV`
Chancriform syndrome
Primary cutaneous coccidioidomycosis
DEF: Acute, self-limiting *Coccidioides immitis* infection in nonpulmonary site.
CC Excl: 114.0-114.9

114.2 Coccidioidal meningitis   `MCC` `HIV`
DEF: *Coccidioides immitis* infection of the lining of the brain and/or spinal cord.
CC Excl: 003.21, 013.00-013.16, 036.0, 047.0-047.9, 049.0-049.1, 053.0, 054.72, 072.1, 090.42, 091.81, 094.2, 098.89, 100.81, 112.83, 114.2-114.3, 114.9, 115.01, 115.11, 115.91, 117.9, 130.0, 139.8, 320.0-322.9, 349.89-349.9, 357.0

114.3 Other forms of progressive coccidioidomycosis   `CC` `HIV`
Coccidioidal granuloma
Disseminated coccidioidomycosis
CC Excl: 114.3, 114.9, 117.9, 139.8

114.4 Chronic pulmonary coccidioidomycosis   `CC` `HIV`
CC Excl: 114.0-115.99

114.5 Pulmonary coccidioidomycosis, unspecified   `CC` `HIV`
CC Excl: See code: 114.4

114.9 Coccidioidomycosis, unspecified   `CC` `HIV`
CC Excl: See code: 114.3

√4ᵗʰ **115 Histoplasmosis**

The following fifth-digit subclassification is for use with category 115:
  0 **without mention of manifestation**
  1 **meningitis**
  2 **retinitis**
  3 **pericarditis**
  4 **endocarditis**
  5 **pneumonia**
  9 **other**

§ √5ᵗʰ **115.0 Infection by Histoplasma capsulatum**   `CC 2,9` `HIV` `MCC 1, 3-5`
[0-5, 9]   American histoplasmosis
Darling's disease
Reticuloendothelial cytomycosis
Small form histoplasmosis
CC Excl: For code 115.01: 003.21, 013.00-013.16, 036.0, 047.0-047.9, 049.0-049.1, 053.0, 054.72, 072.1, 090.42, 091.81, 094.2, 098.89, 100.81, 112.83, 114.2, 115.00-115.01, 115.09, 115.11, 115.90-115.91, 115.99, 117.9, 130.0, 139.8, 320.0-322.9, 349.89-349.9, 357.0; **For code 115.02:** 115.00, 115.02, 115.09, 115.90, 115.92, 115.99, 117.9, 139.8; **For code 115.03:** 115.00, 115.03, 115.09, 115.90, 115.93, 115.99, 117.9, 139.8; **For code 115.04:**115.00, 115.04, 115.09, 115.90, 115.94, 115.99, 117.9, 139.8; **For code 115.05:** 115.00, 115.05-115.09, 115.90, 115.95-115.99, 117.9, 139.8, 480.0-480.2, 480.8-487.1, 488.01-488.02, 488.11-488.12, 494.0-508.9, 517.1, 518.89; **For code 115.09:** 114.0-115.09

§ √5ᵗʰ **115.1 Infection by Histoplasma duboisii**   `CC 2,9` `HIV` `MCC 1, 3-5`
[0-5, 9]   African histoplasmosis
Large form histoplasmosis
CC Excl: For code 115.11: 003.21, 013.00-013.16, 036.0, 047.0-047.9, 049.0-049.1, 053.0, 054.72, 072.1, 090.42, 091.81, 094.2, 098.89, 100.81, 112.83, 114.2, 115.00-115.01, 115.09, 115.11, 115.90-115.91, 115.99, 117.9, 130.0, 139.8, 320.0-322.9, 349.89-349.9, 357.0; **For code 115.12:** 115.10, 115.12, 115.19-115.90, 115.92, 115.99, 117.9, 139.8; **For code 115.13:** 115.10, 115.13, 115.19-115.90, 115.93, 115.99, 117.9, 139.8; **For code 115.14:**115.10, 115.14, 115.19-115.90, 115.94, 115.99, 117.9, 139.8; **For code 115.15:** 115.05, 115.10, 115.15-115.90, 115.95-115.99, 117.9, 139.8, 480.0-480.2, 480.8-487.1, 488.01-488.02, 488.11-488.12, 494.0-508.9, 517.1, 518.89; **For code 115.19:**115.10, 115.19-115.90, 115.99, 117.9, 139.8

§ √5ᵗʰ **115.9 Histoplasmosis, unspecified**   `CC 2` `HIV` `MCC 1, 3-5`
[0-5, 9]   Histoplasmosis NOS
CC Excl: For code 115.91: 003.21, 013.00-013.16, 036.0, 047.0-047.9, 049.0-049.1, 053.0, 054.72, 072.1, 090.42, 091.81, 094.2, 098.89, 100.81, 112.83, 114.2, 115.01, 115.11, 115.91, 115.99, 117.9, 130.0, 139.8, 320.0-322.9, 349.89-349.9, 357.0; **For code 115.92:**115.92, 115.99, 117.9, 139.8; **For code 115.93:** 115.93, 115.99, 117.9, 139.8; **For code 115.94:** 115.94, 115.99, 117.9, 139.8; **For code 115.95:**115.05, 115.15, 115.95-115.99, 117.9, 139.8

√4ᵗʰ **116 Blastomycotic infection**

116.0 Blastomycosis   `CC`
Blastomycotic dermatitis
Chicago disease
Cutaneous blastomycosis
Disseminated blastomycosis
Gilchrist's disease
Infection by Blastomyces [Ajellomyces] dermatitidis
North American blastomycosis
Primary pulmonary blastomycosis
CC Excl: 116.0, 117.9, 139.8

---

[8] CC/MCC except when in combination with 996.64 and POA = N
§ Requires fifth digit. Valid digits are in [brackets] under each code. See category 115 for codes and definitions.

`N` Newborn Age: 0   `P` Pediatric Age: 0-17   `M` Maternity Age: 12-55   `A` Adult Age: 15-124   `MCC` Major CC Condition   `CC` CC Condition   `HIV` HIV Related Dx

116.1 Paracoccidioidomycosis `CC`
    Brazilian blastomycosis
    Infection by Paracoccidioides [Blastomyces] brasiliensis
    Lutz-Splendore-Almeida disease
    Mucocutaneous-lymphangitic paracoccidioidomycosis
    Pulmonary paracoccidioidomycosis
    South American blastomycosis
    Visceral paracoccidioidomycosis
    CC Exd: 116.1, 117.9, 139.8

116.2 Lobomycosis
    Infections by Loboa [Blastomyces] loboi
    Keloidal blastomycosis
    Lobo's disease

√4th **117 Other mycoses**

117.0 Rhinosporidiosis
    Infection by Rhinosporidium seeberi

117.1 Sporotrichosis
    Cutaneous sporotrichosis
    Disseminated sporotrichosis
    Infection by Sporothrix [Sporotrichum] schenckii
    Lymphocutaneous sporotrichosis
    Pulmonary sporotrichosis
    Sporotrichosis of the bones

117.2 Chromoblastomycosis
    Chromomycosis
    Infection by Cladosporidium carrionii, Fonsecaea compactum, Fonsecaea pedrosoi, Phialophora verrucosa

117.3 Aspergillosis `CC`
    Infection by Aspergillus species, mainly A. fumigatus, A. flavus group, A. terreus group
    CC Exd: 117.3, 117.9, 139.8
    AHA: 4Q, '97, 40

117.4 Mycotic mycetomas `CC`
    Infection by various genera and species of Ascomycetes and Deuteromycetes, such as Acremonium [Cephalosporium] falciforme, Neotestudina rosatii, Madurella grisea, Madurella mycetomii, Pyrenochaeta romeroi, Zopfia [Leptosphaeria] senegalensis
    Madura foot, mycotic
    Maduromycosis, mycotic
    EXCLUDES *actinomycotic mycetomas (039.0-039.9)*
    CC Exd: 117.4, 117.9, 139.8

117.5 Cryptococcosis `CC` `HIV`
    Busse-Buschke's disease
    European cryptococcosis
    Infection by Cryptococcus neoformans
    Pulmonary cryptococcosis
    Systemic cryptococcosis
    Torula
    CC Exd: 117.5, 117.9, 139.8

117.6 Allescheriosis [Petriellidosis] `CC`
    Infections by Allescheria [Petriellidium] boydii [Monosporium apiospermum]
    EXCLUDES *mycotic mycetoma (117.4)*
    CC Exd: 117.6, 117.9, 139.8

117.7 Zygomycosis [Phycomycosis or Mucormycosis] `MCC`
    Infection by species of Absidia, Basidiobolus, Conidiobolus, Cunninghamella, Entomophthora, Mucor, Rhizopus, Saksenaea
    CC Exd: 117.7, 117.9, 139.8

117.8 Infection by dematiacious fungi, [Phaephyphomycosis] `CC`
    Infection by dematiacious fungi, such as Cladosporium trichoides [bantianum], Dreschlera hawaiiensis, Phialophora gougerotii, Phialophora jeanselmi
    CC Exd: 117.8-117.9

117.9 Other and unspecified mycoses `CC`
    CC Exd: See code: 117.8

118 Opportunistic mycoses `CC` `HIV`
    Infection of skin, subcutaneous tissues, and/or organs by a wide variety of fungi generally considered to be pathogenic to compromised hosts only (e.g., infection by species of Alternaria, Dreschlera, Fusarium)
    Use additional code to identify manifestation, such as:
        keratitis (370.8)
    CC Exd: 117.9-118, 139.8

Helminthiases (120-129)

√4th **120 Schistosomiasis [bilharziasis]**
    DEF: Infection caused by *Schistosoma*, a genus of flukes or trematode parasites.

120.0 Schistosoma haematobium `CC`
    Vesical schistosomiasis NOS
    CC Exd: 120.0-120.9

120.1 Schistosoma mansoni `CC`
    Intestinal schistosomiasis NOS
    CC Exd: See code: 120.0

120.2 Schistosoma japonicum `CC`
    Asiatic schistosomiasis NOS
    Katayama disease or fever
    CC Exd: See code: 120.0

120.3 Cutaneous `CC`
    Cercarial dermatitis
    Infection by cercariae of Schistosoma
    Schistosome dermatitis
    Swimmers' itch
    CC Exd: See code: 120.0

120.8 Other specified schistosomiasis `CC`
    Infection by Schistosoma:
        bovis
        intercalatum
        mattheii
        spindale
    Schistosomiasis chestermani
    CC Exd: See code: 120.0

120.9 Schistosomiasis, unspecified `CC`
    Blood flukes NOS
    Hemic distomiasis
    CC Exd: See code: 120.0

√4th **121 Other trematode infections**

121.0 Opisthorchiasis `CC`
    Infection by:
        cat liver fluke
        Opisthorchis (felineus) (tenuicollis) (viverrini)
    CC Exd: 121.0-121.9

121.1 Clonorchiasis `CC`
    Biliary cirrhosis due to clonorchiasis
    Chinese liver fluke disease
    Hepatic distomiasis due to Clonorchis sinensis
    Oriental liver fluke disease
    CC Exd: See code: 121.0

121.2 Paragonimiasis `CC`
    Infection by Paragonimus
    Lung fluke disease (oriental)
    Pulmonary distomiasis
    CC Exd: See code: 121.0

121.3 Fascioliasis `CC`
    Infection by Fasciola:
        gigantica
        hepatica
    Liver flukes NOS
    Sheep liver fluke infection
    CC Exd: See code: 121.0

121.4 Fasciolopsiasis `CC`
    Infection by Fasciolopsis (buski)
    Intestinal distomiasis
    CC Exd: See code: 121.0

121.5 Metagonimiasis `CC`
    Infection by Metagonimus yokogawai
    CC Exd: See code: 121.0

4th / 5th Additional Digit Required   Unacceptable PDx   Manifestation Code   Hospital Acquired Condition   ►◄ Revised Text   ● New Code   ▲ Revised Code Title

2014 ICD-9-CM   **Volume 1 – 27**

Infectious and Parasitic Diseases

121.6–125.9

121.6 Heterophyiasis `CC`
Infection by:
Heterophyes heterophyes
Stellantchasmus falcatus
CC Excl: See code: 121.0

121.8 Other specified trematode infections `CC`
Infection by:
Dicrocoelium dendriticum
Echinostoma ilocanum
Gastrodiscoides hominis
CC Excl: See code: 121.0

121.9 Trematode infection, unspecified
Distomiasis NOS
Fluke disease NOS

✓4ᵗʰ **122 Echinococcosis**
INCLUDES echinococciasis
hydatid disease
hydatidosis
DEF: Infection caused by larval forms of tapeworms of the genus *Echinococcus.*

122.0 Echinococcus granulosus infection of liver `CC`
CC Excl: 122.0, 122.8-122.9

122.1 Echinococcus granulosus infection of lung `CC`
CC Excl: 122.1, 122.8-122.9, 480.3

122.2 Echinococcus granulosus infection of thyroid `CC`
CC Excl: 122.2, 122.8-122.9

122.3 Echinococcus granulosus infection, other `CC`
CC Excl: 122.3, 122.8-122.9

122.4 Echinococcus granulosus infection, unspecified `CC`
CC Excl: 122.4, 122.8-122.9

122.5 Echinococcus multilocularis infection of liver `CC`
CC Excl: 122.5, 122.8-122.9

122.6 Echinococcus multilocularis infection, other `CC`
CC Excl: 122.6, 122.8-122.9

122.7 Echinococcus multilocularis infection, unspecified `CC`
CC Excl: 122.7-122.9

122.8 Echinococcosis, unspecified, of liver `CC`
CC Excl: 122.8-122.9

122.9 Echinococcosis, other and unspecified `CC`
CC Excl: See code: 122.8

✓4ᵗʰ **123 Other cestode infection**

123.0 Taenia solium infection, intestinal form `CC`
Pork tapeworm (adult) (infection)
CC Excl: 001.1, 002.0, 002.9-003.0, 004.9-005.2, 006.0-006.2, 006.9,
007.1-009.0, 014.80-014.86, 040.41-040.42, 112.85, 123.0-123.9, 129,
487.8, 488.09, 488.19, 536.3, 536.8, 558.2-558.9, 564.1,
777.50-777.53, 777.8

123.1 Cysticercosis `CC`
Cysticerciasis
Infection by Cysticercus cellulosae [larval form of Taenia solium]
CC Excl: 123.0-123.9
AHA: 2Q, '97, 8

123.2 Taenia saginata infection `CC`
Beef tapeworm (infection)
Infection by Taeniarhynchus saginatus
CC Excl: See code: 123.1

123.3 Taeniasis, unspecified `CC`
CC Excl: See code: 123.1

123.4 Diphyllobothriasis, intestinal `CC`
Diphyllobothrium (adult) (latum) (pacificum) infection
Fish tapeworm (infection)
CC Excl: See code: 123.1

123.5 Sparganosis [larval diphyllobothriasis] `CC`
Infection by:
Diphyllobothrium larvae
Sparganum (mansoni) (proliferum)
Spirometra larvae
CC Excl: See code: 123.1

123.6 Hymenolepiasis `CC`
Dwarf tapeworm (infection)
Hymenolepis (diminuta) (nana) infection
Rat tapeworm (infection)
CC Excl: See code: 123.1

123.8 Other specified cestode infection `CC`
Diplogonoporus (grandis) ⎫
Dipylidium (caninum) ⎬ infection
Dog tapeworm (infection) ⎭
CC Excl: See code: 123.1

123.9 Cestode infection, unspecified
Tapeworm (infection) NOS

124 Trichinosis `CC`
Trichinella spiralis infection
Trichinellosis
Trichiniasis
DEF: Infection by *Trichinella spiralis,* the smallest of the parasitic nematodes.
CC Excl: 013.60-013.66, 046.2, 046.71-046.8, 048-049.0, 049.8, 052.0, 052.2,
054.3, 054.74, 056.01, 057.8-058.29, 059.00-059.9, 062.0-064, 066.2-066.49,
072.2, 073.7, 079.82, 079.99, 081.9, 083.9, 090.41, 094.81, 117.5, 124, 130.0,
290.12, 323.01-323.9, 341.1, 487.8, 488.09, 488.19, 771.2, 984.9

✓4ᵗʰ **125 Filarial infection and dracontiasis**

125.0 Bancroftian filariasis `CC`
Chyluria ⎫
Elephantiasis ⎪
Infection ⎬ due to Wuchereria bancrofti
Lymphadenitis ⎪
Lymphangitis ⎭
Wuchereriasis
CC Excl: 125.0-125.9

125.1 Malayan filariasis `CC`
Brugia filariasis ⎫
Chyluria ⎪
Elephantiasis ⎪
Infection ⎬ due to Wuchereria bancrofti
Lymphadenitis ⎪
Lymphangitis ⎭
CC Excl: See code: 125.0

125.2 Loiasis `CC`
Eyeworm disease of Africa
Loa loa infection
CC Excl: See code: 125.0

125.3 Onchocerciasis `CC`
Onchocerca volvulus infection
Onchocercosis
CC Excl: See code: 125.0

125.4 Dipetalonemiasis `CC`
Infection by:
Acanthocheilonema perstans
Dipetalonema perstans
CC Excl: See code: 125.0

125.5 Mansonella ozzardi infection `CC`
Filariasis ozzardi
CC Excl: See code: 125.0

125.6 Other specified filariasis `CC`
Dirofilaria infection
Infection by:
Acanthocheilonema streptocerca
Dipetalonema streptocerca
CC Excl: See code: 125.0

125.7 Dracontiasis `CC`
Guinea-worm infection
Infection by Dracunculus medinensis
CC Excl: See code: 125.0

125.9 Unspecified filariasis `CC`
CC Excl: See code: 125.0

N Newborn Age: 0   **P** Pediatric Age: 0-17   **M** Maternity Age: 12-55   **A** Adult Age: 15-124   **MCC** Major CC Condition   **CC** CC Condition   **HIV** HIV Related Dx

28 – Volume 1   2014 ICD-9-CM

√4ᵗʰ **126 Ancylostomiasis and necatoriasis**

> INCLUDES   cutaneous larva migrans due to Ancylostoma
> hookworm (disease) (infection)
> uncinariasis

126.0 Ancylostoma duodenale   CC
    CC Exd: 126.0-126.9

126.1 Necator americanus   CC
    CC Exd: See code: 126.0

126.2 Ancylostoma braziliense   CC
    CC Exd: See code: 126.0

126.3 Ancylostoma ceylanicum   CC
    CC Exd: See code: 126.0

126.8 Other specified Ancylostoma   CC
    CC Exd: See code: 126.0

126.9 Ancylostomiasis and necatoriasis, unspecified   CC
    Creeping eruption NOS
    Cutaneous larva migrans NOS
    CC Exd: See code: 126.0

√4ᵗʰ **127 Other intestinal helminthiases**

127.0 Ascariasis   CC
    Ascaridiasis
    Infection by Ascaris lumbricoides
    Roundworm infection
    CC Exd: 127.0-127.9

127.1 Anisakiasis   CC
    Infection by Anisakis larva
    CC Exd: See code: 127.0

127.2 Strongyloidiasis   CC HIV
    Infection by Strongyloides stercoralis
    EXCLUDES   *trichostrongyliasis (127.6)*
    CC Exd: See code: 127.0

127.3 Trichuriasis   CC
    Infection by Trichuris trichiuria
    Trichocephaliasis
    Whipworm (disease) (infection)
    CC Exd: See code: 127.0

127.4 Enterobiasis   CC
    Infection by Enterobius vermicularis
    Oxyuriasis
    Oxyuris vermicularis infection
    Pinworm (disease) (infection)
    Threadworm infection
    CC Exd: See code: 127.0

127.5 Capillariasis   CC
    Infection by Capillaria philippinensis
    EXCLUDES   *infection by Capillaria hepatica (128.8)*
    CC Exd: See code: 127.0

127.6 Trichostrongyliasis   CC
    Infection by Trichostrongylus species
    CC Exd: See code: 127.0

127.7 Other specified intestinal helminthiasis   CC
    Infection by:
      Oesophagostomum apiostomum and related species
      Ternidens diminutus
      other specified intestinal helminth
      Physalopteriasis
    CC Exd: 127.0-129

127.8 Mixed intestinal helminthiasis   CC
    Infection by intestinal helminths classified to more than one
      of the categories 120.0-127.7
    Mixed helminthiasis NOS
    CC Exd: See code: 127.7

127.9 Intestinal helminthiasis, unspecified   CC
    CC Exd: See code: 127.7

√4ᵗʰ **128 Other and unspecified helminthiases**

128.0 Toxocariasis
    Larva migrans visceralis
    Toxocara (canis) (cati) infection
    Visceral larva migrans syndrome

128.1 Gnathostomiasis
    Infection by Gnathostoma spinigerum and related species

128.8 Other specified helminthiasis
    Infection by:
      Angiostrongylus cantonensis
      Capillaria hepatica
      other specified helminth

128.9 Helminth infection, unspecified
    Helminthiasis NOS
    Worms NOS

129 Intestinal parasitism, unspecified

Other Infectious and Parasitic Diseases (130–136)

√4ᵗʰ **130 Toxoplasmosis**

> INCLUDES   infection by toxoplasma gondii
> toxoplasmosis (acquired)
> EXCLUDES   *congenital toxoplasmosis (771.2)*

130.0 Meningoencephalitis due to toxoplasmosis   MCC HIV
    Encephalitis due to acquired toxoplasmosis
    CC Exd: 130.0, 130.7-130.9, 139.8

130.1 Conjunctivitis due to toxoplasmosis   CC HIV
    CC Exd: 130.1, 130.7-130.9, 139.8

130.2 Chorioretinitis due to toxoplasmosis   CC HIV
    Focal retinochoroiditis due to acquired toxoplasmosis
    CC Exd: 130.2, 130.7-130.9, 139.8

130.3 Myocarditis due to toxoplasmosis   MCC HIV
    CC Exd: 130.3, 130.7-130.9, 139.8

130.4 Pneumonitis due to toxoplasmosis   MCC HIV
    CC Exd: 130.4, 130.7-130.9, 139.8, 480.0-480.2, 480.8-487.1,
      488.01-488.02, 488.11-488.12, 494.0-508.9, 517.1, 518.89

130.5 Hepatitis due to toxoplasmosis   CC HIV
    CC Exd: 130.5-130.9, 139.8

130.7 Toxoplasmosis of other specified sites   CC HIV
    CC Exd: 130.7-130.9, 139.8

130.8 Multisystemic disseminated toxoplasmosis   MCC HIV
    Toxoplasmosis of multiple sites
    CC Exd: See code: 130.7

130.9 Toxoplasmosis, unspecified   CC HIV
    CC Exd: 130.9

√4ᵗʰ **131 Trichomoniasis**

> INCLUDES   infection due to Trichomonas (vaginalis)

√5ᵗʰ **131.0 Urogenital trichomoniasis**

131.00 Urogenital trichomoniasis, unspecified
    Fluor (vaginalis)   ⎫ trichomonal or due to
    Leukorrhea   ⎬   Trichomonas
      (vaginalis)   ⎭   (vaginalis)
    DEF: *Trichomonas vaginalis* infection of reproductive and
    urinary organs, transmitted through coitus.

131.01 Trichomonal vulvovaginitis   ♀
    Vaginitis, trichomonal or due to Trichomonas
      (vaginalis)
    DEF: *Trichomonas vaginalis* infection of vulva and vagina;
    often asymptomatic, transmitted through coitus.

131.02 Trichomonal urethritis
    DEF: *Trichomonas vaginalis* infection of the urethra.

131.03 Trichomonal prostatitis   ♂
    DEF: *Trichomonas vaginalis* infection of the prostate.

131.09 Other

131.8 Other specified sites
    EXCLUDES   *intestinal (007.3)*

131.9 Trichomoniasis, unspecified

√4ᵗʰ **132 Pediculosis and phthirus infestation**

132.0 Pediculus capitis [head louse]

132.1 Pediculus corporis [body louse]

132.2 Phthirus pubis [pubic louse]
    Pediculus pubis

132.3 Mixed infestation
    Infestation classifiable to more than one of the categories
      132.0-132.2

Additional Digit Required   Unacceptable PDx   Manifestation Code   Hospital Acquired Condition   ▶◀ Revised Text   ● New Code   ▲ Revised Code Title

2014 ICD-9-CM   Volume 1 – 29

Infectious and Parasitic Diseases

132.9–139.8

132.9 **Pediculosis, unspecified**

√4ᵗʰ 133 **Acariasis**

133.0 **Scabies**
Infestation by Sarcoptes scabiei
Norwegian scabies
Sarcoptic itch

133.8 **Other acariasis**
Chiggers
Infestation by:
Demodex folliculorum
Trombicula

133.9 **Acariasis, unspecified**
Infestation by mites NOS

√4ᵗʰ 134 **Other infestation**

134.0 **Myiasis**
Infestation by:
Dermatobia (hominis)
fly larvae
Gasterophilus (intestinalis)
maggots
Oestrus ovis

134.1 **Other arthropod infestation**
Infestation by:
chigoe
sand flea
Tunga penetrans
Jigger disease
Scarabiasis
Tungiasis

134.2 **Hirudiniasis**
Hirudiniasis (external) (internal)
Leeches (aquatic) (land)

134.8 **Other specified infestations**

134.9 **Infestation, unspecified**
Infestation (skin) NOS
Skin parasites NOS

135 **Sarcoidosis**
Besnier-Boeck-Schaumann disease
Lupoid (miliary) of Boeck
Lupus pernio (Besnier)
Lymphogranulomatosis, benign (Schaumann's)
Sarcoid (any site):
NOS
Boeck
Darier-Roussy
Uveoparotid fever
DEF: A chronic, granulomatous reticulosis (abnormal increase in cells), affecting any organ or tissue; acute form has high rate of remission; chronic form is progressive.
D86.9 Sarcoidosis unspecified   I-10

√4ᵗʰ 136 **Other and unspecified infectious and parasitic diseases**

136.0 **Ainhum**
Dactylolysis spontanea
DEF: A disease affecting the toes, especially the fifth digit, the fingers, mostly seen in black adult males; it is characterized by a linear constriction around the affected digit leading to spontaneous amputation of the distal part of the digit.

136.1 **Behçet's syndrome**
DEF: A chronic inflammatory disorder of unknown etiology involving the small blood vessels; characterized by recurrent aphthous ulceration of the oral and pharyngeal mucous membranes and the genitalia; skin lesions, severe uveitis, retinal vasculitis and optic atrophy.

√5ᵗʰ 136.2 **Specific infections by free-living amebae**
AHA: 4Q, '08, 79-81

136.21 **Specific infection due to acanthamoeba**
Use additional code to identify manifestation, such as:
keratitis (370.8)
AHA: 4Q, '08, 81

136.29 **Other specific infections by free-living amebae**   CC
Meningoencephalitis due to Naegleria
CC Excl: 136.0-136.9

136.3 **Pneumocystosis**   MCC H
Pneumonia due to Pneumocystis carinii
Pneumonia due to Pneumocystis jiroveci
DEF: *Pneumocystis carinii* fungus causing pneumonia in immunocompromised patients; a leading cause of death among AIDS patients.
CC Excl: 136.3, 139.8, 480.0-480.2, 480.8-487.1, 488.01-488.02, 488.11-488.12, 494.0-508.9, 517.1, 518.89
AHA: 1Q, '05, 7; 1Q, '03, 15; N-D, '87, 5-6

136.4 **Psorospermiasis**   C
CC Excl: See code: 136.2

136.5 **Sarcosporidiosis**   C
Infection by Sarcocystis lindemanni
DEF: *Sarcocystis* infection causing muscle cysts of intestinal inflammation.
CC Excl: See code: 136.2

136.8 **Other specified infectious and parasitic diseases**   H
Candiru infestation

136.9 **Unspecified infectious and parasitic diseases**
Infectious disease NOS
Parasitic disease NOS
AHA: 2Q, '91, 8

Late Effects of Infectious and Parasitic Diseases (137-139)

√4ᵗʰ 137 **Late effects of tuberculosis**
NOTE This category is to be used to indicate conditions classifiable t 010-018 as the cause of late effects, which are themselves classified elsewhere. The "late effects" include those specifie as such, as sequelae, or as due to old or inactive tuberculosis, without evidence of active disease.

137.0 **Late effects of respiratory or unspecified tuberculosis**

137.1 **Late effects of central nervous system tuberculosis**

137.2 **Late effects of genitourinary tuberculosis**

137.3 **Late effects of tuberculosis of bones and joints**

137.4 **Late effects of tuberculosis of other specified organs**

138 **Late effects of acute poliomyelitis**
NOTE This category is to be used to indicate conditions classifiable t 045 as the cause of late effects, which are themselves classifie elsewhere. The "late effects" include conditions specified as such, or as sequelae, or as due to old or inactive poliomyeliti without evidence of active disease.
B91 Sequelae of poliomyelitis   I-

√4ᵗʰ 139 **Late effects of other infectious and parasitic diseases**
NOTE This category is to be used to indicate conditions classifiable t categories 001-009, 020-041, 046-136 as the cause of late effects, which are themselves classified elsewhere. The "late effects" include conditions specified as such; they also includ sequela of diseases classifiable to the above categories if ther is evidence that the disease itself is no longer present.

139.0 **Late effects of viral encephalitis**
Late effects of conditions classifiable to 049.8-049.9, 062-06

139.1 **Late effects of trachoma**
Late effects of conditions classifiable to 076

139.8 **Late effects of other and unspecified infectious and parasitic diseases**
AHA: 2Q, '06, 17; 4Q, '91, 15; 3Q, '90, 14; M-A, '87, 8

N Newborn Age: 0   P Pediatric Age: 0-17   M Maternity Age: 12-55   A Adult Age: 15-124   MCC Major CC Condition   CC CC Condition   HIV HIV Related F

30 – Volume 1   2014 ICD-9-C

2. Neoplasms (140-239)

NOTES

1. Content

   This chapter contains the following broad groups:

   140-195 Malignant neoplasms, stated or presumed to be primary, of specified sites, except of lymphatic and hematopoietic tissue

   196-198 Malignant neoplasms, stated or presumed to be secondary, of specified sites

   199 Malignant neoplasms, without specification of site

   200-208 Malignant neoplasms, stated or presumed to be primary, of lymphatic and hematopoietic tissue

   209 Neuroendocrine tumors

   210-229 Benign neoplasms

   230-234 Carcinoma in situ

   235-238 Neoplasms of uncertain behavior [see Note, above category 235]

   239 Neoplasms of unspecified nature

2. Functional activity

   All neoplasms are classified in this chapter, whether or not functionally active. An additional code from Chapter 3 may be used to identify such functional activity associated with any neoplasm, e.g.:

        catecholamine-producing malignant pheochromocytoma of adrenal:

            code 194.0, additional code 255.6

        basophil adenoma of pituitary with Cushing's syndrome:

            code 227.3, additional code 255.0

3. Morphology [Histology]

   For those wishing to identify the histological type of neoplasms, a comprehensive coded nomenclature, which comprises the morphology rubrics of the ICD-Oncology, is given in Appendix A.

4. Malignant neoplasms overlapping site boundaries

   Categories 140-195 are for the classification of primary malignant neoplasms according to their point of origin. A malignant neoplasm that overlaps two or more subcategories within a three-digit rubric and whose point of origin cannot be determined should be classified to the subcategory .8 "Other."

   For example, "carcinoma involving tip and ventral surface of tongue" should be assigned to 141.8. On the other hand, "carcinoma of tip of tongue, extending to involve the ventral surface" should be coded to 141.2, as the point of origin, the tip, is known. Three subcategories (149.8, 159.8, 165.8) have been provided for malignant neoplasms that overlap the boundaries of three-digit rubrics within certain systems.

   Overlapping malignant neoplasms that cannot be classified as indicated above should be assigned to the appropriate subdivision of category 195 (Malignant neoplasm of other and ill-defined sites).

   > **DEF:** An abnormal growth; morphology determines behavior, i.e., whether it will remain intact (benign) or spread to adjacent tissue (malignant). The term mass is not synonymous with neoplasm, as it is often used to describe cysts and thickenings such as those occurring with hematoma or infection.
   > **AHA:** 2Q, '90, 7

Malignant Neoplasm of Lip, Oral Cavity, and Pharynx (140-149)

EXCLUDES *carcinoma in situ (230.0)*

140 Malignant neoplasm of lip

     EXCLUDES *malignant melanoma of skin of lip (172.0)*
                        malignant neoplasm of skin of lip (173.00-173.09)

     140.0 Upper lip, vermilion border
         Upper lip:
            NOS
            external
            lipstick area

     140.1 Lower lip, vermilion border
         Lower lip:
            NOS
            external
            lipstick area

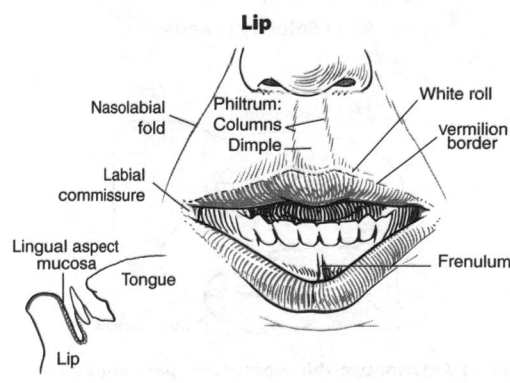

Lip

140.3 Upper lip, inner aspect
     Upper lip:
         buccal aspect
         frenulum
         mucosa
         oral aspect

140.4 Lower lip, inner aspect
     Lower lip:
         buccal aspect
         frenulum
         mucosa
         oral aspect

140.5 Lip, unspecified, inner aspect
     Lip, not specified whether upper or lower:
         buccal aspect
         frenulum
         mucosa
         oral aspect

140.6 Commissure of lip
     Labial commissure

140.8 Other sites of lip
     Malignant neoplasm of contiguous or overlapping sites of lip whose point of origin cannot be determined

140.9 Lip, unspecified, vermilion border
     Lip, not specified as upper or lower:
         NOS
         external
         lipstick area

✓4ᵗʰ 141 Malignant neoplasm of tongue

     141.0 Base of tongue
         Dorsal surface of base of tongue
         Fixed part of tongue NOS
         AHA: 4Q, '06, 90

     141.1 Dorsal surface of tongue
         Anterior two-thirds of tongue, dorsal surface
         Dorsal tongue NOS
         Midline of tongue
         EXCLUDES *dorsal surface of base of tongue (141.0)*

     141.2 Tip and lateral border of tongue

     141.3 Ventral surface of tongue
         Anterior two-thirds of tongue, ventral surface
         Frenulum linguae

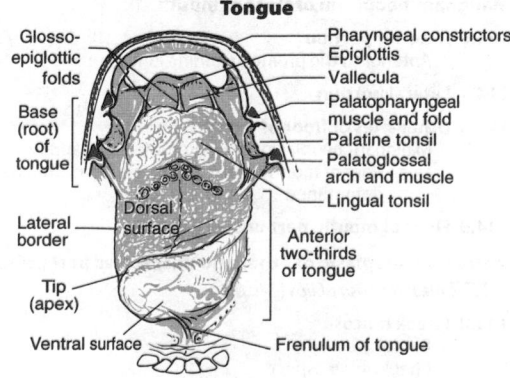

Tongue

Additional Digit Required   **Unacceptable PDx**   **Manifestation Code**   **Hospital Acquired Condition**   ▶◀ Revised Text   ● New Code   ▲ Revised Code Title

4 **ICD-9-CM**   **Volume 1 – 31**

Main Salivary Glands

Mouth

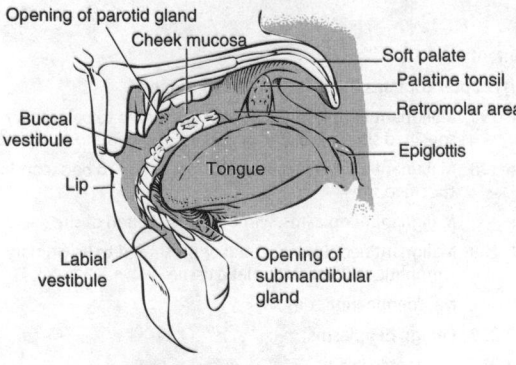

141.4 Anterior two-thirds of tongue, part unspecified
Mobile part of tongue NOS

141.5 Junctional zone
Border of tongue at junction of fixed and mobile parts at insertion of anterior tonsillar pillar

141.6 Lingual tonsil

141.8 Other sites of tongue
Malignant neoplasm of contiguous or overlapping sites of tongue whose point of origin cannot be determined

141.9 Tongue, unspecified
Tongue NOS

☑4ᵗʰ **142 Malignant neoplasm of major salivary glands**
INCLUDES salivary ducts
EXCLUDES *malignant neoplasm of minor salivary glands:*
NOS (145.9)
buccal mucosa (145.0)
soft palate (145.3)
tongue (141.0-141.9)
tonsil, palatine (146.0)

142.0 Parotid gland

142.1 Submandibular gland
Submaxillary gland

142.2 Sublingual gland

142.8 Other major salivary glands
Malignant neoplasm of contiguous or overlapping sites of salivary glands and ducts whose point of origin cannot be determined

142.9 Salivary gland, unspecified
Salivary gland (major) NOS

☑4ᵗʰ **143 Malignant neoplasm of gum**
INCLUDES alveolar (ridge) mucosa
gingiva (alveolar) (marginal)
interdental papillae
EXCLUDES *malignant odontogenic neoplasms (170.0-170.1)*

143.0 Upper gum

143.1 Lower gum

143.8 Other sites of gum
Malignant neoplasm of contiguous or overlapping sites of gum whose point of origin cannot be determined

143.9 Gum, unspecified

☑4ᵗʰ **144 Malignant neoplasm of floor of mouth**

144.0 Anterior portion
Anterior to the premolar-canine junction

144.1 Lateral portion

144.8 Other sites of floor of mouth
Malignant neoplasm of contiguous or overlapping sites of floor of mouth whose point of origin cannot be determined

144.9 Floor of mouth, part unspecified

☑4ᵗʰ **145 Malignant neoplasm of other and unspecified parts of mouth**
EXCLUDES *mucosa of lips (140.0-140.9)*

145.0 Cheek mucosa
Buccal mucosa
Cheek, inner aspect

145.1 Vestibule of mouth
Buccal sulcus (upper) (lower)
Labial sulcus (upper) (lower)

145.2 Hard palate

145.3 Soft palate
EXCLUDES *nasopharyngeal [posterior] [superior] surface of soft palate (147.3)*

145.4 Uvula

145.5 Palate, unspecified
Junction of hard and soft palate
Roof of mouth

145.6 Retromolar area

145.8 Other specified parts of mouth
Malignant neoplasm of contiguous or overlapping sites of mouth whose point of origin cannot be determined

145.9 Mouth, unspecified
Buccal cavity NOS
Minor salivary gland, unspecified site
Oral cavity NOS

Oropharynx

Nasopharynx

N Newborn Age: 0   P Pediatric Age: 0-17   M Maternity Age: 12-55   A Adult Age: 15-124   MCC Major CC Condition   CC CC Condition   HIV HIV Related

32 – Volume 1   2014 ICD-9-

Neoplasms

√4ᵗʰ **146 Malignant neoplasm of oropharynx**

146.0 Tonsil
Tonsil:
  NOS
  faucial
  palatine
  EXCLUDES *lingual tonsil (141.6)*
                  pharyngeal tonsil (147.1)
  AHA: S-O, '87, 8

146.1 Tonsillar fossa

146.2 Tonsillar pillars (anterior) (posterior)
Faucial pillar
Glossopalatine fold
Palatoglossal arch
Palatopharyngeal arch

146.3 Vallecula
Anterior and medial surface of the pharyngoepiglottic fold

146.4 Anterior aspect of epiglottis
Epiglottis, free border [margin]
Glossoepiglottic fold(s)
  EXCLUDES *epiglottis:*
      NOS (161.1)
      suprahyoid portion (161.1)

146.5 Junctional region
Junction of the free margin of the epiglottis, the aryepiglottic fold, and the pharyngoepiglottic fold

146.6 Lateral wall of oropharynx

146.7 Posterior wall of oropharynx

146.8 Other specified sites of oropharynx
Branchial cleft
Malignant neoplasm of contiguous or overlapping sites of oropharynx whose point of origin cannot be determined

146.9 Oropharynx, unspecified
  AHA: 2Q, '02, 6

√4ᵗʰ **147 Malignant neoplasm of nasopharynx**

147.0 Superior wall
Roof of nasopharynx

147.1 Posterior wall
Adenoid
Pharyngeal tonsil

147.2 Lateral wall
Fossa of Rosenmüller
Opening of auditory tube
Pharyngeal recess

147.3 Anterior wall
Floor of nasopharynx
Nasopharyngeal [posterior] [superior] surface of soft palate
Posterior margin of nasal septum and choanae

147.8 Other specified sites of nasopharynx
Malignant neoplasm of contiguous or overlapping sites of nasopharynx whose point of origin cannot be determined

147.9 Nasopharynx, unspecified
Nasopharyngeal wall NOS

√4ᵗʰ **148 Malignant neoplasm of hypopharynx**

148.0 Postcricoid region

148.1 Pyriform sinus
Pyriform fossa

148.2 Aryepiglottic fold, hypopharyngeal aspect
Aryepiglottic fold or interarytenoid fold:
  NOS
  marginal zone
  EXCLUDES *aryepiglottic fold or interarytenoid fold, laryngeal aspect (161.1)*

148.3 Posterior hypopharyngeal wall

Hypopharynx

Skull base from behind

Nasopharynx — Choanae
Oropharynx — Soft palate
Hypopharynx — Uvula — Tongue
To trachea — Epiglottis junctional zone
Esophagus — Aryepiglottic fold — Piriform sinus (fossa) — Posterior cricoid region

148.8 Other specified sites of hypopharynx
Malignant neoplasm of contiguous or overlapping sites of hypopharynx whose point of origin cannot be determined

148.9 Hypopharynx, unspecified
Hypopharyngeal wall NOS
Hypopharynx NOS

√4ᵗʰ **149 Malignant neoplasm of other and ill-defined sites within the lip, oral cavity, and pharynx**

149.0 Pharynx, unspecified

149.1 Waldeyer's ring

149.8 Other
Malignant neoplasms of lip, oral cavity, and pharynx whose point of origin cannot be assigned to any one of the categories 140-148
  EXCLUDES *"book leaf" neoplasm [ventral surface of tongue and floor of mouth] (145.8)*

149.9 Ill-defined

Malignant Neoplasm of Digestive Organs and Peritoneum (150-159)

  EXCLUDES *carcinoma in situ (230.1-230.9)*

√4ᵗʰ **150 Malignant neoplasm of esophagus**

150.0 Cervical esophagus   CC
  CC Excl: 150.0-150.9, 159.0, 159.8-159.9, 176.3, 195.8, 199.0-199.2, 209.20, 209.29-209.30, 209.70, 209.75, 239.0, 239.81-239.9

150.1 Thoracic esophagus   CC
  CC Excl: See code: 150.0

150.2 Abdominal esophagus   CC
  EXCLUDES *adenocarcinoma (151.0)*
                cardio-esophageal junction (151.0)
  CC Excl: See code 150.0

150.3 Upper third of esophagus   CC
Proximal third of esophagus
  CC Excl: See code 150.0

150.4 Middle third of esophagus   CC
  CC Excl: See code 150.0

150.5 Lower third of esophagus   CC
Distal third of esophagus
  EXCLUDES *adenocarcinoma (151.0)*
                cardio-esophageal junction (151.0)
  CC Excl: See code 150.0

150.8 Other specified part   CC
Malignant neoplasm of contiguous or overlapping sites of esophagus whose point of origin cannot be determined
  CC Excl: See code 150.0

150.9 Esophagus, unspecified   CC
  CC Excl: See code 150.0

Additional Digit Required   Unacceptable PDx   Manifestation Code   Hospital Acquired Condition   ►◄ Revised Text   ● New Code   ▲ Revised Code Title

146–150.9

Neoplasms

151–153.9

☑4ᵗʰ **151 Malignant neoplasm of stomach**

> EXCLUDES   *benign carcinoid tumor of stomach (209.63)*
> *malignant carcinoid tumor of stomach (209.23)*

151.0 Cardia   `CC`
Cardiac orifice
Cardio-esophageal junction

> EXCLUDES   *squamous cell carcinoma (150.2, 150.5)*

CC Exd: 151.0-151.9, 159.0, 159.8-159.9, 176.3, 195.8, 199.0-199.2, 209.20, 209.23, 209.25-209.30, 209.70, 209.75, 239.0, 239.81-239.9

151.1 Pylorus   `CC`
Prepylorus
Pyloric canal
CC Exd: See code 151.0

151.2 Pyloric antrum   `CC`
Antrum of stomach NOS
CC Exd: See code 151.0

151.3 Fundus of stomach   `CC`
CC Exd: See code 151.0

151.4 Body of stomach   `CC`
CC Exd: See code 151.0

151.5 Lesser curvature, unspecified   `CC`
Lesser curvature, not classifiable to 151.1-151.4
CC Exd: See code 151.0

151.6 Greater curvature, unspecified   `CC`
Greater curvature, not classifiable to 151.0-151.4
CC Exd: See code 151.0

151.8 Other specified sites of stomach   `CC`
Anterior wall, not classifiable to 151.0-151.4
Posterior wall, not classifiable to 151.0-151.4
Malignant neoplasm of contiguous or overlapping sites of stomach whose point of origin cannot be determined
CC Exd: See code 151.0

151.9 Stomach, unspecified   `CC`
Carcinoma ventriculi
Gastric cancer
CC Exd: See code 151.0
AHA: 2Q, '01, 17

☑4ᵗʰ **152 Malignant neoplasm of small intestine, including duodenum**

> EXCLUDES   *benign carcinoid tumor of small intestine and duodenum (209.40-209.43)*
> *malignant carcinoid tumor of small intestine and duodenum (209.00-209.03)*

152.0 Duodenum   `CC`
CC Exd: 152.0, 152.8-152.9, 159.0, 159.8-159.9, 176.3, 195.8, 199.0-199.2, 209.00-209.01, 209.20, 209.29-209.30, 209.70, 209.75, 239.0, 239.81-239.9

152.1 Jejunum   `CC`
CC Exd: 152.1, 152.8-152.9, 159.0, 159.8-159.9, 176.3, 195.8, 199.0-199.2, 209.00, 209.02, 209.20, 209.29-209.30, 209.70, 209.75, 239.0, 239.81-239.9

152.2 Ileum   `CC`

> EXCLUDES   *ileocecal valve (153.4)*

CC Exd: 152.2, 152.8-152.9, 159.0, 159.8-159.9, 176.3, 195.8, 199.0-199.2, 209.00, 209.03, 209.20, 209.29-209.30, 209.70, 209.75, 239.0, 239.81-239.9

152.3 Meckel's diverticulum   `CC`
CC Exd: 152.3-152.9, 159.0, 159.8-159.9, 176.3, 195.8, 199.0-199.2, 209.00, 209.20, 209.29-209.30, 209.70, 209.75, 239.0, 239.81-239.9

152.8 Other specified sites of small intestine   `CC`
Duodenojejunal junction
Malignant neoplasm of contiguous or overlapping sites of small intestine whose point of origin cannot be determined
CC Exd: 152.8-152.9, 159.0, 159.8-159.9, 176.3, 195.8, 199.0-199.2, 209.00, 209.20, 209.29-209.30, 209.70, 209.75, 239.0, 239.81-239.9

152.9 Small intestine, unspecified   `CC`
CC Exd: See code 152.8

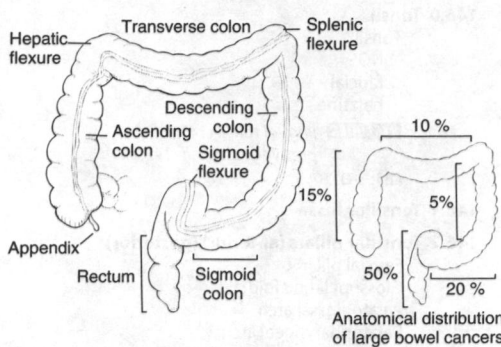

Colon

Anatomical distribution of large bowel cancers

☑4ᵗʰ **153 Malignant neoplasm of colon**

> EXCLUDES   *benign carcinoid tumor of colon (209.50-209.56)*
> *malignant carcinoid tumor of colon (209.10-209.16)*

153.0 Hepatic flexure
CC Exd: 153.0, 153.8-153.9, 159.0, 159.8-159.9, 176.3, 195.8, 199.0-199.2, 209.10, 209.20, 209.29-209.30, 209.70, 209.75, 239.0, 239.81-239.9

153.1 Transverse colon
CC Exd: 153.1, 153.8-153.9, 159.0, 159.8-159.9, 176.3, 195.8, 199.0-199.2, 209.10, 209.14, 209.20, 209.29-209.30, 209.70, 209.7... 239.0, 239.81-239.9

153.2 Descending colon
Left colon
CC Exd: 153.2, 153.8-153.9, 159.0, 159.8-159.9, 176.3, 195.8, 199.0-199.2, 209.10, 209.15, 209.20, 209.29-209.30, 209.70, 209.7... 239.0, 239.81-239.9

153.3 Sigmoid colon
Sigmoid (flexure)

> EXCLUDES   *rectosigmoid junction (154.0)*

CC Exd: 153.3, 153.8-153.9, 159.0, 159.8-159.9, 176.3, 195.8, 199.0-199.2, 209.10, 209.16, 209.20, 209.29-209.30, 209.70, 209.7... 239.0, 239.81-239.9

153.4 Cecum
Ileocecal valve
CC Exd: 153.4, 153.8-153.9, 159.0, 159.8-159.9, 176.3, 195.8, 199.0-199.2, 209.10, 209.12, 209.20, 209.29-209.30, 209.70, 209.7... 239.0, 239.81-239.9
C18.0 Malignant neoplasm of cecum

153.5 Appendix
CC Exd: 153.5, 153.8-153.9, 159.0, 159.8-159.9, 176.3, 195.8, 199.0-199.2, 209.10-209.11, 209.20, 209.29-209.30, 209.70, 209.7... 239.0, 239.81-239.9

153.6 Ascending colon
Right colon
CC Exd: 153.6, 153.8-153.9, 159.0, 159.8-159.9, 176.3, 195.8, 199.0-199.2, 209.10, 209.13, 209.20, 209.29-209.30, 209.70, 209.7... 239.0, 239.81-239.9
C18.2 Malignant neoplasm of ascending colon

153.7 Splenic flexure
CC Exd: 153.7-153.9, 159.0, 159.8-159.9, 176.3, 195.8, 199.0-199.2, 209.10, 209.20, 209.29-209.30, 209.70, 209.75, 239.0, 239.81-239.

153.8 Other specified sites of large intestine
Malignant neoplasm of contiguous or overlapping sites of colon whose point of origin cannot be determined

> EXCLUDES   *ileocecal valve (153.4)*
> *rectosigmoid junction (154.0)*

CC Exd: 153.8-153.9, 159.0, 159.8-159.9, 176.3, 195.8, 199.0-199.2, 209.10, 209.20, 209.29-209.30, 209.70, 209.75, 239.0, 239.81-239.

153.9 Colon, unspecified
Large intestine NOS
CC Exd: See code: 153.8
AHA: 2Q, '10, 12
C18.9 Malignant neoplasm of colon unspecified

Ⓝ Newborn Age: 0   Ⓟ Pediatric Age: 0-17   Ⓜ Maternity Age: 12-55   Ⓐ Adult Age: 15-124   `MCC` Major CC Condition   `CC` CC Condition   `HIV` HIV Related

34 – Volume 1   2014 ICD-9

√4ᵗʰ **154 Malignant neoplasm of rectum, rectosigmoid junction, and anus**

> *EXCLUDES* benign carcinoid tumor of rectum (209.57)
>   malignant carcinoid tumor of rectum (209.17)

154.0 Rectosigmoid junction   `CC`
Colon with rectum
Rectosigmoid (colon)
CC Exd: 154.0, 154.8, 159.0, 159.8-159.9, 176.3, 195.8, 199.0-199.2, 209.20, 209.29-209.30, 209.70, 209.75, 239.0, 239.81-239.9

154.1 Rectum   `CC`
Rectal ampulla
CC Exd: 154.1, 154.8, 159.0, 159.8-159.9, 176.3, 195.8, 199.0-199.2, 209.17-209.20, 209.29-209.30, 209.70, 209.75, 239.0, 239.81-239.9
C20 Malignant neoplasm of rectum   `I-10`

154.2 Anal canal   `CC`
Anal sphincter
> *EXCLUDES* malignant melanoma of skin of anus (172.5)
>   malignant neoplasm of skin of anus (173.50-173.59)

CC Exd: 154.2-154.8, 159.0, 159.8-159.9, 176.3, 195.8, 199.0-199.2, 209.20, 209.29-209.30, 209.70, 209.75, 239.0, 239.81-239.9
AHA: 1Q, '01, 8

154.3 Anus, unspecified   `CC`
> *EXCLUDES* malignant melanoma of:
>   anus:
>   margin (172.5)
>   skin (172.5)
>   perianal skin (172.5)
>   malignant neoplasm of:
>   anus:
>   margin (173.50-173.59)
>   skin (173.50-173.59)
>   perianal skin (173.50-173.59)

CC Exd: See code: 154.2

154.8 Other   `CC`
Anorectum
Cloacogenic zone
Malignant neoplasm of contiguous or overlapping sites of rectum, rectosigmoid junction, and anus whose point of origin cannot be determined
CC Exd: 154.8, 159.0, 159.8-159.9, 176.3, 195.8, 199.0-199.2, 209.20, 209.29-209.30, 209.70, 209.75, 239.0, 239.81-239.9

√4ᵗʰ **155 Malignant neoplasm of liver and intrahepatic bile ducts**

155.0 Liver, primary   `CC`
Carcinoma:
  liver, specified as primary
  hepatocellular
  liver cell
Hepatoblastoma
CC Exd: 155.0-155.2, 159.0, 159.8-159.9, 176.3, 195.8, 199.0-199.2, 209.20, 209.29-209.30, 209.70, 209.75, 239.0, 239.81-239.9
AHA: 4Q, '08, 82
C22.0 Liver cell carcinoma   `I-10`

155.1 Intrahepatic bile ducts   `CC`
Canaliculi biliferi   Intrahepatic:
Interlobular: biliary passages
  bile ducts   canaliculi
  biliary canals   gall duct
> *EXCLUDES* hepatic duct (156.1)

CC Exd: See code 155.0

155.2 Liver, not specified as primary or secondary   `CC`
CC Exd: See code 155.0

√4ᵗʰ **156 Malignant neoplasm of gallbladder and extrahepatic bile ducts**

156.0 Gallbladder   `CC`
CC Exd: 156.0, 156.8-156.9, 159.0, 159.8-159.9, 176.3, 195.8, 199.0-199.2, 209.20, 209.29-209.30, 209.70, 209.75, 239.0, 239.81-239.9

156.1 Extrahepatic bile ducts   `CC`
Biliary duct or passage NOS
Common bile duct
Cystic duct
Hepatic duct
Sphincter of Oddi
CC Exd: 156.1, 156.8-156.9, 159.0, 159.8-159.9, 176.3, 195.8, 199.0-199.2, 209.20, 209.29-209.30, 209.70, 209.75, 239.0, 239.81-239.9

156.2 Ampulla of Vater   `CC`
DEF: Malignant neoplasm in the area of dilation at the juncture of the common bile and pancreatic ducts near the opening into the lumen of the duodenum.
CC Exd: 156.2-156.9, 159.0, 159.8-159.9, 176.3, 195.8, 199.0-199.2, 209.20, 209.29-209.30, 209.70, 209.75, 239.0, 239.81-239.9

156.8 Other specified sites of gallbladder and extrahepatic bile ducts   `CC`
Malignant neoplasm of contiguous or overlapping sites of gallbladder and extrahepatic bile ducts whose point of origin cannot be determined
CC Exd: 156.8-156.9, 159.0, 159.8-159.9, 176.3, 195.8, 199.0-199.2, 209.20, 209.29-209.30, 209.70, 209.75, 239.0, 239.81-239.9

156.9 Biliary tract, part unspecified   `CC`
Malignant neoplasm involving both intrahepatic and extrahepatic bile ducts
CC Exd: See code: 156.8

√4ᵗʰ **157 Malignant neoplasm of pancreas**
AHA: 4Q, '07, 72

157.0 Head of pancreas   `CC`
CC Exd: 157.0-157.9, 159.0, 159.8-159.9, 176.3, 195.8, 199.0-199.2, 209.20, 209.29-209.30, 209.70, 209.75, 239.0, 239.81-239.9
AHA: 2Q, '05, 9; 4Q, '00, 40

157.1 Body of pancreas   `CC`
CC Exd: See code 157.0

157.2 Tail of pancreas   `CC`
CC Exd: See code 157.0

157.3 Pancreatic duct   `CC`
Duct of:
  Santorini
  Wirsung
CC Exd: See code 157.0

157.4 Islets of Langerhans   `CC`
Islets of Langerhans, any part of pancreas
Use additional code to identify any functional activity
DEF: Malignant neoplasm within the structures of the pancreas that produce insulin, somatostatin and glucagon.
CC Exd: See code 157.0

157.8 Other specified sites of pancreas   `CC`
Ectopic pancreatic tissue
Malignant neoplasm of contiguous or overlapping sites of pancreas whose point of origin cannot be determined
CC Exd: See code 157.0

157.9 Pancreas, part unspecified   `CC`
CC Exd: See code 157.0
AHA: 4Q, '89, 11
C25.9 Malignant neoplasm of pancreas unspecified   `I-10`

√4ᵗʰ **158 Malignant neoplasm of retroperitoneum and peritoneum**

158.0 Retroperitoneum   `CC`
Periadrenal tissue   Perirenal tissue
Perinephric tissue   Retrocecal tissue
CC Exd: 158.0, V58.0

158.8 Specified parts of peritoneum   `CC`
Cul-de-sac (of Douglas)
Malignant neoplasm of contiguous or overlapping sites of retroperitoneum and peritoneum whose point of origin cannot be determined
Mesentery
Mesocolon
Omentum
Peritoneum:
  parietal
  pelvic
Rectouterine pouch
CC Exd: 158.0-158.9, V58.0

158.9 Peritoneum, unspecified   `CC`
CC Exd: See code: 158.8

Additional Digit Required   Unacceptable PDx   Manifestation Code   Hospital Acquired Condition   ►◄ Revised Text   ● New Code   ▲ Revised Code Title

Retroperitoneum and Peritoneum

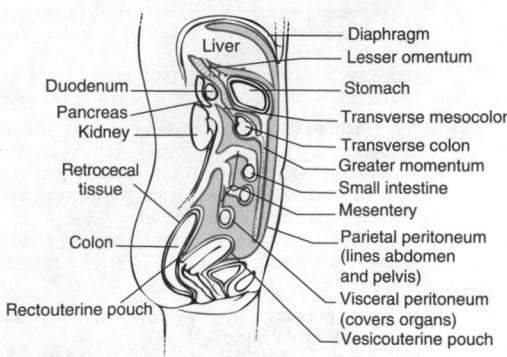

- Liver
- Duodenum
- Pancreas
- Kidney
- Retrocecal tissue
- Colon
- Rectouterine pouch
- Diaphragm
- Lesser omentum
- Stomach
- Transverse mesocolon
- Transverse colon
- Greater momentum
- Small intestine
- Mesentery
- Parietal peritoneum (lines abdomen and pelvis)
- Visceral peritoneum (covers organs)
- Vesicouterine pouch

159 Malignant neoplasm of other and ill-defined sites within the digestive organs and peritoneum

159.0 Intestinal tract, part unspecified
Intestine NOS

159.1 Spleen, not elsewhere classified
Angiosarcoma ⎱ of spleen
Fibrosarcoma ⎰
EXCLUDES   *Hodgkin's disease (201.0-201.9)*
          lymphosarcoma (200.1)
          reticulosarcoma (200.0)

159.8 Other sites of digestive system and intra-abdominal organs
Malignant neoplasm of digestive organs and peritoneum whose point of origin cannot be assigned to any one of the categories 150-158
EXCLUDES   *anus and rectum (154.8)*
          cardio-esophageal junction (151.0)
          colon and rectum (154.0)

159.9 Ill-defined
Alimentary canal or tract NOS
Gastrointestinal tract NOS
EXCLUDES   *abdominal NOS (195.2)*
          intra-abdominal NOS (195.2)

Neoplasm of Respiratory and Intrathoracic Organs (160-165)

EXCLUDES   *carcinoma in situ (231.0-231.9)*

160 Malignant neoplasm of nasal cavities, middle ear, and accessory sinuses

160.0 Nasal cavities
Cartilage of nose   Septum of nose
Conchae, nasal   Vestibule of nose
Internal nose
EXCLUDES   *malignant melanoma of skin of nose (172.3)*
          malignant neoplasm of skin of nose (173.30-173.39)
          nasal bone (170.0)
          nose NOS (195.0)
          olfactory bulb (192.0)
          posterior margin of septum and choanae (147.3)
          turbinates (170.0)

160.1 Auditory tube, middle ear, and mastoid air cells
Antrum tympanicum
Eustachian tube
Tympanic cavity
EXCLUDES   *bone of ear (meatus) (170.0)*
          cartilage of ear (171.0)
          malignant melanoma of:
            auditory canal (external) (172.2)
            ear (external) (skin) (172.2)
          malignant neoplasm of:
            auditory canal (external) (173.20-173.29)
            ear (external) (skin) (173.20-173.29)

160.2 Maxillary sinus
Antrum (Highmore) (maxillary)

160.3 Ethmoidal sinus

160.4 Frontal sinus

160.5 Sphenoidal sinus

160.8 Other
Malignant neoplasm of contiguous or overlapping sites of nasal cavities, middle ear, and accessory sinuses whose point of origin cannot be determined

160.9 Accessory sinus, unspecified

161 Malignant neoplasm of larynx

161.0 Glottis
Intrinsic larynx
Laryngeal commissure (anterior) (posterior)
True vocal cord
Vocal cord NOS

161.1 Supraglottis
Aryepiglottic fold or interarytenoid fold, laryngeal aspect
Epiglottis (suprahyoid portion) NOS
Extrinsic larynx
False vocal cords
Posterior (laryngeal) surface of epiglottis
Ventricular bands
EXCLUDES   *anterior aspect of epiglottis (146.4)*
          aryepiglottic fold or interarytenoid fold:
            NOS (148.2)
            hypopharyngeal aspect (148.2)
            marginal zone (148.2)

161.2 Subglottis

161.3 Laryngeal cartilages
Cartilage:
   arytenoid
   cricoid
   cuneiform
   thyroid

161.8 Other specified sites of larynx
Malignant neoplasm of contiguous or overlapping sites of larynx whose point of origin cannot be determined
AHA: 3Q, '07, 7

161.9 Larynx, unspecified

162 Malignant neoplasm of trachea, bronchus, and lung
EXCLUDES   *benign carcinoid tumor of bronchus (209.61)*
          malignant carcinoid tumor of bronchus (209.21)

162.0 Trachea
Cartilage ⎱ of trachea
Mucosa ⎰
CC Excl: 162.0-162.9, 165.8-165.9, 176.4, 195.1, 195.8, 197.0-197.1, 197.3, 199.0-199.2, 209.20-209.21, 209.29-209.30, 209.70, 209.75, 239.1, 239.81-239.9

162.2 Main bronchus
Carina
Hilus of lung
CC Excl: 162.2, 162.8-162.9, 165.8-165.9, 176.4, 195.8, 199.0-199.2, 209.20-209.21, 209.29-209.30, 209.70, 209.75, 239.1, 239.81-239.9

162.3 Upper lobe, bronchus or lung
CC Excl: 162.3, 162.8-162.9, 165.8-165.9, 176.4, 195.8, 199.0-199.2, 209.20-209.21, 209.29-209.30, 209.70, 209.75, 239.1, 239.81-239.9
AHA: 1Q, '04, 4
C34.10 Malig neoplasm upper lobe unspec bronchus/lung

162.4 Middle lobe, bronchus or lung
CC Excl: 162.4, 162.8-162.9, 165.8-165.9, 176.4, 195.8, 199.0-199.2, 209.20-209.21, 209.29-209.30, 209.70, 209.75, 239.1, 239.81-239.9

162.5 Lower lobe, bronchus or lung
CC Excl: 162.5-162.9, 165.8-165.9, 176.4, 195.8, 199.0-199.2, 209.20-209.21, 209.29-209.30, 209.70, 209.75, 239.1, 239.81-239.9
AHA: 3Q, '10, 3

162.8 Other parts of bronchus or lung
Malignant neoplasm of contiguous or overlapping sites of bronchus or lung whose point of origin cannot be determined
CC Excl: 162.8-162.9, 165.8-165.9, 176.4, 195.8, 199.0-199.2, 209.20-209.21, 209.29-209.30, 209.70, 209.75, 239.1, 239.81-239.9
AHA: 3Q, '06, 7

162.9 Bronchus and lung, unspecified
CC Excl: See code: 162.8
AHA: 2Q, '10, 14; 3Q, '06, 14-15; 2Q, '97, 3; 4Q, '96, 48
C34.90 Malig neoplasm unspec part of unspec bronchus/lung

N Newborn Age: 0   P Pediatric Age: 0-17   M Maternity Age: 12-55   A Adult Age: 15-124   MCC Major CC Condition   CC CC Condition   HIV HIV Related

36 – Volume 1   **2014 ICD-9-**

√4ᵗʰ **163 Malignant neoplasm of pleura**

163.0 Parietal pleura   `CC`
  CC Excl: 163.0-163.9, 165.8-165.9, 195.8, 199.0-199.2, 209.20,
  209.29-209.30, 209.70, 209.75, 239.1, 239.81-239.9

163.1 Visceral pleura   `CC`
  CC Excl: See code 163.0

163.8 Other specified sites of pleura   `CC`
  Malignant neoplasm of contiguous or overlapping sites of
  pleura whose point of origin cannot be determined
  CC Excl: See code 163.0

163.9 Pleura, unspecified   `CC`
  CC Excl: See code 163.0

√4ᵗʰ **164 Malignant neoplasm of thymus, heart, and mediastinum**

164.0 Thymus   `CC`
  EXCLUDES benign carcinoid tumor of the thymus (209.62)
           malignant carcinoid tumor of the thymus (209.22)
  CC Excl: 164.0, 209.22

164.1 Heart   `CC`
  Endocardium
  Epicardium
  Myocardium
  Pericardium
  EXCLUDES great vessels (171.4)
  CC Excl: 164.1

164.2 Anterior mediastinum   `CC`
  CC Excl: 164.2-164.9, 165.8-165.9, 195.8, 199.0-199.2, 209.20,
  209.29-209.30, 209.70, 209.75, 239.1, 239.81-239.9

164.3 Posterior mediastinum   `CC`
  CC Excl: See code 164.2

164.8 Other   `CC`
  Malignant neoplasm of contiguous or overlapping sites of
  thymus, heart, and mediastinum whose point of origin
  cannot be determined
  CC Excl: See code 164.2

164.9 Mediastinum, part unspecified   `CC`
  CC Excl: See code 164.2

√4ᵗʰ **165 Malignant neoplasm of other and ill-defined sites within the
respiratory system and intrathoracic organs**

165.0 Upper respiratory tract, part unspecified

165.8 Other
  Malignant neoplasm of respiratory and intrathoracic organs
  whose point of origin cannot be assigned to any one of
  the categories 160-164

165.9 Ill-defined sites within the respiratory system
  Respiratory tract NOS
  EXCLUDES intrathoracic NOS (195.1)
           thoracic NOS (195.1)

Malignant Neoplasm of Bone, Connective Tissue, Skin, and Breast (170-176)

EXCLUDES carcinoma in situ:
     breast (233.0)
     skin (232.0-232.9)

√4ᵗʰ **170 Malignant neoplasm of bone and articular cartilage**
  INCLUDES cartilage (articular) (joint)
           periosteum
  EXCLUDES bone marrow NOS (202.9)
       cartilage:
         ear (171.0)
         eyelid (171.0)
         larynx (161.3)
         nose (160.0)
         synovia (171.0-171.9)
  AHA: 4Q, '06, 103
  TIP: Do not assign for bone metastasis; see instead code 198.5.

Skull

Orbital rim, Roof, Ethmoid, Lacrimal, Nasal, Maxilla, Palate, Alveolar margins, Mandible, Symphysis, Frontal, Zygoma (malar), Zygomatic arch, Condylar process, Coronoid process, Ramus, Body, Angle

170.0 Bones of skull and face, except mandible   `CC`

Bone:	Bone:
ethmoid	sphenoid
frontal	temporal
malar	zygomatic
nasal	Maxilla (superior)
occipital	Turbinate
orbital	Upper jaw bone
parietal	Vomer

  EXCLUDES carcinoma, any type except intraosseous or
         odontogenic:
         maxilla, maxillary (sinus) (160.2)
         upper jaw bone (143.0)
         jaw bone (lower) (170.1)
  CC Excl: 170.0, 170.9, V58.0

170.1 Mandible   `CC`
  Inferior maxilla
  Jaw bone NOS
  Lower jaw bone
  EXCLUDES carcinoma, any type except intraosseous or
         odontogenic:
         jaw bone NOS (143.9)
         lower (143.1)
         upper jaw bone (170.0)
  CC Excl: 170.1, 170.9, V58.0

170.2 Vertebral column, excluding sacrum and coccyx   `CC`
  Spinal column
  Spine
  Vertebra
  EXCLUDES sacrum and coccyx (170.6)
  CC Excl: 170.2, 170.9, V58.0

170.3 Ribs, sternum, and clavicle   `CC`
  Costal cartilage
  Costovertebral joint
  Xiphoid process
  CC Excl: 170.3, 170.9, V58.0

170.4 Scapula and long bones of upper limb   `CC`
  Acromion
  Bones NOS of upper limb
  Humerus
  Radius
  Ulna
  CC Excl: 170.4, 170.9, V58.0
  AHA: 2Q, '99, 9

170.5 Short bones of upper limb   `CC`

Carpal	Scaphoid (of hand)
Cuneiform, wrist	Semilunar or lunate
Metacarpal	Trapezium
Navicular, of hand	Trapezoid
Phalanges of hand	Unciform
Pisiform	

  CC Excl: 170.5, 170.9, V58.0

170.6 Pelvic bones, sacrum, and coccyx   `CC`
  Coccygeal vertebra
  Ilium
  Ischium
  Pubic bone
  Sacral vertebra
  CC Excl: 170.6, 170.9, V58.0

Additional Digit Required   Unacceptable PDx   Manifestation Code   Hospital Acquired Condition   ►◄ Revised Text   ● New Code   ▲ Revised Code Title

2014 ICD-9-CM   Volume 1 – 37

170.7 Long bones of lower limb `CC`
  Bones NOS of lower limb
  Femur
  Fibula
  Tibia
  CC Exd: 170.7, 170.9, V58.0

170.8 Short bones of lower limb `CC`
  Astragalus [talus]   Navicular (of ankle)
  Calcaneus   Patella
  Cuboid   Phalanges of foot
  Cuneiform, ankle   Tarsal
  Metatarsal
  CC Exd: 170.8-170.9, V58.0

170.9 Bone and articular cartilage, site unspecified `CC`
  CC Exd: 170.0-170.9, V58.0

√4ᵗʰ **171 Malignant neoplasm of connective and other soft tissue**
  `INCLUDES` blood vessel
            bursa
            fascia
            fat
            ligament, except uterine
            muscle
            peripheral, sympathetic, and parasympathetic nerves and
                ganglia
            synovia
            tendon (sheath)
  `EXCLUDES` cartilage (of):
                articular (170.0-170.9)
                larynx (161.3)
                nose (160.0)
             connective tissue:
                breast (174.0-175.9)
                internal organs — code to malignant neoplasm of the site
                    [e.g., leiomyosarcoma of stomach, 151.9]
             heart (164.1)
             uterine ligament (183.4)

171.0 Head, face, and neck `CC`
  Cartilage of:
    ear
    eyelid
  CC Exd: V58.0
  AHA: 2Q, '99, 6

171.2 Upper limb, including shoulder `CC`
  Arm
  Finger
  Forearm
  Hand
  CC Exd: See code: 171.0

171.3 Lower limb, including hip `CC`
  Foot
  Leg
  Popliteal space
  Thigh
  Toe
  CC Exd: See code: 171.0
  AHA: ▶3Q, '12, 7-8◀

171.4 Thorax `CC`
  Axilla
  Diaphragm
  Great vessels
  `EXCLUDES` heart (164.1)
             mediastinum (164.2-164.9)
             thymus (164.0)
  CC Exd: See code: 171.0

171.5 Abdomen `CC`
  Abdominal wall
  Hypochondrium
  `EXCLUDES` peritoneum (158.8)
             retroperitoneum (158.0)
  CC Exd: See code: 171.0

171.6 Pelvis `CC`
  Buttock
  Groin
  Inguinal region
  Perineum
  `EXCLUDES` pelvic peritoneum (158.8)
             retroperitoneum (158.0)
             uterine ligament, any (183.3-183.5)
  CC Exd: See code: 171.0

171.7 Trunk, unspecified `CC`
  Back NOS
  Flank NOS
  CC Exd: See code: 171.0

171.8 Other specified sites of connective and other soft tissue `CC`
  Malignant neoplasm of contiguous or overlapping sites of
      connective tissue whose point of origin cannot be
      determined
  CC Exd: See code: 171.0

171.9 Connective and other soft tissue, site unspecified `CC`
  CC Exd: See code: 171.0

√4ᵗʰ **172 Malignant melanoma of skin**
  `INCLUDES` melanocarcinoma
            melanoma (skin) NOS
            melanoma in situ of skin
  `EXCLUDES` skin of genital organs (184.0-184.9, 187.1-187.9)
             sites other than skin — code to malignant neoplasm of the
                 site
  DEF: Malignant neoplasm of melanocytes; most common in skin, may
  involve oral cavity, esophagus, anal canal, vagina, leptomeninges, or
  conjunctiva.

172.0 Lip
  `EXCLUDES` vermilion border of lip (140.0-140.1, 140.9)

172.1 Eyelid, including canthus

172.2 Ear and external auditory canal
  Auricle (ear)
  Auricular canal, external
  External [acoustic] meatus
  Pinna

172.3 Other and unspecified parts of face
  Cheek (external)
  Chin
  Eyebrow
  Forehead
  Nose, external
  Temple

172.4 Scalp and neck

172.5 Trunk, except scrotum
  Axilla   Perianal skin
  Breast   Perineum
  Buttock   Umbilicus
  Groin
  `EXCLUDES` anal canal (154.2)
             anus NOS (154.3)
             scrotum (187.7)

172.6 Upper limb, including shoulder
  Arm   Forearm
  Finger   Hand

172.7 Lower limb, including hip
  Ankle   Leg
  Foot   Popliteal area
  Heel   Thigh
  Knee   Toe

172.8 Other specified sites of skin
  Malignant melanoma of contiguous or overlapping sites of
      skin whose point of origin cannot be determined

172.9 Melanoma of skin, site unspecified

N Newborn Age: 0   P Pediatric Age: 0-17   M Maternity Age: 12-55   A Adult Age: 15-124   `MCC` Major CC Condition   `CC` CC Condition   `HIV` HIV Related D:

√4ᵗʰ **173 Other and unspecified malignant neoplasm of skin**

INCLUDES malignant neoplasm of:
  sebaceous glands
  sudoriferous, sudoriparous glands
  sweat glands

EXCLUDES *Kaposi's sarcoma (176.0-176.9)*
  malignant melanoma of skin (172.0-172.9)
  Merkel cell carcinoma of skin (209.31-209.36)
  skin of genital organs (184.0-184.9, 187.1-187.9)

AHA: 4Q, '11, 83-87; 1Q, '00, 18; 2Q, '96, 12

TIP: Do not assign for malignant neoplasm of skin documented as melanoma; see instead category 172.

√5ᵗʰ **173.0 Other and unspecified malignant neoplasm of skin of lip**

EXCLUDES *vermilion border of lip (140.0-140.1, 140.9)*

173.00 Unspecified malignant neoplasm of skin of lip

173.01 Basal cell carcinoma of skin of lip

173.02 Squamous cell carcinoma of skin of lip

173.09 Other specified malignant neoplasm of skin of lip

√5ᵗʰ **173.1 Other and unspecified malignant neoplasm of skin of eyelid, including canthus**

EXCLUDES *cartilage of eyelid (171.0)*

173.10 Unspecified malignant neoplasm of eyelid, including canthus

173.11 Basal cell carcinoma of eyelid, including canthus

173.12 Squamous cell carcinoma of eyelid, including canthus

173.19 Other specified malignant neoplasm of eyelid, including canthus

√5ᵗʰ **173.2 Other and unspecified malignant neoplasm of skin of ear and external auditory canal**

  Auricle (ear)
  Auricular canal, external
  External meatus
  Pinna

EXCLUDES *cartilage of ear (171.0)*

173.20 Unspecified malignant neoplasm of skin of ear and external auditory canal

173.21 Basal cell carcinoma of skin of ear and external auditory canal

173.22 Squamous cell carcinoma of skin of ear and external auditory canal

173.29 Other specified malignant neoplasm of skin of ear and external auditory canal

√5ᵗʰ **173.3 Other and unspecified malignant neoplasm of skin of other and unspecified parts of face**

  Cheek, external   Forehead
  Chin   Nose, external
  Eyebrow   Temple

AHA: 1Q, '00, 3

173.30 Unspecified malignant neoplasm of skin of other and unspecified parts of face

173.31 Basal cell carcinoma of skin of other and unspecified parts of face

173.32 Squamous cell carcinoma of skin of other and unspecified parts of face

173.39 Other specified malignant neoplasm of skin of other and unspecified parts of face

√5ᵗʰ **173.4 Other and unspecified malignant neoplasm of scalp and skin of neck**

173.40 Unspecified malignant neoplasm of scalp and skin of neck

173.41 Basal cell carcinoma of scalp and skin of neck

173.42 Squamous cell carcinoma of scalp and skin of neck

173.49 Other specified malignant neoplasm of scalp and skin of neck

√5ᵗʰ **173.5 Other and unspecified malignant neoplasm of skin of trunk, except scrotum**

  Axillary fold   Skin of:
  Perianal skin   buttock
  Skin of: chest wall
    abdominal wall   groin
    anus   perineum
    back   umbilicus
    breast

EXCLUDES *anal canal (154.2)*
  anus NOS (154.3)
  skin of scrotum (187.7)

AHA: 1Q, '01, 8

173.50 Unspecified malignant neoplasm of skin of trunk, except scrotum

173.51 Basal cell carcinoma of skin of trunk, except scrotum

173.52 Squamous cell carcinoma of skin of trunk, except scrotum

173.59 Other specified malignant neoplasm of skin of trunk, except scrotum

√5ᵗʰ **173.6 Other and unspecified malignant neoplasm of skin of upper limb, including shoulder**

  Arm   Forearm
  Finger   Hand

173.60 Unspecified malignant neoplasm of skin of upper limb, including shoulder

173.61 Basal cell carcinoma of skin of upper limb, including shoulder

173.62 Squamous cell carcinoma of skin of upper limb, including shoulder

173.69 Other specified malignant neoplasm of skin of upper limb, including shoulder

√5ᵗʰ **173.7 Other and unspecified malignant neoplasm of skin of lower limb, including hip**

  Ankle   Leg
  Foot   Popliteal area
  Heel   Thigh
  Knee   Toe

173.70 Unspecified malignant neoplasm of skin of lower limb, including hip

173.71 Basal cell carcinoma of skin of lower limb, including hip

173.72 Squamous cell carcinoma of skin of lower limb, including hip

173.79 Other specified malignant neoplasm of skin of lower limb, including hip

√5ᵗʰ **173.8 Other and unspecified malignant neoplasm of other specified sites of skin**

  Malignant neoplasm of contiguous or overlapping sites of skin whose point of origin cannot be determined

173.80 Unspecified malignant neoplasm of other specified sites of skin

173.81 Basal cell carcinoma of other specified sites of skin

173.82 Squamous cell carcinoma of other specified sites of skin

173.89 Other specified malignant neoplasm of other specified sites of skin

√5ᵗʰ **173.9 Other and unspecified malignant neoplasm of skin, site unspecified**

173.90 Unspecified malignant neoplasm of skin, site unspecified
  Malignant neoplasm of skin NOS

173.91 Basal cell carcinoma of skin, site unspecified

173.92 Squamous cell carcinoma of skin, site unspecified

173.99 Other specified malignant neoplasm of skin, site unspecified

Neoplasms

174–182.8

Female Breast

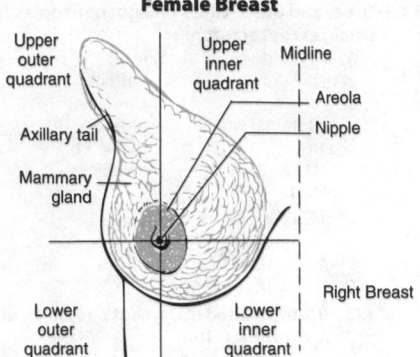

Upper outer quadrant   Upper inner quadrant   Midline   Areola   Nipple   Axillary tail   Mammary gland   Lower outer quadrant   Lower inner quadrant   Right Breast

√4ᵗʰ **174 Malignant neoplasm of female breast**

     INCLUDES breast (female)
         connective tissue
         soft parts
         Paget's disease of:
         breast
         nipple

     Use additional code to identify estrogen receptor status (V86.0, V86.1)

     EXCLUDES *malignant melanoma of skin of breast (172.5)*
         malignant neoplasm of skin of breast (173.50-173.59)

     AHA: 3Q, '97, 8; 4Q, '89, 11

     TIP: For bilateral breast malignancy, do not assign two codes unless documentation indicates separate sites (i.e., different fourth digits).

     174.0 Nipple and areola ♀
     174.1 Central portion ♀
     174.2 Upper-inner quadrant ♀
     174.3 Lower-inner quadrant ♀
     174.4 Upper-outer quadrant ♀
         AHA: 4Q, '08, 155; 1Q, '04, 3; '3Q, '97, 8
     174.5 Lower-outer quadrant ♀
     174.6 Axillary tail ♀
     174.8 Other specified sites of female breast ♀
         Ectopic sites
         Inner breast
         Lower breast
         Midline of breast
         Outer breast
         Upper breast
         Malignant neoplasm of contiguous or overlapping sites of breast whose point of origin cannot be determined

     174.9 Breast (female), unspecified ♀
         AHA: 3Q, '09, 3; 3Q, '05, 11; 2Q, '94, 10; 4Q, '89, 11
         C50.911 Malig neoplasm of uns site of rt female breast   `I-10`

√4ᵗʰ **175 Malignant neoplasm of male breast**
     Use additional code to identify estrogen receptor status (V86.0, V86.1)

     EXCLUDES *malignant melanoma of skin of breast (172.5)*
         malignant neoplasm of skin of breast (173.50-173.59)

     175.0 Nipple and areola ♂
     175.9 Other and unspecified sites of male breast ♂
         Ectopic breast tissue, male

√4ᵗʰ **176 Kaposi's sarcoma**
     AHA: 4Q, '91, 24

     176.0 Skin   `CC` `HIV`
         CC Exd: 176.0, 176.8-176.9, V58.0
         AHA: 4Q, '07, 63; 4Q, '94, 29; 4Q, '91, 24

     176.1 Soft tissue   `CC` `HIV`
         Blood vessel
         Connective tissue
         Fascia
         Ligament
         Lymphatic(s) NEC
         Muscle
         EXCLUDES *lymph glands and nodes (176.5)*
         CC Exd: 176.1, 176.8-176.9, V58.0

     176.2 Palate   `CC` `HIV`
         CC Exd: 176.2, 176.8-176.9, V58.0

     176.3 Gastrointestinal sites   `CC` `HIV`
         CC Exd: 176.3, 176.8-176.9, V58.0

     176.4 Lung   `CC` `HIV`
         CC Exd: 162.8-162.9, 165.8-165.9, 176.4, 195.8, 199.0-199.2, 209.20-209.21, 209.29-209.30, 209.70, 239.1, 239.81-239.9

     176.5 Lymph nodes   `CC` `HIV`
         CC Exd: 176.5, 195.8-196.9, 199.0-199.2, 209.20, 209.29-209.30, 209.70-209.71, 209.75, 239.81-239.9

     176.8 Other specified sites   `CC` `HIV`
         Oral cavity NEC
         CC Exd: 176.0-176.9, V58.0

     176.9 Unspecified   `CC` `HIV`
         Viscera NOS
         CC Exd: 176.0-192.9, 195.0-199.2, 209.20, 209.24, 209.29-209.30, 209.70-209.79, 230.0-237.6, 237.9-238.3, 238.8-239.9, V58.0

Malignant Neoplasm of Genitourinary Organs (179-189)

     EXCLUDES *carcinoma in situ (233.1-233.9)*

   179 Malignant neoplasm of uterus, part unspecified ♀

√4ᵗʰ **180 Malignant neoplasm of cervix uteri**
     INCLUDES invasive malignancy [carcinoma]
     EXCLUDES *carcinoma in situ (233.1)*

     180.0 Endocervix ♀
         Cervical canal NOS
         Endocervical canal
         Endocervical gland

     180.1 Exocervix ♀

     180.8 Other specified sites of cervix ♀
         Cervical stump
         Squamocolumnar junction of cervix
         Malignant neoplasm of contiguous or overlapping sites of cervix uteri whose point of origin cannot be determined

     180.9 Cervix uteri, unspecified ♀

   181 Malignant neoplasm of placenta ♀
     Choriocarcinoma NOS
     Chorioepithelioma NOS
     EXCLUDES *chorioadenoma (destruens) (236.1)*
         hydatidiform mole (630)
            malignant (236.1)
         invasive mole (236.1)
         male choriocarcinoma NOS (186.0-186.9)

√4ᵗʰ **182 Malignant neoplasm of body of uterus**
     EXCLUDES *carcinoma in situ (233.2)*

     182.0 Corpus uteri, except isthmus ♀
         Cornu
         Endometrium
         Fundus
         Myometrium
         AHA: 3Q, '09, 5
         C54.9 Malignant neoplasm of corpus uteri unspecified   `I-10`

     182.1 Isthmus ♀
         Lower uterine segment

     182.8 Other specified sites of body of uterus ♀
         Malignant neoplasm of contiguous or overlapping sites of body of uterus whose point of origin cannot be determined
         EXCLUDES *uterus NOS (179)*

`N` Newborn Age: 0   `P` Pediatric Age: 0-17   `M` Maternity Age: 12-55   `A` Adult Age: 15-124   `MCC` Major CC Condition   `CC` CC Condition   `HIV` HIV Related Dx

40 – Volume 1   **2014 ICD-9-CM**

Neoplasms

☑4ᵗʰ **183 Malignant neoplasm of ovary and other uterine adnexa**

    EXCLUDES Douglas' cul-de-sac (158.8)

  183.0 Ovary   cc ♀
       Use additional code to identify any functional activity
       CC Excl: 183.0-183.9, 195.3, 198.6, 199.0-199.2, 209.20, 209.29-209.30, 209.70, 209.75
       AHA: 4Q, '07, 96
       C56.9 Malignant neoplasm of unspec ovary   I-10

  183.2 Fallopian tube   ♀
       Oviduct
       Uterine tube

  183.3 Broad ligament   ♀
       Mesovarium
       Parovarian region

  183.4 Parametrium   ♀
       Uterine ligament NOS
       Uterosacral ligament

  183.5 Round ligament   ♀
       AHA: 3Q, '99, 5

  183.8 Other specified sites of uterine adnexa   ♀
       Tubo-ovarian
       Utero-ovarian
       Malignant neoplasm of contiguous or overlapping sites of ovary and other uterine adnexa whose point of origin cannot be determined

  183.9 Uterine adnexa, unspecified   ♀

☑4ᵗʰ **184 Malignant neoplasm of other and unspecified female genital organs**

    EXCLUDES carcinoma in situ (233.30-233.39)

  184.0 Vagina   ♀
       Gartner's duct
       Vaginal vault

  184.1 Labia majora   ♀
       Greater vestibular [Bartholin's] gland

  184.2 Labia minora   ♀

  184.3 Clitoris   ♀

  184.4 Vulva, unspecified   ♀
       External female genitalia NOS
       Pudendum

  184.8 Other specified sites of female genital organs   ♀
       Malignant neoplasm of contiguous or overlapping sites of female genital organs whose point of origin cannot be determined

  184.9 Female genital organ, site unspecified   ♀
       Female genitourinary tract NOS

185 Malignant neoplasm of prostate   ♂

    EXCLUDES seminal vesicles (187.8)
     AHA: 2Q, '10, 3; 3Q, '03, 13; 3Q, '99, 5; 3Q, '92, 7
     TIP: Assign as a secondary diagnosis if patient treated for BPH and incidental finding of carcinoma of the prostate is made.
     C61 Malignant neoplasm of prostate   I-10

☑4ᵗʰ **186 Malignant neoplasm of testis**

     Use additional code to identify any functional activity

  186.0 Undescended testis   ♂
       Ectopic testis
       Retained testis

  186.9 Other and unspecified testis   ♂
       Testis:
         NOS
         descended
         scrotal

☑4ᵗʰ **187 Malignant neoplasm of penis and other male genital organs**

  187.1 Prepuce   ♂
       Foreskin

  187.2 Glans penis   ♂

  187.3 Body of penis   ♂
       Corpus cavernosum

  187.4 Penis, part unspecified   ♂
       Skin of penis NOS

  187.5 Epididymis   ♂

  187.6 Spermatic cord   ♂
       Vas deferens

  187.7 Scrotum   ♂
       Skin of scrotum

  187.8 Other specified sites of male genital organs   ♂
       Seminal vesicle
       Tunica vaginalis
       Malignant neoplasm of contiguous or overlapping sites of penis and other male genital organs whose point of origin cannot be determined

  187.9 Male genital organ, site unspecified   ♂
       Male genital organ or tract NOS

☑4ᵗʰ **188 Malignant neoplasm of bladder**

    EXCLUDES carcinoma in situ (233.7)

  188.0 Trigone of urinary bladder

  188.1 Dome of urinary bladder

  188.2 Lateral wall of urinary bladder

  188.3 Anterior wall of urinary bladder

  188.4 Posterior wall of urinary bladder

  188.5 Bladder neck
       Internal urethral orifice

  188.6 Ureteric orifice

  188.7 Urachus

  188.8 Other specified sites of bladder
       Malignant neoplasm of contiguous or overlapping sites of bladder whose point of origin cannot be determined

  188.9 Bladder, part unspecified
       Bladder wall NOS
       AHA: 1Q, '00, 5
       C67.9 Malignant neoplasm of bladder unspecified   I-10

☑4ᵗʰ **189 Malignant neoplasm of kidney and other and unspecified urinary organs**

    EXCLUDES benign carcinoid tumor of kidney (209.64)
             malignant carcinoid tumor of kidney (209.24)

  189.0 Kidney, except pelvis   cc
       Kidney NOS
       Kidney parenchyma
       CC Excl: 189.0-189.1, 189.8-189.9, 195.8, 199.0-199.2, 209.20, 209.24, 209.29-209.30, 209.70, 209.75, 239.5, 239.81-239.9
       AHA: 2Q, '05, 4; 2Q, '04, 4
       C64.9 Malig neoplasm unspec kidney no renal pelvis   I-10

  189.1 Renal pelvis   cc
       Renal calyces   Ureteropelvic junction
       CC Excl: See code: 189.0

  189.2 Ureter   cc
       EXCLUDES ureteric orifice of bladder (188.6)
       CC Excl: 189.2, 189.8-189.9, 195.8, 199.0-199.2, 209.20, 209.29-209.30, 209.70, 209.75, 239.5, 239.81-239.9

  189.3 Urethra   cc
       EXCLUDES urethral orifice of bladder (188.5)
       CC Excl: 189.3-189.9, 198.82

  189.4 Paraurethral glands   cc
       CC Excl: See code: 189.3

  189.8 Other specified sites of urinary organs   cc
       Malignant neoplasm of contiguous or overlapping sites of kidney and other urinary organs whose point of origin cannot be determined
       CC Excl: 189.0-189.9, 195.3, 198.0-198.1, 209.24

  189.9 Urinary organ, site unspecified   cc
       Urinary system NOS
       CC Excl: See code: 189.8

Additional Digit Required   Unacceptable PDx   Manifestation Code   Hospital Acquired Condition   ▶◀ Revised Text   ● New Code   ▲ Revised Code Title

4 ICD-9-CM   **Volume 1 – 41**

Malignant Neoplasm of Other and Unspecified Sites (190-199)

EXCLUDES carcinoma in situ (234.0-234.9)

✓4ᵗʰ **190 Malignant neoplasm of eye**

EXCLUDES carcinoma in situ (234.0)
dark area on retina and choroid (239.81)
cartilage (171.0)
malignant melanoma of eyelid (skin) (172.1)
malignant neoplasm of eyelid (skin) (173.10-173.19)
optic nerve (192.0)
orbital bone (170.0)
retinal freckle (239.81)

190.0 Eyeball, except conjunctiva, cornea, retina, and choroid
Ciliary body   Sclera
Crystalline lens   Uveal tract
Iris

190.1 Orbit
Connective tissue of orbit
Extraocular muscle
Retrobulbar
EXCLUDES bone of orbit (170.0)

190.2 Lacrimal gland

190.3 Conjunctiva

190.4 Cornea

190.5 Retina

190.6 Choroid

190.7 Lacrimal duct
Lacrimal sac
Nasolacrimal duct

190.8 Other specified sites of eye
Malignant neoplasm of contiguous or overlapping sites of eye whose point of origin cannot be determined

190.9 Eye, part unspecified

✓4ᵗʰ **191 Malignant neoplasm of brain**

EXCLUDES cranial nerves (192.0)
retrobulbar area (190.1)

AHA: 4Q, '07, 104

191.0 Cerebrum, except lobes and ventricles   CC
Basal ganglia   Globus pallidus
Cerebral cortex   Hypothalamus
Corpus striatum   Thalamus
CC Exd: 191.0-192.1, 192.8-192.9, 195.8, 199.0-199.2, 209.20, 209.29-209.30, 209.70, 209.75, 239.6-239.9

191.1 Frontal lobe   CC
CC Exd: See code 191.0
AHA: 4Q, '05, 118

191.2 Temporal lobe   CC
Hippocampus   Uncus
CC Exd: See code 191.0
AHA: 3Q, '09, 8; 4Q, '06, 123

191.3 Parietal lobe   CC
CC Exd: See code 191.0

191.4 Occipital lobe   CC
CC Exd: See code 191.0

Brain and Meninges

Fourth ventricle
Cerebrum
Corpus callosum
Thalamus
Hypothalamus
Hypophysis
Cerebellum
Pons
Medulla oblongata
Midsagittal Section (between hemispheres)

191.5 Ventricles
Choroid plexus
Floor of ventricle
CC Exd: See code 191.0

191.6 Cerebellum NOS
Cerebellopontine angle
CC Exd: See code 191.0

191.7 Brain stem
Cerebral peduncle
Medulla oblongata
Midbrain
Pons
CC Exd: See code 191.0

191.8 Other parts of brain
Corpus callosum
Tapetum
Malignant neoplasm of contiguous or overlapping sites of brain whose point of origin cannot be determined
CC Exd: See code 191.0

191.9 Brain, unspecified
Cranial fossa NOS
CC Exd: See code 191.0
AHA: 4Q, '09, 143

✓4ᵗʰ **192 Malignant neoplasm of other and unspecified parts of nervo system**

EXCLUDES peripheral, sympathetic, and parasympathetic nerves an ganglia (171.0-171.9)

192.0 Cranial nerves
Olfactory bulb
CC Exd: 192.0, 192.8-192.9, 195.8, 199.0-199.2, 209.20, 209.29-209.30, 209.70, 209.75, 239.6-239.9

192.1 Cerebral meninges
Dura (mater)   Meninges NOS
Falx (cerebelli) (cerebri)   Tentorium
CC Exd: 192.1, 192.8-192.9, 195.8, 199.0-199.2, 209.20, 209.29-209 209.70, 209.75, 239.6-239.9

192.2 Spinal cord
Cauda equina
CC Exd: 192.2, 192.8-192.9, 195.8, 199.0-199.2, 209.20, 209.29-209 209.70, 209.75, 239.6-239.9

192.3 Spinal meninges
CC Exd: 192.3-192.9, 195.8, 199.0-199.2, 209.20, 209.29-209.30, 209.70, 209.75, 239.6-239.9

192.8 Other specified sites of nervous system
Malignant neoplasm of contiguous or overlapping sites of other parts of nervous system whose point of origin cannot be determined
CC Exd: 191.0-192.9, 195.8, 199.0-199.2, 209.20, 209.29-209.30, 209.70, 209.75, 239.6-239.9

192.9 Nervous system, part unspecified
Nervous system (central) NOS
EXCLUDES meninges NOS (192.1)
CC Exd: 191.0-192.9, 195.8, 198.3-198.4, 199.0-199.2, 209.20, 209.29-209.30, 209.70, 209.75, 239.6-239.9

193 Malignant neoplasm of thyroid gland
Thyroglossal duct
Use additional code to identify any functional activity
C73 Malignant neoplasm of thyroid gland

✓4ᵗʰ **194 Malignant neoplasm of other endocrine glands and related structures**

EXCLUDES islets of Langerhans (157.4)
neuroendocrine tumors (209.00-209.69)
ovary (183.0)
testis (186.0-186.9)
thymus (164.0)

194.0 Adrenal gland
Adrenal cortex   Suprarenal gland
Adrenal medulla
CC Exd: 194.0, 194.9, 195.2, 195.8, 198.7, 199.0-199.2, 209.20, 209.29-209.30, 209.70, 209.75

194.1 Parathyroid gland
CC Exd: 194.1, 194.8-194.9

194.3 Pituitary gland and craniopharyngeal duct `cc`
Craniobuccal pouch   Rathke's pouch
Hypophysis   Sella turcica
CC Excl: 194.3, V58.0
AHA: J-A, '85, 9

194.4 Pineal gland `cc`
CC Excl: 194.4, V58.0

194.5 Carotid body `cc`
CC Excl: 194.5, 194.8-194.9

194.6 Aortic body and other paraganglia `cc`
Coccygeal body   Para-aortic body
Glomus jugulare
CC Excl: 194.5-194.9

194.8 Other `cc`
Pluriglandular involvement NOS
NOTE If the sites of multiple involvements are known, they should be coded separately.
CC Excl: 194.0-194.9

194.9 Endocrine gland, site unspecified `cc`
CC Excl: See code: 194.8

✓4ᵗʰ **195 Malignant neoplasm of other and ill-defined sites**
INCLUDES malignant neoplasms of contiguous sites, not elsewhere classified, whose point of origin cannot be determined
EXCLUDES malignant neoplasm:
lymphatic and hematopoietic tissue (200.0-208.9)
secondary sites (196.0-198.8)
unspecified site (199.0-199.1)

195.0 Head, face, and neck
Cheek NOS   Nose NOS
Jaw NOS   Supraclavicular region NOS
AHA: 4Q, '03, 107

195.1 Thorax
Axilla   Intrathoracic NOS
Chest (wall) NOS

195.2 Abdomen
Intra-abdominal NOS
AHA: 2Q, '97, 3

195.3 Pelvis
Groin
Inguinal region NOS
Presacral region
Sacrococcygeal region
Sites overlapping systems within pelvis, as:
rectovaginal (septum)
rectovesical (septum)

195.4 Upper limb

195.5 Lower limb

195.8 Other specified sites
Back NOS   Trunk NOS
Flank NOS

Lymph Nodes

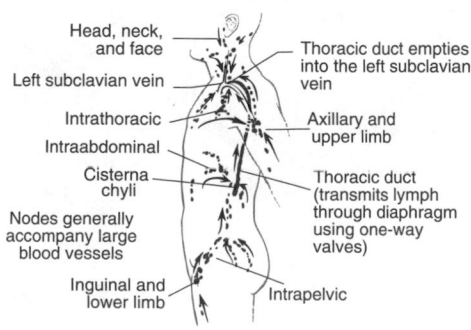

Head, neck, and face
Left subclavian vein
Intrathoracic
Intraabdominal
Cisterna chyli
Nodes generally accompany large blood vessels
Inguinal and lower limb
Thoracic duct empties into the left subclavian vein
Axillary and upper limb
Thoracic duct (transmits lymph through diaphragm using one-way valves)
Intrapelvic

✓4ᵗʰ **196 Secondary and unspecified malignant neoplasm of lymph nodes**
EXCLUDES any malignant neoplasm of lymph nodes, specified as primary (200.0-202.9)
Hodgkin's disease (201.0-201.9)
lymphosarcoma (200.1)
other forms of lymphoma (202.0-202.9)
reticulosarcoma (200.0)
secondary neuroendocrine tumor of (distant) lymph nodes (209.71)

196.0 Lymph nodes of head, face, and neck `cc`
Cervical   Scalene
Cervicofacial   Supraclavicular
CC Excl: 176.5, 195.8-196.9, 199.0-199.2, 209.20, 209.29-209.30, 209.70-209.71, 239.81-239.9
AHA: 3Q, '07, 7
C77.0 Sec & uns malig neo lymph nodes head face & neck   `I-10`

196.1 Intrathoracic lymph nodes `cc`
Bronchopulmonary   Mediastinal
Intercostal   Tracheobronchial
CC Excl: See code 196.0
AHA: 3Q, '06, 7

196.2 Intra-abdominal lymph nodes `cc`
Intestinal   Retroperitoneal
Mesenteric
CC Excl: See code 196.0
AHA: 4Q, '03, 111
C77.2 Sec & uns malig neoplasm intra-abd lymph nodes   `I-10`

196.3 Lymph nodes of axilla and upper limb `cc`
Brachial   Infraclavicular
Epitrochlear   Pectoral
CC Excl: See code 196.0

196.5 Lymph nodes of inguinal region and lower limb `cc`
Femoral   Popliteal
Groin   Tibial
CC Excl: See code 196.0

196.6 Intrapelvic lymph nodes `cc`
Hypogastric   Obturator
Iliac   Parametrial
CC Excl: See code 196.0
AHA: ▶2Q, '12, 9◀

196.8 Lymph nodes of multiple sites `cc`
CC Excl: See code 196.0

196.9 Site unspecified `cc`
Lymph nodes NOS
CC Excl: See code 196.0

✓4ᵗʰ **197 Secondary malignant neoplasm of respiratory and digestive systems**
EXCLUDES lymph node metastasis (196.0-196.9)
secondary neuroendocrine tumor of liver (209.72)
secondary neuroendocrine tumor of respiratory organs (209.79)
AHA: M-J, '85, 3

197.0 Lung `cc`
Bronchus
CC Excl: 195.8, 197.0, 197.3, 198.89-199.2, 209.20, 209.29-209.30, 209.70, 209.75-209.79, 239.81-239.9
AHA: 3Q, '10, 3; 1Q, '06, 4; 2Q, '99, 9
C78.00 Secondary malignant neoplasm of unspec lung   `I-10`

197.1 Mediastinum `cc`
CC Excl: 195.8, 197.1, 197.3, 198.89-199.2, 209.20, 209.29-209.30, 209.70, 209.75-209.79, 239.81-239.9
AHA: 3Q, '06, 7

197.2 Pleura `cc`
CC Excl: 195.8, 197.2-197.3, 198.89-199.2, 209.20, 209.29-209.30, 209.70, 209.75-209.79, 239.81-239.9, 511.81
AHA: 1Q, '08, 16; 3Q, '07, 3; 4Q, '03, 110; 4Q, '89, 11
TIP: Do not assign for malignant pleural effusion; see instead code 511.81.
C78.2 Secondary malignant neoplasm of pleura   `I-10`

197.3 Other respiratory organs `cc`
Trachea
CC Excl: 195.8, 197.0-197.3, 198.89-199.2, 209.20, 209.29-209.30, 209.70, 209.75-209.79, 239.81-239.9

| Additional Digit Required | Unacceptable PDx | Manifestation Code | Hospital Acquired Condition | ▶◀ Revised Text | ● New Code | ▲ Revised Code Title |

14 ICD-9-CM

February 2013 • Volume 1 – 43

197.4 Small intestine, including duodenum `CC`
  CC Excl: 195.8, 197.4, 197.8, 198.89-199.2, 209.20, 209.29-209.30,
  209.70, 209.75-209.79, 239.81-239.9

197.5 Large intestine and rectum `CC`
  CC Excl: 195.8, 197.5, 197.8, 198.89-199.2, 209.20, 209.29-209.30,
  209.70, 209.75-209.79, 239.81-239.9

197.6 Retroperitoneum and peritoneum `CC`
  CC Excl: 195.8, 197.6, 197.8, 198.89-199.2, 209.20, 209.29-209.30,
  209.70, 209.74-209.79, 239.81-239.9
  AHA: 3Q, '10, 3; 2Q, '04, 4; 4Q, '89, 11
  C78.6 Sec malignant neoplasm of retroperiton & periton `I-10`

197.7 Liver, specified as secondary `CC`
  CC Excl: 195.8, 197.7-197.8, 198.89-199.2, 209.20, 209.29-209.30,
  209.70, 209.72, 209.75-209.79, 239.81-239.9
  AHA: 3Q, '10, 3; 1Q, '06, 4; 2Q, '05, 9
  C78.7 Secondary malignant neoplasm of liver `I-10`

197.8 Other digestive organs and spleen `CC`
  CC Excl: 195.8, 197.4-197.8, 198.89-199.2, 209.20, 209.29-209.30,
  209.70, 209.72, 209.74-209.79, 239.81-239.9
  AHA: 2Q, '97, 3; 2Q, '92, 3

✓4th **198 Secondary malignant neoplasm of other specified sites**
  EXCLUDES lymph node metastasis (196.0-196.9)
            secondary neuroendocrine tumor of other specified sites
            (209.79)
  AHA: M-J, '85, 3

198.0 Kidney `CC`
  CC Excl: 195.8, 198.0-198.1, 198.89-199.2, 209.20, 209.29-209.30,
  209.70, 209.75-209.79, 239.81-239.9

198.1 Other urinary organs `CC`
  CC Excl: See code: 198.0

198.2 Skin `CC`
  Skin of breast
  CC Excl: 195.8, 198.2, 198.89-199.2, 209.20, 209.29-209.30, 209.70,
  209.75-209.79, 239.81-239.9

198.3 Brain and spinal cord `CC`
  CC Excl: 195.8, 198.3, 198.89-199.2, 209.20, 209.29-209.30, 209.70,
  209.75-209.79, 239.81-239.9
  AHA: 3Q, '07, 4; 3Q, '99, 7
  C79.31 Secondary malignant neoplasm of brain `I-10`

198.4 Other parts of nervous system `CC`
  Meninges (cerebral) (spinal)
  CC Excl: 195.8, 198.4, 198.89-199.2, 209.20, 209.29-209.30, 209.70,
  209.75-209.79, 239.81-239.9
  AHA: J-F, '87, 7

198.5 Bone and bone marrow `CC`
  CC Excl: 195.8, 198.5, 198.89-199.2, 209.20, 209.29-209.30, 209.70,
  209.73, 209.75-209.79, 239.81-239.9
  AHA: 1Q, '07, 6; 4Q, '03, 110; 3Q, '99, 5; 2Q, '92, 3; 1Q, '91, 16;
  4Q, '89, 10
  C79.51 Secondary malignant neoplasm of bone `I-10`

198.6 Ovary `CC` ♀
  CC Excl: 195.8, 198.6, 198.89-199.2, 209.20, 209.29-209.30, 209.70,
  209.75-209.79, 239.81-239.9

198.7 Adrenal gland `CC`
  Suprarenal gland
  CC Excl: 195.8, 198.7, 198.89-199.2, 209.20, 209.29-209.30, 209.70,
  209.75-209.79, 239.81-239.9
  C79.70 Sec malignant neoplasm of unspec adrenal gland `I-10`

✓5th **198.8 Other specified sites**

198.81 Breast `CC`
  EXCLUDES skin of breast (198.2)
  CC Excl: 195.8, 198.81, 198.89-199.2, 209.20, 209.29-209.30,
  209.70, 209.75-209.79, 239.81-239.9

198.82 Genital organs `CC`
  CC Excl: 195.8, 198.82-199.2, 209.20, 209.29-209.30, 209.70,
  209.75-209.79, 239.81-239.9

198.89 Other `CC`
  EXCLUDES retroperitoneal lymph nodes (196.2)
  CC Excl: 195.8, 198.89-199.2, 209.20, 209.29-209.30, 209.70,
  209.75-209.79, 239.81-239.9
  AHA: 2Q, '05, 4; 2Q, '97, 4
  TIP: Assign for intra-abdominal metastasis when no further
  specificity of site is documented.
  C79.89 Secondary malignant neoplasm of other spec `I-10`
  sites

✓4th **199 Malignant neoplasm without specification of site**
  EXCLUDES malignant carcinoid tumor of unknown primary site (209.20)
            malignant (poorly differentiated) neuroendocrine
            carcinoma, any site (209.30)
            malignant (poorly differentiated) neuroendocrine tumor,
            any site (209.30)
            neuroendocrine carcinoma (high grade), any site (209.30)

199.0 Disseminated `CC`
  Carcinomatosis
  Generalized: } unspecified site (primary)
    cancer   (secondary)
    malignancy
  Multiple cancer
  CC Excl: 195.8, 198.89-199.2, 209.20, 209.29-209.30, 209.70, 209.79,
  239.81-239.9
  AHA: 4Q, '89, 10

199.1 Other
  Cancer   } unspecified site (primary)
  Carcinoma   (secondary)
  Malignancy
  AHA: 3Q, '06, 14-15; 1Q, '06, 4
  TIP: Assign if patient is assessed for a metastatic tumor but primary
  site is unknown.
  C80.1 Malignant neoplasm unspecified `I-1`

199.2 Malignant neoplasm associated with `CC`
transplanted organ
  Code first complication of transplanted organ (996.80-996.89)
  Use additional code for specific malignancy
  CC Excl: 195.8, 198.89-199.2, 209.20, 209.29-209.30, 209.70, 209.79,
  239.81-239.9
  AHA: 4Q, '08, 82-83
  TIP: Assign first the appropriate code from subcategory 996.8,
  Complications of transplanted organ; use additional code for the
  specific malignancy.

Malignant Neoplasm of Lymphatic and Hematopoietic Tissue (200-208)

EXCLUDES *autoimmune lymphoproliferative syndrome (279.41)*
secondary and unspecified neoplasm of lymph nodes (196.0-196.9)
secondary neoplasm of:
bone marrow (198.5)
spleen (197.8)

The following fifth-digit subclassification is for use with categories 200-202:
0 unspecified site, extranodal and solid organ sites
1 lymph nodes of head, face, and neck
2 intrathoracic lymph nodes
3 intra-abdominal lymph nodes
4 lymph nodes of axilla and upper limb
5 lymph nodes of inguinal region and lower limb
6 intrapelvic lymph nodes
7 spleen
8 lymph nodes of multiple sites

√4ᵗʰ **200 Lymphosarcoma and reticulosarcoma and other specified malignant tumors of lymphatic tissue**
AHA: 4Q, '07, 65; 2Q, '92, 3; N-D, '86, 5

§ √5ᵗʰ **200.0 Reticulosarcoma**   CC HIV
[0-8]   Lymphoma (malignant):   Reticulum cell sarcoma:
   histiocytic (diffuse):   NOS
     nodular   pleomorphic cell type
     pleomorphic cell type
     reticulum cell type

DEF: Malignant lymphoma of primarily histolytic cells; commonly originates in reticuloendothelium of lymph nodes.
CC Excl: For code 200.00: 200.00-200.08, 239.81-239.9; For code 200.01: 200.00-200.01, 200.08, 239.81-239.9; For code 200.02: 200.00, 200.02, 200.08, 239.81-239.9; For code 200.03: 200.00, 200.03, 200.08, 239.81-239.9; For code 200.04: 200.00, 200.04, 200.08, 239.81-239.9; For code 200.05: 200.00, 200.05, 200.08, 239.81-239.9; For code 200.06: 200.00, 200.06, 200.08, 239.81-239.9; For code 200.07: 200.00, 200.07-200.08, 239.81-239.9; For code 200.08: 200.00-200.08, 239.81-239.9
AHA: For Code 200.03: 3Q, '01, 12

§ √5ᵗʰ **200.1 Lymphosarcoma**   CC
[0-8]   Lymphoblastoma (diffuse)
   Lymphoma (malignant):
    lymphoblastic (diffuse)
    lymphocytic (cell type) (diffuse)
    lymphosarcoma type
    prolymphocytic
   Lymphosarcoma:
    NOS
    diffuse NOS
    lymphoblastic (diffuse)
    lymphocytic (diffuse)
    prolymphocytic

EXCLUDES *lymphosarcoma:*
    follicular or nodular (202.0)
    mixed cell type (200.8)
    lymphosarcoma cell leukemia (207.8)

DEF: Malignant lymphoma created from anaplastic lymphoid cells resembling lymphocytes or lymphoblasts.
CC Excl: For code 200.10: 200.10-200.18, 239.81-239.9; For code 200.11: 200.10-200.11, 200.18, 239.81-239.9; For code 200.12: 200.10, 200.12, 200.18, 239.81-239.9; For code 200.13: 200.10, 200.13, 200.18, 239.81-239.9; For code 200.14: 200.10, 200.14, 200.18, 239.81-239.9; For code 200.15: 200.10, 200.15, 200.18, 239.81-239.9; For code 200.16: 200.10, 200.16, 200.18, 239.81-239.9; For code 200.17: 200.10, 200.17-200.18, 239.81-239.9; For code 200.18: 200.10-200.18, 239.81-239.9

§ √5ᵗʰ **200.2 Burkitt's tumor or lymphoma**   CC HIV
[0-8]   Malignant lymphoma, Burkitt's type
DEF: Large osteolytic lesion most common in jaw or as abdominal mass; usually found in central Africa but reported elsewhere.
CC Excl: For code 200.20: 200.20-200.28, 239.81-239.9; For code 200.21: 200.20-200.21, 200.28, 239.81-239.9; For code 200.22: 200.20, 200.22, 200.28, 239.81-239.9; For code 200.23: 200.20, 200.23, 200.28, 239.81-239.9; For code 200.24: 200.20, 200.24, 200.28, 239.81-239.9; For code 200.25: 200.20, 200.25, 200.28, 239.81-239.9; For code 200.26: 200.20, 200.26, 200.28, 239.81-239.9; For code 200.27: 200.20, 200.27-200.28, 239.81-239.9; For code 200.28: 200.20-200.28, 239.81-239.9

§ √5ᵗʰ **200.3 Marginal zone lymphoma**   CC HIV
[0-8]   Extranodal marginal zone B-cell lymphoma
   Mucosa associated lymphoid tissue [MALT]
   Nodal marginal zone B-cell lymphoma
   Splenic marginal zone B-cell lymphoma
CC Excl: For code 200.30: 200.30-200.78, 202.70-202.90, 239.81-239.9; For code 200.31: 200.30-200.31, 200.38-200.41, 200.48-200.51, 200.58-200.61, 200.68-200.71, 200.78, 202.70-202.71, 202.78-202.81, 202.88, 202.91, 239.81-239.9; For code 200.32: 200.30, 200.32, 200.38-200.40, 200.42, 200.48-200.50, 200.52, 200.58-200.60, 200.62, 200.68-200.70, 200.72, 200.78, 202.70, 202.72, 202.78-202.80, 202.82, 202.88, 202.92, 239.81-239.9; For code 200.33: 200.30, 200.33, 200.38-200.40, 200.43, 200.48-200.50, 200.53, 200.58-200.60, 200.63, 200.68-200.70, 200.73, 200.78, 202.70, 202.73, 202.78-202.80, 202.83, 202.88, 202.93, 239.81-239.9; For code 200.34: 200.30, 200.34, 200.38-200.40, 200.44, 200.48-200.50, 200.54, 200.58-200.60, 200.64, 200.68-200.70, 200.74, 200.78, 202.70, 202.74, 202.78-202.80, 202.84, 202.88, 202.94, 239.81-239.9; For code 200.35: 200.30, 200.35, 200.38-200.40, 200.45, 200.48-200.50, 200.55, 200.58-200.60, 200.65, 200.68-200.70, 200.75, 200.78, 202.70, 202.75, 202.78-202.80, 202.85, 202.88, 202.95, 239.81-239.9; For code 200.36: 200.30, 200.36, 200.38-200.40, 200.46, 200.48-200.50, 200.56, 200.58-200.60, 200.66, 200.68-200.70, 200.76, 200.78, 202.70, 202.76, 202.78-202.80, 202.86, 202.88, 202.96, 239.81-239.9; For code 200.37: 200.30, 200.37-200.40, 200.47-200.50, 200.57-200.60, 200.67-200.70, 200.77-200.78, 202.70, 202.77-202.80, 202.87-202.88, 202.97, 239.81-239.9; For code 200.38: 200.30-200.78, 202.70-202.88, 202.98, 239.81-239.9
AHA: 4Q, '07, 65

§ √5ᵗʰ **200.4 Mantle cell lymphoma**   CC HIV
[0-8]   CC Excl: For code 200.40: 200.30-200.78, 202.70-202.90, 239.81-239.9; For code 200.41: 200.30-200.31, 200.38-200.41, 200.48-200.51, 200.58-200.61, 200.68-200.71, 200.78, 202.70-202.71, 202.78-202.81, 202.88, 202.91, 239.81-239.9; For code 200.42: 200.30, 200.32, 200.38-200.40, 200.42, 200.48-200.50, 200.52, 200.58-200.60, 200.62, 200.68-200.70, 200.72, 200.78, 202.70, 202.72, 202.78-202.80, 202.82, 202.88, 202.92, 239.81-239.9; For code 200.43: 200.30, 200.33, 200.38-200.40, 200.43, 200.48-200.50, 200.53, 200.58-200.60, 200.63, 200.68-200.70, 200.73, 200.78, 202.70, 202.73, 202.78-202.80, 202.83, 202.88, 202.93, 239.81-239.9; For code 200.44: 200.30, 200.34, 200.38-200.40, 200.44, 200.48-200.50, 200.54, 200.58-200.60, 200.64, 200.68-200.70, 200.74, 200.78, 202.70, 202.74, 202.78-202.80, 202.84, 202.88, 202.94, 239.81-239.9; For code 200.45: 200.30, 200.35, 200.38-200.40, 200.45, 200.48-200.50, 200.55, 200.58-200.60, 200.65, 200.68-200.70, 200.75, 200.78, 202.70, 202.75, 202.78-202.80, 202.85, 202.88, 202.95, 239.81-239.9; For code 200.46: 200.30, 200.36, 200.38-200.40, 200.46, 200.48-200.50, 200.56, 200.58-200.60, 200.66, 200.68-200.70, 200.76, 200.78, 202.70, 202.76, 202.78-202.80, 202.86, 202.88, 202.96, 239.81-239.9; For code 200.47: 200.30, 200.37-200.40, 200.47-200.50, 200.57-200.60, 200.67-200.70, 200.77-200.78, 202.70, 202.77-202.80, 202.87-202.88, 202.97, 239.81-239.9; For code 200.48: 200.30-200.78, 202.70-202.88, 202.98, 239.81-239.9
AHA: 4Q, '07, 65

§ √5ᵗʰ **200.5 Primary central nervous system lymphoma**   CC HIV
[0-8]   CC Excl: For code 200.50: 200.30-200.78, 202.70-202.90, 239.81-239.9; For code 200.51: 200.30-200.31, 200.38-200.41, 200.48-200.51, 200.58-200.61, 200.68-200.71, 200.78, 202.70-202.71, 202.78-202.81, 202.88, 202.91, 239.81-239.9; For code 200.52: 200.30, 200.32, 200.38-200.40, 200.42, 200.48-200.50, 200.52, 200.58-200.60, 200.62, 200.68-200.70, 200.72, 200.78, 202.70, 202.72, 202.78-202.80, 202.82, 202.88, 202.92, 239.81-239.9; For code 200.53: 200.30, 200.33, 200.38-200.40, 200.43, 200.48-200.50, 200.53, 200.58-200.60, 200.63, 200.68-200.70, 200.73, 200.78, 202.70, 202.73, 202.78-202.80, 202.83, 202.88, 202.93, 239.81-239.9; For code 200.54: 200.30, 200.34, 200.38-200.40, 200.44, 200.48-200.50, 200.54, 200.58-200.60, 200.64, 200.68-200.70, 200.74, 200.78, 202.70, 202.74, 202.78-202.80, 202.84, 202.88, 202.94, 239.81-239.9; For code 200.55: 200.30, 200.35, 200.38-200.40, 200.45, 200.48-200.50, 200.55, 200.58-200.60, 200.65, 200.68-200.70, 200.75, 200.78, 202.70, 202.75, 202.78-202.80, 202.85, 202.88, 202.95, 239.81-239.9; For code 200.56: 200.30, 200.36, 200.38-200.40, 200.46, 200.48-200.50, 200.56, 200.58-200.60, 200.66, 200.68-200.70, 200.76, 200.78, 202.70, 202.76, 202.78-202.80, 202.86, 202.88, 202.96, 239.81-239.9; For code 200.57: 200.30, 200.37-200.40, 200.47-200.50, 200.57-200.60, 200.67-200.70, 200.77-200.78, 202.70, 202.77-202.80, 202.87-202.88, 202.97, 239.81-239.9; For code 200.58: 200.30-200.78, 202.70-202.88, 202.98, 239.81-239.9
AHA: 4Q, '07, 66

---

* Requires fifth digit. Valid digits are in [brackets] under each code. See beginning of section 200-208 for codes and definitions.

4ᵗʰ 5ᵗʰ Additional Digit Required   Unacceptable PDx   Manifestation Code   Hospital Acquired Condition   ►◄ Revised Text   ● New Code   ▲ Revised Code Title

Neoplasms

200.6–201.7

§ √5ᵗʰ **200.6 Anaplastic large cell lymphoma**   CC HIV
[0-8]
  CC Excl: For code 200.60: 200.30-200.78, 202.70-202.90, 239.81-239.9;
  For code 200.61: 200.30-200.31, 200.38-200.41, 200.48-200.51,
  200.58-200.61, 200.68-200.71, 200.78, 202.70-202.71,
  202.78-202.81, 202.88, 202.91, 239.81-239.9; For code 200.62: 200.30,
  200.32, 200.38-200.40, 200.42, 200.48-200.50, 200.52,
  200.58-200.60, 200.62, 200.68-200.70, 200.72, 200.78, 202.70,
  202.72, 202.78-202.80, 202.82, 202.88, 202.92, 239.81-239.9; For code
  200.63: 200.30, 200.33, 200.38-200.40, 200.43, 200.48-200.50, 200.53,
  200.58-200.60, 200.63, 200.68-200.70, 200.73, 200.78, 202.70,
  202.73, 202.78-202.80, 202.83, 202.88, 202.93, 239.81-239.9; For code
  200.64: 200.30, 200.34, 200.38-200.40, 200.44, 200.48-200.50, 200.54,
  200.58-200.60, 200.64, 200.68-200.70, 200.74, 200.78, 202.70,
  202.74, 202.78-202.80, 202.84, 202.88, 202.94, 239.81-239.9; For code
  200.65: 200.30, 200.35, 200.38-200.40, 200.45, 200.48-200.50, 200.55,
  200.58-200.60, 200.65, 200.68-200.70, 200.75, 200.78, 202.70,
  202.75, 202.78-202.80, 202.85, 202.88, 202.95, 239.81-239.9; For code
  200.66: 200.30, 200.36, 200.38-200.40, 200.46, 200.48-200.50, 200.56,
  200.58-200.60, 200.66, 200.68-200.70, 200.76, 200.78, 202.70,
  202.76, 202.78-202.80, 202.86, 202.88, 202.96, 239.81-239.9; For code
  200.67: 200.30, 200.37-200.40, 200.47-200.50, 200.57-200.60,
  200.67-200.70, 200.77-200.78, 202.70, 202.77-202.80,
  202.87-202.88, 202.97, 239.81-239.9; For code 200.68: 200.30-200.78,
  202.70-202.88, 202.98, 239.81-239.9

  AHA: 4Q, '07, 66

§ √5ᵗʰ **200.7 Large cell lymphoma**   CC HIV
[0-8]
  CC Excl: For code 200.70: 200.30-200.78, 202.70-202.90, 239.81-239.9;
  For code 200.71: 200.30-200.31, 200.38-200.41, 200.48-200.51,
  200.58-200.61, 200.68-200.71, 200.78, 202.70-202.71,
  202.78-202.81, 202.88, 202.91, 239.81-239.9; For code 200.72: 200.30,
  200.32, 200.38-200.40, 200.42, 200.48-200.50, 200.52,
  200.58-200.60, 200.62, 200.68-200.70, 200.72, 200.78, 202.70,
  202.72, 202.78-202.80, 202.82, 202.88, 202.92, 239.81-239.9; For code
  200.73: 200.30, 200.33, 200.38-200.40, 200.43, 200.48-200.50, 200.53,
  200.58-200.60, 200.63, 200.68-200.70, 200.73, 200.78, 202.70,
  202.73, 202.78-202.80, 202.83, 202.88, 202.93, 239.81-239.9; For code
  200.74: 200.30, 200.34, 200.38-200.40, 200.44, 200.48-200.50, 200.54,
  200.58-200.60, 200.64, 200.68-200.70, 200.74, 200.78, 202.70,
  202.74, 202.78-202.80, 202.84, 202.88, 202.94, 239.81-239.9; For code
  200.75: 200.30, 200.35, 200.38-200.40, 200.45, 200.48-200.50, 200.55,
  200.58-200.60, 200.65, 200.68-200.70, 200.75, 200.78, 202.70,
  202.75, 202.78-202.80, 202.85, 202.88, 202.95, 239.81-239.9; For code
  200.76: 200.30, 200.36, 200.38-200.40, 200.46, 200.48-200.50, 200.56,
  200.58-200.60, 200.66, 200.68-200.70, 200.76, 200.78, 202.70,
  202.76, 202.78-202.80, 202.86, 202.88, 202.96, 239.81-239.9; For code
  200.77: 200.30, 200.37-200.40, 200.47-200.50, 200.57-200.60,
  200.67-200.70, 200.77-200.78, 202.70, 202.77-202.80,
  202.87-202.88, 202.97, 239.81-239.9; For code 200.78: 200.30-200.78,
  202.70-202.88, 202.98, 239.81-239.9

  AHA: 4Q, '07, 66

§ √5ᵗʰ **200.8 Other named variants**   CC HIV
[0-8]
  Lymphoma (malignant):
    lymphoplasmacytoid type
    mixed lymphocytic-histiocytic (diffuse)
  Lymphosarcoma, mixed cell type (diffuse)
  Reticulolymphosarcoma (diffuse)
  CC Excl: For code 200.80: 200.80-200.88, 239.81-239.9; For code 200.81:
  200.80-200.81, 200.88, 239.81-239.9; For code 200.82: 200.80, 200.82,
  200.88, 239.81-239.9; For code 200.83: 200.80, 200.83, 200.88,
  239.81-239.9; For code 200.84: 200.80, 200.84, 200.88, 239.81-239.9;
  For code 200.85: 200.80, 200.85, 200.88, 239.81-239.9; For code 200.86:
  200.80, 200.86, 200.88, 239.81-239.9; For code 200.87: 200.80,
  200.87-200.88, 239.81-239.9; For code 200.88: 200.80-200.88,
  239.81-239.9

√4ᵗʰ **201 Hodgkin's disease**

  DEF: Painless, progressive enlargement of lymph nodes, spleen and general
  lymph tissue; symptoms include anorexia, lassitude, weight loss, fever,
  pruritis, night sweats, anemia.
  AHA: 2Q, '92, 3; N-D, '86, 5

§ √5ᵗʰ **201.0 Hodgkin's paragranuloma**   CC
[0-8]
  CC Excl: For code 201.00: 201.00-201.08, 201.90, 239.81-239.9; For code
  201.01: 201.00-201.01, 201.08, 201.90-201.91, 239.81-239.9; For code
  201.02: 201.00, 201.02, 201.08, 201.90, 201.92, 239.81-239.9; For code
  201.03: 201.00, 201.03, 201.08, 201.90, 201.93, 239.81-239.9; For code
  201.04: 201.00, 201.04, 201.08, 201.90, 201.94, 239.81-239.9; For code
  201.05: 201.00, 201.05, 201.08, 201.90, 201.95, 239.81-239.9; For code
  201.06: 201.00, 201.06, 201.08, 201.90, 201.96, 239.81-239.9; For code
  201.07: 201.00, 201.07-201.08, 201.90, 201.97, 239.81-239.9; For code
  201.08: 201.00-201.08, 201.90, 201.98, 239.81-239.9

§ √5ᵗʰ **201.1 Hodgkin's granuloma**   CC
[0-8]
  CC Excl: For code 201.10: 201.10-201.18, 201.90, 201.98, 239.81-239.9;
  For code 201.11: 201.10-201.11, 201.18, 201.90-201.91, 201.98,
  239.81-239.9; For code 201.12: 201.10-201.11, 201.18, 201.90-201.91,
  201.98, 239.81-239.9; For code 201.13: 201.10, 201.13, 201.18, 201.90,
  201.93, 201.98, 239.81-239.9; For code 201.14: 201.10, 201.14, 201.18,
  201.90, 201.94, 201.98, 239.81-239.9; For code 201.15: 201.10, 201.15,
  201.18, 201.90, 201.95, 201.98, 239.81-239.9; For code 201.16: 201.10,
  201.16, 201.18, 201.90, 201.96, 201.98, 239.81-239.9; For code 201.17:
  201.10, 201.17-201.18, 201.90, 201.97-201.98, 239.81-239.9; For code
  201.18: 201.10-201.18, 201.90, 201.98, 239.81-239.9

  AHA: 2Q, '99, 7

§ √5ᵗʰ **201.2 Hodgkin's sarcoma**   CC
[0-8]
  CC Excl: For code 201.20: 201.20-201.28, 201.90, 201.98, 239.81-239.9;
  For code 201.21: 201.20-201.21, 201.28, 201.90-201.91, 201.98,
  239.81-239.9; For code 201.22: 201.20, 201.22, 201.28, 201.90, 201.92,
  201.98, 239.81-239.9; For code 201.23: 201.20, 201.23, 201.28, 201.90,
  201.93, 201.98, 239.81-239.9; For code 201.24: 201.20, 201.24, 201.28,
  201.90, 201.94, 201.98, 239.81-239.9; For code 201.25: 201.20, 201.25,
  201.28, 201.90, 201.95, 201.98, 239.81-239.9; For code 201.26: 201.20,
  201.26, 201.28, 201.90, 201.96, 201.98, 239.81-239.9; For code 201.27:
  201.20, 201.27-201.28, 201.90, 201.97-201.98, 239.81-239.9; For code
  201.28: 201.20-201.28, 201.90, 201.98, 239.81-239.9

§ √5ᵗʰ **201.4 Lymphocytic-histiocytic predominance**   CC
[0-8]
  CC Excl: For code 201.40: 201.40-201.48, 201.90, 201.98, 239.81-239.9;
  For code 201.41: 201.40-201.41, 201.48, 201.90-201.91, 201.98,
  239.81-239.9; For code 201.42: 201.40, 201.42, 201.48, 201.90, 201.92,
  201.98, 239.81-239.9; For code 201.43: 201.40, 201.43, 201.48, 201.90,
  201.93, 201.98, 239.81-239.9; For code 201.44: 201.40, 201.44, 201.48,
  201.90, 201.94, 201.98, 239.81-239.9; For code 201.45: 201.40, 201.45,
  201.48, 201.90, 201.95, 201.98, 239.81-239.9; For code 201.46: 201.40,
  201.46, 201.48, 201.90, 201.96, 201.98, 239.81-239.9; For code 201.47:
  201.40, 201.47-201.48, 201.90, 201.97-201.98, 239.81-239.9; For code
  201.48: 201.40-201.48, 201.90, 201.98, 239.81-239.9

§ √5ᵗʰ **201.5 Nodular sclerosis**   CC
[0-8]
  Hodgkin's disease, nodular sclerosis:
    NOS
    cellular phase
  CC Excl: For code 201.50: 201.50-201.58, 201.90, 201.98, 239.81-239.9;
  For code 201.51: 201.50-201.51, 201.58, 201.90-201.91, 201.98,
  239.81-239.9; For code 201.52: 201.50, 201.52, 201.58, 201.90, 201.92,
  201.98, 239.81-239.9; For code 201.53: 201.50, 201.53, 201.58, 201.90,
  201.93, 201.98, 239.81-239.9; For code 201.54: 201.50, 201.54, 201.58,
  201.90, 201.94, 201.98, 239.81-239.9; For code 201.55: 201.50, 201.55,
  201.58, 201.90, 201.95, 201.98, 239.81-239.9; For code 201.56: 201.50,
  201.56, 201.58, 201.90, 201.96, 201.98, 239.81-239.9; For code 201.57:
  201.50, 201.57-201.58, 201.90, 201.97-201.98, 239.81-239.9; For code
  201.58: 201.50-201.58, 201.90, 201.98, 239.81-239.9

§ √5ᵗʰ **201.6 Mixed cellularity**   CC
[0-8]
  CC Excl: For code 201.60: 201.60-201.68, 201.90, 201.98, 239.81-239.9;
  For code 201.61: 201.60-201.61, 201.68, 201.90-201.91, 201.98,
  239.81-239.9; For code 201.62: 201.60, 201.62, 201.68, 201.90, 201.92,
  201.98, 239.81-239.9; For code 201.63: 201.60, 201.63, 201.68, 201.90,
  201.93, 201.98, 239.81-239.9; For code 201.64: 201.60, 201.64, 201.68,
  201.90, 201.94, 201.98, 239.81-239.9; For code 201.65: 201.60, 201.65,
  201.68, 201.90, 201.95, 201.98, 239.81-239.9; For code 201.66: 201.60,
  201.66, 201.68, 201.90, 201.96, 201.98, 239.81-239.9; For code 201.67:
  201.60, 201.67-201.68, 201.90, 201.97-201.98, 239.81-239.9; For code
  201.68: 201.60-201.68, 201.90, 201.98, 239.81-239.9

§ √5ᵗʰ **201.7 Lymphocytic depletion**   CC
[0-8]
  Hodgkin's disease, lymphocytic depletion:
    NOS
    diffuse fibrosis
    reticular type
  CC Excl: For code 201.70:201.70-201.90, 201.98, 239.81-239.9; For code
  201.71: 201.70-201.71, 201.78, 201.91, 201.98, 239.81-239.9; For code
  201.72: 201.70, 201.72, 201.78, 201.92, 201.98, 239.81-239.9; For code
  201.73: 201.70, 201.73, 201.78, 201.93, 201.98, 239.81-239.9; For code
  201.74: 201.70, 201.74, 201.78, 201.94, 201.98, 239.81-239.9; For code
  201.75: 201.70, 201.75, 201.78, 201.95, 201.98, 239.81-239.9; For code
  201.76: 201.70, 201.76, 201.78, 201.96, 201.98, 239.81-239.9; For code
  201.77: 201.70, 201.77-201.78, 201.97-201.98, 239.81-239.9; For code
  201.78: 201.70-201.78, 201.98, 239.81-239.9

---

§ Requires fifth digit. Valid digits are in [brackets] under each code. See beginning of section 200-208 for codes and definitions.

N Newborn Age: 0   P Pediatric Age: 0-17   M Maternity Age: 12-55   A Adult Age: 15-124   MCC Major CC Condition   CC CC Condition   HIV HIV Related Dx

46 – Volume 1   2014 ICD-9-CM

§ ☑5ᵗʰ **201.9 Hodgkin's disease, unspecified** `CC`

[0-8]   Hodgkin's: Malignant:
          disease NOS   lymphogranuloma
          lymphoma NOS   lymphogranulomatosis

CC Excl: For code 201.90: 201.90-201.98, 239.81-239.9; **For code 201.91**: 201.90-201.91, 201.98, 239.81-239.9; **For code 201.92**: 201.90, 201.92, 201.98, 239.81-239.9; **For code 201.93**: 201.90, 201.93, 201.98, 239.81-239.9; **For code 201.94**: 201.90, 201.94, 201.98, 239.81-239.9; **For code 201.95**: 201.90, 201.95, 201.98, 239.81-239.9; **For code 201.96**: 201.90, 201.96, 201.98, 239.81-239.9; **For code 201.97**: 201.90, 201.97-201.98, 239.81-239.9; **For code 201.98**: 201.90-201.98, 239.81-239.9

☑4ᵗʰ **202 Other malignant neoplasms of lymphoid and histiocytic tissue**

AHA: 2Q, '92, 3; N-D, '86, 5

§ ☑5ᵗʰ **202.0 Nodular lymphoma** `CC`

[0-8]   Brill-Symmers disease   Lymphosarcoma:
          Lymphoma: follicular (giant)
            follicular (giant) (large cell)   nodular
            lymphocytic, nodular

DEF: Lymphomatous cells clustered into nodules within the lymph node; usually occurs in older adults and may involve all nodes and possibly extranodal sites.

CC Excl: For code 202.00: 200.30, 200.40, 200.50, 200.60, 200.70,202.00-202.08, 202.70, 202.80, 202.90, 239.8-239.9; **For code 202.01**: 200.31, 200.41, 200.51, 200.61, 200.71,202.00-202.01, 202.08, 202.71, 202.81, 202.91, 239.8-239.9; **For code 202.02**: 200.32, 200.42, 200.52, 200.62, 200.72, 202.00, 202.02, 202.08, 202.72, 202.82, 202.92, 239.8-239.9; **For code 202.03**: 200.33, 200.43, 200.53, 200.63, 200.73, 202.00, 202.03, 202.08, 202.73, 202.83, 202.93, 239.8-239.9; ; **For code 202.04**: 3Q, '09, 4; 200.34, 200.44, 200.54, 200.64, 200.74, 202.00, 202.04, 202.08, 202.74, 202.84, 202.94, 239.8-239.9; ; **For code 202.05**: 200.35, 200.45, 200.55, 200.65, 200.75, 202.00, 202.05, 202.08, 202.75, 202.85, 202.95, 239.8-239.9; **For code 202.06**: 200.36, 200.46, 200.56, 200.66, 200.76, 202.00, 202.06, 202.08, 202.76, 202.86, 202.96, 239.8-239.9; **For code 202.07**: 200.37, 200.47, 200.57, 200.67, 200.77, 202.00,202.07-202.08, 202.77, 202.87, 202.97, 239.8-239.9; **For code 202.08**: 200.38, 200.48, 200.58, 200.68, 200.78,202.00-202.08, 202.78, 202.88, 202.98, 239.8-239.9

§ ☑5ᵗʰ **202.1 Mycosis fungoides** `CC`

[0-8]   *EXCLUDES*   *peripheral T-cell lymphoma (202.7)*

DEF: Type of cutaneous T-cell lymphoma; may evolve into generalized lymphoma; formerly thought to be of fungoid origin.

CC Excl: For code 202.10: 200.30, 200.40, 200.50, 200.60, 200.70, 202.10-202.18, 202.70, 202.80, 202.90, 239.81-239.9; **For code 202.11**: 200.31, 200.41, 200.51, 200.61, 200.71, 202.10-202.11, 202.18, 202.71, 202.81, 202.91, 239.81-239.9; **For code 202.12**: 200.32, 200.42, 200.52, 200.62, 200.72, 202.10, 202.12, 202.18, 202.72, 202.82, 202.92, 239.81-239.9; **For code 202.13**: 200.33, 200.43, 200.53, 200.63, 200.73, 202.10, 202.13, 202.18, 202.73, 202.83, 202.93, 239.81-239.9; **For code 202.14**: 200.34, 200.44, 200.54, 200.64, 200.74, 202.10, 202.14, 202.18, 202.74, 202.84, 202.94, 239.81-239.9; **For code 202.15**: 200.35, 200.45, 200.55, 200.65, 200.75, 202.10, 202.15, 202.18, 202.75, 202.85, 202.95, 239.81-239.9; **For code 202.16**: 200.36, 200.46, 200.56, 200.66, 200.76, 202.10, 202.16, 202.18, 202.76, 202.86, 202.96, 239.81-239.9; **For code 202.17**: 200.37, 200.47, 200.57, 200.67, 200.77, 202.10, 202.17-202.18, 202.77, 202.87, 202.97, 239.81-239.9; **For code 202.18**: 200.38, 200.48, 200.58, 200.68, 200.78, 202.10-202.18, 202.78, 202.88, 202.98, 239.81-239.9

AHA: 2Q, '92, 4

§ ☑5ᵗʰ **202.2 Sézary's disease** `CC`

[0-8]   **DEF:** Type of cutaneous T-cell lymphoma with erythroderma, intense pruritus, peripheral lymphadenopathy, abnormal hyperchromatic mononuclear cells in skin, lymph nodes and peripheral blood.

CC Excl: For code 202.20: 200.30, 200.40, 200.50, 200.60, 200.70, 202.20-202.28, 202.70, 202.80, 202.90, 239.81-239.9; **For code 202.21**: 200.31, 200.41, 200.51, 200.61, 200.71, 202.20-202.21, 202.28, 202.71, 202.81, 202.91, 239.81-239.9; **For code 202.22**: 200.32, 200.42, 200.52, 200.62, 200.72, 202.20, 202.22, 202.28, 202.72, 202.82, 202.92, 239.81-239.9; **For code 202.23**: 200.33, 200.43, 200.53, 200.63, 200.73, 202.20, 202.23, 202.28, 202.73, 202.83, 202.93, 239.81-239.9; **For code 202.24**: 200.34, 200.44, 200.54, 200.64, 200.74, 202.20, 202.24, 202.28, 202.74, 202.84, 202.94, 239.81-239.9; **For code 202.25**: 200.35, 200.45, 200.55, 200.65, 200.75, 202.20, 202.25, 202.28, 202.75, 202.85, 202.95, 239.81-239.9; **For code 202.26**: 200.36, 200.46, 200.56, 200.66, 200.76, 202.20, 202.26, 202.28, 202.76, 202.86, 202.96, 239.81-239.9; **For code 202.27**: 200.37, 200.47, 200.57, 200.67, 200.77, 202.20, 202.27-202.28, 202.77, 202.87, 202.97, 239.81-239.9; **For code 202.28**: 200.38, 200.48, 200.58, 200.68, 200.78, 202.20-202.28, 202.78, 202.88, 202.98, 239.81-239.9

AHA: 2Q, '99, 7

§ ☑5ᵗʰ **202.3 Malignant histiocytosis** `CC`

[0-8]   Histiocytic medullary reticulosis
          Malignant:
            reticuloendotheliosis
            reticulosis

CC Excl: For code 202.30: 200.30, 200.40, 200.50, 200.60, 200.70, 202.30-202.38, 202.70, 202.80, 202.90, 239.81-239.9; **For code 202.31**: 200.31, 200.41, 200.51, 200.61, 200.71, 202.30-202.31, 202.38, 202.71, 202.81, 202.91, 239.81-239.9; **For code 202.32**: 200.32, 200.42, 200.52, 200.62, 200.72, 202.30, 202.32, 202.38, 202.72, 202.82, 202.92, 239.81-239.9; **For code 202.33**: 200.33, 200.43, 200.53, 200.63, 200.73, 202.30, 202.33, 202.38, 202.73, 202.83, 202.93, 239.81-239.9; **For code 202.34**: 200.34, 200.44, 200.54, 200.64, 200.74, 202.30, 202.34, 202.38, 202.74, 202.84, 202.94, 239.81-239.9; **For code 202.35**: 200.35, 200.45, 200.55, 200.65, 200.75, 202.30, 202.35, 202.38, 202.75, 202.85, 202.95, 239.81-239.9; **For code 202.36**: 200.36, 200.46, 200.56, 200.66, 200.76, 202.30, 202.36, 202.38, 202.76, 202.86, 202.96, 239.81-239.9; **For code 202.37**: 200.37, 200.47, 200.57, 200.67, 200.77, 202.30, 202.37-202.38, 202.77, 202.87, 202.97, 239.81-239.9; **For code 202.38**: 200.38, 200.48, 200.58, 200.68, 200.78, 202.30-202.38, 202.78, 202.88, 202.98, 239.81-239.9

§ ☑5ᵗʰ **202.4 Leukemic reticuloendotheliosis** `CC`

[0-8]   Hairy-cell leukemia

DEF: Chronic leukemia with large, mononuclear cells with "hairy" appearance in marrow, spleen, liver, blood.

CC Excl: For code 202.40: 200.30, 200.40, 200.50, 200.60, 200.70, 202.40-202.48, 202.70, 202.80, 202.90, 239.81-239.9; **For code 202.41**: 200.31, 200.41, 200.51, 200.61, 200.71, 202.40-202.41, 202.48, 202.71, 202.81, 202.91, 239.81-239.9; **For code 202.42**: 200.32, 200.42, 200.52, 200.62, 200.72, 202.40, 202.42, 202.48, 202.72, 202.82, 202.92, 239.81-239.9; **For code 202.43**: 200.33, 200.43, 200.53, 200.63, 200.73, 202.40, 202.43, 202.48, 202.73, 202.83, 202.93, 239.81-239.9; **For code 202.44**: 200.34, 200.44, 200.54, 200.64, 200.74, 202.40, 202.44, 202.48, 202.74, 202.84, 202.94, 239.81-239.9; **For code 202.45**: 200.35, 200.45, 200.55, 200.65, 200.75, 202.40, 202.45, 202.48, 202.75, 202.85, 202.95, 239.81-239.9; **For code 202.46**: 200.36, 200.46, 200.56, 200.66, 200.76, 202.40, 202.46, 202.48, 202.76, 202.86, 202.96, 239.81-239.9; **For code 202.47**: 200.37, 200.47, 200.57, 200.67, 200.77, 202.40, 202.47-202.48, 202.77, 202.87, 202.97, 239.81-239.9; **For code 202.48**: 200.38, 200.48, 200.58, 200.68, 200.78, 202.40-202.48, 202.78, 202.88, 202.98, 239.81-239.9

§ ☑5ᵗʰ **202.5 Letterer-Siwe disease** `CC`

[0-8]   Acute:
            differentiated progressive histiocytosis
            histiocytosis X (progressive)
            infantile reticuloendotheliosis
            reticulosis of infancy

       EXCLUDES   *adult pulmonary Langerhans cell histiocytosis (516.5)*
                   Hand-Schüller-Christian disease (277.89)
                   histiocytosis (acute) (chronic) (277.89)
                   histiocytosis X (chronic) (277.89)

DEF: A recessive reticuloendotheliosis of early childhood, with a hemorrhagic tendency, eczema-like skin eruption, hepatosplenomegaly, lymph node enlargement, and progressive anemia; often a fatal disease with no established cause.

CC Excl: For code 202.50: 200.30, 200.40, 200.50, 200.60, 200.70, 202.50-202.58, 202.70, 202.80, 202.90, 239.81-239.9; **For code 202.51**: 200.31, 200.41, 200.51, 200.61, 200.71, 202.50-202.51, 202.58, 202.71, 202.81, 202.91, 239.81-239.9; **For code 202.52**: 200.32, 200.42, 200.52, 200.62, 200.72, 202.50, 202.52, 202.58, 202.72, 202.82, 202.92, 239.81-239.9; **For code 202.53**: 200.33, 200.43, 200.53, 200.63, 200.73, 202.50, 202.53, 202.58, 202.73, 202.83, 202.93, 239.81-239.9; **For code 202.54**: 200.34, 200.44, 200.54, 200.64, 200.74, 202.50, 202.54, 202.58, 202.74, 202.84, 202.94, 239.81-239.9; **For code 202.55**: 200.35, 200.45, 200.55, 200.65, 200.75, 202.50, 202.55, 202.58, 202.75, 202.85, 202.95, 239.81-239.9; **For code 202.56**: 200.36, 200.46, 200.56, 200.66, 200.76, 202.50, 202.56, 202.58, 202.76, 202.86, 202.96, 239.81-239.9; **For code 202.57**: 200.37, 200.47, 200.57, 200.67, 200.77, 202.50, 202.57-202.58, 202.77, 202.87, 202.97, 239.81-239.9; **For code 202.58**: 200.38, 200.48, 200.58, 200.68, 200.78, 202.50-202.58, 202.78, 202.88, 202.98, 239.81-239.9

---

§   Requires fifth digit. Valid digits are in [brackets] under each code. See beginning of section 200-208 for codes and definitions.

☑4ᵗʰ ☑5ᵗʰ Additional Digit Required   Unacceptable PDx   Manifestation Code   Hospital Acquired Condition   ►◄ Revised Text   ● New Code   ▲ Revised Code Title

Neoplasms

202.6–204.9

§ ✓5ᵗʰ **202.6 Malignant mast cell tumors**   `CC`
[0-8]   Malignant: Mast cell sarcoma
     mastocytoma   Systemic tissue mast cell disease
     mastocytosis

     EXCLUDES *mast cell leukemia (207.8)*

     CC Excl: For code 202.60: 200.30, 200.40, 200.50, 200.60, 200.70,
202.60-202.70, 202.80, 202.90, 239.81-239.9; For code 202.61: 200.31,
200.41, 200.51, 200.61, 200.71, 202.60-202.61, 202.68, 202.71,
202.81, 202.91, 239.81-239.9; For code 202.62: 200.32, 200.42, 200.52,
200.62, 200.72, 202.60, 202.62, 202.68, 202.72, 202.82, 202.92,
239.81-239.9; For code 202.63: 200.33, 200.43, 200.53, 200.63, 200.73,
202.60, 202.63, 202.68, 202.73, 202.83, 202.93, 239.81-239.9; For code
202.64: 200.34, 200.44, 200.54, 200.64, 200.74, 202.60, 202.64,
202.68, 202.74, 202.84, 202.94, 239.81-239.9; For code 202.65: 200.35,
200.45, 200.55, 200.65, 200.75, 202.60, 202.65, 202.68, 202.75,
202.85, 202.95, 239.81-239.9; For code 202.66: 200.36, 200.46, 200.56,
200.66, 200.76, 202.60, 202.66, 202.68, 202.76, 202.86, 202.96,
239.81-239.9; For code 202.67: 200.37, 200.47, 200.57, 200.67, 200.77,
202.60, 202.67-202.68, 202.77, 202.87, 202.97, 239.81-239.9; For code
202.68: 200.38, 200.48, 200.58, 200.68, 200.78, 202.60-202.68,
202.78, 202.88, 202.98, 239.81-239.9

§ ✓5ᵗʰ **202.7 Peripheral T-cell lymphoma**   `CC` `HIV`
[0-8]   CC Excl: For code 202.70: 200.30, 200.78, 202.70-202.90, 239.81-239.9;
For code 202.71: 200.30-200.31, 200.38-200.41, 200.48-200.51,
200.58-200.61, 200.68-200.71, 200.78, 202.70-202.71,
202.78-202.81, 202.88, 202.91, 239.81-239.9; For code 202.72: 200.30,
200.32, 200.38-200.40, 200.42, 200.48-200.50, 200.52,
200.58-200.60, 200.62, 200.68-200.70, 200.72, 200.78, 202.70,
202.72, 202.78-202.80, 202.82, 202.88, 202.92, 239.81-239.9; For code
202.73: 200.30, 200.33, 200.38-200.40, 200.43, 200.48-200.50, 200.53,
200.58-200.60, 200.63, 200.68-200.70, 200.73, 200.78, 202.70,
202.73, 202.78-202.80, 202.83, 202.88, 202.93, 239.81-239.9; For code
202.74: 200.30, 200.34, 200.38-200.40, 200.44, 200.48-200.50, 200.54,
200.58-200.60, 200.64, 200.68-200.70, 200.74, 200.78, 202.70,
202.74, 202.78-202.80, 202.84, 202.88, 202.94, 239.81-239.9; For code
202.75: 200.30, 200.35, 200.38-200.40, 200.45, 200.48-200.50, 200.55,
200.58-200.60, 200.65, 200.68-200.70, 200.75, 200.78, 202.70,
202.75, 202.78-202.80, 202.85, 202.88, 202.95, 239.81-239.9; For code
202.76: 200.30, 200.36, 200.38-200.40, 200.46, 200.48-200.50, 200.56,
200.58-200.60, 200.66, 200.68-200.70, 200.76, 200.78, 202.70,
202.76, 202.78-202.80, 202.86, 202.88, 202.96, 239.81-239.9; For code
202.77: 200.30, 200.37-200.40, 200.47-200.50, 200.57-200.60,
200.67-200.70, 200.77-200.78, 202.70, 202.77-202.80,
202.87-202.88, 202.97, 239.81-239.9; For code 202.78: 200.30-200.78,
202.70-202.88, 202.98, 239.81-239.9

     AHA: 4Q, '07, 66

§ ✓5ᵗʰ **202.8 Other lymphomas**   `CC` `HIV`
[0-8]   Lymphoma (malignant):
       NOS
       diffuse

     EXCLUDES *benign lymphoma (229.0)*

     CC Excl: For code 202.80: 200.30-200.78, 202.70-202.90, 239.81-239.9;
For code 202.81: 200.30-200.31, 200.38-200.41, 200.48-200.51,
200.58-200.61, 200.68-200.71, 200.78, 202.70-202.71,
202.78-202.81, 202.88, 202.91, 239.81-239.9; For code 202.82: 200.30,
200.32, 200.38-200.40, 200.42, 200.48-200.50, 200.52,
200.58-200.60, 200.62, 200.68-200.70, 200.72, 200.78, 202.70,
202.72, 202.78-202.80, 202.82, 202.88, 202.92, 239.81-239.9; For code
202.83: 200.30, 200.33, 200.38-200.40, 200.43, 200.48-200.50, 200.53,
200.58-200.60, 200.63, 200.68-200.70, 200.73, 200.78, 202.70,
202.73, 202.78-202.80, 202.83, 202.88, 202.93, 239.81-239.9; For code
202.84: 200.30, 200.34, 200.38-200.40, 200.44, 200.48-200.50, 200.54,
200.58-200.60, 200.64, 200.68-200.70, 200.74, 200.78, 202.70,
202.74, 202.78-202.80, 202.84, 202.88, 202.94, 239.81-239.9; For code
202.85: 200.30, 200.35, 200.38-200.40, 200.45, 200.48-200.50, 200.55,
200.58-200.60, 200.65, 200.68-200.70, 200.75, 200.78, 202.70,
202.75, 202.78-202.80, 202.85, 202.88, 202.95, 239.81-239.9; For code
202.86: 200.30, 200.36, 200.38-200.40, 200.46, 200.48-200.50, 200.56,
200.58-200.60, 200.66, 200.68-200.70, 200.76, 200.78, 202.70,
202.76, 202.78-202.80, 202.86, 202.88, 202.96, 239.81-239.9; For code
202.87: 200.30, 200.37-200.40, 200.47-200.50, 200.57-200.60,
200.67-200.70, 200.77-200.78, 202.70, 202.77-202.80,
202.87-202.88, 202.97, 239.81-239.9; For code 202.88: 200.30-200.78,
202.70-202.88, 202.98, 239.81-239.9

     AHA: 4Q, '06, 135; 2Q, '06, 20-21; 2Q, '92, 4; For code 202.80: 4Q, '08, 83;
1Q, '08, 16; 3Q, '07, 3

     C85.80 Oth spec types non-Hodgkins lymphoma unspec site   `I-10`

§ ✓5ᵗʰ **202.9 Other and unspecified malignant neoplasms**   `CC`
[0-8]   **of lymphoid and histiocytic tissue**
     Follicular dendritic cell sarcoma
     Interdigitating dendritic cell sarcoma
     Langerhans cell sarcoma
     Malignant neoplasm of bone marrow NOS

     CC Excl: For code 202.90: 202.90-202.98, 239.81-239.9; For code 202.91:
202.90-202.91, 202.98, 239.81-239.9; For code 202.92: 202.90, 202.92,
202.98, 239.81-239.9; For code 202.93: 202.90, 202.93, 202.98,
239.81-239.9; For code 202.94: 202.90, 202.94, 202.98, 239.81-239.9;
For code 202.95: 202.90, 202.95, 202.98, 239.81-239.9; For code 202.96:
202.90, 202.96, 202.98, 239.81-239.9; For code 202.97: 202.90,
202.97-202.98, 239.81-239.9; For code 202.98: 202.90-202.98,
239.81-239.9

✓4ᵗʰ **203 Multiple myeloma and immunoproliferative neoplasms**
     AHA: 4Q, '08, 83-84; 4Q, '91, 26

     The following fifth-digit subclassification is for use with category 203:
      0 without mention of having achieved remission
       Failed remission
      1 in remission
      2 in relapse

§ ✓5ᵗʰ **203.0 Multiple myeloma**   `CC`
[0-2]   Kahler's disease   Myelomatosis

     EXCLUDES *solitary myeloma (238.6)*

     CC Excl: 203.00-208.92, 239.81-239.9
     AHA: 1Q, '96, 16; 4Q, '89, 10; For code 203.00: ▶3Q, '12,16;◀ 2Q, '10, 6;
2Q, '07, 8; For code 203.01: 4Q, '08, 91
     C90.00 Multiple myeloma not in remission   `I-10`

§ ✓5ᵗʰ **203.1 Plasma cell leukemia**   `CC`
[0-2]   Plasmacytic leukemia

     CC Excl: See code 203.0
     AHA: 4Q, '91, 26

§ ✓5ᵗʰ **203.8 Other immunoproliferative neoplasms**   `CC`
[0-2]   CC Excl: See code 203.0
     AHA: 4Q, '90, 26; S-O, '86, 12

✓4ᵗʰ **204 Lymphoid leukemia**
     INCLUDES leukemia:
       lymphatic
       lymphoblastic
       lymphocytic
       lymphogenous

     AHA: 4Q, '08, 83-84; 3Q, '93, 4

     The following fifth-digit subclassification is for use with category 204:
      0 without mention of having achieved remission
       Failed remission
      1 in remission
      2 in relapse

§ ✓5ᵗʰ **204.0 Acute**   `CC`
[0-2]   **EXCLUDES** *acute exacerbation of chronic lymphoid leukemia*
                (204.1)

     CC Excl: 203.00-208.92, 239.81-239.9
     AHA: 3Q, '99, 6; For code 204.02: 1Q, '12, 13
     For code 204.00: 2Q, '11, 4

§ ✓5ᵗʰ **204.1 Chronic**   `CC`
[0-2]   CC Excl: See code: 204.0
     C91.10 Chronic lymphocytic leukemia not in remission   `I-10`

§ ✓5ᵗʰ **204.2 Subacute**   `CC`
[0-2]   CC Excl: See code: 204.0

§ ✓5ᵗʰ **204.8 Other lymphoid leukemia**   `CC`
[0-2]   Aleukemic leukemia: Aleukemic leukemia:
     lymphatic   lymphoid
     lymphocytic

     CC Excl: See code: 204.0
     AHA: 3Q, '09, 4
     TIP: Assign for T-cell large granular lymphocytic leukemia.

§ ✓5ᵗʰ **204.9 Unspecified lymphoid leukemia**   `CC`
[0-2]   CC Excl: See code: 204.0

---

§   Requires fifth digit. Valid digits are in [brackets] under each code. See appropriate category for codes and definitions.

`N` Newborn Age: 0   `P` Pediatric Age: 0-17   `M` Maternity Age: 12-55   `A` Adult Age: 15-124   `MCC` Major CC Condition   `CC` CC Condition   `HIV` HIV Related Dx

48 – Volume 1 · February 2013   2014 ICD-9-CM

√4ᵗʰ **205 Myeloid leukemia**

INCLUDES leukemia:
    granulocytic
    myeloblastic
    myelocytic
    myelogenous
    myelomonocytic
    myelosclerotic
    myelosis

AHA: 4Q, '08, 83-84; 3Q, '93, 3; 4Q, '91, 26; 4Q, '90, 3; M-J, '85, 18

The following fifth-digit subclassification is for use with category 205:
  0 without mention of having achieved remission
    Failed remission
  1 in remission
  2 in relapse

§ √5ᵗʰ **205.0 Acute**   CC
[0-2]   Acute promyelocytic leukemia
    EXCLUDES *acute exacerbation of chronic myeloid leukemia*
        (205.1)
    CC Excl: 203.00-208.92, 239.81-239.9
    AHA: For code 205.00: 4Q, '09, 79; 2Q, '06, 20-21; For code 205.01: ▶2Q, '12, 16◀
    C92.00 Acute myeloid leukemia not in remission   I-10

§ √5ᵗʰ **205.1 Chronic**   CC
[0-2]   Eosinophilic leukemia   Neutrophilic leukemia
    CC Excl: See code: 205.0
    AHA: 1Q, '00, 6; J-A, '85, 13; For code 205.10: 4Q, '08, 142

§ √5ᵗʰ **205.2 Subacute**   CC
[0-2]   CC Excl: See code: 205.0

§ √5ᵗʰ **205.3 Myeloid sarcoma**   CC
[0-2]   Chloroma   Granulocytic sarcoma
    CC Excl: See code: 205.0

§ √5ᵗʰ **205.8 Other myeloid leukemia**   CC
[0-2]   Aleukemic leukemia: Aleukemic leukemia:
     granulocytic   myeloid
     myelogenous   Aleukemic myelosis
    CC Excl: See code: 205.0

§ √5ᵗʰ **205.9 Unspecified myeloid leukemia**   CC
[0-2]   CC Excl: See code: 205.0

√4ᵗʰ **206 Monocytic leukemia**

INCLUDES leukemia:
    histiocytic
    monoblastic
    monocytoid

AHA: 4Q,, '08, 83-84

The following fifth-digit subclassification is for use with category 206:
  0 without mention of having achieved remission
    Failed remission
  1 in remission
  2 in relapse

§ √5ᵗʰ **206.0 Acute**   CC
[0-2]   EXCLUDES *acute exacerbation of chronic monocytic leukemia*
        (206.1)
    CC Excl: 203.00-208.92, 239.81-239.9

§ √5ᵗʰ **206.1 Chronic**   CC
[0-2]   CC Excl: See code: 206.0

§ √5ᵗʰ **206.2 Subacute**   CC
[0-2]   CC Excl: See code: 206.0

§ √5ᵗʰ **206.8 Other monocytic leukemia**   CC
[0-2]   Aleukemic: Aleukemic:
     monocytic leukemia   monocytoid leukemia
    CC Excl: See code: 206.0

§ √5ᵗʰ **206.9 Unspecified monocytic leukemia**   CC
[0-2]   CC Excl: See code: 206.0

√4ᵗʰ **207 Other specified leukemia**

EXCLUDES *leukemic reticuloendotheliosis (202.4)*
      plasma cell leukemia (203.1)
AHA: 4Q, '08, 83-85

The following fifth-digit subclassification is for use with category 207:
  0 without mention of having achieved remission
    Failed remission
  1 in remission
  2 in relapse

§ √5ᵗʰ **207.0 Acute erythremia and erythroleukemia**   CC
[0-2]   Acute erythremic myelosis   Erythremic myelosis
    Di Guglielmo's disease
    DEF: Erythremia: polycythemia vera.
    DEF: Erythroleukemia: a malignant blood dyscrasia (a
    myeloproliferative disorder).
    CC Excl: 203.00-208.92, 239.81-239.9

§ √5ᵗʰ **207.1 Chronic erythremia**   CC
[0-2]   Heilmeyer-Schöner disease
    CC Excl: See code: 207.0

§ √5ᵗʰ **207.2 Megakaryocytic leukemia**   CC
[0-2]   Megakaryocytic myelosis   Thrombocytic leukemia
    CC Excl: See code: 207.0

§ √5ᵗʰ **207.8 Other specified leukemia**   CC
[0-2]   Lymphosarcoma cell leukemia
    CC Excl: See code: 207.0

√4ᵗʰ **208 Leukemia of unspecified cell type**

AHA: 4Q, '08, 83-85

The following fifth-digit subclassification is for use with category 208:
  0 without mention of having achieved remission
    Failed remission
  1 in remission
  2 in relapse

§ √5ᵗʰ **208.0 Acute**   CC
[0-2]   Acute leukemia NOS   Stem cell leukemia
    Blast cell leukemia
    EXCLUDES *acute exacerbation of chronic unspecified leukemia*
        (208.1)
    CC Excl: 203.00-208.92, 239.81-239.9

§ √5ᵗʰ **208.1 Chronic**   CC
[0-2]   Chronic leukemia NOS
    CC Excl: See code: 208.0

§ √5ᵗʰ **208.2 Subacute**   CC
[0-2]   Subacute leukemia NOS
    CC Excl: See code: 208.0

§ √5ᵗʰ **208.8 Other leukemia of unspecified cell type**   CC
[0-2]   CC Excl: See code: 208.0

§ √5ᵗʰ **208.9 Unspecified leukemia**   CC
[0-2]   Leukemia NOS
    CC Excl: See code: 208.0
    AHA: For code 208.90: 4Q, '11, 148

Neuroendocrine Tumors (209)

√4ᵗʰ **209 Neuroendocrine tumors**

Code first any associated multiple endocrine neoplasia syndrome (258.01-258.03)
Use additional code to identify associated endocrine syndrome, such as:
    carcinoid syndrome (259.2)
EXCLUDES *benign pancreatic islet cell tumors (211.7)*
      malignant pancreatic islet cell tumors (157.4)
AHA: 4Q, '09, 150; 4Q, '08, 85 89

√5ᵗʰ **209.0 Malignant carcinoid tumors of the small intestine**

    209.00 Malignant carcinoid tumor of the small   CC
        intestine, unspecified portion
        CC Excl: 152.8-152.9, 159.0, 159.8-159.9, 176.3, 195.8, 199.0-199.2, 209.00-209.30, 209.70, 209.75, 239.0, 239.81-239.9

---

§ Requires fifth digit. Valid digits are in [brackets] under each code. See appropriate category for codes and definitions.

⁴ᵗʰ/₅ᵗʰ Additional Digit Required   Unacceptable PDx   Manifestation Code   Hospital Acquired Condition   ▶◀ Revised Text   ● New Code   ▲ Revised Code Title

2014 ICD-9-CM   February 2013 · Volume 1 – 49

Neoplasms

209.01 **Malignant carcinoid tumor of the duodenum** `CC`
CC Excl: 152.0, 152.8-152.9, 159.0, 159.8-159.9, 176.3, 195.8, 199.0-199.2, 209.00-209.30, 209.70, 209.75, 239.0, 239.81-239.9 .

209.02 **Malignant carcinoid tumor of the jejunum** `CC`
CC Excl: 152.1, 152.8-152.9, 159.0, 159.8-159.9, 176.3, 195.8, 199.0-199.2, 209.00-209.30, 209.70, 209.75, 239.0, 239.81-239.9

209.03 **Malignant carcinoid tumor of the ileum** `CC`
CC Excl: 152.2, 152.8-152.9, 159.0, 159.8-159.9, 176.3, 195.8, 199.0-199.2, 209.00-209.30, 209.70, 209.75, 239.0, 239.81-239.9

√5ᵗʰ **209.1** **Malignant carcinoid tumors of the appendix, large intestine, and rectum**

209.10 **Malignant carcinoid tumor of the large intestine,** `CC` **unspecified portion**
Malignant carcinoid tumor of the colon NOS
CC Excl: 153.8-153.9, 159.0, 159.8-159.9, 176.3, 195.8, 199.0-199.2, 209.00-209.30, 209.70, 209.75, 239.0, 239.81-239.9

209.11 **Malignant carcinoid tumor of the appendix** `CC`
CC Excl: 153.5, 153.8-153.9, 159.0, 159.8-159.9, 176.3, 195.8, 199.0-199.2, 209.00-209.30, 209.70, 209.75, 239.0, 239.81-239.9

209.12 **Malignant carcinoid tumor of the cecum** `CC`
CC Excl: 153.4, 153.8-153.9, 159.0, 159.8-159.9, 176.3, 195.8, 199.0-199.2, 209.00-209.30, 209.70, 209.75, 239.0, 239.81-239.9

209.13 **Malignant carcinoid tumor of the ascending colon** `CC`
CC Excl: 153.6, 153.8-153.9, 159.0, 159.8-159.9, 176.3, 195.8, 199.0-199.2, 209.00-209.30, 209.70, 209.75, 239.0, 239.81-239.9

209.14 **Malignant carcinoid tumor of the transverse colon** `CC`
CC Excl: 153.1, 153.8-153.9, 159.0, 159.8-159.9, 176.3, 195.8, 199.0-199.2, 209.00-209.30, 209.70, 209.75, 239.0, 239.81-239.9

209.15 **Malignant carcinoid tumor of the descending colon** `CC`
CC Excl: 153.2, 153.8-153.9, 159.0, 159.8-159.9, 176.3, 195.8, 199.0-199.2, 209.00-209.30, 209.70, 209.75, 239.0, 239.81-239.9

209.16 **Malignant carcinoid tumor of the sigmoid colon** `CC`
CC Excl: 153.3, 153.8-153.9, 159.0, 159.8-159.9, 176.3, 195.8, 199.0-199.2, 209.00-209.30, 209.70, 209.75, 239.0, 239.81-239.9

209.17 **Malignant carcinoid tumor of the rectum** `CC`
CC Excl: 154.1, 154.8, 159.0, 159.8-159.9, 176.3, 195.8, 199.0-199.2, 209.00-209.30, 209.70, 209.75, 239.0, 239.81-239.9

√5ᵗʰ **209.2** **Malignant carcinoid tumors of other and unspecified sites**

209.20 **Malignant carcinoid tumor of unknown** `CC` **primary site**
CC Excl: 195.8, 198.89-199.2, 209.00-209.30, 209.70, 209.75-209.79, 239.81-239.9

209.21 **Malignant carcinoid tumor of the bronchus and** `CC` **lung**
CC Excl: 162.8-162.9, 165.8-165.9, 176.4, 195.8, 199.0-199.2, 209.00-209.30, 209.70, 209.75, 239.1, 239.81-239.9

209.22 **Malignant carcinoid tumor of the thymus** `CC`
CC Excl: 164.0, 209.00-209.30

209.23 **Malignant carcinoid tumor of the stomach** `CC`
CC Excl: 151.0-151.9, 159.0, 159.8-159.9, 176.3, 195.8, 199.0-199.2, 209.00-209.30, 209.70, 209.75, 239.0, 239.81-239.9
AHA: 4Q, '08, 89

209.24 **Malignant carcinoid tumor of the kidney** `CC`
CC Excl: 189.0-189.1, 189.8-189.9, 195.8, 199.0-199.2, 209.00-209.30, 209.70, 209.75, 239.5, 239.81-239.9

209.25 **Malignant carcinoid tumor of the foregut NOS** `CC`
CC Excl: 151.0-151.9, 159.0, 159.8-159.9, 176.3, 195.8, 199.0-199.2, 209.00-209.30, 209.70, 239.0, 239.81-239.9

209.26 **Malignant carcinoid tumor of the midgut NOS** `CC`
CC Excl: 151.0-151.9, 159.0, 159.8-159.9, 176.3, 195.8, 199.0-199.2, 209.00-209.30, 209.70, 239.0, 239.81-239.9

209.27 **Malignant carcinoid tumor of the hindgut NOS** `CC`
CC Excl: 151.0-151.9, 159.0, 159.8-159.9, 176.3, 195.8, 199.0-199.2, 209.00-209.30, 209.70, 239.0, 239.81-239.9

209.29 **Malignant carcinoid tumor of the other sites** `CC`
CC Excl: 195.8, 198.89-199.2, 209.00-209.30, 209.70, 209.79, 239.81-239.9

√5ᵗʰ **209.3** **Malignant poorly differentiated neuroendocrine tumors**
AHA: 4Q, '09, 73,74

209.30 **Malignant poorly differentiated neuroendocrine** `CC` **carcinoma, any site**
High grade neuroendocrine carcinoma, any site
Malignant poorly differentiated neuroendocrine tumor NOS
EXCLUDES *Merkel cell carcinoma (209.31-209.36)*
CC Excl: 195.8, 198.89-199.2, 209.00-209.30, 209.70, 209.79, 239.81-239.9

209.31 **Merkel cell carcinoma of the face**
Merkel cell carcinoma of the ear
Merkel cell carcinoma of the eyelid, including canthus
Merkel cell carcinoma of the lip

209.32 **Merkel cell carcinoma of the scalp and neck**

209.33 **Merkel cell carcinoma of the upper limb**

209.34 **Merkel cell carcinoma of the lower limb**

209.35 **Merkel cell carcinoma of the trunk**

209.36 **Merkel cell carcinoma of other sites**
Merkel cell carcinoma of the buttock
Merkel cell carcinoma of the genitals
Merkel cell carcinoma NOS
AHA: 4Q, '09, 74

√5ᵗʰ **209.4** **Benign carcinoid tumors of the small intestine**

209.40 **Benign carcinoid tumor of the small intestine, unspecified portion**

209.41 **Benign carcinoid tumor of the duodenum**

209.42 **Benign carcinoid tumor of the jejunum**

209.43 **Benign carcinoid tumor of the ileum**

√5ᵗʰ **209.5** **Benign carcinoid tumors of the appendix, large intestine, and rectum**

209.50 **Benign carcinoid tumor of the large intestine, unspecified portion**
Benign carcinoid tumor of the colon NOS

209.51 **Benign carcinoid tumor of the appendix**

209.52 **Benign carcinoid tumor of the cecum**

209.53 **Benign carcinoid tumor of the ascending colon**

209.54 **Benign carcinoid tumor of the transverse colon**

209.55 **Benign carcinoid tumor of the descending colon**

209.56 **Benign carcinoid tumor of the sigmoid colon**

209.57 **Benign carcinoid tumor of the rectum**

√5ᵗʰ **209.6** **Benign carcinoid tumors of other and unspecified sites**

209.60 **Benign carcinoid tumor of unknown primary site**
Carcinoid tumor NOS
Neuroendocrine tumor NOS

209.61 **Benign carcinoid tumor of the bronchus and lung**
AHA: 4Q, '09, 151

209.62 **Benign carcinoid tumor of the thymus**

209.63 **Benign carcinoid tumor of the stomach**

209.64 **Benign carcinoid tumor of the kidney**

209.65 **Benign carcinoid tumor of the foregut NOS**

209.66 **Benign carcinoid tumor of the midgut NOS**

209.67 **Benign carcinoid tumor of the hindgut NOS**

209.69 **Benign carcinoid tumors of other sites**

Neoplasms

√5ᵗʰ **209.7 Secondary neuroendocrine tumors**
Secondary carcinoid tumors
AHA: 4Q, '09, 74

209.70 Secondary neuroendocrine tumor, unspecified site

209.71 Secondary neuroendocrine tumor of distant CC
lymph nodes
CC Excl: 176.5, 195.8-196.9, 199.0-199.2, 209.20,
209.29-209.30, 209.70-209.79, 239.81-239.9

209.72 Secondary neuroendocrine tumor of liver CC
CC Excl: 195.8, 197.7-197.8, 198.89-199.2, 209.20,
209.29-209.30, 209.70-209.79, 239.81-239.9

209.73 Secondary neuroendocrine tumor of bone CC
CC Excl: 195.8, 198.5, 198.89-199.2, 209.20, 209.29-209.30,
209.70-209.79, 239.81-239.9

209.74 Secondary neuroendocrine tumor of peritoneum CC
Mesentery metastasis of neuroendocrine tumor
CC Excl: 195.8, 197.6, 197.8, 198.89-199.2, 209.20,
209.29-209.30, 209.70-209.79, 239.81-239.9
AHA: 4Q, '11, 181; 4Q, '09, 150

209.75 Secondary Merkel cell carcinoma
Merkel cell carcinoma nodal presentation
Merkel cell carcinoma visceral metastatic
presentation
Secondary Merkel cell carcinoma, any site

209.79 Secondary neuroendocrine tumor of other sites CC
CC Excl: 195.8, 198.89-199.2, 209.20, 209.29-209.30,
209.70-209.79, 239.81-239.9

Benign Neoplasms (210-229)

√4ᵗʰ **210 Benign neoplasm of lip, oral cavity, and pharynx**
EXCLUDES *cyst (of):*
jaw (526.0-526.2, 526.89)
oral soft tissue (528.4)
radicular (522.8)

210.0 Lip
Frenulum labii
Lip (inner aspect) (mucosa) (vermilion border)
EXCLUDES *labial commissure (210.4)*
skin of lip (216.0)

210.1 Tongue
Lingual tonsil

210.2 Major salivary glands
Gland: Gland:
   parotid   submandibular
   sublingual
EXCLUDES *benign neoplasms of minor salivary glands:*
NOS (210.4)
buccal mucosa (210.4)
lips (210.0)
palate (hard) (soft) (210.4)
tongue (210.1)
tonsil, palatine (210.5)

210.3 Floor of mouth

210.4 Other and unspecified parts of mouth
Gingiva   Oral mucosa
Gum (upper) (lower)   Palate (hard) (soft)
Labial commissure   Uvula
Oral cavity NOS
EXCLUDES *benign odontogenic neoplasms of bone (213.0-213.1)*
developmental odontogenic cysts (526.0)
mucosa of lips (210.0)
nasopharyngeal [posterior] [superior] surface of soft
palate (210.7)

210.5 Tonsil
Tonsil (faucial) (palatine)
EXCLUDES *lingual tonsil (210.1)*
pharyngeal tonsil (210.7)
tonsillar:
fossa (210.6)
pillars (210.6)

210.6 Other parts of oropharynx
Branchial cleft or vestiges   Tonsillar:
Epiglottis, anterior aspect   fossa
Fauces NOS   pillars
Mesopharynx NOS   Vallecula
EXCLUDES *epiglottis:*
NOS (212.1)
suprahyoid portion (212.1)

210.7 Nasopharynx
Adenoid tissue   Pharyngeal tonsil
Lymphadenoid tissue   Posterior nasal septum

210.8 Hypopharynx
Arytenoid fold   Postcricoid region
Laryngopharynx   Pyriform fossa

210.9 Pharynx, unspecified
Throat NOS

√4ᵗʰ **211 Benign neoplasm of other parts of digestive system**
EXCLUDES *benign stromal tumors of digestive system (215.5)*

211.0 Esophagus

211.1 Stomach
Body
Cardia   } of stomach
Fundus
Cardiac orifice
Pylorus
EXCLUDES *benign carcinoid tumors of the stomach (209.63)*
D13.1 Benign neoplasm of stomach   I-10

211.2 Duodenum, jejunum, and ileum
Small intestine NOS
EXCLUDES *ampulla of Vater (211.5)*
benign carcinoid tumors of the small intestine
(209.40-209.43)
ileocecal valve (211.3)

211.3 Colon
Appendix   Ileocecal valve
Cecum   Large intestine NOS
EXCLUDES *benign carcinoid tumors of the large intestine*
(209.50-209.56)
rectosigmoid junction (211.4)
AHA: 2Q, '11, 9; 3Q, '05, 17; 2Q, '05, 16; 4Q, '01, 56
D12.6 Benign neoplasm of colon unspecified   I-10

211.4 Rectum and anal canal
Anal canal or sphincter   Rectosigmoid junction
Anus NOS
EXCLUDES *anus:*
margin (216.5)
skin (216.5)
benign carcinoid tumors of the rectum (209.57)
perianal skin (216.5)
AHA: 2Q, '11, 9

211.5 Liver and biliary passages
Ampulla of Vater   Gallbladder
Common bile duct   Hepatic duct
Cystic duct   Sphincter of Oddi

211.6 Pancreas, except islets of Langerhans

211.7 Islets of Langerhans
Islet cell tumor
Use additional code to identify any functional activity

211.8 Retroperitoneum and peritoneum
Mesentery   Omentum
Mesocolon   Retroperitoneal tissue

211.9 Other and unspecified site
Alimentary tract NOS
Digestive system NOS
Gastrointestinal tract NOS
Intestinal tract NOS
Intestine NOS
Spleen, not elsewhere classified

☑4ᵗʰ **212 Benign neoplasm of respiratory and intrathoracic organs**

212.0 Nasal cavities, middle ear, and accessory sinuses
Cartilage of nose   Sinus:
Eustachian tube   ethmoidal
Nares   frontal
Septum of nose   maxillary
                           sphenoidal

EXCLUDES auditory canal (external) (216.2)
bone of:
ear (213.0)
nose [turbinates] (213.0)
cartilage of ear (215.0)
ear (external) (skin) (216.2)
nose NOS (229.8)
skin (216.3)
olfactory bulb (225.1)
polyp of:
accessory sinus (471.8)
ear (385.30-385.35)
nasal cavity (471.0)
posterior margin of septum and choanae (210.7)

212.1 Larynx
Cartilage: Epiglottis (suprahyoid portion) NOS
arytenoid   Glottis
cricoid   Vocal cords (false)(true)
cuneiform
thyroid

EXCLUDES epiglottis, anterior aspect (210.6)
polyp of vocal cord or larynx (478.4)

212.2 Trachea

212.3 Bronchus and lung
Carina
Hilus of lung

EXCLUDES benign carcinoid tumors of bronchus and lung
(209.61)

212.4 Pleura

212.5 Mediastinum

212.6 Thymus
EXCLUDES benign carcinoid tumors of thymus (209.62)

212.7 Heart
EXCLUDES great vessels (215.4)

212.8 Other specified sites

212.9 Site unspecified
Respiratory organ NOS
Upper respiratory tract NOS
EXCLUDES intrathoracic NOS (229.8)
thoracic NOS (229.8)

☑4ᵗʰ **213 Benign neoplasm of bone and articular cartilage**
INCLUDES cartilage (articular) (joint)
periosteum
EXCLUDES cartilage of:
ear (215.0)
eyelid (215.0))
larynx (212.1)
nose (212.0)
exostosis NOS (726.91
synovia (215.0-215.9)

213.0 Bones of skull and face
EXCLUDES lower jaw bone (213.1)

213.1 Lower jaw bone

213.2 Vertebral column, excluding sacrum and coccyx

213.3 Ribs, sternum, and clavicle

213.4 Scapula and long bones of upper limb

213.5 Short bones of upper limb

213.6 Pelvic bones, sacrum, and coccyx

213.7 Long bones of lower limb

213.8 Short bones of lower limb

213.9 Bone and articular cartilage, site unspecified

☑4ᵗʰ **214 Lipoma**
INCLUDES angiolipoma
fibrolipoma
hibernoma
lipoma (fetal) (infiltrating) (intramuscular)
myelolipoma
myxolipoma
DEF: Benign tumor frequently composed of mature fat cells; may
occasionally be composed of fetal fat cells.

214.0 Skin and subcutaneous tissue of face

214.1 Other skin and subcutaneous tissue

214.2 Intrathoracic organs

214.3 Intra-abdominal organs

214.4 Spermatic cord   ♂

214.8 Other specified sites
AHA: 3Q, '94, 7

214.9 Lipoma, unspecified site

☑4ᵗʰ **215 Other benign neoplasm of connective and other soft tissue**
INCLUDES blood vessel
bursa
fascia
ligament
muscle
peripheral, sympathetic, and parasympathetic nerves and
ganglia
synovia
tendon (sheath)
EXCLUDES cartilage:
articular (213.0-213.9)
larynx (212.1)
nose (212.0)
connective tissue of:
breast (217)
internal organ, except lipoma and hemangioma — code
to benign neoplasm of the site
lipoma (214.0-214.9)

215.0 Head, face, and neck

215.2 Upper limb, including shoulder

215.3 Lower limb, including hip

215.4 Thorax
EXCLUDES heart (212.7)
mediastinum (212.5)
thymus (212.6)

215.5 Abdomen
Abdominal wall
Benign stromal tumors of abdomen
Hypochondrium

215.6 Pelvis
Buttock   Inguinal region
Groin   Perineum
EXCLUDES uterine:
leiomyoma (218.0-218.9)
ligament, any (221.0)

215.7 Trunk, unspecified
Back NOS   Flank NOS

215.8 Other specified sites

215.9 Site unspecified

☑4ᵗʰ **216 Benign neoplasm of skin**
INCLUDES blue nevus
dermatofibroma
hydrocystoma
pigmented nevus
syringoadenoma
syringoma
EXCLUDES skin of genital organs (221.0-222.9)
AHA: 1Q, '00, 21

216.0 Skin of lip
EXCLUDES vermilion border of lip (210.0)

216.1 Eyelid, including canthus
EXCLUDES cartilage of eyelid (215.0)

N Newborn Age: 0   P Pediatric Age: 0-17   M Maternity Age: 12-55   A Adult Age: 15-124   MCC Major CC Condition   CC CC Condition   HIV HIV Related Dx

52 – Volume 1   2014 ICD-9-CM

216.2 Ear and external auditory canal
Auricle (ear)   External meatus
Auricular canal, external Pinna
EXCLUDES *cartilage of ear (215.0)*

216.3 Skin of other and unspecified parts of face
Cheek, external   Nose, external
Eyebrow   Temple

216.4 Scalp and skin of neck
AHA: 3Q, '91, 12

216.5 Skin of trunk, except scrotum
Axillary fold   Skin of:
Perianal skin   buttock
Skin of: chest wall
   abdominal wall   groin
   anus   perineum
   back   Umbilicus
   breast
EXCLUDES *anal canal (211.4)*
anus NOS (211.4)
skin of scrotum (222.4)

216.6 Skin of upper limb, including shoulder

216.7 Skin of lower limb, including hip

216.8 Other specified sites of skin

216.9 Skin, site unspecified

217 Benign neoplasm of breast
Breast (male) (female):   Breast (male) (female):
   connective tissue   soft parts
   glandular tissue
EXCLUDES *adenofibrosis (610.2)*
benign cyst of breast (610.0)
fibrocystic disease (610.1)
skin of breast (216.5)
AHA: 1Q, '00, 4

✓4ᵗʰ 218 Uterine leiomyoma
INCLUDES fibroid (bleeding) (uterine)
uterine:
   fibromyoma
   myoma
DEF: Benign tumor primarily derived from uterine smooth muscle tissue; may contain fibrous, fatty, or epithelial tissue; also called uterine fibroid or myoma.

218.0 Submucous leiomyoma of uterus ♀

218.1 Intramural leiomyoma of uterus ♀
Interstitial leiomyoma of uterus
D25.1 Intramural leiomyoma of uterus   I-10

218.2 Subserous leiomyoma of uterus ♀

218.9 Leiomyoma of uterus, unspecified ♀
AHA: 1Q, '03, 4
D25.9 Leiomyoma of uterus unspecified   I-10

✓4ᵗʰ 219 Other benign neoplasm of uterus

219.0 Cervix uteri ♀

219.1 Corpus uteri ♀
Endometrium   Myometrium
Fundus

219.8 Other specified parts of uterus ♀

219.9 Uterus, part unspecified ♀

220 Benign neoplasm of ovary ♀
Use additional code to identify any functional activity (256.0-256.1)
EXCLUDES *cyst:*
corpus albicans (620.2)
corpus luteum (620.1)
endometrial (617.1)
follicular (atretic) (620.0)
graafian follicle (620.0)
ovarian NOS (620.2)
retention (620.2)
D27.9 Benign neoplasm of unspec ovary   I-10

Types of Uterine Fibroids

✓4ᵗʰ 221 Benign neoplasm of other female genital organs
INCLUDES adenomatous polyp
benign teratoma
EXCLUDES *cyst:*
epoophoron (752.11)
fimbrial (752.11)
Gartner's duct (752.11)
parovarian (752.11)

221.0 Fallopian tube and uterine ligaments ♀
Oviduct
Parametruim
Uterine ligament (broad) (round) (uterosacral)
Uterine tube

221.1 Vagina ♀

221.2 Vulva ♀
Clitoris
External female genitalia NOS
Greater vestibular [Bartholin's] gland
Labia (majora) (minora)
Pudendum
EXCLUDES *Bartholin's (duct) (gland) cyst (616.2)*

221.8 Other specified sites of female genital organs ♀

221.9 Female genital organ, site unspecified ♀
Female genitourinary tract NOS

✓4ᵗʰ 222 Benign neoplasm of male genital organs

222.0 Testis ♂
Use additional code to identify any functional activity

222.1 Penis ♂
Corpus cavernosum   Prepuce
Glans penis

222.2 Prostate ♂
EXCLUDES *adenomatous hyperplasia of prostate*
(600.20-600.21)
prostatic:
adenoma (600.20-600.21)
enlargement (600.00-600.01)
hypertrophy (600.00-600.01)

222.3 Epididymis ♂

222.4 Scrotum ♂
Skin of scrotum

222.8 Other specified sites of male genital organs ♂
Seminal vesicle   Spermatic cord

222.9 Male genital organ, site unspecified ♂
Male genitourinary tract NOS

✓4ᵗʰ 223 Benign neoplasm of kidney and other urinary organs

223.0 Kidney, except pelvis
Kidney NOS
EXCLUDES *benign carcinoid tumors of kidney (209.64)*
renal:
calyces (223.1)
pelvis (223.1)

223.1 Renal pelvis

223.2 Ureter
EXCLUDES *ureteric orifice of bladder (223.3)*

4ᵗʰ/5ᵗʰ Additional Digit Required   Unacceptable PDx   Manifestation Code   Hospital Acquired Condition   ▶◀ Revised Text   ● New Code   ▲ Revised Code Title

2014 ICD-9-CM   Volume 1 – 53

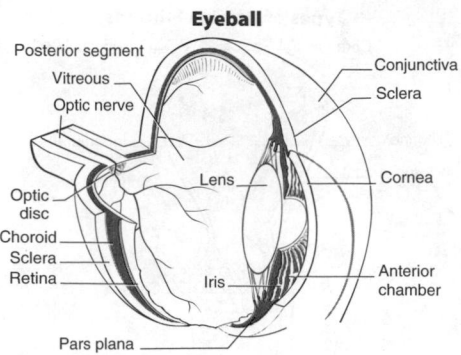

Eyeball

Posterior segment
Vitreous
Optic nerve
Conjunctiva
Sclera
Optic disc
Choroid
Sclera
Retina
Lens
Cornea
Iris
Anterior chamber
Pars plana

223.3 Bladder

✓5ᵗʰ **223.8 Other specified sites of urinary organs**

223.81 Urethra
EXCLUDES *urethral orifice of bladder (223.3)*

223.89 Other
Paraurethral glands

223.9 Urinary organ, site unspecified
Urinary system NOS

✓4ᵗʰ **224 Benign neoplasm of eye**
EXCLUDES *cartilage of eyelid (215.0)*
eyelid (skin) (216.1)
optic nerve (225.1)
orbital bone (213.0)

224.0 Eyeball, except conjunctiva, cornea, retina, and choroid
Ciliary body   Sclera
Iris   Uveal tract

224.1 Orbit
EXCLUDES *bone of orbit (213.0)*

224.2 Lacrimal gland

224.3 Conjunctiva

224.4 Cornea

224.5 Retina
EXCLUDES *hemangioma of retina (228.03)*

224.6 Choroid

224.7 Lacrimal duct
Lacrimal sac   Nasolacrimal duct

224.8 Other specified parts of eye

224.9 Eye, part unspecified

✓4ᵗʰ **225 Benign neoplasm of brain and other parts of nervous system**
EXCLUDES *hemangioma (228.02)*
neurofibromatosis (237.70-237.79)
peripheral, sympathetic, and parasympathetic nerves and ganglia (215.0-215.9)
retrobulbar (224.1)

225.0 Brain

225.1 Cranial nerves
Acoustic neuroma
AHA: 4Q, '04, 113

225.2 Cerebral meninges
Meninges NOS   Meningioma (cerebral)
D32.0 Benign neoplasm of cerebral meninges   I-10

225.3 Spinal cord
Cauda equina

225.4 Spinal meninges
Spinal meningioma

225.8 Other specified sites of nervous system

225.9 Nervous system, part unspecified
Nervous system (central) NOS
EXCLUDES *meninges NOS (225.2)*

226 Benign neoplasm of thyroid glands
Use additional code to identify any functional activity

✓4ᵗʰ **227 Benign neoplasm of other endocrine glands and related structures**
Use additional code to identify any functional activity
EXCLUDES *ovary (220)*
pancreas (211.6)
testis (222.0)

227.0 Adrenal gland
Suprarenal gland

227.1 Parathyroid gland

227.3 Pituitary gland and craniopharyngeal duct (pouch)
Craniobuccal pouch   Rathke's pouch
Hypophysis   Sella turcica

227.4 Pineal gland
Pineal body

227.5 Carotid body

227.6 Aortic body and other paraganglia
Coccygeal body   Para-aortic body
Glomus jugulare
AHA: N-D, '84, 17

227.8 Other

227.9 Endocrine gland, site unspecified

✓4ᵗʰ **228 Hemangioma and lymphangioma, any site**
INCLUDES angioma (benign) (cavernous) (congenital) NOS
cavernous nevus
glomus tumor
hemangioma (benign) (congenital)
EXCLUDES *benign neoplasm of spleen, except hemangioma and lymphangioma (211.9)*
glomus jugulare (227.6)
nevus:
NOS (216.0-216.9)
blue or pigmented (216.0-216.9)
vascular (757.32)
AHA: 1Q, '00, 21

✓5ᵗʰ **228.0 Hemangioma, any site**
DEF: A common benign tumor usually occurring in infancy; composed of newly formed blood vessels due to malformation of angioblastic tissue.
AHA: J-F, '85, 19

228.00 Of unspecified site

228.01 Of skin and subcutaneous tissue
AHA: 3Q, '10, 16

228.02 Of intracranial structures

228.03 Of retina

228.04 Of intra-abdominal structures
Peritoneum
Retroperitoneal tissue

228.09 Of other sites
Systemic angiomatosis
AHA: 3Q, '91, 20

228.1 Lymphangioma, any site
Congenital lymphangioma
Lymphatic nevus

✓4ᵗʰ **229 Benign neoplasm of other and unspecified sites**

229.0 Lymph nodes
EXCLUDES *lymphangioma (228.1)*

229.8 Other specified sites
Intrathoracic NOS
Thoracic NOS

229.9 Site unspecified

N Newborn Age: 0   P Pediatric Age: 0-17   M Maternity Age: 12-55   A Adult Age: 15-124   MCC Major CC Condition   CC CC Condition   HIV HIV Related D

Carcinoma In Situ (230-234)

INCLUDES Bowen's disease
erythroplasia
Queyrat's erythroplasia

EXCLUDES *leukoplakia — see Alphabetic Index*

DEF: A neoplastic type; with tumor cells confined to epithelium of origin; without further invasion.

4ᵗʰ 230 Carcinoma in situ of digestive organs

230.0 Lip, oral cavity, and pharynx

Gingiva	Oropharynx
Hypopharynx	Salivary gland or duct
Mouth [any part]	Tongue
Nasopharynx	

EXCLUDES *aryepiglottic fold or interarytenoid fold, laryngeal aspect (231.0)*
epiglottis:
NOS (231.0)
suprahyoid portion (231.0)
skin of lip (232.0)

230.1 Esophagus

230.2 Stomach

Body
Cardia } of stomach
Fundus
Cardiac orifice
Pylorus

230.3 Colon

Appendix
Cecum
Ileocecal valve
Large intestine NOS

EXCLUDES *rectosigmoid junction (230.4)*

230.4 Rectum

Rectosigmoid junction

230.5 Anal canal

Anal sphincter

230.6 Anus, unspecified

EXCLUDES *anus:*
margin (232.5)
skin (232.5)
perianal skin (232.5)

230.7 Other and unspecified parts of intestine

Duodenum
Ileum
Jejunum
Small intestine NOS

EXCLUDES *ampulla of Vater (230.8)*

230.8 Liver and biliary system

Ampulla of Vater
Common bile duct
Cystic duct
Gallbladder
Hepatic duct
Sphincter of Oddi

230.9 Other and unspecified digestive organs

Digestive organ NOS
Gastrointestinal tract NOS
Pancreas
Spleen

4ᵗʰ 231 Carcinoma in situ of respiratory system

231.0 Larynx

Cartilage:	Epiglottis:
arytenoid	NOS
cricoid	posterior surface
cuneiform	suprahyoid portion
thyroid	Vocal cords (false)(true)

EXCLUDES *aryepiglottic fold or interarytenoid fold:*
NOS (230.0)
hypopharyngeal aspect (230.0)
marginal zone (230.0)

231.1 Trachea

231.2 Bronchus and lung

Carina   Hilus of lung

231.8 Other specified parts of respiratory system

Accessory sinuses
Middle ear
Nasal cavities
Pleura

EXCLUDES *ear (external) (skin) (232.2)*
nose NOS (234.8)
skin (232.3)

231.9 Respiratory system, part unspecified

Respiratory organ NOS

✓4ᵗʰ 232 Carcinoma in situ of skin

INCLUDES pigment cells

EXCLUDES *melanoma in situ of skin (172.0-172.9)*

232.0 Skin of lip

EXCLUDES *vermilion border of lip (230.0)*

232.1 Eyelid, including canthus

232.2 Ear and external auditory canal

232.3 Skin of other and unspecified parts of face

232.4 Scalp and skin of neck

232.5 Skin of trunk, except scrotum

Anus, margin	Skin of:
Axillary fold	breast
Perianal skin	buttock
Skin of:	chest wall
abdominal wall	groin
anus	perineum
back	Umbilicus

EXCLUDES *anal canal (230.5)*
anus NOS (230.6)
skin of genital organs (233.30-233.39, 233.5-233.6)

232.6 Skin of upper limb, including shoulder

232.7 Skin of lower limb, including hip

232.8 Other specified sites of skin

232.9 Skin, site unspecified

✓4ᵗʰ 233 Carcinoma in situ of breast and genitourinary system

TIP: For patients with carcinoma in situ found incidentally when admitted for treatment of another condition, sequence the 233 code as a secondary condition.

233.0 Breast

EXCLUDES *Paget's disease (174.0-174.9)*
skin of breast (232.5)

TIP: Assign for tumors specified as intraductal carcinoma.

233.1 Cervix uteri ♀

Adenocarcinoma in situ of cervix
Cervical intraepithelial glandular neoplasia, grade III
Cervical intraepithelial neoplasia III [CIN III]
Severe dysplasia of cervix

EXCLUDES *cervical intraepithelial neoplasia II [CIN II] (622.12)*
cytologic evidence of malignancy without histologic confirmation (795.06)
high grade squamous intraepithelial lesion (HGSIL) (795.04)
moderate dysplasia of cervix (622.12)

AHA: 3Q, '92, 7; 3Q, '92, 8; 1Q, '91, 11

233.2 Other and unspecified parts of uterus ♀

✓5ᵗʰ 233.3 Other and unspecified female genital organs

AHA: 4Q, '07, 67

233.30 Unspecified female genital organ ♀

233.31 Vagina ♀

Severe dysplasia of vagina
Vaginal intraepithelial neoplasia III [VAIN III]

233.32 Vulva ♀

Severe dysplasia of vulva
Vulvar intraepithelial neoplasia III [VIN III]

233.39 Other female genital organ ♀

233.4 Prostate ♂

Additional Digit Required   Unacceptable PDx   Manifestation Code   Hospital Acquired Condition   ▶◀ Revised Text   ● New Code   ▲ Revised Code Title

4 ICD-9-CM   Volume 1 – 55

Neoplasms

233.5–237.79

233.5 Penis   ♂

233.6 Other and unspecified male genital organs   ♂

233.7 Bladder
     AHA: ▶2Q, '12, 10◀

233.9 Other and unspecified urinary organs

√4ᵗʰ **234 Carcinoma in situ of other and unspecified sites**

234.0 Eye
     EXCLUDES   *cartilage of eyelid (234.8)*
               eyelid (skin) (232.1)
               optic nerve (234.8)
               orbital bone (234.8)

234.8 Other specified sites
     Endocrine gland [any]

234.9 Site unspecified
     Carcinoma in situ NOS

Neoplasms Of Uncertain Behavior (235-238)

NOTE   Categories 235–238 classify by site certain histomorphologically well-defined neoplasms, the subsequent behavior of which cannot be predicted from the present appearance.

TIP: Typically assigned for cases in which the tumor is in transition and may be undergoing malignant transformation, but continued study is required for accurate classification.

√4ᵗʰ **235 Neoplasm of uncertain behavior of digestive and respiratory systems**
     EXCLUDES   *stromal tumors of uncertain behavior of digestive system (238.1)*

235.0 Major salivary glands
     Gland:
       parotid
       sublingual
       submandibular
     EXCLUDES   *minor salivary glands (235.1)*

235.1 Lip, oral cavity, and pharynx
     Gingiva   Nasopharynx
     Hypopharynx   Oropharynx
     Minor salivary glands   Tongue
     Mouth
     EXCLUDES   *aryepiglottic fold or interarytenoid fold, laryngeal*
                 aspect (235.6)
               epiglottis:
                 NOS (235.6)
                 suprahyoid portion (235.6)
               skin of lip (238.2)

235.2 Stomach, intestines, and rectum

235.3 Liver and biliary passages
     Ampulla of Vater
     Bile ducts [any]
     Gallbladder
     Liver

235.4 Retroperitoneum and peritoneum

235.5 Other and unspecified digestive organs
     Anal: Esophagus
       canal   Pancreas
       sphincter   Spleen
     Anus NOS
     EXCLUDES   *anus:*
                 margin (238.2)
                 skin (238.2)
               perianal skin (238.2)

235.6 Larynx
     EXCLUDES   *aryepiglottic fold or interarytenoid fold:*
                 NOS (235.1)
                 hypopharyngeal aspect (235.1)
                 marginal zone (235.1)

235.7 Trachea, bronchus, and lung

235.8 Pleura, thymus, and mediastinum

235.9 Other and unspecified respiratory organs
     Accessory sinuses   Nasal cavities
     Middle ear   Respiratory organ NOS
     EXCLUDES   *ear (external) (skin) (238.2)*
                 nose (238.8)
                 skin (238.2)

√4ᵗʰ **236 Neoplasm of uncertain behavior of genitourinary organs**

236.0 Uterus

236.1 Placenta
     Chorioadenoma (destruens)
     Invasive mole
     Malignant hydatid mole
     Malignant hydatidiform mole

236.2 Ovary
     Use additional code to identify any functional activity

236.3 Other and unspecified female genital organs

236.4 Testis
     Use additional code to identify any functional activity

236.5 Prostate

236.6 Other and unspecified male genital organs

236.7 Bladder

√5ᵗʰ **236.9 Other and unspecified urinary organs**

     236.90 Urinary organ, unspecified

     236.91 Kidney and ureter

     236.99 Other

√4ᵗʰ **237 Neoplasm of uncertain behavior of endocrine glands and nervous system**

237.0 Pituitary gland and craniopharyngeal duct
     Use additional code to identify any functional activity

237.1 Pineal gland

237.2 Adrenal gland
     Suprarenal gland
     Use additional code to identify any functional activity

237.3 Paraganglia
     Aortic body   Coccygeal body
     Carotid body   Glomus jugulare
     AHA: N-D, '84, 17

237.4 Other and unspecified endocrine glands
     Parathyroid gland   Thyroid gland

237.5 Brain and spinal cord

237.6 Meninges
     Meninges:
       NOS
       cerebral
       spinal

√5ᵗʰ **237.7 Neurofibromatosis**
     DEF: An inherited condition with developmental changes in the nervous system, muscles, bones and skin; multiple soft tumors (neurofibromas) distributed over the entire body.

     237.70 Neurofibromatosis, unspecified

     237.71 Neurofibromatosis, type 1 [von Recklinghausen's disease]
         AHA: 4Q, '10, 76

     237.72 Neurofibromatosis, type 2 [acoustic neurofibromatosis]
         DEF: Inherited condition with cutaneous lesions, benign tumors of peripheral nerves and bilateral 8th nerve masse
         AHA: 4Q, '10, 76

     237.73 Schwannomatosis
         DEF: A genetic mutation (SMARCB1/INI1) causing multipl benign tumors along nerve pathways, characterized by th exception of 8th cranial nerve involvement.
         AHA: 4Q, '10, 76-77

     237.79 Other neurofibromatosis
         AHA: 4Q, '10, 76-77

N Newborn Age: 0   P Pediatric Age: 0-17   M Maternity Age: 12-55   A Adult Age: 15-124   MCC Major CC Condition   CC CC Condition   HIV HIV Related C

56 – Volume 1 · February 2013   **2014 ICD-9-C**

237.9 Other and unspecified parts of nervous system
Cranial nerves
EXCLUDES *peripheral, sympathetic, and parasympathetic nerves and ganglia (238.1)*

√4ᵗʰ **238 Neoplasm of uncertain behavior of other and unspecified sites and tissues**

238.0 Bone and articular cartilage
EXCLUDES *cartilage:*
ear (238.1)
eyelid (238.1)
larynx (235.6)
nose (235.9)
synovia (238.1)
AHA: 4Q, '04, 128

238.1 Connective and other soft tissue
Peripheral, sympathetic, and parasympathetic nerves and ganglia
Stromal tumors of digestive system
EXCLUDES *cartilage (of):*
articular (238.0)
larynx (235.6)
nose (235.9)
connective tissue of breast (238.3)

238.2 Skin
EXCLUDES *anus NOS (235.5)*
skin of genital organs (236.3, 236.6)
vermilion border of lip (235.1)
TIP: Assign when documentation indicates keratocanthoma only.

238.3 Breast
EXCLUDES *skin of breast (238.2)*

238.4 Polycythemia vera
DEF: Abnormal proliferation of all bone marrow elements, increased red cell mass and total blood volume; unknown etiology, frequently associated with splenomegaly, leukocytosis, and thrombocythemia.
D45 Polycythemia vera   I-10

238.5 Histiocytic and mast cells   CC
Mast cell tumor NOS
Mastocytoma NOS
CC Excl: 238.4-238.76, 238.79, 289.83, V58.0

238.6 Plasma cells   CC
Plasmacytoma NOS
Solitary myeloma
CC Excl: See code: 238.5

√5ᵗʰ **238.7 Other lymphatic and hematopoietic tissues**
EXCLUDES *acute myelogenous leukemia (205.0)*
chronic myelomonocytic leukemia (205.1)
myelosclerosis NOS (289.89)
myelosis:
NOS (205.9)
megakaryocytic (207.2)
AHA: 3Q, '01, 13; 1Q, '97, 5; 2Q, '89, 8

238.71 Essential thrombocythemia
Essential hemorrhagic thrombocythemia
Essential thrombocytosis
Idiopathic (hemorrhagic) thrombocythemia
Primary thrombocytosis
AHA: 4Q, '06, 63-66
D47.3 Essential (hemorrhagic) thrombocythemia   I-10

238.72 Low grade myelodysplastic syndrome lesions
Refractory anemia (RA)
Refractory anemia with excess blasts-1 (RAEB-1)
Refractory anemia with ringed sideroblasts (RARS)
Refractory cytopenia with multilineage dysplasia (RCMD)
Refractory cytopenia with multilineage dysplasia and ringed sideroblasts (RCMD-RS)
DEF: Refractory anemia (RA): Form of bone marrow disorder (myelodysplastic syndrome) that interferes with red blood cell production in the bone marrow; unresponsive to hematinics; characteristic normal or hypercellular marrow with abnormal erythrocyte development and reticulocytopenia.
AHA: 4Q, '06, 63-66

238.73 High grade myelodysplastic syndrome lesions   CC
Refractory anemia with excess blasts-2 (RAEB-2)
CC Excl: 202.40-202.48, 203.10-203.11, 203.80-203.81, 204.00-208.92, 238.4-238.76, 238.79-238.9
AHA: 4Q, '06, 63-66

238.74 Myelodysplastic syndrome with 5q deletion   CC
5q minus syndrome NOS
EXCLUDES *constitutional 5q deletion (758.39)*
high grade myelodysplastic syndrome with 5q deletion (238.73)
CC Excl: See code: 238.73
AHA: 4Q, '06, 63-66

238.75 Myelodysplastic syndrome, unspecified
AHA: 4Q, '06, 63-66
D46.9 Myelodysplastic syndrome unspecified   I-10

238.76 Myelofibrosis with myeloid metaplasia   CC
Agnogenic myeloid metaplasia
Idiopathic myelofibrosis (chronic)
Myelosclerosis with myeloid metaplasia
Primary myelofibrosis
EXCLUDES *myelofibrosis NOS (289.83)*
myelophthisic anemia (284.2)
myelophthisis (284.2)
secondary myelofibrosis (289.83)
CC Excl: See code: 238.73
AHA: 4Q, '06, 63-66

238.77 Post-transplant lymphoproliferative disorder [PTLD]   CC
Code first complications of transplant (996.80-996.89)
DEF: Excessive proliferation of B-cell lymphocytes following Epstein-Barr virus infection in organ transplant patients; may progress to non-Hodgkins lymphoma.
CC Excl: 238.77, 996.80, 996.87, 997.91-997.99
AHA: 4Q, '08, 90-91

238.79 Other lymphatic and hematopoietic tissues   CC
Lymphoproliferative disease (chronic) NOS
Megakaryocytic myelosclerosis
Myeloproliferative disease (chronic) NOS
Panmyelosis (acute)
CC Excl: 202.40-202.48, 203.10-203.11, 203.80-203.81, 204.00-208.92, 238.4-238.76, 238.79-238.9
AHA: 4Q, '06, 63-66

238.8 Other specified sites
Eye
Heart
EXCLUDES *eyelid (skin) (238.2)*
cartilage (238.1)

238.9 Site unspecified

Neoplasms of Unspecified Nature (239)

√4ᵗʰ **239 Neoplasms of unspecified nature**
NOTE Category 239 classifies by site neoplasms of unspecified morphology and behavior. The term "mass," unless otherwise stated, is not to be regarded as a neoplastic growth.
INCLUDES "growth" NOS
neoplasm NOS
new growth NOS
tumor NOS
TIP: Do not assign for inpatient cases; more information should be available.

239.0 Digestive system
EXCLUDES *anus:*
margin (239.2)
skin (239.2)
perianal skin (239.2)

239.1 Respiratory system

239.2 Bone, soft tissue, and skin

> EXCLUDES   anal canal (239.0)
>   anus NOS (239.0)
>   bone marrow (202.9)
>   cartilage:
>   larynx (239.1)
>   nose (239.1)
>   connective tissue of breast (239.3)
>   skin of genital organs (239.5)
>   vermilion border of lip (239.0)

239.3 Breast

> EXCLUDES   skin of breast (239.2)

239.4 Bladder

239.5 Other genitourinary organs

239.6 Brain

> EXCLUDES   cerebral meninges (239.7)
>   cranial nerves (239.7)

239.7 Endocrine glands and other parts of nervous system

> EXCLUDES   peripheral, sympathetic, and parasympathetic nerves
>   and ganglia (239.2)

√5th **239.8 Other specified sites**

> EXCLUDES   eyelid (skin) (239.2)
>   cartilage (239.2)
>   great vessels (239.2)
>   optic nerve (239.7)

AHA: 4Q, '09, 75

239.81 Retina and choroid
Dark area on retina
Retinal freckle

TIP: Assign for documentation of retinal "freckles" or spots that may be indicative of malignant melanoma. Histologic confirmation not required.

239.89 Other specified sites

239.9 Site unspecified

N Newborn Age: 0   P Pediatric Age: 0-17   M Maternity Age: 12-55   A Adult Age: 15-124   MCC Major CC Condition   CC CC Condition   HIV HIV Related Dx

58 – Volume 1   **2014 ICD-9-CM**

3. Endocrine, Nutritional and Metabolic Diseases, and Immunity Disorders (240-279)

EXCLUDES *endocrine and metabolic disturbances specific to the fetus and newborn (775.0-775.9)*

NOTE All neoplasms, whether functionally active or not, are classified in Chapter 2. Codes in Chapter 3 (i.e., 242.8, 246.0, 251-253, 255-259) may be used to identify such functional activity associated with any neoplasm, or by ectopic endocrine tissue.

Disorders of Thyroid Gland (240-246)

✓4ᵗʰ **240 Simple and unspecified goiter**

DEF: An enlarged thyroid gland often caused by an inadequate dietary intake of iodine.

240.0 Goiter, specified as simple

Any condition classifiable to 240.9, specified as simple

240.9 Goiter, unspecified

Enlargement of thyroid
Goiter or struma:
  NOS
  diffuse colloid
  endemic

Goiter or struma:
  hyperplastic
  nontoxic (diffuse)
  parenchymatous
  sporadic

EXCLUDES *congenital (dyshormonogenic) goiter (246.1)*

✓4ᵗʰ **241 Nontoxic nodular goiter**

EXCLUDES *adenoma of thyroid (226)*
cystadenoma of thyroid (226)

241.0 Nontoxic uninodular goiter

Thyroid nodule   Uninodular goiter (nontoxic)

DEF: Enlarged thyroid, commonly due to decreased thyroid production, with single nodule; no clinical hypothyroidism.

E04.1 Nontoxic single thyroid nodule   **I-10**

241.1 Nontoxic multinodular goiter

Multinodular goiter (nontoxic)

DEF: Enlarged thyroid, commonly due to decreased thyroid production with multiple nodules; no clinical hypothyroidism.

241.9 Unspecified nontoxic nodular goiter

Adenomatous goiter
Nodular goiter (nontoxic) NOS
Struma nodosa (simplex)

✓4ᵗʰ **242 Thyrotoxicosis with or without goiter**

EXCLUDES *neonatal thyrotoxicosis (775.3)*

DEF: A condition caused by excess quantities of thyroid hormones being introduced into the tissues

The following fifth-digit subclassification is for use with categories 242:
  0 without mention of thyrotoxic crisis or storm
  1 with mention of thyrotoxic crisis or storm

§ ✓5ᵗʰ **242.0 Toxic diffuse goiter**   **MCC 1**
[0-1]

Basedow's disease
Exophthalmic or toxic goiter NOS
Graves' disease
Primary thyroid hyperplasia

DEF: Diffuse thyroid enlargement accompanied by hyperthyroidism, bulging eyes, and dermopathy.

CC Excl: For code 242.01: 017.50-017.56, 017.90-017.96, 240.0-246.9, 259.50-259.9

§ ✓5ᵗʰ **242.1 Toxic uninodular goiter**   **MCC 1**
[0-1]

Thyroid nodule
Uninodular goiter } toxic or with hyperthyroidism

DEF: Symptomatic hyperthyroidism with a single nodule on the enlarged thyroid gland. Abrupt onset of symptoms; including extreme nervousness, insomnia, weight loss, tremors, and psychosis or coma.

CC Excl: See code 242.0

§ ✓5ᵗʰ **242.2 Toxic multinodular goiter**   **MCC 1**
[0-1]

Secondary thyroid hyperplasia

DEF: Symptomatic hyperthyroidism with multiple nodules on the enlarged thyroid gland. Abrupt onset of symptoms; including extreme nervousness, insomnia, weight loss, tremors, and psychosis or coma.

CC Excl: See code 242.0

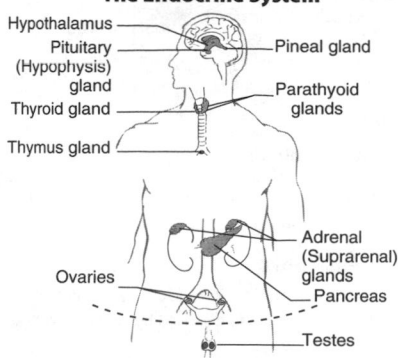

The Endocrine System

Hypothalamus
Pituitary (Hypophysis) gland
Thyroid gland
Thymus gland
Pineal gland
Parathyoid glands
Adrenal (Suprarenal) glands
Pancreas
Ovaries
Testes

§ ✓5ᵗʰ **242.3 Toxic nodular goiter, unspecified**   **MCC 1**
[0-1]

Adenomatous goiter
Nodular goiter } toxic or with hyperthyroidism
Struma nodosa

Any condition classifiable to 241.9 specified as toxic or with hyperthyroidism

CC Excl: See code 242.0

§ ✓5ᵗʰ **242.4 Thyrotoxicosis from ectopic thyroid nodule**   **MCC 1**
[0-1]   **CC Excl:** See code 242.0

§ ✓5ᵗʰ **242.8 Thyrotoxicosis of other specified origin**   **MCC 1**
[0-1]

Overproduction of thyroid-stimulating hormone [TSH]
Thyrotoxicosis:
  factitia from ingestion of excessive thyroid material

Use additional E code to identify cause, if drug-induced

CC Excl: See code 242.0

§ ✓5ᵗʰ **242.9 Thyrotoxicosis without mention of goiter**   **MCC 1**
[0-1] **or other cause**

Hyperthyroidism NOS
Thyrotoxicosis NOS

CC Excl: See code 242.0

E05.90 Thyrotoxicosis uns w/o thyrotoxic crisis or storm   **I-10**

243 Congenital hypothyroidism

Congenital thyroid insufficiency
Cretinism (athyrotic) (endemic)

Use additional code to identify associated intellectual disabilities

EXCLUDES *congenital (dyshormonogenic) goiter (246.1)*

DEF: Underproduction of thyroid hormone present from birth.

✓4ᵗʰ **244 Acquired hypothyroidism**

INCLUDES athyroidism (acquired)
hypothyroidism (acquired)
myxedema (adult) (juvenile)
thyroid (gland) insufficiency (acquired)

244.0 Postsurgical hypothyroidism

DEF: Underproduction of thyroid hormone due to surgical removal of all or part of the thyroid gland.

E89.0 Postprocedural hypothyroidism   **I-10**

244.1 Other postablative hypothyroidism

Hypothyroidism following therapy, such as irradiation

244.2 Iodine hypothyroidism

Hypothyroidism resulting from administration or ingestion of iodide

Use additional E code to identify drug

EXCLUDES *hypothyroidism resulting from administration of radioactive iodine (244.1)*

244.3 Other iatrogenic hypothyroidism

Hypothyroidism resulting from:
  P-aminosalicylic acid [PAS]
  Phenylbutazone
  Resorcinol
Iatrogenic hypothyroidism NOS

Use additional E code to identify drug

244.8 Other specified acquired hypothyroidism

Secondary hypothyroidism NEC

AHA: J-A, '85, 9

Requires fifth digit. Valid digits are in [brackets] under each code. See category 242 for codes and definitions.

✓4ᵗʰ **Additional Digit Required**   **Unacceptable PDx**   **Manifestation Code**   Hospital Acquired Condition   ▶◀ Revised Text   ● New Code   ▲ Revised Code Title

Endocrine, Nutritional and Metabolic Diseases, and Immunity

244.9–249.6

244.9 Unspecified hypothyroidism
Hypothyroidism
Myxedema   } primary or NOS
AHA: 3Q, '99, 19; 4Q, '96, 29
E03.9 Hypothyroidism unspecified   I-10

✓4ᵗʰ **245 Thyroiditis**

245.0 Acute thyroiditis   CC
Abscess of thyroid
Thyroiditis:
nonsuppurative, acute
pyogenic
suppurative
Use additional code to identify organism
DEF: Inflamed thyroid caused by infection, with abscess and liquid
puris.
CC Excl: 245.0-245.9

245.1 Subacute thyroiditis
Thyroiditis:
de Quervain's
giant cell
granulomatous
viral
DEF: Inflammation of the thyroid, characterized by fever and painful
enlargement of the thyroid gland, with granulomas in the gland.

245.2 Chronic lymphocytic thyroiditis
Hashimoto's disease
Struma lymphomatosa
Thyroiditis:
autoimmune
lymphocytic (chronic)
DEF: Autoimmune disease of thyroid; lymphocytes infiltrate the
gland and thyroid antibodies are produced; women more often
affected.

245.3 Chronic fibrous thyroiditis
Struma fibrosa
Thyroiditis:
invasive (fibrous)
ligneous
Riedel's
DEF: Persistent fibrosing inflammation of thyroid with adhesions to
nearby structures; rare condition

245.4 Iatrogenic thyroiditis
Use additional code to identify cause
DEF: Thyroiditis resulting from treatment or intervention by
physician or in a patient intervention setting.

245.8 Other and unspecified chronic thyroiditis
Chronic thyroiditis:
NOS
nonspecific

245.9 Thyroiditis, unspecified
Thyroiditis NOS

✓4ᵗʰ **246 Other disorders of thyroid**

246.0 Disorders of thyrocalcitonin secretion
Hypersecretion of calcitonin or thyrocalcitonin

246.1 Dyshormonogenic goiter
Congenital (dyshormonogenic) goiter
Goiter due to enzyme defect in synthesis of thyroid hormone
Goitrous cretinism (sporadic)

246.2 Cyst of thyroid
EXCLUDES cystadenoma of thyroid (226)

246.3 Hemorrhage and infarction of thyroid   CC
CC Excl: 246.3

246.8 Other specified disorders of thyroid
Abnormality of thyroid-binding globulin
Atrophy of thyroid
Hyper-TBG-nemia
Hypo-TBG-nemia
AHA: 2Q, '06, 5

246.9 Unspecified disorder of thyroid
E07.9 Disorder of thyroid unspecified   I-10

Diseases of Other Endocrine Glands (249-259)

✓4ᵗʰ **249 Secondary diabetes mellitus**
INCLUDES diabetes mellitus (due to) (in) (secondary) (with):
drug-induced or chemical induced
infection
Use additional code to identify any associated insulin use (V58.67)
EXCLUDES gestational diabetes (648.8)
hyperglycemia NOS (790.29)
neonatal diabetes mellitus (775.1)
nonclinical diabetes (790.29)
Type I diabetes — see category 250
Type II diabetes — see category 250
AHA: 4Q, '08, 91-95
TIP: If the secondary DM is due to pancreatectomy, code first 251.3 Postsurgi-
cal hypoinsulinemia; also assign a code from category 249 and any manifestations, and code V88.1x Acquired absence of pancreas.
The following fifth-digit subclassification is for use with category 249:
    0 not stated as uncontrolled, or unspecified
    1 uncontrolled

§ ✓5ᵗʰ **249.0 Secondary diabetes mellitus without mention**
[0-1] **of complication**
Secondary diabetes mellitus without mention of complication
or manifestation classifiable to 249.1-249.9
Secondary diabetes mellitus NOS
E09.9 Drug/chemical induced diabetes mellitus w/o comp   I-10

§ ✓5ᵗʰ **249.1 Secondary diabetes mellitus with ketoacidosis**   MCC
[0-1] Secondary diabetes mellitus with diabetic acidosis
without mention of coma
Secondary diabetes mellitus with diabetic ketosis
without mention of coma
CC Excl: 249.00-251.3, 259.8-259.9

§ ✓5ᵗʰ **249.2 Secondary diabetes mellitus with hyperosmolarity**   MCC
[0-1] Secondary diabetes mellitus with hyperosmolar
(nonketotic) coma
CC Excl: See code: 249.1

§ ✓5ᵗʰ **249.3 Secondary diabetes mellitus with other coma**   MCC
[0-1] Secondary diabetes mellitus with diabetic coma (with
ketoacidosis)
Secondary diabetes mellitus with diabetic
hypoglycemic coma
Secondary diabetes mellitus with insulin coma NOS
EXCLUDES secondary diabetes mellitus with hyperosmolar coma
(249.2)
CC Excl: See code: 249.1

§ ✓5ᵗʰ **249.4 Secondary diabetes mellitus with renal manifestations**
[0-1] Use additional code to identify manifestation, as:
chronic kidney disease (585.1-585.9)
diabetic nephropathy NOS (583.81)
diabetic nephrosis (581.81)
intercapillary glomerulosclerosis (581.81)
Kimmelstiel-Wilson syndrome (581.81)

§ ✓5ᵗʰ **249.5 Secondary diabetes mellitus with ophthalmic**
[0-1] **manifestations**
Use additional code to identify manifestation, as:
diabetic blindness (369.00-369.9)
diabetic cataract (366.41)
diabetic glaucoma (365.44)
diabetic macular edema (362.07)
diabetic retinal edema (362.07)
diabetic retinopathy (362.01-362.07)

§ ✓5ᵗʰ **249.6 Secondary diabetes mellitus with neurological**
[0-1] **manifestations**
Use additional code to identify manifestation, as:
diabetic amyotrophy (353.5)
diabetic gastroparalysis (536.3)
diabetic gastroparesis (536.3)
diabetic mononeuropathy (354.0-355.9)
diabetic neurogenic arthropathy (713.5)
diabetic peripheral autonomic neuropathy (337.1)
diabetic polyneuropathy (357.2)
AHA: For code 249.60: 4Q, '08, 94

---

§ Requires fifth digit. Valid digits are in [brackets] under each code. See category 249 for codes and definitions.

§ ✓5ᵗʰ **249.7 Secondary diabetes mellitus with peripheral**
[0-1]   **circulatory disorders**
    Use additional code to identify manifestation, as:
       diabetic gangrene (785.4)
       diabetic peripheral angiopathy (443.81)

§ ✓5ᵗʰ **249.8 Secondary diabetes mellitus with other**
[0-1]   **specified manifestations**
    Secondary diabetic hypoglycemia in diabetes mellitus
    Secondary hypoglycemic shock in diabetes mellitus
    Use additional code to identify manifestation, as:
       any associated ulceration (707.10-707.19, 707.8, 707.9)
       diabetic bone changes (731.8)

§ ✓5ᵗʰ **249.9 Secondary diabetes mellitus with unspecified complication**
[0-1]

✓4ᵗʰ § **250 Diabetes mellitus**
    EXCLUDES *gestational diabetes (648.8)*
        hyperglycemia NOS (790.29)
        neonatal diabetes mellitus (775.1)
        nonclinical diabetes (790.29)
        secondary diabetes (249.0-249.9)

The following fifth-digit subclassification is for use with category 250:
0 type II or unspecified type, not state as uncontrolled
    Fifth-digit 0 is for use for type II patients, even if the patient requires insulin
    Use additional code, if applicable, for associated long-term (current) insulin use (V58.67)
1 type I [juvenile type], not stated as uncontrolled
2 type II or unspecified type, uncontrolled
    Fifth-digit 2 is for use for type II patients, even if the patient requires insulin
    Use additional code, if applicable, for associated long-term (current) insulin use (V58.67)
3 type I [juvenile type], uncontrolled

DEF: Diabetes mellitus: Inability to metabolize carbohydrates, proteins, and fats due to insufficient secretion of insulin. Symptoms may be unremarkable, with long-term complications, involving kidneys, nerves, blood vessels, and eyes.
DEF: Uncontrolled diabetes: A nonspecific term indicating that the current treatment regimen does not keep the blood sugar level of a patient within acceptable levels.
AHA: 1Q, '11, 9; 4Q, '04, 56; 2Q, '04, 17; 2Q, '02, 13; 2Q,'01, 16; 2Q,'98, 15; 4Q, '97, 32; 2Q, '97, 14; 3Q, '96, 5; 4Q, '93, 19; 2Q, '92, 5; 3Q, '91, 3; 2Q, '90, 22; N-D, '85, 11
TIP: Use of insulin does not ensure type I DM; if patient is on routine insulin, assign also V58.67 Long-term (current) use of insulin.

⁷ § ✓5ᵗʰ **250.0 Diabetes mellitus without mention of complication**
[0-3]   Diabetes mellitus without mention of complication or manifestation classifiable to 250.1-250.9
    Diabetes (mellitus) NOS
    AHA: 1Q, '06, 14; 4Q, '97, 32; 3Q, '91, 3, 12; N-D, '85, 11; **For code 250.00:** ▶2Q, '12, 19;◀ 4Q, '09, 77; 1Q, '05, 15; 4Q, '04, 55; 4Q, '03, 105, 108; 2Q, '03, 16; 1Q, '02, 7, 11; **For code 250.01:** 4Q, '04, 55; 4Q, '03, 110; 2Q, '03, 6; **For code 250.02:** 1Q, '03, 5
    E11.9 Type 2 diabetes mellitus w/o comp   I-10

§ ✓5ᵗʰ **250.1 Diabetes with ketoacidosis**   MCC
[0-3]   Diabetic:
    acidosis ⎫
    ketosis ⎬ without mention of coma
    DEF: Diabetic hyperglycemic crisis causing ketone presence in body fluids.
    CC Excl: For code 250.10: 249.00-251.3, 259.8-259.9; **For code 250.11-250.13:** 249.00-251.3, 259.50-259.9
    AHA: 3Q, '91, 6; **For code 250.11:** 2Q, '06, 19-20; 4Q, '03, 82; **For code 250.13:** 2Q, '06, 19-20
    E10.10 Type 1 diabetes mellitus w/ketoacidosis w/o coma   I-10

§ ✓5ᵗʰ **250.2 Diabetes with hyperosmolarity**   MCC
[0-3]   Hyperosmolar (nonketotic) coma
    CC Excl: For code 250.20: 249.00-251.3, 259.8-259.9; **For code 250.21-250.23:** 249.00-251.3, 259.50-259.9
    AHA: 4Q, '93, 19; 3Q, '91, 7

§ ✓5ᵗʰ **250.3 Diabetes with other coma**   MCC
[0-3]   ·Diabetic coma (with ketoacidosis)
    Diabetic hypoglycemic coma
    Insulin coma NOS
    EXCLUDES *diabetes with hyperosmolar coma (250.2)*
    DEF: Coma (not hyperosmolar) caused by hyperglycemia or hypoglycemia as complication of diabetes.
    CC Excl: For code 250.30: 249.00-251.3, 259.8-259.9; **For code 250.31-250.33:** 249.00-251.3, 259.50-259.9
    AHA: 3Q, '91, 7, 12

§ ✓5ᵗʰ **250.4 Diabetes with renal manifestations**
[0-3]   Use additional code to identify manifestation, as:
    chronic kidney disease (585.1-585.9)
    diabetic:
      nephropathy NOS (583.81)
      nephrosis (581.81)
    intercapillary glomerulosclerosis (581.81)
    Kimmelstiel-Wilson syndrome (581.81)
    AHA: 3Q, '91, 8, 12; S-O, '87, 9; S-O, '84, 3; **For code 250.40:** ▶2Q, '12, 19;◀ 1Q, '03, 20
    E11.22 Type 2 diabetes mellitus w/diabetic ckd   I-10

§ ✓5ᵗʰ **250.5 Diabetes with ophthalmic manifestations**
[0-3]   Use additional code to identify manifestation, as:
    diabetic:
      blindness (369.00-369.9)
      cataract (366.41)
      glaucoma (365.44)
      macular edema (362.07)
      retinal edema (362.07)
      retinopathy (362.01-362.07)
    AHA: 4Q, '05, 65; 3Q, '91, 8; S-O, '85, 11; **For code 250.50:** 4Q, '05, 67
    E10.36 Type 1 diabetes mellitus with diabetic cataract   I-10

§ ✓5ᵗʰ **250.6 Diabetes with neurological manifestations**
[0-3]   Use additional code to identify manifestation, as:
    diabetic:
      amyotrophy (353.5)
      gastroparalysis (536.3)
      gastroparesis (536.3)
      mononeuropathy (354.0-355.9)
      neurogenic arthropathy (713.5)
      peripheral autonomic neuropathy (337.1)
      polyneuropathy (357.2)
    AHA: 4Q, '09, 151; 2Q, '09, 13, 15; 3Q, '08, 5; 2Q, '93, 6; 2Q, '92, 15; 3Q, '91, 9; N-D, '84, 9; **For code 250.60:** 4Q, '03, 105; **For code 250.61:** 2Q, '04, 7
    E11.40 Type 2 diabetes mellitus w/diab neuropathy   I-10

§ ✓5ᵗʰ **250.7 Diabetes with peripheral circulatory disorders**
[0-3]   Use additional code to identify manifestation, as:
    diabetic:
      gangrene (785.4)
      peripheral angiopathy (443.81)
    DEF: Blood vessel damage or disease, usually in the feet, legs, or hands, as a complication of diabetes.
    AHA: 1Q, '96, 10; 3Q, '94, 5; 2Q, '94, 17; 3Q, '91, 10, 12; 3Q, '90, 15; **For code 250.70:** 1Q, '04, 14
    E10.51 Type 1 DM w/diab periph angiopathy w/o gangrene   I-10

§ ✓5ᵗʰ **250.8 Diabetes with other specified manifestations**
[0-3]   Diabetic hypoglycemia NOS
    Hypoglycemic shock NOS
    Use additional code to identify manifestation, as:
      any associated ulceration (707.10-707.19, 707.8, 707.9)
      diabetic bone changes (731.8)
    AHA: 4Q, '00, 44; 4Q, '97, 43; 2Q, '97, 16; 4Q, '93, 20; 3Q, '91, 10; **For code 250.80:** 1Q, '04, 14
    TIP: Assign for diabetic osteomyelitis, along with code 731.8 and the appropriate code from category 730.
    E11.618 Type 2 DM with other diabetic arthropathy   I-10

§ ✓5ᵗʰ **250.9 Diabetes with unspecified complication**
[0-3]   **AHA:** 2Q, '92, 15; 3Q, '91, 7, 12
    TIP: Do not assign with any other code in category 250.
    E10.8 Type 1 diabetes mellitus with unspecified comp   I-10

Requires fifth digit. Valid digits are in [brackets] under each code. See appropriate category for codes and definitions.
Questionable admission when fifth-digit = 0

✓4ᵗʰ 251   Other disorders of pancreatic internal secretion

251.0   Hypoglycemic coma   `CC`
Iatrogenic hyperinsulinism
Non-diabetic insulin coma

Use additional E code to identify cause, if drug-induced

EXCLUDES *hypoglycemic coma in diabetes mellitus (249.3, 250.3)*

DEF: Coma induced by low blood sugar in non-diabetic patient.
CC Excl: 2249.00-251.3, 259.50-259.9
AHA: M-A, '85, 8

251.1   Other specified hypoglycemia
Hyperinsulinism:
  NOS
  ectopic
  functional
Hyperplasia of pancreatic
  islet beta cells NOS

Use additional E code to identify cause, if drug-induced

EXCLUDES *hypoglycemia:*
    in diabetes mellitus (249.8, 250.8)
    in infant of diabetic mother (775.0)
    hypoglycemic coma (251.0)
    neonatal hypoglycemia (775.6)

DEF: Excessive production of insulin by the pancreas; associated with obesity and insulin-producing tumors.
AHA: 1Q, '03, 10

251.2   Hypoglycemia, unspecified
Hypoglycemia: Hypoglycemia:
  NOS   spontaneous
  reactive

EXCLUDES *hypoglycemia:*
    with coma (251.0)
    in diabetes mellitus (249.8, 250.8)
    leucine-induced (270.3)

AHA: M-A, '85, 8
E16.2 Hypoglycemia unspecified   `I-10`

251.3   Postsurgical hypoinsulinemia   `CC`
Hypoinsulinemia following complete or partial
    pancreatectomy
Postpancreatectomy hyperglycemia

Use additional code to identify (any associated):
  acquired absence of pancreas (V88.11-V88.12)
  insulin use (V58.67)
  secondary diabetes mellitus (249.00-249.91)

EXCLUDES *transient hyperglycemia post procedure (790.29)*
    transient hypoglycemia post procedure (251.2)

CC Excl: See code: 251.0
AHA: 3Q, '91, 6

251.4   Abnormality of secretion of glucagon
Hyperplasia of pancreatic islet alpha cells with glucagon
    excess

DEF: Production malfunction of a pancreatic hormone secreted by cells of the islets of Langerhans.

251.5   Abnormality of secretion of gastrin
Hyperplasia of pancreatic alpha cells with gastrin excess
Zollinger-Ellison syndrome

251.8   Other specified disorders of pancreatic internal secretion
AHA: 2Q, '98, 15; 3Q, '91, 6
E16.8 Oth spec d/o of pancreatic internal secretion   `I-10`

251.9   Unspecified disorder of pancreatic internal secretion
Islet cell hyperplasia NOS

✓4ᵗʰ 252   Disorders of parathyroid gland
EXCLUDES *hungry bone syndrome (275.5)*

✓5ᵗʰ 252.0   Hyperparathyroidism
EXCLUDES *ectopic hyperparathyroidism (259.3)*
DEF: Abnormally high secretion of parathyroid hormones causing bone deterioration, reduced renal function, kidney stones.

252.00   Hyperparathyroidism, unspecified
E21.3 Hyperparathyroidism unspecified   `I-10`

Dorsal View of Parathyroid Glands

252.01   Primary hyperparathyroidism
Hyperplasia of parathyroid

DEF: Parathyroid dysfunction commonly caused by hyperplasia of two or more glands; characteristic hypercalcemia and increased parathyroid hormone levels.

252.02   Secondary hyperparathyroidism, non-renal
EXCLUDES *secondary hyperparathyroidism (of renal origin) (588.81)*

DEF: Underlying disease of nonrenal origin decreases bloo levels of calcium causing the parathyroid to release increased levels of parathyroid hormone; parathyroid hormone levels return to normal once underlying condition is treated and blood calcium levels are normal.
AHA: 4Q, '04, 57-59

252.08   Other hyperparathyroidism
Tertiary hyperparathyroidism

DEF: Tertiary hyperparathyroidism: chronic secondary hyperparathyroidism with adenomatous parathyroid causing irreversible abnormal production of parathyroid hormone (PTH); PTH remains high after the serum calcium levels are brought under control.

252.1   Hypoparathyroidism
Parathyroiditis (autoimmune)
Tetany:
  parathyroid
  parathyroprival

EXCLUDES *pseudohypoparathyroidism (275.4)*
    pseudopseudohypoparathyroidism (275.4)
    tetany NOS (781.7)
    transitory neonatal hypoparathyroidism (775.4)

DEF: Abnormally low secretion of parathyroid hormones which causes decreased calcium and increased phosphorus in the blood, resulting in muscle cramps, tetany, urinary frequency and cataracts

252.8   Other specified disorders of parathyroid gland
Cyst   } of parathyroid
Hemorrhage

252.9   Unspecified disorder of parathyroid gland

✓4ᵗʰ 253   Disorders of the pituitary gland and its hypothalamic control
INCLUDES the listed conditions whether the disorder is in the pituitary or the hypothalamus
EXCLUDES *Cushing's syndrome (255.0)*

253.0   Acromegaly and gigantism
Overproduction of growth hormone

DEF: Acromegaly: chronic, middle age condition; caused by hypersecretion of the pituitary growth hormone; enlarged parts of skeleton, especially the nose, ears, jaws, fingers and toes.
DEF: Gigantism: pituitary gigantism caused by excess growth of shor flat bones; men may grow 78 to 80 inches tall.

253.1   Other and unspecified anterior pituitary hyperfunction   `C`
Forbes-Albright syndrome

EXCLUDES *overproduction of:*
    ACTH (255.3)
    thyroid-stimulating hormone [TSH] (242.8)

DEF: Spontaneous galactorrhea-amenorrhea syndrome unrelated t pregnancy; usually related to presence of pituitary tumor.
CC Excl: 253.1, 253.4, 253.6
AHA: J-A, '85, 9

`N` Newborn Age: 0   `P` Pediatric Age: 0-17   `M` Maternity Age: 12-55   `A` Adult Age: 15-124   `MCC` Major CC Condition   `CC` CC Condition   `HIV` HIV Related D

62 – Volume 1   **2014 ICD-9-C**

253.2 Panhypopituitarism `CC`
    Cachexia, pituitary
    Necrosis of pituitary
    Pituitary insufficiency NOS
    Simmonds' disease
    Sheehan's syndrome (postpartum)
    EXCLUDES iatrogenic hypopituitarism (253.7)
    DEF: Damage to or absence of pituitary gland leading to impaired sexual function, weight loss, fatigue, bradycardia, hypotension, pallor, depression, and impaired growth in children; called Simmonds' disease if cachexia is prominent.
    CC Exd: 253.0-253.9, 259.50-259.9

253.3 Pituitary dwarfism
    Isolated deficiency of (human) growth hormone [HGH]
    Lorain-Levi dwarfism
    DEF: Dwarfism with infantile physical characteristics due to abnormally low secretion of growth hormone and gonadotropin deficiency.

253.4 Other anterior pituitary disorders
    Isolated or partial deficiency of an anterior pituitary hormone, other than growth hormone
    Prolactin deficiency
    AHA: J-A, '85, 9

253.5 Diabetes insipidus `CC`
    Vasopressin deficiency
    EXCLUDES nephrogenic diabetes insipidus (588.1)
    DEF: Metabolic disorder causing insufficient antidiuretic hormone release; symptoms include frequent urination, thirst, ravenous hunger, loss of weight, fatigue.
    CC Exd: 253.1-253.2, 253.4-253.9, 259.50-259.9

253.6 Other disorders of neurohypophysis `CC`
    Syndrome of inappropriate secretion of antidiuretic hormone [ADH]
    EXCLUDES ectopic antidiuretic hormone secretion (259.3)
    CC Exd: 253.0-253.9, 259.8-259.9
    E22.2 Synd inappropriate secrectn antidiuretic hormone `I-10`

253.7 Iatrogenic pituitary disorders
    Hypopituitarism:
        hormone-induced
        hypophysectomy-induced
        postablative
        radiotherapy-induced
    Use additional E code to identify cause
    DEF: Pituitary dysfunction that results from drug therapy, radiation therapy, or surgery, causing mild to severe symptoms.

253.8 Other disorders of the pituitary and other syndromes of diencephalohypophyseal origin
    Abscess of pituitary
    Adiposogenital dystrophy
    Cyst of Rathke's pouch
    Fröhlich's syndrome
    EXCLUDES craniopharyngioma (237.0)

253.9 Unspecified
    Dyspituitarism

√4ᵗʰ **254 Diseases of thymus gland**
    EXCLUDES aplasia or dysplasia with immunodeficiency (279.2)
    hypoplasia with immunodeficiency (279.2)
    myasthenia gravis (358.00-358.01)

254.0 Persistent hyperplasia of thymus
    Hypertrophy of thymus
    DEF: Continued abnormal growth of the twin lymphoid lobes that produce T lymphocytes.

254.1 Abscess of thymus `CC`
    CC Exd: 254.0-254.9, 259.50-259.9

254.8 Other specified diseases of thymus gland
    Astrophy }
    Cyst   } of thymus
    EXCLUDES thymoma (212.6)

254.9 Unspecified disease of thymus gland

√4ᵗʰ **255 Disorders of adrenal glands**
    INCLUDES the listed conditions whether the basic disorder is in the adrenals or is pituitary-induced

255.0 Cushing's syndrome `CC`
    Adrenal hyperplasia due to excess ACTH
    Cushing's syndrome:
        NOS
        iatrogenic
        idiopathic
        pituitary-dependent
    Ectopic ACTH syndrome
    Iatrogenic syndrome of excess cortisol
    Overproduction of cortisol
    Use additional E code to identify cause, if drug-induced
    EXCLUDES congenital adrenal hyperplasia (255.2)
    DEF: Due to adrenal cortisol oversecretion or glucocorticoid medications; may cause excess fatty tissue of the face, neck and body; osteoporosis and curvature of spine, hypertension, diabetes mellitus, female genitourinary problems, male impotence, degeneration of muscle tissues, weakness.
    CC Exd: 255.0-255.2, 259.50-259.9

√5ᵗʰ **255.1 Hyperaldosteronism**
    DEF: Oversecretion of aldosterone causing fluid retention, hypertension.
    AHA: 4Q, '03, 48

    255.10 Hyperaldosteronism, unspecified
        Aldosteronism NOS
        Primary aldosteronism, unspecified
        EXCLUDES Conn's syndrome (255.12)

    255.11 Glucocorticoid-remediable aldosteronism
        Familial aldosteronism type I
        EXCLUDES Conn's syndrome (255.12)
        DEF: Rare autosomal dominant familial form of primary aldosteronism in which the secretion of aldosterone is under the influence of adrenocortiotrophic hormone (ACTH) rather than the renin-angiotensin mechanism; moderate hypersecretion of aldosterone and suppressed plasma renin activity rapidly reversed by administration of glucosteroids; symptoms include hypertension and mild hypokalemia.

    255.12 Conn's syndrome
        DEF: A type of primary aldosteronism caused by an adenoma of the glomerulosa cells in the adrenal cortex; presence of hypertension.

    255.13 Bartter's syndrome
        DEF: A cluster of symptoms caused by a defect in the ability of the kidney to reabsorb potassium; signs include alkalosis (hypokalemic alkalosis), increased aldosterone, increased plasma renin, and normal blood pressure; symptoms include muscle cramping, weakness, constipation, frequency of urination, and failure to grow; also known as urinary potassium wasting or juxtaglomerular cell hyperplasia.

    255.14 Other secondary aldosteronism
        AHA: 3Q, '06, 24

255.2 Adrenogenital disorders
    Achard-Thiers syndrome
    Adrenogenital syndromes, virilizing or feminizing, whether acquired or associated with congenital adrenal hyperplasia consequent on inborn enzyme defects in hormone synthesis
    Congenital adrenal hyperplasia
    Female adrenal pseudohermaphroditism
    Male:
        macrogenitosomia praecox
        sexual precocity with adrenal hyperplasia
    Virilization (female) (suprarenal)
    EXCLUDES adrenal hyperplasia due to excess ACTH (255.0)
    isosexual virilization (256.4)

255.3 Other corticoadrenal overactivity `CC`
    Acquired benign adrenal androgenic overactivity
    Overproduction of ACTH
    CC Exd: 017.60-017.66, 017.90-017.96, 255.3-255.9, 259.50-259.9

Additional Digit Required   Unacceptable PDx   Manifestation Code   Hospital Acquired Condition   ▶◀ Revised Text   ● New Code   ▲ Revised Code Title

4 ICD-9-CM   **Volume 1 – 63**

Endocrine, Nutritional and Metabolic Diseases, and Immunity

255.4–259.1

√5ᵗʰ **255.4 Corticoadrenal insufficiency**

EXCLUDES *tuberculous Addison's disease (017.6)*

DEF: Underproduction of adrenal hormones causing low blood pressure.

AHA: 4Q, '07, 68; 3Q, '06, 24

255.41 Glucocorticoid deficiency CC
Addisonian crisis
Addison's disease NOS
Adrenal atrophy (autoimmune)
Adrenal calcification
Adrenal crisis
Adrenal hemorrhage
Adrenal infarction
Adrenal insufficiency NOS
Combined glucocorticoid and mineralocorticoid deficiency
Corticoadrenal insufficiency NOS

DEF: Decreased function of the adrenal cortex resulting in insufficient production of glucocorticoid, the hormone regulating carbohydrate, fat, and protein metabolism; manifestations: hyponatremia, hyperpigmentation, orthostatic hypotension, anemia, loss of appetite, and malaise.

CC Excl: See code: 255.3

AHA: 4Q, '07, 68, 69

E27.1 Primary adrenocortical insufficiency   I-10

255.42 Mineralocorticoid deficiency CC
Hypoaldosteronism

EXCLUDES *combined glucocorticoid and mineralocorticoid deficiency (255.41)*

DEF: Decreased function of the adrenal cortex resulting in insufficient production of mineralocorticoid, which regulates electrolyte and water balance; manifestations: hyponatremia, hyperkalemia, and mild acidosis.

CC Excl: See code: 255.3

255.5 Other adrenal hypofunction CC
Adrenal medullary insufficiency

EXCLUDES *Waterhouse-Friderichsen syndrome (meningococcal) (036.3)*

CC Excl: See code 255.3

255.6 Medulloadrenal hyperfunction CC
Catecholamine secretion by pheochromocytoma

CC Excl: See code 255.3

255.8 Other specified disorders of adrenal glands
Abnormality of cortisol-binding globulin

255.9 Unspecified disorder of adrenal glands

√4ᵗʰ **256 Ovarian dysfunction**
AHA: 4Q, '00, 51

256.0 Hyperestrogenism ♀
DEF: Excess secretion of estrogen by the ovaries; characterized by ovaries containing multiple follicular cysts filled with serous fluid.

256.1 Other ovarian hyperfunction ♀
Hypersecretion of ovarian androgens
AHA: 3Q, '95, 15

256.2 Postablative ovarian failure ♀
Ovarian failure: Ovarian failure:
   iatrogenic   postsurgical
   postirradiation

Use additional code for states associated with artificial menopause (627.4)

EXCLUDES *acquired absence of ovary (V45.77)*
asymptomatic age-related (natural) postmenopausal status (V49.81)

DEF: Failed ovarian function after medical or surgical intervention.

AHA: 2Q, '02, 12

√5ᵗʰ **256.3 Other ovarian failure**
Use additional code for states associated with natural menopause (627.2)

EXCLUDES *asymptomatic age-related (natural) postmenopausal status (V49.81)*

AHA: 4Q, '01, 41

256.31 Premature menopause A ♀
DEF: Permanent cessation of ovarian function before the age of 40 occuring naturally of unknown cause.

256.39 Other ovarian failure
Delayed menarche
Ovarian hypofunction
Primary ovarian failure NOS

256.4 Polycystic ovaries
Isosexual virilization
Stein-Leventhal syndrome

DEF: Multiple serous filled cysts of ovary; symptoms of infertility, hirsutism, oligomenorrhea or amenorrhea.

E28.2 Polycystic ovarian syndrome

256.8 Other ovarian dysfunction

256.9 Unspecified ovarian dysfunction

√4ᵗʰ **257 Testicular dysfunction**

257.0 Testicular hyperfunction
Hypersecretion of testicular hormones

257.1 Postablative testicular hypofunction
Testicular hypofunction:
   iatrogenic
   postirradiation
   postsurgical

257.2 Other testicular hypofunction
Defective biosynthesis of testicular androgen
Eunuchoidism:
   NOS
   hypogonadotropic
Failure:
   Leydig's cell, adult
   seminiferous tubule, adult
Testicular hypogonadism

EXCLUDES *azoospermia (606.0)*

257.8 Other testicular dysfunction

EXCLUDES *androgen insensitivity syndromes (259.50-259.52)*

257.9 Unspecified testicular dysfunction

√4ᵗʰ **258 Polyglandular dysfunction and related disorders**

√5ᵗʰ **258.0 Polyglandular activity in multiple endocrine adenomatos**
Multiple endocrine neoplasia [MEN] syndromes

Use additional codes to identify any malignancies and other conditions associated with the syndromes

AHA: 4Q, '09, 150; 4Q, '07, 70

258.01 Multiple endocrine neoplasia [MEN] type I
Wermer's syndrome

DEF: Wermer's syndrome: A rare hereditary condition characterized by the presence of adenomas or hyperplas in more than one endocrine gland causing premature aging.

AHA: 4Q, '08, 86, 89; 4Q, '07, 70, 72

258.02 Multiple endocrine neoplasia [MEN] type IIA
Sipple's syndrome

DEF: Sipple's syndrome: A hereditary disorder caused by a defect in the RET gene causing overactivity of the thyroid adrenal, and parathyroid glands, resulting in adrenal pheochromocytoma and thyroid medullary carcinoma.

258.03 Multiple endocrine neoplasia [MEN] type IIB

258.1 Other combinations of endocrine dysfunction
Lloyd's syndrome
Schmidt's syndrome

258.8 Other specified polyglandular dysfunction

258.9 Polyglandular dysfunction, unspecified

√4ᵗʰ **259 Other endocrine disorders**

259.0 Delay in sexual development and puberty, not elsewhere classified
Delayed puberty

259.1 Precocious sexual development and puberty, not elsewhere classified
Sexual precocity: Sexual precocity:
   NOS   cryptogenic
   constitutional   idiopathic

N Newborn Age: 0   P Pediatric Age: 0-17   M Maternity Age: 12-55   A Adult Age: 15-124   MCC Major CC Condition   CC CC Condition   HIV HIV Related

64 – Volume 1   2014 ICD-9-

259.2 Carcinoid syndrome `CC`
Hormone secretion by carcinoid tumors
DEF: Presence of carcinoid tumors that spread to liver; characterized by cyanotic flushing of skin, diarrhea, bronchospasm, acquired tricuspid and pulmonary stenosis, sudden drops in blood pressure, edema, ascites.
CC Exd: 259.2-259.3, 259.50-259.9
AHA: 4Q, '08, 85-86, 89

259.3 Ectopic hormone secretion, not elsewhere classified
Ectopic:
antidiuretic hormone secretion [ADH]
hyperparathyroidism
EXCLUDES ectopic ACTH syndrome (255.0)
AHA: N-D, '85, 4

259.4 Dwarfism, not elsewhere classified
Dwarfism:
NOS
constitutional
EXCLUDES dwarfism:
achondroplastic (756.4)
intrauterine (759.7)
nutritional (263.2)
pituitary (253.3)
renal (588.0)
progeria (259.8)

√5ᵗʰ **259.5 Androgen insensitivity syndrome**
DEF: X chromosome abnormality that prohibits the body from recognizing androgen; XY genotype with ambiguous genitalia.
AHA: 4Q, '08, 95-96; 4Q, '05, 53

  259.50 Androgen insensitivity, unspecified

  259.51 Androgen insensitivity syndrome
Complete androgen insensitivity
de Quervain's syndrome
Goldberg-Maxwell Syndrome

  259.52 Partial androgen insensitivity
Partial androgen insensitivity syndrome
Reifenstein syndrome

259.8 Other specified endocrine disorders
Pineal gland dysfunction
Progeria
Werner's syndrome

259.9 Unspecified endocrine disorder
Disturbance:
endocrine NOS
hormone NOS
Infantilism NOS

Nutritional Deficiencies (260-269)

EXCLUDES deficiency anemias (280.0-281.9)
TIP: Assign first a code for the underlying condition (e.g., anorexia nervosa) if specified.

260 Kwashiorkor `MCC`
Nutritional edema with dyspigmentation of skin and hair
DEF: Syndrome, particularly of children; excessive carbohydrate with inadequate protein intake, inhibited growth potential, anomalies in skin and hair pigmentation, edema and liver disease.
CC Exd: 260-263.9
AHA: 3Q, '09, 6
TIP: Do not assign when documentation indicates "mild or moderate protein malnutrition" only. Kwashiorkor is a rare severe protein deficiency.
E40 Kwashiorkor `I-10`

261 Nutritional marasmus `MCC`
Nutritional atrophy
Severe calorie deficiency
Severe malnutrition NOS
DEF: Protein-calorie malabsorption or malnutrition in children; characterized by tissue wasting, dehydration, and subcutaneous fat depletion; may occur with infectious disease; also called infantile atrophy.
CC Exd: See code 260
AHA: ▶3Q, '12, 10;◄4Q, '07, 97; 3Q, '06, 14; 2Q, '06, 12
E41 Nutritional marasmus `I-10`

262 Other severe, protein-calorie malnutrition `MCC`
Nutritional edema without mention of dyspigmentation of skin and hair
CC Exd: See code 260
AHA: 4Q, '92, 24; J-A, '85, 12

√4ᵗʰ **263 Other and unspecified protein-calorie malnutrition**
AHA: 4Q, '92, 24

263.0 Malnutrition of moderate degree `CC`
DEF: Malnutrition characterized by biochemical changes in electrolytes, lipids, blood plasma.
CC Exd: See code 260
AHA: ▶3Q, '12, 10;◄3Q, '09, 6; J-A, '85, 1

263.1 Malnutrition of mild degree `CC`
CC Exd: See code 260
AHA: J-A, '85, 1

263.2 Arrested development following protein-calorie malnutrition `CC`
Nutritional dwarfism
Physical retardation due to malnutrition
CC Exd: See code 260

263.8 Other protein-calorie malnutrition `CC`
CC Exd: See code 260

263.9 Unspecified protein-calorie malnutrition `CC`
Dystrophy due to malnutrition
Malnutrition (calorie) NOS
EXCLUDES nutritional deficiency NOS (269.9)
CC Exd: See code 260
AHA: ▶3Q, '12, 9;◄4Q '03, 109; N-D, '84, 19
E46 Unspecified protein-calorie malnutrition `I-10`

√4ᵗʰ **264 Vitamin A deficiency**

264.0 With conjunctival xerosis
DEF: Vitamin A deficiency with conjunctival dryness.

264.1 With conjunctival xerosis and Bitot's spot
Bitot's spot in the young child
DEF: Vitamin A deficiency with conjunctival dryness, superficial spots of keratinized epithelium.

264.2 With corneal xerosis
DEF: Vitamin A deficiency with corneal dryness.

264.3 With corneal ulceration and xerosis
DEF: Vitamin A deficiency with corneal dryness, epithelial ulceration.

264.4 With keratomalacia
DEF: Vitamin A deficiency creating corneal dryness; progresses to corneal insensitivity, softness, necrosis; usually bilateral.

264.5 With night blindness
DEF: Vitamin A deficiency causing vision failure in dim light.

264.6 With xerophthalmic scars of cornea
DEF: Vitamin A deficiency with corneal scars from dryness.

264.7 Other ocular manifestations of vitamin A deficiency
Xerophthalmia due to vitamin A deficiency

264.8 Other manifestations of vitamin A deficiency
Follicular keratosis
Xeroderma } due to vitamin A deficiency

264.9 Unspecified vitamin A deficiency
Hypovitaminosis A NOS

√4ᵗʰ **265 Thiamine and niacin deficiency states**

265.0 Beriberi `CC`
DEF: Inadequate vitamin B_1 (thiamine) intake, affects heart and peripheral nerves; individual may become edematous and develop cardiac disease due to the excess fluid; affects alcoholics and people with a diet of excessive polished rice.
CC Exd: 265.0-266.9, 269.1-269.9

265.1 Other and unspecified manifestations of thiamine deficiency `CC`
Other vitamin B_1 deficiency states
CC Exd: See code: 265.0

265.2 Pellagra
Deficiency:
niacin (-tryptophan)
nicotinamide
nicotinic acid
vitamin PP
Pellagra (alcoholic)
DEF: Niacin deficiency causing dermatitis, inflammation of mucous membranes, diarrhea, and psychic disturbances.

Additional Digit Required · Unacceptable PDx · Manifestation Code · Hospital Acquired Condition · ▶◄ Revised Text · ● New Code · ▲ Revised Code Title

14 ICD-9-CM · February 2013 · Volume 1 – 65

✓4ᵗʰ **266 Deficiency of B-complex components**

266.0 Ariboflavinosis   `CC`
Riboflavin [vitamin B_2] deficiency
DEF: Vitamin B_2 (riboflavin) deficiency marked by swollen lips and tongue fissures, corneal vascularization, scaling lesions, and anemia.
CC Excl: See code: 265.0
AHA: S-O, '86, 10

266.1 Vitamin B_6 deficiency
Deficiency:
  pyridoxal
  pyridoxamine
  pyridoxine
Vitamin B_6 deficiency syndrome
  EXCLUDES *vitamin B_6-responsive sideroblastic anemia (285.0)*
DEF: Vitamin B_6 deficiency causing skin, lip, and tongue disturbances, peripheral neuropathy; and convulsions in infants.

266.2 Other B-complex deficiencies
Deficiency:
  cyanocobalamin
  folic acid
  vitamin B_{12}
  EXCLUDES *combined system disease with anemia (281.0-281.1)*
    deficiency anemias (281.0-281.9)
    subacute degeneration of spinal cord with anemia (281.0-281.1)
  E53.8 Deficiency of other specified B group vitamins   `I-10`

266.9 Unspecified vitamin B deficiency

267 Ascorbic acid deficiency
Deficiency of vitamin C
Scurvy
  EXCLUDES *scorbutic anemia (281.8)*
DEF: Vitamin C deficiency causing swollen gums, myalgia, weight loss, and weakness.

✓4ᵗʰ **268 Vitamin D deficiency**
  EXCLUDES *vitamin D-resistant:*
    osteomalacia (275.3)
    rickets (275.3)

268.0 Rickets, active   `CC`
  EXCLUDES *celiac rickets (579.0)*
    renal rickets (588.0)
DEF: Inadequate vitamin D intake, usually in pediatrics, that affects bones most involved with muscular action; may cause nodules on ends and sides of bones; delayed closure of fontanels in infants; symptoms may include muscle soreness, and profuse sweating.
CC Excl: 268.0-269.9

268.1 Rickets, late effect
Any condition specified as due to rickets and stated to be a late effect or sequela of rickets
Code first the nature of late effect
DEF: Distorted or demineralized bones as a result of vitamin D deficiency.

268.2 Osteomalacia, unspecified
DEF: Softening of bones due to decrease in calcium; marked by pain, tenderness, muscular weakness, anorexia, and weight loss.

268.9 Unspecified vitamin D deficiency
Avitaminosis D

✓4ᵗʰ **269 Other nutritional deficiencies**

269.0 Deficiency of vitamin K
  EXCLUDES *deficiency of coagulation factor due to vitamin K deficiency (286.7)*
    vitamin K deficiency of newborn (776.0)

269.1 Deficiency of other vitamins
Deficiency:
  vitamin E
  vitamin P

269.2 Unspecified vitamin deficiency
Multiple vitamin deficiency NOS

269.3 Mineral deficiency, not elsewhere classified
Deficiency:
  calcium, dietary
  iodine
  EXCLUDES *deficiency:*
    calcium NOS (275.4)
    potassium (276.8)
    sodium (276.1)

269.8 Other nutritional deficiency
  EXCLUDES *adult failure to thrive (783.7)*
    failure to thrive in childhood (783.41)
    feeding problems (783.3)
    newborn (779.31-779.34)

269.9 Unspecified nutritional deficiency

Other Metabolic and Immunity Disorders (270-279)

Use additional code to identify any associated intellectual disabiliti

✓4ᵗʰ **270 Disorders of amino-acid transport and metabolism**
  EXCLUDES *abnormal findings without manifest disease (790.0-796.9)*
    disorders of purine and pyrimidine metabolism (277.1-277.
    gout (274.00-274.9)

270.0 Disturbances of amino-acid transport   `C`
Cystinosis
Cystinuria
Fanconi (-de Toni) (-Debré) syndrome
Glycinuria (renal)
Hartnup disease
CC Excl: 270.0-273.3, 273.8-273.9

270.1 Phenylketonuria [PKU]   `C`
Hyperphenylalaninemia
DEF: Inherited metabolic condition causing excess phenylpyruvic and other acids in urine; results in mental retardation, neurological manifestations, including spasticity and tremors, light pigmentatio eczema, and mousy odor.
CC Excl: See code: 270.0

270.2 Other disturbances of aromatic amino-acid metabolism   `C`
Albinism
Alkaptonuria
Alkaptonuric ochronosis
Disturbances of metabolism of tyrosine and tryptophan
Homogentisic acid defects
Hydroxykynureninuria
Hypertyrosinemia
Indicanuria
Kynureninase defects
Oasthouse urine disease
Ochronosis
Tyrosinosis
Tyrosinuria
Waardenburg syndrome
  EXCLUDES *vitamin B_6-deficiency syndrome (266.1)*
CC Excl: See code: 270.0
AHA: 3Q, '99, 20

270.3 Disturbances of branched-chain amino-acid metabolism   `C`
Disturbances of metabolism of leucine, isoleucine, and valin
Hypervalinemia
Intermittent branched-chain ketonuria
Leucine-induced hypoglycemia
Leucinosis
Maple syrup urine disease
CC Excl: See code: 270.0
AHA: 3Q, '00, 8

270.4 Disturbances of sulphur-bearing amino-acid metabolism   `C`
Cystathioninemia
Cystathioninuria
Disturbances of metabolism of methionine, homocystine, an cystathionine
Homocystinuria
Hypermethioninemia
Methioninemia
CC Excl: See code: 270.0
AHA: 2Q, '07, 7;1Q, '04, 6

`N` Newborn Age: 0   `P` Pediatric Age: 0-17   `M` Maternity Age: 12-55   `A` Adult Age: 15-124   `MCC` Major CC Condition   `CC` CC Condition   `HIV` HIV Related D

66 – Volume 1   2014 ICD-9-C

270.5 Disturbances of histidine metabolism `CC`
Carnosinemia
Histidinemia
Hyperhistidinemia
Imidazole aminoaciduria
CC Excl: See code: 270.0

270.6 Disorders of urea cycle metabolism `CC`
Argininosuccinic aciduria
Citrullinemia
Disorders of metabolism of ornithine, citrulline,
   argininosuccinic acid, arginine, and ammonia
Hyperammonemia
Hyperomithinemia
CC Excl: See code: 270.0

270.7 Other disturbances of straight-chain amino-acid `CC`
metabolism
Glucoglycinuria
Glycinemia (with methylmalonic acidemia)
Hyperglycinemia
Hyperlysinemia
Other disturbances of metabolism of glycine, threonine,
   serine, glutamine, and lysine
Pipecolic acidemia
Saccharopinuria
CC Excl: See code: 270.0
AHA: 3Q, '00, 8

270.8 Other specified disorders of amino-acid metabolism `CC`
Alaninemia   Iminoacidopathy
Ethanolaminuria   Prolinemia
Glycoprolinuria   Prolinuria
Hydroxyprolinemia   Sarcosinemia
Hyperprolinemia
CC Excl: See code: 270.0

270.9 Unspecified disorder of amino-acid metabolism `CC`
CC Excl: See code: 270.0

✓4ᵗʰ **271 Disorders of carbohydrate transport and metabolism**
   EXCLUDES *abnormality of secretion of glucagon (251.4)*
               diabetes mellitus (249.0-249.9, 250.0-250.9)
               hypoglycemia NOS (251.2)
               mucopolysaccharidosis (277.5)

271.0 Glycogenosis `CC`
Amylopectinosis
Glucose-6-phosphatase deficiency
Glycogen storage disease
McArdle's disease
Pompe's disease
von Gierke's disease
CC Excl: 270.0-273.3, 273.8-273.9
AHA: 1Q, '98, 5

271.1 Galactosemia `CC`
Galactose-1-phosphate uridyl transferase deficiency
Galactosuria
DEF: Any of three genetic disorders due to defective galactose
metabolism; symptoms include failure to thrive in infancy, jaundice,
liver and spleen damage, cataracts, and mental retardation.
CC Excl: See code: 271.0

271.2 Hereditary fructose intolerance
Essential benign fructosuria
Fructosemia
DEF: Chromosome recessive disorder of carbohydrate metabolism; in
infants, occurs after dietary sugar introduced; characterized by
enlarged spleen, yellowish cast to skin, and progressive inability to
thrive.

271.3 Intestinal disaccharidase deficiencies and disaccharide
malabsorption
Intolerance or malabsorption (congenital) (of):
   glucose-galactose
   lactose
   sucrose-isomaltose
E73.9 Lactose intolerance unspecified `I-10`

271.4 Renal glycosuria
Renal diabetes
DEF: Persistent abnormal levels of glucose in urine, with normal
blood glucose levels; caused by failure of the renal tubules to
reabsorb glucose.

271.8 Other specified disorders of carbohydrate `CC`
transport and metabolism
Essential benign pentosuria   Mannosidosis
Fucosidosis   Oxalosis
Glycolic aciduria   Xylosuria
Hyperoxaluria (primary)   Xylulosuria
CC Excl: See code: 271.0

271.9 Unspecified disorder of carbohydrate transport and
metabolism

✓4ᵗʰ **272 Disorders of lipid metabolism**
   EXCLUDES *localized cerebral lipidoses (330.1)*

272.0 Pure hypercholesterolemia
Familial hypercholesterolemia
Fredrickson Type IIa hyperlipoproteinemia
Hyperbetalipoproteinemia
Hyperlipidemia, Group A
Low-density-lipoid-type [LDL] hyperlipoproteinemia
AHA: 4Q, '05, 71
E78.0 Pure hypercholesterolemia `I-10`

272.1 Pure hyperglyceridemia
Endogenous hyperglyceridemia
Fredrickson Type IV hyperlipoproteinemia
Hyperlipidemia, Group B
Hyperprebetalipoproteinemia
Hypertriglyceridemia, essential
Very-low-density-lipoid-type [VLDL] hyperlipoproteinemia

272.2 Mixed hyperlipidemia
Broad- or floating-betalipoproteinemia
Combined hyperlipidemia
Elevated cholesterol with elevated triglycerides NEC
Fredrickson Type IIb or III hyperlipoproteinemia
Hypercholesterolemia with endogenous hyperglyceridemia
Hyperbetalipoproteinemia with prebetalipoproteinemia
Tubo-eruptive xanthoma
Xanthoma tuberosum
DEF: Elevated levels of lipoprotein, a complex of fats and proteins, in
blood due to inherited metabolic disorder.

272.3 Hyperchylomicronemia
Bürger-Grütz syndrome
Fredrickson type I or V hyperlipoproteinemia
Hyperlipidemia, Group D
Mixed hyperglyceridemia

272.4 Other and unspecified hyperlipidemia
Alpha-lipoproteinemia
Hyperlipidemia NOS
Hyperlipoproteinemia NOS
DEF: Hyperlipoproteinemia: elevated levels of transient chylomicrons
in the blood which are a form of lipoproteins that transport dietary
cholesterol and triglycerides from the small intestine to the blood.
AHA: 1Q, '05, 17
E78.4 Other hyperlipidemia `I-10`

272.5 Lipoprotein deficiencies
Abetalipoproteinemia
Bassen-Kornzweig syndrome
High-density lipid deficiency
Hypoalphalipoproteinemia
Hypobetalipoproteinemia (familial)
DEF: Abnormally low levels of lipoprotein, a complex of fats and
protein, in the blood.

Lipid Metabolism

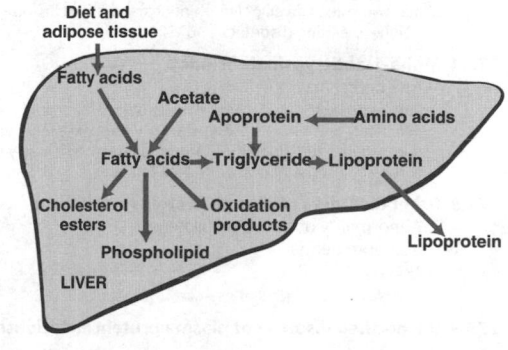

Endocrine, Nutritional and Metabolic Diseases, and Immunity

272.6–275.09

272.6 Lipodystrophy
Barraquer-Simons disease
Progressive lipodystrophy
Use additional E code to identify cause, if iatrogenic
EXCLUDES   *intestinal lipodystrophy (040.2)*
DEF: Disturbance of fat metabolism resulting in loss of fatty tissue in some areas of the body.

272.7 Lipidoses
Chemically-induced lipidosis
Disease:
   Anderson's
   Fabry's
   Gaucher's
   I cell [mucolipidosis I]
   lipoid storage NOS
   Niemann-Pick
   pseudo-Hurler's or mucolipdosis III
   triglyceride storage, Type I or II
   Wolman's or triglyceride storage, Type III
Mucolipidosis II
Primary familial xanthomatosis
EXCLUDES   *cerebral lipidoses (330.1)*
         Tay-Sachs disease (330.1)
DEF: Lysosomal storage diseases marked by an abnormal amount of lipids in reticuloendothelial cells.

272.8 Other disorders of lipoid metabolism
Hoffa's disease or liposynovitis prepatellaris
Launois-Bensaude's lipomatosis
Lipoid dermatoarthritis

272.9 Unspecified disorder of lipoid metabolism

√4th **273 Disorders of plasma protein metabolism**
EXCLUDES   *agammaglobulinemia and*
        hypogammaglobulinemia (279.0-279.2)
      coagulation defects (286.0-286.9)
      hereditary hemolytic anemias (282.0-282.9)

273.0 Polyclonal hypergammaglobulinemia
Hypergammaglobulinemic purpura:
   benign primary
   Waldenström's
DEF: Elevated blood levels of gamma globulins, frequently found in patients with chronic infectious diseases.

273.1 Monoclonal paraproteinemia
Benign monoclonal hypergammaglobulinemia [BMH]
Monoclonal gammopathy:
   NOS
   associated with lymphoplasmacytic dyscrasias
   benign
Paraproteinemia:
   benign (familial)
   secondary to malignant or inflammatory disease

273.2 Other paraproteinemias
Cryoglobulinemic:
   purpura
   vasculitis
Mixed cryoglobulinemia
AHA: 2Q, '08, 17

273.3 Macroglobulinemia
Macroglobulinemia (idiopathic) (primary)
Waldenström's macroglobulinemia
DEF: Elevated blood levels of macroglobulins (plasma globulins of high weight); characterized by malignant neoplasms of bone marrow, spleen, liver, or lymph nodes; symptoms include weakness, fatigue, bleeding disorders, and vision problems.

273.4 Alpha-1-antitrypsin deficiency
AAT deficiency
DEF: Disorder of plasma protein metabolism that results in a deficiency of Alpha-1-antitrypsin, an acute-phase reactive protein, released into the blood in response to infection or injury to protect tissue against the harmful effect of enzymes.

273.8 Other disorders of plasma protein metabolism
Abnormality of transport protein
Bisalbuminemia
AHA: 2Q, '98, 11
E88.09 Other disorders of plasma-protein metablolis NEC   I-10

273.9 Unspecified disorder of plasma protein metabolism

√4th **274 Gout**
EXCLUDES   *lead gout (984.0-984.9)*
DEF: Purine and pyrimidine metabolic disorders; manifested by hyperuricemia and recurrent acute inflammatory arthritis; monosodium urate or monohydrate crystals may be deposited in and around the joints, leading to joint destruction, and severe crippling.
AHA: 2Q, '95, 4

√5th **274.0 Gouty arthropathy**
AHA: 4Q, '09, 76-77

274.00 Gouty arthropathy, unspecified
M10.00 Idiopathic gout unspecified site

274.01 Acute gouty arthropathy
Acute gout   Gout flare
Gout attack   Podagra

274.02 Chronic gouty arthropathy without mention of tophus (tophi)
Chronic gout

274.03 Chronic gouty arthropathy with tophus (tophi)
Chronic tophaceous gout   Gout with tophi NOS
AHA: 4Q, '09, 77

√5th **274.1 Gouty nephropathy**

274.10 Gouty nephropathy, unspecified
AHA: N-D, '85, 15

274.11 Uric acid nephrolithiasis   C
DEF: Sodium urate stones in the kidney.
CC Excl: 016.00-016.06, 016.30-016.36, 016.90-016.96, 017.90-017.96, 078.6, 098.10, 098.19, 098.30-098.31, 098.89, 112.2, 131.00, 131.8-131.9, 249.40-249.41, 249.80-249.91, 250.40-250.43, 250.80-250.93, 274.10-274.19, 274.89, 580.0-584.9, 586-588.1, 588.9-591, 593.0-593.2, 593.89-593.9, 599.60-599.9

274.19 Other

√5th **274.8 Gout with other specified manifestations**

274.81 Gouty tophi of ear
DEF: Chalky sodium urate deposit in the ear due to gout; produces chronic inflammation of external ear.

274.82 Gouty tophi of other sites
Gouty tophi of heart
EXCLUDES   *gout with tophi NOS (274.03)*
      gouty arthropathy with tophi (274.03)

274.89 Other
Use additional code to identify manifestations, as:
   gouty:
      iritis (364.11)
      neuritis (357.4)

274.9 Gout, unspecified
M10.9 Gout unspecified

√4th **275 Disorders of mineral metabolism**
EXCLUDES   *abnormal findings without manifest disease (790.0-796.9)*

√5th **275.0 Disorders of iron metabolism**
EXCLUDES   *anemia:*
        iron deficiency (280.0-280.9)
        sideroblastic (285.0)
AHA: 4Q, '10, 77-78; 2Q, '97, 11

275.01 Hereditary hemochromatosis
Bronzed diabetes
Pigmentary cirrhosis (of liver)
Primary (hereditary) hemochromatosis
E83.110 Hereditary hemochromatosis

275.02 Hemochromatosis due to repeated red blood cell transfusions
Iron overload due to repeated red blood cell transfusions
Transfusion (red blood cell) associated hemochromatosis
AHA: 4Q, '10, 77-78
E83.111 Hemochromatosis due to repeated red blood cell transfusions

275.03 Other hemochromatosis
Hemochromatosis NOS
E83.118 Other hemochromatosis

275.09 Other disorders of iron metabolism
E83.10 Disorder of iron-metabolism unspecified

N Newborn Age: 0   P Pediatric Age: 0-17   M Maternity Age: 12-55   A Adult Age: 15-124   MCC Major CC Condition   CC CC Condition   HIV HIV Related D

68 – Volume 1   2014 ICD-9-C

275.1 Disorders of copper metabolism
Hepatolenticular degeneration
Wilson's disease

275.2 Disorders of magnesium metabolism
Hypermagnesemia   Hypomagnesemia
AHA: 1Q, '10, 14; 3Q, '09, 21
E83.40 Disorders of magnesium metabolism unspecified   [I-10]

275.3 Disorders of phosphorus metabolism
Familial hypophosphatemia
Hypophosphatasia
Vitamin D-resistant:
   osteomalacia
   rickets

√5ᵗʰ **275.4 Disorders of calcium metabolism**
EXCLUDES   *hungry bone syndrome (275.5)*
parathyroid disorders (252.00-252.9)
vitamin D deficiency (268.0-268.9)
AHA: 4Q, '97, 33

275.40 Unspecified disorder of calcium metabolism

275.41 Hypocalcemia
DEF: Abnormally decreased blood calcium level; symptoms include hyperactive deep tendon reflexes, muscle, abdominal cramps, and carpopedal spasm.
AHA: 3Q, '07, 5
E83.51 Hypocalcemia   [I-10]

275.42 Hypercalcemia
DEF: Abnormally increased blood calcium level; symptoms include muscle weakness, fatigue, nausea, depression, and constipation.
AHA: ▶3Q, '12,16;◀ 4Q, '03, 110

275.49 Other disorders of calcium metabolism
Nephrocalcinosis
Pseudohypoparathyroidism
Pseudopseudohypoparathyroidism
DEF: Nephrocalcinosis: calcium phosphate deposits in the tubules of the kidney with resultant renal insufficiency.
DEF: Pseudohypoparathyroidism: inherited hypoparathyroidism disorder; caused by inadequate response to parathyroid hormone, not hormonal deficiency; includes muscle cramps, tetany, urinary frequency, blurred vision due to cataracts, and dry scaly skin.
DEF: Pseudopseudohypoparathyroidism: clinical manifestations of hypoparathyroidism without affecting blood calcium levels.

275.5 Hungry bone syndrome
DEF: Marked and prolonged hypocalcemia; usually involves an extended history of elevated levels of parathyroid hormone, related bone demineralization causing the bone to sequester calcium.
AHA: 4Q, '08, 96-97

275.8 Other specified disorders of mineral metabolism

275.9 Unspecified disorder of mineral metabolism

√4ᵗʰ **276 Disorders of fluid, electrolyte, and acid-base balance**
EXCLUDES   *diabetes insipidus (253.5)*
familial periodic paralysis (359.3)

276.0 Hyperosmolality and/or hypernatremia   [CC]
Sodium [Na] excess
Sodium [Na] overload
CC Excl: 276.0-276.52, 276.61-276.9

276.1 Hyposmolality and/or hyponatremia   [CC]
Sodium [Na] deficiency
CC Excl: See code: 276.0
E87.1 Hypo-osmolality and hyponatremia   [I-10]

276.2 Acidosis   [CC]
Acidosis: Acidosis:
   NOS   metabolic
   lactic   respiratory
EXCLUDES   *diabetic acidosis (249.1, 250.1)*
DEF: Disorder involves decrease of pH (hydrogen ion) concentration in blood and cellular tissues; caused by increase in acid and decrease in bicarbonate.
CC Excl: 276.0-276.9
AHA: J-F, '87, 15
E87.2 Acidosis   [I-10]

276.3 Alkalosis   [CC]
Alkalosis:
   NOS
   metabolic
   respiratory
DEF: Increased blood alkalinity (base) without relative loss of base in body fluids; caused by increased arterial plasma bicarbonate concentration or loss of carbon dioxide due to hyperventilation.
CC Excl: See code: 276.0

276.4 Mixed acid-base balance disorder   [CC]
Hypercapnia with mixed acid-base disorder
CC Excl: See code 276.0

√5ᵗʰ **276.5 Volume depletion**
EXCLUDES   *hypovolemic shock:*
postoperative (998.09)
traumatic (958.4)
AHA: 4Q, '05, 54; 2Q, '05, 9; 1Q, '03, 5, 22; 3Q, '02, 21; 4Q, '97, 30; 2Q, '88, 9

276.50 Volume depletion, unspecified
DEF: Depletion of total body water (dehydration) and/or contraction of total intravascular plasma (hypovolemia).
E86.9 Volume depletion unspecified   [I-10]

276.51 Dehydration
DEF: Depletion of total body water; blood volume may be normal while fluid is pulled from other tissues.
AHA: 1Q, '08, 10
E86.0 Dehydration   [I-10]

276.52 Hypovolemia
Depletion of volume of plasma
DEF: Depletion of volume plasma; depletion of total blood volume.

√5ᵗʰ **276.6 Fluid overload**
EXCLUDES   *ascites (789.51-789.59)*
localized edema (782.3)
AHA: 4Q, '10, 79; 3Q, '07, 9; 4Q, '06, 136

276.61 Transfusion associated circulatory overload
Fluid overload due to transfusion (blood) (blood components)
TACO
AHA: 4Q, '10, 79-80
E87.71 Transfusion associated circulatory overload   [I-10]

276.69 Other fluid overload
Fluid retention
E87.79 Other fluid overload   [I-10]

276.7 Hyperpotassemia
Hyperkalemia
Potassium [K]:
   excess
   intoxication
   overload
DEF: Elevated blood levels of potassium; symptoms include abnormal EKG readings, weakness; related to defective renal excretion.
AHA: 2Q, '11, 6; 1Q, '05, 9; 2Q,'01, 12
E87.5 Hyperkalemia   [I-10]

276.8 Hypopotassemia
Hypokalemia
Potassium [K] deficiency
DEF: Decreased blood levels of potassium; symptoms include neuromuscular disorders.
E87.6 Hypokalemia   [I-10]

276.9 Electrolyte and fluid disorders not elsewhere classified
Electrolyte imbalance
Hyperchloremia
Hypochloremia
EXCLUDES   *electrolyte imbalance:*
associated with hyperemesis gravidarum (643.1)
complicating labor and delivery (669.0)
following abortion and ectopic or molar pregnancy (634-638 with .4, 639.4)
AHA: J-F, '87, 15
E87.8 Oth disorders of electrolyte & fluid balance NEC   [I-10]

Additional Digit Required   Unacceptable PDx   Manifestation Code   Hospital Acquired Condition   ▶◀ Revised Text   ● New Code   ▲ Revised Code Title

✓4ᵗʰ **277 Other and unspecified disorders of metabolism**

✓5ᵗʰ **277.0 Cystic fibrosis**
Fibrocystic disease of the pancreas
Mucoviscidosis

DEF: Genetic disorder of infants, children, and young adults marked by exocrine gland dysfunction; characterized by chronic pulmonary disease with excess mucus production, pancreatic deficiency, and high levels of electrolytes in the sweat.

AHA: 4Q, '90, 16; 3Q, '90, 18

TIP: Sequencing of CF is determined by circumstances of admission. If a patient is admitted for CF, sequence the CF first. If admitted for a complication of CF (e.g., pneumothorax, acute bronchitis, or acute cor pulmonale), sequence the complication first.

277.00 Without mention of meconium ileus `CC`
Cystic fibrosis NOS
CC Excl: 277.00-277.09
AHA: 2Q, '03, 12
E84.9 Cystic fibrosis unspecified `I-10`

277.01 With meconium ileus `MCC` `N`
Meconium:
ileus (of newborn)
obstruction of intestine in mucoviscidosis
CC Excl: See code 277.00

277.02 With pulmonary manifestations `MCC`
Cystic fibrosis with pulmonary exacerbation
Use additional code to identify any infectious organism present, such as:
pseudomonas (041.7)
CC Excl: See code 277.00

277.03 With gastrointestinal manifestations `CC`
EXCLUDES with meconium ileus (277.01)
CC Excl: See code 277.00
AHA: 4Q, '02, 45

277.09 With other manifestations `CC`
CC Excl: See code 277.00

277.1 Disorders of porphyrin metabolism `CC`
Hematoporphyria
Hematoporphyrinuria
Hereditary coproporphyria
Porphyria
Porphyrinuria
Protocoproporphyria
Protoporphyria
Pyrroloporphyria
CC Excl: 277.1-277.2, 277.4-277.7

277.2 Other disorders of purine and pyrimidine metabolism `CC`
Hypoxanthine-guanine-phosphoribosyltransferase deficiency [HG-PRT deficiency]
Lesch-Nyhan syndrome
Xanthinuria
EXCLUDES gout (274.00-274.9)
orotic aciduric anemia (281.4)
CC Excl: See code: 277.1

✓5ᵗʰ **277.3 Amyloidosis**
DEF: Conditions of diverse etiologies characterized by the accumulation of insoluble fibrillar proteins (amyloid) in various organs and tissues of the body, compromising vital functions.
AHA: 1Q, '96, 16

277.30 Amyloidosis, unspecified `CC`
Amyloidosis NOS
CC Excl: 277.30-277.39, 277.7
AHA: 4Q, '06, 66

277.31 Familial Mediterranean fever `CC`
Benign paroxysmal peritonitis
Hereditary amyloid nephropathy
Periodic familial polyserositis
Recurrent polyserositis
DEF: Early-life onset of recurrent attacks characterized by high fevers with pain and inflammation of chest and abdominal cavities, skin and joints, also rash or vasculitis. Etiology unknown, possibly genetic, but may be precipitated by stress, trauma or exertion.
CC Excl: See code: 277.30
AHA: ▶2Q, '12, 18;◀ 4Q, '06, 66

277.39 Other amyloidosis `CC`
Hereditary cardiac amyloidosis
Inherited systemic amyloidosis
Neuropathic (Portuguese) (Swiss) amyloidosis
Secondary amyloidosis
CC Excl: See code: 277.30
AHA: 1Q, '09, 9; 2Q, '08, 8; 4Q, '06, 66

277.4 Disorders of bilirubin excretion
Hyperbilirubinemia:
congenital
constitutional
Syndrome:
Crigler-Najjar
Dubin-Johnson
Gilbert's
Rotor's
EXCLUDES hyperbilirubinemias specific to the perinatal period (774.0-774.7)

277.5 Mucopolysaccharidosis `CC`
Gargoylism
Hunter's syndrome
Hurler's syndrome
Lipochondrodystrophy
Maroteaux-Lamy syndrome
Morquio-Brailsford disease
Osteochondrodystrophy
Sanfilippo's syndrome
Scheie's syndrome
DEF: Metabolic disorders evidenced by excretion of various mucopolysaccharides in urine and infiltration of these substances into connective tissue, with resulting defects of bone, cartilage and connective tissue.
CC Excl: 277.1-277.31, 277.4-277.7

277.6 Other deficiencies of circulating enzymes
Hereditary angioedema
AHA: 2Q, '10, 12

277.7 Dysmetabolic syndrome X
Use additional code for associated manifestation, such as:
cardiovascular disease (414.00-414.07)
obesity (278.00-278.03)
DEF: A specific group of metabolic disorders that are related to the state of insulin resistance (decreased cellular response to insulin) without elevated blood sugars; often related to elevated cholesterol and triglycerides, obesity, cardiovascular disease, and high blood pressure.
AHA: 4Q, '01, 42

✓5ᵗʰ **277.8 Other specified disorders of metabolism**
AHA: 4Q, '03, 50; 2Q, '01, 18; S-O, '87, 9

277.81 Primary carnitine deficiency

277.82 Carnitine deficiency due to inborn errors of metabolism

277.83 Iatrogenic carnitine deficiency
Carnitine deficiency due to:
hemodialysis
valproic acid therapy

277.84 Other secondary carnitine deficiency

277.85 Disorders of fatty acid oxidation `CC`
Carnitine palmitoyltransferase deficiencies (CPT1, CPT2)
Glutaric aciduria type II (type IIA, IIB, IIC)
Long chain 3-hydroxyacyl CoA dehydrogenase deficiency (LCHAD)
Long chain/very long chain acyl CoA dehydrogenase deficiency (LCAD, VLCAD)
Medium chain acyl CoA dehydrogenase deficiency (MCAD)
Short chain acyl CoA dehydrogenase deficiency (SCAD)
EXCLUDES primary carnitine deficiency (277.81)
CC Excl: 277.81-277.84, 277.86-277.87, 277.89

`N` Newborn Age: 0   `P` Pediatric Age: 0-17   `M` Maternity Age: 12-55   `A` Adult Age: 15-124   `MCC` Major CC Condition   `CC` CC Condition   `HIV` HIV Related D

70 – Volume 1 · February 2013   **2014 ICD-9-C**

277.86 Peroxisomal disorders `CC`
Adrenomyeloneuropathy
Neonatal adrenoleukodystrophy
Rhizomelic chrondrodysplasia punctata
X-linked adrenoleukodystrophy
Zellweger syndrome
> *EXCLUDES* *infantile Refsum disease (356.3)*
CC Excl: 277.4, 277.81-277.85, 277.87, 277.89

277.87 Disorders of mitochondrial metabolism `CC`
Kearns-Sayre syndrome
Mitochondrial Encephalopathy, Lactic Acidosis and Stroke-like episodes (MELAS syndrome)
Mitochondrial Neurogastrointestinal Encephalopathy syndrome (MNGIE)
Myoclonus with Epilepsy and with Ragged Red Fibers (MERRF syndrome)
Neuropathy, Ataxia and Retinitis Pigmentosa (NARP syndrome)
Use additional code for associated conditions
> *EXCLUDES* *disorders of pyruvate metabolism (271.8)*
> *Leber's optic atrophy (377.16)*
> *Leigh's subacute necrotizing encephalopathy (330.8)*
> *Reye's syndrome (331.81)*
CC Excl: 277.4, 277.81-277.86, 277.89
AHA: 4Q, '04, 62

277.88 Tumor lysis syndrome `MCC`
Spontaneous tumor lysis syndrome
Tumor lysis syndrome following antineoplastic drug therapy
Use additional E code to identify cause, if drug-induced
DEF: A potentially fatal metabolic complication of tumor necrosis caused by either spontaneous or treatment-related accumulation of byproducts from dying cancer cells; symptoms include hyperkalemia, hyperphosphatemia, hypocalcemia, hyperuricemia, and hyperuricosuria.
CC Excl: 277.88, 580.0-581.0, 581.81-581.9, 583.4-584.9
AHA: 4Q, '09, 78-79

277.89 Other specified disorders of metabolism `CC`
Hand-Schüller-Christian disease
Histiocytosis (acute) (chronic)
Histiocytosis X (chronic)
> *EXCLUDES* *histiocytosis:*
> *acute differentiated progressive (202.5)*
> *adult pulmonary Langerhans cell (516.5)*
> *X, acute (progressive) (202.5)*
CC Excl: 277.4, 277.81-277.87

277.9 Unspecified disorder of metabolism
Enzymopathy NOS

√4ᵗʰ **278 Overweight, obesity and other hyperalimentation**
> *EXCLUDES* *hyperalimentation NOS (783.6)*
> *poisoning by vitamins NOS (963.5)*
> *polyphagia (783.6)*

√5ᵗʰ **278.0 Overweight and obesity**
Use additional code to identify Body Mass Index (BMI), if known (V85.0-V85.54)
> *EXCLUDES* *adiposogenital dystrophy (253.8)*
> *obesity of endocrine origin NOS (259.9)*
AHA: 3Q, '11, 4; 4Q, '05, 97

278.00 Obesity, unspecified
Obesity NOS
DEF: BMI (body mass index) between 30.0 and 39.9.
AHA: 4Q, '01, 42; 1Q, '99, 5, 6

278.01 Morbid obesity
Severe obesity
DEF: BMI (body mass index) 40 or greater.
AHA: 4Q, '10, 81; 2Q, '09, 11; 2Q, '06, 5-6; 3Q, '03, 6-8
E66.01 Morbid (severe) obesity due to excess calories `I-10`

278.02 Overweight
DEF: BMI (body mass index) between 25 and 29.9.
AHA: 4Q, '05, 55
E66.3 Overweight `I-10`

278.03 Obesity hypoventilation syndrome `CC`
Pickwickian syndrome
DEF: Hypoventilation, somnolence and erythrocytosis due to excessive weight against the chest wall.
CC Excl: 278.03, 416.0-416.1, 416.8-416.9
AHA: 4Q, '10, 80-81
E66.2 Morbid obesity w/ alveolar hyperventilation `I-10`

278.1 Localized adiposity
Fat pad
AHA: 2Q, '06, 10

278.2 Hypervitaminosis A

278.3 Hypercarotinemia
DEF: Elevated blood carotene level due to ingesting excess carotenoids or the inability to convert carotenoids to vitamin A.

278.4 Hypervitaminosis D
DEF: Weakness, fatigue, loss of weight, and other symptoms resulting from ingesting excessive amounts of vitamin D.

278.8 Other hyperalimentation
AHA: 2Q, '09, 11

√4ᵗʰ **279 Disorders involving the immune mechanism**
Use additional code for associated manifestations

√5ᵗʰ **279.0 Deficiency of humoral immunity**
DEF: Inadequate immune response to bacterial infections with potential reinfection by viruses due to lack of circulating immunoglobulins (acquired antibodies).

279.00 Hypogammaglobulinemia, unspecified `CC`
Agammaglobulinemia NOS
CC Excl: 279.00-279.49, 279.8-279.9

279.01 Selective IgA immunodeficiency `CC`
CC Excl: See code: 279.00

279.02 Selective IgM immunodeficiency `CC`
CC Excl: 279.02-279.49, 279.8-279.9

279.03 Other selective immunoglobulin deficiencies `CC`
Selective deficiency of IgG
CC Excl: See code: 279.02

279.04 Congenital hypogammaglobulinemia `CC`
Agammaglobulinemia:
Bruton's type
X-linked
CC Excl: See code 279.02

279.05 Immunodeficiency with increased IgM `CC`
Immunodeficiency with hyper-IgM:
autosomal recessive
X-linked
CC Excl: See code 279.02

279.06 Common variable immunodeficiency `CC`
Dysgammaglobulinemia (acquired) (congenital) (primary)
Hypogammaglobulinemia:
acquired primary
congenital non-sex-linked
sporadic
CC Excl: See code 279.02

279.09 Other `CC`
Transient hypogammaglobulinemia of infancy
CC Excl: See code 279.02

√5ᵗʰ **279.1 Deficiency of cell-mediated immunity**

279.10 Immunodeficiency with predominant T-cell defect, unspecified `CC`
CC Excl: See code 279.02
AHA: S-O, '87, 10

279.11 DiGeorge's syndrome `CC`
Pharyngeal pouch syndrome
Thymic hypoplasia
DEF: Congenital hypoplasia or aplasia of the thymus, parathyroid glands; related heart defects, anomalies of the great vessels, esophageal atresia, and abnormalities of facial structures.
CC Excl: See code 279.02

Endocrine, Nutritional and Metabolic Diseases, and Immunity

279.12–279.9

279.12 Wiskott-Aldrich syndrome `CC`

DEF: A disease characterized by chronic conditions, such as eczema, suppurative otitis media and anemia; results from an X-linked recessive gene and is classified as an immune deficiency syndrome.
CC Excl: See code 279.02

279.13 Nezelof's syndrome `CC`

Cellular immunodeficiency with abnormal immunoglobulin deficiency

DEF: Immune system disorder characterized by a pathological deficiency in cellular immunity and humoral antibodies resulting in inability to fight infectious diseases.
CC Excl: See code 279.02

279.19 Other `CC`

EXCLUDES ataxia-telangiectasia (334.8)
CC Excl: See code 279.02

279.2 Combined immunity deficiency `CC`

Agammaglobulinemia:
    autosomal recessive
    Swiss-type
    x-linked recessive
Severe combined immunodeficiency [SCID]
Thymic:
    alymphoplasia
    aplasia or dysplasia with immunodeficiency

EXCLUDES thymic hypoplasia (279.11)

DEF: Agammaglobulinemia: No immunoglobulins in the blood.
DEF: Thymic alymphoplasia: Severe combined immunodeficiency; result of failed lymphoid tissue development.
CC Excl: See code 279.02
AHA: 4Q, '11, 148

279.3 Unspecified immunity deficiency `CC`

CC Excl: See code 279.02

√5ᵗʰ **279.4 Autoimmune disease, not elsewhere classified**

EXCLUDES transplant failure or rejection (996.80-996.89)
AHA: 4Q, '09, 80; 3Q, 08, 5

279.41 Autoimmune lymphoproliferative syndrome
ALPS

DEF: Rare genetic alteration of the Fas protein; impairs normal cellular apoptosis (normal cell death), causing abnormal accumulation of lymphocytes in the lymph glands, liver, and spleen; symptoms include neutropenia, anemia, and thrombocytopenia.

279.49 Autoimmune disease, not elsewhere classified
Autoimmune disease NOS

AHA: ▶3Q, '12, 8;◄ 2Q, '11, 15
TIP: ▶Assign for pediatric autoimmune neuropsychiatric disorder associated with streptococcal infection (PANDAS), with additional codes to report specific neurological or psychiatric manifestations.◄

√5ᵗʰ **279.5 Graft-versus-host disease**

Code first underlying cause, such as:
    complication of blood transfusion (999.89)
    complication of transplanted organ (996.80-996.89)
Use additional code to identify associated manifestations, such as:
    desquamative dermatitis (695.89)
    diarrhea (787.91)
    elevated bilirubin (782.4)
    hair loss (704.09)

DEF: A complication of transplantation, most commonly bone marrow; may involve skin, GI tract, liver and cause increased susceptibility to infection; results when donor cells responsible for immune response attack the cells of the transplant recipient.
AHA:4Q, '08, 97-99, 154

279.50 Graft-versus-host disease, unspecified `CC`

CC Excl: 279.50-279.53, 996.85, 997.91-997.99
AHA: 4Q, '08, 99

279.51 Acute graft-versus-host disease `CC`

CC Excl: See code 279.50
AHA: 4Q, '11, 148; 4Q, '08, 99

279.52 Chronic graft-versus-host disease `CC`

CC Excl: See code 279.50

279.53 Acute on chronic graft-versus-host disease `CC`

CC Excl: See code 279.50

279.8 Other specified disorders involving the immune mechanism

Single complement [C_1-C_9] deficiency or dysfunction

279.9 Unspecified disorder of immune mechanism

AHA: 3Q, '92, 13

N Newborn Age: 0   P Pediatric Age: 0-17   M Maternity Age: 12-55   A Adult Age: 15-124   MCC Major CC Condition   CC CC Condition   HIV HIV Related D

72 – Volume 1 • February 2013
2014 ICD-9-CM

4. Diseases of the Blood and Blood-Forming Organs (280-289)

EXCLUDES *anemia complicating pregnancy or the puerperium (648.2)*

√4th **280 Iron deficiency anemias**

INCLUDES anemia:
asiderotic
hypochromic-microcytic
sideropenic

EXCLUDES *familial microcytic anemia (282.49)*

280.0 Secondary to blood loss (chronic)
Normocytic anemia due to blood loss
EXCLUDES *acute posthemorrhagic anemia (285.1)*
AHA: 4Q, '93, 34

280.1 Secondary to inadequate dietary iron intake

280.8 Other specified iron deficiency anemias
Paterson-Kelly syndrome
Plummer-Vinson syndrome
Sideropenic dysphagia

280.9 Iron deficiency anemia, unspecified
Anemia:
achlorhydric
chlorotic
idiopathic hypochromic
iron [Fe] deficiency NOS

√4th **281 Other deficiency anemias**

281.0 Pernicious anemia
Anemia:
Addison's
Biermer's
congenital pernicious
Congenital intrinsic factor [Castle's] deficiency
EXCLUDES *combined system disease without mention of anemia (266.2)*
subacute degeneration of spinal cord without mention of anemia (266.2)
DEF: Chronic progressive anemia due to Vitamin B12 malabsorption; caused by lack of a secretion of intrinsic factor, which is produced by the gastric mucosa of the stomach.
AHA: N-D, '84, 1; S-O, '84, 16

281.1 Other vitamin B$_{12}$ deficiency anemia
Anemia:
vegan's
vitamin B$_{12}$ deficiency (dietary)
due to selective vitamin B$_{12}$ malabsorption with proteinuria
Syndrome:
Imerslund's
Imerslund-Gräsbeck
EXCLUDES *combined system disease without mention of anemia (266.2)*
subacute degeneration of spinal cord without mention of anemia (266.2)

281.2 Folate-deficiency anemia
Congenital folate malabsorption
Folate or folic acid deficiency anemia:
NOS
dietary
drug-induced
Goat's milk anemia
Nutritional megaloblastic anemia (of infancy)
Use additional E code to identify drug
DEF: Macrocytic anemia resembles pernicious anemia but without absence of hydrochloric acid secretions; responsive to folic acid therapy.

281.3 Other specified megaloblastic anemias not elsewhere classified
Combined B$_{12}$ and folate-deficiency anemia
Refractory megaloblastic anemia
DEF: Megaloblasts predominant in bone marrow with few normoblasts; rare familial type associated with proteinuria and genitourinary tract anomalies.

281.4 Protein-deficiency anemia
Amino-acid-deficiency anemia

281.8 Anemia associated with other specified nutritional deficiency
Scorbutic anemia

281.9 Unspecified deficiency anemia
Anemia: Anemia:
dimorphic   nutritional NOS
macrocytic   simple chronic
megaloblastic NOS

√4th **282 Hereditary hemolytic anemias**
DEF: Escalated rate of erythrocyte destruction; similar to all anemias, occurs when imbalance exists between blood loss and blood production.

282.0 Hereditary spherocytosis
Acholuric (familial) jaundice
Congenital hemolytic anemia (spherocytic)
Congenital spherocytosis
Minkowski-Chauffard syndrome
Spherocytosis (familial)
EXCLUDES *hemolytic anemia of newborn (773.0-773.5)*
DEF: Hereditary, chronic illness marked by abnormal red blood cell membrane; symptoms include enlarged spleen, jaundice; and anemia in severe cases.

282.1 Hereditary elliptocytosis
Elliptocytosis (congenital)
Ovalocytosis (congenital) (hereditary)
DEF: Genetic hemolytic anemia characterized by malformed, elliptical erythrocytes; there is increased destruction of red cells with resulting anemia.

282.2 Anemias due to disorders of glutathione metabolism
Anemia:
6-phosphogluconic dehydrogenase deficiency
enzyme deficiency, drug-induced
erythrocytic glutathione deficiency
glucose-6-phosphate dehydrogenase [G-6-PD] deficiency
glutathione-reductase deficiency
hemolytic nonspherocytic (hereditary), type I
Disorder of pentose phosphate pathway
Favism

282.3 Other hemolytic anemias due to enzyme deficiency
Anemia:
hemolytic nonspherocytic (hereditary), type II
hexokinase deficiency
pyruvate kinase [PK] deficiency
triosephosphate isomerase deficiency

√5th **282.4 Thalassemias**
EXCLUDES *sickle-cell:*
disease (282.60-282.69)
trait (282.5)
DEF: Inherited hemolytic disorders characterized by decreased production of at least one polypeptide globin chain results in defective hemoglobin synthesis; symptoms include severe anemia, expanded marrow spaces, transfusional and absorptive iron overload, impaired growth rate, thickened cranial bones, and pathologic fractures.
AHA: 4Q, '03, 51

282.40 Thalassemia, unspecified
Thalassemia NOS
AHA: 4Q, '11, 87-91

282.41 Sickle-cell thalassemia without crisis
Microdrepanocytosis
Sickle-cell thalassemia NOS
Thalassemia Hb-S disease without crisis

282.42 Sickle-cell thalassemia with crisis   MCC
Sickle-cell thalassemia with vaso-occlusive pain
Thalassemia Hb-S disease with crisis
Use additional code for type of crisis, such as:
acute chest syndrome (517.3)
splenic sequestration (289.52)
CC Exc: 280.0-285.9, 286.53, 289.81-289.83, 289.89-289.9, 517.3

Diseases of the Blood and Blood-Forming Organs

282.43–282.69

282.43 Alpha thalassemia
Alpha thalassemia major
Hemoglobin H Constant Spring
Hemoglobin H disease
Hydrops fetalis due to alpha thalassemia
Severe alpha thalassemia
Triple gene defect alpha thalassemia

> **EXCLUDES**   *alpha thalassemia trait or minor (282.46)*
> *hydrops fetalis due to isoimmunization (773.3)*
> *hydrops fetalis not due to immune hemolysis (778.0)*

DEF: HBA1 and HBA2 genetic variant of chromosome 16 prevalent among Western African and South Asian descent; associated with a wide spectrum of anemic presentation, includes hemoglobin H disease subtypes.
AHA: 4Q, '11, 87-91

282.44 Beta thalassemia
Beta thalassemia major
Cooley's anemia
Homozygous beta thalassemia
Severe beta thalassemia
Thalassemia intermedia
Thalassemia major

> **EXCLUDES**   *beta thalassemia minor (282.46)*
> *beta thalassemia trait (282.46)*
> *delta-beta thalassemia (282.45)*
> *hemoglobin E-beta thalassemia (282.47)*
> *sickle-cell beta thalassemia (282.41, 282.42)*

DEF: Diversity of mutations of HBB gene on chromosome 11 prevalent among Mediterranean and certain South Asian descent with significant cellular damage, can result in toxicity and increased disease severity (e.g., severe beta thalassemia, thalassemia major).
AHA: 4Q, '11, 87-91

282.45 Delta-beta thalassemia
Homozygous delta-beta thalassemia

> **EXCLUDES**   *delta-beta thalassemia trait (282.46)*

AHA: 4Q, '11, 87-91

282.46 Thalassemia minor
Alpha thalassemia minor
Alpha thalassemia trait
Alpha thalassemia silent carrier
Beta thalassemia minor
Beta thalassemia trait
Delta-beta thalassemia trait
Thalassemia trait NOS

> **EXCLUDES**   *alpha thalassemia (282.43)*
> *beta thalassemia (282.44)*
> *delta-beta thalassemia (282.45)*
> *hemoglobin E-beta thalassemia (282.47)*
> *sickle-cell trait (282.5)*

DEF: Solitary abnormal gene that identifies a carrier of the disease, yet with an absence of symptoms or a clinically mild anemic presentation.
AHA: 4Q, '11, 87-91

282.47 Hemoglobin E-beta thalassemia

> **EXCLUDES**   *beta thalassemia (282.44)*
> *beta thalassemia minor (282.46)*
> *beta thalassemia trait (282.46)*
> *delta-beta thalassemia (282.45)*
> *delta-beta thalassemia trait (282.46)*
> *hemoglobin E disease (282.7)*
> *other hemoglobinopathies (282.7)*
> *sickle-cell beta thalassemia (282.41, 282.42)*

DEF: Clinically similar phenotype to B thalassemia major prevalent among Southeast Asian and certain Indian descent; results in severe transfusion-dependent anemia when present with certain B mutations.
AHA: 4Q, '11, 87-91

282.49 Other thalassemia
Dominant thalassemia
Hemoglobin C thalassemia
Hereditary leptocytosis
Mediterranean anemia (with other hemoglobinopathy)
Mixed thalassemia
Thalassemia with other hemoglobinopathy

> **EXCLUDES**   *hemoglobin C disease (282.7)*
> *hemoglobin E disease (282.7)*
> *other hemoglobinopathies (282.7)*
> *sickle-cell anemias (282.60-282.69)*
> *sickle-cell beta thalassemia (282.41-282.42)*

282.5 Sickle-cell trait
Hb-AS genotype   Heterozygous:
Hemoglobin S [Hb-S] trait   hemoglobin S
                              Hb-S

> **EXCLUDES**   *that with other hemoglobinopathy (282.60-282.69)*
> *that with thalassemia (282.41-282.42)*

DEF: Heterozygous genetic makeup characterized by one gene for normal hemoglobin and one for sickle-cell hemoglobin; clinical disease rarely present.
AHA: ▶3Q, '12, 5◀
TIP: ▶ Report in addition to the appropriate code for the live birth (V30–V39) for a newborn with sickle cell trait.◀
TIP: Do not assign along with another code for sickle-cell disease o thalassemia.

√5th 282.6 Sickle-cell disease
Sickle-cell anemia

> **EXCLUDES**   *sickle-cell thalassemia (282.41-282.42)*
> *sickle-cell trait (282.5)*

DEF: Inherited blood disorder; sickle-shaped red blood cells are ha and pointed, clogging blood flow; anemia characterized by perioc episodes of pain, acute abdominal discomfort, skin ulcerations of the legs, increased infections.

282.60 Sickle-cell disease, unspecified
Sickle-cell anemia NOS
AHA: 2Q, '97, 11

282.61 Hb-SS disease without crisis

282.62 Hb-SS disease with crisis   M
Hb-SS disease with vaso-occlusive pain
Sickle-cell crisis NOS

Use additional code for type of crisis, such as:
     acute chest syndrome (517.3)
     splenic sequestration (289.52)
CC Exd: See code: 282.42
AHA: 4Q, '10, 78; 4Q, '03, 56; 2Q, '98, 8; 2Q, '91, 15

282.63 Sickle-cell/Hb-C disease without crisis
Hb-S/Hb-C disease without crisis

282.64 Sickle-cell/Hb-C disease with crisis   M
Hb-S/Hb-C disease with crisis
Sickle-cell/Hb-C disease with vaso-occlusive pain

Use additional code for type of crisis, such as:
     acute chest syndrome (517.3)
     splenic sequestration (289.52)
CC Exd: See code: 282.42
AHA: 4Q, '03, 51

282.68 Other sickle-cell disease without crisis
Hb-S/Hb-D
Hb-S/Hb-E   } diseases without
Sickle-cell/Hb-D   crisis
Sickle-cell/Hb-E
AHA: 4Q, '03, 51

282.69 Other sickle-cell disease with crisis   M
Hb-S/Hb-D
Hb-S/Hb-E   } diseases with crisis
Sickle-cell/Hb-D
Sickle-cell/Hb-E

Other sickle-cell disease with vaso-occlusive pain

Use additional code for type of crisis, such as:
     acute chest syndrome (517.3)
     splenic sequestration (289.52)
CC Exd: 280.0-285.9, 286.53, 289.81-289.83, 289.89-289.9 517.3

N Newborn Age: 0   P Pediatric Age: 0-17   M Maternity Age: 12-55   A Adult Age: 15-124   MCC Major CC Condition   CC CC Condition   HIV HIV Related

282.7 Other hemoglobinopathies
Abnormal hemoglobin NOS
Congenital Heinz-body anemia
Disease:
    hemoglobin C [Hb-C]
    hemoglobin D [Hb-D]
    hemoglobin E [Hb-E]
    hemoglobin Zurich [Hb-Zurich]
Hemoglobinopathy NOS
Hereditary persistence of fetal hemoglobin [HPFH]
Unstable hemoglobin hemolytic disease

EXCLUDES *familial polycythemia (289.6)*
    hemoglobin E-beta thalassemia (282.47)
    hemoglobin M [Hb-M] disease (289.7)
    high-oxygen-affinity hemoglobin (289.0)
    other hemoglobinopathies with thalassemia (282.49)

DEF: Any disorder of hemoglobin due to alteration of molecular structure; may include overt anemia.

282.8 Other specified hereditary hemolytic anemias   `CC`
Stomatocytosis
CC Exd: 280.0-284.2, 284.81-285.9, 289.9, 517.3, 776.5-776.6

282.9 Hereditary hemolytic anemia, unspecified   `CC`
Hereditary hemolytic anemia NOS
CC Exd: See code: 282.8

✓4ᵗʰ 283 Acquired hemolytic anemias
DEF: Non-hereditary anemia characterized by premature destruction of red blood cells; caused by infectious organisms, poisons, and physical agents.
AHA: N-D, '84, 1

283.0 Autoimmune hemolytic anemias   `CC`
Autoimmune hemolytic disease (cold type) (warm type)
Chronic cold hemagglutinin disease
Cold agglutinin disease or hemoglobinuria
Hemolytic anemia:
    cold type (secondary) (symptomatic)
    drug-induced
    warm type (secondary) (symptomatic)
Use additional E code to identify cause, if drug-induced

EXCLUDES *Evans' syndrome (287.32)*
    hemolytic disease of newborn (773.0-773.5)

CC Exd: 280.0-285.9, 286.53, 289.81-289.83, 289.89-289.9, 517.3
AHA: 3Q, '08, 5

✓5ᵗʰ 283.1 Non-autoimmune hemolytic anemias
Use additional E code to identify cause
DEF: Hemolytic anemia and thrombocytopenia with acute renal failure; relatively rare condition; 50 percent of patients require renal dialysis.
AHA: 4Q, '93, 25

283.10 Non-autoimmune hemolytic anemia, unspecified   `CC`
CC Exd: See code: 283.0

283.11 Hemolytic-uremic syndrome   `MCC`
Use additional code to identify associated:
    E. coli infection (041.41-041.49)
    Pneumococcal pnemonia (481)
    Shigella dysenteriae (004.0)
CC Exd: See code: 283.0

283.19 Other non-autoimmune hemolytic anemias   `CC`
Hemolytic anemia:
    mechanical
    microangiopathic
    toxic
CC Exd: See code: 283.0

283.2 Hemoglobinuria due to hemolysis from external causes
Acute intravascular hemolysis
Hemoglobinuria:
    due to other hemolysis
    from exertion
    march
    paroxysmal (cold) (nocturnal)
Marchiafava-Micheli syndrome
Use additional E code to identify cause

283.9 Acquired hemolytic anemia, unspecified   `CC`
Acquired hemolytic anemia NOS
Chronic idiopathic hemolytic anemia
CC Exd: See code: 283.0

✓4ᵗʰ 284 Aplastic anemia and other bone marrow failure syndromes
DEF: Bone marrow failure to produce the normal amount of blood components; generally non-responsive to usual therapy.
AHA: 1Q, '91, 14; N-D, '84, 1; S-0, '84, 16

✓5ᵗʰ 284.0 Constitutional aplastic anemia
AHA: 1Q, '91, 14

284.01 Constitutional red blood cell aplasia   `CC`
Aplasia, (pure) red cell:
    congenital
    of infants
    primary
Blackfan-Diamond syndrome
Familial hypoplastic anemia
CC Exd: 280.0-284.09, 284.81-285.9, 289.9, 776.5-776.6
AHA: 4Q, '06, 67-69

284.09 Other constitutional aplastic anemia   `CC`
Fanconi's anemia
Pancytopenia with malformations
CC Exd: 280.0-284.09, 284.81-285.9, 287.30-287.39, 289.9, 776.5-776.6
AHA: 4Q, '06, 67-69

✓5ᵗʰ 284.1 Pancytopenia
EXCLUDES *pancytopenia (due to) (with):*
    aplastic anemia NOS (284.9)
    bone marrow infiltration (284.2)
    constitutional red blood cell aplasia (284.01)
    hairy cell leukemia (202.4)
    human immunodeficiency virus disease (042)
    leukoerythroblastic anemia (284.2)
    malformations (284.09)
    myelodysplastic syndromes (238.72-238.75)
    myeloproliferative disease (238.79)
    other constitutional aplastic anemia (284.09)
AHA: 4Q, '11, 91-92; 4Q, '06, 67-69

284.11 Antineoplastic chemotherapy induced pancytopenia   `MCC`
EXCLUDES *aplastic anemia due to antineoplastic chemotherapy (284.89)*
CC Exd: 284.11-285.9, 288.00-288.09, 288.4-288.62, 288.66-288.69, 289.9, 776.6
AHA: 4Q, '11, 92

284.12 Other drug-induced pancytopenia   `MCC`
EXCLUDES *aplastic anemia due to drugs (284.89)*
CC Exd: see Code: 284.11

284.19 Other pancytopenia   `CC`
CC Exd: see Code: 284.11

284.2 *Myelophthisis*   `CC`
Leukoerythroblastic anemia
Myelophthisic anemia

Code first the underlying disorder, such as:
    malignant neoplasm of breast (174.0-174.9, 175.0-175.9)
    tuberculosis (015.0-015.9)

EXCLUDES *idiopathic myelofibrosis (238.76)*
    myelofibrosis NOS (289.83)
    myelofibrosis with myeloid metaplasia (238.76)
    primary myelofibrosis (238.76)
    secondary myelofibrosis (289.83)

DEF: A secondary disease process involving replacement of normal hematopoeitic tissue in the bone marrow with abnormal tissue, such as fibrous tissue or tumors. Occurs with advanced-stage neoplasms, granulomatous diseases such as miliary tuberculosis, and other inflammatory diseases.
CC Exd: 284.1-284.2, 284.81-285.9, 288.00-288.09, 288.4-288.62, 288.66-288.69, 289.9, 776.6
AHA: 4Q, '06, 67-69

✓5ᵗʰ 284.8 Other specified aplastic anemias
AHA: 4Q, '07, 72; 3Q, '05, 11; 1Q, '97, 5; 1Q, '92, 15; 1Q, '91, 14

284.81 Red cell aplasia (acquired) (adult) (with thymoma)   `MCC`
Red cell aplasia NOS
CC Exd: 280.0-285.9, 286.53, 289.81-289.83, 289.89-289.9, 517.3

Additional Digit Required   Unacceptable PDx   Manifestation Code   Hospital Acquired Condition   ▶◀ Revised Text   ● New Code   ▲ Revised Code Title

14 ICD-9-CM   Volume 1 – 75

Diseases of the Blood and Blood-Forming Organs

284.89 Other specified aplastic anemias   `MCC`
Aplastic anemia (due to):
chronic systemic disease
drugs
infection
radiation
toxic (paralytic)
Use additional E code to identify cause
CC Excl: See code: 284.81
AHA: 1Q, '11, 6; 1Q, '09, 20; 2Q, '08, 6

284.9 Aplastic anemia, unspecified   `CC`
Anemia:
aplastic (idiopathic) NOS
aregenerative
hypoplastic NOS
nonregenerative
Medullary hypoplasia
EXCLUDES   *refractory anemia (238.72)*
CC Excl: See code: 284.81

✓4ᵗʰ 285   Other and unspecified anemias
AHA: 1Q, '91, 14; N-D, '84, 1

285.0 Sideroblastic anemia
Anemia:
hypochromic with iron loading
sideroachrestic
sideroblastic:
acquired
congenital
hereditary
primary
secondary (drug-induced) (due to disease)
sex-linked hypochromic
vitamin B6-responsive
Pyridoxine-responsive (hypochromic) anemia
Use additional E code to identify cause, if drug induced
EXCLUDES   *refractory sideroblastic anemia (238.72)*
DEF: Characterized by a disruption of final heme synthesis; results in iron overload of reticuloendothelial tissues.

285.1 Acute posthemorrhagic anemia   `CC`
Anemia due to acute blood loss
EXCLUDES   *anemia due to chronic blood loss (280.0)*
blood loss anemia NOS (280.0)
CC Excl: 280.0-285.9, 286.53, 289.81-289.83, 289.89-289.9, 517.3, 958.2
AHA: 4Q, '11, 146; 1Q, '07, 19; 2Q, '92, 15

✓5ᵗʰ 285.2 Anemia of chronic disease
Anemia in (due to) (with) chronic illness
AHA: 4Q, '00, 39

285.21 Anemia in chronic kidney disease
Anemia in end stage renal disease
Erythropoietin-resistant anemia (EPO resistant anemia)
TIP: Assign also a code for the chronic kidney disease (585.X).

285.22 Anemia in neoplastic disease
EXCLUDES   *anemia due to antineoplastic chemotherapy (285.3)*
aplastic anemia due to antineoplastic chemotherapy (284.89)
AHA: 4Q, '09, 81
TIP: Assign also a code for the neoplasm causing the anemia. Do not assign if anemia is caused by chemotherapy drugs, which is instead reported with 285.3.
D63.0 Anemia in neoplastic disease   `I-10`

285.29 Anemia of other chronic disease
Anemia in other chronic illness

285.3 Antineoplastic chemotherapy induced anemia
Anemia due to antineoplastic chemotherapy
EXCLUDES   *anemia due to drug NEC — code to type of anemia*
anemia in neoplastic disease (285.22)
aplastic anemia due to antineoplastic chemotherapy (284.89)
DEF: Reversible adverse effect of chemotherapy, causing inhibition of bone marrow production; decrease in red blood cell production prevents adequate oxygenation of the tissues and organs causing fatigue, SOB, and exacerbation of other medical conditions.
AHA: 4Q, '09, 80-82

285.8 Other specified anemias
Anemia:
dyserythropoietic (congenital)
dyshematopoietic (congenital)
von Jaksch's
Infantile pseudoleukemia
AHA: 1Q, '91, 16

285.9 Anemia, unspecified
Anemia: Anemia:
NOS   profound
essential   progressive
normocytic, not due   secondary
to blood loss   Oligocythemia
EXCLUDES   *anemia (due to):*
blood loss:
acute (285.1)
chronic or unspecified (280.0)
iron deficiency (280.0-280.9)
AHA: 1Q, '11, 16; 1Q, '09, 17, 20; 1Q, '07, 19; 1Q, '02, 14; 2Q, '92, 16; M-A, '85, 13; N-D, '84, 1
TIP: Assign for "postoperative anemia" if there is no mention of blood loss.

✓4ᵗʰ 286   Coagulation defects
AHA: 2Q, '06, 17

286.0 Congenital factor VIII disorder   `MCC`
Antihemophilic globulin [AHG] deficiency
Factor VIII (functional)deficiency
Hemophilia:
NOS
A
classical
familial
hereditary
Subhemophilia
EXCLUDES   *factor VIII deficiency with vascular defect (286.4)*
DEF: Hereditary, sex-linked, results in missing antihemophilic globulin (AHG) (factor VIII); causes abnormal coagulation characterized by increased bleeding, large bruises of skin, bleeding in mouth, nose, gastrointestinal tract; hemorrhages into joints, resulting in swelling and impaired function.
CC Excl: 286.0-286.4, 286.52-287.9, 289.81-289.9

286.1 Congenital factor IX disorder   `MC`
Christmas disease
Deficiency:
factor IX (functional)
plasma thromboplastin component [PTC]
Hemophilia B
DEF: Deficiency of plasma thromboplastin component (PTC) (factor IX) and plasma thromboplastin antecedent (PTA); PTC deficiency clinically indistinguishable from classical hemophilia.
CC Excl: See code: 286.0

286.2 Congenital factor XI deficiency   `C`
Hemophilia C
Plasma thromboplastin antecedent [PTA] deficiency
Rosenthal's disease
CC Excl: See code: 286.0

`N` Newborn Age: 0   `P` Pediatric Age: 0-17   `M` Maternity Age: 12-55   `A` Adult Age: 15-124   `MCC` Major CC Condition   `CC` CC Condition   `HIV` HIV Related D

76 – Volume 1   2014 ICD-9-C

286.3 Congenital deficiency of other clotting factors `CC`
Congenital afibrinogenemia
Deficiency:
  AC globulin factor:
    I [fibrinogen]
    II [prothrombin]
    V [labile]
    VII [stable]
    X [Stuart-Prower]
    XII [Hageman]
    XIII [fibrin stabilizing]
  Laki-Lorand factor
  proaccelerin
Disease:
  Owren's
  Stuart-Prower
Dysfibrinogenemia (congenital)
Dysprothrombinemia (constitutional)
Hypoproconvertinemia
Hypoprothrombinemia (hereditary)
Parahemophilia
CC Excl: See code: 286.0

286.4 von Willebrand's disease `CC`
Angiohemophilia (A) (B)
Constitutional thrombopathy
Factor VIII deficiency with vascular defect
Pseudohemophilia type B
Vascular hemophilia
von Willebrand's (-Jürgens') disease
  EXCLUDES factor VIII deficiency:
    NOS (286.0)
    with functional defect (286.0)
    hereditary capillary fragility (287.8)
DEF: Abnormal blood coagulation caused by deficient blood Factor VII; congenital; symptoms include excess or prolonged bleeding.
CC Excl: See code: 286.0

√5ᵗʰ **286.5 Hemorrhagic disorder due to intrinsic circulating anticoagulants, antibodies, or inhibitors**
AHA: 4Q, '11, 93-95; 3Q, '04, 7; No.5, '93, 16; 3Q, '92, 15; 3Q, '90, 14
TIP: Do not assign a code from subcategory 286.5 for Coumadin/warfarin toxicity, poisoning or adverse effect. Follow coding guidelines for poisoning and adverse reactions.

286.52 Acquired hemophilia `CC`
Autoimmune hemophilia
Autoimmune inhibitors to clotting factors
Secondary hemophilia
CC Excl: 286.0-286.4, 286.52-287.9, 289.81, 289.82, 289.84-289.9

286.53 Antiphospholipid antibody with hemorrhagic disorder `CC`
Lupus anticoagulant [LAC] with hemorrhagic disorder
Systemic lupus erythematosus [SLE] inhibitor with hemorrhagic disorder
  EXCLUDES anti-phospholipid antibody, finding without diagnosis (795.79)
    anti-phospholipid antibody syndrome (289.81)
    anti-phospholipid antibody with hypercoagulable state (289.81)
    lupus anticoagulant [LAC] finding without diagnosis (795.79)
    lupus anticoagulant [LAC] with hypercoagulable state (289.81)
    systemic lupus erythematosus [SLE] inhibitor finding without diagnosis (795.79)
    systemic lupus erythematosus [SLE] inhibitor with hypercoagulable state (289.81)
CC Excl: 286.52-286.59, 288.00-288.51, 288.59-289.9
TIP: When a resulting associated hypercoagulable state is present, assign code 289.81.

286.59 Other hemorrhagic disorder due to intrinsic circulating anticoagulants, antibodies, or inhibitors `CC`
Antithrombinemia
Antithromboplastinemia
Antithromboplastinogenemia
Increase in:
  anti-II (prothrombin)
  anti-VIIIa
  anti-IXa
  anti-XIa
CC Excl: See code: 286.52

286.6 Defibrination syndrome `MCC`
Afibrinogenemia, acquired
Consumption coagulopathy
Diffuse or disseminated intravascular coagulation [DIC syndrome]
Fibrinolytic hemorrhage, acquired
Hemorrhagic fibrinogenolysis
Pathologic fibrinolysis
Purpura:
  fibrinolytic
  fulminans
  EXCLUDES that complicating:
    abortion (634-638 with .1, 639.1)
    pregnancy or the puerperium (641.3, 666.3)
    disseminated intravascular coagulation in newborn (776.2)
DEF: Characterized by destruction of circulating fibrinogen; often precipitated by other conditions, such as injury, causing release of thromboplastic particles in blood stream.
CC Excl: See code: 286.0
AHA: 4Q, '93, 29

286.7 Acquired coagulation factor deficiency `CC`
Deficiency of coagulation factor due to:
  liver disease
  vitamin K deficiency
Hypoprothrombinemia, acquired
Use additional E code to identify cause, if drug induced
  EXCLUDES vitamin K deficiency of newborn (776.0)
CC Excl: See code: 286.0
AHA: 4Q, '93, 29

286.9 Other and unspecified coagulation defects `CC`
Defective coagulation NOS   Disorder:
Deficiency, coagulation   coagulation
  factor NOS   hemostasis
Delay, coagulation
  EXCLUDES abnormal coagulation profile (790.92)
    hemorrhagic disease of newborn (776.0)
    that complicating:
      abortion (634-638 with .1, 639.1)
      pregnancy or the puerperium (641.3, 666.3)
CC Excl: See code: 286.0
AHA: 4Q, '99, 22; 4Q, '93, 29

√4ᵗʰ **287 Purpura and other hemorrhagic conditions**
  EXCLUDES hemorrhagic thrombocythemia (238.71)
    purpura fulminans (286.6)
AHA: 1Q, '91, 14

287.0 Allergic purpura `CC`
Peliosis rheumatica   Purpura:
Purpura: nonthrombocytopenic:
  anaphylactoid   idiopathic
  autoimmune   rheumatica
  Henoch's   Schönlein-Henoch
  nonthrombocytopenic: vascular
    hemorrhagic   Vasculitis, allergic
  EXCLUDES hemorrhagic purpura (287.39)
    purpura annularis telangiectodes (709.1)
DEF: Any hemorrhagic condition, thrombocytic or nonthrombocytopenic in origin, caused by a presumed allergic reaction.
CC Excl: See code: 286.0

Diseases of the Blood and Blood-Forming Organs

287.1–288.3

287.1 Qualitative platelet defects
Thrombasthenia (hemorrhagic) (hereditary)
Thrombocytasthenia
Thrombocytopathy (dystrophic)
Thrombopathy (Bernard-Soulier)
EXCLUDES *von Willebrand's disease (286.4)*

287.2 Other nonthrombocytopenic purpuras
Purpura:
  NOS
  senile
  simplex

√6th **287.3 Primary thrombocytopenia**
EXCLUDES *thrombotic thrombocytopenic purpura (446.6)*
  transient thrombocytopenia of newborn (776.1)
DEF: Decrease in number of blood platelets in circulating blood and purpural skin hemorrhages.
AHA: 4Q, '05, 56

  287.30 Primary thrombocytopenia, unspecified
  Megakaryocytic hypoplasia

  287.31 Immune thrombocytopenic purpura   CC
  Idiopathic thrombocytopenic purpura
  Tidal platelet dysgenesis
  DEF: Tidal platelet dysgenesis: Platelet counts fluctuate from normal to very low within periods of 20 to 40 days and may involve autoimmune platelet destruction.
  CC Excl: See code: 286.0
  AHA: 4Q, '05, 57

  287.32 Evans' syndrome   CC
  DEF: Combination of immunohemolytic anemia and autoimmune hemolytic anemia, sometimes with neutropenia.
  CC Excl: See code: 286.0

  287.33 Congenital and hereditary thrombocytopenic   CC
  purpura
  Congenital and hereditary thrombocytopenia
  Thrombocytopenia with absent radii (TAR) syndrome
  EXCLUDES *Wiskott-Aldrich syndrome (279.12)*
  DEF: Thrombocytopenia with absent radii (TAR) syndrome: autosomal recessive syndrome characterized by thrombocytopenia and bilateral radial aplasia; manifestations include skeletal, gastrointestinal, hematologic, and cardiac system abnormalities.
  CC Excl: See code: 286.0

  287.39 Other primary thrombocytopenia

√5th **287.4 Secondary thrombocytopenia**
Use additional E code to identify cause
EXCLUDES *heparin-induced thrombocytopenia (HIT) (289.84)*
  transient thrombocytopenia of newborn (776.1)
AHA: 4Q, '10, 81-82; M-A, '85, 14

  287.41 Posttransfusion purpura
  Posttransfusion purpura from whole blood (fresh) or
    blood products
  PTP
  DEF: A potentially fatal transfusion complication characterized by sudden onset of severe thrombocytopenia, fever, chills, and cutaneous hemorrhaging.

  287.49 Other secondary thrombocytopenia
  Thrombocytopenia (due to):
    dilutional
    drugs
    extracorporeal circulation of blood
    massive blood transfusion
    platelet alloimmunization
    secondary NOS
  DEF: Reduced number of platelets in circulating blood as consequence of an underlying disease or condition.

287.5 Thrombocytopenia, unspecified

287.8 Other specified hemorrhagic conditions
Capillary fragility (hereditary)
Vascular pseudohemophilia

287.9 Unspecified hemorrhagic conditions
Hemorrhagic diathesis (familial)

√4th **288 Diseases of white blood cells**
EXCLUDES *leukemia (204.0-208.9)*
AHA: 4Q, '06, 69; 1Q, '91, 14

√5th **288.0 Neutropenia**
Decreased absolute neutrophil count [ANC]
Use additional code for any associated:
  fever (780.61)
  mucositis (478.11, 528.00-528.09, 538, 616.81)
EXCLUDES *neutropenic splenomegaly (289.53)*
  transitory neonatal neutropenia (776.7)
DEF: Sudden, severe condition characterized by reduced number of white blood cells; results in sores in the throat, stomach or skin; symptoms include chills, fever.
AHA: 4Q, '06, 69-73; 3Q, '05, 11; 3Q, '99, 6; 2Q, '99, 9; 3Q, '96, 16; 2Q, '96, 6

  288.00 Neutropenia, unspecified
  AHA: 4Q, '06, 69-73

  288.01 Congenital neutropenia
  Congenital agranulocytosis
  Infantile genetic agranulocytosis
  Kostmann's syndrome
  AHA: 4Q, '06, 69-73

  288.02 Cyclic neutropenia
  Cyclic hematopoiesis   Periodic neutropenia
  AHA: 4Q, '06, 69-73

  288.03 Drug induced neutropenia
  Use additional E code to identify drug
  AHA: 4Q, '06, 69-73
  TIP: Assign for neutropenic fever due to chemotherapy drugs, along with codes for the fever, adverse effect, and the underlying malignancy.

  288.04 Neutropenia due to infection
  AHA: 4Q, '06, 69-73

  288.09 Other neutropenia
  Agranulocytosis
  Neutropenia:
    immune
    toxic
  AHA: 4Q, '06, 69-73

288.1 Functional disorders of polymorphonuclear neutrophils
Chronic (childhood) granulomatous disease
Congenital dysphagocytosis
Job's syndrome
Lipochrome histiocytosis (familial)
Progressive septic granulomatosis

288.2 Genetic anomalies of leukocytes
Anomaly (granulation) (granulocyte) or syndrome:
  Alder's (-Reilly)
  Chédiak-Steinbrinck (-Higashi)
  Jordan's
  May-Hegglin
  Pelger-Huet
Hereditary:
  hypersegmentation
  hyposegmentation
  leukomelanopathy

288.3 Eosinophilia
Eosinophilia:
  allergic
  hereditary
  idiopathic
  secondary
Eosinophilic leukocytosis
EXCLUDES *Löffler's syndrome (518.3)*
  pulmonary eosinophilia (518.3)
DEF: Elevated number of eosinophils in the blood; characteristic of allergic states and various parasitic infections.
AHA: 3Q, '00, 11

N Newborn Age: 0   P Pediatric Age: 0-17   M Maternity Age: 12-55   A Adult Age: 15-124   MCC Major CC Condition   CC CC Condition   HIV HIV Related D

78 — Volume 1   2014 ICD-9-C

288.4 Hemophagocytic syndromes   `CC`
     Familial hemophagocytic lymphohistiocytosis
     Familial hemophagocytic reticulosis
     Hemophagocytic syndrome, infection-associated
     Histiocytic syndromes
     Macrophage activation syndrome
     CC Excl: 284.1-284.9, 286.6, 287.30-287.39, 287.41-288.09, 288.50,
     288.59, 289.84, 289.9
     AHA: 4Q, '06, 69-73

√5ᵗʰ 288.5 Decreased white blood cell count
     EXCLUDES neutropenia (288.01-288.09)

     288.50 Leukocytopenia, unspecified
          Decreased leukocytes, unspecified
          Decreased white blood cell count, unspecified
          Leukopenia NOS
          AHA: 4Q, '06, 69-73

     288.51 Lymphocytopenia
          Decreased lymphocytes
          AHA: 4Q, '06, 69-73

     288.59 Other decreased white blood cell count
          Basophilic leukopenia
          Eosinophilic leukopenia
          Monocytopenia
          Plasmacytopenia
          AHA: 4Q, '06, 69-73

√5ᵗʰ 288.6 Elevated white blood cell count
     EXCLUDES eosinophilia (288.3)

     288.60 Leukocytosis, unspecified
          Elevated leukocytes, unspecified
          Elevated white blood cell count, unspecified
          AHA: 4Q, '06, 69-73

     288.61 Lymphocytosis (symptomatic)
          Elevated lymphocytes
          AHA: 4Q, '06, 69-73

     288.62 Leukemoid reaction
          Basophilic leukemoid reaction
          Lymphocytic leukemoid reaction
          Monocytic leukemoid reaction
          Myelocytic leukemoid reaction
          Neutrophilic leukemoid reaction
          AHA: 4Q, '06, 69-73

     288.63 Monocytosis (symptomatic)
          EXCLUDES infectious mononucleosis (075)
          AHA: 4Q, '06, 69-73

     288.64 Plasmacytosis
          AHA: 4Q, '06, 69-73

     288.65 Basophilia
          AHA: 4Q, '06, 69-73

     288.66 Bandemia
          Bandemia without diagnosis of specific infection
          EXCLUDES confirmed infection — code to infection
                    leukemia (204.00-208.9)
          DEF: Increase in early neutrophil cells, called band cells; may
          indicate infection.
          AHA: 4Q, '07, 73
          TIP: Do not assign based on lab values alone; physician
          must substantiate bandemia without evidence of
          corresponding infection.

     288.69 Other elevated white blood cell count
          AHA: 4Q, '06, 69-73

288.8 Other specified disease of white blood cells
     EXCLUDES decreased white blood cell counts (288.50-288.59)
               elevated white blood cell counts (288.60-288.69)
               immunity disorders (279.0-279.9)
     AHA: M-A, '87, 12

288.9 Unspecified disease of white blood cells

√4ᵗʰ 289 Other diseases of blood and blood-forming organs

289.0 Polycythemia, secondary
     High-oxygen-affinity hemoglobin   Polycythemia:
     Polycythemia: erythropoietin
          acquired   hypoxemic
          benign   nephrogenous
          due to: relative
               fall in plasma volume   spurious
               high altitude   stress
          emotional
     EXCLUDES polycythemia:
               neonatal (776.4)
               primary (238.4)
               vera (238.4)
     DEF: Elevated number of red cells in circulating blood as result
     of reduced oxygen supply to the tissues.
     D75.1 Secondary polycythemia   `I-10`

289.1 Chronic lymphadenitis
     Chronic:
          adenitis   } any lymph node, except
          lymphadenitis   }   mesenteric
     EXCLUDES acute lymphadenitis (683)
               mesenteric (289.2)
               enlarged glands NOS (785.6)
     DEF: Persistent inflammation of lymph node tissue; origin of
     infection is usually elsewhere.
     I88.1 Chronic lymphadenitis except mesenteric   `I-10`

289.2 Nonspecific mesenteric lymphadenitis
     Mesenteric lymphadenitis (acute) (chronic)
     DEF: Inflammation of the lymph nodes in peritoneal fold that encases
     abdominal organs; disease resembles acute appendicitis; unknown
     etiology.
     I88.0 Nonspecific mesenteric lymphadenitis   `I-10`

289.3 Lymphadenitis, unspecified, except mesenteric
     AHA: ▶2Q, '12, 18;◀ 2Q, '92, 8
     I88.9 Nonspecific lymphadenitis unspecified   `I-10`

289.4 Hypersplenism
     "Big spleen" syndrome   Hypersplenia
     Dyssplenism
     EXCLUDES primary splenic neutropenia (289.53)
     DEF: An overactive spleen causing a deficiency of the peripheral
     blood components, an increase in bone marrow cells and sometimes
     a notable increase in the size of the spleen.
     D73.1 Hypersplenism   `I-10`

√5ᵗʰ 289.5 Other diseases of spleen

     289.50 Disease of spleen, unspecified
          D73.9 Disease of spleen unspecified   `I-10`

     289.51 Chronic congestive splenomegaly
          D73.2 Chronic congestive splenomegaly   `I-10`

     289.52 Splenic sequestration
          *Code first sickle-cell disease in crisis (282.42, 282.62,
               282.64, 282.69)*
          DEF: Blood is entrapped in the spleen due to vessel
          occlusion; most often associated with sickle-cell disease;
          spleen becomes enlarged and there is a sharp drop in
          hemoglobin.
          AHA: 4Q, '03, 51

     289.53 Neutropenic splenomegaly
          AHA: 4Q, '06, 73
          D73.81 Neutropenic splenomegaly   `I-10`

     289.59 Other
          Lien migrans   Splenic:
          Perisplenitis   fibrosis
          Splenic: infarction
               abscess   rupture, nontraumatic
               atrophy   Splenitis
               cyst   Wandering spleen
          EXCLUDES bilharzial splenic fibrosis (120.0-120.9)
                    hepatolienal fibrosis (571.5)
                    splenomegaly NOS (789.2)
          D73.89 Other diseases of spleen   `I-10`

289.6 Familial polycythemia
     Familial: Familial:
          benign polycythemia   erythrocytosis
     DEF: Elevated number of red blood cells.

Diseases of the Blood and Blood-Forming Organs

289.7–289.9

289.7   Methemoglobinemia   `CC`

Congenital NADH [DPNH]-methemoglobin-
reductase deficiency
Hemoglobin M [Hb-M] disease
Methemoglobinemia:
   NOS
   acquired (with sulfhemoglobinemia)
   hereditary
   toxic
Stokvis' disease
Sulfhemoglobinemia
Use additional E code to identify cause

DEF: Presence of blood methemoglobin, a chemically altered form of
hemoglobin; causes cyanosis, headache, ataxia, dyspnea,
tachycardia, nausea, stupor, and coma.

CC Excl: 282.7-283.10, 283.19-283.9, 285.3-285.9, 289.7, 289.9

D74.0 Congenital methemoglobinemia   `I-10`

✓5ᵗʰ 289.8   Other specified diseases of blood and blood-forming organs

DEF: Hypercoagulable states: a group of inherited or acquired
abnormalities of specific proteins and anticoagulant factors; also
called thromboembolic states or thrombotic disorders, result in
abnormal development of blood clots.

AHA: 4Q, '03, 56; 1Q, '02, 16; 2Q, '89, 8; M-A, '87, 12

289.81   Primary hypercoagulable state   `CC`

Activated protein C resistance
Antiphospholipid antibody syndrome
Antithrombin III deficiency
Factor V Leiden mutation
Lupus anticoagulant with hypercoagulable state
Protein C deficiency
Protein S deficiency
Prothrombin gene mutation
Systemic lupus erythematosus [SLE] inhibitor with
   hypercoagulable state

EXCLUDES   *anti-phospholipid antibody, finding without*
     diagnosis (795.79)
   anti-phospholipid antibody with
     hemorrhagic disorder (286.53)
   lupus anticoagulant [LAC] finding without
     diagnosis (795.79)
   lupus anticoagulant [LAC] with hemorrhagic
     disorder (286.53)
   secondary activated protein C resistance
     (289.82)
   secondary antiphospholipid antibody
     syndrome (289.82)
   secondary lupus anticoagulant with
     hypercoagulable state (289.82)
   secondary systemic lupus erythematosus
     [SLE] inhibitor with hypercoagulable
     state (289.82)
   systemic lupus erythematosus [SLE] inhibitor
     finding without diagnosis (795.79)
   systemic lupus erythematosus [SLE] inhibitor
     with hypercoagulable state (286.53)

DEF: Activated protein C resistance: decreased effectiveness
of protein C to degrade factor V, necessary to inhibit
clotting cascade; also called Factor V Leiden mutation.

DEF: Antithrombin III deficiency: deficiency in plasma
antithrombin III one of six naturally occurring
antithrombins that limit coagulation.

DEF: Factor V Leiden mutation: also called activated protein
C resistance.

DEF: Lupus anticoagulant: autoimmune deficiency in a
circulating anticoagulant that inhibits the conversion of
prothrombin into thrombin; also called anti-phospholipid
syndrome.

DEF: Protein C deficiency: deficiency of activated protein C
which functions to bring the blood-clotting process into
balance; same outcome as factor V Leiden mutation.

DEF: Protein S deficiency: similar to protein C deficiency;
protein S is a vitamin K dependent cofactor in the
activation of protein C.

DEF: Prothrombin gene mutation: increased levels of
prothrombin, or factor II, a plasma protein that is converted
to thrombin, which acts upon fibrinogen to form the fibrin.

CC Excl: 286.53, 288.00-288.9, 289.53, 289.81-289.83,
289.89-289.9

AHA: 4Q, '11, 93

D68.59 Other primary thrombophilia   `I-10`

289.82   Secondary hypercoagulable state   `CC`

EXCLUDES   *heparin-induced thrombocytopenia (HIT)*
     (289.84)

CC Excl: See code: 289.81

D68.69 Other thrombophilia   `I-10`

289.83   Myelofibrosis   `CC`

Myelofibrosis NOS
Secondary myelofibrosis

Code first the underlying disorder, such as:
   malignant neoplasm of breast (174.0-174.9,
     175.0-175.9)

Use additional code for associated therapy-related
   myelodysplastic syndrome, if applicable
   (238.72, 238.73)

Use additional external cause code if due to
   anti-neoplastic chemotherapy (E933.1)

EXCLUDES   *idiopathic myelofibrosis (238.76)*
   leukoerythroblastic anemia (284.2)
   myelofibrosis with myeloid metaplasia
     (238.76)
   myelophthisic anemia (284.2)
   myelophthisis (284.2)
   primary myelofibrosis (238.76)

DEF: A progressive bone marrow disease characterized by
the replacement of bone marrow with the overgrowth of
neoplastic stem cells and fibrotic tissue, also progressive
anemia and enlarged spleen.

CC Excl: 202.40-202.48, 203.10-203.11, 203.80-203.81,
204.00-208.92, 238.4-238.76, 238.79-238.9

AHA: 4Q, '06, 73

D75.81 Myelofibrosis   `I-10`

289.84   Heparin-induced thrombocytopenia [HIT]

DEF: Immune-mediated reaction to heparin therapy
causing an abrupt fall in platelet count and serious
complications such as pulmonary embolism, stroke, AMI or
DVT.

AHA: 4Q, '08, 100-101

289.89   Other specified diseases of blood and blood-forming organs

Hypergammaglobulinemia
Pseudocholinesterase deficiency

D75.89 Oth specified dz of blood & blood-forming   `I-10`
organs

289.9   Unspecified diseases of blood and blood-forming organs

Blood dyscrasia NOS
Erythroid hyperplasia

AHA: M-A, '85, 14

D75.9 Disease of blood and blood-forming organs unspec   `I-10`

`N` Newborn Age: 0   `P` Pediatric Age: 0-17   `M` Maternity Age: 12-55   `A` Adult Age: 15-124   `MCC` Major CC Condition   `CC` CC Condition   `HIV` HIV Related Dx

80 – Volume 1   2014 ICD-9-CM

5. Mental, Behavioral and Neurodevelopmental Disorders (290-319)

Psychoses (290-299)

EXCLUDES *intellectual disabilities (317-319)*

Organic Psychotic Conditions (290-294)

INCLUDES psychotic organic brain syndrome

EXCLUDES *nonpsychotic syndromes of organic etiology (310.0-310.9)*
psychoses classifiable to 295-298 and without impairment of orientation, comprehension, calculation, learning capacity, and judgment, but associated with physical disease, injury, or condition affecting the brain [eg., following childbirth] (295.0-298.8)

√4th 290 Dementias

Code first the associated neurological condition

EXCLUDES *dementia due to alcohol (291.0-291.2)*
dementia due to drugs (292.82)
dementia not classified as senile, presenile, or arteriosclerotic (294.10-294.11)
psychoses classifiable to 295-298 occurring in the senium without dementia or delirium (295.0-298.8)
senility with mental changes of nonpsychotic severity (310.1)
transient organic psychotic conditions (293.0-293.9)

290.0 Senile dementia, uncomplicated　A

Senile dementia:　　　Senile dementia:
NOS　　　　　　　　　simple type

EXCLUDES *mild memory disturbances, not amounting to dementia, associated with senile brain disease (310.89)*
senile dementia with:
delirium or confusion (290.3)
delusional [paranoid] features (290.20)
depressive features (290.21)

AHA: 4Q, '99, 4

F03.90 Unspecif dementia w/o behavioral disturbance　I-10

√5th 290.1 Presenile dementia

Brain syndrome with presenile brain disease

EXCLUDES *arteriosclerotic dementia (290.40-290.43)*
dementia associated with other cerebral conditions (294.10-294.11)

AHA: N-D, '84, 20

290.10 Presenile dementia, uncomplicated　A HIV

Presenile dementia:
NOS
simple type

290.11 Presenile dementia with delirium　CC A HIV

Presenile dementia with acute confusional state

CC Excl: 290.0-290.12, 290.20-290.3, 290.8-290.9, 292.81, 293.0, V62.84

AHA: 1Q, '88, 3

290.12 Presenile dementia with delusional features　CC A HIV

Presenile dementia, paranoid type

CC Excl: 079.82, 290.0-290.12, 290.20-290.3, 290.8-290.9, 292.81, 293.0

290.13 Presenile dementia with depressive features　CC A HIV

Presenile dementia, depressed type

CC Excl: 290.0, 290.13-290.3, 296.21-296.24, 296.30-296.34, 296.43-296.44, 296.53-296.54, 296.63-296.64

√5th 290.2 Senile dementia with delusional or depressive features

EXCLUDES *senile dementia:*
NOS (290.0)
with delirium and/or confusion (290.3)

290.20 Senile dementia with delusional features　CC A

Senile dementia, paranoid type
Senile psychosis NOS

CC Excl: 290.0-290.20, 290.3

290.21 Senile dementia with depressive features　CC A

CC Excl: 290.13, 290.21

290.3 Senile dementia with delirium　CC A

Senile dementia with acute confusional state

EXCLUDES *senile:*
dementia NOS (290.0)
psychosis NOS (290.20)

CC Excl: 290.10-290.20, 290.3, V62.84

AHA: 3Q, '09, 11

√5th 290.4 Vascular dementia

Multi-infarct dementia or psychosis

Use additional code to identify cerebral atherosclerosis (437.0)

EXCLUDES *suspected cases with no clear evidence of arteriosclerosis (290.9)*

AHA: 1Q, '88, 3

290.40 Vascular dementia, uncomplicated　A

Arteriosclerotic dementia:
NOS
simple type

F01.50 Vascular dementia without behavioral disturbance　I-10

290.41 Vascular dementia with delirium　CC A

Arteriosclerotic dementia with acute confusional state

CC Excl: 290.11-290.12, 290.20, 290.3, 290.41

290.42 Vascular dementia with delusions　CC A

Arteriosclerotic dementia, paranoid type

CC Excl: 290.42

290.43 Vascular dementia with depressed mood　CC A

Arteriosclerotic dementia, depressed type

CC Excl: 290.43

290.8 Other specified senile psychotic conditions　CC

Presbyophrenic psychosis

CC Excl: 290.8-291.0, 292.11, 292.81-292.82, 295.00-295.04, 295.10-295.14, 295.21-295.24, 295.31, 295.33-295.34, 295.40-295.44, 295.53-295.54, 295.63-295.64, 295.71, 295.73-295.74, 295.80-295.84, 295.91, 295.93-295.94, 296.21-296.24, 296.30-296.34

290.9 Unspecified senile psychotic condition　CC A

CC Excl: See code: 290.8

√4th 291 Alcohol induced mental disorders

EXCLUDES *alcoholism without psychosis (303.0-303.9)*

AHA: 1Q, '88, 3; S-O, '86, 3

291.0 Alcohol withdrawal delirium　CC

Alcoholic delirium
Delirium tremens

EXCLUDES *alcohol withdrawal (291.81)*

CC Excl: 291.0-294.9, 303.00-305.03, 305.20-305.93, 790.3

AHA: 2Q, '91, 11

F10.921 Alcohol use unsp w/intox delirium　I-10

291.1 Alcohol induced persisting amnestic disorder

Alcoholic polyneuritic psychosis
Korsakoff's psychosis, alcoholic
Wernicke-Korsakoff syndrome (alcoholic)

DEF: Prominent and lasting reduced memory span, disordered time appreciation and confabulation, occurring in alcoholics, as sequel to acute alcoholic psychosis.

AHA: 1Q, '88, 3

291.2 Alcohol induced persisting dementia　CC

Alcoholic dementia NOS
Alcoholism associated with dementia NOS
Chronic alcoholic brain syndrome

CC Excl: See code: 291.0

F10.27 Alcohol depend alcohol-induced persist dementia　I-10

291.3 Alcohol induced psychotic disorder with hallucinations `CC`

Alcoholic:
  hallucinosis (acute)
  psychosis with hallucinosis

  EXCLUDES   *alcohol withdrawal with delirium (291.0)*
  schizophrenia (295.0-295.9) and paranoid states
  (297.0-297.9) taking the form of chronic
  hallucinosis with clear consciousness in an
  alcoholic

DEF: Psychosis lasting less than six months with slight or no clouding of consciousness in which auditory hallucinations predominate.

CC Exd: See code: 291.0
AHA: 2Q, '91, 11

291.4 Idiosyncratic alcohol intoxication

Pathologic: Pathologic:
  alcohol intoxication   drunkenness

  EXCLUDES   *acute alcohol intoxication (305.0)*
  in alcoholism (303.0)
  simple drunkenness (305.0)

DEF: Unique behavioral patterns, like belligerence, after intake of relatively small amounts of alcohol; behavior not due to excess consumption.

291.5 Alcohol induced psychotic disorder with delusions

Alcoholic: Alcoholic:
  paranoia   psychosis, paranoid type

  EXCLUDES   *nonalcoholic paranoid states (297.0-297.9)*
  schizophrenia, paranoid type (295.3)

√5ᵗʰ **291.8 Other specified alcohol induced mental disorders**

AHA: 3Q, '94, 13; J-A, '85, 10

291.81 Alcohol withdrawal `CC`

Alcohol:
  abstinence syndrome or symptoms
  withdrawal syndrome or symptoms

  EXCLUDES   *alcohol withdrawal:*
  delirium (291.0)
  hallucinosis (291.3)
  delirium tremens (291.0)

CC Exd: See code: 291.0
AHA: ▶2Q, '12, 9;◀4Q, '96, 28; 2Q, '91, 11
F10.239 Alcohol dependence with withdrawal unspec `I-10`

291.82 Alcohol induced sleep disorders

Alcohol induced circadian rhythm sleep disorders
Alcohol induced hypersomnia
Alcohol induced insomnia
Alcohol induced parasomnia

291.89 Other `CC`

Alcohol induced anxiety disorder
Alcohol induced mood disorder
Alcohol induced sexual dysfunction

CC Exd: See code: 291.0

291.9 Unspecified alcohol induced mental disorders `CC`

Alcoholic:
  mania NOS
  psychosis NOS
Alcoholism (chronic) with psychosis
Alcohol related disorder NOS

CC Exd: See code: 291.0

√4ᵗʰ **292 Drug induced mental disorders**

INCLUDES   organic brain syndrome associated with consumption of drugs

Use additional code for any associated drug dependence (304.0-304.9)
Use additional E code to identify drug
AHA: 3Q, '04, 8; 2Q, '91, 11; S-O, '86, 3

292.0 Drug withdrawal `CC`

Drug:
  abstinence syndrome or symptoms
  withdrawal syndrome or symptoms

CC Exd: See code: 291.0
AHA: 1Q, '97, 12; 1Q, '88, 3

TIP: Assign only for patients who suffer mental or behavioral disturbances due to drug withdrawal, regardless of the circumstances.

F19.939 Oth psychoactive sbstnc use uns w/withdrawal uns `I-10`

√5ᵗʰ **292.1 Drug induced psychotic disorders**

292.11 Drug induced psychotic disorder with delusions `CC`

Paranoid state induced by drugs
CC Exd: See code: 291.0

292.12 Drug induced psychotic disorder with hallucinations `CC`

Hallucinatory state induced by drugs

  EXCLUDES   *states following LSD or other hallucinogens,*
  lasting only a few days or less ["bad
  trips"] (305.3)

CC Exd: See code: 291.0

292.2 Pathological drug intoxication

Drug reaction:
  NOS
  idiosyncratic } resulting in brief psychotic
  pathologic   states

  EXCLUDES   *expected brief psychotic reactions to hallucinogens*
  ["bad trips"] (305.3)
  physiological side-effects of drugs (e.g., dystonias)

√5ᵗʰ **292.8 Other specified drug induced mental disorders**

292.81 Drug induced delirium `CC`

CC Exd: 291.0-294.9, 303.00-305.03, 305.20-305.93, 790.3
AHA: 1Q, '88, 3
F19.921 Oth psychoactv sbstnc use uns intoxcatn `I-10`
delirium

292.82 Drug induced persisting dementia `CC`

CC Exd: See code: 292.81

292.83 Drug induced persisting amnestic disorder

292.84 Drug induced mood disorder

Depressive state induced by drugs

292.85 Drug induced sleep disorders

Drug induced circadian rhythm sleep disorder
Drug induced hypersomnia
Drug induced insomnia
Drug induced parasomnia

292.89 Other

Drug induced anxiety disorder
Drug induced organic personality syndrome
Drug induced sexual dysfunction
Drug intoxication

292.9 Unspecified drug induced mental disorder

Drug related disorder NOS
Organic psychosis NOS due to or associated with drugs

√4ᵗʰ **293 Transient mental disorders due to conditions classified elsewhere**

INCLUDES   transient organic mental disorders not associated with alcohol or drugs

Code first the associated physical or neurological condition

  EXCLUDES   *confusional state or delirium superimposed on senile*
  dementia (290.3)
  dementia due to:
  alcohol (291.0-291.9)
  arteriosclerosis (290.40-290.43)
  drugs (292.82)
  senility (290.0)

293.0 Delirium due to conditions classified elsewhere `CC`

Acute:
  confusional state
  infective psychosis
  organic reaction
  posttraumatic organic psychosis
  psycho-organic syndrome
Acute psychosis associated with endocrine, metabolic, or cerebrovascular disorder
Epileptic:
  confusional state
  twilight state

CC Exd: 290.11, 290.3, 293.0, V62.84
AHA: 1Q, '88, 3
F05 Delirium due to known physiological condition `I-10`

`N` Newborn Age: 0   `P` Pediatric Age: 0-17   `M` Maternity Age: 12-55   `A` Adult Age: 15-124   `MCC` Major CC Condition   `CC` CC Condition   `HIV` HIV Related Dx

82 – Volume 1 · February 2013   **2014 ICD-9-CM**

293.1 Subacute delirium   `CC`
Subacute:
confusional state
infective psychosis
organic reaction
posttraumatic organic psychosis
psycho-organic syndrome
psychosis associated with endocrine or metabolic disorder
CC Excl: 293.0-293.1, 293.89-293.9

✓5ᵗʰ **293.8 Other specified transient mental disorders due to conditions classified elsewhere**

293.81 Psychotic disorder with delusions in conditions classified elsewhere   `CC`
Transient organic psychotic condition, paranoid type
CC Excl: 291.0-294.9, 303.00-305.03, 305.20-305.93, 790.3
AHA: 1Q, '11, 12

293.82 Psychotic disorder with hallucinations in conditions classified elsewhere   `CC`
Transient organic psychotic condition, hallucinatory type
CC Excl: See code: 293.81

293.83 Mood disorder in conditions classified elsewhere
Transient organic psychotic condition, depressive type

293.84 Anxiety disorder in conditions classified elsewhere
AHA: 4Q, '96, 29

293.89 Other
Catatonic disorder in conditions classified elsewhere

293.9 Unspecified transient mental disorder in conditions classified elsewhere   `CC`
Organic psychosis:
infective NOS
posttraumatic NOS
transient NOS
Psycho-organic syndrome
CC Excl: See code: 293.81

✓4ᵗʰ **294 Persistent mental disorders due to conditions classified elsewhere**
INCLUDES organic psychotic brain syndromes (chronic), not elsewhere classified
AHA: M-A, '85, 12

294.0 Amnestic disorder in conditions classified elsewhere
Korsakoff's psychosis or syndrome (nonalcoholic)
Code first underlying condition
EXCLUDES alcoholic:
amnestic syndrome (291.1)
Korsakoff's psychosis (291.1)

✓5ᵗʰ **294.1 Dementia in conditions classified elsewhere**
Dementia of the Alzheimer's type
Code first any underlying physical condition, as:
Alzheimer's disease (331.0)
cerebral lipidoses (330.1)
dementia with Lewy bodies (331.82)
dementia with Parkinsonism (331.82)
epilepsy (345.0-345.9)
frontal dementia (331.19)
frontotemporal dementia (331.19)
general paresis [syphilis] (094.1)
hepatolenticular degeneration (275.1)
Huntington's chorea (333.4)
Jakob-Creutzfeldt disease (046.11-046.19)
multiple sclerosis (340)
Parkinson's disease (332.0)
Pick's disease of the brain (331.11)
polyarteritis nodosa (446.0)
syphilis (094.1)
EXCLUDES dementia:
arteriosclerotic (290.40-290.43)
presenile (290.10-290.13)
senile (290.0)
epileptic psychosis NOS (294.8)
AHA: 4Q, '00, 40; 1Q, '99, 14; N-D, '85, 5

294.10 *Dementia in conditions classified elsewhere without behavioral disturbance*
Dementia in conditions classified elsewhere NOS
F02.80 Dementia in oth dz class elsw w/o behavrl disturb   `I-10`

294.11 *Dementia in conditions classified elsewhere with behavioral disturbance*   `CC`
Aggressive behavior   Violent behavior
Combative behavior
Use additional code, where applicable, to identify: wandering in conditions classified elsewhere (V40.31)
CC Excl: 294.11, 294.21
AHA: 4Q, '00, 41
TIP: Review entire medical record for documentation of behavioral disturbance (aggressive, combative, violent behavior, wandering off); requires physician substantiation.

✓5ᵗʰ **294.2 Dementia, unspecified**
EXCLUDES mild memory disturbances, not amounting to dementia (310.89)
AHA: 4Q, '11, 95-96

294.20 Dementia, unspecified, without behavioral disturbance
Dementia NOS

294.21 Dementia, unspecified, with behavioral disturbance   `CC`
Aggressive behavior   Violent behavior
Combative behavior
Use additional code, where applicable, to identify: wandering in conditions classified elsewhere (V40.31)
CC Excl: see Code: 294.11
AHA: 4Q, '11, 95

294.8 Other persistent mental disorders due to conditions classified elsewhere
Amnestic disorder NOS
Epileptic psychosis NOS
Mixed paranoid and affective organic psychotic states
Use additional code for associated epilepsy (345.0-345.9)
EXCLUDES mild memory disturbances, not amounting to dementia (310.89)
AHA: 3Q, '09, 11; 3Q, '03, 14; 1Q, '88, 5
F06.8 Oth spec mental disord d/t known physiol cond   `I-10`

294.9 Unspecified persistent mental disorders due to conditions classified elsewhere   `HIV`
Cognitive disorder NOS   Organic psychosis (chronic)
AHA: 2Q, '07, 4

Other Psychoses (295-299)

Use additional code to identify any associated physical disease, injury, or condition affecting the brain with psychoses classifiable to 295-298

✓4ᵗʰ **295 Schizophrenic disorders**
INCLUDES schizophrenia of the types described in 295.0-295.9 occurring in children
EXCLUDES childhood type schizophrenia (299.9)
infantile autism (299.0)

The following fifth-digit subclassification is for use with category 295:
0 unspecified
1 subchronic
2 chronic
3 subchronic with acute exacerbation
4 chronic with acute exacerbation
5 in remission

DEF: Group of disorders with disturbances in thought (delusions, hallucinations), mood (blunted, flattened, inappropriate affect), sense of self; also bizarre, purposeless behavior, repetitive activity, or inactivity.

§ ✓5ᵗʰ **295.0 Simple type**   `CC 0-4`
[0-5]   Schizophrenia simplex
EXCLUDES latent schizophrenia (295.5)
CC Excl: For codes 295.00-295.04: 295.00-301.9, 306.0-310.2, 310.9-315.34, 315.39-319, 339.10-339.12, 388.45, 799.23-799.24

---

§ Requires fifth digit. Valid digits are in [brackets] under each code. See category 295 for codes and definitions.

§ ✓5ᵗʰ **295.1 Disorganized type**   CC 0-4
[0-5]   Hebephrenia
Hebephrenic type schizophrenia
DEF: Inappropriate behavior; results in extreme incoherence and disorganization of time, place and sense of social appropriateness; withdrawal from routine social interaction may occur.
CC Excl: For codes 295.10-295.14: 295.00-301.9, 306.0-319, 339.10-339.12, 388.45, 799.23-799.24

§ ✓5ᵗʰ **295.2 Catatonic type**   CC 0-4
[0-5]   Catatonic (schizophrenia):
     agitation
     excitation
     excited type
     stupor
     withdrawn type
Schizophrenic:
     catalepsy
     catatonia
     flexibilitas cerea
DEF: Extreme changes in motor activity; one extreme is decreased response or reaction to the environment and the other is spontaneous activity.
CC Excl: For codes 295.20-295.24: 295.00-301.9, 306.0-319, 339.10-339.12, 388.45, 799.23-799.24

§ ✓5ᵗʰ **295.3 Paranoid type**   CC 0-4
[0-5]   Paraphrenic schizophrenia
     EXCLUDES   *involutional paranoid state (297.2)*
          paranoia (297.1)
          paraphrenia (297.2)
DEF: Preoccupied with delusional suspicions and auditory hallucinations related to single theme; usually hostile, grandiose, overly religious, occasionally hypochondriacal.
CC Excl: For codes 295.30-295.34: 295.00-301.9, 306.0-319, 339.10-339.12, 388.45, 799.23-799.24
F20.0 Paranoid schizophrenia   I-10

§ ✓5ᵗʰ **295.4 Schizophreniform disorder**   CC 0-4
[0-5]   Oneirophrenia   Schizophreniform:
Schizophreniform: psychosis, confusional type
     attack
     EXCLUDES   *acute forms of schizophrenia of:*
          catatonic type (295.2)
          hebephrenic type (295.1)
          paranoid type (295.3)
          simple type (295.0)
          undifferentiated type (295.8)
CC Excl: For codes 295.40-295.44: 295.00-301.9, 306.0-319, 339.10-339.12, 388.45, 799.23-799.24

§ ✓5ᵗʰ **295.5 Latent schizophrenia**   CC 3-4
[0-5]   Latent schizophrenic reaction
Schizophrenia:
     borderline
     incipient
     prepsychotic
     prodromal
     pseudoneurotic
     pseudopsychopathic
     EXCLUDES   *schizoid personality (301.20-301.22)*
CC Excl: For code 295.53-295.54: 295.00-295.04, 295.10-295.14, 295.21-295.24, 295.31, 295.33-295.34, 295.40-295.44, 295.53-295.54, 295.63-295.64, 295.71, 295.73-295.74, 295.80-295.84, 295.91, 295.93-295.94
AHA: For code 295.50: 1Q, '06, 10

§ ✓5ᵗʰ **295.6 Residual type**   CC 0-4
[0-5]   Chronic undifferentiated schizophrenia
Restzustand (schizophrenic)
Schizophrenic residual state
CC Excl: For codes 295.60-295.64: 295.00-301.9, 306.0-319, 339.10-339.12, 388.45, 799.23-799.24
AHA: For code 295.62: 4Q, '06, 78

§ ✓5ᵗʰ **295.7 Schizoaffective disorder**   CC 1-4
[0-5]   Cyclic schizophrenia
Mixed schizophrenic and affective psychosis
Schizo-affective psychosis
Schizophreniform psychosis, affective type
CC Excl: For codes 295.71-295.74: 295.00-301.9, 306.0-319, 339.10-339.12, 388.45, 799.23-799.24
F25.9 Schizoaffective disorder unspecified   I-10

§ ✓5ᵗʰ **295.8 Other specified types of schizophrenia**   CC 0-4
[0-5]   Acute (undifferentiated) schizophrenia
Atypical schizophrenia
Cenesthopathic schizophrenia
     EXCLUDES   *infantile autism (299.0)*
CC Excl: For codes 295.80-295.84: 295.00-301.9, 306.0-319, 339.10-339.12, 388.45, 799.23-799.24

§ ✓5ᵗʰ **295.9 Unspecified schizophrenia**   CC 1-4
[0-5]   Schizophrenia:
     NOS
     mixed NOS
     undifferentiated NOS
     undifferentiated type
Schizophrenic reaction NOS
Schizophreniform psychosis NOS
CC Excl: For codes 295.91-295.94: 295.00-301.9, 306.0-319, 339.10-339.12, 388.45, 799.23-799.24
AHA: 3Q, '95, 6
F20.9 Schizophrenia unspecified   I-10

✓4ᵗʰ **296 Episodic mood disorders**
     INCLUDES   episodic affective disorders
     EXCLUDES   *neurotic depression (300.4)*
          reactive depressive psychosis (298.0)
          reactive excitation (298.1)

The following fifth-digit subclassification is for use with categories 296.0-296.6:
   0 unspecified
   1 mild
   2 moderate
   3 severe, without mention of psychotic behavior
   4 severe, specified as with psychotic behavior
   5 in partial or unspecified remission
   6 in full remission
AHA: M-A, '85, 14

§ ✓5ᵗʰ **296.0 Bipolar I disorder, single manic episode**   CC 0-4
[0-6]   Hypomania (mild) NOS
Hypomanic psychosis
Mania (monopolar) NOS
Manic-depressive psychosis or } single episode or
   reaction: unspecified
     hypomanic
     manic
     EXCLUDES   *circular type, if there was a previous attack of depression (296.4)*
DEF: Mood disorder identified by hyperactivity; may show extreme agitation or exaggerated excitability; speech and thought processes may be accelerated.
CC Excl: For codes 296.00-296.02: 295.00-301.9, 306.0-319, 388.45; **For codes 296.03:** 296.03-296.04, 296.13-296.14, 296.43-296.44, 296.53-296.54, 296.63-296.64; **For codes 296.04:** 295.00-301.9, 306.0-319, 388.45

§ ✓5ᵗʰ **296.1 Manic disorder, recurrent episode**   CC 0-4
[0-6]   Any condition classifiable to 296.0, stated to be recurrent
     EXCLUDES   *circular type, if there was a previous attack of depression (296.4)*
CC Excl: For codes 296.10-296.12: 295.00-301.9, 306.0-319, 339.10-339.12, 388.45; **For codes 296.13:** 296.13-296.14, 296.43-296.44, 296.53-296.54, 296.63-296.64; **For codes 296.14:** 295.00-301.9, 306.0-319, 339.10-339.12, 388.45

---

§   Requires fifth digit. Valid digits are in [brackets] under each code. See appropriate category for codes and definitions.

§ ✓5ᵗʰ **296.2 Major depressive disorder, single episode** `CC 0-4`
[0-6]

Depressive psychosis	
Endogenous depression	
Involutional melancholia	
Manic-depressive psychosis or reaction, depressed type	single episode or unspecified
Monopolar depression	
Psychotic depression	

EXCLUDES circular type, if previous attack was of manic type (296.5)
depression NOS (311)
reactive depression (neurotic) (300.4)
psychotic (298.0)

DEF: Mood disorder that produces depression; may exhibit as sadness, low self-esteem, or guilt feelings; other manifestations may be withdrawal from friends and family; interrupted sleep.
CC Excl: For code 296.20: 295.00-301.9, 306.0-319, 339.10-339.12, 388.45; **For codes 296.21-296.24:** 296.21-296.24, 296.30-296.34
AHA: For code 296.20: 3Q, '09, 18
F32.9 Major depressive disorder single episode uns   I-10

§ ✓5ᵗʰ **296.3 Major depressive disorder, recurrent episode** `CC 0-4`
[0-6]   Any condition classifiable to 296.2, stated to be recurrent

EXCLUDES circular type, if previous attack was of manic type (296.5)
depression NOS (311)
reactive depression (neurotic) (300.4)
psychotic (298.0)

CC Excl: For codes 296.30-296.33: 296.21-296.24, 296.30-296.34; **For codes 296.34:** 295.00-301.9, 306.0-319, 339.10-339.12, 388.45
F33.2 Maj dprsv disord recur sev w/o psychot features   I-10

§ ✓5ᵗʰ **296.4 Bipolar I disorder, most recent episode** `CC 0-4`
[0-6]   **(or current) manic**
Bipolar disorder, now manic
Manic-depressive psychosis, circular type but currently manic

EXCLUDES brief compensatory or rebound mood swings (296.99)

CC Excl: For codes 296.40-296.42 and 296.44: 295.00-301.9, 306.0-319, 339.10-339.12, 388.45; **For code 296.43:** 296.43-296.44, 296.63-296.64, 339.10-339.12
F31.2 Bipolar d/o currnt epis mnic sev w/psychotc features   I-10

§ ✓5ᵗʰ **296.5 Bipolar I disorder, most recent episode** `CC 0-4`
[0-6]   **(or current) depressed**
Bipolar disorder, now depressed
Manic-depressive psychosis, circular type but currently depressed

EXCLUDES brief compensatory or rebound mood swings (296.99)

CC Excl: For codes 296.50-296.52 and 296.54: 295.00-301.9, 306.0-319, 339.10-339.12, 388.45; **For code 296.53:** 296.43-296.44, 296.53-296.54, 296.63-296.64
F31.30 Bipol disord currnt epis dprsd mild/mod sev uns   I-10

§ ✓5ᵗʰ **296.6 Bipolar I disorder, most recent episode** `CC 0-4`
[0-6]   **(or current) mixed**
Manic-depressive psychosis, circular type, mixed

CC Excl: For codes 296.60-296.62 and 296.64: 295.00-301.9, 306.0-319, 339.10-339.12, 388.45; **For code 296.63:** 296.43-296.44, 296.53-296.54, 296.63-296.64

296.7 Bipolar I disorder, most recent episode (or current) unspecified
Atypical bipolar affective disorder NOS
Manic-depressive psychosis, circular type, current condition not specified as either manic or depressive
DEF: Manic-depressive disorder referred to as bipolar because of the mood range from manic to depressive.

✓5ᵗʰ **296.8 Other and unspecified bipolar disorders**

296.80 Bipolar disorder, unspecified
Bipolar disorder NOS
Manic-depressive:
reaction NOS
syndrome NOS
F31.9 Bipolar disorder unspecified   I-10

296.81 Atypical manic disorder

296.82 Atypical depressive disorder

296.89 Other `CC`
Bipolar II disorder
Manic-depressive psychosis, mixed type
CC Excl: 295.00-301.9, 306.0-319, 339.10-339.12, 388.45
F31.81 Bipolar II disorder   I-10

✓5ᵗʰ **296.9 Other and unspecified episodic mood disorder**
EXCLUDES psychogenic affective psychoses (298.0-298.8)

296.90 Unspecified episodic mood disorder
Affective psychosis NOS
Melancholia NOS
Mood disorder NOS
AHA: M-A, '85, 14
F39 Unspecified mood [affective] disorder   I-10

296.99 Other specified episodic mood disorder `CC`
Mood swings:
brief compensatory
rebound
CC Excl: 295.00-301.9, 306.0-319, 339.10-339.12, 388.45

✓4ᵗʰ **297 Delusional disorders**
INCLUDES paranoid disorders
EXCLUDES acute paranoid reaction (298.3)
alcoholic jealousy or paranoid state (291.5)
paranoid schizophrenia (295.3)

297.0 Paranoid state, simple

297.1 Delusional disorder
Chronic paranoid psychosis
Sander's disease
Systematized delusions
EXCLUDES paranoid personality disorder (301.0)
F22 Delusional disorders   I-10

297.2 Paraphrenia
Involutional paranoid state
Late paraphrenia
Paraphrenia (involutional)
DEF: Paranoid schizophrenic disorder that persists over a prolonged period but does not distort personality despite persistent delusions.

297.3 Shared psychotic disorder
Folie à deux
Induced psychosis or paranoid disorder
DEF: Mental disorder two people share; first person with the delusional disorder convinces second person because of a close relationship and shared experiences to accept the delusions.

297.8 Other specified paranoid states
Paranoia querulans
Sensitiver Beziehungswahn
EXCLUDES acute paranoid reaction or state (298.3)
senile paranoid state (290.20)

297.9 Unspecified paranoid state
Paranoid:
disorder NOS
psychosis NOS
reaction NOS
state NOS
AHA: J-A, '85, 9

✓4ᵗʰ **298 Other nonorganic psychoses**
INCLUDES psychotic conditions due to or provoked by:
emotional stress
environmental factors as major part of etiology

298.0 Depressive type psychosis `CC`
Psychogenic depressive psychosis
Psychotic reactive depression
Reactive depressive psychosis
EXCLUDES manic-depressive psychosis, depressed type (296.2-296.3)
neurotic depression (300.4)
reactive depression NOS (300.4)
CC Excl: 295.00-301.9, 306.0-319, 339.10-339.12, 388.45

• Requires fifth digit. Valid digits are in [brackets] under each code. See category 296 for codes and definitions.

4ᵗʰ 5ᵗʰ Additional Digit Required	Unacceptable PDx	Manifestation Code	Hospital Acquired Condition	►◄ Revised Text	● New Code	▲ Revised Code Title

298.1 Excitative type psychosis `CC`
Acute hysterical psychosis
Psychogenic excitation
Reactive excitation
EXCLUDES *manic-depressive psychosis, manic type (296.0-296.1)*
DEF: Affective disorder similar to manic-depressive psychosis, in the manic phase, seemingly brought on by stress.
CC Excl: See code: 298.0

298.2 Reactive confusion
Psychogenic confusion   Psychogenic twilight state
EXCLUDES *acute confusional state (293.0)*
DEF: Confusion, disorientation, cloudiness in consciousness; brought on by severe emotional upheaval.

298.3 Acute paranoid reaction `CC`
Acute psychogenic paranoid psychosis
Bouffée délirante
EXCLUDES *paranoid states (297.0-297.9)*
CC Excl: See code: 298.0

298.4 Psychogenic paranoid psychosis `CC`
Protracted reactive paranoid psychosis
CC Excl: See code: 298.0

298.8 Other and unspecified reactive psychosis
Brief psychotic disorder
Brief reactive psychosis NOS
Hysterical psychosis
Psychogenic psychosis NOS
Psychogenic stupor
EXCLUDES *acute hysterical psychosis (298.1)*

298.9 Unspecified psychosis `HIV`
Atypical psychosis   Psychotic disorder NOS
Psychosis NOS
AHA: 3Q, '06, 22
F28 Oth psych d/o not d/t sbstnc/knwn physiolog cond `I-10`

√4ᵗʰ 299 Pervasive developmental disorders
EXCLUDES *adult type psychoses occurring in childhood, as:*
affective disorders (296.0-296.9)
manic-depressive disorders (296.0-296.9)
schizophrenia (295.0-295.9)

The following fifth-digit subclassification is for use with category 299:
0 current or active state
1 residual state

§ √5ᵗʰ 299.0 Autistic disorder `CC`
[0-1]   Childhood autism
Infantile psychosis
Kanner's syndrome
EXCLUDES *disintegrative psychosis (299.1)*
Heller's syndrome (299.1)
schizophrenic syndrome of childhood (299.9)
DEF: Severe mental disorder of children, results in impaired social behavior; abnormal development of communicative skills, appears to be unaware of the need for emotional support and little emotional response to family members.
CC Excl: 295.00-301.9, 306.0-319, 339.10-339.12, 388.45
AHA: For code 299.00: ▶3Q, '12, 19-20◄

§ √5ᵗʰ 299.1 Childhood disintegrative disorder `CC`
[0-1]   Heller's syndrome
Use additional code to identify any associated neurological disorder
EXCLUDES *infantile autism (299.0)*
schizophrenic syndrome of childhood (299.9)
DEF: Mental disease of children identified by impaired development of reciprocal social skills, verbal and nonverbal communication skills, imaginative play.
CC Excl: See code: 299.0

§ √5ᵗʰ 299.8 Other specified pervasive developmental disorders `CC`
[0-1]   Asperger's disorder
Atypical childhood psychosis
Borderline psychosis of childhood
EXCLUDES *simple stereotypes without psychotic disturbance (307.3)*
CC Excl: See code: 299.0

§ √5ᵗʰ 299.9 Unspecified pervasive developmental disorder `CC`
[0-1]   Child psychosis NOS
Pervasive developmental disorder NOS
Schizophrenia, childhood type NOS
Schizophrenic syndrome of childhood NOS
EXCLUDES *schizophrenia of adult type occurring in childhood (295.0-295.9)*
CC Excl: See code: 299.0

Neurotic Disorders, Personality Disorders, and Other Nonpsychotic Mental Disorders (300-316)

√4ᵗʰ 300 Anxiety, dissociative and somatoform disorders

√5ᵗʰ 300.0 Anxiety states
EXCLUDES *anxiety in:*
acute stress reaction (308.0)
transient adjustment reaction (309.24)
neurasthenia (300.5)
psychophysiological disorders (306.0-306.9)
separation anxiety (309.21)
DEF: Mental disorder characterized by anxiety and avoidance behavior not particularly related to any specific situation or stimulus; symptoms include emotional instability, apprehension, fatigue.

300.00 Anxiety state, unspecified
Anxiety:
neurosis
reaction
state (neurotic)
Atypical anxiety disorder
AHA: 3Q, '11, 6; 2Q, '11, 5; 1Q, '02, 6
TIP: For chest pain due to anxiety, assign chest pain code first, because chest pain is not integral to the diagnosis of anxiety.
F41.9 Anxiety disorder unspecified `I-10`

300.01 Panic disorder without agoraphobia
Panic:
attack
state
EXCLUDES *panic disorder with agoraphobia (300.21)*
DEF: Neurotic disorder characterized by recurrent panic or anxiety, apprehension, fear or terror; symptoms include shortness of breath, palpitations, dizziness, shakiness; fear of dying may persist.
F41.0 Panic d/o [epis paroxysmal anxiety] w/o agoraphobia `I-10`

300.02 Generalized anxiety disorder

300.09 Other

√5ᵗʰ 300.1 Dissociative, conversion and factitious disorders
EXCLUDES *adjustment reaction (309.0-309.9)*
anorexia nervosa (307.1)
gross stress reaction (308.0-308.9)
hysterical personality (301.50-301.59)
psychophysiologic disorders (306.0-306.9)

300.10 Hysteria, unspecified

300.11 Conversion disorder
Astasia-abasia, hysterical
Conversion hysteria or reaction
Hysterical:
blindness
deafness
paralysis
DEF: Mental disorder that impairs physical functions with no physiological basis; sensory motor symptoms include seizures, paralysis, temporary blindness; increase in stress or avoidance of unpleasant responsibilities may precipitate onset of symptoms.
AHA: 2Q, '11, 5; N-D, '85, 15

300.12 Dissociative amnesia
Hysterical amnesia

300.13 Dissociative fugue
Hysterical fugue
DEF: Dissociative hysteria; identified by loss of memory, flight from familiar surroundings; conscious activity is not associated with perception of surroundings, no later memory of episode.

---

§ Requires fifth digit. Valid digits are in [brackets] under each code. See category 299 for codes and definitions.

`N` Newborn Age: 0   `P` Pediatric Age: 0-17   `M` Maternity Age: 12-55   `A` Adult Age: 15-124   `MCC` Major CC Condition   `CC` CC Condition   `HIV` HIV Related Dx

300.14 Dissociative identity disorder

300.15 Dissociative disorder or reaction, unspecified

> **DEF:** Hysterical neurotic episode; sudden but temporary changes in perceived identity, memory, consciousness, segregated memory patterns exist separate from dominant personality.

300.16 Factitious disorder with predominantly psychological signs and symptoms
Compensation neurosis
Ganser's syndrome, hysterical

> **DEF:** A disorder characterized by the purposeful assumption of mental illness symptoms; which are acted out more often when another person is present.

300.19 Other and unspecified factitious illness
Factitious disorder (with combined psychological and physical signs and symptoms) (with predominantly physical signs and symptoms) NOS

> **EXCLUDES** multiple operations or hospital addiction syndrome (301.51)

√5ᵗʰ 300.2 Phobic disorders

> **EXCLUDES** anxiety state not associated with a specific situation or object (300.00-300.09)
> obsessional phobias (300.3)

300.20 Phobia, unspecified
Anxiety-hysteria NOS
Phobia NOS

300.21 Agoraphobia with panic disorder
Fear of:
  open spaces
  streets   } with panic attacks
  travel
Panic disorder with agoraphobia

> **EXCLUDES** agoraphobia without panic disorder (300.22)
> panic disorder without agoraphobia (300.01)

300.22 Agoraphobia without mention of panic attacks
Any condition classifiable to 300.21 without mention of panic attacks

300.23 Social phobia
Fear of:
  eating in public
  public speaking
  washing in public

300.29 Other isolated or specific phobias
Acrophobia
Animal phobias
Claustrophobia
Fear of crowds

300.3 Obsessive-compulsive disorders
Anancastic neurosis
Compulsive neurosis
Obsessional phobia [any]

> **EXCLUDES** obsessive-compulsive symptoms occurring in:
> endogenous depression (296.2-296.3)
> organic states (eg., encephalitis)
> schizophrenia (295.0-295.9)

300.4 Dysthymic disorder
Anxiety depression
Depression with anxiety
Depressive reaction
Neurotic depressive state
Reactive depression

> **EXCLUDES** adjustment reaction with depressive symptoms (309.0-309.1)
> depression NOS (311)
> manic-depressive psychosis, depressed type (296.2-296.3)
> reactive depressive psychosis (298.0)

> **DEF:** Depression without psychosis; less severe depression related to personal change or unexpected circumstances; also referred to as "reactional depression."

AHA: 3Q, '11, 6

F34.1 Dysthymic disorder   **I-10**

300.5 Neurasthenia
Fatigue neurosis
Nervous debility
Psychogenic:
  asthenia
  general fatigue
Use additional code to identify any associated physical disorder

> **EXCLUDES** anxiety state (300.00-300.09)
> neurotic depression (300.4)
> psychophysiological disorders (306.0-306.9)
> specific nonpsychotic mental disorders following organic brain damage (310.0-310.9)

> **DEF:** Physical and mental symptoms caused primarily by what is known as mental exhaustion; symptoms include chronic weakness, fatigue.

300.6 Depersonalization disorder
Derealization (neurotic)
Neurotic state with depersonalization episode

> **EXCLUDES** depersonalization associated with:
> anxiety (300.00-300.09)
> depression (300.4)
> manic-depressive disorder or psychosis (296.0-296.9)
> schizophrenia (295.0-295.9)

> **DEF:** Dissociative disorder characterized by feelings of strangeness about self or body image; symptoms include dizziness, anxiety, fear of insanity, loss of reality of surroundings.

300.7 Hypochondriasis
Body dysmorphic disorder

> **EXCLUDES** hypochondriasis in:
> hysteria (300.10-300.19)
> manic-depressive psychosis, depressed type (296.2-296.3)
> neurasthenia (300.5)
> obsessional disorder (300.3)
> schizophrenia (295.0-295.9)

√5ᵗʰ 300.8 Somatoform disorders

300.81 Somatization disorder
Briquet's disorder
Severe somatoform disorder

300.82 Undifferentiated somatoform disorder
Atypical somatoform disorder
Somatoform disorder NOS

> **DEF:** Disorders in which patients have symptoms that suggest an organic disease but no evidence of physical disorder after repeated testing.

AHA: 4Q, '96, 29

300.89 Other somatoform disorders
Occupational neurosis, including writers' cramp
Psychasthenia
Psychasthenic neurosis

300.9 Unspecified nonpsychotic mental disorder
Psychoneurosis NOS

√4ᵗʰ 301 Personality disorders

> **INCLUDES** character neurosis

Use additional code to identify any associated neurosis or psychosis, or physical condition

> **EXCLUDES** nonpsychotic personality disorder associated with organic brain syndromes (310.0-310.9)

301.0 Paranoid personality disorder
Fanatic personality
Paranoid personality (disorder)
Paranoid traits

> **EXCLUDES** acute paranoid reaction (298.3)
> alcoholic paranoia (291.5)
> paranoid schizophrenia (295.3)
> paranoid states (297.0-297.9)

AHA: J-A, '85, 9

√5ᵗʰ 301.1 Affective personality disorder

> **EXCLUDES** affective psychotic disorders (296.0-296.9)
> neurasthenia (300.5)
> neurotic depression (300.4)

301.10 Affective personality disorder, unspecified

Additional Digit Required   Unacceptable PDx   Manifestation Code   Hospital Acquired Condition   ▶◀ Revised Text   ● New Code   ▲ Revised Code Title

14 ICD-9-CM   Volume 1 – 87

301.11 Chronic hypomanic personality disorder
Chronic hypomanic disorder
Hypomanic personality

301.12 Chronic depressive personality disorder
Chronic depressive disorder
Depressive character or personality

301.13 Cyclothymic disorder
Cycloid personality
Cyclothymia
Cyclothymic personality

√5ᵗʰ **301.2 Schizoid personality disorder**
> EXCLUDES *schizophrenia (295.0-295.9)*

301.20 Schizoid personality disorder, unspecified

301.21 Introverted personality

301.22 Schizotypal personality disorder

301.3 Explosive personality disorder
Aggressive:
  personality
  reaction
Aggressiveness
Emotional instability (excessive)
Pathological emotionality
Quarrelsomeness
> EXCLUDES *dyssocial personality (301.7)*
> *hysterical neurosis (300.10-300.19)*

301.4 Obsessive-compulsive personality disorder
Anancastic personality
Obsessional personality
> EXCLUDES *obsessive-compulsive disorder (300.3)*
> *phobic state (300.20-300.29)*

√5ᵗʰ **301.5 Histrionic personality disorder**
> EXCLUDES *hysterical neurosis (300.10-300.19)*

DEF: Extreme emotional behavior, often theatrical; often concerned about own appeal; may demand attention, exhibit seductive behavior.

301.50 Histrionic personality disorder, unspecified
Hysterical personality NOS

301.51 Chronic factitious illness with physical symptoms   CC
Hospital addiction syndrome
Multiple operations syndrome
Munchausen syndrome
CC Excl: 295.00-301.9, 306.0-319, 339.10-339.12, 388.45

301.59 Other histrionic personality disorder
Personality:
  emotionally unstable
  labile
  psychoinfantile

301.6 Dependent personality disorder
Asthenic personality
Inadequate personality
Passive personality
> EXCLUDES *neurasthenia (300.5)*
> *passive-aggressive personality (301.84)*

DEF: Overwhelming feeling of helplessness; fears of abandonment may persist; difficulty in making personal decisions without confirmation by others; low self-esteem due to irrational sensitivity to criticism.

301.7 Antisocial personality disorder
Amoral personality
Asocial personality
Dyssocial personality
Personality disorder with predominantly sociopathic or asocial manifestation
> EXCLUDES *disturbance of conduct without specifiable*
> *personality disorder (312.0-312.9)*
> *explosive personality (301.3)*

DEF: Continuous antisocial behavior that violates rights of others; social traits include extreme aggression, total disregard for traditional social rules.
AHA: S-0, '84, 16

√5ᵗʰ **301.8 Other personality disorders**

301.81 Narcissistic personality disorder
DEF: Grandiose fantasy or behavior, lack of social empathy hypersensitive to the lack of others' judgment, exploits others; need for continual admiration.

301.82 Avoidant personality disorder
DEF: Personality disorder marked by feelings of social inferiority; sensitivity to criticism, emotionally restrained due to fear of rejection.

301.83 Borderline personality disorder
DEF: Personality disorder characterized by unstable mood self-image, and interpersonal relationships; uncontrolled anger, impulsive and self-destructive acts, fears of abandonment, feelings of emptiness and boredom, recurrent suicide threats or self-mutilation.
F60.3 Borderline personality disorder

301.84 Passive-aggressive personality
DEF: Pattern of procrastination and refusal to meet standards; introduce own obstacles to success and exploi failure.

301.89 Other
Personality:
  eccentric
  "haltlose" type
  immature
  masochistic
  psychoneurotic
> EXCLUDES *psychoinfantile personality (301.59)*

301.9 Unspecified personality disorder
Pathological personality NOS
Personality disorder NOS
Psychopathic:
  constitutional state
  personality (disorder)

√4ᵗʰ **302 Sexual and gender identity disorders**
> EXCLUDES *sexual disorder manifest in:*
> *organic brain syndrome (290.0-294.9, 310.0-310.9)*
> *psychosis (295.0-298.9)*

302.0 Ego-dystonic sexual orientation
Ego-dystonic lesbianism
Sexual orientation conflict disorder
> EXCLUDES *homosexual pedophilia (302.2)*

302.1 Zoophilia
Bestiality
DEF: A sociodeviant disorder marked by engaging in sexual intercourse with animals.

302.2 Pedophilia
DEF: A sociodeviant condition of adults characterized by sexual activity with children.

302.3 Transvestic fetishism
> EXCLUDES *trans-sexualism (302.5)*

DEF: The desire to dress in clothing of opposite sex.

302.4 Exhibitionism
DEF: Sexual deviant behavior; exposure of genitals to strangers; behavior prompted by intense sexual urges and fantasies.

√5ᵗʰ **302.5 Trans-sexualism**
Sex reassignment surgery status
> EXCLUDES *transvestism (302.3)*

DEF: Gender identity disturbance; overwhelming desire to change anatomic sex, due to belief that individual is a member of the opposite sex.

302.50 With unspecified sexual history

302.51 With asexual history

302.52 With homosexual history

302.53 With heterosexual history

302.6 Gender identity disorder in children
Feminism in boys
Gender identity disorder NOS
> EXCLUDES *gender identity disorder in adult (302.85)*
> *trans-sexualism (302.50-302.53)*
> *transvestism (302.3)*

N Newborn Age: 0   P Pediatric Age: 0-17   M Maternity Age: 12-55   A Adult Age: 15-124   MCC Major CC Condition   CC CC Condition   HIV HIV Related D

88 – Volume 1   2014 ICD-9-C

√5ᵗʰ **302.7 Psychosexual dysfunction**

> *EXCLUDES*   *impotence of organic origin (607.84)*
> *normal transient symptoms from ruptured hymen*
> *transient or occasional failures of erection due to*
> *fatigue, anxiety, alcohol, or drugs*

302.70 Psychosexual dysfunction, unspecified
Sexual dysfunction NOS

302.71 Hypoactive sexual desire disorder
> *EXCLUDES*   *decreased sexual desire NOS (799.81)*

302.72 With inhibited sexual excitement
Female sexual arousal disorder
Frigidity
Impotence
Male erectile disorder

302.73 Female orgasmic disorder   ♀

302.74 Male orgasmic disorder   ♂

302.75 Premature ejaculation   ♂

302.76 Dyspareunia, psychogenic   ♀
DEF: Difficult or painful sex due to psychosomatic state.

302.79 With other specified psychosexual dysfunctions
Sexual aversion disorder

√5ᵗʰ **302.8 Other specified psychosexual disorders**

302.81 Fetishism
DEF: Psychosexual disorder noted for intense sexual urges and arousal precipitated by fantasies; use of inanimate objects, such as clothing, to stimulate sexual arousal, orgasm.

302.82 Voyeurism
DEF: Psychosexual disorder characterized by uncontrollable impulse to observe others, without their knowledge, who are nude or engaged in sexual activity.

302.83 Sexual masochism
DEF: Psychosexual disorder noted for need to achieve sexual gratification through humiliating or hurtful acts inflicted on self.

302.84 Sexual sadism
DEF: Psychosexual disorder noted for need to achieve sexual gratification through humiliating or hurtful acts inflicted on someone else.

302.85 Gender identity disorder in adolescents or adults
Use additional code to identify sex reassignment surgery status (302.5)
> *EXCLUDES*   *gender identity disorder NOS (302.6)*
> *gender identity disorder in children (302.6)*

302.89 Other
Frotteurism
Nymphomania
Satyriasis

302.9 Unspecified psychosexual disorder
Paraphilia NOS
Pathologic sexuality NOS
Sexual deviation NOS
Sexual disorder NOS

√4ᵗʰ **303 Alcohol dependence syndrome**
Use additional code to identify any associated condition, as:
alcoholic psychoses (291.0-291.9)
drug dependence (304.0-304.9)
physical complications of alcohol, such as:
  cerebral degeneration (331.7)
  cirrhosis of liver (571.2)
  epilepsy (345.0-345.9)
  gastritis (535.3)
  hepatitis (571.1)
  liver damage NOS (571.3)
> *EXCLUDES*   *drunkenness NOS (305.0)*

The following fifth-digit subclassification is for use with category 303:
  0 unspecified
  1 continuous
  2 episodic
  3 in remission

AHA: 1Q, '10, 20-21; 3Q, '95, 6; 2Q, '91, 9; 4Q, '88, 8; S-O, '86, 3
TIP: The patient has become physically addicted to alcohol and often experiences withdrawal symptoms when not drinking. Do not assign both 303.0X and 303.9X on the same encounter.

§ √5ᵗʰ **303.0 Acute alcoholic intoxication**
[0-3]   Acute drunkenness in alcoholism

§ √5ᵗʰ **303.9 Other and unspecified alcohol dependence**
[0-3]   Chronic alcoholism
     Dipsomania
AHA: 2Q, '02, 4; 2Q, '89, 9 ; For code 303.90: ▶2Q, '12, 9;◀ 2Q, '07, 6
F10.20 Alcohol dependence uncomplicated   I-10
F10.21 Alcohol dependence in remission   I-10

√4ᵗʰ **304 Drug dependence**
> *EXCLUDES*   *nondependent abuse of drugs (305.1-305.9)*

The following fifth-digit subclassification is for use with category 304:
  0 unspecified
  1 continuous
  2 episodic
  3 in remission

AHA: 1Q, '10, 20-21; 2Q, '91, 10; 4Q, '88, 8; S-O, '86, 3

§ √5ᵗʰ **304.0 Opioid type dependence**   CC 1
[0-3]   Heroin
     Meperidine
     Methadone
     Morphine
     Opium
     Opium alkaloids and their derivatives
     Synthetics with morphine-like effects
CC Excl: For code 304.01: 291.0-292.9, 303.00-305.03, 305.20-305.93, 790.3
AHA: 2Q, '06, 7; For code 304.00: 1Q, '11, 15: 2Q, '10, 13

§ √5ᵗʰ **304.1 Sedative, hypnotic or anxiolytic dependence**   CC 1
[0-3]   Barbiturates
     Nonbarbiturate sedatives and tranquilizers with a similar effect:
       chlordiazepoxide
       diazepam
       glutethimide
       meprobamate
       methaqualone
CC Excl: For code 304.11: 291.0-292.9, 303.00-305.03, 305.20-305.93, 790.3

§ √5ᵗʰ **304.2 Cocaine dependence**   CC 1
[0-3]   Coca leaves and derivatives
CC Excl: For code 304.21: 291.0-292.9, 303.00-305.03, 305.20-305.93, 790.3
F14.20 Cocaine dependence uncomplicated   I-10

§ √5ᵗʰ **304.3 Cannabis dependence**
[0-3]   Hashish   Marihuana
     Hemp

§ √5ᵗʰ **304.4 Amphetamine and other psychostimulant dependence**   CC 1
[0-3]   Methylphenidate   Phenmetrazine
CC Excl: For code 304.41: 291.0-292.9, 303.00-305.03, 305.20-305.93, 790.3

Mental, Behavioral and Neurodevelopmental Disorders

304.5–306.3

§ ✓5ᵗʰ **304.5 Hallucinogen dependence**   CC 1
[0-3]   Dimethyltryptamine [DMT]
Lysergic acid diethylamide [LSD] and derivatives
Mescaline
Psilocybin
CC Excl: For code 304.51: 291.0-292.9, 303.00-305.03, 305.20-305.93, 790.3

§ ✓5ᵗʰ **304.6 Other specified drug dependence**   CC 1
[0-3]   Absinthe addiction
Glue sniffing
Inhalant dependence
Phencyclidine dependence
> **EXCLUDES** tobacco dependence (305.1)

CC Excl: For code 304.61: 291.0-292.9, 303.00-305.03, 305.20-305.93, 790.3

§ ✓5ᵗʰ **304.7 Combinations of opioid type drug with any other**   CC 1
[0-3]   **CC Excl:** For code 304.71: 291.0-292.9, 303.00-305.03, 305.20-305.93, 790.3
AHA: M-A, '86, 12

§ ✓5ᵗʰ **304.8 Combinations of drug dependence excluding opioid type drug**   CC 1
[0-3]   **CC Excl:** For code 304.81: 291.0-292.9, 303.00-305.03, 305.20-305.93, 790.3
AHA: M-A, '86, 12

§ ✓5ᵗʰ **304.9 Unspecified drug dependence**   CC 1
[0-3]   Drug addiction NOS
Drug dependence NOS
CC Excl: For code 304.91: 291.0-292.9, 303.00-305.03, 305.20-305.93, 790.3
AHA: For code 304.90: ▶2Q, '12, 16;◀ 4Q, '03, 103

✓4ᵗʰ **305 Nondependent abuse of drugs**

> **NOTE** Includes cases where a person, for whom no other diagnosis is possible, has come under medical care because of the maladaptive effect of a drug on which he is not dependent and that he has taken on his own initiative to the detriment of his health or social functioning.

> **EXCLUDES** alcohol dependence syndrome (303.0-303.9)
> drug dependence (304.0-304.9)
> drug withdrawal syndrome (292.0)
> poisoning by drugs or medicinal substances (960.0-979.9)

The following fifth-digit subclassification is for use with codes 305.0, 305.2-305.9:
   0 unspecified
   1 continuous
   2 episodic
   3 in remission

AHA: 1Q, '10, 20-21; 2Q, '91, 10; 4Q, '88, 8; S-O, '86, 3

§ ✓5ᵗʰ **305.0 Alcohol abuse**
[0-3]   Drunkenness NOS
Excessive drinking of alcohol NOS
"Hangover" (alcohol)
Inebriety NOS
> **EXCLUDES** acute alcohol intoxication in alcoholism (303.0)
> alcoholic psychoses (291.0-291.9)

AHA: 3Q, '96, 16; For code 305.00: 4Q, '09, 112
F10.10 Alcohol abuse uncomplicated   I-10

305.1 Tobacco use disorder
Tobacco dependence
> **EXCLUDES** history of tobacco use (V15.82)
> smoking complicating pregnancy (649.0)
> tobacco use disorder complicating pregnancy (649.0)

AHA: 1Q, '09, 16; 2Q, '96, 10; N-D, '84, 12
F17.210 Nicotine dependence cigarettes uncomplicated   I-10

§ ✓5ᵗʰ **305.2 Cannabis abuse**
[0-3]   F12.10 Cannabis abuse uncomplicated   I-10

§ ✓5ᵗʰ **305.3 Hallucinogen abuse**
[0-3]   Acute intoxication from hallucinogens ["bad trips"]
LSD reaction

§ ✓5ᵗʰ **305.4 Sedative, hypnotic or anxiolytic abuse**
[0-3]

§ ✓5ᵗʰ **305.5 Opioid abuse**
[0-3]

§ ✓5ᵗʰ **305.6 Cocaine abuse**
[0-3]   **AHA:** For code 305.60: 1Q, '05, 6; 1Q, '93, 25
F14.10 Cocaine abuse uncomplicated   I

§ ✓5ᵗʰ **305.7 Amphetamine or related acting sympathomimetic abuse**
[0-3]   **AHA:** For code 305.70: 2Q, '03, 10–11

§ ✓5ᵗʰ **305.8 Antidepressant type abuse**
[0-3]

§ ✓5ᵗʰ **305.9 Other, mixed, or unspecified drug abuse**
[0-3]   Caffeine intoxication
Inhalant abuse
"Laxative habit"
Misuse of drugs NOS
Nonprescribed use of drugs or patent medicinals
Phencyclidine abuse
AHA: 3Q, '99, 20

✓4ᵗʰ **306 Physiological malfunction arising from mental factors**

> **INCLUDES** psychogenic:
>   physical symptoms
>   physiological } not involving tissue damage
>   manifestations

> **EXCLUDES** hysteria (300.11-300.19)
> physical symptoms secondary to a psychiatric disorder classified elsewhere
> psychic factors associated with physical conditions involvin tissue damage classified elsewhere (316)
> specific nonpsychotic mental disorders following organic brain damage (310.0-310.9)

DEF: Functional disturbances or interruptions due to mental or psychologic causes; no tissue damage sustained in these conditions.

306.0 Musculoskeletal
Psychogenic paralysis
Psychogenic torticollis
> **EXCLUDES** Gilles de la Tourette's syndrome (307.23)
> paralysis as hysterical or conversion reaction (300.1
> tics (307.20-307.22)

306.1 Respiratory
Psychogenic: Psychogenic:
air hunger   hyperventilation
cough   yawning
hiccough
> **EXCLUDES** psychogenic asthma (316 and 493.9)

306.2 Cardiovascular
Cardiac neurosis
Cardiovascular neurosis
Neurocirculatory asthenia
Psychogenic cardiovascular disorder
> **EXCLUDES** psychogenic paroxysmal tachycardia (316 and 427.

DEF: Neurocirculatory asthenia: functional nervous and circulatory irregularities with palpitations, dyspnea, fatigue, rapid pulse, precordial pain, fear of effort, discomfort during exercise, anxiety; also called DaCosta's syndrome, Effort syndrome, Irritable or Soldie Heart.

AHA: J-A, '85, 14

306.3 Skin
Psychogenic pruritus
> **EXCLUDES** psychogenic:
> alopecia (316 and 704.00)
> dermatitis (316 and 692.9)
> eczema (316 and 691.8 or 692.9)
> urticaria (316 and 708.0-708.9)

---

§   Requires fifth digit. Valid digits are in [brackets] under each code. See appropriate category for codes and definitions.

N Newborn Age: 0   P Pediatric Age: 0-17   M Maternity Age: 12-55   A Adult Age: 15-124   MCC Major CC Condition   CC CC Condition   HIV HIV Related I

306.4 Gastrointestinal
Aerophagy
Cyclical vomiting, psychogenic
Diarrhea, psychogenic
Nervous gastritis
Psychogenic dyspepsia

EXCLUDES   cyclical vomiting NOS (536.2)
     associated with migraine (346.2)
globus hystericus (300.11)
mucous colitis (316 and 564.9)
psychogenic:
     cardiospasm (316 and 530.0)
     duodenal ulcer (316 and 532.0-532.9)
     gastric ulcer (316 and 531.0-531.9)
     peptic ulcer NOS (316 and 533.0-533.9)
     vomiting NOS (307.54)

DEF: Aerophagy: excess swallowing of air, usually unconscious; related to anxiety; results in distended abdomen or belching, often interpreted by the patient as a physical disorder.

AHA: 2Q, '89, 11

√5th 306.5 Genitourinary
EXCLUDES   enuresis, psychogenic (307.6)
frigidity (302.72)
impotence (302.72)
psychogenic dyspareunia (302.76)

306.50 Psychogenic genitourinary malfunction, unspecified

306.51 Psychogenic vaginismus   ♀
Functional vaginismus
DEF: Psychogenic response resulting in painful contractions of vaginal canal muscles; can be severe enough to prevent sexual intercourse.

306.52 Psychogenic dysmenorrhea   ♀

306.53 Psychogenic dysuria

306.59 Other
AHA: M-A, '87, 11

306.6 Endocrine

306.7 Organs of special sense
EXCLUDES   hysterical blindness or deafness (300.11)
psychophysical visual disturbances (368.16)

306.8 Other specified psychophysiological malfunction
Bruxism
Teeth grinding

306.9 Unspecified psychophysiological malfunction
Psychophysiologic disorder NOS
Psychosomatic disorder NOS

√4th 307 Special symptoms or syndromes, not elsewhere classified
NOTE This category is intended for use if the psychopathology is manifested by a single specific symptom or group of symptoms which is not part of an organic illness or other mental disorder classifiable elsewhere.

EXCLUDES   those due to mental disorders classified elsewhere
those of organic origin

307.0 Adult onset fluency disorder
EXCLUDES   childhood onset fluency disorder (315.35)
dysphasia (784.59)
fluency disorder due to late effect of cerebrovascular accident (438.14)
fluency disorder in conditions classified elsewhere (784.52)
lisping or lalling (307.9)
retarded development of speech (315.31-315.39)

AHA: 4Q, '10, 83

307.1 Anorexia nervosa   CC
EXCLUDES   eating disturbance NOS (307.50)
feeding problem (783.3)
of nonorganic origin (307.59)
loss of appetite (783.0)
of nonorganic origin (307.59)

CC Excl: 306.4, 306.8-306.9, 307.1, 307.50-307.59, 309.22
AHA: 2Q, '06, 12; 4Q, '89, 11
TIP: Assign an additional code for any associated malnutrition.

√5th 307.2 Tics
EXCLUDES   nail-biting or thumb-sucking (307.9)
stereotypes occurring in isolation (307.3)
tics of organic origin (333.3)

DEF: Involuntary muscle response usually confined to the face, shoulders.

307.20 Tic disorder, unspecified
Tic disorder NOS

307.21 Transient tic disorder

307.22 Chronic motor or vocal tic disorder

307.23 Tourette's disorder
Motor-verbal tic disorder
DEF: Syndrome of facial and vocal tics in childhood; progresses to spontaneous or involuntary jerking, obscene utterances, other uncontrollable actions considered inappropriate.

307.3 Stereotypic movement disorder
Body-rocking
Head banging
Spasmus nutans
Stereotypes NOS
EXCLUDES   tics (307.20-307.23)
of organic origin (333.3)

√5th 307.4 Specific disorders of sleep of nonorganic origin
EXCLUDES   narcolepsy (347.00-347.11)
organic hypersomnia (327.10-327.19)
organic insomnia (327.00-327.09)
those of unspecified cause (780.50-780.59)

307.40 Nonorganic sleep disorder, unspecified

307.41 Transient disorder of initiating or maintaining sleep
Adjustment insomnia
Hyposomnia ⎫ associated with intermittent
Insomnia   ⎬ emotional reactions
Sleeplessness ⎭ or conflicts

307.42 Persistent disorder of initiating or maintaining sleep
Hyposomnia, insomnia, or sleeplessness associated with:
     anxiety
     conditioned arousal
     depression (major) (minor)
     psychosis
Idiopathic insomnia
Paradoxical insomnia
Primary insomnia
Psychophysiological insomnia

307.43 Transient disorder of initiating or maintaining wakefulness
Hypersomnia associated with acute or intermittent emotional reactions or conflicts

307.44 Persistent disorder of initiating or maintaining wakefulness
Hypersomnia associated with depression (major) (minor)
Insufficient sleep syndrome
Primary hypersomnia
EXCLUDES   sleep deprivation (V69.4)

307.45 Circadian rhythm sleep disorder of nonorganic origin

307.46 Sleep arousal disorder
Night terror disorder
Night terrors
Sleep terror disorder
Sleepwalking
Somnambulism
DEF: Sleepwalking marked by extreme terror, panic, screaming, confusion; no recall of event upon arousal; term may refer to simply the act of sleepwalking.

Additional Digit Required   Unacceptable PDx   Manifestation Code   Hospital Acquired Condition   ▶◀ Revised Text   ● New Code   ▲ Revised Code Title

2014 ICD-9-CM   Volume 1 – 91

Mental, Behavioral and Neurodevelopmental Disorders

307.47–309.29

307.47 Other dysfunctions of sleep stages or arousal from sleep
Nightmare disorder
Nightmares:
    NOS
    REM-sleep type
    Sleep drunkenness

307.48 Repetitive intrusions of sleep
Repetitive intrusion of sleep with:
    atypical polysomnographic features
    environmental disturbances
    repeated REM-sleep interruptions

307.49 Other
"Short-sleeper"   Subjective insomnia complaint

✓5ᵗʰ 307.5 Other and unspecified disorders of eating
EXCLUDES   *anorexia:*
    nervosa (307.1)
    of unspecified cause (783.0)
    overeating, of unspecified cause (783.6)
    vomiting:
        NOS (787.03)
        cyclical (536.2)
            associated with migraine (346.2)
            psychogenic (306.4)

307.50 Eating disorder, unspecified
Eating disorder NOS

307.51 Bulimia nervosa   **CC**
Overeating of nonorganic origin
DEF: Mental disorder commonly characterized by binge eating followed by self-induced vomiting; perceptions of being fat; and fear the inability to stop eating voluntarily.
CC Excl: 307.1, 307.50-307.51, 307.53-307.59
AHA: ▶3Q, '12, 9◀

307.52 Pica
Perverted appetite of nonorganic origin
DEF: Compulsive eating disorder characterized by craving for substances other than food, such as paint chips or dirt.

307.53 Rumination disorder
Regurgitation, of nonorganic origin, of food with reswallowing
EXCLUDES   *obsessional rumination (300.3)*

307.54 Psychogenic vomiting

307.59 Other
Feeding disorder of infancy or early childhood of nonorganic origin
Infantile feeding
    disturbances   } of nonorganic
Loss of appetite   origin

307.6 Enuresis
Enuresis (primary) (secondary) of nonorganic origin
EXCLUDES   *enuresis of unspecified cause (788.3)*
DEF: Involuntary urination past age of normal control; also called bedwetting; no trace to biological problem; focus on psychological issues.

307.7 Encopresis
Encopresis (continuous) (discontinuous) of nonorganic origin
EXCLUDES   *encopresis of unspecified cause (787.60-787.63)*
DEF: Inability to control bowel movements; cause traced to psychological, not biological, problems.

✓5ᵗʰ 307.8 Pain disorders related to psychological factors

307.80 Psychogenic pain, site unspecified

307.81 Tension headache
EXCLUDES   *headache:*
    NOS (784.0)
    migraine (346.0-346.9)
    syndromes (339.00-339.89)
    tension type (339.10-339.12)
AHA: 4Q, '08, 103; N-D, '85, 16

307.89 Other
Code first to type or site of pain
EXCLUDES   *pain disorder exclusively attributed to psychological factors (307.80)*
    psychogenic pain (307.80)

307.9 Other and unspecified special symptoms or syndromes, not elsewhere classified
Communication disorder NOS   Masturbation
Hair plucking   Nail-biting
Lalling   Thumb-sucking
Lisping

✓4ᵗʰ 308 Acute reaction to stress
INCLUDES   catastrophic stress
    combat and operational stress reaction
    combat fatigue
    gross stress reaction (acute)
    transient disorders in response to exceptional physical or mental stress which usually subside within hours or days
EXCLUDES   *adjustment reaction or disorder (309.0-309.9)*
    chronic stress reaction (309.1-309.9)

308.0 Predominant disturbance of emotions
Anxiety
Emotional crisis   } as acute reaction to exceptional
Panic state   [gross] stress

308.1 Predominant disturbance of consciousness
Fugues as acute reaction to exceptional [gross] stress

308.2 Predominant psychomotor disturbance
Agitation states   } as acute reaction to exceptional
Stupor   [gross] stress

308.3 Other acute reactions to stress
Acute situational disturbance
Acute stress disorder
EXCLUDES   *prolonged posttraumatic emotional disturbance (309.81)*

308.4 Mixed disorders as reaction to stress

308.9 Unspecified acute reaction to stress

✓4ᵗʰ 309 Adjustment reaction
INCLUDES   adjustment disorders
    reaction (adjustment) to chronic stress
EXCLUDES   *acute reaction to major stress (308.0-308.9)*
    neurotic disorders (300.0-300.9)

309.0 Adjustment disorder with depressed mood
Grief reaction
EXCLUDES   *affective psychoses (296.0-296.9)*
    neurotic depression (300.4)
    prolonged depressive reaction (309.1)
    psychogenic depressive psychosis (298.0)
F43.21 Adjustment disorder with depressed mood   **I-10**

309.1 Prolonged depressive reaction
EXCLUDES   *affective psychoses (296.0-296.9)*
    brief depressive reaction (309.0)
    neurotic depression (300.4)
    psychogenic depressive psychosis (298.0)

✓5ᵗʰ 309.2 With predominant disturbance of other emotions

309.21 Separation anxiety disorder
DEF: Abnormal apprehension by a child when physically separated from support environment; byproduct of abnormal symbiotic child-parent relationship.

309.22 Emancipation disorder of adolescence and early adult life
DEF: Adjustment reaction of late adolescence; conflict over independence from parental supervision; symptoms include difficulty in making decisions, increased reliance on parental advice, deliberate adoption of values in opposition of parents.

309.23 Specific academic or work inhibition

309.24 Adjustment disorder with anxiety

309.28 Adjustment disorder with mixed anxiety and depressed mood
Adjustment reaction with anxiety and depression
F43.23 Adjustment d/o w/mixed anxiety & depressed mood   **I-10**

309.29 Other
Culture shock

N Newborn Age: 0   **P** Pediatric Age: 0-17   **M** Maternity Age: 12-55   **A** Adult Age: 15-124   **MCC** Major CC Condition   **CC** CC Condition   **HIV** HIV Related Dx

92 – Volume 1 • February 2013   2014 ICD-9-CM

309.3 Adjustment disorder with disturbance of conduct
Conduct disturbance ⎱
Destructiveness   ⎰ as adjustment reaction

> EXCLUDES *destructiveness in child (312.9)*
> *disturbance of conduct NOS (312.9)*
> *dyssocial behavior without manifest psychiatric*
> *disorder (V71.01-V71.02)*
> *personality disorder with predominantly sociopathic*
> *or asocial manifestations (301.7)*

309.4 Adjustment disorder with mixed disturbance of emotions and conduct

√5ᵗʰ **309.8 Other specified adjustment reactions**

309.81 Posttraumatic stress disorder
Chronic posttraumatic stress disorder
Concentration camp syndrome
Posttraumatic stress disorder NOS
Post-traumatic stress disorder (PTSD)

> EXCLUDES *acute stress disorder (308.3)*
> *posttraumatic brain syndrome:*
> *nonpsychotic (310.2)*
> *psychotic (293.0-293.9)*

> DEF: Preoccupation with traumatic events beyond normal experience; i.e., rape, personal assault, etc.; also recurring flashbacks of trauma; symptoms include difficulty remembering, sleeping, or concentrating, and guilt feelings for surviving.
> AHA: 2Q, '11, 5

309.82 Adjustment reaction with physical symptoms

309.83 Adjustment reaction with withdrawal
Elective mutism as adjustment reaction
Hospitalism (in children) NOS

309.89 Other

309.9 Unspecified adjustment reaction
Adaptation reaction NOS
Adjustment reaction NOS

√4ᵗʰ **310 Specific nonpsychotic mental disorders due to brain damage**

> EXCLUDES *neuroses, personality disorders, or other nonpsychotic conditions occurring in a form similar to that seen with functional disorders but in association with a physical condition (300.0-300.9, 301.0-301.9)*

310.0 Frontal lobe syndrome
Lobotomy syndrome
Postleucotomy syndrome [state]

> EXCLUDES *postcontusion syndrome (310.2)*

310.1 Personality change due to conditions classified elsewhere
Cognitive or personality change of other type, of nonpsychotic severity
Organic psychosyndrome of nonpsychotic severity
Presbyophrenia NOS
Senility with mental changes of nonpsychotic severity

> EXCLUDES *mild cognitive impairment (331.83)*
> *postconcussion syndrome (310.2)*
> *signs and symptoms involving emotional state (799.21-799.29)*

> DEF: Personality disorder caused by organic factors, such as brain lesions, head trauma, or cerebrovascular accident (CVA).
> AHA: 2Q, '05, 6

310.2 Postconcussion syndrome
Postcontusion syndrome or encephalopathy
Posttraumatic brain syndrome, nonpsychotic
Status postcommotio cerebri
Use additional code to identify associated post-traumatic headache, if applicable (339.20-339.22)

> EXCLUDES *any organic psychotic conditions following head injury (293.0-294.0)*
> *frontal lobe syndrome (310.0)*
> *postencephalitic syndrome (310.89)*

> DEF: Nonpsychotic disorder due to brain trauma, causes symptoms unrelated to any disease process; symptoms include amnesia, serial headaches, rapid heartbeat, fatigue, disrupted sleep patterns, inability to concentrate.
> AHA: 4Q, '90, 24

> TIP: For treatment within 24 to 48 hours of the concussion, clarify with physician whether the concussion is still in the acute phase; if so, assign instead a code from 850.X subcategory.

√5ᵗʰ **310.8 Other specified nonpsychotic mental disorders following organic brain damage**
AHA: 4Q, '11, 96-97

310.81 Pseudobulbar affect
Involuntary emotional expression disorder
Code first underlying cause, if known, such as:
amyotrophic lateral sclerosis (335.20)
late effect of cerebrovascular accident (438.89)
late effect of traumatic brain injury (907.0)
mutiple sclerosis (340)
AHA: 4Q, '11, 97

310.89 Other specified nonpsychotic mental disorders following organic brain damage
Mild memory disturbance
Other focal (partial) organic psychosyndromes
Postencephalitic syndrome

> EXCLUDES *memory loss of unknown cause (780.93)*

310.9 Unspecified nonpsychotic mental disorder   HIV
following organic brain damage
AHA: 4Q, '03, 103

311 Depressive disorder, not elsewhere classified
Depressive disorder NOS   Depression NOS
Depressive state NOS

> EXCLUDES *acute reaction to major stress with depressive symptoms (308.0)*
> *affective personality disorder (301.10-301.13)*
> *affective psychoses (296.0-296.9)*
> *brief depressive reaction (309.0)*
> *depressive states associated with stressful events (309.0-309.1)*
> *disturbance of emotions specific to childhood and adolescence, with misery and unhappiness (313.1)*
> *mixed adjustment reaction with depressive symptoms (309.4)*
> *neurotic depression (300.4)*
> *prolonged depressive adjustment reaction (309.1)*
> *psychogenic depressive psychosis (298.0)*

> AHA: 3Q, '11, 6; 4Q, '03, 75

√4ᵗʰ **312 Disturbance of conduct, not elsewhere classified**

> EXCLUDES *adjustment reaction with disturbance of conduct (309.3)*
> *drug dependence (304.0-304.9)*
> *dyssocial behavior without manifest psychiatric disorder (V71.01-V71.02)*
> *personality disorder with predominantly sociopathic or asocial manifestations (301.7)*
> *sexual deviations (302.0-302.9)*

The following fifth-digit subclassification is for use with categories 312.0-312.2

| 0 unspecified | 2 moderate |
| 1 mild | 3 severe |

§ √5ᵗʰ **312.0 Undersocialized conduct disorder, aggressive type**
[0-3]   Aggressive outburst   Unsocialized aggressive disorder
Anger reaction

> DEF: Mental condition identified by behaviors disrespectful of others' rights and of age-appropriate social norms or rules; symptoms include bullying, vandalism, verbal and physical abusiveness, lying, stealing, defiance.

Requires fifth digit. Valid digits are in [brackets] under each code. See category 312 for codes and definitions.

| Additional Digit Required | Unacceptable PDx | Manifestation Code | Hospital Acquired Condition | ▶◀ Revised Text | ● New Code | ▲ Revised Code Title |

Mental, Behavioral and Neurodevelopmental Disorders

312.1–315.2

§ ✓5ᵗʰ **312.1 Undersocialized conduct disorder, unaggressive type**
[0-3]   Childhood truancy, unsocialized
       Solitary stealing
       Tantrums

§ ✓5ᵗʰ **312.2 Socialized conduct disorder**
[0-3]   Childhood truancy, socialized
       Group delinquency
       EXCLUDES *gang activity without manifest psychiatric disorder (V71.01)*

✓5ᵗʰ **312.3 Disorders of impulse control, not elsewhere classified**

    312.30 Impulse control disorder, unspecified

    312.31 Pathological gambling

    312.32 Kleptomania

    312.33 Pyromania

    312.34 Intermittent explosive disorder

    312.35 Isolated explosive disorder

    312.39 Other
       Trichotillomania

312.4 Mixed disturbance of conduct and emotions
    Neurotic delinquency
    EXCLUDES *compulsive conduct disorder (312.3)*

✓5ᵗʰ **312.8 Other specified disturbances of conduct, not elsewhere classified**

    312.81 Conduct disorder, childhood onset type

    312.82 Conduct disorder, adolescent onset type

    312.89 Other conduct disorder
       Conduct disorder of unspecified onset

312.9 Unspecified disturbance of conduct
    Delinquency (juvenile)
    Disruptive behavior disorder NOS
    AHA: 2Q, '11, 5

✓4ᵗʰ **313 Disturbance of emotions specific to childhood and adolescence**
    EXCLUDES *adjustment reaction (309.0-309.9)*
       emotional disorder of neurotic type (300.0-300.9)
       masturbation, nail-biting, thumbsucking, and other isolated symptoms (307.0-307.9)

313.0 Overanxious disorder
    Anxiety and fearfulness } of childhood and
    Overanxious disorder } adolescence
    EXCLUDES *abnormal separation anxiety (309.21)*
       anxiety states (300.00-300.09)
       hospitalism in children (309.83)
       phobic state (300.20-300.29)

313.1 Misery and unhappiness disorder
    EXCLUDES *depressive neurosis (300.4)*

✓5ᵗʰ **313.2 Sensitivity, shyness, and social withdrawal disorder**
    EXCLUDES *infantile autism (299.0)*
       schizoid personality (301.20-301.22)
       schizophrenia (295.0-295.9)

    313.21 Shyness disorder of childhood
       Sensitivity reaction of childhood or adolescence

    313.22 Introverted disorder of childhood
       Social withdrawal } of childhood and
       Withdrawal reaction } adolescence

    313.23 Selective mutism
       EXCLUDES *elective mutism as adjustment reaction (309.83)*

313.3 Relationship problems
    Sibling jealousy
    EXCLUDES *relationship problems associated with aggression, destruction, or other forms of conduct disturbance (312.0-312.9)*

✓5ᵗʰ **313.8 Other or mixed emotional disturbances of childhood or adolescence**

    313.81 Oppositional defiant disorder
       DEF: Mental disorder of children noted for pervasive opposition, defiance of authority.

    313.82 Identity disorder
       Identity problem
       DEF: Distress of adolescents caused by inability to form acceptable self-identity; uncertainty about career choice, sexual orientation, moral values.

    313.83 Academic underachievement disorder

    313.89 Other
       Reactive attachment disorder of infancy or early childhood

313.9 Unspecified emotional disturbance of childhood or adolescence
    Mental disorder of infancy, childhood or adolescence NOS

✓4ᵗʰ **314 Hyperkinetic syndrome of childhood**
    EXCLUDES *hyperkinesis as symptom of underlying disorder — code the underlying disorder*
    TIP: These codes may be assigned for patients of any age.

✓5ᵗʰ **314.0 Attention deficit disorder**
    Adult   Child
    DEF: A behavioral disorder usually diagnosed at an early age; characterized by the inability to focus attention for a normal period of time.

    314.00 Without mention of hyperactivity
       Predominantly inattentive type
       AHA: 1Q, '97, 8

    314.01 With hyperactivity
       Combined type
       Overactivity NOS
       Predominantly hyperactive/impulsive type
       Simple disturbance of attention with overactivity
       AHA: ▶3Q, '12, 19;◀ 2Q, '11, 5; 1Q, '97, 8
       F90.1 ADHD predominantly hyperactive type

314.1 Hyperkinesis with developmental delay
    Developmental disorder of hyperkinesis
    Use additional code to identify any associated neurological disorder

314.2 Hyperkinetic conduct disorder
    Hyperkinetic conduct disorder without developmental delay
    EXCLUDES *hyperkinesis with significant delays in specific skills (314.1)*

314.8 Other specified manifestations of hyperkinetic syndrome

314.9 Unspecified hyperkinetic syndrome
    Hyperkinetic reaction of childhood or adolescence NOS
    Hyperkinetic syndrome NOS

✓4ᵗʰ **315 Specific delays in development**
    EXCLUDES *that due to a neurological disorder (320.0-389.9)*

✓5ᵗʰ **315.0 Specific reading disorder**

    315.00 Reading disorder, unspecified

    315.01 Alexia
       DEF: Lack of ability to understand written language; manifestation of aphasia.

    315.02 Developmental dyslexia
       DEF: Serious impairment of reading skills unexplained in relation to general intelligence and teaching processes.

    315.09 Other
       Specific spelling difficulty

315.1 Mathematics disorder
    Dyscalculia

315.2 Other specific learning difficulties
    Disorder of written expression
    EXCLUDES *specific arithmetical disorder (315.1)*
       specific reading disorder (315.00-315.09)

---

§   Requires fifth digit. Valid digits are in [brackets] under each code. See category 312 for codes and definitions.

Ⓝ Newborn Age: 0   Ⓟ Pediatric Age: 0-17   Ⓜ Maternity Age: 12-55   Ⓐ Adult Age: 15-124   ᴹᶜᶜ Major CC Condition   ᶜᶜ CC Condition   ᴴᴵⱽ HIV Related D

√5ᵗʰ **315.3 Developmental speech or language disorder**

315.31 Expressive language disorder
Developmental aphasia
Word deafness
EXCLUDES *acquired aphasia (784.3)*
elective mutism (309.83, 313.0, 313.23)

315.32 Mixed receptive-expressive language disorder
Central auditory processing disorder
EXCLUDES *acquired auditory processing disorder (388.45)*
AHA: 2Q, '05, 5; 4Q, '96, 30

315.34 Speech and language developmental delay due to hearing loss
AHA: 4Q, '07, 80, 81

315.35 Childhood onset fluency disorder
Cluttering NOS
Stuttering NOS
EXCLUDES *adult onset fluency disorder (307.0)*
fluency disorder due to late effect of cerebrovascular accident (438.14)
fluency disorder in conditions classified elsewhere (784.52)
AHA: 4Q, '10, 83-84
F80.81 Child onset fluency disorder [I-10]

315.39 Other
Developmental articulation disorder
Dyslalia
Phonological disorder
EXCLUDES *lisping and lalling (307.9)*
AHA: 3Q, '07, 7

315.4 Developmental coordination disorder
Clumsiness syndrome
Dyspraxia syndrome
Specific motor development disorder

315.5 Mixed development disorder
AHA: 2Q, '02, 11

315.8 Other specified delays in development
F88 Other disorders of psychological development [I-10]

315.9 Unspecified delay in development
Developmental disorder NOS
Learning disorder NOS

316 Psychic factors associated with diseases classified elsewhere
Psychologic factors in physical conditions classified elsewhere
Use additional code to identify the associated physical condition, as:
psychogenic:
asthma (493.9)
dermatitis (692.9)
duodenal ulcer (532.0-532.9)
eczema (691.8, 692.9)
gastric ulcer (531.0-531.9)
mucous colitis (564.9)
paroxysmal tachycardia (427.2)
ulcerative colitis (556)
urticaria (708.0-708.9)
psychosocial dwarfism (259.4)
EXCLUDES *physical symptoms and physiological malfunctions, not involving tissue damage, of mental origin (306.0-306.9)*

Intellectual Disabilities (317-319)

Use additional code(s) to identify any associated psychiatric or physical condition(s)
AHA: 4Q, '11, 98

317 Mild intellectual disabilities
High-grade defect
IQ 50-70
Mild mental subnormality
F70 Mild intellectual disabilities [I-10]

√4ᵗʰ **318 Other specified intellectual disabilities**

318.0 Moderate intellectual disabilities
IQ 35-49
Moderate mental subnormality

318.1 Severe intellectual disabilities [CC]
IQ 20-34
Severe mental subnormality
CC Exd: 318.1-318.2

318.2 Profound intellectual disabilities [CC]
IQ under 20
Profound mental subnormality
CC Exd: See code: 318.1

319 Unspecified intellectual disabilities
Mental deficiency NOS
Mental subnormality NOS
F79 Unspecified intellectual disabilities [I-10]

6. Diseases of the Nervous System and Sense Organs (320-389)

Inflammatory Diseases of the Central Nervous System (320-326)

√4ᵗʰ **320 Bacterial meningitis**

INCLUDES arachnoiditis
leptomeningitis
meningitis
meningoencephalitis   } bacterial
meningomyelitis
pachymeningitis

DEF: Bacterial infection causing inflammation of the lining of the brain and/or spinal cord.
AHA: J-F, '87, 6

320.0 Hemophilus meningitis   MCC
Meningitis due to Hemophilus influenzae [H. influenzae]
CC Excl: 003.21, 013.00-013.16, 036.0, 047.0-047.9, 049.0-049.1, 053.0, 054.72, 072.1, 090.42, 091.81, 094.2, 098.89, 100.81, 112.83, 114.2, 115.01, 115.11, 115.91, 130.0, 249.60-249.61, 249.80-249.91, 250.60-250.63, 250.80-250.93, 320.0-322.9, 349.89-349.9, 357.0

320.1 Pneumococcal meningitis   MCC
CC Excl: See code: 320.0

320.2 Streptococcal meningitis   MCC
CC Excl: See code: 320.0

320.3 Staphylococcal meningitis   MCC
CC Excl: See code: 320.0

320.7 *Meningitis in other bacterial diseases classified elsewhere*   MCC
Code first underlying disease, as:
actinomycosis (039.8)
listeriosis (027.0)
typhoid fever (002.0)
whooping cough (033.0-033.9)
EXCLUDES *meningitis (in):*
epidemic (036.0)
gonococcal (098.82)
meningococcal (036.0)
salmonellosis (003.21)
syphilis:
NOS (094.2)
congenital (090.42)
meningovascular (094.2)
secondary (091.81)
tuberculous (013.0)
CC Excl: See code: 320.0

√5ᵗʰ **320.8 Meningitis due to other specified bacteria**

320.81 Anaerobic meningitis   MCC
Bacteroides (fragilis)
Gram-negative anaerobes
CC Excl: See code 320.0

320.82 Meningitis due to gram-negative bacteria, not elsewhere classified   MCC
Aerobacter aerogenes pneumoniae
Escherichia coli [E. coli]
Friedländer bacillus
Klebsiella
Proteus morganii
Pseudomonas
EXCLUDES *gram-negative anaerobes (320.81)*
CC Excl: See code: 320.0
AHA: 4Q, '11, 155

320.89 Meningitis due to other specified bacteria   MCC
Bacillus pyocyaneus
CC Excl: See code: 320.0

320.9 Meningitis due to unspecified bacterium   MCC
Meningitis: Meningitis:
bacterial NOS   pyogenic NOS
purulent NOS   suppurative NOS
CC Excl: See code: 320.0

√4ᵗʰ **321 Meningitis due to other organisms**

INCLUDES arachnoiditis
leptomeningitis   } due to organisms other
meningitis   than bacterial
pachymeningitis

DEF: Infection causing inflammation of the lining of the brain and/or spinal cord, due to organisms other than bacteria.
AHA: J-F, '87, 6

321.0 *Cryptococcal meningitis*   MCC
Code first underlying disease (117.5)
CC Excl: See code: 320.0

321.1 *Meningitis in other fungal diseases*   MCC
Code first underlying disease (110.0-118)
EXCLUDES *meningitis in:*
candidiasis (112.83)
coccidioidomycosis (114.2)
histoplasmosis (115.01, 115.11, 115.91)
CC Excl: See code: 320.0

321.2 *Meningitis due to viruses not elsewhere classified*   MCC
Code first underlying disease, as:
meningitis due to arbovirus (060.0-066.9)
EXCLUDES *meningitis (due to):*
abacterial (047.0-047.9)
adenovirus (049.1)
aseptic NOS (047.9)
Coxsackie (virus)(047.0)
ECHO virus (047.1)
enterovirus (047.0-047.9)
herpes simplex virus (054.72)
herpes zoster virus (053.0)
lymphocytic choriomeningitis virus (049.0)
mumps (072.1)
viral NOS (047.9)
meningo-eruptive syndrome (047.1)
CC Excl: 003.21, 013.00-013.16, 036.0, 047.0-047.9, 049.0-049.1, 053.0, 054.72, 072.1, 090.42, 091.81, 094.2, 098.89, 100.81, 112.83, 114.2, 115.01, 115.11, 115.91, 130.0, 320.0-322.9, 349.89-349.9, 357.0
AHA: 4Q, '04, 51

321.3 *Meningitis due to trypanosomiasis*   MCC
Code first underlying disease (086.0-086.9)
CC Excl: See code: 320.0

321.4 *Meningitis in sarcoidosis*   MCC
Code first underlying disease (135)
CC Excl: See code: 320.0

321.8 *Meningitis due to other nonbacterial organisms classified elsewhere*   MCC
Code first underlying disease
EXCLUDES *leptospiral meningitis (100.81)*
CC Excl: See code: 320.0

√4ᵗʰ **322 Meningitis of unspecified cause**

INCLUDES arachnoiditis
leptomeningitis   } with no organism
meningitis   specified as cause
pachymeningitis

AHA: J-F, '87, 6
DEF: Infection causing inflammation of the lining of the brain and/or spinal cord, due to unspecified cause.

322.0 Nonpyogenic meningitis   MCC
Meningitis with clear cerebrospinal fluid
CC Excl: See code: 320.0

322.1 Eosinophilic meningitis   MCC
CC Excl: See code: 320.0

322.2 Chronic meningitis   CC
CC Excl: See code: 320.0

322.9 Meningitis, unspecified   MCC
CC Excl: See code: 320.0

Diseases of the Nervous System and Sense Organs

323–323.63

√4ᵗʰ **323 Encephalitis, myelitis, and encephalomyelitis**

INCLUDES   acute disseminated encephalomyelitis
meningoencephalitis, except bacterial
meningomyelitis, except bacterial
myelitis:
    ascending
    transverse

EXCLUDES   acute transverse myelitis NOS (341.20)
acute transverse myelitis in conditions classified elsewhere
     (341.21)
bacterial:
    meningoencephalitis (320.0-320.9)
    meningomyelitis (320.0-320.9)
idiopathic transverse myelitis (341.22)

DEF: Encephalitis: inflammation of brain tissues.
DEF: Myelitis: inflammation of the spinal cord.
DEF: Encephalomyelitis: inflammation of brain and spinal cord.

√5ᵗʰ **323.0 Encephalitis, myelitis, and encephalomyelitis in viral diseases classified elsewhere**

Code first underlying disease, as:
    cat-scratch disease (078.3)
    human immunodeficiency virus [HIV] disease (042)
    infectious mononucleosis (075)
    ornithosis (073.7)

323.01 Encephalitis and encephalomyelitis in viral diseases classified elsewhere   MCC

EXCLUDES   encephalitis (in):
    arthropod-borne viral (062.0-064)
    herpes simplex (054.3)
    mumps (072.2)
    other viral diseases of central nervous
      system (049.8-049.9)
    poliomyelitis (045.0-045.9)
    rubella (056.01)
    slow virus infections of central nervous
      system (046.0-046.9)
    viral NOS (049.9)
    West Nile (066.41)

CC Excl: 003.21, 013.00-013.16, 013.60-013.66, 036.0, 046.2, 046.71-046.8, 047.0-049.8, 051.9-052.0, 052.7-053.13, 053.19, 053.79-053.9, 054.3, 054.72, 054.79-054.9, 056.01, 057.8-059.9, 062.0-064, 066.2-066.49, 072.1-072.2, 073.7, 075, 078.89, 079.81-079.82, 079.89, 079.99, 090.41-090.42, 091.81, 094.2, 094.81, 098.89, 100.81, 112.83, 114.2, 115.01, 115.11, 115.91, 130.0, 139.8, 290.12, 320.0-323.9, 341.1, 349.89-349.9, 357.0, 487.8, 488.09, 488.19, 771.2
AHA: 3Q, '10, 13; 4Q, '06, 58-63

323.02 Myelitis in viral diseases classified elsewhere   MCC

EXCLUDES   myelitis (in):
    herpes simplex (054.74)
    herpes zoster (053.14)
    poliomyelitis (045.0-045.9)
    rubella (056.01)
    other viral diseases of central nervous
      system (049.8-049.9)

CC Excl: See code: 323.01
AHA: 4Q, '06, 58-63

323.1 Encephalitis, myelitis, and encephalomyelitis in rickettsial diseases classified elsewhere   MCC

Code first underlying disease (080-083.9)
DEF: Inflammation of the brain caused by rickettsial disease carried by louse, tick, or mite.
CC Excl: 013.60-013.66, 046.2, 046.71-046.8, 048-049.0, 049.8, 052.0, 052.2, 054.3, 054.74, 056.01, 057.8-058.29, 059.00-059.9, 062.0-064, 066.2-066.49, 072.2, 073.7, 079.82, 079.99, 081.9, 083.9, 090.41, 094.81, 117.5, 124, 130.0, 290.12, 323.01-323.9, 341.1, 487.8, 771.2, 984.9

323.2 Encephalitis, myelitis, and encephalomyelitis in protozoal diseases classified elsewhere   MCC

Code first underlying disease, as:
    malaria (084.0-084.9)
    trypanosomiasis (086.0-086.9)
DEF: Inflammation of the brain caused by protozoal disease carried by mosquitoes and flies.
CC Excl: 013.60-013.66, 046.2, 046.71-046.8, 048-049.0, 049.8, 052.0, 052.2, 054.3, 054.74, 056.01, 057.8-058.29, 059.00-059.9, 062.0-064, 066.2-066.49, 072.2, 073.7, 079.82, 079.99, 081.9, 083.9, 084.6, 090.41, 094.81, 117.5, 124, 130.0, 290.12, 323.01-323.9, 341.1, 487.8, 488.09, 488.19, 771.2, 984.9

√5ᵗʰ **323.4 Other encephalitis, myelitis, and encephalomyelitis due to other infections classified elsewhere**

Code first underlying disease

323.41 Other encephalitis and encephalomyelitis due to other infections classified elsewhere   MCC

EXCLUDES   encephalitis (in):
    meningococcal (036.1)
    syphilis:
      NOS (094.81)
      congenital (090.41)
    toxoplasmosis (130.0)
    tuberculosis (013.6)
    meningoencephalitis due to free-living
      ameba [Naegleria] (136.29)

CC Excl: See code: 323.01
AHA: 4Q, '06, 58-63

323.42 Other myelitis due to other infections classified elsewhere   MCC

EXCLUDES   myelitis (in):
    syphilis (094.89)
    tuberculosis (013.6)

CC Excl: See code: 323.01
AHA: 4Q, '06, 58-63

√5ᵗʰ **323.5 Encephalitis, myelitis, and encephalomyelitis following immunization procedures**

Use additional E code to identify vaccine

323.51 Encephalitis and encephalomyelitis following immunization procedures   MCC
Encephalitis postimmunization or postvaccinal
Encephalomyelitis postimmunization or postvaccinal
CC Excl: See code: 323.01
AHA: 4Q, '06, 58-63

323.52 Myelitis following immunization procedures   MCC
Myelitis postimmunization or postvaccinal
CC Excl: See code: 323.01
AHA: 4Q, '06, 58-63

√5ᵗʰ **323.6 Postinfectious encephalitis, myelitis, and encephalomyelitis**

Code first underlying disease
DEF: Infection, inflammation of brain several weeks following the outbreak of a systemic infection.

323.61 Infectious acute disseminated encephalomyelitis [ADEM]   MCC
Acute necrotizing hemorrhagic encephalopathy
EXCLUDES   noninfectious acute disseminated
      encephalo- myelitis (ADEM) (323.81)
CC Excl: See code: 323.01
AHA: 4Q, '06, 58-63

323.62 Other postinfectious encephalitis and encephalomyelitis   MCC
EXCLUDES   encephalitis:
    postchickenpox (052.0)
    postmeasles (055.0)
CC Excl: See code: 323.01
AHA: 4Q, '06, 58-63

323.63 Postinfectious myelitis   MCC
EXCLUDES   postchickenpox myelitis (052.2)
    herpes simplex myelitis (054.74)
    herpes zoster myelitis (053.14)
CC Excl: See code: 323.01
AHA: 4Q, '06, 58-63

N Newborn Age: 0   P Pediatric Age: 0-17   M Maternity Age: 12-55   A Adult Age: 15-124   MCC Major CC Condition   CC CC Condition   HIV HIV Related Dx

√5ᵗʰ **323.7 Toxic encephalitis, myelitis, and encephalomyelitis**

Code first underlying cause, as:
carbon tetrachloride (982.1)
hydroxyquinoline derivatives (961.3)
lead (984.0-984.9)
mercury (985.0)
thallium (985.8)
AHA: 2Q, '97, 8

    323.71 Toxic encephalitis and encephalomyelitis   `MCC`

       CC Excl: See code: 323.01
       AHA: 4Q, '06, 58-63

    323.72 Toxic myelitis   `MCC`

       CC Excl: See code: 323.01
       AHA: 4Q, '06, 58-63

√5ᵗʰ **323.8 Other causes of encephalitis, myelitis, and encephalomyelitis**

    323.81 Other causes of encephalitis and encephalomyelitis   `MCC` `HIV`

       Noninfectious acute disseminated encephalomyelitis (ADEM)
       CC Excl: See code: 323.01
       AHA: 1Q, '11, 12; 3Q, '10, 15; 4Q, '06, 58-63

    323.82 Other causes of myelitis   `MCC` `HIV`

       Transverse myelitis NOS
       CC Excl: See code: 323.01
       AHA: 4Q, '06, 58-63

323.9 Unspecified cause of encephalitis, myelitis, and encephalomyelitis   `MCC` `HIV`

    CC Excl: 013.60-013.66, 046.2, 046.71-046.8, 048-049.0, 049.8, 052.0,
    052.2, 054.3, 054.74, 056.01, 057.8-058.29, 059.00-059.9, 062.0-064,
    066.2-066.49, 072.2, 073.7, 075, 078.3, 079.82, 079.99, 081.9, 083.9,
    084.6, 090.41, 094.81, 117.5, 124, 130.0, 290.12, 323.01-323.9, 341.1,
    382.4, 487.8, 488.09, 488.19, 710.0, 771.2, 984.9
    AHA: 1Q, '06, 8

√4ᵗʰ **324 Intracranial and intraspinal abscess**

324.0 Intracranial abscess   `MCC`

    Abscess (embolic):
       cerebellar
       cerebral
    Abscess (embolic) of brain [any part]:
       epidural
       extradural
       otogenic
       subdural
    EXCLUDES   tuberculous (013.3)
    CC Excl: 006.5, 013.20-013.36, 249.60-249.61, 249.80-249.91,
    250.60-250.63, 250.80-250.93, 324.0-325, 348.81-348.9

324.1 Intraspinal abscess   `MCC`

    Abscess (embolic) of spinal cord [any part]:
       epidural
       extradural
       subdural
    EXCLUDES   tuberculous (013.5)
    CC Excl: 0006.5, 013.20-013.36, 249.60-249.61, 249.80-249.91,
    250.60-250.63, 250.80-250.93, 324.1

324.9 Of unspecified site   `MCC`

    Extradural or subdural abscess NOS
    CC Excl: 006.5, 013.20-013.36, 249.60-249.61, 249.80-249.91,
    250.60-250.63, 250.80-250.93, 324.0-325

325 Phlebitis and thrombophlebitis of intracranial venous sinuses   `MCC`

    Embolism
    Endophlebitis   } of cavernous, lateral or
    Phlebitis, septic or suppurative   other intracranial or
    Thrombophlebitis   unspecified
    Thrombosis   intracranial venous sinus

    EXCLUDES   that specified as:
       complicating pregnancy, childbirth, or the puerperium (671.5)
       of nonpyogenic origin (437.6)
    DEF: Inflammation and formation of blood clot in a vein within the brain or its lining.
    CC Excl: See code: 324.9

326 Late effects of intracranial abscess or pyogenic infection

    NOTE This category is to be used to indicate conditions whose primary classification is to 320-325 [excluding 320.7, 321.0-321.8, 323.01-323.42, 323.6-323.7] as the cause of late effects, themselves classifiable elsewhere. The "late effects" include conditions specified as such, or as sequelae, which may occur at any time after the resolution of the causal condition.

    Use additional code to identify condition, as:
    hydrocephalus (331.4)
    paralysis (342.0-342.9, 344.0-344.9)

Organic Sleep Disorders (327)

TIP: If the sleep disorder is not documented with the etiology related to an organic disease process, see instead subcategory 307.4.

√4ᵗʰ **327 Organic sleep disorders**

    AHA: 4Q, '05, 59-64

√5ᵗʰ **327.0 Organic disorders of initiating and maintaining sleep [Organic insomnia]**

    EXCLUDES   insomnia NOS (780.52)
       insomnia not due to a substance or known physiological condition (307.41-307.42)
       insomnia with sleep apnea NOS (780.51)

    327.00 Organic insomnia, unspecified

    327.01 Insomnia due to medical condition classified elsewhere

       Code first underlying condition
       EXCLUDES   insomnia due to mental disorder (327.02)

    327.02 Insomnia due to mental disorder

       Code first mental disorder
       EXCLUDES   alcohol induced insomnia (291.82)
           drug induced insomnia (292.85)

    327.09 Other organic insomnia

√5ᵗʰ **327.1 Organic disorder of excessive somnolence [Organic hypersomnia]**

    EXCLUDES   hypersomnia NOS (780.54)
       hypersomnia not due to a substance or known physiological condition (307.43-307.44)
       hypersomnia with sleep apnea NOS (780.53)

    327.10 Organic hypersomnia, unspecified

    327.11 Idiopathic hypersomnia with long sleep time

    327.12 Idiopathic hypersomnia without long sleep time

    327.13 Recurrent hypersomnia

       Kleine-Levin syndrome
       Menstrual related hypersomnia

    327.14 Hypersomnia due to medical condition classified elsewhere

       Code first underlying condition
       EXCLUDES   hypersomnia due to mental disorder (327.15)

    327.15 Hypersomnia due to mental disorder

       Code first mental disorder
       EXCLUDES   alcohol induced hypersomnia (291.82)
           drug induced hypersomnia (292.85)

    327.19 Other organic hypersomnia

√5ᵗʰ **327.2 Organic sleep apnea**

    EXCLUDES   Cheyne-Stokes breathing (786.04)
       hypersomnia with sleep apnea NOS (780.53)
       insomnia with sleep apnea NOS (780.51)
       sleep apnea in newborn (770.81-770.82)
       sleep apnea NOS (780.57)

    327.20 Organic sleep apnea, unspecified

    327.21 Primary central sleep apnea

    327.22 High altitude periodic breathing

    327.23 Obstructive sleep apnea (adult) (pediatric)

       G47.33 Obstructive sleep apnea (adult) (pediatric)   `I-10`

    327.24 Idiopathic sleep related nonobstructive alveolar hypoventilation

       Sleep related hypoxia

Additional Digit Required   Unacceptable PDx   Manifestation Code   Hospital Acquired Condition   ►◄ Revised Text   ● New Code   ▲ Revised Code Title

327.25 Congenital central alveolar hypoventilation syndrome

327.26 *Sleep related hypoventilation/ hypoxemia in conditions classifiable elsewhere*

Code first underlying condition

327.27 *Central sleep apnea in conditions classified elsewhere*

Code first underlying condition

327.29 Other organic sleep apnea

√5ᵗʰ **327.3 Circadian rhythm sleep disorder**

Organic disorder of sleep wake cycle
Organic disorder of sleep wake schedule

EXCLUDES   *alcohol induced circadian rhythm sleep disorder (291.82)*
circadian rhythm sleep disorder of nonorganic origin (307.45)
disruption of 24 hour sleep wake cycle NOS (780.55)
drug induced circadian rhythm sleep disorder (292.85)

327.30 Circadian rhythm sleep disorder, unspecified

327.31 Circadian rhythm sleep disorder, delayed sleep phase type

327.32 Circadian rhythm sleep disorder, advanced sleep phase type

327.33 Circadian rhythm sleep disorder, irregular sleep-wake type

327.34 Circadian rhythm sleep disorder, free-running type

327.35 Circadian rhythm sleep disorder, jet lag type

327.36 Circadian rhythm sleep disorder, shift work type

327.37 *Circadian rhythm sleep disorder in conditions classified elsewhere*

Code first underlying condition

327.39 Other circadian rhythm sleep disorder

√5ᵗʰ **327.4 Organic parasomnia**

EXCLUDES   *alcohol induced parasomnia (291.82)*
drug induced parasomnia (292.85)
parasomnia not due to a known physiological condition (307.47)

327.40 Organic parasomnia, unspecified

327.41 Confusional arousals

327.42 REM sleep behavior disorder

327.43 Recurrent isolated sleep paralysis

327.44 *Parasomnia in conditions classified elsewhere*

Code first underlying condition

327.49 Other organic parasomnia

√5ᵗʰ **327.5 Organic sleep related movement disorders**

EXCLUDES   *restless legs syndrome (333.94)*
sleep related movement disorder NOS (780.58)

327.51 Periodic limb movement disorder

Periodic limb movement sleep disorder

327.52 Sleep related leg cramps

327.53 Sleep related bruxism

327.59 Other organic sleep related movement disorders

327.8 Other organic sleep disorders

AHA: 2Q, '07, 6

Hereditary and Degenerative Diseases of the Central Nervous System (330-337)

EXCLUDES   *hepatolenticular degeneration (275.1)*
multiple sclerosis (340)
other demyelinating diseases of central nervous system (341.0-341.9)

√4ᵗʰ **330 Cerebral degenerations usually manifest in childhood**

Use additional code to identify associated intellectual disabilities

330.0 Leukodystrophy   C⁴

Krabbe's disease
Leukodystrophy:
  NOS
  globoid cell
  metachromatic
Leukodystrophy:
  sudanophilic
  Pelizaeus-Merzbacher disease
  Sulfatide lipidosis

DEF: Hereditary disease of arylsulfatase or cerebroside sulfatase; characterized by a diffuse loss of myelin in CNS; infantile form causes blindness, motor disturbances, rigidity, mental deterioration and, occasionally, convulsions.

CC Exd: 330.0-330.9, 331.7, 348.81-348.9, 349.89-349.9

330.1 Cerebral lipidoses   C⁴

Amaurotic (familial) idiocy
Disease:
  Batten
  Jansky-Bielschowsky
  Kufs'
Disease:
  Spielmeyer-Vogt
  Tay-Sachs
  Gangliosidosis

DEF: Genetic disorder causing abnormal lipid accumulation in the reticuloendothelial cells of the brain.

CC Exd: 330.1-331.2, 331.6, 331.7, 331.83-331.9

330.2 *Cerebral degeneration in generalized lipidoses*   C

Code first underlying disease, as:
  Fabry's disease (272.7)
  Gaucher's disease (272.7)
  Niemann-Pick disease (272.7)
  sphingolipidosis (272.7)

CC Exd: See code: 330.1

330.3 *Cerebral degeneration of childhood in other diseases classified elsewhere*   C

Code first underlying disease, as:
  Hunter's disease (277.5)
  mucopolysaccharidosis (277.5)

CC Exd: See code: 330.1

330.8 Other specified cerebral degenerations in childhood   C

Alpers' disease or gray-matter degeneration
Infantile necrotizing encephalomyelopathy
Leigh's disease
Subacute necrotizing encephalopathy or encephalomyelopathy

CC Exd: See code: 330.1
AHA: N-D, '85, 5

330.9 Unspecified cerebral degeneration in childhood   C

CC Exd: See code: 330.1

√4ᵗʰ **331 Other cerebral degenerations**

Use additional code, where applicable, to identify dementia:
  with behavioral disturbance (294.11)
  without behavioral disturbance (294.10)

331.0 Alzheimer's disease

DEF: Diffuse atrophy of cerebral cortex; causing a progressive decline in intellectual and physical functions, including memory loss, personality changes and profound dementia.
AHA: 4Q, '00, 41; 4Q, '99, 7; N-D, '84, 20
G30.9 Alzheimer's disease unspecified   I⁻

√5ᵗʰ **331.1 Frontotemporal dementia**

DEF: Rare, progressive degenerative brain disease, similar to Alzheimer's; cortical atrophy affects the frontal and temporal lobes.
AHA: 4Q, '03, 57

331.11 Pick's disease

DEF: A progressive frontotemporal dementia with asymmetrical atrophy of the frontal and temporal regions of the cerebral cortex, abnormal rounded brain cells called Pick cells with the presence of abnormal staining of protein (called tau); symptoms include prominent apathy, behavioral changes such as disinhibition and restlessness, echolalia, impairment of language, memory, and intellect, increased carelessness, poor personal hygiene, and decreased attention span.

N Newborn Age: 0   P Pediatric Age: 0-17   M Maternity Age: 12-55   A Adult Age: 15-124   MCC Major CC Condition   CC CC Condition   HIV HIV Related D

100 – Volume 1   2014 ICD-9-C

331.19 Other frontotemporal dementia
Frontal dementia

331.2 Senile degeneration of brain
EXCLUDES *senility NOS (797)*

331.3 Communicating hydrocephalus CC
Secondary normal pressure hydrocephalus
EXCLUDES *congenital hydrocephalus (742.3)*
idiopathic normal pressure hydrocephalus (331.5)
normal pressure hydrocephalus (331.5)
spina bifida with hydrocephalus (741.0)
DEF: Subarachnoid hemorrhage and meningitis causing excess buildup of cerebrospinal fluid in cavities due to nonabsorption of fluid back through fluid pathways.
CC Excl: 331.3-331.5
AHA: S-O, '85, 12

331.4 Obstructive hydrocephalus CC
Acquired hydrocephalus NOS
EXCLUDES *congenital hydrocephalus (742.3)*
idiopathic normal pressure hydrocephalus (331.5)
normal pressure hydrocephalus (331.5)
spina bifida with hydrocephalus (741.0)
DEF: Obstruction of cerebrospinal fluid passage from brain into spinal canal.
CC Excl: 249.60-249.61, 249.80-249.91, 250.60-250.63, 250.80-250.93, 331.3-331.7, 331.82-331.9, 348.81, 348.89-348.9, 741.00-741.03, 742.3-742.4, 742.59-742.9
AHA: 4Q, '03, 106; 1Q, '99, 9
G91.1 Obstructive hydrocephalus I-10

331.5 Idiopathic normal pressure hydrocephalus [INPH] CC
Normal pressure hydrocephalus NOS
EXCLUDES *congenital hydrocephalus (742.3)*
secondary normal pressure hydrocephalus (331.3)
spina bifida with hydrocephalus (741.0)
DEF: Abnormal increase of cerebrospinal fluid in the brain's ventricles; results in dementia, progressive mental impairment, gait disturbance, and impaired bladder control.
CC Excl: See code: 331.3
AHA: 4Q, '07, 74

331.6 Corticobasal degeneration
AHA: 4Q, '11, 98

331.7 Cerebral degeneration in diseases classified elsewhere
Code first underlying disease, as:
alcoholism (303.0-303.9)
beriberi (265.0)
cerebrovascular disease (430-438)
congenital hydrocephalus (741.0, 742.3)
myxedema (244.0-244.9)
neoplastic disease (140.0-239.9)
vitamin B12 deficiency (266.2)
EXCLUDES *cerebral degeneration in:*
Jakob-Creutzfeldt disease (046.11-046.19)
progressive multifocal leukoencephalopathy (046.3)
subacute spongiform encephalopathy (046.1)

√5ᵗʰ **331.8 Other cerebral degeneration**

331.81 Reye's syndrome MCC P
DEF: Rare childhood illness, often developed after a viral upper respiratory infection; characterized by vomiting, elevated serum transaminase, changes in liver and other viscera; brain swelling, disturbances of consciousness and seizures; can be fatal.
CC Excl: 331.81

331.82 Dementia with Lewy bodies
Dementia with Parkinsonism
Lewy body dementia
Lewy body disease
DEF: A cerebral dementia with neurophysiologic changes, increased hippocampal volume, hypoperfusion in the occipital lobes, and beta amyloid deposits with neurofibrillarity tangles, atrophy of cortex and brainstem, hallmark neuropsychologic characteristics are fluctuating cognition with pronounced variation in attention and alertness; recurrent hallucinations; and parkinsonism.
AHA: 4Q, '03, 57
G31.83 Dementia with Lewy bodies I-10

331.83 Mild cognitive impairment, so stated
EXCLUDES *altered mental status (780.97)*
cerebral degeneration (331.0-331.9)
change in mental status (780.97)
cognitive deficits following (late effects of) cerebral hemorrhage or infarction (438.0)
cognitive impairment due to intracranial or head injury (850-854, 959.01)
cognitive impairment due to late effect of intracranial injury (907.0)
cognitive impairment due to skull fracture (800-801, 803-804)
dementia (290.0-290.43, 294.20-294.21)
mild memory disturbance (310.89)
neurologic neglect syndrome (781.8)
personality change, nonpsychotic (310.1)
AHA: 4Q, '06, 75

331.89 Other
Cerebral ataxia

331.9 Cerebral degeneration, unspecified

√4ᵗʰ **332 Parkinson's disease**
EXCLUDES *dementia with Parkinsonism (331.82)*

332.0 Paralysis agitans
Parkinsonism or Parkinson's disease:
NOS
idiopathic
primary
DEF: Form of progressive parkinsonism characterized by mask-like facial expressions, inability to stand or walk smoothly, muscle weakness, and involuntary trembling movement.
AHA: M-A, '87, 7
G20 Parkinson's disease I-10

332.1 Secondary Parkinsonism CC
Neuroleptic-induced Parkinsonism
Parkinsonism due to drugs
Use additional E code to identify drug, if drug-induced
EXCLUDES *Parkinsonism (in):*
Huntington's disease (333.4)
progressive supranuclear palsy (333.0)
Shy-Drager syndrome (333.0)
syphilitic (094.82)
CC Excl: 332.0-332.1

√4ᵗʰ **333 Other extrapyramidal disease and abnormal movement disorders**
INCLUDES other forms of extrapyramidal, basal ganglia, or striatopallidal disease
EXCLUDES *abnormal movements of head NOS (781.0)*
sleep related movement disorders (327.51-327.59)

333.0 Other degenerative diseases of the basal ganglia CC
Atrophy or degeneration:
olivopontocerebellar [Déjérine-Thomas syndrome]
pigmentary pallidal [Hallervorden-Spatz disease]
striatonigral
Parkinsonian syndrome associated with:
idiopathic orthostatic hypotension
symptomatic orthostatic hypotension
Progressive supranuclear ophthalmoplegia
Shy-Drager syndrome
CC Excl: 332.0-332.1, 335.23, 337.00-337.09, 348.30-348.39
AHA: 3Q, '96, 8

333.1 Essential and other specified forms of tremor
Benign essential tremor
Familial tremor
Medication-induced postural tremor
Use additional E code to identify drug, if drug-induced
EXCLUDES *tremor NOS (781.0)*

333.2 Myoclonus
Familial essential myoclonus
Palatal myoclonus
EXCLUDES *progressive myoclonic epilepsy (345.1)*
Unverricht-Lundborg disease (345.1)
Use additional E code to identify drug, if drug-induced
DEF: Spontaneous movements or contractions of muscles.
AHA: 3Q, '97, 4; M-A, '87, 12

Diseases of the Nervous System and Sense Organs

333.3–334.8

333.3 Tics of organic origin
Use additional E code to identify drug, if drug-induced
EXCLUDES *Gilles de la Tourette's syndrome (307.23)*
habit spasm (307.22)
tic NOS (307.20)

333.4 Huntington's chorea   CC
DEF: Genetic disease characterized by chronic progressive mental deterioration; dementia and death within 15 years of onset.
CC Excl: 332.0-332.1, 340-341.1, 341.8-341.9, 343.0-344.2, 348.1, 348.30-348.9, 349.1, 349.82-349.9, 780.72

333.5 Other choreas
Hemiballism(us)
Paroxysmal choreo-athetosis
Use additional E code to identify drug, if drug-induced
EXCLUDES *Sydenham's or rheumatic chorea (392.0-392.9)*

333.6 Genetic torsion dystonia
Dystonia:
deformans progressiva
musculorum deformans
(Schwalbe-) Ziehen-Oppenheim disease
DEF: Sustained muscular contractions, causing twisting and repetitive movements that result in abnormal postures of trunk and limbs; etiology unknown.

√5ᵗʰ **333.7 Acquired torsion dystonia**

333.71 Athetoid cerebral palsy   CC
Double athetosis (syndrome)
Vogt's disease
EXCLUDES *infantile cerebral palsy (343.0-343.9)*
CC Excl: 332.0-332.1, 333.71, 333.90, 333.99, 343.0-343.9, 348.30-348.39
AHA: 4Q, '06, 76-78

333.72 Acute dystonia due to drugs   CC
Acute dystonic reaction due to drugs
Neuroleptic induced acute dystonia
Use additional E code to identify drug
EXCLUDES *blepharospasm due to drugs (333.85)*
orofacial dyskinesia due to drugs (333.85)
secondary Parkinsonism (332.1)
subacute dyskinesia due to drugs (333.85)
tardive dyskinesia (333.85)
CC Excl: 332.0-332.1, 333.71, 333.90, 333.99, 348.30-348.39
AHA: 4Q, '06, 76-78

333.79 Other acquired torsion dystonia   CC
CC Excl: See code: 333.72
AHA: 4Q, '06, 76-78

√5ᵗʰ **333.8 Fragments of torsion dystonia**
Use additional E code to identify drug, if drug-induced

333.81 Blepharospasm
EXCLUDES *blepharospasm due to drugs (333.85)*
DEF: Uncontrolled winking or blinking due to orbicularis oculi muscle spasm.

333.82 Orofacial dyskinesia
EXCLUDES *orofacial dyskinesia due to drugs (333.85)*
DEF: Uncontrolled movement of mouth or facial muscles.

333.83 Spasmodic torticollis
EXCLUDES *torticollis:*
NOS (723.5)
hysterical (300.11)
psychogenic (306.0)
DEF: Uncontrolled movement of head due to spasms of neck muscle.

333.84 Organic writers' cramp
EXCLUDES *pychogenic (300.89)*

333.85 Subacute dyskinesia due to drugs
Blepharospasm due to drugs
Orofacial dyskinesia due to drugs
Tardive dyskinesia
Use additional E code to identify drug
EXCLUDES *acute dystonia due to drugs (333.72)*
acute dystonic reaction due to drugs (333.72)
secondary Parkinsonism (332.1)
AHA: 4Q, '06, 76-78

333.89 Other

√5ᵗʰ **333.9 Other and unspecified extrapyramidal diseases and abnormal movement disorders**

333.90 Unspecified extrapyramidal disease and abnormal movement disorder   CC
Medication-induced movement disorders NOS
Use additional E code to identify drug, if drug-induced
CC Excl: 332.0-332.1, 333.1-333.83, 333.85-333.93, 333.99, 335.22-335.23, 340-341.1, 341.8-341.9, 343.0-344.2, 348.1, 348.30-348.9, 349.1, 349.82-349.9, 780.72

333.91 Stiff-man syndrome   CC
CC Excl: See code: 333.90

333.92 Neuroleptic malignant syndrome   MCC
Use additional E code to identify drug
EXCLUDES *neuroleptic induced Parkinsonism (332.1)*
CC Excl: 333.0-333.93, 333.99, 342.00-342.92, 348.2-348.39
AHA: 4Q, '94, 37

333.93 Benign shuddering attacks
AHA: 4Q, '94, 37

333.94 Restless legs syndrome [RLS]
DEF: Neurological disorder of unknown etiology with an irresistible urge to move the legs, which may temporarily relieve the symptoms, is accompanied by motor restlessness and sensations of pain, burning, prickling, or tingling.
AHA: 4Q, '06, 79
TIP: Assign an additional code if the underlying cause of the RLS is specified (e.g., iron deficiency anemia).
G25.81 Restless legs syndrome   I-10

333.99 Other
Neuroleptic-induced acute akathisia
Use additional E code to identify drug, if drug-induced
AHA: 4Q, '04, 95; 2Q, '04, 12; 4Q, '94, 37

√4ᵗʰ **334 Spinocerebellar disease**
EXCLUDES *olivopontocerebellar degeneration (333.0)*
peroneal muscular atrophy (356.1)

334.0 Friedreich's ataxia   CC
DEF: Genetic recessive disease of children; sclerosis of dorsal, lateral spinal cord columns; characterized by ataxia, speech impairment, swaying and irregular movements, with muscle paralysis, especially of lower limbs.
CC Excl: 334.0-334.9, 348.30-348.39

334.1 Hereditary spastic paraplegia   CC
CC Excl: 333.0-333.93, 333.99-337.9, 340-344.9, 348.1, 348.30-348.39, 348.81-349.2, 349.82-349.9, 780.72

334.2 Primary cerebellar degeneration   CC
Cerebellar ataxia:
Marie's
Sanger-Brown
Dyssynergia cerebellaris myoclonica
Primary cerebellar degeneration:
NOS
hereditary
sporadic
CC Excl: 333.0-333.93, 333.99-337.9, 340-344.9, 348.0-348.1, 348.30-348.39, 348.81-348.9, 349.82-349.9, 780.72
AHA: M-A, '87, 9

334.3 Other cerebellar ataxia   CC
Cerebellar ataxia NOS
Use additional E code to identify drug, if drug-induced
CC Excl: See code: 334.2

334.4 *Cerebellar ataxia in diseases classified elsewhere*   CC
Code first underlying disease, as:
alcoholism (303.0-303.9)
myxedema (244.0-244.9)
neoplastic disease (140.0-239.9)
CC Excl: See code: 334.2

334.8 Other spinocerebellar diseases   CC
Ataxia-telangiectasia [Louis-Bar syndrome]
Corticostriatal-spinal degeneration
CC Excl: See code: 334.2

N Newborn Age: 0   P Pediatric Age: 0-17   M Maternity Age: 12-55   A Adult Age: 15-124   MCC Major CC Condition   CC CC Condition   HIV HIV Related Dx

102 – Volume 1   **2014 ICD-9-CM**

334.9 Spinocerebellar disease, unspecified `CC`
CC Excl: 334.0-334.9

✓4ᵗʰ 335 Anterior horn cell disease

335.0 Werdnig-Hoffmann disease `CC`
Infantile spinal muscular atrophy
Progressive muscular atrophy of infancy
DEF: Spinal muscle atrophy manifested in prenatal period or shortly after birth; symptoms include hypotonia, atrophy of skeletal muscle; death occurs in infancy.
CC Excl: 249.60-249.61, 249.80-249.91, 250.60-250.63, 250.80-250.93, 334.8-337.9, 349.89-349.9

✓5ᵗʰ 335.1 Spinal muscular atrophy

335.10 Spinal muscular atrophy, unspecified `CC`
CC Excl: See code: 335.0

335.11 Kugelberg-Welander disease `CC`
Spinal muscular atrophy:
  familial
  juvenile
DEF: Hereditary; juvenile muscle atrophy; appears during first two decades of life; due to lesions of anterior horns of spinal cord; includes wasting, diminution of lower body muscles and twitching.
CC Excl: See code: 335.0

335.19 Other `CC`
Adult spinal muscular atrophy
CC Excl: See code: 335.0

✓5ᵗʰ 335.2 Motor neuron disease

335.20 Amyotrophic lateral sclerosis `CC` `A`
Motor neuron disease (bulbar) (mixed type)
CC Excl: See code: 335.0
AHA: 4Q, '95, 81

335.21 Progressive muscular atrophy `CC`
Duchenne-Aran muscular atrophy
Progressive muscular atrophy (pure)
CC Excl: See code: 335.0

335.22 Progressive bulbar palsy `CC`
CC Excl: See code: 335.0

335.23 Pseudobulbar palsy `CC`
CC Excl: See code: 335.0

335.24 Primary lateral sclerosis `CC`
CC Excl: See code: 335.0

335.29 Other `CC`
CC Excl: See code: 335.0

335.8 Other anterior horn cell diseases `CC`
CC Excl: See code: 335.0

335.9 Anterior horn cell disease, unspecified `CC`
CC Excl: See code: 335.0

✓4ᵗʰ 336 Other diseases of spinal cord

336.0 Syringomyelia and syringobulbia `CC`
CC Excl: 334.8-337.9, 340-344.9, 348.30-348.39, 348.81-349.2, 349.89-349.9, 780.72
AHA: 1Q, '89, 10

336.1 Vascular myelopathies `MCC`
Acute infarction of spinal cord (embolic) (nonembolic)
Arterial thrombosis of spinal cord
Edema of spinal cord
Hematomyelia
Subacute necrotic myelopathy
CC Excl: 249.60-249.61, 250.60-250.63, 334.8-337.9, 340-344.9, 348.1, 348.30-348.39, 349.0-349.2, 349.89-349.9, 780.72

336.2 Subacute combined degeneration of spinal cord in diseases classified elsewhere `CC`
Code first underlying disease, as:
  pernicious anemia (281.0)
  other vitamin B$_{12}$ deficiency anemia (281.1)
  vitamin B$_{12}$ deficiency (266.2)
CC Excl: 334.8-337.9, 340-344.9, 348.1, 348.30-348.39, 349.0-349.2, 349.89-349.9, 780.72

336.3 Myelopathy in other diseases classified elsewhere `CC`
Code first underlying disease, as:
  myelopathy in neoplastic disease (140.0-239.9)
EXCLUDES myelopathy in:
  intervertebral disc disorder (722.70-722.73)
  spondylosis (721.1, 721.41-721.42, 721.91)
CC Excl: See code: 336.1
AHA: 3Q, '99, 5

336.8 Other myelopathy `CC`
Myelopathy: Myelopathy:
  drug-induced   radiation-induced
Use additonal E code to identify cause
CC Excl: See code: 336.1

336.9 Unspecified disease of spinal cord `CC` `HIV`
Cord compression NOS
Myelopathy NOS
EXCLUDES myelitis (323.02, 323.1, 323.2, 323.42, 323.52, 323.63, 323.72, 323.82, 323.9)
  spinal (canal) stenosis (723.0, 724.00-724.09)
CC Excl: 249.60-249.61, 250.60-250.63, 334.1, 334.8-337.9, 340-344.9, 348.1, 348.30-348.39, 349.0-349.2, 349.89-349.9, 780.72

✓4ᵗʰ 337 Disorders of the autonomic nervous system

INCLUDES disorders of peripheral autonomic, sympathetic, parasympathetic, or vegetative system
EXCLUDES familial dysautonomia [Riley-Day syndrome] (742.8)

✓5ᵗʰ 337.0 Idiopathic peripheral autonomic neuropathy

337.00 Idiopathic peripheral autonomic neuropathy, unspecified

337.01 Carotid sinus syndrome
Carotid sinus syncope
DEF: Vagal activation caused by pressure on the carotid sinus baroreceptors; sympathetic nerve impulses may cause sinus arrest or AV block.
AHA: 4Q, '08, 101-102

337.09 Other idiopathic peripheral autonomic neuropathy
Cervical sympathetic dystrophy or paralysis

337.1 Peripheral autonomic neuropathy in disorders classified elsewhere `CC`
Code first underlying disease, as:
  amyloidosis (277.30-277.39)
  diabetes (249.6, 250.6)
CC Excl: 337.00-337.29, 337.9, 348.30-348.39
AHA: 2Q, '09, 13; 2Q, '93, 6; 3Q, '91, 9; N-D, '84, 9

✓5ᵗʰ 337.2 Reflex sympathetic dystrophy

DEF: Disturbance of the sympathetic nervous system evidenced by sweating, pain, pallor and edema following injury to nerves or blood vessels.
AHA: 4Q, '93, 24

337.20 Reflex sympathetic dystrophy, unspecified `CC`
Complex regional pain syndrome type I, unspecified
CC Excl: 337.20-337.29

337.21 Reflex sympathetic dystrophy of the upper limb `CC`
Complex regional pain syndrome type I of the upper limb
CC Excl: 249.60-249.61, 250.60-250.63, 334.8-337.9, 340-344.9, 348.1, 348.30-348.39, 349.0-349.2, 349.89-349.9, 780.72

337.22 Reflex sympathetic dystrophy of the lower limb `CC`
Complex regional pain syndrome type I of the lower limb
CC Excl: See code: 337.21

337.29 Reflex sympathetic dystrophy of other specified site `CC`
Complex regional pain syndrome type I of other specified site
CC Excl: See code: 337.21

Additional Digit Required   Unacceptable PDx   Manifestation Code   Hospital Acquired Condition   ▶◀ Revised Text   ● New Code   ▲ Revised Code Title

337.3 Autonomic dysreflexia

Use additional code to identify the cause, such as:
- fecal impaction (560.32)
- pressure ulcer (707.00-707.09)
- urinary tract infection (599.0)

DEF: Noxious stimuli evokes paroxysmal hypertension, bradycardia, excess sweating, headache, pilomotor responses, facial flushing, and nasal congestion due to uncontrolled parasympathetic nerve response; occurs in patients with spinal cord injury above sympathetic outflow tract (T_6).

AHA: 4Q, '98, 37

337.9 Unspecified disorder of autonomic nervous system

Pain (338)

✓4ᵗʰ 338 Pain, not elsewhere classified

Use additional code to identify:
- pain associated with psychological factors (307.89)

EXCLUDES   generalized pain (780.96)
    headache syndromes (339.00-339.89)
    localized pain, unspecified type — code to pain by site
    migraines (346.0-346.9)
    pain disorder exclusively attributed to psychological factors
      (307.80)
    vulvar vestibulitis (625.71)
    vulvodynia (625.70-625.79)

AHA: 2Q, '07, 12

TIP: Do not assign a 338 code if the pain is not specified as acute or chronic, unless post-thoracotomy, postoperative, neoplasm related or central pain syndrome.

338.0 Central pain syndrome
Déjérine-Roussy syndrome
Myelopathic pain syndrome
Thalamic pain syndrome (hyperesthetic)
AHA: 4Q, '06, 79-81

✓5ᵗʰ 338.1 Acute pain

338.11 Acute pain due to trauma
AHA: 1Q, '07, 7; 4Q, '06, 79-81

338.12 Acute post-thoracotomy pain
Post-thoracotomy pain NOS
AHA: 4Q, '06, 79-81

338.18 Other acute postoperative pain
Postoperative pain NOS
AHA: 4Q, '06, 79-81
G89.18 Other acute postprocedural pain   I-10

338.19 Other acute pain
EXCLUDES neoplasm related acute pain (338.3)
AHA: 2Q, '07, 11; 4Q, '06, 79-81

✓5ᵗʰ 338.2 Chronic pain

EXCLUDES   causalgia (355.9)
     lower limb (355.71)
     upper limb (354.4)
   chronic pain syndrome (338.4)
   myofascial pain syndrome (729.1)
   neoplasm related chronic pain (338.3)
   reflex sympathetic dystrophy (337.20-337.29)

338.21 Chronic pain due to trauma
AHA: 4Q, '06, 79-81

338.22 Chronic post-thoracotomy pain
AHA: 4Q, '06, 79-81

338.28 Other chronic postoperative pain
AHA: 4Q, '06, 79-81
G89.28 Other chronic postprocedural pain   I-10

338.29 Other chronic pain
AHA: 4Q, '06, 79-81

✳ 338.3 Neoplasm related pain (acute) (chronic)
Cancer associated pain
Pain due to malignancy (primary) (secondary)
Tumor associated pain
AHA: 2Q, '07, 11; 4Q, '06, 79-81
G89.3 Neoplasm related pain (acute) (chronic)   I-10

338.4 Chronic pain syndrome
Chronic pain associated with significant psychosocial dysfunction
AHA: 2Q, '07, 11; 4Q, '06, 79-81
G89.4 Chronic pain syndrome

Other Headache Syndromes (339)

✓4ᵗʰ 339 Other headache syndromes
EXCLUDES   headache:
    NOS (784.0)
    due to lumbar puncture (349.0)
    migraine (346.0-346.9)
AHA: 4Q, '08, 102-105

✓5ᵗʰ 339.0 Cluster headaches and other trigeminal autonomic cephalgias
TACS

339.00 Cluster headache syndrome, unspecified
Ciliary neuralgia   Lower half migraine
Cluster headache NOS   Migrainous neuralgia
Histamine cephalgia

339.01 Episodic cluster headache

339.02 Chronic cluster headache

339.03 Episodic paroxysmal hemicrania
Paroxysmal hemicrania NOS

339.04 Chronic paroxysmal hemicrania

339.05 Short lasting unilateral neuralgiform headache with conjunctival injection and tearing
SUNCT

339.09 Other trigeminal autonomic cephalgias

✓5ᵗʰ 339.1 Tension type headache
EXCLUDES tension headache NOS (307.81)
    tension headache related to psychological factors
      (307.81)
AHA: 4Q, '08, 103

339.10 Tension type headache, unspecified

339.11 Episodic tension type headache

339.12 Chronic tension type headache

✓5ᵗʰ 339.2 Post-traumatic headache
TIP: Do not assign during the acute phase of the trauma (e.g., hea injury). When assigning 339.2X, report also a late effect code (e.g. 907.0 for intracranial injury).

339.20 Post-traumatic headache, unspecified
AHA: 4Q, '08, 108

339.21 Acute post-traumatic headache

339.22 Chronic post-traumatic headache

339.3 Drug induced headache, not elsewhere classified
Medication overuse headache
Rebound headache

✓5ᵗʰ 339.4 Complicated headache syndromes

339.41 Hemicrania continua

339.42 New daily persistent headache
NDPH

339.43 Primary thunderclap headache

339.44 Other complicated headache syndrome

✓5ᵗʰ 339.8 Other specified headache syndromes

339.81 Hypnic headache

339.82 Headache associated with sexual activity
Orgasmic headache
Preorgasmic headache

339.83 Primary cough headache

339.84 Primary exertional headache

339.85 Primary stabbing headache

339.89 Other specified headache syndromes

N Newborn Age: 0   P Pediatric Age: 0-17   M Maternity Age: 12-55   A Adult Age: 15-124   MCC Major CC Condition   CC CC Condition   HIV HIV Related

104 – Volume 1   2014 ICD-9

Other Disorders of the Central Nervous System (340-349)

340 Multiple sclerosis
Disseminated or multiple sclerosis:
NOS
brain stem
cord
generalized
CC Exd: 250.60-250.63, 250.80-250.93, 340, 341.8-341.9
G35 Multiple sclerosis   **I-10**

✓4ᵗʰ 341 Other demyelinating diseases of central nervous system

341.0 Neuromyelitis optica   **CC**
CC Exd: 341.0, 348.30-348.39

341.1 Schilder's disease   **CC**
Baló's concentric sclerosis   Encephalitis periaxialis:
Encephalitis periaxialis: diffusa [Schilder's]
   concentrica [Baló's]
DEF: Chronic leukoencephalopathy of children and adolescents;
symptoms include blindness, deafness, bilateral spasticity and
progressive mental deterioration.
CC Exd: 066.40-066.49, 079.82, 348.30-348.39

✓5ᵗʰ 341.2 Acute (transverse) myelitis
EXCLUDES *acute (transverse) myelitis (in) (due to):*
following immunization procedures (323.52)
infection classified elsewhere (323.42)
postinfectious (323.63)
protozoal diseases classified elsewhere (323.2)
rickettsial diseases classified elsewhere (323.1)
toxic (323.72)
viral diseases classified elsewhere (323.02)
transverse myelitis NOS (323.82)

341.20 Acute (transverse) myelitis NOS   **CC**
CC Exd: 003.21, 013.00-013.16, 036.0, 047.0-047.9,
049.0-049.1, 053.0-053.13, 053.19, 053.79-053.9, 054.72,
054.79-054.9, 058.81-058.89, 072.1, 078.89, 079.81, 079.89,
079.99, 090.42, 091.81, 094.2, 098.89, 100.81, 112.83, 114.2,
115.01, 115.11, 115.91, 130.0, 139.8, 249.60-249.61,
250.60-250.63, 320.0-322.9, 334.8-337.9, 340-341.1,
341.8-344.9, 348.1, 348.30-348.39, 349.0-349.2,
349.89-349.9, 357.0, 780.72
AHA: 4Q, '06, 58-63

341.21 *Acute (transverse) myelitis in conditions classified elsewhere*   **CC**
Code first underlying condition
CC Exd: See code: 341.20
AHA: 4Q, '06, 58-63

341.22 Idiopathic transverse myelitis   **CC**
CC Exd: See code: 341.20
AHA: 4Q, '06, 58-63

341.8 Other demyelinating diseases of central nervous system   **CC**
Central demyelination of corpus callosum
Central pontine myelinosis
Marchiafava (-Bignami) disease
CC Exd: 333.1-333.93, 333.99-337.9, 340-344.9, 348.30-348.39,
348.81-348.9, 349.82-349.9, 780.72
AHA: N-D, '87, 6

341.9 Demyelinating disease of central nervous system, unspecified   **CC HIV**
CC Exd: See code: 341.8

✓4ᵗʰ 342 Hemiplegia and hemiparesis
NOTE This category is to be used when hemiplegia (complete)
(incomplete) is reported without further specification, or is
stated to be old or long-standing but of unspecified cause. The
category is also for use in multiple coding to identify these
types of hemiplegia resulting from any cause.
EXCLUDES *congenital (343.1)*
hemiplegia due to late effect of cerebrovascular accident
(438.20-438.22)
infantile NOS (343.4)

The following fifth-dits are for use with codes 342.0-342.9:
0 affecting unspecified side
1 affecting dominant side
2 affecting nondominant side

AHA: 4Q, '94, 38

§ ✓5ᵗʰ 342.0 Flaccid hemiplegia   **CC**
[0-2]   **CC Exd:** 334.0-337.9, 340-344.9, 348.30-348.39, 348.81-348.9,
349.82-349.9, 780.72

§ ✓5ᵗʰ 342.1 Spastic hemiplegia   **CC**
[0-2]   **CC Exd:** See code: 342.0

§ ✓5ᵗʰ 342.8 Other specified hemiplegia   **CC**
[0-2]   **CC Exd:** See code: 342.0

§ ✓5ᵗʰ 342.9 Hemiplegia, unspecified   **CC**
[0-2]   **CC Exd:** See code: 342.0
AHA: 3Q, '06, 5; 4Q, '98, 87
G81.90 Hemiplegia unspecified affect unspecified side   **I-10**

✓4ᵗʰ 343 Infantile cerebral palsy
INCLUDES cerebral:
palsy NOS
spastic infantile paralysis
congenital spastic paralysis (cerebral)
Little's disease
paralysis (spastic) due to birth injury:
intracranial
spinal
EXCLUDES *athetoid cerebral palsy (333.71)*
hereditary cerebral paralysis, such as:
hereditary spastic paraplegia (334.1)
Vogt's disease (333.71)
spastic paralysis specified as noncongenital or noninfantile
(344.0-344.9)

343.0 Diplegic   **CC**
Congenital diplegiaCongenital paraplegia
DEF: Paralysis affecting both sides of the body simultaneously.
CC Exd: 343.0, 348.30-348.39

343.1 Hemiplegic   **CC**
Congenital hemiplegia
EXCLUDES *infantile hemiplegia NOS (343.4)*
CC Exd: 343.1, 348.30-348.39

343.2 Quadriplegic   **MCC**
Tetraplegic
CC Exd: 249.60-249.61, 249.80-249.91, 250.60-250.63, 250.80-250.93,
342.00-344.9, 348.81-348.9, 349.89-349.9,742.59-742.9, 780.72

343.3 Monoplegic

343.4 Infantile hemiplegia   **CC**
Infantile hemiplegia (postnatal) NOS
CC Exd: See code: 342.0

343.8 Other specified infantile cerebral palsy

343.9 Infantile cerebral palsy, unspecified
Cerebral palsy NOS
AHA: 4Q, '05, 89
G80.9 Cerebral palsy unspecified   **I-10**

✓4ᵗʰ 344 Other paralytic syndromes
NOTE This category is to be used when the listed conditions are
reported without further specification or are stated to be old or
long-standing but of unspecified cause. The category is also for
use in multiple coding to identify these conditions resulting
from any cause.
INCLUDES paralysis (complete) (incomplete), except as classifiable to
342 and 343
EXCLUDES *congenital or infantile cerebral palsy (343.0-343.9)*
hemiplegia (342.0-342.9)
congenital or infantile (343.1, 343.4)

✓5ᵗʰ 344.0 Quadriplegia and quadriparesis
TIP: Assign also a code from subcategory 438.5 if late effect of CVA.

344.00 Quadriplegia unspecified   **MCC**
CC Exd: See code: 343.2
AHA: 4Q, '03, 103; 4Q, '98, 38
G82.50 Quadriplegia unspecified   **I-10**

344.01 C₁-C₄ complete   **MCC**
CC Exd: See code: 343.2

344.02 C₁-C₄ incomplete   **MCC**
CC Exd: See code: 343.2

344.03 C₅-C₇ complete   **MCC**
CC Exd: See code: 343.2

---

§   Requires fifth digit. Valid digits are in [brackets] under each code. See category 342 for codes and definitions.

✓4ᵗʰ/5ᵗʰ Additional Digit Required	Unacceptable PDx	Manifestation Code	Hospital Acquired Condition	►◄ Revised Text	● New Code ▲ Revised Code Title

Diseases of the Nervous System and Sense Organs

344.04–345.3

344.04 C₅-C₇ incomplete `MCC`
CC Excl: See code: 343.2

344.09 Other `MCC`
CC Excl: See code: 343.2
AHA: 1Q, '01, 12; 4Q, '98, 39

344.1 Paraplegia `CC`
Paralysis of both lower limbs
Paraplegia (lower)
CC Excl: 334.0-337.9, 340-344.9, 348.30-348.39, 348.8-348.9, 349.82-349.9, 780.72
AHA: 4Q, '03, 110;M-A, '87, 10
G82.20 Paraplegia unspecified `I-10`

344.2 Diplegia of upper limbs `CC`
Diplegia (upper)
Paralysis of both upper limbs
CC Excl: 344.00-344.09, 344.2, 344.81-344.9, 349.89-349.9, 780.72

√5ᵗʰ **344.3 Monoplegia of lower limb**
Paralysis of lower limb
EXCLUDES monoplegia of lower limb due to late effect of cerebrovascular accident (438.40-438.42)

344.30 Affecting unspecified side

344.31 Affecting dominant side

344.32 Affecting nondominant side

√5ᵗʰ **344.4 Monoplegia of upper limb**
Paralysis of upper limb
EXCLUDES monoplegia of upper limb due to late effect of cerebrovascular accident (438.30-438.32)

344.40 Affecting unspecified side

344.41 Affecting dominant side

344.42 Affecting nondominant side

344.5 Unspecified monoplegia

√5ᵗʰ **344.6 Cauda equina syndrome**
DEF: Dull pain and paresthesias in sacrum, perineum and bladder due to compression of spinal nerve roots; pain radiates down buttocks, back of thigh, calf of leg and into foot with prickling, burning sensations.

344.60 Without mention of neurogenic bladder `CC`
CC Excl: 344.00-344.1, 344.30-344.32, 344.60-344.9, 349.89-349.9, 780.72

344.61 With neurogenic bladder `CC`
Acontractile bladder
Autonomic hyperreflexia of bladder
Cord bladder
Detrusor hyperreflexia
CC Excl: 334.0-337.9, 340-344.9, 348.30-348.39, 348.81-348.9, 349.82-349.9, 599.60-599.69, 780.72
AHA: M-J, '87, 12; M-A, '87, 10

√5ᵗʰ **344.8 Other specified paralytic syndromes**

344.81 Locked-in state `MCC`
DEF: State of consciousness where patients are paralyzed and unable to respond to environmental stimuli; patients have eye movements, and stimuli can enter the brain but patients unable to respond.
CC Excl: 342.00-344.9, 348.30-348.39, 348.81-348.9, 349.82-349.9, 780.72
AHA: 4Q, '93, 24

344.89 Other specified paralytic syndrome
AHA: 2Q, '99, 4

344.9 Paralysis, unspecified

√4ᵗʰ **345 Epilepsy and recurrent seizures**
The following fifth-digit subclassification is for use with categories 345.0, .1, .4-.9:
0 without mention of intractable epilepsy
1 with intractable epilepsy
pharmacoresistant (pharmacologically resistant)
poorly controlled
refractory (medically)
treatment resistant

EXCLUDES hippocampal sclerosis (348.81)
mesial temporal sclerosis (348.81)
temporal sclerosis (348.81)
DEF: Brain disorder characterized by electrical-like disturbances; may include occasional impairment or loss of consciousness, abnormal motor phenomena and psychic or sensory disturbances.
AHA: 4Q, '09, 82; 1Q, '93, 24; 2Q, '92, 8; 4Q, '92, 23

§ √5ᵗʰ **345.0 Generalized nonconvulsive epilepsy** `CC 1`
[0-1] Absences:　　　　Pykno-epilepsy
　　　atonic　　　　Seizures:
　　　typical　　　　akinetic
　　Minor epilepsy　　atonic
　　Petit mal
CC Excl: 249.60-249.61, 250.60-250.63, 345.00-345.91, 348.81-348.9, 349.89-349.9; For code 345.01: 249.60-249.61, 250.60-250.63, 345.00-345.91, 348.81, 348.89-348.9, 349.89-349.9, 780.33
AHA: For code 345.00: 1Q, '04, 18

§ √5ᵗʰ **345.1 Generalized convulsive epilepsy** `CC 1`
[0-1] Epileptic seizures:
　　clonic
　　myoclonic
　　tonic
　　tonic-clonic
　Grand mal
　Major epilepsy
　Progressive myoclonic epilepsy
　Unverricht-Lundborg disease
EXCLUDES convulsions:
　　NOS (780.39)
　　infantile (780.39)
　　newborn (779.0)
　infantile spasms (345.6)
DEF: Convulsive seizures with tension of limbs (tonic) or rhythmic contractions (clonic).
CC Excl: For code 345.11: 249.60-249.61, 250.60-250.63, 345.00-345.91, 348.81-348.9, 349.89-349.9
AHA: 3Q, '97, 4

345.2 Petit mal status `MCC`
Epileptic absence status
DEF: Minor myoclonic spasms and sudden momentary loss of consciousness in epilepsy.
CC Excl: 249.60-249.61, 249.80-249.91, 250.60-250.63, 250.80-250.93, 345.00-345.91, 348.81, 348.89-348.9, 349.89-349.9, 780.33

345.3 Grand mal status `MCC`
Status epilepticus NOS
EXCLUDES epilepsia partialis continua (345.7)
status:
　psychomotor (345.7)
　temporal lobe (345.7)
DEF: Sudden loss of consciousness followed by generalized convulsions in epilepsy.
CC Excl: See code: 345.2
AHA: 3Q, '05, 12
G40.301 Gen idiopath epilep&epi syn not intractabl w/se `I-10`

---

§ Requires fifth digit. Valid digits are in [brackets] under each code. See category 345 for codes and definitions.

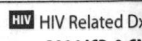

§ ✓5ᵗʰ **345.4 Localization-related (focal) (partial) epilepsy**   CC
[0-1]   **and epileptic syndromes with complex partial seizures**
     Epilepsy:
        limbic system
        partial:
           secondarily generalized
           with impairment of consciousness
           with memory and ideational disturbances
        psychomotor
        psychosensory
        temporal lobe
     Epileptic automatism
     CC Excl: For code 345.40: 345.00-345.91, 348.30-348.39, 348.9,
     349.89-349.9, 780.33; **For code 345.41:** 249.60-249.61, 250.60-250.63,
     345.00-345.91, 348.81-348.9, 349.89-349.9
     AHA: For code 345.41: 4Q, '09, 83

§ ✓5ᵗʰ **345.5 Localization-related (focal) (partial) epilepsy**   CC
[0-1]   **and epileptic syndromes with simple partial seizures**
     Epilepsy:
        Bravais-Jacksonian NOS
        focal (motor) NOS
        Jacksonian NOS
        motor partial
        partial NOS:
           without impairment of consciousness
        sensory-induced
        somatomotor
        somatosensory
        visceral
        visual
     CC Excl: For code 345.50: 345.00-345.91, 348.30-348.39, 348.9,
     349.89-349.9; **For code 345.51:** 249.60-249.61, 250.60-250.63,
     345.00-345.91, 348.81-348.9, 349.89-349.9

§ ✓5ᵗʰ **345.6 Infantile spasms**   CC
[0-1]   Hypsarrhythmia
     Lightning spasms
     Salaam attacks
     EXCLUDES salaam tic (781.0)
     CC Excl: For code 345.60: 345.00-345.91, 348.30-348.39, 348.9,
     349.89-349.9; **For code 345.61:** 249.60-249.61, 250.60-250.63,
     345.00-345.91, 348.81-348.9, 349.89-349.9
     AHA: N-D, '84, 12

§ ✓5ᵗʰ **345.7 Epilepsia partialis continua**   CC 0   MCC 1
[0-1]   Kojevnikov's epilepsy
     DEF: Continuous muscle contractions and relaxation; result of
     abnormal neural discharge.
     CC Excl: 249.60-249.61, 250.60-250.63, 345.00-345.91, 348.81-348.9,
     349.89-349.9

§ ✓5ᵗʰ **345.8 Other forms of epilepsy and recurrent seizures**   CC
[0-1]   Epilepsy: Epilepsy:
        cursive [running]   gelastic
     CC Excl: 249.60-249.61, 250.60-250.63, 345.00-345.91, 348.81-348.9,
     349.89-349.9

§ ✓5ᵗʰ **345.9 Epilepsy, unspecified**   CC 1
[0-1]   Epileptic convulsions, fits, or seizures NOS
     Seizure disorder NOS
     EXCLUDES convulsion (convulsive) disorder (780.39)
           convulsive seizure or fit NOS (780.39)
           recurrent convulsions (780.39)
     CC Excl: For code 345.91: 249.60-249.61, 250.60-250.63, 345.00-345.91,
     348.81-348.9, 349.89-349.9
     AHA: 1Q, '08, 17; N-D, '87, 12; **For code 345.90:** ▶2Q, '12, 9;◀ 2Q, '09, 10
     TIP: ▶Code also alcohol withdrawal seizure with epileptic seizure
     when both conditions are documented by the provider. Assign a
     separate code for the alcohol dependence.◀
     G40.909 Epilepsy uns not intractbl w/o status epilepticus   I-10

✓4ᵗʰ **346 Migraine**
     EXCLUDES headache:
           NOS (784.0)
           syndromes (339.00-339.89)
     AHA: 4Q, '08, 103, 105-107

     The following fifth-digit subclassification is for use with category 346:
     **0 without mention of intractable migraine without mention of
        status migrainosus**
        without mention of refractory migraine without mention of status
        migrainosus
     **1 with intractable migraine, so stated, without mention of
        status migrainosus**
        with refractory migraine, so stated, without mention of status
        migrainosus
     **2 without mention of intractable migraine with status
        migrainosus**
        without mention of refractory migraine with status migrainosus
     3 with intractable migraine, so stated, with status migrainosus
        with refractory migraine, so stated, with status migrainosus

     DEF: Benign vascular headache of extreme pain; commonly associated with
     irritability, nausea, vomiting and often photophobia; premonitory visual
     hallucination of a crescent in the visual field (scotoma).

§ ✓5ᵗʰ **346.0 Migraine with aura**
[0-3]   Basilar migraine
     Classic migraine
     Migraine preceded or accompanied by transient focal
        neurological phenomena
     Migraine triggered seizures
     Migraine with acute-onset aura
     Migraine with aura without headache (migraine
        equivalents)
     Migraine with prolonged aura
     Migraine with typical aura
     Retinal migraine
     EXCLUDES persistent migraine aura (346.5, 346.6)

§ ✓5ᵗʰ **346.1 Migraine without aura**
[0-3]   Common migraine

§ ✓5ᵗʰ **346.2 Variants of migraine, not elsewhere classified**
[0-3]   Abdominal migraine
     Cyclical vomiting associated with migraine
     Ophthalmoplegic migraine
     Periodic headache syndromes in child or adolescent
     EXCLUDES cyclical vomiting NOS (536.2)
           psychogenic cyclical vomiting (306.4)

§ ✓5ᵗʰ **346.3 Hemiplegic migraine**
[0-3]   Familial migraine
     Sporadic migraine

§ ✓5ᵗʰ **346.4 Menstrual migraine**   ♀
[0-3]   Menstrual headache   Premenstrual migraine
     Menstrually related migraine   Pure menstrual migraine
     Premenstrual headache

§ ✓5ᵗʰ **346.5 Persistent migraine aura without cerebral infarction**
[0-3]   Persistent migraine aura NOS

§ ✓5ᵗʰ **346.6 Persistent migraine aura with cerebral infarction**   CC
[0-3]   **CC Excl: For code 346.60:** 346.60-346.63, 433.00-434.91; **For code 346.61,**
     346.62, 346.63: 346.60-346.63, 433.00-434.91, 436
     AHA: For code 346.60: 4Q, '08, 108
     TIP: Assign also a code for the specific type of cerebral infarction.

§ ✓5ᵗʰ **346.7 Chronic migraine without aura**
[0-3]   Transformed migraine without aura

§ ✓5ᵗʰ **346.8 Other forms of migraine**
[0-3]

§ ✓5ᵗʰ **346.9 Migraine, unspecified**
[0-3]   **AHA:** N-D, '85, 16
     G43.909 Migraine unspecified not intract w/o stat migran   I-10

✓4ᵗʰ **347 Cataplexy and narcolepsy**
     DEF: Cataplexy: Sudden onset of muscle weakness with loss of tone and
     strength; caused by aggressive or spontaneous emotions.
     DEF: Narcolepsy: Brief, recurrent, uncontrollable episodes of sound sleep.

  ✓5ᵗʰ **347.0 Narcolepsy**

       347.00 Without cataplexy
          Narcolepsy NOS

Requires fifth digit. Valid digits are in [brackets] under each code. See appropriate category for codes and definitions.

Additional Digit Required   Unacceptable PDx   Manifestation Code   Hospital Acquired Condition   ▶◀ Revised Text   ● New Code   ▲ Revised Code Title

2014 ICD-9-CM   February 2013 · Volume 1 – 107

347.01 With cataplexy

☑5ᵗʰ **347.1 Narcolepsy in conditions classified elsewhere**
Code first underlying condition

347.10 Without cataplexy

347.11 With cataplexy

☑4ᵗʰ **348 Other conditions of brain**

348.0 Cerebral cysts
Arachnoid cyst   Porencephaly, acquired
Porencephalic cyst   Pseudoporencephaly
EXCLUDES porencephaly (congenital) (742.4)

348.1 Anoxic brain damage `CC`
Use additional E code to identify cause
EXCLUDES that occurring in:
abortion (634-638 with .7, 639.8)
ectopic or molar pregnancy (639.8)
labor or delivery (668.2, 669.4)
that of newborn (767.0, 768.0-768.9, 772.1-772.2)
DEF: Brain injury due to lack of oxygen, other than birth trauma.
CC Excl: 249.60-249.61, 249.80-249.91, 250.60-250.63, 250.80-250.93, 348.1-348.2, 349.89-349.9
G93.1 Anoxic brain damage not elsewhere classified `I-10`

348.2 Benign intracranial hypertension
Pseudotumor cerebri
EXCLUDES hypertensive encephalopathy (437.2)
DEF: Elevated pressure in brain due to fluid retention in brain cavities.

☑5ᵗʰ **348.3 Encephalopathy, not elsewhere classified**
AHA: 4Q, '03, 58; 3Q, '97, 4

348.30 Encephalopathy, unspecified `MCC` `HIV`
CC Excl: 333.92, 344.81, 348.31-348.39
G93.40 Encephalopathy unspecified `I-10`

348.31 Metabolic encephalopathy `MCC` `HIV`
Septic encephalopathy
EXCLUDES toxic metabolic encephalopathy (349.82)
CC Excl: 333.92, 344.81, 348.30, 348.39
TIP: Physician documentation of "acute confusional state" denotes delirium inherent to the encephalopathy. Do not report an additional code for the delirium

348.39 Other encephalopathy `MCC` `HIV`
EXCLUDES encephalopathy:
alcoholic (291.2)
hepatic (572.2)
hypertensive (437.2)
toxic (349.82)
CC Excl: 333.92, 344.81, 348.30-348.31

348.4 Compression of brain `MCC`
Compression ⎫
Herniation ⎬ brain (stem)
Posterior fossa compression syndrome
DEF: Elevated pressure in brain due to blood clot, tumor, fracture, abscess, other condition.
CC Excl: 342.90, 348.82
AHA: 3Q, '11, 11;4Q, '94, 37
TIP: Assign for Arnold-Chiari syndrome, Type I. For Type II, III, or IV, refer to categories 741 and 742.

348.5 Cerebral edema `MCC`
DEF: Elevated pressure in the brain due to fluid retention in brain tissues.
CC Excl: 348.5, 348.82
AHA: 4Q, '11, 99; 1Q, '10, 8; 3Q, '09, 8
G93.6 Cerebral edema `I-10`

☑5ᵗʰ **348.8 Other conditions of brain**
AHA: S-O, '87, 9

348.81 Temporal sclerosis
Hippocampal sclerosis
Mesial temporal sclerosis
DEF: Abnormal hardening or scarring of frontal lobe tissues due to injury, tumor, congenital anomaly, or hypoxia, resulting in loss of functional neurons; commonly associated with temporal lobe epilepsy.
AHA: 4Q, '09, 83

348.82 Brain death `MCC`
CC Excl: 070.0-070.9, 249.00-249.91, 250.00-250.93, 251.0-251.3, 338.0-338.4, 348.81-349.9,.430-432.9, 572.2, 780.01-780.09, 780.2, 780.4, 780.64-780.65, 780.91-780.99, 799.81-799.89, 800.00-801.99, 803.00-804.96, 850.0-854.19
AHA: 4Q, '11, 99-100

348.89 Other conditions of brain
Cerebral:
calcification
fungus
EXCLUDES brain death (348.82)

348.9 Unspecified condition of brain `HIV`

☑4ᵗʰ **349 Other and unspecified disorders of the nervous system**
AHA: 4Q, '08, 109

349.0 Reaction to spinal or lumbar puncture
Headache following lumbar puncture
AHA: 2Q, '99, 9; 3Q, '90, 18
G97.1 Other reaction to spinal and lumbar puncture `I-10`

349.1 Nervous system complications from surgically implanted device `CC`
EXCLUDES immediate postoperative complications (997.00-997.09)
mechanical complications of nervous system device (996.2)
CC Excl: 2249.60-249.61, 249.80-249.91, 250.60-250.63, 250.80-250.93, 349.1, 349.89-349.9

349.2 Disorders of meninges, not elsewhere classified
Adhesions, meningeal (cerebral) (spinal)
Cyst, spinal meninges
Meningocele, acquired
Pseudomeningocele, acquired
AHA: 1Q, '06, 15; 2Q, '98, 18; 3Q, '94, 4

☑5ᵗʰ **349.3 Dural tear**

349.31 Accidental puncture or laceration of dura during a procedure `CC`
Incidental (inadvertent) durotomy
CC Excl: 349.31-349.39, 997.91-997.99, 998.2, 998.81, 998.83-998.9
AHA: 4Q, '08, 109-110
TIP: Do not assign code 998.2 Accidental puncture or laceration during a procedure, for an incidental dural tear.

349.39 Other dural tear `CC`
CC Excl: 349.31-349.39, 997.91-997.99, 998.2, 998.81, 998.83-998.9

☑5ᵗʰ **349.8 Other specified disorders of nervous system**

349.81 Cerebrospinal fluid rhinorrhea `CC`
EXCLUDES cerebrospinal fluid otorrhea (388.61)
DEF: Cerebrospinal fluid discharging from the nose; caused by fracture of frontal bone with tearing of dura mater and arachnoid.
CC Excl: 249.60-249.61, 249.80-249.91, 250.60-250.63, 250.80-250.93, 349.81, 349.89-349.9

349.82 Toxic encephalopathy `MCC`
Toxic metabolic encephalopathy
Use additional E code to identify cause
DEF: Brain tissue degeneration due to toxic substance.
CC Excl: 013.60-013.66, 017.90-017.96, 036.1, 049.8-049.9, 052.0, 054.3, 058.21-058.29, 062.0-063.9, 072.2, 090.41, 094.81, 130.0, 249.60-249.61, 249.80-249.91, 250.60-250.63, 250.80-250.93, 323.01-323.9, 341.20-341.22, 348.30-348.39, 348.81-348.9, 349.82-349.9
AHA: 4Q, '93, 29
G92 Toxic encephalopathy `I-1`

349.89 Other

349.9 Unspecified disorders of nervous system
Disorder of nervous system (central) NOS
AHA: ▶3Q, '12, 4◄

`N` Newborn Age: 0   `P` Pediatric Age: 0-17   `M` Maternity Age: 12-55   `A` Adult Age: 15-124   `MCC` Major CC Condition   `CC` CC Condition   `HIV` HIV Related D

108 – Volume 1 • February 2013   **2014 ICD-9-C**

Disorders of the Peripheral Nervous System (350-359)

EXCLUDES diseases of:
  acoustic [8th] nerve (388.5)
  oculomotor [3rd, 4th, 6th] nerves (378.0-378.9)
  optic [2nd] nerve (377.0-377.9)
  peripheral autonomic nerves (337.0-337.9)
  neuralgia
  neuritis   } NOS or "rheumatic" (729.2)
  radiculitis
  peripheral neuritis in pregnancy (646.4)

✓4ᵗʰ 350 Trigeminal nerve disorders

  INCLUDES disorders of 5th cranial nerve

350.1 Trigeminal neuralgia
  Tic douloureux   Trigeminal neuralgia NOS
  Trifacial neuralgia
  EXCLUDES postherpetic (053.12)
  G50.0 Trigeminal neuralgia   I-10

350.2 Atypical face pain

350.8 Other specified trigeminal nerve disorders

350.9 Trigeminal nerve disorder, unspecified

✓4ᵗʰ 351 Facial nerve disorders

  INCLUDES disorders of 7th cranial nerve
  EXCLUDES that in newborn (767.5)

351.0 Bell's palsy
  Facial palsy
  DEF: Unilateral paralysis of face due to lesion on facial nerve; produces facial distortion.
  G51.0 Bell's palsy   I-10

351.1 Geniculate ganglionitis
  Geniculate ganglionitis NOS
  EXCLUDES herpetic (053.11)
  DEF: Inflammation of tissue at bend in facial nerve.

351.8 Other facial nerve disorders
  Facial myokymia   Melkersson's syndrome
  AHA: 3Q, '02, 13

351.9 Facial nerve disorder, unspecified

✓4ᵗʰ 352 Disorders of other cranial nerves

352.0 Disorders of olfactory [lst] nerve

352.1 Glossopharyngeal neuralgia
  DEF: Pain between throat and ear along petrosal and jugular ganglia.
  AHA: 2Q, '02, 8

352.2 Other disorders of glossopharyngeal [9th] nerve

352.3 Disorders of pneumogastric [10th] nerve
  Disorders of vagal nerve
  EXCLUDES paralysis of vocal cords or larynx (478.30-478.34)
  DEF: Nerve disorder affecting ear, tongue, pharynx, larynx, esophagus, viscera and thorax.

352.4 Disorders of accessory [11th] nerve
  DEF: Nerve disorder affecting palate, pharynx, larynx, thoracic viscera, sternocleidomastoid and trapezius muscles.

352.5 Disorders of hypoglossal [12th] nerve
  DEF: Nerve disorder affecting tongue muscles.

Cranial Nerves

Olfactory bulb (I)
Optic nerve (II)
Oculomotor nerve (III)
Trochlear nerve (IV)
Trigeminal nerve (V)
Abducens nerve (VI)
Facial nerve (VII)
Vestibulocochlear nerve (VIII)
Glossopharyngeal nerve (IX)
Vagus nerve (X)
Accessory nerve (XI)
Hypoglossal nerve (XII)
Pons

Peripheral Nervous System

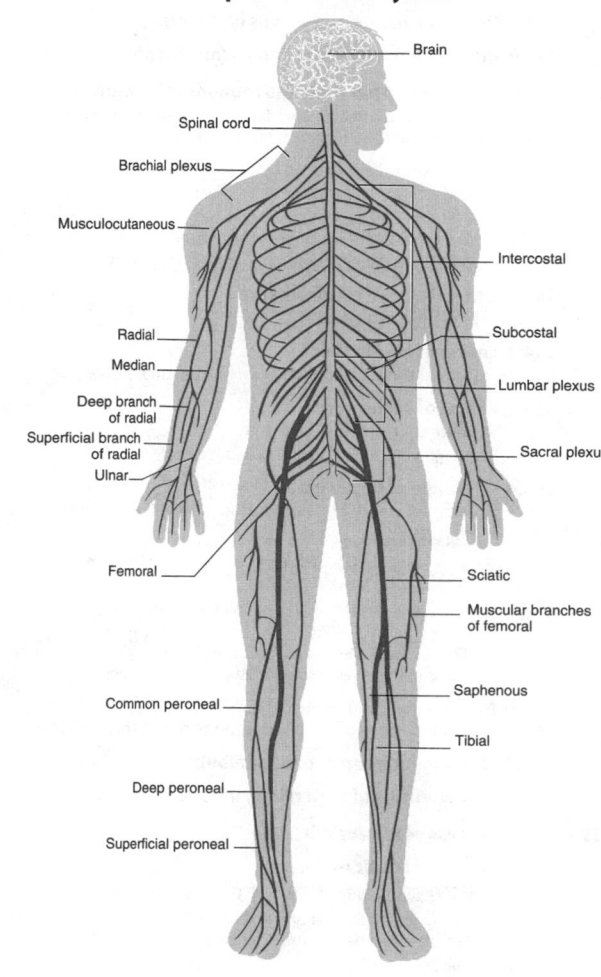

Brain
Spinal cord
Brachial plexus
Musculocutaneous
Intercostal
Radial
Subcostal
Median
Lumbar plexus
Deep branch of radial
Superficial branch of radial
Sacral plexus
Ulnar
Femoral
Sciatic
Muscular branches of femoral
Common peroneal
Saphenous
Tibial
Deep peroneal
Superficial peroneal

352.6 Multiple cranial nerve palsies
  Collet-Sicard syndrome
  Polyneuritis cranialis

352.9 Unspecified disorder of cranial nerves

✓4ᵗʰ 353 Nerve root and plexus disorders

  EXCLUDES conditions due to:
    intervertebral disc disorders (722.0-722.9)
    spondylosis (720.0-721.9)
    vertebrogenic disorders (723.0-724.9)

353.0 Brachial plexus lesions
  Cervical rib syndrome
  Costoclavicular syndrome
  Scalenus anticus syndrome
  Thoracic outlet syndrome
  EXCLUDES brachial neuritis or radiculitis NOS (723.4)
    that in newborn (767.6)
  DEF: Acquired disorder in tissue along nerves in shoulder; causes corresponding motor and sensory dysfunction.
  AHA: 3Q, '06, 12

Trigeminal and Facial Nerve Branches

Temporal branches
Zygomatic branches
Buccal branches
Mandibular branch
Cervical branch
Branches of Facial Nerve (above)
Divisions of Trigeminal Nerve (below)
Ophthalmic (V1)
Trigeminal nerve (CN V)
Maxillary (V2)
Mandibulary (V3)

✓4ᵗʰ Additional Digit Required   Unacceptable PDx   Manifestation Code   Hospital Acquired Condition   ▶◀ Revised Text   ● New Code   ▲ Revised Code Title

014 ICD-9-CM   **Volume 1 – 109**

353.1 Lumbosacral plexus lesions
> **DEF:** Acquired disorder in tissue along nerves in lower back; causes corresponding motor and sensory dysfunction.

353.2 Cervical root lesions, not elsewhere classified

353.3 Thoracic root lesions, not elsewhere classified

353.4 Lumbosacral root lesions, not elsewhere classified

353.5 Neuralgic amyotrophy
> Parsonage-Aldren-Turner syndrome
>
> Code first any associated underlying disease, such as:
>   diabetes mellitus (249.6, 250.6)

353.6 Phantom limb (syndrome)
> **DEF:** Abnormal tingling or a burning sensation, transient aches, and intermittent or continuous pain perceived as originating in the absent limb.

353.8 Other nerve root and plexus disorders

353.9 Unspecified nerve root and plexus disorder

√4ᵗʰ **354 Mononeuritis of upper limb and mononeuritis multiplex**
> **DEF:** Inflammation of a single nerve; known as mononeuritis multiplex when several nerves in unrelated body areas are affected.

354.0 Carpal tunnel syndrome
> Median nerve entrapment   Partial thenar atrophy
> **DEF:** Compression of median nerve by tendons; causes pain, tingling, numbness and burning sensation in hand.
> G56.00 Carpal tunnel syndrome unspec upper limb   I-10

354.1 Other lesion of median nerve
> Median nerve neuritis

354.2 Lesion of ulnar nerve
> Cubital tunnel syndrome   Tardy ulnar nerve palsy

354.3 Lesion of radial nerve
> Acute radial nerve palsy
> **AHA:** N-D, '87, 6

354.4 Causalgia of upper limb
> Complex regional pain syndrome type II of the upper limb
> **EXCLUDES** causalgia:
>   NOS (355.9)
>   lower limb (355.71)
>   complex regional pain syndrome type II of the lower limb (355.71)
> **DEF:** Peripheral nerve damage, upper limb; usually due to injury; causes burning sensation and trophic skin changes.

354.5 Mononeuritis multiplex
> Combinations of single conditions classifiable to 354 or 355

354.8 Other mononeuritis of upper limb

354.9 Mononeuritis of upper limb, unspecified

√4ᵗʰ **355 Mononeuritis of lower limb**

355.0 Lesion of sciatic nerve
> **EXCLUDES** sciatica NOS (724.3)
> **DEF:** Acquired disorder of sciatic nerve; causes motor and sensory dysfunction in back, buttock and leg.
> **AHA:** 2Q, '89, 12

355.1 Meralgia paresthetica
> Lateral cutaneous femoral nerve of thigh compression or syndrome
> **DEF:** Inguinal ligament entraps lateral femoral cutaneous nerve; causes tingling, pain and numbness along outer thigh.

355.2 Other lesion of femoral nerve

355.3 Lesion of lateral popliteal nerve
> Lesion of common peroneal nerve

355.4 Lesion of medial popliteal nerve

355.5 Tarsal tunnel syndrome
> **DEF:** Compressed, entrapped posterior tibial nerve; causes tingling, pain and numbness in sole of foot.

355.6 Lesion of plantar nerve
> Morton's metatarsalgia, neuralgia, or neuroma

√5ᵗʰ **355.7 Other mononeuritis of lower limb**

355.71 Causalgia of lower limb
> **EXCLUDES** causalgia:
>   NOS (355.9)
>   upper limb (354.4)
>   complex regional pain syndrome type II of upper limb (354.4)
> **DEF:** Dysfunction of lower limb peripheral nerve, usually due to injury; causes burning pain and trophic skin changes.

355.79 Other mononeuritis of lower limb

355.8 Mononeuritis of lower limb, unspecified

355.9 Mononeuritis of unspecified site
> Causalgia NOS   Complex regional pain syndrome NOS
> **EXCLUDES** causalgia:
>   lower limb (355.71)
>   upper limb (354.4)
>   complex regional pain syndrome:
>   lower limb (355.71)
>   upper limb (354.4)
> G58.9 Mononeuropathy unspecified   I-10

√4ᵗʰ **356 Hereditary and idiopathic peripheral neuropathy**

356.0 Hereditary peripheral neuropathy
> Déjérine-Sottas disease

356.1 Peroneal muscular atrophy
> Charcôt-Marie-Tooth disease
> Neuropathic muscular atrophy
> **DEF:** Genetic disorder, in muscles innervated by peroneal nerves; symptoms include muscle wasting in lower limbs and locomotor difficulties.

356.2 Hereditary sensory neuropathy
> **DEF:** Inherited disorder in dorsal root ganglia, optic nerve, and cerebellum, causing sensory losses, shooting pains, and foot ulcers.

356.3 Refsum's disease   CC
> Heredopathia atactica polyneuritiformis
> **DEF:** Genetic disorder of lipid metabolism; causes persistent, painful inflammation of nerves and retinitis pigmentosa.
> **CC Exd:** 350.1-357.9

356.4 Idiopathic progressive polyneuropathy

356.8 Other specified idiopathic peripheral neuropathy
> Supranuclear paralysis

356.9 Unspecified
> G60.9 Hereditary & idiopathic neuropathy unspecified   I-10

√4ᵗʰ **357 Inflammatory and toxic neuropathy**

357.0 Acute infective polyneuritis   CC
> Guillain-Barré syndrome
> Postinfectious polyneuritis
> **DEF:** Guillain-Barré syndrome: acute demyelinating polyneuropathy preceded by viral illness (i.e., herpes, cytomegalovirus [CMV], Epstein-Barr virus [EBV]) or a bacterial illness; areflexic motor paralysis with mild sensory disturbance and acellular rise in spinal fluid protein.
> **CC Exd:** 003.21, 013.00-013.16, 036.0, 036.89-036.9, 041.81-041.9, 047.0-047.9, 049.0-049.1, 053.0, 054.72, 072.1, 090.42, 091.81, 094.2, 098.89, 100.81, 112.83, 114.2, 115.01, 115.11, 115.91, 130.0, 139.8, 320.0-322.9, 349.89-349.9, 357.0
> **AHA:** 2Q, '98, 12

357.1 Polyneuropathy in collagen vascular disease
> Code first underlying disease, as:
>   disseminated lupus erythematosus (710.0)
>   polyarteritis nodosa (446.0)
>   rheumatoid arthritis (714.0)

357.2 Polyneuropathy in diabetes
> Code first underlying disease (249.6, 250.6)
> **AHA:** 4Q, '09, 151; 2Q, '09, 13, 15; 3Q, '08, 5; 4Q, '03, 105; 2Q, '92, 15; 3Q, '91, 9

357.3 Polyneuropathy in malignant disease
> Code first underlying disease (140.0-208.9)

Ⓝ Newborn Age: 0   Ⓟ Pediatric Age: 0-17   Ⓜ Maternity Age: 12-55   Ⓐ Adult Age: 15-124   MCC Major CC Condition   CC CC Condition   HIV HIV Related Dx

110 – Volume 1   **2014 ICD-9-CM**

357.4 Polyneuropathy in other diseases classified elsewhere

Code first underlying disease, as:
amyloidosis (277.30-277.39)
beriberi (265.0)
chronic uremia (585.9)
deficiency of B vitamins (266.0-266.9)
diphtheria (032.0-032.9)
hypoglycemia (251.2)
pellagra (265.2)
porphyria (277.1)
sarcoidosis (135)
uremia NOS (586)

EXCLUDES polyneuropathy in:
herpes zoster (053.13)
mumps (072.72)

AHA: 2Q, '08, 8; 2Q, '98, 15
G63 Polyneuropathy in diseases classified elsewhere   I-10

357.5 Alcoholic polyneuropathy

357.6 Polyneuropathy due to drugs

Use additional E code to identify drug

357.7 Polyneuropathy due to other toxic agents

Use additional E code to identify toxic agent

√5ᵗʰ 357.8 Other

AHA: 4Q, '02, 47; 2Q, '98, 12

357.81 Chronic inflammatory demyelinating   CC
polyneuritis

DEF: Inflammation of peripheral nerves resulting in
destruction of myelin sheath; associated with diabetes
mellitus, dysproteinemia, renal failure and malnutrition;
symptoms include tingling, numbness, burning pain,
diminished tendon reflexes, weakness, of lower
extremities.
CC Excl: 351.0-353.5, 353.8-356.9, 357.81-357.89

357.82 Critical illness polyneuropathy   CC
Acute motor neuropathy

DEF: An acute axonal neuropathy, both sensory and motor,
that is associated with Systemic Inflammatory Response
Syndrome (SIRS).
CC Excl: 351.0-353.5, 353.8-356.9, 357.81-357.9
AHA: 4Q, '03, 111

357.89 Other inflammatory and toxic neuropathy

357.9 Unspecified

√4ᵗʰ 358 Myoneural disorders

√5ᵗʰ 358.0 Myasthenia gravis

DEF: Autoimmune disorder of acetylcholine at neuromuscular
junction; causing fatigue of voluntary muscles.
AHA: 4Q, '03, 59

358.00 Myasthenia gravis without (acute) exacerbation
Myasthenia gravis NOS
G70.00 Myathenia gravis without (acute)   I-10
exacerbation

358.01 Myasthenia gravis with (acute) exacerbation   MCC
Myasthenia gravis in crisis
CC Excl: 249.60-249.61, 249.80-249.91, 250.60-250.63,
250.80-250.93, 349.89-349.9, 358.00-358.1, 358.30-358.39
AHA: 4Q, '07, 109; 1Q, '05, 4; 4Q, '04, 139

358.1 Myasthenic syndromes in diseases classified elsewhere   CC

Code first underlying disease, as:
botulism (005.1, 040.41-040.42)
hypothyroidism (244.0-244.9)
malignant neoplasm (140.0-208.9)
pernicious anemia (281.0)
thyrotoxicosis (242.0-242.9)
CC Excl: See code: 358.01

358.2 Toxic myoneural disorders

Use additional E code to identify toxic agent

√5ᵗʰ 358.3 Lambert-Eaton syndrome
Eaton-Lambert syndrome
AHA: 4Q, '11, 100-101

358.30 Lambert-Eaton syndrome, unspecified   CC
Lambert-Eaton syndrome NOS
CC Excl: 249.60-249.61, 249.80-249.81, 249.90-249.91,
250.60-250.63, 250.80-250.83, 250.90-250.93,
349.89-349.9, 358.00-358.1, 358.30-358.39, 359.4, 359.6,
359.81
AHA: 4Q, '11, 101

358.31 Lambert-Eaton syndrome in neoplastic disease   CC
Code first the underlying neoplastic disease
CC Excl: See code: 358.30

358.39 Lambert-Eaton syndrome in other diseases   CC
classified elsewhere

Code first the underlying condition
CC Excl: See code: 358.30

358.8 Other specified myoneural disorders

358.9 Myoneural disorders, unspecified
AHA: 2Q, '02, 16

√4ᵗʰ 359 Muscular dystrophies and other myopathies

EXCLUDES idiopathic polymyositis (710.4)

359.0 Congenital hereditary muscular dystrophy   CC
Benign congenital myopathy
Central core disease
Centronuclear myopathy
Myotubular myopathy
Nemaline body disease

EXCLUDES arthrogryposis multiplex congenita (754.89)

DEF: Genetic disorder; causing progressive or nonprogressive muscle
weakness.
CC Excl: 249.60-249.61, 249.80-249.91, 250.60-250.63, 250.80-250.93,
349.89-349.9, 359.0-359.1

359.1 Hereditary progressive muscular dystrophy   CC

Muscular dystrophy:	Muscular dystrophy:
NOS	Gower's
distal	Landouzy-Déjérine
Duchenne	limb-girdle
Erb's	ocular
fascioscapulohumeral	oculopharyngeal

DEF: Genetic degenerative, muscle disease; causes progressive
weakness, wasting of muscle with no nerve involvement.
CC Excl: See code: 359.0

√5ᵗʰ 359.2 Myotonic disorders

EXCLUDES periodic paralysis (359.3)

DEF: Impaired movement due to spasmatic, rigid muscles.
AHA: 4Q, '07, 75

359.21 Myotonic muscular dystrophy
Dystrophia myotonica
Myotonia atrophica
Myotonic dystrophy
Proximal myotonic myopathy [PROMM]
Steinert's disease

359.22 Myotonia congenita
Acetazolamide responsive myotonia congenita
Dominant form [Thomsen's disease]
Myotonia levior
Recessive form [Becker's disease]

359.23 Myotonic chondrodystrophy
Congenital myotonic chondrodystrophy
Schwartz-Jampel disease

359.24 Drug induced myotonia
Use additional E code to identify drug

359.29 Other specified myotonic disorder
Myotonia fluctuans
Myotonia permanens
Paramyotonia congenita (of von Eulenburg)

Additional Digit Required   Unacceptable PDx   Manifestation Code   Hospital Acquired Condition   ►◄ Revised Text   ● New Code   ▲ Revised Code Title

14 ICD-9-CM   **Volume 1 – 111**

359.3 Periodic paralysis
Familial periodic paralysis
Hypokalemic familial periodic paralysis
Hyperkalemic periodic paralysis
Hypokalemic periodic paralysis
Potassium sensitive periodic paralysis
EXCLUDES *paramyotonia congenita (of von Eulenburg) (359.29)*
DEF: Genetic disorder; characterized by rapidly progressive flaccid paralysis; attacks often occur after exercise or exposure to cold or dietary changes.

359.4 Toxic myopathy   `CC`
Use additional E code to identify toxic agent
DEF: Muscle disorder caused by toxic agent.
CC Excl: 349.89-349.9, 358.00-359.6, 359.81-359.9
AHA: 1Q, '88, 5

359.5 Myopathy in endocrine diseases classified elsewhere
Code first underlying disease, as:
Addison's disease (255.41)
Cushing's syndrome (255.0)
hypopituitarism (253.2)
myxedema (244.0-244.9)
thyrotoxicosis (242.0-242.9)
DEF: Muscle disorder secondary to dysfunction in hormone secretion.

359.6 Symptomatic inflammatory myopathy in diseases classified elsewhere   `CC`
Code first underlying disease, as:
amyloidosis (277.30-277.39)
disseminated lupus erythematosus (710.0)
malignant neoplasm (140.0-208.9)
polyarteritis nodosa (446.0)
rheumatoid arthritis (714.0)
sarcoidosis (135)
scleroderma (710.1)
Sjögren's disease (710.2)
CC Excl: 249.60-249.61, 249.80-249.91, 250.60-250.63, 250.80-250.93, 349.89-349.9, 358.00-359.6, 359.81-359.9

✓5th 359.7 Inflammatory and immune myopathies, NEC

359.71 Inclusion body myositis
IBM
DEF: Progressive, debilitating inflammatory muscle disease characterized by dysphagia, chronic muscle swelling, weakness, and atrophy (wasting); impairs fine motor functions.
AHA: 4Q, '09, 84

359.79 Other inflammatory and immune myopathies, NEC
Inflammatory myopathy NOS

✓5th 359.8 Other myopathies
AHA: 4Q, '02, 47; 3Q, '90, 17

359.81 Critical illness myopathy   `CC`
Acute necrotizing myopathy
Acute quadriplegic myopathy
Intensive care (ICU) myopathy
Myopathy of critical illness
CC Excl: 358.1-359.6, 359.81-359.9

359.89 Other myopathies

359.9 Myopathy, unspecified

Disorders of the Eye and Adnexa (360-379)
Use additional external cause code, if applicable, to identify the cause of the eye condition

✓4th 360 Disorders of the globe
INCLUDES disorders affecting multiple structures of eye

✓5th 360.0 Purulent endophthalmitis
EXCLUDES *bleb associated endophthalmitis (379.63)*

360.00 Purulent endophthalmitis, unspecified   `CC`
CC Excl: 360.00-360.04, 360.13, 360.19, 364.05

360.01 Acute endophthalmitis   `CC`
CC Excl: See code 360.00

360.02 Panophthalmitis   `CC`
CC Excl: See code 360.00

360.03 Chronic endophthalmitis

Eye

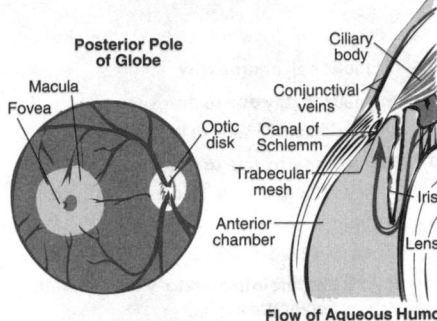

Posterior Pole of Globe

Flow of Aqueous Humor

360.04 Vitreous abscess
CC Excl: 360.00-360.19

✓5th 360.1 Other endophthalmitis
EXCLUDES *bleb associated endophthalmitis (379.63)*

360.11 Sympathetic uveitis
DEF: Inflammation of vascular layer of uninjured eye; follows injury to other eye.
CC Excl: 360.11-360.12

360.12 Panuveitis
DEF: Inflammation of entire vascular layer of eye, including choroid, iris and ciliary body.
CC Excl: 360.11-360.12

360.13 Parasitic endophthalmitis NOS
DEF: Parasitic infection causing inflammation of the entire eye.
CC Excl: 360.00-360.04, 360.13, 360.19, 364.05

360.14 Ophthalmia nodosa
DEF: Conjunctival inflammation caused by embedded hair

360.19 Other
Phacoanaphylactic endophthalmitis
CC Excl: 360.00-360.04, 360.13, 360.19, 364.05

✓5th 360.2 Degenerative disorders of globe
AHA: 3Q, '91, 3

360.20 Degenerative disorder of globe, unspecified

360.21 Progressive high (degenerative) myopia
Malignant myopia
DEF: Severe, progressive nearsightedness in adults, complicated by serious disease of the choroid; leads to retinal detachment and blindness.

360.23 Siderosis
DEF: Iron pigment deposits within tissue of eyeball; cause by high iron content of blood.

360.24 Other metallosis
Chalcosis
DEF: Metal deposits, other than iron, within eyeball tissue

360.29 Other
EXCLUDES *xerophthalmia (264.7)*

✓5th 360.3 Hypotony of eye

360.30 Hypotony, unspecified
DEF: Low osmotic pressure causing lack of tone, tension a strength.

360.31 Primary hypotony

N Newborn Age: 0   P Pediatric Age: 0-17   M Maternity Age: 12-55   A Adult Age: 15-124   MCC Major CC Condition   CC CC Condition   HIV HIV Related

112 – Volume 1   2014 ICD-9-

Adnexa

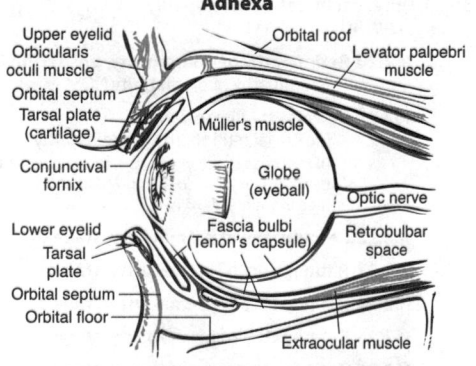

Upper eyelid
Orbicularis oculi muscle
Orbital septum
Tarsal plate (cartilage)
Conjunctival fornix
Lower eyelid
Tarsal plate
Orbital septum
Orbital floor

Orbital roof
Levator palpebri muscle
Müller's muscle
Globe (eyeball)
Fascia bulbi (Tenon's capsule)
Optic nerve
Retrobulbar space
Extraocular muscle

360.32 Ocular fistula causing hypotony
DEF: Low intraocular pressure due to leak through abnormal passage.

360.33 Hypotony associated with other ocular disorders

360.34 Flat anterior chamber
DEF: Low pressure behind cornea, causing compression.

√5ᵗʰ **360.4 Degenerated conditions of globe**

360.40 Degenerated globe or eye, unspecified

360.41 Blind hypotensive eye
Atrophy of globe   Phthisis bulbi
DEF: Vision loss due to extremely low intraocular pressure.

360.42 Blind hypertensive eye
Absolute glaucoma
DEF: Vision loss due to painful, high intraocular pressure.

360.43 Hemophthalmos, except current injury
EXCLUDES traumatic (871.0-871.9, 921.0-921.9)
DEF: Pool of blood within eyeball, not from current injury.

360.44 Leucocoria
DEF: Whitish mass or reflex in the pupil behind lens; also called cat's eye reflex; often indicative of retinoblastoma.

√5ᵗʰ **360.5 Retained (old) intraocular foreign body, magnetic**
Use additional code to identify foreign body (V90.11)
EXCLUDES current penetrating injury with magnetic foreign body (871.5)
retained (old) foreign body of orbit (376.6)

360.50 Foreign body, magnetic, intraocular, unspecified

360.51 Foreign body, magnetic, in anterior chamber

360.52 Foreign body, magnetic, in iris or ciliary body

360.53 Foreign body, magnetic, in lens

360.54 Foreign body, magnetic, in vitreous

360.55 Foreign body, magnetic, in posterior wall

360.59 Foreign body, magnetic, in other or multiple sites

√5ᵗʰ **360.6 Retained (old) intraocular foreign body, nonmagnetic**
Retained (old) foreign body:
NOS
nonmagnetic
Use additional code to identify foreign body (V90.01-V90.10, V90.12, V90.2-V90.9)
EXCLUDES current penetrating injury with (nonmagnetic) foreign body (871.6)
retained (old) foreign body in orbit (376.6)

360.60 Foreign body, intraocular, unspecified

360.61 Foreign body in anterior chamber

360.62 Foreign body in iris or ciliary body

360.63 Foreign body in lens

360.64 Foreign body in vitreous

360.65 Foreign body in posterior wall

360.69 Foreign body in other or multiple sites

√5ᵗʰ **360.8 Other disorders of globe**

360.81 Luxation of globe
DEF: Displacement of eyeball.

360.89 Other

360.9 Unspecified disorder of globe

√4ᵗʰ **361 Retinal detachments and defects**
DEF: Disorders of light-sensitive layer at back of eye, which separates from blood supply, disrupting vision.

√5ᵗʰ **361.0 Retinal detachment with retinal defect**
Rhegmatogenous retinal detachment
EXCLUDES detachment of retinal pigment epithelium (362.42-362.43)
retinal detachment (serous) (without defect) (361.2)

361.00 Retinal detachment with retinal defect, unspecified

361.01 Recent detachment, partial, with single defect

361.02 Recent detachment, partial, with multiple defects

361.03 Recent detachment, partial, with giant tear

361.04 Recent detachment, partial, with retinal dialysis
Dialysis (juvenile) of retina (with detachment)

361.05 Recent detachment, total or subtotal

361.06 Old detachment, partial
Delimited old retinal detachment

361.07 Old detachment, total or subtotal

√5ᵗʰ **361.1 Retinoschisis and retinal cysts**
EXCLUDES juvenile retinoschisis (362.73)
microcystoid degeneration of retina (362.62)
parasitic cyst of retina (360.13)

361.10 Retinoschisis, unspecified
DEF: Separation of retina due to degenerative process of aging; should not be confused with acute retinal detachment.

361.11 Flat retinoschisis
DEF: Slow, progressive split of retinal sensory layers.

361.12 Bullous retinoschisis
DEF: Fluid retention between split retinal sensory layers.

361.13 Primary retinal cysts

361.14 Secondary retinal cysts

361.19 Other
Pseudocyst of retina

361.2 Serous retinal detachment   CC
Retinal detachment without retinal defect
EXCLUDES central serous retinopathy (362.41)
retinal pigment epithelium detachment (362.42-362.43)
CC Excl: 361.00-361.9, 362.40-362.43

√5ᵗʰ **361.3 Retinal defects without detachment**
EXCLUDES chorioretinal scars after surgery for detachment (363.30-363.35)
peripheral retinal degeneration without defect (362.60-362.66)

361.30 Retinal defect, unspecified
Retinal break(s) NOS

361.31 Round hole of retina without detachment

361.32 Horseshoe tear of retina without detachment
Operculum of retina without mention of detachment

361.33 Multiple defects of retina without detachment

√5ᵗʰ **361.8 Other forms of retinal detachment**

361.81 Traction detachment of retina   CC
Traction detachment with vitreoretinal organization
CC Excl: 361.00-361.9, 362.40-362.43

361.89 Other   CC
CC Excl: 361.00-361.9, 362.40-362.43
AHA: 3Q, '99, 12

361.9 Unspecified retinal detachment   CC
CC Excl: 361.00-361.9, 362.40-362.43
AHA: N-D, '87, 10

Additional Digit Required   Unacceptable PDx   Manifestation Code   Hospital Acquired Condition   ►◄ Revised Text   ● New Code   ▲ Revised Code Title

14 ICD-9-CM   Volume 1 – 113

Diseases of the Nervous System and Sense Organs

362–362.50

√4ᵗʰ **362 Other retinal disorders**

EXCLUDES chorioretinal scars (363.30-363.35)
chorioretinitis (363.0-363.2)

√5ᵗʰ **362.0 Diabetic retinopathy**
Code first diabetes (249.5, 250.5)
DEF: Retinal changes in diabetes of long duration; causes hemorrhages, microaneurysms, waxy deposits and proliferative noninflammatory degenerative disease of retina.
AHA: 4Q, '05, 65; 3Q, '91, 8

362.01 Background diabetic retinopathy
Diabetic retinal microaneurysms
Diabetic retinopathy NOS

362.02 Proliferative diabetic retinopathy
DEF: Occurrence of the ischemic effects of vessel blockages result in neovascularization; new blood vessels begin to form to compensate for restricted blood flow; multiple areas of the retina and inner vitreous may be affected.
AHA: 3Q, '96, 5

362.03 Nonproliferative diabetic retinopathy NOS

362.04 Mild nonproliferative diabetic retinopathy
DEF: Early stages of degenerative condition of the retina due to diabetes; microaneurysm formation; small balloon-like swelling of the retinal vessels.

362.05 Moderate nonproliferative diabetic retinopathy
DEF: Stage of degenerative condition of the retina due to diabetes with pronounced microaneurysms; vessel blockages can occur.

362.06 Severe nonproliferative diabetic retinopathy
DEF: Stage of degenerative condition of the retina due to diabetes in which vascular breakdown in the retina results in multiple vascular blockages, or "beadings," with intraretinal hemorrhages.
AHA: 4Q, '05, 67

362.07 Diabetic macular edema
NOTE Code 362.07 must be used with a code for diabetic retinopathy (362.01-362.06)
Diabetic retinal edema
DEF: Leakage from retinal blood vessels causes swelling of the macula and impaired vision; exudates or plaques may develop in the posterior pole of the retina due to the breakdown of retinal vasculature.

√5ᵗʰ **362.1 Other background retinopathy and retinal vascular changes**

362.10 Background retinopathy, unspecified
AHA: 1Q, '06, 12

362.11 Hypertensive retinopathy
DEF: Retinal irregularities caused by systemic hypertension.
AHA: 3Q, '90, 3

362.12 Exudative retinopathy
Coats' syndrome
AHA: 3Q, '99, 12

362.13 Changes in vascular appearance
Vascular sheathing of retina
Use additional code for any associated atherosclerosis (440.8)

362.14 Retinal microaneurysms NOS
DEF: Microscopic dilation of retinal vessels in nondiabetic.

362.15 Retinal telangiectasia
DEF: Dilation of blood vessels of the retina.

362.16 Retinal neovascularization NOS
Neovascularization: Neovascularization:
choroidal   subretinal
DEF: New and abnormal vascular growth in the retina.

362.17 Other intraretinal microvascular abnormalities
Retinal sclerosis   Retinal varices

362.18 Retinal vasculitis
Eales' disease   Retinal:
Retinal: perivasculitis
arteritis   phlebitis
endarteritis
DEF: Inflammation of retinal blood vessels.

√5ᵗʰ **362.2 Other proliferative retinopathy**
AHA: 4Q, '08, 110-111

362.20 Retinopathy of prematurity, unspecified
Retinopathy of prematurity NOS

362.21 Retrolental fibroplasia
Cicatricial retinopathy of prematurity
DEF: Fibrous tissue in vitreous, from retina to lens, causing blindness; associated with premature infants requiring high amounts of oxygen.

362.22 Retinopathy of prematurity, stage 0

362.23 Retinopathy of prematurity, stage 1

362.24 Retinopathy of prematurity, stage 2

362.25 Retinopathy of prematurity, stage 3

362.26 Retinopathy of prematurity, stage 4

362.27 Retinopathy of prematurity, stage 5

362.29 Other nondiabetic proliferative retinopathy
AHA: 3Q, '96, 5

√5ᵗʰ **362.3 Retinal vascular occlusion**
DEF: Obstructed blood flow to and from retina.

362.30 Retinal vascular occlusion, unspecified
CC Exd: 362.30-362.37

362.31 Central retinal artery occlusion
CC Exd: See code: 362.30

362.32 Arterial branch occlusion
CC Exd: See code: 362.30

362.33 Partial arterial occlusion
Hollenhorst plaque
Retinal microembolism
CC Exd: See code: 362.30

362.34 Transient arterial occlusion
Amaurosis fugax
CC Exd: See code: 362.30
AHA: 1Q, '00, 16

362.35 Central retinal vein occlusion
CC Exd: See code: 362.30
AHA: 2Q, '93, 6

362.36 Venous tributary (branch) occlusion

362.37 Venous engorgement
Occlusion:
incipient   } of retinal vein
partial

√5ᵗʰ **362.4 Separation of retinal layers**
EXCLUDES retinal detachment (serous) (361.2)
rhegmatogenous (361.00-361.07)

362.40 Retinal layer separation, unspecified
CC Exd: 361.00-361.9, 362.40-362.43

362.41 Central serous retinopathy
DEF: Serous-filled blister causing detachment of retina fro pigment epithelium.

362.42 Serous detachment of retinal pigment epithelium
Exudative detachment of retinal pigment epithelium
CC Exd: See code: 362.40
DEF: Blister of fatty fluid causing detachment of retina fro pigment epithelium.

362.43 Hemorrhagic detachment of retinal pigment epithelium
CC Exd: See code: 362.40
DEF: Blood-filled blister causing detachment of retina fro pigment epithelium.

√5ᵗʰ **362.5 Degeneration of macula and posterior pole**
EXCLUDES degeneration of optic disc (377.21-377.24)
hereditary retinal degeneration [dystrophy] (362.70-362.77)

362.50 Macular degeneration (senile), unspecified

N Newborn Age: 0   P Pediatric Age: 0-17   M Maternity Age: 12-55   A Adult Age: 15-124   MCC Major CC Condition   CC CC Condition   HIV HIV Related I

114 – Volume 1   2014 ICD-9-C

362.51 Nonexudative senile macular degeneration
Senile macular degeneration:
atrophic
dry

362.52 Exudative senile macular degeneration
Kuhnt-Junius degeneration
Senile macular degeneration:
disciform
wet
DEF: Leakage in macular blood vessels with loss of visual acuity.

362.53 Cystoid macular degeneration
Cystoid macular edema
DEF: Retinal swelling and cyst formation in macula.

362.54 Macular cyst, hole, or pseudohole
AHA: 4Q, '11, 106

362.55 Toxic maculopathy
Use additional E code to identify drug, if drug induced

362.56 Macular puckering
Preretinal fibrosis

362.57 Drusen (degenerative)
DEF: White, hyaline deposits on Bruch's membrane (lamina basalis choroideae).

√5ᵗʰ **362.6 Peripheral retinal degenerations**
EXCLUDES *hereditary retinal degeneration [dystrophy] (362.70-362.77)*
retinal degeneration with retinal defect (361.00-361.07)

362.60 Peripheral retinal degeneration, unspecified

362.61 Paving stone degeneration
DEF: Degeneration of peripheral retina; causes thinning through which choroid is visible.

362.62 Microcystoid degeneration
Blessig's cysts   Iwanoff's cysts

362.63 Lattice degeneration
Palisade degeneration of retina
DEF: Degeneration of retina; often bilateral, usually benign; characterized by lines intersecting at irregular intervals in peripheral retina; retinal thinning and retinal holes may occur.

362.64 Senile reticular degeneration
DEF: Net-like appearance of retina; sign of degeneration.

362.65 Secondary pigmentary degeneration
Pseudoretinitis pigmentosa

362.66 Secondary vitreoretinal degenerations

√5ᵗʰ **362.7 Hereditary retinal dystrophies**
DEF: Genetically induced progressive changes in retina.

362.70 Hereditary retinal dystrophy, unspecified

362.71 Retinal dystrophy in systemic or cerebroretinal lipidoses
Code first underlying disease, as:
cerebroretinal lipidoses (330.1)
systemic lipidoses (272.7)

362.72 Retinal dystrophy in other systemic disorders and syndromes
Code first underlying disease, as:
Bassen-Kornzweig syndrome (272.5)
Refsum's disease (356.3)

362.73 Vitreoretinal dystrophies
Juvenile retinoschisis

362.74 Pigmentary retinal dystrophy
Retinal dystrophy, albipunctate
Retinitis pigmentosa

362.75 Other dystrophies primarily involving the sensory retina
Progressive cone(-rod) dystrophy
Stargardt's disease

362.76 Dystrophies primarily involving the retinal pigment epithelium
Fundus flavimaculatus   Vitelliform dystrophy

362.77 Dystrophies primarily involving Bruch's membrane
Dystrophy:
hyaline
pseudoinflammatory foveal
Hereditary drusen

√5ᵗʰ **362.8 Other retinal disorders**
EXCLUDES *chorioretinal inflammations (363.0-363.2)*
chorioretinal scars (363.30-363.35)

362.81 Retinal hemorrhage
Hemorrhage:
preretinal
retinal (deep) (superficial)
subretinal
AHA: 4Q, '96, 43

362.82 Retinal exudates and deposits

362.83 Retinal edema
Retinal:
cotton wool spots
edema (localized) (macular) (peripheral)
DEF: Retinal swelling due to fluid accumulation.

362.84 Retinal ischemia   CC
CC Excl: 362.81-362.89
DEF: Reduced retinal blood supply.

362.85 Retinal nerve fiber bundle defects

362.89 Other retinal disorders

362.9 Unspecified retinal disorder

√4ᵗʰ **363 Chorioretinal inflammations, scars, and other disorders of choroid**

√5ᵗʰ **363.0 Focal chorioretinitis and focal retinochoroiditis**
EXCLUDES *focal chorioretinitis or retinochoroiditis in:*
histoplasmosis (115.02, 115.12, 115.92)
toxoplasmosis (130.2)
congenital infection (771.2)

363.00 Focal chorioretinitis, unspecified
Focal:
choroiditis or chorioretinitis NOS
retinitis or retinochoroiditis NOS

363.01 Focal choroiditis and chorioretinitis, juxtapapillary

363.03 Focal choroiditis and chorioretinitis of other posterior pole

363.04 Focal choroiditis and chorioretinitis, peripheral

363.05 Focal retinitis and retinochoroiditis, juxtapapillary
Neuroretinitis

363.06 Focal retinitis and retinochoroiditis, macular or paramacular

363.07 Focal retinitis and retinochoroiditis of other posterior pole

363.08 Focal retinitis and retinochoroiditis, peripheral

√5ᵗʰ **363.1 Disseminated chorioretinitis and disseminated retinochoroiditis**
EXCLUDES *disseminated choroiditis or chorioretinitis in:*
secondary syphilis (091.51)
neurosyphilitic disseminated retinitis or retinochoroiditis (094.83)
retinal (peri)vasculitis (362.18)

363.10 Disseminated chorioretinitis, unspecified   CC
Disseminated:
choroiditis or chorioretinitis NOS
retinitis or retinochoroiditis NOS
CC Excl: 363.00-363.22

363.11 Disseminated choroiditis and chorioretinitis, posterior pole   CC
CC Excl: See code: 363.10

363.12 Disseminated choroiditis and chorioretinitis, peripheral   CC
CC Excl: See code: 363.10

√4ᵗʰ √5ᵗʰ Additional Digit Required   Unacceptable PDx   Manifestation Code   Hospital Acquired Condition   ►◄ Revised Text   ● New Code   ▲ Revised Code Title

2014 ICD-9-CM   **Volume 1 – 115**

Diseases of the Nervous System and Sense Organs

363.13–364.11

363.13 Disseminated choroiditis and chorioretinitis, generalized `CC`
Code first any underlying disease, as:
tuberculosis (017.3)
CC Exd: See code: 363.10

363.14 Disseminated retinitis and retinochoroiditis, metastatic `CC`
CC Exd: See code: 363.10

363.15 Disseminated retinitis and retinochoroiditis, pigment epitheliopathy `CC`
Acute posterior multifocal placoid pigment epitheliopathy
DEF: Widespread inflammation of retina and choroid; characterized by pigmented epithelium involvement.
CC Exd: See code: 363.10

√5ᵗʰ **363.2 Other and unspecified forms of chorioretinitis and retinochoroiditis**
EXCLUDES   panophthalmitis (360.02)
sympathetic uveitis (360.11)
uveitis NOS (364.3)

363.20 Chorioretinitis, unspecified `CC`
Choroiditis NOS
Retinitis NOS
Uveitis, posterior NOS
CC Exd: See code: 363.10

363.21 Pars planitis
Posterior cyclitis
DEF: Inflammation of peripheral retina and ciliary body; characterized by bands of white cells.

363.22 Harada's disease
DEF: Retinal detachment and bilateral widespread exudative choroiditis; symptoms include headache, vomiting, increased lymphocytes in cerebrospinal fluid; with temporary or permanent deafness.

√5ᵗʰ **363.3 Chorioretinal scars**
Scar (postinflammatory) (postsurgical) (posttraumatic):
choroid
retina

363.30 Chorioretinal scar, unspecified

363.31 Solar retinopathy
DEF: Retinal scarring caused by solar radiation.

363.32 Other macular scars

363.33 Other scars of posterior pole

363.34 Peripheral scars

363.35 Disseminated scars

√5ᵗʰ **363.4 Choroidal degenerations**

363.40 Choroidal degeneration, unspecified
Choroidal sclerosis NOS

363.41 Senile atrophy of choroid
DEF: Wasting away of choroid; due to aging.

363.42 Diffuse secondary atrophy of choroid
DEF: Wasting away of choroid in systemic disease.

363.43 Angioid streaks of choroid
DEF: Degeneration of choroid; characterized by dark brown steaks radiating from optic disc; occurs with pseudoxanthoma, elasticum or Paget's disease.

√5ᵗʰ **363.5 Hereditary choroidal dystrophies**
Hereditary choroidal atrophy:
partial [choriocapillaris]
total [all vessels]

363.50 Hereditary choroidal dystrophy or atrophy, unspecified

363.51 Circumpapillary dystrophy of choroid, partial

363.52 Circumpapillary dystrophy of choroid, total
Helicoid dystrophy of choroid

363.53 Central dystrophy of choroid, partial
Dystrophy, choroidal:
central areolar
circinate

363.54 Central choroidal atrophy, total
Dystrophy, choroidal: Dystrophy, choroidal:
central gyrate   serpiginous

363.55 Choroideremia
DEF: Hereditary choroid degeneration, occurs in first decade; characterized by constricted visual field and ultimately blindness in males; less debilitating in females.

363.56 Other diffuse or generalized dystrophy, partial
Diffuse choroidal sclerosis

363.57 Other diffuse or generalized dystrophy, total
Generalized gyrate atrophy, choroid

√5ᵗʰ **363.6 Choroidal hemorrhage and rupture**

363.61 Choroidal hemorrhage, unspecified

363.62 Expulsive choroidal hemorrhage

363.63 Choroidal rupture `CC`
CC Exd: 363.61-363.9

√5ᵗʰ **363.7 Choroidal detachment**

363.70 Choroidal detachment, unspecified `CC`
CC Exd: See code: 363.63

363.71 Serous choroidal detachment `CC`
DEF: Detachment of choroid from sclera; due to blister of serous fluid.
CC Exd: See code: 363.63

363.72 Hemorrhagic choroidal detachment `CC`
DEF: Detachment of choroid from sclera; due to blood-filled blister.
CC Exd: See code: 363.63

363.8 Other disorders of choroid
AHA: 1Q, '06, 12

363.9 Unspecified disorder of choroid

√4ᵗʰ **364 Disorders of iris and ciliary body**

√5ᵗʰ **364.0 Acute and subacute iridocyclitis**
Anterior uveitis
Cylitis
Iridocyclitis   } acute, subacute
Iritis
EXCLUDES   gonococcal (098.41)
herpes simplex (054.44)
herpes zoster (053.22)

364.00 Acute and subacute iridocyclitis, unspecified `CC`
CC Exd: 364.00-364.3

364.01 Primary iridocyclitis `CC`
CC Exd: See code: 364.00

364.02 Recurrent iridocyclitis `CC`
CC Exd: See code: 364.00

364.03 Secondary iridocyclitis, infectious `CC`
CC Exd: See code: 364.00

364.04 Secondary iridocyclitis, noninfectious
Aqueous: Aqueous:
cells   flare
fibrin

364.05 Hypopyon
DEF: Accumulation of white blood cells between cornea and lens.

√5ᵗʰ **364.1 Chronic iridocyclitis**
EXCLUDES   posterior cyclitis (363.21)

364.10 Chronic iridocyclitis, unspecified

364.11 Chronic iridocyclitis in diseases classified elsewhere
Code first underlying disease, as:
sarcoidosis (135)
tuberculosis (017.3)
EXCLUDES   syphilitic iridocyclitis (091.52)
DEF: Persistent inflammation of iris and ciliary body; due to underlying disease or condition.

√5ᵗʰ **364.2 Certain types of iridocyclitis**
> **EXCLUDES** posterior cyclitis (363.21)
> sympathetic uveitis (360.11)

364.21 Fuchs' heterochromic cyclitis
> **DEF:** Chronic cyclitis characterized by differences in the color of the two irises; the lighter iris appears in the inflamed eye.

364.22 Glaucomatocyclitic crises   CC
> **DEF:** An uncommon inflammatory unilateral eye condition, characteristic recurrent episodes of high intraocular pressure accompanied by mild inflammation.
> **CC Excl:** See code: 364.00

364.23 Lens-induced iridocyclitis
> **DEF:** Inflammation of iris; due to immune reaction to proteins in lens following trauma or other lens abnormality.

364.24 Vogt-Koyanagi syndrome
> **DEF:** Uveomeningitis with exudative iridocyclitis and choroiditis; causes depigmentation of hair and skin, detached retina; tinnitus and loss of hearing.

364.3 Unspecified iridocyclitis   CC
> Uveitis NOS
> **CC Excl:** See code: 364.00-364.3

√5ᵗʰ **364.4 Vascular disorders of iris and ciliary body**

364.41 Hyphema
> Hemorrhage of iris or ciliary body
> **DEF:** Hemorrhage in anterior chamber; also called hyphemia or "blood shot" eyes.

364.42 Rubeosis iridis
> Neovascularization of iris or ciliary body
> **DEF:** Blood vessel and connective tissue formation on surface of iris; symptomatic of diabetic retinopathy, central retinal vein occlusion and retinal detachment.

√5ᵗʰ **364.5 Degenerations of iris and ciliary body**

364.51 Essential or progressive iris atrophy

364.52 Iridoschisis
> **DEF:** Splitting of the iris into two layers.

364.53 Pigmentary iris degeneration
> Acquired heterochromia
> Pigment dispersion syndrome } of iris
> Translucency

364.54 Degeneration of pupillary margin
> Atrophy of sphincter
> Ectropion of pigment epithelium } of iris

364.55 Miotic cysts of pupillary margin
> **DEF:** Serous-filled sacs in pupillary margin of iris.

364.56 Degenerative changes of chamber angle

364.57 Degenerative changes of ciliary body

364.59 Other iris atrophy
> Iris atrophy (generalized) (sector shaped)

√5ᵗʰ **364.6 Cysts of iris, ciliary body, and anterior chamber**
> **EXCLUDES** miotic pupillary cyst (364.55)
> parasitic cyst (360.13)

364.60 Idiopathic cysts
> **DEF:** Fluid-filled sacs in iris or ciliary body; unknown etiology.

364.61 Implantation cysts
> Epithelial down-growth, anterior chamber
> Implantation cysts (surgical) (traumatic)

364.62 Exudative cysts of iris or anterior chamber

364.63 Primary cyst of pars plana
> **DEF:** Fluid-filled sacs of outermost ciliary ring.

364.64 Exudative cyst of pars plana
> **DEF:** Protein, fatty-filled sacs of outermost ciliary ring; due to fluid leak from blood vessels.

√5ᵗʰ **364.7 Adhesions and disruptions of iris and ciliary body**
> **EXCLUDES** flat anterior chamber (360.34)

364.70 Adhesions of iris, unspecified
> Synechiae (iris) NOS

Plateau Iris Syndrome

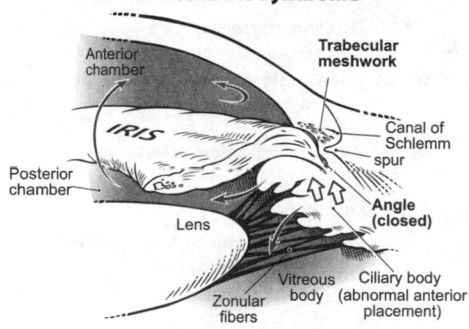

364.71 Posterior synechiae
> **DEF:** Adhesion binding iris to lens.

364.72 Anterior synechiae
> **DEF:** Adhesion binding the iris to cornea.

364.73 Goniosynechiae
> Peripheral anterior synechiae
> **DEF:** Adhesion binding the iris to cornea at the angle of the anterior chamber.

364.74 Pupillary membranes
> Iris bombé   Pupillary:
> Pupillary: seclusion
>   occlusion
> **DEF:** Membrane traversing the pupil and blocking vision.

364.75 Pupillary abnormalities
> Deformed pupil   Rupture of sphincter, pupil
> Ectopic pupil

364.76 Iridodialysis
> **DEF:** Separation of the iris from the ciliary body base; due to trauma or surgical accident.

364.77 Recession of chamber angle
> **DEF:** Receding of anterior chamber angle of the eye; restricts vision.

√5ᵗʰ **364.8 Other disorders of iris and ciliary body**
> **AHA:** 2Q, '07, 9

364.81 Floppy iris syndrome
> Intraoperative floppy iris syndrome [IFIS]
> Use additional E code to identify cause, such as: sympatholytics [antiadrenergics] causing adverse effect in therapeutic use (E941.3)
> **DEF:** Condition complicating cataract surgery for patients who have received alpha blocker treatment for urinary retention problems; iris dilator muscle fails to dilate, and the iris may billow or flap.
> **AHA:** 4Q, '07, 77, 79

364.82 Plateau iris syndrome
> **DEF:** A postoperative chronic angle-closure glaucoma characterized by closing of the anterior chamber angle secondary to a large or anteriorly positioned ciliary body that impairs the normal flow of aqueous fluid.
> **AHA:** 4Q, '08, 112

364.89 Other disorders of iris and ciliary body
> Prolapse of iris NOS
> **EXCLUDES** prolapse of iris in recent wound (871.1)

364.9 Unspecified disorder of iris and ciliary body

√4ᵗʰ **365 Glaucoma**
> **EXCLUDES** blind hypertensive eye [absolute glaucoma] (360.42)
> congenital glaucoma (743.20-743.22)
> **DEF:** Rise in intraocular pressure restricting blood flow; multiple causes.

√5ᵗʰ **365.0 Borderline glaucoma [glaucoma suspect]**
> **AHA:** 1Q, '90, 8

365.00 Preglaucoma, unspecified

365.01 Open angle with borderline findings, low risk
> Open angle, low risk
> **DEF:** Minor block of aqueous outflow from eye.
> **AHA:** 4Q, '11, 102

365.02 Anatomical narrow angle
> Primary angle closure suspect

Diseases of the Nervous System and Sense Organs   **365.03–365.71**

365.03 Steroid responders

365.04 Ocular hypertension
DEF: High fluid pressure within eye; no clear cause.

365.05 Open angle with borderline findings, high risk
Open angle, high risk
AHA: 4Q, '11, 102-103

365.06 Primary angle closure without glaucoma damage
AHA: 4Q, '11, 102-103

√5ᵗʰ **365.1 Open-angle glaucoma**

365.10 Open-angle glaucoma, unspecified
Wide-angle glaucoma NOS
Use additional code to identify glaucoma stage (365.70-365.74)

365.11 Primary open angle glaucoma
Chronic simple glaucoma
Use additional code to identify glaucoma stage (365.70-365.74)
DEF: High intraocular pressure, despite free flow of aqueous.

365.12 Low tension glaucoma
Use additional code to identify glaucoma stage (365.70-365.74)

365.13 Pigmentary glaucoma
Use additional code to identify glaucoma stage (365.70-365.74)
DEF: High intraocular pressure; due to iris pigment granules blocking aqueous flow.

365.14 Glaucoma of childhood
Infantile or juvenile glaucoma

365.15 Residual stage of open angle glaucoma

√5ᵗʰ **365.2 Primary angle-closure glaucoma**
DEF: Glaucoma caused by a shift in the position of the iris of the eye that blocks the surface of the trabecular meshwork causing impairment of the normal flow of aqueous fluid.

365.20 Primary angle-closure glaucoma, unspecified
Use additional code to identify glaucoma stage (365.70-365.74)

365.21 Intermittent angle-closure glaucoma
Angle-closure glaucoma:
   interval
   subacute
DEF: Recurring attacks of high intraocular pressure; due to blocked aqueous flow.

365.22 Acute angle-closure glaucoma   CC
Acute angle-closure glaucoma attack
Acute angle-closure glaucoma crisis
DEF: Sudden, severe rise in intraocular pressure due to blockage in aqueous drainage.
CC Exd: See code: 365.22

365.23 Chronic angle-closure glaucoma
Chronic primary angle closure glaucoma
Use additional code to identify glaucoma stage (365.70-365.74)
AHA: 2Q, '98, 16

365.24 Residual stage of angle-closure glaucoma

√5ᵗʰ **365.3 Corticosteroid-induced glaucoma**
DEF: Elevated intraocular pressure; due to long-term corticosteroid therapy.

365.31 Glaucomatous stage
Use additional code to identify glaucoma stage (365.70-365.74)

365.32 Residual stage

√5ᵗʰ **365.4 Glaucoma associated with congenital anomalies, dystrophies, and systemic syndromes**

365.41 Glaucoma associated with chamber angle anomalies

365.42 Glaucoma associated with anomalies of iris

365.43 Glaucoma associated with other anterior segment anomalies

Normal Aqueous Flow

Angle-Closure Glaucoma

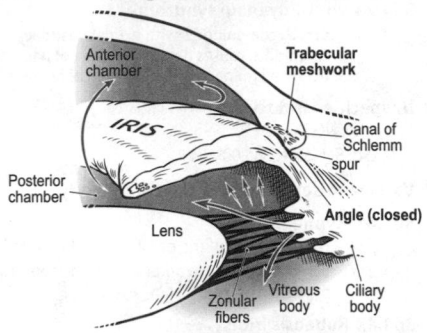

365.44 *Glaucoma associated with systemic syndromes*
Code first associated disease, as
   neurofibromatosis (237.70-237.79)
   Sturge-Weber (-Dimitri) syndrome (759.6)

√5ᵗʰ **365.5 Glaucoma associated with disorders of the lens**

365.51 Phacolytic glaucoma
DEF: Elevated intraocular pressure; due to lens protein blocking aqueous flow.

365.52 Pseudoexfoliation glaucoma
Use additional code to identify glaucoma stage (365.70-365.74)
DEF: Glaucoma characterized by small grayish particles deposited on the lens.

365.59 Glaucoma associated with other lens disorders

√5ᵗʰ **365.6 Glaucoma associated with other ocular disorders**

365.60 Glaucoma associated with unspecified ocular disorder

365.61 Glaucoma associated with pupillary block
DEF: Acute, open-angle glaucoma caused by mature cataract; aqueous flow is blocked by lens material and macrophages.

365.62 Glaucoma associated with ocular inflammations
Use additional code to identify glaucoma stage (365.70-365.74)

365.63 Glaucoma associated with vascular disorders
Use additional code to identify glaucoma stage (365.70-365.74)

365.64 Glaucoma associated with tumors or cysts

365.65 Glaucoma associated with ocular trauma
Use additional code to identify glaucoma stage (365.70-365.74)

√5ᵗʰ **365.7 Glaucoma stage**
Code first associated type of glaucoma (365.10-365.13, 365.20, 365.23, 365.31, 365.52, 365.62-365.63, 365.65)
AHA: 4Q, '11, 101-105
TIP: If a patient has bilateral glaucoma with different stages or the stage evolves during the encounter from one stage to another, assign one code for the highest stage documented.

365.70 Glaucoma stage, unspecified
Glaucoma stage NOS

365.71 Mild stage glaucoma
Early stage glaucoma

N Newborn Age: 0   P Pediatric Age: 0-17   M Maternity Age: 12-55   A Adult Age: 15-124   MCC Major CC Condition   CC CC Condition   HIV HIV Related Dx

118 – Volume 1   **2014 ICD-9-CM**

Cataract

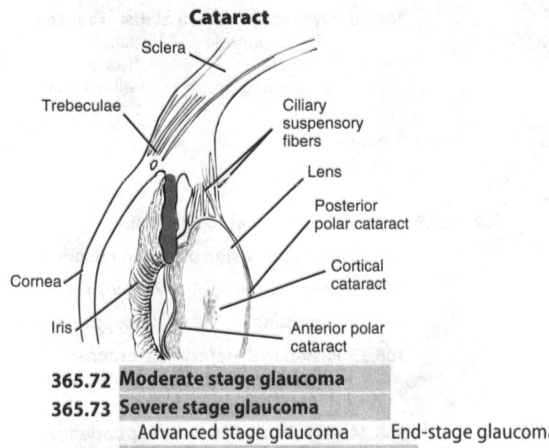

Sclera
Trebeculae
Ciliary suspensory fibers
Lens
Posterior polar cataract
Cortical cataract
Cornea
Iris
Anterior polar cataract

365.72 Moderate stage glaucoma

365.73 Severe stage glaucoma
Advanced stage glaucoma   End-stage glaucoma

365.74 Indeterminate stage glaucoma

√5ᵗʰ **365.8 Other specified forms of glaucoma**

365.81 Hypersecretion glaucoma

365.82 Glaucoma with increased episcleral venous pressure

365.83 Aqueous misdirection
Malignant glaucoma
DEF: A form of secondary angle-closure glaucoma that occurs when aqueous humor flows into the posterior chamber of the eye (vitreous) rather than through the normal recycling channels.
AHA: 4Q, '02, 48

365.89 Other specified glaucoma
AHA: 2Q, '98, 16

365.9 Unspecified glaucoma
AHA: 3Q, '03, 14; 2Q, '01, 16
H40.9 Unspecified glaucoma   I-10

√4ᵗʰ **366 Cataract**
EXCLUDES congenital cataract (743.30-743.34)
DEF: A variety of conditions that create a cloudy, or calcified lens that obstructs vision.

√5ᵗʰ **366.0 Infantile, juvenile, and presenile cataract**

366.00 Nonsenile cataract, unspecified

366.01 Anterior subcapsular polar cataract
DEF: Defect within the front, center lens surface.

366.02 Posterior subcapsular polar cataract
DEF: Defect within the rear, center lens surface.

366.03 Cortical, lamellar, or zonular cataract
DEF: Opacities radiating from center to edge of lens; appear as thin, concentric layers of lens.

366.04 Nuclear cataract

366.09 Other and combined forms of nonsenile cataract

√5ᵗʰ **366.1 Senile cataract**
AHA: 3Q, '91, 9; S-0, '85, 10

366.10 Senile cataract, unspecified   A
AHA: 1Q, '03, 5

366.11 Pseudoexfoliation of lens capsule   A

366.12 Incipient cataract   A
Cataract: Cataract:
  coronary   punctate
  immature NOS   Water clefts
DEF: Minor disorders of lens not affecting vision; due to aging.

366.13 Anterior subcapsular polar senile cataract   A

366.14 Posterior subcapsular polar senile cataract   A

366.15 Cortical senile cataract   A

366.16 Nuclear sclerosis   A
Cataracta brunescens   Nuclear cataract
AHA: 4Q, '07, 79

366.17 Total or mature cataract   A

366.18 Hypermature cataract   A
Morgagni cataract

366.19 Other and combined forms of senile cataract   A

√5ᵗʰ **366.2 Traumatic cataract**

366.20 Traumatic cataract, unspecified

366.21 Localized traumatic opacities
Vossius' ring

366.22 Total traumatic cataract

366.23 Partially resolved traumatic cataract

√5ᵗʰ **366.3 Cataract secondary to ocular disorders**

366.30 Cataracta complicata, unspecified

366.31 Glaucomatous flecks (subcapsular)
Code first underlying glaucoma (365.0-365.9)

366.32 Cataract in inflammatory disorders
Code first underlying condition, as:
  chronic choroiditis (363.0-363.2)

366.33 Cataract with neovascularization
Code first underlying condition, as:
  chronic iridocyclitis (364.10)

366.34 Cataract in degenerative disorders
Sunflower cataract
Code first underlying condition, as:
  chalcosis (360.24)
  degenerative myopia (360.21)
  pigmentary retinal dystrophy (362.74)

√5ᵗʰ **366.4 Cataract associated with other disorders**

366.41 *Diabetic cataract*
Code first diabetes (249.5, 250.5)
AHA: 3Q, '91, 9; S-0, '85, 11

366.42 *Tetanic cataract*
Code first underlying disease, as:
  calcinosis (275.4)
  hypoparathyroidism (252.1)

366.43 *Myotonic cataract*
Code first underlying disorder (359.21, 359.23)

366.44 *Cataract associated with other syndromes*
Code first underlying condition, as:
  craniofacial dysostosis (756.0)
  galactosemia (271.1)

366.45 Toxic cataract
Drug-induced cataract
Use additional E code to identify drug or other toxic substance

366.46 Cataract associated with radiation and other physical influences
Use additional E code to identify cause

√5ᵗʰ **366.5 After-cataract**

366.50 After-cataract, unspecified
Secondary cataract NOS

366.51 Soemmering's ring
DEF: A donut-shaped lens remnant and a capsule behind the pupil as a result of cataract surgery or trauma.

366.52 Other after-cataract, not obscuring vision

366.53 After-cataract, obscuring vision

366.8 Other cataract
Calcification of lens

366.9 Unspecified cataract
AHA: 4Q, '09, 131
H26.9 Unspecified cataract   I-10

√4ᵗʰ **367 Disorders of refraction and accommodation**

367.0 Hypermetropia
Far-sightedness   Hyperopia
DEF: Refraction error, called also hyperopia, focal point is posterior to retina; abnormally short anteroposterior diameter or subnormal refractive power; causes farsightedness.

Diseases of the Nervous System and Sense Organs

367.1–368.59

367.1 Myopia
Near-sightedness
DEF: Refraction error, focal point is anterior to retina; causes near-sightedness.

√5ᵗʰ **367.2 Astigmatism**

367.20 Astigmatism, unspecified

367.21 Regular astigmatism

367.22 Irregular astigmatism

√5ᵗʰ **367.3 Anisometropia and aniseikonia**

367.31 Anisometropia
DEF: Eyes with refractive powers that differ by at least one diopter.

367.32 Aniseikonia
DEF: Eyes with unequal retinal imaging; usually due to refractive error.

367.4 Presbyopia
DEF: Loss of crystalline lens elasticity; causes errors of accommodation; due to aging.

√5ᵗʰ **367.5 Disorders of accommodation**

367.51 Paresis of accommodation
Cycloplegia
DEF: Partial paralysis of ciliary muscle, causing focus problems.

367.52 Total or complete internal ophthalmoplegia
DEF: Total paralysis of ciliary muscle; large pupil incapable of focus.

367.53 Spasm of accommodation
DEF: Abnormal contraction of ciliary muscle; causes focus problems.

√5ᵗʰ **367.8 Other disorders of refraction and accommodation**

367.81 Transient refractive change

367.89 Other
Drug-induced ⎫ disorders of refraction and
Toxic   ⎭   accommodation

367.9 Unspecified disorder of refraction and accommodation

√4ᵗʰ **368 Visual disturbances**
EXCLUDES *electrophysiological disturbances (794.11-794.14)*

√5ᵗʰ **368.0 Amblyopia ex anopsia**
DEF: Vision impaired due to disuse; esotropia often cause.

368.00 Amblyopia, unspecified

368.01 Strabismic amblyopia
Suppression amblyopia

368.02 Deprivation amblyopia
DEF: Decreased vision associated with suppressed retinal image of one eye.

368.03 Refractive amblyopia

√5ᵗʰ **368.1 Subjective visual disturbances**

368.10 Subjective visual disturbance, unspecified

368.11 Sudden visual loss   `CC`
CC Exd: 368.10-368.12, 368.16

368.12 Transient visual loss   `CC`
Concentric fadingScintillating scotoma
CC Exd: See code: 368.11

368.13 Visual discomfort
Asthenopia   Photophobia
Eye strain

368.14 Visual distortions of shape and size
Macropsia   Micropsia
Metamorphopsia

368.15 Other visual distortions and entoptic phenomena
Photopsia   Refractive:
Refractive: polyopia
  diplopia   Visual halos

368.16 Psychophysical visual disturbances
Prosopagnosia   Visual:
Visual: disorientation syndrome
  agnosia   hallucinations
               object agnosia

368.2 Diplopia
Double vision
H53.2 Diplopia   `I-10`

√5ᵗʰ **368.3 Other disorders of binocular vision**

368.30 Binocular vision disorder, unspecified

368.31 Suppression of binocular vision

368.32 Simultaneous visual perception without fusion

368.33 Fusion with defective stereopsis
DEF: Faulty depth perception though normal ability to focus.

368.34 Abnormal retinal correspondence

√5ᵗʰ **368.4 Visual field defects**

368.40 Visual field defect, unspecified

368.41 Scotoma involving central area
Scotoma: Scotoma:
  central   paracentral
  centrocecal
DEF: Vision loss (blind spot) in central five degrees of visual field.

368.42 Scotoma of blind spot area
Enlarged: Paracecal scotoma
  angioscotoma
  blind spot

368.43 Sector or arcuate defects
Scotoma: Scotoma:
  arcuate   Seidel
  Bjerrum
DEF: Arc-shaped blind spot caused by retinal nerve damage.

368.44 Other localized visual field defect
Scotoma: Visual field defect:
  NOS   nasal step
  ring   peripheral

368.45 Generalized contraction or constriction

368.46 Homonymous bilateral field defects
Hemianopsia (altitudinal) (homonymous)
Quadrant anopia
DEF: Disorders found in the corresponding vertical halves of the visual fields of both eyes.

368.47 Heteronymous bilateral field defects
Hemianopsia: Hemianopsia:
  binasal   bitemporal
DEF: Disorders in the opposite halves of the visual fields of both eyes.

√5ᵗʰ **368.5 Color vision deficiencies**
Color blindness

368.51 Protan defect
Protanomaly   Protanopia
DEF: Mild difficulty distinguishing green and red hues with shortened spectrum; sex-linked affecting one percent of males.

368.52 Deutan defect
Deuteranomaly   Deuteranopia
DEF: Male-only disorder; difficulty in distinguishing green and red, no shortened spectrum.

368.53 Tritan defect
Tritanomaly   Tritanopia
DEF: Difficulty in distinguishing blue and yellow; occurs often due to drugs, retinal detachment and central nervous system diseases.

368.54 Achromatopsia
Monochromatism (cone) (rod)
DEF: Complete color blindness; caused by disease, injury to retina, optic nerve or pathway.

368.55 Acquired color vision deficiencies

368.59 Other color vision deficiencies

`N` Newborn Age: 0   `P` Pediatric Age: 0-17   `M` Maternity Age: 12-55   `A` Adult Age: 15-124   `MCC` Major CC Condition   `CC` CC Condition   `HIV` HIV Related Dx

120 – Volume 1   2014 ICD-9-CM

√5ᵗʰ **368.6 Night blindness**
Nyctalopia
DEF: Nyctalopia: disorder of vision in dim light or night blindness.

368.60 Night blindness, unspecified

368.61 Congenital night blindness
Hereditary night blindness   Oguchi's disease

368.62 Acquired night blindness
EXCLUDES *that due to vitamin A deficiency (264.5)*

368.63 Abnormal dark adaptation curve
Abnormal threshold
Delayed adaptation } of cones or rods

368.69 Other night blindness

368.8 Other specified visual disturbances
Blurred vision NOS
AHA: 4Q, '02, 56

368.9 Unspecified visual disturbance
AHA: 3Q, '06, 22; 1Q, '04, 15

√4ᵗʰ **369 Blindness and low vision**
NOTE Visual impairment refers to a functional limitation of the eye (e.g., limited visual acuity or visual field). It should be distinguished from visual disability, indicating a limitation of the abilities of the individual (e.g., limited reading skills, vocational skills), and from visual handicap, indicating a limitation of personal and socioeconomic indepen- dence (e.g., limited mobility, limited employability).

The levels of impairment defined in the table on the next page are based on the recommendations of the WHO Study Group on Prevention of Blindness (Geneva, November 6-10, 1972; WHO Technical Report Series 518), and of the International Council of Ophthalmology (1976).

Note that definitions of blindness vary in different settings.

For international reporting WHO defines blindness as profound impairment. This definition can be applied to blindness of one eye (369.1, 369.6) and to blindness of the individual (369.0).

For determination of benefits in the U.S.A., the definition of legal blindness as severe impairment is often used. This definition applies to blindness of the individual only.

EXCLUDES *correctable impaired vision due to refractive errors (367.0-367.9)*

√5ᵗʰ **369.0 Profound impairment, both eyes**

369.00 Impairment level not further specified
Blindness:
NOS according to WHO definition
both eyes

369.01 Better eye: total impairment; lesser eye: total impairment

369.02 Better eye: near-total impairment; lesser eye: not further specified

369.03 Better eye: near-total impairment; lesser eye: total impairment

369.04 Better eye: near-total impairment; lesser eye: near-total impairment

369.05 Better eye: profound impairment; lesser eye: not further specified

369.06 Better eye: profound impairment; lesser eye: total impairment

369.07 Better eye: profound impairment; lesser eye: near-total impairment

369.08 Better eye: profound impairment; lesser eye: profound impairment

√4ᵗʰ **369.1 Moderate or severe impairment, better eye, profound impairment lesser eye**

369.10 Impairment level not further specified
Blindness, one eye, low vision other eye

369.11 Better eye: severe impairment; lesser eye: blind, not further specified

369.12 Better eye: severe impairment; lesser eye: total impairment

369.13 Better eye: severe impairment; lesser eye: near-total impairment

369.14 Better eye: severe impairment; lesser eye: profound impairment

369.15 Better eye: moderate impairment; lesser eye: blind, not further specified

369.16 Better eye: moderate impairment; lesser eye: total impairment

369.17 Better eye: moderate impairment; lesser eye: near-total impairment

369.18 Better eye: moderate impairment; lesser eye: profound impairment

√5ᵗʰ **369.2 Moderate or severe impairment, both eyes**

369.20 Impairment level not further specified
Low vision, both eyes NOS

369.21 Better eye: severe impairment; lesser eye: not further specified

369.22 Better eye: severe impairment; lesser eye: severe impairment

369.23 Better eye: moderate impairment; lesser eye: not further specified

369.24 Better eye: moderate impairment; lesser eye: severe impairment

369.25 Better eye: moderate impairment; lesser eye: moderate impairment

369.3 Unqualified visual loss, both eyes
EXCLUDES *blindness NOS:*
legal [U.S.A. definition] (369.4)
WHO definition (369.00)

369.4 Legal blindness, as defined in U.S.A.
Blindness NOS according to U.S.A. definition
EXCLUDES *legal blindness with specification of impairment level (369.01-369.08, 369.11-369.14, 369.21-369.22)*
H54.8 Legal blindness as defined in USA   I-10

√5ᵗʰ **369.6 Profound impairment, one eye**

369.60 Impairment level not further specified
Blindness, one eye

369.61 One eye: total impairment; other eye: not specified

369.62 One eye: total impairment; other eye: near normal vision

369.63 One eye: total impairment; other eye: normal vision

369.64 One eye: near-total impairment; other eye: not specified

369.65 One eye: near-total impairment; other eye: near-normal vision

369.66 One eye: near-total impairment; other eye: normal vision

369.67 One eye: profound impairment; other eye: not specified

369.68 One eye: profound impairment; other eye: near-normal vision

369.69 One eye: profound impairment; other eye: normal vision

√5ᵗʰ **369.7 Moderate or severe impairment, one eye**

369.70 Impairment level not further specified
Low vision, one eye

369.71 One eye: severe impairment; other eye: not specified

369.72 One eye: severe impairment; other eye: near-normal vision

369.73 One eye: severe impairment; other eye: normal vision

369.74 One eye: moderate impairment; other eye: not specified

369.75 One eye: moderate impairment; other eye: near-normal vision

---

4ᵗʰ/5ᵗʰ Additional Digit Required   Unacceptable PDx   Manifestation Code   Hospital Acquired Condition   ▶◀ Revised Text   ● New Code   ▲ Revised Code Title

Diseases of the Nervous System and Sense Organs

369.76–370.64

Classification		LEVELS OF VISUAL IMPAIRMENT	Additional descriptors which may be encountered
"legal"	WHO	Visual acuity and/or visual field limitation (whichever is worse)	
	(NEAR-) NORMAL VISION	RANGE OF NORMAL VISION 20/10 20/13 20/16 20/20 20/25 2.0 1.6 1.25 1.0 0.8	
		NEAR-NORMAL VISION 20/30 20/40 20/50 20/60 0.7 0.6 0.5 0.4 0.3	
	LOW VISION	MODERATE VISUAL IMPAIRMENT 20/70 20/80 20/100 20/125 20/160 0.25 0.20 0.16 0.12	Moderate low vision
		SEVERE VISUAL IMPAIRMENT 20/200 20/250 20/320 20/400 0.10 0.08 0.06 0.05 Visual field: 20 degrees or less	Severe low vision, "Legal" blindness
LEGAL BLINDNESS (U.S.A.) both eyes	BLINDNESS (WHO) one or both eyes	PROFOUND VISUAL IMPAIRMENT 20/500 20/630 20/800 20/1000 0.04 0.03 0.025 0.02 Count fingers at: less than 3m (10 ft.) Visual field: 10 degrees or less	Profound low vision, Moderate blindness
		NEAR-TOTAL VISUAL IMPAIRMENT Visual acuity: less than 0.02 (20/1000) Count fingers at: 1m (3 ft.) or less Hand movements: 5m (15 ft.) or less Light projection, light perception Visual field: 5 degrees or less	Severe blindness Near-total blindness
		TOTAL VISUAL IMPAIRMENT No light perception (NLP)	Total blindness

Visual acuity refers to best achievable acuity with correction.
Non-listed Snellen fractions may be classified by converting to the nearest decimal equivalent, e.g. 10/200 = 0.05, 6/30 = 0.20.
CF (count fingers) without designation of distance, may be classified to profound impairment.
HM (hand motion) without designation of distance, may be classified to near-total impairment.
Visual field measurements refer to the largest field diameter for a 1/100 white test object.

369.76 One eye: moderate impairment; other eye: normal vision

369.8 Unqualified visual loss, one eye

369.9 Unspecified visual loss
    AHA: 4Q, '02, 114; 3Q, '02, 20

√4ᵗʰ **370 Keratitis**

√5ᵗʰ **370.0 Corneal ulcer**
    EXCLUDES *that due to vitamin A deficiency (264.3)*

370.00 Corneal ulcer, unspecified

370.01 Marginal corneal ulcer

370.02 Ring corneal ulcer

370.03 Central corneal ulcer

370.04 Hypopyon ulcer
    Serpiginous ulcer
    DEF: Corneal ulcer with an accumulation of pus in the eye's anterior chamber.

370.05 Mycotic corneal ulcer
    DEF: Fungal infection causing corneal tissue loss.

370.06 Perforated corneal ulcer
    DEF: Tissue loss through all layers of cornea.

370.07 Mooren's ulcer
    DEF: Tissue loss, with chronic inflammation, at junction of cornea and sclera; seen in elderly.

√5ᵗʰ **370.2 Superficial keratitis without conjunctivitis**
    EXCLUDES *dendritic [herpes simplex] keratitis (054.42)*

370.20 Superficial keratitis, unspecified

370.21 Punctate keratitis
    Thygeson's superficial punctate keratitis
    DEF: Formation of cellular and fibrinous deposits (keratic precipitates) on posterior surface; deposits develop after injury or iridocyclitis.

370.22 Macular keratitis
    Keratitis: Keratitis:
    areolar   stellate
    nummular   striate

370.23 Filamentary keratitis
    DEF: Keratitis characterized by twisted filaments of mucoid material on the cornea's surface.

370.24 Photokeratitis
    Snow blindness   Welders' keratitis
    DEF: Painful, inflamed cornea; due to extended exposure to ultraviolet light.
    AHA: 3Q, '96, 6

√5ᵗʰ **370.3 Certain types of keratoconjunctivitis**

370.31 Phlyctenular keratoconjunctivitis
    Phlyctenulosis
    Use additional code for any associated tuberculosis (017.3)
    DEF: Miniature blister on conjunctiva or cornea; associated with tuberculosis and malnutrition disorders.

370.32 Limbar and corneal involvement in vernal conjunctivitis
    Use additional code for vernal conjunctivitis (372.13)
    DEF: Corneal itching and inflammation in conjunctivitis; often limited to lining of eyelids.

370.33 Keratoconjunctivitis sicca, not specified as Sjögren's
    EXCLUDES *Sjögren's syndrome (710.2)*
    DEF: Inflammation of conjunctiva and cornea; characterized by "horny" looking tissue and excess blood in these areas; decreased flow of lacrimal (tear) is a contributing factor.

370.34 Exposure keratoconjunctivitis
    DEF: Incomplete closure of eyelid causing dry, inflamed eye.
    AHA: 3Q, '96, 6

370.35 Neurotrophic keratoconjunctivitis

√5ᵗʰ **370.4 Other and unspecified keratoconjunctivitis**

370.40 Keratoconjunctivitis, unspecified
    Superficial keratitis with conjunctivitis NOS

370.44 *Keratitis or keratoconjunctivitis in exanthema*
    Code first underlying condition (050.0-052.9)
    EXCLUDES *herpes simplex (054.43)*
    herpes zoster (053.21)
    measles (055.71)

370.49 Other
    EXCLUDES *epidemic keratoconjunctivitis (077.1)*

√5ᵗʰ **370.5 Interstitial and deep keratitis**

370.50 Interstitial keratitis, unspecified

370.52 Diffuse interstitial keratitis
    Cogan's syndrome
    DEF: Inflammation of cornea; with deposits in middle corneal layers; may obscure vision.

370.54 Sclerosing keratitis
    DEF: Chronic corneal inflammation leading to opaque scarring.

370.55 Corneal abscess
    DEF: Pocket of pus and inflammation on the cornea.

370.59 Other
    EXCLUDES *disciform herpes simplex keratitis (054.43)*
    syphilitic keratitis (090.3)

√5ᵗʰ **370.6 Corneal neovascularization**

370.60 Corneal neovascularization, unspecified

370.61 Localized vascularization of cornea
    DEF: Limited infiltration of cornea by new blood vessels.

370.62 Pannus (corneal)
    DEF: Buildup of superficial vascularization and granulated tissue under epithelium of cornea.
    AHA: 3Q, '02, 20

370.63 Deep vascularization of cornea
    DEF: Deep infiltration of cornea by new blood vessels.

370.64 Ghost vessels (corneal)

Ⓝ Newborn Age: 0   Ⓟ Pediatric Age: 0-17   Ⓜ Maternity Age: 12-55   Ⓐ Adult Age: 15-124   **MCC** Major CC Condition   **CC** CC Condition   **HIV** HIV Related Dx

122 – Volume 1   **2014 ICD-9-CM**

370.8 Other forms of keratitis
Code first underlying condition, such as:
Acanthamoeba (136.21)
Fusarium (118)
AHA: 4Q, '08, 80-81; 3Q, '94, 5

370.9 Unspecified keratitis

√4th 371 Corneal opacity and other disorders of cornea

√5th 371.0 Corneal scars and opacities
EXCLUDES that due to vitamin A deficiency (264.6)

371.00 Corneal opacity, unspecified
Corneal scar NOS

371.01 Minor opacity of cornea
Corneal nebula

371.02 Peripheral opacity of cornea
Corneal macula not interfering with central vision

371.03 Central opacity of cornea
Corneal:
leucoma } interfering with central
macula } vision

371.04 Adherent leucoma
DEF: Dense, opaque corneal growth adhering to the iris; also spelled as leukoma.

371.05 Phthisical cornea
Code first underlying tuberculosis (017.3)

√5th 371.1 Corneal pigmentations and deposits

371.10 Corneal deposit, unspecified

371.11 Anterior pigmentations
Stähli's lines

371.12 Stromal pigmentations
Hematocornea

371.13 Posterior pigmentations
Krukenberg spindle

371.14 Kayser-Fleischer ring
DEF: Copper deposits forming ring at outer edge of cornea; seen in Wilson's disease and other liver disorders.

371.15 Other deposits associated with metabolic disorders

371.16 Argentous deposits
DEF: Silver deposits in cornea.

√5th 371.2 Corneal edema

371.20 Corneal edema, unspecified

371.21 Idiopathic corneal edema
DEF: Corneal swelling and fluid retention of unknown cause.

371.22 Secondary corneal edema
DEF: Corneal swelling and fluid retention caused by an underlying disease, injury, or condition.

371.23 Bullous keratopathy
DEF: Corneal degeneration; characterized by recurring, rupturing epithelial "blisters;" ruptured blebs expose corneal nerves; occurs in glaucoma, iridocyclitis and Fuchs' epithelial dystrophy.

371.24 Corneal edema due to wearing of contact lenses

√5th 371.3 Changes of corneal membranes

371.30 Corneal membrane change, unspecified

371.31 Folds and rupture of Bowman's membrane

371.32 Folds in Descemet's membrane

371.33 Rupture in Descemet's membrane

√5th 371.4 Corneal degenerations

371.40 Corneal degeneration, unspecified

371.41 Senile corneal changes
Arcus senilis   Hassall-Henle bodies

371.42 Recurrent erosion of cornea
EXCLUDES Mooren's ulcer (370.07)

371.43 Band-shaped keratopathy
DEF: Horizontal bands of superficial corneal calcium deposits.

371.44 Other calcerous degenerations of cornea

371.45 Keratomalacia NOS
EXCLUDES that due to vitamin A deficiency (264.4)
DEF: Destruction of the cornea by keratinization of the epithelium with ulceration and perforation of the cornea; seen in cases of vitamin A deficiency.

371.46 Nodular degeneration of cornea
Salzmann's nodular dystrophy

371.48 Peripheral degenerations of cornea
Marginal degeneration of cornea [Terrien's]

371.49 Other
Discrete colliquative keratopathy

√5th 371.5 Hereditary corneal dystrophies
DEF: Genetic disorder; leads to opacities, edema or lesions of cornea.

371.50 Corneal dystrophy, unspecified

371.51 Juvenile epithelial corneal dystrophy

371.52 Other anterior corneal dystrophies
Corneal dystrophy: Corneal dystrophy:
microscopic cystic   ring-like

371.53 Granular corneal dystrophy

371.54 Lattice corneal dystrophy

371.55 Macular corneal dystrophy

371.56 Other stromal corneal dystrophies
Crystalline corneal dystrophy

371.57 Endothelial corneal dystrophy
Combined corneal dystrophy   Fuchs' endothelial
Cornea guttata   dystrophy

371.58 Other posterior corneal dystrophies
Polymorphous corneal dystrophy

√5th 371.6 Keratoconus
DEF: Bilateral bulging protrusion of anterior cornea; often due to noninflammatory thinning.

371.60 Keratoconus, unspecified

371.61 Keratoconus, stable condition

371.62 Keratoconus, acute hydrops

√5th 371.7 Other corneal deformities

371.70 Corneal deformity, unspecified

371.71 Corneal ectasia
DEF: Bulging protrusion of thinned, scarred cornea.

371.72 Descemetocele
DEF: Protrusion of Descemet's membrane into cornea.

371.73 Corneal staphyloma
DEF: Protrusion of cornea into adjacent tissue.

√5th 371.8 Other corneal disorders

371.81 Corneal anesthesia and hypoesthesia
DEF: Decreased or absent sensitivity of cornea.

371.82 Corneal disorder due to contact lens
EXCLUDES corneal edema due to contact lens (371.24)
DEF: Contact lens wear causing cornea disorder, excluding swelling.

371.89 Other
AHA: 3Q, '99, 12

371.9 Unspecified corneal disorder

√4th 372 Disorders of conjunctiva
EXCLUDES keratoconjunctivitis (370.3-370.4)

√5th 372.0 Acute conjunctivitis

372.00 Acute conjunctivitis, unspecified

372.01 Serous conjunctivitis, except viral
EXCLUDES viral conjunctivitis NOS (077.9)
AHA: 3Q, '08, 6

4th/5th Additional Digit Required   Unacceptable PDx   Manifestation Code   Hospital Acquired Condition   ►◄ Revised Text   ● New Code   ▲ Revised Code Title

2014 ICD-9-CM   Volume 1 – 123

Diseases of the Nervous System and Sense Organs

372.02–372.9

372.02 Acute follicular conjunctivitis
Conjunctival folliculosis NOS
EXCLUDES conjunctivitis:
adenoviral (acute follicular) (077.3)
epidemic hemorrhagic (077.4)
inclusion (077.0)
Newcastle (077.8)
epidemic keratoconjunctivitis (077.1)
pharyngoconjunctival fever (077.2)
DEF: Severe conjunctival inflammation with dense
infiltrations of lymphoid tissues of inner eyelids; may be
traced to a viral or chlamydial etiology.

372.03 Other mucopurulent conjunctivitis
Catarrhal conjunctivitis
EXCLUDES blennorrhea neonatorum (gonococcal)
(098.40)
neonatal conjunctivitis(771.6)
ophthalmia neonatorum NOS (771.6)

372.04 Pseudomembranous conjunctivitis
Membranous conjunctivitis
EXCLUDES diphtheritic conjunctivitis (032.81)
DEF: Severe inflammation of conjunctiva; false membrane
develops on inner surface of eyelid; membrane can be
removed without harming epithelium, due to bacterial
infections, toxic and allergic factors, and viral infections.

372.05 Acute atopic conjunctivitis
DEF: Sudden, severe conjunctivitis due to allergens.

372.06 Acute chemical conjunctivitis
Acute toxic conjunctivitis
Use additional E code to identify the chemical or toxic
agent
EXCLUDES burn of eye and adnexa (940.0-940.9)
chemical corrosion injury of eye
(940.2-940.3)
AHA: 4Q, '09, 85

√5ᵗʰ 372.1 Chronic conjunctivitis

372.10 Chronic conjunctivitis, unspecified

372.11 Simple chronic conjunctivitis

372.12 Chronic follicular conjunctivitis
DEF: Persistent conjunctival inflammation with dense,
localized infiltrations of lymphoid tissues of inner eyelids.

372.13 Vernal conjunctivitis
AHA: 3Q, '96, 8

372.14 Other chronic allergic conjunctivitis
AHA: 3Q, '96, 8

372.15 Parasitic conjunctivitis
Code first underlying disease, as:
filariasis (125.0-125.9)
mucocutaneous leishmaniasis (085.5)

√5ᵗʰ 372.2 Blepharoconjunctivitis

372.20 Blepharoconjunctivitis, unspecified

372.21 Angular blepharoconjunctivitis
DEF: Inflammation at junction of upper and lower eyelids;
may block lacrimal secretions.

372.22 Contact blepharoconjunctivitis

√5ᵗʰ 372.3 Other and unspecified conjunctivitis

372.30 Conjunctivitis, unspecified
H10.9 Unspecified conjunctivitis   I-10

372.31 Rosacea conjunctivitis
Code first underlying rosacea dermatitis (695.3)

372.33 Conjunctivitis in mucocutaneous disease
Code first underlying disease, as:
erythema multiforme (695.10-695.19)
Reiter's disease (099.3)
EXCLUDES ocular pemphigoid (694.61)

372.34 Pingueculitis
EXCLUDES pinguecula (372.51)
AHA: 4Q, '08, 112-113

372.39 Other
AHA: 2Q, '07, 9

√5ᵗʰ 372.4 Pterygium
EXCLUDES pseudopterygium (372.52)
DEF: Wedge-shaped, conjunctival thickening that advances from the
inner corner of the eye toward the cornea.

372.40 Pterygium, unspecified

372.41 Peripheral pterygium, stationary

372.42 Peripheral pterygium, progressive

372.43 Central pterygium

372.44 Double pterygium

372.45 Recurrent pterygium

√5ᵗʰ 372.5 Conjunctival degenerations and deposits

372.50 Conjunctival degeneration, unspecified

372.51 Pinguecula
EXCLUDES pingueculitis (372.34)
DEF: Proliferative spot on the bulbar conjunctiva located
near the sclerocorneal junction, usually on the nasal side; it
is seen in elderly people.

372.52 Pseudopterygium
DEF: Conjunctival scar joined to the cornea; it looks like a
pterygium but is not attached to the tissue.

372.53 Conjunctival xerosis
EXCLUDES conjunctival xerosis due to vitamin A
deficiency (264.0, 264.1, 264.7)
DEF: Dry conjunctiva due to vitamin A deficiency; related to
Bitot's spots; may develop into xerophthalmia and
keratomalacia.

372.54 Conjunctival concretions
DEF: Calculus or deposit on conjunctiva.

372.55 Conjunctival pigmentations
Conjunctival argyrosis
DEF: Color deposits in conjunctiva.

372.56 Conjunctival deposits

√5ᵗʰ 372.6 Conjunctival scars

372.61 Granuloma of conjunctiva

372.62 Localized adhesions and strands of conjunctiva
DEF: Abnormal fibrous connections in conjunctiva.

372.63 Symblepharon
Extensive adhesions of conjunctiva
DEF: Adhesion of the eyelids to the eyeball.

372.64 Scarring of conjunctiva
Contraction of eye socket (after enucleation)

√5ᵗʰ 372.7 Conjunctival vascular disorders and cysts

372.71 Hyperemia of conjunctiva
DEF: Conjunctival blood vessel congestion causing eye
redness.

372.72 Conjunctival hemorrhage
Hyposphagma   Subconjunctival hemorrhage

372.73 Conjunctival edema
Chemosis of conjunctiva
Subconjunctival edema
DEF: Fluid retention and swelling in conjunctival tissue.

372.74 Vascular abnormalities of conjunctiva
Aneurysm(ata) of conjunctiva

372.75 Conjunctival cysts
DEF: Abnormal sacs of fluid in conjunctiva.

√5ᵗʰ 372.8 Other disorders of conjunctiva

372.81 Conjunctivochalasis
AHA: 4Q, '00, 41
DEF: Bilateral condition of redundant conjunctival tissue
between globe and lower eyelid margin; may cover lower
punctum, interfering with normal tearing.

372.89 Other disorders of conjunctiva

372.9 Unspecified disorder of conjunctiva

N Newborn Age: 0   P Pediatric Age: 0-17   M Maternity Age: 12-55   A Adult Age: 15-124   MCC Major CC Condition   CC CC Condition   HIV HIV Related Dx

☑4ᵗʰ **373 Inflammation of eyelids**

  ☑5ᵗʰ **373.0 Blepharitis**

    EXCLUDES *blepharoconjunctivitis (372.20-372.22)*

    373.00 Blepharitis, unspecified

    373.01 Ulcerative blepharitis

    373.02 Squamous blepharitis

  ☑5ᵗʰ **373.1 Hordeolum and other deep inflammation of eyelid**

    DEF: Purulent, localized, staphylococcal infection in sebaceous glands of eyelids.

    373.11 Hordeolum externum

      Hordeolum NOS   Stye

      DEF: Infection of the oil glands in the eyelash follicles.

    373.12 Hordeolum internum

      Infection of meibomian gland

      DEF: Infection of the oil gland of the eyelid margin.

    373.13 Abscess of eyelid

      Furuncle of eyelid

      DEF: Inflamed pocket of pus on the eyelid.

  373.2 Chalazion

    Meibomian (gland) cyst

    EXCLUDES *infected meibomian gland (373.12)*

    DEF: Chronic inflammation of the meibomian gland, causing an eyelid mass.

  ☑5ᵗʰ **373.3 Noninfectious dermatoses of eyelid**

    373.31 Eczematous dermatitis of eyelid

    373.32 Contact and allergic dermatitis of eyelid

    373.33 Xeroderma of eyelid

    373.34 Discoid lupus erythematosus of eyelid

  373.4 *Infective dermatitis of eyelid of types resulting in deformity*

    Code first underlying disease, as:

    leprosy (030.0-030.9)

    lupus vulgaris (tuberculous) (017.0)

    yaws (102.0-102.9)

  373.5 *Other infective dermatitis of eyelid*

    Code first underlying disease, as:

    actinomycosis (039.3)

    impetigo (684)

    mycotic dermatitis (110.0-111.9)

    vaccinia (051.0)

      postvaccination (999.0)

    EXCLUDES *herpes:*

      simplex (054.41)

      zoster (053.20)

  373.6 *Parasitic infestation of eyelid*

    Code first underlying disease, as:

    leishmaniasis (085.0-085.9)

    loiasis (125.2)

    onchocerciasis (125.3)

    pediculosis (132.0)

  373.8 Other inflammations of eyelids

  373.9 Unspecified inflammation of eyelid

☑4ᵗʰ **374 Other disorders of eyelids**

  ☑5ᵗʰ **374.0 Entropion and trichiasis of eyelid**

    DEF: Entropion: turning inward of eyelid edge toward eyeball.

    DEF: Trichiasis: ingrowing eyelashes marked by irritation with possible distortion of sight.

    374.00 Entropion, unspecified

    374.01 Senile entropion   Ⓐ

    374.02 Mechanical entropion

    374.03 Spastic entropion

    374.04 Cicatricial entropion

    374.05 Trichiasis without entropion

  ☑5ᵗʰ **374.1 Ectropion**

    DEF: Turning outward (eversion) of eyelid edge; exposes palpebral conjunctiva; dryness irritation result.

    374.10 Ectropion, unspecified

Entropion and Ectropion

Normal eyelashes   Entropion   Ectropion

  374.11 Senile ectropion   Ⓐ

  374.12 Mechanical ectropion

  374.13 Spastic ectropion

  374.14 Cicatricial ectropion

☑5ᵗʰ **374.2 Lagophthalmos**

  DEF: Incomplete closure of eyes; causes dry eye and other complications.

  374.20 Lagophthalmos, unspecified

  374.21 Paralytic lagophthalmos

  374.22 Mechanical lagophthalmos

  374.23 Cicatricial lagophthalmos

☑5ᵗʰ **374.3 Ptosis of eyelid**

  374.30 Ptosis of eyelid, unspecified

    AHA: 2Q, '96, 11

  374.31 Paralytic ptosis

    DEF: Drooping of upper eyelid due to nerve disorder.

  374.32 Myogenic ptosis

    DEF: Drooping of upper eyelid due to muscle disorder.

  374.33 Mechanical ptosis

    DEF: Outside force causes drooping of upper eyelid.

  374.34 Blepharochalasis

    Pseudoptosis

    DEF: Loss of elasticity, thickened or indurated skin of eyelids associated with recurrent episodes of idiopathic edema causing intracellular tissue atrophy.

☑5ᵗʰ **374.4 Other disorders affecting eyelid function**

  EXCLUDES *blepharoclonus (333.81)*

    blepharospasm (333.81)

    facial nerve palsy (351.0)

    third nerve palsy or paralysis (378.51-378.52)

    tic (psychogenic) (307.20-307.23)

    organic (333.3)

  374.41 Lid retraction or lag

  374.43 Abnormal innervation syndrome

    Jaw-blinking   Paradoxical facial movements

  374.44 Sensory disorders

  374.45 Other sensorimotor disorders

    Deficient blink reflex

  374.46 Blepharophimosis

    Ankyloblepharon

    DEF: Narrowing of palpebral fissure horizontally; caused by laterally displaced inner canthi; either acquired or congenital.

☑5ᵗʰ **374.5 Degenerative disorders of eyelid and periocular area**

  374.50 Degenerative disorder of eyelid, unspecified

  374.51 *Xanthelasma*

    Xanthoma (planum) (tuberosum) of eyelid

    Code first underlying condition (272.0-272.9)

    DEF: Fatty tumors of the eyelid linked to high fat content of blood.

  374.52 Hyperpigmentation of eyelid

    Chloasma   Dyspigmentation

    DEF: Excess pigment of eyelid.

---

⁴ᵗʰ ⁵ᵗʰ Additional Digit Required   Unacceptable PDx   Manifestation Code   Hospital Acquired Condition   ▶◀ Revised Text   ● New Code   ▲ Revised Code Title

2014 ICD-9-CM   Volume 1 – 125

Lacrimal System

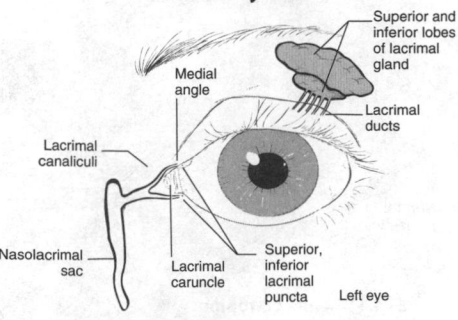

374.53 Hypopigmentation of eyelid
Vitiligo of eyelid
DEF: Lack of color pigment of the eyelid.

374.54 Hypertrichosis of eyelid
DEF: Excessive eyelash growth.

374.55 Hypotrichosis of eyelid
Madarosis of eyelid
DEF: Less than normal, or absent, eyelashes.

374.56 Other degenerative disorders of skin affecting eyelid

√5ᵗʰ **374.8 Other disorders of eyelid**

374.81 Hemorrhage of eyelid
EXCLUDES black eye (921.0)

374.82 Edema of eyelid
Hyperemia of eyelid
DEF: Swelling and fluid retention in eyelid.
AHA: 4Q, '08, 131

374.83 Elephantiasis of eyelid
DEF: Filarial disease causing dermatitis and enlargement of eyelid.

374.84 Cysts of eyelids
Sebaceous cyst of eyelid

374.85 Vascular anomalies of eyelid

374.86 Retained foreign body of eyelid
Use additional code to identify foreign body (V90.01-V90.9)

374.87 Dermatochalasis
DEF: Acquired form of connective tissue disorder associated with decreased elastic tissue and abnormal elastin formation resulting in loss of elasticity of the skin of the eyelid, generally associated with aging.

374.89 Other disorders of eyelid

374.9 Unspecified disorder of eyelid

√4ᵗʰ **375 Disorders of lacrimal system**

√5ᵗʰ **375.0 Dacryoadenitis**

375.00 Dacryoadenitis, unspecified

375.01 Acute dacryoadenitis
DEF: Severe, sudden inflammation of the lacrimal gland.

375.02 Chronic dacryoadenitis
DEF: Persistent inflammation of the lacrimal gland.

375.03 Chronic enlargement of lacrimal gland

√5ᵗʰ **375.1 Other disorders of lacrimal gland**

375.11 Dacryops
DEF: Overproduction and constant flow of tears; may cause distended lacrimal duct.

375.12 Other lacrimal cysts and cystic degeneration

375.13 Primary lacrimal atrophy

375.14 Secondary lacrimal atrophy
DEF: Wasting away of the lacrimal gland due to another disease.

375.15 Tear film insufficiency, unspecified
Dry eye syndrome
AHA: 3Q, '96, 6
DEF: Eye dryness and irritation from insufficient tear production.

375.16 Dislocation of lacrimal gland

√5ᵗʰ **375.2 Epiphora**
DEF: Abnormal development of tears due to stricture of lacrimal passages.

375.20 Epiphora, unspecified as to cause

375.21 Epiphora due to excess lacrimation
DEF: Tear overflow due to overproduction.

375.22 Epiphora due to insufficient drainage
DEF: Tear overflow due to blocked drainage.

√5ᵗʰ **375.3 Acute and unspecified inflammation of lacrimal passages**
EXCLUDES neonatal dacryocystitis (771.6)

375.30 Dacryocystitis, unspecified

375.31 Acute canaliculitis, lacrimal

375.32 Acute dacryocystitis
Acute peridacryocystitis

375.33 Phlegmonous dacryocystitis
DEF: Infection of the tear sac with pockets of pus.

√5ᵗʰ **375.4 Chronic inflammation of lacrimal passages**

375.41 Chronic canaliculitis

375.42 Chronic dacryocystitis

375.43 Lacrimal mucocele

√5ᵗʰ **375.5 Stenosis and insufficiency of lacrimal passages**

375.51 Eversion of lacrimal punctum
DEF: Abnormal turning outward of the tear duct.

375.52 Stenosis of lacrimal punctum
DEF: Abnormal narrowing of the tear duct.

375.53 Stenosis of lacrimal canaliculi

375.54 Stenosis of lacrimal sac
DEF: Abnormal narrowing of the tear sac.

375.55 Obstruction of nasolacrimal duct, neonatal
EXCLUDES congenital anomaly of nasola- crimal duct (743.65)
DEF: Acquired, abnormal obstruction of tear drainage system from the eye to the nose; in an infant.

375.56 Stenosis of nasolacrimal duct, acquired

375.57 Dacryolith
DEF: Concretion or stone anywhere in lacrimal system.

√5ᵗʰ **375.6 Other changes of lacrimal passages**

375.61 Lacrimal fistula
DEF: Abnormal communication from the lacrimal system.

375.69 Other

√5ᵗʰ **375.8 Other disorders of lacrimal system**

375.81 Granuloma of lacrimal passages
DEF: Abnormal nodules within lacrimal system.

375.89 Other

375.9 Unspecified disorder of lacrimal system

√4ᵗʰ **376 Disorders of the orbit**

√5ᵗʰ **376.0 Acute inflammation of orbit**

376.00 Acute inflammation of orbit, unspecified

376.01 Orbital cellulitis   CC
Abscess of orbit
DEF: Infection of tissue between the orbital bone and eyeball.
CC Exd: 376.00-376.04

376.02 Orbital periostitis   CC
DEF: Inflammation of connective tissue covering the orbital bone.
CC Exd: 003.24, 015.50-015.56, 015.70-015.76, 015.90-015.96, 017.90-017.96, 376.02, 730.00-730.39, 730.80-730.99

N Newborn Age: 0   P Pediatric Age: 0-17   M Maternity Age: 12-55   A Adult Age: 15-124   MCC Major CC Condition   CC CC Condition   HIV HIV Related Dx

126 – Volume 1   2014 ICD-9-CM

376.03 Orbital osteomyelitis   `CC`
DEF: Inflammation of the orbital bone.
CC Excl: 003.24, 015.50-015.56, 015.70-015.76, 015.90-015.96, 017.90-017.96, 376.03, 730.00-730.39, 730.80-730.99

376.04 Tenonitis

√5ᵗʰ **376.1 Chronic inflammatory disorders of orbit**

376.10 Chronic inflammation of orbit, unspecified

376.11 Orbital granuloma
Pseudotumor (inflammatory) of orbit
DEF: Abnormal nodule between orbital bone and eyeball.

376.12 Orbital myositis
DEF: Painful inflammation of the muscles of the eye.

376.13 Parasitic infestation of orbit
Code first underlying disease, as:
hydatid infestation of orbit (122.3, 122.6, 122.9)
myiasis of orbit (134.0)

√5ᵗʰ **376.2 Endocrine exophthalmos**
Code first underlying thyroid disorder (242.0-242.9)

376.21 Thyrotoxic exophthalmos
DEF: Painful inflammation of eye muscles.

376.22 Exophthalmic ophthalmoplegia
DEF: Inability to rotate eye as a result of bulging eyes.

√5ᵗʰ **376.3 Other exophthalmic conditions**

376.30 Exophthalmos, unspecified
DEF: Abnormal protrusion of eyeball.

376.31 Constant exophthalmos
DEF: Continuous, abnormal protrusion or bulging of eyeball.

376.32 Orbital hemorrhage
DEF: Bleeding behind the eyeball, causing it to bulge.

376.33 Orbital edema or congestion
DEF: Fluid retention behind eyeball, causing forward bulge.

376.34 Intermittent exophthalmos

376.35 Pulsating exophthalmos
DEF: Bulge or protrusion; associated with a carotid-cavernous fistula.

376.36 Lateral displacement of globe
DEF: Abnormal displacement of the eyeball away from nose, toward temple.

√5ᵗʰ **376.4 Deformity of orbit**

376.40 Deformity of orbit, unspecified

376.41 Hypertelorism of orbit
DEF: Abnormal increase in interorbital distance; associated with congenital facial deformities; may be accompanied by mental deficiency.

376.42 Exostosis of orbit
DEF: Abnormal bony growth of orbit.

376.43 Local deformities due to bone disease
DEF: Acquired abnormalities of orbit; due to bone disease.

376.44 Orbital deformities associated with craniofacial deformities

376.45 Atrophy of orbit
DEF: Wasting away of bone tissue of orbit.

376.46 Enlargement of orbit

376.47 Deformity due to trauma or surgery

√5ᵗʰ **376.5 Enophthalmos**
DEF: Recession of eyeball deep into eye socket.

376.50 Enophthalmos, unspecified as to cause

376.51 Enophthalmos due to atrophy of orbital tissue

376.52 Enophthalmos due to trauma or surgery

376.6 Retained (old) foreign body following penetrating wound of orbit
Retrobulbar foreign body
Use additional code to identify foreign body (V90.01-V90.9)

√5ᵗʰ **376.8 Other orbital disorders**

376.81 Orbital cysts
Encephalocele of orbit
AHA: 3Q, '99, 13

376.82 Myopathy of extraocular muscles
DEF: Disease in the muscles that control eyeball movement.

376.89 Other

376.9 Unspecified disorder of orbit

√4ᵗʰ **377 Disorders of optic nerve and visual pathways**

√5ᵗʰ **377.0 Papilledema**

377.00 Papilledema, unspecified   `CC`
CC Excl: 017.30-017.36, 017.90-017.96, 036.81, 249.50-249.51, 249.80-249.91, 250.50-250.53, 250.80-250.93, 377.00-377.03, 377.14, 377.24, 379.60-379.90, 379.99, 743.8-743.9

377.01 Papilledema associated with increased intracranial pressure   `CC`
CC Excl: See code: 377.00

377.02 Papilledema associated with decreased ocular pressure

377.03 Papilledema associated with retinal disorder

377.04 Foster-Kennedy syndrome
DEF: Retrobulbar optic neuritis, central scotoma and optic atrophy; caused by tumors in frontal lobe of brain that press downward.

√5ᵗʰ **377.1 Optic atrophy**

377.10 Optic atrophy, unspecified

377.11 Primary optic atrophy
EXCLUDES neurosyphilitic optic atrophy (094.84)

377.12 Postinflammatory optic atrophy
DEF: : Adverse effect of inflammation causing wasting away of eye.

377.13 Optic atrophy associated with retinal dystrophies
DEF: Progressive changes in retinal tissue due to metabolic disorder causing wasting away of eye.

377.14 Glaucomatous atrophy [cupping] of optic disc

377.15 Partial optic atrophy
Temporal pallor of optic disc

377.16 Hereditary optic atrophy
Optic atrophy: Optic atrophy:
dominant hereditary   Leber's

√5ᵗʰ **377.2 Other disorders of optic disc**

377.21 Drusen of optic disc

377.22 Crater-like holes of optic disc

377.23 Coloboma of optic disc
DEF: Ocular malformation caused by the failure of fetal fissure of optic stalk to close.

377.24 Pseudopapilledema

√5ᵗʰ **377.3 Optic neuritis**
EXCLUDES meningococcal optic neuritis (036.81)

377.30 Optic neuritis, unspecified   `CC`
CC Excl: 377.30-377.39

377.31 Optic papillitis   `CC`
CC Excl: See code: 377.30
DEF: Swelling and inflammation of the optic disc.

377.32 Retrobulbar neuritis (acute)   `CC`
EXCLUDES syphilitic retrobulbar neuritis (094.85)
CC Excl: See code: 377.30
DEF: Inflammation of optic nerve immediately behind the eyeball.

377.33 Nutritional optic neuropathy
DEF: Malnutrition causing optic nerve disorder.

377.34 Toxic optic neuropathy
Toxic amblyopia
DEF: Toxic substance causing optic nerve disorder.

377.39 Other   `CC`
     EXCLUDES ischemic optic neuropathy (377.41)
     CC Excl: See code: 377.30

√5ᵗʰ **377.4 Other disorders of optic nerve**

     377.41 Ischemic optic neuropathy
       DEF: Decreased blood flow affecting optic nerve.

     377.42 Hemorrhage in optic nerve sheaths
       DEF: Bleeding in meningeal lining of optic nerve.

     377.43 Optic nerve hypoplasia
       AHA: 4Q, '06, 81

     377.49 Other
       Compression of optic nerve

√5ᵗʰ **377.5 Disorders of optic chiasm**

     377.51 Associated with pituitary neoplasms and   `CC`
     disorders
       CC Excl: 377.51-377.63
       DEF: Abnormal pituitary growth causing disruption in nerve chain from retina to brain.

     377.52 Associated with other neoplasms   `CC`
       CC Excl: See code: 377.51
       DEF: Abnormal growth, other than pituitary, causing disruption in nerve chain from retina to brain.

     377.53 Associated with vascular disorders   `CC`
       CC Excl: See code: 377.51
       DEF: Vascular disorder causing disruption in nerve chain from retina to brain.

     377.54 Associated with inflammatory disorders   `CC`
       CC Excl: See code: 377.51
       DEF: Inflammatory disease causing disruption in nerve chain from retina to brain.

√5ᵗʰ **377.6 Disorders of other visual pathways**

     377.61 Associated with neoplasms   `CC`
       CC Excl: See code: 377.51

     377.62 Associated with vascular disorders   `CC`
       CC Excl: See code: 377.51

     377.63 Associated with inflammatory disorders   `CC`
       CC Excl: See code: 377.51

√5ᵗʰ **377.7 Disorders of visual cortex**
     EXCLUDES visual:
         agnosia (368.16)
         hallucinations (368.16)
         halos (368.15)

     377.71 Associated with neoplasms   `CC`
       CC Excl: 377.71-377.9

     377.72 Associated with vascular disorders   `CC`
       CC Excl: See code: 377.71

     377.73 Associated with inflammatory disorders   `CC`
       CC Excl: See code: 377.71

     377.75 Cortical blindness
       DEF: Blindness due to brain disorder, rather than eye disorder.

     377.9 Unspecified disorder of optic nerve and visual pathways

√4ᵗʰ **378 Strabismus and other disorders of binocular eye movements**
     EXCLUDES nystagmus and other irregular eye movements
         (379.50-379.59)
     DEF: Misalignment of the eyes due to imbalance in extraocular muscles.

√5ᵗʰ **378.0 Esotropia**
     Convergent concomitant strabismus
     EXCLUDES intermittent esotropia (378.20-378.22)
     DEF: Visual axis deviation created by one eye fixing upon an image and the other eye deviating inward.

     378.00 Esotropia, unspecified

     378.01 Monocular esotropia

     378.02 Monocular esotropia with A pattern

     378.03 Monocular esotropia with V pattern

     378.04 Monocular esotropia with other noncomitancies
       Monocular esotropia with X or Y pattern

Eye Musculature

Superior rectus   Superior oblique   R.   L.
Lateral rectus   Medial rectus
Monocular (one eye only) esotropia (inward)
Inferior oblique   Inferior rectus
Monocular exotropia (outward)
Muscles and actions (right eye)
Monocular hypertropia (upward)

     378.05 Alternating esotropia

     378.06 Alternating esotropia with A pattern

     378.07 Alternating esotropia with V pattern

     378.08 Alternating esotropia with other noncomitancies
       Alternating esotropia with X or Y pattern

√5ᵗʰ **378.1 Exotropia**
     Divergent concomitant strabismus
     EXCLUDES intermittent exotropia (378.20, 378.23-378.24)
     DEF: Visual axis deviation created by one eye fixing upon an image and the other eye deviating outward.

     378.10 Exotropia, unspecified

     378.11 Monocular exotropia

     378.12 Monocular exotropia with A pattern

     378.13 Monocular exotropia with V pattern

     378.14 Monocular exotropia with other noncomitancies
       Monocular exotropia with X or Y pattern

     378.15 Alternating exotropia

     378.16 Alternating exotropia with A pattern

     378.17 Alternating exotropia with V pattern

     378.18 Alternating exotropia with other noncomitancies
       Alternating exotropia with X or Y pattern

√5ᵗʰ **378.2 Intermittent heterotropia**
     EXCLUDES vertical heterotropia (intermittent) (378.31)
     DEF: Deviation of eyes seen only at intervals; it is also called strabismus.

     378.20 Intermittent heterotropia, unspecified
       Intermittent: Intermittent:
         esotropia NOS   exotropia NOS

     378.21 Intermittent esotropia, monocular

     378.22 Intermittent esotropia, alternating

     378.23 Intermittent exotropia, monocular

     378.24 Intermittent exotropia, alternating

√5ᵗʰ **378.3 Other and unspecified heterotropia**

     378.30 Heterotropia, unspecified

     378.31 Hypertropia
       Vertical heterotropia (constant) (intermittent)

     378.32 Hypotropia

     378.33 Cyclotropia

     378.34 Monofixation syndrome
       Microtropia

     378.35 Accommodative component in esotropia

√5ᵗʰ **378.4 Heterophoria**
     DEF: Deviation occurring only when the other eye is covered.

     378.40 Heterophoria, unspecified

     378.41 Esophoria

     378.42 Exophoria

     378.43 Vertical heterophoria

     378.44 Cyclophoria

     378.45 Alternating hyperphoria

`N` Newborn Age: 0   `P` Pediatric Age: 0-17   `M` Maternity Age: 12-55   `A` Adult Age: 15-124   `MCC` Major CC Condition   `CC` CC Condition   `HIV` HIV Related Dx

√5ᵗʰ **378.5 Paralytic strabismus**
> **DEF:** Deviation of the eye due to nerve paralysis affecting muscle.

    378.50 Paralytic strabismus, unspecified

    378.51 Third or oculomotor nerve palsy, partial
> AHA: 3Q, '91, 9

    378.52 Third or oculomotor nerve palsy, total
> AHA: 2Q, '89, 12

    378.53 Fourth or trochlear nerve palsy
> AHA: 2Q, '01, 21

    378.54 Sixth or abducens nerve palsy
> AHA: 2Q, '89, 12

    378.55 External ophthalmoplegia

    378.56 Total ophthalmoplegia

√5ᵗʰ **378.6 Mechanical strabismus**
> **DEF:** Deviation of the eye due to an outside force upon the extraocular muscles.

    378.60 Mechanical strabismus, unspecified

    378.61 Brown's (tendon) sheath syndrome
> **DEF:** Congenital or acquired shortening of the anter- ior sheath of superior oblique muscle; eye is unable to move upward and inward; usually unilateral.

    378.62 Mechanical strabismus from other musculofascial disorders

    378.63 Limited duction associated with other conditions

√5ᵗʰ **378.7 Other specified strabismus**

    378.71 Duane's syndrome
> **DEF:** Congenital, affects one eye; due to abnormal fibrous bands attached to rectus muscle; inability to abduct affected eye with retraction of globe.

    378.72 Progressive external ophthalmoplegia
> **DEF:** Paralysis progressing from one eye muscle to another.

    378.73 Strabismus in other neuromuscular disorders

√5ᵗʰ **378.8 Other disorders of binocular eye movements**
> *EXCLUDES* nystagmus (379.50-379.56)

    378.81 Palsy of conjugate gaze
> **DEF:** Paralysis progressing from one eye muscle to another.

    378.82 Spasm of conjugate gaze
> **DEF:** Muscle contractions impairing parallel movement of eye.

    378.83 Convergence insufficiency or palsy

    378.84 Convergence excess or spasm

    378.85 Anomalies of divergence

    378.86 Internuclear ophthalmoplegia
> **DEF:** Eye movement anomaly due to brainstem lesion.

    378.87 Other dissociated deviation of eye movements
> Skew deviation

    378.9 Unspecified disorder of eye movements
> Ophthalmoplegia NOS   Strabismus NOS
> AHA: 2Q, '01, 21

√4ᵗʰ **379 Other disorders of eye**

√5ᵗʰ **379.0 Scleritis and episcleritis**
> *EXCLUDES* syphilitic episcleritis (095.0)

    379.00 Scleritis, unspecified
> Episcleritis NOS

    379.01 Episcleritis periodica fugax
> **DEF:** Hyperemia (engorgement) of the sclera and overlying conjunctiva characterized by a sudden onset and short duration.

    379.02 Nodular episcleritis
> **DEF:** Inflammation of the outermost layer of the sclera, with formation of nodules.

    379.03 Anterior scleritis

    379.04 Scleromalacia perforans
> **DEF:** Scleral thinning, softening and degeneration; seen with rheumatoid arthritis.

    379.05 Scleritis with corneal involvement
> Scleroperikeratitis

    379.06 Brawny scleritis
> **DEF:** Severe scleral inflammation with thickening corneal margins.

    379.07 Posterior scleritis
> Sclerotenonitis

    379.09 Other
> Scleral abscess

√5ᵗʰ **379.1 Other disorders of sclera**
> *EXCLUDES* blue sclera (743.47)

    379.11 Scleral ectasia
> Scleral staphyloma NOS
> **DEF:** Protrusion of the contents of the eyeball where the sclera has thinned.

    379.12 Staphyloma posticum
> **DEF:** Ring-shaped protrusion or bulging of sclera and uveal tissue at posterior pole of eye.

    379.13 Equatorial staphyloma
> **DEF:** Ring-shaped protrusion or bulging of sclera and uveal tissue midway between front and back of eye.

    379.14 Anterior staphyloma, localized

    379.15 Ring staphyloma

    379.16 Other degenerative disorders of sclera

    379.19 Other

√5ᵗʰ **379.2 Disorders of vitreous body**
> **DEF:** Disorder of clear gel that fills space between retina and lens.

    379.21 Vitreous degeneration
> Vitreous: Vitreous:
> cavitation   liquefaction
> detachment

    379.22 Crystalline deposits in vitreous
> Asteroid hyalitis   Synchysis scintillans

    379.23 Vitreous hemorrhage
> AHA: 3Q, '91, 15

    379.24 Other vitreous opacities
> Vitreous floaters

    379.25 Vitreous membranes and strands

    379.26 Vitreous prolapse
> **DEF:** Slipping of vitreous from normal position.

    379.27 Vitreomacular adhesion   Ⓐ
> Vitreomacular traction
> *EXCLUDES* traction detachment with vitreoretinal organization (361.81)
> AHA: 4Q, '11, 105-106

    379.29 Other disorders of vitreous
> *EXCLUDES* vitreous abscess (360.04)
> AHA: 1Q, '99, 11

√5ᵗʰ **379.3 Aphakia and other disorders of lens**
> *EXCLUDES* after-cataract (366.50-366.53)

    379.31 Aphakia
> *EXCLUDES* cataract extraction status (V45.61)
> **DEF:** Absence of eye's crystalline lens.

    379.32 Subluxation of lens

    379.33 Anterior dislocation of lens
> **DEF:** Lens displaced toward iris.

    379.34 Posterior dislocation of lens
> **DEF:** Lens displaced backward toward vitreous.

    379.39 Other disorders of lens

√5ᵗʰ **379.4 Anomalies of pupillary function**

    379.40 Abnormal pupillary function, unspecified

    379.41 Anisocoria
> **DEF:** Unequal pupil diameter.

    379.42 Miosis (persistent), not due to miotics
> **DEF:** Abnormal contraction of pupil less than 2 mil.

√4ᵗʰ/√5ᵗʰ Additional Digit Required   Unacceptable PDx   Manifestation Code   Hospital Acquired Condition   ►◄ Revised Text   ● New Code   ▲ Revised Code Title

2014 ICD-9-CM   **Volume 1 – 129**

Diseases of the Nervous System and Sense Organs

379.43–380.39

379.43 Mydriasis (persistent), not due to mydriatics
DEF: Morbid dilation of pupil.

379.45 Argyll Robertson pupil, atypical
Argyll Robertson phenomenon or pupil, nonsyphilitic
EXCLUDES *Argyll Robertson pupil (syphilitic) (094.89)*
DEF: Failure of pupil to respond to light; affects both eyes; may be caused by diseases such as syphilis of the central nervous system or miosis.

379.46 Tonic pupillary reaction
Adie's pupil or syndrome

379.49 Other
Hippus   Pupillary paralysis

√5ᵗʰ **379.5 Nystagmus and other irregular eye movements**

379.50 Nystagmus, unspecified
AHA: 4Q, '02, 68; 2Q, '01, 21
DEF: Involuntary, rapid, rhythmic movement of eyeball; vertical, horizontal, rotatory or mixed; cause may be congenital, acquired, physiological, neurological, myopathic, or due to ocular diseases.

379.51 Congenital nystagmus

379.52 Latent nystagmus

379.53 Visual deprivation nystagmus

379.54 Nystagmus associated with disorders of the vestibular system

379.55 Dissociated nystagmus

379.56 Other forms of nystagmus

379.57 Deficiencies of saccadic eye movements
Abnormal optokinetic response
DEF: Saccadic eye movements; small, rapid, involuntary movements by both eyes simultaneously, due to changing point of fixation on visualized object.

379.58 Deficiencies of smooth pursuit movements

379.59 Other irregularities of eye movements
Opsoclonus

√5ᵗʰ **379.6 Inflammation (infection) of postprocedural bleb**
Postprocedural blebitis

379.60 Inflammation (infection) of postprocedural bleb, unspecified
AHA: 4Q, '06, 82

379.61 Inflammation (infection) of postprocedural bleb, stage 1
AHA: 4Q, '06, 82

379.62 Inflammation (infection) of postprocedural bleb, stage 2
AHA: 4Q, '06, 82

379.63 Inflammation (infection) of postprocedural bleb, stage 3
Bleb associated endophthalmitis
AHA: 4Q, '06, 82

379.8 Other specified disorders of eye and adnexa

√5ᵗʰ **379.9 Unspecified disorder of eye and adnexa**

379.90 Disorder of eye, unspecified

379.91 Pain in or around eye

379.92 Swelling or mass of eye

379.93 Redness or discharge of eye

379.99 Other ill-defined disorders of eye
EXCLUDES *blurred vision NOS (368.8)*

Diseases of the Ear and Mastoid Process (380-389)
Use additional external cause code, if applicable, to identify the cause of the ear condition

√4ᵗʰ **380 Disorders of external ear**

√5ᵗʰ **380.0 Perichondritis and chondritis of pinna**
Chondritis of auricle   Perichondritis of auricle

380.00 Perichondritis of pinna, unspecified

380.01 Acute perichondritis of pinna

Ear and Mastoid Process

Helix — External auditory meatus
Antihelix — Concha
Tragus
Mastoid process — Antitragus

380.02 Chronic perichondritis of pinna

380.03 Chondritis of pinna
AHA: 4Q, '04, 76
DEF: Infection that has progressed into the cartilage; presents as indurated and edematous skin over the pinna; vascular compromise occurs with tissue necrosis and deformity.

√5ᵗʰ **380.1 Infective otitis externa**

380.10 Infective otitis externa, unspecified
Otitis externa (acute):   Otitis externa (acute):
NOS   hemorrhagica
circumscribed   infective NOS
diffuse

380.11 Acute infection of pinna
EXCLUDES *furuncular otitis externa (680.0)*

380.12 Acute swimmers' ear
Beach ear   Tank ear
DEF: Otitis externa due to swimming.

380.13 *Other acute infections of external ear*
Code first underlying disease, as:
erysipelas (035)
impetigo (684)
seborrheic dermatitis (690.10-690.18)
EXCLUDES *herpes simplex (054.73)*
herpes zoster (053.71)

380.14 Malignant otitis externa   CC
CC Exd: 380.14, 383.00-383.1
DEF: Severe necrotic otitis externa; due to bacteria.

380.15 *Chronic mycotic otitis externa*
Code first underlying disease, as:
aspergillosis (117.3)
otomycosis NOS (111.9)
EXCLUDES *candidal otitis externa (112.82)*

380.16 Other chronic infective otitis externa
Chronic infective otitis externa NOS

√5ᵗʰ **380.2 Other otitis externa**

380.21 Cholesteatoma of external ear
Keratosis obturans of external ear (canal)
EXCLUDES *cholesteatoma NOS (385.30-385.35)*
postmastoidectomy (383.32)
DEF: Cystlike mass filled with debris, including cholesterol; rare, congenital condition.

380.22 Other acute otitis externa
Acute otitis externa: Acute otitis externa:
actinic   eczematoid
chemical   reactive
contact

380.23 Other chronic otitis externa
Chronic otitis externa NOS

√5ᵗʰ **380.3 Noninfectious disorders of pinna**

380.30 Disorder of pinna, unspecified

380.31 Hematoma of auricle or pinna

380.32 Acquired deformities of auricle or pinna
EXCLUDES *cauliflower ear (738.7)*
AHA: 3Q, '03, 12

380.39 Other
EXCLUDES *gouty tophi of ear (274.81)*

N Newborn Age: 0   P Pediatric Age: 0-17   M Maternity Age: 12-55   A Adult Age: 15-124   MCC Major CC Condition   CC CC Condition   HIV HIV Related Dx

130 – Volume 1   2014 ICD-9-CM

380.4 Impacted cerumen
Wax in ear

√5ᵗʰ **380.5 Acquired stenosis of external ear canal**
Collapse of external ear canal

380.50 Acquired stenosis of external ear canal, unspecified as to cause

380.51 Secondary to trauma
DEF: Narrowing of the external ear canal; due to trauma.

380.52 Secondary to surgery
DEF: Postsurgical narrowing of the external ear canal.

380.53 Secondary to inflammation
DEF: Narrowing of the external ear canal; due to chronic inflammation.

√5ᵗʰ **380.8 Other disorders of external ear**

380.81 Exostosis of external ear canal

380.89 Other

380.9 Unspecified disorder of external ear

√4ᵗʰ **381 Nonsuppurative otitis media and Eustachian tube disorders**

√5ᵗʰ **381.0 Acute nonsuppurative otitis media**
Acute tubotympanic catarrh
Otitis media, acute or subacute:
catarrhal
exudative
transudative
with effusion
EXCLUDES otitic barotrauma (993.0)

381.00 Acute nonsuppurative otitis media, unspecified

381.01 Acute serous otitis media
Acute or subacute secretory otitis media
DEF: Sudden, severe infection of the middle ear.

381.02 Acute mucoid otitis media
Acute or subacute seromucinous otitis media
Blue drum syndrome
DEF: Sudden, severe infection of the middle ear, with mucous.

381.03 Acute sanguinous otitis media
DEF: Sudden, severe infection of the middle ear, with blood.

381.04 Acute allergic serous otitis media

381.05 Acute allergic mucoid otitis media

381.06 Acute allergic sanguinous otitis media

√5ᵗʰ **381.1 Chronic serous otitis media**
Chronic tubotympanic catarrh

381.10 Chronic serous otitis media, simple or unspecified
DEF: Persistent infection of the middle ear, without pus.

381.19 Other
Serosanguinous chronic otitis media

√5ᵗʰ **381.2 Chronic mucoid otitis media**
Glue ear
EXCLUDES adhesive middle ear disease (385.10-385.19)
DEF: Chronic condition; characterized by viscous fluid in middle ear; due to obstructed Eustachian tube.

381.20 Chronic mucoid otitis media, simple or unspecified

381.29 Other
Mucosanguinous chronic otitis media

381.3 Other and unspecified chronic nonsuppurative otitis media
Otitis media, chronic: Otitis media, chronic:
allergic   seromucinous
exudative   transudative
secretory   /   with effusion

381.4 Nonsuppurative otitis media, not specified as acute or chronic
Otitis media: Otitis media:
allergic   secretory
catarrhal   seromucinous
exudative   serous
mucoid   transudative
                 with effusion

√5ᵗʰ **381.5 Eustachian salpingitis**

381.50 Eustachian salpingitis, unspecified

381.51 Acute Eustachian salpingitis
DEF: Sudden, severe inflammation of the Eustachian tube.

381.52 Chronic Eustachian salpingitis
DEF: Persistent inflammation of the Eustachian tube.

√5ᵗʰ **381.6 Obstruction of Eustachian tube**
Stenosis
Stricture } of Eustachian tube

381.60 Obstruction of Eustachian tube, unspecified

381.61 Osseous obstruction of Eustachian tube
Obstruction of Eustachian tube from cholesteatoma, polyp, or other osseous lesion

381.62 Intrinsic cartilaginous obstruction of Eustachian tube
DEF: Blockage of Eustachian tube; due to cartilage overgrowth.

381.63 Extrinsic cartilaginous obstruction of Eustachian tube
Compression of Eustachian tube

381.7 Patulous Eustachian tube
DEF: Distended, oversized Eustachian tube.

√5ᵗʰ **381.8 Other disorders of Eustachian tube**

381.81 Dysfunction of Eustachian tube

381.89 Other

381.9 Unspecified Eustachian tube disorder

√4ᵗʰ **382 Suppurative and unspecified otitis media**

√5ᵗʰ **382.0 Acute suppurative otitis media**
Otitis media, acute: Otitis media, acute:
necrotizing NOS   purulent

382.00 Acute suppurative otitis media without spontaneous rupture of ear drum
DEF: Sudden, severe inflammation of middle ear, with pus.

382.01 Acute suppurative otitis media with spontaneous rupture of ear drum
DEF: Sudden, severe inflammation of middle ear, with pressure tearing ear drum tissue.

382.02 Acute suppurative otitis media in diseases classified elsewhere
Code first underlying disease, as:
influenza (487.8, 488.09, 488.19)
scarlet fever (034.1)
EXCLUDES postmeasles otitis (055.2)

382.1 Chronic tubotympanic suppurative otitis media
Benign chronic suppurative   } (with anterior
    ottis media   perforation of
Chronic tubotympanic disease } ear drum)
DEF: Inflammation of tympanic cavity and auditory tube; with pus formation.

382.2 Chronic atticoantral suppurative otitis media
Chronic atticoantral disease } (with posterior or superior
Persistent mucosal disease }   maginal perforation of
                            ear drum)
DEF: Inflammation of upper tympanic membrane and mastoid antrum with pus formation.

382.3 Unspecified chronic suppurative otitis media
Chronic purulent otitis media
EXCLUDES tuberculous otitis media (017.4)

382.4 Unspecified suppurative otitis media
Purulent otitis media NOS

382.9 Unspecified otitis media
Otitis media: Otitis media:
NOS   chronic NOS
acute NOS
AHA: N-D, '84, 16
H66.93 Otitis media unspecified bilateral

I-10

4ᵗʰ/5ᵗʰ Additional Digit Required   Unacceptable PDx   Manifestation Code   Hospital Acquired Condition   ▶◀ Revised Text   ● New Code   ▲ Revised Code Title

2014 ICD-9-CM   Volume 1 – 131

Diseases of the Nervous System and Sense Organs

383–385.12

√4th **383 Mastoiditis and related conditions**

√5th **383.0 Acute mastoiditis**
Abscess of mastoid   Empyema of mastoid

383.00 Acute mastoiditis without complications `CC`
DEF: Sudden, severe inflammation of mastoid air cells. .
CC Excl: 015.60-015.66, 017.40-017.46, 017.90-017.96, 383.00-383.9, 388.71-388.9, 744.00, 744.02, 744.09, 744.29-744.3

383.01 Subperiosteal abscess of mastoid `CC`
DEF: Pocket of pus within the mastoid bone.
CC Excl: See code: 383.00

383.02 Acute mastoiditis with other complications `CC`
Gradenigo's syndrome
CC Excl: See code: 383.00

383.1 Chronic mastoiditis
Caries of mastoid   Fistula of mastoid
EXCLUDES tuberculous mastoiditis (015.6)
DEF: Persistent inflammation of the mastoid air cells.

√5th **383.2 Petrositis**
Coalescing osteitis
Inflammation   } of petrous bone
Osteomyelitis

383.20 Petrositis, unspecified

383.21 Acute petrositis
DEF: Sudden, severe inflammation of dense bone behind the ear.

383.22 Chronic petrositis
DEF: Persistent inflammation of dense bone behind the ear.

√5th **383.3 Complications following mastoidectomy**

383.30 Postmastoidectomy complication, unspecified

383.31 Mucosal cyst of postmastoidectomy cavity
DEF: Mucous-lined cyst cavity following removal of mastoid bone.

383.32 Recurrent cholesteatoma of postmastoidectomy cavity
DEF: Cystlike mass of cell debris in cavity following removal of mastoid bone.

383.33 Granulations of postmastoidectomy cavity
Chronic inflammation of postmastoidectomy cavity
DEF: Granular tissue in cavity following removal of mastoid bone.

√5th **383.8 Other disorders of mastoid**

383.81 Postauricular fistula
DEF: Abnormal passage behind mastoid cavity.

383.89 Other

383.9 Unspecified mastoiditis

√4th **384 Other disorders of tympanic membrane**

√5th **384.0 Acute myringitis without mention of otitis media**

384.00 Acute myringitis, unspecified
Acute tympanitis NOS
DEF: Sudden, severe inflammation of ear drum.

384.01 Bullous myringitis
Myringitis bullosa hemorrhagica
DEF: Type of viral otitis media characterized by the appearance of serous or hemorrhagic blebs on the tympanic membrane.

384.09 Other

384.1 Chronic myringitis without mention of otitis media
Chronic tympanitis
DEF: Persistent inflammation of ear drum; with no evidence of middle ear infection.

√5th **384.2 Perforation of tympanic membrane**
Perforation of ear drum:
NOS
persistent posttraumatic
postinflammatory
EXCLUDES otitis media with perforation of tympanic membrane (382.00-382.9)
traumatic perforation [current injury] (872.61)

Middle and Inner Ear

Osseus labyrinth, Semicircular canals, Auditory ossicles: Stapes, Incus, Malleus, Utricle and saccule, CN VIII, Cochlea in bone, Eustachian tube, External auditory canal, Cochlea (round window), Pharynx

Exposed view of middle and inner ear

Cholesteatoma

Middle ear chamber

Cholesteatoma sac   Ear drum

384.20 Perforation of tympanic membrane, unspecified

384.21 Central perforation of tympanic membrane

384.22 Attic perforation of tympanic membrane
Pars flaccida

384.23 Other marginal perforation of tympanic membrane

384.24 Multiple perforations of tympanic membrane

384.25 Total perforation of tympanic membrane

√5th **384.8 Other specified disorders of tympanic membrane**

384.81 Atrophic flaccid tympanic membrane
Healed perforation of ear drum

384.82 Atrophic nonflaccid tympanic membrane

384.9 Unspecified disorder of tympanic membrane

√4th **385 Other disorders of middle ear and mastoid**
EXCLUDES mastoiditis (383.0-383.9)

√5th **385.0 Tympanosclerosis**

385.00 Tympanosclerosis, unspecified as to involvement

385.01 Tympanosclerosis involving tympanic membrane only
DEF: Tough, fibrous tissue impeding functions of ear drum.

385.02 Tympanosclerosis involving tympanic membrane and ear ossicles
DEF: Tough, fibrous tissue impeding functions of middle ear bones (stapes, malleus, incus).

385.03 Tympanosclerosis involving tympanic membrane, ear ossicles, and middle ear
DEF: Tough, fibrous tissue impeding functions of ear drum, middle ear bones and middle ear canal.

385.09 Tympanosclerosis involving other combination of structures

√5th **385.1 Adhesive middle ear disease**
Adhesive otitis   Otitis media:
Otitis media: fibrotic
chronic adhesive
EXCLUDES glue ear (381.20-381.29)
DEF: Adhesions of middle ear structures.

385.10 Adhesive middle ear disease, unspecified as to involvement

385.11 Adhesions of drum head to incus

385.12 Adhesions of drum head to stapes

`N` Newborn Age: 0   `P` Pediatric Age: 0-17   `M` Maternity Age: 12-55   `A` Adult Age: 15-124   `MCC` Major CC Condition   `CC` CC Condition   `HIV` HIV Related Dx

132 – Volume 1   2014 ICD-9-CM

385.13 Adhesions of drum head to promontorium

385.19 Other adhesions and combinations

√5ᵗʰ **385.2 Other acquired abnormality of ear ossicles**

385.21 Impaired mobility of malleus
Ankylosis of malleus

385.22 Impaired mobility of other ear ossicles
Ankylosis of ear ossicles, except malleus

385.23 Discontinuity or dislocation of ear ossicles
DEF: Disruption in auditory chain; created by malleus, incus and stapes.

385.24 Partial loss or necrosis of ear ossicles
DEF: Tissue loss in malleus, incus and stapes.

√5ᵗʰ **385.3 Cholesteatoma of middle ear and mastoid**

Cholesterosis
Epidermosis
Keratosis
Polyp
} of (middle) ear

EXCLUDES cholesteatoma:
external ear canal (380.21)
recurrent of postmastoidectomy cavity (383.32)
DEF: Cystlike mass of middle ear and mastoid antrum filled with debris, including cholesterol.

385.30 Cholesteatoma, unspecified

385.31 Cholesteatoma of attic

385.32 Cholesteatoma of middle ear

385.33 Cholesteatoma of middle ear and mastoid
DEF: Cystlike mass of cell debris in middle ear and mastoid air cells behind ear.
AHA: 3Q, '00, 10

385.35 Diffuse cholesteatosis

√5ᵗʰ **385.8 Other disorders of middle ear and mastoid**

385.82 Cholesterin granuloma
DEF: Granuloma formed of fibrotic tissue; contains cholesterol crystals surrounded by foreign-body cells; found in the middle ear and mastoid area.

385.83 Retained foreign body of middle ear
Use additional code to identify foreign body (V90.01-V90.9)
AHA: 3Q, '94, 7; N-D, '87, 9

385.89 Other

385.9 Unspecified disorder of middle ear and mastoid

√4ᵗʰ **386 Vertiginous syndromes and other disorders of vestibular system**
EXCLUDES vertigo NOS (780.4)
AHA: M-A, '85, 12

√5ᵗʰ **386.0 Ménière's disease**
Endolymphatic hydrops
Lermoyez's syndrome
Ménière's syndrome or vertigo
DEF: Distended membranous labyrinth of middle ear from endolymphatic hydrops; causes ischemia, failure of nerve function; hearing and balance dysfunction; symptoms include fluctuating deafness, ringing in ears and dizziness.

386.00 Ménière's disease, unspecified
Ménière's disease (active)
H81.03 Ménière's disease bilateral   I-10

386.01 Active Ménière's disease, cochleovestibular

386.02 Active Ménière's disease, cochlear

386.03 Active Ménière's disease, vestibular

386.04 Inactive Ménière's disease
Ménière's disease in remission

√5ᵗʰ **386.1 Other and unspecified peripheral vertigo**
EXCLUDES epidemic vertigo (078.81)

386.10 Peripheral vertigo, unspecified

386.11 Benign paroxysmal positional vertigo
Benign paroxysmal positional nystagmus

386.12 Vestibular neuronitis
Acute (and recurrent) peripheral vestibulopathy
DEF: Transient benign vertigo, unknown cause; characterized by response to caloric stimulation on one side, nystagmus with rhythmic movement of eyes; normal auditory function present.

386.19 Other
Aural vertigo   Otogenic vertigo

386.2 Vertigo of central origin
Central positional nystagmus   Malignant positional vertigo

√5ᵗʰ **386.3 Labyrinthitis**

386.30 Labyrinthitis, unspecified

386.31 Serous labyrinthitis
Diffuse labyrinthitis
DEF: Inflammation of labyrinth; with fluid buildup.

386.32 Circumscribed labyrinthitis
Focal labyrinthitis

386.33 Suppurative labyrinthitis
Purulent labyrinthitis
DEF: Inflammation of labyrinth; with pus.

386.34 Toxic labyrinthitis
DEF: Inflammation of labyrinth; due to toxic reaction.

386.35 Viral labyrinthitis

√5ᵗʰ **386.4 Labyrinthine fistula**

386.40 Labyrinthine fistula, unspecified

386.41 Round window fistula

386.42 Oval window fistula

386.43 Semicircular canal fistula

386.48 Labyrinthine fistula of combined sites

√5ᵗʰ **386.5 Labyrinthine dysfunction**

386.50 Labyrinthine dysfunction, unspecified

386.51 Hyperactive labyrinth, unilateral
DEF: Abnormal increased sensitivity of labyrinth to stimuli such as sound, pressure or gravitational change, affecting one ear.

386.52 Hyperactive labyrinth, bilateral
DEF: Abnormal increased sensitivity of labyrinth to stimuli such as sound, pressure or gravitational change, affecting both ears.

386.53 Hypoactive labyrinth, unilateral
DEF: Abnormal decreased sensitivity of labyrinth to stimuli such as sound, pressure or gravitational change, affecting one ear.

386.54 Hypoactive labyrinth, bilateral
DEF: Abnormal decreased sensitivity of labyrinth to stimuli such as sound, pressure or gravitational change, affecting both ears.

386.55 Loss of labyrinthine reactivity, unilateral
DEF: Decreased function of the labyrinth sensors, affecting one ear

386.56 Loss of labyrinthine reactivity, bilateral
DEF: Decreased function of the labyrinth sensors, affecting both ears

386.58 Other forms and combinations

386.8 Other disorders of labyrinth
AHA: 1Q, '11, 6

386.9 Unspecified vertiginous syndromes and labyrinthine disorders

√4ᵗʰ **387 Otosclerosis**
INCLUDES otospongiosis
DEF: Synonym for otospongiosis, spongy bone formation in the labyrinth bones of the ear; it causes progressive hearing impairment.

387.0 Otosclerosis involving oval window, nonobliterative
DEF: Tough, fibrous tissue impeding functions of oval window.

387.1 Otosclerosis involving oval window, obliterative
DEF: Tough, fibrous tissue blocking oval window.

Additional Digit Required   Unacceptable PDx   Manifestation Code   Hospital Acquired Condition   ▶◀ Revised Text   ● New Code   ▲ Revised Code Title

Diseases of the Nervous System and Sense Organs

387.2–389.9

387.2 Cochlear otosclerosis
Otosclerosis involving: Otosclerosis involving:
    otic capsule   round window
DEF: Tough, fibrous tissue impeding functions of cochlea.

387.8 Other otosclerosis

387.9 Otosclerosis, unspecified

√4ᵗʰ **388 Other disorders of ear**

√5ᵗʰ **388.0 Degenerative and vascular disorders of ear**

388.00 Degenerative and vascular disorders, unspecified

388.01 Presbyacusis
DEF: Progressive, bilateral perceptive hearing loss caused by advancing age; it is also known as presbycusis.

388.02 Transient ischemic deafness
DEF: Restricted blood flow to auditory organs causing temporary hearing loss.

√5ᵗʰ **388.1 Noise effects on inner ear**

388.10 Noise effects on inner ear, unspecified

388.11 Acoustic trauma (explosive) to ear
Otitic blast injury

388.12 Noise-induced hearing loss

388.2 Sudden hearing loss, unspecified

√5ᵗʰ **388.3 Tinnitus**
DEF: Abnormal noises in ear; may be heard by others beside the affected individual; noises include ringing, clicking, roaring and buzzing.

388.30 Tinnitus, unspecified

388.31 Subjective tinnitus

388.32 Objective tinnitus

√5ᵗʰ **388.4 Other abnormal auditory perception**

388.40 Abnormal auditory perception, unspecified

388.41 Diplacusis
DEF: Perception of a single auditory sound as two sounds at two different levels of intensity.

388.42 Hyperacusis
DEF: Exceptionally acute sense of hearing caused by such conditions as Bell's palsy; this term may also refer to painful sensitivity to sounds.

388.43 Impairment of auditory discrimination
DEF: Impaired ability to distinguish tone of sound.

388.44 Recruitment
DEF: Perception of abnormally increased loudness caused by a slight increase in sound intensity; it is a term used in audiology.

388.45 Acquired auditory processing disorder
Auditory processing disorder NOS
EXCLUDES central auditory processing disorder (315.32)
DEF: Difficulty in recognizing and interpreting sounds; a failure of the brain to process auditory information; due to neurological problems due to injury, infection, and degenerative conditions.
AHA: 4Q, '07, 79

388.5 Disorders of acoustic nerve
Acoustic neuritis
Degeneration   } of acoustic or eighth nerve
Disorder
EXCLUDES acoustic neuroma (225.1)
syphilitic acoustic neuritis (094.86)
AHA: M-A, '87, 8

√5ᵗʰ **388.6 Otorrhea**

388.60 Otorrhea, unspecified
Discharging ear NOS

388.61 Cerebrospinal fluid otorrhea   CC
EXCLUDES cerebrospinal fluid rhinorrhea (349.81)
CC Exd: 388.61-388.69
DEF: Spinal fluid leakage from ear.

388.69 Other
Otorrhagia

√5ᵗʰ **388.7 Otalgia**

388.70 Otalgia, unspecified
Earache NOS

388.71 Otogenic pain

388.72 Referred pain

388.8 Other disorders of ear

388.9 Unspecified disorder of ear

√4ᵗʰ **389 Hearing loss**

√5ᵗʰ **389.0 Conductive hearing loss**
Conductive deafness
EXCLUDES mixed conductive and sensorineural hearing loss (389.20-389.22)
DEF: Dysfunction in sound-conducting structures of external or middle ear causing hearing loss.
AHA: 4Q, '07, 80; 4Q, '89, 5

389.00 Conductive hearing loss, unspecified

389.01 Conductive hearing loss, external ear

389.02 Conductive hearing loss, tympanic membrane

389.03 Conductive hearing loss, middle ear

389.04 Conductive hearing loss, inner ear

389.05 Conductive hearing loss, unilateral

389.06 Conductive hearing loss, bilateral
AHA: 4Q, '07, 81

389.08 Conductive hearing loss of combined types

√5ᵗʰ **389.1 Sensorineural hearing loss**
Perceptive hearing loss or deafness
EXCLUDES abnormal auditory perception (388.40-388.44)
mixed conductive and sensorineural hearing loss (389.20-389.22)
psychogenic deafness (306.7)
DEF: Nerve conduction causing hearing loss.
AHA: 4Q, '07, 80; 4Q, '89, 5

389.10 Sensorineural hearing loss, unspecified
AHA: 1Q, '93, 29

389.11 Sensory hearing loss, bilateral

389.12 Neural hearing loss, bilateral

389.13 Neural hearing loss, unilateral

389.14 Central hearing loss

389.15 Sensorineural hearing loss, unilateral
AHA: 4Q, '06, 84

389.16 Sensorineural hearing loss, asymmetrical
AHA: 4Q, '06, 84

389.17 Sensory hearing loss, unilateral

389.18 Sensorineural hearing loss, bilateral
AHA: 4Q, '06, 84

√5ᵗʰ **389.2 Mixed conductive and sensorineural hearing loss**
Deafness or hearing loss of type classifiable to 389.00-389.08 with type classifiable to 389.10-389.18
AHA: 4Q, '07, 80

389.20 Mixed hearing loss, unspecified

389.21 Mixed hearing loss, unilateral

389.22 Mixed hearing loss, bilateral

389.7 Deaf, non-speaking, not elsewhere classifiable

389.8 Other specified forms of hearing loss

389.9 Unspecified hearing loss
Deafness NOS
AHA: 1Q, '04, 15
H91.93 Unspecified hearing loss bilateral

N Newborn Age: 0   P Pediatric Age: 0-17   M Maternity Age: 12-55   A Adult Age: 15-124   MCC Major CC Condition   CC CC Condition   HIV HIV Related D:

134 – Volume 1   **2014 ICD-9-CN**

7. Diseases of the Circulatory System (390-459)

Acute Rheumatic Fever (390-392)

DEF: Febrile disease occurs mainly in children or young adults following throat infection by group A streptococci; symptoms include fever, joint pain, lesions of heart, blood vessels and joint connective tissue, abdominal pain, skin changes, and chorea.

390 Rheumatic fever without mention of heart involvement
Arthritis, rheumatic, acute or subacute
Rheumatic fever (active) (acute)
Rheumatism, articular, acute or subacute
EXCLUDES that with heart involvement (391.0-391.9)

√4ᵗʰ 391 Rheumatic fever with heart involvement
EXCLUDES chronic heart diseases of rheumatic origin (393-398.99) unless rheumatic fever is also present or there is evidence of recrudescence or activity of the rheumatic process

391.0 Acute rheumatic pericarditis   `CC`
Rheumatic:
    fever (active) (acute) with pericarditis
    pericarditis (acute)
Any condition classifiable to 390 with pericarditis
EXCLUDES that not specified as rheumatic (420.0-420.9)
DEF: Sudden, severe inflammation of heart lining due to rheumatic fever.
CC Exd: 074.21, 093.81, 391.0, 393, 420.0-420.99, 423.3-423.9, 459.89-459.9

391.1 Acute rheumatic endocarditis   `CC`
Rheumatic:
    endocarditis, acute
    fever (active) (acute) with endocarditis or valvulitis
    valvulitis acute
Any condition classifiable to 390 with endocarditis or valvulitis
DEF: Sudden, severe inflammation of heart cavities due to rheumatic fever.
CC Exd: 002.0, 036.42, 074.22, 083.0, 093.20-093.24, 098.84, 112.81, 115.94, 390, 391.1, 391.8-392.0, 394.0-395.9, 396.9-397.9, 398.90, 398.99, 421.0-421.9, 424.0-424.99, 425.3, 459.89-459.9, 746.09, 746.89, 996.61

391.2 Acute rheumatic myocarditis   `CC`
Rheumatic fever (active) (acute) with myocarditis
Any condition classifiable to 390 with myocarditis
DEF: Sudden, severe inflammation of heart muscles due to rheumatic fever.
CC Exd: 074.20, 074.22-074.23, 093.82, 390, 391.2-391.9, 398.0-398.90, 398.99, 422.0-422.99, 429.0, 429.71-429.79, 459.89-459.9

391.8 Other acute rheumatic heart disease   `CC`
Rheumatic:
    fever (active) (acute) with other or multiple types of heart involvement
    pancarditis, acute
Any condition classifiable to 390 with other or multiple types of heart involvement
CC Exd: 391.0-398.99, 428.20-428.43

391.9 Acute rheumatic heart disease, unspecified   `CC`
Rheumatic:
    carditis, acute
    fever (active) (acute) with unspecified type of heart involvement
    heart disease, active or acute
Any condition classifiable to 390 with unspecified type of heart involvement
CC Exd: 391.0-398.99

√4ᵗʰ 392 Rheumatic chorea
INCLUDES Sydenham's chorea
EXCLUDES chorea:
    NOS (333.5)
    Huntington's (333.4)
DEF: Childhood disease linked with rheumatic fever and streptococcal infections; symptoms include spasmodic, involuntary movements of limbs or facial muscles, psychic symptoms, and irritability.

392.0 With heart involvement   `CC`
Rheumatic chorea with heart involvement of any type classifiable to 391
CC Exd: See code: 391.8

392.9 Without mention of heart involvement   `CC`
CC Exd: See code: 391.9

Chronic Rheumatic Heart Disease (393-398)

393 Chronic rheumatic pericarditis   `CC`
Adherent pericardium, rheumatic
Chronic rheumatic:
    mediastinopericarditis
    myopericarditis
EXCLUDES pericarditis NOS or not specified as rheumatic (423.0-423.9)
DEF: Persistent inflammation of heart lining due to rheumatic heart disease.
CC Exd: 074.21, 093.81, 391.0, 393, 420.0-420.99, 423.3-423.9, 459.89-459.9

√4ᵗʰ 394 Diseases of mitral valve
EXCLUDES that with aortic valve involvement (396.0-396.9)

394.0 Mitral stenosis
Mitral (valve):
    obstruction (rheumatic)
    stenosis NOS
DEF: Narrowing, of mitral valve between left atrium and left ventricle; due to rheumatic heart disease.
TIP: Assign when documentation indicates mitral valve stenosis or obstruction with no further specification of cause.

394.1 Rheumatic mitral insufficiency
Rheumatic mitral:
    incompetence
    regurgitation
EXCLUDES that not specified as rheumatic (424.0)
DEF: Malfunction of mitral valve between left atrium and left ventricle; due to rheumatic heart disease.
AHA: 2Q, '05, 14

394.2 Mitral stenosis with insufficiency
Mitral stenosis with incompetence or regurgitation
DEF: A narrowing or stricture of the mitral valve situated between the left atrium and left ventricle; valve does not completely close, is insufficient (inadequate) in preventing regurgitation into the atrium; also called incompetence.
AHA: 1Q, '07, 11

394.9 Other and unspecified mitral valve diseases
Mitral (valve):
    disease (chronic)
    failure

√4ᵗʰ 395 Diseases of aortic valve
EXCLUDES that not specified as rheumatic (424.1)
    that with mitral valve involvement (396.0-396.9)

395.0 Rheumatic aortic stenosis
Rheumatic aortic (valve) obstruction
DEF: Narrowing of the aortic valve; results in backflow into ventricle; due to rheumatic heart disease.
AHA: 4Q, '88, 8

395.1 Rheumatic aortic insufficiency
Rheumatic aortic:
    incompetence
    regurgitation
DEF: Malfunction of the aortic valve; results in backflow into left ventricle; due to rheumatic heart disease.

395.2 Rheumatic aortic stenosis with insufficiency
Rheumatic aortic stenosis with incompetence or regurgitation
DEF: Malfunction and narrowing, of the aortic valve; results in backflow into left ventricle; due to rheumatic heart disease.

395.9 Other and unspecified rheumatic aortic diseases
Rheumatic aortic (valve) disease

▲ Additional Digit Required   Unacceptable PDx   Manifestation Code   Hospital Acquired Condition   ►◄ Revised Text   ● New Code   ▲ Revised Code Title

Diseases of the Circulatory System

396–402.91

√4ᵗʰ **396 Diseases of mitral and aortic valves**
     INCLUDES involvement of both mitral and aortic valves, whether specified as rheumatic or not
     AHA: N-D, '87, 8

     396.0 Mitral valve stenosis and aortic valve stenosis
         Atypical aortic (valve) stenosis
         Mitral and aortic (valve) obstruction (rheumatic)

     396.1 Mitral valve stenosis and aortic valve insufficiency

     396.2 Mitral valve insufficiency and aortic valve stenosis
         AHA: 2Q, '09, 17; 1Q, '09, 18; 2Q, '00, 16

     396.3 Mitral valve insufficiency and aortic valve insufficiency
         Mitral and aortic (valve):
            incompetence
            regurgitation
         I08.0 Rheumatic d/o of both mitral & aortic valves   I-10

     396.8 Multiple involvement of mitral and aortic valves
         Stenosis and insufficiency of mitral or aortic valve with stenosis or insufficiency, or both, of the other valve

     396.9 Mitral and aortic valve diseases, unspecified

√4ᵗʰ **397 Diseases of other endocardial structures**

     397.0 Diseases of tricuspid valve
         Tricuspid (valve) (rheumatic):
            disease
            insufficiency
            obstruction
            regurgitation
            stenosis
         DEF: Malfunction of the valve between right atrium and right ventricle; due to rheumatic heart disease.
         AHA: 3Q, '06, 7; 2Q, '00, 16
         I07.2 Rheumatic tricuspid stenosis and insufficiency   I-10

     397.1 Rheumatic diseases of pulmonary valve
         EXCLUDES that not specified as rheumatic (424.3)

     397.9 Rheumatic diseases of endocardium, valve unspecified
         Rheumatic:
            endocarditis (chronic)
            valvulitis (chronic)
         EXCLUDES that not specified as rheumatic (424.90-424.99)

√4ᵗʰ **398 Other rheumatic heart disease**

     398.0 Rheumatic myocarditis   CC
         Rheumatic degeneration of myocardium
         EXCLUDES myocarditis not specified as rheumatic (429.0)
         DEF: Chronic inflammation of heart muscle; due to rheumatic heart disease.
         CC Exd: 390, 391.2-391.9, 398.0-398.90, 398.99, 422.0-422.99, 429.0, 429.71-429.79, 459.89-459.9

√5ᵗʰ **398.9 Other and unspecified rheumatic heart diseases**

         398.90 Rheumatic heart disease, unspecified
            Rheumatic: Rheumatic:
            carditis   heart disease NOS
            EXCLUDES carditis not specified as rheumatic (429.89)
                   heart disease NOS not specified as rheumatic (429.9)

         398.91 Rheumatic heart failure (congestive)   CC
            Rheumatic left ventricular failure
            DEF: Decreased cardiac output, edema and hypertension; due to rheumatic heart disease.
            CC Exd: 398.90-398.99, 402.01, 402.11, 402.91, 428.0-428.9, 459.89-459.9
            AHA: 2Q, '05, 14; 1Q, '95, 6; 3Q, '88, 3
            I09.81 Rheumatic heart failure   I-10

         398.99 Other

Hypertensive Disease (401-405)

     EXCLUDES that complicating pregnancy, childbirth, or the puerperium (642.0-642.9)
                 that involving coronary vessels (410.00-414.9)
     AHA: 3Q, '90, 3; 2Q, '89, 12; S-O, '87, 9; J-A, '84, 11

√4ᵗʰ **401 Essential hypertension**
     INCLUDES high blood pressure
                 hyperpiesia
                 hyperpiesis
                 hypertension (arterial) (essential) (primary) (systemic)
                 hypertensive vascular:
                     degeneration
                     disease
     EXCLUDES elevated blood pressure without diagnosis of hypertension (796.2)
                 pulmonary hypertension (416.0-416.9)
                 that involving vessels of:
                     brain (430-438)
                     eye (362.11)
     DEF: Hypertension that occurs without apparent organic cause; idiopathic.
     AHA: 2Q, '92, 5

     401.0 Malignant   CC
         DEF: Severe high arterial blood pressure; results in necrosis in kidney, retina, etc.; hemorrhages occur and death commonly due to uremia or rupture of cerebral vessel.
         CC Exd: 401.0-405.99, 459.89-459.9
         AHA: M-J, '85, 19

     401.1 Benign
         DEF: Mildly elevated arterial blood pressure.

     401.9 Unspecified
         AHA: 1Q, '12, 14; 4Q, '10,124,125, 135; 4Q, '09, 77, 129; 1Q, '09, 16; 2Q, '08, 16; 4Q, '05, 71; 3Q, '05, 8; 4Q, '04, 78; 4Q, '03, 105, 108, 111; 3Q, '03, 14; 2Q, '03, 16; 4Q, '97, 37
         I10 Essential (primary) hypertension   I-10

√4ᵗʰ **402 Hypertensive heart disease**
     INCLUDES hypertensive:
                 cardiomegaly
                 cardiopathy
                 cardiovascular disease
                 heart (disease) (failure)
                 any condition classifiable to 429.0-429.3, 429.8, 429.9 due to hypertension
     Use additional code to specify type of heart failure (428.0-428.43), if known
     AHA: 4Q, '02, 49; 2Q, '93, 9; N-D, '84, 18
     TIP: Assign when a cardiac condition is stated (due to hypertension) or implied (hypertensive).

√5ᵗʰ **402.0 Malignant**

         402.00 Without heart failure   CC
            CC Exd: See code: 401.0

         402.01 With heart failure   CC
            CC Exd: 398.91, 401.0-405.99, 428.0-428.9, 459.89-459.9
            AHA: 4Q, '08, 180

√5ᵗʰ **402.1 Benign**

         402.10 Without heart failure

         402.11 With heart failure

√5ᵗʰ **402.9 Unspecified**

         402.90 Without heart failure
            I11.9 Hypertensive heart disease without heart failure   I-10

         402.91 With heart failure
            AHA: 4Q, '02, 52; 1Q, '93, 19; 2Q, '89, 12

N Newborn Age: 0   **P** Pediatric Age: 0-17   **M** Maternity Age: 12-55   **A** Adult Age: 15-124   **MCC** Major CC Condition   **CC** CC Condition   **HIV** HIV Related D

136 – Volume 1   2014 ICD-9-C

√4ᵗʰ **403 Hypertensive chronic kidney disease**

INCLUDES arteriolar nephritis
arteriosclerosis of:
   kidney
   renal arterioles
arteriosclerotic nephritis (chronic) (interstitial)
hypertensive:
   nephropathy
   renal failure
   uremia (chronic)
nephrosclerosis
renal sclerosis with hypertension

any condition classifiable to 585 and 587 with any condition classifiable to 401

EXCLUDES *acute kidney failure (584.5-584.9)*
renal disease stated as not due to hypertension
renovascular hypertension (405.0-405.9 with fifth-digit 1)

The following fifth-digit subclassification is for use with category 403:
  0 with chronic kidney disease stage I through stage IV, or unspecified
    Use additional code to identify the stage of chronic kidney disease (585.1-585.4, 585.9)
  1 with chronic kidney disease stage V or end stage renal disease
    Use additional code to identify the stage of chronic kidney disease (585.5, 585.6)

AHA: 4Q, '06, 84-86; 4Q, '05, 68; 4Q, '92, 22; 2Q, '92, 5
TIP: Assign whenever a patient has both chronic kidney disease and hypertension (presumed cause-and-effect relationship).

§ √5ᵗʰ **403.0 Malignant**   CC
  [0-1]   CC Exd: 401.0-405.99, 459.89-459.9

§ √5ᵗʰ **403.1 Benign**   CC 1
  [0-1]   CC Exd: For code 403.11: See code 403.0
      AHA: For code 403.11: 3Q,'10, 12

§ √5ᵗʰ **403.9 Unspecified**   CC 1
  [0-1]   CC Exd: For code 403.91: 401.0-405.99, 459.89-459.9, 585.6
      AHA: For code 403.90: 4Q, '10, 137; 1Q, '08, 10; 2Q, '07, 3; 4Q, '06, 86;
      For code 403.91: 4Q, '10, 137; 1Q, '08, 7; 4Q, '05, 69; 1Q, '04, 14; 1Q, '03, 20; 2Q, '01, 11; 3Q, '91, 8
      I12.9 HTN CKD w/stage I thru IV CKD/UNS CKD   I-10

√4ᵗʰ **404 Hypertensive heart and chronic kidney disease**

INCLUDES disease:
   cardiorenal
   cardiovascular renal

any condition classifiable to 402 with any condition classifiable to 403

Use additional code to specify type of heart failure (428.0-428.43), if known

The following fifth-digit subclassification is for use with category 404:
  0 without heart failure and with chronic kidney disease stage I through stage IV, or unspecified
    Use additional code to identify the stage of chronic kidney disease (585.1-585.4, 585.9)
  1 with heart failure and with chronic kidney disease stage I through stage IV, or unspecified
    Use additional code to identify the stage of chronic kidney disease (585.1-585.4, 585.9)
  2 without heart failure and with chronic kidney disease stage V or end stage renal disease
    Use additional code to identify the stage of chronic kidney disease (585.5, 585.6)
  3 with heart failure and chronic kidney disease stage V or end stage renal disease
    Use additional code to identify the stage of chronic kidney disease (585.5, 585.6)

AHA: 4Q, '06, 84-86; 4Q, '05, 68; 4Q, '02, 49; 3Q, '90, 3; J-A, '84, 14

§ √5ᵗʰ **404.0 Malignant**   CC
  [0-3]   CC Exd: 401.0-405.99, 459.89-459.9

§ √5ᵗʰ **404.1 Benign**   CC 1-3
  [0-3]   CC Exd: For codes 404.11-404.13: 401.0-405.99, 459.89-459.9

§ √5ᵗʰ **404.9 Unspecified**   CC 1-3
  [0-3]   CC Exd: For codes 404.91-404.93: 401.0-405.99, 459.89-459.9
      I13.0 HTN heart & CKD HF & stage I thru IV CKD/UNS CKD   I-10

√4ᵗʰ **405 Secondary hypertension**

DEF: High arterial blood pressure due to or with a variety of primary diseases, such as renal disorders, CNS disorders, endocrine, and vascular diseases.
AHA: 3Q, '90, 3; S-O, '87, 9, 11; J-A, '84, 14

√5ᵗʰ **405.0 Malignant**

  405.01 Renovascular   CC
    CC Exd: See code: 404.0

  405.09 Other   CC
    CC Exd: See code: 404.0

√5ᵗʰ **405.1 Benign**

  405.11 Renovascular

  405.19 Other

√5ᵗʰ **405.9 Unspecified**

  405.91 Renovascular

  405.99 Other
    AHA: 3Q, '00, 4

Ischemic Heart Disease (410-414)

INCLUDES that with mention of hypertension
Use additional code to identify presence of hypertension (401.0-405.9)
AHA: 3Q, '91, 10; J-A, '84, 5

√4ᵗʰ **410 Acute myocardial infarction**

INCLUDES cardiac infarction
coronary (artery):
   embolism
   occlusion
   rupture
   thrombosis
infarction of heart, myocardium, or ventricle
rupture of heart, myocardium, or ventricle
ST elevation (STEMI) and non-ST elevation (NSTEMI) myocardial infarction

any condition classifiable to 414.1-414.9 specified as acute or with a stated duration of 8 weeks or less

The following fifth-digit subclassification is for use with category 410:
  0 episode of care unspecified
    Use when the source document does not contain sufficient information for the assigment of fifth-digit 1 or 2.
  1 initial episode of care
    Use fifth-digit 1 to designate the first episode of care (regardless of facility site) for a newly diagnosed myocardial infarction. The fifth-digit 1 is assigned regardless of the number of times a patient may be transferred during the initial episode of care.
  2 subsequent episode of care
    Use fifth-digit 2 to designate an episode of care following the initial episode when the patient is admitted for further observation, evaluation or treatment for a myocardial infarction that has received initial treatment, but is still less than 8 weeks old.

DEF: A sudden insufficiency of blood supply to an area of the heart muscle; usually due to a coronary artery occlusion.
AHA: 1Q, '12, 7; 2Q, '06, 9; 4Q, '05, 69; 3Q, '01, 21; 3Q, '98, 15; 4Q, '97, 37; 3Q, '95, 9; 4Q, 92, 24; 1Q, '92, 10; 3Q, '91, 18; 1Q, '91, 14; 3Q, '89, 3
TIP: Assign an acute MI code with a fifth digit of "1," initial episode of care, for all care before the AMI has resolved, regardless of type or number of transfers between facilities.

§ √5ᵗʰ **410.0 Of anterolateral wall**   MCC 1
  [0-2]   ST elevation myocardial infarction (STEMI) of anterolateral wall
    CC Exd: For code 410.01 410.00-410.92, 459.89-459.9
    AHA: For code 410.01: 4Q, '09, 129; 4Q, '08, 72

§ √5ᵗʰ **410.1 Of other anterior wall**   MCC 1
  [0-2]   Infarction:
    anterior (wall) NOS } (with contiguous portion of
    anteroapical   intraventricular
    anteroseptal   septum)
    ST elevation myocardial infarction (STEMI) of other anterior wall
    CC Exd: For code 410.11: See code 410.0
    AHA: For code 410.11: 3Q, '03, 10

Requires fifth digit. Valid digits are in [brackets] under each code. See appropriate category for codes and definitions.

Additional Digit Required	Unacceptable PDx	Manifestation Code	Hospital Acquired Condition	▶◀ Revised Text	● New Code	▲ Revised Code Title

Acute Myocardial Infarction

Anatomic Sites

Anterolateral 410.0
Other lateral 410.5
Posterobasal 410.6
Postero-lateral 410.5
Anteroseptal 410.1
Atrium only 410.8
Inferoposterior 410.3
Septum only
Apical 410.1
Other and septum 410.4
Papillary muscle

§ ✔5ᵗʰ **410.2 Of inferolateral wall**   `MCC 1`
[0-2]   ST elevation myocardial infarction (STEMI) of inferolateral wall
      CC Excl: For code 410.21: See code 410.0

§ ✔5ᵗʰ **410.3 Of inferoposterior wall**   `MCC 1`
[0-2]   ST elevation myocardial infarction (STEMI) of inferoposterior wall
      CC Excl: For code 410.31: See code 410.0

§ ✔5ᵗʰ **410.4 Of other inferior wall**   `MCC 1`
[0-2]   Infarction:
        diaphragmatic wall NOS ⎱ (with contiguous portion of
        inferior (wall) NOS   ⎰ intraventricular septum)
      ST elevation myocardial infarction (STEMI) of other inferior wall
      CC Excl: For code 410.41: See code 410.0
      AHA: 1Q, '00, 7, 26; 4Q, '99, 9; 3Q, '97, 10; **For code 410.41:** 3Q, '09,10; 2Q, '01, 8, 9
      I21.19 STEMI invlv oth coronary artery of inferior wall   `I-10`

§ ✔5ᵗʰ **410.5 Of other lateral wall**   `MCC 1`
[0-2]   Infarction:
        apical-lateral
        basal-lateral
        high lateral
        posterolateral
      ST elevation myocardial infarction (STEMI) of other lateral wall
      CC Excl: For code 410.51: See code 410.0
      AHA: For code 410.51: 3Q, '09,9

§ ✔5ᵗʰ **410.6 True posterior wall infarction**   `MCC 1`
[0-2]   Infarction:
        posterobasal
        strictly posterior
      ST elevation myocardial infarction (STEMI) of true posterior wall
      CC Excl: For code 410.61: See code 410.0

§ ✔5ᵗʰ **410.7 Subendocardial infarction**   `MCC 1`
[0-2]   Non-ST elevation myocardial infarction (NSTEMI)
      Nontransmural infarction
      CC Excl: For code 410.71: See code 410.0
      AHA: 1Q, '00, 7; **For code 410.71:** 2Q, '10, 8-9; 4Q, '05, 71; 2Q, '05, 19
      I21.4 Non-ST elevation (NSTEMI) myocardial infarction   `I-10`

§ ✔5ᵗʰ **410.8 Of other specified sites**   `MCC 1`
[0-2]   Infarction of:
        atrium
        papillary muscle
        septum alone
      ST elevation myocardial infarction (STEMI) of other specified sites
      CC Excl: For code 410.81: See code 410.0

§ ✔5ᵗʰ **410.9 Unspecified site**   `MCC 1`
[0-2]   Acute myocardial infarction NOS
      Coronary occlusion NOS
      Myocardial infarction NOS
      CC Excl: For code 410.91: See code 410.0
      AHA: 1Q, '96, 17; 1Q, '92, 9; **For code 410.91:** 2Q, '05, 18; 3Q, '02, 5
      I21.3 ST elevation myocardial infarction of uns site   `I-10`

✔4ᵗʰ **411 Other acute and subacute forms of ischemic heart disease**
     AHA: 4Q, '94, 55; 3Q, '91, 24

411.0 Postmyocardial infarction syndrome   `CC`
     Dressler's syndrome
     DEF: Complication developing several days/weeks after myocardial infarction; symptoms include fever, leukocytosis, chest pain, pericarditis, pleurisy, and pneumonitis; tendency to recur.
     CC Excl: 411.0, 411.81-411.89, 459.89-459.9

411.1 Intermediate coronary syndrome   `CC`
     Impending infarction
     Preinfarction angina
     Preinfarction syndrome
     Unstable angina
     EXCLUDES *angina (pectoris) (413.9)*
                decubitus (413.0)
     DEF: A condition representing an intermediate stage between angina of effort and acute myocardial infarction. It is often documented by the physician as "unstable angina."
     CC Excl: 398.91, 402.01, 402.11, 402.91, 404.01, 404.03, 404.11, 404.13, 404.91, 404.93, 410.00-410.92, 411.1-411.89, 413.0-414.00, 414.2-414.9, 428.0-428.1, 428.9, 459.89-459.9, 785.50-785.51
     AHA: 3Q, '07, 9; 4Q, '05, 105; 2Q, '04, 3; 1Q, '03, 12; 3Q, '01, 15; 2Q, '01, 7, 9; 4Q, '98, 86; 2Q, '96, 10; 3Q, '91, 24; 1Q, '91, 14; 3Q, '90, 6; 4Q, '89, 10
     TIP: Do not assign code 411.1 on the same episode of care as an acute myocardial infarction (category 410). Assign 411.1 for accelerated angina.
     I20.0 Unstable angina   `I-10`

✔5ᵗʰ **411.8 Other**
     AHA: 3Q, '91, 18; 3Q, '89, 4

411.81 Acute coronary occlusion without myocardial infarction   `CC`
     Acute coronary (artery):
        embolism   ⎱
        obstruction   ⎰ without or not resulting in
        occlusion   myocardial infarction
        thrombosis ⎰
     EXCLUDES *obstruction without infarction due to atherosclerosis (414.00-414.07)*
                occlusion without infarction due to atherosclerosis (414.00-414.07)
     DEF: Interrupted blood flow to a portion of the heart; without tissue death.
     CC Excl: 410.00-411.89, 413.0-413.9, 414.8-414.9, 459.89-459.9
     AHA: 3Q, '91, 24; 1Q, '91, 14

411.89 Other   `CC`
     Coronary insufficiency (acute)
     Subendocardial ischemia
     CC Excl: See code: 411.81
     AHA: 3Q, '01, 14; 1Q, '92, 9

412 Old myocardial infarction
     Healed myocardial infarction
     Past myocardial infarction diagnosed on ECG [EKG] or other special investigation, but currently presenting no symptoms
     AHA: 2Q, '03, 10; 2Q, '01, 9; 3Q, '98, 15; 2Q, '91, 22; 3Q, '90, 7
     TIP: Assign for any acute myocardial infarction stated to be older than 8 weeks.
     I25.2 Old myocardial infarction   `I-10`

✔4ᵗʰ **413 Angina pectoris**
     DEF: Severe constricting pain in the chest, often radiating from the precordium to the left shoulder and down the arm, due to ischemia of the heart muscle; usually caused by coronary disease; pain is often precipitated by effort or excitement.

413.0 Angina decubitus   `CC`
     Nocturnal angina
     DEF: Angina occurring only in the recumbent position.
     CC Excl: 410.00-410.92, 411.1-411.89, 413.0-413.9, 414.8-414.9, 459.89-459.9

413.1 Prinzmetal angina   `CC`
     Variant angina pectoris
     DEF: Angina occurring when patient is recumbent; associated with ST-segment elevations.
     CC Excl: See code: 413.0
     AHA: 3Q, '06, 23

---

§ Requires fifth digit. Valid digits are in [brackets] under each code. See category 410 for codes and definitions.

N Newborn Age: 0   **P** Pediatric Age: 0-17   **M** Maternity Age: 12-55   **A** Adult Age: 15-124   `MCC` Major CC Condition   `CC` CC Condition   `HIV` HIV Related Dx

138 – Volume 1   **2014 ICD-9-CM**

413.9 Other and unspecified angina pectoris

Angina:
    NOS
    cardiac
    equivalent
    of effort

Anginal syndrome
Status anginosus
Stenocardia
Syncope anginosa

Use additional code(s) for symptoms associated with angina equivalent

EXCLUDES *preinfarction angina (411.1)*

AHA: 2Q, '08, 16; 3Q, '02, 4; 3Q, '91, 16; 3Q, '90, 6

TIP: For patients with both angina and coronary artery disease, sequence the CAD (subcategory 414.0) code first.

I20.9 Angina pectoris unspecified   `I-10`

✔4ᵗʰ **414 Other forms of chronic ischemic heart disease**

EXCLUDES *arteriosclerotic cardiovascular disease [ASCVD] (429.2)*
    cardiovascular:
        arteriosclerosis or sclerosis (429.2)
        degeneration or disease (429.2)

✔5ᵗʰ **414.0 Coronary atherosclerosis**

Arteriosclerotic heart disease [ASHD]
Atherosclerotic heart disease
Coronary (artery):
    arteriosclerosis
    arteritis or endarteritis
    atheroma
    sclerosis
    stricture

Use additional code, if applicable, to identify chronic total occlusion of coronary artery (414.2)

EXCLUDES *embolism of graft (996.72)*
    occlusion NOS of graft (996.72)
    thrombus of graft (996.72)

DEF: A chronic condition marked by thickening and loss of elasticity of the coronary artery; caused by deposits of plaque containing cholesterol, lipoid material and lipophages.

AHA: 2Q, '97, 13; 2Q, '95, 17; 4Q, '94, 49; 2Q, '94, 13; 1Q, '94, 6; 3Q, '90, 7

414.00 Of unspecified type of vessel, native or graft `A`

AHA: 1Q, '04, 24; 2Q, '03, 16; 3Q, '01, 15; 4Q, '99, 4; 3Q, '97, 15; 4Q, '96, 31

414.01 Of native coronary artery `A`

DEF: Plaque deposits in natural heart vessels.

AHA: ▶3Q, '12, 17;◀3Q, '09, 9, 10; 3Q, '08, 10; 2Q, '08, 16; 3Q, '06, 25; 4Q, '05, 71; 2Q, '04, 3; 4Q, '03, 108; 3Q, '03, 9, 14; 3Q, '02, 4-9; 2Q, '01, 8, 9; 3Q, '97, 15; 2Q, '96, 10; 4Q, '96, 31

TIP: Assign for documentation of CAD NOS in a patient with no history of coronary artery bypass procedure.

I25.10 ASHD of native cor artery w/o angina pectoris `I-10`

414.02 Of autologous vein bypass graft `CC` `A`

DEF: Plaque deposit in grafted vein originating within patient.

AHA: 2Q, '10, 8-9

CC Exd: 414.00-414.05, 414.07, 414.2-414.3

414.03 Of nonautologous biological bypass graft `CC` `A`

DEF: Plaque deposits in grafted vessel originating outside patient.

CC Exd: See code: 414.02

414.04 Of artery bypass graft `CC` `A`

Internal mammary artery

DEF: Plaque deposits in grafted artery originating within patient.

CC Exd: See code: 414.02

AHA: 4Q, '96, 31

414.05 Of unspecified type of bypass graft `A`

Bypass graft NOS

AHA: 3Q, '97, 15; 4Q, '96, 31

414.06 Of native coronary artery of transplanted heart `CC`

CC Exd: 414.00-414.07, 414.2-414.3

AHA: 4Q, '03, 60; 4Q, '02, 53

414.07 Of bypass graft (artery) (vein) of transplanted heart `CC` `A`

CC Exd: 414.00-414.06, 414.2-414.3

Arteries of the Heart

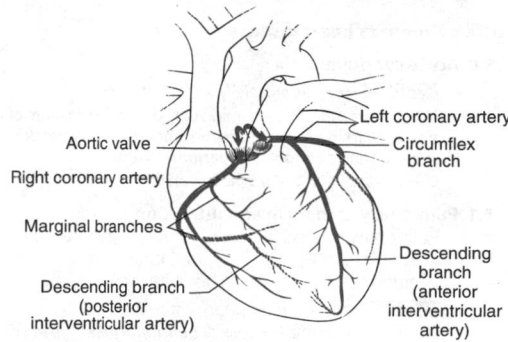

Aortic valve
Right coronary artery
Marginal branches
Descending branch (posterior interventricular artery)
Left coronary artery
Circumflex branch
Descending branch (anterior interventricular artery)

✔5ᵗʰ **414.1 Aneurysm and dissection of heart**

AHA: 4Q, '02, 54

414.10 Aneurysm of heart (wall) `CC`

Aneurysm (arteriovenous):
    mural
    ventricular

CC Exd: 414.10-414.11, 414.19

414.11 Aneurysm of coronary vessels

Aneurysm (arteriovenous) of coronary vessels

DEF: Dilatation of all three-vessel wall layers forming a sac filled with blood.

AHA: 2Q, '10, 8-9; 3Q, '03, 10; 1Q, '99, 17

414.12 Dissection of coronary artery `MCC`

DEF: A tear in the intimal arterial wall of a coronary artery resulting in the sudden intrusion of blood within the layers of the wall.

CC Exd: 414.12, 443.29, 447.2, 447.5-447.6, 447.8-447.9

AHA: 1Q, '11, 3-4

414.19 Other aneurysm of heart `CC`

Arteriovenous fistula, acquired, of heart

CC Exd: See code: 414.10

414.2 Chronic total occlusion of coronary artery

Complete occlusion of coronary artery
Total occlusion of coronary artery

Code first coronary atherosclerosis (414.00-414.07)

EXCLUDES *acute coronary occlusion with myocardial infarction (410.00-410.92)*
    acute coronary occlusion without myocardial infarction (411.81)

DEF: Complete blockage of coronary artery due to plaque accumulation over an extended period of time; results in substantial reduction of blood flow.

AHA: 4Q, '07, 82

414.3 Coronary atherosclerosis due to lipid rich plaque `A`

Code first coronary atherosclerosis (414.00-414.07)

AHA: 4Q, '08, 113

414.4 Coronary atherosclerosis due to calcified coronary lesion

Coronary atherosclerosis due to severely calcified coronary lesion

Code first coronary atherosclerosis (414.00-414.07)

AHA: 4Q, '11, 107

414.8 Other specified forms of chronic ischemic heart disease

Chronic coronary insufficiency
Ischemia, myocardial (chronic)

Any condition classifiable to 410 specified as chronic, or presenting with symptoms after 8 weeks from date of infarction

EXCLUDES *coronary insufficiency (acute) (411.89)*

AHA: 3Q, '01, 15; 1Q, '92, 10; 3Q, '90, 7, 15; 2Q, '90, 19

I25.89 Other forms of chronic ischemic heart disease `I-10`

414.9 Chronic ischemic heart disease, unspecified

Ischemic heart disease NOS

4ᵗʰ 5ᵗʰ Additional Digit Required   Unacceptable PDx   Manifestation Code   Hospital Acquired Condition   ▶◀ Revised Text   ● New Code   ▲ Revised Code Title

014 ICD-9-CM   February 2013 · Volume 1 – 139

Diseases of Pulmonary Circulation (415-417)

✓4ᵗʰ 415   Acute pulmonary heart disease

415.0   Acute cor pulmonale   `MCC`

> **EXCLUDES**   *cor pulmonale NOS (416.9)*
>
> **DEF:** A heart-lung disease marked by dilation and failure of the right side of heart; due to pulmonary embolism; ventilatory function is impaired and pulmonary hypertension results.
>
> **CC Excl:** 415.0, 416.8-416.9, 459.89-459.9

✓5ᵗʰ 415.1   Pulmonary embolism and infarction

> Pulmonary (artery) (vein):   Pulmonary (artery) (vein):
>   apoplexy   infarction (hemorrhagic)
>   embolism   thrombosis
>
> **EXCLUDES**   *chronic pulmonary embolism (416.2)*
> *personal history of pulmonary embolism (V12.55)*
> *that complicating:*
>   *abortion (634-638 with .6, 639.6)*
>   *ectopic or molar pregnancy (639.6)*
>   *pregnancy, childbirth, or the puerperium*
>   *(673.0-673.8)*
>
> **DEF:** Embolism: Closure of the pulmonary artery or branch; due to thrombosis (blood clot).
>
> **DEF:** Infarction: Necrosis of lung tissue; due to obstructed arterial blood supply, most often by pulmonary embolism.
>
> **AHA:** 4Q, '90, 25

¹¹415.11   Iatrogenic pulmonary embolism and infarction   `MCC`

> Use additional code for associated septic pulmonary embolism, if applicable, 415.12
>
> **CC Excl:** 415.11-415.19, 416.2, 444.01-444.09, 459.89-459.9
>
> **AHA:** 4Q, '95, 58
>
> **TIP:** Do not report code 997.39 Other respiratory complications, with code 415.11.

415.12   Septic pulmonary embolism   `MCC`

> Septic embolism NOS
>
> Code first underlying infection, such as:
>   septicemia (038.0-038.9)
>
> **EXCLUDES**   *septic arterial embolism (449)*
>
> **CC Excl:** See code: 415.11
>
> **AHA:** 4Q, '07, 84-86

¹¹415.13   Saddle embolus of pulmonary artery   `MCC`

> **CC Excl:** See code 415.11
>
> **AHA:** 4Q, '11, 107-108

¹¹415.19   Other   `MCC`

> **CC Excl:** See code: 415.11
>
> **AHA:** 3Q, '10, 10; 4Q, '09, 86
>
> I26.99 Other pulmonary emb w/o acute cor pulmonale   `I-10`

✓4ᵗʰ 416   Chronic pulmonary heart disease

416.0   Primary pulmonary hypertension   `CC`

> Idiopathic pulmonary arteriosclerosis
> Pulmonary hypertension (essential) (idiopathic) (primary)
>
> **EXCLUDES**   *pulmonary hypertension NOS (416.8)*
> *secondary pulmonary hypertension (416.8)*
>
> **DEF:** A rare increase in pulmonary circulation, often resulting in right ventricular failure or fatal syncope.
>
> **CC Excl:** 278.03, 416.0, 416.8-416.9, 417.8-417.9, 459.89-459.9
>
> I27.0 Primary pulmonary hypertension   `I-10`

416.1   Kyphoscoliotic heart disease   `CC`

> **DEF:** High blood pressure within the lungs as a result of curvature of the spine.
>
> **CC Excl:** 278.03, 416.0-416.1, 416.8-416.9

416.2   Chronic pulmonary embolism   `CC`

> Use additional code, if applicable, for associated long-term (current) use of anticoagulants (V58.61)
>
> **EXCLUDES**   *personal history of pulmonary embolism (V12.55)*
>
> **DEF:** A long-standing condition commonly associated with pulmonary hypertension in which small blood clots travel to the lungs repeatedly over many weeks, months, or years, requiring continuation of established anticoagulant or thrombolytic therapy.
>
> **CC Excl:** 415.11-415.19, 416.2, 444.01-444.09, 459.89-459.9
>
> **AHA:** 4Q, '09, 85, 86

416.8   Other chronic pulmonary heart diseases

> Pulmonary hypertension NOS
> Pulmonary hypertension, secondary
>
> **AHA:** 1Q, '12, 17; 1Q, '11, 10; 2Q, '10,10
>
> I27.89 Other specified pulmonary heart diseases   `I-10`

416.9   Chronic pulmonary heart disease, unspecified

> Chronic cardiopulmonary disease
> Cor pulmonale (chronic) NOS

✓4ᵗʰ 417   Other diseases of pulmonary circulation

417.0   Arteriovenous fistula of pulmonary vessels   `CC`

> **EXCLUDES**   *congenital arteriovenous fistula (747.32)*
>
> **DEF:** Abnormal communication between blood vessels within lung.
>
> **CC Excl:** 417.0-417.9

417.1   Aneurysm of pulmonary artery   `CC`

> **EXCLUDES**   *congenital aneurysm (747.39)*
> *congenital arteriovenous aneurysm (747.32)*
>
> **CC Excl:** See code: 417.0

417.8   Other specified diseases of pulmonary circulation

> Pulmonary: Pulmonary:
>   arteritis   endarteritis
>
> Rupture } of pulmonary vessel
> Stricture

417.9   Unspecified disease of pulmonary circulation

Other Forms of Heart Disease (420-429)

✓4ᵗʰ 420   Acute pericarditis

> **INCLUDES**   acute:
>   mediastinopericarditis
>   myopericarditis
>   pericardial effusion
>   pleuropericarditis
>   pneumopericarditis
>
> **EXCLUDES**   *acute rheumatic pericarditis (391.0)*
> *postmyocardial infarction syndrome [Dressler's] (411.0)*
>
> **DEF:** Inflammation of the pericardium (heart sac); pericardial friction rub results from this inflammation and is heard as a scratchy or leathery sound.

420.0   *Acute pericarditis in diseases classified elsewhere*   `CC`

> *Code first underlying disease, as:*
>   actinomycosis (039.8)
>   amebiasis (006.8)
>   chronic uremia (585.9)
>   nocardiosis (039.8)
>   tuberculosis (017.9)
>   uremia NOS (586)
>
> **EXCLUDES**   *pericarditis (acute) (in):*
>   *Coxsackie (virus) (074.21)*
>   *gonococcal (098.83)*
>   *histoplasmosis (115.0-115.9 with fifth-digit 3)*
>   *meningococcal infection (036.41)*
>   *syphilitic (093.81)*
>
> **CC Excl:** 391.0, 393, 420.0-420.99, 423.3-423.9, 459.89-459.9

✓5ᵗʰ 420.9   Other and unspecified acute pericarditis

420.90   Acute pericarditis, unspecified   `CC`

> Pericarditis (acute):   Pericarditis (acute):
>   NOS   sicca
>   infective NOS
>
> **CC Excl:** See code: 420.0
>
> **AHA:** 2Q, '89, 12

420.91   Acute idiopathic pericarditis   `CC`

> Pericarditis, acute: Pericarditis, acute:
>   benign   viral
>   nonspecific
>
> **CC Excl:** See code: 420.0

---

¹¹ HAC when reported with procedure codes 00.85-00.87, 81.51, 81.52, 81.54 and POA = N

`N` Newborn Age: 0   `P` Pediatric Age: 0-17   `M` Maternity Age: 12-55   `A` Adult Age: 15-124   `MCC` Major CC Condition   `CC` CC Condition   `HIV` HIV Related Dx

140 – Volume 1   2014 ICD-9-CM

Anatomy

Blood Flow

420.99 Other `CC`
Pericarditis (acute):
  pneumococcal
  purulent
  staphylococcal
  streptococcal
  suppurative
Pneumopyopericardium
Pyopericardium
> *EXCLUDES*   *pericarditis in diseases classified elsewhere (420.0)*

CC Exd: See code: 420.0

✓4th 421   Acute and subacute endocarditis
DEF: Bacterial inflammation of the endocardium (intracardiac area); major symptoms include fever, fatigue, heart murmurs, splenomegaly, embolic episodes and areas of infarction.

421.0   Acute and subacute bacterial endocarditis `MCC` `HIV`
Endocarditis (acute)(chronic) (subacute):
  bacterial
  infective NOS
  lenta
  malignant
  purulent
  septic
  ulcerative
  vegetative
Infective aneurysm
Subacute bacterial endocarditis [SBE]

Use additional code to identify infectious organism [e.g., Streptococcus 041.0, Staphylococcus 041.1]

CC Exd: 391.1, 397.9, 421.0-421.9, 424.90-424.99, 459.89-459.9
AHA: 4Q, '08, 73; 1Q, '99, 12; 1Q, '91, 15
I33.0 Acute and subacute infective endocarditis `I-10`

421.1   *Acute and subacute infective endocarditis in diseases classified elsewhere* `MCC`
Code first underlying disease, as:
  blastomycosis (116.0)
  Q fever (083.0)
  typhoid (fever) (002.0)
> *EXCLUDES*   *endocarditis (in):*
>   *Coxsackie (virus) (074.22)*
>   *gonococcal (098.84)*
>   *histoplasmosis (115.0-115.9 with fifth-digit 4)*
>   *meningococcal infection (036.42)*
>   *monilial (112.81)*

CC Exd: See code: 421.0

421.9   Acute endocarditis, unspecified `MCC` `HIV`
Endocarditis }
Myoendocarditis } acute or subacute
Periendocarditis }
> *EXCLUDES*   *acute rheumatic endocarditis (391.1)*

CC Exd: See code: 421.0

✓4th 422   Acute myocarditis
> *EXCLUDES*   *acute rheumatic myocarditis (391.2)*

DEF: Acute inflammation of the muscular walls of the heart (myocardium).

422.0   *Acute myocarditis in diseases classified elsewhere* `MCC`
Code first underlying disease, as:
  myocarditis (acute):
    influenzal (487.8, 488.09, 488.19)
    tuberculous (017.9)
> *EXCLUDES*   *myocarditis (acute) (due to):*
>   *aseptic, of newborn (074.23)*
>   *Coxsackie (virus) (074.23)*
>   *diphtheritic (032.82)*
>   *meningococcal infection (036.43)*
>   *syphilitic (093.82)*
>   *toxoplasmosis (130.3)*

CC Exd: 391.2, 398.0, 422.0-422.99, 429.0, 429.71-429.79, 459.89-459.9

✓5th 422.9   Other and unspecified acute myocarditis

422.90   Acute myocarditis, unspecified `MCC` `HIV`
Acute or subacute (interstitial) myocarditis
CC Exd: See code: 422.0

422.91   Idiopathic myocarditis `MCC` `HIV`
Myocarditis (acute or subacute):
  Fiedler's
  giant cell
  isolated (diffuse) (granulomatous)
  nonspecific granulomatous
CC Exd: See code: 422.0

422.92   Septic myocarditis `MCC` `HIV`
Myocarditis, acute or subacute:
  pneumococcal
  staphylococcal

Use additional code to identify infectious organism [e.g., Staphylococcus 041.1]
> *EXCLUDES*   *myocarditis, acute or subacute:*
>   *in bacterial diseases classified elsewhere (422.0)*
>   *streptococcal (391.2)*

CC Exd: See code 422.0

422.93   Toxic myocarditis `MCC` `HIV`
DEF: Inflammation of the heart muscle due to an adverse reaction to certain drugs or chemicals reaching the heart through the bloodstream.
CC Exd: See code: 422.0

422.99   Other `MCC` `HIV`
CC Exd: See code: 422.0

✓4th 423   Other diseases of pericardium
> *EXCLUDES*   *that specified as rheumatic (393)*

423.0   Hemopericardium `CC`
DEF: Blood in the pericardial sac (pericardium).
CC Exd: 423.0-423.9, 459.89-459.9

423.1   Adhesive pericarditis `CC`
Adherent pericarditis   Pericarditis:
Fibrosis of pericardium   adhesive
Milk spots   obliterative
              Soldiers' patches
DEF: Two layers of serous pericardium adhere to each other by fibrous adhesions.
CC Exd: See code: 423.0

423.2   Constrictive pericarditis `CC`
Concato's disease   Pick's disease of heart (and liver)
DEF: Inflammation identified by a rigid, thickened and sometimes calcified pericardium; ventricles of the heart not adequately filled; congestive heart failure may result.
CC Exd: See code: 423.0

Additional Digit Required   Unacceptable PDx   Manifestation Code   Hospital Acquired Condition   ►◄ Revised Text   ● New Code   ▲ Revised Code Title

Diseases of the Circulatory System

423.3–425.0

Cardiac Tamponade

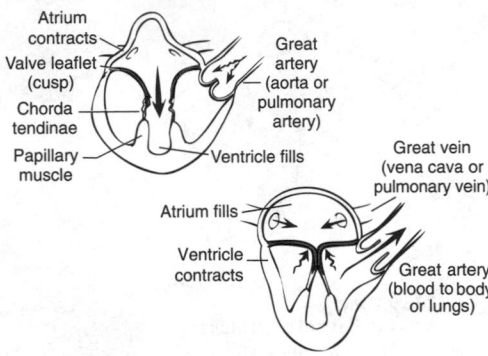

Normal   Cardiac Tamponade

Serous pericardium (visceral layer)

Excessive fluid in pericardial space

Fibrous pericardium

Pericardial space (potential)

Serous pericardium (parietal layer)

⊞ --constricted areas

423.3 Cardiac tamponade   `CC`

Code first the underlying cause

DEF: Life-threatening condition in which fluid or blood accumulates between the muscle of the heart (myocardium) and the outer sac (pericardium), resulting in compression of the heart, which decreases cardiac output.

CC Excl: 074.21, 093.81, 391.0, 393, 420.0-420.99, 423.3-423.9, 459.89-459.9

AHA: 4Q, '07, 86, 87

423.8 Other specified diseases of pericardium   `CC`

Calcification
Fistula } of pericardium

CC Excl: See code: 423.3

AHA: 2Q, '89, 12

423.9 Unspecified disease of pericardium   `CC`

CC Excl: See code: 423.3

AHA: 1Q, '07, 11

✓4ᵗʰ 424 Other diseases of endocardium

EXCLUDES   bacterial endocarditis (421.0-421.9)
       rheumatic endocarditis (391.1, 394.0-397.9)
       syphilitic endocarditis (093.20-093.24)

424.0 Mitral valve disorders

Mitral (valve):

incompetence
insufficiency } NOS of specified cause,
regurgitation   except rheumatic

EXCLUDES   mitral (valve):
       disease (394.9)
       failure (394.9)
       stenosis (394.0)
       the listed conditions:
         specified as rheumatic (394.1)
         unspecified as to cause but with mention of:
           diseases of aortic valve (396.0-396.9)
           mitral stenosis or obstruction (394.2)

AHA: 3Q, '06, 7; 2Q, '00, 16; 3Q, '98, 11; N-D, '87, 8; N-D, '84, 8

I34.8 Other nonrheumatic mitral valve disorders   `I-10`

424.1 Aortic valve disorders

Aortic (valve):

incompetence
insufficiency } NOS of specified cause,
regurgitation   except rheumatic
stenosis

EXCLUDES   hypertrophic subaortic stenosis (425.11)
       that specified as rheumatic (395.0-395.9)
       that of unspecified cause but with mention of diseases
         of mitral valve (396.0-396.9)

AHA: 4Q, '11, 152; 4Q, '08, 179; 4Q, '88, 8; N-D, '87, 8

424.2 Tricuspid valve disorders, specified as nonrheumatic

Tricuspid valve:

incompetence
insufficiency } of specified cause, except
regurgitation   rheumatic
stenosis

EXCLUDES   rheumatic or of unspecified cause (397.0)

Heart Valve Disorders

Incompetent valve (trouble closing)

causes regurgitation (backflow of blood)

Valve stenosis (trouble opening)

Insufficient valve (unable to close completely)

Shortened, fused chorda tendinae

Ventricular hypertrophy

Normal Heart Valve Function

Atrium contracts

Valve leaflet (cusp)

Chorda tendinae

Papillary muscle

Great artery (aorta or pulmonary artery)

Ventricle fills

Great vein (vena cava or pulmonary vein)

Atrium fills

Ventricle contracts

Great artery (blood to body or lungs)

424.3 Pulmonary valve disorders

Pulmonic: Pulmonic:
  incompetence NOS   regurgitation NOS
  insufficiency NOS   stenosis NOS

EXCLUDES   that specified as rheumatic (397.1)

✓5ᵗʰ 424.9 Endocarditis, valve unspecified

424.90 Endocarditis, valve unspecified, unspecified cause   `CC`

Endocarditis (chronic):
  NOS
  nonbacterial thrombotic
Valvular:
  incompetence
  insufficiency } of unspecified valve,
  regurgitation   unspecified
  stenosis   cause
Valvulitis (chronic)

CC Excl: 424.90-424.99, 459.89-459.9

I38 Endocarditis valve unspecified   `I-1`

424.91 Endocarditis in diseases classified elsewhere

Code first underlying disease as:
  atypical verrucous endocarditis [Libman-Sacks] (710.0)
  disseminated lupus erythematosus (710.0)
  tuberculosis (017.9)

EXCLUDES   syphilitic (093.20-093.24)

CC Excl: See code: 424.90

424.99 Other   `C`

Any condition classifiable to 424.90 with specified cause, except rheumatic

EXCLUDES   endocardial fibroelastosis (425.3)
       that specified as rheumatic (397.9)

CC Excl: See code: 424.90

✓4ᵗʰ 425 Cardiomyopathy

INCLUDES   myocardiopathy

AHA: J-A, '85, 15

425.0 Endomyocardial fibrosis   `C`

CC Excl: 398.91, 402.01, 402.11, 402.91, 404.01, 404.03, 404.11, 404.13, 404.91, 404.93, 414.00-414.07, 414.2-414.9, 425.0-425.9, 426.10-426.13, 426.50-426.54, 426.81-426.89, 427.31-427.42, 427.60-427.89, 428.0-428.1, 428.9, 459.89-459.9, 746.86, 785.0-785.1, 785.50-785.51

`N` Newborn Age: 0   `P` Pediatric Age: 0-17   `M` Maternity Age: 12-55   `A` Adult Age: 15-124   `MCC` Major CC Condition   `CC` CC Condition   `HIV` HIV Related D

142 – Volume 1   2014 ICD-9-C

√5ᵗʰ **425.1 Hypertrophic cardiomyopathy**

    EXCLUDES *ventricular hypertrophy (429.3)*

    DEF: Cardiomyopathy marked by left ventricle hypertrophy, enlarged septum; results in obstructed blood flow.

    AHA: 4Q, '11, 109-110

    425.11 Hypertrophic obstructive cardiomyopathy `CC`

        Hypertrophic subaortic stenosis (idiopathic)

        CC Excd: see Code: 425.0

    425.18 Other hypertrophic cardiomyopathy `CC`

        Nonobstructive hypertrophic cardiomyopathy

        CC Excd: see Code: 425.0

425.2 Obscure cardiomyopathy of Africa `CC`

    Becker's disease

    Idiopathic mural endomyocardial disease

    CC Excd: See code: 425.0

425.3 Endocardial fibroelastosis `CC`

    Elastomyofibrosis

    DEF: A condition marked by left ventricle hypertrophy and conversion of the endocardium into a thick fibroelastic coat; capacity of the ventricle may be reduced, but is often increased.

    CC Excd: See code: 425.0

425.4 Other primary cardiomyopathies `CC`

Cardiomyopathy:	Cardiomyopathy:
NOS	idiopathic
congestive	obstructive
constrictive	restrictive
familial	Cardiovascular collagenosis

    CC Excd: See code: 425.0

    AHA: 4Q, '11, 109-110; 4Q, '09, 141; 1Q, '07, 20; 2Q, '05, 14; 1Q, '00, 22; 4Q, '97, 55; 2Q, '90, 19

    TIP: For congestive cardiomyopathy, assign first a code for the CHF (category 428) if the treatment is directed toward the CHF.

    I42.8 Other cardiomyopathies `I-10`

425.5 Alcoholic cardiomyopathy `CC`

    DEF: Heart disease as result of excess alcohol consumption.

    CC Excd: See code: 425.0

    AHA: S-O, '85, 15

425.7 *Nutritional and metabolic cardiomyopathy* `CC`

    Code first underlying disease, as:

        amyloidosis (277.30-277.39)

        beriberi (265.0)

        cardiac glycogenosis (271.0)

        mucopolysaccharidosis (277.5)

        thyrotoxicosis (242.0-242.9)

    EXCLUDES *gouty tophi of heart (274.82)*

    CC Excd: See code 425.0

425.8 *Cardiomyopathy in other diseases classified elsewhere* `CC`

    Code first underlying disease, as:

        Friedreich's ataxia (334.0)

        myotonia atrophica (359.21)

        progressive muscular dystrophy (359.1)

        sarcoidosis (135)

    EXCLUDES *cardiomyopathy in Chagas' disease (086.0)*

    CC Excd: See code 425.0

    AHA: 2Q, '93, 9

    I43 Cardiomyopathy in diseases classified elsewhere `I-10`

425.9 Secondary cardiomyopathy, unspecified `CC`

    CC Excd: See code: 425.0

√4ᵗʰ **426 Conduction disorders**

    DEF: Disruption or disturbance in the electrical impulses that regulate heartbeats.

426.0 Atrioventricular block, complete `CC`

    Third degree atrioventricular block

    CC Excd: 426.0-427.5, 427.89, 459.89-459.9

    AHA: 2Q, '06, 14

    TIP: Assign if documentation indicates intermittent complete heart block.

√5ᵗʰ **426.1 Atrioventricular block, other and unspecified**

    TIP: Assign separate codes for each type of AV block documented.

    426.10 Atrioventricular block, unspecified

        Atrioventricular [AV] block (incomplete) (partial)

        AHA: 2Q, '06, 14

Nerve Conduction of the Heart

    426.11 First degree atrioventricular block

        Incomplete atrioventricular block, first degree

        Prolonged P-R interval NOS

        I44.0 Atrioventricular block first degree `I-10`

    426.12 Mobitz (type) II atrioventricular block `CC`

        Incomplete atrioventricular block:

            Mobitz (type) II

            second degree, Mobitz (type) II

        DEF: Impaired conduction of excitatory impulse from cardiac atrium to ventricle through AV node.

        CC Excd: See code: 426.0

    426.13 Other second degree atrioventricular block

        Incomplete atrioventricular block:

            Mobitz (type) I [Wenckebach's]

            second degree:

                NOS

                Mobitz (type) I

            with 2:1 atrioventricular response [block]

        Wenckebach's phenomenon

        DEF: Wenckebach's phenomenon: impulses generated at constant rate to sinus node, P-R interval lengthens; results in cycle of ventricular inadequacy and shortened P-R interval; second-degree A-V block commonly called "Mobitz type 1."

426.2 Left bundle branch hemiblock

    Block:

        left anterior fascicular

        left posterior fascicular

426.3 Other left bundle branch block

    Left bundle branch block:

        NOS

        anterior fascicular with posterior fascicular

        complete

        main stem

    I44.7 Left bundle-branch block unspecified `I-10`

426.4 Right bundle branch block

    AHA: 3Q, '00, 3

    I45.10 Unspecified right bundle-branch block `I-10`

√5ᵗʰ **426.5 Bundle branch block, other and unspecified**

    426.50 Bundle branch block, unspecified

    426.51 Right bundle branch block and left posterior fascicular block

    426.52 Right bundle branch block and left anterior fascicular block

    426.53 Other bilateral bundle branch block `CC`

        Bifascicular block NOS

        Bilateral bundle branch block NOS

        Right bundle branch with left bundle branch block (incomplete) (main stem)

        CC Excd: 426.0-427.5, 427.89, 459.89-459.9

    426.54 Trifascicular block `CC`

        CC Excd: 426.0-427.5, 427.89, 459.89-459.9

426.6 Other heart block

Intraventricular block:	Sinoatrial block
NOS	Sinoauricular block
diffuse	
myofibrillar	

Additional Digit Required   Unacceptable PDx   Manifestation Code   Hospital Acquired Condition   ▶◀ Revised Text   ● New Code   ▲ Revised Code Title

2014 ICD-9-CM   Volume 1 – 143

Diseases of the Circulatory System

426.7–427.9

Normal and Long QT Electrocardiogram

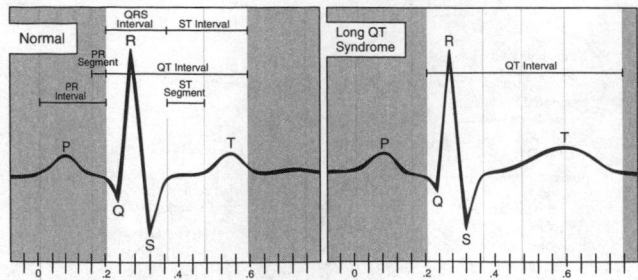

426.7 Anomalous atrioventricular excitation
Atrioventricular conduction:
  accelerated
  accessory
  pre-excitation
Ventricular pre-excitation
Wolff-Parkinson-White syndrome
DEF: Wolff-Parkinson-White: normal conduction pathway is bypassed; results in short P-R interval on EKG; tendency to supraventricular tachycardia.

✓5ᵗʰ 426.8 Other specified conduction disorders

426.81 Lown-Ganong-Levine syndrome
Syndrome of short P-R interval, normal QRS
     complexes, and supraventricular tachycardias

426.82 Long QT syndrome
DEF: Condition characterized by recurrent syncope, malignant arrhythmias, and sudden death; characteristic prolonged Q-T interval on electrocardiogram.
AHA: 4Q, '05, 72

426.89 Other   `CC`
Dissociation:
  atrioventricular [AV]
  interference
  isorhythmic
Nonparoxysmal AV nodal tachycardia
CC Excl: 426.0-426.5, 427.89, 459.89-459.9

426.9 Conduction disorder, unspecified
Heart block NOS
Stokes-Adams syndrome

✓4ᵗʰ 427 Cardiac dysrhythmias
EXCLUDES *that complicating:*
    abortion (634-638 with .7, 639.8)
    ectopic or molar pregnancy (639.8)
    labor or delivery (668.1, 669.4)
DEF: Disruption or disturbance in the rhythm of heartbeats.
AHA: J-A, '85, 15

427.0 Paroxysmal supraventricular tachycardia   `CC`
Paroxysmal tachycardia: Paroxysmal tachycardia:
  atrial [PAT]   junctional
  atrioventricular [AV]   nodal
DEF: Rapid atrial rhythm.
CC Excl: See code: 426.89

427.1 Paroxysmal ventricular tachycardia   `CC`
Ventricular tachycardia (paroxysmal)
DEF: Rapid ventricular rhythm.
CC Excl: See code: 426.89
AHA: 2Q, '09, 14; 1Q, '08, 14; 2Q, '06, 15-16; 3Q, '95, 9; M-A, '86, 11
TIP: If a ventricular tachycardia is documented as sustained or nonsustained but is induced during an EP study, assign 427.1.
I47.2 Ventricular tachycardia   `I-10`

427.2 Paroxysmal tachycardia, unspecified
Bouveret-Hoffmann syndrome
Paroxysmal tachycardia:
  essential
  NOS

✓5ᵗʰ 427.3 Atrial fibrillation and flutter
TIP: Assign V58.61 Long-term (current) use of anticoagulants, as a secondary diagnosis if the patient is maintained on Coumadin.

427.31 Atrial fibrillation
DEF: Irregular, rapid atrial contractions.
AHA: 1Q, '12, 7; 4Q, '08, 135; 3Q, '05, 8; 4Q, '04, 78, 121; 3Q, '04, 7; 4Q, '03, 95, 105; 1Q, '03, 8; 2Q, '99, 17; 3Q '95, 8
I48.0 Atrial fibrillation   `I-10`

427.32 Atrial flutter   `CC`
DEF: Regular, rapid atrial contractions.
CC Excl: See code: 426.89
AHA: 4Q, '03, 94
I48.1 Atrial flutter   `I-10`

✓5ᵗʰ 427.4 Ventricular fibrillation and flutter

¹ 427.41 Ventricular fibrillation   `MCC`
DEF: Irregular, rapid ventricular contractions.
CC Excl: See code: 426.89
AHA: 2Q, '09, 14-15; 3Q, '02, 5

427.42 Ventricular flutter   `MCC`
DEF: Regular, rapid, ventricular contractions.
CC Excl: See code: 426.89

¹ 427.5 Cardiac arrest   `MCC`
Cardiorespiratory arrest
CC Excl: 427.0-427.5, 459.89-459.9
AHA: 3Q '02, 5; 2Q, '00, 12; 3Q, '95, 8; 2Q, '88, 8
I46.9 Cardiac arrest cause unspecified   `I-10`

✓5ᵗʰ 427.6 Premature beats

427.60 Premature beats, unspecified
Ectopic beats
Extrasystoles
Extrasystolic arrhythmia
Premature contractions or systoles NOS

427.61 Supraventricular premature beats
Atrial premature beats, contractions, or systoles

427.69 Other
Ventricular premature beats, contractions, or systoles
AHA: 4Q, '93, 42

✓5ᵗʰ 427.8 Other specified cardiac dysrhythmias

427.81 Sinoatrial node dysfunction
Sinus bradycardia:
  persistent
  severe
Syndrome:
  sick sinus
  tachycardia-bradycardia
EXCLUDES *sinus bradycardia NOS (427.89)*
DEF: Complex cardiac arrhythmia; appears as severe sinus bradycardia, sinus bradycardia with tachycardia, or sinus bradycardia with atrioventricular block.
AHA: 4Q, '11, 168; 3Q, '10, 9; 3Q, '00, 8
I49.5 Sick sinus syndrome   `I-1`

427.89 Other
Rhythm disorder:
  coronary sinus
  ectopic
  nodal
Wandering (atrial) pacemaker
EXCLUDES *carotid sinus syncope (337.0)*
    neonatal bradycardia (779.81)
    neonatal tachycardia (779.82)
    reflex bradycardia (337.0)
    tachycardia NOS (785.0)
AHA: ▶3Q, '12, 9◄
I49.8 Other specified cardiac arrhythmias   `I-1`

427.9 Cardiac dysrhythmia, unspecified
Arrhythmia (cardiac) NOS
AHA: 2Q, '89, 10

---

¹ MCC = Only if patient is discharged alive.

`N` Newborn Age: 0   `P` Pediatric Age: 0-17   `M` Maternity Age: 12-55   `A` Adult Age: 15-124   `MCC` Major CC Condition   `CC` CC Condition   `HIV` HIV Related D

144 – Volume 1 • February 2013   **2014 ICD-9-C**

Diseases of the Circulatory System

✓4ᵗʰ 428 Heart failure

Code, if applicable, heart failure due to hypertension first (402.0-402.9, with fifth-digit 1 or 404.0-404.9 with fifth-digit 1 or 3)

EXCLUDES *following cardiac surgery (429.4)*
rheumatic (398.91)
that complicating:
abortion (634-638 with .7, 639.8)
ectopic or molar pregnancy (639.8)
labor or delivery (668.1, 669.4)

AHA: 4Q, '02, 49; 3Q, '98, 5; 2Q, '90, 16; 2Q, '90, 19; 2Q, '89, 10; 3Q, '88, 3

428.0 Congestive heart failure, unspecified

Congestive heart disease
Right heart failure (secondary to left heart failure)

EXCLUDES *fluid overload NOS (276.69)*

DEF: Mechanical inadequacy; caused by inability of heart to pump and circulate blood; results in fluid collection in lungs, hypertension, congestion and edema of tissue.

AHA: ▶3Q, '12, 9;◀4Q, '09, 141; 1Q, '09, 8, 18; 4Q, '08, 72, 180, 182; 3Q, '08, 12; 3Q, '07, 9; 1Q, 07, 20; 3Q, '06, 7; 4Q, '05, 120; 3Q, '05, 8; 1Q, '05, 5, 9; 1Q, '05, 5, 9; 4Q, '04, 140; 3Q, '04, 7;4Q, '03, 109; 1Q, '03, 9; 4Q, '02, 52; 2Q, '01, 13; 4Q, '00, 48; 2Q, '00, 16; 1Q, '00, 22; 4Q, '99, 4; 1Q, '99, 11; 4Q, '97, 55; 3Q, '97, 10; 3Q, '96, 9; 3Q, '91, 18; 3Q, '91, 19; 2Q, '89, 12

TIP: Assign additional code(s) from subcategory 428.2, 428.3, or 428.4 to specify the type of heart failure.

I50.9 Heart failure unspecified [I-10]

428.1 Left heart failure [cc]

Acute edema of lung ⎱ with heart disease NOS or
Acute pulmonary edema ⎰ heart failure
Cardiac asthma
Left ventricular failure

DEF: Mechanical inadequacy of left ventricle; causing fluid in lungs.
CC Exd: 398.91, 402.01, 402.11, 402.91, 428.0-428.9, 459.89-459.9

✓5ᵗʰ 428.2 Systolic heart failure

EXCLUDES *combined systolic and diastolic heart failure (428.40-428.43)*

DEF: Heart failure due to a defect in expulsion of blood caused by an abnormality in systolic function, or ventricular contractile dysfunction.

428.20 Unspecified [cc]

CC Exd: 398.91, 402.01, 402.11, 402.91, 428.0-428.9, 459.89-459.9, 518.4

I50.20 Unspecified systolic congestive heart failure [I-10]

428.21 Acute [MCC]

CC Exd: See code: 428.20

I50.21 Acute systolic congestive heart failure [I-10]

428.22 Chronic [cc]

CC Exd: See code: 428.20
AHA: 4Q, '05, 120

428.23 Acute on chronic [MCC]

CC Exd: See code: 428.20
AHA: 1Q, '09, 8, 18; 1Q, '03, 9

Echocardiography of Heart Failure

Systolic dysfunction
with dilated LV

Diastolic dysfunction
with LV hypertrophy

Four-chamber echocardiograms, two-dimensional views.
LV: Left ventricle
RV: Right ventricle
RA: Right atrium
LA: Left atrium

✓5ᵗʰ 428.3 Diastolic heart failure

EXCLUDES *combined systolic and diastolic heart failure (428.40-428.43)*

DEF: Heart failure due to resistance to ventricular filling caused by an abnormality in the diastolic function.

AHA: 1Q, '12, 7

428.30 Unspecified [cc]

CC Exd: See code: 428.20
AHA: 4Q, '02, 52

I50.30 Unspecified diastolic congestive heart failure [I-10]

428.31 Acute [MCC]

CC Exd: See code: 428.20

428.32 Chronic [cc]

CC Exd: See code: 428.20
AHA: 3Q, '08, 12

I50.32 Chronic diastolic congestive heart failure [I-10]

428.33 Acute on chronic [MCC]

CC Exd: See code: 428.20
AHA: 4Q, '09, 141; 3Q, '08, 12;1Q, '07, 20

I50.33 Acute on chronic diastolic heart failure [I-10]

✓5ᵗʰ 428.4 Combined systolic and diastolic heart failure

428.40 Unspecified [cc]

CC Exd: See code: 428.20

428.41 Acute [MCC]

CC Exd: See code: 428.20
AHA: 4Q, '04, 140

428.42 Chronic [cc]

CC Exd: See code: 428.20

428.43 Acute on chronic [MCC]

CC Exd: See code: 428.20
AHA: 3Q, '06, 7; 4Q, '02, 52

428.9 Heart failure, unspecified

Cardiac failure NOS
Heart failure NOS
Myocardial failure NOS
Weak heart

AHA: 2Q, '89, 10; N-D, '85, 14

✓4ᵗʰ 429 Ill-defined descriptions and complications of heart disease

429.0 Myocarditis, unspecified

Myocarditis:
NOS
chronic (interstitial ⎱ (with mention of
fibroid ⎰ arteriosclerosis)
senile

Use additional code to identify presence of arteriosclerosis

EXCLUDES *acute or subacute (422.0-422.9)*
rheumatic (398.0)
acute (391.2)
that due to hypertension (402.0-402.9)

429.1 Myocardial degeneration

Degeneration of heart or
myocardium:
fatty
mural ⎱ (with mention of
muscular ⎰ arteriosclerosis)
Myocardial:
degeneration
disease

Use additional code to identify presence of arteriosclerosis

EXCLUDES *that due to hypertension (402.0-402.9)*

429.2 Cardiovascular disease, unspecified

Arteriosclerotic cardiovascular disease [ASCVD]
Cardiovascular arteriosclerosis
Cardiovascular:
degeneration ⎱ (with mention of
disease ⎰ arteriosclerosis)
sclerosis

Use additional code to identify presence of arteriosclerosis

EXCLUDES *that due to hypertension (402.0-402.9)*

AHA: ▶3Q, '12, 17◀

Additional Digit Required | Unacceptable PDx | Manifestation Code | Hospital Acquired Condition | ▶◀ Revised Text | ● New Code | ▲ Revised Code Title

2014 ICD-9-CM | February 2013 • Volume 1 – 145

429.3 Cardiomegaly
Cardiac:
  dilatation
  hypertrophy
Ventricular dilatation
> **EXCLUDES** *that due to hypertension (402.0-402.9)*

I51.7 Cardiomegaly   `I-10`

429.4 Functional disturbances following cardiac surgery
Cardiac insufficiency   } following cardiac surgery or
Heart failure   } due to prosthesis
Postcardiotomy syndrome
Postvalvulotomy syndrome
> **EXCLUDES** *cardiac failure in the immediate postoperative period (997.1)*

AHA: 2Q, '02, 12; N-D, '85, 6

429.5 Rupture of chordae tendineae   `MCC`
> **DEF:** Torn tissue, between heart valves and papillary muscles.
> **CC Excl:** 429.5, 429.71-429.79, 459.89-459.9

429.6 Rupture of papillary muscle   `MCC`
> **DEF:** Torn muscle, between chordae tendineae and heart wall.
> **CC Excl:** 429.6-429.81, 459.89-459.9

√5ᵗʰ 429.7 Certain sequelae of myocardial infarction, not elsewhere classified
Use additional code to identify the associated myocardial infarction:
  with onset of 8 weeks or less (410.00-410.92)
  with onset of more than 8 weeks (414.8)
> **EXCLUDES** *congenital defects of heart (745, 746)*
> *coronary aneurysm (414.11)*
> *disorders of papillary muscle (429.6, 429.81)*
> *postmyocardial infarction syndrome (411.0)*
> *rupture of chordae tendineae (429.5)*

AHA: 3Q, '89, 5

429.71 Acquired cardiac septal defect   `CC` `A`
> **EXCLUDES** *acute septal infarction (410.00-410.92)*
> **DEF:** Abnormal communication, between opposite heart chambers; due to defect of septum; not present at birth.
> **CC Excl:** 422.0-422.99, 429.0, 429.4-429.82, 459.89-459.9, 745.0-745.9, 746.89-746.9, 747.83-747.9, 759.7-759.89

429.79 Other   `CC` `A`
Mural thrombus (atrial) (ventricular), acquired, following myocardial infarction
> **CC Excl:** See code: 429.71
> **AHA:** 1Q, '92, 10

√5ᵗʰ 429.8 Other ill-defined heart diseases

429.81 Other disorders of papillary muscle   `CC`
Papillary muscle:
  atrophy
  degeneration
  dysfunction
  incompetence
  incoordination
  scarring
> **CC Excl:** 429.6-429.81, 459.89-459.9

429.82 Hyperkinetic heart disease   `CC`
> **DEF:** Condition of unknown origin in young adults; marked by increased cardiac output at rest, increased rate of ventricular ejection; may lead to heart failure.
> **CC Excl:** 429.71-429.79, 429.82, 459.89-459.9

429.83 Takotsubo syndrome   `CC`
Broken heart syndrome
Reversible left ventricular dysfunction following sudden emotional stress
Stress induced cardiomyopathy
Transient left ventricular apical ballooning syndrome
> **CC Excl:** 398.91, 402.01, 402.11, 402.91, 428.0-428.9, 429.83, 429.9, 459.89-459.9
> **AHA:** 4Q, '06, 87

429.89 Other
Carditis
> **EXCLUDES** *that due to hypertension (402.0-402.9)*
> **AHA:** 2Q, '06, 18; 3Q, '05, 14; 1Q, '92, 10

Berry Aneurysms

429.9 Heart disease, unspecified
Heart disease (organic) NOS
Morbus cordis NOS
> **EXCLUDES** *that due to hypertension (402.0-402.9)*
> **AHA:** 1Q, '09, 7; 1Q, '93, 19

I51.9 Heart disease unspecified   `I-1`

Cerebrovascular Disease (430-438)

> **INCLUDES** with mention of hypertension (conditions classifiable to 401-405)

Use additional code to identify presence of hypertension
> **EXCLUDES** *any condition classifiable to 430-434, 436, 437 occurring during pregnancy, childbirth, or the puerperium, or specified as puerperal (674.0)*
> *iatrogenic cerebrovascular infarction or hemorrhage (997.02)*

AHA: 1Q, '93, 27; 3Q, '91, 10; 3Q, '90, 3; 2Q, '89, 8; M-A, '85, 6

430 Subarachnoid hemorrhage   `MC`
Meningeal hemorrhage
Ruptured:
  berry aneurysm
  (congenital) cerebral aneurysm NOS
> **EXCLUDES** *berry aneurysm, nonruptured (437.3)*
> *syphilitic ruptured cerebral aneurysm (094.87)*
> **DEF:** Bleeding in space between brain and lining.
> **CC Excl:** 348.82, 430-432.9, 459.89-459.9, 780.01-780.09, 800.00-801.99, 803.00-804.96, 850.0-852.19, 852.21-854.19
> **AHA:** 4Q, '04, 77

431 Intracerebral hemorrhage   `MC`
Hemorrhage (of):	Hemorrhage (of):
basilar	internal capsule
bulbar	intrapontine
cerebellar	pontine
cerebral	subcortical
cerebromeningeal	ventricular
cortical	Rupture of blood vessel in brain

> **DEF:** Bleeding within the brain.
> **CC Excl:** See code: 430
> **AHA:** 1Q, '12, 14; 3Q, '10, 5-6; 1Q, '10, 8; 3Q, '07, 4; 4Q, '04, 77

I61.9 Nontraumatic intracerebral hemorrhage unspec   `I-`

√4ᵗʰ 432 Other and unspecified intracranial hemorrhage
AHA: 4Q, '04, 7

432.0 Nontraumatic extradural hemorrhage   `MC`
Nontraumatic epidural hemorrhage
> **DEF:** Bleeding, nontraumatic, between skull and brain lining.
> **CC Excl:** See code: 430

432.1 Subdural hemorrhage   `MC`
Subdural hematoma, nontraumatic
> **DEF:** Bleeding, between outermost and other layers of brain lining.
> **CC Excl:** See code: 430

432.9 Unspecified intracranial hemorrhage   `C`
Intracranial hemorrhage NOS
> **CC Excl:** See code: 430

`N` Newborn Age: 0   `P` Pediatric Age: 0-17   `M` Maternity Age: 12-55   `A` Adult Age: 15-124   `MCC` Major CC Condition   `CC` CC Condition   `HIV` HIV Related D

146 – Volume 1   **2014 ICD-9-C**

Cerebrovascular Arteries

- Posterior parietal
- Parietal-occipital
- Calcarine
- Posterior cerebral
- Anterior inferior cerebellar
- Posterior inferior cerebellar
- Basilar
- Vertebral
- Callosal-marginal
- Pericallosal
- Anterior cerebral
- Anterior communicating
- Middle cerebral
- Ophthalmic
- Posterior communicating
- External carotid
- Internal carotid
- Aorta

√4ᵗʰ 433 Occlusion and stenosis of precerebral arteries

INCLUDES embolism, narrowing, obstruction, thrombosis } of basilar, carotid, and vertebral arteries

Use additional code, if applicable, to identify status post administration of tPA (rtPA) in a different facility within the last 24 hours prior to admission to current facility (V45.88)

EXCLUDES insufficiency NOS of precerebral arteries (435.0-435.9)

The following fifth-digit subclassification is for use with category 433:
0 without mention of cerebral infarction
1 with cerebral infarction

DEF: Blockage, stricture, arteries branching into brain.
AHA: 2Q, '95, 14; 3Q, '90, 16

§ √5ᵗʰ **433.0 Basilar artery** MCC 1
[0-1] CC Excl: For code 433.01: 249.70-249.91, 250.70-250.93, 346.60-346.63, 433.00-433.91, 435.0, 459.89-459.9

§ √5ᵗʰ **433.1 Carotid artery** MCC 1
[0-1] CC Excl: For code 433.11: 249.70-249.91, 250.70-250.93, 346.60-346.63, 433.00-433.91, 459.89-459.9
AHA: 1Q, '00, 16; For code 433.10: 1Q, '06, 17; 1Q, '02, 7, 10
I65.29 Occlusion and stenosis of unspec carotid artery I-10

§ √5ᵗʰ **433.2 Vertebral artery** MCC 1
[0-1] CC Excl: For code 433.21: 249.70-249.91, 250.70-250.93, 346.60-346.63, 433.00-433.91, 435.1, 459.89-459.9

§ √5ᵗʰ **433.3 Multiple and bilateral** MCC 1
[0-1] CC Excl: For code 433.31: 249.70-249.91, 250.70-250.93, 346.60-346.63, 433.00-433.91, 459.89-459.9
AHA: 2Q, '02, 19

§ √5ᵗʰ **433.8 Other specified precerebral artery** MCC 1
[0-1] CC Excl: For code 433.81: 249.70-249.91, 250.70-250.93, 346.60-346.63, 433.00-433.91, 435.0, 459.89-459.9

§ √5ᵗʰ **433.9 Unspecified precerebral artery** MCC 1
[0-1] Precerebral artery NOS
CC Excl: For code 433.91: 249.70-249.91, 250.70-250.93, 346.60-346.63, 433.00-433.91, 435.0, 459.89-459.9

√4ᵗʰ 434 Occlusion of cerebral arteries

Use additional code, if applicable, to identify status post administration of tPA (rtPA) in a different facility within the last 24 hours prior to admission to current facility (V45.88)

The following fifth-digit subclassification is for use with category 434:
0 without mention of cerebral infarction
1 with cerebral infarction

AHA: 2Q, '95, 14

§§ √5ᵗʰ **434.0 Cerebral thrombosis** MCC 1
[0-1] Thrombosis of cerebral arteries
CC Excl: For code 434.01: 249.70-249.91, 250.70-250.93, 346.60-346.63, 434.00-434.91, 436, 459.89-459.9
AHA: For code 434.01: 4Q, '04, 77

§§ √5ᵗʰ **434.1 Cerebral embolism** MCC 1
[0-1] CC Excl: For code 434.11: 249.70-249.91, 250.70-250.93, 346.60-346.63, 433.00-433.91, 435.0, 459.89-459.9
AHA: For code 434.11: 4Q, '04, 77; 3Q, '97, 11
I63.449 Cerbral infarct d/t embo of uns cerebellar art I-10

§§ √5ᵗʰ 434.9 Cerebral artery occlusion, unspecified MCC 1
[0-1] CC Excl: For code 434.91: 249.70-249.91, 250.70-250.93, 346.60-346.63, 433.00-433.91, 435.0, 459.89-459.9
AHA: For code 434.91: 3Q, '10, 5-6; 4Q, '08, 108; 3Q, '07, 9; 1Q, '07, 23; 4Q, '04, 77-78; 4Q, '98, 87

√4ᵗʰ 435 Transient cerebral ischemia

INCLUDES cerebrovascular insufficiency (acute) with trans- ient focal neurological signs and symptoms
insufficiency of basilar, carotid, and vertebral arteries
spasm of cerebral arteries

EXCLUDES acute cerebrovascular insufficiency NOS (437.1)
that due to any condition classifiable to 433 (433.0-433.9)

435.0 Basilar artery syndrome CC
CC Excl: 249.70-249.91, 250.70-250.93, 433.00-433.91, 435.0-435.9, 459.89-459.9

435.1 Vertebral artery syndrome CC
CC Excl: See code: 435.0

435.2 Subclavian steal syndrome CC
DEF: Cerebrovascular insufficiency, due to occluded subclavian artery; symptoms include pain in mastoid and posterior head regions, flaccid paralysis of arm and diminished or absent radial pulse on affected side.
CC Excl: See code: 435.0

435.3 Vertebrobasilar artery syndrome CC
DEF: Transient ischemic attack; due to brainstem dysfunction; symptoms include confusion, vertigo, binocular blindness, diplopia, unilateral or bilateral weakness and paresthesis of extremities.
CC Excl: See code: 435.0
AHA: 4Q, '95, 60

435.8 Other specified transient cerebral ischemias CC
CC Excl: See code: 435.0

435.9 Unspecified transient cerebral ischemia CC
Impending cerebrovascular accident
Intermittent cerebral ischemia
Transient ischemic attack [TIA]
DEF: Temporary restriction of blood flow to arteries branching into brain.
CC Excl: See code: 435.0
AHA: N-D, '85, 12
G45.9 Transient cerebral ischemic attack unspecified I-10

436 Acute, but ill-defined, cerebrovascular disease CC
Apoplexy, apoplectic:
  NOS
  attack
  cerebral
  seizure
Cerebral seizure

EXCLUDES any condition classifiable to categories 430-435
cerebrovascular accident (434.91)
CVA (ischemic) (434.91)
  embolic (434.11)
  hemorrhagic (430, 431, 432.0-432.9)
  thrombotic (434.01)
postoperative cerebrovascular accident (997.02)
stroke (ischemic) (434.91)
  embolic (434.11)
  hemorrhagic (430, 431, 432.0-432.9)
  thrombotic (434.01)

CC Excl: 249.70-249.91, 250.70-250.93, 346.60-346.63, 348.82, 430-432.9, 434.00-434.91, 436, 459.89-459.9, 780.01-780.09, 800.00-801.99, 803.00-804.96, 850.0-852.19, 852.21-854.19
AHA: 4Q, '04, 77; 4Q, '99, 3
TIP: Do not assign when documentation indicates "CVA, stroke, or cerebral infarction." See instead default code 434.91.

√4ᵗʰ 437 Other and ill-defined cerebrovascular disease

437.0 Cerebral atherosclerosis A
Atheroma of cerebral arteries
Cerebral arteriosclerosis
AHA: 3Q, '10, 15
I67.2 Cerebral atherosclerosis I-10

---

§ Requires fifth digit. Valid digits are in [brackets] under each code. See category 433 for codes and definitions.
§§ Requires fifth digit. Valid digits are in [brackets] under each code. See category 434 for codes and definitions.

| ⁴ᵗʰ⁄⁵ᵗʰ Additional Digit Required | Unacceptable PDx | Manifestation Code | Hospital Acquired Condition | ►◄ Revised Text | ● New Code | ▲ Revised Code Title |

Diseases of the Circulatory System

437.1–438.83

437.1 Other generalized ischemic cerebrovascular disease `CC`
Acute cerebrovascular insufficiency NOS
Cerebral ischemia (chronic)
CC Excl: 249.70-249.91, 250.70-250.93, 430-432.9, 434.00-436, 437.1, 459.89-459.9
AHA: 1Q, '09, 8

437.2 Hypertensive encephalopathy `CC`
DEF: Cerebral manifestations (such as visual disturbances and headache) due to high blood pressure.
CC Excl: 249.70-249.91, 250.70-250.93, 437.2, 459.89-459.9
AHA: J-A, '84, 14

437.3 Cerebral aneurysm, nonruptured
Internal carotid artery, intracranial portion
Internal carotid artery NOS
EXCLUDES   *congenital cerebral aneurysm, nonruptured (747.81)*
internal carotid artery, extracranial portion (442.81)
AHA: 2Q, '09, 12

437.4 Cerebral arteritis `CC`
DEF: Inflammation of a cerebral artery or arteries.
CC Excl: 249.70-249.91, 250.70-250.93, 437.4, 459.89-459.9
AHA: 4Q, '99, 21

437.5 Moyamoya disease `CC`
DEF: Cerebrovascular ischemia; vessels occlude and rupture causing tiny hemorrhages at base of brain; predominantly affects Japanese.
CC Excl: 249.70-249.91, 250.70-250.93, 437.5, 459.89-459.9

437.6 Nonpyogenic thrombosis of intracranial venous sinus `CC`
EXCLUDES   *pyogenic (325)*
CC Excl: 249.70-249.91, 250.70-250.93, 437.6, 459.89-459.9

437.7 Transient global amnesia
DEF: Episode of short-term memory loss, not often recurrent; pathogenesis unknown; with no signs or symptoms of neurological disorder.
AHA: 4Q, '92, 20

437.8 Other

437.9 Unspecified
Cerebrovascular disease or lesion NOS
AHA: 1Q, '09, 9

√4ᵗʰ **438 Late effects of cerebrovascular disease**
NOTE This category is to be used to indicate conditions in 430-437 as the cause of late effects. The "late effects" include conditions specified as such, as sequelae, which may occur at any time after the onset of the causal condition.
EXCLUDES   *personal history of:*
cerebral infarction without residual deficits (V12.54)
PRIND [Prolonged reversible ischemic neurologic deficit] (V12.54)
RIND [Reversible ischemic neurological deficit] (V12.54)
transient ischemic attack [TIA] (V12.54)
AHA: 3Q, '06, 3-4, 6; 4Q, '99, 4, 6, 7; 4Q, '98, 39, 88; 4Q, '97, 35, 37; 4Q, '92, 21;N-D,'86, 12; M-A, '86, 7
TIP: Assign instead code V12.54 TIA and cerebral infarction without residual effects, if no residual deficits are present.

438.0 Cognitive deficits

√5ᵗʰ **438.1 Speech and language deficits**

     438.10 Speech and language deficit, unspecified

     438.11 Aphasia
DEF: Impairment or absence of the ability to communicate by speech, writing or signs or to comprehend the spoken or written language due to disease or injury to the brain.
AHA: 4Q, '03, 105; 4Q, '97, 36

     438.12 Dysphasia
DEF: Impaired speech; marked by inability to sequence language.
AHA: 4Q, '99, 3, 9

     438.13 Dysarthria
DEF: Speech disorder caused by paralysis, spasticity, or other nerve damage resulting in difficulty expressing words or sounds; characterized by slurring, interrupted rhythm of speech, or distorted vowel sounds.
AHA: 4Q, '09, 87-88
TIP: If dysarthria or other speech disturbances are not due to underlying cerebrovascular disease, see subcategory 784.5 codes.

     438.14 Fluency disorder
Stuttering due to late effect of cerebrovascular accident
DEF: Interruption in the flow of speech that significantly interferes with communication; characterized by primary sound and syllable repetitions, articulatory fixations, and abnormal prolongation of speech sounds.
AHA: 4Q, '10, 83; 4Q, '09, 87-88

     438.19 Other speech and language deficits

√5ᵗʰ **438.2 Hemiplegia/hemiparesis**
DEF: Paralysis of one side of the body.
AHA: 1Q, '10, 5

     438.20 Hemiplegia affecting unspecified side `CC`
CC Excl: 438.20
AHA: 4Q, '07, 94; 4Q, '03, 105; 4Q, '99, 3, 9
I69.959 Hemipl & hemiparesis flw uns CVD affect uns side   `I-10`

     438.21 Hemiplegia affecting dominant side `CC`
CC Excl: 438.21

     438.22 Hemiplegia affecting nondominant side `CC`
CC Excl: 438.22
AHA: 4Q, '03, 105; 1Q, '02, 16

√5ᵗʰ **438.3 Monoplegia of upper limb**
DEF: Paralysis of one limb or one muscle group.

     438.30 Monoplegia of upper limb affecting unspecified side

     438.31 Monoplegia of upper limb affecting dominant side

     438.32 Monoplegia of upper limb affecting nondominant side

√5ᵗʰ **438.4 Monoplegia of lower limb**

     438.40 Monoplegia of lower limb affecting unspecified side

     438.41 Monoplegia of lower limb affecting dominant side

     438.42 Monoplegia of lower limb affecting nondominant side

√5ᵗʰ **438.5 Other paralytic syndrome**
Use additional code to identify type of paralytic syndrome, such as:
locked-in state (344.81)
quadriplegia (344.00-344.09)
EXCLUDES   *late effects of cerebrovascular accident with:*
hemiplegia/hemiparesis (438.20-438.22)
monoplegia of lower limb (438.40-438.42)
monoplegia of upper limb (438.30-438.32)

     438.50 Other paralytic syndrome affecting unspecified side

     438.51 Other paralytic syndrome affecting dominant side

     438.52 Other paralytic syndrome affecting nondominant side

     438.53 Other paralytic syndrome, bilateral
AHA: 4Q, '98, 39

438.6 Alterations of sensations
Use additional code to identify the altered sensation

438.7 Disturbances of vision
Use additional code to identify the visual disturbance
AHA: 4Q, '02, 56

√5ᵗʰ **438.8 Other late effects of cerebrovascular disease**

     438.81 Apraxia
DEF: Inability to activate learned movements; no known sensory or motor impairment.

     438.82 Dysphagia
Use additional code to identify the type of dysphagia, if known (787.20-787.29)
DEF: Inability or difficulty in swallowing.
AHA: 4Q, '07, 94
I69.991 Dysphagia following uns cerebrovascular disease   `I-10`

     438.83 Facial weakness
Facial droop

N Newborn Age: 0   P Pediatric Age: 0-17   M Maternity Age: 12-55   A Adult Age: 15-124   MCC Major CC Condition   CC CC Condition   HIV HIV Related Dx

148 – Volume 1   2014 ICD-9-CM

438.84 Ataxia

AHA: 4Q, '02, 56

438.85 Vertigo

438.89 Other late effects of cerebrovascular disease

Use additional code to identify the late effect

AHA: 2Q, '09, 10; 1Q, '05, 13; 4Q, '98, 39

TIP: Assign 438.89 and 728.87 Muscle weakness, for residual weakness secondary to late effect of CVA.

169.998 Other sequelae flw uns cerebrovascular disease   I-10

438.9 Unspecified late effects of cerebrovascular disease

Diseases of Arteries, Arterioles, and Capillaries (440-449)

√4ᵗʰ 440 Atherosclerosis

INCLUDES arteriolosclerosis
arteriosclerosis (obliterans) (senile)
arteriosclerotic vascular disease
atheroma
degeneration:
    arterial
    arteriovascular
    vascular
endarteritis deformans or obliterans
senile:
    arteritis
    endarteritis

EXCLUDES atheroembolism (445.01-445.89)
atherosclerosis of bypass graft of the extremities (440.30-440.32)

DEF: Stricture and reduced elasticity of an artery; due to plaque deposits.

440.0 Of aorta   A

AHA: 2Q, '93, 7; 2Q, '93, 8; 4Q, '88, 8

440.1 Of renal artery   A

EXCLUDES atherosclerosis of renal arterioles (403.00-403.91)

√5ᵗʰ 440.2 Of native arteries of the extremities

Use additional code, if applicable, to identify chronic total occlusion of artery of the extremities (440.4)

EXCLUDES atherosclerosis of bypass graft of the extremities (440.30-440.32)

AHA: 4Q, '94, 49; 4Q, '93, 27; 4Q, '92, 25; 3Q, '90, 15; M-A, '87, 6

TIP: Codes are listed in order of increasing severity; all patients who have gangrene (regardless of whether ulceration, rest pain, and/or intermittent claudication are present) are coded to 440.24. Patients without gangrene, but with ulceration (regardless of whether they also suffer from rest pain or intermittent claudication) are coded to 440.23.

440.20 Atherosclerosis of the extremities, unspecified   A

170.209 Uns atherosclero natv art of extrem uns extrem   I-10

440.21 Atherosclerosis of the extremities with intermittent claudication   A

DEF: Atherosclerosis; marked by pain, tension and weakness after walking; no symptoms while at rest.

170.219 Atherosclerosis native arteries ext w/interm claud uns ext   I-10

440.22 Atherosclerosis of the extremities with rest pain   A

INCLUDES any condition classifiable to 440.21

DEF: Atherosclerosis, marked by pain, tension and weakness while at rest.

440.23 Atherosclerosis of the extremities with ulceration   A

INCLUDES any condition classifiable to 440.21 and 440.22

Use additional code for any associated ulceration (707.10-707.19, 707.8, 707.9)

AHA: 4Q, '00, 44

170.249 Atherosclero natv art lt leg ulceration uns site   I-10

440.24 Atherosclerosis of the extremities with gangrene CC

INCLUDES any condition classifiable to 440.21, 440.22, and 440.23 with ischemic gangrene 785.4

Use additional code for any associated ulceration (707.10-707.19, 707.8, 707.9)

EXCLUDES gas gangrene (040.0)

CC Excl: 338.0-338.4, 440.24, 780.64-780.65, 780.91-780.99, 785.4, 799.81-799.89

AHA: 4Q, '03, 109; 3Q, '03, 14; 4Q, '95, 54; 1Q, '95, 11

440.29 Other   A

√5ᵗʰ 440.3 Of bypass graft of extremities

EXCLUDES atherosclerosis of native arteries of the extremities (440.21-440.24)
embolism [occlusion NOS] [thrombus] of graft (996.74)

AHA: 4Q, '94, 49

440.30 Of unspecified graft   A

440.31 Of autologous vein bypass graft   A

440.32 Of nonautologous biological bypass graft   A

440.4 Chronic total occlusion of artery of the extremities   CC
Complete occlusion of artery of the extremities
Total occlusion of artery of the extremities

Code first atherosclerosis of arteries of the extremities (440.20-440.29, 440.30-440.32)

EXCLUDES acute occlusion of artery of extremity (444.21-444.22)

CC Excl: 440.4, 443.81-443.89, 447.0-447.2, 447.5-447.73, 449

440.8 Of other specified arteries   A

EXCLUDES basilar (433.0)
carotid (433.1)
cerebral (437.0)
coronary (414.00-414.07)
mesenteric (557.1)
precerebral (433.0-433.9)
pulmonary (416.0)
vertebral (433.2)

AHA: 3Q, '09, 9

TIP: Assign for arteriosclerosis of the iliac artery.

440.9 Generalized and unspecified atherosclerosis   A
Arteriosclerotic vascular disease NOS

EXCLUDES arteriosclerotic cardiovascular disease [ASCVD] (429.2)

170.91 Generalized atherosclerosis   I-10

√4ᵗʰ/5ᵗʰ Additional Digit Required   Unacceptable PDx   Manifestation Code   Hospital Acquired Condition   ▶◀ Revised Text   ● New Code   ▲ Revised Code Title

2014 ICD-9-CM   Volume 1 – 149

Diseases of the Circulatory System

Map of Major Arteries

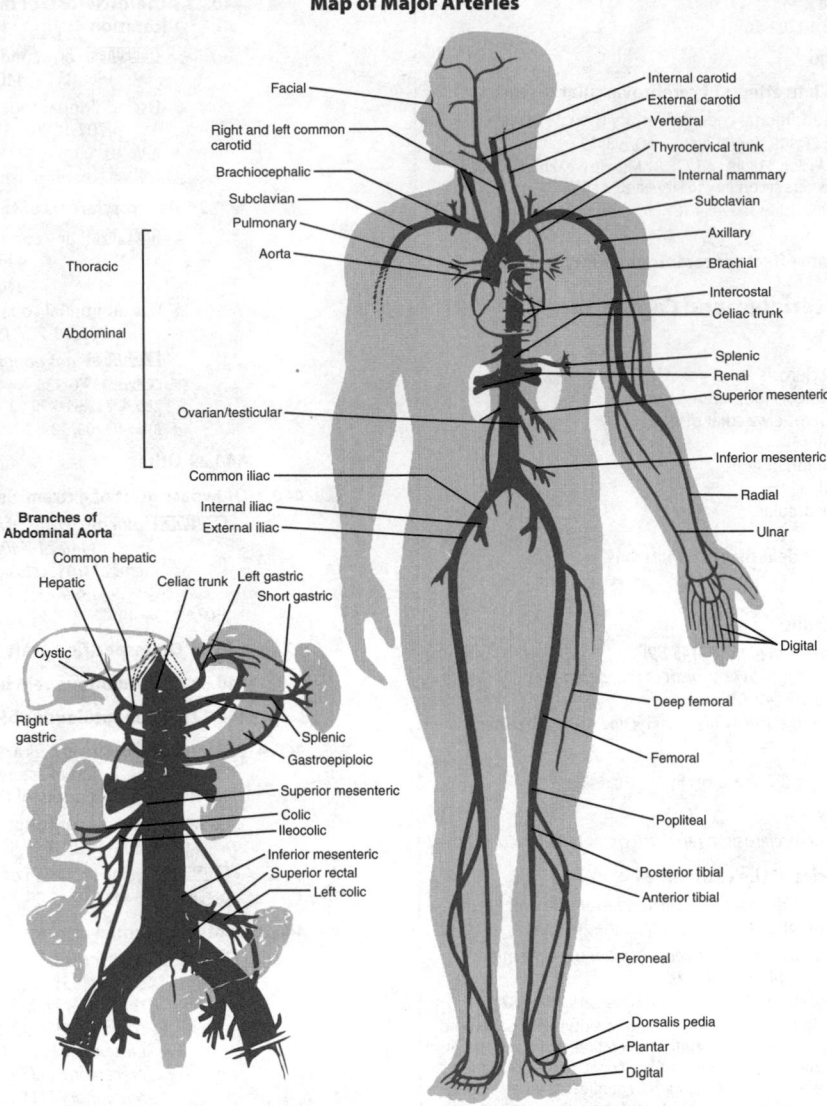

441 **Aortic aneurysm and dissection**

> EXCLUDES   aortic ectasia (447.70-447.73)
>   syphilitic aortic aneurysm (093.0)
>   traumatic aortic aneurysm (901.0, 902.0)

441.0 **Dissection of aorta**

> AHA: 4Q, '89, 10
> DEF: Dissection or splitting of wall of the aorta; due to blood entering through intimal tear or interstitial hemorrhage.

441.00 **Unspecified site**   `MCC`

> CC Excl: 249.70-249.91, 250.70-250.93, 441.00-441.9, 447.70-447.73, 459.89-459.9

441.01 **Thoracic**   `MCC`

> CC Excl: See code: 441.00
> AHA: 1Q, '09, 16; 4Q, '07, 87

441.02 **Abdominal**   `MCC`

> CC Excl: See code: 441.00

441.03 **Thoracoabdominal**   `MCC`

> CC Excl: See code: 441.00

441.1 **Thoracic aneurysm, ruptured**   `MCC`

> CC Excl: See code: 441.00

441.2 **Thoracic aneurysm without mention of rupture**

> AHA: 3Q, '92, 10
> 171.2 Thoracic aortic aneurysm without rupture   `I-10`

441.3 **Abdominal aneurysm, ruptured**   `MCC`

> CC Excl: See code: 441.00
> 171.3 Abdominal aortic aneurysm, ruptured   `I-10`

441.4 **Abdominal aneurysm without mention of rupture**

> AHA: 4Q, '00, 64; 1Q, '99, 15, 16, 17; 3Q, '92, 10
> 171.4 Abdominal aortic aneurysm without rupture   `I-10`

441.5 **Aortic aneurysm of unspecified site, ruptured**   `MCC`
Rupture of aorta NOS

> CC Excl: See code: 441.00

441.6 **Thoracoabdominal aneurysm, ruptured**   `MCC`

> CC Excl: See code: 441.00

441.7 **Thoracoabdominal aneurysm, without mention of rupture**

> AHA: 2Q, '06, 16

441.9 **Aortic aneurysm of unspecified site without mention of rupture**
Aneurysm
Dilatation } of aorta
Hyaline necrosis

> AHA: 4Q, '10, 84

`N` Newborn Age: 0   `P` Pediatric Age: 0-17   `M` Maternity Age: 12-55   `A` Adult Age: 15-124   `MCC` Major CC Condition   `CC` CC Condition   `HIV` HIV Related Dx

150 – Volume 1   **2014 ICD-9-CM**

Thoracic and Abdominal Aortic Aneurysm

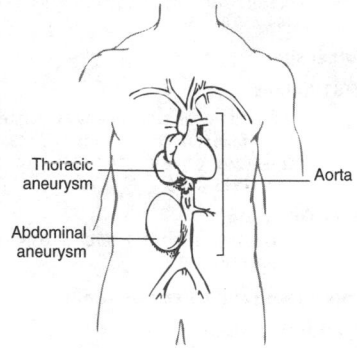

Thoracic aneurysm

Abdominal aneurysm

Aorta

√4ᵗʰ **442　Other aneurysm**

INCLUDES　aneurysm (ruptured) (cirsoid) (false) (varicose)
　　　　　aneurysmal varix

EXCLUDES　arteriovenous aneurysm or fistula:
　　　　　acquired (447.0)
　　　　　congenital (747.60-747.69)
　　　　　traumatic (900.0-904.9)

DEF: Dissection or splitting of arterial wall; due to blood entering through intimal tear or interstitial hemorrhage.

442.0　Of artery of upper extremity

442.1　Of renal artery

442.2　Of iliac artery
　　　　AHA: 1Q, '99, 16, 17

442.3　Of artery of lower extremity
　　　　Aneurysm:
　　　　　femoral artery
　　　　　popliteal artery
　　　　AHA: 2Q, '08, 13; 3Q, '02, 24-26; 1Q, '99, 16

√5ᵗʰ **442.8　Of other specified artery**

442.81　Artery of neck
　　　　Aneurysm of carotid artery (common) (external)
　　　　　(internal, extracranial portion)
　　　　EXCLUDES　internal carotid artery, intracranial portion
　　　　　　　　　(437.3)

442.82　Subclavian artery

442.83　Splenic artery

442.84　Other visceral artery
　　　　Aneurysm:
　　　　　celiac
　　　　　gastroduodenal
　　　　　gastroepiploic　　　} artery
　　　　　hepatic
　　　　　pancreaticoduodenal
　　　　　superior mesenteric

442.89　Other
　　　　Aneurysm:
　　　　　mediastinal artery
　　　　　spinal artery
　　　　EXCLUDES　cerebral (nonruptured) (437.3)
　　　　　　　　　congenital (747.81)
　　　　　　　　　ruptured (430)
　　　　　　　　　coronary (414.11)
　　　　　　　　　heart (414.10)
　　　　　　　　　pulmonary (417.1)

442.9　Of unspecified site

√4ᵗʰ **443　Other peripheral vascular disease**

443.0　Raynaud's syndrome
　　　　Raynaud's:
　　　　　disease
　　　　　phenomenon (secondary)
　　　　Use additional code to identify gangrene (785.4)
　　　　DEF: Constriction of the arteries, due to cold or stress; bilateral ischemic attacks of fingers, toes, nose or ears; symptoms include pallor, paresthesia and pain.
　　　　I73.00 Raynaud's syndrome without gangrene　　I-10

443.1　Thromboangiitis obliterans [Buerger's disease]
　　　　Presenile gangrene
　　　　DEF: Inflammatory disease of extremity blood vessels, mainly the lower; occurs primarily in young men and leads to tissue ischemia and gangrene.

√5ᵗʰ **443.2　Other arterial dissection**
　　　　EXCLUDES　dissection of aorta (441.00-441.03)
　　　　　　　　　dissection of coronary arteries (414.12)
　　　　AHA: 4Q, '02, 54

443.21　Dissection of carotid artery　　MCC
　　　　CC Excl: 447.2, 447.5-447.6, 447.8-447.9

443.22　Dissection of iliac artery　　MCC
　　　　CC Excl: See code: 443.21

443.23　Dissection of renal artery　　MCC
　　　　CC Excl: See code: 443.21

443.24　Dissection of vertebral artery　　MCC
　　　　CC Excl: See code: 443.21

443.29　Dissection of other artery　　MCC
　　　　CC Excl: See code: 443.21

√5ᵗʰ **443.8　Other specified peripheral vascular diseases**

443.81　*Peripheral angiopathy in diseases classified elsewhere*
　　　　Code first underlying disease, as:
　　　　　diabetes mellitus (249.7, 250.7)
　　　　AHA: 1Q, '04, 14; 3Q, '91, 10
　　　　I79.8 Oth d/o art arterioles & cap in dz class elsw　　I-10

443.82　Erythromelalgia
　　　　DEF: Rare syndrome of paroxysmal vasodilation; maldistribution of blood flow causes redness, pain, increased skin temperature, and burning sensations in various parts of the body.
　　　　AHA: 4Q, '05, 73

443.89　Other
　　　　Acrocyanosis
　　　　Acroparesthesia:
　　　　　simple [Schultze's type]
　　　　　vasomotor [Nothnagel's type]
　　　　Erythrocyanosis
　　　　EXCLUDES　chilblains (991.5)
　　　　　　　　　frostbite (991.0-991.3)
　　　　　　　　　immersion foot (991.4)
　　　　AHA: 4Q, '07, 124
　　　　I73.89 Other specified peripheral vascular disease　　I-10

443.9　Peripheral vascular disease, unspecified
　　　　Intermittent claudication NOS
　　　　Peripheral:
　　　　　angiopathy NOS
　　　　　vascular disease NOS
　　　　Spasm of artery
　　　　EXCLUDES　atherosclerosis of the arteries of the extremities
　　　　　　　　　(440.20-440.22)
　　　　　　　　　spasm of cerebral artery (435.0-435.9)
　　　　AHA: 4Q, '92, 25; 3Q, '91, 10
　　　　I73.9 Peripheral vascular disease unspecified　　I-10

Arterial Diseases and Disorders

Lipids
Calcium deposits
Intimal proliferation
Atherosclerosis narrowing lumen
Thrombus (clot) forming in lumen
Organization of thrombus and recanalization
Embolus (from elsewhere) occluding lumen
Aneurysm bypasses lumen or...
...bulges from arterial wall
Arteriovenous fistula

Additional Digit Required　　Unacceptable PDx　　Manifestation Code　　Hospital Acquired Condition　　▶◀ Revised Text　　● New Code　　▲ Revised Code Title

2014 ICD-9-CM　　　　　　　　　　　　　　　　　　　　　　　　　　　　　　**Volume 1 – 151**

✓4ᵗʰ **444 Arterial embolism and thrombosis**

INCLUDES infarction:
  embolic
  thrombotic
  occlusion

EXCLUDES atheroembolism (445.01-445.89)
  that complicating:
  abortion (634-638 with .6, 639.6)
  ectopic or molar pregnancy (639.6)
  pregnancy, childbirth, or the pueperium (673.0-673.8)
  septic arterial embolism (449)

AHA: 2Q, '92, 11; 4Q, '90, 27

✓5ᵗʰ **444.0 Of abdominal aorta**
CC Excl: 249.70-249.91, 250.70-250.93, 444.0, 444.89-444.9, 449, 459.89-459.9
AHA: 4Q, '11, 107-109; 2Q, '93, 7; 4Q, '90, 27

444.01 Saddle embolus of abdominal aorta   MCC
CC Excl: 415.11-415.19, 416.2, 444.01-444.09, 459.89-459.9
AHA: 4Q, '11, 108

444.09 Other arterial embolism and thrombosis of abdominal aorta   CC
Aortic bifurcation syndrome
Aortoiliac obstruction
Leriche's syndrome
CC Excl: See code 444.01

444.1 Of thoracic aorta   CC
Embolism or thrombosis of aorta (thoracic)
CC Excl: 249.70-249.91, 250.70-250.93, 444.1, 444.89-444.9, 449, 459.89-459.9

✓5ᵗʰ **444.2 Of arteries of the extremities**
AHA: M-A, '87, 6

444.21 Upper extremity   CC
CC Excl: 249.70-249.91, 250.70-250.93, 444.21, 444.89-444.9, 449, 459.89-459.9

444.22 Lower extremity   CC
Arterial embolism or thrombosis:
  femoral
  peripheral NOS
  popliteal
EXCLUDES iliofemoral (444.81)
CC Excl: 249.70-249.91, 250.70-250.93, 444.22, 444.89-444.9, 449, 459.89-459.9
AHA: 2Q, '11, 8; 4Q, '07, 85; 3Q, '03, 10; 1Q, '03, 17; 3Q, '90, 16
I74.3 Embo & thromb of arteries of the low extremities   I-10

✓5ᵗʰ **444.8 Of other specified artery**

444.81 Iliac artery   CC
CC Excl: 249.70-249.91, 250.70-250.93, 444.81-444.9, 449, 459.89-459.9
AHA: 1Q, '03, 16

444.89 Other   CC
EXCLUDES basilar (433.0)
  carotid (433.1)
  cerebral (434.0-434.9)
  coronary (410.00-410.92)
  mesenteric (557.0)
  ophthalmic (362.30-362.34)
  precerebral (433.0-433.9)
  pulmonary (415.11-415.19)
  renal (593.81)
  retinal (362.30-362.34)
  vertebral (433.2)
CC Excl: 249.70-249.91, 250.70-250.93, 444.89-444.9, 449, 459.89-459.9

444.9 Of unspecified artery   CC
CC Excl: See code 444.89

✓4ᵗʰ **445 Atheroembolism**

INCLUDES atherothrombotic microembolism
  cholesterol embolism

AHA: 4Q, '02, 57

✓5ᵗʰ **445.0 Of extremities**

445.01 Upper extremity   CC
CC Excl: 249.70-249.91, 250.70-250.93, 444.89-445.01, 449, 459.89-459.9

445.02 Lower extremity   CC
CC Excl: 249.70-249.91, 250.70-250.93, 444.89-444.9, 445.02, 449, 459.89-459.9

✓5ᵗʰ **445.8 Of other sites**

445.81 Kidney   CC
Use additional code for any associated acute kidney failure or chronic kidney disease (584, 585)
CC Excl: 249.70-249.91, 250.70-250.93, 444.89-444.9, 445.81, 449, 459.89-459.9

445.89 Other site   CC
CC Excl: 249.70-249.91, 250.70-250.93, 444.89-444.9, 445.89, 449, 459.89-459.9

✓4ᵗʰ **446 Polyarteritis nodosa and allied conditions**

446.0 Polyarteritis nodosa   CC
Disseminated necrotizing periarteritis
Necrotizing angiitis
Panarteritis (nodosa)
Periarteritis (nodosa)
DEF: Inflammation of small and mid-size arteries; symptoms related to involved arteries in kidneys, muscles, gastrointestinal tract and heart; results in tissue death.
CC Excl: 249.70-249.91, 250.70-250.93, 446.0-446.7, 459.89-459.9

446.1 Acute febrile mucocutaneous lymph node syndrome [MCLS]   CC
Kawasaki disease
DEF: Acute febrile disease of children; marked by erythema of conjunctiva and mucous membranes of upper respiratory tract, skin eruptions and edema.
CC Excl: 446.0-446.29, 446.4-446.7, 459.89-459.9

✓5ᵗʰ **446.2 Hypersensitivity angiitis**
EXCLUDES antiglomerular basement membrane disease without pulmonary hemorrhage (583.89)

446.20 Hypersensitivity angiitis, unspecified   CC
CC Excl: See code: 446.0

446.21 Goodpasture's syndrome   CC
Antiglomerular basement membrane antibody-mediated nephritis with pulmonary hemorrhage
Use additional code to identify renal disease (583.81)
DEF: Glomerulonephritis associated with hematuria, progresses rapidly; results in death from renal failure.
CC Excl: See code: 446.0

446.29 Other specified hypersensitivity angiitis   CC
CC Excl: See code: 446.0
AHA: 1Q, '95, 3

446.3 Lethal midline granuloma   CC
Malignant granuloma of face
DEF: Granulomatous lesion; in nose or paranasal sinuses; often fatal; occurs chiefly in males.
CC Excl: See code: 446.0

446.4 Wegener's granulomatosis   CC
Necrotizing respiratory granulomatosis
Wegener's syndrome
DEF: A disease occurring mainly in men; marked by necrotizing granulomas and ulceration of the upper respiratory tract; cause is a vasculitis affecting small vessels due to an immune disorder.
CC Excl: See code: 446.0
AHA: 3Q, '00, 11

446.5 Giant cell arteritis
Bagratuni's syndrome   Horton's disease
Cranial arteritis   Temporal arteritis
DEF: Inflammation of arteries; due to giant cells affecting carotid artery branches, resulting in occlusion; symptoms include fever, headache and neurological problems.
M31.6 Other giant cell arteritis   I-1

446.6 Thrombotic microangiopathy   MC●
Moschcowitz's syndrome
Thrombotic thrombocytopenic purpura
DEF: Blockage of small blood vessels; due to hyaline deposits; symptoms include purpura, CNS disorders; results in protracted disease or rapid death.
CC Excl: See code: 446.0

N Newborn Age: 0   P Pediatric Age: 0-17   M Maternity Age: 12-55   A Adult Age: 15-124   MCC Major CC Condition   CC CC Condition   HIV HIV Related D

446.7 Takayasu's disease `CC`
Aortic arch arteritis   Pulseless disease
DEF: Progressive obliterative arteritis of brachiocephalic trunk, left subclavian, and left common carotid arteries above aortic arch; results in ischemia in brain, heart and arm.
CC Exd: See code: 446.0

√4ᵗʰ 447 Other disorders of arteries and arterioles

447.0 Arteriovenous fistula, acquired
Arteriovenous aneurysm, acquired
EXCLUDES *cerebrovascular (437.3)*
coronary (414.19)
pulmonary (417.0)
surgically created arteriovenous shunt or fistula:
complication (996.1, 996.61-996.62)
status or presence (V45.11)
traumatic (900.0-904.9)
DEF: Communication between an artery and vein caused by error in healing.

447.1 Stricture of artery
AHA: 2Q, '93, 8; M-A, '87, 6
I77.1 Stricture of artery   `I-10`

447.2 Rupture of artery `CC`
Erosion
Fistula, except arteriovenous } of artery
Ulcer
EXCLUDES *traumatic rupture of artery (900.0-904.9)*
CC Exd: 249.70-249.91, 250.70-250.93, 446.0-446.7, 459.89-459.9

447.3 Hyperplasia of renal artery
Fibromuscular hyperplasia of renal artery
DEF: Overgrowth of cells in muscular lining of renal artery.

447.4 Celiac artery compression syndrome `CC`
Celiac axis syndrome   Marable's syndrome
CC Exd: 447.4

447.5 Necrosis of artery `CC`
CC Exd: 447.5

447.6 Arteritis, unspecified
Aortitis NOS   Endarteritis NOS
EXCLUDES *arteritis, endarteritis:*
aortic arch (446.7)
cerebral (437.4)
coronary (414.00-414.07)
deformans (440.0-440.9)
obliterans (440.0-440.9)
pulmonary (417.8)
senile (440.0-440.9)
polyarteritis NOS (446.0)
syphilitic aortitis (093.1)
AHA: 1Q, '95, 3

√5ᵗʰ 447.7 Aortic ectasia
Ectasis aorta
EXCLUDES *aortic aneurysm and dissection (441.00-441.9)*
DEF: A diffuse, irregular dilation of the aorta less than 3 cm in diameter; increases the patient's risk of developing an aortic aneurysm.
AHA: 4Q, '10, 84-85

447.70 Aortic ectasia, unspecified site

447.71 Thoracic aortic ectasia

447.72 Abdominal aortic ectasia

447.73 Thoracoabdominal aortic ectasia

447.8 Other specified disorders of arteries and arterioles
Fibromuscular hyperplasia of arteries, except renal

447.9 Unspecified disorders of arteries and arterioles

√4ᵗʰ 448 Disease of capillaries

448.0 Hereditary hemorrhagic telangiectasia
Rendu-Osler-Weber disease
DEF: Genetic disease with onset after puberty; results in multiple telangiectases, dilated venules on skin and mucous membranes; recurrent bleeding may occur.

448.1 Nevus, non-neoplastic
Nevus: Nevus:
araneus   spider
senile   stellar
EXCLUDES *neoplastic (216.0-216.9)*
port wine (757.32)
strawberry (757.32)
DEF: Enlarged or malformed blood vessels of skin; results in reddish swelling, skin patch, or birthmark.

448.9 Other and unspecified capillary diseases
Capillary:
hemorrhage
hyperpermeability
thrombosis
EXCLUDES *capillary fragility (hereditary) (287.8)*

449 Septic arterial embolism `CC`
Code first underlying infection, such as:
infective endocarditis (421.0)
lung abscess (513.0)
Use additional code to identify the site of the embolism (433.0-433.9, 444.01-444.9)
EXCLUDES *septic pulmonary embolism (415.12)*
CC Exd: 249.70-249.91, 250.70-250.93, 444.89-444.9, 449, 459.89-459.9
AHA: 4Q, '07, 84-85

Diseases of Veins And Lymphatics, and Other Diseases of Circulatory System (451-459)

√4ᵗʰ 451 Phlebitis and thrombophlebitis
INCLUDES endophlebitis
inflammation, vein
periphlebitis
suppurative phlebitis
Use additional E code to identify drug, if drug-induced
EXCLUDES *that complicating:*
abortion (634-638 with .7, 639.8)
ectopic or molar pregnancy (639.8)
pregnancy, childbirth, or the puerperium (671.0-671.9)
that due to or following:
implant or catheter device (996.61-996.62)
infusion, perfusion, or transfusion (999.2)
DEF: Inflammation of a vein (phlebitis) with formation of a thrombus (thrombophlebitis).
AHA: 1Q, '11, 19; 1Q, '92, 16
TIP: Assign an additional code from category 453 for thrombosis; if both conditions are present, assign codes from categories 451 and 453.

451.0 Of superficial vessels of lower extremities
Saphenous vein (greater) (lesser)
AHA: 3Q, '91, 16

√5ᵗʰ 451.1 Of deep vessels of lower extremities
AHA: 3Q, '91, 16

451.11 Femoral vein (deep) (superficial) `CC`
CC Exd: 249.70-249.91, 250.70-250.93, 451.0-451.9, 459.89-459.9

451.19 Other `CC`
Femoropopliteal vein
Popliteal vein
Tibial vein
CC Exd: 249.70-249.91, 250.70-250.93, 451.0-451.9, 459.89-459.9

451.2 Of lower extremities, unspecified
AHA: 4Q, '04, 80

√5ᵗʰ 451.8 Of other sites
EXCLUDES *intracranial venous sinus (325)*
nonpyogenic (437.6)
portal (vein) (572.1)

451.81 Iliac vein `CC`
CC Exd: See code: 451.19

451.82 Of superficial veins of upper extremities
Antecubital vein
Basilic vein
Cephalic vein

⁴ᵗʰ ⁵ᵗʰ Additional Digit Required   Unacceptable PDx   Manifestation Code   Hospital Acquired Condition   ▶◀ Revised Text   ● New Code   ▲ Revised Code Title

2014 ICD-9-CM   **Volume 1 – 153**

Diseases of the Circulatory System

451.83–453.40

451.83 Of deep veins of upper extremities   `CC`
Brachial vein   Ulnar vein
Radial vein
CC Excl: 451.0-451.2, 451.83, 451.89-451.9

451.84 Of upper extremities, unspecified

451.89 Other   `CC`
Axillary vein
Jugular vein
Subclavian vein
Thrombophlebitis of breast (Mondor's disease)
CC Excl: 451.0-451.2, 451.89-451.9

451.9 Of unspecified site

452 Portal vein thrombosis   `MCC`
Portal (vein) obstruction
EXCLUDES hepatic vein thrombosis (453.0)
phlebitis of portal vein (572.1)
DEF: Formation of a blood clot in main vein of liver.
CC Excl: 249.70-249.91, 250.70-250.93, 452, 453.40-453.9, 459.89-459.9

✓4ᵗʰ **453 Other venous embolism and thrombosis**
EXCLUDES that complicating:
abortion (634-638 with .7, 639.8)
ectopic or molar pregnancy (639.8)
pregnancy, childbirth, or the puerperium (671.0-671.9)
AHA: 1Q, '11, 19-21; 1Q, '92, 16

453.0 Budd-Chiari syndrome   `MCC`
Hepatic vein thrombosis
DEF: Thrombosis or other obstruction of hepatic vein; symptoms include enlarged liver, extensive collateral vessels, intractable ascites and severe portal hypertension.
CC Excl: 249.70-249.91, 250.70-250.93, 453.0, 453.40-453.9, 459.89-459.9

453.1 Thrombophlebitis migrans   `CC`
DEF: Slow, advancing thrombophlebitis; appearing first in one vein then another.
CC Excl: 249.70-249.91, 250.70-250.93, 453.1, 453.40-453.9, 459.89-459.9

453.2 Of inferior vena cava   `MCC`
CC Excl: 249.70-249.91, 250.70-250.93, 453.2, 453.40-453.9, 459.89-459.9

453.3 Of renal vein   `CC`
CC Excl: 249.70-249.91, 250.70-250.93, 453.3-453.9, 459.89-459.9

✓5ᵗʰ **453.4 Acute venous embolism and thrombosis of deep vessels of lower extremity**
AHA: 4Q, '09, 88-92; 3Q, '08, 16

¹¹ **453.40 Acute venous embolism and thrombosis of unspecified deep vessels of lower extremity**   `CC`
Deep vein thrombosis NOS   DVT NOS
CC Excl: 249.70-249.91, 250.70-250.93, 453.40-453.9, 459.89-459.9
AHA: 1Q, '12, 18
TIP: Assign as the default code for "deep vein thrombosis," whether documented as acute or subacute.
I82.409 Ac embo & thrombo of uns deep veins of unsp lower ext   `I-10`

Map of Major Veins

External jugular
Internal jugular
Subclavian
Axillary
Brachial
Cephalic
Medial cubital
Cephalic
Basilic
Digital
Femoral
Great saphenous
Popliteal
Posterior tibial
Anterior tibial
Dorsal venous arch
Digital
Plantar

Brachiocephalic
Internal mammary
Superior vena cava
Azygos
Inferior vena cava
Hepatic
Renal
Ovarian/testicular
Portal
Common iliac
Internal iliac
External iliac
Hypogastric
Common femoral
Superficial femoral
Deep femoral
Femoral

Portal Venous Circulation
Inferior vena cava
Gastric
Portal
Splenic
Superior mesenteric
Right colic
Ileocolic
Inferior mesenteric
Left colic

¹¹ HAC when reported with procedure codes 00.85-00.87, 81.51, 81.52, 81.54 and POA = N

`N` Newborn Age: 0   `P` Pediatric Age: 0-17   `M` Maternity Age: 12-55   `A` Adult Age: 15-124   `MCC` Major CC Condition   `CC` CC Condition   `HIV` HIV Related Dx

154 – Volume 1   **2014 ICD-9-CM**

[11]**453.41 Acute venous embolism and thrombosis of deep vessels of proximal lower extremity** `CC`
Femoral
Iliac
Popliteal
Thigh
Upper leg NOS
CC Excl: See code: 453.40
AHA: 4Q, '04, 79

[11]**453.42 Acute venous embolism and thrombosis of deep vessels of distal lower extremity** `CC`
Calf
Lower leg NOS
Peroneal
Tibial
CC Excl: See code: 453.40

√5ᵗʰ **453.5 Chronic venous embolism and thrombosis of deep vessels of lower extremity**
Use additional code, if applicable, for associated long-term (current) use of anticoagulants (V58.61)
EXCLUDES personal history of venous thrombosis and embolism (V12.51)
AHA: 4Q, '09, 88-92

453.50 Chronic venous embolism and thrombosis of unspecified deep vessels of lower extremity `CC`
CC Excl: See code: 453.40

453.51 Chronic venous embolism and thrombosis of deep vessels of proximal lower extremity `CC`
Femoral   Thigh
Iliac   Upper leg NOS
Popliteal
CC Excl: See code: 453.40

453.52 Chronic venous embolism and thrombosis of deep vessels of distal lower extremity `CC`
Calf   Peroneal
Lower leg NOS   Tibial
CC Excl: See code: 453.40

453.6 Venous embolism and thrombosis of superficial vessels of lower extremity `CC`
Saphenous vein (greater) (lesser)
Use additional code, if applicable, for associated long-term (current) use of anticoagulants (V58.61)
CC Excl: See code: 453.40
AHA: 4Q, '09, 88-92

√5ᵗʰ **453.7 Chronic venous embolism and thrombosis of other specified vessels**
Use additional code, if applicable, for associated long-term (current) use of anticoagulants (V58.61)
EXCLUDES personal history of venous thrombosis and embolism (V12.51)
AHA: 4Q, '09, 88-92

453.71 Chronic venous embolism and thrombosis of superficial veins of upper extremity `CC`
Antecubital vein Cephalic vein
Basilic vein
CC Excl: See code: 453.40

Veins of the Head and Neck

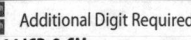

453.72 Chronic venous embolism and thrombosis of deep veins of upper extremity `CC`
Brachial vein
Radial vein
Ulnar vein
CC Excl: 249.70-249.91, 250.70-250.93, 453.40-453.79, 453.81-453.9, 459.89-459.9

453.73 Chronic venous embolism and thrombosis of upper extremity, unspecified `CC`
CC Excl: See code: 453.72

453.74 Chronic venous embolism and thrombosis of axillary veins `CC`
CC Excl: See code: 453.72

453.75 Chronic venous embolism and thrombosis of subclavian veins `CC`
CC Excl: See code: 453.72

453.76 Chronic venous embolism and thrombosis of internal jugular veins `CC`
CC Excl: See code: 453.72

453.77 Chronic venous embolism and thrombosis of other thoracic veins `CC`
Brachiocephalic (innominate)
Superior vena cava
CC Excl: See code: 453.72

453.79 Chronic venous embolism and thrombosis of other specified veins `CC`
CC Excl: See code: 453.72

√5ᵗʰ **453.8 Acute venous embolism and thrombosis of other specified veins**
EXCLUDES cerebral (434.0-434.9)
coronary (410.00-410.92)
intracranial venous sinus (325)
nonpyogenic (437.6)
mesenteric (557.0)
portal (452)
precerebral (433.0-433.9)
pulmonary (415.19)
AHA: 4Q, '09, 88-92; 3Q, '91, 16; M-A, '87, 6

453.81 Acute venous embolism and thrombosis of superficial veins of upper extremity `CC`
Antecubital vein
Basilic vein
Cephalic vein
CC Excl: 249.70-249.91, 250.70-250.93, 453.40-453.79, 453.81-453.9, 459.89-459.9

453.82 Acute venous embolism and thrombosis of deep veins of upper extremity `CC`
Brachial vein
Radial vein
Ulnar vein
CC Excl: See code: 453.81

453.83 Acute venous embolism and thrombosis of upper extremity, unspecified `CC`
CC Excl: See code: 453.81

453.84 Acute venous embolism and thrombosis of axillary veins `CC`
CC Excl: See code: 453.81

453.85 Acute venous embolism and thrombosis of subclavian veins `CC`
CC Excl: See code: 453.81

453.86 Acute venous embolism and thrombosis of internal jugular veins `CC`
CC Excl: See code: 453.81

453.87 Acute venous embolism and thrombosis of other thoracic veins `CC`
Brachiocephalic (innominate)
Superior vena cava
CC Excl: See code: 453.81

453.89 Acute venous embolism and thrombosis of other specified veins `CC`
CC Excl: See code: 453.81
I82.890 Ac embolism and thrombosis of unspec deep vein of unspec lower ext `I-10`

---

¹ HAC when reported with procedure codes 00.85-00.87, 81.51, 81.52, 81.54 and POA = N

4ᵗʰ 5ᵗʰ Additional Digit Required   Unacceptable PDx   Manifestation Code   Hospital Acquired Condition   ►◄ Revised Text   ● New Code   ▲ Revised Code Title

014 ICD-9-CM   Volume 1 – 155

Diseases of the Circulatory System

453.9–457.0

453.9 Of unspecified site   `CC`
Embolism of vein
Thrombosis (vein)
CC Excl: See code: 453.81
AHA: 1Q, '12, 18

√4th 454 Varicose veins of lower extremities
EXCLUDES *that complicating pregnancy, childbirth, or the puerperium (671.0)*
DEF: Dilated leg veins; due to incompetent vein valves that allow reversed blood flow and cause tissue erosion or weakness of wall; may be painful.
AHA: 2Q, '91, 20

454.0 With ulcer   `A`
Varicose ulcer (lower extremity, any part)
Varicose veins with ulcer of lower extremity [any part] or of unspecified site
Any condition classifiable to 454.9 with ulcer or specified as ulcerated
AHA: 4Q, '99, 18

454.1 With inflammation   `A`
Stasis dermatitis
Varicose veins with inflammation of lower extremity [any part] or of unspecified site
Any condition classifiable to 454.9 with inflammation or specified as inflamed

454.2 With ulcer and inflammation   `CC` `A`
Varicose veins with ulcer and inflammation of lower extremity [any part] or of unspecified site
Any condition classifiable to 454.9 with ulcer and inflammation
CC Excl: 454.0-454.2, 454.9

454.8 With other complications
Edema
Pain
Swelling
AHA: 4Q, '02, 58

454.9 Asymptomatic varicose veins   `A`
Phlebectasia
Varicose veins } of lower extremity [any part] or of unspecified site
Varix
Varicose veins NOS
AHA: 4Q, '02, 58
TIP: Do not assign if patient seen for surgical treatment of varicose veins; query physician for specific symptom (inflammation, pain, edema, swelling).

√4th 455 Hemorrhoids
INCLUDES hemorrhoids (anus) (rectum)
     piles
     varicose veins, anus or rectum
EXCLUDES *that complicating pregnancy, childbirth, or the puerperium (671.8)*
DEF: Varicose condition of external hemorrhoidal veins causing painful swellings at the anus.

455.0 Internal hemorrhoids without mention of complication
AHA: 3Q, '05, 17
K64.0 First degree hemorrhoids   `I-10`

455.1 Internal thrombosed hemorrhoids

455.2 Internal hemorrhoids with other complication
Internal hemorrhoids:
     bleeding
     prolapsed
     strangulated
     ulcerated
AHA: 3Q, '05, 17; 1Q, '03, 8
K64.2 Third degree hemorrhoid   `I-10`

455.3 External hemorrhoids without mention of complication
AHA: 1Q, '07, 13; 3Q, '05, 17
K64.4 Residual hemorrhoidal skin tags   `I-10`

455.4 External thrombosed hemorrhoids

455.5 External hemorrhoids with other complication
External hemorrhoids:
     bleeding
     prolapsed
     strangulated
     ulcerated
AHA: 3Q, '05, 17; 1Q, '03, 8

455.6 Unspecified hemorrhoids without mention of complication
Hemorrhoids NOS

455.7 Unspecified thrombosed hemorrhoids
Thrombosed hemorrhoids, unspecified whether internal or external

455.8 Unspecified hemorrhoids with other complication
Hemorrhoids, unspecified whether internal or external:
     bleeding
     prolapsed
     strangulated
     ulcerated

455.9 Residual hemorrhoidal skin tags
Skin tags, anus or rectum

√4th 456 Varicose veins of other sites

456.0 Esophageal varices with bleeding   `MCC`
DEF: Distended, tortuous, veins of lower esophagus, usually due to portal hypertension.
CC Excl: 251.5, 456.0, 456.20, 459.89-459.9, 530.20-530.21, 530.7, 530.82, 530.85, 531.00-534.91, 535.01, 535.11, 535.21, 535.31, 535.41, 535.51, 535.61, 535.71, 537.83, 562.02-562.03, 562.12-562.13, 569.3, 569.85, 578.0-578.9

456.1 Esophageal varices without mention of bleeding   `CC`
CC Excl: 251.5, 456.0-456.20, 459.89-459.9, 530.7, 530.82, 531.00-534.91, 535.01, 535.11, 535.21, 535.31, 535.41, 535.51, 535.61, 535.71, 537.83, 578.0-578.9

√5th 456.2 Esophageal varices in diseases classified elsewhere
Code first underlying cause, as:
     cirrhosis of liver (571.0-571.9)
     portal hypertension (572.3)

456.20 *With bleeding*   `MCC`
CC Excl: 456.0, 456.20, 459.89-459.9, 530.82
AHA: N-D, '85, 14
I85.11 Secondary esophageal varices with bleeding   `I-10`

456.21 *Without mention of bleeding*   `CC`
CC Excl: 251.5, 456.0, 456.20-456.21, 459.89-459.9, 530.7, 530.82, 531.00-534.91, 535.01, 535.11, 535.21, 535.31, 535.41, 535.51, 535.61, 535.71, 537.83, 578.0-578.9
AHA: 3Q, '05, 15; 2Q, '02, 4

456.3 Sublingual varices
DEF: Distended, tortuous veins beneath tongue.

456.4 Scrotal varices   ♂
Varicocele

456.5 Pelvic varices
Varices of broad ligament

456.6 Vulval varices   ♀
Varices of perineum
EXCLUDES *that complicating pregnancy, childbirth, or the puerperium (671.1)*

456.8 Varices of other sites
Varicose veins of nasal septum (with ulcer)
EXCLUDES *placental varices (656.7)*
     retinal varices (362.17)
     varicose ulcer of unspecified site (454.0)
     varicose veins of unspecified site (454.9)
AHA: 2Q, '02, 4

√4th 457 Noninfectious disorders of lymphatic channels

457.0 Postmastectomy lymphedema syndrome   `A`
Elephantiasis
Obliteration of lymphatic vessel } due to mastectomy
DEF: Reduced lymphatic circulation following mastectomy; symptoms include swelling of the arm on the operative side.
AHA: 2Q, '02, 12

`N` Newborn Age: 0   `P` Pediatric Age: 0-17   `M` Maternity Age: 12-55   `A` Adult Age: 15-124   `MCC` Major CC Condition   `CC` CC Condition   `HIV` HIV Related Dx

156 – Volume 1   2014 ICD-9-CM

457.1 Other lymphedema
Elephantiasis (nonfilarial) NOS
Lymphangiectasis
Lymphedema:
   acquired (chronic)
   praecox
   secondary
Obliteration, lymphatic vessel
> **EXCLUDES** *elephantiasis (nonfilarial):*
>   *congenital (757.0)*
>   *eyelid (374.83)*
>   *vulva (624.8)*

DEF: Fluid retention due to reduced lymphatic circulation; due to other than mastectomy.
AHA: 3Q, '04, 5
I89.0 Lymphedema not elsewhere classified   `I-10`

457.2 Lymphangitis
Lymphangitis:
   NOS
   chronic
   subacute
> **EXCLUDES** *acute lymphangitis (682.0-682.9)*

457.8 Other noninfectious disorders of lymphatic channels
Chylocele (nonfilarial)   Lymph node or vessel:
Chylous: fistula
   ascites   infarction
   cyst   rupture
> **EXCLUDES** *chylocele:*
>   *filarial (125.0-125.9)*
>   *tunica vaginalis (nonfilarial) (608.84)*

AHA: 1Q, '04, 5; 3Q, '03, 17

457.9 Unspecified noninfectious disorder of lymphatic channels

`✓4ᵗʰ` **458 Hypotension**
> **INCLUDES** hypopiesis
> **EXCLUDES** *cardiovascular collapse (785.50)*
>   *maternal hypotension syndrome (669.2)*
>   *shock (785.50-785.59)*
>   *Shy-Drager syndrome (333.0)*

458.0 Orthostatic hypotension
Hypotension:
   orthostatic (chronic)
   postural
DEF: Low blood pressure; occurs when standing.
AHA: 3Q, '00, 8; 3Q, '91, 9
I95.1 Orthostatic hypotension   `I-10`

458.1 Chronic hypotension
Permanent idiopathic hypotension
DEF: Persistent low blood pressure.

`✓5ᵗʰ` **458.2 Iatrogenic hypotension**
DEF: Abnormally low blood pressure; due to medical treatment.
AHA: 4Q, '03, 60; 3Q, '02, 12; 4Q, '95, 57

   458.21 Hypotension of hemodialysis
   Intra-dialytic hypotension
   AHA: 4Q, '03, 61

   458.29 Other iatrogenic hypotension
   Postoperative hypotension
   I95.81 Postprocedural hypotension   `I-10`

458.8 Other specified hypotension
AHA: 4Q, '97, 37

458.9 Hypotension, unspecified
Hypotension (arterial) NOS
I95.9 Hypotension unspecified   `I-10`

`✓4ᵗʰ` **459 Other disorders of circulatory system**

459.0 Hemorrhage, unspecified
Rupture of blood vessel NOS
Spontaneous hemorrhage NEC
> **EXCLUDES** *hemorrhage:*
>   *gastrointestinal NOS (578.9)*
>   *in newborn NOS (772.9)*
>   *secondary or recurrent following trauma (958.2)*
>   *traumatic rupture of blood vessel (900.0-904.9)*
>   *nontraumatic hematoma of soft tissue (729.92)*

AHA: 4Q, '90, 26
R58 Hemorrhage not elsewhere classified   `I-10`

`✓5ᵗʰ` **459.1 Postphlebitic syndrome**
Chronic venous hypertension due to deep vein thrombosis
> **EXCLUDES** *chronic venous hypertension without deep vein thrombosis (459.30-459.39)*

DEF: Various conditions following deep vein thrombosis; including edema, pain, stasis dermatitis, cellulitis, varicose veins and ulceration of the lower leg.
AHA: 4Q, '02, 58; 2Q, '91, 20

   459.10 Postphlebitic syndrome without complications
   Asymptomatic postphlebitic syndrome
   Postphlebitic syndrome NOS

   459.11 Postphlebitic syndrome with ulcer   `CC`
   CC Exd: 451.0-451.9

   459.12 Postphlebitic syndrome with inflammation

   459.13 Postphlebitic syndrome with ulcer and inflammation   `CC`
   CC Exd: See code: 459.11

   459.19 Postphlebitic syndrome with other complication

459.2 Compression of vein   `CC`
Stricture of vein
Vena cava syndrome (inferior) (superior)
CC Exd: 459.2

`✓5ᵗʰ` **459.3 Chronic venous hypertension (idiopathic)**
Stasis edema
> **EXCLUDES** *chronic venous hypertension due to deep vein thrombosis (459.10-459.9)*
>   *varicose veins (454.0-454.9)*

AHA: 4Q, '02, 59

   459.30 Chronic venous hypertension without complications
   Asymptomatic chronic venous hypertension
   Chronic venous hypertension NOS

   459.31 Chronic venous hypertension with ulcer   `CC`
   CC Exd: 454.0-454.2, 454.9, 459.81-459.9
   AHA: 4Q, '02, 43

   459.32 Chronic venous hypertension with inflammation

   459.33 Chronic venous hypertension with ulcer and inflammation   `CC`
   CC Exd: See code: 459.31

   459.39 Chronic venous hypertension with other complication

`✓5ᵗʰ` **459.8 Other specified disorders of circulatory system**

   459.81 Venous (peripheral) insufficiency, unspecified
   Chronic venous insufficiency NOS
   Use additional code for any associated ulceration (707.10-707.19, 707.8, 707.9)
   DEF: Insufficient drainage, venous blood, any part of body, results in edema or dermatosis.
   AHA: 3Q, '04, 5; 2Q, '91, 20; M-A, '87, 6
   TIP: Assign for stasis dermatitis without varicose veins or past DVT.
   I87.2 Venous insufficiency (chronic) (peripheral)   `I-10`

   459.89 Other
   Collateral circulation (venous), any site
   Phlebosclerosis
   Venofibrosis

459.9 Unspecified circulatory system disorder

`4ᵗʰ` `5ᵗʰ` Additional Digit Required   Unacceptable PDx   Manifestation Code   Hospital Acquired Condition   ►◄ Revised Text   ● New Code   ▲ Revised Code Title

²014 ICD-9-CM   **Volume 1 – 157**

Diseases of the Circulatory System   **457.1–459.9**

8. Diseases of the Respiratory System (460-519)

Use additional code to identify infectious organism

Acute Respiratory Infections (460-466)

> **EXCLUDES** *pneumonia and influenza (480.0-488.19)*

460 Acute nasopharyngitis [common cold]
Coryza (acute)
Nasal catarrh, acute
Nasopharyngitis:
  NOS
  acute
  infective NOS
Rhinitis:
  acute
  infective

> **EXCLUDES** *nasopharyngitis, chronic (472.2)*
>   *pharyngitis:*
>   *acute or unspecified (462)*
>   *chronic (472.1)*
>   *rhinitis:*
>   *allergic (477.0-477.9)*
>   *chronic or unspecified (472.0)*
>   *sore throat:*
>   *acute or unspecified (462)*
>   *chronic (472.1)*

DEF: Acute inflammation of mucous membranes; extends from nares to pharynx.
AHA: 1Q, '88, 12

☑4ᵗʰ 461 Acute sinusitis
> **INCLUDES** abscess   ⎫
> empyema   ⎪ acute, of sinus
> infection   ⎬ (accessory) (nasal)
> inflammation   ⎪
> suppuration   ⎭

> **EXCLUDES** *chronic or unspecified sinusitis (473.0-473.9)*

461.0 Maxillary
Acute antritis

461.1 Frontal

461.2 Ethmoidal

461.3 Sphenoidal

461.8 Other acute sinusitis
Acute pansinusitis

461.9 Acute sinusitis, unspecified
Acute sinusitis NOS
J01.90 Acute sinusitis unspecified   `I-10`

462 Acute pharyngitis
Acute sore throat NOS   Pharyngitis (acute):
Pharyngitis (acute):   staphylococcal
  NOS   suppurative
  gangrenous   ulcerative
  infective   Sore throat (viral) NOS
  phlegmonous   Viral pharyngitis
  pneumococcal

> **EXCLUDES** *abscess:*
>   *peritonsillar [quinsy] (475)*
>   *pharyngeal NOS (478.29)*
>   *retropharyngeal (478.24)*
> *chronic pharyngitis (472.1)*
> *infectious mononucleosis (075)*
> *that specified as (due to):*
>   *Coxsackie (virus) (074.0)*
>   *gonococcus (098.6)*
>   *herpes simplex (054.79)*
>   *influenza (487.1, 488.02, 488.12)*
>   *septic (034.0)*
>   *streptococcal (034.0)*

AHA: ▶2Q, '12, 18;◀ 4Q, '99, 26; S-O, '85, 8
J02.9 Acute pharyngitis unspecified   `I-10`

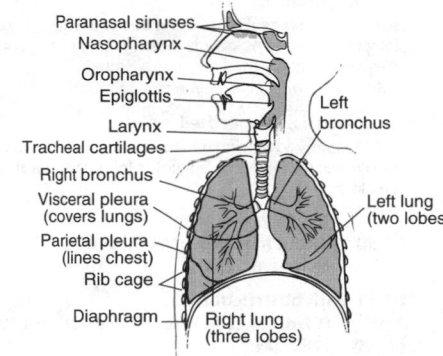

Respiratory System

Paranasal sinuses
Nasopharynx
Oropharynx
Epiglottis
Larynx
Tracheal cartilages
Right bronchus
Visceral pleura (covers lungs)
Parietal pleura (lines chest)
Rib cage
Diaphragm
Left bronchus
Left lung (two lobes)
Right lung (three lobes)

463 Acute tonsillitis
Tonsillitis (acute):   Tonsillitis (acute):
  NOS   septic
  follicular   staphylococcal
  gangrenous   suppurative
  infective   ulcerative
  pneumococcal   viral

> **EXCLUDES** *chronic tonsillitis (474.0)*
> *hypertrophy of tonsils (474.1)*
> *peritonsillar abscess [quinsy] (475)*
> *sore throat:*
>   *acute or NOS (462)*
>   *septic (034.0)*
> *streptococcal tonsillitis (034.0)*

AHA: N-D, '84, 16

☑4ᵗʰ 464 Acute laryngitis and tracheitis
> **EXCLUDES** *that associated with influenza (487.1, 488.02, 488.12)*
> *that due to Streptococcus (034.0)*

☑5ᵗʰ 464.0 Acute laryngitis
Laryngitis (acute):
  NOS
  edematous
  Hemophilus influenzae [H. influenzae]
  pneumococcal
  septic
  suppurative
  ulcerative

> **EXCLUDES** *chronic laryngitis (476.0-476.1)*
> *influenzal laryngitis (487.1, 488.02, 488.12)*

464.00 Without mention of obstruction

464.01 With obstruction   `MCC`
  CC Exd: 012.20-012.86, 464.00-464.31, 579.8-519.9

☑5ᵗʰ 464.1 Acute tracheitis
Tracheitis (acute):   Tracheitis (acute):
  NOS   viral
  catarrhal

> **EXCLUDES** *chronic tracheitis (491.8)*

464.10 Without mention of obstruction

464.11 With obstruction   `MCC`
  CC Exd: 012.20-012.86, 017.90-017.96, 464.00-464.31, 519.8-519.9

☑5ᵗʰ 464.2 Acute laryngotracheitis
Laryngotracheitis (acute)
Tracheitis (acute) with laryngitis (acute)
> **EXCLUDES** *chronic laryngotracheitis (476.1)*

464.20 Without mention of obstruction

464.21 With obstruction   `MCC`
  CC Exd: See code 464.11

☑5ᵗʰ 464.3 Acute epiglottitis
Viral epiglottitis
> **EXCLUDES** *epiglottitis, chronic (476.1)*

464.30 Without mention of obstruction   `CC`
  CC Exd: 464.01, 464.30-464.31, 464.51

464.31 With obstruction   `MCC`
  CC Exd: See code 464.11

4ᵗʰ 5ᵗʰ Additional Digit Required   Unacceptable PDx   Manifestation Code   Hospital Acquired Condition   ▶◀ Revised Text   ● New Code   ▲ Revised Code Title

014 ICD-9-CM   **February 2013 · Volume 1 – 159**

Diseases of the Respiratory System

464.4–472.2

464.4 Croup
Croup syndrome
DEF: Acute laryngeal obstruction due to allergy, foreign body or infection; symptoms include barking cough, hoarseness and harsh, persistent high-pitched respiratory sound.
J05.0 Acute obstructive laryngitis [croup]   I-10

√5th **464.5 Supraglottitis, unspecified**
DEF: A rapidly advancing generalized upper respiratory infection of the lingual tonsillar area, epiglottic folds, false vocal cords, and the epiglottis.
AHA: 4Q, '01, 42

     464.50 Without mention of obstruction
     AHA: 4Q, '01, 43

     464.51 With obstruction   MCC
     CC Excl: 012.20-012.86, 017.90-017.96, 464.00-464.31, 519.8-519.9

√4th **465 Acute upper respiratory infections of multiple or unspecified sites**
     EXCLUDES   upper respiratory infection due to:
         influenza (487.1, 488.02, 488.12)
         Streptococcus (034.0)

465.0 Acute laryngopharyngitis
DEF: Acute infection of the vocal cords and pharynx.

465.8 Other multiple sites
Multiple URI
AHA: 4Q, '07, 85

465.9 Unspecified site
Acute URI NOS
Upper respiratory infection (acute)
J06.9 Acute upper respiratory infection unspecified   I-10

√4th **466 Acute bronchitis and bronchiolitis**
     INCLUDES   that with:
         bronchospasm
         obstruction

466.0 Acute bronchitis
Bronchitis, acute or subacute:
   fibrinous
   membranous
   pneumococcal
   purulent
   septic
   viral
   with tracheitis
Croupous bronchitis
Tracheobronchitis, acute
     EXCLUDES   acute bronchitis with chronic obstructive pulmonary disease (491.22)
DEF: Acute inflammation of main branches of bronchial tree due to infectious or irritant agents; symptoms include cough with a varied production of sputum, fever, substernal soreness, and lung rales.
AHA: 4Q, '04, 137; 1Q, '04, 3; 4Q, '02, 46; 4Q, '96, 28; 4Q, '91, 24; 1Q, '88, 12
TIP: If documented with COPD, assign only 491.22 Obstructive chronic bronchitis with acute bronchitis.
J20.9 Acute bronchitis unspecified   I-10

√5th **466.1 Acute bronchiolitis**
Bronchiolitis (acute)   Capillary pneumonia
     EXCLUDES   respiratory bronchiolitis interstitial lung disease (516.34)
DEF: Acute inflammation of the smallest branches of bronchial tree due to infectious or irritant agents; symptoms include cough, tachycardia, labored breathing, and lung crackles.

     466.11 Acute bronchiolitis due to respiratory syncytial   CC
     virus (RSV)
     CC Excl: 466.11
     AHA: 1Q, '05, 10; 4Q, '96, 27
     J21.0 Acute bronchiolitis d/t resp syncytial virus   I-10

     466.19 Acute bronchiolitis due to other infectious   CC
     organisms
     Use additional code to identify organism
     CC Excl: 466.0-466.19
     J21.8 Acute bronchiolitis d/t oth specified organisms   I-10

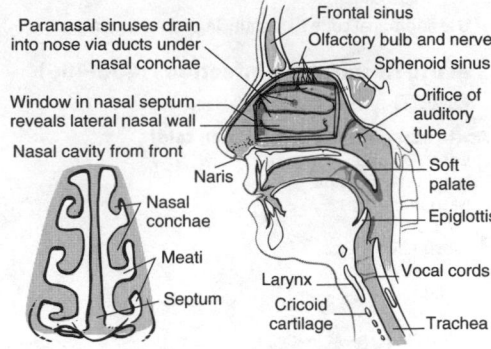

Upper Respiratory System

Paranasal sinuses drain into nose via ducts under nasal conchae
Window in nasal septum reveals lateral nasal wall
Nasal cavity from front
Frontal sinus
Olfactory bulb and nerves
Sphenoid sinus
Orifice of auditory tube
Naris
Nasal conchae
Meati
Septum
Soft palate
Epiglottis
Vocal cords
Larynx
Cricoid cartilage
Trachea

Other Diseases of the Upper Respiratory Tract (470-478)

470 Deviated nasal septum
Deflected septum (nasal) (acquired)
     EXCLUDES   congenital (754.0)

√4th **471 Nasal polyps**
     EXCLUDES   adenomatous polyps (212.0)

471.0 Polyp of nasal cavity
Polyp:
   choanal
   nasopharyngeal

471.1 Polypoid sinus degeneration
Woakes' syndrome or ethmoiditis

471.8 Other polyp of sinus
Polyp of sinus:
   accessory
   ethmoidal
   maxillary
   sphenoidal

471.9 Unspecified nasal polyp
Nasal polyp NOS

√4th **472 Chronic pharyngitis and nasopharyngitis**
472.0 Chronic rhinitis
Ozena   Rhinitis:
Rhinitis: hypertrophic
   NOS   obstructive
   atrophic   purulent
   granulomatous   ulcerative
     EXCLUDES   allergic rhinitis (477.0-477.9)
DEF: Persistent inflammation of mucous membranes of nose.

472.1 Chronic pharyngitis
Chronic sore throat   Pharyngitis:
Pharyngitis: granular (chronic)
   atrophic   hypertrophic

472.2 Chronic nasopharyngitis
     EXCLUDES   acute or unspecified nasopharyngitis (460)
DEF: Persistent inflammation of mucous membranes extending from nares to pharynx.

Paranasal Sinuses

Frontal
Ethmoid
Sphenoid
Maxillary
Frontal
Ethmoid
Sphenoid
Maxillary

✓4ᵗʰ **473 Chronic sinusitis**

INCLUDES abscess
empyema   (chronic) of sinus (accessory)
infection   (nasal)
suppuration

EXCLUDES *acute sinusitis (461.0-461.9)*

473.0 Maxillary
Antritis (chronic)
J32.0 Chronic maxillary sinusitis   I-10

473.1 Frontal

473.2 Ethmoidal
EXCLUDES *Woakes' ethmoiditis (471.1)*

473.3 Sphenoidal

473.8 Other chronic sinusitis
Pansinusitis (chronic)

473.9 Unspecified sinusitis (chronic)
Sinusitis (chronic) NOS
J32.9 Chronic sinusitis unspecified   I-10

✓4ᵗʰ **474 Chronic disease of tonsils and adenoids**

✓5ᵗʰ **474.0 Chronic tonsillitis and adenoiditis**
EXCLUDES *acute or unspecified tonsillitis (463)*
AHA: 4Q, '97, 38

474.00 Chronic tonsillitis

474.01 Chronic adenoiditis

474.02 Chronic tonsillitis and adenoiditis

✓5ᵗʰ **474.1 Hypertrophy of tonsils and adenoids**
Enlargement
Hyperplasia   } of tonsils or adenoids
Hypertrophy

EXCLUDES *that with:*
adenoiditis (474.01)
adenoiditis and tonsillitis (474.02)
tonsillitis (474.00)

474.10 Tonsils with adenoids
AHA: 2Q, '05, 16

474.11 Tonsils alone

474.12 Adenoids alone

474.2 Adenoid vegetations
DEF: Fungus-like growth of lymph tissue between the nares and pharynx.

474.8 Other chronic disease of tonsils and adenoids
Amygdalolith   Tonsillar tag
Calculus, tonsil   Ulcer, tonsil
Cicatrix of tonsil (and adenoid)

474.9 Unspecified chronic disease of tonsils and adenoids
Disease (chronic) of tonsils (and adenoids)

475 Peritonsillar abscess   CC
Abscess of tonsil   Quinsy
Peritonsillar cellulitis

EXCLUDES *tonsillitis:*
acute or NOS (463)
chronic (474.0)
CC Exd: 475, 519.8-519.9
J36 Peritonsillar abscess   I-10

✓4ᵗʰ **476 Chronic laryngitis and laryngotracheitis**

476.0 Chronic laryngitis
Laryngitis:
catarrhal
hypertrophic
sicca

476.1 Chronic laryngotracheitis
Laryngitis, chronic, with tracheitis (chronic)
Tracheitis, chronic, with laryngitis
EXCLUDES *chronic tracheitis (491.8)*
laryngitis and tracheitis, acute or unspecified (464.00-464.51)

✓4ᵗʰ **477 Allergic rhinitis**

INCLUDES allergic rhinitis (nonseasonal) (seasonal)
hay fever
spasmodic rhinorrhea

EXCLUDES *allergic rhinitis with asthma (bronchial) (493.0)*
DEF: True immunoglobulin E (IgE)-mediated allergic reaction of nasal mucosa; seasonal (typical hay fever) or perennial (year-round allergens; dust, food, dander).

477.0 Due to pollen
Pollinosis

477.1 Due to food
AHA: 4Q, '00, 42

477.2 Due to animal (cat) (dog) hair and dander

477.8 Due to other allergen

477.9 Cause unspecified
AHA: 2Q, '97, 9
J30.9 Allergic rhinitis unspecified   I-10

✓4ᵗʰ **478 Other diseases of upper respiratory tract**

478.0 Hypertrophy of nasal turbinates
DEF: Overgrowth, enlargement of shell-shaped bones in nasal cavity.

✓5ᵗʰ **478.1 Other diseases of nasal cavity and sinuses**
EXCLUDES *varicose ulcer of nasal septum (456.8)*

478.11 Nasal mucositis (ulcerative)
Use additional E code to identify adverse effects of therapy, such as:
antineoplastic and immunosuppressive drugs (E930.7, E933.1)
radiation therapy (E879.2)
AHA: 4Q, '06, 88-90

478.19 Other diseases of nasal cavity and sinuses
Abscess
Necrosis } of nose (septum)
Ulcer

Cyst or mucocele of sinus (nasal)
Rhinolith
AHA: 4Q, '06, 88-90
J34.1 Cyst and mucocele of nose and nasal sinus   I-10

✓5ᵗʰ **478.2 Other diseases of pharynx, not elsewhere classified**

478.20 Unspecified disease of pharynx

478.21 Cellulitis of pharynx or nasopharynx   CC
CC Exd: 478.20-478.24, 519.8-519.9

478.22 Parapharyngeal abscess   CC
CC Exd: See code: 478.21

478.24 Retropharyngeal abscess   CC
DEF: Purulent infection, behind pharynx and front of precerebral fascia.
CC Exd: See code 478.21

478.25 Edema of pharynx or nasopharynx

478.26 Cyst of pharynx or nasopharynx

478.29 Other
Abscess of pharynx or nasopharynx
EXCLUDES *ulcerative pharyngitis (462)*

✓5ᵗʰ **478.3 Paralysis of vocal cords or larynx**
DEF: Loss of motor ability of vocal cords or larynx; due to nerve or muscle damage.

478.30 Paralysis, unspecified
Laryngoplegia Paralysis of glottis

478.31 Unilateral, partial

478.32 Unilateral, complete

478.33 Bilateral, partial

478.34 Bilateral, complete   CC
CC Exd: 478.30-478.34, 478.5, 478.70, 519.8-519.9

478.4 Polyp of vocal cord or larynx
EXCLUDES *adenomatous polyps (212.1)*

4ᵗʰ/5ᵗʰ Additional Digit Required   Unacceptable PDx   Manifestation Code   Hospital Acquired Condition   ►◄ Revised Text   ● New Code   ▲ Revised Code Title

2014 ICD-9-CM   **Volume 1 – 161**

Diseases of the Respiratory System *(side tab)*

478.5   Other diseases of vocal cords

Abscess
Cellulitis
Granuloma   } of vocal cords
Leukoplakia

Chorditis (fibrinous) (nodosa) (tuberosa)
Singers' nodes

478.6   Edema of larynx

Edema (of):   Edema (of):
   glottis   supraglottic
   subglottic

√5ᵗʰ **478.7   Other diseases of larynx, not elsewhere classified**

478.70   Unspecified disease of larynx

478.71   Cellulitis and perichondritis of larynx `CC`

DEF: Inflammation of deep soft tissues or lining of bone of the larynx.
CC Excl: 478.70-478.71, 478.79

478.74   Stenosis of larynx

478.75   Laryngeal spasm

Laryngismus (stridulus)
DEF: Involuntary muscle contraction of the larynx.

478.79   Other

Abscess
Necrosis
Obstruction   } of larynx
Pachyderma
Ulcer

EXCLUDES   *ulcerative laryngitis (464.00-464.01)*
AHA: 3Q, '91, 20

478.8   Upper respiratory tract hypersensitivity reaction, site unspecified

EXCLUDES   *hypersensitivity reaction of lower respiratory tract, as:*
     extrinsic allergic alveolitis (495.0-495.9)
     pneumoconiosis (500-505)

478.9   Other and unspecified diseases of upper respiratory tract

Abscess
Cicatrix   } of trachea

Pneumonia and Influenza (480-488)

EXCLUDES   *pneumonia:*
     allergic or eosinophilic (518.3)
     aspiration:
        NOS (507.0)
        newborn (770.18)
        solids and liquids (507.0-507.8)
     congenital (770.0)
     lipoid (507.1)
     passive (514)
     rheumatic (390)
     ventilator-associated (997.31)

√4ᵗʰ **480   Viral pneumonia**

480.0   Pneumonia due to adenovirus `MCC`

CC Excl: 011.00-012.16, 012.80-012.86, 017.90-017.96, 020.3-020.5, 021.3, 022.1, 031.0, 039.1, 073.0, 115.05, 115.15, 115.95, 122.1, 130.4, 136.3, 480.0-487.1, 488.01-488.02, 488.11-488.12, 495.0-495.9, 500-508.9, 517.1, 517.8, 518.89, 519.8-519.9

480.1   Pneumonia due to respiratory syncytial virus `MCC`

CC Excl: See code: 480.0
AHA: 4Q, '10, 98; 4Q, '96, 28; 1Q, '88, 12

480.2   Pneumonia due to parainfluenza virus `MCC`

CC Excl: See code: 480.0

480.3   Pneumonia due to SARS-associated coronavirus `MCC` `HIV`

DEF: A severe adult respiratory syndrome caused by the coronavirus, specified as inflammation of the lungs with consolidation.
CC Excl: 011.00-012.16, 012.80-012.86, 017.90-017.96, 021.2, 031.0, 039.1, 115.05, 115.15, 115.95, 122.1, 130.4, 136.3, 480.0-487.1, 488.01-488.02, 488.11-488.12, 494.0-508.9, 517.1, 517.8, 518.89, 519.8-519.9, 748.61
AHA: 4Q, '03, 46-47

Lungs

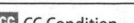

Right Lung (Three Lobes)   Trachea   **Left Lung (Two Lobes)**
Bronchopulmonary segments: Primary bronchus   Secondary bronchus
Upper lobe   S1   S3   S1,2   Upper lobe
S2   S3   S4   S5
Middle lobe   S5   S6
S4   S7,8
Lower lobe   S8   Lower lobe   S9
Diaphragm   S9   S10   S7   S10

480.8   Pneumonia due to other virus not elsewhere classified `MCC` `HIV`

EXCLUDES   *congenital rubella pneumonitis (771.0)*
     pneumonia complicating viral diseases classified elsewhere (484.1-484.8)
CC Excl: See code: 480.0

480.9   Viral pneumonia, unspecified `MCC` `HIV`

CC Excl: See code: 480.0
AHA: 3Q, '98, 5

481   Pneumococcal pneumonia [Streptococcus pneumoniae pneumonia] `MCC` `HIV`

Lobar pneumonia, organism unspecified
CC Excl: 011.00-012.16, 012.80-012.86, 017.90-017.96, 021.2, 031.0, 039.1, 115.05, 115.15, 115.95, 122.1, 130.4, 136.3, 480.0-480.2, 480.8-487.1, 488.01-488.02, 488.11-488.12, 494.0-508.9, 517.1, 517.8, 518.89, 519.8-519.9, 748.61
AHA: 2Q, '98, 7; 4Q, '92, 19; 1Q, '92, 18; 1Q, '91, 13; 1Q, '88, 13; M-A, '85, 6

√4ᵗʰ **482   Other bacterial pneumonia**

AHA: 4Q, '93, 39

482.0   Pneumonia due to Klebsiella pneumoniae `MCC` `HIV`

CC Excl: See code 481

482.1   Pneumonia due to Pseudomonas `MCC` `HIV`

CC Excl: See code 481

482.2   Pneumonia due to Hemophilus influenzae [H. influenzae] `MCC` `HIV`

CC Excl: See code 481
AHA: 2Q, '05, 19

√5ᵗʰ **482.3   Pneumonia due to Streptococcus**

EXCLUDES   *Streptococcus pneumoniae (481)*
AHA: 1Q, '88, 13

482.30   Streptococcus, unspecified `MCC` `HIV`

CC Excl: See code 481

482.31   Group A `MCC` `HIV`

CC Excl: See code 481

482.32   Group B `MCC` `HIV`

CC Excl: See code 481

482.39   Other Streptococcus `MCC` `HIV`

CC Excl: See code 481

√5ᵗʰ **482.4   Pneumonia due to Staphylococcus**

AHA: 3Q, '91, 16

482.40   Pneumonia due to Staphylococcus, unspecified `MCC` `HIV`

CC Excl: See code 481

482.41   Methicillin susceptible pneumonia due to Staphylococcus aureus `MCC` `HIV`

Staphylococcus aureus
MSSA pneumonia
Pneumonia due to Staphylococcus aureus NOS
CC Excl: See code 481
J15.211 Pneumonia d/t methicillin suscep staph `I-10`

482.42   Methicillin resistant pneumonia due to Staphylococcus aureus `MCC` `HIV`

CC Excl: See code 481
AHA: 4Q, '08, 69, 71, 72

482.49   Other Staphylococcus pneumonia `MCC` `HIV`

CC Excl: See code 481

`N` Newborn Age: 0   `P` Pediatric Age: 0-17   `M` Maternity Age: 12-55   `A` Adult Age: 15-124   `MCC` Major CC Condition   `CC` CC Condition   `HIV` HIV Related Dx

162 – Volume 1   2014 ICD-9-CM

√5ᵗʰ **482.8 Pneumonia due to other specified bacteria**

EXCLUDES pneumonia, complicating infectious disease classified elsewhere (484.1-484.8)

AHA: 3Q, '88, 11

482.81 Anaerobes MCC HIV

Bacteroides (melaninogenicus)
Gram-negative anaerobes

CC Exd: See code 481

482.82 Escherichia coli [E. coli] MCC HIV

CC Exd: See code 481

482.83 Other gram-negative bacteria MCC HIV

Gram-negative pneumonia   Proteus
   NOS   Serratia marcescens

EXCLUDES gram-negative anaerobes (482.81)
Legionnaires' disease (482.84)

CC Exd: See code 481

AHA: 2Q, '98, 5; 3Q, '94, 9

TIP: Do not assign based solely on laboratory findings of gram-negative bacteria on gram-stain. Physician substantiation is required.

J15.6 Pneumonia d/t oth aerobic Gram-negative bacteria   I-10

482.84 Legionnaires' disease MCC HIV

DEF: Severe and often fatal infection by Legionella pneumophilia; symptoms include high fever, gastrointestinal pain, headache, myalgia, dry cough, and pneumonia; usually transmitted airborne via air conditioning systems.

CC Exd: See code 481

AHA: 4Q, '97, 38

482.89 Other specified bacteria MCC HIV

CC Exd: See code 481

AHA: 2Q, '97, 6

TIP: Do not assign based on documentation of "mixed bacterial pneumonia" or "gram-positive pneumonia." See instead 482.9.

482.9 Bacterial pneumonia unspecified MCC HIV

CC Exd: See code 481

AHA: 2Q, '98, 6; 2Q, '97, 6; 1Q, '94, 17

J15.9 Unspecified bacterial pneumonia   I-10

√4ᵗʰ **483 Pneumonia due to other specified organism**

AHA: N-D, '87, 5

TIP: Do not assign if pneumonia due to candidiasis; see instead code 112.4.

483.0 Mycoplasma pneumoniae MCC

Eaton's agent   Pleuropneumonia-like organism [PPLO]

CC Exd: See code 481

483.1 Chlamydia MCC

CC Exd: See code 481

AHA: 4Q, '96, 31

483.8 Other specified organism MCC

CC Exd: See code 481

√4ᵗʰ **484 Pneumonia in infectious diseases classified elsewhere**

484.1 Pneumonia in cytomegalic inclusion disease MCC

Code first underlying disease (078.5)

CC Exd: See code 481

484.3 Pneumonia in whooping cough MCC

Code first underlying disease (033.0-033.9)

CC Exd: See code 481

484.5 Pneumonia in anthrax MCC

Code first underlying disease (022.1)

CC Exd: See code 481

484.6 Pneumonia in aspergillosis MCC

Code first underlying disease (117.3)

CC Exd: See code 481

AHA: 4Q, '97, 40

484.7 Pneumonia in other systemic mycoses MCC

Code first underlying disease

EXCLUDES pneumonia in:
candidiasis (112.4)
coccidioidomycosis (114.0)
histoplasmosis (115.0-115.9 with fifth-digit 5)

CC Exd: See code 481

484.8 Pneumonia in other infectious diseases classified elsewhere MCC

Code first underlying disease, as:
Q fever (083.0)
typhoid fever (002.0)

EXCLUDES pneumonia in:
actinomycosis (039.1)
measles (055.1)
nocardiosis (039.1)
ornithosis (073.0)
Pneumocystis carinii (136.3)
salmonellosis (003.22)
toxoplasmosis (130.4)
tuberculosis (011.6)
tularemia (021.2)
varicella (052.1)

CC Exd: See code 481

485 Bronchopneumonia, organism unspecified MCC

Bronchopneumonia: Pneumonia:
  hemorrhagic   lobular
  terminal   segmental
Pleurobronchopneumonia

EXCLUDES bronchiolitis (acute) (466.11-466.19)
chronic (491.8)
lipoid pneumonia (507.1)

CC Exd: See code 481

486 Pneumonia, organism unspecified MCC HIV

EXCLUDES hypostatic or passive pneumonia (514)
inhalation or aspiration pneumonia due to foreign materials (507.0-507.8)
pneumonitis due to fumes and vapors (506.0)

CC Exd: 011.00-012.16, 012.80-012.86, 017.90-017.96, 021.2, 031.0, 039.1, 115.05, 115.15, 115.95, 122.1, 130.4, 136.3, 480.0-480.2, 480.8-487.1, 488, 494.0-508.9, 517.1, 517.8, 518.89, 519.8-519.9, 748.61

AHA: 4Q, '10, 135; 1Q, '10, 3, 12; 3Q, '09, 16; 4Q, '08, 142; 4Q, '99, 6; 3Q, '99, 9; 3Q, '98, 7; 2Q, '98, 4, 5; 1Q, '98, 8; 3Q, '97, 9; 3Q, '94, 10; 3Q, '88, 11

TIP: Never assume a causal organism based on laboratory or radiology findings alone.

J18.9 Pneumonia unspecified organism   I-10

√4ᵗʰ **487 Influenza**

Influenza caused by unspecified influenza virus

EXCLUDES Hemophilus influenzae [H. influenzae]:
infection NOS (041.5)
influenza due to identified avian influenza virus (488.01-488.09)
influenza due to 2009 H1N1 [swine] influenza virus (488.11-488.19)
influenza due to identified (novel) 2009 H1N1 influenza virus (488.11-488.19)
laryngitis (464.00-464.01)
meningitis (320.0)

487.0 With pneumonia MCC

Influenza with pneumonia,   Influenzal:
  any form   pneumonia
                         bronchopneumonia

Use additional code to identify the type of pneumonia (480.0-480.9, 481, 482.0-482.9, 483.0-483.8, 485)

CC Exd: See code 486

AHA: 1Q, '06, 18; 2Q, '05, 18

TIP: Selection of the principal diagnosis will be dependent on the circumstances of admission.

487.1 With other respiratory manifestations

Influenza NEC   Influenzal:
Influenza NOS   pharyngitis
Influenzal: respiratory infection (upper) (acute)
  laryngitis

AHA: 4Q, '11, 114; 1Q, '10, 4; 1Q, '06, 18; 2Q, '05, 18; 4Q, '99, 26

J10.1 Influenza d/t oth influenza virus w/resp manifestations   I-10

487.8 With other manifestations

Encephalopathy due to influenza
Influenza with involvement of gastrointestinal tract

EXCLUDES "intestinal flu" [viral gastroenteritis] (008.8)

◢◣ Additional Digit Required   Unacceptable PDx   Manifestation Code   Hospital Acquired Condition   ►◄ Revised Text   ● New Code   ▲ Revised Code Title

2014 ICD-9-CM   Volume 1 – 163

√4ᵗʰ **488   Influenza due to certain identified influenza viruses**

EXCLUDES *influenza caused by unspecified or seasonal influenza viruses (487.0-487.8)*

AHA: 4Q, '09, 92-93

TIP: Do not assign a code from this category unless the specified influenza virus is confirmed.

√5ᵗʰ **488.0   Influenza due to identified avian influenza virus**

Avian influenza   Influenza A/H5N1
Bird flu

DEF: Infection caused by contact with bird influenza viruses; results in flu-like symptoms that may progress to other severe and life-threatening complications.

AHA: 4Q, '10, 85-87; 4Q, '07, 87

488.01   Influenza due to identified avian influenza MCC HIV
virus with pneumonia

Avian influenzal:
    bronchopneumonia
    pneumonia
Influenza due to identified avian influenza virus with pneumonia, any form

Use additional code to identify the type of pneumonia (480.0- 480.9, 481, 482.0-482.9, 483.0-483.8, 485)

CC Excl: 011.00-012.16, 012.80-012.86, 017.90-017.96, 021.2, 031.0, 039.1, 115.05, 115.15, 115.95, 122.1, 130.4, 136.3, 480.0-480.2, 480.8-487.1, 488.01-488.19, 491.21-491.22, 493.01-493.02, 493.11-493.12, 493.21-493.22, 493.91-508.9, 517.1, 517.8, 518.89, 519.8-519.9, 748.61

J09.X1 Influenza d/t ident novel influenza A virus   I-10
w/pneumonia

488.02   Influenza due to identified avian influenza virus CC
with other respiratory manifestations

Avian influenzal:
    laryngitis
    pharyngitis
    respiratory infection (acute) (upper)
Identified avian influenza NOS

CC Excl: 488.01-488.19, 491.21-491.22, 493.01-493.02, 493.11-493.12, 493.21-493.22, 493.91-493.92, 494.1

J09.X2 Flu d/t ident novel influenza A virus   I-10
w/oth resp manifest

488.09   Influenza due to identified avian influenza virus CC
virus with other manifestations

Avian influenza with involvement of gastrointestinal tract
Encephalopathy due to identified avian influenza

EXCLUDES *"intestinal flu" [viral gastroenteritis] (008.8)*

CC Excl: 488.01-488.19, 491.21-491.22, 493.01-493.02, 493.11-493.12, 493.21-493.22, 493.91-493.92, 494.1

√5ᵗʰ **488.1   Influenza due to identified 2009 H1N1 influenza virus**

2009 H1N1 swine influenza virus
(Novel) 2009 influenza H1N1
Novel H1N1 influenza
Novel influenza A/H1N1

EXCLUDES *bird influenza virus infection (488.01-488.09)*
influenza A/H5N1 (488.01-488.09)
other human infection with influenza virus of animal origin (488.81-488.89)
swine influenza virus infection (488.81-488.89)

AHA: 4Q, '11, 110-112, 114; 4Q, '10, 85-87; 1Q, '10, 3-4

488.11   Influenza due to identified 2009 H1N1   MCC
influenza virus with pneumonia

Influenza due to identified (novel) 2009 H1N1 with pneumonia, any form
(Novel) 2009 H1N1 influenzal:
    bronchopneumonia
    pneumonia

Use additional code to identify the type of pneumonia (480.0- 480.9, 481, 482.0-482.9, 483.0-483.8, 485)

CC Excl: 011.00-012.16, 012.80-012.86, 017.90-017.96, 021.2, 031.0, 039.1, 115.05, 115.15, 115.95, 122.1, 130.4, 136.3, 480.0-480.2, 480.8-487.1, 488.01-488.19, 491.21-491.22, 493.01-493.02, 493.11-493.12, 493.21-493.22, 493.91-508.9, 517.1, 517.8, 518.89, 519.8-519.9, 748.61

J10.08 Influenza d/t oth ident influenza virus   I-10
w/oth pneumonia

488.12   Influenza due to identified 2009 H1N1 influenza
virus with other respiratory manifestations

(Novel) 2009 H1N1 influenza NOS
(Novel) 2009 H1N1 influenzal:
    laryngitis
    pharyngitis
    respiratory infection (acute) (upper)

J10.1 Flu d/t oth ident influenza virus w/oth   I-10
resp manifest

488.19   Influenza due to identified 2009 H1N1 influenza
virus with other manifestations

Encephalopathy due to identified (novel) 2009 H1N1 influenza
(Novel) 2009 H1N1 influenza with involvement of gastrointestinal tract

EXCLUDES *"intestinal flu" [viral gastroenteritis] (008.8)*

√5ᵗʰ **488.8   Influenza due to novel influenza A**

Influenza due to animal origin influenza virus
Infection with influenza viruses occurring in pigs or other animals
Other novel influenza A viruses not previously found in humans

EXCLUDES *bird influenza virus infection (488.01-488.09)*
influenza A/H5N1 (488.01-488.09)
influenza due to identified 2009 H1N1 influenza virus (488.11- 488.19)

AHA: 4Q, '11, 110-114

488.81   Influenza due to identified novel influenza A   MCC
virus with pneumonia

Influenza due to animal origin influenza virus with pneumonia, any form
Novel influenza A:
    bronchopneumonia
    pneumonia

Use additional code to identify the type of pneumonia (480.0-480.9, 481, 482.0-482.9, 483.0-483.8, 485)

CC Excl: 011.00-012.16, 012.80-012.86, 017.90-017.96, 021.2, 031.0, 039.1, 115.05, 115.15, 115.95, 122.1, 130.4, 136.3, 480.0-480.2, 480.8-487.1, 488.01-488.02, 488.11-488.12, 488.81-488.82, 494.0-508.1, 508.8-508.9, 517.1, 517.8, 518.89, 519.8-519.9, 748.61, 793.11

488.82   Influenza due to identified novel influenza A virus
with other respiratory manifestations

Influenza due to animal origin influenza A virus with other respiratory manifestations
Novel influenza A:
    laryngitis
    pharyngitis
    respiratory infection (acute) (upper)

488.89   Influenza due to identified novel influenza A virus
with other manifestations

Encephalopathy due to novel influenza A
Influenza due to animal origin influenza virus with encephalopathy
Influenza due to animal origin influenza virus with involvement of gastrointestinal tract
Novel influenza A with involvement of gastrointestinal tract

EXCLUDES *"intestinal flu" [viral gastroenteritis] (008.8)*

Bronchioli and Alveoli

To trachea
Terminal bronchiolus
Elastic fibers
Pulmonary arteriole
Capillary network over all alveoli
Alveoli
Alveolus

N Newborn Age: 0   P Pediatric Age: 0-17   M Maternity Age: 12-55   A Adult Age: 15-124   MCC Major CC Condition   CC CC Condition   HIV HIV Related D.

164 – Volume 1   **2014 ICD-9-CM**

Diseases of the Respiratory System

Interrelationship Between Chronic Airway Obstruction, Chronic Bronchitis, and Emphysema

Chronic Airway Obstruction (COPD, NOS) 496

Chronic Bronchitis 491

Emphysema 492

Shaded area: Obstructive Chronic Bronchitis (Chronic Bronchitis with COPD) 491.20-491.21

Chronic Obstructive Pulmonary Disease and Allied Conditions (490-496)

AHA: 3Q, '88, 5

TIP: Due to the overlapping nature of conditions that make up COPD, it's essential that the coder review all instructional notes carefully.

490 Bronchitis, not specified as acute or chronic

Bronchitis NOS: Tracheobronchitis NOS
   catarrhal
   with tracheitis NOS

EXCLUDES bronchitis:
    allergic NOS (493.9)
    asthmatic NOS (493.9)
    due to fumes and vapors (506.0)

J40 Bronchitis not specified as acute or chronic   `I-10`

√4ᵗʰ 491 Chronic bronchitis

EXCLUDES chronic obstructive asthma (493.2)

491.0 Simple chronic bronchitis

Catarrhal bronchitis, chronic
Smokers' cough

J41.0 Simple chronic bronchitis   `I-10`

491.1 Mucopurulent chronic bronchitis

Bronchitis (chronic) (recurrent):
   fetid
   mucopurulent
   purulent

DEF: Chronic bronchial infection characterized by both mucus and pus secretions in the bronchial tree; recurs after asymptomatic periods; signs are coughing, expectoration and secondary changes in the lung.

AHA: 3Q, '88, 12

√5ᵗʰ 491.2 Obstructive chronic bronchitis

Bronchitis: Bronchitis with:
  emphysematous   chronic airway obstruction
  obstructive (chronic)   emphysema
   (diffuse)

EXCLUDES asthmatic bronchitis (acute) NOS (493.9)
    chronic obstructive asthma (493.2)

AHA: 3Q, '97, 9; 4Q, '91, 25; 2Q, '91, 21

491.20 Without exacerbation

Emphysema with chronic bronchitis

AHA: 3Q, '97, 9

J44.9 Chronic obst pulmonary disease, unspecified   `I-10`

491.21 With (acute) exacerbation   `CC`

Acute exacerbation of chronic obstructive pulmonary disease [COPD]
Decompensated chronic obstructive pulmonary disease [COPD]
Decompensated chronic obstructive pulmonary disease [COPD] with exacerbation

EXCLUDES chronic obstructive asthma with acute exacerbation (493.22)

CC Exd: 488.01-488.11, 491.1-491.9, 493.20-493.21

AHA: 1Q, '10, 12; 1Q, '04, 3; 3Q, '02, 18, 19; 4Q, '01, 43; 2Q, '96, 10

J44.1 Chronic obst pulmonary disease with exacerbation   `I-10`

491.22 With acute bronchitis   `CC`

CC Exd: See code 491.21

AHA: 3Q, '06, 20; 4Q, '04, 82

J44.0 Chronic obst pulm dz acute lower respiratory inf   `I-10`

491.8 Other chronic bronchitis

Chronic: Chronic:
  tracheitis   tracheobronchitis

491.9 Unspecified chronic bronchitis

J42 Unspecified chronic bronchitis   `I-10`

√4ᵗʰ 492 Emphysema

AHA: 2Q, '91, 21

492.0 Emphysematous bleb

Giant bullous emphysema   Tension pneumatocele
Ruptured emphysematous bleb   Vanishing lung

DEF: Formation of vesicle or bulla in emphysematous lung, more than one millimeter; contains serum or blood.

AHA: 2Q, '93, 3

492.8 Other emphysema

Emphysema (lung or pulmonary):   MacLeod's syndrome
  NOS   Swyer-James syndrome
  centriacinar   Unilateral hyperlucent
  centrilobular   lung
  obstructive
  panacinar
  panlobular
  unilateral
  vesicular

EXCLUDES emphysema:
    with chronic bronchitis (491.20-491.22)
    compensatory (518.2)
    due to fumes and vapors (506.4)
    interstitial (518.1)
      newborn (770.2)
    mediastinal (518.1)
    surgical (subcutaneous) (998.81)
    traumatic (958.7)

AHA: 4Q, '08, 175; 1Q, '05, 4; 4Q, '93, 41; J-A, '84, 17

J43.9 Emphysema unspecified   `I-10`

√4ᵗʰ 493 Asthma

EXCLUDES wheezing NOS (786.07)

The following fifth-digit subclassification is for use with codes 493.0-493.2, 493.9:
  0 unspecified
  1 with status asthmaticus
  2 with (acute) exacerbation

DEF: Status asthmaticus: severe, intractable episode of asthma unresponsive to normal therapeutic measures.

AHA: 4Q, '04, 137; 4Q, '03, 62; 4Q, '01, 43; 4Q, '00, 42; 1Q, '91, 13; 3Q, '88, 9; J-A, '85, 8; N-D, '84, 17

TIP: If documentation indicates both exacerbation and status asthmaticus, assign only the code for status asthmaticus.

§ √5ᵗʰ 493.0 Extrinsic asthma   `CC 1-2`

[0-2]   Asthma: Asthma:
      allergic with stated cause   hay
      atopic   platinum
      childhood   Hay fever with asthma

EXCLUDES asthma:
    allergic NOS (493.9)
    detergent (507.8)
    miners' (500)
    wood (495.8)

DEF: Transient stricture of airway diameters of bronchi; due to environmental factor; also called allergic (bronchial) asthma.

CC Exd: For code 493.01 and 493.02: 488.01-488.11, 493.00-493.92, 517.8, 518.89, 519.8-519.9

J45.20 Mild intermittent asthma uncomplicated   `I-10`

§ √5ᵗʰ 493.1 Intrinsic asthma   `CC 1-2`

[0-2]   Late-onset asthma

DEF: Transient stricture of airway diameters of bronchi; due to pathophysiological disturbances.

CC Exd: For code 493.11 and 493.12: See code 493.01

AHA: 3Q, '88, 9; M-A, '85, 7

---

§ Requires fifth digit. Valid digits are in [brackets] under each code. See category 493 for codes and definitions.

√4ᵗʰ/√5ᵗʰ Additional Digit Required   Unacceptable PDx   Manifestation Code   Hospital Acquired Condition   ►◄ Revised Text   ● New Code   ▲ Revised Code Title

2014 ICD-9-CM   **Volume 1 – 165**

Diseases of the Respiratory System

493.2–506.0

§ ✓5ᵗʰ **493.2 Chronic obstructive asthma** `CC 1-2`
[0-2]   Asthma with chronic obstructive pulmonary disease [COPD]
   Chronic asthmatic bronchitis
   EXCLUDES *acute bronchitis (466.0)*
           chronic obstructive bronchitis (491.20-491.22)
   DEF: Persistent narrowing of airway diameters in the bronchial tree, restricting airflow and causing constant labored breathing.
   CC Excl: For code 493.21: 488.01-488.11, 491.1-493.92, 517.8, 518.89, 519.8-519.9; **For code 493.22:** 493.00-493.92, 517.8, 518.89, 519.8-519.9
   AHA: 2Q, '91, 21; 2Q, '90, 20; **For code 493.20:** 4Q, '03, 108; **For code 493.22:** 1Q, '09, 17; 3Q, '06, 20

✓5ᵗʰ **493.8 Other forms of asthma**
   AHA: 4Q, '03, 62

     493.81 Exercise induced bronchospasm

     493.82 Cough variant asthma

§ ✓5ᵗʰ **493.9 Asthma, unspecified** `CC 1-2`
[0-2]   Asthma (bronchial) (allergic NOS)   Bronchitis:
   Bronchitis: asthmatic
     allergic
   CC Excl: For code 493.91 and 493.92: 493.00-493.92, 517.8, 518.89, 519.8-519.9
   AHA: 4Q, '97, 40, **For code 493.90:** 4Q, '04, 137; 4Q, '03, 108; 4Q, '99, 25; 1Q, '97, 7; **For code 493.91:** 1Q, '05, 5; **For code 493.92:** 1Q, '03, 9
   J45.909 Unspecified asthma uncomplicated `I-10`
   J45.901 Unspecified asthma with acute exacerbation `I-10`

✓4ᵗʰ **494 Bronchiectasis**
   Bronchiectasis (fusiform) (postinfectious) (recurrent)
   Bronchiolectasis
   EXCLUDES *congenital (748.61)*
           tuberculous bronchiectasis (current disease) (011.5)
   DEF: Dilation of bronchi; due to infection or chronic conditions; causes decreased lung capacity and recurrent infections of lungs.
   AHA: 4Q, '00, 42
   J47.9 Bronchiectasis uncomplicated `I-10`

   494.0 Bronchiectasis without acute exacerbation
     J47.9 Bronchiectasis uncomplicated `I-10`

   494.1 Bronchiectasis with acute exacerbation `CC`
     CC Excl: 017.90-017.96, 487.1, 488.01-488.12, 494.1, 496, 506.1, 506.4-506.9, 748.61

✓4ᵗʰ **495 Extrinsic allergic alveolitis**
   INCLUDES allergic alveolitis and pneumonitis due to inhaled organic dust particles of fungal, thermophilic actinomycete, or other origin
   DEF: Pneumonitis due to particles inhaled into lung, often at workplace; symptoms include cough, chills, fever, increased heart and respiratory rates; develops within hours of exposure.

   495.0 Farmers' lung

   495.1 Bagassosis

   495.2 Bird-fanciers' lung
     Budgerigar-fanciers' disease or lung
     Pigeon-fanciers' disease or lung

   495.3 Suberosis
     Cork-handlers' disease or lung

   495.4 Malt workers' lung
     Alveolitis due to Aspergillus clavatus

   495.5 Mushroom workers' lung

   495.6 Maple bark-strippers' lung
     Alveolitis due to Cryptostroma corticale

   495.7 "Ventilation" pneumonitis `CC`
     Allergic alveolitis due to fungal, thermophilic actinomycete, and other organisms growing in ventilation [air conditioning] systems
     CC Excl: 011.00-012.16, 012.80-012.86, 017.90-017.96, 021.2, 031.0, 039.1, 115.05, 115.15, 115.95, 122.1, 130.4, 136.3, 480.0-480.2, 480.8-487.1, 488, 494.0-508.9, 517.1, 517.8, 518.89, 519.8-519.9, 748.61

495.8 Other specified allergic alveolitis and pneumonitis `CC`
   Cheese-washers' lung   Pituitary snuff-takers' disease
   Coffee workers' lung   Sequoiosis or red-cedar
   Fish-meal workers' lung   asthma
   Furriers' lung   Wood asthma
   Grain-handlers' disease or lung
   CC Excl: See code 495.7

495.9 Unspecified allergic alveolitis and pneumonitis `CC`
   Alveolitis, allergic (extrinsic)
   Hypersensitivity pneumonitis
   CC Excl: See code 495.7

496 Chronic airway obstruction, not elsewhere classified
   NOTE This code is not to be used with any code from categories 491-493
   Chronic: Chronic:
     nonspecific lung disease   obstructive pulmonary disease
     obstructive lung disease   [COPD] NOS
   EXCLUDES *chronic obstructive lung disease [COPD] specified (as) (with):*
       allergic alveolitis (495.0-495.9)
       asthma (493.20-493.22)
       bronchiectasis (494.0-494.1)
       bronchitis (491.20-491.22)
          with emphysema (491.20-491.22)
       decompensated (491.21)
       emphysema (492.0-492.8)
   AHA: 1Q, '10, 5, 18; 1Q, '09, 16; 3Q, '07, 10; 4Q, '03, 109; 2Q, '00, 15; 2Q, '92, 16; 2Q, '91, 21; 3Q, '88, 56
   TIP: COPD is a nonspecific term that encompasses many different respiratory conditions; review medical record and query physician for more specific documentation of emphysema, bronchitis, asthma, etc.
   J44.9 Chronic obstructive pulmonary disease unspec `I-10`

Pneumoconioses and Other Lung Diseases Due to External Agents (500-508)

   DEF: Permanent deposits of particulate matter, within lungs; due to occupational or environmental exposure; results in chronic induration and fibrosis. (See specific listings in 500-508 code range)

500 Coal workers' pneumoconiosis `A`
   Anthracosilicosis   Coal workers' lung
   Anthracosis   Miner's asthma
   Black lung disease

501 Asbestosis `A`

502 Pneumoconiosis due to other silica or silicates
   Pneumoconiosis due to talc   Silicosis (simple) (complicated)
   Silicotic fibrosis (massive) of lung

503 Pneumoconiosis due to other inorganic dust
   Aluminosis (of lung)   Graphite fibrosis (of lung)
   Baritosis   Siderosis
   Bauxite fibrosis (of lung)   Stannosis
   Berylliosis

504 Pneumonopathy due to inhalation of other dust
   Byssinosis   Flax-dressers' disease
   Cannabinosis
   EXCLUDES *allergic alveolitis (495.0-495.9)*
       asbestosis (501)
       bagassosis (495.1)
       farmers' lung (495.0)

505 Pneumoconiosis, unspecified

✓4ᵗʰ **506 Respiratory conditions due to chemical fumes and vapors**
   Use additional E code to identify cause
   Use additional code to identify associated respiratory conditions, such as:
   acute respiratory failure (518.81)

   506.0 Bronchitis and pneumonitis due to fumes and vapors `CC`
     Chemical bronchitis (acute)
     CC Excl: 011.00-012.16, 012.80-012.86, 017.90-017.96, 021.2, 031.0, 039.1, 115.05, 115.15, 115.95, 122.1, 130.4, 136.3, 480.0-480.2, 480.8-487.1, 488, 494.0-508.9, 517.1, 517.8, 518.89, 519.8-519.9, 748.61
     AHA: 3Q, '10, 19; 3Q, '08, 7

---

§   Requires fifth digit. Valid digits are in [brackets] under each code. See category 493 for codes and definitions.

N Newborn Age: 0   **P** Pediatric Age: 0-17   **M** Maternity Age: 12-55   **A** Adult Age: 15-124   **MCC** Major CC Condition   **CC** CC Condition   **HIV** HIV Related Dx

166 – Volume 1   **2014 ICD-9-CM**

506.1 Acute pulmonary edema due to fumes and vapors `MCC`
Chemical pulmonary edema (acute)
EXCLUDES acute pulmonary edema NOS (518.4)
chronic or unspecified pulmonary edema (514)
CC Excl: See code 506.0
AHA: 3Q, '88, 4

506.2 Upper respiratory inflammation due to fumes and vapors
AHA: 3Q, '05, 10

506.3 Other acute and subacute respiratory conditions due to fumes and vapors
AHA: 3Q. '10, 19

506.4 Chronic respiratory conditions due to fumes and vapors
Emphysema (diffuse) (chronic)   ⎫ due to inhalation of
Obliterative bronchiolitis   ⎬ chemical fumes and
   (chronic) (subacute)   ⎪ vapors
Pulmonary fibrosis (chronic)   ⎭

506.9 Unspecified respiratory conditions due to fumes and vapors
Silo-fillers' disease

√4ᵗʰ **507 Pneumonitis due to solids and liquids**
EXCLUDES fetal aspiration pneumonitis (770.18)
postprocedural pneumonitis (997.32)
AHA: 3Q, '91, 16

507.0 Due to inhalation of food or vomitus `MCC`
Aspiration pneumonia (due to):
NOS
food (regurgitated)
gastric secretions
milk
saliva
vomitus
CC Excl: See code 506.0
AHA: 4Q, '11, 150; 1Q, '11, 16; 1Q, '08, 18;1Q, '89, 10
TIP: If postprocedural or postoperative aspiration pneumonia is specified, assign instead 997.32.
J69.0 Pneumonitis due to inhalation of food and vomit `I-10`

507.1 Due to inhalation of oils and essences `MCC`
Lipoid pneumonia (exogenous)
EXCLUDES endogenous lipoid pneumonia (516.8)
CC Excl: See code 506.0

507.8 Due to other solids and liquids `MCC`
Detergent asthma
CC Excl: See code 506.0

√4ᵗʰ **508 Respiratory conditions due to other and unspecified external agents**
Use additional E code to identify cause
Use additional code to identify associated respiratory conditions, such as:
acute respiratory failure (518.81)

508.0 Acute pulmonary manifestations due to radiation `CC`
Radiation pneumonitis
CC Excl: See code 506.0
AHA: 2Q, '88, 4

508.1 Chronic and other pulmonary manifestations due to radiation `CC`
Fibrosis of lung following radiation
CC Excl: See code 506.0

508.2 Respiratory conditions due to smoke inhalation `CC`
Smoke inhalation NOS
EXCLUDES smoke inhalation due to chemical fumes and vapors (506.9)
AHA: 4Q, '11, 114-115
TIP: Assign for smoke inhalation, along with the appropriate E code describing the source of the smoke and fumes.

508.8 Respiratory conditions due to other specified external agents

508.9 Respiratory conditions due to unspecified external agent

Other Diseases of Respiratory System (510-519)

√4ᵗʰ **510 Empyema**
Use additional code to identify infectious organism (041.0-041.9)
EXCLUDES abscess of lung (513.0)
DEF: Purulent infection within pleural space.

510.0 With fistula `MCC`
Fistula: Fistula:
  bronchocutaneous   mediastinal
  bronchopleural   pleural
  hepatopleural   thoracic
Any condition classifiable to 510.9 with fistula
DEF: Purulent infection of respiratory cavity, with communication from cavity to another structure.
CC Excl: 510.0-510.9, 517.8, 518.89, 519.8-519.9

510.9 Without mention of fistula `MCC`
Abscess: Pleurisy:
  pleura   septic
  thorax   seropurulent
Empyema (chest) (lung) (pleura)   suppurative
Fibrinopurulent pleurisy   Pyopneumothorax
Pleurisy: Pyothorax
  purulent
CC Excl: See code: 510.0
AHA: 4Q, '07, 113; 3Q, '94, 6
J86.9 Pyothorax without fistula `I-10`

√4ᵗʰ **511 Pleurisy**
EXCLUDES pleurisy with mention of tuberculosis, current disease (012.0)
DEF: Inflammation of serous membrane of lungs and lining of thoracic cavity; causes exudation in cavity or membrane surface.

511.0 Without mention of effusion or current tuberculosis
Adhesion, lung or pleura   Pleurisy:
Calcification of pleura   NOS
Pleurisy (acute) (sterile):   pneumococcal
  diaphragmatic   staphylococcal
  fibrinous   streptococcal
  interlobar   Thickening of pleura
AHA: 3Q, '94, 5

511.1 With effusion, with mention of a bacterial cause other than tuberculosis `MCC`
Pleurisy with effusion (exudative) (serous):
  other specified nontuberculous bacterial cause
  pneumococcal
  staphylococcal
  streptococcal
CC Excl: 011.00-012.16, 012.80-012.86, 017.90-017.96, 511.0-511.9, 517.8, 518.89, 519.8-519.9

√5ᵗʰ **511.8 Other specified forms of effusion, except tuberculous**
EXCLUDES traumatic (860.2-860.5, 862.29, 862.39)
AHA: 4Q, '08, 113-114;1Q, '97, 10

511.81 Malignant pleural effusion `CC`
Code first malignant neoplasm, if known
CC Excl: 195.8, 197.2-197.3, 198.89-199.2, 209.20, 209.29-209.30, 209.70, 209.75-209.79, 239.81-239.9, 511.81-511.89
J91.0 Malignant pleural effusion `I-10`

511.89 Other specified forms of effusion, except tuberculous `CC`
Encysted pleurisy   Hydropneumothorax
Hemopneumothorax   Hydrothorax
Hemothorax
CC Excl: 011.00-012.16, 012.80-012.86, 017.90-017.96, 511.0-511.9, 517.8, 518.89, 519.8-519.9

511.9 Unspecified pleural effusion `CC`
Pleural effusion NOS   Pleurisy:
Pleurisy: serous
  exudative   with effusion NOS
  serofibrinous
CC Excl: 011.00-012.16, 012.80-012.86, 017.90-017.96, 511.0-511.9, 517.8, 518.89, 519.8-519.9
AHA: 2Q, '03, 7; 3Q, '91, 19; 4Q, '89, 11
TIP: Do not assign when the pleural effusion is a symptom of CHF and no therapeutic treatment (e.g., thoracentesis) is directed towards the pleural effusion.
J90 Pleural effusion not elsewhere classified `I-10`

⁴ᵗʰ ⁵ᵗʰ   Additional Digit Required | Unacceptable PDx | | Manifestation Code | Hospital Acquired Condition   ▶◀ Revised Text   ● New Code   ▲ Revised Code Title

2014 ICD-9-CM   **Volume 1 – 167**

Diseases of the Respiratory System

512–516.37

√4ᵗʰ **512 Pneumothorax and air leak**
> **DEF:** Collapsed lung; due to gas or air in pleural space.
> **AHA:** 4Q, '11, 115-116

512.0 Spontaneous tension pneumothorax `MCC`
> **DEF:** Leaking air from lung into lining causing collapse.
> **CC Excl:** 512.0-512.89, 517.8, 518.89, 519.8-519.9, 793.11
> **AHA:** 3Q, '94, 5

16 **512.1 Iatrogenic pneumothorax** `CC`
> Postoperative pneumothorax
> **DEF:** Air trapped in the lining of the lung following surgery.
> **CC Excl:** See code 512.0
> **AHA:** 1Q, '11, 14; 4Q, '94, 40
> **TIP:** Pneumothorax is a known risk associated with most thoracic surgery; do not assign based on radiology findings alone, without physician substantiation.
> J95.811 Postprocedural pneumothorax `I-10`

512.2 Postoperative air leak `CC`
> **CC Excl:** see Code: 512.0
> **AHA:** 4Q, '11, 115-117

√5ᵗʰ **512.8 Other pneumothorax and air leak**
> *EXCLUDES* pneumothorax:
> > *congenital (770.2)*
> > *traumatic (860.0-860.1, 860.4-860.5)*
> > *tuberculous, current disease (011.7)*
> **AHA:** 4Q, '11, 115-117; 2Q, '93, 3

512.81 Primary spontaneous pneumothorax `CC`
> **CC Excl:** see Code: 512.0
> J93.11 Primary spontaneous pneumothorax `I-10`

512.82 Secondary spontaneous pneumothorax `CC`
> Code first underlying condition, such as:
> > cancer metastatic to lung (197.0)
> > catamenial pneumothorax due to endometriosis (617.8)
> > cystic fibrosis (277.02)
> > eosinophilic pneumonia (518.3)
> > lymphangioleiomyomatosis (516.4)
> > Marfan syndrome (759.82)
> > pneumocystis carinii pneumonia (136.3)
> > primary lung cancer (162.3-162.9)
> > spontaneous rupture of the esophagus (530.4)
> **CC Excl:** see Code: 512.0

512.83 Chronic pneumothorax `CC`
> **CC Excl:** see Code: 512.0

512.84 Other air leak `CC`
> Persistent air leak
> **CC Excl:** see Code: 512.0

512.89 Other pneumothorax `CC`
> Acute pneumothorax
> Pneumothorax NOS
> Spontaneous pneumothorax NOS
> **CC Excl:** see Code: 512.0
> J93.9 Pneumothorax unspecified `I-10`

√4ᵗʰ **513 Abscess of lung and mediastinum**

513.0 Abscess of lung `MCC`
> Abscess (multiple) of lung
> Gangrenous or necrotic pneumonia
> Pulmonary gangrene or necrosis
> **CC Excl:** 006.4, 011.00-012.16, 012.80-012.86, 017.90-017.96, 513.0, 519.8-519.9
> **AHA:** 4Q, '07, 85; 2Q, '98, 7

513.1 Abscess of mediastinum `MCC`
> **CC Excl:** 513.1, 519.8-519.9

---

514 Pulmonary congestion and hypostasis `CC`
> Hypostatic: Pulmonary edema:
> > bronchopneumonia   NOS
> > pneumonia   chronic
> Passive pneumonia
> Pulmonary congestion (chronic) (passive)
> *EXCLUDES* acute pulmonary edema:
> > NOS (518.4)
> > with mention of heart disease or failure (428.1)
> > hypostatic pneumonia due to or specified as a specific type of pneumonia — code to the type of pneumonia (480.0-480.9, 481, 482.0-482.9, 483.0-483.8, 487.0, 488.01, 488.11)
> **DEF:** Excessive retention of interstitial fluid in the lungs and pulmonary vessels due to poor circulation.
> **CC Excl:** 514, 517.8, 518.89, 519.8-519.9
> **AHA:** 2Q, '98, 6; 3Q, '88, 5
> J81.1 Chronic pulmonary edema `I-10`

515 Postinflammatory pulmonary fibrosis
> Cirrhosis of lung
> Fibrosis of lung (atrophic)
> > (confluent) (massive)   } chronic or unspecified
> > (perialveolar) (peribronchial)
> Induration of lung
> **DEF:** Fibrosis and scarring of the lungs due to inflammatory reaction.
> J84.10 Pulmonary fibrosis, unspecified `I-10`

√4ᵗʰ **516 Other alveolar and parietoalveolar pneumonopathy**

516.0 Pulmonary alveolar proteinosis `CC`
> **DEF:** Reduced ventilation due to proteinaceous deposits on alveoli; symptoms include dyspnea, cough, chest pain, and hemoptysis.
> **CC Excl:** 011.00-012.16, 012.80-012.86, 017.90-017.96, 494.0-508.1, 508.8-508.9, 515-516.2, 516.30-516.5, 516.8-516.9, 517.2, 517.8, 518.89, 519.8-519.9, 748.61, 793.11

516.1 Idiopathic pulmonary hemosiderosis `CC`
> Code first underlying disease (275.01-275.09)
> Essential brown induration of lung
> *EXCLUDES* acute idiopathic pulmonary hemorrhage in infants [AIPHI] (786.31)
> **DEF:** Fibrosis of alveolar walls; marked by abnormal amounts hemosiderin in lungs; primarily affects children; symptoms include anemia, fluid in lungs, and blood in sputum; etiology unknown.
> **CC Excl:** See code: 516.0

516.2 Pulmonary alveolar microlithiasis `CC`
> **DEF:** Small calculi in pulmonary alveoli resembling sand-like particles on x-ray.
> **CC Excl:** See code: 516.0

√5ᵗʰ **516.3 Idiopathic interstitial pneumonia**
> **AHA:** 4Q, '11, 117-119

516.30 Idiopathic interstitial pneumonia, not otherwise specified
> Idiopathic fibrosing alveolitis

516.31 Idiopathic pulmonary fibrosis
> Cryptogenic fibrosing alveolitis
> **DEF:** Chronic disease of unknown causation characterized by scarring and thickening of the lungs.

516.32 Idiopathic non-specific interstitial pneumonitis
> *EXCLUDES* non-specific interstitial pneumonia NOS, or due to known underlying cause (516.8)

516.33 Acute interstitial pneumonitis `CC`
> Hamman Rich syndrome
> *EXCLUDES* pneumocystis pneumonia (136.3)
> **CC Excl:** see Code: 516.0

516.34 Respiratory bronchiolitis interstitial lung disease

516.35 Idiopathic lymphoid interstitial pneumonia `CC`
> Idiopathic lymphocytic interstitial pneumonitis
> *EXCLUDES* lymphoid interstitial pneumonia NOS, or due to known underlying cause (516.8) pneumocystis pneumonia (136.3)
> **CC Excl:** See code 516.0

516.36 Cryptogenic organizing pneumonia `CC`
> *EXCLUDES* organizing pneumonia NOS, or due to known underlying cause (516.8)
> **CC Excl:** See code 516.0

516.37 Desquamative interstitial pneumonia `CC`
> **CC Excl:** See code 516.0

---

16 HAC when reported with procedure code 38.93 and POA = N.

N Newborn Age: 0   P Pediatric Age: 0-17   M Maternity Age: 12-55   A Adult Age: 15-124   MCC Major CC Condition   CC CC Condition   HIV HIV Related Dx

168 – Volume 1   **2014 ICD-9-CM**

516.4 Lymphangioleiomyomatosis ♀ MCC
Lymphangiomyomatosis
CC Excl: See Code: 516.0
AHA: 4Q, '11, 119

516.5 Adult pulmonary Langerhans cell histiocytosis A CC
Adult PLCH
CC Excl: See code 516.0
AHA: 4Q, '11, 119

√5th **516.6 Interstitial lung diseases of childhood**
AHA: 4Q, '11, 120-123

516.61 Neuroendocrine cell hyperplasia of infancy MCC
CC Excl: 516.61-516.69, 768.5-768.9, 769-770.9,
779.81-779.89

516.62 Pulmonary interstitial glycogenosis MCC
CC Excl: see code 516.61

516.63 Surfactant mutations of the lung MCC
CC Excl: see code 516.61
DEF: Group of genetic disorders resulting in potentially fatal
pediatric lung disease with onset typically within the
perinatal period; leading indication for pediatric lung
transplantation.

516.64 Alveolar capillary dysplasia with vein MCC
misalignment
CC Excl: see code 516.61

516.69 Other interstitial lung diseases of childhood MCC
CC Excl: see code 516.61

516.8 Other specified alveolar and parietoalveolar CC
pneumonopathies
Endogenous lipoid pneumonia
Interstitial pneumonia
Lymphoid interstitial pneumonia due to known underlying
cause
Lymphoid interstitial pneumonia NOS
Non-specific interstitial pneumonia due to known underlying
cause
Non-specific interstitial pneumonia NOS
Organizing pneumonia due to known underlying cause
Organizing pneumonia NOS
Code first, if applicable, underlying cause of pneumonopathy,
if known
Use additional E code, if applicable, for drug-induced or toxic
pneumonopathy
EXCLUDES cryptogenic organizing pneumonia (516.36)
idiopathic lymphoid interstitial pneumonia (516.35)
idiopathic non-specific interstitial pneumonitis
(516.32)
lipoid pneumonia, exogenous or unspecified (507.1)
CC Excl: 011.00-012.16, 012.80-012.86, 017.90-017.96, 494.0-508.9,
515-516.9, 517.2, 517.8, 518.89, 519.8-519.9, 748.61
AHA: 1Q, '11, 16; 1Q, '10, 6; 2Q, '06, 20; 1Q, '92, 12

516.9 Unspecified alveolar and parietoalveolar CC
pneumonopathy
CC Excl: See code: 516.0

√4th **517 Lung involvement in conditions classified elsewhere**
EXCLUDES rheumatoid lung (714.81)

517.1 Rheumatic pneumonia CC
Code first underlying disease (390)
CC Excl: 011.00-012.16, 012.80-012.86, 017.90-017.96, 480.0-480.2,
480.8-487.1, 488.01-488.02, 488.11-488.12, 494.0-508.9, 515-516.2,
516.30-516.5, 516.8-517.2, 517.8, 518.89, 519.8-519.9, 748.61

517.2 Lung involvement in systemic sclerosis CC
Code first underlying disease (710.1)
CC Excl: 011.00-012.16, 012.80-012.86, 017.90-017.96, 494.0- 508.9,
515-516.9, 517.2, 517.8, 518.89, 519.8-519.9, 748.61

517.3 Acute chest syndrome CC
Code first sickle-cell disease in crisis (282.42, 282.62, 282.64,
282.69)
CC Excl: 280.0-282.3, 282.5-282.63, 282.69-284.2, 284.81-285.9, 289.9,
776.5-776.6
AHA: 4Q, '03, 51, 56

517.8 Lung involvement in other diseases classified elsewhere
Code first underlying disease, as:
amyloidosis (277.30-277.39)
polymyositis (710.4)
sarcoidosis (135)
Sjögren's disease (710.2)
systemic lupus erythematosus (710.0)
EXCLUDES syphilis (095.1)
AHA: 2Q, '03, 7

√4th **518 Other diseases of lung**

518.0 Pulmonary collapse CC
Atelectasis   Middle lobe syndrome
Collapse of lung
EXCLUDES atelectasis:
congenital (partial) (770.5)
primary (770.4)
tuberculous, current disease (011.8)
CC Excl: 518.0, 519.8-519.9
AHA: 4Q, '90, 25
J98.11 Atelectasis I-10

518.1 Interstitial emphysema
Mediastinal emphysema
EXCLUDES surgical (subcutaneous) emphysema (998.81)
that in fetus or newborn (770.2)
traumatic emphysema (958.7)
DEF: Escaped air from the alveoli trapped in the interstices of the
lung; trauma or cough may cause the disease.

518.2 Compensatory emphysema
DEF: Distention of all or part of the lung due to disease processes or
surgical intervention that decreased volume in other parts of lung.

518.3 Pulmonary eosinophilia CC
Eosinophilic asthma   Pneumonia:
Löffler's syndrome   eosinophilic
Pneumonia: Tropical eosinophilia
allergic
EXCLUDES pulmonary infiltrate NOS (793.19)
DEF: Infiltration, into pulmonary parenchyma of eosinophils; results
in cough, fever, and dyspnea.
CC Excl: 011.00-012.16, 012.80-012.86, 017.90-017.96, 020.3-020.5,
021.3, 022.1, 031.0, 039.1, 073.0, 115.05, 115.15, 115.95, 122.1, 130.4,
136.3, 480.0-480.2, 480.8-487.1, 488.01-488.02, 488.11-488.12,
494.0-495.9, 500-508.9, 517.1, 517.8, 518.3, 518.89, 519.8-519.9,
748.61
AHA: 4Q, '11, 139

518.4 Acute edema of lung, unspecified MCC
Acute pulmonary edema NOS
Pulmonary edema, postoperative
EXCLUDES pulmonary edema:
acute, with mention of heart disease or failure
(428.1)
chronic or unspecified (514)
due to external agents (506.0-508.9)
DEF: Severe, sudden fluid retention within lung tissues.
CC Excl: 398.91, 428.0-428.9, 518.4, 519.8-519.9
TIP: Do not assign separately if associated with CHF or heart disease;
it is incorporated into those codes.

√5th **518.5 Pulmonary insufficiency following trauma and surgery**
EXCLUDES adult respiratory distress syndrome associated with
other conditions (518.82)
pneumonia:
aspiration (507.0)
hypostatic (514)
respiratory failure in other conditions (518.81,
518.83-518.84)
AHA: 4Q, '11, 123-125; 3Q, '10, 19; 4Q, '04, 139; 3Q, '88, 3; 3Q, '88, 7;
S-O, '87, 1

518.51 Acute respiratory failure following trauma MCC
and surgery
Respiratory failure, not otherwise specified, following
trauma and surgery
EXCLUDES acute respiratory failure in other conditions
(518.81)
CC Excl: 518.5, 519.8-519.9
J95.821 Acute postprocedural respiratory failure I-10

Diseases of the Respiratory System

518.52–519.9

518.52 Other pulmonary insufficiency, not elsewhere classified, following trauma and surgery `MCC`

Adult respiratory distress syndrome
Pulmonary insufficiency following surgery
Pulmonary insufficiency following trauma
Shock lung related to trauma and surgery

EXCLUDES   adult respiratory distress syndrome associated with other conditions (518.82)
     aspiration pneumonia (507.0)
     hypostatic pneumonia (514)
     shock lung, not related to trauma or surgery (518.82)

CC Excl: see code 518.51

518.53 Acute and chronic respiratory failure following trauma and surgery `MCC`

EXCLUDES   acute and chronic respiratory failure in other conditions (518.84)

CC Excl: see code 518.51

518.6 Allergic bronchopulmonary aspergillosis `CC`

DEF: Noninvasive hypersensitive reaction; due to allergic reaction to *Aspergillus fumigatus* (mold).
CC Excl: 518.6, 519.8-519.9
AHA: 4Q, '97, 39

518.7 Transfusion related acute lung injury [TRALI] `CC`

DEF: A relatively rare, but serious pulmonary complication of blood transfusion, with acute respiratory distress, noncardiogenic pulmonary edema, cyanosis, hypoxemia, hypotension, fever and chills.
CC Excl: 518.7, 997.31-997.39, 997.91-997.99, 998.81, 998.83-998.9
AHA: 4Q, '06, 91

√5ᵗʰ **518.8 Other diseases of lung**

518.81 Acute respiratory failure `MCC`

Respiratory failure NOS

EXCLUDES   acute and chronic respiratory failure (518.84)
     acute respiratory distress (518.82)
     acute respiratory failure following trauma and surgery (518.51)
     chronic respiratory failure (518.83)
     respiratory arrest (799.1)
     respiratory failure, newborn (770.84)

CC Excl: 518.81-518.84, 519.8-519.9, 799.1
AHA: ►3Q, '12, 21-22;◄ 4Q, '10, 80; 1Q, '10, 18-19; 3Q, '09, 14; 2Q, '09, 11; 1Q, '08, 18; 3Q, '07, 6; 2Q, '06, 25; 4Q, '05, 96; 2Q, '05, 19; 1Q, '05, 3-8; 1Q, '05, 3-8; 4Q, '04, 139; 1Q, '03, 15; 4Q, '98, 41; 3Q, '91, 14; 2Q, '91, 3; 4Q, '90, 25; 2Q, '90, 20; 3Q, '88, 7; 3Q, '88, 10; S-O, '87, 1
TIP: If both respiratory failure and another acute condition are equally responsible for admission, either may be sequenced as principal diagnosis in the absence of chapter-specific guidelines to the contrary.
J96.01 Acute respiratory failure with hypoxia   `I-10`

518.82 Other pulmonary insufficiency, not elsewhere classified `CC`

Acute respiratory distress
Acute respiratory insufficiency
Adult respiratory distress syndrome NEC

EXCLUDES   acute interstitial pneumonitis (516.33)
     adult respiratory distress syndrome associated with trauma or surgery (518.52)
     pulmonary insufficiency following trauma or surgery (518.52)
     respiratory distress:
       NOS (786.09)
       newborn (770.89)
       syndrome, newborn (769)

CC Excl: See code: 518.81
AHA: 4Q, '03, 105; 2Q, '91, 21; 3Q, '88, 7
J80 Acute respiratory distress syndrome   `I-10`

518.83 Chronic respiratory failure `CC`

CC Excl: See code: 518.81
AHA: 4Q, '05, 96; 4Q, '03, 103, 111
J96.10 Chronic respiratory failure, unsp whth w/hypox or hypercap   `I-10`

518.84 Acute and chronic respiratory failure `MCC`

Acute on chronic respiratory failure

EXCLUDES   acute and chronic respiratory failure following trauma or surgery (518.53)

CC Excl: See code: 518.81
AHA: 2Q, '11, 7
J96.20 Ac & chr resp failure unsp whth w/hypox or hypercap   `I-10`

518.89 Other diseases of lung, not elsewhere classified

Broncholithiasis   Lung disease NOS
Calcification of lung   Pulmolithiasis
DEF: Broncholithiasis: calculi in lumen of transbronchial tree.
DEF: Pulmolithiasis: calculi in lung.
AHA: 3Q, '90, 18; 4Q, '88, 6
TIP: Do not assign for solitary lung nodule; see instead code 793.11.
J98.4 Other disorders of lung   `I-10`

√4ᵗʰ **519 Other diseases of respiratory system**

√5ᵗʰ **519.0 Tracheostomy complications**

519.00 Tracheostomy complication, unspecified `CC`

CC Excl: 519.00-519.19, 519.8-519.9

519.01 Infection of tracheostomy `CC`

Use additional code to identify type of infection, such as:
     abscess or cellulitis of neck (682.1)
     septicemia (038.0-038.9)
Use additional code to identify organism (041.00-041.9)
CC Excl: See code 519.00
AHA:4Q, '98, 41

519.02 Mechanical complication of tracheostomy `CC`

Tracheal stenosis due to tracheostomy
CC Excl: See code 519.00

519.09 Other tracheostomy complications `CC`

Hemorrhage due to tracheostomy
Tracheoesophageal fistula due to tracheostomy
CC Excl: See code 519.00

√5ᵗʰ **519.1 Other diseases of trachea and bronchus, not elsewhere classified**

AHA: 3Q, '02, 18; 3Q, '88, 6

519.11 Acute bronchospasm

Bronchospasm NOS

EXCLUDES   acute bronchitis with bronchospasm (466.0)
     asthma (493.00-493.92)
     exercise induced bronchospasm (493.81)

AHA: 4Q, '06, 92

519.19 Other diseases of trachea and bronchus

Calcification
Stenosis } of bronchus or trachea
Ulcer
AHA: 4Q, '06, 92

⁹ **519.2 Mediastinitis** `MCC`

DEF: Inflammation of tissue between organs behind sternum.
CC Excl: 519.2-519.3, 519.8-519.9

519.3 Other diseases of mediastinum, not elsewhere classified

Fibrosis
Hernia } of mediastinum
Retraction

519.4 Disorders of diaphragm

Diaphragmitis   Relaxation of diaphragm
Paralysis of diaphragm

EXCLUDES   congenital defect of diaphragm (756.6)
     diaphragmatic hernia (551-553 with .3)
     congenital (756.6)

519.8 Other diseases of respiratory system, not elsewhere classified

AHA: 4Q, '89, 12

519.9 Unspecified disease of respiratory system

Respiratory disease (chronic) NOS

---

⁹ HAC = when in combination with a procedure code from 36.10-36.19.

N Newborn Age: 0   P Pediatric Age: 0-17   M Maternity Age: 12-55   A Adult Age: 15-124   MCC Major CC Condition   CC CC Condition   HIV HIV Related D

170 – Volume 1 • February 2013   2014 ICD-9-C

9. Diseases of the Digestive System (520-579)

Diseases of Oral Cavity, Salivary Glands, and Jaws (520-529)

✓4ᵗʰ 520 Disorders of tooth development and eruption

520.0 Anodontia
Absence of teeth (complete) (congenital) (partial)
Hypodontia
Oligodontia
EXCLUDES *acquired absence of teeth (525.10-525.19)*

520.1 Supernumerary teeth
Distomolar   Paramolar
Fourth molar   Supplemental teeth
Mesiodens
EXCLUDES *supernumerary roots (520.2)*

520.2 Abnormalities of size and form
Concrescence ⎫
Fusion   ⎬ of teeth
Gemination ⎭

Dens evaginatus
Dens in dente
Dens invaginatus
Enamel pearls
Macrodontia
Microdontia
Peg-shaped [conical] teeth
Supernumerary roots
Taurodontism
Tuberculum paramolare
EXCLUDES *that due to congenital syphilis (090.5)*
tuberculum Carabelli, which is regarded as a normal variation

520.3 Mottled teeth
Mottling of enamel
Dental fluorosis
Nonfluoride enamel opacities

Digestive System

The Oral Cavity

Teeth

Maxillary view

Mandibulary view

520.4 Disturbances of tooth formation
Aplasia and hypoplasia of cementum
Dilaceration of tooth
Enamel hypoplasia (neonatal) (postnatal) (prenatal)
Horner's teeth
Hypocalcification of teeth
Regional odontodysplasia
Turner's tooth
EXCLUDES *Hutchinson's teeth and mulberry molars in congenital syphilis (090.5)*
mottled teeth (520.3)

520.5 Hereditary disturbances in tooth structure, not elsewhere classified
Amelogensis ⎫
Dentinogenesis ⎬ imperfecta
Odontogenesis ⎭

Dentinal dysplasia
Shell teeth

520.6 Disturbances in tooth eruption
Teeth: Tooth eruption:
  embedded   late
  impacted   obstructed
  natal   premature
  neonatal
  prenatal
  primary [deciduous]:
    persistent
    shedding, premature
EXCLUDES *exfoliation of teeth (attributable to disease of surrounding tissues) (525.0-525.19)*
AHA: 1Q, '06, 18; 2Q, '05, 15

520.7 Teething syndrome

520.8 Other specified disorders of tooth development and eruption
Color changes during tooth formation
Pre-eruptive color changes
EXCLUDES *posteruptive color changes (521.7)*

520.9 Unspecified disorder of tooth development and eruption

✓4ᵗʰ 521 Diseases of hard tissues of teeth

✓5ᵗʰ 521.0 Dental caries
AHA: 4Q, '01, 44

521.00 Dental caries, unspecified

4ᵗʰ / 5ᵗʰ   Additional Digit Required   Unacceptable PDx   Manifestation Code   Hospital Acquired Condition   ▶◀ Revised Text   ● New Code   ▲ Revised Code Title

2014 ICD-9-CM   **Volume 1 – 171**

Diseases of the Digestive System

521.01 Dental caries limited to enamel
Initial caries   White spot lesion

521.02 Dental caries extending into dentine

521.03 Dental caries extending into pulp

521.04 Arrested dental caries

521.05 Odontoclasia
Infantile melanodontia   Melanodontoclasia
EXCLUDES *internal and external resorption of teeth (521.40-521.49)*
DEF: A pathological dental condition described as stained areas, loss of tooth substance, and hypoplasia linked to nutritional deficiencies during tooth development and to cariogenic oral conditions.

521.06 Dental caries pit and fissure
Primary dental caries, pit and fissure origin

521.07 Dental caries of smooth surface
Primary dental caries, smooth surface origin

521.08 Dental caries of root surface
Primary dental caries, root surface

521.09 Other dental caries
AHA: 3Q, '02, 14

√5ᵗʰ **521.1 Excessive attrition (approximal wear) (occlusal wear)**

521.10 Excessive attrition, unspecified

521.11 Excessive attrition, limited to enamel

521.12 Excessive attrition, extending into dentine

521.13 Excessive attrition, extending into pulp

521.14 Excessive attrition, localized

521.15 Excessive attrition, generalized

√5ᵗʰ **521.2 Abrasion**
Abrasion:
dentifrice
habitual
occupational   } of teeth
ritual
traditional
Wedge defect NOS

521.20 Abrasion, unspecified

521.21 Abrasion, limited to enamel

521.22 Abrasion, extending into dentine

521.23 Abrasion, extending into pulp

521.24 Abrasion, localized

521.25 Abrasion, generalized

√5ᵗʰ **521.3 Erosion**
Erosion of teeth:
NOS
due to:
medicine
persistent vomiting
idiopathic
occupational

521.30 Erosion, unspecified

521.31 Erosion, limited to enamel

521.32 Erosion, extending into dentine

521.33 Erosion, extending into pulp

521.34 Erosion, localized

521.35 Erosion, generalized

√5ᵗʰ **521.4 Pathological resorption**
DEF: Loss of dentin and cementum due to disease process.

521.40 Pathological resorption, unspecified

521.41 Pathological resorption, internal

521.42 Pathological resorption, external

521.49 Other pathological resorption
Internal granuloma of pulp

521.5 Hypercementosis
Cementation hyperplasia
DEF: Excess deposits of cementum, on tooth root.

521.6 Ankylosis of teeth
DEF: Adhesion of tooth to surrounding bone.

521.7 Intrinsic posteruptive color changes
Staining [discoloration] of teeth:
NOS
due to:
drugs
metals
pulpal bleeding
EXCLUDES *accretions [deposits] on teeth (523.6)*
extrinsic color changes (523.6)
pre-eruptive color changes (520.8)

√5ᵗʰ **521.8 Other specified diseases of hard tissues of teeth**

521.81 Cracked tooth
EXCLUDES *asymptomatic craze lines in enamel — omit code*
broken tooth due to trauma (873.63, 873.73)
fractured tooth due to trauma (873.63, 873.73)

521.89 Other specified diseases of hard tissues of teeth
Irradiated enamel
Sensitive dentin

521.9 Unspecified disease of hard tissues of teeth

√4ᵗʰ **522 Diseases of pulp and periapical tissues**

522.0 Pulpitis   CC
Pulpal:
abscess
polyp
Pulpitis:
acute
chronic (hyperplastic) (ulcerative)
suppurative
CC Excl: 520.0-525.9

522.1 Necrosis of the pulp
Pulp gangrene
DEF: Death of pulp tissue.

522.2 Pulp degeneration
Denticles
Pulp calcifications
Pulp stones

522.3 Abnormal hard tissue formation in pulp
Secondary or irregular dentin

522.4 Acute apical periodontitis of pulpal origin   CC
DEF: Severe inflammation of periodontal ligament due to pulpal inflammation or necrosis.
CC Excl: See code: 522.0

522.5 Periapical abscess without sinus
Abscess:
dental
dentoalveolar
EXCLUDES *periapical abscess with sinus (522.7)*

522.6 Chronic apical periodontitis
Apical or periapical granuloma
Apical periodontitis NOS

522.7 Periapical abscess with sinus
Fistula:
alveolar process
dental

522.8 Radicular cyst
Cyst:
apical (periodontal)
periapical
radiculodental
residual radicular
EXCLUDES *lateral developmental or lateral periodontal cyst (526.0)*
DEF: Cyst in tissue around tooth apex due to chronic infection of granuloma around root.

N   Newborn Age: 0   P   Pediatric Age: 0-17   M   Maternity Age: 12-55   A   Adult Age: 15-124   MCC   Major CC Condition   CC   CC Condition   HIV   HIV Related Dx

172 – Volume 1   2014 ICD-9-CM

522.9 Other and unspecified diseases of pulp and periapical tissues

✓4ᵗʰ **523 Gingival and periodontal diseases**

✓5ᵗʰ **523.0 Acute gingivitis**

> EXCLUDES *acute necrotizing ulcerative gingivitis (101)*
> *herpetic gingivostomatitis (054.2)*

523.00 Acute gingivitis, plaque induced
Acute gingivitis NOS

523.01 Acute gingivitis, non-plaque induced

✓5ᵗʰ **523.1 Chronic gingivitis**
Gingivitis (chronic):
desquamative
hyperplastic
simple marginal
ulcerative

> EXCLUDES *herpetic gingivostomatitis (054.2)*

523.10 Chronic gingivitis, plaque induced
Chronic gingivitis NOS
Gingivitis NOS

523.11 Chronic gingivitis, non-plaque induced

✓5ᵗʰ **523.2 Gingival recession**
Gingival recession (postinfective) (postoperative)

523.20 Gingival recession, unspecified

523.21 Gingival recession, minimal

523.22 Gingival recession, moderate

523.23 Gingival recession, severe

523.24 Gingival recession, localized

523.25 Gingival recession, generalized

✓5ᵗʰ **523.3 Aggressive and acute periodontitis**
Acute:
pericementitis
pericoronitis

> EXCLUDES *acute apical periodontitis (522.4)*
> *periapical abscess (522.5, 522.7)*

DEF: Severe inflammation of tissues supporting teeth.

523.30 Aggressive periodontitis, unspecified

523.31 Aggressive periodontitis, localized
Periodontal abscess

523.32 Aggressive periodontitis, generalized

523.33 Acute periodontitis

✓5ᵗʰ **523.4 Chronic periodontitis**
Chronic pericoronitis
Pericementitis (chronic)
Periodontitis:
complex
simplex
NOS

> EXCLUDES *chronic apical periodontitis (522.6)*

523.40 Chronic periodontitis, unspecified

523.41 Chronic periodontitis, localized

523.42 Chronic periodontitis, generalized

523.5 Periodontosis

523.6 Accretions on teeth
Dental calculus:
subgingival
supragingival
Deposits on teeth:
betel
materia alba
soft
tartar
tobacco
Extrinsic discoloration of teeth

> EXCLUDES *intrinsic discoloration of teeth (521.7)*

DEF: Foreign material on tooth surface, usually plaque or calculus.

523.8 Other specified periodontal diseases
Giant cell:
epulis
peripheral granuloma
Gingival:
cysts
enlargement NOS
fibromatosis
Gingival polyp
Periodontal lesions due to traumatic occlusion
Peripheral giant cell granuloma

> EXCLUDES *leukoplakia of gingiva (528.6)*

523.9 Unspecified gingival and periodontal disease
AHA: 3Q, '02, 14

✓4ᵗʰ **524 Dentofacial anomalies, including malocclusion**

✓5ᵗʰ **524.0 Major anomalies of jaw size**

> EXCLUDES *hemifacial atrophy or hypertrophy (754.0)*
> *unilateral condylar hyperplasia or hypoplasia of mandible (526.89)*

524.00 Unspecified anomaly
DEF: Unspecified deformity of jaw size.

524.01 Maxillary hyperplasia
DEF: Overgrowth or over development of upper jaw bone.

524.02 Mandibular hyperplasia
DEF: Overgrowth or over development of lower jaw bone.

524.03 Maxillary hypoplasia
DEF: Incomplete or underdeveloped upper jaw bone.

524.04 Mandibular hypoplasia
DEF: Incomplete or underdeveloped lower jaw bone.
AHA: ▶2Q, '12, 17◀

524.05 Macrogenia
DEF: Enlarged jaw, especially chin; affects bone, soft tissue, or both.

524.06 Microgenia
DEF: Underdeveloped mandible, characterized by an extremely small chin.

524.07 Excessive tuberosity of jaw
Entire maxillary tuberosity

524.09 Other specified anomaly

✓5ᵗʰ **524.1 Anomalies of relationship of jaw to cranial base**

524.10 Unspecified anomaly
Prognathism
Retrognathism
DEF: Prognathism: protrusion of lower jaw.
DEF: Retrognathism: jaw is located posteriorly to a normally positioned jaw; backward position of mandible.

524.11 Maxillary asymmetry
DEF: Absence of symmetry of maxilla.

524.12 Other jaw asymmetry

524.19 Other specified anomaly

✓5ᵗʰ **524.2 Anomalies of dental arch relationship**
Anomaly of dental arch

> EXCLUDES *hemifacial atrophy or hypertrophy (754.0)*
> *soft tissue impingement (524.81-524.82)*
> *unilateral condylar hyperplasia or hypoplasia of mandible (526.89)*

524.20 Unspecified anomaly of dental arch relationship

524.21 Malocclusion, Angle's class I
Neutro-occlusion

524.22 Malocclusion, Angle's class II
Disto-occlusion Division I
Disto-occlusion Division II

524.23 Malocclusion, Angle's class III
Mesio-occlusion

524.24 Open anterior occlusal relationship
Anterior open bite

524.25 Open posterior occlusal relationship
Posterior open bite

¹ˢᵗ ₅ᵗʰ Additional Digit Required   Unacceptable PDx   Manifestation Code   Hospital Acquired Condition   ▶◀ Revised Text   ● New Code   ▲ Revised Code Title

014 ICD-9-CM   **February 2013 • Volume 1 – 173**

Angle's Classification of Malocclusion

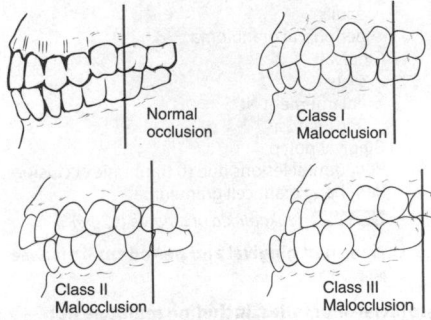

Normal occlusion

Class I Malocclusion

Class II Malocclusion

Class III Malocclusion

524.26 Excessive horizontal overlap
Excessive horizontal overjet

524.27 Reverse articulation
Anterior articulation   Posterior articulation
Crossbite

524.28 Anomalies of interarch distance
Excessive interarch distance
Inadequate interarch distance

524.29 Other anomalies of dental arch relationship
Other anomalies of dental arch

√5ᵗʰ **524.3 Anomalies of tooth position of fully erupted teeth**
EXCLUDES impacted or embedded teeth with abnormal position of such teeth or adjacent teeth (520.6)

524.30 Unspecified anomaly of tooth position
Diastema of teeth NOS
Displacement of teeth NOS
Transposition of teeth NOS

524.31 Crowding of teeth

524.32 Excessive spacing of teeth

524.33 Horizontal displacement of teeth
Tipped teeth   Tipping of teeth

524.34 Vertical displacement of teeth
Extruded tooth   Intruded tooth
Infraeruption of teeth   Supraeruption of teeth

524.35 Rotation of tooth/teeth

524.36 Insufficient interocclusal distance of teeth (ridge)
Lack of adequate intermaxillary vertical dimension

524.37 Excessive interocclusal distance of teeth
Excessive intermaxillary vertical dimension
Loss of occlusal vertical dimension

524.39 Other anomalies of tooth position

524.4 Malocclusion, unspecified
DEF: Malposition of top and bottom teeth; interferes with chewing.

√5ᵗʰ **524.5 Dentofacial functional abnormalities**

524.50 Dentofacial functional abnormality, unspecified

524.51 Abnormal jaw closure

524.52 Limited mandibular range of motion

524.53 Deviation in opening and closing of the mandible

524.54 Insufficient anterior guidance
Insufficient anterior occlusal guidance

524.55 Centric occlusion maximum intercuspation discrepancy
Centric occlusion of teeth discrepancy

524.56 Non-working side interference
Balancing side interference

524.57 Lack of posterior occlusal support

524.59 Other dentofacial functional abnormalities
Abnormal swallowing
Mouth breathing
Sleep postures
Tongue, lip, or finger habits

√5ᵗʰ **524.6 Temporomandibular joint disorders**
EXCLUDES current temporomandibular joint:
dislocation (830.0-830.1)
strain (848.1)

524.60 Temporomandibular joint disorders, unspecified
Temporomandibular joint-pain-dysfunction syndrome [TMJ]

524.61 Adhesions and ankylosis (bony or fibrous)
DEF: Stiffening or union of temporomandibular joint due to bony or fibrous union across joint.

524.62 Arthralgia of temporomandibular joint
DEF: Pain in temporomandibular joint; not inflammatory in nature.

524.63 Articular disc disorder (reducing or non-reducing)

524.64 Temporomandibular joint sounds on opening and/or closing the jaw

524.69 Other specified temporomandibular joint disorders

√5ᵗʰ **524.7 Dental alveolar anomalies**

524.70 Unspecified alveolar anomaly

524.71 Alveolar maxillary hyperplasia
DEF: Excessive tissue formation in the dental alveoli of upper jaw.

524.72 Alveolar mandibular hyperplasia
DEF: Excessive tissue formation in the dental alveoli of lower jaw.

524.73 Alveolar maxillary hypoplasia
DEF: Incomplete or underdeveloped alveolar tissue of upper jaw.

524.74 Alveolar mandibular hypoplasia
DEF: Incomplete or underdeveloped alveolar tissue of lower jaw.

524.75 Vertical displacement of alveolus and teeth
Extrusion of alveolus and teeth

524.76 Occlusal plane deviation

524.79 Other specified alveolar anomaly

√5ᵗʰ **524.8 Other specified dentofacial anomalies**

524.81 Anterior soft tissue impingement

524.82 Posterior soft tissue impingement

524.89 Other specified dentofacial anomalies

524.9 Unspecified dentofacial anomalies

√4ᵗʰ **525 Other diseases and conditions of the teeth and supporting structures**

525.0 Exfoliation of teeth due to systemic causes
DEF: Deterioration of teeth and surrounding structures due to systemic disease.

√5ᵗʰ **525.1 Loss of teeth due to trauma, extraction, or periodontal disease**
Code first class of edentulism (525.40-525.44, 525.50-525.54)
AHA: 4Q, '05, 74; 4Q, '01, 44

525.10 *Acquired absence of teeth, unspecified*
Tooth extraction status, NOS

525.11 *Loss of teeth due to trauma*

525.12 *Loss of teeth due to periodontal disease*

525.13 *Loss of teeth due to caries*

525.19 *Other loss of teeth*

√5ᵗʰ **525.2 Atrophy of edentulous alveolar ridge**

525.20 Unspecified atrophy of edentulous alveolar ridge
Atrophy of the mandible NOS
Atrophy of the maxilla NOS

525.21 Minimal atrophy of the mandible

525.22 Moderate atrophy of the mandible

525.23 Severe atrophy of the mandible

525.24 Minimal atrophy of the maxilla

525.25 Moderate atrophy of the maxilla

N Newborn Age: 0   P Pediatric Age: 0-17   M Maternity Age: 12-55   A Adult Age: 15-124   MCC Major CC Condition   CC CC Condition   HIV HIV Related Dx

174 – Volume 1   2014 ICD-9-CM

525.26 Severe atrophy of the maxilla

525.3 Retained dental root

√5ᵗʰ **525.4 Complete edentulism**
Use additional code to identify cause of edentulism (525.10-525.19)
AHA: 4Q, '05, 74

525.40 Complete edentulism, unspecified
Edentulism NOS

525.41 Complete edentulism, class I

525.42 Complete edentulism, class II

525.43 Complete edentulism, class III

525.44 Complete edentulism, class IV

√5ᵗʰ **525.5 Partial edentulism**
Use additional code to identify cause of edentulism (525.10-525.19)
AHA: 4Q, '05, 74

525.50 Partial edentulism, unspecified

525.51 Partial edentulism, class I

525.52 Partial edentulism, class II

525.53 Partial edentulism, class III

525.54 Partial edentulism, class IV

√5ᵗʰ **525.6 Unsatisfactory restoration of tooth**
Defective bridge, crown, fillings
Defective dental restoration
EXCLUDES dental restoration status (V45.84)
unsatisfactory endodontic treatment (526.61-526.69)

525.60 Unspecified unsatisfactory restoration of tooth
Unspecified defective dental restoration

525.61 Open restoration margins
Dental restoration failure of marginal integrity
Open margin on tooth restoration

525.62 Unrepairable overhanging of dental restorative materials
Overhanging of tooth restoration

525.63 Fractured dental restorative material without loss of material
EXCLUDES cracked tooth (521.81)
fractured tooth (873.63, 873.73)

525.64 Fractured dental restorative material with loss of material
EXCLUDES cracked tooth (521.81)
fractured tooth (873.63, 873.73)

525.65 Contour of existing restoration of tooth biologically incompatible with oral health
Dental restoration failure of periodontal anatomical integrity
Unacceptable contours of existing restoration
Unacceptable morphology of existing restoration

525.66 Allergy to existing dental restorative material
Use additional code to identify the specific type of allergy

525.67 Poor aesthetics of existing restoration
Dental restoration aesthetically inadequate or displeasing

525.69 Other unsatisfactory restoration of existing tooth

√5ᵗʰ **525.7 Endosseous dental implant failure**

525.71 Osseointegration failure of dental implant
Failure of dental implant due to infection
Failure of dental implant due to unintentional loading
Failure of dental implant osseointegration due to premature loading
Failure of dental implant to osseointegrate prior to intentional prosthetic loading
Hemorrhagic complications of dental Implant placement
Iatrogenic osseointegration failure of dental implant
Osseointegration failure of dental implant due to complications of systemic disease
Osseointegration failure of dental implant due to poor bone quality
Pre-integration failure of dental implant NOS
Pre-osseointegration failure of dental implant

525.72 Post-osseointegration biological failure of dental implant
Failure of dental implant due to lack of attached gingiva
Failure of dental implant due to occlusal trauma (caused by poor prosthetic design)
Failure of dental implant due to parafunctional habits
Failure of dental implant due to periodontal infection (peri-implantitis)
Failure of dental implant due to poor oral hygiene
Failure of dental implant to osseointegrate following intentional prosthetic loading
Iatrogenic post-osseointegration failure of dental implant
Post-osseointegration failure of dental implant due to complications of systemic disease

525.73 Post-osseointegration mechanic failure of dental implant
Failure of dental prosthesis causing loss of dental implant
Fracture of dental implant
Mechanical failure of dental implant NOS
EXCLUDES cracked tooth (521.81)
fractured dental restorative material with loss of material (525.64)
fractured dental restorative material without loss of material (525.63)
fractured tooth (873.63, 873.73)

525.79 Other endosseous dental implant failure
Dental implant failure NOS

525.8 Other specified disorders of the teeth and supporting structures
Enlargement of alveolar ridge NOS
Irregular alveolar process

525.9 Unspecified disorder of the teeth and supporting structures

√4ᵗʰ **526 Diseases of the jaws**

526.0 Developmental odontogenic cysts
Cyst: Cyst:
dentigerous   lateral periodontal
eruption   primordial
follicular   Keratocyst
lateral developmental
EXCLUDES radicular cyst (522.8)

526.1 Fissural cysts of jaw
Cyst: Cyst:
globulomaxillary   median palatal
incisor canal   nasopalatine
median anterior maxillary   palatine of papilla
EXCLUDES cysts of oral soft tissues (528.4)

526.2 Other cysts of jaws
Cyst of jaw: Cyst of jaw:
NOS   hemorrhagic
aneurysmal   traumatic

526.3 Central giant cell (reparative) granuloma
EXCLUDES peripheral giant cell granuloma (523.8)

4ᵗʰ 5ᵗʰ Additional Digit Required   Unacceptable PDx   Manifestation Code   Hospital Acquired Condition   ►◄ Revised Text   ● New Code   ▲ Revised Code Title

2014 ICD-9-CM   Volume 1 – 175

526.4 Inflammatory conditions

Abscess
Osteitis
Osteomyelitis (neonatal) } of jaw (acute) (chronic)
Periostitis (suppurative)

Sequestrum of jaw bone
EXCLUDES alveolar osteitis (526.5)
osteonecrosis of jaw (733.45)

526.5 Alveolitis of jaw

Alveolar osteitis　　Dry socket
DEF: Inflammation of alveoli or tooth socket.

√5ᵗʰ 526.6 Periradicular pathology associated with previous endodontic treatment

526.61 Perforation of root canal space

526.62 Endodontic overfill

526.63 Endodontic underfill

526.69 Other periradicular pathology associated with previous endodontic treatment

√5ᵗʰ 526.8 Other specified diseases of the jaws

526.81 Exostosis of jaw
Torus mandibularis　　Torus palatinus
DEF: Spur or bony outgrowth on the jaw.

526.89 Other
Cherubism
Fibrous dysplasia } of jaw(s)
Latent bone cyst
Osteoradionecrosis

Unilateral condylar hyperplasia or hypoplasia of mandible

526.9 Unspecified disease of the jaws
AHA: 4Q, '10, 93-94

√4ᵗʰ 527 Diseases of the salivary glands

527.0 Atrophy
DEF: Wasting away, necrosis of salivary gland tissue.

527.1 Hypertrophy
DEF: Overgrowth or overdeveloped salivary gland tissue.

527.2 Sialoadenitis
Parotitis:　　　　　Sialoangitis
NOS　　　　　　　Sialodochitis
allergic
toxic
EXCLUDES epidemic or infectious parotitis (072.0-072.9)
uveoparotid fever (135)
DEF: Inflammation of salivary gland.

527.3 Abscess `CC`
CC Excl: 527.0-527.9, 537.89-538

527.4 Fistula `CC`
EXCLUDES congenital fistula of salivary gland (750.24)
CC Excl: See code: 527.3

527.5 Sialolithiasis
Calculus
Stone } of salivary gland or duct
Sialodocholithiasis

527.6 Mucocele
Mucous:
extravasation cyst of salivary gland
retention cyst of salivary gland
Ranula
DEF: Dilated salivary gland cavity filled with mucous.

527.7 Disturbance of salivary secretion
Hyposecretion　　Sialorrhea
Ptyalism　　　　　Xerostomia

527.8 Other specified diseases of the salivary glands
Benign lymphoepithelial lesion of salivary gland
Sialectasia
Sialosis
Stenosis } of salivary duct
Stricture

527.9 Unspecified disease of the salivary glands

√4ᵗʰ 528 Diseases of the oral soft tissues, excluding lesions specific for gingiva and tongue

√5ᵗʰ 528.0 Stomatitis and mucositis (ulcerative)
EXCLUDES cellulitis and abscess of mouth (528.3)
diphtheritic stomatitis (032.0)
epizootic stomatitis (078.4)
gingivitis (523.0-523.1)
oral thrush (112.0)
Stevens-Johnson syndrome (695.13)
stomatitis:
acute necrotizing ulcerative (101)
aphthous (528.2)
gangrenous (528.1)
herpetic (054.2)
Vincent's (101)
DEF: Stomatitis: Inflammation of oral mucosa; labial and buccal mucosa, tongue, palate, floor of the mouth, and gingivae.
AHA: 2Q, '99, 9
TIP: Do not assign if documented as fungal oral thrush, or as due to candidiasis. See instead 112.0.

528.00 Stomatitis and mucositis, unspecified
Mucositis NOS
Ulcerative mucositis NOS
Ulcerative stomatitis NOS
Vesicular stomatitis NOS
AHA: 4Q, '06, 88-90

528.01 Mucositis (ulcerative) due to antineoplastic therapy
Use additional E code to identify adverse effects of therapy, such as:
antineoplastic and immunosuppressive drugs (E930.7, E933.1)
radiation therapy (E879.2)
AHA: 4Q, '06, 88-90

528.02 Mucositis (ulcerative) due to other drugs
Use additional E code to identify drug
AHA: 4Q, '06, 88-90

528.09 Other stomatitis and mucositis (ulcerative)
AHA: 4Q, '06, 88-90

528.1 Cancrum oris
Gangrenous stomatitis　　　　Noma
DEF: A severely gangrenous lesion of mouth due to fusospirochetal infection; destroys buccal, labial and facial tissues; can be fatal; found primarily in debilitated and malnourished children.

528.2 Oral aphthae
Aphthous stomatitis
Canker sore
Periadenitis mucosa necrotica recurrens
Recurrent aphthous ulcer
Stomatitis herpetiformis
EXCLUDES herpetic stomatitis (054.2)
DEF: Small oval or round ulcers of the mouth marked by a grayish exudate and a red halo effect.
AHA: ▶2Q, '12, 18◄

528.3 Cellulitis and abscess `CC`
Cellulitis of mouth (floor)　　　　Oral fistula
Ludwig's angina
EXCLUDES abscess of tongue (529.0)
cellulitis or abscess of lip (528.5)
fistula (of):
dental (522.7)
lip (528.5)
gingivitis (523.00-523.11)
CC Excl: 528.00-528.09, 528.3, 529.0, 529.2

528.4 Cysts
Dermoid cyst
Epidermoid cyst
Epstein's pearl } or mouth
Lymphoepithelial cyst
Nasoalveolar cyst
Nasolabial cyst

EXCLUDES cyst:
gingiva (523.8)
tongue (529.8)

 Newborn Age: 0　　 Pediatric Age: 0-17　　M Maternity Age: 12-55　　A Adult Age: 15-124　　MCC Major CC Condition　　CC CC Condition　　HIV HIV Related D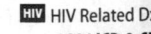

176 – Volume 1 • February 2013　　　　　　　　　　　　　　　　　　　　　　　　　　　　　2014 ICD-9-CM

528.5 Diseases of lips

Abscess
Cellulitis
Fistula } of lips
Hypertrophy

Cheilitis:
  NOS
  angular
Cheilodynia
Cheilosis

EXCLUDES actinic cheilitis (692.79)
  congenital fistula of lip (750.25)
  leukoplakia of lips (528.6)

AHA: S-O, '86, 10

528.6 Leukoplakia of oral mucosa, including tongue

Leukokeratosis of oral mucosa   Leukoplakia of:
Leukoplakia of: lips
  gingiva   tongue

EXCLUDES carcinoma in situ (230.0, 232.0)
  leukokeratosis nicotina palati (528.79)

DEF: Thickened white patches of epithelium on mucous membranes of mouth.

√5ᵗʰ **528.7 Other disturbances of oral epithelium, including tongue**

EXCLUDES carcinoma in situ (230.0, 232.0)
  leukokeratosis NOS (702.8)

528.71 Minimal keratinized residual ridge mucosa
Minimal keratinization of alveolar ridge mucosa

528.72 Excessive keratinized residual ridge mucosa
Excessive keratinization of alveolar ridge mucosa

528.79 Other disturbances of oral epithelium, including tongue
Erythroplakia of mouth or tongue
Focal epithelial hyperplasia of mouth or tongue
Leukoedema of mouth or tongue
Leukokeratosis nicotina palate
Other oral epithelium disturbances

528.8 Oral submucosal fibrosis, including of tongue

528.9 Other and unspecified diseases of the oral soft tissues
Cheek and lip biting
Denture sore mouth
Denture stomatitis
Melanoplakia
Papillary hyperplasia of palate

Eosinophilic granuloma
Irritative hyperplasisa } of oral mucosa
Pyogenic granuloma
Ulcer (traumatic)

√4ᵗʰ **529 Diseases and other conditions of the tongue**

529.0 Glossitis

Abscess
Ulceration (traumatic) } of tongue

EXCLUDES glossitis:
  benign migratory (529.1)
  Hunter's (529.4)
  median rhomboid (529.2)
  Moeller's (529.4)

529.1 Geographic tongue
Benign migratory glossitis   Glossitis areata exfoliativa
DEF: Chronic glossitis; marked by filiform papillae atrophy and inflammation; no known etiology.

529.2 Median rhomboid glossitis
DEF: A noninflammatory, congenital disease characterized by rhomboid-like lesions at the middle third of the tongue's dorsal surface.

529.3 Hypertrophy of tongue papillae
Black hairy tongue   Hypertrophy of foliate papillae
Coated tongue   Lingua villosa nigra

529.4 Atrophy of tongue papillae
Bald tongue   Glossitis:
Glazed tongue   Moeller's
Glossitis: Glossodynia exfoliativa
  Hunter's   Smooth atrophic tongue

529.5 Plicated tongue

Fissured
Furrowed } tongue
Scrotal

EXCLUDES fissure of tongue, congenital (750.13)
DEF: Cracks, fissures or furrows, on dorsal surface of tongue.

529.6 Glossodynia
Glossopyrosis
Painful tongue
EXCLUDES glossodynia exfoliativa (529.4)

529.8 Other specified conditions of the tongue

Atrophy
Crenated
Enlargement } (of) tongue
Hypertrophy

Glossocele
Glossoptosis

EXCLUDES erythroplasia of tongue (528.79)
  leukoplakia of tongue (528.6)
  macroglossia (congenital) (750.15)
  microglossia (congenital) (750.16)
  oral submucosal fibrosis (528.8)

529.9 Unspecified condition of the tongue

Diseases of Esophagus, Stomach, and Duodenum (530-539)

√4ᵗʰ **530 Diseases of esophagus**
EXCLUDES esophageal varices (456.0-456.2)

530.0 Achalasia and cardiospasm
Achalasia (of cardia)   Megaesophagus
Aperistalsis of esophagus
EXCLUDES congenital cardiospasm (750.7)
DEF: Failure of smooth muscle fibers to relax at gastrointestinal junctures; such as esophagogastric sphincter when swallowing.

√5ᵗʰ **530.1 Esophagitis**

Esophagitis: Esophagitis:
  chemical   postoperative
  peptic   regurgitant

Use additional E code to identify cause, if induced by chemical
EXCLUDES tuberculous esophagitis (017.8)
AHA: 4Q, '93, 27; 1Q, '92, 17; 3Q, '91, 20
TIP: Do not assign if esophagitis due to candidiasis; see instead code 112.84.

530.10 Esophagitis, unspecified
Esophagitis NOS
AHA: 3Q, '05, 17

530.11 Reflux esophagitis
DEF: Inflammation of lower esophagus; due to regurgitated gastric acid.
AHA: 4Q, '95, 82
K21.0 Gastro-esophageal reflux disease w/esophagitis I-10

530.12 Acute esophagitis CC
DEF: An acute inflammation of the mucous lining or submucosal coat of the esophagus.
CC Excl: 530.10-530.21, 530.4, 530.7, 530.82, 530.85-530.89
AHA: 4Q, '01, 45

530.13 Eosinophilic esophagitis
AHA: 4Q, '08, 115-116

Esophagus

Pharyngeal constrictors
Front view
Epiglottis
Cricoid cartilage
Trachea
C6
Pharyngoesophageal sphincter
Side view
Gastroesophageal sphincter
Diaphragm
Stomach

4ᵗʰ 5ᵗʰ Additional Digit Required   Unacceptable PDx   Manifestation Code   Hospital Acquired Condition   ▶◀ Revised Text   ● New Code   ▲ Revised Code Title

2014 ICD-9-CM   Volume 1 – 177

Diseases of the Digestive System

530.19–531.7

530.19 Other esophagitis
Abscess of esophagus
AHA: 3Q, '01, 10
K20.8 Other esophagitis   `I-10`

√5th 530.2 Ulcer of esophagus
Ulcer of esophagus:
  fungal
  peptic
Ulcer of esophagus due to ingestion of:
  aspirin
  chemicals
  medicines
Use additional E code to identify cause, if induced by chemical or drug
AHA: 4Q, '03, 63

530.20 Ulcer of esophagus without bleeding   `CC`
Ulcer of esophagus NOS
CC Excl: 530.21, 530.89-530.9, 537.84

530.21 Ulcer of esophagus with bleeding   `MCC`
EXCLUDES bleeding esophageal varices (456.0, 456.20)
CC Excl: 251.5, 456.0, 530.20-530.21, 530.7, 530.82, 530.85, 531.00-534.91, 535.01, 535.11, 535.21, 535.31, 535.41, 535.51, 535.61, 535.71, 537.83, 537.89-538, 562.02-562.03, 562.12-562.13, 569.3, 569.85, 578.0-578.9

530.3 Stricture and stenosis of esophagus
Compression of esophagus   Obstruction of esophagus
EXCLUDES congenital stricture of esophagus (750.3)
AHA: 1Q, '12, 15; 2Q, '01, 4; 2Q, '97, 3; 1Q, '88, 13
TIP: If esophageal obstruction is due to impacted foreign body, such as meat or other substance, assign instead code 935.1.
K22.2 Esophageal obstruction   `I-10`

530.4 Perforation of esophagus   `MCC`
Rupture of esophagus
EXCLUDES traumatic perforation of esophagus (862.22, 862.32, 874.4-874.5)
CC Excl: 530.4, 530.7-530.81, 530.83-530.84, 530.89-530.9

530.5 Dyskinesia of esophagus
Corkscrew esophagus   Esophagospasm
Curling esophagus   Spasm of esophagus
EXCLUDES cardiospasm (530.0)
DEF: Difficulty performing voluntary esophageal movements.
AHA: 1Q, '88, 13; N-D, '84, 19

530.6 Diverticulum of esophagus, acquired
Diverticulum, acquired: Diverticulum, acquired:
  epiphrenic   traction
  pharyngoesophageal   Zenker's (hypopharyngeal)
  pulsion   Esophageal pouch, acquired
  subdiaphragmatic   Esophagocele, acquired
EXCLUDES congenital diverticulum of esophagus (750.4)
AHA: J-F, '85, 3

530.7 Gastroesophageal laceration-hemorrhage syndrome   `MCC`
Mallory-Weiss syndrome
DEF: Laceration of distal esophagus and proximal stomach due to vomiting, hiccups or other sustained activity.
CC Excl: 251.5, 456.0, 530.20-530.21, 530.4, 530.7-530.85, 530.89-534.91, 535.01, 535.11, 535.21, 535.31, 535.41, 535.51, 535.61, 535.71, 537.83, 562.02-562.03, 562.12-562.13, 569.3, 569.85, 578.0-578.9

√5th 530.8 Other specified disorders of esophagus

530.81 Esophageal reflux
Gastroesophageal reflux
EXCLUDES reflux esophagitis (530.11)
DEF: Regurgitation of the gastric contents into esophagus and possibly pharynx.
AHA: 4Q, '10, 97; 2Q, '01, 4; 1Q, '95, 7; 4Q, '92, 27
K21.9 Gastro-esophageal reflux dz w/o esophagitis   `I-10`

530.82 Esophageal hemorrhage   `MCC`
EXCLUDES hemorrhage due to esophageal varices (456.0-456.2)
CC Excl: 251.5, 456.0, 456.20, 459.89-459.9, 530.20-530.21, 530.7, 530.82, 530.85, 531.00-534.91, 535.01, 535.11, 535.21, 535.31, 535.41, 535.51, 535.61, 537.83, 562.02-562.03, 562.12-562.13, 569.3, 569.85, 578.0-578.9
AHA: 1Q, '05, 17

530.83 Esophageal leukoplakia

530.84 Tracheoesophageal fistula   `MCC`
EXCLUDES congenital tracheoesophageal fistula (750.3)
CC Excl: 530.4, 530.7-530.81, 530.83-530.84, 530.89-530.9

530.85 Barrett's esophagus
DEF: A metaplastic disorder in which specialized columnar epithelial cells replace the normal squamous epithelial cells; secondary to chronic gastroesophageal reflux damage to the mucosa; increases risk of developing adenocarcinoma.
AHA: 4Q, '03, 63
K22.70 Barrett's esophagus w/o dysphagia   `I-10`

530.86 Infection of esophagostomy   `CC`
Use additional code to specify infection
CC Excl: 530.86-530.87, 536.40-536.49, 539.01-539.89, 569.71-569.79, 997.41-997.49, 997.71, 997.91-997.99, 998.81, 998.83-998.9

530.87 Mechanical complication of esophagostomy   `CC`
Malfunction of esophagostomy
CC Excl: See code: 530.86

530.89 Other
EXCLUDES Paterson-Kelly syndrome (280.8)

530.9 Unspecified disorder of esophagus

√4th 531 Gastric ulcer
INCLUDES ulcer (peptic):
  prepyloric
  pylorus
  stomach
Use additional E code to identify drug, if drug-induced
EXCLUDES peptic ulcer NOS (533.0-533.9)

The following fifth-digit subclassification is for use with category 531:
  0 without mention of obstruction
  1 with obstruction

DEF: Destruction of tissue in lumen of stomach due to action of gastric acid and pepsin on gastric mucosa decreasing resistance to ulcers.
AHA: 1Q, '91, 15; 4Q, '90, 27

§ √5th 531.0 Acute with hemorrhage   `MCC`
[0-1]   **CC Excl:** 251.5, 456.0, 530.20-530.21, 530.7, 530.82, 530.85, 531.00-534.91, 535.01, 535.11, 535.21, 535.31, 535.41, 535.51, 535.61, 537.83, 537.89-538, 562.02-562.03, 562.12-562.13, 569.3, 569.85, 578.0-578.9
  AHA: N-D, '84, 15

§ √5th 531.1 Acute with perforation   `MCC`
[0-1]   **CC Excl:** See code 531.0

§ √5th 531.2 Acute with hemorrhage and perforation   `MCC`
[0-1]   **CC Excl:** See code 531.0

§ √5th 531.3 Acute without mention of hemorrhage or perforation   `MCC 1` `CC 0`
[0-1]   **CC Excl:** See code 531.0

§ √5th 531.4 Chronic or unspecified with hemorrhage   `MCC`
[0-1]   **CC Excl:** See code 531.0
  AHA: 4Q, '90, 22
  K25.4 Chronic/unspecified gastric ulcer w/hemorrhage   `I-10`

§ √5th 531.5 Chronic or unspecified with perforation   `MCC`
[0-1]   **CC Excl:** See code 531.0

§ √5th 531.6 Chronic or unspecified with hemorrhage and perforation   `MCC`
[0-1]   **CC Excl:** See code 531.0

§ √5th 531.7 Chronic without mention of hemorrhage or perforation   `MCC`
[0-1]   **CC Excl:** For code 531.71: see code 531.0

---

§   Requires fifth digit. Valid digits are in [brackets] under each code. See category 531 for codes and definitions.

`N` Newborn Age: 0   `P` Pediatric Age: 0-17   `M` Maternity Age: 12-55   `A` Adult Age: 15-124   `MCC` Major CC Condition   `CC` CC Condition   `HIV` HIV Related Dx

178 – Volume 1   **2014 ICD-9-CM**

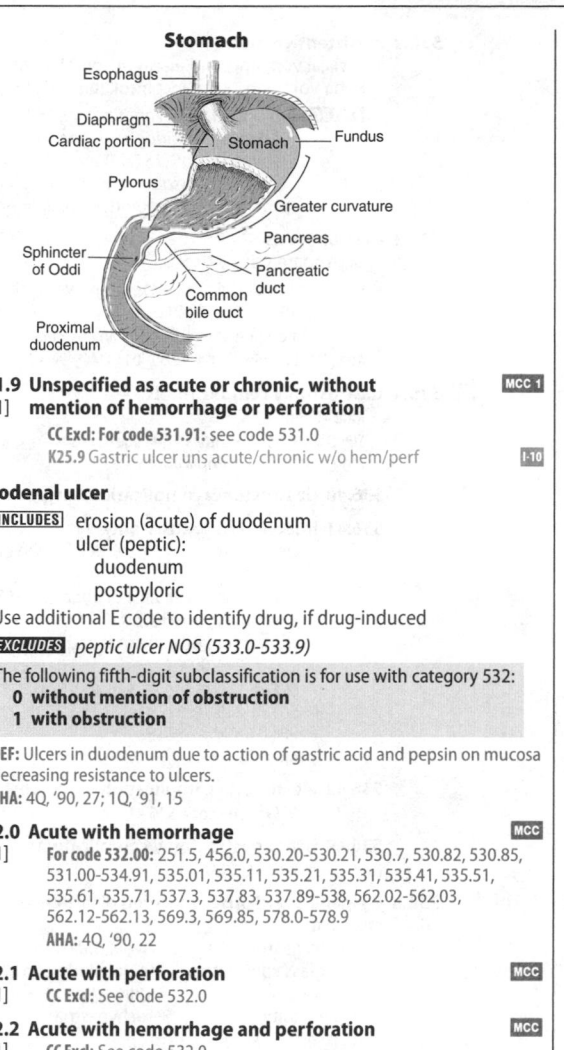

Stomach

§ ✓5ᵗʰ **531.9 Unspecified as acute or chronic, without**   `MCC 1`
[0-1]   **mention of hemorrhage or perforation**
          CC Excl: For code 531.91: see code 531.0
          K25.9 Gastric ulcer uns acute/chronic w/o hem/perf   `I-10`

✓4ᵗʰ **532 Duodenal ulcer**
    `INCLUDES`   erosion (acute) of duodenum
                ulcer (peptic):
                    duodenum
                    postpyloric
    Use additional E code to identify drug, if drug-induced
    `EXCLUDES` *peptic ulcer NOS (533.0-533.9)*

> The following fifth-digit subclassification is for use with category 532:
> **0 without mention of obstruction**
> **1 with obstruction**

    DEF: Ulcers in duodenum due to action of gastric acid and pepsin on mucosa decreasing resistance to ulcers.
    AHA: 4Q, '90, 27; 1Q, '91, 15

§ ✓5ᵗʰ **532.0 Acute with hemorrhage**   `MCC`
[0-1]   **For code 532.00:** 251.5, 456.0, 530.20-530.21, 530.7, 530.82, 530.85, 531.00-534.91, 535.01, 535.11, 535.21, 535.31, 535.41, 535.51, 535.61, 535.71, 537.3, 537.83, 537.89-538, 562.02-562.03, 562.12-562.13, 569.3, 569.85, 578.0-578.9
          AHA: 4Q, '90, 22

§ ✓5ᵗʰ **532.1 Acute with perforation**   `MCC`
[0-1]   **CC Excl:** See code 532.0

§ ✓5ᵗʰ **532.2 Acute with hemorrhage and perforation**   `MCC`
[0-1]   **CC Excl:** See code 532.0

§ ✓5ᵗʰ **532.3 Acute without mention of hemorrhage or**   `MCC 1` `CC 0`
[0-1]   **perforation**
          For code 532.30: 251.5, 456.0, 530.7, 530.82, 531.00-534.91, 535.01, 535.11, 535.21, 535.31, 535.41, 535.51, 535.61, 535.71, 537.3, 537.83-538, 562.02-562.03, 562.12-562.13, 569.3, 569.85, 578.0-578.9; **For code 532.31:** 251.5, 456.0, 530.20-530.21, 530.7, 530.82, 530.85, 531.00-534.91, 535.01, 535.11, 535.21, 535.31, 535.41, 535.51, 535.61, 537.3, 537.83, 537.89-538, 562.02-562.03, 562.12-562.13, 569.3, 569.85, 578.0-578.9

§ ✓5ᵗʰ **532.4 Chronic or unspecified with hemorrhage**   `MCC`
[0-1]   **CC Excl:** See code 532.0
          K26.4 Chronic/unspecified duodenal ulcer w/hemorrhage   `I-10`

§ ✓5ᵗʰ **532.5 Chronic or unspecified with perforation**   `MCC`
[0-1]   **CC Excl:** See code 532.0

§ ✓5ᵗʰ **532.6 Chronic or unspecified with hemorrhage and**   `MCC`
[0-1]   **perforation**
          CC Excl: See code 532.0

§ ✓5ᵗʰ **532.7 Chronic without mention of hemorrhage or**   `MCC 1`
[0-1]   **peforation**
          CC Excl: For code 532.71: See code 532.0

§ ✓5ᵗʰ **532.9 Unspecified as acute or chronic, without mention of**   `MCC 1`
[0-1]   **hemorrhage or perforation**
          CC Excl: For code 532.91: See code 532.0
          K26.9 Duodenal ulcer uns acute/chronic w/o hem/perf   `I-10`

✓4ᵗʰ **533 Peptic ulcer, site unspecified**
    `INCLUDES`   gastroduodenal ulcer NOS
                peptic ulcer NOS
                stress ulcer NOS
    Use additional E code to identify drug, if drug-induced
    `EXCLUDES` *peptic ulcer:*
                duodenal (532.0-532.9)
                gastric (531.0-531.9)

> The following fifth-digit subclassification is for use with category 533:
> **0 without mention of obstruction**
> **1 with obstruction**

    DEF: Ulcer of mucous membrane of esophagus, stomach or duodenum due to gastric acid secretion.
    AHA: 1Q, '91, 15; 4Q, '90, 27

§ ✓5ᵗʰ **533.0 Acute with hemorrhage**   `MCC`
[0-1]   **CC Excl:** See code 532.0

§ ✓5ᵗʰ **533.1 Acute with perforation**   `MCC`
[0-1]   **CC Excl:** See code 533.0

§ ✓5ᵗʰ **533.2 Acute with hemorrhage and perforation**   `MCC`
[0-1]   **CC Excl:** See code 533.0

§ ✓5ᵗʰ **533.3 Acute without mention of hemorrhage**   `MCC 1` `CC 0`
[0-1]   **and perforation**
          CC Excl: See: 533.0

§ ✓5ᵗʰ **533.4 Chronic or unspecified with hemorrhage**   `MCC`
[0-1]   **CC Excl:** See code 533.0

§ ✓5ᵗʰ **533.5 Chronic or unspecified with perforation**   `MCC`
[0-1]   **CC Excl:** See code 533.0

§ ✓5ᵗʰ **533.6 Chronic or unspecified with hemorrhage**   `MCC`
[0-1]   **and perforation**
          CC Excl: See code 533.0

§ ✓5ᵗʰ **533.7 Chronic without mention of hemorrhage or**   `MCC 1`
[0-1]   **perforation**
          CC Excl: For code 533.71: See code 533.0
          AHA: 2Q, '89, 16

§ ✓5ᵗʰ **533.9 Unspecified as acute or chronic, without**   `MCC 1`
[0-1]   **mention of hemorrhage or perforation**
          CC Excl: For code 533.91: See code 533.0

✓4ᵗʰ **534 Gastrojejunal ulcer**
    `INCLUDES`   ulcer (peptic) or erosion:
                anastomotic
                gastrocolic
                gastrointestinal
                gastrojejunal
                jejunal
                marginal
                stomal
    `EXCLUDES` *primary ulcer of small intestine (569.82)*

> The following fifth-digit subclassification is for use with category 534:
> **0 without mention of obstruction**
> **1 with obstruction**

    AHA: 1Q, '91, 15; 4Q, '90, 27

§ ✓5ᵗʰ **534.0 Acute with hemorrhage**   `MCC`
[0-1]   **CC Excl:** 251.5, 456.0, 530.20-530.21, 530.7, 530.82, 530.85, 531.00-534.91, 535.01, 535.11, 535.21, 535.31, 535.41, 535.51, 535.61, 537.83, 537.89-538, 562.02-562.03, 562.12-562.13, 569.3, 569.85, 578.0-578.9

§ ✓5ᵗʰ **534.1 Acute with perforation**   `MCC`
[0-1]   **CC Excl:** See code 534.0

§ ✓5ᵗʰ **534.2 Acute with hemorrhage and perforation**   `MCC`
[0-1]   **CC Excl:** See code 534.0

§ ✓5ᵗʰ **534.3 Acute without mention of hemorrhage**   `MCC 1` `CC 0`
[0-1]   **or perforation**
          CC Excl:: See code 534.0

§ ✓5ᵗʰ **534.4 Chronic or unspecified with hemorrhage**   `MCC`
[0-1]   **CC Excl:** See code 534.0

§ ✓5ᵗʰ **534.5 Chronic or unspecified with perforation**   `MCC`
[0-1]   **CC Excl:** See code 534.0

---

§   Requires fifth digit. Valid digits are in [brackets] under each code. See appropriate category for codes and definitions.

✓4ᵗʰ
✓5ᵗʰ Additional Digit Required   Unacceptable PDx   Manifestation Code   Hospital Acquired Condition   ▶◀ Revised Text   ● New Code   ▲ Revised Code Title

Diseases of the Digestive System

534.6–537.3

§ ✓5ᵗʰ **534.6 Chronic or unspecified with hemorrhage** `MCC`
[0-1] **and perforation**
     CC Excl: See code 534.0

§ ✓5ᵗʰ **534.7 Chronic without mention of hemorrhage or** `MCC 1`
[0-1] **perforation**
     CC Excl: For code 534.71: See code 534.0

§ ✓5ᵗʰ **534.9 Unspecified as acute or chronic, without** `MCC 1`
[0-1] **mention of hemorrhage or perforation**
     CC Excl: For code 534.91: See code 534.0

✓4ᵗʰ **535 Gastritis and duodenitis**
     The following fifth-digit subclassification is for use with category 535:
       0 without mention of hemorrhage
       1 with hemorrhage

     AHA: 2Q, '92, 9; 4Q, '91, 25

§ ✓5ᵗʰ **535.0 Acute gastritis** `MCC 1`
[0-1]   **For code 532.01:** 251.5, 456.0, 530.20-530.21, 530.7, 530.82, 530.85,
       531.00-534.91, 535.01, 535.11, 535.21, 535.31, 535.41, 535.51,
       535.61, 535.71, 537.83, 562.02-562.03, 562.12-562.13, 569.3, 569.85,
       578.0-578.9
     AHA: 2Q, '92, 8; N-D, '86, 9

§ ✓5ᵗʰ **535.1 Atrophic gastritis** `MCC 1`
[0-1]   Gastritis: Gastritis:
       atrophic-hyperplastic   chronic (atrophic)
     DEF: Inflammation of stomach, with mucous membrane atrophy and
     peptic gland destruction.
     CC Excl: For code 535.11: See code 535.01
     AHA: 1Q, '94, 18
     K29.50 Unspecified chronic gastritis without bleeding   `I-10`

§ ✓5ᵗʰ **535.2 Gastric mucosal hypertrophy** `MCC 1`
[0-1]   Hypertrophic gastritis
     CC Excl: For code 535.21: See code 535.01

§ ✓5ᵗʰ **535.3 Alcoholic gastritis** `MCC 1`
[0-1]   CC Excl: For code 535.31: See code 535.01

§ ✓5ᵗʰ **535.4 Other specified gastritis** `MCC 1`
[0-1]   Gastritis: Gastritis:
       allergic   superficial
       bile induced   toxic
       irritant
     EXCLUDES eosinophilic gastritis (535.7)
     CC Excl: For code 535.41: See code 535.01
     AHA: 4Q, '90, 27

§ ✓5ᵗʰ **535.5 Unspecified gastritis and gastroduodenitis** `MCC 1`
[0-1]   CC Excl: For code 535.51: See code 535.01
     AHA: For code 535.50: 3Q, '05, 17; 4Q, '99, 25

§ ✓5ᵗʰ **535.6 Duodenitis** `MCC 1`
[0-1]   **DEF:** Inflammation of intestine, between pylorus and jejunum.
     CC Excl: For code 535.61: See code 535.01
     AHA: For code 535.60: 3Q, '05, 17
     K29.80 Duodenitis without bleeding   `I-10`

§ ✓5ᵗʰ **535.7 Eosinophilic gastritis** `MCC 1`
[0-1]   CC Excl: For code 535.71: 251.5, 456.0, 530.20-530.21, 530.7, 530.82,
       530.85, 531.00-534.91, 535.01, 535.11, 535.21, 535.31, 535.41,
       535.51, 535.61-535.71, 537.83, 558.41, 562.02-562.03,
       562.12-562.13, 569.3, 569.85, 578.0-578.9
     AHA: 4Q, '08, 115-116

✓4ᵗʰ **536 Disorders of function of stomach**
     EXCLUDES functional disorders of stomach specified as psychogenic
         (306.4)

     536.0 Achlorhydria
       DEF: Absence of gastric acid due to gastric mucosa atrophy;
       unresponsive to histamines; also known as gastric anacidity.

     536.1 Acute dilatation of stomach `CC`
       Acute distention of stomach
       CC Excl: 536.1

     536.2 Persistent vomiting
       Cyclical vomiting   Persistent vomiting [not of pregnancy]
       Habit vomiting   Uncontrollable vomiting
       EXCLUDES bilious emesis (vomiting) (787.04)
          excessive vomiting in pregnancy (643.0-643.9)
          vomiting NOS (787.03)
            cyclical, associated with migraine (346.2)
          vomiting of fecal matter (569.87)

     536.3 Gastroparesis
       Gastroparalysis
       Code first underlying disease, if known, such as:
         diabetes mellitus (249.6, 250.6)
       DEF: Slight degree of paralysis within muscular coat of stomach.
       AHA: 4Q, '08, 94; 2Q, '04, 7; 2Q, '01, 4; 4Q, '94, 42

✓5ᵗʰ **536.4 Gastrostomy complications**
     AHA: 4Q, '98, 42
     TIP: Do not assign code 997.4 Digestive system complications, for
     any gastrostomy complications.

     536.40 Gastrostomy complication, unspecified

     536.41 Infection of gastrostomy `CC`
       Use additional code to specify type of infection, such
         as:
       abscess or cellulitis of abdomen (682.2)
       septicemia (038.0-038.9)
       Use additional code to identify organism
         (041.00-041.9)
       CC Excl: 530.86-530.87, 536.40-536.49, 539.01-539.89,
       569.71-569.79, 997.41-997.49, 997.71, 997.91-997.99,
       998.81, 998.83-998.9
       AHA: 4Q, '98, 42

     536.42 Mechanical complication of gastrostomy `CC`
       CC Excl: See code 536.41

     536.49 Other gastrostomy complications
       AHA: 4Q, '98, 42

     536.8 Dyspepsia and other specified disorders of function of
     stomach
       Achylia gastrica   Hyperchlorhydria
       Hourglass contraction   Hypochlorhydria
         of stomach   Indigestion
       Hyperacidity   Tachygastria
       EXCLUDES achlorhydria (536.0)
          heartburn (787.1)
       AHA: 2Q, '93, 6; 2Q, '89, 16; N-D, '84, 9
       K30 Functional dyspepsia   `I-10`

     536.9 Unspecified functional disorder of stomach
       Functional gastrointestinal: Functional gastrointestinal:
         disorder   irritation
         disturbance

✓4ᵗʰ **537 Other disorders of stomach and duodenum**

     537.0 Acquired hypertrophic pyloric stenosis `CC`
       Constriction
       Obstruction   } of pylorus, acquired or adult
       Stricture
       EXCLUDES congenital or infantile pyloric stenosis (750.5)
       CC Excl: 536.3, 536.8-537.0, 537.3, 750.5, 750.8-750.9, 751.1, 751.5
       AHA: 2Q, '01, 4; J-F, '85, 14

     537 .1 Gastric diverticulum
       EXCLUDES congenital diverticulum of stomach (750.7)
       DEF: Herniated sac or pouch within stomach or duodenum.
       AHA: J-F, '85, 4

     537.2 Chronic duodenal ileus
       DEF: Persistent obstruction between pylorus and jejunum.

     537.3 Other obstruction of duodenum `CC`
       Cicatrix
       Stenosis
       Stricture   } of duodenum
       Volvulus
       EXCLUDES congenital obstruction of duodenum (751.1)
       CC Excl: 537.3, 750.8-750.9, 751.1, 751.5

---

§   Requires fifth digit. Valid digits are in [brackets] under each code. See appropriate category for codes and definitions.

| `N` Newborn Age: 0 | `P` Pediatric Age: 0-17 | `M` Maternity Age: 12-55 | `A` Adult Age: 15-124 | `MCC` Major CC Condition | `CC` CC Condition | `HIV` HIV Related Dx |

Duodenum

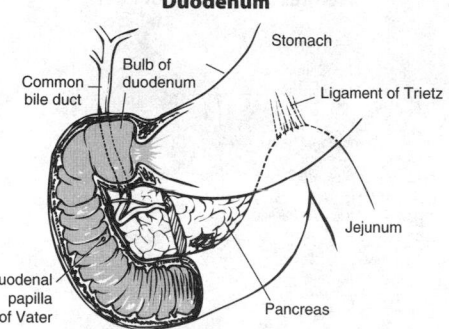

Common bile duct
Bulb of duodenum
Stomach
Ligament of Trietz
Jejunum
Pancreas
Duodenal papilla of Vater

537.4 Fistula of stomach or duodenum   [CC]
Gastrocolic fistula   Gastrojejunocolic fistula
CC Exd: 537.4, 750.8-750.9, 751.5
AHA: 1Q, '12, 10
TIP: Assign when a previous G-tube site has failed to spontaneously close and requires further treatment.

537.5 Gastroptosis
DEF: Downward displacement of stomach.

537.6 Hourglass stricture or stenosis of stomach
Cascade stomach
> *EXCLUDES*   *congenital hourglass stomach (750.7)*
>   *hourglass contraction of stomach (536.8)*

✓5ᵗʰ 537.8 Other specified disorders of stomach and duodenum
AHA: 4Q, '91, 25

537.81 Pylorospasm
> *EXCLUDES*   *congenital pylorospasm (750.5)*
DEF: Spasm of the pyloric sphincter.

537.82 Angiodysplasia of stomach and duodenum (without mention of hemorrhage)
AHA: 2Q, '07, 7; 3Q, '96, 10; 4Q, '90, 4

537.83 Angiodysplasia of stomach and duodenum with hemorrhage   [MCC]
CC Exd: 251.5, 456.0, 530.20-530.21, 530.7, 530.82, 530.85, 531.00-534.91, 535.01, 535.11, 535.21, 535.31, 535.41, 535.51, 535.61, 537.83, 562.02- 562.03, 562.12-562.13, 569.3, 569.85, 578.0-578.9
DEF: Bleeding of stomach and duodenum due to vascular abnormalities.
AHA: 2Q, '07, 7

537.84 Dieulafoy lesion (hemorrhagic) of stomach and duodenum   [MCC]
CC Exd: 251.5, 456.0, 530.20-530.21, 530.7, 530.82, 530.85, 531.00-534.91, 535.01, 535.11, 535.21, 535.31, 535.41, 535.51, 535.61, 535.71, 537.83-537.84, 562.02-562.03, 562.12-562.13, 569.3, 569.85, 578.0-578.9
DEF: An abnormally large and convoluted submucosal artery protruding through a defect in the mucosa in the stomach or intestines that can erode the epithelium causing hemorrhaging.
AHA: 4Q, '02, 60

537.89 Other
Gastric or duodenal:
     prolapse
     rupture
Intestinal metaplasia of gastric mucosa
Passive congestion of stomach
> *EXCLUDES*   *diverticula of duodenum (562.00-562.01)*
>   *gastrointestinal hemorrhage (578.0-578.9)*
AHA: 1Q, '11, 10-11; 3Q, '05, 15; N-D, '84, 7
TIP: Assign for congestive portal gastropathy or portal hypertensive gastropathy.

537.9 Unspecified disorder of stomach and duodenum

---

538 Gastrointestinal mucositis (ulcerative)   [CC]
Use additional E code to identify adverse effects of therapy, such as:
antineoplastic and immunosuppressive drugs (E930.7, E933.1)
radiation therapy (E879.2)
> *EXCLUDES*   *mucositis (ulcerative) of mouth and oral soft tissue (528.00-528.09)*
CC Exd: 251.5, 456.0, 530.20-530.21, 530.7, 530.82, 530.85, 531.00-534.91, 535.01, 535.11, 535.21, 535.31, 535.41, 535.51, 535.61, 537.83, 537.89-538, 562.02-562.03, 562.12-562.13, 569.3, 569.85, 578.0-578.9
AHA: 4Q, '06, 88-90

✓4ᵗʰ 539 Complications of bariatric procedures
TIP: If associated dumping syndrome is documented, assign also code 564.2.

✓5ᵗʰ 539.0 Complications of gastric band procedure
AHA: 4Q, '11, 125-127

¹⁴539.01 Infection due to gastric band procedure   [CC]
Use additional code to specify type of infection, such as:
     abscess or cellulitis of abdomen (682.2)
     septicemia (038.0-038.9)
Use additional code to identify organism (041.00-041.9)
CC Exd: 530.86-530.87, 536.40-536.49, 539.01-539.89, 569.71-569.79, 997.41-997.49, 997.71, 997.91-997.99, 998.81, 998.83-998.9
AHA: 4Q, '11, 127

539.09 Other complications of gastric band procedure   [CC]
Use additional code(s) to further specify the complication
CC Exd: See code 539.01

✓5ᵗʰ 539.8 Complications of other bariatric procedure
> *EXCLUDES*   *complications of gastric band procedure (539.01-539.09)*
AHA: 4Q, '11, 125-127

¹⁴539.81 Infection due to other bariatric procedure   [CC]
Use additional code to specify type of infection, such as:
     abscess or cellulitis of abdomen (682.2)
     septicemia (038.0-038.9)
Use additional code to identify organism (041.00-041.9)
CC Exd: 530.86-530.87, 536.40-536.49, 539.01-539.89, 569.71-569.79, 997.41-997.49, 997.71, 997.91-997.99, 998.81, 998.83-998.9

539.89 Other complications of other bariatric procedure   [CC]
Use additional code(s) to further specify the complication
CC Exd: See code 539.81

Appendicitis (540-543)

✓4ᵗʰ 540 Acute appendicitis
DEF: Inflammation of vermiform appendix due to fecal obstruction, neoplasm or foreign body of appendiceal lumen; causes infection, edema and infarction of appendiceal wall; may result in mural necrosis, and perforation.
AHA: N-D, '84, 19

540.0 With generalized peritonitis   [MCC]
Appendicitis (acute) with: { perforation / peritonitis (generalized) / rupture } { fulminating / gangrenous / obstructive }
Cecitis (acute) with perforation, peritonitis (generalized), rupture
Rupture of appendix
> *EXCLUDES*   *acute appendicitis with peritoneal abscess (540.1)*
CC Exd: 537.89-543.9
K35.2 Acute appendicitis w/generalized peritonitis   [I-10]

540.1 With peritoneal abscess   [MCC]
Abscess of appendix   With generalized peritonitis
CC Exd: See code 540.0
AHA: N-D, '84, 19

---

⁴ HAC = when in combination with principal diagnosis 278.01 and procedure code 44.38, 44.39, or 44.95.

| ⁴ᵗʰ/⁵ᵗʰ Additional Digit Required | Unacceptable PDx | Manifestation Code | Hospital Acquired Condition | ►◄ Revised Text | ● New Code | ▲ Revised Code Title |

2014 ICD-9-CM   **Volume 1 – 181**

Diseases of the Digestive System

540.9–551.9

Appendix

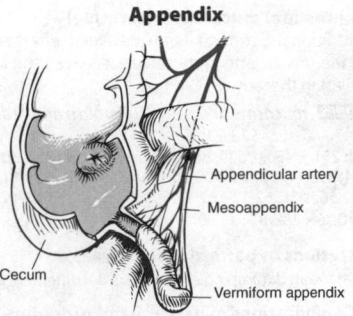

Appendicular artery

Mesoappendix

Cecum

Vermiform appendix

540.9 Without mention of peritonitis   `CC`
Acute appendicitis without mention of perforation, peritonitis, or rupture:
fulminating
gangrenous
inflamed
obstructive
Acute cecitis without mention of perforation, peritonitis, or rupture
CC Excl: See code 540.0
AHA: 1Q, '01, 15; 4Q, '97, 52
K35.80 Unspecified acute appendicitis   `I-10`

541 Appendicitis, unqualified
AHA: 2Q, '90, 26
TIP: Do not assign for normal appendix found at appendectomy. Assign instead symptom code (e.g., abdominal pain).

542 Other appendicitis
Appendicitis: Appendicitis:
chronic   relapsing
recurrent   subacute
EXCLUDES hyperplasia (lymphoid) of appendix (543.0)
AHA: 1Q, '01, 15

✓4ᵗʰ 543 Other diseases of appendix

543.0 Hyperplasia of appendix (lymphoid)
DEF: Proliferation of cells in appendix tissue.

543.9 Other and unspecified diseases of appendix
Appendicular or appendiceal:
colic
concretion
fistula
Diverticulum ⎫
Fecalith   ⎪
Intussusception ⎬ of appendix
Mucocele   ⎪
Stercolith   ⎭

Hernia of Abdominal Cavity (550-553)

INCLUDES hernia:
acquired
congenital, except diaphragmatic or hiatal

✓4ᵗʰ 550 Inguinal hernia
INCLUDES bubonocele
inguinal hernia (direct) (double) (indirect) (oblique) (sliding)
scrotal hernia

The following fifth-digit subclassification is for use with category 550:
0 unilateral or unspecified (not specified as recurrent)
Unilateral NOS
1 unilateral or unspecified, recurrent
2 bilateral (not specified as recurrent)
Bilateral NOS
3 bilateral, recurrent

DEF: Hernia protrusion of an abdominal organ or tissue through inguinal canal.
DEF: Indirect inguinal hernia: (external or oblique) leaves abdomen through deep inguinal ring, passes through inguinal canal lateral to the inferior epigastric artery.
DEF: Direct inguinal hernia: (internal) emerges between inferior epigastric artery and rectus muscle edge.
AHA: N-D, '85, 12

Hernias of Abdominal Cavity

Hiatal hernia
Diaphragm
Epigastric hernia
Incisional hernia
Umbilical hernia
Inguinal hernia

§ ✓5ᵗʰ 550.0 Inguinal hernia, with gangrene   `MCC`
[0-3]   Inguinal hernia with gangrene (and obstruction)
CC Excl: 537.89-538, 550.00-550.93, 552.8-552.9, 553.8-553.9

§ ✓5ᵗʰ 550.1 Inguinal hernia, with obstruction, without   `CC`
[0-3]   **mention of gangrene**
Inguinal hernia with mention of incarceration, irreducibility, or strangulation
CC Excl: See code 550.0

§ ✓5ᵗʰ 550.9 Inguinal hernia, without mention of obstruction or
[0-3]   **gangrene**
Inguinal hernia NOS
AHA: For code 550.91: 3Q, '03, 10; 1Q, '03, 4
K40.90 Uni ingin hernia w/o obst/gangrene not spec recur   `I-10`

✓4ᵗʰ 551 Other hernia of abdominal cavity, with gangrene
INCLUDES that with gangrene (and obstruction)

✓5ᵗʰ 551.0 Femoral hernia with gangrene

551.00 Unilateral or unspecified (not specified   `MCC`
as recurrent)
Femoral hernia NOS with gangrene
CC Excl: 537.89-538, 551.00-551.03, 552.8-553.03, 553.8-553.9

551.01 Unilateral or unspecified, recurrent   `MCC`
CC Excl: See code 551.00

551.02 Bilateral (not specified as recurrent)   `MCC`
CC Excl: See code 551.00

551.03 Bilateral, recurrent   `MCC`
CC Excl: See code 551.00

551.1 Umbilical hernia with gangrene   `MCC`
Parumbilical hernia specified as gangrenous
CC Excl: 537.89-538, 551.1-551.29, 552.1-552.29, 552.8-552.9, 553.1-553.29, 553.8-553.9

✓5ᵗʰ 551.2 Ventral hernia with gangrene

551.20 Ventral, unspecified, with gangrene   `MCC`
CC Excl: See code 551.1

551.21 Incisional, with gangrene   `MCC`
Hernia:
postoperative ⎫ specified as
recurrent, ventral ⎬ gangrenous
CC Excl: See code 551.1

551.29 Other   `MCC`
Epigastric hernia specified as gangrenous
CC Excl: See code 551.1

551.3 Diaphragmatic hernia with gangrene   `MCC`
Hernia:
hiatal (esophageal) (sliding) ⎫ specified as
paraesophageal   ⎬ gangrenous
Thoracic stomach   ⎭
EXCLUDES congenital diaphragmatic hernia (756.6)
CC Excl: 551.3, 552.3-552.9, 553.3-553.9

551.8 Hernia of other specified sites, with gangrene   `MCC`
Any condition classifiable to 553.8 if specified as gangrenous
CC Excl: 537.89-538, 550.00-553.9

551.9 Hernia of unspecified site, with gangrene   `MCC`
Any condition classifiable to 553.9 if specified as gangrenous
CC Excl: See code 551.8

---

§   Requires fifth digit. Valid digits are in [brackets] under each code. See category 550 for codes and definitions.

`N` Newborn Age: 0   `P` Pediatric Age: 0-17   `M` Maternity Age: 12-55   `A` Adult Age: 15-124   `MCC` Major CC Condition   `CC` CC Condition   `HIV` HIV Related Dx

182 – Volume 1   **2014 ICD-9-CM**

Inguinal Hernias

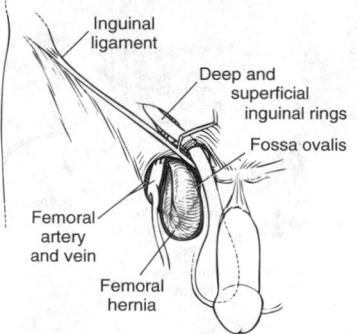

Abdominal wall

Spermatic cord

Inguinal ligament

Internal inguinal ring

Deep inferior epigastric artery and vein

Indirect hernia (internal inguinal ring)

Direct inguinal hernia (between deep inferior epigastric vessels and rectus fascia)

Incarcerated hernia

Femoral Hernia

Inguinal ligament

Deep and superficial inguinal rings

Fossa ovalis

Femoral artery and vein

Femoral hernia

552.3 Diaphragmatic hernia with obstruction   `CC`
Hernia:
hiatal (esophageal) ⎫ specified as caracerated,
(sliding)   ⎬ irreducible,
paraesophageal   ⎪ strangulated, or
Thoracic stomach ⎭ causing obstruction
    EXCLUDES congenital diaphragmatic hernia (756.6)
    CC Excl: 551.3, 552.3-552.9, 553.3-553.9

552.8 Hernia of other specified sites, with obstruction   `CC`
Any condition classifiable to 553.8 if specified as incarcerated, irreducible, strangulated, or causing obstruction
    CC Excl: 550.00-553.9
    AHA: 1Q, '04, 10

552.9 Hernia of unspecified site, with obstruction   `CC`
Any condition classifiable to 553.9 if specified as incarcerated, irreducible, strangulated, or causing obstruction
    CC Excl: See code: 552.8

√4ᵗʰ **553 Other hernia of abdominal cavity without mention of obstruction or gangrene**
    EXCLUDES the listed conditions with mention of:
        gangrene (and obstruction) (551.0-551.9)
        obstruction (552.0-552.9)

√5ᵗʰ **553.0 Femoral hernia**

    553.00 Unilateral or unspecified (not specified as recurrent)
        Femoral hernia NOS

    553.01 Unilateral or unspecified, recurrent

    553.02 Bilateral (not specified as recurrent)

    553.03 Bilateral, recurrent

553.1 Umbilical hernia
Parumbilical hernia
    K42.9 Umbilical hernia without obstruction/gangrene   `I-10`

√5ᵗʰ **553.2 Ventral hernia**

    553.20 Ventral, unspecified
        AHA: 2Q, '06, 10; 3Q, '03, 6

    553.21 Incisional
        Hernia:
          postoperative
          recurrent, ventral
        AHA: 3Q, '03, 6
        K43.2 Incisional hernia w/o obstruction or gangrene   `I-10`

    553.29 Other
        Hernia:
          epigastric
          spigelian

√4ᵗʰ **552 Other hernia of abdominal cavity, with obstruction, but without mention of gangrene**
    EXCLUDES that with mention of gangrene (551.0-551.9)

√5ᵗʰ **552.0 Femoral hernia with obstruction**
Femoral hernia specified as incarcerated, irreducible, strangulated, or causing obstruction

    552.00 Unilateral or unspecified (not specified as recurrent)   `CC`
        CC Excl: 537.89-538, 551.00-551.03, 552.00-552.03, 552.8-553.03, 553.8-553.9

    552.01 Unilateral or unspecified, recurrent   `CC`
        CC Excl: See code 552.00

    552.02 Bilateral (not specified as recurrent)   `CC`
        CC Excl: See code 552.00

    552.03 Bilateral, recurrent   `CC`
        CC Excl: See code 552.00

552.1 Umbilical hernia with obstruction   `CC`
Parumbilical hernia specified as incarcerated, irreducible, strangulated, or causing obstruction
    CC Excl: 551.1-551.29, 552.1-552.29, 552.8-552.9, 553.8-553.9

√5ᵗʰ **552.2 Ventral hernia with obstruction**
Ventral hernia specified as incarcerated, irreducible, strangulated, or causing obstruction

    552.20 Ventral, unspecified, with obstruction   `CC`
        CC Excl: See code 552.1
        AHA: 2Q, '11, 18

    552.21 Incisional, with obstruction   `CC`
        Hernia:
          postoperative ⎫ specified as incarcerated,
          recurrent,   ⎬ irreducible, strangulated,
          ventral   ⎭ or causing obstruction
        CC Excl: See code 552.1
        AHA: 1Q, '12, 8; 3Q, '03, 11

    552.29 Other   `CC`
        Epigastric hernia specified as incarcerated, irreducible, strangulated, or causing obstruction
        CC Excl: See code 552.1

4ᵗʰ
5ᵗʰ
Additional Digit Required   Unacceptable PDx   Manifestation Code   Hospital Acquired Condition   ►◄ Revised Text   ● New Code   ▲ Revised Code Title

2014 ICD-9-CM   **Volume 1 – 183**

Diseases of the Digestive System

553.3–557.1

Diaphragmatic Hernias

553.3 Diaphragmatic hernia

Hernia:
    hiatal (esophageal) (sliding)   Thoracic stomach
    paraesophageal

EXCLUDES *congenital:*
       diaphragmatic hernia (756.6)
       hiatal hernia (750.6)
       esophagocele (530.6)

AHA: 2Q, '01, 6; 1Q, '00, 6

K44.9 Diaphragmatic hernia w/o obstruction/gangrene   **I-10**

553.8 Hernia of other specified sites

Hernia: Hernia:
    ischiatic   pudendal
    ischiorectal   retroperitoneal
    lumbar   sciatic
    obturator
Other abdominal hernia of specified site

EXCLUDES *vaginal enterocele (618.6)*

553.9 Hernia of unspecified site

Enterocele   Hernia:
Epiplocele   intestinal
Hernia: intra-abdominal
    NOS   Rupture (nontraumatic)
    interstitial   Sarcoepiplocele

Noninfectious Enteritis and Colitis (555-558)

√4ᵗʰ 555 Regional enteritis

INCLUDES Crohn's disease
           granulomatous enteritis

EXCLUDES *ulcerative colitis (556)*

DEF: Inflammation of intestine; classified to site.

TIP: Assign separate code for fistula, if present. Sequence 555 code as first-listed/principal diagnosis (if underlying cause of fistula).

555.0 Small intestine   **CC**

Ileitis: Regional enteritis or Crohn's disease of:
    regional   duodenum
    segmental   ileum
    terminal   jejunum
CC Exd: 555.0-556.9

555.1 Large intestine   **CC**

Colitis: Regional enteritis or Crohn's disease of:
    granulmatous   colon
    regional   large bowel
    transmural   rectum
CC Exd: See code: 555.0
AHA: 3Q, '99, 8

Large Intestine

555.2 Small intestine with large intestine   **CC**

Regional ileocolitis
CC Exd: See code: 555.0
AHA: 1Q, '03, 18

555.9 Unspecified site   **CC**

Crohn's disease NOS   Regional enteritis NOS
CC Exd: 555.9-555.9
AHA: 1Q, '09, 5; 2Q, '05, 11; 3Q, '99, 8; 4Q, '97, 42; 2Q, '97, 3

K50.90 Crohns disease unspecified w/o complications   **I-10**

√4ᵗʰ 556 Ulcerative colitis

DEF: Chronic inflammation of mucosal lining of intestinal tract; may be single area or entire colon.
AHA: 3Q, '99, 8

556.0 Ulcerative (chronic) enterocolitis   **CC**

CC Exd: 555.0-556.9

556.1 Ulcerative (chronic) ileocolitis   **CC**

CC Exd: 555.0-556.9

556.2 Ulcerative (chronic) proctitis   **CC**

CC Exd: 555.0-556.9

556.3 Ulcerative (chronic) proctosigmoiditis   **CC**

CC Exd: 555.0-556.9

556.4 Pseudopolyposis of colon   **CC**

CC Exd: 555.0-556.9

556.5 Left-sided ulcerative (chronic) colitis   **CC**

CC Exd: 555.0-556.9

556.6 Universal ulcerative (chronic) colitis   **CC**

Pancolitis
CC Exd: 555.0-556.9

556.8 Other ulcerative colitis   **CC**

CC Exd: 555.0-556.9

556.9 Ulcerative colitis, unspecified   **CC**

Ulcerative enteritis NOS
CC Exd: 555.0-556.9
AHA: 1Q, '03, 10

K51.90 Ulcerative colitis unspecified w/o complications   **I-10**

√4ᵗʰ 557 Vascular insufficiency of intestine

EXCLUDES *necrotizing enterocolitis of the newborn (777.50-777.53)*
DEF: Inadequacy of intestinal vessels.

557.0 Acute vascular insufficiency of intestine   **MCC**

Acute:
    hemorrhagic enterocolitis
    ischemic colitis, enteritis, or enterocolitis
    massive necrosis of intestine
Bowel infarction
Embolism of mesenteric artery
Fulminant enterocolitis
Hemorrhagic necrosis of intestine
Infarction of appendices epiploicae
Intestinal gangrene
Intestinal infarction (acute) (agnogenic) (hemorrhagic)
    (nonocclusive)
Mesenteric infarction (embolic) (thrombotic)
Necrosis of intestine
Terminal hemorrhagic enteropathy
Thrombosis of mesenteric artery
CC Exd: 557.0-557.1
AHA: 3Q, '11, 11; 2Q, '08, 15; 4Q, '01, 53
TIP: Do not assign an additional code for GI bleeding; it is inherent in 557.0.

K55.0 Acute vascular disorders of intestine   **I-10**

557.1 Chronic vascular insufficiency of intestine   **CC**

Angina, abdominal
Chronic ischemic colitis, enteritis, or enterocolitis
Ischemic stricture of intestine
Mesenteric:
    angina
    artery syndrome (superior)
    vascular insufficiency
CC Exd: 557.0-557.9
AHA: 3Q, '96, 9; 4Q, '90, 4; N-D, '86, 11; N-D, '84, 7

N Newborn Age: 0   **P** Pediatric Age: 0-17   **M** Maternity Age: 12-55   **A** Adult Age: 15-124   **MCC** Major CC Condition   **CC** CC Condition   **HIV** HIV Related Dx

184 – Volume 1   **2014 ICD-9-CM**

557.9 Unspecified vascular insufficiency of intestine `CC`
Alimentary pain due to vascular insufficiency
Ischemic colitis, enteritis, or enterocolitis NOS
CC Excl: 557.0-557.9
K55.9 Vascular disorder of intestine unspecified `I-10`

`√4ᵗʰ` **558 Other and unspecified noninfectious gastroenteritis and colitis**
EXCLUDES infectious:
colitis, enteritis, or gastroenteritis (009.0-009.1)
diarrhea (009.2-009.3)

558.1 Gastroenteritis and colitis due to radiation `CC`
Radiation enterocolitis
CC Excl: 558.1

558.2 Toxic gastroenteritis and colitis `CC`
Use additional E code to identify cause
CC Excl: 558.2

558.3 Allergic gastroenteritis and colitis
Use additional code to identify type of food allergy
(V15.01-V15.05)
DEF: True immunoglobulin E (IgE)-mediated allergic reaction of the
lining of the stomach, intestines, or colon to food proteins; causes
nausea, vomiting, diarrhea, and abdominal cramping.
AHA: 4Q, '08, 116; 1Q, '03, 12; 4Q, '00, 42

`√5ᵗʰ` **558.4 Eosinophilic gastroenteritis and colitis**
AHA: 4Q, '08, 115-116

558.41 Eosinophilic gastroenteritis
Eosinophilic enteritis

558.42 Eosinophilic colitis

558.9 Other and unspecified noninfectious gastroenteritis and colitis
Colitis
Enteritis
Gastroenteritis } NOS, dietetic, or
Ileitis   noninfectious
Jejunitis
Sigmoiditis
AHA: 3Q, '11, 11; 2Q, '08, 10; 1Q, '08, 10; 3Q, '99, 4, 6; N-D, '87, 7
K52.9 Noninfective gastroenteritis & colitis unspec `I-10`

Other Diseases of Intestines and Peritoneum (560-569)

`√4ᵗʰ` **560 Intestinal obstruction without mention of hernia**
EXCLUDES duodenum (537.2-537.3)
inguinal hernia with obstruction (550.1)
intestinal obstruction complicating hernia (552.0-552.9)
mesenteric:
embolism (557.0)
infarction (557.0)
thrombosis (557.0)
neonatal intestinal obstruction (277.01, 777.1-777.2, 777.4)
TIP: If intestinal obstruction is due to abdominal carcinomatosis or Crohn's
disease, sequence that condition first.

560.0 Intussusception `CC`
Intussusception (colon) (intestine) (rectum)
Invagination of intestine or colon
EXCLUDES intussusception of appendix (543.9)
CC Excl: 560.0-560.31, 560.39-560.9, 569.87-569.9
AHA: 4Q, '98, 82

560.1 Paralytic ileus `CC`
Adynamic ileus
Ileus (of intestine) (of bowel) (of colon)
Paralysis of intestine or colon
EXCLUDES gallstone ileus (560.31)
DEF: Obstruction of ileus due to inhibited bowel motility.
CC Excl: See code 560.0
AHA: 1Q, '12, 6; J-F, '87, 13
K56.0 Paralytic ileus `I-10`

560.2 Volvulus `MCC`
Knotting
Strangulation } if intestine, bowel, or colon
Torsion
Twist
DEF: Entanglement of bowel; causes obstruction; may compromise
bowel circulation.
CC Excl: See code 560.0

`√5ᵗʰ` **560.3 Impaction of intestine**

560.30 Impaction of intestine, unspecified `CC`
Impaction of colon
CC Excl: See code 560.0

560.31 Gallstone ileus `CC`
Obstruction of intestine by gallstone
CC Excl: See code 560.0

560.32 Fecal impaction
EXCLUDES constipation (564.00-564.09)
incomplete defecation (787.61)
AHA: 4Q, '10, 87-89
K56.41 Fecal impaction `I-10`

560.39 Other `CC`
Concretion of intestine
Enterolith
CC Excl: See code 560.0
AHA: 4Q, '98, 38
K56.49 Other impaction of intestine `I-10`

`√5ᵗʰ` **560.8 Other specified intestinal obstruction**

560.81 Intestinal or peritoneal adhesions with obstruction (postoperative) (postinfection) `CC`
EXCLUDES adhesions without obstruction (568.0)
DEF: Obstruction of peritoneum or intestine due to
abnormal union of tissues.
CC Excl: See code 560.0
AHA: 1Q, '10, 11; 4Q, '95, 55; 3Q, '95, 6; N-D, '87, 9
TIP: Do not assign additional code 997.4 Digestive system
complications.
K56.5 Intestinal adhes [bands] w/obst (postproc)
(postinfec) `I-10`

560.89 Other `CC`
Acute pseudo-obstruction of intestine
Mural thickening causing obstruction
EXCLUDES ischemic stricture of intestine (557.1)
CC Excl: See code 560.0
AHA: 2Q, '97, 3; 1Q, '88, 6

560.9 Unspecified intestinal obstruction `CC`
Enterostenosis
Obstruction
Occlusion } of intestine or colon
Stenosis
Stricture
EXCLUDES congenital stricture or stenosis of intestine
(751.1-751.2)
CC Excl: See code 560.0
K56.60 Unspecified intestinal obstruction `I-10`

`√4ᵗʰ` **562 Diverticula of intestine**
Use additional code to identify any associated:
peritonitis (567.0-567.9)
EXCLUDES congenital diverticulum of colon (751.5)
diverticulum of appendix (543.9)
Meckel's diverticulum (751.0)
AHA: 4Q, '91, 25; J-F, '85, 1

`√5ᵗʰ` **562.0 Small intestine**

562.00 Diverticulosis of small intestine (without mention of hemorrhage)
Diverticulosis:
duodenum
ileum } without mention of
jejunum   diverticulitis
DEF: Saclike herniations of mucous lining of small intestine.

562.01 Diverticulitis of small intestine (without mention of hemorrhage) `CC`
Diverticulitis (with diverticulosis):
duodenum
ileum
jejunum
small intestine
DEF: Inflamed saclike herniations of mucous lining of small
intestine
CC Excl: 562.00-562.03

Additional Digit Required   Unacceptable PDx   Manifestation Code   Hospital Acquired Condition   ▶◀ Revised Text   ● New Code   ▲ Revised Code Title

Diseases of the Digestive System

562.02–566

562.02 Diverticulosis of small intestine with hemorrhage `MCC`
CC Exd: 251.5, 456.0, 530.20-530.21, 530.7, 530.82, 530.85, 531.00-534.91, 535.01, 535.11, 535.21, 535.31, 535.41, 535.51, 535.61, 537.83, 562.02-562.03, 562.12-562.13, 569.3, 569.85, 578.0-578.9

562.03 Diverticulitis of small intestine with hemorrhage `MCC`
CC Exd: See code 562.02

☑5ᵗʰ **562.1 Colon**

562.10 Diverticulosis of colon (without mention of hemorrhage)
Diverticulosis:
  NOS   } without mention of
  intestine (large)   } diverticulitis
Diverticular disease (colon) without mention of diverticulitis
DEF: Saclike herniations of mucous lining of large intestine.
AHA: 3Q, '05, 17; 3Q, '02, 15; 4Q, '90, 21; J-F, '85, 5
K57.30 Divrticulos lg intest uns w/o perf/absc w/o bldg `I-10`

562.11 Diverticulitis of colon (without mention of hemorrhage) `CC`
Diverticulitis (with diverticulosis):
  NOS
  colon
  intestine (large)
DEF: Inflamed saclike herniations of mucosal lining of large intestine.
CC Exd: 562.10-562.13
AHA: 1Q, '96, 14; J-F, '85, 5
K57.32 Divrticulit lg intest uns w/o perf/absc w/o bldg `I-10`

562.12 Diverticulosis of colon with hemorrhage `MCC`
CC Exd: See code 562.02

562.13 Diverticulitis of colon with hemorrhage `MCC`
CC Exd: See code 562.02

☑4ᵗʰ **564 Functional digestive disorders, not elsewhere classified**
EXCLUDES functional disorders of stomach (536.0-536.9)
those specified as psychogenic (306.4)

☑5ᵗʰ **564.0 Constipation**
EXCLUDES fecal impaction (560.32)
incomplete defecation (787.61)
AHA: 4Q, '01, 45

564.00 Constipation, unspecified
K59.00 Constipation unspecified `I-10`

564.01 Slow transit constipation
DEF: Delay in the transit of fecal material through the colon secondary to smooth muscle dysfunction or decreased peristaltic contractions along the colon; also called colonic inertia or delayed transit.

564.02 Outlet dysfunction constipation
DEF: Failure to relax the paradoxical contractions of the striated pelvic floor muscles during the attempted defecation.

564.09 Other constipation

564.1 Irritable bowel syndrome
Irritable colon   Spastic colon
DEF: Functional gastrointestinal disorder (FGID); symptoms include diarrhea, constipation, abdominal pain, gas, distended abdomen, nausea, vomiting, emotional distress, and depression.
AHA: 1Q, '88, 6
K58.9 Irritable bowel syndrome without diarrhea `I-10`

564.2 Postgastric surgery syndromes
Dumping syndrome   Postgastrectomy syndrome
Jejunal syndrome   Postvagotomy syndrome
EXCLUDES malnutrition following gastrointestinal surgery (579.3)
postgastrojejunostomy ulcer (534.0-534.9)
AHA: 1Q, '95, 11

564.3 Vomiting following gastrointestinal surgery
Vomiting (bilious) following gastrointestinal surgery

564.4 Other postoperative functional disorders
Diarrhea following gastrointestinal surgery
EXCLUDES colostomy and enterostomy complications (569.60-569.69)

564.5 Functional diarrhea
EXCLUDES diarrhea:
  NOS (787.91)
  psychogenic (306.4)
DEF: Diarrhea with no detectable organic cause.

564.6 Anal spasm
Proctalgia fugax

564.7 Megacolon, other than Hirschsprung's `C`
Dilatation of colon
EXCLUDES megacolon:
  congenital [Hirschsprung's] (751.3)
  toxic (556)
DEF: Enlarged colon; congenital or acquired; can occur acutely or become chronic.
CC Exd: 564.1-564.9

☑5ᵗʰ **564.8 Other specified functional disorders of intestine**
EXCLUDES malabsorption (579.0-579.9)
AHA: 1Q, '88, 6

564.81 Neurogenic bowel `C`
DEF: Disorder of bowel due to spinal cord lesion above conus medullaris; symptoms include precipitous micturition, nocturia, headache, sweating, nasal obstruction and spastic contractions.
CC Exd: See code: 564.7
AHA: 1Q, '01, 12; 4Q, '98, 45

564.89 Other functional disorders of intestine
Atony of colon
AHA: ▶3Q, '12, 22◀
TIP: ▶Assign for visceral hypersensitivity; an overstimulation response causing extreme pain.◀

564.9 Unspecified functional disorder of intestine

☑4ᵗʰ **565 Anal fissure and fistula**

565.0 Anal fissure
EXCLUDES anal sphincter tear (healed) (non-traumatic) (old) (569.43)
traumatic (863.89, 863.99)
DEF: Ulceration of cleft at anal mucosa; causes pain, itching, bleeding, infection, and sphincter spasm; may occur with hemorrhoids.

565.1 Anal fistula
Fistula: Fistula:
  anorectal   rectum to skin
  rectal
EXCLUDES fistula of rectum to internal organs—see Alphabetic Index
ischiorectal fistula (566)
rectovaginal fistula (619.1)
DEF: Abnormal opening on cutaneous surface near anus; may lack connection with rectum.
AHA: 1Q, '07, 13

566 Abscess of anal and rectal regions `C`
Abscess: Cellulitis:
  ischiorectal   anal
  perianal   perirectal
  perirectal   rectal
                  Ischiorectal fistula
CC Exd: 566

Anal Fistula and Abscess

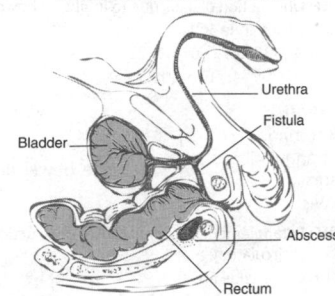

Urethra
Fistula
Bladder
Abscess
Rectum

N Newborn Age: 0   P Pediatric Age: 0-17   M Maternity Age: 12-55   A Adult Age: 15-124   `MCC` Major CC Condition   `CC` CC Condition   `HIV` HIV Related D

186 – Volume 1 · February 2013   2014 ICD-9-C

√4ᵗʰ **567 Peritonitis and retroperitoneal infections**

EXCLUDES *peritonitis:*
    benign paroxysmal (277.31)
    pelvic, female (614.5, 614.7)
    periodic familial (277.31)
    puerperal (670.8)
    with or following:
        abortion (634-638 with .0, 639.0)
        appendicitis (540.0-540.1)
        ectopic or molar pregnancy (639.0)
DEF: Inflammation of the peritoneal cavity.

567.0 Peritonitis in infectious diseases classified elsewhere MCC
    Code first underlying disease
    EXCLUDES *peritonitis:*
        gonococcal (098.86)
        syphilitic (095.2)
        tuberculous (014.0)
    CC Excl: 567.0-567.29, 567.38-567.9, 569.87-569.9

567.1 Pneumococcal peritonitis MCC
    CC Excl: See code: 567.0

√5ᵗʰ **567.2 Other suppurative peritonitis**
    AHA: 4Q, '05, 74; 2Q, '01, 11, 12; 3Q, '99, 9; 2Q, '98, 19

    567.21 Peritonitis (acute) generalized MCC
        Pelvic peritonitis, male
        CC Excl: See code 567.0
        TIP: For pelvic peritonitis in a female patient, refer to code 614.5.

    567.22 Peritoneal abscess MCC
        Abscess (of):   Abscess (of):
           abdominopelvic   retrocecal
           mesenteric   subdiaphragmatic
           omentum   subhepatic
           peritoneum   subphrenic
        CC Excl: See code 567.0
        K65.1 Peritoneal abscess   I-10

    567.23 Spontaneous bacterial peritonitis MCC
        EXCLUDES *bacterial peritonitis NOS (567.29)*
        CC Excl: See code 567.0

    567.29 Other suppurative peritonitis MCC
        Subphrenic peritonitis
        AHA: 2Q, '10, 4
        CC Excl: See code 567.0

√5ᵗʰ **567.3 Retroperitoneal infections**
    AHA: 4Q, '05, 74

    567.31 Psoas muscle abscess MCC
        DEF: Infection that extends into or around the psoas muscle that connects the lumbar vertebrae to the femur.
        CC Excl: 567.31, 728.0, 728.11-728.3, 728.81, 728.86

    567.38 Other retroperitoneal abscess MCC
        AHA: 4Q, '05, 77
        CC Excl: See code 567.0

    567.39 Other retroperitoneal infections MCC
        CC Excl: See code 567.0

Psoas Muscle Abscess

Psoas minor muscle
Psoas major muscle
Small intestine (ilium)
Peritoneal cavity
Small intestine (jejunum)
Abscess
Ascending colon
Ascending colon
Pelvic bone
Psoas major muscle
Psoas major muscle
Spinous process of L4
Erector spinae muscles

√5ᵗʰ **567.8 Other specified peritonitis**
    AHA: 4Q, '05, 74

    567.81 Choleperitonitis MCC
        Peritonitis due to bile
        DEF: Inflammation or infection due to presence of bile in the peritoneum resulting from rupture of the bile passages or gallbladder.
        CC Excl: See code 567.0

    567.82 Sclerosing mesenteritis CC
        Fat necrosis of peritoneum
        (Idiopathic) sclerosing mesenteric fibrosis
        Mesenteric lipodystrophy
        Mesenteric panniculitis
        Retractile mesenteritis
        DEF: Inflammatory processes involving the mesenteric fat; progresses to fibrosis and necrosis of tissue.
        CC Excl: See code 567.0
        AHA: 4Q, '05, 77

    567.89 Other specified peritonitis MCC
        Chronic proliferative peritonitis
        Mesenteric saponification
        Peritonitis due to urine
        CC Excl: See code 567.0

567.9 Unspecified peritonitis MCC
    Peritonitis NOS   Peritonitis of unspecified cause
    CC Excl: See code 567.0
    AHA: 1Q, '04, 10

√4ᵗʰ **568 Other disorders of peritoneum**

568.0 Peritoneal adhesions (postoperative) (postinfection)
    Adhesions (of):   Adhesions (of):
        abdominal (wall)   mesenteric
        diaphragm   omentum
        intestine   stomach
        male pelvis   Adhesive bands
    EXCLUDES *adhesions:*
        pelvic, female (614.6)
        with obstruction:
            duodenum (537.3)
            intestine (560.81)
    DEF: Abnormal union of tissues in peritoneum.
    AHA: 1Q, '12, 8; 2Q, '11, 18; 3Q, '03, 7, 11; 4Q, '95, 55; 3Q, '95, 7; S-O, '85, 11
    TIP: Do not assign additional code from subcategory 997.4 Digestive system complications.
    K66.0 Peritoneal adhesns (postprocedural) (postinfection)   I-10

√5ᵗʰ **568.8 Other specified disorders of peritoneum**

    568.81 Hemoperitoneum (nontraumatic) MCC
        CC Excl: 568.81

    568.82 Peritoneal effusion (chronic) CC
        EXCLUDES *ascites NOS (789.51-789.59)*
        DEF: Persistent leakage of fluid within peritoneal cavity.
        CC Excl: 568.82

    568.89 Other
        Peritoneal: Peritoneal:
           cyst   granuloma

568.9 Unspecified disorder of peritoneum

√4ᵗʰ **569 Other disorders of intestine**

569.0 Anal and rectal polyp
    Anal and rectal polyp NOS
    EXCLUDES *adenomatous anal and rectal polyp (211.4)*

569.1 Rectal prolapse
    Procidentia: Prolapse:
        anus (sphincter)   anal canal
        rectum (sphincter)   rectal mucosa
    Proctoptosis
    EXCLUDES *prolapsed hemorrhoids (455.2, 455.5)*

Additional Digit Required   Unacceptable PDx   Manifestation Code   Hospital Acquired Condition   ▶◀ Revised Text   ● New Code   ▲ Revised Code Title

014 ICD-9-CM   Volume 1 – 187

Diseases of the Digestive System

569.2–569.84

Rectum and Anus

569.2 Stenosis of rectum and anus
Stricture of anus (sphincter)

569.3 Hemorrhage of rectum and anus   `CC`
> **EXCLUDES** gastrointestinal bleeding NOS (578.9)
> melena (578.1)

CC Excl: 251.5, 456.0, 530.20-530.21, 530.7, 530.82, 530.85, 531.00-534.91, 535.01, 535.11, 535.21, 535.31, 535.41, 535.51, 535.61, 537.83, 562.02-562.03, 562.12-562.13, 569.3, 569.85, 578.0-578.9

AHA: 3Q, '05, 17

K62.5 Hemorrhage of anus and rectum   `I-10`

✓5ᵗʰ 569.4 Other specified disorders of rectum and anus

569.41 Ulcer of anus and rectum   `CC`
Solitary ulcer } of anus (sphincter) or
Stercoral ulcer } rectum (sphincter)
CC Excl: 569.41

569.42 Anal or rectal pain
AHA: 1Q, '03, 8; 1Q, '96, 13

569.43 Anal sphincter tear (healed) (old)
Tear of anus, nontraumatic
Use additional code for any associated fecal incontinence (787.60-787.63)
> **EXCLUDES** anal fissure (565.0)
> anal sphincter tear (healed) (old)
> complicating delivery (654.8)

AHA: 4Q, '07, 88

569.44 Dysplasia of anus
Anal intraepithelial neoplasia I and II (AIN I and II) (histologically confirmed)
Dysplasia of anus NOS
Mild and moderate dysplasia of anus (histologically confirmed)
> **EXCLUDES** abnormal results from anal cytologic
> examination without histologic
> confirmation (796.70-796.79)
> anal intraepithelial neoplasia III (230.5, 230.6)
> carcinoma in situ of anus (230.5, 230.6)
> HGSIL of anus (796.74)
> severe dysplasia of anus (230.5, 230.6)

AHA: 4Q, '08, 117

569.49 Other
Granuloma } of rectum (sphincter)
Rupture }
Hypertrophy of anal papillae
Proctitis NOS
Use additional code for any associated fecal incontinence (787.60-787.63)
> **EXCLUDES** fistula of rectum to:
> internal organs — see Alphabetic Index
> skin (565.1)
> hemorrhoids (455.0-455.9)

569.5 Abscess of intestine   `CC`
> **EXCLUDES** appendiceal abscess (540.1)

CC Excl: 569.5

K63.0 Abscess of intestine   `I-10`

✓5ᵗʰ 569.6 Colostomy and enterostomy complications
DEF: Complication in a surgically created opening, from intestine to surface skin.
AHA: 4Q, '95, 58
TIP: Do not assign additional code from subcategory 997.4 Digestive system complications.

569.60 Colostomy and enterostomy complication, unspecified

569.61 Infection of colostomy or enterostomy   `CC`
Use additional code to identify organism (041.00-041.9)
Use additional code to specify type of infection, such as:
  abscess or cellulitis of abdomen (682.2)
  septicemia (038.0-038.9)
CC Excl: 569.60-569.69

569.62 Mechanical complication of colostomy and enterostomy   `CC`
Malfunction of colostomy and enterostomy
CC Excl: 530.86-530.87, 536.40-536.49, 539.01-539.89, 569.60-569.79, 997.41-997.49, 997.71, 997.91-997.99, 998.81, 998.83-998.9
AHA: 2Q, '05, 11 ; 1Q, '03, 10; 4Q, '98, 44

569.69 Other complication   `CC`
Fistula   Prolapse
Hernia
CC Excl: See code: 569.61
AHA: 3Q, '98, 16

✓5ᵗʰ 569.7 Complications of intestinal pouch
TIP: Do not assign code from subcategory 997.4 Digestive system complications in addition to a code from this subcategory.

569.71 Pouchitis   `CC`
Inflammation of internal ileoanal pouch
DEF: Inflammatory complication of an existing surgically created ileoanal pouch, resulting in multiple GI complaints including diarrhea, abdominal pain, rectal bleeding, fecal urgency, or incontinence.
CC Excl: 530.86-530.87, 536.40-536.49, 539.01-539.89, 569.60-569.79, 997.41-997.49, 997.71, 997.91-997.99, 998.81, 998.83-998.9
AHA: 4Q, '09, 94

569.79 Other complications of intestinal pouch   `CC`
CC Excl: See code: 569.71

✓5ᵗʰ 569.8 Other specified disorders of intestine
AHA: 4Q, '91, 25

569.81 Fistula of intestine, excluding rectum and anus   `CC`
Fistula: Fistula:
  abdominal wall   enteroenteric
  enterocolic   ileorectal
> **EXCLUDES** fistula of intestine to internal organs — see
> Alphabetic Index
> persistent postoperative fistula (998.6)

CC Excl: 569.81
AHA: 3Q, '99, 8

569.82 Ulceration of intestine   `CC`
Primary ulcer of intestine   Ulceration of colon
> **EXCLUDES** that with perforation (569.83)

CC Excl: 569.82

569.83 Perforation of intestine   `MCC`
CC Excl: 569.83
AHA: ▶2Q, '12, 5◄

569.84 Angiodysplasia of intestine (without mention of hemorrhage)
DEF: Small vascular abnormalities of the intestinal tract without bleeding problems.
AHA: 3Q, '96, 10; 4Q, '90, 4; 4Q, '90, 21
TIP: Assign code 569.84 or 569.85 for documentation of either intestinal arteriovenous (AV) malformation or angiodysplasia.

`N` Newborn Age: 0   `P` Pediatric Age: 0-17   `M` Maternity Age: 12-55   `A` Adult Age: 15-124   `MCC` Major CC Condition   `CC` CC Condition   `HIV` HIV Related D

188 – Volume 1 • February 2013   2014 ICD-9-C

569.85 Angiodysplasia of intestine with hemorrhage `MCC`
> **DEF:** Small vascular abnormalities of the intestinal tract with bleeding problems.
> **CC Excl:** 251.5, 456.0, 530.20-530.21, 530.7, 530.82, 530.85, 531.00-534.91, 535.01, 535.11, 535.21, 535.31, 535.41, 535.51, 535.61, 537.83, 562.02-562.03, 562.12-562.13, 569.3, 569.85, 578.0-578.9
> **AHA:** 3Q, '96, 9

569.86 Dieulafoy lesion (hemorrhagic) of intestine `MCC`
> **CC Excl:** 251.5, 456.0, 530.20-530.21, 530.7, 530.82, 530.85, 531.00-534.91, 535.01, 535.11, 535.21, 535.31, 535.41, 535.51, 535.61, 535.71, 537.83, 562.02-562.03, 562.12-562.13, 569.3, 569.85-569.86, 578.0-578.9
> **AHA:** 4Q, '02, 60-61

569.87 Vomiting of fecal matter
> **DEF:** Spasmodic expulsion of partially digested substance with similar odor to fecal matter; often suggestive of bowel obstruction or other underlying causal pathology.
> **AHA:** 4Q, '09, 105

569.89 Other
> Enteroptosis
> Granuloma ⎫
> Prolapse   ⎬ of intestine
> Pericolitis
> Perisigmoiditis
> Visceroptosis
> **EXCLUDES** *gangrene of intestine, mesentery, or*
>   *omentum (557.0)*
>   *hemorrhage of intestine NOS (578.9)*
>   *obstruction of intestine (560.0-560.9)*
> **AHA:** 3Q, '96, 9

569.9 Unspecified disorder of intestine

Other Diseases of Digestive System (570-579)

570 Acute and subacute necrosis of liver `MCC`
> Acute hepatic failure
> Acute or subacute hepatitis, not specified as infective
> Necrosis of liver (acute) (diffuse) (massive) (subacute)
> Parenchymatous degeneration of liver
> Yellow atrophy (liver) (acute) (subacute)
> **EXCLUDES** *icterus gravis of newborn (773.0-773.2)*
>   *serum hepatitis (070.2-070.3)*
>   *that with:*
>   *abortion (634-638 with .7, 639.8)*
>   *ectopic or molar pregnancy (639.8)*
>   *pregnancy, childbirth, or the puerperium (646.7)*
>   *viral hepatitis (070.0-070.9)*
> **CC Excl:** 570, 573.4-573.9
> **AHA:** 2Q, '05, 9; 1Q, '00, 22
> `K72.00` Acute and subacute hepatic failure without coma `I-10`

✓4ᵗʰ 571 Chronic liver disease and cirrhosis

571.0 Alcoholic fatty liver `A`

571.1 Acute alcoholic hepatitis `A`
> Acute alcoholic liver disease
> **AHA:** 2Q, '02, 4

Liver

Inferior vena cava — Hepatic veins
Diaphragm —
— Caudate lobe
Gallbladder — Portal vein
Common bile duct — Medial segment — Lateral segment
Right lobe — Left lobe

571.2 Alcoholic cirrhosis of liver `A`
> Florid cirrhosis   Laennec's cirrhosis (alcoholic)
> **DEF:** Fibrosis and dysfunction of liver; due to alcoholic liver disease.
> **AHA:** 1Q, '11, 23; 3Q, '07, 7; 2Q, '07, 6; 2Q, '02, 4; 1Q, '02, 3; N-D, '85, 14
> **TIP:** For a patient admitted for bleeding esophageal varices due to alcoholic liver cirrhosis, sequence the liver cirrhosis first.
> `K70.30` Alcoholic cirrhosis of liver without ascites `I-10`

571.3 Alcoholic liver damage, unspecified `A`

✓5ᵗʰ 571.4 Chronic hepatitis
> **EXCLUDES** *viral hepatitis (acute) (chronic) (070.0-070.9)*

571.40 Chronic hepatitis, unspecified

571.41 Chronic persistent hepatitis

571.42 Autoimmune hepatitis
> **AHA:** 4Q, '08, 120

571.49 Other
> Chronic hepatitis: Recurrent hepatitis
>   active
>   aggressive
> **AHA:** 3Q, '99, 19; N-D, '85, 14

571.5 Cirrhosis of liver without mention of alcohol
> Cirrhosis of liver: Cirrhosis of liver:
>   NOS   posthepatitic
>   cryptogenic   postnecrotic
>   macronodular   Healed yellow atrophy (liver)
>   micronodular   Portal cirrhosis
> Code first, if applicable, viral hepatitis (acute) (chronic) (070.0-070.9)
> **DEF:** Fibrosis and dysfunction of liver; not alcohol related.
> **AHA:** 1Q, '11, 23: 3Q, '07, 7; 2Q, '07, 5
> **TIP:** For a patient admitted for bleeding esophageal varices due to liver cirrhosis, sequence the liver cirrhosis first.

571.6 Biliary cirrhosis
> Chronic nonsuppurative   Cirrhosis:
>   destructive cholangitis   cholangitic
>   cholestatic

571.8 Other chronic nonalcoholic liver disease
> Chronic yellow atrophy (liver)
> Fatty liver, without mention of alcohol
> **AHA:** 2Q, '96, 12

571.9 Unspecified chronic liver disease without mention of alcohol

✓4ᵗʰ 572 Liver abscess and sequelae of chronic liver disease

572.0 Abscess of liver `MCC`
> **EXCLUDES** *amebic liver abscess (006.3)*
> **CC Excl:** 006.3, 572.0-572.1, 573.8-573.9

572.1 Portal pyemia `MCC`
> Phlebitis of portal vein   Pylephlebitis
> Portal thrombophlebitis   Pylethrombophlebitis
> **DEF:** Inflammation of portal vein or branches; may be due to intestinal disease; symptoms include fever, chills, jaundice, sweating, and abscess in various body parts.
> **CC Excl:** See code 572.0

572.2 Hepatic encephalopathy `MCC`
> Hepatic coma   Portal-systemic encephalopathy
> Hepatocerebral intoxication
> **EXCLUDES** *hepatic coma associated with viral hepatitis — see*
>   *category 070*
> **CC Excl:** 572.2, 573.8-573.9
> **AHA:** 2Q, '07, 5; 2Q, '05, 9; 1Q, '02, 3; 3Q, '95, 14
> **TIP:** Do not assign if hepatic coma is documented with viral hepatitis; see category 070 with fourth digit indicating hepatic coma.
> `K72.91` Hepatic failure unspecified with coma `I-10`

572.3 Portal hypertension `CC`
> Use additional code for any associated complications, such as:
>   portal hypertensive gastropathy (537.89)
> **DEF:** Abnormally high blood pressure in the portal vein.
> **CC Excl:** 572.2-572.3, 573.8-573.9
> **AHA:** 3Q, '05, 15
> `K76.6` Portal hypertension `I-10`

✓4ᵗʰ / ✓5ᵗʰ   Additional Digit Required   Unacceptable PDx   Manifestation Code   Hospital Acquired Condition   ►◄ Revised Text   ● New Code   ▲ Revised Code Title

2014 ICD-9-CM   **Volume 1 – 189**

Diseases of the Digestive System

572.4–574.8

572.4 Hepatorenal syndrome `MCC`

> *EXCLUDES*   *that following delivery (674.8)*
>
> **DEF:** Hepatic and renal failure characterized by cirrhosis with ascites or obstructive jaundice, oliguria, and low sodium concentration.
>
> **CC Excl:** 572.4, 573.8-573.9
>
> **AHA:** 3Q, '93, 15

572.8 Other sequelae of chronic liver disease

> *EXCLUDES*   *hepatopulmonary syndrome (573.5)*

√4ᵗʰ **573 Other disorders of liver**

> *EXCLUDES*   *amyloid or lardaceous degeneration of liver (277.39)*
> *congenital cystic disease of liver (751.62)*
> *glycogen infiltration of liver (271.0)*
> *hepatomegaly NOS (789.1)*
> *portal vein obstruction (452)*

573.0 Chronic passive congestion of liver

> **DEF:** Blood accumulation in liver tissue.

573.1 Hepatitis in viral diseases classified elsewhere `CC`

> Code first underlying disease as:
> Coxsackie virus disease (074.8)
> cytomegalic inclusion virus disease (078.5)
> infectious mononucleosis (075)
>
> *EXCLUDES*   *hepatitis (in):*
> *mumps (072.71)*
> *viral (070.0-070.9)*
> *yellow fever (060.0-060.9)*
>
> **CC Excl:** 573.1-573.3, 573.8-573.9

573.2 Hepatitis in other infectious diseases classified elsewhere `CC`

> Code first underlying disease, as:
> malaria (084.9)
>
> *EXCLUDES*   *hepatitis in:*
> *late syphilis (095.3)*
> *secondary syphilis (091.62)*
> *toxoplasmosis (130.5)*
>
> **CC Excl:** See code: 573.1

573.3 Hepatitis, unspecified

> Toxic (noninfectious) hepatitis
> Use additional E code to identify cause
>
> **AHA:** 3Q, '98, 3, 4; 4Q, '90, 26
>
> K75.9 Inflammatory liver disease unspecified   `I-10`

573.4 Hepatic infarction `MCC`

> **CC Excl:** 570, 573.4-573.9

573.5 Hepatopulmonary syndrome

> Code first underlying liver disease, such as:
> alcoholic cirrhosis of liver (571.2)
> cirrhosis of liver without mention of alcohol (571.5)
>
> **AHA:** 4Q, '11, 127-128

573.8 Other specified disorders of liver

> Hepatoptosis

573.9 Unspecified disorder of liver

√4ᵗʰ **574 Cholelithiasis**

> The following fifth-digit subclassification is for use with category 574:
> **0 without mention of obstruction**
> **1 with obstruction**
>
> *EXCLUDES*   *retained cholelithiasis following cholecystectomy (997.41)*

§ √5ᵗʰ **574.0 Calculus of gallbladder with acute cholecystitis** `CC`
[0-1]

> Biliary calculus
> Calculus of cystic duct } with acute cholecystitis
> Cholelithiasis
>
> Any condition classifiable to 574.2 with acute cholecystitis
>
> **CC Excl: For code 574.00:** 574.00-574.21, 574.40, 574.60-574.61, 574.80-574.81, 575.0-575.12, 575.9, 576.8-576.9; **For code 574.01:** 574.00-574.21, 574.60-574.61, 574.80-574.81, 575.0-575.12, 575.9, 576.8-576.9
>
> **AHA:** 4Q, '96, 32
>
> K80.00 Calculus of GB w/acute cholecystitis w/o obst   `I-10`

Gallbladder and Bile Ducts

Right hepatic artery — Right and left bile ducts
Cystic artery — Triangle of Calot
— Common hepatic artery
— Portal vein
Cystic duct
Gallstone in fundus
Hartmann's pouch (infundibulum) — Common bile duct empties into Duodenum

§ √5ᵗʰ **574.1 Calculus of gallbladder with other cholecystitis** `CC`
[0-1]

> Biliary calculus
> Calculus of cystic duct } with cholecystitis
> Choleithiasis
>
> Cholecystitis with cholelithiasis NOS
>
> Any condition classifiable to 574.2 with cholecystitis (chronic)
>
> **CC Excl:** See code 574.01
>
> **AHA:** 3Q, '99, 9; 4Q, '96, 32, 69; 2Q, '96, 13; **For code 574.10:** 1Q, '03, 5
>
> K80.10 Calculus of GB w/chronic cholecystitis w/o obst   `I-10`

§ √5ᵗʰ **574.2 Calculus of gallbladder without mention of** `CC 1`
[0-1] **cholecystitis**

> Biliary: Cholelithiasis NOS
> calculus NOS   Colic (recurrent) of gallbladder
> colic NOS   Gallstone (impacted)
> Calculus of cystic duct
>
> **CC Excl: For code 574.21:** See code 574.01
>
> **AHA: For code 574.20:** 1Q, '88, 14
>
> K80.20 Calculus of GB w/o cholecystitis w/o obst   `I-10`

§ √5ᵗʰ **574.3 Calculus of bile duct with acute cholecystitis** `CC`
[0-1]

> Calculus of bile duct (any) } with acute cholecystitis
> Choledocholithiasis
>
> Any condition classifiable to 574.5 with acute cholecystitis
>
> **CC Excl:** 574.30-575.12, 576.8-576.9

§ √5ᵗʰ **574.4 Calculus of bile duct with other cholecystitis** `CC`
[0-1]

> Calculus of bile duct (any) } with cholecystitis (chronic)
> Choledocholithiasis
>
> Any condition classifiable to 574.5 with cholecystitis (chronic)
>
> **CC Excl:** See code 574.3

§ √5ᵗʰ **574.5 Calculus of bile duct without mention of cholecystitis** `CC 1`
[0-1]

> Calculus of: Choledocholithiasis
> bile duct [any]   Hepatic:
> common duct   colic (recurrent)
> hepatic duct   lithiasis
>
> **CC Excl: For code 574.51:** 574.30-575.12, 576.8-576.9
>
> **AHA:** 3Q, '94, 11

§ √5ᵗʰ **574.6 Calculus of gallbladder and bile duct with** `CC`
[0-1] **acute cholecystitis**

> Any condition classifiable to 574.0 and 574.3
>
> **CC Excl:** 574.60-574.61, 575.0-575.12, 575.9, 576.8-576.9
>
> **AHA:** 4Q, '96, 32

§ √5ᵗʰ **574.7 Calculus of gallbladder and bile duct with** `CC`
[0-1] **other cholecystitis**

> Any condition classifiable to 574.1 and 574.4
>
> **CC Excl:** 574.30-575.12, 576.8-576.9
>
> **AHA:** 4Q, '96, 32

§ √5ᵗʰ **574.8 Calculus of gallbladder and bile duct** `MCC 1 CC 0`
[0-1] **with acute and chronic cholecystitis**

> Any condition classifiable to 574.6 and 574.7
>
> **CC Excl:** 574.80-574.81, 575.0-575.12, 575.9, 576.8-576.9
>
> **AHA:** 4Q, '96, 32

---

§   Requires fifth digit. Valid digits are in [brackets] under each code. See category 574 for codes and definitions.

N Newborn Age: 0   **P** Pediatric Age: 0-17   **M** Maternity Age: 12-55   **A** Adult Age: 15-124   `MCC` Major CC Condition   `CC` CC Condition   **HIV** HIV Related Dx

190 – Volume 1   **2014 ICD-9-CM**

§ ✓5th **574.9 Calculus of gallbladder and bile duct** `CC 1`
[0-1] **without cholecystitis**
Any condition classifiable to 574.2 and 574.5
CC Exd: For code 574.91: 574.30-575.12, 576.8-576.9
AHA: 4Q, '96, 32

✓4th **575 Other disorders of gallbladder**
TIP: Do not assign a separate cholecystitis code from category 575 with a code from category 574.

575.0 Acute cholecystitis `CC`
Abscess of gallbladder
Angiocholecystitis
Cholecystitis:
   emphysematous (acute)
   gangrenous   } without mention of
   suppurative   calculus
Empyema of gallbladder
Gangrene of gallbladder

EXCLUDES that with:
   acute and chronic cholecystitis (575.12)
   choledocholithiasis (574.3)
   choledocholithiasis and cholelithiasis (574.6)
   cholelithiasis (574.0)
CC Exd: 574.60-574.61, 574.80-574.81, 575.0-575.12, 575.9, 576.8-576.9
AHA: 3Q, '91, 17
K81.0 Acute cholecystitis `I-10`

✓5th **575.1 Other cholecystitis**
Cholecystitis:
   NOS   } without mention of calculus
   chronic

EXCLUDES that with:
   choledocholithiasis (574.4)
   choledocholithiasis and cholelithiasis (574.8)
   cholelithiasis (574.1)
AHA: 4Q, '96, 32

575.10 Cholecystitis, unspecified
Cholecystitis NOS

575.11 Chronic cholecystitis
K81.1 Chronic cholecystitis `I-10`

575.12 Acute and chronic cholecystitis `CC`
CC Exd: 575.0-575.12, 575.9, 576.8-576.9
AHA: 4Q, '97, 52; 4Q, '96, 32

575.2 Obstruction of gallbladder `CC`
Occlusion
Stenosis   } of cystic duct or gallbladder without
Stricture   mention of calculus

EXCLUDES that with calculus (574.0-574.2 with fifth-digit 1)
CC Exd: 575.2-575.9, 576.8-576.9

575.3 Hydrops of gallbladder `CC`
Mucocele of gallbladder
DEF: Serous fluid accumulation in bladder.
CC Exd: See code 575.2
AHA: 2Q, '89, 13

575.4 Perforation of gallbladder `MCC`
Rupture of cystic duct or gallbladder
CC Exd: See code 575.2

575.5 Fistula of gallbladder `CC`
Fistula: Fistula:
   cholecystoduodenal   cholecystoenteric
CC Exd: See code 575.2

575.6 Cholesterolosis of gallbladder
Strawberry gallbladder
DEF: Cholesterol deposits in gallbladder tissue.
AHA: 4Q, '90, 17

575.8 Other specified disorders of gallbladder
Adhesions
Atrophy
Cyst
Hypertrophy   } of cystic duct or gallbladder
Nonfunctioning
Ulcer

Biliary dyskinesia
EXCLUDES Hartmann's pouch of intestine (V44.3)
   nonvisualization of gallbladder (793.3)
AHA: 4Q, '90, 26; 2Q, '89, 13

575.9 Unspecified disorder of gallbladder

✓4th **576 Other disorders of biliary tract**
EXCLUDES that involving the:
   cystic duct (575.0-575.9)
   gallbladder (575.0-575.9)

576.0 Postcholecystectomy syndrome
DEF: Jaundice or abdominal pain following cholecystectomy.
AHA: 1Q, '88, 10
TIP: Do not assign additional code from subcategory 997.4 Digestive system complications.

576.1 Cholangitis `CC`
Cholangitis: Cholangitis:
   NOS   recurrent
   acute   sclerosing
   ascending   secondary
   chronic   stenosing
   primary   suppurative
CC Exd: 576.1, 576.8-576.9
AHA: 2Q, '99, 13
K83.0 Cholangitis `I-10`

576.2 Obstruction of bile duct `MCC`
Occlusion
Stenosis   } of bile duct, except cystic duct, without
Stricture   mention of calculus

EXCLUDES congenital (751.61)
   that with calculus (574.3-574.5 with fifth-digit 1)
CC Exd: 574.31, 574.41, 574.51, 576.2, 576.8-576.9, 751.61
AHA: 3Q, '03, 17-18; 1Q, '01, 8; 2Q, '99, 13
K83.1 Obstruction of bile duct `I-10`

576.3 Perforation of bile duct `MCC`
Rupture of bile duct, except cystic duct
CC Exd: 576.3-576.4, 576.8-576.9

576.4 Fistula of bile duct `CC`
Choledochoduodenal fistula
CC Exd: See code: 576.3

576.5 Spasm of sphincter of Oddi

576.8 Other specified disorders of biliary tract
Adhesions
Atrophy
Cyst
Hypertrophy   } of bile duct (any)
Nonfunctioning
Ulcer

EXCLUDES congenital choledochal cyst (751.69)
AHA: 3Q, '03, 17; 2Q, '99, 14

576.9 Unspecified disorder of biliary tract

§ Requires fifth digit. Valid digits are in [brackets] under each code. See category 574 for codes and definitions.

 Additional Digit Required   Unacceptable PDx   Manifestation Code   Hospital Acquired Condition   ►◄ Revised Text   ● New Code   ▲ Revised Code Title

2014 ICD-9-CM   **Volume 1 – 191**

Diseases of the Digestive System

577–579.9

Pancreas

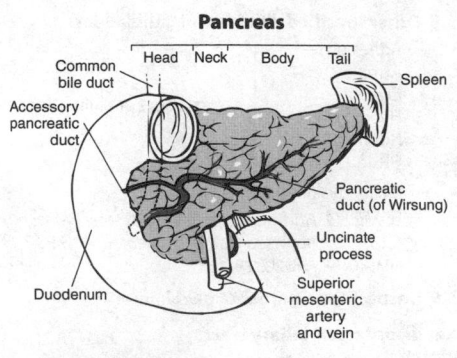

Common bile duct
Accessory pancreatic duct
Head Neck Body Tail
Spleen
Pancreatic duct (of Wirsung)
Uncinate process
Duodenum
Superior mesenteric artery and vein

✓4ᵗʰ **577 Diseases of pancreas**

577.0 Acute pancreatitis `MCC`

Abscess of pancreas	Pancreatitis:
Necrosis of pancreas:	acute (recurrent)
acute	apoplectic
infective	hemorrhagic
Pancreatitis:	subacute
NOS	suppurative

EXCLUDES *mumps pancreatitis (072.3)*
CC Excl: 577.0-577.1, 577.8-577.9
AHA: 3Q, '99, 9; 2Q, '98, 19; 2Q, '96, 13; 2Q, '89, 9
K85.0 Idiopathic acute pancreatitis `I-10`

577.1 Chronic pancreatitis `CC`

Chronic pancreatitis:	Pancreatitis:
NOS	painless
infectious	recurrent
interstitial	relapsing

CC Excl: 251.8, 577.0-577.9
AHA: 1Q, '01, 8; 2Q, '96, 13; 3Q, '94, 11
K86.1 Other chronic pancreatitis `I-10`

577.2 Cyst and pseudocyst of pancreas `CC`
CC Excl: 577.2-577.9
K86.2 Cyst of pancreas `I-10`

577.8 Other specified diseases of pancreas

Atrophy
Calculus
Cirrhosis   } of pancreas
Fibrosis

Pancreatic:	Pancreatolithiasis
infantilism	
necrosis:	
NOS	
aseptic	
fat	

EXCLUDES *fibrocystic disease of pancreas(277.00-277.09)*
islet cell tumor of pancreas (211.7)
pancreatic steatorrhea (579.4)
AHA: 1Q, '01, 8

577.9 Unspecified disease of pancreas

✓4ᵗʰ **578 Gastrointestinal hemorrhage**

EXCLUDES *that with mention of:*
angiodysplasia of stomach and duodenum (537.83)
angiodysplasia of intestine (569.85)
diverticulitis, intestine:
large (562.13)
small (562.03)
diverticulosis, intestine:
large (562.12)
small (562.02)
gastritis and duodenitis (535.0-535.6)
ulcer:
duodenal, gastric, gastrojejunal or peptic (531.00-534.91)
AHA: 2Q, '92, 9; 4Q, '90, 20

578.0 Hematemesis `CC`
Vomiting of blood
CC Excl: 251.5, 456.0, 530.20-530.21, 530.7, 530.82, 530.85, 531.00-534.91, 535.01, 535.11, 535.21, 535.31, 535.41, 535.51, 535.61, 537.83, 562.02-562.03, 562.12-562.13, 569.3, 569.85, 578.0-578.9
AHA: 2Q, '02, 4

578.1 Blood in stool `CC`
Melena
EXCLUDES *melena of the newborn (772.4, 777.3)*
occult blood (792.1)
CC Excl: See code 578.0
AHA: 2Q, '06, 17; 2Q, '92, 8
K92.1 Melena `I-10`

578.9 Hemorrhage of gastrointestinal tract, unspecified `CC`
Gastric hemorrhage   Intestinal hemorrhage
CC Excl: See code 578.0
AHA: 4Q, '06, 91; 3Q, '05, 17; N-D, '86, 9
TIP: Assign 578.9 if the physician does not establish a causal link between GI bleeding and any possible causes found on endoscopy.
K92.2 Gastrointestinal hemorrhage unspecified `I-10`

✓4ᵗʰ **579 Intestinal malabsorption**

579.0 Celiac disease

Celiac:	Gee (-Herter) disease
crisis	Gluten enteropathy
infantilism	Idiopathic steatorrhea
rickets	Nontropical sprue

DEF: Malabsorption syndrome due to gluten consumption; symptoms include fetid, bulky, frothy, oily stools, distended abdomen, gas, asthenia, electrolyte depletion and vitamin B, D and K deficiency.

579.1 Tropical sprue `CC`

Sprue:	Tropical steatorrhea
NOS	
tropical	

DEF: Diarrhea, occurs in tropics; may be due to enteric infection and malnutrition.
CC Excl: 277.03, 579.0-579.9

579.2 Blind loop syndrome `CC`
Postoperative blind loop syndrome
DEF: Obstruction or impaired passage in small intestine due to alterations, from strictures or surgery; causes stasis, abnormal bacterial flora, diarrhea, weight loss, multiple vitamin deficiency, and megaloblastic anemia.
CC Excl: See code: 579.1
TIP: Do not assign additional code from subcategory 997.4 Digestive system complications.

579.3 Other and unspecified postsurgical nonabsorption `CC`
Hypoglycemia   } following gastrointestinal
Malnutrition   }   surgery
CC Excl: 579.3-579.9
AHA: 4Q, '03, 104

579.4 Pancreatic steatorrhea `CC`
DEF: Excess fat in feces due to absence of pancreatic secretions in intestine.
CC Excl: See code: 579.1

579.8 Other specified intestinal malabsorption `CC`
Enteropathy: Steatorrhea (chronic)
exudative
protein-losing
CC Excl: See code: 579.1
AHA: 1Q, '88, 6

579.9 Unspecified intestinal malabsorption `CC`
Malabsorption syndrome NOS
CC Excl: See code: 579.1
AHA: 2Q, '11, 15; 4Q, '04, 59

`N` Newborn Age: 0   `P` Pediatric Age: 0-17   `M` Maternity Age: 12-55   `A` Adult Age: 15-124   `MCC` Major CC Condition   `CC` CC Condition   `HIV` HIV Related Dx

192 – Volume 1   **2014 ICD-9-CM**

10. Diseases of the Genitourinary System (580-629)

Nephritis, Nephrotic Syndrome, and Nephrosis (580-589)

EXCLUDES hypertensive chronic kidney disease (403.00-403.91, 404.00-404.93)

✓4ᵗʰ 580 Acute glomerulonephritis

INCLUDES acute nephritis

DEF: Acute, severe inflammation in tuft of capillaries that filter the kidneys.

580.0 With lesion of proliferative glomerulonephritis `MCC`

Acute (diffuse) proliferative glomerulonephritis

Acute poststreptococcal glomerulonephritis

CC Excl: 016.00-016.06, 016.30-016.36, 016.90-016.96, 017.90-017.96, 098.10, 098.19, 098.30-098.31, 098.89, 112.2, 131.00, 131.8-131.9, 249.40-249.41, 249.80-249.91, 250.40-250.43, 250.80-250.93, 274.10, 274.19, 277.88, 580.0-591, 593.0-593.2, 593.89-593.9, 599.70-599.9

580.4 With lesion of rapidly progressive glomerulonephritis `MCC`

Acute nephritis with lesion of necrotizing glomerulitis

DEF: Acute glomerulonephritis; progresses to ESRD with diffuse epithelial proliferation.

CC Excl: See code 580.0

✓5ᵗʰ 580.8 With other specified pathological lesion in kidney

580.81 Acute glomerulonephritis in diseases classified elsewhere `MCC`

Code first underlying disease, as:

infectious hepatitis (070.0-070.9)

mumps (072.79)

subacute bacterial endocarditis (421.0)

typhoid fever (002.0)

CC Excl: See code 580.0

580.89 Other `MCC`

Glomerulonephritis, acute, with lesion of:

exudative nephritis

interstitial (diffuse) (focal) nephritis

CC Excl: 016.00-016.06, 016.30-016.36, 016.90-016.96, 017.90-017.96, 098.10, 098.19, 098.30-098.31, 098.89, 112.2, 131.00, 131.8-131.9, 274.10, 274.19, 277.88, 580.0-591, 593.0-593.2, 593.89-593.9, 599.70-599.9

580.9 Acute glomerulonephritis with unspecified pathological lesion in kidney `MCC`

Glomerulonephritis

NOS

hemorrhagic   } specified as acute

Nephritis

Nephropathy

CC Excl: See code 580.0

✓4ᵗʰ 581 Nephrotic syndrome

DEF: Disease process marked by symptoms such as extensive edema, notable proteinuria, hypoalbuminemia, and susceptibility to intercurrent infections.

581.0 With lesion of proliferative glomerulonephritis `CC`

CC Excl: 016.00-016.06, 016.30-016.36, 016.90-016.96, 017.90-017.96, 098.10, 098.19, 098.30-098.31, 098.89, 112.2, 131.00, 131.8-131.9, 249.40-249.41, 249.80-249.91, 250.40-250.43, 250.80-250.93, 274.10, 274.19, 277.88, 580.0-591, 593.0-593.2, 593.89-593.9, 599.70-599.9

Nephron

Kidney

581.1 With lesion of membranous glomerulonephritis `CC`

Epimembranous nephritis

Idiopathic membranous glomerular disease

Nephrotic syndrome with lesion of:

focal glomerulosclerosis

sclerosing membranous glomerulonephritis

segmental hyalinosis

CC Excl: See code 581.0

581.2 With lesion of membranoproliferative glomerulonephritis `CC`

Nephrotic syndrome with lesion (of):

endothelial

hypocomplementemic persistent

lobular   } glomerulonephritis

mesangiocapillary

mixed membranous and proliferative

DEF: Glomerulonephritis combined with clinical features of nephrotic syndrome; characterized by uneven thickening of glomerular capillary walls and mesangial cell increase; slowly progresses to ESRD.

CC Excl: See code 581.0

581.3 With lesion of minimal change glomerulonephritis `CC`

Foot process disease

Lipoid nephrosis

Minimal change:

glomerular disease

glomerulitis

nephrotic syndrome

CC Excl: See code 581.0

AHA: 1Q, '07, 23

✓5ᵗʰ 581.8 With other specified pathological lesion in kidney

581.81 Nephrotic syndrome in diseases classified elsewhere `CC`

Code first underlying disease, as:

amyloidosis (277.30-277.39)

diabetes mellitus (249.4, 250.4)

malaria (084.9)

polyarteritis (446.0)

systemic lupus erythematosus (710.0)

EXCLUDES nephrosis in epidemic hemorrhagic fever (078.6)

CC Excl: See code 581.0

AHA: 3Q, '91, 8, 12; S-O, '85, 3

581.89 Other `CC`

Glomerulonephritis with edema and lesion of:

exudative nephritis

interstitial (diffuse) (focal) nephritis

CC Excl: See code 581.0

581.9 Nephrotic syndrome with unspecified pathological lesion in kidney `CC`

Glomerulonephritis with edema NOS

Nephritis:

nephrotic NOS

with edema NOS

Nephrosis NOS

Renal disease with edema NOS

CC Excl: See code 581.0

✓4ᵗʰ ✓5ᵗʰ Additional Digit Required   Unacceptable PDx   Manifestation Code   Hospital Acquired Condition   ▶◀ Revised Text   ● New Code   ▲ Revised Code Title

2014 ICD-9-CM   **Volume 1 – 193**

Diseases of the Genitourinary System

582–583.9

✓4ᵗʰ 582 Chronic glomerulonephritis

> **INCLUDES** chronic nephritis
>
> **DEF:** Slow progressive type of nephritis characterized by inflammation of the capillary loops in the glomeruli of the kidney, which leads to renal failure.

582.0 With lesion of proliferative glomerulonephritis **CC**

> Chronic (diffuse) proliferative glomerulonephritis
>
> **CC Excl:** 016.00-016.06, 016.30-016.36, 016.90-016.96, 017.90-017.96, 078.6, 098.10, 098.19, 098.30-098.31, 098.89, 112.2, 131.00, 131.8-131.9, 249.40-249.41, 249.80-249.91, 250.40-250.43, 250.80-250.93, 274.10, 274.19, 580.0-584.9, 586-591, 593.0-593.2, 593.89-593.9, 599.70-599.9

582.1 With lesion of membranous glomerulonephritis **CC**

> Chronic glomerulonephritis:
>   membranous
>   sclerosing
> Focal glomerulosclerosis
> Segmental hyalinosis
>
> **CC Excl:** See code: 582.0
>
> **AHA:** S-O, '84, 16

582.2 With lesion of membranoproliferative glomerulonephritis **CC**

> Chronic glomerulonephritis:
>   endothelial
>   hypocomplementemic persistent
>   lobular
>   membranoproliferative
>   mesangiocapillary
>   mixed membranous and proliferative
>
> **DEF:** Chronic glomerulonephritis with mesangial cell proliferation.
>
> **CC Excl:** See code: 582.0

582.4 With lesion of rapidly progressive glomerulonephritis **CC**

> Chronic nephritis with lesion of necrotizing glomerulitis
>
> **DEF:** Chronic glomerulonephritisrapidly progresses to ESRD; marked by diffuse epithelial proliferation.
>
> **CC Excl:** See code: 582.0

✓5ᵗʰ 582.8 With other specified pathological lesion in kidney

> **582.81 _Chronic glomerulonephritis in diseases classified elsewhere_** **CC**
>
> > Code first underlying disease, as:
> >   amyloidosis (277.30-277.39)
> >   systemic lupus erythematosus (710.0)
> >
> > **CC Excl:** See code: 582.0
>
> **582.89 Other** **CC**
>
> > Chronic glomerulonephritis with lesion of:
> >   exudative nephritis
> >   interstitial (diffuse) (focal) nephritis
> >
> > **CC Excl:** See code: 582.0

582.9 Chronic glomerulonephritis with unspecified pathological lesion in kidney **CC**

> Glomerulonephritis: ⎫
>   NOS   ⎬ specified as chronic
>   hemorrhagic ⎪
> Nephritis ⎪
> Nephropathy ⎭
>
> **CC Excl:** See code: 582.0
>
> **AHA:** 2Q, '01, 12

✓4ᵗʰ 583 Nephritis and nephropathy, not specified as acute or chronic

> **INCLUDES** "renal disease" so stated, not specified as acute or chronic but with stated pathology or cause

583.0 With lesion of proliferative glomerulonephritis **CC**

> Proliferative:
>   glomerulonephritis (diffuse) NOS
>   nephritis NOS
>   nephropathy NOS
>
> **CC Excl:** See code: 582.0

583.1 With lesion of membranous glomerulonephritis **CC**

> Membranous:
>   glomerulonephritis NOS
>   nephritis NOS
> Membranous nephropathy NOS
>
> **DEF:** Kidney inflammation or dysfunction with deposits on glomerular capillary basement membranes.
>
> **CC Excl:** See code: 582.0
>
> **N05.2** Uns nephritic syndr w/ diffuse membranous gln   **I-10**

583.2 With lesion of membranoproliferative glomerulonephritis **CC**

> Membranoproliferative:
>   glomerulonephritis NOS
>   nephritis NOS
>   nephropathy NOS
> Nephritis NOS, with lesion of:
>   hypocomplementemic ⎫
>   persistent   ⎪
>   lobular   ⎬ glomerulonephritis
>   mesangiocapillary   ⎪
>   mixed membranous and ⎪
>   proliferative   ⎭
>
> **DEF:** Kidney inflammation or dysfunction with mesangial cell proliferation.
>
> **CC Excl:** See code: 582.0

583.4 With lesion of rapidly progressive glomerulonephritis **MCC**

> Necrotizing or rapidly progressive:
>   glomerulitis NOS
>   glomerulonephritis NOS
>   nephritis NOS
>   nephropathy NOS
> Nephritis, unspecified, with lesion of necrotizing glomerulitis
>
> **DEF:** Kidney inflammation or dysfunction; rapidly progresses to ESRD marked by diffuse epithelial proliferation.
>
> **CC Excl:** 016.00-016.06, 016.30-016.36, 016.90-016.96, 017.90-017.96, 098.10, 098.19, 098.30-098.31, 098.89, 112.2, 131.00, 131.8-131.9, 249.40-249.41, 249.80-249.91, 250.40-250.43, 250.80-250.93, 274.10, 274.19, 277.88, 580.0-591, 593.0-593.2, 593.89-593.9, 599.70-599.9

583.6 With lesion of renal cortical necrosis **MCC**

> Nephritis, NOS   ⎫ with (renal) cortical necrosis
> Nephropathy NOS ⎭
>
> Renal cortical necrosis NOS
>
> **CC Excl:** 277.88, 583.6, 588.81-588.89

583.7 With lesion of renal medullary necrosis **CC**

> Nephritis, NOS   ⎫ with (renal) medullary
> Nephropathy NOS ⎭   [papillary] necrosis
>
> **CC Excl:** 277.88, 583.7, 588.81-588.89

✓5ᵗʰ 583.8 With other specified pathological lesion in kidney

> **583.81 _Nephritis and nephropathy, not specified as acute or chronic, in diseases classified elsewhere_**
>
> > Code first underlying disease, as:
> >   amyloidosis (277.30-277.39)
> >   diabetes mellitus (249.4, 250.4)
> >   gonococcal infection (098.19)
> >   Goodpasture's syndrome (446.21)
> >   systemic lupus erythematosus (710.0)
> >   tuberculosis (016.0)
> >
> > **EXCLUDES** gouty nephropathy (274.10)
> >   syphilitic nephritis (095.4)
> >
> > **AHA:** ▶2Q, '12, 19;◀ 2Q, '03, 7; 3Q, '91, 8; S-O, '85, 3
>
> **583.89 Other**
>
> > Glomerulitis   ⎫
> > Glomerulonephritis ⎪ with lesions of:
> > Nephritis   ⎬   exudative nephritis
> > Nephropathy   ⎪   interstitial nephritis
> > Renal disease   ⎭

583.9 With unspecified pathological lesion in kidney

> Glomerulitis   ⎫
> Glomerulonephritis ⎬ NOS
> Nephritis   ⎪
> Nephropathy   ⎭
>
> **EXCLUDES** nephropathy complicating pregnancy, labor, or the puerperium (642.0-642.9, 646.2)
>   renal disease NOS with no stated cause (593.9)

N Newborn Age: 0   **P** Pediatric Age: 0-17   **M** Maternity Age: 12-55   **A** Adult Age: 15-124   **MCC** Major CC Condition   **CC** CC Condition   **HIV** HIV Related Dx

✓4ᵗʰ 584 Acute kidney failure

> **INCLUDES** acute renal failure
>
> **EXCLUDES** *following labor and delivery (669.3)*
> *posttraumatic (958.5)*
> *that complicating:*
> *abortion (634-638 with .3, 639.3)*
> *ectopic or molar pregnancy (639.3)*
>
> **DEF:** State resulting from increasing urea and related substances from the blood (azotemia), often with urine output of less than 500 ml per day.
> **AHA:** 2Q, '11, 15; 3Q. '10, 15; 1Q, '93, 18; 2Q, '92, 5; 4Q, '92, 22
> **TIP:** Report acute renal failure separately when documented in addition to or association with hypertensive renal disease.

584.5 Acute kidney failure with lesion of tubular necrosis   `MCC`

> Lower nephron nephrosis
> Renal failure with (acute) tubular necrosis
> Tubular necrosis:
>   NOS
>   acute
> **DEF:** Acute decline in kidney efficiency with destruction of tubules.
> **CC Excl:** 249.40-249.41, 249.80-249.91, 250.40-250.43, 250.80-250.93, 274.10, 274.19, 277.88, 580.0-591, 593.0-593.2, 593.89-593.9, 599.70-599.9, 753.0-753.3, 753.9
> N17.0 Acute renal failure with tubular necrosis   `I-10`

584.6 Acute kidney failure with lesion of renal cortical necrosis   `MCC`

> **DEF:** Acute decline in kidney efficiency with destruction of renal tissues that filter blood.
> **CC Excl:** See code: 584.5

584.7 Acute kidney failure with lesion of renal medullary [papillary] necrosis   `MCC`

> Necrotizing renal papillitis
> **DEF:** Acute decline in kidney efficiency with destruction of renal tissues that collect urine.
> **CC Excl:** See code: 584.5

584.8 Acute kidney failure with other specified pathological lesion in kidney   `CC`

> **CC Excl:** 249.40-249.41, 249.80-249.91, 250.40-250.43, 250.80-250.93, 274.10, 274.19, 277.88, 580.0-591, 593.0-593.2, 593.89-593.9, 599.70-599.9
> **AHA:** 3Q, '11, 16-17; N-D, '85, 1

584.9 Acute kidney failure, unspecified   `CC`

> Acute kidney injury (nontraumatic)
> **EXCLUDES** *traumatic kidney injury (866.00-866.13)*
> **CC Excl:** See code: 584.5
> **AHA:** 3Q, '11, 16-17; 4Q, '09, 98; 4Q, '08, 192; 4Q, '07, 97; 2Q, '05, 18; 2Q, '03, 7; 1Q, '03, 22; 3Q, '02, 21, 28; 2Q, '01, 14; 1Q, '00, 22; 3Q, '96, 9; 4Q, '88, 1
> N17.9 Acute renal failure unspecified   `I-10`

✓4ᵗʰ 585 Chronic kidney disease [CKD]

> Chronic uremia
>
> Code first hypertensive chronic kidney disease, if applicable, (403.00-403.91, 404.00-404.93)
> Use additional code to identify kidney transplant status, if applicable (V42.0)
> Use additional code to identify manifestation as:
>   uremic:
>   neuropathy (357.4)
>   pericarditis (420.0)
> **AHA:** 4Q, '06, 84-86; 4Q, '05, 68, 77; 1Q, '04, 5; 4Q, '03, 61, 111; 2Q, '03, 7; 2Q, '01, 12, 13; 1Q, '01, 3; 4Q, '98, 55; 3Q, '98, 6, 7; 2Q, '98, 20; 3Q, '96, 9; 1Q, '93, 18; 3Q, '91, 8; 4Q, '89, 1; N-D, '85, 15; S-O, '84, 3

585.1 Chronic kidney disease, Stage I

> **DEF:** Some kidney damage; normal or slightly increased GFR (> 90).

585.2 Chronic kidney disease, Stage II (mild)

> **DEF:** Kidney damage with mild decrease in GFR (60–89).

585.3 Chronic kidney disease, Stage III (moderate)

> **DEF:** Kidney damage with moderate decrease in GFR (30–59).
> **AHA:** 4Q, '05, 69
> N18.3 Chronic kidney disease stage 3 (moderate)   `I-10`

585.4 Chronic kidney disease, Stage IV (severe)   `CC`

> **DEF:** Kidney damage with severe decrease in GFR (15–29).
> **CC Excl:** See code: 584.5
> N18.4 Chronic kidney disease stage 4 (severe)   `I-10`

585.5 Chronic kidney disease, Stage V   `CC`

> **EXCLUDES** *chronic kidney disease, stage V requiring chronic dialysis (585.6)*
> **DEF:** Kidney failure with GFR value of less than 15.
> **AHA:** 4Q, '10, 137
> **CC Excl:** See code 584.5

585.6 End stage renal disease   `MCC`

> Chronic kidney disease requiring chronic dialysis
> **DEF:** Federal government indicator of a stage V CKD patient undergoing treatment by dialysis or transplantation.
> **CC Excl:** 249.40-249.41, 249.80-249.91, 250.40-250.43, 250.80-250.93, 274.10, 274.19, 403.90, 580.0-591, 593.0-593.2, 593.89-593.9, 599.70-599.9, 753.0-753.3, 753.9
> **AHA:** 3Q, '11,15; 2Q, '11, 6; 3Q '10, 12, 15; 4Q, '08, 193; 1Q, '08, 7; 4Q, '07, 86; 3Q, '07, 5, 9; 4Q, '06, 136; 4Q, '05, 79
> N18.6 End stage renal disease   `I-10`

585.9 Chronic kidney disease, unspecified

> Chronic renal disease
> Chronic renal failure NOS
> Chronic renal insufficiency
> **AHA:** 1Q, '08, 10; 2Q, '07, 3; 4Q, '06, 86; 4Q, '05, 79
> N18.9 Chronic kidney disease unspecified   `I-10`

586 Renal failure, unspecified

> Uremia NOS
> **EXCLUDES** *following labor and delivery (669.3)*
> *posttraumatic renal failure (958.5)*
> *that complicating:*
> *abortion (634-638 with .3, 639.3)*
> *ectopic or molar pregnancy (639.3)*
> *uremia:*
> *extrarenal (788.9)*
> *prerenal (788.9)*
> **DEF:** Renal failure: kidney functions cease; malfunction may be due to inability to excrete metabolized substances or retain level of electrolytes.
> **DEF:** Uremia: excess urea, creatinine and other nitrogenous products of protein and amino acid metabolism in blood due to reduced excretory function in bilateral kidney disease; also called azotemia.
> **AHA:** 3Q, '98, 6; 1Q, '93, 18; 1Q, '88, 3
> N19 Unspecified renal failure   `I-10`

587 Renal sclerosis, unspecified

> Atrophy of kidney
> Contracted kidney
> Renal:
>   cirrhosis
>   fibrosis
> **AHA:** 4Q, '10, 137

✓4ᵗʰ 588 Disorders resulting from impaired renal function

588.0 Renal osteodystrophy

> Azotemic osteodystrophy
> Phosphate-losing tubular disorders
> Renal:
>   dwarfism
>   infantilism
>   rickets
> **DEF:** Condition resulting from chronic renal failure results in osteomalacia, osteoporosis or osteosclerosis; an abnormal level of phosphorus in the blood and impaired stimulation of the parathyroid.

588.1 Nephrogenic diabetes insipidus   `CC`

> **EXCLUDES** *diabetes insipidus NOS (253.5)*
> **DEF:** Type of diabetes due to renal tubules inability to reabsorb water; not responsive to vasopressin; may develop into chronic renal insufficiency.
> **CC Excl:** 016.00-016.06, 016.30-016.36, 016.90-016.96, 017.90-017.96, 078.6, 098.10, 098.19, 098.30-098.31, 098.89, 112.2, 131.00, 131.8 131.9, 249.40-249.41, 249.80-249.91, 250.40-250.43, 250.80-250.93, 274.10, 274.19, 580.0-584.9, 585.3-585.6, 586-591, 593.0-593.2, 593.89-593.9, 599.70-599.9

4ᵗʰ/5ᵗʰ Additional Digit Required   Unacceptable PDx   Manifestation Code   Hospital Acquired Condition   ►◄ Revised Text   ● New Code   ▲ Revised Code Title

2014 ICD-9-CM   Volume 1 – 195

Diseases of the Genitourinary System

588.8–593.1

✓5ᵗʰ **588.8 Other specified disorders resulting from impaired renal function**

> EXCLUDES *secondary hypertension (405.0-405.9)*

588.81 Secondary hyperparathyroidism (of CC **renal origin)**

Secondary hyperparathyroidism NOS

DEF: Parathyroid dysfunction caused by chronic renal failure; phosphate clearance is impaired, phosphate is released from bone, vitamin D is not produced, intestinal calcium absorption is low, and blood levels of calcium are lowered causing excessive production of parathyroid hormone.

CC Excl: 016.00-016.06, 016.30-016.36, 016.90-016.96, 017.90-017.96, 078.6, 098.10, 098.19, 098.30-098.31, 098.89, 112.2, 131.00, 131.8-131.9, 249.40-249.41, 249.80-249.91, 250.40-250.43, 250.80-250.93, 274.10, 274.19, 580.0-584.9, 586-588.1, 588.89-591, 593.0-593.2, 593.89-593.9, 599.70-599.9

AHA: 4Q, '04, 58-59

N25.81 Secondary hyperparathyroidism of   I-10 renal origin

588.89 Other specified disorders resulting from impaired renal function

Hypokalemic nephropathy

588.9 Unspecified disorder resulting from impaired renal function

✓4ᵗʰ **589 Small kidney of unknown cause**

589.0 Unilateral small kidney

589.1 Bilateral small kidneys

589.9 Small kidney, unspecified

Other Diseases of Urinary System (590-599)

✓4ᵗʰ **590 Infections of kidney**

Use additional code to identify organism, such as Escherichia coli [E. coli] (041.41-041.49)

✓5ᵗʰ **590.0 Chronic pyelonephritis**

Chronic pyelitis

Chronic pyonephrosis

Code if applicable, any casual condition first

590.00 Without lesion of renal medullary necrosis

590.01 With lesion of renal medullary necrosis CC

CC Excl: 016.00-016.06, 016.30-016.36, 016.90-016.96, 017.90-017.96, 078.6, 098.10, 098.19, 098.30-098.31, 098.89, 112.2, 131.00, 131.8-131.9, 249.40-249.41, 249.80-249.91, 250.40-250.43, 250.80-250.93, 274.10, 274.19, 580.0-584.9, 586-591, 593.0-593.2, 593.89-593.9, 599.70-599.9, 646.61-646.64

✓5ᵗʰ **590.1 Acute pyelonephritis**

Acute pyelitis

Acute pyonephrosis

⁸ **590.10 Without lesion of renal medullary necrosis** CC

CC Excl: 016.00-016.06, 016.30-016.36, 016.90-016.96, 017.90-017.96, 098.10, 098.19, 098.30-098.31, 098.89, 112.2, 131.00, 131.8-131.9, 249.40-249.41, 249.80-249.91, 250.40-250.43, 250.80-250.93, 274.10, 274.19, 580.0-591, 593.0-593.2, 593.89-593.9, 599.0, 599.70-599.9

Genitourinary System

Inferior vena cava —   — Aorta

Right kidney —   — Left kidney

Anterior division of internal iliac artery —   — Ureter

— Ovarian or testicular artery and vein

Superior and Inferior vesicular arteries —

— Urinary bladder

Ureteral orifice —   — Urogenital diaphragm

Urethra —

⁸ **590.11 With lesion of renal medullary necrosis** MCC

CC Excl: See code 590.10

⁸ **590.2 Renal and perinephric abscess** MCC

Abscess: Carbuncle of kidney

kidney

nephritic

perirenal

CC Excl: See code 590.10

⁸ **590.3 Pyeloureteritis cystica** CC

Infection of renal pelvis and ureter

Ureteritis cystica

DEF: Inflammation and formation of submucosal cysts in the kidney, pelvis, and ureter.

CC Excl: 016.00-016.06, 016.30-016.36, 016.90-016.96, 017.90-017.96, 098.10, 098.19, 098.30-098.31, 098.89, 112.2, 131.00, 131.8-131.9, 274.10, 274.19, 580.0-591, 593.0-593.2, 593.89-593.9, 599.0, 599.70-599.9

✓5ᵗʰ **590.8 Other pyelonephritis or pyonephrosis, not specified as acute or chronic**

⁸ **590.80 Pyelonephritis, unspecified** CC

Pyelitis NOS

Pyelonephritis NOS

CC Excl: See code 590.3

AHA: 1Q, '98, 10; 4Q, '97, 40

N11.9 Chronic tubulo-interstitial nephritis uns   I-10

⁸ **590.81 *Pyelitis or pyelonephritis in diseases classified elsewhere*** CC

Code first underlying disease, as:

tuberculosis (016.0)

CC Excl: See code 590.3

590.9 Infection of kidney, unspecified

> EXCLUDES *urinary tract infection NOS (599.0)*

591 Hydronephrosis CC

Hydrocalycosis   Hydroureteronephrosis

Hydronephrosis

> EXCLUDES *congenital hydronephrosis (753.29)*
> *hydroureter (593.5)*

DEF: Distention of kidney and pelvis, with urine build-up due to ureteral obstruction; pyonephrosis may result.

CC Excl: See code 590.3

AHA: ▶3Q, '12, 11-12;◀ 2Q, '98, 9

TIP: Hydronephrosis is not inherent in urinary obstructions and should be coded separately.

N13.30 Unspecified hydronephrosis   I-10

✓4ᵗʰ **592 Calculus of kidney and ureter**

> EXCLUDES *nephrocalcinosis (275.4)*

592.0 Calculus of kidney

Nephrolithiasis NOS   Staghorn calculus

Renal calculus or stone   Stone in kidney

> EXCLUDES *uric acid nephrolithiasis (274.11)*

AHA: ▶3Q, '12, 11-12;◀1Q, '00, 4

N20.0 Calculus of kidney   I-10

592.1 Calculus of ureter CC

Ureteric stone

Ureterolithiasis

CC Excl: 592.0-592.9, 593.3-593.5, 593.89-594.9, 599.60-599.9

AHA: 2Q, '98, 9; 1Q, '98, 10; 1Q, '91, 11

N20.1 Calculus of ureter   I-10

592.9 Urinary calculus, unspecified

AHA: 1Q, '98, 10; 4Q, '97, 40

✓4ᵗʰ **593 Other disorders of kidney and ureter**

593.0 Nephroptosis

Floating kidney

Mobile kidney

593.1 Hypertrophy of kidney

---

⁸ CC/MCC except when in combination with 996.64 and POA = N

N Newborn Age: 0   P Pediatric Age: 0-17   M Maternity Age: 12-55   A Adult Age: 15-124   MCC Major CC Condition   CC CC Condition   HIV HIV Related Dx

196 – Volume 1 • February 2013   2014 ICD-9-CM

593.2 Cyst of kidney, acquired
Cyst (multiple) (solitary) of kidney, not congenital
Peripelvic (lymphatic) cyst
> **EXCLUDES** *calyceal or pyelogenic cyst of kidney (591)*
> *congenital cyst of kidney (753.1)*
> *polycystic (disease of) kidney (753.1)*

DEF: Abnormal, fluid-filled sac in the kidney, not present at birth.
AHA: 4Q, '90, 3
N28.1 Cyst of kidney acquired   `I-10`

593.3 Stricture or kinking of ureter
Angulation
Constriction   } of ureter (post-operative)
Stricture of pelviureteric junction
DEF: Stricture or knot in tube connecting kidney to bladder.
AHA: 2Q, '98, 9

593.4 Other ureteric obstruction   `CC`
Idiopathic retroperitoneal fibrosis
Occlusion NOS of ureter
> **EXCLUDES** *that due to calculus (592.1)*

CC Exd: 593.3-593.5, 593.89-593.9, 595.0-595.9, 596.89-596.9, 599.0, 599.60-599.9, 753.4-753.5, 753.9, V45.74
AHA: 1Q, '10, 9; 2Q, '97, 4

593.5 Hydroureter   `CC`
> **EXCLUDES** *congenital hydroureter (753.22)*
> *hydroureteronephrosis (591)*

CC Exd: 593.3-593.5, 593.89-593.9, 595.0-595.9, 596.89-596.9, 599.0, 599.60-599.9, 753.4-753.5, 753.9

593.6 Postural proteinuria
Benign postural proteinuria
Orthostatic proteinuria
> **EXCLUDES** *proteinuria NOS (791.0)*

DEF: Excessive amounts of serum protein in the urine caused by the body position, e.g., orthostatic and lordotic.

√5ᵗʰ 593.7 Vesicoureteral reflux
DEF: Backflow of urine, from bladder into ureter due to obstructed bladder neck.
AHA: 4Q, '94, 42

593.70 Unspecified or without reflux nephropathy

593.71 With reflux nephropathy, unilateral

593.72 With reflux nephropathy, bilateral

593.73 With reflux nephropathy NOS

√5ᵗʰ 593.8 Other specified disorders of kidney and ureter

593.81 Vascular disorders of kidney   `CC`
Renal (artery):   Renal (artery):
embolism   thrombosis
hemorrhage   Renal infarction
CC Exd: 593.70-593.81, 593.9

593.82 Ureteral fistula   `CC`
Intestinoureteral fistula
> **EXCLUDES** *fistula between ureter and female genital tract (619.0)*

DEF: Abnormal communication, between tube connecting kidney to bladder and another structure.
CC Exd: 593.82-593.9

593.89 Other
Adhesions, kidney or ureter
Periureteritis
Polyp of ureter
Pyelectasia
Ureterocele
> **EXCLUDES** *tuberculosis of ureter (016.2)*
> *ureteritis cystica (590.3)*

593.9 Unspecified disorder of kidney and ureter
Acute renal disease   Renal disease NOS
Acute renal insufficiency   Salt-losing nephritis or syndrome
> **EXCLUDES** *chronic renal insufficiency (585.9)*
> *cystic kidney disease (753.1)*
> *nephropathy, so stated (583.0-583.9)*
> *renal disease:*
> *arising in pregnancy or the puerperium*
> *(642.1-642.2, 642.4-642.7, 646.2)*
> *not specified as acute or chronic, but with stated*
> *pathology or cause (583.0-583.9)*

AHA: 4Q, '05, 79; 1Q, '93, 17
N28.9 Disorder of kidney and ureter unspecified   `I-10`

√4ᵗʰ 594 Calculus of lower urinary tract

594.0 Calculus in diverticulum of bladder
DEF: Stone or mineral deposit in abnormal sac on the bladder wall.

594.1 Other calculus in bladder
Urinary bladder stone
> **EXCLUDES** *staghorn calculus (592.0)*

DEF: Stone or mineral deposit in bladder.

594.2 Calculus in urethra
DEF: Stone or mineral deposit in tube that empties urine from bladder.

594.8 Other lower urinary tract calculus
AHA: J-F, '85, 16

594.9 Calculus of lower urinary tract, unspecified
> **EXCLUDES** *calculus of urinary tract NOS (592.9)*

√4ᵗʰ 595 Cystitis
Use additional code to identify organism, such as Escherichia coli [E. coli] (041.41-041.49)
> **EXCLUDES** *prostatocystitis (601.3)*

8 595.0 Acute cystitis   `CC`
> **EXCLUDES** *trigonitis (595.3)*

DEF: Acute inflammation of bladder.
CC Exd: 016.10-016.16, 016.30-016.36, 016.90-016.96, 017.90-017.96, 098.0, 098.11, 098.2, 098.39, 098.89, 112.2, 131.00, 131.8-131.9, 593.3-593.5, 593.89-593.9, 595.0-595.9, 596.89-596.9, 599.0, 599.60-599.9
AHA: 2Q, '99, 15
N30.00 Acute cystitis without hematuria   `I-10`

595.1 Chronic interstitial cystitis
Hunner's ulcer   Submucous cystitis
Panmural fibrosis of bladder
DEF: Inflamed lesion affecting bladder wall; symptoms include urinary frequency, pain on bladder filling, nocturia, and distended bladder.

595.2 Other chronic cystitis
Chronic cystitis NOSSubacute cystitis
> **EXCLUDES** *trigonitis (595.3)*

DEF: Persistent inflammation of bladder.

595.3 Trigonitis
Follicular cystitis   Urethrotrigonitis
Trigonitis (acute) (chronic)
DEF: Inflammation of the triangular area of the bladder called the trigonum vesicae.

595.4 *Cystitis in diseases classified elsewhere*
Code first underlying disease, as:
actinomycosis (039.8)
amebiasis (006.8)
bilharziasis (120.0-120.9)
Echinococcus infestation (122.3, 122.6)
> **EXCLUDES** *cystitis:*
> *diphtheritic (032.84)*
> *gonococcal (098.11, 098.31)*
> *monilial (112.2)*
> *trichomonal (131.09)*
> *tuberculous (016.1)*

√5ᵗʰ 595.8 Other specified types of cystitis

595.81 Cystitis cystica
DEF: Inflammation of the bladder characterized by formation of multiple cysts.

CC/MCC except when in combination with 996.64 and POA = N

Additional Digit Required   Unacceptable PDx   Manifestation Code   Hospital Acquired Condition   ▶◀ Revised Text   ● New Code   ▲ Revised Code Title

14 ICD-9-CM   **Volume 1 – 197**

Diseases of the Genitourinary System

595.82 Irradiation cystitis `CC`
Use additional E code to identify cause
DEF: Inflammation of the bladder due to effects of radiation.
CC Exd: see code 595.0

595.89 Other
Abscess of bladder
Cystitis:
   bullous

Cystitis:
   emphysematous
   glandularis

595.9 Cystitis, unspecified

√4ᵗʰ **596 Other disorders of bladder**
Use additional code to identify urinary incontinence (625.6, 788.30-788.39)
AHA: M-A, '87, 10

596.0 Bladder neck obstruction
Contracture (acquired)
Obstruction (acquired) ⎫ of bladder neck or
Stenosis (acquired) ⎭ vesicourethral orifice

EXCLUDES congenital (753.6)
DEF: Bladder outlet and vesicourethral obstruction; occurs as a consequence of benign prostatic hypertrophy or prostatic cancer; may also occur in either sex due to strictures, following radiation, cystoscopy, catheterization, injury, infection, blood clots, bladder cancer, impaction or disease compressing bladder neck.
AHA: 3Q, '02, 28; 2Q, '01, 14; N-D, '86, 10
N32.0 Bladder-neck obstruction   `I-10`

596.1 Intestinovesical fistula `CC`
Fistula:
   enterovesical
   vesicocolic

Fistula:
   vesicoenteric
   vesicorectal

DEF: Abnormal communication, between intestine and bladder.
CC Exd: 098.0, 098.2, 098.39, 098.89, 596.1-596.2, 596.89-596.9, 599.70-599.9, 788.1

596.2 Vesical fistula, not elsewhere classified `CC`
Fistula:
   bladder NOS
   urethrovesical

Fistula:
   vesicocutaneous
   vesicoperineal

EXCLUDES fistula between bladder and female genital tract (619.0)
DEF: Abnormal communication between bladder and another structure.
CC Exd: See code: 596.1

596.3 Diverticulum of bladder
Diverticulitis
Diverticulum (acquired) (false) ⎭ of bladder

EXCLUDES that with calculus in diverticulum of bladder (594.0)
DEF: Abnormal pouch in bladder wall.

Bladder

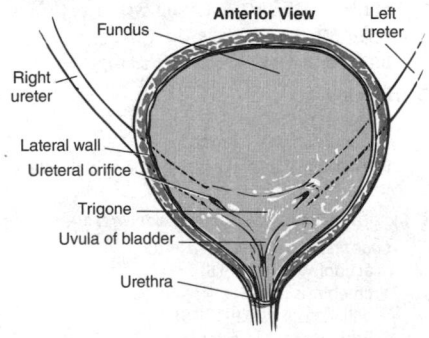

Anterior View

Fundus — Left ureter
Right ureter
Lateral wall
Ureteral orifice
Trigone
Uvula of bladder
Urethra

Lateral View

Urachus
Left ureter
Peritoneum
Pubic bone
Urogenital diaphragm

596.4 Atony of bladder
High compliance bladder
Hypotonicity ⎫ of bladder
Inertia ⎭

EXCLUDES neurogenic bladder (596.54)
DEF: Distended, bladder with loss of expulsive force; linked to CNS disease.

√5ᵗʰ **596.5 Other functional disorders of bladder**
EXCLUDES cauda equina syndrome with neurogenic bladder (344.61)

596.51 Hypertonicity of bladder
Hyperactivity   Overactive bladder
DEF: Abnormal tension of muscular wall of bladder; may appear after surgery of voluntary nerve.
N32.81 Overactive bladder   `I-`

596.52 Low bladder compliance
DEF: Low bladder capacity; causes increased pressure and frequent urination.

596.53 Paralysis of bladder
DEF: Impaired bladder motor function due to nerve or muscle damage.

596.54 Neurogenic bladder NOS
DEF: Unspecified dysfunctional bladder due to lesion of central, peripheral nervous system; may result in incontinence, residual urine retention, urinary infection, stones and renal failure.
AHA: 1Q, '01, 12
N31.9 Neuromuscular dysfunction of bladder unspecified   `I-`

596.55 Detrusor sphincter dyssynergia
DEF: Instability of the urinary bladder sphincter muscle associated with urinary incontinence.

596.59 Other functional disorder of bladder
Detrusor instability
DEF: Detrusor instability: instability of bladder; marked by uninhibited contractions often leading to incontinence.

596.6 Rupture of bladder, nontraumatic `MC`
CC Exd: 596.6-596.7, 596.89-596.9, 599.70-599.9, 788.1

596.7 Hemorrhage into bladder wall `C`
Hyperemia of bladder
EXCLUDES acute hemorrhagic cystitis (595.0)
CC Exd: See code: 596.6

√5ᵗʰ **596.8 Other specified disorders of bladder**
EXCLUDES cystocele, female (618.01-618.02, 618.09, 618.2-618.4)
hernia or prolapse of bladder, female (618.01-618.0, 618.09, 618.2-618.4)
AHA: 4Q, '11, 128-129; J-F, '85, 8

596.81 Infection of cystostomy `C`
Use additional code to specify type of infection, such as:
   abscess or cellulitis of abdomen (682.2)
   septicemia (038.0-038.9)
Use additional code to identify organism (041.00-041.9)
CC Exd: 596.81-596.89, 599.0, 996.30, 996.39, 996.56-996.6 996.64-996.65, 996.68-996.70, 996.76, 996.79, 997.91-997.99, 998.81, 998.83-998.9
AHA: 4Q, '11, 129

596.82 Mechanical complication of cystostomy `C`
Malfunction of cystostomy
CC Exd: 596.81-596.89, 996.39, 996.64-996.65, 996.76, 997.91-997.99, 998.81, 998.83-998.9

596.83 Other complication of cystostomy `C`
Fistula
Hernia
Prolapse
CC Exd: 596.81-596.89, 996.30, 996.39, 996.52, 996.55-996.60, 996.64-996.65, 996.68-996.70, 996.76, 996.79, 997.91-997.99, 998.81, 998.83-998.9

596.89 Other specified disorders of bladder
Bladder hemorrhage   Calcified bladder
Bladder hypertrophy   Contracted bladder

596.9 Unspecified disorder of bladder
AHA: J-F, '85, 8

√4ᵗʰ **597 Urethritis, not sexually transmitted, and urethral syndrome**
  EXCLUDES *nonspecific urethritis, so stated (099.4)*

  ⁸ **597.0 Urethral abscess**   CC
    Abscess: Abscess of:
     periurethral   Cowper's gland
     urethral (gland)   Littré's gland
    Abscess of: Periurethral cellulitis
     bulbourethral gland
    EXCLUDES *urethral caruncle (599.3)*
    DEF: Pocket of pus in tube that empties urine from the bladder.
    CC Excl: 098.0, 098.2, 098.39, 098.89, 099.40-099.49, 112.2, 131.00, 131.02, 131.8-131.9, 597.0-598.01, 598.8-599.0, 599.60-599.9, 607.1-607.83, 607.85-607.9, 608.4-608.81, 608.85, 608.87-608.89, 752.61-752.69, 752.81-752.9, 753.6-753.9, 788.1

  √5ᵗʰ **597.8 Other urethritis**
    597.80 Urethritis, unspecified
    597.81 Urethral syndrome NOS
    597.89 Other
      Adenitis, Skene's glands   Ulcer, urethra (meatus)
      Cowperitis   Verumontanitis
      Meatitis, urethral
      EXCLUDES *trichomonal (131.02)*

√4ᵗʰ **598 Urethral stricture**
  Use additional code to identify urinary incontinence (625.6, 788.30-788.39)
  INCLUDES pinhole meatus
    stricture of urinary meatus
  EXCLUDES *congenital stricture of urethra and urinary meatus (753.6)*
  DEF: Narrowing of tube that empties urine from bladder.

  √5ᵗʰ **598.0 Urethral stricture due to infection**
    598.00 Due to unspecified infection
    598.01 Due to infective diseases classified elsewhere
      Code first underlying disease, as:
       gonococcal infection (098.2)
       schistosomiasis (120.0-120.9)
       syphilis (095.8)

  598.1 Traumatic urethral stricture
    Stricture of urethra:
     late effect of injury
     postobstetric
    EXCLUDES *postoperative following surgery on genitourinary tract (598.2)*

  598.2 Postoperative urethral stricture
    Postcatheterization stricture of urethra
    AHA: 3Q, '97, 6

  598.8 Other specified causes of urethral stricture
    AHA: N-D, '84, 9

  598.9 Urethral stricture, unspecified

√4ᵗʰ **599 Other disorders of urethra and urinary tract**
  ⁸ **599.0 Urinary tract infection, site not specified**   CC
    Use additional code to identify organism, such as Escherichia coli [E. coli] (041.41-041.49)
    EXCLUDES *candidiasis of urinary tract (112.2)*
      urinary tract infection of newborn (771.82)
    CC Excl: 098.2, 098.39, 098.89, 099.40-099.49, 112.2, 131.00, 131.8-131.9, 590.10-591, 593.89-593.9, 595.0-595.9, 596.81, 599.0, 599.60-599.9, 788.1, 996.64
    AHA: ▶2Q, '12, 20;◀1Q, '12, 11;4Q, '11, 129; 1Q, '10, 9; 3Q, '09, 10-11; 3Q, '05, 12; 2Q, '04, 13; 4Q, '03, 79; 4Q, '99, 6; 2Q, '99, 15;1Q, '98, 5; 2Q, '96, 7; 4Q, '96, 33; 2Q, '95, 7; 1Q, '92, 13
    N39.0 Urinary tract infection site not specified   I-10

599.1 Urethral fistula   CC
  Fistula: Urinary fistula NOS
   urethroperineal
   urethrorectal
  EXCLUDES *fistula:*
    urethroscrotal (608.89)
    urethrovaginal (619.0)
    urethrovesicovaginal (619.0)
  CC Excl: 597.0-598.9, 599.1-599.9, 607.1-607.83, 607.85-607.9, 608.4-608.81, 608.85, 608.87-608.89, 752.61-752.69, 752.81-752.9, 753.9, 788.1
  AHA: 2Q, '11, 13; 3Q, '97, 6

599.2 Urethral diverticulum
  DEF: Abnormal pouch in urethral wall.

599.3 Urethral caruncle
  Polyp of urethra

599.4 Urethral false passage
  DEF: Abnormal opening in urethra due to surgery; trauma or disease.

599.5 Prolapsed urethral mucosa
  Prolapse of urethra   Urethrocele
  EXCLUDES *urethrocele, female (618.03, 618.09, 618.2-618.4)*

√5ᵗʰ **599.6 Urinary obstruction**
  Use additional code to identify urinary incontinence (625.6, 788.30-788.39)
  EXCLUDES *obstructive nephropathy NOS (593.89)*
  AHA: 4Q, '05, 80
  599.60 Urinary obstruction, unspecified
    Obstructive uropathy NOS
    Urinary (tract) obstruction NOS
    N13.9 Obstructive and reflux uropathy unspec   I-10
  599.69 Urinary obstruction, not elsewhere classified
    Code, if applicable, any causal condition first, such as: hyperplasia of prostate (600.0-600.9 with fifth-digit 1)
    AHA: 4Q, '06, 93

√5ᵗʰ **599.7 Hematuria**
  Hematuria (benign) (essential)
  EXCLUDES *hemoglobinuria (791.2)*
  AHA: 4Q, '08, 121; 1Q, '00, 5; 3Q, '95, 8
  599.70 Hematuria, unspecified
    R31.9 Hematuria unspecified   I-10
  599.71 Gross hematuria
    AHA: 2Q, '10, 3
  599.72 Microscopic hematuria

√5ᵗʰ **599.8 Other specified disorders of urethra and urinary tract**
  Use additional code to identify urinary incontinence (625.6, 788.30-788.39), if present
  EXCLUDES *symptoms and other conditions classifiable to 788.0-788.2, 788.4-788.9, 791.0-791.9*
  599.81 Urethral hypermobility
    DEF: Hyperactive urethra.
  599.82 Intrinsic (urethral) sphincter deficiency [ISD]
    DEF: Malfunctioning urethral sphincter.
    AHA: 2Q, '96, 15
  599.83 Urethral instability
    DEF: Inconsistent functioning of urethra.
  599.84 Other specified disorders of urethra
    Rupture of urethra   Urethral:
     (nontraumatic)   cyst
                  granuloma
    DEF: Rupture of urethra due to herniation or breaking down of tissue; not due to trauma.
    DEF: Urethral cyst: abnormal sac in urethra; usually fluid filled.
    DEF: Granuloma: inflammatory cells forming small nodules in urethra.
    AHA: 1Q, '09, 15
  599.89 Other specified disorders of urinary tract
599.9 Unspecified disorder of urethra and urinary tract

CC/MCC except when in combination with 996.64 and POA = N

Diseases of the Genitourinary System

600–601.9

Male Pelvic Organs

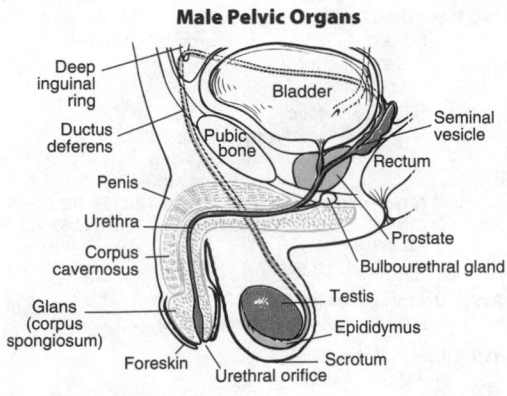

Deep inguinal ring
Ductus deferens
Penis
Urethra
Corpus cavernosus
Glans (corpus spongiosum)
Foreskin
Bladder
Pubic bone
Seminal vesicle
Rectum
Prostate
Bulbourethral gland
Testis
Epididymus
Scrotum
Urethral orifice

Diseases of Male Genital Organs (600-608)

√4ᵗʰ 600 Hyperplasia of prostate
     INCLUDES enlarged prostate
     DEF: Fibrostromal proliferation in periurethral glands, causes blood in urine; etiology unknown.
     AHA: 3Q, '05, 20; 4Q, '00, 43; 3Q, '94, 12; 3Q, '92, 7; N-D, '86, 10

√5ᵗʰ 600.0 Hypertrophy (benign) of prostate
     Benign prostatic hypertrophy   Smooth enlarged prostate
     Enlargement of prostate   Soft enlarged prostate
     AHA: 4Q, '06, 93-95; 3Q, '05, 20; 4Q, '03, 63; 1Q, '03, 6; 3Q, '02, 28; 2Q, '01, 14

600.00 Hypertrophy (benign) of prostate without urinary obstruction and other lower urinary tract symptoms [LUTS]   A ♂
     Hypertrophy (benign) of prostate NOS
     N40.0 Enlarged prostate without LUTS   I-10

600.01 Hypertrophy (benign) of prostate with urinary obstruction and other lower urinary tract symptoms [LUTS]   A ♂
     Hypertrophy (benign) of prostate with urinary retention
     Use additional code to identify symptoms:
       incomplete bladder emptying (788.21)
       nocturia (788.43)
       straining on urination (788.65)
       urinary frequency (788.41)
       urinary hesitancy (788.64)
       urinary incontinence (788.30-788.39)
       urinary obstruction (599.69)
       urinary retention (788.20)
       urinary urgency (788.63)
       weak urinary stream (788.62)
     AHA: 4Q, '06, 93-95; 4Q, '03, 64

√5ᵗʰ 600.1 Nodular prostate
     Hard, firm prostate
     Multinodular prostate
     EXCLUDES malignant neoplasm of prostate (185)
     DEF: Hard, firm nodule in prostate.
     AHA: 4Q, '03, 63

600.10 Nodular prostate without urinary obstruction   A ♂
     Nodular prostate NOS

600.11 Nodular prostate with urinary obstruction   A ♂
     Nodular prostate with urinary retention

√5ᵗʰ 600.2 Benign localized hyperplasia of prostate
     Adenofibromatous hypertrophy of prostate
     Adenoma of prostate
     Fibroadenoma of prostate
     Fibroma of prostate
     Myoma of prostate
     Polyp of prostate
     EXCLUDES benign neoplasms of prostate (222.2)
       hypertrophy of prostate (600.00-600.01)
       malignant neoplasm of prostate (185)
     DEF: Benign localized hyperplasia clearly defined epithelial tumor.
     AHA: 4Q, '06, 93-95; 4Q, '03, 63

600.20 Benign localized hyperplasia of prostate without urinary obstruction and other lower urinary tract symptoms [LUTS]   A
     Benign localized hyperplasia of prostate NOS

600.21 Benign localized hyperplasia of prostate with urinary obstruction and other lower urinary tract symptoms [LUTS]   A
     Benign localized hyperplasia of prostate with urinary retention
     Use additional code to identify symptoms:
       incomplete bladder emptying (788.21)
       nocturia (788.43)
       straining on urination (788.65)
       urinary frequency (788.41)
       urinary hesitancy (788.64)
       urinary incontinence (788.30-788.39)
       urinary obstruction (599.69)
       urinary retention (788.20)
       urinary urgency (788.63)
       weak urinary stream (788.62)

600.3 Cyst of prostate   A
     DEF: Sacs of fluid, which differentiate this from either nodular or adenomatous tumors.

√5ᵗʰ 600.9 Hyperplasia of prostate, unspecified
     Median bar
     Prostatic obstruction NOS
     AHA: 4Q, '06, 93-95; 4Q, '03, 63

600.90 Hyperplasia of prostate, unspecified, without urinary obstruction and other lower urinary tract symptoms [LUTS]   A
     Hyperplasia of prostate NOS

600.91 Hyperplasia of prostate, unspecified with urinary obstruction and other lower urinary tract symptoms [LUTS]   A
     Hyperplasia of prostate, unspecified, with urinary retention
     Use additional code to identify symptoms:
       incomplete bladder emptying (788.21)
       nocturia (788.43)
       straining on urination (788.65)
       urinary frequency (788.41)
       urinary hesitancy (788.64)
       urinary incontinence (788.30-788.39)
       urinary obstruction (599.69)
       urinary retention (788.20)
       urinary urgency (788.63)
       weak urinary stream (788.62)

√4ᵗʰ 601 Inflammatory diseases of prostate
     Use additional code to identify organism, such as Staphylococcus (041.1), or Streptococcus (041.0)

601.0 Acute prostatitis   CC A
     CC Excl: 098.12, 098.32, 098.89, 112.2, 131.00, 131.03, 131.8-131.9, 600.00-602.9

601.1 Chronic prostatitis   A

601.2 Abscess of prostate   CC A
     CC Excl: See code: 601.0

601.3 Prostatocystitis   A

601.4 *Prostatitis in diseases classified elsewhere*   A
     Code first underlying disease, as:
       actinomycosis (039.8)
       blastomycosis (116.0)
       syphilis (095.8)
       tuberculosis (016.5)
     EXCLUDES prostatitis:
       gonococcal (098.12, 098.32)
       monilial (112.2)
       trichomonal (131.03)

601.8 Other specified inflammatory diseases of prostate   A
     Prostatitis:
       cavitary
       diverticular
       granulomatous

601.9 Prostatitis, unspecified   A
     Prostatitis NOS

N Newborn Age: 0   **P** Pediatric Age: 0-17   **M** Maternity Age: 12-55   **A** Adult Age: 15-124   **MCC** Major CC Condition   **CC** CC Condition   **HIV** HIV Related

200 – Volume 1   **2014 ICD-9-**

Common Inguinal Canal Anomalies

Peritoneal cavity — Normal anatomy — Obliterated process vaginalis — Tunica vaginalis — Vas deferens — Testis — Scrotal hernia — Inguinal hernia — Hydrocele of the cord — Communicating hydrocele — Hydrocele of tunica vaginalis

602 Other disorders of prostate

602.0 Calculus of prostate
Prostatic stone
DEF: Stone or mineral deposit in prostate.

602.1 Congestion or hemorrhage of prostate
DEF: Bleeding or fluid collection in prostate.

602.2 Atrophy of prostate

602.3 Dysplasia of prostate
Prostatic intraepithelial neoplasia I (PIN I)
Prostatic intraepithelial neoplasia II (PIN II)
EXCLUDES *prostatic intraepithelial neoplasia III (PIN III) (233.4)*
DEF: Abnormality of shape and size of the intraepithelial tissues of the prostate; premalignant condition characterized by stalks and absence of a basilar cell layer; synonyms are intraductal dysplasia, large acinar atypical hyperplasia, atypical primary hyperplasia, hyperplasia with malignant changes, marked atypia, or duct-acinar dysplasia.
AHA: 4Q, '01, 46

602.8 Other specified disorders of prostate
Fistula
Infarction ⎱ of prostate
Stricture
Periprostatic adhesions

602.9 Unspecified disorder of prostate

603 Hydrocele
INCLUDES hydrocele of spermatic cord, testis or tunica vaginalis
EXCLUDES *congenital (778.6)*
DEF: Circumscribed collection of fluid in tunica vaginalis, spermatic cord or testis.

603.0 Encysted hydrocele

603.1 Infected hydrocele
Use additional code to identify organism
CC Exd: 112.2, 131.00, 131.8-131.9, 603.0-603.9

603.8 Other specified types of hydrocele

603.9 Hydrocele, unspecified

604 Orchitis and epididymitis
Use additional code to identify organism, such as:
Escherichia coli [E. coli] (041.41-041.49)
Staphylococcus (041.10-041.19)
Streptococcus (041.00-041.09)

604.0 Orchitis, epididymitis, and epididymoorchitis, with abscess
Abscess of epididymis or testis
CC Exd: 072.0, 098.13-098.14, 098.33-098.34, 098.89, 112.2, 131.00, 131.8-131.9, 604.0-604.99

604.9 Other orchitis, epididymitis, and epididymo-orchitis, without mention of abscess

604.90 Orchitis and epididymitis, unspecified

604.91 Orchitis and epididymitis in diseases classified elsewhere
Code first underlying disease, as:
diphtheria (032.89)
filariasis (125.0-125.9)
syphilis (095.8)
EXCLUDES *orchitis:*
gonococcal (098.13, 098.33)
mumps (072.0)
tuberculous (016.5)
tuberculous epididymitis (016.4)

604.99 Other

605 Redundant prepuce and phimosis
Adherent prepuce   Phimosis (congenital)
Paraphimosis   Tight foreskin
DEF: Constriction of preputial orifice causing inability of the prepuce to be drawn back over the glans; it may be congenital or caused by infection.
AHA: 3Q, '08, 9

606 Infertility, male
AHA: 2Q, '96, 9

606.0 Azoospermia
Absolute infertility
Infertility due to:
germinal (cell) aplasia
spermatogenic arrest (complete)
DEF: Absence of spermatozoa in the semen or inability to produce spermatozoa.

606.1 Oligospermia
Infertility due to:
germinal cell desquamation
hypospermatogenesis
incomplete spermatogenic arrest
DEF: Insufficient number of sperm in semen.

606.8 Infertility due to extratesticular causes
Infertility due to:
drug therapy
infection
obstruction of efferent ducts
radiation
systemic disease

606.9 Male infertility, unspecified

607 Disorders of penis
EXCLUDES *phimosis (605)*

607.0 Leukoplakia of penis
Kraurosis of penis
EXCLUDES *carcinoma in situ of penis (233.5)*
erythroplasia of Queyrat (233.5)
DEF: White, thickened patches on glans penis.

607.1 Balanoposthitis
Balanitis
Use additional code to identify organism
DEF: Inflammation of glans penis and prepuce.

607.2 Other inflammatory disorders of penis
Abscess
Boil ⎱ of corpus cavernosum or
Carbuncle ⎰ penis
Cellulitis
Cavernitis (penis)
Use additional code to identify organism
EXCLUDES *herpetic infection (054.13)*

607.3 Priapism
Painful erection
DEF: Prolonged penile erection without sexual stimulation.
CC Exd: 607.0-607.9

607.8 Other specified disorders of penis

607.81 Balanitis xerotica obliterans
Induratio penis plastica
DEF: Inflammation of the glans penis, caused by stricture of the opening of the prepuce.

Additional Digit Required   Unacceptable PDx   Manifestation Code   Hospital Acquired Condition   ►◄ Revised Text   ● New Code   ▲ Revised Code Title

014 ICD-9-CM   **Volume 1 – 201**

607.82 Vascular disorders of penis   `CC` ♂

Embolisim
Hematoma
(nontraumatic)   } of corpus
Hemorrhage   cavernosum
Thrombosis   or penis
CC Excl: 607.82-607.83

607.83 Edema of penis   ♂
DEF: Fluid retention within penile tissues.

607.84 Impotence of organic origin   `A` ♂
EXCLUDES nonorganic (302.72)
DEF: Physiological cause interfering with erection.
AHA: 3Q, '91, 11
TIP: If impotence is a result of previous radical prostatectomy, report code 997.99 first.

607.85 Peyronie's disease   ♂
DEF: A severe curvature of the erect penis due to fibrosis of the cavernous sheaths.
AHA: 4Q, '03, 64

607.89 Other   ♂
Atrophy
Fibrosis   } of corpus
Hypertrophy   cavernosum
Ulcer (chronic)   or penis

607.9 Unspecified disorder of penis   ♂

√4ᵗʰ **608 Other disorders of male genital organs**

608.0 Seminal vesiculitis   ♂
Abscess
Cellulitis   } of seminal vesicle

Vesiculitis (seminal)
Use additional code to identify organism
EXCLUDES gonococcal infection (098.14, 098.34)
DEF: Inflammation of seminal vesicle.

608.1 Spermatocele   ♂
DEF: Cystic enlargement of the epididymis or the testis; the cysts contain spermatozoa.

√5ᵗʰ **608.2 Torsion of testis**
DEF: Twisted or rotated testis; may compromise blood flow.

608.20 Torsion of testis, unspecified   `CC` ♂
CC Excl: 608.20-608.24
AHA: 4Q, '06, 95

608.21 Extravaginal torsion of spermatic cord   `CC` ♂
DEF: Torsion of the spermatic cord just below the tunica vaginalis attachments.
CC Excl: See code: 608.20
AHA: 4Q, '06, 95

608.22 Intravaginal torsion of spermatic cord   `CC` ♂
Torsion of spermatic cord NOS
DEF: Torsion within the tunica vaginalis also called the "bell-clapper" anomaly. It usually occurs in older children.
CC Excl: See code: 608.20
AHA: 4Q, '06, 95

608.23 Torsion of appendix testis   `CC` ♂
DEF: Torsion of small solid projection of tissue on the upper outer surface of the testis (hydatid of Morgagni); a remnant of the embryologic Müllerian duct.
CC Excl: See code: 608.20
AHA: 4Q, '06, 95

608.24 Torsion of appendix epididymis   `CC` ♂
DEF: Torsion of small stalked appendage of the head of the epididymis (pedunculated hydatid); a detached embryologic efferent duct.
CC Excl: See code: 608.20
AHA: 4Q, '06, 95

608.3 Atrophy of testis   ♂

608.4 Other inflammatory disorders of male genital organs   ♂
Abscess
Boil   of scrotum, spermatic cord, testis
Carbuncle   [except abscess], tunica
Cellulitis   vaginalis, or vas deferens
Vasitis
Use additional code to identify organism
EXCLUDES abscess of testis (604.0)

√5ᵗʰ **608.8 Other specified disorders of male genital organs**

608.81 Disorders of male genital organs in diseases classified elsewhere   ♂
Code first underlying disease, as:
filariasis (125.0-125.9)
tuberculosis (016.5)

608.82 Hematospermia   ♂
DEF: Presence of blood in the ejaculate; relatively common, affecting men of any age after puberty; cause is often the result of a viral or bacterial infection and inflammation.
AHA: 4Q, '01, 46

608.83 Vascular disorders   ♂
Hematoma (non-
traumatic)   of seminal vessel, spermatic
Hemorrhage   cord, testis, scrotum,
Thrombosis   tunica vaginalis, or vas
deferens

Hematocele NOS, male
AHA: 4Q, '03, 110
TIP: Assign for Fournier's gangrene, which is a result of an infection in the genital area.

608.84 Chylocele of tunica vaginalis   ♂
DEF: Chylous effusion into tunica vaginalis; due to infusion of lymphatic fluids.

608.85 Stricture   ♂
Stricture of: Stricture of:
spermatic cord   vas deferens
tunica vaginalis

608.86 Edema   ♂

608.87 Retrograde ejaculation   ♂
DEF: Condition where the semen travels to the bladder rather than out through the urethra due to damaged nerves causing the bladder neck to remain open during ejaculation.
AHA: 4Q, '01, 46

608.89 Other   ♂
Atrophy   } of seminal vessel, spermatic
Fibrosis   cord, testis, scrotum,
Hypertrophy   tunica vaginalis, or vas
Ulcer   deferens
EXCLUDES atrophy of testis (608.3)

608.9 Unspecified disorder of male genital organs   ♂

Disorders of Breast (610-612)

√4ᵗʰ **610 Benign mammary dysplasias**

610.0 Solitary cyst of breast
Cyst (solitary) of breast

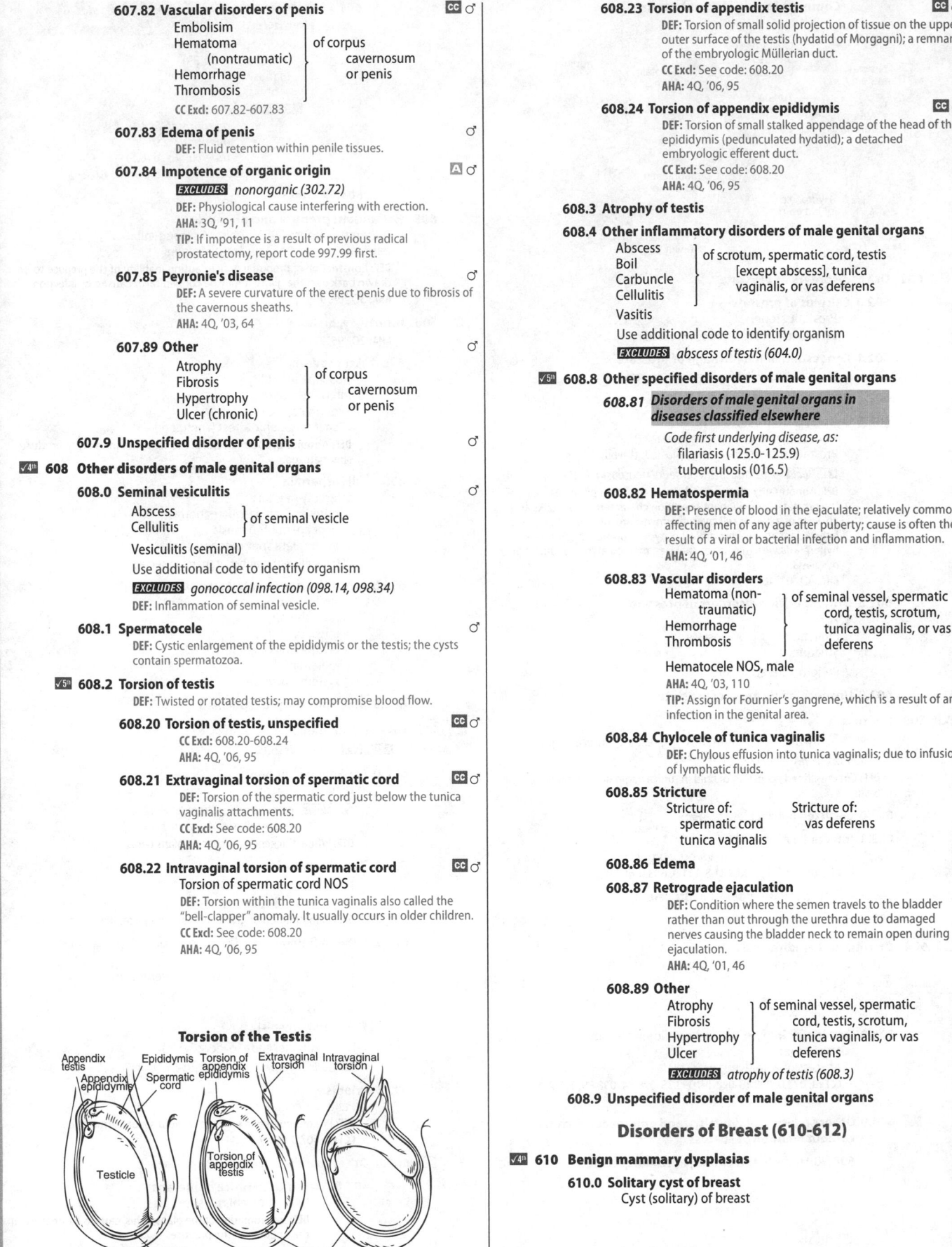

Torsion of the Testis

Appendix testis
Appendix epididymis
Epididymis
Spermatic cord
Torsion of appendix epididymis
Extravaginal torsion
Intravaginal torsion
Testicle
Torsion of appendix testis
Tunica vaginalis
Tunica vaginalis

`N` Newborn Age: 0   `P` Pediatric Age: 0-17   `M` Maternity Age: 12-55   `A` Adult Age: 15-124   `MCC` Major CC Condition   `CC` CC Condition   `HIV` HIV Related Dx

202 – Volume 1   2014 ICD-9-CM

610.1 Diffuse cystic mastopathy   A

Chronic cystic mastitis
Cystic breast
Fibrocystic disease of
breast

DEF: Extensive formation of nodular cysts in breast tissue; symptoms include tenderness, change in size and hyperplasia of ductal epithelium.

AHA: 2Q, '06, 10

TIP: Assign in addition to screening mammography V code; is a normal variant, commonly found in normal breasts and not a pathological condition.

610.2 Fibroadenosis of breast

Fibroadenosis of breast: Fibroadenosis of breast:
NOS   diffuse
chronic   periodic
cystic   segmental

DEF: Non-neoplastic nodular condition of breast.

610.3 Fibrosclerosis of breast

DEF: Fibrous tissue in breast.

610.4 Mammary duct ectasia

Comedomastitis   Mastitis:
Duct ectasia   periductal
                 plasma cell

DEF: Atrophy of duct epithelium; causes distended collecting ducts of mammary gland, drying up of breast secretion, intraductal inflammation and periductal and interstitial chronic inflammatory reaction.

610.8 Other specified benign mammary dysplasias

Mazoplasia   Sebaceous cyst of breast

AHA: 2Q, '09, 9

610.9 Benign mammary dysplasia, unspecified

√4ᵗʰ **611 Other disorders of breast**

EXCLUDES *that associated with lactation or the puerperium (675.0-676.9)*

611.0 Inflammatory disease of breast

Abscess (acute) (chronic) (nonpuerperal) of:
areola
breast
Mammillary fistula
Mastitis (acute) (subacute) (nonpuerperal):
NOS
infective
retromammary
submammary

EXCLUDES *carbuncle of breast (680.2)*
chronic cystic mastitis (610.1)
neonatal infective mastitis (771.5)
thrombophlebitis of breast [Mondor's disease] (451.89)

611.1 Hypertrophy of breast

Gynecomastia
Hypertrophy of breast:
NOS
massive pubertal

EXCLUDES *breast engorgement in newborn (778.7)*
disproportion of reconstructed breast (612.1)

611.2 Fissure of nipple

611.3 Fat necrosis of breast

Fat necrosis (segmental) of breast

Code first breast necrosis due to breast graft (996.79)

DEF: Splitting of neutral fats in adipose tissue cells as a result of trauma; a firm circumscribed mass is then formed in the breast.

611.4 Atrophy of breast

611.5 Galactocele

DEF: Milk-filled cyst in breast due to blocked duct.

611.6 Galactorrhea not associated with childbirth

DEF: Flow of milk not associated with childbirth or pregnancy.

√5ᵗʰ **611.7 Signs and symptoms in breast**

611.71 Mastodynia

Pain in breast

611.72 Lump or mass in breast

AHA: 4Q, '09, 106; 2Q, '03, 4-5

TIP: Do not assign if the underlying cause of the breast lump or mass is determined and documented during the episode of care.

611.79 Other

Induration of breast
Inversion of nipple
Nipple discharge
Retraction of nipple

√5ᵗʰ **611.8 Other specified disorders of breast**

AHA: 4Q, '08, 121-122

611.81 Ptosis of breast   A

EXCLUDES *ptosis of native breast in relation to reconstructed breast (612.1)*

611.82 Hypoplasia of breast   A

Micromastia

EXCLUDES *congenital absence of breast (757.6)*
hypoplasia of native breast in relation to reconstructed breast (612.1)

611.83 Capsular contracture of breast implant   A

TIP: Do not assign additional code from category 996 Complications peculiar to certain specified procedures.

611.89 Other specified disorders of breast

Hematoma (nontraumatic) of breast
Infarction of breast
Occlusion of breast duct
Subinvolution of breast (postlactational) (postpartum)

611.9 Unspecified breast disorder

√4ᵗʰ **612 Deformity and disproportion of reconstructed breast**

AHA: 4Q, '08, 123

612.0 Deformity of reconstructed breast   A

Contour irregularity in reconstructed breast
Excess tissue in reconstructed breast
Misshapen reconstructed breast

612.1 Disproportion of reconstructed breast   A

Breast asymmetry between native breast and reconstructed breast
Disproportion between native breast and reconstructed breast

Inflammatory Disease of Female Pelvic Organs (614-616)

Use additional code to identify organism, such as Staphylococcus (041.1), or Streptococcus (041.0)

EXCLUDES *that associated with pregnancy, abortion, childbirth, or the puerperium (630-676.9)*

√4ᵗʰ **614 Inflammatory disease of ovary, fallopian tube, pelvic cellular tissue, and peritoneum**

EXCLUDES *endometritis (615.0-615.9)*
major infection following delivery (670.0-670.8)
that complicating:
abortion (634-638 with .0, 639.0)
ectopic or molar pregnancy (639.0)
pregnancy or labor (646.6)

614.0 Acute salpingitis and oophoritis   CC ♀

Any condition classifiable to 614.2, specified as acute or subacute

DEF: Acute inflammation of ovary and fallopian tube.

CC Excl: 016.60-016.96, 017.90-017.96, 098.15-098.17, 098.35-098.37, 098.89, 112.2, 131.00, 131.8-131.9, 614.0-615.9, 616.81-616.9, 625.70, 625.79-625.9, 629.20-629.9, 752.81-752.9

614.1 Chronic salpingitis and oophoritis   ♀

Hydrosalpinx
Salpingitis:
follicularis
isthmica nodosa
Any condition classifiable to 614.2, specified as chronic

DEF: Persistent inflammation of ovary and fallopian tube.

▲
⁴ᵗʰ
⁵ᵗʰ   Additional Digit Required   Unacceptable PDx   Manifestation Code   Hospital Acquired Condition   ▶◀ Revised Text   ● New Code   ▲ Revised Code Title

2014 ICD-9-CM   **Volume 1 – 203**

Diseases of the Genitourinary System

614.2–616.51

614.2 Salpingitis and oophoritis not specified as acute, subacute, or chronic ♀

Abscess (of):
fallopian tube
ovary
tubo-ovarian
Oophoritis
Perioophoritis
Perisalpingitis
Pyosalpinx
Salpingitis
Salpingo-oophoritis
Tubo-ovarian inflammatory disease

EXCLUDES gonococcal infection (chronic) (098.37)
acute (098.17)
tuberculous (016.6)

AHA: 2Q, '91, 5

614.3 Acute parametritis and pelvic cellulitis CC ♀

Acute inflammatory pelvic disease
Any condition classifiable to 614.4, specified as acute

DEF: Parametritis: inflammation of the parametrium; pelvic cellulitis is a synonym for parametritis.

CC Excl: See code 614.0

614.4 Chronic or unspecified parametritis and pelvic cellulitis ♀

Abscess (of):
broad ligament
parametrium
pelvis, femal
pouch of Douglas } chronic or NOS

Chronic inflammatory pelvic disease
Pelvic cellulitis, female

EXCLUDES tuberculous (016.7)

614.5 Acute or unspecified pelvic peritonitis, female MCC ♀

CC Excl: See code 614.0

AHA: 4Q, '05, 74

TIP: For pelvic peritonitis in a male patient, refer to code 567.21.

614.6 Pelvic peritoneal adhesions, female (postoperative) (postinfection) ♀

Adhesions:
peritubal
tubo-ovarian

Use additional code to identify any associated infertility (628.2)

DEF: Fibrous scarring abnormally joining structures within abdomen.

AHA: 2Q, '11, 19; 3Q, '03, 6; 1Q, '03, 4; 3Q, '95, 7; 3Q, '94, 12

N73.6 Female pelvic peritoneal adhesions (postinfective)   I-10

614.7 Other chronic pelvic peritonitis, female CC ♀

EXCLUDES tuberculous (016.7)

CC Excl: See code: 614.0

614.8 Other specified inflammatory disease of female pelvic organs and tissues ♀

614.9 Unspecified inflammatory disease of female pelvic organs and tissues ♀

Pelvic infection or inflammation, female NOS
Pelvic inflammatory disease [PID]

√4ʰ 615 Inflammatory diseases of uterus, except cervix

EXCLUDES following delivery (670.0-670.8)
hyperplastic endometritis (621.30-621.35)
that complicating:
abortion (634-638 with .0, 639.0)
ectopic or molar pregnancy (639.0)
pregnancy or labor (646.6)

615.0 Acute CC ♀

Any condition classifiable to 615.9, specified as acute or subacute

CC Excl: 016.60-016.96, 017.90-017.96, 098.15-098.17, 098.35-098.37, 098.89, 112.2, 131.00, 131.8-131.9, 614.0-616.0, 616.81-616.9, 621.8-621.9, 625.70, 625.79-625.9, 629.20-629.9, 752.81-752.9

615.1 Chronic ♀

Any condition classifiable to 615.9, specified as chronic

615.9 Unspecified inflammatory disease of uterus ♀

Endometritis
Endomyometritis
Intrauterine infection
Metritis
Myometritis
Perimetritis
Pyometra
Uterine abscess

N71.9 Inflammatory disease of uterus unspecified   I-10

√4ʰ 616 Inflammatory disease of cervix, vagina, and vulva

EXCLUDES that complicating:
abortion (634-638 with .0, 639.0)
ectopic or molar pregnancy (639.0)
pregnancy, childbirth, or the puerperium (646.6)

616.0 Cervicitis and endocervicitis

Cervicitis
Endocervicitis } with or without mention of erosion or ectropion

Nabothian (gland) cyst or follicle

EXCLUDES erosion or ectropion without mention of cervicitis (622.0)

N72 Inflammatory disease of cervix uteri   I-10

√5ʰ 616.1 Vaginitis and vulvovaginitis

EXCLUDES vulvar vestibulitis (625.71)

DEF: Inflammation or infection of vagina or external female genitalia.

616.10 Vaginitis and vulvovaginitis, unspecified ♀

Vaginitis:
NOS
postirradiation
Vulvitis NOS
Vulvovaginitis NOS

Use additional code to identify organism, such as:
Escherichia coli [E. coli] (041.41-041.49)
Staphylococcus (041.10-041.19)
Streptococcus (041.00-041.09)

EXCLUDES noninfective leukorrhea (623.5)
postmenopausal or senile vaginitis (627.3)

616.11 Vaginitis and vulvovaginitis in diseases classified elsewhere ♀

Code first underlying disease, as:
pinworm vaginitis (127.4)

EXCLUDES herpetic vulvovaginitis (054.11)
monilial vulvovaginitis (112.1)
trichomonal vaginitis or vulvovaginitis (131.01)

616.2 Cyst of Bartholin's gland ♀

Bartholin's duct cyst

DEF: Fluid-filled sac within gland of vaginal orifice.

616.3 Abscess of Bartholin's gland CC ♀

Vulvovaginal gland abscess

CC Excl: 016.70-016.96, 017.90-017.96, 112.1-112.2, 131.00-131.01, 131.8-131.9, 616.10-616.9, 624.3-624.9, 625.70-625.9, 629.20-629.9, 752.81-752.9

616.4 Other abscess of vulva CC ♀

Abscess
Carbuncle } of vulva
Furuncle

CC Excl: See code 616.3

√5ʰ 616.5 Ulceration of vulva

616.50 Ulceration of vulva, unspecified ♀

Ulcer NOS of vulva

616.51 Ulceration of vulva in diseases classified elsewhere ♀

Code first underlying disease, as:
Behçet's syndrome (136.1)
tuberculosis (016.7)

EXCLUDES vulvar ulcer (in):
gonococcal (098.0)
herpes simplex (054.12)
syphilitic (091.0)

Female Genitourinary System

Uterine (fallopian) tube
Ovary
Rectouterine pouch (of Douglas)
Uterus (fundus)
Cervix
Pubic bone
Bladder
Rectum
Clitoris
Urogenital diaphragm
Urethral orifice (meatus)
Labia minora
Labia majora
Anus
Vaginal canal

 Newborn Age: 0   Pediatric Age: 0-17   M Maternity Age: 12-55   A Adult Age: 15-124   MCC Major CC Condition   CC CC Condition   HIV HIV Related Dx

204 – Volume 1   **2014 ICD-9-CM**

Common Sites of Endometriosis

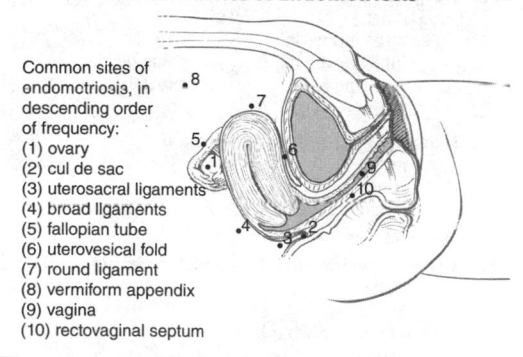

Common sites of
ondometriosis, in
descending order
of frequency:
(1) ovary
(2) cul de sac
(3) uterosacral ligaments
(4) broad ligaments
(5) fallopian tube
(6) uterovesical fold
(7) round ligament
(8) vermiform appendix
(9) vagina
(10) rectovaginal septum

√5ᵗʰ 616.8 Other specified inflammatory diseases of cervix, vagina, and vulva

> **EXCLUDES** noninflammatory disorders of:
> cervix (622.0-622.9)
> vagina (623.0-623.9)
> vulva (624.0-624.9)

616.81 Mucositis (ulcerative) of cervix, vagina, and vulva   **CC** ♀

> Use additional E code to identify adverse effects of therapy, such as:
> antineoplastic and immunosuppressive drugs (E930.7, E933.1)
> radiation therapy (E879.2)
>
> **CC Exd:** 616.0, 616.81-616.9
> **AHA:** 4Q, '06, 88-90

616.89 Other inflammatory disease of cervix, vagina, and vulva   ♀

> Caruncle, vagina or labium
> Ulcer, vagina
>
> **AHA:** 4Q, '06, 88-90

616.9 Unspecified inflammatory disease of cervix, vagina, and vulva   ♀

Other Disorders of Female Genital Tract (617-629)

√4ᵗʰ 617 Endometriosis

617.0 Endometriosis of uterus   ♀

> Adenomyosis   Endometriosis:
> Endometriosis: internal
>   cervix   myometrium
>
> **EXCLUDES** stromal endometriosis (236.0)
>
> **DEF:** Aberrant uterine mucosal tissue; creating products of menses and inflamed uterine tissues.
> **AHA:** 3Q, '92, 7
> **N80.0** Endometriosis of uterus   **I-10**

617.1 Endometriosis of ovary   ♀

> Chocolate cyst of ovary
> Endometrial cystoma of ovary
>
> **DEF:** Aberrant uterine tissue; creating products of menses and inflamed ovarian tissues.
> **N80.1** Endometriosis of ovary   **I-10**

617.2 Endometriosis of fallopian tube   ♀

> **DEF:** Aberrant uterine tissue; creating products of menses and inflamed tissues of fallopian tubes.

Vaginal Midline Cystocele

Uterus
Pubocervical fascia
Bladder
Rectum
Urethra
Rectovaginal fascia
Vaginal epithelium
Uterus
Normal vaginal support
Bladder
Midline cystocele
Urethra
Defect of pubocervical fascia

Vaginal Lateral Cystocele

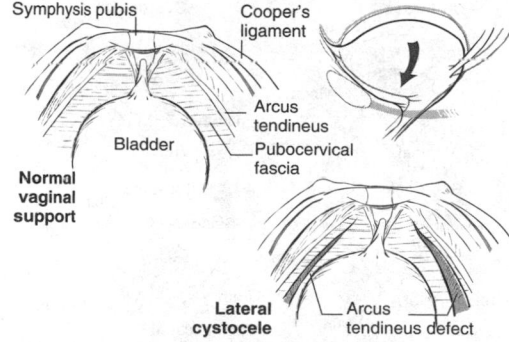

Symphysis pubis
Cooper's ligament
Arcus tendineus
Bladder
Pubocervical fascia
Normal vaginal support
Lateral cystocele
Arcus tendineus defect

617.3 Endometriosis of pelvic peritoneum   ♀

> Endometriosis:
> broad ligament
> cul-de-sac (Douglas')
> parametrium
> round ligament
>
> **DEF:** Aberrant uterine tissue; creating products of menses and inflamed peritoneum tissues.

617.4 Endometriosis of rectovaginal septum and vagina   ♀

> **DEF:** Aberrant uterine tissue; creating products of menses and inflamed tissues in and behind vagina.

617.5 Endometriosis of intestine   ♀

> Endometriosis: Endometriosis:
> appendix   rectum
> colon
>
> **DEF:** Aberrant uterine tissue; creating products of menses and inflamed intestinal tissues.

617.6 Endometriosis in scar of skin   ♀

617.8 Endometriosis of other specified sites   ♀

> Endometriosis:
> bladder
> lung
> umbilicus
> vulva

617.9 Endometriosis, site unspecified   ♀

√4ᵗʰ 618 Genital prolapse

> Use additional code to identify urinary incontinence (625.6, 788.31, 788.33-788.39)
>
> **EXCLUDES** that complicating pregnancy, labor, or delivery (654.4)

√5ᵗʰ 618.0 Prolapse of vaginal walls without mention of uterine prolapse

> **EXCLUDES** that with uterine prolapse (618.2-618.4)
> enterocele (618.6)
> vaginal vault prolapse following hysterectomy (618.5)

618.00 Unspecified prolapse of vaginal walls   ♀

> Vaginal prolapse NOS

618.01 Cystocele, midline   ♀

> Cystocele NOS
>
> **DEF:** Defect in the pubocervical fascia, the supportive layer of the bladder, causing bladder drop and herniated into the vagina along the midline.
> **N81.11** Cystocele midline   **I-10**

618.02 Cystocele, lateral   ♀

> Paravaginal
>
> **DEF:** Loss of support of the lateral attachment of the vagina at the arcus tendinous results in bladder drop; bladder herniates into the vagina laterally.

618.03 Urethrocele   ♀

618.04 Rectocele   ♀

> Proctocele
>
> Use additional code for any associated fecal incontinence (787.60-787.63)
> **N81.6** Rectocele   **I-10**

618.05 Perineocele   ♀

Additional Digit Required   Unacceptable PDx   Manifestation Code   Hospital Acquired Condition   ▶◀ Revised Text   ● New Code   ▲ Revised Code Title

2014 ICD-9-CM   Volume 1 – 205

Diseases of the Genitourinary System

618.09–620.4

Types of Vaginal Hernias

Urethrocele

Uterus
Bladder
Rectum
Urethra
Urethrocele
Vaginal canal

Cystocele

Uterus
Bladder
Rectum
Urethra
Cystocele
Vaginal canal

Rectocele

Uterus
Bladder
Rectum
Urethra
Rectocele
Vaginal canal

Enterocele

Uterus
Bladder
Rectum
Urethra
Terminal ileum
Vaginal canal

618.09 Other prolapse of vaginal walls without mention of uterine prolapse ♀
Cystourethrocele

618.1 Uterine prolapse without mention of vaginal wall prolapse ♀
Descensus uteri
Uterine prolapse:
  NOS
  complete
  first degree
  second degree
  third degree
  EXCLUDES that with mention of cystocele, urethrocele, or rectocele (618.2-618.4)

618.2 Uterovaginal prolapse, incomplete ♀
DEF: Downward displacement of uterus downward into vagina.
N81.2 Incomplete uterovaginal prolapse   [I-10]

618.3 Uterovaginal prolapse, complete ♀
DEF: Downward displacement of uterus exposed within external genitalia.

618.4 Uterovaginal prolapse, unspecified ♀
N81.4 Uterovaginal prolapse unspecified   [I-10]

618.5 Prolapse of vaginal vault after hysterectomy ♀
N99.3 Prolapse of vaginal vault after hysterectomy   [I-10]

618.6 Vaginal enterocele, congenital or acquired ♀
Pelvic enterocele, congenital or acquired
DEF: Vaginal vault hernia formed by the loop of the small intestine protruding into the rectal vaginal pouch; can also accompany uterine prolapse or follow hysterectomy.
N81.5 Vaginal enterocele   [I-10]

618.7 Old laceration of muscles of pelvic floor ♀

√5ᵗʰ **618.8 Other specified genital prolapse**

618.81 Incompetence or weakening of pubocervical tissue ♀

618.82 Incompetence or weakening of rectovaginal tissue ♀

618.83 Pelvic muscle wasting ♀
Disuse atrophy of pelvic muscles and anal sphincter

618.84 Cervical stump prolapse ♀
AHA: 4Q, '06, 97

618.89 Other specified genital prolapse ♀

618.9 Unspecified genital prolapse ♀

√4ᵗʰ **619 Fistula involving female genital tract**
EXCLUDES vesicorectal and intestinovesical fistula (596.1)

619.0 Urinary-genital tract fistula, female [CC] ♀
Fistula: Fistula:
  cervicovesical   uteroureteric
  ureterovaginal   uterovesical
  urethrovaginal   vesicocervicovaginal
  urethrovesicovaginal   vesicovaginal
CC Exd: 619.0-619.9

619.1 Digestive-genital tract fistula, female [CC] ♀
Fistula: Fistula:
  intestinouterine   rectovulval
  intestinovaginal   sigmoidovaginal
  rectovaginal   uterorectal
CC Exd: See code: 619.0

619.2 Genital tract-skin fistula, female [CC] ♀
Fistula:
  uterus to abdominal wall
  vaginoperineal
CC Exd: See code: 619.0

619.8 Other specified fistulas involving female genital tract [CC] ♀
Fistula:
  cervix
  cul-de-sac (Douglas')
  uterus
  vagina
CC Exd: See code: 619.0

619.9 Unspecified fistula involving female genital tract [CC] ♀
CC Exd: see code 619.0

√4ᵗʰ **620 Noninflammatory disorders of ovary, fallopian tube, and broad ligament**
EXCLUDES hydrosalpinx (614.1)

620.0 Follicular cyst of ovary ♀
Cyst of graafian follicle
DEF: Fluid-filled, encapsulated cyst due to occluded follicle duct that secretes hormones into ovaries.
N83.0 Follicular cyst of ovary   [I-1]

620.1 Corpus luteum cyst or hematoma ♀
Corpus luteum hemorrhage or rupture
Lutein cyst
DEF: Fluid-filled cyst due to serous developing from corpus luteum or clotted blood.
N83.1 Corpus luteum cyst   [I-]

620.2 Other and unspecified ovarian cyst ♀
Cyst:
  NOS
  corpus albicans
  retention NOS } of ovary
  serous
  theca-lutein
Simple cystoma of ovary
EXCLUDES cystadenoma (benign) (serous) (220)
    developmental cysts (752.0)
    neoplastic cysts (220)
    polycystic ovaries (256.4)
    Stein-Leventhal syndrome (256.4)
N83.20 Unspecified ovarian cysts   [I-]

620.3 Acquired atrophy of ovary and fallopian tube ♀
Senile involution of ovary

620.4 Prolapse or hernia of ovary and fallopian tube ♀
Displacement of ovary and fallopian tube
Salpingocele

Uterus and Ovaries

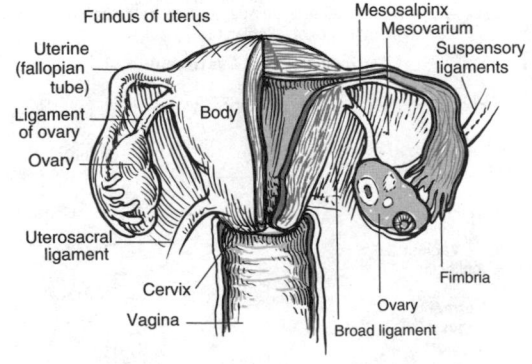

Fundus of uterus
Uterine (fallopian tube)
Ligament of ovary
Ovary
Uterosacral ligament
Cervix
Vagina
Body
Mesosalpinx
Mesovarium
Suspensory ligaments
Fimbria
Ovary
Broad ligament

 Newborn Age: 0   Pediatric Age: 0-17   [M] Maternity Age: 12-55   [A] Adult Age: 15-124   [MCC] Major CC Condition   [CC] CC Condition   [HIV] HIV Related

206 – Volume 1   **2014 ICD-9-**

620.5 Torsion of ovary, ovarian pedicle, or fallopian tube `CC` ♀
Torsion:
    accessory tube
    hydatid of Morgagni
CC Excl: 620.0-620.9

620.6 Broad ligament laceration syndrome ♀
Masters-Allen syndrome

620.7 Hematoma of broad ligament ♀
Hematocele, broad ligament
DEF: Blood within peritoneal fold that supports uterus.

620.8 Other noninflammatory disorders of ovary, fallopian tube, and broad ligament ♀
Cyst } of broad ligament or
Polyp } fallopian tube

Infarction } of ovary or fallopian tube
Rupture }
Hematosalpinx
EXCLUDES *hematosalpinx in ectopic pregnancy (639.2)*
peritubal adhesions (614.6)
torsion of ovary, ovarian pedicle, or fallopian tube (620.5)

620.9 Unspecified noninflammatory disorder of ovary, fallopian tube, and broad ligament ♀

√4th **621 Disorders of uterus, not elsewhere classified**

621.0 Polyp of corpus uteri ♀
Polyp: Polyp:
  endometrium   uterus NOS
EXCLUDES *cervical polyp NOS (622.7)*
N84.0 Polyp of corpus uteri   `I-10`

621.1 Chronic subinvolution of uterus ♀
EXCLUDES *puerperal (674.8)*
DEF: Abnormal size of uterus after delivery; the uterus does not return to its normal size after the birth of a child.
AHA: 1Q, '91, 11

621.2 Hypertrophy of uterus ♀
Bulky or enlarged uterus
EXCLUDES *puerperal (674.8)*

√5th **621.3 Endometrial hyperplasia**
DEF: Abnormal cystic overgrowth of endometrial tissue.

621.30 Endometrial hyperplasia, unspecified ♀
Endometrial hyperplasia NOS
Hyperplasia (adenomatous) (cystic) (glandular) of endometrium
Hyperplastic endometritis

621.31 Simple endometrial hyperplasia without atypia ♀
EXCLUDES *benign endometrial hyperplasia (621.34)*

621.32 Complex endometrial hyperplasia without atypia ♀
EXCLUDES *benign endometrial hyperplasia (621.34)*

621.33 Endometrial hyperplasia with atypia ♀
EXCLUDES *endometrial intraepithelial neoplasia [EIN] (621.35)*

621.34 Benign endometrial hyperplasia ♀
DEF: Excessive cell growth of the endometrium due to primary hormonal changes (menopause) that result in secondary effects to the endometrial stroma and associated structures.
AHA: 4Q, '09, 95-96

621.35 Endometrial intraepithelial neoplasia [EIN] ♀
EXCLUDES *malignant neoplasm of endometrium with endometrial intraepithelial neoplasia [EIN] (182.0)*
DEF: Abnormal premalignant neoplastic changes of the endometrial glands prone to malignant transformation.
AHA: 4Q, '09, 95-96
TIP: Do not confuse (EIN) with unrelated serous intraepithelial carcinoma (serous EIC), which is an early phase of (Type II) papillary serous adenocarcinoma of the endometrium.

621.4 Hematometra ♀
Hemometra
EXCLUDES *that in congenital anomaly (752.2-752.39)*
DEF: Accumulated blood in uterus.

621.5 Intrauterine synechiae ♀
Adhesions of uterus
Band(s) of uterus

621.6 Malposition of uterus ♀
Anteversion
Retroflexion } of uterus
Retroversion
EXCLUDES *malposition complicating pregnancy, labor, or delivery (654.3-654.4)*

621.7 Chronic inversion of uterus ♀
EXCLUDES *current obstetrical trauma (665.2)*
prolapse of uterus (618.1-618.4)

621.8 Other specified disorders of uterus, not elsewhere classified ♀
Atrophy, acquired
Cyst
Fibrosis NOS } of uterus
Old laceration (postpartum)
Ulcer
EXCLUDES *bilharzial fibrosis (120.0-120.9)*
endometriosis (617.0)
fistulas (619.0-619.8)
inflammatory diseases (615.0-615.9)

621.9 Unspecified disorder of uterus ♀

√4th **622 Noninflammatory disorders of cervix**
EXCLUDES *abnormality of cervix complicating pregnancy, labor, or delivery (654.5-654.6)*
fistula (619.0-619.8)

622.0 Erosion and ectropion of cervix ♀
Eversion } of cervix
Ulcer }
EXCLUDES *that in chronic cervicitis (616.0)*
DEF: Ulceration or turning outward of uterine cervix.

√5th **622.1 Dysplasia of cervix (uteri)**
EXCLUDES *abnormal results from cervical cytologic examination without histologic confirmation (795.00-795.09)*
carcinoma in situ of cervix (233.1)
cervical intraepithelial neoplasia III [CIN III] (233.1)
HGSIL of cervix (795.04)
DEF: Abnormal cell structures in portal between uterus and vagina.
AHA: 1Q, '91, 11

622.10 Dysplasia of cervix, unspecified ♀
Anaplasia of cervix
Cervical atypism
Cervical dysplasia NOS

622.11 Mild dysplasia of cervix ♀
Cervical intraepithelial neoplasia I [CIN I]

622.12 Moderate dysplasia of cervix ♀
Cervical intraepithelial neoplasia II [CIN II]
EXCLUDES *carcinoma in situ of cervix (233.1)*
cervical intraepithelial neoplasia III [CIN III] (233.1)
severe dysplasia (233.1)

622.2 Leukoplakia of cervix (uteri) ♀
EXCLUDES *carcinoma in situ of cervix (233.1)*
DEF: Thickened, white patches on portal between uterus and vagina.

622.3 Old laceration of cervix ♀
Adhesions
Band(s) } of cervix
Cicatrix (postpartum)
EXCLUDES *current obstetrical trauma (665.3)*
DEF: Scarring or other evidence of old wound on cervix.

Diseases of the Genitourinary System

622.4–625.4

622.4 Stricture and stenosis of cervix ♀

Atresia (acquired)
Contracture } of cervix
Occlusion

Pinpoint os uteri

EXCLUDES congenital (752.49)
that complicating labor (654.6)

622.5 Incompetence of cervix ♀

EXCLUDES complicating pregnancy (654.5)
that affecting fetus or newborn (761.0)

DEF: Inadequate functioning of cervix; marked by abnormal widening during pregnancy; causing miscarriage.

622.6 Hypertrophic elongation of cervix ♀

DEF: Overgrowth of cervix tissues extending down into vagina.

622.7 Mucous polyp of cervix ♀

Polyp NOS of cervix

EXCLUDES adenomatous polyp of cervix (219.0)

622.8 Other specified noninflammatory disorders of cervix ♀

Atrophy (senile)
Cyst } of cervix
Fibrosis
Hemorrhage

EXCLUDES endometriosis (617.0)
fistula (619.0-619.8)
inflammatory diseases (616.0)

622.9 Unspecified noninflammatory disorder of cervix ♀

√4ᵗʰ **623 Noninflammatory disorders of vagina**

EXCLUDES abnormality of vagina complicating pregnancy, labor, or delivery (654.7)
congenital absence of vagina (752.49)
congenital diaphragm or bands (752.49)
fistulas involving vagina (619.0-619.8)

623.0 Dysplasia of vagina ♀

Mild and moderate dysplasia of vagina
Vaginal intraepithelial neoplasia I and II [VAIN I and II]

EXCLUDES abnormal results from vaginal cytological examination without histologic confirmation (795.10-795.19)
carcinoma in situ of vagina (233.31)
HGSIL of vagina (795.14)
severe dysplasia of vagina (233.31)
vaginal intraepithelial neoplasia III [VAIN III] (233.31)

623.1 Leukoplakia of vagina ♀

DEF: Thickened white patches on vaginal canal.

623.2 Stricture or atresia of vagina ♀

Adhesions (postoperative) (postradiation) of vagina
Occlusion of vagina
Stenosis, vagina

Use additional E code to identify any external cause

EXCLUDES congenital atresia or stricture (752.49)

623.3 Tight hymenal ring ♀

Rigid hymen
Tight hymenal ring } acquired or congenital
Tight introitus

EXCLUDES imperforate hymen (752.42)

623.4 Old vaginal laceration ♀

EXCLUDES old laceration involving muscles of pelvic floor (618.7)

DEF: Scarring or other evidence of old wound on vagina.

623.5 Leukorrhea, not specified as infective ♀

Leukorrhea NOS of vagina
Vaginal discharge NOS

EXCLUDES trichomonal (131.00)

DEF: Viscid whitish discharge from vagina.

623.6 Vaginal hematoma ♀

EXCLUDES current obstetrical trauma (665.7)

623.7 Polyp of vagina ♀

623.8 Other specified noninflammatory disorders of vagina ♀

Cyst } of vagina
Hemorrhage

623.9 Unspecified noninflammatory disorder of vagina ♀

√4ᵗʰ **624 Noninflammatory disorders of vulva and perineum**

EXCLUDES abnormality of vulva and perineum complicating pregnanc
labor, or delivery (654.8)
condyloma acuminatum (078.11)
fistulas involving:
perineum — see Alphabetic Index
vulva (619.0-619.8)
vulval varices (456.6)
vulvar involvement in skin conditions (690-709.9)

√5ᵗʰ **624.0 Dystrophy of vulva**

EXCLUDES carcinoma in situ of vulva (233.32)
severe dysplasia of vulva (233.32)
vulvar intraepithelial neoplasia III [VIN III] (233.32)

AHA: 4Q, '07, 90

624.01 Vulvar intraepithelial neoplasia I [VIN I]

Mild dysplasia of vulva

624.02 Vulvar intraepithelial neoplasia II [VIN II]

Moderate dysplasia of vulva

AHA: 4Q, '07, 91

624.09 Other dystrophy of vulva

Kraurosis of vulva
Leukoplakia of vulva

624.1 Atrophy of vulva

624.2 Hypertrophy of clitoris

EXCLUDES that in endocrine disorders (255.2, 256.1)

624.3 Hypertrophy of labia

Hypertrophy of vulva NOS

DEF: Overgrowth of fleshy folds on either side of vagina.

624.4 Old laceration or scarring of vulva

DEF: Scarring or other evidence of old wound on external female genitalia.

624.5 Hematoma of vulva

EXCLUDES that complicating delivery (664.5)

DEF: Blood in tissue of external genitalia.

624.6 Polyp of labia and vulva

624.8 Other specified noninflammatory disorders of vulva and perineum

Cyst
Edema } of vulva
Stricture

AHA: 1Q, '03, 13; 1Q, '95, 8

624.9 Unspecified noninflammatory disorder of vulva and perineum

√4ᵗʰ **625 Pain and other symptoms associated with female genital orga**

625.0 Dyspareunia

EXCLUDES psychogenic dyspareunia (302.76)

DEF: Difficult or painful sexual intercourse.

625.1 Vaginismus

Colpospasm
Vulvismus

EXCLUDES psychogenic vaginismus (306.51)

DEF: Vaginal spasms; due to involuntary contraction of musculatu prevents intercourse.

625.2 Mittelschmerz

Intermenstrual pain
Ovulation pain

DEF: Pain occurring between menstrual periods.

625.3 Dysmenorrhea

Painful menstruation

EXCLUDES psychogenic dysmenorrhea (306.52)

AHA: 2Q, '94, 12

N94.6 Dysmenorrhea unspecified

625.4 Premenstrual tension syndromes

Menstrual molimen
Premenstrual dysphoric disorder
Premenstrual syndrome
Premenstrual tension NOS

EXCLUDES menstrual migraine (346.4)

AHA: 4Q, '03, 116

N Newborn Age: 0   P Pediatric Age: 0-17   M Maternity Age: 12-55   A Adult Age: 15-124   MCC Major CC Condition   CC CC Condition   HIV HIV Related

208 – Volume 1   **2014 ICD-9**

625.5 Pelvic congestion syndrome ♀
Congestion-fibrosis syndrome
Taylor's syndrome
DEF: Excessive accumulation of blood in vessels of pelvis; may occur after orgasm; causes abnormal menstruation, lower back pain and vaginal discharge.

625.6 Stress incontinence, female ♀
EXCLUDES mixed incontinence (788.33)
stress incontinence, male (788.32)
DEF: Involuntary leakage of urine due to insufficient sphincter control; occurs upon sneezing, laughing, coughing, sudden movement or lifting.
N39.3 Stress incontinence (female) (male) `I-10`

√5ᵗʰ **625.7 Vulvodynia**
DEF: Vulvar pain without an identifiable cause that persists for three months or longer.
AHA: 4Q, '08, 124

625.70 Vulvodynia, unspecified ♀
Vulvodynia NOS

625.71 Vulvar vestibulitis ♀

625.79 Other vulvodynia ♀

625.8 Other specified symptoms associated with female genital organs ♀
AHA: N-D, '85, 16

625.9 Unspecified symptom associated with female genital organs ♀
AHA: 4Q, '06, 110
R10.2 Pelvic and perineal pain `I-10`

√4ᵗʰ **626 Disorders of menstruation and other abnormal bleeding from female genital tract**
EXCLUDES menopausal and premenopausal bleeding (627.0)
pain and other symptoms associated with menstrual cycle (625.2-625.4)
postmenopausal bleeding (627.1)
precocious puberty (259.1)

626.0 Absence of menstruation ♀
Amenorrhea (primary) (secondary)

626.1 Scanty or infrequent menstruation ♀
Hypomenorrhea　Oligomenorrhea

626.2 Excessive or frequent menstruation ♀
Heavy periods
Menometrorrhagia
Menorrhagia
Plymenorrhea
EXCLUDES premenopausal (627.0)
that in puberty (626.3)
AHA: 4Q, '11, 146
N92.0 Excess & frequent menstruation w/regular cycle `I-10`

626.3 Puberty bleeding ♀
Excessive bleeding associated with onset of menstrual periods
Pubertal menorrhagia

626.4 Irregular menstrual cycle ♀
Irregular:
bleeding NOS
menstruation
periods

626.5 Ovulation bleeding ♀
Regular intermenstrual bleeding

626.6 Metrorrhagia ♀
Bleeding unrelated to menstrual cycle
Irregular intermenstrual bleeding

626.7 Postcoital bleeding ♀
DEF: Bleeding from vagina after sexual intercourse.

626.8 Other ♀
Dysfunctional or functional uterine hemorrhage NOS
Menstruation:
retained
suppression of
N92.5 Other specified irregular menstruation `I-10`

626.9 Unspecified ♀

√4ᵗʰ **627 Menopausal and postmenopausal disorders**
EXCLUDES asymptomatic age-related (natural) postmenopausal status (V49.81)

627.0 Premenopausal menorrhagia ♀
Excessive bleeding associated with onset of menopause
Menorrhagia:
climacteric
menopausal
preclimacteric

627.1 Postmenopausal bleeding ♀
N95.0 Postmenopausal bleeding `I-10`

627.2 Symptomatic menopausal or female climacteric states ♀
Symptoms, such as flushing, sleeplessness, headache, lack of concentration, associated with the menopause

627.3 Postmenopausal atrophic vaginitis ♀
Senile (atrophic) vaginitis

627.4 Symptomatic states associated with artificial menopause ♀
Postartificial menopause syndromes
Any condition classifiable to 627.1, 627.2, or 627.3 which follows induced menopause
DEF: Conditions arising after hysterectomy.

627.8 Other specified menopausal and postmenopausal disorders ♀
EXCLUDES premature menopause NOS (256.31)

627.9 Unspecified menopausal and postmenopausal disorder ♀

√4ᵗʰ **628 Infertility, female**
INCLUDES primary and secondary sterility
DEF: Infertility: inability to conceive for at least one year with regular intercourse.
DEF: Primary infertility: occurring in patients who have never conceived.
DEF: Secondary infertility: occurring in patients who have previously conceived.
AHA: 2Q, '96, 9; 1Q, '95, 7

628.0 Associated with anovulation ♀
Anovulatory cycle
Use additional code for any associated Stein-Leventhal syndrome (256.4)

628.1 *Of pituitary-hypothalamic origin* ♀
Code first underlying cause, as:
adiposogenital dystrophy (253.8)
anterior pituitary disorder (253.0-253.4)

628.2 Of tubal origin ♀
Infertility associated with congenital anomaly of tube
Tubal:
block
occlusion
stenosis
Use additional code for any associated peritubal adhesions (614.6)

628.3 Of uterine origin ♀
Infertility associated with congenital anomaly of uterus
Nonimplantation
Use additional code for any associated tuberculous endometritis (016.7)

628.4 Of cervical or vaginal origin ♀
Infertility associated with:
anomaly of cervical mucus
congenital structural anomaly
dysmucorrhea

628.8 Of other specified origin ♀

628.9 Of unspecified origin ♀

√4ᵗʰ **629 Other disorders of female genital organs**

629.0 Hematocele, female, not elsewhere classified ♀
EXCLUDES hematocele or hematoma:
broad ligament (620.7)
fallopian tube (620.8)
that associated with ectopic pregnancy (633.00-633.91)
uterus (621.4)
vagina (623.6)
vulva (624.5)

Diseases of the Genitourinary System

629.1 Hydrocele, canal of Nuck ♀
     Cyst of canal of Nuck (acquired)
     EXCLUDES *congenital (752.41)*

√5ᵗʰ **629.2 Female genital mutilation status**
     Female circumcision status
     Female genital cutting
     AHA: 4Q, '04, 88

     629.20 Female genital mutilation status, unspecified ♀
        Female genital cutting status, unspecified
        Female genital mutilation status NOS

     629.21 Female genital mutilation Type I status ♀
        Clitorectomy status
        Female genital cutting Type I status
        DEF: Female genital mutilation involving clitorectomy, with
        part or all of the clitoris removed.

     629.22 Female genital mutilation Type II status ♀
        Clitorectomy with excision of labia minora status
        Female genital cutting Type II status
        DEF: Female genital mutilation involving clitoris and the
        labia minora amputation.
        AHA: 4Q, '04, 90

     629.23 Female genital mutilation Type III status ♀
        Female genital cutting Type III status
        Infibulation status
        DEF: Female genital mutilation involving removal, most or
        all of the labia minora excised, labia majora incised which is
        then made into a hood of skin over the urethral and vaginal
        opening.
        AHA: 4Q, '04, 90

     629.29 Other female genital mutilation status ♀
        Female genital cutting Type IV status
        Female genital mutilation Type IV status
        Other female genital cutting status
        AHA: 4Q, '06, 97

√5ᵗʰ **629.3 Complication of implanted vaginal mesh and other prosthetic materials**
     AHA: 4Q, '11, 130-131

     629.31 Erosion of implanted vaginal mesh and other prosthetic materials to surrounding organ or tissu
        Erosion of implanted vaginal mesh and other
        prosthetic materials into pelvic floor muscles

     629.32 Exposure of implanted vaginal mesh and other prosthetic materials into vagina
        Exposure of vaginal mesh and other prosthetic
        materials through vaginal wall

√5ᵗʰ **629.8 Other specified disorders of female genital organs**

     629.81 Recurrent pregnancy loss without current pregnancy
        EXCLUDES *recurrent pregnancy loss with current*
        pregnancy (646.3)
        AHA: 4Q, '06, 98

     629.89 Other specified disorders of female genital organs
        AHA: 4Q, '06, 98

629.9 Unspecified disorder of female genital organs

Ⓝ Newborn Age: 0   Ⓟ Pediatric Age: 0-17   Ⓜ Maternity Age: 12-55   Ⓐ Adult Age: 15-124   **MCC** Major CC Condition   **CC** CC Condition   **HIV** HIV Related

210 – Volume 1   **2014 ICD-9-**

11. Complications of Pregnancy, Childbirth, and the Puerperium (630-679)

Ectopic and Molar Pregnancy (630-633)
Use additional code from category 639 to identify any complications

630 Hydatidiform mole   Ⓜ♀
Trophoblastic disease NOS   Vesicular mole

EXCLUDES chorioadenoma (destruens) (236.1)
chorionepithelioma (181)
malignant hydatidiform mole (236.1)

DEF: Abnormal product of pregnancy; marked by mass of cysts resembling bunch of grapes due to chorionic villi proliferation, and dissolution; must be surgically removed.

✓4ᵗʰ 631 Other abnormal product of conception
AHA: 4Q, '11, 131-132

631.0 Inappropriate change in quantitative human chorionic gonadotropin (hCG) in early pregnancy   Ⓜ♀
Biochemical pregnancy
Chemical pregnancy
Inappropriate level of quantitative human chorionic gonadotropin (hCG) for gestational age in early pregnancy

EXCLUDES blighted ovum (631.8)
molar pregnancy (631.8)

631.8 Other abnormal products of conception   Ⓜ♀
Blighted ovum

632 Missed abortion   Ⓜ♀
Early fetal death before completion of 22 weeks' gestation with retention of dead fetus
Retained products of conception, not following spontaneous or induced abortion or delivery

EXCLUDES failed induced abortion (638.0-638.9)
fetal death (intrauterine) (late) (656.4)
missed delivery (656.4)
that with hydatidiform mole (630)
that with other abnormal products of conception (631.8)

AHA: 1Q, '01, 5
002.1 Missed abortion   I-10

✓4ᵗʰ 633 Ectopic pregnancy
INCLUDES ruptured ectopic pregnancy
DEF: Fertilized egg develops outside uterus.
AHA: 4Q, '02, 61

✓5ᵗʰ 633.0 Abdominal pregnancy
Intraperitoneal pregnancy

633.00 Abdominal pregnancy without intrauterine pregnancy   CC Ⓜ♀
CC Excl: 633.01, 633.11-633.91

633.01 Abdominal pregnancy with intrauterine pregnancy   CC Ⓜ♀
CC Excl: 633.00-633.91

✓5ᵗʰ 633.1 Tubal pregnancy
Fallopian pregnancy
Rupture of (fallopian) tube due to pregnancy
Tubal abortion
AHA: 2Q, '90, 27

633.10 Tubal pregnancy without intrauterine pregnancy   CC Ⓜ♀
CC Excl: See code: 633.01
000.1 Tubal pregnancy   I-10

633.11 Tubal pregnancy with intrauterine pregnancy   CC Ⓜ♀
CC Excl: See code: 633.01

✓5ᵗʰ 633.2 Ovarian pregnancy

633.20 Ovarian pregnancy without intrauterine pregnancy   CC Ⓜ♀
CC Excl: See code: 633.01

633.21 Ovarian pregnancy with intrauterine pregnancy   CC Ⓜ♀
CC Excl: See code: 633.01

✓5ᵗʰ 633.8 Other ectopic pregnancy
Pregnancy: Pregnancy:
cervical   intraligamentous
combined   mesometric
cornual   mural

633.80 Other ectopic pregnancy without intrauterine pregnancy   CC Ⓜ♀
CC Excl: See code: 633.01

633.81 Other ectopic pregnancy with intrauterine pregnancy   CC Ⓜ♀
CC Excl: See code: 633.01

✓5ᵗʰ 633.9 Unspecified ectopic pregnancy

633.90 Unspecified ectopic pregnancy without intrauterine pregnancy   CC Ⓜ♀
CC Excl: See code: 633.01

633.91 Unspecified ectopic pregnancy with intrauterine pregnancy   CC Ⓜ♀
CC Excl: See code: 633.01

Other Pregnancy with Abortive Outcome (634-639)

The following fourth-digit subdivisions are for use with categories 634-638:
.0 Complicated by genital tract and pelvic infection
Endometritis
Salpingo-oophoritis
Sepsis NOS
Septicemia NOS
Any condition classifiable to 639.0 with condition classifiable to 634-638
EXCLUDES urinary tract infection (634-638 with .7)
.1 Complicated by delayed or excessive hemorrhage
Afibrinogenemia
Defibrination syndrome
Intravascular hemolysis
Any condition classifiable to 639.1 with condition classifiable to 634-638
.2 Complicated by damage to pelvic organs and tissues
Laceration, perforation, or tear of:
bladder
uterus
Any condition classifiable to 639.2 with condition classifiable to 634-638
.3 Complicated by renal failure
Oliguria   Uremia
Any condition classifiable to 639.3, with condition classifiable to 634-638
.4 Complicated by metabolic disorder
Electrolyte imbalance with conditions classfiable to 634-638
.5 Complicated by shock
Circulatory collapse
Shock (postoperative) (septic)
Any condition classifiable to 639.5 with condition classifiable to 634-638
.6 Complicated by embolism
Embolism: Embolism:
NOS   pulmonary
amniotic fluid
Any condition classifiable to 639.6, with condition classifiable to 634-638
.7 With other specified complications
Cardiac arrest or failure
Urinary tract infection
Any condition classiable to 639.8 with condition classifiable to 634-638
.8 With unspecified complication
.9 Without mention of complication

§ ✓4ᵗʰ 634 Spontaneous abortion
Requires fifth digit to identify stage:
  0 unspecified
  1 incomplete
  2 complete

INCLUDES miscarriage
spontaneous abortion
DEF: Spontaneous premature expulsion of the products of conception from the uterus.
AHA: 4Q, '11, 181; 2Q, '91, 16

§§ ✓5ᵗʰ 634.0 Complicated by genital tract and pelvic infection   CC Ⓜ♀
[0-2]   CC Excl: 634.00-638.9, 640.00-641.23, 646.80-646.93, 648.90-649.64, 650, 669.40-669.44, 669.80-669.94, 679.00-679.04, 679.12, 679.14

See beginning of section 634-639 for fourth-digit definitions.
§ Requires fifth digit. Valid digits are in [brackets] under each code. See appropriate category for codes and definitions.

Additional Digit Required   Unacceptable PDx   Manifestation Code   Hospital Acquired Condition   ►◄ Revised Text   ● New Code   ▲ Revised Code Title

2014 ICD-9-CM   Volume 1 – 211

Ectopic Pregnancy Sites

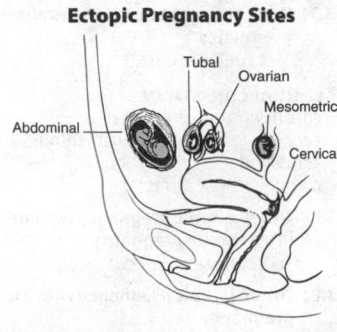

§§ ✓5ᵗʰ **634.1 Complicated by delayed or excessive hemorrhage** M♀
[0-2] AHA: For Code 634.11: 1Q, '03, 6

§§ ✓5ᵗʰ **634.2 Complicated by damage to pelvic organs** CC M♀
[0-2] **or tissues**
  CC Excl: See code: 634.0

§§ ✓5ᵗʰ **634.3 Complicated by renal failure** MCC M♀
[0-2] CC Excl: See code: 634.0

§§ ✓5ᵗʰ **634.4 Complicated by metabolic disorder** CC M♀
[0-2] CC Excl: See code: 634.0

§§ ✓5ᵗʰ **634.5 Complicated by shock** MCC M♀
[0-2] CC Excl: See code: 634.0

§§ ✓5ᵗʰ **634.6 Complicated by embolism** MCC 1-2 CC 0 M♀
[0-2] CC Excl: See code: 634.0

§§ ✓5ᵗʰ **634.7 With other specified complications** CC M♀
[0-2] CC Excl: See code: 634.0

§§ ✓5ᵗʰ **634.8 With unspecified complication** CC M♀
[0-2] CC Excl: See code: 634.0

§§ ✓5ᵗʰ **634.9 Without mention of complication** M♀
[0-2]

§ ✓4ᵗʰ **635 Legally induced abortion**

Requires fifth digit to identify stage:
  0 unspecified
  1 incomplete
  2 complete

INCLUDES abortion or termination of pregnancy:
  elective
  legal
  therapeutic

EXCLUDES menstrual extraction or regulation (V25.3)
DEF: Intentional expulsion of products of conception from uterus performed by medical professionals inside boundaries of law.
AHA: 4Q, '11, 181; 2Q, '94, 14

§§ ✓5ᵗʰ **635.0 Complicated by genital tract and pelvic infection** CC M♀
[0-2] CC Excl: 634.00-635.02, 635.20-635.22, 635.70-638.9, 640.00-641.23, 646.80-646.93, 648.90-649.64, 650, 669.40-669.44, 669.80-669.94, 679.00-679.04, 679.12, 679.14

§§ ✓5ᵗʰ **635.1 Complicated by delayed or excessive hemorrhage** M♀
[0-2]

§§ ✓5ᵗʰ **635.2 Complicated by damage to pelvic organs or tissues** CC M♀
[0-2] CC Excl: For code 635.20: 634.00-638.9, 640.00-641.23, 646.80-646.93, 648.90-649.64, 650, 669.40-669.44, 669.80-669.94, 679.00-679.04, 679.12, 679.14; For code 635.21: 634.00-635.62, 638.5-638.9, 640.00-641.00; For code 635.22: 635.22

§§ ✓5ᵗʰ **635.3 Complicated by renal failure** MCC M♀
[0-2] CC Excl: For code 635.30: 635.30-635.32; For code 635.31: 635.30-635.32, 637.11-638.9, 640.00-641.23, 646.80-646.93, 648.90-649.64, 650, 669.40-669.44, 669.80-669.94, 679.00-679.04, 679.12, 679.14; For code 635.32: 634.00-634.92, 635.30-635.32, 635.70-638.9, 640.00-641.23, 646.80-646.93, 648.90-649.64, 650, 669.40-669.44, 669.80-669.94, 679.00-679.04, 679.12, 679.144

§§ ✓5ᵗʰ **635.4 Complicated by metabolic disorder** CC M♀
[0-2] CC Excl: 634.00-638.9, 640.00-641.23, 646.80-646.93, 648.90-649.64, 650, 669.40-669.44, 669.80-669.94, 679.00-679.04, 679.12, 679.14

§§ ✓5ᵗʰ **635.5 Complicated by shock** MCC M♀
[0-2] CC Excl: 634.00-634.92, 635.50-635.52, 635.70-638.9, 640.00-641.23, 646.80-646.93, 648.90-649.64, 650, 669.40-669.44, 669.80-669.94, 679.00-679.04, 679.12, 679.14

§§ ✓5ᵗʰ **635.6 Complicated by embolism** MCC M♀
[0-2] CC Excl: 634.00-634.92, 635.60-638.9, 640.00-641.23, 646.80-646.93, 648.90-649.64, 650, 669.40-669.44, 669.80-669.94, 679.00-679.04, 679.12, 679.14

§§ ✓5ᵗʰ **635.7 With other specified complications** CC M♀
[0-2] CC Excl: 634.00-638.9, 640.00-641.23, 646.80-646.93, 648.90-649.64, 650, 669.40-669.44, 669.80-669.94, 679.00-679.04, 679.12, 679.14

§§ ✓5ᵗʰ **635.8 With unspecified complication** CC M♀
[0-2] CC Excl: 634.00-638.9, 640.00-641.23, 646.80-646.93, 648.90-649.64, 650, 669.40-669.44, 669.80-669.94, 679.00-679.04, 679.12, 679.14

§§ ✓5ᵗʰ **635.9 Without mention of complication** M♀
[0-2] AHA: For code 635.92: 2Q, '10, 6-7; 2Q, '94, 14

§ ✓4ᵗʰ **636 Illegally induced abortion**

Requires fifth digit to identify stage:
  0 unspecified
  1 incomplete
  2 complete

INCLUDES abortion:
  criminal
  illegal
  self-induced

DEF: Intentional expulsion of products of conception from uterus; outside boundaries of law.
AHA: 4Q, '11, 181

§§ ✓5ᵗʰ **636.0 Complicated by genital tract and pelvic infection** CC M♀
[0-2] CC Excl: 634.00-636.02, 636.70-638.9, 640.00-641.23, 646.80-646.93, 648.90-649.64, 650, 669.40-669.44, 669.80-669.94, 679.00-679.04, 679.12, 679.14

§§ ✓5ᵗʰ **636.1 Complicated by delayed or excessive hemorrhage** M♀
[0-2]

§§ ✓5ᵗʰ **636.2 Complicated by damage to pelvic organs or tissues** CC M♀
[0-2] CC Excl: 634.00-638.9, 640.00-641.23, 646.80-646.93, 648.90-649.64, 650, 669.40-669.44, 669.80-669.94, 679.00-679.04, 679.12, 679.14

§§ ✓5ᵗʰ **636.3 Complicated by renal failure** MCC M♀
[0-2] CC Excl: 634.00-635.92, 636.30-636.32, 636.70-638.9, 640.00-641.23, 646.80-646.93, 648.90-649.64, 650, 669.40-669.44, 669.80-669.94, 679.00-679.04, 679.12, 679.14

§§ ✓5ᵗʰ **636.4 Complicated by metabolic disorder** CC M♀
[0-2] CC Excl: 634.00-635.92, 636.30-636.32, 636.70-638.9, 640.00-641.23, 646.80-646.93, 648.90-649.64, 650, 669.40-669.44, 669.80-669.94, 679.00-679.04, 679.12, 679.14

§§ ✓5ᵗʰ **636.5 Complicated by shock** MCC M♀
[0-2] CC Excl: For codes 636.50 and 636.51: 634.00-635.92, 636.50-636.52, 636.70-638.9, 640.00-641.23, 646.80-646.93, 648.90-649.64, 650, 669.40-669.44, 669.80-669.94, 679.00-679.04, 679.12, 679.14; For code 636.52: 634.00-635.92, 636.50-636.52, 636.70-636.92, 637.50-637.52, 637.70-637.92, 638.5, 638.7-638.9, 640.00-641.23, 646.80-646.93, 648.90- 649.64, 650, 669.40-669.44, 669.80-669.94, 679.00-679.04, 679.12, 679.14

§§ ✓5ᵗʰ **636.6 Complicated by embolism** MCC M♀
[0-2] CC Excl: 634.00-635.92, 636.60-638.9, 640.00-641.23, 646.80-646.93, 648.90-649.64, 650, 669.40-669.44, 669.80-669.94, 679.00-679.04, 679.12, 679.14

§§ ✓5ᵗʰ **636.7 With other specified complications** CC M♀
[0-2] CC Excl: 634.00-638.9, 640.00-641.23, 646.80-646.93, 648.90-649.64, 650, 669.40-669.44, 669.80-669.94, 679.00-679.04, 679.12, 679.14

§§ ✓5ᵗʰ **636.8 With unspecified complication** CC M♀
[0-2] CC Excl: See code: 636.2

§§ ✓5ᵗʰ **636.9 Without mention of complication** M♀
[0-2]

§ ✓4ᵗʰ **637 Unspecified abortion**

Requires fifth digit to identify stage:
  0 unspecified
  1 incomplete
  2 complete

INCLUDES abortion NOS
  retained products of conception following abortion, not classifiable elsewhere

AHA: 4Q, '11, 181

---

§ See beginning of section 634-639 for fourth-digit definitions.
§§ Requires fifth digit. Valid digits are in [brackets] under each code. See appropriate category for codes and definitions.

§§ ✓5ᵗʰ **637.0 Complicated by genital tract and pelvic infection** `CC` `M` ♀
[0-2]   **CC Excl:** 634.00-637.02, 637.70-638.9, 640.00-641.23, 646.80-646.93, 648.90-649.64, 650, 669.40-669.44, 669.80-669.94, 679.00-679.04, 679.12, 679.14

§§ ✓5ᵗʰ **637.1 Complicated by delayed or excessive hemorrhage** `M` ♀
[0-2]

§§ ✓5ᵗʰ **637.2 Complicated by damage to pelvic organs or tissues** `CC` `M` ♀
[0-2]   **CC Excl:** 634.00-636.92, 637.30-637.32, 637.70-638.9, 640.00-641.23, 646.80-646.93, 648.90-649.64, 650, 669.40-669.44, 669.80-669.94, 679.00-679.04, 679.12, 679.14

§§ ✓5ᵗʰ **637.3 Complicated by renal failure** `MCC` `M` ♀
[0-2]   **CC Excl:** 634.00-636.92, 637.30-637.32, 637.70-638.9, 640.00-641.23, 646.80-646.93, 648.90-649.64, 650, 669.40-669.44, 669.80-669.94, 679.00-679.04, 679.12, 679.14

§§ ✓5ᵗʰ **637.4 Complicated by metabolic disorder** `CC` `M` ♀
[0-2]   **CC Excl:** See code: 637.2

§§ ✓5ᵗʰ **637.5 Complicated by shock** `MCC` `M` ♀
[0-2]   **CC Excl:** 634.00-636.92, 637.50-637.52, 637.70-638.9, 640.00-641.23, 646.80-646.93, 648.90-649.64, 650, 669.40-669.44, 669.80-669.94, 679.00-679.04, 679.12, 679.14

§§ ✓5ᵗʰ **637.6 Complicated by embolism** `MCC` `M` ♀
[0-2]   **CC Excl: For codes 637.60 and 637.61:** 634.00-636.92, 637.60-638.9, 640.00-641.23, 646.80-646.93, 648.90-649.64, 650, 669.40-669.44, 669.80-669.94, 679.00-679.04, 679.12, 679.14; **For code 637.62:** 634.00-636.92, 637.60-638.9, 640.00-641.23, 646.80-646.93, 648.90-649.64, 650, 669.40-669.44, 669.80-669.94, 679.00-679.04, 679.12, 679.14

§§ ✓5ᵗʰ **637.7 With other specified complications** `CC` `M` ♀
[0-2]   **CC Excl:** See code: 637.2

§§ ✓5ᵗʰ **637.8 With unspecified complication** `CC` `M` ♀
[0-2]   **CC Excl: For codes 637.80 and 637.82:** 634.00-638.9, 640.00-641.23, 646.80-646.93, 648.90-649.64, 650, 669.40-669.44, 669.80-669.94, 679.00-679.04, 679.12, 679.14; **For code 637.81:** 634.00-635.32, 635.41-638.9, 640.00-641.23, 646.80-646.93, 648.90-649.64, 650, 669.40-669.44, 669.80-669.94, 679.00-679.04, 679.12, 679.14

§§ ✓5ᵗʰ **637.9 Without mention of complication** `M` ♀
[0-2]

§ ✓4ᵗʰ **638 Failed attempted abortion**
INCLUDES failure of attempted induction of (legal) abortion
EXCLUDES *incomplete abortion (634.0-637.9)*
DEF: Continued pregnancy despite an attempted legal abortion.

638.0 Complicated by genital tract and pelvic infection `CC` `M` ♀
CC Excl: 634.00-638.0, 638.7-638.9, 640.00-641.23, 646.80-646.93, 648.90-649.64, 650, 669.40-669.44, 669.80-669.94, 679.00-679.04, 679.12, 679.14

638.1 Complicated by delayed or excessive hemorrhage `CC` `M` ♀
CC Excl: 634.00-637.92, 638.1, 638.7-638.9, 640.00-641.23, 646.80-646.93, 648.90-649.64, 650, 669.40-669.44, 669.80-669.94, 679.00-679.04, 679.12, 679.14

638.2 Complicated by damage to pelvic organs or tissues `CC` `M` ♀
CC Excl: 634.00-637.92, 638.2, 638.7-638.9, 640.00-641.23, 646.80-646.93, 648.90-649.64, 650, 669.40-669.44, 669.80-669.94, 679.00-679.04, 679.12, 679.14

638.3 Complicated by renal failure `MCC` `M` ♀
CC Excl: 634.00-637.92, 638.3, 638.7-638.9, 640.00-641.23, 646.80-646.93, 648.90-649.64, 650, 669.40-669.44, 669.80-669.94, 679.00-679.04, 679.12, 679.14

638.4 Complicated by metabolic disorder `CC` `M` ♀
CC Excl: 634.00-638.9, 640.00-641.23, 646.80-646.93, 648.90-649.64, 650, 669.40-669.44, 669.80-669.94, 679.00-679.04, 679.12, 679.14

638.5 Complicated by shock `MCC` `M` ♀
CC Excl: 634.00-637.12, 637.21-637.92, 638.4-638.5, 638.7-638.9, 640.00-641.23, 646.80-646.93, 648.90-649.64, 650, 669.40-669.44, 669.80-669.94, 679.00-679.04, 679.12, 679.14

638.6 Complicated by embolism `MCC` `M` ♀
CC Excl: 634.00-637.92, 638.6-638.9, 640.00-641.23, 646.80-646.93, 648.90-649.64, 650, 669.40-669.44, 669.80-669.94, 679.00-679.04, 679.12, 679.14

638.7 With other specified complications `CC` `M` ♀
CC Excl: See code: 638.4

638.8 With unspecified complication `CC` `M` ♀
CC Excl: See code: 638.4

638.9 Without mention of complication `M` ♀

✓4ᵗʰ **639 Complications following abortion and ectopic and molar pregnancies**
NOTE This category is provided for use when it is required to classify separately the complications classifiable to the fourth-digit level in categories 634-638; for example:
a) when the complication itself was responsible for an episode of medical care, the abortion, ectopic or molar pregnancy itself having been dealt with at a previous episode
b) when these conditions are immediate complications of ectopic or molar pregnancies classifiable to 630-633 where they cannot be identified at fourth-digit level.

639.0 Genital tract and pelvic infection `CC` `M` ♀
Endometritis
Parametritis
Pelvic peritonitis
Salpingitis   } following conditions classifiable to 630-638
Salpingo-oophoritis
Sepsis NOS
Septicemia NOS

   EXCLUDES *urinary tract infection (639.8)*
CC Excl: 639.0, 639.2-641.23, 646.80-646.93, 648.90-649.64, 650, 669.40-669.44, 669.80-669.94, 679.00-679.04, 679.12, 679.14

639.1 Delayed or excessive hemorrhage `CC` ♀
Afibrinogenemia
Defibrination syndrome   } following conditions classfiable to 630-638
Intravascular
CC Excl: 639.1-641.23, 646.80-646.93, 648.90-649.64, 650, 669.40-669.44, 669.80-669.94, 679.00-679.04, 679.12, 679.14

639.2 Damage to pelvic organs and tissues `CC` `M` ♀
Laceration, perforation, or tear of:
   bladder
   bowel
   broad ligament
   cervix   } following conditions classifiable to 630-638
   periurethral tissue
   uterus
   vagina
CC Excl: 639.2-641.23, 646.80-646.93, 648.90-649.64, 650, 669.40-669.44, 669.80-669.94, 679.00-679.04, 679.12, 679.14

639.3 Kidney failure `MCC` ♀
Oliguria
Renal (kidney):
   failure (acute)
   shutdown   } following conditions classifiable to 630-638
   tubular necrosis
Uremia
CC Excl: See code: 639.2

639.4 Metabolic disorders `CC` ♀
Electrolyte imbalance following conditions classifiable to 630-638
CC Excl: See code: 639.2

639.5 Shock `MCC` `M` ♀
Circulatory collapse
Shock (postoperative) (septic)   } following conditions classifiable to 630-638
CC Excl: See code: 639.2

639.6 Embolism `MCC` `M` ♀
Embolism:
   NOS
   air
   amniotic fluid
   blood-clot
   fat   } following conditions classifiable to 630-638
   pulmonary
   pyemic
   septic
   soap
CC Excl: See code: 639.2

§   See beginning of section 634-639 for fourth-digit definitions.
§§ Requires fifth digit. Valid digits are in [brackets] under each code. See appropriate category for codes and definitions.

✓4ᵗʰ / ✓5ᵗʰ Additional Digit Required   `Unacceptable PDx`   `Manifestation Code`   `Hospital Acquired Condition`   ►◄ Revised Text   ● New Code   ▲ Revised Code Title

639.8 Other specified complications following abortion or ectopic and molar pregnancy CC M ♀

Acute yellow atrophy or necrosis of liver
Cardiac arrest or failure
Cerebral anoxia
Urinary tract infection
} following conditons classifiable to 630-638

CC Excl: See code: 639.2

639.9 Unspecified complication following abortion or ectopic and molar pregnancy CC M ♀

Complication(s) not further specified following conditions classifiable to 630-638

CC Excl: See code: 639.2

Complications Mainly Related to Pregnancy (640-649)

INCLUDES the listed conditions even if they arose or were present during labor, delivery, or the puerperium

AHA: 2Q, '90, 11

The following fifth-digit subclassification is for use with categories 640-649 to denote the current episode of care. Valid fifth-digits are in [brackets] under each code.

0 unspecified as to episode of care or not applicable
1 delivered, with or without mention of antepartum condition
Antepartum condition with delivery
Delivery NOS (with mention of antepartum complication during current episode of care)
Intrapartum obstetric condition (with mention of antepartum complication during current episode of care)
Pregnancy, delivered (with mention of antepartum complication during current episode of care)
2 delivered, with mention of postpartum complication
Delivery with mention of puerperal complication during current episode of care
3 antepartum condition or complication
Antepartum obstetric condtion, not delivered during the current episode of care
4 postpartum condition or complication
Postpartum or puerperal obstetric condition or complication following delivery that occurred:
during previous episode of care
outside hospital, with subsequent admission for observation or care

✓4ᵗʰ **640 Hemorrhage in early pregnancy**

INCLUDES hemorrhage before completion of 22 weeks' gestation

§ ✓5ᵗʰ **640.0 Threatened abortion** CC 1,3 M ♀
[0,1,3] DEF: Bloody discharge during pregnancy; cervix may be dilated and pregnancy is threatened, but the pregnancy is not terminated.
CC Excl: For codes 640.01 and 640.03: 640.00-641.13, 646.80-646.93, 648.90-649.64, 650, 669.40-669.44, 669.80-669.94, 679.00-679.04, 679.12, 679.14

§ ✓5ᵗʰ **640.8 Other specified hemorrhage in early pregnancy** M ♀
[0,1,3]

§ ✓5ᵗʰ **640.9 Unspecified hemorrhage in early pregnancy** CC 3 M ♀
[0,1,3] CC Excl: For code 640.93: 640.00-641.13, 646.80-646.93, 648.90-649.64, 650, 669.40-669.44, 669.80-669.94, 679.00-679.04, 679.12, 679.14

✓4ᵗʰ **641 Antepartum hemorrhage, abruptio placentae, and placenta previa**

§ ✓5ᵗʰ **641.0 Placenta previa without hemorrhage** CC 1,3 M ♀
[0,1,3]
Low implantation of placenta
Placenta previa noted:
during pregnancy
before labor (and delivered by caesarean delivery)
} without hemorrhage

DEF: Placenta implanted in lower segment of uterus; commonly causes hemorrhage in the last trimester of pregnancy.
CC Excl: For codes 641.01 and 641.03: 640.00-641.13, 646.80-646.93, 648.90-649.64, 650, 669.40-669.44, 669.80-669.94, 679.00-679.04, 679.12, 679.14

Placenta Previa

Low (marginal) implantation | Partial placenta previa | Total placenta previa

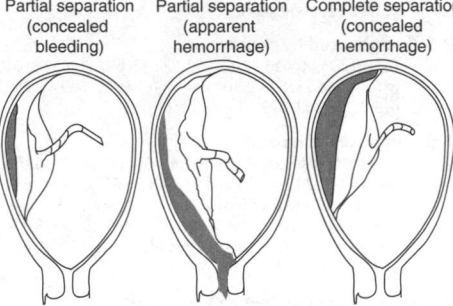

Abruptio Placentae

Partial separation (concealed bleeding) | Partial separation (apparent hemorrhage) | Complete separation (concealed hemorrhage)

§ ✓5ᵗʰ **641.1 Hemorrhage from placenta previa** MCC 1,3 M ♀
[0,1,3]
Low-lying placenta
Placenta previa
incomplete
marginal
partial
total
} NOS or with hemorrhage (intrapartum)

EXCLUDES hemorrhage from vasa previa (663.5)
CC Excl: For codes 641.11 and 641.13: 640.00-641.13, 646.80-646.93, 648.90-649.64, 650, 669.40-669.44, 669.80-669.94, 679.00-679.04, 679.12, 679.14

§ ✓5ᵗʰ **641.2 Premature separation of placenta** MCC 1 CC 3 M ♀
[0,1,3]
Ablatio placentae
Abruptio placentae
Accidental antepartum hemorrhage
Couvelaire uterus
Detachment of placenta (premature)
Premature separation of normally implanted placenta
DEF: Abruptio placentae: premature detachment of the placenta, characterized by shock, oliguria and decreased fibrinogen.
CC Excl: For code 641.21: 640.00-641.13, 641.21, 646.80-646.93, 648.90-649.64, 650, 669.40-669.44, 669.80-669.94, 679.00-679.04, 679.12, 679.14; For code 641.23: 640.00-641.13, 641.23, 646.80-646.93, 648.90-649.64, 650, 669.40-669.44, 669.80-669.94, 679.00-679.04, 679.12, 679.14
045.90 Premature sep of placenta unspec, uns trimester I-10

§ ✓5ᵗʰ **641.3 Antepartum hemorrhage associated** MCC 1,3 M ♀
[0,1,3] **with coagulation defects**
Antepartum or intrapartum hemorrhage associated with:
afibrinogenemia
hyperfibrinolysis
hypofibrinogenemia
EXCLUDES coagulation defects not associated with antepartum hemorrhage (649.3)
DEF: Uterine hemorrhage prior to delivery.
CC Excl: For codes 641.31 and 641.33: 641.30-641.93, 646.80-646.93, 648.90-649.64, 650, 669.40-669.44, 669.80-669.94, 679.00-679.04, 679.12, 679.14

§ ✓5ᵗʰ **641.8 Other antepartum hemorrhage** M ♀
[0,1,3]
Antepartum or intrapartum hemorrhage associated with:
trauma
uterine leiomyoma

§ ✓5ᵗʰ **641.9 Unspecified antepartum hemorrhage** M ♀
[0,1,3]
Hemorrhage: Hemorrhage:
antepartum NOS   of pregnancy NOS
intrapartum NOS

---

§ Requires fifth digit. Valid digits are in [brackets] under each code. See beginning of section 640-649 for codes and definitions.

N Newborn Age: 0 | P Pediatric Age: 0-17 | M Maternity Age: 12-55 | A Adult Age: 15-124 | MCC Major CC Condition | CC CC Condition | HIV HIV Related Dx

214 – Volume 1   2014 ICD-9-CM

✓4th **642 Hypertension complicating pregnancy, childbirth, and the puerperium**

§ ✓5th **642.0 Benign essential hypertension complicating** `CC 1-3` M♀
[0-4] **pregnancy, childbirth, and the puerperium**

Hypertension } specified as complicating, or as
benign essential } reason for obstetric care
chronic NOS } during pregnancy,
essential } childbirth, or the
pre-existing NOS } puerperium

CC Excl: For codes 642.01, 642.02, 642.03: 642.00-642.94, 646.10-646.14, 646.80-646.93, 648.90-649.64, 650, 669.40-669.44, 669.80-669.94, 679.00-679.04, 679.12, 679.14
010.02 Pre-exist essential hypertension comp childbirth `I-10`

§ ✓5th **642.1 Hypertension secondary to renal disease,** `MCC 1-2` `CC 3-4` M♀
[0-4] **complicating pregnancy, childbirth, and the puerperium**

Hypertension secondary to renal disease, specified as complicating, or as a reason for obstetric care during pregnancy, childbirth, or the puerperium

CC Excl: For codes 642.11-642.14: See code: 642.01

§ ✓5th **642.2 Other pre-existing hypertension complicating** M♀
[0-4] **pregnancy, childbirth, and the puerperium**

Hypertensive } specified as complicating,
chronic kidney disease } or as a reason for
heart and chronic } obstetric care
kidney disease } during pregnancy,
heart disease } childbirth, or the
Malignant hypertension } puerperium

§ ✓5th **642.3 Transient hypertension of pregnancy** `CC 1-2` M♀
[0-4] Gestational hypertension
Transient hypertension, so described, in pregnancy, childbirth, or the puerperium

CC Excl: For codes 642.31, 642.32: See code: 642.01
AHA: 3Q, '90, 4
013.9 Gestatnl pg-inducd HTN w/o sig protnuria uns tri `I-10`

§ ✓5th **642.4 Mild or unspecified pre-eclampsia** `MCC 2` `CC 1, 3, 4` M♀
[0-4] Hypertension in pregnancy, childbirth, or the puerperium, not specified as pre-existing, with either albuminuria or edema, or both; mild or unspecified

Pre-eclampsia:
NOS
mild
Toxemia (pre-eclamptic):
NOS
mild

EXCLUDES albuminuria in pregnancy, without mention of hypertension (646.2)
edema in pregnancy, without mention of hypertension (646.1)

CC Excl: For codes 642.41-642.44: See code: 642.01
AHA: For code 642.41: 4Q, '09, 153
014.00 Mild to moderate pre-eclampsia unspec trimester `I-10`

§ ✓5th **642.5 Severe pre-eclampsia** `MCC 1-4` M♀
[0-4] Hypertension in pregnancy, childbirth, or the puerperium, not specified as pre-existing, with either albuminuria or edema, or both; specified as severe

Pre-eclampsia, severe
Toxemia (pre-eclamptic), severe

CC Excl: For codes 642.51-642.54: See code: 642.01
AHA: N-D, '85, 3

§ ✓5th **642.6 Eclampsia** `MCC 1-4` M♀
[0-4] Toxemia:
eclamptic
with convulsions

CC Excl: For codes 642.61-642.64: See code: 642.01

§ ✓5th **642.7 Pre-eclampsia or eclampsia superimposed** `MCC 1-4` M♀
[0-4] **on pre-existing hypertension**
Conditions classifiable to 642.4-642.6, with conditions classifiable to 642.0-642.2

CC Excl: For codes 642.71-642.74: See code: 642.01

§ ✓5th **642.9 Unspecified hypertension complicating** `CC 1-4` M♀
[0-4] **pregnancy, childbirth, or the puerperium**
Hypertension NOS, without mention of albuminuria or edema, complicating pregnancy, childbirth, or the puerperium

CC Excl: For codes 642.91, 642.92: 640.00-641.13, 646.80-646.93, 648.90-649.64, 650, 669.40-669.44, 669.80-669.94, 679.00-679.04, 679.12, 679.14; For codes 642.93, 642.94: 642.01-642.44, 642.61-642.94
AHA: For code 642.94: 1Q, '09, 17

✓4th **643 Excessive vomiting in pregnancy**
`INCLUDES` hyperemesis }
vomiting: }
persistent } arising during pregnancy
vicious }
hyperemesis gravidarum

§ ✓5th **643.0 Mild hyperemesis gravidarum** M♀
[0,1,3] Hyperemesis gravidarum, mild or unspecified, starting before the end of the 22nd week of gestation
DEF: Detrimental vomiting and nausea.

§ ✓5th **643.1 Hyperemesis gravidarum with metabolic disturbance** M♀
[0,1,3] Hyperemesis gravidarum, starting before the end of the 22nd week of gestation, with metabolic disturbance, such as:
carbohydrate depletion
dehydration
electrolyte imbalance

§ ✓5th **643.2 Late vomiting of pregnancy** M♀
[0,1,3] Excessive vomiting starting after 22 completed weeks of gestation

§ ✓5th **643.8 Other vomiting complicating pregnancy** M♀
[0,1,3] Vomiting due to organic disease or other cause, specified as complicating pregnancy, or as a reason for obstetric care during pregnancy
Use additional code to specify cause

§ ✓5th **643.9 Unspecified vomiting of pregnancy** M♀
[0,1,3] Vomiting as a reason for care during pregnancy, length of gestation unspecified

✓4th **644 Early or threatened labor**

§ ✓5th **644.0 Threatened premature labor** `MCC 3` M♀
[0,3] Premature labor after 22 weeks, but before 37 completed weeks of gestation without delivery

EXCLUDES that occurring before 22 completed weeks of gestation (640.0)

CC Excl: For code 644.03: 644.00-644.21, 646.80-646.93, 648.90-649.64, 650, 669.40-669.44, 669.80-669.94, 679.00-679.04, 679.12, 679.14
060.00 Preterm labor without delivery unspec trimester `I-10`

§ ✓5th **644.1 Other threatened labor** `CC 3` M♀
[0,3] False labor:
NOS }
after 37 completed weeks } without delivery
of gestation }
Threatened labor NOS }

CC Excl: For code 644.13: See code 644.03

§ ✓5th **644.2 Early onset of delivery** `MCC 1` `CC 0` M♀
[0,1] Onset (spontaneous) of delivery } before 37 completed
Premature labor with onset of } weeks of
delivery } gestation

CC Excl: See code: 644.03
AHA: For code 644.21: 3Q, '11, 3; 2Q, '91, 16
TIP: Assign if an attempted termination of pregnancy results in a liveborn fetus.
060.14x0 Pt labor 3rd tri w/pt del 3rd tri not applic/uns `I-10`

✓4th **645 Late pregnancy**
AHA: 4Q, '00, 43; 4Q, '91, 26

§ ✓5th **645.1 Post term pregnancy** M♀
[0,1,3] Pregnancy over 40 completed weeks to 42 completed weeks gestation
048.0 Post-term pregnancy `I-10`

§ ✓5th **645.2 Prolonged pregnancy** M♀
[0,1,3] Pregnancy which has advanced beyond 42 completed weeks gestation

§ Requires fifth digit. Valid digits are in [brackets] under each code. See beginning of section 640-649 for codes and definitions.

Complications of Pregnancy, Childbirth, and the Puerperium

646–648.4

√4ᵗʰ **646 Other complications of pregnancy, not elsewhere classified**
Use additional code(s) to further specify complication
AHA: 4Q, '95, 59

§ √5ᵗʰ **646.0 Papyraceous fetus** M♀
[0,1,3]   **DEF:** Fetus that dies in the second trimester of pregnancy and is retained in the uterus, with subsequent atrophy and mummification; commonly occurs in twin pregnancy, nonviable fetus becomes compressed by growth of living twin.

§ √5ᵗʰ **646.1 Edema or excessive weight gain in pregnancy, without** M♀
[0-4]   **mention of hypertension**
Gestational edema
Maternal obesity syndrome
EXCLUDES *that with mention of hypertension (642.0-642.9)*

§ √5ᵗʰ **646.2 Unspecified renal disease in pregnancy,** CC 1-4 M♀
[0-4]   **without mention of hypertension**
Albuminuria ⎫ in pregnancy or the
Nephropathy NOS ⎬ puerperium, without
Renal disease NOS ⎪ mention of
Uremia ⎭ hypertension

Gestational proteinuria
EXCLUDES *that with mention of hypertension (642.0-642.9)*
CC Excl: For codes 646.21- 646.24: 646.21-646.24

§ √5ᵗʰ **646.3 Recurrent pregnancy loss** CC 1 M♀
[0,1,3]   **EXCLUDES** *with current abortion (634.0-634.9)*
without current pregnancy (629.81)
DEF: Treatment Site Three or more consecutive spontaneous abortions.
CC Excl: For code 646.31: 646.31

§ √5ᵗʰ **646.4 Peripheral neuritis in pregnancy** M♀
[0-4]

§ √5ᵗʰ **646.5 Asymptomatic bacteriuria in pregnancy** M♀
[0-4]

§ √5ᵗʰ **646.6 Infections of genitourinary tract in pregnancy** CC 1-4 M♀
[0-4]   Conditions classifiable to 590, 595, 597, 599.0, 616
complicating pregnancy, childbirth, or the puerperium
Conditions classifiable to 614.0-614.5, 614.7-614.9, 615
complicating pregnancy or labor
EXCLUDES *major puerperal infection (670.0-670.8)*
CC Excl: For code 646.61-646.64: 646.60-646.64, 646.80-646.93, 648.90-649.64, 650, 669.40-669.44, 669.80-669.94, 679.00-679.04, 679.12, 679.14
AHA: For code 646.63: 4Q, '04, 90
023.90 Unspec GU tract infection in pregnancy uns tri   I-10

§ √5ᵗʰ **646.7 Liver and biliary tract disorders in pregnancy** CC 1,3 ♀
[0,1,3]   Acute yellow atrophy of liver ⎫
(obstetric) (true) ⎬ of pregnancy
Icterus gravis ⎪
Necrosis of liver ⎭

EXCLUDES *hepatorenal syndrome following delivery (674.8)*
viral hepatitis (647.6)
CC Excl: For code 646.71, 646.73: 646.70-646.93, 648.90-649.64, 650, 669.40-669.44, 669.80-669.94, 679.00-679.04, 679.12, 679.14

§ √5ᵗʰ **646.8 Other specified complications of pregnancy** M♀
[0-4]   Fatigue during pregnancy
Herpes gestationis
Insufficient weight gain of pregnancy
AHA: 3Q, '98, 16; J-F, '85, 15

§ √5ᵗʰ **646.9 Unspecified complication of pregnancy** M♀
[0,1,3]

√4ᵗʰ **647 Infectious and parasitic conditions in the mother classifiable elsewhere, but complicating pregnancy, childbirth, or the puerperium**
INCLUDES the listed conditions when complicating the pregnant state, aggravated by the pregnancy, or when a main reason for obstetric care
EXCLUDES *those conditions in the mother known or suspected to have affected the fetus (655.0-655.9)*
Use additional code(s) to further specify complication

§ √5ᵗʰ **647.0 Syphilis** CC 1-4 M♀
[0-4]   Conditions classifiable to 090-097
CC Excl: For code 647.01- 647.04: 646.81-647.24, 679.12, 679.14

§ √5ᵗʰ **647.1 Gonorrhea** CC 1-4 M♀
[0-4]   Conditions classifiable to 098
CC Excl: For code 647.11-647.14: See code: 647.01

§ √5ᵗʰ **647.2 Other venereal diseases** CC 1-4 M♀
[0-4]   Conditions classifiable to 099
CC Excl: For code 647.21-647.24: See code: 647.01

§ √5ᵗʰ **647.3 Tuberculosis** CC 1-4 M♀
[0-4]   Conditions classifiable to 010-018
CC Excl: For code 647.31-647.34: 646.80-646.93, 647.30-647.34, 648.90-649.64, 650, 669.40-669.44, 669.80-669.94, 679.00-679.04, 679.12, 679.14

§ √5ᵗʰ **647.4 Malaria** CC 1-4 M♀
[0-4]   Conditions classifiable to 084
CC Excl: For code 647.41-647.44: 646.80-646.93, 647.40-647.44, 648.90-649.64, 650, 669.40-669.44, 669.80-669.94, 679.00-679.04, 679.12, 679.14

§ √5ᵗʰ **647.5 Rubella** CC 1-4 M♀
[0-4]   Conditions classifiable to 056
CC Excl: For code 647.51-647.54: 647.51-647.94

§ √5ᵗʰ **647.6 Other viral diseases** CC 1-4 M♀
[0-4]   Conditions classifiable to 042, 050-055, 057-079, 795.05, 795.15, 796.75
CC Excl: For code 647.61-647.64: See code 647.51
AHA: J-F, '85, 15; **For code 647.61:** 2Q, '10, 10
TIP: Assign when pregnant patient has any HIV-related condition or is stated to have an asymptomatic HIV infection.
098.52 Other viral diseases complicating childbirth   I-10

§ √5ᵗʰ **647.8 Other specified infectious and parasitic diseases** CC 1-4 M♀
[0-4]   **CC Excl: For code 647.81-647.84:** See code 647.51

§ √5ᵗʰ **647.9 Unspecified infection or infestation** CC 1-4 M♀
[0-4]   **CC Excl: For code 647.91-647.94:** See code 647.51

√4ᵗʰ **648 Other current conditions in the mother classifiable elsewhere, but complicating pregnancy, childbirth, or the puerperium**
INCLUDES the listed conditions when complicating the pregnant state, aggravated by the pregnancy, or when a main reason for obstetric care
Use additional code(s) to identify the condition
EXCLUDES *those conditions in the mother known or suspected to have affected the fetus (655.0-655.9)*

§ √5ᵗʰ **648.0 Diabetes mellitus** MCC 1-2 CC 0, 3, 4 M♀
[0-4]   Conditions classifiable to 249, 250
EXCLUDES *gestational diabetes (648.8)*
CC Excl: 646.80-646.93, 648.00-648.04, 648.90-649.64, 650, 669.40-669.44, 669.80-669.94, 679.00-679.04, 679.12, 679.14
AHA: 3Q, '91, 5, 11
024.32 Uns pre-existing diabetes mellitus in childbirth   I-10

§ √5ᵗʰ **648.1 Thyroid dysfunction** M♀
[0-4]   Conditions classifiable to 240-246

§ √5ᵗʰ **648.2 Anemia** M♀
[0-4]   Conditions classifiable to 280-285
AHA: For Code 648.22: 1Q, '02, 14; **For code 648.24:** 1Q, '09, 17
TIP: Assign with fifth digit 2 for postpartum anemia.
099.013 Anemia complicating pregnancy third trimester   I-10

§ √5ᵗʰ **648.3 Drug dependence** CC 1-4 M♀
[0-4]   Conditions classifiable to 304
CC Excl: For code 648.31-648.34: 646.80-646.93, 648.30-648.34, 648.90-649.64, 650, 669.40-669.44, 669.80-669.94, 679.00-679.04, 679.12, 679.14
AHA: 2Q, '98, 13; 4Q, '88, 8

§ √5ᵗʰ **648.4 Mental disorders** M♀
[0-4]   Conditions classifiable to 290-303, 305.0, 305.2-305.9, 306-316, 317-319
AHA: 2Q, '98, 13; 4Q, '95, 63
099.314 Alcohol use complicating childbirth   I-10

---

§   Requires fifth digit. Valid digits are in [brackets] under each code. See beginning of section 640-649 for codes and definitions.

Ⓝ Newborn Age: 0   Ⓟ Pediatric Age: 0-17   Ⓜ Maternity Age: 12-55   Ⓐ Adult Age: 15-124   MCC Major CC Condition   CC CC Condition   HIV HIV Related Dx

§ ✓5ᵗʰ **648.5 Congenital cardiovascular disorders**   CC 1-4 M♀
[0-4]   Conditions classifiable to 745-747
CC Excl: For code 648.51, 648.52, 648.53, 648.54: 646.80-646.93,
648.50-648.64, 648.90-649.64, 650, 669.40-669.44, 669.80-669.94,
679.00-679.04, 679.12, 679.14

§ ✓5ᵗʰ **648.6 Other cardiovascular diseases**   CC 1-4 M♀
[0-4]   Conditions classifiable to 390-398, 410-429

> *EXCLUDES*   *cerebrovascular disorders in the puerperium (674.0)*
> *peripartum cardiomyopathy (674.5)*
> *venous complications (671.0-671.9)*

CC Excl: For code 648.61, 648.62, 648.63, 648.64: 646.80-646.93,
648.50-648.64, 648.90-649.64, 650, 669.40-669.44, 669.80-669.94,
679.00-679.04, 679.12, 679.14
AHA: 3Q, '98, 11; For code 648.64: ▶3Q, '12, 9◀

§ ✓5ᵗʰ **648.7 Bone and joint disorders of back, pelvis, and**   CC 1-4 M♀
[0-4]   **lower limbs**
Conditions classifiable to 720-724, and those classifiable to
711-719 or 725-738, specified as affecting the lower
limbs
CC Excl: For code 648.71, 648.72, 648.73, 648.74: 648.71-648.74

§ ✓5ᵗʰ **648.8 Abnormal glucose tolerance**   M♀
[0-4]   Conditions classifiable to 790.21-790.29
Gestational diabetes

Use additional code, if applicable, for associated long-term
(current) insulin use (V58.67)
DEF: Glucose intolerance arising in pregnancy, resolving at end of
pregnancy.
AHA: 3Q, '91, 5; For code 648.83: 4Q, '04, 56
TIP: Do not assign if patient was diabetic before becoming pregnant;
should never be assigned in combination with code 648.0x.
024.429 Gestational diab mellitus childbirth uns cntrl   I-10

§ ✓5ᵗʰ **648.9 Other current conditions classifiable elsewhere**   M♀
[0-4]   Conditions classifiable to 440-459, 795.01-795.04, 795.06,
795.10-795.14, 795.16, 796.70-796.74, 796.76
Nutritional deficiencies [conditions classifiable to 260-269]
AHA: 3Q, '06, 14; 4Q, '04, 88; N-D, '87, 10; For code 648.91: 1Q, '02, 14;
For code 648.93: 4Q, '04, 90; For code 648.94: 1Q, '09, 17
TIP: Assign for group B streptococcus carrier patients, along with
code V02.51 Carrier or suspected carrier of infectious diseases.

✓4ᵗʰ **649 Other conditions or status of the mother complicating
pregnancy, childbirth, or the puerperium**
AHA: 4Q, '06, 99

§ ✓5ᵗʰ **649.0 Tobacco use disorder complicating pregnancy,**   M♀
[0-4]   **childbirth, or the puerperium**
Smoking complicating pregnancy, childbirth, or the
puerperium
AHA: 4Q, '06, 99
099.334 Smoking tobacco complicating childbirth   I-10

§ ✓5ᵗʰ **649.1 Obesity complicating pregnancy, childbirth, or the**   M♀
[0-4]   **puerperium**
Use additional code to identify the obesity (278.00- 278.03)
AHA: 4Q, '06, 99
099.214 Obesity complicating childbirth   I-10

§ ✓5ᵗʰ **649.2 Bariatric surgery status complicating pregnancy,**   M♀
[0-4]   **childbirth, or the puerperium**
Gastric banding status complicating pregnancy, childbirth, or
the puerperium
Gastric bypass status for obesity complicating pregnancy,
childbirth, or the puerperium
Obesity surgery status complicating pregnancy, childbirth, or
the puerperium
AHA: 4Q, '06, 99, 118

§ ✓5ᵗʰ **649.3 Coagulation defects complicating pregnancy,**   CC M♀
[0-4]   **childbirth, or the puerperium**
Conditions classifiable to 286, 287, 289

Use additional code to identify the specific coagulation defect
(286.0-286.9, 287.0-287.9, 289.0-289.9)

> *EXCLUDES*   *coagulation defects causing antepartum*
> *hemorrhage (641.3)*
> *postpartum coagulation defects (666.3)*

CC Excl: For code 649.30: 648.90; For codes 649.31, 649.32, 649.33, 649.34:
648.91-648.94
AHA: 4Q, '06, 99

§ ✓5ᵗʰ **649.4 Epilepsy complicating pregnancy, childbirth, or**   CC 1-4 M♀
[0-4]   **the puerperium**
Conditions classifiable to 345

Use additional code to identify specific type of epilepsy
(345.00-345.91)

> *EXCLUDES*   *eclampsia (642.6)*

CC Excl: For codes 649.41, 649.42, 649.43, 649.44: 648.91-648.94
AHA: 4Q, '06, 99

§ ✓5ᵗʰ **649.5 Spotting complicating pregnancy**   M♀
[0,1,3]   *EXCLUDES*   *antepartum hemorrhage (641.0-641.9)*
hemorrhage in early pregnancy (640.0-640.9)
AHA: 4Q, '06, 99

§ ✓5ᵗʰ **649.6 Uterine size date discrepancy**   M♀
[0-4]   *EXCLUDES*   *suspected problem with fetal growth not found
(V89.04)*
AHA: 4Q, '06, 99

§ ✓5ᵗʰ **649.7 Cervical shortening**   M CC
[0,1,3]   *EXCLUDES*   *suspected cervical shortening not found (V89.05)*
DEF: A cervix that has shortened to < 25 mm in length by the 16th
week of pregnancy; warning sign for impending premature delivery;
treated by cervical cerclage placement or progesterone.
CC Excl: For code 649.70, 649.71, 649.73: 649.70-649.73, 654.51-654.54
AHA: 4Q, '08, 124-125; For Code 649.73: 4Q '08, 125

§ ✓5ᵗʰ **649.8 Onset (spontaneous) of labor after 37 completed**   M♀
[1,2]   **weeks of gestation but before 39 completed weeks
gestation, with delivery by (planned) cesarean section**
Delivery by (planned) cesarean section occurring after 37
completed weeks of gestation but before 39 completed
weeks gestation due to (spontaneous) onset of labor

Use additional code to specify reason for planned cesarean
section such as:
cephalopelvic disproportion (normally formed fetus)
(653.4)
previous cesarean delivery (654.2)
AHA: 4Q, '11, 132-133; For code 649.81: 4Q, '11, 133

Normal Delivery, and Other Indications for Care in Pregnancy, Labor, and Delivery (650-659)

> The following fifth-digit subclassification is for use with categories
> 651-659 to denote the current episode of care. Valid fifth-digits are in
> [brackets] under each code.
> 0   unspecified as to episode of care or not applicable
> 1   delivered, with or without mention of antepartum condition
> 2   delivered, with mention of postpartum complication
> 3   antepartum condition or complication
> 4   postpartum condition or complication

650 Normal delivery   M♀
NOTE Delivery requiring minimal or no assistance, with or without
episiotomy, without fetal manipulation [e.g., rotation version]
or instrumentation [forceps] of spontaneous, cephalic, vaginal,
full-term, single, live-born infant. This code is for use as a single
diagnosis code and is not to be used with any other code in the
range 630-676.

Use additional code to indicate outcome of delivery (V27.0)

> *EXCLUDES*   *breech delivery (assisted) (spontaneous) NOS (652.2)*
> *delivery by vacuum extractor, forceps, cesarean section, or
> breech extraction, without specified complication
> (669.5-669.7)*

AHA: 2Q, '02, 10; 3Q, '01, 12; 3Q, '00, 5; 4Q, '95, 28, 59
TIP: Code 650 is to be assigned only for the episode of care during which the
patient delivers and may be assigned if the patient is admitted for induction
of labor.
080 Encounter for full-term uncomplicated delivery   I-10

✓4ᵗʰ **651 Multiple gestation**
Use additional code to specify placenta status (V91.00-V91.99)

§ ✓5ᵗʰ **651.0 Twin pregnancy**   CC 1 M♀
[0,1,3]   *EXCLUDES*   *fetal conjoined twins (678.1)*
CC Excl: For code 651.01: 650-651.63, 651.71-652.20, 652.23-652.93
AHA: 3Q, '06, 16
030.009 Twin preg unspec numb of placenta & unspec   I-10
numb amniotic sacs unspec tri

Requires fifth digit. Valid digits are in [brackets] under each code. See beginning of section 640-649 for codes and definitions.

Additional Digit Required   Unacceptable PDx   Manifestation Code   Hospital Acquired Condition   ▶◀ Revised Text   ● New Code   ▲ Revised Code Title

Complications of Pregnancy, Childbirth, and the Puerperium

651.1–654.2

Malposition and Malpresentation

Breech

Mother's pelvis

Face (mentum)

Shoulder (arm prolapse)

Compound (extremity together with head)

Oblique

§ ✓5ᵗʰ **651.1 Triplet pregnancy**   CC 1,3 M♀
[0,1,3]   **CC Excl:** For code 651.11, 651.13: 650-651.63, 651.71-652.93

§ ✓5ᵗʰ **651.2 Quadruplet pregnancy**   CC 1,3 M♀
[0,1,3]   **CC Excl:** For code 651.21, 651.23: See code 651.11

§ ✓5ᵗʰ **651.3 Twin pregnancy with fetal loss and retention of one** M♀
[0,1,3] **fetus**
    Vanishing twin syndrome (651.33)

§ ✓5ᵗʰ **651.4 Triplet pregnancy with fetal loss and retention of** CC 1,3 M♀
[0,1,3] **one or more fetus(es)**
    CC Excl: For code 651.41, 651.43: See code 651.11

§ ✓5ᵗʰ **651.5 Quadruplet pregnancy with fetal loss and** CC 1,3 M♀
[0,1,3] **retention of one or more fetus(es)**
    CC Excl: For code 651.51, 651.53: See code 651.11

§ ✓5ᵗʰ **651.6 Other multiple pregnancy with fetal loss and retention** M♀
[0,1,3] **of one or more fetus(es)**

§ ✓5ᵗʰ **651.7 Multiple gestation following (elective) fetal reduction** M♀
[0,1,3]   Fetal reduction of multiple fetuses reduced to single fetus
    AHA: 3Q, '06, 18; For code 651.71: 4Q, '05, 81

§ ✓5ᵗʰ **651.8 Other specified multiple gestation**   CC 1,3 M♀
[0,1,3]   **CC Excl:** For code 651.81, 651.83: See code 651.11

§ ✓5ᵗʰ **651.9 Unspecified multiple gestation** M♀
[0,1,3]

✓4ᵗʰ **652 Malposition and malpresentation of fetus**
    Code first any associated obstructed labor (660.0)

§ ✓5ᵗʰ **652.0 Unstable lie** M♀
[0,1,3] **DEF:** Changing fetal position.

§ ✓5ᵗʰ **652.1 Breech or other malpresentation successfully** M♀
[0,1,3] **converted to cephalic presentation**
    Cephalic version NOS

§ ✓5ᵗʰ **652.2 Breech presentation without mention of version** M♀
[0,1,3]   Breech delivery (assisted) (spontaneous) NOS
    Buttocks presentation
    Complete breech
    Frank breech
    EXCLUDES footling presentation (652.8)
                incomplete breech (652.8)
    DEF: Fetal presentation of buttocks or feet at birth canal.
    032.1xx0 Maternal care breech presentation not applic/uns   I-10

§ ✓5ᵗʰ **652.3 Transverse or oblique presentation** M♀
[0,1,3]   Oblique lie   Transverse lie
    EXCLUDES transverse arrest of fetal head (660.3)
    DEF: Delivery of fetus, shoulder first.

§ ✓5ᵗʰ **652.4 Face or brow presentation** M♀
[0,1,3]   Mentum presentation

§ ✓5ᵗʰ **652.5 High head at term** M♀
[0,1,3]   Failure of head to enter pelvic brim
    032.4xx0 Maternal care high head at term not applic/uns   I-10

§ ✓5ᵗʰ **652.6 Multiple gestation with malpresentation of one** M♀
[0,1,3] **fetus or more**

§ ✓5ᵗʰ **652.7 Prolapsed arm** M♀
[0,1,3]

Cephalopelvic Disproportion

Pubic symphysis

Ischial tuberosity

Contraction of pelvic outlet (from below)

Cephalopelvic disproportion due to: Contraction of pelvic inlet, or large fetus, or hydrocephalus

Pubic symphysis

Pelvic inlet from above

§ ✓5ᵗʰ **652.8 Other specified malposition or malpresentation** M♀
[0,1,3]   Compound presentation

§ ✓5ᵗʰ **652.9 Unspecified malposition or malpresentation** M♀
[0,1,3]

✓4ᵗʰ **653 Disproportion**
    Code first any associated obstructed labor (660.1)

§ ✓5ᵗʰ **653.0 Major abnormality of bony pelvis, not further** M♀
[0,1,3] **specified**
    Pelvic deformity NOS

§ ✓5ᵗʰ **653.1 Generally contracted pelvis** M♀
[0,1,3]   Contracted pelvis NOS

§ ✓5ᵗʰ **653.2 Inlet contraction of pelvis** M♀
[0,1,3]   Inlet contraction (pelvis)

§ ✓5ᵗʰ **653.3 Outlet contraction of pelvis** M♀
[0,1,3]   Outlet contraction (pelvis)

§ ✓5ᵗʰ **653.4 Fetopelvic disproportion** M♀
[0,1,3]   Cephalopelvic disproportion NOS
    Disproportion of mixed maternal and fetal origin, with
       normally formed fetus
    033.4xx0 Mtrn care dispropor mtrn&fetal orig not applic   I-10

§ ✓5ᵗʰ **653.5 Unusually large fetus causing disproportion** M♀
[0,1,3]   Disproportion of fetal origin with normally formed fetus
    Fetal disproportion NOS
    EXCLUDES that when the reason for medical care was concern
              for the fetus (656.6)

§ ✓5ᵗʰ **653.6 Hydrocephalic fetus causing disproportion** M♀
[0,1,3]   **EXCLUDES** that when the reason for medical care was concern
              for the fetus (655.0)

§ ✓5ᵗʰ **653.7 Other fetal abnormality causing disproportion** M♀
[0,1,3]   Fetal: Fetal:
       ascites   sacral teratoma
       hydrops   tumor
       myelomeningocele
    EXCLUDES conjoined twins causing disproportion (678.1)

§ ✓5ᵗʰ **653.8 Disproportion of other origin** M♀
[0,1,3]   **EXCLUDES** shoulder (girdle) dystocia (660.4)

§ ✓5ᵗʰ **653.9 Unspecified disproportion** M♀
[0,1,3]

✓4ᵗʰ **654 Abnormality of organs and soft tissues of pelvis**
    INCLUDES the listed conditions during pregnancy, childbirth, or the
               puerperium
    Code first any associated obstructed labor (660.2)
    EXCLUDES trauma to perineum and vulva complicating current delivery
              (664.0-664.9)

§ ✓5ᵗʰ **654.0 Congenital abnormalities of uterus** M♀
[0-4]   Double uterus
    Uterus bicornis

§ ✓5ᵗʰ **654.1 Tumors of body of uterus** M♀
[0-4]   Uterine fibroids

§ ✓5ᵗʰ **654.2 Previous cesarean delivery** M♀
[0,1,3]   Uterine scar from previous cesarean delivery
    AHA: 1Q, '92, 8; For code 654.21: 4Q, '11, 133
    034.21 Maternal care for scar from prev cesarean del

---

§ · Requires fifth digit. Valid digits are in [brackets] under each code. See beginning of section 640-649 for codes and definitions.

N Newborn Age: 0   P Pediatric Age: 0-17   M Maternity Age: 12-55   A Adult Age: 15-124   MCC Major CC Condition   CC CC Condition   HIV HIV Related Dx

218 – Volume 1   2014 ICD-9-CM

§ ✓5ᵗʰ **654.3 Retroverted and incarcerated gravid uterus**   Ⓜ♀
[0-4]   **DEF:** Treatment Site Retroverted: tilted back uterus; no change in
angle of longitudinal axis.
    DEF: Treatment Site Incarcerated: immobile, fixed uterus.

§ ✓5ᵗʰ **654.4 Other abnormalities in shape or position**   Ⓜ♀
[0-4]   **of gravid uterus and of neighboring structures**
    Cystocele   Prolapse of gravid uterus
    Pelvic floor repair   Rectocele
    Pendulous abdomen   Rigid pelvic floor
    Prolapse of gravid uterus

§ ✓5ᵗʰ **654.5 Cervical incompetence**   MCC 1-4 Ⓜ♀
[0-4]   Presence of Shirodkar suture with or without mention of
cervical incompetence
    DEF: Abnormal cervix; tendency to dilate in second trimester; causes
premature fetal expulsion.
    DEF: Shirodkar suture: purse-string suture used to artificially close
incompetent cervix.
    CC Excl: For code 654.51-654.54: 649.70-649.73, 654.51-654.54

§ ✓5ᵗʰ **654.6 Other congenital or acquired abnormality**   Ⓜ♀
[0-4]   **of cervix**
    Cicatricial cervix
    Polyp of cervix
    Previous surgery to cervix
    Rigid cervix (uteri)
    Stenosis or stricture of cervix
    Tumor of cervix

§ ✓5ᵗʰ **654.7 Congenital or acquired abnormality of vagina**   Ⓜ♀
[0-4]   Previous surgery to vagina
    Septate vagina
    Stenosis of vagina (acquired) (congenital)
    Stricture of vagina
    Tumor of vagina

§ ✓5ᵗʰ **654.8 Congenital or acquired abnormality of vulva**   Ⓜ♀
[0-4]   Anal sphincter tear (healed) (old) complicating delivery
    Fibrosis of perineum
    Persistent hymen
    Previous surgery to perineum or vulva
    Rigid perineum
    Tumor of vulva
    EXCLUDES *anal sphincter tear (healed) (old) not associated with*
*   delivery (569.43)*
*   varicose veins of vulva (671.1)*
    AHA: 1Q, '03, 14

§ ✓5ᵗʰ **654.9 Other and unspecified**   Ⓜ♀
[0-4]   Uterine scar NEC

✓4ᵗʰ **655 Known or suspected fetal abnormality affecting management**
of mother
    INCLUDES   the listed conditions in the fetus as a reason for
               observation or obstetrical care of the mother, or for
               termination of pregnancy
    AHA: 3Q, '90, 4
    TIP: Only assign when the fetal condition affects the management of the
mother. Assign on mother's chart when in utero procedures are performed
on the fetus.

§ ✓5ᵗʰ **655.0 Central nervous system malformation in fetus**   Ⓜ♀
[0,1,3]   Fetal or suspected fetal:
      anencephaly
      hydrocephalus
      spina bifida (with myelomeningocele)

§ ✓5ᵗʰ **655.1 Chromosomal abnormality in fetus**   Ⓜ♀
[0,1,3]

§ ✓5ᵗʰ **655.2 Hereditary disease in family possibly affecting fetus**   Ⓜ♀
[0,1,3]

§ ✓5ᵗʰ **655.3 Suspected damage to fetus from viral disease in**   Ⓜ♀
[0,1,3] **the mother**
    Suspected damage to fetus from maternal rubella

§ ✓5ᵗʰ **655.4 Suspected damage to fetus from other disease in**   Ⓜ♀
[0,1,3] **the mother**
    Suspected damage to fetus from maternal:
      alcohol addiction
      listeriosis
      toxoplasmosis

§ ✓5ᵗʰ **655.5 Suspected damage to fetus from drugs**   Ⓜ♀
[0,1,3]

§ ✓5ᵗʰ **655.6 Suspected damage to fetus from radiation**   Ⓜ♀
[0,1,3]

§ ✓5ᵗʰ **655.7 Decreased fetal movements**   Ⓜ♀
[0,1,3]   **AHA:** 4Q, '97, 41

§ ✓5ᵗʰ **655.8 Other known or suspected fetal abnormality, not**   Ⓜ♀
[0,1,3] **elsewhere classified**
    Suspected damage to fetus from:
      environmental toxins
      intrauterine contraceptive device
    AHA: 3Q, '06, 16, 18

§ ✓5ᵗʰ **655.9 Unspecified**   Ⓜ♀
[0,1,3]   **AHA:** For code 655.93: 2Q, '10, 6-7

✓4ᵗʰ **656 Other known or suspected fetal and placental problems**
affecting management of mother
    EXCLUDES *fetal hematologic conditions (678.0)*
*   suspected placental problems not found (V89.02)*

§ ✓5ᵗʰ **656.0 Fetal-maternal hemorrhage**   Ⓜ♀
[0,1,3]   Leakage (microscopic) of fetal blood into maternal circulation

§ ✓5ᵗʰ **656.1 Rhesus isoimmunization**   CC 3 Ⓜ♀
[0,1,3]   Anti-D [Rh] antibodies
    Rh incompatibility
    DEF: Antibodies developing against Rh factor; mother with Rh
negative develops antibodies against Rh positive fetus.
    CC Excl: For code 656.13: 656.11-656.13
    036.0190 Mtrn care anti-D Rh antibods uns tri not applic   I-10

§ ✓5ᵗʰ **656.2 Isoimmunization from other and unspecified blood-**   Ⓜ♀
[0,1,3] **group incompatibility**
    ABO isoimmunization
    AHA: 4Q, '06, 135

§ ✓5ᵗʰ **656.3 Fetal distress**   CC 1 Ⓜ♀
[0,1,3]   Fetal metabolic acidemia
    EXCLUDES *abnormal fetal acid-base balance (656.8)*
*   abnormality in fetal heart rate or rhythm (659.7)*
*   fetal bradycardia (659.7)*
*   fetal tachycardia (659.7)*
*   meconium in liquor (656.8)*
    DEF: Life-threatening disorder; fetal anoxia, hemolytic disease and
other miscellaneous diseases cause fetal distress.
    CC Excl: For code 656.31: 656.31-656.33, 659.71, 763.82
    AHA: N-D, '86, 4

§ ✓5ᵗʰ **656.4 Intrauterine death**   CC 1,3 Ⓜ♀
[0,1,3]   Fetal death:
      NOS
      after completion of 22 weeks' gestation
      late
    Missed delivery
    EXCLUDES *missed abortion (632)*
    CC Excl: For code 656.41: 656.41-656.43; For code 656.43: 656.43

§ ✓5ᵗʰ **656.5 Poor fetal growth**   CC 1 Ⓜ♀
[0,1,3]   "Light-for-dates"
    "Placental insufficiency"
    "Small-for-dates"
    CC Excl: For code 656.51: 656.51-656.53
    036.5190 Mtrn care known/spct placental insuff uns tri   I-10

§ ✓5ᵗʰ **656.6 Excessive fetal growth**   Ⓜ♀
[0,1,3]   "Large-for-dates"
    036.60x0 Mtrn care excess fetl grwth uns tri not applic   I-10

§ ✓5ᵗʰ **656.7 Other placental conditions**   Ⓜ♀
[0,1,3]   Abnormal placenta
    Placental infarct
    EXCLUDES *placental polyp (674.4)*
*   placentitis (658.4)*

---

§   Requires fifth digit. Valid digits are in [brackets] under each code. See beginning of section 640-649 for codes and definitions.

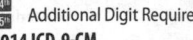

✓4ᵗʰ/✓5ᵗʰ Additional Digit Required   Unacceptable PDx   Manifestation Code   Hospital Acquired Condition   ►◄ Revised Text   ● New Code   ▲ Revised Code Title

§ ✓5ᵗʰ **656.8 Other specified fetal and placental problems**　Ｍ♀
　　[0,1,3]　　Abnormal acid-base balance
　　　　　　Intrauterine acidosis
　　　　　　Lithopedian
　　　　　　Meconium in liquor
　　　　　　Subchorionic hematoma
　　　　　DEF: Lithopedion: Calcified fetus; not expelled by mother.
　　　　　036.20x0 Mtrn care hydrops fetalis uns tri not applic/uns　I-10

§ ✓5ᵗʰ **656.9 Unspecified fetal and placental problem**　Ｍ♀
　　[0,1,3]

✓4ᵗʰ **657 Polyhydramnios**　CC 1　Ｍ♀
　　[0,1,3]

§ ✓5ᵗʰ　Use 0 as fourth-digit for this category
　　　　Hydramnios
　　　　EXCLUDES suspected polyhydramnios not found (V89.01)
　　　　DEF: Excess amniotic fluid.
　　　　CC Excl: For code 657.01: 657.01-657.03
　　　　AHA: 3Q, '06, 16; 4Q, '91, 26
　　　　040.9xx0 Polyhydraminos uns trimester not applicable/uns　I-10

✓4ᵗʰ **658 Other problems associated with amniotic cavity and membranes**
　　　　EXCLUDES amniotic fluid embolism (673.1)
　　　　　　　suspected problems with amniotic cavity and membranes not found (V89.01)

§ ✓5ᵗʰ **658.0 Oligohydramnios**　CC 1,3　Ｍ♀
　　[0,1,3]　Oligohydramnios without mention of rupture of membranes
　　　　　DEF: Deficient amount of amniotic fluid.
　　　　　CC Excl: For code 658.01, 658.03: 658.01-658.03
　　　　　AHA: 3Q, '06, 16
　　　　　041.00x0 Oligohydraminos uns trimester not applicable/uns　I-10

§ ✓5ᵗʰ **658.1 Premature rupture of membranes**　Ｍ♀
　　[0,1,3]　Rupture of amniotic sac less than 24 hours prior to the onset of labor
　　　　　AHA: For code 658.13: 1Q, '01, 5; 4Q, '98, 77
　　　　　042.00 Prmat rom ool w/in 24 hrs of rup uns wks gestatn　I-10

§ ✓5ᵗʰ **658.2 Delayed delivery after spontaneous or unspecified**　Ｍ♀
　　[0,1,3] **rupture of membranes**
　　　　　Prolonged rupture of membranes NOS
　　　　　Rupture of amniotic sac 24 hours or more prior to the onset of labor

§ ✓5ᵗʰ **658.3 Delayed delivery after artificial rupture**　Ｍ♀
　　[0,1,3] **of membranes**

§ ✓5ᵗʰ **658.4 Infection of amniotic cavity**　MCC 1,3　Ｍ♀
　　[0,1,3]　Amnionitis
　　　　　　Chorioamnionitis
　　　　　　Membranitis
　　　　　　Placentitis
　　　　　CC Excl: For code 658.41, 658.43: 658.41-658.43
　　　　　041.1090 Inf amniotic sac & memb uns, uns tri not applic/uns　I-10

§ ✓5ᵗʰ **658.8 Other**　CC 1　Ｍ♀
　　[0,1,3]　Amnion nodosum
　　　　　　Amniotic cyst
　　　　　CC Excl: For code 658.81: 658.81

§ ✓5ᵗʰ **658.9 Unspecified**　Ｍ♀
　　[0,1,3]

✓4ᵗʰ **659 Other indications for care or intervention related to labor and delivery, not elsewhere classified**

§ ✓5ᵗʰ **659.0 Failed mechanical induction**　Ｍ♀
　　[0,1,3]　Failure of induction of labor by surgical or other instrumental methods

§ ✓5ᵗʰ **659.1 Failed medical or unspecified induction**　Ｍ♀
　　[0,1,3]　Failed induction NOS
　　　　　　Failure of induction of labor by medical methods, such as oxytocic drugs
　　　　　061.9 Failed induction of labor unspecified　I-10

§ ✓5ᵗʰ **659.2 Maternal pyrexia during labor, unspecified**　CC 1　Ｍ♀
　　[0,1,3]　**DEF:** Fever during labor.
　　　　　CC Excl: For code 659.21: 659.21-659.23
　　　　　075.2 Pyrexia during labor not elsewhere classified　I-10

§ ✓5ᵗʰ **659.3 Generalized infection during labor**　MCC 1, 3　Ｍ♀
　　[0,1,3]　Septicemia during labor
　　　　　CC Excl: For code 659.31, 659.33: 646.80-646.93, 648.90-649.64, 650, 659.30-659.33, 669.40-669.44, 669.80-669.94, 679.00-679.04, 679.12, 679.14

§ ✓5ᵗʰ **659.4 Grand multiparity**　Ｍ♀
　　[0,1,3]　**EXCLUDES** supervision only, in pregnancy (V23.3)
　　　　　　　　　without current pregnancy (V61.5)
　　　　　DEF: Having borne six or more children previously.

§ ✓5ᵗʰ **659.5 Elderly primigravida**　Ｍ♀
　　[0,1,3]　First pregnancy in a woman who will be 35 years of age or older at expected date of delivery
　　　　　EXCLUDES supervision only, in pregnancy (V23.81)
　　　　　AHA: 3Q, '01, 12
　　　　　009.519 Supervisn of elderly primigravida uns trimester　I-10

§ ✓5ᵗʰ **659.6 Elderly multigravida**　Ｍ♀
　　[0,1,3]　Second or more pregnancy in a woman who will be 35 years of age or older at expected date of delivery
　　　　　EXCLUDES elderly primigravida 659.5
　　　　　　　　　supervision only, in pregnancy (V23.82)
　　　　　AHA: 3Q, '01, 12
　　　　　009.529 Supervisn of elderly multigravida uns trimester　I-10

§ ✓5ᵗʰ **659.7 Abnormality in fetal heart rate or rhythm**　Ｍ♀
　　[0,1,3]　Depressed fetal heart tones
　　　　　　Fetal:
　　　　　　　bradycardia
　　　　　　　tachycardia
　　　　　　Fetal heart rate decelerations
　　　　　　Non-reassuring fetal heart rate or rhythm
　　　　　AHA: 4Q, '98, 48
　　　　　076 Abn in fetal heart rate & rhythm comp L&D　I-10

§ ✓5ᵗʰ **659.8 Other specified indications for care or intervention**　Ｍ♀
　　[0,1,3] **related to labor and delivery**
　　　　　　Pregnancy in a female less than 16 years old at expected date of delivery
　　　　　　Very young maternal age
　　　　　AHA: 3Q, '01, 12

§ ✓5ᵗʰ **659.9 Unspecified indication for care or**　Ｍ♀
　　[0,1,3] **intervention related to labor and delivery**

Complications Occurring Mainly in the Course of Labor and Delivery (660-669)

The following fifth-digit subclassification is for use with categories 660-669 to denote the current episode of care. Valid fifth-digits are in [brackets] under each code.
　0 unspecified as to episode of care or not applicable
　1 delivered, with or without mention of antepartum condition
　2 delivered, with mention of postpartum complication
　3 antepartum condition or complication
　4 postpartum condition or complication

✓4ᵗʰ **660 Obstructed labor**
　　AHA: 3Q, '95, 10

§ ✓5ᵗʰ **660.0 Obstruction caused by malposition of fetus at**　CC 3　Ｍ♀
　　[0,1,3] **onset of labor**
　　　　　　Any condition classifiable to 652, causing obstruction during labor
　　　　　　Use additional code from 652.0-652.9 to identify condition
　　　　　CC Excl: For code 660.03: 646.80-646.93, 648.90-649.64, 650, 655.70-655.73, 660.03, 665.00-665.11, 665.50-665.54, 665.80-665.94, 669.40-669.44, 669.80-669.94, 679.00-679.04, 679.12, 679.14

§ ✓5ᵗʰ **660.1 Obstruction by bony pelvis**　Ｍ♀
　　[0,1,3]　Any condition classifiable to 653, causing obstruction during labor
　　　　　　Use additional code from 653.0-653.9 to identify condition

§ ✓5ᵗʰ **660.2 Obstruction by abnormal pelvic soft tissues**　Ｍ♀
　　[0,1,3]　Prolapse of anterior lip of cervix
　　　　　　Any condition classifiable to 654, causing obstruction during labor
　　　　　　Use additional code from 654.0-654.9 to identify condition

---

§　Requires fifth digit. Valid digits are in [brackets] under each code. See beginning of section 640-649 for codes and definitions.

§ ✓5ᵗʰ **660.3 Deep transverse arrest and persistent** Ⓜ♀
[0,1,3] **occipitoposterior position**
     O64.0xx0 Obst labor incpl rotat of fetal head not applic   I-10

§ ✓5ᵗʰ **660.4 Shoulder (girdle) dystocia** Ⓜ♀
[0,1,3]   Impacted shoulders
     DEF: Obstructed labor due to impacted fetal shoulders.
     O66.0 Obstructed labor due to shoulder dystocia   I-10

§ ✓5ᵗʰ **660.5 Locked twins** Ⓜ♀
[0,1,3]

§ ✓5ᵗʰ **660.6 Failed trial of labor, unspecified** Ⓜ♀
[0,1,3]   Failed trial of labor, without mention of
         condition or suspected condition

§ ✓5ᵗʰ **660.7 Failed forceps or vacuum extractor, unspecified** Ⓜ♀
[0,1,3]   Application of ventouse or forceps, without mention of
         condition

§ ✓5ᵗʰ **660.8 Other causes of obstructed labor** Ⓜ♀
[0,1,3]   Use additional code to identify condition
     AHA: 4Q, '04, 88

§ ✓5ᵗʰ **660.9 Unspecified obstructed labor** Ⓜ♀
[0,1,3]   Dystocia:
       NOS
       fetal NOS
       maternal NOS

✓4ᵗʰ **661 Abnormality of forces of labor**

§ ✓5ᵗʰ **661.0 Primary uterine inertia** Ⓜ♀
[0,1,3]   Failure of cervical dilation
     Hypotonic uterine dysfunction, primary
     Prolonged latent phase of labor
     DEF: Lack of efficient contractions during labor causing prolonged
     labor.
     O62.0 Primary inadequate contractions   I-10

§ ✓5ᵗʰ **661.1 Secondary uterine inertia** Ⓜ♀
[0,1,3]   Arrested active phase of labor
     Hypotonic uterine dysfunction, secondary
     O62.1 Secondary uterine inertia   I-10

§ ✓5ᵗʰ **661.2 Other and unspecified uterine inertia** Ⓜ♀
[0,1,3]   Atony of uterus without hemorrhage
     Desultory labor
     Irregular labor
     Poor contractions
     Slow slope active phase of labor
     EXCLUDES atony of uterus with hemorrhage (666.1)
         postpartum atony of uterus without hemorrhage
         (669.8)

§ ✓5ᵗʰ **661.3 Precipitate labor** Ⓜ♀
[0,1,3]   **DEF:** Rapid labor and delivery.

§ ✓5ᵗʰ **661.4 Hypertonic, incoordinate, or prolonged** Ⓜ♀
[0,1,3] **uterine contractions**
     Cervical spasm
     Contraction ring (dystocia)
     Dyscoordinate labor
     Hourglass contraction of uterus
     Hypertonic uterine dysfunction
     Incoordinate uterine action
     Retraction ring (Bandl's) (pathological)
     Tetanic contractions
     Uterine dystocia NOS
     Uterine spasm

§ ✓5ᵗʰ **661.9 Unspecified abnormality of labor** Ⓜ♀
[0,1,3]

✓4ᵗʰ **662 Long labor**

§ ✓5ᵗʰ **662.0 Prolonged first stage** Ⓜ♀
[0,1,3]

§ ✓5ᵗʰ **662.1 Prolonged labor, unspecified** CC1 Ⓜ♀
[0,1,3]   **CC Excl: For code 662.11:** 646.80-646.93, 648.90-649.64, 650,
     655.70-655.73, 662.11, 665.00-665.11, 665.50-665.54,
     665.80-665.94, 669.40-669.44, 669.80-669.94, 679.00-679.04,
     679.12, 679.14

Perineal Lacerations

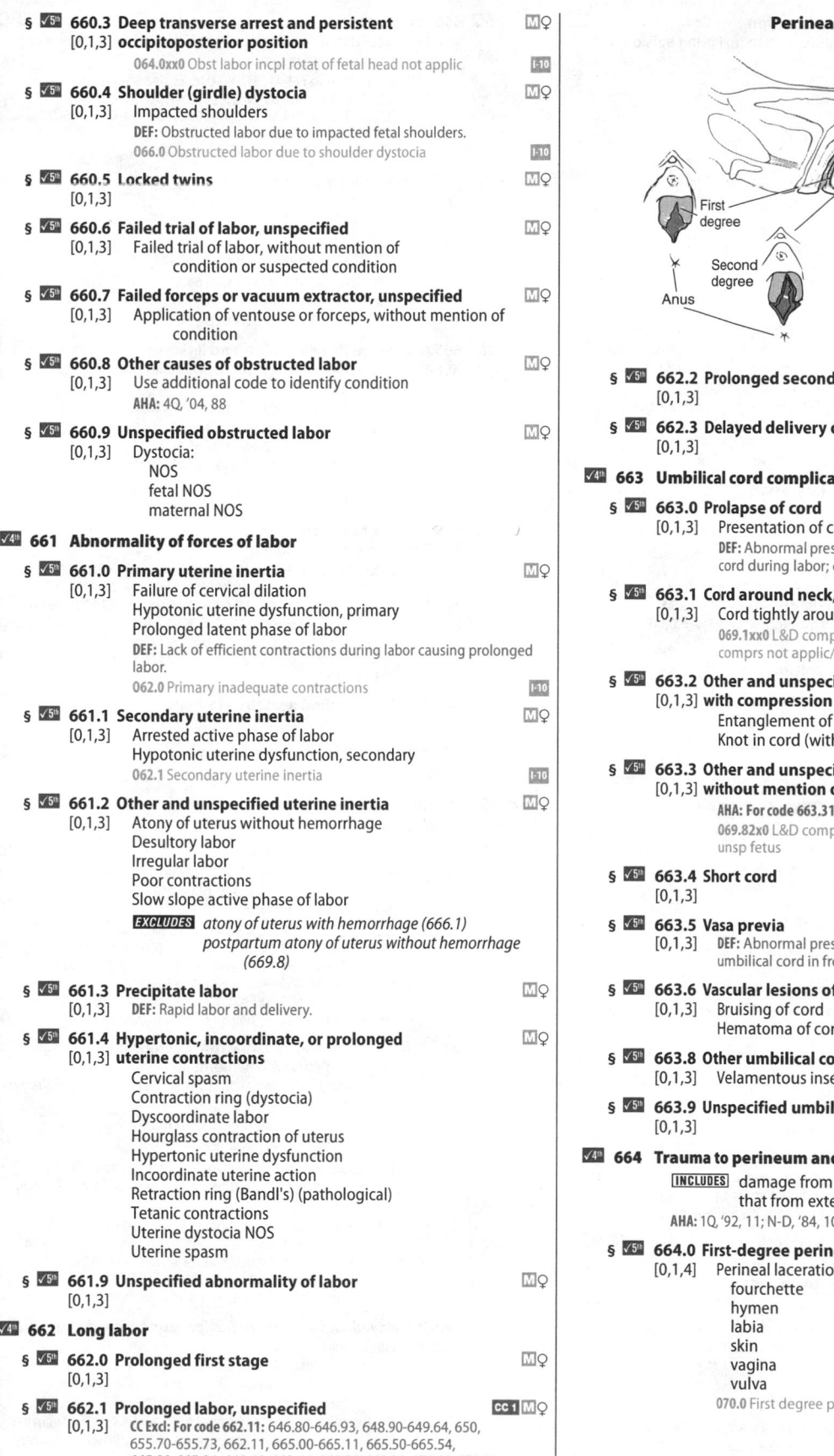

§ ✓5ᵗʰ **662.2 Prolonged second stage** Ⓜ♀
[0,1,3]

§ ✓5ᵗʰ **662.3 Delayed delivery of second twin, triplet, etc.** Ⓜ♀
[0,1,3]

✓4ᵗʰ **663 Umbilical cord complications**

§ ✓5ᵗʰ **663.0 Prolapse of cord** Ⓜ♀
[0,1,3]   Presentation of cord
     DEF: Abnormal presentation of fetus; marked by protruding umbilical
     cord during labor; can cause fetal death.

§ ✓5ᵗʰ **663.1 Cord around neck, with compression** Ⓜ♀
[0,1,3]   Cord tightly around neck
     O69.1xx0 L&D comp by cord arnd neck with   I-10
     comprs not applic/uns

§ ✓5ᵗʰ **663.2 Other and unspecified cord entanglement,** Ⓜ♀
[0,1,3] **with compression**
     Entanglement of cords of twins in mono-amniotic sac
     Knot in cord (with compression)

§ ✓5ᵗʰ **663.3 Other and unspecified cord entanglement,** Ⓜ♀
[0,1,3] **without mention of compression**
     AHA: For code 663.31: 2Q, '03, 9
     O69.82x0 L&D comp by oth cord entanglement w/o comprs   I-10
     unsp fetus

§ ✓5ᵗʰ **663.4 Short cord** Ⓜ♀
[0,1,3]

§ ✓5ᵗʰ **663.5 Vasa previa** Ⓜ♀
[0,1,3]   **DEF:** Abnormal presentation of fetus marked by blood vessels of
     umbilical cord in front of fetal head.

§ ✓5ᵗʰ **663.6 Vascular lesions of cord** Ⓜ♀
[0,1,3]   Bruising of cord   Thrombosis of vessels of cord
     Hematoma of cord

§ ✓5ᵗʰ **663.8 Other umbilical cord complications** Ⓜ♀
[0,1,3]   Velamentous insertion of umbilical cord

§ ✓5ᵗʰ **663.9 Unspecified umbilical cord complication** Ⓜ♀
[0,1,3]

✓4ᵗʰ **664 Trauma to perineum and vulva during delivery**
     INCLUDES damage from instruments
         that from extension of episiotomy
     AHA: 1Q, '92, 11; N-D, '84, 10

§ ✓5ᵗʰ **664.0 First-degree perineal laceration** Ⓜ♀
[0,1,4]   Perineal laceration, rupture, or tear involving:
       fourchette
       hymen
       labia
       skin
       vagina
       vulva
     O70.0 First degree perineal laceration during delivery   I-10

Requires fifth digit. Valid digits are in [brackets] under each code. See beginning of section 640-649 for codes and definitions.

Additional Digit Required   Unacceptable PDx   Manifestation Code   Hospital Acquired Condition   ►◄ Revised Text   ● New Code   ▲ Revised Code Title

2014 ICD-9-CM   Volume 1 – 221

Complications of Pregnancy, Childbirth, and the Puerperium

664.1–666.2

§ √5ᵗʰ **664.1 Second-degree perineal laceration**   M♀
[0,1,4]   Perineal laceration, rupture, or tear (following episiotomy) involving:
    pelvic floor
    perineal muscles
    vaginal muscles
   EXCLUDES *that involving anal sphincter (664.2)*
   AHA: For code 664.11: 4Q, '08, 192
   070.1 Second degree perineal laceration dur delivery   I-10

§ √5ᵗʰ **664.2 Third-degree perineal laceration**   CC 1 M♀
[0,1,4]   Perineal laceration, rupture, or tear
    (following episiotomy) involving:
    anal sphincter
    rectovaginal septum
    sphincter NOS
   EXCLUDES *anal sphincter tear during delivery not associated with third-degree perineal laceration (664.6)*
     that with anal or rectal mucosal laceration (664.3)
   CC Excl: For code 664.21: 646.80-646.93, 648.90-649.64, 650, 655.70-655.73, 664.21, 664.61, 665.00-665.11, 665.50-665.54, 665.80- 665.94, 669.40-669.44, 669.80-669.94, 679.00-679.04, 679.12, 679.14
   070.2 Third degree perineal laceration during delivery   I-10

§ √5ᵗʰ **664.3 Fourth-degree perineal laceration**   CC 1 M♀
[0,1,4]   Perineal laceration, rupture, or tear as classifiable to 664.2 and involving also:
    anal mucosa
    rectal mucosa
   CC Excl: For code 664.31: 646.80-646.93, 648.90-649.64, 650, 655.70-655.73, 664.31, 665.00-665.11, 665.50-665.54, 665.80-665.94, 669.40-669.44, 669.80-669.94, 679.00-679.04, 679.12, 679.14

§ √5ᵗʰ **664.4 Unspecified perineal laceration**   M♀
[0,1,4]   Central laceration
   AHA: 1Q, '92, 8

§ √5ᵗʰ **664.5 Vulval and perineal hematoma**   M♀
[0,1,4]   **AHA:** N-D, '84, 10

§ √5ᵗʰ **664.6 Anal sphincter tear complicating delivery,**   CC 1,4 M♀
[0,1,4] **not associated with third-degree perineal laceration**
   EXCLUDES *third-degree perineal laceration (664.2)*
   CC Excl: For code 664.61, 664.64: 646.80-646.93, 648.90-649.64, 650, 655.70-655.73, 664.21, 664.60-664.64, 665.00-665.11, 665.50-665.54, 665.80-665.94, 669.40-669.44, 669.80-669.94, 679.00-679.04, 679.12, 679.14
   AHA: For code 664.61: 4Q, '07, 88, 90

§ √5ᵗʰ **664.8 Other specified trauma to perineum and vulva**   M♀
[0,1,4]   Periurethral trauma
   AHA: For code 664.81: 4Q, '07, 125
   TIP: Assign when documentation indicates periurethral laceration only.

§ √5ᵗʰ **664.9 Unspecified trauma to perineum and vulva**   M♀
[0,1,4]

√4ᵗʰ **665 Other obstetrical trauma**
   INCLUDES damage from instruments

§ √5ᵗʰ **665.0 Rupture of uterus before onset of labor**   MCC 1,3 M♀
[0,1,3]   **CC Excl:** For code 665.01, 665.03: 646.80-646.93, 648.90-649.64, 650, 655.70-655.73, 665.00-665.11, 665.50-665.54, 665.80-665.94, 669.40-669.44, 669.80-669.94, 679.00-679.04, 679.12, 679.14

§ √5ᵗʰ **665.1 Rupture of uterus during labor**   MCC 1 M♀
[0,1]   Rupture of uterus NOS
   CC Excl: For code 665.11: See code 665.01

§ √5ᵗʰ **665.2 Inversion of uterus**   CC 2 ♀
[0,2,4]   **CC Excl:** For code 665.22: 646.80-646.93, 648.90-649.64, 650, 655.70-655.73, 665.00-665.11, 665.22, 665.50-665.54, 665.80-665.94, 669.40-669.44, 669.80-669.94, 679.00-679.04, 679.12, 679.14

§ √5ᵗʰ **665.3 Laceration of cervix**   CC 1 M♀
[0,1,4]   **CC Excl:** For code 665.31: 646.80-646.93, 648.90-649.64, 650, 655.70-655.73, 665.00-665.11, 665.31, 665.50-665.54, 665.80-665.94, 669.40-669.44, 669.80-669.94, 679.00-679.04, 679.12, 679.14

§ √5ᵗʰ **665.4 High vaginal laceration**   CC 1 M♀
[0,1,4]   Laceration of vaginal wall or sulcus without mention of perineal laceration
   CC Excl: For code 665.41: 646.80-646.93, 648.90-649.64, 650, 655.70-655.73, 665.00-665.11, 665.41, 665.50-665.54, 665.80-665.94, 669.40-669.44, 669.80-669.94, 679.00-679.04, 679.12, 679.14
   071.4 Obstetric high vaginal laceration alone   I-1

§ √5ᵗʰ **665.5 Other injury to pelvic organs**   CC 1 M♀
[0,1,4]   Injury to:
    bladder
    urethra
   EXCLUDES *periurethral trauma (664.8)*
   CC Excl: For code 665.51: See code 665.01
   AHA: M-A, '87, 10
   071.5 Other obstetric injury to pelvic organs   I-1

§ √5ᵗʰ **665.6 Damage to pelvic joints and ligaments**   CC 1 M♀
[0,1,4]   Avulsion of inner symphyseal cartilage
    Damage to coccyx
    Separation of symphysis (pubis)
   CC Excl: For code 665.61: 646.80-646.93, 648.90-649.64, 650, 655.70-655.73, 665.00-665.11, 665.50-665.54, 665.61, 665.80-665.94, 669.40-669.44, 669.80-669.94, 679.00-679.04, 679.12, 679.14
   AHA: N-D, '84, 12

§ √5ᵗʰ **665.7 Pelvic hematoma**   CC 1-2 M♀
[0,1,2,4]   Hematoma of vagina
   CC Excl: For code 665.71: 646.80-646.93, 648.90-649.64, 650, 655.70-655.73, 665.00-665.11, 665.50-665.54, 665.71, 665.80-665.94, 669.40-669.44, 669.80-669.94, 679.00-679.04, 679.12, 679.14; For code 665.72: 646.80-646.93, 648.90-649.64, 650, 655.70-655.73, 665.00-665.11, 665.50-665.54, 665.72, 665.80-665.94, 669.40-669.44, 669.80-669.94, 679.00-679.04, 679.12, 679.14

§ √5ᵗʰ **665.8 Other specified obstetrical trauma**   M
[0-4]

§ √5ᵗʰ **665.9 Unspecified obstetrical trauma**   M
[0-4]

√4ᵗʰ **666 Postpartum hemorrhage**
   AHA: 1Q, '88, 14

§ √5ᵗʰ **666.0 Third-stage hemorrhage**   CC 2,4 M
[0,2,4]   Hemorrhage associated with retained, trapped, or adherent placenta
    Retained placenta NOS
   CC Excl: For code 666.02: 646.80-646.93, 648.90-649.64, 650, 655.70-655.73, 665.00-665.11, 665.50-665.54, 665.80-665.94, 666.02, 669.40-669.44, 669.80-669.94, 679.00-679.04, 679.12, 679.14; For code 666.04: 646.80-646.93, 648.90-649.64, 650, 655.70-655.73, 665.00-665.11, 665.50-665.54, 665.80-665.94, 666.04, 669.40-669.44, 669.80-669.94, 679.00-679.04, 679.12, 679.1

§ √5ᵗʰ **666.1 Other immediate postpartum hemorrhage**   CC 2,4 M
[0,2,4]   Atony of uterus with hemorrhage
    Hemorrhage within the first 24 hours following delivery of placenta
    Postpartum atony of uterus with hemorrhage
    Postpartum hemorrhage (atonic) NOS
   EXCLUDES *atony of uterus without hemorrhage (661.2)*
     postpartum atony of uterus without hemorrhage (669.8)
   CC Excl: For code 666.12: 646.80-646.93, 648.90-649.64, 650, 655.70-655.73, 665.00-665.11, 665.50-665.54, 665.80- 665.94, 666.12, 669.40-669.44, 669.80-669.94, 679.00-679.04, 679.12, 679.14; For code 666.14: 666.10-666.14
   072.1 Other immediate postpartum hemorrhage   I-1

§ √5ᵗʰ **666.2 Delayed and secondary postpartum hemorrhage**   CC 2,4 M
[0,2,4]   Hemorrhage:
    after the first 24 hours following delivery
    associated with retained portions of placenta or membranes
    Postpartum hemorrhage specified as delayed or secondary
    Retained products of conception NOS, following delivery
   CC Excl: For code 666.22: 646.80-646.93, 648.90-649.64, 650, 655.70-655.73, 665.00-665.11, 665.50-665.54, 665.80- 665.94, 666.22, 669.40-669.44, 669.80-669.94, 679.00-679.04, 679.12, 679.14; For code 666.24: 666.20-666.24

---

§   Requires fifth digit. Valid digits are in [brackets] under each code. See beginning of section 640-649 for codes and definitions.

Ⓝ Newborn Age: 0   Ⓟ Pediatric Age: 0-17   Ⓜ Maternity Age: 12-55   Ⓐ Adult Age: 15-124   **MCC** Major CC Condition   **CC** CC Condition   **HIV** HIV Related D

222 – Volume 1   2014 ICD-9-C

§ ✓5ᵗʰ **666.3 Postpartum coagulation defects**   CC2 M♀
  [0,2,4]   Postpartum:
      afibrinogenemia
      fibrinolysis
    CC Excl: For code 666.32: 646.80-646.93, 648.90-649.64, 650,
    666.00-666.34, 669.40-669.44, 669.80-669.94, 679.00-679.04,
    679.12, 679.14

✓4ᵗʰ **667 Retained placenta or membranes, without hemorrhage**
  DEF: Postpartum condition resulting from failure to expel placental
  membrane tissues due to failed contractions of uterine wall.
  AHA: 1Q, '88, 14
  TIP: A retained placenta is one that has not separated or been expelled
  within one hour after completion of the second stage of labor (birth of the
  fetus).

§ ✓5ᵗʰ **667.0 Retained placenta without hemorrhage**   M♀
  [0,2,4]   Placenta accreta
      Retained placenta:
        NOS   } without hemorrhage
        total
    073.0 Retained placenta without hemorrhage   I-10

§ ✓5ᵗʰ **667.1 Retained portions of placenta or membranes,**   M♀
  [0,2,4]   **without hemorrhage**
      Retained products of conception following delivery, without
      hemorrhage

✓4ᵗʰ **668 Complications of the administration of anesthetic or other**
  sedation in labor and delivery
    INCLUDES complications arising from the administration of a general
        or local anesthetic, analgesic, or other sedation in
        labor and delivery
    Use additional code(s) to further specify complication
    EXCLUDES reaction to spinal or lumbar puncture (349.0)
        spinal headache (349.0)

§ ✓5ᵗʰ **668.0 Pulmonary complications**   M♀
  [0-4]   Inhalation (aspiration) of
        stomach contents or   } following anesthesia or
        secretions   other sedation in
      Mendelson's syndrome   labor or delivery
      Pressure collapse of lung

§ ✓5ᵗʰ **668.1 Cardiac complications**   M♀
  [0-4]   Cardiac arrest or failure following anesthesia
      or other sedation in labor and delivery

§ ✓5ᵗʰ **668.2 Central nervous system complications**   M♀
  [0-4]   Cerebral anoxia following anesthesia or other sedation in
      labor and delivery

§ ✓5ᵗʰ **668.8 Other complications of anesthesia or other**   M♀
  [0-4]   **sedation in labor and delivery**
      AHA: 2Q, '99, 9

§ ✓5ᵗʰ **668.9 Unspecified complication of anesthesia**   M♀
  [0-4]   **and other sedation**

✓4ᵗʰ **669 Other complications of labor and delivery, not elsewhere**
  classified

§ ✓5ᵗʰ **669.0 Maternal distress**   M♀
  [0-4]   Metabolic disturbance in labor and delivery

§ ✓5ᵗʰ **669.1 Shock during or following labor and delivery**   MCC 1-4 M♀
  [0-4]   Obstetric shock
    CC Excl: For codes 669.11-669.14: 646.80-646.93, 648.90-649.64, 650,
    669.10-669.14, 669.40-669.44, 669.80-669.94, 679.00-679.04,
    679.12, 679.14

§ ✓5ᵗʰ **669.2 Maternal hypotension syndrome**   MCC 1-2 CC4 M♀
  [0-4]   **DEF:** Low arterial blood pressure in mother during labor and delivery.
    CC Excl: For code 669.21: 646.80-646.93, 648.90-649.64, 650,
    669.10-669.14, 669.21, 669.40-669.44, 669.80-669.94,
    679.00-679.04, 679.12, 679.14; **For code 669.22:** 646.80-646.93,
    648.90-649.64, 650, 669.10-669.14, 669.22, 669.40-669.44,
    669.80-669.94, 679.00-679.04, 679.12, 679.14; **For code 669.24:**
    646.80-646.93, 648.90-649.64, 650, 669.10-669.14, 669.24,
    669.40-669.44, 669.80-669.94, 679.00-679.04, 679.12, 679.14

§ ✓5ᵗʰ **669.3 Acute kidney failure following labor**   MCC 2,4 M♀
  [0,2,4]   **and delivery**
    CC Excl: For codes 669.32, 669.34: 646.80-646.93, 648.90-649.64, 650,
    669.30-669.44, 669.80-669.94, 679.00-679.04, 679.12, 679.14

§ ✓5ᵗʰ **669.4 Other complications of obstetrical surgery**   M♀
  [0-4]   **and procedures**
      Cardiac:
        arrest   } following cesarean or other
        failure   obstetrical surgery or
      Cerebral   procedure, including
        anoxia   } delivery NOS
    EXCLUDES complications of obstetrical surgical wounds
        (674.1-674.3)

§ ✓5ᵗʰ **669.5 Forceps or vacuum extractor delivery**   M♀
  [0,1]   **without mention of indication**
      Delivery by ventouse, without mention of indication

§ ✓5ᵗʰ **669.6 Breech extraction, without mention of indication**   M♀
  [0,1]   **EXCLUDES** breech delivery NOS (652.2)

§ ✓5ᵗʰ **669.7 Cesarean delivery, without mention of indication**   M♀
  [0,1]   **AHA: For code 669.71:** 1Q, '01, 11
    082 Encounter for cesarean delivery w/o indication   I-10

§ ✓5ᵗʰ **669.8 Other complications of labor and delivery**   M♀
  [0-4]   **AHA:** 4Q, '06, 135

§ ✓5ᵗʰ **669.9 Unspecified complication of labor and delivery**   M♀
  [0-4]

Complications of the Puerperium (670-677)

  NOTE Categories 671 and 673-676 include the listed conditions even
    if they occur during pregnancy or childbirth.

The following fifth-digit subclassification is for use with categories 670-676 to denote
the current episode of care. Valid fifth-digits are in [brackets] under each code.
  0 unspecified as to episode of care or not applicable
  1 delivered, with or without mention of antepartum condition
  2 delivered, with mention of postpartum complication
  3 antepartum condition or complication
  4 postpartum condition or complication

✓4ᵗʰ **670 Major puerperal infection**
    EXCLUDES infection following abortion (639.0)
        minor genital tract infection following delivery (646.6)
        puerperal pyrexia NOS (672)
        puerperal fever NOS (672)
        puerperal pyrexia of unknown origin (672)
        urinary tract infection following delivery (646.6)
  DEF: Infection and inflammation following childbirth.
  AHA: 4Q, '91, 26; 2Q, '91, 7

§ ✓5ᵗʰ **670.0 Major puerperal infection, unspecified**   MCC 2,4 M♀
  [0,2,4]   **AHA: For code 670.02:** 3Q, '07, 8
    CC Excl: 646.80-646.93, 648.90-649.64, 650, 669.40-669.44,
    669.80-670.84, 679.00-679.04, 679.12, 679.14

§ ✓5ᵗʰ **670.1 Puerperal endometritis**   CC M♀
  [0,2,4]   **CC Excl:** See code: 670.0

§ ✓5ᵗʰ **670.2 Puerperal sepsis**   CC0 MCC 2,4 M♀
  [0,2,4]   Puerperal pyemia
      Use additional code to identify severe sepsis (995.92) and any
        associated acute organ dysfunction, if applicable
    CC Excl: See code: 670.0
    AHA: For code 670.24: 4Q, '09, 98
    TIP: Do not assign a code from category 038 or 995.91 Sepsis, along
    with a code from this subcategory. If applicable, assign additional
    codes to indicate severe sepsis (995.92), and any associated acute
    organ dysfunction.

§ ✓5ᵗʰ **670.3 Puerperal septic thrombophlebitis**   CC0 MCC 2,4 M♀
  [0,2,4]   **CC Excl:** See code: 670.0

§ ✓5ᵗʰ **670.8 Other major puerperal infection**   MCC M♀
  [0,2,4]   Puerperal:
      pelvic cellulitis
      peritonitis
      salpingitis
    CC Excl: See code: 670.0

---

§ Requires fifth digit. Valid digits are in [brackets] under each code. See beginning of section 640-649 for codes and definitions.

✓4ᵗʰ / ✓5ᵗʰ Additional Digit Required   Unacceptable PDx   Manifestation Code   Hospital Acquired Condition   ▶◀ Revised Text   ● New Code   ▲ Revised Code Title

2014 ICD-9-CM   **Volume 1 – 223**

Complications of Pregnancy, Childbirth, and the Puerperium

671–675.0

√4th **671 Venous complications in pregnancy and the puerperium**

EXCLUDES *personal history of venous complications prior to pregnancy, such as:*
thrombophlebitis (V12.52)
thrombosis and embolism (V12.51)

§ √5th **671.0 Varicose veins of legs**   M♀
[0–4]   Varicose veins NOS
    DEF: Distended, tortuous veins on legs associated with pregnancy.

§ √5th **671.1 Varicose veins of vulva and perineum**   M♀
[0–4]   DEF: Distended, tortuous veins on external female genitalia associated with pregnancy.

§ √5th **671.2 Superficial thrombophlebitis**   CC M♀
[0–4]   Phlebitis NOS
    Thrombophlebitis (superficial)
    Thrombosis NOS

    Use additional code to identify the superficial thrombophlebitis (453.6, 453.71, 453.81)
    CC Exd: 646.80-646.93, 648.90-669.64, 650, 669.40-669.44, 669.80-669.94, 671.20-671.94, 679.00-679.04, 679.12, 679.14

§ √5th **671.3 Deep phlebothrombosis, antepartum**   MCC 1,3 CC 0 M♀
[0,1,3]   Deep vein thrombosis antepartum

    Use additional code to identify the deep vein thrombosis (453.40-453.42, 453.50-453.52, 453.72-453.79, 453.82-453.89)
    Use additional code for long term (current) use of anticoagulants, if applicable (V58.61)
    CC Exd: See code: 671.2

§ √5th **671.4 Deep phlebothrombosis, postpartum**   MCC 2,4 CC 0 M♀
[0,2,4]   Deep-vein thrombosis, postpartum
    Pelvic thrombophlebitis, postpartum
    Phlegmasia alba dolens (puerperal)

    Use additional code to identify the deep vein thrombosis (453.40-453.42, 453.50-453.52, 453.72-453.79, 453.82-453.89)
    Use additional code for long term (current) use of anticoagulants, if applicable (V58.61)
    CC Exd: See code: 671.2

§ √5th **671.5 Other phlebitis and thrombosis**   CC M♀
[0–4]   Cerebral venous thrombosis
    Thrombosis of intracranial venous sinus
    CC Exd: See code: 671.2

§ √5th **671.8 Other venous complications**   CC M♀
[0–4]   Hemorrhoids
    CC Exd: For codes 671.80-671.83: 646.80-646.93, 648.90-649.64, 650, 669.40-669.44, 669.80-669.94, 671.20-671.94, 679.00-679.04, 679.12, 679.14; For code 671.84: 671.80-671.84

§ √5th **671.9 Unspecified venous complication**   CC 0-2 M♀
[0–4]   CC Exd: For code 671.90-671.92: 646.80-646.93, 648.90-649.64, 650, 669.40-669.44, 669.80-669.94, 671.20-671.94, 679.00-679.04, 679.12, 679.14

√4th **672 Pyrexia of unknown origin during the puerperium**   CC 2,4 M♀
[0,2,4]

§ √5th   Use 0 as fourth-digit for this category

    Postpartum fever NOS
    Puerperal fever NOS
    Puerperal pyrexia NOS
    DEF: Fever of unknown origin experienced by the mother after childbirth.
    CC Exd: For code 672.02: 646.80-646.93, 648.90-649.64, 650, 669.40-669.44, 669.80-669.94, 671.20, 671.23-671.30, 671.33-671.40, 671.50, 671.53-671.80, 671.83-671.90, 671.93-671.94, 672.02, 679.00-679.04, 679.12, 679.14; For code 672.04: 672.02-672.04
    AHA: 4Q, '91, 26
    086.4 Pyrexia of unknown origin following delivery   I-10

√4th **673 Obstetrical pulmonary embolism**

INCLUDES *pulmonary emboli in pregnancy, childbirth, or the puerperium, or specified as puerperal*
EXCLUDES *embolism following abortion (639.6)*

§ √5th **673.0 Obstetrical air embolism**   MCC 1-4 M♀
[0–4]   DEF: Sudden blocking of pulmonary artery with air or nitrogen bubbles during puerperium.
    CC Exd: 646.80-646.93, 648.90-649.64, 650, 669.40-669.44, 669.80-669.94, 673.00-673.84, 679.00-679.04, 679.12, 679.14

§ √5th **673.1 Amniotic fluid embolism**   MCC 1-4 M♀
[0–4]   DEF: Sudden onset of pulmonary artery blockage from amniotic fluid entering the mother's circulation near the end of pregnancy due to strong uterine contractions.
    CC Exd: For code 673.11-673.14: See code: 673.0

§ √5th **673.2 Obstetrical blood-clot embolism**   MCC 1-4 M♀
[0–4]   Puerperal pulmonary embolism NOS
    DEF: Blood clot blocking artery in the lung; associated with pregnancy.
    CC Exd: For code 673.21-673.24: See code: 673.0
    AHA: For code 673.24: 1Q, '05, 6
    TIP: If a pregnant or postpartum patient develops a pulmonary embolism that progresses to acute respiratory failure, the code for the pregnancy/delivery complication (673.2x) should be sequenced first.

§ √5th **673.3 Obstetrical pyemic and septic embolism**   MCC 1-4 CC 0 M♀
[0–4]   CC Exd: See code: 673.0

§ √5th **673.8 Other pulmonary embolism**   MCC 1-4 M♀
[0–4]   Fat embolism
    CC Exd: For code 673.81-673.84: See code: 673.0

√4th **674 Other and unspecified complications of the puerperium, not elsewhere classified**

§ √5th **674.0 Cerebrovascular disorders in the**   MCC 1 CC 2-4 M♀
[0–4]   **puerperium**
    Any condition classifiable to 430-434, 436-437 occurring during pregnancy, childbirth, or the puerperium, or specified as puerperal

    EXCLUDES *intracranial venous sinus thrombosis (671.5)*
    CC Exd: For code 674.01-674.04: 646.80-646.93, 648.90-649.64, 650, 669.40-669.44, 669.80-669.94, 674.00-674.04, 674.50-674.54, 679.00-679.04, 679.12, 679.14

§ √5th **674.1 Disruption of cesarean wound**   M♀
[0,2,4]   Dehiscence or disruption of uterine wound

    EXCLUDES *uterine rupture before onset of labor (665.0)*
    uterine rupture during labor (665.1)

§ √5th **674.2 Disruption of perineal wound**   M♀
[0,2,4]   Breakdown of perineum
    Disruption of wound of:
     episiotomy
     perineal laceration
    Secondary perineal tear
    AHA: For code 674.24: 1Q, '97, 9

§ √5th **674.3 Other complications of obstetrical surgical wounds**   M♀
[0,2,4]   Hematoma ⎫
    Hemorrhage ⎬ of cesarean section or perineal wound
    Infection ⎭

    EXCLUDES *damage from instruments in delivery (664.0-665.9)*
    AHA: For code 674.32: 2Q, '91, 7; For code 674.34: 4Q, '09, 98

§ √5th **674.4 Placental polyp**   M♀
[0,2,4]

§ √5th **674.5 Peripartum cardiomyopathy**   MCC M♀
[0–4]   Postpartum cardiomyopathy
    DEF: Any structural or functional abnormality of the ventricular myocardium, non-inflammatory disease of obscure or unknown etiology with onset during the postpartum period.
    CC Exd: See code: 674.01
    AHA: 4Q, '03, 65; For code 674.54: ▶3Q, '12, 9◀

§ √5th **674.8 Other**   M♀
[0,2,4]   Hepatorenal syndrome, following delivery
    Postpartum:
     subinvolution of uterus
     uterine hypertrophy
    AHA: 3Q, '98, 16

§ √5th **674.9 Unspecified**   M♀
[0,2,4]   Sudden death of unknown cause during the puerperium

√4th **675 Infections of the breast and nipple associated with childbirth**

INCLUDES *the listed conditions during pregnancy, childbirth, or the puerperium*

§ √5th **675.0 Infections of nipple**   M♀
[0–4]   Abscess of nipple

---

§   Requires fifth digit. Valid digits are in [brackets] under each code. See beginning of section 640-649 for codes and definitions.

N Newborn Age: 0   P Pediatric Age: 0-17   M Maternity Age: 12-55   A Adult Age: 15-124   MCC Major CC Condition   CC CC Condition   HIV HIV Related Dx

§ ✓5ᵗʰ **675.1 Abscess of breast**   CC 1-2 M♀
[0-4]   Abscess:
       mammary
       subareolar
       submammary
       purulent
       retromammary
       submammary
    CC Excl: For codes 675.11-675.12: 646.80-646.93, 648.90-649.64, 650, 669.40-669.44, 669.80-669.94, 675.00-675.94, 679.00-679.04, 679.12, 679.14

§ ✓5ᵗʰ **675.2 Nonpurulent mastitis**   M♀
[0-4]   Lymphangitis of breast
    Mastitis:
       NOS
       interstitial
       parenchymatous

§ ✓5ᵗʰ **675.8 Other specified infections of the breast and nipple**   M♀
[0-4]

§ ✓5ᵗʰ **675.9 Unspecified infection of the breast and nipple**   M♀
[0-4]

✓4ᵗʰ **676 Other disorders of the breast associated with childbirth and disorders of lactation**
    INCLUDES the listed conditions during pregnancy, the puerperium, or lactation

§ ✓5ᵗʰ **676.0 Retracted nipple**   M♀
[0-4]

§ ✓5ᵗʰ **676.1 Cracked nipple**   M♀
[0-4]   Fissure of nipple

§ ✓5ᵗʰ **676.2 Engorgement of breasts**   M♀
[0-4]   **DEF:** Abnormal accumulation of milk in ducts of breast.

§ ✓5ᵗʰ **676.3 Other and unspecified disorder of breast**   M♀
[0-4]

§ ✓5ᵗʰ **676.4 Failure of lactation**   M♀
[0-4]   Agalactia
    DEF: Abrupt ceasing of milk secretion by breast.

§ ✓5ᵗʰ **676.5 Suppressed lactation**   M♀
[0-4]

§ ✓5ᵗʰ **676.6 Galactorrhea**   M♀
[0-4]   **EXCLUDES** *galactorrhea not associated with childbirth (611.6)*
    DEF: Excessive or persistent milk secretion by breast; may be in absence of nursing.

§ ✓5ᵗʰ **676.8 Other disorders of lactation**   M♀
[0-4]   Galactocele
    DEF: Galactocele: Obstructed mammary gland, creating retention cyst, results in milk-filled cysts enlarging mammary gland.
    AHA: ▶3Q, '12, 7◀

§ ✓5ᵗʰ **676.9 Unspecified disorder of lactation**   M♀
[0-4]

Lactation Process: Ejection Reflex Arc

---

677 **Late effect of complication of pregnancy, childbirth, and the puerperium**   ♀
    NOTE This category is to be used to indicate conditions in 632-648.9 and 651-676.9 as the cause of the late effect, themselves classifiable elsewhere. The "late effects" include conditions specified as such, or as sequelae, which may occur at any time after puerperium.
    Code first any sequelae
    AHA: 1Q, '97, 9; 4Q, '94, 42
    TIP: Sequence as a secondary diagnosis, after the code for the late effect complication. May be assigned at any time after the initial postpartum period (six weeks following delivery).

Other Maternal and Fetal Complications (678-679)

The following fifth-digit subclassification is for use with categories 678-679 to denote the current episode of care. Valid fifth-digits are in [brackets] under each code.
    0 unspecified as to episode of care or not applicable
    1 delivered, with or without mention of antepartum condition
    2 delivered, with mention of postpartum complication
    3 antepartum condition or complication
    4 postpartum condition or complication

✓4ᵗʰ **678 Other fetal conditions**

§ ✓5ᵗʰ **678.0 Fetal hematologic conditions**   M♀
[0,1,3]   Fetal anemia
    Fetal thrombocytopenia
    Fetal twin to twin transfusion
    EXCLUDES *fetal and neonatal hemorrhage (772.0-772.9)*
       fetal hematologic disorders affecting newborn (776.0-776.9)
       fetal-maternal hemorrhage (656.00-656.03)
       isoimmunization incompatibility (656.10-656.13, 656.20-656.23)
    AHA: 4Q, '08, 125-127

§ ✓5ᵗʰ **678.1 Fetal conjoined twins**   M♀
[0,1,3]   **AHA:** 4Q, '08, 125-127

✓4ᵗʰ **679 Complications of in utero procedures**
    AHA: 4Q, '08, 127-128, 158

§ ✓5ᵗʰ **679.0 Maternal complications from in utero procedure**   M♀
[0-4]   **EXCLUDES** *maternal history of in utero procedure during previous pregnancy (V23.86)*

§ ✓5ᵗʰ **679.1 Fetal complications from in utero procedure**   M♀
[0-4]   Fetal complications from amniocentesis
    EXCLUDES *newborn affected by in utero procedure (760.61-760.64)*
    TIP: Assign only on the mother's record. Although there is a fetal complication, it affects the mother's pregnancy.

---

§   Requires fifth digit. Valid digits are in [brackets] under each code. See beginning of section 640-649 for codes and definitions.

✓4ᵗʰ ✓5ᵗʰ Additional Digit Required   Unacceptable PDx   Manifestation Code   Hospital Acquired Condition   ▶◀ Revised Text   ● New Code   ▲ Revised Code Title

2014 ICD-9-CM   **February 2013 · Volume 1 – 225**

12. Diseases of the Skin and Subcutaneous Tissue (680-709)

Infections of Skin and Subcutaneous Tissue (680-686)

EXCLUDES *certain infections of skin classified under "Infectious and Parasitic Diseases," such as:*
erysipelas (035)
erysipeloid of Rosenbach (027.1)
herpes:
    simplex (054.0-054.9)
    zoster (053.0-053.9)
molluscum contagiosum (078.0)
viral warts (078.10-078.19)

✓4ᵗʰ 680 Carbuncle and furuncle

INCLUDES boil
    furunculosis

DEF: Carbuncle: necrotic boils in skin and subcutaneous tissue of neck or back mainly due to staphylococcal infection.
DEF: Furuncle: circumscribed inflammation of corium and subcutaneous tissue due to staphylococcal infection.

680.0 Face

Ear [any part]
Face [any part, except eye]
Nose (septum)
Temple (region)

EXCLUDES *eyelid (373.13)*
lacrimal apparatus (375.31)
orbit (376.01)

680.1 Neck

680.2 Trunk

Abdominal wall
Back [any part, except buttocks]
Breast
Chest wall
Flank
Groin
Pectoral region
Perineum
Umbilicus

EXCLUDES *buttocks (680.5)*
external genital organs:
    female (616.4)
    male (607.2, 608.4)

680.3 Upper arm and forearm

Arm [any part, except hand]
Axilla
Shoulder

680.4 Hand

Finger [any]
Thumb
Wrist

680.5 Buttock

Anus
Gluteal region

680.6 Leg, except foot

Ankle
Hip
Knee
Thigh

680.7 Foot

Heel
Toe

680.8 Other specified sites

Head [any part, except face]
Scalp

EXCLUDES *external genital organs:*
female (616.4)
male (607.2, 608.4)

680.9 Unspecified site

Boil NOS
Carbuncle NOS
Furuncle NOS

Skin and Subcutaneous Layer

Hair follicle
Epidermis
Dermis
Hypodermis (subcutaneous layer)
Bulb
Sebaceous gland
Arrector pili muscle
Thick-skin epidermis
Hair shaft
Pacinian corpuscle
Hair matrix
Sweat (eccrine gland)
Sensory nerve
Blood vessels

✓4ᵗʰ 681 Cellulitis and abscess of finger and toe

INCLUDES that with lymphangitis

Use additional code to identify organism, such as Staphylococcus (041.1)

DEF: Acute suppurative inflammation and edema in subcutaneous tissue or muscle of finger or toe.
AHA: 2Q, '91, 5; J-F, '87, 12
TIP: Coding of cellulitis due to superficial injury, burn, or frostbite requires two codes, one for the injury and one for the cellulitis. Sequencing depends on the circumstances of the admission.

✓5ᵗʰ 681.0 Finger

681.00 Cellulitis and abscess, unspecified
L03.019 Cellulitis of unspecified finger   I-10

681.01 Felon
Pulp abscess
Whitlow
EXCLUDES *herpetic whitlow (054.6)*
DEF: Painful abscess of fingertips caused by infection in the closed space of terminal phalanx.

681.02 Onychia and paronychia of finger
Panaritium ⎫
Perionychia ⎬ of finger
DEF: Onychia: inflammation of nail matrix; causes nail loss.
DEF: Paronychia: inflammation of tissue folds around nail.

✓5ᵗʰ 681.1 Toe

681.10 Cellulitis and abscess, unspecified
AHA: 1Q, '05, 14
L03.039 Cellulitis of unspecified toe   I-10

681.11 Onychia and paronychia of toe
Panaritium ⎫
Perionychia ⎬ of toe

681.9 Cellulitis and abscess of unspecified digit
Infection of nail NOS

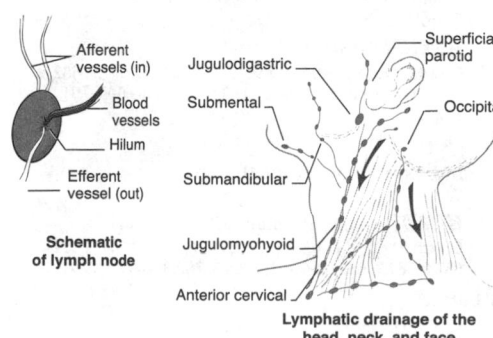

Lymphatic System of Head and Neck

Afferent vessels (in)
Blood vessels
Hilum
Efferent vessel (out)
Schematic of lymph node
Jugulodigastric
Submental
Submandibular
Jugulomyohyoid
Anterior cervical
Superficial parotid
Occipital

Lymphatic drainage of the head, neck, and face

Diseases of the Skin and Subcutaneous Tissue

682–685.1

√4ᵗʰ **682 Other cellulitis and abscess**

> **INCLUDES** abscess (acute)
> cellulitis (diffuse) }(with lymphangitis) except
> lymphangitis, acute } of finger or toe

Use additional code to identify organism, such as Staphylococcus (041.1)

> **EXCLUDES** *lymphangitis (chronic) (subacute) (457.2)*

DEF: Cellulitis: Acute suppurative inflammation of deep subcutaneous tissue and sometimes muscle due to infection of wound, burn or other lesion.

AHA: 2Q, '91, 5; J-F, '87, 12; S-O, '85, 10

TIP: Coding of cellulitis due to superficial injury, burn, or frostbite requires two codes, one for the injury and one for the cellulitis. Sequencing depends on the circumstances of the admission.

682.0 Face   **CC**

Cheek, external	Nose, external
Chin	Submandibular
Forehead	Temple (region)

> **EXCLUDES** *ear [any part] (380.10-380.16)*
> *eyelid (373.13)*
> *lacrimal apparatus (375.31)*
> *lip (528.5)*
> *mouth (528.3)*
> *nose (internal) (478.1)*
> *orbit (376.01)*

CC Exd: 017.00-017.06, 017.90-017.96, 040.82-041.9, 682.0, 682.8-682.9, 686.00-686.9, 705.83, 709.8, V09.0-V09.91

L03.211 Cellulitis of face   I-10

682.1 Neck   **CC**

CC Exd: 017.00-017.06, 017.90-017.96, 040.82-041.9, 682.1, 682.8-682.9, 686.00-686.9, 705.83, 709.8, V09.0-V09.91

L03.221 Cellulitis of neck   I-10

682.2 Trunk   **CC**

Abdominal wall
Back [any part, except buttock]
Chest wall
Flank
Groin
Pectoral region
Perineum
Umbilicus, except newborn

> **EXCLUDES** *anal and rectal regions (566)*
> *breast:*
> *NOS (611.0)*
> *puerperal (675.1)*
> *external genital organs:*
> *female (616.3-616.4)*
> *male (604.0, 607.2, 608.4)*
> *umbilicus, newborn (771.4)*

CC Exd: 017.00-017.06, 017.90-017.96, 040.82-041.9, 682.2, 682.8-682.9, 686.00-686.9, 705.83, 709.8, V09.0-V09.91

AHA: 4Q, '98, 42

L03.319 Cellulitis of trunk unspecified   I-10

682.3 Upper arm and forearm   **CC**

Arm [any part, except hand]
Axilla
Shoulder

> **EXCLUDES** *hand (682.4)*

CC Exd: 017.00-017.06, 017.90-017.96, 040.82-041.9, 682.3, 682.8-682.9, 686.00-686.9, 705.83, 709.8, V09.0-V09.91

AHA: 2Q, '03, 7

L03.113 Cellulitis of right upper limb   I-10

682.4 Hand, except fingers and thumb   **CC**

Wrist

> **EXCLUDES** *finger and thumb (681.00-681.02)*

CC Exd: 017.00-017.06, 017.90-017.96, 040.82-041.9, 682.4, 682.8-682.9, 686.00-686.9, 705.83, 709.8, V09.0-V09.91

682.5 Buttock   **CC**

Gluteal region

> **EXCLUDES** *anal and rectal regions (566)*

CC Exd: 017.00-017.06, 017.90-017.96, 040.82-041.9, 682.5, 682.8-682.9, 686.00-686.9, 705.83, 709.8, V09.0-V09.91

L03.317 Cellulitis of buttock   I-10

682.6 Leg, except foot   **CC**

Ankle
Hip
Knee
Thigh

CC Exd: 017.00-017.06, 017.90-017.96, 040.82-041.9, 682.6, 682.8-682.9, 686.00-686.9, 705.83, 709.8, V09.0-V09.91

AHA: ▶3Q, '12, 13;◄ 1Q, '09, 10; 3Q, '04, 5; 4Q, '03, 108

L03.115 Cellulitis of right lower limb   I-1

682.7 Foot, except toes   **CC**

Heel

> **EXCLUDES** *toe (681.10-681.11)*

CC Exd: 017.00-017.06, 017.90-017.96, 040.82-041.9, 682.7-682.9, 686.00-686.9, 705.83, 709.8, V09.0-V09.91

682.8 Other specified sites   **CC**

Head [except face]
Scalp

> **EXCLUDES** *face (682.0)*

CC Exd: 017.00-017.06, 017.90-017.96, 040.82-041.9, 682.8-682.9, 686.00-686.9, 705.83, 709.8, V09.0-V09.91

682.9 Unspecified site   **CC**

Abscess NOS
Cellulitis NOS
Lymphangitis, acute NOS

> **EXCLUDES** *lymphangitis NOS (457.2)*

CC Exd: See code: 682.8

683 Acute lymphadenitis

> Abscess (acute)
> Adenitis, acute } lymph gland or node,
> Lymphadenitis, acute } except mesenteric

Use additional code to identify organism, such as Staphylococcus (041.1)

> **EXCLUDES** *enlarged glands NOS (785.6)*
> *lymphadenitis:*
> *chronic or subacute, except mesenteric (289.1)*
> *mesenteric (acute) (chronic) (subacute) (289.2)*
> *unspecified (289.3)*

DEF: Acute inflammation of lymph nodes due to primary infection located elsewhere in the body.

684 Impetigo

Impetiginization of other dermatoses
Impetigo (contagiosa) [any site] [any organism]:
bullous
circinate
neonatorum
simplex
Pemphigus neonatorum

> **EXCLUDES** *impetigo herpetiformis (694.3)*

DEF: Infectious skin disease commonly occurring in children; caused by group A streptococci or *Staphylococcus aureus;* skin lesions usually appear on the face and consist of subcorneal vesicles and bullae that burst and form yellow crusts.

√4ᵗʰ **685 Pilonidal cyst**

> **INCLUDES** fistula }coccygeal or pilonidal
> sinus }

DEF: Hair-containing cyst or sinus in the tissues of the sacrococcygeal area; often drains through opening at the postanal dimple.

685.0 With abscess   **C**

CC Exd: 685.0-685.1, 709.8

685.1 Without mention of abscess

AHA: 3Q, '11, 9

Stages of Pilonidal Disease

Normal follicle
Stretched follicle
Infected follicle
Acute abscess
Chronic abscess
Epithelial tube

N Newborn Age: 0   **P** Pediatric Age: 0-17   **M** Maternity Age: 12-55   **A** Adult Age: 15-124   **MCC** Major CC Condition   **CC** CC Condition   **HIV** HIV Related

228 – Volume 1 · February 2013   2014 ICD-9-C

√4th **686 Other local infections of skin and subcutaneous tissue**

Use additional code to identify any infectious organism (041.0-041.8)

√5th **686.0 Pyoderma**

Dermatitis:
  purulent
  septic
  suppurative

DEF: Nonspecific purulent skin disease related most to furuncles, pustules, or possibly carbuncles.

686.00 Pyoderma, unspecified

686.01 Pyoderma gangrenosum   CC

DEF: Persistent debilitating skin disease, characterized by irregular, boggy, blue-red ulcerations, with central healing and undermined edges.

CC Exd: 686.00-686.09

AHA: 4Q, '97, 42

686.09 Other pyoderma

686.1 Pyogenic granuloma

Granuloma:
  septic
  suppurative
  telangiectaticum

EXCLUDES *pyogenic granuloma of oral mucosa (528.9)*

DEF: Solitary polypoid capillary hemangioma often associated with local irritation, trauma, and superimposed inflammation; located on the skin and gingival or oral mucosa.

686.8 Other specified local infections of skin and subcutaneous tissue

Bacterid (pustular)
Dermatitis vegetans
Ecthyma
Perlèche

EXCLUDES *dermatitis infectiosa eczematoides (690.8)*
panniculitis (729.30-729.39)

686.9 Unspecified local infection of skin and subcutaneous tissue

Fistula of skin NOS
Skin infection NOS

EXCLUDES *fistula to skin from internal organs — see Alphabetic Index*

Other Inflammatory Conditions of Skin and Subcutaneous Tissue (690-698)

EXCLUDES *panniculitis (729.30-729.39)*

√4th **690 Erythematosquamous dermatosis**

EXCLUDES *eczematous dermatitis of eyelid (373.31)*
parakeratosis variegata (696.2)
psoriasis (696.0-696.1)
seborrheic keratosis (702.11-702.19)

√5th **690.1 Seborrheic dermatitis**

AHA: 4Q, '95, 58

690.10 Seborrheic dermatitis, unspecified

Seborrheic dermatitis NOS

L21.9 Seborrheic dermatitis unspecified   I-10

690.11 Seborrhea capitis   P

Cradle cap

690.12 Seborrheic infantile dermatitis   P

690.18 Other seborrheic dermatitis

690.8 Other erythematosquamous dermatosis

√4th **691 Atopic dermatitis and related conditions**

DEF: Atopic dermatitis: chronic, pruritic, inflammatory skin disorder found on the face and antecubital and popliteal fossae; often accompanied by allergic rhinitis, hay fever, asthma, and extreme itching; also called allergic dermatitis, or disseminated neurodermatitis.

691.0 Diaper or napkin rash

Ammonia dermatitis
Diaper or napkin:
  dermatitis
  erythema
  rash
Psoriasiform napkin eruption

691.8 Other atopic dermatitis and related conditions

Atopic dermatitis
Besnier's prurigo
Eczema:
  atopic
  flexural
  intrinsic (allergic)
Neurodermatitis:
  atopic
  diffuse (of Brocq)

√4th **692 Contact dermatitis and other eczema**

INCLUDES dermatitis:
  NOS
  contact
  occupational
  venenata
eczema (acute) (chronic):
  NOS
  allergic
  erythematous
  occupational

EXCLUDES *allergy NOS (995.3)*
contact dermatitis of eyelids (373.32)
dermatitis due to substances taken internally (693.0-693.9)
eczema of external ear (380.22)
perioral dermatitis (695.3)
urticarial reactions (708.0-708.9, 995.1)

DEF: Contact dermatitis: acute or chronic dermatitis caused by initial irritant effect of a substance, or by prior sensitization to a substance coming once again in contact with skin.

692.0 Due to detergents

692.1 Due to oils and greases

692.2 Due to solvents

Dermatitis due to solvents of:
  chlorocompound ⎫
  cyclohexane ⎬
  ester   ⎬ group
  glycol   ⎬
  hydrocarbon ⎬
  ketone   ⎭

692.3 Due to drugs and medicines in contact with skin

Dermatitis (allergic) (contact) due to:
  arnica
  fungicides
  iodine
  keratolytics
  mercurials
  neomycin
  pediculocides
  phenols
  scabicides
  any drug applied to skin
Dermatitis medicamentosa due to drug applied to skin

Use additional E code to identify drug

EXCLUDES *allergy NOS due to drugs (995.27)*
dermatitis due to ingested drugs (693.0)
dermatitis medicamentosa NOS (693.0)

692.4 Due to other chemical products

Dermatitis due to:
  acids
  adhesive plaster
  alkalis
  caustics
  dichromate
  insecticide
  nylon
  plastic
  rubber

AHA: 3Q, '08, 6-7; 2Q, '89, 16

4th / 5th Additional Digit Required   Unacceptable PDx   Manifestation Code   Hospital Acquired Condition   ▶◀ Revised Text   ● New Code   ▲ Revised Code Title

2014 ICD-9-CM   **Volume 1 – 229**

692.5 Due to food in contact with skin
Dermatitis, contact, due to:
cereals
fish
flour
fruit
meat
milk

EXCLUDES dermatitis due to:
dyes (692.89)
ingested foods (693.1)
preservatives (692.89)

692.6 Due to plants [except food]
Dermatitis due to:
lacquer tree [Rhus verniciflua]
poison:
ivy [Rhus toxicodendron]
oak [Rhus diversiloba]
sumac [Rhus venenata]
vine [Rhus radicans]
primrose [Primula]
ragweed [Senecio jacobae]
other plants in contact with the skin

EXCLUDES allergy NOS due to pollen (477.0)
nettle rash (708.8)

✓5ᵗʰ 692.7 Due to solar radiation

EXCLUDES sunburn due to other ultraviolet radiation exposure
(692.82)

692.70 Unspecified dermatitis due to sun

692.71 Sunburn
First degree sunburn
Sunburn NOS
AHA: 4Q, '01, 47
TIP: Do not assign if sunburn is due to tanning bed use; see instead code 692.82.

692.72 Acute dermatitis due to solar radiation
Acute solar skin damage NOS
Berlogue dermatitis
Photoallergic response
Phototoxic response
Polymorphus light eruption
Use additional E code to identify drug, if drug induced

EXCLUDES sunburn (692.71, 692.76-692.77)

DEF: Berloque dermatitis: Phytophotodermatitis due to sun exposure after use of a product containing bergamot oil; causes red patches, that turn brown.
DEF: Photoallergic response: Dermatitis due to hypersensitivity to the sun; causes papulovesicular, eczematous or exudative eruptions.
DEF: Phototoxic response: Chemically induced sensitivity to sun causes burn-like reaction, occasionally vesiculation and subsequent hyperpigmentation.
DEF: Polymorphous light eruption: Inflammatory skin eruptions due to sunlight exposure; eruptions differ in size and shape.
DEF: Acute solar skin damage (NOS): Rapid, unspecified injury to skin from sun.

692.73 Actinic reticuloid and actinic granuloma
DEF: Actinic reticuloid: Dermatosis aggravated by light, causes chronic eczema-like eruption on exposed skin which extends to other unexposed surfaces; occurs in the elderly.
DEF: Actinic granuloma: Inflammatory response of skin to sun causing small nodule of microphages.

692.74 Other chronic dermatitis due to solar radiation
Chronic solar skin damage NOS
Solar elastosis

EXCLUDES actinic [solar] keratosis (702.0)

DEF: Solar elastosis: Premature aging of skin of light-skinned people; causes inelasticity, thinning or thickening, wrinkling, dryness, scaling and hyperpigmentation.
DEF: Chronic solar skin damage (NOS): Chronic skin impairment due to exposure to the sun, not otherwise specified.

692.75 Disseminated superficial actinic porokeratosis [DSAP]
DEF: Autosomal dominant skin condition occurring in skin that has been overexposed to the sun; characterized by superficial annular, keratotic, brownish-red spots or thickenings with depressed centers and sharp, ridged borders, may evolve into squamous cell carcinoma.
AHA: 4Q, '00, 43

692.76 Sunburn of second degree
AHA: 4Q, '01, 47
TIP: Do not assign if sunburn is due to tanning bed use; see instead code 692.82.

692.77 Sunburn of third degree
AHA: 4Q, '01, 47
TIP: Do not assign if sunburn is due to tanning bed use; see instead code 692.82.

692.79 Other dermatitis due to solar radiation
Hydroa aestivale
Photodermatitis
Photosensitiveness } (due to sun)
Solar skin damage NOS

✓5ᵗʰ 692.8 Due to other specified agents

692.81 Dermatitis due to cosmetics

692.82 Dermatitis due to other radiation
Infrared rays
Light, except from sun
Radiation NOS
Tanning bed
Ultraviolet rays, except from sun
X-rays

EXCLUDES solar radiation (692.70-692.79)

AHA: 4Q, '01, 47; 3Q, '00, 5

692.83 Dermatitis due to metals
Jewelry

692.84 Due to animal (cat) (dog) dander
Due to animal (cat) (dog) hair

692.89 Other
Dermatitis due to: Dermatitis due to:
cold weather   hot weather
dyes   preservatives

EXCLUDES allergy (NOS) (rhinitis) due to animal hair or dander (477.2)
allergy to dust (477.8)
sunburn (692.71, 692.76-692.77)

692.9 Unspecified cause
Dermatitis:
NOS
contact NOS
venenata NOS
Eczema NOS

L23.9 Allergic contact dermatitis unspecified cause   I-10

✓4ᵗʰ 693 Dermatitis due to substances taken internally

EXCLUDES adverse effect NOS of drugs and medicines (995.20)
allergy NOS (995.3)
contact dermatitis (692.0-692.9)
urticarial reactions (708.0-708.9, 995.1)

DEF: Inflammation of skin due to ingested substance.

693.0 Due to drugs and medicines
Dermatitis medicamentosa NOS
Use additional E code to identify drug

EXCLUDES that due to drugs in contact with skin (692.3)

AHA: 2Q, '07, 8
TIP: Assign for palmar plantar erythrodysesthesia (PPE) or hand-foot syndrome due to chemotherapy drugs.

L27.0 Gen skin eruption d/t Rx & med taken internally   I-10

693.1 Due to food

693.8 Due to other specified substances taken internally

693.9 Due to unspecified substance taken internally

EXCLUDES dermatitis NOS (692.9)

N Newborn Age: 0   P Pediatric Age: 0-17   M Maternity Age: 12-55   A Adult Age: 15-124   MCC Major CC Condition   CC CC Condition   HIV HIV Related Dx

230 – Volume 1   2014 ICD-9-CM

√4th **694 Bullous dermatoses**

694.0 Dermatitis herpetiformis
Dermatosis herpetiformisHydroa herpetiformis
Duhring's disease

  EXCLUDES *herpes gestationis (646.8)*
      dermatitis herpetiformis:
        juvenile (694.2)
        senile (694.5)

  DEF: Chronic, multisystem disease manifested in the cutaneous system; seen as an extremely pruritic eruption of various lesions that frequently heal leaving hyperpigmentation or hypopigmentation and occasionally scarring; usually associated with an asymptomatic gluten-sensitive enteropathy, and immunogenic factors .

694.1 Subcorneal pustular dermatosis
Sneddon-Wilkinson disease or syndrome

  DEF: Chronic relapses of sterile pustular blebs beneath the horny skin layer of the trunk and skin folds; resembles dermatitis herpetiformis.

694.2 Juvenile dermatitis herpetiformis
Juvenile pemphigoid

694.3 Impetigo herpetiformis

  DEF: Rare dermatosis associated with pregnancy; marked by itching pustules in third trimester, hypocalcemia, tetany, fever and lethargy; may result in maternal or fetal death.

694.4 Pemphigus   `CC`
Pemphigus: Pemphigus:
  NOS   malignant
  erythematosus   vegetans
  foliaceus   vulgaris

  EXCLUDES *pemphigus neonatorum (684)*
  CC Excl: 694.4-694.9, 709.8

  DEF: Chronic, relapsing, sometimes fatal skin diseases; causes vesicles, bullae; autoantibodies against intracellular connections cause acantholysis.

694.5 Pemphigoid   `CC`
Benign pemphigus NOS
Bullous pemphigoid
Herpes circinatus bullosus
Senile dermatitis herpetiformis

  CC Excl: See code 694.4

√5th **694.6 Benign mucous membrane pemphigoid**
Cicatricial pemphigoid
Mucosynechial atrophic bullous dermatitis

  694.60 Without mention of ocular involvement

  694.61 With ocular involvement
    Ocular pemphigus

    DEF: Mild self-limiting, subepidermal blistering of mucosa including the conjunctiva, seen predominantly in the elderly, produces adhesions and scarring.

694.8 Other specified bullous dermatoses
  EXCLUDES *herpes gestationis (646.8)*

694.9 Unspecified bullous dermatoses

√4th **695 Erythematous conditions**

695.0 Toxic erythema   `CC`
Erythema venenatum
  CC Excl: 695.0-695.4, 709.8

√5th **695.1 Erythema multiforme**
Use additional code to identify associated manifestations, such as:
  arthropathy associated with dermatological disorders (713.3)
  conjunctival edema (372.73)
  conjunctivitis (372.04, 372.33)
  corneal scars and opacities (371.00-371.05)
  corneal ulcer (370.00-370.07)
  edema of eyelid (374.82)
  inflammation of eyelid (373.8)
  keratoconjunctivitis sicca (370.33)
  mechanical lagophthalmos (374.22)
  mucositis (478.11, 528.00, 538, 616.81)
  stomatitis (528.00)
  symblepharon (372.63)

Use additional E code to identify drug, if drug-induced

Use additional code to identify percentage of skin exfoliation (695.50-695.59)

  EXCLUDES *(Staphylococcal) scalded skin syndrome (695.81)*

  DEF: Symptom complex with varied skin eruption pattern of macular, bullous, papular, nodose, or vesicular lesions on the neck, face, and legs; gastritis and rheumatic pains; secondary to number of factors, including infections, ingestants, physical agents, malignancy and pregnancy.

  AHA: 4Q, '08, 128-130

  695.10 Erythema multiforme, unspecified
    Erythema iris
    Herpes iris

  695.11 Erythema multiforme minor

  695.12 Erythema multiforme major   `CC`
    CC Excl: 695.0-695.4, 695.81-695.9, 709.8

  695.13 Stevens-Johnson syndrome   `CC`
    CC Excl: See code 695.12

  695.14 Stevens-Johnson syndrome-toxic epidermal   `CC`
    necrolysis overlap syndrome
    SJS-TEN overlap syndrome
    CC Excl: See code 695.12
    AHA: 4Q, '08, 131

  695.15 Toxic epidermal necrolysis   `CC`
    Lyell's syndrome
    CC Excl: See code 695.12

  695.19 Other erythema multiforme

695.2 Erythema nodosum
  EXCLUDES *tuberculous erythema nodosum (017.1)*

  DEF: Panniculitis (an inflammatory reaction of the subcutaneous fat) of women, usually seen as a hypersensitivity reaction to infections, drugs, sarcoidosis, and specific enteropathies; the acute stage associated with fever, malaise, and arthralgia; the lesions are pink to blue in color as tender nodules found on the front of the legs below the knees.

695.3 Rosacea
Acne: Perioral dermatitis
  erythematosa   Rhinophyma
  rosacea

  DEF: Chronic skin disease, usually of the face, characterized by persistent erythema and telangiectasis with acute episodes of edema, engorgement papules, and pustules.

695.4 Lupus erythematosus
Lupus:
  erythematodes (discoid)
  erythematosus (discoid), not disseminated

  EXCLUDES *lupus (vulgaris) NOS (017.0)*
        systemic [disseminated] lupus erythematosus (710.0)

  DEF: Group of connective tissue disorders occurring as various cutaneous diseases of unknown origin; it primarily affects women between the ages of 20 and 40.

Diseases of the Skin and Subcutaneous Tissue

694–695.4

Additional Digit Required   Unacceptable PDx   Manifestation Code   Hospital Acquired Condition   ►◄ Revised Text   ● New Code   ▲ Revised Code Title

14 ICD-9-CM   Volume 1 – 231

Diseases of the Skin and Subcutaneous Tissue

695.5–698.2

√5ᵗʰ **695.5 Exfoliation due to erythematous conditions according to extent of body surface involved**
Code first erythematous condition causing exfoliation, such as:
Ritter's disease (695.81)
(Staphylococcal) scalded skin syndrome (695.81)
Stevens-Johnson syndrome (695.13)
Stevens-Johnson syndrome-toxic epidermal necrolysis overlap syndrome (695.14)
toxic epidermal necrolysis (695.15)
AHA: 4Q, '08, 128-131

695.50 Exfoliation due to erythematous condition involving less than 10 percent of body surface
Exfoliation due to erythematous condition NOS

695.51 Exfoliation due to erythematous condition involving 10-19 percent of body surface

695.52 Exfoliation due to erythematous condition involving 20-29 percent of body surface

695.53 Exfoliation due to erythematous condition involving 30-39 percent of body surface `CC`
CC Excl: 695.53
AHA: 4Q, '08, 131

695.54 Exfoliation due to erythematous condition involving 40-49 percent of body surface `CC`
CC Excl: 695.54

695.55 Exfoliation due to erythematous condition involving 50-59 percent of body surface `CC`
CC Excl: 695.55

695.56 Exfoliation due to erythematous condition involving 60-69 percent of body surface `CC`
CC Excl: 695.56

695.57 Exfoliation due to erythematous condition involving 70-79 percent of body surface `CC`
CC Excl: 695.57

695.58 Exfoliation due to erythematous condition involving 80-89 percent of body surface `CC`
CC Excl: 695.58

695.59 Exfoliation due to erythematous condition involving 90 percent or more of body surface `CC`
CC Excl: 695.59

√5ᵗʰ **695.8 Other specified erythematous conditions**

695.81 Ritter's disease
Dermatitis exfoliativa neonatorum
(Staphylococcal) Scalded skin syndrome
Use additional code to identify percentage of skin exfoliation (695.50-695.59)
DEF: Infectious skin disease of young children marked by eruptions ranging from a localized bullous to widespread easily ruptured fine vesicles and bullae; results in exfoliation of large planes of skin and leaves raw areas.

695.89 Other
Erythema intertrigo
Intertrigo
Pityriasis rubra (Hebra)
EXCLUDES mycotic intertrigo (111.0-111.9)
AHA: S-O, '86, 10

695.9 Unspecified erythematous condition
Erythema NOS   Erythroderma (secondary)

√4ᵗʰ **696 Psoriasis and similar disorders**

696.0 Psoriatic arthropathy
DEF: Psoriasis associated with inflammatory arthritis; often involves interphalangeal joints.

696.1 Other psoriasis
Acrodermatitis continua   Psoriasis:
Dermatitis repens   NOS
Psoriasis: any type, except arthropathic
EXCLUDES psoriatic arthropathy (696.0)
L40.9 Psoriasis unspecified   `I-10`

696.2 Parapsoriasis
Parakeratosis variegata
Parapsoriasis lichenoides chronica
Pityriasis lichenoides et varioliformis
DEF: Erythrodermas similar to lichen, planus and psoriasis; symptom include redness and itching; resistant to treatment.

696.3 Pityriasis rosea
Pityriasis circinata (et maculata)
DEF: Common, self-limited rash of unknown etiology marked by a solitary erythematous, salmon or fawn-colored herald plaque on the trunk, arms or thighs; followed by development of papular or macular lesions that tend to peel and form a scaly collarette.

696.4 Pityriasis rubra pilaris
Devergie's disease   Lichen ruber acuminatus
EXCLUDES pityriasis rubra (Hebra) (695.89)
DEF: Inflammatory disease of hair follicles; marked by firm, red lesions topped by horny plugs; may form patches; occurs on fingers elbows, knees.

696.5 Other and unspecified pityriasis
Pityriasis: Pityriasis:
NOS   streptogenes
alba
EXCLUDES pityriasis:
simplex (690.18)
versicolor (111.0)

696.8 Other

√4ᵗʰ **697 Lichen**
EXCLUDES lichen:
obtusus corneus (698.3)
pilaris (congenital) (757.39)
ruber acuminatus (696.4)
sclerosus et atrophicus (701.0)
scrofulosus (017.0)
simplex chronicus (698.3)
spinulosus (congenital) (757.39)
urticatus (698.2)

697.0 Lichen planus
Lichen: Lichen:
planopilaris   ruber planus
DEF: Inflammatory, pruritic skin disease; marked by angular, flat-top violet-colored papules; may be acute and widespread or chronic an localized.

697.1 Lichen nitidus
Pinkus' disease
DEF: Chronic, inflammatory, asymptomatic skin disorder, characterized by numerous glistening, flat-topped, discrete, skin-colored micropapules most often on penis, lower abdomen, inner thighs, wrists, forearms, breasts and buttocks.

697.8 Other lichen, not elsewhere classified
Lichen: Lichen:
ruber moniliforme   striata

697.9 Lichen, unspecified

√4ᵗʰ **698 Pruritus and related conditions**
EXCLUDES pruritus specified as psychogenic (306.3)
DEF: Pruritus: Intense, persistent itching due to irritation of sensory nerve endings from organic or psychogenic causes.

698.0 Pruritus ani
Perianal itch

698.1 Pruritus of genital organs

698.2 Prurigo
Lichen urticatus   Prurigo:
Prurigo: mitis
NOS   simplex
Hebra's   Urticaria papulosa (Hebra)
EXCLUDES prurigo nodularis (698.3)

N Newborn Age: 0   P Pediatric Age: 0-17   M Maternity Age: 12-55   A Adult Age: 15-124   MCC Major CC Condition   CC CC Condition   HIV HIV Related

232 – Volume 1   2014 ICD-9-C

698.3 Lichenification and lichen simplex chronicus
Hyde's disease
Neurodermatitis (circumscripta) (local)
Prurigo nodularis

EXCLUDES　*neurodermatitis, diffuse (of Brocq) (691.8)*

DEF: Lichenification: thickening of skin due to prolonged rubbing or scratching.

DEF: Lichen simplex chronicus: eczematous dermatitis, of face, neck, extremities, scrotum, vulva, and perianal region due to repeated itching, rubbing and scratching; spontaneous or evolves with other dermatoses.

698.4 Dermatitis factitia [artefacta]
Dermatitis ficta　　Neurotic excoriation

Use additional code to identify any associated mental disorder

DEF: Various types of self-inflicted skin lesions characterized in appearance as an erythema to a gangrene.

698.8 Other specified pruritic conditions
Pruritus:　　　　　　Winter itch
　hiemalis
　senilis

698.9 Unspecified pruritic disorder
Itch NOS　　　　Pruritus NOS

L29.9 Pruritus unspecified　　　　　　　　　　I-10

Other Diseases of Skin and Subcutaneous Tissue (700-709)

EXCLUDES　*conditions confined to eyelids (373.0-374.9)*
congenital conditions of skin, hair, and nails (757.0-757.9)

700　Corns and callosities
Callus
Clavus

DEF: Corns: Conical or horny thickening of skin on toes, due to friction, pressure from shoes and hosiery; pain and inflammation may develop.

DEF: Callosities: Localized overgrowth (hyperplasia) of the horny epidermal layer due to pressure or friction.

✓4ᵗʰ 701　Other hypertrophic and atrophic conditions of skin

EXCLUDES　*dermatomyositis (710.3)*
hereditary edema of legs (757.0)
scleroderma (generalized) (710.1)

701.0　Circumscribed scleroderma
Addison's keloid
Dermatosclerosis, localized
Lichen sclerosus et atrophicus
Morphea
Scleroderma, circumscribed or localized

DEF: Thickened, hardened, skin and subcutaneous tissue; may involve musculoskeletal system.

701.1　Keratoderma, acquired
Acquired:
　ichthyosis
　keratoderma palmaris et plantaris
Elastosis perforans serpiginosa
Hyperkeratosis:
　NOS
　follicularis in cutem penetrans
　palmoplantaris climacterica
Keratoderma:
　climactericum
　tylodes, progressive
Keratosis (blennorrhagica)

EXCLUDES　*Darier's disease [keratosis follicularis] (congenital)*
(757.39)
keratosis:
arsenical (692.4)
gonococcal (098.81)

AHA:4Q, '94, 48

701.2　Acquired acanthosis nigricans
Keratosis nigricans

DEF: Diffuse velvety hyperplasia of the spinous skin layer of the axilla and other body folds marked by gray, brown, or black pigmentation; in adult form often associated with malignant acanthosis nigricans in a benign, nevoid form relatively generalized.

701.3　Striae atrophicae
Atrophic spots of skin
Atrophoderma maculatum
Atrophy blanche (of Milian)
Degenerative colloid atrophy
Senile degenerative atrophy
Striae distensae

DEF: Bands of atrophic, depressed, wrinkled skin associated with stretching of skin from pregnancy, obesity, or rapid growth during puberty.

701.4　Keloid scar
Cheloid
Hypertrophic scar
Keloid

DEF: Overgrowth of scar tissue due to excess amounts of collagen during connective tissue repair; occurs mainly on upper trunk, face.

701.5　Other abnormal granulation tissue
Excessive granulation

701.8　Other specified hypertrophic and atrophic conditions of skin
Acrodermatitis atrophicans chronica
Atrophia cutis senilis
Atrophoderma neuriticum
Confluent and reticulate papillomatosis
Cutis laxa senilis
Elastosis senilis
Folliculitis ulerythematosa reticulata
Gougerot-Carteaud syndrome or disease

AHA: 1Q, '08, 7

TIP: Assign for nephrogenic fibrosing dermopathy (NFD) or nephrogenic systemic dermopathy (NSD), a systemic condition occurring only in patients with kidney disease.

701.9　Unspecified hypertrophic and atrophic conditions of skin
Atrophoderma
Skin tag

✓4ᵗʰ 702　Other dermatoses

EXCLUDES　*carcinoma in situ (232.0-232.9)*

702.0　Actinic keratosis
DEF: Wart-like growth, red or skin-colored; may form a cutaneous horn.
AHA: 1Q, '92, 18

✓5ᵗʰ 702.1　Seborrheic keratosis
DEF: Common, benign, lightly pigmented, warty growth composed of basaloid cells.

702.11　Inflamed seborrheic keratosis
AHA: 4Q, '94, 48

702.19　Other seborrheic keratosis
Seborrheic keratosis NOS

702.8　Other specified dermatoses

✓4ᵗʰ 703　Diseases of nail

EXCLUDES　*congenital anomalies (757.5)*
onychia and paronychia (681.02, 681.11)

703.0　Ingrowing nail
Ingrowing nail with infection
Unguis incarnatus

EXCLUDES　*infection, nail NOS (681.9)*

703.8　Other specified diseases of nail
Dystrophia unguium
Hypertrophy of nail
Koilonychia
Leukonychia (punctata) (striata)
Onychauxis
Onychogryposis
Onycholysis

703.9　Unspecified disease of nail

Additional Digit Required　　Unacceptable PDx　　Manifestation Code　　Hospital Acquired Condition　　▶◀ Revised Text　　● New Code　　▲ Revised Code Title

014 ICD-9-CM　　　　　　　　　　　　　　　　　　　　　　　　　　　　　　　　　　　　　　　**Volume 1 – 233**

Diseases of the Skin and Subcutaneous Tissue

704–706.0

√4ᵗʰ **704 Diseases of hair and hair follicles**
     EXCLUDES *congenital anomalies (757.4)*

√5ᵗʰ **704.0 Alopecia**
     EXCLUDES *madarosis (374.55)*
               syphilitic alopecia (091.82)
     DEF: Lack of hair, especially on scalp; often called baldness; may be partial or total; occurs at any age.

     704.00 Alopecia, unspecified
         Baldness
         Loss of hair

     704.01 Alopecia areata
         Ophiasis
         DEF: Alopecia areata: usually reversible, inflammatory, patchy hair loss found in beard or scalp.
         DEF: Ophiasis: alopecia areata of children; marked by band around temporal and occipital scalp margins.

     704.02 Telogen effluvium
         DEF: Shedding of hair from premature telogen development in follicles due to stress, including shock, childbirth, surgery, drugs or weight loss.

     704.09 Other
         Folliculitis decalvans
         Hypotrichosis:
            NOS
            postinfectional NOS
         Pseudopelade

704.1 Hirsutism
     Hypertrichosis:
         NOS
         lanuginosa, acquired
     Polytrichia
     EXCLUDES *hypertrichosis of eyelid (374.54)*
     DEF: Excess hair growth; often in unexpected places and amounts.

704.2 Abnormalities of the hair
     Atrophic hair
     Clastothrix
     Fragilitas crinium
     Trichiasis:
         NOS
         cicatrical
     Trichorrhexis (nodosa)
     EXCLUDES *trichiasis of eyelid (374.05)*

704.3 Variations in hair color
     Canities (premature)
     Grayness, hair (premature)
     Heterochromia of hair
     Poliosis:
         NOS
         circumscripta, acquired

√5ᵗʰ **704.4 Pilar and trichilemmal cysts**
     AHA: 4Q, '11, 134-135

     704.41 Pilar cyst

     704.42 Trichilemmal cyst
         Trichilemmal proliferating cyst
         AHA: 4Q, '11, 135

704.8 Other specified diseases of hair and hair follicles
     Folliculitis:
         NOS
         abscedens et suffodiens
         pustular
     Perifolliculitis:
         NOS
         capitis abscedens et suffodiens
         scalp
     Sycosis:
         NOS
         barbae [not parasitic]
         lupoid
         vulgaris
     AHA: 1Q, '11, 8

704.9 Unspecified disease of hair and hair follicles

√4ᵗʰ **705 Disorders of sweat glands**

705.0 Anhidrosis
     Hypohidrosis
     Oligohidrosis
     DEF: Lack or deficiency of ability to sweat.

705.1 Prickly heat
     Heat rash
     Miliaria rubra (tropicalis)
     Sudamina

√5ᵗʰ **705.2 Focal hyperhidrosis**
     EXCLUDES *generalized (secondary) hyperhidrosis (780.8)*

     705.21 Primary focal hyperhidrosis
         Focal hyperhidrosis NOS
         Hyperhidrosis NOS
         Hyperhidrosis of:
            axilla
            face
            palms
            soles
         DEF: A rare disorder of the sweat glands resulting in excessive production of sweat; occurs in the absence of any underlying condition, almost always focal, confined to one or more specific areas of the body.
         AHA: 4Q, '04, 91

     705.22 Secondary focal hyperhidrosis
         Frey's syndrome
         DEF: Secondary focal hyperhidrosis: a symptom of an underlying disease process resulting in excessive sweating beyond what the body requires to maintain thermal control, confined to one or more specific areas of the body.
         DEF: Frey's syndrome: an auriculotemporal syndrome due to lesion on the parotid gland; characteristic redness and excessive sweating on the cheek in connection with eating
         AHA: 4Q, '04, 91

√5ᵗʰ **705.8 Other specified disorders of sweat glands**

     705.81 Dyshidrosis
         Cheiropompholyx
         Pompholyx
         DEF: Vesicular eruption, on hands, feet causing itching and burning.

     705.82 Fox-Fordyce disease
         DEF: Chronic, usually pruritic disease evidenced by small follicular papular eruptions, especially in the axillary and pubic areas; develops from the closure and rupture of the affected apocrine glands' intraepidermal portion of the ducts.

     705.83 Hidradenitis
         Hidradenitis suppurativa
         DEF: Inflamed sweat glands.

     705.89 Other
         Bromhidrosis
         Chromhidrosis
         Granulosis rubra nasi
         Urhidrosis
         EXCLUDES *generalized hyperhidrosis (780.8)*
                  hidrocystoma (216.0-216.9)
         DEF: Bromhidrosis: foul-smelling axillary sweat due to decomposed bacteria.
         DEF: Chromhidrosis: secretion of colored sweat.
         DEF: Granulosis rubra nasi: idiopathic condition of children causes redness, sweating around nose, face and chin; tends to end by puberty.
         DEF: Urhidrosis: urinous substance, such as uric acid, in sweat; occurs in uremia.

705.9 Unspecified disorder of sweat glands
     Disorder of sweat glands NOS

√4ᵗʰ **706 Diseases of sebaceous glands**

706.0 Acne varioliformis
     Acne: Acne:
         frontalis   necrotica
     DEF: Rare form of acne characterized by persistent brown papulo-pustules usually on the brow and temporoparietal part of the scalp.

N Newborn Age: 0   **P** Pediatric Age: 0-17   **M** Maternity Age: 12-55   **A** Adult Age: 15-124   **MCC** Major CC Condition   **CC** CC Condition   **HIV** HIV Related D

234 – Volume 1   2014 ICD-9-C

706.1 Other acne
Acne: Blackhead
   NOS   Comedo
   conglobata
   cystic
   pustular
   vulgaris
   EXCLUDES   acne rosacea (695.3)

706.2 Sebaceous cyst
Atheroma, skin
Keratin cyst
Wen
   EXCLUDES   pilar cyst (704.41)
           trichilemmal (proliferating) cyst (704.42)
DEF: Benign epidermal cyst, contains sebum and keratin; presents as firm, circumscribed nodule.

706.3 Seborrhea
   EXCLUDES   seborrhea:
           capitis (690.11)
           sicca (690.18)
        seborrheic
           dermatitis (690.10)
           keratosis (702.11-702.19)
DEF: Seborrheic dermatitis marked by excessive secretion of sebum; the sebum forms an oily coating, crusts, or scales on the skin; it is also called hypersteatosis.

706.8 Other specified diseases of sebaceous glands
Asteatosis (cutis)
Xerosis cutis

706.9 Unspecified disease of sebaceous glands

✓4ᵗʰ 707 Chronic ulcer of skin
   INCLUDES   non-infected sinus of skin
           non-healing ulcer
   EXCLUDES   varicose ulcer (454.0, 454.2)
   AHA: 4Q, '04, 92

✓5ᵗʰ 707.0 Pressure ulcer
Bed sore   Plaster ulcer
Decubitus ulcer
Use additional code to identify pressure ulcer stage (707.20-707.25)
AHA: 4Q, '08, 132-133; 1Q, '04, 14; 4Q, '03, 110; 4Q, '99, 20; 1Q, '96, 15; 3Q, '90, 15; N-D, '87, 9

707.00 Unspecified site

707.01 Elbow

707.02 Upper back
Shoulder blades

707.03 Lower back
Coccyx
Sacrum
AHA: 3Q, '08, 17; 1Q, '05, 16
L89.159 Pressure ulcer of sacral region uns stage   I-10

707.04 Hip
L89.209 Pressure ulcer of unspecified hip uns stage   I-10

707.05 Buttock
AHA: ▶2Q, '12, 3◀
L89.309 Pressure ulcer of unspecified buttock uns stage   I-10

707.06 Ankle

Four Stages of Pressure Ulcers

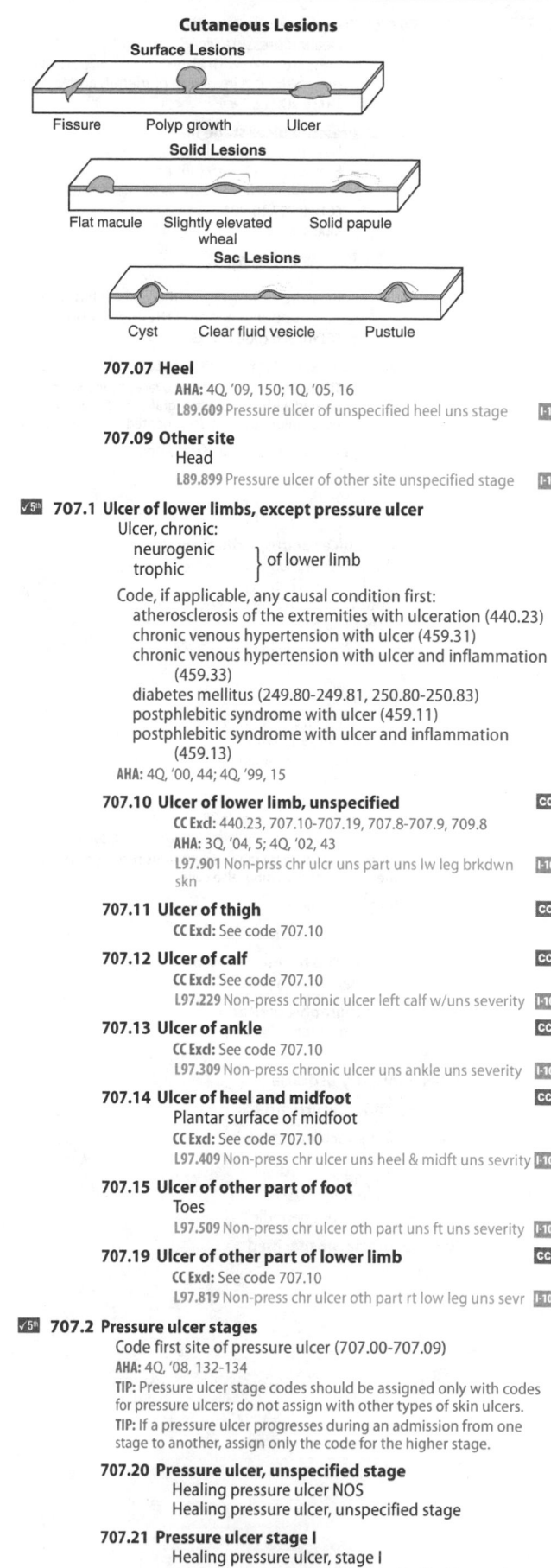

First Stage
Persistent focal erythema

Second Stage
Partial thickness skin loss involving epidermis, dermis, or both

Third Stage
Full thickness skin loss extending through subcutaneous tissue

Fourth Stage
Necrosis of soft tissue extending to muscle and bone

Cutaneous Lesions
Surface Lesions

Fissure   Polyp growth   Ulcer

Solid Lesions

Flat macule   Slightly elevated   Solid papule
          wheal

Sac Lesions

Cyst   Clear fluid vesicle   Pustule

707.07 Heel
AHA: 4Q, '09, 150; 1Q, '05, 16
L89.609 Pressure ulcer of unspecified heel uns stage   I-10

707.09 Other site
Head
L89.899 Pressure ulcer of other site unspecified stage   I-10

✓5ᵗʰ 707.1 Ulcer of lower limbs, except pressure ulcer
Ulcer, chronic:
    neurogenic
    trophic   } of lower limb

Code, if applicable, any causal condition first:
   atherosclerosis of the extremities with ulceration (440.23)
   chronic venous hypertension with ulcer (459.31)
   chronic venous hypertension with ulcer and inflammation (459.33)
   diabetes mellitus (249.80-249.81, 250.80-250.83)
   postphlebitic syndrome with ulcer (459.11)
   postphlebitic syndrome with ulcer and inflammation (459.13)
AHA: 4Q, '00, 44; 4Q, '99, 15

707.10 Ulcer of lower limb, unspecified   CC
CC Excl: 440.23, 707.10-707.19, 707.8-707.9, 709.8
AHA: 3Q, '04, 5; 4Q, '02, 43
L97.901 Non-prss chr ulcr uns part uns lw leg brkdwn skn   I-10

707.11 Ulcer of thigh   CC
CC Excl: See code 707.10

707.12 Ulcer of calf   CC
CC Excl: See code 707.10
L97.229 Non-press chronic ulcer left calf w/uns severity   I-10

707.13 Ulcer of ankle   CC
CC Excl: See code 707.10
L97.309 Non-press chronic ulcer uns ankle uns severity   I-10

707.14 Ulcer of heel and midfoot   CC
Plantar surface of midfoot
CC Excl: See code 707.10
L97.409 Non-press chr ulcer uns heel & midft uns sevrity   I-10

707.15 Ulcer of other part of foot
Toes
L97.509 Non-press chr ulcer oth part uns ft uns severity   I-10

707.19 Ulcer of other part of lower limb   CC
CC Excl: See code 707.10
L97.819 Non-press chr ulcer oth part rt low leg uns sevr   I-10

✓5ᵗʰ 707.2 Pressure ulcer stages
Code first site of pressure ulcer (707.00-707.09)
AHA: 4Q, '08, 132-134
TIP: Pressure ulcer stage codes should be assigned only with codes for pressure ulcers; do not assign with other types of skin ulcers.
TIP: If a pressure ulcer progresses during an admission from one stage to another, assign only the code for the higher stage.

707.20 Pressure ulcer, unspecified stage
Healing pressure ulcer NOS
Healing pressure ulcer, unspecified stage

707.21 Pressure ulcer stage I
Healing pressure ulcer, stage I
Pressure pre-ulcer skin changes limited to persistent focal erythema

▲ Additional Digit Required   Unacceptable PDx   Manifestation Code   Hospital Acquired Condition   ▶◀ Revised Text   ● New Code   ▲ Revised Code Title

14 ICD-9-CM   February 2013 · Volume 1 – 235

Diseases of the Skin and Subcutaneous Tissue

707.22–709.9

707.22 Pressure ulcer stage II
Healing pressure ulcer, stage II
Pressure ulcer with abrasion, blister, partial thickness
skin loss involving epidermis and/or dermis
AHA: ►2Q, '12, 3◄

707.23 Pressure ulcer stage III   `MCC`
Healing pressure ulcer, stage III
Pressure ulcer with full thickness skin loss involving
damage or necrosis of subcutaneous tissue
CC Exd: 707.10-707.9
AHA: 4Q, '09, 150

707.24 Pressure ulcer stage IV   `MCC`
Healing pressure ulcer, stage IV
Pressure ulcer with necrosis of soft tissues through to
underlying muscle, tendon, or bone
CC Exd: See code 707.23

707.25 Pressure ulcer, unstageable
TIP: Assign only if ulcer is covered by eschar, has been
treated with skin or other graft, or is documented as a deep
tissue injury but not documented as due to trauma.

707.8 Chronic ulcer of other specified sites
Ulcer, chronic:
neurogenic   } of other specified sites
trophic

707.9 Chronic ulcer of unspecified site
Chronic ulcer NOS
Trophic ulcer NOS
Tropical ulcer NOS
Ulcer of skin NOS
L98.499 Non-press chr ulcer skin oth sites uns severity   `I-10`

`√4ᵗʰ` **708 Urticaria**
`EXCLUDES` *edema:*
angioneurotic (995.1)
Quincke's (995.1)
hereditary angioedema (277.6)
urticaria:
giant (995.1)
papulosa (Hebra) (698.2)
pigmentosa (juvenile) (congenital) (757.33)
DEF: Skin disorder marked by raised edematous patches of skin or mucous
membrane with intense itching; also called hives.

708.0 Allergic urticaria

708.1 Idiopathic urticaria

708.2 Urticaria due to cold and heat
Thermal urticaria

708.3 Dermatographic urticaria
Dermatographia
Factitial urticaria

708.4 Vibratory urticaria

708.5 Cholinergic urticaria

708.8 Other specified urticaria
Nettle rash
Urticaria:
chronic
recurrent periodic

708.9 Urticaria, unspecified
Hives NOS

`√4ᵗʰ` **709 Other disorders of skin and subcutaneous tissue**

`√5ᵗʰ` **709.0 Dyschromia**
`EXCLUDES` *albinism (270.2)*
pigmented nevus (216.0-216.9)
that of eyelid (374.52-374.53)
DEF: Pigment disorder of skin or hair.

709.00 Dyschromia, unspecified

709.01 Vitiligo
DEF: Persistent, progressive development of nonpigmented
white patches on otherwise normal skin.

709.09 Other

709.1 Vascular disorders of skin
Angioma serpiginosum
Purpura (primary)annularis telangiectodes

709.2 Scar conditions and fibrosis of skin
Adherent scar (skin)
Cicatrix
Disfigurement (due to scar)
Fibrosis, skin NOS
Scar NOS
`EXCLUDES` *keloid scar (701.4)*
AHA: N-D, '84, 19

709.3 Degenerative skin disorders
Calcinosis:
circumscripta
cutis
Colloid milium
Degeneration, skin
Deposits, skin
Senile dermatosis NOS
Subcutaneous calcification

709.4 Foreign body granuloma of skin and subcutaneous tissue
Use additional code to identify foreign body (V90.01-V90.9)
`EXCLUDES` *residual foreign body without granuloma of skin and*
subcutaneous tissue (729.6)
that of muscle (728.82)

709.8 Other specified disorders of skin
Epithelial hyperplasia
Menstrual dermatosis
Vesicular eruption
DEF: Epithelial hyperplasia: increased number of epithelial cells.
DEF: Vesicular eruption: liquid-filled structures appearing through
skin.
AHA: 4Q, '08, 99; N-D, '87, 6
L98.8 Other spec disorders skin & subcutaneous tissue   `I-?`

709.9 Unspecified disorder of skin and subcutaneous tissue
Dermatosis NOS

`N` Newborn Age: 0   `P` Pediatric Age: 0-17   `M` Maternity Age: 12-55   `A` Adult Age: 15-124   `MCC` Major CC Condition   `CC` CC Condition   `HIV` HIV Related D

236 – Volume 1 · February 2013   2014 ICD-9-C

13. Diseases of the Musculoskeletal System and Connective Tissue (710-739)

Use additional external cause code, if applicable, to identify the cause of the musculoskeletal condition

The following fifth-digit subclassification is for use with categories 711-712, 715-716, 718-719, and 730:

0 site unspecified
1 shoulder region
  Acromioclavicular joint(s)
  Clavicle
  Glenohumeral joint(s)
  Scapula
  Sternoclavicular joint(s)
2 upper arm
  Elbow joint
  Humerus
3 forearm
  Radius
  Ulna
  Wrist joint
4 hand
  Carpus
  Metacarpus
  Phalanges [fingers]
5 pelvic region and thigh
  Buttock
  Femur
  Hip (joint)

6 lower leg
  Fibula
  Knee joint
  Patella
  Tibia
7 ankle and foot
  Ankle joint
  Digits [toes]
  Metatarsus
  Phalanges, foot
  Tarsus
  Other joints in foot
8 other specified sites
  Head
  Neck
  Ribs
  Skull
  Trunk
  Vertebral column
9 multiple sites

Arthropathies and Related Disorders (710-719)

EXCLUDES *disorders of spine (720.0-724.9)*

✓4ᵗʰ 710 Diffuse diseases of connective tissue

INCLUDES all collagen diseases whose effects are not mainly confined to a single system

EXCLUDES *those affecting mainly the cardiovascular system, i.e., polyarteritis nodosa and allied conditions (446.0-446.7)*

710.0 Systemic lupus erythematosus
Disseminated lupus erythematosus   Libman-Sacks disease

Use additional code to identify manifestation, as:
  endocarditis (424.91)
  nephritis (583.81)
    chronic (582.81)
  nephrotic syndrome (581.81)

EXCLUDES *lupus erythematosus (discoid) NOS (695.4)*

DEF: A chronic multisystemic inflammatory disease affecting connective tissue; marked by anemia, leukopenia, muscle and joint pains, fever, rash of a butterfly pattern around cheeks and forehead area; of unknown etiology.
AHA: 2Q, '03, 7-8; 2Q, '97, 8
M32.9 Systemic lupus erythematosus unspecified   I-10

710.1 Systemic sclerosis
Acrosclerosis   Progressive systemic sclerosis
CRST syndrome   Scleroderma

Use additional code to identify manifestation, as:
  lung involvement (517.2)
  myopathy (359.6)

EXCLUDES *circumscribed scleroderma (701.0)*

DEF: Systemic disease, involving excess fibrotic collagen build-up; symptoms include thickened skin, fibrotic degenerative changes in various organs, and vascular abnormalities; condition occurs more often in females.
AHA: 1Q, '88, 6

710.2 Sicca syndrome
Keratoconjunctivitis sicca   Sjögren's disease
DEF: Autoimmune disease; associated with keratoconjunctivitis, laryngopharyngitis, rhinitis, dry mouth, enlarged parotid gland, and chronic polyarthritis.

710.3 Dermatomyositis   CC
Poikilodermatomyositis   Polymyositis with skin involvement
DEF: Polymyositis characterized by flat-top purple papules on knuckles; upper eyelid rash, edema of eyelids and orbit area, red rash on forehead, neck, shoulders, trunk and arms; symptoms include fever, weight loss, aching muscles; visceral cancer.
CC Excl: 710.3

710.4 Polymyositis   CC
DEF: Chronic, progressive, inflammatory skeletal muscle disease; causes weakness of limb girdles, neck, pharynx; may precede or follow scleroderma, Sjogren's disease, systemic lupus erythematosus, arthritis, or malignancy.
CC Excl: 710.4

710.5 Eosinophilia myalgia syndrome   CC
Toxic oil syndrome

Use additional E code to identify drug, if drug induced
DEF: Eosinophilia myalgia syndrome (EMS): inflammatory, multisystem fibrosis; associated with ingesting elementary L-tryptophan; symptoms include myalgia, weak limbs and bulbar muscles, distal sensory loss, areflexia, arthralgia, cough, fever, fatigue, skin rashes, myopathy, and eosinophil counts greater than 1000/microliter.
DEF: Toxic oil syndrome: syndrome similar to EMS due to ingesting contaminated cooking oil.
CC Excl: 292.0-293.9, 710.5
AHA: 4Q, '92, 21

710.8 Other specified diffuse diseases of connective tissue   CC
Multifocal fibrosclerosis (idiopathic) NEC
Systemic fibrosclerosing syndrome
CC Excl: 359.71-359.79, 710.8
AHA: M-A, '87, 12

710.9 Unspecified diffuse connective tissue disease
Collagen disease NOS

✓4ᵗʰ 711 Arthropathy associated with infections

INCLUDES arthritis
  arthropathy } associated with conditions
  polyarthritis } classifiable below
  polyarthropathy

EXCLUDES *rheumatic fever (390)*

The following fifth-digit subclassification is for use with category 711; valid digits are in [brackets] under each code. See list at beginning of chapter for definitions.
  0 site unspecified
  1 shoulder region
  2 upper arm
  3 forearm
  4 hand
  5 pelvic region and thigh
  6 lower leg
  7 ankle and foot
  8 other specified sites
  9 multiple sites

AHA: 1Q, '92, 17

§ ✓5ᵗʰ 711.0 Pyogenic arthritis   CC
[0-9] Arthritis or polyarthritis (due to):
  coliform [Escherichia coli]
  Hemophilus influenzae [H. influenzae]
  pneumococcal
  Pseudomonas
  staphylococcal
  streptococcal
  Pyarthrosis

Use additional code to identify infectious organism (041.0-041.8)
DEF: Infectious arthritis caused by various bacteria; marked by inflamed synovial membranes, and purulent effusion in joints.
CC Excl: For codes 711.00, 711.08-711.09: 015.80-015.96, 017.90-017.96, 036.82, 056.71, 098.50-098.51, 098.59, 098.89, 711.00-714.0, 715.00, 715.09-715.10, 715.18-716.99, 718.00-718.08, 719.00-719.10, 719.18-719.99; **For code 711.01:** 015.80-015.96, 017.90-017.96, 036.82, 056.71, 098.50-098.51, 098.59, 098.89, 711.00-711.01, 711.08-711.11, 711.18-711.21, 711.28-711.31, 711.38-711.41, 711.48-

Requires fifth digit. Valid digits are in [brackets] under each code. See beginning of section 710-739 for codes and defintions.

Additional Digit Required   Unacceptable PDx   Manifestation Code   Hospital Acquired Condition   ►◄ Revised Text   ● New Code   ▲ Revised Code Title

2014 ICD-9-CM   Volume 1 – 237

711.51, 711.58-711.61, 711.68-711.71, 711.78-711.81, 711.88-
711.91, 711.98-712.11, 712.18-712.21, 712.28-712.31, 712.38-
712.81, 712.88-712.91, 712.98-714.0, 715.00, 715.09-715.11, 715.18-
715.21, 715.28-715.31, 715.38-715.91, 715.98-716.01,
716.08-716.11, 716.18-716.21, 716.28-716.31, 716.38-716.41,
716.48-716.51, 716.58-716.61, 716.68-716.81, 716.88-716.91,
716.98-716.99, 718.00-718.01, 718.08, 719.00-719.01, 719.08-
719.11, 719.18-719.21, 719.28-719.31, 719.38-719.41, 719.48-
719.51, 719.58-719.61, 719.68-719.81, 719.88-719.91, 719.98-
719.99; **For code 711.02:** 015.80-015.96, 017.90-017.96, 036.82,
056.71, 098.50-098.51, 098.59, 098.89, 711.00, 711.02, 711.08-
711.10, 711.12, 711.18-711.20, 711.22, 711.28-711.30, 711.32,
711.38-711.40, 711.42, 711.48-711.50, 711.52, 711.58-711.60,
711.62, 711.68-711.70, 711.72, 711.78-711.80, 711.82, 711.88-
711.90, 711.92, 711.98-712.10, 712.12, 712.18-712.20, 712.22,
712.28-712.30, 712.32, 712.38-712.80, 712.82, 712.88-712.90,
712.92, 712.98-714.0, 715.00, 715.09-715.10, 715.12, 715.18-715.20,
715.22, 715.28-715.30, 715.32, 715.38-715.90, 715.92, 715.98-
716.00, 716.02, 716.08-716.10, 716.12, 716.18-716.20, 716.22,
716.28-716.30, 716.32, 716.38-716.40, 716.42, 716.48-716.50,
716.52, 716.58-716.60, 716.62, 716.68-716.80, 716.82, 716.88-
716.90, 716.92, 716.98-716.99, 718.00, 718.02, 718.08, 719.00,
719.02, 719.08-719.10, 719.12, 719.18-719.20, 719.22, 719.28-
719.30, 719.32, 719.38-719.40, 719.42, 719.48-719.50, 719.52,
719.58-719.60, 719.62, 719.68-719.80, 719.82, 719.88-719.90,
719.92, 719.98-719.99; **For code 711.03:** 015.80-015.96, 017.90-017.96,
036.82, 056.71, 098.50-098.51, 098.59, 098.89, 711.00, 711.03,
711.08-711.10, 711.13, 711.18-711.20, 711.23, 711.28-711.30,
711.33, 711.38-711.40, 711.43, 711.48-711.50, 711.53, 711.58-
711.60, 711.63, 711.68-711.70, 711.73, 711.78-711.80, 711.83,
711.88-711.90, 711.93, 711.98-712.10, 712.13, 712.18-712.20,
712.23, 712.28-712.30, 712.33, 712.38-712.80, 712.83, 712.88-
712.90, 712.93, 712.98-714.0, 715.00, 715.09-715.10, 715.13, 715.18-
715.20, 715.23, 715.28-715.30, 715.33, 715.38-715.90, 715.93,
715.98-716.00, 716.03, 716.08-716.10, 716.13, 716.18-716.20,
716.23, 716.28-716.30, 716.33, 716.38-716.40, 716.43, 716.48-
716.50, 716.53, 716.58-716.60, 716.63, 716.68-716.80, 716.83,
716.88-716.90, 716.93, 716.98-716.99, 718.00, 718.03, 718.08,
719.00, 719.03, 719.08-719.10, 719.13, 719.18-719.20, 719.23,
719.28-719.30, 719.33, 719.38-719.40, 719.43, 719.48-719.50,
719.53, 719.58-719.60, 719.63, 719.68-719.80, 719.83, 719.88-
719.90, 719.93, 719.98-719.99; **For code 711.04:** 015.80-015.96,
017.90-017.96, 036.82, 056.71, 098.50-098.51, 098.59, 098.89,
711.00, 711.04, 711.08-711.10, 711.14, 711.18-711.20, 711.24,
711.28-711.30, 711.34, 711.38-711.40, 711.44, 711.48-711.50,
711.54, 711.58-711.60, 711.64, 711.68-711.70, 711.74, 711.78-
711.80, 711.84, 711.88-711.90, 711.94, 711.98-712.10, 712.14,
712.18-712.20, 712.24, 712.28-712.30, 712.34, 712.38-712.80,
712.84, 712.88-712.90, 712.94, 712.98-714.0, 715.00-715.10, 715.14,
715.18-715.20, 715.24, 715.28-715.30, 715.34, 715.38-715.90,
715.94, 715.98-716.00, 716.04, 716.08-716.10, 716.14, 716.18-
716.20, 716.24, 716.28-716.30, 716.34, 716.38-716.40, 716.44,
716.48-716.50, 716.54, 716.58-716.60, 716.64, 716.68-716.80,
716.84, 716.88-716.90, 716.94, 716.98-716.99, 718.00, 718.04,
718.08, 719.00, 719.04, 719.08-719.10, 719.14, 719.18-719.20,
719.24, 719.28-719.30, 719.34, 719.38-719.40, 719.44, 719.48-
719.50, 719.54, 719.58-719.60, 719.64, 719.68-719.80, 719.84,
719.88-719.90, 719.94, 719.98-719.99; **For code 711.05:** 015.80-015.96,
017.90-017.96, 036.82, 056.71, 098.50-098.51, 098.59, 098.89,
711.00, 711.05, 711.08-711.10, 711.15, 711.18-711.20, 711.25,
711.28-711.30, 711.35, 711.38-711.40, 711.45, 711.48-711.50,
711.55, 711.58-711.60, 711.65, 711.68-711.70, 711.75, 711.78-
711.80, 711.85, 711.88-711.90, 711.95, 711.98-712.10, 712.15,
712.18-712.20, 712.25, 712.28-712.30, 712.35, 712.38-712.80,
712.85, 712.88-712.90, 712.95, 712.98-714.0,
715.00, 715.09-715.10, 715.15, 715.18-715.20, 715.25, 715.28-
715.30, 715.35, 715.38-715.90, 715.95, 715.98-716.00, 716.05,
716.08-716.10, 716.15, 716.18-716.20, 716.25, 716.28-716.30,
716.35, 716.38-716.40, 716.45, 716.48-716.50, 716.55, 716.58-
716.60, 716.65, 716.68-716.80, 716.85, 716.88-716.90, 716.95,
716.98-716.99, 718.00, 718.05, 718.08, 719.00, 719.05, 719.08-
719.10, 719.15, 719.18-719.20, 719.25, 719.28-719.30, 719.35,
719.38-719.40, 719.45, 719.48-719.50, 719.55, 719.58-719.60,
719.65, 719.68-719.80, 719.85, 719.88-719.90, 719.95, 719.98-
719.99; **For code 711.06:** 015.80-015.96, 017.90-017.96, 036.82,
056.71, 098.50-098.51, 098.59, 098.89, 711.00, 711.06, 711.08-
711.10, 711.16, 711.18-711.20, 711.26, 711.28-711.30, 711.36,
711.38-711.40, 711.46, 711.48-711.50, 711.56, 711.58-711.60,
711.66, 711.68-711.70, 711.76, 711.78-711.80, 711.86, 711.88-
711.90, 711.96, 711.98-712.10, 712.16, 712.18-712.20, 712.26,
712.28-712.30, 712.36, 712.38-712.80, 712.86, 712.88-712.90,
712.96, 712.98-714.0, 715.00, 715.09-715.10, 715.16, 715.18-715.20,
715.26, 715.28-715.30, 715.36, 715.38-715.90, 715.96, 715.98-
716.00, 716.06, 716.08-716.10, 716.16, 716.18-716.20, 716.26,
716.28-716.30, 716.36, 716.38-716.40, 716.46, 716.48-716.50,
716.56, 716.58-716.60, 716.66, 716.68-716.80, 716.86, 716.88-
716.90, 716.96, 716.98-716.99, 718.00, 718.08, 719.00, 719.06,

719.08-719.10, 719.16, 719.18-719.20, 719.26, 719.28-719.30,
719.36, 719.38-719.40, 719.46, 719.48-719.50, 719.56, 719.58-
719.60, 719.66, 719.68-719.80, 719.86, 719.88-719.90, 719.96,
719.98-719.99; **For code 711.07:** 015.80-015.96, 017.90-017.96, 036.82,
056.71, 098.50-098.51, 098.59, 098.89, 711.00, 711.07-711.10,
711.17-711.20, 711.27-711.30, 711.37-711.40, 711.47-711.50,
711.57-711.60, 711.67-711.70, 711.77-711.80, 711.87-711.90,
711.97-712.10, 712.17-712.20, 712.27-712.30, 712.37-712.80,
712.87-712.90, 712.97-714.0, 715.00, 715.09-715.10, 715.17-715.20,
715.27-715.30, 715.37-715.90, 715.97-716.00, 716.07-716.10,
716.17-716.20, 716.27-716.30, 716.37-716.40, 716.47-716.50,
716.57-716.60, 716.67-716.80, 716.87-716.90, 716.97-716.99,
718.00, 718.07-718.08, 719.00, 719.07-719.10, 719.17-719.20,
719.27-719.30, 719.37-719.40, 719.47-719.50, 719.57-719.60,
719.67-719.80, 719.87-719.90, 719.97-719.99

AHA: 1Q, '92, 16; 1Q, '91, 15

M00.869 Arthritis due to other bacteria unspecified knee   `I-10`

§ ✓5ᵗʰ **711.1** **Arthropathy associated with Reiter's disease and**   `CC`
[0-9]   **nonspecific urethritis**

   Code first underlying disease as:
    nonspecific urethritis (099.4)
    Reiter's disease (099.3)

   DEF: Reiter's disease: joint disease marked by diarrhea, urethritis,
   conjunctivitis, keratosis and arthritis; of unknown etiology; affects
   young males.

   DEF: Urethritis: inflamed urethra.

   CC Excl: 003.23, 015.80-015.96, 017.90-017.96, 036.82, 056.71, 098.50-
   098.51, 098.59, 098.89, 711.00-714.0, 715.00, 715.09-715.10, 715.18-
   716.99, 718.00-718.08, 719.00-719.10, 719.18-719.69, 719.80-719.99

§ ✓5ᵗʰ **711.2** **Arthropathy in Behçet's syndrome**   `CC`
[0-9]   *Code first underlying disease (136.1)*

   DEF: Behçet's syndrome: Chronic inflammatory disorder, of unknown
   etiology; affects small blood vessels; causes ulcers of oral and
   pharyngeal mucous membranes and genitalia, skin lesions, retinal
   vasculitis, optic atrophy and severe uveitis.

   CC Excl: 003.23, 015.80-015.96, 017.90-017.96, 036.82, 056.71, 098.50-
   098.51, 098.59, 098.89, 711.00-714.0, 715.00, 715.09-715.10, 715.18-
   716.99, 718.00-718.08, 719.00-719.10, 719.18-719.69, 719.80-719.99

§ ✓5ᵗʰ **711.3** **Postdysenteric arthropathy**   `CC`
[0-9]   *Code first underlying disease as:*
    dysentery (009.0)
    enteritis, infectious (008.0-009.3)
    paratyphoid fever (002.1-002.9)
    typhoid fever (002.0)

   EXCLUDES   salmonella arthritis (003.23)

   CC Excl: For codes 711.30-711.35, 711.37, and 711.39: 003.23, 015.80-
   015.96, 017.90-017.96, 036.82, 056.71, 098.50-098.51, 098.59,
   098.89, 711.00-714.0, 715.00, 715.09-715.10, 715.18-716.99, 718.00-
   718.08, 719.00-719.10, 719.18-719.69, 719.80-719.99; **For code 711.36:**
   003.23, 015.80-015.96, 017.90-017.96, 036.82, 056.71, 098.50-
   098.51, 098.59, 098.89, 711.00-714.0, 715.00, 715.09-715.10, 715.18-
   716.07, 716.09-716.99, 718.00-718.08, 719.00-719.10, 719.18-
   719.69, 719.80-719.99; **For code 711.38:** 003.23, 015.80-015.96,
   017.90-017.96, 036.82, 056.71, 098.50-098.51, 098.59, 098.89,
   711.00-714.0, 715.00, 715.09-715.10, 715.18-716.57, 716.59-716.99,
   718.00-718.08, 719.00-719.10, 719.18-719.69, 719.80-719.99

§ ✓5ᵗʰ **711.4** **Arthropathy associated with other bacterial diseases**   `CC`
[0-9]   *Code first underlying disease as:*
    diseases classifiable to 010-040, 090-099, except as in 711.1,
     711.3, and 713.5
    leprosy (030.0-030.9)
    tuberculosis (015.0-015.9)

   EXCLUDES   gonococcal arthritis (098.50)
           meningococcal arthritis (036.82)

   CC Excl: For codes 711.40, 711.42-711.49: 003.23, 015.80-015.96, 017.90-
   017.96, 036.82, 056.71, 098.50-098.51, 098.59, 098.89, 711.00-714.0,
   715.00, 715.09-715.10, 715.18-716.99, 718.00-718.08, 719.00-
   719.10, 719.18-719.69, 719.80-719.99; **For code 711.41:** 003.23,
   015.80-015.96, 017.90-017.96, 036.82, 056.71, 098.50-098.51,
   098.59, 098.89, 711.00-714.0, 715.00, 715.09-715.10, 715.18-716.99,
   718.00-718.08, 719.00-719.10, 719.18-719.39, 719.41-719.69,
   719.80-719.99

---

§ Requires fifth digit. Valid digits are in [brackets] under each code. See beginning of section 710-739 for codes and defintions.

`N` Newborn Age: 0   `P` Pediatric Age: 0-17   `M` Maternity Age: 12-55   `A` Adult Age: 15-124   `MCC` Major CC Condition   `CC` CC Condition   `HIV` HIV Related Dx

238 – Volume 1   2014 ICD-9-CM

Joint Structures

Muscle
Periosteum (covers bone)
Cortical bone
Medullary bone
Fascia over Muscle
Sesamoid bone
Bursa (with synovial fluid)
Tendon (muscle to bone)
Muscle insertion into bone (crosses one or more joints)

Retinaculum
Tendon sheath around
Tendon
Synovium lines
Joint capsule around
Synovial cavity (with fluid)
Articular cartilage
Ligament (bone to bone)
Bursa
Bone covered with periosteum

§ ✓5ᵗʰ **711.5 Arthropathy associated with other viral diseases**   CC
[0-9]
Code first underlying disease as:
diseases classifiable to 045-049, 050-079, 480, 487
O'nyong nyong (066.3)

EXCLUDES that due to rubella (056.71)

CC Excl: 003.23, 015.80-015.96, 017.90-017.96, 036.82, 056.71, 098.50-098.51, 098.59, 098.89, 711.00-714.0, 715.00, 715.09-715.10, 715.18-716.99, 718.00-718.08, 719.00-719.10, 719.18-719.69, 719.80-719.99

§ ✓5ᵗʰ **711.6 Arthropathy associated with mycoses**   CC
[0-9]
Code first underlying disease (110.0-118)

CC Excl: For codes 711.60, 711.68-711.69: 015.80-015.96, 017.90-017.96, 036.82, 056.71, 098.50-098.51, 098.59, 098.89, 711.00-714.0, 715.00, 715.09-715.10, 715.18-716.99, 718.00-718.08, 719.00-719.10, 719.18-719.99; For code 711.61: 015.80-015.96, 017.90-017.96, 036.82, 056.71, 098.50-098.51, 098.59, 098.89, 711.00-714.0, 715.00, 715.09-715.10, 715.18-716.99, 718.00-718.08, 719.00-719.10, 719.18-719.99; For code 711.62: 015.80-015.96, 017.90-017.96, 036.82, 056.71, 098.50-098.51, 098.59, 098.89, 711.00-711.01, 711.11, 711.18-711.21, 711.28-711.31, 711.38-711.41, 711.48-711.51, 711.58-711.61, 711.68-711.71, 711.78-711.81, 711.88-711.91, 711.98-712.11, 712.18-712.21, 712.28-712.31, 712.38-712.81, 712.88-712.91, 712.98-714.0, 715.00, 715.09-715.11, 715.18-715.21, 715.28-715.31, 715.38-715.91, 715.98-716.01, 716.08-716.11, 716.18-716.21, 716.28-716.31, 716.38-716.41, 716.48-716.51, 716.58-716.61, 716.68-716.81, 716.88-716.91, 716.98-716.99, 718.00-718.01, 718.08, 719.00-719.01, 719.08-719.11, 719.18-719.21, 719.28-719.31, 719.38-719.41, 719.48-719.51, 719.58-719.61, 719.68-719.81, 719.88-719.91, 719.98-719.99; For code 711.63: 015.80-015.96, 017.90-017.96, 036.82, 056.71, 098.50-098.51, 098.59, 098.89, 711.00, 711.02, 711.08-711.10, 711.12, 711.18-711.20, 711.22, 711.28-711.30, 711.32, 711.38-711.40, 711.42, 711.48-711.50, 711.52, 711.58-711.60, 711.62, 711.68-711.70, 711.72, 711.78-711.80, 711.82, 711.88-711.90, 711.92, 711.98-712.10, 712.12, 712.18-712.20, 712.22, 712.28-712.30, 712.32, 712.38-712.80, 712.82, 712.88-712.90, 712.92, 712.98-714.0, 715.00, 715.09-715.10, 715.12, 715.18-715.20, 715.22, 715.28-715.30, 715.32, 715.38-715.90, 715.92, 715.98-716.00, 716.02, 716.08-716.10, 716.12, 716.18-716.20, 716.22, 716.28-716.30, 716.32, 716.38-716.40, 716.42, 716.48-716.50, 716.52, 716.58-716.60, 716.62, 716.68-716.80, 716.82, 716.88-716.90, 716.92, 716.98-716.99, 718.00, 718.02, 718.08, 719.00, 719.02, 719.08-719.10, 719.12, 719.18-719.20, 719.22, 719.28-719.30, 719.32, 719.38-719.40, 719.42, 719.48-719.50, 719.52, 719.58-719.60, 719.62, 719.68-719.80, 719.82, 719.88-719.90, 719.92, 719.98-719.99; For code 711.64: 015.80-015.96, 017.90-017.96, 036.82, 056.71, 098.50-098.51, 098.59, 098.89, 711.00, 711.03, 711.08-711.10, 711.13, 711.18-711.20, 711.23, 711.28-711.30, 711.33, 711.38-711.40, 711.43, 711.48-711.50, 711.53, 711.58-711.60, 711.63, 711.68-711.70, 711.73, 711.78-711.80, 711.83, 711.88-711.90, 711.93, 711.98-712.10, 712.13, 712.18-712.20, 712.23, 712.28-712.30, 712.33, 712.38-712.80, 712.83, 712.88-712.90, 712.93, 712.98-714.0, 715.00, 715.09-715.10, 715.13, 715.18-715.20, 715.23, 715.28-715.30, 715.33, 715.38-715.90, 715.93, 715.98-716.00, 716.03, 716.08-716.10, 716.13, 716.18-716.20, 716.23, 716.28-716.30, 716.33, 716.38-716.40, 716.43, 716.48-716.50, 716.53, 716.58-716.60, 716.63, 716.68-716.80, 716.83, 716.88-716.90, 716.93, 716.98-716.99, 718.00, 718.03, 718.08, 719.00, 719.03, 719.08-719.10, 719.13, 719.18-719.20, 719.23, 719.28-719.30, 719.33, 719.38-719.40, 719.43, 719.48-719.50, 719.53, 719.58-719.60, 719.63, 719.68-719.80, 719.83, 719.88-719.90, 719.93, 719.98-719.99; For code 711.65: 015.80-015.96, 017.90-017.96, 036.82, 056.71, 098.50-098.51, 098.59, 098.89, 711.00, 711.04, 711.08-711.10, 711.14, 711.18-711.20, 711.24, 711.28-711.30, 711.34, 711.38-711.40, 711.44, 711.48-711.50, 711.54, 711.58-711.60, 711.64, 711.68-711.70, 711.74, 711.78-711.80, 711.84, 711.88-711.90, 711.94, 711.98-712.10, 712.14, 712.18-712.20, 712.24, 712.28-712.30, 712.34, 712.38-712.80, 712.84, 712.88-

712.90, 712.94, 712.98-714.0, 715.00-715.10, 715.14, 715.18-715.20, 715.24, 715.28-715.30, 715.34, 715.38-715.90, 715.94, 715.98-716.00, 716.04, 716.08-716.10, 716.14, 716.18-716.20, 716.24, 716.28-716.30, 716.34, 716.38-716.40, 716.44, 716.48-716.50, 716.54, 716.58-716.60, 716.64, 716.68-716.80, 716.84, 716.88-716.90, 716.94, 716.98-716.99, 718.00, 718.04, 718.08, 719.00, 719.04, 719.08-719.10, 719.14, 719.18-719.20, 719.24, 719.28-719.30, 719.34, 719.38-719.40, 719.44, 719.48-719.50, 719.54, 719.58-719.60, 719.64, 719.68-719.80, 719.84, 719.88-719.90, 719.94, 719.98-719.99; For code 711.66: 015.80-015.96, 017.90-017.96, 036.82, 056.71, 098.50-098.51, 098.59, 098.89, 711.00, 711.05, 711.08-711.10, 711.15, 711.18-711.20, 711.25, 711.28-711.30, 711.35, 711.38-711.40, 711.45, 711.48-711.50, 711.55, 711.58-711.60, 711.65, 711.68-711.70, 711.75, 711.78-711.80, 711.85, 711.88-711.90, 711.98-712.10, 712.15, 712.18-712.20, 712.25, 712.28-712.30, 712.35, 712.38-712.80, 712.85, 712.88-712.90, 712.95, 712.98-714.0, 715.00, 715.09-715.10, 715.15, 715.18-715.20, 715.25, 715.28-715.30, 715.35, 715.38-715.90, 715.95, 715.98-716.00, 716.15,

716.18-716.20, 716.25, 716.28-716.30, 716.35, 716.38-716.40, 716.45, 716.48-716.50, 716.55, 716.58-716.60, 716.65, 716.68-716.80, 716.85, 716.88-716.90, 716.95, 716.98-716.99, 718.00, 718.05, 718.08, 719.00, 719.05, 719.08-719.10, 719.15, 719.18-719.20, 719.25, 719.28-719.30, 719.35, 719.38-719.40, 719.45, 719.48-719.50, 719.55, 719.58-719.60, 719.65, 719.68-719.80, 719.85, 719.88-719.90, 719.95, 719.98-719.99; For code 711.67: 015.80-015.96, 017.90-017.96, 036.82, 056.71, 098.50-098.51, 098.59, 098.89, 711.00, 711.06, 711.08-711.10, 711.16, 711.18-711.20, 711.26, 711.28-711.30, 711.36, 711.38-711.40, 711.46, 711.48-711.50, 711.56, 711.58-711.60, 711.66, 711.68-711.70, 711.76, 711.78-711.80, 711.86, 711.88-711.90, 711.96, 711.98-712.10, 712.16, 712.18-712.20, 712.26, 712.28-712.30, 712.36, 712.38-712.80, 712.86, 712.88-712.90, 712.96, 712.98-714.0, 715.00, 715.09-715.10, 715.16, 715.18-715.20, 715.26, 715.28-715.30, 715.36, 715.38-715.90, 715.96, 715.98-716.00, 716.06, 716.08-716.10, 716.16, 716.18-716.20, 716.26, 716.28-716.30, 716.36, 716.38-716.40, 716.46, 716.48-716.50, 716.56, 716.58-716.60, 716.66, 716.68-716.80, 716.86, 716.88-716.90, 716.96, 716.98-716.99, 718.00, 718.08, 719.00, 719.06, 719.08-719.10, 719.16, 719.18-719.20, 719.26, 719.28-719.30, 719.36, 719.38-719.40, 719.46, 719.48-719.50, 719.56, 719.58-719.60, 719.66, 719.68-719.80, 719.86, 719.88-719.90, 719.96, 719.98-719.99 For code 711.68: 015.80-015.96, 017.90-017.96, 036.82, 056.71, 098.50-098.51, 098.59, 098.89, 711.00-711.99, 712.10-712.99, 713.0-713.8, 714.0, 715.00, 715.09-715.10, 715.18-715.98, 716.00-716.99, 718.00-718.08, 719.00-719.10, 719.18-719.99 For code 711.69: See code 711.68

§ ✓5ᵗʰ **711.7 Arthropathy associated with helminthiasis**   CC
[0-9]
Code first underlying disease as:
filariasis (125.0-125.9)

CC Excl: For codes 711.70-711.74, 711.76, 711.78-711.79: 003.23, 015.80-015.96, 017.90-017.96, 036.82, 056.71, 098.50-098.51, 098.59, 098.89, 711.00-714.0, 715.00, 715.09-715.10, 715.18-716.99, 718.00-718.08, 719.00-719.10, 719.18-719.69, 719.80-719.99; For code 711.75: 003.23, 015.80-015.96, 017.90-017.96, 036.82, 056.71, 098.50-098.51, 098.59, 098.89, 711.00-714.0, 715.00, 715.09-715.10, 715.18-716.99, 718.00-718.08, 719.00-719.10, 719.18-719.43, 719.45-719.69, 719.80-719.99; For code 711.77: 003.23, 015.80-015.96, 017.90-017.96, 036.82, 056.71, 098.50-098.51, 098.59, 098.89, 711.00-714.0, 715.00, 715.09-715.10, 715.18-716.99, 718.00-718.08, 719.00-719.10, 719.18-719.69, 719.80-719.97, 719.99

§ ✓5ᵗʰ **711.8 Arthropathy associated with other infectious and parasitic diseases**   CC
[0-9]

Code first underlying disease as:
diseases classifiable to 080-088, 100-104, 130-136

EXCLUDES arthropathy associated with sarcoidosis (713.7)

CC Excl: For codes 711.80, 711.82-711.89: 003.23, 015.80-015.96, 017.90-017.96, 036.82, 056.71, 098.50-098.51, 098.59, 098.89, 711.00-714.0, 715.00, 715.09-715.10, 715.18-716.99, 718.00-718.08, 719.00-719.10, 719.18-719.69, 719.80-719.99; For code 711.81: 003.23, 015.80-015.96, 017.90-017.96, 036.82, 056.71, 098.50-098.51, 098.59, 098.89, 711.00-711.41, 711.43-714.0, 715.00, 715.09-715.10, 715.18-716.99, 718.00-718.08, 719.00-719.10, 719.18 719.69, 719.80-719.99

AHA: 4Q, '91, 15; 3Q, '90, 14

§ ✓5ᵗʰ **711.9 Unspecified infective arthritis**   CC
[0-9]
Infective arthritis or polyarthritis (acute) (chronic) (subacute) NOS

CC Excl: 003.23, 015.80-015.96, 017.90-017.96, 036.82, 056.71, 098.50-098.51, 098.59, 098.89, 711.00-714.0, 715.00, 715.09-715.10, 715.18-716.99, 718.00-718.08, 719.00-719.10, 719.18-719.69, 719.80-719.99

Requires fifth digit. Valid digits are in [brackets] under each code. See beginning of section 710-739 for codes and defintions.

Additional Digit Required   Unacceptable PDx   Manifestation Code   Hospital Acquired Condition   ►◄ Revised Text   ● New Code   ▲ Revised Code Title

Diseases of the Musculoskeletal System and Connective Tissue

712–714.32

✓4ᵗʰ 712 Crystal arthropathies
INCLUDES   crystal-induced arthritis and synovitis
EXCLUDES   *gouty arthropathy (274.00-274.03)*
DEF: Joint disease due to urate crystal deposit in joints or synovial membranes.

The following fifth-digit subclassification is for use with category 712; valid digits are in [brackets] under each code. See list at beginning of chapter for definitions.
  0 site unspecified
  1 shoulder region
  2 upper arm
  3 forearm
  4 hand
  5 pelvic region and thigh
  6 lower leg
  7 ankle and foot
  8 other specified sites
  9 multiple sites

§ ✓5ᵗʰ **712.1 Chondrocalcinosis due to dicalcium phosphate crystals**
[0-9]   Chondrocalcinosis due to dicalcium phosphate crystals (with other crystals)
    Code first underlying disease (275.4)

§ ✓5ᵗʰ **712.2 Chondrocalcinosis due to pyrophosphate crystals**
[0-9]   *Code first underlying disease (275.4)*

§ ✓5ᵗʰ **712.3 Chondrocalcinosis, unspecified**
[0-9]   *Code first underlying disease (275.4)*

§ ✓5ᵗʰ **712.8 Other specified crystal arthropathies**
[0-9]

§ ✓5ᵗʰ **712.9 Unspecified crystal arthropathy**
[0-9]

✓4ᵗʰ 713 Arthropathy associated with other disorders classified elsewhere
INCLUDES   arthritis
    arthropathy   associated with conditions
    polyarthritis   classifiable below
    polyarthropathy

713.0 Arthropathy associated with other endocrine and metabolic disorders
    Code first underlying disease as:
      acromegaly (253.0)
      hemochromatosis (275.01-275.09)
      hyperparathyroidism (252.00-252.08)
      hypogammaglobulinemia (279.00-279.09)
      hypothyroidism (243-244.9)
      lipoid metabolism disorder (272.0-272.9)
      ochronosis (270.2)
    EXCLUDES   *arthropathy associated with:*
      amyloidosis (713.7)
      crystal deposition disorders, except gout (712.1-712.9)
      diabetic neuropathy (713.5)
      gout (274.00-274.03)

713.1 Arthropathy associated with gastrointestinal conditions other than infections
    Code first underlying disease as:
      regional enteritis (555.0-555.9)
      ulcerative colitis (556)

713.2 Arthropathy associated with hematological disorders
    Code first underlying disease as:
      hemoglobinopathy (282.4-282.7)
      hemophilia (286.0-286.2)
      leukemia (204.0-208.9)
      malignant reticulosis (202.3)
      multiple myelomatosis (203.0)
    EXCLUDES   *arthropathy associated with Henoch-Schönlein purpura (713.6)*

713.3 Arthropathy associated with dermatological disorders
    Code first underlying disease as:
      erythema multiforme (695.10-695.19)
      erythema nodosum (695.2)
    EXCLUDES   *psoriatic arthropathy (696.0)*

713.4 Arthropathy associated with respiratory disorders
    Code first underlying disease as:
      diseases classifiable to 490-519
    EXCLUDES   *arthropathy associated with respiratory infections (711.0, 711.4-711.8)*

713.5 Arthropathy associated with neurological disorders
    Charcôt's arthropathy } associated with diseases
    Neuropathic arthritis } classifiable elsewhere
    Code first underlying disease as:
      neuropathic joint disease [Charcôt's joints]:
       NOS (094.0)
       diabetic (249.6, 250.6)
       syringomyelic (336.0)
       tabetic [syphilitic] (094.0)
    AHA: ▶3Q, '12, 4◄

713.6 Arthropathy associated with hypersensitivity reaction
    Code first underlying disease as:
      Henoch (-Schönlein) purpura (287.0)
      serum sickness (999.51-999.59)
    EXCLUDES   *allergic arthritis NOS (716.2)*

713.7 Other general diseases with articular involvement
    Code first underlying disease as:
      amyloidosis (277.30-277.39)
      familial Mediterranean fever (277.31)
      sarcoidosis (135)
    AHA: 2Q, '97, 12

713.8 Arthropathy associated with other condition classifiable elsewhere
    Code first underlying disease as:
      conditions classifiable elsewhere except as in 711.1-711.8, 712, and 713.0-713.7

✓4ᵗʰ 714 Rheumatoid arthritis and other inflammatory polyarthropathies
EXCLUDES   *rheumatic fever (390)*
       rheumatoid arthritis of spine NOS (720.0)
AHA: 2Q, '95, 3

714.0 Rheumatoid arthritis
    Arthritis or polyarthritis: Arthritis or polyarthritis:
      atrophic   rheumatic (chronic)
    Use additional code to identify manifestation, as:
      myopathy (359.6)
      polyneuropathy (357.1)
    EXCLUDES   *juvenile rheumatoid arthritis NOS (714.30)*
    DEF: Chronic systemic disease principally of joints, manifested by inflammatory changes in articular structures and synovial membranes, atrophy, and loss in bone density.
    AHA: 2Q, '06, 20; 1Q, '90, 5
    M06.9 Rheumatoid arthritis unspecified

714.1 Felty's syndrome
    Rheumatoid arthritis with splenoadenomegaly and leukopenia
    DEF: Syndrome marked by rheumatoid arthritis, splenomegaly, leukopenia, pigmented spots on lower extremity skin, anemia, an thrombocytopenia.

714.2 Other rheumatoid arthritis with visceral or systemic involvement
    Rheumatoid carditis

✓5ᵗʰ 714.3 Juvenile chronic polyarthritis
    DEF: Rheumatoid arthritis of more than one joint; lasts longer than six weeks in age 17 or younger; symptoms include fever, erythematous rash, weight loss, lymphadenopathy, hepatosplenomegaly and pericarditis.

714.30 Polyarticular juvenile rheumatoid arthritis, chron or unspecified
    Juvenile rheumatoid arthritis NOS
    Still's disease

714.31 Polyarticular juvenile rheumatoid arthritis, acute
    CC Excl: 036.82, 056.71, 711.00-714.4, 715.00, 715.09-715., 715.18-716.99, 718.00-718.08, 719.00-719.10, 719.18-719.99

714.32 Pauciarticular juvenile rheumatoid arthritis

---

§   Requires fifth digit. Valid digits are in [brackets] under each code. See beginning of section 710-739 for codes and defintions.

714.33 Monoarticular juvenile rheumatoid arthritis

714.4 Chronic postrheumatic arthropathy
Chronic rheumatic nodular fibrositis
Jaccoud's syndrome
DEF: Persistent joint disorder; follows previous rheumatic infection.

√5ᵗʰ 714.8 Other specified inflammatory polyarthropathies

714.81 Rheumatoid lung
Caplan's syndrome
Diffuse interstitial rheumatoid disease of lung
Fibrosing alveolitis, rheumatoid
DEF: Lung disorders associated with rheumatoid arthritis.

714.89 Other

714.9 Unspecified inflammatory polyarthropathy
Inflammatory polyarthropathy or polyarthritis NOS
EXCLUDES polyarthropathy NOS (716.5)

√4ᵗʰ 715 Osteoarthrosis and allied disorders
NOTE Localized, in the subcategories below, includes bilateral involvement of the same site.
INCLUDES arthritis or polyarthritis:
    degenerative
    hypertrophic
    degenerative joint disease
    osteoarthritis
EXCLUDES Marie-Strümpell spondylitis (720.0)
    osteoarthrosis [osteoarthritis] of spine (721.0-721.9)

The following fifth-digit subclassification is for use with category 715; valid digits are in [brackets] under each code. See list at beginning of chapter for definitions.
  0 site unspecified
  1 shoulder region
  2 upper arm
  3 forearm
  4 hand
  5 pelvic region and thigh
  6 lower leg
  7 ankle and foot
  8 other specified sites
  9 multiple sites

§ √5ᵗʰ 715.0 Osteoarthrosis, generalized
[0,4,9] Degenerative joint disease, involving multiple joints
Primary generalized hypertrophic osteoarthrosis
DEF: Chronic noninflammatory arthritis; marked by degenerated articular cartilage and enlarged bone; symptoms include pain and stiffness with activity.

§ √5ᵗʰ 715.1 Osteoarthrosis, localized, primary
[0-8] Localized osteoarthropathy, idiopathic
M17.0 Bilateral primary osteoarthritis of knee   I-10

§ √5ᵗʰ 715.2 Osteoarthrosis, localized, secondary
[0-8] Coxae malum senilis

§ √5ᵗʰ 715.3 Osteoarthrosis, localized, not specified whether
[0-8] **primary or secondary**
Otto's pelvis
AHA: For code 715.35: 3Q, '04, 12; 2Q, '04, 15; **For code 715.36:** 4Q, '03, 118; 2Q, '95, 5
M16.9 Osteoarthritis of hip unspecified   I-10

§ √5ᵗʰ 715.8 Osteoarthrosis involving, or with mention of
[0,9] **more than one site, but not specified as generalized**

§ √5ᵗʰ 715.9 Osteoarthrosis, unspecified whether generalized or
[0-8] **localized**
AHA: For code 715.90: 2Q, '97, 12
M19.90 Unspecified osteoarthritis unspecified site   I-10
M17.9 Osteoarthritis of knee unspecified   I-10

√4ᵗʰ 716 Other and unspecified arthropathies
EXCLUDES cricoarytenoid arthropathy (478.79)
The following fifth-digit subclassification is for use with category 716; valid digits are in [brackets] under each code. See list at beginning of chapter for definitions.
  0 site unspecified
  1 shoulder region
  2 upper arm
  3 forearm
  4 hand
  5 pelvic region and thigh
  6 lower leg
  7 ankle and foot
  8 other specified sites
  9 multiple sites
AHA: 2Q, '95, 3

§ √5ᵗʰ 716.0 Kaschin-Beck disease
[0-9] Endemic polyarthritis
DEF: Chronic degenerative disease of spine and peripheral joints; occurs in eastern Siberian, northern Chinese, and Korean youth; may be a mycotoxicosis caused by eating cereals infected with fungus.

§ √5ᵗʰ 716.1 Traumatic arthropathy
[0-9] **AHA: For Code 716.11:** 1Q, '02, 9; **For Code 716.15:** 2Q, '09, 11

§ √5ᵗʰ 716.2 Allergic arthritis
[0-9] **EXCLUDES** arthritis associated with Henoch-Schönlein purpura or serum sickness (713.6)

§ √5ᵗʰ 716.3 Climacteric arthritis   ♀
[0-9] Menopausal arthritis
DEF: Ovarian hormone deficiency; causes pain in small joints, shoulders, elbows or knees; affects females at menopause; also called arthropathia ovaripriva.

§ √5ᵗʰ 716.4 Transient arthropathy
[0-9] **EXCLUDES** palindromic rheumatism (719.3)

§ √5ᵗʰ 716.5 Unspecified polyarthropathy or polyarthritis
[0-9]

§ √5ᵗʰ 716.6 Unspecified monoarthritis
[0-8] Coxitis

§ √5ᵗʰ 716.8 Other specified arthropathy
[0-9]

§ √5ᵗʰ 716.9 Arthropathy, unspecified
[0-9] Arthritis
   Arthropathy } (acute) (chronic) (subacute)
   Articular rheumatism (chronic)
   Inflammation of joint NOS
M12.9 Arthropathy unspecified   I-10

√4ᵗʰ 717 Internal derangement of knee
INCLUDES degeneration
   rupture, old } of articular cartilage or meniscus of knee
   tear, old
EXCLUDES acute derangement of knee (836.0-836.6)
   ankylosis (718.5)
   contracture (718.4)
   current injury (836.0-836.6)
   deformity (736.4-736.6)
   recurrent dislocation (718.3)

717.0 Old bucket handle tear of medial meniscus
Old bucket handle tear of unspecified cartilage

Disruption and Tears of Meniscus

Bucket-handle   Flap-type   Peripheral / Radial

Horizontal cleavage   Vertical   Congenital discoid meniscus

Requires fifth digit. Valid digits are in [brackets] under each code. See beginning of section 710-739 for codes and definitions.

Additional Digit Required   Unacceptable PDx   Manifestation Code   Hospital Acquired Condition   ►◄ Revised Text   ● New Code   ▲ Revised Code Title

Internal Derangements of Knee

Disruptions of Cruciate Ligament

Anterior

Posterior

Chondromalacia of Patella

"Kissing" lesion of femur

717.1 Derangement of anterior horn of medial meniscus

717.2 Derangement of posterior horn of medial meniscus

717.3 Other and unspecified derangement of medial meniscus
Degeneration of internal semilunar cartilage

√5ᵗʰ 717.4 Derangement of lateral meniscus

    717.40 Derangement of lateral meniscus, unspecified

    717.41 Bucket handle tear of lateral meniscus

    717.42 Derangement of anterior horn of lateral meniscus

    717.43 Derangement of posterior horn of lateral meniscus

    717.49 Other

717.5 Derangement of meniscus, not elsewhere classified
Congenital discoid meniscus
Cyst of semilunar cartilage
Derangement of semilunar cartilage NOS

717.6 Loose body in knee
Joint mice, knee
Rice bodies, knee (joint)
DEF: The presence in the joint synovial area of a small, frequently calcified, loose body created from synovial membrane, organized fibrin fragments of articular cartilage or arthritis osteophytes.

717.7 Chondromalacia of patella
Chondromalacia patellae
Degeneration [softening] of articular cartilage of patella
DEF: Softened patella cartilage.
AHA: M-A, '85, 14; N-D, '84, 9

√5ᵗʰ 717.8 Other internal derangement of knee

    717.81 Old disruption of lateral collateral ligament

    717.82 Old disruption of medial collateral ligament

    717.83 Old disruption of anterior cruciate ligament

    717.84 Old disruption of posterior cruciate ligament

    717.85 Old disruption of other ligaments of knee
        Capsular ligament of knee

    717.89 Other
        Old disruption of ligaments NOS

717.9 Unspecified internal derangement of knee
Derangement NOS of knee

Joint Derangements and Disorders

Loose body in joint

Dislocation of joint

Joint contracture

Ankylosis of joint

Synovial effusion (fluid)

Hemarthrosis (blood)

√4ᵗʰ 718 Other derangement of joint
    EXCLUDES   current injury (830.0-848.9)
              jaw (524.60-524.69)

The following fifth-digit subclassification is for use with category 718; valid digits are in [brackets] under each code. See list at beginning of chapter for definitions.
    0 site unspecified
    1 shoulder region
    2 upper arm
    3 forearm
    4 hand
    5 pelvic region and thigh
    6 lower leg
    7 ankle and foot
    8 other specified sites
    9 multiple sites

§ √5ᵗʰ 718.0 Articular cartilage disorder
[0-5,7-9] Meniscus:
    disorder
    rupture, old
    tear, old
    Old rupture of ligament(s) of joint NOS
    EXCLUDES   articular cartilage disorder:
           in ochronosis (270.2)
           knee (717.0-717.9)
          chondrocalcinosis (275.4)
          metastatic calcification (275.4)

§ √5ᵗʰ 718.1 Loose body in joint
[0-5,7-9] Joint mice
    EXCLUDES   knee (717.6)
    DEF: Calcified loose bodies in synovial fluid; due to arthritic osteophytes.
    AHA: For code 718.17: 2Q, '01, 15

§ √5ᵗʰ 718.2 Pathological dislocation
[0-9]   Dislocation or displacement of joint, not recurrent and not
          current injury
        Spontaneous dislocation (joint)

§ √5ᵗʰ 718.3 Recurrent dislocation of joint
[0-9]   **AHA:** N-D, '87, 7

§ √5ᵗʰ 718.4 Contracture of joint
[0-9]   **AHA:** 4Q, '98, 40
    TIP: Assign an additional code from category 438 if the contracture a result of a CVA.

§ √5ᵗʰ 718.5 Ankylosis of joint
[0-9]   Ankylosis of joint (fibrous) (osseous)
    EXCLUDES   spine (724.9)
              stiffness of joint without mention of ankylosis (719
    DEF: Immobility and solidification of joint; due to disease, injury o surgical procedure.

§ √5ᵗʰ 718.6 Unspecified intrapelvic protrusion of acetabulum
[5]   Protrusio acetabuli, unspecified
    DEF: Sinking of the floor of acetabulum, causing femoral head to protrude, limits hip movement; of unknown etiology.

§ √5ᵗʰ 718.7 Developmental dislocation of joint
[0-9]   *EXCLUDES*   congenital dislocation of joint (754.0-755.8)
               traumatic dislocation of joint (830-839)
    AHA: 4Q, '01, 48

§ √5ᵗʰ 718.8 Other joint derangement, not elsewhere classified
[0-9]   Flail joint (paralytic)Instability of joint
    EXCLUDES   deformities classifiable to 736 (736.0-736.9)
    AHA: For code 718.81: 2Q, '00, 14
    TIP: Assign 718.81 for multidirectional shoulder instability.

§ √5ᵗʰ 718.9 Unspecified derangement of joint
[0-5,7-9] *EXCLUDES*   knee (717.9)

---

§   Requires fifth digit. Valid digits are in [brackets] under each code. See beginning of section 710-739 for codes and defintions.

N Newborn Age: 0   **P** Pediatric Age: 0-17   **M** Maternity Age: 12-55   **A** Adult Age: 15-124   **MCC** Major CC Condition   **CC** CC Condition   **HIV** HIV Related

242 – Volume 1   **2014 ICD-9-**

√4ᵗʰ **719 Other and unspecified disorders of joint**

> *EXCLUDES*   jaw (524.60-524.69)

> The following fifth-digit subclassification is for use with codes 719.0-719.6, 719.8-719.9; valid digits are in [brackets] under each code. See list at beginning of chapter for definitions.
> 0   site unspecified
> 1   shoulder region
> 2   upper arm
> 3   forearm
> 4   hand
> 5   pelvic region and thigh
> 6   lower leg
> 7   ankle and foot
> 8   other specified sites
> 9   multiple sites

§ √5ᵗʰ **719.0 Effusion of joint**
[0-9]   Hydrarthrosis
       Swelling of joint, with or without pain
> *EXCLUDES*   intermittent hydrarthrosis (719.3)
       M25.469 Effusion unspecified knee   **I-10**

§ √5ᵗʰ **719.1 Hemarthrosis**   **CC**
[0-9]   *EXCLUDES*   current injury (840.0-848.9)
       CC Excl: For codes: 719.10, 719.15, 719.18-719.19: 719.10-719.19, 958.91-958.92; **For code 719.11:** 719.10-719.13, 719.18-719.19, 958.91; **For code 719.12:** 719.10-719.12, 719.18-719.19, 958.91; **For code 719.13:** 719.10, 719.12-719.14, 719.18-719.19, 958.91; **For code 719.14:** 719.10, 719.13-719.14, 719.18-719.19, 958.91; **For codes 719.16-719.17:** 719.10, 719.16-719.19, 958.92

§ √5ᵗʰ **719.2 Villonodular synovitis**
[0-9]   **DEF:** Overgrowth of synovial tissue, especially at knee joint; due to macrophage infiltration of giant cells in synovial villi and fibrous nodules.

§ √5ᵗʰ **719.3 Palindromic rheumatism**
[0-9]   Hench-Rosenberg syndrome
       Intermittent hydrarthrosis
       DEF: Recurrent episodes of afebrile arthritis and periarthritis marked by their complete disappearance after a few days or hours; causes swelling, redness, and disability usually affecting only one joint; no known cause.

§ √5ᵗʰ **719.4 Pain in joint**
[0-9]   Arthralgia
       AHA: For code 719.46: 1Q, '01, 3
       TIP: Assign 719.46 for patellofemoral syndrome, a chronic knee pain common among athletes.
       M25.519 Pain in unspecified shoulder   **I-10**
       M25.552 Pain in left hip   **I-10**

§ √5ᵗʰ **719.5 Stiffness of joint, not elsewhere classified**
[0-9]

§ √5ᵗʰ **719.6 Other symptoms referable to joint**
[0-9]   Joint crepitus
       Snapping hip
       AHA: 1Q, '94, 15; **For code 719.66:** 2Q, '07, 6
       TIP: Assign 719.66 for patellar clunk syndrome, which is a fibrous reaction caused by chronic pressure on the patella, S/P knee replacement surgery.

719.7 Difficulty in walking
> *EXCLUDES*   abnormality of gait (781.2)
       AHA: 2Q, '04, 15; 4Q, '03, 66
       R26.2 Difficulty in walking not elsewhere classified   **I-10**

§ √5ᵗʰ **719.8 Other specified disorders of joint**
[0-9]   Calcification of joint
       Fistula of joint
> *EXCLUDES*   temporomandibular joint-pain-dysfunction syndrome [Costen's syndrome] (524.60)

§ √5ᵗʰ **719.9 Unspecified disorder of joint**
[0-9]

Dorsopathies (720-724)

> *EXCLUDES*   curvature of spine (737.0-737.9)
>   osteochondrosis of spine (juvenile) (732.0)
>   adult (732.8)

√4ᵗʰ **720 Ankylosing spondylitis and other inflammatory spondylopathies**

    720.0 Ankylosing spondylitis
       Rheumatoid arthritis of spine NOS
       Spondylitis:
          Marie-Strümpell
          rheumatoid
       DEF: Rheumatoid arthritis of spine and sacroiliac joints; fusion and deformity in spine follows; affects mainly males; cause unknown.

    720.1 Spinal enthesopathy
       Disorder of peripheral ligamentous or muscular attachments of spine
       Romanus lesion
       DEF: Tendinous or muscular vertebral bone attachment abnormality.

    720.2 Sacroiliitis, not elsewhere classified
       Inflammation of sacroiliac joint NOS
       DEF: Pain due to inflammation in joint, at juncture of sacrum and hip.

√5ᵗʰ **720.8 Other inflammatory spondylopathies**

      720.81 Inflammatory spondylopathies in diseases classified elsewhere
          Code first underlying disease as:
          tuberculosis (015.0)

      720.89 Other

    720.9 Unspecified inflammatory spondylopathy
       Spondylitis NOS

√4ᵗʰ **721 Spondylosis and allied disorders**
       DEF: Degenerative changes in spinal joint.
       AHA: 2Q, '89, 14

    721.0 Cervical spondylosis without myelopathy
       Cervical or cervicodorsal:
          arthritis
          osteoarthritis
          spondylarthritis

    721.1 Cervical spondylosis with myelopathy   **CC**
       Anterior spinal artery compression syndrome
       Spondylogenic compression of cervical spinal cord
       Vertebral artery compression syndrome
       CC Excl: 721.0-721.1
       M47.12 Other spondylosis w/myelopathy cervical region   **I-10**

    721.2 Thoracic spondylosis without myelopathy
       Thoracic: Thoracic:
          arthritis   spondylarthritis
          osteoarthritis

    721.3 Lumbosacral spondylosis without myelopathy
       Lumbar or lumbosacral:
          arthritis
          osteoarthritis
          spondylarthritis
       AHA: 4Q, '02, 107
       M47.817 Spondylosis w/o myelopath/radiculopath lumboscrl   **I-10**

√5ᵗʰ **721.4 Thoracic or lumbar spondylosis with myelopathy**

      721.41 Thoracic region   **CC**
          Spondylogenic compression of thoracic spinal cord
          CC Excl: 721.41

      721.42 Lumbar region   **CC**
          CC Excl: 721.3, 721.42, 722.10, 722.2, 722.32, 722.52-722.70, 722.73, 722.83-722.90, 722.93

    721.5 Kissing spine
       Baastrup's syndrome
       DEF: Compression of spinous processes of adjacent vertebrae; due to mutual contact.

    721.6 Ankylosing vertebral hyperostosis

    721.7 Traumatic spondylopathy   **CC**
       Kümmell's disease or spondylitis
       CC Excl: 721.7

---

§   Requires fifth digit. Valid digits are in [brackets] under each code. See beginning of section 710-739 for codes and defintions.

721.8 Other allied disorders of spine

√5ᵗʰ **721.9 Spondylosis of unspecified site**

721.90 Without mention of myelopathy
Spinal:
    arthritis (deformans) (degenerative) (hypertrophic)
osteoarthritis NOS
Spondylarthrosis NOS

721.91 With myelopathy   `CC`
Spondylogenic compression of spinal cord NOS
CC Exd: 721.0-721.91, 724.03

√4ᵗʰ **722 Intervertebral disc disorders**
AHA: 1Q, '88, 10

722.0 Displacement of cervical intervertebral disc without myelopathy
Neuritis (brachial) or radiculitis due to displacement or rupture of cervical intervertebral disc
Any condition classifiable to 722.2 of the cervical or cervicothoracic intervertebral disc
M50.20 Other cerv disc displacement uns cerv region   `I-10`

√5ᵗʰ **722.1 Displacement of thoracic or lumbar intervertebral disc without myelopathy**

722.10 Lumbar intervertebral disc without myelopathy
Lumbago or sciatica due to displacement of intervertebral disc
Neuritis or radiculitis due to displacement or rupture of lumbar intervertebral disc
Any condition classifiable to 722.2 of the lumbar or lumbosacral intervertebral disc
AHA: 4Q, '08, 184; 1Q, '07, 9; 3Q, '03, 12; 1Q, '03, 7; 4Q, '02, 107
M51.26 Oth intervertebral disc displcmnt lumbar region   `I-10`

722.11 Thoracic intervertebral disc without myelopathy
Any condition classifiable to 722.2 of thoracic intervertebral disc

Anatomy of Vertebral Disc

722.2 Displacement of intervertebral disc, site unspecified, without myelopathy
Discogenic syndrome NOS
Herniation of nucleus pulposus NOS
Intervertebral disc NOS:
    extrusion
    prolapse
    protrusion
    rupture
Neuritis or radiculitis due to displacement or rupture of intervertebral disc

√5ᵗʰ **722.3 Schmorl's nodes**
DEF: Irregular bone defect in the margin of the vertebral body; causes herniation into end plate of vertebral body.

722.30 Unspecified region

722.31 Thoracic region

722.32 Lumbar region

722.39 Other

722.4 Degeneration of cervical intervertebral disc
Degeneration of cervicothoracic intervertebral disc
M50.30 Other cerv disc degeneration uns cerv region   `I-10`

√5ᵗʰ **722.5 Degeneration of thoracic or lumbar intervertebral disc**

722.51 Thoracic or thoracolumbar intervertebral disc
AHA: 2Q, '11, 8

722.52 Lumbar or lumbosacral intervertebral disc
AHA: 2Q, '06, 18; 4Q, '04, 133
M51.37 Oth intervertebral disc degen lumbosacral region   `I-10`

722.6 Degeneration of intervertebral disc, site unspecified
Degenerative disc disease NOS
Narrowing of intervertebral disc or space NOS

√5ᵗʰ **722.7 Intervertebral disc disorder with myelopathy**

722.70 Unspecified region

722.71 Cervical region   `CC`
CC Exd: 722.0, 722.71

722.72 Thoracic region   `CC`
CC Exd: 722.11, 722.72

722.73 Lumbar region   `CC`
CC Exd: 722.11, 722.73, 724.03

√5ᵗʰ **722.8 Postlaminectomy syndrome**
DEF: Spinal disorder due to spinal laminectomy surgery.
AHA: J-F, '87, 7
TIP: Assign if documentation indicates that pain is due to scar tissue formation following disc surgery.

722.80 Unspecified region

722.81 Cervical region

722.82 Thoracic region

722.83 Lumbar region
AHA: 2Q, '97, 15
M96.1 Postlaminectomy syndrome NEC   `I-10`

√5ᵗʰ **722.9 Other and unspecified disc disorder**
Calcification of intervertebral cartilage or disc
Discitis

722.90 Unspecified region
AHA: N-D, '84, 19

722.91 Cervical region

722.92 Thoracic region

722.93 Lumbar region
M51.86 Other intervertebral disc disorder lumbar region   `I-10`

√4ᵗʰ **723 Other disorders of cervical region**
EXCLUDES conditions due to:
    intervertebral disc disorders (722.0-722.9)
    spondylosis (721.0-721.9)
AHA: 3Q, '94, 14; 2Q, '89, 14

723.0 Spinal stenosis in cervical region
AHA: 4Q, '03, 101
M48.02 Spinal stenosis cervical region   `I-10`

Derangement of Vertebral Disc

N Newborn Age: 0   P Pediatric Age: 0-17   M Maternity Age: 12-55   A Adult Age: 15-124   MCC Major CC Condition   CC CC Condition   HIV HIV Related Dx

244 – Volume 1   **2014 ICD-9-CM**

723.1 Cervicalgia
Pain in neck
DEF: Pain in cervical spine or neck region.
M54.2 Cervicalgia   `I-10`

723.2 Cervicocranial syndrome
Barré-Liéou syndrome
Posterior cervical sympathetic syndrome
DEF: Neurologic disorder of upper cervical spine and nerve roots.

723.3 Cervicobrachial syndrome (diffuse)
DEF: Complex of symptoms due to scalenus anterior muscle compressing the brachial plexus; pain radiates from shoulder to arm or back of neck.
AHA: N-D, '85, 12

723.4 Brachial neuritis or radiculitis NOS
Cervical radiculitis   Radicular syndrome of upper limbs

723.5 Torticollis, unspecified
Contracture of neck
> EXCLUDES   congenital (754.1)
> due to birth injury (767.8)
> hysterical (300.11)
> ocular torticollis (781.93)
> psychogenic (306.0)
> spasmodic (333.83)
> traumatic, current (847.0)

DEF: Abnormally positioned neck relative to head due to cervical muscle or fascia contractions; also called wryneck.
AHA: 2Q, '01, 21; 1Q, '95, 7

723.6 Panniculitis specified as affecting neck
DEF: Inflammation of the panniculus adiposus (subcutaneous fat) in the neck.

723.7 Ossification of posterior longitudinal ligament in cervical region

723.8 Other syndromes affecting cervical region
Cervical syndrome NEC   Occipital neuralgia
Klippel's disease
AHA: 1Q, '00, 7

723.9 Unspecified musculoskeletal disorders and symptoms referable to neck
Cervical (region) disorder NOS

√4th **724 Other and unspecified disorders of back**
> EXCLUDES   collapsed vertebra (code to cause, e.g., osteoporosis, 733.00-733.09)
> conditions due to:
> intervertebral disc disorders (722.0-722.9)
> spondylosis (721.0-721.9)

AHA: 2Q, '89, 14

√5th **724.0 Spinal stenosis, other than cervical**

724.00 Spinal stenosis, unspecified region
M48.00 Spinal stenosis site unspecified   `I-10`

724.01 Thoracic region

724.02 Lumbar region, without neurogenic claudication
Lumbar region NOS
AHA: 4Q, '08, 109; 4Q, '07, 120; 1Q, '07, 10, 20; 4Q, '99, 13
M48.06 Spinal stenosis lumbar region   `I-10`

724.03 Lumbar region, with neurogenic claudication
DEF: Spinal canal narrowing with nerve root compression causing muscle pain, fatigue, and weakness during extension of the lumbar spine; pain is relieved by sitting or bending.
AHA: 2Q, '11, 10; 4Q, '10, 89

724.09 Other

724.1 Pain in thoracic spine

724.2 Lumbago
Low back pain
Low back syndrome
Lumbalgia
AHA: 2Q, '07, 11; N-D, '85, 12
M54.5 Low back pain   `I-10`

724.3 Sciatica
Neuralgia or neuritis of sciatic nerve
> EXCLUDES   specified lesion of sciatic nerve (355.0)

AHA: 2Q, '89, 12
M54.30 Sciatica unspecified side   `I-10`

Stenosis in Cervical Region

724.4 Thoracic or lumbosacral neuritis or radiculitis, unspecified
Radicular syndrome of lower limbs
AHA: 2Q, '99, 3
M51.14 Intervertebral disc d/o w/radiculopathy thoracic   `I-10`

724.5 Backache, unspecified
Vertebrogenic (pain) syndrome NOS
M54.9 Dorsalgia unspecified   `I-10`

724.6 Disorders of sacrum
Ankylosis
Instability } lumbosacral or sacroiliac (joint)

√5th **724.7 Disorders of coccyx**

724.70 Unspecified disorder of coccyx

724.71 Hypermobility of coccyx

724.79 Other
Coccygodynia

724.8 Other symptoms referable to back
Ossification of posterior longitudinal ligament NOS
Panniculitis specified as sacral or affecting back

724.9 Other unspecified back disorders
Ankylosis of spine NOS
Compression of spinal nerve root NEC
Spinal disorder NOS
> EXCLUDES   sacroiliitis (720.2)

Rheumatism, Excluding the Back (725-729)

> INCLUDES   disorders of muscles and tendons and their attachments, and of other soft tissues

725 Polymyalgia rheumatica
DEF: Joint and muscle pain, pelvis, and shoulder girdle stiffness, high sedimentation rate and temporal arteritis; occurs in elderly.
M35.3 Polymyalgia rheumatica   `I-10`

√4th **726 Peripheral enthesopathies and allied syndromes**
> NOTE   Enthesopathies are disorders of peripheral ligamentous or muscular attachments.
> EXCLUDES   spinal enthesopathy (720.1)

726.0 Adhesive capsulitis of shoulder

√5th **726.1 Rotator cuff syndrome of shoulder and allied disorders**

726.10 Disorders of bursae and tendons in shoulder region, unspecified
Rotator cuff syndrome NOS
Supraspinatus syndrome NOS
AHA: 2Q, '01, 11
M75.50 Bursitis of unspecified shoulder   `I-10`

726.11 Calcifying tendinitis of shoulder

726.12 Bicipital tenosynovitis

726.13 Partial tear of rotator cuff
> EXCLUDES   complete rupture of rotator cuff, nontraumatic (727.61)

AHA: 4Q, '11, 135-136

726.19 Other specified disorders
> EXCLUDES   complete rupture of rotator cuff, nontraumatic (727.61)

4th / 5th   Additional Digit Required   Unacceptable PDx   Manifestation Code   Hospital Acquired Condition   ▶◀ Revised Text   ● New Code   ▲ Revised Code Title

2014 ICD-9-CM   Volume 1 – 245

726.2 Other affections of shoulder region, not elsewhere classified
Periarthritis of shoulder
Scapulohumeral fibrositis

√5ᵗʰ **726.3 Enthesopathy of elbow region**

726.30 Enthesopathy of elbow, unspecified

726.31 Medial epicondylitis

726.32 Lateral epicondylitis
Epicondylitis NOS
Golfers' elbow
Tennis elbow

726.33 Olecranon bursitis
Bursitis of elbow

726.39 Other

726.4 Enthesopathy of wrist and carpus
Bursitis of hand or wrist
Periarthritis of wrist

726.5 Enthesopathy of hip region
Bursitis of hip
Gluteal tendinitis
Iliac crest spur
Psoas tendinitis
Trochanteric tendinitis

√5ᵗʰ **726.6 Enthesopathy of knee**

726.60 Enthesopathy of knee, unspecified
Bursitis of knee NOS

726.61 Pes anserinus tendinitis or bursitis
DEF: Inflamed tendons of sartorius, gracilis and semitendinosus muscles of medial aspect of knee.

726.62 Tibial collateral ligament bursitis
Pellegrini-Stieda syndrome

726.63 Fibular collateral ligament bursitis

726.64 Patellar tendinitis

726.65 Prepatellar bursitis
AHA: 2Q, '06, 15

726.69 Other
Bursitis:
infrapatellar
subpatellar

√5ᵗʰ **726.7 Enthesopathy of ankle and tarsus**

726.70 Enthesopathy of ankle and tarsus, unspecified
Metatarsalgia NOS
EXCLUDES *Morton's metatarsalgia (355.6)*

726.71 Achilles bursitis or tendinitis

726.72 Tibialis tendinitis
Tibialis (anterior) (posterior) tendinitis

726.73 Calcaneal spur
DEF: Overgrowth of calcaneus bone; causes pain on walking; due to chronic avulsion injury of plantar fascia from calcaneus.

726.79 Other
Peroneal tendinitis

726.8 Other peripheral enthesopathies

√5ᵗʰ **726.9 Unspecified enthesopathy**

726.90 Enthesopathy of unspecified site
Capsulitis NOS   Tendinitis NOS
Periarthritis NOS

726.91 Exostosis of unspecified site
Bone spur NOS
AHA: 2Q, '01, 15

√4ᵗʰ **727 Other disorders of synovium, tendon, and bursa**

√5ᵗʰ **727.0 Synovitis and tenosynovitis**

727.00 Synovitis and tenosynovitis, unspecified
Synovitis NOS
Tenosynovitis NOS
M65.9 Synovitis and tenosynovitis unspecified I-10

Bunion

Normal metatarsophalangeal joint

Exostosis

727.01 Synovitis and tenosynovitis in diseases classified elsewhere
Code first underlying disease as:
tuberculosis (015.0-015.9)
EXCLUDES *crystal-induced (275.4)*
gonococcal (098.51)
gout (274.00-274.03)
syphilitic (095.7)

727.02 Giant cell tumor of tendon sheath

727.03 Trigger finger (acquired)
DEF: Stenosing tenosynovitis or nodule in flexor tendon; cessation of flexion or extension movement in finger, followed by snapping into place.

727.04 Radial styloid tenosynovitis
de Quervain's disease

727.05 Other tenosynovitis of hand and wrist

727.06 Tenosynovitis of foot and ankle

727.09 Other

727.1 Bunion
DEF: Enlarged first metatarsal head due to inflamed bursa; results in laterally displaced great toe.

727.2 Specific bursitides often of occupational origin
Beat: Chronic crepitant synovitis of wrist
elbow   Miners':
hand   elbow
knee   knee

727.3 Other bursitis
Bursitis NOS
EXCLUDES *bursitis:*
gonococcal (098.52)
subacromial (726.19)
subcoracoid (726.19)
subdeltoid (726.19)
syphilitic (095.7)
"frozen shoulder" (726.0)

√5ᵗʰ **727.4 Ganglion and cyst of synovium, tendon, and bursa**

727.40 Synovial cyst, unspecified
EXCLUDES *that of popliteal space (727.51)*
AHA: 2Q, '97, 6

727.41 Ganglion of joint

Ganglia

Extensor tendon sheaths

Ganglion of wrist (fluid-filled sac)

Baker's cyst connected to knee joint synovial cavity

N Newborn Age: 0   P Pediatric Age: 0-17   M Maternity Age: 12-55   A Adult Age: 15-124   MCC Major CC Condition   CC CC Condition   HIV HIV Related D

246 – Volume 1   2014 ICD-9-CM

727.42 Ganglion of tendon sheath

727.43 Ganglion, unspecified

727.49 Other
Cyst of bursa

√5ᵗʰ **727.5 Rupture of synovium**

727.50 Rupture of synovium, unspecified

727.51 Synovial cyst of popliteal space
Baker's cyst (knee)

727.59 Other

√5ᵗʰ **727.6 Rupture of tendon, nontraumatic**

727.60 Nontraumatic rupture of unspecified tendon

727.61 Complete rupture of rotator cuff
EXCLUDES *partial tear of rotator cuff (726.13)*
AHA: 4Q, '11, 136

727.62 Tendons of biceps (long head)

727.63 Extensor tendons of hand and wrist

727.64 Flexor tendons of hand and wrist

727.65 Quadriceps tendon

727.66 Patellar tendon

727.67 Achilles tendon

727.68 Other tendons of foot and ankle

727.69 Other

√5ᵗʰ **727.8 Other disorders of synovium, tendon, and bursa**

727.81 Contracture of tendon (sheath)
Short Achilles tendon (acquired)

727.82 Calcium deposits in tendon and bursa
Calcification of tendon NOS
Calcific tendinitis NOS
EXCLUDES *peripheral ligamentous or muscular attachments (726.0-726.9)*

727.83 Plica syndrome
Plica knee
DEF: A fold in the synovial tissue formed before birth, creating a septum between two pockets of synovial tissue; most common are the medial patellar plica and the suprapatellar plica. Plica syndrome, or plica knee, refers to symptomatic plica.
AHA: 4Q, '00, 44

727.89 Other
Abscess of bursa or tendon
EXCLUDES *xanthomatosis localized to tendons (272.7)*
AHA: 2Q, '89, 15

727.9 Unspecified disorder of synovium, tendon, and bursa

√4ᵗʰ **728 Disorders of muscle, ligament, and fascia**
EXCLUDES *enthesopathies (726.0-726.9)*
muscular dystrophies (359.0-359.1)
myoneural disorders (358.00-358.9)
myopathies (359.2-359.9)
nontraumatic hematoma of muscle (729.92)
old disruption of ligaments of knee (717.81-717.89)

728.0 Infective myositis CC
Myositis: Myositis:
purulent   suppurative
EXCLUDES *myositis:*
epidemic (074.1)
interstitial (728.81)
syphilitic (095.6)
tropical (040.81)
CC Excl: 567.31, 728.0, 728.11-728.3, 728.81, 728.86
DEF: Inflamed connective septal tissue of muscle.

√5ᵗʰ **728.1 Muscular calcification and ossification**

728.10 Calcification and ossification, unspecified
Massive calcification (paraplegic)

728.11 Progressive myositis ossificans
DEF: Progressive myositic disease; marked by bony tissue formed by voluntary muscle; occurs among very young.

728.12 Traumatic myositis ossificans
Myositis ossificans (circumscripta)

728.13 Postoperative heterotopic calcification
DEF: Abnormal formation of calcium deposits in muscular tissue after surgery, marked by a corresponding loss of muscle tone and tension.

728.19 Other
Polymyositis ossificans

728.2 Muscular wasting and disuse atrophy, not elsewhere classified
Amyotrophia NOS   Myofibrosis
EXCLUDES *neuralgic amyotrophy (353.5)*
pelvic muscle wasting and disuse atrophy (618.83)
progressive muscular atrophy (335.0-335.9)

728.3 Other specific muscle disorders
Arthrogryposis
Immobility syndrome (paraplegic)
EXCLUDES *arthrogryposis multiplex congenita (754.89)*
stiff-man syndrome (333.91)

728.4 Laxity of ligament

728.5 Hypermobility syndrome

728.6 Contracture of palmar fascia A
Dupuytren's contracture
DEF: Dupuytren's contracture: flexion deformity of finger, due to shortened, thickened fibrosing of palmar fascia; cause unknown; associated with long-standing epilepsy.

√5ᵗʰ **728.7 Other fibromatoses**

728.71 Plantar fascial fibromatosis
Contracture of plantar fascia
Plantar fasciitis (traumatic)
DEF: Plantar fascia fibromatosis; causes nodular swelling and pain; not associated with contractures.

728.79 Other
Garrod's or knuckle pads
Nodular fasciitis
Pseudosarcomatous fibromatosis (proliferative) (subcutaneous)
DEF: Knuckle pads: Pea-size nodules on dorsal surface of interphalangeal joints; new growth of fibrous tissue with thickened dermis and epidermis.

√5ᵗʰ **728.8 Other disorders of muscle, ligament, and fascia**

728.81 Interstitial myositis
DEF: Inflammation of septal connective parts of muscle tissue.

728.82 Foreign body granuloma of muscle
Talc granuloma of muscle
Use additional code to identify foreign body (V90.01-V90.9)

728.83 Rupture of muscle, nontraumatic

728.84 Diastasis of muscle
Diastasis recti (abdomen)
EXCLUDES *diastasis recti complicating pregnancy, labor, and delivery (665.8)*
DEF: Muscle separation, such as recti abdominis after repeated pregnancies.

728.85 Spasm of muscle
M62.838 Other muscle spasm I-10

728.86 Necrotizing fasciitis MCC
Use additional code to identify:
gangrene (785.4), if applicable
infectious organism (041.00-041.89)
DEF: Fulminating infection begins with extensive cellulitis, spreads to superficial and deep fascia; causes thrombosis of subcutaneous vessels, and gangrene of underlying tissue.
CC Excl: 567.31, 728.0, 728.11-728.3, 728.81, 728.86
AHA: 4Q, '95, 54

728.87 Muscle weakness (generalized)
EXCLUDES *generalized weakness (780.79)*
AHA: 1Q, '05, 13; 4Q, '03, 66
TIP: Assign an additional code from category 438 if the weakness is a result of a CVA.

728.88 Rhabdomyolysis `CC`
DEF: A disintegration or destruction of muscle; an acute disease characterized by the excretion of myoglobin into the urine.
CC Excl: 567.31, 728.0, 728.11-728.3, 728.81, 728.86, 728.88
AHA: 4Q, '03, 66

728.89 Other
Eosinophilic fasciitis
Use additional E code to identify drug, if drug induced
DEF: Eosinophilic fasciitis: inflammation of fascia of extremities associated with eosinophilia, edema, and swelling; occurs alone or as part of myalgia syndrome.
AHA: 3Q, '06, 13; 3Q, '02, 28; 2Q, '01, 14, 15

728.9 Unspecified disorder of muscle, ligament, and fascia

✓4ᵗʰ 729 Other disorders of soft tissues
EXCLUDES acroparesthesia (443.89)
carpal tunnel syndrome (354.0)
disorders of the back (720.0-724.9)
entrapment syndromes (354.0-355.9)
palindromic rheumatism (719.3)
periarthritis (726.0-726.9)
psychogenic rheumatism (306.0)

729.0 Rheumatism, unspecified and fibrositis
DEF: General term describes diseases of muscle, tendon, nerve, joint, or bone; symptoms include pain and stiffness.

729.1 Myalgia and myositis, unspecified
Fibromyositis NOS
DEF: Myalgia: muscle pain.
DEF: Myositis: inflamed voluntary muscle.
DEF: Fibromyositis: inflamed fibromuscular tissue.
M79.1 Myalgia `I-10`

729.2 Neuralgia, neuritis, and radiculitis, unspecified
EXCLUDES brachial radiculitis (723.4)
cervical radiculitis (723.4)
lumbosacral radiculitis (724.4)
mononeuritis (354.0-355.9)
radiculitis due to intervertebral disc involvement (722.0-722.2, 722.7)
sciatica (724.3)
DEF: Neuralgia: paroxysmal pain along nerve; symptoms include brief pain and tenderness at point nerve exits.
DEF: Neuritis: inflamed nerve, symptoms include paresthesia, paralysis and loss of reflexes at nerve site.
DEF: Radiculitis: inflamed nerve root.

✓5ᵗʰ 729.3 Panniculitis, unspecified
DEF: Inflammatory reaction of subcutaneous fat; causes nodules; often develops in abdominal region.

729.30 Panniculitis, unspecified site
Weber-Christian disease
DEF: Febrile, nodular, nonsuppurative, relapsing inflammation of subcutaneous fat.

729.31 Hypertrophy of fat pad, knee
Hypertrophy of infrapatellar fat pad

729.39 Other site
EXCLUDES panniculitis specified as (affecting):
back (724.8)
neck (723.6)
sacral (724.8)
AHA: 2Q, '11, 3

729.4 Fasciitis, unspecified
EXCLUDES necrotizing fasciitis (728.86)
nodular fasciitis (728.79)
AHA: 2Q, '94, 13

729.5 Pain in limb
AHA: 2Q, '07, 11
M79.609 Pain in unspecified limb `I-10`

729.6 Residual foreign body in soft tissue
Use additional code to identify foreign body (V90.01-V90.9)
EXCLUDES foreign body granuloma:
muscle (728.82)
skin and subcutaneous tissue (709.4)

✓5ᵗʰ 729.7 Nontraumatic compartment syndrome
Code first, if applicable, postprocedural complication (998.89)
EXCLUDES compartment syndrome NOS (958.90)
traumatic compartment syndrome (958.90-958.99)
DEF: Compression of nerves and blood vessels within an enclosed space, leading to impaired blood flow and muscle and nerve damage.

729.71 Nontraumatic compartment syndrome of upper extremity `CC`
Nontraumatic compartment syndrome of shoulder, arm, forearm, wrist, hand, and fingers
CC Excl: 729.81, 729.89-729.99, 903.8, 904.9
AHA: 4Q, '06, 100-102

729.72 Nontraumatic compartment syndrome of lower extremity `CC`
Nontraumatic compartment syndrome of hip, buttock, thigh, leg, foot, and toes
CC Excl: 729.81, 729.89-729.99, 904.7, 904.9
AHA: 4Q, '06, 100-102

729.73 Nontraumatic compartment syndrome of abdomen `CC`
CC Excl: 863.0-867.3, 867.5-868.14, 869.0-869.1, 879.2-879.9, 929.0-929.9, 958.8, 959.8-959.9
AHA: 4Q, '06, 100-102

729.79 Nontraumatic compartment syndrome of other sites `CC`
CC Excl: 868.03-868.10, 868.13-869.1
AHA: 4Q, '06, 100-102

✓5ᵗʰ 729.8 Other musculoskeletal symptoms referable to limbs

729.81 Swelling of limb
AHA: 4Q, '88, 6
TIP: Assign for hyperalgesic pseudothrombophlebitis, which involves painful swelling of the lower extremity and mimics deep vein thrombosis (DVT).

729.82 Cramp

729.89 Other
EXCLUDES abnormality of gait (781.2)
tetany (781.7)
transient paralysis of limb (781.4)
AHA: 4Q, '88, 12
R29.898 Oth symptoms & signs involv musculoskeletal system `I-10`

✓5ᵗʰ 729.9 Other and unspecified disorders of soft tissue
AHA: 4Q, '08, 134-136

729.90 Disorders of soft tissue, unspecified

729.91 Post-traumatic seroma
EXCLUDES seroma complicating a procedure (998.13)

729.92 Nontraumatic hematoma of soft tissue
Nontraumatic hematoma of muscle
AHA: 4Q, '08, 135
TIP: Assign an additional E code for a drug adverse effect if caused by Coumadin or other anticoagulants.

729.99 Other disorders of soft tissue
Polyalgia

Osteopathies, Chondropathies, and Acquired Musculoskeletal Deformities (730-739)

√4ᵗʰ **730 Osteomyelitis, periostitis, and other infections involving bone**

> EXCLUDES   jaw (526.4-526.5)
>   petrous bone (383.2)

> Use additional code to identify organism, such as Staphylococcus (041.1)

> The following fifth-digit subclassification is for use with category 730; valid digits are in [brackets] under each code. See list at beginning of chapter for definitions.
>   0 site unspecified
>   1 shoulder region
>   2 upper arm
>   3 forearm
>   4 hand
>   5 pelvic region and thigh
>   6 lower leg
>   7 ankle and foot
>   8 other specified sites
>   9 multiple sites

> **DEF:** Osteomyelitis: bacterial inflammation of bone tissue and marrow.
> **DEF:** Periostitis: inflammation of specialized connective tissue; causes swelling of bone and aching pain.
> **AHA:** 4Q, '97, 43

§ √5ᵗʰ **730.0 Acute osteomyelitis**   CC
[0-9]
> Abscess of any bone except accessory sinus, jaw, or mastoid
> Acute or subacute osteomyelitis, with or without mention of periostitis
> Use additional code to identify major osseous defect, if applicable (731.3)
> **CC Excl: For code 730.00:** 015.50-015.56, 015.70-015.76, 015.90-015.96, 017.90-017.96, 730.00-730.39, 730.80-730.99 **For code 730.01:** 015.50-015.56, 015.70-015.76, 015.90-015.96, 017.90-017.96, 730.00, 730.08-730.11, 730.18-730.21, 730.28-730.31, 730.38-730.39, 730.80-730.81, 730.88-730.91, 730.98-730.99 **For code 730.02:** 015.50-015.56, 015.70-015.76, 015.90-015.96, 017.90-017.96, 730.00, 730.08-730.10, 730.12, 730.18-730.20, 730.22, 730.28-730.30, 730.32, 730.38-730.39, 730.80, 730.82, 730.88-730.90, 730.92, 730.98-730.99 **For code 730.03:** 015.50-015.56, 015.70-015.76, 015.90-015.96, 017.90-017.96, 730.00, 730.08-730.10, 730.13, 730.18-730.20, 730.23, 730.28-730.30, 730.33, 730.38-730.39, 730.80, 730.83, 730.88-730.90, 730.93, 730.98-730.99 **For code 730.04:** 015.50-015.56, 015.70-015.76, 015.90-015.96, 017.90-017.96, 730.00, 730.08-730.10, 730.14, 730.18-730.20, 730.24, 730.28-730.30, 730.34, 730.38-730.39, 730.80, 730.84, 730.88-730.90, 730.94, 730.98-730.99 **For code 730.05:** 015.10-015.16, 015.50-015.56, 015.70-015.76, 015.90-015.96, 017.90-017.96, 730.00, 730.08-730.10, 730.15, 730.18-730.20, 730.25, 730.28-730.30, 730.35, 730.38-730.39, 730.80, 730.85, 730.88-730.90, 730.95, 730.98-730.99 **For code 730.06:** 015.20-015.56, 015.70-015.76, 015.90-015.96, 017.90-017.96, 730.00, 730.08-730.10, 730.16, 730.18-730.20, 730.26, 730.28-730.30, 730.36, 730.38-730.39, 730.80, 730.86, 730.88-730.90, 730.96, 730.98-730.99 **For code 730.07:** 015.50-015.56, 015.70-015.76, 015.90-015.96, 017.90-017.96, 730.00, 730.08-730.10, 730.17-730.20, 730.27-730.30, 730.37-730.39, 730.80, 730.87-730.90, 730.97-730.99 **For code 730.08:** 015.00-015.06, 015.50-015.56, 015.70-015.76, 015.90-015.96, 017.90-017.96, 730.00-730.39, 730.80-730.99 **For code 730.09:** 015.50-015.56, 015.70-015.76, 015.90-015.96, 017.90-017.96, 730.00-730.39, 730.80-730.99
> **AHA:** 4Q, '06, 103; **For code 730.06:** 1Q, '02, 4; **For code 730.07:** 1Q, '04, 14

§ √5ᵗʰ **730.1 Chronic osteomyelitis**   CC
[0-9]
> Brodie's abscess
> Chronic or old osteomyelitis, with or without mention of periostitis
> Sclerosing osteomyelitis of Garré
> Sequestrum of bone
> Use additional code to identify major osseous defect, if applicable (731.3)
> EXCLUDES   aseptic necrosis of bone (733.40-733.49)
> **CC Excl: For code 730.10:** 730.10-730.39, 730.80-731.1; **For codes 730.11-730.19:** 003.24, 015.50-015.56, 015.70-015.76, 015.90-015.96, 017.90-017.96, 730.00-730.39, 730.80-730.99
> **AHA:** 4Q, '06, 103; **For code 730.17:** 3Q, '11, 15; 3Q, '00, 4

§ √5ᵗʰ **730.2 Unspecified osteomyelitis**   CC
[0-9]
> Osteitis or osteomyelitis NOS, with or without mention of periostitis
> Use additional code to identify major osseous defect, if applicable (731.3)
> **CC Excl: For code 730.20:** 730.10-730.39, 730.80-731.1; **For codes 730.21-730.29:** 003.24, 015.50-015.56, 015.70-015.76, 015.90-015.96, 017.90-017.96, 730.00-730.39, 730.80-730.99
> **AHA:** 4Q, '06, 103;
> M86.9 Osteomyelitis unspecified   I-10

§ √5ᵗʰ **730.3 Periostitis without mention of osteomyelitis**
[0-9]
> Abscess of periosteum ⎫ without mention of
> Periostosis   ⎬   osteomyelitis
> EXCLUDES   that in secondary syphilis (091.61)

§ √5ᵗʰ **730.7 *Osteopathy resulting from poliomyelitis***
[0-9]
> *Code first underlying disease (045.0-045.9)*

§ √5ᵗʰ **730.8 *Other infections involving bone in diseases classified elsewhere***   CC
[0-9]
> *Code first underlying disease as:*
>   tuberculosis (015.0-015.9)
>   typhoid fever (002.0)
> EXCLUDES   syphilis of bone NOS (095.5)
> **CC Excl: For codes 730.80, 730.89:** 015.50-015.56, 015.70-015.76, 015.90-015.96, 017.90-017.96, 730.00-730.39, 730.80-730.99; **For code 730.81:** 015.50-015.56, 015.70-015.76, 015.90-015.96, 017.90-017.96, 730.00-730.01, 730.08-730.11, 730.18-730.21, 730.28-730.31, 730.38-730.39, 730.80, 730.88-730.91, 730.98-730.99;
> **For code 730.82:** 015.50-015.56, 015.70-015.76, 015.90-015.96, 017.90-017.96, 730.00, 730.02, 730.08-730.10, 730.12, 730.18-730.20, 730.22, 730.28-730.30, 730.32, 730.38-730.39, 730.80, 730.88-730.90, 730.92, 730.98-730.99; **For code 730.83:** 015.50-015.56, 015.70-015.76, 015.90-015.96, 017.90-017.96, 730.00, 730.03, 730.08-730.10, 730.13, 730.18-730.20, 730.23, 730.28-730.30, 730.33, 730.38-730.39, 730.80, 730.88-730.90, 730.93, 730.98-730.99; **For code 730.84:** 015.50-015.56, 015.70-015.76, 015.90-015.96, 017.90-017.96, 730.00, 730.04, 730.08-730.10, 730.14, 730.18-730.20, 730.24, 730.28-730.30, 730.34, 730.38-730.39, 730.80, 730.88-730.90, 730.94, 730.98-730.99; **For code 730.85:** 015.10-015.16, 015.50-015.56, 015.70-015.76, 015.90-015.96, 017.90-017.96, 730.00, 730.05, 730.08-730.10, 730.15, 730.18-730.20, 730.25, 730.28-730.30, 730.35, 730.38-730.39, 730.80, 730.88-730.90, 730.95, 730.98-730.99; **For code 730.86:** 015.20-015.56, 015.70-015.76, 015.90-015.96, 017.90-017.96, 730.00, 730.06, 730.08-730.10, 730.16, 730.18-730.20, 730.26, 730.28-730.30, 730.36, 730.38-730.39, 730.80, 730.88-730.90, 730.96, 730.98-730.99; **For code 730.87:** 015.50-015.56, 015.70-015.76, 015.90-015.96, 017.90-017.96, 730.00, 730.07-730.10, 730.17-730.20, 730.27-730.30, 730.37-730.39, 730.80, 730.88-730.90, 730.97-730.99; **For code 730.88:** 015.00-015.06, 015.50-015.56, 015.70-015.76, 015.90-015.96, 017.90-017.96, 730.00-730.39, 730.80-730.99
> **AHA:** 2Q, '97, 16; 3Q, '91, 10

§ √5ᵗʰ **730.9 Unspecified infection of bone**   CC
[0-9]
> **CC Excl: For codes 730.90, 730.99:** 015.50-015.56, 015.70-015.76, 015.90-015.96, 017.90-017.96, 730.00-730.39, 730.80-730.99; **For code 730.91:** 015.50-015.56, 015.70-015.76, 015.90-015.96, 017.90-017.96, 730.00-730.01, 730.08-730.11, 730.18-730.21, 730.28-730.31, 730.38-730.39, 730.80-730.81, 730.88-730.90, 730.98-730.99; **For code 730.92:** 015.50-015.56, 015.70-015.76, 015.90-015.96, 017.90-017.96, 730.00, 730.02, 730.08-730.10, 730.12, 730.18-730.20, 730.22, 730.28-730.30, 730.32, 730.38-730.39, 730.80, 730.82, 730.88-730.90, 730.98-730.99; **For code 730.93:** 015.50-015.56, 015.70-015.76, 015.90-015.96, 017.90-017.96, 730.00, 730.03, 730.08-730.10, 730.13, 730.18-730.20, 730.23, 730.33, 730.38-730.39, 730.80, 730.83, 730.88-730.90, 730.98-730.99; **For code 730.94:** 015.50-015.56, 015.70-015.76, 015.90-015.96, 017.90-017.96, 730.00, 730.04, 730.08-730.10, 730.14, 730.18-730.20, 730.24, 730.28-730.30, 730.34, 730.38-730.39, 730.80, 730.84, 730.88-730.90, 730.98-730.99; **For code 730.95:** 015.10-015.16, 015.50-015.56, 015.70-015.76, 015.90-015.96, 017.90-017.96, 730.00, 730.05, 730.08-730.10, 730.15, 730.18-730.20, 730.25, 730.28-730.30, 730.35, 730.38-730.39, 730.80, 730.85, 730.88-730.90, 730.98-730.99; **For code 730.96:** 015.20-015.56, 015.70-015.76, 015.90-015.96, 017.90-017.96, 730.00, 730.06, 730.08-730.10, 730.16, 730.18-730.20, 730.26, 730.28-730.30, 730.36, 730.38-730.39, 730.80, 730.86, 730.88-730.90, 730.98-730.99; **For code 730.97:** 015.50-015.56, 015.70-015.76, 015.90-015.96, 017.90-017.96, 730.00, 730.07-730.10, 730.17-730.20, 730.27-730.30, 730.37-730.39, 730.80, 730.87-730.90, 730.98-730.99; **For code 730.98:** 0015.00-015.06, 015.50-015.56, 015.70-015.76, 015.90-015.96, 017.90-017.96, 730.00-730.39, 730.80-730.99

---

§   Requires fifth digit. Valid digits are in [brackets] under each code. See beginning of section 710-739 for codes and defintions.

√4ᵗʰ/√5ᵗʰ Additional Digit Required   Unacceptable PDx   Manifestation Code   Hospital Acquired Condition   ►◄ Revised Text   ● New Code   ▲ Revised Code Title

Diseases of the Musculoskeletal System and Connective Tissue

731–733.09

√4ᵗʰ 731 Osteitis deformans and osteopathies associated with other disorders classified elsewhere

DEF: Osteitis deformans: Bone disease marked by episodes of increased bone loss, excessive repair attempts; causes weakened, deformed bones with increased mass, bowed long bones, deformed flat bones, pain and pathological fractures; may be fatal if associated with congestive heart failure, giant cell tumors or bone sarcoma; also called Paget's disease.

731.0 Osteitis deformans without mention of bone tumor
Paget's disease of bone

731.1 Osteitis deformans in diseases classified elsewhere
Code first underlying disease as:
malignant neoplasm of bone (170.0-170.9)

731.2 Hypertrophic pulmonary osteoarthropathy
Bamberger-Marie disease
DEF: Clubbing of fingers and toes; related to enlarged ends of long bones, due to chronic lung and heart disease.

731.3 Major osseous defects
Code first underlying disease, if known, such as:
aseptic necrosis (733.40-733.49)
malignant neoplasm of bone (170.0-170.9)
osteomyelitis (730.00-730.29)
osteoporosis (733.00-733.09)
peri-prosthetic osteolysis (996.45)
AHA: 4Q, '06, 103

731.8 Other bone involvement in diseases classified elsewhere
Code first underlying disease as:
diabetes mellitus (249.8, 250.8)

Use additional code to specify bone condition, such as:
acute osteomyelitis (730.00-730.09)
AHA: 2Q, '10, 6; 1Q, '04, 14; 4Q, '97, 43; 2Q, '97, 16
TIP: For diabetic osteomyelitis, assign a total of three codes: 250.8X, 731.8, and a code from category 730.
M90.89 Osteopathy dz classified elsewhere multiple site   I-10

√4ᵗʰ 732 Osteochondropathies
DEF: Conditions related to both bone and cartilage, or conditions in which cartilage is converted to bone (enchondral ossification).

732.0 Juvenile osteochondrosis of spine
Juvenile osteochondrosis (of):
marginal or vertebral epiphysis (of Scheuermann)
spine NOS
Vertebral epiphysitis
EXCLUDES *adolescent postural kyphosis (737.0)*

732.1 Juvenile osteochondrosis of hip and pelvis
Coxa plana
Ischiopubic synchondrosis (of van Neck)
Osteochondrosis (juvenile) of:
acetabulum
head of femur (of Legg-Calvé-Perthes)
iliac crest (of Buchanan)
symphysis pubis (of Pierson)
Pseudocoxalgia

732.2 Nontraumatic slipped upper femoral epiphysis
Slipped upper femoral epiphysis NOS

732.3 Juvenile osteochondrosis of upper extremity
Osteochondrosis (juvenile) of:
capitulum of humerus (of Panner)
carpal lunate (of Kienbock)
hand NOS
head of humerus (of Haas)
heads of metacarpals (of Mauclaire)
lower ulna (of Burns)
radial head (of Brailsford)
upper extremity NOS

732.4 Juvenile osteochondrosis of lower extremity, excluding foot
Osteochondrosis (juvenile) of:
lower extremity NOS
primary patellar center (of Köhler)
proximal tibia (of Blount)
secondary patellar center (of Sinding-Larsen)
tibial tubercle (of Osgood-Schlatter)
Tibia vara

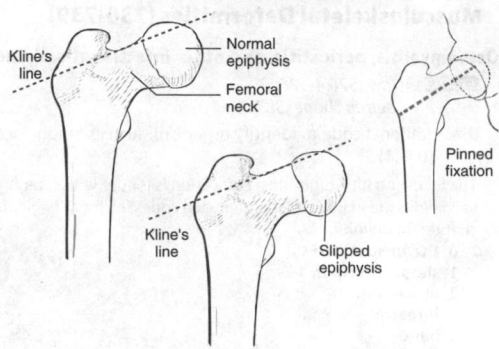

Slipped Femoral Epiphysis

Kline's line — Normal epiphysis — Femoral neck — Pinned fixation — Kline's line — Slipped epiphysis

732.5 Juvenile osteochondrosis of foot
Calcaneal apophysitis
Epiphysitis, os calcis
Osteochondrosis (juvenile) of:
astragalus (of Diaz)
calcaneum (of Sever)
foot NOS
metatarsal
second (of Freiberg)
fifth (of Iselin)
os tibiale externum (of Haglund)
tarsal navicular (of Köhler)

732.6 Other juvenile osteochondrosis
Apophysitis
Epiphysitis } specified as juvenile, of other
Osteochondritis } site, or site NOS
Osteochondrosis

732.7 Osteochondritis dissecans

732.8 Other specified forms of osteochondropathy
Adult osteochondrosis of spine

732.9 Unspecified osteochondropathy
Apophysitis   NOS
Epiphysitis   not specified as adult or
Osteochondritis } juvenile, of unspecified
Osteochondrosis } site

√4ᵗʰ 733 Other disorders of bone and cartilage
EXCLUDES *bone spur (726.91)*
cartilage of, or loose body in, joint (717.0-717.9, 718.0-718.9)
giant cell granuloma of jaw (526.3)
osteitis fibrosa cystica generalisata (252.01)
osteomalacia (268.2)
polyostotic fibrous dysplasia of bone (756.54)
prognathism, retrognathism (524.1)
xanthomatosis localized to bone (272.7)

√5ᵗʰ 733.0 Osteoporosis
Use additional code to identify major osseous defect, if applicable (731.3)
Use additional code to identify personal history of pathologic (healed) fracture (V13.51)
DEF: Bone mass reduction that ultimately results in fractures after minimal trauma; dorsal kyphosis or loss of height often occur.
AHA: 4Q, '06, 103

733.00 Osteoporosis, unspecified
Wedging of vertebra NOS
AHA: 4Q, '07, 92; 1Q, '07, 22; 3Q, '01, 19; 2Q, '98, 12
M81.0 Age-related osteoporosis w/o curr path fx   I-10

733.01 Senile osteoporosis
Postmenopausal osteoporosis
AHA: 1Q, '07, 5, 6

733.02 Idiopathic osteoporosis
M81.8 Other osteoporosis w/o current pathological fx   I-10

733.03 Disuse osteoporosis

733.09 Other
Drug-induced osteoporosis
Use additional E code to identify drug
AHA: 4Q, '03, 108

N Newborn Age: 0   **P** Pediatric Age: 0-17   **M** Maternity Age: 12-55   **A** Adult Age: 15-124   **MCC** Major CC Condition   **CC** CC Condition   **HIV** HIV Related Dx

250 – Volume 1   2014 ICD-9-CM

√5ᵗʰ **733.1 Pathologic fracture**
Chronic fracture
Spontaneous fracture
EXCLUDES *stress fracture (733.93-733.95)*
traumatic fracture (800-829)
DEF: Fracture due to bone structure weakening by pathological processes (e.g., osteoporosis, neoplasms and osteomalacia).
AHA: 4Q, '08, 158; 1Q, '07, 3-4; 4Q, '93, 25; N-D, '86, 10; N-D, '85, 16
TIP: Assign only for newly diagnosed fractures; refer to V code aftercare categories if patient is receiving routine care during healing or recovery phase.

733.10 Pathologic fracture, unspecified site `CC`
CC Exd: 733.10-733.19, 733.93-733.98

733.11 Pathologic fracture of humerus `CC`
CC Exd: See code 733.10
AHA: 2Q, '10, 6

733.12 Pathologic fracture of distal radius and ulna `CC`
Wrist NOS
CC Exd: See code 733.10

733.13 Pathologic fracture of vertebrae `CC`
Collapse of vertebra NOS
CC Exd: See code 733.10
AHA: 3Q, '08, 4; 1Q, '07, 5, 6, 22; 3Q, '99, 5
TIP: Assign for a chronic vertebral pathological fracture for which the patient is receiving medication.
M48.53xA Collasped vertebra NEC cervicothorac initial enc `I-10`

733.14 Pathologic fracture of neck of femur `CC`
Femur NOS
Hip NOS
CC Exd: See code 733.10
AHA: 1Q, '01, 1; 1Q, '96, 16

733.15 Pathologic fracture of other specified part of femur `CC`
CC Exd: See code 733.10
AHA: 2Q, '98, 12

733.16 Pathologic fracture of tibia or fibula `CC`
Ankle NOS
CC Exd: See code 733.10

733.19 Pathologic fracture of other specified site `CC`
CC Exd: See code 733.10

√5ᵗʰ **733.2 Cyst of bone**

733.20 Cyst of bone (localized), unspecified

733.21 Solitary bone cyst
Unicameral bone cyst

733.22 Aneurysmal bone cyst
DEF: Solitary bone lesion, bulges into periosteum; marked by calcified rim.

733.29 Other
Fibrous dysplasia (monostotic)
EXCLUDES *cyst of jaw (526.0-526.2, 526.89)*
osteitis fibrosa cystica (252.01)
polyostotic fibrousdysplasia of bone (756.54)

733.3 Hyperostosis of skull
Hyperostosis interna frontalis
Leontiasis ossium
DEF: Abnormal bone growth on inner aspect of cranial bones.

√5ᵗʰ **733.4 Aseptic necrosis of bone**
Use additional code to identify major osseous defect, if applicable (731.3)
EXCLUDES *osteochondropathies (732.0-732.9)*
DEF: Infarction of bone tissue due to a noninfectious etiology, such as a fracture, ischemic disorder or administration of immunosuppressive drugs; leads to degenerative joint disease or nonunion of fractures.
AHA: 4Q, '06, 103

733.40 Aseptic necrosis of bone, site unspecified `CC`
CC Exd: 733.40-733.49

733.41 Head of humerus `CC`
CC Exd: 733.40-733.41, 733.45-733.49

733.42 Head and neck of femur `CC`
Femur NOS
EXCLUDES *Legg-Calvé-Perthes disease (732.1)*
CC Exd: 733.40, 733.42, 733.45-733.49
M87.256 Osteonecrosis due to previous trauma uns femur `I-10`

733.43 Medial femoral condyle `CC`
CC Exd: 733.40, 733.43, 733.45-733.49

733.44 Talus `CC`
CC Exd: 733.40, 733.44-733.49

733.45 Jaw `CC`
Use additional E code to identify drug, if drug-induced
EXCLUDES *osteoradionecrosis of jaw (526.89)*
CC Exd: See code: 733.40
AHA: 4Q, '07, 91

733.49 Other `CC`
CC Exd: See code: 733.40

733.5 Osteitis condensans
Piriform sclerosis of ilium
DEF: Idiopathic condition marked by low back pain; associated with oval or triangular sclerotic, opaque bone next to sacroiliac joints in the ileum.

733.6 Tietze's disease
Costochondral junction syndrome
Costochondritis
DEF: Painful, idiopathic, nonsuppurative, swollen costal cartilage sometimes confused with cardiac symptoms because the anterior chest pain resembles that of coronary artery disease.
M94.0 Chondrocostal junction syndrome (Tietze dz) `I-10`

733.7 Algoneurodystrophy
Disuse atrophy of bone
Sudeck's atrophy

√5ᵗʰ **733.8 Malunion and nonunion of fracture**
AHA: 2Q, '94, 5

733.81 Malunion of fracture `CC`
CC Exd: 733.81-733.82

733.82 Nonunion of fracture `CC`
Pseudoarthrosis (bone)
CC Exd: See code: 733.81

√5ᵗʰ **733.9 Other unspecified disorders of bone and cartilage**
AHA: 4Q, '08, 136-137

733.90 Disorder of bone and cartilage
M89.9 Disorder of bone, unspecified `I-10`

733.91 Arrest of bone development or growth
Epiphyseal arrest

733.92 Chondromalacia
Chondromalacia: Chondromalacia:
NOS   systemic
localized, except patella   tibial plateau
EXCLUDES *chondromalacia of patella (717.7)*
DEF: Articular cartilage softening.

733.93 Stress fracture of tibia or fibula
Stress reaction of tibia or fibula
Use additional external cause code(s) to identify the cause of the stress fracture
AHA: 4Q, '08, 158; 4Q, '01, 48

733.94 Stress fracture of the metatarsals
Stress reaction of metatarsals
Use additional external cause code(s) to identify the cause of the stress fracture
AHA: 4Q, '08, 158; 4Q, '01, 48

733.95 Stress fracture of other bone

Stress reaction of other bone

Use additional external cause code(s) to identify the cause of the stress fracture

EXCLUDES *stress fracture of:*
femoral neck (733.96)
fibula (733.93)
metatarsals (733.94)
pelvis (733.98)
shaft of femur (733.97)
tibia (733.93)

AHA: 4Q, '08, 158; 4Q, '01, 48

733.96 Stress fracture of femoral neck

Stress reaction of femoral neck

Use additional external cause code(s) to identify the cause of the stress fracture

AHA: 4Q, '08, 158

733.97 Stress fracture of shaft of femur

Stress reaction of shaft of femur

Use additional external cause code(s) to identify the cause of the stress fracture

AHA: 4Q, '08, 158

733.98 Stress fracture of pelvis

Stress reaction of pelvis

Use additional external cause code(s) to identify the cause of the stress fracture

AHA: 4Q, '08, 158

733.99 Other

Diaphysitis   Relapsing polychondritis
Hypertrophy of bone

AHA: 1Q, '11, 6; J-F, '87, 14

734 Flat foot

Pes planus (acquired)
Talipes planus (acquired)

EXCLUDES *congenital (754.61)*
rigid flat foot (754.61)
spastic (everted) flat foot (754.61)

√4ᵗʰ 735 Acquired deformities of toe

EXCLUDES *congenital (754.60-754.69, 755.65-755.66)*

735.0 Hallux valgus (acquired)

DEF: Angled displacement of the great toe, causing it to ride over or under other toes.

Acquired Deformities of Toe

Hallux valgus
Hallux varus
Hallux malleus (hammer of big toe)
Hammertoe

Acquired Deformities of Forearm

Cubitus valgus
Cubitus varus
Varus deformity of wrist
Valgus deformity of wrist
Claw hand
Wrist drop
Club hand

735.1 Hallux varus (acquired)

DEF: Angled displacement of the great toe toward the body midline away from the other toes.

735.2 Hallux rigidus

DEF: Limited flexion movement at metatarsophalangeal joint of great toe; due to degenerative joint disease.

735.3 Hallux malleus

DEF: Extended proximal phalanx, flexed distal phalanges of great toe foot resembles claw or hammer.

735.4 Other hammer toe (acquired)

735.5 Claw toe (acquired)

DEF: Hyperextended proximal phalanges, flexed middle and distal phalanges

735.8 Other acquired deformities of toe

AHA: 4Q, '07, 123

TIP: Assign for hallux limitus, a deformity of the first metatarsophalangeal joint, which restricts the range of motion and can lead to stiffness and pain in the joint.

735.9 Unspecified acquired deformity of toe

√4ᵗʰ 736 Other acquired deformities of limbs

EXCLUDES *congenital (754.3-755.9)*

√5ᵗʰ 736.0 Acquired deformities of forearm, excluding fingers

736.00 Unspecified deformity

Deformity of elbow, forearm, hand, or wrist (acquired) NOS

736.01 Cubitus valgus (acquired)

DEF: Deviation of the elbow away from the body midline upon extension; it occurs when the palm is turning outward.

736.02 Cubitus varus (acquired)

DEF: Elbow joint displacement angled laterally; when the forearm is extended, it is deviated toward the midline of the body; also called "gun stock" deformity.

736.03 Valgus deformity of wrist (acquired)

DEF: Abnormal angulation away from the body midline.

736.04 Varus deformity of wrist (acquired)

DEF: Abnormal angulation toward the body midline.

736.05 Wrist drop (acquired)

DEF: Inability to extend the hand at the wrist due to extensor muscle paralysis.

736.06 Claw hand (acquired)

DEF: Flexion and atrophy of the hand and fingers; found in ulnar nerve lesions, syringomyelia, and leprosy.

736.07 Club hand, acquired

DEF: Twisting of the hand out of shape or position; caused by the congenital absence of the ulna or radius.

736.09 Other

736.1 Mallet finger

DEF: Permanently flexed distal phalanx.

√5ᵗʰ 736.2 Other acquired deformities of finger

736.20 Unspecified deformity

Deformity of finger (acquired) NOS

736.21 Boutonniere deformity

DEF: A deformity of the finger caused by flexion of the proximal interphalangeal joint and hyperextension of the distal joint; also called buttonhole deformity.

736.22 Swan-neck deformity

DEF: Flexed distal and hyperextended proximal interphalangeal joint.

736.29 Other

EXCLUDES *trigger finger (727.03)*

AHA: 2Q, '05, 7; 2Q, '89, 13

√5ᵗʰ 736.3 Acquired deformities of hip

736.30 Unspecified deformity

Deformity of hip (acquired) NOS

736.31 Coxa valga (acquired)

DEF: Increase of at least 140 degrees in the angle formed by the axis of the head and the neck of the femur, and the ax of its shaft.

N Newborn Age: 0   P Pediatric Age: 0-17   M Maternity Age: 12-55   A Adult Age: 15-124   MCC Major CC Condition   CC CC Condition   HIV HIV Related D

252 – Volume 1   2014 ICD-9-C

Deformities of Lower Limb

736.32 Coxa vara (acquired)
DEF: The bending downward of the neck of the femur, causing difficulty in movement; a right angle or less may be formed by the axis of the head and neck of the femur and the axis of its shaft.

736.39 Other
AHA: 2Q, '08, 4; 2Q, '91, 18
TIP: Assign as principal diagnosis for follow-up visit for patient with hip methylmethacrylate cement spacer, following removal of infected joint prosthesis.

√5ᵗʰ 736.4 Genu valgum or varum (acquired)

736.41 Genu valgum (acquired)
DEF: Abnormally close together and an abnormally large space between the ankles; also called "knock-knees."

736.42 Genu varum (acquired)
DEF: Abnormally separated knees and the inward bowing of the legs; it is also called "bowlegs."

736.5 Genu recurvatum (acquired)
DEF: Hyperextended knees; also called "backknee."

736.6 Other acquired deformities of knee
Deformity of knee (acquired) NOS

√5ᵗʰ 736.7 Other acquired deformities of ankle and foot
EXCLUDES deformities of toe (acquired) (735.0-735.9)
pes planus (acquired) (734)

736.70 Unspecified deformity of ankle and foot, acquired

736.71 Acquired equinovarus deformity
Clubfoot, acquired
EXCLUDES clubfoot not specified as acquired (754.5-754.7)

736.72 Equinus deformity of foot, acquired
DEF: A plantar flexion deformity that forces people to walk on their toes.

736.73 Cavus deformity of foot
EXCLUDES that with claw foot (736.74)
DEF: Abnormally high longitudinal arch of the foot.

736.74 Claw foot, acquired
DEF: High foot arch with hyperextended toes at metatarsophalangeal joint and flexed toes at distal joints; also called "main en griffe."

Acquired Deformities of Hip

736.75 Cavovarus deformity of foot, acquired
DEF: Inward turning of the heel from the midline of the leg and an abnormally high longitudinal arch.

736.76 Other calcaneus deformity

736.79 Other
Acquired:
pes
talipes } not elsewhere classified

√5ᵗʰ 736.8 Acquired deformities of other parts of limbs

736.81 Unequal leg length (acquired)

736.89 Other
Deformity (acquired):
arm or leg, not elsewhere classified
shoulder
AHA: 2Q, '08, 5
TIP: Assign as principal diagnosis for follow-up visit for patient with humeral methylmethacrylate cement spacer, following removal of infected joint prosthesis.

736.9 Acquired deformity of limb, site unspecified

√4ᵗʰ 737 Curvature of spine
EXCLUDES congenital (754.2)

737.0 Adolescent postural kyphosis
EXCLUDES osteochondrosis of spine (juvenile) (732.0)
adult (732.8)

√5ᵗʰ 737.1 Kyphosis (acquired)

737.10 Kyphosis (acquired) (postural)
M40.05 Postural kyphosis thoracolumbar region   I-10

737.11 Kyphosis due to radiation

737.12 Kyphosis, postlaminectomy
AHA: J-F, '87, 7
M96.3 Postlaminectomy kyphosis   I-10

737.19 Other
EXCLUDES that associated with conditions classifiable elsewhere (737.41)
AHA: 1Q, '07, 20

Kyphosis and Lordosis

Scoliosis and Kyphoscoliosis

√5ᵗʰ **737.2 Lordosis (acquired)**

> **DEF:** Swayback appearance created by an abnormally increased spinal curvature; it is also referred to as "hollow back" or "saddle back."

737.20 Lordosis (acquired) (postural)

737.21 Lordosis, postlaminectomy

737.22 Other postsurgical lordosis

737.29 Other

> **EXCLUDES** *that associated with conditions classifiable elsewhere (737.42)*

√5ᵗʰ **737.3 Kyphoscoliosis and scoliosis**

> **DEF:** Kyphoscoliosis: backward and lateral curvature of the spinal column; it is found in vertebral osteochondrosis.
> **DEF:** Scoliosis: an abnormal deviation of the spine to the left or right of the midline.

737.30 Scoliosis [and kyphoscoliosis], idiopathic

> **AHA:** 3Q, '03, 19
> **M41.115** Juvenile idiopathic scoliosis thoracolumbar region   I-10

737.31 Resolving infantile idiopathic scoliosis

737.32 Progressive infantile idiopathic scoliosis

> **AHA:** 3Q, '02, 12

737.33 Scoliosis due to radiation

737.34 Thoracogenic scoliosis

737.39 Other

> **EXCLUDES** *that associated with conditions classifiable elsewhere (737.43)*
> *that in kyphoscoliotic heart disease (416.1)*
> **AHA:** 2Q, '02, 16

√5ᵗʰ **737.4 Curvature of spine associated with other conditions**

> *Code first associated condition as:*
> Charcôt-Marie-Tooth disease (356.1)
> mucopolysaccharidosis (277.5)
> neurofibromatosis (237.70-237.79)
> osteitis deformans (731.0)
> osteitis fibrosa cystica (252.01)
> osteoporosis (733.00-733.09)
> poliomyelitis (138)
> tuberculosis [Pott's curvature] (015.0)

737.40 Curvature of spine, unspecified

737.41 Kyphosis

737.42 Lordosis

737.43 Scoliosis

737.8 Other curvatures of spine

737.9 Unspecified curvature of spine

> Curvature of spine (acquired) (idiopathic) NOS
> Hunchback, acquired
> **EXCLUDES** *deformity of spine NOS (738.5)*

√4ᵗʰ **738 Other acquired deformity**

> **EXCLUDES** *congenital (754.0-756.9, 758.0-759.9)*
> *dentofacial anomalies (524.0-524.9)*

738.0 Acquired deformity of nose

> Deformity of nose (acquired)
> Overdevelopment of nasal bones
> **EXCLUDES** *deflected or deviated nasal septum (470)*

√5ᵗʰ **738.1 Other acquired deformity of head**

738.10 Unspecified deformity

738.11 Zygomatic hyperplasia

> **DEF:** Abnormal enlargement of the zygoma (processus zygomaticus temporalis).

738.12 Zygomatic hypoplasia

> **DEF:** Underdevelopment of the zygoma (processus zygomaticus temporalis).

738.19 Other specified deformity

> **AHA:** 1Q, '06, 6; 2Q, '03, 13

738.2 Acquired deformity of neck

738.3 Acquired deformity of chest and rib

> Deformity: Pectus:
>   chest (acquired)   carinatum, acquired
>   rib (acquired)   excavatum, acquired

738.4 Acquired spondylolisthesis

> Degenerative spondylolisthesis
> Spondylolysis, acquired
> **EXCLUDES** *congenital (756.12)*
> **DEF:** Vertebra displaced forward over another; due to bilateral defect in vertebral arch, eroded articular surface of posterior facets and elongated pedicle between fifth lumbar vertebra and sacrum.
> **AHA:** 4Q, '07, 120; 1Q, '07, 10
> **M43.10** Spondylolisthesis site unspecified   I-10

738.5 Other acquired deformity of back or spine

> Deformity of spine NOS
> **EXCLUDES** *curvature of spine (737.0-737.9)*
> **AHA:** 1Q, '08, 11
> **TIP:** Assign for post procedural flat back syndrome, which may be the result of a previous spinal fusion surgery. Do not assign a surgical complication code.

738.6 Acquired deformity of pelvis

> Pelvic obliquity
> **EXCLUDES** *intrapelvic protrusion of acetabulum (718.6)*
> *that in relation to labor and delivery (653.0-653.4, 653.8-653.9)*
> **DEF:** Pelvic obliquity: slanting or inclination of the pelvis at an angle between 55 and 60 degrees between the plane of the pelvis and the horizontal plane.

738.7 Cauliflower ear

> **DEF:** Abnormal external ear; due to injury, subsequent perichondritis.

738.8 Acquired deformity of other specified site

> Deformity of clavicle
> **AHA:** 2Q, '01, 15

738.9 Acquired deformity of unspecified site

√4ᵗʰ **739 Nonallopathic lesions, not elsewhere classified**

> **INCLUDES** segmental dysfunction
> somatic dysfunction
> **DEF:** Disability, loss of function or abnormality of a body part that is neither classifiable to a particular system nor brought about therapeutically to counteract another disease.

739.0 Head region

> Occipitocervical region

739.1 Cervical region

> Cervicothoracic region

739.2 Thoracic region

> Thoracolumbar region

739.3 Lumbar region

> Lumbosacral region

739.4 Sacral region

> Sacrococcygeal region
> Sacroiliac region

739.5 Pelvic region

> Hip region
> Pubic region

739.6 Lower extremities

739.7 Upper extremities

> Acromioclavicular region
> Sternoclavicular region

739.8 Rib cage

> Costochondral region
> Costovertebral region
> Sternochondral region

739.9 Abdomen and other

> **AHA:** 2Q, '89, 14

N Newborn Age: 0   P Pediatric Age: 0-17   M Maternity Age: 12-55   A Adult Age: 15-124   MCC Major CC Condition   CC CC Condition   HIV HIV Related Dx

14. Congenital Anomalies (740-759)

AHA: ▶2Q, '12, 17◀

TIP: Codes from chapter 14 may be assigned throughout the life of the patient, whenever the congenital anomaly is diagnosed.

✓4ᵗʰ **740 Anencephalus and similar anomalies**

740.0 Anencephalus `MCC`
Acrania
Amyelencephalus
Hemicephaly
Hemianencephaly
DEF: Fetus without cerebrum, cerebellum and flat bones of skull.
CC Excl: 740.0-740.2

740.1 Craniorachischisis `MCC`
DEF: Congenital slit in cranium and vertebral column.
CC Excl: See code: 740.0

740.2 Iniencephaly `MCC`
DEF: Spinal cord passes through enlarged occipital bone (foramen magnum); absent vertebral bone layer and spinal processes; resulting in both reduction in number and proper fusion of the vertebrae.
CC Excl: See code: 740.0

✓4ᵗʰ **741 Spina bifida**
EXCLUDES spina bifida occulta (756.17)

The following fifth-digit subclassification is for use with category 741:
 0 unspecified region
 1 cervical region
 2 dorsal [thoracic] region
 3 lumbar region

DEF: Lack of closure of spinal cord's bony encasement; marked by cord protrusion into lumbosacral area; evident by elevated alpha-fetoprotein of amniotic fluid.
AHA: 3Q, '94, 7
TIP: For Arnold-Chiari syndrome, Type I, refer to code 348.4.

§ ✓5ᵗʰ **741.0 With hydrocephalus** `CC`
[0-3] Arnold-Chiari syndrome, type II
Chiari malformation, type II
Any condition classifiable to 741.9 with any condition classifiable to 742.3
CC Excl: 741.00-741.93, 742.59-742.9, 759.7-759.89
AHA: 4Q, '97, 51; 4Q, '94, 37; S-O, '87, 10
Q05.4 Unspecified spina bifida with hydrocephalus `I-10`

§ ✓5ᵗʰ **741.9 Without mention of hydrocephalus**
[0-3] Hydromeningocele (spinal)
Hydromyelocele
Meningocele (spinal)
Meningomyelocele
Myelocele
Myelocystocele
Rachischisis
Spina bifida (aperta)
Syringomyelocele
Q05.8 Sacral spina bifida without hydrocephalus `I-10`

✓4ᵗʰ **742 Other congenital anomalies of nervous system**
EXCLUDES congenital central alveolar hypoventilation syndrome (327.25)

742.0 Encephalocele `CC`
Encephalocystocele
Encephalomyelocele
Hydroencephalocele
Hydromeningocele, cranial
Meningocele, cerebral
Meningoencephalocele
DEF: Brain tissue protrudes through skull defect.
CC Excl: 742.0-742.2, 742.4
AHA: 4Q, '94, 37

742.1 Microcephalus
Hydromicrocephaly
Micrencephaly
DEF: Extremely small head or brain.

Spina Bifida

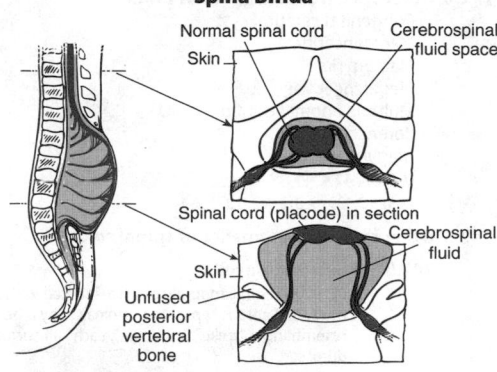

742.2 Reduction deformities of brain `MCC`
Absence
Agenesis
Aplasia
Hypoplasia } of part of brain

Agyria
Arhinencephaly
Holoprosencephaly
Microgyria
CC Excl: See code 742.0
AHA: 3Q, '03, 15; 4Q, '94, 37
TIP: Assign for septo-optic dysplasia.

742.3 Congenital hydrocephalus
Aqueduct of Sylvius:
 anomaly
 obstruction, congenital
 stenosis
Atresia of foramina of Magendie and Luschka
Hydrocephalus in newborn
EXCLUDES hydrocephalus:
 acquired (331.3-331.4)
 due to congenital toxoplasmosis (771.2)
 with any condition classifiable to 741.9 (741.0)
DEF: Fluid accumulation within the skull; involves subarachnoid (external) or ventricular (internal) brain spaces.
AHA: 4Q, '05, 83
Q03.9 Congenital hydrocephalus unspecified `I-10`

Normal Ventricles and Hydrocephalus

---

§ Requires fifth digit. Valid digits are in [brackets] under each code. See category 741 for codes and defintions.

4ᵗʰ 5ᵗʰ Additional Digit Required | Unacceptable PDx | Manifestation Code | Hospital Acquired Condition | ▶◀ Revised Text | ● New Code | ▲ Revised Code Title

2014 ICD-9-CM | February 2013 • Volume 1 – 255

742.4 Other specified anomalies of brain   `CC`
Congenital cerebral cyst
Macroencephaly
Macrogyria
Megalencephaly
Multiple anomalies of brain NOS
Porencephaly
Ulegyria
CC Excl: 742.4
AHA: 1Q, '99, 9; 3Q, '92, 12

√5ᵗʰ **742.5 Other specified anomalies of spinal cord**

742.51 Diastematomyelia
DEF: Congenital anomaly often associated with spina bifida; the spinal cord is separated into halves by a bony tissue resembling a "spike" (a spicule), each half surrounded by a dural sac.

742.53 Hydromyelia
Hydrorhachis
DEF: Dilated central spinal cord canal; characterized by increased fluid accumulation.

742.59 Other
Amyelia
Atelomyelia
Congenital anomaly of spinal meninges
Defective development of cauda equina
Hypoplasia of spinal cord
Myelatelia
Myelodysplasia
AHA: 2Q, '91, 14; 1Q, '89, 10
TIP: Assign for tethered spinal cord syndrome, regardless of when it is diagnosed.

742.8 Other specified anomalies of nervous system
Agenesis of nerve
Displacement of brachial plexus
Familial dysautonomia
Jaw-winking syndrome
Marcus-Gunn syndrome
Riley-Day syndrome
EXCLUDES neurofibromatosis (237.70-237.79)

742.9 Unspecified anomaly of brain, spinal cord, and nervous system
Anomaly
Congenital: brain
    disease   of: nervous system
    lesion   spinal cord
Deformity

√4ᵗʰ **743 Congenital anomalies of eye**

√5ᵗʰ **743.0 Anophthalmos**
DEF: Complete absence of the eyes or the presence of vestigial eyes.

743.00 Clinical anophthalmos, unspecified
Agenesis
Congenital } of eye
   absence
Anophthalmos NOS

743.03 Cystic eyeball, congenital

743.06 Cryptophthalmos
DEF: Skin is continuous over eyeball, results in apparent absence of eyelids.

√5ᵗʰ **743.1 Microphthalmos**
Dysplasia } of eye
Hypoplasia
Rudimentary eye
DEF: Abnormally small eyeballs, may be opacities of cornea and lens, scarring of choroid and retina.

743.10 Microphthalmos, unspecified

743.11 Simple microphthalmos

743.12 Microphthalmos associated with other anomalies of eye and adnexa

√5ᵗʰ **743.2 Buphthalmos**
Glaucoma:
   congenital
   newborn
Hydrophthalmos
EXCLUDES glaucoma of childhood (365.14)
         traumatic glaucoma due to birth injury (767.8)
DEF: Distended, enlarged fibrous coats of eye; due to intraocular pressure of congenital glaucoma.

743.20 Buphthalmos, unspecified

743.21 Simple buphthalmos

743.22 Buphthalmos associated with other ocular anomalies
Keratoglobus, congenital } associated with
Megalocornea   buphthalmos

√5ᵗʰ **743.3 Congenital cataract and lens anomalies**
EXCLUDES infantile cataract (366.00-366.09)
DEF: Opaque eye lens.

743.30 Congenital cataract, unspecified

743.31 Capsular and subcapsular cataract

743.32 Cortical and zonular cataract

743.33 Nuclear cataract

743.34 Total and subtotal cataract, congenital

743.35 Congenital aphakia
Congenital absence of lens

743.36 Anomalies of lens shape
Microphakia
Spherophakia

743.37 Congenital ectopic lens

743.39 Other

√5ᵗʰ **743.4 Coloboma and other anomalies of anterior segment**
DEF: Coloboma: ocular tissue defect associated with defect of ocular fetal intraocular fissure; may cause small pit on optic disk, major defects of iris, ciliary body, choroid, and retina.

743.41 Anomalies of corneal size and shape
Microcornea
EXCLUDES that associated with buphthalmos (743.22)

743.42 Corneal opacities, interfering with vision, congenital

743.43 Other corneal opacities, congenital

743.44 Specified anomalies of anterior chamber, chamber angle, and related structures
Anomaly:
   Axenfeld's
   Peters'
   Rieger's

743.45 Aniridia
DEF: Incompletely formed or absent iris; affects both eyes; dominant trait; also called congenital absence of iris.
AHA: 2Q, '10, 4-5; 3Q, '02, 20

743.46 Other specified anomalies of iris and ciliary body
Anisocoria, congenital   Coloboma of iris
Atresia of pupil   Corectopia

743.47 Specified anomalies of sclera

743.48 Multiple and combined anomalies of anterior segment

743.49 Other

√5ᵗʰ **743.5 Congenital anomalies of posterior segment**

743.51 Vitreous anomalies
Congenital vitreous opacity

743.52 Fundus coloboma
DEF: Absent retinal and choroidal tissue; occurs in lower fundus; a bright white ectatic zone of exposed sclera extends into and changes the optic disk.

743.53 Chorioretinal degeneration, congenital

743.54 Congenital folds and cysts of posterior segment

743.55 Congenital macular changes

N Newborn Age: 0   P Pediatric Age: 0-17   M Maternity Age: 12-55   A Adult Age: 15-124   MCC Major CC Condition   CC CC Condition   HIV HIV Related Dx

256 – Volume 1   **2014 ICD-9-CM**

743.56 Other retinal changes, congenital
AHA: 3Q, '99, 12

743.57 Specified anomalies of optic disc
Coloboma of optic disc (congenital)

743.58 Vascular anomalies
Congenital retinal aneurysm

743.59 Other

√5ᵗʰ **743.6 Congenital anomalies of eyelids, lacrimal system, and orbit**

743.61 Congenital ptosis
DEF: Drooping of eyelid.

743.62 Congenital deformities of eyelids
Ablepharon
Absence of eyelid
Accessory eyelid
Congenital:
ectropion
entropion
AHA: 1Q, '00, 22
TIP: Assign for epiblepharon, in which a redundant horizontal skin fold under the eyelid causes an abnormal vertical orientation of the eyelashes; may result in the eyelashes touching the eyeball.

743.63 Other specified congenital anomalies of eyelid
Absence, agenesis, of cilia

743.64 Specified congenital anomalies of lacrimal gland

743.65 Specified congenital anomalies of lacrimal passages
Absence, agenesis of:
lacrimal apparatus
punctum lacrimale
Accessory lacrimal canal

743.66 Specified congenital anomalies of orbit

743.69 Other
Accessory eye muscles

743.8 Other specified anomalies of eye
EXCLUDES congenital nystagmus (379.51)
ocular albinism (270.2)
optic nerve hypoplasia (377.43)
retinitis pigmentosa (362.74)

743.9 Unspecified anomaly of eye
Congenital:
anomaly NOS ⎱ of eye (any part)
deformity NOS ⎰

√4ᵗʰ **744 Congenital anomalies of ear, face, and neck**
EXCLUDES anomaly of:
cervical spine (754.2, 756.10-756.19)
larynx (748.2-748.3)
nose (748.0-748.1)
parathyroid gland (759.2)
thyroid gland (759.2)
cleft lip (749.10-749.25)

√5ᵗʰ **744.0 Anomalies of ear causing impairment of hearing**
EXCLUDES congenital deafness without mention of cause (389.0-389.9)

744.00 Unspecified anomaly of ear with impairment of hearing

744.01 Absence of external ear
Absence of:
auditory canal (external)
auricle (ear) (with stenosis or atresia of auditory canal)

744.02 Other anomalies of external ear with impairment of hearing
Atresia or stricture of auditory canal (external)

744.03 Anomaly of middle ear, except ossicles
Atresia or stricture of osseous meatus (ear)

744.04 Anomalies of ear ossicles
Fusion of ear ossicles

744.05 Anomalies of inner ear
Congenital anomaly of:
membranous labyrinth
organ of Corti

744.09 Other
Absence of ear, congenital

744.1 Accessory auricle
Accessory tragus
Polyotia
Preauricular appendage
Supernumerary:
ear
lobule
DEF: Redundant tissue or structures of ear.

√5ᵗʰ **744.2 Other specified anomalies of ear**
EXCLUDES that with impairment of hearing (744.00-744.09)

744.21 Absence of ear lobe, congenital

744.22 Macrotia
DEF: Abnormally large pinna of ear.

744.23 Microtia
DEF: Hypoplasia of pinna; associated with absent or closed auditory canal.

744.24 Specified anomalies of Eustachian tube
Absence of Eustachian tube

744.29 Other
Bat ear
Darwin's tubercle
Pointed ear
Prominence of auricle
Ridge ear
EXCLUDES preauricular sinus (744.46)

744.3 Unspecified anomaly of ear
Congenital:
anomaly NOS ⎱ of ear, not elsewhere
deformity NOS ⎰ classified

√5ᵗʰ **744.4 Branchial cleft cyst or fistula; preauricular sinus**

744.41 Branchial cleft sinus or fistula
Branchial:
sinus (external) (internal)
vestige
DEF: Cyst due to failed closure of embryonic branchial cleft.

744.42 Branchial cleft cyst

744.43 Cervical auricle

744.46 Preauricular sinus or fistula

744.47 Preauricular cyst

744.49 Other
Fistula (of):
auricle, congenital
cervicoaural

744.5 Webbing of neck
Pterygium colli
DEF: Thick, triangular skinfold, stretches from lateral side of neck across shoulder; associated with Turner's and Noonan's syndromes.

√5ᵗʰ **744.8 Other specified anomalies of face and neck**

744.81 Macrocheilia
Hypertrophy of lip, congenital
DEF: Abnormally large lips.

744.82 Microcheilia
DEF: Abnormally small lips.

744.83 Macrostomia
DEF: Bilateral or unilateral anomaly of mouth due to malformed maxillary and mandibular processes; results in mouth extending toward ear.

744.84 Microstomia
DEF: Abnormally small mouth.

744.89 Other
EXCLUDES congenital fistula of lip (750.25)
musculoskeletal anomalies (754.0-754.1, 756.0)

Congenital Anomalies

744.9 Unspecified anomalies of face and neck
Congenital:
anomaly NOS ⎫ of face [any part] or neck [any
deformity NOS ⎭ part]

✓4th **745 Bulbus cordis anomalies and anomalies of cardiac septal closure**

745.0 Common truncus `MCC`
Absent septum ⎫ between aorta and
Communication (abnormal) ⎭ pulmonary artery
Aortic septal defect
Common aortopulmonary trunk
Persistent truncus arteriosus
CC Exd: 429.71-429.79, 745.0-745.9, 746.89-746.9, 747.83-747.9, 759.7-759.89

✓5th **745.1 Transposition of great vessels**

745.10 Complete transposition of great vessels `MCC`
Transposition of great vessels:
NOS
classical
CC Exd: See code 745.0

745.11 Double outlet right ventricle `MCC`
Dextratransposition of aorta
Incomplete transposition of great vessels
Origin of both great vessels from right ventricle
Taussig-Bing syndrome or defect
CC Exd: See code 745.0

745.12 Corrected transposition of great vessels `CC`
CC Exd: See code 745.0

745.19 Other `MCC`
CC Exd: See code 745.0

745.2 Tetralogy of Fallot `MCC`
Fallot's pentalogy
Ventricular septal defect with pulmonary stenosis or atresia, dextraposition of aorta, and hypertrophy of right ventricle
EXCLUDES Fallot's triad (746.09)
DEF: Obstructed cardiac outflow causes pulmonary stenosis, interventricular septal defect and right ventricular hypertrophy.
CC Exd: See code 745.0

745.3 Common ventricle `MCC`
Cor triloculare biatriatum
Single ventricle
CC Exd: See code 745.0

745.4 Ventricular septal defect `CC`
Eisenmenger's defect or complex
Gerbo dedefect
Interventricular septal defect
Left ventricular-right atrial communication
Roger's disease
EXCLUDES common atrioventricular canal type (745.69)
single ventricle (745.3)
CC Exd: See code 745.0
Q21.0 Ventricular septal defect `I-10`

Heart Defects

Atrial septal defect
Aortic stenosis
Ventricular septal defect
Patent ductus arteriosus
Pulmonary stenosis
Transposition of the great vessels
Tetralogy of Fallot

745.5 Ostium secundum type atrial septal defect `CC`
Defect:
atrium secundum
fossa ovalis
Lutembacher's syndrome
Patent or persistent:
foramen ovale
ostium secundum
DEF: Opening in atrial septum due to failure of the septum secundum and the endocardial cushions to fuse; there is a rim of septum surrounding the defect.
CC Exd: 429.71-429.79, 745.0-745.3, 745.5-745.9, 746.89-746.9, 747.89-747.9, 759.7, 759.89
AHA: ▶2Q, '12, 3;◀ 3Q, '09, 17
Q21.1 Atrial septal defect `I-10`

✓5th **745.6 Endocardial cushion defects**
DEF: Atrial and/or ventricular septal defects causing abnormal fusion of cushions in atrioventricular canal.

745.60 Endocardial cushion defect, unspecified type `CC`
DEF: Septal defect due to imperfect fusion of endocardial cushions.
CC Exd: See code 745.0

745.61 Ostium primum defect `CC`
Persistent ostium primum
DEF: Opening in low, posterior septum primum; causes cleft in basal portion of atrial septum; associated with cleft mitral valve.
CC Exd: See code: 745.0

745.69 Other `CC`
Absence of atrial septum
Atrioventricular canal type ventricular septal defect
Common atrioventricular canal
Common atrium
CC Exd: See code 745.0

745.7 Cor biloculare `MCC`
Absence of atrial and ventricular septa
DEF: Atrial and ventricular septal defect; marked by heart with two cardiac chambers (one atrium, one ventricle), and one atrioventricular valve.
CC Exd: See code 745.0

745.8 Other

745.9 Unspecified defect of septal closure
Septal defect NOS

✓4th **746 Other congenital anomalies of heart**
EXCLUDES endocardial fibroelastosis (425.3)

✓5th **746.0 Anomalies of pulmonary valve**
EXCLUDES infundibular or subvalvular pulmonic stenosis (746.83)
tetralogy of Fallot (745.2)

746.00 Pulmonary valve anomaly, unspecified `CC`
CC Exd: 746.00-746.09, 746.89-746.9, 747.89-747.9, 759.7, 759.89

746.01 Atresia, congenital `MCC`
Congenital absence of pulmonary valve
CC Exd: 746.00-746.09, 746.89-746.9, 747.89-747.9, 759.7, 759.89

746.02 Stenosis, congenital `CC`
DEF: Stenosis of opening between pulmonary artery and right ventricle; causes obstructed blood outflow from right ventricle.
CC Exd: See code 746.01
AHA: 1Q, '04, 16

746.09 Other `CC`
Congenital insufficiency of pulmonary valve
Fallot's triad or trilogy
CC Exd: See code: 746.00

746.1 Tricuspid atresia and stenosis, congenital `MCC`
Absence of tricuspid valve
CC Exd: 746.1-746.7, 746.89-746.9, 747.83-747.9, 759.7-759.89

N Newborn Age: 0   P Pediatric Age: 0-17   M Maternity Age: 12-55   A Adult Age: 15-124   `MCC` Major CC Condition   `CC` CC Condition   `HIV` HIV Related Dx

258 – Volume 1 • February 2013   2014 ICD-9-CM

746.2 Ebstein's anomaly `MCC`
  DEF: Malformation of the tricuspid valve characterized by septal and posterior leaflets attaching to the wall of the right ventricle; causing the right ventricle to fuse with the atrium into a large right atrium and a small ventricle; causes heart failure and abnormal cardiac rhythm.
  CC Excl: See code 746.1

746.3 Congenital stenosis of aortic valve `CC`
  Congenital aortic stenosis
  EXCLUDES congenital:
      subaortic stenosis (746.81)
      supravalvular aortic stenosis (747.22)
  DEF: Stenosis of orifice of aortic valve; obstructs blood outflow from left ventricle.
  CC Excl: See code 746.1
  AHA: 4Q, '88, 8

746.4 Congenital insufficiency of aortic valve `CC`
  Bicuspid aortic valve
  Congenital aortic insufficiency
  DEF: Impaired functioning of aortic valve due to incomplete closure; causes backflow (regurgitation) of blood from aorta to left ventricle.
  CC Excl: See code 746.1
  Q23.1 Congenital insufficiency of aortic valve `I-10`

746.5 Congenital mitral stenosis `CC`
  Fused commissure
  Parachute deformity } of mitral valve
  Supernumerary cusps
  DEF: Stenosis of left atrioventricular orifice.
  CC Excl: See code 746.1
  AHA: 3Q, '07, 3

746.6 Congenital mitral insufficiency `CC`
  DEF: Impaired functioning of mitral valve due to incomplete closure; causes backflow of blood from left ventricle to left atrium.
  CC Excl: See code 746.1

746.7 Hypoplastic left heart syndrome `MCC`
  Atresia, or marked hypoplasia, of aortic orifice or valve, with hypoplasia of ascending aorta and defective development of left ventricle (with mitral valve atresia)
  CC Excl: See code 746.1

√5ᵗʰ **746.8 Other specified anomalies of heart**

  746.81 Subaortic stenosis `MCC`
    DEF: Stenosis, of left ventricular outflow tract due to fibrous tissue ring or septal hypertrophy below aortic valve.
    CC Excl: 746.81-746.84, 746.89-746.9, 747.83-747.9, 759.7-759.89
    AHA: 3Q, '07, 3

  746.82 Cor triatriatum `MCC`
    DEF: Transverse septum divides left atrium due to failed resorption of embryonic common pulmonary vein; results in three atrial chambers.
    CC Excl: See code 746.81

  746.83 Infundibular pulmonic stenosis `CC`
    Subvalvular pulmonic stenosis
    DEF: Stenosis of right ventricle outflow tract within infundibulum due to fibrous diaphragm below valve or long, narrow fibromuscular channel.
    CC Excl: See code 746.81

  746.84 Obstructive anomalies of heart, not elsewhere classified `MCC`
    Shone's syndrome   Uhl's disease
    Use additional code for associated anomalies, such as:
      coarctation of aorta (747.10)
      congenital mitral stenosis (746.5)
      subaortic stenosis (746.81)
    CC Excl: See code: 746.81
    AHA: ▶2Q, '12, 3◀

  746.85 Coronary artery anomaly `CC`
    Anomalous origin or communication of coronary artery
    Arteriovenous malformation of coronary artery
    Coronary artery:
      absence
      arising from aorta or pulmonary trunk
      single
    CC Excl: 746.85, 746.89-746.9
    AHA: N-D, '85, 3

746.86 Congenital heart block `MCC`
  Complete or incomplete atrioventricular [AV] block
  DEF: Impaired conduction of electrical impulses; due to maldeveloped junctional tissue.
  CC Excl: 746.86, 746.89-746.9, 747.83-747.9, 759.7-759.89

746.87 Malposition of heart and cardiac apex `CC`
  Abdominal heart
  Dextrocardia
  Ectopia cordis
  Levocardia (isolated)
  Mesocardia
  EXCLUDES dextrocardia with complete transposition of viscera (759.3)
  CC Excl: 746.81-746.84, 746.87-746.9, 747.89-747.9, 759.7, 759.89

746.89 Other
  Atresia
  Hypoplasia } of cardiac vein
  Congenital:
    cardiomegaly
    diverticulum, left ventricle
    pericardial defect
  AHA: 3Q, '00, 3; 1Q, '99, 11; J-F, '85, 3
  TIP: Assign for Brugada syndrome. Additional codes may be required.
  Q24.8 Other specified congenital malformations of heart `I-10`

746.9 Unspecified anomaly of heart
  Congenital:
    anomaly of heart NOS
    heart disease NOS

√4ᵗʰ **747 Other congenital anomalies of circulatory system**

  747.0 Patent ductus arteriosus `CC`
    Patent ductus Botalli
    Persistent ductus arteriosus
    DEF: Open lumen in ductus arteriosus causes arterial blood recirculation in lungs; inhibits blood supply to aorta; symptoms such as shortness of breath more noticeable upon activity.
    CC Excl: 747.0, 747.89
    AHA: 3Q, '09, 17
    Q25.0 Patent ductus arteriosus `I-10`

√5ᵗʰ **747.1 Coarctation of aorta**
    DEF: Localized deformity of aortic media seen as a severe constriction of the vessel lumen; major symptom is high blood pressure in the arms and low pressure in the legs; may result in a CVA, rupture of the aorta, bacterial endocarditis or congestive heart failure.

  747.10 Coarctation of aorta (preductal) (postductal) `CC`
    Hypoplasia of aortic arch
    CC Excl: 747.10-747.22, 747.89-747.9, 759.7, 759.89
    AHA: 3Q, '07, 3; 1Q, '99, 11; 4Q, '88, 8

  747.11 Interruption of aortic arch `MCC`
    CC Excl: 747.10-747.22, 747.83-747.9, 759.7-759.89

√5ᵗʰ **747.2 Other anomalies of aorta**

  747.20 Anomaly of aorta, unspecified `CC`
    CC Excl: 747.10-747.22, 747.89-747.9, 759.7, 759.89

  747.21 Anomalies of aortic arch `CC`
    Anomalous origin, right subclavian artery
    Dextraposition of aorta
    Double aortic arch
    Kommerell's diverticulum
    Overriding aorta
    Persistent:
      convolutions, aortic arch
      right aortic arch
    Vascular ring
    EXCLUDES hypoplasia of aortic arch (747.10)
    CC Excl: See code: 747.20
    AHA: 1Q, '03, 15

747.22 Atresia and stenosis of aorta `CC`

Absence
Aplasia } of aorta
Hypoplasia
Stricture

Supra (valvular)-aortic stenosis

EXCLUDES congenital aortic (valvular) stenosis or
stricture, so stated (746.3)
hypoplasia of aorta in hypoplastic left heart
syndrome (746.7)

CC Exd: 747.10-747.22, 747.83-747.9, 759.7-759.89

747.29 Other `CC`

Aneurysm of sinus of Valsalva
Congenital:
aneurysm } of aorta
dilation

CC Exd: 747.10-747.29, 747.89-747.9, 759.7, 759.89

√5ᵗʰ **747.3 Anomalies of pulmonary artery**

AHA: 4Q, '11, 137-138

747.31 Pulmonary artery coarctation and atresia `MCC`

Agenesis of pulmonary artery
Atresia of pulmonary artery
Coarctation of pulmonary artery
Hypoplasia of pulmonary artery
Stenosis of pulmonary artery

CC Exd: 747.31-747.39, 747.89-747.9
AHA: ▶2Q, '12, 3◀

747.32 Pulmonary arteriovenous malformation `MCC`

Pulmonary arteriovenous aneurysm

EXCLUDES acquired pulmonary arteriovenous fistula
(417.0)

CC Exd: See code 747.31
AHA: 4Q, '11, 138

747.39 Other anomalies of pulmonary artery and `MCC`
pulmonary circulation

Anomaly of pulmonary artery

CC Exd: See code 747.31
AHA: 3Q, '10, 9; 3Q, '09, 17, 18; 1Q, '04, 16; 1Q, '94, 15;
4Q, '88, 8
TIP: Assign for peripheral pulmonary stenosis (PPS)
murmur.
Q25.7 Oth congenital malformations pulmonary artery `I-10`

√5ᵗʰ **747.4 Anomalies of great veins**

747.40 Anomaly of great veins, unspecified `CC`

Anomaly NOS of:
pulmonary veins
vena cava

CC Exd: 747.40, 747.89-747.9

747.41 Total anomalous pulmonary venous connection `CC`

Total anomalous pulmonary venous return [TAPVR]:
subdiaphragmatic
supradiaphragmatic

CC Exd: 747.41, 747.89-747.9

747.42 Partial anomalous pulmonary venous `CC`
connection

Partial anomalous pulmonary venous return

CC Exd: 747.42, 747.89-747.9

747.49 Other anomalies of great veins `CC`

Absence } of vena cava (inferior)
Congenital stenosis } (superior)

Persistent:
left posterior cardinal vein
left superior vena cava
Scimitar syndrome
Transposition of pulmonary veins NOS

CC Exd: 747.49, 747.89-747.9

747.5 Absence or hypoplasia of umbilical artery

Single umbilical artery

√5ᵗʰ **747.6 Other anomalies of peripheral vascular system**

Absence
Anomaly } of artery or vein, NEC
Atresia

Arteriovenous aneurysm (peripheral)
Arteriovenous malformation of the peripheral vascular system
Congenital:
aneurysm (peripheral)
phlebectasia
stricture, artery
varix
Multiple renal arteries

EXCLUDES anomalies of:
cerebral vessels (747.81)
pulmonary artery (747.39)
congenital retinal aneurysm (743.58)
hemangioma (228.00-228.09)
lymphangioma (228.1)

747.60 Anomaly of the peripheral vascular system,
unspecified site

747.61 Gastrointestinal vessel anomaly

AHA: 3Q, '96, 10
TIP: Do not assign for gastric or intestinal AV malformation
or angiodysplasia not stated to be congenital. See instead
code 537.82, 537.83, 569.84, or 569.85.

747.62 Renal vessel anomaly

747.63 Upper limb vessel anomaly

747.64 Lower limb vessel anomaly

747.69 Anomalies of other specified sites of peripheral
vascular system

√5ᵗʰ **747.8 Other specified anomalies of circulatory system**

747.81 Anomalies of cerebrovascular system `MCC`

Arteriovenous malformation of brain
Cerebral arteriovenous aneurysm, congenital
Congenital anomalies of cerebral vessels

EXCLUDES ruptured cerebral (arteriovenous) aneurysm
(430)

CC Exd: 747.81, 747.89-747.9
Q28.3 Other malformations of cerebral vessels `I-10`

747.82 Spinal vessel anomaly `CC`

Arteriovenous malformation of spinal vessel

CC Exd: 747.82, 747.89-747.9
AHA: 3Q, '95, 5

747.83 Persistent fetal circulation `MCC` `N`

Persistent pulmonary hypertension
Primary pulmonary hypertension of newborn

DEF: A return to fetal circulation due to constriction of
pulmonary arterioles and opening of the ductus arteriosus
and foramen ovale, right-to-left shunting, oxygenation of
the blood does not occur, and the lungs remain constricted
after birth; is seen in term or post-term infants; causes
include asphyxiation, meconium aspiration syndrome,
acidosis, sepsis, and developmental immaturity.

CC Exd: 416.0, 416.8-416.9
AHA: 4Q, '02, 62

Persistent Fetal Circulation

√5ᵗʰ symbol:

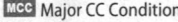

`N` Newborn Age: 0   `P` Pediatric Age: 0-17   `M` Maternity Age: 12-55   `A` Adult Age: 15-124   `MCC` Major CC Condition   `CC` CC Condition   **HIV** HIV Related Dx

260 – Volume 1 • February 2013   2014 ICD-9-CM

747.89 Other   `CC`
Aneurysm, congenital, specified site not elsewhere classified
> **EXCLUDES** congenital aneurysm:
> coronary (746.85)
> peripheral (747.6)
> pulmonary (747.39)
> arteriovenous (747.32)
> retinal (743.58)

CC Excl: 745.0–745.9, 747.89
AHA: 4Q, '02, 63

747.9 Unspecified anomaly of circulatory system   `CC`
CC Excl: 745.0–747.29, 747.31–747.82, 747.89–747.9

√4ᵗʰ **748 Congenital anomalies of respiratory system**
> **EXCLUDES** congenital central alveolar hypoventilation syndrome (327.25)
> congenital defect of diaphragm (756.6)

748.0 Choanal atresia
Atresia
Congenital stenosis } of nares (anterior) (posterior)
DEF: Occluded posterior nares (choana), bony or membranous due to failure of embryonic bucconasal membrane to rupture.

748.1 Other anomalies of nose
Absent nose
Accessory nose
Cleft nose
Congenital:
   deformity of nose
   notching of tip of nose
   perforation of wall of nasal sinus
Deformity of wall of nasal sinus
> **EXCLUDES** congenital deviation of nasal septum (754.0)

748.2 Web of larynx
Web of larynx: Web of larynx:
  NOS   subglottic
  glottic
DEF: Malformed larynx; marked by thin, translucent, or thick, fibrotic spread between vocal folds; affects speech.

748.3 Other anomalies of larynx, trachea, and bronchus   `CC`
Absence or agenesis of: Congenital:
  bronchus   dilation, trachea
  larynx   stenosis:
  trachea   larynx
Anomaly (of):   trachea
  cricoid cartilage   tracheocele
  epiglottis   Diverticulum:
  thyroid cartilage   bronchus
  tracheal cartilage   trachea
Atresia (of):   Fissure of epiglottis
  epiglottis   Laryngocele
  glottis   Posterior cleft of cricoid
  larynx   cartilage (congenital)
  trachea   Rudimentary tracheal bronchus
Cleft thyroid, cartilage,   Stridor, laryngeal, congenital
  congenital
CC Excl: 493.81, 519.19, 748.3, 748.8–748.9
AHA: 1Q, '99, 14
Q32.4 Other congenital malformations of bronchus   `I-10`

748.4 Congenital cystic lung   `CC`
Disease, lung:
  cystic, congenital
  polycystic, congenital
Honeycomb lung, congenital
> **EXCLUDES** acquired or unspecified cystic lung (518.89)
DEF: Enlarged air spaces of lung parenchyma.
CC Excl: 748.4–748.9

748.5 Agenesis, hypoplasia, and dysplasia of lung   `MCC`
Absence of lung (fissures) (lobe) (lobe)
Aplasia of lung
Hypoplasia of lung
Sequestration of lung
CC Excl: See code 748.4

√5ᵗʰ **748.6 Other anomalies of lung**

748.60 Anomaly of lung, unspecified

748.61 Congenital bronchiectasis   `CC`
CC Excl: 494.0–494.1, 496, 506.1,506.4–506.9, 748.61

748.69 Other
Accessory lung (lobe)
Azygos lobe (fissure), lung

748.8 Other specified anomalies of respiratory system
Abnormal communication between pericardial and pleural sacs
Anomaly, pleural folds
Atresia of nasopharynx
Congenital cyst of mediastinum

748.9 Unspecified anomaly of respiratory system
Anomaly of respiratory system NOS

√4ᵗʰ **749 Cleft palate and cleft lip**
AHA: ▶2Q, '12, 17◀

√5ᵗʰ **749.0 Cleft palate**

749.00 Cleft palate, unspecified

749.01 Unilateral, complete

749.02 Unilateral, incomplete
Cleft uvula

749.03 Bilateral, complete

749.04 Bilateral, incomplete

√5ᵗʰ **749.1 Cleft lip**
Cheiloschisis
Congenital fissure of lip
Harelip
Labium leporinum

749.10 Cleft lip, unspecified

749.11 Unilateral, complete

749.12 Unilateral, incomplete

749.13 Bilateral, complete

749.14 Bilateral, incomplete

√5ᵗʰ **749.2 Cleft palate with cleft lip**
Cheilopalatoschisis

749.20 Cleft palate with cleft lip, unspecified

749.21 Unilateral, complete

749.22 Unilateral, incomplete

749.23 Bilateral, complete
AHA: 1Q, '96, 14

749.24 Bilateral, incomplete

749.25 Other combinations

Cleft Lip and Palate

Unilateral cleft lip

No cleft palate

Cleft lip with cleft alveolar ridge
No cleft palate

Unilateral cleft lip and cleft palate

Alveolar ridge
Cleft palate

Prolabium

Bilateral cleft lip and cleft palate

Isolated cleft palate

Congenital Anomalies

750–751.3

✓4ᵗʰ **750 Other congenital anomalies of upper alimentary tract**

EXCLUDES *dentofacial anomalies (524.0-524.9)*

750.0 Tongue tie

Ankyloglossia

DEF: Restricted tongue movement due to lingual frenum extending toward tip of tongue. Tongue may be fused to mouth floor affecting speech.

✓5ᵗʰ **750.1 Other anomalies of tongue**

750.10 Anomaly of tongue, unspecified

750.11 Aglossia

DEF: Absence of tongue.

750.12 Congenital adhesions of tongue

750.13 Fissure of tongue

Bifid tongue

Double tongue

750.15 Macroglossia

Congenital hypertrophy of tongue

750.16 Microglossia

Hypoplasia of tongue

750.19 Other

✓5ᵗʰ **750.2 Other specified anomalies of mouth and pharynx**

750.21 Absence of salivary gland

750.22 Accessory salivary gland

750.23 Atresia, salivary duct

Imperforate salivary duct

750.24 Congenital fistula of salivary gland

750.25 Congenital fistula of lip

Congenital (mucus) lip pits

750.26 Other specified anomalies of mouth

Absence of uvula

750.27 Diverticulum of pharynx

Pharyngeal pouch

750.29 Other specified anomalies of pharynx

Imperforate pharynx

750.3 Tracheoesophageal fistula, esophageal atresia and stenosis   MCC

Absent esophagus

Atresia of esophagus

Congenital:

esophageal ring

stenosis of esophagus

stricture of esophagus

Congenital fistula:

esophagobronchial

esophagotracheal

Imperforate esophagus

Webbed esophagus

CC Exd: 530.84, 750.3-750.4, 751.8-751.9

AHA: 1Q, '12, 15

750.4 Other specified anomalies of esophagus   CC

Dilatation, congenital ⎫

Displacement, congenital ⎪

Diverticulum   ⎬ (of) esophagus

Duplication   ⎪

Giant   ⎭

Esophageal pouch

EXCLUDES *congenital hiatus hernia (750.6)*

CC Exd: 750.4, 751.8-751.9

AHA: J-F, '85, 3

750.5 Congenital hypertrophic pyloric stenosis

Congenital or infantile:

constriction ⎫

hypertrophy ⎪

spasm   ⎬ of pylorus

stenosis   ⎪

stricture   ⎭

DEF: Obstructed pylorus due to overgrowth of pyloric muscle.

Q40.0 Congenital hypertrophic pyloric stenosis   I-10

750.6 Congenital hiatus hernia

Displacement of cardia through esophageal hiatus

EXCLUDES *congenital diaphragmatic hernia (756.6)*

750.7 Other specified anomalies of stomach

Congenital:

cardiospasm

hourglass stomach

Displacement of stomach

Diverticulum of stomach, congenital

Duplication of stomach

Megalogastria

Microgastria

Transposition of stomach

750.8 Other specified anomalies of upper alimentary tract

750.9 Unspecified anomaly of upper alimentary tract

Congenital:

anomaly NOS   ⎫ of upper alimentary tract [any

deformity NOS   ⎬ part, except tongue]

✓4ᵗʰ **751 Other congenital anomalies of digestive system**

751.0 Meckel's diverticulum

Meckel's diverticulum (displaced) (hypertrophic)

Persistent:

omphalomesenteric duct

vitelline duct

DEF: Malformed sacs or appendages of ileum of small intestine; can cause strangulation, volvulus and intussusception.

AHA: 1Q, '04, 10

TIP: Assign for mesodiverticular band, a fibrous band connecting the tip of the diverticulum to the mesentery; can cause small bowel herniation and obstruction.

751.1 Atresia and stenosis of small intestine   C

Atresia of:

duodenum

ileum

intestine NOS

Congenital:

absence   ⎫

obstruction ⎬ of small intestine or intestine

stenosis   ⎪   NOS

stricture   ⎭

Imperforate jejunum

CC Exd: 751.1, 751.8-751.9

751.2 Atresia and stenosis of large intestine rectum, and anal canal   C

Absence:

anus (congenital)

appendix, congenital

large intestine, congenital

rectum

Atresia of:

anus

colon

rectum

Congenital or infantile:

obstruction of large intestine

occlusion of anus

stricture of anus

Imperforate:

anus

rectum

Stricture of rectum, congenital

CC Exd: 751.2, 751.8-751.9

AHA: 2Q, '11, 13; 2Q, '98, 16

751.3 Hirschsprung's disease and other congenital functional disorders of colon   C

Aganglionosis

Congenital dilation of colon

Congenital megacolon

Macrocolon

DEF: Hirschsprung's disease: enlarged or dilated colon (megacolon) with absence of ganglion cells in the narrowed wall distally; causes inability to defecate.

CC Exd: 751.3, 751.8-751.9

Ⓝ Newborn Age: 0   Ⓟ Pediatric Age: 0-17   Ⓜ Maternity Age: 12-55   Ⓐ Adult Age: 15-124   MCC Major CC Condition   CC CC Condition   HIV HIV Related D

751.4 Anomalies of intestinal fixation   `CC`
Congenital adhesions:
omental, anomalous
peritoneal
Jackson's membrane
Malrotation of colon
Rotation of cecum or colon:
failure of
incomplete
insufficient
Universal mesentery
CC Excl: 751.4-751.5

751.5 Other anomalies of intestine   `CC`
Congenital diverticulum, colon   Megaloappendix
Dolichocolon   Megaloduodenum
Duplication of: Microcolon
anus   Persistent cloaca
appendix   Transposition of:
cecum   appendix
intestine   colon
Ectopic anus   intestine
CC Excl: 751.0-751.5
AHA: 2Q, '10, 12; 3Q, '02, 11; 3Q, '01, 8
Q43.9 Congenital malformation of intestine unspecified   `I-10`

`√5ᵗʰ` **751.6 Anomalies of gallbladder, bile ducts, and liver**

751.60 Unspecified anomaly of gallbladder, bile ducts,   `CC`
and liver
CC Excl: 751.60

751.61 Biliary atresia   `MCC`
Congenital:
absence
hypoplasia   } of bile duct (common) of
obstruction   passage
stricture
CC Excl: 751.61, 751.8-751.9
AHA: S-O, '87, 8

751.62 Congenital cystic disease of liver   `CC`
Congenital polycystic disease of liver
Fibrocystic disease of liver
CC Excl: 751.62-751.69

751.69 Other anomalies of gallbladder, bile   `CC`
ducts, and liver
Absence of:
gallbladder, congenital
liver (lobe)
Accessory:
hepatic ducts
liver
Congenital:
choledochal cyst
hepatomegaly
Duplication of:
biliary duct
cystic duct
gallbladder
liver
Floating:
gallbladder
liver
Intrahepatic gallbladder
CC Excl: 751.60-751.69
AHA: S-O, '87, 8

751.7 Anomalies of pancreas   `CC`
Absence
Accessory
Agenesis   } (of) pancreas
Annular
Hypoplasia
Ectopic pancreatic tissue
Pancreatic heterotopia
EXCLUDES *diabetes mellitus (249.0-249.9, 250.0-250.9)*
fibrocystic disease of pancreas (277.00-277.09)
neonatal diabetes mellitus (775.1)
CC Excl: 751.7-751.9

751.8 Other specified anomalies of digestive system
Absence (complete) (partial) of alimentary tract NOS
Duplication   } of digestive organs NOS
Malposition, congenital
EXCLUDES *congenital diaphragmatic hernia (756.6)*
congenital hiatus hernia (750.6)

751.9 Unspecified anomaly of digestive system
Congenital:
anomaly NOS   } of digestive system NOS
deformity NOS

`√4ᵗʰ` **752 Congenital anomalies of genital organs**
EXCLUDES *syndromes associated with anomalies in the number and*
form of chromosomes (758.0-758.9)

752.0 Anomalies of ovaries   ♀
Absence, congenital }
Accessory   } (of) ovary
Ectopic   }
Streak   }

`√5ᵗʰ` **752.1 Anomalies of fallopian tubes and broad ligaments**

752.10 Unspecified anomaly of fallopian tubes and   ♀
broad ligaments

752.11 Embryonic cyst of fallopian tubes and broad   ♀
ligaments
Cyst: Cyst:
epoophoron   parovarian
fimbrial
AHA: S-O, '85, 13

752.19 Other   ♀
Absence   } (of) fallopian tube or broad
Accessory   ligament
Atresia

752.2 Doubling of uterus   ♀
Didelphic uterus
Doubling of uterus [any degree] (associated with doubling of
cervix and vagina)

`√5ᵗʰ` **752.3 Other anomalies of uterus**
AHA: 4Q, '10, 90-91; 3Q, '06, 18

752.31 Agenesis of uterus   ♀
Congenital absence of uterus
Q51.0 Congenital absence of uterus   `I-10`

752.32 Hypoplasia of uterus   ♀
Q51.811 Hypoplasia of uterus   `I-10`

752.33 Unicornuate uterus   ♀
Unicornuate uterus with or without a separate
uterine horn
Uterus with only one functioning horn
Q51.4 Unicornuate uterus   `I-10`

752.34 Bicornuate uterus   ♀
Bicornuate uterus, complete or partial
Q51.3 Bicornuate uterus   `I-10`

752.35 Septate uterus   ♀
Septate uterus, complete or partial

752.36 Arcuate uterus   ♀
Q51.810 Arcuate uterus   `I-10`

752.39 Other anomalies of uterus   ♀
Aplasia of uterus NOS
Müllerian anomaly of the uterus, NEC
EXCLUDES *anomaly of uterus due to exposure to*
diethylstilbestrol [DES] in utero
(760.76)
didelphic uterus (752.2)
doubling of uterus (752.2)
DEF: Müllerian anomalies: The failure or disruption of
female embryonic Müllerian ducts to transform into the
upper vagina, cervix uterus, and oviducts, resulting in
anomalous organ development.

`√5ᵗʰ` **752.4 Anomalies of cervix, vagina, and external female genitalia**

752.40 Unspecified anomaly of cervix, vagina, and   ♀
external female genitalia

752.41 Embryonic cyst of cervix, vagina, and external female genitalia ♀
Cyst of: Cyst of:
canal of Nuck,   vagina, embryonal
congenital   vulva, congenital
Gartner's duct
DEF: Embryonic fluid-filled cysts of cervix, vagina or external female genitalia.

752.42 Imperforate hymen ♀
DEF: Complete closure of membranous fold around external opening of vagina.

752.43 Cervical agenesis ♀
Cervical hypoplasia
AHA: 4Q, '10, 90-92
Q51.5 Agenesis and aplasia of cervix   `I-10`

752.44 Cervical duplication ♀
AHA: 4Q, '10, 90-92

752.45 Vaginal agenesis ♀
Agenesis of vagina, total or partial
AHA: 4Q, '10, 90-92
Q52.0 Congenital absence of vagina   `I-10`

752.46 Transverse vaginal septum ♀
AHA: 4Q, '10, 90-92

752.47 Longitudinal vaginal septum ♀
Longitudinal vaginal septum with or without obstruction
AHA: 4Q, '10, 90-92

752.49 Other anomalies of cervix, vagina, and external female genitalia ♀
Absence of clitoris or vulva
Agenesis of clitoris or vulva
Anomalies of cervix, NEC
Anomalies of hymen, NEC
Congenital stenosis or stricture of:
cervical canal
vagina
Müllerian anomalies of the cervix and vagina, NEC
EXCLUDES double vagina associated with total duplication (752.2)
AHA: 3Q, '06, 18

√5ᵗʰ **752.5 Undescended and retractile testicle**
AHA: 4Q, '96, 33

752.51 Undescended testis ♂
Cryptorchism
Ectopic testis
Q53.20 Undescended testicle unspecified bilateral   `I-10`

752.52 Retractile testis ♂

√5ᵗʰ **752.6 Hypospadias and epispadias and other penile anomalies**
AHA: 4Q, '96, 34, 35

752.61 Hypospadias ♂
DEF: Abnormal opening of urethra on the ventral surface of the penis or perineum.
AHA: 4Q, '03, 67-68; 3Q, '97, 6
Q54.1 Hypospadias penile   `I-10`

752.62 Epispadias ♂
Anaspadias
DEF: Urethra opening on dorsal surface of penis.

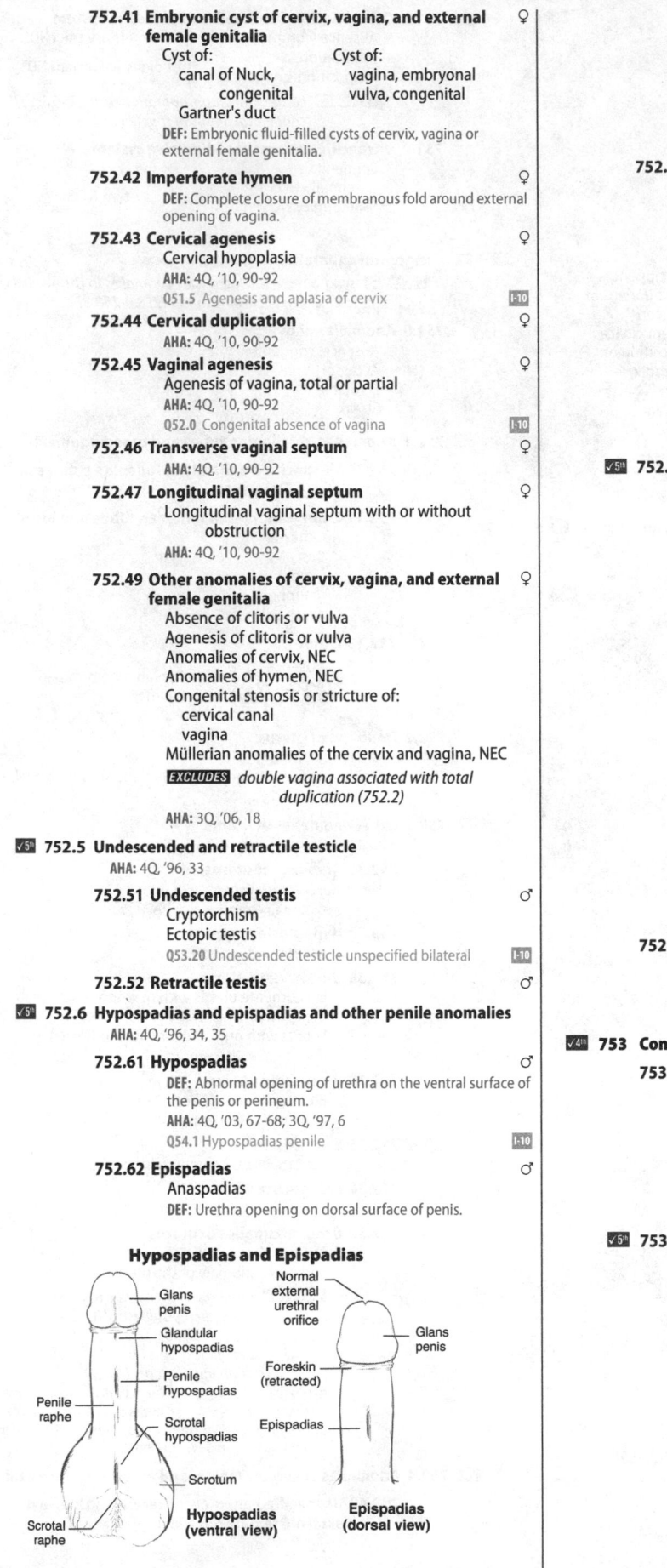

Hypospadias and Epispadias

Glans penis
Glandular hypospadias
Penile hypospadias
Penile raphe
Scrotal hypospadias
Scrotum
Scrotal raphe
Hypospadias (ventral view)

Normal external urethral orifice
Glans penis
Foreskin (retracted)
Epispadias
Epispadias (dorsal view)

752.63 Congenital chordee ♂
DEF: Ventral bowing of penis due to fibrous band along corpus spongiosum; occurs with hypospadias.

752.64 Micropenis ♂

752.65 Hidden penis ♂

752.69 Other penile anomalies ♂

752.7 Indeterminate sex and pseudohermaphroditism
Gynandrism
Hermaphroditism
Ovotestis
Pseudohermaphroditism (male) (female)
Pure gonadal dysgenesis
EXCLUDES androgen insensitivity (259.50-259.52)
pseudohermaphroditism:
female, with adrenocortical disorder (255.2)
male, with gonadal disorder (257.8)
with specified chromosomal anomaly (758.0-758.9)
testicular feminization syndrome (259.50-259.52)
DEF: Pseudohermaphroditism: presence of gonads of one sex and external genitalia of other sex.

√5ᵗʰ **752.8 Other specified anomalies of genital organs**
EXCLUDES congenital hydrocele (778.6)
penile anomalies (752.61-752.69)
phimosis or paraphimosis (605)

752.81 Scrotal transposition ♂
AHA: 4Q, '03, 67-68

752.89 Other specified anomalies of genital organs
Absence of:
prostate
spermatic cord
vas deferens
Anorchism
Aplasia (congenital) of:
prostate
round ligament
testicle
Atresia of:
ejaculatory duct
vas deferens
Fusion of testes
Hypoplasia of testis
Monorchism
Polyorchism

752.9 Unspecified anomaly of genital organs
Congenital:
anomaly NOS } of genital organ, not
deformity NOS } elsewhere classified

√4ᵗʰ **753 Congenital anomalies of urinary system**

753.0 Renal agenesis and dysgenesis `CC`
Atrophy of kidney:
congenital
infantile
Congenital absence of kidney(s)
Hypoplasia of kidney(s)
CC Exd: 599.60-599.69, 753.0
Q60.2 Renal agenesis unspecified   `I-10`

√5ᵗʰ **753.1 Cystic kidney disease**
EXCLUDES acquired cyst of kidney (593.2)
AHA: 4Q, '90, 3

753.10 Cystic kidney disease, unspecified `CC`
CC Exd: 599.60-599.69, 753.10
Q61.9 Cystic kidney disease unspecified   `I-10`

753.11 Congenital single renal cyst `CC`
CC Exd: 599.60-599.69, 753.11

753.12 Polycystic kidney, unspecified type `CC`
CC Exd: 599.60-599.69, 753.12-753.14
Q61.3 Polycystic kidney unspecified   `I-10`

753.13 Polycystic kidney, autosomal dominant `CC`
DEF: Slow progressive disease characterized by bilateral cysts causing increased kidney size and impaired function.
CC Exd: See code: 753.12

`N` Newborn Age: 0   `P` Pediatric Age: 0-17   `M` Maternity Age: 12-55   `A` Adult Age: 15-124   `MCC` Major CC Condition   `CC` CC Condition   `HIV` HIV Related Dx

753.14 Polycystic kidney, autosomal recessive `CC`
DEF: Rare disease characterized by multiple cysts involving kidneys and liver, producing renal and hepatic failure in childhood or adolescence.
CC Exd: See code: 753.12

753.15 Renal dysplasia `CC`
CC Exd: 599.60-599.69, 753.15

753.16 Medullary cystic kidney `CC`
Nephronopthisis
DEF: Diffuse kidney disease results in uremia onset prior to age 20.
CC Exd: 599.60-599.69, 753.16-753.19

753.17 Medullary sponge kidney `CC`
DEF: Dilated collecting tubules; usually asymptomatic but calcinosis in tubules may cause renal insufficiency.
CC Exd: See code: 753.16

753.19 Other specified cystic kidney disease `CC`
Multicystic kidney
CC Exd: See code: 753.16

√5ᵗʰ **753.2 Obstructive defects of renal pelvis and ureter**
AHA: 4Q, '96, 35

753.20 Unspecified obstructive defect of renal pelvis and ureter `CC`
CC Exd: 599.60-599.69, 753.20-753.22, 753.29

753.21 Congenital obstruction of ureteropelvic junction `CC`
DEF: Stricture at junction of ureter and renal pelvis.
CC Exd: See code: 753.20

753.22 Congenital obstruction of ureterovesical junction `CC`
Adynamic ureter
Congenital hydroureter
DEF: Stricture at junction of ureter and bladder.
CC Exd: See code: 753.20

753.23 Congenital ureterocele `CC`
CC Exd: See code: 753.20

753.29 Other `CC`
CC Exd: See code: 753.20
Q62.11 Congen occlusion of ureteropelvic junct `I-10`

753.3 Other specified anomalies of kidney
Accessory kidney
Congenital:
  calculus of kidney
  displaced kidney
Discoid kidney
Double kidney with double pelvis
Ectopic kidney
Fusion of kidneys
Giant kidney
Horseshoe kidney
Hyperplasia of kidney
Lobulation of kidney
Malrotation of kidney
Trifid kidney (pelvis)
AHA: 1Q, '07, 23
TIP: Assign for Finnish-type congenital nephrosis, along with code 581.3 Nephrotic syndrome.
Q63.8 Oth specified congenital malformations of kidney `I-10`

753.4 Other specified anomalies of ureter
Absent ureter
Accessory ureter
Deviation of ureter
Displaced ureteric orifice
Double ureter
Ectopic ureter
Implantation, anomalous of ureter

753.5 Exstrophy of urinary bladder `CC`
Ectopia vesicae
Extroversion of bladder
DEF: Absence of lower abdominal and anterior bladder walls with posterior bladder wall protrusion.
CC Exd: 599.60-599.69, 753.5, 753.9

753.6 Atresia and stenosis of urethra and bladder neck `CC`
Congenital obstruction:
  bladder neck
  urethra
Congenital stricture of:
  urethra (valvular)
  urinary meatus
  vesicourethral orifice
Imperforate urinary meatus
Impervious urethra
Urethral valve formation
CC Exd: 599.60-599.69, 753.6, 753.9

753.7 Anomalies of urachus
Cyst
Fistula   } (of) urachus/sinus
Patent
Persistent umbilical sinus

753.8 Other specified anomalies of bladder and urethra
Absence, congenital of:
  bladder
  urethra
Accessory:
  bladder
  urethra
Congenital:
  diverticulum of bladder
  hernia of bladder
  urethrorectal fistula
  prolapse of:
    bladder (mucosa)
    urethra
Double:
  urethra
  urinary meatus

753.9 Unspecified anomaly of urinary system
Congenital:
  anomaly NOS   } of urinary system [any part,
  deformity NOS   except urachus]
AHA: 2Q, '11, 6

√4ᵗʰ **754 Certain congenital musculoskeletal deformities**
INCLUDES nonteratogenic deformities which are considered to be due to intrauterine malposition and pressure

754.0 Of skull, face, and jaw
Asymmetry of face
Compression facies
Depressions in skull
Deviation of nasal septum, congenital
Dolichocephaly
Plagiocephaly
Potter's facies
Squashed or bent nose, congenital
EXCLUDES dentofacial anomalies (524.0-524.9)
syphilitic saddle nose (090.5)

754.1 Of sternocleidomastoid muscle
Congenital sternomastoid torticollis
Congenital wryneck
Contracture of sternocleidomastoid (muscle)
Sternomastoid tumor

754.2 Of spine `CC`
Congenital postural:
  lordosis
  scoliosis
CC Exd: 754.2

√5ᵗʰ **754.3 Congenital dislocation of hip**

754.30 Congenital dislocation of hip, unilateral
Congenital dislocation of hip NOS

754.31 Congenital dislocation of hip, bilateral

754.32 Congenital subluxation of hip, unilateral
Congenital flexion deformity, hip or thigh
Predislocation status of hip at birth
Preluxation of hip, congenital

754.33 Congenital subluxation of hip, bilateral

754.35 Congenital dislocation of one hip with subluxation of other hip

Additional Digit Required   Unacceptable PDx   Manifestation Code   Hospital Acquired Condition   ►◄ Revised Text   ● New Code   ▲ Revised Code Title
14 ICD-9-CM   **Volume 1 – 265**

753.14–754.35

Congenital Anomalies

754.4–755.29

√5ᵗʰ **754.4 Congenital genu recurvatum and bowing of long bones of leg**

754.40 Genu recurvatum
DEF: Backward curving of knee joint.

754.41 Congenital dislocation of knee (with genu recurvatum)

754.42 Congenital bowing of femur

754.43 Congenital bowing of tibia and fibula

754.44 Congenital bowing of unspecified long bones of leg

√5ᵗʰ **754.5 Varus deformities of feet**
EXCLUDES   acquired (736.71, 736.75, 736.79)

754.50 Talipes varus
Congenital varus deformity of foot, unspecified
Pes varus
DEF: Inverted foot marked by outer sole resting on ground.

754.51 Talipes equinovarus
Equinovarus (congenital)
DEF: Elevated, outward rotation of heel; also called clubfoot.

754.52 Metatarsus primus varus
DEF: Malformed first metatarsal bone, with bone angled toward body.

754.53 Metatarsus varus

754.59 Other
Talipes calcaneovarus

√5ᵗʰ **754.6 Valgus deformities of feet**
EXCLUDES   valgus deformity of foot (acquired) (736.79)

754.60 Talipes valgus
Congenital valgus deformity of foot, unspecified

754.61 Congenital pes planus
Congenital rocker bottom flat foot
Flat foot, congenital
EXCLUDES   pes planus (acquired) (734)

754.62 Talipes calcaneovalgus

754.69 Other
Talipes:
equinovalgus
planovalgus

√5ᵗʰ **754.7 Other deformities of feet**
EXCLUDES   acquired (736.70-736.79)

754.70 Talipes, unspecified
Congenital deformity of foot NOS

754.71 Talipes cavus
Cavus foot (congenital)

754.79 Other
Asymmetric talipes
Talipes:
calcaneus
equinus

√5ᵗʰ **754.8 Other specified nonteratogenic anomalies**

754.81 Pectus excavatum
Congenital funnel chest

754.82 Pectus carinatum
Congenital pigeon chest [breast]

754.89 Other   `CC`
Club hand (congenital)
Congenital:
deformity of chest wall
dislocation of elbow
Generalized flexion contractures of lower limb joints, congenital
Spade-like hand (congenital)
CC Excl: 754.81-754.89

√4ᵗʰ **755 Other congenital anomalies of limbs**
EXCLUDES   those deformities classifiable to 754.0-754.8

√5ᵗʰ **755.0 Polydactyly**

755.00 Polydactyly, unspecified digits
Supernumerary digits

755.01 Of fingers
Accessory fingers

755.02 Of toes
Accessory toes

√5ᵗʰ **755.1 Syndactyly**
Symphalangy
Webbing of digits

755.10 Of multiple and unspecified sites

755.11 Of fingers without fusion of bone

755.12 Of fingers with fusion of bone

755.13 Of toes without fusion of bone

755.14 Of toes with fusion of bone

√5ᵗʰ **755.2 Reduction deformities of upper limb**

755.20 Unspecified reduction deformity of upper limb
Ectromelia NOS ⎫
Hemimelia NOS ⎬ of upper limb
Shortening of arm, congenital

755.21 Transverse deficiency of upper limb
Amelia of upper limb
Congenital absence of:
fingers, all (complete or partial)
forearm, including hand and fingers
upper limb, complete
Congenital amputation of upper limb
Transverse hemimelia of upper limb

755.22 Longitudinal deficiency of upper limb, not elsewhere classified
Phocomelia NOS of upper limb
Rudimentary arm

755.23 Longitudinal deficiency, combined, involving humerus, radius, and ulna (complete or incomplete
Congenital absence of arm and forearm (complete or incomplete) with or without metacarpal deficiency and/or phalangeal deficiency, incomplete
Phocomelia, complete, of upper limb

755.24 Longitudinal deficiency, humeral, complete or partial (with or without distal deficiencies, incomplete)
Congenital absence of humerus (with or without absence of some [but not all] distal elements)
Proximal phocomelia of upper limb

755.25 Longitudinal deficiency, radioulnar, complete or partial (with or without distal deficiencies, incomplete)
Congenital absence of radius and ulna (with or without absence of some [but not all] distal elements)
Distal phocomelia of upper limb

755.26 Longitudinal deficiency, radial, complete or partial (with or without distal deficiencies, incomplete)
Agenesis of radius
Congenital absence of radius (with or without absence of some [but not all] distal elements)

755.27 Longitudinal deficiency, ulnar, complete or partial (with or without distal deficiencies, incomplete)
Agenesis of ulna
Congenital absence of ulna (with or without absence of some [but not all] distal elements)

755.28 Longitudinal deficiency, carpals or metacarpals, complete or partial (with or without incomplete phalangeal deficiency)

755.29 Longitudinal deficiency, phalanges, complete or partial
Absence of finger, congenital
Aphalangia of upper limb, terminal, complete or partial
EXCLUDES   terminal deficiency of all five digits (755.21)
transverse deficiency of phalanges (755.21)

N Newborn Age: 0   P Pediatric Age: 0-17   M Maternity Age: 12-55   A Adult Age: 15-124   MCC Major CC Condition   CC CC Condition   HIV HIV Related D

266 – Volume 1   2014 ICD-9-C

☑5ᵗʰ **755.3 Reduction deformities of lower limb**

755.30 Unspecified reduction deformity of lower limb

Ectromelia NOS
Hemimelia NOS ⎫ of lower limb

Shortening of leg, congenital

755.31 Transverse deficiency of lower limb

Amelia of lower limb
Congenital absence of:
  foot
  leg, including foot and toes
  lower limb, complete
  toes, all, complete
Transverse hemimelia of lower limb

755.32 Longitudinal deficiency of lower limb, not elsewhere classified

Phocomelia NOS of lower limb

755.33 Longitudinal deficiency, combined, involving femur, tibia, and fibula (complete or incomplete)

Congenital absence of thigh and (lower) leg (complete or incomplete) with or without metacarpal deficiency and/or phalangeal deficiency, incomplete
Phocomelia, complete, of lower limb

755.34 Longitudinal deficiency, femoral, complete or partial (with or without distal deficiencies, incomplete)

Congenital absence of femur (with or without absence of some [but not all] distal elements)
Proximal phocomelia of lower limb

755.35 Longitudinal deficiency, tibiofibular, complete or partial (with or without distal deficiencies, incomplete)

Congenital absence of tibia and fibula (with or without absence of some [but not all] distal elements)
Distal phocomelia of lower limb

755.36 Longitudinal deficiency, tibia, complete or partial (with or without distal deficiencies, incomplete)

Agenesis of tibia
Congenital absence of tibia (with or without absence of some [but not all] distal elements)

755.37 Longitudinal deficiency, fibular, complete or partial (with or without distal deficiencies, incomplete)

Agenesis of fibula
Congenital absence of fibula (with or without absence of some [but not all] distal elements)

755.38 Longitudinal deficiency, tarsals or metatarsals, complete or partial (with or without incomplete phalangeal deficiency)

755.39 Longitudinal deficiency, phalanges, complete or partial

Absence of toe, congenital
Aphalangia of lower limb, terminal, complete or partial

  EXCLUDES *terminal deficiency of all five digits (755.31)*
  transverse deficiency of phalanges (755.31)

755.4 Reduction deformities, unspecified limb

Absence, congenital (complete or partial) of limb NOS

Amelia
Ectromelia
Hemimelia ⎫ of unspecified limb
Phocomelia

☑5ᵗʰ **755.5 Other anomalies of upper limb, including shoulder girdle**

755.50 Unspecified anomaly of upper limb

755.51 Congenital deformity of clavicle

755.52 Congenital elevation of scapula

Sprengel's deformity

755.53 Radioulnar synostosis

  DEF: Osseous adhesion of radius and ulna.

755.54 Madelung's deformity

  DEF: Distal ulnar overgrowth or radial shortening; also called carpus curvus.

755.55 Acrocephalosyndactyly MCC

Apert's syndrome

  DEF: Premature cranial suture fusion (craniostenosis); marked by cone-shaped or pointed (acrocephaly) head and webbing of the fingers (syndactyly); similar to craniofacial dysostosis.
  CC Excl: 755.50, 755.55, 755.59

755.56 Accessory carpal bones

755.57 Macrodactylia (fingers)

  DEF: Abnormally large fingers, toes.

755.58 Cleft hand, congenital

Lobster-claw hand

  DEF: Extended separation between fingers into metacarpus; also may refer to large fingers and absent middle fingers of hand.

755.59 Other

Cleidocranial dysostosis
Cubitus:
  valgus, congenital
  varus, congenital

  EXCLUDES *club hand (congenital) (754.89)*
  congenital dislocation of elbow (754.89)

☑5ᵗʰ **755.6 Other anomalies of lower limb, including pelvic girdle**

755.60 Unspecified anomaly of lower limb

755.61 Coxa valga, congenital

  DEF: Abnormally wide angle between the neck and shaft of the femur.

755.62 Coxa vara, congenital

  DEF: Diminished angle between neck and shaft of femur.

755.63 Other congenital deformity of hip (joint)

Congenital anteversion of femur (neck)

  EXCLUDES *congenital dislocation of hip (754.30-754.35)*
  AHA: 1Q, '94, 15; S-O, '84, 15
  Q65.9 Congenital deformity of hip unspecified I-10

755.64 Congenital deformity of knee (joint)

Congenital:
  absence of patella
  genu valgum [knock-knee]
  genu varum [bowleg]
Rudimentary patella

755.65 Macrodactylia of toes

  DEF: Abnormally large toes.

755.66 Other anomalies of toes

Congenital:
  hallux valgus
  hallux varus
  hammer toe

755.67 Anomalies of foot, not elsewhere classified

Astragaloscaphoid synostosis
Calcaneonavicular bar
Coalition of calcaneus
Talonavicular synostosis
Tarsal coalitions

755.69 Other

Congenital:
  angulation of tibia
  deformity (of):
    ankle (joint)
    sacroiliac (joint)
  fusion of sacroiliac joint

755.8 Other specified anomalies of unspecified limb

755.9 Unspecified anomaly of unspecified limb

Congenital:
  anomaly NOS
  deformity NOS ⎫ of unspecified limb

  EXCLUDES *reduction deformity of unspecified limb (755.4)*

Congenital Anomalies

756-756.73

☑4ᵗʰ **756 Other congenital musculoskeletal anomalies**

    EXCLUDES *congenital myotonic chondrodystrophy (359.23)*
        those deformities classifiable to 754.0-754.8

756.0 Anomalies of skull and face bones
Absence of skull bones
Acrocephaly
Congenital deformity of forehead
Craniosynostosis
Crouzon's disease
Hypertelorism
Imperfect fusion of skull
Oxycephaly
Platybasia
Premature closure of cranial sutures
Tower skull
Trigonocephaly

    EXCLUDES *acrocephalosyndactyly [Apert's syndrome] (755.55)*
        dentofacial anomalies (524.0-524.9)
        skull defects associated with brain anomalies, such as:
            anencephalus (740.0)
            encephalocele (742.0)
            hydrocephalus (742.3)
            microcephalus (742.1)

AHA: ▶2Q, '12, 17;◀ 3Q, '98, 9; 3Q, '96, 15

TIP: Assign for Nager syndrome (preaxial acrofacial dysostosis), along with codes for any additional features that are not captured in the code.

Q75.8 Other spec cong malformations skull & face bones   I-10

☑5ᵗʰ ### 756.1 Anomalies of spine

756.10 Anomaly of spine, unspecified

756.11 Spondylolysis, lumbosacral region
Prespondylolisthesis (lumbosacral)

DEF: Bilateral or unilateral defect through the pars interarticularis of a vertebra causes spondylolisthesis.

756.12 Spondylolisthesis
DEF: Downward slipping of lumbar vertebra over next vertebra; usually related to pelvic deformity.

Q76.2 Congenital spondylolisthesis   I-10

756.13 Absence of vertebra, congenital   CC
CC Excl: 756.10-756.19

756.14 Hemivertebra
DEF: Incomplete development of one side of a vertebra.

756.15 Fusion of spine [vertebra], congenital

756.16 Klippel-Feil syndrome
DEF: Short, wide neck; limits range of motion due to abnormal number of cervical vertebra or fused hemivertebrae.

756.17 Spina bifida occulta
    EXCLUDES *spina bifida (aperta) (741.0-741.9)*

DEF: Spina bifida marked by a bony spinal canal defect without a protrusion of the cord or meninges; it is diagnosed by radiography and has no symptoms.

756.19 Other
Platyspondylia
Supernumerary vertebra

756.2 Cervical rib
Supernumerary rib in the cervical region
DEF: Costa cervicalis: extra rib attached to cervical vertebra.

756.3 Other anomalies of ribs and sternum   CC
Congenital absence of:
  rib
  sternum
Congenital:
  fissure of sternum
  fusion of ribs
Sternum bifidum

    EXCLUDES *nonteratogenic deformity of chest wall (754.81-754.89)*

CC Excl: 756.2-756.3

756.4 Chondrodystrophy
Achondroplasia   Enchondromatosis
Chondrodystrophia (fetalis)   Ollier's disease
Dyschondroplasia

    EXCLUDES *congenital myotonic chondrodystrophy (359.23)*
        lipochondrodystrophy [Hurler's syndrome] (277.5)
        Morquio's disease (277.5)

DEF: Abnormal development of cartilage.

AHA: 2Q, '02, 16; S-O, '87, 10

TIP: Assign for Jeune's syndrome, and also for cartilage-hair syndrome (cartilage-hair hypoplasia).

☑5ᵗʰ ### 756.5 Osteodystrophies

756.50 Osteodystrophy, unspecified

756.51 Osteogenesis imperfecta   CC
Fragilitas ossium
Osteopsathyrosis

DEF: A collagen disorder commonly characterized by brittle, osteoporotic, easily fractured bones, hypermobility of joints, blue sclerae, and a tendency to hemorrhage.

CC Excl: 756.50-756.59

756.52 Osteopetrosis   CC
DEF: Abnormally dense bone, optic atrophy, hepatosplenomegaly, deafness; sclerosing depletes bone marrow and nerve foramina of skull; often fatal.

CC Excl: See code: 756.51

756.53 Osteopoikilosis
DEF: Multiple sclerotic foci on ends of long bones, stippling in round, flat bones; identified by x-ray.

756.54 Polyostotic fibrous dysplasia of bone
DEF: Fibrous tissue displaces bone results in segmented ragged-edge café-au-lait spots; occurs in girls of early puberty.

756.55 Chondroectodermal dysplasia
Ellis-van Creveld syndrome

DEF: Inadequate enchondral bone formation; impaired development of hair and teeth, polydactyly, and cardiac septum defects.

756.56 Multiple epiphyseal dysplasia

756.59 Other
Albright (-McCune)-Sternberg syndrome

756.6 Anomalies of diaphragm   MCC
Absence of diaphragm   Eventration of diaphragm
Congenital hernia:
  diaphragmatic
  foramen of Morgagni

    EXCLUDES *congenital hiatus hernia (750.6)*

CC Excl: 750.6, 756.6

☑5ᵗʰ ### 756.7 Anomalies of abdominal wall

756.70 Anomaly of abdominal wall, unspecified   MCC
CC Excl: 756.70-756.79

756.71 Prune belly syndrome   MCC
Eagle-Barrett syndrome
Prolapse of bladder mucosa

DEF: Prune belly syndrome: absence of lower rectus abdominis muscle and lower and medial oblique muscles; results in dilated bladder and ureters, dysplastic kidneys and hydronephrosis; common in male infants with undescended testicles.

CC Excl: See code: 756.70

AHA: 4Q, '97, 44

756.72 Omphalocele   MCC
Exomphalos

DEF: Exomphalos: umbilical hernia prominent navel.
DEF: Omphalocele: hernia of umbilicus due to impaired abdominal wall; results in membrane-covered intestine protruding through peritoneum and amnion.

CC Excl: See code: 756.70

AHA: 4Q, '09, 98-99

756.73 Gastroschisis   MCC
DEF: Fissure of abdominal wall, results in protruding small or large intestine.

CC Excl: See code: 756.70

AHA: 4Q, '09, 98-99

N Newborn Age: 0   P Pediatric Age: 0-17   M Maternity Age: 12-55   A Adult Age: 15-124   MCC Major CC Condition   CC CC Condition   HIV HIV Related Dx

Omphalocele

Gastroschisis

756.79 Other congenital anomalies of abdominal wall MCC

> EXCLUDES *umbilical hernia (551-553 with .1)*
> **CC Excl:** See code: 756.70

√5th **756.8 Other specified anomalies of muscle, tendon, fascia, and connective tissue**

756.81 Absence of muscle and tendon
Absence of muscle (pectoral)
AHA: 1Q, '10, 13

756.82 Accessory muscle

756.83 Ehlers-Danlos syndrome CC
> **DEF:** Danlos syndrome: connective tissue disorder causes hyperextended skin and joints; results in fragile blood vessels with bleeding, poor wound healing and subcutaneous pseudotumors.
> **CC Excl:** 756.83-756.89

756.89 Other
Amyotrophia congenita
Congenital shortening of tendon
AHA: 3Q, '99, 16
TIP: Assign for Stickler's syndrome, a hereditary progressive arthro-ophthalmopathy, along with codes for the specific manifestations.

756.9 Other and unspecified anomalies of musculoskeletal system
Congenital:
 anomaly NOS } of musculoskeletal system,
 deformity NOS } not elsewhere classified

√4th **757 Congenital anomalies of the integument**
> INCLUDES anomalies of skin, subcutaneous tissue, hair, nails, and breast
> EXCLUDES *hemangioma (228.00-228.09)*
> *pigmented nevus (216.0-216.9)*

757.0 Hereditary edema of legs
Congenital lymphedema
Hereditary trophedema
Milroy's disease

757.1 Ichthyosis congenita
Congenital ichthyosis   Ichthyosiform erythroderma
Harlequin fetus
> **DEF:** Overproduction of skin cells causes scaling of skin; may result in stillborn fetus or death soon after birth.

757.2 Dermatoglyphic anomalies
Abnormal palmar creases
> **DEF:** Abnormal skin-line patterns of fingers, palms, toes and soles; initial finding of possible chromosomal abnormalities.

√5th **757.3 Other specified anomalies of skin**

757.31 Congenital ectodermal dysplasia
> **DEF:** Tissues and structures originate in embryonic ectoderm; includes anhidrotic and hidrotic ectodermal dysplasia and EEC syndrome.

757.32 Vascular hamartomas
Birthmarks
Port-wine stain
Strawberry nevus
> **DEF:** Benign tumor of blood vessels; due to malformed angioblastic tissues.
> **AHA:** ▶2Q, '12, 7◀
> **TIP:** ▶Assign for nevus flammeus, which may be associated with increased risk for seizure or glaucoma. Further testing may be required. ◀
> Q82.5 Congenital non-neoplastic nevus   I-10

757.33 Congenital pigmentary anomalies of skin
Congenital poikiloderma
Urticaria pigmentosa
Xeroderma pigmentosum
> EXCLUDES *albinism (270.2)*
> Q82.2 Mastocytosis   I-10

757.39 Other
Accessory skin tags, congenital
Congenital scar
Epidermolysis bullosa
Keratoderma (congenital)
> EXCLUDES *pilonidal cyst (685.0-685.1)*
> Q82.8 Other specified congenital malformations of skin   I-10

757.4 Specified anomalies of hair
Congenital:
 alopecia
 atrichosis
 beaded hair
 hypertrichosis
 monilethrix
Persistent lanugo

757.5 Specified anomalies of nails
Anonychia   Congenital:
Congenital: leukonychia
 clubnail   onychauxis
 koilonychia   pachyonychia

757.6 Specified congenital anomalies of breast
Accessory
Congenital absent } breast or nipple
Supernumerary
> EXCLUDES *absence of pectoral muscle (756.81)*
> *hypoplasia of breast (611.82)*
> *micromastia (611.82)*

757.8 Other specified anomalies of the integument

757.9 Unspecified anomaly of the integument
Congenital:
 anomaly NOS } of integument
 deformity NOS

√4th **758 Chromosomal anomalies**
> INCLUDES syndromes associated with anomalies in the number and form of chromosomes
> Use additional codes for conditions associated with the chromosomal anomalies

758.0 Down's syndrome
Mongolism
Translocation Down's syndrome
Trisomy:
 21 or 22
 G
> Q90.9 Down's syndrome unspecified   I-10

Additional Digit Required   Unacceptable PDx   Manifestation Code   Hospital Acquired Condition   ▶◀ Revised Text   ● New Code   ▲ Revised Code Title

14 ICD-9-CM   February 2013 · Volume 1 – 269

758.1 Patau's syndrome   `CC`
Trisomy:
13
D_1
DEF: Trisomy of 13th chromosome; characteristic failure to thrive, severe mental impairment, seizures, abnormal eyes, low-set ears and sloped forehead.
CC Exd: 758.0-758.9

758.2 Edwards' syndrome   `CC`
Trisomy:
18
E_3
DEF: Trisomy of 18th chromosome; characteristic mental and physical impairments; mainly affects females.
CC Exd: See code: 758.1

√5ᵗʰ **758.3 Autosomal deletion syndromes**

    758.31 Cri-du-chat syndrome   `CC`
Deletion 5p
DEF: Hereditary congenital syndrome caused by a microdeletion of short arm of chromosome 5; characterized by catlike cry in newborn, microencephaly, severe mental deficiency, and hypertelorism.
CC Exd: 758.0-758.2, 758.32-758.9

    758.32 Velo-cardio-facial syndrome   `MCC`
Deletion 22q11.2
DEF: Microdeletion syndrome affecting multiple organs; characteristic cleft palate, heart defects, elongated face with almond-shaped eyes, wide nose, small ears, weak immune systems, weak musculature, hypothyroidism, short stature, and scoliosis; deletion at q11.2 on the long arm of the chromosome 22.
CC Exd: 758.0-758.31, 758.33-758.9

    758.33 Other microdeletions   `CC`
Miller-Dieker syndrome
Smith-Magenis syndrome
DEF: Miller-Dieker syndrome: deletion from the short arm of chromosome 17; characteristic mental retardation, speech and motor development delays, neurological complications, and multiple abnormalities affecting the kidneys, heart, gastrointestinal tract; death in infancy or early childhood.
DEF: Smith-Magenis syndrome: deletion in a certain area of chromosome 17 that results in craniofacial changes, speech delay, hoarse voice, hearing loss, and behavioral problems, such as self-destructive head banging, wrist biting, and tearing at nails.
CC Exd: 758.0-758.32, 758.39-758.9

    758.39 Other autosomal deletions   `CC`
CC Exd: 758.0-758.33, 758.4-758.9

758.4 Balanced autosomal translocation in normal individual

758.5 Other conditions due to autosomal anomalies
Accessory autosomes NEC

758.6 Gonadal dysgenesis
Ovarian dysgenesis
Turner's syndrome
XO syndrome
EXCLUDES pure gonadal dysgenesis (752.7)

758.7 Klinefelter's syndrome   ♂
XXY syndrome
DEF: Impaired embryonic development of seminiferous tubes; results in small testes, azoospermia, infertility and enlarged mammary glands.

√5ᵗʰ **758.8 Other conditions due to chromosome anomalies**

    758.81 Other conditions due to sex chromosome anomalies

    758.89 Other
Q99.8 Other specified chromosome abnormalities   `I-10`

758.9 Conditions due to anomaly of unspecified chromosome

√4ᵗʰ **759 Other and unspecified congenital anomalies**

759.0 Anomalies of spleen   `C`
Aberrant
Absent } spleen
Accessory
Congenital splenomegaly
Ectopic spleen
Lobulation of spleen
CC Exd: 759.0, 759.9

759.1 Anomalies of adrenal gland
Aberrant
Absent } adrenal gland
Accessory
EXCLUDES adrenogenital disorders (255.2)
congenital disorders of steroid metabolism (255.2)

759.2 Anomalies of other endocrine glands
Absent parathyroid gland
Accessory thyroid gland
Persistent thyroglossal or thyrolingual duct
Thyroglossal (duct) cyst
EXCLUDES congenital:
goiter (246.1)
hypothyroidism (243)

759.3 Situs inversus   `C`
Situs inversus or transversus:
abdominalis
thoracis
Transposition of viscera:
abdominal
thoracic
EXCLUDES dextrocardia without mention of complete transposition (746.87)
DEF: Laterally transposed thoracic and abdominal viscera.
CC Exd: 759.3, 759.7, 759.9

759.4 Conjoined twins   `MC`
Craniopagus
Dicephalus
Pygopagus
Thoracopagus
Xiphopagus
CC Exd: 759.4, 759.7, 759.9

759.5 Tuberous sclerosis   `C`
Bourneville's disease
Epiloia
DEF: Hamartomas of brain, retina and viscera, impaired mental ability, seizures and adenoma sebaceum.
CC Exd: 759.5-759.7, 759.9

759.6 Other hamartoses, not elsewhere classified   `C`
Syndrome:
Peutz-Jeghers
Sturge-Weber (-Dimitri)
von Hippel-Lindau
EXCLUDES neurofibromatosis (237.70-237.79)
DEF: Peutz-Jeghers: hereditary syndrome characterized by hamartomas of small intestine.
DEF: Sturge-Weber: congenital syndrome characterized by unilatera port-wine stain over trigeminal nerve, underlying meninges and cerebral cortex.
DEF: von Hipple-Lindau: hereditary syndrome of congenital angiomatosis of the retina and cerebellum.
CC Exd: 759.6, 759.9
AHA: 3Q, '92, 12

759.7 Multiple congenital anomalies, so described   `C`
Congenital:
anomaly, multiple NOS
deformity, multiple NOS
CC Exd: See code: 759.3

N Newborn Age: 0   P Pediatric Age: 0-17   M Maternity Age: 12-55   A Adult Age: 15-124   MCC Major CC Condition   CC CC Condition   HIV HIV Related D

270 – Volume 1   **2014 ICD-9-C**

√5ᵗʰ **759.8 Other specified anomalies**
AHA: S-O, '87, 9; S-O, '85, 11

759.81 Prader-Willi syndrome `cc`
CC Exd: 759.6-759.9

759.82 Marfan syndrome `cc`
CC Exd: See code: 759.81
AHA: 3Q, '93, 11

759.83 Fragile X syndrome
AHA: 4Q, '94, 41

759.89 Other `cc`
Congenital malformation syndromes affecting
multiple systems, not elsewhere classified
Laurence-Moon-Biedl syndrome
CC Exd: 759.81-759.89
AHA: ▶2Q, '12, 3;◀ 3Q, '08, 3; 3Q, '06, 21; 2Q, '05, 17; 2Q, '04,
12; 1Q, '01, 3; 3Q, '99, 17, 18; 3Q, '98, 8
TIP: Assign for the following syndromes:
Alagille s.
Alport's s.
Antley-Bixler s.
branchio-oto-renal ((BOR) s.
Borjeson-Forsmann-Lehmann s.
cardiofaciocutaneous (CFC) s.
Costello s.
fasciocutaneoskeletal (FCS)s.
mutliple pterygium s.
▶Noonan's s.◀
Startle s.
Williams s.
Assign additional codes for any documented
manifestations.

759.9 Congenital anomaly, unspecified

15. Certain Conditions Originating in the Perinatal Period (760-779)

INCLUDES conditions which have their origin in the perinatal period, before birth through the first 28 days after birth, even though death or morbidity occurs later

Use additional code(s) to further specify condition

TIP: A newborn condition is clinically significant when it has implications for the newborn's *future* health care. This is an exception to the UHDDS guidelines.

Maternal Causes of Perinatal Morbidity and Mortality (760-763)

AHA: 2Q, '89, 14; 3Q, '90, 5

√4th **760 Fetus or newborn affected by maternal conditions which may be unrelated to present pregnancy**

INCLUDES the listed maternal conditions only when specified as a cause of mortality or morbidity of the fetus or newborn

EXCLUDES *maternal endocrine and metabolic disorders affecting fetus or newborn (775.0-775.9)*

AHA: 1Q, '94, 8; 2Q, '92, 12; N-D, '84, 11

TIP: Do not assign unless the mother's condition has actually affected the fetus or newborn.

760.0 Maternal hypertensive disorders
Fetus or newborn affected by maternal conditions classifiable to 642

760.1 Maternal renal and urinary tract diseases
Fetus or newborn affected by maternal conditions classifiable to 580-599

760.2 Maternal infections
Fetus or newborn affected by maternal infectious disease classifiable to 001-136 and 487, but fetus or newborn not manifesting that disease

EXCLUDES *congenital infectious diseases (771.0-771.8)*
maternal genital tract and other localized infections (760.8)

760.3 Other chronic maternal circulatory and respiratory diseases
Fetus or newborn affected by chronic maternal conditions classifiable to 390-459, 490-519, 745-748

760.4 Maternal nutritional disorders
Fetus or newborn affected by:
maternal disorders classifiable to 260-269
maternal malnutrition NOS

EXCLUDES *fetal malnutrition (764.10-764.29)*

760.5 Maternal injury
Fetus or newborn affected by maternal conditions classifiable to 800-995

√5th **760.6 Surgical operation on mother and fetus**

EXCLUDES *cesarean section for present delivery (763.4)*
damage to placenta from amniocentesis, cesarean section, or surgical induction (762.1)

AHA: 4Q, '08, 137-138

TIP: These codes include existing conditions present at the time of birth that are related to procedures performed before the time of delivery.

760.61 Newborn affected by amniocentesis

EXCLUDES *fetal complications from amniocentesis (679.1)*

760.62 Newborn affected by other in utero procedure

EXCLUDES *fetal complications of in utero procedure (679.1)*

760.63 Newborn affected by other surgical operations on mother during pregnancy

EXCLUDES *newborn affected by previous surgical procedure on mother not associated with pregnancy (760.64)*

760.64 Newborn affected by previous surgical procedure on mother not associated with pregnancy

√5th **760.7 Noxious influences affecting fetus or newborn via placenta or breast milk**
Fetus or newborn affected by noxious substance transmitted via placenta or breast milk

EXCLUDES *anesthetic and analgesic drugs administered during labor and delivery (763.5)*
drug withdrawal syndrome in newborn (779.5)

AHA: 3Q, '91, 21

760.70 Unspecified noxious substance
Fetus or newborn affected by:
Drug NEC

760.71 Alcohol
Fetal alcohol syndrome

760.72 Narcotics

760.73 Hallucinogenic agents

760.74 Anti-infectives
Antibiotics
Antifungals

760.75 Cocaine
AHA: 3Q, '94, 6; 2Q, '92, 12; 4Q, '91, 26
TIP: If documentation indicates drug withdrawal in the newborn, also assign code 779.5 Drug withdrawal syndrome in newborn.

760.76 Diethylstilbestrol [DES]
AHA: 4Q, '94, 45

760.77 Anticonvulsants   N
Carbamazepine
Phenobarbital
Phenytoin
Valproic acid
AHA: 4Q, '05, 82

760.78 Antimetabolic agents   N
Methotrexate
Retinoic acid
Statins
AHA: 4Q, '05, 82-83

760.79 Other
Fetus or newborn affected by:
immune sera ⎫
medicinal agents NEC ⎬ transmitted via placenta or breast
toxic substance NEC ⎭
AHA: 1Q, '10, 14; 3Q, '09, 21
P04.8 Newborn (suspected) affected by oth   I-10
maternl noxious substnce

760.8 Other specified maternal conditions affecting fetus or newborn
Maternal genital tract and other localized infection affecting fetus or newborn, but fetus or newborn not manifesting that disease

EXCLUDES *maternal urinary tract infection affecting fetus or newborn (760.1)*

760.9 Unspecified maternal condition affecting fetus or newborn

√4th **761 Fetus or newborn affected by maternal complications of pregnancy**

INCLUDES the listed maternal conditions only when specified as a cause of mortality or morbidity of the fetus or newborn

761.0 Incompetent cervix
DEF: Inadequate functioning of uterine cervix.

761.1 Premature rupture of membranes

761.2 Oligohydramnios
EXCLUDES *that due to premature rupture of membranes (761.1)*
DEF: Deficient amniotic fluid.

761.3 Polyhydramnios
Hydramnios (acute) (chronic)
DEF: Excess amniotic fluid.

761.4 Ectopic pregnancy
Pregnancy: Pregnancy:
  abdominal   tubal
  intraperitoneal

Additional Digit Required   Unacceptable PDx   Manifestation Code   Hospital Acquired Condition   ►◄ Revised Text   ● New Code   ▲ Revised Code Title

2014 ICD-9-CM   Volume 1 – 273

761.5 Multiple pregnancy
Triplet (pregnancy)
Twin (pregnancy)

761.6 Maternal death

761.7 Malpresentation before labor
Breech presentation
External version
Oblique lie } before labor
Transverse lie
Unstable lie

761.8 Other specified maternal complications of pregnancy affecting fetus or newborn
Spontaneous abortion, fetus

761.9 Unspecified maternal complication of pregnancy affecting fetus or newborn

√4ᵗʰ **762 Fetus or newborn affected by complications of placenta, cord, and membranes**

INCLUDES the listed maternal conditions only when specified as a cause of mortality or morbidity in the fetus or newborn

AHA: 1Q, '94, 8

762.0 Placenta previa N
DEF: Placenta developed in lower segment of uterus; causes hemorrhaging in last trimester.

762.1 Other forms of placental separation and hemorrhage N
Abruptio placentae
Antepartum hemorrhage
Damage to placenta from amniocentesis, cesarean section, or surgical induction
Maternal blood loss
Premature separation of placenta
Rupture of marginal sinus

762.2 Other and unspecified morphological and functional abnormalities of placenta N
Placental: Placental:
  dysfunction   insufficiency
  infarction

762.3 Placental transfusion syndromes N
Placental and cord abnormality resulting in twin-to-twin or other transplacental transfusion

Use additional code to indicate resultant condition in newborn:
  fetal blood loss (772.0)
  polycythemia neonatorum (776.4)

762.4 Prolapsed cord N
Cord presentation

762.5 Other compression of umbilical cord N
Cord around neck   Knot in cord
Entanglement of cord Torsion of cord
AHA: 2Q, '03, 9
TIP: Assign only if the cord compression or entanglement was documented as having affected the fetus/newborn.
P02.5 Newborn (suspected) affected by oth compression umb cord   I-10

762.6 Other and unspecified conditions of umbilical cord N
Short cord
Thrombosis
Varices
Velamentous insertion } of umbilical cord
Vasa previa

EXCLUDES infection of umbilical cord (771.4)
         single umbilical artery (747.5)
P02.69 Newborn (suspected) affected by oth cond umbili cord   I-10

762.7 Chorioamnionitis N
Amnionitis   Placentitis
Membranitis
DEF: Inflamed fetal membrane.

762.8 Other specified abnormalities of chorion and amnion N

762.9 Unspecified abnormality of chorion and amnion N

√4ᵗʰ **763 Fetus or newborn affected by other complications of labor and delivery**

INCLUDES the listed conditions only when specified as a cause of mortality or morbidity in the fetus or newborn
EXCLUDES newborn affected by surgical procedures on mother (760.61-760.64)

AHA: 1Q, '94, 8

763.0 Breech delivery and extraction N

763.1 Other malpresentation, malposition, and disproportion during labor and delivery N
Fetus or newborn affected by:
  abnormality of bony pelvis
  contracted pelvis
  persistent occipitoposterior position
  shoulder presentation
  transverse lie
Fetus or newborn affected by conditions classifiable to 652, 653, and 660

763.2 Forceps delivery N
Fetus or newborn affected by forceps extraction

763.3 Delivery by vacuum extractor N

763.4 Cesarean delivery N
EXCLUDES placental separation or hemorrhage from cesarean section (762.1)

763.5 Maternal anesthesia and analgesia N
Reactions and intoxications from maternal opiates and tranquilizers during labor and delivery
EXCLUDES drug withdrawal syndrome in newborn (779.5)

763.6 Precipitate delivery N
Rapid second stage

763.7 Abnormal uterine contractions N
Fetus or newborn affected by:
  contraction ring
  hypertonic labor
  hypotonic uterine dysfunction
  uterine inertia or dysfunction
Fetus or newborn affected by conditions classifiable to 661, except 661.3

√5ᵗʰ **763.8 Other specified complications of labor and delivery affecting fetus or newborn**
AHA: 4Q, '98, 46

763.81 Abnormality in fetal heart rate or rhythm before the onset of labor N

763.82 Abnormality in fetal heart rate or rhythm during labor N
AHA: 4Q, '98, 46

763.83 Abnormality in fetal heart rate or rhythm, unspecified as to time of onset N

763.84 Meconium passage during delivery N
EXCLUDES meconium aspiration (770.11, 770.12)
         meconium staining (779.84)
DEF: Fetal intestinal activity that increases in response to a distressed state during delivery; anal sphincter relaxes, and meconium is passed into the amniotic fluid.
AHA: 4Q, '05, 83
TIP: If the meconium was documented as aspirated or had any effect on the newborn, see codes 770.11 and 770.12.

763.89 Other specified complications of labor and delivery affecting fetus or newborn N
Fetus or newborn affected by:
  abnormality of maternal soft tissues
  destructive operation on live fetus to facilitate delivery
  induction of labor (medical)
  other procedures used in labor and delivery
Fetus or newborn affected by other conditions classifiable to 650-699

763.9 Unspecified complication of labor and delivery affecting fetus or newborn N

N Newborn Age: 0   P Pediatric Age: 0-17   M Maternity Age: 12-55   A Adult Age: 15-124   MCC Major CC Condition   CC CC Condition   HIV HIV Related D

274 – Volume 1   2014 ICD-9-CM

Other Conditions Originating in the Perinatal Period (764–779)

The following fifth-digit subclassification is for use with category 764 and codes 765.0-765.1 to denote birthweight:

- 0 unspecified [weight]
- 1 less than 500 grams
- 2 500-749 grams
- 3 750-999 grams
- 4 1,000-1,249 grams
- 5 1,250-1,499 grams
- 6 1,500-1,749 grams
- 7 1,750-1,999 grams
- 8 2,000-2,499 grams
- 9 2,500 grams and over

√4ᵗʰ **764 Slow fetal growth and fetal malnutrition**
AHA: 1Q, '09, 13; 3Q, '04, 4; 4Q, '02, 63; 1Q,'94, 8; 2Q, '91, 19; 2Q, '89, 15

§ √5ᵗʰ **764.0 "Light-for-dates" without mention of fetal** N
[0-9] **malnutrition**
Infants underweight for gestational age
"Small-for-dates"
P05.00 Newborn light for gest age unsp weight   I-10

§ √5ᵗʰ **764.1 "Light-for-dates" with signs of fetal malnutrition** N
[0-9] Infants "light-for-dates" classifiable to 764.0, who in addition show signs of fetal malnutrition, such as dry peeling skin and loss of subcutaneous tissue

§ √5ᵗʰ **764.2 Fetal malnutrition without mention of** N
[0-9] **"light-for-dates"**
Infants, not underweight for gestational age, showing signs of fetal malnutrition, such as dry peeling skin and loss of subcutaneous tissue
Intrauterine malnutrition

§ √5ᵗʰ **764.9 Fetal growth retardation, unspecified** N
[0-9] Intrauterine growth retardation
AHA: For code 764.97: 1Q, '97, 6

√4ᵗʰ **765 Disorders relating to short gestation and low birthweight**
INCLUDES the listed conditions, without further specification, as causes of mortality, morbidity, or additional care, in fetus or newborn
AHA: 1Q, '97, 6; 1Q, '94, 8; 2Q, '91, 19; 2Q, '89, 15

§ √5ᵗʰ **765.0 Extreme immaturity** N
[0-9] NOTE Usually implies a birthweight of less than 1000 grams.
Use additional code for weeks of gestation (765.20-765.29)
AHA: 1Q, '09, 13 3Q, '04, 4; 4Q, '02, 63; For code 765.03: 4Q, '01, 51

§ √5ᵗʰ **765.1 Other preterm infants** N
[0-9] NOTE Usually implies a birthweight of 1000-2499 grams.
Prematurity NOS
Prematurity or small size, not classifiable to 765.0 or as "light-for-dates" in 764
Use additional code for weeks of gestation (765.20-765.29)
AHA: 1Q, '09, 13; 3Q, '04, 4; 4Q, '02, 63; For code 765.10: 1Q, '09, 15; 1Q, '94, 14; For code 765.17: 4Q, '08, 139; 1Q, '97, 6; For code 765.18: 4Q, '02, 64
P07.10 Other low birth weight newborn uns weight   I-10

√5ᵗʰ **765.2 Weeks of gestation**
AHA: 3Q, '04, 4; 4Q, '02, 63
TIP: Assign as an additional code with category 764 and codes from 765.0 and 765.1, as documented by the provider.

765.20 Unspecified weeks of gestation N

765.21 Less than 24 completed weeks of gestation N

765.22 24 completed weeks of gestation N

765.23 25-26 completed weeks of gestation N
AHA: 1Q, '09, 14

765.24 27-28 completed weeks of gestation N

765.25 29-30 completed weeks of gestation N
P07.32 Preterm newborn, gestl age 29 compl wks   I-10

765.26 31-32 completed weeks of gestation N
AHA: 1Q, '09, 14; 4Q, '08, 139

765.27 33-34 completed weeks of gestation N
AHA: 4Q, '10, 97

765.28 35-36 completed weeks of gestation N
AHA: 4Q, '02, 64
P07.38 Preterm newborn, gestl age 35 compl wks   I-10

765.29 37 or more completed weeks of gestation N

√4ᵗʰ **766 Disorders relating to long gestation and high birthweight**
INCLUDES the listed conditions, without further specification, as causes of mortality, morbidity, or additional care, in fetus or newborn

766.0 Exceptionally large baby N
NOTE Usually implies a birthweight of 4500 grams or more.

766.1 Other "heavy-for-dates" infants N
Other fetus or infant "heavy-" or "large-for-dates" regardless of period of gestation
P08.1 Other heavy for gestational age newborn   I-10

√5ᵗʰ **766.2 Late infant, not "heavy-for-dates"**
AHA: 2Q, '06, 12
TIP: May be assigned based on gestational age alone, without documentation of any related specific condition or disorder.

766.21 Post-term infant N
Infant with gestation period over 40 completed weeks to 42 completed weeks
AHA: 1Q, '09, 12; 4Q, '03, 69
P08.21 Post-term newborn   I-10

766.22 Prolonged gestation of infant N
Infant with gestation period over 42 completed weeks
Postmaturity NOS
AHA: 1Q, '09, 12

√4ᵗʰ **767 Birth trauma**

767.0 Subdural and cerebral hemorrhage MCC N
Subdural and cerebral hemorrhage, whether described as due to birth trauma or to intrapartum anoxia or hypoxia
Subdural hematoma (localized)
Tentorial tear
Use additional code to identify cause
EXCLUDES intraventricular hemorrhage (772.10-772.14)
subarachnoid hemorrhage (772.2)
CC Exd: 767.0, 767.8-767.9, 779.81-779.84, 779.89

√5ᵗʰ **767.1 Injuries to scalp**
AHA: 4Q, '03, 69

767.11 Epicranial subaponeurotic hemorrhage CC N
(massive)
Subgaleal hemorrhage
DEF: A hemorrhage that occurs within the space between the galea aponeurotica, or epicranial aponeurosis, a thin tendinous structure that is attached to the skull laterally, and the periosteum of the skull.
CC Exd: 767.0-767.11, 767.8-767.9, 779.81-779.84, 779.89

767.19 Other injuries to scalp N
Caput succedaneum
Cephalhematoma
Chignon (from vacuum extraction)
P12.89 Other birth injuries to scalp   I-10

767.2 Fracture of clavicle N

Epicranial Aponeurosis

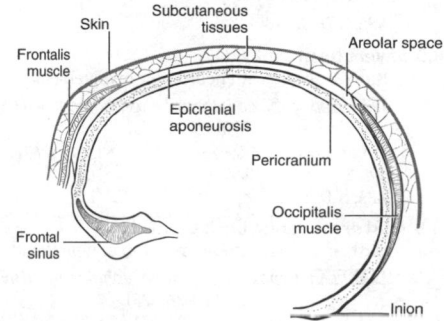

Requires fifth digit. Valid digits are in [brackets] under each code. See beginning of section 764-779 for fifth digit definitions.

| 4ᵗʰ 5ᵗʰ Additional Digit Required | Unacceptable PDx | Manifestation Code | Hospital Acquired Condition | ▶◀ Revised Text | ● New Code | ▲ Revised Code Title |

767.3 Other injuries to skeleton   N
Fracture of:
    long bones
    skull
    EXCLUDES *congenital dislocation of hip (754.30-754.35)*
         fracture of spine, congenital (767.4)

767.4 Injury to spine and spinal cord   N
Dislocation
Fracture   } of spine or spinal cord due to
Laceration   birth trauma
Rupture

767.5 Facial nerve injury   N
Facial palsy

767.6 Injury to brachial plexus   N
Palsy or paralysis:
    brachial
    Erb (-Duchenne)
    Klumpke (-Déjérine)

767.7 Other cranial and peripheral nerve injuries   N
Phrenic nerve paralysis

767.8 Other specified birth trauma   N
Eye damage   Rupture of:
Hematoma of: liver
    liver (subcapsular)   spleen
    testes   Scalpel wound
    vulva   Traumatic glaucoma
    EXCLUDES *hemorrhage classifiable to 772.0-772.9*

767.9 Birth trauma, unspecified   N
Birth injury NOS

√4ᵗʰ 768 Intrauterine hypoxia and birth asphyxia
NOTE Use only when associated with newborn morbidity classifiable elsewhere
EXCLUDES *acidemia NOS of newborn (775.81)*
    acidosis NOS of newborn (775.81)
    cerebral ischemia NOS (779.2)
    hypoxia NOS of newborn (770.88)
    mixed metabolic and respiratory acidosis of newborn
        (775.81)
    respiratory arrest of newborn (770.87)
DEF: Oxygen intake insufficiency due to interrupted placental circulation or premature separation of placenta.
AHA: 4Q, '92, 20

768.0 Fetal death from asphyxia or anoxia before onset of labor or at unspecified time   N

768.1 Fetal death from asphyxia or anoxia during labor   N

768.2 Fetal distress before onset of labor, in liveborn infant   N
Fetal metabolic acidemia before onset of labor, in liveborn infant

768.3 Fetal distress first noted during labor and delivery, in liveborn infant   N
Fetal metabolic acidemia first noted during labor and delivery, in liveborn infant

768.4 Fetal distress, unspecified as to time of onset, in liveborn infant   N
Fetal metabolic acidemia unspecified as to time of onset, in liveborn infant
CC Exd: 516.61-516.69, 768.5-768.6, 768.9-770.86, 770.89-770.9, 779.81-779.84, 779.89
AHA: N-D, '86, 10

768.5 Severe birth asphyxia   MCC N
Birth asphyxia with neurologic involvement
EXCLUDES *hypoxic-ischemic encephalopathy [HIE]*
    (768.70-768.73)
CC Exd: 516.61-516.69, 768.5-768.6, 768.9-770.86, 770.89-770.9, 779.81-779.84, 779.89
AHA: N-D, '86, 3

768.6 Mild or moderate birth asphyxia   N
Birth asphyxia (without mention of neurologic involvement)
EXCLUDES *hypoxic-ischemic encephalopathy [HIE]*
    (768.70-768.73)
AHA: N-D, '86, 3

√5ᵗʰ 768.7 Hypoxic-ischemic encephalopathy [HIE]
AHA: 4Q, '09, 99-101; 4Q, '06, 104

768.70 Hypoxic-ischemic encephalopathy, unspecified   CC N
CC Exd: 768.5-768.9

768.71 Mild hypoxic-ischemic encephalopathy   CC N
CC Exd: See code: 768.70

768.72 Moderate hypoxic-ischemic encephalopathy   CC N
CC Exd: See code: 768.70
AHA: 4Q, '09,101

768.73 Severe hypoxic-ischemic encephalopathy   MCC N
CC Exd: See code: 768.70

768.9 Unspecified birth asphyxia in liveborn infant   N
Anoxia   } NOS, in liveborn infant
Asphyxia

769 Respiratory distress syndrome   MCC N
Cardiorespiratory distress syndrome of newborn
Hyaline membrane disease (pulmonary)
Idiopathic respiratory distress syndrome [IRDS or RDS] of newborn
Pulmonary hypoperfusion syndrome
EXCLUDES *transient tachypnea of newborn (770.6)*
DEF: Severe chest contractions upon air intake and expiratory grunting; infant appears blue due to oxygen deficiency and has rapid respiratory rate; formerly called hyaline membrane disease.
CC Exd: 516.61-516.69, 768.5-768.6, 768.9-770.86, 770.89-770.9, 779.81-779.84, 779.89
AHA: 1Q, '89, 10; N-D, '86, 6
TIP: Do not assign if documentation specifies Type II respiratory distress syndrome, which usually resolves within six to 24 hours after birth; see instead 770.6.
P22.0 Respiratory distress syndrome of newborn   I-10

√4ᵗʰ 770 Other respiratory conditions of fetus and newborn

770.0 Congenital pneumonia   MCC N
Infective pneumonia acquired prenatally
EXCLUDES *pneumonia from infection acquired after birth*
    (480.0-486)
CC Exd: 516.61-516.69, 768.5-768.6, 768.9-770.86, 770.89-770.9, 779.81-779.84, 779.89
AHA: 1Q, '05, 10

√5ᵗʰ 770.1 Fetal and newborn aspiration
EXCLUDES *aspiration of postnatal stomach contents (770.85,*
    770.86)
    meconium passage during delivery (763.84)
    meconium staining (779.84)
AHA: 4Q, '05, 83

770.10 Fetal and newborn aspiration, unspecified   N

770.11 Meconium aspiration without respiratory symptoms   N
Meconium aspiration NOS

770.12 Meconium aspiration with respiratory symptoms   MCC N
Meconium aspiration pneumonia
Meconium aspiration pneumonitis
Meconium aspiration syndrome NOS
Use additional code to identify any secondary pulmonary hypertension (416.8), if applicable
DEF: Meconium aspiration syndrome: aspiration of fetal intestinal material during or prior to delivery, usually a complication of placental insufficiency, causing pneumonitis and bronchial obstruction (inflammatory reaction of lungs).
CC Exd: See code: 770.0

770.13 Aspiration of clear amniotic fluid without respiratory symptoms   N
Aspiration of clear amniotic fluid NOS

770.14 Aspiration of clear amniotic fluid with respiratory symptoms   MCC N
Aspiration of clear amniotic fluid with pneumonia
Aspiration of clear amniotic fluid with pneumonitis
Use additional code to identify any secondary pulmonary hypertension (416.8), if applicable
CC Exd: See code: 770.0

N Newborn Age: 0   P Pediatric Age: 0-17   M Maternity Age: 12-55   A Adult Age: 15-124   MCC Major CC Condition   CC CC Condition   HIV HIV Related Dx

276 – Volume 1   2014 ICD-9-CM

770.15 Aspiration of blood without respiratory symptoms `N`
Aspiration of blood NOS

770.16 Aspiration of blood with respiratory symptoms `MCC` `N`
Aspiration of blood with pneumonia
Aspiration of blood with pneumonitis
Use additional code to identify any secondary pulmonary hypertension (416.8), if applicable
CC Excl: See code: 770.0

770.17 Other fetal and newborn aspiration without respiratory symptoms `N`

770.18 Other fetal and newborn aspiration with respiratory symptoms `MCC` `N`
Other aspiration pneumonia
Other aspiration pneumonitis
Use additional code to identify any secondary pulmonary hypertension (416.8), if applicable
CC Excl: See code: 770.0

770.2 Interstitial emphysema and related conditions `MCC` `N`
Pneumomediastinum
Pneumopericardium } originating in the perinatal period
Pneumothorax
CC Excl: See code: 770.0
P25.0 Interstitial emphysema origin perinatal period `I-10`

770.3 Pulmonary hemorrhage `MCC` `N`
Hemorrhage:
alveolar (lung)
intra-alveolar (lung) } originating in the perinatal period
massive pulmonary
CC Excl: See code: 770.0

770.4 Primary atelectasis `CC` `N`
Pulmonary immaturity NOS
DEF: Alveoli fail to expand causing insufficient air intake by newborn.
CC Excl: See code: 770.0

770.5 Other and unspecified atelectasis `CC` `N`
Atelectasis:
NOS
partial } originating in the perinatal period
secondary
Pulmonary collapse
CC Excl: See code: 770.0

770.6 Transitory tachypnea of newborn `N`
Idiopathic tachypnea of newborn
Wet lung syndrome
EXCLUDES respiratory distress syndrome (769)
DEF: Quick, shallow breathing of newborn; short-term problem.
AHA: 4Q, '95, 4; 1Q, '94, 12; 3Q, '93, 7; 1Q, '89, 10; N-D, '86, 6
P22.1 Transient tachypnea of newborn `I-10`

770.7 Chronic respiratory disease arising in the perinatal period `MCC`
Bronchopulmonary dysplasia
Interstitial pulmonary fibrosis of prematurity
Wilson-Mikity syndrome
CC Excl: See code: 770.0
AHA: 1Q, '11, 16; 2Q, '91, 19; N-D, '86, 11
P27.8 Other chronic resp dz origin perinatal period `I-10`

√5ᵗʰ **770.8 Other respiratory problems after birth**
EXCLUDES mixed metabolic and respiratory acidosis of newborn (775.81)
AHA: 4Q, '02, 65; 2Q, '98, 10; 2Q, '96, 10

770.81 Primary apnea of newborn `CC` `N`
Apneic spells of newborn NOS
Essential apnea of newborn
Sleep apnea of newborn
DEF: Cessation of breathing when a neonate makes no respiratory effort for 15 seconds, resulting in cyanosis and bradycardia.
CC Excl: 770.82-770.83, 770.87-770.9, 786.03
P28.3 Primary sleep apnea of newborn `I-10`

770.82 Other apnea of newborn `CC` `N`
Obstructive apnea of newborn
CC Excl: 770.81-770.83, 770.87-770.9, 786.03

770.83 Cyanotic attacks of newborn `CC` `N`
CC Excl: 770.81-770.83, 770.87-770.9, 782.5, 786.03

770.84 Respiratory failure of newborn `MCC` `N`
EXCLUDES respiratory distress syndrome (769)
CC Excl: 516.61-516.69, 768.5-768.6, 768.9-770.86, 770.89-770.9, 779.81-779.84, 779.89
AHA: 4Q, '08, 99

770.85 Aspiration of postnatal stomach contents without respiratory symptoms `N`
Aspiration of postnatal stomach contents NOS
AHA: 4Q, '05, 83

770.86 Aspiration of postnatal stomach contents with respiratory symptoms `MCC` `N`
Aspiration of postnatal stomach contents with pneumonia
Aspiration of postnatal stomach contents with pneumonitis
Use additional code to identify any secondary pulmonary hypertension (416.8), if applicable
CC Excl: See code: 770.84
AHA: 4Q, '05, 83

770.87 Respiratory arrest of newborn `MCC` `N`
CC Excl: 770.11, 770.13, 770.15, 770.17, 770.6, 770.81-770.85, 770.88-770.9, 779.85, 786.03, 799.1
AHA: 4Q, '06, 104-106

770.88 Hypoxemia of newborn `N`
Hypoxia NOS of newborn
AHA: 4Q, '06, 104-106

770.89 Other respiratory problems after birth `N`
AHA: 3Q, '09, 20
P28.89 Oth specified respiratory conditions of newborn `I-10`

770.9 Unspecified respiratory condition of fetus and newborn `N`

√4ᵗʰ **771 Infections specific to the perinatal period**
INCLUDES infections acquired before or during birth or via the umbilicus or during the first 28 days after birth
EXCLUDES congenital pneumonia (770.0)
congenital syphilis (090.0-090.9)
infant botulism (040.41)
maternal infectious disease as a cause of mortality or morbidity in fetus or newborn, but fetus or newborn not manifesting the disease (760.2)
ophthalmia neonatorum due to gonococcus (098.40)
other infections not specifically classified to this category
AHA: N-D, '85, 4

771.0 Congenital rubella `CC` `N`
Congenital rubella pneumonitis
CC Excl: 771.0-771.2, 779.81-779.84, 779.89

771.1 Congenital cytomegalovirus infection `MCC` `N`
Congenital cytomegalic inclusion disease
CC Excl: See code: 771.0

771.2 Other congenital infections `MCC` `N`
Congenital: Congenital:
herpes simplex   toxoplasmosis
listeriosis   tuberculosis
malaria
CC Excl: 013.60-013.66, 046.2, 046.71-046.8, 048-049.0, 049.8, 052.0, 052.2, 054.3, 054.74, 056.01, 057.8-058.29, 059.00-059.9, 062.0-064, 066.2-066.49, 072.2, 073.7, 075, 078.3, 079.82, 079.99, 081.9, 083.9, 084.6, 090.41, 094.81, 117.5, 124, 130.0, 290.12, 323.01-323.9, 341.1, 382.4, 487.8, 710.0, 771.2, 984.9

771.3 Tetanus neonatorum `MCC` `N`
Tetanus omphalitis
EXCLUDES hypocalcemic tetany (775.4)
DEF: Severe infection of central nervous system; due to exotoxin of tetanus bacillus from navel infection prompted by nonsterile technique during umbilical ligation.
CC Excl: 771.3, 779.81-779.84, 779.89

√4ᵗʰ / √5ᵗʰ Additional Digit Required   Unacceptable PDx   Manifestation Code   Hospital Acquired Condition   ►◄ Revised Text   ● New Code   ▲ Revised Code Title

771.4 Omphalitis of the newborn `CC` `N`
Infection:
  navel cord
  umbilical stump
EXCLUDES *tetanus omphalitis (771.3)*
DEF: Inflamed umbilicus.
CC Excl: 771.89
AHA: 4Q, '09, 102

771.5 Neonatal infective mastitis `CC` `N`
EXCLUDES *noninfective neonatal mastitis (778.7)*
CC Excl: See code: 771.4

771.6 Neonatal conjunctivitis and dacryocystitis `N`
Ophthalmia neonatorum NOS
EXCLUDES *ophthalmia neonatorum due to gonococcus (098.40)*

771.7 Neonatal Candida infection `N`
Neonatal moniliasis
Thrush in newborn

☑5ᵗʰ **771.8 Other infection specific to the perinatal period**
Use additional code to identify organism or specific infection
AHA: 4Q, '02, 66

  771.81 Septicemia [sepsis] of newborn `MCC` `N`
Use additional codes to identify severe sepsis (995.92) and any associated acute organ dysfunction, if applicable
CC Excl: 771.4-771.89, 776.0-776.9, 779.81-779.84, 779.89
AHA: 4Q, '08, 99
P36.9 Bacterial sepsis newborn unspecified   `I-10`

  771.82 Urinary tract infection of newborn `CC` `N`
CC Excl: 041.9, 590.00-590.9, 593.89-593.9, 595.0-595.81, 595.89-595.9, 596.81, 599.0, 599.9, 771.89, 788.1, 996.64

  771.83 Bacteremia of newborn `CC` `N`
CC Excl: See code: 771.81

  771.89 Other infections specific to the perinatal period `CC` `N`
Intra-amniotic infection of fetus NOS
Infection of newborn NOS
CC Excl: 003.1, 020.2, 022.3, 036.2, 038.0-038.9, 040.89-041.3, 041.41-041.9, 054.5, 139.8, 771.82-771.89, 779.9, 790.7

☑4ᵗʰ **772 Fetal and neonatal hemorrhage**
EXCLUDES *fetal hematologic conditions complicating pregnancy (678.0)*
    hematological disorders of fetus and newborn (776.0-776.9)

772.0 Fetal blood loss affecting newborn `N`
Fetal blood loss from:
  cut end of co-twin's cord
  placenta
  ruptured cord
  vasa previa
Fetal exsanguination
Fetal hemorrhage into:
  co-twin
  mother's circulation

☑5ᵗʰ **772.1 Intraventricular hemorrhage**
Intraventricular hemorrhage from any perinatal cause
AHA: 4Q, '01, 49; 3Q, '92, 8; 4Q, '88, 8

  772.10 Unspecified grade `CC` `N`
CC Excl: 772.0-772.2, 772.8-772.9, 776.0-776.9, 779.81-779.84, 779.89

  772.11 Grade I `CC` `N`
Bleeding into germinal matrix
CC Excl: See code: 772.10

  772.12 Grade II `CC` `N`
Bleeding into ventricle
CC Excl: See code 772.10

  772.13 Grade III `MCC` `N`
Bleeding with enlargement of ventricle
CC Excl: See code 772.10
AHA: 4Q, '01, 51

  772.14 Grade IV `MCC` `N`
Bleeding into cerebral cortex
CC Excl: See code 772.10

772.2 Subarachnoid hemorrhage `MCC` `N`
Subarachnoid hemorrhage from any perinatal cause
EXCLUDES *subdural and cerebral hemorrhage (767.0)*
CC Excl: 772.0-772.2, 772.8-772.9, 776.0-776.9, 779.7-779.84, 779.89

772.3 Umbilical hemorrhage after birth `N`
Slipped umbilical ligature

772.4 Gastrointestinal hemorrhage `MCC` `N`
EXCLUDES *swallowed maternal blood (777.3)*
CC Excl: 772.0, 772.4-772.5, 772.8-772.9, 776.0-776.9, 779.81-779.84, 779.89

772.5 Adrenal hemorrhage `CC` `N`
CC Excl: See code: 772.4

772.6 Cutaneous hemorrhage `N`
Bruising
Ecchymoses   } in fetus or newborn
Petechiae
Superficial hematoma
P54.5 Neonatal cutaneous hemorrhage   `I-10`

772.8 Other specified hemorrhage of fetus or newborn `N`
EXCLUDES *hemorrhagic disease of newborn (776.0)*
    pulmonary hemorrhage (770.3)

772.9 Unspecified hemorrhage of newborn `N`

☑4ᵗʰ **773 Hemolytic disease of fetus or newborn, due to isoimmunization**
DEF: Hemolytic anemia of fetus or newborn due to maternal antibody formation against fetal erythrocytes; infant blood contains nonmaternal antigen.
TIP: Do not assign unless the physician substantiates confirmation by a positive Coomb's (direct antibody or direct antiglobulin) test.

773.0 Hemolytic disease due to Rh isoimmunization `N`
Anemia   } due to RH:
Erythroblastosis (fetalis)   antibodies
Hemolytic disease (fetus)   isoimmunization
  (newborn)   maternal/fetal
Jaundice   incompatibility
Rh hemolytic disease
Rh isoimmunization

773.1 Hemolytic disease due to ABO isoimmunization `N`
ABO hemolytic disease
ABO isoimmunization
Anemia   } due to ABO:
Erythroblastosis (fetalis)   antibodies
Hemolytic disease (fetus)   isoimmunization
  (newborn)   maternal/fetal
Jaundice   incompatibility
DEF: Incompatible Rh fetal-maternal blood grouping; prematurely destroys red blood cells; detected by Coombs test.
AHA: 3Q, '92, 8
P55.1 ABO isoimmunization of newborn   `I-10`

773.2 Hemolytic disease due to other and unspecified isoimmunization `N`
Eythroblastosis (fetalis) (neonatorum) NOS
Hemolytic disease (fetus) (newborn) NOS
Jaundice or anemia due to other and unspecified blood-group incompatibility
AHA: 1Q, '94, 13
P55.9 Hemolytic disease of newborn unspecified   `I-10`

773.3 Hydrops fetalis due to isoimmunization `MCC` `N`
Use additional code to identify type of isoimmunization (773.0-773.2)
DEF: Massive edema of entire body and severe anemia; may result in fetal death or stillbirth.
CC Excl: 773.0-773.5, 779.81-779.84, 779.89

773.4 Kernicterus due to isoimmunization `MCC` `N`
Use additional code to identify type of isoimmunization (773.0-773.2)
DEF: Complication of erythroblastosis fetalis associated with severe neural symptoms, high blood bilirubin levels and nerve cell destruction; results in bilirubin-pigmented gray matter of central nervous system.
CC Excl: See code: 773.3

773.5 Late anemia due to isoimmunization `N`

`N` Newborn Age: 0   `P` Pediatric Age: 0-17   `M` Maternity Age: 12-55   `A` Adult Age: 15-124   `MCC` Major CC Condition   `CC` CC Condition   `HIV` HIV Related Dx

278 – Volume 1   **2014 ICD-9-CM**

☑4ᵗʰ **774** **Other perinatal jaundice**

774.0 *Perinatal jaundice from hereditary hemolytic anemias* N
Code first underlying disease (282.0-282.9)

774.1 Perinatal jaundice from other excessive hemolysis N
Fetal or neonatal jaundice from:
bruising
drugs or toxins transmitted from mother
infection
polycythemia
swallowed maternal blood
Use additional code to identify cause
EXCLUDES *jaundice due to isoimmunization (773.0-773.2)*

774.2 Neonatal jaundice associated with preterm delivery N
Hyperbilirubinemia of prematurity
Jaundice due to delayed conjugation associated with preterm
delivery
AHA: 3Q, '91, 21
P59.0 Neonatal jaundice associated w/preterm delivery I-10

☑5ᵗʰ **774.3 Neonatal jaundice due to delayed conjugation from other causes**

774.30 Neonatal jaundice due to delayed N
conjugation, cause unspecified
DEF: Jaundice of newborn with abnormal bilirubin
metabolism; causes excess accumulated unconjugated
bilirubin in blood.

774.31 *Neonatal jaundice due to delayed conjugation* N
in diseases classified elsewhere
Code first underlying diseases as:
congenital hypothyroidism (243)
Crigler-Najjar syndrome (277.4)
Gilbert's syndrome (277.4)

774.39 Other N
Jaundice due to delayed conjugation from causes,
such as:
breast milk inhibitors
delayed development of conjugating system

774.4 Perinatal jaundice due to hepatocellular damage MCC N
Fetal or neonatal hepatitis
Giant cell hepatitis
Inspissated bile syndrome
CC Exd: 774.0-774.7, 779.81-779.84, 779.89

774.5 *Perinatal jaundice from other causes* N
Code first underlying cause as:
congenital obstruction of bile duct (751.61)
galactosemia (271.1)
mucoviscidosis (277.00-277.09)

774.6 Unspecified fetal and neonatal jaundice N
Icterus neonatorum
Neonatal hyperbilirubinemia (transient)
Physiologic jaundice NOS in newborn
EXCLUDES *that in preterm infants (774.2)*
AHA: 1Q, '94, 13; 2Q, '89, 15
P59.9 Neonatal jaundice unspecified I-10

774.7 Kernicterus not due to isoimmunization MCC N
Bilirubin encephalopathy
Kernicterus of newborn NOS
EXCLUDES *kernicterus due to isoimmunization (773.4)*
CC Exd: See code: 774.4

☑4ᵗʰ **775** **Endocrine and metabolic disturbances specific to the fetus and newborn**
INCLUDES transitory endocrine and metabolic disturbances caused
by the infant's response to maternal endocrine and
metabolic factors, its removal from them, or its
adjustment to extrauterine existence

775.0 Syndrome of "infant of a diabetic mother" N
Maternal diabetes mellitus affecting fetus or newborn (with
hypoglycemia)
AHA: 1Q, '04, 7-8; 3Q, '91, 5
TIP: Do not assign if the infant has no manifestations or symptoms of
the syndrome; refer instead to code V18.0 Family history, diabetes
mellitus.
P70.1 Syndrome of infant of diabetic mother I-10

775.1 Neonatal diabetes mellitus CC N
Diabetes mellitus syndrome in newborn infant
CC Exd: 775.0-775.7, 775.9, 779.81-779.84, 779.89
AHA: 3Q, '91, 6

775.2 Neonatal myasthenia gravis CC N
CC Exd: See code: 775.1

775.3 Neonatal thyrotoxicosis CC N
Neonatal hyperthydroidism (transient)
CC Exd: See code 775.1

775.4 Hypocalcemia and hypomagnesemia of newborn CC N
Cow's milk hypocalcemia
Hypocalcemic tetany, neonatal
Neonatal hypoparathyroidism
Phosphate-loading hypocalcemia
CC Exd: See code 775.1

775.5 Other transitory neonatal electrolyte disturbances N
Dehydration, neonatal
AHA: 1Q, '10, 14; 3Q, '09, 21; 1Q, '05, 9
TIP: If the patient has neonatal hyperkalemia, assign also code 276.7
Hyperpotassemia.
P74.1 Dehydration of newborn I-10

775.6 Neonatal hypoglycemia N
EXCLUDES *infant of mother with diabetes mellitus (775.0)*
AHA: 1Q, '94, 8
P70.4 Other neonatal hypoglycemia I-10

775.7 Late metabolic acidosis of newborn MCC N
CC Exd: See code: 775.1

☑5ᵗʰ **775.8 Other neonatal endocrine and metabolic disturbances**

775.81 Other acidosis of newborn CC N
Acidemia NOS of newborn
Acidosis of newborn NOS
Mixed metabolic and respiratory acidosis of newborn
CC Exd: 775.5, 775.7, 775.9
AHA: 4Q, '06, 104-106

775.89 Other neonatal endocrine and metabolic CC N
disturbances
Amino-acid metabolic disorders described as
transitory
CC Exd: 775.0-775.7, 775.9
AHA: 4Q, '06, 104-106

775.9 Unspecified endocrine and metabolic disturbances N
specific to the fetus and newborn

☑4ᵗʰ **776** **Hematological disorders of newborn**
INCLUDES disorders specific to the newborn though possibly
originating in utero
EXCLUDES *fetal hematologic conditions (678.0)*

776.0 Hemorrhagic disease of newborn CC N
Hemorrhagic diathesis of newborn
Vitamin K deficiency of newborn
EXCLUDES *fetal or neonatal hemorrhage (772.0-772.9)*
CC Exd: 776.0-776.9, 779.81-779.84, 779.89

776.1 Transient neonatal thrombocytopenia MCC N
Neonatal thrombocytopenia due to:
exchange transfusion
idiopathic maternal thrombocytopenia
isoimmunization
DEF: Temporary decrease in blood platelets of newborn.
CC Exd: See code 776.0
P61.0 Transient neonatal thrombocytopenia I-10

776.2 Disseminated intravascular coagulation in newborn MCC N
DEF: Disseminated intravascular coagulation of newborn: clotting
disorder due to excess thromboplastic agents in blood as a result of
disease or trauma; causes blood clotting within vessels and reduces
available elements necessary for blood coagulation.
CC Exd: See code 776.0

776.3 Other transient neonatal disorders of coagulation CC N
Transient coagulation defect, newborn
CC Exd: See code 776.0

☑4ᵗʰ Additional Digit Required | Unacceptable PDx | Manifestation Code | Hospital Acquired Condition | ►◄ Revised Text | ● New Code | ▲ Revised Code Title

2014 ICD-9-CM | Volume 1 – 279

776.4 Polycythemia neonatorum `N`
Plethora of newborn
Polycythemia due to:
donor twin transfusion
maternal-fetal transfusion
DEF: Abnormal increase of total red blood cells of newborn.

776.5 Congenital anemia `CC` `N`
Anemia following fetal blood loss
EXCLUDES anemia due to isoimmunization (773.0-773.2, 773.5)
hereditary hemolytic anemias (282.0-282.9)
CC Exd: 280.0-282.3, 282.5-284.2, 284.81-285.9, 289.9, 517.3, 776.5-776.6

776.6 Anemia of prematurity `CC` `N`
CC Exd: See code: 776.5
P61.2 Anemia of prematurity `I-10`

776.7 Transient neonatal neutropenia `MCC` `N`
Isoimmune neutropenia
Maternal transfer neutropenia
EXCLUDES congenital neutropenia (nontransient) (288.01)
DEF: Decreased neutrophilic leukocytes in blood of newborn.
CC Exd: 280.1-281.9, 282.5-282.63, 282.69-282.7, 283.0, 283.11, 284.01-284.2, 284.81-285.0, 285.21-285.9, 289.9, 776.7-776.9

776.8 Other specified transient hematological disorders `N`

776.9 Unspecified hematological disorder specific to newborn `N`

777 Perinatal disorders of digestive system ✓4ᵗʰ
INCLUDES disorders specific to the fetus and newborn
EXCLUDES intestinal obstruction classifiable to 560.0-560.9

777.1 Meconium obstruction `N`
Congenital fecaliths
Delayed passage of meconium
Meconium ileus NOS
Meconium plug syndrome
EXCLUDES meconium ileus in cystic fibrosis (277.01)
DEF: Meconium blocked digestive tract of newborn.

777.2 Intestinal obstruction due to inspissated milk `N`

777.3 Hematemesis and melena due to swallowed maternal blood `N`
Swallowed blood syndrome in newborn
EXCLUDES that not due to swallowed maternal blood (772.4)

777.4 Transitory ileus of newborn `CC` `N`
EXCLUDES Hirschsprung's disease (751.3)
CC Exd: 777.1-777.9

777.5 Necrotizing enterocolitis in newborn ✓5ᵗʰ
DEF: Serious intestinal infection and inflammation in preterm infants; severity is measured by stages and may progress to life-threatening perforation or peritonitis; resection surgical treatment may be necessary.
AHA: 4Q, '08, 138-140

777.50 Necrotizing enterocolitis in newborn, unspecified `MCC` `N`
Necrotizing enterocolitis in newborn, NOS
CC Exd: 777.1-777.9, 779.81-779.84, 779.89

777.51 Stage I necrotizing enterocolitis in newborn `MCC` `N`
Necrotizing enterocolitis without pneumatosis, without perforation
DEF: Broad-spectrum symptoms with non-specific signs including feeding intolerance, sepsis, gastroenteritis, ileus, metabolic abnormalities.
CC Exd: 777.1-777.9, 779.81-779.84, 779.89

777.52 Stage II necrotizing enterocolitis in newborn `MCC` `N`
Necrotizing enterocolitis with pneumatosis, without perforation
DEF: Radiographic confirmation of necrotizing enterocolitis showing intestinal dilatation, fixed loops of bowels, pneumatosis intestinalis, metabolic acidosis, and thrombocytopenia.
CC Exd: 777.1-777.9, 779.81-779.84, 779.89

777.53 Stage III necrotizing enterocolitis in newborn `MCC` `N`
Necrotizing enterocolitis with perforation
Necrotizing enterocolitis with pneumatosis and perforation
DEF: Advanced stage in which infant demonstrates signs of bowel perforation, septic shock, metabolic acidosis, ascites disseminated intravascular coagulopathy, neutropenia.
CC Exd: 777.1-777.9, 779.81-779.84, 779.89
AHA: 4Q, '08, 139

777.6 Perinatal intestinal perforation `MCC` `N`
Meconium peritonitis
CC Exd: See code: 777.50

777.8 Other specified perinatal disorders of digestive system `N`
AHA: 4Q, '10, 97

777.9 Unspecified perinatal disorder of digestive system `N`

778 Conditions involving the integument and temperature regulation of fetus and newborn ✓4ᵗʰ

778.0 Hydrops fetalis not due to isoimmunization `MCC` `N`
Idiopathic hydrops
EXCLUDES hydrops fetalis due to isoimmunization (773.3)
DEF: Edema of entire body, unrelated to immune response.
CC Exd: 778.0, 779.81-779.84, 779.89

778.1 Sclerema neonatorum `CC` `N`
Subcutaneous fat necrosis
DEF: Diffuse, rapidly progressing white, waxy, nonpitting hardening of tissue, usually of legs and feet, life-threatening; found in preterm or debilitated infants; unknown etiology.
CC Exd: 778.1, 778.5

778.2 Cold injury syndrome of newborn `N`

778.3 Other hypothermia of newborn `N`

778.4 Other disturbances of temperature regulation of newborn `N`
Dehydration fever in newborn
Environmentally-induced pyrexia
Hyperthermia in newborn
Transitory fever of newborn
P81.9 Disturbance of temp regulation newborn uns `I-1`

778.5 Other and unspecified edema of newborn `CC` `N`
Edema neonatorum
CC Exd: 778.1-778.5

778.6 Congenital hydrocele
Congenital hydrocele of tunica vaginalis
P83.5 Congenital hydrocele `I-1`

778.7 Breast engorgement in newborn `N`
Noninfective mastitis of newborn
EXCLUDES infective mastitis of newborn (771.5)

778.8 Other specified conditions involving the integument of fetus and newborn `N`
Urticaria neonatorum
EXCLUDES impetigo neonatorum (684)
pemphigus neonatorum (684)
P83.8 Oth spec conditions integument specific to newborn `I-1`

778.9 Unspecified condition involving the integument and temperature regulation of fetus and newborn `N`

779 Other and ill-defined conditions originating in the perinatal period ✓4ᵗʰ

779.0 Convulsions in newborn `MCC` `N`
Fits ⎫
Seizures ⎬ in newborn
CC Exd: 779.0-779.1, 779.81-779.84, 779.89
AHA: N-D, '84, 11
TIP: Clarify with the physician that convulsions are not actually infantile spasms; if so, refer to subcategory 345.6.

779.1 Other and unspecified cerebral irritability in newborn `N`

779.2 Cerebral depression, coma, and other abnormal cerebral signs `MCC` `N`
Cerebral ischemia NOS of newborn
CNS dysfunction in newborn NOS
EXCLUDES cerebral ischemia due to birth trauma (767.0)
intrauterine cerebral ischemia (768.2-768.9)
intraventricular hemorrhage (772.10-772.14)
CC Exd: 779.0-779.2

`N` Newborn Age: 0   `P` Pediatric Age: 0-17   `M` Maternity Age: 12-55   `A` Adult Age: 15-124   `MCC` Major CC Condition   `CC` CC Condition   `HIV` HIV Related D

✓5ᵗʰ 779.3 Disorder of stomach function and feeding problems in newborn
AHA: 2Q, '89, 15

779.31 Feeding problems in newborn ⬛N
Slow feeding in newborn
EXCLUDES feeding problem in child over 28 days old (783.3)

AHA: 4Q, '09, 102
P92.9 Feeding problem of newborn unspecified I-10

779.32 Bilious vomiting in newborn MCC ⬛N
EXCLUDES bilious vomiting in child over 28 days old (787.04)

CC Exd: 779.32-779.33

779.33 Other vomiting in newborn ⬛N
Regurgitation of food in newborn
EXCLUDES vomiting in child over 28 days old (536.2, 787.01-787.04)

779.34 Failure to thrive in newborn ⬛N
EXCLUDES failure to thrive in child over 28 days old (783.41)

779.4 Drug reactions and intoxications specific to newborn CC ⬛N
Gray syndrome from chloramphenicol administration in newborn
EXCLUDES fetal alcohol syndrome (760.71)
reactions and intoxications from maternal opiates and tranquilizers (763.5)

CC Exd: 779.4-779.5

779.5 Drug withdrawal syndrome in newborn CC ⬛N
Drug withdrawal syndrome in infant of dependent mother
EXCLUDES fetal alcohol syndrome (760.71)

CC Exd: See code: 779.4
AHA: 3Q, '94, 6
TIP: If the infant is asymptomatic but has a positive drug screen (e.g., for cocaine), assign instead 760.75.

779.6 Termination of pregnancy (fetus) ⬛N
Fetal death due to:
induced abortion
termination of pregnancy
EXCLUDES spontaneous abortion (fetus) (761.8)

779.7 Periventricular leukomalacia MCC
DEF: Necrosis of white matter adjacent to lateral ventricles with the formation of cysts; cause of PVL has not been firmly established, but thought to be related to inadequate blood flow in certain areas of the brain.
CC Exd: 772.0-772.2, 772.8-772.9, 776.0-776.9, 779.7-779.84, 779.89
AHA: 4Q, '01, 50, 51

✓5ᵗʰ 779.8 Other specified conditions originating in the perinatal period
AHA: 4Q, '02, 67; 1Q, '94, 15

779.81 Neonatal bradycardia ⬛N
EXCLUDES abnormality in fetal heart rate or rhythm complicating labor and delivery (763.81-763.83)
bradycardia due to birth asphyxia (768.5-768.9)

P29.12 Neonatal bradycardia I-10

779.82 Neonatal tachycardia ⬛N
EXCLUDES abnormality in fetal heart rate or rhythm complicating labor and delivery (763.81-763.83)

779.83 Delayed separation of umbilical cord ⬛N
AHA: 4Q, '03, 71

779.84 Meconium staining ⬛N
EXCLUDES meconium aspiration (770.11, 770.12)
meconium passage during delivery (763.84)

AHA: 4Q, '05, 83, 88
P96.83 Meconium staining I-10

779.85 Cardiac arrest of newborn MCC ⬛N
CC Exd: 779.85
AHA: 4Q, '06, 104-106

779.89 Other specified conditions originating in the perinatal period ⬛N
Use additional code to specify condition
AHA: ▶3Q, '12, 5;◀ 3Q, '11, 3-4; 2Q, '11, 13; 1Q, '06, 18; 2Q, '05, 15;
1Q, '05, 9
P96.89 Oth spec conditions originating perinatal period I-10

779.9 Unspecified condition originating in the perinatal period ⬛N
Congenital debility NOS
Stillbirth NEC

| ⁴ᵗʰ ✓ ⁵ᵗʰ Additional Digit Required | Unacceptable PDx | Manifestation Code | Hospital Acquired Condition | ▶◀ Revised Text | ● New Code | ▲ Revised Code Title |

2014 ICD-9-CM

February 2013 • Volume 1 – 281

Certain Conditions Originating in the Perinatal Period — 779.3–779.9

16. Symptoms, Signs, and Ill-Defined Conditions (780-799)

This section includes symptoms, signs, abnormal results of laboratory or other investigative procedures, and ill-defined conditions regarding which no diagnosis classifiable elsewhere is recorded.

Signs and symptoms that point rather definitely to a given diagnosis are assigned to some category in the preceding part of the classification. In general, categories 780-796 include the more ill-defined conditions and symptoms that point with perhaps equal suspicion to two or more diseases or to two or more systems of the body, and without the necessary study of the case to make a final diagnosis. Practically all categories in this group could be designated as "not otherwise specified," or as "unknown etiology," or as "transient." The Alphabetic Index should be consulted to determine which symptoms and signs are to be allocated here and which to more specific sections of the classification; the residual subcategories numbered .9 are provided for other relevant symptoms which cannot be allocated elsewhere in the classification.

The conditions and signs or symptoms included in categories 780-796 consist of: (a) cases for which no more specific diagnosis can be made even after all facts bearing on the case have been investigated; (b) signs or symptoms existing at the time of initial encounter that proved to be transient and whose causes could not be determined; (c) provisional diagnoses in a patient who failed to return for further investigation or care; (d) cases referred elsewhere for investigation or treatment before the diagnosis was made; (e) cases in which a more precise diagnosis was not available for any other reason; (f) certain symptoms which represent important problems in medical care and which it might be desired to classify in addition to a known cause.

AHA: 3Q, '11, 12

Symptoms (780-789)

AHA: 1Q, '91, 12; 2Q, '90, 3; 2Q, '90, 5; 2Q, '90, 15; M-A, '85, 3

√4ᵗʰ **780 General symptoms**

√5ᵗʰ **780.0 Alteration of consciousness**

> EXCLUDES alteration of consciousness due to:
> intracranial injuries (850.0-854.19)
> skull fractures (800.00-801.99, 803.00-804.99)
> coma:
> diabetic (249.2-249.3, 250.2-250.3)
> hepatic (572.2)
> originating in the perinatal period (779.2)
>
> AHA: 4Q, '92, 20

780.01 Coma   MCC

> DEF: State of unconsciousness from which the patient cannot be awakened.
> CC Excl: 070.0-070.9, 249.00-251.3, 338.0-338.4, 348.81-348.9, 349.89-349.9, 430-432.9, 572.2, 780.01-780.09, 780.2, 780.4, 780.64-780.65, 780.91-780.99, 799.81-799.89, 800.00-801.99, 803.00-804.96, 850.0-852.19, 852.21-854.19
> AHA: 1Q, '12, 14; 3Q, '96, 16
> TIP: Although found in the symptoms and signs chapter, coma is not inherent in other conditions and should be reported whenever appropriately documented.

780.02 Transient alteration of awareness

> DEF: Temporary, recurring spells of reduced consciousness.

780.03 Persistent vegetative state   CC

> DEF: Persistent wakefulness without consciousness due to nonfunctioning cerebral cortex.
> CC Excl: See code: 780.01

780.09 Other

> Drowsiness   Stupor
> Semicoma   Unconsciousness
> Somnolence
> R40.1 Stupor   I-10

780.1 Hallucinations   CC

> Hallucinations: Hallucinations:
> NOS   olfactory
> auditory   tactile
> gustatory
>
> EXCLUDES those associated with mental disorders, as functional psychoses (295.0-298.9)
> organic brain syndromes (290.0-294.9, 310.0-310.9)
> visual hallucinations (368.16)
>
> DEF: Perception of external stimulus in absence of stimulus; inability to distinguish between real and imagined.
> CC Excl: 338.0-338.4, 780.1, 780.4, 780.64-780.65, 780.91-780.99, 799.81-799.89

780.2 Syncope and collapse

> Blackout   (Near) (Pre) syncope
> Fainting   Vasovagal attack
>
> EXCLUDES carotid sinus syncope (337.0)
> heat syncope (992.1)
> neurocirculatory asthenia (306.2)
> orthostatic hypotension (458.0)
> shock NOS (785.50)
>
> DEF: Sudden unconsciousness due to reduced blood flow to brain.
> AHA: 1Q, '02, 6; 3Q, '00, 12; 4Q, '95, 42; 3Q, '95, 14; N-D, '85, 12
> R55 Syncope and collapse   I-10

√5ᵗʰ **780.3 Convulsions**

> EXCLUDES convulsions:
> epileptic (345.10-345.91)
> in newborn (779.0)
>
> DEF: Sudden, involuntary contractions of the muscles.
> AHA: ▶2Q, '12, 9;◀ 2Q, '97, 8; 1Q, '97, 12; 3Q, '94, 9; 1Q, '93, 24; 4Q, '92, 23; N-D, '87, 12

780.31 Febrile convulsions (simple), unspecified   CC

> Febrile seizure NOS
> CC Excl: 338.0-338.4, 345.00-345.91, 348.81, 348.89-348.9, 349.89-349.9, 779.0-779.1, 780.31-780.39, 780.64-780.65, 780.91-780.99, 799.81-799.89
> AHA: 4Q, '97, 45

780.32 Complex febrile convulsions   CC

> Febrile seizure:
> atypical
> complex
> complicated
> EXCLUDES status epilepticus (345.3)
> CC Excl: See code: 780.31
> AHA: 4Q, '06, 106

780.33 Post traumatic seizures   CC

> EXCLUDES post traumatic epilepsy (345.00-345.91)
> CC Excl: 249.60-249.61, 250.60-250.63, 345.00-345.91, 348.81-348.9, 349.89-349.9, 780.33
> AHA: 4Q, '10, 92-93

780.39 Other convulsions

> Convulsive disorder NOS
> Fit NOS
> Recurrent convulsions NOS
> Seizure NOS
> AHA: ▶2Q, '12, 9;◀ 2Q, '11, 5; 1Q, '08, 17; 3Q, '06, 22; 4Q, '04, 51; 1Q, '03, 7; 2Q, '99, 17; 4Q, '98, 39
> R56.9 Unspecified convulsions   I-10

780.4 Dizziness and giddiness

> Light-headedness   Vertigo NOS
>
> EXCLUDES Méniére's disease and other specified vertiginous syndromes (386.0-386.9)
> DEF: Whirling sensations in head with feeling of falling.
> AHA: 2Q, '03, 11; 3Q, '00, 12; 2Q, '97, 9; 2Q, '91, 17
> R42 Dizziness and giddiness   I-10

√5ᵗʰ **780.5 Sleep disturbances**

> EXCLUDES circadian rhythm sleep disorders (327.30-327.39)
> organic hypersomnia (327.10-327.19)
> organic insomnia (327.00-327.09)
> organic sleep apnea (327.20-327.29)
> organic sleep related movement disorders (327.51-327.59)
> parasomnias (327.40-327.49)
> that of nonorganic origin (307.40-307.49)
> AHA: 4Q, '05, 59

780.50 Sleep disturbance, unspecified

4ᵗʰ/5ᵗʰ Additional Digit Required   Unacceptable PDx   Manifestation Code   Hospital Acquired Condition   ▶◀ Revised Text   ● New Code   ▲ Revised Code Title

2014 ICD-9-CM   February 2013 · Volume 1 – 283

Symptoms, Signs, and Ill-Defined Conditions

780.51–780.92

780.51 Insomnia with sleep apnea, unspecified
DEF: Transient cessation of breathing disturbing sleep.

780.52 Insomnia, unspecified
DEF: Inability to maintain adequate sleep cycle.
G47.00 Insomnia unspecified　　[I-10]

780.53 Hypersomnia with sleep apnea, unspecified
DEF: Autonomic response inhibited during sleep; causes insufficient oxygen intake, acidosis and pulmonary hypertension.
AHA: 1Q, '93, 28; N-D, '85, 4

780.54 Hypersomnia, unspecified
DEF: Prolonged sleep cycle.

780.55 Disruptions of 24 hour sleep wake cycle, unspecified

780.56 Dysfunctions associated with sleep stages or arousal from sleep

780.57 Unspecified sleep apnea
AHA: 1Q, '01, 6 ; 1Q, '97, 5; 1Q, '93, 28
G47.30 Sleep apnea unspecified　　[I-10]

780.58 Sleep related movement disorder, unspecified
EXCLUDES restless legs syndrome (333.94)
AHA: 4Q, '04, 95

780.59 Other

√5ᵗʰ **780.6 Fever and other physiologic disturbances of temperature regulation**
EXCLUDES effects of reduced environmental temperature (991.0-991.9)
effects of heat and light (992.0-992.9)
fever, chills or hypothermia associated with confirmed infection — code to infection
AHA: 4Q, '08, 140-142; 3Q, '05, 16; 3Q, '00,13; 4Q, '99, 26; 2Q, '91, 8

780.60 Fever, unspecified
Chills with fever
Fever NOS
Fever of unknown origin (FUO)
Hyperpyrexia NOS
Pyrexia NOS
Pyrexia of unknown origin
EXCLUDES chills without fever (780.64)
neonatal fever (778.4)
pyrexia of unknown origin (during):
in newborn (778.4)
labor (659.2)
the puerperium (672)
R50.9 Fever unspecified　　[I-10]

780.61 Fever presenting with conditions classified elsewhere
Code first underlying condition when associated fever is present, such as with:
leukemia (conditions classifiable to 204-208)
neutropenia (288.00-288.09)
sickle-cell disease (282.60-282.69)
AHA: ▶2Q, '12, 18;◀ 4Q, '08, 142

780.62 Postprocedural fever
EXCLUDES posttransfusion fever (780.66)
postvaccination fever (780.63)
TIP: Do not assign a code from category 998 for post-procedural fever.

780.63 Postvaccination fever
Postimmunization fever

780.64 Chills (without fever)
Chills NOS
EXCLUDES chills with fever (780.60)

780.65 Hypothermia not associated with low environmental temperature
EXCLUDES hypothermia:
associated with low environmental temperature (991.6)
due to anesthesia (995.89)
of newborn (778.2, 778.3)

780.66 Febrile nonhemolytic transfusion reaction
FNHTR
Posttransfusion fever
AHA: 4Q, '10, 99-100

√5ᵗʰ **780.7 Malaise and fatigue**
EXCLUDES debility, unspecified (799.3)
fatigue (during):
combat (308.0-308.9)
heat (992.6)
pregnancy (646.8)
neurasthenia (300.5)
senile asthenia (797)
AHA: 4Q, '88, 12; M-A, '87, 8

780.71 Chronic fatigue syndrome
DEF: Persistent fatigue, symptoms include weak muscles, sore throat, lymphadenitis, headache, depression and mild fever; no known cause; also called chronic mononucleosis, benign myalgic encephalomyelitis, Iceland disease and neurosthenia.
AHA: 4Q, '98, 48

780.72 Functional quadriplegia　　MCC
Complete immobility due to severe physical disability or frailty
EXCLUDES hysterical paralysis (300.11)
immobility syndrome (728.3)
neurologic quadriplegia (344.00-344.09)
quadriplegia NOS (344.00)
DEF: Inability to move due to another condition such as dementia, severe contractures, or arthritis, not a physiologic one; no mental ability to move independently; typically found in severely demented patients.
CC Excl: 249.60-249.61, 249.80-249.91, 250.60-250.63, 250.80-250.93, 342.00-344.9, 348.8-348.9, 349.89-349.9, 742.59-742.9, 780.72
AHA: 4Q, '08, 143
TIP: The functional quadriplegic patient typically has severe dementia and the quadriplegia will be due to a nonneurologic condition.

780.79 Other malaise and fatigue
Asthenia NOS
Lethargy
Postviral (asthenic) syndrome
Tiredness
DEF: Asthenia: Any weakness, lack of strength or loss of energy, especially neuromuscular.
DEF: Lethargy: Listlessness, drowsiness, stupor and apathy.
DEF: Malaise: Vague feeling of debility or lack of good health.
DEF: Postviral (asthenic) syndrome: Listlessness, drowsiness, stupor and apathy; follows acute viral infection.
DEF: Tiredness: General exhaustion or fatigue.
AHA: 4Q, '04, 78; 1Q, '00, 6; 4Q, '99, 26
R53.83 Other fatigue　　[I-10]

780.8 Generalized hyperhidrosis
Diaphoresis　　　　Secondary hyperhidrosis
Excessive sweating
EXCLUDES focal (localized) (primary) (secondary) hyperhidrosis (705.21-705.22)
Frey's syndrome (705.22)
DEF: Excessive sweating, appears as droplets on skin; general or localized.

√5ᵗʰ **780.9 Other general symptoms**
EXCLUDES hypothermia:
NOS (accidental) (991.6)
due to anesthesia (995.89)
of newborn (778.2-778.3)
memory disturbance as part of a pattern of mental disorder
AHA: 4Q, '02, 67; 4Q, '99, 10; 3Q, '93, 11; N-D, '85, 12

780.91 Fussy infant (baby)　　P

780.92 Excessive crying of infant (baby)　　N
EXCLUDES excessive crying of child, adolescent or adult (780.95)

N Newborn Age: 0　　P Pediatric Age: 0-17　　M Maternity Age: 12-55　　A Adult Age: 15-124　　MCC Major CC Condition　　CC CC Condition　　HIV HIV Related Dx

284 – Volume 1 · February 2013　　　　　　2014 ICD-9-CM

780.93 Memory loss
Amnesia (retrograde)
Memory loss NOS
EXCLUDES memory loss due to:
intracranial injuries (850.0-854.19)
skull fractures (800.00-801.99,
803.00-804.99)
mild memory disturbance due to organic
brain damage (310.89)
transient global amnesia (437.7)
AHA: 4Q, '03, 71

780.94 Early satiety
DEF: The premature feeling of being full; mechanism of
satiety is multifactorial.
AHA: 4Q, '03, 72

780.95 Excessive crying of child, adolescent, or adult
EXCLUDES excessive crying of infant (baby) (780.92)
AHA: 4Q, '05, 89

780.96 Generalized pain
Pain NOS
AHA: 4Q, '06, 79-81
TIP: For pain syndromes, refer to category 338; if site is
specified, refer to index.

780.97 Altered mental status
Change in mental status
EXCLUDES altered level of consciousness
(780.01-780.09)
altered mental status due to known
condition — code to condition
delirium NOS (780.09)
AHA: 4Q, '06, 107
R41.82 Altered mental status unspecified   I-10

780.99 Other general symptoms
AHA: 4Q, '03, 103

781 Symptoms involving nervous and musculoskeletal systems
EXCLUDES depression NOS (311)
disorders specifically relating to:
back (724.0-724.9)
hearing (388.0-389.9)
joint (718.0-719.9)
limb (729.0-729.9)
neck (723.0-723.9)
vision (368.0-369.9)
pain in limb (729.5)

781.0 Abnormal involuntary movements
Abnormal head movements
Fasciculation
Spasms NOS
Tremor NOS
EXCLUDES abnormal reflex (796.1)
chorea NOS (333.5)
infantile spasms (345.60-345.61)
spastic paralysis (342.1, 343.0-344.9)
specified movement disorders classifiable to 333
(333.0-333.9)
that of nonorganic origin (307.2-307.3)
R25.9 Unspecified abnormal involuntary movements   I-10

781.1 Disturbances of sensation of smell and taste
Anosmia
Parageusia
Parosmia
DEF: Anosmia: loss of sense of smell due to organic factors, including
loss of olfactory nerve conductivity, cerebral disease, nasal fossae
formation and peripheral olfactory nerve diseases; can also be
psychological disorder.
DEF: Parageusia: distorted sense of taste, or bad taste in mouth.
DEF: Parosmia: distorted sense of smell.

781.2 Abnormality of gait
Gait:
ataxic
paralytic
spastic
staggering
EXCLUDES ataxia:
NOS (781.3)
locomotor (progressive) (094.0)
difficulty in walking (719.7)
DEF: Abnormal, asymmetric gait.
AHA: 1Q, '11, 9; 2Q, '05, 6; 2Q, '04, 15
TIP: If the patient's gait abnormality is due to a joint problem, refer to
code 719.7 Difficulty in walking.
R26.9 Unspecified abnormalities of gait and mobility   I-10

781.3 Lack of coordination
Ataxia NOS
Muscular incoordination
EXCLUDES ataxic gait (781.2)
cerebellar ataxia (334.0-334.9)
difficulty in walking (719.7)
vertigo NOS (780.4)
AHA: 4Q, '04, 51; 3Q, '97, 12

781.4 Transient paralysis of limb   CC
Monoplegia, transient NOS
EXCLUDES paralysis (342.0-344.9)
CC Exd: 781.4, 781.94

781.5 Clubbing of fingers
DEF: Enlarged soft tissue of distal fingers.

781.6 Meningismus   CC
Dupré's syndrome
Meningism
DEF: Condition with signs and symptoms that resemble meningeal
irritation; it is associated with febrile illness and dehydration with no
evidence of infection.
CC Exd: 781.4, 781.94
AHA: 3Q, '00,13; J-F, '87, 7

781.7 Tetany   CC
Carpopedal spasm
EXCLUDES tetanus neonatorum (771.3)
tetany:
hysterical (300.11)
newborn (hypocalcemic) (775.4)
parathyroid (252.1)
psychogenic (306.0)
DEF: Nerve and muscle hyperexcitability; symptoms include muscle
spasms, twitching, cramps, laryngospasm with inspiratory stridor,
hyperreflexia and choreiform movements.
CC Exd: 037, 332.0-333.93, 333.99-334.4, 338.0-338.4, 342.10-342.12,
771.3, 780.64-780.65, 780.91-780.99, 781.7, 799.81-799.89

781.8 Neurologic neglect syndrome   CC
Asomatognosia
Hemi-akinesia
Hemi-inattention
Hemispatial neglect
Left-sided neglect
Sensory extinction
Sensory neglect
Visuospatial neglect
EXCLUDES visuospatial deficit (799.53)
CC Exd: 781.8-781.92, 781.94-781.99
AHA: 4Q, '94, 37
TIP: If documented as sequelae of a CVA, assign also a code from
category 438.

**781.9 Other symptoms involving nervous and musculoskeletal
systems**
AHA: 4Q, '00, 45

781.91 Loss of height
EXCLUDES osteoporosis (733.00-733.09)

781.92 Abnormal posture

781.93 Ocular torticollis
DEF: Abnormal head posture as a result of a contracted
state of cervical muscles to correct a visual disturbance;
either double vision or a visual field defect.
AHA: 4Q, '02, 68

781.94 Facial weakness
Facial droop
EXCLUDES *facial weakness due to late effect of*
cerebrovascular accident (438.83)
AHA: 4Q, '03, 72
TIP: Do not assign if facial droop or weakness is due to Bell's
palsy; see instead code 351.0.
R29.810 Facial weakness　　　　[I-10]

**781.99 Other symptoms involving nervous and
musculoskeletal systems**

√4ᵗʰ **782 Symptoms involving skin and other integumentary tissue**
EXCLUDES *symptoms relating to breast (611.71-611.79)*

782.0 Disturbance of skin sensation
Anesthesia of skin
Burning or prickling sensation
Hyperesthesia
Hypoesthesia
Numbness
Paresthesia
Tingling
R20.9 Unspecified disturbances of skin sensation　　[I-10]

782.1 Rash and other nonspecific skin eruption
Exanthem
EXCLUDES *vesicular eruption (709.8)*
AHA: 4Q, '08, 99

782.2 Localized superficial swelling, mass, or lump
Subcutaneous nodules
EXCLUDES *localized adiposity (278.1)*

782.3 Edema
Anasarca　　　　Localized edema NOS
Dropsy
EXCLUDES *ascites (789.51-789.59)*
edema of:
newborn NOS (778.5)
pregnancy (642.0-642.9, 646.1)
fluid retention (276.69)
hydrops fetalis (773.3, 778.0)
hydrothorax (511.81-511.89)
nutritional edema (260, 262)
DEF: Edema: excess fluid in intercellular body tissue.
DEF: Anasarca: massive edema in all body tissues.
DEF: Dropsy: serous fluid accumulated in body cavity or cellular
tissue.
DEF: Localized edema: edema in specific body areas.
AHA: 2Q, '00, 18
R60.9 Edema unspecified　　　　[I-10]

782.4 Jaundice, unspecified, not of newborn　　[CC]
Cholemia NOS
Icterus NOS
EXCLUDES *jaundice in newborn (774.0-774.7)*
due to isoimmunization (773.0-773.2, 773.4)
DEF: Bilirubin deposits of skin, causing yellow cast.
CC Exd: 774.0-774.7, 782.4, 782.9
R17 Unspecified jaundice　　　　[I-10]

782.5 Cyanosis
EXCLUDES *newborn (770.83)*
DEF: Deficient oxygen of blood; causes blue cast to skin.

√5ᵗʰ **782.6 Pallor and flushing**

782.61 Pallor

782.62 Flushing
Excessive blushing

782.7 Spontaneous ecchymoses
Petechiae
EXCLUDES *ecchymosis in fetus or newborn (772.6)*
purpura (287.0-287.9)
DEF: Hemorrhagic spots of skin; resemble freckles.

782.8 Changes in skin texture
Induration ⎫
Thickening ⎬ of skin

782.9 Other symptoms involving skin and integumentary tissues

√4ᵗʰ **783 Symptoms concerning nutrition, metabolism, and development**

783.0 Anorexia
Loss of appetite
EXCLUDES *anorexia nervosa (307.1)*
loss of appetite of nonorganic origin (307.59)
R63.0 Anorexia　　　　[I-10]

783.1 Abnormal weight gain
EXCLUDES *excessive weight gain in pregnancy (646.1)*
obesity (278.00)
morbid (278.01)

√5ᵗʰ **783.2 Abnormal loss of weight and underweight**
Use additional code to identify Body Mass Index (BMI), if
known (V85.0-V85.54)
AHA: 4Q, '00, 45

783.21 Loss of weight
AHA: 4Q, '05, 96
R63.4 Abnormal weight loss　　　　[I-10]

783.22 Underweight
AHA: 4Q, '05, 96

783.3 Feeding difficulties and mismanagement
Feeding problem (elderly) (infant)
EXCLUDES *feeding disturbance or problems:*
in newborn (779.31-779.34)
of nonorganic origin (307.50-307.59)
AHA: 3Q, '97, 12

√5ᵗʰ **783.4 Lack of expected normal physiological development in
childhood**
EXCLUDES *delay in sexual development and puberty (259.0)*
gonadal dysgenesis (758.6)
pituitary dwarfism (253.3)
slow fetal growth and fetal malnutrition
(764.00-764.99)
specific delays in mental development (315.0-315.9)
AHA: 4Q, '00, 45; 3Q, '97, 4

**783.40 Lack of normal physiological development,
unspecified**
Inadequate development
Lack of development

783.41 Failure to thrive　　[P]
Failure to gain weight
EXCLUDES *failure to thrive in newborn (779.34)*
DEF: Organic failure to thrive: acute or chronic illness that
interferes with nutritional intake, absorption, metabolism
excretion and energy requirements. Nonorganic FTT is
symptom of neglect or abuse.
AHA: 1Q, '03, 12

783.42 Delayed milestones　　[P]
Late talker
Late walker

783.43 Short stature
Growth failure
Growth retardation
Lack of growth
Physical retardation
DEF: Constitutional short stature: stature inconsistent with
chronological age. Genetic short stature is when skeletal
maturation matches chronological age.

783.5 Polydipsia
Excessive thirst

783.6 Polyphagia
Excessive eating
Hyperalimentation NOS
EXCLUDES *disorders of eating of nonorganic origin*
(307.50-307.59)

783.7 Adult failure to thrive　　[A]
R62.7 Adult failure to thrive　　　　[I-10]

783.9 Other symptoms concerning nutrition, metabolism, and development
Hypometabolism
EXCLUDES *abnormal basal metabolic rate (794.7)*
dehydration (276.51)
other disorders of fluid, electrolyte, and acid-base balance (276.0-276.9)
AHA: 2Q, '04, 3

✓4ᵗʰ **784 Symptoms involving head and neck**
EXCLUDES *encephalopathy NOS (348.30)*
specific symptoms involving neck classifiable to 723 (723.0-723.9)

784.0 Headache
Facial pain
Pain in head NOS
EXCLUDES *atypical face pain (350.2)*
migraine (346.0-346.9)
tension headache (307.81)
AHA: 3Q, '06, 22; 2Q, '06, 17; 3Q, '00, 13; 1Q, '90, 4; 3Q, '92, 14
TIP: Do not assign if headache syndrome has been diagnosed, refer to category 339.
R51 Headache   I-10

784.1 Throat pain
EXCLUDES *dysphagia (787.20-787.29)*
neck pain (723.1)
sore throat (462)
chronic (472.1)

784.2 Swelling, mass, or lump in head and neck
Space-occupying lesion, intracranial NOS
AHA: 1Q, '03, 8

784.3 Aphasia   CC
EXCLUDES *aphasia due to late effects of cerebrovascular disease (438.11)*
developmental aphasia (315.31)
DEF: Inability to communicate through speech, written word, or sign language.
CC Exd: 315.31, 315.35, 432.0-434.91, 436, 784.3-784.59
AHA: 3Q, '10, 5; 4Q, '04, 78; 4Q, '98, 87; 3Q, '97, 12
R47.01 Aphasia   I-10

✓5ᵗʰ **784.4 Voice and resonance disorders**
AHA: 4Q, '09, 102-103

784.40 Voice and resonance disorder, unspecified

784.41 Aphonia
Loss of voice

784.42 Dysphonia
Hoarseness

784.43 Hypernasality

784.44 Hyponasality

784.49 Other voice and resonance disorders
Change in voice

✓5ᵗʰ **784.5 Other speech disturbance**
EXCLUDES *speech disorder due to late effect of cerebrovascular accident (438.10-438.19)*
stuttering (315.35)
AHA: 4Q, '09, 87-88

784.51 Dysarthria
EXCLUDES *dysarthria due to late effect of cerebrovascular accident (438.13)*

784.52 Fluency disorder in conditions classified elsewhere
Stuttering in conditions classified elsewhere
Code first underlying disease or condition, such as:
Parkinson's disease (332.0)
EXCLUDES *adult onset fluency disorder (307.0)*
childhood onset fluency disorder (315.35)
fluency disorder due to late effect of cerebrovascular accident (438.14)
AHA: 4Q, '10, 83-84

784.59 Other speech disturbance
Dysphasia
Slurred speech
Speech disturbance NOS
R47.89 Other speech disturbances   I-10

✓5ᵗʰ **784.6 Other symbolic dysfunction**
EXCLUDES *developmental learning delays (315.0-315.9)*

784.60 Symbolic dysfunction, unspecified

784.61 Alexia and dyslexia
Alexia (with agraphia)
DEF: Alexia: Inability to understand written word due to central brain lesion.
DEF: Dyslexia: Ability to recognize letters but inability to read, spell, and write words; genetic.

784.69 Other
Acalculia   Agraphia NOS
Agnosia   Apraxia

784.7 Epistaxis
Hemorrhage from nose
Nosebleed
AHA: 3Q, '04, 7
R04.0 Epistaxis   I-10

784.8 Hemorrhage from throat
EXCLUDES *hemoptysis (786.30-786.39)*

✓5ᵗʰ **784.9 Other symptoms involving head and neck**

784.91 Postnasal drip
AHA: 4Q, '06, 108

784.92 Jaw pain
Mandibular pain
Maxilla pain
EXCLUDES *temporomandibular joint arthralgia (524.62)*
AHA: 4Q, '10, 83-84
R68.84 Jaw pain   I-10

784.99 Other symptoms involving head and neck
Choking sensation
Feeling of foreign body in throat
Halitosis
Mouth breathing
Sneezing
EXCLUDES *foreign body in throat (933.0)*
AHA: 4Q, '06, 108

✓4ᵗʰ **785 Symptoms involving cardiovascular system**
EXCLUDES *heart failure NOS (428.9)*

785.0 Tachycardia, unspecified
Rapid heart beat
EXCLUDES *neonatal tachycardia (779.82)*
paroxysmal tachycardia (427.0-427.2)
DEF: Excessively rapid heart rate.
AHA: 2Q, '03, 11
R00.0 Tachycardia unspecified   I-10

785.1 Palpitations
Awareness of heart beat
EXCLUDES *specified dysrhythmias (427.0-427.9)*
R00.2 Palpitations   I-10

785.2 Undiagnosed cardiac murmurs
Heart murmurs NOS
AHA: 4Q, '92, 16
R01.1 Cardiac murmur unspecified   I-10

785.3 Other abnormal heart sounds
Cardiac dullness, increased or decreased
Friction fremitus, cardiac
Precordial friction

785.4 Gangrene   `CC`
Gangrene:
NOS
spreading cutaneous
Gangrenous cellulitis
Phagedena

Code first any associated underlying condition
> *EXCLUDES* gangrene of certain sites — see Alphabetic Index
> gangrene with atherosclerosis of the extremities
> (440.24)
> gas gangrene (040.0)

DEF: Gangrene: necrosis of skin tissue due to bacterial infection,
diabetes, embolus and vascular supply loss.
DEF: Gangrenous cellulitis: group A streptococcal infection; begins
with severe cellulitis, spreads to superficial and deep fascia;
produces gangrene of underlying tissues.
CC Exd: 338.0-338.4, 440.24, 780.91-780.99, 785.4, 799.81-799.89
AHA: 1Q, '04, 14; 3Q, '91, 12; 3Q, '90, 15; M-A, '86, 12
I96 Gangrene not elsewhere classified   `I-10`

√5ᵗʰ 785.5 Shock without mention of trauma

785.50 Shock, unspecified   `CC`
Failure of peripheral circulation
DEF: Peripheral circulatory failure due to heart
insufficiencies.
CC Exd: 338.0-338.4, 780.64-780.65, 780.91-780.99,
785.50-785.59, 785.9, 799.81-799.89
AHA: 2Q, '96, 10

¹ **785.51 Cardiogenic shock**   `MCC`
DEF: Shock syndrome: associated with myocardial
infarction, cardiac tamponade and massive pulmonary
embolism; symptoms include mental confusion, reduced
blood pressure, tachycardia, pallor and cold, clammy skin.
CC Exd: See code: 785.50
AHA: 4Q, '08, 182; 3Q, '05, 14
R57.0 Cardiogenic shock   `I-10`

785.52 Septic shock   `MCC`
Shock:
endotoxic
gram-negative

Code first underlying infection
Use additional code, if applicable, to identify systemic
inflammatory response syndrome due to
infectious process with organ dysfunction
(995.92)
CC Exd: See code 785.50
AHA: 2Q, '10, 4; 4Q, '08, 99; 4Q, '06, 113; 2Q, '05, 18-19; 4Q,
'03, 73, 79
TIP: The diagnosis of septic shock indicates the presence of
severe sepsis; code 785.52 should not be assigned without
first assigning code 995.92.

¹ **785.59 Other**   `MCC`
Shock:
hypovolemic
> *EXCLUDES* shock (due to):
> anesthetic (995.4)
> anaphylactic (995.0)
> due to serum (999.41-999.49)
> electric (994.8)
> following abortion (639.5)
> lightning (994.0)
> obstetrical (669.1)
> postoperative (998.00-998.09)
> traumatic (958.4)

CC Exd: see code 785.50
AHA: 2Q, '00, 3

785.6 Enlargement of lymph nodes
Lymphadenopathy
"Swollen glands"
> *EXCLUDES* lymphadenitis (chronic) (289.1-289.3)
> acute (683)

R59.9 Enlarged lymph nodes unspecified   `I-10`

785.9 Other symptoms involving cardiovascular system
Bruit (arterial)
Weak pulse

√4ᵗʰ 786 Symptoms involving respiratory system and other chest symptoms

√5ᵗʰ 786.0 Dyspnea and respiratory abnormalities

786.00 Respiratory abnormality, unspecified

786.01 Hyperventilation
> *EXCLUDES* hyperventilation, psychogenic (306.1)

DEF: Rapid breathing causes carbon dioxide loss from
blood.

786.02 Orthopnea
DEF: Difficulty breathing except in upright position.

786.03 Apnea
> *EXCLUDES* apnea of newborn (770.81, 770.82)
> sleep apnea (780.51, 780.53, 780.57)

DEF: Cessation of breathing.
AHA: 4Q, '98, 50

786.04 Cheyne-Stokes respiration   `CC`
DEF: Rhythmic increase of depth and frequency of
breathing with apnea; occurs in frontal lobe and
diencephalic dysfunction.
CC Exd: 518.81-518.84, 519.8-519.9, 786.03-786.04, 799.1
AHA: 4Q, '98, 50

786.05 Shortness of breath
DEF: Inability to take in sufficient oxygen.
AHA: 4Q, '99, 25; 1Q, '99, 6; 4Q, '98, 50
R06.02 Shortness of breath   `I-10`

786.06 Tachypnea
> *EXCLUDES* transitory tachypnea of newborn (770.6)

DEF: Abnormal rapid respiratory rate; called
hyperventilation.
AHA: 1Q, '11, 16-17; 4Q, '98, 50

786.07 Wheezing
> *EXCLUDES* asthma (493.00-493.92)

DEF: Stenosis of respiratory passageway; causes whistling
sound; due to asthma, coryza, croup, emphysema, hay
fever, edema, and pleural effusion.
AHA: 4Q, '98, 50

786.09 Other
Respiratory: Respiratory:
distress   insufficiency
> *EXCLUDES* respiratory distress:
> following trauma and surgery (518.52)
> newborn (770.89)
> syndrome (newborn) (769)
> adult (518.52)
> respiratory failure (518.81, 518.83-518.84)
> newborn (770.84)

AHA: 4Q, '05, 90; 2Q, '98, 10; 1Q, '97, 7; 1Q, '90, 9
R06.00 Dyspnea, unspecified   `I-10`

786.1 Stridor
> *EXCLUDES* congenital laryngeal stridor (748.3)

DEF: Obstructed airway causes harsh sound.

786.2 Cough
> *EXCLUDES* cough:
> psychogenic (306.1)
> smokers' (491.0)
> with hemorrhage (786.39)

AHA: 4Q, '99, 26
R05 Cough   `I-10`

√5ᵗʰ 786.3 Hemoptysis
DEF: Coughing up blood or blood-stained sputum. .
AHA: 3Q, '11, 12; 4Q, '10, 94-95; 2Q, '06, 17; 4Q, '90, 26

786.30 Hemoptysis, unspecified   `CC`
Pulmonary hemorrhage NOS
CC Exd: 786.30-786.4, 799.82
R04.2 Hemoptysis   `I-10`

---

¹ MCC = Only if patient discharged alive.

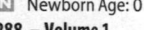 Newborn Age: 0   `P` Pediatric Age: 0-17   `M` Maternity Age: 12-55   `A` Adult Age: 15-124   `MCC` Major CC Condition   `CC` CC Condition   `HIV` HIV Related Dx

288 – Volume 1   **2014 ICD-9-CM**

786.31 Acute idiopathic pulmonary hemorrhage in infants [AIPHI] `CC` `P`
    Acute idiopathic pulmonary hemorrhage in infant over 28 days old
    EXCLUDES pulmonary hemorrhage of newborn under 28 days old (770.3)
               von Willebrand's disease (286.4)
    CC Excl: See code: 786.30
    DEF: An abrupt onset of bleeding or blood in the airway with acute respiratory distress or failure in a patient with no prior history of an identifiable causal condition.
    R04.81 Acute idiopathic pulmonary hemorrhage in infants   `I-10`

786.39 Other hemoptysis `CC`
    Cough with hemorrhage
    CC Excl: See code: 786.30
    R04.89 Hemorrhage from othr site in resp passages   `I-10`

786.4 Abnormal sputum
    Abnormal:
        amount
        color } sputum
        odor
    Excessive septum

✓5ᵗʰ 786.5 Chest pain

786.50 Chest pain, unspecified
    AHA: 1Q, '07, 19; 2Q, '06, 7; 1Q, '03, 6; 1Q, '02, 4; 4Q, '99, 25
    R07.9 Chest pain unspecified   `I-10`

786.51 Precordial pain
    DEF: Chest pain over heart and lower thorax.

786.52 Painful respiration
    Pain: Pleurodynia
        anterior chest wall
        pleuritic
    EXCLUDES epidemic pleurodynia (074.1)
    AHA: N-D, '84, 17
    TIP: Assign for musculoskeletal chest pain with no indication of underlying cause.
    R07.1 Chest pain on breathing   `I-10`

786.59 Other
    Discomfort
    Pressure } in chest
    Tightness
    EXCLUDES pain in breast (611.71)
    AHA: 1Q, '02, 6
    TIP: Assign for chest pain due to anxiety, along with an additional code for anxiety. Chest pain is not integral to the diagnosis of anxiety.
    R07.89 Other chest pain   `I-10`

786.6 Swelling, mass, or lump in chest
    EXCLUDES lump in breast (611.72)
    R22.2 Localized swelling, mass, lump, trunk   `I-10`

786.7 Abnormal chest sounds
    Abnormal percussion, chest   Rales
    Friction sounds, chest   Tympany, chest
    EXCLUDES wheezing (786.07)

786.8 Hiccough
    EXCLUDES psychogenic hiccough (306.1)

786.9 Other symptoms involving respiratory system and chest
    Breath-holding spell

Phases of Swallowing

Oral phase

Oropharyngeal phase

Pharyngeal phase   Pharyngeoesophageal phase

✓4ᵗʰ 787 Symptoms involving digestive system
    EXCLUDES constipation (564.00-564.09)
                pylorospasm (537.81)
                  congenital (750.5)

✓5ᵗʰ 787.0 Nausea and vomiting
    Emesis
    EXCLUDES hematemesis NOS (578.0)
           vomiting:
             bilious, following gastrointestinal surgery (564.3)
             cyclical (536.2)
                 associated with migraine (346.2)
                 psychogenic (306.4)
             excessive, in pregnancy (643.0-643.9)
             fecal matter (569.87)
             habit (536.2)
             of newborn (779.32, 779.33)
             persistent (536.2)
             psychogenic NOS (307.54)
    AHA: M-A, '85, 11

787.01 Nausea with vomiting
    AHA: 1Q, '03, 5
    R11.2 Nausea with vomiting, unspecified   `I-10`

787.02 Nausea alone
    AHA: 3Q, '00, 12; 2Q, '97, 9
    R11.0 Nausea alone   `I-10`

787.03 Vomiting alone

787.04 Bilious emesis
    Bilious vomiting
    EXCLUDES bilious emesis (vomiting) in newborn (779.32)
    AHA: 4Q, '09, 103-104

787.1 Heartburn
    Pyrosis
    Waterbrash
    EXCLUDES dyspepsia or indigestion (536.8)
    AHA: 2Q, '01, 6

✓5ᵗʰ 787.2 Dysphagia
    Code first, if applicable, dysphagia due to late effect of cerebrovascular accident (438.82)
    AHA: 4Q, '07, 92-94; 3Q, '07, 7; 4Q, '03, 103, 109; 2Q, '01, 4

787.20 Dysphagia, unspecified
    Difficulty in swallowing NOS

787.21 Dysphagia, oral phase

787.22 Dysphagia, oropharyngeal phase
    AHA: 4Q, '07, 94

787.23 Dysphagia, pharyngeal phase

787.24 Dysphagia, pharyngoesophageal phase

787.29 Other dysphagia
    Cervical dysphagia
    Neurogenic dysphagia
    R13.19 Other dysphagia   `I-10`

787.3 Flatulence, eructation, and gas pain
    Abdominal distention (gaseous)
    Bloating
    Tympanites (abdominal) (intestinal)
    EXCLUDES aerophagy (306.4)
    DEF: Flatulence: excess air or gas in intestine or stomach.
    DEF: Eructation: belching, expelling gas through mouth.
    DEF: Gas pain: gaseous pressure affecting gastrointestinal system.

787.4 Visible peristalsis
    Hyperperistalsis
    DEF: Increase in involuntary movements of intestines.

787.5 Abnormal bowel sounds
    Absent bowel sounds
    Hyperactive bowel sounds

Symptoms, Signs, and Ill-Defined Conditions

787.6–788.62

√5th **787.6 Incontinence of feces**
Encopresis NOS
Incontinence of sphincter ani
> **EXCLUDES** *that of nonorganic origin (307.7)*
AHA: 4Q, '10, 87-89; 1Q, '97, 9

787.60 Full incontinence of feces
Fecal incontinence NOS
R15.9 Full incontinence of feces   I-10

787.61 Incomplete defecation
> **EXCLUDES** *constipation (564.00-564.09)*
> *fecal impaction (560.32)*

787.62 Fecal smearing
Fecal soiling

787.63 Fecal urgency
R15.2 Fecal urgency   I-10

787.7 Abnormal feces
Bulky stools
> **EXCLUDES** *abnormal stool content (792.1)*
> *melena:*
> *NOS (578.1)*
> *newborn (772.4, 777.3)*

√5th **787.9 Other symptoms involving digestive system**
> **EXCLUDES** *gastrointestinal hemorrhage (578.0-578.9)*
> *intestinal obstruction (560.0-560.9)*
> *specific functional digestive disorders:*
> *esophagus (530.0-530.9)*
> *stomach and duodenum (536.0-536.9)*
> *those not elsewhere classified (564.00-564.9)*

787.91 Diarrhea
Diarrhea NOS
AHA: 2Q, '10, 12; 4Q, '08, 99; 4Q, '95, 54
R19.7 Diarrhea unspecified   I-10

787.99 Other
Change in bowel habits
Tenesmus (rectal)
DEF: Tenesmus: Painful, ineffective straining at the rectum with limited passage of fecal matter.

√4th **788 Symptoms involving urinary system**
> **EXCLUDES** *hematuria (599.70-599.72)*
> *nonspecific findings on examination of the urine (791.0-791.9)*
> *small kidney of unknown cause (589.0-589.9)*
> *uremia NOS (586)*
> *urinary obstruction (599.60, 599.69)*

788.0 Renal colic
Colic (recurrent) of:
kidney
ureter
DEF: Kidney pain.
AHA: 3Q, '04, 8
TIP: Do not assign if renal colic is due to calculus; see category 592.

788.1 Dysuria
Painful urination
Strangury

√5th **788.2 Retention of urine**
Code, if applicable, any causal condition first, such as:
hyperplasia of prostate (600.0-600.9 with fifth-digit 1)
DEF: Accumulation of urine in the bladder due to inability to void.

788.20 Retention of urine, unspecified
AHA: 4Q, '06, 93, 95; 2Q, '04, 18; 3Q, '03, 12-13; 1Q, '03, 6; 3Q, '96, 10
R33.9 Retention of urine unspecified   I-10

788.21 Incomplete bladder emptying
AHA: 4Q, '06, 93

788.29 Other specified retention of urine

√5th **788.3 Urinary incontinence**
Code, if applicable, any causal condition first, such as:
congenital ureterocele (753.23)
genital prolapse (618.00-618.9)
hyperplasia of prostate (600.0-600.9 with fifth-digit 1)
> **EXCLUDES** *functional urinary incontinence (788.91)*
> *that of nonorganic origin (307.6)*
> *urinary incontinence associated with cognitive impairment (788.91)*
AHA: 4Q, '06, 93; 4Q, '92, 22

788.30 Urinary incontinence, unspecified
Enuresis NOS
AHA: 1Q, '09, 15
R32 Unspecified urinary incontinence   I-10

788.31 Urge incontinence
DEF: Inability to control urination, upon urge to urinate.
AHA: 1Q, '00, 19

788.32 Stress incontinence, male   ♂
> **EXCLUDES** *stress incontinence, female (625.6)*
DEF: Inability to control urination associated with weak sphincter in males.

788.33 Mixed incontinence, (male) (female)
Urge and stress
DEF: Urge, stress incontinence: involuntary discharge of urine due to anatomic displacement.

788.34 Incontinence without sensory awareness
DEF: Involuntary discharge of urine without sensory warning.

788.35 Post-void dribbling
DEF: Involuntary discharge of residual urine after voiding.

788.36 Nocturnal enuresis
DEF: Involuntary discharge of urine during the night.

788.37 Continuous leakage
DEF: Continuous, involuntary urine seepage.

788.38 Overflow incontinence
DEF: Leakage caused by pressure of retained urine in the bladder after the bladder has fully contracted due to weakened bladder muscles or an obstruction of the urethra.

788.39 Other urinary incontinence

√5th **788.4 Frequency of urination and polyuria**
Code, if applicable, any causal condition first, such as:
hyperplasia of prostate (600.0-600.9 with fifth-digit 1)

788.41 Urinary frequency
Frequency of micturition
AHA: 4Q, '06, 93

788.42 Polyuria
DEF: Excessive urination.

788.43 Nocturia
DEF: Urination affecting sleep patterns.
AHA: 4Q, '06, 93

788.5 Oliguria and anuria
Deficient secretion of urine
Suppression of urinary secretion
> **EXCLUDES** *that complicating:*
> *abortion (634-638 with .3, 639.3)*
> *ectopic or molar pregnancy (639.3)*
> *pregnancy, childbirth, or the puerperium (642.0-642.9, 646.2)*
DEF: Oliguria: diminished urinary secretion related to fluid intake.
DEF: Anuria: lack of urinary secretion due to renal failure or obstructed urinary tract.

√5th **788.6 Other abnormality of urination**
Code, if applicable, any causal condition first, such as:
hyperplasia of prostate (600.0-600.9 with fifth-digit 1)

788.61 Splitting of urinary stream
Intermittent urinary stream

788.62 Slowing of urinary stream
Weak stream
AHA: 4Q, '06, 93

N Newborn Age: 0   P Pediatric Age: 0-17   M Maternity Age: 12-55   A Adult Age: 15-124   MCC Major CC Condition   CC CC Condition   HIV HIV Related Dx

788.63 **Urgency of urination**

> **EXCLUDES** *urge incontinence (788.31, 788.33)*
> **DEF:** Feeling of intense need to urinate; abrupt sensation of imminent urination.
> **AHA:** 4Q, '06, 93; 4Q, '03, 74

788.64 **Urinary hesitancy**

> **AHA:** 4Q, '06, 93, 109

788.65 **Straining on urination**

> **AHA:** 4Q, '06, 93, 109

788.69 **Other**

788.7 **Urethral discharge**
Penile discharge
Urethrorrhea

788.8 **Extravasation of urine** cc

> **DEF:** Leaking or infiltration of urine into tissues.
> **CC Exd:** 788.8-788.99

√5ᵗʰ 788.9 **Other symptoms involving urinary system**

> **AHA:** 1Q, '05, 12; 4Q, '88, 1

788.91 **Functional urinary incontinence**
Urinary incontinence due to cognitive impairment, or severe physical disability or immobility

> **EXCLUDES** *urinary incontinence due to physiologic condition (788.30-788.39)*
> **AHA:** 4Q, '08, 144-145

788.99 **Other symptoms involving urinary system**

Extrarenal uremia	Vesical:
Vesical:	tenesmus
pain	

√4ᵗʰ 789 **Other symptoms involving abdomen and pelvis**

> **EXCLUDES** *symptoms referable to genital organs:*
> *female (625.0-625.9)*
> *male (607.0-608.9)*
> *psychogenic (302.70-302.79))*

The following fifth-digit subclassification is to be used for codes 789.0, 789.3, 789.4, 789.6:
  0 unspecified site
  1 right upper quadrant
  2 left upper quadrant
  3 right lower quadrant
  4 left lower quadrant
  5 periumbilic
  6 epigastric
  7 generalized
  9 other specified site
     Multiple sites

§ √5ᵗʰ 789.0 **Abdominal pain**
[0-7, 9] Cramps, abdominal

> **AHA:** 1Q, '95, 3; **For code 789.06:** 1Q, '02, 5
> R10.9 Unspecified abdominal pain I-10
> R10.31 Right lower quadrant pain I-10
> R10.13 Epigastric pain I-10
> R10.84 Generalized abdominal pain I-10

789.1 **Hepatomegaly**
Enlargement of liver

789.2 **Splenomegaly**
Enlargement of spleen

§ √5ᵗʰ 789.3 **Abdominal or pelvic swelling, mass, or lump**
[0-7, 9] Diffuse or generalized swelling or mass:
     abdominal NOS
     umbilical

> **EXCLUDES** *abdominal distention (gaseous) (787.3)*
> *ascites (789.51-789.59)*

§ √5ᵗʰ 789.4 **Abdominal rigidity**
[0-7, 9]

√5ᵗʰ 789.5 **Ascites**
Fluid in peritoneal cavity

> **DEF:** Serous fluid effusion and accumulation in abdominal cavity.
> **AHA:** 4Q, '07, 95; 2Q, '05, 8; 4Q, '89, 11

789.51 **Malignant ascites** cc

> *Code first malignancy, such as:*
> *malignant neoplasm of ovary (183.0)*
> *secondary malignant neoplasm of retroperitoneum and peritoneum (197.6)*
> **AHA:** 4Q, '07, 96
> **CC Exd:** 338.0-338.4, 780.64-780.65, 780.91-780.99, 789.30-789.59, 789.9, 799.81-799.89
> R18.0 Malignant ascites I-10

789.59 **Other ascites** cc

> **CC Exd:** See code: 789.51
> **AHA:** 4Q, '08, 99
> R18.8 Other ascites I-10

§ √5ᵗʰ 789.6 **Abdominal tenderness**
[0-7, 9] Rebound tenderness

789.7 **Colic** P
Colic NOS
Infantile colic

> **EXCLUDES** *colic in adult and child over 12 months old (789.0)*
> *renal colic (788.0)*
> **DEF:** Inconsolable crying in an otherwise well-fed and healthy infant for more than three hours a day, three days a week, for more than three weeks.
> **AHA:** 4Q, '09, 104-105

789.9 **Other symptoms involving abdomen and pelvis**
Umbilical:
  bleeding
  discharge

Nonspecific Abnormal Findings (790-796)

> **AHA:** 3Q, '11, 4; 2Q, '90, 16

√4ᵗʰ 790 **Nonspecific findings on examination of blood**

> **EXCLUDES** *abnormality of:*
> *platelets (287.0-287.9)*
> *thrombocytes (287.0-287.9)*
> *white blood cells (288.00-288.9)*

√5ᵗʰ 790.0 **Abnormality of red blood cells**

> **EXCLUDES** *anemia:*
> *congenital (776.5)*
> *newborn, due to isoimmunization (773.0-773.2, 773.5)*
> *of premature infant (776.6)*
> *other specified types (280.0-285.9)*
> *hemoglobin disorders (282.5-282.7)*
> *polycythemia:*
> *familial (289.6)*
> *neonatorum (776.4)*
> *secondary (289.0)*
> *vera (238.4)*
> **AHA:** 4Q, '00, 46

790.01 **Precipitous drop in hematocrit** cc
Drop in hematocrit
Drop in hemoglobin

> **CC Exd:** 285.1, 285.3-285.9
> **TIP:** Typically reported as a reason for encounter at a dialysis center.

790.09 **Other abnormality of red blood cells**
Abnormal red cell morphology NOS
Abnormal red cell volume NOS
Anisocytosis
Poikilocytosis

790.1 **Elevated sedimentation rate**

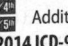 Requires fifth digit. Valid digits are in [brackets] under each code. See category 789 for codes and definitions.

⁴ᵗʰ/⁵ᵗʰ Additional Digit Required   Unacceptable PDx   Manifestation Code   Hospital Acquired Condition   ►◄ Revised Text   ● New Code   ▲ Revised Code Title

2014 ICD-9-CM   **Volume 1 – 291**

Symptoms, Signs, and Ill-Defined Conditions

790.2–791.9

√5th **790.2 Abnormal glucose**

EXCLUDES   *diabetes mellitus (249.00-249.91, 250.00-250.93)*
dysmetabolic syndrome X (277.7)
gestational diabetes (648.8)
glycosuria (791.5)
hypoglycemia (251.2)
that complicating pregnancy, childbirth, or
     puerperium (648.8)

AHA: 1Q, '11, 9; 4Q, '03, 74; 3Q, '91, 5

TIP: These codes are typically assigned on encounters before a patient is diagnosed with diabetes mellitus.

790.21 Impaired fasting glucose
Elevated fasting glucose

790.22 Impaired glucose tolerance test (oral)
Elevated glucose tolerance test

790.29 Other abnormal glucose
Abnormal glucose NOS
Abnormal non-fasting glucose
Hyperglycemia NOS
Pre-diabetes NOS

AHA: 1Q, '12, 17; 3Q, '09, 5; 2Q, '05, 21

TIP: Assign for any stress hyperglycemia for which no causal condition is determined including postoperative hyperglycemia that is not specifically documented as a complication of the procedure.

R73.09 Other abnormal glucose   I-10

790.3 Excessive blood level of alcohol
Elevated blood-alcohol
AHA: S-O, '86, 3

790.4 Nonspecific elevation of levels of transaminase or lactic acid dehydrogenase [LDH]
R74.0 Nonspecific elevation levels transaminase & LDH   I-10

790.5 Other nonspecific abnormal serum enzyme levels
Abnormal serum level of:
acid phosphatase
alkaline phosphatase
amylase
lipase

EXCLUDES   *deficiency of circulating enzymes (277.6)*
R74.8 Abnormal levels of other serum enzymes   I-10

790.6 Other abnormal blood chemistry

Abnormal blood level of:	Abnormal blood level of:
cobalt	lithium
copper	magnesium
iron	mineral
lead	zinc

EXCLUDES   *abnormality of electrolyte or acid-base balance*
    (276.0-276.9)
hypoglycemia NOS (251.2)
lead poisoning (984.0-984.9)
specific finding indicating abnormality of:
    amino-acid transport and metabolism
      (270.0-270.9)
    carbohydrate transport and metabolism
      (271.0-271.9)
    lipid metabolism (272.0-272.9)
uremia NOS (586)

AHA: 4Q, '88, 1

TIP: If only azotemia is documented (indexed to 790.6), clarify with physician; if due to uremia or renal failure, code to those conditions instead.

R78.89 Finding oth spec substances not norm found blood   I-10

790.7 Bacteremia   CC

EXCLUDES   *bacteremia of newborn (771.83)*
septicemia (038)

Use additional code to identify organism (041)

DEF: Laboratory finding of bacteria in the blood in the absence of two or more signs of sepsis; transient in nature, progresses to septicemia with severe infectious process.

CC Excl: 338.0-338.4, 780.64-780.65, 780.91-780.99, 790.7-790.99, 799.81-799.89

AHA: 2Q, '11, 7; 2Q, '03, 7; 4Q, '93, 29; 3Q, '88, 12

TIP: If clinical signs or symptoms indicating systemic disease exist, query physician for the presence of sepsis; code to category 038 if documented.

790.8 Viremia, unspecified
DEF: Presence of a virus in the blood stream.
AHA: 4Q, '88, 10

√5th **790.9 Other nonspecific findings on examination of blood**
AHA: 4Q, '93, 29

790.91 Abnormal arterial blood gases

790.92 Abnormal coagulation profile
Abnormal or prolonged:
bleeding time
coagulation time
partial thromboplastin time [PTT]
prothrombin time [PT]

EXCLUDES   *coagulation (hemorrhagic) disorders*
    (286.0-286.9)

R79.1 Abnormal coagulaton profile   I-10

790.93 Elevated prostate specific antigen, [PSA]   A ♂

790.94 Euthyroid sick syndrome
DEF: Transient alteration of thyroid hormone metabolism due to nonthyroid illness or stress.
AHA: 4Q, '97, 45

790.95 Elevated C-reactive protein [CRP]
DEF: Inflammation in an arterial wall results in elevated C-reactive protein (CRP) in the blood; CRP is a recognized risk factor in cardiovascular disease.

790.99 Other
AHA: ▶3Q, '12, 18;◀ 3Q, '11, 4; 2Q, '03, 14
TIP: ▶Assign for documentation of secondary thrombocytosis as clinically significant but without other reportable underlying cause.◀

√4th **791 Nonspecific findings on examination of urine**

EXCLUDES   *hematuria NOS (599.70-599.72)*
specific findings indicating abnormality of:
    amino-acid transport and metabolism (270.0-270.9)
    carbohydrate transport and metabolism (271.0-271.9)

791.0 Proteinuria
Albuminuria   Bence-Jones proteinuria

EXCLUDES   *postural proteinuria (593.6)*
that arising during pregnancy or the puerperium
    (642.0-642.9, 646.2)

DEF: Excess protein in urine.
AHA: ▶2Q, '12, 19;◀ 3Q, '91, 8

791.1 Chyluria   CC

EXCLUDES   *filarial (125.0-125.9)*
DEF: Excess chyle in urine.
CC Excl: 338.0-338.4, 780.64-780.65, 780.91-780.99, 791.1, 791.9, 799.81-799.89

791.2 Hemoglobinuria
DEF: Free hemoglobin in blood due to rapid hemolysis of red blood cells.

791.3 Myoglobinuria   CC
DEF: Myoglobin (oxygen-transporting pigment) in urine.
CC Excl: 338.0-338.4, 780.64-780.65, 780.91-780.99, 791.2-791.3, 791.9, 799.81-799.89

791.4 Biliuria
DEF: Bile pigments in urine.

791.5 Glycosuria
EXCLUDES   *renal glycosuria (271.4)*
DEF: Sugar in urine.

791.6 Acetonuria
Ketonuria
DEF: Excess acetone in urine.

791.7 Other cells and casts in urine

791.9 Other nonspecific findings on examination of urine

Crystalluria	Elevated urine levels of:
Elevated urine levels of:	indolacetic acid
17-ketosteroids	vanillylmandelic acid [VMA]
catecholamines	Melanuria

AHA: 1Q, '05, 12

N   Newborn Age: 0   P   Pediatric Age: 0-17   M   Maternity Age: 12-55   A   Adult Age: 15-124   MCC   Major CC Condition   CC   CC Condition   HIV   HIV Related Dx

✓4ᵗʰ **792 Nonspecific abnormal findings in other body substances**

     EXCLUDES *that in chromosomal analysis (795.2)*

792.0 Cerebrospinal fluid

792.1 Stool contents
     Abnormal stool color   Occult stool
     Fat in stool   Pus in stool
     Mucus in stool
     EXCLUDES *blood in stool [melena] (578.1)*
                newborn (772.4, 777.3)
     AHA: 2Q, '92, 9

792.2 Semen   ♂
     Abnormal spermatozoa
     EXCLUDES *azoospermia (606.0)*
                oligospermia (606.1)

792.3 Amniotic fluid   Ⓜ ♀
     DEF: Nonspecific abnormal findings in amniotic fluid.
     AHA: N-D, '86, 4

792.4 Saliva
     EXCLUDES *that in chromosomal analysis (795.2)*

792.5 Cloudy (hemodialysis) (peritoneal) dialysis effluent
     AHA: 4Q, '00, 46

792.9 Other nonspecific abnormal findings in body substances
     Peritoneal fluid   Synovial fluid
     Pleural fluid   Vaginal fluids

✓4ᵗʰ **793 Nonspecific (abnormal) findings on radiological and other examination of body structure**

     INCLUDES   nonspecific abnormal findings of:
               thermography
               ultrasound examination [echogram]
               x-ray examination

     EXCLUDES *abnormal results of function studies and radioisotope scans (794.0-794.9)*

793.0 Skull and head
     EXCLUDES *nonspecific abnormal echoencephalogram (794.01)*
     AHA: 3Q, '06, 22

✓5ᵗʰ **793.1 Lung field**
     AHA: 4Q, '11, 138-139

     793.11 Solitary pulmonary nodule
         Coin lesion lung
         Solitary pulmonary nodule, subsegmental branch of the bronchial tree

     793.19 Other nonspecific abnormal finding of lung field
         Pulmonary infiltrate NOS
         Shadow, lung
         AHA: 4Q, '11, 139

793.2 Other intrathoracic organ
     Abnormal:
       echocardiogram
       heart shadow
       ultrasound cardiogram
     Mediastinal shift
     AHA: 1Q, '12, 17

793.3 Biliary tract
     Nonvisualization of gallbladder

793.4 Gastrointestinal tract

793.5 Genitourinary organs
     Filling defect:
       bladder
       kidney
       ureter

793.6 Abdominal area, including retroperitoneum

793.7 Musculoskeletal system

✓5ᵗʰ **793.8 Breast**
     AHA: 4Q, '01, 51

     793.80 Abnormal mammogram, unspecified

     793.81 Mammographic microcalcification
         EXCLUDES *mammographic calcification (793.89)*
                    mammographic calculus (793.89)
         DEF: Calcium and cellular debris deposits in the breast that cannot be felt but can be detected on a mammogram; can be a sign of cancer, benign conditions, or changes in the breast tissue as a result of inflammation, injury, or obstructed duct.

     793.82 Inconclusive mammogram
         Dense breasts NOS
         Inconclusive mammogram NEC
         Inconclusive mammography due to dense breasts
         Inconclusive mammography NEC
         AHA: 4Q, '09, 105-106

     793.89 Other (abnormal) findings on radiological examination of breast
         Mammographic calcification
         Mammographic calculus

✓5ᵗʰ **793.9 Other**
     EXCLUDES *abnormal finding by radioisotope localization of placenta (794.9)*
     TIP: Sequence a code for the sign or symptom that was the reason for the imaging or radiological test first.

     793.91 Image test inconclusive due to excess body fat
         Use additional code to identify Body Mass Index (BMI), if known (V85.0-V85.54)
         AHA: 4Q, '06, 109

     793.99 Other nonspecific (abnormal) findings on radiological and other examinations of body structure
         Abnormal:
           placental finding by x-ray or ultrasound method
           radiological findings in skin and subcutaneous tissue
         AHA: 4Q, '06, 109

✓4ᵗʰ **794 Nonspecific abnormal results of function studies**

     INCLUDES   radioisotope:
               scans
               uptake studies
               scintiphotography

✓5ᵗʰ **794.0 Brain and central nervous system**

     794.00 Abnormal function study, unspecified

     794.01 Abnormal echoencephalogram

     794.02 Abnormal electroencephalogram [EEG]

     794.09 Other
         Abnormal brain scan

✓5ᵗʰ **794.1 Peripheral nervous system and special senses**

     794.10 Abnormal response to nerve stimulation, unspecified

     794.11 Abnormal retinal function studies
         Abnormal electroretinogram [ERG]

     794.12 Abnormal electro-oculogram [EOG]

     794.13 Abnormal visually evoked potential

     794.14 Abnormal oculomotor studies

     794.15 Abnormal auditory function studies
         AHA: 1Q, '04, 15-16
         TIP: If the reason for the encounter was for a hearing examination, sequence a code from subcategory V72.1 first. When nonspecific hearing loss is documented, assign 389.9 instead of 794.15.

     794.16 Abnormal vestibular function studies

     794.17 Abnormal electromyogram [EMG]
         EXCLUDES *that of eye (794.14)*

     794.19 Other

794.2 Pulmonary
     Abnormal lung scan
     Reduced:
       ventilatory capacity
       vital capacity

◨ Additional Digit Required   Unacceptable PDx   Manifestation Code   Hospital Acquired Condition   ▶◀ Revised Text   ● New Code   ▲ Revised Code Title

2014 ICD-9-CM   **Volume 1 – 293**

Symptoms, Signs, and Ill-Defined Conditions

794.3–795.19

√5ᵗʰ **794.3 Cardiovascular**

    794.30 Abnormal function study, unspecified

    794.31 Abnormal electrocardiogram [ECG] [EKG]
        EXCLUDES *long QT syndrome (426.82)*
        R94.31 Abnormal electrocardiogram [ECG]   I-10

    794.39 Other
        Abnormal:
          ballistocardiogram
          phonocardiogram
          vectorcardiogram
        R94.39 Abnormal result oth cardiovasculr function   I-10
        study

794.4 Kidney
    Abnormal renal function test

794.5 Thyroid
    Abnormal thyroid:
      scan
      uptake

794.6 Other endocrine function study

794.7 Basal metabolism
    Abnormal basal metabolic rate [BMR]

794.8 Liver
    Abnormal liver scan
    R94.5 Abnormal results of liver function studies   I-10

794.9 Other
    Bladder   Placenta
    Pancreas   Spleen

√4ᵗʰ **795 Other and nonspecific abnormal cytological, histological, immunological and DNA test findings**
    EXCLUDES *abnormal cytologic smear of anus and anal HPV (796.70-796.79)*
        nonspecific abnormalities of red blood cells (790.01-790.09)

√5ᵗʰ **795.0 Abnormal Papanicolaou smear of cervix and cervical HPV**
    Abnormal thin preparation smear of cervix
    Abnormal cervical cytology
    EXCLUDES *abnormal cytologic smear of vagina and vaginal HPV (795.10-795.19)*
        carcinoma in situ of cervix (233.1)
        cervical intraepithelial neoplasia I (CIN I) (622.11)
        cervical intraepithelial neoplasia II (CIN II) (622.12)
        cervical intraepithelial neoplasia III (CIN III) (233.1)
        dysplasia (histologically confirmed) of cervix (uteri) NOS (622.10)
        mild cervical dysplasia (histologically confirmed) (622.11)
        moderate cervical dysplasia (histologically confirmed) (622.12)
        severe cervical dysplasia (histologically confirmed) (233.1)
    AHA: 4Q, '08, 145-146; 4Q, '02, 69

    795.00 Abnormal glandular Papanicolaou smear of cervix ♀
        Atypical endocervical cells NOS
        Atypical endometrial cells NOS
        Atypical cervical glandular cells NOS

    795.01 Papanicolaou smear of cervix with atypical squamous cells of undetermined significance [ASC-US] ♀
        AHA: 2Q, '06, 4

    795.02 Papanicolaou smear of cervix with atypical squamous cells cannot exclude high grade squamous intraepithelial lesion [ASC-H] ♀

    795.03 Papanicolaou smear of cervix with low grade squamous intraepithelial lesion [LGSIL] ♀

    795.04 Papanicolaou smear of cervix with high grade squamous intraepithelial lesion [HGSIL] ♀

    795.05 Cervical high risk human papillomavirus [HPV] DNA test positive ♀

    795.06 Papanicolaou smear of cervix with cytologic evidence of malignancy ♀
        AHA: 4Q, '06, 110

    795.07 Satisfactory cervical smear but lacking transformation zone ♀

    795.08 Unsatisfactory cervical cytology smear ♀
        Inadequate cervical cytology sample
        AHA: 2Q, '06, 4

    795.09 Other abnormal Papanicolaou smear of cervix and cervical HPV ♀
        Cervical low risk human papillomavirus (HPV) DNA test positive
        Use additional code for associated human papillomavirus (079.4)
        EXCLUDES *encounter for Papanicolaou cervical smear to confirm findings of recent normal smear following initial abnormal smear (V72.32)*

√5ᵗʰ **795.1 Abnormal Papanicolaou smear of vagina and vaginal HPV**
    Abnormal thin preparation smear of vagina NOS
    Abnormal vaginal cytology NOS
    Use additional code to identify acquired absence of uterus and cervix, if applicable (V88.01-V88.03)
    EXCLUDES *abnormal cytologic smear of cervix and cervical HPV (795.00-795.09)*
        carcinoma in situ of vagina (233.31)
        carcinoma in situ of vulva (233.32)
        dysplasia (histologically confirmed) of vagina NOS (623.0, 233.31)
        dysplasia (histologically confirmed) of vulva NOS (624.01, 624.02, 233.32)
        mild vaginal dysplasia (histologically confirmed) (623.0)
        mild vulvar dysplasia (histologically confirmed) (624.01)
        moderate vaginal dysplasia (histologically confirmed) (623.0)
        moderate vulvar dysplasia (histologically confirmed) (624.02)
        severe vaginal dysplasia (histologically confirmed) (233.31)
        severe vulvar dysplasia (histologically confirmed) (233.32)
        vaginal intraepithelial neoplasia I (VAIN I) (623.0)
        vaginal intraepithelial neoplasia II (VAIN II) (623.0)
        vaginal intraepithelial neoplasia III (VAIN III) (233.31)
        vulvar intraepithelial neoplasia I (VIN I) (624.01)
        vulvar intraepithelial neoplasia II (VIN II) (624.02)
        vulvar intraepithelial neoplasia III (VIN III) (233.32)
    AHA: 4Q, '08, 145-148

    795.10 Abnormal glandular Papanicolaou smear of vagina ♀
        Atypical vaginal glandular cells NOS

    795.11 Papanicolaou smear of vagina with atypical squamous cells of undetermined significance [ASC-US] ♀

    795.12 Papanicolaou smear of vagina with atypical squamous cells cannot exclude high grade squamous intraepithelial lesion [ASC-H] ♀

    795.13 Papanicolaou smear of vagina with low grade squamous intraepithelial lesion [LGSIL] ♀

    795.14 Papanicolaou smear of vagina with high grade squamous intraepithelial lesion [HGSIL] ♀

    795.15 Vaginal high risk human papillomavirus [HPV] DNA test positive ♀
        EXCLUDES *condyloma acuminatum (078.11)*
        genital warts (078.11)

    795.16 Papanicolaou smear of vagina with cytologic evidence of malignancy ♀

    795.18 Unsatisfactory vaginal cytology smear ♀
        Inadequate vaginal cytology sample

    795.19 Other abnormal Papanicolaou smear of vagina and vaginal HPV ♀
        Vaginal low risk human papillomavirus (HPV) DNA test positive
        Use additional code for associated human papillomavirus (079.4)

N Newborn Age: 0   P Pediatric Age: 0-17   M Maternity Age: 12-55   A Adult Age: 15-124   MCC Major CC Condition   CC CC Condition   HIV HIV Related D

294 – Volume 1   2014 ICD-9-C

795.2 Nonspecific abnormal findings on chromosomal analysis
Abnormal karyotype

√5ᵗʰ **795.3 Nonspecific positive culture findings**
Positive culture findings in:
    nose
    throat
    sputum
    wound
    EXCLUDES   that of:
        blood (790.7-790.8)
        urine (791.9)

    795.31 Nonspecific positive findings for anthrax
        Positive findings by nasal swab
        AHA: 4Q, '02, 70
        TIP: If the patient has been exposed only to anthrax, assign instead V01.81. If a patient has not been exposed but fears anthrax and tests negative, assign instead V71.82.

    795.39 Other nonspecific positive culture findings
        EXCLUDES   colonization status (V02.0-V02.9)

795.4 Other nonspecific abnormal histological findings

√5ᵗʰ **795.5 Nonspecific reaction to test for tuberculosis**
    AHA: 4Q, '11, 140-141

    795.51 Nonspecific reaction to tuberculin skin test without active tuberculosis
        Abnormal result of Mantoux test
        PPD positive
        Tuberculin (skin test) positive
        Tuberculin (skin test) reactor
        EXCLUDES   nonspecific reaction to cell mediated immunity measurement of gamma interferon antigen response without active tuberculosis (795.52)
        AHA: 4Q, '11, 182
        TIP: Assign when documentation indicates "latent tuberculosis."

    795.52 Nonspecific reaction to cell mediated immunity measurement of gamma interferon antigen response without active tuberculosis
        Nonspecific reaction to QuantiFERON-TB test (QFT) without active tuberculosis
        EXCLUDES   nonspecific reaction to tuberculin skin test without active tuberculosis (795.51)
                positive tuberculin skin test (795.51)

795.6 False positive serological test for syphilis
False positive Wassermann reaction

√5ᵗʰ **795.7 Other nonspecific immunological findings**
    EXCLUDES   abnormal tumor markers (795.81-795.89)
            elevated prostate specific antigen [PSA] (790.93)
            elevated tumor associated antigens (795.81-795.89)
            isoimmunization, in pregnancy (656.1-656.2)
                affecting fetus or newborn (773.0-773.2)
    AHA: 2Q, '93, 6

    795.71 Nonspecific serologic evidence of human immunodeficiency virus [HIV]
        Inclusive human immunodeficiency [HIV] test (adult) (infant)
        NOTE This code is **only** to be used when a test finding is reported as nonspecific. Asymptomatic positive findings are coded to V08. If any HIV infection symptom or condition is present, see code 042. Negative findings are not coded.
        EXCLUDES   acquired immunodeficiency syndrome [AIDS] (042)
            asymptomatic human immunodeficiency virus, [HIV] infection status (V08)
            HIV infection, symptomatic (042)
            human immunodeficiency virus [HIV] disease (042)
            positive (status) NOS (V08)
        AHA: 2Q, '04, 11; 1Q, '93, 21; 1Q, '93, 22; 2Q, '92, 11; J-A, '87, 24

795.79 Other and unspecified nonspecific immunological findings
Raised antibody titer
Raised level of immunoglobulins
AHA: 4Q, '11, 93

√5ᵗʰ **795.8 Abnormal tumor markers**
Elevated tumor associated antigens [TAA]
Elevated tumor specific antigens [TSA]
EXCLUDES   elevated prostate specific antigen [PSA] (790.93)

    795.81 Elevated carcinoembryonic antigen [CEA]
        AHA: 4Q, '06, 111

    795.82 Elevated cancer antigen 125 [CA 125]   ♀
        AHA: 4Q, '06, 111

    795.89 Other abnormal tumor markers
        AHA: 4Q, '06, 111

√4ᵗʰ **796 Other nonspecific abnormal findings**

796.0 Nonspecific abnormal toxicological findings
Abnormal levels of heavy metals or drugs in blood, urine, or other tissue
Use additional code for retained foreign body, if applicable, (V90.01-V90.9)
EXCLUDES   excessive blood level of alcohol (790.3)
AHA: 1Q, '97, 16

796.1 Abnormal reflex

796.2 Elevated blood pressure reading without diagnosis of hypertension
    NOTE This category is to be used to record an episode of elevated blood pressure in a patient in whom no formal diagnosis of hypertension has been made, or as an incidental finding.
    AHA: 2Q, '03, 11; 3Q, '90, 4; J-A, '84, 12
    TIP: Assign an additional E code for poisoning or adverse effect of a drug if the documentation indicates it's the underlying cause of the elevated blood pressure.
    R03.0 Elevated blood-pressure reading without dx HTN   I-10

796.3 Nonspecific low blood pressure reading

796.4 Other abnormal clinical findings
AHA: 1Q, '97, 16

796.5 Abnormal finding on antenatal screening   ♀ Ⓜ
AHA: 4Q, '97, 46

796.6 Abnormal findings on neonatal screening   Ⓝ
EXCLUDES   nonspecific serologic evidence of human immunodeficiency virus [HIV] (795.71)
AHA: 4Q, '04, 99

√5ᵗʰ **796.7 Abnormal cytologic smear of anus and anal HPV**
    EXCLUDES   abnormal cytologic smear of cervix and cervical HPV (795.00-795.09)
            abnormal cytologic smear of vagina and vaginal HPV (795.10-795.19)
            anal intraepithelial neoplasia I (AIN I) (569.44)
            anal intraepithelial neoplasia II (AIN II) (569.44)
            anal intraepithelial neoplasia III (AIN III) (230.5, 230.6)
            carcinoma in situ of anus (230.5, 230.6)
            dysplasia (histologically confirmed) of anus NOS (569.44)
            mild anal dysplasia (histologically confirmed) (569.44)
            moderate anal dysplasia (histologically confirmed) (569.44)
            severe anal dysplasia (histologically confirmed) (230.5, 230.6)
    AHA: 4Q, '08, 117-119

    796.70 Abnormal glandular Papanicolaou smear of anus
        Atypical anal glandular cells NOS

    796.71 Papanicolaou smear of anus with atypical squamous cells of undetermined significance [ASC-US]

    796.72 Papanicolaou smear of anus with atypical squamous cells cannot exclude high grade squamous intraepithelial lesion [ASC-H]

    796.73 Papanicolaou smear of anus with low grade squamous intraepithelial lesion [LGSIL]

796.74 Papanicolaou smear of anus with high grade squamous intraepithelial lesion [HGSIL]

796.75 Anal high risk human papillomavirus [HPV] DNA test positive

796.76 Papanicolaou smear of anus with cytologic evidence of malignancy

796.77 Satisfactory anal smear but lacking transformation zone

796.78 Unsatisfactory anal cytology smear
Inadequate anal cytology sample

796.79 Other abnormal Papanicolaou smear of anus and anal HPV
Anal low risk human papillomavirus (HPV) DNA test positive
Use additional code for associated human papillomavirus (079.4)

796.9 Other

Ill-Defined and Unknown Causes of Morbidity and Mortality (797-799)

797 Senility without mention of psychosis
Frailty
Old age
Senescence
Senile asthenia
Senile:
  debility
  exhaustion
EXCLUDES *senile psychoses (290.0-290.9)*

√4ᵗʰ 798 Sudden death, cause unknown

798.0 Sudden infant death syndrome ▣P
Cot death
Crib death
Sudden death of nonspecific cause in infancy
DEF: Death of infant under age one due to nonspecific cause.

798.1 Instantaneous death

798.2 Death occurring in less than 24 hours from onset of symptoms, not otherwise explained
Death known not to be violent or instantaneous, for which no cause could be discovered
Died without sign of disease

798.9 Unattended death
Death in circumstances where the body of the deceased was found and no cause could be discovered
Found dead

√4ᵗʰ 799 Other ill-defined and unknown causes of morbidity and mortality

√5ᵗʰ 799.0 Asphyxia and hypoxemia
EXCLUDES *asphyxia and hypoxemia (due to):*
  carbon monoxide (986)
  hypercapnia (786.09)
  inhalation of food or foreign body (932-934.9)
  newborn (768.0-768.9)
  traumatic (994.7)

799.01 Asphyxia ▣CC
DEF: Lack of oxygen in inspired air, causing a deficiency of oxygen in tissues (hypoxia) and elevated levels of arterial carbon dioxide (hypercapnia).
CC Exd: 338.0-338.4, 518.81-518.84, 780.64-780.65, 780.91-780.99, 798.0, 799.01-799.1, 799.81-799.89
AHA: 4Q, '05, 90

799.02 Hypoxemia
DEF: Deficient oxygenation of the blood.
AHA: 3Q, '09, 20; 2Q, '06, 24, 25; 4Q, '05, 90
TIP: Hypoxia is not inherent in COPD (496) and may be assigned in addition, if applicable.
R09.02 Hypoxemia ▣I-10

---

¹ 799.1 Respiratory arrest ▣MCC
Cardiorespiratory failure
EXCLUDES *cardiac arrest (427.5)*
  failure of peripheral circulation (785.50)
  respiratory distress:
    NOS (786.09)
    acute (518.82)
    following trauma and surgery (518.52)
    newborn (770.89)
    syndrome (newborn) (769)
      adult (following trauma and surgery) (518.52)
    other (518.82)
  respiratory failure (518.81, 518.83-518.84)
    newborn (770.84)
  respiratory insufficiency (786.09)
    acute (518.82)
CC Exd: See code: 799.01

√5ᵗʰ 799.2 Signs and symptoms involving emotional state
EXCLUDES *anxiety (293.84, 300.00-300.09)*
  depression (311)
AHA: 4Q, '09,107
TIP: If associated with underlying history of traumatic brain injury (TBI), assign in addition to a code for the late effect of TBI (e.g., 905.0 or 907.0).

799.21 Nervousness
Nervous
AHA: 4Q, '09, 108

799.22 Irritability
Irritable
AHA: 4Q, '09, 108

799.23 Impulsiveness
Impulsive
EXCLUDES *impulsive neurosis (300.3)*

799.24 Emotional lability

799.25 Demoralization and apathy
Apathetic

799.29 Other signs and symptoms involving emotional state

799.3 Debility, unspecified
EXCLUDES *asthenia (780.79)*
  nervous debility (300.5)
  neurasthenia (300.5)
  senile asthenia (797)

799.4 Cachexia ▣C
Wasting disease
Code first underlying condition, if known
DEF: General ill health and poor nutrition.
CC Exd: 338.0-338.4, 780.64-780.65, 780.91-780.99, 799.3-799.4, 799.81-799.89
AHA: 3Q, '06, 14, 15; 3Q, '90, 17
TIP: Assign an additional code for any associated malnutrition, if documented.
R64 Cachexia ▣I-1

√5ᵗʰ 799.5 Signs and symptoms involving cognition
EXCLUDES *amnesia (780.93)*
  amnestic syndrome (294.0)
  attention deficit disorder (314.00-314.01)
  late effects of cerebrovascular disease (438.0)
  memory loss (780.93)
  mild cognitive impairment, so stated (331.83)
  specific problems in developmental delay (315.00-315.9)
  transient global amnesia (437.7)
  visuospatial neglect (781.8)
AHA: ▶3Q, '12, 19-20;◀4Q, '10, 95-96
TIP: ▶Report as additional diagnoses not integral to a known condition to describe the nature or type of deficit due to unknown o unrelated cause.◀

799.51 Attention or concentration deficit
AHA: ▶3Q, '12, 20◀

799.52 Cognitive communication deficit
AHA: ▶3Q, '12, 19-21◀

799.53 Visuospatial deficit

---

¹ MCC = Only if patient discharged alive.

▣N Newborn Age: 0   ▣P Pediatric Age: 0-17   ▣M Maternity Age: 12-55   ▣A Adult Age: 15-124   ▣MCC Major CC Condition   ▣CC CC Condition   ▣HIV HIV Related D

296 – Volume 1 · February 2013   2014 ICD-9-C

799.54 Psychomotor deficit
AHA: 4Q, '10, 95-97

799.55 Frontal lobe and executive function deficit
AHA: ▶3Q, '12, 20◀

799.59 Other signs and symptoms involving cognition

√5ᵗʰ **799.8 Other ill-defined conditions**

799.81 Decreased libido   A
Decreased sexual desire
EXCLUDES *psychosexual dysfunction with inhibited sexual desire (302.71)*
AHA: 4Q, '03, 75

799.82 Apparent life threatening event in infant   P
ALTE
Apparent life threatening event in newborn and infant
Code first confirmed diagnosis, if known
Use additional code(s) for associated signs and symptoms if no confirmed diagnosis established, or if signs and symptoms are not associated routinely with confirmed diagnosis, or provide additional information for cause of ALTE
AHA: 4Q, '10, 97-98; 4Q, '09, 109

799.89 Other ill-defined conditions

799.9 Other unknown and unspecified cause
Undiagnosed disease, not specified as to site or system involved
Unknown cause of morbidity or mortality
AHA: 1Q, '98,.4; 1Q, '90, 20

Additional Digit Required   Unacceptable PDx   Manifestation Code   Hospital Acquired Condition   ▶◀ Revised Text   ● New Code   ▲ Revised Code Title

2014 ICD-9-CM   **February 2013 • Volume 1 – 297**

17. Injury and Poisoning (800-999)

Use E code(s) to identify the cause and intent of the injury or poisoning (E800-E999)

Use additional code for retained foreign body, if applicable, (V90.01-V90.9)

NOTE

1. The principle of multiple coding of injuries should be followed wherever possible. Combination categories for multiple injuries are provided for use when there is insufficient detail as to the nature of the individual conditions, or for primary tabulation purposes when it is more convenient to record a single code; otherwise, the component injuries should be coded separately.

   Where multiple sites of injury are specified in the titles, the word "with" indicates involvement of both sites, and the word "and" indicates involvement of either or both sites. The word "finger" includes thumb.

2. Categories for "late effect" of injuries are to be found at 905-909.

Fractures (800-829)

EXCLUDES malunion (733.81)
nonunion (733.82)
pathological or spontaneous fracture (733.10-733.19)
stress fractures (733.93-733.95)

NOTE The terms "condyle," "coronoid process," "ramus," and "symphysis" indicate the portion of the bone fractured, not the name of the bone involved.

The descriptions "closed" and "open" used in the fourth-digit subdivisions include the following terms:

closed (with or without delayed healing):
comminuted	impacted
depressed	linear
elevated	simple
fissured	slipped epiphysis
fracture NOS	spiral
greenstick	

open (with or without delayed healing):
compound	puncture
infected	with foreign body
missile	

A fracture not indicated as closed or open should be classified as closed.

AHA: 4Q, '08, 158;1Q, '07, 3-4; 4Q, '90, 26; 3Q, '90, 5; 3Q, '90, 13; 2Q, '90, 7; 2Q, '89, 15, S-O, '85, 3

TIP: Assign the acute fracture codes only while the patient is receiving active treatment for the fracture, such as during surgical care, an ED encounter, or evaluation and treatment by a new physician. Otherwise, refer to aftercare category V54.

Fracture of Skull (800-804)

INCLUDES traumatic brain injury due to fracture of skull

The following fifth-digit subclassification is for use with the appropriate codes in category 800, 801, 803, and 804:

0 unspecified state of consciousness
1 with no loss of consciousness
2 with brief [less than one hour] loss of consciousness
3 with moderate [1-24 hours] loss of consciousness
4 with prolonged [more than 24 hours] loss of consciousness and return to pre-existing conscious level
5 with prolonged [more than 24 hours] loss of consciousness, without return to pre-existing conscious level
  Use fifth-digit 5 to designate when a patient is unconscious and dies before regaining consciousness, regardless of the duration of the loss of consciousness
6 with loss of consciousness of unspecified duration
9 with concussion, unspecified

✓4ᵗʰ **800** **Fracture of vault of skull**

INCLUDES frontal bone
parietal bone

DEF: Fracture of bone that forms skull dome and protects brain.
AHA: 4Q, '96, 36

§ ✓5ᵗʰ **800.0** **Closed without mention of intracranial** `CC 0-2, 6, 9` `MCC 3-5`
[0-6, 9] **injury**
CC Excl: 800.00-801.99, 803.00-804.99, 829.0-829.1, 850.0-852.19, 852.21-854.19, 873.8-873.9, 879.8-879.9, 905.0, 925.1-925.2, 929.0-929.9, 958.8-959.9

Fractures

§ ✓5ᵗʰ **800.1** **Closed with cerebral laceration and contusion** `MCC`
[0-6, 9] **CC Excl:** See code 800.0

§ ✓5ᵗʰ **800.2** **Closed with subarachnoid, subdural, and** `MCC`
[0-6, 9] **extradural hemorrhage**
CC Excl: See code 800.0

§ ✓5ᵗʰ **800.3** **Closed with other and unspecified** `MCC`
[0-6, 9] **intracranial hemorrhage**
CC Excl: See code 800.0

§ ✓5ᵗʰ **800.4** **Closed with intracranial injury of other** `CC 0-2, 6, 9` `MCC 3-5`
[0-6, 9] **and unspecified nature**
CC Excl: See code 800.0

§ ✓5ᵗʰ **800.5** **Open without mention of intracranial injury** `MCC`
[0-6, 9] **CC Excl:** See code 800.0

§ ✓5ᵗʰ **800.6** **Open with cerebral laceration and contusion** `MCC`
[0-6, 9] **CC Excl:** See code 800.0

§ ✓5ᵗʰ **800.7** **Open with subarachnoid, subdural, and** `MCC`
[0-6, 9] **extradural hemorrhage**
CC Excl: See code 800.0

§ ✓5ᵗʰ **800.8** **Open with other and unspecified intracranial** `MCC`
[0-6, 9] **hemorrhage**
CC Excl: See code 800.0

§ ✓5ᵗʰ **800.9** **Open with intracranial injury of other and** `MCC`
[0-6, 9] **unspecified nature**
CC Excl: See code 800.0

✓4ᵗʰ **801** **Fracture of base of skull**

INCLUDES fossa:
anterior
middle
posterior
occiput bone
orbital roof
sinus:
ethmoid
frontal
sphenoid bone
temporal bone

DEF: Fracture of bone that forms skull floor.
AHA: 4Q, '96, 36

§ ✓5ᵗʰ **801.0** **Closed without mention of intracranial** `CC 0-2, 6, 9` `MCC 3-5`
[0-6, 9] **injury**
CC Excl: 800.00-801.99, 803.00-804.99, 829.0-829.1, 850.0-852.19, 852.21-854.19, 873.8-873.9, 879.8-879.9, 905.0, 925.1-925.2, 929.0-929.9, 958.8-959.9

§ ✓5ᵗʰ **801.1** **Closed with cerebral laceration and contusion** `MCC`
[0-6, 9] **CC Excl:** See code: 801.0
AHA: 4Q, '96, 36

§ ✓5ᵗʰ **801.2** **Closed with subarachnoid, subdural, and** `MCC`
[0-6, 9] **extradural hemorrhage**
CC Excl: See code: 801.0

§ ✓5ᵗʰ **801.3** **Closed with other and unspecified** `MCC`
[0-6, 9] **intracranial hemorrhage**
CC Excl: See code: 801.0

§ ✓5ᵗʰ **801.4** **Closed with intracranial injury of other** `CC 0-2, 6, 9` `MCC 3-5`
[0-6, 9] **and unspecified nature**
CC Excl: See code 801.0

Requires fifth digit. Valid digits are in [brackets] under each code. See beginning of section 800-804 for codes and definitions.

Additional Digit Required   Unacceptable PDx   Manifestation Code   Hospital Acquired Condition   ▶◀ Revised Text   ● New Code   ▲ Revised Code Title

014 ICD-9-CM   **Volume 1 – 299**

Injury and Poisoning

801.5–803.0

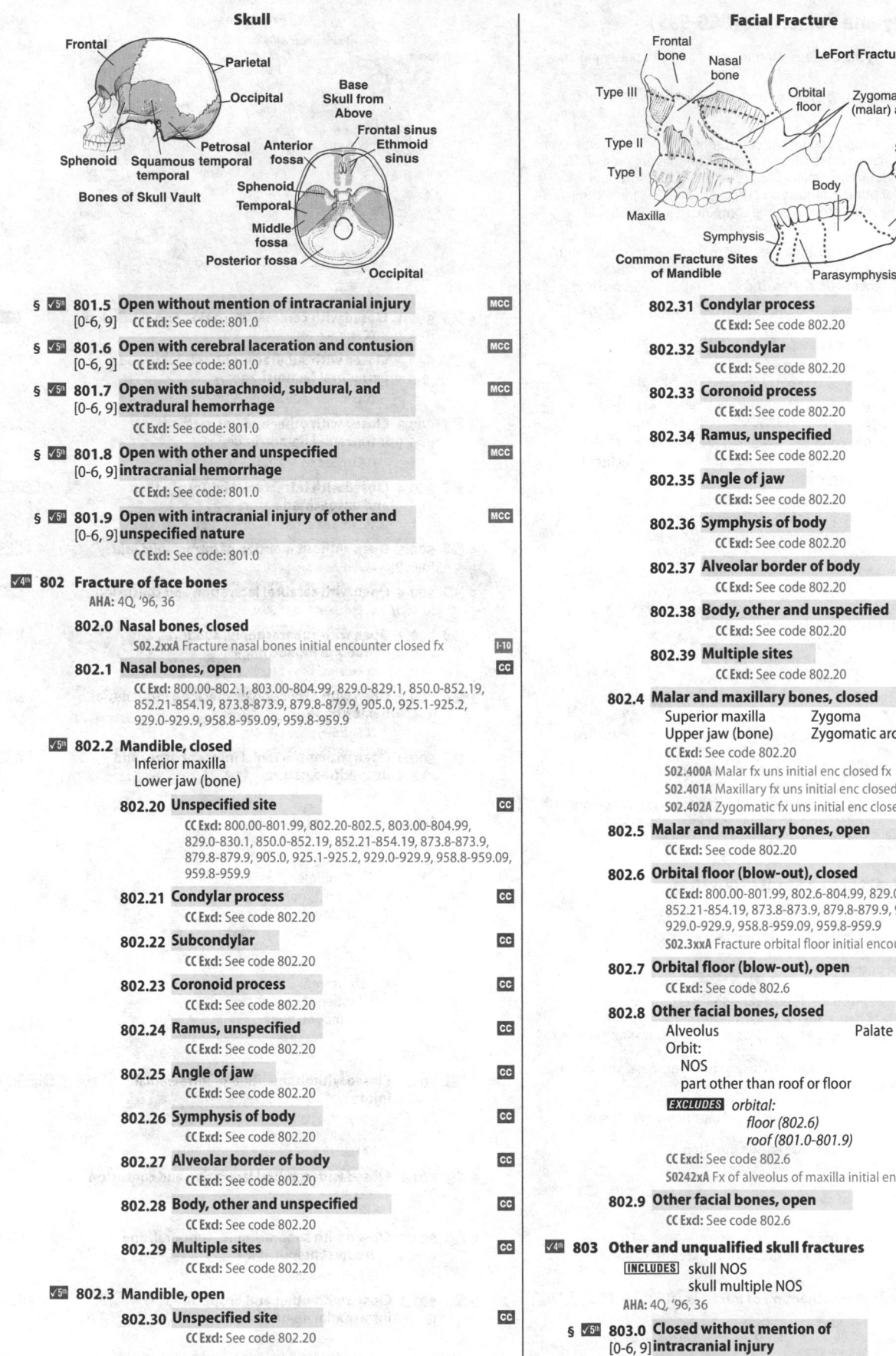

Skull

Facial Fracture

§ ✔5ᵗʰ **801.5 Open without mention of intracranial injury** `MCC`
[0-6, 9] CC Excl: See code: 801.0

§ ✔5ᵗʰ **801.6 Open with cerebral laceration and contusion** `MCC`
[0-6, 9] CC Excl: See code: 801.0

§ ✔5ᵗʰ **801.7 Open with subarachnoid, subdural, and** `MCC`
[0-6, 9] **extradural hemorrhage**
CC Excl: See code: 801.0

§ ✔5ᵗʰ **801.8 Open with other and unspecified** `MCC`
[0-6, 9] **intracranial hemorrhage**
CC Excl: See code: 801.0

§ ✔5ᵗʰ **801.9 Open with intracranial injury of other and** `MCC`
[0-6, 9] **unspecified nature**
CC Excl: See code: 801.0

✔4ᵗʰ **802 Fracture of face bones**
AHA: 4Q, '96, 36

802.0 Nasal bones, closed
S02.2xxA Fracture nasal bones initial encounter closed fx `I-10`

802.1 Nasal bones, open `CC`
CC Excl: 800.00-802.1, 803.00-804.99, 829.0-829.1, 850.0-852.19, 852.21-854.19, 873.8-873.9, 879.8-879.9, 905.0, 925.1-925.2, 929.0-929.9, 958.8-959.09, 959.8-959.9

✔5ᵗʰ **802.2 Mandible, closed**
Inferior maxilla
Lower jaw (bone)

802.20 Unspecified site `CC`
CC Excl: 800.00-801.99, 802.20-802.5, 803.00-804.99, 829.0-830.1, 850.0-852.19, 852.21-854.19, 873.8-873.9, 879.8-879.9, 905.0, 925.1-925.2, 929.0-929.9, 958.8-959.09, 959.8-959.9

802.21 Condylar process `CC`
CC Excl: See code 802.20

802.22 Subcondylar `CC`
CC Excl: See code 802.20

802.23 Coronoid process `CC`
CC Excl: See code 802.20

802.24 Ramus, unspecified `CC`
CC Excl: See code 802.20

802.25 Angle of jaw `CC`
CC Excl: See code 802.20

802.26 Symphysis of body `CC`
CC Excl: See code 802.20

802.27 Alveolar border of body `CC`
CC Excl: See code 802.20

802.28 Body, other and unspecified `CC`
CC Excl: See code 802.20

802.29 Multiple sites `CC`
CC Excl: See code 802.20

✔5ᵗʰ **802.3 Mandible, open**

802.30 Unspecified site `CC`
CC Excl: See code 802.20

802.31 Condylar process `CC`
CC Excl: See code 802.20

802.32 Subcondylar `CC`
CC Excl: See code 802.20

802.33 Coronoid process `CC`
CC Excl: See code 802.20

802.34 Ramus, unspecified `CC`
CC Excl: See code 802.20

802.35 Angle of jaw `CC`
CC Excl: See code 802.20

802.36 Symphysis of body `CC`
CC Excl: See code 802.20

802.37 Alveolar border of body `CC`
CC Excl: See code 802.20

802.38 Body, other and unspecified `CC`
CC Excl: See code 802.20

802.39 Multiple sites `CC`
CC Excl: See code 802.20

802.4 Malar and maxillary bones, closed `CC`
Superior maxilla   Zygoma
Upper jaw (bone)   Zygomatic arch
CC Excl: See code 802.20
S02.400A Malar fx uns initial enc closed fx `I-10`
S02.401A Maxillary fx uns initial enc closed fx `I-10`
S02.402A Zygomatic fx uns initial enc closed fx `I-10`

802.5 Malar and maxillary bones, open `CC`
CC Excl: See code 802.20

802.6 Orbital floor (blow-out), closed `CC`
CC Excl: 800.00-801.99, 802.6-804.99, 829.0-829.1, 850.0-852.19, 852.21-854.19, 873.8-873.9, 879.8-879.9, 905.0, 925.1-925.2, 929.0-929.9, 958.8-959.09, 959.8-959.9
S02.3xxA Fracture orbital floor initial encounter clos fx `I-10`

802.7 Orbital floor (blow-out), open `CC`
CC Excl: See code 802.6

802.8 Other facial bones, closed `CC`
Alveolus   Palate
Orbit:
   NOS
   part other than roof or floor
   `EXCLUDES` orbital:
      floor (802.6)
      roof (801.0-801.9)
CC Excl: See code 802.6
S0242xA Fx of alveolus of maxilla initial enc closed fx `I-10`

802.9 Other facial bones, open `CC`
CC Excl: See code 802.6

✔4ᵗʰ **803 Other and unqualified skull fractures**
`INCLUDES` skull NOS
skull multiple NOS
AHA: 4Q, '96, 36

§ ✔5ᵗʰ **803.0 Closed without mention of** `MCC 3-5` `CC 0-2, 6, 9`
[0-6, 9] **intracranial injury**
CC Excl: 800.00-801.99, 803.00-804.99, 829.0-829.1, 850.0-852.19, 852.21-854.19, 873.8-873.9, 879.8-879.9, 905.0, 925.1-925.2, 929.0-929.9, 958.8-959.09, 959.8-959.9

§ Requires fifth digit. Valid digits are in [brackets] under each code. See beginning of section 800-804 for codes and definitions.

N Newborn Age: 0   P Pediatric Age: 0-17   M Maternity Age: 12-55   A Adult Age: 15-124   `MCC` Major CC Condition   `CC` CC Condition   HIV HIV Related Dx

Vertebral Column

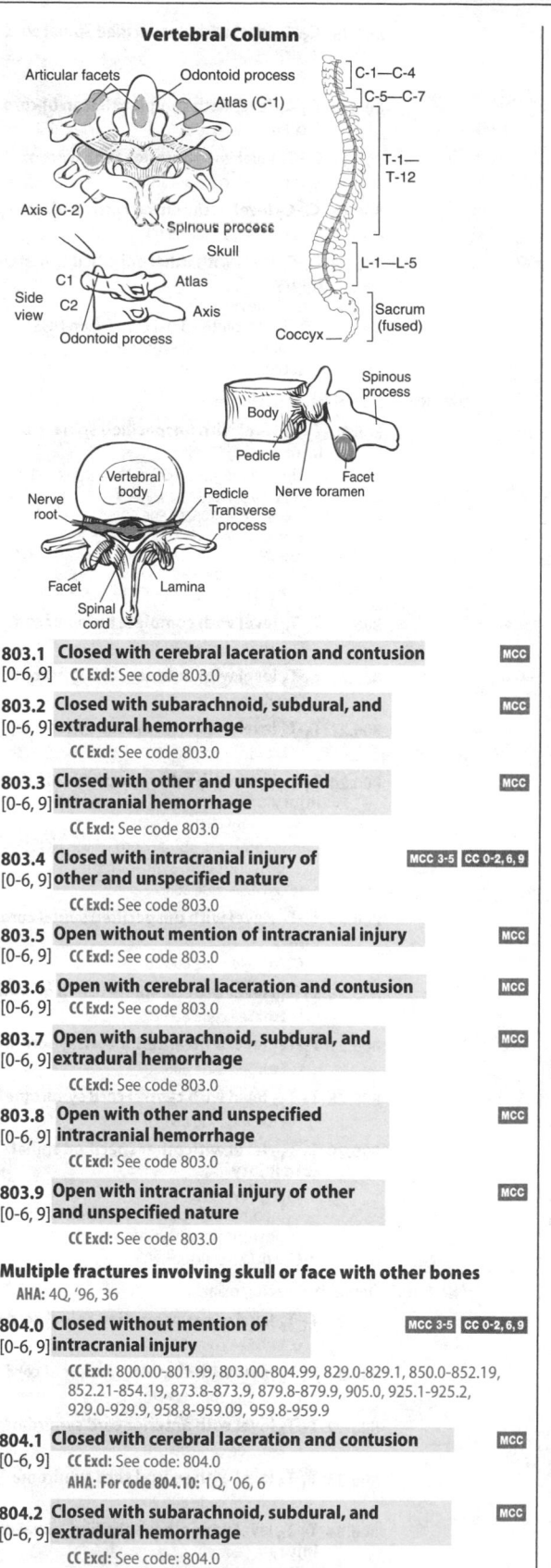

§ ✓5th **803.1 Closed with cerebral laceration and contusion**   MCC
[0-6, 9]   CC Exd: See code 803.0

§ ✓5th **803.2 Closed with subarachnoid, subdural, and**   MCC
[0-6, 9] **extradural hemorrhage**
    CC Exd: See code 803.0

§ ✓5th **803.3 Closed with other and unspecified**   MCC
[0-6, 9] **intracranial hemorrhage**
    CC Exd: See code 803.0

§ ✓5th **803.4 Closed with intracranial injury of**   MCC 3-5   CC 0-2, 6, 9
[0-6, 9] **other and unspecified nature**
    CC Exd: See code 803.0

§ ✓5th **803.5 Open without mention of intracranial injury**   MCC
[0-6, 9]   CC Exd: See code 803.0

§ ✓5th **803.6 Open with cerebral laceration and contusion**   MCC
[0-6, 9]   CC Exd: See code 803.0

§ ✓5th **803.7 Open with subarachnoid, subdural, and**   MCC
[0-6, 9] **extradural hemorrhage**
    CC Exd: See code 803.0

§ ✓5th **803.8 Open with other and unspecified**   MCC
[0-6, 9] **intracranial hemorrhage**
    CC Exd: See code 803.0

§ ✓5th **803.9 Open with intracranial injury of other**   MCC
[0-6, 9] **and unspecified nature**
    CC Exd: See code 803.0

✓4th **804 Multiple fractures involving skull or face with other bones**
    AHA: 4Q, '96, 36

§ ✓5th **804.0 Closed without mention of**   MCC 3-5   CC 0-2, 6, 9
[0-6, 9] **intracranial injury**
    CC Exd: 800.00-801.99, 803.00-804.99, 829.0-829.1, 850.0-852.19,
    852.21-854.19, 873.8-873.9, 879.8-879.9, 905.0, 925.1-925.2,
    929.0-929.9, 958.8-959.9, 959.9

§ ✓5th **804.1 Closed with cerebral laceration and contusion**   MCC
[0-6, 9]   CC Exd: See code 804.0
    AHA: For code 804.10: 1Q, '06, 6

§ ✓5th **804.2 Closed with subarachnoid, subdural, and**   MCC
[0-6, 9] **extradural hemorrhage**
    CC Exd: See code 804.0

§ ✓5th **804.3 Closed with other and unspecified intracranial**   MCC
[0-6, 9] **hemorrhage**
    CC Exd: See code 804.0

§ ✓5th **804.4 Closed with intracranial injury of other**   MCC 3-5   CC 0-2, 6, 9
[0-6, 9] **and unspecified nature**
    CC Exd: See code: 804.0

§ ✓5th **804.5 Open without mention of intracranial**   MCC 3-5   CC 0-2, 6, 9
[0-6, 9] **injury**
    CC Exd: See code: 804.0

§ ✓5th **804.6 Open with cerebral laceration and contusion**   MCC
[0-6, 9]   CC Exd: See code: 804.0

§ ✓5th **804.7 Open with subarachnoid, subdural, and**   MCC
[0-6, 9] **extradural hemorrage**
    CC Exd: See code: 804.0

§ ✓5th **804.8 Open with other and unspecified intracranial**   MCC
[0-6, 9] **hemorrhage**
    CC Exd: See code: 804.0

§ ✓5th **804.9 Open with intracranial injury of other**   MCC 3-5   CC 0-2, 6, 9
[0-6, 9] **and unspecified nature**
    CC Exd: See code: 804.0

Fracture of Neck and Trunk (805-809)

✓4th **805 Fracture of vertebral column without mention of spinal cord injury**

    INCLUDES   neural arch
                 spine
                 spinous process
                 transverse process
                 vertebra

The following fifth-digit subclassification is for use with codes 805.0-805.1:
    0 cervical vertebra, unspecified level
    1 first cervical vertebra
    2 second cervical vertebra
    3 third cervical vertebra
    4 fourth cervical vertebra
    5 fifth cervical vertebra
    6 sixth cervical vertebra
    7 seventh cervical vertebra
    8 multiple cervical vertebrae

§ ✓5th **805.0 Cervical, closed**   CC
[0-8]   Atlas
      Axis
    CC Exd: 805.00-805.18, 805.8-806.19, 806.8-806.9, 829.0-829.1,
    839.00-839.18, 839.40, 839.49-839.50, 839.59, 839.69, 839.79-839.9,
    847.0, 847.9, 848.8-848.9, 879.8-879.9, 905.1, 926.11, 929.0-929.9,
    952.00-952.09, 952.8-952.9, 958.8-958.99, 959.11-959.19,
    959.8-959.9
    S12.101A Uns nondisplcd fx 2nd cerv vert initial enc clos   I-10

§ ✓5th **805.1 Cervical, open**   MCC
[0-8]   CC Exd: See code 805.0

805.2 Dorsal [thoracic], closed   CC
    CC Exd: 805.2-805.3, 805.8-805.9, 806.20-806.39, 806.8-806.9,
    829.0-829.1, 839.21, 839.31-839.40, 839.49-839.50, 839.59, 839.69,
    839.79-839.9, 847.1, 847.9, 848.8-848.9, 879.8-879.9, 905.1, 926.11,
    929.0-929.9, 952.10-952.19, 952.8-952.9, 958.8-958.99,
    959.11-959.19, 959.8-959.9
    S22.008A Oth fx uns thoracic vertebra initial enc clos fx   I-10

805.3 Dorsal [thoracic], open   MCC
    CC Exd: See code 805.2

805.4 Lumbar, closed   CC
    CC Exd: 805.4-805.5, 805.8-805.9, 806.4-806.5, 806.8-806.9,
    829.0-829.1, 839.20, 839.30, 839.40, 839.49-839.50, 839.59, 839.69,
    839.79-839.9, 847.2, 847.9, 848.8-848.9, 879.8-879.9, 905.1, 926.11,
    929.0-929.9, 952.2, 952.8-952.9, 958.8-958.99, 959.11-959.19,
    959.8-959.9
    AHA: 1Q, '07, 7; 4Q, '99, 12
    S32.008A Oth fx uns lumbar vertebra initial enc closed fx   I-10

805.5 Lumbar, open   MCC
    CC Exd: See code 805.4

805.6 Sacrum and coccyx, closed   CC
    CC Exd: 805.6-805.9, 806.60-806.9, 829.0-829.1, 839.40-839.59,
    839.69, 839.79-839.9, 846.0-846.9, 847.3-847.9, 848.5-848.9,
    879.8-879.9, 905.1, 926.11, 929.0-929.9, 952.3-952.9, 958.8-958.99,
    959.11-959.19, 959.8-959.9
    S32.19xA Other fx of sacrum initial encounter closed fx   I-10

Requires fifth digit. Valid digits are in [brackets] under each code. See appropriate category for codes and definitions.

§ Additional Digit Required	Unacceptable PDx	Manifestation Code	Hospital Acquired Condition	▶◀ Revised Text	● New Code	▲ Revised Code Title

Injury and Poisoning

805.7–806.35

805.7 **Sacrum and coccyx, open**   `MCC`
CC Excl: See code 805.6

805.8 **Unspecified, closed**   `CC`
CC Excl: 733.10-733.19, 733.93-733.98, 805.00-806.9, 829.0-829.1,
839.00-839.59, 839.69, 839.79-839.9, 846.0-847.9, 848.5-848.9,
879.8-879.9, 905.1, 926.11, 929.0-929.9, 952.00-952.9, 958.8-958.99,
959.11-959.19, 959.8-959.9

805.9 **Unspecified, open**   `MCC`
CC Excl: See code 805.8

✓4th **806** **Fracture of vertebral column with spinal cord injury**
`INCLUDES` any condition classifiable to 805 with:
complete or incomplete transverse lesion (of cord)
hematomyelia
injury to:
    cauda equina
    nerve
paralysis
paraplegia
quadriplegia
spinal concussion

✓5th **806.0** **Cervical, closed**

806.00 **C_1-C_4 level with unspecified spinal cord injury**   `MCC`
Cervical region NOS with spinal cord injury NOS
CC Excl: 733.10-733.19, 733.93-733.98, 805.00-805.18,
805.8-806.19, 806.8-806.9, 829.0-829.1, 839.00-839.18,
839.40, 839.49-839.50, 839.59, 839.69, 839.79-839.9, 847.9,
848.8-848.9, 879.8-879.9, 905.1, 926.11, 929.0-929.9,
952.00-952.09, 952.8-952.9, 958.8-958.99, 959.11-959.19,
959.8-959.9

806.01 **C_1-C_4 level with complete lesion of cord**   `MCC`
CC Excl: See code 806.00

806.02 **C_1-C_4 level with anterior cord syndrome**   `MCC`
CC Excl: See code 806.00

806.03 **C_1-C_4 level with central cord syndrome**   `MCC`
CC Excl: See code 806.00

806.04 **C_1-C_4 level with other specified spinal cord injury**   `MCC`
C_1-C_4 level with:
    incomplete spinal cord lesion NOS
    posterior cord syndrome
CC Excl: See code 806.00

806.05 **C_5-C_7 level with unspecified spinal cord injury**   `MCC`
CC Excl: See code 806.00

806.06 **C_5-C_7 level with complete lesion of cord**   `MCC`
CC Excl: See code 806.00

806.07 **C_5-C_7 level with anterior cord syndrome**   `MCC`
CC Excl: See code 806.00

806.08 **C_5-C_7 level with central cord syndrome**   `MCC`
CC Excl: See code 806.00

806.09 **C_5-C_7 level with other specified spinal cord injury**   `MCC`
C_5-C_7 level with:
    incomplete spinal cord lesion NOS
    posterior cord syndrome
CC Excl: See code 806.00

✓5th **806.1** **Cervical, open**

806.10 **C_1-C_4 level with unspecified spinal cord injury**   `MCC`
CC Excl: See code 806.00

806.11 **C_1-C_4 level with complete lesion of cord**   `MCC`
CC Excl: See code 806.00

806.12 **C_1-C_4 level with anterior cord syndrome**   `MCC`
CC Excl: See code 806.00

806.13 **C_1-C_4 level with central cord syndrome**   `MCC`
CC Excl: See code 806.00

806.14 **C_1-C_4 level with other specified spinal cord injury**   `MCC`
C_1-C_4 level with:
    incomplete spinal cord lesion NOS
    posterior cord syndrome
CC Excl: See code 806.00

806.15 **C_5-C_7 level with unspecified spinal cord injury**   `MCC`
CC Excl: See code 806.00

806.16 **C_5-C_7 level with complete lesion of cord**   `MCC`
CC Excl: See code 806.00

806.17 **C_5-C_7 level with anterior cord syndrome**   `MCC`
CC Excl: See code 806.00

806.18 **C_5-C_7 level with central cord syndrome**   `MCC`
CC Excl: See code 806.00

806.19 **C_5-C_7 level with other specified spinal cord injury**   `MCC`
C_5-C_7 level with:
    incomplete spinal cord lesion NOS
    posterior cord syndrome
CC Excl: See code 806.00

✓5th **806.2** **Dorsal [thoracic], closed**

806.20 **T_1-T_6 level with unspecified spinal cord injury**   `MCC`
Thoracic region NOS with spinal cord injury NOS
CC Excl: 733.10-733.19, 733.93-733.98, 805.2-805.3,
805.8-805.9, 806.20-806.39, 806.8-806.9, 829.0-829.1,
839.21, 839.31-839.40, 839.49-839.50, 839.59, 839.69,
839.79-839.9, 847.1, 847.9, 848.8-848.9, 879.8-879.9, 905.1,
926.11, 929.0-929.9, 952.10-952.19, 952.8-952.9,
958.8-958.99, 959.11-959.19, 959.8-959.9

806.21 **T_1-T_6 level with complete lesion of cord**   `MCC`
CC Excl: See code 806.20

806.22 **T_1-T_6 level with anterior cord syndrome**   `MCC`
CC Excl: See code 806.20

806.23 **T_1-T_6 level with central cord syndrome**   `MCC`
CC Excl: See code 806.20

806.24 **T_1-T_6 level with other specified spinal cord injury**   `MCC`
T_1-T_6 level with:
    incomplete spinal cord lesion NOS
    posterior cord syndrome
CC Excl: See code 806.20

806.25 **T_7-T_{12} level with unspecified spinal cord injury**   `MCC`
CC Excl: See code 806.20

806.26 **T_7-T_{12} level with complete lesion of cord**   `MCC`
CC Excl: See code 806.20

806.27 **T_7-T_{12} level with anterior cord syndrome**   `MCC`
CC Excl: See code 806.20

806.28 **T_7-T_{12} level with central cord syndrome**   `MCC`
CC Excl: See code 806.20

806.29 **T_7-T_{12} level with other specified spinal cord injury**   `MCC`
T_7-T_{12} level with:
    incomplete spinal cord lesion NOS
    posterior cord syndrome
CC Excl: See code 806.20

✓5th **806.3** **Dorsal [thoracic], open**

806.30 **T_1-T_6 level with unspecified spinal cord injury**   `MCC`
CC Excl: See code 806.20

806.31 **T_1-T_6 level with complete lesion of cord**   `MCC`
CC Excl: See code 806.20

806.32 **T_1-T_6 level with anterior cord syndrome**   `MCC`
CC Excl: See code 806.20

806.33 **T_1-T_6 level with central cord syndrome**   `MCC`
CC Excl: See code 806.20

806.34 **T_1-T_6 level with other specified spinal cord injury**   `MCC`
T_1-T_6 level with:
    incomplete spinal cord lesion NOS
    posterior cord syndrome
CC Excl: See code 806.20

806.35 **T_7-T_{12} level with unspecified spinal cord injury**   `MCC`
CC Excl: See code 806.20

`N` Newborn Age: 0   `P` Pediatric Age: 0-17   `M` Maternity Age: 12-55   `A` Adult Age: 15-124   `MCC` Major CC Condition   `CC` CC Condition   `HIV` HIV Related D

302 – Volume 1   2014 ICD-9-C

806.36 T$_7$-T$_{12}$ level with complete lesion of cord `MCC`
CC Excl: See code 806.20

806.37 T$_7$-T$_{12}$ level with anterior cord syndrome `MCC`
CC Excl: See code 806.20

806.38 T$_7$-T$_{12}$ level with central cord syndrome `MCC`
CC Excl: See code 806.20

806.39 T$_7$-T$_{12}$ level with other specified spinal cord injury `MCC`
T$_7$-T$_{12}$ level with:
incomplete spinal cord lesion NOS
posterior cord syndrome
CC Excl: See code 806.20

806.4 **Lumbar, closed** `MCC`
CC Excl: 733.10-733.19, 733.93-733.98, 805.4-805.5, 805.8-805.9, 806.4-806.5, 806.8-806.9, 829.0-829.1, 839.20, 839.30, 839.40, 839.49-839.50, 839.59, 839.69, 839.79-839.9, 847.2, 847.9, 848.8-848.9, 879.8-879.9, 905.1, 926.11, 929.0-929.9, 952.2, 952.8-952.9, 958.8-958.99, 959.11-959.19, 959.8-959.9
AHA: 4Q, '99, 11, 13

806.5 **Lumbar, open** `MCC`
CC Excl: See code 806.4

√5ᵗʰ 806.6 **Sacrum and coccyx, closed**

806.60 **With unspecified spinal cord injury** `MCC`
CC Excl: 733.10-733.19, 733.93-733.98, 805.6-805.9, 806.60-806.9, 829.0-829.1, 839.40-839.59, 839.69, 839.79-839.9, 846.0-847.0, 847.3-847.9, 848.5-848.9, 879.8-879.9, 905.1, 926.11, 929.0-929.9, 952.3-952.9, 958.8-958.99, 959.11-959.19, 959.8-959.9

806.61 **With complete cauda equina lesion** `MCC`
CC Excl: See code 806.60

806.62 **With other cauda equina injury** `MCC`
CC Excl: See code 806.60

806.69 **With other spinal cord injury** `MCC`
CC Excl: See code 806.60

√5ᵗʰ 806.7 **Sacrum and coccyx, open**

806.70 **With unspecified spinal cord injury** `MCC`
CC Excl: See code 806.60

806.71 **With complete cauda equina lesion** `MCC`
CC Excl: See code 806.60

806.72 **With other cauda equina injury** `MCC`
CC Excl: See code 806.60

806.79 **With other spinal cord injury** `MCC`
CC Excl: See code 806.60

806.8 **Unspecified, closed** `MCC`
CC Excl: 733.10-733.19, 733.93-733.95, 805.00-806.9, 829.0-829.1, 839.00-839.59, 839.69, 839.79-839.9, 846.0-847.9, 848.5-848.9, 879.8-879.9, 905.1, 926.11, 929.0-929.9, 952.00-952.9, 958.8-958.99, 959.11-959.19, 959.8-959.9

806.9 **Unspecified, open** `MCC`
CC Excl: See code 806.

Ribs, Sternum, Larynx, and Trachea

√4ᵗʰ **807 Fracture of rib(s), sternum, larynx, and trachea**
The following fifth-digit subclassification is for use with codes 807.0-807.1:
0 rib(s) unspecifed
1 one rib
2 two ribs
3 three ribs
4 four ribs
5 five ribs
6 six ribs
7 seven ribs
8 eight or more ribs
9 multiple ribs, unspecified

§ √5ᵗʰ 807.0 **Rib(s), closed** `CC`
[0-9] CC Excl: For codes 807.00-807.02: 807.00-807.4, 819.0-819.1, 828.0-829.1, 848.8-848.9, 879.8-879.9, 929.0-929.9, 958.8-958.99, 959.8-959.9; For code 807.03: 807.00-807.19, 807.4, 819.0-819.1, 828.0-829.1, 848.8-848.9, 879.8-879.9, 929.0-929.9, 958.8, 959.8-959.9; For codes 807.04-807.09: 807.00-807.19, 807.4, 819.0-819.1, 828.0-829.1, 848.8-848.9, 879.8-879.9, 929.0-929.9, 958.8-958.99, 959.8-959.9
S22.31xA Fracture one rib right side, initial encounter closed fx `I-10`

§ √5ᵗʰ 807.1 **Rib(s), open** `MCC`
[0-9] CC Excl: 807.00-807.19, 807.4, 819.0-819.1, 828.0-829.1, 848.8-848.9, 879.8-879.9, 929.0-929.9, 958.8-958.99, 959.8-959.9

807.2 **Sternum, closed** `CC`
DEF: Break in flat bone (breast bone) in anterior thorax.
CC Excl: 807.2-807.4, 829.0-829.1, 848.8-848.9, 879.8-879.9, 929.0-929.9, 958.8-958.99, 959.8-959.9

807.3 **Sternum, open** `MCC`
DEF: Break, with open wound, in flat bone in mid anterior thorax.
CC Excl: See code: 807.2

807.4 **Flail chest** `MCC`
CC Excl: 807.00-807.4, 829.0-829.1, 848.8-848.9, 879.8-879.9, 929.0-929.9, 958.8-958.99, 959.8-959.9

807.5 **Larynx and trachea, closed** `MCC`
Hyoid bone
Thyroid cartilage
Trachea
CC Excl: 807.5-807.6, 829.0-829.1, 848.8-848.9, 879.8-879.9, 929.0-929.9, 958.8-958.99, 959.8-959.9

807.6 **Larynx and trachea, open** `MCC`
CC Excl: See code 807.5

√4ᵗʰ **808 Fracture of pelvis**

808.0 **Acetabulum, closed** `MCC`
CC Excl: 733.10-733.19, 733.93-733.98, 808.0-808.1, 808.43-808.49, 808.53-809.1, 829.0-829.1, 835.00-835.13, 843.0-843.9, 846.0-846.9, 848.5-848.9, 879.8-879.9, 929.0-929.9, 958.8-958.99, 959.6, 959.8-959.9

808.1 **Acetabulum, open** `MCC`
CC Excl: 808.0-808.1, 808.43-808.49, 808.53-809.1, 829.0-829.1, 835.00-835.13, 843.0-843.9, 846.0-846.9, 848.5-848.9, 879.8-879.9, 929.0-929.9, 958.8-958.99, 959.6, 959.8-959.9

Pelvis and Pelvic Fractures

Fractures Disrupting Pelvic Circle — Pelvic circle — Stable — Unstable (two-place fracture) — Posterior pillar — Acetabular Fractures — Iliac crest — Ilium — Anterior superior iliac spine — Ischial spine — Acetabulum — Femur — Ischial tuberosity — L5 — Sacrum — Coccyx — Pubis — Pubic symphysis — Transverse — Pelvic Bones

---

Requires fifth digit. Valid digits are in [brackets] under each code. See category 807 for codes and definitions.

Additional Digit Required | Unacceptable PDx | Manifestation Code | Hospital Acquired Condition | ▶◀ Revised Text | ● New Code | ▲ Revised Code Title

Injury and Poisoning

808.2–812.02

808.2 Pubis, closed `CC`

CC Excl: 733.10-733.19, 733.93-733.98, 808.2-808.3, 808.43-808.49, 808.53-809.1, 829.0-829.1, 835.00-835.13, 843.0-843.9, 846.0-846.9, 848.5-848.9, 879.8-879.9, 929.0-929.9, 958.8-958.99, 959.6, 959.8-959.9

AHA: 1Q, '08, 9

S32.509A Unspec fx unspec pubis initial encounter clsd fx `I-10`

808.3 Pubis, open `MCC`

CC Excl: See code 808.2

√5ᵗʰ **808.4 Other specified part, closed**

808.41 Ilium `CC`

CC Excl: 733.10, 733.19, 808.0-809.1, 829.0-829.1, 835.00-835.13, 843.0-843.9, 846.0-846.9, 848.5-848.9, 879.8-879.9, 929.0-929.9, 958.8, 958.99, 959.6, 959.8-959.9

808.42 Ischium `CC`

CC Excl: 808.42

808.43 Multiple closed pelvic fractures with disruption of pelvic circle `CC`

Multiple closed pelvic fractures with disruption of pelvic ring

CC Excl: 733.10-733.19, 733.93-733.98, 808.0-809.1, 829.0-829.1, 835.00-835.13, 843.0-843.9, 846.0-846.9, 848.5-848.9, 879.8-879.9, 929.0-929.9, 958.8-958.99, 959.6, 959.8-959.9

AHA: 1Q, '08, 9

TIP: To assign, documentation must indicate multiple pelvic fractures with complete disruption of the pelvic circle.

808.44 Multiple closed pelvic fractures without disruption of pelvic circle `CC`

Multiple closed pelvic fractures without disruption of pelvic ring

CC Excl: 808.49

AHA: 4Q, '11, 141-142

808.49 Other `CC`

Innominate bone
Pelvic rim
CC Excl: See code: 808.43

√5ᵗʰ **808.5 Other specified part, open**

808.51 Ilium `MCC`

CC Excl: 733.10-733.19, 733.93-733.98, 808.41, 808.43-808.51, 808.53-809.1, 829.0-829.1, 835.00-835.13, 843.0-843.9, 846.0-846.9, 848.5-848.9, 879.8-879.9, 929.0-929.9, 958.8-958.99, 959.6, 959.8-959.9

808.52 Ischium `MCC`

CC Excl: 733.10-733.19, 733.93-733.98, 808.42-808.49, 808.52-809.1, 829.0-829.1, 835.00-835.13, 843.0-843.9, 846.0-846.9, 848.5-848.9, 879.8-879.9, 929.0-929.9, 958.8-958.99, 959.6, 959.8-959.9

808.53 Multiple open pelvic fractures with disruption of pelvic circle `MCC`

Multiple open pelvic fractures with disruption of pelvic ring
CC Excl: See code: 808.43

808.54 Multiple open pelvic fractures without disruption of pelvic circle `MCC`

Multiple open pelvic fractures without disruption of pelvic ring

CC Excl: 808.49

AHA: 4Q, '11, 141-142

808.59 Other `MCC`

CC Excl: See code: 808.43

808.8 Unspecified, closed `CC`

CC Excl: See code: 808.43

808.9 Unspecified, open `MCC`

CC Excl: See code: 808.43

Right Clavicle and Scapula, Anterior View

√4ᵗʰ **809 Ill-defined fractures of bones of trunk**

INCLUDES   bones of trunk with other bones except those of skull an face
multiple bones of trunk

EXCLUDES   *multiple fractures of:*
pelvic bones alone (808.0-808.9)
ribs alone (807.0-807.1, 807.4)
ribs or sternum with limb bones (819.0-819.1, 828.0-828.
skull or face with other bones (804.0-804.9)

809.0 Fracture of bones of trunk, closed

CC Excl: 733.10, 733.19, 808.0-809.1, 829.0-829.1, 835.00-835.13, 843.0-843.9, 846.0-846.9, 848.5-848.9, 879.8-879.9, 929.0-929.9, 958.8, 958.99, 959.6, 959.8-959.9

809.1 Fracture of bones of trunk, open `M`

CC Excl: See code: 809.0

Fracture of Upper Limb (810-819)

√4ᵗʰ **810 Fracture of clavicle**

INCLUDES   collar bone
interligamentous part of clavicle

The following fifth-digit subclassification is for use with category 810:
  0 unspecified part
   Clavicle NOS
  1 sternal end of clavicle
  2 shaft of clavicle
  3 acromial end of clavicle

§ √5ᵗʰ **810.0 Closed**
[0-3]

§ √5ᵗʰ **810.1 Open**
[0-3]   CC Excl: 810.00-810.13, 818.0-819.1

√4ᵗʰ **811 Fracture of scapula**

INCLUDES   shoulder blade

The following fifth-digit subclassification is for use with category 811:
  0 unspecified part
  1 acromial process
   Acromion (process)
  2 coracoid process
  3 glenoid cavity and neck of scapula
  9 other

§ √5ᵗʰ **811.0 Closed**
[0-3, 9]

§ √5ᵗʰ **811.1 Open**
[0-3, 9]   CC Excl: 811.00-811.19, 818.0-819.1

√4ᵗʰ **812 Fracture of humerus**

√5ᵗʰ **812.0 Upper end, closed**

812.00 Upper end, unspecified part
Proximal end   Shoulder
CC Excl: 812.00-812.59, 819.0-819.1

812.01 Surgical neck
Neck of humerus NOS
CC Excl: See code: 812.00
S42.214A Uns nondsplcd fx surg neck rt humerus inital clo fx

812.02 Anatomical neck
CC Excl: See code: 812.00

---

§   Requires fifth digit. Valid digits are in [brackets] under each code. See appropriate category for codes and definitions.

`N` Newborn Age: 0   `P` Pediatric Age: 0-17   `M` Maternity Age: 12-55   `A` Adult Age: 15-124   `MCC` Major CC Condition   `CC` CC Condition   `HIV` HIV Related

304 – Volume 1   **2014 ICD-9-**

Right Humerus, Anterior View

812.03 Greater tuberosity `CC`
CC Excl: See code: 812.00

812.09 Other `CC`
Head
Lesser tuberosity
Upper epiphysis
CC Excl: See code: 812.00
S42.294A Oth nondsplcd fx up end rt humerus initial clos fx `I-10`

√5ᵗʰ **812.1 Upper end, open**

812.10 Upper end, unspecified part `MCC`
CC Excl: 812.10-812.59, 818.0-819.1

812.11 Surgical neck `MCC`
CC Excl: See code: 812.10

812.12 Anatomical neck `MCC`
CC Excl: See code: 812.10

812.13 Greater tuberosity `MCC`
CC Excl: See code: 812.10

812.19 Other `MCC`
CC Excl: See code: 812.10

√5ᵗʰ **812.2 Shaft or unspecified part, closed**

812.20 Unspecified part of humerus `CC`
Humerus NOS
Lesser tuberosity
Upper arm NOS
CC Excl: See code: 812.00

812.21 Shaft of humerus `CC`
CC Excl: 812.21
AHA: 4Q, '05, 129; 3Q, '99, 14

√5ᵗʰ **812.3 Shaft or unspecified part, open**

812.30 Unspecified part of humerus `MCC`
CC Excl: See code: 812.10

812.31 Shaft of humerus `MCC`
CC Excl: See code: 812.10

√5ᵗʰ **812.4 Lower end, closed**
Distal end of humerus   Elbow

812.40 Lower end, unspecified part `CC`
CC Excl: 812.00-812.59, 819.0-819.1

812.41 Supracondylar fracture of humerus `CC`
CC Excl: See code: 812.40

812.42 Lateral condyle `CC`
External condyle
CC Excl: See code: 812.40

812.43 Medial condyle `CC`
Internal epicondyle
CC Excl: See code: 812.40

812.44 Condyle(s), unspecified `CC`
Articular process NOS   Lower epiphysis NOS
CC Excl: See code: 812.40

812.49 Other `CC`
Multiple fractures of lower end
Trochlea
CC Excl: See code: 812.40

√5ᵗʰ **812.5 Lower end, open**

812.50 Lower end, unspecified part `MCC`
CC Excl: 812.00-812.59, 819.0-819.1

812.51 Supracondylar fracture of humerus `MCC`
CC Excl: See code: 812.50

812.52 Lateral condyle `MCC`
CC Excl: See code: 812.50

812.53 Medial condyle `MCC`
CC Excl: See code: 812.50

812.54 Condyle(s), unspecified `MCC`
CC Excl: See code: 812.50

812.59 Other `MCC`
CC Excl: See code: 812.50

√4ᵗʰ **813 Fracture of radius and ulna**

√5ᵗʰ **813.0 Upper end, closed**
Proximal end

813.00 Upper end of forearm, unspecified

813.01 Olecranon process of ulna

813.02 Coronoid process of ulna

813.03 Monteggia's fracture
DEF: Fracture near the head of the ulnar shaft, causing dislocation of the radial head.

813.04 Other and unspecified fractures of proximal end of ulna (alone)
Multiple fractures of ulna, upper end

813.05 Head of radius

813.06 Neck of radius

813.07 Other and unspecified fractures of proximal end of radius (alone)
Multiple fractures of radius, upper end

813.08 Radius with ulna, upper end [any part]

√5ᵗʰ **813.1 Upper end, open**

813.10 Upper end of forearm, unspecified `MCC`
CC Excl: 813.10-813.44, 813.50-813.93, 818.0-819.1

813.11 Olecranon process of ulna `MCC`
CC Excl: 813.10-813.40, 813.42-813.44, 813.50-813.93, 818.0-819.1

813.12 Coronoid process of ulna `MCC`
CC Excl: See code: 813.10

813.13 Monteggia's fracture `MCC`
CC Excl: See code: 813.10

813.14 Other and unspecified fractures of proximal end of ulna `MCC`
CC Excl: See code: 813.10

813.15 Head of radius `MCC`
CC Excl: See code: 813.10

813.16 Neck of radius `MCC`
CC Excl: See code: 813.10

813.17 Other and unspecified fractures of proximal end of radius (alone) `MCC`
CC Excl: See code: 813.10

813.18 Radius with ulna, upper end [any part] `MCC`
CC Excl: See code: 813.10

Right Radius and Ulna, Anterior View

Additional Digit Required   Unacceptable PDx   Manifestation Code   Hospital Acquired Condition   ▶◀ Revised Text   ● New Code   ▲ Revised Code Title

■4 ICD-9-CM   Volume 1 – 305

Injury and Poisoning

813.2–815.1

√5ᵗʰ **813.2 Shaft, closed**

     813.20 Shaft, unspecified   CC
        CC Excl: 813.00-813.93, 819.0-819.1

     813.21 Radius (alone)   CC
        CC Excl: See code: 813.20

     813.22 Ulna (alone)   CC
        CC Excl: See code: 813.20

     813.23 Radius with ulna   CC
        CC Excl: See code: 813.20
        AHA: 4Q, '09, 120

√5ᵗʰ **813.3 Shaft, open**

     813.30 Shaft, unspecified   MCC
        CC Excl: 813.10-813.44, 813.50-813.93, 818.0-819.1

     813.31 Radius (alone)   MCC
        CC Excl: See code: 813.30

     813.32 Ulna (alone)   MCC
        CC Excl: See code: 813.30

     813.33 Radius with ulna   MCC
        CC Excl: See code: 813.30

√5ᵗʰ **813.4 Lower end, closed**
     Distal end

     813.40 Lower end of forearm, unspecified   CC
        CC Excl: 813.00-813.93, 819.0-819.1

     813.41 Colles' fracture   CC
        Smith's fracture
        DEF: Break of lower end of radius; associated with backward
        movement of the radius lower section.
        CC Excl: See code: 813.40

     813.42 Other fractures of distal end of radius (alone)   CC
        Dupuytren's fracture, radius
        Radius, lower end
        DEF: Dupuytren's fracture: fracture and dislocation of the
        forearm; the fracture is of the radius above wrist, and the
        dislocation is of the ulna at lower end.
        CC Excl: See code: 813.40
        S52.501A Uns fx lower end rt radius initial enc closed fx   I-10

     813.43 Distal end of ulna (alone)   CC
        Ulna: Ulna:
          head   lower epiphysis
          lower end   styloid process
        CC Excl: See code: 813.40

     813.44 Radius with ulna, lower end   CC
        CC Excl: See code: 813.40
        AHA: 1Q, '07, 7

     813.45 Torus fracture of radius (alone)   CC
        EXCLUDES   torus fracture of radius and ulna (813.47)
        CC Excl: See code: 813.40
        AHA: 4Q, '02, 70

     813.46 Torus fracture of ulna (alone)   CC
        EXCLUDES   torus fracture of radius and ulna (813.47)
        CC Excl: See code: 813.40
        AHA: 4Q, '09, 110

     813.47 Torus fracture of radius and ulna   CC
        CC Excl: See code: 813.40
        AHA: 4Q, '09, 110

√5ᵗʰ **813.5 Lower end, open**

     813.50 Lower end of forearm, unspecified   MCC
        CC Excl: 813.10-813.44, 813.50-813.93, 818.0-819.1

     813.51 Colles' fracture   MCC
        CC Excl: See code: 813.50

     813.52 Other fractures of distal end of radius (alone)   MCC
        CC Excl: See code: 813.50

     813.53 Distal end of ulna (alone)   MCC
        CC Excl: See code: 813.50

     813.54 Radius with ulna, lower end   MCC
        CC Excl: See code: 813.50

Hand Fractures

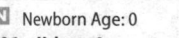

√5ᵗʰ **813.8 Unspecified part, closed**

     813.80 Forearm, unspecified   C
        CC Excl: 813.00-813.93, 819.0-819.1

     813.81 Radius (alone)
        AHA: 2Q, '98, 19

     813.82 Ulna (alone)   C
        CC Excl: See code: 813.80

     813.83 Radius with ulna   C
        CC Excl: See code: 813.80

√5ᵗʰ **813.9 Unspecified part, open**

     813.90 Forearm, unspecified   M
        CC Excl: 813.10-813.44, 813.50-813.93, 818.0-819.1

     813.91 Radius (alone)   M
        CC Excl: See code: 813.90

     813.92 Ulna (alone)   M
        CC Excl: See code: 813.90

     813.93 Radius with ulna   M
        CC Excl: See code: 813.90

√4ᵗʰ **814 Fracture of carpal bone(s)**

     The following fifth-digit subclassification is for use with category 814:
      0 carpal bone, unspecified
        Wrist NOS
      1 navicular [scaphoid] of wrist
      2 lunate [semilunar] bone of wrist
      3 triquetral [cuneiform] bone of wrist
      4 pisiform
      5 trapezium bone [larger multangular]
      6 trapezoid bone [smaller multangular]
      7 capitate bone [os magnum]
      8 hamate [unciform] bone
      9 other

§ √5ᵗʰ **814.0 Closed**
     [0-9]

§ √5ᵗʰ **814.1 Open**
     [0-9]   CC Excl: 814.00-814.19, 819.0-819.1

√4ᵗʰ **815 Fracture of metacarpal bone(s)**

     INCLUDES   hand [except finger]
            metacarpus

     The following fifth-digit subclassification is for use with category 815:
      0 metacarpal bone(s), site unspecified
      1 base of thumb [first] metacarpal
        Bennett's fracture
      2 base of other metacarpal bone(s)
      3 shaft of metacarpal bone(s)
      4 neck of metacarpal bone(s)
      9 multiple sites of metacarpus

§ √5ᵗʰ **815.0 Closed**
     [0-4, 9]

§ √5ᵗʰ **815.1 Open**
     [0-4, 9]   CC Excl: 815.00-815.19, 817.0-817.1

---

§   Requires fifth digit. Valid digits are in [brackets] under each code. See appropriate category for codes and definitions.

N Newborn Age: 0   P Pediatric Age: 0-17   M Maternity Age: 12-55   A Adult Age: 15-124   MCC Major CC Condition   CC CC Condition   HIV HIV Related

306 – Volume 1   **2014 ICD-9-**

✓4ᵗʰ **816 Fracture of one or more phalanges of hand**

INCLUDES finger(s)
thumb

The following fifth-digit subclassification is for use with category 816:
0 phalanx or phalanges, unspecified
1 middle or proximal phalanx or phalanges
2 distal phalanx or phalanges
3 multiple sites

TIP: If phalangeal fracture(s) are due to crushing injury, sequence that code (927.3) first.

§ ✓5ᵗʰ **816.0 Closed**
[0-3]

§ ✓5ᵗʰ **816.1 Open** CC
[0-3]
CC Excl: For codes 816.10-816.12: 816.00-817.1; For code 816.13: 816.00-816.13, 818.0-819.1
AHA: For code 816.12: 4Q, '03, 77

✓4ᵗʰ **817 Multiple fractures of hand bones**

INCLUDES metacarpal bone(s) with phalanx or phalanges of same hand

817.0 Closed

817.1 Open CC
CC Excl: 814.00-819.1

✓4ᵗʰ **818 Ill-defined fractures of upper limb**

INCLUDES arm NOS
multiple bones of same upper limb

EXCLUDES multiple fractures of:
metacarpal bone(s) with phalanx or phalanges (817.0-817.1)
phalanges of hand alone (816.0-816.1)
radius with ulna (813.0-813.9)

818.0 Closed

818.1 Open CC
CC Excl: 812.00-813.44, 813.50-819.1

✓4ᵗʰ **819 Multiple fractures involving both upper limbs, and upper limb with rib(s) and sternum**

INCLUDES arm(s) with rib(s) or sternum
both arms [any bones]

819.0 Closed CC
CC Excl: 807.00-807.4, 812.00-813.44, 813.50-819.1

819.1 Open CC
CC Excl: See code: 819.0

Fracture of Lower Limb (820-829)

✓4ᵗʰ **820 Fracture of neck of femur**

✓5ᵗʰ **820.0 Transcervical fracture, closed**

820.00 Intracapsular section, unspecified MCC
CC Excl: 733.10-733.19, 733.93-733.98, 820.00-821.39, 827.0-829.1, 843.0-843.9, 848.8-848.9, 879.8-879.9, 929.0-929.9, 958.8-958.99, 959.6, 959.8-959.9

820.01 Epiphysis (separation) (upper) MCC
Transepiphyseal
CC Excl: See code 820.00

820.02 Midcervical section MCC
Transcervical NOS
CC Excl: See code 820.00
AHA: 3Q, '03, 12

820.03 Base of neck MCC
Cervicotrochanteric section
CC Excl: See code 820.00

820.09 Other MCC
Head of femur
Subcapital
CC Excl: See code 820.00
S72.064A Nondsplcd art fx head rt femur initial enc clos fx I-10

✓5ᵗʰ **820.1 Transcervical fracture, open**

820.10 Intracapsular section, unspecified MCC
CC Excl: See code 820.00

820.11 Epiphysis (separation) (upper) MCC
CC Excl: See code 820.00

820.12 Midcervical section MCC
CC Excl: See code 820.00

820.13 Base of neck MCC
CC Excl: See code 820.00

820.19 Other MCC
CC Excl: See code 820.00

✓5ᵗʰ **820.2 Pertrochanteric fracture, closed**

820.20 Trochanteric section, unspecified MCC
Trochanter: Trochanter:
NOS   lesser
greater
CC Excl: See code 820.00

820.21 Intertrochanteric section MCC
CC Excl: See code 820.00

820.22 Subtrochanteric section MCC
CC Excl: See code 820.00
S72.25xA Nondsplcd subtrochant fx lt femur inital enc clo fx I-10

✓5ᵗʰ **820.3 Pertrochanteric fracture, open**

820.30 Trochanteric section, unspecified MCC
CC Excl: See code 820.00

820.31 Intertrochanteric section MCC
CC Excl: See code 820.00

820.32 Subtrochanteric section MCC
CC Excl: See code 820.00

820.8 Unspecified part of neck of femur, closed MCC
Hip NOS   Neck of femur NOS
CC Excl: See code 820.00
S72.002A Fx uns part neck left femur initial enc clos fx I-10

820.9 Unspecified part of neck of femur, open MCC
CC Excl: See code 820.00

✓4ᵗʰ **821 Fracture of other and unspecified parts of femur**

✓5ᵗʰ **821.0 Shaft or unspecified part, closed**

821.00 Unspecified part of femur MCC
Thigh
Upper leg
EXCLUDES hip NOS (820.8)
CC Excl: 733.10-733.19, 733.93-733.95, 820.00-821.39, 827.0-829.1, 843.0-843.9, 848.8-848.9, 879.8-879.9, 929.0-929.9, 958.8-958.99, 959.6, 959.8-959.9

821.01 Shaft MCC
CC Excl: See code: 821.00
AHA: 1Q, '07, 4; 1Q, '99, 5
S72.331A Displaced obl fx shaft rt femur initl enc clos fx I-10

✓5ᵗʰ **821.1 Shaft or unspecified part, open**

821.10 Unspecified part of femur MCC
CC Excl: See code: 821.00

821.11 Shaft MCC
CC Excl: See code: 821.00

Right Femur, Anterior View

Greater trochanter
Intertrochanteric line
Lesser trochanter
Head
Neck
Shaft
Medial epicondyle
Lateral epicondyle
Articular cartilage

§ Requires fifth digit. Valid digits are in [brackets] under each code. See appropriate category for codes and definitions.

4ᵗʰ/5ᵗʰ Additional Digit Required   Unacceptable PDx   Manifestation Code   Hospital Acquired Condition   ►◄ Revised Text   ● New Code   ▲ Revised Code Title

2014 ICD-9-CM   Volume 1 – 307

Right Tibia and Fibula, Anterior View

Patella
Tibial plateau
Tibial tubercle
Shaft of fibula
Tibia
Lateral (fibular) malleolus
Medial (tibial) malleolus
Pott's fracture

√5ᵗʰ 821.2 Lower end, closed
Distal end

821.20 Lower end, unspecified part `CC`
CC Excl: 733.10, 733.14-733.15, 733.19, 820.00-821.39,
827.0-829.1, 843.0-843.9, 848.8-848.9, 879.8-879.9,
929.0-929.9, 958.8, 958.99, 959.6, 959.8-959.9

821.21 Condyle, femoral `CC`
CC Excl: See code: 821.20

821.22 Epiphysis, lower (separation) `CC`
CC Excl: See code: 821.20

821.23 Supracondylar fracture of femur `CC`
CC Excl: See code: 821.20

821.29 Other `CC`
Multiple fractures of lower end
CC Excl: See code: 821.20

√5ᵗʰ 821.3 Lower end, open

821.30 Lower end, unspecified part `MCC`
CC Excl: See code: 821.20

821.31 Condyle, femoral `MCC`
CC Excl: See code: 821.20

821.32 Epiphysis, lower (separation) `MCC`
CC Excl: See code: 821.20

821.33 Supracondylar fracture of femur `MCC`
CC Excl: See code: 821.20

821.39 Other `MCC`
CC Excl: 733.10, 733.14-733.15, 733.19, 821.39-822.1,
827.0-829.1, 843.0-843.9, 848.8-848.9, 879.8-879.9,
929.0-929.9, 958.8, 958.99, 959.6, 959.8-959.9

√4ᵗʰ 822 Fracture of patella

822.0 Closed `CC`
CC Excl: 822.0-822.1, 828.0-828.1
S82.001A Uns fx right patella initial encounter closed fx `I-10`

822.1 Open `CC`
CC Excl: 733.10, 733.19, 822.1-823.32, 823.80-823.92, 827.0-829.1,
843.0-843.9, 848.8-848.9, 879.8-879.9, 929.0-929.9, 958.8, 958.99,
959.6, 959.8-959.9

Torus Fracture

Fibula
Tibia
Diaphysis
Direction of force
Torus, bulging, fracture

Anterior views of torus compression fracture

√4ᵗʰ 823 Fracture of tibia and fibula
EXCLUDES Dupuytren's fracture (824.4-824.5)
ankle (824.4-824.5)
radius (813.42, 813.52)
Pott's fracture (824.4-824.5)
that involving ankle (824.0-824.9)

The following fifth-digit subclassification is for use with category 823:
0 tibia alone
1 fibula alone
2 fibula with tibia

10 § √5ᵗʰ 823.0 Upper end, closed `CC 0,2`
[0-2] Head   Tibia:
Proximal end   condyles
tuberosity
CC Excl: For codes 823.00, 823.02: 733.10, 733.16-733.19, 823.00-823.32,
823.80-823.92, 827.0-829.1, 843.0-843.9, 848.8-848.9, 879.8-879.9,
929.0-929.9, 958.8, 958.99, 959.6, 959.8-959.9
S82.121A Displcd fx lat condyle rt tibia initial enc clos fx `I-10`

§ √5ᵗʰ 823.1 Upper end, open `MCC`
[0-2] CC Excl: See code: 823.00

10 § √5ᵗʰ 823.2 Shaft, closed `CC 0,2`
[0-2] CC Excl: See code: 823.00

§ √5ᵗʰ 823.3 Shaft, open `MCC`
[0-2] CC Excl: See code: 823.00

10 § √5ᵗʰ 823.4 Torus fracture `CC 0,2`
[0-2] DEF: A bone deformity in children, occurring commonly in the tibia
and fibula, in which the bone bends and buckles but does not
fracture.
CC Excl: See code: 823.00
AHA: 4Q, '02, 70

10 § √5ᵗʰ 823.8 Unspecified part, closed `CC 0,2`
[0-2] Lower leg NOS
CC Excl: For code 823.80: 823.00-823.92; For code 823.82: 733.10,
733.16-733.19, 823.00-823.32, 823.80-823.92, 827.0-829.1,
843.0-843.9, 848.8-848.9, 879.8-879.9, 929.0-929.9, 958.8, 958.99,
959.6, 959.8-959.9
AHA: For code 823.82: 1Q, '97, 8

§ √5ᵗʰ 823.9 Unspecified part, open `MCC`
[0-2] CC Excl: See code: 823.00\

√4ᵗʰ 824 Fracture of ankle
TIP: If ankle fracture also includes syndesmotic injury, assign also code
845.03 Sprains and strains of tibiofibular (ligament), distal.

824.0 Medial malleolus, closed
Tibia involving: Tibia involving:
ankle   malleolus
AHA: 1Q, '04, 9

824.1 Medial malleolus, open `CC`
CC Excl: 733.10, 733.16-733.19, 824.1-824.9, 827.0-829.1, 843.0-843.9,
848.8-848.9, 879.8-879.9, 929.0-929.9, 958.8, 958.99, 959.6,
959.8-959.9

824.2 Lateral malleolus, closed
Fibula involving: Fibula involving:
ankle   malleolus
AHA: 2Q, '02, 3

824.3 Lateral malleolus, open `CC`
CC Excl: See code: 824.1

824.4 Bimalleolar, closed
Dupuytren's fracture, fibula   Pott's fracture
DEF: Bimalleolar, closed: Breaking of both nodules (malleoli) on
either side of ankle joint, without an open wound.
DEF: Dupuytren's fracture (Pott's fracture): The breaking of the
farthest end of the lower leg bone (fibula), with injury to the farthest
end joint of the other lower leg bone (tibia).
AHA: ▶2Q, '12, 11◀
S82.841A Displcd bimalleolar fx rt lw leg intial enc clos fx `I-10`

824.5 Bimalleolar, open `CC`
CC Excl: See code: 824.1

824.6 Trimalleolar, closed
Lateral and medial malleolus with anterior or posterior lip of
tibia
S82.855A Nondispl trimalleolar fx of left lower leg, init `I-10`

---

10 HAC = only for valid CC or MCC codes.
§ Requires fifth digit. Valid digits are in [brackets] under each code. See category 823 for codes and definitions.

N Newborn Age: 0   **P** Pediatric Age: 0-17   **M** Maternity Age: 12-55   **A** Adult Age: 15-124   **MCC** Major CC Condition   **CC** CC Condition   **HIV** HIV Related Dx

308 – Volume 1 · February 2013   2014 ICD-9-CM

Right Foot, Dorsal

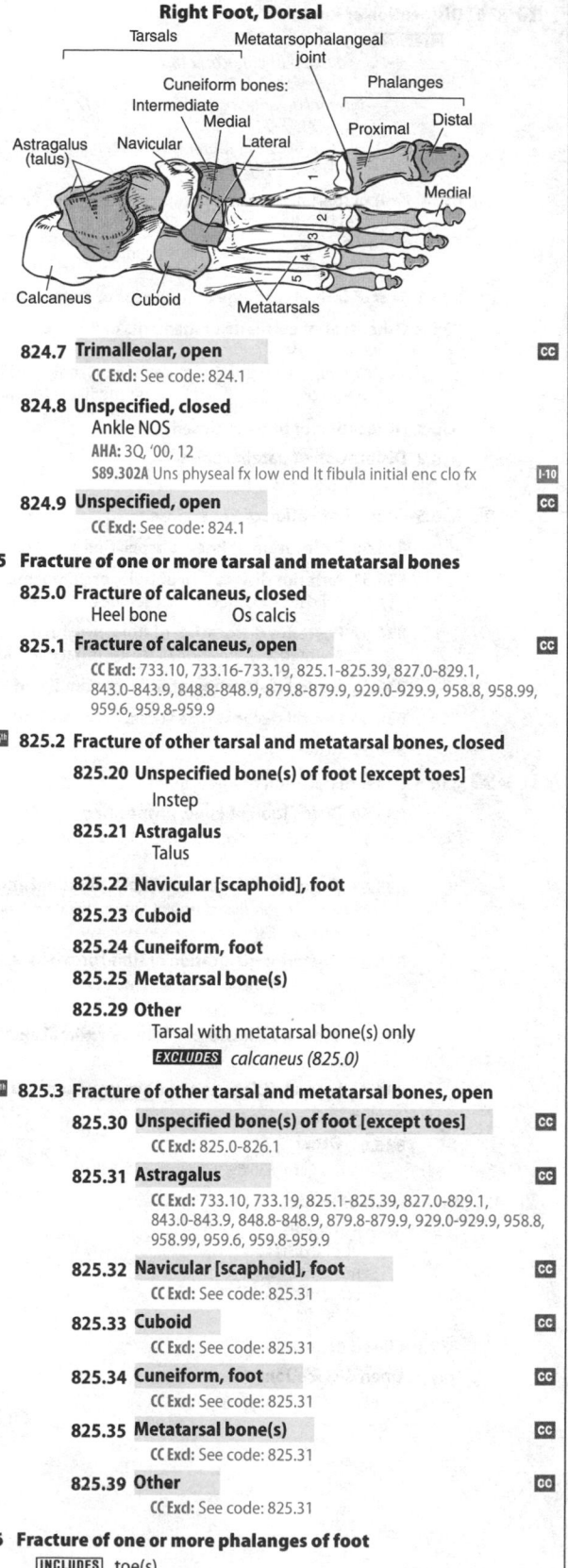

824.7 Trimalleolar, open `CC`
CC Exd: See code: 824.1

824.8 Unspecified, closed
Ankle NOS
AHA: 3Q, '00, 12
S89.302A Uns physeal fx low end lt fibula initial enc clo fx `I-10`

824.9 Unspecified, open `CC`
CC Exd: See code: 824.1

✓4ᵗʰ 825 Fracture of one or more tarsal and metatarsal bones

825.0 Fracture of calcaneus, closed
Heel bone   Os calcis

825.1 Fracture of calcaneus, open `CC`
CC Exd: 733.10, 733.16-733.19, 825.1-825.39, 827.0-829.1,
843.0-843.9, 848.8-848.9, 879.8-879.9, 929.0-929.9, 958.8, 958.99,
959.6, 959.8-959.9

✓5ᵗʰ 825.2 Fracture of other tarsal and metatarsal bones, closed

    825.20 Unspecified bone(s) of foot [except toes]
        Instep

    825.21 Astragalus
        Talus

    825.22 Navicular [scaphoid], foot

    825.23 Cuboid

    825.24 Cuneiform, foot

    825.25 Metatarsal bone(s)

    825.29 Other
        Tarsal with metatarsal bone(s) only
        EXCLUDES calcaneus (825.0)

✓5ᵗʰ 825.3 Fracture of other tarsal and metatarsal bones, open

    825.30 Unspecified bone(s) of foot [except toes] `CC`
        CC Exd: 825.0-826.1

    825.31 Astragalus `CC`
        CC Exd: 733.10, 733.19, 825.1-825.39, 827.0-829.1,
        843.0-843.9, 848.8-848.9, 879.8-879.9, 929.0-929.9, 958.8,
        958.99, 959.6, 959.8-959.9

    825.32 Navicular [scaphoid], foot `CC`
        CC Exd: See code: 825.31

    825.33 Cuboid `CC`
        CC Exd: See code: 825.31

    825.34 Cuneiform, foot `CC`
        CC Exd: See code: 825.31

    825.35 Metatarsal bone(s) `CC`
        CC Exd: See code: 825.31

    825.39 Other `CC`
        CC Exd: See code: 825.31

✓4ᵗʰ 826 Fracture of one or more phalanges of foot
    INCLUDES toe(s)

826.0 Closed

826.1 Open

✓4ᵗʰ 827 Other, multiple, and ill-defined fractures of lower limb

    INCLUDES leg NOS
        multiple bones of same lower limb

    EXCLUDES multiple fractures of:
        ankle bones alone (824.4-824.9)
        phalanges of foot alone (826.0-826.1)
        tarsal with metatarsal bones (825.29, 825.39)
        tibia with fibula (823.0-823.9 with fifth-digit 2)

827.0 Closed

827.1 Open `CC`
CC Exd: 820.00-823.32, 823.80-829.1

✓4ᵗʰ 828 Multiple fractures involving both lower limbs, lower with upper limb, and lower limb(s) with rib(s) and sternum
    INCLUDES arm(s) with leg(s) [any bones]
        both legs [any bones]
        leg(s) with rib(s) or sternum

828.0 Closed `MCC`
CC Exd: See code: 827.1

828.1 Open `MCC`
CC Exd: See code: 827.1

✓4ᵗʰ 829 Fracture of unspecified bones

829.0 Unspecified bone, closed

829.1 Unspecified bone, open

Dislocation (830-839)

    INCLUDES displacement
        subluxation

    EXCLUDES congenital dislocation (754.0-755.8)
        pathological dislocation (718.2)
        recurrent dislocation (718.3)

NOTE The descriptions "closed" and "open," used in the fourth-digit
    subdivisions, include the following terms:

closed:	open:
complete	compound
dislocation NOS	infected
partial	with foreign body
simple	
uncomplicated	

A dislocation not indicated as closed or open should be classified as
    closed.

AHA: 3Q, '90, 12

TIP: Do not assign if documentation indicates developmental dislocation;
see instead subcategory 718.7.

Unless otherwise directed, dislocations that occur with fractures of the same
site should not be coded separately; assign only the fracture code.

✓4ᵗʰ 830 Dislocation of jaw
    INCLUDES jaw (cartilage) (meniscus)
        mandible
        maxilla (inferior)
        temporomandibular (joint)

830.0 Closed dislocation

830.1 Open dislocation `CC`
CC Exd: 830.0-830.1, 839.69, 839.79-839.9

✓4ᵗʰ 831 Dislocation of shoulder
    EXCLUDES sternoclavicular joint (839.61, 839.71)
        sternum (839.61, 839.71)

The following fifth-digit subclassification is for use with category 831:
    0 shoulder, unspecified
        Humerus NOS
    1 anterior dislocation of humerus
    2 posterior dislocation of humerus
    3 inferior dislocation of humerus
    4 acromioclavicular (joint)
        Clavicle
    9 other
        Scapula

TIP: Do not assign if documentation indicates recurrent shoulder dislocation;
see instead code 718.31.

§ ✓5ᵗʰ 831.0 Closed dislocation
    [0-4, 9]

§ Requires fifth digit. Valid digits are in [brackets] under each code. See category 831 for codes and definitions.

Additional Digit Required   Unacceptable PDx   Manifestation Code   Hospital Acquired Condition   ▶◀ Revised Text   ● New Code   ▲ Revised Code Title

2014 ICD-9-CM   Volume 1 – 309

Injury and Poisoning

831.1–837.1

§ ✓5ᵗʰ **831.1 Open dislocation**   CC
[0-4, 9]   CC Excl: For code 831.10: 831.10, 839.69, 839.79-839.9; For code 831.11: 831.11, 839.69, 839.79-839.9; For code 831.12: 831.12, 839.69, 839.79-839.9; For code 831.13: 831.13, 839.69, 839.79-839.9; For code 831.14: 831.14, 839.69, 839.79-839.9; For code 831.19: 831.19, 839.69, 839.79-839.9

✓4ᵗʰ **832 Dislocation of elbow**

The following fifth-digit subclassification is for use with subcategories 832.0 and 832.1:
  0   elbow, unspecified
  1   anterior dislocation of elbow
  2   posterior dislocation of elbow
  3   medial dislocation of elbow
  4   lateral dislocation of elbow
  9   other

§ ✓5ᵗʰ **832.0 Closed dislocation**
[0-4, 9]

§ ✓5ᵗʰ **832.1 Open dislocation**   CC
[0-4, 9]   CC Excl: For code 832.10: 832.10; For code 832.11: 832.11; For code 832.12: 832.12; For code 832.13: 832.13; For code 832.14: 832.14; For code 832.19: 832.19

832.2 Nursemaid's elbow
Subluxation of radial head
AHA: 4Q, '09, 110-111

✓4ᵗʰ **833 Dislocation of wrist**

The following fifth-digit subclassification is for use with category 833:
  0   wrist unspecified part
    Carpal (bone)
    Radius, distal end
  1   radioulnar (joint), distal
  2   radiocarpal (joint)
  3   midcarpal (joint)
  4   carpometacarpal (joint)
  5   metacarpal (bone), proximal end
  9   other
    Ulna, distal end

§ ✓5ᵗʰ **833.0 Closed dislocation**
[0-5, 9]

§ ✓5ᵗʰ **833.1 Open dislocation**   CC
[0-5, 9]   CC Excl: For codes 833.10, 833.13-833.19: 833.00-833.19; For code 833.11: 833.11; For code 833.12: 833.12

✓4ᵗʰ **834 Dislocation of finger**
INCLUDES   finger(s)
  phalanx of hand
  thumb

The following fifth-digit subclassification is for use with category 834:
  0   finger unspecified part
  1   metacarpophalangeal (joint)
    Metacarpal (bone), distal end
  2   interphalangeal (joint), hand

§ ✓5ᵗʰ **834.0 Closed dislocation**
[0-2]

§ ✓5ᵗʰ **834.1 Open dislocation**
[0-2]

✓4ᵗʰ **835 Dislocation of hip**

The following fifth-digit subclassification is for use with category 835:
  0   dislocation of hip, unspecified
  1   posterior dislocation
  2   obturator dislocation
  3   other anterior dislocation

§ ✓5ᵗʰ **835.0 Closed dislocation**   CC
[0-3]   CC Excl: For code 835.00: 835.00, 839.69, 839.79-839.9; For code 835.01: 835.01, 839.69, 839.79-839.9; For code 835.02: 835.02, 839.69, 839.79-839.9; For code 835.03: 835.03, 839.69, 839.79-839.9

§ ✓5ᵗʰ **835.1 Open dislocation**   MCC
[0-3]   CC Excl: For code 835.10: 835.10, 839.69, 839.79-839.9; For code 835.11: 835.11, 839.69, 839.79-839.9; For code 835.12: 835.12, 839.69, 839.79-839.9; For code 835.13: 835.13, 839.69, 839.79-839.9

✓4ᵗʰ **836 Dislocation of knee**
EXCLUDES   dislocation of knee:
    old or pathological (718.2)
    recurrent (718.3)
  internal derangement of knee joint (717.0-717.5, 717.8-717.9)
  old tear of cartilage or meniscus of knee (717.0-717.5, 717.8-717.9)

836.0 Tear of medial cartilage or meniscus of knee, current
Bucket handle tear:
  NOS }
  medial meniscus } current injury

836.1 Tear of lateral cartilage or meniscus of knee, current

836.2 Other tear of cartilage or meniscus of knee, current
Tear of:
  cartilage (semilunar) } current injury, not specified
  meniscus }   as medial or lateral

836.3 Dislocation of patella, closed

836.4 Dislocation of patella, open   CC
CC Excl: 836.3-836.4

✓5ᵗʰ **836.5 Other dislocation of knee, closed**

836.50 Dislocation of knee, unspecified

836.51 Anterior dislocation of tibia, proximal end
Posterior dislocation of femur, distal end, closed

836.52 Posterior dislocation of tibia, proximal end
Anterior dislocation of femur, distal end, closed

836.53 Medial dislocation of tibia, proximal end

836.54 Lateral dislocation of tibia, proximal end

836.59 Other

✓5ᵗʰ **836.6 Other dislocation of knee, open**

836.60 Dislocation of knee, unspecified   CC
CC Excl: 717.0-717.9, 718.26, 718.36, 836.60, 839.69, 839.79-839.9

836.61 Anterior dislocation of tibia, proximal end   CC
Posterior dislocation of femur, distal end, open
CC Excl: 836.61, 839.69, 839.79-839.9

836.62 Posterior dislocation of tibia, proximal end   CC
Anterior dislocation of femur, distal end, open
CC Excl: 836.62, 839.69, 839.79-839.9

836.63 Medial dislocation of tibia, proximal end   CC
CC Excl: 836.63, 839.69, 839.79-839.9

836.64 Lateral dislocation of tibia, proximal end   CC
CC Excl: 836.64, 839.69, 839.79-839.9

836.69 Other   CC
CC Excl: 836.69, 839.69, 839.79-839.9

✓4ᵗʰ **837 Dislocation of ankle**
INCLUDES   astragalus
  fibula, distal end
  navicular, foot
  scaphoid, foot
  tibia, distal end

837.0 Closed dislocation

837.1 Open dislocation   CC
CC Excl: 837.1, 839.69, 839.79-839.9

---

§   Requires fifth digit. Valid digits are in [brackets] under each code. See appropriate category for codes and definitions.

 Newborn Age: 0   Pediatric Age: 0-17   Maternity Age: 12-55   Adult Age: 15-124   MCC Major CC Condition   CC CC Condition   HIV HIV Related Dx

310 – Volume 1   2014 ICD-9-CM

Injury and Poisoning

√4ᵗʰ **838 Dislocation of foot**

The following fifth-digit subclassification is for use with category 838:

0 foot unspecified
1 tarsal (bone), joint unspecified
2 midtarsal (joint)
3 tarsometatarsal (joint)
4 metatarsal (bone), joint unspecified
5 metatarsophalangeal (joint)
6 interphalangeal (joint), foot
9 other
    Phalanx of foot
    Toe(s)

§ √5ᵗʰ **838.0 Closed dislocation**
[0-6, 9]

§ √5ᵗʰ **838.1 Open dislocation**
[0-6, 9]

√4ᵗʰ **839 Other, multiple, and ill-defined dislocations**

√5ᵗʰ **839.0 Cervical vertebra, closed**
Cervical spine
Neck

839.00 Cervical vertebra, unspecified   CC
CC Excl: 805.00-805.18, 806.00-806.19, 806.8-806.9,
839.00-839.18, 847.0, 848.8-848.9, 879.8-879.9,
929.0-929.9, 952.00-952.09, 958.8-958.99, 959.8-959.9

839.01 First cervical vertebra   CC
CC Excl: See code 839.00

839.02 Second cervical vertebra   CC
CC Excl: See code 839.00

839.03 Third cervical vertebra   CC
CC Excl: See code 839.00

839.04 Fourth cervical vertebra   CC
CC Excl: See code 839.00

839.05 Fifth cervical vertebra   CC
CC Excl: See code 839.00

839.06 Sixth cervical vertebra   CC
CC Excl: See code 839.00

839.07 Seventh cervical vertebra   CC
CC Excl: See code 839.00

839.08 Multiple cervical vertebrae   CC
CC Excl: See code 839.00

√5ᵗʰ **839.1 Cervical vertebra, open**

839.10 Cervical vertebra, unspecified   MCC
CC Excl: See code 839.00

839.11 First cervical vertebra   MCC
CC Excl: See code 839.00

839.12 Second cervical vertebra   MCC
CC Excl: See code 839.00

839.13 Third cervical vertebra   MCC
CC Excl: See code 839.00

839.14 Fourth cervical vertebra   MCC
CC Excl: See code 839.00

839.15 Fifth cervical vertebra   MCC
CC Excl: See code 839.00

839.16 Sixth cervical vertebra   MCC
CC Excl: See code 839.00

839.17 Seventh cervical vertebra   MCC
CC Excl: See code 839.00

839.18 Multiple cervical vertebrae   MCC
CC Excl: See code 839.00

√5ᵗʰ **839.2 Thoracic and lumbar vertebra, closed**

839.20 Lumbar vertebra

839.21 Thoracic vertebra
Dorsal [thoracic] vertebra

√5ᵗʰ **839.3 Thoracic and lumbar vertebra, open**

839.30 Lumbar vertebra   MCC
CC Excl: 839.30

839.31 Thoracic vertebra   MCC
CC Excl: 839.21, 839.31

√5ᵗʰ **839.4 Other vertebra, closed**

839.40 Vertebra, unspecified site
Spine NOS

839.41 Coccyx

839.42 Sacrum
Sacroiliac (joint)

839.49 Other

√5ᵗʰ **839.5 Other vertebra, open**

839.50 Vertebra, unspecified site   MCC
CC Excl: 839.10-839.18, 839.30-839.31, 839.50-839.59,
839.79, 839.9

839.51 Coccyx   CC
CC Excl: 839.51

839.52 Sacrum   CC
CC Excl: 839.52

839.59 Other   MCC
CC Excl: See code: 839.50

√5ᵗʰ **839.6 Other location, closed**

839.61 Sternum   CC
Sternoclavicular joint
CC Excl: 839.61, 839.71

839.69 Other
Pelvis

√6ᵗʰ **839.7 Other location, open**

839.71 Sternum   MCC
CC Excl: See code: 839.61

839.79 Other   CC
CC Excl: 830.1, 831.10-831.19, 832.10-832.19, 833.10-833.19,
834.10-834.12, 835.10-835.13, 836.4, 836.60-836.69, 837.1,
838.10-838.19, 839.10-839.18, 839.30-839.31,
839.50-839.59, 839.71-839.79, 839.9

839.8 Multiple and ill-defined, closed
Arm
Back
Hand
Multiple locations, except fingers or toes alone
Other ill-defined locations
Unspecified location

839.9 Multiple and ill-defined, open   CC
CC Excl: See code: 839.79

Sprains and Strains of Joints and Adjacent Muscles (840-848)

INCLUDES
avulsion	
hemarthrosis	of:
laceration	joint capsule
rupture	ligament
sprain	muscle
strain	tendon
tear	

EXCLUDES *laceration of tendon in open wounds (880-884 and 890-894 with .2)*

√4ᵗʰ **840 Sprains and strains of shoulder and upper arm**

840.0 Acromioclavicular (joint) (ligament)

840.1 Coracoclavicular (ligament)

840.2 Coracohumeral (ligament)

840.3 Infraspinatus (muscle) (tendon)

840.4 Rotator cuff (capsule)
EXCLUDES *complete rupture of rotator cuff, nontraumatic (727.61)*

840.5 Subscapularis (muscle)

840.6 Supraspinatus (muscle) (tendon)

838–840.6

---

§ Requires fifth digit. Valid digits are in [brackets] under each code. See appropriate category for codes and definitions.

√4ᵗʰ
√5ᵗʰ Additional Digit Required   Unacceptable PDx   Manifestation Code   Hospital Acquired Condition   ▶◀ Revised Text   ● New Code   ▲ Revised Code Title

Injury and Poisoning

840.7–848.9

840.7 **Superior glenoid labrum lesion**
SLAP lesion
DEF: Detachment injury of the superior aspect of the glenoid labrum which is the ring of fibrocartilage attached to the rim of the glenoid cavity of the scapula.
AHA: ▶2Q, '12, 15;◀ 4Q, '01, 52

840.8 **Other specified sites of shoulder and upper arm**

840.9 **Unspecified site of shoulder and upper arm**
Arm NOS   Shoulder NOS

√4ᵗʰ 841 **Sprains and strains of elbow and forearm**

841.0 **Radial collateral ligament**

841.1 **Ulnar collateral ligament**

841.2 **Radiohumeral (joint)**

841.3 **Ulnohumeral (joint)**

841.8 **Other specified sites of elbow and forearm**

841.9 **Unspecified site of elbow and forearm**
Elbow NOS

√4ᵗʰ 842 **Sprains and strains of wrist and hand**

√5ᵗʰ 842.0 **Wrist**

842.00 **Unspecified site**

842.01 **Carpal (joint)**

842.02 **Radiocarpal (joint) (ligament)**

842.09 **Other**
Radioulnar joint, distal

√5ᵗʰ 842.1 **Hand**

842.10 **Unspecified site**

842.11 **Carpometacarpal (joint)**

842.12 **Metacarpophalangeal (joint)**

842.13 **Interphalangeal (joint)**

842.19 **Other**
Midcarpal (joint)

√4ᵗʰ 843 **Sprains and strains of hip and thigh**

843.0 **Iliofemoral (ligament)**

843.1 **Ischiocapsular (ligament)**

843.8 **Other specified sites of hip and thigh**

843.9 **Unspecified site of hip and thigh**
Hip NOS   Thigh NOS

√4ᵗʰ 844 **Sprains and strains of knee and leg**

844.0 **Lateral collateral ligament of knee**

844.1 **Medial collateral ligament of knee**

844.2 **Cruciate ligament of knee**

844.3 **Tibiofibular (joint) (ligament), superior**

844.8 **Other specified sites of knee and leg**

844.9 **Unspecified site of knee and leg**
Knee NOS   Leg NOS

√4ᵗʰ 845 **Sprains and strains of ankle and foot**

√5ᵗʰ 845.0 **Ankle**

845.00 **Unspecified site**
AHA: 2Q, '02, 3

845.01 **Deltoid (ligament), ankle**
Internal collateral (ligament), ankle

845.02 **Calcaneofibular (ligament)**

845.03 **Tibiofibular (ligament), distal**
AHA: 1Q, '04, 9

845.09 **Other**
Achilles tendon

√5ᵗʰ 845.1 **Foot**

845.10 **Unspecified site**

845.11 **Tarsometatarsal (joint) (ligament)**

845.12 **Metatarsophalangeal (joint)**

845.13 **Interphalangeal (joint), toe**

845.19 **Other**

√4ᵗʰ 846 **Sprains and strains of sacroiliac region**

846.0 **Lumbosacral (joint) (ligament)**

846.1 **Sacroiliac ligament**

846.2 **Sacrospinatus (ligament)**

846.3 **Sacrotuberous (ligament)**

846.8 **Other specified sites of sacroiliac region**

846.9 **Unspecified site of sacroiliac region**

√4ᵗʰ 847 **Sprains and strains of other and unspecified parts of back**
EXCLUDES *lumbosacral (846.0)*

847.0 **Neck**
Anterior longitudinal (ligament), cervical
Atlanto-axial (joints)
Atlanto-occipital (joints)
Whiplash injury
EXCLUDES *neck injury NOS (959.0)*
thyroid region (848.2)
S13.4xxA Sprain ligaments cervical spine initial encounter   I-10

847.1 **Thoracic**

847.2 **Lumbar**

847.3 **Sacrum**
Sacrococcygeal (ligament)

847.4 **Coccyx**

847.9 **Unspecified site of back**
Back NOS

√4ᵗʰ 848 **Other and ill-defined sprains and strains**

848.0 **Septal cartilage of nose**

848.1 **Jaw**
Temporomandibular (joint) (ligament)

848.2 **Thyroid region**
Cricoarytenoid (joint) (ligament)
Cricothyroid (joint) (ligament)
Thyroid cartilage

848.3 **Ribs**
Chondrocostal (joint)   } without mention of injury
Costal cartilage   }   to sternum

√5ᵗʰ 848.4 **Sternum**

848.40 **Unspecified site**

848.41 **Sternoclavicular (joint) (ligament)**

848.42 **Chondrosternal (joint)**

848.49 **Other**
Xiphoid cartilage

848.5 **Pelvis**
Symphysis pubis
EXCLUDES *that in childbirth (665.6)*

848.8 **Other specified sites of sprains and strains**

848.9 **Unspecified site of sprain and strain**

N Newborn Age: 0   P Pediatric Age: 0-17   M Maternity Age: 12-55   A Adult Age: 15-124   MCC Major CC Condition   CC CC Condition   HIV HIV Related Dx

312 – Volume 1 • February 2013   2014 ICD-9-CM

Intracranial Injury, Excluding Those With Skull Fracture (850-854)

INCLUDES traumatic brain injury without skull fracture
open wound of head without intracranial injury (870.0-873.9)
skull fracture alone (800-801 and 803-804 with .0, .5)

EXCLUDES *intracranial injury with skull fracture (800-801 and 803-804, except .0 and .5)*

NOTE The description "with open intracranial wound," used in the fourth-digit subdivisions, includes those specified as open or with mention of infection or foreign body.

The following fifth-digit subclassification is for use with categories 851-854:
0 unspecified state of consciousness
1 with no loss of consciousness
2 with brief [less than one hour] loss of consciousness
3 with moderate [1-24 hours] loss of consciousness
4 with prolonged [more than 24 hours] loss of consciousness and return to pre-existing conscious level
5 with prolonged [more than 24 hours] loss of consciousness without return to pre-existing conscious level
   Use fifth-digit 5 to designate when a patient is unconscious and dies before regaining consciousness, regardless of the duration of the loss of consciousness
6 with loss of consciousness of unspecified duration
9 with concussion, unspecified

AHA: 1Q, '93, 22

TIP: If documentation specifies only "head injury," with no further specificity, and is self-limiting, assign instead code 959.01 Head injury, unspecified.

850 Concussion

INCLUDES commotio cerebri

EXCLUDES concussion with:
cerebral laceration or contusion (851.0-851.9)
cerebral hemorrhage (852-853)
head injury NOS (959.01)

AHA: 2Q, '96, 6; 4Q, '90, 24

TIP: When a patient is treated for symptoms within 24 to 48 hours of the concussion, clarify with the physician whether the concussion is still in the acute phase or is a postconcussion syndrome; if so, assign instead code 310.2.

850.0 With no loss of consciousness
Concussion with mental confusion or disorientation, without loss of consciousness

✓5ᵗʰ 850.1 With brief loss of consciousness
Loss of consciousness for less than one hour
AHA: 4Q, '03, 76; 1Q, '99, 10; 2Q, '92, 5

850.11 With loss of consciousness of 30 minutes or less **CC**
CC Excl: 800.00-801.99, 803.00-804.99, 850.0-852.19, 852.21-854.19, 873.8-873.9, 879.8-879.9, 905.0, 925.1-925.2, 929.0-929.9, 958.8-959.09, 959.8-959.9
S06.0x1A Concussion w/loc 30 min/less initial encounter **I-10**

850.12 With loss of consciousness from 31 to 59 minutes **CC**
CC Excl: See code: 850.11
AHA: 4Q, '10, 111

850.2 With moderate loss of consciousness **CC**
Loss of consciousness for 1-24 hours
CC Excl: See code: 850.11

850.3 With prolonged loss of consciousness and return to pre-existing conscious level **CC**
Loss of consciousness for more than 24 hours with complete recovery
CC Excl: See code: 850.11

850.4 With prolonged loss of consciousness, without return to pre-existing conscious level **MCC**
CC Excl: See code: 850.11

850.5 With loss of consciousness of unspecified duration **CC**
CC Excl: See code: 850.11
S06.0x9A Concussion w/loc uns duration initial encounter **I-10**

850.9 Concussion, unspecified

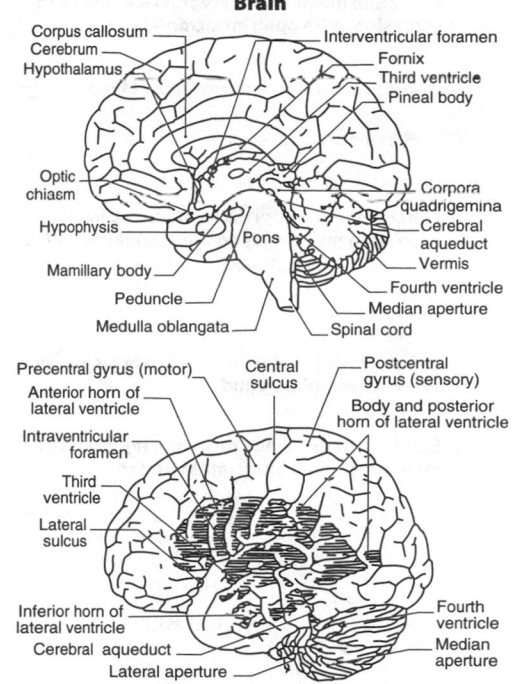

Brain

851 Cerebral laceration and contusion
AHA: 4Q, '96, 36; 1Q, '93, 22; 4Q, '90, 24

¹⁰§ ✓5ᵗʰ 851.0 Cortex (cerebral) contusion without mention of open intracranial wound   **MCC 5** **CC 2-4, 6**
[0-6, 9]
CC Excl: For codes 851.02-851.06: 800.00-801.99, 803.00-804.99, 850.0-852.19, 852.21-854.19, 873.8-873.9, 879.8-879.9, 905.0, 925.1-925.2, 929.0-929.9, 958.8-959.09, 959.8-959.9
AHA: For code 851.00: 4Q, '10, 93

§ ✓5ᵗʰ 851.1 Cortex (cerebral) contusion with open intracranial wound   **MCC**
[0-6, 9]
CC Excl: 800.00-801.99, 803.00-804.99, 850.0-852.19, 852.21-854.19, 873.8-873.9, 879.8-879.9, 905.0, 925.1-925.2, 929.0-929.9, 958.8-959.09, 959.8-959.9
AHA: 1Q, '92, 9

§ ✓5ᵗʰ 851.2 Cortex (cerebral) laceration without mention of open intracranial wound   **MCC**
[0-6, 9]
CC Excl: See code: 851.1
S06.330A Contus/lac cereb, w/o loss of consciousness, init **I-10**

§ ✓5ᵗʰ 851.3 Cortex (cerebral) laceration with open intracranial wound   **MCC**
[0-6, 9]
CC Excl: See code: 851.1

¹⁰§ ✓5ᵗʰ 851.4 Cerebellar or brain stem contusion without mention of open intracranial wound   **MCC 5** **CC 2-4, 6**
CC Excl: For codes 851.42-851.46: 800.00-801.99, 803.00-804.99, 850.0-852.19, 852.21-854.19, 873.8-873.9, 879.8-879.9, 905.0, 925.1-925.2, 929.0-929.9, 958.8-959.09, 959.8-959.9

§ ✓5ᵗʰ 851.5 Cerebellar or brain stem contusion with open intracranial wound   **MCC**
[0-6, 9]
CC Excl: See code: 851.1

§ ✓5ᵗʰ 851.6 Cerebellar or brain stem laceration without mention of open intracranial wound   **MCC**
[0-6, 9]
CC Excl: See code: 851.1

§ ✓5ᵗʰ 851.7 Cerebellar or brain stem laceration with open intracranial wound   **MCC**
[0-6, 9]
CC Excl: See code: 851.1

§ ✓5ᵗʰ 851.8 Other and unspecified cerebral laceration and contusion, without mention of open intracranial wound   **MCC**
[0-6, 9]
Brain (membrane) NOS
CC Excl: See code: 851.1
AHA: 4Q, '96, 37

---

¹⁰ HAC = only for valid CC or MCC codes.
§ Requires fifth digit. Valid digits are in [brackets] under each code. See beginning of section 850–854 for codes and definitions.

✓4ᵗʰ ✓5ᵗʰ Additional Digit Required   Unacceptable PDx   Manifestation Code   Hospital Acquired Condition   ►◄ Revised Text   ● New Code   ▲ Revised Code Title

2014 ICD-9-CM   **Volume 1 – 313**

Injury and Poisoning

851.9–861.11

§ ✓5ᵗʰ **851.9 Other and unspecified cerebral laceration and contusion, with open intracranial wound**   MCC
[0-6, 9]
CC Excl: See code: 851.1

✓4ᵗʰ **852 Subarachnoid, subdural, and extradural hemorrhage, following injury**
EXCLUDES *cerebral contusion or laceration (with hemorrhage) (851.0-851.9)*
DEF: Bleeding from lining of brain; due to injury.

§ ✓5ᵗʰ **852.0 Subarachnoid hemorrhage following injury without mention of open intracranial wound**   MCC
[0-6, 9]
Middle meningeal hemorrhage following injury
CC Excl: 800.0-801.99, 803.00-804.99, 850.0-852.19, 852.21-854.19, 873.8-873.9, 879.8-879.9, 905.0, 925.1-925.2, 929.0-929.9, 958.8-959.09, 959.8-959.9

§ ✓5ᵗʰ **852.1 Subarachnoid hemorrhage following injury with open intracranial wound**   MCC
[0-6, 9]
CC Excl: See code: 852.0

§ ✓5ᵗʰ **852.2 Subdural hemorrhage following injury without mention of open intracranial wound**   MCC
[0-6, 9]
CC Excl: For code 852.20: 800.00-801.99, 803.00-804.99, 850.0-854.19, 873.8-873.9, 879.8-879.9, 905.0, 925.1-925.2, 929.0-929.9, 958.8-959.09, 959.8-959.9; For codes 852.21-852.29: 800.0-801.99, 803.00-804.99, 850.0-852.19, 852.21-854.19, 873.8-873.9, 879.8-879.9, 905.0, 925.1-925.2, 929.0-929.9, 958.8-959.09, 959.8-959.9
AHA: 4Q, '96, 43; For codes 852.21-852.29: 4Q, '07, 107; For code 852.25: 4Q, '11, 99
S06.5x0A Traumatic subdurl hemorrhage w/o loc initial enc   I-10

§ ✓5ᵗʰ **852.3 Subdural hemorrhage following injury with open intracranial wound**   MCC
[0-6, 9]
CC Excl: See code: 852.0

§ ✓5ᵗʰ **852.4 Extradural hemorrhage following injury without mention of open intracranial wound**   MCC
[0-6, 9]
Epidural hematoma following injury
CC Excl: See code: 852.0

§ ✓5ᵗʰ **852.5 Extradural hemorrhage following injury with open intracranial wound**   MCC
[0-6, 9]
CC Excl: See code: 852.0

✓4ᵗʰ **853 Other and unspecified intracranial hemorrhage following injury**

§ ✓5ᵗʰ **853.0 Without mention of open intracranial wound**   MCC
[0-6, 9]
Cerebral compression due to injury
Intracranial hematoma following injury
Traumatic cerebral hemorrhage
CC Excl: 800.00-801.99, 803.00-804.99, 850.0-852.19, 852.21-854.19, 873.8-873.9, 879.8-879.9, 905.0, 925.1-925.2, 929.0-929.9, 958.8-959.09, 959.8-959.9
AHA: 3Q, '90, 14

§ ✓5ᵗʰ **853.1 With open intracranial wound**   MCC
[0-6, 9] CC Excl: See code: 853.0

✓4ᵗʰ **854 Intracranial injury of other and unspecified nature**
INCLUDES injury:
    brain NOS
    cavernous sinus
    intracranial
    traumatic brain NOS
EXCLUDES *any condition classifiable to 850-853 head injury NOS (959.01)*
AHA: 1Q, '99, 10; 2Q, '92, 6
TIP: Assign a code from category 854 for traumatic brain injury (TBI) with diffuse axonal injury (DAI), also known as a shear injury.

¹⁰ § ✓5ᵗʰ **854.0 Without mention of open intracranial wound**   MCC 5   CC 2-4, 6
[0-6, 9]
CC Excl: For codes 854.02-854.06: 800.00-801.99, 803.00-804.99, 850.0-852.19, 852.21-854.19, 873.8-873.9, 879.8-879.9, 905.0, 925.1-925.2, 929.0-929.9, 958.8-959.09, 959.8-959.9
AHA: For code 854.00: 4Q, '09, 108; 2Q, '05, 6

§ ✓5ᵗʰ **854.1 With open intracranial wound**   MCC
[0-6, 9] CC Excl: 800.0-801.99, 803.00-804.99, 850.0-852.19, 852.21-854.19, 873.8-873.9, 879.8-879.9, 905.0, 925.1-925.2, 929.0-929.9, 958.8-959.09, 959.8-959.9

Internal Injury of Thorax, Abdomen, and Pelvis (860-869)

INCLUDES   blast injuries
    blunt trauma
    bruise
    concussion injuries (except cerebral)
    crushing   } of internal
    hematoma   organs
    laceration
    puncture
    tear
    traumatic rupture

EXCLUDES *concussion NOS (850.0-850.9)*
flail chest (807.4)
foreign body entering through orifice (930.0-939.9)
injury to blood vessels (901.0-902.9)

NOTE The description "with open wound," used in the fourth-digit subdivisions, includes those with mention of infection or foreign body.

✓4ᵗʰ **860 Traumatic pneumothorax and hemothorax**
DEF: Traumatic pneumothorax: air or gas leaking into pleural space of lung due to trauma.
DEF: Traumatic hemothorax: blood buildup in pleural space of lung due to trauma.
AHA: 2Q, '93, 4
TIP: If there's no mention of trauma associated with pneumothorax, see instead category 512.

860.0 Pneumothorax without mention of open wound into thorax   CC
CC Excl: 860.0-860.5, 861.20-861.32, 862.29, 862.39-862.9, 875.0-875.1, 879.8-879.9, 929.0-929.9, 958.7-958.99, 959.8-959.9
S27.0xxA Traumatic pneumothorax initial encounter   I-10

860.1 Pneumothorax with open wound into thorax   MCC
CC Excl: See code 860.0

860.2 Hemothorax without mention of open wound into thorax   MCC
CC Excl: See code 860.0

860.3 Hemothorax with open wound into thorax   MCC
CC Excl: See code 860.0

860.4 Pneumohemothorax without mention of open wound into thorax   MCC
CC Excl: See code 860.0

860.5 Pneumohemothorax with open wound into thorax   MCC
CC Excl: See code 860.0

✓4ᵗʰ **861 Injury to heart and lung**
EXCLUDES *injury to blood vessels of thorax (901.0-901.9)*

✓5ᵗʰ **861.0 Heart, without mention of open wound into thorax**
AHA: 1Q, '92, 9

    861.00 Unspecified injury   CC
    CC Excl: 861.00-861.13, 862.29, 862.39-862.9, 959.9

    861.01 Contusion   CC
    Cardiac contusion
    Myocardial contusion
    DEF: Bruising within the pericardium with no mention of open wound.
    CC Excl: 861.00-861.13, 862.29, 862.39-862.9, 875.0-875.1, 879.8-879.9, 929.0-929.9, 958.7-958.99, 959.8-959.9

    861.02 Laceration without penetration of heart chambers   MCC
    DEF: Tearing injury of heart tissue, without penetration of chambers; no open wound.
    CC Excl: See code 861.01

    861.03 Laceration with penetration of heart chambers   MCC
    CC Excl: See code 861.01

✓5ᵗʰ **861.1 Heart, with open wound into thorax**

    861.10 Unspecified injury   MCC
    CC Excl: See code 861.01

    861.11 Contusion   MCC
    CC Excl: See code 861.01

---

¹⁰   HAC = only for valid CC or MCC codes.
§   Requires fifth digit. Valid digits are in [brackets] under each code. See beginning of section 850–854 for codes and definitions.

N Newborn Age: 0   P Pediatric Age: 0-17   M Maternity Age: 12-55   A Adult Age: 15-124   MCC Major CC Condition   CC CC Condition   HIV HIV Related Dx

314 – Volume 1   2014 ICD-9-CM

861.12 Laceration without penetration of heart chambers `MCC`
CC Exd: See code 861.01

861.13 Laceration with penetration of heart chambers `MCC`
CC Exd: See code 861.01

√5ᵗʰ **861.2 Lung, without mention of open wound into thorax**

861.20 Unspecified injury `CC`
CC Exd: 861.20-861.32, 862.29, 862.39-862.9, 875.0-875.1, 879.8-879.9, 929.0-929.9, 958.7-958.8, 958.99, 959.8-959.9

861.21 Contusion `CC`
DEF: Bruising of lung without mention of open wound.
CC Exd: See code: 861.20
S27.321A Contusion of lung unilateral initial encounter `I-10`

861.22 Laceration `MCC`
CC Exd: 861.20-861.32, 862.29, 862.39-862.9, 875.0-875.1, 879.8-879.9, 929.0-929.9, 958.7-958.99, 959.8-959.9

√5ᵗʰ **861.3 Lung, with open wound into thorax**

861.30 Unspecified injury `MCC`
CC Exd: See code 861.22

861.31 Contusion `MCC`
CC Exd: See code 861.22

861.32 Laceration `MCC`
CC Exd: See code 861.22

√4ᵗʰ **862 Injury to other and unspecified intrathoracic organs**
EXCLUDES injury to blood vessels of thorax (901.0-901.9)

862.0 Diaphragm, without mention of open wound into cavity `CC`
CC Exd: 862.0-862.1, 862.29, 862.39-862.9, 875.0-875.1, 879.8-879.9, 929.0-929.9, 958.7-958.8, 958.99, 959.8-959.9

862.1 Diaphragm, with open wound into cavity `MCC`
CC Exd: 862.0-862.1, 862.29, 862.39-862.9, 875.0-875.1, 879.8-879.9, 929.0-929.9, 958.7-958.99, 959.8-959.9

862.2 Other specified intrathoracic organs, without mention of open wound into cavity

862.21 Bronchus `MCC`
CC Exd: 862.21, 862.29-862.31, 862.39-862.9, 875.0-875.1, 879.8-879.9, 929.0-929.9, 958.7-958.8, 959.8-959.9

862.22 Esophagus `MCC`
CC Exd: 862.22-862.29, 862.32-862.9, 875.0-875.1, 879.8-879.9, 929.0-929.9, 958.7-958.99, 959.8-959.9

862.29 Other `CC`
Pleura   Thymus gland
CC Exd: 862.29, 862.39-862.9, 875.0-875.1, 879.8-879.9, 929.0-929.9, 958.7-958.99, 959.8-959.9

√5ᵗʰ **862.3 Other specified intrathoracic organs, with open wound into cavity**

862.31 Bronchus `MCC`
CC Exd: See code: 862.21

862.32 Esophagus `MCC`
CC Exd: See code: 862.22

862.39 Other `MCC`
CC Exd: See code: 862.29

862.8 Multiple and unspecified intrathoracic organs, without mention of open wound into cavity `CC`
Crushed chest
Multiple intrathoracic organs
CC Exd: 862.29, 862.39-862.9, 875.0-875.1, 879.8-879.9, 929.0-929.9, 958.7-958.8, 958.93-958.99, 959.8-959.9

862.9 Multiple and unspecified intrathoracic organs, with open wound into cavity `MCC`
CC Exd: See code: 862.29

√4ᵗʰ **863 Injury to gastrointestinal tract**
EXCLUDES anal sphincter laceration during delivery (664.2)
bile duct (868.0-868.1 with fifth-digit 2)
gallbladder (868.0-868.1 with fifth-digit 2)

863.0 Stomach, without mention of open wound into cavity `CC`
CC Exd: 729.73, 863.0-863.1, 863.80, 863.89-863.90, 863.99, 868.00, 868.03-868.10, 868.13-869.1, 879.2-879.9, 929.0-929.9, 958.8, 958.93-958.99, 959.8-959.9

863.1 Stomach, with open wound into cavity `MCC`
CC Exd: 863.0-863.1, 863.80, 863.89-863.90, 863.99, 868.00, 868.03-868.10, 868.13-869.1, 879.2-879.9, 929.0-929.9, 958.8-958.99, 959.8-959.9

√5ᵗʰ **863.2 Small intestine, without mention of open wound into cavity**

863.20 Small intestine, unspecified site `CC`
CC Exd: 729.73, 863.20-863.39, 863.80, 863.89-863.90, 863.99, 868.00, 868.03-868.10, 868.13-869.1, 879.2-879.9, 929.0-929.9, 958.8, 958.93-958.99, 959.8-959.9

863.21 Duodenum `CC`
CC Exd: See code: 863.20

863.29 Other `CC`
CC Exd: See code: 863.20

√5ᵗʰ **863.3 Small intestine, with open wound into cavity**

863.30 Small intestine, unspecified site `MCC`
CC Exd: 863.20-863.39, 863.80, 863.89-863.90, 863.99, 868.00, 868.03-868.10, 868.13-869.1, 879.2-879.9, 929.0-929.9, 958.8-958.99, 959.8-959.9

863.31 Duodenum `MCC`
CC Exd: 863.21, 863.31-863.39, 863.80, 863.89-863.90, 863.99, 868.00, 868.03-868.10, 868.13-869.1, 879.2-879.9, 929.0-929.9, 958.8-958.99, 959.8-959.9

863.39 Other `MCC`
CC Exd: See code: 863.30

√5ᵗʰ **863.4 Colon or rectum, without mention of open wound into cavity**

863.40 Colon, unspecified site `CC`
CC Exd: 729.73, 863.40-863.80, 863.89-863.90, 863.99, 868.00, 868.03-868.10, 868.13-869.1, 879.2-879.9, 929.0-929.9, 958.8, 958.93-958.99, 959.8-959.9

863.41 Ascending [right] colon `CC`
CC Exd: See code: 863.40

863.42 Transverse colon `CC`
CC Exd: See code: 863.40

863.43 Descending [left] colon `CC`
CC Exd: See code: 863.40

863.44 Sigmoid colon `CC`
CC Exd: See code: 863.40

863.45 Rectum `CC`
CC Exd: See code: 863.40

863.46 Multiple sites in colon and rectum `CC`
CC Exd: See code: 863.40

863.49 Other `CC`
CC Exd: See code: 863.40

√5ᵗʰ **863.5 Colon or rectum, with open wound into cavity**

863.50 Colon, unspecified site `MCC`
CC Exd: 863.40-863.80, 863.89-863.90, 863.99, 868.00, 868.03-868.10, 868.13-869.1, 879.2-879.9, 929.0-929.9, 958.8-958.99, 959.8-959.9

863.51 Ascending [right] colon `MCC`
CC Exd: See code 863.50

863.52 Transverse colon `MCC`
CC Exd: See code 863.50

863.53 Descending [left] colon `MCC`
CC Exd: See code 863.50

863.54 Sigmoid colon `MCC`
CC Exd: See code 863.50

863.55 Rectum `MCC`
CC Exd: See code 863.50

863.56 Multiple sites in colon and rectum `MCC`
CC Exd: See code 863.50

█ Additional Digit Required   Unacceptable PDx   Manifestation Code   Hospital Acquired Condition   ▶◀ Revised Text   ● New Code   ▲ Revised Code Title

863.59 Other `MCC`
CC Excl: See code 863.50

√5ᵗʰ **863.8 Other and unspecified gastrointestinal sites, without mention of open wound into cavity**

863.80 Gastrointestinal tract, unspecified site `CC`
CC Excl: 729.73, 863.0-863.80, 863.89-863.90, 863.99, 868.00, 868.03-868.10, 868.13-869.1, 879.2-879.9, 929.0-929.9, 958.8, 958.93-958.99, 959.8-959.9

863.81 Pancreas, head `CC`
CC Excl: 729.73, 863.80-863.84, 863.91-863.94, 863.99, 868.00, 868.03-868.10, 868.13-869.1, 879.2-879.9, 929.0-929.9, 958.8, 958.93-958.99, 959.8-959.9

863.82 Pancreas, body `CC`
CC Excl: See code: 863.81

863.83 Pancreas, tail `CC`
CC Excl: See code: 863.81

863.84 Pancreas, multiple and unspecified sites `CC`
CC Excl: See code: 863.81

863.85 Appendix `CC`
CC Excl: 729.73, 863.40-863.80, 863.85-863.90, 863.99, 868.00, 868.03-868.10, 868.13-869.1, 879.2-879.9, 929.0-929.9, 958.8, 958.93-958.99, 959.8-959.9

863.89 Other `CC`
Intestine NOS
CC Excl: 729.73, 863.0-863.84, 863.89-863.94, 863.99, 868.00, 868.03-868.10, 868.13-869.1, 879.2-879.9, 929.0-929.9, 958.8, 958.93-958.90, 958.93-958.99, 959.8-959.9

√5ᵗʰ **863.9 Other and unspecified gastrointestinal sites, with open wound into cavity**

863.90 Gastrointestinal tract, unspecified site `MCC`
CC Excl: 863.80-863.84, 863.89-863.94, 863.99, 868.00, 868.03-868.10, 868.13-869.1, 879.2-879.9, 929.0-929.9, 958.8-958.99, 959.8-959.9

863.91 Pancreas, head `MCC`
CC Excl: 863.80-863.84, 863.91-863.94, 863.99, 868.00, 868.03-868.10, 868.13-869.1, 879.2-879.9, 929.0-929.9, 958.8-958.99, 959.8-959.9

863.92 Pancreas, body `MCC`
CC Excl: See code 863.91

863.93 Pancreas, tail `MCC`
CC Excl: See code 863.91

863.94 Pancreas, multiple and unspecified sites `MCC`
CC Excl: See code 863.91

863.95 Appendix `MCC`
CC Excl: 863.80, 863.85, 863.95-863.99, 868.00, 868.03-868.10, 868.13-869.1, 879.2-879.9, 929.0-929.9, 958.8-958.99, 959.8-959.9

863.99 Other `MCC`
CC Excl: 863.80, 863.99, 868.00, 868.03-868.10, 868.13-869.1, 879.2-879.9, 929.0-929.9, 958.8-958.99, 959.8-959.9

√4ᵗʰ **864 Injury to liver**

The following fifth-digit subclassification is for use with category 864:
0 **unspecified injury**
1 **hematoma and contusion**
2 **laceration, minor**
Laceration involving capsule only, or without significant involvement of hepatic parenchyma [i.e., less than 1 cm deep]
3 **laceration, moderate**
Laceration involving parenchyma but without major disruption of parenchyma [i.e., less than 10 cm long and less than 3 cm deep]
4 **laceration, major**
Laceration with significant disruption of hepatic parenchyma [i.e., 10 cm long and 3 cm deep]
Multiple moderate lacerations, with or without hematoma
Stellate lacerations of liver
5 **laceration, unspecified**
9 **other**

§ √5ᵗʰ **864.0 Without mention of open wound** `MCC 3-4` `CC 0-2, 5, 9`
[0-5, 9] **into cavity**
CC Excl: 863.80, 863.99-864.19, 868.00, 868.03-868.10, 868.13-869.1, 879.2-879.9, 929.0-929.9, 958.8-958.99, 959.8-959.9

§ √5ᵗʰ **864.1 With open wound into cavity** `MCC`
[0-5, 9] CC Excl: See code 864.0

√4ᵗʰ **865 Injury to spleen**

The following fifth-digit subclassification is for use with category 865:
0 **unspecified injury**
1 **hematoma without rupture of capsule**
2 **capsular tears, without major disruption of parenchyma**
3 **laceration extending into parenchyma**
4 **massive parenchymal disruption**
9 **other**

§ √5ᵗʰ **865.0 Without mention of wound into** `MCC 3-4` `CC 0-2, 9`
[0-4, 9] **cavity**
CC Excl: 865.00-865.19, 868.00, 868.03-868.10, 868.13-869.1, 879.2-879.9, 929.0-929.9, 958.8-958.99, 959.8-959.9

§ √5ᵗʰ **865.1 With open wound into cavity** `MCC`
[0-4, 9] CC Excl: See code 865.0

√4ᵗʰ **866 Injury to kidney**
EXCLUDES acute kidney injury (nontraumatic) (584.9)
AHA: 4Q, '08, 192

The following fifth-digit subclassification is for use with category 866:
0 **unspecified injury**
1 **hematoma without rupture of capsule**
2 **laceration**
3 **complete disruption of kidney parenchyma**

§ √5ᵗʰ **866.0 Without mention of open wound** `MCC 3` `CC 0-2`
[0-3] **into cavity**
CC Excl: 866.00-866.13, 868.00, 868.03-868.10, 868.13-869.1, 879.2-879.9, 929.0-929.9, 958.8-958.99, 959.8-959.9

§ √5ᵗʰ **866.1 With open wound into cavity** `MCC`
[0-3] CC Excl: See code 866.0

√4ᵗʰ **867 Injury to pelvic organs**
EXCLUDES injury during delivery (664.0-665.9)

867.0 Bladder and urethra, without mention of open wound `CC`
into cavity
CC Excl: 867.0-867.1, 867.6-868.00, 868.03-868.10, 868.13- 869.1, 879.2-879.9, 929.0-929.9, 958.8-958.99, 959.8-959.9
AHA: N-D, '85, 15
TIP: Assign for urethral injury due to senile patient's pulling out indwelling urinary catheter.
S37.20xA Unspecified injury of bladder initial encounter `I-10`

867.1 Bladder and urethra, with open wound into cavity `MCC`
CC Excl: See code 867.0

867.2 Ureter, without mention of open wound into cavity `CC`
CC Excl: 867.2-867.3, 867.6-868.00, 868.03-868.10, 868.13- 869.1, 879.2-879.9, 929.0-929.9, 958.8-958.99, 959.8-959.9

867.3 Ureter, with open wound into cavity `MCC`
CC Excl: See code 867.2

867.4 Uterus, without mention of open wound into cavity `CC` `♀`
CC Excl: 867.4-868.00, 868.03-868.10, 868.13-869.1, 879.2-879.9, 929.0-929.9, 958.8-958.99, 959.8-959.9

867.5 Uterus, with open wound into cavity `MCC` `♀`
CC Excl: See code 867.4

867.6 Other specified pelvic organs, without mention of open `CC`
wound into cavity
Fallopian tube   Seminal vesicle
Ovary   Vas deferens
Prostate
CC Excl: 867.6-868.00, 868.03-868.10, 868.13-869.1, 879.2-879.9, 929.0-929.9, 958.8-958.99, 959.8-959.9

867.7 Other specified pelvic organs, with open `MCC`
wound into cavity
CC Excl: See code 867.6

867.8 Unspecified pelvic organ, without mention `CC`
of open wound into cavity
CC Excl: See code 867.6

867.9 Unspecified pelvic organ, with open wound into cavity `MCC`
CC Excl: See code 867.6

---

§   Requires fifth digit. Valid digits are in [brackets] under each code. See appropriate category for codes and definitions.

`N` Newborn Age: 0   `P` Pediatric Age: 0-17   `M` Maternity Age: 12-55   `A` Adult Age: 15-124   `MCC` Major CC Condition   `CC` CC Condition   `HIV` HIV Related Dx

316 – Volume 1   **2014 ICD-9-CM**

☑4ᵗʰ **868 Injury to other intra-abdominal organs**

The following fifth-digit subclassification is for use with category 868:
- **0** unspecified intra-abdominal organ
- **1** adrenal gland
- **2** bile duct and gallbladder
- **3** peritoneum
- **4** retroperitoneum
- **9** other and multiple intra-abdominal organs

§ ☑5ᵗʰ **868.0 Without mention of open wound into cavity** `CC`
[0-4, 9] CC Excl: For codes 868.00, 868.03-863.09: 868.00, 868.03-868.10, 868.13-869.1, 879.2-879.9, 929.0-929.9, 958.8-958.99, 959.8-959.9; For code 868.01: 868.00-868.01, 868.03-868.11, 868.13-869.1, 879.2-879.9, 929.0-929.9, 958.8-958.99, 959.8- 959.9; For code 868.02: 868.00, 868.02-868.10, 868.13-869.1, 879.2-879.9, 929.0-929.9, 958.8-958.99, 959.8-959.9

§ ☑5ᵗʰ **868.1 With open wound into cavity** `MCC`
[0-4, 9] CC Excl: For codes 868.10, 868.13-868.19: 868.00, 868.03-868.10, 868.13-869.1, 879.2-879.9, 929.0-929.9, 958.8-958.99, 959.8-959.9; For code 868.11: 868.00-868.01, 868.03-868.11, 868.13-869.1, 879.2-879.9, 929.0-929.9, 958.8-958.99, 959.8- 959.9; For code 868.12: 868.00, 868.03-868.10, 868.12-869.1, 879.2-879.9, 929.0-929.9, 958.8-958.99, 959.8-959.9

☑4ᵗʰ **869 Internal injury to unspecified or ill-defined organs**

INCLUDES internal injury NOS
multiple internal injury NOS

869.0 Without mention of open wound into cavity `CC`
CC Excl: 868.00, 868.03-868.10, 868.13-869.1, 879.2-879.9, 929.0-929.9, 958.8-958.99, 959.8-959.9

869.1 With open wound into cavity `MCC`
CC Excl: See code: 869.0
AHA: 2Q, '89, 15

Open Wound (870-897)

INCLUDES animal bite
avulsion
cut
laceration
puncture wound
traumatic amputation

EXCLUDES *burn (940.0-949.5)*
crushing (925.0-929.9)
puncture of internal organs (860.0-869.1)
superficial injury (910.0-919.9)
that incidental to:
dislocation (830.0-839.9)
fracture (800.0-829.1)
internal injury (860.0-869.1)
intracranial injury (851.0-854.1)

NOTE The description "complicated" used in the fourth-digit subdivisions includes those with mention of delayed healing, delayed treatment, foreign body, or infection.
AHA: 4Q, '01, 52

TIP: Do not assign a code designated as "complicated" based only on physician documentation of complicated. For coding purposes, there must be indications of delayed healing, delayed treatment, infection, or foreign body.

Open Wound of Head, Neck, and Trunk (870-879)

☑4ᵗʰ **870 Open wound of ocular adnexa**

870.0 Laceration of skin of eyelid and periocular area

870.1 Laceration of eyelid, full-thickness, not involving lacrimal passages

870.2 Laceration of eyelid involving lacrimal passages `CC`
CC Excl: 870.0-871.9, 879.8-879.9, 929.0-929.9, 958.8, 959.8-959.9

870.3 Penetrating wound of orbit, without mention of foreign body `CC`
CC Excl: 870.0-871.9, 879.8-879.9, 929.0-929.9, 958.8-958.99, 959.8-959.9

870.4 Penetrating wound of orbit with foreign body `CC`
EXCLUDES *retained (old) foreign body in orbit (376.6)*
CC Excl: See code 870.3

870.8 Other specified open wounds of ocular adnexa `CC`
CC Excl: See code 870.3

870.9 Unspecified open wound of ocular adnexa `CC`
CC Excl: See code 870.3

☑4ᵗʰ **871 Open wound of eyeball**
EXCLUDES *2nd cranial nerve [optic] injury (950.0-950.9)*
3rd cranial nerve [oculomotor] injury (951.0)

871.0 Ocular laceration without prolapse of intraocular tissue `CC`
DEF: Tear in ocular tissue without displacing structures.
CC Excl: See code 870.3
AHA: 3Q, '96, 7

871.1 Ocular laceration with prolapse or exposure of intraocular tissue `CC`
CC Excl: See code 870.3

871.2 Rupture of eye with partial loss of intraocular tissue `CC`
DEF: Forcible tearing of eyeball, with tissue loss.
CC Excl: See code 870.3

871.3 Avulsion of eye `CC`
Traumatic enucleation
DEF: Traumatic extraction of eyeball from socket.
CC Excl: See code 870.3

871.4 Unspecified laceration of eye

871.5 Penetration of eyeball with magnetic foreign body `CC`
EXCLUDES *retained (old) magnetic foreign body in globe (360.50-360.59)*
CC Excl: 870.0-871.9, 879.8-879.9, 929.0-929.9, 958.8, 959.8-959.9

871.6 Penetration of eyeball with (nonmagnetic) foreign body `CC`
EXCLUDES *retained (old) (nonmagnetic) foreign body in globe (360.60-360.69)*
CC Excl: 870.0-871.9, 879.8-879.9, 929.0-929.9, 958.8, 959.8-959.9

871.7 Unspecified ocular penetration

871.9 Unspecified open wound of eyeball `CC`
CC Excl: See code: 870.3

☑4ᵗʰ **872 Open wound of ear**

☑5ᵗʰ **872.0 External ear, without mention of complication**

872.00 External ear, unspecified site

872.01 Auricle, ear
Pinna
DEF: Open wound of fleshy, outer ear.

872.02 Auditory canal
DEF: Open wound of passage from external ear to eardrum.

☑5ᵗʰ **872.1 External ear, complicated**

872.10 External ear, unspecified site

872.11 Auricle, ear

872.12 Auditory canal `CC`
CC Excl: 872.00-872.9, 879.8-879.9, 929.0-929.9, 958.8, 959.8-959.9

☑5ᵗʰ **872.6 Other specified parts of ear, without mention of complication**

872.61 Ear drum `CC`
Drumhead
Tympanic membrane
CC Excl: See code: 872.12

872.62 Ossicles `CC`
CC Excl: See code: 872.12

872.63 Eustachian tube `CC`
DEF: Open wound of channel between nasopharynx and tympanic cavity.
CC Excl: See code: 872.12

872.64 Cochlea `CC`
DEF: Open wound of snail shell shaped tube of inner ear.
CC Excl: See code: 872.12

872.69 Other and multiple sites `CC`
CC Excl: See code 872.12

☑5ᵗʰ **872.7 Other specified parts of ear, complicated**

872.71 Ear drum `CC`
CC Excl: See code: 872.12

⚹ Requires fifth digit. Valid digits are in [brackets] under each code. See category 868 for codes and definitions.

| 4ᵗʰ 5ᵗʰ Additional Digit Required | Unacceptable PDx | Manifestation Code | Hospital Acquired Condition | ►◄ Revised Text | ● New Code | ▲ Revised Code Title |

Injury and Poisoning

872.72–875.1

872.72 Ossicles `CC`
CC Exd: 872.00-872.9, 879.8-879.9, 929.0-929.9, 958.8-958.99, 959.8-959.9

872.73 Eustachian tube `CC`
CC Exd: See code 872.72

872.74 Cochlea `CC`
CC Exd: See code 872.72

872.79 Other and multiple sites `CC`
CC Exd: See code: 872.12

872.8 Ear, part unspecified, without mention of complication
Ear NOS

872.9 Ear, part unspecified, complicated

√4ᵗʰ **873 Other open wound of head**

873.0 Scalp, without mention of complication
S01.01xA Laceration w/o foreign body scalp initial enc `I-10`

873.1 Scalp, complicated

√6ᵗʰ **873.2 Nose, without mention of complication**

873.20 Nose, unspecified site

873.21 Nasal septum
DEF: Open wound between nasal passages.

873.22 Nasal cavity
DEF: Open wound of nostrils.

873.23 Nasal sinus `CC`
DEF: Open wound of mucous-lined respiratory cavities.
CC Exd: 873.20-873.39, 879.8-879.9, 929.0-929.9, 958.8, 959.8-959.9

873.29 Multiple sites

√5ᵗʰ **873.3 Nose, complicated**

873.30 Nose, unspecified site

873.31 Nasal septum

873.32 Nasal cavity

873.33 Nasal sinus `CC`
CC Exd: 873.20-873.39, 879.8-879.9, 929.0-929.9, 958.8-958.99, 959.8-959.9

873.39 Multiple sites

√6ᵗʰ **873.4 Face, without mention of complication**

873.40 Face, unspecified site

873.41 Cheek

873.42 Forehead
Eyebrow
AHA: 4Q, '96, 43
S01.81xA Laceration w/o FB other part head initial enc `I-10`

873.43 Lip

873.44 Jaw

873.49 Other and multiple sites

√6ᵗʰ **873.5 Face, complicated**

873.50 Face, unspecified site

873.51 Cheek

873.52 Forehead

873.53 Lip

873.54 Jaw

873.59 Other and multiple sites

√6ᵗʰ **873.6 Internal structures of mouth, without mention of complication**

873.60 Mouth, unspecified site

873.61 Buccal mucosa
DEF: Open wound of inside of cheek.

873.62 Gum (alveolar process)

873.63 Tooth (broken) (fractured) (due to trauma)
EXCLUDES cracked tooth (521.81)
AHA: 1Q, '04, 17

873.64 Tongue and floor of mouth

873.65 Palate
DEF: Open wound of roof of mouth.

873.69 Other and multiple sites

√5ᵗʰ **873.7 Internal structures of mouth, complicated**

873.70 Mouth, unspecified site

873.71 Buccal mucosa

873.72 Gum (alveolar process)

873.73 Tooth (broken) (fractured) (due to trauma)
EXCLUDES cracked tooth (521.81)
AHA: 1Q, '04, 17

873.74 Tongue and floor of mouth

873.75 Palate

873.79 Other and multiple sites

873.8 Other and unspecified open wound of head without mention of complication
Head NOS

873.9 Other and unspecified open wound of head, complicated

√4ᵗʰ **874 Open wound of neck**

√5ᵗʰ **874.0 Larynx and trachea, without mention of complication**

874.00 Larynx with trachea `MCC`
CC Exd: 847.0, 874.00-874.12, 874.8-874.9, 879.8-879.9, 929.0-929.9, 958.8-958.99, 959.8-959.9

874.01 Larynx `MCC`
CC Exd: See code 874.00

874.02 Trachea `MCC`
CC Exd: See code 874.00

√5ᵗʰ **874.1 Larynx and trachea, complicated**

874.10 Larynx with trachea `MCC`
CC Exd: See code 874.00

874.11 Larynx `MCC`
CC Exd: See code 874.00

874.12 Trachea `MCC`
CC Exd: See code 874.00

874.2 Thyroid gland, without mention of complication `CC`
CC Exd: 847.0, 874.2-874.3, 874.8-874.9, 879.8-879.9, 929.0-929.9, 958.8, 959.8-959.9

874.3 Thyroid gland, complicated `CC`
CC Exd: 847.0, 874.2-874.3, 874.8-874.9, 879.8-879.9, 929.0-929.9, 958.8-958.99, 959.8-959.9

874.4 Pharynx, without mention of complication `CC`
Cervical esophagus
CC Exd: 847.0, 874.4-874.9, 879.8-879.9, 929.0-929.9, 958.8, 959.8-959.9

874.5 Pharynx, complicated `CC`
CC Exd: 847.0, 874.4-874.9, 879.8-879.9, 929.0-929.9, 958.8-958.99, 959.8-959.9

874.8 Other and unspecified parts, without mention of complication
Nape of neck
Supraclavicular region
Throat NOS

874.9 Other and unspecified parts, complicated

√4ᵗʰ **875 Open wound of chest (wall)**
EXCLUDES open wound into thoracic cavity (860.0-862.9)
traumatic pneumothorax and hemothorax (860.1, 860.3, 860.5)
AHA: 3Q, '95, 17; 3Q, '93, 17

875.0 Without mention of complication `CC`
CC Exd: 847.1, 862.29, 862.39-862.9, 875.0-875.1, 879.8-879.9, 929.0-929.9, 958.7-958.99, 959.8-959.9

875.1 Complicated `CC`
CC Exd: See code 875.0

`N` Newborn Age: 0   `P` Pediatric Age: 0-17   `M` Maternity Age: 12-55   `A` Adult Age: 15-124   `MCC` Major CC Condition   `CC` CC Condition   `HIV` HIV Related Dx

318 – Volume 1   2014 ICD-9-CM

☑4ᵗʰ **876 Open wound of back**

    INCLUDES loin
                 lumbar region
    EXCLUDES open wound into thoracic cavity (860.0-862.9)
                 traumatic pneumothorax and hemothorax (860.1, 860.3,
                     860.5)

    876.0 Without mention of complication

    876.1 Complicated

☑4ᵗʰ **877 Open wound of buttock**

    INCLUDES sacroiliac region

    877.0 Without mention of complication

    877.1 Complicated

☑4ᵗʰ **878 Open wound of genital organs (external), including traumatic amputation**

    EXCLUDES injury during delivery (664.0-665.9)
                 internal genital organs (867.0-867.9)

    878.0 Penis, without mention of complication ♂

    878.1 Penis, complicated ♂

    878.2 Scrotum and testes, without mention of complication ♂

    878.3 Scrotum and testes, complicated ♂

    878.4 Vulva, without mention of complication ♀
        Labium (majus) (minus)

    878.5 Vulva, complicated ♀

    878.6 Vagina, without mention of complication ♀

    878.7 Vagina, complicated ♀

    878.8 Other and unspecified parts, without mention of complication

    878.9 Other and unspecified parts, complicated

☑4ᵗʰ **879 Open wound of other and unspecified sites, except limbs**

    879.0 Breast, without mention of complication

    879.1 Breast, complicated

    879.2 Abdominal wall, anterior, without mention of complication
        Abdominal wall NOS
        Epigastric region
        Hypogastric region
        Pubic region
        Umbilical region
        AHA: 2Q, '91, 22; 3Q, '90, 5
        TIP: If the abdominal wall open wound results in aortic rupture, sequence code 902.0 first.

    879.3 Abdominal wall, anterior, complicated

    879.4 Abdominal wall, lateral, without mention of complication
        Flank
        Groin
        Hypochondrium
        Iliac (region)
        Inguinal region

    879.5 Abdominal wall, lateral, complicated

    879.6 Other and unspecified parts of trunk, without mention of complication
        Pelvic region
        Perineum
        Trunk NOS

    879.7 Other and unspecified parts of trunk, complicated

    879.8 Open wound(s) (multiple) of unspecified site(s) without mention of complication
        Multiple open wounds NOS
        Open wound NOS

    879.9 Open wound(s) (multiple) of unspecified site(s), complicated

Open Wound of Upper Limb (880-887)

AHA: N-D, '85, 5
TIP: For degloving injuries, assign code for open wound of the specified site, most often involving extremities.

☑4ᵗʰ **880 Open wound of shoulder and upper arm**

    The following fifth-digit subclassification is for use with category 880:
        0 shoulder region
        1 scapular region
        2 axillary region
        3 upper arm
        9 multiple sites

§ ☑5ᵗʰ **880.0 Without mention of complication**
        [0-3,9]

§ ☑5ᵗʰ **880.1 Complicated**
        [0-3,9]   AHA: For code 880.13: 2Q, '06, 7

§ ☑5ᵗʰ **880.2 With tendon involvement**   CC
        [0-3,9]   CC Excl: 880.00-880.29

☑4ᵗʰ **881 Open wound of elbow, forearm, and wrist**

    The following fifth-digit subclassification is for use with category 881:
        0 forearm
        1 elbow
        2 wrist

§ ☑5ᵗʰ **881.0 Without mention of complication**
        [0-2]

§ ☑5ᵗʰ **881.1 Complicated**
        [0-2]

§ ☑5ᵗʰ **881.2 With tendon involvement**   CC
        [0-2]   CC Excl: 881.00-881.22

☑4ᵗʰ **882 Open wound of hand except finger(s) alone**

    882.0 Without mention of complication

    882.1 Complicated
        AHA: 4Q, '08, 152

    882.2 With tendon involvement   CC
        CC Excl: 882.0-882.2

☑4ᵗʰ **883 Open wound of finger(s)**

    INCLUDES fingernail
                 thumb (nail)

    883.0 Without mention of complication

    883.1 Complicated

    883.2 With tendon involvement   CC
        CC Excl: 883.0-883.2

☑4ᵗʰ **884 Multiple and unspecified open wound of upper limb**

    INCLUDES arm NOS
                 multiple sites of one upper limb
                 upper limb NOS

    884.0 Without mention of complication

    884.1 Complicated

    884.2 With tendon involvement   CC
        CC Excl: 884.0-884.2

☑4ᵗʰ **885 Traumatic amputation of thumb (complete) (partial)**

    INCLUDES thumb(s) (with finger(s) of either hand)

    885.0 Without mention of complication
        AHA: 1Q, '03, 7

    885.1 Complicated

☑4ᵗʰ **886 Traumatic amputation of other finger(s) (complete) (partial)**

    INCLUDES finger(s) of one or both hands, without mention of
                   thumb(s)

    886.0 Without mention of complication

    886.1 Complicated

☑4ᵗʰ **887 Traumatic amputation of arm and hand (complete) (partial)**

    887.0 Unilateral, below elbow, without mention   CC
        of complication
        CC Excl: 880.00-887.7, 929.0-929.9, 958.8-958.99, 959.8-959.9

§ Requires fifth digit. Valid digits are in [brackets] under each code. See appropriate category for codes and definitions.

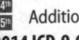

4ᵗʰ 5ᵗʰ Additional Digit Required	Unacceptable PDx	Manifestation Code	Hospital Acquired Condition	►◄ Revised Text	● New Code	▲ Revised Code Title

Injury and Poisoning

887.1 Unilateral, below elbow, complicated `CC`
CC Excd: See code 887.0

887.2 Unilateral, at or above elbow, without mention of complication `CC`
CC Excd: See code 887.0

887.3 Unilateral, at or above elbow, complicated `CC`
CC Excd: See code 887.0

887.4 Unilateral, level not specified, without mention of complication `CC`
CC Excd: See code 887.0

887.5 Unilateral, level not specified, complicated `CC`
CC Excd: See code 887.0

887.6 Bilateral [any level], without mention of complication `MCC`
One hand and other arm
CC Excd: See code 887.0

887.7 Bilateral [any level], complicated `MCC`
CC Excd: See code 887.0

Open Wound of Lower Limb (890-897)
AHA: N-D, '85, 5

√4th **890 Open wound of hip and thigh**

890.0 Without mention of complication

890.1 Complicated

890.2 With tendon involvement `CC`
CC Excd: 890.0-890.2

√4th **891 Open wound of knee, leg [except thigh], and ankle**
INCLUDES leg NOS
multiple sites of leg, except thigh
EXCLUDES that of thigh (890.0-890.2)
with multiple sites of lower limb (894.0-894.2)

891.0 Without mention of complication
S81.031A Puncture wound w/o FB rt knee initial encounter `I-10`

891.1 Complicated

891.2 With tendon involvement `CC`
CC Excd: 891.0-891.2

√4th **892 Open wound of foot except toe(s) alone**
INCLUDES heel

892.0 Without mention of complication

892.1 Complicated

892.2 With tendon involvement `CC`
CC Excd: 892.0-892.2

√4th **893 Open wound of toe(s)**
INCLUDES toenail

893.0 Without mention of complication

893.1 Complicated
AHA: 4Q, '08, 73

893.2 With tendon involvement `CC`
CC Excd: 893.0-893.2

√4th **894 Multiple and unspecified open wound of lower limb**
INCLUDES lower limb NOS
multiple sites of one lower limb, with thigh

894.0 Without mention of complication

894.1 Complicated

894.2 With tendon involvement `CC`
CC Excd: 894.0-894.2

√4th **895 Traumatic amputation of toe(s) (complete) (partial)**
INCLUDES toe(s) of one or both feet

895.0 Without mention of complication

895.1 Complicated

√4th **896 Traumatic amputation of foot (complete) (partial)**

896.0 Unilateral, without mention of complication `CC`
CC Excd: 890.0-897.7, 929.0-929.9, 958.8-958.99, 959.8-959.9

896.1 Unilateral, complicated `CC`
CC Excd: See code 896.0

896.2 Bilateral, without mention of complication `MCC`
EXCLUDES one foot and other leg (897.6-897.7)
CC Excd: See code 896.0

896.3 Bilateral, complicated `MCC`
CC Excd: See code 896.0

√4th **897 Traumatic amputation of leg(s) (complete) (partial)**

897.0 Unilateral, below knee, without mention of complication `CC`
CC Excd: See code 896.0

897.1 Unilateral, below knee, complicated `CC`
CC Excd: See code 896.0

897.2 Unilateral, at or above knee, without mention of complication `CC`
CC Excd: See code 896.0

897.3 Unilateral, at or above knee, complicated `CC`
CC Excd: See code 896.0

897.4 Unilateral, level not specified, without mention of complication `CC`
CC Excd: See code 896.0

897.5 Unilateral, level not specified, complicated `CC`
CC Excd: See code 896.0

897.6 Bilateral [any level], without mention of complication `MCC`
One foot and other leg
CC Excd: See code 896.0

897.7 Bilateral [any level], complicated `MCC`
CC Excd: See code 896.0
AHA: 3Q, '90, 5

Injury to Blood Vessels (900-904)
INCLUDES arterial hematoma
avulsion
cut   of blood vessel
laceration   secondary to other
rupture   injuries, e.g.;
traumatic aneurysm or fistula   fracture or open
(arteriovenous)   wound

EXCLUDES accidental puncture or laceration during medical procedure (998.2)
intracranial hemorrhage following injury (851.0-854.1)
AHA: 3Q, '90, 5

√4th **900 Injury to blood vessels of head and neck**

√5th **900.0 Carotid artery**

900.00 Carotid artery, unspecified `CC`
CC Excd: 900.00, 900.82-900.9, 904.9, 929.0-929.9, 958.8-958.99, 959.8-959.9

900.01 Common carotid artery `CC`
CC Excd: See code 900.00

900.02 External carotid artery `CC`
CC Excd: See code 900.00

900.03 Internal carotid artery `CC`
CC Excd: See code 900.00

900.1 Internal jugular vein `CC`
CC Excd: 900.82-900.9, 904.9, 929.0-929.9, 958.8-958.99, 959.8-959.9

√5th **900.8 Other specified blood vessels of head and neck**

900.81 External jugular vein `CC`
Jugular vein NOS
CC Excd: See code 900.1

900.82 Multiple blood vessels of head and neck `CC`
CC Excd: See code 900.1

900.89 Other `CC`
CC Excd: See code 900.1

900.9 Unspecified blood vessel of head and neck `CC`
CC Excd: See code 900.1

Injury and Poisoning

✓4ᵗʰ **901 Injury to blood vessels of thorax**

> EXCLUDES *traumatic hemothorax (860.2-860.5)*

901.0 Thoracic aorta   `MCC`
CC Exd: 901.0, 904.9, 929.0-929.9, 958.8-958.99, 959.8-959.9

901.1 Innominate and subclavian arteries   `MCC`
CC Exd: 901.1, 904.9, 929.0-929.9, 958.8-958.99, 959.8-959.9

901.2 Superior vena cava   `MCC`
CC Exd: 901.2, 904.9, 929.0-929.9, 958.8-958.99, 959.8-959.9

901.3 Innominate and subclavian veins   `MCC`
CC Exd: 901.3, 904.9, 929.0-929.9, 958.8-958.99, 959.8-959.9

✓5ᵗʰ **901.4 Pulmonary blood vessels**

901.40 Pulmonary vessel(s), unspecified   `MCC`
CC Exd: 901.40-901.41, 904.9, 929.0-929.9, 958.8-958.90, 958.99, 959.8-959.9

901.41 Pulmonary artery   `MCC`
CC Exd: 901.40-901.41, 904.9, 929.0-929.9, 958.8-958.99, 959.8-959.9

901.42 Pulmonary vein   `MCC`
CC Exd: 901.40, 901.42, 904.9, 929.0-929.9, 958.8-958.99, 959.8-959.9

✓5ᵗʰ **901.8 Other specified blood vessels of thorax**

901.81 Intercostal artery or vein   `CC`
CC Exd: 901.81, 901.83-901.89

901.82 Internal mammary artery or vein   `CC`
CC Exd: 901.82-901.89

901.83 Multiple blood vessels of thorax   `MCC`
CC Exd: 904.9, 929.0-929.9, 958.8-958.99, 959.8-959.9

901.89 Other   `CC`
Azygos vein
Hemiazygos vein
CC Exd: 901.0-901.9

901.9 Unspecified blood vessel of thorax   `CC`
CC Exd: See code: 901.89

✓4ᵗʰ **902 Injury to blood vessels of abdomen and pelvis**

902.0 Abdominal aorta   `MCC`
CC Exd: 902.0, 902.87-902.9, 904.9, 929.0-929.9, 958.8-958.99, 959.8-959.9

✓5ᵗʰ **902.1 Inferior vena cava**

902.10 Inferior vena cava, unspecified   `MCC`
CC Exd: 902.10, 902.87-902.9, 904.9, 929.0-929.9, 958.8-958.99, 959.8-959.9

902.11 Hepatic veins   `MCC`
CC Exd: 902.11, 902.87-902.9, 904.9, 929.0-929.9, 958.8-958.99, 959.8-959.9

902.19 Other   `MCC`
CC Exd: 902.19, 902.87-902.9, 904.9, 929.0-929.9, 958.8-958.99, 959.8-959.9

✓5ᵗʰ **902.2 Celiac and mesenteric arteries**

902.20 Celiac and mesenteric arteries, unspecified   `MCC`
CC Exd: 902.20, 902.87-902.9, 904.9, 929.0-929.9, 958.8-958.99, 959.8-959.9

902.21 Gastric artery   `MCC`
CC Exd: 902.21, 902.87-902.9, 904.9, 929.0-929.9, 958.8-958.90, 958.93-958.99, 959.8-959.9

902.22 Hepatic artery   `MCC`
CC Exd: 902.22, 902.87-902.9, 904.9, 929.0-929.9, 958.8-958.99, 959.8-959.9

902.23 Splenic artery   `MCC`
CC Exd: 902.23, 902.87-902.9, 904.9, 929.0-929.9, 958.8-958.90, 958.93-958.99, 959.8-959.9

902.24 Other specified branches of celiac axis   `MCC`
CC Exd: 902.24, 902.87-902.9, 904.9, 929.0-929.9, 958.8-958.99, 959.8-959.9

902.25 Superior mesenteric artery (trunk)   `MCC`
CC Exd: 902.25, 902.87-902.9, 904.9, 929.0-929.9, 958.8-958.99, 959.8-959.9

902.26 Primary branches of superior mesenteric artery   `MCC`
Ileocolic artery
CC Exd: 902.26, 902.87-902.9, 904.9, 929.0-929.9, 958.8-958.99, 959.8-959.9

902.27 Inferior mesenteric artery   `MCC`
CC Exd: 902.27, 902.87-902.9, 904.9, 929.0-929.9, 958.8-958.99, 959.8-959.9

902.29 Other   `MCC`
CC Exd: 902.29, 902.87-902.9, 904.9, 929.0-929.9, 958.8-958.99, 959.8-959.9

✓5ᵗʰ **902.3 Portal and splenic veins**

902.31 Superior mesenteric vein and primary subdivisions   `MCC`
Ileocolic vein
CC Exd: 902.31, 902.87-902.9, 904.9, 929.0-929.9, 958.8-958.99, 959.8-959.9

902.32 Inferior mesenteric vein   `MCC`
CC Exd: 902.32, 902.87-902.9, 904.9, 929.0-929.9, 958.8-958.99, 959.8-959.9

902.33 Portal vein   `MCC`
CC Exd: 902.33, 902.87-902.9, 904.9, 929.0-929.9, 958.8-958.99, 959.8-959.9

902.34 Splenic vein   `MCC`
CC Exd: 902.34, 902.87-902.9, 904.9, 929.0-929.9, 958.8-958.99, 959.8-959.9

902.39 Other   `MCC`
Cystic vein
Gastric vein
CC Exd: 902.39, 902.87-902.9, 904.9, 929.0-929.9, 958.8-958.99, 959.8-959.9

✓5ᵗʰ **902.4 Renal blood vessels**

902.40 Renal vessel(s), unspecified   `MCC`
CC Exd: 902.40, 902.87-902.9, 904.9, 929.0-929.9, 958.8-958.99, 959.8-959.9

902.41 Renal artery   `MCC`
CC Exd: 902.41, 902.87-902.9, 904.9, 929.0-929.9, 958.8-958.99, 959.8-959.9

902.42 Renal vein   `MCC`
CC Exd: 902.42, 902.87-902.9, 904.9, 929.0-929.9, 958.8-958.99, 959.8-959.9

902.49 Other   `MCC`
Suprarenal arteries
CC Exd: 902.49, 902.87-902.9, 904.9, 929.0-929.9, 958.8-958.99, 959.8-959.9

✓5ᵗʰ **902.5 Iliac blood vessels**

902.50 Iliac vessel(s), unspecified   `MCC`
CC Exd: 902.50, 902.53-902.54, 902.59, 902.87-902.9, 904.9, 929.0-929.9, 958.8-958.99, 959.8-959.9

902.51 Hypogastric artery   `MCC`
CC Exd: 902.51, 902.87-902.9, 904.9, 929.0-929.9, 958.8-958.99, 959.8-959.9

902.52 Hypogastric vein   `MCC`
CC Exd: 902.52, 902.87-902.9, 904.9, 929.0-929.9, 958.8-958.99, 959.8-959.9

902.53 Iliac artery   `MCC`
CC Exd: 902.50, 902.53, 902.59, 902.87-902.9, 904.9, 929.0-929.9, 958.8-958.99, 959.8-959.9

902.54 Iliac vein   `MCC`
CC Exd: 902.50, 902.54, 902.59, 902.87-902.9, 904.9, 929.0-929.9, 958.8-958.99, 959.8-959.9

902.55 Uterine artery   `CC` ♀
CC Exd: 902.55, 902.59, 902.87-902.9, 904.9, 929.0-929.9, 958.8-958.90, 958.93-958.99, 959.8-959.9

902.56 Uterine vein   `CC` ♀
CC Exd: 902.56-902.59, 902.87-902.9, 904.9, 929.0-929.9, 958.8-958.90, 958.93-958.99, 959.8-959.9

902.59 Other   `MCC`
CC Exd: See code: 902.50

4ᵗʰ
5ᵗʰ
Additional Digit Required   Unacceptable PDx   Manifestation Code   Hospital Acquired Condition   ▶◀ Revised Text   ● New Code   ▲ Revised Code Title

2014 ICD-9-CM   **Volume 1 – 321**

Injury and Poisoning

902.8–906.5

√5ᵗʰ **902.8 Other specified blood vessels of abdomen and pelvis**

     902.81 Ovarian artery   CC ♀
         CC Exd: 902.81, 902.87-902.9, 904.9, 929.0-929.9, 958.8-958.90, 958.93-958.99, 959.8-959.9

     902.82 Ovarian vein   CC ♀
         CC Exd: 902.82-902.9, 904.9, 929.0-929.9, 958.8-958.90, 958.93-958.99, 959.8-959.9

     902.87 Multiple blood vessels of abdomen and pelvis   MCC
         CC Exd: 902.87-902.9, 904.9, 929.0-929.9, 958.8-958.99, 959.8-959.9

     902.89 Other   CC
         CC Exd: 902.87-902.9, 904.9, 929.0-929.9, 958.8-958.90, 958.93-958.99, 959.8-959.9

   902.9 Unspecified blood vessel of abdomen and pelvis   CC
         CC Exd: 902.0-902.9, 904.9, 929.0-929.9, 958.8-958.90, 958.93-958.99, 959.8-959.9

√4ᵗʰ **903 Injury to blood vessels of upper extremity**

√5ᵗʰ **903.0 Axillary blood vessels**

     903.00 Axillary vessel(s), unspecified   MCC
         CC Exd: 903.00-903.02, 903.8-903.9, 904.9

     903.01 Axillary artery   MCC
         CC Exd: 903.00-903.01, 903.8-903.9, 904.9

     903.02 Axillary vein   MCC
         CC Exd: 903.00, 903.02, 903.8-903.9, 904.9

   903.1 Brachial blood vessels   CC
         CC Exd: 903.1, 903.8-903.9, 904.9

   903.2 Radial blood vessels   CC
         CC Exd: 903.2, 903.8-903.9, 904.9

   903.3 Ulnar blood vessels   CC
         CC Exd: 903.3, 903.8-903.9, 904.9

   903.4 Palmar artery   CC
         CC Exd: 903.4, 903.8-903.9, 904.9

   903.5 Digital blood vessels   CC
         CC Exd: 903.5-903.9, 904.9

   903.8 Other specified blood vessels of upper extremity   CC
         Multiple blood vessels of upper extremity
         CC Exd: 903.3-903.9, 904.9

   903.9 Unspecified blood vessel of upper extremity   CC
         CC Exd: See code: 903.8

√4ᵗʰ **904 Injury to blood vessels of lower extremity and unspecified sites**

   904.0 Common femoral artery   MCC
         Femoral artery above profunda origin
         CC Exd: 904.0, 904.7-904.9

   904.1 Superficial femoral artery   MCC
         CC Exd: 904.1, 904.7-904.9

   904.2 Femoral veins   MCC
         CC Exd: 904.2, 904.7-904.9

   904.3 Saphenous veins   CC
         Saphenous vein (greater) (lesser)
         CC Exd: 904.3, 904.7-904.9

√5ᵗʰ **904.4 Popliteal blood vessels**

     904.40 Popliteal vessel(s), unspecified   MCC
         CC Exd: 904.40, 904.7-904.9

     904.41 Popliteal artery   MCC
         CC Exd: 904.41, 904.7-904.9

     904.42 Popliteal vein   MCC
         CC Exd: 904.42, 904.7-904.9

√5ᵗʰ **904.5 Tibial blood vessels**

     904.50 Tibial vessel(s), unspecified   CC
         CC Exd: 904.50, 904.7-904.9

     904.51 Anterior tibial artery   CC
         CC Exd: 904.51, 904.7-904.9

     904.52 Anterior tibial vein   CC
         CC Exd: 904.52, 904.7-904.9

     904.53 Posterior tibial artery   CC
         CC Exd: 904.53, 904.7-904.9

     904.54 Posterior tibial vein   CC
         CC Exd: 904.54, 904.7-904.9

   904.6 Deep plantar blood vessels   CC
         CC Exd: 904.6-904.9

   904.7 Other specified blood vessels of lower extremity   CC
         Multiple blood vessels of lower extremity
         CC Exd: 729.72, 904.0-904.9

   904.8 Unspecified blood vessel of lower extremity   CC
         CC Exd: See code: 904.7

   904.9 Unspecified site   CC
         Injury to blood vessel NOS
         CC Exd: 729.71-729.72, 900.00-904.9

Late Effects Of Injuries, Poisonings, Toxic Effects, and Other External Causes (905-909)

NOTE These categories are to be used to indicate conditions classifiable to 800-999 as the cause of late effects, which are themselves classified elsewhere. The "late effects" include those specified as such, or as sequelae, which may occur at any time after the acute injury.

√4ᵗʰ **905 Late effects of musculoskeletal and connective tissue injuries**
     AHA: 1Q, '95, 10; 2Q, '94, 3

   905.0 Late effect of fracture of skull and face bones
         Late effect of injury classifiable to 800-804
         AHA: 3Q, '97, 12

   905.1 Late effect of fracture of spine and trunk without mention of spinal cord lesion
         Late effect of injury classifiable to 805, 807-809
         AHA: 1Q, '07, 20

   905.2 Late effect of fracture of upper extremities
         Late effect of injury classifiable to 810-819

   905.3 Late effect of fracture of neck of femur
         Late effect of injury classifiable to 820

   905.4 Late effect of fracture of lower extremities
         Late effect of injury classifiable to 821-827
         S79.001S Uns physeal fx upper end right femur sequela   I-10

   905.5 Late effect of fracture of multiple and unspecified bones
         Late effect of injury classifiable to 828-829

   905.6 Late effect of dislocation
         Late effect of injury classifiable to 830-839

   905.7 Late effect of sprain and strain without mention of tendon injury
         Late effect of injury classifiable to 840-848, except tendon injury

   905.8 Late effect of tendon injury
         Late effect of tendon injury due to:
            open wound [injury classifiable to 880-884 with .2, 890-894 with .2]
            sprain and strain [injury classifiable to 840-848]
         AHA: 2Q, '89, 13; 2Q, '89, 15

   905.9 Late effect of traumatic amputation
         Late effect of injury classifiable to 885-887, 895-897
         EXCLUDES late amputation stump complication (997.60-997.69)

√4ᵗʰ **906 Late effects of injuries to skin and subcutaneous tissues**

   906.0 Late effect of open wound of head, neck, and trunk
         Late effect of injury classifiable to 870-879

   906.1 Late effect of open wound of extremities without mention of tendon injury
         Late effect of injury classifiable to 880-884, 890-894 except .2

   906.2 Late effect of superficial injury
         Late effect of injury classifiable to 910-919

   906.3 Late effect of contusion
         Late effect of injury classifiable to 920-924

   906.4 Late effect of crushing
         Late effect of injury classifiable to 925-929

   906.5 Late effect of burn of eye, face, head, and neck
         Late effect of injury classifiable to 940-941
         AHA: 4Q, '04, 76

N Newborn Age: 0   P Pediatric Age: 0-17   M Maternity Age: 12-55   A Adult Age: 15-124   MCC Major CC Condition   CC CC Condition   HIV HIV Related Dx

322 – Volume 1   2014 ICD-9-CM

906.6 Late effect of burn of wrist and hand
Late effect of injury classifiable to 944
AHA: 4Q, '94, 22

906.7 Late effect of burn of other extremities
Late effect of injury classifiable to 943 or 945
AHA: 4Q, '94, 22

906.8 Late effect of burns of other specified sites
Late effect of injury classifiable to 942, 946-947
AHA: 4Q, '94, 22

906.9 Late effect of burn of unspecified site
Late effect of injury classifiable to 948-949
AHA: 4Q, '94, 22

√4ᵗʰ **907 Late effects of injuries to the nervous system**

907.0 Late effect of intracranial injury without mention of skull fracture
Late effect of injury classifiable to 850-854
AHA: ▶3Q, '12, 20;◀ 4Q, '11, 97; 4Q, '10, 96; 4Q, '09, 108; 4Q, '08, 108; 4Q, '03, 103; 3Q, '90, 14
S06.2x1S Diffuse traumatic brain inj loc 30 min/less seq   I-10

907.1 Late effect of injury to cranial nerve
Late effect of injury classifiable to 950-951

907.2 Late effect of spinal cord injury
Late effect of injury classifiable to 806, 952
AHA: 4Q, '03, 103; 4Q, '98, 38
S34.114S Complete lesion L4 of lumbar spinal cord sequela   I-10

907.3 Late effect of injury to nerve root(s), spinal plexus(es), and other nerves of trunk
Late effect of injury classifiable to 953-954
AHA: 2Q, '07, 11

907.4 Late effect of injury to peripheral nerve of shoulder girdle and upper limb
Late effect of injury classifiable to 955

907.5 Late effect of injury to peripheral nerve of pelvic girdle and lower limb
Late effect of injury classifiable to 956

907.9 Late effect of injury to other and unspecified nerve
Late effect of injury classifiable to 957

√4ᵗʰ **908 Late effects of other and unspecified injuries**

908.0 Late effect of internal injury to chest
Late effect of injury classifiable to 860-862

908.1 Late effect of internal injury to intra-abdominal organs
Late effect of injury classifiable to 863-866, 868

908.2 Late effect of internal injury to other internal organs
Late effect of injury classifiable to 867 or 869

908.3 Late effect of injury to blood vessel of head, neck, and extremities
Late effect of injury classifiable to 900, 903-904

908.4 Late effect of injury to blood vessel of thorax, abdomen, and pelvis
Late effect of injury classifiable to 901-902

908.5 Late effect of foreign body in orifice
Late effect of injury classifiable to 930-939

908.6 Late effect of certain complications of trauma
Late effect of complications classifiable to 958

908.9 Late effect of unspecified injury
Late effect of injury classifiable to 959
AHA: 3Q, '00, 4

√4ᵗʰ **909 Late effects of other and unspecified external causes**

909.0 Late effect of poisoning due to drug, medicinal or biological substance
Late effect of conditions classifiable to 960-979
EXCLUDES *late effect of adverse effect of drug, medicinal or biological substance (909.5)*
AHA: 4Q, '03, 103

909.1 Late effect of toxic effects of nonmedical substances
Late effect of conditions classifiable to 980-989

909.2 Late effect of radiation
Late effect of conditions classifiable to 990

909.3 Late effect of complications of surgical and medical care
Late effect of conditions classifiable to 996-999
AHA: 1Q, '93, 29

909.4 Late effect of certain other external causes
Late effect of conditions classifiable to 991-994

909.5 Late effect of adverse effect of drug, medical or biological substance
EXCLUDES *late effect of poisoning due to drug, medicinal or biological substance (909.0)*
AHA: 4Q, '94, 48

909.9 Late effect of other and unspecified external causes

Superficial Injury (910-919)

EXCLUDES *burn (blisters) (940.0-949.5)*
contusion (920-924.9)
foreign body:
    granuloma (728.82)
    inadvertently left in operative wound (998.4)
    residual in soft tissue (729.6)
insect bite, venomous (989.5)
open wound with incidental foreign body (870.0-897.7)
AHA: 2Q, '89, 15
TIP: Do not code separately when associated with more severe injuries of the same site.

√4ᵗʰ **910 Superficial injury of face, neck, and scalp except eye**
INCLUDES cheek
ear
gum
lip
nose
throat
EXCLUDES *eye and adnexa (918.0-918.9)*

910.0 Abrasion or friction burn without mention of infection
S00.01xA Abrasion of scalp initial encounter   I-10

910.1 Abrasion or friction burn, infected

910.2 Blister without mention of infection

910.3 Blister, infected

910.4 Insect bite, nonvenomous, without mention of infection

910.5 Insect bite, nonvenomous, infected

910.6 Superficial foreign body (splinter) without major open wound and without mention of infection

910.7 Superficial foreign body (splinter) without major open wound, infected

910.8 Other and unspecified superficial injury of face, neck, and scalp without mention of infection

910.9 Other and unspecified superficial injury of face, neck, and scalp, infected

√4ᵗʰ **911 Superficial injury of trunk**
INCLUDES abdominal wall   interscapular region
anus   labium (majus) (minus)
back   penis
breast   perineum
buttock   scrotum
chest wall   testis
flank   vagina
groin   vulva
EXCLUDES *hip (916.0-916.9)*
scapular region (912.0-912.9)

911.0 Abrasion or friction burn without mention of infection
AHA: 3Q, '01, 10

911.1 Abrasion or friction burn, infected

911.2 Blister without mention of infection

911.3 Blister, infected

911.4 Insect bite, nonvenomous, without mention of infection

911.5 Insect bite, nonvenomous, infected

911.6 Superficial foreign body (splinter) without major open wound and without mention of infection

911.7 Superficial foreign body (splinter) without major open wound, infected

4ᵗʰ/5ᵗʰ Additional Digit Required   Unacceptable PDx   Manifestation Code   Hospital Acquired Condition   ▶◀ Revised Text   ● New Code   ▲ Revised Code Title

2014 ICD-9-CM   February 2013 · Volume 1 – 323

911.8 Other and unspecified superficial injury of trunk without mention of infection

911.9 Other and unspecified superficial injury of trunk, infected

☑4ᵗʰ **912 Superficial injury of shoulder and upper arm**

INCLUDES   axilla
scapular region

912.0 Abrasion or friction burn without mention of infection

912.1 Abrasion or friction burn, infected

912.2 Blister without mention of infection

912.3 Blister, infected

912.4 Insect bite, nonvenomous, without mention of infection

912.5 Insect bite, nonvenomous, infected

912.6 Superficial foreign body (splinter) without major open wound and without mention of infection

912.7 Superficial foreign body (splinter) without major open wound, infected

912.8 Other and unspecified superficial injury of shoulder and upper arm without mention of infection

912.9 Other and unspecified superficial injury of shoulder and upper arm, infected

☑4ᵗʰ **913 Superficial injury of elbow, forearm, and wrist**

913.0 Abrasion or friction burn without mention of infection

913.1 Abrasion or friction burn, infected

913.2 Blister without mention of infection

913.3 Blister, infected

913.4 Insect bite, nonvenomous, without mention of infection

913.5 Insect bite, nonvenomous, infected

913.6 Superficial foreign body (splinter) without major open wound and without mention of infection

913.7 Superficial foreign body (splinter) without major open wound, infected

913.8 Other and unspecified superficial injury of elbow, forearm, and wrist without mention of infection

913.9 Other and unspecified superficial injury of elbow, forearm, and wrist, infected

☑4ᵗʰ **914 Superficial injury of hand(s) except finger(s) alone**

914.0 Abrasion or friction burn without mention of infection

914.1 Abrasion or friction burn, infected

914.2 Blister without mention of infection

914.3 Blister, infected

914.4 Insect bite, nonvenomous, without mention of infection

914.5 Insect bite, nonvenomous, infected

914.6 Superficial foreign body (splinter) without major open wound and without mention of infection

914.7 Superficial foreign body (splinter) without major open wound, infected

914.8 Other and unspecified superficial injury of hand without mention of infection

914.9 Other and unspecified superficial injury of hand, infected

☑4ᵗʰ **915 Superficial injury of finger(s)**

INCLUDES   fingernail
thumb (nail)

915.0 Abrasion or friction burn without mention of infection

915.1 Abrasion or friction burn, infected

915.2 Blister without mention of infection

915.3 Blister, infected

915.4 Insect bite, nonvenomous, without mention of infection

915.5 Insect bite, nonvenomous, infected

915.6 Superficial foreign body (splinter) without major open wound and without mention of infection

915.7 Superficial foreign body (splinter) without major open wound, infected

915.8 Other and unspecified superficial injury of fingers without mention of infection
AHA: 3Q, '01, 10

915.9 Other and unspecified superficial injury of fingers, infected

☑4ᵗʰ **916 Superficial injury of hip, thigh, leg, and ankle**

916.0 Abrasion or friction burn without mention of infection
S80.812A Abrasion left lower leg initial encounter   I-10

916.1 Abrasion or friction burn, infected

916.2 Blister without mention of infection

916.3 Blister, infected

916.4 Insect bite, nonvenomous, without mention of infection

916.5 Insect bite, nonvenomous, infected

916.6 Superficial foreign body (splinter) without major open wound and without mention of infection

916.7 Superficial foreign body (splinter) without major open wound, infected

916.8 Other and unspecified superficial injury of hip, thigh, leg, and ankle without mention of infection

916.9 Other and unspecified superficial injury of hip, thigh, leg, and ankle, infected

☑4ᵗʰ **917 Superficial injury of foot and toe(s)**

INCLUDES   heel
toenail

917.0 Abrasion or friction burn without mention of infection

917.1 Abrasion or friction burn, infected

917.2 Blister without mention of infection

917.3 Blister, infected

917.4 Insect bite, nonvenomous, without mention of infection

917.5 Insect bite, nonvenomous, infected

917.6 Superficial foreign body (splinter) without major open wound and without mention of infection

917.7 Superficial foreign body (splinter) without major open wound, infected

917.8 Other and unspecified superficial injury of foot and toes without mention of infection
AHA: 1Q, '03, 13

917.9 Other and unspecified superficial injury of foot and toes, infected
AHA: 1Q, '03, 13
TIP: Assign for hair strangulation of toe, with infection.

☑4ᵗʰ **918 Superficial injury of eye and adnexa**

EXCLUDES   *burn (940.0-940.9)*
foreign body on external eye (930.0-930.9)

918.0 Eyelids and periocular area
Abrasion
Insect bite
Superficial foreign body (splinter)

918.1 Cornea
Corneal abrasion
Superficial laceration
EXCLUDES   *corneal injury due to contact lens (371.82)*

918.2 Conjunctiva

918.9 Other and unspecified superficial injuries of eye
Eye (ball) NOS

☑4ᵗʰ **919 Superficial injury of other, multiple, and unspecified sites**

EXCLUDES   *multiple sites classifiable to the same three-digit category (910.0-918.9)*

919.0 Abrasion or friction burn without mention of infection

919.1 Abrasion or friction burn, infected

919.2 Blister without mention of infection

919.3 Blister, infected

Ⓝ Newborn Age: 0   Ⓟ Pediatric Age: 0-17   Ⓜ Maternity Age: 12-55   Ⓐ Adult Age: 15-124   MCC Major CC Condition   CC CC Condition   HIV HIV Related D:

324 – Volume 1   2014 ICD-9-CM

919.4 **Insect bite, nonvenomous, without mention of infection**

919.5 **Insect bite, nonvenomous, infected**

919.6 **Superficial foreign body (splinter) without major open wound and without mention of infection**

919.7 **Superficial foreign body (splinter) without major open wound, infected**

919.8 **Other and unspecified superficial injury without mention of infection**

919.9 **Other and unspecified superficial injury, infected**

Contusion with Intact Skin Surface (920-924)

INCLUDES   bruise   } without fracture or open
          hematoma }   wound

EXCLUDES   *concussion (850.0-850.9)*
      hemarthrosis (840.0-848.9)
      internal organs (860.0-869.1)
      that incidental to:
        crushing injury (925-929.9)
        dislocation (830.0-839.9)
        fracture (800.0-829.1)
        internal injury (860.0-869.1)
        intracranial injury (850.0-854.1)
        nerve injury (950.0-957.9)
        open wound (870.0-897.7)

920 **Contusion of face, scalp, and neck except eye(s)**

Cheek	Mandibular joint area
Ear (auricle)	Nose
Gum	Throat
Lip	

   S00.33xA Contusion of nose initial encounter   I-10

✓4ᵗʰ 921 **Contusion of eye and adnexa**

921.0 **Black eye, not otherwise specified**

921.1 **Contusion of eyelids and periocular area**

921.2 **Contusion of orbital tissues**

921.3 **Contusion of eyeball**
   AHA: J-A, '85, 16
   TIP: If iridodialysis (rupture of the root of the iris) is present and is due to the eyeball contusion, assign also code 364.76.

921.9 **Unspecified contusion of eye**
   Injury of eye NOS

✓4ᵗʰ 922 **Contusion of trunk**

922.0 **Breast**

922.1 **Chest wall**
   S20.212A Contusion left front wall thorax initial enc   I-10

922.2 **Abdominal wall**
   Flank
   Groin

✓5ᵗʰ 922.3 **Back**
   AHA: 4Q, '96, 39

   922.31 **Back**
     EXCLUDES   *interscapular region (922.33)*
     AHA: 3Q, '99, 14

   922.32 **Buttock**

   922.33 **Interscapular region**

922.4 **Genital organs**

Labium (majus) (minus)	Testis
Penis	Vagina
Perineum	Vulva
Scrotum	

922.8 **Multiple sites of trunk**

922.9 **Unspecified part**
   Trunk NOS

✓4ᵗʰ 923 **Contusion of upper limb**

✓5ᵗʰ 923.0 **Shoulder and upper arm**

   923.00 **Shoulder region**

   923.01 **Scapular region**

   923.02 **Axillary region**

   923.03 **Upper arm**

   923.09 **Multiple sites**

✓5ᵗʰ 923.1 **Elbow and forearm**

   923.10 **Forearm**

   923.11 **Elbow**

✓5ᵗʰ 923.2 **Wrist and hand(s), except finger(s) alone**

   923.20 **Hand(s)**

   923.21 **Wrist**

923.3 **Finger**
   Fingernail
   Thumb (nail)

923.8 **Multiple sites of upper limb**

923.9 **Unspecified part of upper limb**
   Arm NOS

✓4ᵗʰ 924 **Contusion of lower limb and of other and unspecified sites**

✓5ᵗʰ 924.0 **Hip and thigh**

   924.00 **Thigh**
     AHA: 1Q, '09, 10

   924.01 **Hip**
     S70.02xA Contusion of left hip initial encounter   I-10

✓5ᵗʰ 924.1 **Knee and lower leg**

   924.10 **Lower leg**

   924.11 **Knee**

✓5ᵗʰ 924.2 **Ankle and foot, excluding toe(s)**

   924.20 **Foot**
     Heel

   924.21 **Ankle**

924.3 **Toe**
   Toenail

924.4 **Multiple sites of lower limb**

924.5 **Unspecified part of lower limb**
   Leg NOS

924.8 **Multiple sites, not elsewhere classified**
   AHA: 1Q, '03, 7
   S70.10xA Contusion of unspecified thigh initial encounter   I-10

924.9 **Unspecified site**

Crushing Injury (925-929)

Use additional code to identify any associated injuries, such as:
   fractures (800-829)
   internal injuries (860.0-869.1)
   intracranial injuries (850.0-854.1)
AHA: 4Q, '03, 77; 2Q, '93, 7

✓4ᵗʰ 925 **Crushing injury of face, scalp, and neck**

Cheek	Pharynx
Ear	Throat
Larynx	

   925.1 **Crushing injury of face and scalp**   CC
     Cheek
     Ear
     CC Excl: 873.8-873.9, 905.0, 925.1-925.2, 929.0-929.9, 958.8-959.09, 959.8-959.9

   925.2 **Crushing injury of neck**   CC
     Larynx   Throat
     Pharynx
     CC Excl: See code: 925.1

✓4ᵗʰ 926 **Crushing injury of trunk**

   926.0 **External genitalia**

Labium (majus) (minus)	Testis
Penis	Vulva
Scrotum	

✓5ᵗʰ 926.1 **Other specified sites**

   926.11 **Back**

   926.12 **Buttock**

✓ Additional Digit Required	Unacceptable PDx	Manifestation Code	Hospital Acquired Condition	▶◀ Revised Text	● New Code ▲ Revised Code Title

Injury and Poisoning

926.19–939.9

926.19 Other
Breast

926.8 Multiple sites of trunk

926.9 Unspecified site
Trunk NOS

✓4ʰ **927 Crushing injury of upper limb**

✓5ʰ **927.0 Shoulder and upper arm**

927.00 Shoulder region

927.01 Scapular region

927.02 Axillary region

927.03 Upper arm

927.09 Multiple sites

✓5ʰ **927.1 Elbow and forearm**

927.10 Forearm

927.11 Elbow

✓5ʰ **927.2 Wrist and hand(s), except finger(s) alone**

927.20 Hand(s)

927.21 Wrist

927.3 Finger(s)
AHA: 4Q, '03, 77

927.8 Multiple sites of upper limb

927.9 Unspecified site
Arm NOS

✓4ʰ **928 Crushing injury of lower limb**

✓5ʰ **928.0 Hip and thigh**

928.00 Thigh   CC
CC Exd: 928.00, 928.8-929.9

928.01 Hip   CC
CC Exd: 928.01, 928.8-929.9

✓5ʰ **928.1 Knee and lower leg**

928.10 Lower leg

928.11 Knee

✓5ʰ **928.2 Ankle and foot, excluding toe(s) alone**

928.20 Foot
Heel

928.21 Ankle

928.3 Toe(s)

928.8 Multiple sites of lower limb

928.9 Unspecified site
Leg NOS

✓4ʰ **929 Crushing injury of multiple and unspecified sites**

929.0 Multiple sites, not elsewhere classified

929.9 Unspecified site

Effects of Foreign Body Entering Through Orifice (930-939)

EXCLUDES *foreign body:*
granuloma (728.82)
inadvertently left in operative wound (998.4, 998.7)
in open wound (800-839, 851-897)
residual in soft tissues (729.6)
superficial without major open wound (910-919
with .6 or .7)

✓4ʰ **930 Foreign body on external eye**
EXCLUDES *foreign body in penetrating wound of:*
eyeball (871.5-871.6)
retained (old) (360.5-360.6)
ocular adnexa (870.4)
retained (old) (376.6)

930.0 Corneal foreign body

930.1 Foreign body in conjunctival sac

930.2 Foreign body in lacrimal punctum

930.8 Other and combined sites

930.9 Unspecified site
External eye NOS

931 Foreign body in ear
Auditory canal
Auricle

932 Foreign body in nose
Nasal sinus
Nostril

✓4ʰ **933 Foreign body in pharynx and larynx**

933.0 Pharynx
Nasopharynx
Throat NOS

933.1 Larynx
Asphyxia due to foreign body
Choking due to:
food (regurgitated)
phlegm
TIP: Assign for mucous plug causing asphyxia; otherwise, for tracheobronchial, refer to code 519.19 Other diseases of trachea and bronchus.

✓4ʰ **934 Foreign body in trachea, bronchus, and lung**

934.0 Trachea   CC
CC Exd: 934.0

934.1 Main bronchus   CC
CC Exd: 934.0-934.9
AHA: 3Q, '02, 18

934.8 Other specified parts   CC
Bronchioles
Lung
CC Exd: See code: 934.1

934.9 Respiratory tree, unspecified
Inhalation of liquid or vomitus, lower respiratory tract NOS

✓4ʰ **935 Foreign body in mouth, esophagus, and stomach**

935.0 Mouth

935.1 Esophagus
AHA: 1Q, '88, 13
TIP: If esophageal obstruction is due to stenosis, caustic stricture (e.g., lye ingestion), or tumor, assign instead code 530.3.

935.2 Stomach

936 Foreign body in intestine and colon

937 Foreign body in anus and rectum
Rectosigmoid (junction)

938 Foreign body in digestive system, unspecified
Alimentary tract NOS
Swallowed foreign body

✓4ʰ **939 Foreign body in genitourinary tract**

939.0 Bladder and urethra

939.1 Uterus, any part
EXCLUDES *intrauterine contraceptive device:*
complications from (996.32, 996.65)
presence of (V45.51)

939.2 Vulva and vagina

939.3 Penis

939.9 Unspecified site

N Newborn Age: 0   **P** Pediatric Age: 0-17   **M** Maternity Age: 12-55   **A** Adult Age: 15-124   **MCC** Major CC Condition   **CC** CC Condition   **HIV** HIV Related D

326 – Volume 1   2014 ICD-9-C

Burns (940-949)

INCLUDES burns from:
electrical heating appliance
electricity
flame
hot object
lightning
radiation
chemical burns (external) (internal)
scalds

EXCLUDES friction burns (910-919 with .0, .1)
sunburn (692.71, 692.76-692.77)

AHA: 4Q, 94, 22; 2Q, '90, 7; 4Q, '88, 3; M-A, '86, 9

TIP: Nonhealing burns are coded as acute burns, as is necrosis of burned skin.
Assign code 958.3 for any documented infected burn site.

√4ᵗʰ **940 Burn confined to eye and adnexa**

940.0 Chemical burn of eyelids and periocular area

940.1 Other burns of eyelids and periocular area

940.2 Alkaline chemical burn of cornea and conjunctival sac

940.3 Acid chemical burn of cornea and conjunctival sac

940.4 Other burn of cornea and conjunctival sac

940.5 Burn with resulting rupture and destruction of eyeball CC
CC Excl: No exclusion

940.9 Unspecified burn of eye and adnexa

√4ᵗʰ **941 Burn of face, head, and neck**

EXCLUDES mouth (947.0)

The following fifth-digit subclassification is for use with category 941:
0 face and head, unspecified site
1 ear [any part]
2 eye (with other parts of face, head, and neck)
3 lip(s)
4 chin
5 nose (septum)
6 scalp [any part]
   Temple (region)
7 forehead and cheek
8 neck
9 multiple sites [except with eye] of face, head, and neck

AHA: 4Q, '94, 22; M-A, '86, 9

§ √5ᵗʰ **941.0 Unspecified degree**
[0-9]

§ √5ᵗʰ **941.1 Erythema [first degree]**
[0-9] AHA: For code 941.19: 3Q. '10, 19; 3Q, '05, 10

§ √5ᵗʰ **941.2 Blisters, epidermal loss [second degree]**
[0-9]

§ √5ᵗʰ **941.3 Full-thickness skin loss [third degree NOS]** CC
[0-9] CC Excl: For code 941.30: 941.30, 941.39; For code 941.31: 941.31, 941.39;
For code 941.32: 941.32, 941.39; For code 941.33: 941.33, 941.39; For
code 941.34: 941.34, 941.39; For code 941.35: 941.35, 941.39; For code
941.36: 941.36, 941.39; For code 941.37: 941.37, 941.39; For code 941.38:
941.38-941.39; For code 941.39: 941.30-941.39

§ √5ᵗʰ **941.4 Deep necrosis of underlying tissues [deep third** CC
[0-9] **degree] without mention of loss of a body part**
CC Excl: For code 941.40, 941.49: 941.40, 941.49; For code 941.41:
941.40-941.41, 941.49; For code 941.42: 941.40, 941.42, 941.49; For
code 941.43: 941.40, 941.43, 941.49; For code 941.44: 941.40, 941.44,
941.49; For code 941.45: 941.40, 941.45, 941.49; For code 941.46:
941.40, 941.46, 941.49; For code 941.47: 941.40, 941.47, 941.49; For
code 941.48: 941.40, 941.48-941.49

§ √5ᵗʰ **941.5 Deep necrosis of underlying tissues [deep** CC
[0-9] **third degree] with loss of a body part**
CC Excl: For code 941.50, 941.59: 941.50, 941.59; For code 941.51:
941.50-941.51, 941.59; For code 941.52: 941.50, 941.52, 941.59; For
code 941.53: 941.50, 941.53, 941.59; For code 941.54: 941.50, 941.54,
941.59; For code 941.55: 941.50, 941.55, 941.59; For code 941.56:
941.50, 941.56, 941.59; For code 941.57: 941.50, 941.57, 941.59; For
code 941.58: 941.50, 941.58-941.59

√4ᵗʰ **942 Burn of trunk**

EXCLUDES scapular region (943.0-943.5 with fifth-digit 6)

The following fifth-digit subclassificaiton is for use with category 942:
0 trunk, unspecified
1 breast
2 chest wall, excluding breast and nipple
3 abdominal wall
   Flank
   Groin
4 back [any part]
   Buttock
   Interscapular region
5 genitalia
   Labium (majus) (minus
   Penis
   Perineum
   Scrotum
   Testis
   Vulva
9 other and multiple sites of trunk

AHA: 4Q, '94, 22; M-A, '86, 9

§ √5ᵗʰ **942.0 Unspecified degree**
[0-5, 9]

§ √5ᵗʰ **942.1 Erythema [first degree]**
[0-5, 9]

§ √5ᵗʰ **942.2 Blisters, epidermal loss [second degree]**
[0-5, 9]

§ √5ᵗʰ **942.3 Full-thickness skin loss [third degree NOS]** CC
[0-5, 9] CC Excl: For code 942.30, 942.39: 942.30, 942.39; For code 942.31:
942.30-942.31, 942.39; For code 942.32: 942.30, 942.32, 942.39; For
code 942.33: 942.30, 942.33, 942.39; For code 942.34: 942.30, 942.34,
942.39; For code 942.35: 942.30, 942.35-942.39

§ √5ᵗʰ **942.4 Deep necrosis of underlying tissues [deep third** CC
[0-5, 9] **degree] without mention of loss of a body part**
CC Excl: For code 942.40: 942.40, 942.49; For code 942.41: 942.40-942.41,
942.49; For code 942.42: 942.40, 942.42, 942.49; For code 942.43:
942.40, 942.43, 942.49; For code 942.44: 942.40, 942.44, 942.49; For
code 942.45: 942.40, 942.45-942.49; For code 942.49: 942.40-942.49

§ √5ᵗʰ **942.5 Deep necrosis of underlying tissues [deep** CC
[0-5, 9] **third degree] with loss of a body part**
CC Excl: For code 942.50: 942.50, 942.59; For code 942.51: 942.50-942.51,
942.59; For code 942.52: 942.50, 942.52, 942.59; For code 942.53:
942.50, 942.53, 942.59; For code 942.54: 942.50, 942.54, 942.59; For
code 942.55: 942.50, 942.55-942.59; For code 942.59: 942.50, 942.59

√4ᵗʰ **943 Burn of upper limb, except wrist and hand**

The following fifth-digit subclassificaiton is for use with category 943:
0 upper limb, unspecified site
1 forearm
2 elbow
3 upper arm
4 axilla
5 shoulder
6 scapular region
9 multiple sites of upper limb, except wrist and hand

AHA: 4Q, '94, 22; M-A, '86, 9

§ √5ᵗʰ **943.0 Unspecified degree**
[0-6, 9] AHA: For code 943.00: 3Q. '10, 19

§ √5ᵗʰ **943.1 Erythema [first degree]**
[0-6, 9]

§ √5ᵗʰ **943.2 Blisters, epidermal loss [second degree]**
[0-6, 9]

§ √5ᵗʰ **943.3 Full-thickness skin loss [third degree NOS]** CC
[0-6, 9] CC Excl: For code 943.30, 943.39: 943.30, 943.39; For code 943.31:
943.30-943.31, 943.39; For code 943.32: 943.30, 943.32, 943.39; For
code 943.33: 943.30, 943.33, 943.39; For code 943.34: 943.30, 943.34,
943.39; For code 943.35: 943.30, 943.35, 943.39; For code 943.36:
943.30, 943.36-943.39

§ √5ᵗʰ **943.4 Deep necrosis of underlying tissues [deep third** CC
[0-6, 9] **degree] without mention of loss of a body part**
CC Excl: For code 943.40, 943.49: 943.40, 943.49; For code 943.41:
943.40-943.41, 943.49; For code 943.42: 943.40, 943.42, 943.49; For
code 943.43: 943.40, 943.43, 943.49; For code 943.44: 943.40, 943.44,
943.49; For code 943.45: 943.40, 943.45, 943.49; For code 943.46:
943.40, 943.46-943.49

§ Requires fifth digit. Valid digits are in [brackets] under each code. See appropriate category for codes and definitions.

4ᵗʰ/5ᵗʰ Additional Digit Required Unacceptable PDx Manifestation Code Hospital Acquired Condition ►◄ Revised Text ● New Code ▲ Revised Code Title

2014 ICD-9-CM Volume 1 – 327

Injury and Poisoning

943.5–948.0

§ ✓5ᵗʰ **943.5 Deep necrosis of underlying tissues [deep third degree] with loss of a body part** [0-6, 9]   **CC**

CC Excl: For code 943.50, 943.59: 943.50, 943.59; For code 943.51: 943.50-943.51, 943.59; For code 943.52: 943.50, 943.52, 943.59; For code 943.53: 943.50, 943.53, 943.59; For code 943.54: 943.50, 943.54, 943.59; For code 943.55: 943.50, 943.55, 943.59; For code 943.56: 943.50, 943.56-943.59

✓4ᵗʰ **944 Burn of wrist(s) and hand(s)**

The following fifth-digit subclassification is for use with category 944:
- **0 hand, unspecified site**
- **1 single digit [finger (nail)] other than thumb**
- **2 thumb (nail)**
- **3 two or more digits, not including thumb**
- **4 two or more digits including thumb**
- **5 palm**
- **6 back of hand**
- **7 wrist**
- **8 multiple sites of wrist(s) and hand(s)**

§ ✓5ᵗʰ **944.0 Unspecified degree**
[0-8]

§ ✓5ᵗʰ **944.1 Erythema [first degree]**
[0-8]

§ ✓5ᵗʰ **944.2 Blisters, epidermal loss [second degree]**
[0-8]

§ ✓5ᵗʰ **944.3 Full-thickness skin loss [third degree NOS]**   **CC**
[0-8]   CC Excl: For code 944.30, 944.38: 944.30, 944.38; For code 944.31: 944.30-944.31, 944.38; For code 944.32: 944.30, 944.32, 944.38; For code 944.33: 944.30, 944.33, 944.38; For code 944.34: 944.30, 944.34, 944.38; For code 944.35: 944.30, 944.35, 944.38; For code 944.36: 944.30, 944.36, 944.38; For code 944.37: 944.30, 944.37-944.38

§ ✓5ᵗʰ **944.4 Deep necrosis of underlying tissues [deep third degree] without mention of loss of a body part**   **CC**
[0-8]   CC Excl: For code 944.40, 944.48: 944.40, 944.48; For code 944.41: 944.40-944.41, 944.48; For code 944.42: 944.40, 944.42, 944.48; For code 944.43: 944.40, 944.43, 944.48; For code 944.44: 944.40, 944.44, 944.48; For code 944.45: 944.40, 944.45, 944.48; For code 944.46: 944.40, 944.46, 944.48; For code 944.47: 944.40, 944.47-944.48

§ ✓5ᵗʰ **944.5 Deep necrosis of underlying tissues [deep third degree] with loss of a body part**   **CC**
[0-8]   CC Excl: For code 944.50, 944.58: 944.50, 944.58; For code 944.51: 944.50-944.51, 944.58; For code 944.52: 944.50, 944.52, 944.58; For code 944.53: 944.50, 944.53, 944.58; For code 944.54: 944.50, 944.54, 944.58; For code 944.55: 944.50, 944.55, 944.58; For code 944.56: 944.50, 944.56, 944.58; For code 944.57: 944.50, 944.57-944.58

✓4ᵗʰ **945 Burn of lower limb(s)**

The following fifth-digit subclassification is for use with category 945:
- **0 lower limb [leg], unspecified site**
- **1 toe(s) (nail)**
- **2 foot**
- **3 ankle**
- **4 lower leg**
- **5 knee**
- **6 thigh [any part]**
- **9 multiple sites of lower limb(s)**

AHA: 4Q, '94, 22; M-A, '86, 9

§ ✓5ᵗʰ **945.0 Unspecified degree**
[0-6, 9]

§ ✓5ᵗʰ **945.1 Erythema [first degree]**
[0-6, 9]

§ ✓5ᵗʰ **945.2 Blisters, epidermal loss [second degree]**
[0-6, 9]

§ ✓5ᵗʰ **945.3 Full-thickness skin loss [third degree NOS]**   **CC**
[0-6, 9]   CC Excl: For code 945.30, 945.39: 945.30, 945.39; For code 945.31: 945.30-945.31, 945.39; For code 945.32: 945.30, 945.32, 945.39; For code 945.33: 945.30, 945.33, 945.39; For code 945.34: 945.30, 945.34, 945.39; For code 945.35: 945.30, 945.35, 945.39; For code 945.36: 945.30, 945.36-945.39

§ ✓5ᵗʰ **945.4 Deep necrosis of underlying tissues [deep third degree] without mention of loss of a body part**   **CC**
[0-6, 9]   CC Excl: For code 945.40, 945.49: 945.40, 945.49; For code 945.41: 945.40-945.41, 945.49; For code 945.42: 945.40, 945.42, 945.49; For code 945.43: 945.40, 945.43, 945.49; For code 945.44: 945.40, 945.44, 945.49; For code 945.45: 945.40, 945.45, 945.49; For code 945.46: 945.40, 945.46-945.49

§ ✓5ᵗʰ **945.5 Deep necrosis of underlying tissues [deep third degree] with loss of a body part** [0-6, 9]   **CC**

CC Excl: For code 945.50, 945.59: 945.50, 945.59; For code 945.51: 945.50-945.51, 945.59; For code 945.52: 945.50, 945.52, 945.59; For code 945.53: 945.50, 945.53, 945.59; For code 945.54: 945.50, 945.54, 945.59; For code 945.55: 945.50, 945.55, 945.59; For code 945.56: 945.50, 945.56-945.59

✓4ᵗʰ **946 Burns of multiple specified sites**

INCLUDES burns of sites classifiable to more than one three-digit category in 940-945

EXCLUDES multiple burns NOS (949.0-949.5)

AHA: 4Q, '94, 22; M-A, '86, 9

TIP: Only assign if the specific sites of the multiple burns are not specified.

946.0 Unspecified degree

946.1 Erythema [first degree]

946.2 Blisters, epidermal loss [second degree]

946.3 Full-thickness skin loss [third degree NOS]   **CC**
CC Excl: 946.3

946.4 Deep necrosis of underlying tissues [deep third degree] without mention of loss of a body part   **CC**
CC Excl: 946.4

946.5 Deep necrosis of underlying tissues [deep third degree] with loss of a body part   **CC**
CC Excl: 946.5

✓4ᵗʰ **947 Burn of internal organs**

INCLUDES burns from chemical agents (ingested)

AHA: 4Q, '94, 22; M-A, '86, 9

947.0 Mouth and pharynx
Gum   Tongue

947.1 Larynx, trachea, and lung   **CC**
CC Excl: 947.1, 947.8-947.9

947.2 Esophagus   **CC**
CC Excl: 947.2, 947.8-947.9

947.3 Gastrointestinal tract   **CC**
Colon   Small intestine
Rectum   Stomach
CC Excl: 947.3, 947.8-947.9
AHA: ▶2Q, '12, 8◀

947.4 Vagina and uterus   **CC** ♀
CC Excl: 947.4-947.9

947.8 Other specified sites

947.9 Unspecified site

✓4ᵗʰ **948 Burns classified according to extent of body surface involved**

NOTE This category is to be used when the site of the burn is unspecified, or with categories 940-947 when the site is specified.

EXCLUDES sunburn (692.71, 692.76-692.77)

The following fifth-digit subclassification is for use with category 948 to indicate the percent of body surface with third degree burn; valid digits are in [brackets] under each code:
- **0 less than 10 percent or unspecified**
- **1 10-19%**
- **2 20-29%**
- **3 30-39%**
- **4 40-49%**
- **5 50-59%**
- **6 60-69%**
- **7 70-79%**
- **8 80-89%**
- **9 90% or more of body surface**

AHA: 4Q, '94, 22; 4Q, '88, 3; M-A, '86, 9; N-D, '84, 13

§ ✓5ᵗʰ **948.0 Burn [any degree] involving less than 10 percent of body surface**
[0]   T31.0 Burns involving less than 10% of body surface   I-10

---

§ Requires fifth digit. Valid digits are in [brackets] under each code. See appropriate category for codes and definitions.

N Newborn Age: 0   P Pediatric Age: 0-17   M Maternity Age: 12-55   A Adult Age: 15-124   MCC Major CC Condition   CC CC Condition   HIV HIV Related Dx

328 – Volume 1 • February 2013   2014 ICD-9-CM

Burns
Degrees of Burns

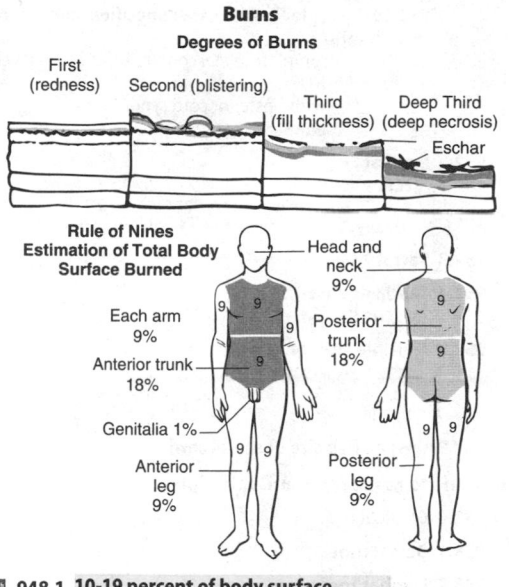

First (redness)
Second (blistering)
Third (fill thickness)
Deep Third (deep necrosis)
Eschar

Rule of Nines
Estimation of Total Body Surface Burned

Head and neck 9%

Each arm 9%

Posterior trunk 18%

Anterior trunk 18%

Genitalia 1%

Anterior leg 9%

Posterior leg 9%

---

10 § √5ᵗʰ **948.1 10-19 percent of body surface**   CC 0-1
[0-1]   CC Excl: 948.00-948.99

10 § √5ᵗʰ **948.2 20-29 percent of body surface**   MCC 1-2   CC 0
[0-2]   CC Excl: See code: 948.1

10 § √5ᵗʰ **948.3 30-39 percent of body surface**   MCC 1-3   CC 0
[0-3]   CC Excl: See code: 948.1

10 § √5ᵗʰ **948.4 40-49 percent of body surface**   MCC 1-4   CC 0
[0-4]   CC Excl: See code: 948.1

10 § √5ᵗʰ **948.5 50-59 percent of body surface**   MCC 1-5   CC 0
[0-5]   CC Excl: See code: 948.1

10 § √5ᵗʰ **948.6 60-69 percent of body surface**   MCC 1-6   CC 0
[0-6]   CC Excl: See code: 948.1

10 § √5ᵗʰ **948.7 70-79 percent of body surface**   MCC 1-7   CC 0
[0-7]   CC Excl: See code: 948.1

10 § √5ᵗʰ **948.8 80-89 percent of body surface**   MCC 1-8   CC 0
[0-8]   CC Excl: See code: 948.1

10 § √5ᵗʰ **948.9 90 percent or more of body surface**   MCC 1-9   CC 0
[0-9]   CC Excl: See code: 948.1

√4ᵗʰ **949 Burn, unspecified**

INCLUDES   burn NOS
multiple burns NOS

EXCLUDES   *burn of unspecified site but with statement of the extent of body surface involved (948.0-948.9)*

AHA: 4Q, '94, 22; M-A, '86, 9

949.0 Unspecified degree

949.1 Erythema [first degree]

949.2 Blisters, epidermal loss [second degree]

949.3 Full-thickness skin loss [third degree NOS]   CC
CC Excl: 941.30-941.39, 942.30-942.39, 944.30-944.38, 945.30-945.39, 946.3, 949.3

949.4 Deep necrosis of underlying tissues [deep third degree] without mention of loss of a body part   CC
CC Excl: 941.40-941.49, 942.40-942.49, 944.40-944.48, 945.40-945.49, 946.4, 949.4

949.5 Deep necrosis of underlying tissues [deep third degree] with loss of a body part   CC
CC Excl: 946.5, 949.5

Injury to Nerves and Spinal Cord (950-957)

INCLUDES   division of nerve
lesion in continuity   } (with open
traumatic neuroma   wound)
traumatic transient paralysis

EXCLUDES   *accidental puncture or laceration during medical procedure (998.2)*

√4ᵗʰ **950 Injury to optic nerve and pathways**

950.0 Optic nerve injury   CC
Second cranial nerve
CC Excl: 950.0-950.9, 951.8-951.9

950.1 Injury to optic chiasm   CC
CC Excl: See code: 950.0

950.2 Injury to optic pathways   CC
CC Excl: See code: 950.0

950.3 Injury to visual cortex   CC
CC Excl: See code: 950.0

950.9 Unspecified   CC
Traumatic blindness NOS
CC Excl: See code: 950.0

√4ᵗʰ **951 Injury to other cranial nerve(s)**

951.0 Injury to oculomotor nerve   CC
Third cranial nerve
CC Excl: 951.0, 951.8-951.9

951.1 Injury to trochlear nerve   CC
Fourth cranial nerve
CC Excl: 951.1, 951.8-951.9

951.2 Injury to trigeminal nerve   CC
Fifth cranial nerve
CC Excl: 951.2, 951.8-951.9

951.3 Injury to abducens nerve   CC
Sixth cranial nerve
CC Excl: 951.3, 951.8-951.9

951.4 Injury to facial nerve   CC
Seventh cranial nerve
CC Excl: 951.4, 951.8-951.9

951.5 Injury to acoustic nerve   CC
Auditory nerve
Eighth cranial nerve
Traumatic deafness NOS
CC Excl: 951.5, 951.8-951.9

951.6 Injury to accessory nerve   CC
Eleventh cranial nerve
CC Excl: 951.6, 951.8-951.9

951.7 Injury to hypoglossal nerve   CC
Twelfth cranial nerve
CC Excl: 951.7-951.9

951.8 Injury to other specified cranial nerves   CC
Glossopharyngeal [9th] nerve
Olfactory [1st cranial] nerve
Pneumogastric [10th cranial] nerve
Traumatic anosmia NOS
Vagus [10th cranial] nerve
CC Excl: 951.8-951.9

951.9 Injury to unspecified cranial nerve   CC
CC Excl: See code: 951.8

√4ᵗʰ **952 Spinal cord injury without evidence of spinal bone injury**

√5ᵗʰ **952.0 Cervical**

952.00 C₁-C₄ level with unspecified spinal cord injury   MCC
Spinal cord injury, cervical region NOS
CC Excl: 805.00-805.18, 805.8-806.19, 806.8-806.9, 839.00-839.18, 839.40, 839.49-839.50, 839.59, 839.69, 839.79-839.9, 847.9, 905.1, 926.11, 952.00-952.09, 952.8-952.9, 958.8-958.99, 959.11-959.19, 959.8-959.9

952.01 C₁-C₄ level with complete lesion of spinal cord   MCC
CC Excl: See code 952.00

HAC = only for valid CC or MCC codes.
Requires fifth digit. Valid digits are in [brackets] under each code. See appropriate category for codes and definitions.

| Additional Digit Required | Unacceptable PDx | Manifestation Code | Hospital Acquired Condition | ▶◀ Revised Text | ● New Code | ▲ Revised Code Title |

952.02 C_1-C_4 level with anterior cord syndrome   `MCC`
CC Excl: See code 952.00

952.03 C_1-C_4 level with central cord syndrome   `MCC`
CC Excl: See code 952.00

952.04 C_1-C_4 level with other specified spinal cord injury   `MCC`
Incomplete spinal cord lesion at C_1-C_4 level:
NOS
with posterior cord syndrome
CC Excl: See code 952.00

952.05 C_5-C_7 level with unspecified spinal cord injury   `MCC`
CC Excl: See code 952.00

952.06 C_5-C_7 level with complete lesion of spinal cord   `MCC`
CC Excl: See code 952.00

952.07 C_5-C_7 level with anterior cord syndrome   `MCC`
CC Excl: See code 952.00

952.08 C_5-C_7 level with central cord syndrome   `MCC`
CC Excl: See code 952.00

952.09 C_5-C_7 level with other specified spinal cord injury   `MCC`
Incomplete spinal cord lesion at C_5-C_7 level:
NOS
with posterior cord syndrome
CC Excl: See code 952.00

√5th **952.1 Dorsal [thoracic]**

952.10 T_1-T_6 level with unspecified spinal cord injury   `MCC`
Spinal cord injury, thoracic region NOS
CC Excl: 805.8-805.9, 806.20-806.39, 839.40, 839.49-839.50,
839.59, 839.69, 839.79-839.9, 847.9, 905.1, 926.11,
952.10-952.19, 952.8-952.9, 958.8-958.99, 959.11-959.19,
959.8-959.9

952.11 T_1-T_6 level with complete lesion of spinal cord   `MCC`
CC Excl: See code 952.10

952.12 T_1-T_6 level with anterior cord syndrome   `MCC`
CC Excl: See code 952.10

952.13 T_1-T_6 level with central cord syndrome   `MCC`
CC Excl: See code 952.10

952.14 T_1-T_6 level with other specified spinal cord injury   `MCC`
Incomplete spinal cord lesion at T_1-T_6 level:
NOS
with posterior cord syndrome
CC Excl: See code 952.10

952.15 T_7-T_{12} level with unspecified spinal cord injury   `MCC`
CC Excl: See code 952.10

952.16 T_7-T_{12} level with complete lesion of spinal cord   `MCC`
CC Excl: See code 952.10

952.17 T_7-T_{12} level with anterior cord syndrome   `MCC`
CC Excl: See code 952.10

952.18 T_7-T_{12} level with central cord syndrome   `MCC`
CC Excl: See code 952.10

952.19 T_1-T_{12} level with other specified spinal cord injury   `MCC`
Incomplete spinal cord lesion at T_7-T_{12} level:
NOS
with posterior cord syndrome
CC Excl: See code 952.10

952.2 Lumbar   `MCC`
CC Excl: 805.8-805.9, 806.4-806.5, 839.40, 839.49-839.50, 839.59,
839.69, 839.79-839.9, 847.9, 905.1, 926.11, 952.2,
952.8-952.9,958.8-958.99, 959.11-959.19, 959.8-959.9

952.3 Sacral   `MCC`

952.4 Cauda equina   `MCC`
CC Excl: See code 952.3

952.8 Multiple sites of spinal cord   `MCC`
CC Excl: 805.8-805.9, 839.40, 839.49-839.50, 839.59, 839.69,
839.79-839.9, 847.9, 905.1, 926.11, 952.8-952.9, 958.8-958.99,
959.11-959.19, 959.8-959.9

952.9 Unspecified site of spinal cord

√4th **953 Injury to nerve roots and spinal plexus**

953.0 Cervical root

953.1 Dorsal root

953.2 Lumbar root

953.3 Sacral root

953.4 Brachial plexus

953.5 Lumbosacral plexus

953.8 Multiple sites

953.9 Unspecified site

√4th **954 Injury to other nerve(s) of trunk, excluding shoulder and pelvic girdles**

954.0 Cervical sympathetic

954.1 Other sympathetic
Celiac ganglion or plexus
Inferior mesenteric plexus
Splanchnic nerve(s)
Stellate ganglion

954.8 Other specified nerve(s) of trunk

954.9 Unspecified nerve of trunk

√4th **955 Injury to peripheral nerve(s) of shoulder girdle and upper limb**

955.0 Axillary nerve

955.1 Median nerve

955.2 Ulnar nerve

955.3 Radial nerve

955.4 Musculocutaneous nerve

955.5 Cutaneous sensory nerve, upper limb

955.6 Digital nerve

955.7 Other specified nerve(s) of shoulder girdle and upper limb

955.8 Multiple nerves of shoulder girdle and upper limb

955.9 Unspecified nerve of shoulder girdle and upper limb

√4th **956 Injury to peripheral nerve(s) of pelvic girdle and lower limb**

956.0 Sciatic nerve

956.1 Femoral nerve

956.2 Posterior tibial nerve

956.3 Peroneal nerve

956.4 Cutaneous sensory nerve, lower limb

956.5 Other specified nerve(s) of pelvic girdle and lower limb

956.8 Multiple nerves of pelvic girdle and lower limb

956.9 Unspecified nerve of pelvic girdle and lower limb

√4th **957 Injury to other and unspecified nerves**

957.0 Superficial nerves of head and neck

957.1 Other specified nerve(s)

Spinal Nerve Roots

Gray matter
White matter
Anterior (ventral) root
Rootlets
Rami communicantes
Dorsal root ganglion
Posterior primary ramus
Posterior (dorsal) root

C_1
C_7
T_1 Cervical Nerve Roots
T_{12} Thoracic Nerve Roots
L_1
Cauda equina
L_5 Lumbar Nerve Roots
Sacrum
Filum terminale

N Newborn Age: 0   P Pediatric Age: 0-17   M Maternity Age: 12-55   A Adult Age: 15-124   `MCC` Major CC Condition   `CC` CC Condition   `HIV` HIV Related

330 – Volume 1   2014 ICD-9-

957.8 Multiple nerves in several parts
Multiple nerve injury NOS

957.9 Unspecified site
Nerve injury NOS

Certain Traumatic Complications and Unspecified Injuries (958-959)

√4ᵗʰ **958 Certain early complications of trauma**
EXCLUDES adult respiratory distress syndrome (518.52)
flail chest (807.4)
post-traumatic seroma (729.91)
shock lung related to trauma and surgery (518.52)
that occurring during or following medical procedures (996.0-999.9)

958.0 Air embolism   MCC
Pneumathemia
EXCLUDES that complicating:
abortion (634-638 with .6, 639.6)
ectopic or molar pregnancy (639.6)
pregnancy, childbirth, or the puerperium (673.0)
DEF: Arterial obstruction due to introduction of air bubbles into the veins following surgery or trauma.
CC Exd: 958.0, 958.8-958.99, 959.8-959.9, 997.91-997.99, 998.81, 998.83-998.9, 999.1

958.1 Fat embolism   MCC
EXCLUDES that complicating:
abortion (634-638 with .6, 639.6)
pregnancy, childbirth, or the puerperium (673.8)
DEF: Arterial blockage due to the entrance of fat in circulatory system, after fracture of large bones or administration of corticosteroids.
CC Exd: 958.1, 958.8-958.99, 959.8-959.9, 997.91-997.99, 998.81, 998.83-998.9

958.2 Secondary and recurrent hemorrhage   CC
CC Exd: 958.2, 958.8-958.99, 959.8-959.9, 997.91-997.99, 998.81, 998.83-998.9

958.3 Posttraumatic wound infection, not elsewhere classified CC
EXCLUDES infected open wounds — code to complicated open wound of site
CC Exd: 958.3, 958.8-958.99, 959.8-959.9, 997.91-997.99, 998.81, 998.83-998.9
AHA: 4Q, '01, 53; S-O, '85, 10
TIP: Do not assign if the infection is documented as due to cellulitis; see instead categories 681 and 682 and complicated wound codes.

958.4 Traumatic shock   MCC
Shock (immediate) (delayed) following injury
EXCLUDES shock:
anaphylactic (995.0)
due to serum (999.41-999.49)
anesthetic (995.4)
electric (994.8)
following abortion (639.5)
lightning (994.0)
nontraumatic NOS (785.50)
obstetric (669.1)
postoperative (998.00-998.09)
DEF: Shock, immediate or delayed following injury.
CC Exd: 958.4, 958.8-958.99, 959.8-959.9, 997.91-997.99, 998.81, 998.83-998.9

958.5 Traumatic anuria   MCC
Crush syndrome
Renal failure following crushing
EXCLUDES that due to a medical procedure (997.5)
DEF: Complete suppression of urinary secretion by kidneys due to trauma.
CC Exd: 958.5, 958.8-958.99, 959.8-959.9, 995.4, 997.91-998.13, 998.81, 998.83-998.9

958.6 Volkmann's ischemic contracture
Posttraumatic muscle contracture
DEF: Muscle deterioration due to loss of blood supply from injury or tourniquet; causes muscle contraction and results in inability to extend the muscles fully.

958.7 Traumatic subcutaneous emphysema   CC
EXCLUDES subcutaneous emphysema resulting from a procedure (998.81)
CC Exd: 860.0-860.5, 861.20-862.1, 862.29-862.9, 875.0-875.1, 958.7-958.99, 959.8-959.9, 997.91-997.99, 998.81, 998.83-998.9

958.8 Other early complications of trauma
AHA: 2Q, '92, 13

√5ᵗʰ **958.9 Traumatic compartment syndrome**
EXCLUDES nontraumatic compartment syndrome (729.71-729.79)
DEF: Compression of nerves and blood vessels within an enclosed space due to previous trauma, which leads to impaired blood flow and muscle and nerve damage.
TIP: If the compartment syndrome is specified as chronic or exercise-induced, see instead subcategory 729.7.

958.90 Compartment syndrome, unspecified   CC
CC Exd: 868.03-868.10, 868.13-869.1
AHA: 4Q, '06, 100-102

958.91 Traumatic compartment syndrome of upper extremity   CC
Traumatic compartment syndrome of shoulder, arm, forearm, wrist, hand, and fingers
CC Exd: 729.81, 729.89-729.99
AHA: 4Q, '06, 100-102

958.92 Traumatic compartment syndrome of lower extremity   CC
Traumatic compartment syndrome of hip, buttock, thigh, leg, foot, and toes
CC Exd: See code: 958.91
AHA: 4Q, '06, 100-102

958.93 Traumatic compartment syndrome of abdomen   CC
CC Exd: 863.0-867.3, 867.5-869.1, 879.2-879.9, 929.0-929.9, 958.8, 959.8-959.9
AHA: 4Q, '06, 100-102

958.99 Traumatic compartment syndrome of other sites   CC
CC Exd: 868.03-868.10, 868.13-869.1
AHA: 4Q, '06, 100-102

√4ᵗʰ **959 Injury, other and unspecified**
INCLUDES injury NOS
EXCLUDES injury NOS of:
blood vessels (900.0-904.9)
eye (921.0-921.9)
internal organs (860.0-869.1)
intracranial sites (854.0-854.1)
nerves (950.0-951.9, 953.0-957.9)
spinal cord (952.0-952.9)

√5ᵗʰ **959.0 Head, face and neck**

959.01 Head injury, unspecified
EXCLUDES concussion (850.1-850.9)
with head injury NOS (850.1-850.9)
head injury NOS with loss of consciousness (850.1-850.5)
specified intracranial injuries (850.0-854.1)
AHA: 4Q, '08, 108; 4Q, '97, 46
S09.90xA Unspecified injury of head initial encounter   I-10

959.09 Injury of face and neck

Cheek	Mouth
Ear	Nose
Eyebrow	Throat
Lip	

AHA: 4Q, '97, 46

√5ᵗʰ **959.1 Trunk**
EXCLUDES scapular region (959.2)
AHA: 4Q, '03, 78; 1Q, '99, 10

959.11 Other injury of chest wall

959.12 Other injury of abdomen

959.13 Fracture of corpus cavernosum penis   ♂

959.14 Other injury of external genitals

959.19 Other injury of other sites of trunk
Injury of trunk NOS

Additional Digit Required   Unacceptable PDx   Manifestation Code   Hospital Acquired Condition   ▶◀ Revised Text   ● New Code   ▲ Revised Code Title

2014 ICD-9-CM   Volume 1 – 331

Injury and Poisoning *(left margin)*

959.2 Shoulder and upper arm
 Axilla
 Scapular region

959.3 Elbow, forearm, and wrist
 AHA: 1Q, '97, 8

959.4 Hand, except finger

959.5 Finger
 Fingernail
 Thumb (nail)

959.6 Hip and thigh
 Upper leg

959.7 Knee, leg, ankle, and foot

959.8 Other specified sites, including multiple
 EXCLUDES *multiple sites classifiable to the same four-digit*
 category (959.0-959.7)

959.9 Unspecified site

Poisoning by Drugs, Medicinal and Biological Substances (960-979)

 INCLUDES overdose of these substances
 wrong substance given or taken in error
 Use additional code to specify the effects of the poisoning
 EXCLUDES *adverse effects ["hypersensitivity," "reaction," etc.] of correct*
 substance properly administered. Such cases are to be
 classified according to the nature of the adverse effect,
 such as:
 adverse effect NOS (995.20)
 allergic lymphadenitis (289.3)
 aspirin gastritis (535.4)
 blood disorders (280.0-289.9)
 dermatitis:
 contact (692.0-692.9)
 due to ingestion (693.0-693.9)
 nephropathy (583.9)
 [The drug giving rise to the adverse effect may be identified
 by use of categories E930-E949.]
 drug dependence (304.0-304.9)
 drug reaction and poisoning affecting the newborn
 (760.0-779.9)
 nondependent abuse of drugs (305.0-305.9)
 pathological drug intoxication (292.2)

 AHA: 2Q, '90, 11

 TIP: Assign a poisoning code for interaction between prescribed drug and
 alcohol or prescribed drug and other nonprescribed drug or medicinal
 agent. Sequence poisoning code first, then code for manifestation of poisoning.
 If respiratory failure is due to a poisoning, the poisoning code must be
 sequenced first.

√4ᵗʰ 960 Poisoning by antibiotics
 EXCLUDES *antibiotics:*
 ear, nose, and throat (976.6)
 eye (976.5)
 local (976.0)

960.0 Penicillins
 Ampicillin   Cloxacillin
 Carbenicillin   Penicillin G

960.1 Antifungal antibiotics
 Amphotericin B   Nystatin
 Griseofulvin   Trichomycin
 EXCLUDES *preparations intended for topical use (976.0-976.9)*

960.2 Chloramphenicol group
 Chloramphenicol
 Thiamphenicol

960.3 Erythromycin and other macrolides
 Oleandomycin
 Spiramycin

960.4 Tetracycline group
 Doxycycline   Oxytetracycline
 Minocycline

960.5 Cephalosporin group
 Cephalexin   Cephaloridine
 Cephaloglycin   Cephalothin

960.6 Antimycobacterial antibiotics
 Cycloserine   Rifampin
 Kanamycin   Streptomycin

960.7 Antineoplastic antibiotics
 Actinomycin such as: Actinomycin such as:
 Bleomycin   Daunorubicin
 Cactinomycin   Mitomycin
 Dactinomycin

960.8 Other specified antibiotics

960.9 Unspecified antibiotic

√4ᵗʰ 961 Poisoning by other anti-infectives
 EXCLUDES *anti-infectives:*
 ear, nose, and throat (976.6)
 eye (976.5)
 local (976.0)

961.0 Sulfonamides
 Sulfadiazine   Sulfamethoxazole
 Sulfafurazole

961.1 Arsenical anti-infectives

961.2 Heavy metal anti-infectives
 Compounds of: Compounds of:
 antimony   lead
 bismuth   mercury
 EXCLUDES *mercurial diuretics (974.0)*

961.3 Quinoline and hydroxyquinoline derivatives
 Chiniofon
 Diiodohydroxyquin
 EXCLUDES *antimalarial drugs (961.4)*

961.4 Antimalarials and drugs acting on other blood protozoa
 Chloroquine   Proguanil [chloroguanide]
 Cycloguanil   Pyrimethamine
 Primaquine   Quinine

961.5 Other antiprotozoal drugs
 Emetine

961.6 Anthelmintics
 Hexylresorcinol   Thiabendazole
 Piperazine

961.7 Antiviral drugs
 Methisazone
 EXCLUDES *amantadine (966.4)*
 cytarabine (963.1)
 idoxuridine (976.5)

961.8 Other antimycobacterial drugs
 Ethambutol
 Ethionamide
 Isoniazid
 Para-aminosalicylic acid derivatives
 Sulfones

961.9 Other and unspecified anti-infectives
 Flucytosine
 Nitrofuran derivatives

√4ᵗʰ 962 Poisoning by hormones and synthetic substitutes
 EXCLUDES *oxytocic hormones (975.0)*

962.0 Adrenal cortical steroids
 Cortisone derivatives
 Desoxycorticosterone derivatives
 Fluorinated corticosteroids

962.1 Androgens and anabolic congeners
 Methandriol   Oxymetholone
 Nandrolone   Testosterone

962.2 Ovarian hormones and synthetic substitutes
 Contraceptives, oral
 Estrogens
 Estrogens and progestogens, combined
 Progestogens

Ⓝ Newborn Age: 0   Ⓟ Pediatric Age: 0-17   Ⓜ Maternity Age: 12-55   Ⓐ Adult Age: 15-124   MCC Major CC Condition   CC CC Condition   HIV HIV Related Dx

332 – Volume 1   2014 ICD-9-CM

962.3 Insulins and antidiabetic agents
Acetohexamide
Biguanide derivatives, oral
Chlorpropamide
Glucagon
Insulin
Phenformin
Sulfonylurea derivatives, oral
Tolbutamide
AHA: 4Q, '93, 19; M-A, '85, 8
TIP: Assign only if documentation indicates overdose of insulin; if due to diabetic adjusting dosage, assign instead 250.8x or 249.8x and E932.3 for adverse reaction to insulin, if applicable.

962.4 Anterior pituitary hormones
Corticotropin
Gonadotropin
Somatotropin [growth hormone]

962.5 Posterior pituitary hormones
Vasopressin
EXCLUDES   oxytocic hormones (975.0)

962.6 Parathyroid and parathyroid derivatives

962.7 Thyroid and thyroid derivatives
Dextrothyroxin   Liothyronine
Levothyroxine sodium   Thyroglobulin

962.8 Antithyroid agents
Iodides
Thiouracil
Thiourea

962.9 Other and unspecified hormones and synthetic substitutes

✓4ᵗʰ **963 Poisoning by primarily systemic agents**

963.0 Antiallergic and antiemetic drugs
Antihistamines   Diphenylpyraline
Chlorpheniramine   Thonzylamine
Diphenhydramine   Tripelennamine
EXCLUDES   phenothiazine-based tranquilizers (969.1)

963.1 Antineoplastic and immunosuppressive drugs
Azathioprine   Cytarabine
Busulfan   Fluorouracil
Chlorambucil   Mercaptopurine
Cyclophosphamidethio-TEPA
EXCLUDES   antineoplastic antibiotics (960.7)

963.2 Acidifying agents

963.3 Alkalizing agents

963.4 Enzymes, not elsewhere classified
Penicillinase

963.5 Vitamins, not elsewhere classified
Vitamin A
Vitamin D
EXCLUDES   nicotinic acid (972.2)
            vitamin K (964.3)

963.8 Other specified systemic agents
Heavy metal antagonists

963.9 Unspecified systemic agent

✓4ᵗʰ **964 Poisoning by agents primarily affecting blood constituents**

964.0 Iron and its compounds
Ferric salts
Ferrous sulfate and other ferrous salts

964.1 Liver preparations and other antianemic agents
Folic acid

964.2 Anticoagulants
Coumarin   Phenindione
Heparin   Warfarin sodium
AHA: 1Q, '94, 22
TIP: If documentation indicates an adverse reaction to Coumadin, assign instead manifestation (e.g., hematuria or epistaxis), code 790.92 if abnormal coagulation profile is documented, and E934.2.

964.3 Vitamin K [phytonadione]

964.4 Fibrinolysis-affecting drugs
Aminocaproic acid   Streptokinase
Streptodornase   Urokinase

964.5 Anticoagulant antagonists and other coagulants
Hexadimethrine
Protamine sulfate

964.6 Gamma globulin

964.7 Natural blood and blood products
Blood plasma   Packed red cells
Human fibrinogen   Whole blood
EXCLUDES   transfusion reactions (999.41-999.8)

964.8 Other specified agents affecting blood constituents
Macromolecular blood substitutes
Plasma expanders

964.9 Unspecified agent affecting blood constituents

✓4ᵗʰ **965 Poisoning by analgesics, antipyretics, and antirheumatics**
EXCLUDES   drug dependence (304.0-304.9)
            nondependent abuse (305.0-305.9)

✓5ᵗʰ **965.0 Opiates and related narcotics**

     965.00 Opium (alkaloids), unspecified
        AHA: 3Q, '07, 6

     965.01 Heroin
        Diacetylmorphine

     965.02 Methadone

     965.09 Other
        Codeine [methylmorphine]
        Meperidine [pethidine]
        Morphine
        AHA: 3Q, '07, 6
        T40.4x1A Poisoning oth synthetic narc accidnt initial enc I-10

965.1 Salicylates
Acetylsalicylic acid [aspirin]
Salicylic acid salts
AHA: N-D, '94, 15

965.4 Aromatic analgesics, not elsewhere classified
Acetanilid
Paracetamol [acetaminophen]
Phenacetin [acetophenetidin]

965.5 Pyrazole derivatives
Aminophenazone [aminopyrine]
Phenylbutazone

✓5ᵗʰ **965.6 Antirheumatics [antiphlogistics]**
EXCLUDES   salicylates (965.1)
            steroids (962.0-962.9)
AHA: 4Q, '98, 50

     965.61 Propionic acid derivatives
        Fenoprofen   Ketoprofen
        Flurbiprofen   Naproxen
        Ibuprofen   Oxaprozin
        AHA: 4Q, '98, 50

     965.69 Other antirheumatics
        Gold salts
        Indomethacin

965.7 Other non-narcotic analgesics
Pyrabital

965.8 Other specified analgesics and antipyretics
Pentazocine

965.9 Unspecified analgesic and antipyretic

✓4ᵗʰ **966 Poisoning by anticonvulsants and anti-Parkinsonism drugs**

966.0 Oxazolidine derivatives
Paramethadione
Trimethadione

966.1 Hydantoin derivatives
Phenytoin

966.2 Succinimides
Ethosuximide
Phensuximide

966.3 Other and unspecified anticonvulsants
Primidone
EXCLUDES   barbiturates (967.0)
            sulfonamides (961.0)

Additional Digit Required   Unacceptable PDx   Manifestation Code   Hospital Acquired Condition   ▶◀ Revised Text   ● New Code   ▲ Revised Code Title

2014 ICD-9-CM   Volume 1 – 333

Injury and Poisoning

966.4–970.9

966.4 Anti-Parkinsonism drugs
Amantadine
Ethopropazine [profenamine]
Levodopa [L-dopa]

√4th **967 Poisoning by sedatives and hypnotics**
EXCLUDES   drug dependence (304.0-304.9)
         nondependent abuse (305.0-305.9)

967.0 Barbiturates
Amobarbital [amylobarbitone]
Barbital [barbitone]
Butabarbital [butabarbitone]
Pentobarbital [pentobarbitone]
Phenobarbital [phenobarbitone]
Secobarbital [quinalbarbitone]
EXCLUDES   thiobarbiturate anesthetics (968.3)

967.1 Chloral hydrate group

967.2 Paraldehyde

967.3 Bromine compounds
Bromide
Carbromal (derivatives)

967.4 Methaqualone compounds

967.5 Glutethimide group

967.6 Mixed sedatives, not elsewhere classified

967.8 Other sedatives and hypnotics

967.9 Unspecified sedative or hypnotic
Sleeping:
   drug
   pill   } NOS
   tablet

√4th **968 Poisoning by other central nervous system depressants and anesthetics**
EXCLUDES   drug dependence (304.0-304.9)
         nondependent abuse (305.0-305.9)

968.0 Central nervous system muscle-tone depressants
Chlorphenesin (carbamate)
Mephenesin
Methocarbamol

968.1 Halothane

968.2 Other gaseous anesthetics
Ether
Halogenated hydrocarbon derivatives, except halothane
Nitrous oxide

968.3 Intravenous anesthetics
Ketamine
Methohexital [methohexitone]
Thiobarbiturates, such as thiopental sodium

968.4 Other and unspecified general anesthetics

968.5 Surface (topical) and infiltration anesthetics
Cocaine (topical)
Lidocaine (lignocaine)
Procaine
Tetracaine
EXCLUDES   poisoning by cocaine used as a central nervous
         system stimulant (970.81)
AHA: 1Q, '93, 25

968.6 Peripheral nerve- and plexus-blocking anesthetics

968.7 Spinal anesthetics

968.9 Other and unspecified local anesthetics
T41.44xA Poisoning uns anesthetic undetermind initial enc   I-10

√4th **969 Poisoning by psychotropic agents**
EXCLUDES   drug dependence (304.0-304.9)
         nondependent abuse (305.0-305.9)

√5th **969.0 Antidepressants**
AHA: 4Q, '09, 111-112

969.00 Antidepressant, unspecified
AHA: 3Q, '07, 6; #5, '94, 9; 3Q, '91, 14; N-D, '84, 14

969.01 Monoamine oxidase inhibitors
MAOI

969.02 Selective serotonin and norepinephrine reuptake inhibitors
SSNRI antidepressants
TIP: Assign for serotonin syndrome due to poisoning, along with 333.99 and E854.0, for accidental poisoning.

969.03 Selective serotonin reuptake inhibitors
SSRI antidepressants
TIP: Assign for serotonin syndrome due to poisoning, along with 333.99 and E854.0, for accidental poisoning.

969.04 Tetracyclic antidepressants

969.05 Tricyclic antidepressants
AHA: 4Q, '09, 112

969.09 Other antidepressants

969.1 Phenothiazine-based tranquilizers
Chlorpromazine   Prochlorperazine
Fluphenazine   Promazine

969.2 Butyrophenone-based tranquilizers
Haloperidol
Spiperone
Trifluperidol

969.3 Other antipsychotics, neuroleptics, and major tranquilizers

969.4 Benzodiazepine-based tranquilizers
Chlordiazepoxide
Diazepam
Flurazepam
Lorazepam
Medazepam
Nitrazepam
AHA: 4Q, '09, 112
T42.4X1A Poisoning by benzodiazepines, accidental, init   I-10

969.5 Other tranquilizers
Hydroxyzine
Meprobamate

969.6 Psychodysleptics [hallucinogens]
Cannabis (derivatives)
Lysergide [LSD]
Marihuana (derivatives)
Mescaline
Psilocin
Psilocybin

√5th **969.7 Psychostimulants**
EXCLUDES   central appetite depressants (977.0)
AHA: 4Q, '09, 113-114

969.70 Psychostimulant, unspecified
AHA: 2Q, '03, 11

969.71 Caffeine

969.72 Amphetamines
Methamphetamines
TIP: Assign for overdose and poisoning by the club drug ecstasy.

969.73 Methylphenidate

969.79 Other psychostimulants

969.8 Other specified psychotropic agents

969.9 Unspecified psychotropic agent

√4th **970 Poisoning by central nervous system stimulants**

970.0 Analeptics
Lobeline
Nikethamide

970.1 Opiate antagonists
Levallorphan
Nalorphine
Naloxone

√5th **970.8 Other specified central nervous system stimulants**
AHA: 1Q, '05, 6

970.81 Cocaine
Crack

970.89 Other central nervous system stimulants

970.9 Unspecified central nervous system stimulant

N Newborn Age: 0   P Pediatric Age: 0-17   M Maternity Age: 12-55   A Adult Age: 15-124   MCC Major CC Condition   CC CC Condition   HIV HIV Related D

334 – Volume 1   2014 ICD-9-C

√4ᵗʰ **971 Poisoning by drugs primarily affecting the autonomic nervous system**

971.0 Parasympathomimetics [cholinergics]
Acetylcholine
Anticholinesterase:
  organophosphorus
  reversible
Pilocarpine

971.1 Parasympatholytics [anticholinergics and antimuscarinics] and spasmolytics
Atropine
Homatropine
Hyoscine [scopolamine]
Quaternary ammonium derivatives
EXCLUDES *papaverine (972.5)*

971.2 Sympathomimetics [adrenergics]
Epinephrine [adrenalin]
Levarterenol [noradrenalin]

971.3 Sympatholytics [antiadrenergics]
Phenoxybenzamine
Tolazoline hydrochloride

971.9 Unspecified drug primarily affecting autonomic nervous system

√4ᵗʰ **972 Poisoning by agents primarily affecting the cardiovascular system**

972.0 Cardiac rhythm regulators
Practolol
Procainamide
Propranolol
Quinidine
EXCLUDES *lidocaine (968.5)*

972.1 Cardiotonic glycosides and drugs of similar action
Digitalis glycosides
Digoxin
Strophanthins

972.2 Antilipemic and antiarteriosclerotic drugs
Clofibrate
Nicotinic acid derivatives

972.3 Ganglion-blocking agents
Pentamethonium bromide

972.4 Coronary vasodilators
Dipyridamole
Nitrates [nitroglycerin]
Nitrites

972.5 Other vasodilators
Cyclandelate
Diazoxide
Papaverine
EXCLUDES *nicotinic acid (972.2)*

972.6 Other antihypertensive agents
Clonidine
Guanethidine
Rauwolfia alkaloids
Reserpine

972.7 Antivaricose drugs, including sclerosing agents
Sodium morrhuate
Zinc salts

972.8 Capillary-active drugs
Adrenochrome derivatives
Metaraminol

972.9 Other and unspecified agents primarily affecting the cardiovascular system

√4ᵗʰ **973 Poisoning by agents primarily affecting the gastrointestinal system**

973.0 Antacids and antigastric secretion drugs
Aluminum hydroxide
Magnesium trisilicate
AHA: 1Q, '03, 19

973.1 Irritant cathartics
Bisacodyl
Castor oil
Phenolphthalein

973.2 Emollient cathartics
Dioctyl sulfosuccinates

973.3 Other cathartics, including intestinal atonia drugs
Magnesium sulfate

973.4 Digestants
Pancreatin
Papain
Pepsin

973.5 Antidiarrheal drugs
Kaolin
Pectin
EXCLUDES *anti-infectives (960.0-961.9)*

973.6 Emetics

973.8 Other specified agents primarily affecting the gastrointestinal system

973.9 Unspecified agent primarily affecting the gastrointestinal system

√4ᵗʰ **974 Poisoning by water, mineral, and uric acid metabolism drugs**

974.0 Mercurial diuretics
Chlormerodrin   Mersalyl
Mercaptomerin

974.1 Purine derivative diuretics
Theobromine
Theophylline
EXCLUDES *aminophylline [theophylline ethylenediamine]*
    (975.7)
    caffeine (969.71)

974.2 Carbonic acid anhydrase inhibitors
Acetazolamide

974.3 Saluretics
Benzothiadiazides
Chlorothiazide group

974.4 Other diuretics
Ethacrynic acid
Furosemide

974.5 Electrolytic, caloric, and water-balance agents

974.6 Other mineral salts, not elsewhere classified

974.7 Uric acid metabolism drugs
Allopurinol   Probenecid
Colchicine

√4ᵗʰ **975 Poisoning by agents primarily acting on the smooth and skeletal muscles and respiratory system**

975.0 Oxytocic agents
Ergot alkaloids
Oxytocin
Prostaglandins

975.1 Smooth muscle relaxants
Adiphenine
Metaproterenol [orciprenaline]
EXCLUDES *papaverine (972.5)*

975.2 Skeletal muscle relaxants

975.3 Other and unspecified drugs acting on muscles

975.4 Antitussives
Dextromethorphan
Pipazethate

975.5 Expectorants
Acetylcysteine
Guaifenesin
Terpin hydrate

975.6 Anti-common cold drugs

975.7 Antiasthmatics
Aminophylline [theophylline ethylenediamine]

975.8 Other and unspecified respiratory drugs

Additional Digit Required   Unacceptable PDx   Manifestation Code   Hospital Acquired Condition   ▶◀ Revised Text   ● New Code   ▲ Revised Code Title

2014 ICD-9-CM   **Volume 1 – 335**

Injury and Poisoning

976–983.1

√4ᵗʰ **976 Poisoning by agents primarily affecting skin and mucous membrane, ophthalmological, otorhinolaryngological, and dental drugs**

976.0 Local anti-infectives and anti-inflammatory drugs

976.1 Antipruritics

976.2 Local astringents and local detergents

976.3 Emollients, demulcents, and protectants

976.4 Keratolytics, keratoplastics, other hair treatment drugs and preparations

976.5 Eye anti-infectives and other eye drugs
Idoxuridine

976.6 Anti-infectives and other drugs and preparations for ear, nose, and throat

976.7 Dental drugs topically applied
EXCLUDES *anti-infectives (976.0)*
local anesthetics (968.5)

976.8 Other agents primarily affecting skin and mucous membrane
Spermicides [vaginal contraceptives]

976.9 Unspecified agent primarily affecting skin and mucous membrane

√4ᵗʰ **977 Poisoning by other and unspecified drugs and medicinal substances**

977.0 Dietetics
Central appetite depressants

977.1 Lipotropic drugs

977.2 Antidotes and chelating agents, not elsewhere classified

977.3 Alcohol deterrents

977.4 Pharmaceutical excipients
Pharmaceutical adjuncts

977.8 Other specified drugs and medicinal substances
Contrast media used for diagnostic x-ray procedures
Diagnostic agents and kits

977.9 Unspecified drug or medicinal substance

√4ᵗʰ **978 Poisoning by bacterial vaccines**

978.0 BCG

978.1 Typhoid and paratyphoid

978.2 Cholera

978.3 Plague

978.4 Tetanus

978.5 Diphtheria

978.6 Pertussis vaccine, including combinations with a pertussis component

978.8 Other and unspecified bacterial vaccines

978.9 Mixed bacterial vaccines, except combinations with a pertussis component

√4ᵗʰ **979 Poisoning by other vaccines and biological substances**
EXCLUDES *gamma globulin (964.6)*

979.0 Smallpox vaccine

979.1 Rabies vaccine

979.2 Typhus vaccine

979.3 Yellow fever vaccine

979.4 Measles vaccine

979.5 Poliomyelitis vaccine

979.6 Other and unspecified viral and rickettsial vaccines
Mumps vaccine

979.7 Mixed viral-rickettsial and bacterial vaccines, except combinations with a pertussis component
EXCLUDES *combinations with a pertussis component (978.6)*

979.9 Other and unspecified vaccines and biological substances

Toxic Effects of Substances Chiefly Nonmedicinal as to Source (980-989)

Use additional code to identify:
personal history of retained foreign body fully removed (V15.53)
retained foreign body status, if applicable, (V90.01-V90.9)

Use additional code to specify the nature of the toxic effect

EXCLUDES *burns from chemical agents (ingested) (947.0-947.9)*
localized toxic effects indexed elsewhere (001.0-799.9)
respiratory conditions due to external agents (506.0-508.9)
respiratory conditions due to smoke inhalation NOS (508.2)

AHA: 3Q, '10, 19

√4ᵗʰ **980 Toxic effect of alcohol**

980.0 Ethyl alcohol
Denatured alcohol   Grain alcohol
Ethanol

Use additional code to identify any associated:
acute alcohol intoxication (305.0)
in alcoholism (303.0)
drunkenness (simple) (305.0)
pathological (291.4)

AHA: 4Q, '09, 112; 3Q, '96, 16

T51.0x1A Toxic effect ethanol accidental initial encountr   I-10

980.1 Methyl alcohol
Methanol
Wood alcohol

980.2 Isopropyl alcohol
Dimethyl carbinol
Isopropanol
Rubbing alcohol

980.3 Fusel oil
Alcohol:
amyl
butyl
propyl

980.8 Other specified alcohols

980.9 Unspecified alcohol

981 Toxic effect of petroleum products
Benzine
Gasoline
Kerosene
Paraffin wax
Petroleum:
ether
naphtha
spirit

√4ᵗʰ **982 Toxic effect of solvents other than petroleum-based**

982.0 Benzene and homologues

982.1 Carbon tetrachloride

982.2 Carbon disulfide
Carbon bisulfide

982.3 Other chlorinated hydrocarbon solvents
Tetrachloroethylene
Trichloroethylene
EXCLUDES *chlorinated hydrocarbon preparations other than solvents (989.2)*

AHA: 3Q, '08, 6-7

982.4 Nitroglycol

982.8 Other nonpetroleum-based solvents
Acetone

√4ᵗʰ **983 Toxic effect of corrosive aromatics, acids, and caustic alkalis**

983.0 Corrosive aromatics
Carbolic acid or phenol   Cresol

983.1 Acids
Acid:
hydrochloric
nitric
sulfuric

N Newborn Age: 0   P Pediatric Age: 0-17   M Maternity Age: 12-55   A Adult Age: 15-124   MCC Major CC Condition   CC CC Condition   HIV HIV Related Da

336 – Volume 1   2014 ICD-9-CM

983.2 Caustic alkalis
Lye
Potassium hydroxide
Sodium hydroxide

983.9 Caustic, unspecified

√4ᵗʰ **984 Toxic effect of lead and its compounds (including fumes)**
INCLUDES that from all sources except medicinal substances

984.0 Inorganic lead compounds
Lead dioxide
Lead salts

984.1 Organic lead compounds
Lead acetate
Tetraethyl lead

984.8 Other lead compounds

984.9 Unspecified lead compound

√4ᵗʰ **985 Toxic effect of other metals**
INCLUDES that from all sources except medicinal substances

985.0 Mercury and its compounds
Minamata disease

985.1 Arsenic and its compounds

985.2 Manganese and its compounds

985.3 Beryllium and its compounds

985.4 Antimony and its compounds

985.5 Cadmium and its compounds

985.6 Chromium

985.8 Other specified metals
Brass fumes   Iron compounds
Copper salts   Nickel compounds
AHA: 1Q, '88, 5
TIP: Assign for aluminum overloading or excessive concentration of aluminum in the body, along with E879.1 if due to renal dialysis and E879.8 if due to total parenteral nutrition.

985.9 Unspecified metal

986 Toxic effect of carbon monoxide
Carbon monoxide from any source

√4ᵗʰ **987 Toxic effect of other gases, fumes, or vapors**

987.0 Liquefied petroleum gases
Butane
Propane

987.1 Other hydrocarbon gas

987.2 Nitrogen oxides
Nitrogen dioxide
Nitrous fumes

987.3 Sulfur dioxide

987.4 Freon
Dichloromonofluoromethane

987.5 Lacrimogenic gas
Bromobenzyl cyanide
Chloroacetophenone
Ethyliodoacetate

987.6 Chlorine gas

987.7 Hydrocyanic acid gas

987.8 Other specified gases, fumes, or vapors
Phosgene
Polyester fumes

987.9 Unspecified gas, fume, or vapor
AHA: 4Q, '11, 114; 3Q, '05, 10
TIP: Do not assign for conditions due to smoke inhalation; assign instead code 508.2.

√4ᵗʰ **988 Toxic effect of noxious substances eaten as food**
EXCLUDES *allergic reaction to food, such as:*
gastroenteritis (558.3)
rash (692.5, 693.1)
food poisoning (bacterial) (005.0-005.9)
toxic effects of food contaminants, such as:
aflatoxin and other mycotoxin (989.7)
mercury (985.0)

988.0 Fish and shellfish

988.1 Mushrooms

988.2 Berries and other plants

988.8 Other specified noxious substances eaten as food

988.9 Unspecified noxious substance eaten as food

√4ᵗʰ **989 Toxic effect of other substances, chiefly nonmedicinal as to source**

989.0 Hydrocyanic acid and cyanides
Potassium cyanide
Sodium cyanide
EXCLUDES *gas and fumes (987.7)*

989.1 Strychnine and salts

989.2 Chlorinated hydrocarbons
Aldrin
Chlordane
DDT
Dieldrin
EXCLUDES *chlorinated hydrocarbon solvents (982.0-982.3)*

989.3 Organophosphate and carbamate
Carbaryl
Dichlorvos
Malathion
Parathion
Phorate
Phosdrin

989.4 Other pesticides, not elsewhere classified
Mixtures of insecticides

989.5 Venom
Bites of venomous snakes, lizards, and spiders
Tick paralysis

989.6 Soaps and detergents

989.7 Aflatoxin and other mycotoxin [food contaminants]

√5ᵗʰ **989.8 Other substances, chiefly nonmedicinal as to source**
AHA: 4Q, '95, 60

    989.81 Asbestos
      EXCLUDES *asbestosis (501)*
exposure to asbestos (V15.84)

    989.82 Latex

    989.83 Silicone
      EXCLUDES *silicone used in medical devices, implants and grafts (996.00-996.79)*

    989.84 Tobacco

    989.89 Other

989.9 Unspecified substance, chiefly nonmedicinal as to source

Other and Unspecified Effects of External Causes (990-995)

990 Effects of radiation, unspecified
Complication of:
phototherapy
radiation therapy
Radiation sickness
[The type of radiation giving rise to the adverse effect may be identified by use of the E codes.]
EXCLUDES *specified adverse effects of radiation. Such conditions are to be classified according to the nature of the adverse effect, as:*
burns (940.0-949.5)
dermatitis (692.7-692.8)
leukemia (204.0-208.9)
pneumonia (508.0)
sunburn (692.71, 692.76-692.77)

Additional Digit Required   Unacceptable PDx   Manifestation Code   Hospital Acquired Condition   ►◄ Revised Text   ● New Code   ▲ Revised Code Title

014 ICD-9-CM   Volume 1 – 337

Injury and Poisoning

991–994.9

√4th **991 Effects of reduced temperature**

991.0 Frostbite of face   CC
     CC Exd: 991.0, 991.3

991.1 Frostbite of hand   CC
     CC Exd: 991.1, 991.3

991.2 Frostbite of foot   CC
     CC Exd: 991.2-991.3

991.3 Frostbite of other and unspecified sites   CC
     CC Exd: 991.0-991.4

991.4 Immersion foot   CC
     Trench foot
     DEF: Paresthesia, edema, blotchy cyanosis of foot, the skin is soft (macerated), pale and wrinkled, and the sole is swollen with surface ridging and following sustained immersion in water.
     CC Exd: 991.3-991.4

991.5 Chilblains
     Erythema pernio
     Perniosis
     DEF: Red, swollen, itchy skin; follows damp cold exposure; also associated with pruritus and a burning feeling in hands, feet, ears, and face in children, legs and toes in women, and hands and fingers in men.

991.6 Hypothermia
     Hypothermia (accidental)
     EXCLUDES   *hypothermia following anesthesia (995.89)*
         hypothermia not associated with low environmental temperature (780.65)
     DEF: Reduced body temperature due to low environmental temperatures.

991.8 Other specified effects of reduced temperature

991.9 Unspecified effect of reduced temperature
     Effects of freezing or excessive cold NOS

√4th **992 Effects of heat and light**
     EXCLUDES   *burns (940.0-949.5)*
         diseases of sweat glands due to heat (705.0-705.9)
         malignant hyperpyrexia following anesthesia (995.86)
         sunburn (692.71, 692.76-692.77)

992.0 Heat stroke and sunstroke   CC
     Heat apoplexy
     Heat pyrexia
     Ictus solaris
     Siriasis
     Thermoplegia
     Use additional code(s) to identify any associated complication of heat stroke, such as:
         alterations of consciousness (780.01-780.09)
         systemic inflammatory response syndrome (995.93-995.94)
     DEF: Headache, vertigo, cramps and elevated body temperature due to high environmental temperatures.
     CC Exd: 992.0-992.9

992.1 Heat syncope
     Heat collapse

992.2 Heat cramps

992.3 Heat exhaustion, anhydrotic
     Heat prostration due to water depletion
     EXCLUDES   *that associated with salt depletion (992.4)*

992.4 Heat exhaustion due to salt depletion
     Heat prostration due to salt (and water) depletion

992.5 Heat exhaustion, unspecified
     Heat prostration NOS

992.6 Heat fatigue, transient

992.7 Heat edema
     DEF: Fluid retention due to high environmental temperatures.

992.8 Other specified heat effects

992.9 Unspecified

√4th **993 Effects of air pressure**

993.0 Barotrauma, otitic
     Aero-otitis media
     Effects of high altitude on ears
     DEF: Ringing ears, deafness, pain and vertigo due to air pressure changes.

993.1 Barotrauma, sinus
     Aerosinusitis
     Effects of high altitude on sinuses

993.2 Other and unspecified effects of high altitude
     Alpine sickness
     Andes disease
     Anoxia due to high altitude
     Hypobaropathy
     Mountain sickness
     AHA: 3Q, '88, 4

993.3 Caisson disease   CC
     Bends
     Compressed-air disease
     Decompression sickness
     Divers' palsy or paralysis
     DEF: Rapid reduction in air pressure while breathing compressed air; symptoms include skin lesions, joint pains, respiratory and neurological problems.
     CC Exd: 993.3-993.9

993.4 Effects of air pressure caused by explosion

993.8 Other specified effects of air pressure

993.9 Unspecified effect of air pressure

√4th **994 Effects of other external causes**
     EXCLUDES   *certain adverse effects not elsewhere classified (995.0-995.8)*

994.0 Effects of lightning
     Shock from lightning
     Struck by lightning NOS
     EXCLUDES   *burns (940.0-949.5)*

994.1 Drowning and nonfatal submersion   CC
     Bathing cramp
     Immersion
     CC Exd: 994.1
     AHA: 3Q, '09, 14; 3Q, '88, 4
     TIP: When near-drowning results in acute respiratory edema, assign also code 518.5 Post-traumatic pulmonary insufficiency.

994.2 Effects of hunger
     Deprivation of food
     Starvation

994.3 Effects of thirst
     Deprivation of water

994.4 Exhaustion due to exposure

994.5 Exhaustion due to excessive exertion
     Exhaustion due to overexertion

994.6 Motion sickness
     Air sickness
     Seasickness
     Travel sickness

994.7 Asphyxiation and strangulation   CC
     Suffocation (by):   Suffocation (by):
       bedclothes   plastic bag
       cave-in   pressure
       constriction   strangulation
       mechanical
     EXCLUDES   *asphyxia from:*
         carbon monoxide (986)
         inhalation of food or foreign body (932-934.9)
         other gases, fumes, and vapors (987.0-987.9)
     CC Exd: 994.7

994.8 Electrocution and nonfatal effects of electric current
     Shock from electric current
     Shock from electroshock gun (taser)
     EXCLUDES   *electric burns (940.0-949.5)*

994.9 Other effects of external causes
     Effects of:
         abnormal gravitational [G] forces or states
         weightlessness

N Newborn Age: 0   P Pediatric Age: 0-17   M Maternity Age: 12-55   A Adult Age: 15-124   MCC Major CC Condition   CC CC Condition   HIV HIV Related Dx

338 – Volume 1   2014 ICD-9-CM

√4ᵗʰ 995 Certain adverse effects not elsewhere classified

> *EXCLUDES* *complications of surgical and medical care (996.0-999.9)*

995.0 Other anaphylactic reaction `cc`

Allergic shock
Anaphylactic reaction
Anaphylactic shock NOS or due to adverse effect of correct medicinal substance properly administered
Anaphylactoid reaction, NOS
Anaphylaxis

Use additional E code to identify external cause, such as: adverse effects of correct medicinal substance properly administered [E930-E949]

> *EXCLUDES* *anaphylactic reaction to serum (999.41-999.49)*
> *anaphylactic shock or reaction due to adverse food reaction (995.60-995.69)*

DEF: Immediate sensitivity response after exposure to specific antigen; results in life-threatening respiratory distress; usually followed by vascular collapse, shock, urticaria, angioedema and pruritus.
CC Excl: 995.60-995.69
AHA: 4Q, '93, 30

995.1 Angioneurotic edema

Allergic angioedema
Giant urticaria

> *EXCLUDES* *urticaria:*
> *due to serum (999.51-999.59)*
> *other specified (698.2, 708.0-708.9, 757.33)*

DEF: Circulatory response of deep dermis, subcutaneous or submucosal tissues; causes localized edema and wheals.

√5ᵗʰ 995.2 Other and unspecified adverse effect of drug, medicinal and biological substance

> *EXCLUDES* *pathological drug intoxication (292.2)*
> **AHA:** 2Q, '97, 12; 3Q, '95, 13; 3Q, '92, 16
> **TIP:** Codes from this subcategory should not be assigned for inpatient cases; their use is limited to certain outpatient cases in which there is no documentation of specific symptoms associated with the adverse effect.

995.20 Unspecified adverse effect of unspecified drug, medicinal and biological substance
Unspecified adverse effect of unspecified medicinal substance properly administered
AHA: 4Q, '06, 112

995.21 Arthus phenomenon
Arthus reaction
AHA: 4Q, '06, 112

995.22 Unspecified adverse effect of anesthesia
AHA: 4Q, '06, 112

995.23 Unspecified adverse effect of insulin
AHA: 4Q, '06, 112

995.24 Failed moderate sedation during procedure
Failed conscious sedation during procedure
AHA: 4Q, '09, 114
TIP: If documentation indicates a personal history of failed moderate sedation, assign instead code V15.80 History of failed moderate sedation.

995.27 Other drug allergy
Allergic reaction NEC (due) to correct medical substance properly administered
Drug allergy NOS
Drug hypersensitivity NOS
Hypersensitivity (due) to correct medical substance properly administered
AHA: 4Q, '06, 112

995.29 Unspecified adverse effect of other drug, medicinal and biological substance
Unspecified adverse effect of medicinal substance NEC properly administered
AHA: 4Q, '06, 112

995.3 Allergy, unspecified

Allergic reaction NOS   Idiosyncrasy NOS
Hypersensitivity NOS

> *EXCLUDES* *allergic reaction NOS to correct medicinal substance properly administered (995.27)*
> *allergy to existing dental restorative materials (525.66)*
> *specific types of allergic reaction, such as:*
> *allergic diarrhea (558.3)*
> *dermatitis (691.0-693.9)*
> *hayfever (477.0-477.9)*

995.4 Shock due to anesthesia `cc`
Shock due to anesthesia in which the correct substance was properly administered

> *EXCLUDES* *complications of anesthesia in labor or delivery (668.0-668.9)*
> *overdose or wrong substance given (968.0-969.9)*
> *postoperative shock NOS (998.00)*
> *specified adverse effects of anesthesia classified elsewhere, such as:*
> *anoxic brain damage (348.1)*
> *hepatitis (070.0-070.9), etc.*
> *unspecified adverse effect of anesthesia (995.22)*

CC Excl: 958.4, 995.4, 997.91-998.13, 998.81, 998.83-998.9

√5ᵗʰ 995.5 Child maltreatment syndrome
Use additional code(s), if applicable, to identify any associated injuries

Use additional E code to identify:
nature of abuse (E960-E968)
perpetrator (E967.0-E967.9)
AHA: ►2Q, '12, 12;◄ 1Q, '98, 11
TIP: Although separate codes for any associated injuries should be assigned, codes from this subcategory may be assigned alone if there are no documented injuries or associated conditions.

995.50 Child abuse, unspecified `cc` `P`
CC Excl: 995.50-995.59, 995.80-995.85

995.51 Child emotional/psychological abuse `cc` `P`
CC Excl: See code: 995.50
AHA: 4Q, '96, 38, 40

995.52 Child neglect (nutritional) `cc` `P`
CC Excl: See code: 995.50
AHA: 4Q, '96, 38, 40

995.53 Child sexual abuse `cc` `P`
CC Excl: See code: 995.50
AHA: 4Q, '96, 39, 40

995.54 Child physical abuse `cc` `P`
Battered baby or child syndrome

> *EXCLUDES* *shaken infant syndrome (995.55)*

CC Excl: See code: 995.50
AHA: 3Q, '99, 14; 4Q, '96, 39, 40

995.55 Shaken infant syndrome `cc` `P`
Use additional code(s) to identify any associated injuries
CC Excl: See code: 995.50
AHA: 4Q, '96, 40, 43

995.59 Other child abuse and neglect `cc` `P`
Multiple forms of abuse
CC Excl: See code: 995.50

√5ᵗʰ 995.6 Anaphylactic reaction due to food
Anaphylactic reaction due to adverse food reaction
Anaphylactic shock or reaction due to nonpoisonous foods
Anaphylactoid reaction due to food
AHA: 4Q, '11, 142-145; 4Q, '93, 30
TIP: Codes from this subcategory may be assigned not only for anaphylactic shock, but also for any documentation of anaphylactic reaction to food.

995.60 Anaphylactic reaction due to unspecified food `cc`
CC Excl: 995.60-995.69

995.61 Anaphylactic reaction due to peanuts `cc`
CC Excl: See code: 995.60

995.62 Anaphylactic reaction due to crustaceans `cc`
CC Excl: See code: 995.60

Injury and Poisoning

995.63–995.92

995.63 Anaphylactic reaction due to fruits and vegetables `CC`
CC Excl: See code: 995.60

995.64 Anaphylactic reaction due to tree nuts and seeds `CC`
AHA: 1Q, '08, 12
CC Excl: See code: 995.60

995.65 Anaphylactic reaction due to fish `CC`
CC Excl: See code: 995.60

995.66 Anaphylactic reaction due to food additives `CC`
CC Excl: See code: 995.60

995.67 Anaphylactic reaction due to milk products `CC`
CC Excl: See code: 995.60

995.68 Anaphylactic reaction due to eggs `CC`
CC Excl: See code: 995.60

995.69 Anaphylactic reaction due to other specified food `CC`
CC Excl: See code: 995.60

995.7 Other adverse food reactions, not elsewhere classified
Use additional code to identify the type of reaction, such as:
hives (708.0)
wheezing (786.07)

> **EXCLUDES** *anaphylactic reaction or shock due to adverse food reaction (995.60-995.69)*
> *asthma (493.0, 493.9)*
> *dermatitis due to food (693.1)*
> *in contact with skin (692.5)*
> *gastroenteritis and colitis due to food (558.3)*
> *rhinitis due to food (477.1)*

√5ᵗʰ 995.8 Other specified adverse effects, not elsewhere classified

995.80 Adult maltreatment, unspecified `CC` `A`
Abused person NOS

Use additional code to identify:
any associated injury
perpetrator (E967.0-E967.9)
CC Excl: 995.80
AHA: ▶2Q, '12, 12;◀ 4Q, '96, 41, 43

995.81 Adult physical abuse `CC` `A`
Battered: Battered:
person syndrome NEC   spouse
man   woman

Use additional code to identify:
any association injury
nature of abuse (E960-E968)
perpetrator (E967.0-E967.9)
CC Excl: 995.50-995.59, 995.80-995.85
AHA: ▶2Q, '12, 12;◀ 4Q, '96, 42, 43

995.82 Adult emotional/psychological abuse `A`
Use additional E code to identify perpetrator (E967.0-E967.9)
AHA: ▶2Q, '12, 12◀

995.83 Adult sexual abuse `CC` `A`
Use additional code(s) to identify:
any associated injury
perpetrator (E967.0-E967.9)
CC Excl: See code: 995.81
AHA: ▶2Q, '12, 12◀

995.84 Adult neglect (nutritional) `CC` `A`
Use additional code(s) to identify:
intent of neglect (E904.0, E968.4)
perpetrator (E967.0-E967.9)
CC Excl: See code: 995.81
AHA: ▶2Q, '12, 12◀

995.85 Other adult abuse and neglect `CC` `A`
Multiple forms of abuse and neglect

Use additional code(s) to identify
any associated injury
intent of neglect (E904.0, E968.4)
nature of abuse (E960-E968)
perpetrator (E967.0-E967.9)
CC Excl: See code: 995.81
AHA: ▶2Q, '12, 12◀

Continuum of Illness Due to Infection

Bacteremia ➡ Septicemia ➡ Sepsis
Severe Sepsis with Septic Shock ⬅ Severe Sepsis ⬅
⬇
MODS (Multiple Organ Dysfunction Syndrome) ➡ Death

995.86 Malignant hyperthermia `CC`
Malignant hyperpyrexia due to anesthesia
CC Excl: 958.4, 995.4, 995.86, 997.91-998.13, 998.81, 998.83-998.9
AHA: 4Q, '98, 51

995.89 Other
Hypothermia due to anesthesia
AHA: 2Q, '04, 18; 3Q, '03, 12

√5ᵗʰ 995.9 Systemic inflammatory response syndrome (SIRS)
DEF: Clinical response to infection or trauma that can trigger an acute inflammatory reaction and progresses to coagulation, impaired fibrinolysis, and organ failure; manifested by two or more of the following symptoms: fever, tachycardia, tachypnea, leukocytosis or leukopenia.
AHA: 4Q, '06, 113-116; 2Q, '04, 16; 4Q, '02, 71
TIP: Coding these conditions requires a minimum of two codes: the underlying cause (e.g., Infection or trauma) is sequenced first, followed by a code from subcategory 995.9.

995.90 Systemic inflammatory response syndrome, unspecified `CC`
SIRS NOS
CC Excl: 003.1, 020.2, 036.2, 038.0-038.9, 040.82-041.9, 054.5, 139.8, 995.90-995.94, V09.0-V09.91

995.91 Sepsis `MCC`
Systemic inflammatory response syndrome due to infectious process without acute organ dysfunction

Code first underlying infection
> **EXCLUDES** *sepsis with acute organ dysfunction (995.92)*
> *sepsis with multiple organ dysfunction (995.92)*
> *severe sepsis (995.92)*

CC Excl: See code 995.90
AHA: ▶3Q, '12, 11,13; 2Q, '12, 21;◀ 3Q, '11, 15;4Q, '08, 72; 4Q, '07, 86; 4Q, '06, 113-116; 2Q, '04, 16; 4Q, '03, 79

995.92 Severe sepsis `MCC`
Sepsis with acute organ dysfunction
Sepsis with multiple organ dysfunction (MOD)
Systemic inflammatory response syndrome due to infectious process with acute organ dysfunction

Code first underlying infection

Use additional code to specify acute organ dysfunction, such as:
acute kidney failure (584.5-584.9)
acute respiratory failure (518.81)
critical illness myopathy (359.81)
critical illness polyneuropathy (357.82)
disseminated intravascular coagulopathy [DIC] (286.6)
encephalopathy (348.31)
hepatic failure (570)
septic shock (785.52)
CC Excl: See code 995.90
AHA: ▶3Q, '12, 11;◀ 4Q, '11, 153; 2Q, '10, 4; 4Q, '09, 98; 4Q, '08, 99; 4Q, '07, 97; 4Q, '06, 113-116; 2Q, '05, 18-19; 1Q, '05, 7; 1Q, '05, 7; 2Q, '04, 16; 4Q, '03, 73, 79
R65.21 Severe sepsis with septic shock `I-10`

`N` Newborn Age: 0   `P` Pediatric Age: 0-17   `M` Maternity Age: 12-55   `A` Adult Age: 15-124   `MCC` Major CC Condition   `CC` CC Condition   `HIV` HIV Related Dx

995.93 Systemic inflammatory response syndrome due to noninfectious process without acute organ dysfunction `CC`

Code first underlying conditions, such as:
  acute pancreatitis (577.0)
  trauma

EXCLUDES *systemic inflammatory response syndrome due to noninfectious process with acute organ dysfunction (995.94)*

CC Excl: See code 995.90

AHA: 1Q, '11, 22; 1Q, '10, 10-11; 4Q, '06, 113-116

995.94 Systemic inflammatory response syndrome due to noninfectious process with acute organ dysfunction `MCC`

Code first underlying conditions, such as:
  acute pancreatitis (577.0)
  heat stroke (992.0)
  trauma

Use additional code to specify acute organ dysfunction, such as:
  acute kidney failure (584.5-584.9)
  acute respiratory failure (518.81)
  critical illness myopathy (359.81)
  critical illness polyneuropathy (357.82)
  disseminated intravascular coagulopathy [DIC] syndrome (286.6)
  encephalopathy (348.31)
  hepatic failure (570)

EXCLUDES *severe sepsis (995.92)*

CC Excl: See code 995.90

AHA: 1Q, '10, 10; 4Q, '06, 113-116; 4Q, '03, 79

Complications of Surgical and Medical Care, Not Elsewhere Classified (996-999)

EXCLUDES *adverse effects of medicinal agents (001.0-799.9, 995.0-995.8)*
burns from local applications and irradiation (940.0-949.5)
complications of:
  conditions for which the procedure was performed
  surgical procedures during abortion, labor, and delivery (630-676.9)
poisoning and toxic effects of drugs and chemicals (960.0-989.9)
postoperative conditions in which no complications are present, such as:
  artificial opening status (V44.0-V44.9)
  closure of external stoma (V55.0-V55.9)
  fitting of prosthetic device (V52.0-V52.9)
specified complications classified elsewhere
  anesthetic shock (995.4)
  electrolyte imbalance (276.0-276.9)
  postlaminectomy syndrome (722.80-722.83)
  postmastectomy lymphedema syndrome (457.0)
  postoperative psychosis (293.0-293.9)
  any other condition classified elsewhere in the Alphabetic Index when described as due to a procedure

AHA: ▶2Q, '12, 5, 8◀

TIP: ▶Assign additional codes to further specify the nature of the complication unless the complication code provides a complete description of the condition.◀

✓4ᵗʰ 996 Complications peculiar to certain specified procedures

INCLUDES complications, not elsewhere classified, in the use of artificial substitutes [e.g., Dacron, metal, Silastic, Teflon] or natural sources [e.g., bone] involving:
  anastomosis (internal)
  graft (bypass) (patch)
  implant
  internal device:
    catheter
    electronic
    fixation
    prosthetic
  reimplant
  transplant

EXCLUDES *accidental puncture or laceration during procedure (998.2)*
capsular contracture of breast implant (611.83)
complications of internal anastomosis of:
  gastrointestinal tract (997.49)
  urinary tract (997.5)
endosseous dental implant failures (525.71-525.79)
intraoperative floppy iris syndrome [IFIS] (364.81)
mechanical complication of respirator (V46.14)
other specified complications classified elsewhere, such as:
  hemolytic anemia (283.1)
  functional cardiac disturbances (429.4)
  serum hepatitis (070.2-070.3)

AHA: 1Q, '94, 3

✓5ᵗʰ 996.0 Mechanical complication of cardiac device, implant, and graft

Breakdown (mechanical)   Obstruction, mechanical
Displacement   Perforation
Leakage   Protrusion

AHA: 2Q, '08, 9; 2Q, '93, 9

TIP: If the documentation indicates that the cardiac device (e.g., pacemaker, heart valve prosthesis) has reached its normally occurring end of life, do not assign a complication code; see instead subcategory V53.3.

996.00 Unspecified device, implant, and graft `CC`
CC Excl: 996.00, 996.04, 996.61-996.62, 996.70-996.74, 997.91-997.99, 998.81, 998.83-998.9

996.01 Due to cardiac pacemaker (electrode) `CC`
CC Excl: 996.01, 997.91-997.99, 998.81, 998.83-998.9
AHA: 2Q, '06, 15; 2Q, '99, 11
T82.120A Displacement cardiac electrode initial encounter `I-10`

996.02 Due to heart valve prosthesis `CC`
CC Excl: 996.02, 997.91-997.99, 998.81, 998.83-998.9

996.03 Due to coronary bypass graft `CC`
EXCLUDES *atherosclerosis of graft (414.02, 414.03)*
embolism [occlusion NOS] [thrombus] of graft (996.72)
CC Excl: 996.03, 997.91-997.99, 998.81, 998.83-998.9
AHA: 2Q, '95, 17; N-D, '86, 5

996.04 Due to automatic implantable cardiac defibrillator `CC`
CC Excl: 996.04, 997.91-997.99, 998.81, 998.83-998.9
AHA: 2Q, '05, 3

996.09 Other `CC`
CC Excl: 996.09, 997.91-997.99, 998.81, 998.83-998.9
AHA: 2Q, '93, 9

✓4ᵗʰ / ✓5ᵗʰ Additional Digit Required   Unacceptable PDx   Manifestation Code   Hospital Acquired Condition   ▶◀ Revised Text   ● New Code   ▲ Revised Code Title

2014 ICD-9-CM   **February 2013 • Volume 1 – 341**

Injury and Poisoning

996.1–996.54

996.1 Mechanical complication of other vascular device, implant, and graft `CC`
　　Mechanical complications involving:
　　　aortic (bifurcation) graft (replacement)
　　　arteriovenous:
　　　　dialysis catheter
　　　　fistula } surgically created
　　　　shunt
　　　balloon (counterpulsation) device, intra-aortic
　　　carotid artery bypass graft
　　　femoral-popliteal bypass graft
　　　umbrella device, vena cava
　　　　EXCLUDES *atherosclerosis of biological graft (440.30-440.32)*
　　　　　　embolism [occlusion NOS] [thrombus] of (biological) (synthetic) graft (996.74)
　　　　　　peritoneal dialysis catheter (996.56)
　　CC Excl: 996.1, 997.91-997.99, 998.81, 998.83-998.9
　　AHA: 1Q, '12, 18;1Q, '11, 5; 1Q, '06, 10; 2Q, '05, 8; 1Q, '02, 13; 1Q, '95, 3
　　TIP: Assign for a nonmaturing AV fistula and also for postprocedural reduction in transjugular intrahepatic portosystemic shunt flow in a patient with a TIPS catheter.
　　T82.330A Leakage aortic bifurcation graft initial enc `I-10`

996.2 Mechanical complication of nervous system device, implant, and graft `CC`
　　Mechanical complications involving:
　　　dorsal column stimulator
　　　electrodes implanted in brain [brain "pacemaker"]
　　　peripheral nerve graft
　　　ventricular (communicating) shunt
　　CC Excl: 996.2, 996.63, 996.75, 997.91-997.99, 998.81, 998.83-998.9
　　AHA: 2Q, '99, 4; S-O, '87, 10

√5ᵗʰ 996.3 Mechanical complication of genitourinary device, implant, and graft
　　AHA: 3Q, '01, 13; S-O, '85, 3

996.30 Unspecified device, implant, and graft `CC`
　　CC Excl: 596.81, 596.83, 996.30, 996.64-996.65, 996.76, 997.91-997.99, 998.81, 998.83-998.9

996.31 Due to urethral [indwelling] catheter

996.32 Due to intrauterine contraceptive device ♀

996.39 Other `CC`
　　Prosthetic reconstruction of vas deferens
　　Repair (graft) of ureter without mention of resection
　　EXCLUDES *complications due to:*
　　　　external stoma of urinary tract (596.81-596.83)
　　　　internal anastomosis of urinary tract (997.5)
　　CC Excl: 596.81-596.83, 996.39, 996.64-996.65, 996.76, 997.91-997.99, 998.81, 998.83-998.9

√5ᵗʰ 996.4 Mechanical complication of internal orthopedic device, implant, and graft
　　Mechanical complications involving:
　　　external (fixation) device utilizing internal screw(s), pin(s) or other methods of fixation
　　　grafts of bone, cartilage, muscle, or tendon
　　　internal (fixation) device such as nail, plate, rod, etc.
　　Use additional code to identify prosthetic joint with mechanical complication (V43.60-V43.69)
　　EXCLUDES *complications of external orthopedic device, such as: pressure ulcer due to cast (707.00-707.09)*
　　AHA: 4Q, '05, 91; 2Q, '99, 10; 2Q, '98, 19; 2Q, '96, 11; 3Q, '95, 16; N-D, '85, 11
　　TIP: Since these codes may be used for any joint device complications, assign an additional code from subcategory V43.6 to specify the joint involved.

996.40 Unspecified mechanical complication of internal orthopedic device, implant, and graft `CC`
　　CC Excl: 996.40-996.49, 996.66-996.67, 996.77-996.78, 997.91-997.99, 998.81, 998.83-998.9

996.41 Mechanical loosening of prosthetic joint `CC`
　　Aseptic loosening
　　CC Excl: See code: 996.40
　　AHA: 4Q, '05, 112
　　T84.031A Mech loosening int lt hip prosth jnt initial enc `I-10`

996.42 Dislocation of prosthetic joint `CC`
　　Instability of prosthetic joint
　　Subluxation of prosthetic joint
　　CC Excl: See code 996.40
　　T84.020A Disloc of internal rt hip prosthesis, init encntr `I-10`

996.43 Broken prosthetic joint implant `CC`
　　Breakage (fracture) of prosthetic joint
　　CC Excl: See code 996.40

996.44 Peri-prosthetic fracture around prosthetic joint `CC`
　　CC Excl: See code 996.40
　　AHA: 4Q, '05, 93

996.45 Peri-prosthetic osteolysis `CC`
　　Use additional code to identify major osseous defect, if applicable (731.3)
　　CC Excl: See code 996.40
　　AHA: 4Q, '06, 103

996.46 Articular bearing surface wear of prosthetic joint `CC`
　　CC Excl: See code 996.40

996.47 Other mechanical complication of prosthetic joint implant `CC`
　　Mechanical complication of prosthetic joint NOS
　　Prosthetic joint implant failure NOS
　　CC Excl: See code 996.40

996.49 Other mechanical complication of other internal orthopedic device, implant, and graft `CC`
　　Breakage of internal fixation device in bone
　　Dislocation of internal fixation device in bone
　　EXCLUDES *mechanical complication of prosthetic joint implant (996.41-996.47)*
　　CC Excl: See code 996.40
　　AHA: 1Q, '10, 7

√5ᵗʰ 996.5 Mechanical complication of other specified prosthetic device, implant, and graft
　　Mechanical complications involving:
　　　nonabsorbable surgical material NOS
　　　other graft, implant, and internal device, not elsewhere classified
　　　prosthetic implant in:
　　　　bile duct
　　　　breast
　　　　chin
　　　　orbit of eye
　　AHA: 1Q, '98, 11

996.51 Due to corneal graft `CC`
　　CC Excl: 996.51, 997.91-997.99
　　AHA: 2Q, '10, 4-5

996.52 Due to graft of other tissue, not elsewhere classified `CC`
　　Skin graft failure or rejection
　　EXCLUDES *failure of artificial skin graft (996.55)*
　　　　failure of decellularized allodermis (996.55)
　　　　sloughing of temporary skin allografts or xenografts (pigskin) — omit code
　　CC Excl: 996.52, 996.55, 997.91-997.99
　　AHA: ►3Q, '12, 6;◄1Q, '96, 10
　　TIP: ►Assign for failure of living biological wound care materials used to treat nonhealing wounds recalcitrant to conventional therapy (e.g., Apligraft, CelTx, Dermagraft).◄

996.53 Due to ocular lens prosthesis `CC`
　　EXCLUDES *contact lenses — code to condition*
　　CC Excl: 996.53, 997.91-997.99
　　AHA: 1Q, '00, 9

996.54 Due to breast prosthesis `CC`
　　Breast capsule (prosthesis)
　　Mammary implant
　　CC Excl: 996.54, 997.91-997.99
　　AHA: 2Q, '98, 14; 3Q, '92, 4
　　TIP: If documentation indicates capsular contracture of breast implant, see instead code 611.83.

996.55 Due to artificial skin graft and decellularized allodermis `CC`
Dislodgement
Displacement
Failure
Non-adherence
Poor incorporation
Shearing
CC Excl: 996.52, 996.55-996.60, 996.68-996.70, 996.79, 997.91-997.99
AHA: 4Q, '98, 52

996.56 Due to peritoneal dialysis catheter `CC`
EXCLUDES *mechanical complication of arteriovenous dialysis catheter (996.1)*
CC Excl: 996.56-996.60, 996.68-996.70, 996.79, 997.91-997.99
AHA: 4Q, '98, 54

996.57 Due to insulin pump `CC`
CC Excl: 596.81-596.83, 996.00-996.30, 996.39-996.79, 997.91-997.99, 998.81, 998.83-998.9
AHA: 4Q, '03, 81-82

996.59 Due to other implant and internal device, not elsewhere classified `CC`
Nonabsorbable surgical material NOS
Prosthetic implant in:
 bile duct
 chin
 orbit of eye
CC Excl: See code: 996.56
AHA: 1Q, '11, 10-11; 2Q, '99, 13; 3Q, '94, 7
TIP: Assign for clogged biliary stent and also for nonfunctioning pressure equalization (PE) tubes.

✓5ᵗʰ **996.6 Infection and inflammatory reaction due to internal prosthetic device, implant, and graft**
Infection (causing obstruction) ⎤ due to (presence of) any device,
Inflammation ⎦ implant, and graft classifiable to 996.0-996.5
Use additional code to identify specified infections
AHA: 2Q, '89, 16; J-F, '87, 14

996.60 Due to unspecified device, implant, and graft `CC`
CC Excl: 596.81-596.83, 996.00-996.79, 997.91-997.99, 998.81, 998.83-998.9

¹⁵ **996.61 Due to cardiac device, implant, and graft** `CC`
Cardiac pacemaker or defibrillator:
 electrode(s), lead(s)
 pulse generator
 subcutaneous pocket
Coronary artery bypass graft
Heart valve prosthesis
CC Excl: 996.00-996.1, 996.52, 996.55-996.62, 996.68-996.74, 996.79, 997.91-997.99, 998.81, 998.83-998.9

996.62 Due to other vascular device, implant, and graft `CC`
Arterial graft
Arteriovenous fistula or shunt
Infusion pump
Vascular catheter (arterial) (dialysis) (peripheral venous)
EXCLUDES *infection due to:*
  central venous catheter (999.31-999.32)
  Hickman catheter (999.31-999.32)
  peripherally inserted central catheter [PICC] (999.31-999.32)
  portacath (port-a-cath) (999.31-999.32)
  triple lumen catheter (999.31-999.32)
  umbilical venous catheter (999.31-999.32)
CC Excl: See code 996.61
AHA: 2Q, '10, 8; 4Q, '07, 86; 2Q, '04, 16; 1Q, '04, 5; 4Q, '03, 107, 111; 2Q, '03, 7; 2Q, '94, 13
T82.7xxA Inf & inflam react oth card vasc dev gft initial enc `I-10`

996.63 Due to nervous system device, implant, and graft `CC`
Electrodes implanted in brain
Peripheral nerve graft
Spinal canal catheter
Ventricular (communicating) shunt (catheter)
CC Excl: 996.2, 996.52, 996.55-996.60, 996.63, 996.68-996.69, 996.70, 996.75, 996.79, 997.91-997.99, 998.81, 998.83-998.9

996.64 Due to indwelling urinary catheter `CC`
Use additional code to identify specified infections, such as:
 cystitis (595.0-595.9)
 sepsis (038.0-038.9)
EXCLUDES *complications due to:*
  external stoma of urinary tract (596.81-596.83)
CC Excl: 596.81-596.83, 599.0, 996.30, 996.39, 996.56-996.59, 996.60, 996.64, 996.65, 996.68, 996.69, 996.70, 996.76, 996.79, 998.81, 998.83-998.9
AHA: ▶2Q, '12, 20;◀ 1Q, '12, 11; 3Q, '09,10-11; 3Q, '93, 6
TIP: Assign for documented infection due to the presence of an indwelling urinary catheter, whether Foley, suprapubic, or other type.
T83.51XA Infect/inflm reaction d/t indwell urinary catheter, init `I-10`

996.65 Due to other genitourinary device, implant, and graft `CC`
Intrauterine contraceptive device
CC Excl: 596.81-596.83, 996.30, 996.39, 996.52, 996.55-996.59, 996.60, 996.64, 996.65, 996.68, 996.69, 996.70, 996.76, 996.79, 998.81, 998.83-998.9
AHA: 1Q, '00, 15

996.66 Due to internal joint prosthesis `CC`
Use additional code to identify infected prosthetic joint (V43.60-V43.69)
CC Excl: 996.40-996.49, 996.52, 996.55-996.59, 996.60, 996.66-996.69, 996.70, 996.77-996.79, 997.91-997.99, 998.81, 998.83-998.9
AHA: 2Q, '08, 3-5; 2Q, '07, 7; 4Q, '05, 91, 113; 2Q, '91, 18
TIP: Do not assign for the second admission of a staged procedure whereby the infected prosthesis has been previously removed and the patient now returns for placement of a new prosthesis; see instead codes from category 736.
T84.51xA Inf & inflam reaction int rt hip pros initial enc `I-10`

¹² **996.67 Due to other internal orthopedic device, implant, and graft** `CC`
Bone growth stimulator (electrode)
Internal fixation device (pin) (rod) (screw)
CC Excl: 996.40-996.49, 996.52, 996.55-996.59, 996.60, 996.66-996.69, 996.70, 996.77-996.79, 997.91-997.99, 998.81, 998.83-998.9

996.68 Due to peritoneal dialysis catheter `CC`
Exit-site infection or inflammation
CC Excl: 996.56-996.59, 996.60, 996.68, 996.69, 996.70, 996.79, 997.91-997.99
AHA: 4Q, '98, 54

996.69 Due to other internal prosthetic device, implant, and graft `CC`
Breast prosthesis
Ocular lens prosthesis
Prosthetic orbital implant
CC Excl: See code 996.60
AHA: 1Q, '11, 10; 2Q, '08, 11; 4Q, '03, 108; 4Q, '98, 52

---

² HAC when reported with procedure codes 81.01-81.08, 81.23-81.24, 81.31-81.38, 81.83, or 81.85 and POA = N
⁵ HAC when reported with procedure codes 00.50-00.54, 37.74-37.77, 37.79, 37.80-37.89, 37.94, 37.96, or 37.98 and POA = N

Injury and Poisoning

996.7–996.94

√5ᵗʰ 996.7 Other complications of internal (biological) (synthetic) prosthetic device, implant, and graft

Complication NOS
Occlusion NOS
Embolism
Fibrosis   due to (presence of) any device,
Hemorrhage   implant, and graft
Pain   classifiable to 996.0-996.5
Stenosis
Thrombus

Use additional code to identify complication, such as:
   pain due to presence of device, implant or graft (338.18-338.19, 338.28-338.29)
   venous embolism and thrombosis (453.2-453.9)

EXCLUDES disruption (dehiscence) of internal suture material (998.31)
        transplant rejection (996.80-996.89)

AHA: ▶2Q, '12, 5;◀ 2Q, '07, 12; 4Q, '05, 94; 1Q, '89, 9; N-D, '86, 5

996.70 Due to unspecified device, implant, and graft

996.71 Due to heart valve prosthesis `CC`
CC Exd: 996.00, 996.02, 996.09-996.1, 996.52, 996.55-996.62, 996.68-996.74, 996.79, 997.91-997.99, 998.81, 998.83-998.9

996.72 Due to other cardiac device, implant, and graft `CC`
Cardiac pacemaker or defibrillator:
   electrode(s), lead(s)
   subcutaneous pocket
Coronary artery bypass (graft)
EXCLUDES occlusion due to atherosclerosis (414.02-414.06)
CC Exd: 996.00-996.02, 996.04-996.1, 996.52, 996.55-996.62, 996.68-996.74, 996.79, 997.91-997.99, 998.81, 998.83-998.9
AHA: 2Q, '10, 8-9; 3Q, '08, 10; 3Q, '06, 8, 25; 3Q, '01, 20
TIP: Assign for in-stent stenosis of previously placed coronary artery stent.
T82.847A Pain cardiac prosth devc impl graft initial enc `I-10`

996.73 Due to renal dialysis device, implant, and graft `CC`
CC Exd: 996.1, 996.52, 996.55-996.60, 996.68-996.70, 996.73, 996.79, 997.91-997.99, 998.81, 998.83-998.9
AHA: 2Q, '91, 18
T82.858A Stenosis vasc prosth devc impl graft initial enc `I-10`

996.74 Due to other vascular device, implant, and graft `CC`
EXCLUDES occlusion of biological graft due to atherosclerosis (440.30-440.32)
CC Exd: 996.00-996.1, 996.52, 996.55-996.62, 996.68-996.74, 996.79, 997.91-997.99, 998.81, 998.83-998.9
AHA: 1Q, '12, 18; 2Q, '11, 8; 1Q, '03, 16, 17
TIP: Assign for clotted peripherally inserted central catheter (PICC) line.

996.75 Due to nervous system device, implant, and graft `CC`
CC Exd: 996.2, 996.52, 996.55-996.60, 996.63, 996.68-996.70, 996.75, 996.79, 997.91-997.99, 998.81, 998.83-998.9

996.76 Due to genitourinary device, implant, and graft `CC`
EXCLUDES complications of implanted vaginal mesh (629.31-629.32)
CC Exd: 596.81-596.83, 996.30, 996.39, 996.52, 996.55-996.59, 996.60, 996.64-996.65, 996.68-996.69, 996.70, 996.76, 996.79, 998.81, 998.83-998.9
AHA: 1Q, '09, 15; 1Q, '00, 15
T83.83xA Hemorrhage GU prosth devc impl graft initial enc `I-10`

996.77 Due to internal joint prosthesis `CC`
Use additional code to identify prosthetic joint (V43.60-V43.69)
CC Exd: 996.40-996.49, 996.52, 996.55-996.60, 996.66-996.70, 996.77-996.79, 997.91-997.99, 998.81, 998.83-998.9
AHA: 4Q, '05, 91
T84.84xA Pain int ortho prosth devc impl gft initial enc `I-10`

996.78 Due to other internal orthopedic device, implant, and graft `CC`
CC Exd: 996.40-996.49, 996.52, 996.55-996.60, 996.66-996.70, 996.77-996.79, 997.91-997.99, 998.81, 998.83-998.9
AHA: 2Q, '03, 14

996.79 Due to other internal prosthetic device, implant, and graft `CC`
CC Exd: 596.81-596.83, 996.00- 996.79, 997.91-997.99, 998.81, 998.83-998.9
AHA: 2Q, '04, 7; 1Q,'01, 8; 3Q, '95, 14; 3Q, '92, 4

√5ᵗʰ 996.8 Complications of transplanted organ
Transplant failure or rejection
Use additional code to identify nature of complication, such as:
   cytomegalovirus (CMV) infection (078.5)
   graft-versus-host disease (279.50-279.53)
   malignancy associated with organ transplant (199.2)
   post-transplant lymphoproliferative disorder (PTLD) (238.77)
AHA: 4Q, '08, 82-83; 3Q, '01, 12; 3Q, '93, 3, 4; 2Q, '93, 11; 1Q, '93, 24
TIP: Assign only if the complication affects the function of the transplanted organ. Assign also a code for the specific complication

996.80 Transplanted organ, unspecified `C`
CC Exd: 238.77, 996.80, 996.87, 997.91-997.99

996.81 Kidney `C`
CC Exd: 996.81, 997.91-997.99
AHA: ▶2Q, '12, 6;◀ 2Q, '11, 6; 1Q, '10, 9; 4Q, '08, 83; 3Q, '03, 16; 3Q, '98, 6, 7; 3Q, '94, 8; 2Q, '94, 9; 1Q, '93, 24
TIP: Do not assign for chronic kidney disease (CKD) status following kidney transplant. The provider must indicate transplant failure, rejection, or other complication to support assignment of this code.
T86.11 Kidney transplant rejection `I-1`

996.82 Liver `C`
CC Exd: 996.82, 997.91-997.99
AHA: 4Q, '08, 82, 99; 3Q, '03, 17; 3Q, '98, 3, 4

996.83 Heart `C`
CC Exd: 996.83, 997.91-997.99
AHA: 3Q, '03, 16; 4Q, '02, 53; 3Q, '98, 5

996.84 Lung `C`
CC Exd: 996.84, 997.91-997.99
AHA: 2Q, '03, 12; 3Q, '98, 5

996.85 Bone marrow `C`
CC Exd: 279.50-279.53, 996.85, 997.91-997.99
AHA: 1Q, '12, 13;4Q, '08, 91x; 4Q, '90, 4
TIP: Do not assign for recurrence or relapse of hematopoietic or lymphatic malignancy following bone marrow/stem cell transplant.

996.86 Pancreas `C`
CC Exd: 996.86, 997.91-997.99

996.87 Intestine `C`
CC Exd: 238.77, 996.80, 996.87, 997.91-997.99

996.88 Stem cell `C`
Complications from stem cells from:
   peripheral blood
   umbilical cord
CC Exd: 996.88-996.89, 997.91- 997.99
AHA: 4Q, '11, 147-148

996.89 Other specified transplanted organ `C`
CC Exd: 996.88-996.89, 997.91- 997.99
AHA: 1Q, '11, 8; 3Q, '94, 5

√5ᵗʰ 996.9 Complications of reattached extremity or body part

996.90 Unspecified extremity `C`
CC Exd: 996.90, 997.91-997.99, 998.81, 998.83-998.9

996.91 Forearm `C`
CC Exd: 996.91, 997.91-997.99, 998.81, 998.83-998.9

996.92 Hand `C`
CC Exd: 996.92, 997.91-997.99, 998.81, 998.83-998.9

996.93 Finger(s) `C`
CC Exd: 996.93, 997.91-997.99, 998.81, 998.83-998.9

996.94 Upper extremity, other and unspecified `C`
CC Exd: 996.94, 997.91-997.99, 998.81, 998.83-998.9

N Newborn Age: 0   **P** Pediatric Age: 0-17   **M** Maternity Age: 12-55   **A** Adult Age: 15-124   **MCC** Major CC Condition   **CC** CC Condition   **HIV** HIV Related D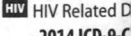

344 – Volume 1 • February 2013   2014 ICD-9-C

996.95 Foot and toe(s) `CC`
    CC Exd: 996.95, 997.91-997.99, 998.81, 998.83-998.9

996.96 Lower extremity, other and unspecified `CC`
    CC Exd: 996.96, 997.91-997.99, 998.81, 998.83-998.9

996.99 Other specified body part `CC`
    CC Exd: 996.99, 997.91-997.99, 998.81, 998.83-998.9

☑4ᵗʰ **997 Complications affecting specified body systems, not elsewhere classified**
    Use additional code to identify complications
    EXCLUDES *the listed conditions when specified as:*
        causing shock (998.00-998.09)
        complications of:
          anesthesia:
            adverse effect (001.0-799.9, 995.0-995.8)
            in labor or delivery (668.0-668.9)
            poisoning (968.0-969.9)
          implanted device or graft (996.0-996.9)
          obstetrical procedures (669.0-669.4)
          reattached extremity (996.90-996.96)
          transplanted organ (996.80-996.89)
    AHA: 1Q, '94, 4; 1Q, '93, 26

☑5ᵗʰ **997.0 Nervous system complications**

997.00 Nervous system complication, unspecified

997.01 Central nervous system complication `CC`
    Anoxic brain damage
    Cerebral hypoxia
    EXCLUDES *cerebrovascular hemorrhage or infarction (997.02)*
    CC Exd: 997.00-997.09, 997.91-997.99, 998.81, 998.83-998.9
    AHA: 1Q, '07, 22; 1Q, '06, 15
    TIP: Assign for hyperperfusion syndrome, a complication of carotid endarterectomy.

997.02 Iatrogenic cerebrovascular infarction or hemorrhage `CC`
    Postoperative stroke
    CC Exd: See code: 997.01
    AHA: 3Q, '10, 5; 3Q, '06, 6; 2Q, '04, 8; 4Q, '95, 57
    TIP: Assign an additional code to specify the type of postoperative stroke involved.
    I97.810 Intraop cerebrvascular infarct during card surg `I-10`

997.09 Other nervous system complications `CC`
    CC Exd: See code: 997.01
    G97.0 Cerebrospinal fluid leak from spinal puncture `I-10`

997.1 Cardiac complications `CC`
    Cardiac:
      arrest
      insufficiency   } during or resulting from a procedure
    Cardiorespiratory failure
    Heart failure
    EXCLUDES *the listed conditions as long-term effects of cardiac surgery or due to the presence of cardiac prosthetic device (429.4)*
    CC Exd: 997.1, 997.91-997.99, 998.81, 998.83-998.9
    AHA: 1Q, '11, 3-4; 4Q, '08, 179; 2Q, '02, 12
    I97.711 Intraoperative cardiac arrest during oth surgery `I-10`

997.2 Peripheral vascular complications `CC`
    Phlebitis or thrombophlebitis during or resulting from a procedure
    EXCLUDES *the listed conditions due to:*
        implant or catheter device (996.62)
        infusion, perfusion, or transfusion (999.2)
        complications affecting blood vessels (997.71-997.79)
    CC Exd: 997.2, 997.79-997.99, 998.81, 998.83-998.9
    AHA: 1Q, '03, 6; 3Q, '02, 24-26
    T81.72xA Complication of vein following a procedure NEC intl enc `I-10`

☑5ᵗʰ **997.3 Respiratory complications**
    EXCLUDES *iatrogenic [postoperative] pneumothorax (512.1)*
        iatrogenic pulmonary embolism (415.11)
        specified complications classified elsewhere, such as:
          adult respiratory distress syndrome (518.52)
          pulmonary edema, postoperative (518.4)
          respiratory insufficiency, acute, postoperative (518.52)
          shock lung related to trauma and surgery (518.52)
          tracheostomy complications (519.00-519.09)
          transfusion related acute lung injury [TRALI] (518.7)
    AHA: 4Q, '11, 148-150; 1Q, '97, 10; 2Q, '93, 3; 2Q, '93, 9; 4Q, '90, 25

997.31 Ventilator associated pneumonia `CC`
    Ventilator associated pneumonitis
    Use additional code to identify organism
    CC Exd: 518.7, 997.31-997.39, 997.91-997.99, 998.81, 998.83-998.9
    AHA: 4Q, '08, 148-149
    TIP: Do not assign unless the provider has documented the relationship between the pneumonia and ventilation status.

997.32 Postprocedural aspiration pneumonia `CC`
    Chemical pneumonitis resulting from a procedure
    Mendelson's syndrome resulting from a procedure
    EXCLUDES *aspiration pneumonia during labor and delivery (668.0)*
    CC Exd: See code 997.31
    DEF: Mendelson's syndrome: acid pneumonitis due to aspiration of gastric acids, may occur after anesthesia or sedation.
    AHA: 4Q, '11, 150
    TIP: Do not assign code 507.0 in addittion to 997.32; aspiration pneumonia due to a procedure is fully captured with this code.

997.39 Other respiratory complications `CC`
    CC Exd: See code 997.31
    AHA: 1Q, '11, 16
    J95.4 Chem pneumonitis d/t anesthesia [Mendelson's syndrm] `I-10`

☑5ᵗʰ **997.4 Digestive system complications**
    Complications of:
      intestinal (internal) anastomosis and bypass, not elsewhere classified, except that involving urinary tract
    Hepatic failure
    Hepatorenal syndrome } specified as due to a procedure
    Intestinal obstruction NOS
    EXCLUDES *complications of gastric band procedure (539.01-539.09)*
        complications of other bariatric procedure (539.81-539.89)
        gastrostomy complications (536.40-536.49)
        specified gastrointestinal complications classified elsewhere, such as:
          blind loop syndrome (579.2)
          colostomy and enterostomy complications (569.60-569.69)
          complications of intestinal pouch (569.71-569.79)
          gastrojejunal ulcer (534.0-534.9)
          infection of esophagostomy (530.86)
          infection of external stoma (569.61)
          mechanical complication of esophagostomy (530.87)
          pelvic peritoneal adhesions, female (614.6)
          peritoneal adhesions (568.0)
          peritoneal adhesions with obstruction (560.81)
          postcholecystectomy syndrome (576.0)
          postgastric surgery syndromes (564.2)
          pouchitis (569.71)
          vomiting following gastrointestinal surgery (564.3)
    AHA: 4Q, '11, 125, 148-150; 2Q, '01, 4-6; 3Q, '99, 4; 2Q, '99, 14; 3Q, '97, 7; 1Q, '97, 11; 2Q, '95, 7; 1Q, '93, 26; 3Q, '92, 15; 2Q, '89, 15; 1Q, '88, 14

997.41 Retained cholelithiasis following cholecystectomy `CC`
    CC Exd: 530.86-530.87, 536.40-536.49, 539.01-539.89, 569.62, 569.71-569.79, 997.41-997.49, 997.71, 997.91-997.99, 998.81, 998.83-998.9

4ᵗʰ 5ᵗʰ Additional Digit Required   Unacceptable PDx   Manifestation Code   Hospital Acquired Condition   ▶◀ Revised Text   ● New Code   ▲ Revised Code Title

2014 ICD-9-CM   Volume 1 – 345

997.49 Other digestive system complications `CC`
CC Exd: See code 997.41
AHA: 1Q, '12, 6
TIP: Assign for ileus following gastrointestinal surgery; physician documentation of the cause-and-effect relationship is not required.
K91.89 Oth postproc comp & disorder of digest syst `I-10`

997.5 Urinary complications
Complications of:
internal anastomosis and bypass of urinary tract, including that involving intestinal tract
Oliguria or anuria
Renal (kidney):
  failure (acute)
  insufficiency (acute)
Tubular necrosis (acute)
} specified as due to procedure

EXCLUDES complications of cystostomy (596.81-596.83)
complications of external stoma of urinary tract (596.81-596.83)
specified complications classified elsewhere, such as:
postoperative stricture of:
ureter (593.3)
urethra (598.2)
AHA: 1Q, '12, 11; 3Q, '03, 13; 3Q, '96, 10, 15; 4Q, '95, 73; 1Q, '92, 13; 2Q, '89, 16; M-A, '87, 10; S-O, '85, 3
TIP: If a urinary tract infection is specified as a postoperative complication, assign both 997.5 and 599.0.
TIP: Assign for a urostomy-associated urinary tract infection with poor self-catheterization technique/hygiene.
N99.0 Postprocedural (acute) (chronic) renal failure `I-10`

√5ᵗʰ 997.6 Amputation stump complication
EXCLUDES admission for treatment for a current traumatic amputation — code to complicated traumatic amputation
phantom limb (syndrome) (353.6)
AHA: 4Q, '95, 82

997.60 Unspecified complication

997.61 Neuroma of amputation stump
DEF: Hyperplasia generated nerve cell mass following amputation.

997.62 Infection (chronic) `CC`
Use additional code to identify the organism
CC Exd: 997.60, 997.62-997.69, 997.91-997.99, 998.81, 998.83-998.9
AHA: 1Q, '05, 15 4Q, '96, 46
TIP: If cellulitis is specified as a manifestation of the infection, assign an additional code from category 681 or 682.
T87.43 Infection amputation stump right lower extremity `I-10`

997.69 Other
AHA: 1Q, '05, 15

√5ᵗʰ 997.7 Vascular complications of other vessels
EXCLUDES peripheral vascular complications (997.2)

997.71 Vascular complications of mesenteric artery `CC`
CC Exd: 997.2, 997.71-997.99, 998.81, 998.83-998.9
AHA: 4Q, '01, 53
TIP: For postoperative mesenteric artery embolism, assign also code 557.0 Acute vascular insufficiency of intestine.

997.72 Vascular complications of renal artery `CC`
CC Exd: See code 997.71

997.79 Vascular complications of other vessels `CC`
CC Exd: See code 997.71

√5ᵗʰ 997.9 Complications affecting other specified body systems, not elsewhere classified
EXCLUDES specified complications classified elsewhere, such as:
broad ligament laceration syndrome (620.6)
postartificial menopause syndrome (627.4)
postoperative stricture of vagina (623.2)

997.91 Hypertension
EXCLUDES essential hypertension (401.0-401.9)
AHA: 4Q, '95, 57

997.99 Other `CC`
Vitreous touch syndrome
DEF: Vitreous touch syndrome: vitreous protruding through pupil and attaches to corneal epithelium; causes aqueous fluid in vitreous body; marked by corneal edema, loss of lucidity; complication of cataract surgery.
CC Exd: 997.91-997.99, 998.81, 998.83-998.9
AHA: 2Q, '94, 12; 1Q, '94, 17

√4ᵗʰ 998 Other complications of procedures, not elsewhere classified
EXCLUDES fluid overload due to transfusion (blood) (276.61)
TACO (276.61)
transfusion associated circulatory overload (276.61)
AHA: 1Q, '94, 4

√5ᵗʰ 998.0 Postoperative shock
Shock during or resulting from a surgical procedure
EXCLUDES shock:
anaphylactic due to serum (999.41-999.49)
anesthetic (995.4)
electric (994.8)
following abortion (639.5)
obstetric (669.1)
traumatic (958.4)
AHA: 4Q, '11, 150-153

998.00 Postoperative shock, unspecified `CC`
Collapse, not otherwise specified, during or resulting from a surgical procedure
Failure of peripheral circulation, postoperative
CC Exd: 958.4, 995.4, 997.91-998.13, 998.81, 998.83-998.9

998.01 Postoperative shock, cardiogenic `MCC`
CC Exd: see Code: 998.00
AHA: 4Q, '11, 152

998.02 Postoperative shock, septic `MCC`
Postoperative endotoxic shock
Postoperative gram-negative shock
Code first underlying infection
Use additional code, to identify severe sepsis (995.92) and any associated acute organ dysfunction, if applicable
CC Exd: see Code: 998.00
AHA: 4Q, '11, 153

998.09 Postoperative shock, other `MCC`
Postoperative hypovolemic shock
CC Exd: see Code: 998.00

√5ᵗʰ 998.1 Hemorrhage or hematoma or seroma complicating a procedure
EXCLUDES hemorrhage, hematoma, or seroma:
complicating cesarean section or puerperal perineal wound (674.3)
due to implanted device or graft (996.70-996.79)

998.11 Hemorrhage complicating a procedure `CC`
CC Exd: 456.0, 456.20, 530.81-530.83, 530.89, 531.00-531.01, 531.20-531.21, 531.40-531.41, 531.60-531.61, 532.00-532.01, 532.20-532.21, 532.40-532.41, 532.60-532.61, 533.00-533.01, 533.20-533.21, 533.40-533.41, 533.60-533.61, 534.00-534.01, 534.20-534.21, 534.40-534.41, 534.60-534.61, 535.01, 535.11, 535.21, 535.31, 535.41, 535.51, 535.61, 535.71, 537.83, 562.02-562.03, 562.12-562.13, 569.3, 569.85, 578.0-578.9, 772.4, 997.91-998.13, 998.81, 998.89-998.9
AHA: 1Q, '11, 13; 3Q, '03, 13; 1Q, '03, 4; 4Q, '97, 52; 1Q, '97, 10
I97.410 Intraop hemorrhage circ sys organ comp card cath `I-10`

998.12 Hematoma complicating a procedure `CC`
CC Exd: see code 998.11
AHA: 1Q, '11, 13; 3Q, '06, 12; 1Q, '03, 6; 3Q, '02, 24, 26

998.13 Seroma complicating a procedure `CC`
CC Exd: See code 998.11
AHA: 4Q, '96, 46; 1Q, '93, 26; 2Q, '92, 15; S-O, '87, 8

`N` Newborn Age: 0   `P` Pediatric Age: 0-17   `M` Maternity Age: 12-55   `A` Adult Age: 15-124   `MCC` Major CC Condition   `CC` CC Condition   `HIV` HIV Related Dx

346 – Volume 1   2014 ICD-9-CM

998.2 Accidental puncture or laceration during a procedure `CC`

Accidental perforation by catheter or other instrument during a procedure on:

blood vessel   organ
nerve

> *EXCLUDES* *iatrogenic [postoperative] pneumothorax (512.1)*
> *puncture or laceration caused by implanted device intentionally left in operation wound (996.0-996.5)*
> *specified complications classified elsewhere, such as:*
> *broad ligament laceration syndrome (620.6)*
> *dural tear (349.31)*
> *incidental durotomy (349.31)*
> *trauma from instruments during delivery (664.0-665.9)*

CC Excl: 349.31-349.39, 997.91-997.99, 998.2, 998.81, 998.83-998.9
AHA: ▶2Q, '12, 5;◀ 1Q, '10, 8, 11; 2Q, '07, 9; 1Q, '06, 15; 3Q, '02, 24, 26; 3Q, '94, 6; 3Q, '90, 17; 3Q, '90, 18
TIP: ▶Assign an additional code to describe the nature or site (e.g., organ) of the perforation.◀
I97.51 Accidentl punct lac circ sys organ dur circ proc `I-10`

✓5ᵗʰ 998.3 Disruption of wound

Dehiscence } of operation wound
Rupture

Disruption of any suture materials or other closure method

> *EXCLUDES* *disruption of:*
> *cesarean wound (674.1)*
> *perineal wound, puerperal (674.2)*

AHA: 4Q, '08,149-152; 4Q, '02, 73; 1Q, '93, 19

998.30 Disruption of wound, unspecified `CC`

Disruption of wound NOS

CC Excl: 997.91-997.99, 998.30-998.33, 998.81, 998.83-998.9

998.31 Disruption of internal operation (surgical) wound `CC`

Disruption or dehiscence of closure of:
fascia, superficial or muscular
internal organ
muscle or muscle flap
ribs or rib cage
skull or craniotomy
sternum or sternotomy
tendon or ligament
Deep disruption or dehiscence of operation wound NOS

> *EXCLUDES* *complications of internal anastomosis of:*
> *gastrointestinal tract (997.49)*
> *urinary tract (997.5)*

CC Excl: See code 998.30
AHA: 4Q, '10, 131

998.32 Disruption of external operation (surgical) wound `CC`

Disruption of operation wound NOS
Disruption or dehiscence of closure of:
cornea
mucosa
skin
subcutaneous tissue
Full-thickness skin disruption or dehiscence
Superficial disruption or dehiscence of operation wound

CC Excl: See code 998.30
AHA: 2Q, '06, 8; 1Q, '05, 11; 4Q, '03, 104, 106
T81.31xA Disruption ext operation wound NEC initial enc `I-10`

998.33 Disruption of traumatic injury wound repair `CC`

Disruption or dehiscence of closure of traumatic laceration (external) (internal)

CC Excl: See code 998.30
AHA: 4Q, '08, 151, 152

998.4 Foreign body accidentally left during a procedure `CC`

Adhesions ⎫ due to foreign body accidentally left in
Obstruction ⎬ operative wound or body cavity
Perforation ⎭ during a procedure

> *EXCLUDES* *obstruction or perforation caused by implanted device intentionally left in body (996.0-996.5)*

CC Excl: 997.91-997.99, 998.4, 998.81, 998.83-998.9
AHA: 1Q, '12, 12; 1Q, '11, 5-6; 1Q, '09,18 1Q, '89, 9
TIP: Report for an unintended retention of a foreign object following any type of procedure, in any type of setting.

✓5ᵗʰ 998.5 Postoperative infection

> *EXCLUDES* *bleb associated endophthalmitis (379.63)*
> *infection due to:*
> *implanted device (996.60-996.69)*
> *infusion, perfusion, or transfusion (999.31-999.39)*
> *postoperative obstetrical wound infection (674.3)*

998.51 Infected postoperative seroma `CC`

Use additional code to identify organism

CC Excl: 997.91-997.99, 998.51-998.59, 998.81, 998.89-998.9
AHA: 4Q, '96, 46

¹³,¹⁴,¹⁵ 998.59 Other postoperative infection `CC`

Abscess:
intra-abdominal
stitch
subphrenic ⎬ postoperative
wound
Septicemia

Use additional code to identify infection

CC Excl: See code: 998.51
AHA: 4Q, '11, 153; 2Q, '06, 23; 4Q, '04, 76; 4Q, '03, 104, 106-107; 3Q, '98, 3; 3Q, '95, 5; 2Q, '95, 7; 3Q, '94, 6; 1Q, '93, 19; J-F, '87, 14
TIP: Do not assign if the infection is related to an internal prosthetic device, implant, or graft; see instead subcategory 996.6.
T81.4xxA Infection following procedure initial encounter `I-10`

998.6 Persistent postoperative fistula `CC`

CC Excl: 997.91-997.99, 998.6, 998.81, 998.83-998.9
AHA: J-F, '87, 14
T81.83XA Persistent postprocedural fistula, init encntr `I-10`

998.7 Acute reaction to foreign substance accidentally left during a procedure `CC`

Peritonitis:
aseptic
chemical

CC Excl: 997.91-997.99, 998.7-998.81, 998.83-998.9

✓5ᵗʰ 998.8 Other specified complications of procedures, not elsewhere classified

AHA: 4Q, '94, 46; 1Q, '89, 9

998.81 Emphysema (subcutaneous) (surgical) resulting from a procedure

998.82 Cataract fragments in eye following cataract surgery

998.83 Non-healing surgical wound `CC`

CC Excl: 997.91-997.99, 998.81, 998.83-998.9
AHA: 4Q, '96, 47

998.89 Other specified complications

AHA: ▶2Q, '12, 8;◀ 2Q, '09, 11; 3Q, '06, 9; 3Q, '05, 16; 3Q, '99, 13; 2Q, '98, 16
TIP: Assign for cases in which a procedure is performed on the wrong body site (e.g., right leg versus left leg), along with E876.5-E876.7.
T81.89xA Other complications of procedures NEC, init enc `I-10`

998.9 Unspecified complication of procedure, not elsewhere classified

Postoperative complication NOS

> *EXCLUDES* *complication NOS of obstetrical, surgery or procedure (669.4)*

AHA: 4Q, '93, 37

---

³ HAC when reported with procedure codes 81.01-81.08, 81.23-81.24, 81.31-81.38, 81.83, 81.85, and POA = N
⁴ HAC when reported with principal diagnosis 278.01 and with procedure code 44.38, 44.39, or 44.95 and POA = N
⁵ HAC when reported with procedure codes 00.50-00.54, 37.74-37.77, 37.79, 37.80-37.89, 37.94, 37.96, or 37.98 and POA = N

| ⁴ Additional Digit Required | Unacceptable PDx | Manifestation Code | Hospital Acquired Condition | ▶◀ Revised Text | ● New Code | ▲ Revised Code Title |

Injury and Poisoning

999–999.41

√4ᵗʰ **999 Complications of medical care, not elsewhere classified**

INCLUDES   complications, not elsewhere classified, of:
    dialysis (hemodialysis) (peritoneal) (renal)
    extracorporeal circulation
    hyperalimentation therapy
    immunization
    infusion
    inhalation therapy
    injection
    inoculation
    perfusion
    transfusion
    vaccination
    ventilation therapy

Use additional code, where applicable, to identify specific complication

EXCLUDES   *specified complications classified elsewhere such as:*
    complications of implanted device (996.0-996.9)
    contact dermatitis due to drugs (692.3)
    dementia dialysis (294.8)
    transient (293.9)
    dialysis disequilibrium syndrome (276.0-276.9)
    poisoning and toxic effects of drugs and chemicals
        (960.0-989.9)
    postvaccinal encephalitis (323.51)
    water and electrolyte imbalance (276.0-276.9)

999.0 Generalized vaccinia   CC

EXCLUDES   *vaccinia not from vaccine (051.02)*

DEF: Skin eruption, self-limiting; follows vaccination; due to transient viremia with virus localized in skin.

CC Exd: 999.0

999.1 Air embolism   MCC

Air embolism to any site following infusion, perfusion, or transfusion

EXCLUDES   *embolism specified as:*
    complicating:
        abortion (634-638 with .6, 639.6)
        ectopic or molar pregnancy (639.6)
        pregnancy, childbirth, or the puerperium
            (673.0)
    due to implanted device (996.7)
    traumatic (958.0)

CC Exd: 958.0, 999.1

999.2 Other vascular complications   CC

Phlebitis
Thromboembolism   }   following infusion, perfusion,
Thrombophlebitis   or transfusion

EXCLUDES   *extravasation of vesicant drugs (999.81, 999.82)*
    the listed conditions when specified as:
        due to implanted device (996.61-996.62.
            996.72-996.74)
        postoperative NOS (997.2, 997.71-997.79)

CC Exd: 999.2, 999.81-999.82, 999.88

AHA: 2Q, '97, 5

TIP: Do not assign for IV infiltration; if the infiltration is severe enough to cause other complications, a code for the specific complication should be assigned. For chemotherapy extravasation, see code 999.81.

T80.1xxA Vasc comp follw inf transfusn tx inj initial enc   I-10

√5ᵗʰ **999.3 Other infection**

Infection   }   following infusion, injection,
Sepsis   transfusion, or
Septicemia   vaccination

Use additional code to identify the specified infection, such as:
    septicemia (038.0-038.9)

EXCLUDES   *the listed conditions when specified as:*
    due to implanted device (996.60-996.69)
    postoperative NOS (998.51-998.59)

AHA: 4Q, '07, 96; 2Q, '01, 11, 12; 2Q, '97, 5; J-F, '87, 14

999.31 Other and unspecified infection due to central venous catheter   CC

Central line-associated infection
Infection due to:
    central venous catheter NOS
    Hickman catheter
    peripherally inserted central catheter (PICC)
    triple lumen catheter
    umbilical venous catheter

EXCLUDES   *infection due to:*
    arterial catheter (996.62)
    catheter NOS (996.69)
    peripheral venous catheter (996.62)
    urinary catheter (996.64)

CC Exd: 996.62, 999.31-999.39

AHA: ▶2Q, '12, 16;◀ 2Q, '11, 7; 2Q, '10, 8; 4Q, '08, 72, 193; 4Q, '07, 97

999.32 Bloodstream infection due to central venous catheter   CC

Bloodstream infection due to:
    Hickman catheter
    peripherally inserted central catheter (PICC)
    portacath (port-a-cath)
    triple lumen catheter
    umbilical venous catheter
Catheter-related bloodstream infection (CRBSI) NOS
Central line-associated bloodstream infection (CLABSI)

CC Exd: See code 999.31

AHA: 4Q, '11, 153-155

999.33 Local infection due to central venous catheter   CC

Local infection due to:
    Hickman catheter
    peripherally inserted central catheter (PICC)
    portacath (port-a-cath)
    triple lumen catheter
    umbilical venous catheter
Port or reservoir infection
Tunnel infection

CC Exd: See code 999.31

AHA: 4Q, '11, 153-155

999.34 Acute infection following transfusion, infusion, or injection of blood and blood products   CC

CC Exd: See code 999.31

AHA: 4Q, '11, 153-155

TIP: If the acute infection transmitted via transfusion, infusion, or injection is HIV, sequence code 042 first.

999.39 Infection following other infusion, injection, transfusion, or vaccination   CC

CC Exd: 996.62, 999.31-999.39

AHA: 4Q, '08, 99

√5ᵗʰ **999.4 Anaphylactic reaction due to serum**

Allergic shock
Anaphylactic shock due to serum
Anaphylactoid reaction due to serum
Anaphylaxis

EXCLUDES   *ABO incompatibility reaction due to transfusion of*
        blood or blood products (999.60-999.69)
    reaction:
        allergic NOS (995.0)
        anaphylactic:
            NOS (995.0)
            due to drugs and chemicals (995.0)
        other serum (999.51-999.59)
    shock:
        allergic NOS (995.0)
        anaphylactic:
            NOS (995.0)
            due to drugs and chemicals (995.0)

DEF: Life-threatening hypersensitivity to foreign serum; causes respiratory distress, vascular collapse, and shock.

AHA: 4Q, '11, 142-147

999.41 Anaphylactic reaction due to administration of blood and blood products   CC

CC Exd: 999.41-999.49, 999.51-999.59

AHA: 4Q, '11, 146

N Newborn Age: 0   P Pediatric Age: 0-17   M Maternity Age: 12-55   A Adult Age: 15-124   MCC Major CC Condition   CC CC Condition   HIV HIV Related Dx

348 – Volume 1 • February 2013   2014 ICD-9-CM

999.42 Anaphylactic reaction due to vaccination `CC`
CC Excl: See code 999.41

999.49 Anaphylactic reaction due to other serum `CC`
CC Excl: See code 999.41

√5th 999.5 Other serum reaction
Intoxication by serum
Protein sickness
Serum rash
Serum sickness
Urticaria due to serum
EXCLUDES serum hepatitis (070.2-070.3)
DEF: Serum sickness: Hypersensitivity to foreign serum; causes fever, hives, swelling, and lymphadenopathy.
AHA: 4Q, '11, 142-146

999.51 Other serum reaction due to administration of blood and blood products `CC`
CC Excl: 999.41-999.49, 999.51-999.59

999.52 Other serum reaction due to vaccination `CC`
CC Excl: See code 999.51

999.59 Other serum reaction `CC`
CC Excl: 999.51-999.59

√5th 999.6 ABO incompatibility reaction due to transfusion of blood or blood products
EXCLUDES minor blood group antigens reactions (Duffy) (E) (K(ell)) (Kidd) (Lewis) (M) (N) (P) (S) (999.75-999.79)

999.60 ABO incompatibility reaction, unspecified `CC`
ABO incompatible blood transfusion NOS
Reaction to ABO incompatibility from transfusion NOS
CC Excl: 999.60-999.69, 999.70-999.80, 999.83-999.85, 999.89

999.61 ABO incompatibility with hemolytic transfusion reaction not specified as acute or delayed `CC`
ABO incompatibility with hemolytic transfusion reaction at unspecified time after transfusion
Hemolytic transfusion reaction (HTR) due to ABO incompatibility
CC Excl: See code: 999.60

999.62 ABO incompatibility with acute hemolytic transfusion reaction `CC`
ABO incompatibility with hemolytic transfusion reaction less than 24 hours after transfusion
Acute hemolytic transfusion reaction (AHTR) due to ABO incompatibility
CC Excl: See code: 999.60

999.63 ABO incompatibility with delayed hemolytic transfusion reaction `CC`
ABO incompatibility with hemolytic transfusion reaction 24 hours or more after transfusion
Delayed hemolytic transfusion reaction (DHTR) due to ABO incompatibility
CC Excl: See code: 999.60

999.69 Other ABO incompatibility reaction `CC`
Delayed serologic transfusion reaction (DSTR) from ABO incompatibility
Other ABO incompatible blood transfusion
Other reaction to ABO incompatibility from transfusion
CC Excl: See code: 999.60

√5th 999.7 Rh and other non-ABO incompatibility reaction due to transfusion of blood or blood products
Elevation of Rh titer
AHA: 4Q, '10, 99-100,102-105

999.70 Rh incompatibility reaction, unspecified `CC`
Reaction due to Rh factor in transfusion NOS
Rh incompatible blood transfusion NOS
Unspecified reaction due to incompatibility related to Rh antigens (C) (c) (D) (E) (e)
Unspecified reaction to Rh incompatibility
CC Excl: See code: 999.60

999.71 Rh incompatibility with hemolytic transfusion reaction not specified as acute or delayed `CC`
Hemolytic transfusion reaction (HTR) due to Rh incompatibility
HTR due to incompatibility related to Rh antigens (C) (c) (D) (E) (e), not specified as acute or delayed
Rh incompatibility with hemolytic transfusion reaction at unspecified time after transfusion
CC Excl: See code: 999.60

999.72 Rh incompatibility with acute hemolytic transfusion reaction `CC`
Acute hemolytic transfusion reaction (AHTR) due to Rh incompatibility
AHTR due to incompatibility related to Rh antigens (C) (c) (D) (E) (e)
Rh incompatibility with hemolytic transfusion reaction less than 24 hours after transfusion
CC Excl: See code: 999.60

999.73 Rh incompatibility with delayed hemolytic transfusion reaction `CC`
Delayed hemolytic transfusion reaction (DHTR) due to Rh incompatibility
DHTR due to incompatibility related to Rh antigens (C) (c) (D) (E) (e)
Rh incompatibility with hemolytic transfusion reaction 24 hours or more after transfusion
CC Excl: See code: 999.60

999.74 Other Rh incompatibility reaction `CC`
Delayed serologic transfusion reaction (DSTR) from Rh incompatibility
Other reaction due to incompatibility related to Rh antigens (C) (c) (D) (E) (e)
Other reaction to Rh incompatible blood transfusion
CC Excl: 999.60-999.69, 999.70-999.73, 999.79-999.80, 999.83-999.85, 999.89

999.75 Non-ABO incompatibility reaction, unspecified `CC`
Non-ABO incompatible blood transfusion NOS
Reaction to non-ABO antigen incompatibility from transfusion NOS
Unspecified reaction due to incompatibility related to minor antigens (Duffy) (Kell) (Kidd) (Lewis) (M) (N) (P) (S)
CC Excl: See code: 999.74

999.76 Non-ABO incompatibility with hemolytic transfusion reaction not specified as acute or delayed `CC`
Hemolytic transfusion reaction (HTR) due to non-ABO incompatibility
HTR from incompatibility related to minor antigens (Duffy) (Kell) (Kidd) (Lewis) (M) (N) (P) (S)
Non-ABO incompatibility with hemolytic transfusion reaction at unspecified time after transfusion
CC Excl: See code: 999.74

999.77 Non-ABO incompatibility with acute hemolytic transfusion reaction `CC`
Acute hemolytic transfusion reaction (AHTR) due to non-ABO incompatibility
AHTR from incompatibility related to minor antigens (Duffy) (Kell) (Kidd) (Lewis) (M) (N) (P) (S)
Non-ABO incompatibility with hemolytic transfusion reaction less than 24 hours after transfusion
CC Excl: See code: 999.74

999.78 Non-ABO incompatibility with delayed hemolytic transfusion reaction `CC`
Delayed hemolytic transfusion reaction (DHTR) due to non-ABO incompatibility
DHTR from incompatibility related to minor antigens (Duffy) (Kell) (Kidd) (Lewis) (M) (N) (P) (S)
Non-ABO incompatibility with hemolytic transfusion reaction 24 hours or more after transfusion
CC Excl: See code: 999.74

Injury and Poisoning

999.79 Other non-ABO incompatibility reaction   `CC`

Delayed serologic transfusion reaction (DSTR) from non-ABO incompatibility

Other non-ABO incompatible blood transfusion

Other reaction due to incompatibility related to minor antigens (Duffy) (Kell) (Kidd) (Lewis) (M) (N) (P) (S)

Other reaction to non-ABO incompatibility from transfusion

CC Excl: 999.60-999.69, 999.70-999.80, 999.83-999.85, 999.89

√5ᵗʰ **999.8 Other and unspecified infusion and transfusion reaction**

EXCLUDES *ABO incompatibility reactions (999.60-999.69)*

febrile nonhemolytic transfusion reaction (FNHTR) (780.66)

hemochromatosis due to repeated red blood cell transfusions (275.02)

non-ABO incompatibility reactions (999.70-999.79)

postoperative shock (998.00-998.09)

posttransfusion purpura (287.41)

Rh incompatibility reactions (999.70-999.74)

transfusion associated circulatory overload (TACO) (276.61)

transfusion related acute lung injury [TRALI] (518.7)

AHA: 4Q, '08, 152-155; 3Q, '00, 9

999.80 Transfusion reaction, unspecified

Incompatible blood transfusion NOS

Reaction to blood group incompatibility in infusion or transfusion NOS

AHA: 4Q, '10, 99-100, 106-107

999.81 Extravasation of vesicant chemotherapy   `CC`

Infiltration of vesicant chemotherapy

CC Excl: 999.2, 999.81-999.88

AHA: 4Q, '08, 155

999.82 Extravasation of other vesicant agent   `CC`

Infiltration of other vesicant agent

CC Excl: 999.2, 999.81-999.88

999.83 Hemolytic transfusion reaction, incompatibility unspecified   `CC`

Hemolytic transfusion reaction (HTR) with antigen incompatibility unspecified, not specified as acute or delayed

HTR with incompatibility unspecified at unspecified time after transfusion

CC Excl: 999.60-999.69, 999.70-999.80, 999.83-999.85, 999.89

AHA: 4Q, '10, 99-100, 106-107

999.84 Acute hemolytic transfusion reaction, incompatibility unspecified   `CC`

Acute hemolytic transfusion reaction (AHTR) with antigen incompatibility unspecified

AHTR, incompatibility unspecified

CC Excl: 999.60-999.69, 999.70-999.80, 999.83-999.85, 999.89

AHA: 4Q, '10, 99-100, 106-107

999.85 Delayed hemolytic transfusion reaction, incompatibility unspecified   `CC`

Delayed hemolytic transfusion reaction (DHTR) with antigen incompatibility unspecified

DHTR, incompatibility unspecified

CC Excl: 999.60-999.69, 999.70-999.80, 999.83-999.85, 999.89

AHA: 4Q, '10, 99-100, 106-107

999.88 Other infusion reaction

999.89 Other transfusion reaction

Delayed serologic transfusion reaction (DSTR), incompatibility unspecified

Use additional code to identify graft-versus-host reaction (279.5)

AHA: 4Q, '08, 99, 154

999.9 Other and unspecified complications of medical care, not elsewhere classified

Complications, not elsewhere classified, of:

electroshock

inhalation

ultrasound   } therapy

ventilation

Unspecified misadventure of medical care

EXCLUDES *unspecified complication of:*

phototherapy (990)

radiation therapy (999)

ventilator associated pneumonia (997.31)

AHA: 3Q, '06, 25; 1Q, '03, 19; 2Q, '97, 5

`N` Newborn Age: 0   `P` Pediatric Age: 0-17   `M` Maternity Age: 12-55   `A` Adult Age: 15-124   `MCC` Major CC Condition   `CC` CC Condition   `HIV` HIV Related Dx

350 – Volume 1   **2014 ICD-9-CM**

Supplementary Classification of Factors Influencing Health Status and Contact with Health Services (V01-V91)

This classification is provided to deal with occasions when circumstances other than a disease or injury classifiable to categories 001-999 (the main part of ICD) are recorded as "diagnoses" or "problems." This can arise mainly in three ways:

a) When a person who is not currently sick encounters the health services for some specific purpose, such as to act as a donor of an organ or tissue, to receive prophylactic vaccination, or to discuss a problem which is in itself not a disease or injury. This will be a fairly rare occurrence among hospital inpatients, but will be relatively more common among hospital outpatients and patients of family practitioners, health clinics, etc.

b) When a person with a known disease or injury, whether it is current or resolving, encounters the health care system for a specific treatment of that disease or injury (e.g., dialysis for renal disease; chemotherapy for malignancy; cast change).

c) When some circumstance or problem is present which influences the person's health status but is not in itself a current illness or injury. Such factors may be elicited during population surveys, when the person may or may not be currently sick, or be recorded as an additional factor to be borne in mind when the person is receiving care for some current illness or injury classifiable to categories 001-999.

In the latter circumstances the V code should be used only as a supplementary code and should not be the one selected for use in primary, single cause tabulations. Examples of these circumstances are a personal history of certain diseases, or a person with an artificial heart valve in situ.

AHA: J-F, '87, 8

Persons with Potential Health Hazards Related to Communicable Diseases (V01-V06)

EXCLUDES *family history of infectious and parasitic diseases (V18.8)*
personal history of infectious and parasitic diseases (V12.0)

√4ᵗʰ **V01 Contact with or exposure to communicable diseases**

TIP: Do not assign if the patient shows signs or symptoms of the disease to which he or she was exposed.

V01.0 **Cholera**
Conditions classifiable to 001

V01.1 **Tuberculosis**
Conditions classifiable to 010-018

V01.2 **Poliomyelitis**
Conditions classifiable to 045

V01.3 **Smallpox**
Conditions classifiable to 050

V01.4 **Rubella**
Conditions classifiable to 056

V01.5 **Rabies**
Conditions classifiable to 071

V01.6 **Venereal diseases**
Conditions classifiable to 090-099
AHA: 4Q, '07, 125

√5ᵗʰ V01.7 **Other viral diseases**
Conditions classifiable to 042-078 and V08, except as above
AHA: 2Q, '92, 11

² V01.71 **Varicella**

² V01.79 **Other viral diseases**

√5ᵗʰ V01.8 **Other communicable diseases**
Conditions classifiable to 001-136, except as above
AHA: J-A, '87, 24

V01.81 **Anthrax**
AHA: 4Q, '02, 70, 78

² V01.82 **Exposure to SARS-associated coronavirus**
AHA: 4Q, '03, 46-47

² V01.83 **Escherichia coli (E. coli)**

² V01.84 **Meningococcus**
Z20.811 Contact with and exposure to meningococcus   I-10

V01.89 **Other communicable diseases**

V01.9 **Unspecified communicable diseases**

√4ᵗʰ **V02 Carrier or suspected carrier of infectious diseases**
INCLUDES colonization status
AHA: 3Q, '95, 18; 3Q, '94, 4

V02.0 **Cholera**

V02.1 **Typhoid**

V02.2 **Amebiasis**

V02.3 **Other gastrointestinal pathogens**

V02.4 **Diphtheria**

√5ᵗʰ V02.5 **Other specified bacterial diseases**

V02.51 **Group B streptococcus**
AHA: 3Q, '06, 14; 1Q, '02, 14; 4Q, '98, 56

V02.52 **Other streptococcus**

V02.53 **Methicillin susceptible Staphylococcus aureus**
MSSA colonization
AHA: 4Q, '08, 69, 71, 156

V02.54 **Methicillin resistant Staphylococcus aureus**
MRSA colonization
AHA: 4Q, '08, 69, 71, 72, 156

V02.59 **Other specified bacterial diseases**
Meningococcal   Staphylococcal

√5ᵗʰ V02.6 **Viral hepatitis**
Hepatitis Australian-antigen [HAA] [SH] carrier
Serum hepatitis carrier

V02.60 **Viral hepatitis carrier, unspecfied**
AHA: 4Q, '97, 47

V02.61 **Hepatitis B carrier**
AHA: 4Q, '97, 47
Z22.51 Carrier of viral hepatitis B   I-10

V02.62 **Hepatitis C carrier**
AHA: 4Q, '97, 47

V02.69 **Other viral hepatitis carrier**
AHA: 4Q, '97, 47

V02.7 **Gonorrhea**

V02.8 **Other veneral diseases**

V02.9 **Other specified infectious organism**
AHA: 3Q, '95, 18; 1Q, '93, 22; J-A, '87, 24

√4ᵗʰ **V03 Need for prophylactic vaccination and inoculation against bacterial diseases**
EXCLUDES *vaccination not carried out (V64.00-V64.09)*
vaccines against combinations of diseases (V06.0-V06.9)

V03.0 **Cholera alone**

V03.1 **Typhoid-paratyphoid alone [TAB]**

V03.2 **Tuberculosis [BCG]**

V03.3 **Plague**

V03.4 **Tularemia**

V03.5 **Diphtheria alone**

V03.6 **Pertussis alone**

V03.7 **Tetanus toxoid alone**

√5ᵗʰ V03.8 **Other specified vaccinations against single bacterial diseases**

V03.81 **Hemophilus influenza, type B [Hib]**

V03.82 **Streptococcus pneumoniae [pneumococcus]**

V03.89 **Other specified vaccination**
AHA: 2Q, '00, 9
TIP: Assign for vaccination against Lyme disease.

V03.9 **Unspecified single bacterial disease**

√4ᵗʰ **V04 Need for prophylactic vaccination and inoculation against certain viral diseases**
EXCLUDES *vaccines against combinations of diseases (V06.0-V06.9)*

V04.0 **Poliomyelitis**

---

² These V codes may be used as principal diagnosis on Medicare patients.

4ᵗʰ/5ᵗʰ Additional Digit Required	Unacceptable PDx	Manifestation Code	Hospital Acquired Condition	►◄ Revised Text	● New Code	▲ Revised Code Title

V04.1 Smallpox

V04.2 Measles alone

V04.3 Rubella alone

V04.4 Yellow fever

V04.5 Rabies

V04.6 Mumps alone

V04.7 Common cold

✓5ᵗʰ **V04.8 Other viral diseases**
AHA: 4Q, '03, 83

V04.81 Influenza

V04.82 Respiratory syncytial virus (RSV)
AHA: 1Q, '09, 14

V04.89 Other viral diseases
AHA: 2Q, '07, 9
TIP: Assign for vaccination against human papilloma virus (HPV).

✓4ᵗʰ **V05 Need for other prophylactic vaccination and inoculation against single diseases**
EXCLUDES *vaccines against combinations of diseases (V06.0-V06.9)*

V05.0 Athropod-borne viral encephalitis

V05.1 Other arthropod-borne viral diseases

V05.2 Leshmaniasis

V05.3 Viral hepatitis

V05.4 Varicella
Chickenpox

V05.8 Other specified disease
AHA: 1Q, '01, 4; 3Q, '91, 20

V05.9 Unspecified single disease

✓4ᵗʰ **V06 Need for prophylactic vaccination and inoculation against combinations of diseases**
NOTE Use additional single vaccination codes from categories V03-V05 to identify any vaccinations not included in a combination code.

V06.0 Cholera with typhoid-paratyphoid [cholera+TAB]

V06.1 Diphtheria-tetanus-pertussis, combined [DTP] [DTaP]
AHA: 4Q, '03, 83; 3Q, '98, 13

V06.2 Diphtheria-tetanus-pertussis with typhoid-paratyphoid [DTP+TAB]

V06.3 Diphtheria-tetanus-pertussis with poliomyelitis [DTP+polio]

V06.4 Measles-mumps-rubella [MMR]

V06.5 Tetanus-diphtheria [Td] [DT]
AHA: 4Q, '03, 83

V06.6 Streptococcus pneumoniae [pneumococcus] and influenza

V06.8 Other combinations
EXCLUDES *multiple single vaccination codes (V03.0-V05.9)*
AHA: 1Q, '12, 11; 1Q, '94, 19

V06.9 Unspecified combined vaccine

Persons with Need for Isolation, Other Potential Health Hazards and Prophylactic Measures (V07-V09)

✓4ᵗʰ **V07 Need for isolation and other prophylactic or treatment measures**
EXCLUDES *long-term (current) (prophylactic) use of certain specific drugs (V58.61-V58.69)*
prophylactic organ removal (V50.41-V50.49)

² **V07.0 Isolation**
Admission to protect the individual from his surroundings or for isolation of individual after contact with infectious diseases

V07.1 Desensitization to allergens

V07.2 Prophylactic immunotherapy
Administration of:
antivenin
immune sera [gamma globulin]
RhoGAM
tetanus antitoxin

✓5ᵗʰ **V07.3 Other prophylactic chemotherapy**

V07.31 Prophylactic fluoride administration

² **V07.39 Other prophylactic chemotherapy**
EXCLUDES *maintenance chemotherapy following disease (V58.11)*

V07.4 Hormone replacement therapy (postmenopausal) ♀
Z79.890 Hormone replacement therapy postmenopausal   I-10

✓5ᵗʰ **V07.5 Use of agents affecting estrogen receptors and estrogen levels**
Code first, if applicable:
malignant neoplasm of breast (174.0-174.9, 175.0-175.9)
malignant neoplasm of prostate (185)

Use additional code, if applicable, to identify:
estrogen receptor positive status (V86.0)
family history of breast cancer (V16.3)
genetic susceptibility to cancer (V84.01-V84.09)
personal history of breast cancer (V10.3)
personal history of prostate cancer (V10.46)
postmenopausal status (V49.81)

EXCLUDES *hormone replacement therapy (postmenopausal) (V07.4)*
AHA: 4Q, '10, 108; 4Q, '08, 156

V07.51 Use of selective estrogen receptor modulators [SERMs]
Use of:
raloxifene (Evista)
tamoxifen (Nolvadex)
toremifene (Fareston)
Z79.810 Lng term sel estrogen receptor modulators SERMS   I-10

V07.52 Use of aromatase inhibitors
Use of:
anastrozole (Arimidex)
exemestane (Aromasin)
letrozole (Femara)

V07.59 Use of other agents affecting estrogen receptors and estrogen levels
Use of:
estrogen receptor downregulators
fulvestrant (Faslodex)
gonadotropin-releasing hormone (GnRH) agonist
goserelin acetate (Zoladex)
leuprolide acetate (leuprorelin) (Lupron)
megestrol acetate (Megace)

² **V07.8 Other specified prophylactic or treatment measure**
AHA: 2Q, '10, 6, 14; 1Q, '92, 11
TIP: Assign for patients having prophylactic breast removal because of a strong family history of breast cancer, along with code V16.3 Family history of breast cancer.

V07.9 Unspecified prophylactic or treatment measure

V08 Asymptomatic human immunodeficiency virus [HIV] infection status
HIV positive NOS
NOTE This code is only to be used when no HIV infection symptoms or conditions are present. If any HIV infection symptoms or conditions are present, see code 042.
EXCLUDES *AIDS (042)*
human immunodeficiency virus [HIV] disease (042)
exposure to HIV (V01.79)
nonspecific serologic evidence of HIV (795.71)
symptomatic human immunodeficiency virus [HIV] infection (042)
AHA: 2Q, '04, 11; 2Q, '99, 8; 3Q, '95, 18
Z21 Asymptomatic HIV infection status   I-10

---

² These V codes may be used as principal diagnosis on Medicare patients.

N Newborn Age: 0   P Pediatric Age: 0-17   M Maternity Age: 12-55   A Adult Age: 15-124   MCC Major CC Condition   CC CC Condition   HIV HIV Related Dx

352 – Volume 1   2014 ICD-9-CM

☑4ᵗʰ **V09 Infection with drug-resistant microorganisms**

> **NOTE** This category is intended for use as an additional code for infectious conditions classified elsewhere to indicate the presence of drug-resistance of the infectious organism.
> AHA: 3Q, '94, 4; 4Q, '93, 22

V09.0 Infection with microorganisms resistant to penicillins
> AHA: 2Q, '06, 16; 4Q, '03, 104, 106

V09.1 Infection with microorganisms resistant to cephalosporins and other B-lactam antibiotics

V09.2 Infection with microorganisms resistant to macrolides

V09.3 Infection with microorganisms resistant to tetracyclines

V09.4 Infection with microorganisms resistant to aminoglycosides

☑5ᵗʰ **V09.5 Infection with microorganisms resistant to quinolones and fluoroquinolones**

V09.50 Without mention of resistance to multiple quinolones and fluoroquinoles

V09.51 With resistance to multiple quinolones and fluoroquinoles

V09.6 Infection with microorganisms resistant to sulfonamides

☑5ᵗʰ **V09.7 Infection with microorganisms resistant to other specified antimycobacterial agents**

> **EXCLUDES** Amikacin (V09.4)
> Kanamycin (V09.4)
> Streptomycin [SM] (V09.4)

V09.70 Without mention of resistance to multiple antimycobacterial agents

V09.71 With resistance to multiple antimycobacterial agents

☑5ᵗʰ **V09.8 Infection with microorganisms resistant to other specified drugs**
> Vancomycin (glycopeptide) intermediate staphylococcus aureus (VISA/GISA)
> Vancomycin (glycopeptide) resistant enterococcus (VRE)
> Vancomycin (glycopeptide) resistant staphylococcus aureus (VRSA/GRSA)

V09.80 Without mention of resistance to multiple drugs

V09.81 With resistance to multiple drugs

☑5ᵗʰ **V09.9 Infection with drug-resistant microorganisms, unspecified**
> Drug resistance, NOS

V09.90 Without mention of multiple drug resistance
> Z16.30 Resist to unspec antimicrobial drugs I-10

V09.91 With multiple drug resistance
> Multiple drug resistance NOS

Persons with Potential Health Hazards Related to Personal and Family History (V10-V19)

> **EXCLUDES** obstetric patients where the possibility that the fetus might be affected is the reason for observation or management during pregnancy (655.0-655.9)
> AHA: J-F, '87, 1

☑4ᵗʰ **V10 Personal history of malignant neoplasm**
> AHA: 4Q, '02, 80; 4Q, '98, 69; 1Q, '95, 4; 3Q, '92, 5; M-J, '85, 10; 2Q, '90, 9
> **TIP:** Assign the codes in this category only for a personal history of primary malignancy (not metastatic malignancies).

☑5ᵗʰ **V10.0 Gastrointestinal tract**
> History of conditions classifiable to 140-159
> **EXCLUDES** personal history of malignant carcinoid tumor (V10.91)
> personal history of malignant neuroendocrine tumor (V10.91)

V10.00 Gastrointestinal tract, unspecified

V10.01 Tongue

V10.02 Other and unspecified oral cavity and pharynx

V10.03 Esophagus

V10.04 Stomach

V10.05 Large intestine
> AHA: 3Q, '99, 7; 1Q, '95, 4
> Z85.038 Personal hx othr malig neoplasm lrg intestine I-10

V10.06 Rectum, rectosigmoid junction, and anus

V10.07 Liver

V10.09 Other
> AHA: 4Q, '03, 111

☑5ᵗʰ **V10.1 Trachea, bronchus, and lung**
> History of conditions classifiable to 162
> **EXCLUDES** personal history of malignant carcinoid tumor (V10.91)
> personal history of malignant neuroendocrine tumor (V10.91)

V10.11 Bronchus and lung

V10.12 Trachea

☑5ᵗʰ **V10.2 Other respiratory and intrathoracic organs**
> History of conditions classifiable to 160, 161, 163-165

V10.20 Respiratory organ, unspecified

V10.21 Larynx
> AHA: 4Q, '03, 108, 110

V10.22 Nasal cavities, middle ear, and accessory sinuses

V10.29 Other

V10.3 Breast
> History of conditions classifiable to 174 and 175
> AHA: 1Q, '12, 11; 2Q, '11, 12; 3Q, '07, 4; 1Q, '07, 6; 2Q, '03, 5; 4Q, '01, 66; 4Q, '98, 65; 4Q, '97, 50; 1Q, '91, 16; 1Q, '90, 21
> **TIP:** Do not assign for personal history of ductal carcinoma in situ (DCIS); assign code V13.89.
> Z85.3 Personal history primary malig neoplasm breast I-10

☑5ᵗʰ **V10.4 Genital organs**
> History of conditions classifiable to 179-187

V10.40 Female genital organ, unspecfied ♀

V10.41 Cervix uteri ♀
> AHA: 4Q, '07, 99

V10.42 Other parts of uterus ♀

V10.43 Ovary ♀

V10.44 Other female genital organs ♀

V10.45 Male genital organ, unspecfied ♂

V10.46 Prostate ♂
> AHA: 1Q, '09,15

V10.47 Testis ♂
> Z85.47 Personal history primary malig neoplasm testis I-10

V10.48 Epididymis ♂

V10.49 Other male genital organs ♂

☑5ᵗʰ **V10.5 Urinary organs**
> History of conditions classifiable to 188 and 189
> **EXCLUDES** personal history of malignant carcinoid tumor (V10.91)
> personal history of malignant neuroendocrine tumor (V10.91)

V10.50 Urinary organ, unspecified

V10.51 Bladder

V10.52 Kidney
> AHA: 2Q, '04, 4
> **EXCLUDES** renal pelvis (V10.53)

V10.53 Renal pelvis
> AHA: 4Q, '01, 55

V10.59 Other

☑5ᵗʰ **V10.6 Leukemia**
> Conditions classifiable to 204-208
> **EXCLUDES** leukemia in remission (204-208)
> AHA: 2Q, '92, 13; 4Q, '91, 26; 4Q, '90, 3

V10.60 Leukemia, unspecified

V10.61 Lymphoid leukemia

☑4ᵗʰ / ☑5ᵗʰ Additional Digit Required | Unacceptable PDx | Manifestation Code | Hospital Acquired Condition | ▶◀ Revised Text | ● New Code | ▲ Revised Code Title
2014 ICD-9-CM | Volume 1 – 353

V09–V10.61

V10.62 **Myeloid leukemia**

V10.63 **Monocytic leukemia**

V10.69 **Other**

√5th V10.7 **Other lymphatic and hematopoietic neoplasms**
Conditions classifiable to 200-203
EXCLUDES *listed conditions in 200-203 in remission*
AHA: M-J, '85, 18

V10.71 **Lymphosarcoma and reticulosarcoma**

V10.72 **Hodgkin's disease**

V10.79 **Other**

√5th V10.8 **Personal history of malignant neoplasm of other sites**
History of conditions classifiable to 170-173, 190-195
EXCLUDES *personal history of malignant carcinoid tumor*
(V10.91)
personal history of malignant neuroendocrine tumor
(V10.91)

V10.81 **Bone**
AHA: 2Q, '03, 13

V10.82 **Malignant melanoma of skin**

V10.83 **Other malignant neoplasm of skin**

V10.84 **Eye**

V10.85 **Brain**
AHA: 1Q, '01, 6

V10.86 **Other parts of the nervous system**
EXCLUDES *peripheral sympathetic, and*
parasympathetic nerves (V10.89)

V10.87 **Thyroid**

V10.88 **Other endocrine glands and related**
structures

V10.89 **Other**

√5th V10.9 **Other and unspecified personal history of malignant**
neoplasm
AHA: 4Q, '09, 115

V10.90 **Personal history of unspecified**
malignant neoplasm
Personal history of malignant neoplasm NOS
EXCLUDES *personal history of malignant carcinoid*
tumor (V10.91)
personal history of malignant
neuroendocrine tumor (V10.91)
personal history of Merkel cell carcinoma
(V10.91)

V10.91 **Personal history of malignant**
neuroendocrine tumor
Personal history of malignant carcinoid tumor NOS
Personal history of malignant neuroendocrine tumor
NOS
Personal history of Merkel cell carcinoma NOS
Code first any continuing functional activity, such as:
carcinoid syndrome (259.2)

√4th V11 **Personal history of mental disorder**

V11.0 **Schizophrenia**
EXCLUDES *that in remission (295.0-295.9 with fifth-digit 5)*

V11.1 **Affective disorders**
Personal history of manic-depressive psychosis
EXCLUDES *that in remission (296.0-296.6 with fifth-digit 5, 6)*

V11.2 **Neurosis**

V11.3 **Alcoholism**

V11.4 **Combat and operational stress reaction**   A
AHA: 4Q, '10, 108

V11.8 **Other mental disorders**

V11.9 **Unspecified mental disorder**

√4th V12 **Personal history of certain other diseases**
AHA: 3Q, '92, 11

√5th V12.0 **Infectious and parasitic diseases**
EXCLUDES *personal history of infectious diseases specific to a*
body system

V12.00 **Unspecified infectious and parasitic disease**

V12.01 **Tuberculosis**

V12.02 **Poliomyelitis**
Z86.12 Personal history of poliomyelitis   I-10

V12.03 **Malaria**

V12.04 **Methicillin resistant Staphylococcus aureus**
MRSA
AHA: 4Q, '08, 69, 71

V12.09 **Other**

V12.1 **Nutritional deficiency**

√5th V12.2 **Endocrine, metabolic, and immunity disorders**
AHA: 4Q, '11, 156

V12.21 **Gestational diabetes**   ♀

V12.29 **Other endocrine, metabolic, and immunity**
disorders

V12.3 **Diseases of blood and blood-forming organs**

√5th V12.4 **Disorders of nervous system and sense organs**

V12.40 **Unspecified disorder of nervous**
system and sense organs

V12.41 **Benign neoplasm of the brain**
AHA: 4Q, '97, 48
TIP: Benign neoplasms of the brain are tracked separately
because, besides being potentially life-threatening, they
often recur and can be difficult to treat.

V12.42 **Infections of the central nervous system**
Encephalitis Meningitis
AHA: 4Q, '05, 95

V12.49 **Other disorders of nervous**
system and sense organs
AHA: 4Q, '98, 59

√5th V12.5 **Diseases of circulatory system**
EXCLUDES *history of anaphylactic shock (V13.81)*
old myocardial infarction (412)
postmyocardial infarction syndrome (411.0)
AHA: 4Q, '95, 61

V12.50 **Unspecified circulatory disease**

V12.51 **Venous thrombosis and embolism**
EXCLUDES *pulmonary embolism (V12.55)*
AHA: 1Q, '11, 20; 3Q, '06, 12; 4Q, '03, 108; 1Q, '02, 15

V12.52 **Thrombophlebitis**

V12.53 **Sudden cardiac arrest**
Sudden cardiac death successfully resuscitated
AHA: 4Q, '07, 98

V12.54 **Transient ischemic attack [TIA], and**
cerebral infarction without residual deficits
Prolonged reversible ischemic neurological deficit
[PRIND]
Reversible ischemic neurologic deficit [RIND]
Stroke NOS without residual deficits
EXCLUDES *history of traumatic brain injury (V15.52)*
late effects of cerebrovascular disease
(438.0-438.9)
AHA: 4Q, '07, 98
TIP: Assign for old CVA for which the patient has no residual
deficits; if deficits are present, see category 438.
Z86.73 Personal hx TIA & cerebral infarct w/o deficits   I-10

V12.55 **Pulmonary embolism**
AHA: 4Q, '11, 156

V12.59 **Other**
AHA: 2Q, '07, 3; 4Q, '99, 4; 4Q, '98, 88; 4Q, '97, 37

N Newborn Age: 0   P Pediatric Age: 0-17   M Maternity Age: 12-55   A Adult Age: 15-124   MCC Major CC Condition   CC CC Condition   HIV HIV Related Dx

354 – Volume 1   2014 ICD-9-CM

✓5ᵗʰ **V12.6 Diseases of respiratory system**
    EXCLUDES *tuberculosis (V12.01)*

    V12.60 Unspecified disease of respiratory system

    V12.61 Pneumonia (recurrent)
        AHA: 4Q, '05, 95

    V12.69 Other diseases of respiratory system

✓5ᵗʰ **V12.7 Diseases of digestive system**
    AHA: 1Q, '95, 3; 2Q, '89, 16

    V12.70 Unspecified digestive disease

    V12.71 Peptic ulcer disease

    V12.72 Colonic polyps
        AHA: 3Q, '02, 15
        Z86.010 Personal history of colonic polyps   I-10

    V12.79 Other

✓4ᵗʰ **V13 Personal history of other diseases**

   ✓5ᵗʰ **V13.0 Disorders of urinary system**

    V13.00 Unspecified urinary disorder

    V13.01 Urinary calculi

    V13.02 Urinary (tract) infection
        AHA: 4Q, '05, 95

    V13.03 Nephrotic syndrome
        AHA: 4Q, '05, 95

    V13.09 Other

   V13.1 Trophoblastic disease   ♀
    EXCLUDES *supervision during a current pregnancy (V23.1)*

   ✓5ᵗʰ **V13.2 Other genital system and obstetric disorders**
    EXCLUDES *recurrent pregnancy loss (646.3)*
          without current pregnancy (629.81)
          supervision during a current pregnancy of a woman
          with poor obstetric history (V23.0-V23.9)

    V13.21 Personal history of pre-term labor   ♀
      EXCLUDES *current pregnancy with history of pre-term*
          labor (V23.41)
      AHA: 4Q, '02, 78

    V13.22 Personal history of cervical dysplasia   ♀
      Personal history of conditions classifiable to
        622.10-622.12
      EXCLUDES *personal history of malignant neoplasm of*
          cervix uteri (V10.41)
      AHA: 4Q, '07, 98

    V13.23 Personal history of vaginal dysplasia   ♀
      Personal history of conditions classifiable to 623.0
      EXCLUDES *personal history of malignant neoplasm of*
          vagina (V10.44)
      AHA: 4Q, '10, 108

    V13.24 Personal history of vulvar dysplasia   ♀
      Personal history of conditions classifiable to
        624.01-624.02
      EXCLUDES *personal history of malignant neoplasm of*
          vulva (V10.44)
      AHA: 4Q, '10, 108

    V13.29 Other genital system and obstetric disorders   ♀

   V13.3 Diseases of skin and subcutaneous tissue

   V13.4 Arthritis

   ✓5ᵗʰ **V13.5 Other musculoskeletal disorders**
    AHA: 4Q, '08, 158
    TIP: Personal histories of pathological, stress, or traumatic fractures
    are separately classified because a patient with such a history is at
    much higher risk of refracture of the same site.

    V13.51 Pathologic fracture
      Healed pathologic fracture
      EXCLUDES *personal history of traumatic fracture*
          (V15.51)

    V13.52 Stress fracture
      Healed stress fracture
      EXCLUDES *personal history of traumatic fracture*
          (V15.51)

    V13.59 Other musculoskeletal disorders

   ✓5ᵗʰ **V13.6 Congenital (corrected) malformations**
    AHA: 4Q, '10, 108, 136; 4Q, '98, 63

    V13.61 Personal history of (corrected) hypospadias   ♂

    V13.62 Personal history of other (corrected) congenital malformations of genitourinary system

    V13.63 Personal history of (corrected) congenital malformations of nervous system

    V13.64 Personal history of (corrected) congenital malformations of eye, ear, face and neck
      Corrected cleft lip and palate

    V13.65 Personal history of (corrected) congenital malformations of heart and circulatory system

    V13.66 Personal history of (corrected) congenital malformations of respiratory system

    V13.67 Personal history of (corrected) congenital malformations of digestive system

    V13.68 Personal history of (corrected) congenital malformations of integument, limbs, and musculoskeletal systems

    V13.69 Personal history of other (corrected) congenital malformations
      AHA: 4Q, '10, 108; 1Q, '04, 16

   V13.7 Perinatal problems
    EXCLUDES *low birth weight status (V21.30-V21.35)*

   ✓5ᵗʰ **V13.8 Other specified diseases**
    AHA: 4Q, '11, 156

    V13.81 Anaphylaxis

    V13.89 Other specified diseases
      AHA: 1Q, '12, 11

   V13.9 Unspecified disease
    AHA: 4Q, '06, 117

✓4ᵗʰ **V14 Personal history of allergy to medicinal agents**

   V14.0 Penicillin
    Z88.0 Allergy status to penicillin   I-10

   V14.1 Other antibiotic agent

   V14.2 Sulfonamides

   V14.3 Other anti-infective agent

   V14.4 Anesthetic agent

   V14.5 Narcotic agent

   V14.6 Analgesic agent

   V14.7 Serum or vaccine

   V14.8 Other specified medicinal agents

   V14.9 Unspecified medicinal agent

✓4ᵗʰ **V15 Other personal history presenting hazards to health**
    EXCLUDES *personal history of drug therapy (V87.41-V87.49)*

   ✓5ᵗʰ **V15.0 Allergy, other than to medicinal agents**
    EXCLUDES *allergy to food substance used as base for medicinal*
          agent (V14.0-V14.9)
    AHA: 4Q, '00, 42, 49
    TIP: A person who has had an allergic episode to a substance in the
    past should always be considered allergic to the substance.

    V15.01 Allergy to peanuts
      Z91.010 Allergy to peanuts   I-10

    V15.02 Allergy to milk products
      EXCLUDES *lactose intolerance (271.3)*
      AHA: 1Q, '03, 12

    V15.03 Allergy to eggs

    V15.04 Allergy to seafood
      Seafood (octopus) (squid) ink   Shellfish

Additional Digit Required   Unacceptable PDx   Manifestation Code   Hospital Acquired Condition   ►◄ Revised Text   ● New Code   ▲ Revised Code Title

V Codes

V15.05–V16.43

V15.05 Allergy to other foods
Food additives　　　Nuts other than peanuts

V15.06 Allergy to insects and arachnids
Bugs
Insect bites and stings
Spiders

V15.07 Allergy to latex
Latex sensitivity

V15.08 Allergy to radiographic dye
Contrast media used for diagnostic x-ray procedures

V15.09 Other allergy, other than to medicinal agents

V15.1 Surgery to heart and great vessels
EXCLUDES　replacement by transplant or other means
(V42.1-V42.2, V43.2-V43.4)
AHA: 1Q, '04, 16

√5ᵗʰ **V15.2 Surgery to other organs**
EXCLUDES　replacement by transplant or other means
(V42.0-V43.8)
AHA: 4Q, '08, 158

V15.21 Personal history of undergoing in utero procedure during pregnancy ♀
AHA: 4Q, '08, 158

V15.22 Personal history of undergoing in utero procedure while a fetus
AHA: 4Q, '08, 158

V15.29 Surgery to other organs

V15.3 Irradiation
Previous exposure to therapeutic or other ionizing radiation
AHA: 2Q, '11, 12;

√5ᵗʰ **V15.4 Psychological trauma**
EXCLUDES　history of condition classifiable to 290-316
(V11.0-V11.9)

V15.41 History of physical abuse
Rape
AHA: 3Q, '99, 15

V15.42 History of emotional abuse
Neglect
AHA: 3Q, '99, 15

V15.49 Other
AHA: 3Q, '99, 15

√5ᵗʰ **V15.5 Injury**
AHA: 4Q, '08, 158

V15.51 Traumatic fracture
Healed traumatic fracture
EXCLUDES　personal history of pathologic and stress
fracture (V13.51, V13.52)
TIP: Personal histories of pathological, stress, or traumatic fractures are separately classified because a patient with such a history is at much higher risk of refracture of the same site.

V15.52 History of traumatic brain injury
EXCLUDES　personal history of cerebrovascular accident
(cerebral infarction) without residual
deficits (V12.54)
AHA: 4Q, '09, 115

V15.53 Personal history of retained foreign body fully removed
AHA: 4Q, '10, 108

V15.59 Other injury

V15.6 Poisoning

V15.7 Contraception
EXCLUDES　current contraceptive management (V25.0-V25.4)
presence of intrauterine contraceptive device as
incidental finding (V45.5)

√5ᵗʰ **V15.8 Other specified personal history presenting hazards to health**
EXCLUDES　contact with and (suspected) exposure to:
aromatic compounds and dyes (V87.11-V87.19)
arsenic and other metals (V87.01-V87.09)
molds (V87.31)
AHA: 4Q, '95, 62

V15.80 History of failed moderate sedation
History of failed conscious sedation
AHA: 4Q, '09, 115

V15.81 Noncompliance with medical treatment
EXCLUDES　noncompliance with renal dialysis (V45.12)
AHA: ▶2Q, '12, 16;◀ 3Q, '07, 9; 4Q, '06, 136; 2Q, '03, 7; 2Q,
'01, 11, 12, 13; 2Q, '99, 17; 2Q, '97, 11; 1Q, '97, 12; 3Q, '96, 9

V15.82 History of tobacco use
EXCLUDES　tobacco dependence (305.1)
AHA: 1Q, '09, 17
Z87.891 Personal history of nicotine dependence　I-10

V15.83 Underimmunization status
Delinquent immunization status
Lapsed immunization schedule status
AHA: 4Q, '09, 115

V15.84 Contact with and (suspected) exposure to asbestos
AHA: 4Q, '09, 116

V15.85 Contact with and (suspected) exposure to potentially hazardous body fluids
AHA: 4Q, '09, 116

V15.86 Contact with and (suspected) exposure to lead
AHA: 4Q, '09, 116

V15.87 History of extracorporeal membrane oxygenation [ECMO]
AHA: 4Q, '03, 84

V15.88 History of fall
At risk for falling
AHA: 4Q, '05, 95
Z91.81 History of falling　I-10

V15.89 Other
EXCLUDES　contact with and (suspected) exposure to
other potentially hazardous:
chemicals (V87.2)
substances (V87.39)
AHA: 3Q, '08, 7; 3Q, '07, 5; 1Q, '90, 21; N-D, '84, 12

V15.9 Unspecified personal history presenting hazards to health

√4ᵗʰ **V16 Family history of malignant neoplasm**

V16.0 Gastrointestinal tract
Family history of condition classifiable to 140-159
AHA: 1Q, '99, 4
TIP: Family history of colon cancer is a condition that meets the criteria of "high risk" for a screening colonoscopy.

V16.1 Trachea, bronchus, and lung
Family history of condition classifiable to 162

V16.2 Other respiratory and intrathoracic organs
Family history of condition classifiable to 160-161, 163-165

V16.3 Breast
Family history of condition classifiable to 174
AHA: 4Q, '04, 107; 2Q, '03, 4; 2Q, '00, 8; 1Q, '92, 11
Z80.3 Family history of malignant neoplasm of breast　I-10

√5ᵗʰ **V16.4 Genital organs**
Family history of condition classifiable to 179-187
AHA: 4Q, '97, 48

V16.40 Genital organ, unspecified

V16.41 Ovary
AHA: 3Q, '09, 5

V16.42 Prostate
Z80.42 Family history of malignant neoplasm of
prostate　I-10

V16.43 Testis

N　Newborn Age: 0　　P　Pediatric Age: 0-17　　M　Maternity Age: 12-55　　A　Adult Age: 15-124　　MCC　Major CC Condition　　CC　CC Condition　　HIV　HIV Related Dx

356 – Volume 1 · February 2013
2014 ICD-9-CM

V16.49 Other

    AHA: 2Q, '06, 2

✓5ᵗʰ **V16.5 Urinary organs**

    Family history of condition classifiable to 188-189

V16.51 Kidney

V16.52 Bladder

    AHA: 4Q, '07, 98

V16.59 Other

V16.6 Leukemia

    Family history of condition classifiable to 204-208

V16.7 Other lymphatic and hematopoietic neoplasms

    Family history of condition classifiable to 200-203

V16.8 Other specified malignant neoplasm

    Family history of other condition classifiable to 140-199

V16.9 Unspecified malignant neoplasm

✓4ᵗʰ **V17 Family history of certain chronic disabling diseases**

V17.0 Psychiatric condition

    EXCLUDES *family history of intellectual disabilities (V18.4)*

V17.1 Stroke (cerebrovascular)

    Z82.3 Family history of stroke   I-10

V17.2 Other neurological diseases

    Epilepsy   Huntington's chorea

V17.3 Ischemic heart disease

✓5ᵗʰ **V17.4 Other cardiovascular diseases**

    AHA: 1Q, '04, 6

V17.41 Family history of sudden cardiac death [SCD]

    EXCLUDES *family history of ischemic heart disease (V17.3)*
          family history of myocardial infarction (V17.3)

    AHA: 4Q, '07, 98

V17.49 Family history of other cardiovascular diseases

    Family history of cardiovascular disease NOS

V17.5 Asthma

V17.6 Other chronic respiratory conditions

V17.7 Arthritis

✓5ᵗʰ **V17.8 Other musculoskeletal diseases**

V17.81 Osteoporosis

    AHA: 4Q, '05, 95

V17.89 Other musculoskeletal diseases

✓4ᵗʰ **V18 Family history of certain other specific conditions**

V18.0 Diabetes mellitus

    AHA: 1Q, '04, 8

    TIP: Assign for a normal infant born to a diabetic mother who presents with no manifestations of the syndrome.

✓5ᵗʰ **V18.1 Other endocrine and metabolic diseases**

V18.11 Multiple endocrine neoplasia [MEN] syndrome

    AHA: 4Q, '07, 98, 100

V18.19 Other endocrine and metabolic diseases

V18.2 Anemia

V18.3 Other blood disorders

V18.4 Intellectual disabilities

✓5ᵗʰ **V18.5 Digestive disorders**

V18.51 Colonic polyps

    EXCLUDES *family history of malignant neoplasm of gastrointestinal tract (V16.0)*

    AHA: 4Q, '06, 117

    Z83.71 Family history of colonic polyps   I-10

V18.59 Other digestive disorders

✓5ᵗʰ **V18.6 Kidney diseases**

V18.61 Polycystic kidney

V18.69 Other kidney diseases

V18.7 Other genitourinary diseases

V18.8 Infectious and parasitic diseases

V18.9 Genetic disease carrier

    AHA: 4Q, '05, 95

✓4ᵗʰ **V19 Family history of other conditions**

V19.0 Blindness or visual loss

✓5ᵗʰ **V19.1 Other eye disorders**

    AHA: 4Q, '11, 156

V19.11 Glaucoma

V19.19 Other specified eye disorder

V19.2 Deafness or hearing loss

V19.3 Other ear disorders

V19.4 Skin conditions

V19.5 Congenital anomalies

V19.6 Allergic disorders

V19.7 Consanguinity

V19.8 Other condition

Persons Encountering Health Services in Circumstances Related to Reproduction and Development (V20-V29)

✓4ᵗʰ **V20 Health supervision of infant or child**

² **V20.0** Foundling   P

V20.1 Other healthy infant or child receiving care   P

    Medical or nursing care supervision of healthy infant in cases of:
        maternal illness, physical or psychiatric
        socioeconomic adverse condition at home
        too many children at home preventing or interfering with normal care

    AHA: 1Q, '00, 25; 3Q, '89, 14

V20.2 Routine infant or child health check   P

    Developmental testing of infant or child
    Health check for child over 28 days old
    Immunizations appropriate for age
    Routine vision and hearing testing

    Use additional code(s) to identify:
        special screening examination(s) performed (V73.0-V82.9)

    EXCLUDES *health check for child under 29 days old (V20.31-V20.32)*
        newborn health supervision (V20.31-V20.32)
        special screening for developmental handicaps (V79.3)

    AHA: 4Q, '09, 115; 1Q, '09, 15; 1Q, '04, 15

✓5ᵗʰ **V20.3 Newborn health supervision**

    Health check for child under 29 days old

    EXCLUDES *health check for child over 28 days old (V20.2)*

    AHA: 4Q, '09, 117

V20.31 Health supervision for newborn under 8 days old   N

    Health check for newborn under 8 days old

V20.32 Health supervision for newborn 8 to 28 days old   N

    Health check for newborn 8 to 28 days old
    Newborn weight check

    AHA: 4Q, '09, 102,117

✓4ᵗʰ **V21 Constitutional states in development**

V21.0 Period of rapid growth in childhood

V21.1 Puberty

V21.2 Other adolecsence

✓5ᵗʰ **V21.3 Low birth weight status**

    EXCLUDES *history of perinatal problems*

    AHA: 4Q, '00, 51

    TIP: There are no age restrictions on these V codes after the perinatal period; assign for patients without the initial condition who may continue to manifest the consequences of it.

V21.30 Low birth weight status, unspecified

These V codes may be used as principal diagnosis on Medicare patients.

Additional Digit Required   Unacceptable PDx   Manifestation Code   Hospital Acquired Condition   ▶◀ Revised Text   ● New Code   ▲ Revised Code Title

V Codes

V21.31–V25.2

V21.31 **Low birth weight status, less than 500 grams**

V21.32 **Low birth weight status, 500-999 grams**

V21.33 **Low birth weight status, 1000-1499 grams**

V21.34 **Low birth weight status, 1500-1999 grams**

V21.35 **Low birth weight status, 2000-2500 grams**

V21.8 **Other specified constitutional states in development**

V21.9 **Unspecified constitutional state in development**

☑4th V22 **Normal pregnancy**
  EXCLUDES *pregnancy examination or test, pregnancy unconfirmed (V72.40)*
  AHA: 1Q, '12, 10;4Q, '07, 125
  TIP: Do not assign with any code from chapter 11, "Complications of Pregnancy, Childbirth, and the Puerperium."

V22.0 **Supervision of normal first pregnancy** ♀
  AHA: 3Q, '99, 16
  Z34.00 Encounter suprvisn norm 1 pregnancy uns trimestr   I-10

V22.1 **Supervision of other normal pregnancy** ♀
  AHA: 3Q, '99, 16

V22.2 **Pregnant state, incidental** ♀
  Pregnant state NOS

☑4th V23 **Supervision of high-risk pregnancy**
  AHA: 1Q, '12, 10;1Q, '90, 10

V23.0 **Pregnancy with history of infertility** M ♀

V23.1 **Pregnancy with history of trophoblastic disease** M ♀
  Pregnancy with history of:
    hydatidiform mole
    vesicular mole
  EXCLUDES *that without current pregnancy (V13.1)*

V23.2 **Pregnancy with history of abortion** M ♀
  Pregnancy with history of conditions classifiable to 634-638
  EXCLUDES *recurrent pregnancy loss:*
    care during pregnancy (646.3)
    that without current pregnancy (629.81)

V23.3 **Grand multiparity** M ♀
  EXCLUDES *care in relation to labor and delivery (659.4)*
    that without current pregnancy (V61.5)

☑5th V23.4 **Pregnancy with other poor obstetric history**
  Pregnancy with history of other conditions classifiable to 630-676

  V23.41 **Pregnancy with history of pre-term labor** M ♀
    AHA: 4Q, '02, 79

  V23.42 **Pregnancy with history of ectopic pregnancy** M ♀
    AHA: 4Q, '11, 157

  V23.49 **Pregnancy with other poor obstetric history** M ♀

V23.5 **Pregnancy with other poor reproductive history** M ♀
  Pregnancy with history of stillbirth or neonatal death

V23.7 **Insufficient prenatal care** M ♀
  History of little or no prenatal care

☑5th V23.8 **Other high-risk pregnancy**
  AHA: 4Q, '08, 158; 4Q, '98, 56, 63

  V23.81 **Elderly primigravida** M ♀
    First pregnancy in a woman who will be 35 years of age or older at expected date of delivery
    EXCLUDES *elderly primigravida complicating pregnancy (659.5)*

  V23.82 **Elderly multigravida** M ♀
    Second or more pregnancy in a woman who will be 35 years of age or older at expected date of delivery
    EXCLUDES *elderly multigravida complicating pregnancy (659.6)*
    AHA: 4Q, '11, 133

V23.83 **Young primigravida** M ♀
  First pregnancy in a female less than 16 years old at expected date of delivery
  EXCLUDES *young primigravida complicating pregnancy (659.8)*

V23.84 **Young multigravida** M ♀
  Second or more pregnancy in a female less than 16 years old at expected date of delivery
  EXCLUDES *young multigravida complicating pregnancy (659.8)*

V23.85 **Pregnancy resulting from assisted reproductive technology** A M ♀
  Pregnancy resulting from in vitro fertilization
  AHA: 4Q, '08, 160

V23.86 **Pregnancy with history of in utero procedure during previous pregnancy** M ♀
  EXCLUDES *management of pregnancy affected by in utero procedure during current pregnancy (679.0-679.1)*
  AHA: 4Q, '08, 158, 160

V23.87 **Pregnancy with inconclusive fetal viability** M ♀
  Encounter to determine fetal viability of pregnancy
  AHA: 4Q, '11, 157

V23.89 **Other high-risk pregnancy** M ♀
  AHA: 3Q, '06, 14

V23.9 **Unspecified high-risk pregnancy** M ♀

☑4th V24 **Postpartum care and examination**

[2] V24.0 **Immediately after delivery** M ♀
  Care and observation in uncomplicated cases
  AHA: 3Q, '06, 11

V24.1 **Lactating mother** ♀
  Supervision of lactation
  AHA: ▶3Q, '12, 7◀

V24.2 **Routine postpartum follow-up** ♀

☑4th V25 **Encounter for contraceptive management**
  AHA: 4Q, '92, 24

☑5th V25.0 **General counseling and advice**

  V25.01 **Prescription of oral contraceptives** ♀

  V25.02 **Initiation of other contraceptive measures**
    Fitting of diaphragm
    Prescription of foams, creams, or other agents
    AHA: 3Q, '97, 7

  V25.03 **Encounter for emergency contraceptive counseling and prescription**
    Encounter for postcoital contraceptive counseling and prescription
    AHA: 4Q, '03, 84

  V25.04 **Counseling and instruction in natural family planning to avoid pregnancy**
    AHA: 4Q, '07, 99
    Z30.02 Counsel & instruct natural family plan avoid pg   I-1

  V25.09 **Other**
    Family planning advice

☑5th V25.1 **Encounter for insertion or removal of intrauterine contraceptive device**
  EXCLUDES *encounter for routine checking of intrauterine contraceptive device (V25.42)*
  AHA: 4Q, '10, 109

  V25.11 **Encounter for insertion of intrauterine contraceptive device**

  V25.12 **Encounter for removal of intrauterine contraceptive device**

  V25.13 **Encounter for removal and reinsertion of intrauterine contraceptive device**
    Encounter for replacement of intrauterine contraceptive device

[2] V25.2 **Sterilization**
  Admission for interruption of fallopian tubes or vas deferens

---

[2] These V codes may be used as principal diagnosis on Medicare patients.

N Newborn Age: 0   P Pediatric Age: 0-17   M Maternity Age: 12-55   A Adult Age: 15-124   MCC Major CC Condition   CC CC Condition   HIV HIV Related D

358 – Volume 1 · February 2013   2014 ICD-9-CM

² **V25.3 Menstrual extraction** ♀
Menstrual regulation

V25.4 Surveillance of previously prescribed contraceptive methods
Checking, reinsertion, or removal of contraceptive device
Repeat prescription for contraceptive method
Routine examination in connection with contraceptive maintenance

V25.40 Contraceptive surveillance, unspecified

V25.41 Contraceptive pill ♀

V25.42 Intrauterine contraceptive device ♀
Checking of intrauterine device
EXCLUDES *insertion or removal of intrauterine contraceptive device (V25.11-V25.13)*
presence of intrauterine contraceptive device as incidental finding (V45.51)
AHA: 4Q, '10, 109-110;

V25.43 Implantable subdermal contraceptive ♀

V25.49 Other contraceptive method
AHA: 3Q, '97, 7

V25.5 Insertion of implantable subdermal contraceptive ♀
AHA: 3Q, '92, 9

V25.8 Other specified contraceptive management
Postvasectomy sperm count
EXCLUDES *sperm count following sterilization reversal (V26.22)*
sperm count for fertility testing (V26.21)
AHA: 3Q, '96, 9

V25.9 Unspecified contraceptive management

V26 Procreative management

² **V26.0 Tuboplasty or vasoplasty after previous sterilization**
AHA: 2Q, '95, 10
TIP: Assign for encounters for tubal ligation or vasectomy reversal procedures.

V26.1 Artificial insemination ♀

V26.2 Investigation and testing
EXCLUDES *postvasectomy sperm count (V25.8)*
AHA: 4Q, '00, 56

V26.21 Fertility testing
Fallopian insufflation
Sperm count for fertility testing
EXCLUDES *genetic counseling and testing (V26.31-V26.39)*

V26.22 Aftercare following sterilization reversal
Fallopian insufflation following sterilization reversal
Sperm count following sterilization reversal

V26.29 Other investigation and testing
AHA: 2Q, '96, 9; N-D, '85, 15

V26.3 Genetic counseling and testing
EXCLUDES *fertility testing (V26.21)*
nonprocreative genetic screening (V82.71, V82.79)
AHA: 4Q, '05, 96

V26.31 Testing of female for genetic disease carrier status ♀
AHA: 4Q, '06, 117

V26.32 Other genetic testing of female ♀
Use additional code to identify recurrent pregnancy loss (629.81, 646.3)
AHA: 4Q, '06, 117
Z31.438 Encounter oth genetic test female procreative mngmnt I-10

V26.33 Genetic counseling

V26.34 Testing of male for genetic disease carrier status ♂
AHA: 4Q, '06, 117

V26.35 Encounter for testing of male partner of female with recurrent pregnancy loss ♂
AHA: 4Q, '06, 117

V26.39 Other genetic testing of male ♂
AHA: 4Q, '06, 117

V26.4 General counseling and advice

V26.41 Procreative counseling and advice using natural family planning
AHA: 4Q, '07, 99

V26.42 Encounter for fertility preservation counseling
Encounter for fertility preservation counseling prior to cancer therapy
Encounter for fertility preservation counseling prior to surgical removal of gonads
AHA: 4Q, '09, 117

V26.49 Other procreative management, counseling and advice

V26.5 Sterilization status

V26.51 Tubal ligation status ♀
EXCLUDES *infertility not due to previous tubal ligation (628.0-628.9)*
Z98.51 Tubal ligation status I-10

V26.52 Vasectomy status ♂

V26.8 Other specified procreative management

V26.81 Encounter for assisted reproductive fertility procedure cycle ♀
Patient undergoing in vitro fertilization cycle
Use additional code to identify the type of infertility
EXCLUDES *pre-cycle diagnosis and testing — code to reason for encounter*
AHA: 4Q, '07, 99

V26.82 Encounter for fertility preservation procedure
Encounter for fertility preservation procedure prior to cancer therapy
Encounter for fertility preservation procedure prior to surgical removal of gonads
AHA: 4Q, '09, 117

V26.89 Other specified procreative management

V26.9 Unspecified procreative management

V27 Outcome of delivery
NOTE This category is intended for the coding of the outcome of delivery on the mother's record.
AHA: 2Q, '91, 16
TIP: Assign on the maternal chart for every admission during which a delivery occurs.

V27.0 Single liveborn M ♀
AHA: 4Q, '11, 133; 4Q, '08, 192; 4Q, '05, 81; 2Q, '03, 9; 2Q, '02, 10; 1Q, '01, 10; 3Q, '00, 5; 4Q, '98, 77; 4Q, '95, 59; 1Q, '92, 9
Z37.0 Single live birth I-10

V27.1 Single stillborn M ♀

V27.2 Twins, both liveborn M ♀
Z37.2 Twins both liveborn I-10

V27.3 Twins, one liveborn and one stillborn M ♀

V27.4 Twins, both stillborn M ♀

V27.5 Other multiple birth, all liveborn M ♀

V27.6 Other multiple birth, some liveborn M ♀

V27.7 Other multiple birth, all stillborn M ♀

V27.9 Unspecified outcome of delivery M ♀
Single birth
Multiple birth } outcome to infant unspecified

V28 Encounter for antenatal screening of mother
EXCLUDES *abnormal findings on screening — code to findings*
routine prenatal care (V22.0-V23.9)
suspected fetal conditions affecting management of pregnancy (655.00-655.93, 656.00-656.93, 657.00-657.03, 658.00, 658.93)
suspected fetal conditions not found (V89.01-V89.09)
AHA: 4Q, '06, 117; 1Q, '04, 11

V28.0 Screening for chromosomal anomalies by amniocentesis M ♀

These V codes may be used as principal diagnosis on Medicare patients.

Additional Digit Required   Unacceptable PDx   Manifestation Code   Hospital Acquired Condition   ►◄ Revised Text   ● New Code   ▲ Revised Code Title

V Codes

V28.1–V42.0

V28.1 Screening for raised alpha-fetoprotein levels in amniotic fluid   M ♀

V28.2 Other screening based on amniocentesis   M ♀

V28.3 Encounter for routine screening for malformation using ultrasonics   ♀

    Encounter for routine fetal ultrasound NOS

    EXCLUDES *encounter for fetal anatomic survey (V28.81)*
      genetic counseling and testing (V26.31-V26.39)

V28.4 Screening for fetal growth retardation using ultrasonics   ♀

V28.5 Screening for isoimmunization   ♀

V28.6 Screening for Streptococcus B   M ♀
    AHA: 4Q, '97, 46

√5ᵗʰ **V28.8** Other specified antenatal screening
    AHA: 4Q, '08, 159; 3Q, '99, 16

    V28.81 Encounter for fetal anatomic survey   M ♀

    V28.82 Encounter for screening for risk of pre-term labor   M ♀

    V28.89 Other specified antenatal screening   M ♀
      Chorionic villus sampling
      Genomic screening
      Nuchal translucency testing
      Proteomic screening

V28.9 Unspecified antenatal screening   ♀

√4ᵗʰ **V29** Observation and evaluation of newborns and infants for suspected condition not found

    NOTE This category is to be used for newborns, within the neonatal period, (the first 28 days of life) who are suspected of having an abnormal condition resulting from exposure from the mother or the birth process, but without signs or symptoms, and, which after examination and observation, is found not to exist.

    EXCLUDES *suspected fetal conditions not found (V89.01-V89.09)*
    AHA: 1Q, '00, 25; 4Q, '94, 47; 1Q, '94, 9; 4Q, '92, 21
    TIP: Do not assign if the infant shows any signs or symptoms.

² **V29.0** Observation for suspected infectious condition   N
    AHA: 1Q, '01, 10

² **V29.1** Observation for suspected neurological condition   N

² **V29.2** Observation for suspected respiratory condition   N

V29.3 Observation for suspected genetic or metabolic condition   N
    AHA: 2Q, '05, 21; 4Q, '98, 59, 68

² **V29.8** Observation for other specified suspected condition   N
    AHA: 2Q, '03, 15

V29.9 Observation for unspecified suspected condition   N
    AHA: 1Q, '02, 6

Liveborn Infants According to Type of Birth (V30-V39)

NOTE These categories are intended for the coding of liveborn infants who are consuming health care [e.g., crib or bassinet occupancy].

The following fourth digit subdivisions are for use with categories V30-V39

√5ᵗʰ   0   **Born in hospital**   N
     1   Born before admission to hospital   N
     2   Born outside hospital and not hospitalized

The following two fifth digits are for use with the fourth digit .0, Born in hospital:

     0   delivered without mention of cesarean delivery
     1   delivered by cesarean delivery

AHA: 1Q, '01, 10

³ §√4ᵗʰ **V30** Single liveborn
    AHA: ▶2Q, '12, 17;◀ 2Q, '03, 9; 4Q, '98, 46, 59; 1Q, '94, 9; For code V30.00: ▶3Q, '12, 5;◀ 1Q, '04, 8, 16; 4Q, '03, 68; For code V30.01: 4Q, '09, 101; 4Q, '05, 88; For code V30.10: 3Q, '06, 10
    Z38.00 Single liveborn infant delivered vaginally   I-10

³ §√4ᵗʰ **V31** Twin, mate liveborn
    AHA: 3Q, '92, 10
    Z38.31 Twin liveborn infant delivered by cesarean   I-10

³ §√4ᵗʰ **V32** Twin, mate stillborn

³ §√4ᵗʰ **V33** Twin, unspecified

³ §√4ᵗʰ **V34** Other multiple, mates all liveborn

³ §√4ᵗʰ **V35** Other multiple, mates all stillborn

³ §√4ᵗʰ **V36** Other multiple, mates live and stillborn

³ §√4ᵗʰ **V37** Other multiple, unspecified

⁴ §√4ᵗʰ **V39** Unspecified

Persons with a Condition Influencing their Health Status (V40-V49)

NOTE These categories are intended for use when these conditions are recorded as "diagnoses" or "problems."

TIP: Includes patients with a carrier status or who have sequelae or residual of a past condition or disease, which may affect current or future treatment

√4ᵗʰ **V40** Mental and behavioral problems

V40.0 Problems with learning

V40.1 Problems with communication [including speech]

V40.2 Other mental problems

√5ᵗʰ **V40.3** Other behavioral problems
    AHA: 4Q, '11, 158

    V40.31 *Wandering in diseases classified elsewhere*

      Code first underlying disorder such as:
       Alzheimer's disease (331.0)
       autism or pervasive developmental disorder (299.0-299.9)
       dementia, unspecified, with behavioral disturbance (294.21)
       intellectual disabilities (317-319)

    V40.39 Other specified behavioral problem

V40.9 Unspecified mental or behavioral problem

√4ᵗʰ **V41** Problems with special senses and other special functions

V41.0 Problems with sight

V41.1 Other eye problems

V41.2 Problems with hearing

V41.3 Other ear problems

V41.4 Problems with voice production

V41.5 Problems with smell and taste

V41.6 Problems with swallowing and mastication

V41.7 Problems with sexual function
    EXCLUDES *marital problems (V61.10)*
      psychosexual disorders (302.0-302.9)

V41.8 Other problems with special functions

V41.9 Unspecified problem with special functions

√4ᵗʰ **V42** Organ or tissue replaced by transplant
    INCLUDES *homologous or heterologous (animal) (human) transplant organ status*
    AHA: 3Q, '11, 5; 3Q, '98, 3, 4
    TIP: Do not assign if the patient has a complication of the transplanted organ; the code from subcategory 996.8 provides the information.

V42.0 Kidney   C
    CC Excl: 238.77, 996.80-996.81, 996.87, V42.0, V42.89-V42.9
    AHA: 1Q, '08, 10; 1Q, '03, 10; 3Q, '01, 12
    Z94.0 Kidney transplant status   I-10

---

² These V codes may be used as principal diagnosis on Medicare patients.
³ These codes with a fourth digit of 0 or 1 may be used as a principal diagnosis for Medicare patients
⁴ These codes with a fourth digit of 0 may be used as a principal diagnosis for Medicare patients
§ Requires fourth and fifth digit. See beginning of section V30-V39 for codes and definitions.

N Newborn Age: 0   P Pediatric Age: 0-17   M Maternity Age: 12-55   A Adult Age: 15-124   MCC Major CC Condition   CC CC Condition   HIV HIV Related D

V42.1 Heart `CC`
    CC Excl: 238.77, 996.80, 996.83, 996.87, V42.1, V42.89-V42.9
    AHA: 3Q, '03, 16; 3Q, '01, 13

V42.2 Heart valve

V42.3 Skin

V42.4 Bone

V42.5 Cornea

V42.6 Lung `CC`
    CC Excl: 238.77, 996.80, 996.84, 996.87, V42.6, V42.89-V42.9

V42.7 Liver `CC`
    CC Excl: 238.77, 996.80, 996.82, 996.87, V42.7, V42.89-V42.9
    AHA: 3Q, '11, 5
    Z94.4 Liver transplant status `I-10`

√5ᵗʰ **V42.8 Other specified organ or tissue**
    AHA: 4Q, '98, 64; 4Q, '97, 49

    V42.81 Bone marrow `CC`
      CC Excl: 238.77, 279.50-279.53, 996.80, 996.85, 996.87, V42.9
      AHA: 1Q, '12, 13

    V42.82 Peripheral stem cells `CC`
      CC Excl: 238.77, 996.80, 996.87, V42.9

    V42.83 Pancreas `CC`
      CC Excl: 238.77, 996.80, 996.86-996.87, V42.83, V42.9
      AHA: 1Q, '03, 10; 2Q, '01, 16

    V42.84 Intestines `CC`
      CC Excl: 238.77, 996.80, 996.89, V42.84-V42.9
      AHA: 4Q, '00, 48, 50

    V42.89 Other

V42.9 Unspecified organ or tissue

√4ᵗʰ **V43 Organ or tissue replaced by other means**
    INCLUDES organ or tissue assisted by other means
    replacement of organ by:
      artificial device
      mechanical device
      prosthesis
    EXCLUDES cardiac pacemaker in situ (V45.01)
      fitting and adjustment of prosthetic device (V52.0-V52.9)
      renal dialysis status (V45.11)

V43.0 Eye globe

V43.1 Lens
    Pseudophakos
    AHA: 4Q, '98, 65

√5ᵗʰ **V43.2 Heart**
    AHA: 4Q, '03, 85

    V43.21 Heart assist device `CC`
      CC Excl: 238.77, 996.80, 996.83, 996.87, V42.1, V43.21-V43.22

    V43.22 Fully implantable artificial heart `CC`
      CC Excl: See code: V43.21

V43.3 Heart valve
    AHA: 3Q, '06, 7; 3Q, '02, 13, 14
    TIP: If the status post heart valve replacement information includes "porcine" or mention of other homologous or heterologous tissue, assign instead V42.2.
    Z95.2 Presence of prosthetic heart valve `I-10`

V43.4 Blood vessel

V43.5 Bladder

√5ᵗʰ **V43.6 Joint**
    AHA: 4Q, '05, 91

    V43.60 Unspecified joint

    V43.61 Shoulder

    V43.62 Elbow

    V43.63 Wrist

    V43.64 Hip
      AHA: 1Q, '09, 6; 2Q, '08, 3-5; 3Q, '06, 4, 5; 4Q, '05, 93, 112; 2Q, '04, 15
      Z96.641 Presence of right artificial hip joint `I-10`

    V43.65 Knee
      AHA: 3Q, '06, 5

    V43.66 Ankle

    V43.69 Other

V43.7 Limb

√5ᵗʰ **V43.8 Other organ or tissue**

    V43.81 Larynx
      AHA: 4Q, '95, 55

    V43.82 Breast
      AHA: 4Q, '95, 55
      Z98.82 Breast implant status `I-10`

    V43.83 Artificial skin

    V43.89 Other

√4ᵗʰ **V44 Artificial opening status**
    EXCLUDES artificial openings requiring attention or management (V55.0-V55.9)
    TIP: Do not assign if the patient has a complication of the artificial opening, such as infection or obstruction; assign only the complication code.

V44.0 Tracheostomy
    AHA: 4Q, '03, 103, 107, 111; 1Q, '01, 6

V44.1 Gastrostomy
    AHA: 4Q, '03, 103, 107-108, 110; 1Q, '01, 12; 3Q, '97, 12; 1Q, '93, 26

V44.2 Ileostomy

V44.3 Colostomy
    AHA: 4Q, '03, 110
    Z93.3 Colostomy status `I-10`

V44.4 Other artificial opening of gastrointestinal tract

√5ᵗʰ **V44.5 Cystostomy**

    V44.50 Cystostomy, unspecified

    V44.51 Cutaneous-vesicostomy

    V44.52 Appendico-vesicostomy

    V44.59 Other cystostomy

V44.6 Other artificial opening of urinary tract
    Nephrostomy   Urethrostomy
    Ureterostomy
    AHA: ▶3Q, '12, 11-12◀

V44.7 Artificial vagina

V44.8 Other artificial opening status

V44.9 Unspecified artificial opening status

√4ᵗʰ **V45 Other postprocedural states**
    EXCLUDES aftercare management (V51-V58.9)
      malfunction or other complication — code to condition
    AHA: 4Q, '03, 85

√5ᵗʰ **V45.0 Cardiac device in situ**
    EXCLUDES artificial heart (V43.22)
      heart assist device (V43.21)

    V45.00 Unspecified cardiac device

    V45.01 Cardiac pacemaker
      EXCLUDES cardiac defibrillator with synchronous cardiac pacemaker (V45.02)

    V45.02 Automatic implantable cardiac defibrillator
      With synchronous cardiac pacemaker
      Z95.810 Presence auto implantable cardiac defibrillator `I-10`

    V45.09 Other specified cardiac device
      Carotid sinus pacemaker in situ

√5ᵗʰ **V45.1 Renal dialysis status**
    EXCLUDES admission for dialysis treatment or session (V56.0)
    AHA: 4Q, '08, 157; 1Q, '08, 10; 4Q, '07, 86; 3Q, '07, 9; 4Q, '06, 136; 4Q, '05, 96; 2Q, '03, 7; 2Q, '01, 12, 13

    V45.11 Renal dialysis status
      Hemodialysis status
      Patient requiring intermittent renal dialysis
      Peritoneal dialysis status
      Presence of arterial-venous shunt (for dialysis)
      AHA: 3Q, '11, 15; 4Q, '08, 157, 193
      Z99.2 Dependence on renal dialysis `I-10`

    V45.12 Noncompliance with renal dialysis

Additional Digit Required   Unacceptable PDx   Manifestation Code   Hospital Acquired Condition   ▶◀ Revised Text   ● New Code   ▲ Revised Code Title

2014 ICD-9-CM   February 2013 · Volume 1 — 361

V Codes

V45.2–V46.2

V45.2 Presence of cerebrospinal fluid drainage device
Cerebral ventricle (communicating) shunt, valve, or device in situ
EXCLUDES malfunction (996.2)
AHA: 4Q, '03, 106

V45.3 Intestinal bypass or anastomosis status
EXCLUDES bariatric surgery status (V45.86)
gastric bypass status (V45.86)
obesity surgery status (V45.86)

V45.4 Arthrodesis status
AHA: N-D, '84, 18
TIP: If there is a complication of the fusion graft site that requires refusion or revision, assign instead a code from subcategory 996.4.

√5ᵗʰ **V45.5 Presence of contraceptive device**

V45.51 Intrauterine contraceptive device ♀
EXCLUDES checking of device (V25.42)
complication from device (996.32)
insertion and removal of device (V25.11-V25.13)
Z97.5 Presence of intrauterine contraceptive device   I-10

V45.52 Subdermal contraceptive implant

V45.59 Other

√5ᵗʰ **V45.6 States following surgery of eye and adnexa**
Cataract extraction ⎫
Filtering bleb ⎬ state following eye surgery
Surgical eyelid adhesion ⎭
EXCLUDES aphakia (379.31)
artificial eye globe (V43.0)
AHA: 4Q, '98, 65; 4Q, '97, 49

V45.61 Cataract extraction status
Use additional code for associated artificial lens status (V43.1)

V45.69 Other states following surgery of eye and adnexa
AHA: 2Q, '01, 16; 1Q, '98, 10; 4Q, '97, 19

√5ᵗʰ **V45.7 Acquired absence of organ**
AHA: 4Q, '98, 65; 4Q, '97, 50

[2] **V45.71 Acquired absence of breast and nipple**
EXCLUDES congenital absence of breast and nipple (757.6)
AHA: 4Q, '08, 159; 4Q, '01, 66; 4Q, '97, 50

V45.72 Acquired absence of intestine (large) (small)

V45.73 Acquired absence of kidney

V45.74 Other parts of urinary tract
Bladder
AHA: 4Q, '00, 51

V45.75 Stomach
AHA: 4Q, '00, 51

V45.76 Lung
AHA: 4Q, '00, 51

V45.77 Genital organs
EXCLUDES acquired absence of cervix and uterus (V88.01-V88.03)
female genital mutilation status (629.20-629.29)
AHA: 1Q, '03, 13, 14; 4Q, '00, 51

V45.78 Eye
AHA: 4Q, '00, 51

V45.79 Other acquired absence of organ
EXCLUDES acquired absence of pancreas (V88.11-V88.12)
AHA: 4Q, '00, 51

√5ᵗʰ **V45.8 Other postprocedural status**

V45.81 Aortocoronary bypass status
AHA: 4Q, '11, 153; 4Q, '10, 131; 4Q, '03, 105; 3Q, '01, 15; 3Q, '97, 16

V45.82 Percutaneous transluminal coronary angioplasty status

V45.83 Breast implant removal status
AHA: 4Q, '95, 55

V45.84 Dental restoration status
Dental crowns status
Dental fillings status
AHA: 4Q, '01, 54

V45.85 Insulin pump status

V45.86 Bariatric surgery status
Gastric banding status
Gastric bypass status for obesity
Obesity surgery status
EXCLUDES bariatric surgery status complicating pregnancy, childbirth or the puerperium (649.2)
intestinal bypass or anastomosis status (V45.3)
AHA: 2Q, '09, 10; 4Q, '06, 118
Z98.84 Bariatric surgery status   I-10

V45.87 Transplanted organ removal status
Transplanted organ previously removed due to complication, failure, rejection or infection
EXCLUDES encounter for removal of transplanted organ — code to complication of transplanted organ (996.80-996.89)
AHA: 4Q, '08, 157

V45.88 Status post administration of tPA (rtPA) in a different facility within the last 24 hours prior to admission to current facility
Code first condition requiring tPA administration, such as:
acute cerebral infarction (433.0-433.9 with fifth-digit 1, 434.0-434.9 with fifth digit 1)
acute myocardial infarction (410.00-410.92)
AHA: 4Q, '08, 157
TIP: Assign only on receiving facility record; assign even if the patient is still receiving tPA at the time of transfer.

V45.89 Other
Presence of neuropacemaker or other electronic device
EXCLUDES artificial heart valve in situ (V43.3)
vascular prosthesis in situ (V43.4)
AHA: 1Q, '95, 11

√4ᵗʰ **V46 Other dependence on machines and devices**

V46.0 Aspirator

√5ᵗʰ **V46.1 Respirator [Ventilator]**
Iron lung
AHA: 4Q, '05, 96; 4Q, '03, 103; 1Q, '01, 12; J-F, '87, 7 3

[2] **V46.11 Dependence on respirator, status** CC
CC Excl: V46.0-V46.2, V46.8-V46.9
AHA: 4Q, '04, 100
Z99.11 Dependence on respirator ventilator status   I-10

[2] **V46.12 Encounter for respirator dependence during power failure** CC
CC Excl: See code V46.11
AHA: 4Q, '04, 100

[2] **V46.13 Encounter for weaning from respirator [ventilator]** CC
CC Excl: See code V46.11

[2] **V46.14 Mechanical complication of respirator [ventilator]** CC
Mechanical failure of respirator [ventilator]
CC Excl: See code V46.11

V46.2 Supplemental oxygen
Long-term oxygen therapy
AHA: 4Q, '03, 108; 4Q, '02, 79

---

[2] These V codes may be used as principal diagnosis on Medicare patients.

V46.3 Wheelchair dependence
Wheelchair confinement status
Code first cause of dependence, such as:
   muscular dystrophy (359.1)
   obesity (278.00-278.03)
AHA: 4Q, '08, 157

V46.8 Other enabling machines
Hyperbaric chamber
Possum [Patient-Operated-Selector-Mechanism]
EXCLUDES *cardiac pacemaker (V45.0)*
           kidney dialysis machine (V45.11)

V46.9 Unspecified machine dependence
AHA: 4Q, '06, 117

✓4ᵗʰ V47 Other problems with internal organs

V47.0 Deficiencies of internal organs

V47.1 Mechanical and motor problems with internal organs

V47.2 Other cardiorespiratory problems
Cardiovascular exercise intolerance with pain (with):
   at rest
   less than ordinary activity
   ordinary activity

V47.3 Other digestive problems

V47.4 Other urinary problems

V47.5 Other genital problems

V47.9 Unspecified

✓4ᵗʰ V48 Problems with head, neck, and trunk

V48.0 Deficiencies of head
EXCLUDES *deficiencies of ears, eyelids, and nose (V48.8)*

V48.1 Deficiencies of neck and trunk

V48.2 Mechanical and motor problems with head

V48.3 Mechanical and motor problems with neck and trunk

V48.4 Sensory problem with head

V48.5 Sensory problem with neck and trunk

V48.6 Disfigurements of head

V48.7 Disfigurements of neck and trunk

V48.8 Other problems with head, neck, and trunk

V48.9 Unspecified problem with head, neck, or trunk

✓4ᵗʰ V49 Other conditions influencing health status

V49.0 Deficiencies of limbs

V49.1 Mechanical problems with limbs

V49.2 Motor problems with limbs

V49.3 Sensory problems with limbs

V49.4 Disfigurements of limbs

V49.5 Other problems of limbs

✓5ᵗʰ V49.6 Upper limb amputation status
AHA: 4Q, '05, 94; 4Q, '98; 42; 4Q, '94, 39

  V49.60 Unspecified level
     Z89.201 Acquired absence of right upper limb uns level **I-10**

  V49.61 Thumb

  V49.62 Other finger(s)
     AHA: 2Q, '05, 7

  V49.63 Hand

  V49.64 Wrist
     Disarticulation of wrist

  V49.65 Below elbow

  V49.66 Above elbow
     Disarticulation of elbow

  V49.67 Shoulder
     Disarticulation of shoulder

✓5ᵗʰ V49.7 Lower limb amputation status
AHA: 3Q, '06, 5; 4Q, '05, 94; 4Q, '98, 42; 4Q, '94, 39

  V49.70 Unspecified level

  V49.71 Great toe

  V49.72 Other toe(s)

  V49.73 Foot

  V49.74 Ankle
     Disarticulation of ankle

  V49.75 Below knee
     Z89.512 Acq absence of lt leg below knee **I-10**

  V49.76 Above knee
     Disarticulation of knee
     AHA: 2Q, '05, 14

  V49.77 Hip
     Disarticulation of hip

✓5ᵗʰ V49.8 Other specified conditions influencing health status
AHA: 4Q, '00, 51

  V49.81 Asymptomatic postmenopausal status (age-related) (natural) **A ♀**
     EXCLUDES *menopausal and premenopausal disorder (627.0-627.9)*
             postsurgical menopause (256.2)
             premature menopause (256.31)
             symptomatic menopause (627.0-627.9)
     AHA: 4Q, '09,106; 4Q, '02, 79; 4Q, '00, 54

  V49.82 Dental sealant status
     AHA: 4Q, '01, 54

  V49.83 Awaiting organ transplant status

  V49.84 Bed confinement status
     AHA: 4Q, '05, 96

  V49.85 Dual sensory impairment
     Blindness with deafness
     Combined visual hearing impairment
     Code first:
       hearing impairment (389.00-389.9)
       visual impairment (369.00-369.9)
     AHA: 4Q, '07, 100

  V49.86 Do not resuscitate status
     AHA: 1Q, '12, 14; 4Q, '10, 108
     Z66 Do not resuscitate **I-10**

  V49.87 Physical restraints status
     AHA: 4Q, '10, 108-109
     EXCLUDES *restraint due to a procedure – omit code*

  V49.89 Other specified conditions influencing health status
     AHA: 4Q, '05, 94

V49.9 Unspecified

Persons Encountering Health Services for Specific Procedures and Aftercare (V50-V59)

NOTE Categories V51-V59 are intended for use to indicate a reason for care in patients who may have already been treated for some disease or injury not now present, or who are receiving care to consolidate the treatment, to deal with residual states, or to prevent recurrence.

EXCLUDES *follow-up examination for medical surveillance following treatment (V67.0-V67.9)*

✓4ᵗʰ V50 Elective surgery for purposes other than remedying health states

  ² V50.0 Hair transplant

  ² V50.1 Other plastic surgery for unacceptable cosmetic appearance
     Breast augmentation or reduction
     Face-lift
     EXCLUDES *encounter for breast reduction (611.1)*
             plastic surgery following healed injury or operation (V51.0-V51.8)

These V codes may be used as principal diagnosis on Medicare patients.

4ᵗʰ ⁵ᵗʰ Additional Digit Required   Unacceptable PDx   Manifestation Code   Hospital Acquired Condition   ►◄ Revised Text   ● New Code   ▲ Revised Code Title

2014 ICD-9-CM   Volume 1 – 363

[2] **V50.2 Routine or ritual circumcision** ♂
Circumcision in the absence of significant medical indication

V50.3 Ear piercing

✓5th **V50.4 Prophylactic organ removal**
EXCLUDES *organ donations (V59.0-V59.9)*
therapeutic organ removal — code to condition
AHA: 4Q, '94, 44
TIP: Assign an additional code, such as one from category V16 Family history of malignant neoplasm, to indicate the reason for the prophylactic organ removal.

[2] **V50.41 Breast**
AHA: 2Q, '11, 12; 4Q, '04, 107

[2] **V50.42 Ovary** ♀
AHA: 3Q, '09, 5

[2] **V50.49 Other**
AHA: 3Q, '09, 5

V50.8 Other
Z40.8 Encounter for other prophylactic surgery [I-10]

V50.9 Unspecified

✓4th **V51 Aftercare involving the use of plastic surgery**
Plastic surgery following healed injury or operation
EXCLUDES *cosmetic plastic surgery (V50.1)*
plastic surgery as treatment for current condtion or injury — code to condition or injury
repair of scarred tissue — code to scar
AHA: 4Q, '08, 159

[2] **V51.0 Encounter for breast reconstruction following mastectomy** [A]
EXCLUDES *deformity and disproportion of reconstructed breast (612.0-612.1)*
AHA: 4Q, '08, 159-160

[2] **V51.8 Other aftercare involving the use of plastic surgery**

✓4th **V52 Fitting and adjustment of prosthetic device and implant**
INCLUDES removal of device
EXCLUDES *malfunction or complication of prosthetic device (996.0-996.7)*
status only, without need for care (V43.0-V43.8)
AHA: 4Q, '05, 94; 4Q, '95, 55 ; 1Q, '90, 7

[2] **V52.0 Artificial arm (complete) (partial)**

[2] **V52.1 Artificial leg (complete) (partial)**

[2] **V52.2 Artificial eye**

[2] **V52.3 Dental prosthetic device**

[2] **V52.4 Breast prosthesis and implant** ♀
Elective implant exchange (different material) (different size)
Removal of tissue expander without synchronous insertion of permanent implant
EXCLUDES *admission for initial breast implant insertion for breast augmentation (V50.1)*
complications of breast implant (996.54, 996.69, 996.79)
encounter for breast reconstruction following mastectomy (V51.0)
AHA: 4Q, '95, 80, 81

[2] **V52.8 Other specified prosthetic device**
AHA: 2Q, '02, 12, 16

V52.9 Unspecified prosthetic device

✓4th **V53 Fitting and adjustment of other device**
INCLUDES removal of device
replacement of device
EXCLUDES *status only, without need for care (V45.0-V45.8)*

✓5th **V53.0 Devices related to nervous system and special senses**
AHA: 4Q, '98, 66; 4Q, '97, 51

[2] **V53.01 Fitting and adjustment of cerebral ventricular (communicating) shunt**
AHA: 4Q, '97, 51

[2] **V53.02 Neuropacemaker (brain) (peripheral nerve) (spinal cord)**

[2] **V53.09 Fitting and adjustment of other devices related to nervous system and special senses**
Auditory substitution device
Visual substitution device
AHA: 2Q, '99, 4

V53.1 Spectacles and contact lenses

V53.2 Hearing aid

✓5th **V53.3 Cardiac device**
Reprogramming
AHA: 3Q, '92, 3; 1Q, '90, 7; M-J, '87, 8 ; N-D, '84, 18
TIP: Assign for cardiac device replacement when the device has reached normal end-of-life parameters.

V53.31 Cardiac pacemaker
EXCLUDES *automatic implantable cardiac defibrillator with synchronous cardiac pacemaker (V53.32)*
mechanical complication of cardiac pacemaker (996.01)
AHA: 3Q, '10, 9; 1Q, '02, 3

V53.32 Automatic implantable cardiac defibrillator
With synchronous cardiac pacemaker
AHA: 3Q, '05, 8

V53.39 Other cardiac device
AHA: 4Q, '10, 124,125; 2Q, '08, 9; 1Q, '07, 20

V53.4 Orthodontic devices

✓5th **V53.5 Other gastrointestinal appliance and device**
EXCLUDES *colostomy (V55.3)*
ileostomy (V55.2)
other artificial opening of digestive tract (V55.4)
AHA: 4Q, '09, 116

V53.50 Fitting and adjustment of intestinal appliance and device

V53.51 Fitting and adjustment of gastric lap band

V53.59 Fitting and adjustment of other gastrointestinal appliance and device

V53.6 Urinary devices
Urinary catheter
EXCLUDES *cystostomy (V55.5)*
nephrostomy (V55.6)
ureterostomy (V55.6)
urethrostomy (V55.6)

V53.7 Orthopedic devices
Orthopedic: Orthopedic:
brace   corset
cast   shoes
EXCLUDES *other orthopedic aftercare (V54)*

V53.8 Wheelchair

✓5th **V53.9 Other and unspecified device**
AHA: 2Q, '03, 6

V53.90 Unspecified device

V53.91 Fitting and adjustment of insulin pump
Insulin pump titration

V53.99 Other device
AHA: 2Q, '09, 10

✓4th **V54 Other orthopedic aftercare**
EXCLUDES *fitting and adjustment of orthopedic devices (V53.7)*
malfunction of internal orthopedic device (996.40-996.49)
other complication of nonmechanical nature (996.60-996.79)
AHA: 4Q, '08, 158; 1Q, '07, 3-4; 3Q, '95, 3

✓5th **V54.0 Aftercare involving internal fixation device**
EXCLUDES *malfunction of internal orthopedic device (996.40-996.49)*
other complication of nonmechanical nature (996.60-996.79)
removal of external fixation device (V54.89)
AHA: 4Q, '03, 87

[2] **V54.01 Encounter for removal of internal fixation device**

---

[2] These V codes may be used as principal diagnosis on Medicare patients.

[N] Newborn Age: 0   [P] Pediatric Age: 0-17   [M] Maternity Age: 12-55   [A] Adult Age: 15-124   [MCC] Major CC Condition   [CC] CC Condition   [HIV] HIV Related Dx

364 – Volume 1   2014 ICD-9-CM

V Codes

² **V54.02 Encounter for lengthening/adjustment of growth rod**

² **V54.09 Other aftercare involving internal fixation device**

✓5ᵗʰ **V54.1 Aftercare for healing traumatic fracture**

     EXCLUDES   *aftercare following joint replacement (V54.81)*
                  aftercare for amputation stump (V54.89)

     AHA: 4Q, '02, 80

     TIP: Assign for follow-up and treatment during the healing phase of the fracture; an aftercare code should be used for all subsequent encounters after the initial encounter for care of a fracture.

² **V54.10 Aftercare for healing traumatic fracture of arm, unspecified**

² **V54.11 Aftercare for healing traumatic fracture of upper arm**

² **V54.12 Aftercare for healing traumatic fracture of lower arm**

     AHA: 1Q, '07, 7

² **V54.13 Aftercare for healing traumatic fracture of hip**

     AHA: 1Q, '09, 6; 4Q, '03, 103, 105; 2Q, '03, 16

² **V54.14 Aftercare for healing traumatic fracture of leg, unspecified**

² **V54.15 Aftercare for healing traumatic fracture of upper leg**

     EXCLUDES   *aftercare for healing traumatic fracture of hip (V54.13)*

     AHA: 3Q, '06, 6

² **V54.16 Aftercare for healing traumatic fracture of lower leg**

² **V54.17 Aftercare for healing traumatic fracture of vertebrae**

² **V54.19 Aftercare for healing traumatic fracture of other bone**

     AHA: 1Q, '05, 13; 4Q, '02, 80

✓5ᵗʰ **V54.2 Aftercare for healing pathologic fracture**

     EXCLUDES   *aftercare following joint replacement (V54.81)*

     AHA: 4Q, '02, 80

² **V54.20 Aftercare for healing pathologic fracture of arm, unspecified**

² **V54.21 Aftercare for healing pathologic fracture of upper arm**

² **V54.22 Aftercare for healing pathologic fracture of lower arm**

² **V54.23 Aftercare for healing pathologic fracture of hip**

² **V54.24 Aftercare for healing pathologic fracture of leg, unspecified**

² **V54.25 Aftercare for healing pathologic fracture of upper leg**

     EXCLUDES   *aftercare for healing pathologic fracture of hip (V54.23)*

² **V54.26 Aftercare for healing pathologic fracture of lower leg**

² **V54.27 Aftercare for healing pathologic fracture of vertebrae**

     AHA: 1Q, '07, 6; 4Q, '03, 108

² **V54.29 Aftercare for healing pathologic fracture of other bone**

     AHA: 4Q, '02, 80

✓5ᵗʰ **V54.8 Other orthopedic aftercare**

     AHA: 3Q, '01, 19; 4Q, '99, 5

² **V54.81 Aftercare following joint replacement**

     Use additional code to identify joint replacement site (V43.60-V43.69)

     AHA: 1Q, '11, 9; 1Q, '09, 6; 3Q, '06, 4; 2Q, '04, 15; 4Q, '02, 80

² **V54.82 Aftercare following explantation of joint prosthesis**

     Aftercare following explantation of joint prosthesis, staged procedure

     Encounter for joint prosthesis insertion following prior explantation of joint prosthesis

     AHA: 4Q, '11, 156

     TIP: Assign also a code from subcategory V88.2 to identify the specific joint.

² **V54.89 Other orthopedic aftercare**

     Aftercare for healing fracture NOS

V54.9 Unspecified orthopedic aftercare

✓4ᵗʰ **V55 Attention to artificial openings**

     INCLUDES   adjustment or repositioning of catheter
                  closure
                  passage of sounds or bougies
                  reforming
                  removal or replacement of catheter
                  toilet or cleansing

     EXCLUDES   *complications of external stoma (519.00-519.09, 569.60-569.69, 596.81-596.83, 997.49)*
                  status only, without need for care (V44.0-V44.9)

² **V55.0 Tracheostomy**

² **V55.1 Gastrostomy**   CC

     CC Excl: V55.1

     AHA: 4Q, '99, 9; 3Q, '97, 7, 8; 1Q, '96, 14; 3Q, '95, 13

     TIP: Assign for gastrostomy or PEG tube that has been dislodged or clogged, for which simple irrigation or replacement is performed.

² **V55.2 Ileostomy**

² **V55.3 Colostomy**

     AHA: 1Q, '09, 5; 2Q, '05, 4; 3Q, '97, 9

     Z43.3 Encounter for attention to colostomy   I-10

² **V55.4 Other artificial opening of digestive tract**

     AHA: 2Q, '05, 14; 1Q, '03, 10

² **V55.5 Cystostomy**

² **V55.6 Other artificial opening of urinary tract**

     Nephrostomy   Urethrostomy
     Ureterostomy

² **V55.7 Artificial vagina**

² **V55.8 Other specified artificial opening**

V55.9 Unspecified artificial opening

✓4ᵗʰ **V56 Encounter for dialysis and dialysis catheter care**

     Use additional code to identify the associated condition

     EXCLUDES   *dialysis preparation — code to condition*

     AHA: 4Q, '98, 66; 1Q, '93, 29

² **V56.0 Extracorporeal dialysis**

     Dialysis (renal) NOS

     EXCLUDES   *dialysis status (V45.11)*

     AHA: 4Q, '05, 79; 1Q, '04, 23; 4Q, '00, 40; 3Q, '98, 6; 2Q, '98, 20

² **V56.1 Fitting and adjustment of extracorporeal dialysis catheter**

     Removal or replacement of catheter
     Toilet or cleansing
     Use additional code for any concurrent extracorporeal dialysis (V56.0)

     AHA: 2Q, '98, 20

V56.2 Fitting and adjustment of peritoneal dialysis catheter

     Use additional code for any concurrent peritoneal dialysis (V56.8)

     AHA: 4Q, '98, 55

✓5ᵗʰ **V56.3 Encounter for adequacy testing for dialysis**

     AHA: 4Q, '00, 55

V56.31 Encounter for adequacy testing for hemodialysis

V56.32 Encounter for adequacy testing for peritoneal dialysis

     Peritoneal equilibration test

² **V56.8 Other dialysis**

     Peritoneal dialysis

     AHA: 4Q, '98, 55

These V codes may be used as principal diagnosis on Medicare patients.

Additional Digit Required   Unacceptable PDx   Manifestation Code   Hospital Acquired Condition   ►◄ Revised Text   ● New Code   ▲ Revised Code Title

☑4ᵗʰ **V57 Care involving use of rehabilitation procedures**
Use additional code to identify underlying condition
AHA: 3Q, '06, 3; 1Q, '02, 19; 3Q, '97, 12; 1Q, '90, 6; S-O, '86, 3
TIP: Assign codes from V57 for episodes of care related to rehabilitation.

V57.0 Breathing exercises

⁵ **V57.1 Other physical therapy**
Therapeutic and remedial exercises, except breathing
AHA: 3Q, '06, 4; 2Q, '04, 15; 4Q, '02, 56; 4Q, '99, 5

☑5ᵗʰ **V57.2 Occupational therapy and vocational rehabilitation**

⁵ **V57.21 Encounter for occupational therapy**
AHA: 4Q, '99, 7

⁵ **V57.22 Encounter for vocational therapy**

⁵ **V57.3 Speech-language therapy**
AHA: 4Q, '97, 36

V57.4 Orthoptic training

☑5ᵗʰ **V57.8 Other specified rehabilitation procedure**

V57.81 Orthotic training
Gait training in the use of artificial limbs

⁵ **V57.89 Other**
Multiple training or therapy
AHA: 4Q, '07, 94; 3Q, '06, 6; 4Q, '03, 105-106, 108; 2Q, '03, 16; 1Q '02, 16; 3Q, '01, 21; 3Q, '97, 11, 12; S-O, '86, 4

⁵ **V57.9 Unspecified rehabilitation procedure**

☑4ᵗʰ **V58 Encounter for other and unspecified procedures and aftercare**
EXCLUDES convalescence and palliative care (V66)
TIP: If a patient is admitted for both radiation therapy and chemotherapy, either code V58.0 or V58.11 may be sequenced as the principal diagnosis.

² **V58.0 Radiotherapy**
Encounter or admission for radiotherapy
EXCLUDES encounter for radioactive implant — code to condition
radioactive iodine therapy — code to condition
AHA: 3Q, '92, 5; 2Q, '90, 7; J-F, '87, 13
Z51.0 Encounter for antineoplastic radiation therapy   I-10

☑5ᵗʰ **V58.1 Encounter for antineoplastic chemotherapy and immunotherapy**
Encounter or admission for chemotherapy
EXCLUDES chemotherapy and immunotherapy for nonneoplastic conditions — code to condition
AHA: 1Q, '04, 13; 2Q, '03, 16; 3Q, '93, 4; 2Q, '92, 6; 2Q, '91, 17; 2Q, '90, 7; S-O, '84, 5

² **V58.11 Encounter for antineoplastic chemotherapy**
AHA: 1Q, '12, 13; 2Q, '11, 4; 4Q, '09, 79; 4Q, '08, 82, 155; 4Q, '07, 104; 2Q, '06, 20-21; 4Q, '05, 98
Z51.11 Encounter for antineoplastic chemotherapy   I-10

² **V58.12 Encounter for antineoplastic immunotherapy**
AHA: 4Q, '05, 98

V58.2 Blood transfusion, without reported diagnosis

☑5ᵗʰ **V58.3 Attention to dressings and sutures**
Change or removal of wound packing
EXCLUDES attention to drains (V58.49)
planned postoperative wound closure (V58.41)
AHA: 2Q, '05, 14

V58.30 Encounter for change or removal of nonsurgical wound dressing
Encounter for change or removal of wound dressing NOS
AHA: 4Q, '09, 150; 4Q, '06, 117

V58.31 Encounter for change or removal of surgical wound dressing
AHA: 4Q, '06, 117
Z48.01 Encounter change/removal surgical wound dress   I-10

V58.32 Encounter for removal of sutures
Encounter for removal of staples
AHA: 4Q, '06, 117
Z48.02 Encounter for removal of sutures   I-10

☑5ᵗʰ **V58.4 Other aftercare following surgery**
NOTE Codes from this subcategory should be used in conjunction with other aftercare codes to fully identify the reason for the aftercare encounter
EXCLUDES aftercare following sterilization reversal surgery (V26.22)
attention to artificial openings (V55.0-V55.9)
orthopedic aftercare (V54.0-V54.9)
AHA: 4Q, '99, 9; N-D, '87, 9

⁶ **V58.41 Encounter for planned postoperative wound closure**
EXCLUDES disruption of operative wound (998.31-998.32)
encounter for dressings and suture aftercare (V58.30-V58.32)
AHA: 4Q, '99, 15

⁶ **V58.42 Aftercare following surgery for neoplasm**
Conditions classifiable to 140-239
AHA: 4Q, '02, 80

⁶ **V58.43 Aftercare following surgery for injury and trauma**
Conditions classifiable to 800-999
EXCLUDES aftercare for healing traumatic fracture (V54.10-V54.19)
AHA: 4Q, '02, 80

⁶ **V58.44 Aftercare following organ transplant**
Use additional code to identify the organ transplanted (V42.0-V42.9)
AHA: 3Q, '11, 5; 4Q, '04, 101

⁶ **V58.49 Other specified aftercare following surgery**
Change or removal of drains
AHA: 1Q, '96, 8, 9

⁶ **V58.5 Orthodontics**
EXCLUDES fitting and adjustment of orthodontic device (V53.4)

☑5ᵗʰ **V58.6 Long-term (current) drug use**
Long-term (current) prophylactic drug use
EXCLUDES drug abuse and dependence complicating pregnancy (648.3-648.4)
drug abuse (305.00-305.93)
drug dependence (304.00-304.93)
hormone replacement therapy (postmenopausal) (V07.4)
use of agents affecting estrogen receptors and estrogen levels (V07.51-V07.59)
AHA: 1Q, '11, 15; 4Q, '08, 159; 4Q, '03, 85; 4Q, '02, 84; 3Q, '02, 15; 4Q, '95, 61
TIP: Do not assign for patients on detoxification drugs or maintenance programs to prevent withdrawal symptoms related to drug dependence; assign instead drug dependence code(s).

⁶ **V58.61 Long-term (current) use of anticoagulants**
EXCLUDES long-term (current) use of aspirin (V58.66)
AHA: 4Q, '08, 135; 3Q, '06, 13; 3Q, '04, 7; 4Q, '03, 108; 3Q, '02, 13-16; 1Q, '02, 15, 16
Z79.01 Long term (current) use of anticoagulants   I-10

V58.62 Long-term (current) use of antibiotics
AHA: 4Q, '98, 59

V58.63 Long-term (current) use of antiplatelets/antithrombotics
EXCLUDES long-term (current) use of aspirin (V58.66)

V58.64 Long-term (current) use of non-steroidal anti-inflammatories (NSAID)
EXCLUDES long-term (current) use of aspirin (V58.66)

V58.65 Long-term (current) use of steroids
Z79.52 Long term (current) use of systemic steroids   I-1

⁶ **V58.66 Long-term (current) use of aspirin**
AHA: 4Q, '04, 102

⁶ **V58.67 Long-term (current) use of insulin**
AHA: 4Q, '04, 55-56, 103
Z79.4 Long term (current) use of insulin   I-1

V58.68 Long term (current) use of bisphosphonates
AHA: 4Q, '11, 157

---

² These V codes may be used as principal diagnosis on Medicare patients.
⁵ Rehabilitation codes acceptable as a principal diagnosis when accompanied by a secondary diagnosis reflecting the condition treated.
⁶ These V codes are acceptable as principal diagnosis and group to DRGs 949-950.

N Newborn Age: 0   P Pediatric Age: 0-17   M Maternity Age: 12-55   A Adult Age: 15-124   MCC Major CC Condition   CC CC Condition   HIV HIV Related D

6 V58.69 Long-term (current) use of other medications
  Other high-risk medications
  Long term current use of methadone for pain control
  Long term current use of opiate analgesic
  EXCLUDES *methadone maintenance NOS (304.00)*
  methadone use NOS (304.00)
  AHA: 2Q, '11, 7; 2Q, '10, 10, 13; 4Q, '09, 83; 3Q, '09, 3;
  4Q, '08, 156; 2Q, '04, 10; 1Q, '04, 13; 1Q, '03, 11; 2Q, '00, 8;
  3Q, '99, 13; 2Q, '99, 17; 1Q, '97, 12; 2Q, '96, 7

√5ᵗʰ V58.7 Aftercare following surgery to specified body systems, not elsewhere classified
  NOTE Codes from this subcategory should be used in conjunction with other aftercare codes to fully identify the reason for the aftercare encounter
  EXCLUDES *aftercare following organ transplant (V58.44)*
  aftercare following surgery for neoplasm (V58.42)
  AHA: 4Q, '03, 104; 4Q, '02, 80

6 V58.71 Aftercare following surgery of the sense organs, NEC
  Conditions classifiable to 360-379, 380-389

6 V58.72 Aftercare following surgery of the nervous system, NEC
  Conditions classifiable to 320-359
  EXCLUDES *aftercare following surgery of the sense organs, NEC (V58.71)*

6 V58.73 Aftercare following surgery of the circulatory system, NEC
  Conditions classifiable to 390-459
  AHA: 2Q, '09, 12; 4Q, '03, 105

6 V58.74 Aftercare following surgery of the respiratory system, NEC
  Conditions classifiable to 460-519

6 V58.75 Aftercare following surgery of the teeth, oral cavity and digestive system, NEC
  Conditions classifiable to 520-579
  AHA: 2Q, '05, 14

6 V58.76 Aftercare following surgery of the genitourinary system, NEC
  Conditions classifiable to 580-629
  EXCLUDES *aftercare following sterilization reversal (V26.22)*
  AHA: 1Q, '05, 11-12

6 V58.77 Aftercare following surgery of the skin and subcutaneous tissue, NEC
  Conditions classifiable to 680-709

6 V58.78 Aftercare following surgery of the musculoskeletal system, NEC
  Conditions classifiable to 710-739
  EXCLUDES *orthopedic aftercare (V54.01-V54.9)*

√5ᵗʰ V58.8 Other specified procedures and aftercare
  AHA: 4Q, '94, 45; 2Q, '94, 8

6 V58.81 Fitting and adjustment of vascular catheter
  Removal or replacement of catheter
  Toilet or cleansing
  EXCLUDES *complication of renal dialysis (996.73)*
  complication of vascular catheter (996.74)
  dialysis preparation — code to condition
  encounter for dialysis (V56.0-V56.8)
  fitting and adjustment of dialysis catheter (V56.1)
  AHA: 2Q, '11, 4

6 V58.82 Fitting and adjustment of nonvascular catheter, NEC
  Removal or replacement of catheter
  Toilet or cleansing
  EXCLUDES *fitting and adjustment of peritoneal dialysis catheter (V56.2)*
  fitting and adjustment of urinary catheter (V53.6)

6 V58.83 Encounter for therapeutic drug monitoring
  Use additional code for any associated long- term (current) drug use (V58.61-V58.69)
  EXCLUDES *blood-drug testing for medicolegal reasons (V70.4)*
  DEF: Drug monitoring: Measurement of the level of a specific drug in the body or measurement of a specific function to assess effectiveness of a drug.
  AHA: 4Q, '08, 156; 2Q, '04, 10; 1Q, '04, 13;4Q, '03, 85; 4Q, '02, 84; 3Q, '02, 13-16

6 V58.89 Other specified aftercare
  AHA: 4Q, '98, 59

6 V58.9 Unspecified aftercare

√4ᵗʰ V59 Donors
  EXCLUDES *examination of potential donor (V70.8)*
  self-donation of organ or tissue — code to condition
  AHA: 4Q, '95, 62; 1Q, '90, 10; N-D, '84, 8
  TIP: Assign only for living donations to other individuals, not for self-donation or for cadaveric donations.

√5ᵗʰ V59.0 Blood

  V59.01 Whole blood

  V59.02 Stem cells

  V59.09 Other

2 V59.1 Skin

2 V59.2 Bone

2 V59.3 Bone marrow

2 V59.4 Kidney

2 V59.5 Cornea

2 V59.6 Liver

√5ᵗʰ V59.7 Egg (oocyte) (ovum)
  AHA: 4Q, '05, 99

  V59.70 Egg (oocyte) (ovum) donor, unspecified   ♀

  V59.71 Egg (oocyte) (ovum) donor, under age 35, anonymous recipient   ♀
    Egg donor, under age 35 NOS

  V59.72 Egg (oocyte) (ovum) donor, under age 35, designated recipient   ♀

  V59.73 Egg (oocyte) (ovum) donor, age 35 and over, anonymous recipient   ♀
    Egg donor, age 35 and over NOS

  V59.74 Egg (oocyte) (ovum) donor, age 35 and over, designated recipient   ♀

2 V59.8 Other specified organ or tissue
  AHA: 3Q, '02, 20

2 V59.9 Unspecified organ or tissue

Persons Encountering Health Services in Other Circumstances (V60-V69)

√4ᵗʰ V60 Housing, household, and economic circumstances

  V60.0 Lack of housing
    Hobos   Transients
    Social migrants   Vagabonds
    Tramps

  V60.1 Inadequate housing
    Lack of heating
    Restriction of space
    Technical defects in home preventing adequate care

  V60.2 Inadequate material resources
    Economic problem
    Poverty NOS

  V60.3 Person living alone

These V codes may be used as principal diagnosis on Medicare patients.
These V codes are acceptable as principal diagnosis and group to DRGs 949-950.

| ✔ Additional Digit Required | Unacceptable PDx | Manifestation Code | Hospital Acquired Condition | ►◄ Revised Text | ● New Code | ▲ Revised Code Title |

V Codes

V60.4–V62.1

V60.4 No other household member able to render care

Person requiring care (has) (is):
    family member too handicapped, ill, or otherwise unsuited to render care
    partner temporarily away from home
    temporarily away from usual place of abode

EXCLUDES *holiday relief care (V60.5)*

V60.5 Holiday relief care

Provision of health care facilities to a person normally cared for at home, to enable relatives to take a vacation

V60.6 Person living in residential institution

Boarding school resident

√5ᵗʰ **V60.8 Other specified housing or economic circumstances**

AHA: 4Q, '09, 118

V60.81 Foster care (status)

V60.89 Other specified housing or economic circumstances

V60.9 Unspecified housing or economic circumstance

√4ᵗʰ **V61 Other family circumstances**

INCLUDES when these circumstances or fear of them, affecting the person directly involved or others, are mentioned as the reason, justified or not, for seeking or receiving medical advice or care

AHA: 1Q, '90, 9

√5ᵗʰ **V61.0 Family disruption**

AHA: 4Q, '08, 160

V61.01 Family disruption due to family member on military deployment

Individual or family affected by other family member being on deployment

EXCLUDES *family disruption due to family member on non-military extended absence from home (V61.08)*

V61.02 Family disruption due to return of family member from military deployment

Individual or family affected by other family member having returned from deployment (current or past conflict)

V61.03 Family disruption due to divorce or legal separation

V61.04 Family disruption due to parent-child estrangement

EXCLUDES *other family estrangement (V61.09)*

V61.05 Family disruption due to child in welfare custody

V61.06 Family disruption due to child in foster care or in care of non-parental family member

V61.07 Family disruption due to death of family member

EXCLUDES *bereavement (V62.82)*

AHA: 4Q, '09, 117

V61.08 Family disruption due to other extended absence of family member

EXCLUDES *family disruption due to family member on military deployment (V61.01)*

AHA: 4Q, '09, 117

V61.09 Other family disruption

Family estrangement NOS

√5ᵗʰ **V61.1 Counseling for marital and partner problems**

EXCLUDES *problems related to:*
    psychosexual disorders (302.0-302.9)
    sexual function (V41.7)

V61.10 Counseling for marital and partner problems, unspecified

Marital conflict
Marital relationship problem
Partner conflict
Partner relationship problem

V61.11 Counseling for victim of spousal and partner abuse

EXCLUDES *encounter for treatment of current injuries due to abuse (995.80-995.85)*

V61.12 Counseling for perpetrator of spousal and partner abuse

√5ᵗʰ **V61.2 Parent-child problems**

V61.20 Counseling for parent-child problem, unspecified

Concern about behavior of child
Parent-child conflict
Parent-child relationship problem

² **V61.21 Counseling for victim of child abuse**

Child battering
Child neglect

EXCLUDES *current injuries due to abuse (995.50-995.59)*

V61.22 Counseling for perpetrator of parental child abuse

EXCLUDES *counseling for non-parental abuser (V62.83)*

V61.23 Counseling for parent-biological child problem

Concern about behavior of biological child
Parent-biological child conflict
Parent-biological child relationship problem

AHA: 4Q, '09, 117

V61.24 Counseling for parent-adopted child problem

Concern about behavior of adopted child
Parent-adopted child conflict
Parent-adopted child relationship problem

AHA: 4Q, '09, 117

V61.25 Counseling for parent (guardian)-foster child problem

Concern about behavior of foster child
Parent (guardian)-foster child conflict
Parent (guardian)-foster child relationship problem

AHA: 4Q, '09, 117

V61.29 Other parent-child problems

AHA: 3Q, '99, 16

V61.3 Problems with aged parents or in-laws

√5ᵗʰ **V61.4 Health problems within family**

V61.41 Alcoholism in family

V61.42 Substance abuse in family

AHA: 4Q, '09, 117

V61.49 Other

Care of   } sick or handicapped person
Presence of } in family or household

V61.5 Multiparity

V61.6 Illegitimacy or illegitimate pregnancy   M

V61.7 Other unwanted pregnancy   M

V61.8 Other specified family circumstances

Problems with family members NEC
Sibling relationship problem

V61.9 Unspecified family circumstance

√4ᵗʰ **V62 Other psychosocial circumstances**

INCLUDES those circumstances or fear of them, affecting the person directly involved or others, mentioned as the reason, justified or not, for seeking or receiving medical advice or care

EXCLUDES *previous psychological trauma (V15.41-V15.49)*

V62.0 Unemployment

EXCLUDES *circumstances when main problem is economic inadequacy or poverty (V60.2)*

V62.1 Adverse effects of work environment

N Newborn Age: 0   P Pediatric Age: 0-17   M Maternity Age: 12-55   A Adult Age: 15-124   MCC Major CC Condition   CC CC Condition   HIV HIV Related

√5ᵗʰ **V62.2 Other occupational circumstances or maladjustment**
AHA: 4Q, '08, 160

V62.21 Personal current military deployment status A
Individual (civilian or military) currently deployed in theater or in support of military war, peacekeeping and humanitarian operations

V62.22 Personal history of return from military deployment A
Individual (civilian or military) with past history of military war, peacekeeping and humanitarian deployment (current or past conflict)

V62.29 Other occupational circumstances or maladjustment A
Career choice problem
Dissatisfaction with employment
Occupational problem

V62.3 Educational circumstances
Academic problem
Dissatisfaction with school environment
Educational handicap

V62.4 Social maladjustment
Acculturation problem
Cultural deprivation
Political, religious, or sex discrimination
Social: isolation   persecution

V62.5 Legal circumstances
Imprisonment   Litigation
Legal investigation   Prosecution

V62.6 Refusal of treatment for reasons of religion or conscience

√5ᵗʰ **V62.8 Other psychological or physical stress, not elsewhere classified**

V62.81 Interpersonal problems, not elsewhere classified
Relational problem NOS

V62.82 Bereavement, uncomplicated
EXCLUDES *family disruption due to death of family member (V61.07)*

V62.83 Counseling for perpetrator of physical/sexual abuse
EXCLUDES *counseling for perpetrator of parental child abuse (V61.22)*
counseling for perpetrator of spousal and partner abuse (V61.12)

² **V62.84 Suicidal ideation** CC
EXCLUDES *suicidal tendencies (300.9)*
DEF: Thoughts of committing suicide; no actual attempt of suicide has been made.
CC Excl: 290.11, 290.3, 293.0
AHA: 4Q, '05, 96
TIP: Assign patients who have not attempted suicide, and who may not be considered a suicide risk, but who have indicated thoughts about suicide.
R45.851 Suicidal ideations I-10

V62.85 Homicidal ideation
AHA: 4Q, '10, 110
R45.850 Homicidal ideations I-10

V62.89 Other
Borderline intellectual functioning
Life circumstance problems
Phase of life problems
Religious or spiritual problem

V62.9 Unspecified psychosocial circumstance

√4ᵗʰ **V63 Unavailability of other medical facilities for care**
AHA: 1Q, '91, 21

V63.0 Residence remote from hospital or other health care facility

V63.1 Medical services in home not available
EXCLUDES *no other household member able to render care (V60.4)*
AHA: 4Q, '01, 67; 1Q, '01, 12

V63.2 Person awaiting admission to adequate facility elsewhere

V63.8 Other specified reasons for unavailability of medical facilities
Person on waiting list undergoing social agency investigation

V63.9 Unspecified reason for unavailability of medical facilities

√4ᵗʰ **V64 Persons encountering health services for specific procedures, not carried out**

√5ᵗʰ **V64.0 Vaccination not carried out**
AHA: 4Q, '05, 99

V64.00 Vaccination not carried out, unspecified reason

V64.01 Vaccination not carried out because of acute illness

V64.02 Vaccination not carried out because of chronic illness or condition

V64.03 Vaccination not carried out because of immune compromised state

V64.04 Vaccination not carried out because of allergy to vaccine or component
Z28.04 Immunization not carried out pt allergy vaccine I-10

V64.05 Vaccination not carried out because of caregiver refusal
Guardian refusal   Parent refusal
EXCLUDES *vaccination not carried out because of caregiver refusal for religious reasons (V64.07)*
AHA: 4Q, '09, 115; 1Q, '07, 12

V64.06 Vaccination not carried out because of patient refusal

V64.07 Vaccination not carried out for religious reasons

V64.08 Vaccination not carried out because patient had disease being vaccinated against

V64.09 Vaccination not carried out for other reason

V64.1 Surgical or other procedure not carried out because of contraindication
TIP: Assign an additional code to indicate the contraindication (reason the surgery or other procedure was canceled).

V64.2 Surgical or other procedure not carried out because of patient's decision
AHA: 2Q, '01, 8

V64.3 Procedure not carried out for other reasons

√5ᵗʰ **V64.4 Closed surgical procedure converted to open procedure**
AHA: 4Q, '03, 87; 4Q, '98, 68; 4Q, '97, 52

V64.41 Laparoscopic surgical procedure converted to open procedure
AHA: 1Q, '11, 14-15

V64.42 Thoracoscopic surgical procedure converted to open procedure

V64.43 Arthroscopic surgical procedure converted to open procedure

√4ᵗʰ **V65 Other persons seeking consultation**

² **V65.0 Healthy person accompanying sick person**
Boarder

√5ᵗʰ **V65.1 Person consulting on behalf of another person**
Advice or treatment for nottending third party
EXCLUDES *concern (normal) about sick person in family (V61.41-V61.49)*
AHA: 4Q, '03, 84

V65.11 Pediatric pre-birth visit for expectant parent(s)
Pre-adoption visit for adoptive parent(s)

V65.19 Other person consulting on behalf of another person

These V codes may be used as principal diagnosis on Medicare patients.

| Additional Digit Required | Unacceptable PDx | Manifestation Code | Hospital Acquired Condition | ►◄ Revised Text | ● New Code | ▲ Revised Code Title |

[2] **V65.2 Person feigning illness**

Malingerer   Peregrinating patient

AHA: 3Q, '99, 20

TIP: Assign for patients engaged in what is documented as "drug- seeking behavior."

V65.3 Dietary surveillance and counseling

Dietary surveillance and counseling (in):

NOS

colitis

diabetes mellitus

food allergies or intolerance

gastritis

hypercholesterolemia

hypoglycemia

obesity

Use additional code to identify Body Mass Index (BMI), if known (V85.0-V85.54)

AHA: 4Q, '05, 96

√5th **V65.4 Other counseling, not elsewhere classified**

Health: Health:

advice   instruction

education

EXCLUDES *counseling (for):*

contraception (V25.40-V25.49)

genetic (V26.31-V26.39)

on behalf of third party (V65.11-V65.19)

procreative management (V26.41-V26.49)

V65.40 Counseling NOS

V65.41 Exercise counseling

V65.42 Counseling on substance use and abuse

Z71.6 Tobacco abuse counseling   I-10

V65.43 Counseling on injury prevention

V65.44 Human immunodeficiency virus [HIV] counseling

V65.45 Counseling on other sexually transmitted diseases

V65.46 Encounter for insulin pump training

Z46.81 Encounter for fitting & adjustment insulin pump   I-10

V65.49 Other specified counseling

AHA: 4Q, '08, 156; 2Q, '00, 8

V65.5 Person with feared complaint in whom no diagnosis was made

Feared condition not demonstrated

Problem was normal state

"Worried well"

V65.8 Other reasons for seeking consultation

EXCLUDES *specified symptoms*

AHA: 3Q, '92, 4

V65.9 Unspecified reason for consultation

√4th **V66 Convalescence and palliative care**

[2] **V66.0 Following surgery**

[2] **V66.1 Following radiotherapy**

[2] **V66.2 Following chemotherapy**

[2] **V66.3 Following psychotherapy and other treatment for mental disorder**

[2] **V66.4 Following treatment of fracture**

V66.5 Following other treatment

[2] **V66.6 Following combined treatment**

V66.7 Encounter for palliative care

End of life care   Terminal care

Hospice care

Code first underlying disease

AHA: ▶3Q, '12, 16;◀ 1Q, '12, 14; 3Q, '10, 18; 3Q, '08, 13; 2Q, '05, 9; 4Q, '03, 107; 1Q, '98, 11; 4Q, '96, 47, 48

TIP: Assign as secondary diagnosis when treatment is focused on management of pain and symptoms in a patient with an incurable disease.

Z51.5 Encounter for palliative care   I-10

V66.9 Unspecified convalescence

AHA: 4Q, '99, 8

√4th **V67 Follow-up examination**

INCLUDES surveillance only following completed treatment

EXCLUDES *surveillance of contraception (V25.40-V25.49)*

AHA: 4Q, '08, 157; 2Q, '03, 5

√5th **V67.0 Following surgery**

AHA: 4Q, '00, 56; 4Q, '98, 69; 4Q, '97, 50; 2Q, '95, 8;1Q, '95, 4; 3Q, '92, 11

[6] **V67.00 Following surgery, unspecified**

[6] **V67.01 Follow-up vaginal pap smear**

Vaginal pap-smear, status-post hysterectomy for malignant condition

Use additional code to identify:

acquired absence of uterus (V88.01-V88.03)

personal history of malignant neoplasm (V10.40-V10.44)

EXCLUDES *vaginal pap smear status-post hysterectom for non-malignant condition (V76.47*

AHA: 4Q, '08, 157

[6] **V67.09 Following other surgery**

EXCLUDES *sperm count following sterilization reversal (V26.22)*

sperm count for fertility testing (V26.21)

AHA: 3Q, '08, 6; 3Q, '03, 16; 3Q, '02, 15

[2] **V67.1 Following radiotherapy**

[2] **V67.2 Following chemotherapy**

Cancer chemotherapy follow-up

[2] **V67.3 Following psychotherapy and other treatment for mental disorder**

[6] **V67.4 Following treatment of healed fracture**

EXCLUDES *current (healing) fracture aftercare (V54.0-V54.9)*

AHA: 1Q, '09, 6; 1Q, '90, 7

√5th **V67.5 Following other treatment**

[2] **V67.51 Following completed treatment with high-risk medications, not elsewhere classified**

EXCLUDES *long-term (current) drug use (V58.61-V58.69)*

AHA: 1Q, '99, 5, 6; 4Q, '95, 61; 1Q, '90, 18

[2] **V67.59 Other**

[2] **V67.6 Following combined treatment**

V67.9 Unspecified follow-up examination

√4th **V68 Encounters for administrative purposes**

√5th **V68.0 Issue of medical certificates**

EXCLUDES *encounter for general medical examination (V70.0-V70.9)*

V68.01 Disability examination

Use additional code(s) to identify specific examination(s), screening and testing performed (V72.0-V82.9)

AHA: 4Q, '07, 101

V68.09 Other issue of medical certificates

V68.1 Issue of repeat prescriptions

Issue of repeat prescription for:

appliance

glasses

medications

EXCLUDES *repeat prescription for contraceptives (V25.41-V25.49)*

V68.2 Request for expert evidence

√5th **V68.8 Other specified administrative purpose**

V68.81 Referral of patient without examination or treatment

V68.89 Other

V68.9 Unspecified administrative purpose

---

[2] These V codes may be used as principal diagnosis on Medicare patients.

[6] These V codes are acceptable as principal diagnosis and group to DRGs 949-950.

N Newborn Age: 0   P Pediatric Age: 0-17   M Maternity Age: 12-55   A Adult Age: 15-124   MCC Major CC Condition   CC CC Condition   HIV HIV Related I

370 – Volume 1 · February 2013   **2014 ICD-9-C**

V Codes

☑4ᵗʰ **V69 Problems related to lifestyle**
AHA: 4Q, '94, 48

V69.0 Lack of physical exercise

V69.1 Inappropriate diet and eating habits
EXCLUDES   *anorexia nervosa (307.1)*
           bulimia (783.6)
           malnutrition and other nutritional deficiencies
              (260-269.9)
           other and unspecified eating disorders
              (307.50-307.59)

V69.2 High-risk sexual behavior

V69.3 Gambling and betting
EXCLUDES   *pathological gambling (312.31)*

² **V69.4 Lack of adequate sleep**
Sleep deprivation
EXCLUDES   *insomnia (780.52)*

V69.5 Behavioral insomnia of childhood   Ⓟ
DEF: Behaviors on the part of the child or caregivers that cause
negative compliance with a child's sleep schedule; results in lack of
adequate sleep.
AHA: 4Q, '05, 99

V69.8 Other problems related to lifestyle
Self-damaging behavior

V69.9 Problem related to lifestyle, unspecified

Persons Without Reported Diagnosis Encountered During Examination and Investigation of Individuals and Populations (V70-V82)

NOTE Nonspecific abnormal findings disclosed at the time of these
examinations are classifiable to categories 790-796.

☑4ᵗʰ **V70 General medical examination**
Use additional code(s) to identify any special screening
examination(s) performed (V73.0-V82.9)

**V70.0 Routine general medical examination at a health
care facility**
Health checkup
EXCLUDES   *health checkup of infant or child over 28 days old*
              (V20.2)
           health supervision of newborn 8 to 28 days old
              (V20.32)
           health supervision of newborn under 8 days old
              (V20.31)
           pre-procedural general physical examination
              (V72.83)

² **V70.1 General psychiatric examination, requested by
the authority**

**V70.2 General psychiatric examination, other and
unspecified**

**V70.3 Other medical examination for administrative
purposes**
General medical examination for:
     admission to old age home
     adoption
     camp
     driving license
     immigration and naturalization
     insurance certification
     marriage
     prison
     school admission
     sports competition
EXCLUDES   *attendance for issue of medical certificates (V68.0)*
           pre-employment screening (V70.5)
AHA: 3Q, '08, 6; 1Q, '90, 6
Z02.6 Encounter for exam for insurance purposes   I-10

² **V70.4 Examination for medicolegal reasons**
Blood-alcohol tests   Paternity testing
Blood-drug tests
EXCLUDES   *examination and observation following:*
           accidents (V71.3, V71.4)
           assault (V71.6)
           rape (V71.5)

² **V70.5 Health examination of defined subpopulations**
Armed forces personnel   Prisoners
Inhabitants of institutions   Prostitutes
Occupational health examinations   Refugees
Pre-employment screening   School children
Preschool children   Students

V70.6 Health examination in population surveys
EXCLUDES   *special screening (V73.0-V82.9)*

² **V70.7 Examination of participant in clinical trial**
Examination of participant or control in clinical research
AHA: 2Q, '06, 5-6; 4Q, '01, 55

V70.8 Other specified general medical examinations
Examination of potential donor of organ or tissue

V70.9 Unspecified general medical examination

☑4ᵗʰ **V71 Observation and evaluation for suspected conditions not found**
INCLUDES   This category is to be used when persons without a
diagnosis are suspected of having an abnormal
condition, without signs or symptoms, which
requires study, but after examination and
observation, is found not to exist. This category is
also for use for administrative and legal observation
status.
EXCLUDES   *suspected maternal and fetal conditions not found*
           (V89.01-V89.09)
AHA: 4Q, '94, 47; 2Q, '90, 5; M-A, '87, 1
TIP: Assign observation codes only as principal/first-listed diagnosis and only
if there is no documentation of any signs or symptoms.

☑5ᵗʰ **V71.0 Observation for suspected mental condition**
² **V71.01 Adult antisocial behavior**   Ⓐ
Dyssocial behavior or gang activity in adult without
manifest psychiatric disorder

² **V71.02 Childhood or adolescent antisocial behavior**
Dyssocial behavior or gang activity in child or
adolescent without manifest psychiatric
disorder

² **V71.09 Other suspected mental condition**

² **V71.1 Observation for suspected malignant neoplasm**

² **V71.2 Observation for suspected tuberculosis**

² **V71.3 Observation following accident at work**

² **V71.4 Observation following other accident**
Examination of individual involved in motor vehicle traffic
accident
AHA: 1Q, '06, 9

² **V71.5 Observation following alleged rape or seduction**
Examination of victim or culprit

² **V71.6 Observation following other inflicted injury**
Examination of victim or culprit

² **V71.7 Observation for suspected cardiovascular disease**
AHA: 1Q, '04, 6; 3Q, '90, 10; S-O, '87, 10

☑5ᵗʰ **V71.8 Observation and evaluation for other specified suspected
conditions**
EXCLUDES   *contact with and (suspected) exposure to*
           (potentially) hazardous substances
           (V15.84-V15.86, V87.0-V87.31)
AHA: 4Q, '00, 54 ; 1Q, '90, 19

² **V71.81 Abuse and neglect**
EXCLUDES   *adult abuse and neglect (995.80-995.85)*
           child abuse and neglect (995.50-995.59)
AHA: 4Q, '00, 55

² **V71.82 Observation and evaluation for suspected exposure
to anthrax**
AHA: 4Q, '02, 70, 85

---

²   These V codes may be used as principal diagnosis on Medicare patients.

☑4ᵗʰ/5ᵗʰ Additional Digit Required   Unacceptable PDx   Manifestation Code   Hospital Acquired Condition   ▶◀ Revised Text   ● New Code   ▲ Revised Code Title

2014 ICD-9-CM   **Volume 1 – 371**

V Codes

V71.83–V74.1

² **V71.83 Observation and evaluation for suspected exposure to other biological agent**
AHA: 4Q, '03, 47

² **V71.89 Other specified suspected conditions**
AHA: 2Q, '11, 4; 3Q, '08, 7; 2Q, '03, 15

V71.9 Observation for unspecified suspected condition
AHA: 1Q, '02, 6

√4ᵗʰ **V72 Special investigations and examinations**
INCLUDES   routine examination of specific system
Use additional code(s) to identify any special screening examination(s) performed (V73.0-V82.9)
EXCLUDES   *general medical examination (V70.0-V70.4)*
general screening examination of defined population groups (V70.5, V70.6, V70.7)
health supervision of newborn 8 to 28 days old (V20.32)
health supervision of newborn under 8 days old (V20.31)
routine examination of infant or child over 28 days old (V20.2)

² **V72.0 Examination of eyes and vision**
AHA: 1Q, '04, 15

√5ᵗʰ **V72.1 Examination of ears and hearing**
AHA: 1Q, '04, 15

V72.11 Encounter for hearing examination following failed hearing screening
AHA: 3Q, '11, 3; 4Q, '06, 118
Z01.110 Encounter hearing exam follow failed hearing scr   I-10

V72.12 Encounter for hearing conservation and treatment
AHA: 4Q, '07, 100

V72.19 Other examination of ears and hearing

V72.2 Dental examination

√5ᵗʰ **V72.3 Gynecological examination**
EXCLUDES   *cervical Papanicolaou smear without general gynecological examination (V76.2)*
routine examination in contraceptive management (V25.40-V25.49)

² **V72.31 Routine gynecological examination**   ♀
General gynecological examination with or without Papanicolaou cervical smear
Pelvic examination (annual) (periodic)
Use additional code to identify:
human papillomavirus (HPV) screening (V73.81)
routine vaginal Papanicolaou smear (V76.47)
AHA: 2Q, '06, 2-3; 4Q, '05, 9

² **V72.32 Encounter for Papanicolaou cervical smear to confirm findings of recent normal smear following initial abnormal smear**   ♀
AHA: 2Q, '06, 4

√5ᵗʰ **V72.4 Pregnancy examination or test**
AHA: 4Q, '05, 98

² **V72.40 Pregnancy examination or test, pregnancy unconfirmed**   ♀
Possible pregnancy, not (yet) confirmed

² **V72.41 Pregnancy examination or test, negative result**   ♀

² **V72.42 Pregnancy examination or test, positive result**   ♀ M

V72.5 Radiological examination, not elsewhere classified
Routine chest x-ray
EXCLUDES   *radiologic examinations as part of pre-procedural testing (V72.81-V72.84)*
AHA: 1Q, '90, 19

√5ᵗʰ **V72.6 Laboratory examination**
Encounters for blood and urine testing
AHA: 4Q, '09, 117-118; 2Q, '06, 4; 1Q, '90, 22

V72.60 Laboratory examination, unspecified

V72.61 Antibody response examination
Immunity status testing
EXCLUDES   *encounter for allergy testing (V72.7)*

V72.62 Laboratory examination ordered as part of a routine general medical examination
Blood tests for routine general physical examination

V72.63 Pre-procedural laboratory examination
Blood tests prior to treatment or procedure
Pre-operative laboratory examination

V72.69 Other laboratory examination

V72.7 Diagnostic skin and sensitization tests
Allergy tests
Skin tests for hypersensitivity
EXCLUDES   *diagnostic skin tests for bacterial diseases (V74.0-V74.9)*

√5ᵗʰ **V72.8 Other specified examinations**
EXCLUDES   *pre-procedural laboratory examinations (V72.63)*

² **V72.81 Pre-operative cardiovascular examination**
Pre-procedural cardiovascular examination
Z01.810 Encounter for preprocedural cardiovascular exam   I-10

² **V72.82 Pre-operative respiratory examination**
Pre-procedural respiratory examination
AHA: 3Q, '96, 14

² **V72.83 Other specified pre-operative examination**
Examination prior to chemotherapy
Other pre-procedural examination
Pre-procedural general physical examination
EXCLUDES   *routine general medical examination (V70.0)*
AHA: 3Q, '96, 14

V72.84 Pre-operative examination, unspecified
Pre-procedural examination, unspecified

V72.85 Other specified examination
AHA: 1Q, '12, 10; 4Q, '05, 96; 1Q, '04, 12

V72.86 Encounter for blood typing

V72.9 Unspecified examination
AHA: 4Q, '06, 117

√4ᵗʰ **V73 Special screening examination for viral and chlamydial diseases**
AHA: 1Q, '04, 11

V73.0 Poliomyelitis

V73.1 Smallpox

V73.2 Measles

V73.3 Rubella

V73.4 Yellow fever

V73.5 Other arthropod-borne viral diseases
Dengue fever   Viral encephalitis:
Hemorrhagic fever   tick-borne
Viral encephalitis:
mosquito-borne

V73.6 Trachoma

√5ᵗʰ **V73.8 Other specified viral and chlamydial diseases**

V73.81 Human papillomavirus [HPV]
AHA: 4Q, '07, 100

V73.88 Other specified chlamydial diseases
AHA: 4Q, '07, 124

V73.89 Other specified viral diseases

√5ᵗʰ **V73.9 Unspecified viral and chlamydial disease**

V73.98 Unspecified chlamydial disease

V73.99 Unspecified viral disease

√4ᵗʰ **V74 Special screening examination for bacterial and spirochetal diseases**
INCLUDES   diagnostic skin tests for these diseases
AHA: 1Q, '04, 11

V74.0 Cholera

V74.1 Pulmonary tuberculosis

---

²   These V codes may be used as principal diagnosis on Medicare patients.

V74.2 Leprosy [Hansen's disease]

V74.3 Diphtheria

V74.4 Bacterial conjunctivitis

V74.5 Venereal disease
Screening for bacterial and spirochetal sexually transmitted diseases
Screening for sexually transmitted diseases NOS
EXCLUDES *special screening for nonbacterial sexually transmitted diseases (V73.81-V73.89, V75.4, V75.8)*
AHA: 4Q, '07, 124

V74.6 Yaws

V74.8 Other specified bacterial and spirochetal diseases
Brucellosis   Tetanus
Leptospirosis   Whooping cough
Plague

V74.9 Unspecified bacterial and spirochetal disease

V75 Special screening examination for other infectious diseases
AHA: 1Q, '04, 11

V75.0 Rickettsial diseases

V75.1 Malaria

V75.2 Leishmaniasis

V75.3 Trypanosomiasis
Chagas' disease
Sleeping sickness

V75.4 Mycotic infections

V75.5 Schistosomiasis

V75.6 Filariasis

V75.7 Intestinal helminthiasis

V75.8 Other specified parasitic infections

V75.9 Unspecified infectious disease

V76 Special screening for malignant neoplasms
AHA: 1Q, '04, 11
TIP: Whenever a screening examination is performed, the screening code is the first-listed code, regardless of the findings or any procedure that is performed as a result of the findings.

V76.0 Respiratory organs

V76.1 Breast
AHA: 4Q, '98, 67

V76.10 Breast screening, unspecified

V76.11 Screening mammogram for high-risk patient ♀
AHA: 2Q, '03, 4

V76.12 Other screening mammogram
AHA: 4Q, '09, 106; 2Q, '06, 10; 2Q, '03, 3-4

V76.19 Other screening breast examination

V76.2 Cervix ♀
Routine cervical Papanicolaou smear
EXCLUDES *special screening for human papillomavirus (V73.81) that as part of a general gynecological examination (V72.31)*

V76.3 Bladder

V76.4 Other sites

V76.41 Rectum

V76.42 Oral cavity

V76.43 Skin

[2] **V76.44 Prostate** ♂
Z12.5 Encounter screening malignant neoplasm prostate [I-10]

V76.45 Testis ♂

V76.46 Ovary ♀
AHA: 4Q, '00, 52

V76.47 Vagina ♀
Vaginal pap smear status-post hysterectomy for non-malignant condition
Use additional code to identify acquired absence of uterus (V88.01-V88.03)
EXCLUDES *vaginal pap smear status-post hysterectomy for malignant condition (V67.01)*
AHA: 4Q, '08, 157; 4Q, '00, 52

V76.49 Other sites
AHA: 1Q, '99, 4

V76.5 Intestine
AHA: 4Q, '00, 52

V76.50 Intestine, unspecified

V76.51 Colon
Screening colonoscopy NOS
EXCLUDES *rectum (V76.41)*
AHA: 4Q, '01, 56
Z12.11 Enc screening malignant neoplasm of colon [I-10]

V76.52 Small intestine

V76.8 Other neoplasm
AHA: 4Q, '00, 52

V76.81 Nervous system

V76.89 Other neoplasm

V76.9 Unspecified

V77 Special screening for endocrine, nutritional, metabolic, and immunity disorders
AHA: 1Q, '04, 11

V77.0 Thyroid disorders

V77.1 Diabetes mellitus

V77.2 Malnutrition

V77.3 Phenylketonuria [PKU]

V77.4 Galactosemia

V77.5 Gout

V77.6 Cystic fibrosis
Screening for mucoviscidosis

V77.7 Other inborn errors of metabolism

V77.8 Obesity

V77.9 Other and unspecified endocrine, nutritional, metabolic, and immunity disorders
AHA: 4Q, '00, 53

V77.91 Screening for lipoid disorders
Screening for cholesterol level
Screening for hypercholesterolemia
Screening for hyperlipidemia

V77.99 Other and unspecified endocrine, nutritional, metabolic, and immunity disorders

V78 Special screening for disorders of blood and blood-forming organs
AHA: 1Q, '04, 11

V78.0 Iron deficiency anemia

V78.1 Other and unspecified deficiency anemia

V78.2 Sickle cell disease or trait

V78.3 Other hemoglobinopathies

V78.8 Other disorders of blood and blood-forming organs

V78.9 Unspecified disorder of blood and blood-forming organs

V79 Special screening for mental disorders and developmental handicaps
AHA: 1Q, '04, 11

V79.0 Depression

V79.1 Alcoholism

V79.2 Intellectual disabilities

---

[2] These V codes may be used as principal diagnosis on Medicare patients.

Additional Digit Required | Unacceptable PDx | Manifestation Code | Hospital Acquired Condition | ►◄ Revised Text | ● New Code | ▲ Revised Code Title

V79.3 Developmental handicaps in early childhood

V79.8 Other specified mental disorders and developmental handicaps

V79.9 Unspecified mental disorder and developmental handicap

√4th V80 Special screening for neurological, eye, and ear diseases
AHA: 1Q, '04, 11

√5th V80.0 Neurological conditions
AHA: 4Q, '09, 116

V80.01 Traumatic brain injury

V80.09 Other neurological conditions

V80.1 Glaucoma

V80.2 Other eye conditions
Screening for: Screening for:
   cataract   senile macular
   congenital anomaly of eye   lesions
EXCLUDES general vision examination (V72.0)

V80.3 Ear diseases
EXCLUDES general hearing examination (V72.11-V72.19)

√4th V81 Special screening for cardiovascular, respiratory, and genitourinary diseases
AHA: 1Q, '04, 11

V81.0 Ischemic heart disease

V81.1 Hypertension

V81.2 Other and unspecified cardiovascular conditions

V81.3 Chronic bronchitis and emphysema

V81.4 Other and unspecified respiratory conditions
EXCLUDES screening for:
   lung neoplasm (V76.0)
   pulmonary tuberculosis (V74.1)

V81.5 Nephropathy
Screening for asymptomatic bacteriuria

V81.6 Other and unspecified genitourinary conditions

√4th V82 Special screening for other conditions
AHA: 1Q, '04, 11

V82.0 Skin conditions

V82.1 Rheumatoid arthritis

V82.2 Other rheumatic disorders

V82.3 Congenital dislocation of hip

V82.4 Maternal postnatal screening for chromosomal anomalies ♀
EXCLUDES antenatal screening by amniocentesis (V28.0)

V82.5 Chemical poisoning and other contamination
Screening for:
   heavy metal poisoning
   ingestion of radioactive substance
   poisoning from contaminated water supply
   radiation exposure

V82.6 Multiphasic screening

√5th V82.7 Genetic screening
EXCLUDES genetic testing for procreative management (V26.31-V26.39)

V82.71 Screening for genetic disease carrier status
AHA: 4Q, '06, 118

V82.79 Other genetic screening
AHA: 4Q, '06, 118

√5th V82.8 Other specified conditions
AHA: 4Q, '00, 53

V82.81 Osteoporosis
Use additional code to identify:
   hormone replacement therapy (postmenopausal) status (V07.4)
   postmenopausal (age-related) (natural) status (V49.81)
AHA: 4Q, '00, 54

V82.89 Other specified conditions

V82.9 Unspecified condition

Genetics (V83-V84)

√4th V83 Genetic carrier status
AHA: 4Q, '02, 79; 4Q, '01, 54
TIP: The patient does not have the disease or carry a risk of developing it, but may genetically pass it to offspring who then may develop it.

√5th V83.0 Hemophilia A carrier

V83.01 Asymptomatic hemophilia A carrier

V83.02 Symptomatic hemophilia A carrier

√5th V83.8 Other genetic carrier status

V83.81 Cystic fibrosis gene carrier

V83.89 Other genetic carrier status

√4th V84 Genetic susceptibility to disease
INCLUDES confirmed abnormal gene
EXCLUDES chromosomal anomalies (758.0-758.9)
Use additional code, if applicable, for any associated family history of the disease (V16-V19)
AHA: 4Q, '04, 106
TIP: The patient has a gene that increases the risk of developing a specific disease; assign only as a secondary condition.

√5th V84.0 Genetic susceptibility to malignant neoplasm
Code first, if applicable, any current malignant neoplasms (140.0-195.8, 200.0-208.9, 230.0-234.9)
Use additional code, if applicable, for any personal history of malignant neoplasm (V10.0-V10.9)

V84.01 Genetic susceptibility to malignant neoplasm of breast
AHA: 2Q, '11, 12; 4Q, '04, 107
Z15.01 Genetic susceptibility malignant neoplasm breast   I-10

V84.02 Genetic susceptibility to malignant neoplasm of ovary ♀

V84.03 Genetic susceptibility to malignant neoplasm of prostate ♂

V84.04 Genetic susceptibility to malignant neoplasm of endometrium ♀

V84.09 Genetic susceptibility to other malignant neoplasm

√5th V84.8 Genetic susceptibility to other disease

V84.81 Genetic susceptibility to multiple endocrine neoplasia [MEN]
EXCLUDES multiple endocrine neoplasia [MEN] syndromes (258.01-258.03)
AHA: 4Q, '07, 100

V84.89 Genetic susceptibility to other disease

Body Mass Index (V85)

√4th V85 Body Mass Index [BMI]
Kilograms per meters squared
NOTE BMI adult codes are for use for persons over 20 years old
AHA: 3Q, '11, 4-5; 2Q, '10, 15; 4Q, '08, 191; 4Q, '05, 97
TIP: While BMI may be coded from dietician or other caregiver documentation, the diagnosis of being overweight or obese must be coded from physician documentation.

V85.0 Body Mass Index less than 19, adult   CC A
CC Excl: 278.00-278.01, 278.03, V77.8, V85.0-V85.39, V85.41-V85.54

V85.1 Body Mass Index between 19-24, adult   A

√5th V85.2 Body Mass Index between 25-29, adult

V85.21 Body Mass Index 25.0-25.9, adult   A

V85.22 Body Mass Index 26.0-26.9, adult   A

V85.23 Body Mass Index 27.0-27.9, adult   A

V85.24 Body Mass Index 28.0-28.9, adult   A

V85.25 Body Mass Index 29.0-29.9, adult   A

N Newborn Age: 0   **P** Pediatric Age: 0-17   **M** Maternity Age: 12-55   **A** Adult Age: 15-124   **MCC** Major CC Condition   **CC** CC Condition   **HIV** HIV Related Dx

374 – Volume 1   2014 ICD-9-CM

✓5ᵗʰ **V85.3 Body Mass Index between 30-39, adult**

V85.30 Body Mass Index 30.0-30.9, adult	A
V85.31 Body Mass Index 31.0-31.9, adult	A
V85.32 Body Mass Index 32.0-32.9, adult	A
V85.33 Body Mass Index 33.0-33.9, adult	A
V85.34 Body Mass Index 34.0-34.9, adult	A
V85.35 Body Mass Index 35.0-35.9, adult	A
V85.36 Body Mass Index 36.0-36.9, adult	A
V85.37 Body Mass Index 37.0-37.9, adult	A
V85.38 Body Mass Index 38.0-38.9, adult	A
V85.39 Body Mass Index 39.0-39.9, adult	A

✓5ᵗʰ **V85.4 Body Mass Index 40 and over, adult**
AHA: 4Q, '10, 81, 109

V85.41 Body Mass Index 40.0-44.9, adult　CC A
CC Exd: 278.00-278.01, 278.1, V85.0-V85.39, V85.41-V85.54
AHA: 4Q, '10, 109

V85.42 Body Mass Index 45.0-49.9, adult　CC A
CC Exd: See code: V85.41

V85.43 Body Mass Index 50.0-59.9, adult　CC A
CC Exd: See code: V85.41

V85.44 Body Mass Index 60.0-69.9, adult　CC A
CC Exd: See code: V85.41

V85.45 Body Mass Index 70 and over, adult　CC A
CC Exd: See code: V85.41

✓5ᵗʰ **V85.5 Body Mass Index, pediatric**
NOTE BMI pediatric codes are for use for persons age 2-20
years old. These percentiles are based on the growth
charts published by the Centers for Disease Control and
Prevention (CDC)
AHA: 4Q, '06, 118

**V85.51 Body Mass Index, pediatric, less than 5th
percentile for age**　P

**V85.52 Body Mass Index, pediatric, 5th percentile to
less than 85th percentile for age**　P

**V85.53 Body Mass Index, pediatric, 85th percentile
to less than 95th percentile for age**　P

**V85.54 Body Mass Index, pediatric, greater than or
equal to 95th percentile for age**　P
Z68.54 Body mass index ped >/equal to 95th % for age　I-10

Estrogen Receptor Status (V86)

✓4ᵗʰ **V86 Estrogen receptor status**
Code first malignant neoplasm of breast (174.0-174.9, 175.0-175.9)
AHA: 4Q, '06, 118

V86.0 Estrogen receptor positive status [ER+]

V86.1 Estrogen receptor negative status [ER-]

Other Specified Personal Exposures and History Presenting Hazards To Health (V87)

✓4ᵗʰ **V87 Other specified personal exposures and history presenting
hazards to health**

✓5ᵗʰ **V87.0 Contact with and (suspected) exposure to hazardous
metals**
EXCLUDES exposure to lead (V15.86)
toxic effect of metals (984.0-985.9)
AHA: 4Q, '08, 158

V87.01 Arsenic

V87.02 Contact with and (suspected) exposure to uranium
EXCLUDES retained depleted uranium fragments
(V90.01)
AHA: 4Q, '11, 156

V87.09 Other hazardous metals
Chromium compounds
Nickel dust

✓5ᵗʰ **V87.1 Contact with and (suspected) exposure to hazardous
aromatic compounds**
EXCLUDES toxic effects of aromatic compounds (982.0, 983.0)
AHA: 4Q, '08, 158

V87.11 Aromatic amines

V87.12 Benzene

V87.19 Other hazardous aromatic compounds
Aromatic dyes NOS
Polycyclic aromatic hydrocarbons

**V87.2 Contact with and (suspected) exposure to other
potentially hazardous chemicals**
Dyes NOS
EXCLUDES exposure to asbestos (V15.84)
toxic effect of chemicals (980-989)
AHA: 4Q, '08, 158

✓5ᵗʰ **V87.3 Contact with and (suspected) exposure to other potentially
hazardous substances**
EXCLUDES contact with and (suspected) exposure to potentially
hazardous body fluids (V15.85)
personal history of retained foreign body fully
removed (V15.53)
toxic effect of substances (980-989)

V87.31 Exposure to mold

**V87.32 Contact with and (suspected) exposure
to algae bloom**
AHA: 4Q, '09, 116

**V87.39 Contact with and (suspected) exposure to
other potentially hazardous substances**

✓5ᵗʰ **V87.4 Personal history of drug therapy**
EXCLUDES long-term (current) drug use (V58.61-V58.69)
AHA: 4Q, '09, 116; 4Q, '08, 159

**V87.41 Personal history of antineoplastic
chemotherapy**
Z92.21 Personal hx antineoplastic chemotherapy　I-10

V87.42 Personal history of monoclonal drug therapy

V87.43 Personal history of estrogen therapy

V87.44 Personal history of inhaled steroid therapy

V87.45 Personal history of systemic steroid therapy
Personal history of steroid therapy NOS

V87.46 Personal history of immunosuppression therapy
EXCLUDES personal history of steroid therapy (V87.44,
V87.45)

V87.49 Personal history of other drug therapy

Acquired Absence of Other Organs and Tissue (V88)

✓4ᵗʰ **V88 Acquired absence of other organs and tissue**

✓5ᵗʰ **V88.0 Acquired absence of cervix and uterus**
AHA: 4Q, '08, 157

V88.01 Acquired absence of both cervix and uterus　♀
Acquired absence of uterus NOS
Status post total hysterectomy

**V88.02 Acquired absence of uterus with
remaining cervical stump**　♀
Status post partial hysterectomy with remaining
cervical stump

**V88.03 Acquired absence of cervix with
remaining uterus**　♀

✓5ᵗʰ **V88.1 Acquired absence of pancreas**
Use additional code to identify any associated:
insulin use (V58.67)
secondary diabetes mellitus (249.00-249.91)
AHA: 4Q, '10, 109

V88.11 Acquired total absence of pancreas
Acquired absence of pancreas NOS

V88.12 Acquired partial absence of pancreas

√5ᵗʰ **V88.2 Acquired absence of joint**
Acquired absence of joint following prior explantation of joint prosthesis
Joint prosthesis explantation status
AHA: 4Q, '11, 156-157

V88.21 Acquired absence of hip joint
Acquired absence of hip joint following explantation of joint prosthesis, with or without presence of antibiotic-impregnated cement spacer

V88.22 Acquired absence of knee joint
Acquired absence of knee joint following explantation of joint prosthesis, with or without presence of antibiotic-impregnated cement spacer

V88.29 Acquired absence of other joint
Acquired absence of other joint following explantation of joint prosthesis, with or without presence of antibiotic-impregnated cement spacer

Other Suspected Conditions Not Found (V89)

√4ᵗʰ **V89 Other suspected conditions not found**

√5ᵗʰ **V89.0 Suspected maternal and fetal conditions not found**
EXCLUDES known or suspected fetal anomalies affecting management of mother, not ruled out (655.00, 655.93, 656.00-656.93, 657.00-657.03, 658.00-658.93)
newborn and perinatal conditions — code to condition
AHA: 4Q, '08, 159
TIP: These investigations are performed while the fetus is in utero; the codes should be assigned only on the mother's medical record.

V89.01 Suspected problem with amniotic cavity and membrane not found Ⓜ♀
Suspected oligohydramnios not found
Suspected polyhydramnios not found

V89.02 Suspected placental problem not found Ⓜ♀

V89.03 Suspected fetal anomaly not found Ⓜ♀

V89.04 Suspected problem with fetal growth not found Ⓜ♀

V89.05 Suspected cervical shortening not found Ⓜ♀

V89.09 Other suspected maternal and fetal condition not found Ⓜ♀

Retained Foreign Body (V90)

√4ᵗʰ **V90 Retained foreign body**
Embedded fragment (status)   Retained foreign body status
Embedded splinter (status)
EXCLUDES artificial joint prosthesis status (V43.60-V43.69)
foreign body accidentally left during a procedure (998.4)
foreign body entering through orifice (930.0-939.9)
in situ cardiac devices (V45.00-V45.09)
organ or tissue replaced by other means (V43.0-V43.89)
organ or tissue replaced by transplant (V42.0-V42.9)
personal history of retained foreign body removed (V15.53)
superficial foreign body (splinter) (categories 910-917 and 919 with 4ᵗʰ character 6 or 7, 918.0)
AHA: 4Q, '10, 109

√5ᵗʰ **V90.0 Retained radioactive fragment**
V90.01 Retained depleted uranium fragments
V90.09 Other retained radioactive fragments
Other retained depleted isotope fragments
Retained nontherapeutic radioactive fragments

√5ᵗʰ **V90.1 Retained metal fragments**
EXCLUDES retained radioactive metal fragments (V90.01-V90.09)
V90.10 Retained metal fragments, unspecified
Retained metal fragment NOS
V90.11 Retained magnetic metal fragments
V90.12 Retained nonmagnetic metal fragments

V90.2 Retained plastic fragments
Acrylics fragments
Diethylhexylphthalates fragments
Isocyanate fragments

√5ᵗʰ **V90.3 Retained organic fragments**
V90.31 Retained animal quills or spines
V90.32 Retained tooth
V90.33 Retained wood fragments
V90.39 Other retained organic fragments

√5ᵗʰ **V90.8 Other specified retained foreign body**
V90.81 Retained glass fragments
V90.83 Retained stone or crystalline fragments
Retained concrete or cement fragments
V90.89 Other specified retained foreign body

V90.9 Retained foreign body, unspecified material

Multiple Gestation Placenta Status (V91)

√4ᵗʰ **V91 Multiple gestation placenta status**
Code first multiple gestation (651.0-651.9)
AHA: 4Q, '10, 110

√5ᵗʰ **V91.0 Twin gestation placenta status**
V91.00 Twin gestation, unspecified number of placenta, unspecified number of amniotic sacs Ⓜ♀
V91.01 Twin gestation, monochorionic/monoamniotic (one placenta, one amniotic sac) Ⓜ♀
V91.02 Twin gestation, monochorionic/diamniotic (one placenta, two amniotic sacs) Ⓜ♀
V91.03 Twin gestation, dichorionic/diamniotic (two placentae, two amniotic sacs) Ⓜ♀
V91.09 Twin gestation, unable to determine number of placenta and number of amniotic sacs Ⓜ♀

√5ᵗʰ **V91.1 Triplet gestation placenta status**
V91.10 Triplet gestation, unspecified number of placenta and unspecified number of amniotic sacs Ⓜ♀
V91.11 Triplet gestation, with two or more monochorionic fetuses Ⓜ♀
V91.12 Triplet gestation, with two or more monoamniotic fetuses Ⓜ♀
V91.19 Triplet gestation, unable to determine number of placenta and number of amniotic sacs Ⓜ♀

√5ᵗʰ **V91.2 Quadruplet gestation placenta status**
V91.20 Quadruplet gestation, unspecified number of placenta and unspecified number of amniotic sacs Ⓜ♀
V91.21 Quadruplet gestation, with two or more monochorionic fetuses Ⓜ♀
V91.22 Quadruplet gestation, with two or more monoamniotic fetuses Ⓜ♀
V91.29 Quadruplet gestation, unable to determine number of placenta and number of amniotic sacs Ⓜ♀

√5ᵗʰ **V91.9 Other specified multiple gestation placenta status**
Placenta status for multiple gestations greater than quadruplets
V91.90 Other specified multiple gestation, unspecified number of placenta and unspecified number of amniotic sacs Ⓜ♀
V91.91 Other specified multiple gestation, with two or more monochorionic fetuses Ⓜ♀
V91.92 Other specified multiple gestation, with two or more monoamniotic fetuses Ⓜ♀
V91.99 Other specified multiple gestation, unable to determine number of placenta and number of amniotic sacs Ⓜ♀

Ⓝ Newborn Age: 0   Ⓟ Pediatric Age: 0-17   Ⓜ Maternity Age: 12-55   Ⓐ Adult Age: 15-124   **MCC** Major CC Condition   **CC** CC Condition   **HIV** HIV Related Dx

376 – Volume 1   **2014 ICD-9-CM**

Supplementary Classification of External Causes of Injury and Poisoning (E000-E999)

This section is provided to permit the classification of environmental events, circumstances, and conditions as the cause of injury, poisoning, and other adverse effects. Where a code from this section is applicable, it is intended that it shall be used in addition to a code from one of the main chapters of ICD-9-CM, indicating the nature of the condition. Certain other conditions which may be stated to be due to external causes are classified in Chapters 1 to 16 of ICD-9-CM. For these, the "E" code classification should be used as an additional code for more detailed analysis.

Machinery accidents [other than those connected with transport] are classifiable to category E919, in which the fourth digit allows a broad classification of the type of machinery involved.

Categories for "late effects" of accidents and other external causes are to be found at E929, E959, E969, E977, E989, and E999.

External Cause Status (E000)

NOTE A code from category E000 may be used in conjunction with the external cause code(s) assigned to a record to indicate the status of the person at the time the event occurred. A single code from category E000 should be assigned for an encounter.

√4ᵗʰ **E000   External cause status**

E000.0 Civilian activity done for income or pay
Civilian activity done for financial or other compensation
EXCLUDES *military activity (E000.1)*

E000.2 Volunteer activity
EXCLUDES *activity of child or other family member assisting in compensated work of other family member (E000.8)*

E000.1 Military activity
EXCLUDES *activity of off-duty military personnel (E000.8)*

E000.8 Other external cause status
Activity of child or other family member assisting in compensated work of other family member
Activity NEC
Hobby not done for income
Leisure activity
Off-duty activity of military personnel
Recreation or sport not for income or while a student
Student activity
EXCLUDES *civilian activity done for income or compensation (E000.0)*
military activity (E000.1)

E000.9 Unspecified external cause status

Activity (E001-E030)

NOTE Categories E001 to E030 are provided for use to indicate the activity of the person seeking healthcare for an injury or health condition, such as a heart attack while shoveling snow, which resulted from, or was contributed to, by the activity. These codes are appropriate for use for both acute injuries, such as those from chapter 17, and conditions that are due to the long-term, cumulative affects of an activity, such as those from chapter 13. They are also appropriate for use with external cause codes for cause and intent if identifying the activity provides additional information on the event.

These codes should be used in conjunction with other external cause codes for external cause status (E000) and place of occurrence (E849).

This section contains the following broad activity categories:

E001   Activities involving walking and running
E002   Activities involving water and water craft
E003   Activities involving ice and snow
E004   Activities involving climbing, rappelling, and jumping off
E005   Activities involving dancing and other rhythmic movement
E006   Activities involving other sports and athletics played individually
E007   Activities involving other sports and athletics played as a team or group
E008   Activities involving other specified sports and athletics
E009   Activity involving other cardiorespiratory exercise
E010   Activity involving other muscle strengthening exercises
E011   Activities involving computer technology and electronic devices
E012   Activities involving arts and handcrafts
E013   Activities involving personal hygiene and household maintenance
E014   Activities involving person providing caregiving
E015   Activities involving food preparation, cooking and grilling
E016   Activities involving property and land maintenance, building and construction
E017   Activities involving roller coasters and other types of external motion
E018   Activities involving playing musical instrument
E019   Activities involving animal care
E029   Other activity
E030   Unspecified activity

√4ᵗʰ **E001   Activities involving walking and running**
EXCLUDES *walking an animal (E019.0)*
walking or running on a treadmill (E009.0)

E001.0 Walking, marching and hiking
Walking, marching and hiking on level or elevated terrain
EXCLUDES *mountain climbing (E004.0)*

E001.1 Running

√4ᵗʰ **E002   Activities involving water and water craft**
EXCLUDES *activities involving ice (E003.0-E003.9)*
boating and other watercraft transport accidents (E830-E838)

E002.0 Swimming

E002.1 Springboard and platform diving

E002.2 Water polo

E002.3 Water aerobics and water exercise

E002.4 Underwater diving and snorkeling
SCUBA diving

E002.5 Rowing, canoeing, kayaking, rafting and tubing
Canoeing, kayaking, rafting and tubing in calm and turbulent water

E002.6 Water skiing and wake boarding

E002.7 Surfing, windsurfing and boogie boarding

E002.8 Water sliding

E002.9 Other activity involving water and watercraft
Activity involving water NOS
Parasailing
Water survival training and testing

√4ᵗʰ **E003   Activities involving ice and snow**
EXCLUDES *shoveling ice and snow (E016.0)*

E003.0 Ice skating
Figure skating (singles) (pairs)
Ice dancing
EXCLUDES *ice hockey (E003.1)*

E003.1 Ice hockey

E003.2 Snow (alpine) (downhill) skiing, snow boarding, sledding, tobogganing and snow tubing
EXCLUDES *cross country skiing (E003.3)*

E003.3 Cross country skiing
Nordic skiing

E003.9 Other activity involving ice and snow
Activity involving ice and snow NOS

√4ᵗʰ **E004   Activities involving climbing, rappelling, and jumping off**
EXCLUDES *hiking on level or elevated terrain (E001.0)*
jumping rope (E006.5)
sky diving (E840-E844)
trampoline jumping (E005.3)

E004.0 Mountain climbing, rock climbing and wall climbing

E004.1 Rappelling

E004.2 BASE jumping
Building, Antenna, Span, Earth jumping

E004.3 Bungee jumping

E004.4 Hang gliding

E004.9 Other activity involving climbing, rappelling and jumping off

√4ᵗʰ **E005 Activities involving dancing and other rhythmic movement**
   EXCLUDES *martial arts (E008.4)*

E005.0 Dancing

E005.1 Yoga

E005.2 Gymnastics
   Rhythmic gymnastics
   EXCLUDES *trampoline (E005.3)*

E005.3 Trampoline

E005.4 Cheerleading

E005.9 Other activity involving dancing and other rhythmic movements

√4ᵗʰ **E006 Activities involving other sports and athletics played individually**
   EXCLUDES *dancing (E005.0)*
     gymnastic (E005.2)
     trampoline (E005.3)
     yoga (E005.1)

E006.0 Roller skating (inline) and skateboarding

E006.1 Horseback riding

E006.2 Golf

E006.3 Bowling

E006.4 Bike riding
   EXCLUDES *transport accident involving bike riding (E800-E829)*

E006.5 Jumping rope

E006.6 Non-running track and field events
   EXCLUDES *running (any form) (E001.1)*

E006.9 Other activity involving other sports and athletics played individually
   EXCLUDES *activities involving climbing, rappelling, and jumping (E004.0-E004.9)*
     activities involving ice and snow (E003.0-E003.9)
     activities involving walking and running (E001.0-E001.9)
     activities involving water and watercraft (E002.0-E002.9)

√4ᵗʰ **E007 Activities involving other sports and athletics played as a team or group**
   EXCLUDES *ice hockey (E003.1)*
     water polo (E002.2)

E007.0 American tackle football
   Football NOS

E007.1 American flag or touch football

E007.2 Rugby

E007.3 Baseball
   Softball

E007.4 Lacrosse and field hockey

E007.5 Soccer

E007.6 Basketball

E007.7 Volleyball (beach) (court)

E007.8 Physical games generally associated with school recess, summer camp and children
   Capture the flag   Four square
   Dodge ball   Kickball

E007.9 Other activity involving other sports and athletics played as a team or group
   Cricket

√4ᵗʰ **E008 Activities involving other specified sports and athletics**

E008.0 Boxing

E008.1 Wrestling

E008.2 Racquet and hand sports
   Handball   Squash
   Racquetball   Tennis

E008.3 Frisbee
   Ultimate frisbee

E008.4 Martial arts
   Combatives

E008.9 Other specified sports and athletics activity
   EXCLUDES *sports and athletics activities specified in categories E001-E007*

√4ᵗʰ **E009 Activity involving other cardiorespiratory exercise**
   Activity involving physical training

E009.0 Exercise machines primarily for cardiorespiratory conditioning
   Elliptical and stepper machines
   Stationary bike
   Treadmill

E009.1 Calisthenics
   Jumping jacks   Warm up and cool down

E009.2 Aerobic and step exercise

E009.3 Circuit training

E009.4 Obstacle course
   Challenge course   Confidence course

E009.5 Grass drills
   Guerilla drills

E009.9 Other activity involving cardiorespiratory exercise
   EXCLUDES *activities involving cardiorespiratory exercise specified in categories E001-E008*

√4ᵗʰ **E010 Activity involving other muscle strengthening exercises**

E010.0 Exercise machines primarily for muscle strengthening

E010.1 Push-ups, pull-ups, sit-ups

E010.2 Free weights
   Barbells
   Dumbbells

E010.3 Pilates

E010.9 Other activity involving other muscle strengthening exercises
   EXCLUDES *activities involving muscle strengthening specified in categories E001-E009*

√4ᵗʰ **E011 Activities involving computer technology and electronic devices**
   EXCLUDES *electronic musical keyboard or instruments (E018.0)*

E011.0 Computer keyboarding
   Electronic game playing using keyboard or other stationary device

E011.1 Hand held interactive electronic device
   Cellular telephone and communication device
   Electronic game playing using interactive device
   EXCLUDES *electronic game playing using keyboard or other stationary device (E011.0)*

E011.9 Other activity involving computer technology and electronic devices

√4ᵗʰ **E012 Activities involving arts and handcrafts**
   EXCLUDES *activities involving playing musical instrument (E018.0-E018.3)*

E012.0 Knitting and crocheting

E012.1 Sewing

E012.2 Furniture building and finishing
   Furniture repair

E012.9 Activity involving other arts and handcrafts

√4ᵗʰ **E013 Activities involving personal hygiene and household maintenance**
   EXCLUDES *activities involving cooking and grilling (E015.0-E015.9)*
     activities involving property and land maintenance, building and construction (E016.0-E016.9)
     activity involving persons providing caregiving (E014.0-E014.9)
     dishwashing (E015.0)
     food preparation (E015.0)
     gardening (E016.1)

E013.0 Personal bathing and showering

√4ᵗʰ Fourth-digit Required   ▶◀ Revised Text   ● New Code   ▲ Revised Code TitleDx

E013.1 Laundry

E013.2 Vacuuming

E013.3 Ironing

E013.4 Floor mopping and cleaning

E013.5 Residential relocation
Packing up and unpacking involved in moving to a new residence

E013.8 Other personal hygiene activity

E013.9 Other household maintenance

☑4ᵗʰ **E014 Activities involving person providing caregiving**

E014.0 Caregiving involving bathing

E014.1 Caregiving involving lifting

E014.9 Other activity involving person providing caregiving

☑4ᵗʰ **E015 Activities involving food preparation, cooking and grilling**

E015.0 Food preparation and clean up
Dishwasing

E015.1 Grilling and smoking food

E015.2 Cooking and baking
Use of stove, oven and microwave oven

E015.9 Other activity involving cooking and grilling

☑4ᵗʰ **E016 Activities involving property and land maintenance, building and construction**

E016.0 Digging, shoveling and raking
Dirt digging
Raking leaves
Snow shoveling

E016.1 Gardening and landscaping
Pruning, trimming shrubs, weeding

E016.2 Building and construction

E016.9 Other activity involving property and land maintenance, building and construction

☑4ᵗʰ **E017 Activities involving roller coasters and other types of external motion**

E017.0 Roller coaster riding

E017.9 Other activity involving external motion

☑4ᵗʰ **E018 Activities involving playing musical instrument**
Activity involving playing electric musical instrument

E018.0 Piano playing
Musical keyboard (electronic) playing

E018.1 Drum and other percussion instrument playing

E018.2 String instrument playing

E018.3 Wind and brass instrument playing

☑4ᵗʰ **E019 Activities involving animal care**
EXCLUDES horseback riding (E006.1)

E019.0 Walking an animal

E019.1 Milking an animal

E019.2 Grooming and shearing an animal

E019.9 Other activity involving animal care

☑4ᵗʰ **E029 Other activity**

E029.0 Refereeing a sports activity

E029.1 Spectator at an event

E029.2 Rough housing and horseplay

E029.9 Other activity

E030 Unspecified activity

Transport Accidents (E800-E848)

Definitions and Examples Related to Transport Accidents

(a) A **transport accident** (E800-E848) is any accident involving a device designed primarily for, or being used at the time primarily for, conveying persons or goods from one place to another.

INCLUDES accidents involving:
    aircraft and spacecraft (E840-E845)
    watercraft (E830-E838)
    motor vehicle (E810-E825)
    railway (E800-E807)
    other road vehicles (E826-E829)

In classifying accidents which involve more than one kind of transport, the above order of precedence of transport accidents should be used.

Accidents involving agricultural and construction machines, such as tractors, cranes, and bulldozers, are regarded as transport accidents only when these vehicles are under their own power on a highway [otherwise the vehicles are regarded as machinery]. Vehicles which can travel on land and water, such as hovercraft and other amphibious vehicles, are regarded as watercraft when on the water, as motor vehicles when on the highway, and as off-road motor vehicles when on land, but off the highway.

EXCLUDES accidents:
    in sports which involve the use of transport but where the transport vehicle itself was not involved in the accident
    involving vehicles which are part of industrial equipment used entirely on industrial premises
    occurring during transportation but unrelated to the hazards associated with the means of transportation [e.g., injuries received in a fight on board ship; transport vehicle involved in a cataclysm such as an earthquake]
    to persons engaged in the maintenance or repair of transport equipment or vehicle not in motion, unlesss injured by another vehicle in motion

(b) A **railway accident** is a transport accident involving a railway train or other railway vehicle operated on rails, whether in motion or not.

EXCLUDES accidents:
    in repair shops
    in roundhouse or on turntable
    on railway premises but not involving a train or other railway vehicle

(c) A **railway train** or **railway vehicle** is any device with or without cars coupled to it, desiged for traffic on a railway.

INCLUDES interurban:
    electric car   (operated chiefly on its own
    street car   right-of-way, not open to
                         other traffic)
    railway train, any power [diesel] [electric] [steam]:
        funicular
        monorail or two-rail
        subterranean or elevated
    other vehicle designed to run on a railway track

EXCLUDES interurban electric cars [streetcars] specified to be operating on a right-of-way that forms part of the public street or highway [definition (h)]

(d) A **railway** or **railroad** is a right-of-way designed for traffic on rails, which is used by carriages or wagons transporting passengers or freight, and by other rolling stock, and which is not open to other public vehicular traffic.

(e) A **motor vehicle accident** is a transport accident involving a motor vehicle. It is defined as a motor vehicle traffic accident or as a motor vehicle nontraffic accident according to whether the accident occurs on a public highway or elsewhere.

EXCLUDES injury or damage due to cataclysm
    injury or damage while a motor vehicle, not under its own power, is being loaded on, or unloaded from, another conveyance

(f) A **motor vehicle traffic accident** is any motor vehicle accident occurring on a public highway [i.e., originating, terminating, or involving a vehicle partially on the highway]. A motor vehicle accident is assumed to have occurred on the highway unless another place is specified, except in the case of accidents involving only off-road motor vehicles which are classified as nontraffic accidents unless the contrary is stated.

(g) A **motor vehicle nontraffic accident** is any motor vehicle accident which occurs entirely in any place other than a public highway.

(h) A **public highway [trafficway]** or **street** is the entire width between property lines [or other boundary lines] of every way or place, of which any part is open to the use of the public for purposes of vehicular traffic as a matter of right or custom. A **roadway** is that part of the public highway designed, improved, and ordinarily used, for vehicular travel.

INCLUDES approaches (public) to:
     docks
     public building
     station

EXCLUDES *driveway (private)*
     parking lot
     ramp
     roads in:
        airfield
        farm
        industrial premises
        mine
        private grounds
        quarry

(i) A **motor vehicle** is any mechanically or electrically powered device, not operated on rails, upon which any person or property may be transported or drawn upon a highway. Any object such as a trailer, coaster, sled, or wagon being towed by a motor vehicle is considered a part of the motor vehicle.

INCLUDES automobile [any type]
     bus
     construction machinery, farm and industrial machinery, steam roller, tractor, army tank, highway grader, or similar vehicle on wheels or treads, while in transport under own power
     fire engine (motorized)
     motorcycle
     motorized bicycle [moped] or scooter
     trolley bus not operating on rails
     truck
     van

EXCLUDES *devices used solely to move persons or materials within the confines of a building and its premises, such as:*
        building elevator
        coal car in mine
        electric baggage or mail truck used solely within a railroad station
        electric truck used solely within an industrial plant
        moving overhead crane

(j) A **motorcycle** is a two-wheeled motor vehicle having one or two riding saddles and sometimes having a third wheel for the support of a sidecar. The sidecar is considered part of the motorcycle.

INCLUDES motorized:
     bicycle [moped]
     scooter
     tricycle

(k) An **off-road motor vehicle** is a motor vehicle of special design, to enable it to negotiate rough or soft terrain or snow. Examples of special design are high construction, special wheels and tires, driven by treads, or support on a cushion of air.

INCLUDES all terrain vehicle [ATV]
     army tank
     hovercraft, on land or swamp
     snowmobile

(l) A **driver** of a motor vehicle is the occupant of the motor vehicle operating it or intending to operate it. A **motorcyclist** is the driver of a motorcycle. Other authorized occupants of a motor vehicle are **passengers**.

(m) An **other road vehicle** is any device, except a motor vehicle, in, on, or by which any person or property may be transported on a highway.

INCLUDES animal carrying a person or goods
     animal-drawn vehicles
     animal harnessed to conveyance
     bicycle [pedal cycle]
     streetcar
     tricycle (pedal)

EXCLUDES *pedestrian conveyance [definition (q)]*

(n) A **streetcar** is a device designed and used primarily for transporting persons within a municipality, running on rails, usually subject to normal traffic control signals, and operated principally on a right-of-way that forms part of the traffic way. A trailer being towed by a streetcar is considered a part of the streetcar.

INCLUDES interurban or intraurban electric or streetcar, when specified to be operating on a street or public highway
     tram (car)
     trolley (car)

(o) A **pedal cycle** is any road transport vehicle operated solely by pedals.

INCLUDES bicycle
     pedal cycle
     tricycle

EXCLUDES *motorized bicycle [definition (j)]*

(p) A **pedal cyclist** is any person riding on a pedal cycle or in a sidecar attached to such a vehicle.

(q) A **pedestrian conveyance** is any human powered device by which a pedestrian may move other than by walking or by which a walking person may move another pedestrian.

INCLUDES baby carriage
     coaster wagon
     heelies, wheelies
     ice skates
     motorized mobility scooter
     perambulator
     pushcart
     pushchair
     roller skates
     scooter
     skateboard
     skis
     sled
     wheelchair (electric)

(r) A **pedestrian** is any person involved in an accident who was not at the time of the accident riding in or on a motor vehicle, railroad train, streetcar, animal-drawn or other vehicle, or on a bicycle or animal.

INCLUDES person:
     changing tire of vehicle
     in or operating a pedestrian conveyance
     making adjustment to motor of vehicle
     on foot

(s) A **watercraft** is any device for transporting passengers or goods on the water.

(t) A **small boat** is any watercraft propelled by paddle, oars, or small motor, with a passenger capacity of less than ten.

INCLUDES boat NOS
     canoe
     coble
     dinghy
     punt
     raft
     rowboat
     rowing shell
     scull
     skiff
     small motorboat

EXCLUDES *barge*
     lifeboat (used after abandoning ship)
     raft (anchored) being used as a diving platform
     yacht

(u) An **aircraft** is any device for transporting passengers or goods in the air.

INCLUDES airplane [any type]
     balloon
     bomber
     dirigible
     glider (hang)
     military aircraft
     parachute

(v) A **commercial transport aircraft** is any device for collective passenger or freight transportation by air, whether run on commercial lines for profit or by government authorities, with the exception of military craft.

☑ Fourth-digit Required   ▶◀ Revised Text   ● New Code   ▲ Revised Code TitleDx

Railway Accidents (E800-E807)

NOTE For definitions of railway accident and related terms see definitions (a) to (d).

EXCLUDES accidents involving railway train and:
   aircraft (E840.0-E845.9)
   motor vehicle (E810.0-E825.9)
   watercraft (E830.0-E838.9)

The following fourth digit subdivisions are for use with categories E800-E807 to identify the injured person:

.0 Railway employee
   Any person who by virtue of his employment in connection with a railway, whether by the railway company or not, is at increased risk of involvement in a railway accident, such as:
      catering staff of train
      driver
      guard
      porter
      postal staff on train
      railway fireman
      shunter
      sleeping car attendant

.1 Passenger on railway
   Any authorized person traveling on a train, except a railway employee.
   EXCLUDES intending passenger waiting at station (.8)
      unauthorized rider on railway vehicle (.8)

.2 Pedestrian
   See definition (r)

.3 Pedal cyclist
   See definition (p)

.8 Other specified person
   Intending passenger or bystander waiting at station
   Unauthorized rider on railway vehicle

.9 Unspecified person

§ ☑4ᵗʰ **E800   Railway accident involving collision with rolling stock**
   INCLUDES collision between railway trains or railway vehicles, any kind
      collision NOS on railway
      derailment with antecedent collision with rolling stock or NOS

§ ☑4ᵗʰ **E801   Railway accident involving collision with other object**
   INCLUDES collision of railway train with:
      buffers
      fallen tree on railway
      gates
      platform
      rock on railway
      streetcar
      other nonmotor vehicle
      other object
   EXCLUDES collision with:
      aircraft (E840.0-E842.9)
      motor vehicle (E810.0-E810.9, E820.0-E822.9)

§ ☑4ᵗʰ **E802   Railway accident involving derailment without antecedent collision**

§ ☑4ᵗʰ **E803   Railway accident involving explosion, fire, or burning**
   EXCLUDES explosion or fire, with antecedent derailment (E802.0-E802.9)
      explosion or fire, with mention of antecedent collision (E800.0-E801.9)

§ ☑4ᵗʰ **E804   Fall in, on, or from railway train**
   INCLUDES fall while alighting from or boarding railway train
   EXCLUDES fall related to collision, derailment, or explosion of railway train (E800.0-E803.9)

§ ☑4ᵗʰ **E805   Hit by rolling stock**
   INCLUDES crushed
      injured
      killed
      knocked down
      run over   } by railway train or part
   EXCLUDES pedestrian hit by object set in motion by railway train (E806.0-E806.9)

§ ☑4ᵗʰ **E806   Other specified railway accident**
   INCLUDES hit by object falling in railway train
      injured by door or window on railway train
      nonmotor road vehicle or pedestrian hit by object set in motion by railway train
      railway train hit by falling:
         earth NOS
         rock
         tree
         other object
   EXCLUDES railway accident due to cataclysm (E908-E909)

§ ☑4ᵗʰ **E807   Railway accident of unspecified nature**
   INCLUDES found dead
      injured   } on railway right-of-way NOS
      railway accident NOS

Motor Vehicle Traffic Accidents (E810-E819)

NOTE For definitions of motor vehicle traffic accident, and related terms, see definitions (e) to (k).

EXCLUDES accidents involving motor vehicle and aircraft (E840.0-E845.9)

The following fourth digit subdivisions are for use with categories E810-E819 to identify the injured person:

.0 Driver of motor vehicle other than motorcycle
   See definition (l)

.1 Passenger in motor vehicle other than motorcycle
   See definition (l)

.2 Motorcyclist
   See definition (l)

.3 Passenger on motorcycle
   See definition (l)

.4 Occupant of streetcar

.5 Rider of animal; occupant of animal-drawn vehicle

.6 Pedal cyclist
   See definition (p)

.7 Pedestrian
   See definition (r)

.8 Other specified person
   Occupant of vehicle other than above
   Person in railway train involved in accident
   Unauthorized rider of motor vehicle

.9 Unspecified person

§ ☑4ᵗʰ **E810   Motor vehicle traffic accident involving collision with train**
   EXCLUDES motor vehicle collision with object set in motion by railway train (E815.0-E815.9)
      railway train hit by object set in motion by motor vehicle (E818.0-E818.9)

§ ☑4ᵗʰ **E811   Motor vehicle traffic accident involving re-entrant collision with another motor vehicle**
   INCLUDES collision between motor vehicle which accidentally leaves the roadway then re-enters the same roadway, or the opposite roadway on a divided highway, and another motor vehicle
   EXCLUDES collision on the same roadway when none of the motor vehicles involved have left and re-entered the highway (E812.0-E812.9)

§ ☑4ᵗʰ **E812   Other motor vehicle traffic accident involving collision with motor vehicle**
   INCLUDES collision with another motor vehicle parked, stopped, stalled, disabled, or abandoned on the highway
      motor vehicle collision NOS
   EXCLUDES collision with object set in motion by another motor vehicle (E815.0-E815.9)
      re-entrant collision with another motor vehicle (E811.0-E811.9)

_____
§ Requires fourth digit. See beginning of appropriate section for codes and definitions.

§ ✓4ᵗʰ **E813　Motor vehicle traffic accident involving collision with other vehicle**

INCLUDES　collision between motor vehicle, any kind, and:
other road (nonmotor transport) vehicle, such as:
animal carrying a person
animal-drawn vehicle
pedal cycle
streetcar

EXCLUDES　*collision with:*
object set in motion by nonmotor road vehicle (E815.0-E815.9)
pedestrian (E814.0-E814.9)
nonmotor road vehicle hit by object set in motion by motor vehicle (E818.0-E818.9)

§ ✓4ᵗʰ **E814　Motor vehicle traffic accident involving collision with pedestrian**

INCLUDES　collision between motor vehicle, any kind, and pedestrian
pedestrian dragged, hit, or run over by motor vehicle, any kind

EXCLUDES　*pedestrian hit by object set in motion by motor vehicle (E818.0-E818.9)*

§ ✓4ᵗʰ **E815　Other motor vehicle traffic accident involving collision on the highway**

INCLUDES　collision (due to loss of control) (on highway) between motor vehicle, any kind, and:
abutment (bridge) (overpass)
animal (herded) (unattended)
fallen stone, traffic sign, tree, utility pole
guard rail or boundary fence
interhighway divider
landslide (not moving)
object set in motion by railway train or road vehicle (motor) (nonmotor)
object thrown in front of motor vehicle
other object, fixed, movable, or moving
safety island
temporary traffic sign or marker
wall of cut made for road

EXCLUDES　*collision with:*
any object off the highway (resulting from loss of control) (E816.0-E816.9)
any object which normally would have been off the highway and is not stated to have been on it (E816.0-E816.9)
motor vehicle parked, stopped, stalled, disabled, or abandoned on highway (E812.0-E812.9)
moving landslide (E909)
motor vehicle hit by object:
set in motion by railway train or road vehicle (motor) (nonmotor) (E818.0-E818.9)
thrown into or on vehicle (E818.0-E818.9)

§ ✓4ᵗʰ **E816　Motor vehicle traffic accident due to loss of control, without collision on the highway**

INCLUDES　motor vehicle:
failing to make curve
going out of control (due to):　　and:
blowout　　　　　　　　　coliding with object off the highway
burst tire　　　　　　　　overturning
driver falling asleep　　　stopping abruptly off the highway
drive inattention
excessive speed
failure of mechanical part

EXCLUDES　*collision on highway following loss of control (E810.0-E815.9)*
loss of control of motor vehicle following collision on the highway (E810.0-E815.9)

§ ✓4ᵗʰ **E817　Noncollision motor vehicle traffic accident while boarding or alighting**

INCLUDES　fall down stairs of motor bus
fall from car in street　　　　　} while boarding or alighting
injured by moving part of the vehicle
trapped by door of motor bus

§ ✓4ᵗʰ **E818　Other noncollision motor vehicle traffic accident**

INCLUDES　accidental poisoning from exhaust gas generated by
breakage of any part of
explosion of any part of
fall, jump, or being accidentally pushed from　　　　　} motor vehicle while in motion
fire starting in
hit by object thrown into or on
injured by being thrown against some part of, or object in
injury from moving part of
object falling in or on
object thrown on

collision of railway train or road vehicle except motor vehicle, with object set in motion by motor vehicle
motor vehicle hit by object set in motion by railway train or road vehicle (motor) (nonmotor)
pedestrian, railway train, or road vehicle (motor) (nonmotor) hit by object set in motion by motor vehicle

EXCLUDES　*collision between motor vehicle and:*
object set in motion by railway train or road vehicle (motor) (nonmotor) (E815.0-E815.9)
object thrown towards the motor vehicle (E815.0-E815.9)
person overcome by carbon monoxide generated by stationary motor vehicle off the roadway with motor running (E868.2)

§ ✓4ᵗʰ **E819　Motor vehicle traffic accident of unspecified nature**

INCLUDES　motor vehicle traffic accident NOS
traffic accident NOS

Motor Vehicle Nontraffic Accidents (E820-E825)

NOTE　For definitions of motor vehicle nontraffic accident and related terms see definition (a) to (k).

INCLUDES　accidents involving motor vehicles being used in recreational or sporting activities off the highway
collision and noncollision motor vehicle accidents occurring entirely off the highway

EXCLUDES　*accidents involving motor vehicle and:*
aircraft (E840.0-E845.9)
watercraft (E830.0-E838.9)
accidents, not on the public highway, involving agricultural and construction machinery but not involving another motor vehicle (E919.0, E919.2, E919.7)

The following fourth digit subdivisions are for use with categories E820-E825 to identify the injured person:
.0 Driver of motor vehicle other than motorcycle
See definition (l)
.1 Passenger in motor vehicle other than motorcycle
See definition (l)
.2 Motorcyclist
See definition (l)
.3 Passenger on motorcycle
See definition (l)
.4 Occupant of streetcar
.5 Rider of animal; occupant of animal-drawn vehicle
.6 Pedal cyclist
See definition (p)
.7 Pedestrian
See definition (r)
.8 Other specified person
Occupant of vehicle other than above
Person in railway train involved in accident
Unauthorized rider of motor vehicle
.9 Unspecified person

§　Requires fourth digit. See beginning of appropriate section for codes and definitions.

✓4ᵗʰ Fourth-digit Required　　►◄ Revised Text　　● New Code　　▲ Revised Code TitleDx

§ ✓4ᵗʰ **E820 Nontraffic accident involving motor-driven snow vehicle**

INCLUDES breakage of part of
fall from
hit by ⎱ motor-driven snow
overturning of ⎰ vehicle (not on
run over or dragged by public highway)

collision of motor-driven snow vehicle with:
animal (being ridden) (-drawn vehicle)
another off-road motor vehicle
other motor vehicle, not on public highway
railway train
other object, fixed or movable
injury caused by rough landing of motor-driven snow
vehicle (after leaving ground on rough terrain)

EXCLUDES *accident on the public highway involving motor driven*
snow vehicle (E810.0-E819.9)

§ ✓4ᵗʰ **E821 Nontraffic accident involving other off-road motor vehicle**

INCLUDES breakage of part of
fall from
hit by ⎫ off-road motor vehicle
overturning of ⎬ except snow
run over or dragged by vehicle (not on
thrown against some part ⎭ public highway
of or object in

collision with:
animal (being ridden) (-drawn vehicle)
another off-road motor vehicle, except snow vehicle
other motor vehicle, not on public highway
other object, fixed or movable

EXCLUDES *accident on public highway involving off-road motor*
vehicle (E810.0-E819.9)
collision between motor driven snow vehicle and other
off-road motor vehicle (E820.0-E820.9)
hovercraft accident on water (E830.0-E838.9)

✓4ᵗʰ **E822 Other motor vehicle nontraffic accident involving collision with moving object**

INCLUDES collision, not on public highway, between motor vehicle,
except off-road motor vehicle and:
animal
nonmotor vehicle
other motor vehicle, except off-road motor vehicle
pedestrian
railway train
other moving object

EXCLUDES *collision with:*
motor-driven snow vehicle (E820.0-E820.9)
other off-road motor vehicle (E821.0-E821.9)

✓4ᵗʰ **E823 Other motor vehicle nontraffic accident involving collision with stationary object**

INCLUDES collision, not on public highway, between motor vehicle,
except off-road motor vehicle, and any object,
fixed or movable, but not in motion

✓4ᵗʰ **E824 Other motor vehicle nontraffic accident while boarding and alighting**

INCLUDES fall
injury from oving part ⎫ while boarding or alighting
of motor ⎬ from motor vehicle,
vehicle except off-road motor
trapped by door of ⎭ vehicle, not on public
motor vehhicle highway

§ ✓4ᵗʰ **E825 Other motor vehicle nontraffic accident of other and unspecified nature**

INCLUDES accidental poisoning from carbon
monoxide generated by
breakage of any part of
explosion of any part of
fall, jump, or being accidentally ⎫ motor vehicle
pushed from ⎬ while in
fire starting in motion, not
hit by object thrown into, towards, on public
or on ⎭ highway
injured by being thrown against
some part of, or object in
injury from moving part of
object falling in or on
motor vehicle nontraffic accident NOS

EXCLUDES *fall from or in stationary motor vehicle (E884.9, E885.9)*
overcome by carbon monoxide or exhaust gas generated by
stationary motor vehicle off the roadway with motor
running (E868.2)
struck by falling object from or in stationary motor vehicle
(E916)

Other Road Vehicle Accidents (E826-E829)

NOTE Other road vehicle accidents are transport accidents involving road
vehicles other than motor vehicles. For definitions of other road
vehicle and related terms see definitions (m) to (o).

INCLUDES accidents involving other road vehicles being used in recreational
or sporting activities

EXCLUDES *collision of other road vehicle [any] with:*
aircraft (E840.0-E845.9)
motor vehicle (E813.0-E813.9, E820.0-E822.9)
railway train (E801.0-E801.9))

The following fourth digit subdivisions are for use with categories E826-E829
to identify the injured person:
.0 Pedestrian
See definition (r)
.1 Pedal cyclist
See definition (p)
.2 Rider of animal
.3 Occupant of animal-drawn vehicle
.4 Occupant of streetcar
.8 Other specified person
.9 Unspecified person

§ ✓4ᵗʰ **E826 Pedal cycle accident**

[0-9] INCLUDES breakage of any part of pedal cycle
collision between pedal cycle and:
animal (being ridden) (herded) (unattended)
another pedal cycle
any pedestrian
nonmotor road vehicle
other object, fixed, movable, or moving, not set in
motion by motor vehicle, railway train, or aircraft
entanglement in wheel of pedal cycle
fall from pedal cycle
hit by object falling or thrown on the pedal cycle
pedal cycle accident NOS
pedal cycle overturned

§ ✓4ᵗʰ **E827 Animal-drawn vehicle accident**

[0,2,4,8,9] INCLUDES breakage of any part of vehicle
collision between animal-drawn vehicle and:
animal (being ridden) (herded) (unattended)
nonmotor road vehicle, except pedal cycle
pedestrian, pedestrian conveyance, or pedestrian
vehicle
other object, fixed, movable, or moving, not set in
motion by motor vehicle, railway train, or aircraft

fall from
knocked down by ⎫
overturning of ⎬ animal drawn vehicle
running over by
thrown from ⎭

EXCLUDES *collision of animal-drawn vehicle with pedal cycle*
(E826.0-E826.9)

Requires fourth digit. See beginning of appropriate section for codes and definitions.

✓4ᵗʰ Fourth-digit Required ▶◀ Revised Text ● New Code ▲ Revised Code TitleDx

E Codes

E828–E838

§ ✓4ᵗʰ **E828 Accident involving animal being ridden**

[0,2,4,8,9] INCLUDES collision between animal being ridden and:
  another animal
  nonmotor road vehicle, except pedal cycle, and animal-drawn vehicle
  pedestrian, pedestrian conveyance, or pedestrian vehicle
  other object, fixed, movable, or moving, not set in motion by motor vehicle, railway train, or aircraft

  fall from
  knocked down by
  thrown from   } animal being ridden
  trampled by

  ridden animal stumbled and fell

EXCLUDES collision of animal being ridden with:
  animal-drawn vehicle (E827.0-E827.9)
  pedal cycle (E826.0-E826.9)

§ ✓4ᵗʰ **E829 Other road vehicle accidents**

[0,4,8,9] INCLUDES accident while boarding or alighting from
  blow from object in
  breakage of any part of   streetcar
  caught in door of   nonmotor road vehicle
  derailment of   not classifiable to
  fall in, on, or from   E826-E828
  fire in

  collision between streetcar or nonmotor road vehicle, except as in E826-E828, and:
  animal (not being ridden)
  another nonmotor road vehicle not classifiable to E826-E828
  pedestrian
  other object, fixed, movable, or moving, not set in motion by motor vehicle, railway train, or aircraft
  nonmotor road vehicle accident NOS
  streetcar accident NOS

EXCLUDES collision with:
  animal being ridden (E828.0-E828.9)
  animal-drawn vehicle (E827.0-E827.9)
  pedal cycle (E826.0-E826.9)

Water Transport Accidents (E830-E838)

NOTE For definitions of water transport accident and related terms see definitions (a), (s), and (t).

INCLUDES watercraft accidents in the course of recreational activities

EXCLUDES accidents involving both aircraft, including objects set in motion by aircraft, and watercraft (E840.0-E845.9)

The following fourth digit subdivisions are for use with categories E830-E838 to identify the injured person:

.0 Occupant of small boat, unpowered
.1 Occupant of small boat, powered
  See definition (t)
  EXCLUDES water skier (.4)
.2 Occupant of other watercraft — crew
  Persons:
  engaged in operation of watercraft
  providing passenger services [cabin attendants, ship's physician, catering personnel]
  working on ship during voyage in other capacity [musician in band, operators of shops and beauty parlors]
.3 Occupant of other watercraft — other than crew
  Passenger
  Occupant of lifeboat, other than crew, after abandoning ship
.4 Water skier
.5 Swimmer
.6 Dockers, stevedores
  Longshoreman employed on the dock in loading and unloading ships
.7 Occupant of military watercraft, any type
.8 Other specified person
  Immigration and custom officials on board ship
  Person:
  accompanying passenger or member of crew visiting boat
  Pilot (guiding ship into port)
.9 Unspecified person

§ ✓4ᵗʰ **E830 Accident to watercraft causing submersion**

INCLUDES submersion and drowning due to:
  boat overturning
  boat submerging
  falling or jumping from burning ship
  falling or jumping from crushed watercraft
  ship sinking
  other accident to watercraft

§ ✓4ᵗʰ **E831 Accident to watercraft causing other injury**

INCLUDES any injury, except submersion and drowning, as a result of an accident to watercraft
  burned while ship on fire
  crushed between ships in collision
  crushed by lifeboat after abandoning ship
  fall due to collision or other accident to watercraft
  hit by falling object due to accident to watercraft
  injured in watercraft accident involving collision
  struck by boat or part thereof after fall or jump from damaged boat

EXCLUDES burns from localized fire or explosion on board ship (E837.0-E837.9)

§ ✓4ᵗʰ **E832 Other accidental submersion or drowning in water transport accident**

INCLUDES submersion or drowning as a result of an accident other than accident to the watercraft, such as:
  fall:
  from gangplank
  from ship
  overboard
  thrown overboard by motion of ship
  washed overboard

EXCLUDES submersion or drowning of swimmer or diver who voluntarily jumps from boat not involved in an accident (E910.0-E910.9)

§ ✓4ᵗʰ **E833 Fall on stairs or ladders in water transport**

EXCLUDES fall due to accident to watercraft (E831.0-E831.9)

§ ✓4ᵗʰ **E834 Other fall from one level to another in water transport**

EXCLUDES fall due to accident to watercraft (E831.0-E831.9)

§ ✓4ᵗʰ **E835 Other and unspecified fall in water transport**

EXCLUDES fall due to accident to watercraft (E831.0-E831.9)

§ ✓4ᵗʰ **E836 Machinery accident in water transport**

INCLUDES injuries in water transport caused by:
  deck
  engine room
  galley   } machinery
  laundry
  loading

§ ✓4ᵗʰ **E837 Explosion, fire, or burning in watercraft**

INCLUDES explosion of boiler on steamship
  localized fire on ship

EXCLUDES burning ship (due to collision or explosion) resulting in:
  submersion or drowning (E830.0-E830.9)
  other injury (E831.0-E831.9)

§ ✓4ᵗʰ **E838 Other and unspecified water transport accident**

INCLUDES accidental poisoning by gases or fumes on ship
  atomic power plant malfunction in watercraft
  crushed between ship and stationary object [wharf]
  crushed between ships without accident to watercraft
  crushed by falling object on ship or while loading or unloading
  hit by boat while water skiing
  struck by boat or part thereof (after fall from boat)
  watercraft accident NOS

---

§   Requires fourth digit. Valid digits are in [brackets] under each code. See beginning of appropriate section for codes and definitions.

✓4ᵗʰ Fourth-digit Required   ▶◀ Revised Text   ● New Code   ▲ Revised Code TitleDx

8 – E Codes   2014 ICD-9-CM

Air and Space Transport Accidents (E840-E845)

NOTE For definition of aircraft and related terms see definitions (u) and (v).

The following fourth digit subdivisions are for use with categories E840-E845 to identify the injured person. Valid fourth digits are in [brackets] under codes E842-E845:

.0 Occupant of spacecraft

.1 Occupant of military aircraft, any
Crew in military aircraft [air force] [army] [national guard] [navy]
Passenger (civilian) (military) in military aircraft [air force] [army] [national guard] [navy]
Troops in military aircraft [air force] [army] [national guard] [navy]
EXCLUDES occupants of aircraft operated under jurisdiction of police departments (.5)
parachutist (.7)

.2 Crew of commercial aircraft (powered) in surface to surface transport

.3 Other occupant of commercial aircraft (powered) in surface to surface transport
Flight personnel:
not part of crew
on familiarization flight
Passenger on aircraft (powered) NOS

.4 Occupant of commercial aircraft (powered) in surface to air transport
Occupant [crew] [passenger] of aircraft (powered) engaged in activities, such as:
aerial spraying (crops) (fire retardants)
air drops of emergency supplies
air drops of parachutists, except from military craft
crop dusting
lowering of construction material [bridge or telephone pole]
sky writing

.5 Occupant of other powered aircraft
Occupant [crew] [passenger] of aircraft (powered) engaged in activities, such as:
aerobatic flying
aircraft racing
rescue operation
storm surveillance
traffic surveillance
Occupant of private plane NOS

.6 Occupant of unpowered aircraft, except parachutist
Occupant of aircraft classifiable to E842

.7 Parachutist (military) (other)
Person making voluntary descent
EXCLUDES person making descent after accident to aircraft (.1-.6)

.8 Ground crew, airline employee
Persons employed at airfields (civil) (military) or launching pads, not occupants of aircraft

.9 Other person

✓4ᵗʰ **E840 Accident to powered aircraft at takeoff or landing**
INCLUDES collision of aircraft with any object, fixed, movable, or moving } while taking off or landing
crash
explosion on aircraft
fire on aircraft
forced landing

✓4ᵗʰ **E841 Accident to powered aircraft, other and unspecified**
INCLUDES aircraft accident NOS
aircraft crash or wreck NOS
any accident to powered aircraft while in transit or when not specified whether in transit, taking off, or landing
collision of aircraft with another aircraft, bird, or any object, while in transit
explosion on aircraft while in transit
fire on aircraft while in transit

✓4ᵗʰ **E842 Accident to unpowered aircraft**
[6-9] **INCLUDES** any accident, except collision with powered aircraft, to:
balloon
glider
hang glider
kite carrying a person
hit by object falling from unpowered aircraft

§ ✓4ᵗʰ **E843 Fall in, on, or from aircraft**
[0-9] **INCLUDES** accident in boarding or alighting from aircraft, any kind
fall in, on, or from aircraft [any kind], while in transit, taking off, or landing, except when as a result of an accident to aircraft

§ ✓4ᵗʰ **E844 Other specified air transport accidents**
[0-9] **INCLUDES** hit by:
aircraft
object falling from aircraft
injury by or from:
machinery of aircraft } without
rotating propeller } accident
voluntary parachute descent } to aircraft
poisoning by carbon monoxide from aircraft while in transit
sucked into jet
any accident involving other transport vehicle (motor) (nonmotor) due to being hit by object set in motion by aircraft (powered)
EXCLUDES air sickness (E903)
effects of:
high altitude (E902.0-E902.1)
pressure change (E902.0-E902.1)
injury in parachute descent due to accident to aircraft (E840.0-E842-9)

§ ✓4ᵗʰ **E845 Accident involving spacecraft**
[0,8,9] **INCLUDES** launching pad accident
EXCLUDES effects of weightlessness in spacecraft (E928.0)

Vehicle Accidents Not Elsewhere Classifiable (E846-E848)

E846 Accidents involving powered vehicles used solely within the buildings and premises of industrial or commercial establishment
Accident to, on, or involving:
battery powered airport passenger vehicle
battery powered trucks (baggage) (mail)
coal car in mine
logging car
self propelled truck, industrial
station baggage truck (powered)
tram, truck, or tub (powered) in mine or quarry
Collision with:
pedestrian
other vehicle or object within premises
Explosion of
Fall from } powered vehicle, industrial or
Overturning of } commercial
Struck by
EXCLUDES accidental poisoning by exhaust gas from vehicle not elsewhere classifiable (E868.2)
injury by crane, lift (fork), or elevator (E919.2)

E847 Accidents involving cable cars not running on rails
Accident to, on, or involving:
cable car, not on rails
ski chair-lift
ski-lift with gondola
téléférique
Breakage of cable
Caught or dragged by
Fall or jump from } cable car, not on rails
Object thrown from or in

E848 Accidents involving other vehicles, not elsewhere classifiable
Accident to, on, or involving:
ice yacht
land yacht
nonmotor, nonroad vehicle NOS

Requires fourth digit. See beginning of appropriate section for codes and definitions.

E Codes

E849–E851

Place of Occurrence (E849)

☑4ᵗʰ **E849 Place of Occurrence**

NOTE The following category is for use to denote the place where the injury or poisoning occurred.

E849.0 Home

Apartment	Private:
Boarding house	garage
Farm house	garden
Home premises	home
House (residential)	walk
Noninstitutional place	Swimming pool in private
of residence	house or garden
Private:	Yard of home
driveway	

EXCLUDES home under construction but not yet occupied (E849.3)

institutional place of residence (E849.7)

E849.1 Farm

Farm:
  buildings
  land under cultivation

EXCLUDES farm house and home premises of farm (E849.0)

E849.2 Mine and quarry

Gravel pit	Tunnel under construction
Sand pit	

E849.3 Industrial place and premises

Building under construction	Industrial yard
Dockyard	Loading platform (factory)
Dry dock	(store)
Factory	Plant, industrial
building	Railway yard
premises	Shop (place of work)
Garage (place of work)	Warehouse
	Workhouse

E849.4 Place for recreation and sport

Amusement park	Playground, including school
Baseball field	playground
Basketball court	Public park
Beach resort	Racecourse
Cricket ground	Resort NOS
Fives court	Riding school
Football field	Rifle range
Golf course	Seashore resort
Gymnasium	Skating rink
Hockey field	Sports palace
Holiday camp	Stadium
Ice palace	Swimming pool, public
Lake resort	Tennis court
Mountain resort	Vacation resort

EXCLUDES that in private house or garden (E849.0)

E849.5 Street and highway

E849.6 Public building

Building (including adjacent grounds) used by the general public or by a particular group of the public, such as:

airport	music hall
bank	nightclub
café	office
casino	office building
church	opera house
cinema	post office
clubhouse	public hall
courthouse	radio broadcasting station
dance hall	restaurant
garage building	school (state) (public) (private)
(for car storage)	shop, commercial
hotel	station (bus) (railway)
market (grocery or	store
other commodity)	theater
movie house	

EXCLUDES home garage (E849.0)

industrial building or workplace (E849.3)

E849.7 Residential institution

Children's home	Old people's home
Dormitory	Orphanage
Hospital	Prison
Jail	Reform school

E849.8 Other specified places

Beach NOS	Pond or pool (natural)
Canal	Prairie
Caravan site NOS	Public place NOS
Derelict house	Railway line
Desert	Reservoir
Dock	River
Forest	Sea
Harbor	Seashore NOS
Hill	Stream
Lake NOS	Swamp
Mountain	Trailer court
Parking lot	Woods
Parking place	

E849.9 Unspecified place

Accidental Poisoning by Drugs, Medicinal Substances, and Biologicals (E850-E858)

INCLUDES accidental overdose of drug, wrong drug given or taken in error, and drug taken inadvertently

accidents in the use of drugs and biologicals in medical and surgical procedures

EXCLUDES administration with suicidal or homicidal intent or intent to harm, or in circumstances classifiable to E980-E989 (E950.0-E950.5, E962.0, E980.0-E980.5)

correct drug properly administered in therapeutic or prophylactic dosage, as the cause of adverse effect (E930.0-E949.9)

NOTE See Alphabetic Index for more complete list of specific drugs to be classified under the fourth digit subdivisions. The American Hospital Formulary numbers can be used to classify new drugs listed by the American Hospital Formulary Service (AHFS). See Appendix C.

☑4ᵗʰ **E850 Accidental poisoning by analgesics, antipyretics, and antirheumatics**

E850.0 Heroin
Diacetylmorphine

E850.1 Methadone

E850.2 Other opiates and related narcotics
Codeine [methylmorphine]
Meperidine [pethidine]
Morphine
Opium (alkaloids)

E850.3 Salicylates
Acetylsalicylic acid [aspirin]
Amino derivatives of salicylic acid
Salicylic acid salts

E850.4 Aromatic analgesics, not elsewhere classified
Acetanilid
Paracetamol [acetaminophen]
Phenacetin [acetophenetidin]

E850.5 Pyrazole derivatives
Aminophenazone [amidopyrine]
Phenylbutazone

E850.6 Antirheumatics [antiphlogistics]
Gold salts
Indomethacin
EXCLUDES salicylates (E850.3)
steroids (E858.0)

E850.7 Other non-narcotic analgesics
Pyrabital

E850.8 Other specified analgesics and antipyretics
Pentazocine

E850.9 Unspecified analgesic or antipyretic

E851 Accidental poisoning by barbiturates
Amobarbital [amylobarbitone]
Barbital [barbitone]
Butabarbital [butabarbitone]
Pentobarbital [pentobarbitone]
Phenobarbital [phenobarbitone]
Secobarbital [quinalbarbitone]
EXCLUDES thiobarbiturates (E855.1)

☑4ᵗʰ Fourth-digit Required   ▶◀ Revised Text   ● New Code   ▲ Revised Code TitleDx

☑️4ᵗʰ **E852 Accidental poisoning by other sedatives and hypnotics**

E852.0 Chloral hydrate group

E852.1 Paraldehyde

E852.2 Bromine compounds
Bromides
Carbromal (derivatives)

E852.3 Methaqualone compounds

E852.4 Glutethimide group

E852.5 Mixed sedatives, not elsewhere classified

E852.8 Other specified sedatives and hypnotics

E852.9 Unspecified sedative or hypnotic
Sleeping:
drug ⎫
pill ⎬ NOS
tablet ⎭

☑️4ᵗʰ **E853 Accidental poisoning by tranquilizers**

E853.0 Phenothiazine-based tranquilizers
Chlorpromazine   Prochlorperazine
Fluphenazine   Promazine

E853.1 Butyrophenone-based tranquilizers
Haloperidol   Trifluperidol
Spiperone

E853.2 Benzodiazepine-based tranquilizers
Chlordiazepoxide Lorazepam
Diazepam   Medazepam
Flurazepam   Nitrazepam

E853.8 Other specified tranquilizers
Hydroxyzine   Meprobamate

E853.9 Unspecified tranquilizer

☑️4ᵗʰ **E854 Accidental poisoning by other psychotropic agents**

E854.0 Antidepressants
Amitriptyline
Imipramine
Monoamine oxidase [MAO] inhibitors

E854.1 Psychodysleptics [hallucinogens]
Cannabis derivatives   Mescaline
Lysergide [LSD]   Psilocin
Marihuana (derivatives) Psilocybin

E854.2 Psychostimulants
Amphetamine
Caffeine

EXCLUDES *central appetite depressants (E858.8)*

E854.3 Central nervous system stimulants
Analeptics
Opiate antagonists

E854.8 Other psychotropic agents

☑️4ᵗʰ **E855 Accidental poisoning by other drugs acting on central and autonomic nervous system**

E855.0 Anticonvulsant and anti-Parkinsonism drugs
Amantadine
Hydantoin derivatives
Levodopa [L-dopa]
Oxazolidine derivatives [paramethadione] [trimethadione]
Succinimides

E855.1 Other central nervous system depressants
Ether
Gaseous anesthetics
Halogenated hydrocarbon derivatives
Intravenous anesthetics
Thiobarbiturates, such as thiopental sodium

E855.2 Local anesthetics
Cocaine   Procaine
Lidocaine [lignocaine] Tetracaine

E855.3 Parasympathomimetics [cholinergics]
Acetylcholine   Anticholinesterase:
Anticholinesterase: reversible
  organophosphorus Pilocarpine

E855.4 Parasympatholytics [anticholinergics and antimuscarinics] and spasmolytics
Atropine   Hyoscine [scopamine]
Homatropine   Quaternary ammonium derivatives

E855.5 Sympathomimetics [adrenergics]
Epinephrine [adrenalin]
Levarterenol [noradrenalin]

E855.6 Sympatholytics [antiadrenergics]
Phenoxybenzamine
Tolazoline hydrochloride

E855.8 Other specified drugs acting on central and autonomic nervous systems

E855.9 Unspecified drug acting on central and autonomic nervous systems

E856 Accidental poisoning by antibiotics

E857 Accidental poisoning by other anti-infectives

☑️4ᵗʰ **E858 Accidental poisoning by other drugs**

E858.0 Hormones and synthetic substitutes

E858.1 Primarily systemic agents

E858.2 Agents primarily affecting blood constituents

E858.3 Agents primarily affecting cardiovascular system

E858.4 Agents primarily affecting gastrointestinal system

E858.5 Water, mineral, and uric acid metabolism drugs

E858.6 Agents primarily acting on the smooth and skeletal muscles and respiratory system

E858.7 Agents primarily affecting skin and mucous membrane, ophthalmological, otorhinolaryngological, and dental drugs

E858.8 Other specified drugs
Central appetite depressants

E858.9 Unspecified drug

Accidental Poisoning by Other Solid and Liquid Substances, Gases, and Vapors (E860-E869)

NOTE Categories in this section are intended primarily to indicate the external cause of poisoning states classifiable to 980-989. They may also be used to indicate external causes of localized effects classifiable to 001-799.

☑️4ᵗʰ **E860 Accidental poisoning by alcohol, not elsewhere classified**

E860.0 Alcoholic beverages
Alcohol in preparations intended for consumption

E860.1 Other and unspecified ethyl alcohol and its products
Denatured alcohol   Grain alcohol NOS
Ethanol NOS   Methylated spirit

E860.2 Methyl alcohol
Methanol   Wood alcohol

E860.3 Isopropyl alcohol
Dimethyl carbinol   Rubbing alcohol subsitute
Isopropanol   Secondary propyl alcohol

E860.4 Fusel oil
Alcohol: Alcohol:
amyl   propyl
butyl

E860.8 Other specified alcohols

E860.9 Unspecified alcohol

☑️4ᵗʰ **E861 Accidental poisoning by cleansing and polishing agents, disinfectants, paints, and varnishes**

E861.0 Synthetic detergents and shampoos

E861.1 Soap products

E861.2 Polishes

E861.3 Other cleansing and polishing agents
Scouring powders

E861.4 Disinfectants
Household and other disinfectants not ordinarily used on the person
EXCLUDES   *carbolic acid or phenol (E864.0)*

E861.5 Lead paints

E861.6 Other paints and varnishes
Lacquers	Paints, other than lead
Oil colors	White washes

E861.9 Unspecified

☑4ᵗʰ **E862 Accidental poisoning by petroleum products, other solvents and their vapors, not elsewhere classified**

E862.0 Petroleum solvents
Petroleum:	Petroleum:
ether	naphtha
benzine	

E862.1 Petroleum fuels and cleaners
Antiknock additives to petroleum fuels
Gas oils
Gasoline or petrol
Kerosene
EXCLUDES   *kerosene insecticides (E863.4)*

E862.2 Lubricating oils

E862.3 Petroleum solids
Paraffin wax

E862.4 Other specified solvents
Benzene

E862.9 Unspecified solvent

☑4ᵗʰ **E863 Accidental poisoning by agricultural and horticultural chemical and pharmaceutical preparations other than plant foods and fertilizers**
EXCLUDES   *plant foods and fertilizers (E866.5)*

E863.0 Insecticides of organochlorine compounds
Benzene hexachloride	Dieldrin
Chlordane	Endrine
DDT	Toxaphene

E863.1 Insecticides of organophosphorus compounds
Demeton	Parathion
Diazinon	Phenylsulphthion
Dichlorvos	Phorate
Malathion	Phosdrin
Methyl parathion	

E863.2 Carbamates
Aldicarb	Propoxur
Carbaryl	

E863.3 Mixtures of insecticides

E863.4 Other and unspecified insecticides
Kerosene insecticides

E863.5 Herbicides
2, 4-Dichlorophenoxyacetic acid [2, 4-D]
2, 4, 5-Trichlorophenoxyacetic acid [2, 4, 5-T]
Chlorates
Diquat
Mixtures of plant foods and fertilizers with herbicides
Paraquat

E863.6 Fungicides
Organic mercurials (used in seed dressing)
Pentachlorophenols

E863.7 Rodenticides
Fluoroacetates	Warfarin
Squill and derivatives	Zinc phosphide
Thallium	

E863.8 Fumigants
Cyanides	Phosphine
Methyl bromide	

E863.9 Other and unspecified

☑4ᵗʰ **E864 Accidental poisoning by corrosives and caustics, not elsewhere classified**
EXCLUDES   *those as components of disinfectants (E861.4)*

E864.0 Corrosive aromatics
Carbolic acid or phenol

E864.1 Acids
Acid:
  hydrochloric
  nitric
  sulfuric

E864.2 Caustic alkalis
Lye

E864.3 Other specified corrosives and caustics

E864.4 Unspecified corrosives and caustics

☑4ᵗʰ **E865 Accidental poisoning from poisonous foodstuffs and poisonous plants**
INCLUDES   any meat, fish, or shellfish
           plants, berries, and fungi eaten as, or in mistake for, food, or by a child
EXCLUDES   *anaphylactic shock due to adverse food reaction (995.60-995.69)*
           food poisoning (bacterial) (005.0-005.9)
           poisoning and toxic reactions to venomous plants (E905.6-E905.7)

E865.0 Meat

E865.1 Shellfish

E865.2 Other fish

E865.3 Berries and seeds

E865.4 Other specified plants

E865.5 Mushrooms and other fungi

E865.8 Other specified foods

E865.9 Unspecified foodstuff or poisonous plant

☑4ᵗʰ **E866 Accidental poisoning by other and unspecified solid and liquid substances**
EXCLUDES   *these substances as a component of:*
           medicines (E850.0-E858.9)
           paints (E861.5-E861.6)
           pesticides (E863.0-E863.9)
           petroleum fuels (E862.1)

E866.0 Lead and its compounds and fumes

E866.1 Mercury and its compounds and fumes

E866.2 Antimony and its compounds and fumes

E866.3 Arsenic and its compounds and fumes

E866.4 Other metals and their compounds and fumes
Beryllium (compounds)	Iron (compounds)
Brass fumes	Manganese (compounds)
Cadmium (compounds)	Nickel (compounds)
Copper salts	Thallium (compounds)

E866.5 Plant foods and fertilizers
EXCLUDES   *mixtures with herbicides (E863.5)*

E866.6 Glues and adhesives

E866.7 Cosmetics

E866.8 Other specified solid or liquid substances

E866.9 Unspecified solid or liquid substance

E867 Accidental poisoning by gas distributed by pipeline
Carbon monoxide from incomplete combustion of piped gas
Coal gas NOS
Liquefied petroleum gas distributed through pipes (pure or mixed with air)
Piped gas (natural) (manufactured)

☑4ᵗʰ Fourth-digit Required   ▶◀ Revised Text   ● New Code   ▲ Revised Code TitleDx

✓4ᵗʰ **E868 Accidental poisoning by other utility gas and other carbon monoxide**

E868.0 Liquefied petroleum gas distributed in mobile containers

Butane	} or carbon monoxide
Liquefied hydrocarbon gas	from incomplete
NOS	conbustion of
Propane	these gases

E868.1 Other and unspecified utility gas

Acetylene	} or carbon monoxide
Gas NOS used for lighting,	from incomplete
heating, or cooking	conbustion of
Water gas	these gases

E868.2 Motor vehicle exhaust gas

Exhaust gas from:
any type of combustion engine not in watercraft
farm tractor, not in transit
gas engine
motor pump
motor vehicle, not in transit

EXCLUDES poisoning by carbon monoxide from:
aircraft while in transit (E844.0-E844.9)
motor vehicle while in transit (E818.0-E818.9)
watercraft whether or not in transit
(E838.0-E838.9)

E868.3 Carbon monoxide from incomplete combustion of other domestic fuels

Carbon monoxide from incomplete combustion of:

coal	}
coke	in domestic stove or fireplace
kerosene	
wood	

EXCLUDES carbon monoxide from smoke and fumes due to conflagration (E890.0-E893.9)

E868.8 Carbon monoxide from other sources

Carbon monoxide from:
blast furnace gas
incomplete combustion of fuels in industrial use
kiln vapor

E868.9 Unspecified carbon monoxide

✓4ᵗʰ **E869 Accidental poisoning by other gases and vapors**

EXCLUDES effects of gases used as anesthetics (E855.1, E938.2)
fumes from heavy metals (E866.0-E866.4)
smoke and fumes due to conflagration or explosion (E890.0-E899)

E869.0 Nitrogen oxides

E869.1 Sulfur dioxide

E869.2 Freon

E869.3 Lacrimogenic gas [tear gas]
Bromobenzyl cyanide
Chloroacetophenone
Ethyliodoacetate

E869.4 Second-hand tobacco smoke

E869.8 Other specified gases and vapors
Chlorine
Hydrocyanic acid gas

E869.9 Unspecified gases and vapors

Misadventures to Patients During Surgical and Medical Care (E870-E876)

EXCLUDES accidental overdose of drug and wrong drug given in error
(E850.0-E858.9)
surgical and medical procedures as the cause of abnormal reaction by
the patient, without mention of misadventure at the time of
procedure (E878.0-E879.9)

✓4ᵗʰ **E870 Accidental cut, puncture, perforation, or hemorrhage during medical care**

E870.0 Surgical operation

E870.1 Infusion or transfusion

E870.2 Kidney dialysis or other perfusion

E870.3 Injection or vaccination

E870.4 Endoscopic examination

E870.5 Aspiration of fluid or tissue, puncture, and catheterization
Abdominal paracentesis
Aspirating needle biopsy
Blood sampling
Lumbar puncture
Thoracentesis
EXCLUDES heart catheterization (E870.6)

E870.6 Heart catheterization

E870.7 Administration of enema

E870.8 Other specified medical care

E870.9 Unspecified medical care

✓4ᵗʰ **E871 Foreign object left in body during procedure**

E871.0 Surgical operation

E871.1 Infusion or transfusion

E871.2 Kidney dialysis or other perfusion

E871.3 Injection or vaccination

E871.4 Endoscopic examination

E871.5 Aspiration of fluid or tissue, puncture, and catheterization
Abdominal paracentesis
Aspiration needle biopsy
Blood sampling
Lumbar puncture
Thoracentesis
EXCLUDES heart catheterization (E871.6)

E871.6 Heart catheterization

E871.7 Removal of catheter or packing

E871.8 Other specified procedures

E871.9 Unspecified procedure

✓4ᵗʰ **E872 Failure of sterile precautions during procedure**

E872.0 Surgical operation

E872.1 Infusion or transfusion

E872.2 Kidney dialysis and other perfusion

E872.3 Injection or vaccination

E872.4 Endoscopic examination

E872.5 Aspiration of fluid or tissue, puncture, and catheterization

Abdominal paracentesis	Lumbar puncture
Aspiration needle biopsy	Thoracentesis
Blood sampling	

EXCLUDES heart catheterization (E872.6)

E872.6 Heart catheterization

E872.8 Other specified procedures

E872.9 Unspecified procedure

✓4ᵗʰ **E873 Failure in dosage**

EXCLUDES accidental overdose of drug, medicinal or biological substance (E850.0-E858.9)

E873.0 Excessive amount of blood or other fluid during transfusion or infusion

E873.1 Incorrect dilution of fluid during infusion

E873.2 Overdose of radiation in therapy

E873.3 Inadvertent exposure of patient to radiation during medical care

E873.4 Failure in dosage in electroshock or insulin-shock therapy

E873.5 Inappropriate [too hot or too cold] temperature in local application and packing

E873.6 Nonadministration of necessary drug or medicinal substance

E873.8 Other specified failure in dosage

E873.9 Unspecified failure in dosage

E Codes

E874–E879.9

☑4ᵗʰ **E874 Mechanical failure of instrument or apparatus during procedure**

E874.0 Surgical operation

E874.1 Infusion and transfusion
    Air in system

E874.2 Kidney dialysis and other perfusion

E874.3 Endoscopic examination

E874.4 Aspiration of fluid or tissue, puncture, and catheterization
    Abdominal paracentesis   Lumbar puncture
    Aspiration needle biopsy   Thoracentesis
    Blood sampling
    EXCLUDES heart catheterization (E874.5)

E874.5 Heart catheterization

E874.8 Other specified procedures

E874.9 Unspecified procedure

☑4ᵗʰ **E875 Contaminated or infected blood, other fluid, drug, or biological substance**
    INCLUDES presence of:
        bacterial pyrogens
        endotoxin-producing bacteria
        serum hepatitis-producing agent

E875.0 Contaminated substance transfused or infused

E875.1 Contaminated substance injected or used for vaccination

E875.2 Contaminated drug or biological substance administered by other means

E875.8 Other

E875.9 Unspecified

☑4ᵗʰ **E876 Other and unspecified misadventures during medical care**

E876.0 Mismatched blood in transfusion

E876.1 Wrong fluid in infusion

E876.2 Failure in suture and ligature during surgical operation

E876.3 Endotracheal tube wrongly placed during anesthetic procedure

E876.4 Failure to introduce or to remove other tube or instrument
    EXCLUDES foreign object left in body during procedure (E871.0-E871.9)

* **E876.5 Performance of wrong operation (procedure) on correct patient**
    Wrong device implanted into correct surgical site
    EXCLUDES correct operation (procedure) performed on wrong body part (E876.7)

* **E876.6 Performance of operation (procedure) on patient not scheduled for surgery**
    Performance of operation (procedure) intended for another patient
    Performance of operation (procedure) on wrong patient

* **E876.7 Performance of correct operation (procedure) on wrong side/body part**
    Performance of correct operation (procedure) on wrong side
    Performance of correct operation (procedure) on wrong site

E876.8 Other specified misadventures during medical care
    Performance of inappropriate treatment NEC

E876.9 Unspecified misadventure during medical care

Surgical and Medical Procedures as the Cause of Abnormal Reaction of Patient or Later Complication, Without Mention of Misadventure at the Time of Procedure (E878-E879)

    INCLUDES procedures as the cause of abnormal reaction, such as:
        displacement or malfunction of prosthetic device
        hepatorenal failure, postoperative
        malfunction of external stoma
        postoperative intestinal obstruction
        rejection of transplanted organ
    EXCLUDES anesthetic management properly carried out as the cause of adverse effect (E937.0-E938.9)
    infusion and transfusion, without mention of misadventure in the technique of procedure (E930.0-E949.9)

☑4ᵗʰ **E878 Surgical operation and other surgical procedures as the cause of abnormal reaction of patient, or of later complication, without mention of misadventure at the time of operation**

E878.0 Surgical operation with transplant of whole organ
    Transplantation of:
        heart
        kidney
        liver

E878.1 Surgical operation with implant of artificial internal device
    Cardiac pacemaker
    Electrodes implanted in brain
    Heart valve prosthesis
    Internal orthopedic device

E878.2 Surgical operation with anastomosis, bypass, or graft, with natural or artificial tissues used as implant
    Anastomosis:
        arteriovenous
        gastrojejunal
    Graft of blood vessel, tendon, or skin
    EXCLUDES external stoma (E878.3)

E878.3 Surgical operation with formation of external stoma
    Colostomy   Gastrostomy
    Cystostomy   Ureterostomy
    Duodenostomy

E878.4 Other restorative surgery

E878.5 Amputation of limb(s)

E878.6 Removal of other organ (partial) (total)

E878.8 Other specified surgical operations and procedures

E878.9 Unspecified surgical operations and procedures

☑4ᵗʰ **E879 Other procedures, without mention of misadventure at the time of procedure, as the cause of abnormal reaction of patient, or of later complication**

E879.0 Cardiac catheterization

E879.1 Kidney dialysis

E879.2 Radiological procedure and radiotherapy
    EXCLUDES radio-opaque dyes for diagnostic x-ray procedures (E947.8)

E879.3 Shock therapy
    Electroshock therapy
    Insulin-shock therapy

E879.4 Aspiration of fluid
    Lumbar puncture
    Thoracentesis

E879.5 Insertion of gastric or duodenal sound

E879.6 Urinary catheterization

E879.7 Blood sampling

E879.8 Other specified procedures
    Blood transfusion

E879.9 Unspecified procedure

---

* Wrong surgery edit applies.

☑4ᵗʰ Fourth-digit Required   ►◄ Revised Text   ● New Code   ▲ Revised Code TitleDx

Accidental Falls (E880-E888)

EXCLUDES *falls (in or from):*
　burning building (E890.8, E891.8)
　into fire (E890.0-E899)
　into water (with submersion or drowning)
　　(E910.0-E910.9)
　machinery (in operation) (E919.0-E919.9)
　on edged, pointed, or sharp object (E920.0-E920.9)
　transport vehicle (E800.0-E845.9)
　vehicle not elsewhere classifiable (E846-E848)

✓4th **E880　Fall on or from stairs or steps**

E880.0　Escalator

E880.1　Fall on or from sidewalk curb
　EXCLUDES *fall from moving sidewalk (E885.9)*

E880.9　Other stairs or steps

✓4th **E881　Fall on or from ladders or scaffolding**

E881.0　Fall from ladder

E881.1　Fall from scaffolding

E882　Fall from or out of building or other structure
　Fall from:　　　　　Fall from:
　　balcony　　　　　　turret
　　bridge　　　　　　viaduct
　　building　　　　　wall
　　flagpole　　　　　window
　　tower　　　　　　　Fall through roof
　EXCLUDES *collapse of a building or structure (E916)*
　　　　　fall or jump from burning building (E890.8, E891.8)

✓4th **E883　Fall into hole or other opening in surface**
　INCLUDES fall into:　　　　fall into:
　　　　cavity　　　　　shaft
　　　　dock　　　　　　swimming pool
　　　　hole　　　　　　tank
　　　　pit　　　　　　　well
　　　　quarry
　EXCLUDES *fall into water NOS (E910.9)*
　　　　that resulting in drowning or submersion without mention
　　　　of injury (E910.0-E910.9)

E883.0　Accident from diving or jumping into water [swimming pool]
　Strike or hit:
　　against bottom when jumping or diving into water
　　wall or board of swimming pool
　　water surface
　EXCLUDES *diving with insufficient air supply (E913.2)*
　　　　effects of air pressure from diving (E902.2)

E883.1　Accidental fall into well

E883.2　Accidental fall into storm drain or manhole

E883.9　Fall into other hole or other opening in surface

✓4th **E884　Other fall from one level to another**

E884.0　Fall from playground equipment
　EXCLUDES *recreational machinery (E919.8)*

E884.1　Fall from cliff

E884.2　Fall from chair

E884.3　Fall from wheelchair
　Fall from motorized mobility scooter
　Fall from motorized wheelchair

E884.4　Fall from bed

E884.5　Fall from other furniture

E884.6　Fall from commode
　Toilet

E884.9　Other fall from one level to another
　Fall from:　　　Fall from:
　　embankment　　stationary vehicle
　　haystack　　　　tree

✓4th **E885　Fall on same level from slipping, tripping, or stumbling**

E885.0　Fall from (nonmotorized) scooter
　EXCLUDES *fall from motorized mobility scooter (E884.3)*

E885.1　Fall from roller skates
　Heelies　　　　　Wheelies
　In-line skates

E885.2　Fall from skateboard

E885.3　Fall from skis

E885.4　Fall from snowboard

E885.9　Fall from other slipping, tripping, or stumbling
　Fall on moving sidewalk

✓4th **E886　Fall on same level from collision, pushing, or shoving, by or with other person**
　EXCLUDES *crushed or pushed by a crowd or human stampede (E917.1, E917.6)*

E886.0　In sports
　Tackles in sports
　EXCLUDES *kicked, stepped on, struck by object, in sports*
　　　　(E917.0, E917.5)

E886.9　Other and unspecified
　Fall from collision of pedestrian (conveyance) with another
　　pedestrian (conveyance)

E887　Fracture, cause unspecified

✓4th **E888　Other and unspecified fall**
　Accidental fall NOS
　Fall on same level NOS

E888.0　Fall resulting in striking against sharp object
　Use additional external cause code to identify object (E920)

E888.1　Fall resulting in striking against other object

E888.8　Other fall

E888.9　Unspecified fall
　Fall NOS

Accidents Caused by Fire and Flames (E890-E899)

INCLUDES asphyxia or poisoning due to conflagration or ignition
　burning by fire
　secondary fires resulting from explosion
EXCLUDES *arson (E968.0)*
　fire in or on:
　　machinery (in operation) (E919.0-E919.9)
　　transport vehicle other than stationary vehicle
　　　(E800.0-E845.9)
　　vehicle not elsewhere classifiable (E846-E848)

✓4th **E890　Conflagration in private dwelling**
　INCLUDES conflagration in:
　　　apartment
　　　boarding house
　　　camping place
　　　caravan
　　　farmhouse
　　　house
　　　lodging house
　　　mobile home
　　　private garage
　　　rooming house
　　　tenement
　　conflagration originating from sources classifiable to
　　　E893-E898 in the above buildings

E890.0　Explosion caused by conflagration

E890.1　Fumes from combustion of polyvinylchloride [PVC] and similar material in conflagration

E890.2　Other smoke and fumes from conflagration
　Carbon monoxide ⎫
　Fumes NOS　　　⎬ from conflagration in private
　Smoke NOS　　　⎭　　building

E890.3　Burning caused by conflagration

E890.8　Other accident resulting from conflagration
　Collapse of　　　　⎫
　Fall from　　　　　⎬ burning private
　Hit by object falling from　　building
　Jump from　　　　⎭

E890.9　Unspecified accident resulting from conflagration in private dwelling

E Codes

E891–E899

✓4ᵗʰ **E891 Conflagration in other and unspecified building or structure**
Conflagration in:
- barn
- church
- convalescent and other residential home
- dormitory of educational institution
- factory
- farm outbuildings
- hospital
- hotel
- school
- store
- theater

Conflagration originating from sources classifiable to E893-E898, in the above buildings

E891.0 Explosion caused by conflagration

E891.1 Fumes from combustion of polyvinylchloride [PVC] and similar material in conflagration

E891.2 Other smoke and fumes from conflagration
Carbon monoxide }
Fumes NOS } from conflagration in private
Smoke NOS } building or structure

E891.3 Burning caused by conflagration

E891.8 Other accident resulting from conflagration
Collapse of }
Fall from } burning private
Hit by object falling from } building or
Jump from } structure

E891.9 Unspecified accident resulting from conflagration of other and unspecified building or structure

E892 Conflagration not in building or structure
Fire (uncontrolled) (in) (of):   Fire (uncontrolled) (in) (of):
- forest   prairie
- grass   transport vehicle [any],
- hay   except while in transit
- lumber   tunnel
- mine

✓4ᵗʰ **E893 Accident caused by ignition of clothing**
EXCLUDES *ignition of clothing:*
from highly inflammable material (E894)
with conflagration (E890.0-E892)

E893.0 From controlled fire in private dwelling
Ignition of clothing from:
normal fire (charcoal) (coal) }
(electric) (gas) (wood) in: } in private dwelling
brazier } (as listed in
fireplace } E890)
furnace }
stove }

E893.1 From controlled fire in other building or structure
Ignition of clothing from:
normal fire (charcoal) (coal) }
(electric) (gas) (wood) in: } in other building or
brazier } structure (as
fireplace } listed in E891)
furnace }
stove }

E893.2 From controlled fire not in building or structure
Ignition of clothing from:
- bonfire (controlled)
- brazier fire (controlled), not in building or structure
- trash fire (controlled)

EXCLUDES *conflagration not in building (E892)*
trash fire out of control (E892)

E893.8 From other specified sources
Ignition of clothing from: Ignition of clothing from:
- blowlamp   cigarette
- blowtorch   lighter
- burning bedspread   matches
- candle   pipe
- cigar   welding torch

E893.9 Unspecified source
Ignition of clothing (from controlled fire NOS) (in building NOS) NOS

E894 Ignition of highly inflammable material
Ignition of:
- benzine }
- gasoline }
- fat } (with ignition of clothing)
- kerosene }
- paraffin }
- petrol }

EXCLUDES *ignition of highly inflammable material with:*
conflagration (E890.0-E892)
explosion (E923.0-E923.9)

E895 Accident caused by controlled fire in private dwelling
Burning by (flame of) normal fire (charcoal) (coal) (electric) (gas) (wood) in:
- brazier }
- fireplace } in private dwelling (as listed in E890)
- furnace }
- stove }

EXCLUDES *burning by hot objects not producing fire or flames (E924.0-E924.9)*
ignition of clothing from these sources (E893.0)
poisoning by carbon monoxide from incomplete combustion of fuel (E867-E868.9)
that with conflagration (E890.0-E890.9)

E896 Accident caused by controlled fire in other and unspecified building or structure
Burning by (flame of) normal fire (charcoal) (coal)(electric)(gas)(wood) in:
- brazier }
- fireplace } in other building or structure (as
- furnace } listed in E891)
- stove }

EXCLUDES *burning by hot objects not producing fire or flames (E924.0-E924.9)*
ignition of clothing from these sources (E893.1)
poisoning by carbon monoxide from incomplete combustion of fuel (E867-E868.9)
that with conflagration (E891.0-E891.9)

E897 Accident caused by controlled fire not in building or structure
Burns from flame of:
- bonfire }
- brazier fire, not in building or structure } controlled
- trash fire }

EXCLUDES *ignition of clothing from these sources (E893.2)*
trash fire out of control (E892)
that with conflagration (E892)

✓4ᵗʰ **E898 Accident caused by other specified fire and flames**
EXCLUDES *conflagration (E890.0-E892)*
that with ignition of:
clothing (E893.0-E893.9)
highly inflammable material (E894)

E898.0 Burning bedclothes
Bed set on fire NOS

E898.1 Other
Burning by: Burning by:
- blowlamp   lamp
- blowtorch   lighter
- candle   matches
- cigar   pipe
- cigarette   welding torch
- fire in room NOS

E899 Accident caused by unspecified fire
Burning NOS

Accidents Due to Natural and Environmental Factors (E900-E909)

√4ᵗʰ E900 Excessive heat

E900.0 Due to weather conditions
Excessive heat as the external cause of:
   ictus solaris
   siriasis
   sunstroke

E900.1 Of man-made origin

Heat (in):	Heat (in):
boiler room	furnace room
drying room	generated in transport vehicle
factory	kitchen

E900.9 Of unspecified origin

√4ᵗʰ E901 Excessive cold

E901.0 Due to weather conditions
Excessive cold as the cause of:
   chilblains NOS
   immersion foot

E901.1 Of man-made origin

Contact with or inhalation of:	Prolonged exposure in:
dry ice	deep freeze unit
liquid air	refrigerator
liquid hydrogen	
liquid nitrogen	

E901.8 Other specified origin

E901.9 Of unspecified origin

√4ᵗʰ E902 High and low air pressure and changes in air pressure

E902.0 Residence or prolonged visit at high altitude
Residence or prolonged visit at high altitude as the cause of:
   Acosta syndrome
   Alpine sickness
   altitude sickness
   Andes disease
   anoxia, hypoxia
   barotitis, barodontalgia, barosinusitis, otitic barotrauma
   hypobarism, hypobaropathy
   mountain sickness
   range disease

E902.1 In aircraft
Sudden change in air pressure in aircraft during ascent or descent as the cause of:
   aeroneurosis
   aviators' disease

E902.2 Due to diving

High air pressure from rapid descent in water	as the cause of:
Reduction in atmospheric pressure while surfacing from deep water diving	caisson disease divers' disease divers' palsy or paralysis

E902.8 Due to other specified causes
Reduction in atmospheric pressure while surfacing from underground

E902.9 Unspecified cause

E903 Travel and motion

√4ᵗʰ E904 Hunger, thirst, exposure, and neglect
EXCLUDES *any condition resulting from homicidal intent (E968.0-E968.9)*
hunger, thirst, and exposure resulting from accidents connected with transport (E800.0-E848)

E904.0 Abandonment or neglect of infants and helpless persons

Exposure to weather conditions	resulting from abandonment or neglect
Hunger or thirst	

Desertion of newborn
Inattention at or after birth
Lack of care (helpless person) (infant)
EXCLUDES *criminal [purposeful] neglect (E968.4)*

E904.1 Lack of food
Lack of food as the cause of:
   inanition
   insufficient nourishment
   starvation
EXCLUDES *hunger resulting from abandonment or neglect (E904.0)*

E904.2 Lack of water
Lack of water as the cause of:
   dehydration
   inanition
EXCLUDES *dehydration due to acute fluid loss (276.51)*

E904.3 Exposure (to weather conditions), not elsewhere classifiable

Exposure NOS	Struck by hailstones
Humidity	

EXCLUDES *struck by lightning (E907)*

E904.9 Privation, unqualified
Destitution

√4ᵗʰ E905 Venomous animals and plants as the cause of poisoning and toxic reactions
INCLUDES chemical released by animal
insects
release of venom through fangs, hairs, spines, tentacles, and other venom apparatus
EXCLUDES *eating of poisonous animals or plants (E865.0-E865.9)*

E905.0 Venomous snakes and lizards

Cobra	Mamba
Copperhead snake	Rattlesnake
Coral snake	Sea snake
Fer de lance	Snake (venomous)
Gila monster	Viper
Krait	Water moccasin

EXCLUDES *bites of snakes and lizards known to be nonvenomous (E906.2)*

E905.1 Venomous spiders

Black widow spider	Tarantula (venomous)
Brown spider	

E905.2 Scorpion

E905.3 Hornets, wasps, and bees
Yellow jacket

E905.4 Centipede and venomous millipede (tropical)

E905.5 Other venomous arthropods
Sting of:
   ant
   caterpillar

E905.6 Venomous marine animals and plants

Puncture by sea urchin spine	Sting of:
Sting of:	sea anemone
coral	sea cucumber
jelly fish	other marine animal
nematocysts	or plant

EXCLUDES *bites and other injuries caused by nonvenomous marine animal (E906.2-E906.8)*
bite of sea snake (venomous) (E905.0)

E905.7 Poisoning and toxic reactions caused by other plants
Injection of poisons or toxins into or through skin by plant thorns, spines, or other mechanisms
EXCLUDES *puncture wound NOS by plant thorns or spines (E920.8)*

E905.8 Other specified

E905.9 Unspecified
Sting NOS
Venomous bite NOS

√4ᵗʰ E906 Other injury caused by animals
EXCLUDES *poisoning and toxic reactions caused by venomous animals and insects (E905.0-E905.9)*
road vehicle accident involving animals (E827.0-E828.9)
tripping or falling over an animal (E885.9)

E906.0 Dog bite

E906.1 Rat bite

E906.2 Bite of nonvenomous snakes and lizards

E906.3 Bite of other animal except arthropod
Cats
Moray eel
Rodents, except rats
Shark

E906.4 Bite of nonvenomous arthropod
Insect bite NOS

E906.5 Bite by unspecified animal
Animal bite NOS

E906.8 Other specified injury caused by animal
Butted by animal
Fallen on by horse or other animal, not being ridden
Gored by animal
Implantation of quills of porcupine
Pecked by bird
Run over by animal, not being ridden
Stepped on by animal, not being ridden
EXCLUDES injury by animal being ridden (E828.0-E828.9)

E906.9 Unspecified injury caused by animal

E907 Lightning
EXCLUDES injury from:
fall of tree or other object caused by lightning (E916)
fire caused by lightning (E890.0-E892)

✓4ᵗʰ E908 Cataclysmic storms, and floods resulting from storms
EXCLUDES collapse of dam or man-made structure causing flood (E909.3)

E908.0 Hurricane
Storm surge
"Tidal wave" caused by storm action
Typhoon

E908.1 Tornado
Cyclone
Twisters

E908.2 Floods
Torrential rainfall
Flash flood
EXCLUDES collapse of dam or man-made structure causing flood (E909.3)

E908.3 Blizzard (snow)(ice)

E908.4 Dust storm

E908.8 Other cataclysmic storms
Cloudburst

E908.9 Unspecified cataclysmic storms, and floods resulting from storms
Storm NOS

✓4ᵗʰ E909 Cataclysmic earth surface movements and eruptions

E909.0 Earthquakes

E909.1 Volcanic eruptions
Burns from lava
Ash inhalation

E909.2 Avalanche, landslide, or mudslide

E909.3 Collapse of dam or man-made structure

E909.4 Tidalwave caused by earthquake
Tidalwave NOS
Tsunami
EXCLUDES tidalwave caused by tropical storm (E908.0)

E909.8 Other cataclysmic earth surface movements and eruptions

E909.9 Unspecified cataclysmic earth surface movements and eruptions

Accidents Caused by Submersion, Suffocation, and Foreign Bodies (E910-E915)

✓4ᵗʰ E910 Accidental drowning and submersion
INCLUDES immersion
swimmers' cramp
EXCLUDES diving accident (NOS) (resulting in injury except drowning (E883.0)
diving with insufficient air supply (E913.2)
drowning and submersion due to:
cataclysm (E908-E909)
machinery accident (E919.0-E919.9)
transport accident (E800.0-E845.9)
effect of high and low air pressure (E902.2)
injury from striking against objects while in running water (E917.2)

E910.0 While water-skiing
Fall from water skis with submersion or drowning
EXCLUDES accident to water-skier involving a watercraft and resulting in submersion or other injury (E830.4, E831.4)

E910.1 While engaged in other sport or recreational activity wit diving equipment
Scuba diving NOS
Skin diving NOS
Underwater spear fishing NOS

E910.2 While engaged in other sport or recreational activity without diving equipment
Fishing or hunting, except from boat or with diving equipment
Ice skating
Playing in water
Surfboarding
Swimming NOS
Voluntarily jumping from boat, not involved in accident, f swim NOS
Wading in water
EXCLUDES jumping into water to rescue another person (E910.3)

E910.3 While swimming or diving for purposes other than recreation or sport
Marine salvage
Pearl diving
Placement of fishing nets
Rescue (attempt) of another person
Underwater construction or repairs
} (with diving equipment)

E910.4 In bathtub

E910.8 Other accidental drowning or submersion
Drowning in:
quenching tank
swimming pool

E910.9 Unspecified accidental drowning or submersion
Accidental fall into water NOS
Drowning NOS

E911 Inhalation and ingestion of food causing obstruction of respiratory tract or suffocation
Aspiration and inhalation of food [any] (into respiratory tract) NOS
Asphyxia by
Choked on
Suffocation by
} food [including bone, seed in food, regurgitated food]
Compression of trachea
Interruption of respiration
Obstruction of respiration
} by food lodged in esophagus
Obstruction of pharynx by food (bolus)
EXCLUDES injury, except asphyxia and obstruction of respiratory passage, caused by food (E915)
obstruction of esophagus by food without mention of asphyxia or obstruction of respiratory passage (E9

E912 Inhalation and ingestion of other object causing obstruction of respiratory tract or suffocation

Aspiration and inhalation of foreign body except food (into respiratory tract) NOS

Foreign object [bean] [marble] in nose

Obstruction of pharynx by foreign body

Compression

Interruption of respiration } by foreign body in esophagus

Obstruction of respiration

EXCLUDES *injury, except asphyxia and obstruction of respiratory passage, caused by foreign body (E915)*
obstruction of esophagus by foreign body without mention of asphyxia or obstruction in respiratory passage (E915)

✓4ᵗʰ E913 Accidental mechanical suffocation

EXCLUDES *mechanical suffocation from or by:*
accidental inhalation or ingestion of:
food (E911)
foreign object (E912)
cataclysm (E908-E909)
explosion (E921.0-E921.9, E923.0-E923.9)
machinery accident (E919.0-E919.9)

E913.0 In bed or cradle

EXCLUDES *suffocation by plastic bag (E913.1)*

E913.1 By plastic bag

E913.2 Due to lack of air (in closed place)

Accidentally closed up in refrigerator or other airtight enclosed space

Diving with insufficient air supply

EXCLUDES *suffocation by plastic bag (E913.1)*

E913.3 By falling earth or other substance

Cave-in NOS

EXCLUDES *cave-in caused by cataclysmic earth surface movements and eruptions (E909)*
struck by cave-in without asphyxiation or suffocation (E916)

E913.8 Other specified means

Accidental hanging, except in bed or cradle

E913.9 Unspecified means

Asphyxia, mechanical NOS

Strangulation NOS

Suffocation NOS

E914 Foreign body accidentally entering eye and adnexa

EXCLUDES *corrosive liquid (E924.1)*

E915 Foreign body accidentally entering other orifice

EXCLUDES *aspiration and inhalation of foreign body, any, (into respiratory tract) NOS (E911-E912)*

Other Accidents (E916-E928)

E916 Struck accidentally by falling object

Collapse of building, except on fire

Falling:
rock
snowslide NOS
stone
tree

Object falling from:
machine, not in operation
stationary vehicle

Code first:
collapse of building on fire (E890.0-E891.9)
falling object in:
cataclysm (E908-E909)
machinery accidents (E919.0-E919.9)
transport accidents (E800.0-E845.9)
vehicle accidents not elsewhere classifiable (E846-E848)
object set in motion by:
explosion (E921.0-E921.9, E923.0-E923.9)
firearm (E922.0-E922.9)
projected object (E917.0-E917.9)

✓4ᵗʰ E917 Striking against or struck accidentally by objects or persons

INCLUDES bumping into or against
colliding with
kicking against
stepping on
struck by

} object (moving) (projected) (stationary)
pedestrian conveyance
person

EXCLUDES *fall from:*
collision with another person, except when caused by a crowd (E886.0-E886.9)
stumbling over object (E885.9)
fall resulting in striking against object (E888.0, E888.1)
injury caused by:
assault (E960.0-E960.1, E967.0-E967.9)
cutting or piercing instrument (E920.0-E920.9)
explosion (E921.0-E921.9, E923.0-E923.9)
firearm (E922.0-E922.9)
machinery (E919.0-E919.9)
transport vehicle (E800.0-E845.9)
vehicle not elsewhere classifiable (E846-E848)

E917.0 In sports without subsequent fall

Kicked or stepped on during game (football) (rugby)

Struck by hit or thrown ball

Struck by hockey stick or puck

E917.1 Caused by a crowd, by collective fear or panic without subsequent fall

Crushed
Pushed
Stepped on
} by crowd or human stampede

E917.2 In running water without subsequent fall

EXCLUDES *drowning or submersion (E910.0-E910.9)*
that in sports (E917.0, E917.5)

E917.3 Furniture without subsequent fall

EXCLUDES *fall from furniture (E884.2, E884.4-E884.5)*

E917.4 Other stationary object without subsequent fall

Bath tub
Fence
Lamp-post

E917.5 Object in sports with subsequent fall

Knocked down while boxing

E917.6 Caused by a crowd, by collective fear or panic with subsequent fall

E917.7 Furniture with subsequent fall

EXCLUDES *fall from furniture (E884.2, E884.4-E884.5)*

E917.8 Other stationary object with subsequent fall

Bath tub
Fence
Lamp-post

E917.9 Other striking against with or without subsequent fall

E918 Caught accidentally in or between objects

Caught, crushed, jammed, or pinched in or between moving or stationary objects, such as:
escalator
folding object
hand tools, appliances, or implements
sliding door and door frame
under packing crate
washing machine wringer

EXCLUDES *injury caused by:*
cutting or piercing instrument (E920.0-E920.9)
machinery (E919.0-E919.9)
mechanism or component of firearm and air gun (E928.7)
transport vehicle (E800.0-E845.9)
vehicle not elsewhere classifiable (E846-E848)
struck accidentally by:
falling object (E916)
object (moving) (projected) (E917.0-E917.9)

☑4ᵗʰ **E919 Accidents caused by machinery**

INCLUDES

burned by
caught in (moving parts of)
collapse of
crushed by
cut or pierced by
drowning or submersion caused by
explosion of, on, in
fall from or into moving part of
fire starting in or on   machinery
mechanical suffocation caused by   (accident)
object falling from, on, in motion
     by
overturning of
pinned under
run over by
struck by
thrown from

caught between machinery and other object
machinery accident NOS

EXCLUDES   accidents involving machinery, not in operation (E884.9,
            E916-E918)
          injury caused by:
            electric current in connection with machinery
               (E925.0-E925.9)
            escalator (E880.0, E918)
            explosion of pressure vessel in connection with
               machinery (E921.0-E921.9)
            mechanism or component of firearm and air gun
               (E928.7)
            moving sidewalk (E885.9)
            powered hand tools, appliances, and implements
               (E916-E918, E920.0-E921.9, E923.0-E926.9)
            transport vehicle accidents involving machinery
               (E800.0-E848)
          poisoning by carbon monoxide generated by machine
               (E868.8)

E919.0 Agricultural machines

Animal-powered	Farm tractor
agricultural machine	Harvester
Combine	Hay mower or rake
Derrick, hay	Reaper
Farm machinery NOS	Thresher

EXCLUDES   that in transport under own power on the highway
            (E810.0-E819.9)
          that being towed by another vehicle on the
            highway (E810.0-E819.9, E827.0-E827.9,
            E829.0-E829.9)
          that involved in accident classifiable to E820-E829
            (E820.0-E829.9)

E919.1 Mining and earth-drilling machinery

Bore or drill (land) (seabed)
Shaft hoist
Shaft lift
Under-cutter

EXCLUDES   coal car, tram, truck, and tub in mine (E846)

E919.2 Lifting machines and appliances

Chain hoist
Crane
Derrick
Elevator (building) (grain)   except in agricultural
Forklift truck   or mining
Lift   operations
Pulley block
Winch

EXCLUDES   that being towed by another vehicle on the
            highway (E810.0-E819.9, E827.0-E827.9,
            E829.0-829.9)
          that in transport under own power on the highway
            (E810.0-E819.9)
          that involved in accident classifiable to E820-E829
            (E820.0-E829.9)

E919.3 Metalworking machines

Abrasive wheel	Metal:
Forging machine	milling machine
Lathe	power press
Mechanical shears	rolling-mill
Metal:	sawing machine
drilling machine	

E919.4 Woodworking and forming machines

Band saw	Overhead plane
Bench saw	Powered saw
Circular saw	Radial saw
Molding machine	Sander

EXCLUDES   hand saw (E920.1)

E919.5 Prime movers, except electrical motors

Gas turbine
Internal combustion engine
Steam engine
Water driven turbine

EXCLUDES   that being towed by other vehicle on the highway
            (E810.0-E819.9, E827.0-E827.9,
            E829.0-E829.9)
          that in transport under own power on the highway
            (E810.0-E819.9)

E919.6 Transmission machinery

Transmission:	Transmission:
belt	pinion
cable	pulley
chain	shaft
gear	

E919.7 Earth moving, scraping, and other excavating machines

Bulldozer	Steam shovel
Road scraper	

EXCLUDES   that being towed by other vehicle on the highway
            (E810.0-E819.9, E827.0-E827.9,
            E829.0-E829.9)
          that in transport under own power on the highway
            (E810.0-E819.9)

E919.8 Other specified machinery

Machines for manufacture of:
   clothing
   foodstuffs and beverages
   paper
Printing machine
Recreational machinery
Spinning, weaving, and textile machines

E919.9 Unspecified machinery

☑4ᵗʰ **E920 Accidents caused by cutting and piercing instruments or objects**

INCLUDES

                                  edged
accidental injury (by) object   pointed
                                  sharp

EXCLUDES   injury caused by mechanism or component of firearm and
            air gun (E928.7)

E920.0 Powered lawn mower

E920.1 Other powered hand tools

Any powered hand tool [compressed air] [electric]
     [explosive cartridge] [hydraulic power], such as:
     drill
     hand saw
     hedge clipper
     rivet gun
     snow blower
     staple gun

EXCLUDES   band saw (E919.4)
          bench saw (E919.4)

E920.2 Powered household appliances and implements

Blender	Electric:
Electric:	knife
beater or mixer	sewing machine
can opener	Garbage disposal appliance
fan	

E920.3 Knives, swords, and daggers

E920.4 Other hand tools and implements

Axe	Paper cutter
Can opener NOS	Pitchfork
Chisel	Rake
Fork	Scissors
Hand saw	Screwdriver
Hoe	Sewing machine, not powered
Ice pick	Shovel
Needle (sewing)	

E920.5 Hypodermic needle
Contaminated needle
Needle stick

E920.8 Other specified cutting and piercing instruments or objects

Arrow	Nail
Broken glass	Plant thorn
Dart	Splinter
Edge of stiff paper	Tin can lid
Lathe turnings	

EXCLUDES *animal spines or quills (E906.8)*
flying glass due to explosion (E921.0-E923.9)

E920.9 Unspecified cutting and piercing instrument or object

E921 Accident caused by explosion of pressure vessel

INCLUDES accidental explosion of pressure vessels, whether or not part of machinery

EXCLUDES *explosion of pressure vessel on transport vehicle (E800.0-E845.9)*

E921.0 Boilers

E921.1 Gas cylinders
Air tank   Pressure gas tank

E921.8 Other specified pressure vessels
Aerosol can   Tin can lid
Automobile tire

E921.9 Unspecified pressure vessel

E922 Accident caused by firearm, and air gun missile

EXCLUDES *injury caused by mechanism or component of firearm and air gun (E928.7)*

E922.0 Handgun
Pistol   Revolver
EXCLUDES *Verey pistol (E922.8)*

E922.1 Shotgun (automatic)

E922.2 Hunting rifle

E922.3 Military firearms
Army rifle   Machine gun

E922.4 Air gun
BB gun   Pellet gun

E922.5 Paintball gun

E922.8 Other specified firearm missile
Verey pistol [flare]

E922.9 Unspecified firearm missile
Gunshot wound NOS
Shot NOS

E923 Accident caused by explosive material

INCLUDES flash burns and other injuries resulting from explosion of explosive material
ignition of highly explosive material with explosion

EXCLUDES *explosion:*
in or on machinery (E919.0-E919.9)
on any transport vehicle, except stationary motor vehicle (E800.0-E848)
with conflagration (E890.0, E891.0,E892)
injury caused by mechanism or component of firearm and air gun (E928.7)
secondary fires resulting from explosion (E890.0-E899)

E923.0 Fireworks

E923.1 Blasting materials

Blasting cap	Dynamite
Detonator	Explosive [any] used in blasting operations

E923.2 Explosive gases

Acetylene	Fire damp
Butane	Gasoline fumes
Coal gas	Methane
Explosion in mine NOS	Propane

E923.8 Other explosive materials

Bomb	Torpedo
Explosive missile	Explosion in munitions:
Grenade	dump
Mine	factory
Shell	

E923.9 Unspecified explosive material
Explosion NOS

E924 Accident caused by hot substance or object, caustic or corrosive material, and steam

EXCLUDES *burning NOS (E899)*
chemical burn resulting from swallowing a corrosive substance (E860.0-E864.4)
fire caused by these substances and objects (E890.0-E894)
radiation burns (E926.0-E926.9)
therapeutic misadventures (E870.0-E876.9)

E924.0 Hot liquids and vapors, including steam
Burning or scalding by:
boiling water
hot or boiling liquids not primarily caustic or corrosive
liquid metal
steam
other hot vapor
EXCLUDES *hot (boiling) tap water (E924.2)*

E924.1 Caustic and corrosive substances
Burning by:
acid [any kind]
ammonia
caustic oven cleaner or other substance
corrosive substance
lye
vitriol

E924.2 Hot (boiling) tap water

E924.8 Other
Burning by:
heat from electric heating appliance
hot object NOS
light bulb
steam pipe

E924.9 Unspecified

E925 Accident caused by electric current

INCLUDES electric current from exposed wire, faulty appliance, high voltage cable, live rail, or open electric socket as the cause of:
burn
cardiac fibrillation
convulsion
electric shock
electrocution
puncture wound
respiratory paralysis

EXCLUDES *burn by heat from electrical appliance (E924.8)*
lightning (E907)

E925.0 Domestic wiring and appliances

E925.1 Electric power generating plants, distribution stations, transmission lines
Broken power line

E925.2 Industrial wiring, appliances, and electrical machinery
Conductors
Control apparatus
Electrical equipment and machinery
Transformers

E925.8 Other electric current
Wiring and appliances in or on:
farm [not farmhouse]
outdoors
public building
residential institutions
schools

E925.9 Unspecified electric current
Burns or other injury from electric current NOS
Electric shock NOS
Electrocution NOS

✓4ᵗʰ **E926 Exposure to radiation**
EXCLUDES *abnormal reaction to or complication of treatment without mention of misadventure (E879.2)*
atomic power plant malfunction in water transport (E838.0-E838.9)
misadventure to patient in surgical and medical procedures (E873.2-E873.3)
use of radiation in war operations (E996-E997.9)

E926.0 Radiofrequency radiation

Overexposure to:	from:
microwave radiation	high-powered radio and
radar radiation	television transmitters
radiofrequency	industrial radiofrequency
radiofrequency	induction heaters
radiation [any]	radar installations

E926.1 Infrared heaters and lamps
Exposure to infrared radiation from heaters and lamps as the cause of:
blistering
burning
charring
inflammatory change
EXCLUDES *physical contact with heater or lamp (E924.8)*

E926.2 Visible and ultraviolet light sources
Arc lamps
Black light sources
Electrical welding arc
Oxygas welding torch
Sun rays
Tanning bed
EXCLUDES *excessive heat from these sources (E900.1-E900.9)*

E926.3 X-rays and other electromagnetic ionizing radiation
Gamma rays
X-rays (hard) (soft)

E926.4 Lasers

E926.5 Radioactive isotopes
Radiobiologicals
Radiopharmaceuticals

E926.8 Other specified radiation
Artificially accelerated beams of ionized particles generated by:
betatrons
synchrotrons

E926.9 Unspecified radiation
Radiation NOS

✓4ᵗʰ **E927 Overexertion and strenuous and repetitive movements or loads**
Use additional code to identify activity (E001-E030)

E927.0 Overexertion from sudden strenuous movement
Sudden trauma from strenuous movement

E927.1 Overexertion from prolonged static position
Overexertion from maintaining prolonged positions, such as:
holding
sitting
standing

E927.2 Excessive physical exertion from prolonged activity

E927.3 Cumulative trauma from repetitive motion
Cumulative trauma from repetitive movements

E927.4 Cumulative trauma from repetitive impact

E927.8 Other overexertion and strenuous and repetitive movements or loads

E927.9 Unspecified overexertion and strenuous and repetitive movements or loads

✓4ᵗʰ **E928 Other and unspecified environmental and accidental causes**

E928.0 Prolonged stay in weightless environment
Weightlessness in spacecraft (simulator)

E928.1 Exposure to noise
Noise (pollution)
Sound waves
Supersonic waves

E928.2 Vibration

E928.3 Human bite

E928.4 External constriction caused by hair

E928.5 External constriction caused by other object

E928.6 Environmental exposure to harmful algae and toxins
Algae bloom NOS   Florida red tide
Blue-green algae bloom   Harmful algae bloom
Brown tide   Pfiesteria piscicida
Cyanobacteria bloom   Red tide

E928.7 Mechanism or component of firearm and air gun
Injury due to:
explosion of gun parts
recoil
Pierced, cut, crushed, or pinched by slide, trigger mechanism, scope, or other gun part
Powder burn from firearm or air gun
EXCLUDES *accident caused by firearm and air gun missile (E922.0-E922.9)*

E928.8 Other

E928.9 Unspecified accident

Accident NOS	
Blow NOS	stated as accidentally
Casualty (not due to war)	inflicted
Decapitation	

Knocked down	
Killed	stated as accidentally
Injury [any part of body, or unspecified]	inflicted, but not otherwise specified
Mangled	
Wound	

EXCLUDES *fracture, cause unspecified (E887)*
injuries undetermined whether accidentally or purposely inflicted (E980.0-E989)

Late Effects Of Accidental Injury (E929)

NOTE This category is to be used to indicate accidental injury as the cause of death or disability from late effects, which are themselves classifiable elsewhere. The "late effects" include conditions reported as such, or as sequelae which may occur at any time after the attempted suicide or self-inflicted injury.

✓4ᵗʰ **E929 Late effects of accidental injury**
EXCLUDES *late effects of:*
surgical and medical procedures (E870.0-E879.9)
therapeutic use of drugs and medicines (E930.0-E949.9)

E929.0 Late effects of motor vehicle accident
Late effects of accidents classifiable to E810-E825

E929.1 Late effects of other transport accident
Late effects of accidents classifiable to E800-E807, E826-E838, E840-E848

E929.2 Late effects of accidental poisoning
Late effects of accidents classifiable to E850-E858, E860-E869

E929.3 Late effects of accidental fall
Late effects of accidents classifiable to E880-E888

E929.4 Late effects of accident caused by fire
Late effects of accidents classifiable to E890-E899

E929.5 Late effects of accident due to natural and environmental factors
Late effects of accidents classifiable to E900-E909

E929.8 Late effects of other accidents
Late effects of accidents classifiable to E910-E928.8

E929.9 Late effects of unspecified accident
Late effects of accidents classifiable to E928.9

✓4ᵗʰ Fourth-digit Required   ▶◀ Revised Text   ● New Code   ▲ Revised Code TitleDx

Drugs, Medicinal And Biological Substances Causing Adverse Effects In Therapeutic Use (E930-E949)

INCLUDES correct drug properly administered in therapeutic or prophylactic dosage, as the cause of any adverse effect including allergic or hypersensitivity reactions

EXCLUDES *accidental overdose of drug and wrong drug given or taken in error (E850.0-E858.9)*

accidents in the technique of administration of drug or biological substance, such as accidental puncture during injection, or contamination of drug (E870.0-E876.9)

administration with suicidal or homicidal intent or intent to harm, or in circumstances classifiable to E950.0-E950.5, E962.0, E980.0-E980.5

NOTE See Alphabetic Index for more complete list of specific drugs to be classified under the fourth digit subdivisions. The American Hospital Formulary numbers can be used to classify new drugs listed by the American Hospital Formulary Service (AHFS). See Appendix C.

✓4ᵗʰ E930 Antibiotics

EXCLUDES *that used as eye, ear, nose, and throat [ENT], and local anti-infectives (E946.0-E946.9)*

E930.0 Penicillins
Natural
Synthetic
Semisynthetic, such as:
 ampicillin
Semisynthetic, such as:
 cloxacillin
 nafcillin
 oxacillin

E930.1 Antifungal antibiotics
Amphotericin B
Griseofulvin
Hachimycin [trichomycin]
Nystatin

E930.2 Chloramphenicol group
Chloramphenicol
Thiamphenicol

E930.3 Erythromycin and other macrolides
Oleandomycin
Spiramycin

E930.4 Tetracycline group
Doxycycline
Minocycline
Oxytetracycline

E930.5 Cephalosporin group
Cephalexin
Cephaloglycin
Cephaloridine
Cephalothin

E930.6 Antimycobacterial antibiotics
Cycloserine
Kanamycin
Rifampin
Streptomycin

E930.7 Antineoplastic antibiotics
Actinomycins, such as:
 Bleomycin
 Cactinomycin
 Dactinomycin
Actinomycins, such as:
 Daunorubicin
 Mitomycin

EXCLUDES *other antineoplastic drugs (E933.1)*

E930.8 Other specified antibiotics

E930.9 Unspecified antibiotic

✓4ᵗʰ E931 Other anti-infectives

EXCLUDES *ENT, and local anti-infectives (E946.0-E946.9)*

E931.0 Sulfonamides
Sulfadiazine
Sulfafurazole
Sulfamethoxazole

E931.1 Arsenical anti-infectives

E931.2 Heavy metal anti-infectives
Compounds of:
 antimony
 bismuth
Compounds of:
 lead
 mercury

EXCLUDES *mercurial diuretics (E944.0)*

E931.3 Quinoline and hydroxyquinoline derivatives
Chiniofon
Diiodohydroxyquin

EXCLUDES *antimalarial drugs (E931.4)*

E931.4 Antimalarials and drugs acting on other blood protozoa
Chloroquine phosphate
Cycloguanil
Primaquine
Proguanil [chloroguanide]
Pyrimethamine
Quinine (sulphate)

E931.5 Other antiprotozoal drugs
Emetine

E931.6 Anthelmintics
Hexylresorcinol
Male fern oleoresin
Piperazine
Thiabendazole

E931.7 Antiviral drugs
Methisazone

EXCLUDES *amantadine (E936.4)*
cytarabine (E933.1)
idoxuridine (E946.5)

E931.8 Other antimycobacterial drugs
Ethambutol
Ethionamide
Isoniazid
Para-aminosalicylic acid derivatives
Sulfones

E931.9 Other and unspecified anti-infectives
Flucytosine
Nitrofuranderivatives

✓4ᵗʰ E932 Hormones and synthetic substitutes

E932.0 Adrenal cortical steroids
Cortisone derivatives
Desoxycorticosterone derivatives
Fluorinated corticosteroid

E932.1 Androgens and anabolic congeners
Nandrolone phenpropionate
Oxymetholone
Testosterone and preparations

E932.2 Ovarian hormones and synthetic substitutes
Contraceptives, oral
Estrogens
Estrogens and progestogens combined
Progestogens

E932.3 Insulins and antidiabetic agents
Acetohexamide
Biguanide derivatives, oral
Chlorpropamide
Glucagon
Insulin
Phenformin
Sulfonylurea derivatives, oral
Tolbutamide

EXCLUDES *adverse effect of insulin administered for shock therapy (E879.3)*

E932.4 Anterior pituitary hormones
Corticotropin
Gonadotropin
Somatotropin [growth hormone]

E932.5 Posterior pituitary hormones
Vasopressin

EXCLUDES *oxytocic agents (E945.0)*

E932.6 Parathyroid and parathyroid derivatives

E932.7 Thyroid and thyroid derivatives
Dextrothyroxine
Levothyroxine sodium
Liothyronine
Thyroglobulin

E932.8 Antithyroid agents
Iodides
Thiouracil
Thiourea

E932.9 Other and unspecified hormones and synthetic substitutes

✓4ᵗʰ E933 Primarily systemic agents

E933.0 Antiallergic and antiemetic drugs
Antihistamines
Chlorpheniramine
Diphenhydramine
Diphenylpyraline
Thonzylamine
Tripelennamine

EXCLUDES *phenothiazine-based tranquilizers (E939.1)*

E933.1 Antineoplastic and immunosuppressive drugs
Azathioprine
Busulfan
Chlorambucil
Cyclophosphamide
Cytarabine
Fluorouracil
Mechlorethamine hydrochloride
Mercaptopurine
Triethylenethiophosphoramide [thio-TEPA]

EXCLUDES *antineoplastic antibiotics (E930.7)*

E933.2 Acidifying agents

E933.3 Alkalizing agents

E933.4 Enzymes, not elsewhere classified
Penicillinase

✓4ᵗʰ Fourth-digit Required ►◄ Revised Text ● New Code ▲ Revised Code TitleDx

E933.5 Vitamins, not elsewhere classified
Vitamin A
Vitamin D
EXCLUDES nicotinic acid (E942.2)
vitamin K (E934.3)

E933.6 Oral bisphosphonates

E933.7 Intravenous bisphosphonates

E933.8 Other systemic agents, not elsewhere classified
Heavy metal antagonists

E933.9 Unspecified systemic agent

☑4ᵗʰ E934 Agents primarily affecting blood constituents

E934.0 Iron and its compounds
Ferric salts
Ferrous sulphate and other ferrous salts

E934.1 Liver preparations and other antianemic agents
Folic acid

E934.2 Anticoagulants
Coumarin   Prothrombin synthesis inhibitor
Heparin   Warfarin sodium
Phenindione

E934.3 Vitamin K [phytonadione]

E934.4 Fibrinolysis-affecting drugs
Aminocaproic acid   Streptokinase
Streptodornase   Urokinase

E934.5 Anticoagulant antagonists and other coagulants
Hexadimethrine bromide
Protamine sulfate

E934.6 Gamma globulin

E934.7 Natural blood and blood products
Blood plasma   Packed red cells
Human fibrinogen   Whole blood

E934.8 Other agents affecting blood constituents
Macromolecular blood substitutes

E934.9 Unspecified agent affecting blood constituents

☑4ᵗʰ E935 Analgesics, antipyretics, and antirheumatics

E935.0 Heroin
Diacetylmorphine

E935.1 Methadone

E935.2 Other opiates and related narcotics
Codeine [methylmorphine]
Meperidine [pethidine]
Morphine
Opium (alkaloids)

E935.3 Salicylates
Acetylsalicylic acid [aspirin]
Amino derivatives of salicylic acid
Salicylic acid salts

E935.4 Aromatic analgesics, not elsewhere classified
Acetanilid
Paracetamol [acetaminophen]
Phenacetin [acetophenetidin]

E935.5 Pyrazole derivatives
Aminophenazone [aminopyrine]
Phenylbutazone

E935.6 Antirheumatics [antiphlogistics]
Gold salts   Indomethacin
EXCLUDES salicylates (E935.3)
steroids (E932.0)

E935.7 Other non-narcotic analgesics
Pyrabital

E935.8 Other specified analgesics and antipyretics
Pentazocine

E935.9 Unspecified analgesic and antipyretic

☑4ᵗʰ E936 Anticonvulsants and anti-Parkinsonism drugs

E936.0 Oxazolidine derivatives
Paramethadione   Trimethadione

E936.1 Hydantoin derivatives
Phenytoin

E936.2 Succinimides
Ethosuximide   Phensuximide

E936.3 Other and unspecified anticonvulsants
Beclamide
Primidone

E936.4 Anti-Parkinsonism drugs
Amantadine
Ethopropazine [profenamine]
Levodopa [L-dopa]

☑4ᵗʰ E937 Sedatives and hypnotics

E937.0 Barbiturates
Amobarbital [amylobarbitone]
Barbital [barbitone]
Butabarbital [butabarbitone]
Pentobarbital [pentobarbitone]
Phenobarbital [phenobarbitone]
Secobarbital [quinalbarbitone]
EXCLUDES thiobarbiturates (E938.3)

E937.1 Chloral hydrate group

E937.2 Paraldehyde

E937.3 Bromine compounds
Bromide
Carbromal (derivatives)

E937.4 Methaqualone compounds

E937.5 Glutethimide group

E937.6 Mixed sedatives, not elsewhere classified

E937.8 Other sedatives and hypnotics

E937.9 Unspecified
Sleeping:
drug
pill   } NOS
tablet

☑4ᵗʰ E938 Other central nervous system depressants and anesthetics

E938.0 Central nervous system muscle-tone depressants
Chlorphenesin (carbamate)
Mephenesin
Methocarbamol

E938.1 Halothane

E938.2 Other gaseous anesthetics
Ether
Halogenated hydrocarbon derivatives, except halothane
Nitrous oxide

E938.3 Intravenous anesthetics
Ketamine
Methohexital [methohexitone]
Thiobarbiturates, such as thiopental sodium

E938.4 Other and unspecified general anesthetics

E938.5 Surface and infiltration anesthetics
Cocaine
Lidocaine [lignocaine]
Procaine
Tetracaine

E938.6 Peripheral nerve- and plexus-blocking anesthetics

E938.7 Spinal anesthetics

E938.9 Other and unspecified local anesthetics

☑4ᵗʰ E939 Psychotropic agents

E939.0 Antidepressants
Amitriptyline   Monoamine oxidase
Imipramine   [MAO] inhibitors

E939.1 Phenothiazine-based tranquilizers
Chlorpromazine   Prochlorperazine
Fluphenazine   Promazine
Phenothiazine

E939.2 Butyrophenone-based tranquilizers
Haloperidol   Trifluperidol
Spiperone

☑4ᵗʰ Fourth-digit Required   ▶◀ Revised Text   ● New Code   ▲ Revised Code TitleDx

E939.3 Other antipsychotics, neuroleptics, and major tranquilizers

E939.4 Benzodiazepine-based tranquilizers

Chlordiazepoxide	Lorazepam
Diazepam	Medazepam
Flurazepam	Nitrazepam

E939.5 Other tranquilizers

Hydroxyzine	Meprobamate

E939.6 Psychodysleptics [hallucinogens]

Cannabis (derivatives)	Mescaline
Lysergide [LSD]	Psilocin
Marihuana (derivatives)	Psilocybin

E939.7 Psychostimulants

Amphetamine	Caffeine

EXCLUDES *central appetite depressants (E947.0)*

E939.8 Other psychotropic agents

E939.9 Unspecified psychotropic agent

✓4ᵗʰ **E940 Central nervous system stimulants**

E940.0 Analeptics

Lobeline	Nikethamide

E940.1 Opiate antagonists

Levallorphan	Naloxone
Nalorphine	

E940.8 Other specified central nervous system stimulants

E940.9 Unspecified central nervous system stimulant

✓4ᵗʰ **E941 Drugs primarily affecting the autonomic nervous system**

E941.0 Parasympathomimetics [cholinergics]

Acetylcholine
Anticholinesterase:
  organophosphorus
  reversible
Pilocarpine

E941.1 Parasympatholytics [anticholinergics and antimuscarinics] and spasmolytics

Atropine	Hyoscine [scopolamine]
Homatropine	Quaternary ammonium derivatives

EXCLUDES *papaverine (E942.5)*

E941.2 Sympathomimetics [adrenergics]

Epinephrine [adrenalin]
Levarterenol [noradrenalin]

E941.3 Sympatholytics [antiadrenergics]

Phenoxybenzamine
Tolazolinehydrochloride

E941.9 Unspecified drug primarily affecting the autonomic nervous system

✓4ᵗʰ **E942 Agents primarily affecting the cardiovascular system**

E942.0 Cardiac rhythm regulators

Practolol	Propranolol
Procainamide	Quinidine

E942.1 Cardiotonic glycosides and drugs of similar action

Digitalis glycosides	Strophanthins
Digoxin	

E942.2 Antilipemic and antiarteriosclerotic drugs

Cholestyramine	Nicotinic acid derivatives
Clofibrate	Sitosterols

EXCLUDES *dextrothyroxine (E932.7)*

E942.3 Ganglion-blocking agents

Pentamethonium bromide

E942.4 Coronary vasodilators

Dipyridamole	Nitrites
Nitrates [nitroglycerin]	Prenylamine

E942.5 Other vasodilators

Cyclandelate	Hydralazine
Diazoxide	Papaverine

E942.6 Other antihypertensive agents

Clonidine	Rauwolfia alkaloids
Guanethidine	Reserpine

E942.7 Antivaricose drugs, including sclerosing agents

Monoethanolamine	Zinc salts

E942.8 Capillary-active drugs

Adrenochrome derivatives	Metaraminol
Bioflavonoids	

E942.9 Other and unspecified agents primarily affecting the cardiovascular system

✓4ᵗʰ **E943 Agents primarily affecting gastrointestinal system**

E943.0 Antacids and antigastric secretion drugs

Aluminum hydroxide	Magnesium trisilicate

E943.1 Irritant cathartics

Bisacodyl	Phenolphthalein
Castor oil	

E943.2 Emollient cathartics

Sodium dioctyl sulfosuccinate

E943.3 Other cathartics, including intestinal atonia drugs

Magnesium sulfate

E943.4 Digestants

Pancreatin	Pepsin
Papain	

E943.5 Antidiarrheal drugs

Bismuth subcarbonate	Kaolin
Pectin	

EXCLUDES *anti-infectives (E930.0-E931.9)*

E943.6 Emetics

E943.8 Other specified agents primarily affecting the gastrointestinal system

E943.9 Unspecified agent primarily affecting the gastrointestinal system

✓4ᵗʰ **E944 Water, mineral, and uric acid metabolism drugs**

E944.0 Mercurial diuretics

Chlormerodrin	Mercurophylline
Mercaptomerin	Mersalyl

E944.1 Purine derivative diuretics

Theobromine
Theophylline

EXCLUDES *aminophylline [theophylline ethylenediamine]*
      (E945.7)

E944.2 Carbonic acid anhydrase inhibitors

Acetazolamide

E944.3 Saluretics

Benzothiadiazides	Chlorothiazide group

E944.4 Other diuretics

Ethacrynic acid	Furosemide

E944.5 Electrolytic, caloric, and water-balance agents

E944.6 Other mineral salts, not elsewhere classified

E944.7 Uric acid metabolism drugs

Cinchophen and congeners	Phenoquin
Colchicine	Probenecid

✓4ᵗʰ **E945 Agents primarily acting on the smooth and skeletal muscles and respiratory system**

E945.0 Oxytocic agents

Ergot alkaloids	Prostaglandins

E945.1 Smooth muscle relaxants

Adiphenine
Metaproterenol [orciprenaline]

EXCLUDES *papaverine (E942.5)*

E945.2 Skeletal muscle relaxants

Alcuronium chloride
Suxamethonium chloride

E945.3 Other and unspecified drugs acting on muscles

E945.4 Antitussives

Dextromethorphan
Pipazethate hydrochloride

✓4ᵗʰ Fourth-digit Required   ▶◀ Revised Text   ● New Code   ▲ Revised Code TitleDx

E945.5 Expectorants
Acetylcysteine
Cocillana
Guaifenesin [glyceryl guaiacolate]
Ipecacuanha
Terpin hydrate

E945.6 Anti-common cold drugs

E945.7 Antiasthmatics
Aminophylline [theophylline ethylenediamine]

E945.8 Other and unspecified respiratory drugs

☑4ᵗʰ **E946 Agents primarily affecting skin and mucous membrane, ophthalmological, otorhinolaryngological, and dental drugs**

E946.0 Local anti-infectives and anti-inflammatory drugs

E946.1 Antipruritics

E946.2 Local astringents and local detergents

E946.3 Emollients, demulcents, and protectants

E946.4 Keratolytics, kerstoplastics, other hair treatment drugs and preparations

E946.5 Eye anti-infectives and other eye drugs
Idoxuridine

E946.6 Anti-infectives and other drugs and preparations for ear, nose, and throat

E946.7 Dental drugs topically applied

E946.8 Other agents primarily affecting skin and mucous membrane
Spermicides

E946.9 Unspecified agent primarily affecting skin and mucous membrane

☑4ᵗʰ **E947 Other and unspecified drugs and medicinal substances**

E947.0 Dietetics

E947.1 Lipotropic drugs

E947.2 Antidotes and chelating agents, not elsewhere classified

E947.3 Alcohol deterrents

E947.4 Pharmaceutical excipients

E947.8 Other drugs and medicinal substances
Contrast media used for diagnostic x-ray procedures
Diagnostic agents and kits

E947.9 Unspecified drug or medicinal substance

☑4ᵗʰ **E948 Bacterial vaccines**

E948.0 BCG vaccine

E948.1 Typhoid and paratyphoid

E948.2 Cholera

E948.3 Plague

E948.4 Tetanus

E948.5 Diphtheria

E948.6 Pertussis vaccine, including combinations with a pertussis component

E948.8 Other and unspecified bacterial vaccines

E948.9 Mixed bacterial vaccines, except combinations with a pertussis component

☑4ᵗʰ **E949 Other vaccines and biological substances**
EXCLUDES *gamma globulin (E934.6)*

E949.0 Smallpox vaccine

E949.1 Rabies vaccine

E949.2 Typhus vaccine

E949.3 Yellow fever vaccine

E949.4 Measles vaccine

E949.5 Poliomyelitis vaccine

E949.6 Other and unspecified viral and rickettsial vaccines
Mumps vaccine

E949.7 Mixed viral-rickettsial and bacterial vaccines, except combinations with a pertussis component
EXCLUDES *combinations with a pertussis component (E948.6)*

E949.9 Other and unspecified vaccines and biological substances

Suicide and Self-inflicted Injury (E950-E959)

INCLUDES injuries in suicide and attempted suicide
self-inflicted injuries specified as intentional

☑4ᵗʰ **E950 Suicide and self-inflicted poisoning by solid or liquid substances**

E950.0 Analgesics, antipyretics, and antirheumatics

E950.1 Barbiturates

E950.2 Other sedatives and hypnotics

E950.3 Tranquilizers and other psychotropic agents

E950.4 Other specified drugs and medicinal substances

E950.5 Unspecified drug or medicinal substance

E950.6 Agricultural and horticultural chemical and pharmaceutical preparations other than plant foods and fertilizers

E950.7 Corrosive and caustic substances
Suicide and self-inflicted poisoning by substances classifiable to E864

E950.8 Arsenic and its compounds

E950.9 Other and unspecified solid and liquid substances

☑4ᵗʰ **E951 Suicide and self-inflicted poisoning by gases in domestic use**

E951.0 Gas distributed by pipeline

E951.1 Liquefied petroleum gas distributed in mobile containers

E951.8 Other utility gas

☑4ᵗʰ **E952 Suicide and self-inflicted poisoning by other gases and vapors**

E952.0 Motor vehicle exhaust gas

E952.1 Other carbon monoxide

E952.8 Other specified gases and vapors

E952.9 Unspecified gases and vapors

☑4ᵗʰ **E953 Suicide and self-inflicted injury by hanging, strangulation, and suffocation**

E953.0 Hanging

E953.1 Suffocation by plastic bag

E953.8 Other specified means

E953.9 Unspecified means

E954 Suicide and self-inflicted injury by submersion [drowning]

☑4ᵗʰ **E955 Suicide and self-inflicted injury by firearms, air guns and explosives**

E955.0 Handgun

E955.1 Shotgun

E955.2 Hunting rifle

E955.3 Military firearms

E955.4 Other and unspecified firearm
Gunshot NOS
Shot NOS

E955.5 Explosives

E955.6 Air gun
BB gun
Pellet gun

E955.7 Paintball gun

E955.9 Unspecified

E956 Suicide and self-inflicted injury by cutting and piercing instrument

☑4ᵗʰ **E957 Suicide and self-inflicted injuries by jumping from high place**

E957.0 Residential premises

☑4ᵗʰ Fourth-digit Required   ►◄ Revised Text   ● New Code   ▲ Revised Code TitleDx

E957.1 **Other man-made structures**

E957.2 **Natural sites**

E957.9 **Unspecified**

☑4ᵗʰ E958 **Suicide and self-inflicted injury by other and unspecified means**

E958.0 **Jumping or lying before moving object**

E958.1 **Burns, fire**

E958.2 **Scald**

E958.3 **Extremes of cold**

E958.4 **Electrocution**

E958.5 **Crashing of motor vehicle**

E958.6 **Crashing of aircraft**

E958.7 **Caustic substances, except poisoning**

> EXCLUDES *poisoning by caustic substance (E950.7)*

E958.8 **Other specified means**

E958.9 **Unspecified means**

E959 **Late effects of self-inflicted injury**

> NOTE This category is to be used to indicate circumstances classifiable to E950-E958 as the cause of death or disability from late effects, which are themselves classifiable elsewhere. The "late effects" include conditions reported as such, or as sequelae which may occur at any time after the attempted suicide or self-inflicted injury.

Homicide and Injury Purposely Inflicted by Other Persons (E960-E969)

> INCLUDES injuries inflicted by another person with intent to injure or kill, by any means

> EXCLUDES *injuries due to:*
> *legal intervention (E970-E978)*
> *operations of war (E990-E999)*
> *terrorism (E979)*

☑4ᵗʰ E960 **Fight, brawl, rape**

E960.0 **Unarmed fight or brawl**
Beatings NOS
Brawl or fight with hands, fists, feet
Injured or killed in fight NOS

> EXCLUDES *homicidal:*
> *injury by weapons (E965.0-E966, E969)*
> *strangulation (E963)*
> *submersion (E964)*

E960.1 **Rape**

E961 **Assault by corrosive or caustic substance, except poisoning**
Injury or death purposely caused by corrosive or caustic substance, such as:
acid [any]
corrosive substance
vitriol

> EXCLUDES *burns from hot liquid (E968.3)*
> *chemical burns from swallowing a corrosive substance (E962.0-E962.9)*

☑4ᵗʰ E962 **Assault by poisoning**

E962.0 **Drugs and medicinal substances**
Homicidal poisoning by any drug or medicinal substance

E962.1 **Other solid and liquid substances**

E962.2 **Other gases and vapors**

E962.9 **Unspecified poisoning**

E963 **Assault by hanging and strangulation**
Homicidal (attempt):   Homicidal (attempt):
garrotting or ligature   strangulation
hanging   suffocation

E964 **Assault by submersion [drowning]**

☑4ᵗʰ E965 **Assault by firearms and explosives**

E965.0 **Handgun**
Pistol   Revolver

E965.1 **Shotgun**

E965.2 **Hunting rifle**

E965.3 **Military firearms**

E965.4 **Other and unspecified firearm**

E965.5 **Antipersonnel bomb**

E965.6 **Gasoline bomb**

E965.7 **Letter bomb**

E965.8 **Other specified explosive**
Bomb NOS (placed in):
car
house
Dynamite

E965.9 **Unspecified explosive**

E966 **Assault by cutting and piercing instrument**
Assassination (attempt), homicide (attempt) by any instrument classifiable under E920
Homicidal:
cut
puncture ⎫ any part of the body
stab ⎭
Stabbed any part of the body

☑4ᵗʰ E967 **Perpetrator of child and adult abuse**

> NOTE Selection of the correct perpetrator code is based on the relationship between the perpetrator and the victim

E967.0 **By father, stepfather, or boyfriend**
Male partner of child's parent or guardian

E967.1 **By other specified person**

E967.2 **By mother, stepmother, or girlfriend**
Female partner of child's parent or guardian

E967.3 **By spouse or partner**
Abuse of spouse or partner by ex-spouse or ex-partner

E967.4 **By child**

E967.5 **By sibling**

E967.6 **By grandparent**

E967.7 **By other relative**

E967.8 **By non-related caregiver**

E967.9 **By unspecified person**

☑4ᵗʰ E968 **Assault by other and unspecified means**

E968.0 **Fire**
Arson   Homicidal burns NOS
> EXCLUDES *burns from hot liquid (E968.3)*

E968.1 **Pushing from a high place**

E968.2 **Striking by blunt or thrown object**

E968.3 **Hot liquid**
Homicidal burns by scalding

E968.4 **Criminal neglect**
Abandonment of child, infant, or other helpless person with intent to injure or kill

E968.5 **Transport vehicle**
Being struck by other vehicle or run down with intent to injure
Pushed in front of, thrown from, or dragged by moving vehicle with intent to injure

E968.6 **Air gun**
BB gun
Pellet gun

E968.7 **Human bite**

E968.8 **Other specified means**

E968.9 **Unspecified means**
Assassination (attempt) NOS
Homicidal (attempt):
injury NOS
wound NOS
Manslaughter (nonaccidental)
Murder (attempt) NOS
Violence, non-accidental

☑4ᵗʰ Fourth-digit Required   ▶◀ Revised Text   ● New Code   ▲ Revised Code TitleDx

E Codes

E969–E980.8

E969 Late effects of injury purposely inflicted by other person

> **NOTE** This category is to be used to indicate circumstances classifiable to E960-E968 as the cause of death or disability from late effects, which are themselves classifiable elsewhere. The "late effects" include conditions reported as such, or as sequelae which may occur at any time after injury purposely inflicted by another person.

Legal Intervention (E970-E978)

> **INCLUDES** injuries inflicted by the police or other law-enforcing agents, including military on duty, in the course of arresting or attempting to arrest lawbreakers, suppressing disturbances, maintaining order, and other legal action
>
> legal execution

> **EXCLUDES** injuries caused by civil insurrections (E990.0-E999)

E970 Injury due to legal intervention by firearms

Gunshot wound
Injury by:
  machine gun
  revolver
Injury by:
  rifle pellet or rubber bullet
  shot NOS

E971 Injury due to legal intervention by explosives

Injury by:
  dynamite
  explosive shell
Injury by:
  grenade
  mortar bomb

E972 Injury due to legal intervention by gas

Asphyxiation by gas
Injury by tear gas
Poisoning by gas

E973 Injury due to legal intervention by blunt object

Hit, struck by:
  baton (nightstick)
  blunt object
Hit, struck by:
  stave

E974 Injury due to legal intervention by cutting and piercing instrument

Cut
Incised wound
Injured by bayonet
Stab wound

E975 Injury due to legal intervention by other specified means

Blow
Manhandling

E976 Injury due to legal intervention by unspecified means

E977 Late effects of injuries due to legal intervention

> **NOTE** This category is to be used to indicate circumstances classifiable to E970-E976 as the cause of death or disability from late effects, which are themselves classifiable elsewhere. The "late effects" include conditions reported as such, or as sequelae, which may occur at any time after the injury due to legal intervention.

E978 Legal execution

All executions performed at the behest of the judiciary or ruling authority [whether permanent or temporary] as:

asphyxiation by gas
beheading, decapitation (by guillotine)
capital punishment
electrocution
hanging
poisoning
shooting
other specified means

Terrorism (E979)

√4ᵗʰ **E979 Terrorism**

Injuries resulting from the unlawful use of force or violence against persons or property to intimidate or coerce a Government, the civilian population, or any segment thereof, in furtherance of political or social objective

E979.0 Terrorism involving explosion of marine weapons

Depth-charge
Marine mine
Mine NOS, at sea or in harbour
Sea-based artillery shell
Torpedo
Underwater blast

E979.1 Terrorism involving destruction of aircraft

Aircraft used as a weapon
Aircraft:
  burned
  exploded
Aircraft:
  shot down
Crushed by falling aircraft

E979.2 Terrorism involving other explosions and fragments

Antipersonnel bomb
  (fragments)
Blast NOS
Explosion (of):
  artillery shell
  breech-block
  cannon block
  mortar bomb
  munitions being used
    in terrorism
NOS
Fragments from:
  artillery shell
  bomb
  grenade
  guided missile
  land-mine
  rocket
  shell
  shrapnel
Mine NOS

E979.3 Terrorism involving fires, conflagration and hot substances

Burning building or
  structure:
  collapse of
  fall from
  hit by falling object in
  jump from
Conflagration NOS
Fire (causing):
  Asphyxia
  Burns
Fire (causing):
  NOS
  Other injury
Melting of fittings and
  furniture in burning
Petrol bomb
Smouldering building
  or structure

E979.4 Terrorism involving firearms

Bullet:
  carbine
  machine gun
  pistol
Bullet:
  rifle
  rubber (rifle)
Pellets (shotgun)

E979.5 Terrorism involving nuclear weapons

Blast effects
Exposure to ionizing radiation from nuclear weapon
Fireball effects
Heat from nuclear weapon
Other direct and secondary effects of nuclear weapons

E979.6 Terrorism involving biological weapons

Anthrax
Cholera
Smallpox

E979.7 Terrorism involving chemical weapons

Gases, fumes, chemicals
Hydrogen cyanide
Phosgene
Sarin

E979.8 Terrorism involving other means

Drowning and submersion
Lasers
Piercing or stabbing instruments
Terrorism NOS

E979.9 Terrorism, secondary effects

> **NOTE** This code is for use to identify conditions occurring subsequent to a terrorist attack not those that are due to the initial terrorist act

> **EXCLUDES** late effect of terrorist attack (E999.1)

Injury Undetermined Whether Accidentally or Purposely Inflicted (E980-E989)

> **NOTE** Categories E980-E989 are for use when it is unspecified or it cannot be determined whether the injuries are accidental (unintentional), suicide (attempted), or assault.

√4ᵗʰ **E980 Poisoning by solid or liquid substances, undetermined whether accidentally or purposely inflicted**

E980.0 Analgesics, antipyretics, and antirheumatics

E980.1 Barbiturates

E980.2 Other sedatives and hypnotics

E980.3 Tranquilizers and other psychotropic agents

E980.4 Other specified drugs and medicinal substances

E980.5 Unspecified drug or medicinal substance

E980.6 Corrosive and caustic substances

Poisoning, undetermined whether accidental or purposeful, by substances classifiable to E864

E980.7 Agricultural and horticultural chemical and pharmaceutical preparations other than plant foods and fertilizers

E980.8 Arsenic and its compounds

√4ᵗʰ Fourth-digit Required   ▶◀ Revised Text   ● New Code   ▲ Revised Code TitleDx

E980.9 Other and unspecified solid and liquid substances

☑4ᵗʰ **E981 Poisoning by gases in domestic use, undetermined whether accidentally or purposely inflicted**

E981.0 Gas distributed by pipeline

E981.1 Liquefied petroleum gas distributed in mobile containers

E981.8 Other utility gas

☑4ᵗʰ **E982 Poisoning by other gases, undetermined whether accidentally or purposely inflicted**

E982.0 Motor vehicle exhaust gas

E982.1 Other carbon monoxide

E982.8 Other specified gases and vapors

E982.9 Unspecified gases and vapors

☑4ᵗʰ **E983 Hanging, strangulation, or suffocation, undetermined whether accidentally or purposely inflicted**

E983.0 Hanging

E983.1 Suffocation by plastic bag

E983.8 Other specified means

E983.9 Unspecified means

E984 Submersion [drowning], undetermined whether accidentally or purposely inflicted

☑4ᵗʰ **E985 Injury by firearms, air guns and explosives, undetermined whether accidentally or purposely inflicted**

E985.0 Handgun

E985.1 Shotgun

E985.2 Hunting rifle

E985.3 Military firearms

E985.4 Other and unspecified firearm

E985.5 Explosives

E985.6 Air gun
    BB gun   Pellet gun

E985.7 Paintball gun

E986 Injury by cutting and piercing instruments, undetermined whether accidentally or purposely inflicted

☑4ᵗʰ **E987 Falling from high place, undetermined whether accidentally or purposely inflicted**

E987.0 Residential premises

E987.1 Other man-made structures

E987.2 Natural sites

E987.9 Unspecified site

☑4ᵗʰ **E988 Injury by other and unspecified means, undetermined whether accidentally or purposely inflicted**

E988.0 Jumping or lying before moving object

E988.1 Burns, fire

E988.2 Scald

E988.3 Extremes of cold

E988.4 Electrocution

E988.5 Crashing of motor vehicle

E988.6 Crashing of aircraft

E988.7 Caustic substances, except poisoning

E988.8 Other specified means

E988.9 Unspecified means

E989 Late effects of injury, undetermined whether accidentally or purposely inflicted

> **NOTE** This category is to be used to indicate circumstances classifiable to E980-E988 as the cause of death or disability from late effects, which are themselves classifiable elsewhere. The "late effects" include conditions reported as such, or as sequelae, which may occur at any time after injury, undetermined whether accidentally or purposely inflicted.

Injury Resulting from Operations of War (E990-E999)

> **INCLUDES** injuries to military personnel and civilians caused by war and civil insurrections and occurring during the time of war and insurrection, and peacekeeping missions
>
> **EXCLUDES** *accidents during training of military personnel manufacture of war material and transport, unless attributable to enemy action*

☑4ᵗʰ **E990 Injury due to war operations by fires and conflagrations**

> **INCLUDES** asphyxia, burns, or other injury originating from fire caused by a fire-producing device or indirectly by any conventional weapon

E990.0 From gasoline bomb
    Incendiary bomb

E990.1 From flamethrower

E990.2 From incendiary bullet

E990.3 From fire caused indirectly from conventional weapon
> **EXCLUDES** *fire aboard military aircraft (E994.3)*

E990.9 From other and unspecified source

☑4ᵗʰ **E991 Injury due to war operations by bullets and fragments**

> **EXCLUDES** *injury due to bullets and fragments due to war operations, but occurring after cessation of hostilities (E998.0)*
> *injury due to explosion of artillery shells and mortars (E993.2)*
> *injury due to explosion of improvised explosive device [IED] (E993.3-E993.5)*
> *injury due to sea-based artillery shell (E992.3)*

E991.0 Rubber bullets (rifle)

E991.1 Pellets (rifle)

E991.2 Other bullets
    Bullet [any, except rubber bullets and pellets]:
      carbine
      machine gun
      pistol
      rifle
      shotgun

E991.3 Antipersonnel bomb (fragments)

E991.4 Fragments from munitions

Fragments from:	Fragments from:
artillery shell	guided missile
bombs, except antipersonnel	land mine
detonation of unexploded ordnance [UXO]	rockets
grenade	shell

E991.5 Fragments from person-borne improvised explosive device [IED]

E991.6 Fragments from vehicle-borne improvised explosive device [IED]
    IED borne by land, air, or water transport vehicle

E991.7 Fragments from other improvised explosive device [IED]
    Roadside IED

E991.8 Fragments from weapons

Fragments from:	Fragments from:
artillery	missile launchers
autocannons	mortars
automatic grenade launchers	small arms

E991.9 Other and unspecified fragments
    Shrapnel NOS

☑4ᵗʰ **E992 Injury due to war operations by explosion of marine weapons**

E992.0 Torpedo

E992.1 Depth charge

E992.2 Marine mines
    Marine mines at sea or in harbor

E992.3 Sea-based artillery shell

E992.8 Other marine weapons

E992.9 Unspecified marine weapon
    Underwater blast NOS

E Codes

E993–E999.1

☑️4ᵗʰ **E993 Injury due to war operations by other explosion**

Injuries due to direct or indirect pressure or air blast of an explosion occurring during war operations

EXCLUDES *injury due to fragments resulting from an explosion (E991.0-E991.9)*

injury due to detonation of unexploded ordnance but occurring after cessation of hostilities (E998.0-E998.9)

injury due to nuclear weapons (E996.0-E996.9)

E993.0 Aerial bomb

E993.1 Guided missile

E993.2 Mortar
Artillery shell

E993.3 Person-borne improvised explosive device [IED]

E993.4 Vehicle-borne improvised explosive device [IED]
IED borne by land, air, or water transport vehicle

E993.5 Other improvised explosive device [IED]
Roadside IED

E993.6 Unintentional detonation of own munitions
Unintentional detonation of own ammunition (artillery) (mortars)

E993.7 Unintentional discharge of own munitions launch device
Unintentional explosion of own:
autocannons
automatic grenade launchers
missile launchers
small arms

E993.8 Other specified explosion
Bomb   Land mine
Grenade

E993.9 Unspecified explosion
Air blast NOS   Blast wind NOS
Blast NOS   Explosion NOS
Blast wave NOS

☑️4ᵗʰ **E994 Injury due to war operations by destruction of aircraft**

E994.0 Destruction of aircraft due to enemy fire or explosives
Air to air missile   Rocket propelled grenade [RPG]
Explosive device placed   Small arms fire
on aircraft   Surface to air missile

E994.1 Unintentional destruction of aircraft due to own onboard explosives

E994.2 Destruction of aircraft due to collision with other aircraft

E994.3 Destruction of aircraft due to onboard fire

E994.8 Other destruction of aircraft

E994.9 Unspecified destruction of aircraft

☑️4ᵗʰ **E995 Injury due to war operations by other and unspecified forms of conventional warfare**

E995.0 Unarmed hand-to-hand combat
EXCLUDES *intentional restriction of airway (E995.3)*

E995.1 Struck by blunt object
Baton (nightstick)
Stave

E995.2 Piercing object
Bayonet
Knife
Sword

E995.3 Intentional restriction of air and airway
Intentional submersion
Strangulation
Suffocation

E995.4 Unintentional drowning due to inability to surface or obtain air
Submersion

E995.8 Other forms of conventional warfare

E995.9 Unspecified form of conventional warfare

☑️4ᵗʰ **E996 Injury due to war operations by nuclear weapons**
Dirty bomb NOS
EXCLUDES *late effects of injury due to nuclear weapons (E999.0, E999.1)*

E996.0 Direct blast effect of nuclear weapon
Injury to bodily organs due to blast pressure

E996.1 Indirect blast effect of nuclear weapon
Injury due to being thrown by blast
Injury due to being struck or crushed by blast debris

E996.2 Thermal radiation effect of nuclear weapon
Burns due to thermal radiation
Fireball effects
Flash burns
Heat effects

E996.3 Nuclear radiation effects
Acute radiation exposure
Beta burns
Fallout exposure
Radiation sickness
Secondary effects of nuclear weapons

E996.8 Other effects of nuclear weapons

E996.9 Unspecified effect of nuclear weapon

☑️4ᵗʰ **E997 Injury due to war operations by other forms of unconventional warfare**

E997.0 Lasers

E997.1 Biological warfare

E997.2 Gases, fumes, and chemicals

E997.3 Weapon of mass destruction [WMD], unspecified

E997.8 Other specified forms of unconventional warfare

E997.9 Unspecified form of unconventional warfare

☑️4ᵗʰ **E998 Injury due to war operations but occurring after cessation of hostilities**
Injuries due to operations of war but occurring after cessation of hostilities by any means classifiable under E990-E997
Injuries by explosion of bombs or mines placed in the course of operations of war, if the explosion occurred after cessation of hostilities

E998.0 Explosion of mines

E998.1 Explosion of bombs

E998.8 Injury due to other war operations but occurring after cessation of hostilities

E998.9 Injury due to unspecified war operations but occurring after cessation of hostilities

☑️4ᵗʰ **E999 Late effect of injury due to war operations and terrorism**
NOTE This category is to be used to indicate circumstances classifiable to E979, E990-E998 as the cause of death or disability from late effects, which are themselves classifiable elsewhere. The "late effects" include conditions reported as such, or as sequelae, which may occur at any time after the injury, resulting from operations of war or terrorism

E999.0 Late effect of injury due to war operations

E999.1 Late effect of injury due to terrorism

☑️4ᵗʰ Fourth-digit Required   ►◄ Revised Text   ● New Code   ▲ Revised Code TitleDx

Appendix A: Morphology of Neoplasms

The World Health Organization has published an adaptation of the International Classification of Diseases for oncology (ICD-O). It contains a coded nomenclature for the morphology of neoplasms, which is reproduced here for those who wish to use it in conjunction with Chapter 2 of the International Classification of Diseases, 9th Revision, Clinical Modification.

The morphology code numbers consist of five digits; the first four identify the histological type of the neoplasm and the fifth indicates its behavior. The one-digit behavior code is as follows:

0   Benign
1   Uncertain whether benign or malignant
     Borderline malignancy
2   Carcinoma in situ
     Intraepithelial
     Noninfiltrating
     Noninvasive
3   Malignant, primary site
6   Malignant, metastatic site
     Secondary site
9   Malignant, uncertain whether primary or metastatic site

In the nomenclature below, the morphology code numbers include the behavior code appropriate to the histological type of neoplasm, but this behavior code should be changed if other reported information makes this necessary. For example, "chordoma (M9370/3)" is assumed to be malignant; the term "benign chordoma" should be coded M9370/0. Similarly, "superficial spreading adenocarcinoma (M8143/3)" described as "noninvasive" should be coded M8143/2 and "melanoma (M8720/3)" described as "secondary" should be coded M8720/6.

The following table shows the correspondence between the morphology code and the different sections of Chapter 2:

Morphology Code Histology/Behavior		ICD-9-CM Chapter 2	
Any	0	210-229	Benign neoplasms
M8000-M8004	1	239	Neoplasms of unspecified nature
M8010+	1	235-238	Neoplasms of uncertain behavior
Any	2	230-234	Carcinoma in situ
Any	3	140-195, 200-208	Malignant neoplasms, stated or presumed to be primary
Any	6	196-198	Malignant neoplasms, stated or presumed to be secondary

The ICD-O behavior digit /9 is inapplicable in an ICD context, since all malignant neoplasms are presumed to be primary (/3) or secondary (/6) according to other information on the medical record. the first-listed term of the full ICD-O morphology nomenclature appears against each code number in the list below. The ICD-9-CM Alphabetical Index (Volume 2), however, includes all the ICD-O synonyms as well as a number of other morphological names still likely to be encountered on medical records but omitted from ICD-O as outdated or otherwise undesirable.

A coding difficulty sometimes arises where a morphological diagnosis contains two qualifying adjectives that have different code numbers. An example is "transitional cell epidermoid carcinoma." "Transitional cell carcinoma NOS" is M8120/3 and "epidermoid carcinoma NOS" is M8070/3. In such circumstances, the higher number (M8120/3 in this example) should be used, as it is usually more specific.

Coded Nomenclature for Morphology of Neoplasms

M800	Neoplasms NOS
M8000/0	Neoplasm, benign
M8000/1	Neoplasm, uncertain whether benign or malignant
M8000/3	Neoplasm, malignant
M8000/6	Neoplasm, metastatic
M8000/9	Neoplasm, malignant, uncertain whether primary or metastatic
M8001/0	Tumor cells, benign
M8001/1	Tumor cells, uncertain whether benign or malignant
M8001/3	Tumor cells, malignant
M8002/3	Malignant tumor, small cell type
M8003/3	Malignant tumor, giant cell type
M8004/3	Malignant tumor, fusiform cell type

M801-M804	Epithelial neoplasms NOS
M8010/0	Epithelial tumor, benign
M8010/2	Carcinoma in situ NOS
M8010/3	Carcinoma NOS
M8010/6	Carcinoma, metastatic NOS
M8010/9	Carcinomatosis
M8011/0	Epithelioma, benign
M8011/3	Epithelioma, malignant
M8012/3	Large cell carcinoma NOS
M8020/3	Carcinoma, undifferentiated type NOS
M8021/3	Carcinoma, anaplastic type NOS
M8022/3	Pleomorphic carcinoma
M8030/3	Giant cell and spindle cell carcinoma
M8031/3	Giant cell carcinoma
M8032/3	Spindle cell carcinoma
M8033/3	Pseudosarcomatous carcinoma
M8034/3	Polygonal cell carcinoma
M8035/3	Spheroidal cell carcinoma
M8040/1	Tumorlet
M8041/3	Small cell carcinoma NOS
M8042/3	Oat cell carcinoma
M8043/3	Small cell carcinoma, fusiform cell type

M805-M808	Papillary and squamous cell neoplasms
M8050/0	Papilloma NOS (except Papilloma of urinary bladder M8120/1)
M8050/2	Papillary carcinoma in situ
M8050/3	Papillary carcinoma NOS
M8051/0	Verrucous papilloma
M8051/3	Verrucous carcinoma NOS
M8052/0	Squamous cell papilloma
M8052/3	Papillary squamous cell carcinoma
M8053/0	Inverted papilloma
M8060/0	Papillomatosis NOS
M8070/2	Squamous cell carcinoma in situ NOS
M8070/3	Squamous cell carcinoma NOS
M8070/6	Squamous cell carcinoma, metastatic NOS
M8071/3	Squamous cell carcinoma, keratinizing type NOS
M8072/3	Squamous cell carcinoma, large cell, nonkeratinizing type
M8073/3	Squamous cell carcinoma, small cell, nonkeratinizing type
M8074/3	Squamous cell carcinoma, spindle cell type
M8075/3	Adenoid squamous cell carcinoma
M8076/2	Squamous cell carcinoma in situ with questionable stromal invasion
M8076/3	Squamous cell carcinoma, microinvasive
M8080/2	Queyrat's erythroplasia
M8081/2	Bowen's disease
M8082/3	Lymphoepithelial carcinoma

M809-M811	Basal cell neoplasms
M8090/1	Basal cell tumor
M8090/3	Basal cell carcinoma NOS
M8091/3	Multicentric basal cell carcinoma
M8092/3	Basal cell carcinoma, morphea type
M8093/3	Basal cell carcinoma, fibroepithelial type
M8094/3	Basosquamous carcinoma
M8095/3	Metatypical carcinoma
M8096/0	Intraepidermal epithelioma of Jadassohn
M8100/0	Trichoepithelioma
M8101/0	Trichofolliculoma
M8102/0	Tricholemmoma
M8110/0	Pilomatrixoma

M812-M813	Transitional cell papillomas and carcinomas
M8120/0	Transitional cell papilloma NOS
M8120/1	Urothelial papilloma
M8120/2	Transitional cell carcinoma in situ
M8120/3	Transitional cell carcinoma NOS
M8121/0	Schneiderian papilloma
M8121/1	Transitional cell papilloma, inverted type
M8121/3	Schneiderian carcinoma
M8122/3	Transitional cell carcinoma, spindle cell type
M8123/3	Basaloid carcinoma
M8124/3	Cloacogenic carcinoma
M8130/3	Papillary transitional cell carcinoma

M814-M838	Adenomas and adenocarcinomas
M8140/0	Adenoma NOS
M8140/1	Bronchial adenoma NOS
M8140/2	Adenocarcinoma in situ
M8140/3	Adenocarcinoma NOS
M8140/6	Adenocarcinoma, metastatic NOS
M8141/3	Scirrhous adenocarcinoma
M8142/3	Linitis plastica
M8143/3	Superficial spreading adenocarcinoma
M8144/3	Adenocarcinoma, intestinal type
M8145/3	Carcinoma, diffuse type
M8146/0	Monomorphic adenoma
M8147/0	Basal cell adenoma
M8150/0	Islet cell adenoma
M8150/3	Islet cell carcinoma
M8151/0	Insulinoma NOS
M8151/3	Insulinoma, malignant
M8152/0	Glucagonoma NOS
M8152/3	Glucagonoma, malignant
M8153/1	Gastrinoma NOS
M8153/3	Gastrinoma, malignant
M8154/3	Mixed islet cell and exocrine adenocarcinoma
M8160/0	Bile duct adenoma
M8160/3	Cholangiocarcinoma

Appendix A: Morphology of Neoplasms

M8161/0	Bile duct cystadenoma
M8161/3	Bile duct cystadenocarcinoma
M8170/0	Liver cell adenoma
M8170/3	Hepatocellular carcinoma NOS
M8180/0	Hepatocholangioma, benign
M8180/3	Combined hepatocellular carcinoma and cholangiocarcinoma
M8190/0	Trabecular adenoma
M8190/3	Trabecular adenocarcinoma
M8191/0	Embryonal adenoma
M8200/0	Eccrine dermal cylindroma
M8200/3	Adenoid cystic carcinoma
M8201/3	Cribriform carcinoma
M8210/0	Adenomatous polyp NOS
M8210/3	Adenocarcinoma in adenomatous polyp
M8211/0	Tubular adenoma NOS
M8211/3	Tubular adenocarcinoma
M8220/0	Adenomatous polyposis coli
M8220/3	Adenocarcinoma in adenomatous polyposis coli
M8221/0	Multiple adenomatous polyps
M8230/3	Solid carcinoma NOS
M8231/3	Carcinoma simplex
M8240/1	Carcinoid tumor NOS
M8240/3	Carcinoid tumor, malignant
M8241/1	Carcinoid tumor, argentaffin NOS
M8241/3	Carcinoid tumor, argentaffin, malignant
M8242/1	Carcinoid tumor, nonargentaffin NOS
M8242/3	Carcinoid tumor, nonargentaffin, malignant
M8243/3	Mucocarcinoid tumor, malignant
M8244/3	Composite carcinoid
M8250/1	Pulmonary adenomatosis
M8250/3	Bronchiolo-alveolar adenocarcinoma
M8251/0	Alveolar adenoma
M8251/3	Alveolar adenocarcinoma
M8260/0	Papillary adenoma NOS
M8260/3	Papillary adenocarcinoma NOS
M8261/1	Villous adenoma NOS
M8261/3	Adenocarcinoma in villous adenoma
M8262/3	Villous adenocarcinoma
M8263/0	Tubulovillous adenoma
M8270/0	Chromophobe adenoma
M8270/3	Chromophobe carcinoma
M8280/0	Acidophil adenoma
M8280/3	Acidophil carcinoma
M8281/0	Mixed acidophil-basophil adenoma
M8281/3	Mixed acidophil-basophil carcinoma
M8290/0	Oxyphilic adenoma
M8290/3	Oxyphilic adenocarcinoma
M8300/0	Basophil adenoma
M8300/3	Basophil carcinoma
M8310/0	Clear cell adenoma
M8310/3	Clear cell adenocarcinoma NOS
M8311/1	Hypernephroid tumor
M8312/3	Renal cell carcinoma
M8313/0	Clear cell adenofibroma
M8320/3	Granular cell carcinoma
M8321/0	Chief cell adenoma
M8322/0	Water-clear cell adenoma
M8322/3	Water-clear cell adenocarcinoma
M8323/0	Mixed cell adenoma
M8323/3	Mixed cell adenocarcinoma
M8324/0	Lipoadenoma
M8330/0	Follicular adenoma
M8330/3	Follicular adenocarcinoma NOS
M8331/3	Follicular adenocarcinoma, well differentiated type
M8332/3	Follicular adenocarcinoma, trabecular type

M8333/0	Microfollicular adenoma
M8334/0	Macrofollicular adenoma
M8340/3	Papillary and follicular adenocarcinoma
M8350/3	Nonencapsulated sclerosing carcinoma
M8360/1	Multiple endocrine adenomas
M8361/1	Juxtaglomerular tumor
M8370/0	Adrenal cortical adenoma NOS
M8370/3	Adrenal cortical carcinoma
M8371/0	Adrenal cortical adenoma, compact cell type
M8372/0	Adrenal cortical adenoma, heavily pigmented variant
M8373/0	Adrenal cortical adenoma, clear cell type
M8374/0	Adrenal cortical adenoma, glomerulosa cell type
M8375/0	Adrenal cortical adenoma, mixed cell type
M8380/0	Endometrioid adenoma NOS
M8380/1	Endometrioid adenoma, borderline malignancy
M8380/3	Endometrioid carcinoma
M8381/0	Endometrioid adenofibroma NOS
M8381/1	Endometrioid adenofibroma, borderline malignancy
M8381/3	Endometrioid adenofibroma, malignant

M839-M842   Adnexal and skin appendage neoplasms

M8390/0	Skin appendage adenoma
M8390/3	Skin appendage carcinoma
M8400/0	Sweat gland adenoma
M8400/1	Sweat gland tumor NOS
M8400/3	Sweat gland adenocarcinoma
M8401/0	Apocrine adenoma
M8401/3	Apocrine adenocarcinoma
M8402/0	Eccrine acrospiroma
M8403/0	Eccrine spiradenoma
M8404/0	Hidrocystoma
M8405/0	Papillary hydradenoma
M8406/0	Papillary syringadenoma
M8407/0	Syringoma NOS
M8410/0	Sebaceous adenoma
M8410/3	Sebaceous adenocarcinoma
M8420/0	Ceruminous adenoma
M8420/3	Ceruminous adenocarcinoma

M843   Mucoepidermoid neoplasms

M8430/1	Mucoepidermoid tumor
M8430/3	Mucoepidermoid carcinoma

M844-M849   Cystic, mucinous, and serous neoplasms

M8440/0	Cystadenoma NOS
M8440/3	Cystadenocarcinoma NOS
M8441/0	Serous cystadenoma NOS
M8441/1	Serous cystadenoma, borderline malignancy
M8441/3	Serous cystadenocarcinoma NOS
M8450/0	Papillary cystadenoma NOS
M8450/1	Papillary cystadenoma, borderline malignancy
M8450/3	Papillary cystadenocarcinoma NOS
M8460/0	Papillary serous cystadenoma NOS
M8460/1	Papillary serous cystadenoma, borderline malignancy
M8460/3	Papillary serous cystadenocarcinoma
M8461/0	Serous surface papilloma NOS
M8461/1	Serous surface papilloma, borderline malignancy
M8461/3	Serous surface papillary carcinoma
M8470/0	Mucinous cystadenoma NOS
M8470/1	Mucinous cystadenoma, borderline malignancy

M8470/3	Mucinous cystadenocarcinoma NOS
M8471/0	Papillary mucinous cystadenoma NOS
M8471/1	Papillary mucinous cystadenoma, borderline malignancy
M8471/3	Papillary mucinous cystadenocarcinoma
M8480/0	Mucinous adenoma
M8480/3	Mucinous adenocarcinoma
M8480/6	Pseudomyxoma peritonei
M8481/3	Mucin-producing adenocarcinoma
M8490/3	Signet ring cell carcinoma
M8490/6	Metastatic signet ring cell carcinoma

M850-M854   Ductal, lobular, and medullary neoplasms

M8500/2	Intraductal carcinoma, noninfiltrating NOS
M8500/3	Infiltrating duct carcinoma
M8501/2	Comedocarcinoma, noninfiltrating
M8501/3	Comedocarcinoma NOS
M8502/3	Juvenile carcinoma of the breast
M8503/0	Intraductal papilloma
M8503/2	Noninfiltrating intraductal papillary adenocarcinoma
M8504/0	Intracystic papillary adenoma
M8504/2	Noninfiltrating intracystic carcinoma
M8505/0	Intraductal papillomatosis NOS
M8506/0	Subareolar duct papillomatosis
M8510/3	Medullary carcinoma NOS
M8511/3	Medullary carcinoma with amyloid stroma
M8512/3	Medullary carcinoma with lymphoid stroma
M8520/2	Lobular carcinoma in situ
M8520/3	Lobular carcinoma NOS
M8521/3	Infiltrating ductular carcinoma
M8530/3	Inflammatory carcinoma
M8540/3	Paget's disease, mammary
M8541/3	Paget's disease and infiltrating duct carcinoma of breast
M8542/3	Paget's disease, extramammary (except Paget's disease of bone)

M855   Acinar cell neoplasms

M8550/0	Acinar cell adenoma
M8550/1	Acinar cell tumor
M8550/3	Acinar cell carcinoma

M856-M858   Complex epithelial neoplasms

M8560/3	Adenosquamous carcinoma
M8561/0	Adenolymphoma
M8570/3	Adenocarcinoma with squamous metaplasia
M8571/3	Adenocarcinoma with cartilaginous and osseous metaplasia
M8572/3	Adenocarcinoma with spindle cell metaplasia
M8573/3	Adenocarcinoma with apocrine metaplasia
M8580/0	Thymoma, benign
M8580/3	Thymoma, malignant

M859-M867   Specialized gonadal neoplasms

M8590/1	Sex cord-stromal tumor
M8600/0	Thecoma NOS
M8600/3	Theca cell carcinoma
M8610/0	Luteoma NOS
M8620/1	Granulosa cell tumor NOS
M8620/3	Granulosa cell tumor, malignant
M8621/1	Granulosa cell-theca cell tumor
M8630/0	Androblastoma, benign
M8630/1	Androblastoma NOS
M8630/3	Androblastoma, malignant
M8631/0	Sertoli-Leydig cell tumor

M8632/1	Gynandroblastoma	
M8640/0	Tubular androblastoma NOS	
M8640/3	Sertoli cell carcinoma	
M8641/0	Tubular androblastoma with lipid storage	
M8650/0	Leydig cell tumor, benign	
M8650/1	Leydig cell tumor NOS	
M8650/3	Leydig cell tumor, malignant	
M8660/0	Hilar cell tumor	
M8670/0	Lipid cell tumor of ovary	
M8671/0	Adrenal rest tumor	

M868-M871   Paragangliomas and glomus tumors

M8680/1	Paraganglioma NOS
M8680/3	Paraganglioma, malignant
M8681/1	Sympathetic paraganglioma
M8682/1	Parasympathetic paraganglioma
M8690/1	Glomus jugulare tumor
M8691/1	Aortic body tumor
M8692/1	Carotid body tumor
M8693/1	Extra-adrenal paraganglioma NOS
M8693/3	Extra-adrenal paraganglioma, malignant
M8700/0	Pheochromocytoma NOS
M8700/3	Pheochromocytoma, malignant
M8710/3	Glomangiosarcoma
M8711/0	Glomus tumor
M8712/0	Glomangioma

M872-M879   Nevi and melanomas

M8720/0	Pigmented nevus NOS
M8720/3	Malignant melanoma NOS
M8721/3	Nodular melanoma
M8722/0	Balloon cell nevus
M8722/3	Balloon cell melanoma
M8723/0	Halo nevus
M8724/0	Fibrous papule of the nose
M8725/0	Neuronevus
M8726/0	Magnocellular nevus
M8730/0	Nonpigmented nevus
M8730/3	Amelanotic melanoma
M8740/0	Junctional nevus
M8740/3	Malignant melanoma in junctional nevus
M8741/2	Precancerous melanosis NOS
M8741/3	Malignant melanoma in precancerous melanosis
M8742/2	Hutchinson's melanotic freckle
M8742/3	Malignant melanoma in Hutchinson's melanotic freckle
M8743/3	Superficial spreading melanoma
M8750/0	Intradermal nevus
M8760/0	Compound nevus
M8761/1	Giant pigmented nevus
M8761/3	Malignant melanoma in giant pigmented nevus
M8770/0	Epithelioid and spindle cell nevus
M8771/3	Epithelioid cell melanoma
M8772/3	Spindle cell melanoma NOS
M8773/3	Spindle cell melanoma, type A
M8774/3	Spindle cell melanoma, type B
M8775/3	Mixed epithelioid and spindle cell melanoma
M8780/0	Blue nevus NOS
M8780/3	Blue nevus, malignant
M8790/0	Cellular blue nevus

M880   Soft tissue tumors and sarcomas NOS

M8800/0	Soft tissue tumor, benign
M8800/3	Sarcoma NOS
M8800/9	Sarcomatosis NOS
M8801/3	Spindle cell sarcoma
M8802/3	Giant cell sarcoma (except of bone M9250/3)

M8803/3	Small cell sarcoma
M8804/3	Epithelioid cell sarcoma

M881-M883   Fibromatous neoplasms

M8810/0	Fibroma NOS
M8810/3	Fibrosarcoma NOS
M8811/0	Fibromyxoma
M8811/3	Fibromyxosarcoma
M8812/0	Periosteal fibroma
M8812/3	Periosteal fibrosarcoma
M8813/0	Fascial fibroma
M8813/3	Fascial fibrosarcoma
M8814/3	Infantile fibrosarcoma
M8820/0	Elastofibroma
M8821/1	Aggressive fibromatosis
M8822/1	Abdominal fibromatosis
M8823/1	Desmoplastic fibroma
M8830/0	Fibrous histiocytoma NOS
M8830/1	Atypical fibrous histiocytoma
M8830/3	Fibrous histiocytoma, malignant
M8831/0	Fibroxanthoma NOS
M8831/1	Atypical fibroxanthoma
M8831/3	Fibroxanthoma, malignant
M8832/0	Dermatofibroma NOS
M8832/1	Dermatofibroma protuberans
M8832/3	Dermatofibrosarcoma NOS

M884   Myxomatous neoplasms

M8840/0	Myxoma NOS
M8840/3	Myxosarcoma

M885-M888   Lipomatous neoplasms

M8850/0	Lipoma NOS
M8850/3	Liposarcoma NOS
M8851/0	Fibrolipoma
M8851/3	Liposarcoma, well differentiated type
M8852/0	Fibromyxolipoma
M8852/3	Myxoid liposarcoma
M8853/3	Round cell liposarcoma
M8854/3	Pleomorphic liposarcoma
M8855/3	Mixed type liposarcoma
M8856/0	Intramuscular lipoma
M8857/0	Spindle cell lipoma
M8860/0	Angiomyolipoma
M8860/3	Angiomyoliposarcoma
M8861/0	Angiolipoma NOS
M8861/1	Angiolipoma, infiltrating
M8870/0	Myelolipoma
M8880/0	Hibernoma
M8881/0	Lipoblastomatosis

M889-M892   Myomatous neoplasms

M8890/0	Leiomyoma NOS
M8890/1	Intravascular leiomyomatosis
M8890/3	Leiomyosarcoma NOS
M8891/1	Epithelioid leiomyoma
M8891/3	Epithelioid leiomyosarcoma
M8892/1	Cellular leiomyoma
M8893/0	Bizarre leiomyoma
M8894/0	Angiomyoma
M8894/3	Angiomyosarcoma
M8895/0	Myoma
M8895/3	Myosarcoma
M8900/0	Rhabdomyoma NOS
M8900/3	Rhabdomyosarcoma NOS
M8901/3	Pleomorphic rhabdomyosarcoma
M8902/3	Mixed type rhabdomyosarcoma
M8903/0	Fetal rhabdomyoma
M8904/0	Adult rhabdomyoma
M8910/3	Embryonal rhabdomyosarcoma
M8920/3	Alveolar rhabdomyosarcoma

M893-M899   Complex mixed and stromal neoplasms

M8930/3	Endometrial stromal sarcoma
M8931/1	Endolymphatic stromal myosis
M8932/0	Adenomyoma
M8940/0	Pleomorphic adenoma
M8940/3	Mixed tumor, malignant NOS
M8950/3	Mullerian mixed tumor
M8951/3	Mesodermal mixed tumor
M8960/1	Mesoblastic nephroma
M8960/3	Nephroblastoma NOS
M8961/3	Epithelial nephroblastoma
M8962/3	Mesenchymal nephroblastoma
M8970/3	Hepatoblastoma
M8980/3	Carcinosarcoma NOS
M8981/3	Carcinosarcoma, embryonal type
M8982/0	Myoepithelioma
M8990/0	Mesenchymoma, benign
M8990/1	Mesenchymoma NOS
M8990/3	Mesenchymoma, malignant
M8991/3	Embryonal sarcoma

M900-M903   Fibroepithelial neoplasms

M9000/0	Brenner tumor NOS
M9000/1	Brenner tumor, borderline malignancy
M9000/3	Brenner tumor, malignant
M9010/0	Fibroadenoma NOS
M9011/0	Intracanalicular fibroadenoma NOS
M9012/0	Pericanalicular fibroadenoma
M9013/0	Adenofibroma NOS
M9014/0	Serous adenofibroma
M9015/0	Mucinous adenofibroma
M9020/0	Cellular intracanalicular fibroadenoma
M9020/1	Cystosarcoma phyllodes NOS
M9020/3	Cystosarcoma phyllodes, malignant
M9030/0	Juvenile fibroadenoma

M904   Synovial neoplasms

M9040/0	Synovioma, benign
M9040/3	Synovial sarcoma NOS
M9041/3	Synovial sarcoma, spindle cell type
M9042/3	Synovial sarcoma, epithelioid cell type
M9043/3	Synovial sarcoma, biphasic type
M9044/3	Clear cell sarcoma of tendons and aponeuroses

M905   Mesothelial neoplasms

M9050/0	Mesothelioma, benign
M9050/3	Mesothelioma, malignant
M9051/0	Fibrous mesothelioma, benign
M9051/3	Fibrous mesothelioma, malignant
M9052/0	Epithelioid mesothelioma, benign
M9052/3	Epithelioid mesothelioma, malignant
M9053/0	Mesothelioma, biphasic type, benign
M9053/3	Mesothelioma, biphasic type, malignant
M9054/0	Adenomatoid tumor NOS

M906-M909   Germ cell neoplasms

M9060/3	Dysgerminoma
M9061/3	Seminoma NOS
M9062/3	Seminoma, anaplastic type
M9063/3	Spermatocytic seminoma
M9064/3	Germinoma
M9070/3	Embryonal carcinoma NOS
M9071/3	Endodermal sinus tumor
M9072/3	Polyembryoma
M9073/1	Gonadoblastoma
M9080/0	Teratoma, benign
M9080/1	Teratoma NOS
M9080/3	Teratoma, malignant NOS
M9081/3	Teratocarcinoma

M9082/3	Malignant teratoma, undifferentiated type
M9083/3	Malignant teratoma, intermediate type
M9084/0	Dermoid cyst
M9084/3	Dermoid cyst with malignant transformation
M9090/0	Struma ovarii NOS
M9090/3	Struma ovarii, malignant
M9091/1	Strumal carcinoid

M910 Trophoblastic neoplasms

M9100/0	Hydatidiform mole NOS
M9100/1	Invasive hydatidiform mole
M9100/3	Choriocarcinoma
M9101/3	Choriocarcinoma combined with teratoma
M9102/3	Malignant teratoma, trophoblastic

M911 Mesonephromas

M9110/0	Mesonephroma, benign
M9110/1	Mesonephric tumor
M9110/3	Mesonephroma, malignant
M9111/1	Endosalpingioma

M912-M916 Blood vessel tumors

M9120/0	Hemangioma NOS
M9120/3	Hemangiosarcoma
M9121/0	Cavernous hemangioma
M9122/0	Venous hemangioma
M9123/0	Racemose hemangioma
M9124/3	Kupffer cell sarcoma
M9130/0	Hemangioendothelioma, benign
M9130/1	Hemangioendothelioma NOS
M9130/3	Hemangioendothelioma, malignant
M9131/0	Capillary hemangioma
M9132/0	Intramuscular hemangioma
M9140/3	Kaposi's sarcoma
M9141/0	Angiokeratoma
M9142/0	Verrucous keratotic hemangioma
M9150/0	Hemangiopericytoma, benign
M9150/1	Hemangiopericytoma NOS
M9150/3	Hemangiopericytoma, malignant
M9160/0	Angiofibroma NOS
M9161/1	Hemangioblastoma

M917 Lymphatic vessel tumors

M9170/0	Lymphangioma NOS
M9170/3	Lymphangiosarcoma
M9171/0	Capillary lymphangioma
M9172/0	Cavernous lymphangioma
M9173/0	Cystic lymphangioma
M9174/0	Lymphangiomyoma
M9174/1	Lymphangiomyomatosis
M9175/0	Hemolymphangioma

M918-M920 Osteomas and osteosarcomas

M9180/0	Osteoma NOS
M9180/3	Osteosarcoma NOS
M9181/3	Chondroblastic osteosarcoma
M9182/3	Fibroblastic osteosarcoma
M9183/3	Telangiectatic osteosarcoma
M9184/3	Osteosarcoma in Paget's disease of bone
M9190/3	Juxtacortical osteosarcoma
M9191/0	Osteoid osteoma NOS
M9200/0	Osteoblastoma

M921-M924 Chondromatous neoplasms

M9210/0	Osteochondroma
M9210/1	Osteochondromatosis NOS
M9220/0	Chondroma NOS
M9220/1	Chondromatosis NOS
M9220/3	Chondrosarcoma NOS
M9221/0	Juxtacortical chondroma

M9221/3	Juxtacortical chondrosarcoma
M9230/0	Chondroblastoma NOS
M9230/3	Chondroblastoma, malignant
M9240/3	Mesenchymal chondrosarcoma
M9241/0	Chondromyxoid fibroma

M925 Giant cell tumors

M9250/1	Giant cell tumor of bone NOS
M9250/3	Giant cell tumor of bone, malignant
M9251/1	Giant cell tumor of soft parts NOS
M9251/3	Malignant giant cell tumor of soft parts

M926 Miscellaneous bone tumors

M9260/3	Ewing's sarcoma
M9261/3	Adamantinoma of long bones
M9262/0	Ossifying fibroma

M927-M934 Odontogenic tumors

M9270/0	Odontogenic tumor, benign
M9270/1	Odontogenic tumor NOS
M9270/3	Odontogenic tumor, malignant
M9271/0	Dentinoma
M9272/0	Cementoma NOS
M9273/0	Cementoblastoma, benign
M9274/0	Cementifying fibroma
M9275/0	Gigantiform cementoma
M9280/0	Odontoma NOS
M9281/0	Compound odontoma
M9282/0	Complex odontoma
M9290/0	Ameloblastic fibro-odontoma
M9290/3	Ameloblastic odontosarcoma
M9300/0	Adenomatoid odontogenic tumor
M9301/0	Calcifying odontogenic cyst
M9310/0	Ameloblastoma NOS
M9310/3	Ameloblastoma, malignant
M9311/0	Odontoameloblastoma
M9312/0	Squamous odontogenic tumor
M9320/0	Odontogenic myxoma
M9321/0	Odontogenic fibroma NOS
M9330/0	Ameloblastic fibroma
M9330/3	Ameloblastic fibrosarcoma
M9340/0	Calcifying epithelial odontogenic tumor

M935-M937 Miscellaneous tumors

M9350/1	Craniopharyngioma
M9360/1	Pinealoma
M9361/1	Pineocytoma
M9362/3	Pineoblastoma
M9363/0	Melanotic neuroectodermal tumor
M9370/3	Chordoma

M938-M948 Gliomas

M9380/3	Glioma, malignant
M9381/3	Gliomatosis cerebri
M9382/3	Mixed glioma
M9383/1	Subependymal glioma
M9384/1	Subependymal giant cell astrocytoma
M9390/0	Choroid plexus papilloma NOS
M9390/3	Choroid plexus papilloma, malignant
M9391/3	Ependymoma NOS
M9392/3	Ependymoma, anaplastic type
M9393/1	Papillary ependymoma
M9394/1	Myxopapillary ependymoma
M9400/3	Astrocytoma NOS
M9401/3	Astrocytoma, anaplastic type
M9410/3	Protoplasmic astrocytoma
M9411/3	Gemistocytic astrocytoma
M9420/3	Fibrillary astrocytoma
M9421/3	Pilocytic astrocytoma
M9422/3	Spongioblastoma NOS
M9423/3	Spongioblastoma polare
M9430/3	Astroblastoma

M9440/3	Glioblastoma NOS
M9441/3	Giant cell glioblastoma
M9442/3	Glioblastoma with sarcomatous component
M9443/3	Primitive polar spongioblastoma
M9450/3	Oligodendroglioma NOS
M9451/3	Oligodendroglioma, anaplastic type
M9460/3	Oligodendroblastoma
M9470/3	Medulloblastoma NOS
M9471/3	Desmoplastic medulloblastoma
M9472/3	Medullomyoblastoma
M9480/3	Cerebellar sarcoma NOS
M9481/3	Monstrocellular sarcoma

M949-M952 Neuroepitheliomatous neoplasms

M9490/0	Ganglioneuroma
M9490/3	Ganglioneuroblastoma
M9491/0	Ganglioneuromatosis
M9500/3	Neuroblastoma NOS
M9501/3	Medulloepithelioma NOS
M9502/3	Teratoid medulloepithelioma
M9503/3	Neuroepithelioma NOS
M9504/3	Spongioneuroblastoma
M9505/1	Ganglioglioma
M9506/0	Neurocytoma
M9507/0	Pacinian tumor
M9510/3	Retinoblastoma NOS
M9511/3	Retinoblastoma, differentiated type
M9512/3	Retinoblastoma, undifferentiated type
M9520/3	Olfactory neurogenic tumor
M9521/3	Esthesioneurocytoma
M9522/3	Esthesioneuroblastoma
M9523/3	Esthesioneuroepithelioma

M953 Meningiomas

M9530/0	Meningioma NOS
M9530/1	Meningiomatosis NOS
M9530/3	Meningioma, malignant
M9531/0	Meningotheliomatous meningioma
M9532/0	Fibrous meningioma
M9533/0	Psammomatous meningioma
M9534/0	Angiomatous meningioma
M9535/0	Hemangioblastic meningioma
M9536/0	Hemangiopericytic meningioma
M9537/0	Transitional meningioma
M9538/1	Papillary meningioma
M9539/3	Meningeal sarcomatosis

M954-M957 Nerve sheath tumor

M9540/0	Neurofibroma NOS
M9540/1	Neurofibromatosis NOS
M9540/3	Neurofibrosarcoma
M9541/0	Melanotic neurofibroma
M9550/0	Plexiform neurofibroma
M9560/0	Neurilemmoma NOS
M9560/1	Neurinomatosis
M9560/3	Neurilemmoma, malignant
M9570/0	Neuroma NOS

M958 Granular cell tumors and alveolar soft part sarcoma

M9580/0	Granular cell tumor NOS
M9580/3	Granular cell tumor, malignant
M9581/3	Alveolar soft part sarcoma

M959-M963 Lymphomas, NOS or diffuse

M9590/0	Lymphomatous tumor, benign
M9590/3	Malignant lymphoma NOS
M9591/3	Malignant lymphoma, non Hodgkin's type
M9600/3	Malignant lymphoma, undifferentiated cell type NOS
M9601/3	Malignant lymphoma, stem cell type

M9602/3	Malignant lymphoma, convoluted cell type NOS	
M9610/3	Lymphosarcoma NOS	
M9611/3	Malignant lymphoma, lymphoplasmacytoid type	
M9612/3	Malignant lymphoma, immunoblastic type	
M9613/3	Malignant lymphoma, mixed lymphocytic-histiocytic NOS	
M9614/3	Malignant lymphoma, centroblastic-centrocytic, diffuse	
M9615/3	Malignant lymphoma, follicular center cell NOS	
M9620/3	Malignant lymphoma, lymphocytic, well differentiated NOS	
M9621/3	Malignant lymphoma, lymphocytic, intermediate differentiation NOS	
M9622/3	Malignant lymphoma, centrocytic	
M9623/3	Malignant lymphoma, follicular center cell, cleaved NOS	
M9630/3	Malignant lymphoma, lymphocytic, poorly differentiated NOS	
M9631/3	Prolymphocytic lymphosarcoma	
M9632/3	Malignant lymphoma, centroblastic type NOS	
M9633/3	Malignant lymphoma, follicular center cell, noncleaved NOS	

M964 **Reticulosarcomas**
M9640/3	Reticulosarcoma NOS
M9641/3	Reticulosarcoma, pleomorphic cell type
M9642/3	Reticulosarcoma, nodular

M965-M966 **Hodgkin's disease**
M9650/3	Hodgkin's disease NOS
M9651/3	Hodgkin's disease, lymphocytic predominance
M9652/3	Hodgkin's disease, mixed cellularity
M9653/3	Hodgkin's disease, lymphocytic depletion NOS
M9654/3	Hodgkin's disease, lymphocytic depletion, diffuse fibrosis
M9655/3	Hodgkin's disease, lymphocytic depletion, reticular type
M9656/3	Hodgkin's disease, nodular sclerosis NOS
M9657/3	Hodgkin's disease, nodular sclerosis, cellular phase
M9660/3	Hodgkin's paragranuloma
M9661/3	Hodgkin's granuloma
M9662/3	Hodgkin's sarcoma

M969 **Lymphomas, nodular or follicular**
M9690/3	Malignant lymphoma, nodular NOS

M9691/3	Malignant lymphoma, mixed lymphocytic-histiocytic, nodular
M9692/3	Malignant lymphoma, centroblastic-centrocytic, follicular
M9693/3	Malignant lymphoma, lymphocytic, well differentiated, nodular
M9694/3	Malignant lymphoma, lymphocytic, intermediate differentiation, nodular
M9695/3	Malignant lymphoma, follicular center cell, cleaved, follicular
M9696/3	Malignant lymphoma, lymphocytic, poorly differentiated, nodular
M9697/3	Malignant lymphoma, centroblastic type, follicular
M9698/3	Malignant lymphoma, follicular center cell, noncleaved, follicular

M970 **Mycosis fungoides**
M9700/3	Mycosis fungoides
M9701/3	Sezary's disease

M971-M972 **Miscellaneous reticuloendothelial neoplasms**
M9710/3	Microglioma
M9720/3	Malignant histiocytosis
M9721/3	Histiocytic medullary reticulosis
M9722/3	Letterer-Siwe's disease

M973 **Plasma cell tumors**
M9730/3	Plasma cell myeloma
M9731/0	Plasma cell tumor, benign
M9731/1	Plasmacytoma NOS
M9731/3	Plasma cell tumor, malignant

M974 **Mast cell tumors**
M9740/1	Mastocytoma NOS
M9740/3	Mast cell sarcoma
M9741/3	Malignant mastocytosis

M975 **Burkitt's tumor**
M9750/3	Burkitt's tumor

M980-M994 **Leukemias NOS**
M9800/3	Leukemias NOS
M9800/3	Leukemia NOS
M9801/3	Acute leukemia NOS
M9802/3	Subacute leukemia NOS
M9803/3	Chronic leukemia NOS
M9804/3	Aleukemic leukemia NOS

M981 **Compound leukemias**
M9810/3	Compound leukemia

M982 **Lymphoid leukemias**
M9820/3	Lymphoid leukemia NOS

M9821/3	Acute lymphoid leukemia
M9822/3	Subacute lymphoid leukemia
M9823/3	Chronic lymphoid leukemia
M9824/3	Aleukemic lymphoid leukemia
M9825/3	Prolymphocytic leukemia

M983 **Plasma cell leukemias**
M9830/3	Plasma cell leukemia

M984 **Erythroleukemias**
M9840/3	Erythroleukemia
M9841/3	Acute erythremia
M9842/3	Chronic erythremia

M985 **Lymphosarcoma cell leukemias**
M9850/3	Lymphosarcoma cell leukemia

M986 **Myeloid leukemias**
M9860/3	Myeloid leukemia NOS
M9861/3	Acute myeloid leukemia
M9862/3	Subacute myeloid leukemia
M9863/3	Chronic myeloid leukemia
M9864/3	Aleukemic myeloid leukemia
M9865/3	Neutrophilic leukemia
M9866/3	Acute promyelocytic leukemia

M987 **Basophilic leukemias**
M9870/3	Basophilic leukemia

M988 **Eosinophilic leukemias**
M9880/3	Eosinophilic leukemia

M989 **Monocytic leukemias**
M9890/3	Monocytic leukemia NOS
M9891/3	Acute monocytic leukemia
M9892/3	Subacute monocytic leukemia
M9893/3	Chronic monocytic leukemia
M9894/3	Aleukemic monocytic leukemia

M990-M994 **Miscellaneous leukemias**
M9900/3	Mast cell leukemia
M9910/3	Megakaryocytic leukemia
M9920/3	Megakaryocytic myelosis
M9930/3	Myeloid sarcoma
M9940/3	Hairy cell leukemia

M995-M997 **Miscellaneous myeloproliferative and lymphoproliferative disorders**
M9950/1	Polycythemia vera
M9951/1	Acute panmyelosis
M9960/1	Chronic myeloproliferative disease
M9961/1	Myelosclerosis with myeloid metaplasia
M9962/1	Idiopathic thrombocythemia
M9970/1	Chronic lymphoproliferative disease

Appendix B: Glossary of Mental Disorders

was officially deleted October 1, 2004

Appendix C: Classification of Drugs by American Hospital Formulary Service List Number and Their ICD-9-CM Equivalents

The coding of adverse effects of drugs is keyed to the continually revised Hospital Formulary of the American Hospital Formulary Service (AHFS) published under the direction of the American Society of Hospital Pharmacists.

The following section gives the ICD-9-CM diagnosis code for each AHFS list.

	AHFS* List	ICD-9-CM Dx Code
4:00	ANTIHISTAMINE DRUGS	963.0
8:00	ANTI-INFECTIVE AGENTS	
8:04	Amebacides	961.5
	hydroxyquinoline derivatives	961.3
	arsenical anti-infectives	961.1
	quinoline derivatives	961.3
8:12.04	Antifungal Antibiotics	960.1
	nonantibiotics	961.9
8:12.06	Cephalosporins	960.5
8:12.08	Chloramphenicol	960.2
8:12.12	The Erythromycins	960.3
8:12.16	The Penicillins	960.0
8:12.20	The Streptomycins	960.6
8:12.24	The Tetracyclines	960.4
8:12.28	Other Antibiotics	960.8
	antimycobacterial antibiotics	960.6
	macrolides	960.3
8:16	Antituberculars	961.8
	antibiotics	960.6
8:18	Antivirals	961.7
8:20	Plasmodicides (antimalarials)	961.4
8:24	Sulfonamides	961.0
8:26	The Sulfones	961.8
8:28	Treponemicides	961.2
8:32	Trichomonacides	961.5
	hydroxyquinoline derivatives	961.3
	nitrofuran derivatives	961.9
8:36	Urinary Germicides	961.9
	quinoline derivatives	961.3
8:40	Other Anti-Infectives	961.9
10:00	ANTINEOPLASTIC AGENTS	963.1
	antibiotics	960.7
	progestogens	962.2
12:00	AUTONOMIC DRUGS	
12:04	Parasympathomimetic (Cholinergic) Agents	971.0
12:08	Parasympatholytic (Cholinergic Blocking Agents	971.1
12:12	Sympathomimetic (Adrenergic) Agents	971.2
12:16	Sympatholytic (Adrenergic Blocking) Agents	971.3
12:20	Skeletal Muscle Relaxants	975.2
	central nervous system	
	muscle-tone depressants	968.0
16:00	BLOOD DERIVATIVES	964.7
20:00	BLOOD FORMATION AND COAGULATION	
20:04	Antianemia Drugs	964.1
20:04.04	Iron Preparations	964.0
20:04.08	Liver and Stomach Preparations	964.1
20:12.04	Anticoagulants	964.2
20:12.08	Antiheparin Agents	964.5
20:12.12	Coagulants	964.5
20:12.16	Hemostatics	964.5
	capillary-active drugs	972.8
	fibrinolysis-affecting agents	964.4
	natural products	964.7
24:00	CARDIOVASCULAR DRUGS	
24:04	Cardiac Drugs	972.9
	cardiotonic agents	972.1
	rhythm regulators	972.0
24:06	Antilipemic Agents	972.2
	thyroid derivatives	962.7

	AHFS* List	ICD-9-CM Dx Code
24:08	Hypotensive Agents	972.6
	adrenergic blocking agents	971.3
	ganglion-blocking agents	972.3
	vasodilators	972.5
24:12	Vasodilating Agents	972.5
	coronary	972.4
	nicotinic acid derivatives	972.2
24:16	Sclerosing Agents	972.7
28:00	CENTRAL NERVOUS SYSTEM DRUGS	
28:04	General Anesthetics	968.4
	gaseous anesthetics	968.2
	halothane	968.1
	intravenous anesthetics	968.3
28:08	Analgesics and Antipyretics	965.9
	antirheumatics	965.61-965.69
	aromatic analgesics	965.4
	non-narcotics NEC	965.7
	opium alkaloids	965.00
	heroin	965.01
	methadone	965.02
	specified type NEC	965.09
	pyrazole derivatives	965.5
	salicylates	965.1
	specified type NEC	965.8
28:10	Narcotic Antagonists	970.1
28:12	Anticonvulsants	966.3
	barbiturates	967.0
	benzodiazepine-based tranquilizers	969.4
	bromides	967.3
	hydantoin derivatives	966.1
	oxazolidine derivative	966.0
	succinimides	966.2
28:16.04	Antidepressants	969.00-969.09
28:16.08	Tranquilizers	969.5
	benzodiazepine-based	969.4
	butyrophenone-based	969.2
	major NEC	969.3
	phenothiazine-based	969.1
28:16.12	Other Psychotherapeutic Agents	969.8
28:20	Respiratory and Cerebral Stimulants	970.9
	analeptics	970.0
	anorexigenic agents	977.0
	psychostimulants	969.70-969.79
	specified type NEC	970.81-970.89
28:24	Sedatives and Hypnotics	967.9
	barbiturates	967.0
	benzodiazepine-based tranquilizers	969.4
	chloral hydrate group	967.1
	glutethamide group	967.5
	intravenous anesthetics	968.3
	methaqualone	967.4
	paraldehyde	967.2
	phenothiazine-based tranquilizers	969.1
	specified type NEC	967.8
	thiobarbiturates	968.3
	tranquilizer NEC	969.5
36:00	DIAGNOSTIC AGENTS	977.8
40:00	ELECTROLYTE, CALORIC, AND WATER BALANCE AGENTS NEC	974.5
40:04	Acidifying Agents	963.2
40:08	Alkalinizing Agents	963.3
40:10	Ammonia Detoxicants	974.5
40:12	Replacement Solutions NEC	974.5
	plasma volume expanders	964.8
40:16	Sodium-Removing Resins	974.5
40:18	Potassium-Removing Resins	974.5
40:20	Caloric Agents	974.5
40:24	Salt and Sugar Substitutes	974.5
40:28	Diuretics NEC	974.4
	carbonic acid anhydrase inhibitors	974.2
	mercurials	974.0
	purine derivatives	974.1
	saluretics	974.3

AHFS* List	ICD-9-CM Dx Code
40:36 Irrigating Solutions	974.5
40:40 Uricosuric Agents	974.7
44:00 ENZYMES NEC	963.4
fibrinolysis-affecting agents	964.4
gastric agents	973.4
48:00 EXPECTORANTS AND COUGH PREPARATIONS	
antihistamine agents	963.0
antitussives	975.4
codeine derivatives	965.09
expectorants	975.5
narcotic agents NEC	965.09
52:00 EYE, EAR, NOSE, AND THROAT PREPARATIONS	
52:04 Anti-Infectives	
ENT	976.6
ophthalmic	976.5
52:04.04 Antibiotics	
ENT	976.6
ophthalmic	976.5
52:04.06 Antivirals	
ENT	976.6
ophthalmic	976.5
52:04.08 Sulfonamides	
ENT	976.6
ophthalmic	976.5
52:04.12 Miscellaneous Anti-Infectives	
ENT	976.6
ophthalmic	976.5
52:08 Anti-Inflammatory Agents	
ENT	976.6
ophthalmic	976.5
52:10 Carbonic Anhydrase Inhibitors	974.2
52:12 Contact Lens Solutions	976.5
52:16 Local Anesthetics	968.5
52:20 Miotics	971.0
52:24 Mydriatics	
adrenergics	971.2
anticholinergics	971.1
antimuscarinics	971.1
parasympatholytics	971.1
spasmolytics	971.1
sympathomimetics	971.2
52:28 Mouth Washes and Gargles	976.6
52:32 Vasoconstrictors	971.2
52:36 Unclassified Agents	
ENT	976.6
ophthalmic	976.5
56:00 GASTROINTESTINAL DRUGS	
56:04 Antacids and Absorbents	973.0
56:08 Anti-Diarrhea Agents	973.5
56:10 Antiflatulents	973.8
56:12 Cathartics NEC	973.3
emollients	973.2
irritants	973.1
56:16 Digestants	973.4
56:20 Emetics and Antiemetics	
antiemetics	963.0
emetics	973.6
56:24 Lipotropic Agents	977.1
60:00 GOLD COMPOUNDS	965.69
64:00 HEAVY METAL ANTAGONISTS	963.8
68:00 HORMONES AND SYNTHETIC SUBSTITUTES	
68:04 Adrenals	962.0
68:08 Androgens	962.1
68:12 Contraceptives	962.2
68:16 Estrogens	962.2
68:18 Gonadotropins	962.4
68:20 Insulins and Antidiabetic Agents	962.3
68:20.08 Insulins	962.3
68:24 Parathyroid	962.6
68:28 Pituitary	
anterior	962.4
posterior	962.5
68:32 Progestogens	962.2

AHFS* List	ICD-9-CM Dx Code
68:34 Other Corpus Luteum Hormones	962.2
68:36 Thyroid and Antithyroid	
antithyroid	962.8
thyroid	962.7
72:00 LOCAL ANESTHETICS NEC	968.9
topical (surface) agents	968.5
infiltrating agents (intradermal) (subcutaneous) (submucosal)	968.5
nerve blocking agents (peripheral) (plexus) (regional)	968.6
spinal	968.7
76:00 OXYTOCICS	975.0
78:00 RADIOACTIVE AGENTS	990
80:00 SERUMS, TOXOIDS, AND VACCINES	
80:04 Serums	979.9
immune globulin (gamma) (human)	964.6
80:08 Toxoids NEC	978.8
diphtheria	978.5
and tetanus	978.9
with pertussis component	978.6
tetanus	978.4
and diphtheria	978.9
with pertussis component	978.6
80:12 Vaccines NEC	979.9
bacterial NEC	978.8
with other bacterial component	978.9
pertussis component	978.6
viral and rickettsial component	979.7
rickettsial NEC	979.6
with bacterial component	979.7
pertussis component	978.6
viral component	979.7
viral NEC	979.6
with bacterial component	979.7
pertussis component	978.6
rickettsial component	979.7
84:00 SKIN AND MUCOUS MEMBRANE PREPARATIONS	
84:04 Anti-Infectives	976.0
84:04.04 Antibiotics	976.0
84:04.08 Fungicides	976.0
84:04.12 Scabicides and Pediculicides	976.0
84:04.16 Miscellaneous Local Anti-Infectives	976.0
84:06 Anti-Inflammatory Agents	976.0
84:08 Antipruritics and Local Anesthetics	
antipruritics	976.1
local anesthetics	968.5
84:12 Astringents	976.2
84:16 Cell Stimulants and Proliferants	976.8
84:20 Detergents	976.2
84:24 Emollients, Demulcents, and Protectants	976.3
84:28 Keratolytic Agents	976.4
84:32 Keratoplastic Agents	976.4
84:36 Miscellaneous Agents	976.8
86:00 SPASMOLYTIC AGENTS	975.1
antiasthmatics	975.7
papaverine	972.5
theophyllin	974.1
88:00 VITAMINS	
88:04 Vitamin A	963.5
88:08 Vitamin B Complex	963.5
hematopoietic vitamin	964.1
nicotinic acid derivatives	972.2
88:12 Vitamin C	963.5
88:16 Vitamin D	963.5
88:20 Vitamin E	963.5
88:24 Vitamin K Activity	964.3
88:28 Multivitamin Preparations	963.5
92:00 UNCLASSIFIED THERAPEUTIC AGENTS	977.8

* American Hospital Formulary Service

Appendix D: Classification of Industrial Accidents According to Agency

Annex B to the Resolution concerning Statistics of Employment Injuries adopted by the Tenth International Conference of Labor Statisticians on 12 October 1962

1 Machines

11	Prime-Movers, except Electrical Motors
111	Steam engines
112	Internal combustion engines
119	Others
12	Transmission Machinery
121	Transmission shafts
122	Transmission belts, cables, pulleys, pinions, chains, gears
129	Others
13	Metalworking Machines
131	Power presses
132	Lathes
133	Milling machines
134	Abrasive wheels
135	Mechanical shears
136	Forging machines
137	Rolling-mills
139	Others
14	Wood and Assimilated Machines
141	Circular saws
142	Other saws
143	Molding machines
144	Overhand planes
149	Others
15	Agricultural Machines
151	Reapers (including combine reapers)
152	Threshers
159	Others
16	Mining Machinery
161	Under-cutters
169	Others
19	Other Machines Not Elsewhere Classified
191	Earth-moving machines, excavating and scraping machines, except means of transport
192	Spinning, weaving and other textile machines
193	Machines for the manufacture of food- stuffs and beverages
194	Machines for the manufacture of paper
195	Printing machines
199	Others

2 Means of Transport and Lifting Equipment

21	Lifting Machines and Appliances
211	Cranes
212	Lifts and elevators
213	Winches
214	Pulley blocks
219	Others
22	Means of Rail Transport
221	Inter-urban railways
222	Rail transport in mines, tunnels, quarries, industrial establishments, docks, etc.
229	Others
23	Other Wheeled Means of Transport, Excluding Rail Transport
231	Tractors
232	Lorries
233	Trucks
234	Motor vehicles, not elsewhere classified
235	Animal-drawn vehicles
236	Hand-drawn vehicles
239	Others
24	Means of Air Transport
25	Means of Water Transport
251	Motorized means of water transport
252	Non-motorized means of water transport
26	Other Means of Transport
261	Cable-cars
262	Mechanical conveyors, except cable-cars
269	Others

3 Other Equipment

31	Pressure Vessels
311	Boilers
312	Pressurized containers
313	Pressurized piping and accessories
314	Gas cylinders
315	Caissons, diving equipment
319	Others
32	Furnaces, Ovens, Kilns
321	Blast furnaces
322	Refining furnaces
323	Other furnaces
324	Kilns
325	Ovens
33	Refrigerating Plants
34	Electrical Installations, Including Electric Motors, but Excluding Electric Hand Tools
341	Rotating machines
342	Conductors
343	Transformers
344	Control apparatus
349	Others
35	Electric Hand Tools
36	Tools, Implements, and Appliances, Except Electric Hand Tools
361	Power-driven hand tools, except electrichand tools
362	Hand tools, not power-driven
369	Others
37	Ladders, Mobile Ramps
38	Scaffolding
39	Other Equipment, Not Elsewhere Classified

4 Materials, Substances and Radiations

41	Explosives
42	Dusts, Gases, Liquids and Chemicals, Excluding Explosives
421	Dusts
422	Gases, vapors, fumes
423	Liquids, not elsewhere classified
424	Chemicals, not elsewhere classified
43	Flying Fragments
44	Radiations
441	Ionizing radiations
449	Others
49	Other Materials and Substances Not Elsewhere Classified

5 Working Environment

51	Outdoor
511	Weather
512	Traffic and working surfaces
513	Water
519	Others
52	Indoor
521	Floors
522	Confined quarters
523	Stairs
524	Other traffic and working surfaces
525	Floor openings and wall openings
526	Environmental factors (lighting, ventilation, temperature, noise, etc.)
529	Others
53	Underground
531	Roofs and faces of mine roads and tunnels, etc.
532	Floors of mine roads and tunnels, etc.
533	Working-faces of mines, tunnels, etc.
534	Mine shafts
535	Fire
536	Water
539	Others

6 Other Agencies, Not Elsewhere Classified

61	Animals
611	Live animals
612	Animal products
69	Other Agencies, Not Elsewhere Classified

7 Agencies Not Classified for Lack of Sufficient Data

Appendix E: List of Three-digit Categories

1. Infectious and Parasitic Diseases

Intestinal infectious diseases (001-009)
001   Cholera
002   Typhoid and paratyphoid fevers
003   Other salmonella infections
004   Shigellosis
005   Other food poisoning (bacterial)
006   Amebiasis
007   Other protozoal intestinal diseases
008   Intestinal infections due to other organisms
009   Ill-defined intestinal infections

Tuberculosis (010-018)
010   Primary tuberculous infection
011   Pulmonary tuberculosis
012   Other respiratory tuberculosis
013   Tuberculosis of meninges and central nervous system
014   Tuberculosis of intestines, peritoneum, and mesenteric glands
015   Tuberculosis of bones and joints
016   Tuberculosis of genitourinary system
017   Tuberculosis of other organs
018   Miliary tuberculosis

Zoonotic bacterial diseases (020-027)
020   Plague
021   Tularemia
022   Anthrax
023   Brucellosis
024   Glanders
025   Melioidosis
026   Rat-bite fever
027   Other zoonotic bacterial diseases

Other bacterial diseases (030-041)
030   Leprosy
031   Diseases due to other mycobacteria
032   Diphtheria
033   Whooping cough
034   Streptococcal sore throat and scarlet fever
035   Erysipelas
036   Meningococcal infection
037   Tetanus
038   Septicemia
039   Actinomycotic infections
040   Other bacterial diseases
041   Bacterial infection in conditions classified elsewhere and of unspecified site

Human immunodeficiency virus (042)
042   Human immunodeficiency virus [HIV] disease

Poliomyelitis and other non-arthropod-borne viral diseases and prion diseases of central nervous system (045-049)
045   Acute poliomyelitis
046   Slow virus infections and prion diseases of central nervous system
047   Meningitis due to enterovirus
048   Other enterovirus diseases of central nervous system
049   Other non-arthropod-borne viral diseases of central nervous system

Viral diseases generally accompanied by exanthem (050-059)
050   Smallpox
051   Cowpox and paravaccinia
052   Chickenpox
053   Herpes zoster
054   Herpes simplex
055   Measles
056   Rubella
057   Other viral exanthemata
058   Other human herpesvirus
059   Other poxvirus infections

Arthropod-borne viral diseases (060-066)
060   Yellow fever
061   Dengue
062   Mosquito-borne viral encephalitis
063   Tick-borne viral encephalitis
064   Viral encephalitis transmitted by other and unspecified arthropods
065   Arthropod-borne hemorrhagic fever
066   Other arthropod-borne viral diseases

Other diseases due to viruses and Chlamydiae (070-079)
070   Viral hepatitis
071   Rabies
072   Mumps
073   Ornithosis
074   Specific diseases due to Coxsackie virus
075   Infectious mononucleosis
076   Trachoma
077   Other diseases of conjunctiva due to viruses and Chlamydiae
078   Other diseases due to viruses and Chlamydiae
079   Viral and chlamydial infection in conditions classified elsewhere and of unspecified site

Rickettsioses and other arthropod-borne diseases (080-088)
080   Louse-borne [epidemic] typhus
081   Other typhus
082   Tick-borne rickettsioses
083   Other rickettsioses
084   Malaria
085   Leishmaniasis
086   Trypanosomiasis
087   Relapsing fever
088   Other arthropod-borne diseases

Syphilis and other venereal diseases (090-099)
090   Congenital syphilis
091   Early syphilis, symptomatic
092   Early syphilis, latent
093   Cardiovascular syphilis
094   Neurosyphilis
095   Other forms of late syphilis, with symptoms
096   Late syphilis, latent
097   Other and unspecified syphilis
098   Gonococcal infections
099   Other venereal diseases

Other spirochetal diseases (100-104)
100   Leptospirosis
101   Vincent's angina
102   Yaws
103   Pinta
104   Other spirochetal infection

Mycoses (110-118)
110   Dermatophytosis
111   Dermatomycosis, other and unspecified
112   Candidiasis
114   Coccidioidomycosis
115   Histoplasmosis
116   Blastomycotic infection
117   Other mycoses
118   Opportunistic mycoses

Helminthiases (120-129)
120   Schistosomiasis [bilharziasis]
121   Other trematode infections
122   Echinococcosis
123   Other cestode infection
124   Trichinosis
125   Filarial infection and dracontiasis
126   Ancylostomiasis and necatoriasis
127   Other intestinal helminthiases
128   Other and unspecified helminthiases
129   Intestinal parasitism, unspecified

Other infectious and parasitic diseases (130-136)
130   Toxoplasmosis
131   Trichomoniasis
132   Pediculosis and phthirus infestation
133   Acariasis
134   Other infestation
135   Sarcoidosis
136   Other and unspecified infectious and parasitic diseases

Late effects of infectious and parasitic diseases (137-139)
137   Late effects of tuberculosis
138   Late effects of acute poliomyelitis
139   Late effects of other infectious and parasitic diseases

2. Neoplasms

Malignant neoplasm of lip, oral cavity, and pharynx (140-149)
140   Malignant neoplasm of lip
141   Malignant neoplasm of tongue
142   Malignant neoplasm of major salivary glands
143   Malignant neoplasm of gum
144   Malignant neoplasm of floor of mouth
145   Malignant neoplasm of other and unspecified parts of mouth
146   Malignant neoplasm of oropharynx
147   Malignant neoplasm of nasopharynx
148   Malignant neoplasm of hypopharynx
149   Malignant neoplasm of other and ill-defined sites within the lip, oral cavity, and pharynx

Malignant neoplasm of digestive organs and peritoneum (150-159)
150   Malignant neoplasm of esophagus
151   Malignant neoplasm of stomach
152   Malignant neoplasm of small intestine, including duodenum
153   Malignant neoplasm of colon
154   Malignant neoplasm of rectum, rectosigmoid junction, and anus
155   Malignant neoplasm of liver and intrahepatic bile ducts
156   Malignant neoplasm of gallbladder and extrahepatic bile ducts
157   Malignant neoplasm of pancreas
158   Malignant neoplasm of retroperitoneum and peritoneum
159   Malignant neoplasm of other and ill-defined sites within the digestive organs and peritoneum

Malignant neoplasm of respiratory and intrathoracic organs (160-165)
160   Malignant neoplasm of nasal cavities, middle ear, and accessory sinuses
161   Malignant neoplasm of larynx
162   Malignant neoplasm of trachea, bronchus, and lung
163   Malignant neoplasm of pleura
164   Malignant neoplasm of thymus, heart, and mediastinum
165   Malignant neoplasm of other and ill-defined sites within the respiratory system and intrathoracic organs

Malignant neoplasm of bone, connective tissue, skin, and breast (170-176)
170   Malignant neoplasm of bone and articular cartilage
171   Malignant neoplasm of connective and other soft tissue
172   Malignant melanoma of skin
173   Other and unspecified malignant neoplasm of skin
174   Malignant neoplasm of female breast
175   Malignant neoplasm of male breast
176   Kaposi's sarcoma

Malignant neoplasm of genitourinary organs (179-189)
179 Malignant neoplasm of uterus, part unspecified
180 Malignant neoplasm of cervix uteri
181 Malignant neoplasm of placenta
182 Malignant neoplasm of body of uterus
183 Malignant neoplasm of ovary and other uterine adnexa
184 Malignant neoplasm of other and unspecified female genital organs
185 Malignant neoplasm of prostate
186 Malignant neoplasm of testis
187 Malignant neoplasm of penis and other male genital organs
188 Malignant neoplasm of bladder
189 Malignant neoplasm of kidney and other unspecified urinary organs

Malignant neoplasm of other and unspecified sites (190-199)
190 Malignant neoplasm of eye
191 Malignant neoplasm of brain
192 Malignant neoplasm of other and unspecified parts of nervous system
193 Malignant neoplasm of thyroid gland
194 Malignant neoplasm of other endocrine glands and related structures
195 Malignant neoplasm of other and ill-defined sites
196 Secondary and unspecified malignant neoplasm of lymph nodes
197 Secondary malignant neoplasm of respiratory and digestive systems
198 Secondary malignant neoplasm of other specified sites
199 Malignant neoplasm without specification of site

Malignant neoplasm of lymphatic and hematopoietic tissue (200-208)
200 Lymphosarcoma and reticulosarcoma and other specified malignant tumors of lymphatic tissue
201 Hodgkin's disease
202 Other malignant neoplasm of lymphoid and histiocytic tissue
203 Multiple myeloma and immunoproliferative neoplasms
204 Lymphoid leukemia
205 Myeloid leukemia
206 Monocytic leukemia
207 Other specified leukemia
208 Leukemia of unspecified cell type

Neuroendocrine tumors (209)
209 Neuroendocrine tumors

Benign neoplasms (210-229)
210 Benign neoplasm of lip, oral cavity, and pharynx
211 Benign neoplasm of other parts of digestive system
212 Benign neoplasm of respiratory and intrathoracic organs
213 Benign neoplasm of bone and articular cartilage
214 Lipoma
215 Other benign neoplasm of connective and other soft tissue
216 Benign neoplasm of skin
217 Benign neoplasm of breast
218 Uterine leiomyoma
219 Other benign neoplasm of uterus
220 Benign neoplasm of ovary
221 Benign neoplasm of other female genital organs
222 Benign neoplasm of male genital organs
223 Benign neoplasm of kidney and other urinary organs
224 Benign neoplasm of eye
225 Benign neoplasm of brain and other parts of nervous system
226 Benign neoplasm of thyroid gland

227 Benign neoplasm of other endocrine glands and related structures
228 Hemangioma and lymphangioma, any site
229 Benign neoplasm of other and unspecified sites

Carcinoma in situ (230-234)
230 Carcinoma in situ of digestive organs
231 Carcinoma in situ of respiratory system
232 Carcinoma in situ of skin
233 Carcinoma in situ of breast and genitourinary system
234 Carcinoma in situ of other and unspecified sites

Neoplasms of uncertain behavior (235-238)
235 Neoplasm of uncertain behavior of digestive and respiratory systems
236 Neoplasm of uncertain behavior of genitourinary organs
237 Neoplasm of uncertain behavior of endocrine glands and nervous system
238 Neoplasm of uncertain behavior of other and unspecified sites and tissues

Neoplasms of unspecified nature (239)
239 Neoplasm of unspecified nature

3. Endocrine, Nutritional and Metabolic Diseases, and Immunity Disorders

Disorders of thyroid gland (240-246)
240 Simple and unspecified goiter
241 Nontoxic nodular goiter
242 Thyrotoxicosis with or without goiter
243 Congenital hypothyroidism
244 Acquired hypothyroidism
245 Thyroiditis
246 Other disorders of thyroid

Diseases of other endocrine glands (249-259)
249 Secondary diabetes mellitus
250 Diabetes mellitus
251 Other disorders of pancreatic internal secretion
252 Disorders of parathyroid gland
253 Disorders of the pituitary gland and its hypothalamic control
254 Diseases of thymus gland
255 Disorders of adrenal glands
256 Ovarian dysfunction
257 Testicular dysfunction
258 Polyglandular dysfunction and related disorders
259 Other endocrine disorders

Nutritional deficiencies (260-269)
260 Kwashiorkor
261 Nutritional marasmus
262 Other severe protein-calorie malnutrition
263 Other and unspecified protein-calorie malnutrition
264 Vitamin A deficiency
265 Thiamine and niacin deficiency states
266 Deficiency of B-complex components
267 Ascorbic acid deficiency
268 Vitamin D deficiency
269 Other nutritional deficiencies

Other metabolic disorders and immnity disorders (270-279)
270 Disorders of amino-acid transport and metabolism
271 Disorders of carbohydrate transport and metabolism
272 Disorders of lipoid metabolism
273 Disorders of plasma protein metabolism
274 Gout
275 Disorders of mineral metabolism
276 Disorders of fluid, electrolyte, and acid-base balance
277 Other and unspecified disorders of metabolism

278 Overweight, obesity and other hyperalimentation
279 Disorders involving the immune mechanism

4. Diseases of Blood and Blood-forming Organs (280-289)
280 Iron deficiency anemias
281 Other deficiency anemias
282 Hereditary hemolytic anemias
283 Acquired hemolytic anemias
284 Aplastic anemia and other bone marrow failure syndromes
285 Other and unspecified anemias
286 Coagulation defects
287 Purpura and other hemorrhagic conditions
288 Diseases of white blood cells
289 Other diseases of blood and blood-forming organs

5. Mental, Behavioral and Neurodevelopmental Disorders

Organic psychotic conditions (290-294)
290 Dementias
291 Alcoholic induced mental disorders
292 Drug induced mental disorders
293 Transient mental disorders due to conditions classified elsewhere
294 Persistent mental disorders due to conditions classified elsewhere

Other psychoses (295-299)
295 Schizophrenic disorders
296 Episodic mood disorders
297 Delusional disorders
298 Other nonorganic psychoses
299 Pervasive developmental disorders

Neurotic disorders, personality disorders, and other nonpsychotic mental disorders (300-316)
300 Anxiety, dissociative and somatoform disorders
301 Personality disorders
302 Sexual and gender identity disorders
303 Alcohol dependence syndrome
304 Drug dependence
305 Nondependent abuse of drugs
306 Physiological malfunction arising from mental factors
307 Special symptoms or syndromes, not elsewhere classified
308 Acute reaction to stress
309 Adjustment reaction
310 Specific nonpsychotic mental disorders due to brain damage
311 Depressive disorder, not elsewhere classified
312 Disturbance of conduct, not elsewhere classified
313 Disturbance of emotions specific to childhood and adolescence
314 Hyperkinetic syndrome of childhood
315 Specific delays in development
316 Psychic factors associated with diseases classified elsewhere

Intellectual Disabilities (317-319)
317 Mild intellectual disabilities
318 Other specified intellectual disabilities
319 Unspecified intellectual disabilities

6. Diseases of the Nervous System and Sense Organs

Inflammatory diseases of the central nervous system (320-326)
320 Bacterial meningitis
321 Meningitis due to other organisms
322 Meningitis of unspecified cause
323 Encephalitis, myelitis, and encephalomyelitis

324 Intracranial and intraspinal abscess
325 Phlebitis and thrombophlebitis of intracranial venous sinuses
326 Late effects of intracranial abscess or pyogenic infection

Organic Sleep Disorders (327)
327 Organic sleep disorders

Hereditary and degenerative diseases of the central nervous system (330-337)
330 Cerebral degenerations usually manifest in childhood
331 Other cerebral degenerations
332 Parkinson's disease
333 Other extrapyramidal diseases and abnormal movement disorders
334 Spinocerebellar disease
335 Anterior horn cell disease
336 Other diseases of spinal cord
337 Disorders of the autonomic nervous system

Pain (338)
338 Pain, not elsewhere classified

Other headache syndromes (339)
339 Other headache syndromes

Other disorders of the central nervous system (340-349)
340 Multiple sclerosis
341 Other demyelinating diseases of central nervous system
342 Hemiplegia and hemiparesis
343 Infantile cerebral palsy
344 Other paralytic syndromes
345 Epilepsy and recurrent seizures
346 Migraine
347 Cataplexy and narcolepsy
348 Other conditions of brain
349 Other and unspecified disorders of the nervous system

Disorders of the peripheral nervous system (350-359)
350 Trigeminal nerve disorders
351 Facial nerve disorders
352 Disorders of other cranial nerves
353 Nerve root and plexus disorders
354 Mononeuritis of upper limb and mononeuritis multiplex
355 Mononeuritis of lower limb
356 Hereditary and idiopathic peripheral neuropathy
357 Inflammatory and toxic neuropathy
358 Myoneural disorders
359 Muscular dystrophies and other myopathies

Disorders of the eye and adnexa (360-379)
360 Disorders of the globe
361 Retinal detachments and defects
362 Other retinal disorders
363 Chorioretinal inflammations and scars and other disorders of choroid
364 Disorders of iris and ciliary body
365 Glaucoma
366 Cataract
367 Disorders of refraction and accommodation
368 Visual disturbances
369 Blindness and low vision
370 Keratitis
371 Corneal opacity and other disorders of cornea
372 Disorders of conjunctiva
373 Inflammation of eyelids
374 Other disorders of eyelids
375 Disorders of lacrimal system
376 Disorders of the orbit
377 Disorders of optic nerve and visual pathways
378 Strabismus and other disorders of binocular eye movements
379 Other disorders of eye

Diseases of the ear and mastoid process (380-389)
380 Disorders of external ear
381 Nonsuppurative otitis media and Eustachian tube disorders
382 Suppurative and unspecified otitis media
383 Mastoiditis and related conditions
384 Other disorders of tympanic membrane
385 Other disorders of middle ear and mastoid
386 Vertiginous syndromes and other disorders of vestibular system
387 Otosclerosis
388 Other disorders of ear
389 Hearing loss

7. Diseases of the Circulatory System

Acute rheumatic fever (390-392)
390 Rheumatic fever without mention of heart involvement
391 Rheumatic fever with heart involvement
392 Rheumatic chorea

Chronic rheumatic heart disease (393-398)
393 Chronic rheumatic pericarditis
394 Diseases of mitral valve
395 Diseases of aortic valve
396 Diseases of mitral and aortic valves
397 Diseases of other endocardial structures
398 Other rheumatic heart disease

Hypertensive disease (401-405)
401 Essential hypertension
402 Hypertensive heart disease
403 Hypertensive chronic kidney disease
404 Hypertensive heart and chronic kidney disease
405 Secondary hypertension

Ischemic heart disease (410-414)
410 Acute myocardial infarction
411 Other acute and subacute forms of ischemic heart disease
412 Old myocardial infarction
413 Angina pectoris
414 Other forms of chronic ischemic heart disease

Diseases of pulmonary circulation (415-417)
415 Acute pulmonary heart disease
416 Chronic pulmonary heart disease
417 Other diseases of pulmonary circulation

Other forms of heart disease (420-429)
420 Acute pericarditis
421 Acute and subacute endocarditis
422 Acute myocarditis
423 Other diseases of pericardium
424 Other diseases of endocardium
425 Cardiomyopathy
426 Conduction disorders
427 Cardiac dysrhythmias
428 Heart failure
429 Ill-defined descriptions and complications of heart disease

Cerebrovascular disease (430-438)
430 Subarachnoid hemorrhage
431 Intracerebral hemorrhage
432 Other and unspecified intracranial hemorrhage
433 Occlusion and stenosis of precerebral arteries
434 Occlusion of cerebral arteries
435 Transient cerebral ischemia
436 Acute, but ill-defined, cerebrovascular disease
437 Other and ill-defined cerebrovascular disease
438 Late effects of cerebrovascular disease

Diseases of arteries, arterioles, and capillaries (440-449)
440 Atherosclerosis
441 Aortic aneurysm and dissection
442 Other aneurysm
443 Other peripheral vascular disease
444 Arterial embolism and thrombosis
445 Atheroembolism
446 Polyarteritis nodosa and allied conditions
447 Other disorders of arteries and arterioles
448 Diseases of capillaries
449 Septic arterial embolism

Diseases of veins and lymphatics, and other diseases of circulatory system (451-459)
451 Phlebitis and thrombophlebitis
452 Portal vein thrombosis
453 Other venous embolism and thrombosis
454 Varicose veins of lower extremities
455 Hemorrhoids
456 Varicose veins of other sites
457 Noninfectious disorders of lymphatic channels
458 Hypotension
459 Other disorders of circulatory system

8. Diseases of the Respiratory System

Acute respiratory infections (460-466)
460 Acute nasopharyngitis [common cold]
461 Acute sinusitis
462 Acute pharyngitis
463 Acute tonsillitis
464 Acute laryngitis and tracheitis
465 Acute upper respiratory infections of multiple or unspecified sites
466 Acute bronchitis and bronchiolitis

Other diseases of upper respiratory tract (470-478)
470 Deviated nasal septum
471 Nasal polyps
472 Chronic pharyngitis and nasopharyngitis
473 Chronic sinusitis
474 Chronic disease of tonsils and adenoids
475 Peritonsillar abscess
476 Chronic laryngitis and laryngotracheitis
477 Allergic rhinitis
478 Other diseases of upper respiratory tract

Pneumonia and influenza (480-488)
480 Viral pneumonia
481 Pneumococcal pneumonia [Streptococcus pneumoniae pneumonia]
482 Other bacterial pneumonia
483 Pneumonia due to other specified organism
484 Pneumonia in infectious diseases classified elsewhere
485 Bronchopneumonia, organism unspecified
486 Pneumonia, organism unspecified
487 Influenza
488 Influenza due to certain identified influenza viruses

Chronic obstructive pulmonary disease and allied conditions (490-496)
490 Bronchitis, not specified as acute or chronic
491 Chronic bronchitis
492 Emphysema
493 Asthma
494 Bronchiectasis
495 Extrinsic allergic alveolitis
496 Chronic airways obstruction, not elsewhere classified

Pneumoconioses and other lung diseases due to external agents (500-508)
500 Coal workers' pneumoconiosis
501 Asbestosis
502 Pneumoconiosis due to other silica or silicates
503 Pneumoconiosis due to other inorganic dust
504 Pneumopathy due to inhalation of other dust
505 Pneumoconiosis, unspecified
506 Respiratory conditions due to chemical fumes and vapors
507 Pneumonitis due to solids and liquids
508 Respiratory conditions due to other and unspecified external agents

Other diseases of respiratory system (510-519)
510 Empyema
511 Pleurisy
512 Pneumothorax and air leak
513 Abscess of lung and mediastinum
514 Pulmonary congestion and hypostasis
515 Postinflammatory pulmonary fibrosis
516 Other alveolar and parietoalveolar pneumopathy
517 Lung involvement in conditions classified elsewhere
518 Other diseases of lung
519 Other diseases of respiratory system

9. Diseases of the Digestive System

Diseases of oral cavity, salivary glands, and jaws (520-529)
520 Disorders of tooth development and eruption
521 Diseases of hard tissues of teeth
522 Diseases of pulp and periapical tissues
523 Gingival and periodontal diseases
524 Dentofacial anomalies, including malocclusion
525 Other diseases and conditions of the teeth and supporting structures
526 Diseases of the jaws
527 Diseases of the salivary glands
528 Diseases of the oral soft tissues, excluding lesions specific for gingiva and tongue
529 Diseases and other conditions of the tongue

Diseases of esophagus, stomach, and duodenum (530-539)
530 Diseases of esophagus
531 Gastric ulcer
532 Duodenal ulcer
533 Peptic ulcer, site unspecified
534 Gastrojejunal ulcer
535 Gastritis and duodenitis
536 Disorders of function of stomach
537 Other disorders of stomach and duodenum
538 Gastrointestinal mucositis (ulcerative)
539 Complications of bariatric procedures

Appendicitis (540-543)
540 Acute appendicitis
541 Appendicitis, unqualified
542 Other appendicitis
543 Other diseases of appendix

Hernia of abdominal cavity (550-553)
550 Inguinal hernia
551 Other hernia of abdominal cavity, with gangrene
552 Other hernia of abdominal cavity, with obstruction, but without mention of gangrene
553 Other hernia of abdominal cavity without mention of obstruction or gangrene

Noninfective enteritis and colitis (555-558)
555 Regional enteritis
556 Ulcerative colitis
557 Vascular insufficiency of intestine
558 Other noninfective gastroenteritis and colitis

Other diseases of intestines and peritoneum (560-569)
560 Intestinal obstruction without mention of hernia
562 Diverticula of intestine
564 Functional digestive disorders, not elsewhere classified
565 Anal fissure and fistula
566 Abscess of anal and rectal regions
567 Peritonitis and retroperitoneal infections
568 Other disorders of peritoneum
569 Other disorders of intestine

Other diseases of digestive system (570-579)
570 Acute and subacute necrosis of liver
571 Chronic liver disease and cirrhosis
572 Liver abscess and sequelae of chronic liver disease
573 Other disorders of liver
574 Cholelithiasis
575 Other disorders of gallbladder
576 Other disorders of biliary tract
577 Diseases of pancreas
578 Gastrointestinal hemorrhage
579 Intestinal Malabsorption

10. Diseases of the Genitourinary System

Nephritis, nephrotic syndrome, and nephrosis (580-589)
580 Acute gloerulonephritis
581 Nephrotic syndrome
582 Chronic glomerulonephritis
583 Nephritis and nephropathy, not specified as acute or chronic
584 Acute kidney failure
585 Chronic kidney disease (CKD)
586 Renal failure, unspecified
587 Renal sclerosis, unspecified
588 Disorders resulting from impaired renal function
589 Small kidney of unknown cause

Other diseases of urinary system (590-599)
590 Infections of kidney
591 Hydronephrosis
592 Calculus of kidney and ureter
593 Other disorders of kidney and ureter
594 Calculus of lower urinary tract
595 Cystitis
596 Other disorders of bladder
597 Urethritis, not sexually transmitted, and urethral syndrome
598 Urethral stricture
599 Other disorders of urethra and urinary tract

Diseases of male genital organs (600-608)
600 Hyperplasia of prostate
601 Inflammatory diseases of prostate
602 Other disorders of prostate
603 Hydrocele
604 Orchitis and epididymitis
605 Redundant prepuce and phimosis
606 Infertility, male
607 Disorders of penis
608 Other disorders of male genital organs

Disorders of breast (610-612)
610 Benign mammary dysplasias
611 Other disorders of breast
612 Deformity and disproportion of reconstructed breast

Inflammatory disease of female pelvic organs (614-616)
614 Inflammatory disease of ovary, fallopian tube, pelvic cellular tissue, and peritoneum
615 Inflammatory diseases of uterus, except cervix
616 Inflammatory disease of cervix, vagina, and vulva

Other disorders of female genital tract (617-629)
617 Endometriosis
618 Genital prolapse
619 Fistula involving female genital tract
620 Noninflammatory disorders of ovary, fallopian tube, and broad ligament
621 Disorders of uterus, not elsewhere classified
622 Noninflammatory disorders of cervix
623 Noninflammatory disorders of vagina
624 Noninflammatory disorders of vulva and perineum
625 Pain and other symptoms associated with female genital organs
626 Disorders of menstruation and other abnormal bleeding from female genital tract
627 Menopausal and postmenopausal disorders
628 Infertility, female
629 Other disorders of female genital organs

11. Complications of Pregnancy, Childbirth and the Puerperium

Ectopic and molar pregnancy (630-633)
630 Hydatidiform mole
631 Other abnormal product of conception
632 Missed abortion
633 Ectopic pregnancy

Other pregnancy with abortive outcome (634-639)
634 Spontaneous abortion
635 Legally induced abortion
636 Illegally induced abortion
637 Unspecified abortion
638 Failed attempted abortion
639 Complications following abortion and ectopic and molar pregnancies

Complications mainly related to pregnancy (640-649)
640 Hemorrhage in early pregnancy
641 Antepartum hemorrhage, abruptio placentae, and placenta previa
642 Hypertension complicating pregnancy, childbirth, and the puerperium
643 Excessive vomiting in pregnancy
644 Early or threatened labor
645 Late pregnancy
646 Other complications of pregnancy, not elsewhere classified
647 Infectious and parasitic conditions in the mother classifiable elsewhere, but complicating pregnancy, childbirth, and the puerperium
648 Other current conditions in the mother classifiable elsewhere, but complicating pregnancy, childbirth, and the puerperium
649 Other conditions or status of the mother complicating pregnancy, childbirth, or the puerperium

Normal delivery, and other indications for care in pregnancy, labor, and delivery (650-659)
650 Normal delivery
651 Multiple gestation
652 Malposition and malpresentation of fetus
653 Disproportion
654 Abnormality of organs and soft tissues of pelvis
655 Known or suspected fetal abnormality affecting management of mother
656 Other known or suspected fetal and placental problems affecting management of mother
657 Polyhydramnios
658 Other problems associated with amniotic cavity and membranes
659 Other indications for care or intervention related to labor and delivery, not elsewhere classified

Complications occurring mainly in the course of labor and delivery (660-669)
660 Obstructed labor
661 Abnormality of forces of labor
662 Long labor
663 Umbilical cord complications
664 Trauma to perineum and vulva during delivery
665 Other obstetrical trauma
666 Postpartum hemorrhage
667 Retained placenta or membranes, without hemorrhage
668 Complications of the administration of anesthetic or other sedation in labor and delivery
669 Other complications of labor and delivery, not elsewhere classified

Complications of the puerperium (670-677)
670 Major puerperal infection

671   Venous complications in pregnancy and the puerperium
672   Pyrexia of unknown origin during the puerperium
673   Obstetrical pulmonary embolism
674   Other and unspecified complications of the puerperium, not elsewhere classified
675   Infections of the breast and nipple associated with childbirth
676   Other disorders of the breast associated with childbirth, and disorders of lactation
677   Late effect of complication of pregnancy, childbirth, and the puerperium

Other maternal and fetal complications (678-679)
678   Other fetal conditions
679   Complications of in utero procedures

12. Diseases of the Skin and Subcutaneous Tissue

Infections of skin and subcutaneous tissue (680-686)
680   Carbuncle and furuncle
681   Cellulitis and abscess of finger and toe
682   Other cellulitis and abscess
683   Acute lymphadenitis
684   Impetigo
685   Pilonidal cyst
686   Other local infections of skin and subcutaneous tissue

Other inflammatory conditions of skin and subcutaneous tissue (690-698)
690   Erythematosquamous dermatosis
691   Atopic dermatitis and related conditions
692   Contact dermatitis and other eczema
693   Dermatitis due to substances taken internally
694   Bullous dermatoses
695   Erythematous conditions
696   Psoriasis and similar disorders
697   Lichen
698   Pruritus and related conditions

Other diseases of skin and subcutaneous tissue (700-709)
700   Corns and callosities
701   Other hypertrophic and atrophic conditions of skin
702   Other dermatoses
703   Diseases of nail
704   Diseases of hair and hair follicles
705   Disorders of sweat glands
706   Diseases of sebaceous glands
707   Chronic ulcer of skin
708   Urticaria
709   Other disorders of skin and subcutaneous tissue

13. Diseases of the Musculoskeletal System and Connective Tissue

Arthropathies and related disorders (710-719)
710   Diffuse diseases of connective tissue
711   Arthropathy associated with infections
712   Crystal arthropathies
713   Arthropathy associated with other disorders classified elsewhere
714   Rheumatoid arthritis and other inflammatory polyarthropathies
715   Osteoarthrosis and allied disorders
716   Other and unspecified arthropathies
717   Internal derangement of knee
718   Other derangement of joint
719   Other and unspecified disorder of joint

Dorsopathies (720-724)
720   Ankylosing spondylitis and other inflammatory spondylopathies
721   Spondylosis and allied disorders

722   Intervertebral disc disorders
723   Other disorders of cervical region
724   Other and unspecified disorders of back

Rheumatism, excluding the back (725-729)
725   Polymyalgia rheumatica
726   Peripheral enthesopathies and allied syndromes
727   Other disorders of synovium, tendon, and bursa
728   Disorders of muscle, ligament, and fascia
729   Other disorders of soft tissues

Osteopathies, chondropathies, and acquired musculoskeletal deformities (730-739)
730   Osteomyelitis, periostitis, and other infections involving bone
731   Osteitis deformans and osteopathies associated with other disorders classified elsewhere
732   Osteochondropathies
733   Other disorders of bone and cartilage
734   Flat foot
735   Acquired deformities of toe
736   Other acquired deformities of limbs
737   Curvature of spine
738   Other acquired deformity
739   Nonallopathic lesions, not elsewhere classified

14. Congenital Anomalies

740   Anencephalus and similar anomalies
741   Spina bifida
742   Other congenital anomalies of nervous system
743   Congenital anomalies of eye
744   Congenital anomalies of ear, face, and neck
745   Bulbus cordis anomalies and anomalies of cardiac septal closure
746   Other congenital anomalies of heart
747   Other congenital anomalies of circulatory system
748   Congenital anomalies of respiratory system
749   Cleft palate and cleft lip
750   Other congenital anomalies of upper alimentary tract
751   Other congenital anomalies of digestive system
752   Congenital anomalies of genital organs
753   Congenital anomalies of urinary system
754   Certain congenital musculoskeletal deformities
755   Other congenital anomalies of limbs
756   Other congenital musculoskeletal anomalies
757   Congenital anomalies of the integument
758   Chromosomal anomalies
759   Other and unspecified congenital anomalies

15. Certain Conditions Originating in the Perinatal Period

Maternal causes of perinatal morbidity and mortality (760-763)
760   Fetus or newborn affected by maternal conditions which may be unrelated to present pregnancy
761   Fetus or newborn affected by maternal complications of pregnancy
762   Fetus or newborn affected by complications of placenta, cord, and membranes
763   Fetus or newborn affected by other complications of labor and delivery

Other conditions originating in the perinatal period (764-779)
764   Slow fetal growth and fetal malnutrition
765   Disorders relating to short gestation and unspecified low birthweight
766   Disorders relating to long gestation and high birthweight
767   Birth trauma
768   Intrauterine hypoxia and birth asphyxia
769   Respiratory distress syndrome
770   Other respiratory conditions of fetus and newborn

771   Infections specific to the perinatal period
772   Fetal and neonatal hemorrhage
773   Hemolytic disease of fetus or newborn, due to isoimmunization
774   Other perinatal jaundice
775   Endocrine and metabolic disturbances specific to the fetus and newborn
776   Hematological disorders of newborn
777   Perinatal disorders of digestive system
778   Conditions involving the integument and temperature regulation of fetus and newborn
779   Other and ill-defined conditions originating in the perinatal period

16. Symptoms, Signs, and Ill-defined Conditions

Symptoms (780-789)
780   General symptoms
781   Symptoms involving nervous and musculoskeletal systems
782   Symptoms involving skin and other integumentary tissue
783   Symptoms concerning nutrition, metabolism, and development
784   Symptoms involving head and neck
785   Symptoms involving cardiovascular system
786   Symptoms involving respiratory system and other chest symptoms
787   Symptoms involving digestive system
788   Symptoms involving urinary system
789   Other symptoms involving abdomen and pelvis

Nonspecific abnormal findings (790-796)
790   Nonspecific findings on examination of blood
791   Nonspecific findings on examination of urine
792   Nonspecific abnormal findings in other body substances
793   Nonspecific (abnormal) findings on radiological and other examination of body structure
794   Nonspecific abnormal results of function studies
795   Other and nonspecific abnormal cystological, histological, immunological and DNA test findings
796   Other nonspecific abnormal findings

Ill-defined and unknown causes of morbidity and mortality (797-799)
797   Senility without mention of psychosis
798   Sudden death, cause unknown
799   Other ill-defined and unknown causes of morbidity and mortality

17. Injury and Poisoning

Fracture of skull (800-804)
800   Fracture of vault of skull
801   Fracture of base of skull
802   Fracture of face bones
803   Other and unqualified skull fractures
804   Multiple fractures involving skull or face with other bones

Fracture of spine and trunk (805-809)
805   Fracture of vertebral column without mention of spinal cord injury
806   Fracture of vertebral column with spinal cord injury
807   Fracture of rib(s), sternum, larynx, and trachea
808   Fracture of pelvis
809   Ill-defined fractures of bones of trunk

Fracture of upper limb (810-819)
810   Fracture of clavicle
811   Fracture of scapula
812   Fracture of humerus
813   Fracture of radius and ulna
814   Fracture of carpal bone(s)
815   Fracture of metacarpal bone(s)

816 Fracture of one or more phalanges of hand
817 Multiple fractures of hand bones
818 Ill-defined fractures of upper limb
819 Multiple fractures involving both upper limbs, and upper limb with rib(s) and sternum

Fracture of lower limb (820-829)
820 Fracture of neck of femur
821 Fracture of other and unspecified parts of femur
822 Fracture of patella
823 Fracture of tibia and fibula
824 Fracture of ankle
825 Fracture of one or more tarsal and metatarsal bones
826 Fracture of one or more phalanges of foot
827 Other, multiple, and ill-defined fractures of lower limb
828 Multiple fractures involving both lower limbs, lower with upper limb, and lower limb(s) with rib(s) and sternum
829 Fracture of unspecified bones

Dislocation (830-839)
830 Dislocation of jaw
831 Dislocation of shoulder
832 Dislocation of elbow
833 Dislocation of wrist
834 Dislocation of finger
835 Dislocation of hip
836 Dislocation of knee
837 Dislocation of ankle
838 Dislocation of foot
839 Other, multiple, and ill-defined dislocations

Sprains and strains of joints and adjacent muscles (840-848)
840 Sprains and strains of shoulder and upper arm
841 Sprains and strains of elbow and forearm
842 Sprains and strains of wrist and hand
843 Sprains and strains of hip and thigh
844 Sprains and strains of knee and leg
845 Sprains and strains of ankle and foot
846 Sprains and strains of sacroiliac region
847 Sprains and strains of other and unspecified parts of back
848 Other and ill-defined sprains and strains

Intracranial injury, excluding those with skull fracture (850-854)
850 Concussion
851 Cerebral laceration and contusion
852 Subarachnoid, subdural, and extradural hemorrhage, following injury
853 Other and unspecified intracranial hemorrhage following injury
854 Intracranial injury of other and unspecified nature

Internal injury of thorax, abdomen, and pelvis (860-869)
860 Traumatic pneumothorax and hemothorax
861 Injury to heart and lung
862 Injury to other and unspecified intrathoracic organs
863 Injury to gastrointestinal tract
864 Injury to liver
865 Injury to spleen
866 Injury to kidney
867 Injury to pelvic organs
868 Injury to other intra-abdominal organs
869 Internal injury to unspecified or ill-defined organs

Open wound of head, neck, and trunk (870-879)
870 Open wound of ocular adnexa
871 Open wound of eyeball
872 Open wound of ear
873 Other open wound of head
874 Open wound of neck
875 Open wound of chest (wall)

876 Open wound of back
877 Open wound of buttock
878 Open wound of genital organs (external), including traumatic amputation
879 Open wound of other and unspecified sites, except limbs

Open wound of upper limb (880-887)
880 Open wound of shoulder and upper arm
881 Open wound of elbow, forearm, and wrist
882 Open wound of hand except finger(s) alone
883 Open wound of finger(s)
884 Multiple and unspecified open wound of upper limb
885 Traumatic amputation of thumb (complete) (partial)
886 Traumatic amputation of other finger(s) (complete) (partial)
887 Traumatic amputation of arm and hand (complete) (partial)

Open wound of lower limb (890-897)
890 Open wound of hip and thigh
891 Open wound of knee, leg [except thigh], and ankle
892 Open wound of foot except toe(s) alone
893 Open wound of toe(s)
894 Multiple and unspecified open wound of lower limb
895 Traumatic amputation of toe(s) (complete) (partial)
896 Traumatic amputation of foot (complete) (partial)
897 Traumatic amputation of leg(s) (complete) (partial)

Injury to blood vessels (900-904)
900 Injury to blood vessels of head and neck
901 Injury to blood vessels of thorax
902 Injury to blood vessels of abdomen and pelvis
903 Injury to blood vessels of upper extremity
904 Injury to blood vessels of lower extremity and unspecified sites

Late effects of injuries, poisonings, toxic effects, and other external causes (905-909)
905 Late effects of musculoskeletal and connective tissue injuries
906 Late effects of injuries to skin and subcutaneous tissues
907 Late effects of injuries to the nervous system
908 Late effects of other and unspecified injuries
909 Late effects of other and unspecified external causes

Superficial injury (910-919)
910 Superficial injury of face, neck, and scalp except eye
911 Superficial injury of trunk
912 Superficial injury of shoulder and upper arm
913 Superficial injury of elbow, forearm, and wrist
914 Superficial injury of hand(s) except finger(s) alone
915 Superficial injury of finger(s)
916 Superficial injury of hip, thigh, leg, and ankle
917 Superficial injury of foot and toe(s)
918 Superficial injury of eye and adnexa
919 Superficial injury of other, multiple, and unspecified sites

Contusion with intact skin surface (920-924)
920 Contusion of face, scalp, and neck except eye(s)
921 Contusion of eye and adnexa
922 Contusion of trunk
923 Contusion of upper limb
924 Contusion of lower limb and of other and unspecified sites

Crushing injury (925-929)
925 Crushing injury of face, scalp, and neck
926 Crushing injury of trunk

927 Crushing injury of upper limb
928 Crushing injury of lower limb
929 Crushing injury of multiple and unspecified sites

Effects of foreign body entering through orifice (930-939)
930 Foreign body on external eye
931 Foreign body in ear
932 Foreign body in nose
933 Foreign body in pharynx and larynx
934 Foreign body in trachea, bronchus, and lung
935 Foreign body in mouth, esophagus, and stomach
936 Foreign body in intestine and colon
937 Foreign body in anus and rectum
938 Foreign body in digestive system, unspecified
939 Foreign body in genitourinary tract

Burns (940-949)
940 Burn confined to eye and adnexa
941 Burn of face, head, and neck
942 Burn of trunk
943 Burn of upper limb, except wrist and hand
944 Burn of wrist(s) and hand(s)
945 Burn of lower limb(s)
946 Burns of multiple specified sites
947 Burn of internal organs
948 Burns classified according to extent of body surface involved
949 Burn, unspecified

Injury to nerves and spinal cord (950-957)
950 Injury to optic nerve and pathways
951 Injury to other cranial nerve(s)
952 Spinal cord injury without evidence of spinal bone injury
953 Injury to nerve roots and spinal plexus
954 Injury to other nerve(s) of trunk excluding shoulder and pelvic girdles
955 Injury to peripheral nerve(s) of shoulder girdle and upper limb
956 Injury to peripheral nerve(s) of pelvic girdle and lower limb
957 Injury to other and unspecified nerves

Certain traumatic complications and unspecified injuries (958-959)
958 Certain early complications of trauma
959 Injury, other and unspecified

Poisoning by drugs, medicinals and biological substances (960-979)
960 Poisoning by antibiotics
961 Poisoning by other anti-infectives
962 Poisoning by hormones and synthetic substitutes
963 Poisoning by primarily systemic agents
964 Poisoning by agents primarily affecting blood constituents
965 Poisoning by analgesics, antipyretics, and antirheumatics
966 Poisoning by anticonvulsants and anti-Parkinsonism drugs
967 Poisoning by sedatives and hypnotics
968 Poisoning by other central nervous system depressants and anesthetics
969 Poisoning by psychotropic agents
970 Poisoning by central nervous system stimulants
971 Poisoning by drugs primarily affecting the autonomic nervous system
972 Poisoning by agents primarily affecting the cardiovascular system
973 Poisoning by agents primarily affecting the gastrointestinal system
974 Poisoning by water, mineral, and uric acid metabolism drugs
975 Poisoning by agents primarily acting on the smooth and skeletal muscles and respiratory system

976   Poisoning by agents primarily affecting skin and mucous membrane, ophthalmological, otorhinolaryngological, and dental drugs
977   Poisoning by other and unspecified drugs and medicinals
978   Poisoning by bacterial vaccines
979   Poisoning by other vaccines and biological substances

Toxic effects of substances chiefly nonmedicinal as to source (980-989)
980   Toxic effect of alcohol
981   Toxic effect of petroleum products
982   Toxic effect of solvents other than petroleum-based
983   Toxic effect of corrosive aromatics, acids, and caustic alkalis
984   Toxic effect of lead and its compounds (including fumes)
985   Toxic effect of other metals
986   Toxic effect of carbon monoxide
987   Toxic effect of other gases, fumes, or vapors
988   Effect of noxious substances eaten as food
989   Toxic effect of other substances, chiefly nonmedicinal as to source

Other and unspecified effects of external causes (990-995)
990   Effects of radiation, unspecified
991   Effects of reduced temperature
992   Effects of heat and light
993   Effects of air pressure
994   Effects of other external causes
995   Certain adverse effects, not elsewhere classified

Complications of surgical and medical care, not elsewhere classified (996-999)
996   Complications peculiar to certain specified procedures
997   Complications affecting specified body systems, not elsewhere classified
998   Other complications of procedures, not elsewhere classified
999   Complications of medical care, not elsewhere classified

Supplementary Classification of Factors Influencing Health Status and Contact With Health Services

Persons with potential health hazards related to communicable diseases (V01-V06)
V01   Contact with or exposure to communicable diseases
V02   Carrier or suspected carrier of infectious diseases
V03   Need for prophylactic vaccination and inoculation against bacterial diseases
V04   Need for prophylactic vaccination and inoculation against certain viral diseases
V05   Need for other prophylactic vaccination and inoculation against single diseases
V06   Need for prophylactic vaccination and inoculation against combinations of diseases

Persons with need for isolation, other potential health hazards, and prophylactic measures (V07-V09)
V07   Need for isolation and other prophylactic or treatment measures
V08   Asymptomatic human immunodeficiency virus [HIV] infection status
V09   Infection with drug-resistant microorganisms

Persons with potential health hazards related to personal and family history (V10-V19)
V10   Personal history of malignant neoplasm
V11   Personal history of mental disorder
V12   Personal history of certain other diseases

V13   Personal history of other diseases
V14   Personal history of allergy to medicinal agents
V15   Other personal history presenting hazards to health
V16   Family history of malignant neoplasm
V17   Family history of certain chronic disabling diseases
V18   Family history of certain other specific conditions
V19   Family history of other conditions

Persons encountering health services in circumstances related to reproduction and development (V20-V29)
V20   Health supervision of infant or child
V21   Constitutional states in development
V22   Normal pregnancy
V23   Supervision of high-risk pregnancy
V24   Postpartum care and examination
V25   Encounter for contraceptive management
V26   Procreative management
V27   Outcome of delivery
V28   Encounter for antenatal screening of mother
V29   Observation and evaluation of newborns and infants for suspected condition not found

Liveborn infants according to type of birth (V30-V39)
V30   Single liveborn
V31   Twin, mate liveborn
V32   Twin, mate stillborn
V33   Twin, unspecified
V34   Other multiple, mates all liveborn
V35   Other multiple, mates all stillborn
V36   Other multiple, mates live and stillborn
V37   Other multiple, unspecified
V39   Unspecified

Persons with a condition influencing their health status (V40-V49)
V40   Mental and behavioral problems
V41   Problems with special senses and other special functions
V42   Organ or tissue replaced by transplant
V43   Organ or tissue replaced by other means
V44   Artificial opening status
V45   Other postprocedural states
V46   Other dependence on machines and devices
V47   Other problems with internal organs
V48   Problems with head, neck, and trunk
V49   Other conditions influencing health status

Persons encountering health services for specific procedures and aftercare (V50-V59)
V50   Elective surgery for purposes other than remedying health states
V51   Aftercare involving the use of plastic surgery
V52   Fitting and adjustment of prosthetic device and implant
V53   Fitting and adjustment of other device
V54   Other orthopedic aftercare
V55   Attention to artificial openings
V56   Encounter for dialysis and dialysis catheter care
V57   Care involving use of rehabilitation procedures
V58   Encounter for other and unspecified procedures and aftercare
V59   Donors

Persons encountering health services in other circumstances (V60-V69)
V60   Housing, household, and economic circumstances
V61   Other family circumstances
V62   Other psychosocial circumstances
V63   Unavailability of other medical facilities for care
V64   Persons encountering health services for specific procedures, not carried out
V65   Other persons seeking consultation
V66   Convalescence and palliative care
V67   Follow-up examination

V68   Encounters for administrative purposes
V69   Problems related to lifestyle

Persons without reported diagnosis encountered during examination and investigation of individuals and populations (V70-V82)
V70   General medical examination
V71   Observation and evaluation for suspected conditions not found
V72   Special investigations and examinations
V73   Special screening examination for viral and chlamydial diseases
V74   Special screening examination for bacterial and spirochetal diseases
V75   Special screening examination for other infectious diseases
V76   Special screening for malignant neoplasms
V77   Special screening for endocrine, nutritional, metabolic, and immunity disorders
V78   Special screening for disorders of blood and blood-forming organs
V79   Special screening for mental disorders and developmental handicaps
V80   Special screening for neurological, eye, and ear diseases
V81   Special screening for cardiovascular, respiratory, and genitourinary diseases
V82   Special screening for other conditions

Genetics (V83-V84)
V83   Genetic carrier status
V84   Genetic susceptibility to disease

Body mass index (V85)
V85   Body Mass Index [BMI]

Estrogen receptor status (V86)
V86   Estrogen receptor status

Other specified personal exposures and history presenting hazards to health (V87)
V87   Other specified personal exposures and history presenting hazards to health

Acquired absence of other organs and tissue (V88)
V88   Acquired absence of other organs and tissue

Other suspected conditions not found (V89)
V89   Other suspected conditions not found

Retained Foreign Body (V90)
V90   Retained foreign body

Multiple Gestation Placenta Status (V91)
V91   Multiple gestation placenta status

Supplementary Classification of External Causes of Injury and Poisoning

External Cause Status (E000)
E000   External cause status

Activity (E001-E030)
E001   Activities involving walking and running
E002   Activities involving water and water craft
E003   Activities involving ice and snow
E004   Activities involving climbing, rappelling, and jumping off
E005   Activities involving dancing and other rhythmic movement
E006   Activities involving other sports and athletics played individually
E007   Activities involving other sports and athletics played as a team or group
E008   Activities involving other specified sports and athletics
E009   Activity involving other cardiorespiratory exercise
E010   Activity involving other muscle strengthening exercises

11   Activities involving computer technology and electronic devices
12   Activities involving arts and handcrafts
13   Activities involving personal hygiene and household maintenance
14   Activities involving person providing caregiving
15   Activities involving food preparation, cooking and grilling
16   Activities involving property and land maintenance, building and construction
17   Activities involving roller coasters and other types of external motion
18   Activities involving playing musical instrument
19   Activities involving animal care
29   Other activity
30   Unspecified activity

Transport Accidents (E800-E848)

Railway accidents (E800-E807)
00   Railway accident involving collision with roling stock
01   Railway accident involving collision with other object
02   Railway accident involving derailment without antecedent collision
03   Railway accident involving explosion, fire, or burning
04   Fall in, on, or from railway train
05   Hit by rolling stock
06   Other specified railway accident
07   Railway accident of unspecified nature

Motor vehicle traffic accidents (E810-E819)
10   Motor vehicle traffic accident involving collision with train
11   Motor vehicle traffic accident involving re-entrant collision with another motor vehicle
12   Other motor vehicle traffic accident involving collision with another motor vehicle
13   Motor vehicle traffic accident involving collision with other vehicle
14   Motor vehicle traffic accident involving collision with pedestrian
15   Other motor vehicle traffic accident involving collision on the highway
16   Motor vehicle traffic accident due to loss of control, without collision on the highway
17   Noncollision motor vehicle traffic accident while boarding or alighting
18   Other noncollision motor vehicle traffic accident
19   Motor vehicle traffic accident of unspecified nature

Motor vehicle nontraffic accidents (E820-E825)
20   Nontraffic accident involving motor-driven snow vehicle
21   Nontraffic accident involving other off-road motor vehicle
22   Other motor vehicle nontraffic accident involving collision with moving object
23   Other motor vehicle nontraffic accident involving collision with stationary object
24   Other motor vehicle nontraffic accident while boarding and alighting
25   Other motor vehicle nontraffic accident of other and unspecified nature

Other road vehicle accidents (E826-E829)
26   Pedal cycle accident
27   Animal-drawn vehicle accident
28   Accident involving animal being ridden
29   Other road vehicle accidents

Water transport accidents (E830-E838)
30   Accident to watercraft causing submersion
31   Accident to watercraft causing other injury
32   Other accidental submersion or drowning in water transport accident
E833   Fall on stairs or ladders in water transport
E834   Other fall from one level to another in water transport
E835   Other and unspecified fall in water transport
E836   Machinery accident in water transport
E837   Explosion, fire, or burning in watercraft
E838   Other and unspecified water transport accident

Air and space transport accidents (E840-E845)
E840   Accident to powered aircraft at takeoff or landing
E841   Accident to powered aircraft, other and unspecified
E842   Accident to unpowered aircraft
E843   Fall in, on, or from aircraft
E844   Other specified air transport accidents
E845   Accident involving spacecraft

Vehicle accidents, not elsewhere classfiable (E846-E849)
E846   Accidents involving powered vehicles used solely within the buildings and premises of an industrial or commercial establishment
E847   Accidents involving cable cars not running on rails
E848   Accidents involving other vehicles, not elsewhere classifiable
E849   Place of occurrence

Accidental poisoning by drugs, medicinal substances, and biologicals (E850-E858)
E850   Accidental poisoning by analgesics, antipyretics, and antirheumatics
E851   Accidental poisoning by barbiturates
E852   Accidental poisoning by other sedatives and hypnotics
E853   Accidental poisoning by tranquilizers
E854   Accidental poisoning by other psychotropic agents
E855   Accidental poisoning by other drugs acting on central and autonomic nervous systems
E856   Accidental poisoning by antibiotics
E857   Accidental poisoning by anti-infectives
E858   Accidental poisoning by other drugs

Accidental poisoning by other solid and liquid substances, gases, and vapors (E860-E869)
E860   Accidental poisoning by alcohol, not elsewhere classified
E861   Accidental poisoning by cleansing and polishing agents, disinfectants, paints, and varnishes
E862   Accidental poisoning by petroleum products, other solvents and their vapors, not elsewhere classified
E863   Accidental poisoning by agricultural and horticultural chemical and pharmaceutical preparations other than plant foods and fertilizers
E864   Accidental poisoning by corrosives and caustics, not elsewhere classified
E865   Accidental poisoning from poisonous foodstuffs and poisonous plants
E866   Accidental poisoning by other and unspecified solid and liquid substances
E867   Accidental poisoning by gas distributed by pipeline
E868   Accidental poisoning by other utility gas and other carbon monoxide
E869   Accidental poisoning by other gases and vapors

Misadventures to patients during surgical and medical care (E870-E876)
E870   Accidental cut, puncture, perforation, or hemorrhage during medical care
E871   Foreign object left in body during procedure
E872   Failure of sterile precautions during procedure
E873   Failure in dosage
E874   Mechanical failure of instrument or apparatus during procedure
E875   Contaminated or infected blood, other fluid, drug, or biological substance
E876   Other and unspecified misadventures during medical care

Surgical and medical procedures as the cause of abnormal reaction of patient or later complication, without mention of misadventure at the time of procedure (E878-E879)
E878   Surgical operation and other surgical procedures as the cause of abnormal reaction of patient, or of later complication, without mention of misadventure at the time of operation
E879   Other procedures, without mention of misadventure at the time of procedure, as the cause of abnormal reaction of patient, or of later complication

Accidental falls (E880-E888)
E880   Fall on or from stairs or steps
E881   Fall on or from ladders or scaffolding
E882   Fall from or out of building or other structure
E883   Fall into hole or other opening in surface
E884   Other fall from one level to another
E885   Fall on same level from slipping, tripping, or stumbling
E886   Fall on same level from collision, pushing or shoving, by or with other person
E887   Fracture, cause unspecified
E888   Other and unspecified fall

Accidents caused by fire and flames (E890-E899)
E890   Conflagration in private dwelling
E891   Conflagration in other and unspecified building or structure
E892   Conflagration not in building or structure
E893   Accident caused by ignition of clothing
E894   Ignition of highly inflammable material
E895   Accident caused by controlled fire in private dwelling
E896   Accident caused by controlled fire in other and unspecified building or structure
E897   Accident caused by controlled fire not in building or structure
E898   Accident caused by other specified fire and flames
E899   Accident caused by unspecified fire

Accidents due to natural and environmental factors (E900-E909)
E900   Excessive heat
E901   Excessive cold
E902   High and low air pressure and changes in air pressure
E903   Travel and motion
E904   Hunger, thirst, exposure, and neglect
E905   Venomous animals and plants as the cause of poisoning and toxic reactions
E906   Other injury caused by animals
E907   Lightning
E908   Cataclysmic storms, and floods resulting from storms
E909   Cataclysmic earth surface movements and eruptions

Accidents caused by submersion, suffocation, and foreign bodies (E910-E915)
E910   Accidental drowning and submersion
E911   Inhalation and ingestion of food causing obstruction of respiratory tract or suffocation
E912   Inhalation and ingestion of other object causing obstruction of respiratory tract or suffocation
E913   Accidental mechanical suffocation
E914   Foreign body accidentally entering eye and adnexa
E915   Foreign body accidentally entering other orifice

Other accidents (E916-E928)
E916   Struck accidentally by falling object

E917 Striking against or struck accidentally by objects or persons
E918 Caught accidentally in or between objects
E919 Accidents caused by machinery
E920 Accidents caused by cutting and piercing instruments or objects
E921 Accident caused by explosion of pressure vessel
E922 Accident caused by firearm and air gun missile
E923 Accident caused by explosive material
E924 Accident caused by hot substance or object, caustic or corrosive material, and steam
E925 Accident caused by electric current
E926 Exposure to radiation
E927 Overexertion and strenuous and repetitive movements or loads
E928 Other and unspecified environmental and accidental causes

Late effects of accidental injury (E929)
E929 Late effects of accidental injury

Drugs, medicinal and biological substances causing adverse effects in therapeutic use (E930-E949)
E930 Antibiotics
E931 Other anti-infectives
E932 Hormones and synthetic substitutes
E933 Primarily systemic agents
E934 Agents primarily affecting blood constituents
E935 Analgesics, antipyretics, and antirheumatics
E936 Anticonvulsants and anti-Parkinsonism drugs
E937 Sedatives and hypnotics
E938 Other central nervous system depressants and anesthetics
E939 Psychotropic agents
E940 Central nervous system stimulants
E941 Drugs primarily affecting the autonomic nervous system
E942 Agents primarily affecting the cardiovascular system
E943 Agents primarily affecting gastrointestinal system
E944 Water, mineral, and uric acid metabolism drugs
E945 Agents primarily acting on the smooth and skeletal muscles and respiratory system
E946 Agents primarily affecting skin and mucous membrane, ophthalmological, otorhinolaryngological, and dental drugs
E947 Other and unspecified drugs and medicinal substances
E948 Bacterial vaccines
E949 Other vaccines and biological substances

Suicide and self-inflicted injury (E950-E959)
E950 Suicide and self-inflicted poisoning by solid or liquid substances
E951 Suicide and self-inflicted poisoning by gases in domestic use
E952 Suicide and self-inflicted poisoning by other gases and vapors
E953 Suicide and self-inflicted injury by hanging, strangulation, and suffocation
E954 Suicide and self-inflicted injury by submersion [drowning]
E955 Suicide and self-inflicted injury by firearms, air guns and explosives
E956 Suicide and self-inflicted injury by cutting and piercing instruments
E957 Suicide and self-inflicted injuries by jumping from high place
E958 Suicide and self-inflicted injury by other and unspecified means
E959 Late effects of self-inflicted injury

Homicide and injury purposely inflicted by other persons (E960-E969)
E960 Fight, brawl, and rape
E961 Assault by corrosive or caustic substance, except poisoning
E962 Assault by poisoning
E963 Assault by hanging and strangulation
E964 Assault by submersion [drowning]
E965 Assault by firearms and explosives
E966 Assault by cutting and piercing instrument
E967 Perpetrator of child and adult abuse
E968 Assault by other and unspecified means
E969 Late effects of injury purposely inflicted by other person

Legal intervention (E970-E978)
E970 Injury due to legal intervention by firearms
E971 Injury due to legal intervention by explosives
E972 Injury due to legal intervention by gas
E973 Injury due to legal intervention by blunt object
E974 Injury due to legal intervention by cutting and piercing instruments
E975 Injury due to legal intervention by other specified means
E976 Injury due to legal intervention by unspecified means
E977 Late effects of injuries due to legal intervention
E978 Legal execution

Terrorism (E979)
E979 Terrorism

Injury undetermined whether accidentally or purposely inflicted (E980-E989)
E980 Poisoning by solid or liquid substances, undetermined whether accidentally or purposely inflicted
E981 Poisoning by gases in domestic use, undetermined whether accidentally or purposely inflicted
E982 Poisoning by other gases, undetermined whether accidentally or purposely inflicted
E983 Hanging, strangulation, or suffocation, undetermined whether accidentally or purposely inflicted
E984 Submersion [drowning], undetermined whether accidentally or purposely inflicted
E985 Injury by firearms and explosives, undetermined whether accidentally or purposely inflicted
E986 Injury by cutting and piercing instruments, undetermined whether accidentally or purposely inflicted
E987 Falling from high place, undetermined whether accidentally or purposely inflicted
E988 Injury by other and unspecified means, undetermined whether accidentally or purposely inflicted
E989 Late effects of injury, undetermined whether accidentally or purposely inflicted

Injury resulting from operations of war (E990-E999)
E990 Injury due to war operations by fires and conflagrations
E991 Injury due to war operations by bullets and fragments
E992 Injury due to war operations by explosion of marine weapons
E993 Injury due to war operations by other explosion
E994 Injury due to war operations by destruction of aircraft
E995 Injury due to war operations by other and unspecified forms of conventional warfare
E996 Injury due to war operations by nuclear weapons
E997 Injury due to war operations by other forms of unconventional warfare
E998 Injury due to war operations but occurring after cessation of hostilities
E999 Late effects of injury due to war operations and terrorism

A

Abbe operation
  construction of vagina 70.61
    with graft or prosthesis 70.63
  intestinal anastomosis — see Anastomosis, intestine
Abciximab, infusion 99.20
Abdominocentesis 54.91
Abdominohysterectomy 68.49
  laparoscopic 68.41
Abdominoplasty 86.83
Abdominoscopy 54.21
Abdominouterotomy 68.0
  obstetrical 74.99
Abduction, arytenoid 31.69
AbioCor® total replacement heart 37.52
Ablation
  biliary tract (lesion) by ERCP 51.64
  endometrial (hysteroscopic) 68.23
  inner ear (cryosurgery) (ultrasound) 20.79
    by injection 20.72
  lesion
    esophagus 42.39
      endoscopic 42.33
    heart
      by peripherally inserted catheter 37.34
      endovascular approach 37.34
      maze procedure (Cox-maze)
        endovascular approach 37.34
        open approach 37.33
        thoracoscopic approach 37.37
      thoracoscopic approach 37.37
    intestine
      large 45.49
        endoscopic 45.43
    large intestine 45.49
      endoscopic 45.43
    liver 50.26
      laparoscopic 50.25
      open 50.23
      percutaneous 50.24
    lung 32.26
      bronchoscopic thermoplasty 32.27
      open 32.23
      percutaneous 32.24
      thoracoscopic 32.25
    renal 55.35
      laparoscopic 55.34
      open 55.32
      percutaneous 55.33
  pituitary 07.69
    by
      Cobalt 60 92.32
      implantation (strontium-yttrium) (Y) NEC 07.68
        transfrontal approach 07.64
        transphenoidal approach 07.65
      proton beam (Bragg peak) 92.33
  prostate
    by
      cryoablation 60.62
      laser, transurethral 60.21
      radical cryosurgical ablation (RCSA) 60.62
      radiofrequency thermotherapy 60.97
      transurethral needle ablation (TUNA) 60.97
  tissue
    heart — see Ablation, lesion, heart
    liver — see Ablation, lesion, liver
    lung — see Ablation, lesion, lung
    renal — see Ablation, lesion, renal
Abortion, therapeutic 69.51
  by
    aspiration curettage 69.51
    dilation and curettage 69.01
    hysterectomy — see Hysterectomy
    hysterotomy 74.91
    insertion
      laminaria 69.93
      prostaglandin suppository 96.49
    intra-amniotic injection (saline) 75.0
Abrasion
  corneal epithelium 11.41
    for smear or culture 11.21

Abrasion — continued
  epicardial surface 36.39
  pleural 34.6
  skin 86.25
Abscission, cornea 11.49
Absorptiometry
  photon (dual) (single) 88.98
Aburel operation (intra-amniotic injection for abortion) 75.0
Accouchement forcé 73.99
Acetabulectomy 77.85
Acetabuloplasty NEC 81.40
  with prosthetic implant 81.52
Achillorrhaphy 83.64
  delayed 83.62
Achillotenotomy 83.11
  plastic 83.85
Achillotomy 83.11
  plastic 83.85
Acid peel, skin 86.24
Acromionectomy 77.81
Acromioplasty 81.83
  for recurrent dislocation of shoulder 81.82
  partial replacement 81.81
  total replacement, NEC 81.80
    other 81.80
    reverse 81.88
Actinotherapy 99.82
Activities of daily living (ADL)
  therapy 93.83
  training for the blind 93.78
Acupuncture 99.92
  with smouldering moxa 93.35
  for anesthesia 99.91
Adams operation
  advancement of round ligament 69.22
  crushing of nasal septum 21.88
  excision of palmar fascia 82.35
Adenectomy — see also Excision, by site
  prostate NEC 60.69
    retropubic 60.4
Adenoidectomy (without tonsillectomy) 28.6
  with tonsillectomy 28.3
Adhesiolysis — see also Lysis, adhesions
  for collapse of lung 33.39
  middle ear 20.23
Adipectomy 86.83
Adjustment
  cardiac pacemaker program (reprogramming) — omit code
  cochlear prosthetic device (external components) 95.49
  dental 99.97
  gastric restrictive device (laparoscopic) 44.98
  occlusal 24.8
  orthopedic device (noninvasive)
    external fixator — omit code
  spectacles 95.31
Administration (of) — see also Injection
  Activase® 99.10
  adhesion barrier substance 99.77
  Alteplase (tPA, generic) 99.10
  Anistreplase (tPA, generic) 99.10
  antitoxins NEC 99.58
    botulism 99.57
    diphtheria 99.58
    gas gangrene 99.58
    scarlet fever 99.58
    tetanus 99.56
  Bender Visual-Motor Gestalt test 94.02
  Benton Visual Retention test 94.02
  DrotAA 00.11
  Eminase® 99.10
  Inhaled nitric oxide 00.12
  intelligence test or scale (Stanford-Binet) (Wechsler) (adult) (children) 94.01
  Minnesota Multiphasic Personality Inventory (MMPI) 94.02
  MMPI (Minnesota Multiphasic Personality Inventory) 94.02
  neuroprotective agent 99.75
  Proleukin® (low-dose) 99.28
    high-dose 00.15
  psychologic test 94.02
  Retavase® 99.10

Administration — see also Injection — continued
  Reteplase (tPA, generic) 99.10
  Stanford-Binet test 94.01
  Streptase® 99.10
  Streptokinase (tPA, generic) 99.10
  Tenecteplase (tPA, generic) 99.10
  TNKase™ 99.10
  toxoid
    diphtheria 99.36
      with tetanus and pertussis, combined (DTP) 99.39
    tetanus 99.38
      with diphtheria and pertussis, combined (DTP) 99.39
  vaccine (see also Vaccination)
    BCG 99.33
    measles-mumps-rubella (MMR) 99.48
    poliomyelitis 99.41
    TAB 99.32
  Wechsler
    Intelligence Scale (adult) (children) 94.01
    Memory Scale 94.02
  Xigris® 00.11
Adrenalectomy (unilateral) 07.22
  with partial removal of remaining gland 07.29
  bilateral 07.3
    partial 07.29
    subtotal 07.29
  complete 07.3
  partial NEC 07.29
  remaining gland 07.3
  subtotal NEC 07.29
  total 07.3
Adrenalorrhaphy 07.44
Adrenalotomy (with drainage) 07.41
Advancement
  extraocular muscle 15.12
    multiple (with resection or recession) 15.3
  eyelid muscle 08.59
  eye muscle 15.12
    multiple (with resection or recession) 15.3
  graft — see Graft
  leaflet (heart) 35.10
  pedicle (flap) 86.72
  profundus tendon (Wagner) 82.51
  round ligament 69.22
  tendon 83.71
    hand 82.51
    profundus (Wagner) 82.51
  Wagner (profundus tendon) 82.51
AESOP® (Automated Endoscopic System for Optimal Positioning) — see category 17.4 ☑
Albee operation
  bone peg, femoral neck 78.05
  graft for slipping patella 78.06
  sliding inlay graft, tibia 78.07
Albert operation (arthrodesis of knee) 81.22
Aldridge (-Studdiford) operation (urethral sling) 59.5
Alexander-Adams operation (shortening of round ligaments) 69.22
Alexander operation
  prostatectomy
    perineal 60.62
    suprapubic 60.3
  shortening of round ligaments 69.22
Alimentation, parenteral 99.29
Allograft — see Graft
Almoor operation (extrapetrosal drainage) 20.22
Altemeier operation (perineal rectal pull-through) 48.49
Alveolectomy (interradicular) (intraseptal) (radical) (simple) (with graft) (with implant) 24.5
Alveoloplasty (with graft or implant) 24.5
Alveolotomy (apical) 24.0
Ambulatory cardiac monitoring (ACM) 89.50
Ammon operation (dacryocystotomy) 09.53
Amniocentesis (transuterine) (diagnostic) 75.1
  with intra-amniotic injection of saline 75.0

Amniography 87.81
Amnioinfusion 75.37
Amnioscopy, internal 75.31
Amniotomy 73.09
  to induce labor 73.01
Amputation (cineplastic) (closed flap) (guillotine) (kineplastic) (open) 84.91
  abdominopelvic 84.19
  above-elbow 84.07
  above-knee (AK) 84.17
  ankle (disarticulation) 84.13
    through malleoli of tibia and fibula 84.14
  arm NEC 84.00
    through
      carpals 84.03
      elbow (disarticulation) 84.06
      forearm 84.05
      humerus 84.07
      shoulder (disarticulation) 84.08
      wrist (disarticulation) 84.04
    upper 84.07
  Batch-Spittler-McFaddin (knee disarticulation) 84.16
  below-knee (BK) NEC 84.15
    conversion into above-knee amputation 84.17
  Boyd (hip disarticulation) 84.18
  Burgess operation (amputation of ankle) 84.14
  Callander's (knee disarticulation) 84.16
  carpals 84.03
  cervix 67.4
  Chopart's (midtarsal) 84.12
  clitoris 71.4
  Dieffenbach (hip disarticulation) 84.18
  Dupuytren's (shoulder disarticulation) 84.08
  ear, external 18.39
  elbow (disarticulation) 84.06
  finger, except thumb 84.01
    thumb 84.02
  foot (middle) 84.12
  forearm 84.05
  forefoot 84.12
  forequarter 84.09
  Gordon-Taylor (hindquarter) 84.19
  Gritti-Stokes (knee disarticulation) 84.16
  Guyon (ankle) 84.13
  hallux 84.11
  hand 84.03
  Hey's (foot) 84.12
  hindquarter 84.19
  hip (disarticulation) 84.18
  humerus 84.07
  interscapulothoracic 84.09
  interthoracoscapular 84.09
  King-Steelquist (hindquarter) 84.19
  Kirk (thigh) 84.17
  knee (disarticulation) 84.16
  Kutler (revision of current traumatic amputation of finger) 84.01
  Larry (shoulder disarticulation) 84.08
  leg NEC 84.10
    above knee (AK) 84.17
    below knee (BK) 84.15
    through
      ankle (disarticulation) 84.13
      femur (AK) 84.17
      foot 84.12
      hip (disarticulation) 84.18
      tibia and fibula (BK) 84.15
  Lisfranc
    foot 84.12
    shoulder (disarticulation) 84.08
  Littlewood (forequarter) 84.09
  lower limb NEC (see also Amputation, leg) 84.10
  Mazet (knee disarticulation) 84.16
  metacarpal 84.03
  metatarsal 84.11
    head (bunionectomy) 77.59
  metatarsophalangeal (joint) 84.11
  midtarsal 84.12
  nose 21.4
  penis (circle) (complete) (flap) (partial) (radical) 64.3

☑ Additional Digit Required — Refer to the Tabular List for Digit Selection   ▽ Subterms under main terms may continue to next column or page

2014 ICD-9-CM   ▶◀ Revised Text   ● New Line   ▲ Revised Code   Volume 3 — 1

Abbe operation — Amputation

Amputation — *continued*
  Pirogoff's (ankle amputation through malleoli of tibia and fibula) 84.14
  ray
    finger 84.01
    foot 84.11
    toe (metatarsal head) 84.11
  root (tooth) (apex) 23.73
    with root canal therapy 23.72
  shoulder (disarticulation) 84.08
  Sorondo-Ferré (hindquarter) 84.19
  S.P. Rogers (knee disarticulation) 84.16
  supracondyler, above-knee 84.17
  supramalleolar, foot 84.14
  Syme's (ankle amputation through malleoli of tibia and fibula) 84.14
  thigh 84.17
  thumb 84.02
  toe (through metatarsophalangeal joint) 84.11
  transcarpal 84.03
  transmetatarsal 84.12
  upper limb NEC (*see also* Amputation, arm) 84.00
  wrist (disarticulation) 84.04
Amygdalohippocampectomy 01.59
Amygdalohippocampotomy 01.39
Amygdalotomy 01.39
Analysis
  cardiac rhythm device (CRT-D) (CRT-P) (AICD) (pacemaker) — *see* Interrogation
  character 94.03
  gastric 89.39
  psychologic 94.31
  transactional
    group 94.44
    individual 94.39
Anastomosis
  abdominal artery to coronary artery 36.17
  accessory-facial nerve 04.72
  accessory-hypoglossal nerve 04.73
  anus (with formation of endorectal ileal pouch) 45.95
  aorta (descending)-pulmonary (artery) 39.0
  aorta-renal artery 39.24
  aorta-subclavian artery 39.22
  aortoceliac 39.26
  aorto(ilio)femoral 39.25
  aortomesenteric 39.26
  appendix 47.99
  arteriovenous NEC 39.29
    for renal dialysis 39.27
  artery (suture of distal to proximal end) 39.31
    with
      bypass graft 39.29
        extracranial-intracranial [EC-IC] 39.28
      excision or resection of vessel — *see* Arteriectomy, with anastomosis, by site
    revision 39.49
  bile ducts 51.39
  bladder NEC 57.88
    with
      isolated segment of intestine 57.87 *[45.50]*
        colon (sigmoid) 57.87 *[45.52]*
        ileum 57.87 *[45.51]*
        open loop of ileum 57.87 *[45.51]*
      to intestine 57.88
        ileum 57.87 *[45.51]*
  bowel (*see also* Anastomosis, intestine) 45.90
  bronchotracheal 33.48
  bronchus 33.48
  carotid-subclavian artery 39.22
  caval-mesenteric vein 39.1
  caval-pulmonary artery 39.21
  cervicoesophageal 42.59
  colohypopharyngeal (intrathoracic) 42.55
    antesternal or antethoracic 42.65
  common bile duct 51.39
  common pulmonary trunk and left atrium (posterior wall) 35.82

Anastomosis — *continued*
  cystic bile duct 51.39
  cystocolic 57.88
  epididymis to vas deferens 63.83
  esophagocolic (intrathoracic) NEC 42.56
    with interposition 42.55
    antesternal or antethoracic NEC 42.66
      with interposition 42.65
  esophagocologastric (intrathoracic) 42.55
    antesternal or antethoracic 42.65
  esophagoduodenal (intrathoracic) NEC 42.54
    with interposition 42.53
  esophagoenteric (intrathoracic) NEC (*see also* Anastomosis, esophagus, to intestinal segment) 42.54
    antesternal or antethoracic NEC (*see also* Anastomosis, esophagus, antesternal, to intestinal segment) 42.64
  esophagoesophageal (intrathoracic) 42.51
    antesternal or antethoracic 42.61
  esophagogastric (intrathoracic) 42.52
    antesternal or antethoracic 42.62
  esophagus (intrapleural) (intrathoracic) (retrosternal) NEC 42.59
    with
      gastrectomy (partial) 43.5
        complete or total 43.99
      interposition (of) NEC 42.58
        colon 42.55
        jejunum 42.53
        small bowel 42.53
    antesternal or antethoracic NEC 42.69
      with
        interposition (of) NEC 42.68
          colon 42.65
          jejunal loop 42.63
          small bowel 42.63
        rubber tube 42.68
      to intestinal segment NEC 42.64
        with interposition 42.68
        colon NEC 42.66
          with interposition 42.65
        small bowel NEC 42.64
          with interposition 42.63
    to intestinal segment (intrathoracic) NEC 42.54
      with interposition 42.58
      antesternal or antethoracic NEC 42.64
        with interposition 42.68
      colon (intrathoracic) NEC 42.56
        with interposition 42.55
        antesternal or antethoracic 42.66
          with interposition 42.65
      small bowel NEC 42.54
        with interposition 42.53
        antesternal or antethoracic 42.64
          with interposition 42.63
  facial-accessory nerve 04.72
  facial-hypoglossal nerve 04.71
  fallopian tube 66.73
    by reanastomosis 66.79
  gallbladder 51.35
    to
      hepatic ducts 51.31
      intestine 51.32
      pancreas 51.33
      stomach 51.34
  gastroepiploic artery to coronary artery 36.17
  hepatic duct 51.39
  hypoglossal-accessory nerve 04.73
  hypoglossal-facial nerve 04.71
  ileal loop to bladder 57.87 *[45.51]*
  ileoanal 45.95
  ileorectal 45.93
  inferior vena cava and portal vein 39.1
  internal mammary artery (to)
    coronary artery (single vessel) 36.15
      double vessel 36.16
    myocardium 36.2
  intestine 45.90
    large-to-anus 45.95
    large-to-large 45.94
    large-to-rectum 45.94

Anastomosis — *continued*
  intestine — *continued*
    large-to-small 45.93
    small-to-anus 45.95
    small-to-large 45.93
    small-to-rectal stump 45.92
    small-to-small 45.91
  intrahepatic 51.79
  intrathoracic vessel NEC 39.23
  kidney (pelvis) 55.86
  lacrimal sac to conjunctiva 09.82
  left-to-right (systemic-pulmonary artery) 39.0
  lymphatic (channel) (peripheral) 40.9
  mesenteric-caval 39.1
  mesocaval 39.1
  nasolacrimal 09.81
  nerve (cranial) (peripheral) NEC 04.74
    accessory-facial 04.72
    accessory-hypoglossal 04.73
    hypoglossal-facial 04.71
  pancreas (duct) (to) 52.96
    bile duct 51.39
    gall bladder 51.33
    intestine 52.96
    jejunum 52.96
    stomach 52.96
  pleurothecal (with valve) 03.79
  portacaval 39.1
  portal vein to inferior vena cava 39.1
  pulmonary-aortic (Pott's) 39.0
  pulmonary-innominate artery (Blalock) 39.0
  pulmonary-subclavian artery (Blalock-Taussig) 39.0
  pulmonary artery and superior vena cava 39.21
  pulmonary vein and azygos vein 39.23
  pyeloileocutaneous 56.51
  pyeloureterovesical 55.86
  radial artery 36.19
  rectum, rectal NEC 48.74
    stump to small intestine 45.92
  renal (pelvis) 55.86
    vein and splenic vein 39.1
  renoportal 39.1
  salpingothecal (with valve) 03.79
  splenic to renal veins 39.1
  splenorenal (venous) 39.1
    arterial 39.26
  subarachnoid-peritoneal (with valve) 03.71
  subarachnoid-ureteral (with valve) 03.72
  subclavian-aortic 39.22
  superior vena cava to pulmonary artery 39.21
  systemic-pulmonary artery 39.0
  thoracic artery (to)
    coronary artery (single) 36.15
      double 36.16
    myocardium 36.2
  ureterocalyceal 55.86
  ureterocolic 56.71
  ureterovesical 56.74
  ureter (to) NEC 56.79
    bladder 56.74
    colon 56.71
    ileal pouch (bladder) 56.51
    ileum 56.71
    intestine 56.71
    skin 56.61
  urethra (end-to-end) 58.44
  vas deferens 63.82
  veins (suture of proximal to distal end) (with bypass graft) 39.29
    with excision or resection of vessel — *see* Phlebectomy, with anastomosis, by site
    mesenteric to vena cava 39.1
    portal to inferior vena cava 39.1
    revision 39.49
    splenic and renal 39.1
  ventricle, ventricular (intracerebral) (with valve) (*see also* Shunt, ventricular) 02.22
  ventriculoatrial (with valve) 02.32
  ventriculocaval (with valve) 02.32
  ventriculomastoid (with valve) 02.31

Anastomosis — *continued*
  ventriculopleural (with valve) 02.33
  vesicle — *see* Anastomosis, bladder
Anderson operation (tibial lengthening) 78.37
Anel operation (dilation of lacrimal duct) 09.42
Anesthesia
  acupuncture for 99.91
  cryoanalgesia, nerve (cranial) (peripheral) 04.2
  spinal — *omit code*
Aneurysmectomy 38.60
  with
    anastomosis 38.30
      abdominal
        artery 38.36
        vein 38.37
      aorta (arch) (ascending) (descending) 38.34
      head and neck NEC 38.32
      intracranial NEC 38.31
      lower limb
        artery 38.38
        vein 38.39
      thoracic NEC 38.35
      upper limb (artery) (vein) 38.33
    graft replacement (interposition) 38.40
      abdominal
        aorta
          endovascular approach 39.71
            fenestrated (branching) graft 39.78
          open approach 38.44
            Zenith® Renu™ AAA graft 39.71
        artery 38.46
        vein 38.47
      aorta (arch) (ascending) (descending thoracic)
        abdominal 38.44
        thoracic 38.45
        thoracoabdominal 38.45 *[38.44]*
      head and neck NEC 38.42
      intracranial NEC 38.41
      lower limb
        artery 38.48
        vein 38.49
      thoracic NEC 38.45
      upper limb (artery) (vein) 38.43
  abdominal
    artery 38.66
    vein 38.67
  aorta (arch) (ascending) (descending) 38.64
  atrial, auricular 37.32
  head and neck NEC 38.62
  heart 37.32
  intracranial NEC 38.61
  lower limb
    artery 38.68
    vein 38.69
  sinus of Valsalva 35.39
  thoracic NEC 38.65
  upper limb (artery) (vein) 38.63
  ventricle (myocardium) 37.32
Aneurysmoplasty — *see* Aneurysmorrhaphy
Aneurysmorrhaphy NEC 39.52
  by or with
    anastomosis — *see* Aneurysmectomy, with anastomosis, by site
    clipping 39.51
    coagulation 39.52
    electrocoagulation 39.52
    endovascular graft
      abdominal aorta 39.71
        fenestrated (branching) graft 39.78
      lower extremity artery(s) 39.79
      thoracic aorta 39.73
      upper extremity artery(s) 39.79
    excision or resection (*see also* Aneurysmectomy, by site)
      with
        anastomosis — *see* Aneurysmectomy, with anastomosis, by site

☑ **Additional Digit Required** — Refer to the Tabular List for Digit Selection   ▽ **Subterms under main terms may continue to next column or page**

2 — Volume 3   ►◄ Revised Text   ● New Line   ▲ Revised Code   2014 ICD-9-CM

Application — continued
  strapping (non-traction) 93.59
  substance, adhesion barrier 99.77
  Thomas collar 93.52
    with reduction of fracture or dislocation
      — see Reduction, fracture and
      Reduction, dislocation
  traction
    with reduction of fracture or dislocation
      — see Reduction, fracture and
      Reduction, dislocation
    adhesive tape (skin) 93.46
    boot 93.46
    Bryant's 93.44
    Buck's 93.46
    Cotrel's 93.42
    Dunlop's 93.44
    gallows 93.46
    Lyman Smith 93.44
    Russell's 93.44
    skeletal NEC 93.44
      intermittent 93.43
    skin, limbs NEC 93.46
    spinal NEC 93.42
      with skull device (halo) (caliper)
        (Crutchfield) (Gardner-Wells)
        (Vinke) (tongs) 93.41
        with synchronous insertion 02.94
    Thomas' splint 93.45
  Unna's paste boot 93.53
  vasopneumatic device 93.58
  Velpeau dressing 93.59
  Vinke tongs (skull) (with synchronous
    skeletal traction) 02.94
  wound dressing NEC 93.57
Aquapheresis 99.78
Arc lamp — see Photocoagulation
Arcuplasty 81.66
Arrest
  bone growth (epiphyseal) 78.20
    by stapling — see Stapling, epiphyseal
      plate
    femur 78.25
    fibula 78.27
    humerus 78.22
    radius 78.23
    tibia 78.27
    ulna 78.23
  cardiac, induced (anoxic) (circulatory) 39.63
  circulatory, induced (anoxic) 39.63
  hemorrhage — see Control, hemorrhage
Arslan operation (fenestration of inner ear)
  20.61
Arteriectomy 38.60
  with
    anastomosis 38.30
      abdominal 38.36
      aorta (arch) (ascending) (descending
        thoracic) 38.34
      head and neck NEC 38.32
      intracranial NEC 38.31
      lower limb 38.38
      thoracic NEC 38.35
      upper limb 38.33
    graft replacement (interposition) 38.40
      abdominal
        aorta 38.44
      aorta (arch) (ascending) (descending
        thoracic)
        abdominal 38.44
        thoracic 38.45
        thoracoabdominal 38.45 [38.44]
      head and neck NEC 38.42
      intracranial NEC 38.41
      lower limb 38.48
      thoracic NEC 38.45
      upper limb 38.43
  abdominal 38.66
  aorta (arch) (ascending) (descending) 38.64
  head and neck NEC 38.62
  intracranial NEC 38.61
  lower limb 38.68
  thoracic NEC 38.65
  upper limb 38.63
Arteriography (contrast) (fluoroscopic) (retrograde) 88.40

Arteriography — continued
  by
    radioisotope — see Scan, radioisotope
    ultrasound (Doppler) — see Ultrasonog-
      raphy, by site
  aorta (arch) (ascending) (descending) 88.42
  basilar 88.41
  brachial 88.49
  carotid (internal) 88.41
  cerebral (posterior circulation) 88.41
  coronary (direct) (selective) NEC 88.57
    double catheter technique (Judkins)
      (Ricketts and Abrams) 88.56
    intra-operative fluorescence vascular
      88.59
    single catheter technique (Sones) 88.55
  Doppler (ultrasonic) — see Ultrasonography,
    by site
  femoral 88.48
  head and neck 88.41
  intra-abdominal NEC 88.47
  intrathoracic NEC 88.44
  lower extremity 88.48
  placenta 88.46
  pulmonary 88.43
  radioisotope — see Scan, radioisotope
  renal 88.45
  specified site NEC 88.49
  SPY, coronary 88.59
  superior mesenteric artery 88.47
  transfemoral 88.48
  ultrasound — see Ultrasonography, by site
  upper extremity 88.49
Arterioplasty — see Repair, artery
Arteriorrhaphy 39.31
Arteriotomy 38.00
  abdominal 38.06
  aorta (arch) (ascending) (descending) 38.04
  head and neck NEC 38.02
  intracranial NEC 38.01
  lower limb 38.08
  thoracic NEC 38.05
  upper limb 38.03
Arteriovenostomy 39.29
  for renal dialysis 39.27
Arthrectomy 80.90
  ankle 80.97
  elbow 80.92
  foot and toe 80.98
  hand and finger 80.94
  hip 80.95
  intervertebral disc — see category 80.5 ☑
  knee 80.96
    semilunar cartilage 80.6
  shoulder 80.91
  specified site NEC 80.99
  spine NEC 80.99
  wrist 80.93
Arthrocentesis 81.91
  for arthrography — see Arthrogram
Arthrodesis (compression) (extra-articular)
  (intra-articular) (with bone graft) (with
  fixation device) 81.20
  ankle 81.11
  carporadial 81.25
  cricoarytenoid 31.69
  elbow 81.24
  finger 81.28
  foot NEC 81.17
  hip 81.21
  interphalangeal
    finger 81.28
    toe NEC 77.58
      claw toe repair 77.57
      hammer toe repair 77.56
  ischiofemoral 81.21
  knee 81.22
  lumbosacral, lumbar NEC 81.08
    ALIF (anterior lumbar interbody fusion)
      81.06
    anterior column (interbody)
      anterolateral (anterior) technique
        81.06
      posterior technique 81.08
    axial lumbar interbody fusion (AxiaLIF®)
      81.08

Arthrodesis — continued
  lumbosacral, lumbar — continued
    direct lateral interbody fusion (DLIF)
      81.06
    extreme lateral interbody fusion (XLIF®)
      81.06
    facet 81.07
    lateral transverse process technique
      81.07
    PLIF (posterior lumbar interbody fusion)
      81.08
    TLIF (transforaminal lumbar interbody
      fusion) 81.08
  McKeever (metatarsophalangeal) 81.16
  metacarpocarpal 81.26
  metacarpophalangeal 81.27
  metatarsophalangeal 81.16
  midtarsal 81.14
  pantalar 81.11
  sacroiliac 81.08
  shoulder 81.23
  specified joint NEC 81.29
  spinal (see also Fusion, spinal) 81.00
  subtalar 81.13
  tarsometatarsal 81.15
  tibiotalar 81.11
  toe NEC 77.58
    claw toe repair 77.57
    hammer toe repair 77.56
  triple 81.12
  wrist 81.26
Arthroendoscopy — see Arthroscopy
Arthroereisis, subtalar joint 81.18
Arthrogram, arthrography 88.32
  temporomandibular 87.13
Arthrolysis 93.26
Arthroplasty (with fixation device) (with traction) 81.96
  ankle 81.49
  carpals 81.75
    with prosthetic implant 81.74
  carpocarpal, carpometacarpal 81.75
    with prosthetic implant 81.74
  Carroll and Taber (proximal interphalangeal
    joint) 81.72
  cup (partial hip) 81.52
  Curtis (interphalangeal joint) 81.72
  elbow 81.85
    with prosthetic replacement (partial)
      (total) 81.84
  femoral head NEC 81.40
    with prosthetic implant 81.52
  finger(s) 81.72
    with prosthetic implant 81.71
  foot (metatarsal) with joint replacement
    81.57
  Fowler (metacarpophalangeal joint) 81.72
  hand (metacarpophalangeal) (interpha-
    langeal) 81.72
    with prosthetic implant 81.71
  hip (with bone graft) 81.40
    cup (partial hip) 81.52
    femoral head NEC 81.40
      with prosthetic implant 81.52
        with total replacement 81.51
    partial replacement 81.52
    total replacement 81.51
  interphalangeal joint 81.72
    with prosthetic implant 81.71
  Kessler (carpometacarpal joint) 81.74
  knee (see also Repair, knee) 81.47
    prosthetic replacement (bicompartmen-
      tal) (hemijoint) (partial) (total)
      (tricompartmental) (unicompart-
      mental) 81.54
    revision 81.55
  metacarpophalangeal joint 81.72
    with prosthetic implant 81.71
  shoulder 81.83
    for recurrent dislocation 81.82
    prosthetic replacement (partial) 81.81
      total, NEC 81.80
      other 81.80
      reverse 81.88
  temporomandibular 76.5
  toe NEC 77.58

Arthroplasty — continued
  toe — continued
    with prosthetic replacement 81.57
    for hallux valgus repair 77.59
  wrist 81.75
    with prosthetic implant 81.74
    total replacement 81.73
Arthroscopy 80.20
  ankle 80.27
  elbow 80.22
  finger 80.24
  foot 80.28
  hand 80.24
  hip 80.25
  knee 80.26
  shoulder 80.21
  specified site NEC 80.29
  toe 80.28
  wrist 80.23
Arthrostomy — see also Arthrotomy 80.10
Arthrotomy 80.10
  as operative approach — omit code
  with
    arthrography — see Arthrogram
    arthroscopy — see Arthroscopy
    injection of drug 81.92
    removal of prosthesis without replace-
      ment (see Removal, prosthesis,
      joint structures)
  ankle 80.17
  elbow 80.12
  foot and toe 80.18
  hand and finger 80.14
  hip 80.15
  knee 80.16
  shoulder 80.11
  specified site NEC 80.19
  spine 80.19
  wrist 80.13
Artificial
  heart 37.52
    AbioCor® 37.52
    CardioWest™ (TAH-t) 37.52
  insemination 69.92
  kidney 39.95
  rupture of membranes 73.09
Arytenoidectomy 30.29
Arytenoidopexy 31.69
Asai operation (larynx) 31.75
Aspiration
  abscess — see Aspiration, by site
  anterior chamber, eye (therapeutic) 12.91
    diagnostic 12.21
  aqueous (eye) (humor) (therapeutic) 12.91
    diagnostic 12.21
  ascites 54.91
  Bartholin's gland (cyst) (percutaneous) 71.21
  biopsy — see Biopsy, by site
  bladder (catheter) 57.0
    percutaneous (needle) 57.11
  bone marrow (for biopsy) 41.31
    from donor for transplant 41.91
    stem cell 99.79
  branchial cleft cyst 29.0
  breast 85.91
  bronchus 96.05
    with lavage 96.56
  bursa (percutaneous) 83.94
    hand 82.92
  calculus, bladder 57.0
  cataract 13.3
    with
      phacoemulsification 13.41
      phacofragmentation 13.43
      posterior route 13.42
  chest 34.91
  cisternal 01.01
  cranial (puncture) 01.09
  craniobuccal pouch 07.72
  craniopharyngioma 07.72
  cul-de-sac (abscess) 70.0
  curettage, uterus 69.59
    after abortion or delivery 69.52
    diagnostic 69.59
    to terminate pregnancy 69.51
  cyst — see Aspiration, by site

☑ **Additional Digit Required** — Refer to the Tabular List for Digit Selection   �触 **Subterms under main terms may continue to next column or page**

4 — Volume 3   ▶◀ Revised Text   ● New Line   ▲ Revised Code   2014 ICD-9-CM

☑ **Additional Digit Required** — Refer to the Tabular List for Digit Selection
▽ **Subterms under main terms may continue to next column or page**
2014 ICD-9-CM
▶◀ **Revised Text**
● **New Line**
▲ **Revised Code**
Volume 3 — 5

☑ Additional Digit Required — Refer to the Tabular List for Digit Selection   ⁧ Subterms under main terms may continue to next column or page

6 — Volume 3   ▶◀ Revised Text   ● New Line   ▲ Revised Code   2014 ICD-9-CM

Index

Biopsy — Blood

C

⚃ Additional Digit Required — Refer to the Tabular List for Digit Selection　　　　　　　　　　▽ Subterms under main terms may continue to next column or page

2014 ICD-9-CM　　　　▶◀ Revised Text　　　　● New Line　　　　▲ Revised Code　　　　**Volume 3 — 7**

Blood — Catheterization

☑ **Additional Digit Required** — Refer to the Tabular List for Digit Selection

▽ **Subterms under main terms may continue to next column or page**

8 — Volume 3

►◄ Revised Text

● New Line

▲ Revised Code

2014 ICD-9-CM

Closure — *see also* Repair — *continued*
  stoma
    bile duct 51.79
    bladder 57.82
    bronchus 33.42
    common duct 51.72
    esophagus 42.83
    gallbladder 51.92
    hepatic duct 51.79
    intestine 46.50
      large 46.52
      small 46.51
    kidney 55.82
    larynx 31.62
    rectum 48.72
    stomach 44.62
    thorax 34.72
    trachea 31.72
    ureter 56.83
    urethra 58.42
  thoracostomy 34.72
  tracheostomy 31.72
  ulcer (bleeding) (peptic) (perforated) 44.40
    duodenum 44.42
    gastric 44.41
    intestine (perforated) 46.79
    skin 86.59
    stomach 44.41
  ureterostomy 56.83
  urethrostomy 58.42
  vagina 70.8
  vascular
    percutaneous puncture — *omit code*
  vesicostomy 57.22
  wound (*see also* Suture, by site)
    with graft — *see* Graft
    with tissue adhesive 86.59
Coagulation, electrocoagulation — *see also*
  Destruction, lesion, by site
  aneurysm (cerebral) (peripheral vessel)
    39.52
  arteriovenous fistula 39.53
  brain tissue (incremental) (radio-frequency)
    01.59
  broad ligament 69.19
  cervix 67.32
  ear
    external 18.29
    inner 20.79
    middle 20.51
  fallopian tube 66.61
  gasserian ganglion 04.05
  nose for epistaxis (with packing) 21.03
  ovary 65.29
    laparoscopic 65.25
  pharynx (by diathermy) 29.39
  prostatic bed 60.94
  rectum (polyp) 48.32
    radical 48.31
  retina (for)
    destruction of lesion 14.21
    reattachment 14.51
    repair of tear 14.31
  round ligament 69.19
  semicircular canals 20.79
  spinal cord (lesion) 03.4
  urethrovesical junction, transurethral 57.49
  uterosacral ligament 69.19
  uterus 68.29
  vagina 70.33
  vulva 71.3
Coating, aneurysm of brain 39.52
Cobalt-60 therapy (treatment) 92.23
Coccygectomy (partial) 77.89
  total 77.99
Coccygotomy 77.39
"Cocked hat" procedure (metacarpal lengthening and transfer of local flap) 82.69
Cockett operation (varicose vein)
  lower limb 38.59
  upper limb 38.53
Cody tack (perforation of footplate) 19.0
Coffey operation (uterine suspension) (Meig's
  modification) 69.22

Colectomy (partial) (segmental) (subtotal)
  cecum (with terminal ileum)
    laparoscopic 17.32
    open and other 45.72
  laparoscopic 17.39
  left (Hartmann) (lower) (radical)
    laparoscopic 17.35
    open and other 45.75
  multiple segmental
    laparoscopic 17.31
    open and other 45.71
  open and other 45.79
  right (radical)
    laparoscopic 17.33
    open and other 45.73
  sigmoid
    laparoscopic 17.36
    open and other 45.76
  terminal ileum with cecum
    laparoscopic 17.32
    open and other 45.72
  total
    laparoscopic 45.81
    open 45.82
    other 45.83
    unspecified 45.83
  transverse
    laparoscopic 17.34
    open and other 45.74
Cole operation (anterior tarsal wedge osteotomy) 77.28
Collapse, lung, surgical 33.39
  by
    destruction of phrenic nerve 33.31
    pneumoperitoneum 33.33
    pneumothorax, artificially-induced 33.32
    thoracoplasty 33.34
Collection, sperm for artificial insemination
  99.96
Collis-Nissen operation (hiatal hernia repair
  with esophagogastroplasty) 53.80
Colocentesis 45.03
Colocolostomy 45.94
  proximal to distal segment 45.79
Colocystoplasty 57.87 [45.52]
Colofixation 46.64
Coloileotomy 45.00
Colonna operation
  adductor tenotomy (first stage) 83.12
  hip arthroplasty (second stage) 81.40
  reconstruction of hip (second stage) 81.40
Colonoscopy 45.23
  with
    biopsy 45.25
      rectum 48.24
    stent — *see* Insertion, stent, colon
  fiberoptic (flexible) 45.23
  intraoperative 45.21
  through stoma (artificial) 45.22
  transabdominal 45.21
Colopexy 46.63
Coloplication 46.64
Coloproctostomy 45.94
Colorectosigmoidostomy 45.94
Colorectostomy 45.94
Colorrhaphy 46.75
Coloscopy — *see* Colonoscopy
Colosigmoidostomy 45.94
Colostomy (ileo-ascending) (ileo-transverse)
  (perineal) (transverse) 46.10
  with anterior rectal resection 48.62
  delayed opening 46.14
  loop 46.03
  permanent (magnetic) 46.13
  temporary 46.11
Colotomy 45.03
Colpectomy 70.4
Colpoceliocentesis 70.0
Colpocentesis 70.0
Colpocleisis (complete) (partial) 70.8
Colpohysterectomy 68.59
  laparoscopically assisted (LAVH) 68.51
Colpoperineoplasty 70.79
  with repair of urethrocele 70.51
    with graft or prosthesis 70.53
Colpoperineorrhaphy 70.71

Colpoperineorrhaphy — *continued*
  following delivery 75.69
Colpopexy 70.77
  with graft or prosthesis 70.78
Colpoplasty 70.79
Colpopoiesis 70.61
  vaginal construction 70.61
    with graft or prosthesis 70.63
Colporrhaphy 70.71
  anterior (cystocele repair) 70.51
    with graft or prosthesis 70.54
  for repair of
    cystocele 70.51
      with rectocele 70.50
        with graft or prosthesis 70.53
      enterocele 70.92
        with graft or prosthesis 70.93
      rectocele 70.52
        with cystocele 70.50
          with graft or prosthesis 70.53
      urethrocele 70.51
        with graft or prosthesis 70.54
    posterior (rectocele repair) 70.52
      with graft or prosthesis 70.55
Colposcopy 70.21
Colpotomy 70.14
  for pelvic peritoneal drainage 70.12
Commando operation (radical glossectomy)
  25.4
Commissurotomy
  closed heart technique — *see* Valvulotomy,
    heart
  open heart technique — *see* Valvuloplasty,
    heart
Compression, trigeminal nerve 04.02
Conchectomy 21.69
Conchotomy 21.1
Conduction study, nerve 89.15
Conduitogram, ileum 87.78
Condylectomy — *see* category 77.8 ☑
  mandible 76.5
Condylotomy NEC — *see also* Division, joint
  capsule 80.40
  mandible (open) 76.62
    closed 76.61
Conization
  cervix (knife) (sharp) (biopsy) 67.2
    by
      cryosurgery 67.33
      electroconization 67.32
Conjunctivocystorhinostomy 09.82
  with insertion of tube or stent 09.83
Conjunctivodacryocystorhinostomy (CDCR)
  09.82
  with insertion of tube or stent 09.83
Conjunctivodacryocystostomy 09.82
  with insertion of tube or stent 09.83
Conjunctivoplasty 10.49
Conjunctivorhinostomy 09.82
  with insertion of tube or stent 09.83
Constriction of globe, for scleral buckling
  — *see also* Buckling, scleral 14.49
Construction
  auricle, ear (with graft) (with implant) 18.71
  ear
    auricle (with graft) (with implant) 18.71
    meatus (osseous) (skin-lined) 18.6
  endorectal ileal pouch (J-pouch) (H-pouch)
    (S-pouch) (with anastomosis to anus)
    45.95
  esophagus, artificial — *see* Anastomosis,
    esophagus
  ileal bladder (open) 56.51
    closed 57.87 [45.51]
  ileal conduit 56.51
  larynx, artificial 31.75
  patent meatus (ear) 18.6
  penis (rib graft) (skin graft) (myocutaneous
    flap) 64.43
  pharyngeal valve, artificial 31.75
  urethra 58.46
  vagina, artificial 70.61
    with graft or prosthesis 70.63
  venous valves (peripheral) 39.59
Consultation 89.09
  comprehensive 89.07

Consultation — *continued*
  limited (single organ system) 89.06
  specified type NEC 89.08
Continuous positive airway pressure [CPAP]
  (non-invasive) 93.90
  delivered by
    endotracheal tube — *see* category
      96.7 ☑
    tracheostomy — *see* category 96.7 ☑
Control
  atmospheric pressure and composition NEC
    93.98
    antigen-free air conditioning 93.98
    decompression chamber 93.97
    mountain sanatorium 93.98
  epistaxis 21.00
    by
      cauterization (and packing) 21.03
      coagulation (with packing) 21.03
      electrocoagulation (with packing)
        21.03
      excision of nasal mucosa with graft-
        ing 21.07
      ligation of artery 21.09
        ethmoidal 21.04
        external carotid 21.06
        maxillary (transantral) 21.05
    packing (nasal) (anterior) 21.01
      posterior (and anterior) 21.02
    specified means NEC 21.09
  hemorrhage 39.98
    abdominal cavity 54.19
    adenoids (postoperative) 28.7
    anus (postoperative) 49.95
    bladder (postoperative) 57.93
    chest 34.09
    colon 45.49
      endoscopic 45.43
    duodenum (ulcer) 44.49
      by
        embolization (transcatheter)
          44.44
        suture (ligation) 44.42
      endoscopic 44.43
    esophagus 42.39
      endoscopic 42.33
    gastric (ulcer) 44.49
      by
        embolization (transcatheter)
          44.44
        suture (ligation) 44.41
      endoscopic 44.43
    intrapleural 34.09
      postoperative (recurrent) 34.03
    laparotomy site 54.12
    nose (*see also* Control, epistaxis) 21.00
    peptic (ulcer) 44.49
      by
        embolization (transcatheter)
          44.44
        suture (ligation) 44.40
      endoscopic 44.43
    pleura, pleural cavity 34.09
      postoperative (recurrent) 34.03
    postoperative NEC 39.98
    postvascular surgery 39.41
    prostate 60.94
    specified site NEC 39.98
    stomach — *see* Control, hemorrhage,
      gastric
    thorax NEC 34.09
      postoperative (recurrent) 34.03
    thyroid (postoperative) 06.02
    tonsils (postoperative) 28.7
Conversion
  anastomosis — *see* Revision, anastomosis
  atrial rhythm (to sinus rhythm) 99.61
  cardiac rhythm NEC 99.69
    to sinus rhythm 99.62
  gastrostomy to jejunostomy (endoscopic)
    for feeding tube placement 46.32
  obstetrical position — *see* Version
Cooling, gastric 96.31
CorCap™ 37.41
Cordectomy, vocal 30.22
Cordopexy, vocal 31.69

☑ Additional Digit Required — Refer to the Tabular List for Digit Selection   Subterms under main terms may continue to next column or page

10 — Volume 3   ►◄ Revised Text   ● New Line   ▲ Revised Code   2014 ICD-9-CM

Cordotomy
spinal (bilateral) NEC 03.29
percutaneous 03.21
vocal 31.3
Corectomy 12.12
Corelysis 12.35
Coreoplasty 12.35
Corneoconjunctivoplasty 11.53
Corpectomy, (vertebral) 80.99
with diskectomy 80.99
Correction — *see also* Repair
atresia
esophageal 42.85
by magnetic forces 42.99
external meatus (ear) 18.6
nasopharynx, nasopharyngeal 29.4
rectum 48.0
tricuspid 35.94
atrial septal defect (*see also* Repair, atrial
septal defect) 35.71
combined with repair of valvular and
ventricular septal defects — *see*
Repair, endocardial cushion defect
blepharoptosis (*see also* Repair, blepharoptosis) 08.36
bunionette (with osteotomy) 77.54
chordee 64.42
claw toe 77.57
cleft
lip 27.54
palate 27.62
clubfoot NEC 83.84
coarctation of aorta
with
anastomosis 38.34
graft replacement 38.44
cornea NEC 11.59
refractive NEC 11.79
epikeratophakia 11.76
keratomileusis 11.71
keratophakia 11.72
radial keratotomy 11.75
esophageal atresia 42.85
by magnetic forces 42.99
everted lacrimal punctum 09.71
eyelid
ptosis (*see also* Repair, blepharoptosis)
08.36
retraction 08.38
fetal defect 75.36
forcible, of musculoskeletal deformity NEC
93.29
hammer toe 77.56
hydraulic pressure, open surgery for penile
inflatable prosthesis 64.99
urinary artificial sphincter 58.99
intestinal malrotation 46.80
large 46.82
small 46.81
inverted uterus — *see* Repair, inverted
uterus
lymphedema (of limb) 40.9
excision with graft 40.9
obliteration of lymphatics 40.9
transplantation of autogenous lymphatics 40.9
nasopharyngeal atresia 29.4
overlapping toes 77.58
palate (cleft) 27.62
prognathism NEC 76.64
prominent ear 18.5
punctum (everted) 09.71
spinal pseudarthrosis — *see* Refusion, spinal
syndactyly 86.85
tetralogy of Fallot
one-stage 35.81
partial — *see* specific procedure
total 35.81
total anomalous pulmonary venous connection
one-stage 35.82
partial — *see* specific procedure
total 35.82
transposition, great arteries, total 35.84
tricuspid atresia 35.94

Correction — *see also* Repair — *continued*
truncus arteriosus
one-stage 35.83
partial — *see* specific procedure
total 35.83
ureteropelvic junction 55.87
ventricular septal defect (*see also* Repair,
ventricular septal defect) 35.72
combined with repair of valvular and
atrial septal defects — *see* Repair,
endocardial cushion defect
Costectomy 77.91
with lung excision — *see* Excision, lung
associated with thoracic operation — *omit
code*
Costochondrectomy 77.91
associated with thoracic operation — *omit
code*
Costosternoplasty (pectus excavatum repair)
34.74
Costotomy 77.31
Costotransectomy 77.91
associated with thoracic operation — *omit
code*
Counseling (for) NEC 94.49
alcoholism 94.46
drug addiction 94.45
employers 94.49
family (medical) (social) 94.49
marriage 94.49
ophthalmologic (with instruction) 95.36
pastoral 94.49
Countershock, cardiac NEC 99.62
Coventry operation (tibial wedge osteotomy)
77.27
CPAP (continuous positive airway pressure)
93.90
delivered by
endotracheal tube — *see* category
96.7 ☑
tracheostomy — *see* category 96.7 ☑
Craniectomy 01.25
linear (opening of cranial suture) 02.01
reopening of site 01.23
strip (opening of cranial suture) 02.01
Cranioclasis, fetal 73.8
Cranioplasty 02.06
with synchronous repair of encephalocele
02.12
Craniotomy 01.24
as operative approach — *omit code*
fetal 73.8
for decompression of fracture 02.02
reopening of site 01.23
Craterization, bone — *see also* Excision, lesion,
bone 77.60
Crawford operation (tarso-frontalis sling of
eyelid) 08.32
Creation — *see also* Formation
cardiac device (defibrillator) (pacemaker)
pocket
with initial insertion of cardiac device —
omit code
new site (skin) (subcutaneous) 37.79
conduit
apical-aortic (AAC) 35.93
ileal (urinary) 56.51
left ventricle and aorta 35.93
right atrium and pulmonary artery 35.94
right ventricle and pulmonary (distal)
artery 35.92
in repair of
pulmonary artery atresia 35.92
transposition of great vessels
35.92
truncus arteriosus 35.83
endorectal ileal pouch (J-pouch) (H-pouch)
(S-pouch) (with anastomosis to anus)
45.95
esophagogastric sphincteric competence
NEC 44.66
laparoscopic 44.67
Hartmann pouch — *see* Colectomy, by site
interatrial fistula 35.42
pericardial window 37.12
pleural window, for drainage 34.09

Creation — *see also* Formation —
continued
pocket
cardiac device (defibrillator) (pacemaker)
with initial insertion of cardiac device
— *omit code*
new site (skin) (subcutaneous) 37.79
loop recorder 37.79
thalamic stimulator pulse generator
with initial insertion of battery package — *omit code*
new site (skin) (subcutaneous) 86.09
shunt (*see also* Shunt)
arteriovenous fistula, for dialysis 39.93
left-to-right (systemic to pulmonary circulation) 39.0
subcutaneous tunnel for esophageal anastomosis 42.86
with anastomosis — *see* Anastomosis,
esophagus, antesternal
syndactyly (finger) (toe) 86.89
thalamic stimulator pulse generator pocket
with initial insrtion of battery package
— *omit code*
new site (skin) (subcutaneous) 86.09
tracheoesophageal fistula 31.95
window
pericardial 37.12
pleura, for drainage 34.09
Credé maneuver 73.59
Cricoidectomy 30.29
Cricothyreotomy (for assistance in breathing)
31.1
Cricothyroidectomy 30.29
Cricothyrostomy 31.1
Cricothyrotomy (for assistance in breathing)
31.1
Cricotomy (for assistance in breathing) 31.1
Cricotracheotomy (for assistance in breathing)
31.1
Crisis intervention 94.35
Croupette, croup tent 93.94
Crown, dental (ceramic) (gold) 23.41
Crushing
bone — *see* category 78.4 ☑
calculus
bile (hepatic) passage 51.49
endoscopic 51.88
bladder (urinary) 57.0
pancreatic duct 52.09
endoscopic 52.94
fallopian tube — *see* Ligation, fallopian
tube) 66.39
ganglion — *see* Crushing, nerve
hemorrhoids 49.45
nasal septum 21.88
nerve (cranial) (peripheral) NEC 04.03
acoustic 04.01
auditory 04.01
phrenic 04.03
for collapse of lung 33.31
sympathetic 05.0
trigeminal 04.02
vestibular 04.01
vas deferens 63.71
Cryoablation — *see* Ablation
Cryoanalgesia
nerve (cranial) (peripheral) 04.2
Cryoconization, cervix 67.33
Cryodestruction — *see* Destruction, lesion, by
site
Cryoextraction, lens — *see also* Extraction,
cataract, intracapsular 13.19
Cryohypophysectomy (complete) (total) —
see also Hypophysectomy 07.69
Cryoleucotomy 01.32
Cryopexy, retinal — *see* Cryotherapy, retina
Cryoprostatectomy 60.62
Cryoretinopexy (for)
reattachment 14.52
repair of tear or defect 14.32
Cryosurgery — *see* Cryotherapy
Cryothalamectomy 01.41
Cryotherapy — *see also* Destruction, lesion,
by site
bladder 57.59

Cryotherapy — *see also* Destruction, lesion, by
site — *continued*
brain 01.59
cataract 13.19
cervix 67.33
choroid — *see* Cryotherapy, retina
ciliary body 12.72
corneal lesion (ulcer) 11.43
to reshape cornea 11.79
ear
external 18.29
inner 20.79
esophagus 42.39
endoscopic 42.33
eyelid 08.25
hemorrhoids 49.44
iris 12.41
nasal turbinates 21.61
palate (bony) 27.31
prostate 60.62
retina (for)
destruction of lesion 14.22
reattachment 14.52
repair of tear 14.32
skin 86.3
stomach 43.49
endoscopic 43.41
subcutaneous tissue 86.3
turbinates (nasal) 21.61
warts 86.3
genital 71.3
Cryptectomy (anus) 49.39
endoscopic 49.31
Cryptorchidectomy (unilateral) 62.3
bilateral 62.41
Cryptotomy (anus) 49.39
endoscopic 49.31
Cuirass 93.99
Culdocentesis 70.0
Culdoplasty 70.92
with graft or prosthesis 70.93
Culdoscopy (exploration) (removal of foreign
body or lesion) 70.22
Culdotomy 70.12
Culp-Deweerd operation (spiral flap pyeloplasty) 55.87
Culp-Scardino operation (ureteral flap
pyeloplasty) 55.87
Culture (and sensitivity) — *see* Examination,
microscopic
Curettage (with packing) (with secondary closure) — *see also* Dilation and curettage
adenoids 28.6
anus 49.39
endoscopic 49.31
bladder 57.59
transurethral 57.49
bone (*see also* Excision, lesion, bone) 77.60
brain 01.59
bursa 83.39
hand 82.29
cartilage (*see also* Excision, lesion, joint)
80.80
cerebral meninges 01.51
chalazion 08.25
conjunctiva (trachoma follicles) 10.33
corneal epithelium 11.41
for smear or culture 11.21
ear, external 18.29
eyelid 08.25
joint (*see also* Excision, lesion, joint) 80.80
meninges (cerebral) 01.51
spinal 03.4
muscle 83.32
hand 82.22
nerve (peripheral) 04.07
sympathetic 05.29
sclera 12.84
skin 86.3
spinal cord (meninges) 03.4
subgingival 24.31
tendon 83.39
sheath 83.31
hand 82.21
uterus (with dilation) 69.09
aspiration (diagnostic) NEC 69.59

☑ **Additional Digit Required** — Refer to the Tabular List for Digit Selection   ▽ **Subterms under main terms may continue to next column or page**

2014 ICD-9-CM   ▶◀ **Revised Text**   ● **New Line**   ▲ **Revised Code**   Volume 3 — 11

Curettage — see also Dilation and curettage — continued
  uterus — continued
    aspiration — continued
      after abortion or delivery 69.52
      to terminate pregnancy 69.51
      following delivery or abortion 69.02
Curette evacuation, lens 13.2
Curtis operation (interphalangeal joint arthroplasty) 81.72
Cutaneolipectomy 86.83
Cutdown, venous 38.94
Cutting
  nerve (cranial) (peripheral) NEC 04.03
    acoustic 04.01
    auditory 04.01
    root, spinal 03.1
    sympathetic 05.0
    trigeminal 04.02
    vestibular 04.01
  pedicle (flap) graft 86.71
  pylorus (with wedge resection) 43.3
  spinal nerve root 03.1
  ureterovesical orifice 56.1
  urethral sphincter 58.5
CVP (central venous pressure monitoring) 89.62
Cyclectomy (ciliary body) 12.44
  eyelid margin 08.20
Cyclicotomy 12.55
Cycloanemization 12.74
Cyclocryotherapy 12.72
Cyclodialysis (initial) (subsequent) 12.55
Cyclodiathermy (penetrating) (surface) 12.71
Cycloelectrolysis 12.71
Cyclophotocoagulation 12.73
Cyclotomy 12.55
Cystectomy — see also Excision, lesion, by site
  gallbladder — see Cholecystectomy
  urinary (partial) (subtotal) 57.6
    complete (with urethrectomy) 57.79
    radical 57.71
      with pelvic exenteration (female) 68.8
    total (with urethrectomy) 57.79
Cystocolostomy 57.88
Cystogram, cystography NEC 87.77
Cystolitholapaxy 57.0
Cystolithotomy 57.19
Cystometrogram 89.22
Cystopexy NEC 57.89
Cystoplasty NEC 57.89
Cystoproctostomy 57.88
Cystoprostatectomy, radical 57.71
Cystopyelography 87.74
Cystorrhaphy 57.81
Cystoscopy (transurethral) 57.32
  for
    control of hemorrhage
      bladder 57.93
      prostate 60.94
    retrograde pyelography 87.74
  with biopsy 57.33
  ileal conduit 56.35
  through stoma (artificial) 57.31
Cystostomy
  closed (suprapubic) (percutaneous) 57.17
  open (suprapubic) 57.18
  percutaneous (closed) (suprapubic) 57.17
  suprapubic
    closed 57.17
    open 57.18
Cystotomy (open) (for removal of calculi) 57.19
Cystourethrogram (retrograde) (voiding) 87.76
Cystourethropexy (by) 59.79
  levator muscle sling 59.71
  retropubic suspension 59.5
  suprapubic suspension 59.4
Cystourethroplasty 57.85
Cystourethroscopy 57.32
  with biopsy
    bladder 57.33
    ureter 56.33
Cytology — see Examination, microscopic

D

Dacryoadenectomy 09.20
  partial 09.22
  total 09.23
Dacryoadenotomy 09.0
Dacryocystectomy (complete) (partial) 09.6
Dacryocystogram 87.05
Dacryocystorhinostomy (DCR) (by intubation) (external) (intranasal) 09.81
Dacryocystostomy 09.53
Dacryocystosyringotomy 09.53
Dacryocystotomy 09.53
Dahlman operation (excision of esophageal diverticulum) 42.31
Dana operation (posterior rhizotomy) 03.1
Danforth operation (fetal) 73.8
Darrach operation (ulnar resection) 77.83
da Vinci® (S HD) Surgical System — see category 17.4 ☑
Davis operation (intubated ureterotomy) 56.2
Deaf training 95.49
Debridement, NOS 86.28
  excisional, NOS 86.22
    abdominal wall 54.3
    bone (see also Excision, lesion, bone) 77.60
      fracture — see Debridement, open fracture
    brain 01.59
    burn (skin) 86.22
    bursa 83.5
    cerebral meninges 01.51
    fascia 83.44
    flap graft 86.75
    graft (flap) (pedicle) 86.75
    heart valve (calcified) — see Valvuloplasty, heart
    infection (skin) 86.22
      nail bed or fold 86.27
    joint — see Excision, lesion, joint
    meninges (cerebral) 01.51
      spinal 03.4
    muscle 83.45
      hand 82.36
    nail 86.27
    nerve (peripheral) 04.07
    open fracture (compound) 79.60
      arm NEC 79.62
      carpal, metacarpal 79.63
      facial bone 76.2
      femur 79.65
      fibula 79.66
      foot NEC 79.67
      hand NEC 79.63
      humerus 79.61
      leg NEC 79.66
      phalanges
        foot 79.68
        hand 79.64
      radius 79.62
      specified site NEC 79.69
      tarsal, metatarsal 79.67
      tibia 79.66
      ulna 79.62
    patella 77.66
    pedicle graft 86.75
    skin or subcutaneous tissue (burn) (infection) (wound) 86.22
      cardioverter/defibrillator (automatic) pocket 37.79
      graft 86.75
      nail, nail bed, nail fold 86.27
      pacemaker pocket 37.79
      pocket
        cardiac device NEC 37.79
        cardiac pacemaker 37.79
        cardioverter/defibrillator (automatic) 37.79
    skull 01.25
      compound fracture 02.02
    spinal cord (meninges) 03.4
    tendon 83.39
    wound (skin) 86.22
  nonexcisional, NOS 86.28
    burn (skin) 86.28
    dental 96.54

Debridement, — continued
  nonexcisional, — continued
    infection (skin) 86.28
    skin or subcutaneous tissue (burn) (infection) (wound) 86.28
    ultrasonic, ultrasound 86.28
    VersaJet™ 86.28
    wound (skin) 86.28
Decapitation, fetal 73.8
Decapsulation, kidney 55.91
Declotting — see also Removal, thrombus
  arteriovenous cannula or shunt 39.49
Decompression
  anus (imperforate) 48.0
  biliary tract 51.49
    by intubation 51.43
      endoscopic 51.87
      percutaneous 51.98
  brain 01.24
  carpal tunnel 04.43
  cauda equina 03.09
  chamber 93.97
  colon 96.08
    by incision 45.03
    endoscopic (balloon) 46.85
  common bile duct 51.42
    by intubation 51.43
      endoscopic 51.87
      percutaneous 51.98
  cranial 01.24
    for skull fracture 02.02
  endolymphatic sac 20.79
  ganglion (peripheral) NEC 04.49
    cranial NEC 04.42
  gastric 96.07
  heart 37.0
  intestine 96.08
    by incision 45.00
    endoscopic (balloon) 46.85
  intracranial 01.24
  labyrinth 20.79
  laminectomy 03.09
  laminotomy 03.09
  median nerve 04.43
  muscle 83.02
    hand 82.02
  nerve (peripheral) NEC 04.49
    auditory 04.42
    cranial NEC 04.42
    median 04.43
    trigeminal (root) 04.41
  orbit (see also Orbitotomy) 16.09
  pancreatic duct 52.92
    endoscopic 52.93
  pericardium 37.0
  rectum 48.0
  skull fracture 02.02
  spinal cord (canal) 03.09
  tarsal tunnel 04.44
  tendon (sheath) 83.01
    hand 82.01
  thoracic outlet
    by
      myotomy (division of scalenus anticus muscle) 83.19
      tenotomy 83.13
  trigeminal (nerve root) 04.41
Decortication
  arterial 05.25
  brain 01.51
  cerebral meninges 01.51
  heart 37.31
  kidney 55.91
  lung (partial) (total) 34.51
    thoracoscopic 34.52
  nasal turbinates — see Turbinectomy
  nose 21.89
  ovary 65.29
    laparoscopic 65.25
  periarterial 05.25
  pericardium 37.31
  ventricle, heart (complete) 37.31
Decoy, E2F 00.16
Deepening
  alveolar ridge 24.5
  buccolabial sulcus 24.91

Deepening — continued
  lingual sulcus 24.91
Defatting, flap or pedicle graft 86.75
Defibrillation, electric (external) (internal) 99.62
  automatic cardioverter/defibrillator — see category 37.9 ☑
de Grandmont operation (tarsectomy) 08.35
Delaying of pedicle graft 86.71
Delivery (with)
  assisted spontaneous 73.59
  breech extraction (assisted) 72.52
    partial 72.52
      with forceps to aftercoming head 72.51
    total 72.54
      with forceps to aftercoming head 72.53
    unassisted (spontaneous delivery) — omit code
  cesarean section — see Cesarean section
  Credé maneuver 73.59
  De Lee maneuver 72.4
  forceps 72.9
    application to aftercoming head (Piper) 72.6
    with breech extraction
      partial 72.51
      total 72.53
    Barton's 72.4
    failed 73.3
    high 72.39
      with episiotomy 72.31
    low (outlet) 72.0
      with episiotomy 72.1
    mid 72.29
      with episiotomy 72.21
    outlet (low) 72.0
      with episiotomy 72.1
    rotation of fetal head 72.4
    trial 73.3
  instrumental NEC 72.9
    specified NEC 72.8
  key-in-lock rotation 72.4
  Kielland rotation 72.4
  Malström's extraction 72.79
    with episiotomy 72.71
  manually assisted (spontaneous) 73.59
  spontaneous (unassisted) 73.59
    assisted 73.59
  vacuum extraction 72.79
    with episiotomy 72.71
Delorme operation
  pericardiectomy 37.31
  proctopexy 48.76
  repair of prolapsed rectum 48.76
  thoracoplasty 33.34
Denervation
  aortic body 39.89
  carotid body 39.89
  facet, percutaneous (radiofrequency) 03.96
  ovarian 65.94
  paracervical uterine 69.3
  uterosacral 69.3
Denker operation (radical maxillary antrotomy) 22.31
Dennis-Barco operation — see Repair, hernia, femoral
Denonvillier operation (limited rhinoplasty) 21.86
Densitometry, bone (serial) (radiographic) 88.98
Depilation, skin 86.92
Derlacki operation (tympanoplasty) 19.4
Dermabond 86.59
Dermabrasion (laser) 86.25
  for wound debridement 86.28
Derotation — see Reduction, torsion
Desensitization
  allergy 99.12
  psychologic 94.33
Desmotomy — see also Division, ligament 80.40
Destruction
  breast 85.20

☑ **Additional Digit Required** — Refer to the Tabular List for Digit Selection   ▽ **Subterms under main terms may continue to next column or page**

12 — Volume 3   ▶◀ **Revised Text**   ● **New Line**   ▲ **Revised Code**   2014 ICD-9-CM

Destruction — *continued*
chorioretinopathy (*see also* Destruction, lesion, choroid) 14.29
ciliary body 12.74
epithelial downgrowth, anterior chamber 12.93
fallopian tube 66.39
with
crushing (and ligation) 66.31
by endoscopy (laparoscopy) 66.21
division (and ligation) 66.32
by endoscopy (culdoscopy) (hysteroscopy) (laparoscopy) (peritoneoscopy) 66.22
ligation 66.39
with
crushing 66.31
by endoscopy (laparoscopy) 66.21
division 66.32
by endoscopy (culdoscopy) (hysteroscopy) (laparoscopy) (peritoneoscopy) 66.22
fetus 73.8
hemorrhoids 49.49
by
cryotherapy 49.44
sclerotherapy 49.42
inner ear NEC 20.79
by injection 20.72
intervertebral disc (NOS) 80.50
by injection 80.52
by other specified method 80.59
herniated (nucleus pulposus) 80.51
LAA 37.36
lacrimal sac 09.6
left atrial appendage 37.36
lesion (local)
anus 49.39
endoscopic 49.31
Bartholin's gland 71.24
by
aspiration 71.21
excision 71.24
incision 71.22
marsupialization 71.23
biliary ducts 51.69
endoscopic 51.64
bladder 57.59
transurethral 57.49
bone — *see* Excision, lesion, bone
bowel — *see* Destruction, lesion, intestine
brain (transtemporal approach) NEC 01.59
by stereotactic radiosurgery 92.30
cobalt 60 92.32
linear accelerator (LINAC) 92.31
multi-source 92.32
particle beam 92.33
particulate 92.33
radiosurgery NEC 92.39
single source photon 92.31
breast NEC 85.20
bronchus NEC 32.09
endoscopic 32.01
cerebral NEC 01.59
meninges 01.51
cervix 67.39
by
cauterization 67.32
cryosurgery, cryoconization 67.33
electroconization 67.32
choroid 14.29
by
cryotherapy 14.22
diathermy 14.21
implantation of radiation source 14.27
photocoagulation 14.25
laser 14.24
xenon arc 14.23
radiation therapy 14.26

Destruction — *continued*
lesion — *continued*
ciliary body (nonexcisional) 12.43
by excision 12.44
conjunctiva 10.32
by excision 10.31
cornea NEC 11.49
by
cryotherapy 11.43
electrocauterization 11.42
thermocauterization 11.42
cul-de-sac 70.32
duodenum NEC 45.32
by excision 45.31
endoscopic 45.30
endoscopic 45.30
esophagus (chemosurgery) (cryosurgery) (electroresection) (fulguration) NEC 42.39
by excision 42.32
endoscopic 42.33
endoscopic 42.33
eyebrow 08.25
eyelid 08.25
excisional — *see* Excision, lesion, eyelid
eye NEC 16.93
heart
by catheter ablation 37.34
by endovascular approach 37.34
by open approach 37.33
by thoracoscopic approach 37.37
left atrial appendage 37.36
intestine (large) 45.49
by excision 45.41
endoscopic 45.43
polypectomy 45.42
endoscopic 45.43
polypectomy 45.42
small 45.34
by excision 45.33
intranasal 21.31
iris (nonexcisional) NEC 12.41
by excision 12.42
kidney 55.39
by marsupialization 55.31
lacrimal sac 09.6
larynx 30.09
liver 50.29
lung 32.29
endoscopic 32.28
meninges (cerebral) 01.51
spinal 03.4
nerve (peripheral) 04.07
sympathetic 05.29
nose 21.30
intranasal 21.31
specified NEC 21.32
ovary
by
aspiration 65.91
excision 65.29
laparoscopic 65.25
cyst by rupture (manual) 65.93
palate (bony) (local) 27.31
wide 27.32
pancreas 52.22
by marsupialization 52.3
endoscopic 52.21
pancreatic duct 52.22
endoscopic 52.21
penis 64.2
pharynx (excisional) NEC 29.39
pituitary gland
by stereotactic radiosurgery 92.30
cobalt 60 92.32
linear accelerator (LINAC) 92.31
multi-source 92.32
particle beam 92.33
particulate 92.33
radiosurgery NEC 92.39
single source photon 92.31
rectum (local) 48.32
by
cryosurgery 48.34
electrocoagulation 48.32

Destruction — *continued*
lesion — *continued*
rectum — *continued*
by — *continued*
excision 48.35
fulguration 48.32
laser (Argon) 48.33
polyp 48.36
radical 48.31
retina 14.29
by
cryotherapy 14.22
diathermy 14.21
implantation of radiation source 14.27
photocoagulation 14.25
laser 14.24
xenon arc 14.23
radiation therapy 14.26
salivary gland NEC 26.29
by marsupialization 26.21
sclera 12.84
scrotum 61.3
skin NEC 86.3
sphincter of Oddi 51.69
endoscopic 51.64
spinal cord (meninges) 03.4
spleen 41.42
by marsupialization 41.41
stomach NEC 43.49
by excision 43.42
endoscopic 43.41
endoscopic 43.41
subcutaneous tissue NEC 86.3
testis 62.2
tongue 25.1
urethra (excisional) 58.39
endoscopic 58.31
uterus 68.29
nerve (cranial) (peripheral) (by cryoanalgesia) by radiofrequency 04.2
sympathetic, by injection of neurolytic agent 05.32
neuroma
acoustic 04.01
by craniotomy 04.01
by stereotactic radiosurgery 92.30
cobalt 60 92.32
linear accelerator (LINAC) 92.31
multi-source 92.32
particle beam 92.33
particulate 92.33
radiosurgery NEC 92.39
single source photon 92.31
cranial 04.07
Morton's 04.07
peripheral
Morton's 04.07
prostate (prostatic tissue)
by
cryotherapy 60.62
microwave 60.96
radiofrequency 60.97
transurethral microwave thermotherapy (TUMT) 60.96
transurethral needle ablation (TUNA) 60.97
TULIP (transurethral (ultrasound) guided laser induced prostatectomy) 60.21
TUMT (transurethral microwave thermotherapy) 60.96
TUNA (transurethral needle ablation) 60.97
semicircular canals, by injection 20.72
tissue of heart — *see* Excision, lesion, heart
vestibule, by injection 20.72
Detachment, uterosacral ligaments 69.3
Determination
mental status (clinical) (medicolegal) (psychiatric) NEC 94.11
psychologic NEC 94.09
vital capacity (pulmonary) 89.37
Detorsion
intestine (twisted) (volvulus) 46.80
large 46.82

Detorsion — *continued*
intestine — *continued*
large — *continued*
endoscopic (balloon) 46.85
small 46.81
kidney 55.84
ovary 65.95
spermatic cord 63.52
with orchiopexy 62.5
testis 63.52
with orchiopexy 62.5
volvulus 46.80
endoscopic (balloon) 46.85
Detoxification therapy 94.25
alcohol 94.62
with rehabilitation 94.63
combined alcohol and drug 94.68
with rehabilitation 94.69
drug 94.65
with rehabilitation 94.66
combined alcohol and drug 94.68
with rehabilitation 94.69
Devascularization, stomach 44.99
Device
CorCap™ 37.41
external fixator — *see* Fixator, external
Dewebbing
esophagus 42.01
syndactyly (fingers) (toes) 86.85
Dextrorotation — *see* Reduction, torsion
Dialysis
hemodiafiltration, hemofiltration (extracorporeal) 39.95
kidney (extracorporeal) 39.95
liver 50.92
peritoneal 54.98
renal (extracorporeal) 39.95
Diaphanoscopy
nasal sinuses 89.35
skull (newborn) 89.16
Diaphysectomy — *see* category 77.8 ☑
Diathermy 93.34
choroid — *see* Diathermy, retina
nasal turbinates 21.61
retina
for
destruction of lesion 14.21
reattachment 14.51
repair of tear 14.31
surgical — *see* Destruction, lesion, by site
turbinates (nasal) 21.61
Dickson-Diveley operation (tendon transfer and arthrodesis to correct claw toe) 77.57
Dickson operation (fascial transplant) 83.82
Dieffenbach operation (hip disarticulation) 84.18
Dilation
achalasia 42.92
ampulla of Vater 51.81
endoscopic 51.84
anus, anal (sphincter) 96.23
biliary duct
endoscopic 51.84
pancreatic duct 52.99
endoscopic 52.98
percutaneous (endoscopy) 51.98
sphincter
of Oddi 51.81
endoscopic 51.84
pancreatic 51.82
endoscopic 51.85
bladder 96.25
neck 57.92
bronchus 33.91
cervix (canal) 67.0
obstetrical 73.1
to assist delivery 73.1
choanae (nasopharynx) 29.91
colon (endoscopic) (balloon) 46.85
with insertion of colonic stent
endoscopic 46.86
other 46.87
colostomy stoma 96.24
duodenum (endoscopic) (balloon) 46.85

Destruction — Dilation

☑ **Additional Digit Required — Refer to the Tabular List for Digit Selection**   ▽ **Subterms under main terms may continue to next column or page**

2014 ICD-9-CM   ▶◀ **Revised Text**   ● **New Line**   ▲ **Revised Code**   **Volume 3 — 13**

☑ **Additional Digit Required** — Refer to the Tabular List for Digit Selection   ▽ **Subterms under main terms may continue to next column or page**

14 — Volume 3   ▶◀ Revised Text   ● New Line   ▲ Revised Code   **2014 ICD-9-CM**

Dilation — Division

Division — *continued*
  vein — *continued*
    head and neck NEC 38.82
    intracranial NEC 38.81
    lower limb 38.89
      varicose 38.59
    thoracic NEC 38.85
    upper limb 38.83
    varicose 38.50
      abdominal 38.57
      head and neck NEC 38.52
      intracranial NEC 38.51
      lower limb 38.59
      thoracic NEC 38.55
      upper limb 38.53
    vitreous, cicatricial bands (posterior approach) 14.74
      anterior approach 14.73
Doleris operation (shortening of round ligaments) 69.22
D'Ombrain operation (excision of pterygium with corneal graft) 11.32
Domestic tasks therapy 93.83
Dopplergram, Doppler flow mapping — *see also* Ultrasonography
  aortic arch 88.73
  head and neck 88.71
  heart 88.72
  intraoperative transcranial 00.94
  thorax NEC 88.73
Dorrance operation (push-back operation for cleft palate) 27.62
Dotter operation (transluminal angioplasty) 39.59
Douche, vaginal 96.44
Douglas' operation (suture of tongue to lip for micrognathia) 25.59
Downstream® System (AO therapy) (aqueous oxygen) 00.49
Doyle operation (paracervical uterine denervation) 69.3
Drainage
  by
    anastomosis — *see* Anastomosis
    aspiration — *see* Aspiration
    incision — *see* Incision
  abdomen 54.19
    percutaneous 54.91
  abscess (*see also* Drainage, by site *and* Incision, by site)
    appendix 47.2
      with appendectomy 47.09
        laparoscopic 47.01
    parapharyngeal (oral) (transcervical) 28.0
    peritonsillar (oral) (transcervical) 28.0
    retropharyngeal (oral) (transcervical) 28.0
    thyroid (field) (gland) 06.09
      percutaneous (needle) 06.01
      postoperative 06.02
    tonsil, tonsillar (oral) (transcervical) 28.0
  antecubital fossa 86.04
  appendix 47.91
    with appendectomy 47.09
      laparoscopic 47.01
    abscess 47.2
      with appendectomy 47.09
        laparoscopic 47.01
  axilla 86.04
  bladder (without incision) 57.0
    by indwelling catheter 57.94
      percutaneous suprapubic (closed) 57.17
      suprapubic NEC 57.18
  buccal space 27.0
  bursa 83.03
    by aspiration 83.94
      hand 82.92
    hand 82.03
      by aspiration 82.92
    radial 82.03
    ulnar 82.03
  cerebrum, cerebral (meninges) (ventricle) (incision) (trephination) 01.39
    by
      anastomosis — *see* Shunt, ventricular

Drainage — *continued*
  cerebrum, cerebral — *continued*
    by — *continued*
      aspiration 01.09
        through previously implanted catheter 01.02
  chest (closed) 34.04
    open (by incision) 34.09
    thoracoscopic 34.06
  cranial sinus (incision) (trephination) 01.21
    by aspiration 01.09
  cul-de-sac 70.12
    by aspiration 70.0
  cyst (*see also* Drainage, by site and Incision, by site)
    pancreas (by catheter) 52.01
      by marsupialization 52.3
      internal (anastomosis) 52.4
    pilonidal 86.03
    spleen, splenic (by marsupialization) 41.41
  duodenum (tube) 46.39
    by incision 45.01
  ear
    external 18.09
    inner 20.79
    middle (by myringotomy) 20.09
      with intubation 20.01
  epidural space, cerebral (incision) (trephination) 01.24
    by aspiration 01.09
  extradural space, cerebral (incision) (trephination) 01.24
    by aspiration 01.09
  extraperitoneal 54.0
  facial region 27.0
  fascial compartments, head and neck 27.0
  fetal hydrocephalic head (needling) (trocar) 73.8
  fluid (blood) (cerebrospinal) (CSF)
    by
      external ventricular drain (EVD) placement 02.21
  gallbladder 51.04
    by
      anastomosis 51.35
      aspiration 51.01
      incision 51.04
  groin region (abdominal wall) (inguinal) 54.0
    skin 86.04
    subcutaneous tissue 86.04
  hematoma — *see* Drainage, by site and Incision, by site
  hydrocephalic head (needling) (trocar) 73.8
  hypochondrium 54.0
    intra-abdominal 54.19
  iliac fossa 54.0
  infratemporal fossa 27.0
  intracranial space (epidural) (extradural) (incision) (trephination) 01.24
    by aspiration 01.09
    subarachnoid or subdural (incision) (trephination) 01.31
      by aspiration 01.09
  intraperitoneal 54.19
    percutaneous 54.91
  kidney (by incision) 55.01
    by
      anastomosis 55.86
      catheter 59.8
    pelvis (by incision) 55.11
  liver 50.0
    by aspiration 50.91
  Ludwig's angina 27.0
  lung (by incision) 33.1
    by punch (needle) (trocar) 33.93
  midpalmar space 82.04
  mouth floor 27.0
  mucocele, nasal sinus 22.00
    by puncture 22.01
    through natural ostium 22.02
  omentum 54.19
    percutaneous 54.91
  ovary (aspiration) 65.91
    by incision 65.09

Drainage — *continued*
  ovary — *continued*
    laparoscopic 65.01
  palmar space (middle) 82.04
  pancreas (by catheter) 52.01
    by anastomosis 52.96
  parapharyngeal 28.0
  paronychia 86.04
  parotid space 27.0
  pelvic peritoneum (female) 70.12
    male 54.19
  pericardium 37.0
  perigastric 54.19
    percutaneous 54.91
  perineum
    female 71.09
    male 86.04
  perisplenic tissue 54.19
    percutaneous 54.91
  peritoneum 54.19
    pelvic (female) 70.12
    percutaneous 54.91
  peritonsillar 28.0
  pharyngeal space, lateral 27.0
  pilonidal cyst or sinus 86.03
  pleura (closed) 34.04
    open (by incision) 34.09
    thoracoscopic 34.06
  popliteal space 86.04
  postural 93.99
  postzygomatic space 27.0
  pseudocyst, pancreas 52.3
    by anastomosis 52.4
  pterygopalatine fossa 27.0
  retropharyngeal 28.0
  scrotum 61.0
  skin 86.04
  spinal (canal) (cord) 03.09
    by anastomosis — *see* Shunt, spinal
    diagnostic 03.31
  spleen 41.2
    cyst (by marsupialization) 41.41
  subarachnoid space, cerebral (incision) (trephination) 01.31
    by aspiration 01.09
  subcutaneous tissue 86.04
  subdiaphragmatic 54.19
    percutaneous 54.91
  subdural space, cerebral (incision) (trephination) 01.31
    by aspiration 01.09
  subhepatic space 54.19
    percutaneous 54.91
  sublingual space 27.0
  submental space 27.0
  subphrenic space 54.19
    percutaneous 54.91
  supraclavicular fossa 86.04
  temporal pouches 27.0
  tendon (sheath) 83.01
    hand 82.01
  thenar space 82.04
  thorax (closed) 34.04
    open (by incision) 34.09
    thoracoscopic 34.06
  thyroglossal tract (by incision) 06.09
    by aspiration 06.01
  thyroid (field) (gland) (by incision) 06.09
    by aspiration 06.01
    postoperative 06.02
  tonsil 28.0
  tunica vaginalis 61.0
  ureter (by catheter) 59.8
    by
      anastomosis NEC (*see also* Anastomosis, ureter) 56.79
      incision 56.2
  ventricle (cerebral) (incision)
    by
      anastomosis — *see* Shunt, ventricular
      aspiration 01.09
        through previously implanted catheter 01.02
      extracranial ventricular shunt — *see* category 02.3
  vertebral column 03.09

Drawing test 94.08
Dressing
  burn 93.57
  ulcer 93.56
  wound 93.57
Drilling
  bone (*see also* Incision, bone) 77.10
  ovary 65.99
Drotrecogin alfa (activated), infusion 00.11
Ductogram, mammary 87.35
Duhamel operation (abdominoperineal pull-through) 48.65
Dührssen's
  incisions (cervix, to assist delivery) 73.93
  operation (vaginofixation of uterus) 69.22
Dunn operation (triple arthrodesis) 81.12
Duodenectomy 45.62
  with
    gastrectomy — *see* Gastrectomy
    pancreatectomy — *see* Pancreatectomy
Duodenocholedochotomy 51.51
Duodenoduodenostomy 45.91
  proximal to distal segment 45.62
Duodenoileostomy 45.91
Duodenojejunostomy 45.91
Duodenoplasty 46.79
Duodenorrhaphy 46.71
Duodenoscopy 45.13
  through stoma (artificial) 45.12
  transabdominal (operative) 45.11
Duodenostomy 46.39
Duodenotomy 45.01
Dupuytren operation
  fasciectomy 82.35
  fasciotomy 82.12
    with excision 82.35
  shoulder disarticulation 84.08
Durabond 86.59
Duraplasty 02.12
Durham (-Caldwell) operation (transfer of biceps femoris tendon) 83.75
DuToit and Roux operation (staple capsulorrhaphy of shoulder) 81.82
DuVries operation (tenoplasty) 83.88
Dwyer operation
  fasciotomy 83.14
  soft tissue release NEC 83.84
  wedge osteotomy, calcaneus 77.28

E

E2F decoy 00.16
Eagleton operation (extrapetrosal drainage) 20.22
EC-IC vascular bypass 39.28
ECG — *see* Electrocardiogram
Echocardiography 88.72
  intracardiac (heart chambers) (ICE) 37.28
  intravascular (coronary vessels) 00.24
  transesophageal 88.72
    monitoring (Doppler) (ultrasound) 89.68
Echoencephalography 88.71
Echography — *see* Ultrasonography
Echogynography 88.79
Echoplacentogram 88.78
ECMO (extracorporeal membrane oxygenation) 39.65
Eden-Hybinette operation (glenoid bone block) 78.01
Educational therapy (bed-bound children) (handicapped) 93.82
EEG (electroencephalogram) 89.14
  monitoring (radiographic) (video) 89.19
Effler operation (heart) 36.2
Effleurage 93.39
EGD (esophagogastroduodenoscopy) 45.13
  with closed biopsy 45.16
Eggers operation
  tendon release (patellar retinacula) 83.13
  tendon transfer (biceps femoris tendon) (hamstring tendon) 83.75
EKG — *see also* Electrocardiogram 89.52
Elastic hosiery 93.59
Electro-oculogram (EOG) 95.22
Electrocardiogram (with 12 or more leads) 89.52
  with vectorcardiogram 89.53

☑ Additional Digit Required — Refer to the Tabular List for Digit Selection   ⧫ Subterms under main terms may continue to next column or page

2014 ICD-9-CM   ►◄ Revised Text   ● New Line   ▲ Revised Code   Volume 3 — 15

Division — Electrocardiogram

Electrocardiogram — *continued*
  fetal (scalp), intrauterine 75.32
  rhythm (with one to three leads) 89.51
Electrocautery — *see also* Cauterization
  cervix 67.32
  corneal lesion (ulcer) 11.42
  esophagus 42.39
    endoscopic 42.33
Electrocoagulation — *see also* Destruction, lesion, by site
  aneurysm (cerebral) (peripheral vessels) 39.52
  cervix 67.32
  cystoscopic 57.49
  ear
    external 18.29
    inner 20.79
    middle 20.51
  fallopian tube (lesion) 66.61
    for tubal ligation — *see* Ligation, fallopian tube
  gasserian ganglion 04.02
  nasal turbinates 21.61
  nose, for epistaxis (with packing) 21.03
  ovary 65.29
    laparoscopic 65.25
  prostatic bed 60.94
  rectum (polyp) 48.32
    radical 48.31
  retina (for)
    destruction of lesion 14.21
    reattachment 14.51
    repair of tear 14.31
  round ligament 69.19
  semicircular canals 20.79
  urethrovesical junction, transurethral 57.49
  uterine ligament 69.19
  uterosacral ligament 69.19
  uterus 68.29
  vagina 70.33
  vulva 71.3
Electrocochleography 20.31
Electroconization, cervix 67.32
Electroconvulsive therapy (ECT) 94.27
Electroencephalogram (EEG) 89.14
  monitoring (radiographic) (video) 89.19
    intraoperative 00.94
Electrogastrogram 44.19
Electrokeratotomy 11.49
Electrolysis
  ciliary body 12.71
  hair follicle 86.92
  retina (for)
    destruction of lesion 14.21
    reattachment 14.51
    repair of tear 14.31
  skin 86.92
  subcutaneous tissue 86.92
Electromyogram, electromyography (EMG) (muscle) 93.08
  eye 95.25
  urethral sphincter 89.23
Electronarcosis 94.29
Electronic gaiter 93.59
Electronystagmogram (ENG) 95.24
Electroresection — *see also* Destruction, lesion, by site
  bladder neck (transurethral) 57.49
  esophagus 42.39
    endoscopic 42.33
  prostate (transurethral) 60.29
  stomach 43.49
    endoscopic 43.41
Electroretinogram (ERG) 95.21
Electroshock therapy (EST) 94.27
  subconvulsive 94.26
Elevation
  bone fragments (fractured)
    orbit 76.79
    sinus (nasal)
      frontal 22.79
      maxillary 22.79
    skull (with debridement) 02.02
    spinal 03.53
  pedicle graft 86.71

Elliot operation (scleral trephination with iridectomy) 12.61
Ellis Jones operation (repair of peroneal tendon) 83.88
Ellison operation (reinforcement of collateral ligament) 81.44
Elmslie-Cholmeley operation (tarsal wedge osteotomy) 77.28
Eloesser operation
  thoracoplasty 33.34
  thoracostomy 34.09
Elongation — *see* Lengthening
Embolectomy 38.00
  with endarterectomy — *see* Endarterectomy
  abdominal
    artery 38.06
    vein 38.07
  aorta (arch) (ascending) (descending) 38.04
  arteriovenous shunt or cannula 39.49
  bovine graft 39.49
  head and neck NEC 38.02
  intracranial NEC 38.01
  lower limb
    artery 38.08
    vein 38.09
  mechanical
    endovascular
      head and neck 39.74
  pulmonary (artery) (vein) 38.05
  thoracic NEC 38.05
  upper limb (artery) (vein) 38.03
Embolization (transcatheter)
  adhesive (glue) 39.79
    head and neck 39.72
  arteriovenous fistula 39.53
    endovascular 39.72
  artery (selective) 38.80
    by
      endovascular approach 39.79
        head and neck vessels
          bare coils 39.75
          bioactive coils 39.76
          partial occlusion (balloon) (temporary) 39.77
      percutaneous transcatheter infusion 99.29
    abdominal NEC 38.86
      duodenal (transcatheter) 44.44
      gastric (transcatheter) 44.44
      renal (transcatheter) 38.86
    aorta (arch) (ascending) (descending) 38.84
      temporary therapeutic endovascular (balloon) (partial occlusion) 39.77
    duodenal (transcatheter) 44.44
    gastric (transcatheter) 44.44
    head and neck NEC 38.82
    intracranial NEC 38.81
    lower limb 38.88
    renal (transcatheter) 38.86
    thoracic NEC 38.85
    upper limb 38.83
    uterine (gelatin sponge) (gelfoam) (microspheres) (PVA) (spherical embolics) (without coil(s)) 68.25
  AVM, intracranial, endovascular approach 39.72
  carotid cavernous fistula 39.53
  chemoembolization 99.25
  coil, endovascular 39.79
    head and neck 39.75
      bare coils 39.75
      bioactive coils 39.76
    uterine artery 68.24
  vein (selective) 38.80
    by
      endovascular approach 39.79
        head and neck 39.72
        partial occlusion (balloon) (temporary) 39.77
    abdominal NEC 38.87
      duodenal (transcatheter) 44.44
      gastric (transcatheter) 44.44
    duodenal (transcatheter) 44.44
    gastric (transcatheter) 44.44

Embryotomy 73.8
EMG — *see* Electromyogram
Emmet operation (cervix) 67.61
Encephalocentesis — *see also* Puncture 01.09
  fetal head, transabdominal 73.8
Encephalography (cisternal puncture) (fractional) (lumbar) (pneumoencephalogram) 87.01
Encephalopuncture 01.09
Encircling procedure — *see also* Cerclage
  sclera, for buckling 14.49
    with implant 14.41
Endarterectomy (gas) (with patch graft) 38.10
  abdominal 38.16
  aorta (arch) (ascending) (descending) 38.14
  coronary artery — *see* category 36.0 ☑
    open chest approach 36.03
  head and neck (open) NEC 38.12

Note — Also use 00.40, 00.41, 00.42, or 00.43 to show the total number of vessels treated. Use code 00.44 once to show procedure on a bifurcated vessel. In addition, use 00.45, 00.46, 00.47, or 00.48 to show the number of vascular stents inserted.

    percutaneous approach, extracranial vessel(s) 00.61
    percutaneous approach, intracranial vessel(s) 00.62
  intracranial (open) NEC 38.11

Note — Also use 00.40, 00.41, 00.42, or 00.43 to show the total number of vessels treated. Use code 00.44 once to show procedure on a bifurcated vessel. In addition, use 00.45, 00.46, 00.47, or 00.48 to show the number of vascular stents inserted.

    percutaneous approach, intracranial vessel(s) 00.62
  lower limb 38.18
  thoracic NEC 38.15
  upper limb 38.13
Endoaneurysmorrhaphy — *see also*
  Aneurysmorrhaphy 39.52
  by or with
    endovascular graft
      abdominal aorta 39.71
        fenestrated (branching) graft 39.78
      lower extremity artery(s) 39.79
      thoracic aorta 39.73
      upper extremity artery(s) 39.79
Endolymphatic (-subarachnoid) shunt 20.71
Endometrectomy (uterine) (internal) 68.29
  bladder 57.59
  cul-de-sac 70.32
Endoprosthesis
  bile duct 51.87
  femoral head (bipolar) 81.52
Endoscopy
  with biopsy — *see* Biopsy, by site, closed
  anus 49.21
  biliary tract (operative) 51.11
    by retrograde cholangiography (ERC) 51.11
    by retrograde cholangiopancreatography (ERCP) 51.10
    intraoperative 51.11
    percutaneous (via T-tube or other tract) 51.98
      with removal of common duct stones 51.96
  bladder 57.32
    through stoma (artificial) 57.31
  bronchus NEC 33.23
    with biopsy 33.24
    fiberoptic 33.22
    through stoma (artificial) 33.21
  colon 45.23
    through stoma (artificial) 45.22
    transabdominal (operative) 45.21
  cul-de-sac 70.22
  ear 18.11
  esophagus NEC 42.23
    through stoma (artificial) 42.22

Endoscopy — *continued*
  esophagus — *continued*
    transabdominal (operative) 42.21
    ileum 45.13
      through stoma (artificial) 45.12
      transabdominal (operative) 45.11
    intestine NEC 45.24
      large 45.24
        fiberoptic (flexible) 45.23
        through stoma (artificial) 45.22
        transabdominal (intraoperative) 45.21
      small 45.13
        esophagogastroduodenoscopy (EGD) 45.13
          with closed biopsy 45.16
        through stoma (artificial) 45.12
        transabdominal (operative) 45.11
    jejunum 45.13
      through stoma (artificial) 45.12
      transabdominal (operative) 45.11
    kidney 55.21
    larynx 31.42
      through stoma (artificial) 31.41
    lung — *see* Bronchoscopy
    mediastinum (transpleural) 34.22
    nasal sinus 22.19
    nose 21.21
    pancreatic duct 52.13
    pelvis 55.22
    peritoneum 54.21
    pharynx 29.11
    rectum 48.23
      through stoma (artificial) 48.22
      transabdominal (operative) 48.21
    sinus, nasal 22.19
    stomach NEC 44.13
      through stoma (artificial) 44.12
      transabdominal (operative) 44.11
    thorax (transpleural) 34.21
    trachea NEC 31.42
      through stoma (artificial) 31.41
    transpleural
      mediastinum 34.22
      thorax 34.21
    ureter 56.31
    urethra 58.22
    uterus 68.12
    vagina 70.21
Enema (transanal) NEC 96.39
  for removal of impacted feces 96.38
ENG (electronystagmogram) 95.24
Enlargement
  aortic lumen, thoracic 38.14
  atrial septal defect (pre-existing) 35.41
    in repair of total anomalous pulmonary venous connection 35.82
  eye socket 16.64
  foramen ovale (pre-existing) 35.41
    in repair of total anomalous pulmonary venous connection 35.82
  intestinal stoma 46.40
    large intestine 46.43
    small intestine 46.41
  introitus 96.16
  orbit (eye) 16.64
  palpebral fissure 08.51
  punctum 09.41
  sinus tract (skin) 86.89
Enterectomy NEC 45.63
Enteroanastomosis
  large-to-large intestine 45.94
  small-to-large intestine 45.93
  small-to-small intestine 45.91
Enterocelectomy 53.9
  female 70.92
    with graft or prosthesis 70.93
  vaginal 70.92
    with graft or prosthesis 70.93
Enterocentesis 45.00
  duodenum 45.01
  large intestine 45.03
  small intestine NEC 45.02
Enterocholecystostomy 51.32
Enteroclysis (small bowel) 96.43
Enterocolectomy NEC 45.79

☑ **Additional Digit Required** — Refer to the Tabular List for Digit Selection   ▼ **Subterms under main terms may continue to next column or page**

16 — Volume 3   ▶◀ **Revised Text**   ● **New Line**   ▲ **Revised Code**   2014 ICD-9-CM

Enterocolostomy 45.93
Enteroentectropy 46.99
Enteroenterostomy 45.90
  small-to-large intestine 45.93
  small-to-small intestine 45.91
Enterogastrostomy 44.39
  laparoscopic 44.38
Enterolithotomy 45.00
Enterolysis 54.59
  laparoscopic 54.51
Enteropancreatostomy 52.96
Enterorrhaphy 46.79
  large intestine 46.75
  small intestine 46.73
Enterostomy NEC 46.39
  cecum (see also Colostomy) 46.10
  colon (transverse) (see also Colostomy) 46.10
    loop 46.03
  delayed opening 46.31
  duodenum 46.39
    loop 46.01
  feeding NEC 46.39
    percutaneous (endoscopic) 46.32
  ileum (Brooke) (Dragstedt) 46.20
    loop 46.01
  jejunum (feeding) 46.39
    loop 46.01
    percutaneous (endoscopic) 46.32
  sigmoid colon (see also Colostomy) 46.10
    loop 46.03
  transverse colon (see also Colostomy) 46.10
    loop 46.03
Enterotomy 45.00
  large intestine 45.03
  small intestine 45.02
Enucleation — see also Excision, lesion, by site
  cyst
    broad ligament 69.19
    dental 24.4
    liver 50.29
    ovarian 65.29
      laparoscopic 65.25
    parotid gland 26.29
    salivary gland 26.29
    skin 86.3
    subcutaneous tissue 86.3
  eyeball 16.49
    with implant (into Tenon's capsule) 16.42
      with attachment of muscles 16.41
EOG (electro-oculogram) 95.22
Epicardiectomy 36.39
Epididymectomy 63.4
  with orchidectomy (unilateral) 62.3
    bilateral 62.41
Epididymogram 87.93
Epididymoplasty 63.59
Epididymorrhaphy 63.81
Epididymotomy 63.92
Epididymovasostomy 63.83
Epiglottidectomy 30.21
Epikeratophakia 11.76
Epilation
  eyebrow (forceps) 08.93
    cryosurgical 08.92
    electrosurgical 08.91
  eyelid (forceps) NEC 08.93
    cryosurgical 08.92
    electrosurgical 08.91
  skin 86.92
Epiphysiodesis — see also Arrest, bone growth
  — see category 78.2 ☑
Epiphysiolysis — see also Arrest, bone growth
  — see category 78.2 ☑
Epiploectomy 54.4
Epiplopexy 54.74
Epiplorrhaphy 54.74
Episioperineoplasty 71.79
Episioperineorrhaphy 71.71
  obstetrical 75.69
Episioplasty 71.79
Episioproctotomy 73.6
Episiorrhaphy 71.71
  following episiotomy — see Episiotomy
  for obstetrical laceration 75.69

Episiotomy (with subsequent episiorrhaphy) 73.6
  high forceps 72.31
  low forceps 72.1
  mid forceps 72.21
  nonobstetrical 71.09
  outlet forceps 72.1
EPS (electrophysiologic stimulation)
  as part of intraoperative testing — omit code
  catheter based invasive electrophysiologic testing 37.26
  device interrogation only without arrhythmia induction (bedside check) 89.45-89.49
  noninvasive programmed electrical stimulation (NIPS) 37.20
Eptifibatide, infusion 99.20
Equalization, leg
  lengthening — see category 78.3 ☑
  shortening — see category 78.2 ☑
Equilibration (occlusal) 24.8
Equiloudness balance 95.43
ERC (endoscopic retrograde cholangiography) 51.11
ERCP (endoscopic retrograde cholangiopancreatography) 51.10
  cannulation of pancreatic duct 52.93
ERG (electroretinogram) 95.21
ERP (endoscopic retrograde pancreatography) 52.13
Eruption, tooth, surgical 24.6
Erythrocytapheresis, therapeutic 99.73
Escharectomy 86.22
Escharotomy 86.09
Esophageal voice training (post-laryngectomy) 93.73
Esophagectomy 42.40
  abdominothoracocervical (combined) (synchronous) 42.42
  partial or subtotal 42.41
  total 42.42
Esophagocologastrostomy (intrathoracic) 42.55
  antesternal or antethoracic 42.65
Esophagocolostomy (intrathoracic) NEC 42.56
  with interposition of colon 42.55
  antesternal or antethoracic NEC 42.66
    with interposition of colon 42.65
Esophagoduodenostomy (intrathoracic) NEC 42.54
  with
    complete gastrectomy 43.99
    interposition of small bowel 42.53
Esophagoenterostomy (intrathoracic) NEC — see also Anastomosis, esophagus, to intestinal segment 42.54
  antesternal or antethoracic (see also Anastomosis, esophagus, antesternal, to intestinal segment) 42.64
Esophagoesophagostomy (intrathoracic) 42.51
  antesternal or antethoracic 42.61
Esophagogastrectomy 43.99
Esophagogastroduodenoscopy (EGD) 45.13
  with closed biopsy 45.16
  through stoma (artificial) 45.12
  transabdominal (operative) 45.11
Esophagogastromyotomy 42.7
Esophagogastropexy 44.65
Esophagogastroplasty 44.65
Esophagogastroscopy NEC 44.13
  through stoma (artificial) 44.12
  transabdominal (operative) 44.11
Esophagogastrostomy (intrathoracic) 42.52
  with partial gastrectomy 43.5
  antesternal or antethoracic 42.62
Esophagoileostomy (intrathoracic) NEC 42.54
  with interposition of small bowel 42.53
  antesternal or antethoracic NEC 42.64
    with interposition of small bowel 42.63
Esophagojejunostomy (intrathoracic) NEC 42.54
  with
    complete gastrectomy 43.99
    interposition of small bowel 42.53

Esophagojejunostomy — continued
  antesternal or antethoracic NEC 42.64
    with interposition of small bowel 42.63
Esophagomyotomy 42.7
Esophagoplasty NEC 42.89
Esophagorrhaphy 42.82
Esophagoscopy NEC 42.23
  by incision (operative) 42.21
  with closed biopsy 42.24
  through stoma (artificial) 42.22
  transabdominal (operative) 42.21
Esophagostomy 42.10
  cervical 42.11
  thoracic 42.19
Esophagotomy NEC 42.09
Estes operation (ovary) 65.72
  laparoscopic 65.75
Estlander operation (thoracoplasty) 33.34
ESWL (extracorporeal shockwave lithotripsy) NEC 98.59
  bile duct 98.52
  bladder 98.51
  gallbladder 98.52
  kidney 98.51
  Kock pouch (urinary diversion) 98.51
  renal pelvis 98.51
  specified site NEC 98.59
  ureter 98.51
Ethmoidectomy 22.63
Ethmoidotomy 22.51
Evacuation
  abscess — see Drainage, by site
  anterior chamber (eye) (aqueous) (hyphema) 12.91
  cyst (see also Excision, lesion, by site)
    breast 85.91
    kidney 55.01
    liver 50.29
  hematoma (see also Incision, hematoma)
    obstetrical 75.92
    incisional 75.91
  hemorrhoids (thrombosed) 49.47
  pelvic blood clot (by incision) 54.19
    by
      culdocentesis 70.0
      culdoscopy 70.22
  retained placenta
    with curettage 69.02
    manual 75.4
  streptothrix from lacrimal duct 09.42
Evaluation (of)
  audiological 95.43
  cardiac rhythm device (CRT-D) (CRT-P) (AICD) (pacemaker) — see Interrogation
  criminal responsibility, psychiatric 94.11
  functional (physical therapy) 93.01
  hearing NEC 95.49
  orthotic (for brace fitting) 93.02
  prosthetic (for artificial limb fitting) 93.03
  psychiatric NEC 94.19
    commitment 94.13
  psychologic NEC 94.08
  testimentary capacity, psychiatric 94.11
Evans operation (release of clubfoot) 83.84
Evisceration
  eyeball 16.39
    with implant (into scleral shell) 16.31
  ocular contents 16.39
    with implant (into scleral shell) 16.31
  orbit (see also Exenteration, orbit) 16.59
  pelvic (anterior) (posterior) (partial) (total) (female) 68.8
    male 57.71
Evulsion
  nail (bed) (fold) 86.23
  skin 86.3
  subcutaneous tissue 86.3
Examination (for)
  breast
    manual 89.36
    radiographic NEC 87.37
    thermographic 88.85
    ultrasonic 88.73
  cervical rib (by x-ray) 87.43
  colostomy stoma (digital) 89.33

Examination — continued
  dental (oral mucosa) (peridontal) 89.31
    radiographic NEC 87.12
  enterostomy stoma (digital) 89.33
  eye 95.09
    color vision 95.06
    comprehensive 95.02
    dark adaptation 95.07
    limited (with prescription of spectacles) 95.01
    under anesthesia 95.04
  fetus, intrauterine 75.35
  general physical 89.7
  glaucoma 95.03
  gynecological 89.26
  hearing 95.47
  microscopic (specimen) (of) 91.9 ☑

> Note — Use the following fourth-digit subclassification with categories 90–91 to identify type of examination:
> 1 bacterial smear
> 2 culture
> 3 culture and sensitivity
> 4 parasitology
> 5 toxicology
> 6 cell block and Papanicolaou smear
> 9 other microsopic examination

  adenoid 90.3 ☑
  adrenal gland 90.1 ☑
  amnion 91.4 ☑
  anus 90.9 ☑
  appendix 90.9 ☑
  bile ducts 91.0 ☑
  bladder 91.3 ☑
  blood 90.5 ☑
  bone 91.5 ☑
    marrow 90.6 ☑
  brain 90.0 ☑
  breast 91.6 ☑
  bronchus 90.4 ☑
  bursa 91.5 ☑
  cartilage 91.5 ☑
  cervix 91.4 ☑
  chest wall 90.4 ☑
  chorion 91.4 ☑
  colon 90.9 ☑
  cul-de-sac 91.1 ☑
  dental 90.8 ☑
  diaphragm 90.4 ☑
  duodenum 90.8 ☑
  ear 90.3 ☑
  endocrine gland NEC 90.1 ☑
  esophagus 90.8 ☑
  eye 90.2 ☑
  fallopian tube 91.4 ☑
  fascia 91.5 ☑
  female genital tract 91.4 ☑
  fetus 91.4 ☑
  gallbladder 91.0 ☑
  hair 91.6 ☑
  ileum 90.9 ☑
  jejunum 90.9 ☑
  joint fluid 91.5 ☑
  kidney 91.2 ☑
  large intestine 90.9 ☑
  larynx 90.3 ☑
  ligament 91.5 ☑
  liver 91.0 ☑
  lung 90.4 ☑
  lymph (node) 90.7 ☑
  meninges 90.0 ☑
  mesentery 91.1 ☑
  mouth 90.8 ☑
  muscle 91.5 ☑
  musculoskeletal system 91.5 ☑
  nails 91.6 ☑
  nerve 90.0 ☑
  nervous system 90.0 ☑
  nose 90.3 ☑

☑ Additional Digit Required — Refer to the Tabular List for Digit Selection   Subterms under main terms may continue to next column or page

2014 ICD-9-CM   ▶◀ Revised Text   ● New Line   ▲ Revised Code   Volume 3 — 17

Examination — *continued*
  microscopic — *continued*
    omentum 91.1 ☑
    operative wound 91.7 ☑
    ovary 91.4 ☑
    pancreas 91.0 ☑
    parathyroid gland 90.1 ☑
    penis 91.3 ☑
    perirenal tissue 91.2 ☑
    peritoneum (fluid) 91.1 ☑
    periureteral tissue 91.2 ☑
    perivesical (tissue) 91.3 ☑
    pharynx 90.3 ☑
    pineal gland 90.1 ☑
    pituitary gland 90.1 ☑
    placenta 91.4 ☑
    pleura (fluid) 90.4 ☑
    prostate 91.3 ☑
    rectum 90.9 ☑
    retroperitoneum 91.1 ☑
    semen 91.3 ☑
    seminal vesicle 91.3 ☑
    sigmoid 90.9 ☑
    skin 91.6 ☑
    small intestine 90.9 ☑
    specified site NEC 91.8 ☑
    spinal fluid 90.0 ☑
    spleen 90.6 ☑
    sputum 90.4 ☑
    stomach 90.8 ☑
    stool 90.9 ☑
    synovial membrane 91.5 ☑
    tendon 91.5 ☑
    thorax NEC 90.4 ☑
    throat 90.3 ☑
    thymus 90.1 ☑
    thyroid gland 90.1 ☑
    tonsil 90.3 ☑
    trachea 90.4 ☑
    ureter 91.2 ☑
    urethra 91.3 ☑
    urine 91.3 ☑
    uterus 91.4 ☑
    vagina 91.4 ☑
    vas deferens 91.3 ☑
    vomitus 90.8 ☑
    vulva 91.4 ☑
  neuro-ophthalmology 95.03
  neurologic 89.13
  ophthalmoscopic 16.21
  panorex, mandible 87.12
  pelvic (manual) 89.26
    instrumental (by pelvimeter) 88.25
    pelvimetric 88.25
  physical, general 89.7
  postmortem 89.8
  rectum (digital) 89.34
    endoscopic 48.23
      through stoma (artificial) 48.22
      transabdominal 48.21
  retinal disease 95.03
  specified type (manual) NEC 89.39
  thyroid field, postoperative 06.02
  uterus (digital) 68.11
    endoscopic 68.12
  vagina 89.26
    endoscopic 70.21
  visual field 95.05
Exchange transfusion 99.01
  intrauterine 75.2
Excision
  aberrant tissue — *see* Excision, lesion, by site of tissue origin
  abscess — *see* Excision, lesion, by site
  accessory tissue (*see also* Excision, lesion, by site of tissue origin)
    lung 32.29
      endoscopic 32.28
      thoracoscopic 32.20
    spleen 41.93
  adenoids (tag) 28.6
    with tonsillectomy 28.3
  adenoma — *see* Excision, lesion, by site
  adrenal gland (*see also* Adrenalectomy) 07.22

Excision — *continued*
  ampulla of Vater (with reimplantation of common duct) 51.62
  anal papilla 49.39
    endoscopic 49.31
  aneurysm (arteriovenous) (*see also* Aneurysmectomy) 38.60
    coronary artery 36.91
    heart 37.32
    myocardium 37.32
    sinus of Valsalva 35.39
    ventricle (heart) 37.32
  anus (complete) (partial) 49.6
  aortic subvalvular ring 35.35
  apocrine gland 86.3
  aponeurosis 83.42
    hand 82.33
  appendage, left atrial 37.36
  appendiceal stump 47.09
    laparoscopic 47.01
  appendices epiploicae 54.4
  appendix (*see also* Appendectomy) 47.01, 47.09
    epididymis 63.3
    testis 62.2
  arcuate ligament (spine) — omit code
  arteriovenous fistula (*see also* Aneurysmectomy) 38.60
  artery (*see also* Arteriectomy) 38.60
  Baker's cyst, knee 83.39
  Bartholin's gland 71.24
  basal ganglion 01.59
  bile duct 51.69
    endoscopic 51.64
  bladder (*see also* Cystectomy)
  bleb (emphysematous), lung 32.29
    endoscopic 32.28
    thoracoscopic 32.20
  blood vessel (*see also* Angiectomy) 38.60
  bone (ends) (partial), except facial — *see* category 77.8 ☑
    facial NEC 76.39
      total 76.45
        with reconstruction 76.44
    for graft (autograft) (homograft) — *see* category 77.7 ☑
    fragments (chips) (*see also* Incision, bone) 77.10
    joint (*see also* Arthrotomy) 80.10
    necrotic (*see also* Sequestrectomy, bone) 77.00
    heterotopic, from
      muscle 83.32
        hand 82.22
      skin 86.3
      tendon 83.31
        hand 82.21
    mandible 76.31
      with arthrodesis — *see* Arthrodesis
      total 76.42
        with reconstruction 76.41
    spur — *see* Excision, lesion, bone
    total, except facial — *see* category 77.9 ☑
      facial NEC 76.45
        with reconstruction 76.44
      mandible 76.42
        with reconstruction 76.41
  brain 01.59
    hemisphere 01.52
    lobe 01.53
  branchial cleft cyst or vestige 29.2
  breast (*see also* Mastectomy) 85.41
    aberrant tissue 85.24
    accessory 85.24
    ectopic 85.24
    nipple 85.25
      accessory 85.24
    segmental 85.23
    supernumerary 85.24
    wedge 85.21
  broad ligament 69.19
  bronchogenic cyst 32.09
    endoscopic 32.01
  bronchus (wide sleeve) NEC 32.1
  buccal mucosa 27.49

Excision — *continued*
  bulbourethral gland 58.92
  bulbous tuberosities (mandible) (maxilla) (fibrous) (osseous) 24.31
  bunion (*see also* Bunionectomy) 77.59
  bunionette (with osteotomy) 77.54
  bursa 83.5
    hand 82.31
  canal of Nuck 69.19
  cardioma 37.33
  carotid body (lesion) (partial) (total) 39.89
  cartilage (*see also* Chondrectomy) 80.90
    intervertebral — *see* category 80.5 ☑
    knee (semilunar) 80.6
    larynx 30.29
    nasal (submucous) 21.5
  caruncle, urethra 58.39
    endoscopic 58.31
  cataract (*see also* Extraction, cataract) 13.19
    secondary membrane (after cataract) 13.65
  cervical
    rib 77.91
    stump 67.4
  cervix (stump) NEC 67.4
    cold (knife) 67.2
    conization 67.2
    cryoconization 67.33
    electroconizaton 67.32
  chalazion (multiple) (single) 08.21
  cholesteatoma — *see* Excision, lesion, by site
  choroid plexus 02.14
  cicatrix (skin) 86.3
  cilia base 08.20
  ciliary body, prolapsed 12.98
  clavicle (head) (partial) 77.81
    total (complete) 77.91
  clitoris 71.4
  coarctation of aorta (end-to-end anastomosis) 38.64
    with
      graft replacement (interposition)
        abdominal 38.44
        thoracic 38.45
        thoracoabdominal 38.45 *[38.44]*
  common
    duct 51.63
    wall between posterior and coronary sinus (with roofing of resultant defect with patch graft) 35.82
  condyle — *see* category 77.8 ☑
    mandible 76.5
  conjunctival ring 10.31
  cornea 11.49
    epithelium (with chemocauterization) 11.41
    for smear or culture 11.21
  costal cartilage 80.99
  cul-de-sac (Douglas') 70.92
    with graft or prosthesis 70.93
  cusp, heart valve 35.10
    aortic 35.11
    mitral 35.12
    tricuspid 35.14
  cyst (*see also* Excision, lesion, by site)
    apical (tooth) 23.73
      with root canal therapy 23.72
    Baker's (popliteal) 83.39
    breast 85.21
    broad ligament 69.19
    bronchogenic 32.09
      endoscopic 32.01
    cervix 67.39
    dental 24.4
    dentigerous 24.4
    epididymis 63.2
    fallopian tube 66.61
    Gartner's duct 70.33
    hand 82.29
    labia 71.3
    lung 32.29
      endoscopic 32.28
      thoracoscopic 32.20
    mesonephric duct 69.19

Excision — *continued*
  cyst (*see also* Excision, lesion, by site) — *continued*
    Morgagni
      female 66.61
      male 62.2
    Müllerian duct 60.73
    nasolabial 27.49
    nasopalatine 27.31
      by wide excision 27.32
    ovary 65.29
      laparoscopic 65.25
    parovarian 69.19
    pericardium 37.31
    periodontal (apical) (lateral) 24.4
    popliteal (Baker's), knee 83.39
    radicular 24.4
    spleen 41.42
    synovial (membrane) 83.39
    thyroglossal (with resection of hyoid bone) 06.7
    urachal (bladder) 57.51
      abdominal wall 54.3
    vagina (Gartner's duct) 70.33
  cystic
    duct remnant 51.61
    hygroma 40.29
  dentinoma 24.4
  diaphragm 34.81
  disc, intervertebral (NOS) 80.50
    herniated (nucleus pulposus) 80.51
    other specified (diskectomy) 80.51
  diverticulum
    ampulla of Vater 51.62
    anus 49.39
      endoscopic 49.31
    bladder 57.59
      transurethral 57.49
    duodenum 45.31
      endoscopic 45.30
    esophagus (local) 42.31
      endoscopic 42.33
    hypopharyngeal (by cricopharyngeal myotomy) 29.32
    intestine
      large 45.41
        endoscopic 45.43
      small NEC 45.33
    Meckel's 45.33
    pharyngeal (by cricopharyngeal myotomy) 29.32
    pharyngoesophageal (by cricopharyngeal myotomy) 29.32
    stomach 43.42
      endoscopic 43.41
    urethra 58.39
      endoscopic 58.31
    ventricle, heart 37.33
  duct
    Müllerian 69.19
    paramesonephric 69.19
    thyroglossal (with resection of hyoid bone) 06.7
  ear, external (complete) NEC 18.39
    partial 18.29
    radical 18.31
  ectopic
    abdominal fetus 74.3
    tissue (*see also* Excision, lesion, by site of tissue origin)
      bone, from muscle 83.32
      breast 85.24
      lung 32.29
        endoscopic 32.28
        thoracoscopic 32.20
      spleen 41.93
  empyema pocket, lung 34.09
  epididymis 63.4
  epiglottis 30.21
  epithelial downgrowth, anterior chamber (eye) 12.93
  epulis (gingiva) 24.31
  esophagus (*see also* Esophagectomy) 42.40
  exostosis (*see also* Excision, lesion, bone) 77.60
    auditory canal, external 18.29

☑ **Additional Digit Required — Refer to the Tabular List for Digit Selection**
▼ **Subterms under main terms may continue to next column or page**

18 — Volume 3   ▶◀ **Revised Text**   ● **New Line**   ▲ **Revised Code**   **2014 ICD-9-CM**

☑ **Additional Digit Required** — Refer to the Tabular List for Digit Selection   ▼ **Subterms under main terms may continue to next column or page**

2014 ICD-9-CM   ▶◀ Revised Text   ● New Line   ▲ Revised Code   **Volume 3 — 19**

Excision — continued
  lesion — continued
    nose — continued
      polyp 21.31
      skin 21.32
        specified site NEC 21.32
    odontogenic 24.4
    omentum 54.4
    orbit 16.92
    ovary 65.29
      by wedge resection 65.22
        laparoscopic 65.24
      that by laparoscope 65.25
    palate (bony) 27.31
      by wide excision 27.32
      soft 27.49
    pancreas (local) 52.22
      endoscopic 52.21
    parathyroid 06.89
    parotid gland or duct NEC 26.29
    pelvic wall 54.3
    pelvirectal tissue 48.82
    penis 64.2
    pericardium 37.31
    perineum (female) 71.3
      male 86.3
    periprostatic tissue 60.82
    perirectal tissue 48.82
    perirenal tissue 59.91
    peritoneum 54.4
    perivesical tissue 59.91
    pharynx 29.39
      diverticulum 29.32
    pineal gland 07.53
    pinna 18.29
      radical 18.31
    pituitary (gland) (see also Hypophysecto-
        my, partial) 07.63
      by stereotactic radiosurgery 92.30
        cobalt 60 92.32
        linear accelerator (LINAC) 92.31
        multi-source 92.32
        particle beam 92.33
        particulate 92.33
        radiosurgery NEC 92.39
        single source photon 92.31
    pleura 34.59
    pouch of Douglas 70.32
    preauricular (ear) 18.21
    presacral 54.4
    prostate (transurethral) 60.61
    pulmonary (fibrosis) 32.29
      endoscopic 32.28
      thoracoscopic 32.20
    rectovaginal septum 48.82
    rectum 48.35
      polyp (endoscopic) 48.36
    retroperitoneum 54.4
    salivary gland or duct NEC 26.29
      en bloc 26.32
    sclera 12.84
    scrotum 61.3
    sinus (nasal) — see Excision, lesion, nasal
        sinus
    Skene's gland 71.3
    skin 86.3
      breast 85.21
      nose 21.32
      radical (wide) (involving underlying
          or adjacent structure) (with
          flap closure) 86.4
      scrotum 61.3
    skull 01.6
    soft tissue NEC 83.39
      hand 82.29
    spermatic cord 63.3
    sphincter of Oddi 51.62
      endoscopic 51.64
    spinal cord (meninges) 03.4
    spleen (cyst) 41.42
    stomach NEC 43.42
      endoscopic 43.41
        polyp 43.41
      polyp (endoscopic) 43.41
    subcutaneous tissue 86.3
      breast 85.21

Excision — continued
  lesion — continued
    subgingival 24.31
    sweat gland 86.3
    tendon 83.39
      hand 82.29
      ocular 15.13
      sheath 83.31
        hand 82.21
    testis 62.2
    thorax 34.4
    thymus
      partial (open) (other) 07.81
        thoracoscopic 07.83
      total (open) (other) 07.82
        thoracoscopic 07.84
    thyroid 06.31
      substernal or transsternal route 06.51
    tongue 25.1
    tonsil 28.92
    trachea 31.5
    tunica vaginalis 61.92
    ureter 56.41
    urethra 58.39
      endoscopic 58.31
    uterine ligament 69.19
    uterosacral ligament 69.19
    uterus 68.29
    vagina 70.33
    vein 38.60
      abdominal 38.67
      head and neck NEC 38.62
      intracranial NEC 38.61
      lower limb 38.69
      thoracic NEC 38.65
      upper limb 38.63
      ventricle (heart) 37.33
    vocal cords 30.09
    vulva 71.3
  ligament (see also Arthrectomy) 80.90
    broad 69.19
    round 69.19
    uterine 69.19
    uterosacral 69.19
  ligamentum flavum (spine) — omit code
  lingual tonsil 28.5
  lip 27.43
  liver (partial) 50.22
  loose body
    bone — see Sequestrectomy, bone
    joint 80.10
  lung (with mediastinal dissection) 32.59
    accessory or ectopic tissue 32.29
      endoscopic 32.28
      thoracoscopic 32.20
    segmental 32.39
      thoracoscopic 32.30
    specified type NEC 32.29
      endoscopic 32.28
      thoracoscopic 32.20
    thoracoscopic 32.50
    volume reduction surgery 32.22
      biologic lung volume reduction
          (BLVR) — see category
          33.7 ☑
    wedge 32.29
      thoracoscopic 32.20
  lymphangioma (simple) (see also Excision,
      lymph, lymphatic node) 40.29
  lymph, lymphatic
    drainage area 40.29
      radical — see Excision, lymph, node,
          radical
      regional (with lymph node, skin,
          subcutaneous tissue, and fat)
          40.3
    node (simple) NEC 40.29
      with
        lymphatic drainage area (includ-
            ing skin, subcutaneous tis-
            sue, and fat) 40.3
        mastectomy — see Mastectomy,
            radical
        muscle and deep fascia — see
            Excision, lymph, node,
            radical

Excision — continued
  lymph, lymphatic — continued
    node — continued
      axillary 40.23
        radical 40.51
        regional (extended) 40.3
      cervical (deep) (with excision of sca-
          lene fat pad) 40.21
        with laryngectomy 30.4
        radical (including muscle and
            deep fascia) 40.40
          bilateral 40.42
          unilateral 40.41
        regional (extended) 40.3
        superficial 40.29
      groin 40.24
        radical 40.54
        regional (extended) 40.3
      iliac 40.29
        radical 40.53
        regional (extended) 40.3
      inguinal (deep) (superficial) 40.24
        radical 40.54
        regional (extended) 40.3
      jugular — see Excision, lymph, node,
          cervical
      mammary (internal) 40.22
        external 40.29
          radical 40.59
          regional (extended) 40.3
        radical 40.59
          regional (extended) 40.3
      paratracheal — see Excision, lymph,
          node, cervical
      periaortic 40.29
        radical 40.52
        regional (extended) 40.3
      radical 40.50
        with mastectomy — see Mastec-
            tomy, radical
        specified site NEC 40.59
      regional (extended) 40.3
      sternal — see Excision, lymph, node,
          mammary
      structure(s) (simple) NEC 40.29
        radical 40.59
        regional (extended) 40.3
    lymphocele 40.29
    mastoid (see also Mastoidectomy) 20.49
    median bar, transurethral approach 60.29
    meibomian gland 08.20
    meniscus (knee) 80.6
      acromioclavicular 80.91
      jaw 76.5
      sternoclavicular 80.91
      temporomandibular (joint) 76.5
      wrist 80.93
    müllerian duct cyst 60.73
    muscle 83.45
      for graft 83.43
      hand 82.34
      hand 82.36
        for graft 82.34
    myositis ossificans 83.32
      hand 82.22
    nail (bed) (fold) 86.23
    nasolabial cyst 27.49
    nasopalatine cyst 27.31
      by wide excision 27.32
    neoplasm — see Excision, lesion, by site
    nerve (cranial) (peripheral) NEC 04.07
      sympathetic 05.29
    neuroma (Morton's) (peripheral nerve) 04.07
      acoustic
        by craniotomy 04.01
        by stereotactic radiosurgery 92.30
          cobalt 60 92.32
          linear accelerator (LINAC) 92.31
          multi-source 92.32
          particle beam 92.33
          particulate 92.33
          radiosurgery NEC 92.39
          single source photon 92.31
      sympathetic nerve 05.29
    nipple 85.25
      accessory 85.24

Excision — continued
  odontoma 24.4
  orbital contents (see also Exenteration, orbit)
      16.59
  osteochondritis dissecans (see also Excision,
      lesion, joint) 80.80
  ovary (see also Oophorectomy)
    partial 65.29
      by wedge resection 65.22
        laparoscopic 65.24
      that by laparoscope 65.25
  Pancoast tumor (lung) 32.6
  pancreas (total) (with synchronous duo-
      denectomy) 52.6
    partial NEC 52.59
      distal (tail) (with part of body) 52.52
      proximal (head) (with part of body)
          (with synchronous duodenec-
          tomy) 52.51
      radical subtotal 52.53
    radical (one-stage) (two-stage) 52.7
    subtotal 52.53
  paramesonephric duct 69.19
  parathyroid gland (partial) (subtotal) NEC
      (see also Parathyroidectomy) 06.89
  parotid gland (see also Excision, salivary
      gland) 26.30
  parovarian cyst 69.19
  patella (complete) 77.96
    partial 77.86
  pelvirectal tissue 48.82
  perianal tissue 49.04
    skin tags 49.03
  pericardial adhesions 37.31
  periprostatic tissue 60.82
  perirectal tissue 48.82
  perirenal tissue 59.91
  periurethral tissue 58.92
  perivesical tissue 59.91
  petrous apex cells 20.59
  pharyngeal bands 29.54
  pharynx (partial) 29.33
  pilonidal cyst or sinus (open) (with partial
      closure) 86.21
  pineal gland (complete) (total) 07.54
    partial 07.53
  pituitary gland (complete) (total) (see also
      Hypophysectomy) 07.69
  pleura NEC 34.59
  polyp (see also Excision, lesion, by site)
    esophagus 42.32
      endoscopic 42.33
    large intestine 45.41
      endoscopic 45.42
    nose 21.31
    rectum (endoscopic) 48.36
    stomach (endoscopic) 43.41
  preauricular
    appendage (remnant) 18.29
    cyst, fistula, or sinus (congenital) 18.21
    remnant 18.29
  prolapsed iris (in wound) 12.13
  prostate — see Prostatectomy
  pterygium (simple) 11.39
    with corneal graft 11.32
  radius (head) (partial) 77.83
    total 77.93
  ranula, salivary gland NEC 26.29
  rectal mucosa 48.35
  rectum — see Resection, rectum
  redundant mucosa
    colostomy 45.41
      endoscopic 45.43
    duodenostomy 45.31
      endoscopic 45.30
    ileostomy 45.33
    jejunostomy 45.33
    perineum 71.3
    rectum 48.35
    vulva 71.3
  renal vessel, aberrant 38.66
  rib (cervical) 77.91
  ring of conjunctiva around cornea 10.31
  round ligament 69.19
  salivary gland 26.30
    complete 26.32

☑ Additional Digit Required — Refer to the Tabular List for Digit Selection   ▽ Subterms under main terms may continue to next column or page

20 — Volume 3   ▶◀ Revised Text   ● New Line   ▲ Revised Code   2014 ICD-9-CM

Excision — Exploration

☑ **Additional Digit Required** — Refer to the Tabular List for Digit Selection   ▼ **Subterms under main terms may continue to next column or page**

2014 ICD-9-CM   ▶◀ **Revised Text**   ● **New Line**   ▲ **Revised Code**   **Volume 3 — 21**

Exploration — *see also* Incision — *continued*
  spinal (canal) (nerve root) 03.09
  spleen 41.2
  stomach (by incision) 43.0
    endoscopic — *see* Gastroscopy
  subcutaneous tissue 86.09
  subdiaphragmatic space 54.11
  superficial fossa 86.09
  tarsal tunnel 04.44
  tendon (sheath) 83.01
    hand 82.01
  testes 62.0
  thymus (gland) 07.92
    field 07.91
    thoracoscopic 07.95
  thyroid (field) (gland) (by incision) 06.09
    postoperative 06.02
  trachea (by incision) 31.3
    endoscopic — *see* Tracheoscopy
  tunica vaginalis 61.0
  tympanum 20.09
    transtympanic route 20.23
  ureter (by incision) 56.2
    endoscopic 56.31
  urethra (by incision) 58.0
    endoscopic 58.22
  uterus (corpus) 68.0
    cervix 69.95
    digital 68.11
    postpartal, manual 75.7
  vagina (by incision) 70.14
    endoscopic 70.21
  vas deferens 63.6
  vein 38.00
    abdominal 38.07
    head and neck NEC 38.02
    intracranial NEC 38.01
    lower limb 38.09
    thoracic NEC 38.05
    upper limb 38.03
  vulva (by incision) 71.09
Exposure — *see also* Incision, by site
  tooth (for orthodontic treatment) 24.6
Expression, trachoma follicles 10.33
Exsanguination transfusion 99.01
Extension
  buccolabial sulcus 24.91
  limb, forced 93.25
  lingual sulcus 24.91
  mandibular ridge 76.43
Exteriorization
  esophageal pouch 42.12
  intestine 46.03
    large 46.03
    small 46.01
  maxillary sinus 22.9
  pilonidal cyst or sinus (open excision) (with partial closure) 86.21
Extirpation — *see also* Excision, by site
  aneurysm — *see* Aneurysmectomy
  arteriovenous fistula — *see* Aneurysmectomy
  lacrimal sac 09.6
  larynx 30.3
    with radical neck dissection (with synchronous thyroidectomy) (with synchronous tracheostomy) 30.4
  nerve, tooth (*see also* Therapy, root canal) 23.70
  varicose vein (peripheral) (lower limb) 38.59
    upper limb 38.53
Extracorporeal
  circulation (regional), except hepatic 39.61
    hepatic 50.92
    percutaneous 39.66
  hemodialysis 39.95
  membrane oxygenation (ECMO) 39.65
  photopheresis, therapeutic 99.88
  shockwave lithotripsy (ESWL) NEC 98.59
    bile duct 98.52
    bladder 98.51
    gallbladder 98.52
    kidney 98.51
    renal pelvis 98.51
    specified site NEC 98.59

Extracorporeal — *continued*
  shockwave lithotripsy — *continued*
    ureter 98.51
Extracranial-intracranial bypass [EC-IC] 39.28
Extraction
  breech (partial) 72.52
    with forceps to aftercoming head 72.51
    total 72.54
      with forceps to aftercoming head 72.53
  cataract 13.19
    after cataract (by)
      capsulectomy 13.65
      capsulotomy 13.64
      discission 13.64
      excision 13.65
      iridocapsulectomy 13.65
      mechanical fragmentation 13.66
      needling 13.64
      phacofragmentation (mechanical) 13.66
    aspiration (simple) (with irrigation) 13.3
    cryoextraction (intracapsular approach) 13.19
      temporal inferior route (in presence of fistulization bleb) 13.11
    curette evacuation (extracapsular approach) 13.2
    emulsification (and aspiration) 13.41
    erysiphake (intracapsular approach) 13.19
      temporal inferior route (in presence of fistulization bleb) 13.11
    extracapsular approach (with iridectomy) NEC 13.59
      by temporal inferior route (in presence of fistulization bleb) 13.51
      aspiration (simple) (with irrigation) 13.3
      curette evacuation 13.2
      emulsification (and aspiration) 13.41
      linear extraction 13.2
      mechanical fragmentation with aspiration by
        posterior route 13.42
        specified route NEC 13.43
      phacoemulsification (ultrasonic) (with aspiration) 13.41
      phacofragmentation (mechanical)
        with aspiration by
          posterior route 13.42
          specified route NEC 13.43
        ultrasonic (with aspiration) 13.41
      rotoextraction (mechanical) with aspiration by
        posterior route 13.42
        specified route NEC 13.43
    intracapsular (combined) (simple) (with iridectomy) (with suction) (with zonulolysis) 13.19
      by temporal inferior route (in presence of fistulization bleb) 13.11
    linear extraction (extracapsular approach) 13.2
    phacoemulsification (and aspiration) 13.41
    phacofragmentation (mechanical)
      with aspiration by
        posterior route 13.42
        specified route NEC 13.43
      ultrasonic 13.41
    rotoextraction (mechanical)
      with aspiration by
        posterior route 13.42
        specified route NEC 13.43
    secondary membranous (after cataract) (by)
      capsulectomy 13.65
      capsulotomy 13.64
      discission 13.64
      excision 13.65
      iridocapsulectomy 13.65
      mechanical fragmentation 13.66
      needling 13.64

Extraction — *continued*
  cataract — *continued*
    secondary membranous — *continued*
      phacofragmentation (mechanical) 13.66
  common duct stones (percutaneous) (through sinus tract) (with basket) 51.96
  fat for graft or banking 86.90
  foreign body — *see* Removal, foreign body
  kidney stone(s), percutaneous 55.03
    with fragmentation procedure 55.04
  lens (eye) (*see also* Extraction, cataract) 13.19
  Malström's 72.79
    with episiotomy 72.71
  menstrual, menses 69.6
  milk from lactating breast (manual) (pump) 99.98
  tooth (by forceps) (multiple) (single) NEC 23.09
    with mucoperiosteal flap elevation 23.19
    deciduous 23.01
    surgical NEC (*see also* Removal, tooth, surgical) 23.19
  vacuum, fetus 72.79
    with episiotomy 72.71
  vitreous (*see also* Removal, vitreous) 14.72

F

Face lift 86.82
Facetectomy 77.89
Facilitation, intraocular circulation NEC 12.59
Failed (trial) forceps 73.3
Family
  counselling (medical) (social) 94.49
  therapy 94.42
Farabeuf operation (ischiopubiotomy) 77.39
Fasanella-Servatt operation (blepharoptosis repair) 08.35
Fasciaplasty — *see* Fascioplasty
Fascia sling operation — *see* Operation, sling
Fasciectomy 83.44
  for graft 83.43
    hand 82.34
  hand 82.35
    for graft 82.34
  palmar (release of Dupuytren's contracture) 82.35
Fasciodesis 83.89
  hand 82.89
Fascioplasty — *see also* Repair, fascia 83.89
  hand (*see also* Repair, fascia, hand) 82.89
Fasciorrhaphy — *see* Suture, fascia
Fasciotomy 83.14
  Dupuytren's 82.12
    with excision 82.35
  Dwyer 83.14
  hand 82.12
  Ober-Yount 83.14
  orbital (*see also* Orbitotomy) 16.09
  palmar (release of Dupuytren's contracture) 82.12
    with excision 82.35
Fenestration
  aneurysm (dissecting), thoracic aorta 39.54
  aortic aneurysm 39.54
  cardiac valve 35.10
  chest wall 34.01
  ear
    inner (with graft) 20.61
      revision 20.62
    tympanic 19.55
  labyrinth (with graft) 20.61
  Lempert's (endaural) 19.9
  operation (aorta) 39.54
  oval window, ear canal 19.55
  palate 27.1
  pericardium 37.12
  semicircular canals (with graft) 20.61
  stapes foot plate (with vein graft) 19.19
    with incus replacement 19.11
  tympanic membrane 19.55
  vestibule (with graft) 20.61
Ferguson operation (hernia repair) 53.00

Fetography 87.81
Fetoscopy 75.31
Fiberoscopy — *see* Endoscopy, by site
Fibroidectomy, uterine 68.29
Fick operation (perforation of foot plate) 19.0
Filipuncture (aneurysm) (cerebral) 39.52
Filleting
  hammer toe 77.56
  pancreas 52.3
Filling, tooth (amalgam) (plastic) (silicate) 23.2
  root canal (*see also* therapy, root canal) 23.70
Fimbriectomy — *see also* Salpingectomy, partial 66.69
  Uchida (with tubal ligation) 66.32
Finney operation (pyloroplasty) 44.29
Fissurectomy, anal 49.39
  endoscopic 49.31
  skin (subcutaneous tissue) 49.04
Fistulectomy — *see also* Closure, fistula, by site
  abdominothoracic 34.83
  abdominouterine 69.42
  anus 49.12
  appendix 47.92
  bile duct 51.79
  biliary tract NEC 51.79
  bladder (transurethral approach) 57.84
  bone (*see also* Excision, lesion, bone) 77.60
  branchial cleft 29.52
  bronchocutaneous 33.42
  bronchoesophageal 33.42
  bronchomediastinal 34.73
  bronchopleural 34.73
  bronchopleurocutaneous 34.73
  bronchopleuromediastinal 34.73
  bronchovisceral 33.42
  cervicosigmoidal 67.62
  cholecystogastroenteric 51.93
  cornea 11.49
  diaphragm 34.83
  enterouterine 69.42
  esophagopleurocutaneous 34.73
  esophagus NEC 42.84
  fallopian tube 66.73
  gallbladder 51.93
  gastric NEC 44.63
  hepatic duct 51.79
  hepatopleural 34.73
  hepatopulmonary 34.73
  intestine
    large 46.76
    small 46.74
  intestinouterine 69.42
  joint (*see also* Excision, lesion, joint) 80.80
  lacrimal
    gland 09.21
    sac 09.6
  laryngotracheal 31.62
  larynx 31.62
  mediastinocutaneous 34.73
  mouth NEC 27.53
  nasal 21.82
    sinus 22.71
  nasolabial 21.82
  nasopharyngeal 21.82
  oroantral 22.71
  oronasal 21.82
  pancreas 52.95
  perineorectal 71.72
  perineosigmoidal 71.72
  perirectal, not opening into rectum 48.93
  pharyngoesophageal 29.53
  pharynx NEC 29.53
  pleura 34.73
  rectolabial 71.72
  rectourethral 58.43
  rectouterine 69.42
  rectovaginal 70.73
  rectovesical 57.83
  rectovulvar 71.72
  rectum 48.73
  salivary (duct) (gland) 26.42
  scrotum 61.42
  skin 86.3
  stomach NEC 44.63

☑ Additional Digit Required — Refer to the Tabular List for Digit Selection   ▽ Subterms under main terms may continue to next column or page

22 — Volume 3   ▶◀ Revised Text   ● New Line   ▲ Revised Code   2014 ICD-9-CM

☑ Additional Digit Required — Refer to the Tabular List for Digit Selection   ▽ Subterms under main terms may continue to next column or page

2014 ICD-9-CM   ▶◀ Revised Text   ● New Line   ▲ Revised Code   Volume 3 — 23

☑ Additional Digit Required — Refer to the Tabular List for Digit Selection   ▽ Subterms under main terms may continue to next column or page

24 — Volume 3   ▶◀ Revised Text   ● New Line   ▲ Revised Code   2014 ICD-9-CM

☑ Additional Digit Required — Refer to the Tabular List for Digit Selection
▽ Subterms under main terms may continue to next column or page
2014 ICD-9-CM
▶◀ Revised Text
● New Line
▲ Revised Code
Volume 3 — 25

Girdlestone operation — Grice operation

☑ **Additional Digit Required** — Refer to the Tabular List for Digit Selection

▽ **Subterms under main terms may continue to next column or page**

26 — Volume 3

▶◀ **Revised Text**

● **New Line**

▲ **Revised Code**

2014 ICD-9-CM

Imaging — *continued*
  intravascular ultrasound — *continued*
    coronary vessel 00.24
    intrathoracic vessel 00.22
    other specified vessel 00.28
    peripheral vessel 00.23
    renal vessel 00.25
    vena cava (inferior) (superior) 00.22
  magnetic resonance (nuclear) (proton) NEC 88.97
    abdomen 88.97
    bladder (urinary) 88.95
    bone marrow blood supply 88.94
    brain (brain stem) 88.91
      intraoperative (iMRI) 88.96
      real-time 88.96
    chest (hilar) (mediastinal) 88.92
    computer assisted surgery (CAS) with MR/MRA 00.32
    extremity (upper) (lower) 88.94
    eye orbit 88.97
    face 88.97
    head NEC 88.97
    musculoskeletal 88.94
    myocardium 88.92
    neck 88.97
    orbit of eye 88.97
    prostate 88.95
    specified site NEC 88.97
    spinal canal (cord) (spine) 88.93
  VH™-IVUS — *see* Imaging (diagnostic), intravascular ultrasound (IVUS), by site
  virtual histology intravascular ultrasound — *see* Imaging (diagnostic), intravascular ultrasound (IVUS), by site

Immobilization (by)
  with fracture-reduction — *see* Reduction, fracture
  bandage 93.59
  bone 93.53
  cast NEC 93.53
    with reduction of fracture or dislocation — *see* Reduction, fracture, *and* Reduction, dislocation
  device NEC 93.59
  pressure dressing 93.56
  splint (plaster) (tray) 93.54
    with reduction of fracture or dislocation — *see* Reduction, fracture, *and* Reduction, dislocation
  stereotactic head frame 93.59
  strapping (non-traction) 93.59

Immunization — *see also* Vaccination
  allergy 99.12
  autoimmune disease 99.13
  BCG 99.33
  brucellosis 99.55
  cholera 99.31
  diphtheria 99.36
  DPT 99.39
  epidemic parotitis 99.46
  German measles 99.47
  Hemophilus influenzae 99.52
  influenza 99.52
  measles 99.45
  meningococcus 99.55
  mumps 99.46
  pertussis 99.37
  plague 99.34
  poliomyelitis 99.41
  rabies 99.44
  rubella 99.47
  salmonella 99.55
  smallpox 99.42
  staphylococcus 99.55
  TAB 99.32
  tetanus 99.38
  triple vaccine 99.48
  tuberculosis 99.33
  tularemia 99.35
  typhoid-paratyphoid 99.32
  typhus 99.55
  viral NEC 99.55
  whooping cough 99.37
  yellow fever 99.43

Immunoadsorption
  extracorporeal (ECI) 99.76
Immunotherapy, antineoplastic 99.28
  C-Parvum 99.28
  Interferon 99.28
  interleukin-2 (low-dose) 99.28
    high-dose 00.15
  Levamisole 99.28
  Proleukin (low-dose) 99.28
    high-dose 00.15
  Thymosin 99.28
Impella® percutaneous external heart assist device 37.68
Implant, implantation
  abdominal artery to coronary artery 36.17
  artery
    aortic branches to heart muscle 36.2
    mammary to ventricular wall (Vineberg) 36.2
  baffle, atrial or interatrial 35.91
  biliary fistulous tract into stomach or intestine 51.39
  bipolar endoprosthesis (femoral head) 81.52
  bladder sphincter, artificial (inflatable) 58.93
  blood vessels to myocardium 36.2
  bone growth stimulator (invasive) (percutaneous) (semi-invasive) — *see* category 78.9 ☑
  bone morphogenetic protein (Infuse™) (OP-1™) (recombinant) (rhBMP) 84.52
  bone void filler 84.55
    that with percutaneous vertebral augmentation 81.66
    that with percutaneous vertebroplasty 81.65
  breast (for augmentation) (bilateral) 85.54
    unilateral 85.53
  cardiac contractility modulation (CCM)
    rechargeable pulse generator only 17.52
    total system 17.51
  cardiac resynchronization device
    defibrillator (biventricular) (BiV ICD) (BiV pacemaker with defibrillator) (BiV pacing with defibrillator) (CRT-D) (device and one or more leads) (total system) 00.51
      left ventricular coronary venous lead only 00.52
      pulse generator only 00.54
    pacemaker (BiV) (biventricular) (CRT-P) (device and one or more leads) (total system) 00.50
      left ventricular coronary venous lead only 00.52
      pulse generator only 00.53
  cardiac support device (CSD) 37.41
  cardiomyostimulation system 37.67
  cardioverter/defibrillator (automatic) 37.94
    leads only (patch electrodes) (sensing) (pacing) 37.95
    pulse generator only 37.96
    total system 37.94
  CCM (cardiac contractility modulation)
    rechargeable pulse generator only 17.52
    total system 17.51
  chemotherapeutic agent 00.10
  chest wall (mesh) (silastic) 34.79
  chin (polyethylene) (silastic) 76.68
  cochlear (electrode) 20.96
    prosthetic device (electrode and receiver) 20.96
      channel (single) 20.97
        multiple 20.98
      electrode only 20.99
      internal coil only 20.99
  coil(s), endovascular 39.79
    head or neck vessels
      bare metal 39.75
      bioactive 39.76
  CorCap™ 37.41
  cornea 11.73
  CRT-D (biventricular defibrillator) (BiV ICD) (BiV pacemaker with defibrillator) (BiV pacing with defibrillator) (cardiac resynchronization defibrillator) (device and one or more leads) 00.51

Implant, implantation — *continued*
  CRT-D — *continued*
    left ventricular coronary venous lead only 00.52
    pulse generator only 00.54
  CRT-P (biventricular pacemaker) (BiV pacemaker) (cardiac resynchronization pacemaker) (device and one or more leads) 00.50
    left ventricular coronary venous lead only 00.52
    pulse generator only 00.53
  custodis eye 14.41
  dental (endosseous) (prosthetic) 23.6
  device
    adjustable gastric band and port 44.95
    bronchial device NOS 33.79
    bronchial substance NOS 33.79
    bronchial valve(s)
      multiple lobes 33.73
      single lobe 33.71
    cardiac support device (CSD) 37.41
    CorCap™ 37.41
    epicardial support device 37.41
    Lap-Band™ 44.95
    left atrial appendage 37.90
    left atrial filter 37.90
    left atrial occluder 37.90
    MitraClip® percutaneous mitral valve leaflet clip 35.97
    prosthetic cardiac support device 37.41
    sternal fixation device with rigid plates 84.94
    subcutaneous for intracardiac or great vessel hemodynamic monitoring 00.57
    vascular access 86.07
    ventricular support device 37.41
  diaphragmatic pacemaker 34.85
  Dynesys® 84.82
  electrode(s)
    brain 02.93
      depth 02.93
      foramen ovale 02.93
      sphenoidal 02.93
    cardiac (initial) (transvenous) 37.70
      atrium (initial) 37.73
        replacement 37.76
      atrium and ventricle (initial) 37.72
        replacement 37.76
      epicardium (sternotomy or thoracotomy approach) 37.74
      left ventricular coronary venous system 00.52
      temporary transvenous pacemaker system 37.78
        during and immediately following cardiac surgery 39.64
      ventricle (initial) 37.71
        replacement 37.76
    carotid sinus 39.82
      with synchronous pulse generator implantation (total system) 39.81
    depth 02.93
    foramen ovale 02.96
    gastric 04.92
    heart (*see also* Implant, electrode(s), cardiac) 37.70
    intracranial 02.93
    osteogenic (invasive) for bone growth stimulation — *see* category 78.9 ☑
    peripheral nerve 04.92
    sacral nerve 04.92
    sphenoidal 02.96
    spine 03.93
  electroencephalographic receiver
    brain 02.93
    intracranial 02.93
  electronic stimulator
    anus (subcutaneous) 49.92
    bladder 57.96
    bone growth (invasive) (percutaneous) (semi-invasive) 78.9 ☑

Implant, implantation — *continued*
  electronic stimulator — *continued*
    brain — *see* Implant, neurostimulator, brain
    carotid sinus 39.83
      with synchronous lead(s) implantation (total system) 39.81
    cochlear 20.96
      channel (single) 20.97
        multiple 20.98
    gastric 04.92
    intracranial — *see* Implant, neurostimulator, intracranial
    peripheral nerve — *see* Implant, neurostimulator, peripheral nerve
    phrenic nerve 34.85
    skeletal muscle 83.92
    spine — *see* Implant, neurostimulator, spine
    ureter 56.92
  electrostimulator — *see* Implant, electronic stimulator, by site
  endoprosthesis
    bile duct 51.87
    femoral head (bipolar) 81.52
    pancreatic duct 52.93
  endosseous (dental) 23.6
  epidural pegs 02.93
  epikeratoprosthesis 11.73
  epiretinal visual prosthesis 14.81 ●
  estradiol (pellet) 99.23
  eye (Iowa type) 16.61
    integrated 16.41
  facial bone, synthetic (alloplastic) 76.92
  fallopian tube (Mulligan hood) (silastic tube) (stent) 66.93
    into uterus 66.74
  gastroepiploic artery to coronary artery 36.17
  hearing device, electromagnetic 20.95
  heart
    artificial 37.52
      total internal biventricular replacement system 37.52
        AbioCor® 37.52
        CardioWest™ (TAH-t) 37.52
    assist system
      CentriMag® — *see* Insertion, circulatory support device
      external heart assist device, percutaneous — *see* Insertion, circulatory support device
      external heart assist system, open approach 37.65
      extrinsic 37.68
      HeartMate® II left ventricular assist system [LVAS] 37.66
      HeartMate® implantable heart assist system 37.66
      Impella® percutaneous external circulatory assist device — *see* Insertion, circulatory support device
      implantable 37.66
      non-implantable — *see* Insertion, circulatory support device
      percutaneous external circulatory assist device — *see* Insertion, circulatory support device
      pulsation balloon 37.61
      pVAD (percutaneous VAD) — *see* Insertion, circulatory support device
      TandemHeart® — *see* Insertion, circulatory support device
      temporary non-implantable circulatory assist device — *see* Insertion, circulatory support device
      that for destination therapy (DT) 37.66
    auxiliary ventricle 37.62
    cardiac support device (CSD) 37.41
    circulatory assist system — *see* Implant, heart, assist system
    CorCap™ 37.41

☑ **Additional Digit Required — Refer to the Tabular List for Digit Selection**   ▽ **Subterms under main terms may continue to next column or page**

2014 ICD-9-CM   ▶◀ **Revised Text**   ● **New Line**   ▲ **Revised Code**   October 2013 · Volume 3 — 27

☑ Additional Digit Required — Refer to the Tabular List for Digit Selection   ▽ Subterms under main terms may continue to next column or page

28 — Volume 3 · October 2013   ▶◀ Revised Text   ● New Line   ▲ Revised Code   2014 ICD-9-CM

Implant, implantation — *continued*
  prosthesis, prosthetic device — *continued*
    penis — *continued*
      inflatable (internal) 64.97
    skin (dermal regenerative) (matrix) 86.67
    testicular (bilateral) (unilateral) 62.7
  pulsation balloon (phase-shift) 37.61
  pump, infusion 86.06
  radial artery 36.19
  radioactive isotope 92.27
  radium (radon) 92.27
  retinal attachment 14.41
    with buckling 14.41
  Rheos™ carotid sinus baroreflex activation device 39.81
  Rickham reservoir 02.22
  silicone
    breast (bilateral) 85.54
      unilateral 85.53
    skin (for filling of defect) 86.02
      for augmentation NEC 86.89
  spine NEC 84.59
    facet replacement device(s) 84.84
    interspinous process decompression device 84.80
    pedicle-based dynamic stabilization device(s) 84.82
    posterior motion preservation device(s) — *see* category 84.8
  stimoceiver — *see* Implant, neurostimulator, by site
  stimulator
    electrodes
      carotid sinus (baroflex activation device) 39.82
        with synchronous pulse generator implantation (total system) 39.81
    pulse generator
      carotid sinus (baroreflex activation device) 39.83
        with synchronous electrode(s) implantation (total system) 39.81
  subdural
    grids 02.93
    strips 02.93
  Swanson prosthesis (joint) (silastic) NEC 81.96
    carpocarpal, carpometacarpal 81.74
    finger 81.71
    hand (metacarpophalangeal) (interphalangeal) 81.71
    interphalangeal 81.71
    knee (partial) (total) 81.54
      revision 81.55
    metacarpophalangeal 81.71
    toe 81.57
      for hallux valgus repair 77.59
    wrist (partial) 81.74
      total 81.73
  systemic arteries into myocardium (Vineberg type operation) 36.2
  Tandem™ heart 37.68
  telescope (IMT) (miniature) 13.91
  testicular prosthesis (bilateral) (unilateral) 62.7
  tissue expander (skin) NEC 86.93
    breast 85.95
  tissue mandril (for vascular graft) 39.99
    with
      blood vessel repair 39.56
      vascular bypass or shunt — *see* Bypass, vascular
  tooth (bud) (germ) 23.5
    prosthetic 23.6
  umbrella, vena cava 38.7
  ureters into
    bladder 56.74
    intestine 56.71
      external diversion 56.51
    skin 56.61
  urethra
    for repair of urinary stress incontinence
      collagen 59.72

Implant, implantation — *continued*
  urethra — *continued*
    for repair of urinary stress incontinence — *continued*
      fat 59.72
      polytef 59.72
  urethral sphincter, artificial (inflatable) 58.93
  urinary sphincter, artificial (inflatable) 58.93
  valve(s)
    endovascular — *see* Replacement, heart valve, by site
  vascular access device 86.07
  vitreous (silicone) 14.75
    for retinal reattachment 14.41
      with buckling 14.41
  vocal cord(s) (paraglottic) 31.98
  X Stop™ 84.80
Implosion (psychologic desensitization) 94.33
Incision (and drainage)
  with
    exploration — *see* Exploration
    removal of foreign body — *see* Removal, foreign body
  abdominal wall 54.0
    as operative approach — *omit code*
  abscess (*see also* Incision, by site)
    antecubital fossa 86.04
    appendix 47.2
      with appendectomy 47.09
        laparoscopic 47.01
    axilla 86.04
    cheek 86.04
    extraperitoneal 54.0
    face 86.04
    gluteal 86.04
    groin region (abdominal wall) (inguinal) 54.0
      skin 86.04
      subcutaneous tissue 86.04
    hair follicle 86.04
    ischiorectal 49.01
    lip 27.0
    nailbed or nailfold 86.04
    neck 86.04
    omental 54.19
    paronychia 86.04
    perianal 49.01
    perigastric 54.19
    perineum (female) 71.09
      male 86.04
    perisplenic 54.19
    peritoneal NEC 54.19
      pelvic (female) 70.12
    popliteal space 86.04
    retroperitoneal 54.0
    sclera 12.89
    skin 86.04
    subcutaneous tissue 86.04
    subdiaphragmatic 54.19
    subhepatic 54.19
    submaxillary 86.04
    subphrenic 54.19
    supraclavicular fossa 86.04
    vas deferens 63.6
  adrenal gland 07.41
  alveolus, alveolar bone 24.0
  antecubital fossa 86.09
  anus NEC 49.93
    fistula 49.11
    septum 49.91
  appendix 47.2
  artery 38.00
    abdominal 38.06
      aorta (arch) (ascending) (descending) 38.04
    head and neck NEC 38.02
    intracranial NEC 38.01
    lower limb 38.08
    thoracic NEC 38.05
    upper limb 38.03
  atrium (heart) 37.11
  auditory canal or meatus, external 18.02
  auricle 18.09
  axilla 86.09
  Bartholin's gland or cyst 71.22

Incision — *continued*
  bile duct (with T or Y tube insertion) NEC 51.59
    for
      exploration 51.59
      relief of obstruction 51.49
    common (exploratory) 51.51
      for
        relief of obstruction NEC 51.42
        removal of calculus 51.41
  bladder 57.19
    neck (transurethral) 57.91
    percutaneous suprapubic (closed) 57.17
    suprapubic NEC 57.18
  blood vessel (*see also* Angiotomy) 38.00
  bone 77.10
    alveolus, alveolar 24.0
    carpals, metacarpals 77.14
    clavicle 77.11
    facial 76.09
    femur 77.15
    fibula 77.17
    humerus 77.12
    patella 77.16
    pelvic 77.19
    phalanges (foot) (hand) 77.19
    radius 77.13
    scapula 77.11
    skull 01.24
    specified site NEC 77.19
    tarsals, metatarsals 77.18
    thorax (ribs) (sternum) 77.11
    tibia 77.17
    ulna 77.13
    vertebrae 77.19
  brain 01.39
    cortical adhesions 02.91
  breast (skin) 85.0
    with removal of tissue expander 85.96
  bronchus 33.0
  buccal space 27.0
  bulbourethral gland 58.91
  bursa 83.03
    hand 82.03
    pharynx 29.0
  carotid body 39.89
  cerebral (meninges) 01.39
    epidural or extradural space 01.24
    subarachnoid or subdural space 01.31
  cerebrum 01.39
  cervix 69.95
    to
      assist delivery 73.93
      replace inverted uterus 75.93
  chalazion 08.09
    with removal of capsule 08.21
  cheek 86.09
  chest wall (for extrapleural drainage) (for removal of foreign body) 34.01
    as operative approach — *omit code*
  common bile duct (for exploration) 51.51
    for
      relief of obstruction 51.42
      removal of calculus 51.41
  common wall between posterior left atrium and coronary sinus (with roofing of resultant defect with patch graft) 35.82
  conjunctiva 10.1
  cornea 11.1
    radial (refractive) 11.75
  cranial sinus 01.21
  craniobuccal pouch 07.72
  cul-de-sac 70.12
  cyst
    dentigerous 24.0
    radicular (apical) (periapical) 24.0
  Dührssen's (cervix, to assist delivery) 73.93
  duodenum 45.01
  ear
    external 18.09
    inner 20.79
    middle 20.23
  endocardium 37.11
  endolymphatic sac 20.79
  epididymis 63.92

Incision — *continued*
  epidural space, cerebral 01.24
  epigastric region 54.0
    intra-abdominal 54.19
  esophagus, esophageal NEC 42.09
    web 42.01
  exploratory — *see* Exploration
  extradural space (cerebral) 01.24
  extrapleural 34.01
  eyebrow 08.09
  eyelid 08.09
    margin (trichiasis) 08.01
  face 86.09
  fallopian tube 66.01
  fascia 83.09
    with division 83.14
      hand 82.12
    hand 82.09
      with division 82.12
  fascial compartments, head and neck 27.0
  fistula, anal 49.11
  flank 54.0
  furuncle — *see* Incision, by site
  gallbladder 51.04
  gingiva 24.0
  gluteal 86.09
  groin region (abdominal wall) (inguinal) 54.0
    skin 86.09
    subcutaneous tissue 86.09
  gum 24.0
  hair follicles 86.09
  heart 37.10
    valve — *see* Valvulotomy
  hematoma (*see also* Incision, by site)
    axilla 86.04
    broad ligament 69.98
    ear 18.09
    episiotomy site 75.91
    fossa (superficial) NEC 86.04
    groin region (abdominal wall) (inguinal) 54.0
      skin 86.04
      subcutaneous tissue 86.04
    laparotomy site 54.12
    mediastinum 34.1
    perineum (female) 71.09
      male 86.04
    popliteal space 86.04
    scrotum 61.0
    skin 86.04
    space of Retzius 59.19
    subcutaneous tissue 86.04
    vagina (cuff) 70.14
      episiotomy site 75.91
      obstetrical NEC 75.92
  hepatic ducts 51.59
  hordeolum 08.09
  hygroma (*see also* Incision, by site)
    cystic 40.0
  hymen 70.11
  hypochondrium 54.0
    intra-abdominal 54.19
  hypophysis 07.72
  iliac fossa 54.0
  infratemporal fossa 27.0
  ingrown nail 86.09
  intestine 45.00
    large 45.03
    small 45.02
  intracerebral 01.39
  intracranial (epidural space) (extradural space) 01.24
    subarachnoid or subdural space 01.31
  intraperitoneal 54.19
  ischiorectal tissue 49.02
    abscess 49.01
  joint structures (*see also* Arthrotomy) 80.10
  kidney 55.01
    pelvis 55.11
  labia 71.09
  lacrimal
    canaliculus 09.52
    gland 09.0
    passage NEC 09.59
    punctum 09.51

☑ **Additional Digit Required** — Refer to the Tabular List for Digit Selection   🔻 **Subterms under main terms may continue to next column or page**

2014 ICD-9-CM   ▶◀ **Revised Text**   ● **New Line**   ▲ **Revised Code**   **Volume 3 — 29**

Incision — continued
  lacrimal — continued
    sac 09.53
  larynx NEC 31.3
  ligamentum flavum (spine) — omit code
  liver 50.0
  lung 33.1
  lymphangioma 40.0
  lymphatic structure (channel) (node) (vessel)
    40.0
  mastoid 20.21
  mediastinum 34.1
  meibomian gland 08.09
  meninges (cerebral) 01.31
    spinal 03.09
  midpalmar space 82.04
  mouth NEC 27.92
    floor 27.0
  muscle 83.02
    with division 83.19
      hand 82.19
    hand 82.02
      with division 82.19
  myocardium 37.11
  nailbed or nailfold 86.09
  nasolacrimal duct (stricture) 09.59
  neck 86.09
  nerve (cranial) (peripheral) NEC 04.04
    root (spinal) 03.1
  nose 21.1
  omentum 54.19
  orbit (see also Orbitotomy) 16.09
  ovary 65.09
    laparoscopic 65.01
  palate 27.1
  palmar space (middle) 82.04
  pancreas 52.09
  pancreatic sphincter 51.82
    endoscopic 51.85
  parapharyngeal (oral) (transcervical) 28.0
  paronychia 86.09
  parotid
    gland or duct 26.0
    space 27.0
  pelvirectal tissue 48.81
  penis 64.92
  perianal (skin) (tissue) 49.02
    abscess 49.01
  perigastric 54.19
  perineum (female) 71.09
    male 86.09
  peripheral vessels
    lower limb
      artery 38.08
      vein 38.09
    upper limb (artery) (vein) 38.03
  periprostatic tissue 60.81
  perirectal tissue 48.81
  perirenal tissue 59.09
  perisplenic 54.19
  peritoneum 54.95
    by laparotomy 54.19
    pelvic (female) 70.12
      male 54.19
  periureteral tissue 59.09
  periurethral tissue 58.91
  perivesical tissue 59.19
  petrous pyramid (air cells) (apex) (mastoid)
    20.22
  pharynx, pharyngeal (bursa) 29.0
    space, lateral 27.0
  pilonidal sinus (cyst) 86.03
  pineal gland 07.52
  pituitary (gland) 07.72
  pleura NEC 34.09
  popliteal space 86.09
  postzygomatic space 27.0
  pouch of Douglas 70.12
  prostate (perineal approach) (transurethral
    approach) 60.0
  pterygopalatine fossa 27.0
  pulp canal (tooth) 24.0
  Rathke's pouch 07.72
  rectovaginal septum 48.81
  rectum 48.0
    stricture 48.91

Incision — continued
  renal pelvis 55.11
  retroperitoneum 54.0
  retropharyngeal (oral) (transcervical) 28.0
  salivary gland or duct 26.0
  sclera 12.89
  scrotum 61.0
  sebaceous cyst 86.04
  seminal vesicle 60.72
  sinus — see Sinusotomy
  Skene's duct or gland 71.09
  skin 86.09
    with drainage 86.04
    breast 85.0
    cardiac pacemaker pocket, new site
      37.79
    ear 18.09
    nose 21.1
    subcutaneous tunnel for pulse generator
      lead wire 86.99
      with initial procedure — omit code
    thalamic stimulator pulse generator
      pocket, new site 86.99
      with initial insertion of battery pack-
        age — omit code
    tunnel, subcutaneous for pulse genera-
      tor lead wire 86.99
      with initial procedure — omit code
  skull (bone) 01.24
  soft tissue NEC 83.09
    with division 83.19
      hand 82.19
    hand 82.09
      with division 82.19
  space of Retzius 59.19
  spermatic cord 63.93
  sphincter of Oddi 51.82
    endoscopic 51.85
  spinal
    cord 03.09
    nerve root 03.1
  spleen 41.2
  stomach 43.0
  stye 08.09
  subarachnoid space, cerebral 01.31
  subcutaneous tissue 86.09
    with drainage 86.04
    tunnel
      esophageal 42.86
        with anastomosis — see Anasto-
          mosis, esophagus, an-
          testernal
      pulse generator lead wire 86.99
        with initial procedure — omit
          code
  subdiaphragmatic space 54.19
  subdural space, cerebral 01.31
  sublingual space 27.0
  submandibular space 27.0
  submaxillary 86.09
    with drainage 86.04
  submental space 27.0
  subphrenic space 54.19
  supraclavicular fossa 86.09
    with drainage 86.04
  sweat glands, skin 86.04
  temporal pouches 27.0
  tendon (sheath) 83.01
    with division 83.13
      hand 82.11
    hand 82.01
      with division 82.11
  testis 62.0
  thenar space 82.04
  thymus (open) (other) 07.92
    thoracoscopic 07.95
  thyroid (field) (gland) NEC 06.09
    postoperative 06.02
  tongue NEC 25.94
    for tongue tie 25.91
  tonsil 28.0
  trachea NEC 31.3
  tunica vaginalis 61.0
  umbilicus 54.0
  urachal cyst 54.0
  ureter 56.2

Incision — continued
  urethra 58.0
  uterus (corpus) 68.0
    cervix 69.95
    for termination of pregnancy 74.91
    septum (congenital) 68.22
  uvula 27.71
  vagina (cuff) (septum) (stenosis) 70.14
    for
      incisional hematoma (episiotomy)
        75.91
      obstetrical hematoma NEC 75.92
      pelvic abscess 70.12
  vas deferens 63.6
  vein 38.00
    abdominal 38.07
    head and neck NEC 38.02
    intracranial NEC 38.01
    lower limb 38.09
    thoracic NEC 38.05
    upper limb 38.03
  vertebral column 03.09
  vulva 71.09
    obstetrical 75.92
  web, esophageal 42.01
Incudectomy NEC 19.3
  with
    stapedectomy (see also Stapedectomy)
      19.19
    tympanoplasty — see Tympanoplasty
Incudopexy 19.19
Incudostapediopexy 19.19
  with incus replacement 19.11
Indentation, sclera, for buckling — see also
  Buckling, scleral 14.49
Indicator dilution flow measurement 89.68
Induction
  abortion
    by
      D and C 69.01
      insertion of prostaglandin supposito-
        ry 96.49
      intra-amniotic injection
        (prostaglandin) (saline) 75.0
  labor
    medical 73.4
    surgical 73.01
      intra- and extra-amniotic injection
        73.1
    stripping of membranes 73.1
Inflation
  belt wrap 93.99
  Eustachian tube 20.8
  fallopian tube 66.8
    with injection of therapeutic agent 66.95
Infolding, sclera, for buckling — see also
  Buckling, scleral 14.49
Infraction, turbinates (nasal) 21.62
Infundibulectomy
  hypophyseal (see also Hypophysectomy,
    partial) 07.63
  ventricle (heart) (right) 35.34
    in total repair of tetralogy of Fallot 35.81
Infusion (intra-arterial) (intravenous)
  with
    disruption of blood brain barrier [BBBD]
      00.19
  4-Factor Prothrombin Complex Concen- ●
    trate 00.96
  Abciximab 99.20
  antibiotic
    oxazolidinone class 00.14
  antineoplastic agent (chemotherapeutic)
    99.25
    biological response modifier [BRM] 99.28
    cintredekin besudotox 99.28
    CLO 17.70
    clofarabine 17.70
    CLOLAR® 17.70
    high-dose interleukin-2 00.15
    low-dose interleukin-2 99.28
  biological response modifier [BRM], antineo-
    plastic agent 99.28
    cintredekin besudotox 99.28
    high-dose interleukin-2 00.15
    low-dose interleukin-2 99.28

Infusion — continued
  cancer chemotherapy agent NEC 99.25
  cintredekin besudotox 99.28
  CLO 17.70
  clofarabine 17.70
  CLOLAR® 17.70
  drotrecogin alfa (activated) 00.11
  electrolytes 99.18
  enzymes, thrombolytic (streptokinase) (tis-
    sue plasminogen activator) (TPA)
    (urokinase)
    direct coronary artery 36.04
    intravenous 99.10
  Eptifibatide 99.20
  gamma globulin 99.14
  glucarpidase 00.95
  GP IIb/IIIa inhibitor 99.20
  hormone substance NEC 99.24
  human B-type natriuretic peptide (hBNP)
    00.13
  IgG (immunoglobulin) 99.14
  immunoglobulin (IgG) (IVIG) (IVIg) 99.14
  immunosuppressive antibody therapy 00.18
  interleukin-2
    high-dose 00.15
    low-dose 99.28
  IVIG (immunoglobulin) (IVIg) 99.14
  Kcentra™ 00.96   ●
  lymphocyte 99.09
  nesiritide 00.13
  neuroprotective agent 99.75
  nimodipine 99.75
  nutritional substance — see Nutrition
  platelet inhibitor
    direct coronary artery 36.04
    intravenous 99.20
  Proleukin (low-dose) 99.28
    high-dose 00.15
  prophylactic substance NEC 99.29
  radioimmunoconjugate 92.28
  radioimmunotherapy 92.28
  radioisotope (liquid brachytherapy) (liquid
    I-125) 92.20
  recombinant protein 00.11
  reteplase 99.10
  therapeutic substance NEC 99.29
  thrombolytic agent (enzyme) (streptoki-
    nase) 99.10
    with percutaneous transluminal angio-
      plasty

> Note: Also use 00.40, 00.41, 00.42, or
> 00.43 to show the total number of ves-
> sels treated.

        coronary 00.66
          non-coronary vessel(s) 39.50
          specified site NEC 39.50
        direct intracoronary artery 36.04
  tirofiban (HCl) 99.20
  vaccine
    tumor 99.28
  vasopressor 00.17
  Voraxaze® 00.95
Injection (into) (hypodermically) (intramuscularly) (intravenously) (acting locally or
  systemically)
  Actinomycin D, for cancer chemotherapy
    99.25
  adhesion barrier substance 99.77
  alcohol
    nerve — see Injection, nerve
    spinal 03.8
  anterior chamber, eye (air) (liquid) (medica-
    tion) 12.92
  anti-D (Rhesus) globulin 99.11
  anti-infective NEC 99.22
  antibiotic 99.21
    oxazolidinone class 00.14
  anticoagulant 99.19
  antidote NEC 99.16
  antineoplastic agent (chemotherapeutic)
    NEC 99.25
    biological response modifier [BRM] 99.28
    cintredekin besudotox 99.28
    high-dose interleukin-2 00.15
    low-dose interleukin-2 99.28
  antivenin 99.16

Injection — Insertion

☑ **Additional Digit Required** — Refer to the Tabular List for Digit Selection   ▽ **Subterms under main terms may continue to next column or page**

2014 ICD-9-CM   ►◄ Revised Text   ● New Line   ▲ Revised Code   Volume 3 — 31

☑ Additional Digit Required — Refer to the Tabular List for Digit Selection   ▽ Subterms under main terms may continue to next column or page

32 — Volume 3   ▶◀ Revised Text   ● New Line   ▲ Revised Code   2014 ICD-9-CM

Insertion — Insertion

☑ **Additional Digit Required** — Refer to the Tabular List for Digit Selection   ▽ **Subterms under main terms may continue to next column or page**

2014 ICD-9-CM   ▶◀ Revised Text   ● New Line   ▲ Revised Code   **Volume 3 — 33**

Insertion — *continued*
  stent(s) — *continued*
    peripheral vessel 39.90

Note — Also use 00.40, 00.41, 00.42, or 00.43 to show the total number of vessels treated. Use code 00.44 once to show procedure on a bifurcated vessel. In addition, use 00.45, 00.46, 00.47, or 00.48 to show the number of vascular stents inserted.

        bare, drug-coated 39.90
        drug-eluting 00.55
        femoral artery, superficial, drug-eluting 00.60
        precerebral 00.64

Note — Also use 00.40, 00.41, 00.42, or 00.43 to show the total number of vessels treated. Use code 00.44 once to show procedure on a bifurcated vessel. In addition, use 00.45, 00.46, 00.47, or 00.48 to show the number of vascular stents inserted.

    renal 39.90
        bare, drug-coated 39.90
        drug-eluting 00.55
    subclavian 39.90

Note — Also use 00.40, 00.41, 00.42, or 00.43 to show the total number of vessels treated. Use code 00.44 once to show procedure on a bifurcated vessel In addition, use 00.45, 00.46, 00.47, or 00.48 to show the number of vascular stents inserted.

        bare, drug-coated 39.90
        drug-eluting 00.55
    tracheobronchial 96.05
    vertebral 00.64

Note — Also use 00.40, 00.41, 00.42, or 00.43 to show the total number of vessels treated. Use code 00.44 once to show procedure on a bifurcated vessel. In addition, use 00.45, 00.46, 00.47, or 00.48 to show the number of vascular stents inserted.

  sternal fixation device with rigid plates 84.94
  stimoceiver — *see* Implant, neurostimulator, by site
  stimulator for bone growth — *see* category 78.9 ☑
  subdural
    grids 02.93
    strips 02.93
  suppository
    prostaglandin (for abortion) 96.49
    vagina 96.49
  Swan-Ganz catheter (pulmonary) 89.64
  tampon
    esophagus 96.06
    uterus 69.91
    vagina 96.14
      after delivery or abortion 75.8
  Tandem™ heart 37.68
  telescope (IMT) (miniature) 13.91
  testicular prosthesis (bilateral) (unilateral) 62.7
  tissue expander (skin) NEC 86.93
    breast 85.95
  tissue mandril (peripheral vessel) (Dacron) (Spark's type) 39.99
    with
      blood vessel repair 39.56
      vascular bypass or shunt — *see* Bypass, vascular
  tongs, skull (with synchronous skeletal traction) 02.94
  totally implanted device for bone growth (invasive) — *see* category 78.9 ☑
  tube (see also Catheterization and Intubation)
    bile duct 51.43
      endoscopic 51.87
    chest 34.04

Insertion — *continued*
  tube (see also Catheterization and Intubation) — *continued*
    chest — *continued*
      revision (with lysis of adhesions) 34.04
        thoracoscopic 34.06
      thoracoscopic 34.06
    endotracheal 96.04
    esophagus (nonoperative) (Sengstaken) 96.06
      permanent (silicone) (Souttar) 42.81
    feeding
      esophageal 42.81
      gastric 96.6
      nasogastric 96.6
    gastric
      by gastrostomy — *see* category 43.1 ☑
      for
        decompression, intestinal 96.07
        feeding 96.6
    intercostal catheter (with water seal), for drainage 34.04
      revision (with lysis of adhe-sions) 34.04
        thoracoscopic 34.06
      thoracoscopic 34.06
    Miller-Abbott (for intestinal decompression) 96.08
    naso-intestinal 96.08
    nasobiliary (drainage) 51.86
    nasogastric (for intestinal decompression) NEC 96.07
    nasopancreatic drainage (endoscopic) 52.97
    pancreatic duct 52.92
      endoscopic 52.93
    rectum 96.09
    stomach (nasogastric) (for intestinal de-compression) NEC 96.07
      for feeding 96.6
    tracheobronchial 96.05
  umbrella device
    atrial septum (King-Mills) 35.52
    vena cava (Mobitz-Uddin) 38.7
  ureteral stent (transurethral) 59.8
    with ureterotomy 59.8 *[56.2]*
  urinary sphincter, artificial (AUS) (inflatable) 58.93
  vaginal mold 96.15
  valve(s)
    bronchus
      multiple lobes 33.73
      single lobe 33.71
    Holter 02.22
    Hufnagel — *see* Replacement, heart valve
    pharyngeal (artificial) 31.75
    Spitz-Holter 02.22
    vas deferens 63.95
  vascular access device, totally implantable 86.07
  vena cava sieve or umbrella 38.7
  Vinke tongs (skull) (with synchronous skeletal traction) 02.94
  X Stop™ 84.80
Instillation
  bladder 96.49
  digestive tract, except gastric gavage 96.43
  genitourinary NEC 96.49
  radioisotope (intracavitary) (intravenous) 92.28
  thoracic cavity 34.92
Insufflation
  Eustachian tube 20.8
  fallopian tube (air) (dye) (gas) (saline) 66.8
    for radiography — *see* Hysterosalpingography
    therapeutic substance 66.95
  lumbar retroperitoneal, bilateral 88.15
Intercricothyroidotomy (for assistance in breathing) 31.1
Interleukin-2, infusion
  high-dose 00.15
  low-dose 99.28

Intermittent positive pressure breathing (IPPB) 93.91
Interposition operation
  antesternal or antethoracic NEC (see also Anastomosis, esophagus, antesternal, with, interposition) 42.68
  esophageal reconstruction (intrathoracic) (retrosternal) NEC (see also Anastomosis, esophagus, with, interposition) 42.58
  uterine suspension 69.21
Interrogation
  cardioverter-defibrillator, automatic (AICD)
    with catheter based invasive electrophysiologic testing 37.26
    with NIPS (arrhythmia induction) 37.20
    interrogation only (bedside device check) 89.49
  CRT-D (cardiac resynchronization defibrillator)
    with catheter based invasive electrophysiologic testing 37.26
    with NIPS (arrhythmia induction) 37.20
    interrogation only (bedside device check) 89.49
  CRT-P (cardiac resynchronization pacemaker)
    with catheter based invasive electrophysiologic testing 37.26
    with NIPS (arrhythmia induction) 37.20
    interrogation only (bedside device check) 89.45
  pacemaker
    with catheter based invasive electrophysiologic testing 37.26
    with NIPS (arrhythmia induction) 37.20
    interrogation only (bedside device check) 89.45
Interruption
  vena cava (inferior) (superior) 38.7
Interview (evaluation) (diagnostic)
  medical, except psychiatric 89.05
    brief (abbreviated history) 89.01
    comprehensive (history and evaluation of new problem) 89.03
    limited (interval history) 89.02
    specified type NEC 89.04
  psychiatric NEC 94.19
    follow-up 94.19
    initial 94.19
    pre-commitment 94.13
Intimectomy 38.10
  abdominal 38.16
  aorta (arch) (ascending) (descending) 38.14
  head and neck NEC 38.12
  intracranial NEC 38.11
  lower limb 38.18
  thoracic NEC 38.15
  upper limb 38.13
Intraoperative anesthetic effect monitoring and titration (IAEMT) 00.94 *[89.14]*
Introduction
  orthodontic appliance 24.7
  therapeutic substance (acting locally or systemically) NEC 99.29
    bursa 83.96
      hand 82.94
    fascia 83.98
      hand 82.96
    heart 37.92
    joint 81.92
      temporomandibular 76.96
    ligament (joint) 81.92
    pericardium 37.93
    soft tissue NEC 83.98
      hand 82.96
    tendon 83.97
      hand 82.95
    vein 39.92
Intubation — *see also* Catheterization and Insertion
  bile duct(s) 51.59
    common 51.51
      endoscopic 51.87
    endoscopic 51.87

Intubation — *see also* Catheterization and Insertion — *continued*
  esophagus (nonoperative) (Sengstaken) 96.06
    permanent tube (silicone) (Souttar) 42.81
  Eustachian tube 20.8
  intestine (for decompression) 96.08
  lacrimal for
    dilation 09.42
    tear drainage, intranasal 09.81
  larynx 96.05
  naso-intestinal 96.08
  nasobiliary (drainage) 51.86
  nasogastric
    for
      decompression, intestinal 96.07
      feeding 96.6
  nasolacrimal (duct) (with irrigation) 09.44
  nasopancreatic drainage (endoscopic) 52.97
  respiratory tract NEC 96.05
  small intestine (Miller-Abbott) 96.08
  stomach (nasogastric) (for intestinal decompression) NEC 96.07
    for feeding 96.6
  trachea 96.04
  ventriculocisternal 02.22
Invagination, diverticulum
  gastric 44.69
    laparoscopic 44.68
  pharynx 29.59
  stomach 44.69
    laparoscopic 44.68
Inversion
  appendix 47.99
  diverticulum
    gastric 44.69
      laparoscopic 44.68
    intestine
      large 45.49
        endoscopic 45.43
      small 45.34
    stomach 44.69
      laparoscopic 44.68
  tunica vaginalis 61.49
IOERT (intra-operative electron radiation therapy) 92.41
IOM (intra-operative neurophysiologic monitoring) 00.94
Ionization, medical 99.27
Iontherapy 99.27
Iontophoresis 99.27
Iridectomy (basal) (buttonhole) (optical) (peripheral) (total) 12.14
  with
    capsulectomy 13.65
    cataract extraction — *see* Extraction, cataract
    filtering operation (for glaucoma) NEC 12.65
    scleral
      fistulization 12.65
      thermocauterization 12.62
      trephination 12.61
Iridencleisis 12.63
Iridesis 12.63
Irido-capsulectomy 13.65
Iridocyclectomy 12.44
Iridocystectomy 12.42
Iridodesis 12.63
Iridoplasty NEC 12.39
Iridosclerectomy 12.65
Iridosclerotomy 12.69
Iridotasis 12.63
Iridotomy 12.12
  by photocoagulation 12.12
  with transfixion 12.11
  for iris bombé 12.11
  specified type NEC 12.12
Iron lung 93.99
Irradiation
  gamma, stereotactic 92.32
Irrigation
  anterior chamber (eye) 12.91
  bronchus NEC 96.56
  canaliculus 09.42

☑ Additional Digit Required — Refer to the Tabular List for Digit Selection   ⩗ Subterms under main terms may continue to next column or page

34 — Volume 3   ►◄ Revised Text   ● New Line   ▲ Revised Code   2014 ICD-9-CM

Irrigation — *continued*
  catheter
    ureter 96.46
    urinary, indwelling NEC 96.48
    vascular 96.57
    ventricular 02.41
    wound 96.58
  cholecystostomy 96.41
  cornea 96.51
    with removal of foreign body 98.21
  corpus cavernosum 64.98
  cystostomy 96.47
  ear (removal of cerumen) 96.52
  enterostomy 96.36
  eye 96.51
    with removal of foreign body 98.21
  gastrostomy 96.36
  lacrimal
    canaliculi 09.42
    punctum 09.41
  muscle 83.02
    hand 82.02
  nasal
    passages 96.53
    sinus 22.00
  nasolacrimal duct 09.43
    with insertion of tube or stent 09.44
  nephrostomy 96.45
  peritoneal 54.25
  pyelostomy 96.45
  rectal 96.39
  stomach 96.33
  tendon (sheath) 83.01
    hand 82.01
  trachea NEC 96.56
  traumatic cataract 13.3
  tube
    biliary NEC 96.41
    nasogastric NEC 96.34
    pancreatic 96.42
  ureterostomy 96.46
  ventricular shunt 02.41
  wound (cleaning) NEC 96.59
Irving operation (tubal ligation) 66.32
Irwin operation — *see also* Osteotomy 77.30
Ischiectomy (partial) 77.89
  total 77.99
Ischiopubiotomy 77.39
Isolation
  after contact with infectious disease 99.84
  ileal loop 45.51
  intestinal segment or pedicle flap
    large 45.52
    small 45.51
Isthmectomy, thyroid — *see also* Thyroidectomy, partial 06.39
IVUS — *see* Ultrasound, intravascular, by site

J

Jaboulay operation (gastroduodenostomy) 44.39
  laparoscopic 44.38
Janeway operation (permanent gastrostomy) 43.19
Jatene operation (arterial switch) 35.84
Jejunectomy 45.62
Jejunocecostomy 45.93
Jejunocholecystostomy 51.32
Jejunocolostomy 45.93
Jejunoileostomy 45.91
Jejunojejunostomy 45.91
Jejunopexy 46.61
Jejunorrhaphy 46.73
Jejunostomy (feeding) 46.39
  delayed opening 46.31
  loop 46.01
  percutaneous (endoscopic) (PEJ) 46.32
  revision 46.41
Jejunotomy 45.02
Johanson operation (urethral reconstruction) 58.46
Jones operation
  claw toe (transfer of extensor hallucis longus tendon) 77.57
    modified (with arthrodesis) 77.57
  dacryocystorhinostomy 09.81

Jones operation — *continued*
  hammer toe (interphalangeal fusion) 77.56
    modified (tendon transfer with arthrodesis) 77.57
  repair of peroneal tendon 83.88
Joplin operation (exostectomy with tendon transfer) 77.53

K

Kader operation (temporary gastrostomy) 43.19
Kasai portoenterostomy 51.37
Kaufman operation (for urinary stress incontinence) 59.79
Kazanjiian operation (buccal vestibular sulcus extension) 24.91
Kehr operation (hepatopexy) 50.69
Keller operation (bunionectomy) 77.59
Kelly-Stoeckel operation (urethrovesical plication) 59.3
Kelly (-Kennedy) operation (urethrovesical plication) 59.3
Kelotomy 53.9
Keratectomy (complete) (partial) (superficial) 11.49
  for pterygium 11.39
    with corneal graft 11.32
Keratocentesis (for hyphema) 12.91
Keratomileusis 11.71
Keratophakia 11.72
Keratoplasty (tectonic) (with autograft) (with homograft) 11.60
  lamellar (nonpenetrating) (with homograft) 11.62
    with autograft 11.61
  penetrating (full-thickness) (with homograft) 11.64
    with autograft 11.63
  perforating — *see* Keratoplasty, penetrating
  refractive 11.71
  specified type NEC 11.69
Keratoprosthesis 11.73
Keratotomy (delimiting) (posterior) 11.1
  radial (refractive) 11.75
Kerr operation (low cervical cesarean section) 74.1
Kessler operation (arthroplasty, carpometacarpal joint) 81.74
Kidner operation (excision of accessory navicular bone) (with tendon transfer) 77.98
Killian operation (frontal sinusotomy) 22.41
Kineplasty — *see* Cineplasty
King-Steelquist operation (hind-quarter amputation) 84.19
Kirk operation (amputation through thigh) 84.17
Kockogram (ileal conduitogram) 87.78
Kockoscopy 45.12
Kock pouch
  bowel anastomosis — *omit code*
  continent ileostomy 46.22
  cutaneous uretero-ileostomy 56.51
  ESWL (extracorporeal shockwave lithotripsy) 98.51
  removal, calculus 57.19
  revision, cutaneous uretero-ileostomy 56.52
  urinary diversion procedure 56.51
Kondoleon operation (correction of lymphedema) 40.9
Krause operation (sympathetic denervation) 05.29
Kroener operation (partial salpingectomy) 66.69
Kroenlein operation (lateral orbitotomy) 16.01
Krönig operation (low cervical cesarean section) 74.1
Krukenberg operation (reconstruction of below-elbow amputation) 82.89
Kuhnt-Szymanowski operation (ectropion repair with lid reconstruction) 08.44
Kyphoplasty 81.66

L

Labbe operation (gastrotomy) 43.0
Labiectomy (bilateral) 71.62

Labiectomy — *continued*
  unilateral 71.61
Labyrinthectomy (transtympanic) 20.79
Labyrinthotomy (transtympanic) 20.79
Ladd operation (mobilization of intestine) 54.95
Lagrange operation (iridosclerectomy) 12.65
Lambrinudi operation (triple arthrodesis) 81.12
Laminectomy (decompression) (for exploration) 03.09
  as operative approach — *omit code*
  with
    excision of herniated intervertebral disc (nucleus pulposus) 80.51
    excision of other intraspinal lesion (tumor) 03.4
  reopening of site 03.02
Laminography — *see* Radiography
Laminoplasty, expansile 03.09
Laminotomy (decompression) (for exploration) 03.09
  as operative approach — *omit code*
  reopening of site 03.02
Langenbeck operation (cleft palate repair) 27.62
Laparoamnioscopy 75.31
Laparorrhaphy 54.63
Laparoscopy 54.21
  with
    biopsy (intra-abdominal) 54.24
      uterine ligaments 68.15
      uterus 68.16
    destruction of fallopian tubes — *see* Destruction, fallopian tube
Laparotomy NEC 54.19
  as operative approach — *omit code*
  exploratory (pelvic) 54.11
  reopening of recent operative site (for control of hemorrhage) (for exploration) (for incision of hematoma) 54.12
Laparotrachelotomy 74.1
Lapidus operation (bunionectomy with metatarsal osteotomy) 77.51
Larry operation (shoulder disarticulation) 84.08
Laryngectomy
  with radical neck dissection (with synchronous thyroidectomy) (with synchronous tracheostomy) 30.4
  complete (with partial laryngectomy) (with synchronous tracheostomy) 30.3
    with radical neck dissection (with synchronous thyroidectomy) (with synchronous tracheostomy) 30.4
  frontolateral partial (extended) 30.29
  glottosupraglottic partial 30.29
  lateral partial 30.29
  partial (frontolateral) (glottosupraglottic) (lateral) (submucous) (supraglottic) (vertical) 30.29
  radical (with synchronous thyroidectomy) (with synchronous tracheostomy) 30.4
  submucous (partial) 30.29
  supraglottic partial 30.29
  total (with partial pharyngectomy) (with synchronous tracheostomy) 30.3
    with radical neck dissection (with synchronous thyroidectomy) (with synchronous tracheostomy) 30.4
  vertical partial 30.29
  wide field 30.3
Laryngocentesis 31.3
Laryngoesophagectomy 30.4
Laryngofissure 30.29
Laryngogram 87.09
  contrast 87.07
Laryngopharyngectomy (with synchronous tracheostomy) 30.3
  radical (with synchronous thyroidectomy) 30.4
Laryngopharyngoesophagectomy (with synchronous tracheostomy) 30.3
  with radical neck dissection (with synchronous thyroidectomy) 30.4

Laryngoplasty 31.69
Laryngorrhaphy 31.61
Laryngoscopy (suspension) (through artificial stoma) 31.42
Laryngostomy (permanent) 31.29
  revision 31.63
  temporary (emergency) 31.1
Laryngotomy 31.3
Laryngotracheobronchoscopy 33.23
  with biopsy 33.24
Laryngotracheoscopy 31.42
Laryngotracheostomy (permanent) 31.29
  temporary (emergency) 31.1
Laryngotracheotomy (temporary) 31.1
  permanent 31.29
Laser — *see also* Coagulation, Destruction, and Photocoagulation by site
  angioplasty, percutaneous transluminal 39.59
  coronary — *see* Angioplasty, coronary
Laser interstitial thermal therapy (LITT) **under guidance**
  lesion
    brain 17.61
    breast 17.69
    head and neck 17.62
    liver 17.63
    lung 17.69
    prostate 17.69
    thyroid 17.62
Lash operation
  internal cervical os repair 67.59
  laparoscopic supracervical hysterectomy 68.31
LASIK (laser-assisted in situ keratomileusis) 11.71
Latzko operation
  cesarean section 74.2
  colpocleisis 70.8
Lavage
  antral 22.00
  bronchus NEC 96.56
    diagnostic (endoscopic) bronchoalveolar lavage (BAL) (Mini-BAL) 33.24
  endotracheal 96.56
  gastric 96.33
  lung (total) (whole) 33.99
    diagnostic (endoscopic) bronchoalveolar lavage (BAL) 33.24
  nasal sinus(es) 22.00
    by puncture 22.01
    through natural ostium 22.02
  peritoneal (diagnostic) 54.25
  trachea NEC 96.56
Leadbetter-Politano operation (ureteroneocystostomy) 56.74
Leadbetter operation (urethral reconstruction) 58.46
LEEP (loop electrosurgical excision procedure) of cervix 67.32
Le Fort operation (colpocleisis) 70.8
LeMesurier operation (cleft lip repair) 27.54
Lengthening
  bone (with bone graft) 78.30
    femur 78.35
    for reconstruction of thumb 82.69
    specified site NEC (*see also* category 78.3 ☑)
    tibia 78.37
    ulna 78.33
  extraocular muscle NEC 15.21
    multiple (two or more muscles) 15.4
  fascia 83.89
    hand 82.89
  hamstring NEC 83.85
  heel cord 83.85
  leg
    femur 78.35
    tibia 78.37
  levator palpebrae muscle 08.38
  muscle 83.85
    extraocular 15.21
      multiple (two or more muscles) 15.4
    hand 82.55
  palate 27.62
    secondary or subsequent 27.63

☑ **Additional Digit Required** — Refer to the Tabular List for Digit Selection

▽ **Subterms under main terms may continue to next column or page**

Lengthening — continued
  tendon 83.85
    for claw toe repair 77.57
    hand 82.55
Leriche operation (periarterial sympathectomy) 05.25
Leucotomy, leukotomy 01.32
Leukopheresis, therapeutic 99.72
Lid suture operation (blepharoptosis) 08.31
Ligation
  adrenal vessel (artery) (vein) 07.43
  aneurysm 39.52
  appendages, dermal 86.26
  arteriovenous fistula 39.53
    coronary artery 36.99
  artery 38.80
    abdominal 38.86
    adrenal 07.43
    aorta (arch) (ascending) (descending) 38.84
    coronary (anomalous) 36.99
    ethmoidal 21.04
    external carotid 21.06
    for control of epistaxis — see Control, epistaxis
    head and neck NEC 38.82
    intracranial NEC 38.81
    lower limb 38.88
    maxillary (transantral) 21.05
    middle meningeal 02.13
    thoracic NEC 38.85
    thyroid 06.92
    upper limb 38.83
  atrium, heart 37.99
  auricle, heart 37.99
  bleeding vessel — see Control, hemorrhage
  blood vessel 38.80
    abdominal
      artery 38.86
      vein 38.87
    adrenal 07.43
    aorta (arch) (ascending) (descending) 38.84
    esophagus 42.91
      endoscopic 42.33
    head and neck NEC 38.82
    intracranial NEC 38.81
    lower limb
      artery 38.88
      vein 38.89
    meningeal (artery) (longitudinal sinus) 02.13
    thoracic NEC 38.85
    thyroid 06.92
    upper limb (artery) (vein) 38.83
  bronchus 33.92
  cisterna chyli 40.64
  coronary
    artery (anomalous) 36.99
    sinus 36.39
  dermal appendage 86.26
  ductus arteriosus, patent 38.85
  esophageal vessel 42.91
    endoscopic 42.33
  ethmoidal artery 21.04
  external carotid artery 21.06
  fallopian tube (bilateral) (remaining) (solitary) 66.39
    by endoscopy (culdoscopy) (hysteroscopy) (laparoscopy) (peritoneoscopy) 66.29
    with
      crushing 66.31
        by endoscopy (laparoscopy) 66.21
      division 66.32
        by endoscopy (culdoscopy) (laparoscopy) (peritoneoscopy) 66.22
      Falope ring 66.39
        by endoscopy (laparoscopy) 66.29
    unilateral 66.92
  fistula, arteriovenous 39.53
    coronary artery 36.99

Ligation — continued
  gastric
    artery 38.86
    varices 44.91
      endoscopic 43.41
  hemorrhoids 49.45
  longitudinal sinus (superior) 02.13
  lymphatic (channel) (peripheral) 40.9
    thoracic duct 40.64
  maxillary artery 21.05
  meningeal vessel 02.13
  spermatic
    cord 63.72
      varicocele 63.1
    vein (high) 63.1
  splenic vessels 38.86
  subclavian artery 38.85
  superior longitudinal sinus 02.13
  supernumerary digit 86.26
  thoracic duct 40.64
  thyroid vessel (artery) (vein) 06.92
  toes (supernumerary) 86.26
  tooth 93.55
    impacted 24.6
  ulcer (peptic) (base) (bed) (bleeding vessel) 44.40
    duodenal 44.42
    gastric 44.41
  ureter 56.95
  varices
    esophageal 42.91
      endoscopic 42.33
    gastric 44.91
      endoscopic 43.41
    peripheral vein (lower limb) 38.59
    upper limb 38.53
  varicocele 63.1
  vas deferens 63.71
  vein 38.80
    abdominal 38.87
    adrenal 07.43
    head and neck NEC 38.82
    intracranial NEC 38.81
    lower limb 38.89
    spermatic, high 63.1
    thoracic NEC 38.85
    thyroid 06.92
    upper limb 38.83
    varicose 38.50
      abdominal 38.57
      esophagus 42.91
        endoscopic 42.33
      gastric 44.91
        endoscopic 43.41
      head and neck NEC 38.52
      intracranial NEC 38.51
      lower limb 38.59
      stomach 44.91
      thoracic NEC 38.55
      upper limb 38.53
  vena cava, inferior 38.7
  venous connection between anomalous vein to
    left innominate vein 35.82
    superior vena cava 35.82
  wart 86.26
Light coagulation — see Photocoagulation
Lindholm operation (repair of ruptured tendon) 83.88
Lingulectomy, lung 32.39
Linton operation (varicose vein) 38.59
Lipectomy (subcutaneous tissue) (abdominal) (submental) 86.83
Liposuction 86.83
Lip reading training 95.49
Lip shave 27.43
Lisfranc operation
  foot amputation 84.12
  shoulder disarticulation 84.08
Litholapaxy, bladder 57.0
  by incision 57.19
Lithotomy
  bile passage 51.49
  bladder (urinary) 57.19
  common duct 51.41
    percutaneous 51.96

Lithotomy — continued
  gallbladder 51.04
  hepatic duct 51.49
  kidney 55.01
    percutaneous 55.03
  ureter 56.2
Lithotripsy
  bile duct NEC 51.49
    extracorporeal shockwave (ESWL) 98.52
  bladder 57.0
    with ultrasonic fragmentation 57.0 [59.95]
    extracorporeal shockwave (ESWL) 98.51
  extracorporeal shockwave (ESWL) NEC 98.59
    bile duct 98.52
    bladder (urinary) 98.51
    gallbladder 98.52
    kidney 98.51
    Kock pouch 98.51
    renal pelvis 98.51
    specified site NEC 98.59
    ureter 98.51
  gallbladder NEC 51.04
    endoscopic 51.88
    extracorporeal shockwave (ESWL) 98.52
  kidney 56.0
    extracorporeal shockwave (ESWL) 98.51
    percutaneous nephrostomy with fragmentation (laser) (ultrasound) 55.04
  renal pelvis 56.0
    extracorporeal shockwave (ESWL) 98.51
    percutaneous nephrostomy with fragmentation (laser) (ultrasound) 55.04
  ureter 56.0
    extracorporeal shockwave (ESWL) 98.51
Littlewood operation (forequarter amputation) 84.09
LITT (laser interstitial thermal therapy) **under guidance**
  lesion
    brain 17.61
    breast 17.69
    head and neck 17.62
    liver 17.63
    lung 17.69
    prostate 17.69
    thyroid 17.62
LLETZ (large loop excision of the transformation zone) of cervix 67.32
Lloyd-Davies operation (abdominoperineal resection), NOS 48.50
  laparoscopic 48.51
  open 48.52
  other 48.59
Lobectomy
  brain 01.53
    partial 01.59
  liver (with partial excision of adjacent lobes) 50.3
  lung (complete) 32.49
    partial 32.39
      thoracoscopic 32.30
    segmental (with resection of adjacent lobes) 32.49
      thoracoscopic 32.41
    thoracoscopic 32.41
  thyroid (total) (unilateral) (with removal of isthmus) (with removal of portion of remaining lobe) 06.2
    partial (see also Thyroidectomy, partial) 06.39
    substernal 06.51
    subtotal (see also Thyroidectomy, partial) 06.39
Lobotomy, brain 01.32
Localization, placenta 88.78
  by RISA injection 92.17
Longmire operation (bile duct anastomosis) 51.39
Loop ileal stoma — see also Ileostomy 46.01
Loopogram 87.78
Looposcopy (ileal conduit) 56.35

Lord operation
  dilation of anal canal for hemorrhoids 49.49
  hemorrhoidectomy 49.49
  orchidopexy 62.5
Lower GI series (x-ray) 87.64
Lucas and Murray operation (knee arthrodesis with plate) 81.22
Lumpectomy
  breast 85.21
  specified site — see Excision, lesion, by site
Lymphadenectomy (simple) — see also Excision, lymph, node 40.29
Lymphadenotomy 40.0
Lymphangiectomy (radical) — see also Excision, lymph, node, by site, radical 40.50
Lymphangiogram
  abdominal 88.04
  cervical 87.08
  intrathoracic 87.34
  lower limb 88.36
  pelvic 88.04
  upper limb 88.34
Lymphangioplasty 40.9
Lymphangiorrhaphy 40.9
Lymphangiotomy 40.0
Lymphaticostomy 40.9
  thoracic duct 40.62
Lysis
  adhesions

> **Note:**
> blunt — omit code
> digital — omit code
> manual — omit code
> mechanical — omit code
> without instrumentation — omit code

    abdominal 54.59
      laparoscopic 54.51
    appendiceal 54.59
      laparoscopic 54.51
    artery-vein-nerve bundle 39.91
    biliary tract 54.59
      laparoscopic 54.51
    bladder (neck) (intraluminal) 57.12
      external 59.11
        laparoscopic 59.12
      transurethral 57.41
    blood vessels 39.91
    bone — see category 78.4 ☑
    bursa 83.91
      by stretching or manipulation 93.28
      hand 82.91
    cartilage of joint 93.26
    chest wall 33.99
    choanae (nasopharynx) 29.54
    conjunctiva 10.5
    corneovitreal 12.34
    cortical (brain) 02.91
    ear, middle 20.23
    Eustachean tube 20.8
    extraocular muscle 15.7
    extrauterine 54.59
      laparoscopic 54.51
    eyelid 08.09
      and conjunctiva 10.5
    eye muscle 15.7
    fallopian tube 65.89
      laparoscopic 65.81
    fascia 83.91
      hand 82.91
        by stretching or manipulation 93.26
    gallbladder 54.59
      laparoscopic 54.51
    ganglion (peripheral) NEC 04.49
      cranial NEC 04.42
    hand 82.91
      by stretching or manipulation 93.26
    heart 37.10
    intestines 54.59
      laparoscopic 54.51
    iris (posterior) 12.33
      anterior 12.32
    joint (capsule) (structure) (see also Division, joint capsule) 80.40
    kidney 59.02
      laparoscopic 59.03

☑ Additional Digit Required — Refer to the Tabular List for Digit Selection   ▽ Subterms under main terms may continue to next column or page

36 — Volume 3   ▶◀ Revised Text   ● New Line   ▲ Revised Code   2014 ICD-9-CM

Lysis — *continued*
adhesions — *continued*
labia (vulva) 71.01
larynx 31.92
liver 54.59
laparoscopic 54.51
lung (for collapse of lung) 33.39
mediastinum 34.99
meninges (spinal) 03.6
cortical 02.91
middle ear 20.23
muscle 83.91
by stretching or manipulation 93.27
extraocular 15.7
hand 82.91
by stretching or manipulation 93.26
nasopharynx 29.54
nerve (peripheral) NEC 04.49
cranial NEC 04.42
roots, spinal 03.6
trigeminal 04.41
nose, nasal 21.91
ocular muscle 15.7
ovary 65.89
laparoscopic 65.81
pelvic 54.59
laparoscopic 54.51
penile 64.93
pericardium 37.12
perineal (female) 71.01
peripheral vessels 39.91
perirectal 48.81
perirenal 59.02
laparoscopic 59.03
peritoneum (pelvic) 54.59
laparoscopic 54.51
periureteral 59.02
laparoscopic 59.03
perivesical 59.11
laparoscopic 59.12
pharynx 29.54
pleura (for collapse of lung) 33.39
spermatic cord 63.94
spinal (cord) (meninges) (nerve roots) 03.6
spleen 54.59
laparoscopic 54.51
tendon 83.91
by stretching or manipulation 93.27
hand 82.91
by stretching or manipulation 93.26
thorax 34.99
tongue 25.93
trachea 31.92
tubo-ovarian 65.89
laparoscopic 65.81
ureter 59.02
with freeing or repositioning of ureter 59.02
intraluminal 56.81
laparoscopic 59.03
urethra (intraluminal) 58.5
uterus 54.59
intraluminal 68.21
laparoscopic 54.51
peritoneal 54.59
laparoscopic 54.51
vagina (intraluminal) 70.13
vitreous (posterior approach) 14.74
anterior approach 14.73
vulva 71.01
goniosynechiae (with injection of air or liquid) 12.31
synechiae (posterior) 12.33
anterior (with injection of air or liquid) 12.32

M

Madlener operation (tubal ligation) 66.31
Magnet extraction
foreign body
anterior chamber, eye 12.01
choroid 14.01
ciliary body 12.01

Magnet extraction — *continued*
foreign body — *continued*
conjunctiva 98.22
cornea 11.0
eye, eyeball NEC 98.21
anterior segment 12.01
posterior segment 14.01
intraocular (anterior segment) 12.01
iris 12.01
lens 13.01
orbit 98.21
retina 14.01
sclera 12.01
vitreous 14.01
Magnetic resonance imaging (nuclear) — *see* Imaging, magnetic resonance
Magnuson (-Stack) operation (arthroplasty for recurrent shoulder dislocation) 81.82
Mako Tactile Guidance System™ [TSG] — *see* category 17.4 ☑
Malleostapediopexy 19.19
with incus replacement 19.11
Malström's vacuum extraction 72.79
with episiotomy 72.71
Mammaplasty — *see* Mammoplasty
Mammectomy — *see also* Mastectomy
subcutaneous (unilateral) 85.34
with synchronous implant 85.35
bilateral 85.36
Mammilliplasty 85.87
Mammography NEC 87.37
Mammoplasty 85.89
with
full-thickness graft 85.83
muscle flap 85.85
pedicle graft 85.84
split-thickness graft 85.82
amputative (reduction) (bilateral) 85.32
unilateral 85.31
augmentation 85.50
with
breast implant (bilateral) 85.54
unilateral 85.53
injection into breast (bilateral) 85.52
unilateral 85.51
reduction (bilateral) 85.32
unilateral 85.31
revision 85.89
size reduction (gynecomastia) (bilateral) 85.32
unilateral 85.31
Mammotomy 85.0
Manchester (-Donald) (-Fothergill) operation (uterine suspension) 69.22
Mandibulectomy (partial) 76.31
total 76.42
with reconstruction 76.41
Maneuver (method)
Bracht 72.52
Credé 73.59
De Lee (key-in-lock) 72.4
Kristeller 72.54
Loveset's (extraction of arms in breech birth) 72.52
Mauriceau (-Smellie-Veit) 72.52
Pinard (total breech extraction) 72.54
Prague 72.52
Ritgen 73.59
Scanzoni (rotation) 72.4
Van Hoorn 72.52
Wigand-Martin 72.52
Manipulation
with reduction of fracture or dislocation — *see* Reduction, fracture *and* Reduction, dislocation
enterostomy stoma (with dilation) 96.24
intestine (intra-abdominal) 46.80
large 46.82
small 46.81
joint
adhesions 93.26
temporomandibular 76.95
dislocation — *see* Reduction, dislocation
lacrimal passage (tract) NEC 09.49
muscle structures 93.27

Manipulation — *continued*
musculoskeletal (physical therapy) NEC 93.29
nasal septum, displaced 21.88
osteopathic NEC 93.67
for general mobilization (general articulation) 93.61
high-velocity, low-amplitude forces (thrusting) 93.62
indirect forces 93.65
isotonic, isometric forces 93.64
low-velocity, high-amplitude forces (springing) 93.63
to move tissue fluids 93.66
rectum 96.22
salivary duct 26.91
stomach, intraoperative 44.92
temporomandibular joint NEC 76.95
ureteral calculus by catheter
with removal 56.0
without removal 59.8
uterus NEC 69.98
gravid 75.99
inverted
manual replacement (following delivery) 75.94
surgical — *see* Repair, inverted uterus
Manometry
esophageal 89.32
spinal fluid 89.15
urinary 89.21
Manual arts therapy 93.81
Mapping
cardiac (electrophysiologic) 37.27
doppler (flow) 88.72
electrocardiogram only 89.52
Marckwald operation (cervical os repair) 67.59
Marshall-Marchetti (-Krantz) operation (retropubic urethral suspension) 59.5
Marsupialization — *see also* Destruction, lesion, by site
cyst
Bartholin's 71.23
brain 01.59
cervical (nabothian) 67.31
dental 24.4
dentigerous 24.4
kidney 55.31
larynx 30.01
liver 50.21
ovary 65.21
laparoscopic 65.23
pancreas 52.3
pilonidal (open excision) (with partial closure) 86.21
salivary gland 26.21
spinal (intraspinal) (meninges) 03.4
spleen, splenic 41.41
lesion
brain 01.59
cerebral 01.59
liver 50.21
pilonidal cyst or sinus (open excision) (with partial closure) 86.21
pseudocyst, pancreas 52.3
ranula, salivary gland 26.21
Massage
cardiac (external) (manual) (closed) 99.63
open 37.91
prostatic 99.94
rectal (for levator spasm) 99.93
MAST (military anti-shock trousers) 93.58
Mastectomy (complete) (prophylactic) (simple) (unilateral) 85.41
with
excision of regional lymph nodes 85.43
bilateral 85.44
preservation of skin and nipple 85.34
with synchronous implant 85.33
bilateral 85.36
with synchronous implant 85.35
bilateral 85.42
extended
radical (Urban) (unilateral) 85.47
bilateral 85.48

Mastectomy — *continued*
extended — *continued*
simple (with regional lymphadenectomy) (unilateral) 85.43
bilateral 85.44
modified radical (unilateral) 85.43
bilateral 85.44
partial 85.23
radical (Halsted) (Meyer) (unilateral) 85.45
bilateral 85.46
extended (Urban) (unilateral) 85.47
bilateral 85.48
modified (unilateral) 85.43
bilateral 85.44
subcutaneous 85.34
with synchronous implant 85.33
bilateral 85.36
with synchronous implant 85.35
subtotal 85.23
Masters' stress test (two-step) 89.42
Mastoidectomy (cortical) (conservative) 20.49
complete (simple) 20.41
modified radical 20.49
radical 20.42
modified 20.49
simple (complete) 20.41
Mastoidotomy 20.21
Mastoidotympanectomy 20.42
Mastopexy 85.6
Mastoplasty — *see* Mammoplasty
Mastorrhaphy 85.81
Mastotomy 85.0
Matas operation (aneurysmorrhaphy) 39.52
Mayo operation
bunionectomy 77.59
herniorrhaphy
laparoscopic 53.43
with graft or prosthesis 53.42
other and open with graft or prosthesis 53.41
other open 53.49
vaginal hysterectomy 68.59
laparoscopically assisted (LAVH) 68.51
Maze procedure
Cox-maze, open 37.33
maze, modified, endovascular 37.34
maze, modified, open 37.33
Mazet operation (knee disarticulation) 84.16
McBride operation (bunionectomy with soft tissue correction) 77.53
McBurney operation — *see* Repair, hernia, inguinal
McCall operation (enterocele repair) 70.92
McCauley operation (release of clubfoot) 83.84
McDonald operation (encirclement suture, cervix) 67.59
McIndoe operation (vaginal construction) 70.61
with graft or prosthesis 70.63
McKeever operation (fusion of first metatarsophalangeal joint for hallux valgus repair) 77.52
McKissock operation (breast reduction) 85.33
McReynolds operation (transposition of pterygium) 11.31
McVay operation
femoral hernia — *see* Repair, hernia, femoral
inguinal hernia — *see* Repair, hernia, inguinal
Measurement
airway resistance 89.38
anatomic NEC 89.39
arterial blood gases 89.65
basal metabolic rate (BMR) 89.39
blood gases
arterial 89.65
continuous intra-arterial 89.60
venous 89.66
body 93.07
cardiac output (by)
Fick method 89.67
indicator dilution technique 89.68
oxygen consumption technique 89.67
thermodilution indicator 89.68
cardiovascular NEC 89.59
central venous pressure 89.62

☑ **Additional Digit Required** — Refer to the Tabular List for Digit Selection   ⬆ **Subterms under main terms may continue to next column or page**
2014 ICD-9-CM   ▶◀ **Revised Text**   ● **New Line**   ▲ **Revised Code**   **Volume 3 — 37**

Lysis — Measurement

☑ **Additional Digit Required** — Refer to the Tabular List for Digit Selection ▼ **Subterms under main terms may continue to next column or page**

38 — Volume 3 ▶◀ Revised Text ● New Line ▲ Revised Code **2014 ICD-9-CM**

Operation — continued
cecum NEC 46.99
cerebral (meninges) NEC 02.99
cervix NEC 69.99
Chandler (hip fusion) 81.21
Charles (correction of lymphedema) 40.9
Charnley (compression arthrodesis)
  ankle 81.11
  hip 81.21
  knee 81.22
Cheatle-Henry — *see* Repair, hernia, femoral
chest cavity NEC 34.99
Chevalier-Jackson (partial laryngectomy)
  30.29
Child (radical subtotal pancreatectomy)
  52.53
Chopart (midtarsal amputation) 84.12
chordae tendineae NEC 35.32
choroid NEC 14.9
ciliary body NEC 12.98
cisterna chyli NEC 40.69
Clagett (closure of chest wall following open
  flap drainage) 34.72
Clayton (resection of metatarsal heads and
  bases of phalanges) 77.88
clitoris NEC 71.4
cocked hat (metacarpal lengthening and
  transfer of local flap) 82.69
Cockett (varicose vein)
  lower limb 38.59
  upper limb 38.53
Cody tack (perforation of footplate) 19.0
Coffey (uterine suspension) (Meigs' modification) 69.22
Cole (anterior tarsal wedge osteotomy)
  77.28
Collis-Nissen (hiatal hernia repair) 53.80
Colonna
  adductor tenotomy (first stage) 83.12
  hip arthroplasty (second stage) 81.40
  reconstruction of hip (second stage)
    81.40
colon NEC 46.99
commando (radical glossectomy) 25.4
conjunctiva NEC 10.99
  destructive NEC 10.33
cornea NEC 11.99
Coventry (tibial wedge osteotomy) 77.27
Cox-maze procedure (ablation or destruction of heart tissue) — *see* Operation,
  maze procedure
Crawford (tarso-frontalis sling of eyelid)
  08.32
cul-de-sac NEC 70.92
Culp-Deweerd (spiral flap pyeloplasty) 55.87
Culp-Scardino (ureteral flap pyeloplasty)
  55.87
Curtis (interphalangeal joint arthroplasty)
  81.72
cystocele NEC 70.51
Dahlman (excision of esophageal diverticulum) 42.31
Dana (posterior rhizotomy) 03.1
Danforth (fetal) 73.8
Darrach (ulnar resection) 77.83
Davis (intubated ureterotomy) 56.2
de Grandmont (tarsectomy) 08.35
Delorme
  pericardiectomy 37.31
  proctopexy 48.76
  repair of prolapsed rectum 48.76
  thoracoplasty 33.34
Denker (radical maxillary antrotomy) 22.31
Dennis-Varco (herniorrhaphy) — *see* Repair,
  hernia, femoral
Denonvillier (limited rhinoplasty) 21.86
dental NEC 24.99
  orthodontic NEC 24.8
Derlacki (tympanoplasty) 19.4
diaphragm NEC 34.89
Dickson-Diveley (tendon transfer and
  arthrodesis to correct claw toe) 77.57
Dickson (fascial transplant) 83.82
Dieffenbach (hip disarticulation) 84.18
digestive tract NEC 46.99

Operation — continued
Doléris (shortening of round ligaments)
  69.22
D'Ombrain (excision of pterygium with
  corneal graft) 11.32
Dorrance (push-back operation for cleft
  palate) 27.62
Dotter (transluminal angioplasty) 39.59
Douglas (suture of tongue to lip for micrognathia) 25.59
Doyle (paracervical uterine denervation)
  69.3
Duhamel (abdominoperineal pull-through)
  48.65
Dührssen (vaginofixation of uterus) 69.22
Dunn (triple arthrodesis) 81.12
duodenum NEC 46.99
Dupuytren
  fasciectomy 82.35
  fasciotomy 82.12
    with excision 82.35
  shoulder disarticulation 84.08
Durham (-Caldwell) (transfer of biceps
  femoris tendon) 83.75
DuToit and Roux (staple capsulorrhaphy of
  shoulder) 81.82
DuVries (tenoplasty) 83.88
Dwyer
  fasciotomy 83.14
  soft tissue release NEC 83.84
  wedge osteotomy, calcaneus 77.28
Eagleton (extrapetrosal drainage) 20.22
ear (external) NEC 18.9
  middle or inner NEC 20.99
Eden-Hybinette (glenoid bone block) 78.01
Effler (heart) 36.2
Eggers
  tendon release (patellar retinacula) 83.13
  tendon transfer (biceps femoris tendon)
    (hamstring tendon) 83.75
Elliot (scleral trephination with iridectomy)
  12.61
Ellis Jones (repair of peroneal tendon) 83.88
Ellison (reinforcement of collateral ligament)
  81.44
Elmslie-Cholmeley (tarsal wedge osteotomy) 77.28
Eloesser
  thoracoplasty 33.34
  thoracostomy 34.09
Emmet (cervix) 67.61
endorectal pull-through 48.41
epididymis NEC 63.99
esophagus NEC 42.99
Estes (ovary) 65.72
  laparoscopic 65.75
Estlander (thoracoplasty) 33.34
Evans (release of clubfoot) 83.84
extraocular muscle NEC 15.9
  multiple (two or more muscles) 15.4
    with temporary detachment from
      globe 15.3
  revision 15.6
  single 15.29
    with temporary detachment from
      globe 15.19
eyeball NEC 16.99
eyelid(s) NEC 08.99
face NEC 27.99
facial bone or joint NEC 76.99
fallopian tube NEC 66.99
Farabeuf (ischiopubiotomy) 77.39
Fasanella-Servatt (blepharoptosis repair)
  08.35
fascia NEC 83.99
  hand 82.99
female (genital organs) NEC 71.9
  hysterectomy NEC 68.9
fenestration (aorta) 39.54
Ferguson (hernia repair) 53.00
Fick (perforation of footplate) 19.0
filtering (for glaucoma) 12.79
  with iridectomy 12.65
Finney (pyloroplasty) 44.29
fistulizing, sclera NEC 12.69
Foley (pyeloplasty) 55.87

Operation — continued
Fontan (creation of conduit between right
  atrium and pulmonary artery) 35.94
Fothergill (-Donald) (uterine suspension)
  69.22
Fowler
  arthroplasty of metacarpophalangeal
    joint 81.72
  release (mallet finger repair) 82.84
  tenodesis (hand) 82.85
  thoracoplasty 33.34
Fox (entropion repair with wedge resection)
  08.43
Franco (suprapubic cystotomy) 57.18
Frank (permanent gastrostomy) 43.19
Frazier (-Spiller) (subtemporal trigeminal
  rhizotomy) 04.02
Fredet-Ramstedt (pyloromyotomy) (with
  wedge resection) 43.3
Frenckner (intrapetrosal drainage) 20.22
Frickman (abdominal proctopexy) 48.75
Frommel (shortening of uterosacral ligaments) 69.22
Gabriel (abdominoperineal resection of
  rectum), NOS 48.50
  laparoscopic 48.51
  open 48.52
  other 48.59
gallbladder NEC 51.99
ganglia NEC 04.99
  sympathetic 05.89
Gant (wedge osteotomy of trochanter) 77.25
Garceau (tibial tendon transfer) 83.75
Gardner (spinal meningocele repair) 03.51
gastric NEC 44.99
Gelman (release of clubfoot) 83.84
genital organ NEC
  female 71.9
  male 64.99
Ghormley (hip fusion) 81.21
Gifford
  destruction of lacrimal sac 09.6
  keratotomy (delimiting) 11.1
Gill-Stein (carporadial arthrodesis) 81.25
Gill
  arthrodesis of shoulder 81.23
  laminectomy 03.09
Gilliam (uterine suspension) 69.22
Girdlestone-Taylor (muscle transfer for claw
  toe repair) 77.57
Girdlestone
  laminectomy with spinal fusion 81.00
  muscle transfer for claw toe 77.57
  resection of femoral head and neck
    (without insertion of joint prosthe-
    sis) 77.85
    with replacement prosthesis — *see*
      Implant, joint, hip
  resection of hip prosthesis 80.05
    with replacement prosthesis — *see*
      Implant, joint, hip
glaucoma NEC 12.79
Glenn (anastomosis of superior vena cava
  to right pulmonary artery) 39.21
globus pallidus NEC 01.42
Goebel-Frangenheim-Stoeckel (urethrovesical suspension) 59.4
Goldner (clubfoot release) 80.48
Goldthwait
  ankle stabilization 81.11
  patella stabilization 81.44
  tendon transfer for patella dislocation
    81.44
Goodall-Power (vagina) 70.4
Gordon-Taylor (hindquarter amputation)
  84.19
Graber-Duvernay (drilling femoral head)
  77.15
Green (scapulopexy) 78.41
Grice (subtalar arthrodesis) 81.13
Gritti-Stokes (knee disarticulation) 84.16
Gross (herniorrhaphy)
  laparoscopic 53.43
    with graft or prosthesis 53.42
  other and open with graft or prosthesis
    53.41

Operation — continued
Gross — continued
  other open 53.49
gum NEC 24.39
Guyon (amputation of ankle) 84.13
Hagner (epididymotomy) 63.92
Halsted — *see* Repair, hernia, inguinal
Halsted mastectomy 85.45
Hampton (anastomosis small intestine to
  rectal stump) 45.92
hanging hip (muscle release) 83.19
harelip 27.54
Harrison-Richardson (vaginal suspension)
  70.77
  with graft or prosthesis 70.78
Hartmann — *see* Colectomy, by site
Hauser
  achillotenotomy 83.11
  bunionectomy with adductor tendon
    transfer 77.53
  stabilization of patella 81.44
Heaney (vaginal hysterectomy) 68.59
  laparoscopically assisted (LAVH) 68.51
heart NEC 37.99
  valve NEC 35.99
    adjacent structure NEC 35.39
Hegar (perineorrhaphy) 71.79
Heine (cyclodialysis) 12.55
Heineke-Mikulicz (pyloroplasty) — *see* category 44.2 ☑
Heller (esophagomyotomy) 42.7
Hellström (transplantation of aberrant renal
  vessel) 39.55
hemorrhoids NEC 49.49
Henley (jejunal transposition) 43.81
hepatic NEC 50.99
hernia — *see* Repair, hernia
Hey-Groves (reconstruction of anterior cruciate ligament) 81.45
Hey (amputation of foot) 84.12
Heyman-Herndon (-Strong) (correction of
  metatarsus varus) 80.48
Heyman (soft tissue release for clubfoot)
  83.84
Hibbs (lumbar spinal fusion) — *see* Fusion,
  lumbar
Higgins — *see* Repair, hernia, femoral
Hill-Allison (hiatal hernia repair, transpleural
  approach) 53.80
Hitchcock (anchoring tendon of biceps)
  83.88
Hofmeister (gastrectomy) 43.7
Hoke
  midtarsal fusion 81.14
  triple arthrodesis 81.12
Holth
  iridencleisis 12.63
  sclerectomy 12.65
Homan (correction of lymphedema) 40.9
Hutch (ureteroneocystostomy) 56.74
Hybinette-eden (glenoid bone block) 78.01
hymen NEC 70.91
hypopharynx NEC 29.99
hypophysis NEC 07.79
ileal loop 56.51
ileum NEC 46.99
intestine NEC 46.99
iris NEC 12.97
  inclusion 12.63
Irving (tubal ligation) 66.32
Irwin (*see also* Osteotomy) 77.30
Jaboulay (gastroduodenostomy) 44.39
  laparoscopic 44.38
Janeway (permanent gastrostomy) 43.19
Jatene (arterial switch) 35.84
jejunum NEC 46.99
Johanson (urethral reconstruction) 58.46
joint (capsule) (ligament) (structure) NEC
  81.99
  facial NEC 76.99
Jones
  claw toe (transfer of extensor hallucis
    longus tendon) 77.57
  modified (with arthrodesis) 77.57
  dacryocystorhinostomy 09.81

☑ Additional Digit Required — Refer to the Tabular List for Digit Selection   ▽ Subterms under main terms may continue to next column or page

40 — Volume 3   ▶◀ Revised Text   ● New Line   ▲ Revised Code   2014 ICD-9-CM

Operation — *continued*

Jones — *continued*
hammer toe (interphalangeal fusion) 77.56
modified (tendon transfer with arthrodesis) 77.57
repair of peroneal tendon 83.88
Joplin (exostectomy with tendon transfer) 77.53
Kader (temporary gastrostomy) 43.19
Kaufman (for urinary stress incontinence) 59.79
Kazanjiian (buccal vestibular sulcus extension) 24.91
Kehr (hepatopexy) 50.69
Keller (bunionectomy) 77.59
Kelly-Stoeckel (urethrovesical plication) 59.3
Kelly (-Kennedy) (urethrovesical plication) 59.3
Kerr (cesarean section) 74.1
Kessler (arthroplasty, carpometacarpal joint) 81.74
Kidner (excision of accessory navicular bone) (with tendon transfer) 77.98
kidney NEC 55.99
Killian (frontal sinusotomy) 22.41
King-Steelquist (hindquarter amputation) 84.19
Kirk (amputation through thigh) 84.17
Kock pouch
bowel anastomosis — *omit code*
continent ileostomy 46.22
cutaneous uretero-ileostomy 56.51
ESWL (electrocorporeal shockwave lithotripsy) 98.51
removal, calculus 57.19
revision, cutaneous uretero-ileostomy 56.52
urinary diversion procedure 56.51
Kondoleon (correction of lymphedema) 40.9
Krause (sympathetic denervation) 05.29
Kroener (partial salpingectomy) 66.69
Kroenlein (lateral orbitotomy) 16.01
Krönig (low cervical cesarean section) 74.1
Krukenberg (reconstruction of below-elbow amputation) 82.89
Kuhnt-Szymanowski (ectropion repair with lid reconstruction) 08.44
Labbe (gastrotomy) 43.0
labia NEC 71.8
lacrimal
gland 09.3
system NEC 09.99
Ladd (mobilization of intestine) 54.95
Lagrange (iridosclerectomy) 12.65
Lambrinudi (triple arthrodesis) 81.12
Langenbeck (cleft palate repair) 27.62
Lapidus (bunionectomy with metatarsal osteotomy) 77.51
Larry (shoulder disarticulation) 84.08
larynx NEC 31.98
Lash
internal cervical os repair 67.59
laparoscopic supracervical hysterectomy 68.31
Latzko
cesarean section, extraperitoneal 74.2
colpocleisis 70.8
Leadbetter-Politano (ureteroneocystostomy) 56.74
Leadbetter (urethral reconstruction) 58.46
Le Fort (colpocleisis) 70.8
LeMesurier (cleft lip repair) 27.54
lens NEC 13.90
Leriche (periarterial sympathectomy) 05.25
levator muscle sling
eyelid ptosis repair 08.33
urethrovesical suspension 59.71
urinary stress incontinence 59.71
lid suture (blepharoptosis) 08.31
ligament NEC 81.99
broad NEC 69.98
round NEC 69.98
uterine NEC 69.98
Lindholm (repair of ruptured tendon) 83.88
Linton (varicose vein) 38.59

Operation — *continued*

lip NEC 27.99
Lisfranc
foot amputation 84.12
shoulder disarticulation 84.08
Littlewood (forequarter amputation) 84.09
liver NEC 50.99
Lloyd-Davies (abdominoperineal resection), NOS 48.50
laparoscopic 48.51
open 48.52
other 48.59
Longmire (bile duct anastomosis) 51.39
Lord
dilation of anal canal for hemorrhoids 49.49
hemorrhoidectomy 49.49
orchidopexy 62.5
Lucas and Murray (knee arthrodesis with plate) 81.22
lung volume reduction 32.22
biologic lung volume reduction (BLVR) — *see* category 33.7 ☑
lung NEC 33.99
lymphatic structure(s) NEC 40.9
duct, left (thoracic) NEC 40.69
Madlener (tubal ligation) 66.31
Magnuson (-Stack) (arthroplasty for recurrent shoulder dislocation) 81.82
male genital organs NEC 64.99
Manchester (-Donald) (-Fothergill) (uterine suspension) 69.22
mandible NEC 76.99
orthognathic 76.64
Marckwald operation (cervical os repair) 67.59
Marshall-Marchetti (-Krantz) (retropubic urethral suspension) 59.5
Matas (aneurysmorrhaphy) 39.52
Mayo
bunionectomy 77.59
herniorrhaphy
laparoscopic 53.43
with graft or prosthesis 53.42
other and open with graft or prosthesis 53.41
other open 53.49
vaginal hysterectomy 68.59
laparoscopically assisted (LAVH) 68.51
maze procedure (ablation or destruction of heart tissue)
by incision (open) 37.33
by median sternotomy 37.33
by peripherally inserted catheter 37.34
by thoracotomy without thoracoscope 37.33
endovascular approach 37.34
Mazet (knee disarticulation) 84.16
McBride (bunionectomy with soft tissue correction) 77.53
McBurney — *see* Repair, hernia, inguinal
McCall (enterocele repair) 70.92
with graft or prosthesis 70.93
McCauley (release of clubfoot) 83.84
McDonald (encirclement suture, cervix) 67.59
McIndoe (vaginal construction) 70.61
with graft or prosthesis 70.63
McKeever (fusion of first metatarsophalangeal joint for hallux valgus repair) 77.52
McKissock (breast reduction) 85.33
McReynolds (transposition of pterygium) 11.31
McVay
femoral hernia — *see* Repair, hernia, femoral
inguinal hernia — *see* Repair, hernia, inguinal
meninges (spinal) NEC 03.99
cerebral NEC 02.99
mesentery NEC 54.99
Mikulicz (exteriorization of intestine) (first stage) 46.03
second stage 46.04

Operation — *continued*

Miles (complete proctectomy), NOS 48.50
laparoscopic 48.51
open 48.52
other 48.59
Millard (cheiloplasty) 27.54
Miller
midtarsal arthrodesis 81.14
urethrovesical suspension 59.4
Millin-Read (urethrovesical suspension) 59.4
Mitchell (hallux valgus repair) 77.51
Mohs (chemosurgical excision of skin) 86.24
Moore (arthroplasty) 81.52
Moschowitz
enterocele repair 70.92
with graft or prosthesis 70.93
herniorrhaphy — *see* Repair, hernia, femoral
sigmoidopexy 46.63
mouth NEC 27.99
Muller (banding of pulmonary artery) 38.85
Mumford (partial claviculectomy) 77.81
muscle NEC 83.99
extraocular — *see* Operation, extraocular
hand NEC 82.99
papillary heart NEC 35.31
musculoskeletal system NEC 84.99
Mustard (interatrial transposition of venous return) 35.91
nail (finger) (toe) NEC 86.99
nasal sinus NEC 22.9
nasopharynx NEC 29.99
nerve (cranial) (peripheral) NEC 04.99
adrenal NEC 07.49
sympathetic NEC 05.89
nervous system NEC 05.9
Nicola (tenodesis for recurrent dislocation of shoulder) 81.82
nipple NEC 85.99
Nissen (fundoplication of stomach) 44.66
laparoscopic 44.67
Noble (plication of small intestine) 46.62
node (lymph) NEC 40.9
Norman Miller (vaginopexy) 70.77
with graft or prosthesis 70.78
Norton (extraperitoneal cesarean operation) 74.2
nose, nasal NEC 21.99
sinus NEC 22.9
Ober (-Yount) (gluteal-iliotibial fasciotomy) 83.14
obstetric NEC 75.99
ocular NEC 16.99
muscle — *see* Operation, extraocular muscle
O'Donoghue (triad knee repair) 81.43
Olshausen (uterine suspension) 69.22
omentum NEC 54.99
ophthalmologic NEC 16.99
oral cavity NEC 27.99
orbicularis muscle sling 08.36
orbit NEC 16.98
oropharynx NEC 29.99
orthodontic NEC 24.8
orthognathic NEC 76.69
Oscar Miller (midtarsal arthrodesis) 81.14
Osmond-Clark (soft tissue release with peroneus brevis tendon transfer) 83.75
ovary NEC 65.99
Oxford (for urinary incontinence) 59.4
palate NEC 27.99
palpebral ligament sling 08.36
Panas (linear proctotomy) 48.0
Pancoast (division of trigeminal nerve at foramen ovale) 04.02
pancreas NEC 52.99
pantaloon (revision of gastric anastomosis) 44.5
papillary muscle (heart) NEC 35.31
parathyroid gland(s) NEC 06.99
parotid gland or duct NEC 26.99
Partsch (marsupialization of dental cyst) 24.4
Pattee (auditory canal) 18.6
Peet (splanchnic resection) 05.29

Operation — *continued*

Pemberton
osteotomy of ilium 77.39
rectum (mobilization and fixation for prolapse repair) 48.76
penis NEC 64.98
Pereyra (paraurethral suspension) 59.6
pericardium NEC 37.99
perineum (female) NEC 71.8
male NEC 86.99
perirectal tissue NEC 48.99
perirenal tissue NEC 59.92
peritoneum NEC 54.99
periurethral tissue NEC 58.99
perivesical tissue NEC 59.92
pharyngeal flap (cleft palate repair) 27.62
secondary or subsequent 27.63
pharynx, pharyngeal (pouch) NEC 29.99
pineal gland NEC 07.59
Pinsker (obliteration of nasoseptal telangiectasia) 21.07
Piper (forceps) 72.6
Pirogoff (ankle amputation through malleoli of tibia and fibula) 84.14
pituitary gland NEC 07.79
plastic — *see* Repair, by site
pleural cavity NEC 34.99
Politano-Leadbetter (ureteroneocystostomy) 56.74
pollicization (with nerves and blood supply) 82.61
Polya (gastrectomy) 43.7
Pomeroy (ligation and division of fallopian tubes) 66.32
Poncet
lengthening of Achilles tendon 83.85
urethrostomy, perineal 58.0
Porro (cesarean section) 74.99
posterior chamber (eye) NEC 14.9
Potts-Smith (descending aorta-left pulmonary artery anastomosis) 39.0
Printen and Mason (high gastric bypass) 44.31
prostate NEC (*see also* Prostatectomy) 60.69
specified type 60.99
pterygium 11.39
with corneal graft 11.32
Puestow (pancreaticojejunostomy) 52.96
pull-through NEC 48.49
pulmonary NEC 33.99
push-back (cleft palate repair) 27.62
Putti-Platt (capsulorrhaphy of shoulder for recurrent dislocation) 81.82
pyloric exclusion 44.39
laparoscopic 44.38
pyriform sinus NEC 29.99
"rabbit ear" (anterior urethropexy) (Tudor) 59.79
Ramadier (intrapetrosal drainage) 20.22
Ramstedt (pyloromyotomy) (with wedge resection) 43.3
Rankin
exteriorization of intestine 46.03
proctectomy (complete), NOS 48.50
laparoscopic 48.51
open 48.52
other 48.59
Rashkind (balloon septostomy) 35.41
Rastelli (creation of conduit between right ventricle and pulmonary artery) 35.92
in repair of
pulmonary artery atresia 35.92
transposition of great vessels 35.92
truncus arteriosus 35.83
Raz-Pereyra procedure (bladder neck suspension) 59.79
re-entry (aorta) 39.54
rectal NEC 48.99
rectocele NEC 70.52
renal NEC 55.99
respiratory (tract) NEC 33.99
retina NEC 14.9
Ripstein (repair of rectal prolapse) 48.75
Rodney Smith (radical subtotal pancreatectomy) 52.53

☑ **Additional Digit Required — Refer to the Tabular List for Digit Selection**

▽ **Subterms under main terms may continue to next column or page**

Operation — *continued*
  Roux-en-Y
    bile duct 51.36
    cholecystojejunostomy 51.32
    esophagus (intrathoracic) 42.54
    gastroenterostomy 44.39
      laparoscopic 44.38
    gastrojejunostomy 44.39
      laparoscopic 44.38
    pancreaticojejunostomy 52.96
  Roux-Goldthwait (repair of patellar dislocation) 81.44
  Roux-Herzen-Judine (jejunal loop interposition) 42.63
  Ruiz-Mora (proximal phalangectomy for hammer toe) 77.99
  Russe (bone graft of scaphoid) 78.04
  Saemisch (corneal section) 11.1
  salivary gland or duct NEC 26.99
  Salter (innominate osteotomy) 77.39
  Sauer-Bacon (abdominoperineal resection), NOS 48.50
    laparoscopic 48.51
    open 48.52
    other 48.59
  Schanz (femoral osteotomy) 77.35
  Schauta (-Amreich) (radical vaginal hysterectomy) 68.79
    laparoscopic 68.71
  Schede (thoracoplasty) 33.34
  Scheie
    cautery of sclera 12.62
    sclerostomy 12.62
  Schlatter (total gastrectomy) 43.99
  Schroeder (endocervical excision) 67.39
  Schuchardt (nonobstetrical episiotomy) 71.09
  Schwartze (simple mastoidectomy) 20.41
  sclera NEC 12.89
  Scott
    intestinal bypass for obesity 45.93
    jejunocolostomy (bypass) 45.93
  scrotum NEC 61.99
  Seddon-Brooks (transfer of pectoralis major tendon) 83.75
  Semb (apicolysis of lung) 33.39
  seminal vesicle NEC 60.79
  Senning (correction of transposition of great vessels) 35.91
  Sever (division of soft tissue of arm) 83.19
  Sewell (heart) 36.2
  sex transformation NEC 64.5
  Sharrard (iliopsoas muscle transfer) 83.77
  shelf (hip arthroplasty) 81.40
  Shirodkar (encirclement suture, cervix) 67.59
  sigmoid NEC 46.99
  Silver (bunionectomy) 77.59
  Sistrunk (excision of thyroglossal cyst) 06.7
  Skene's gland NEC 71.8
  skin NEC 86.99
  skull NEC 02.99
  sling
    eyelid
      fascia lata, palpebral 08.36
      frontalis fascial 08.32
      levator muscle 08.33
      orbicularis muscle 08.36
      palpebral ligament, fascia lata 08.36
      tarsus muscle 08.35
    fascial (fascia lata)
      eye 08.32
      for facial weakness (trigeminal nerve paralysis) 86.81
      palpebral ligament 08.36
      tongue 25.59
    tongue (fascial) 25.59
    urethra (suprapubic) 59.4
      retropubic 59.5
    urethrovesical 59.5
  Slocum (pes anserinus transfer) 81.47
  Sluder (tonsillectomy) 28.2
  Smith-Peterson (radiocarpal arthrodesis) 81.25
  Smith (open osteotomy of mandible) 76.62
  Smithwick (sympathectomy) 05.29
  Soave (endorectal pull-through) 48.41

Operation — *continued*
  soft tissue NEC 83.99
    hand 82.99
  Sonneberg (inferior maxillary neurectomy) 04.07
  Sorondo-Ferré (hindquarter amputation) 84.19
  Soutter (iliac crest fasciotomy) 83.14
  Spalding-Richardson (uterine suspension) 69.22
  spermatic cord NEC 63.99
  sphincter of Oddi NEC 51.89
  spinal (canal) (cord) (structures) NEC 03.99
  Spinelli (correction of inverted uterus) 75.93
  Spivack (permanent gastrostomy) 43.19
  spleen NEC 41.99
  S.P. Rogers (knee disarticulation) 84.16
  Ssabanejew-Frank (permanent gastrostomy) 43.19
  Stacke (simple mastoidectomy) 20.41
  Stallard (conjunctivocystorhinostomy) 09.82
    with insertion of tube or stent 09.83
  Stamm (-Kader) (temporary gastrostomy) 43.19
  Steinberg 44.5
  Steindler
    fascia stripping (for cavus deformity) 83.14
    flexorplasty (elbow) 83.77
    muscle transfer 83.77
  sterilization NEC
    female (*see also* specific operation) 66.39
    male (*see also* Ligation, vas deferens) 63.70
  Stewart (renal plication with pyeloplasty) 55.87
  stomach NEC 44.99
  Stone (anoplasty) 49.79
  Strassman (metroplasty) 69.49
    metroplasty (Jones modification) 69.49
    uterus 68.22
  Strayer (gastrocnemius recession) 83.72
  stress incontinence — *see* Repair, stress incontinence
  Stromeyer-Little (hepatotomy) 50.0
  Strong (unbridling of celiac artery axis) 39.91
  Sturmdorf (conization of cervix) 67.2
  subcutaneous tissue NEC 86.99
  sublingual gland or duct NEC 26.99
  submaxillary gland or duct NEC 26.99
  Summerskill (dacryocystorhinostomy by intubation) 09.81
  Surmay (jejunostomy) 46.39
  Swenson
    bladder reconstruction 57.87
    proctectomy 48.49
  Swinney (urethral reconstruction) 58.46
  Syme
    ankle amputation through malleoli of tibia and fibula 84.14
    urethrotomy, external 58.0
  sympathetic nerve NEC 05.89
  Taarnhoj (trigeminal nerve root decompression) 04.41
  Tack (sacculotomy) 20.79
  Talma-Morison (omentopexy) 54.74
  Tanner (devascularization of stomach) 44.99
  TAPVC NEC 35.82
  tarsus NEC 08.99
    muscle sling 08.35
  tendon NEC 83.99
    extraocular NEC 15.9
    hand NEC 82.99
  testis NEC 62.99
  tetralogy of Fallot
    partial repair — *see* specific procedure
    total (one-stage) 35.81
  Thal (repair of esophageal stricture) 42.85
  thalamus 01.41
    by stereotactic radiosurgery 92.32
      cobalt 60 92.32
      linear accelerator (LINAC) 92.31
      multi-source 92.32
      particle beam 92.33
      particulate 92.33
      radiosurgery NEC 92.39

Operation — *continued*
  thalamus — *continued*
    by stereotactic radiosurgery — *continued*
      single source photon 92.31
  Thiersch
    anus 49.79
    skin graft 86.69
      hand 86.62
  Thompson
    cleft lip repair 27.54
    correction of lymphedema 40.9
    quadricepsplasty 83.86
    thumb apposition with bone graft 82.69
  thoracic duct NEC 40.69
  thorax NEC 34.99
  Thorek (partial cholecystectomy) 51.21
  three-snip, punctum 09.51
  thymus NEC 07.99
    thoracoscopic NEC 07.98
  thyroid gland NEC 06.98
  TKP (thermokeratoplasty) 11.74
  Tomkins (metroplasty) 69.49
  tongue NEC 25.99
    flap, palate 27.62
    tie 25.91
  tonsil NEC 28.99
  Torek (-Bevan) (orchidopexy) (first stage) (second stage) 62.5
  Torkildsen (ventriculocisternal shunt) 02.22
  Torpin (cul-de-sac resection) 70.92
  Toti (dacryocystorhinostomy) 09.81
  Touchas 86.83
  Touroff (ligation of subclavian artery) 38.85
  trabeculae corneae cordis (heart) NEC 35.35
  trachea NEC 31.99
  Trauner (lingual sulcus extension) 24.91
  truncus arteriosus NEC 35.83
  Tsuge (macrodactyly repair) 82.83
  Tudor "rabbit ear" (anterior urethropexy) 59.79
  Tuffier
    apicolysis of lung 33.39
    vaginal hysterectomy 68.59
      laparoscopically assisted (LAVH) 68.51
  tunica vaginalis NEC 61.99
  Turco (release of joint capsules in clubfoot) 80.48
  Uchida (tubal ligation with or without fimbriectomy) 66.32
  umbilicus NEC 54.99
  urachus NEC 57.51
  Urban (mastectomy) (unilateral) 85.47
    bilateral 85.48
  ureter NEC 56.99
  urethra NEC 58.99
  urinary system NEC 59.99
  uterus NEC 69.99
    supporting structures NEC 69.98
  uvula NEC 27.79
  vagina NEC 70.91
  vascular NEC 39.99
  vas deferens NEC 63.99
    ligation NEC 63.71
  vein NEC 39.99
  vena cava sieve 38.7
  vertebra NEC 78.49
  vesical (bladder) NEC 57.99
  vessel NEC 39.99
    cardiac NEC 36.99
  Vicq d'Azyr (larynx) 31.1
  Vidal (varicocele ligation) 63.1
  Vineberg (implantation of mammary artery into ventricle) 36.2
  vitreous NEC 14.79
  vocal cord NEC 31.98
  von Kraske (proctectomy) 48.64
  Voss (hanging hip operation) 83.19
  Vulpius (-Compere) (lengthening of gastrocnemius muscle) 83.85
  vulva NEC 71.8
  Ward-Mayo (vaginal hysterectomy) 68.59
    laparoscopically assisted (LAVH) 68.51
  Wardill (cleft palate) 27.62

Operation — *continued*
  Waters (extraperitoneal cesarean section) 74.2
  Waterston (aorta-right pulmonary artery anastomosis) 39.0
  Watkins (-Wertheim) (uterus interposition) 69.21
  Watson-Jones
    hip arthrodesis 81.21
    reconstruction of lateral ligaments, ankle 81.49
    shoulder arthrodesis (extra-articular) 81.23
    tenoplasty 83.88
  Weir
    appendicostomy 47.91
    correction of nostrils 21.86
  Wertheim (radical hysterectomy) 68.69
    laparoscopic 68.61
  West (dacryocystorhinostomy) 09.81
  Wheeler
    entropion repair 08.44
    halving procedure (eyelid) 08.24
  Whipple (radical pancreaticoduodenectomy) 52.7
    Child modification (radical subtotal pancreatectomy) 52.53
    Rodney Smith modification (radical subtotal pancreatectomy) 52.53
  White (lengthening of tendo calcaneus by incomplete tenotomy) 83.11
  Whitehead
    glossectomy, radical 25.4
    hemorrhoidectomy 49.46
  Whitman
    foot stabilization (talectomy) 77.98
    hip reconstruction 81.40
    repair of serratus anterior muscle 83.87
    talectomy 77.98
    trochanter wedge osteotomy 77.25
  Wier (entropion repair) 08.44
  Williams-Richardson (vaginal construction) 70.61
    with graft or prosthesis 70.63
  Wilms (thoracoplasty) 33.34
  Wilson (angulation osteotomy for hallux valgus) 77.51
  window
    antrum (nasal sinus) — *see* Antrotomy, maxillary
    aorticopulmonary 39.59
    bone cortex (*see also* Incision, bone) 77.10
      facial 76.09
    nasoantral — *see* Antrotomy, maxillary
    pericardium 37.12
    pleural 34.09
  Winiwarter (cholecystoenterostomy) 51.32
  Witzel (temporary gastrostomy) 43.19
  Woodward (release of high riding scapula) 81.83
  Young
    epispadias repair 58.45
    tendon transfer (anterior tibialis) (repair of flat foot) 83.75
  Yount (division of iliotibial band) 83.14
  Zancolli
    capsuloplasty 81.72
    tendon transfer (biceps) 82.56
  Ziegler (iridectomy) 12.14
Operculectomy 24.6
Ophthalmectomy 16.49
  with implant (into Tenon's capsule) 16.42
    with attachment of muscles 16.41
Ophthalmoscopy 16.21
Opponensplasty (hand) 82.56
Optical coherence tomography (OCT) (intravascular imaging)
  coronary vessel(s) 38.24
  non-coronary vessel(s) 38.25
Orbitomaxillectomy, radical 16.51
Orbitotomy (anterior) (frontal) (temporofrontal) (transfrontal) NEC 16.09
  with
    bone flap 16.01
    insertion of implant 16.02

Orbitotomy — *continued*
Kroenlein (lateral) 16.01
lateral 16.01
Orchidectomy (with epididymectomy) (unilateral) 62.3
bilateral (radical) 62.41
remaining or solitary testis 62.42
Orchidopexy 62.5
Orchidoplasty 62.69
Orchidorrhaphy 62.61
Orchidotomy 62.0
Orchiectomy (with epididymectomy) (unilateral) 62.3
bilateral (radical) 62.41
remaining or solitary testis 62.42
Orchiopexy 62.5
Orchioplasty 62.69
Orthoroentgenography — *see* Radiography
Oscar Miller operation (midtarsal arthrodesis) 81.14
Osmond-Clark operation (soft tissue release with peroneus brevis tendon transfer) 83.75
Ossiculectomy NEC 19.3
with
stapedectomy (*see also* Stapedectomy) 19.19
stapes mobilization 19.0
tympanoplasty 19.53
revision 19.6
Ossiculotomy NEC 19.3
Ostectomy (partial), except facial — *see also* category 77.8 ☑
facial NEC 76.39
total 76.45
with reconstruction 76.44
first metatarsal head — *see* Bunionectomy
for graft (autograft) (homograft) (*see also* category) 77.7 ☑
mandible 76.31
total 76.42
with reconstruction 76.41
total, except facial (*see also* category) 77.9 ☑
facial NEC 76.45
with reconstruction 76.44
mandible 76.42
with reconstruction 76.41
Osteoarthrotomy — *see also* Osteotomy 77.30
Osteoclasis 78.70
carpal, metacarpal 78.74
clavicle 78.71
ear 20.79
femur 78.75
fibula 78.77
humerus 78.72
patella 78.76
pelvic 78.79
phalanges (foot) (hand) 78.79
radius 78.73
scapula 78.71
specified site NEC 78.79
tarsal, metatarsal 78.78
thorax (ribs) (sternum) 78.71
tibia 78.77
ulna 78.73
vertebrae 78.79
Osteolysis — *see* category 78.4 ☑
Osteopathic manipulation — *see also* Manipulation, osteopathic 93.67
Osteoplasty NEC — *see* category 78.4 ☑
for
bone lengthening — *see* Lengthening, bone
bone shortening — *see* Shortening, bone
repair of malunion or nonunion of fracture — *see* Repair, fracture, malunion or nonunion
with bone graft — *see* Graft, bone
carpal, metacarpal 78.44
clavicle 78.41
cranium NEC 02.06
with
flap (bone) 02.03
graft (bone) 02.04

Osteoplasty — *see* category — *continued*
facial bone NEC 76.69
femur 78.45
fibula 78.47
humerus 78.42
mandible, mandibular NEC 76.64
body 76.63
ramus (open) 76.62
closed 76.61
maxilla (segmental) 76.65
total 76.66
nasal bones 21.89
patella 78.46
pelvic 78.49
phalanges (foot) (hand) 78.49
radius 78.43
scapula 78.41
skull NEC 02.06
with
flap (bone) 02.03
graft (bone) 02.04
specified site NEC 78.49
tarsal, metatarsal 78.48
thorax (ribs) (sternum) 78.41
tibia 78.47
ulna 78.43
vertebrae 78.49
Osteorrhaphy — *see also* Osteoplasty 78.40
Osteosynthesis (fracture) — *see* Reduction, fracture
Osteotomy (adduction) (angulation) (block) (derotational) (displacement) (partial) (rotational) 77.30
carpals, metacarpals 77.34
wedge 77.24
clavicle 77.31
wedge 77.21
facial bone NEC 76.69
femur 77.35
wedge 77.25
fibula 77.37
wedge 77.27
humerus 77.32
wedge 77.22
mandible (segmental) (subapical) 76.64
angle (open) 76.62
closed 76.61
body 76.63
Gigli saw 76.61
ramus (open) 76.62
closed 76.61
maxilla (segmental) 76.65
total 76.66
metatarsal 77.38
wedge 77.28
for hallux valgus repair 77.51
patella 77.36
wedge 77.26
pelvic 77.39
wedge 77.29
phalanges (foot) (hand) 77.39
for repair of
bunion — *see* Bunionectomy
bunionette 77.54
hallux valgus — *see* Bunionectomy
wedge 77.29
for repair of
bunion — *see* Bunionectomy
bunionette 77.54
hallux valgus — *see* Bunionectomy
radius 77.33
wedge 77.23
scapula 77.31
wedge 77.21
specified site NEC 77.39
wedge 77.29
tarsal 77.38
wedge 77.28
thorax (ribs) (sternum) 77.31
wedge 77.21
tibia 77.37
wedge 77.27
toe 77.39
for repair of
bunion — *see* Bunionectomy

Osteotomy — *continued*
toe — *continued*
for repair of — *continued*
bunionette 77.54
hallux valgus — *see* Bunionectomy
wedge 77.29
for repair of
bunion — *see* Bunionectomy
bunionette 77.54
hallux valgus — *see* Bunionectomy
ulna 77.33
wedge 77.23
vertebrae 77.39
wedge 77.29
Otonecrectomy (inner ear) 20.79
Otoplasty (external) 18.79
auditory canal or meatus 18.6
auricle 18.79
cartilage 18.79
reconstruction 18.71
prominent or protruding 18.5
Otoscopy 18.11
Outfolding, sclera, for buckling — *see also* Buckling, scleral 14.49
Outfracture, turbinates (nasal) 21.62
Output and clearance, circulatory 92.05
Overdistension, bladder (therapeutic) 96.25
Overlapping, sclera, for buckling — *see also* Buckling, scleral 14.49
Oversewing
left atrial appendage (LAA) 37.36
pleural bleb 32.21
ulcer crater (peptic) 44.40
duodenum 44.42
stomach 44.41
Oxford operation (for urinary incontinence) 59.4
Oximetry
fetal pulse 75.38
Oxygenation 93.96
extracorporeal membrane (ECMO) 39.65
hyperbaric 93.95
wound 93.59
infusion therapy, Super 00.49
Oxygen therapy (catalytic) (pump) 93.96
hyperbaric 93.95
SuperSaturated 00.49

P

Pacemaker
cardiac (*see also* Insertion, pacemaker, cardiac)
intraoperative (temporary) 39.64
temporary (during and immediately following cardiac surgery) 39.64
Packing — *see also* Insertion, pack
auditory canal 96.11
nose, for epistaxis (anterior) 21.01
posterior (and anterior) 21.02
rectal 96.19
sella turcica 07.79
vaginal 96.14
Palatoplasty 27.69
for cleft palate 27.62
secondary or subsequent 27.63
Palatorrhaphy 27.61
for cleft palate 27.62
Pallidectomy 01.42
Pallidoansotomy 01.42
Pallidotomy 01.42
by stereotactic radiosurgery 92.32
cobalt 60 92.32
linear accelerator (LINAC) 92.31
multi-source 92.32
particle beam 92.33
particulate 92.33
radiosurgery NEC 92.39
single source photon 92.31
Panas operation (linear proctotomy) 48.0
Pancoast operation (division of trigeminal nerve at foramen ovale) 04.02
Pancreatectomy (total) (with synchronous duodenectomy) 52.6
partial NEC 52.59
distal (tail) (with part of body) 52.52

Pancreatectomy — *continued*
partial — *continued*
proximal (head) (with part of body) (with synchronous duodenectomy) 52.51
radical 52.53
subtotal 52.53
radical 52.7
subtotal 52.53
Pancreaticocystoduodenostomy 52.4
Pancreaticocystoenterostomy 52.4
Pancreaticocystogastrostomy 52.4
Pancreaticocystojejunostomy 52.4
Pancreaticoduodenectomy (total) 52.6
partial NEC 52.59
proximal 52.51
radical subtotal 52.53
radical (one-stage) (two-stage) 52.7
subtotal 52.53
Pancreaticoduodenostomy 52.96
Pancreaticoenterostomy 52.96
Pancreaticogastrostomy 52.96
Pancreaticoileostomy 52.96
Pancreaticojejunostomy 52.96
Pancreatoduodenectomy (total) 52.6
partial NEC 52.59
radical (one-stage) (two-stage) 52.7
subtotal 52.53
Pancreatogram 87.66
endoscopic retrograde (ERP) 52.13
Pancreatolithotomy 52.09
endoscopic 52.94
Pancreatotomy 52.09
Pancreolithotomy 52.09
endoscopic 52.94
Panendoscopy 57.32
specified site, other than bladder — *see* Endoscopy, by site
through artificial stoma 57.31
Panhysterectomy (abdominal) 68.49
laparoscopic 68.41
vaginal 68.59
laparoscopically assisted (LAVH) 68.51
Panniculectomy 86.83
Panniculotomy 86.83
Pantaloon operation (revision of gastric anastomosis) 44.5
Papillectomy, anal 49.39
endoscopic 49.31
Papillotomy (pancreas) 51.82
endoscopic 51.85
Paquin operation (ureteroneocystostomy) 56.74
Paracentesis
abdominal (percutaneous) 54.91
anterior chamber, eye 12.91
bladder 57.11
cornea 12.91
eye (anterior chamber) 12.91
thoracic, thoracis 34.91
tympanum 20.09
with intubation 20.01
Parasitology — *see* Examination, microscopic
Parathyroidectomy (partial) (subtotal) NEC 06.89
complete 06.81
ectopic 06.89
global removal 06.81
mediastinal 06.89
total 06.81
Parenteral nutrition, total 99.15
peripheral 99.15
Parotidectomy 26.30
complete 26.32
partial 26.31
radical 26.32
Partsch operation (marsupialization of dental cyst) 24.4
Passage — *see* Insertion and Intubation
Passage of sounds, urethra 58.6
Patch
blood, spinal (epidural) 03.95
graft — *see* Graft
spinal, blood (epidural) 03.95
subdural, brain 02.12
Patellapexy 78.46

Patellaplasty NEC 78.46
Patellectomy 77.96
  partial 77.86
Pattee operation (auditory canal) 18.6
PDT (percutaneous dilatational tracheostomy) — *see* Tracheostomy
Pectenotomy — *see also* Sphincterotomy, anal 49.59
Pedicle flap — *see* Graft, skin, pedicle
Peet operation (splanchnic resection) 05.29
PEG (percutaneous endoscopic gastrostomy) 43.11
PEGJJ (percutaneous [endoscopic] gastroje-junostomy) 44.32
PEJ (percutaneous endoscopic jejunostomy) 46.32
Pelvectomy, kidney (partial) 55.4
Pelvi-ureteroplasty 55.87
Pelvimetry 88.25
  gynecological 89.26
Pelviolithotomy 55.11
Pelvioplasty, kidney 55.87
Pelviostomy 55.12
  closure 55.82
Pelviotomy 77.39
  to assist delivery 73.94
Pemberton operation
  osteotomy of ilium 77.39
  rectum (mobilization and fixation for pro-lapse repair) 48.76
Penectomy 64.3
Pereyra operation (paraurethral suspension) 59.6
Perforation
  stapes footplate 19.0
Perfusion NEC 39.97
  for
    chemotherapy NEC 99.25
    hormone therapy NEC 99.24
  carotid artery 39.97
  coronary artery 39.97
  head 39.97
  hyperthermic (lymphatic), localized region or site 93.35
  intestine (large) (local) 46.96
    small 46.95
  kidney, local 55.95
  limb (lower) (upper) 39.97
  liver, localized 50.93
  neck 39.97
  subarachnoid (spinal cord) (refrigerated saline) 03.92
  total body 39.96
Pericardiectomy 37.31
Pericardiocentesis 37.0
Pericardiolysis 37.12
Pericardioplasty 37.49
Pericardiorrhaphy 37.49
Pericardiostomy (tube) 37.12
Pericardiotomy 37.12
Peridectomy 10.31
Perilimbal suction 89.11
Perimetry 95.05
Perineoplasty 71.79
Perineorrhaphy 71.71
  obstetrical laceration (current) 75.69
Perineotomy (nonobstetrical) 71.09
  to assist delivery — *see* Episiotomy
Periosteotomy — *see also* Incision, bone 77.10
  facial bone 76.09
Perirectofistulectomy 48.93
Peritectomy 10.31
Peritomy 10.1
Peritoneocentesis 54.91
Peritoneoscopy 54.21
Peritoneotomy 54.19
Peritoneumectomy 54.4
Phacoemulsification (ultrasonic) (with aspira-tion) 13.41
Phacofragmentation (mechanical) (with aspi-ration) 13.43
  posterior route 13.42
  ultrasonic 13.41
Phalangectomy (partial) 77.89
  claw toe 77.57
  cockup toe 77.58

Phalangectomy — *continued*
  hammer toe 77.56
  overlapping toe 77.58
  total 77.99
Phalangization (fifth metacarpal) 82.81
Pharyngeal flap operation (cleft palate repair) 27.62
  secondary or subsequent 27.63
Pharyngectomy (partial) 29.33
  with laryngectomy 30.3
Pharyngogram 87.09
  contrast 87.06
Pharyngolaryngectomy 30.3
Pharyngoplasty (with silastic implant) 29.4
  for cleft palate 27.62
    secondary or subsequent 27.63
Pharyngorrhaphy 29.51
  for cleft palate 27.62
Pharyngoscopy 29.11
Pharyngotomy 29.0
Phenopeel (skin) 86.24
Phlebectomy 38.60
  with
    anastomosis 38.30
      abdominal 38.37
      head and neck NEC 38.32
      intracranial NEC 38.31
      lower limb 38.39
      thoracic NEC 38.35
      upper limb 38.33
    graft replacement 38.4 ☑
      abdominal 38.47
      head and neck NEC 38.42
      intracranial NEC 38.41
      lower limb 38.49
      thoracic NEC 38.45
      upper limb 38.43
  abdominal 38.67
  head and neck NEC 38.62
  intracranial NEC 38.61
  lower limb 38.69
  thoracic NEC 38.65
  upper limb 38.63
  varicose 38.50
    abdominal 38.57
    head and neck NEC 38.52
    intracranial NEC 38.51
    lower limb 38.59
    thoracic NEC 38.55
    upper limb 38.53
Phlebogoniostomy 12.52
Phlebography (contrast) (retrograde) 88.60
  by radioisotope — *see* Scan, radioisotope, by site
  adrenal 88.65
  femoral 88.66
  head 88.61
  hepatic 88.64
  impedance 88.68
  intra-abdominal NEC 88.65
  intrathoracic NEC 88.63
  lower extremity NEC 88.66
  neck 88.61
  portal system 88.64
  pulmonary 88.62
  specified site NEC 88.67
  vena cava (inferior) (superior) 88.51
Phleborrhaphy 39.32
Phlebotomy 38.99
Phonocardiogram, with ECG lead 89.55
Photochemotherapy NEC 99.83
  extracorporeal 99.88
Photocoagulation
  ciliary body 12.73
  eye, eyeball 16.99
  iris 12.41
  macular hole — *see* Photocoagulation, retina
  orbital lesion 16.92
  retina
    for
      destruction of lesion 14.25
      reattachment 14.55
      repair of tear or defect 14.35

Photocoagulation — *continued*
  retina — *continued*
    laser (beam)
      for
        destruction of lesion 14.24
        reattachment 14.54
        repair of tear or defect 14.34
    xenon arc
      for
        destruction of lesion 14.23
        reattachment 14.53
        repair of tear or defect 14.33
Photography 89.39
  fundus 95.11
Photopheresis, therapeutic 99.88
Phototherapy NEC 99.83
  newborn 99.83
  ultraviolet 99.82
Phrenemphraxis 04.03
  for collapse of lung 33.31
Phrenicectomy 04.03
  for collapse of lung 33.31
Phrenicoexeresis 04.03
  for collapse of lung 33.31
Phrenicotomy 04.03
  for collapse of lung 33.31
Phrenicotripsy 04.03
  for collapse of lung 33.31
Phrenoplasty 34.84
Physical medicine — *see* Therapy, physical
Physical therapy — *see* Therapy, physical
Physiotherapy, chest 93.99
PICC (peripherally inserted central catheter) 38.93
Piercing ear, external (pinna) 18.01
Pigmenting, skin 86.02
Pilojection (aneurysm) (Gallagher) 39.52
Pinealectomy (complete) (total) 07.54
  partial 07.53
Pinealotomy (with drainage) 07.52
Pinning
  bone — *see* Fixation, bone, internal
  ear 18.5
Pinsker operation (obliteration of nasoseptal telangiectasia) 21.07
Piper operation (forceps) 72.6
Pirogoff operation (ankle amputation through malleoli of tibia and fibula) 84.14
Pituitectomy (complete) (total) — *see also* Hypophysectomy 07.69
Placentogram, placentography 88.46
  with radioisotope (RISA) 92.17
Planing, skin 86.25
Plantation, tooth (bud) (germ) 23.5
  prosthetic 23.6
Plasma exchange 99.07
Plasmapheresis, therapeutic 99.71
Plastic repair — *see* Repair, by site
Plasty — *see also* Repair, by site
  bladder neck (V-Y) 57.85
  skin (without graft) 86.89
  subcutaneous tissue 86.89
Platelet inhibitor (GP IIb/IIIa inhibitor only), infusion 99.20
Plateletpheresis, therapeutic 99.74
Play
  psychotherapy 94.36
  therapy 93.81
Pleating
  eye muscle 15.22
    multiple (two or more muscles) 15.4
  sclera, for buckling (*see also* Buckling, scler-al) 14.49
Plethysmogram (carotid) 89.58
  air-filled (pneumatic) 89.58
  capacitance 89.58
  cerebral 89.58
  differential 89.58
  oculoplethysmogram 89.58
  penile 89.58
  photoelectric 89.58
  regional 89.58
  respiratory function measurement (body) 89.38
  segmental 89.58
  strain-gauge 89.58

Plethysmogram — *continued*
  thoracic impedance 89.38
  venous occlusion 89.58
  water-filled 89.58
Plethysmography
  CaverMap™ 89.58
  penile 89.58
Pleurectomy NEC 34.59
Pleurocentesis 34.91
Pleurodesis 34.6
  chemical 34.92
    with cancer chemotherapy substance 34.92 *[99.25]*
    tetracycline 34.92 *[99.21]*
Pleurolysis (for collapse of lung) 33.39
Pleuropexy 34.99
Pleurosclerosis 34.6
  chemical 34.92
    with cancer chemotherapy substance 34.92 *[99.25]*
    tetracycline 34.92 *[99.21]*
Pleurotomy 34.09
Plexectomy
  choroid 02.14
  hypogastric 05.24
Plication
  aneurysm
    heart 37.32
  annulus, heart valve 35.33
  bleb (emphysematous), lung 32.21
  broad ligament 69.22
  diaphragm (for hernia repair) (thoracic ap-proach) (thoracoabdominal ap-proach) 53.81
  eye muscle (oblique) (rectus) 15.22
    multiple (two or more muscles) 15.4
  fascia 83.89
    hand 82.89
  inferior vena cava 38.7
  intestine (jejunum) (Noble) 46.62
  Kelly (-Stoeckel) (urethrovesical junction) 59.3
  levator, for blepharoptosis 08.34
  ligament (*see also* Arthroplasty) 81.96
    broad 69.22
    round 69.22
    uterosacral 69.22
  mesentery 54.75
  round ligament 69.22
  sphincter, urinary bladder 57.85
  stomach 44.69
    laparoscopic 44.68
  superior vena cava 38.7
  tendon 83.85
    hand 82.55
  tricuspid valve (with repositioning) 35.14
  ureter 56.89
  urethra 58.49
  urethrovesical junction 59.3
  vein (peripheral) 39.59
  vena cava (inferior) (superior) 38.7
  ventricle (heart)
    aneurysm 37.32
Plicotomy, tympanum 20.23
Plombage, lung 33.39
Pneumocentesis 33.93
Pneumocisternogram 87.02
Pneumoencephalogram 87.01
Pneumogram, pneumography
  extraperitoneal 88.15
  mediastinal 87.33
  orbit 87.14
  pelvic 88.13
  peritoneum NEC 88.13
  presacral 88.15
  retroperitoneum 88.15
Pneumogynecography 87.82
Pneumomediastinography 87.33
Pneumonectomy (extended) (radical) (stan-dard) (total) (with mediastinal dissec-tion) 32.59
  partial
    complete excision, one lobe 32.49
    resection (wedge), one lobe 32.39
    thoracoscopic 32.50
Pneumonolysis (for collapse of lung) 33.39

☑ **Additional Digit Required — Refer to the Tabular List for Digit Selection**   ▽ **Subterms under main terms may continue to next column or page**

44 — Volume 3   ▶◀ **Revised Text**   ● **New Line**   ▲ **Revised Code**   **2014 ICD-9-CM**

Index

Pneumonotomy — Pubiotomy

Pneumonotomy (with exploration) 33.1
Pneumoperitoneum (surgically-induced) 54.96
  for collapse of lung 33.33
  pelvic 88.12
Pneumothorax (artificial) (surgical) 33.32
  intrapleural 33.32
Pneumoventriculogram 87.02
Politano-Leadbetter operation (ureteroneo-cystostomy) 56.74
Politerization, Eustachian tube 20.8
Pollicization (with carry over of nerves and blood supply) 82.61
Polya operation (gastrectomy) 43.7
Polypectomy — see also Excision, lesion, by site
  esophageal 42.32
    endoscopic 42.33
  gastric (endoscopic) 43.41
  large intestine (colon) 45.42
  nasal 21.31
  rectum (endoscopic) 48.36
Polysomnogram 89.17
Pomeroy operation (ligation and division of fallopian tubes) 66.32
Poncet operation
  lengthening of Achilles tendon 83.85
  urethrostomy, perineal 58.0
Porro operation (cesarean section) 74.99
Portoenterostomy (Kasai) 51.37
Positrocephalogram 92.11
Positron emission tomography (PET) — see Scan, radioisotope
Postmortem examination 89.8
Potts-Smith operation (descending aorta-left pulmonary artery anastomosis) 39.0
Poudrage
  intrapericardial 36.39
  pleural 34.6
PPN (peripheral parenteral nutrition) 99.15
PPVI (percutaneous pulmonary valve implantation) 35.07
Preparation (cutting) pedicle (flap) graft 86.71
Preputiotomy 64.91
Prescription for glasses 95.31
Pressurized
  graft treatment 00.16
Printen and Mason operation (high gastric bypass) 44.31
Probing
  canaliculus, lacrimal (with irrigation) 09.42
  lacrimal
    canaliculi 09.42
    punctum (with irrigation) 09.41
    nasolacrimal duct (with irrigation) 09.43
     with insertion of tube or stent 09.44
  salivary duct (for dilation of duct) (for removal of calculus) 26.91
    with incision 26.0
Procedure — see also specific procedure
  diagnostic NEC
    abdomen (region) 54.29
    adenoid 28.19
    adrenal gland 07.19
    alveolus 24.19
    amnion 75.35
    anterior chamber, eye 12.29
    anus 49.29
    appendix 45.28
    biliary tract 51.19
    bladder 57.39
    blood vessel (any site) 38.29
    bone 78.80
     carpal, metacarpal 78.84
     clavicle 78.81
     facial 76.19
     femur 78.85
     fibula 78.87
     humerus 78.82
     marrow 41.38
     patella 78.86
     pelvic 78.89
     phalanges (foot) (hand) 78.89
     radius 78.83
     scapula 78.81
     specified site NEC 78.89

Procedure — see also specific procedure — continued
  diagnostic — continued
    bone — continued
     tarsal, metatarsal 78.88
     thorax (ribs) (sternum) 78.81
     tibia 78.87
     ulna 78.83
     vertebrae 78.89
    brain 01.18
    breast 85.19
    bronchus 33.29
    buccal 27.24
    bursa 83.29
    canthus 08.19
    cecum 45.28
    cerebral meninges 01.18
    cervix 67.19
    chest wall 34.28
    choroid 14.19
    ciliary body 12.29
    clitoris 71.19
    colon 45.28
    conjunctiva 10.29
    cornea 11.29
    cul-de-sac 70.29
    dental 24.19
    diaphragm 34.28
    duodenum 45.19
    ear
     external 18.19
     inner and middle 20.39
    epididymis 63.09
    esophagus 42.29
    Eustachian tube 20.39
    extraocular muscle or tendon 15.09
    eye 16.29
     anterior chamber 12.29
     posterior chamber 14.19
    eyeball 16.29
    eyelid 08.19
    fallopian tube 66.19
    fascia (any site) 83.29
    fetus 75.35
    gallbladder 51.19
    ganglion (cranial) (peripheral) 04.19
     sympathetic 05.19
    gastric 44.19
    globus pallidus 01.18
    gum 24.19
    heart 37.29
    hepatic 50.19
    hypophysis 07.19
    ileum 45.19
    intestine 45.29
     large 45.28
     small 45.19
    iris 12.29
    jejunum 45.19
    joint (capsule) (ligament) (structure) NEC 81.98
     facial 76.19
    kidney 55.29
    labia 71.19
    lacrimal (system) 09.19
    large intestine 45.28
    larynx 31.48
    ligament 81.98
     uterine 68.19
    liver 50.19
    lung 33.29
    lymphatic structure (channel) (gland) (node) (vessel) 40.19
    mediastinum 34.29
    meninges (cerebral) 01.18
     spinal 03.39
    mouth 27.29
    muscle 83.29
     extraocular (oblique) (rectus) 15.09
     papillary (heart) 37.29
    nail 86.19
    nasopharynx 29.19
    nerve (cranial) (peripheral) NEC 04.19
     sympathetic 05.19
    nipple 85.19
    nose, nasal 21.29

Procedure — see also specific procedure — continued
  diagnostic — continued
    nose, nasal — continued
     sinus 22.19
    ocular 16.29
     muscle 15.09
    omentum 54.29
    ophthalmologic 16.29
    oral (cavity) 27.29
    orbit 16.29
    orthodontic 24.19
    ovary 65.19
     laparoscopic 65.14
    palate 27.29
    pancreas 52.19
    papillary muscle (heart) 37.29
    parathyroid gland 06.19
    penis 64.19
    perianal tissue 49.29
    pericardium 37.29
    periprostatic tissue 60.18
    perirectal tissue 48.29
    perirenal tissue 59.29
    peritoneum 54.29
    periurethral tissue 58.29
    perivesical tissue 59.29
    pharynx 29.19
    pineal gland 07.19
    pituitary gland 07.19
    pleura 34.28
    posterior chamber, eye 14.19
    prostate 60.18
    pulmonary 33.29
    rectosigmoid 48.29
    rectum 48.29
    renal 55.29
    respiratory 33.29
    retina 14.19
    retroperitoneum 59.29
    salivary gland or duct 26.19
    sclera 12.29
    scrotum 61.19
    seminal vesicle 60.19
    sigmoid 45.28
    sinus, nasal 22.19
    skin 86.19
    skull 87.19
    soft tissue 83.29
    spermatic cord 63.09
    sphincter of Oddi 51.19
    spine, spinal (canal) (cord) (meninges) (structure) 03.39
    spleen 41.39
    stomach 44.19
    subcutaneous tissue 86.19
    sympathetic nerve 05.19
    tarsus 09.19
    tendon NEC 83.29
     extraocular 15.09
    testicle 62.19
    thalamus 01.18
    thoracic duct 40.19
    thorax 34.28
    thymus 07.19
    thyroid gland 06.19
    tongue 25.09
    tonsils 28.19
    tooth 24.19
    trachea 31.49
    tunica vaginalis 61.19
    ureter 56.39
    urethra 58.29
    uterus and supporting structures 68.19
    uvula 27.29
    vagina 70.29
    vas deferens 63.09
    vesical 57.39
    vessel (blood) (any site) 38.29
    vitreous 14.19
    vulva 71.19
  fistulizing, sclera NEC 12.69
  miscellaneous (nonoperative) NEC 99.99
  respiratory (nonoperative) NEC 93.99
  surgical — see Operation
Proctectasis 96.22

Proctectomy (partial) — see also Resection, rectum 48.69
  abdominoperineal, NOS 48.50
    laparoscopic 48.51
    open 48.52
    other 48.59
  complete (Miles) (Rankin), NOS 48.50
    laparoscopic 48.51
    open 48.52
    other 48.59
  pull-through
    laparoscopic 48.42
    not otherwise specified 48.40
    open 48.43
    other 48.49
Proctoclysis 96.37
Proctolysis 48.99
Proctopexy (Delorme) 48.76
  abdominal (Ripstein) 48.75
Proctoplasty 48.79
Proctorrhaphy 48.71
Proctoscopy 48.23
  with biopsy 48.24
  through stoma (artificial) 48.22
  transabdominal approach 48.21
Proctosigmoidectomy — see also Resection, rectum 48.69
Proctosigmoidopexy 48.76
Proctosigmoidoscopy (rigid) 48.23
  with biopsy 48.24
  flexible 45.24
  through stoma (artificial) 48.22
  transabdominal approach 48.21
Proctostomy 48.1
Proctotomy (decompression) (linear) 48.0
Production — see also Formation and Creation
  atrial septal defect 35.42
  subcutaneous tunnel for esophageal anastomosis 42.86
    with anastomosis — see Anastomosis, esophagus, antesternal
Prognathic recession 76.64
Prophylaxis, dental (scaling) (polishing) 96.54
Prostatectomy (complete) (partial) NEC 60.69
  loop 60.29
  perineal 60.62
  radical (any approach) 60.5
  retropubic (punch) (transcapsular) 60.4
  suprapubic (punch) (transvesical) 60.3
  transcapsular NEC 60.69
    retropubic 60.4
  transperineal 60.62
  transurethral 60.29
    ablation (contact) (noncontact) by laser 60.21
    electrovaporization 60.29
    enucleative 60.29
    resection of prostate (TURP) 60.29
    ultrasound guided laser induced (TULIP) 60.21
  transvesical punch (suprapubic) 60.3
Prostatocystotomy 60.0
Prostatolithotomy 60.0
Prostatotomy (perineal) 60.0
Prostatovesiculectomy 60.5
Protection (of)
  individual from his surroundings 99.84
  surroundings from individual 99.84
Psychoanalysis 94.31
Psychodrama 94.43
Psychotherapy NEC 94.39
  biofeedback 94.39
  exploratory verbal 94.37
  group 94.44
    for psychosexual dysfunctions 94.41
  play 94.36
  psychosexual dysfunctions 94.34
  supportive verbal 94.38
PTCA (percutaneous transluminal coronary angioplasty) — see Angioplasty, balloon, coronary
Ptyalectasis 26.91
Ptyalithotomy 26.0
Ptyalolithotomy 26.0
Pubiotomy 77.39
  assisting delivery 73.94

☑ Additional Digit Required — Refer to the Tabular List for Digit Selection   ▽ Subterms under main terms may continue to next column or page

2014 ICD-9-CM   ▶◀ Revised Text   ● New Line   ▲ Revised Code   Volume 3 — 45

☑ **Additional Digit Required** — Refer to the Tabular List for Digit Selection   ▽ **Subterms under main terms may continue to next column or page**

46 — Volume 3   ▶◀ Revised Text   ● New Line   ▲ Revised Code   2014 ICD-9-CM

Index — Pubococcygeoplasty — Reattachment

☑ **Additional Digit Required — Refer to the Tabular List for Digit Selection**

Subterms under main terms may continue to next column or page

2014 ICD-9-CM

▶◀ **Revised Text**

● **New Line**

▲ **Revised Code**

Volume 3 — 47

Reattachment — Reduction

Reduction — *continued*
  fracture — *continued*
    ulna — *continued*
      open — *continued*
        with internal fixation 79.32
    vertebra 03.53
    zygoma, zygomatic arch (closed) 76.71
      open 76.72
  heart volume 37.35
  hemorrhoids (manual) 49.41
  hernia (*see also* Repair, hernia)
    manual 96.27
  intussusception (open) 46.80
    with
      fluoroscopy 96.29
      ionizing radiation enema 96.29
      ultrasonography guidance 96.29
    hydrostatic 96.29
    large intestine 46.82
      endoscopic (balloon) 46.85
    pneumatic 96.29
    small intestine 46.81
  lung volume 32.22
    biologic lung volume reduction (BLVR)
      — *see* category 33.7 ☑
  malrotation, intestine (manual) (surgical)
    46.80
    large 46.82
      endoscopic (balloon) 46.85
    small 46.81
  mammoplasty (bilateral) 85.32
    unilateral 85.31
  prolapse
    anus (operative) 49.94
    colostomy (manual) 96.28
    enterostomy (manual) 96.28
    ileostomy (manual) 96.28
    rectum (manual) 96.26
    uterus
      by pessary 96.18
      surgical 69.22
  ptosis overcorrection 08.37
  retroversion, uterus by pessary 96.18
  separation, epiphysis (with internal fixation)
    (closed) 79.40
    femur (closed) 79.45
      open 79.55
    fibula (closed) 79.46
      open 79.56
    humerus (closed) 79.41
      open 79.51
    open 79.50
    specified site (closed) NEC (*see also* category) 79.4 ☑
      open — *see* category 79.5 ☑
    tibia (closed) 79.46
      open 79.56
  size
    abdominal wall (adipose) (pendulous)
      86.83
    arms (adipose) (batwing) 86.83
    breast (bilateral) 85.32
      unilateral 85.31
    buttocks (adipose) 86.83
    finger (macrodactyly repair) 82.83
    skin 86.83
    subcutaneous tissue 86.83
    thighs (adipose) 86.83
  torsion
    intestine (manual) (surgical) 46.80
      large 46.82
        endoscopic (balloon) 46.85
      small 46.81
    kidney pedicle 55.84
    omentum 54.74
    spermatic cord 63.52
      with orchiopexy 62.5
    testis 63.52
      with orchiopexy 62.5
    uterus NEC 69.98
      gravid 75.99
  ventricular 37.35
  volvulus
    intestine 46.80
      large 46.82
        endoscopic (balloon) 46.85

Reduction — *continued*
  volvulus — *continued*
    intestine — *continued*
      small 46.81
    stomach 44.92
Reefing, joint capsule — *see also* Arthroplasty 81.96
Referral (for)
  psychiatric aftercare (halfway house) (outpatient clinic) 94.52
  psychotherapy 94.51
  rehabilitation
    alcoholism 94.53
    drug addiction 94.54
    psychologic NEC 94.59
    vocational 94.55
Reformation
  cardiac pacemaker pocket, new site (skin) (subcutaneous) 37.79
  cardioverter/defibrillator (automatic) pocket, new site (skin) (subcutaneous) 37.79
  chamber of eye 12.99
Refracture
  bone (for faulty union) (*see also* Osteoclasis) 78.70
  nasal bones 21.88
Refusion
  spinal, NOS 81.30

Note: Also use either 81.62, 81.63, or 81.64 as an additional code to show the total number of vertebrae fused

    atlas-axis (anterior) (transoral) (posterior) 81.31
    axial lumbar interbody fusion (AxiaLIF®) 81.38
    cervical (C₂ level or below) NEC 81.32
      anterior column (interbody), anterolateral (anterior) technique 81.32
      C_1-C_2 level (anterior) (posterior) 81.31
      posterior column, posterolateral (posterior) technique 81.33
    craniocervical (anterior) (transoral) (posterior) 81.31
    direct lateral interbody fusion (DLIF) 81.36
    dorsal, dorsolumbar NEC 81.35
      anterior column (interbody), anterolateral (anterior) (extracavitary) technique 81.34
      posterior column, posterolateral (posterior) technique 81.35
    extreme lateral interbody fusion (XLIF®) 81.36
    facet 81.37
    lumbar, lumbosacral NEC 81.38
      anterior column (interbody)
        anterolateral (anterior) technique 81.36
        posterior technique 81.38
      anterior lumbar interbody fusion (ALIF) 81.36
      lateral transverse process technique 81.37
      posterior column, posterior (posterolateral) (transverse process) technique 81.37
      posterior lumbar interbody fusion (PLIF) 81.38
      posterior (interbody), posterolateral technique 81.38
      transforaminal lumbar interbody fusion (TLIF) 81.38
    number of vertebrae — *see* codes 81.62-81.64
    occiput — C₂ (anterior) (transoral) (posterior) 81.31
    refusion NEC 81.39
Regional blood flow study 92.05
Regulation, menstrual 69.6
Rehabilitation programs NEC 93.89
  alcohol 94.61
    with detoxification 94.63

Rehabilitation programs — *continued*
  alcohol — *continued*
    combined alcohol and drug 94.67
      with detoxification 94.69
  drug 94.64
    with detoxification 94.66
    combined drug and alcohol 94.67
      with detoxification 94.69
  sheltered employment 93.85
  vocational 93.85
Reimplantation
  adrenal tissue (heterotopic) (orthotopic) 07.45
  artery 39.59
    renal, aberrant 39.55
  bile ducts following excision of ampulla of Vater 51.62
  extremity — *see* Reattachment, extremity
  fallopian tube into uterus 66.74
  kidney 55.61
  lung 33.5 ☑
  ovary 65.72
    laparoscopic 65.75
  pancreatic tissue 52.81
  parathyroid tissue (heterotopic) (orthotopic) 06.95
  pulmonary artery for hemitruncus repair 35.83
  renal vessel, aberrant 39.55
  testis in scrotum 62.5
  thyroid tissue (heterotopic) (orthotopic) 06.94
  tooth 23.5
  ureter into bladder 56.74
Reinforcement — *see also* Repair, by site
  sclera NEC 12.88
    with graft 12.87
Reinsertion — *see also* Insertion or Revision
  cystostomy tube 59.94
  fixation device (internal) (*see also* Fixation, bone, internal) 78.50
  heart valve (prosthetic) 35.95
  Holter (-Spitz) valve 02.42
  implant (expelled) (extruded)
    eyeball (with conjunctival graft) 16.62
    orbital 16.62
  nephrostomy tube 55.93
  pyelostomy tube 55.94
  ureteral stent (transurethral) 59.8
    with ureterotomy 59.8 *[56.2]*
  ureterostomy tube 59.93
  valve
    heart (prosthetic) 35.95
    ventricular (cerebral) 02.42
Relaxation — *see also* Release training 94.33
Release
  carpal tunnel (for nerve decompression) 04.43
  celiac artery axis 39.91
  central slip, extensor tendon hand (mallet finger repair) 82.84
  chordee 64.42
  clubfoot NEC 83.84
  de Quervain's tenosynovitis 82.01
  Dupuytren's contracture (by palmar fasciectomy) 82.35
    by fasciotomy (subcutaneous) 82.12
    with excision 82.35
  Fowler (mallet finger repair) 82.84
  joint (capsule) (adherent) (constrictive) (*see also* Division, joint capsule) 80.40
  laryngeal 31.92
  ligament (*see also* Division, ligament) 80.40
    median arcuate 39.91
  median arcuate ligament 39.91
  muscle (division) 83.19
    hand 82.19
  nerve (peripheral) NEC 04.49
    cranial NEC 04.42
    trigeminal 04.41
  pressure, intraocular 12.79
  scar tissue
    skin 86.84
    stoma — *see* Revision, stoma
  tarsal tunnel 04.44
  tendon 83.13

Release — *continued*
  tendon — *continued*
    hand 82.11
      extensor, central slip (repair mallet finger) 82.84
    sheath 83.01
      hand 82.01
    tenosynovitis 83.01
      abductor pollicis longus 82.01
      de Quervain's 82.01
      external pollicis brevis 82.01
      hand 82.01
    torsion
      intestine 46.80
        large 46.82
          endoscopic (balloon) 46.85
        small 46.81
      kidney pedicle 55.84
      ovary 65.95
      testes 63.52
    transverse carpal ligament (for nerve decompression) 04.43
    trigger finger or thumb 82.01
    urethral stricture 58.5
    Volkmann's contracture
      excision of scar, muscle 83.32
      fasciotomy 83.14
      muscle transplantation 83.77
    web contracture (skin) 86.84
Relief — *see* Release
Relocation — *see also* Revision
  cardiac device (CRT-D) (CRT-P) (defibrillator) (pacemaker) pocket, new site (skin) (subcutaneous) 37.79
  CRT-D pocket 37.79
  CRT-P pocket 37.79
  subcutaneous device pocket NEC 86.09
Remobilization
  joint 93.16
  stapes 19.0
Remodel
  ventricle 37.35
Removal — *see also* Excision
  Abrams bar (chest wall) 34.01
  abscess — *see* Incision, by site
  adenoid tag(s) 28.6
  anal sphincter
    with revision 49.75
    without revision 49.76
  arch bars (orthodontic) 24.8
    immobilization device 97.33
  arterial graft or prosthesis 39.49
  arteriovenous shunt (device) 39.43
    with creation of new shunt 39.42
  artificial heart
    internal biventricular replacement system 37.55
  Barton's tongs (skull) 02.95
    with synchronous replacement 02.94
  bladder sphincter, artificial 58.99
    with replacement 58.93
  blood clot (*see also* Incision, by site)
    bladder (by incision) 57.19
      without incision 57.0
    kidney (without incision) 56.0
      by incision 55.01
    ureter
      by incision 56.2
  bone fragment (chip) (*see also* Incision, bone) 77.10
    joint (*see also* Arthrotomy) 80.10
    necrotic (*see also* Sequestrectomy, bone) 77.00
    joint (*see also* Arthrotomy) 80.10
    skull 01.25
      with debridement compound fracture 02.02
  bone growth stimulator — *see* category 78.6 ☑
  bony spicules, spinal canal 03.53
  brace 97.88
  breast implant 85.94
    tissue expander 85.96
  bronchial device or substance
    endoscopic 33.78

☑ **Additional Digit Required — Refer to the Tabular List for Digit Selection**

▽ **Subterms under main terms may continue to next column or page**

☑ **Additional Digit Required** — Refer to the Tabular List for Digit Selection   ▽ **Subterms under main terms may continue to next column or page**

Removal — *see also* Excision — *continued*
foreign body (*see also* Incision, by site) — *continued*
  eye, eyeball — *continued*
    anterior segment (by incision) 12.00
      with use of magnet 12.01
      without use of magnet 12.02
    posterior segment (by incision) 14.00
      with use of magnet 14.01
      without use of magnet 14.02
    superficial 98.21
  eyelid 98.22
    by incision 08.09
  fallopian tube
    by salpingostomy 66.02
    by salpingotomy 66.01
  fascia 83.09
    hand 82.09
  foot 98.28
  gall bladder 51.04
  groin region (abdominal wall) (inguinal) 54.0
  gum 98.22
    by incision 24.0
  hand 98.26
  head and neck NEC 98.22
  heart 37.11
  internal fixation device — *see* Removal, fixation device, internal
  intestine
    by incision 45.00
    large (intraluminal) 98.04
      by incision 45.03
    small (intraluminal) 98.03
      by incision 45.02
  intraocular (by incision) 12.00
    with use of magnet 12.01
    without use of magnet 12.02
  iris (by incision) 12.00
    with use of magnet 12.01
    without use of magnet 12.02
  joint structures (*see also* Arthrotomy) 80.10
  kidney (transurethral) (by endoscopy) 56.0
    by incision 55.01
    pelvis (transurethral) 56.0
      by incision 55.11
  labia 98.23
    by incision 71.09
  lacrimal
    canaliculi 09.42
      by incision 09.52
    gland 09.3
      by incision 09.0
    passage(s) 09.49
      by incision 09.59
    punctum 09.41
      by incision 09.51
    sac 09.49
      by incision 09.53
  large intestine (intraluminal) 98.04
    by incision 45.03
  larynx (intraluminal) 98.14
    by incision 31.3
  lens 13.00
    by incision 13.02
      with use of magnet 13.01
  liver 50.0
  lower limb, except foot 98.29
    foot 98.28
  lung 33.1
  mediastinum 34.1
  meninges (cerebral) 01.31
    spinal 03.01
  mouth (intraluminal) 98.01
    by incision 27.92
  muscle 83.02
    hand 82.02
  nasal sinus 22.50
    antrum 22.2
      with Caldwell-Luc approach 22.39
    ethmoid 22.51
    frontal 22.41
    maxillary 22.2
      with Caldwell-Luc approach 22.39

Removal — *see also* Excision — *continued*
foreign body (*see also* Incision, by site) — *continued*
  nasal sinus — *continued*
    sphenoid 22.52
  nerve (cranial) (peripheral) NEC 04.04
    root 03.01
  nose (intraluminal) 98.12
    by incision 21.1
  oral cavity (intraluminal) 98.01
    by incision 27.92
  orbit (by magnet) 98.21
    by incision 16.1
  palate (penetrating) 98.22
    by incision 27.1
  pancreas 52.09
  penis 98.24
    by incision 64.92
  pericardium 37.12
  perineum (female) 98.23
    by incision 71.09
    male 98.25
      by incision 86.05
  perirenal tissue 59.09
  peritoneal cavity 54.92
  perivesical tissue 59.19
  pharynx (intraluminal) 98.13
    by pharyngotomy 29.0
  pleura (by incision) 34.09
  popliteal space 98.29
    by incision 86.05
  rectum (intraluminal) 98.05
    by incision 48.0
  renal pelvis (transurethral) 56.0
    by incision 56.1
  retina (by incision) 14.00
    with use of magnet 14.01
    without use of magnet 14.02
  retroperitoneum 54.92
  sclera (by incision) 12.00
    with use of magnet 12.01
    without use of magnet 12.02
  scrotum 98.24
    by incision 61.0
  sinus (nasal) 22.50
    antrum 22.2
      with Caldwell-Luc approach 22.39
    ethmoid 22.51
    frontal 22.41
    maxillary 22.2
      with Caldwell-Luc approach 22.39
    sphenoid 22.52
  skin NEC 98.20
    by incision 86.05
  skull 01.24
    with incision into brain 01.39
  small intestine (intraluminal) 98.03
    by incision 45.02
  soft tissue NEC 83.09
    hand 82.09
  spermatic cord 63.93
  spinal (canal) (cord) (meninges) 03.01
  stomach (intraluminal) 98.03
    by incision 43.0
    bubble (balloon) 44.94
  subconjunctival (by magnet) 98.22
    by incision 10.0
  subcutaneous tissue NEC 98.20
    by incision 86.05
  supraclavicular fossa 98.27
    by incision 86.05
  tendon (sheath) 83.01
    hand 82.01
  testis 62.0
  thorax (by incision) 34.09
  thyroid (field) (gland) (by incision) 06.09
  tonsil 98.13
    by incision 28.91
  trachea (intraluminal) 98.15
    by incision 31.3
  trunk NEC 98.25
  tunica vaginalis 98.24
  upper limb, except hand 98.27
    hand 98.26
  ureter (transurethral) 56.0
    by incision 56.2

Removal — *see also* Excision — *continued*
foreign body (*see also* Incision, by site) — *continued*
  urethra (intraluminal) 98.19
    by incision 58.0
  uterus (intraluminal) 98.16
  vagina (intraluminal) 98.17
    by incision 70.14
  vas deferens 63.6
  vitreous (by incision) 14.00
    with use of magnet 14.01
    without use of magnet 14.02
  vulva 98.23
    by incision 71.09
gallstones
  bile duct (by incision) NEC 51.49
    endoscopic 51.88
  common duct (by incision) 51.41
    endoscopic 51.88
    percutaneous 51.96
  duodenum 45.01
  gallbladder 51.04
    endoscopic 51.88
    laparoscopic 51.88
  hepatic ducts 51.49
    endoscopic 51.88
  intestine 45.00
    large 45.03
    small NEC 45.02
  liver 50.0
Gardner Wells tongs (skull) 02.95
  with synchronous replacement 02.94
gastric band (adjustable), laparoscopic 44.97
gastric bubble (balloon) 44.94
granulation tissue (*see also* Excision, lesion, by site)
  with repair — *see* Repair, by site
  cranial 01.6
  skull 01.6
halo traction device (skull) 02.95
  with synchronous replacement 02.94
heart assist system
  with replacement 37.63
  intra-aortic balloon pump (IABP) 97.44
  nonoperative 97.44
  open removal 37.64
  percutaneous external device 97.44
heart replacement system
  internal biventricular 37.55
hematoma — *see* Drainage, by site
Hoffman minifixator device (bone) — *see* category 78.6 ☑
hydatidiform mole 68.0
impacted
  feces (rectum) (by flushing) (manual) 96.38
  tooth 23.19
    from nasal sinus (maxillary) 22.61
implant
  breast 85.94
  cochlear prosthetic device 20.99
  cornea 11.92
  lens (prosthetic) 13.8
  middle ear NEC 20.99
  ocular 16.71
    posterior segment 14.6
  orbit 16.72
  retina 14.6
  tympanum 20.1
implantable hemodynamic sensor (lead) and monitor device 37.79
internal biventricular heart replacement system 37.55
internal fixation device — *see* Removal, fixation device, internal
intra-aortic balloon pump (IABP) 97.44
intrauterine contraceptive device (IUD) 97.71
joint (structure) NOS 80.90
  ankle 80.97
  elbow 80.92
  foot and toe 80.98
  hand and finger 80.94
  hip 80.95
  knee 80.96
  other specified sites 80.99

Removal — *see also* Excision — *continued*
joint — *continued*
  shoulder 80.91
  spine 80.99
  toe 80.98
  wrist 80.93
Kantrowitz heart pump 37.64
  nonoperative 97.44
keel (tantalum plate), larynx 31.98
kidney (*see also* Nephrectomy)
  mechanical 55.98
  transplanted or rejected 55.53
laminaria (tent), uterus 97.79
leads (cardiac) — *see* Removal, electrodes, cardiac pacemaker
lesion — *see* Excision, lesion, by site
ligamentum flavum (spine) — *omit code*
ligature
  fallopian tube 66.79
  ureter 56.86
  vas deferens 63.84
limb lengthening device, internal — *see* category 78.6 ☑
loop recorder 86.05
loose body
  bone — *see* Sequestrectomy, bone
  joint 80.10
  mesh (surgical) — *see* Removal, foreign body, by site
lymph node — *see* Excision, lymph, node
minifixator device (bone) — *see* category 78.6 ☑
  external fixation device 97.88
Mulligan hood, fallopian tube 66.94
  with synchronous replacement 66.93
muscle stimulator (skeletal) 83.93
  with replacement 83.92
myringotomy device or tube 20.1
nail (bed) (fold) 86.23
  internal fixation device — *see* Removal, fixation device, internal
necrosis
  skin 86.28
  excisional 86.22
neuropacemaker — *see* Removal, neurostimulator, by site
neurostimulator
  brain 01.22
    with synchronous replacement 02.93
  electrodes
    brain 01.22
      with synchronous replacement 02.93
    gastric 04.93
      with synchronous replacement 04.92
    intracranial 01.22
      with synchronous replacement 02.93
    peripheral nerve 04.93
      with synchronous replacement 04.92
    sacral nerve 04.93
      with synchronous replacement 04.92
    spinal 03.94
      with synchronous replacement 03.93
  intracranial 01.22
    with synchronous replacement 02.93
  peripheral nerve 04.93
    with synchronous replacement 04.92
  pulse generator (subcutaneous single array, multiple array) 86.05
    with synchronous replacement 86.96
    multiple array 86.95
      rechargeable 86.98
    single array 86.94
      rechargeable 86.97
  cranial 01.29
    with synchronous replacement 01.20
  spinal 03.94
    with synchronous replacement 03.93
nonabsorbable surgical material NEC — *see* Removal, foreign body, by site

---

☑ **Additional Digit Required** — Refer to the Tabular List for Digit Selection
▽ **Subterms under main terms may continue to next column or page**

50 — Volume 3
▶◀ Revised Text
● New Line
▲ Revised Code
2014 ICD-9-CM

☑ **Additional Digit Required** — Refer to the Tabular List for Digit Selection   ▽ **Subterms under main terms may continue to next column or page**

2014 ICD-9-CM   ▶◀ **Revised Text**   ● **New Line**   ▲ **Revised Code**   October 2013 · Volume 3 — 51

Repair — *Repair*

☑ **Additional Digit Required** — Refer to the Tabular List for Digit Selection   ▽ **Subterms under main terms may continue to next column or page**

52 — Volume 3   ▶◀ Revised Text   ● New Line   ▲ Revised Code   2014 ICD-9-CM

Repair — *continued*
epicanthus (fold) 08.59
epididymis (and spermatic cord) NEC 63.59
  with vas deferens 63.89
epiglottis 31.69
episiotomy
  routine following delivery — *see* Episiotomy
  secondary 75.69
epispadias 58.45
esophagus, esophageal NEC 42.89
  fistula NEC 42.84
  stricture 42.85
exstrophy of bladder 57.86
eyebrow 08.89
  linear 08.81
eye, eyeball 16.89
  multiple structures 16.82
  rupture 16.82
  socket 16.64
    with graft 16.63
eyelid 08.89
  full-thickness 08.85
    involving lid margin 08.84
  laceration 08.81
    full-thickness 08.85
      involving lid margin 08.84
    partial-thickness 08.83
      involving lid margin 08.82
    linear 08.81
  partial-thickness 08.83
    involving lid margin 08.82
  retraction 08.38
fallopian tube (with prosthesis) 66.79
  by
    anastomosis 66.73
    reanastomosis 66.79
    reimplantation into
      ovary 66.72
      uterus 66.74
    suture 66.71
false aneurysm — *see* Repair, aneurysm
fascia 83.89
  by or with
    arthroplasty — *see* Arthroplasty
    graft (fascial) (muscle) 83.82
      hand 82.72
      tendon 83.81
        hand 82.79
    suture (direct) 83.65
      hand 82.46
  hand 82.89
    by
      graft NEC 82.79
        fascial 82.72
        muscle 82.72
      suture (direct) 82.46
  joint — *see* Arthroplasty
filtering bleb (corneal) (scleral) (by excision) 12.82
  by
    corneal graft (*see also* Keratoplasty) 11.60
    scleroplasty 12.82
    suture 11.51
      with conjunctival flap 11.53
fistula (*see also* Closure, fistula)
  anovaginal 70.73
  arteriovenous 39.53
    clipping 39.53
    coagulation 39.53
      endovascular approach 39.79
        head and neck 39.72
    division 39.53
    excision or resection (*see also* Aneurysmectomy, by site)
      with
        anastomosis — *see* Aneurysmectomy, with anastomosis, by site
        graft replacement — *see* Aneurysmectomy, with graft replacement, by site
    ligation 39.53
      coronary artery 36.99

Repair — *continued*
fistula (*see also* Closure, fistula) — *continued*
  arteriovenous — *continued*
    occlusion 39.53
      endovascular approach 39.79
        head and neck 39.72
    suture 39.53
  cervicovesical 57.84
  cervix 67.62
  choledochoduodenal 51.72
  colovaginal 70.72
  enterovaginal 70.74
  enterovesical 57.83
  esophagocutaneous 42.84
  ileovesical 57.83
  intestinovaginal 70.74
  intestinovesical 57.83
  oroantral 22.71
  perirectal 48.93
  pleuropericardial 37.49
  rectovaginal 70.73
  rectovesical 57.83
  rectovesicovaginal 57.83
  scrotum 61.42
  sigmoidovaginal 70.74
  sinus
    nasal 22.71
    of Valsalva 35.39
  splenocolic 41.95
  urethroperineovesical 57.84
  urethrovesical 57.84
  urethrovesicovaginal 57.84
  uterovesical 57.84
  vagina NEC 70.75
  vaginocutaneous 70.75
  vaginoenteric NEC 70.74
  vaginoileal 70.74
  vaginoperineal 70.75
  vaginovesical 57.84
  vesicocervicovaginal 57.84
  vesicocolic 57.83
  vesicocutaneous 57.84
  vesicoenteric 57.83
  vesicointestinal 57.83
  vesicometrorectal 57.83
  vesicoperineal 57.84
  vesicorectal 57.83
  vesicosigmoidal 57.83
  vesicosigmoidovaginal 57.83
  vesicourethral 57.84
  vesicourethrorectal 57.83
  vesicouterine 57.84
  vesicovaginal 57.84
  vulva 71.72
  vulvorectal 48.73
foramen ovale (patent) 35.71
  with
    prosthesis (open heart technique) 35.51
    closed heart technique 35.52
    tissue graft 35.61
fracture (*see also* Reduction, fracture)
  larynx 31.64
  malunion or nonunion (delayed) NEC — *see* category 78.4 ☑
    with
      graft — *see* Graft, bone
      insertion (of)
        bone growth stimulator (invasive) — *see* category 78.9 ☑
        internal fixation device 78.5 ☑
      manipulation for realignment — *see* Reduction, fracture, by site, closed
      osteotomy
        with
          correction of alignment — *see* category 77.3 ☑
          with internal fixation device — *see* categories 77.3 ☑ [78.5] ☑

Repair — *continued*
fracture (*see also* Reduction, fracture) — *continued*
  malunion or nonunion — *see* category — *continued*
    with — *continued*
      osteotomy — *continued*
        with — *continued*
          correction of alignment — *see* category — *continued*
            with intramed-ullary rod — *see* categories 77.3 ☑ [78.5] ☑
      replacement arthroplasty — *see* Arthroplasty
      sequestrectomy — *see* category 77.0 ☑
      Sofield type procedure — *see* categories 77.3 ☑ [78.5] ☑
      synostosis technique — *see* Arthrodesis
  vertebra 03.53
funnel chest (with implant) 34.74
gallbladder 51.91
gastroschisis 54.71
great vessels NEC 39.59
  laceration (by suture) 39.30
    artery 39.31
    vein 39.32
hallux valgus NEC 77.59
  resection of joint with prosthetic implant 77.59
hammer toe 77.56
hand 82.89
  with graft or implant 82.79
    fascia 82.72
    muscle 82.72
    tendon 82.79
heart 37.49
  assist system 37.63
  septum 35.70
    with
      prosthesis 35.50
      tissue graft 35.60
    atrial 35.71
      with
        prosthesis (open heart technique) 35.51
        closed heart technique 35.52
        tissue graft 35.61
      combined with repair of valvular and ventricular septal defects — *see* Repair, endocardial cushion defect
      in total repair of
        tetralogy of Fallot 35.81
        total anomalous pulmonary venous connection 35.82
        truncus arteriosus 35.83
    combined with repair of valvular defect — *see* Repair, endocardial cushion defect
    ventricular 35.72
      with
        prosthesis (open heart technique) 35.53
        closed heart technique 35.55
        tissue graft 35.62
      combined with repair of valvular and atrial septal defects — *see* Repair, endocardial cushion defect
      in total repair of
        tetralogy of Fallot 35.81
        total anomalous pulmonary venous connection 35.82
        truncus arteriosus 35.83
  total internal biventricular replacement system 37.52

Repair — *continued*
heart — *continued*
  total internal biventricular replacement system — *continued*
    implantable battery 37.54
    implantable controller 37.54
    thoracic unit 37.53
    transcutaneous energy transfer (TET) device 37.54
  valve (cusps) (open heart technique) 35.10
    aortic (without replacement) 35.11
    combined with repair of atrial and ventricular septal defects — *see* Repair, endocardial cushion defect
    mitral (without replacement) 35.12
      with
        leaflet clip implant 35.97
        MitraClip® 35.97
      balloon, percutaneous 35.96
      endovascular repair with implant 35.97
      percutaneous with leaflet clip implant 35.97
    pulmonary (without replacement) 35.13
      with
        tissue graft 35.25
        in total repair of tetralogy of Fallot 35.81
    tricuspid (without replacement) 35.14
hepatic duct 51.79
hernia NEC 53.9
  anterior abdominal wall NEC (laparoscopic without graft or prosthesis) 53.59
    with prosthesis or graft
      laparoscopic 53.63
      other and open 53.69
  colostomy 46.42
  crural 53.29
  cul-de-sac (Douglas') 70.92
  diaphragmatic
    abdominal approach
      laparoscopic 53.71
      other and open 53.72
      unspecified 53.75
    thoracic, thoracoabdominal approach 53.80
      laparoscopic 53.83
      other and open 53.84
  epigastric 53.59
    with prosthesis or graft 53.69
  esophageal hiatus
    abdominal approach
      laparoscopic 53.71
      other and open 53.72
      unspecified 53.75
    thoracic, thoracoabdominal approach 53.80
  fascia 83.89
    hand 82.89
  femoral (unilateral) 53.29
    with prosthesis or graft 53.21
    bilateral 53.39
      with prosthesis or graft 53.31
  Ferguson 53.00
  Halsted 53.00
  Hill-Allison (hiatal hernia repair, transpleural approach) 53.80
  hypogastric 53.59
    with prosthesis or graft 53.69
  incisional 53.51
    laparoscopic with prosthesis or graft 53.62
    other open with prosthesis or graft 53.61
  inguinal (unilateral) 53.00
    with prosthesis or graft 53.05
    bilateral 53.10
      with prosthesis or graft 53.17
        laparoscopic 17.24

☑ **Additional Digit Required — Refer to the Tabular List for Digit Selection**   🔻 **Subterms under main terms may continue to next column or page**

2014 ICD-9-CM   ▶◀ **Revised Text**   ● **New Line**   ▲ **Revised Code**   **Volume 3 — 53**

Index

Repair — Repair

Repair — *continued*
  hernia — *continued*
    inguinal — *continued*
      bilateral — *continued*
        direct
          laparoscopic with graft or
            prosthesis 17.21
          other and open laparoscopic
            without graft or pros-
            thesis 53.11
          with prosthesis or graft
            53.14
        direct and indirect
          laparoscopic with graft or
            prosthesis 17.23
          other and open (laparoscopic
            without graft or pros-
            thesis) 53.13
          with prosthesis or graft
            53.16
        indirect
          laparoscopic with graft or
            prosthesis 17.22
          other and open (laparoscopic
            without graft or pros-
            thesis) 53.12
          with prosthesis or graft
            53.15
      direct (unilateral)
        with prosthesis or graft 53.03
        and indirect (unilateral)
          laparoscopic with graft or
            prosthesis 17.11
          other and open (laparoscopic
            without graft or pros-
            thesis) 53.01
          with prosthesis or graft
            53.03
        laparoscopic with graft or prosthe-
          sis 17.11
        other and open (laparoscopic
          without graft or prosthe-
          sis) 53.01
        with prosthesis or graft 53.03
      indirect (unilateral)
        laparoscopic with graft or prosthe-
          sis 17.12
        other and open (laparoscopic
          without graft or prosthe-
          sis) 53.02
        with prosthesis or graft 53.04
    internal 53.9
    ischiatic 53.9
    ischiorectal 53.9
    laparoscopic with graft or prosthesis,
      NOS 17.13
    lumbar 53.9
    manual 96.27
    obturator 53.9
    omental 53.9
    paraesophageal
      laparoscopic 53.71
      other and open 53.72
      unspecified 53.75
    parahiatal
      laparoscopic 53.71
      other and open 53.72
      unspecified 53.75
    paraileostomy 46.41
    parasternal 53.82
    paraumbilical
      laparoscopic 53.43
        with graft or prosthesis 53.42
      other and open with graft or prosthe-
        sis 53.41
      other open 53.49
    pericolostomy 46.42
    perineal (enterocele) 53.9
    preperitoneal 53.29
    pudendal 53.9
    retroperitoneal 53.9
    sciatic 53.9
    scrotal — *see* Repair, hernia, inguinal
    spigelian 53.59
      with prosthesis or graft 53.69

Repair — *continued*
  hernia — *continued*
    umbilical
      laparoscopic 53.43
        with graft or prosthesis 53.42
      other and open with graft or prosthe-
        sis 53.41
      other open 53.49
    uveal 12.39
    ventral (laparoscopic without graft or
      prosthesis) 53.59
      with prosthesis or graft
        laparoscopic 53.63
        other and open 53.69
      incisional 53.51
        (laparoscopic without graft or
          prosthesis) 53.59
        other open with prosthesis or
          graft 53.61
  hydrocele
    round ligament 69.19
    spermatic cord 63.1
    tunica vaginalis 61.2
  hymen 70.76
  hypospadias 58.45
  ileostomy 46.41
  ingrown toenail 86.23
  intestine, intestinal NEC 46.79
    fistula — *see* Closure, fistula, intestine
    laceration
      large intestine 46.75
      small intestine NEC 46.73
    stoma — *see* Repair, stoma
  inverted uterus NEC 69.29
    manual
      nonobstetric 69.94
      obstetric 75.94
    obstetrical
      manual 75.94
      surgical 75.93
    vaginal approach 69.23
  iris (rupture) NEC 12.39
  jejunostomy 46.41
  joint (capsule) (cartilage) NEC (*see also*
    Arthroplasty) 81.96
  kidney NEC 55.89
  knee (joint) NEC 81.47
    collateral ligaments 81.46
    cruciate ligaments 81.45
    five-in-one 81.42
    triad 81.43
  labia — *see* Repair, vulva
  laceration — *see* Suture, by site
  lacrimal system NEC 09.99
    canaliculus 09.73
    punctum 09.72
      for eversion 09.71
  laryngostomy 31.62
  laryngotracheal cleft 31.69
  larynx 31.69
    fracture 31.64
    laceration 31.61
  leads (cardiac) NEC 37.75
  ligament (*see also* Arthroplasty) 81.96
    broad 69.29
    collateral, knee NEC 81.46
    cruciate, knee NEC 81.45
    round 69.29
    uterine 69.29
  lip NEC 27.59
    cleft 27.54
    laceration (by suture) 27.51
  liver NEC 50.69
    laceration 50.61
  lop ear 18.79
  lung NEC 33.49
  lymphatic (channel) (peripheral) NEC 40.9
    duct, left (thoracic) NEC 40.69
  macrodactyly 82.83
  mallet finger 82.84
  mandibular ridge 76.64
  mastoid (antrum) (cavity) 19.9
  meninges (cerebral) NEC 02.12
    spinal NEC 03.59
      meningocele 03.51
      myelomeningocele 03.52

Repair — *continued*
  meningocele (spinal) 03.51
    cranial 02.12
  mesentery 54.75
  mouth NEC 27.59
    laceration NEC 27.52
  muscle NEC 83.87
    by
      graft or implant (fascia) (muscle)
        83.82
        hand 82.72
        tendon 83.81
          hand 82.79
      suture (direct) 83.65
        hand 82.46
      transfer or transplantation (muscle)
        83.77
        hand 82.58
    hand 82.89
      by
        graft or implant NEC 82.79
          fascia 82.72
        suture (direct) 82.46
        transfer or transplantation (mus-
          cle) 82.58
  musculotendinous cuff, shoulder 83.63
  myelomeningocele 03.52
  nasal
    septum (perforation) NEC 21.88
    sinus NEC 22.79
      fistula 22.71
  nasolabial flaps (plastic) 21.86
  nasopharyngeal atresia 29.4
  nerve (cranial) (peripheral) NEC 04.79
    old injury 04.76
    revision 04.75
    sympathetic 05.81
  nipple NEC 85.87
  nose (external) (internal) (plastic) NEC (*see
    also* Rhinoplasty) 21.89
    laceration (by suture) 21.81
  notched lip 27.59
  omentum 54.74
  omphalocele
    laparoscopic 53.43
      with graft or prosthesis 53.42
    other and open with graft or prosthesis
      53.41
    other open 53.49
  orbit 16.89
    wound 16.81
  ostium
    primum defect 35.73
      with
        prosthesis 35.54
        tissue graft 35.63
    secundum defect 35.71
      with
        prosthesis (open heart technique)
          35.51
        closed heart technique 35.52
        tissue graft 35.61
  ovary 65.79
    with tube 65.73
      laparoscopic 65.76
  overlapping toe 77.58
  pacemaker
    cardiac
      device (permanent) 37.89
      electrode(s) (leads) NEC 37.75
      pocket (skin) (subcutaneous) 37.79
  palate NEC 27.69
    cleft 27.62
      secondary or subsequent 27.63
    laceration (by suture) 27.61
  pancreas NEC 52.95
    Wirsung's duct 52.99
  papillary muscle (heart) 35.31
  patent ductus arteriosus 38.85
  pectus deformity (chest) (carinatum) (exca-
    vatum) 34.74
  pelvic floor NEC 70.79
    obstetric laceration (current) 75.69
      old 70.79
  penis NEC 64.49
    for epispadias or hypospadias 58.45

Repair — *continued*
  penis — *continued*
    inflatable prosthesis 64.99
    laceration 64.41
  pericardium 37.49
  perineum (female) 71.79
    laceration (by suture) 71.71
      obstetric (current) 75.69
      old 71.79
    male NEC 86.89
      laceration (by suture) 86.59
  peritoneum NEC 54.73
    by suture 54.64
  pharynx NEC 29.59
    laceration (by suture) 29.51
    plastic 29.4
  pleura NEC 34.93
  postcataract wound dehiscence 11.52
    with conjunctival flap 11.53
  pouch of Douglas 70.52
  primum ostium defect 35.73
    with
      prosthesis 35.54
      tissue graft 35.63
  prostate 60.93
  ptosis, eyelid — *see* Repair, blepharoptosis
  punctum, lacrimal NEC 09.72
    for correction of eversion 09.71
  quadriceps (mechanism) 83.86
  rectocele (posterior colporrhaphy) 70.52
    with graft or prosthesis 70.55
    and cystocele 70.50
      with graft or prosthesis 70.53
  rectum NEC 48.79
    laceration (by suture) 48.71
    prolapse NEC 48.76
      abdominal, approach 48.75
    STARR procedure 48.74
  retina, retinal
    detachment 14.59
      by
        cryotherapy 14.52
        diathermy 14.51
        photocoagulation 14.55
          laser 14.54
          xenon arc 14.53
        scleral buckling (*see also* Buckling,
          scleral) 14.49
    tear or defect 14.39
      by
        cryotherapy 14.32
        diathermy 14.31
        photocoagulation 14.35
          laser 14.34
          xenon arc 14.33
  retroperitoneal tissue 54.73
  rotator cuff (graft) (suture) 83.63
  round ligament 69.29
  ruptured tendon NEC 83.88
    hand 82.86
  salivary gland or duct NEC 26.49
  sclera, scleral 12.89
    fistula 12.82
    staphyloma NEC 12.86
      with graft 12.85
  scrotum 61.49
  sinus
    nasal NEC 22.79
    of Valsalva (aneurysm) 35.39
  skin (plastic) (without graft) 86.89
    laceration (by suture) 86.59
  skull NEC 02.06
    with
      flap (bone) 02.03
      graft (bone) 02.04
  spermatic cord NEC 63.59
    laceration (by suture) 63.51
  sphincter ani 49.79
    laceration (by suture) 49.71
      obstetric (current) 75.62
      old 49.79
  spina bifida NEC 03.59
    meningocele 03.51
    myelomeningocele 03.52
  spinal (cord) (meninges) (structures) NEC
    03.59

☑ Additional Digit Required — Refer to the Tabular List for Digit Selection   ▽ Subterms under main terms may continue to next column or page

2014 ICD-9-CM   ►◄ Revised Text   ● New Line   ▲ Revised Code   Volume 3 — 55

Replacement — Resection

Replacement — *continued*
  electrode(s) — *see* Implant, electrode or lead
      by site or name of device — *contin-
      ued*
    foramen ovale 02.93
    gastric 04.92
    intracranial 02.93
    pacemaker — *see* Replacement, pace-
        maker, electrode(s)
    peripheral nerve 04.92
    sacral nerve 04.92
    sphenoidal 02.96
    spine 03.93
  electroencephalographic receiver (brain)
      (intracranial) 02.93
  electronic
    cardioverter/defibrillator — *see* Replace-
        ment, cardioverter/defibrillator
    leads (electrode) (s) — *see* Replacement,
        electrode(s)
    stimulator (*see also* Implant, electronic
        stimulator, by site)
      bladder 57.97
      muscle (skeletal) 83.92
      ureter 56.93
  electrostimulator — *see* Implant, electronic
      stimulator by site
  enterostomy device (tube)
    large intestine 97.04
    small intestine 97.03
  epidural pegs 02.93
  femoral head, by prosthesis 81.52
    revision 81.53
  Gardner Wells tongs (skull) 02.94
  gastric band, laparoscopic 44.96
  gastric port device (subcutaneous) 44.96
  graft — *see* Graft
  halo traction device (skull) 02.94
  Harrington rod (with refusion of spine) —
      see Refusion, spinal
  heart
    artificial
      total internal biventricular replace-
          ment system 37.52
        implantable battery 37.54
        implantable controller 37.54
        thoracic unit 37.53
        transcutaneous energy transfer
            (TET) device 37.54
      total internal biventricular replacement
          system 37.52
        implantable battery 37.54
        implantable controller 37.54
        thoracic unit 37.53
        transcutaneous energy transfer (TET)
            device 37.54
    valve, NOS (with prosthesis) (with tissue
        graft) 35.20
      aortic, NOS 35.22
        with
            prosthesis 35.22
            tissue graft 35.21
              endovascular 35.05
          endovascular (TAVI) (TAVR)
              (transarterial) (tran-
              scatheter) (transfemoral)
              (with tissue graft) 35.05
          transapical (intercostal) (tran-
              scatheter) (transthoracic)
              (transventricular) (with
              tissue graft) 35.06
        endovascular, NOS 35.09
      mitral, NOS 35.24
        with
            prosthesis 35.24
            tissue graft 35.23
        poppet (prosthetic) 35.95
      pulmonary, NOS 35.26
        with
            prosthesis 35.26
            tissue graft 35.25
          endovascular (percutaneous)
              (PPVI) (TPVR) (tran-
              scatheter) (transfemoral)
              (transvenous) 35.07

Replacement — *continued*
  heart — *continued*
    valve, — *continued*
      pulmonary, — *continued*
        in total repair of tetralogy of Fal-
            lot 35.81
        transapical (intercostal) (tran-
            scatheter) (transthoracic)
            (transventricular) 35.08
      tricuspid, NOS 35.28
        with
            prosthesis 35.28
            tissue graft 35.27
  hip (partial) (with fixation device) (with
      prosthesis) (with traction) 81.52
    acetabulum 81.52
      revision 81.53
    femoral head 81.52
      revision 81.53
    total 81.51
      revision 81.53
  intervertebral disc
    artificial, NOS 84.60
      cervical 84.62
        nucleus 84.61
        partial 84.61
        total 84.62
      lumbar, lumbosacral 84.65
        nucleus 84.64
        partial 84.64
        total 84.65
      thoracic (partial) (total) 84.63
  inverted uterus — *see* Repair, inverted
      uterus
  iris NEC 12.39
  kidney, mechanical 55.97
  knee (bicompartmental) (hemijoint) (partial)
      (total) (tricompartmental) (unicom-
      partmental) 81.54
    revision 81.55
  laryngeal stent 31.93
  leads (electrode) (s) — *see* Replacement,
      electrode(s)
  mechanical kidney 55.97
  mitral valve, NOS 35.24
    with
        prosthesis 35.24
        tissue graft 35.23
  Mulligan hood, fallopian tube 66.93
  muscle stimulator (skeletal) 83.92
  nephrostomy tube 55.93
  neuropacemaker — *see* Implant, neurostim-
      ulator, by site
  neurostimulator — *see* Implant, neurostim-
      ulator, by site
  skeletal muscle 83.92
  pacemaker
    brain — *see* Implant, neurostimulator,
        brain
    cardiac device (initial) (permanent)
      dual-chamber device 37.87
      resynchronization — *see* Replace-
          ment, CRT-P
      single-chamber device 37.85
        rate responsive 37.86
    electrode(s), cardiac (atrial) (transve-
        nous) (ventricular) 37.76
      epicardium (myocardium) 37.74
      left ventricular coronary venous sys-
          tem 00.52
    gastric — *see* Implant, neurostimulator,
        gastric
    intracranial — *see* Implant, neurostimu-
        lator, intracranial
    neural — *see* Implant, neurostimulator,
        by site
    peripheral nerve — *see* Implant, neu-
        rostimulator, peripheral nerve
    sacral nerve — *see* Implant, neurostimu-
        lator, sacral nerve
    spine — *see* Implant, neurostimulator,
        spine
    temporary transvenous pacemaker sys-
        tem 37.78
  pack or bag
    nose 97.21

Replacement — *continued*
  pack or bag — *continued*
    teeth, tooth 97.22
    vagina 97.26
    vulva 97.26
    wound 97.16
  pessary, vagina NEC 97.25
  prosthesis
    acetabulum 81.53
    arm (bioelectric) (cineplastic) (kineplas-
        tic) 84.44
    biliary tract 51.99
    channel (single) 20.97
      multiple 20.98
    cochlear 20.96
    elbow 81.97
    epiretinal visual 14.83
    extremity (bioelectric) (cineplastic)
        (kineplastic) 84.40
      lower 84.48
      upper 84.44
    fallopian tube (Mulligan hood) (stent)
        66.93
    femur 81.53
    knee 81.55
    leg (bioelectric) (cineplastic) (kineplastic)
        84.48
    penis (internal) (non-inflatable) 64.95
      inflatable (internal) 64.97
  pulmonary valve, NOS 35.26
    with
        prosthesis 35.26
        tissue graft 35.25
    endovascular (percutaneous) (PPVI)
        (TPVR) (transcatheter) (trans-
        femoral) (transvenous) 35.07
    in total repair of tetralogy of Fallot 35.81
    transapical (intercostal) (transcatheter)
        (transthoracic) (transventricular)
        35.08
  pyelostomy tube 55.94
  rectal tube 96.09
  Rheos™ carotid sinus baroreflex activation
      device 39.81
  sensor (lead)
    intracardiac or great vessel hemodynam-
        ic monitoring 00.56
  shoulder NEC 81.83
    partial 81.81
    total, NEC 81.80
      other 81.80
      reverse 81.88
  skull
    plate 02.05
    tongs 02.94
  spacer (cement) (joint) (methylmethacry-
      late) 84.56
  specified appliance or device NEC 97.29
  spinal motion preservation device
    facet replacement device(s) 84.84
    interspinous process device(s) 84.80
    pedicle-based dynamic stabilization de-
        vice(s) 84.82
  splint 97.14
  stent
    bile duct 97.05
    fallopian tube 66.93
    larynx 31.93
    pancreatic duct 97.05
    trachea 31.93
  stimoceiver — *see* Implant, stimoceiver, by
      site
  stimulator
    electrode(s)
      carotid sinus 39.82
        with synchronous pulse genera-
            tor replacement (total sys-
            tem) 39.81
    pulse generator
      carotid sinus 39.83
        with synchronous electrode(s)
            replacement (total system)
            39.81
  subdural
    grids 02.93
    strips 02.93

Replacement — *continued*
  testis in scrotum 62.5
  tongs, skull 02.94
  tracheal stent 31.93
  tricuspid valve (with prosthesis) 35.28
    with tissue graft 35.27
  tube
    bile duct 97.05
    bladder 57.95
    cystostomy 59.94
    esophagostomy 97.01
    gastrostomy 97.02
    large intestine 97.04
    nasogastric 97.01
    nephrostomy 55.93
    pancreatic duct 97.05
    pyelostomy 55.94
    rectal 96.09
    small intestine 97.03
    tracheostomy 97.23
    ureterostomy 59.93
    ventricular (cerebral) 02.42
  umbilical cord, prolapsed 73.92
  ureter (with)
    bladder flap 56.74
    ileal segment implanted into bladder
        56.89 *[45.51]*
  ureterostomy tube 59.93
  urethral sphincter, artificial 58.93
  urinary sphincter, artificial 58.93
  valve
    heart (*see also* Replacement, heart valve
        poppet (prosthetic) 35.95
    ventricular (cerebral) 02.42
  ventricular shunt (valve) 02.42
  Vinke tongs (skull) 02.94
  vitreous (silicone) 14.75
    for retinal reattachment 14.59
Replant, replantation — *see also* Reattach-
    ment
  extremity — *see* Reattachment, extremity
  penis 64.45
  scalp 86.51
  tooth 23.5
Reposition
  cardiac pacemaker
    electrode(s) (atrial) (transvenous) (ven-
        tricular) 37.75
    pocket 37.79
  cardiac resynchronization defibrillator (CRT
      D) — *see* Revision, cardiac resynchro-
      nization defibrillator
  cardiac resynchronization pacemaker (CRT
      P) — *see* Revision, cardiac resynchro-
      nization pacemaker
  cardioverter/defibrillator (automatic)
    lead(s) (sensing) (pacing) (epicardial
        patch) 37.75
    pocket 37.79
    pulse generator 37.79
  cilia base 08.71
  implantable hemodynamic sensor (lead)
      and monitor device 37.79
  iris 12.39
  neurostimulator
    leads
      subcutaneous, without device re-
          placement 86.09
      within brain 02.93
      within or over gastric nerve 04.92
      within or over peripheral nerve 04.92
      within or over sacral nerve 04.92
      within spine 03.93
    pulse generator
      subcutaneous, without device re-
          placement 86.09
  renal vessel, aberrant 39.55
  subcutaneous device pocket NEC 86.09
  thyroid tissue 06.94
  tricuspid valve (with plication) 35.14
Resection — *see also* Excision, by site
  abdominoendorectal (combined), NOS
      48.50
    laparoscopic 48.51
    open 48.52
    other 48.59

☑ Additional Digit Required — Refer to the Tabular List for Digit Selection   ▽ Subterms under main terms may continue to next column or page

56 — Volume 3 • October 2013   ▶◀ Revised Text   ● New Line   ▲ Revised Code   2014 ICD-9-CM

Resection — *see also* Excision, by site — *continued*
- abdominoperineal (rectum), NOS 48.50
  - pull-through (Altemeier) (Swenson) NEC 48.49
    - Duhamel type 48.65
    - laparoscopic 48.42
    - not otherwise specified 48.40
    - open 48.43
- alveolar process and palate (en bloc) 27.32
- aneurysm — *see* Aneurysmectomy
- aortic valve (for subvalvular stenosis) 35.11
- artery — *see* Arteriectomy
- bile duct NEC 51.69
  - common duct NEC 51.63
- bladder (partial) (segmental) (transvesical) (wedge) 57.6
  - complete or total 57.79
  - lesion NEC 57.59
    - transurethral approach 57.49
  - neck 57.59
    - transurethral approach 57.49
- blood vessel — *see* Angiectomy
- brain 01.59
  - by
    - stereotactic radiosurgery 92.30
      - cobalt 60 92.32
      - linear accelerator (LINAC) 92.31
      - multi-source 92.32
      - particle beam 92.33
      - particulate 92.33
      - radiosurgery NEC 92.39
      - single source photon 92.31
  - hemisphere 01.52
  - lobe 01.53
- breast (*see also* Mastectomy)
  - quadrant 85.22
  - segmental 85.23
- broad ligament 69.19
- bronchus (sleeve) (wide sleeve) 32.1
  - block (en bloc) (with radical dissection of brachial plexus, bronchus, lobe of lung, ribs, and sympathetic nerves) 32.6
- bursa 83.5
  - hand 82.31
- cecum (and terminal ileum)
  - laparoscopic 17.32
  - open and other 45.72
- cerebral meninges 01.51
- chest wall 34.4
- clavicle 77.81
- clitoris 71.4
- colon (partial) (segmental)
  - ascending (cecum and terminal ileum)
    - laparoscopic 17.32
    - open and other 45.72
  - cecum (and terminal ileum)
    - laparoscopic 17.32
    - open and other 45.72
  - complete
    - laparoscopic 45.81
    - open 45.82
    - other 45.83
    - unspecified 45.83
  - descending (sigmoid)
    - laparoscopic 17.36
    - open and other 45.76
  - for interposition 45.52
  - Hartmann
    - laparoscopic 17.35
    - open and other 45.75
  - hepatic flexure
    - laparoscopic 17.33
    - open and other 45.73
  - laparoscopic 17.39
  - left radical (hemicolon)
    - laparoscopic 17.35
    - open and other 45.75
  - multiple segmental
    - laparoscopic 17.31
    - open and other 45.71
  - open and other 45.79
  - right radical (hemicolon) (ileocolectomy)
    - laparoscopic 17.33
    - open and other 45.73

Resection — *see also* Excision, by site — *continued*
- colon — *continued*
  - segmental NEC
    - laparoscopic 17.39
    - multiple
      - laparoscopic 17.31
      - open and other 45.71
    - open and other 45.79
  - sigmoid
    - laparascopic 17.36
    - open and other 45.76
  - splenic flexure
    - laparoscopic 17.35
    - open and other 45.75
  - total
    - laparoscopic 45.81
    - open 45.82
    - other 45.83
    - unspecified 45.83
  - transverse
    - laparoscopic 17.34
    - open and other 45.74
- conjunctiva, for pterygium 11.39
  - corneal graft 11.32
- cornual (fallopian tube) (unilateral) 66.69
  - bilateral 66.63
- diaphragm 34.81
- endaural 20.79
- endorectal (pull-through) (Soave) 48.41
  - combined abdominal, NOS 48.50
    - laparoscopic 48.51
    - open 48.52
    - other 48.59
- esophagus (partial) (subtotal) (*see also* Esophagectomy) 42.41
  - total 42.42
- exteriorized intestine — *see* Resection, intestine, exteriorized
- fascia 83.44
  - for graft 83.43
    - hand 82.34
  - hand 82.35
    - for graft 82.34
- gallbladder (total) 51.22
- gastric (partial) (sleeve) (subtotal) NEC (*see also* Gastrectomy) 43.89
  - with anastomosis NEC 43.89
    - esophagogastric 43.5
    - gastroduodenal 43.6
    - gastrogastric 43.89
    - gastrojejunal 43.7
  - complete or total NEC 43.99
    - with intestinal interposition 43.91
  - laparoscopic 43.82
  - radical NEC 43.99
    - with intestinal interposition 43.91
  - wedge 43.42
    - endoscopic 43.41
- hallux valgus (joint) (*see also* Bunionectomy)
  - with prosthetic implant 77.59
- hepatic
  - duct 51.69
  - flexure (colon)
    - laparoscopic 17.33
    - open and other 45.73
- infundibula, heart (right) 35.34
- intestine (partial) NEC
  - cecum (with terminal ileum)
    - laparoscopic 17.32
    - open and other 45.72
  - exteriorized (large intestine) 46.04
    - small intestine 46.02
  - for interposition 45.50
    - large intestine 45.52
    - small intestine 45.51
  - hepatic flexure
    - laparoscopic 17.33
    - open and other 45.73
  - ileum 45.62
    - with cecum
      - laparoscopic 17.32
      - open and other 45.72
  - laparoscopic 17.39
  - large (partial) (segmental) NEC
    - for interposition 45.52

Resection — *see also* Excision, by site — *continued*
- intestine — *continued*
  - large — *continued*
    - laparoscopic 17.39
    - multiple segmental
      - laparoscopic 17.31
      - open and other 45.71
    - other 45.79
    - total
      - laparoscopic 45.81
      - open 45.82
      - other 45.83
      - unspecified 45.83
    - unspecified 45.79
  - left hemicolon
    - laparoscopic 17.35
    - open and other 45.75
  - multiple segmental (large intestine)
    - laparoscopic 17.31
    - open and other 45.71
    - small intestine 45.61
  - open and other 45.79
  - right hemicolon
    - laparoscopic 17.33
    - open and other 45.73
  - segmental (large intestine)
    - laparoscopic 17.39
    - multiple
      - laparoscopic 17.31
      - open and other 45.71
    - open and other 45.79
    - small intestine 45.62
      - multiple 45.61
  - sigmoid
    - laparoscopic 17.36
    - open and other 45.76
  - small (partial) (segmental) NEC 45.62
    - for interposition 45.51
    - multiple segmental 45.61
    - total 45.63
  - total
    - large intestine
      - laparoscopic 45.81
      - open 45.82
      - other 45.83
      - unspecified 45.83
    - small intestine 45.63
- joint structure NEC (*see also* Arthrectomy) 80.90
- kidney (segmental) (wedge) 55.4
- larynx (*see also* Laryngectomy)
  - submucous 30.29
- lesion — *see* Excision, lesion, by site
- levator palpebrae muscle 08.33
- ligament (*see also* Arthrectomy) 80.90
  - broad 69.19
  - round 69.19
  - uterine 69.19
- lip (wedge) 27.43
- liver (partial) (wedge) 50.22
  - lobe (total) 50.3
  - total 50.4
- lung (wedge) NEC 32.29
  - endoscopic 32.28
  - segmental (any part) 32.39
    - thoracoscopic 32.30
  - thoracoscopic 32.20
  - volume reduction 32.22
    - biologic lung volume reduction (BLVR) — *see* category 33.7 ☑
- meninges (cerebral) 01.51
  - spinal 03.4
- mesentery 54.4
- muscle 83.45
  - extraocular 15.13
    - with
      - advancement or recession of other eye muscle 15.3
      - suture of original insertion 15.13
    - levator palpebrae 08.33
    - Müller's, for blepharoptosis 08.35
    - orbicularis oculi 08.20
    - tarsal, for blepharoptosis 08.35
  - for graft 83.43

Resection — *see also* Excision, by site — *continued*
- muscle — *continued*
  - for graft — *continued*
    - hand 82.34
  - hand 82.36
    - for graft 82.34
  - ocular — *see* Resection, muscle, extraocular
- myocardium 37.33
- nasal septum (submucous) 21.5
- nerve (cranial) (peripheral) NEC 04.07
  - phrenic 04.03
    - for collapse of lung 33.31
  - sympathetic 05.29
  - vagus — *see* Vagotomy
- nose (complete) (extended) (partial) (radical) 21.4
- omentum 54.4
- orbitomaxillary, radical 16.51
- ovary (*see also* Oophorectomy, wedge) 65.22
  - laparoscopic 65.24
- palate (bony) (local) 27.31
  - by wide excision 27.32
  - soft 27.49
- pancreas (total) (with synchronous duodenectomy) 52.6
  - partial NEC 52.59
    - distal (tail) (with part of body) 52.52
    - proximal (head) (with part of body) (with synchronous duodenectomy) 52.51
    - radical subtotal 52.53
  - radical (one-stage) (two-stage) 52.7
  - subtotal 52.53
- pancreaticoduodenal (*see also* Pancreatectomy) 52.6
- pelvic viscera (en masse) (female) 68.8
  - male 57.71
- penis 64.3
- pericardium (partial) (for)
  - chronic constrictive pericarditis 37.31
  - drainage 37.12
  - removal of adhesions 37.31
- peritoneum 54.4
- pharynx (partial) 29.33
- phrenic nerve 04.03
  - for collapse of lung 33.31
- prostate (*see also* Prostatectomy)
  - transurethral (punch) 60.29
- pterygium 11.39
- radial head 77.83
- rectosigmoid (*see also* Resection, rectum) 48.69
- rectum (partial) NEC 48.69
  - with
    - pelvic exenteration 68.8
    - transsacral sigmoidectomy 48.61
  - abdominoendorectal (combined), NOS 48.50
    - laparoscopic 48.51
    - open 48.52
    - other 48.59
  - abdominoperineal, NOS 48.50
    - laparoscopic 48.51
    - open 48.52
    - other 48.59
    - pull-through NEC 48.49
      - Duhamel type 48.65
      - laparoscopic 48.42
      - not otherwise specified 48.40
      - open 48.43
  - anterior 48.63
    - with colostomy (synchronous) 48.62
  - Duhamel 48.65
  - endorectal 48.41
    - combined abdominal, NOS 48.50
      - laparoscopic 48.51
      - open 48.52
      - other 48.59
  - posterior 48.64
  - pull-through NEC 48.49
    - endorectal 48.41
    - laparoscopic 48.42
    - not otherwise specified 48.40
    - open 48.43

☑ **Additional Digit Required — Refer to the Tabular List for Digit Selection**   ▽ **Subterms under main terms may continue to next column or page**

Revision — *continued*
  joint replacement — *continued*
    hip — *continued*
      acetabular and femoral components (total) 00.70
      acetabular component only 00.71
      acetabular liner and/or femoral head only 00.73
      femoral component only 00.72
      femoral head only and/or acetabular liner 00.73
      partial
        acetabular component only 00.71
        acetabular liner and/or femoral head only 00.73
        femoral component only 00.72
        femoral head only and/or acetabular liner 00.73
      total (acetabular and femoral components) 00.70
    knee replacement NOS 81.55
      femoral component 00.82
      partial
        femoral component 00.82
        patellar component 00.83
        tibial component 00.81
        tibial insert 00.84
      patellar component 00.83
      tibial component 00.81
      tibial insert 00.84
      total (all components) 00.80
    lower extremity NEC 81.59
    toe 81.59
    upper extremity 81.97
    wrist 81.97
  knee replacement (prosthesis) NOS 81.55
    femoral component 00.82
    partial
      femoral component 00.82
      patellar component 00.83
      tibial component 00.81
      tibial insert 00.84
    patellar component 00.83
    tibial component 00.81
    tibial insert 00.84
    total (all components) 00.80
  laryngostomy 31.63
  lateral canthus 08.59
  mallet finger 82.84
  mastoid antrum 19.9
  mastoidectomy 20.92
  nephrostomy 55.89
  neuroplasty 04.75
  ocular implant 16.62
  orbital implant 16.62
  pocket
    cardiac device (defibrillator) (pacemaker)
      with initial insertion of cardiac device — *omit code*
    new site (cardiac device pocket) (skin) (subcutaneous) 37.79
    carotid sinus stimulation pulse generator 39.85
      with initial insertion of pulse generator — *omit code*
    intracardiac hemodynamic monitoring 37.79
    subcutaneous device pocket NEC
      with initial insertion of generator or device — *omit code*
    new site 86.09
    thalamic stimulator pulse generator
      with initial insertion of battery package — *omit code*
    new site (skin) (subcutaneous) 86.09
  previous mastectomy site — *see category* 85.0-85.99
  proctostomy 48.79
  prosthesis
    acetabular and femoral components (total) 00.70
    acetabular component only 00.71
    acetabular liner and/or femoral head only 00.73
    ankle 81.59
    breast 85.93

Revision — *continued*
  prosthesis — *continued*
    elbow 81.97
    epiretinal visual 14.83   ●
    femoral component only 00.72
    femoral head only and/or acetabular liner 00.73
    foot 81.59
    hand 81.97
    heart valve (poppet) 35.95
    hip 81.53
      acetabular and femoral components (total) 00.70
      acetabular component only 00.71
      acetabular liner and/or femoral head only 00.73
      femoral component only 00.72
      femoral head only and/or acetabular liner 00.73
      partial
        acetabular component only 00.71
        acetabular liner and/or femoral head only 00.73
        femoral component only 00.72
        femoral head only and/or acetabular liner 00.73
      total (acetabular and femoral components) 00.70
    knee NOS 81.55
      femoral component 00.82
      partial
        femoral component 00.82
        patellar component 00.83
        tibial component 00.81
        tibial insert 00.84
      patellar component 00.83
      tibial component 00.81
      tibial insert 00.84
      total (all components) 00.80
    lower extremity NEC 81.59
    shoulder 81.97
    spine
      facet replacement device(s) 84.85
      interspinous process device(s) 84.81
      pedicle-based dynamic stabilization device(s) 84.83
    toe 81.59
    upper extremity NEC 81.97
    wrist 81.97
  ptosis overcorrection 08.37
  pyelostomy 55.12
  pyloroplasty 44.29
  rhinoplasty 21.84
    scar
      skin 86.84
        with excision 86.3
  scleral fistulization 12.66
  shoulder replacement (prosthesis) 81.97
  shunt
    arteriovenous (cannula) (for dialysis) 39.42
    lumbar-subarachnoid NEC 03.97
    peritoneojugular 54.99
    peritoneovascular 54.99
    pleurothecal 03.97
    salpingothecal 03.97
    spinal (thecal) NEC 03.97
    subarachnoid-peritoneal 03.97
    subarachnoid-ureteral 03.97
    ventricular (cerebral) 02.42
    ventriculoperitoneal
      at peritoneal site 54.95
      at ventricular site 02.42
  stapedectomy NEC 19.29
    with incus replacement (homograft) (prosthesis) 19.21
  stimulator
    electrode(s)
      carotid sinus 39.84
    pulse generator
      carotid sinus 39.85
  stoma
    bile duct 51.79
    bladder (vesicostomy) 57.22
    bronchus 33.42
    common duct 51.72

Revision — *continued*
  stoma — *continued*
    esophagus 42.89
    gallbladder 51.99
    hepatic duct 51.79
    intestine 46.40
      large 46.43
      small 46.41
    kidney 55.89
    larynx 31.63
    rectum 48.79
    stomach 44.69
      laparoscopic 44.68
    thorax 34.79
    trachea 31.74
    ureter 56.62
    urethra 58.49
  tack operation 20.79
  toe replacement (prosthesis) 81.59
  tracheostomy 31.74
  tunnel
    pulse generator lead wire 86.99
      with initial procedure — *omit code*
  tympanoplasty 19.6
  uretero-ileostomy, cutaneous 56.52
  ureterostomy (cutaneous) (stoma) NEC 56.62
    ileal 56.52
  urethrostomy 58.49
  urinary conduit 56.52
  vascular procedure (previous) NEC 39.49
  ventricular shunt (cerebral) 02.42
  vesicostomy stoma 57.22
  wrist replacement (prosthesis) 81.97
Rhinectomy 21.4
Rhinocheiloplasty 27.59
  cleft lip 27.54
Rhinomanometry 89.12
Rhinoplasty (external) (internal) NEC 21.87
  augmentation (with graft) (with synthetic implant) 21.85
  limited 21.86
  revision 21.84
  tip 21.86
  twisted nose 21.84
Rhinorrhaphy (external) (internal) 21.81
  for epistaxis 21.09
Rhinoscopy 21.21
Rhinoseptoplasty 21.84
Rhinotomy 21.1
Rhizotomy (radiofrequency) (spinal) 03.1
  acoustic 04.01
  trigeminal 04.02
Rhytidectomy (facial) 86.82
  eyelid
    lower 08.86
    upper 08.87
Rhytidoplasty (facial) 86.82
Ripstein operation (repair of prolapsed rectum) 48.75
Robotic assisted surgery
  endoscopic 17.44
  laparoscopic 17.42
  open 17.41
  other and unspecified 17.49
  percutaneous 17.43
  thoracoscopic 17.45
Rodney Smith operation (radical subtotal pancreatectomy) 52.53
Roentgenography — *see also* Radiography
  cardiac, negative contrast 88.58
Rolling of conjunctiva 10.33
Root
  canal (tooth) (therapy) 23.70
    with
      apicoectomy 23.72
      irrigation 23.71
      resection (tooth) (apex) 23.73
        with root canal therapy 23.72
      residual or retained 23.11
Rotation of fetal head
  forceps (instrumental) (Kielland) (Scanzoni) (key-in-lock) 72.4
  manual 73.51
Routine
  chest x-ray 87.44

Routine — *continued*
  psychiatric visit 94.12
Roux-en-Y operation
  bile duct 51.36
  cholecystojejunostomy 51.32
  esophagus (intrathoracic) 42.54
  gastroenterostomy 44.39
    laparoscopic 44.38
  gastrojejunostomy 44.39
    laparoscopic 44.38
  pancreaticojejunostomy 52.96
Roux-Goldthwait operation (repair of recurrent patellar dislocation) 81.44
Roux-Herzen-Judine operation (jejunal loop interposition) 42.63
Rubin test (insufflation of fallopian tube) 66.8
Ruiz-Mora operation (proximal phalangectomy for hammer toe) 77.99
Rupture
  esophageal web 42.01
  joint adhesions, manual 93.26
  membranes, artificial 73.09
    for surgical induction of labor 73.01
  ovarian cyst, manual 65.93
Russe operation (bone graft of scaphoid) 78.04

S

Sacculotomy (tack) 20.79
Sacrectomy (partial) 77.89
  total 77.99
Saemisch operation (corneal section) 11.1
Salpingectomy (bilateral) (total) (transvaginal) 66.51
  with oophorectomy 65.61
    laparoscopic 65.63
  partial (unilateral) 66.69
    with removal of tubal pregnancy 66.62
      bilateral 66.63
        for sterilization 66.39
          by endoscopy 66.29
    remaining or solitary tube 66.52
      with ovary 65.62
        laparoscopic 65.64
  unilateral (total) 66.4
    with
      oophorectomy 65.49
        laparoscopic 65.41
      removal of tubal pregnancy 66.62
    partial 66.69
Salpingo-oophorectomy (unilateral) 65.49
  bilateral (same operative episode) 65.61
    laparoscopic 65.63
  remaining or solitary tube and ovary 65.62
    laparoscopic 65.64
  that by laparoscope 65.41
Salpingo-oophoroplasty 65.73
  laparoscopic 65.76
Salpingo-oophororrhaphy 65.79
Salpingo-oophorostomy 66.72
Salpingo-oophorotomy 65.09
  laparoscopic 65.01
Salpingo-uterostomy 66.74
Salpingography 87.85
Salpingohysterostomy 66.74
Salpingoplasty 66.79
Salpingorrhaphy 66.71
Salpingosalpingostomy 66.73
Salpingostomy (for removal of non-ruptured ectopic pregnancy) 66.02
Salpingotomy 66.01
Salter operation (innominate osteotomy) 77.39
Salvage (autologous blood) (intraoperative) (perioperative) (postoperative) 99.00
Sampling, blood for genetic determination of fetus 75.33
Sandpapering (skin) 86.25
Saucerization
  bone (*see also* Excision, lesion, bone) 77.60
  rectum 48.99
Sauer-Bacon operation (abdominoperineal resection), NOS 48.50
  laparoscopic 48.51
  open 48.52
  other 48.59
Scalenectomy 83.45

Revision — Scalenectomy

☑ **Additional Digit Required — Refer to the Tabular List for Digit Selection**   ▽ **Subterms under main terms may continue to next column or page**

2014 ICD-9-CM   ▶◀ **Revised Text**   ● **New Line**   ▲ **Revised Code**   October 2013 · Volume 3 — 59

Scalenotomy 83.19
Scaling and polishing, dental 96.54
Scan, scanning
C.A.T. (computerized axial tomography) 88.38
with computer assisted surgery (CAS) 00.31
abdomen 88.01
bone 88.38
mineral density 88.98
brain 87.03
cardiac 87.41
coronary 87.41
head 87.03
kidney 87.71
skeletal 88.38
mineral density 88.98
thorax 87.41
computerized axial tomography (C.A.T.) (see also Scan, C.A.T.) 88.38
C.T. — see Scan, C.A.T.
gallium — see Scan, radioisotope
liver 92.02
MUGA (multiple gated acquisition) — see Scan, radioisotope
positron emission tomography (PET) — see Scan, radioisotope
radioisotope
adrenal 92.09
bone 92.14
marrow 92.05
bowel 92.04
cardiac output 92.05
cardiovascular 92.05
cerebral 92.11
circulation time 92.05
eye 95.16
gastrointestinal 92.04
head NEC 92.12
hematopoietic 92.05
intestine 92.04
iodine-131 92.01
kidney 92.03
liver 92.02
lung 92.15
lymphatic system 92.16
myocardial infarction 92.05
pancreatic 92.04
parathyroid 92.13
pituitary 92.11
placenta 92.17
protein-bound iodine 92.01
pulmonary 92.15
radio-iodine uptake 92.01
renal 92.03
specified site NEC 92.19
spleen 92.05
thyroid 92.01
total body 92.18
uterus 92.19
renal 92.03
thermal — see Thermography
Scapulectomy (partial) 77.81
total 77.91
Scapulopexy 78.41
Scarification
conjunctiva 10.33
nasal veins (with packing) 21.03
pericardium 36.39
pleura 34.6
chemical 34.92
with cancer chemotherapy substance 34.92 [99.25]
tetracycline 34.92 [99.21]
Schanz operation (femoral osteotomy) 77.35
Schauta (-Amreich) operation (radical vaginal hysterectomy) 68.79
laparoscopic 68.71
Schede operation (thoracoplasty) 33.34
Scheie operation
cautery of sclera 12.62
sclerostomy 12.62
Schlatter operation (total gastrectomy) 43.99
Schroeder operation (endocervical excision) 67.39

Schuchardt operation (nonobstetrical episiotomy) 71.09
Schwartze operation (simple mastoidectomy) 20.41
Scintiphotography — see Scan, radioisotope
Scintiscan — see Scan, radioisotope
Sclerectomy (punch) (scissors) 12.65
for retinal reattachment 14.49
Holth's 12.65
trephine 12.61
with implant 14.41
Scleroplasty 12.89
Sclerosis — see Sclerotherapy
Sclerostomy (Scheie's) 12.62
Sclerotherapy
esophageal varices (endoscopic) 42.33
hemorrhoids 49.42
pleura 34.92
treatment of malignancy (cytotoxic agent) 34.92 [99.25]
with tetracycline 34.92 [99.21]
varicose vein 39.92
vein NEC 39.92
Sclerotomy (exploratory) 12.89
anterior 12.89
with
iridectomy 12.65
removal of vitreous 14.71
posterior 12.89
with
iridectomy 12.65
removal of vitreous 14.72
Scott operation
intestinal bypass for obesity 45.93
jejunocolostomy (bypass) 45.93
Scraping
corneal epithelium 11.41
for smear or culture 11.21
trachoma follicles 10.33
Scrotectomy (partial) 61.3
Scrotoplasty 61.49
Scrotorrhaphy 61.41
Scrototomy 61.0
Scrub, posterior nasal (adhesions) 21.91
Sculpturing, heart valve — see Valvuloplasty, heart
Section — see also Division and Incision
cesarean — see Cesarean section
ganglion, sympathetic 05.0
hypophyseal stalk (see also Hypophysectomy, partial) 07.63
ligamentum flavum (spine) — omit code
nerve (cranial) (peripheral) NEC 04.03
acoustic 04.01
spinal root (posterior) 03.1
sympathetic 05.0
trigeminal tract 04.02
Saemisch (corneal) 11.1
spinal ligament 80.49
arcuate — omit code
flavum — omit code
tooth (impacted) 23.19
Sedden-Brooks operation (transfer of pectoralis major tendon) 83.75
Semb operation (apicolysis of lung) 33.39
Senning operation (correction of transposition of great vessels) 35.91
Separation
twins (attached) (conjoined) (Siamese) 84.93
asymmetrical (unequal) 84.93
symmetrical (equal) 84.92
Septectomy
atrial (closed) 35.41
open 35.42
transvenous method (balloon) 35.41
submucous (nasal) 21.5
Septoplasty NEC 21.88
with submucous resection of septum 21.5
Septorhinoplasty 21.84
Septostomy (atrial) (balloon) 35.41
Septotomy, nasal 21.1
Sequestrectomy
bone 77.00
carpals, metacarpals 77.04
clavicle 77.01
facial 76.01

Sequestrectomy — continued
bone — continued
femur 77.05
fibula 77.07
humerus 77.02
nose 21.32
patella 77.06
pelvic 77.09
phalanges (foot) (hand) 77.09
radius 77.03
scapula 77.01
skull 01.25
specified site NEC 77.09
tarsals, metatarsals 77.08
thorax (ribs) (sternum) 77.01
tibia 77.07
ulna 77.03
vertebrae 77.09
nose 21.32
skull 01.25
Sesamoidectomy 77.98
Setback, ear 18.5
Severing of blepharorrhaphy 08.02
Sever operation (division of soft tissue of arm) 83.19
Sewell operation (heart) 36.2
Sharrard operation (iliopsoas muscle transfer) 83.77
Shaving
bone (see also Excision, lesion, bone) 77.60
cornea (epithelium) 11.41
for smear or culture 11.21
patella 77.66
Shelf operation (hip arthroplasty) 81.40
Shirodkar operation (encirclement suture, cervix) 67.59
Shock therapy
chemical 94.24
electroconvulsive 94.27
electrotonic 94.27
insulin 94.24
subconvulsive 94.26
Shortening
bone (fusion) 78.20
femur 78.25
specified site NEC — see category 78.2 ☑
tibia 78.27
ulna 78.23
endopelvic fascia 69.22
extraocular muscle NEC 15.22
multiple (two or more muscles) 15.4
eyelid margin 08.71
eye muscle NEC 15.22
multiple (two or more muscles) (with lengthening) 15.4
finger (macrodactyly repair) 82.83
heel cord 83.85
levator palpebrae muscle 08.33
ligament (see also Arthroplasty)
round 69.22
uterosacral 69.22
muscle 83.85
extraocular 15.22
multiple (two or more muscles) 15.4
hand 82.55
sclera (for repair of retinal detachment) 14.59
by scleral buckling (see also Buckling, scleral) 14.49
tendon 83.85
hand 82.55
ureter (with reimplantation) 56.41
Shunt — see also Anastomosis and Bypass, vascular
abdominovenous 54.94
aorta-coronary sinus 36.39
aorta (descending)-pulmonary (artery) 39.0
aorto-myocardial (graft) 36.2
aortocarotid 39.22
aortoceliac 39.26
aortofemoral 39.25
aortoiliac 39.25
aortoiliofemoral 39.25
aortomesenteric 39.26
aortorenal 39.24

Shunt — see also Anastomosis and Bypass, vascular — continued
aortosubclavian 39.22
apicoaortic 35.93
aqueous drainage 12.67
arteriovenous NEC 39.29
for renal dialysis (by)
anastomosis 39.27
external cannula 39.93
ascending aorta to pulmonary artery (Waterston) 39.0
axillary-femoral 39.29
carotid-carotid 39.22
carotid-subclavian 39.22
caval-mesenteric 39.1
corpora-saphenous 64.98
corpora cavernosa-corpus spongiosum 64.98
descending aorta to pulmonary artery (Potts-Smith) 39.0
endolymph-perilymph 20.71
endolymphatic (-subarachnoid) 20.71
extracranial-intracranial (EC-IC) 39.28
femoroperoneal 39.29
femoropopliteal 39.29
iliofemoral 39.25
ilioiliac 39.25
intestinal
large-to-large 45.94
small-to-large 45.93
small-to-small 45.91
left-to-right (systemic-pulmonary artery) 39.0
left subclavian to descending aorta (Blalock-Park) 39.0
left ventricle (heart) (apex) and aorta 35.93
lienorenal 39.1
lumbar-subarachnoid (with valve) NEC 03.79
mesocaval 39.1
peritoneal-jugular 54.94
peritoneo-vascular 54.94
peritoneovenous 54.94
pleuroperitoneal 34.05
pleurothecal (with valve) 03.79
portacaval (double) 39.1
portal-systemic 39.1
portal vein to vena cava 39.1
pulmonary-innominate 39.0
pulmonary vein to atrium 35.82
renoportal 39.1
right atrium and pulmonary artery 35.94
right ventricle and pulmonary artery (distal 35.92
in repair of
pulmonary artery atresia 35.92
transposition of great vessels 35.92
truncus arteriosus 35.83
salpingothecal (with valve) 03.79
semicircular-subarachnoid 20.71
spinal (thecal) (with valve) NEC 03.79
subarachnoid-peritoneal 03.71
subarachnoid-ureteral 03.72
splenorenal (venous) 39.1
arterial 39.26
subarachnoid-peritoneal (with valve) 03.71
subarachnoid-ureteral (with valve) 03.72
subclavian-pulmonary 39.0
subdural-peritoneal (with valve) 02.34
superior mesenteric-caval 39.1
systemic-pulmonary artery 39.0
transjugular intrahepatic portosystemic [TIPS] 39.1
vena cava to pulmonary artery (Green) 39.2
ventricular (cerebral) (with valve) 02.22
to
abdominal cavity or organ 02.34
bone marrow 02.39
cervical subarachnoid space 02.22
circulatory system 02.32
cisterna magna 02.22
extracranial site NEC 02.39
gallbladder 02.34
head or neck structure 02.31
intracerebral site NEC 02.22
lumbar site 02.39
mastoid 02.31

☑ Additional Digit Required — Refer to the Tabular List for Digit Selection
▽ Subterms under main terms may continue to next column or page
60 — Volume 3   ▶◀ Revised Text   ● New Line   ▲ Revised Code   2014 ICD-9-CM

Shunt — *see also* Anastomosis and Bypass,
   vascular — *continued*
   ventricular — *continued*
     to — *continued*
       nasopharynx 02.31
       peritoneal 02.34
       thoracic cavity 02.33
       ureter 02.35
       urinary system 02.35
       venous system 02.32
     ventriculoatrial (with valve) 02.32
     ventriculocaval (with valve) 02.32
     ventriculocisternal (with valve) 02.22
     ventriculolumbar (with valve) 02.39
     ventriculomastoid (with valve) 02.31
     ventriculonasopharyngeal 02.31
     ventriculopleural (with valve) 02.33
Sialoadenectomy (parotid) (sublingual) (sub-
   maxillary) 26.30
   complete 26.32
   partial 26.31
   radical 26.32
Sialoadenolithotomy 26.0
Sialoadenotomy 26.0
Sialodochoplasty NEC 26.49
Sialogram 87.09
Sialolithotomy 26.0
Sieve, vena cava 38.7
Sigmoid bladder 57.87 [45.52]
Sigmoidectomy
   laparoscopic 17.36
   open and other 45.76
Sigmoidomyotomy 46.91
Sigmoidopexy (Moschowitz) 46.63
Sigmoidoproctectomy — *see also* Resection,
   rectum 48.69
Sigmoidoproctostomy 45.94
Sigmoidorectostomy 45.94
Sigmoidorrhaphy 46.75
Sigmoidoscopy (rigid) 48.23
   with biopsy 45.25
   flexible 45.24
   through stoma (artificial) 45.22
   transabdominal 45.21
Sigmoidosigmoidostomy 45.94
   proximal to distal segment
     laparoscopic 17.36
     open and other 45.76
Sigmoidostomy — *see also* Colostomy 46.10
Sigmoidotomy 45.03
Sign language 93.75
Silver operation (bunionectomy) 77.59
Sinogram
   abdominal wall 88.03
   chest wall 87.38
   retroperitoneum 88.14
Sinusectomy (nasal) (complete) (partial) (with
   turbinectomy) 22.60
   antrum 22.62
     with Caldwell-Luc approach 22.61
   ethmoid 22.63
   frontal 22.42
   maxillary 22.62
     with Caldwell-Luc approach 22.61
   sphenoid 22.64
Sinusotomy (nasal) 22.50
   antrum (intranasal) 22.2
     with external approach (Caldwell-Luc)
      22.39
      radical (with removal of membrane
       lining) 22.31
   ethmoid 22.51
   frontal 22.41
   maxillary (intranasal) 22.2
     external approach (Caldwell-Luc) 22.39
      radical (with removal of membrane
       lining) 22.31
   multiple 22.53
   perinasal 22.50
   sphenoid 22.52
Sistrunk operation (excision of thyroglossal
   cyst) 06.7
Size reduction
   abdominal wall (adipose) (pendulous) 86.83
   arms (adipose) (batwing) 86.83
   breast (bilateral) 85.32

Size reduction — *continued*
   breast — *continued*
     unilateral 85.31
   buttocks (adipose) 86.83
   skin 86.83
   subcutaneous tissue 86.83
   thighs (adipose) 86.83
Skeletal series (x-ray) 88.31
SKyphoplasty 81.66
Sling — *see also* Operation, sling
   fascial (fascia lata)
     for facial weakness (trigeminal nerve
      paralysis) 86.81
     mouth 86.81
     orbicularis (mouth) 86.81
     tongue 25.59
   levator muscle (urethrocystopexy) 59.71
   pubococcygeal 59.71
   rectum (puborectalis) 48.76
   tongue (fascial) 25.59
Slitting
   canaliculus for
     passage of tube 09.42
     removal of streptothrix 09.42
   lens 13.2
   prepuce (dorsal) (lateral) 64.91
Slocum operation (pes anserinus transfer)
   81.47
Sluder operation (tonsillectomy) 28.2
Small bowel series (x-ray) 87.63
Smith-Peterson operation (radiocarpal
   arthrodesis) 81.25
Smith operation (open osteotomy of
   mandible) 76.62
Smithwick operation (sympathectomy) 05.29
Snaring, polyp, colon (endoscopic) 45.42
Snip, punctum (with dilation) 09.51
Soave operation (endorectal pull-through)
   48.41
Somatotherapy, psychiatric NEC 94.29
Sonneberg operation (inferior maxillary
   neurectomy) 04.07
Sorondo-Ferré operation (hindquarter ampu-
   tation) 84.19
Soutter operation (iliac crest fasciotomy) 83.14
Spaulding-Richardson operation (uterine
   suspension) 69.22
Spectrophotometry NEC 89.39
   blood 89.39
   placenta 89.29
   urine 89.29
Spectroscopy
   intravascular 38.23
   near infrared (NIR) 38.23
Speech therapy NEC 93.75
Spermatocelectomy 63.2
Spermatocystectomy 60.73
Spermatocystotomy 60.72
Sphenoidectomy 22.64
Sphenoidotomy 22.52
Sphincterectomy, anal 49.6
Sphincteroplasty
   anal 49.79
     obstetrical laceration (current) 75.62
     old 49.79
   bladder neck 57.85
   pancreas 51.83
   sphincter of Oddi 51.83
Sphincterorrhaphy, anal 49.71
   obstetrical laceration (current) 75.62
   old 49.79
Sphincterotomy
   anal (external) (internal) 49.59
     left lateral 49.51
     posterior 49.52
   bladder (neck) (transurethral) 57.91
   choledochal 51.82
     endoscopic 51.85
   iris 12.12
   pancreatic 51.82
     endoscopic 51.85
   sphincter of Oddi 51.82
     endoscopic 51.85
   transduodenal ampullary 51.82
     endoscopic 51.85

Spinal anesthesia — *omit code*
Spinelli operation (correction of inverted
   uterus) 75.93
Spineoplasty 81.66
Spirometry (incentive) (respiratory) 89.37
Spivack operation (permanent gastrostomy)
   43.19
Splanchnicectomy 05.29
Splanchnicotomy 05.0
Splenectomy (complete) (total) 41.5
   partial 41.43
Splenogram 88.64
   radioisotope 92.05
Splenolysis 54.59
   laparoscopic 54.51
Splenopexy 41.95
Splenoplasty 41.95
Splenoportogram (by splenic arteriography)
   88.64
Splenorrhaphy 41.95
Splenotomy 41.2
Splinting
   dental (for immobilization) 93.55
     orthodontic 24.7
   musculoskeletal 93.54
   ureteral 56.2
Splitting — *see also* Division
   canaliculus 09.52
   lacrimal papilla 09.51
   spinal cord tracts 03.29
     percutaneous 03.21
   tendon sheath 83.01
     hand 82.01
Spondylosyndesis — *see also* Fusion, spinal
   81.00
S.P. Rogers operation (knee disarticulation)
   84.16
Ssabanejew-Frank operation (permanent
   gastrostomy) 43.19
Stabilization, joint — *see also* Arthrodesis
   patella (for recurrent dislocation) 81.44
Stab, intercostal 34.09
Stacke operation (simple mastoidectomy)
   20.41
Stallard operation (conjunctivocystorhinostomy) 09.82
   with insertion of tube or stent 09.83
Stamm (-Kader) operation (temporary gastrostomy) 43.19
Stapedectomy 19.19
   with incus replacement (homograft) (pros-
     thesis) 19.11
   revision 19.29
     with incus replacement 19.21
Stapediolysis 19.0
Stapling
   artery 39.31
   blebs, lung (emphysematous) 32.21
   diaphysis (*see also* Stapling, epiphyseal
     plate) 78.20
   epiphyseal plate 78.20
     femur 78.25
     fibula 78.27
     humerus 78.22
     radius 78.23
     specified site NEC 78.29
     tibia 78.27
     ulna 78.23
   gastric varices 44.91
   graft — *see* Graft
   left atrial appendage 37.36
   vein 39.32
STARR (stapled transanal rectal resection) 48.74
StaXx® FX Structural Kyphoplasty System
   81.66
Steinberg operation 44.5
Steindler operation
   fascia stripping (for cavus deformity) 83.14
   flexorplasty (elbow) 83.77
   muscle transfer 83.77
Stereotactic head frame application 93.59
Stereotactic radiosurgery 92.30
   cobalt 60 92.32
   linear accelerator (LINAC) 92.31
   multi-source 92.32
   particle beam 92.33

Stereotactic radiosurgery — *continued*
   particulate 92.33
   radiosurgery NEC 92.39
   single source photon 92.31
Sterilization
   female (*see also* specific operation) 66.39
   male NEC (*see also* Ligation, vas deferens)
     63.70
Sternotomy 77.31
   as operative approach — *omit code*
   for bone marrow biopsy 41.31
Stewart operation (renal plication with
   pyeloplasty) 55.87
Stimulation (electronic) — *see also* Implant,
   electronic stimulator
   bone growth (percutaneous) — *see* catego-
     ry 78.9 ☑
     transcutaneous (surface) 99.86
   cardiac (external) 99.62
     internal 37.91
   carotid sinus 99.64
   CaverMap™ 89.58
   defibrillator
     as part of intraoperative testing — *omit*
      code
     catheter based invasive electrophysio-
      logic testing 37.26
     device interrogation only without ar-
      rhythmia induction (bedside
      check) 89.45-89.49
     non-invasive programmed electrical
      stimulation (NIPS) 37.20
   electrophysiologic, cardiac
     as part of intraoperative testing — *omit*
      code
     catheter based invasive electrophysio-
      logic testing 37.26
     device interrogation only without ar-
      rhythmia induction (bedside
      check) 89.45-89.49
     noninvasive programmed electrical
      stimulation (NIPS) 37.20
   nerve
     CaverMap™ 89.58
     penile 89.58
     peripheral or spinal cord, transcutaneous
      93.39
Stitch, Kelly-Stoeckel (urethra) 59.3
Stomatoplasty 27.59
Stomatorrhaphy 27.52
Stone operation (anoplasty) 49.79
Strapping (non-traction) 93.59
Strassman operation (metroplasty) 69.49
Strayer operation (gastrocnemius recession)
   83.72
Stretching
   eyelid (with elongation) 08.71
   fascia 93.28
   foreskin 99.95
   iris 12.63
   muscle 93.27
   nerve (cranial) (peripheral) 04.91
   tendon 93.27
Stripping
   bone (*see also* Incision, bone) 77.10
   carotid sinus 39.89
   cranial suture 02.01
   fascia 83.14
     hand 82.12
   membranes for surgical induction of labor
     73.1
   meninges (cerebral) 01.51
     spinal 03.4
   saphenous vein, varicose 38.59
   subdural membrane (cerebral) 01.51
     spinal 03.4
   varicose veins (lower limb) 38.59
     upper limb 38.53
   vocal cords 30.09
Stromeyer-Little operation (hepatotomy)
   50.0
Strong operation (unbridling of celiac artery
   axis) 39.91
Stryker frame 93.59
Study
   bone mineral density 88.98

Shunt — Study

☑ **Additional Digit Required** — Refer to the Tabular List for Digit Selection   ▽ **Subterms under main terms may continue to next column or page**

2014 ICD-9-CM   ▶◀ **Revised Text**   ● **New Line**   ▲ **Revised Code**   **Volume 3 — 61**

☑ **Additional Digit Required** — Refer to the Tabular List for Digit Selection   ▽ **Subterms under main terms may continue to next column or page**

62 — Volume 3   ▶◀ Revised Text   ● New Line   ▲ Revised Code   2014 ICD-9-CM

Swinney operation (urethral reconstruction) 58.46

Switch, switching
coronary arteries 35.84
great arteries, total 35.84

Syme operation
ankle amputation through malleoli of tibia and fibula 84.14
urethrotomy, external 58.0

Sympathectomy NEC 05.29
cervical 05.22
cervicothoracic 05.22
lumbar 05.23
periarterial 05.25
presacral 05.24
renal 05.29
thoracolumbar 05.23
tympanum 20.91

Sympatheticotripsy 05.0

Symphysiotomy 77.39
assisting delivery (obstetrical) 73.94
kidney (horseshoe) 55.85

Symphysis, pleural 34.6

Synchondrotomy — *see also* Division, cartilage 80.40

Syndactylization 86.89

Syndesmotomy — *see also* Division, ligament 80.40

Synechiotomy
endometrium 68.21
iris (posterior) 12.33
anterior 12.32

Synovectomy (joint) (complete) (partial) 80.70
ankle 80.77
elbow 80.72
foot and toe 80.78
hand and finger 80.74
hip 80.75
knee 80.76
shoulder 80.71
specified site NEC 80.79
spine 80.79
tendon sheath 83.42
hand 82.33
wrist 80.73

Syringing
lacrimal duct or sac 09.43
nasolacrimal duct 09.43
with
dilation 09.43
insertion of tube or stent 09.44

T

Taarnhoj operation (trigeminal nerve root decompression) 04.41

Tack operation (sacculotomy) 20.79

Tactile Guidance System™ [TGS] — *see* category 17.4 ☑

Take-down
anastomosis
arterial 39.49
blood vessel 39.49
gastric, gastrointestinal 44.5
intestine 46.93
stomach 44.5
vascular 39.49
ventricular 02.43
arterial bypass 39.49
arteriovenous shunt 39.43
with creation of new shunt 39.42
cecostomy 46.52
colostomy 46.52
duodenostomy 46.51
enterostomy 46.50
esophagostomy 42.83
gastroduodenostomy 44.5
gastrojejunostomy 44.5
ileostomy 46.51
intestinal stoma 46.50
large 46.52
small 46.51
jejunoileal bypass 46.93
jejunostomy 46.51
laryngostomy 31.62
sigmoidostomy 46.52

Take-down — *continued*
stoma
bile duct 51.79
bladder 57.82
bronchus 33.42
common duct 51.72
esophagus 42.83
gall bladder 51.92
hepatic duct 51.79
intestine 46.50
large 46.52
small 46.51
kidney 55.82
larynx 31.62
rectum 48.72
stomach 44.62
thorax 34.72
trachea 31.72
ureter 56.83
urethra 58.42
systemic-pulmonary artery anastomosis 39.49
in total repair of tetralogy of Fallot 35.81
tracheostomy 31.72
vascular anastomosis or bypass 39.49
ventricular shunt (cerebral) 02.43

Talectomy 77.98

Talma-Morison operation (omentopexy) 54.74

Tamponade
esophageal 96.06
intrauterine (nonobstetric) 69.91
after delivery or abortion 75.8
antepartum 73.1
vagina 96.14
after delivery or abortion 75.8
antepartum 73.1

Tanner operation (devascularization of stomach) 44.99

Tap
abdomen 54.91
chest 34.91
cisternal 01.01
cranial 01.09
joint 81.91
lumbar (diagnostic) (removal of dye) 03.31
perilymphatic 20.79
spinal (diagnostic) 03.31
subdural (through fontanel) 01.09
thorax 34.91

Tarsectomy 08.20
de Grandmont 08.35

Tarsoplasty — *see also* Reconstruction, eyelid 08.70

Tarsorrhaphy (lateral) 08.52
division or severing 08.02

Tattooing
cornea 11.91
skin 86.02

Tautening, eyelid for entropion 08.42

TAVI (transcatheter aortic valve implantation) 35.05

TAVR (transcatheter aortic valve replacement) 35.05

Telemetry (cardiac) 89.54

Teleradiotherapy
beta particles 92.25
intra-operative 92.41
Betatron 92.24
cobalt-60 92.23
electrons 92.25
intra-operative 92.41
iodine-125 92.23
linear accelerator 92.24
neutrons 92.26
particulate radiation NEC 92.26
photons 92.24
protons 92.26
radioactive cesium 92.23
radioisotopes NEC 92.23

Temperament assessment 94.02

Temperature gradient study — *see also* Thermography 88.89

Tendinoplasty — *see* Repair, tendon

Tendinosuture (immediate) (primary) — *see also* Suture, tendon 83.64

Tendinosuture — *see also* Suture, tendon — *continued*
hand (*see also* Suture, tendon, hand) 82.45

Tendolysis 83.91
hand 82.91

Tendoplasty — *see* Repair, tendon

Tenectomy 83.39
eye 15.13
levator palpebrae 08.33
multiple (two or more tendons) 15.3
hand 82.29
levator palpebrae 08.33
tendon sheath 83.31
hand 82.21

Tenodesis (tendon fixation to skeletal attachment) 83.88
Fowler 82.85
hand 82.85

Tenolysis 83.91
hand 82.91

Tenomyoplasty — *see also* Repair, tendon 83.88
hand (*see also* Repair, tendon, hand) 82.86

Tenomyotomy — *see* Tenonectomy

Tenonectomy 83.42
for graft 83.41
hand 82.32
hand 82.33
for graft 82.32

Tenontomyoplasty — *see* Repair, tendon

Tenontoplasty — *see* Repair, tendon

Tenoplasty — *see also* Repair, tendon 83.88
hand (*see also* Repair, tendon, hand) 82.86

Tenorrhaphy — *see also* Suture, tendon 83.64
hand (*see also* Suture, tendon, hand) 82.45
to skeletal attachment 83.88
hand 82.85

Tenosuspension 83.88
hand 82.86

Tenosuture — *see also* Suture, tendon 83.64
hand (*see also* Suture, tendon, hand) 82.45
to skeletal attachment 83.88
hand 82.85

Tenosynovectomy 83.42
hand 82.33

Tenotomy 83.13
Achilles tendon 83.11
adductor (hip) (subcutaneous) 83.12
eye 15.12
levator palpebrae 08.38
multiple (two or more tendons) 15.4
hand 82.11
levator palpebrae 08.38
pectoralis minor tendon (decompression thoracic outlet) 83.13
stapedius 19.0
tensor tympani 19.0

Tenovaginotomy — *see* Tenotomy

Tensing, orbicularis oculi 08.59

Termination of pregnancy
by
aspiration curettage 69.51
dilation and curettage 69.01
hysterectomy — *see* Hysterectomy
hysterotomy 74.91
intra-amniotic injection (saline) 75.0

Test, testing (for)
14 C-Urea breath 89.39
auditory function
NEC 95.46
Bender Visual-Motor Gestalt 94.02
Benton Visual Retention 94.02
cardiac (vascular)
function NEC 89.59
stress 89.44
bicycle ergometer 89.43
Masters' two-step 89.42
treadmill 89.41
Denver developmental (screening) 94.02
fetus, fetal
nonstress (fetal activity acceleration determinations) 75.34
oxytocin challenge (contraction stress) 75.35

Test, testing — *continued*
fetus, fetal — *continued*
sensitivity (to oxytocin) — *omit code*
function
cardiac NEC 89.59
hearing NEC 95.46
muscle (by)
electromyography 93.08
manual 93.04
neurologic NEC 89.15
vestibular 95.46
clinical 95.44
glaucoma NEC 95.26
hearing 95.47
clinical NEC 95.42
intelligence 94.01
internal jugular-subclavian venous reflux 89.62
intracarotid amobarbital (Wada) 89.10
Masters' two-step stress (cardiac) 89.42
muscle function (by)
electromyography 93.08
manual 93.04
neurologic function NEC 89.15
neurophysiologic monitoring
intra-operative 00.94
nocturnal penile tumescence 89.29
provocative, for glaucoma 95.26
psychologic NEC 94.08
psychometric 94.01
radio-cobalt B$_{12}$ Schilling 92.04
range of motion 93.05
rotation (Bárány chair) (hearing) 95.45
sleep disorder function — *see* categories 89.17-89.18
Stanford-Binet 94.01
Thallium stress (transesophageal pacing) 89.44
tuning fork (hearing) 95.42
Urea breath, (14 C) 89.39
vestibular function NEC 95.46
thermal 95.44
Wada (hemispheric function) 89.10
whispered speech (hearing) 95.42

TEVAP (transurethral electrovaporization of prostate) 60.29

Thalamectomy 01.41

Thalamotomy 01.41
by stereotactic radiosurgery 92.32
cobalt 60 92.32
linear accelerator (LINAC) 92.31
multi-source 92.32
particle beam 92.33
particulate 92.33
radiosurgery NEC 92.39
single source photon 92.31

Thal operation (repair of esophageal stricture) 42.85

Theleplasty 85.87

Therapy
Antabuse 94.25
aqueous oxygen (AO) 00.49
art 93.89
aversion 94.33
behavior 94.33
Bennett respirator — *see* category 96.7 ☑
blind rehabilitation NEC 93.78
Byrd respirator — *see* category 96.7 ☑
carbon dioxide 94.25
cobalt-60 92.23
conditioning, psychiatric 94.33
continuous positive airway pressure (CPAP) 93.90
delivered by
endotracheal tube — *see* category 96.7 ☑
tracheostomy — *see* category 96.7 ☑
croupette, croup tent 93.94
daily living activities 93.83
for the blind 93.78
dance 93.89
desensitization 94.33
detoxification 94.25
diversional 93.81
domestic tasks 93.83

☑ **Additional Digit Required** — Refer to the Tabular List for Digit Selection   ▽ **Subterms under main terms may continue to next column or page**

2014 ICD-9-CM   ▶◀ Revised Text   ● New Line   ▲ Revised Code   Volume 3 — 63

Swinney operation — Therapy

Trachelotomy — Transplant, transplantation

◄ Additional Digit Required — Refer to the Tabular List for Digit Selection   ▽ Subterms under main terms may continue to next column or page

2014 ICD-9-CM   ▶◄ Revised Text   ● New Line   ▲ Revised Code   Volume 3 — 65

Transplant, transplantation — *continued*
 toe (replacing absent thumb) (with amputation) 82.69 *[84.11]*
  to finger, except thumb 82.81 *[84.11]*
 tooth 23.5
 ureter to
  bladder 56.74
  ileum (external diversion) 56.51
   internal diversion only 56.71
  intestine 56.71
  skin 56.61
 vein (peripheral) 39.59
  renal, aberrant 39.55
 vitreous 14.72
  anterior approach 14.71
Transposition
 extraocular muscles 15.5
 eyelash flaps 08.63
  eye muscle (oblique) (rectus) 15.5
 finger (replacing absent thumb) (same hand) 82.61
  to
   finger, except thumb 82.81
   opposite hand (with ampu-tation) 82.69 *[84.01]*
 interatrial venous return 35.91
 jejunal (Henley) 43.81
 joint capsule (*see also* Arthroplasty) 81.96
 muscle NEC 83.79
  extraocular 15.5
  hand 82.59
 nerve (cranial) (peripheral) (radial anterior) (ulnar) 04.6
 nipple 85.86
 pterygium 11.31
 tendon NEC 83.76
  hand 82.57
 vocal cords 31.69
Transureteroureterostomy 56.75
Transversostomy — *see also* Colostomy 46.10
Trapping, aneurysm (cerebral) 39.52
Trauner operation (lingual sulcus extension) 24.91
Trephination, trephining
 accessory sinus — *see* Sinusotomy
 corneoscleral 12.89
 cranium 01.24
 nasal sinus — *see* Sinusotomy
 sclera (with iridectomy) 12.61
Trial (failed) forceps 73.3
Trigonectomy 57.6
Trimming, amputation stump 84.3
Triple arthrodesis 81.12
Trochanterplasty 81.40
Tsuge operation (macrodactyly repair) 82.83
Tuck, tucking — *see also* Plication
 eye muscle 15.22
  multiple (two or more muscles) 15.4
 levator palpebrae, for blepharoptosis 08.34
Tudor "rabbit ear" operation (anterior ure-thropexy) 59.79
Tuffier operation
 apicolysis of lung 33.39
 vaginal hysterectomy 68.59
  laparoscopically assisted (LAVH) 68.51
TULIP (transurethral ultrasound guided laser induced prostatectomy) 60.21
TUMT (transurethral microwave thermothera-py) **of prostate** 60.96
TUNA (transurethral needle ablation) **of prostate** 60.97
Tunnel, subcutaneous (antethoracic) 42.86
 with esophageal anastomosis 42.68
 esophageal 42.86
  with anastomosis — *see* Anastomosis, esophagus, antesternal
 pulse generator lead wire 86.99
  with initial procedure — *omit code*
Turbinectomy (complete) (partial) NEC 21.69
 by
  cryosurgery 21.61
  diathermy 21.61
 with sinusectomy — *see* Sinusectomy
Turco operation (release of joint capsules in clubfoot) 80.48
TURP (transurethral resection of prostate) 60.29

Tylectomy (breast) (partial) 85.21
Tympanectomy 20.59
 with tympanoplasty — *see* Tympanoplasty
Tympanogram 95.41
Tympanomastoidectomy 20.42
Tympanoplasty (type I) (with graft) 19.4
 with
  air pocket over round window 19.54
  fenestra in semicircular canal 19.55
  graft against
   incus or malleus 19.52
   mobile and intact stapes 19.53
  incudostapediopexy 19.52
 epitympanic, type I 19.4
 revision 19.6
 type
  II (graft against incus or malleus) 19.52
  III (graft against mobile and intact stapes) 19.53
  IV (air pocket over round window) 19.54
  V (fenestra in semicircular canal) 19.55
Tympanosympathectomy 20.91
Tympanotomy 20.09
 with intubation 20.01

U

UAE (uterine artery embolization), NOS 68.25
 with
  coils 68.24
  particulate agent (gelatin sponge) (gelfoam) (microspheres) (polyvinyl alcohol) (PVA) (spheri-cal embolics) 68.25
Uchida operation (tubal ligation with or without fimbriectomy) 66.32
UFR (uroflowmetry) 89.24
Ultrafiltration 99.78
 hemodiafiltration 39.95
 hemodialysis (kidney) 39.95
 removal, plasma water 99.78
 therapeutic plasmapheresis 99.71
Ultrasonography
 abdomen 88.76
 aortic arch 88.73
 biliary tract 88.74
 breast 88.73
 deep vein thrombosis 88.77
 digestive system 88.74
 eye 95.13
 head and neck 88.71
 heart 88.72
 intestine 88.74
 intravascular — *see* Ultrasound, intravascu-lar (IVUS)
 lung 88.73
 midline shift, brain 88.71
 multiple sites 88.79
 peripheral vascular system 88.77
 retroperitoneum 88.76
 therapeutic — *see* Ultrasound
 thorax NEC 88.73
 total body 88.79
 urinary system 88.75
 uterus 88.79
  gravid 88.78
Ultrasound
 diagnostic — *see* Ultrasonography
 fragmentation (of)
  cataract (with aspiration) 13.41
  urinary calculus, stones (Kock pouch) 59.95
 heart (intravascular) 88.72
  intracardiac (heart chambers) (ICE) 37.28
  intravascular (coronary vessels) (IVUS) 00.24
  non-invasive 88.72
 inner ear 20.79
 intravascular (IVUS) (VH™-IVUS) 00.29
  aorta 00.22
  aortic arch 00.22
  cerebral vessel, extracranial 00.21
  coronary vessel 00.24
  intrathoracic vessel 00.22
  other specified vessel 00.28
  peripheral vessel 00.23
  renal vessel 00.25

Ultrasound — *continued*
 intravascular — *continued*
  vena cava (inferior) (superior) 00.22
 therapeutic
  head 00.01
  heart 00.02
  neck 00.01
  other therapeutic ultrasound 00.09
  peripheral vascular vessels 00.03
  vessels of head and neck 00.01
 therapy 93.35
 VH™-IVUS — *see* Ultrasound, intravascular, by site
 virtual histology intravascular ultrasound — *see* Ultrasound, intravascular, by site
Umbilectomy 54.3
Unbridling
 blood vessel, peripheral 39.91
 celiac artery axis 39.91
Uncovering — *see* Incision, by site
Undercutting
 hair follicle 86.09
 perianal tissue 49.02
Unroofing — *see also* Incision, by site
 external
  auditory canal 18.02
  ear NEC 18.09
 kidney cyst 55.39
UPP (urethral pressure profile) 89.25
Upper GI series (x-ray) 87.62
UPPP (uvulopalatopharyngoplasty) 27.69 *[29.4]*
Uranoplasty (for cleft palate repair) 27.62
Uranorrhaphy (for cleft palate repair) 27.62
Uranostaphylorrhaphy 27.62
Urban operation (mastectomy) (unilateral) 85.47
 bilateral 85.48
Ureterectomy 56.40
 with nephrectomy 55.51
 partial 56.41
 total 56.42
Ureterocecostomy 56.71
Ureterocelectomy 56.41
Ureterocolostomy 56.71
Ureterocystostomy 56.74
Ureteroenterostomy 56.71
Ureteroileostomy (internal diversion) 56.71
 external diversion 56.51
Ureterolithotomy 56.2
Ureterolysis 59.02
 with freeing or repositioning of ureter 59.02
 laparoscopic 59.03
Ureteroneocystostomy 56.74
Ureteropexy 56.85
Ureteroplasty 56.89
Ureteroplication 56.89
Ureteroproctostomy 56.71
Ureteropyelography (intravenous) (diuretic infusion) 87.73
 percutaneous 87.75
 retrograde 87.74
Ureteropyeloplasty 55.87
Ureteropyelostomy 55.86
Ureterorrhaphy 56.82
Ureteroscopy 56.31
 with biopsy 56.33
Ureterosigmoidostomy 56.71
Ureterostomy (cutaneous) (external) (tube) 56.61
 closure 56.83
 ileal 56.51
Ureterotomy 56.2
Ureteroureterostomy (crossed) 56.75
 lumbar 56.41
 resection with end-to-end anastomosis 56.41
 spatulated 56.41
Urethral catheterization, indwelling 57.94
Urethral pressure profile (UPP) 89.25
Urethrectomy (complete) (partial) (radical) 58.39
 with
  complete cystectomy 57.79
  pelvic exenteration 68.8
  radical cystectomy 57.71

Urethrocystography (retrograde) (voiding) 87.76
Urethrocystopexy (by) 59.79
 levator muscle sling 59.71
 retropubic suspension 59.5
 suprapubic suspension 59.4
Urethrolithotomy 58.0
Urethrolysis 58.5
Urethropexy 58.49
 anterior 59.79
Urethroplasty 58.49
 augmentation 59.79
 collagen implant 59.72
 fat implant 59.72
 injection (endoscopic) of implant into ure-thra 59.72
 polytef implant 59.72
Urethrorrhaphy 58.41
Urethroscopy 58.22
 for control of hemorrhage of prostate 60.9─
 perineal 58.21
Urethrostomy (perineal) 58.0
Urethrotomy (external) 58.0
 internal (endoscopic) 58.5
Uroflowmetry (UFR) 89.24
Urography (antegrade) (excretory) (intra-venous) 87.73
 retrograde 87.74
Uteropexy (abdominal approach) (vaginal ap─proach) 69.22
UVP (uvulopalatopharyngoplasty) 27.69 *[29.─*
Uvulectomy 27.72
Uvulopalatopharyngoplasty (UPPP) 27.69 *[29.4]*
Uvulotomy 27.71

V

V-Y operation (repair)
 bladder 57.89
  neck 57.85
 ectropion 08.44
 lip 27.59
 skin (without graft) 86.89
 subcutaneous tissue (without skin graft) 86.89
 tongue 25.59
Vaccination (prophylactic) (against) 99.59
 anthrax 99.55
 brucellosis 99.55
 cholera 99.31
 common cold 99.51
 disease NEC 99.55
  arthropod-borne viral NEC 99.54
 encephalitis, arthropod-borne viral 99.53
 German measles 99.47
 hydrophobia 99.44
 infectious parotitis 99.46
 influenza 99.52
 measles 99.45
 mumps 99.46
 paratyphoid fever 99.32
 pertussis 99.37
 plague 99.34
 poliomyelitis 99.41
 rabies 99.44
 Rocky Mountain spotted fever 99.55
 rubella 99.47
 rubeola 99.45
 smallpox 99.42
 Staphylococcus 99.55
 Streptococcus 99.55
 tuberculosis 99.33
 tularemia 99.35
 tumor 99.28
 typhoid 99.32
 typhus 99.55
 undulant fever 99.55
 yellow fever 99.43
Vacuum extraction, fetal head 72.79
 with episiotomy 72.71
VAD
 vascular access device — *see* Vascular acce─ device, totally implantable
 ventricular assist device — *see* Implant, heart assist system

---

☑ Additional Digit Required — Refer to the Tabular List for Digit Selection   ⟱ Subterms under main terms may continue to next column or page

66 — Volume 3   ▶◀ Revised Text   ● New Line   ▲ Revised Code   2014 ICD-9-CM

Vagectomy (subdiaphragmatic) — *see also*
   Vagotomy 44.00
Vaginal douche 96.44
Vaginectomy 70.4
Vaginofixation 70.77
   with graft or prosthesis 70.78
Vaginoperineotomy 70.14
Vaginoplasty 70.79
Vaginorrhaphy 70.71
   obstetrical 75.69
Vaginoscopy 70.21
Vaginotomy 70.14
   for
      culdocentesis 70.0
      pelvic abscess 70.12
Vagotomy (gastric) 44.00
   parietal cell 44.02
   selective NEC 44.03
      highly 44.02
      Holle's 44.02
      proximal 44.02
   truncal 44.01
Valvotomy — *see* Valvulotomy
Valvulectomy, heart — *see* Valvuloplasty,
   heart
Valvuloplasty
   heart, unspecified (without valve replace-
      ment) 35.10
      with prosthesis or tissue graft — *see*
         Replacement, heart, valve, by site
      aortic valve 35.11
         percutaneous (balloon) 35.96
      balloon, percutaneous 35.96
      combined with repair of atrial and ven-
         tricular septal defects — *see* Re-
         pair, endocardial cushion defect
      mitral valve
         balloon, percutaneous repair 35.96
         endovascular repair with implant
            35.97
         open, without replacement 35.12
         percutaneous repair
            with implant (leaflet clip) 35.97
         transcatheter repair with implant
            35.97
      open heart technique 35.10
      percutaneous (balloon) 35.96
      pulmonary valve 35.13
         in total repair of tetralogy of Fallot
            35.81
         percutaneous (balloon) 35.96
      tricuspid valve 35.14
Valvulotomy
   heart (closed heart technique) (transatrial)
      (transventricular) 35.00
      aortic valve 35.01
      mitral valve 35.02
      open heart technique — *see* Valvuloplas-
        ty, heart
      pulmonary valve 35.03
         in total repair of tetralogy of Fallot
            35.81
      tricuspid valve 35.04
Varicocelectomy, spermatic cord 63.1
Varicotomy, peripheral vessels (lower limb)
   38.59
   upper limb 38.53
Vascular access device, totally implantable
   86.07
Vascular closure, percutaneous puncture —
   omit code
Vascularization — *see* Revascularization
Vasectomy (complete) (partial) 63.73
Vasogram 87.94
Vasoligation 63.71
   gastric 38.86
Vasorrhaphy 63.81
Vasostomy 63.6
Vasotomy 63.6
Vasotripsy 63.71
Vasovasostomy 63.82
Vectorcardiogram (VCG) (with ECG) 89.53
Vectra® vascular access graft 86.07
Venectomy — *see* Phlebectomy
Venipuncture NEC 38.99

Venipuncture — *continued*
   for injection of contrast material — *see*
      Phlebography
Venography — *see* Phlebography
Venorrhaphy 39.32
Venotomy 38.00
   abdominal 38.07
   head and neck NEC 38.02
   intracranial NEC 38.01
   lower limb 38.09
   thoracic NEC 38.05
   upper limb 38.03
Venotripsy 39.98
Venovenostomy 39.29
Ventilation
   bi-level positive airway pressure [BiPAP]
      93.90
      delivered by
         endotracheal tube — *see* category
            96.7 ☑
         tracheostomy — *see* category
            96.7 ☑
   continuous positive airway pressure [CPAP]
      93.90
      delivered by
         endotracheal tube — *see* category
            96.7 ☑
         tracheostomy — *see* category
            96.7 ☑
   endotracheal respiratory assistance — *see*
      category 96.7 ☑
   intermittent positive pressure breathing
      [IPPB] 93.91
   mechanical, NOS 93.90
      by endotracheal tube — *see* category
         96.7 ☑
      by tracheostomy — *see* category 96.7 ☑
      endotracheal respiratory assistance —
         see category 96.7 ☑
      invasive — *see* category 96.7 ☑
      non-invasive [NIPPV] 93.90
      other continuous invasive (unspecified
         duration) 96.70
         for 96 consecutive hours or more
            96.72
         for less than 96 consecutive hours
            96.71
      positive end expiratory pressure [PEEP]
         invasive — *see* category 96.7 ☑
         non-invasive [NIPPV] 93.90
   negative pressure (continuous) [CNP] 93.99
   non-invasive positive pressure (NIPPV) 93.90
Ventriculectomy, heart
   partial 37.35
Ventriculocholecystostomy 02.34
Ventriculocisternostomy 02.22
Ventriculocordectomy 30.29
Ventriculogram, ventriculography (cerebral)
   87.02
   cardiac
      left ventricle (outflow tract) 88.53
         combined with right heart 88.54
      right ventricle (outflow tract) 88.52
         combined with left heart 88.54
      radionuclide cardiac 92.05
Ventriculomyocardiotomy 37.11
Ventriculoperitoneostomy 02.34
Ventriculopuncture 01.09
   through previously implanted catheter or
      reservoir (Ommaya) (Rickham) 01.02
Ventriculoseptopexy — *see also* Repair, ven-
   tricular septal defect 35.72
Ventriculoseptoplasty — *see also* Repair,
   ventricular septal defect 35.72
Ventriculostomy
   for
      external ventricular drainage (EVD) 02.21
      placement of ventricular catheter 02.21
      third (endoscopic) 02.22
Ventriculotomy
   cerebral 02.22
   heart 37.11
Ventriculoureterostomy 02.35
Ventriculovenostomy 02.32
Ventrofixation, uterus 69.22
Ventrohysteropexy 69.22

Ventrosuspension, uterus 69.22
VEP (visual evoked potential) 95.23
Version, obstetrical (bimanual) (cephalic)
   (combined) (internal) (podalic) 73.21
   with extraction 73.22
   Braxton Hicks 73.21
      with extraction 73.22
   external (bipolar) 73.91
   Potter's (podalic) 73.21
      with extraction 73.22
   Wigand's (external) 73.91
   Wright's (cephalic) 73.21
      with extraction 73.22
Vertebroplasty, percutaneous 81.65
Vesicolithotomy (suprapubic) 57.19
Vesicostomy 57.21
Vesicourethroplasty 57.85
Vesiculectomy 60.73
   with radical prostatectomy 60.5
Vesiculogram, seminal 87.92
   contrast 87.91
Vesiculotomy 60.72
Vestibuloplasty (buccolabial) (lingual) 24.91
Vestibulotomy 20.79
VH™-IVUS — *see* Ultrasound, intravascular, by
   site
Vicq D'azyr operation (larynx) 31.1
Vidal operation (varicocele ligation) 63.1
Vidianectomy 05.21
Villusectomy — *see also* Synovectomy 80.70
Vision check 95.09
Visual evoked potential (VEP) 95.23
Vitrectomy (mechanical) (posterior approach)
   14.74
   with scleral buckling 14.49
   anterior approach 14.73
Vocational
   assessment 93.85
   retraining 93.85
   schooling 93.82
Voice training (postlaryngectomy) 93.73
von Kraske operation (proctectomy) 48.64
Voss operation (hanging hip operation) 83.19
Vulpius (-Compere) operation (lengthening
   of gastrocnemius muscle) 83.85
Vulvectomy (bilateral) (simple) 71.62
   partial (unilateral) 71.61
   radical (complete) 71.5
   unilateral 71.61

W

Wada test (hemispheric function) 89.10
Wang needle aspiration biopsy
   bronchus 33.24
   lung 33.27
Ward-Mayo operation (vaginal hysterectomy)
   68.59
   laparoscopically assisted (LAVH) 68.51
Wardill operation 27.62
Washing — *see* Lavage and Irrigation
Waterston operation (aorta-right pulmonary
   artery anastomosis) 39.0
Watkins (-Wertheim) operation (uterus interposition) 69.21
Watson-Jones operation
   hip arthrodesis 81.21
   reconstruction of lateral ligaments, ankle
      81.49
   shoulder arthrodesis (extra-articular) 81.23
   tenoplasty 83.88
Webbing (syndactylization) 86.89
Weir operation
   appendicostomy 47.91
   correction of nostrils 21.86
Wertheim operation (radical hysterectomy)
   68.69
   laparoscopic 68.61
West operation (dacryocystorhinostomy) 09.81
Wheeler operation
   entropion repair 08.44
   halving procedure (eyelid) 08.24
Whipple operation (radical pancreaticoduodenectomy) 52.7
   Child modification (radical subtotal pancre-
      atectomy) 52.53

Whipple operation — *continued*
   Rodney Smith modification (radical subtotal
      pancreatectomy) 52.53
Whitehead operation
   glossectomy, radical 25.4
   hemorrhoidectomy 49.46
White operation (lengthening of tendo calcaneus by incomplete tenotomy) 83.11
Whitman operation
   foot stabilization (talectomy) 77.98
   hip reconstruction 81.40
   repair of serratus anterior muscle 83.87
   talectomy 77.98
   trochanter wedge osteotomy 77.25
Wier operation (entropion repair) 08.44
Williams-Richardson operation (vaginal
   construction) 70.61
   with graft or prosthesis 70.63
Wilms operation (thoracoplasty) 33.34
Wilson operation (angulation osteotomy for
   hallux valgus) 77.51
Window operation
   antrum (nasal sinus) — *see* Antrotomy,
      maxillary
   aorticopulmonary 39.59
   bone cortex (*see also* Incision, bone) 77.10
      facial 76.09
   nasoantral — *see* Antrotomy, maxillary
   pericardium 37.12
   pleura 34.09
Winiwarter operation (cholecystoenterostomy) 51.32
Wiring
   aneurysm 39.52
   dental (for immobilization) 93.55
      with fracture-reduction — *see* Reduc-
         tion, fracture
      orthodontic 24.7
Wirsungojejunostomy 52.96
Witzel operation (temporary gastrostomy)
   43.19
Woodward operation (release of high riding
   scapula) 81.83
Wrapping, aneurysm (gauze) (methyl
   methacrylate) (plastic) 39.52

X

X-ray
   chest (routine) 87.44
      wall NEC 87.39
   contrast — *see* Radiography, contrast
   diagnostic — *see* Radiography
   injection of radio-opaque substance — *see*
      Radiography, contrast
   skeletal series, whole or complete 88.31
   therapeutic — *see* Therapy, radiation
Xenograft 86.65
Xerography, breast 87.36
Xeromammography 87.36
Xiphoidectomy 77.81

Y

Young operation
   epispadias repair 58.45
   tendon transfer (anterior tibialis) (repair of
      flat foot) 83.75
Yount operation (division of iliotibial band)
   83.14

Z

Z-plasty
   epicanthus 08.59
   eyelid (*see also* Reconstruction, eyelid) 08.70
   hypopharynx 29.4
   skin (scar) (web contracture) 86.84
      with excision of lesion 86.3
Zancolli operation
   capsuloplasty 81.72
   tendon transfer (biceps) 82.56
Zeus® Robotic Surgical System — *see* category 17.4
Ziegler operation (iridectomy) 12.14
Zonulolysis (with lens extraction) — *see also*
   Extraction, cataract, intracapsular 13.19

☑ **Additional Digit Required** — Refer to the Tabular List for Digit Selection   ⬹ **Subterms under main terms may continue to next column or page**

0. Procedures and Interventions, Not Elsewhere Classified (00)

✓3ʳᵈ **00 Procedures and interventions, not elsewhere classified**

✓4ᵗʰ **00.0 Therapeutic ultrasound**

EXCLUDES *diagnostic ultrasound (non-invasive) (88.71-88.79)*
intracardiac echocardiography [ICE] (heart chamber(s)) (37.28)
intravascular imaging (adjunctive) (00.21-00.29)

DEF: Interventional treatment modality using lower frequency and higher intensity levels of ultrasound energy than used in diagnostic ultrasound modality for the purpose of limiting intimal hyperplasia, or restenosis, associated with atherosclerotic vascular disease.

AHA: 4Q, '02, 90

00.01 Therapeutic ultrasound of vessels of head and neck
Anti-restenotic ultrasound
Intravascular non-ablative ultrasound
EXCLUDES *diagnostic ultrasound of:*
eye (95.13)
head and neck (88.71)
that of inner ear (20.79)
ultrasonic:
angioplasty of non-coronary vessel (39.50)
embolectomy (38.01, 38.02)
endarterectomy (38.11, 38.12)
thrombectomy (38.01, 38.02)

00.02 Therapeutic ultrasound of heart
Anti-restenotic ultrasound
Intravascular non-ablative ultrasound
EXCLUDES *diagnostic ultrasound of heart (88.72)*
ultrasonic ablation of heart lesion (37.34)
ultrasonic angioplasty of coronary vessels (00.66, 36.09)

00.03 Therapeutic ultrasound of peripheral vascular vessels
Anti-restenotic ultrasound
Intravascular non-ablative ultrasound
EXCLUDES *diagnostic ultrasound of peripheral vascular system (88.77)*
ultrasonic angioplasty of:
non-coronary vessel (39.50)

00.09 Other therapeutic ultrasound
EXCLUDES *ultrasonic:*
fragmentation of urinary stones (59.95)
percutaneous nephrostomy with fragmentation (55.04)
physical therapy (93.35)
transurethral guided laser induced prostatectomy (TULIP) (60.21)

✓4ᵗʰ **00.1 Pharmaceuticals**

00.10 Implantation of chemotherapeutic agent
Brain wafer chemotherapy
Interstitial/intracavitary
EXCLUDES *injection or infusion of cancer chemotherapeutic substance (99.25)*

DEF: Brain wafer chemotherapy: Placement of wafers containing antineoplastic agent against the wall of the resection cavity subsequent to the surgeon completing a tumor excision to deliver chemotherapy directly to the tumor site; used to treat glioblastoma multiforme (GBM).

AHA: 4Q, '02, 93

00.11 Infusion of drotrecogin alfa (activated)
Infusion of recombinant protein
AHA: 4Q, '02, 93
TIP: A recombinant version of naturally occurring activated protein C (APC), required to ensure the control of inflammation and clotting in blood vessels; used for patients with severe sepsis.

00.12 Administration of inhaled nitric oxide
Nitric oxide therapy
AHA: 4Q, '02, 94

00.13 Injection or infusion of nesiritide
Human B-type natriuretic peptide (hBNP)
AHA: 4Q, '02, 94
TIP: Used for the treatment of acutely decompensated congestive heart failure with dyspnea at rest or with minimal activity; is administered intravenously by infusion or bolus.

00.14 Injection or infusion of oxazolidinone class of antibiotics
Linezolid injection
AHA: 4Q, '02, 95

00.15 High-dose infusion interleukin-2 [IL-2]
Infusion (IV bolus, CIV) interleukin
Injection of aldesleukin
EXCLUDES *low-dose infusion interleukin-2 (99.28)*

DEF: A high-dose anti-neoplastic therapy using a biological response modifier (BRM); the body naturally produces substances called interleukins, which are multi-function cytokines in the generation of an immune response.
AHA: 4Q, '03, 92

00.16 Pressurized treatment of venous bypass graft [conduit] with pharmaceutical substance
Ex-vivo treatment of vessel
Hyperbaric pressurized graft [conduit]
DEF: Ex-vivo process of delivering small nucleic acid molecules that block protein transcription factors essential for the expression of genes controlling cell proliferation into graft tissue under nondistending pressure; reduces intimal hyperplasia and vein graft failure.

00.17 Infusion of vasopressor agent

00.18 Infusion of immunosuppressive antibody therapy
Monoclonal antibody therapy
Polyclonal antibody therapy
INCLUDES *during induction phase of solid organ transplantation*
AHA: 4Q, '05, 101

00.19 Disruption of blood brain barrier via infusion [BBBD]
Infusion of substance to disrupt blood brain barrier
Code also chemotherapy (99.25)
EXCLUDES *other perfusion (39.97)*
DEF: Infusion of chemotherapy drug that temporarily allows the transport of materials into the brain through the blood brain barrier (BBB), which is the protective mechanism that limits transport of toxins while allowing necessary nutrients to pass from the blood vessels into the brain tissue; used in the treatment of brain cancers.
AHA: 4Q, '07, 103-104

✓4ᵗʰ **00.2 Intravascular imaging of blood vessels**
NOTE Real-time imaging of lumen of blood vessel(s) using sound waves
Endovascular ultrasonography
Intravascular [ultrasound] imaging of blood vessels
Intravascular ultrasound (IVUS)
Virtual histology intravascular ultrasound [VH-IVUS]
Code also any synchronous diagnostic or therapeutic procedures
EXCLUDES *adjunct vascular system procedures, number of vessels treated (00.40-00.43)*
diagnostic procedures on blood vessels (38.21-38.29)
diagnostic ultrasound of peripheral vascular system (88.77)
intravascular imaging of vessel(s) by OCT (38.24-38.25)
magnetic resonance imaging (MRI) (88.91-88.97)
therapeutic ultrasound (00.01-00.09)

00.21 Intravascular imaging of extracranial cerebral vessels
Common carotid vessels and branches
Intravascular ultrasound (IVUS), extracranial cerebral vessels
EXCLUDES *diagnostic ultrasound (non-invasive) of head and neck (88.71)*

Procedures and Interventions, Not Elsewhere Classified

00.22   Intravascular imaging of intrathoracic vessels
Aorta and aortic arch
Intravascular ultrasound (IVUS), intrathoracic vessels
Vena cava (superior) (inferior)
EXCLUDES   *diagnostic ultrasound (non-invasive) of other sites of thorax (88.73)*

00.23   Intravascular imaging of peripheral vessels
Imaging of:
   vessels of arm(s)
   vessels of leg(s)
Intravascular ultrasound (IVUS), peripheral vessels
EXCLUDES   *diagnostic ultrasound (non-invasive) of peripheral vascular system (88.77)*

00.24   Intravascular imaging of coronary vessels
Intravascular ultrasound (IVUS), coronary vessels
EXCLUDES   *diagnostic ultrasound (non-invasive) of heart (88.72)*
    intracardiac echocardiography [ICE] (ultrasound of heart chamber(s)) (37.28)
AHA: 3Q, '06, 8

00.25   Intravascular imaging of renal vessels
Intravascular ultrasound (IVUS), renal vessels
Renal artery
EXCLUDES   *diagnostic ultrasound (non-invasive) of urinary system (88.75)*

00.28   Intravascular imaging, other specified vessel(s)

00.29   Intravascular imaging, unspecified vessel(s)

√4ᵗʰ **00.3   Computer assisted surgery [CAS]**
CT-free navigation
Image guided navigation (IGN)
Image guided surgery (IGS)
Imageless navigation
That without the use of robotic(s) technology
Code also diagnostic or therapeutic procedure
EXCLUDES   *robotic assisted procedures (17.41-17.49)*
    stereotactic frame application only (93.59)
TIP: CAS includes three key activities: surgical planning, registration, and navigation; typically used in brain; cranial; ear, nose and throat (ENT); spinal; and orthopaedic surgeries.

00.31   Computer assisted surgery with CT/CTA
AHA: 4Q, '04, 113

00.32   Computer assisted surgery with MR/MRA
AHA: 4Q, '04, 113

00.33   Computer assisted surgery with fluoroscopy

00.34   Imageless computer assisted surgery

00.35   Computer assisted surgery with multiple datasets

00.39   Other computer assisted surgery
Computer assisted surgery NOS

√4ᵗʰ **00.4   Adjunct vascular system procedures**
NOTE   These codes can apply to both coronary and peripheral vessels. These codes are to be used in conjunction with other therapeutic procedure codes to provide additional information on the number of vessels upon which a procedure was performed and/or the number of stents inserted. As appropriate, code both the number of vessels operated on (00.40-00.43), and the number of stents inserted (00.45-00.48).
Code also any:
   angioplasty (00.61-00.62, 00.66, 39.50)
   atherectomy (17.53-17.56)
   endarterectomy (38.10-38.18)
   insertion of vascular stent(s) (00.55, 00.63-00.65, 36.06-36.07, 39.90)
   other removal of coronary artery obstruction (36.09)
AHA: 4Q, '05, 101

00.40   Procedure on single vessel
Number of vessels, unspecified
EXCLUDES   *(aorto)coronary bypass (36.10-36.19)*
    intravascular imaging of blood vessels (00.21-00.29)
AHA: ▶2Q, '12, 15;◀ 4Q, '11, 166-167; 4Q, '10, 113; 2Q, '10, 8-9; 3Q, '09, 13; 2Q, '09, 12; 1Q, '07, 17; 3Q, '06, 8; 4Q, '05, 71, 106

Stenting Techniques on Vessel Bifurcation

00.41   Procedure on two vessels
EXCLUDES   *(aorto)coronary bypass (36.10-36.19)*
    intravascular imaging of blood vessels (00.21-00.29)
AHA: ▶3Q, '12, 5;◀ 4Q, '06, 119; 4Q, '05, 105

00.42   Procedure on three vessels
EXCLUDES   *(aorto)coronary bypass (36.10-36.19)*
    intravascular imaging of blood vessels (00.21-00.29)

00.43   Procedure on four or more vessels
EXCLUDES   *(aorto)coronary bypass (36.10-36.19)*
    intravascular imaging of blood vessels (00.21-00.29)

00.44   Procedure on vessel bifurcation
NOTE   This code is to be used to identify the presence of a vessel bifurcation; it does not describe a specific bifurcation stent. Use this code only once per operative episode, irrespective of the number of bifurcations in vessels.
AHA: 4Q, '06, 119

00.45   Insertion of one vascular stent
Number of stents, unspecified
AHA: 4Q, '11, 167; 4Q, '10, 113; 3Q, '09, 13; 4Q, '05, 71

00.46   Insertion of two vascular stents
AHA: ▶3Q, '12, 5;◀ 2Q, '09, 12; 4Q, '05, 105-106

00.47   Insertion of three vascular stents
AHA: 4Q, '06, 119

00.48   Insertion of four or more vascular stents

00.49   SuperSaturated oxygen therapy
Aqueous oxygen (AO) therapy
SSO_2
SuperOxygenation infusion therapy
Code also any:
   injection or infusion of thrombolytic agent (99.10)
   insertion of coronary artery stent(s) (36.06-36.07)
   intracoronary artery thrombolytic infusion (36.04)
   number of vascular stents inserted (00.45-00.48)
   number of vessels treated (00.40-00.43)
   open chest coronary artery angioplasty (36.03)
   other removal of coronary obstruction (36.09)
   percutaneous transluminal coronary angioplasty [PTCA] (00.66)
   procedure on vessel bifurcation (00.44)
   transluminal coronary atherectomy (17.55)
EXCLUDES   *other oxygen enrichment (93.96)*
    other perfusion (39.97)
DEF: Method of reducing myocardial tissue damage via infusion of super-oxygenated blood directly to oxygen-deprived myocardial tissue in MI patients; typically performed as an adjunct procedure during PTCA or stent insertion.
AHA: 4Q, '08, 162

BI   Bilateral Procedure   NC   Non-covered Procedure   LC   Limited Coverage Procedure   ▶◀ Revised Text   ● New Code   ▲ Revised Code Title

70 – Volume 3 • February 2013   2014 ICD-9-CM

☑4ᵗʰ **00.5 Other cardiovascular procedures**
AHA: 4Q, '02, 95

00.50 Implantation of cardiac resynchronization pacemaker without mention of defibrillation, total system [CRT-P]

NOTE Device testing during procedure — *omit code*

Biventricular pacemaker
Biventricular pacing without internal cardiac defibrillator
BiV pacemaker
Implantation of cardiac resynchronization (biventricular) pulse generator pacing device, formation of pocket, transvenous leads including placement of lead into left ventricular coronary venous system, and intraoperative procedures for evaluation of lead signals
That with CRT-P generator and one or more leads

EXCLUDES *implantation of cardiac resynchronization defibrillator, total system [CRT-D] (00.51)*
insertion or replacement of any type pacemaker device (37.80-37.87)
replacement of cardiac resynchronization:
defibrillator, pulse generator only [CRT-D] (00.54)
pacemaker, pulse generator only [CRT-P] (00.53)

DEF: Cardiac resynchronization pacemaker: CRT-P, or bi-ventricular pacing, adds a third lead to traditional pacemaker designs that connects to the left ventricle. The device provides electrical stimulation and coordinates ventricular contractions to improve cardiac output.
AHA: 3Q, '05, 3-9; 4Q, '02, 100

00.51 Implantation of cardiac resynchronization defibrillator, total system [CRT-D]

NOTE Device testing during procedure — *omit code*

BiV defibrillator
Biventricular defibrillator
Biventricular pacing with internal cardiac defibrillator
BiV ICD
BiV pacemaker with defibrillator
BiV pacing with defibrillator
Implantation of cardiac resynchronization (biventricular) pulse generator with defibrillator [AICD], formation of pocket, transvenous leads, including placement of lead into left ventricular coronary venous system, intraoperative procedures for evaluation of lead signals, and obtaining defibrillator threshold measurements
That with CRT-D generator and one or more leads

EXCLUDES *implantation of cardiac resynchronization pacemaker, total system [CRT-P] (00.50)*
implantation or replacement of automatic cardioverter/ defibrillator, total system [AICD] (37.94)
replacement of cardiac resynchronization defibrillator, pulse generator only [CRT-D] (00.54)

AHA: ▶2Q, '12, 14;◀3Q, '08, 18; 1Q, '07, 16, 17; 3Q, '05, 3-9; 4Q, '02, 99, 100
TIP: If an angiogram or a venogram is performed in conjunction with CRT-D placement, it should be coded separately; refer to subcategories 88.5 and 88.6.

00.52 Implantation or replacement of transvenous lead [electrode] into left ventricular coronary venous system

EXCLUDES *implantation of cardiac resynchronization:*
defibrillator, total system [CRT-D] (00.51)
pacemaker, total system [CRT-P] (00.50)
initial insertion of transvenous lead [electrode] (37.70-37.72)
replacement of transvenous atrial and/or ventricular lead(s) [electrodes] (37.76)

00.53 Implantation or replacement of cardiac resynchronization pacemaker, pulse generator only [CRT-P]

NOTE Device testing during procedure — *omit code*

Implantation of CRT-P device with removal of any existing CRT-P or other pacemaker device

EXCLUDES *implantation of cardiac resynchronization pacemaker, total system [CRT-P] (00.50)*
implantation or replacement of cardiac resynchronization defibrillator, pulse generator only [CRT-D] (00.54)
insertion or replacement of any type pacemaker device (37.80-37.87)

AHA: 3Q, '05, 3-9

00.54 Implantation or replacement of cardiac resynchronization defibrillator, pulse generator device only [CRT-D]

NOTE Device testing during procedure — *omit code*

Implantation of CRT-D device with removal of any existing CRT-D, CRT-P, pacemaker, or defibrillator device

EXCLUDES *implantation of automatic cardioverter/defibrillator pulse generator only (37.96)*
implantation of cardiac resynchronization defibrillator, total system [CRT-D] (00.51)
implantation or replacement of cardiac resynchronization pacemaker, pulse generator only [CRT-P] (00.53)

AHA: ▶2Q, '12, 13,14;◀3Q, '05, 3-9; 4Q, '02, 100

00.55 Insertion of drug-eluting stent(s) of other peripheral vessel(s)

Endograft(s)
Endovascular graft(s)
Stent graft(s)
Code also any:
angioplasty of other non-coronary vessel(s) (39.50)
atherectomy of other non-coronary vessel(s) (17.56)
number of vascular stents inserted (00.45-00.48)
number of vessels treated (00.40-00.43)
procedure on vessel bifurcation (00.44)

EXCLUDES *drug-coated peripheral stents, e.g., heparin coated (39.90)*
insertion of cerebrovascular stent(s) (00.63-00.65)
insertion of drug-eluting coronary artery stent (36.07)
insertion of drug-eluting stent(s) of superficial femoral artery (00.60)
insertion of non-drug-eluting stent(s):
coronary artery (36.06)
peripheral vessel (39.90)
that for other endovascular procedure (39.71-39.79)

AHA: ▶3Q, '12, 13;◀4Q, '02, 101
TIP: Drug-eluting stents gradually release a drug, such as Sirolimus, Taxol, or Paclitaxel into the vessel wall tissue over a period of 30 to 45 days to prevent the build-up of scar tissue that can narrow the reopened artery.

00.56 **Insertion or replacement of implantable pressure sensor with lead for intracardiac or great vessel hemodynamic monitoring**

> **NOTE** The sensor is physically connected by a lead to a separately implanted monitor
>
> Code also any associated implantation or replacement of subcutaneous monitor (00.57)
>
> **EXCLUDES** *circulatory monitoring (blood gas, arterial or venous pressure, cardiac output and coronary blood flow) (89.60-89.69)*
>
> *insertion of implantable pressure sensor without lead for intracardiac or great vessel hemodynamic monitoring (38.26)*
>
> **DEF:** Insertion of an implantable device consisting of a data storage system, a single lead with a pressure sensor tip and a wireless antenna that continuously collects data on heart rate, pressures, physical activity and temperature.
>
> **AHA:** 4Q, '06, 119

00.57 **Implantation or replacement of subcutaneous device for intracardiac or great vessel hemodynamic monitoring**

> Implantation of monitoring device with formation of subcutaneous pocket and connection to intracardiac pressure sensor via lead
>
> Code also any associated insertion or replacement of implanted pressure sensor with lead (00.56)
>
> **AHA:** 4Q, '06, 119

00.58 **Insertion of intra-aneurysm sac pressure monitoring device (intraoperative)**

> Insertion of pressure sensor during endovascular repair of abdominal or thoracic aortic aneurysm(s)
>
> **DEF:** Placement of a device in an aortic aneurysm sac during aneurysm repair to evaluate sac pressure before and after stent graft placement; helps detect endoleaks and prevents serious aneurysm complications.
>
> **AHA:** 4Q, '08, 163-165

00.59 **Intravascular pressure measurement of coronary arteries**

> **INCLUDES** fractional flow reserve (FFR)
>
> Code also any synchronous diagnostic or therapeutic procedures
>
> **EXCLUDES** *intravascular pressure meas- urement of intrathoracic arteries (00.67)*
>
> **AHA:** 4Q, '08, 163

√4ᵗʰ **00.6** **Procedures on blood vessels**

00.60 **Insertion of drug-eluting stent(s) of superficial femoral artery**

> Code also any:
>
> angioplasty of other non-coronary vessel(s) (39.50)
> atherectomy of other non-coronary vessel(s) (17.56)
> non-drug-eluting peripheral stents (39.90)
> number of vascular stents inserted (00.45-00.48)
> number of vessels treated (00.40-00.43)
> procedure on vessel bifurcation (00.44)
>
> **EXCLUDES** *insertion of drug-eluting stent(s) of other peripheral vessel (00.55)*
>
> *that for other endovascular procedure (39.71-39.79)*
>
> **DEF:** A self-expanding device made of nitinol, a thin, specialized durable metal coated with pharmacological agents that targets delivery of a drug directly to the arterial lesion to restore blood flow and reduce restenosis.
>
> **AHA:** 4Q, '10, 112-113

00.61 **Percutaneous angioplasty of extracranial vessel(s)**

> Carotid   Vertebral
>
> Code also any:
>
> injection or infusion of thrombolytic agent (99.10)
> number of vascular stents inserted (00.45-00.48)
> number of vessels treated (00.40-00.43)
> percutaneous atherectomy of extracranial vessel(s) (17.53)
> percutaneous insertion of carotid artery stent(s) (00.63)
> percutaneous insertion of other extracranial artery stent(s) (00.64)
> procedure on vessel bifurcation (00.44)
>
> **EXCLUDES** *angioplasty of other non-coronary vessel(s) (39.50)*
>
> *atherectomy of other non-coronary vessel(s) (17.56)*
>
> *removal of cerebrovascular obstruction of vessel(s) by open approach (38.01-38.02, 38.11-38.12, 38.31-38.32, 38.41-38.42)*
>
> **AHA:** 3Q, '10, 17,18

⁷ **00.62** **Percutaneous angioplasty of intracranial vessel(s)**   **NC**

> Basilar artery
> Intracranial portion of vertebral artery
>
> Code also any:
>
> injection or infusion of thrombolytic agent (99.10)
> number of vascular stents inserted (00.45-00.48)
> number of vessels treated (00.40-00.43)
> percutaneous atherectomy of intracranial vessel(s) (17.54)
> percutaneous insertion of intracranial stent(s) (00.65)
> procedure on vessel bifurcation (00.44)
>
> **EXCLUDES** *angioplasty of other non-coronary vessel(s) (39.50)*
>
> *atherectomy of other non-coronary vessel(s) (17.56)*
>
> *removal of cerebrovascular obstruction of vessel(s) by open approach (38.01-38.02, 38.11-38.12, 38.31-38.32, 38.41-38.42)*
>
> **AHA:** 4Q, '11, 166

00.63 **Percutaneous insertion of carotid artery stent(s)**

> Includes the use of any embolic protection device, distal protection device, filter device, or stent delivery system
> Non-drug-eluting stent
>
> Code also any:
>
> number of vascular stents inserted (00.45-00.48)
> number of vessels treated (00.40-00.43)
> percutaneous angioplasty of extracranial vessel(s) (00.61)
> percutaneous atherectomy of extracranial vessel(s) (17.53)
> procedure on vessel bifurcation (00.44)
>
> **EXCLUDES** *angioplasty of other non-coronary vessel(s) (39.50)*
>
> *atherectomy of other non-coronary vessel(s) (17.56)*
>
> *insertion of coil-retention or embolization stent (39.72)*
>
> *insertion of drug-eluting peripheral vessel stent(s) (00.55)*
>
> **AHA:** 3Q, '10, 18

---

⁷ Noncovered except when reported with code 00.65.

BI Bilateral Procedure   **NC** Non-covered Procedure   **LC** Limited Coverage Procedure   ▶◀ Revised Text   ● New Code   ▲ Revised Code Title

72 – Volume 3   2014 ICD-9-CM

00.64 **Percutaneous insertion of other extracranial artery stent(s)**

Includes the use of any embolic protection device, distal protection device, filter device, or stent delivery system

Vertebral stent

Code also any:
number of vascular stents inserted (00.45-00.48)
number of vessels treated (00.40-00.43)
percutaneous angioplasty of extracranial vessel(s) (00.61)
percutaneous atherectomy of extracranial vessel(s) (17.53)
procedure on vessel bifurcation (00.44)

EXCLUDES *angioplasty of other non-coronary vessel(s) (39.50)*
atherectomy of other non-coronary vessel(s) (17.56)
insertion of coil-retention or embolization stent (39.72)
insertion of drug-eluting peripheral vessel stent(s) (00.55)

00.65 **Percutaneous insertion of intracranial vascular stent(s)**

Includes the use of any embolic protection device, distal protection device, filter device, or stent delivery system

Basilar stent

Code also any:
number of vascular stents inserted (00.45-00.48)
number of vessels treated (00.40-00.43)
percutaneous angioplasty of intracranial vessel(s) (00.62)
percutaneous atherectomy of intracranial vessel(s) (17.54)
procedure on vessel bifurcation (00.44)

EXCLUDES *angioplasty of other non-coronary vessel(s) (39.50)*
atherectomy of other non-coronary vessel(s) (17.56)
insertion of coil-retention or embolization stent (39.72)
insertion of drug-eluting peripheral vessel stent(s) (00.55)

00.66 **Percutaneous transluminal coronary angioplasty [PTCA]**

Balloon angioplasty of coronary artery
Percutaneous coronary angioplasty NOS
PTCA NOS

Code also any:
injection or infusion of thrombolytic agent (99.10)
insertion of coronary artery stent(s) (36.06-36.07)
intracoronary artery thrombolytic infusion (36.04)
number of vascular stents inserted (00.45-00.48)
number of vessels treated (00.40-00.43)
procedure on vessel bifurcation (00.44)
SuperSaturated oxygen therapy (00.49)
transluminal coronary atherectomy (17.55)

DEF: Balloon angioplasty: Insertion of catheter with inflation of balloon to flatten plaque and widen vessels.

AHA: ▶4Q, '12, 83, 85; 3Q, '12, 5;◀4Q, '11, 167; 2Q, '10, 8-9; 2Q, '09, 12; 1Q, '07, 17; 3Q, '06, 8; 4Q, '05, 71, 101; **The following references pertain to deleted PTCA codes (36.01, 36.02, 36.05):** 1Q, '04, 10; 3Q, '03, 9; 4Q, '02, 114; 3Q, '02, 19; 1Q, '01, 9; 2Q, '01, 24; 1Q, '00, 11; 1Q, '99, 17; 4Q, '98, 74, 85; 1Q, '97, 3; 1Q, '94, 3; 3Q, '91, 24

PTCA (Balloon Angioplasty)

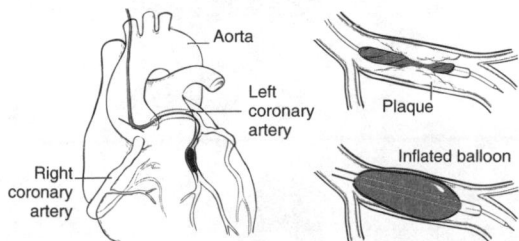

00.67 **Intravascular pressure measurement of intrathoracic arteries**

Assessment of:
aorta and aortic arch
carotid

Code also any synchronous diagnostic or therapeutic procedures

AHA: 4Q, '08, 163-164

00.68 **Intravascular pressure measurement of peripheral arteries**

Assessment of:
other peripheral vessels
vessels of arm(s)
vessels of leg(s)

Code also any synchronous diagnostic or therapeutic procedures

AHA: 4Q, '08, 163-164

00.69 **Intravascular pressure measurement, other specified and unspecified vessels**

Assessment of:
iliac vessels
intra-abdominal vessels
mesenteric vessels
renal vessels

Code also any synchronous diagnostic or therapeutic procedures

EXCLUDES *intravascular pressure measurement of:*
coronary arteries (00.59)
intrathoracic arteries (00.67)
peripheral arteries (00.68)

AHA: 4Q, '08, 163-164

✓4ᵗʰ **00.7** **Other hip procedures**
AHA: 4Q, '05, 106

00.70 **Revision of hip replacement, both acetabular and femoral components** `BI`

Total hip revision

Code also any:
removal of (cement) (joint) spacer (84.57)
type of bearing surface, if known (00.74-00.77)

EXCLUDES *revision of hip replacement, acetabular component only (00.71)*
revision of hip replacement, fem- oral component only (00.72)
revision of hip replacement, not otherwise specified (81.53)
revision with replacement of acetabular liner and/or femoral head only (00.73)

AHA: 2Q, '08, 3, 4; 1Q, '08, 6; 4Q, '05, 113
TIP: Assign for a conversion from a previously placed hip hemiarthroplasty to a total hip joint replacement procedure.

00.71 **Revision of hip replacement, acetabular component**

Partial, acetabular component only
That with:
exchange of acetabular cup and liner
exchange of femoral head

Code also any type of bearing surface, if known (00.74-00.77)

EXCLUDES *revision of hip replacement, both acetabular and femoral components (00.70)*
revision of hip replacement, femoral component (00.72)
revision of hip replacement, not otherwise specified (81.53)
revision with replacement of acetabular liner and/or femoral head only (00.73)

AHA: 4Q, '05, 112

Procedures and Interventions, Not Elsewhere Classified

00.64–00.71

00.72 Revision of hip replacement, femoral component
Partial, femoral component only
That with:
    exchange of acetabular liner
    exchange of femoral stem and head
Code also any type of bearing surface, if known
    (00.74-00.77)
EXCLUDES *revision of hip replacement, acetabular*
                component (00.71)
            revision of hip replacement, both acetabular
                and femoral components (00.70)
            revision of hip replacement, not otherwise
                specified (81.53)
            revision with replacement of acetabular liner
                and/or femoral head only (00.73)

00.73 Revision of hip replacement, acetabular liner and/or femoral head only
Code also any type of bearing surface, if known
    (00.74-00.77)

00.74 Hip bearing surface, metal-on- polyethylene

00.75 Hip bearing surface, metal-on-metal
AHA: 4Q, '06, 121

00.76 Hip bearing surface, ceramic-on-ceramic
AHA: 4Q, '05, 112

00.77 Hip bearing surface, ceramic-on- polyethylene
Hip bearing surface, oxidized
    zirconium-on-polyethylene
AHA: 4Q, '06, 120

✓4ᵗʰ **00.8 Other knee and hip procedures**
NOTE Report up to two components using 00.81-00.83 to
        describe revision of knee replacements. If all three
        components are revised, report 00.80.
AHA: 4Q, '05, 113

00.80 Revision of knee replacement, total (all components) [BI]
Replacement of femoral, tibial, and patellar
    components (all components)
Code also any removal of (cement) (joint) spacer
    (84.57)
EXCLUDES *revision of only one or two components*
                (tibial, femoral or patellar component)
                (00.81-00.84)
AHA: 1Q, '08, 6
TIP: Assign for the revision of a unicompartment knee
replacement to total knee arthroplasty; the procedure is
still considered a revision, even though part of the
component is being replaced for the first time.

00.81 Revision of knee replacement, tibial component
Replacement of tibial baseplate and tibial insert
    (liner)
EXCLUDES *revision of knee replacement, total (all*
                components) (00.80)
AHA: 4Q, '05, 117

00.82 Revision of knee replacement, femoral component
That with replacement of tibial insert (liner)
EXCLUDES *revision of knee replacement, total (all*
                components) (00.80)
AHA: 3Q, '06, 9; 4Q, '05, 117

00.83 Revision of knee replacement, patellar component
EXCLUDES *revision of knee replacement, total (all*
                components) (00.80)

00.84 Revision of total knee replacement, tibial insert (liner)
Replacement of tibial insert (liner)
EXCLUDES *that with replacement of tibial component*
                (tibial base plate and liner) (00.81)

00.85 Resurfacing hip, total, acetabulum and femoral head [BI]
Hip resurfacing arthroplasty, total
AHA: 4Q, '06, 121

00.86 Resurfacing hip, partial, femoral head [BI]
Hip resurfacing arthroplasty, NOS
Hip resurfacing arthroplasty, partial, femoral head
EXCLUDES *that with resurfacing of acetabulum (00.85)*
AHA: 4Q, '06, 121

00.87 Resurfacing hip, partial, acetabulum [BI]
Hip resurfacing arthroplasty, partial, acetabulum
EXCLUDES *that with resurfacing of femoral head (00.85)*
AHA: 4Q, '06, 121

✓4ᵗʰ **00.9 Other procedures and interventions**

00.91 Transplant from live related donor
Code also organ transplant procedure

00.92 Transplant from live non-related donor
Code also organ transplant procedure
AHA: 1Q, '12, 13; 2Q, '08, 8; 4Q, '04, 117
TIP: Assign for a transplant from a patient who is designated
as brain dead but is kept alive for organ harvesting.

00.93 Transplant from cadaver
Code also organ transplant procedure
AHA: 2Q, '11, 6

00.94 Intra-operative neurophysiologic monitoring
INCLUDES cranial nerve, peripheral nerve and spinal
                cord testing performed
                intra-operatively
Intra-operative neurophysiologic testing
IOM
Nerve monitoring
Neuromonitoring
That by:
    brainstem auditory evoked potentials [BAEP]
    electroencephalogram [EEG]
    electromyogram [EMG]
    motor evoked potentials [MEP]
    nerve conduction study
    somatosensory evoked potentials [SSEP]
    transcranial Doppler
EXCLUDES *brain temperature monitoring (01.17)*
                intracranial oxygen monitoring (01.16)
                intracranial pressure monitoring (01.10)
                plethysmogram (89.58)
DEF: Real-time testing techniques used in brain, spinal cord,
and nerve procedures to assist in lesion excision and
provide ongoing neurological functioning information
and/or warning of impending neural structure injury.
AHA:1Q, '11, 7; 2Q, '09, 4; 4Q, '07, 104

00.95 Injection or infusion of glucarpidase
AHA: 4Q, '12, 87

● **00.96 Infusion of 4-Factor Prothrombin Complex Concentrate**
Infusion of 4F-PCC
EXCLUDES *transfusion of coagulation factors (99.06)*
                transfusion of Factor IX complex (99.06)

1. Operations on the Nervous System (01-05)

√3ʳᵈ **01**   **Incision and excision of skull, brain, and cerebral meninges**

√4ᵗʰ   **01.0**   **Cranial puncture**

01.01   **Cisternal puncture**
Cisternal aspiration
Cisternal tap
EXCLUDES   *pneumocisternogram (87.02)*
DEF: Needle insertion through subarachnoid space to withdraw cerebrospinal fluid.

01.02   **Ventriculopuncture through previously implanted catheter**
Puncture of ventricular shunt tubing
DEF: Piercing of artificial, fluid-diverting tubing in the brain for withdrawal of cerebrospinal fluid.

01.09   **Other cranial puncture**
Aspiration of:
  subarachnoid space
  subdural space
Cranial aspiration NOS
Puncture of anterior fontanel
Subdural tap (through fontanel)
AHA: 3Q, '09, 15-16; 4Q, '07, 107
TIP: Assign for aspiration of a subdural hematoma.

√4ᵗʰ   **01.1**   **Diagnostic procedures on skull, brain, and cerebral meninges**

01.10   **Intracranial pressure monitoring**
INCLUDES   insertion of catheter or probe for monitoring
AHA: 3Q, '09, 15-16; 4Q, '07, 105, 107
TIP: Several different devices are available that are connected to a catheter inserted via ventriculostomy, subarachnoid bolt, or screw; used to monitor intracranial pressure in patients with traumatic brain injury (TBI) or other serious brain disorders.

01.11   **Closed [percutaneous] [needle] biopsy of cerebral meninges**
Burr hole approach
DEF: Needle excision of tissue sample through skin into cerebral membranes; no other procedure performed.

01.12   **Open biopsy of cerebral meninges**
DEF: Open surgical excision of tissue sample from cerebral membrane.

01.13   **Closed [percutaneous] [needle] biopsy of brain**
Burr hole approach
Stereotactic method
DEF: Removal by needle of brain tissue sample through skin.
AHA: M-A, '87, 9

01.14   **Open biopsy of brain**
DEF: Open surgical excision of brain tissue sample.
AHA: ▶4Q, '12, 81◀

01.15   **Biopsy of skull**

01.16   **Intracranial oxygen monitoring**
Partial pressure of brain oxygen (PbtO$_2$)
INCLUDES   insertion of catheter or probe for monitoring
AHA: 4Q, '07, 105, 107

01.17   **Brain temperature monitoring**
INCLUDES   insertion of catheter or probe for monitoring
AHA: 4Q, '07, 105

01.18   **Other diagnostic procedures on brain and cerebral meninges**
EXCLUDES   *brain temperature monitoring (01.17)*
  cerebral:
    arteriography (88.41)
    thermography (88.81)
  contrast radiogram of brain (87.01-87.02)
  echoencephalogram (88.71)
  electroencephalogram (89.14)
  intracranial oxygen monitoring (01.16)
  intracranial pressure monitoring (01.10)
  microscopic examination of specimen from nervous system and of spinal fluid (90.01-90.09)
  neurologic examination (89.13)
  phlebography of head and neck (88.61)
  pneumoencephalogram (87.01)
  radioisotope scan:
    cerebral (92.11)
    head NEC (92.12)
  tomography of head:
    C.A.T. scan (87.03)
    other (87.04)
AHA: 3Q, '98, 12

01.19   **Other diagnostic procedures on skull**
EXCLUDES   *transillumination of skull (89.16)*
  x-ray of skull (87.17)

√4ᵗʰ   **01.2**   **Craniotomy and craniectomy**
EXCLUDES   *decompression of skull fracture (02.02)*
  exploration of orbit (16.01-16.09)
  that as operative approach — omit code
DEF: Craniotomy: Incision into skull.
DEF: Craniectomy: Excision of part of skull.
AHA: 1Q, '91, 1

01.20   **Cranial implantation or replacement of neurostimulator pulse generator**
Code also any associated lead implantation (02.93)
EXCLUDES   *implantation or replacement of subcutaneous neurostimulator pulse generator (86.94-86.98)*
DEF: Implantation or replacement of a small neurostimulator pulse generator in the cranium designed to treat medically intractable epilepsy, detect new-onset seizures, and apply stimulation at a seizure focus to suppress the seizure.
AHA: 4Q, '10, 113-114

01.21   **Incision and drainage of cranial sinus**
DEF: Incision for drainage, including drainage of air cavities in skull bones.

01.22   **Removal of intracranial neurostimulator lead(s)**
Code also any removal of neurostimulator pulse generator (86.05)
EXCLUDES   *removal with synchronous replacement (02.93)*

01.23   **Reopening of craniotomy site**
DEF: Reopening of skull incision.

01.24   **Other craniotomy**
Cranial:
  decompression
  exploration
  trephination
Craniotomy NOS
Craniotomy with removal of:
  epidural abscess
  extradural hematoma
  foreign body of skull
EXCLUDES   *removal of foreign body with incision into brain (01.39)*
AHA: 4Q, '10, 93; 2Q, '91, 14

01.25   **Other craniectomy**
Debridement of skull NOS
Sequestrectomy of skull
EXCLUDES   *debridement of compound fracture of skull (02.02)*
  strip craniectomy (02.01)
AHA: 1Q, '06, 6

Operations on the Nervous System

01.26–02.14

01.26   **Insertion of catheter(s) into cranial cavity or tissue**

Code also any concomitant procedure (e.g. resection (01.59))

EXCLUDES *placement of intracerebral catheter(s) via burr hole(s) (01.28)*

AHA: 3Q, '09, 16; 4Q, '05, 117-118
TIP: Assign for balloon catheter placement in brain for infusion of liquid brachytherapy radioisotope for malignancy treatment; see also code 92.20 for infusion procedure.

01.27   **Removal of catheter(s) from cranial cavity or tissue**

AHA: 4Q, '05, 117-118

01.28   **Placement of intracerebral catheter(s) via burr hole(s)**

Convection enhanced delivery
Stereotactic placement of intracerebral catheter(s)

Code also infusion of medication

EXCLUDES *insertion of catheter(s) into cranial cavity or tissue(s) (01.26)*

DEF: The strategic neurosurgical placement of catheters via burr holes into targeted brain tissue, through which therapeutic agents such as antineoplastics are microinfused.

AHA: 3Q, '09, 16; 4Q, '06, 122

01.29   **Removal of cranial neurostimulator pulse generator**

AHA: 4Q, '10, 113-114

01.3   **Incision of brain and cerebral meninges**

01.31   **Incision of cerebral meninges**

Drainage of:
     intracranial hygroma
     subarachnoid abscess (cerebral)
     subdural empyema

01.32   **Lobotomy and tractotomy**

Division of:
     brain tissue
     cerebral tracts
Percutaneous (radiofrequency) cingulotomy

DEF: Lobotomy: Incision of nerve fibers of brain lobe, usually frontal.
DEF: Tractotomy: Severing of a nerve fiber group to relieve pain.

01.39   **Other incision of brain**

Amygdalohippocampotomy
Drainage of intracerebral hematoma
Incision of brain NOS

EXCLUDES *division of cortical adhesions (02.91)*

AHA: 4Q, '09, 83

01.4   **Operations on thalamus and globus pallidus**

01.41   **Operations on thalamus**

Chemothalamectomy
Thalamotomy

EXCLUDES *that by stereotactic radiosurgery (92.30-92.39)*

01.42   **Operations on globus pallidus**

Pallidoansectomy
Pallidotomy

EXCLUDES *that by stereotactic radiosurgery (92.30-92.39)*

01.5   **Other excision or destruction of brain and meninges**

AHA: 4Q, '93, 33

01.51   **Excision of lesion or tissue of cerebral meninges**

Decortication
Resection   } of (cerebral)
Stripping of subdural   meninges
     membrane

EXCLUDES *biopsy of cerebral meninges (01.11-01.12)*

01.52   **Hemispherectomy**

DEF: Removal of one half of the brain. Most often performed for malignant brain tumors or intractable epilepsy.

01.53   **Lobectomy of brain**

DEF: Excision of a brain lobe.

01.59   **Other excision or destruction of lesion or tissue of brain**

Amygdalohippocampectomy
Curettage of brain
Debridement of brain
Marsupialization of brain cyst
Transtemporal (mastoid) excision of brain tumor

EXCLUDES *biopsy of brain (01.13-01.14)*
            laser interstitial thermal therapy [LITT] of lesion or tissue of brain under guidance (17.61)
            that by stereotactic radiosurgery (92.30-92.39)

AHA: 4Q, '05, 118; 3Q, '99, 7; 1Q, '99, 9; 3Q, '98, 12; 1Q, '98, 6

01.6   **Excision of lesion of skull**

Removal of granulation tissue of cranium

EXCLUDES *biopsy of skull (01.15)*
            sequestrectomy (01.25)

02   **Other operations on skull, brain, and cerebral meninges**

02.0   **Cranioplasty**

EXCLUDES *that with synchronous repair of encephalocele (02.12)*

02.01   **Opening of cranial suture**

Linear craniectomy
Strip craniectomy

DEF: Opening of the lines of junction between the bones of the skull for removal of strips of skull bone.

02.02   **Elevation of skull fracture fragments**

Debridement of compound fracture of skull
Decompression of skull fracture
Reduction of skull fracture

Code also any synchronous debridement of brain (01.59)

EXCLUDES *debridement of skull NOS (01.25)*
            removal of granulation tissue of cranium (01.6)

02.03   **Formation of cranial bone flap**

Repair of skull with flap

02.04   **Bone graft to skull**

Pericranial graft (autogenous) (heterogenous)
AHA: 1Q, '11, 7

02.05   **Insertion of skull plate**

Replacement of skull plate

02.06   **Other cranial osteoplasty**

Repair of skull NOS
Revision of bone flap of skull

DEF: Plastic surgery repair of skull bones.
AHA: 1Q, '06, 6; 1Q, '05, 11; 3Q, '98, 9

02.07   **Removal of skull plate**

EXCLUDES *removal with synchronous replacement (02.05)*

02.1   **Repair of cerebral meninges**

EXCLUDES *marsupialization of cerebral lesion (01.59)*

02.11   **Simple suture of dura mater of brain**

02.12   **Other repair of cerebral meninges**

Closure of fistula of cerebrospinal fluid
Dural graft
Repair of encephalocele including synchronous cranioplasty
Repair of meninges NOS
Subdural patch

02.13   **Ligation of meningeal vessel**

Ligation of:
     longitudinal sinus
     middle meningeal artery

02.14   **Choroid plexectomy**

Cauterization of choroid plexus

DEF: Excision or destruction of the ependymal cells that form the membrane lining in the third, fourth, and lateral ventricles of the brain and secrete cerebrospinal fluid.

BI Bilateral Procedure   **NC** Non-covered Procedure   **LC** Limited Coverage Procedure   ►◄ Revised Text   ● New Code   ▲ Revised Code Title

76 – Volume 3   **2014 ICD-9-CM**

Operations on the Nervous System

02.2–02.95

External Ventricular Drain (EVD)

Shunt tubing to reservoir

Ventricles

Cerebellum

✓4ᵗʰ 02.2 Ventriculostomy
AHA: 4Q, '11, 159-161

02.21 Insertion or replacement of external ventricular drain [EVD]
External ventricular drainage [EVD] setup
Replacement of external ventricular drain
Ventricular catheter placement for:
drainage of cerebrospinal fluid [CSF]
injection of medication or other substance
sampling of cerebrospinal fluid [CSF]
EXCLUDES extracranial ventricular shunt (02.31-02.35, 02.39)
intracranial ventricular shunt (02.22)
other cranial puncture (01.09)
ventricular shunt replacement (02.41-02.43)
DEF: Placement of a catheter into the ventricles for external drainage of cerebrospinal fluid into a container outside the body.
AHA: 4Q, '11, 161-162

02.22 Intracranial ventricular shunt or anastomosis
Anastomosis of ventricle to:
cervical subarachnoid space
cistern magna
Insertion of Holter valve into intracranial system
Shunt between two intracranial ventricles
That by endoscopy
Third ventriculostomy
Ventriculocisternostomy
DEF: Surgical creation of an opening of ventricle; often performed to drain cerebrospinal fluid in treating hydrocephalus.

✓4ᵗʰ 02.3 Extracranial ventricular shunt
INCLUDES that with insertion of valve
DEF: Placement of shunt or creation of artificial passage leading from skull cavities to site outside skull to relieve excess cerebrospinal fluid created in the chorioid plexuses of the third and fourth ventricles of the brain.

02.31 Ventricular shunt to structure in head and neck
Ventricle to nasopharynx shunt
Ventriculomastoid anastomosis

02.32 Ventricular shunt to circulatory system
Ventriculoatrial anastomosis
Ventriculocaval shunt

02.33 Ventricular shunt to thoracic cavity
Ventriculopleural anastomosis

Extracranial Ventricular Shunt

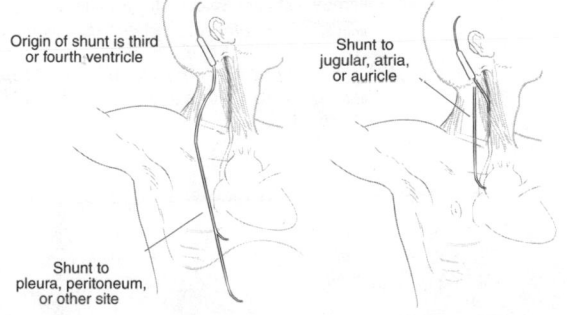

Origin of shunt is third or fourth ventricle

Shunt to jugular, atria, or auricle

Shunt to pleura, peritoneum, or other site

02.34 Ventricular shunt to abdominal cavity and organs
Ventriculocholecystostomy
Ventriculoperitoneostomy

02.35 Ventricular shunt to urinary system
Ventricle to ureter shunt

02.39 Ventricular shunt to extracranial site NEC
Ventricle to bone marrow shunt

✓4ᵗʰ 02.4 Revision, removal, and irrigation of ventricular shunt
EXCLUDES revision of distal catheter of ventricular shunt (54.95)

02.41 Irrigation and exploration of ventricular shunt
Exploration of ventriculoperitoneal shunt at ventricular site
Re-programming of ventriculoperitoneal shunt

02.42 Replacement of ventricular shunt
Reinsertion of Holter valve
Revision of ventriculoperitoneal shunt at ventricular site
AHA: N-D, '86, 8
TIP: If a ventriculoperitoneal shunt is explored or revised at the peritoneal site, assign instead code 54.95.

02.43 Removal of ventricular shunt
AHA: N-D, '86, 8

✓4ᵗʰ 02.9 Other operations on skull, brain, and cerebral meninges
EXCLUDES operations on:
pineal gland (07.17, 07.51-07.59)
pituitary gland [hypophysis] (07.13-07.15, 07.61-07.79)

02.91 Lysis of cortical adhesions
DEF: Breaking up of fibrous structures in brain outer layer.

02.92 Repair of brain

02.93 Implantation or replacement of intracranial neurostimulator lead(s)
Implantation, insertion, placement, or replacement of intracranial:
brain pacemaker [neuropacemaker]
depth electrodes
epidural pegs
electroencephalographic receiver
foramen ovale electrodes
intracranial electrostimulator
subdural grids
subdural strips
Code also any:
insertion of cranial implantation or replacement of neurostimulator pulse generator (01.20)
insertion of subcutaneous neurostimulator pulse generator (86.94-86.98)
AHA: 4Q, '97, 57; 4Q, '92, 28

02.94 Insertion or replacement of skull tongs or halo traction device
DEF: Halo traction device: Metal or plastic band encircles the head or neck secured to the skull with four pins and attached to a metal chest plate by rods; provides support and stability for the head and neck.
DEF: Skull tongs: Device inserted into each side of the skull used to apply parallel traction to the long axis of the cervical spine.
AHA: 3Q, '01, 8; 3Q, '96, 14

02.95 Removal of skull tongs or halo traction device

Operations on the Nervous System

02.96–03.53

Laminotomy with Decompression

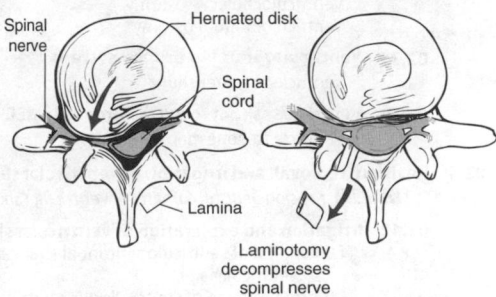

Spinal nerve — Herniated disk — Spinal cord — Lamina — Laminotomy decompresses spinal nerve

Lumbar Spinal Puncture

Cut edge of dura mater — "Cauda equina" (shown cut) — Injection site — Sacrum — Filum terminale — L-4 — L-5

02.96   **Insertion of sphenoidal electrodes**
       AHA: 4Q, '92, 28

02.99   **Other**
       EXCLUDES   *chemical shock therapy (94.24)*
                      electroshock therapy:
                         subconvulsive (94.26)
                         other (94.27)

√3ʳᵈ 03   **Operations on spinal cord and spinal canal structures**
       Code also any application or administration of an adhesion barrier substance (99.77)

     √4ᵗʰ 03.0   **Exploration and decompression of spinal canal structures**

         03.01   **Removal of foreign body from spinal canal**

         03.02   **Reopening of laminectomy site**

         03.09   **Other exploration and decompression of spinal canal**
             Decompression:
               laminectomy
               laminotomy
             Expansile laminoplasty
             Exploration of spinal nerve root
             Foraminotomy
             Code also any synchronous insertion, replacement and revision of posterior spinal motion preservation device(s), if performed (84.80-84.85)
             EXCLUDES   *drainage of spinal fluid by anastomosis (03.71-03.79)*
                        laminectomy with excision of intervertebral disc (80.51)
                        spinal tap (03.31)
                        that as operative approach — omit code
             DEF: Decompression of spinal canal: Excision of bone pieces, hematoma or other lesion to relieve spinal cord pressure.
             DEF: Expansile laminoplasty: Lamina is incised at the level of the pedicle to relieve pressure; no tissue is excised.
             DEF: Foraminotomy: Removal of root opening between vertebrae to relieve nerve root pressure.
             AHA: 2Q, '11, 10; 4Q, '08, 109; 2Q, '08, 12; 4Q, '07, 117, 120; 1Q, '07, 10; 3Q, '04, 6; 4Q, '02, 109; 2Q, '02, 15; 4Q, '99, 14; 2Q, '97, 6; 2Q, '95, 9; 2Q, '95, 10; 2Q, '90, 22; S-Q, '86, 12

     03.1   **Division of intraspinal nerve root**
         Rhizotomy
         DEF: Rhizotomy: Surgical severing of spinal nerve roots within spinal canal for pain relief.

     √4ᵗʰ 03.2   **Chordotomy**
         DEF: Chordotomy: Surgical cutting of lateral spinothalamic tract of spinal cord to relieve pain.

         03.21   **Percutaneous chordotomy**
             Stereotactic chordotomy
             DEF: Percutaneous chordotomy: Insertion of hollow needle through skin to interrupt spinal nerve root.
             DEF: Stereotactic chordotomy: Use of three-dimensional imaging to locate spinal nerve root for surgical interruption.

         03.29   **Other chordotomy**
             Chordotomy NOS
             Tractotomy (one-stage) (two-stage) of spinal cord
             Transection of spinal cord tracts
             DEF: Tractotomy (one stage) (two stages) of the spinal cord: Surgical incision or severing of a nerve tract of spinal cord.
             DEF: Transection of spinal cord tracts: Use of transverse incision to divide spinal nerve root.

     √4ᵗʰ 03.3   **Diagnostic procedures on spinal cord and spinal canal structures**

         03.31   **Spinal tap**
             Lumbar puncture for removal of dye
             EXCLUDES   *lumbar puncture for injection of dye [myelogram] (87.21)*
             DEF: Puncture into lumbar subarachnoid space to tap cerebrospinal fluid.
             AHA: 2Q, '90, 22

         03.32   **Biopsy of spinal cord or spinal meninges**

         03.39   **Other diagnostic procedures on spinal cord and spinal canal structures**
             EXCLUDES   *microscopic examination of specimen from nervous system or of spinal fluid (90.01-90.09)*
                        x-ray of spine (87.21-87.29)

     03.4   **Excision or destruction of lesion of spinal cord or spinal meninges**
         Curettage
         Debridement   } of spinal cord or spinal meninges
         Marsupialization of cyst
         Resection
         EXCLUDES   *biopsy of spinal cord or meninges (03.32)*
         AHA: 2Q, '08, 10; 3Q, '95, 5
         TIP: A laminectomy is inherent to the excision of a spinal cord tumor, do not assign 03.09 separately.

     √4ᵗʰ 03.5   **Plastic operations on spinal cord structures**

         03.51   **Repair of spinal meningocele**
             Repair of meningocele NOS
             DEF: Restoration of hernial protrusion of spinal meninges through defect in vertebral column.

         03.52   **Repair of spinal myelomeningocele**
             DEF: Restoration of hernial protrusion of spinal cord and meninges through defect in vertebral column.

         03.53   **Repair of vertebral fracture**
             Elevation of spinal bone fragments
             Reduction of fracture of vertebrae
             Removal of bony spicules from spinal canal
             EXCLUDES   *percutaneous vertebral augmentation (81.66)*
                        percutaneous vertebroplasty (81.65)
             AHA: 1Q, '07, 20; 4Q, '04, 126; 2Q, '02, 14; 4Q, '99, 11, 12, 13; 3Q, '96, 14

BI Bilateral Procedure   **NC** Non-covered Procedure   **LC** Limited Coverage Procedure   ▶◀ Revised Text   ● New Code   ▲ Revised Code Title

78 – Volume 3   **2014 ICD-9-CM**

03.59 **Other repair and plastic operations on spinal cord structures**

Repair of: Repair of:
    diastematomyelia   spinal meninges NOS
    spina bifida NOS   vertebral arch defect
    spinal cord NOS

AHA: 4Q, '08, 109

TIP: Assign for repair of dural tears occurring during spinal surgery.

03.6 **Lysis of adhesions of spinal cord and nerve roots**

AHA: 2Q, '98, 18

✓4ᵗʰ 03.7 **Shunt of spinal theca**

INCLUDES that with valve

DEF: Surgical passage created from spinal cord dura mater to another channel.

03.71 **Spinal subarachnoid-peritoneal shunt**

03.72 **Spinal subarachnoid-ureteral shunt**

03.79 **Other shunt of spinal theca**

Lumbar-subarachnoid shunt NOS
Pleurothecal anastomosis
Salpingothecal anastomosis

AHA: 1Q, '97, 7

03.8 **Injection of destructive agent into spinal canal**

✓4ᵗʰ 03.9 **Other operations on spinal cord and spinal canal structures**

03.90 **Insertion of catheter into spinal canal for infusion of therapeutic or palliative substances**

Insertion of catheter into epidural, subarachnoid, or subdural space of spine with intermittent or continuous infusion of drug (with creation of any reservoir)

Code also any implantation of infusion pump (86.06)

03.91 **Injection of anesthetic into spinal canal for analgesia**

EXCLUDES that for operative anesthesia — omit code

AHA: 3Q, '00, 15; 1Q, '99, 8; 2Q, '98, 18

03.92 **Injection of other agent into spinal canal**

Intrathecal injection of steroid
Subarachnoid perfusion of refrigerated saline

EXCLUDES injection of:
    contrast material for myelogram (87.21)
    destructive agent into spinal canal (03.8)

AHA: 2Q, '03, 6; 3Q, '00, 15; 2Q, '98, 18

TIP: Assign, along with code 99.23 for a steroid injection into the spinal canal; if both steroid and other anesthetic agent are injected, assign 03.91, 03.92, and 99.23.

03.93 **Implantation or replacement of spinal neurostimulator lead(s)**

Code also any insertion of neurostimulator pulse generator (86.94-86.98)

AHA: 1Q, '00, 19

03.94 **Removal of spinal neurostimulator lead(s)**

Code also any removal of neurostimulator pulse generator (86.05)

03.95 **Spinal blood patch**

DEF: Injection of blood into epidural space to patch hole in outer spinal membrane made by previous spinal puncture; blood clots and fills hole.

03.96 **Percutaneous denervation of facet**

03.97 **Revision of spinal thecal shunt**

AHA: 2Q, '99, 4

03.98 **Removal of spinal thecal shunt**

03.99 **Other**

✓3ʳᵈ 04 **Operations on cranial and peripheral nerves**

✓4ᵗʰ 04.0 **Incision, division, and excision of cranial and peripheral nerves**

EXCLUDES opticociliary neurectomy (12.79)
    sympathetic ganglionectomy (05.21-05.29)

04.01 **Excision of acoustic neuroma**

That by craniotomy

EXCLUDES that by stereotactic radiosurgery (92.3)

AHA: 2Q, '98, 20; 2Q, '95, 8; 4Q, '92, 26

04.02 **Division of trigeminal nerve**

Retrogasserian neurotomy

DEF: Transection of sensory root fibers of trigeminal nerve for relief of trigeminal neuralgia.

04.03 **Division or crushing of other cranial and peripheral nerves**

EXCLUDES that of:
    glossopharyngeal nerve (29.92)
    laryngeal nerve (31.91)
    nerves to adrenal glands (07.42)
    phrenic nerve for collapse of lung (33.31)
    vagus nerve (44.00-44.03)

AHA: 2Q, '98, 20

04.04 **Other incision of cranial and peripheral nerves**

04.05 **Gasserian ganglionectomy**

04.06 **Other cranial or peripheral ganglionectomy**

EXCLUDES sympathetic ganglionectomy (05.21-05.29)

04.07 **Other excision or avulsion of cranial and peripheral nerves**

Curettage
Debridement   } of peripheral nerve
Resection

Excision of peripheral neuroma [Morton's]

EXCLUDES biopsy of cranial or peripheral nerve (04.11-04.12)

AHA: 2Q, '95, 8; 4Q, '92, 26

✓4ᵗʰ 04.1 **Diagnostic procedures on peripheral nervous system**

04.11 **Closed [percutaneous] [needle] biopsy of cranial or peripheral nerve or ganglion**

04.12 **Open biopsy of cranial or peripheral nerve or ganglion**

04.19 **Other diagnostic procedures on cranial and peripheral nerves and ganglia**

EXCLUDES microscopic examination of specimen from nervous system (90.01-90.09)
    neurologic examination (89.13)

04.2 **Destruction of cranial and peripheral nerves**

Destruction of cranial or peripheral nerves by:
    cryoanalgesia
    injection of neurolytic agent
    radiofrequency
Radiofrequency ablation

DEF: Radiofrequency ablation: High frequency radio waves are applied to injure the nerve resulting in interruption of the pain signal.

AHA: 3Q, '02, 10, 11; 4Q, '95, 74

04.3 **Suture of cranial and peripheral nerves**

✓4ᵗʰ 04.4 **Lysis of adhesions and decompression of cranial and peripheral nerves**

04.41 **Decompression of trigeminal nerve root**

04.42 **Other cranial nerve decompression**

AHA: 3Q, '02, 13

04.43 **Release of carpal tunnel**

04.44 **Release of tarsal tunnel**

04.49 **Other peripheral nerve or ganglion decompression or lysis of adhesions**

Peripheral nerve neurolysis NOS

04.5 **Cranial or peripheral nerve graft**

04.6 **Transposition of cranial and peripheral nerves**

Nerve transplantation

DEF: Relocation of cranial or peripheral nerves without detaching or severing them.

✓4ᵗʰ 04.7 **Other cranial or peripheral neuroplasty**

04.71 **Hypoglossal-facial anastomosis**

DEF: Surgical connection of hypoglossal nerve to facial nerve.

Operations on the Nervous System

04.72–05.9

Release of Carpal Tunnel

Median nerve

(Deep) transverse carpal ligament being cut

04.72 Accessory-facial anastomosis
DEF: Surgical connection of accessory nerve to facial nerve.

04.73 Accessory-hypoglossal anastomosis
DEF: Surgical connection of accessory nerve to hypoglossal nerve.

04.74 Other anastomosis of cranial or peripheral nerve

04.75 Revision of previous repair of cranial and peripheral nerves

04.76 Repair of old traumatic injury of cranial and peripheral nerves

04.79 Other neuroplasty
AHA: 1Q, '06, 11
TIP: Assign for application of a NeuraWrap nerve protector, an absorbable collagen implant that provides a nonconstricting encasement for injured peripheral nerves.

√4ᵗʰ 04.8 Injection into peripheral nerve
EXCLUDES destruction of nerve (by injection of neurolytic agent) (04.2)

04.80 Peripheral nerve injection, not otherwise specified

04.81 Injection of anesthetic into peripheral nerve for analgesia
EXCLUDES that for operative anesthesia — omit code
AHA: 1Q, '00, 7

04.89 Injection of other agent, except neurolytic
EXCLUDES injection of neurolytic agent (04.2)

√4ᵗʰ 04.9 Other operations on cranial and peripheral nerves

04.91 Neurectasis
DEF: Surgical stretching of peripheral or cranial nerve.

04.92 Implantation or replacement of peripheral neurostimulator lead(s)
Code also any insertion of neurostimulator pulse generator (86.94-86.98)
EXCLUDES implantation or replacement of carotid sinus stimulation lead(s) (39.82)
DEF: Placement of or removal and replacement of neurostimulator lead(s) during the same episode.
AHA: 2Q, '07, 8; 2Q, '06, 5; 2Q, '04, 7; 3Q, '01, 16; 2Q, '00, 22; 3Q, '96, 12

04.93 Removal of peripheral neurostimulator lead(s)
Code also any removal of neurostimulator pulse generator (86.05)
AHA: 3Q, '01, 16

04.99 Other

√3ʳᵈ 05 Operations on sympathetic nerves or ganglia
EXCLUDES paracervical uterine denervation (69.3)

05.0 Division of sympathetic nerve or ganglion
EXCLUDES that of nerves to adrenal glands (07.42)

√4ᵗʰ 05.1 Diagnostic procedures on sympathetic nerves or ganglia

05.11 Biopsy of sympathetic nerve or ganglion

05.19 Other diagnostic procedures on sympathetic nerves or ganglia

√4ᵗʰ 05.2 Sympathectomy
DEF: Sympathectomy: Division of nerve pathway at a specific site of a sympathetic nerve.

05.21 Sphenopalatine ganglionectomy

05.22 Cervical sympathectomy

05.23 Lumbar sympathectomy
DEF: Excision, resection of lumber chain nerve group to relieve causalgia, Raynaud's disease, or lower extremity thromboangiitis.

05.24 Presacral sympathectomy
DEF: Excision or resection of hypogastric nerve network.

05.25 Periarterial sympathectomy
DEF: Removal of arterial sheath containing sympathetic nerve fibers.

05.29 Other sympathectomy and ganglionectomy
Excision or avulsion of sympathetic nerve NOS
Sympathetic ganglionectomy NOS
EXCLUDES biopsy of sympathetic nerve or ganglion (05.11)
opticociliary neurectomy (12.79)
periarterial sympathectomy (05.25)
tympanosympathectomy (20.91)

√4ᵗʰ 05.3 Injection into sympathetic nerve or ganglion
EXCLUDES injection of ciliary sympathetic ganglion (12.79)

05.31 Injection of anesthetic into sympathetic nerve for analgesia

05.32 Injection of neurolytic agent into sympathetic nerve

05.39 Other injection into sympathetic nerve or ganglion

√4ᵗʰ 05.8 Other operations on sympathetic nerves or ganglia

05.81 Repair of sympathetic nerve or ganglion

05.89 Other

05.9 Other operations on nervous system

BI Bilateral Procedure   NC Non-covered Procedure   LC Limited Coverage Procedure   ▶◀ Revised Text   ● New Code   ▲ Revised Code Title

80 – Volume 3   **2014 ICD-9-CM**

2. Operations on the Endocrine System (06-07)

✓3ʳᵈ 06 Operations on thyroid and parathyroid glands
> **INCLUDES** incidental resection of hyoid bone

✓4ᵗʰ 06.0 Incision of thyroid field
> **EXCLUDES** division of isthmus (06.91)

06.01 Aspiration of thyroid field
> Percutaneous or needle drainage of thyroid field
> **EXCLUDES** aspiration biopsy of thyroid (06.11)
> drainage by incision (06.09)
> postoperative aspiration of field (06.02)

06.02 Reopening of wound of thyroid field
> Reopening of wound of thyroid field for:
> control of (postoperative) hemorrhage
> examination
> exploration
> removal of hematoma

06.09 Other incision of thyroid field
> Drainage of hematoma
> Drainage of thyroglossal tract
> Exploration
> neck
> thyroid (field) } by incision
> Removal of foreign body
> Thyroidotomy NOS
> **EXCLUDES** postoperative exploration (06.02)
> removal of hematoma by aspiration (06.01)

✓4ᵗʰ 06.1 Diagnostic procedures on thyroid and parathyroid glands

06.11 Closed [percutaneous] [needle] biopsy of thyroid gland
> Aspiration biopsy of thyroid
> **DEF:** Insertion of needle-type device for removal of thyroid tissue sample.

06.12 Open biopsy of thyroid gland

06.13 Biopsy of parathyroid gland

06.19 Other diagnostic procedures on thyroid and parathyroid glands
> **EXCLUDES** radioisotope scan of:
> parathyroid (92.13)
> thyroid (92.01)
> soft tissue x-ray of thyroid field (87.09)

06.2 Unilateral thyroid lobectomy
> Complete removal of one lobe of thyroid (with removal of isthmus or portion of other lobe)
> Hemithyroidectomy
> **EXCLUDES** partial substernal thyroidectomy (06.51)
> **DEF:** Excision of thyroid lobe.

✓4ᵗʰ 06.3 Other partial thyroidectomy

06.31 Excision of lesion of thyroid
> **EXCLUDES** biopsy of thyroid (06.11-06.12)
> laser interstitial thermal therapy [LITT] of lesion or tissue of neck under guidance (17.62)
> **DEF:** Removal of growth on thyroid.

Thyroidectomy

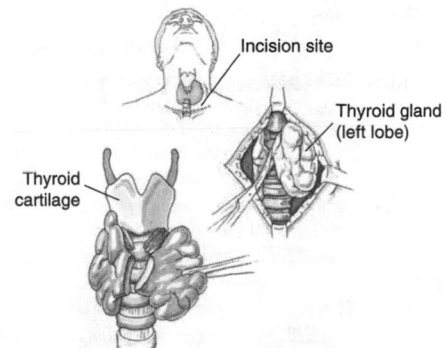

Incision site

Thyroid gland
(left lobe)

Thyroid
cartilage

06.39 Other
> Isthmectomy
> Partial thyroidectomy NOS
> **EXCLUDES** partial substernal thyroidectomy (06.51)

06.4 Complete thyroidectomy
> **EXCLUDES** complete substernal thyroidectomy (06.52)
> that with laryngectomy (30.3-30.4)

✓4ᵗʰ 06.5 Substernal thyroidectomy
> **DEF:** Removal of thyroid tissue below breastbone.

06.50 Substernal thyroidectomy, not otherwise specified

06.51 Partial substernal thyroidectomy

06.52 Complete substernal thyroidectomy

06.6 Excision of lingual thyroid
> Excision of thyroid by: Excision of thyroid by:
> submental route   transoral route
> **DEF:** Excision of thyroid tissue at base of tongue.

06.7 Excision of thyroglossal duct or tract

✓4ᵗʰ 06.8 Parathyroidectomy
> **DEF:** Removal of parathyroid glands.

06.81 Complete parathyroidectomy

06.89 Other parathyroidectomy
> Parathyroidectomy NOS
> Partial parathyroidectomy
> **EXCLUDES** biopsy of parathyroid (06.13)

✓4ᵗʰ 06.9 Other operations on thyroid (region) and parathyroid

06.91 Division of thyroid isthmus
> Transection of thyroid isthmus
> **DEF:** Cutting or division of tissue at narrowest point of thyroid.

06.92 Ligation of thyroid vessels

06.93 Suture of thyroid gland

06.94 Thyroid tissue reimplantation
> Autotransplantation of thyroid tissue
> **DEF:** Placement of thyroid tissue graft into functional site.
> **DEF:** Autotransplantation of thyroid tissue: Tissue graft from patient's own thyroid tissue to another site on thyroid.

06.95 Parathyroid tissue reimplantation
> Autotransplantation of parathyroid tissue
> **DEF:** Placement of parathyroid tissue graft into functional site.
> **DEF:** Autotransplantation of parathyroid tissue: Use of patient's own parathyroid tissue for graft.

06.98 Other operations on thyroid glands

06.99 Other operations on parathyroid glands

✓4ᵗʰ 07 Operations on other endocrine glands
> **INCLUDES** operations on:
> adrenal glands
> pineal gland
> pituitary gland
> thymus
> **EXCLUDES** operations on:
> aortic and carotid bodies (39.81-39.89)
> ovaries (65.0-65.99)
> pancreas (52.01-52.99)
> testes (62.0-62.99)

✓4ᵗʰ 07.0 Exploration of adrenal field
> **EXCLUDES** incision of adrenal (gland) (07.41)

07.00 Exploration of adrenal field, not otherwise specified

07.01 Unilateral exploration of adrenal field
> **DEF:** Investigation of one adrenal gland for diagnostic reasons.

07.02 Bilateral exploration of adrenal field
> **DEF:** Investigation of both adrenal glands for diagnostic reasons.

07.1 Diagnostic procedures on adrenal glands, pituitary gland, pineal gland, and thymus

   07.11 Closed [percutaneous] [needle] biopsy of adrenal gland

   07.12 Open biopsy of adrenal gland

   07.13 Biopsy of pituitary gland, transfrontal approach
     DEF: Excision of pituitary gland tissue for exam through frontal bone.

   07.14 Biopsy of pituitary gland, transsphenoidal approach
     DEF: Excision of pituitary gland tissue for exam through sphenoid bone.

   07.15 Biopsy of pituitary gland, unspecified approach

   07.16 Biopsy of thymus

   07.17 Biopsy of pineal gland

   07.19 Other diagnostic procedures on adrenal glands, pituitary gland, pineal gland, and thymus
     EXCLUDES microscopic examination of specimen from endocrine gland (90.11-90.19)
     radioisotope scan of pituitary gland (92.11)

07.2 Partial adrenalectomy

   07.21 Excision of lesion of adrenal gland
     EXCLUDES biopsy of adrenal gland (07.11-07.12)

   07.22 Unilateral adrenalectomy
     Adrenalectomy NOS
     EXCLUDES excision of remaining adrenal gland (07.3)
     DEF: Excision of one adrenal gland.

   07.29 Other partial adrenalectomy
     Partial adrenalectomy NOS
     AHA: 2Q, '05, 4
     TIP: Assign in addition to a code from subcategory 55.5 if the documentation specifies radical nephrectomy, which includes adrenal gland resection.

07.3 Bilateral adrenalectomy
   Excision of remaining adrenal gland
   EXCLUDES bilateral partial adrenalectomy (07.29)

07.4 Other operations on adrenal glands, nerves, and vessels

   07.41 Incision of adrenal gland
     Adrenalotomy (with drainage)

   07.42 Division of nerves to adrenal glands

   07.43 Ligation of adrenal vessels

   07.44 Repair of adrenal gland

   07.45 Reimplantation of adrenal tissue
     Autotransplantation of adrenal tissue
     DEF: Autotransplantation of adrenal tissue: Use of tissue graft from the patient's own body.

   07.49 Other

07.5 Operations on pineal gland

   07.51 Exploration of pineal field
     EXCLUDES that with incision of pineal gland (07.52)

   07.52 Incision of pineal gland

   07.53 Partial excision of pineal gland
     EXCLUDES biopsy of pineal gland (07.17)

   07.54 Total excision of pineal gland
     Pinealectomy (complete) (total)

   07.59 Other operations on pineal gland

07.6 Hypophysectomy
   DEF: Excision, destruction of pituitary gland.

   07.61 Partial excision of pituitary gland, transfrontal approach
     Cryohypophysectomy, partial
     Division of hypophyseal stalk
     Excision of lesion of pituitary [hypophysis]
     Hypophysectomy subtotal
     Infundibulectomy, hypophyseal
     } transfrontal approach
     EXCLUDES biopsy of pituitary gland, transfrontal approach (07.13)
     DEF: Removal of partial pituitary gland through frontal bone.

   07.62 Partial excision of pituitary gland, transsphenoidal approach
     EXCLUDES biopsy of pituitary gland, transsphenoidal approach (07.14)
     DEF: Removal of partial pituitary gland through sphenoid bone.

   07.63 Partial excision of pituitary gland, unspecified approach
     EXCLUDES biopsy of pituitary gland NOS (07.15)

   07.64 Total excision of pituitary gland, transfrontal approach
     Ablation of pituitary by implantation (strontium-yttrium)(Y)
     Cryohypophysectomy, complete
     } transfrontal approach
     DEF: Removal of total pituitary gland through frontal bone.

   07.65 Total excision of pituitary gland, transsphenoidal approach
     DEF: Removal of total pituitary gland through sphenoid bone.

   07.68 Total excision of pituitary gland, other specified approach
     DEF: Destroy or remove pituitary gland by a specified approach, other than those listed.

   07.69 Total excision of pituitary gland, unspecified approach
     Hypophysectomy NOS
     Pituitectomy NOS

07.7 Other operations on hypophysis

   07.71 Exploration of pituitary fossa
     EXCLUDES exploration with incision of pituitary gland (07.72)
     DEF: Exploration of region of pituitary gland.

   07.72 Incision of pituitary gland
     Aspiration of:
     craniobuccal pouch
     craniopharyngioma
     hypophysis
     pituitary gland
     Rathke's pouch

   07.79 Other
     Insertion of pack into sella turcica

07.8 Thymectomy

   07.80 Thymectomy, not otherwise specified

   07.81 Other partial excision of thymus
     Open partial excision of thymus
     EXCLUDES biopsy of thymus (07.16)
     thoracoscopic partial excision of thymus (07.83)

   07.82 Other total excision of thymus
     Open total excision of thymus
     EXCLUDES thoracoscopic total excision of thymus (07.84)

   07.83 Thoracoscopic partial excision of thymus
     EXCLUDES other partial excision of thymus (07.81)
     AHA: 4Q, '07, 108

BI Bilateral Procedure   NC Non-covered Procedure   LC Limited Coverage Procedure   ►◄ Revised Text   ● New Code   ▲ Revised Code Title

07.84 **Thoracoscopic total excision of**
      EXCLUDES *other total excision of thymus (07.82)*
      AHA: 4Q, '07, 108, 109

√4ᵗʰ 07.9 **Other operations on thymus**

    07.91 **Exploration of thymus field**
      EXCLUDES *exploration with incision of thymus (07.92)*

    07.92 **Other incision of thymus**
      Open incision of thymus
      EXCLUDES *thoracoscopic incision of thymus (07.95)*

    07.93 **Repair of thymus**

07.94 **Transplantation of thymus**
      DEF: Placement of thymus tissue grafts into functional area of gland.

07.95 **Thoracoscopic incision of thymus**
      EXCLUDES *other incision of thymus (07.92)*
      AHA: 4Q, '07, 108

07.98 **Other and unspecified thoracoscopic operations on thymus**
      AHA: 4Q, '07, 108

07.99 **Other and unspecified operations on thymus**
      Transcervical thymectomy
      EXCLUDES *other thoracoscopic operations on thymus (07.98)*

Operations on the Eye

3. Operations on the Eye (08-16)

√3ʳ **08** **Operations on eyelids**
    INCLUDES operations on the eyebrow

√4ᵗʰ **08.0** **Incision of eyelid**

    08.01 **Incision of lid margin**
       DEF: Cutting into eyelid edge.

    08.02 **Severing of blepharorrhaphy**
       DEF: Freeing of eyelids previously sutured shut.

    08.09 **Other incision of eyelid**

√4ᵗʰ **08.1** **Diagnostic procedures on eyelid**

    08.11 **Biopsy of eyelid**

    08.19 **Other diagnostic procedures on eyelid**

√4ᵗʰ **08.2** **Excision or destruction of lesion or tissue of eyelid**
    Code also any synchronous reconstruction (08.61-08.74)
    EXCLUDES *biopsy of eyelid (08.11)*

    08.20 **Removal of lesion of eyelid, not otherwise specified**
       Removal of meibomian gland NOS

    08.21 **Excision of chalazion**

    08.22 **Excision of other minor lesion of eyelid**
       Excision of:
         verruca
         wart

    08.23 **Excision of major lesion of eyelid, partial-thickness**
       Excision involving one-fourth or more of lid margin, partial-thickness
       DEF: Excision of lesion not in all eyelid layers.

    08.24 **Excision of major lesion of eyelid, full-thickness**
       Excision involving one-fourth or more of lid margin, full-thickness
       Wedge resection of eyelid
       DEF: Excision of growth in all eyelid layers, full thickness.
       AHA: 4Q, '11, 135

    08.25 **Destruction of lesion of eyelid**

√4ᵗʰ **08.3** **Repair of blepharoptosis and lid retraction**

    08.31 **Repair of blepharoptosis by frontalis muscle technique with suture**
       DEF: Correction of drooping upper eyelid with suture of frontalis muscle.

    08.32 **Repair of blepharoptosis by frontalis muscle technique with fascial sling**
       DEF: Correction of drooping upper eyelid with fascial tissue sling of frontalis muscle.

    08.33 **Repair of blepharoptosis by resection or advancement of levator muscle or aponeurosis**
       DEF: Correction of drooping upper eyelid with levator muscle, extended, cut, or by expanded tendon.

    08.34 **Repair of blepharoptosis by other levator muscle techniques**

    08.35 **Repair of blepharoptosis by tarsal technique**
       DEF: Correction of drooping upper eyelid with tarsal muscle.

    08.36 **Repair of blepharoptosis by other techniques**
       Correction of eyelid ptosis NOS
       Orbicularis oculi muscle sling for correction of blepharoptosis

    08.37 **Reduction of overcorrection of ptosis**
       DEF: Correction, release of previous plastic repair of drooping eyelid.

    08.38 **Correction of lid retraction**
       DEF: Fixing of withdrawn eyelid into normal position.

√4ᵗʰ **08.4** **Repair of entropion or ectropion**

    08.41 **Repair of entropion or ectropion by thermocauterization**
       DEF: Restoration of eyelid margin to normal position with heat cautery.

    08.42 **Repair of entropion or ectropion by suture technique**
       DEF: Restoration of eyelid margin to normal position by suture.

    08.43 **Repair of entropion or ectropion with wedge resection**
       DEF: Restoration of eyelid margin to normal position by removing tissue.

    08.44 **Repair of entropion or ectropion with lid reconstruction**
       DEF: Reconstruction of eyelid margin.

    08.49 **Other repair of entropion or ectropion**

√4ᵗʰ **08.5** **Other adjustment of lid position**

    08.51 **Canthotomy**
       DEF: Incision into outer canthus of eye.

    08.52 **Blepharorrhaphy**
       Canthorrhaphy   Tarsorrhaphy
       DEF: Eyelids are partially sutured together; done to shorten palpebral fissure or protect cornea.

    08.59 **Other**
       Canthoplasty NOS
       Repair of epicanthal fold

√4ᵗʰ **08.6** **Reconstruction of eyelid with flaps or grafts**
    EXCLUDES *that associated with repair of entropion and ectropion (08.44)*

    08.61 **Reconstruction of eyelid with skin flap or graft**
       DEF: Rebuild of eyelid by graft or flap method.
       AHA: 4Q, '11, 135

    08.62 **Reconstruction of eyelid with mucous membrane flap or graft**
       DEF: Rebuild of eyelid with mucous membrane graft or flap method.

    08.63 **Reconstruction of eyelid with hair follicle graft**
       DEF: Rebuild of eyelid with hair follicle graft.

    08.64 **Reconstruction of eyelid with tarsoconjunctival flap**
       Transfer of tarsoconjunctival flap from opposing lid
       DEF: Recreation of eyelid with tarsoconjunctival tissue.

    08.69 **Other reconstruction of eyelid with flaps or grafts**

√4ᵗʰ **08.7** **Other reconstruction of eyelid**
    EXCLUDES *that associated with repair of entropion and ectropion (08.44)*
    TIP: Assign these codes twice for bilateral blepharoplasty procedures; medical necessity may require documentation of visua field loss.

    08.70 **Reconstruction of eyelid, not otherwise specified**
       AHA: 2Q, '96, 11

    08.71 **Reconstruction of eyelid involving lid margin, partial-thickness**
       DEF: Repair of eyelid margin not using all lid layers.

    08.72 **Other reconstruction of eyelid, partial-thickness**
       DEF: Reshape of eyelid not using all lid layers.

    08.73 **Reconstruction of eyelid involving lid margin, full-thickness**
       DEF: Repair of eyelid and margin using all tissue layers.

    08.74 **Other reconstruction of eyelid, full-thickness**
       DEF: Other repair of eyelid using all tissue layers.

√4ᵗʰ **08.8** **Other repair of eyelid**

    08.81 **Linear repair of laceration of eyelid or eyebrow**

    08.82 **Repair of laceration involving lid margin, partial-thickness**
       DEF: Repair of laceration not involving all layers of eyelid margin.

    08.83 **Other repair of laceration of eyelid, partial thickness**
       DEF: Repair of eyelid tear not involving all eyelid layers.

    08.84 **Repair of laceration involving lid margin, full-thickness**
       DEF: Repair of eyelid margin tear involving all margin layer

---

BI   Bilateral Procedure   NC   Non-covered Procedure   LC   Limited Coverage Procedure   ►◄ Revised Text   ● New Code   ▲ Revised Code Title

08.85 Other repair of laceration of eyelid, full-thickness
DEF: Repair of eyelid tear involving all layers.

08.86 Lower eyelid rhytidectomy
DEF: Removal of wrinkles from lower eyelid.

08.87 Upper eyelid rhytidectomy
DEF: Removal of wrinkles from upper eyelid.
AHA: 2Q, '96, 11

08.89 Other eyelid repair
AHA: 1Q, '00, 22

√4th **08.9 Other operations on eyelids**

08.91 Electrosurgical epilation of eyelid
DEF: Electrical removal of eyelid hair roots.

08.92 Cryosurgical epilation of eyelid
DEF: Removal of eyelid hair roots by freezing.

08.93 Other epilation of eyelid

08.99 Other

√3rd **09 Operations on lacrimal system**

09.0 Incision of lacrimal gland
Incision of lacrimal cyst (with drainage)

√4th **09.1 Diagnostic procedures on lacrimal system**

09.11 Biopsy of lacrimal gland

09.12 Biopsy of lacrimal sac

09.19 Other diagnostic procedures on lacrimal system
EXCLUDES *contrast dacryocystogram (87.05)*
soft tissue x-ray of nasolacrimal duct (87.09)

√4th **09.2 Excision of lesion or tissue of lacrimal gland**

09.20 Excision of lacrimal gland, not otherwise specified

09.21 Excision of lesion of lacrimal gland
EXCLUDES *biopsy of lacrimal gland (09.11)*

09.22 Other partial dacryoadenectomy
EXCLUDES *biopsy of lacrimal gland (09.11)*
DEF: Partial excision of tear gland.

09.23 Total dacryoadenectomy
DEF: Total excision of tear gland.

09.3 Other operations on lacrimal gland

√4th **09.4 Manipulation of lacrimal passage**
INCLUDES removal of calculus
that with dilation
EXCLUDES *contrast dacryocystogram (87.05)*

09.41 Probing of lacrimal punctum
DEF: Exploration of tear duct entrance with flexible rod.

09.42 Probing of lacrimal canaliculi
DEF: Exploration of tear duct with flexible rod.

09.43 Probing of nasolacrimal duct
EXCLUDES *that with insertion of tube or stent (09.44)*
DEF: Exploration of passage between tear sac and nose with flexible rod.

09.44 Intubation of nasolacrimal duct
Insertion of stent into nasolacrimal duct
AHA: 2Q, '94, 11

09.49 Other manipulation of lacrimal passage

√4th **09.5 Incision of lacrimal sac and passages**

09.51 Incision of lacrimal punctum

09.52 Incision of lacrimal canaliculi

09.53 Incision of lacrimal sac
DEF: Cutting into lacrimal pouch of tear gland.

09.59 Other incision of lacrimal passages
Incision (and drainage) of nasolacrimal duct NOS

09.6 Excision of lacrimal sac and passage
EXCLUDES *biopsy of lacrimal sac (09.12)*
DEF: Removal of pouch and passage of tear gland.

√4th **09.7 Repair of canaliculus and punctum**
EXCLUDES *repair of eyelid (08.81-08.89)*

09.71 Correction of everted punctum
DEF: Repair of an outwardly turned tear duct entrance.

09.72 Other repair of punctum

09.73 Repair of canaliculus

√4th **09.8 Fistulization of lacrimal tract to nasal cavity**

09.81 Dacryocystorhinostomy [DCR]
DEF: Creation of entrance between tear gland and nasal passage for tear flow.

09.82 Conjunctivocystorhinostomy
Conjunctivodacryocystorhinostomy [CDCR]
EXCLUDES *that with insertion of tube or stent (09.83)*
DEF: Creation of tear drainage path from lacrimal sac to nasal cavity through conjunctiva.

09.83 Conjunctivorhinostomy with insertion of tube or stent
DEF: Creation of passage between eye sac membrane and nasal cavity with tube or stent.

√4th **09.9 Other operations on lacrimal system**

09.91 Obliteration of lacrimal punctum
DEF: Total destruction of tear gland opening in eyelid.

09.99 Other
AHA: 2Q, '94, 11
TIP: Assign for removal of nasolacrimal stent.

√3rd **10 Operations on conjunctiva**

10.0 Removal of embedded foreign body from conjunctiva by incision
EXCLUDES removal of:
embedded foreign body without incision (98.22)
superficial foreign body (98.21)

10.1 Other incision of conjunctiva

√4th **10.2 Diagnostic procedures on conjunctiva**

10.21 Biopsy of conjunctiva

10.29 Other diagnostic procedures on conjunctiva

√4th **10.3 Excision or destruction of lesion or tissue of conjunctiva**

10.31 Excision of lesion or tissue of conjunctiva
Excision of ring of conjunctiva around cornea
EXCLUDES *biopsy of conjunctiva (10.21)*
DEF: Removal of growth or tissue from eye membrane.
AHA: 4Q, '00, 41; 3Q, '96, 7
TIP: Assign for excision of conjunctivochalasis.

10.32 Destruction of lesion of conjunctiva
EXCLUDES *excision of lesion (10.31)*
thermocauterization for entropion (08.41)
DEF: Destruction of eye membrane growth; not done by excision.

10.33 Other destructive procedures on conjunctiva
Removal of trachoma follicles

√4th **10.4 Conjunctivoplasty**
DEF: Correction of conjunctiva by plastic surgery.

10.41 Repair of symblepharon with free graft
AHA: 3Q, '96, 7

10.42 Reconstruction of conjunctival cul-de-sac with free graft
EXCLUDES *revision of enucleation socket with graft (16.63)*
DEF: Rebuilding of eye membrane fold with graft of unattached tissue.

10.43 Other reconstruction of conjunctival cul-de-sac
EXCLUDES *revision of enucleation socket (16.64)*

10.44 Other free graft to conjunctiva

10.49 Other conjunctivoplasty
EXCLUDES *repair of cornea with conjunctival flap (11.53)*

10.5 Lysis of adhesions of conjunctiva and eyelid
Division of symblepharon (with insertion of conformer)

Operations on the Eye

10.6–12.29

10.6   **Repair of laceration of conjunctiva**
   EXCLUDES   *that with repair of sclera (12.81)*

√4ᵗʰ **10.9**   **Other operations on conjunctiva**

10.91   **Subconjunctival injection**
   AHA: 3Q, '96, 7

10.99   **Other**

√3ʳᵈ **11**   **Operations on cornea**

11.0   **Magnetic removal of embedded foreign body from cornea**
   EXCLUDES   *that with incision (11.1)*

11.1   **Incision of cornea**
   Incision of cornea for removal of foreign body

√4ᵗʰ **11.2**   **Diagnostic procedures on cornea**

11.21   **Scraping of cornea for smear or culture**

11.22   **Biopsy of cornea**

11.29   **Other diagnostic procedures on cornea**

√4ᵗʰ **11.3**   **Excision of pterygium**

11.31   **Transposition of pterygium**
   DEF: Cutting into membranous structure extending from eye membrane to cornea and suturing it in a downward position.

11.32   **Excision of pterygium with corneal graft**
   DEF: Surgical removal and repair of membranous structure extending from eye membrane to cornea using corneal tissue graft.

11.39   **Other excision of pterygium**

√4ᵗʰ **11.4**   **Excision or destruction of tissue or other lesion of cornea**

11.41   **Mechanical removal of corneal epithelium**
   That by chemocauterization
   EXCLUDES   *that for smear or culture (11.21)*
   DEF: Removal of outer layer of cornea by mechanical means.
   AHA: 3Q, '02, 20

11.42   **Thermocauterization of corneal lesion**
   DEF: Destruction of corneal lesion by electrical cautery.

11.43   **Cryotherapy of corneal lesion**
   DEF: Destruction of corneal lesion by freezing.

11.49   **Other removal or destruction of corneal lesion**
   Excision of cornea NOS
   EXCLUDES   *biopsy of cornea (11.22)*

√4ᵗʰ **11.5**   **Repair of cornea**

11.51   **Suture of corneal laceration**
   AHA: 3Q, '96, 7

11.52   **Repair of postoperative wound dehiscence of cornea**
   DEF: Repair of ruptured postoperative corneal wound.

11.53   **Repair of corneal laceration or wound with conjunctival flap**
   DEF: Correction corneal wound or tear with conjunctival tissue.

11.59   **Other repair of cornea**

√4ᵗʰ **11.6**   **Corneal transplant**
   EXCLUDES   *excision of pterygium with corneal graft (11.32)*

11.60   **Corneal transplant, not otherwise specified**
   NOTE   To report donor sources — see codes 00.91-00.93
   Keratoplasty NOS

11.61   **Lamellar keratoplasty with autograft**
   DEF: Restoration of sight using patient's own corneal tissue, partial thickness.

11.62   **Other lamellar keratoplasty**
   DEF: Restoration of sight using donor corneal tissue, partial thickness.
   AHA: S-O, '85, 6

11.63   **Penetrating keratoplasty with autograft**
   Perforating keratoplasty with autograft
   TIP: Penetrating keratoplasty infers a full-thickness corneal transplant grafting procedure.

11.64   **Other penetrating keratoplasty**
   Perforating keratoplasty (with homograft)

11.69   **Other corneal transplant**

√4ᵗʰ **11.7**   **Other reconstructive and refractive surgery on cornea**

11.71   **Keratomileusis**   NC
   DEF: Restoration of corneal shape by removing portion of cornea, freezing, reshaping curve and reattaching it.

11.72   **Keratophakia**   NC
   DEF: Correction of eye lens loss by dissecting the central zone of the cornea and replacing it with a thickened graft of the cornea.

11.73   **Keratoprosthesis**
   DEF: Placement of corneal artificial implant.

11.74   **Thermokeratoplasty**
   DEF: Reshaping and reforming cornea by heat application.

11.75   **Radial keratotomy**   NC
   DEF: Incisions around cornea radius to correct nearsightedness.

11.76   **Epikeratophakia**   NC
   DEF: Repair lens loss by cornea graft sutured to central corneal zone.

11.79   **Other**

√4ᵗʰ **11.9**   **Other operations on cornea**

11.91   **Tattooing of cornea**

11.92   **Removal of artificial implant from cornea**

11.99   **Other**
   AHA: 3Q, '02, 20
   TIP: Assign for keratolimbal stem cell transplant, typically performed for aniridia and decreasing vision with deep vascular pannus of the eye.

√3ʳᵈ **12**   **Operations on iris, ciliary body, sclera, and anterior chamber**
   EXCLUDES   *operations on cornea (11.0-11.99)*

√4ᵗʰ **12.0**   **Removal of intraocular foreign body from anterior segment of eye**

12.00   **Removal of intraocular foreign body from anterior segment of eye, not otherwise specified**

12.01   **Removal of intraocular foreign body from anterior segment of eye with use of magnet**

12.02   **Removal of intraocular foreign body from anterior segment of eye without use of magnet**

√4ᵗʰ **12.1**   **Iridotomy and simple iridectomy**
   EXCLUDES   *iridectomy associated with:*
     cataract extraction (13.11-13.69)
     removal of lesion (12.41-12.42)
     scleral fistulization (12.61-12.69)

12.11   **Iridotomy with transfixion**

12.12   **Other iridotomy**
   Corectomy
   Discission of iris
   Iridotomy NOS
   DEF: Corectomy: Incision into iris (also called iridectomy).

12.13   **Excision of prolapsed iris**
   DEF: Removal of downwardly placed portion of iris.

12.14   **Other iridectomy**
   Iridectomy (basal) (peripheral) (total)
   DEF: Partial or total removal of iris.

√4ᵗʰ **12.2**   **Diagnostic procedures on iris, ciliary body, sclera, and anterior chamber**

12.21   **Diagnostic aspiration of anterior chamber of eye**
   DEF: Suction withdrawal of fluid from anterior eye chamber for diagnostic reasons.

12.22   **Biopsy of iris**

12.29   **Other diagnostic procedures on iris, ciliary body, sclera, and anterior chamber**

BI Bilateral Procedure   **NC** Non-covered Procedure   **LC** Limited Coverage Procedure   ►◄ Revised Text   ● New Code   ▲ Revised Code Title

86 – Volume 3   **2014 ICD-9-CM**

✓4ᵗʰ **12.3**   **Iridoplasty and coreoplasty**
DEF: Correction of abnormal iris or pupil by plastic surgery.

12.31   **Lysis of goniosynechiae**
Lysis of goniosynechiae by injection of air or liquid
DEF: Freeing of fibrous structures between cornea and iris by injecting air or liquid.

12.32   **Lysis of other anterior synechiae**
Lysis of anterior synechiae:
    NOS
    by injection of air or liquid

12.33   **Lysis of posterior synechiae**
Lysis of iris adhesions NOS

12.34   **Lysis of corneovitreal adhesions**
DEF: Release of adhesions of cornea and vitreous body.

12.35   **Coreoplasty**
Needling of pupillary membrane
DEF: Correction of an iris defect.

12.39   **Other iridoplasty**

✓4ᵗʰ **12.4**   **Excision or destruction of lesion of iris and ciliary body**

12.40   **Removal of lesion of anterior segment of eye, not otherwise specified**

12.41   **Destruction of lesion of iris, nonexcisional**
Destruction of lesion of iris by:
    cauterization
    cryotherapy
    photocoagulation

12.42   **Excision of lesion of iris**
EXCLUDES   *biopsy of iris (12.22)*

12.43   **Destruction of lesion of ciliary body, nonexcisional**

12.44   **Excision of lesion of ciliary body**

✓4ᵗʰ **12.5**   **Facilitation of intraocular circulation**

12.51   **Goniopuncture without goniotomy**
DEF: Stab incision into anterior chamber of eye to relieve optic pressure.

12.52   **Goniotomy without goniopuncture**
DEF: Incision into Schlemm's canal to drain aqueous and relieve pressure.

12.53   **Goniotomy with goniopuncture**

12.54   **Trabeculotomy ab externo**
DEF: Incision into supporting connective tissue strands of eye capsule, via exterior approach.

12.55   **Cyclodialysis**
DEF: Creation of passage between anterior chamber and suprachoroidal space.

12.59   **Other facilitation of intraocular circulation**

✓4ᵗʰ **12.6**   **Scleral fistulization**
EXCLUDES   *exploratory sclerotomy (12.89)*

12.61   **Trephination of sclera with iridectomy**
DEF: Cut around sclerocornea to remove part of the iris.

12.62   **Thermocauterization of sclera with iridectomy**
DEF: Destruction of outer eyeball layer with partial excision of iris using heat.

Trabeculectomy Ab Externo

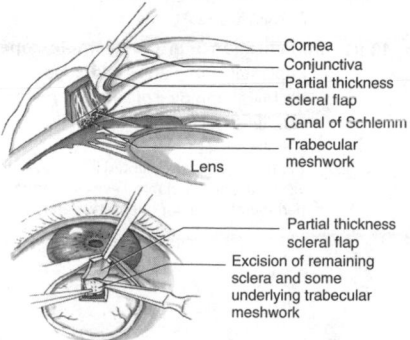

- Cornea
- Conjunctiva
- Partial thickness scleral flap
- Canal of Schlemm
- Trabecular meshwork
- Lens
- Partial thickness scleral flap
- Excision of remaining sclera and some underlying trabecular meshwork

12.63   **Iridencleisis and iridotasis**
DEF: Creation of permanent drain in iris by transposing or stretching iris tissue.

12.64   **Trabeculectomy ab externo**
DEF: Excision of supporting connective tissue strands of eye capsule, via exterior approach.

12.65   **Other scleral fistulization with iridectomy**
Holth's sclerectomy
DEF: Creation of outer eyeball layer passage with partial excision of iris.

12.66   **Postoperative revision of scleral fistulization procedure**
Revision of filtering bleb
EXCLUDES   *repair of fistula (12.82)*
AHA: 2Q, '01, 16

12.67   **Insertion of aqueous drainage device**
Anterior chamber drainage device
Aqueous drainage shunt or stent
Eye valve implant
Filtration canal shunt or device
DEF: Placement of glaucoma drainage devices, shunts or valves that shunt aqueous fluid from the anterior chamber of the eye for absorption into the lymph and blood vessels around the eye.
AHA: 4Q, '11, 162
TIP: This procedure is typically for patients who have failed medical therapy and trabeculectomy.

12.69   **Other fistulizing procedure**

✓4ᵗʰ **12.7**   **Other procedures for relief of elevated intraocular pressure**

12.71   **Cyclodiathermy**
DEF: Destruction of ciliary body tissue with heat.

12.72   **Cyclocryotherapy**
DEF: Destruction of ciliary body tissue by freezing.

12.73   **Cyclophotocoagulation**
DEF: Destruction of ciliary body tissue by high energy light source.

12.74   **Diminution of ciliary body, not otherwise specified**

12.79   **Other glaucoma procedures**
AHA: 2Q, '98, 16
TIP: Assign for suture lysis performed for elevated intraocular pressure status post trabeculectomy.

✓4ᵗʰ **12.8**   **Operations on sclera**
EXCLUDES   *those associated with:*
    retinal reattachment (14.41-14.59)
    scleral fistulization (12.61-12.69)

12.81   **Suture of laceration of sclera**
Suture of sclera with synchronous repair of conjunctiva

12.82   **Repair of scleral fistula**
EXCLUDES   *postoperative revision of scleral fistulization procedure (12.66)*

12.83   **Revision of operative wound of anterior segment, not elsewhere classified**
EXCLUDES   *postoperative revision of scleral fistulization procedure (12.66)*

12.84   **Excision or destruction of lesion of sclera**

12.85   **Repair of scleral staphyloma with graft**
DEF: Repair of protruding outer eyeball layer with a graft.

12.86   **Other repair of scleral staphyloma**

12.87   **Scleral reinforcement with graft**
DEF: Restoration of outer eyeball shape with tissue graft.

12.88   **Other scleral reinforcement**

12.89   **Other operations on sclera**
Exploratory sclerotomy

✓4ᵗʰ **12.9**   **Other operations on iris, ciliary body, and anterior chamber**

12.91   **Therapeutic evacuation of anterior chamber**
Paracentesis of anterior chamber
EXCLUDES   *diagnostic aspiration (12.21)*

12.92   **Injection into anterior chamber**

Injection of:
air
liquid   } into anterior chamber
medication

AHA: J-A, '84, 1

12.93   **Removal or destruction of epithelial downgrowth from anterior chamber**

EXCLUDES *that with iridectomy (12.41-12.42)*

DEF: Excision or destruction of epithelial overgrowth in anterior eye chamber.

12.97   **Other operations on iris**

12.98   **Other operations on ciliary body**

12.99   **Other operations on anterior chamber**

✓3ʳᵈ **13**   **Operations on lens**

✓4ᵗʰ **13.0**   **Removal of foreign body from lens**

EXCLUDES *removal of pseudophakos (13.8)*

13.00   **Removal of foreign body from lens, not otherwise specified**

13.01   **Removal of foreign body from lens with use of magnet**

13.02   **Removal of foreign body from lens without use of magnet**

✓4ᵗʰ **13.1**   **Intracapsular extraction of lens**

Code also any synchronous insertion of pseudophakos (13.71)

AHA: S-O, '85, 6

13.11   **Intracapsular extraction of lens by temporal inferior route**

DEF: Extraction of lens and capsule via anterior approach through outer side of eyeball.

13.19   **Other intracapsular extraction of lens**

Cataract extraction NOS
Cryoextraction of lens
Erysiphake extraction of cataract
Extraction of lens NOS

13.2   **Extracapsular extraction of lens by linear extraction technique**

Code also any synchronous insertion of pseudophakos (13.71)

DEF: Excision of lens without the posterior capsule at junction between the cornea and outer eyeball layer by means of a linear incision.

AHA: S-O, '85, 6

13.3   **Extracapsular extraction of lens by simple aspiration (and irrigation) technique**

Irrigation of traumatic cataract

Code also any synchronous insertion of pseudophakos (13.71)

DEF: Removal of lens without the posterior capsule by suctioning and flushing out the area.

AHA: S-O, '85, 6

✓4ᵗʰ **13.4**   **Extracapsular extraction of lens by fragmentation and aspiration technique**

Code also any synchronous insertion of pseudophakos (13.71)

DEF: Removal of lens after division into smaller pieces with posterior capsule left intact.

AHA: S-O, '85, 6

TIP: Assign an additional code from subcategory 14.7 if a vitrectomy procedure is also performed with cataract extraction procedures.

13.41   **Phacoemulsification and aspiration of cataract**

AHA: 3Q, '96, 4; 1Q, '94, 16

13.42   **Mechanical phacofragmentation and aspiration of cataract by posterior route**

Code also any synchronous vitrectomy (14.74)

13.43   **Mechanical phacofragmentation and other aspiration of cataract**

Extraction of Lens (with insertion of intraocular lens prosthesis)

Iris

Lens cataract removed

Iris

Lens

Intraocular lens insertion

✓4ᵗʰ **13.5**   **Other extracapsular extraction of lens**

Code also any synchronous insertion of pseudophakos (13.71)

AHA: S-O, '85, 6

13.51   **Extracapsular extraction of lens by temporal inferior route**

DEF: Removal of lens through outer eyeball with posterior capsule left intact.

13.59   **Other extracapsular extraction of lens**

✓4ᵗʰ **13.6**   **Other cataract extraction**

Code also any synchronous insertion of pseudophakos (13.71)

AHA: S-O, '85, 6

13.64   **Discission of secondary membrane [after cataract]**

DEF: Breaking up of fibrotic lens capsule developed after previous lens extraction.

13.65   **Excision of secondary membrane [after cataract]**

Capsulectomy

DEF: Capsulectomy: Excision of lens capsule membrane after previous lens extraction.

13.66   **Mechanical fragmentation of secondary membrane [after cataract]**

DEF: Breaking up and removal of fibrotic lens capsule developed after previous lens extraction.

13.69   **Other cataract extraction**

✓4ᵗʰ **13.7**   **Insertion of prosthetic lens [pseudophakos]**

EXCLUDES *implantation of intraocular telescope prosthesis (13.91)*

DEF: Insertion of ocular implant, following lens extraction.

AHA: J-A, '84, 1

13.70   **Insertion of pseudophakos, not otherwise specified**

13.71   **Insertion of intraocular lens prosthesis at time of cataract extraction, one-stage**

Code also synchronous extraction of cataract (13.11-13.69)

AHA: 3Q, '96, 4

13.72   **Secondary insertion of intraocular lens prosthesis**

13.8   **Removal of implanted lens**

Removal of pseudophakos

✓4ᵗʰ **13.9**   **Other operations on lens**

AHA: 1Q, '00, 9

13.90   **Operation on lens, not elsewhere classified**

AHA: 4Q, '06, 123

13.91   **Implantation of intraocular telescope prosthesis**

Implantable miniature telescope

INCLUDES removal of lens, any method

EXCLUDES *secondary insertion of ocular implant (16.61)*

AHA: 4Q, '06, 123

TIP: This device is implanted in one eye, providing central vision; the nonimplanted eye can continue to provide peripheral vision for orientation and mobility.

BI Bilateral Procedure   **NC** Non-covered Procedure   **LC** Limited Coverage Procedure   ▶◀ Revised Text   ● New Code   ▲ Revised Code Title

88 – Volume 3   **2014 ICD-9-C**

Laser Surgery (YAG)

Scleral Buckling with Implant

√3ʳᵈ **14 Operations on retina, choroid, vitreous, and posterior chamber**

√4ᵗʰ **14.0 Removal of foreign body from posterior segment of eye**
    EXCLUDES *removal of surgically implanted material (14.6)*

  14.00 Removal of foreign body from posterior segment of eye, not otherwise specified

  14.01 Removal of foreign body from posterior segment of eye with use of magnet

  14.02 Removal of foreign body from posterior segment of eye without use of magnet

√4ᵗʰ **14.1 Diagnostic procedures on retina, choroid, vitreous, and posterior chamber**

  14.11 Diagnostic aspiration of vitreous

  14.19 Other diagnostic procedures on retina, choroid, vitreous, and posterior chamber

√4ᵗʰ **14.2 Destruction of lesion of retina and choroid**
  INCLUDES destruction of chorioretinopathy or isolated chorioretinal lesion
  EXCLUDES *that for repair of retina (14.31-14.59)*
  DEF: Destruction of damaged retina and choroid tissue.

  14.21 Destruction of chorioretinal lesion by diathermy

  14.22 Destruction of chorioretinal lesion by cryotherapy

  14.23 Destruction of chorioretinal lesion by xenon arc photocoagulation

  14.24 Destruction of chorioretinal lesion by laser photocoagulation

  14.25 Destruction of chorioretinal lesion by photocoagulation of unspecified type

  14.26 Destruction of chorioretinal lesion by radiation therapy

  14.27 Destruction of chorioretinal lesion by implantation of radiation source

  14.29 Other destruction of chorioretinal lesion
    Destruction of lesion of retina and choroid NOS

√4ᵗʰ **14.3 Repair of retinal tear**
  INCLUDES repair of retinal defect
  EXCLUDES *repair of retinal detachment (14.41-14.59)*

  14.31 Repair of retinal tear by diathermy

  14.32 Repair of retinal tear by cryotherapy

  14.33 Repair of retinal tear by xenon arc photocoagulation

  14.34 Repair of retinal tear by laser photocoagulation
    AHA: 1Q, '94, 17

  14.35 Repair of retinal tear by photocoagulation of unspecified type

  14.39 Other repair of retinal tear

√4ᵗʰ **14.4 Repair of retinal detachment with scleral buckling and implant**
  DEF: Placement of material around eye to indent sclera and close a hole or tear or to reduce vitreous traction.

  14.41 Scleral buckling with implant
    AHA: 3Q, '96, 6

  14.49 Other scleral buckling
    Scleral buckling with:
      air tamponade
      resection of sclera
      vitrectomy
    AHA: 1Q, '94, 16

√4ᵗʰ **14.5 Other repair of retinal detachment**
  INCLUDES that with drainage

  14.51 Repair of retinal detachment with diathermy

  14.52 Repair of retinal detachment with cryotherapy

  14.53 Repair of retinal detachment with xenon arc photocoagulation

  14.54 Repair of retinal detachment with laser photocoagulation
    AHA: N-D, '87, 10

  14.55 Repair of retinal detachment with photocoagulation of unspecified type

  14.59 Other

14.6 Removal of surgically implanted material from posterior segment of eye

√4ᵗʰ **14.7 Operations on vitreous**

  14.71 Removal of vitreous, anterior approach
    Open sky technique
    Removal of vitreous, anterior approach (with replacement)
    DEF: Removal of all or part of the eyeball fluid via the anterior segment of the eyeball.

  14.72 Other removal of vitreous
    Aspiration of vitreous by posterior sclerotomy

  14.73 Mechanical vitrectomy by anterior approach
    DEF: Removal of abnormal tissue in eyeball fluid to control fibrotic overgrowth in severe intraocular injury.
    AHA: 3Q, '96, 4, 5

  14.74 Other mechanical vitrectomy
    Posterior approach
    AHA: 4Q, '11, 106; 2Q, '10, 4-5; 3Q, '96, 4, 5

  14.75 Injection of vitreous substitute
    EXCLUDES *that associated with removal (14.71-14.72)*
    AHA: 1Q, '98, 6; 3Q, '96, 4, 5; 1Q, '94, 17

  14.79 Other operations on vitreous
    AHA: 3Q, '99, 12; 1Q, '99, 11; 1Q, '98, 6
    TIP: Assign for an endoscopic vitreous washout and reinjection of silicone oil.

● √4ᵗʰ **14.8 Implantation of epiretinal visual prosthesis**

●   **14.81 Implantation of epiretinal visual prosthesis**
    NOTE Includes lens removal, if present, scleral buckling, vitrectomy, epiretinal membrane peeling and pericardial grafting
    EXCLUDES *implantation of intraocular telescope prosthesis (13.91)*
      other operations on retina, choroid, and posterior chamber (14.9)
      replacement of epiretinal visual prosthesis (14.83)

Operations on the Eye

14.82–16.42

● **14.82** **Removal of epiretinal visual prosthesis**

> **NOTE** Includes 360-degree limbal peritomy and vitrectomy, if performed, and device extraction
> **EXCLUDES** *removal of eye prosthesis (97.31)*

● **14.83** **Revision or replacement of epiretinal visual prosthesis**

> **NOTE** Includes tack replacement, device relocation, and replacement of pericardial grafting, if needed
> **EXCLUDES** *implantation of epiretinal visual prosthesis (14.81)*

14.9 **Other operations on retina, choroid, and posterior chamber**

> AHA: 3Q, '96, 5
> TIP: Assign for epiretinal membrane peeling, which is typically performed with vitrectomy but is not an inherent component.

√3rd **15** **Operations on extraocular muscles**

> TIP: If a procedure is performed on the same muscle in both eyes, assign the appropriate code twice from subcategory 15.1 or 15.2.

√4th **15.0** **Diagnostic procedures on extraocular muscles or tendons**

15.01 **Biopsy of extraocular muscle or tendon**

15.09 **Other diagnostic procedures on extraocular muscles and tendons**

√4th **15.1** **Operations on one extraocular muscle involving temporary detachment from globe**

15.11 **Recession of one extraocular muscle**

> **DEF:** Detachment of exterior eye muscle with posterior reattachment to correct strabismus.
> AHA: 3Q, '96, 3

15.12 **Advancement of one extraocular muscle**

> **DEF:** Detachment of exterior eye muscle with forward reattachment to correct strabismus.

15.13 **Resection of one extraocular muscle**

15.19 **Other operations on one extraocular muscle involving temporary detachment from globe**

> **EXCLUDES** *transposition of muscle (15.5)*

√4th **15.2** **Other operations on one extraocular muscle**

15.21 **Lengthening procedure on one extraocular muscle**

> **DEF:** Extension of exterior eye muscle length.

Lengthening Procedure on One Extraocular Muscle

Proposed second cut

Lengthened muscle

Extraocular muscle

Shortening Procedure on One Extraocular Muscle

To be resected

Muscle advanced and reattached

Iris

15.22 **Shortening procedure on one extraocular muscle**

> **DEF:** Shortening of exterior eye muscle.

15.29 **Other**

15.3 **Operations on two or more extraocular muscles involving temporary detachment from globe, one or both eyes**

> AHA: 3Q, '96, 3

15.4 **Other operations on two or more extraocular muscles, one or both eyes**

15.5 **Transposition of extraocular muscles**

> **EXCLUDES** *that for correction of ptosis (08.31-08.36)*
> **DEF:** Relocation of exterior eye muscle to a more functional site.

15.6 **Revision of extraocular muscle surgery**

> **DEF:** Repair of previous exterior eye muscle surgery.

15.7 **Repair of injury of extraocular muscle**

> Freeing of entrapped extraocular muscle
> Lysis of adhesions of extraocular muscle
> Repair of laceration of extraocular muscle, tendon, or Tenon' capsule

15.9 **Other operations on extraocular muscles and tendons**

√3rd **16** **Operations on orbit and eyeball**

> **EXCLUDES** *reduction of fracture of orbit (76.78-76.79)*

√4th **16.0** **Orbitotomy**

16.01 **Orbitotomy with bone flap**

> Orbitotomy with lateral approach
> **DEF:** Incision into orbital bone with insertion of small bone piece.

16.02 **Orbitotomy with insertion of orbital implant**

> **EXCLUDES** *that with bone flap (16.01)*

16.09 **Other orbitotomy**

16.1 **Removal of penetrating foreign body from eye, not otherwise specified**

> **EXCLUDES** *removal of nonpenetrating foreign body (98.21)*
> **DEF:** Removal of foreign body from an unspecified site in eye.

√4th **16.2** **Diagnostic procedures on orbit and eyeball**

16.21 **Ophthalmoscopy**

16.22 **Diagnostic aspiration of orbit**

16.23 **Biopsy of eyeball and orbit**

16.29 **Other diagnostic procedures on orbit and eyeball**

> **EXCLUDES** *examination of form and structure of eye (95.11-95.16)*
> *general and subjective eye examination (95.01-95.09)*
> *microscopic examination of specimen from eye (90.21-90.29)*
> *objective functional tests of eye (95.21-95.26)*
> *ocular thermography (88.82)*
> *tonometry (89.11)*
> *x-ray of orbit (87.14, 87.16)*

√4th **16.3** **Evisceration of eyeball**

> **DEF:** Removal of eyeball, leaving sclera and occasionally cornea.

16.31 **Removal of ocular contents with synchronous implant into scleral shell**

> **DEF:** Removal of eyeball leaving outer eyeball layer with ocular implant into shell.

16.39 **Other evisceration of eyeball**

√4th **16.4** **Enucleation of eyeball**

> **DEF:** Removal of entire eyeball after severing eye muscles and optic nerves.

16.41 **Enucleation of eyeball with synchronous implant into Tenon's capsule with attachment of muscles**

> Integrated implant of eyeball
> **DEF:** Removal of eyeball with insertion of ocular implant and muscle attachment.

16.42 **Enucleation of eyeball with other synchronous implant**

BI Bilateral Procedure   **NC** Non-covered Procedure   **LC** Limited Coverage Procedure   ►◄ Revised Text   ● New Code   ▲ Revised Code Titl

90 – Volume 3 · October 2013   **2014 ICD-9-C**

16.49   **Other enucleation of eyeball**
> Removal of eyeball NOS

✓4ᵗʰ   **16.5**   **Exenteration of orbital contents**

16.51   **Exenteration of orbit with removal of adjacent structures**
> Radical orbitomaxillectomy
>
> **DEF:** Removal of contents of bony cavity of eye as well as related tissues and structures.
>
> **DEF:** Radical orbitomaxillectomy: Removal of contents of bony cavity of eye, related tissues and structures, and a portion of maxillary bone.

16.52   **Exenteration of orbit with therapeutic removal of orbital bone**

16.59   **Other exenteration of orbit**
> Evisceration of orbit NOS
> Exenteration of orbit with temporalis muscle transplant

✓4ᵗʰ   **16.6**   **Secondary procedures after removal of eyeball**
> **EXCLUDES** *that with synchronous:*
> > *enucleation of eyeball (16.41-16.42)*
> > *evisceration of eyeball (16.31)*

16.61   **Secondary insertion of ocular implant**
> **DEF:** Insertion of ocular implant after previous eye removal.

16.62   **Revision and reinsertion of ocular implant**
> **DEF:** Reimplant or correction of ocular implant.

16.63   **Revision of enucleation socket with graft**
> **DEF:** Implant of tissue to correct socket after eye removal.

16.64   **Other revision of enucleation socket**

16.65   **Secondary graft to exenteration cavity**
> **DEF:** Implant of tissue in place of eye after removal.

16.66   **Other revision of exenteration cavity**

16.69   **Other secondary procedures after removal of eyeball**

✓4ᵗʰ   **16.7**   **Removal of ocular or orbital implant**

16.71   **Removal of ocular implant**

16.72   **Removal of orbital implant**

✓4ᵗʰ   **16.8**   **Repair of injury of eyeball and orbit**

16.81   **Repair of wound of orbit**
> **EXCLUDES** *reduction of orbital fracture (76.78-76.79)*
> > *repair of extraocular muscles (15.7)*

16.82   **Repair of rupture of eyeball**
> Repair of multiple structures of eye
> **EXCLUDES** *repair of laceration of:*
> > *cornea (11.51-11.59)*
> > *sclera (12.81)*

16.89   **Other repair of injury of eyeball or orbit**

✓4ᵗʰ   **16.9**   **Other operations on orbit and eyeball**
> **EXCLUDES** *irrigation of eye (96.51)*
> > *prescription and fitting of low vision aids (95.31-95.33)*
> > *removal of:*
> > > *eye prosthesis NEC (97.31)*
> > > *nonpenetrating foreign body from eye without incision (98.21)*

16.91   **Retrobulbar injection of therapeutic agent**
> **EXCLUDES** *injection of radiographic contrast material (87.14)*
> > *opticociliary injection (12.79)*

16.92   **Excision of lesion of orbit**
> **EXCLUDES** *biopsy of orbit (16.23)*

16.93   **Excision of lesion of eye, unspecified structure**
> **EXCLUDES** *biopsy of eye NOS (16.23)*

16.98   **Other operations on orbit**

16.99   **Other operations on eyeball**

Other Miscellaneous Diagnostic and Therapeutic Procedures

3A. Other Miscellaneous Diagnostic and Therapeutic Procedures (17)

✓3rd 17　Other miscellaneous procedures

✓4th 17.1　Laparoscopic unilateral repair of inguinal hernia
> EXCLUDES *other and open unilateral repair of hernia (53.00-53.05)*
> AHA: 4Q, '08, 165-166

17.11　Laparoscopic repair of direct inguinal hernia with graft or prosthesis
> Laparoscopic repair of direct and indirect inguinal hernia with graft or prosthesis

17.12　Laparoscopic repair of indirect inguinal hernia with graft or prosthesis

17.13　Laparoscopic repair of inguinal hernia with graft or prosthesis, not otherwise specified

✓4th 17.2　Laparoscopic bilateral repair of inguinal hernia
> EXCLUDES *other and open bilateral repair of hernia (53.10-53.17)*
> AHA: 4Q, '08, 165-166

17.21　Laparoscopic bilateral repair of direct inguinal hernia with graft or prosthesis

17.22　Laparoscopic bilateral repair of indirect inguinal hernia with graft or prosthesis

17.23　Laparoscopic bilateral repair of inguinal hernia, one direct and one indirect, with graft or prosthesis

17.24　Laparoscopic bilateral repair of inguinal hernia with graft or prosthesis, not otherwise specified

17.3　Laparoscopic partial excision of large intestine
> EXCLUDES *other and open partial excision of large intestine (45.71-45.79)*
> AHA: 4Q, '08, 169-170

17.31　Laparoscopic multiple segmental resection of large intestine

17.32　Laparoscopic cecectomy

17.33　Laparoscopic right hemicolectomy

17.34　Laparoscopic resection of transverse colon

17.35　Laparoscopic left hemicolectomy

17.36　Laparoscopic sigmoidectomy

17.39　Other laparoscopic partial excision of large intestine

✓4th 17.4　Robotic assisted procedures
> NOTE This category includes use of a computer console with (3-D) imaging, software, camera(s), visualization and instrumentation *combined* with the use of robotic arms, device(s), or system(s) at the time of the procedure.
> Computer assisted robotic surgery
> Computer-enhanced robotic surgery
> Robotic procedure with computer assistance
> Surgeon-controlled robotic surgery
> Code first primary procedure
> EXCLUDES *computer assisted surgery (00.31-00.35, 00.39)*
> AHA: 4Q, '08, 172-174

17.41　Open robotic assisted procedure
> Robotic assistance in open procedure

17.42　Laparoscopic robotic assisted procedure
> Robotic assistance in laparoscopic procedure
> AHA: 3Q, '09, 5; 4Q, '08, 174

17.43　Percutaneous robotic assisted procedure
> Robotic assistance in percutaneous procedure

17.44　Endoscopic robotic assisted procedure
> Robotic assistance in endoscopic procedure

17.45　Thoracoscopic robotic assisted procedure
> Robotic assistance in thoracoscopic procedure

17.49　Other and unspecified robotic assisted procedure
> Robotic assistance in other and unspecified procedure
> EXCLUDES *endoscopic robotic assisted procedure (17.44)*
> *laparoscopic robotic assisted procedure (17.42)*
> *open robotic assisted procedure (17.41)*
> *percutaneous robotic assisted procedure (17.43)*
> *thoracoscopic robotic assisted procedure (17.45)*

✓4th 17.5　Additional cardiovascular procedures
> AHA: ▶3Q, '12, 13;◄4Q, '09, 139-140

17.51　Implantation of rechargeable cardiac contractility modulation [CCM], total system
> NOTE Device testing during procedure — *omit code*
> Implantation of CCM system includes formation of pocket, transvenous leads, including placement of leads, placement of catheter into left ventricle, intraoperative procedures for evaluation of lead signals, obtaining sensing threshold measurements, obtaining defibrillator threshold measurements.
> Includes implantation of device with removal of existing device
> Code also any concomitant:
> coronary bypass (36.10-36.19)
> extracorporeal circulation (39.61)
> insertion or replacement of automatic cardioverter/defibrillator, total system [AICD] 37.94
> EXCLUDES *implantation of CCM pulse generator only (17.52)*
> AHA: 4Q, '09, 141
> DEF: Device that delivers nonexcitatory impulses to the right ventricular septum during the absolute refractory period and signals that enhance myocardial strength and performance.

17.52　Implantation or replacement of cardiac contractility modulation [CCM] rechargeable pulse generator only
> NOTE Device testing during procedure — *omit code*
> Implantation of CCM device with removal of any existing CCM device
> Code also any concomitant:
> revision of device pocket (37.79)
> revision of lead [electrode] (37.75)

17.53　Percutaneous atherectomy of extracranial vessel(s)
> Directional atherectomy
> Excimer laser atherectomy
> Rotational atherectomy
> That by laser
> That by transluminal extraction
> Code also any:
> injection or infusion of thrombolytic agent (99.10)
> number of vascular stents inserted (00.45-00.48)
> number of vessels treated (00.40-00.43)
> percutaneous insertion of carotid artery stent(s) (00.63)
> percutaneous insertion of other extracranial artery stent(s) (00.64)
> procedure on vessel bifurcation (00.44)
> EXCLUDES *angioplasty of other non-coronary vessel(s) (39.50)*
> *atherectomy of intracranial vessel(s) (17.54)◄*
> *atherectomy of other non-coronary vessel(s) (17.56)*
> *removal of cerebrovascular obstruction of vessel(s) by open approach (38.01-38.02, 38.11-38.12, 38.31-38.32, 38.41-38.42)*
> AHA: 4Q, '11, 163-167
> TIP: This procedure may be performed instead of or in addition to angioplasty. If angioplasty is also performed, report it separately.

BI Bilateral Procedure　　NC Non-covered Procedure　　LC Limited Coverage Procedure　　▶◀ Revised Text　　● New Code　　▲ Revised Code Title

92 – Volume 3 • February 2013　　　　　　　　　　　　　　　　　　　　2014 ICD-9-CM

17.54 Percutaneous atherectomy of intracranial vessel(s)

Directional atherectomy   That by laser
Excimer laser atherectomy   That by transluminal
Rotational atherectomy   extraction

Code also any:
   injection or infusion of thrombolytic agent (99.10)
   number of vascular stents inserted (00.45-00.48)
   number of vessels treated (00.40-00.43)
   percutaneous insertion of intracranial vascular
      stent(s) (00.65)
   procedure on vessel bifurcation (00.44)

EXCLUDES *angioplasty of other non-coronary vessel(s) (39.50)*
    atherectomy of extracranial vessel(s) (17.53)
    atherectomy of other non-coronary vessel(s) (17.56)
    removal of cerebrovascular obstruction of
      vessel(s) by open approach
      (38.01-38.02, 38.11-38.12,
      38.31-38.32, 38.41-38.42)

AHA: 4Q, '11, 163-167
TIP: See tip under code 17.53

17.55 Transluminal coronary atherectomy

Directional atherectomy   That by percutaneous
Excimer laser atherectomy   approach
Rotational atherectomy   That by transluminal
That by laser   extraction

Code also any:
   injection or infusion of thrombolytic agent (99.10)
   insertion of coronary artery stent (36.06-36.07)
   intracoronary artery thrombolytic infusion (36.04)
   number of vascular stents inserted (00.45-00.48)
   number of vessels treated (00.40-00.43)
   procedure on vessel bifurcation (00.44)
   SuperSaturated oxygen therapy (00.49)
   transluminal coronary angioplasty (00.66)

AHA: 4Q, '11, 163-167
TIP: See tip under code 17.53

17.56 Atherectomy of other non-coronary vessel(s)

INCLUDES directional atherectomy
    excimer laser atherectomy
    rotational atherectomy
    that by laser
    that by transluminal extraction

Percutaneous transluminal angioplasty of:
   lower extremity vessels
   mesenteric artery
   renal artery
   upper extremity vessels

Code also any:
   injection or infusion of thrombolytic agent (99.10)
   insertion of drug-eluting peripheral vessel stent
      (00.55)
   insertion of non-drug-eluting peripheral vessel
      stent(s) or stent graft(s) (39.90)
   number of vascular stents inserted (00.45-00.48)
   number of vessels treated (00.40-00.43)
   procedure on vessel bifurcation (00.44)

EXCLUDES *percutaneous angioplasty of extracranial or*
    intracranial vessel(s) (00.61-00.62)
    percutaneous angioplasty of other
    non-coronary vessel(s) (39.50)
    percutaneous atherectomy of extracranial
    vessel(s) (17.53)
    percutaneous atherectomy of intracranial
    vessel(s) (17.54)

AHA: 4Q, '11, 163-167
TIP: See tip under code 17.53

Laser Interstitial Thermal Therapy

MRI-compatible laser probe
tumor
Radial laser thermal energy

✓4th 17.6 Laser interstitial thermal therapy [LITT] under guidance

Focused laser interstitial thermal therapy [f-LITT] under MRI
   guidance
MRI-guided LITT

AHA: 4Q, '09, 141-143
DEF: Selective, real-time thermal ablation of tumors using a laser
probe placed directly into the tumor.

17.61 Laser interstitial thermal therapy [LITT] of lesion or tissue of brain under guidance

Focused laser interstitial thermal therapy [f-LITT]
   under MRI guidance
MRI-guided LITT of lesion or tissue of brain

EXCLUDES *laser interstitial thermal therapy [LITT] of*
    lesion or tissue of head under guidance
    (17.62)

AHA: 4Q, '09, 143

17.62 Laser interstitial thermal therapy [LITT] of lesion or tissue of head and neck under guidance

Focused laser interstitial thermal therapy [f-LITT]
   under MRI guidance
MRI-guided LITT of lesion or tissue of head and neck

EXCLUDES *laser interstitial thermal therapy [LITT] of*
    lesion or tissue of brain under
    guidance (17.61)

17.63 Laser interstitial thermal therapy [LITT] of lesion or tissue of liver under guidance

Focused laser interstitial thermal therapy [f-LITT]
   under MRI guidance
MRI-guided LITT of lesion or tissue of liver

17.69 Laser interstitial thermal therapy [LITT] of lesion or tissue of other and unspecified site under guidance

Focused laser interstitial thermal therapy [f-LITT]
   under MRI guidance
MRI-guided LITT of lesion or tissue of breast
MRI-guided LITT of lesion or tissue of lung
MRI-guided LITT of lesion or tissue of prostate

EXCLUDES *laser interstitial thermal therapy [LITT] of*
    lesion or tissue of brain under
    guidance (17.61)
    laser interstitial thermal therapy [LITT] of
    lesion or tissue of head and neck under
    guidance (17.62)
    laser interstitial thermal therapy [LITT] of
    lesion or tissue of liver under guidance
    (17.63)

✓4th 17.7 Other diagnostic and therapeutic procedures

17.70 Intravenous infusion of clofarabine

EXCLUDES *injection or infusion of cancer*
    chemotherapeutic substance (99.25)

AHA: 4Q, '09, 144

17.71 Non-coronary intra-operative fluorescence vascular angiography [IFVA]

Intraoperative laser arteriogram
SPY arteriogram
SPY arteriography

EXCLUDES *intra-operative coronary fluorescence*
    vascular angiography (88.59)

AHA: 4Q, '10,114-115

✓4th 17.8 Other adjunct procedures

NOTE These codes are to be used in conjunction with other
therapeutic procedure codes to provide additional
information on devices used as part of a procedure.

17.81 Insertion of antimicrobial envelope

Use of anti-microbial (mesh) (prophylactic antibiotics
   embedded) envelope with the insertion of
   cardiovascular implantable electronic devices
   [CIED]

Code first primary procedure:
   insertion of cardiovascular implantable electronic
     device(s) [CIED] (00.51, 00.53, 00.54, 37.94,
     37.96, 37.98)

AHA: 4Q, '11, 167-168
TIP: The envelope holds the device and releases
antimicrobial agents to reduce postoperative infections.

4. Operations on the Ear (18-20)

√3ʳᵈ **18 Operations on external ear**
    INCLUDES operations on:
        external auditory canal
        skin and cartilage of:
           auricle
           meatus

√4ᵗʰ **18.0 Incision of external ear**
    EXCLUDES *removal of intraluminal foreign body (98.11)*

    18.01 Piercing of ear lobe
        Piercing of pinna

    18.02 Incision of external auditory canal

    18.09 Other incision of external ear

√4ᵗʰ **18.1 Diagnostic procedures on external ear**

    18.11 Otoscopy
        DEF: Exam of the ear with instrument designed for visualization.

    18.12 Biopsy of external ear

    18.19 Other diagnostic procedures on external ear
        EXCLUDES *microscopic examination of specimen from ear (90.31-90.39)*

√4ᵗʰ **18.2 Excision or destruction of lesion of external ear**

    18.21 Excision of preauricular sinus
        Radical excision of preauricular sinus or cyst
        EXCLUDES *excision of preauricular remnant [appendage] (18.29)*
        DEF: Excision of preauricular sinus or cyst with adjacent tissues.

    18.29 Excision or destruction of other lesion of external ear
        Cauterization
        Coagulation
        Cryosurgery   } of external ear
        Curettage
        Electrocoagulation
        Enucleation
        Excision of:
           exostosis of external auditory canal
           preauricular remnant [appendage]
        Partial excision of ear
        EXCLUDES *biopsy of external ear (18.12)*
                 radical excision of lesion (18.31)
                 removal of cerumen (96.52)

√4ᵗʰ **18.3 Other excision of external ear**
    EXCLUDES *biopsy of external ear (18.12)*

    18.31 Radical excision of lesion of external ear
        EXCLUDES *radical excision of preauricular sinus (18.21)*
        DEF: Removal of damaged, diseased ear and adjacent tissue.

    18.39 Other
        Amputation of external ear
        EXCLUDES *excision of lesion (18.21-18.29, 18.31)*

    18.4 Suture of laceration of external ear

    18.5 Surgical correction of prominent ear
        Ear: Ear:
          pinning   setback
        DEF: Reformation of protruding outer ear.

    18.6 Reconstruction of external auditory canal
        Canaloplasty of external auditory meatus
        Construction [reconstruction] of external meatus of ear:
          osseous portion
          skin-lined portion (with skin graft)
        DEF: Repair of outer ear canal.

√4ᵗʰ **18.7 Other plastic repair of external ear**

    18.71 Construction of auricle of ear ▲
        Prosthetic appliance for absent ear
        Reconstruction:
          auricle
          ear
        DEF: Reformation or repair of external ear flap.

    18.72 Reattachment of amputated ear

    18.79 Other plastic repair of external ear
        Otoplasty NOS
        Postauricular skin graft
        Repair of lop ear
        DEF: Postauricular skin graft: Graft repair behind ear.
        DEF: Repair of lop ear: Reconstruction of ear that is at right angle to head.
        AHA: 3Q, '03, 12

    18.9 Other operations on external ear
        EXCLUDES *Irrigation of ear (96.52)*
                packing of external auditory canal (96.11)
                removal of:
                   cerumen (96.52)
                   foreign body (without incision) (98.11)

√3ʳᵈ **19 Reconstructive operations on middle ear**

    19.0 Stapes mobilization
        Division, otosclerotic: Remobilization of stapes
          material   Stapediolysis
          process   Transcrural stapes mobilization
        EXCLUDES *that with synchronous stapedectomy (19.11-19.19)*
        DEF: Repair of innermost bone of middle ear to enable movement and response to sound.

√4ᵗʰ **19.1 Stapedectomy**
    EXCLUDES *revision of previous stapedectomy (19.21-19.29)*
                stapes mobilization only (19.0)
    DEF: Removal of innermost bone of middle ear.

    19.11 Stapedectomy with incus replacement
        Stapedectomy with incus:
          homograft
          prosthesis
        DEF: Removal of innermost bone of middle ear with autograft or prosthesis replacement.

    19.19 Other stapedectomy

√4ᵗʰ **19.2 Revision of stapedectomy**

    19.21 Revision of stapedectomy with incus replacement

    19.29 Other revision of stapedectomy

    19.3 Other operations on ossicular chain
        Incudectomy NOS
        Ossiculectomy NOS
        Reconstruction of ossicles, second stage
        DEF: Incudectomy: Excision of middle bone of middle ear, not otherwise specified.
        DEF: Ossiculectomy: Excision of middle ear bones, not otherwise specified.
        DEF: Reconstruction of ossicles, second stage: Repair of middle ear bones following previous surgery.

Stapedectomy with Incus Replacement

Incus — Stapes with footplate in oval window — Malleus — Handle of malleus — Tympanic membrane — Cochlea — Wire piston — Tissue seal on oval window

▪ Area excised

BI Bilateral Procedure   NC Non-covered Procedure   LC Limited Coverage Procedure   ▶◀ Revised Text   ● New Code   ▲ Revised Code Title

94 – Volume 3   2014 ICD-9-CM

19.4 Myringoplasty

Epitympanic, type I

Myringoplasty by:
  cauterization
  graft

Tympanoplasty (type I)

DEF: Epitympanic, type I: Repair over or upon eardrum.

DEF: Myringoplasty by cauterization: Plastic repair of tympanic membrane of eardrum by heat.

DEF: Graft: Plastic repair using implanted tissue.

DEF: Tympanoplasty (type I): Reconstruction of eardrum to restore hearing.

✓4ᵗʰ 19.5 Other tympanoplasty

19.52 Type II tympanoplasty

Closure of perforation with graft against incus or malleus

19.53 Type III tympanoplasty

Graft placed in contact with mobile and intact stapes

AHA: M-A, '85, 15

TIP: Assign for a total ossicular replacement prosthesis (TORP) procedure.

19.54 Type IV tympanoplasty

Mobile footplate left exposed with air pocket between round window and graft

19.55 Type V tympanoplasty

Fenestra in horizontal semicircular canal covered by graft

19.6 Revision of tympanoplasty

DEF: Repair or correction of previous plastic surgery on eardrum.

19.9 Other repair of middle ear

Closure of mastoid fistula

Mastoid myoplasty

Obliteration of tympanomastoid cavity

DEF: Closure of mastoid fistula: Closing of abnormal channel in mastoid.

DEF: Mastoid myoplasty: Restoration or repair of mastoid muscle.

DEF: Obliteration of tympanomastoid cavity: Removal, total, of functional elements of middle ear.

✓3ʳᵈ 20 Other operations on middle and inner ear

✓4ᵗʰ 20.0 Myringotomy

DEF: Myringotomy: Puncture of tympanic membrane or eardrum, also called tympanocentesis

20.01 Myringotomy with insertion of tube

Myringostomy

20.09 Other myringotomy

Aspiration of middle ear NOS

20.1 Removal of tympanostomy tube

✓4ᵗʰ 20.2 Incision of mastoid and middle ear

20.21 Incision of mastoid

20.22 Incision of petrous pyramid air cells

20.23 Incision of middle ear

Atticotomy

Division of tympanum

Lysis of adhesions of middle ear

EXCLUDES division of otosclerotic process (19.0)
    stapediolysis (19.0)
    that with stapedectomy (19.11-19.19)

✓4ᵗʰ 20.3 Diagnostic procedures on middle and inner ear

20.31 Electrocochleography

DEF: Measure of electric potential of eighth cranial nerve by electrode applied sound.

20.32 Biopsy of middle and inner ear

20.39 Other diagnostic procedures on middle and inner ear

EXCLUDES auditory and vestibular function tests (89.13, 95.41-95.49)
    microscopic examination of specimen from ear (90.31-90.39)

✓4ᵗʰ 20.4 Mastoidectomy

Code also any:
  skin graft (18.79)
  tympanoplasty (19.4-19.55)

EXCLUDES that with implantation of cochlear prosthetic device (20.96-20.98)

DEF: Mastoidectomy: Excision of bony protrusion behind ear.

20.41 Simple mastoidectomy

20.42 Radical mastoidectomy

20.49 Other mastoidectomy

Atticoantrostomy

Mastoidectomy:
  NOS
  modified radical

DEF: Atticoantrotomy: Opening of cavity of mastoid bone and middle ear.

✓4ᵗʰ 20.5 Other excision of middle ear

EXCLUDES that with synchronous mastoidectomy (20.41-20.49)

20.51 Excision of lesion of middle ear

EXCLUDES biopsy of middle ear (20.32)

20.59 Other

Apicectomy of petrous pyramid

Tympanectomy

✓4ᵗʰ 20.6 Fenestration of inner ear

20.61 Fenestration of inner ear (initial)

Fenestration of:
  labyrinth
  semicircular canals   } with graft (skin)
  vestibule   (vein)

EXCLUDES that with tympanoplasty, type V (19.55)

DEF: Creation of inner ear opening.

20.62 Revision of fenestration of inner ear

✓4ᵗʰ 20.7 Incision, excision, and destruction of inner ear

20.71 Endolymphatic shunt

DEF: Insertion of tube to drain fluid in inner ear cavities.

20.72 Injection into inner ear

Destruction by injection (alcohol):
  inner ear
  semicircular canals
  vestibule

20.79 Other incision, excision, and destruction of inner ear

Decompression of labyrinth

Drainage of inner ear

Fistulization:
  endolymphatic sac
  labyrinth

Incision of endolymphatic sac

Labyrinthectomy (transtympanic)

Opening of bony labyrinth

Perilymphatic tap

EXCLUDES biopsy of inner ear (20.32)

DEF: Decompression of labyrinth: Controlled relief of pressure in cavities of inner ear.

DEF: Drainage of inner ear: Removal of fluid from inner ear.

DEF: Fistulization of endolymphatic sac: Creation of passage to fluid sac in inner ear cavities.

DEF: Fistulization of labyrinth: Creation of passage to inner ear cavities.

DEF: Incision of endolymphatic sac: Cutting into fluid sac in inner ear cavities.

DEF: Labyrinthectomy (transtympanic): Excision of cavities across eardrum.

DEF: Opening of bony labyrinth: Cutting into inner ear bony cavities.

DEF: Perilymphatic tap: Puncture or incision into fluid sac of inner ear cavities.

20.8   Operations on Eustachian tube

Catheterization
Inflation
Injection (Teflon paste)
Insufflation (boric
     acid-salicylic acid) } of Eustachian tube
Intubation
Politzerization

DEF: Catheterization: Passing catheter into passage between pharynx and middle ear.
DEF: Inflation: Blowing air, gas or liquid into passage between pharynx and middle ear to inflate.
DEF: Injection (Teflon paste): Forcing fluid (Teflon paste) into passage between pharynx and middle ear.
DEF: Insufflation (boric acid-salicylic acid): Blowing gas or liquid into passage between pharynx and middle ear.
DEF: Intubation: Placing tube into passage between pharynx and middle ear.
DEF: Politzerization: Inflating passage between pharynx and middle ear with Politzer bag.

√4ᵗʰ   20.9   Other operations on inner and middle ear

⁎20.91   Tympanosympathectomy

DEF: Excision or chemical suppression of impulses of middle ear nerves.

20.92   Revision of mastoidectomy

AHA: 2Q, '98, 20

DEF: Correction of previous removal of mastoid cells from temporal or mastoid bone.

20.93   Repair of oval and round windows

Closure of fistula:
    oval window
    perilymph
    round window

DEF: Restoration of middle ear openings.

20.94   Injection of tympanum

20.95   Implantation of electromagnetic hearing device

Bone conduction hearing device
EXCLUDES *cochlear prosthetic device (20.96-20.98)*
AHA: 3Q, '07, 4; 4Q, '89, 5

20.96   Implantation or replacement of cochlear prosthetic device, not otherwise specified

Implantation of receiver (within skull) and insertion of electrode(s) in the cochlea
INCLUDES mastoidectomy
EXCLUDES *electromagnetic hearing device (20.95)*
AHA: 4Q, '89, 5

20.97   Implantation or replacement of cochlear prosthetic device, single channel

Implantation of receiver (within skull) and insertion of electrode in the cochlea
INCLUDES mastoidectomy
EXCLUDES *electromagnetic hearing device (20.95)*
AHA: 4Q, '89, 5

20.98   Implantation or replacement of cochlear prosthetic device, multiple channel

Implantation of receiver (within skull) and insertion of electrodes in the cochlea
INCLUDES mastoidectomy
EXCLUDES *electromagnetic hearing device (20.95)*
AHA: 4Q, '89, 5

20.99   Other operations on middle and inner ear

Attachment of percutaneous abutment (screw) for prosthetic device
Repair or removal of cochlear prosthetic device (receiver) (electrode)
EXCLUDES *adjustment (external components) of cochlear prosthetic device (95.49)*
           fitting of hearing aid (95.48)
AHA: 3Q, '07, 4; 4Q, '89, 7

BI Bilateral Procedure   **NC** Non-covered Procedure   **LC** Limited Coverage Procedure   ►◄ Revised Text   ● New Code   ▲ Revised Code Title

96 – Volume 3   2014 ICD-9-C

5. Operations on the Nose, Mouth, and Pharynx (21-29)

☑3ʳᵈ **21 Operations on nose**

INCLUDES operations on:
bone ⎫
skin ⎭ of nose

AHA: 1Q, '94, 5

☑4ᵗʰ **21.0 Control of epistaxis**

21.00 Control of epistaxis, not otherwise specified

21.01 Control of epistaxis by anterior nasal packing

21.02 Control of epistaxis by posterior (and anterior) packing

21.03 Control of epistaxis by cauterization (and packing)

21.04 Control of epistaxis by ligation of ethmoidal arteries

21.05 Control of epistaxis by (transantral) ligation of the maxillary artery

21.06 Control of epistaxis by ligation of the external carotid artery

21.07 Control of epistaxis by excision of nasal mucosa and skin grafting of septum and lateral nasal wall

21.09 Control of epistaxis by other means

21.1 Incision of nose

Chondrotomy
Incision of skin of nose
Nasal septotomy
DEF: Chondrotomy: Incision or division of nasal cartilage.
DEF: Nasal septotomy: Incision into bone dividing nose into two chambers.

☑4ᵗʰ **21.2 Diagnostic procedures on nose**

21.21 Rhinoscopy
DEF: Visualization of nasal passage with nasal speculum.

21.22 Biopsy of nose

21.29 Other diagnostic procedures on nose
EXCLUDES microscopic examination of specimen from nose (90.31-90.39)
nasal:
function study (89.12)
x-ray (87.16)
rhinomanometry (89.12)

☑4ᵗʰ **21.3 Local excision or destruction of lesion of nose**
EXCLUDES biopsy of nose (21.22)
nasal fistulectomy (21.82)

21.30 Excision or destruction of lesion of nose, not otherwise specified

21.31 Local excision or destruction of intranasal lesion
Nasal polypectomy

21.32 Local excision or destruction of other lesion of nose
AHA: 2Q, '89, 16

21.4 Resection of nose
Amputation of nose

21.5 Submucous resection of nasal septum
DEF: Partial resection of nasal septum with mucosa reimplanted after excision.

☑4ᵗʰ **21.6 Turbinectomy**
DEF: Partial or total removal of turbinate bones; inferior turbinate is most often excised.

21.61 Turbinectomy by diathermy or cryosurgery
DEF: Destruction of turbinate bone by heat or freezing.

21.62 Fracture of the turbinates
DEF: Surgical breaking of turbinate bones.

21.69 Other turbinectomy
EXCLUDES turbinectomy associated with sinusectomy (22.31-22.39, 22.42, 22.60-22.64)

Excision of Turbinate

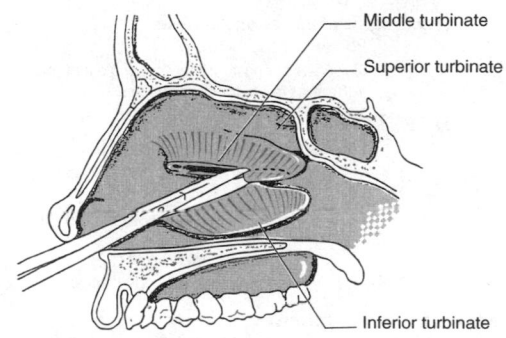
- Middle turbinate
- Superior turbinate
- Inferior turbinate

☑4ᵗʰ **21.7 Reduction of nasal fracture**

21.71 Closed reduction of nasal fracture

21.72 Open reduction of nasal fracture

☑4ᵗʰ **21.8 Repair and plastic operations on the nose**

21.81 Suture of laceration of nose

21.82 Closure of nasal fistula
Nasolabial ⎫
Nasopharyngeal ⎬ fistulectomy
Oronasal ⎭
DEF: Sealing off crack or hole between nose and lip, nose and pharynx, or nose and mouth.

21.83 Total nasal reconstruction
Reconstruction of nose with:
arm flap
forehead flap
DEF: Plastic reformation of nasal structure with tissue flap from arm or forehead.

21.84 Revision rhinoplasty
Rhinoseptoplasty
Twisted nose rhinoplasty
DEF: Rhinoseptoplasty: Repair of nose and the bone dividing the nose into two chambers.
DEF: Twisted nose rhinoplasty: Repair of nose alignment following reconstructive surgery.

21.85 Augmentation rhinoplasty
Augmentation rhinoplasty with:
graft
synthetic implant
DEF: Implant of tissue or synthetic graft to enlarge nose.

21.86 Limited rhinoplasty
Plastic repair of nasolabial flaps
Tip rhinoplasty
DEF: Plastic repair of nasolabial flaps: Reconstruction of nasal area above lips.
DEF: Tip rhinoplasty: Reconstruction or restoration of nasal tip.

21.87 Other rhinoplasty
Rhinoplasty NOS

21.88 Other septoplasty
Crushing of nasal septum
Repair of septal perforation
EXCLUDES septoplasty associated with submucous resection of septum (21.5)
DEF: Crushing of nasal septum: Division and reconstruction of defects in bone dividing nasal chambers.
DEF: Repair of septal perforation: Repair of hole in bone dividing nasal chambers with adjacent tissue.

21.89 Other repair and plastic operations on nose
Reattachment of amputated nose

Operations on the Nose, Mouth, and Pharynx

21.9–24.2

√4ᵗʰ **21.9 Other operations on nose**

21.91 Lysis of adhesions of nose
Posterior nasal scrub
DEF: Posterior nasal scrub: Clearing out of abnormal
adhesions in posterior nasal area.

21.99 Other
EXCLUDES *dilation of frontonasal duct (96.21)*
irrigation of nasal passages (96.53)
removal of:
intraluminal foreign body without incision
(98.12)
nasal packing (97.32)
replacement of nasal packing (97.21)

√3ʳᵈ **22 Operations on nasal sinuses**

√4ᵗʰ **22.0 Aspiration and lavage of nasal sinus**

**22.00 Aspiration and lavage of nasal sinus, not otherwise
specified**

22.01 Puncture of nasal sinus for aspiration or lavage

**22.02 Aspiration or lavage of nasal sinus through natural
ostium**
DEF: Withdrawal of fluid and washing of nasal cavity
through natural opening.

√4ᵗʰ **22.1 Diagnostic procedures on nasal sinus**

22.11 Closed [endoscopic] [needle] biopsy of nasal sinus

22.12 Open biopsy of nasal sinus

22.19 Other diagnostic procedures on nasal sinuses
Endoscopy without biopsy
EXCLUDES *transillumination of sinus (89.35)*
x-ray of sinus (87.15-87.16)

22.2 Intranasal antrotomy
EXCLUDES *antrotomy with external approach (22.31-22.39)*
DEF: Incision of intranasal sinus.

√4ᵗʰ **22.3 External maxillary antrotomy**

22.31 Radical maxillary antrotomy
Removal of lining membrane of maxillary sinus using
Caldwell-Luc approach
DEF: Caldwell-Luc approach: Removal of membrane lining
the maxillary cavity through incision above canine teeth.

22.39 Other external maxillary antrotomy
Exploration of maxillary antrum with Caldwell-Luc
approach

√4ᵗʰ **22.4 Frontal sinusotomy and sinusectomy**

22.41 Frontal sinusotomy

22.42 Frontal sinusectomy
Excision of lesion of frontal sinus
Obliteration of frontal sinus (with fat)
EXCLUDES *biopsy of nasal sinus (22.11-22.12)*

√4ᵗʰ **22.5 Other nasal sinusotomy**

22.50 Sinusotomy, not otherwise specified

22.51 Ethmoidotomy

22.52 Sphenoidotomy

22.53 Incision of multiple nasal sinuses

√4ᵗʰ **22.6 Other nasal sinusectomy**
INCLUDES that with incidental turbinectomy
EXCLUDES *biopsy of nasal sinus (22.11-22.12)*

22.60 Sinusectomy, not otherwise specified

**22.61 Excision of lesion of maxillary sinus with
Caldwell-Luc approach**

**22.62 Excision of lesion of maxillary sinus with
other approach**

22.63 Ethmoidectomy
DEF: Removal of ethmoid cells and bone; includes excising
partial or total mucosal lining.

22.64 Sphenoidectomy
DEF: Removal of wedge shaped sphenoid bone at base of
brain.

√4ᵗʰ **22.7 Repair of nasal sinus**

22.71 Closure of nasal sinus fistula
Repair of oro-antral fistula

22.79 Other repair of nasal sinus
Reconstruction of frontonasal duct
Repair of bone of accessory sinus

22.9 Other operations on nasal sinuses
Exteriorization of maxillary sinus
Fistulization of sinus
EXCLUDES *dilation of frontonasal duct (96.21)*
DEF: Exteriorization of maxillary sinus: Creation of external maxillary
cavity opening.
DEF: Fistulization of sinus: Creation of fistula canal in nasal cavity.

√3ʳᵈ **23 Removal and restoration of teeth**

√4ᵗʰ **23.0 Forceps extraction of tooth**

23.01 Extraction of deciduous tooth

23.09 Extraction of other tooth
Extraction of tooth NOS

√4ᵗʰ **23.1 Surgical removal of tooth**

23.11 Removal of residual root

23.19 Other surgical extraction of tooth
Odontectomy NOS
Removal of impacted tooth
Tooth extraction with elevation of mucoperiosteal
flap

23.2 Restoration of tooth by filling

23.3 Restoration of tooth by inlay
DEF: Restoration of tooth by cementing in a molded filling.

√4ᵗʰ **23.4 Other dental restoration**

23.41 Application of crown

23.42 Insertion of fixed bridge

23.43 Insertion of removable bridge

23.49 Other

23.5 Implantation of tooth
DEF: Insertion of a sound tooth to replace extracted tooth.

23.6 Prosthetic dental implant
Endosseous dental implant
DEF: Implant of artificial denture within bone covering tooth socket

√4ᵗʰ **23.7 Apicoectomy and root canal therapy**

23.70 Root canal, not otherwise specified

23.71 Root canal therapy with irrigation

23.72 Root canal therapy with apicoectomy
DEF: Removal of tooth root to treat damaged root canal
tissue.

23.73 Apicoectomy

√3ʳᵈ **24 Other operations on teeth, gums, and alveoli**

24.0 Incision of gum or alveolar bone
Apical alveolotomy

√4ᵗʰ **24.1 Diagnostic procedures on teeth, gums, and alveoli**

24.11 Biopsy of gum

24.12 Biopsy of alveolus

**24.19 Other diagnostic procedures on teeth, gums, and
alveoli**
EXCLUDES *dental:*
examination (89.31)
x-ray:
full-mouth (87.11)
other (87.12)
microscopic examination of dental specimen
(90.81-90.89)

24.2 Gingivoplasty
Gingivoplasty with bone or soft tissue graft
DEF: Repair of gum tissue.

B1 Bilateral Procedure   NC Non-covered Procedure   LC Limited Coverage Procedure   ▶◀ Revised Text   ● New Code   ▲ Revised Code Title

✓4ᵗʰ **24.3   Other operations on gum**

    24.31   Excision of lesion or tissue of gum
        EXCLUDES   *biopsy of gum (24.11)*
                   excision of odontogenic lesion (24.4)

    24.32   Suture of laceration of gum

    24.39   Other

24.4   Excision of dental lesion of jaw
    Excision of odontogenic lesion

24.5   Alveoloplasty
    Alveolectomy (interradicular) (intraseptal) (radical) (simple)
       (with graft or implant)
    EXCLUDES   *biopsy of alveolus (24.12)*
               en bloc resection of alveolar process and palate
                  (27.32)
    DEF: Repair or correction of bony tooth socket.

24.6   Exposure of tooth

24.7   Application of orthodontic appliance
    Application, insertion, or fitting of:
       arch bars
       orthodontic obturator
       orthodontic wiring
       periodontal splint
    EXCLUDES   *nonorthodontic dental wiring (93.55)*

24.8   Other orthodontic operation
    Closure of diastema (alveolar) (dental)
    Occlusal adjustment
    Removal of arch bars
    Repair of dental arch
    EXCLUDES   *removal of nonorthodontic wiring (97.33)*

✓4ᵗʰ **24.9   Other dental operations**

    24.91   Extension or deepening of buccolabial or lingual sulcus

    24.99   Other
        EXCLUDES   *dental:*
                 debridement (96.54)
                 examination (89.31)
                 prophylaxis (96.54)
                 scaling and polishing (96.54)
                 wiring (93.55)
            fitting of dental appliance [denture] (99.97)
            microscopic examination of dental specimen
                 (90.81-90.89)
            removal of dental:
                 packing (97.34)
                 prosthesis (97.35)
                 wiring (97.33)
             replacement of dental packing (97.22)

✓3ʳᵈ **25   Operations on tongue**

✓4ᵗʰ **25.0   Diagnostic procedures on tongue**

    25.01   Closed [needle] biopsy of tongue

    25.02   Open biopsy of tongue
        Wedge biopsy

    25.09   Other diagnostic procedures on tongue

25.1   Excision or destruction of lesion or tissue of tongue
    EXCLUDES   *biopsy of tongue (25.01-25.02)*
               frenumectomy:
                 labial (27.41)
                 lingual (25.92)
    AHA: 2Q, '02, 5
    TIP: Assign for tongue-based somnoplasty procedure, a tempera-ture-controlled radiofrequency-based technology, used for treat-ment of obstructive sleep apnea.

25.2   Partial glossectomy

25.3   Complete glossectomy
    Glossectomy NOS
    Code also any neck dissection (40.40-40.42)

25.4   Radical glossectomy
    Code also any:
       neck dissection (40.40-40.42)
       tracheostomy (31.1-31.29)

✓4ᵗʰ **25.5   Repair of tongue and glossoplasty**

    25.51   Suture of laceration of tongue

    25.59   Other repair and plastic operations on tongue
        Fascial sling of tongue
        Fusion of tongue (to lip)
        Graft of mucosa or skin to tongue
        EXCLUDES   *lysis of adhesions of tongue (25.93)*
        AHA: 1Q, '97, 5
        TIP: Assign for genioglossus advancement, which may be performed in association with uvulopalatopharyngoplasty (UPPP).

✓4ᵗʰ **25.9   Other operations on tongue**

    25.91   Lingual frenotomy
        EXCLUDES   *labial frenotomy (27.91)*
        DEF: Extension of groove between cheek and lips or cheek and tongue.

    25.92   Lingual frenectomy
        EXCLUDES   *labial frenectomy (27.41)*
        DEF: Frenectomy: Removal of vertical membrane attaching tongue to floor of mouth.

    25.93   Lysis of adhesions of tongue

    25.94   Other glossotomy

    25.99   Other

✓3ʳᵈ **26   Operations on salivary glands and ducts**
    INCLUDES   operations on:
          lesser salivary
          parotid   } gland and duct
          sublingual
          submaxillry
    Code also any neck dissection (40.40-40.42)

    26.0   Incision of salivary gland or duct

✓4ᵗʰ **26.1   Diagnostic procedures on salivary glands and ducts**

    26.11   Closed [needle] biopsy of salivary gland or duct

    26.12   Open biopsy of salivary gland or duct

    26.19   Other diagnostic procedures on salivary glands and ducts
        EXCLUDES   *x-ray of salivary gland (87.09)*

✓4ᵗʰ **26.2   Excision of lesion of salivary gland**

    26.21   Marsupialization of salivary gland cyst
        DEF: Creation of pouch of salivary gland cyst to drain and promote healing.

    26.29   Other excision of salivary gland lesion
        EXCLUDES   *biopsy of salivary gland (26.11-26.12)*
               salivary fistulectomy (26.42)

✓4ᵗʰ **26.3   Sialoadenectomy**
    DEF: Removal of salivary gland.

    26.30   Sialoadenectomy, not otherwise specified

    26.31   Partial sialoadenectomy

    26.32   Complete sialoadenectomy
        En bloc excision of salivary gland lesion
        Radical sialoadenectomy

✓4ᵗʰ **26.4   Repair of salivary gland or duct**

    26.41   Suture of laceration of salivary gland

    26.42   Closure of salivary fistula
        DEF: Closing of abnormal opening in salivary gland.

    26.49   Other repair and plastic operations on salivary gland or duct
        Fistulization of salivary gland
        Plastic repair of salivary gland or duct NOS
        Transplantation of salivary duct opening

✓4ᵗʰ **26.9   Other operations on salivary gland or duct**

    26.91   Probing of salivary duct

    26.99   Other

☑3ʳᵈ **27 Other operations on mouth and face**

INCLUDES operations on:
lips
palate
soft tissue of face and mouth, except tongue and
gingiva
EXCLUDES operations on:
gingiva (24.0-24.99)
tongue (25.01-25.99)

27.0 Drainage of face and floor of mouth

Drainage of:
facial region (abscess)
fascial compartment of face
Ludwig's angina
EXCLUDES *drainage of thyroglossal tract (06.09)*

27.1 Incision of palate

☑4ᵗʰ **27.2 Diagnostic procedures on oral cavity**

27.21 Biopsy of bony palate

27.22 Biopsy of uvula and soft palate

27.23 Biopsy of lip

27.24 Biopsy of mouth, unspecified structure

27.29 Other diagnostic procedures on oral cavity
EXCLUDES *soft tissue x-ray (87.09)*

☑4ᵗʰ **27.3 Excision of lesion or tissue of bony palate**

**27.31 Local excision or destruction of lesion or
tissue of bony palate**

Local excision or destruction of palate by:
cautery
chemotherapy
cryotherapy
EXCLUDES *biopsy of bony palate (27.21)*

**27.32 Wide excision or destruction of lesion or
tissue of bony palate**

En bloc resection of alveolar process and palate

☑4ᵗʰ **27.4 Excision of other parts of mouth**

27.41 Labial frenectomy
EXCLUDES *division of labial frenum (27.91)*
DEF: Removal of mucous membrane fold of lip.

27.42 Wide excision of lesion of lip

27.43 Other excision of lesion or tissue of lip

27.49 Other excision of mouth
EXCLUDES *biopsy of mouth NOS (27.24)*
excision of lesion of:
palate (27.31-27.32)
tongue (25.1)
uvula (27.72)
fistulectomy of mouth (27.53)
frenectomy of:
lip (27.41)
tongue (25.92)
AHA: 2Q, '05, 8
TIP: Assign for "composite resection," which includes the
mandible and floor of the mouth, performed for
mandibular carcinoma. Codes for bone and lymph node
resection should also be assigned.

☑4ᵗʰ **27.5 Plastic repair of lip and mouth**
EXCLUDES *palatoplasty (27.61-27.69)*

27.51 Suture of laceration of lip

27.52 Suture of laceration of other part of mouth

27.53 Closure of fistula of mouth
EXCLUDES *fistulectomy:*
nasolabial (21.82)
oro-antral (22.71)
oronasal (21.82)

27.54 Repair of cleft lip

27.55 Full-thickness skin graft to lip and mouth

27.56 Other skin graft to lip and mouth

**27.57 Attachment of pedicle or flap graft to
lip and mouth**
AHA: 1Q, '96, 14
DEF: Repair of lip or mouth with tissue pedicle or flap still
connected to original vascular base.

27.59 Other plastic repair of mouth

☑4ᵗʰ **27.6 Palatoplasty**

27.61 Suture of laceration of palate

27.62 Correction of cleft palate
Correction of cleft palate by push-back operation
EXCLUDES *revision of cleft palate repair (27.63)*

27.63 Revision of cleft palate repair
Secondary:
attachment of pharyngeal flap
lengthening of palate
AHA: 1Q, '96, 14

27.64 Insertion of palatal implant
DEF: Nonabsorbable polyester implants placed into the soft
palate at the back of the roof of the mouth; one implant
placed at the soft palate midline and two are positioned on
either side; used to support and stiffen the palate, reducing
vibration (snoring).

27.69 Other plastic repair of palate
Code also any insertion of palatal implant (27.64)
EXCLUDES *fistulectomy of mouth (27.53)*
AHA: 3Q, '99, 22; 1Q, '97, 14; 3Q, '92, 18
TIP: Assign for uvulopalatopharyngoplasty (UPPP), along
with code 29.4 Plastic operation on pharynx, along with
additional codes for hyoid suspension and genioglossus
advancement, if performed.

☑4ᵗʰ **27.7 Operations on uvula**

27.71 Incision of uvula

27.72 Excision of uvula
EXCLUDES *biopsy of uvula (27.22)*

27.73 Repair of uvula
EXCLUDES *that with synchronous cleft palate repair
(27.62)*
uranostaphylorrhaphy (27.62)

27.79 Other operations on uvula
AHA: 3Q, '92, 18

☑4ᵗʰ **27.9 Other operations on mouth and face**

27.91 Labial frenotomy
Division of labial frenum
EXCLUDES *lingual frenotomy (25.91)*
DEF: Division of labial frenum: Cutting and separating
mucous membrane fold of lip.

27.92 Incision of mouth, unspecified structure
EXCLUDES *incision of:*
gum (24.0)
palate (27.1)
salivary gland or duct (26.0)
tongue (25.94)
uvula (27.71)

27.99 Other operations on oral cavity
Graft of buccal sulcus
EXCLUDES *removal of:*
intraluminal foreign body (98.01)
*penetrating foreign body from mouth
without incision (98.22)*
DEF: Graft of buccal sulcus: Implant of tissue into groove of
interior cheek lining.

☑3ʳᵈ **28 Operations on tonsils and adenoids**

**28.0 Incision and drainage of tonsil and
peritonsillar structures**

Drainage (oral) (transcervical) of:
parapharyngeal
peritonsillar ⎫
retropharyngeal ⎬ abscess
tonsillar ⎭

BI Bilateral Procedure   NC Non-covered Procedure   LC Limited Coverage Procedure   ▶◀ Revised Text   ● New Code   ▲ Revised Code Title

100 — Volume 3   **2014 ICD-9-CM**

☑4th 28.1 Diagnostic procedures on tonsils and adenoids

    28.11 Biopsy of tonsils and adenoids

    28.19 Other diagnostic procedures on tonsils and adenoids

        EXCLUDES *soft tissue x-ray (87.09)*

28.2 Tonsillectomy without adenoidectomy

    AHA: 1Q, '97, 5; 2Q, '90, 23

28.3 Tonsillectomy with adenoidectomy

    AHA: 2Q, '05, 16

28.4 Excision of tonsil tag

28.5 Excision of lingual tonsil

28.6 Adenoidectomy without tonsillectomy

    Excision of adenoid tag

28.7 Control of hemorrhage after tonsillectomy and adenoidectomy

    AHA: 2Q, '05, 16

☑4th 28.9 Other operations on tonsils and adenoids

    28.91 Removal of foreign body from tonsil and adenoid by incision

        EXCLUDES *that without incision (98.13)*

    28.92 Excision of lesion of tonsil and adenoid

        EXCLUDES *biopsy of tonsil and adenoid (28.11)*

    28.99 Other

☑3rd 29 Operations on pharynx

    INCLUDES operations on:
        hypopharynx
        nasopharynx
        oropharynx
        pharyngeal pouch
        pyriform sinus

29.0 Pharyngotomy

    Drainage of pharyngeal bursa

    EXCLUDES *incision and drainage of retropharyngeal abscess (28.0)*
          removal of foreign body (without incision) (98.13)

☑4th 29.1 Diagnostic procedures on pharynx

    29.11 Pharyngoscopy

    29.12 Pharyngeal biopsy

        Biopsy of supraglottic mass

    29.19 Other diagnostic procedures on pharynx

        EXCLUDES *x-ray of nasopharynx:*
            contrast (87.06)
            other (87.09)

29.2 Excision of branchial cleft cyst or vestige

    EXCLUDES *branchial cleft fistulectomy (29.52)*

☑4th 29.3 Excision or destruction of lesion or tissue of pharynx

    AHA: 2Q, '89, 18

    29.31 Cricopharyngeal myotomy

        EXCLUDES *that with pharyngeal diverticulectomy (29.32)*

        DEF: Removal of outward pouching of throat.

    29.32 Pharyngeal diverticulectomy

    29.33 Pharyngectomy (partial)

        EXCLUDES *laryngopharyngectomy (30.3)*

    29.39 Other excision or destruction of lesion or tissue of pharynx

29.4 Plastic operation on pharynx

    Correction of nasopharyngeal atresia

    EXCLUDES *pharyngoplasty associated with cleft palate repair (27.62-27.63)*

    AHA: 3Q, '99, 22; 1Q, '97, 5; 3Q, '92, 18

    DEF: Correction of nasopharyngeal atresia: Construction of normal opening for throat stricture behind nose.

    TIP: Assign for uvulopalatopharyngoplasty (UPPP), secondary to code 27.69 Other plastic repair of the palate. Report additional codes for hyoid suspension and genioglossus advancement, if performed.

☑4th 29.5 Other repair of pharynx

    29.51 Suture of laceration of pharynx

    29.52 Closure of branchial cleft fistula

        DEF: Sealing off an abnormal opening of the branchial fissure in throat.

    29.53 Closure of other fistula of pharynx

        Pharyngoesophageal fistulectomy

    29.54 Lysis of pharyngeal adhesions

    29.59 Other

        AHA: 2Q, '89, 18

☑4th 29.9 Other operations on pharynx

    29.91 Dilation of pharynx

        Dilation of nasopharynx

    29.92 Division of glossopharyngeal nerve

    29.99 Other

        EXCLUDES *insertion of radium into pharynx and nasopharynx (92.27)*
            removal of intraluminal foreign body (98.13)

Operations on the Respiratory System

30–31.74

6. Operations on the Respiratory System (30-34)

√3ʳᵈ **30   Excision of larynx**

√4ᵗʰ   **30.0   Excision or destruction of lesion or tissue of larynx**

     30.01   Marsupialization of laryngeal cyst

       DEF: Incision of cyst of larynx with the edges sutured open to create pouch.

     30.09   Other excision or destruction of lesion or lesion or tissue of larynx

       Stripping of vocal cords

       EXCLUDES   biopsy of larynx (31.43)

                laryngeal fistulectomy (31.62)

                laryngotracheal fistulectomy (31.62)

   30.1   Hemilaryngectomy

       DEF: Excision of one side (half) of larynx.

√4ᵗʰ   **30.2   Other partial laryngectomy**

     30.21   Epiglottidectomy

     30.22   Vocal cordectomy

       Excision of vocal cords

     30.29   Other partial laryngectomy

       Excision of laryngeal cartilage

   30.3   Complete laryngectomy

       Block dissection of larynx (with thyroidectomy) (with synchronous tracheostomy)

       Laryngopharyngectomy

       EXCLUDES   that with radical neck dissection (30.4)

       AHA: 1Q, '12, 9

   30.4   Radical laryngectomy

       Complete [total] laryngectomy with radical neck dissection (with thyroidectomy) (with synchronous tracheostomy)

√3ʳᵈ **31   Other operations on larynx and trachea**

   31.0   Injection of larynx

       Injection of inert material into larynx or vocal cords

   31.1   Temporary tracheostomy

       Temporary percutaneous dilatational tracheostomy [PDT]

       Tracheotomy for assistance in breathing

       Code also any synchronous bronchoscopy, if performed (33.21-33.24, 33.27)

       AHA: 1Q, '97, 6

       TIP: Assign for a procedure described as a mini-tracheostomy.

√4ᵗʰ   **31.2   Permanent tracheostomy**

     31.21   Mediastinal tracheostomy

       DEF: Placement of artificial breathing tube in windpipe through mediastinum, for long-term use.

     31.29   Other permanent tracheostomy

       Permanent percutaneous dilatational tracheostomy [PDT]

       Code also any synchronous bronchoscopy, if performed (33.21-33.24, 33.27)

       EXCLUDES   that with laryngectomy (30.3-30.4)

       AHA: ►4Q, '12, 84;◄ 2Q, '05, 8; 2Q, '02, 6

   31.3   Other incision of larynx or trachea

       EXCLUDES   that for assistance in breathing (31.1-31.29)

Temporary Tracheostomy

Trachea

Tracheostomy tube

In place

Closed Endoscopic Biopsy of Larynx

Laryngoscope

Palate

Trachea

Growth on vocal cord

√4ᵗʰ   **31.4   Diagnostic procedures on larynx and trachea**

     31.41   Tracheoscopy through artificial stoma

       EXCLUDES   that with biopsy (31.43-31.44)

       DEF: Exam of trachea by scope through an artificial opening.

     31.42   Laryngoscopy and other tracheoscopy

       EXCLUDES   that with biopsy (31.43-31.44)

     31.43   Closed [endoscopic] biopsy of larynx

     31.44   Closed [endoscopic] biopsy of trachea

     31.45   Open biopsy of larynx or trachea

     31.48   Other diagnostic procedures on larynx

       EXCLUDES   contrast laryngogram (87.07)

             microscopic examination of specimen from larynx (90.31-90.39)

             soft tissue x-ray of larynx NEC (87.09)

     31.49   Other diagnostic procedures on trachea

       EXCLUDES   microscopic examination of specimen from trachea (90.41-90.49)

             x-ray of trachea (87.49)

   31.5   Local excision or destruction of lesion or tissue of trachea

       EXCLUDES   biopsy of trachea (31.44-31.45)

             laryngotracheal fistulectomy (31.62)

             tracheoesophageal fistulectomy (31.73)

√4ᵗʰ   **31.6   Repair of larynx**

     31.61   Suture of laceration of larynx

     31.62   Closure of fistula of larynx

       Laryngotracheal fistulectomy

       Take-down of laryngostomy

       DEF: Laryngotracheal fistulectomy: Excision and closing of passage between voice box and trachea.

       DEF: Take-down of laryngostomy: Removal of laryngostomy tube and restoration of voice box.

     31.63   Revision of laryngostomy

     31.64   Repair of laryngeal fracture

       DEF: Alignment and positioning of harder structures of larynx such as hyoid bone, following fracture.

     31.69   Other repair of larynx

       Arytenoidopexy   Graft of larynx

       Cordopexy   Transposition of vocal cords

       EXCLUDES   construction of artificial larynx (31.75)

       DEF: Arytenoidopexy: Fixation of pitcher-shaped cartilage in voice box.

       DEF: Graft of larynx: Implant of graft tissue into voice box.

       DEF: Transposition of the vocal cords: Placement of vocal cords into more functional positions.

√4ᵗʰ   **31.7   Repair and plastic operations on trachea**

     31.71   Suture of laceration of trachea

     31.72   Closure of external fistula of trachea

       Closure of tracheotomy

     31.73   Closure of other fistula of trachea

       Tracheoesophageal fistulectomy

       EXCLUDES   laryngotracheal fistulectomy (31.62)

       DEF: Tracheoesophageal fistulectomy: Excision and closure of abnormal opening between windpipe and esophagus.

     31.74   Revision of tracheostomy

BI Bilateral Procedure   **NC** Non-covered Procedure   **LC** Limited Coverage Procedure   ►◄ Revised Text   ● New Code   ▲ Revised Code Title

102 – Volume 3 · February 2013   2014 ICD-9-CM

31.75 Reconstruction of trachea and construction of artificial larynx
Tracheoplasty with artificial larynx

31.79 Other repair and plastic operations on trachea

✓4th **31.9 Other operations on larynx and trachea**

31.91 Division of laryngeal nerve

31.92 Lysis of adhesions of trachea or larynx

31.93 Replacement of laryngeal or tracheal stent
DEF: Removal and substitution of tubed molding into larynx or trachea.

31.94 Injection of locally-acting therapeutic substance into trachea

31.95 Tracheoesophageal fistulization
DEF: Creation of passage between trachea and esophagus.

31.98 Other operations on larynx
Dilation
Division of congenital web } of larynx
Removal of keel or stent
EXCLUDES *removal of intraluminal foreign body from larynx without incision (98.14)*
DEF: Dilation: Increasing larynx size by stretching.
DEF: Division of congenital web: Cutting and separating congenital membranes around larynx.
DEF: Removal of keel or stent: Removal of prosthetic device from larynx.

31.99 Other operations on trachea
EXCLUDES *removal of:*
intraluminal foreign body from trachea without incision (98.15)
tracheostomy tube (97.37)
replacement of tracheostomy tube (97.23)
tracheostomy toilette (96.55)
AHA: 3Q, '10, 6; 1Q, '97, 14
TIP: Assign for tracheal dilation associated with insertion of tracheobronchial endoprosthesis performed for treating benign tracheobronchial strictures or strictures produced by malignant neoplasms.

✓3rd **32 Excision of lung and bronchus**
INCLUDES rib section
sternotomy
sternum-splitting incision } as operative approach
thoracotomy
Code also any synchronous bronchoplasty (33.48)
DEF: Rib resection: Cutting of ribs to access operative field.
DEF: Sternotomy: Cut through breastbone as an operative approach.
DEF: Sternum-splitting incision: Breaking through breastbone to access operative field.

✓4th **32.0 Local excision or destruction of lesion or tissue of bronchus**
EXCLUDES *biopsy of bronchus (33.24-33.25)*
bronchial fistulectomy (33.42)
AHA: 4Q, '88, 11

32.01 Endoscopic excision or destruction of lesion or tissue of bronchus

32.09 Other local excision or destruction of lesion or tissue of bronchus
EXCLUDES *that by endoscopic approach (32.01)*

32.1 Other excision of bronchus
Resection (wide sleeve) of bronchus
EXCLUDES *radical dissection [excision] of bronchus (32.6)*
DEF: Resection (wide sleeve) of bronchus: Excision and partial, lengthwise removal of a lung branch.

✓4th **32.2 Local excision or destruction of lesion or tissue of lung**

32.20 Thoracoscopic excision of lesion or tissue of lung
Thoracoscopic wedge resection
AHA: 4Q, '07, 109, 110

32.21 Plication of emphysematous bleb
DEF: Stitching of a swollen vesicle into folds or tuck.

32.22 Lung volume reduction surgery   LC
DEF: Excision of portion of lung(s) to reduce respiratory effort in moderate to severe emphysema.
AHA: 1Q, '97, 6; 3Q, '96, 20; 4Q, '95, 64

Lung Volume Reduction

Chest wall
Diaphragm (dome-shaped)
Normal lungs
Flattened diaphragm
Lungs with emphysema
Original lung area
Staples
Diaphragm resumes a more domed shape
Lungs after surgery

32.23 Open ablation of lung lesion or tissue
AHA: 4Q, '06, 124

32.24 Percutaneous ablation of lung lesion or tissue
AHA: 4Q, '06, 124

32.25 Thoracoscopic ablation of lung lesion or tissue
EXCLUDES *thoracoscopic excision of lesion or tissue of lung (32.20)*
AHA: 4Q, '06, 124

32.26 Other and unspecified ablation of lung lesion or tissue
EXCLUDES *bronchoscopic bronchial thermoplasty, ablation of smooth airway muscle (32.27)*
AHA: 4Q, '06, 124

32.27 Bronchoscopic bronchial thermoplasty, ablation of airway smooth muscle
DEF: A transcatheter radiofrequency (RF)-based technology for severe asthma in which therapeutic heat is applied to the smooth muscle of the tracheobronchial tree and lungs to reduce bronchoconstriction.
AHA: 4Q, '10, 115-116

32.28 Endoscopic excision or destruction of lesion or tissue of lung
EXCLUDES *ablation of lung lesion or tissue:*
open (32.23)
other (32.26)
percutaneous (32.24)
thoracoscopic (32.25)
biopsy of lung (33.26-33.27)

32.29 Other local excision or destruction of lesion or tissue of lung
Resection of lung: Resection of lung:
NOS   wedge
EXCLUDES *ablation of lung lesion or tissue:*
open (32.23)
other (32.26)
percutaneous (32.24)
thoracoscopic (32.25)
biopsy of lung (33.26-33.27)
laser interstitial thermal therapy [LITT] of lesion or tissue of lung under guidance (17.69)
that by endoscopic approach (32.28)
thoracoscopic excision of lesion or tissue of lung (32.20)
wide excision of lesion of lung (32.3)
AHA: 3Q, '99, 3

✓4th **32.3 Segmental resection of lung**
Partial lobectomy
AHA: 4Q, '07, 109

32.30 Thoracoscopic segmental resection of lung
AHA: 4Q, '07, 110

32.39 Other and unspecified segmental resection of lung
EXCLUDES *thoracoscopic segmental resection of lung (32.30)*

3rd
4th Additional Digit Required   Valid OR Procedure   Non-OR Procedure   Adjunct Code

Operations on the Respiratory System

32.4–33.39

✓4ᵗʰ 32.4 Lobectomy of lung
Lobectomy with segmental resection of adjacent lobes of lung

EXCLUDES *that with radical dissection [excision] of thoracic structures (32.6)*

AHA: 4Q, '07, 109

32.41 Thoracoscopic lobectomy of lung
AHA: 4Q, '07, 110

32.49 Other lobectomy of lung
EXCLUDES *thoracoscopic lobectomy of lung (32.41)*

✓4ᵗʰ 32.5 Pneumonectomy
Excision of lung NOS
Pneumonectomy (with mediastinal dissection)

AHA: 1Q, '99, 6

32.50 Thoracoscopic pneumonectomy
AHA: 4Q, '07, 110

32.59 Other and unspecified pneumonectomy
EXCLUDES *thoracoscopic pneumonectomy (32.50)*

32.6 Radical dissection of thoracic structures
Block [en bloc] dissection of bronchus, lobe of lung, brachial plexus, intercostal structure, ribs (transverse process), and sympathetic nerves

32.9 Other excision of lung
EXCLUDES *biopsy of lung and bronchus (33.24-33.27)*
pulmonary decortication (34.51)

✓3ʳᵈ 33 Other operations on lung and bronchus
INCLUDES rib section
sternotomy
sternum-splitting incision   }   as operative approach
thoracotomy

33.0 Incision of bronchus

33.1 Incision of lung
EXCLUDES *puncture of lung (33.93)*

✓4ᵗʰ 33.2 Diagnostic procedures on lung and bronchus

33.20 Thoracoscopic lung biopsy
EXCLUDES *closed endoscopic biopsy of lung (33.27)*
closed [percutaneous] [needle] biopsy of lung (33.26)
open biopsy of lung (33.28)

AHA: 4Q, '07, 110

33.21 Bronchoscopy through artificial stoma
EXCLUDES *that with biopsy (33.24, 33.27)*

DEF: Visual exam of lung and its branches via tube through artificial opening.

33.22 Fiber-optic bronchoscopy
EXCLUDES *that with biopsy (33.24, 33.27)*

DEF: Exam of lung and bronchus via flexible optical instrument for visualization.

AHA: 1Q, '04, 4

33.23 Other bronchoscopy
EXCLUDES *that for:*
aspiration (96.05)
biopsy (33.24, 33.27)

AHA: 3Q, '02, 18; 1Q, '99, 6

Bronchoscopy with Bite Biopsy

33.24 Closed [endoscopic] biopsy of bronchus
Bronchoscopy (fiberoptic) (rigid) with:
   brush biopsy of "lung"
   brushing or washing for specimen collection
   excision (bite) biopsy
Diagnostic bronchoalveolar lavage [BAL]
Mini-bronchoalveolar lavage [mini-BAL]
Transbronchoscopic needle aspiration [TBNA] of bronchus

EXCLUDES *closed biopsy of lung, other than brush biopsy of "lung" (33.26, 33.27)*
whole lung lavage (33.99)

DEF: Bronchoalveolar lavage (BAL): Saline is introduced into the subsegment of a lobe and retrieved using gentle suction; also called 'liquid biopsy'.
DEF: Brush biopsy: Obtaining cell or tissue samples via bristled instrument without incision.

AHA: 2Q, '09, 9, 16; 2Q, '06, 20; 3Q, '04, 9; 3Q, '02, 16; 4Q, '92, 27; 3Q, '91, 15

33.25 Open biopsy of bronchus
EXCLUDES *open biopsy of lung (33.28)*

33.26 Closed [percutaneous] [needle] biopsy of lung
Fine needle aspiration [FNA] of lung
Transthoracic needle biopsy of lung [TTNB]

EXCLUDES *endoscopic biopsy of lung (33.27)*
thoracoscopic lung biopsy (33.20)

AHA: 3Q, '92, 12

33.27 Closed endoscopic biopsy of lung
Fiber-optic (flexible) bronchoscopy with fluoroscopic guidance with biopsy
Transbronchial lung biopsy
Transbronchoscopic needle aspiration [TBNA] of lung

EXCLUDES *brush biopsy of "lung" (33.24)*
percutaneous biopsy of lung (33.26)
thoracoscopic lung biopsy (33.20)

AHA: 1Q, '11, 18; 2Q, '09, 9, 16; 3Q, '04, 9; 3Q, '02, 16; 4Q, '92, 27; 3Q, '91, 15; S-O, '86, 11
TIP: Transbronchial lung biopsy involves a biopsy taken endoscopically through the bronchus into the lung alveoli if separate biopsies are taken of the bronchial and/or tracheal tissue, assign also 33.24.

33.28 Open biopsy of lung
AHA: 3Q, '99, 3; 3Q, '92, 12

33.29 Other diagnostic procedures on lung and bronchus
EXCLUDES *bronchoalveolar lavage [BAL] (33.24)*
contrast bronchogram:
endotracheal (87.31)
other (87.32)
endoscopic pulmonary airway flow measurement (33.72)
lung scan (92.15)
magnetic resonance imaging (88.92)
microscopic examination of specimen from bronchus or lung (90.41-90.49)
routine chest x-ray (87.44)
ultrasonography of lung (88.73)
vital capacity determination (89.37)
x-ray of bronchus or lung NOS (87.49)

✓4ᵗʰ 33.3 Surgical collapse of lung

33.31 Destruction of phrenic nerve for collapse of lung
DEF: Therapeutic deadening or destruction of diaphragmatic nerve to collapse the lung.

33.32 Artificial pneumothorax for collapse of lung
Thoracotomy for collapse of lung
DEF: Forcing air or gas into diaphragmatic space to achieve therapeutic collapse of lung.
DEF: Thoracotomy for collapse of lung: Incision into chest for therapeutic collapse of lung.

33.33 Pneumoperitoneum for collapse of lung
DEF: Forcing air or gas into abdominal serous membrane to achieve therapeutic collapse of lung.

33.34 Thoracoplasty
DEF: Removal of ribs for therapeutic collapse of lungs.

33.39 Other surgical collapse of lung
Collapse of lung NOS

BI Bilateral Procedure   NC Non-covered Procedure   LC Limited Coverage Procedure   ▶◀ Revised Text   ● New Code   ▲ Revised Code Title

✓4ᵗʰ **33.4** **Repair and plastic operation on lung and bronchus**

33.41 **Suture of laceration of bronchus**

33.42 **Closure of bronchial fistula**
Closure of bronchostomy
Fistulectomy:
bronchocutaneous
bronchoesophageal
bronchovisceral
EXCLUDES *closure of fistula:*
bronchomediastinal (34.73)
bronchopleural (34.73)
bronchopleuromediastinal (34.73)
DEF: Closure of bronchostomy: Removal of bronchostomy tube and repair of surgical wound.
DEF: Fistulectomy: Closure of abnormal passage.
Bronchocutaneous: Between skin and lung branch.
Bronchoesophagus: Between esophagus and lung branch.
Bronchovisceral: Between an internal organ and lung branch.

33.43 **Closure of laceration of lung**

33.48 **Other repair and plastic operations on bronchus**

33.49 **Other repair and plastic operations on lung**
EXCLUDES *closure of pleural fistula (34.73)*

✓4ᵗʰ **33.5** **Lung transplant**
NOTE To report donor source — *see* codes 00.91-00.93
Code also cardiopulmonary bypass [extracorporeal circulation] [heart-lung machine] (39.61)
EXCLUDES *combined heart-lung transplantation (33.6)*
AHA: 4Q, '95, 75

33.50 **Lung transplantation, not otherwise specified** LC

33.51 **Unilateral lung transplantation** LC

33.52 **Bilateral lung transplantation** LC
Double-lung transplantation
En bloc transplantation
DEF: Sequential excision and implant of both lungs.

33.6 **Combined heart-lung transplantation** LC
NOTE To report donor source — *see* codes 00.91-00.93
Code also cardiopulmonary bypass [extracorporeal circulation] [heart-lung machine] (39.61)

✓4ᵗʰ **33.7** **Other endoscopic procedures in bronchus or lung**
EXCLUDES *insertion of tracheobronchial stent (96.05)*

33.71 **Endoscopic insertion or replacement of bronchial valve(s), single lobe**
Endobronchial airflow redirection valve
Intrabronchial airflow redirection valve
EXCLUDES *endoscopic insertion or replacement of bronchial valve(s), multiple lobes (33.73)*
AHA: 4Q, '09, 144, 145; 4Q, '08, 175; 4Q, '06, 126
TIP: Bronchial valve placement is a less invasive treatment than lung volume reduction surgery (LVRS) or lung transplant in a patient with severe or end-stage emphysema or COPD.

33.72 **Endoscopic pulmonary airway flow measurement**
Assessment of pulmonary airway flow
Code also any diagnostic or therapeutic procedure, if performed
AHA: 4Q, '08, 174-175

33.73 **Endoscopic insertion or replacement of bronchial valve(s), multiple lobes**
Endobronchial airflow redirection valve
Intrabronchial airflow redirection valve
EXCLUDES *endoscopic insertion or replacement of bronchial valve(s), single lobe (33.71)*
AHA: 4Q, '09, 144,145
DEF: Minimally invasive treatment of air leaks resulting from disease, injury, or surgical intervention by the endoscopic placement of more than one bronchial valve.

33.78 **Endoscopic removal of bronchial device(s) or substances**
AHA: 4Q, '06, 126

33.79 **Endoscopic insertion of other bronchial device or substances**
Biologic lung volume reduction NOS (BLVR)
AHA: 4Q, '06, 126

✓4ᵗʰ **33.9** **Other operations on lung and bronchus**

33.91 **Bronchial dilation**
AHA: 1Q, '97, 14

33.92 **Ligation of bronchus**
DEF: Tying off of a lung branch.

33.93 **Puncture of lung**
EXCLUDES *needle biopsy (33.26)*
DEF: Piercing of lung with surgical instrument.

33.98 **Other operations on bronchus**
EXCLUDES *bronchial lavage (96.56)*
removal of intraluminal foreign body from bronchus without incision (98.15)

33.99 **Other operations on lung**
Whole lung lavage
EXCLUDES *other continuous mechanical ventilation (96.70-96.72)*
respiratory therapy (93.90-93.99)
AHA: 3Q, '02, 17

✓3ʳᵈ **34** **Operations on chest wall, pleura, mediastinum, and diaphragm**
EXCLUDES *operations on breast (85.0-85.99)*

✓4ᵗʰ **34.0** **Incision of chest wall and pleura**
EXCLUDES *that as operative approach — omit code*

34.01 **Incision of chest wall**
Extrapleural drainage
EXCLUDES *incision of pleura (34.09)*
DEF: Extrapleural drainage: Incision to drain fluid from external pleura.
AHA: 3Q, '00, 12; 1Q, '92, 13
TIP: Assign for removal of a broken sternal wire (S/P CABG procedure) when no replacement is implanted.

34.02 **Exploratory thoracotomy**

34.03 **Reopening of recent thoracotomy site**

34.04 **Insertion of intercostal catheter for drainage**
Chest tube
Closed chest drainage
Revision of intercostal catheter (chest tube) (with lysis of adhesions)
EXCLUDES *thoracoscopic drainage of pleural cavity (34.06)*
DEF: Insertion of catheter between ribs for drainage.
AHA: 2Q, '03, 7; 1Q, '99, 10; 2Q, '99, 12; 1Q, '95, 5; 1Q, '92, 12

34.05 **Creation of pleuroperitoneal shunt**
AHA: 4Q, '94, 50

34.06 **Thoracoscopic drainage of pleural cavity**
Evacuation of empyema
AHA: 4Q, '07, 110, 112

34.09 **Other incision of pleura**
Creation of pleural window for drainage
Intercostal stab
Open chest drainage
EXCLUDES *thoracoscopy (34.21)*
thoracotomy for collapse of lung (33.32)
DEF: Creation of pleural window: Creation of circumscribed drainage hole in serous membrane of chest.
DEF: Intercostal stab: Creation of penetrating stab wound between ribs.
DEF: Open chest drainage: Insertion of tube through ribs and serous membrane of chest for drainage.
AHA: 1Q, '07,14; 3Q, '02, 22; 1Q, '94, 7; 4Q, '94, 50

34.1 **Incision of mediastinum**
Code also any biopsy, if performed
EXCLUDES *mediastinoscopy (34.22)*
mediastinotomy associated with pneumonectomy (32.5)

✓4ᵗʰ **34.2** **Diagnostic procedures on chest wall, pleura, mediastinum, and diaphragm**

34.20 **Thoracoscopic pleural biopsy**
AHA: 4Q, '07, 110

Operations on the Respiratory System

34.21–34.99

34.21 Transpleural thoracoscopy
DEF: Exam of chest through serous membrane using scope.
AHA: 3Q, '02, 27

34.22 Mediastinoscopy
Code also any biopsy, if performed
DEF: Exam of lung cavity and heart using scope.

34.23 Biopsy of chest wall

34.24 Other pleural biopsy
EXCLUDES thoracoscopic pleural biopsy (34.20)
AHA: 3Q, '02, 22, 27; 1Q, '92, 14

34.25 Closed [percutaneous] [needle] biopsy of mediastinum

34.26 Open biopsy of mediastinum

34.27 Biopsy of diaphragm

34.28 Other diagnostic procedures on chest wall, pleura, and diaphragm
EXCLUDES angiocardiography (88.50-88.58)
    aortography (88.42)
    arteriography of:
      intrathoracic vessels NEC (88.44)
      pulmonary arteries (88.43)
    microscopic examination of specimen from chest wall, pleura, and diaphragm (90.41-90.49)
    phlebography of:
      intrathoracic vessels NEC (88.63)
      pulmonary veins (88.62)
    radiological examinations of thorax:
      C.A.T. scan (87.41)
      diaphragmatic x-ray (87.49)
      intrathoracic lymphangiogram (87.34)
      routine chest x-ray (87.44)
      sinogram of chest wall (87.38)
      soft tissue x-ray of chest wall NEC (87.39)
      tomogram of thorax NEC (87.42)
      ultrasonography of thorax (88.73)

34.29 Other diagnostic procedures on mediastinum
EXCLUDES mediastinal:
    pneumogram (87.33)
    x-ray NEC (87.49)

34.3 Excision or destruction of lesion or tissue of mediastinum
EXCLUDES biopsy of mediastinum (34.25-34.26)
    mediastinal fistulectomy (34.73)
AHA: 2Q, '11, 12

34.4 Excision or destruction of lesion of chest wall
Excision of lesion of chest wall NOS (with excision of ribs)
EXCLUDES biopsy of chest wall (34.23)
    costectomy not incidental to thoracic procedure (77.91)
    excision of lesion of:
      breast (85.20-85.25)
      cartilage (80.89)
      skin (86.2-86.3)
      fistulectomy (34.73)

√4th **34.5 Pleurectomy**

34.51 Decortication of lung
EXCLUDES thoracoscopic decortication of lung (34.52)
DEF: Removal of thickened serous membrane for lung expansion.

34.52 Thoracoscopic decortication of lung
AHA: 4Q, '07, 111, 113

34.59 Other excision of pleura
Excision of pleural lesion
EXCLUDES biopsy of pleura (34.24)
    pleural fistulectomy (34.73)

34.6 Scarification of pleura
Pleurosclerosis
EXCLUDES injection of sclerosing agent (34.92)
DEF: Destruction of fluid-secreting serous membrane cells of chest.
AHA: 1Q, '92, 12

√4th **34.7 Repair of chest wall**

34.71 Suture of laceration of chest wall
EXCLUDES suture of skin and subcutaneous tissue alone (86.59)

34.72 Closure of thoracostomy

34.73 Closure of other fistula of thorax
Closure of:
    bronchopleural
    bronchopleurocutaneous } fistula
    bronchopleuromediastinal

34.74 Repair of pectus deformity
Repair of:
    pectus carinatum } (with implant)
    pectus excavatum
DEF: Pectus carinatum repair: Restoration of prominent chest bone defect with implant.
DEF: Pectus excavatum: Restoration of depressed chest bone defect with implant.
AHA: 2Q, '04, 6

34.79 Other repair of chest wall
Repair of chest wall NOS
AHA: 2Q, '04, 6; J-F, '87, 13
TIP: Assign for removal and replacement of broken sternal wires (S/P CABG procedure), along with code 77.61 if sternal bone debridement was also performed.

√4th **34.8 Operations on diaphragm**

34.81 Excision of lesion or tissue of diaphragm
EXCLUDES biopsy of diaphragm (34.27)

34.82 Suture of laceration of diaphragm

34.83 Closure of fistula of diaphragm
Thoracicoabdominal
Thoracicogastric } fistulectomy
Thoracicointestinal
DEF: Fistulectomy: Closure of abnormal passage.

34.84 Other repair of diaphragm
EXCLUDES repair of diaphragmatic hernia (53.7-53.82)

34.85 Implantation of diaphragmatic pacemaker

34.89 Other operations on diaphragm

√4th **34.9 Other operations on thorax**

34.91 Thoracentesis
DEF: Puncture of pleural cavity for fluid aspiration, also called pleurocentesis.
AHA: ▶4Q, '12, 83;◀ S-O, '85, 6

34.92 Injection into thoracic cavity
Chemical pleurodesis
Injection of cytotoxic agent or tetracycline
Instillation into thoracic cavity
Requires additional code for any cancer chemotherapeutic substance (99.25)
EXCLUDES that for collapse of lung (33.32)
DEF: Chemical pleurodesis: Tetracycline hydrochloride injections to create adhesions between parietal and visceral pleura for treatment of pleural effusion.
AHA: ▶3Q, '12, 24;◀ 4Q, '07, 112; 1Q, '07, 14; 1Q, '92, 12; 2Q, '89, 17
TIP: Assign for installation of biological glue and/or talc into the pleural cavity.

34.93 Repair of pleura

34.99 Other
EXCLUDES removal of:
    mediastinal drain (97.42)
    sutures (97.43)
    thoracotomy tube (97.41)
DEF: Pleural tent: Extrapleural mobilization of parietal pleura that allows draping of membrane over visceral pleura to eliminate intrapleural dead space and seal visceral pleura.
AHA: 1Q, '00, 17; 1Q, '88, 9
TIP: Assign for formation of a pleural tent, which involves extrapleural mobilization of the parietal pleura in the apex of the chest cavity.

BI Bilateral Procedure   NC Non-covered Procedure   LC Limited Coverage Procedure   ▶◀ Revised Text   ● New Code   ▲ Revised Code Title

106 – Volume 3 · February 2013   2014 ICD-9-CM

7. Operations on the Cardiovascular System (35-39)

√3ʳᵈ **35   Operations on valves and septa of heart**

INCLUDES sternotomy (median)
(tranverse) } as operative approach
thoracotomy

Code also any cardiopulmonary bypass [extracorporeal circulation] [heart-lung machine] (39.61)

√4ᵗʰ **35.0   Closed heart valvotomy or transcatheter replacement of heart valve**

EXCLUDES *percutaneous (balloon) valvuloplasty (35.96)*

DEF: Incision into valve to restore function.

35.00   Closed heart valvotomy, unspecified valve

35.01   Closed heart valvotomy, aortic valve

35.02   Closed heart valvotomy, mitral valve

35.03   Closed heart valvotomy, pulmonary valve

35.04   Closed heart valvotomy, tricuspid valve

35.05   Endovascular replacement of aortic valve

NOTE Includes that with any balloon valvuloplasty; do not code separately

Implantation of transcatheter aortic valve
Replacement of aortic valve with tissue graft
(autograft) (bioprosthetic) (heterograft)
(homograft):
transarterial approach
transfemoral approach
TAVI (transcatheter aortic valve implantation)
TAVR (transcatheter aortic valve replacement)

EXCLUDES *open and other replacement of heart valve (35.20-35.28)*

AHA: 4Q, '11, 169-175

35.06   Transapical replacement of aortic valve

NOTE Includes that with any balloon valvuloplasty; do not code separately

Implantation of transcatheter aortic valve
Replacement of aortic valve with tissue graft
(autograft) (bioprosthetic) (heterograft)
(homograft):
intercostal approach
transventricular approach
That via transthoracic exposure, i.e. thoracotomy, sternotomy, or subxiphoid approach

EXCLUDES *open and other replacement of heart valve (35.20-35.28)*

AHA: 4Q, '11, 169-175

35.07   Endovascular replacement of pulmonary valve

NOTE Includes that with any balloon valvuloplasty; do not code separately

Implantation of transcatheter pulmonary valve
PPVI (percutaneous pulmonary valve implantation)
Replacement of pulmonary valve:
transfemoral approach
transvenous approach
That within previously created right ventricle to pulmonary artery conduit
TPVI (transcatheter pulmonary valve implantation)

EXCLUDES *open and other replacement of heart valve (35.20-35.28)*

AHA: 4Q, '11, 169-175

35.08   Transapical replacement of pulmonary valve

NOTE Includes that with any balloon valvuloplasty; do not code separately

Implantation of transcatheter pulmonary valve
Replacement of pulmonary valve:
intercostal approach
transventricular approach
That via transthoracic exposure, i.e. thoracotomy, sternotomy, or subxiphoid approach

EXCLUDES *open and other replacement of heart valve (35.20-35.28)*

AHA: 4Q, '11, 169-175

35.09   Endovascular replacement of unspecified heart valve

NOTE Includes that with any balloon valvuloplasty; do not code separately

Replacement of valve via:
intercostal approach
transventricular approach

EXCLUDES *open and other replacement of heart valve (35.20-35.28)*

AHA: 4Q, '11, 169-175

√4ᵗʰ **35.1   Open heart valvuloplasty without replacement**

INCLUDES open heart valvotomy

Code also cardiopulmonary bypass, if performed [extracorporeal circulation] [heart-lung machine] (39.61)

EXCLUDES *that associated with repair of:*
endocardial cushion defect (35.54,35.63,35.73)
percutaneous (balloon) valvuloplasty (35.96)
valvular defect associated with atrial and ventricular septal defects (35.54, 35.63, 35.73)

DEF: Incision into heart for plastic valve repair without replacing valve.

35.10   Open heart valvuloplasty without replacement, unspecified valve

35.11   Open heart valvuloplasty of aortic valve without replacement

AHA: 2Q, '08, 13

TIP: Assign for resuspension of aortic valve, in which 4-0 Prolene sutures are used to lift the valve into correct anatomical position, and a double layer of felt is placed on the inside and outside of the valve.

35.12   Open heart valvuloplasty of mitral valve without replacement

AHA: 3Q, '10, 6; 1Q, '10, 14; 1Q, '97, 13

35.13   Open heart valvuloplasty of pulmonary valve without replacement

35.14   Open heart valvuloplasty of tricuspid valve without replacement

√4ᵗʰ **35.2   Open and other replacement of heart valve**

INCLUDES excision of heart valve with replacement

Code also cardiopulmonary bypass [extracorporeal circulation] [heart-lung machine] (39.61)

EXCLUDES *that associated with repair of:*
endocardial cushion defect (35.54,35.63, 35.73)
valvular defect associated with atrial and ventricular septal defects (35.54, 35.63, 35.73)
transapical replacement of heart valve (35.06, 35.08)
transcatheter replacement of heart valve (35.05, 35.07)

DEF: Removal and replacement of valve with tissue from patient, animal, other human, or prosthetic (synthetic) valve.

35.20   Open and other replacement of unspecified heart valve

That with tissue graft or prosthetic implant

EXCLUDES *endovascular replacement of unspecified heart valve (35.09)*

35.21   Open and other replacement of aortic valve with tissue graft

Includes that by: Includes that by:
autograft   homograft
heterograft

EXCLUDES *endovascular replacement of aortic valve (35.05)*
transapical replacement of aortic valve (35.06)

AHA: 2Q, '97, 8

35.22   Open and other replacement of aortic valve

Replacement of aortic valve, NOS
That with prosthetic (partial) (synthetic) (total)

EXCLUDES *endovascular replacement of aortic valve (35.05)*
transapical replacement of aortic valve (35.06)

AHA: 4Q, '11, 152; 4Q, '08, 179; 1Q, '96, 11

√3ʳᵈ
√4ᵗʰ Additional Digit Required   Valid OR Procedure   Non-OR Procedure   Adjunct Code

Operations on the Cardiovascular System

35–35.22

Operations on the Cardiovascular System

35.23–35.55

35.23 Open and other replacement of mitral valve with tissue graft

Includes that by:
autograft
heterograft
homograft

35.24 Open and other replacement of mitral valve

Replacement of mitral valve, NOS
That with prosthetic (partial) (synthetic) (total)

EXCLUDES   *percutaneous repair with implant or leaflet clip (35.97)*

AHA: 4Q, '97, 55

35.25 Open and other replacement of pulmonary valve with tissue graft

Includes that by:
autograft
heterograft
homograft

EXCLUDES   *endovascular replacement of pulmonary valve (35.07)*
transapical replacement of pulmonary valve (35.08)

AHA: 1Q, '11, 24; 1Q, '07, 14; 1Q, '04, 16; 2Q, '97, 8
TIP: Assign for a Ross procedure, in which a patient's aortic valve is replaced by utilizing the pulmonary valve and the pulmonary valve is replaced with a homograft. Also assign code 35.21 for the aortic valve replacement.

35.26 Open and other replacement of pulmonary valve

Replacement of pulmonary valve, NOS
That with prosthetic (partial) (synthetic) (total)

EXCLUDES   *endovascular replacement of pulmonary valve (35.07)*
transapical replacement of pulmonary valve (35.08)

35.27 Open and other replacement of tricuspid valve with tissue graft

Includes that by:
autograft
heterograft
homograft

35.28 Open and other replacement of tricuspid valve

Replacement of tricuspid valve, NOS
That with prosthetic (partial) (synthetic) (total)

√4ᵗʰ **35.3 Operations on structures adjacent to heart valves**

Code also cardiopulmonary bypass [extracorporeal circulation] [heart-lung machine] (39.61)

35.31 Operations on papillary muscle

Division
Reattachment } of papillary muscle
Repair

35.32 Operations on chordae tendineae

Division } chordae tendineae
Repair

35.33 Annuloplasty

Plication of annulus
DEF: Plication of annulus: Tuck stitched in valvular ring for tightening.
AHA: 1Q, '97, 13; 1Q, '88, 10
TIP: Do not assign unless the annuloplasty is the only procedure performed; if it included an operation on the leaflet as well, refer to valvuloplasty codes, which include the annuloplasty.

35.34 Infundibulectomy

Right ventricular infundibulectomy
DEF: Infundibulectomy: Excision of funnel-shaped heart passage.
DEF: Right ventricular infundibulectomy: Excision of funnel-shaped passage in right upper heart chamber.

35.35 Operations on trabeculae carneae cordis

Division } of trabeculae carneae cordis
Excision

Excision of aortic subvalvular ring

35.39 Operations on other structures adjacent to valves of heart

Repair of sinus of Valsalva (aneurysm)

√4ᵗʰ **35.4 Production of septal defect in heart**

35.41 Enlargement of existing atrial septal defect

Rashkind procedure
Septostomy (atrial) (balloon)
DEF: Enlargement of partition wall defect in lower heart chamber to improve function.
DEF: Rashkind procedure: Enlargement of partition wall defect between the two lower heart chambers by balloon catheter.

35.42 Creation of septal defect in heart

Blalock-Hanlon operation
DEF: Blalock-Hanlon operation: Removal of partition wall defect in lower heart chamber.

√4ᵗʰ **35.5 Repair of atrial and ventricular septa with prosthesis**

INCLUDES   repair of septa with synthetic implant or patch

Code also cardiopulmonary bypass [extracorporeal circulation] [heart-lung machine] (39.61)

35.50 Repair of unspecified septal defect of heart with prosthesis

EXCLUDES   *that associated with repair of:*
endocardial cushion defect (35.54)
septal defect associated with valvular defect (35.54)

35.51 Repair of atrial septal defect with prosthesis, open technique

Atrioseptoplasty
Correction of atrial septal defect
Repair: } with prosthesis
foramen ovale (patent)
ostium secundum defect

EXCLUDES   *that associated with repair of:*
atrial septal defect associated with valvular and ventricular septal defects (35.54)
endocardial cushion defect (35.54)

DEF: Repair of opening or weakening in septum separating the atria; prosthesis implanted through heart incision.

35.52 Repair of atrial septal defect with prosthesis, closed technique

Insertion of atrial septal umbrella [King-Mills]
DEF: Correction of partition wall defect in lower heart chamber with artificial material, without incision into heart.
DEF: Insertion of atrial septal umbrella (King-Mills): Correction of partition wall defect in lower heart chamber with atrial septal umbrella.
AHA: 2Q, '05, 17; 3Q, '98, 11
TIP: Assign for Amplatzer balloon occlusion, used to repair cardiac anomalies; is implanted at the site of the defect via a catheter; typically performed in the cardiac catheterization lab.

35.53 Repair of ventricular septal defect with prosthesis, open technique

Correction of ventricular
    septal defect   } with prosthesis
Repair of supracristal defect

EXCLUDES   *that associated with repair of:*
endocardial cushion defect (35.54)
ventricular defect associated with valvular and atrial septal defects (35.54)

AHA: 1Q, '07, 14

35.54 Repair of endocardial cushion defect with prosthesis

Repair:
atrioventricular canal
ostium primum defect   } with prosthesis
valvular defect associated with } (grafted to
    atrial and ventricular   septa)
    septal defects

EXCLUDES   *repair of isolated:*
atrial septal defect (35.51-35.52)
valvular defect (35.20, 35.22, 35.24, 35.26, 35.28)
ventricular septal defect (35.53)

35.55 Repair of ventricular septal defect with prosthesis, closed technique

BI   Bilateral Procedure   NC   Non-covered Procedure   LC   Limited Coverage Procedure   ►◄ Revised Text   ● New Code   ▲ Revised Code Title

108 – Volume 3   **2014 ICD-9-CM**

✓4ᵗʰ   **35.6**   **Repair of atrial and ventricular septa with tissue graft**
Code also cardiopulmonary bypass [extracorporeal circulation] [heart-lung machine] (39.61)

     35.60   **Repair of unspecified septal defect of heart with tissue graft**
EXCLUDES *that associated with repair of:*
endocardial cushion defect (35.63)
septal defect associated with valvular defect (35.63)

     35.61   **Repair of atrial septal defect with tissue graft**
Atrioseptoplasty
Correction of atrial septal defect
Repair: with tissue graft
   foramen ovale (patent)
   ostium secundum defect
EXCLUDES *that associated with repair of:*
atrial septal defect associated with valvular and ventricular septal defects (35.63)
endocardial cushion defect (35.63)

     35.62   **Repair of ventricular septal defect with tissue graft**
Correction of ventricular
   septal defect   with tissue
Repair of supracristal defect   graft
EXCLUDES *that associated with repair of:*
endocardial cushion defect (35.63)
ventricular defect associated with valvular and atrial septal defects (35.63)

     35.63   **Repair of endocardial cushion defect with tissue graft**
Repair of:
   artrioventricular canal
   ostium primum defect   with tissue
   valvular defect associated with   graft
     atrial and ventricular
     septal defects
EXCLUDES *repair of isolated:*
atrial septal defect (35.61)
valvular defect (35.20-35.21, 35.23, 35.25, 35.27)
ventricular septal defect (35.62)

✓4ᵗʰ   **35.7**   **Other and unspecified repair of atrial and ventricular septa**
Code also cardiopulmonary bypass [extracorporeal circulation] [heart-lung machine] (39.61)

     35.70   **Other and unspecified repair of unspecified septal defect of heart**
Repair of septal defect NOS
EXCLUDES *that associated with repair of:*
endocardial cushion defect (35.73)
septal defect associated with valvular defect (35.73)

     35.71   **Other and unspecified repair of atrial septal defect**
Repair NOS: Repair NOS:
   atrial septum   ostium secundum defect
   foramen ovale (patent)
EXCLUDES *that associated with repair of:*
atrial septal defect associated with valvular and ventricular septal defects (35.73)
endocardial cushion defect (35.73)

     35.72   **Other and unspecified repair of ventricular septal defect**
Repair NOS: Repair NOS:
   supracristal defect   ventricular septum
EXCLUDES *that associated with repair of:*
endocardial cushion defect (35.73)
ventricular septal defect associated with valvular and atrial septal defects (35.73)

     35.73   **Other and unspecified repair of endocardial cushion defect**
Repair NOS:
   atrioventricular canal
   ostium primum defect
   valvular defect associated with atrial and ventricular septal defects
EXCLUDES *repair of isolated:*
atrial septal defect (35.71)
valvular defect (35.20, 35.22, 35.24, 35.26, 35.28)
ventricular septal defect (35.72)

✓4ᵗʰ   **35.8**   **Total repair of certain congenital cardiac anomalies**
NOTE For partial repair of defect [e.g. repair of atrial septal defect in tetralogy of Fallot] — code to specific procedure

     35.81   **Total repair of tetralogy of Fallot**
One-stage total correction of tetralogy of Fallot with or without:
   commissurotomy of pulmonary valve
   infundibulectomy
   outflow tract prosthesis
   patch graft of outflow tract
   prosthetic tube for pulmonary artery
   repair of ventricular septal defect (with prosthesis)
   take-down of previous systemic-pulmonary artery anastomosis

     35.82   **Total repair of total anomalous venous connection**
One-stage total correction of total anomalous pulmonary venous connection with or without:
   anastomosis between (horizontal) common pulmonary trunk and posterior wall of left atrium (side-to-side)
   enlargement of foramen ovale
   incision [excision] of common wall between posterior left atrium and coronary sinus and roofing of resultant defect with patch graft (synthetic)
   ligation of venous connection (descending anomalous vein) (to left innominate vein) (to superior vena cava)
   repair of atrial septal defect (with prosthesis)

     35.83   **Total repair of truncus arteriosus**
One-stage total correction of truncus arteriosus with or without:
   construction (with aortic homograft) (with prosthesis) of a pulmonary artery placed from right ventricle to arteries supplying the lung
   ligation of connections between aorta and pulmonary artery
   repair of ventricular septal defect (with prosthesis)

     35.84   **Total correction of transposition of great vessels, not elsewhere classified**
Arterial switch operation [Jatene]
Total correction of transposition of great arteries at the arterial level by switching the great arteries, including the left or both coronary arteries, implanted in the wall of the pulmonary artery
EXCLUDES *baffle operation [Mustard] [Senning] (35.91)*
creation of shunt between right ventricle and pulmonary artery [Rastelli] (35.92)

3ʳᵈ
4ᵗʰ   Additional Digit Required   Valid OR Procedure   Non-OR Procedure   Adjunct Code

Operations on the Cardiovascular System

35.9–36.06

√4ᵗʰ **35.9 Other operations on valves and septa of heart**

Code also cardiopulmonary bypass, if performed [extracorporeal circulation] [heart-lung machine] (39.61)

35.91 Interatrial transposition of venous return

Baffle:
  atrial
  interatrial
Mustard's operation
Resection of atrial septum and insertion of patch to direct systemic venous return to tricuspid valve and pulmonary venous return to mitral valve

DEF: Atrial baffle: Correction of venous flow of abnormal or deviated lower heart chamber.

DEF: Interatrial baffle: Correction of venous flow between abnormal lower heart chambers.

DEF: Mustard's operation: Creates intra-atrial baffle using pericardial tissue to correct transposition of the great vessels.

35.92 Creation of conduit between right ventricle and pulmonary artery

Creation of shunt between right ventricle and (distal) pulmonary artery

EXCLUDES *that associated with total repair of truncus arteriosus (35.83)*

AHA: 1Q, '07, 14

35.93 Creation of conduit between left ventricle and aorta

Creation of apicoaortic shunt
Shunt between apex of left ventricle and aorta

AHA: 2Q, '09, 8

35.94 Creation of conduit between atrium and pulmonary artery

Fontan procedure

35.95 Revision of corrective procedure on heart

Replacement of prosthetic heart valve poppet
Resuture of prosthesis of:
  septum
  valve

EXCLUDES *complete revision — code to specific procedure*
replacement of prosthesis or graft of:
septum (35.50-35.63)
valve (35.20-35.28)

DEF: Replacement of prosthetic heart valve poppet: Removal and replacement of valve-supporting prosthesis.

DEF: Resuture of prosthesis of septum: Restitching of prosthesis in partition wall.

DEF: Resuture of prosthesis of valve: Restitching of prosthetic valve.

35.96 Percutaneous balloon valvuloplasty

Balloon dilation of valve

EXCLUDES *endovascular replacement of heart valve (35.05, 35.07)*
mitral valve repair with implant (35.97)
transapical replacement of heart valve (35.06, 35.08)

DEF: Percutaneous balloon valvuloplasty: Repair of valve with inflatable catheter.

AHA: 1Q, '11, 24; 3Q, '10, 16; 3Q, '09, 19; 3Q, '04, 10; M-J, '86, 6; N-D, '85, 10

35.97 Percutaneous mitral valve repair with implant

Endovascular mitral valve repair
Implantation of mitral valve leaflet clip
Transcatheter mitral valve repair

Code also any transesophageal echocardiography [TEE] (88.72)

EXCLUDES *percutaneous balloon valvuloplasty (35.96)*

AHA: 4Q, '10, 116-117

TIP: Assign for mitral valve reconstruction by use of the Evalve® Cardiovascular Valve Repair System or MitraClip® implant.

35.98 Other operations on septa of heart

AHA: 1Q, '07, 11

35.99 Other operations on valves of heart

√3ʳᵈ **36 Operations on vessels of heart**

INCLUDES sternotomy (median)
                (transverse)   } as operative approach
           thoracotomy

Code also any:
  injection or infusion of platelet inhibitor (99.20)
  injection or infusion of thrombolytic agent (99.10)
Code also cardiopulmonary bypass, if performed [extra- corporeal circulation] [heart-lung machine] (39.61)

√4ᵗʰ **36.0 Removal of coronary artery obstruction and insertion of stent(s)**

AHA: 4Q, '95, 66; 2Q, '94, 13; 1Q, '94, 3; 2Q, '90, 23; N-D, '86, 8

36.03 Open chest coronary artery angioplasty

Coronary (artery):
  endarterectomy (with patch graft)
  thromboendarterectomy (with patch graft)
Open surgery for direct relief of coronary artery obstruction

Code also any:
  insertion of drug-eluting coronary stent(s) (36.07)
  insertion of non-drug-eluting coronary stent(s) (36.06)
  number of vascular stents inserted (00.45-00.48)
  number of vessels treated (00.40-00.43)
  procedure on vessel bifurcation (00.44)

EXCLUDES *that with coronary artery bypass graft (36.10-36.19)*

DEF: Endarterectomy (with patch graft): Excision of thickened material within coronary artery; repair with patch graft.

DEF: Thromboendarterectomy (with patch graft): Excision o blood clot and thickened material within coronary artery; repair with patch graft.

DEF: Open surgery for direct relief of coronary artery obstruction: Removal of coronary artery obstruction through opening in chest.

AHA: 2Q, '01, 24; 3Q, '93, 7

TIP: Do not assign if the procedure was performed percutaneously; see instead code 00.66.

36.04 Intracoronary artery thrombolytic infusion

Enzyme infusion
Platelet inhibitor
That by direct coronary artery injection, infusion, or catheterization

EXCLUDES *infusion of platelet inhibitor (99.20)*
infusion of thrombolytic agent (99.10)
that associated with any procedure in 36.0:

DEF: Infusion of clot breaking solution into intracoronary artery.

AHA: 4Q, '05, 102; 4Q, '02, 114; 3Q, '02, 20; 2Q, '01, 24; 4Q, '98, 85; 1Q, '97, 3; 4Q, '95, 67

TIP: If tPA infusion was performed in another facility withi the previous 24 hours prior to arrival in the current facility assign also diagnosis code V45.88.

36.06 Insertion of non-drug- eluting coronary artery stent(s)

Bare stent(s)   Endograft(s)
Bonded stent(s)   Endovascular graft(s)
Drug-coated stent(s),e.g.,   Stent graft(s)
  heparin coated

Code also any:
  number of vascular stents inserted (00.45-00.48)
  number of vessels treated (00.40-00.43)
  open chest coronary artery angioplasty (36.03)
  percutaneous transluminal coronary angioplasty [PTCA] (00.66)
  procedure on vessel bifurcation (00.44)
  transluminal coronary atherectomy (17.55)

EXCLUDES *insertion of drug-eluting coronary artery stent(s) (36.07)*

DEF: Percutaneous implant of metal stent via catheter, to enlarge, maintain lumen size of coronary artery.

AHA: 4Q, '11, 167; 2Q, '09, 12; 4Q, '05, 71; 2Q, '04, 3; 4Q, '0: 101; 1Q,'01, 9; 2Q, '01, 24; 1Q, '00, 11; 1Q, '99, 17

BI Bilateral Procedure   NC Non-covered Procedure   LC Limited Coverage Procedure   ▶◀ Revised Text   ● New Code   ▲ Revised Code Titl

110 – Volume 3   2014 ICD-9-C

36.07 Insertion of drug-eluting coronary artery stent(s)

    Endograft(s)   Stent graft(s)

    Endovascular graft(s)

    Code also any:

      number of vascular stents inserted (00.45-00.48)

      number of vessels treated (00.40-00.43)

      open chest coronary artery angioplasty (36.03)

      percutaneous transluminal coronary angioplasty [PTCA] (00.66)

      procedure on vessel bifurcation (00.44)

      transluminal coronary atherectomy (17.55)

      EXCLUDES *drug-coated stents, e.g., heparin coated (36.06)*

                insertion of non-drug-eluting coronary artery stent(s) (36.06)

    DEF: Drug-eluting stent technology developed to prevent the accumulation of scar tissue that can narrow reopened coronary arteries. A special polymer is used to coat the drug onto the stent, which slowly releases into the coronary artery wall tissue.

    AHA: ▶3Q, '12, 5;◀ 4Q, '05, 105-106; 4Q, '02, 101

36.09 Other removal of coronary artery obstruction

    Coronary angioplasty NOS

    Code also any:

      number of vascular stents inserted (00.45-00.48)

      number of vessels treated (00.40-00.43)

      procedure on vessel bifurcation (00.44)

      EXCLUDES *that by open angioplasty (36.03)*

                that by percutaneous transluminal coronary angioplasty [PTCA] (00.66)

                transluminal coronary atherectomy (17.55)

✓4th **36.1 Bypass anastomosis for heart revascularization**

    NOTE Do not assign codes from series 00.40-00.43 with codes from series 36.10-36.19

    Code also:

      cardiopulmonary bypass [extracorporeal circulation] [heart-lung machine] (39.61)

      pressurized treatment of venous bypass graft [conduit] with pharmaceutical substance, if performed (00.16)

    DEF: Insertion of alternate vessel to bypass blocked coronary artery, correct coronary blood flow.

    AHA: 4Q, '07, 121; 2Q, '96, 7; 3Q, '95, 7; 3Q, '93, 8; 1Q, '91, 7; 2Q, '90, 24; 4Q, '89, 3

    TIP: The determining factor for coding an aortocoronary artery bypass graft operation is the number of coronary arteries involved rather than the number of grafts; the use of the sequential technique does not affect the code assignment.

36.10 Aortocoronary bypass for heart revascularization, not otherwise specified

    Direct revascularization:

      cardiac   } with catheter stent,

      coronary   prosthesis, or vein

      hear muscule   graft

      myocardial

    Heart revascularization NOS

    AHA: 2Q, '96, 7

36.11 (Aorto)coronary bypass of one coronary artery

    AHA: 3Q, '02, 4, 9; 4Q, '89, 3

36.12 (Aorto)coronary bypass of two coronary arteries

    AHA: 3Q, '02, 8; 4Q, '99, 15; 2Q, '96, 7; 3Q, '97, 14; 4Q, '89, 3

Coronary Bypass

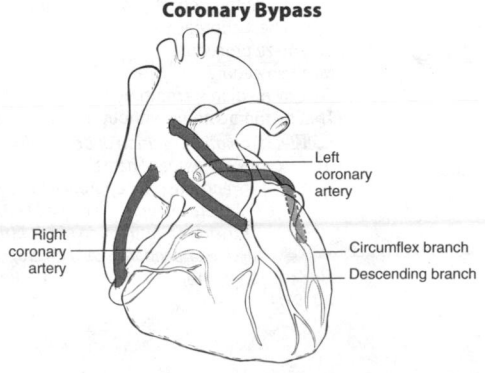

  Right coronary artery

  Left coronary artery

  Circumflex branch

  Descending branch

36.13 (Aorto)coronary bypass of three coronary arteries

    AHA: 3Q, '02, 6, 7, 9; 2Q, '96, 7; 4Q, '89, 3

36.14 (Aorto)coronary bypass of four or more coronary arteries

    AHA: 3Q, '02, 5; 2Q, '96, 7; 4Q, '89, 3

36.15 Single internal mammary-coronary artery bypass

    Anastomosis (single):

      mammary artery to coronary artery

      thoracic artery to coronary artery

    AHA: 3Q, '02, 4-9; 4Q, '99, 15; 3Q, '97, 14; 2Q, '96, 7

36.16 Double internal mammary-coronary artery bypass

    Anastomosis, double:

      mammary artery to coronary artery

      thoracic artery to coronary artery

    AHA: 3Q, '02, 6, 8, 9; 2Q, '96, 7

36.17 Abdominal-coronary artery bypass

    Anastomosis:

      gastroepiploic artery to coronary artery

    AHA: 3Q, '97, 14; 4Q, '96, 64

36.19 Other bypass anastomosis for heart revascularization

    AHA: 2Q, '96, 7

36.2 Heart revascularization by arterial implant

    Implantation of:

      aortic branches [ascending aortic branches] into heart muscle

      blood vessels into myocardium

      internal mammary artery [internal thoracic artery] into:

        heart muscle

        myocardium

        ventricle

        ventricular wall

    Indirect heart revascularization NOS

✓4th **36.3 Other heart revascularization**

36.31 Open chest transmyocardial revascularization

    DEF: Transmyocardial revascularization (TMR): Laser creation of channels through myocardium allows oxygenated blood flow from sinusoids to myocardial tissue.

36.32 Other transmyocardial revascularization

    AHA: 4Q, '98, 74

36.33 Endoscopic transmyocardial revascularization

    Thoracoscopic transmyocardial revascularization

    AIIA: 4Q, '06, 127

36.34 Percutaneous transmyocardial revascularization

    Endovascular transmyocardial revascularization

    AHA: 4Q, '06, 127

36.39 Other heart revascularization

    Abrasion of epicardium   Myocardial graft:

    Cardio-omentopexy   mediastinal fat

    Intrapericardial poudrage   omentum

                                  pectoral muscles

    DEF: Cardio-omentopexy: Suture of omentum segment to heart after drawing segment through incision in diaphragm to improve blood supply.

    DEF: Intrapericardial poudrage: Application of powder to heart lining to promote fusion.

✓4th **36.9 Other operations on vessels of heart**

    Code also cardiopulmonary bypass [extracorporeal circulation] [heart-lung machine] (39.61)

36.91 Repair of aneurysm of coronary vessel

36.99 Other operations on vessels of heart

    Exploration

    Incision   } of coronary artery

    Ligation

    Repair of arteriovenous fistula

    AHA: 3Q, '03, 18; 1Q, '94, 3

Operations on the Cardiovascular System

37–37.33

☑3ʳᵈ **37 Other operations on heart and pericardium**
Code also any injection or infusion of platelet inhibitor (99.20)

37.0 Pericardiocentesis
DEF: Puncture of the heart lining to withdraw fluid.
AHA: 1Q, '07, 11

☑4ᵗʰ **37.1 Cardiotomy and pericardiotomy**
Code also cardiopulmonary bypass [extracorporeal circulation] [heart-lung machine] (39.61)

37.10 Incision of heart, not otherwise specified
Cardiolysis NOS

37.11 Cardiotomy
Incision of: Incision of:
  atrium   myocardium
  endocardium   ventricle

37.12 Pericardiotomy
Pericardial window operation
Pericardiolysis
Pericardiotomy
DEF: Pericardial window operation: Incision into heart lining for drainage.
DEF: Pericardiolysis: Destruction of heart tissue lining.

☑4ᵗʰ **37.2 Diagnostic procedures on heart and pericardium**

37.20 Non-invasive programmed electrical stimulation [NIPS]
EXCLUDES   *catheter based invasive electro- physiologic testing (37.26)*
device interrogation only without arrhythmia induction (bedside check) (89.45-89.49)
that as part of intraoperative testing — omit code
DEF: Non-invasive testing of a previously implanted cardioverter-defibrillator to ensure proper lead placement and system function.
AHA: 4Q, '06, 128

37.21 Right heart cardiac catheterization
Cardiac catheterization NOS
EXCLUDES   *that with catheterization of left heart (37.23)*
AHA: 3Q, '04, 10; 3Q, '03, 9; 2Q, '90, 23; M-J, '87, 11

37.22 Left heart cardiac catheterization
EXCLUDES   *that with catheterization of right heart (37.23)*
AHA: 2Q, '10, 8-9; 4Q, '05, 71; 3Q, '05, 14; 3Q, '04, 10; 2Q, '04, 3; 1Q, '00, 21; 2Q, '90, 23; 4Q, '88, 4; M-J, '87, 11

37.23 Combined right and left heart cardiac catheterization
AHA: 1Q, '07, 11; 2Q, '05, 17; 3Q, '04, 10; 2Q, '01, 8; 1Q, '00, 20; 3Q, '98, 11; 2Q, '90, 23; M-J, '87, 11

37.24 Biopsy of pericardium

37.25 Biopsy of heart
AHA: 3Q, '03, 16; 3Q, '94, 8

37.26 Catheter based invasive electrophysiologic testing
Electrophysiologic studies [EPS]
Code also any concomitant procedure
EXCLUDES   *device interrogation only without arrhythmia induction (bedside check) (89.45-89.49)*
His bundle recording (37.29)
non-invasive programmed electrical stimulation (NIPS) (37.20)
that as part of intraoperative testing — omit code
DEF: Diagnostic mapping and measurement of intracardiac electrical activity; requires inserting three to six catheters into heart blood vessels and positioning catheters under fluoroscopic guidance to determine site of the tachycardia or abnormal impulse pathway; may also be used to terminate arrhythmias.
AHA: 2Q, '11, 13; 3Q, '03, 23; 2Q, '03, 19; 1Q, '02, 8, 9; 1Q, '99, 3; 2Q, '97, 10; 3Q, '90, 11

Intracardiac Echocardiography

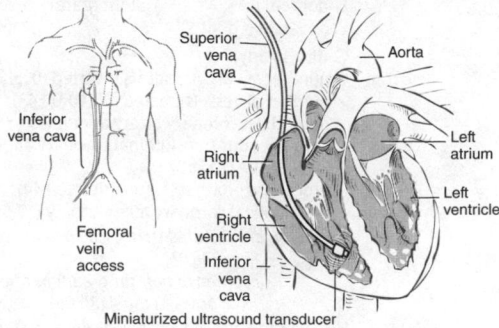

Miniaturized ultrasound transducer

37.27 Cardiac mapping
Code also any concomitant procedure
EXCLUDES   *electrocardiogram (89.52)*
His bundle recording (37.29)
AHA: 2Q, '11, 13

37.28 Intracardiac echocardiography
Echocardiography of heart chambers
ICE
Code also any synchronous Doppler flow mapping (88.72)
EXCLUDES   *intravascular imaging of coronary vessels (intravascular ultra-sound) (IVUS) (00.24)*
DEF: Creation of a two-dimensional graphic of heart using endoscopic echocardiographic equipment.
AHA: 4Q, '01, 62

37.29 Other diagnostic procedures on heart and pericardium
EXCLUDES   *angiocardiography (88.50-88.58)*
cardiac function tests (89.41-89.69)
cardiovascular radioisotopic scan and function study (92.05)
coronary arteriography (88.55-88.57)
diagnostic pericardiocentesis (37.0)
diagnostic ultrasound of heart (88.72)
x-ray of heart (87.49)
AHA: S-O, '87, 3

☑4ᵗʰ **37.3 Pericardiectomy and excision of lesion of heart**
Code also cardiopulmonary bypass [extracorporeal circulation] [heart-lung machine], if performed (39.61)

37.31 Pericardiectomy
Excision of:
  adhesions of pericardium
  constricting scar of:
    epicardium
    pericardium
DEF: Excision of a portion of heart lining.

37.32 Excision of aneurysm of heart
Repair of aneurysm of heart

37.33 Excision or destruction of other lesion or tissue of heart, open approach
Ablation or incision of heart tissue (cryoablation) (electrocurrent) (laser) (microwave) (radiofrequency) (resection) (ultrasound), open chest approach
Cox-maze procedure
Maze procedure
That by median sternotomy
That by thoracotomy without use of thoracoscope
EXCLUDES   *ablation, excision or destruction of lesion or tissue of heart:*
endovascular approach (37.34)
thoracoscopic approach (37.37)
excision or destruction of left atrial appendage (LAA) (37.36)
AHA: 4Q, '10,118-119; 3Q, '10, 6; 3Q, '06, 13; 4Q, '03, 93-94; 2Q, '94, 12

BI Bilateral Procedure   NC Non-covered Procedure   LC Limited Coverage Procedure   ▶◀ Revised Text   ● New Code   ▲ Revised Code Title

112 – Volume 3   **2014 ICD-9-CM**

37.34 Excision or destruction of other lesion or tissue of heart, endovascular approach

Ablation of heart tissue (cryoablation) (electrocurrent) (laser) (microwave) (radiofrequency) (ultrasound), via peripherally inserted catheter

Modified maze procedure, percutaneous approach

EXCLUDES ablation, excision or destruction of lesion of tissue of heart:
     open approach (37.33)
     thoracoscopic approach (37.37)

DEF: Destruction of heart tissue or lesion by freezing or electric current.

AHA: 2Q, '11, 13; 4Q, '10,118-119; 4Q, '03, 93-95; 1Q, '00, 20

TIP: If the ablation is performed via a right and left cardiac catheterization, report also code 37.23 and any associated procedures (e.g., angiography).

37.35 Partial ventriculectomy   NC

Ventricular reduction surgery
Ventricular remodeling

Code also any synchronous:
     mitral valve repair (35.02, 35.12)
     mitral valve replacement (35.23-35.24)

DEF: Removal of elliptical slice of ventricle between anterior and posterior papillary muscle; also called Batiste operation.

AHA: 4Q, '97, 54, 55

37.36 Excision, destruction, or exclusion of left atrial appendage [LAA]

INCLUDES thoracoscopic approach, minithoracotomy approach, percutaneous approach, endovascular approach, or subxiphoid approach

Clipping of left atrial appendage
Oversewing of left atrial appendage
Stapling of left atrial appendage
That by fastener or suture

Code also any:
     concomitant (open) procedure performed
     fluoroscopy (87.49)
     transesophageal echocardiography (TEE) (88.72)

EXCLUDES ablation, excision or destruction of lesion or tissue of heart, endovascular approach (37.34)
     excision or destruction of other lesion or tissue of heart, thoracoscopic approach (37.37)
     insertion of left atrial appendage device (37.90)

DEF: Closure of LAA tissue via use of stapler, clip, or suture; performed for patients with atrial fibrillation for whom traditional anticoagulant therapies are contraindicated; prevents strokes and other embolic events.

AHA: 4Q, '08, 176

37.37 Excision or destruction of other lesion or tissue of heart, thoracoscopic approach

Ablation or incision of heart tissue (cryoablation) (electrocautery) (laser) (microwave) (radiofrequency) (resection) (ultrasound), via thoracoscope

Modified maze procedure, thoracoscopic approach

That via thoracoscopically-assisted approach (without thoracotomy) (with port access) (with subxiphoid incision)

EXCLUDES ablation, excision or destruction of lesion or tissue of heart:
     endovascular approach (37.34)
     open approach (37.33)
     thoracoscopic excision or destruction of left atrial appendage [LAA] (37.36)

AHA: 1Q, '12, 14; 4Q, '10, 118-120

Ventricular Reduction Surgery

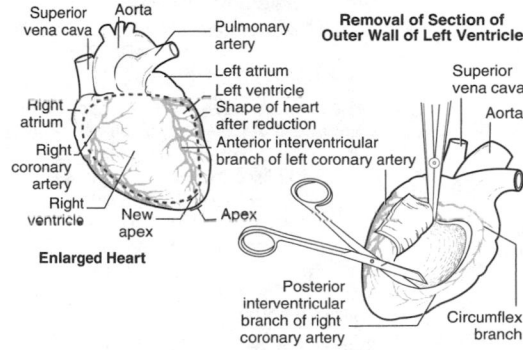

Enlarged Heart

Removal of Section of Outer Wall of Left Ventricle

✓4th 37.4 Repair of heart and pericardium

AHA: 2Q, '90, 24

37.41 Implantation of prosthetic cardiac support device around the heart

Cardiac support device [CSD]
Epicardial support device
Fabric (textile) (mesh) device
Ventricular support device on surface of heart

Code also any:
     cardiopulmonary bypass [extracorporeal circulation] [heart-lung machine] if performed (39.61)
     mitral valve repair (35.02, 35.12)
     mitral valve replacement (35.23-35.24)
     transesophageal echocardiography (88.72)

EXCLUDES circulatory assist systems (37.61-37.68)

DEF: Cardiac support device: any device implanted around the ventricles of the heart for cardiac support

DEF: Fabric (textile) (mesh) device: textile mesh net sutured around the heart for support.

AHA: 4Q, '05, 119-120

37.49 Other repair of heart and pericardium

AHA: 3Q, '08, 9

TIP: Assign for surgical ventricular restoration (SVR), performed to remodel or restore the left ventricle to a more normal size and shape in patients with akinetic parts of the heart.

✓4th 37.5 Heart replacement procedures

AHA: 4Q, '03, 96

37.51 Heart transplantation   LC

EXCLUDES combined heart-lung transplantation (33.6)

AHA: 4Q, '08, 182; 2Q, '05, 14

12 37.52 Implantation of total internal biventricular heart replacement system   LC

NOTE This procedure includes substantial removal of part or all of the biological heart. Both ventricles are resected, and the native heart is no longer intact. Ventriculectomy is included in this procedure; do not code separately.

Artificial heart

EXCLUDES implantation of heart assist system [VAD] (37.62, 37.65, 37.66, 37.68)

AHA: 4Q, '08, 181

Total Internal Biventricular Heart Replacement System

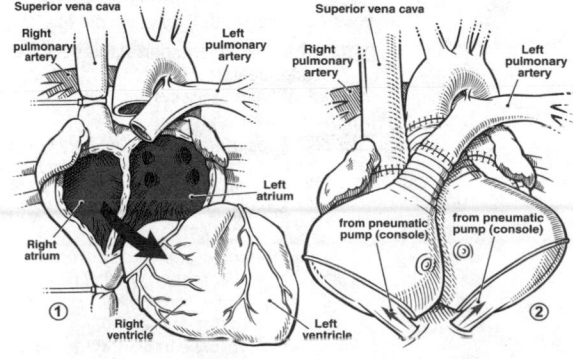

---

² Limited coverage only when reported in combination with diagnosis code V70.7.

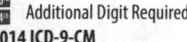 Additional Digit Required   Valid OR Procedure   Non-OR Procedure   Adjunct Code

2014 ICD-9-CM   Volume 3 – 113

Operations on the Cardiovascular System

37.53–37.67

37.53 Replacement or repair of thoracic unit of (total) replacement heart system NC

EXCLUDES   *replacement and repair of heart assist system [VAD] (37.63)*

AHA: 4Q, '08, 181

37.54 Replacement or repair of other implantable component of (total) replacement heart system NC

Implantable battery   Transcutaneous energy
Implantable controller   transfer [TET] device

EXCLUDES   *replacement and repair of heart assist system [VAD] (37.63)*
replacement or repair of thoracic unit of (total) replacement heart system (37.53)

AHA: 4Q, '08, 181

37.55 Removal of internal biventricular heart replacement system

Explantation of artificial heart

Code also any concomitant procedure, such as:
combined heart-lung transplantation (33.6)
heart transplantation (37.51)
implantation of internal biventricular heart replacement system (37.52)

EXCLUDES   *explantation [removal] of external heart assist system (37.64)*
explantation [removal] of percutaneous external heart assist device (97.44)
nonoperative removal of heart assist system (97.44)
that with replacement or repair of heart replacement system (37.53, 37.54)

AHA: 4Q, '08, 180-182

✓4ᵗʰ **37.6 Implantation of heart and circulatory assist system(s)**

EXCLUDES   *implantation of prosthetic cardiac support system (37.41)*

DEF: Implant of device for assisting heart in circulating blood.
AHA: 4Q, '08, 177-179; 4Q, '95, 68

37.60 Implantation or insertion of biventricular external heart assist system

NOTE   Device (outside the body but connected to heart) with external circulation pump. Ventriculotomy is included; do not code separately.

INCLUDES   open chest (sternotomy) procedure for cannulae attachments

Temporary cardiac support for both left and right ventricles, inserted in the same operative episode

EXCLUDES   *implantation of internal biventricular heart replacement system (artificial heart) (37.52)*
implant of pulsation balloon (37.61)
insertion of percutaneous external heart assist device (37.68)
insertion of temporary non-implantable extracorporeal circulatory assist device (37.62)

AHA: 4Q, '08, 179

37.61 Implant of pulsation balloon

AHA: 3Q, '05, 14

37.62 Insertion of temporary non-implantable extracorporeal circulatory assist device

NOTE   Includes explantation of this device; do not code separately.

Insertion of heart assist system, NOS
Insertion of heart pump

EXCLUDES   *implantation of total internal biventricular heart replacement system [artificial heart] (37.52)*
implant of external heart assist system (37.65)
insertion of implantable extracorporeal heart assist system (37.66)
insertion of percutaneous external heart assist device (37.68)
removal of heart assist system (37.64)

AHA: 4Q, '03, 116; 2Q, '90, 25

37.63 Repair of heart assist system

Replacement of parts of an existing ventricular assist device (VAD)

EXCLUDES   *replacement or repair of other implantable component of (total) replacement heart system [artificial heart] (37.54)*
replacement or repair of thoracic unit of (total) replacement heart system [artificial heart] (37.53)

37.64 Removal of external heart assist system(s) or device(s)

Explantation of external device(s) providing left and right ventricular support
Explantation of single external device and cannulae

EXCLUDES   *explantation [removal] of percutaneous external heart assist device (97.44)*
nonoperative removal of heart assist system (97.44)
temporary non implantable extracorporeal circulatory assist device (37.62)
that with replacement of implant (37.63)

AHA: 4Q, '08, 177-178, 180

37.65 Implant of single ventricular (extracorporeal) external heart assist system

NOTE   Device (outside the body but connected to heart) with external circulation and pump

NOTE   Insertion or implantation of one external VAD for left or right heart support

INCLUDES   open chest (sternotomy) procedure for cannulae attachments

Insertion of one device into one ventricle

EXCLUDES   *implantation of total internal biventricular heart replace- ment system (37.52)*
implant of pulsation balloon (37.61)
insertion of implantable heart assist system (37.66)
insertion or implantation of two external VADs for simultaneous right and left heart support (37.60)
insertion of percutaneous external heart assist device (37.68)
that without sternotomy (37.62)

DEF: Insertion of short-term circulatory support device with pump outside body.

37.66 Insertion of implantable heart assist system LC

NOTE   Device directly connected to the heart and implanted in the upper left quadrant of peritoneal cavity.This device can be used for either destination therapy (DT) or bridge-to-transplant (BTT).

Axial flow heart assist system
Diagonal pump heart assist system
Left ventricular assist device (LVAD)
Pulsatile heart assist system
Right ventricular assist device (RVAD)
Rotary pump heart assist system
Transportable, implantable heart assist system
Ventricular assist device (VAD) not otherwise specified

EXCLUDES   *implantation of total internal biventricular heart replacement system [artificial heart] (37.52)*
implant of pulsation balloon (37.61)
insertion of percutaneous external heart assist device (37.68)

DEF: Insertion of long-term circulatory support device with pump in body.

AHA: 4Q, '03, 116; 1Q, '98, 8

37.67 Implantation of cardiomyostimulation system

NOTE   Two-step open procedure consisting of tranfer of one end of the latissimus dorsi muscle; wrapping it around the heart; rib resection; implantation of epicardial cardiac pacing leads into the right ventricle; tunneling and pocket creation for the cardiomyostimulator.

AHA: 4Q, '98, 75; 1Q, '98, 8

BI Bilateral Procedure   NC Non-covered Procedure   LC Limited Coverage Procedure   ►◄ Revised Text   ● New Code   ▲ Revised Code Title

114 – Volume 3   2014 ICD-9-CM

Ventricular Assist Devices

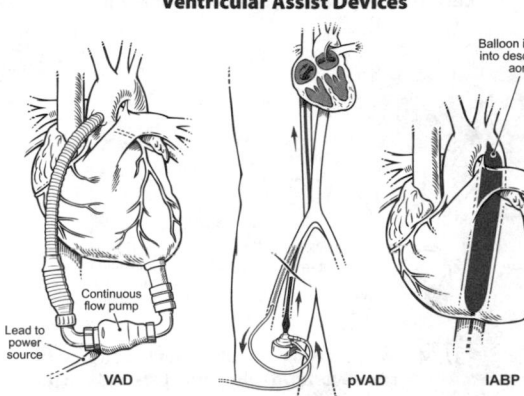

Balloon inserted
into descending
aorta

Continuous
flow pump

Lead to
power
source

VAD   pVAD   IABP

37.68 Insertion of percutaneous external heart assist device

> **INCLUDES** percutaneous [femoral] insertion of cannulae attachments
>
> Circulatory assist device
> Extrinsic heart assist device
> pVAD
> Percutaneous heart assist device
>
> AHA: 3Q, '09, 12; 2Q, '08, 12
> TIP: Assign for placement of the Orqis device, an extracorporeal, minimally invasive cardiac system designed to increase blood velocity down the thoracic aorta; used for patients with CHF who respond poorly to medical treatment.

√4ᵗʰ **37.7 Insertion, revision, replacement, and removal of leads; insertion of temporary pacemaker system; or revision of cardiac device pocket**

> Code also any insertion and replacement of pacemaker device (37.80-37.87)
>
> **EXCLUDES** implantation or replacement of transvenous lead [electrode] into left ventricular cardiac venous system (00.52)
>
> AHA: 1Q, '94, 16; 3Q, '92, 3; M-J, '87, 1

¹ **37.70 Initial insertion of lead [electrode], not otherwise specified**

> **EXCLUDES** insertion of temporary transvenous pacemaker system (37.78)
> replacement of atrial and/or ventricular lead(s) (37.76)

¹ **37.71 Initial insertion of transvenous lead [electrode] into ventricle**

> **EXCLUDES** insertion of temporary transvenous pacemaker system (37.78)
> replacement of atrial and/or ventricular lead(s) (37.76)

² **37.72 Initial insertion of transvenous leads [electrodes] into atrium and ventricle**

> **EXCLUDES** insertion of temporary transvenous pacemaker system (37.78)
> replacement of atrial and/or ventricular lead(s) (37.76)
>
> AHA: 4Q, '11, 168; 4Q, '08, 102; 2Q, '97, 4

¹ **37.73 Initial insertion of transvenous lead [electrode] into atrium**

> **EXCLUDES** insertion of temporary transvenous pacemaker system (37.78)
> replacement of atrial and/or ventricular lead(s) (37.76)

⁴ **37.74 Insertion or replacement of epicardial lead [electrode] into epicardium**

> Insertion or replacement of epicardial lead by:
> sternotomy
> thoracotomy
> **EXCLUDES** replacement of atrial and/or ventricular lead(s) (37.76)
>
> AHA: 1Q, '07, 20; 3Q, '05, 3-9

37.75 Revision of lead [electrode]

> Repair of electrode [removal with re-insertion]
> Repositioning of lead(s) (AICD) (cardiac device) (CRT-D) (CRT-P) (defibrillator) (pacemaker) (pacing) (sensing) [electrode]
> Revision of lead NOS
> **EXCLUDES** repositioning of temporary transvenous pacemaker system — omit code
>
> AHA: ▶4Q, '12, 82, 88; 2Q, '12, 14;◀ 3Q, '05, 8; 2Q, '99, 11

³ **37.76 Replacement of transvenous atrial and/or ventricular lead(s) [electrode]**

> Removal or abandonment of existing transvenous or epicardial lead(s) with transvenous lead(s) replacement
> **EXCLUDES** replacement of epicardial lead [electrode] (37.74)
>
> AHA: 3Q, '05, 3-9

37.77 Removal of lead(s) [electrode] without replacement

> Removal:
> epicardial lead (transthoracic approach)
> transvenous lead(s)
> **EXCLUDES** removal of temporary transvenous pacemaker system — omit code
> that with replacement of:
> atrial and/or ventricular lead(s) [electrode] (37.76)
> epicardial lead [electrode] (37.74)

37.78 Insertion of temporary transvenous pacemaker system

> **EXCLUDES** intraoperative cardiac pacemaker (39.64)
>
> AHA: 3Q, '05, 7; 3Q, '93, 12; 1Q, '89, 2

37.79 Revision or relocation of cardiac device pocket

> Debridement and reforming pocket (skin and subcutaneous tissue)
> Insertion of loop recorder
> Relocation of pocket [creation of new pocket] pacemaker or CRT-P
> Removal of cardiac device/pulse generator without replacement
> Removal of the implantable hemodynamic pressure sensor [lead] and monitor device
> Removal without replacement of cardiac resynchronization defibrillator device
> Repositioning of implantable hemodynamic pressure sensor [lead] and monitor device
> Repositioning of pulse generator
> Revision of cardioverter/defibrillator (automatic) pocket
> Revision of pocket for intracardiac hemodynamic monitoring
> Revision or relocation of CRT-D pocket
> Revision or relocation of pacemaker, defibrillator, or other implanted cardiac device pocket
> **EXCLUDES** removal of loop recorder (86.05)
>
> AHA: ▶4Q, '12, 88;◀ 3Q, '05, 3-9

√4ᵗʰ **37.8 Insertion, replacement, removal, and revision of pacemaker device**

> **NOTE** Device testing during procedure — omit code
> Code also any lead insertion, lead replacement, lead removal and/or lead revision (37.70-37.77)
> **EXCLUDES** implantation of cardiac resynchronization pacemaker, total system [CRT-P] (00.50)
> implantation or replacement of cardiac resynchronization pacemaker pulse generator only [CRT-P] (00.53)
>
> AHA: M-J, '87, 1

37.80 Insertion of permanent pacemaker, initial or replacement, type of device not specified

⁵ **37.81 Initial insertion of single-chamber device, not specified as rate responsive**

> **EXCLUDES** replacement of existing pacemaker device (37.85-37.87)

---

¹ Valid OR procedure code if accompanied by one of the following codes: 37.80, 37.81, 37.82, 37.85, 37.86, 37.87
² Valid OR procedure code if accompanied by one of the following codes: 37.80, 37.83
³ Valid OR procedure code if accompanied by one of the following codes: 37.80, 37.85, 37.86, 37.87
⁴ Valid OR procedure code if accompanied by one of the following codes: 37.80, 37.81, 37.82, 37.83, 37.85, 37.86, 37.87
⁵ Valid OR procedure code if accompanied by one of the following codes: 37.70, 37.71, 37.73, 37.74

Additional Digit Required   **Valid OR Procedure**   Non-OR Procedure   Adjunct Code

Operations on the Cardiovascular System

37.82–37.97

Insertion of Pacemaker

Left Atrial Appendage Device Insertion

5　37.82　Initial insertion of single-chamber device, rate responsive

Rate responsive to physiologic stimuli other than atrial rate

EXCLUDES *replacement of existing pacemaker device (37.85-37.87)*

6　37.83　Initial insertion of dual-chamber device

Atrial ventricular sequential device

EXCLUDES *replacement of existing pacemaker device (37.85-37.87)*

AHA: 4Q, '11, 168; 4Q, '08, 102; 2Q, '97, 4

37.85　Replacement of any type pacemaker device with single-chamber device, not specified as rate responsive

37.86　Replacement of any type pacemaker device with single-chamber device, rate responsive

Rate responsive to physiologic stimuli other than atrial rate

37.87　Replacement of any type pacemaker device with dual-chamber device

Atrial ventricular sequential device

37.89　Revision or removal of pacemaker device

Removal without replacement of cardiac re-synchronization pacemaker device [CRT-P]

Repair of pacemaker device

EXCLUDES *removal of temporary transvenous pacemaker system — omit code*
replacement of existing pacemaker device (37.85-37.87)
replacement of existing pacemaker device with CRT-P pacemaker device (00.53)

AHA: N-D, '86, 1

✓4ᵗʰ　37.9　Other operations on heart and pericardium

AHA: 3Q, '90, 11

37.90　Insertion of left atrial appendage device

Left atrial filter

Left atrial occluder

Transseptal catheter technique

DEF: Implantation of a filtering device within the left atrial appendage (LAA) to block emboli from exiting the LAA causing stroke or systemic thromboembolism.

AHA: 4Q, '04, 121

37.91　Open chest cardiac massage

EXCLUDES *closed chest cardiac massage (99.63)*

DEF: Massage of heart through opening in chest wall to reinstate or maintain circulation.

AHA: 4Q, '88, 12

37.92　Injection of therapeutic substance into heart

37.93　Injection of therapeutic substance into pericardium

37.94　Implantation or replacement of automatic cardioverter/defibrillator, total system [AICD]

NOTE Device testing during procedure — *omit code*

Implantation of defibrillator with leads (epicardial patches), formation of pocket (abdominal fascia) (subcutaneous), any transvenous leads, intra-operative procedures for evaluation of lead signals, and obtaining defibrillator threshold measurements

Techniques:
lateral thoracotomy
medial sternotomy
subxiphoid procedure

Code also extracorporeal circulation, if performed (39.61)

Code also any concomitant procedure [e.g., coronary bypass (36.10-36.19) or CCM, total system (17.51)]

EXCLUDES *implantation of cardiac resynchronization defibrillator, total system [CRT-D] (00.51)*

DEF: Direct insertion of defibrillator/cardioverter system to deliver shock and restore heart rhythm.

AHA: ▶4Q, '12, 88;◀ 4Q, '09, 141; 2Q, '03, 19; 3Q, '01, 5-7; 3Q, '99, 12; 1Q, '99, 3; 3Q, '90, 11; S-O, '87, 5

TIP: Assign for AICD placement, regardless of approach, whether by thoracotomy or by cephalic vein cutdown.

37.95　Implantation of automatic cardioverter/defibrillator lead(s) only

AHA: ▶4Q, '12, 88;◀ 3Q, '90, 11

37.96　Implantation of automatic cardioverter/defibrillator pulse generator only

NOTE Device testing during procedure — *omit code*

EXCLUDES *implantation or replacement of cardiac resynchronization defibrillator, pulse generator device only [CRT-D] (00.54)*

AHA: ▶4Q, '12, 88;◀ 3Q, '90, 11

37.97　Replacement of automatic cardioverter/defibrillator lead(s) only

EXCLUDES *replacement of epicardial lead [electrode] into epicardium (37.74)*
replacement of transvenous lead [electrode] into left ventricular coronary venous system (00.52)

AHA: ▶4Q, '12, 88;◀ 3Q, '05, 3-9; 3Q, '90, 11

Automatic Implantable Cardioverter/Defibrillator

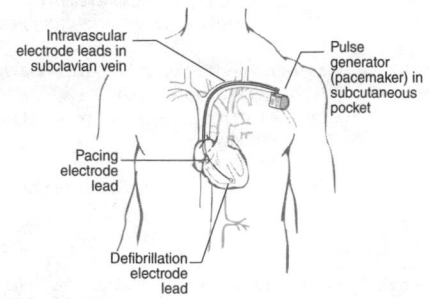

5　Valid OR procedure code if accompanied by one of the following codes: 37.70, 37.71, 37.73, 37.74
6　Valid OR procedure code if accompanied by one of the following codes: 37.72, 37.74

BI Bilateral Procedure　　　**NC** Non-covered Procedure　　　**LC** Limited Coverage Procedure　　　▶◀ Revised Text　　　● New Code　　　▲ Revised Code Title

37.98 Replacement of automatic cardioverter defibrillator pulse generator only

NOTE Device testing during procedure — *omit code*
EXCLUDES *replacement of cardiac resynchronization defibrillator, pulse generator device only [CRT-D] (00.54)*
AHA: ▶4Q, '12, 88;◀ 1Q, '99, 3; 3Q, '90, 11

37.99 Other

EXCLUDES *cardiac retraining (93.36)*
conversion of cardiac rhythm (99.60-99.69)
implantation of prosthetic cardiac support device (37.41)
insertion of left atrial appendage device (37.90)
maze procedure (Cox-maze), open (37.33)
maze procedure, endovascular approach (37.34)
repositioning of pulse generator (37.79)
revision of lead(s) (37.75)
revision or relocation of pacemaker, defibrillator or other implanted cardiac device pocket (37.79)
AHA: 3Q, '05, 5; 2Q, '05, 14; 1Q, '97, 12; 1Q, '94, 19; 3Q, '90, 11; 1Q, '89, 11

✓3rd 38 Incision, excision, and occlusion of vessels

Code also any application or administration of an adhesion barrier substance (99.77)
Code also cardiopulmonary bypass [extracorporeal circulation] [heart-lung machine] (39.61)
EXCLUDES *that of coronary vessels (00.66, 36.03, 36.04, 36.09, 36.10-36.99)*

The following fourth-digit subclassification is for use with appropriate categories in section 38.0, 38.1, 38.3, 38.5, 38.6, and 38.8 according to site. Valid fourth-digits are in [brackets] under each code.

0 unspecified
1 intracranial vessels
 Cerebral (anterior) (middle)
 Circle of Willis
 Posterior communicating artery
2 other vessels of head and neck
 Carotid artery (common) (external) (internal)
 Jugular vein (external) (internal)
3 upper limb vessels
 Axillary Radial
 Brachial Ulnar
4 aorta
5 other thoracic vessels
 Innominate Subclavian
 Pulmonary (artery) (vein) Vena cava, superior
6 abdominal arteries
 Celiac Mesenteric
 Gastric Renal
 Hepatic Splenic
 Iliac Umbilical
 EXCLUDES *abdominal aorta (4)*
7 abdominal veins
 Iliac Splenic
 Portal Vena cava (inferior)
 Renal
8 lower limb arteries
 Femoral (common) Popliteal
  (superficial) Tibial
9 lower limb veins
 Femoral Saphenous
 Popliteal Tibial

Endarterectomy of Aortic Bifurcation

Aorta (shown sectioned)
Plaque
Femoral artery
Plaque removed

§ ✓4th 38.0 Incision of vessel
[0-9] Embolectomy Thrombectomy
EXCLUDES *endovascular removal of obstruction from head and neck vessel(s) (39.74)*
puncture or catheterization of any:
artery (38.91, 38.98)
vein (38.92-38.95, 38.99)
AHA: 2Q, '98, 23; For code 38.04: 4Q, '11, 108;
For code 38.08 and 38.09: 1Q, '03, 17

§ ✓4th 38.1 Endarterectomy
[0-6,8] Endarterectomy with:
 embolectomy
 patch graft
 temporary bypass during procedure
 thrombectomy

Code also any:
 number of vascular stents inserted (00.45-00.48)
 number of vessels treated (00.40-00.43)
 procedure on vessel bifurcation (00.44)
DEF: Excision of tunica intima of artery to relieve arterial walls thickened by plaque or chronic inflammation.
AHA: 1Q, '00, 16; 2Q, '99, 5; 2Q, '95, 16; For code 38.12: 3Q, '06, 20; 1Q, '02, 10

✓4th 38.2 Diagnostic procedures on blood vessels
EXCLUDES *adjunct vascular system procedures (00.40-00.43)*

38.21 Biopsy of blood vessel

38.22 Percutaneous angioscopy
EXCLUDES *angioscopy of eye (95.12)*
DEF: Exam with fiberoptic catheter inserted through peripheral artery to visualize inner lining of blood vessels.

38.23 Intravascular spectroscopy
INCLUDES spectroscopy of both coronary and peripheral vessels
Intravascular chemography
Near infrared (NIR) spectroscopy
EXCLUDES *intravascular imaging of:*
coronary vessels (00.24, 38.24)
peripheral vessels (00.23, 38.25)
DEF: Method of identifying the chemical composition of coronary plaques by shining a near infrared (NIR) light at the plaque and measuring the amount of light reflected at different wavelengths.
AHA: 4Q, '08, 182-183

38.24 Intravascular imaging of coronary vessel(s) by optical coherence tomography [OCT]
DEF: Use of fiberoptic catheter probes that employ near-infrared electromagnetic radiation light to produce cross-sectional and enhanced resolution images of vessel plaque and intraluminal thrombus.
AHA: 1Q, '10, 16-17

38.25 Intravascular imaging of non-coronary vessel(s) by optical coherence tomography [OCT]
EXCLUDES *intravascular imaging of coronary vessel(s) by OCT (38.24)*
DEF: Use of fiberoptic catheter probes that employ near-infrared electromagnetic radiation light to produce cross-sectional and enhanced resolution images of vessel plaque and intraluminal thrombus.
AHA: 1Q, '10, 16-17

§ Requires fourth digit. Valid digits are in [brackets] under each code. See category 38 for definitions.

✓3rd ✓4th Additional Digit Required Valid OR Procedure Non-OR Procedure Adjunct Code
2014 ICD-9-CM February 2013 • Volume 3 – 117

Operations on the Cardiovascular System

38.26–38.6

Methods of Vessel Anastomoses

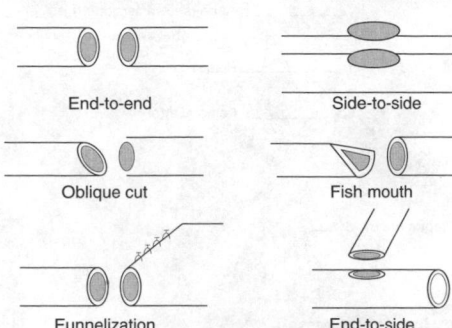

End-to-end   Side-to-side

Oblique cut   Fish mouth

Funnelization   End-to-side

38.26 Insertion of implantable pressure sensor without lead for intracardiac or great vessel hemodynamic monitoring

NOTE The sensor is a standalone device and is not physically connected to a separately implanted monitor.

Leadless pressure sensor not physically connected to a separately implanted monitor

Single device combination leadless pressure sensor with integral monitor for intracardiac or great vessel (or branch thereof) hemodynamic monitoring

With or without internal batteries

Without leads

EXCLUDES circulatory monitoring (blood gas, arterial or venous pressure, cardiac output and coronary blood flow (89.60-89.69)

hemodynamic monitoring system with sensor and separately implanted monitor (00.56-00.57)

insertion or replacement of implantable pressure sensor with lead for intracardiac or great vessel hemodynamic monitoring (00.56)

AHA: 4Q, '11, 175-176

38.29 Other diagnostic procedures on blood vessels

EXCLUDES blood vessel thermography (88.86)
circulatory monitoring (89.61-89.69)
contrast:
    angiocardiography (88.50-88.58)
    arteriography (88.40-88.49)
    phlebography (88.60-88.67)
impedance phlebography (88.68)
peripheral vascular ultrasonography (88.77)
plethysmogram (89.58)

AHA: 3Q, '00, 16; 1Q, '99, 7

TIP: Assign for an artery test occlusion, performed to determine the feasibility of coil occlusion of an aneurysm.

§§ ✓4ᵗʰ #### 38.3 Resection of vessel with anastomosis
[0-9]

Angiectomy
Excision of:
    aneurysm (arteriovenous) } with anastomosis
    blood vessel (lesion)

DEF: Reconstruction and reconnection of vessel after partial excision.

§ ✓4ᵗʰ #### 38.4 Resection of vessel with replacement
[0-9]

Angiectomy
Excision of:
    aneurysm (arteriovenous) or } with replacement
    blood vessel (lesion)

Partial resection with replacement

EXCLUDES endovascular repair of aneurysm (39.71-39.79)

Subcategory 38.4 requires the use of one of the following fourth-digit subclassifications to identify site:

0 unspecified

1 intracranial vessels
Cerebral (anterior) (middle)
Circle of Willis
Posterior communicating artery

2 other vessels of head and neck
Carotid artery (common) (external) (internal)
Jugular vein (external) (internal)

3 upper limb vessels
Axillary   Radial
Brachial   Ulnar

4 aorta, abdominal
Code also any thoracic vessel involvement (thoracoabdominal procedure) (38.45)

5 other thoracic vessels
Aorta (thoracic)   Subclavian
Innominate   Vena cava, superior
Pulmonary (artery) (vein)
Code also any abdominal aorta involvement (thoracoabdominal procedure) (38.44)

6 abdominal arteries
Celiac   Mesenteric
Gastric   Renal
Hepatic   Splenic
Iliac   Umbilical
EXCLUDES abdominal aorta (4)

7 abdominal veins
Iliac   Splenic
Portal   Vena cava (inferior)
Renal

8 lower limb arteries
Femoral (common)(superficial)
Tibial

9 lower limb veins
Femoral   Saphenous
Popliteal   Tibial

DEF: Excision of aneurysm (arteriovenous): Excision and replacement of segment of stretched or bulging blood vessel.

DEF: Excision of blood vessel (lesion): Excision and replacement of segment of vessel containing lesion.

AHA: 2Q, '99, 5, 6; **For code 38.44:** 3Q, '06, 15; **For code 38.45:** 2Q, '08, 13; **For code 38.48:** 2Q, '08, 13

§§ ✓4ᵗʰ #### 38.5 Ligation and stripping of varicose veins
[0-3,5,7,9] EXCLUDES ligation of varices:
    esophageal (42.91)
    gastric (44.91)

DEF: Ligation of varicose veins: Typing off vein with thread or wire to eliminate blood flow; stripping involves excising length of vein.

AHA: **For code 38.59:** 2Q, '97, 7

TIP: Do not assign a separate code for subfascial endoscopic perforator vein interruption, which is an integral part of the procedure.

§§ ✓4ᵗʰ #### 38.6 Other excision of vessels
[0-9]

Excision of blood vessel (lesion) NOS

EXCLUDES excision of vessel for aortocoronary bypass (36.10-36.14)
excision with:
    anastomosis (38.30-38.39)
    graft replacement (38.40-38.49)
    implant (38.40-38.49)

AHA: 3Q, '90, 17

§   Requires fourth digit. Valid digits are in [brackets] under each code. See subcategory 38.4 for definitions
§§   Requires fourth digit. Valid digits are in [brackets] under each code. See category 38 for definitions.

BI Bilateral Procedure   NC Non-covered Procedure   LC Limited Coverage Procedure   ▶◀ Revised Text   ● New Code   ▲ Revised Code Title

118 – Volume 3   **2014 ICD-9-CM**

38.7 Interruption of the vena cava

Insertion of implant or sieve in vena cava
Ligation of vena cava (inferior) (superior)
Plication of vena cava

DEF: Interruption of the blood flow through the venous heart vessels to prevent clots from reaching the chambers of the heart by means of implanting a sieve or implant, separating off a portion or by narrowing the venous blood vessels.

AHA: 2Q, '07, 4; 2Q, '94, 9; S-O, '85, 5

TIP: Assign this code for placement of a vena cava sieve, umbrella, or filter, regardless of the approach (open or percutaneous).

§§ ✓4th **38.8 Other surgical occlusion of vessels**
[0-9]

Clamping ⎫
Division ⎬ of blood vessel
Ligation ⎪
Occlusion ⎭

EXCLUDES   adrenal vessels (07.43)
     esophageal varices (42.91)
     gastric or duodenal vessel for ulcer (44.40-44.49)
     gastric varices (44.91)
     meningeal vessel (02.13)
     percutaneous transcatheter infusion
       embolization (99.29)
     spermatic vein for varicocele (63.1)
     surgical occlusion of vena cava (38.7)
     that for chemoembolization (99.25)
     that for control of (postoperative) hemorrhage:
       anus (49.95)
       bladder (57.93)
       following vascular procedure (39.41)
       nose (21.00-21.09)
       prostate (60.94)
       tonsil (28.7)
       thyroid vessel (06.92)
     transcatheter (infusion) 99.29

AHA: 2Q, '90, 23; M-A, '87, 9; For code 38.85: 1Q, '03, 15; For code 38.86: 1Q, '05, 14; N-D, '87, 4

✓4th **38.9 Puncture of vessel**

EXCLUDES   that for circulatory monitoring (89.60-89.69)

38.91 Arterial catheterization

AHA: 1Q, '05, 14; 1Q, '97, 3; 1Q, '95, 3; 2Q, '91, 15; 2Q, '90, 23

38.92 Umbilical vein catheterization

38.93 Venous catheterization, not elsewhere classified

EXCLUDES   that for cardiac catheterization
       (37.21-37.23)
     that for renal dialysis (38.95)
     that with guidance (electrocardiogram)
       (fluoroscopy) (ultrasound) (38.97)

AHA: 3Q, '10, 14; 3Q, '00, 9, 2Q, '98, 24; 1Q, '96, 3; 2Q, '96, 15; 3Q, '91, 13; 4Q, '90, 14; 2Q, '90, 24; 3Q, '88, 13

38.94 Venous cutdown

DEF: Incision of vein to place needle or catheter.

38.95 Venous catheterization for renal dialysis

EXCLUDES   insertion of totally implantable vascular
       access device [VAD] (86.07)

AHA: ▶3Q, '12, 6;◄ 4Q, '08, 193; 3Q, '98, 13; 2Q, '94, 11

TIP: Do not assign for intravascular vessel-to-vessel cannula to create an external shunt; see instead code 39.93.

TIP: ▶Assign a separate subcategory 88.7 code for guidance by ultrasound.◄

38.97 Central venous catheter placement with guidance

INCLUDES   guidance by:
       electrocardiogram
       fluoroscopy
       ultrasound

38.98 Other puncture of artery

EXCLUDES   that for:
       arteriography (88.40-88.49)
       coronary arteriography (88.55-88.57)

Typical Venous Cutdown

Vein mobilized, opened by oblique cut, catheter inserted

Distal vein tied

Saphenous vein (typical site) accessed by transverse incision

---

38.99 Other puncture of vein

Phlebotomy

EXCLUDES   that for:
       angiography of veins (88.60-88.68)
       extracorporeal circulation (39.61, 50.92)
       injection or infusion of:
       sclerosing solution (39.92)
       therapeutic or prophylactic substance
         (99.11-99.29)
       perfusion (39.96, 39.97)
       phlebography 88.60-88.68)
       transfusion (99.01-99.09)

AHA: 4Q, '94, 50; 1Q, '88, 11

✓3rd **39 Other operations on vessels**

EXCLUDES   those on coronary vessels (36.03-36.99)

39.0 Systemic to pulmonary artery shunt

Descending aorta-pulmonary artery ⎫
Left to right ⎬ anastomosis (graft)
Subclavian-pulmonary ⎭

Code also cardiopulmonary bypass [extracorporeal
     circulation] [heart-lung machine] (39.61)

DEF: Descending aorta-pulmonary artery anastomosis (graft): Connection of descending main heart artery to pulmonary artery.

DEF: Left to right anastomosis (graft): Connection of systemic arterial blood vessel to venous pulmonary system.

DEF: Subclavian-pulmonary anastomosis (graft): Connection of subclavian artery to pulmonary artery

39.1 Intra-abdominal venous shunt

Anastomosis:
   mesocaval
   portacaval
   portal vein to inferior vena cava
   splenic and renal veins
   transjugular intrahepatic portosystemic shunt [TIPS]

EXCLUDES   peritoneovenous shunt (54.94)

DEF: Connection of two venous blood vessels within abdominal cavity.

AHA: 2Q, '02, 4; 4Q, '94, 50; 4Q, '93, 31; 2Q, '93, 8

✓4th **39.2 Other shunt or vascular bypass**

Code also pressurized treatment of venous bypass graft
     [conduit] with pharmaceutical substance,
     if performed (00.16)

DEF: Creation of supplemental blood flow to area with inadequate blood supply due to disease or injury of vessels.

TIP: Assign separate codes for any concomitant procedures performed, such as arterial or venous thrombectomy or arteriography.

39.21 Caval-pulmonary artery anastomosis

Code also cardiopulmonary bypass (39.61)

39.22 Aorta-subclavian-carotid bypass

Bypass (arterial):
   aorta to carotid and brachial
   aorta to subclavian and carotid
   carotid to subclavian

39.23 Other intrathoracic vascular shunt or bypass

Intrathoracic (arterial) bypass graft NOS

EXCLUDES   coronary artery bypass (36.10-36.19)

39.24 Aorta-renal bypass

---

§§ Requires fourth digit. Valid digits are in [brackets] under each code. See category 38 for definitions.

3rd Additional Digit Required   Valid OR Procedure   Non-OR Procedure   Adjunct Code

2014 ICD-9-CM   February 2013 • Volume 3 – 119

Operations on the Cardiovascular System

39.25   **Aorta-iliac-femoral bypass**

Bypass: Bypass:
    aortofemoral   aortopopliteal
    aortoiliac   iliofemoral [iliac-femoral]
    aortoiliac to popliteal

AHA: 1Q, '03, 16; 4Q, '90, 27; 1Q, '88, 10

39.26   **Other intra-abdominal vascular shunt or bypass**

Bypass:
    aortoceliac
    aortic-superior mesenteric
    common hepatic-common iliac-renal
Intra-abdominal arterial bypass graft NOS

EXCLUDES   *peritoneovenous shunt (54.94)*

39.27   **Arteriovenostomy for renal dialysis**

Anastomosis for renal dialysis
Formation of (peripheral) arteriovenous fistula for
    renal [kidney] dialysis

Code also any renal dialysis (39.95)
AHA: 1Q, '07, 18; 1Q, '06, 10
TIP: Assign for creation of an internal shunt by arteriovenostomy for renal dialysis; includes transposition of the basilic vein.

39.28   **Extracranial-intracranial (EC-IC) vascular bypass**   [NC]

AHA: 2Q, '92, 7; 4Q, '91, 22

39.29   **Other (peripheral) vascular shunt or bypass**

Bypass (graft):
    axillary-brachial
    axillary-femoral [axillofemoral] (superficial)
    brachial
    femoral-femoral
    femoroperoneal
    femoropopliteal (arteries)
    femorotibial (anterior) (posterior)
    popliteal
    vascular NOS

EXCLUDES   *peritoneovenous shunt (54.94)*
AHA: 1Q, '03, 17; 2Q, '02, 8; 1Q, '02, 13; S-O, '85, 13

√4ᵗʰ   **39.3**   **Suture of vessel**

Repair of laceration of blood vessel

EXCLUDES   *any other vascular puncture closure device — omit code*
suture of aneurysm (39.52)
that for control of hemorrhage (postoperative):
    anus (49.95)
    bladder (57.93)
    following vascular procedure (39.41)
    nose (21.00-21.09)
    prostate (60.94)
    tonsil (28.7)

39.30   **Suture of unspecified blood vessel**

39.31   **Suture of artery**

AHA: ▶4Q, '12, 81;◄ 3Q, '06, 9

39.32   **Suture of vein**

√4ᵗʰ   **39.4**   **Revision of vascular procedure**

39.41   **Control of hemorrhage following vascular surgery**

EXCLUDES   *that for control of hemorrhage*
    (postoperative):
    anus (49.95)
    bladder (57.93)
    nose (21.00-21.09)
    prostate (60.94)
    tonsil (28.7)

39.42   **Revision of arteriovenous shunt for renal dialysis**

Conversion of renal dialysis:
    end-to-end anastomosis to end-to-side
    end-to-side anastomosis to end-to-end
    vessel-to-vessel cannula to arteriovenous shunt
Removal of old arteriovenous shunt and creation of
    new shunt

EXCLUDES   *replacement of vessel-to-vessel cannula (39.94)*
AHA: 2Q, '94, 15; 4Q, '93, 33

39.43   **Removal of arteriovenous shunt for renal dialysis**

EXCLUDES   *that with replacement [revision] of shunt (39.42)*

39.49   **Other revision of vascular procedure**

Declotting (graft)
Revision of:
    anastomosis of blood vessel
    vascular procedure (previous)

DEF: Declotting (graft): Removal of clot from graft.
AHA: 2Q, '98, 17; 1Q, '97, 3; 2Q, '94, 15
TIP: Do not assign if a declotting procedure of an AV dialysis graft is performed as a component of a revision procedure; see instead code 39.42.

√4ᵗʰ   **39.5**   **Other repair of vessels**

39.50   **Angioplasty of other non-coronary vessel(s)**

Percutaneous transluminal angioplasty (PTA) of
    non-coronary vessels:
    lower extremity vessels
    mesenterlc artery
    renal artery
    upper extremity vessels

Code also any:
    atherectomy of other non-coronary vessels(s)
      (17.56)
    injection or infusion of thrombolytic agent (99.10)
    insertion of drug-eluting peripheral vessel stent
      (00.55)
    insertion of non-drug-eluting peripheral vessel
      stent(s) or stent grafts(s) (39.90)
    number of vascular stents inserted (00.45-00.48)
    number of vessels treated (00.40-00.43)
    procedure on vessel bifurcation (00.44)

EXCLUDES   *percutaneous angioplasty of extracranial or intracranial vessel(s) (00.61-00.62)*
percutaneous atherectomy of extracranial or intracranial vessel(s) (17.53-17.54)
AHA: ▶3Q, '12, 13; 2Q, '12, 15;◄ 3Q, '09, 13; 4Q, '06, 119; 3Q, '03, 10; 1Q, '02, 13; 2Q, '01, 23; 2Q, '00, 10; 1Q, '00, 12; 2Q, '98, 17; 1Q, '97, 3; 4Q, '96, 63; 4Q, '95, 66

39.51   **Clipping of aneurysm**

EXCLUDES   *clipping of arteriovenous fistula (39.53)*

39.52   **Other repair of aneurysm**

Repair of aneurysm by: Repair of aneurysm by:
    coagulation   suture
    electrocoagulation   wiring
    filipuncture   wrapping
    methyl methacrylate

EXCLUDES   *endovascular repair of aneurysm (39.71-39.79)*
re-entry operation (aorta) (39.54)
that with:
    graft replacement (38.40-38.49)
    resection (38.30-38.49, 38.60-38.69)

DEF: Application of device to repair abnormally stretched blood vessel and prevent a hemorrhage from vessel.
DEF: Repair of aneurysm by: Coagulation: Clotting or solidifying. Electrocoagulation: Electrically produced clotting. Filipuncture: Insertion of wire or thread. Methyl methacrylate: Injection or insertion of plastic material. Suture: Stitching. Wiring: Insertion of wire. Wrapping: Compression.
AHA: 3Q, '06, 15-16; 3Q, '02, 25, 26; 1Q, '99, 15, 16, 17; 1Q, '88, 10
TIP: Do not assign if any type of grafting material was used in the aneurysm repair; see instead subcategory 38.4 or endovascular repair subcategory 39.7.

[BI]   Bilateral Procedure   [NC]   Non-covered Procedure   [LC]   Limited Coverage Procedure   ▶◄ Revised Text   ● New Code   ▲ Revised Code Title

39.53 Repair of arteriovenous fistula
Embolization of carotid cavernous fistula
Repair of arteriovenous fistula by:
    clipping
    coagulation
    ligation and division
EXCLUDES *repair of:*
      arteriovenous shunt for renal dialysis
        (39.42)
      head and neck vessels, endovascular
        approach (39.72)
      that with:
        graft replacement (38.40-38.49)
        resection (38.30-38.49, 38.60-38.69)
DEF: Correction of arteriovenous fistula by application of clamps, causing coagulation or by tying off and dividing the connection.
AHA: 1Q, '00, 8
TIP: Do not assign for an embolization procedure performed by interventional radiologists via radiological guidance; it is not considered a surgical procedure; see instead code 99.29.

39.54 Re-entry operation (aorta)
Fenestration of dissecting aneurysm of thoracic aorta
Code also cardiopulmonary bypass [extracorporeal circulation] [heart-lung machine] (39.61)
DEF: Re-entry operation: Creation of passage between stretched wall of the vessel and major arterial channel to heart.
DEF: Fenestration of dissecting aneurysm of thoracic aorta: Creation of passage between stretched arterial heart vessel and functional part of vessel.

39.55 Reimplantation of aberrant renal vessel
DEF: Reimplant of renal vessel into normal position.

39.56 Repair of blood vessel with tissue patch graft
EXCLUDES *that with resection (38.40-38.49)*
AHA: 1Q, '04, 16

39.57 Repair of blood vessel with synthetic patch graft
EXCLUDES *that with resection (38.40-38.49)*

39.58 Repair of blood vessel with unspecified type of patch graft
EXCLUDES *that with resection (38.40-38.49)*

39.59 Other repair of vessel
Aorticopulmonary window operation
Arterioplasty NOS
Construction of venous valves (peripheral)
Plication of vein (peripheral)
Reimplantation of artery
Code also cardiopulmonary bypass [extracorporeal circulation] [heart-lung machine] (39.61)
EXCLUDES *interruption of the vena cava (38.7)*
      reimplantation of renal artery (39.55)
      that with:
        graft (39.56-39.58)
        resection (38.30-38.49, 38.60-38.69)
DEF: Aorticopulmonary window operation: Repair of abnormal opening between major heart arterial vessel above valves and pulmonary artery.
DEF: Construction of venous valves (peripheral): Reconstruction of valves within peripheral veins.
DEF: Plication of vein (peripheral): Shortening of peripheral vein.
DEF: Reimplantation of artery: Reinsertion of artery into its normal position.
AHA: 4Q, '93, 31; 2Q, '89, 17; N-D, '86, 8; S-O, '85, 5; M-A, '85, 15

✓4ᵗʰ 39.6 Extracorporeal circulation and procedures auxiliary to heart surgery
AHA: 1Q, '95, 5

39.61 Extracorporeal circulation auxiliary to open heart surgery
Artificial heart and lung   Pump oxygenator
Cardiopulmonary bypass
EXCLUDES *extracorporeal hepatic assistance (50.92)*
      extracorporeal membrane oxygenation
        [ECMO] (39.65)
      hemodialysis (39.95)
      percutaneous cardiopulmonary bypass
        (39.66)
AHA: 3Q, '10, 6; 1Q, '10, 14; 2Q, '09, 8; 3Q, '08, 9; 2Q, '08, 13; 1Q, '04, 16; 3Q, '02, 5; 4Q, '97, 55; 3Q, '97, 14; 2Q, '97, 8; 2Q, '90, 24

39.62 Hypothermia (systemic) incidental to open heart surgery

39.63 Cardioplegia
Arrest:
    anoxic
    circulatory
DEF: Purposely inducing electromechanical cardiac arrest.

39.64 Intraoperative cardiac pacemaker
Temporary pacemaker used during and immediately following cardiac surgery
AHA: 1Q, '89, 2; M-J, '87, 3

39.65 Extracorporeal membrane oxygenation [ECMO]
EXCLUDES *extracorporeal circulation auxiliary to open heart surgery (39.61)*
      percutaneous cardiopulmonary bypass (39.66)
DEF: Creation of closed-chest, heart-lung bypass or Bard cardiopulmonary assist system with tube insertion.
AHA: 4Q, '11, 152; 2Q, '90, 23; 2Q, '89, 17; 4Q, '88, 5

39.66 Percutaneous cardiopulmonary bypass
Closed chest
EXCLUDES *extracorporeal circulation auxiliary to open heart surgery (39.61)*
      extracorporeal hepatic assistance (50.92)
      extracorporeal membrane oxygenation [ECMO] (39.65)
      hemodialysis (39.95)
DEF: Use of mechanical pump system to oxygenate and pump blood throughout the body via catheter in the femoral artery and vein.
AHA: 3Q, '96, 11

✓4ᵗʰ 39.7 Endovascular procedures on vessel(s)
Embolization   Occlusion
Endoluminal repair   Removal
Implantation   Repair
EXCLUDES *angioplasty of other non-coronary vessel(s) (39.50)*
      atherectomy of other non-coronary vessel(s) (17.56)
      insertion of non-drug-eluting peripheral vessel stent(s) (39.90)
      other repair of aneurysm (39.52)
      percutaneous insertion of carotid artery stent(s) (00.63)
      percutaneous insertion of intracranial stent(s) (00.65)
      percutaneous insertion of other precerebral artery stent(s) (00.64)
      resection of abdominal aorta with replacement (38.44)
      resection of lower limb arteries with replacement (38.48)
      resection of thoracic aorta with replacement (38.45)
      resection of upper limb vessels with replacement (38.43)
      temporary therapeutic partial occlusion of vessel (39.77)

Operations on the Cardiovascular System

39.71–39.78

Endovascular Repair of Abdominal Aortic Aneurysm

Renal arteries

Stent

Abdominal aortic aneurysm

Common iliac arteries

39.71 Endovascular implantation of other graft in abdominal aorta

Endovascular repair of abdominal aortic aneurysm with graft

Stent graft(s)

Code also intra-aneurysm sac pressure monitoring (intraoperative) (00.58)

EXCLUDES   *endovascular implantation of branching or fenestrated graft in aorta (39.78)*

DEF: Replacement of a section of abdominal aorta with mesh graft via catheters inserted through femoral arteries.

AHA: 1Q, '02, 13; 4Q, '00, 63, 64

39.72 Endovascular (total) embolization or occlusion of head and neck vessels

Coil-retention stent

Embolization stent

Endograft(s)

Endovascular graft(s)

Liquid tissue adhesive (glue) embolization or occlusion

Other implant or substance for repair, embolization or occlusion

That for repair of aneurysm, arteriovenous malformation [AVM] or fistula

EXCLUDES   *embolization of head or neck vessels using bare coils (39.75)*
     embolization of head or neck vessels using bioactive coils (39.76)
     mechanical thrombectomy of precerebral and cerebral vessels (39.74)

DEF: Coil embolization or occlusion: Utilizing x-ray guidance a neuro-microcatheter is guided from entry in the femoral artery in the groin to the site of the aneurysm of the head and neck vessels for delivery of micro-coils that stop blood flow to the arteriovenous malfomation (AVM).

AHA: 4Q, '02, 103

39.73 Endovascular implantation of graft in thoracic aorta

Endograft(s)

Endovascular graft(s)

Endovascular repair of defect of thoracic aorta with graft(s) or device(s)

Stent graft(s) or device(s)

That for repair of aneurysm, dissection, or injury

Code also intra-aneurysm sac pressure monitoring (intraoperative) (00.58)

EXCLUDES   *fenestration of dissecting aneurysm of thoracic aorta (39.54)*

DEF: Intravascular transcatheter deployment of an expanding stent-graft for repair of thoracic aortic aneurysm, performed without opening the chest.

AHA: 4Q, '05, 120

39.74 Endovascular removal of obstruction from head and neck vessel(s)

Endovascular embolectomy

Endovascular thrombectomy of pre-cerebral and cerebral vessels

Mechanical embolectomy or thrombectomy

Code also:

any injection or infusion of thrombolytic agent (99.10)

number of vessels treated (00.40-00.43)

procedure on vessel bifurcation (00.44)

EXCLUDES   *endarterectomy of intracranial vessels and other vessels of head and neck (38.11-38.12)*
     occlusive endovascular embolization of hea or neck vessels using bare coils (39.75
     occlusive endovascular embolization of hea or neck vessel(s) using bioactive coils (39.76)
     open embolectomy or thrombectomy (38.01-38.02)

AHA: 4Q, '06, 129

TIP: Mechanical thrombectomy represented by this code may also be documented as mechanical embolus remova in cerebral ischemia (MERCI®) extraction.

39.75 Endovascular embolization or occlusion of vessel(s) of head or neck using bare coils

Bare metal coils

Bare platinum coils [BPC]

That for treatment of aneurysm, arteriovenous malformation [AVM] or fistula

AHA: 4Q, '09, 145-146

39.76 Endovascular embolization or occlusion of vessel(s) of head or neck using bioactive coils

Biodegradable inner luminal polymer coils

Coil embolization or occlusion utilizing bioactive co

Coils containing polyglycolic acid [PGA]

That for treatment of aneurysm, arteriovenous malformation [AVM] or fistula

AHA: 4Q, '09, 145-146

DEF: Enhanced aneurysm treatment by deployment of co packed with novel polyglycol acid (PGA) or other bioactiv substance to improve healing response.

39.77 Temporary (partial) therapeutic endovascular occlusion of vessel

Includes that of aorta

That by balloon catheter

Code also any: diagnostic arteriogram (88.40-88.49)

EXCLUDES   *any endovascular head or neck vessel procedure (39.72, 39.74-39.76)*
     diagnostic procedures on blood vessels (38.21-38.29)
     permanent endovascular procedure (39.79

AHA: 4Q, '11, 176-178

39.78 Endovascular implantation of branching or fenestrated graft(s) in aorta

AHA: 4Q, '11, 176-178

DEF: A tubular, fabric graft with specialized reinforced openings allowing physicians to custom fit and position the stent into vessel branches or bifurcations at complex anatomic sites.

TIP: These grafts provide an option for patients who are n anatomical candidates for traditional AAA grafts.

BI Bilateral Procedure   NC Non-covered Procedure   LC Limited Coverage Procedure   ▶◀ Revised Text   ● New Code   ▲ Revised Code Tit

122 – Volume 3   2014 ICD-9-

39.79   **Other endovascular procedures on other vessels**
Endograft(s)
Endovascular graft(s)
Liquid tissue adhesive (glue) embolization or occlusion
Other coil embolization or occlusion
Other implant or substance for repair, embolization or occlusion
Repair of aneurysm

EXCLUDES   *abdominal aortic aneurysm resection [AAA] (38.44)*
endovascular implantation of graft in abdominal aorta (39.71)
endovascular implantation of graft in thoracic aorta (39.73)
endovascular embolization or occlusion of head and neck vessels, bare metal coils (39.75)
endovascular embolization or occlusion of head and neck vessels, bioactive coils (39.76)
insertion of drug-eluting peripheral vessel stent(s) (00.55)
insertion of non-drug-eluting peripheral vessel stent(s) (for other than aneurysm repair) (39.90)
non-endovascular repair of arteriovenous fistula (39.53)
other surgical occlusion of vessels — see category 38.8
percutaneous transcatheter infusion (99.29)
thoracic aortic aneurysm resection (38.45)
transcatheter embolization for gastric or duodenal bleeding (44.44)
uterine artery embolization with coils (68.24)

AHA: ▶2Q, '12, 15;◀4Q, '11, 138; 2Q, '10, 8-9; 1Q, '10, 21; 2Q, '09, 7-8; 2Q, '06, 22, 23; 4Q, '02, 103; 3Q, '01, 17,18; 4Q, '00, 64

☑4ᵗʰ **39.8**   **Operations on carotid body, carotid sinus and other vascular bodies**
AHA: 4Q, '10,121-124; 2Q, '07, 8

39.81   **Implantation or replacement of carotid sinus stimulation device, total system**
INCLUDES   carotid explorations
Carotid sinus baroreflex activation device
Implantation of carotid sinus stimulator and lead(s)

EXCLUDES   *implantation or replacement of carotid sinus stimulation lead(s) only (39.82)*
implantation or replacement of carotid sinus stimulation pulse generator only (39.83)

DEF: A surgically implantable medical device that electrically activates the baroreflex; the system that helps regulate cardiovascular function to treat primary hypertension and hypertensive heart failure recalcitrant to medical therapy.
TIP: Assign for insertion of the Rheos Baroreflex Hypertension Therapy System.

39.82   **Implantation or replacement of carotid sinus stimulation lead(s) only**
EXCLUDES   *implantation or replacement of carotid sinus stimulation device, total system (39.81)*

39.83   **Implantation or replacement of carotid sinus stimulation pulse generator only**
EXCLUDES   *implantation or replacement of carotid sinus stimulation device, total system (39.81)*

AHA: 4Q, '10, 125

39.84   **Revision of carotid sinus stimulation lead(s) only**
Repair of electrode [removal with re-insertion]
Repositioning of lead(s) [electrode]
AHA: 4Q, '10, 121-124

39.85   **Revision of carotid sinus stimulation pulse generator**
Debridement and reforming pocket (skin and subcutaneous tissue)
Relocation of pocket [creation of new pocket]
Repositioning of pulse generator
Revision of carotid sinus stimulation pulse generator pocket

39.86   **Removal of carotid sinus stimulation device, total system**

39.87   **Removal of carotid sinus stimulation lead(s) only**

39.88   **Removal of carotid sinus stimulation pulse generator only**

39.89   **Other operations on carotid body, carotid sinus and other vascular bodies**
Chemodectomy
Denervation of:
aortic body
carotid body
Glomectomy, carotid
EXCLUDES   *excision of glomus jugulare (20.51)*
DEF: Chemodectomy: Removal of a chemoreceptor vascular body.
DEF: Denervation of aortic body: Destruction of nerves attending the major heart blood vessels.
DEF: Denervation of carotid body: Destruction of nerves of carotid artery.
DEF: Glomectomy, carotid: Removal of the carotid artery framework.

☑4ᵗʰ **39.9**   **Other operations on vessels**

39.90   **Insertion of non-drug-eluting peripheral (non-coronary) vessel stent(s)**
Bare stent(s)
Bonded stent(s)
Drug-coated stent(s), i.e., heparin coated
Endograft(s)
Endovascular graft(s)
Endovascular recanalization techniques
Stent graft(s)
Code also any:
non-coronary angioplasty or atherectomy (39.50)
number of vascular stents inserted (00.45-00.48)
number of vessels treated (00.40-00.43)
procedure on vessel bifurcation (00.44)
EXCLUDES   *insertion of drug-eluting, peripheral vessel stent(s) (00.55)*
percutaneous insertion of carotid artery stent(s) (00.63)
percutaneous insertion of intracranial stent(s) (00.65)
percutaneous insertion of other precerebral artery stent(s) (00.64)
that for aneurysm repair (39.71-39.79)

AHA: ▶3Q, '12, 13;◀3Q, '09, 13; 4Q, '06, 119; 4Q, '02, 101; 1Q, '00, 12; 4Q, '96, 63

39.91   **Freeing of vessel**
Dissection and freeing of adherent tissue:
artery-vein-nerve bundle
vascular bundle
AHA: 3Q, '02, 12

39.92   **Injection of sclerosing agent into vein**
EXCLUDES   *injection:*
esophageal varices (42.33)
hemorrhoids (49.42)
AHA: 2Q, '92, 17

Operations on the Cardiovascular System

39.79-39.92

Operations on the Cardiovascular System

External Arteriovenous Shunt

Cephalic vein

Radial artery

39.93　Insertion of vessel-to-vessel cannula

Formation of:

arteriovenous:
  fistula　　⎫
  shunt　　 ⎬ by external cannula

Code also any renal dialysis (39.95)

AHA: 3Q, '88, 13; S-O, '85, 5, 12

TIP: If the AV fistula or shunt catheter or device is considered totally implantable, assign instead 86.07.

39.94　Replacement of vessel-to-vessel cannula

Revision of vessel-to-vessel cannula

39.95　Hemodialysis

Artificial kidney　　　Hemofiltration
Hemodiafiltration　　Renal dialysis

EXCLUDES *peritoneal dialysis (54.98)*

DEF: Filtration process to treat acute and chronic renal failure by eliminating toxic end products of nitrogen metabolism from blood.

AHA: 2Q, '11, 6; 4Q, '08, 193; 3Q, '07, 9; 1Q, '04, 22; 4Q, '03, 111; 2Q, '01, 2-14; 4Q, '00, 40; 2Q, '98, 20; S-O, '86, 11

39.96　Total body perfusion

Code also substance perfused (99.21-99.29)

39.97　Other perfusion

Perfusion NOS
Perfusion, local [regional] of:
  carotid artery
  coronary artery
  head
  lower limb
  neck
  upper limb

Code also substance perfused (99.21-99.29)

EXCLUDES *perfusion of:*
  kidney (55.95)
  large intestine (46.96)
  liver (50.93)
  small intestine (46.95)
  SuperSaturated oxygen
    therapy (00.49)

AHA: 3Q, '96, 11

39.98　Control of hemorrhage, not otherwise specified

Angiotripsy
Control of postoperative hemorrhage NOS
Venotripsy

EXCLUDES *control of hemorrhage (postoperative):*
  anus (49.95)
  bladder (57.93)
  following vascular procedure (39.41)
  nose (21.00-21.09)
  prostate (60.94)
  tonsil (28.7)
  that by:
    ligation (38.80-38.89)
    suture (39.30-39.32)

DEF: Angiotripsy: Clamping of tissue to stop arterial blood flow.

DEF: Venotripsy: Clamping of tissue to stop venous blood flow.

AHA: ▶2Q, '12, 10◀

39.99　Other operations on vessels

EXCLUDES *injection or infusion of therapeutic or*
    prophylactic substance (99.11-99.29,
  transfusion of blood and blood component
    (99.01-99.09)

AHA: 1Q, '89, 11

TIP: Assign for removal of a vena cava filter via percutaneous transluminal approach via the jugular vein.

BI Bilateral Procedure　　NC Non-covered Procedure　　LC Limited Coverage Procedure　　▶◀ Revised Text　　● New Code　　▲ Revised Code Titl

124 – Volume 3 • February 2013　　　　　　　　　　　　　　　　　　　　　　　　　　　　　　　　　　2014 ICD-9-C

8. Operations on the Hemic and Lymphatic Systems (40-41)

√3rd 40   **Operations on lymphatic system**

40.0   **Incision of lymphatic structures**

√4th 40.1   **Diagnostic procedures on lymphatic structures**

40.11   **Biopsy of lymphatic structure**

Transbronchoscopic needle aspiration [TBNA] of lymph node

AHA: 3Q, '10, 9; 4Q, '09, 74; 4Q, '08, 91

40.19   **Other diagnostic procedures on lymphatic structures**

EXCLUDES   *lymphangiogram:*
    abdominal (88.04)
    cervical (87.08)
    intrathoracic (87.34)
    lower limb (88.36)
    upper limb (88.34)
    microscopic examination of specimen
      (90.71-90.79)
    radioisotope scan (92.16)
    thermography (88.89)

√4th 40.2   **Simple excision of lymphatic structure**

EXCLUDES   *biopsy of lymphatic structure (40.11)*

DEF: Removal of lymphatic structure only.

40.21   **Excision of deep cervical lymph node**

AHA: 4Q, '99, 16

40.22   **Excision of internal mammary lymph node**

40.23   **Excision of axillary lymph node**

AHA: ▶2Q, '12, 4;◀ 2Q, '02, 7

40.24   **Excision of inguinal lymph node**

40.29   **Simple excision of other lymphatic structure**

Excision of:
    cystic hygroma
    lymphangioma
Simple lymphadenectomy

DEF: Lymphangioma: Removal of benign congenital lymphatic malformation.
DEF: Simple lymphadenectomy: Removal of lymph node.
AHA: 1Q, '99, 6

40.3   **Regional lymph node excision**

Extended regional lymph node excision
Regional lymph node excision with excision of lymphatic drainage area including skin, subcutaneous tissue, and fat

DEF: Extended regional lymph node excision: Removal of lymph node group, including area around nodes.
AHA:1Q, '12, 9; 2Q, '92, 7
TIP: Assign for "selective neck dissection."

√4th 40.4   **Radical excision of cervical lymph nodes**

Resection of cervical lymph nodes down to muscle and deep fascia

EXCLUDES   *that associated with radical laryngectomy (30.4)*

TIP: Assign a code from this subcategory for procedures described as modified radical neck dissection.

40.40   **Radical neck dissection, not otherwise specified**

40.41   **Radical neck dissection, unilateral**

AHA: 2Q, '05, 8; 2Q, '99, 6
DEF: Total dissection of cervical lymph nodes on one side of neck.

40.42   **Radical neck dissection, bilateral**

DEF: Total dissection of cervical lymph nodes on both sides of neck.

√4th 40.5   **Radical excision of other lymph nodes**

EXCLUDES   *that associated with radical mastectomy (85.45-85.48)*

40.50   **Radical excision of lymph nodes, not otherwise specified**

Radical (lymph) node dissection NOS

40.51   **Radical excision of axillary lymph nodes**

40.52   **Radical excision of periaortic lymph nodes**

40.53   **Radical excision of iliac lymph nodes**

40.54   **Radical groin dissection**

40.59   **Radical excision of other lymph nodes**

EXCLUDES   *radical neck dissection (40.40-40.42)*

√4th 40.6   **Operations on thoracic duct**

40.61   **Cannulation of thoracic duct**

DEF: Placement of cannula in main lymphatic duct of chest.

40.62   **Fistulization of thoracic duct**

DEF: Creation of passage in main lymphatic duct of chest.

40.63   **Closure of fistula of thoracic duct**

DEF: Closure of fistula in main lymphatic duct of chest.

40.64   **Ligation of thoracic duct**

DEF: Tying off main lymphatic duct of chest.

40.69   **Other operations on thoracic duct**

40.9   **Other operations on lymphatic structures**

Anastomosis
Dilation
Ligation
Obliteration   } of peripheral lymphatics
Reconstruction
Repair
Transplantation

Correction of lymphedema of limb, NOS

EXCLUDES   *reduction of elephantiasis of scrotum (61.3)*

√3rd 41   **Operations on bone marrow and spleen**

√4th 41.0   **Bone marrow or hematopoietic stem cell transplant**

NOTE To report donor source — see codes 00.91-00.93
EXCLUDES   *aspiration of bone marrow from donor (41.91)*
AHA: 4Q, '00, 64; 1Q, '91, 3; 4Q, '91, 26

41.00   **Bone marrow transplant, not otherwise specified**

[8] **41.01**   **Autologous bone marrow transplant without purging**   `NC`

EXCLUDES   *that with purging (41.09)*
DEF: Transplant of patient's own bone marrow.

[9] **41.02**   **Allogeneic bone marrow transplant with purging**   `NC`

Allograft of bone marrow with in vitro removal (purging) of T-cells
DEF: Transplant of bone marrow from donor to patient after donor marrow purged of undesirable cells.

[9] **41.03**   **Allogeneic bone marrow transplant without purging**   `NC`

Allograft of bone marrow NOS

[8] **41.04**   **Autologous hematopoietic stem cell transplant without purging**   `NC`

EXCLUDES   *that with purging (41.07)*
AHA: 4Q, '94, 52

[9] **41.05**   **Allogeneic hematopoietic stem cell transplant without purging**   `NC`

EXCLUDES   *that with purging (41.08)*
AHA: 1Q, '11, 24; 1Q, '09, 9; 4Q, '97, 55

41.06   **Cord blood stem cell transplant**

AHA: 4Q, '97, 56

[8] **41.07**   **Autologous hematopoietic stem cell transplant with purging**   `NC`

Cell depletion
AHA: 2Q, '06, 20-22
TIP: Assign for autologous peripheral blood stem cell boost reinfusion.

[9] **41.08**   **Allogeneic hematopoietic stem cell transplant with purging**   `NC`

Cell depletion

[8] **41.09**   **Autologous bone marrow transplant with purging**   `NC`

With extracorporeal purging of malignant cells from marrow
Cell depletion

---

[8] Noncovered procedure only when the following diagnoses are present as either principal or secondary diagnosis: 204.00, 205.00, 205.10, 205.11, 206.00, 207.00, 208.00
[9] Noncovered procedure only when the following diagnoses are present as either principal or secondary diagnosis: 203.00, 203.01

Additional Digit Required	Valid OR Procedure	Non-OR Procedure	Adjunct Code

Operations on the Hemic and Lymphatic Systems

41.1–41.99

Partial Splenectomy

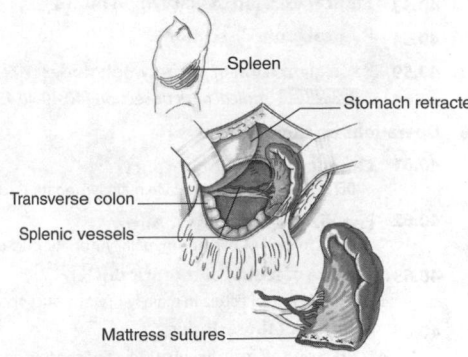

Spleen

Stomach retracted

Transverse colon

Splenic vessels

Mattress sutures

Total Splenectomy

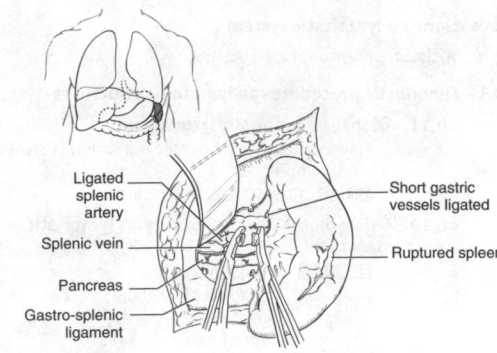

Ligated splenic artery

Splenic vein

Pancreas

Gastro-splenic ligament

Short gastric vessels ligated

Ruptured spleen

41.1   **Puncture of spleen**
> *EXCLUDES*   *aspiration biopsy of spleen (41.32)*

41.2   **Splenotomy**

√4ᵗʰ **41.3**   **Diagnostic procedures on bone marrow and spleen**

    41.31   **Biopsy of bone marrow**

    41.32   **Closed [aspiration] [percutaneous] biopsy of spleen**
       Needle biopsy of spleen

    41.33   **Open biopsy of spleen**

    41.38   **Other diagnostic procedures on bone marrow**
> *EXCLUDES*   *microscopic examination of specimen from bone marrow (90.61-90.69)*
> *radioisotope scan (92.05)*

    41.39   **Other diagnostic procedures on spleen**
> *EXCLUDES*   *microscopic examination of specimen from spleen (90.61-90.69)*
> *radioisotope scan (92.05)*

√4ᵗʰ **41.4**   **Excision or destruction of lesion or tissue of spleen**
     Code also any application or administration of an adhesion barrier substance (99.77)
> *EXCLUDES*   *excision of accessory spleen (41.93)*

    41.41   **Marsupialization of splenic cyst**
       DEF: Incision of cyst of spleen with edges sutured open to create pouch.

    41.42   **Excision of lesion or tissue of spleen**
> *EXCLUDES*   *biopsy of spleen (41.32-41.33)*

    41.43   **Partial splenectomy**
       DEF: Partial removal of spleen.

41.5   **Total splenectomy**
     Splenectomy NOS
     Code also any application or administration of an adhesion barrier substance (99.77)

√4ᵗʰ **41.9**   **Other operations on spleen and bone marrow**
     Code also any application or administration of an adhesion barrier substance (99.77)

    41.91   **Aspiration of bone marrow from donor for transplant**
> *EXCLUDES*   *biopsy of bone marrow (41.31)*
       AHA: 1Q, '91, 3

    41.92   **Injection into bone marrow**
> *EXCLUDES*   *bone marrow transplant (41.00-41.03)*
       AHA: 3Q, '96, 17
       TIP: Assign for intraosseous IV access, performed emergently for a dehydrated infant whose peripheral vein cannot be accessed.

    41.93   **Excision of accessory spleen**

    41.94   **Transplantation of spleen**

    41.95   **Repair and plastic operations on spleen**

    41.98   **Other operations on bone marrow**
       AHA: 2Q, '11, 10; 3Q, '08, 19

    41.99   **Other operations on spleen**

BI Bilateral Procedure   **NC** Non-covered Procedure   **LC** Limited Coverage Procedure   ▶◀ Revised Text   ● New Code   ▲ Revised Code Title

126 – Volume 3   **2014 ICD-9-CM**

9. Operations on the Digestive System (42-54)

✓3rd **42 Operations on esophagus**

✓4th **42.0 Esophagotomy**

42.01 Incision of esophageal web

DEF: Cutting into congenital esophageal membrane.

42.09 Other incision of esophagus

Esophagotomy NOS

EXCLUDES esophagomyotomy (42.7)
esophagostomy (42.10-42.19)

✓4th **42.1 Esophagostomy**

42.10 Esophagostomy, not otherwise specified

42.11 Cervical esophagostomy

DEF: Creation of opening into upper region of esophagus.

42.12 Exteriorization of esophageal pouch

DEF: Transfer of section of esophageal pouch to exterior of the body.

42.19 Other external fistulization of esophagus

Thoracic esophagostomy

Code also any resection (42.40-42.42)

✓4th **42.2 Diagnostic procedures on esophagus**

42.21 Operative esophagoscopy by incision

DEF: Esophageal examination with an endoscope through incision.

42.22 Esophagoscopy through artificial stoma

EXCLUDES that with biopsy (42.24)

42.23 Other esophagoscopy

EXCLUDES that with biopsy (42.24)

AHA: 1Q, '00, 20; 3Q, '98, 11

TIP: Two codes may be assigned to report transesophageal echocardiography (TEE): 88.72 for the diagnostic radiology portion of the procedure and 42.23 for the endoscopic approach.

42.24 Closed [endoscopic] biopsy of esophagus

Brushing or washing for specimen collection
Esophagoscopy with biopsy
Suction biopsy of the esophagus

EXCLUDES esophagogastroduodenoscopy [EGD] with closed biopsy (45.16)

DEF: Scope passed through mouth and throat to obtain biopsy specimen, usually by brushing and swabbing.

42.25 Open biopsy of esophagus

42.29 Other diagnostic procedures on esophagus

EXCLUDES barium swallow (87.61)
esophageal manometry (89.32)
microscopic examination of specimen from esophagus (90.81-90.89)

AHA: 3Q, '96, 12

✓4th **42.3 Local excision or destruction of lesion or tissue of esophagus**

42.31 Local excision of esophageal diverticulum

42.32 Local excision of other lesion or tissue of esophagus

EXCLUDES biopsy of esophagus (42.24-42.25)
esophageal fistulectomy (42.84)

42.33 Endoscopic excision or destruction of lesion or tissue of esophagus

Ablation of esophageal neoplasm
Control of esophageal bleeding } by endoscopic approach
Esophageal polypectomy
Espohageal varices
Injection of esophageal varies

EXCLUDES biopsy of esophagus (42.24-42.25)
fistulectomy (42.84)
open ligation of esophageal varices (42.91)

AHA: ▶4Q, '12, 85◀

TIP: Assign for endoscopic sclerotherapy for bleeding esophageal varices.

42.39 Other destruction of lesion or tissue of esophagus

EXCLUDES that by endoscopic approach (42.33)

✓4th **42.4 Excision of esophagus**

EXCLUDES esophagogastrectomy NOS 43.99)

42.40 Esophagectomy, not otherwise specified

42.41 Partial esophagectomy

Code also any synchronous:
anastomosis other than end-to-end (42.51-42.69)
esophagostomy (42.10-42.19)
gastrostomy (43.11-43.19)

DEF: Surgical removal of any part of esophagus.

42.42 Total esophagectomy

Code also any synchronous:
gastrostomy (43.11-43.19)
interposition or anastomosis other than end-to-end (42.51-42.69)

EXCLUDES esophagogastrectomy (43.99)

AHA: 4Q, '88, 11

DEF: Surgical removal of entire esophagus.

✓4th **42.5 Intrathoracic anastomosis of esophagus**

Code also any synchronous:
esophagectomy (42.40-42.42)
gastrostomy (43.1)

DEF: Connection of esophagus to conduit within chest.

42.51 Intrathoracic esophagoesophagostomy

DEF: Connection of both ends of esophagus within chest cavity.

42.52 Intrathoracic esophagogastrostomy

DEF: Connection of esophagus to stomach within chest; follows esophagogastrectomy.

42.53 Intrathoracic esophageal anastomosis with interposition of small bowel

42.54 Other intrathoracic esophagoenterostomy

Anastomosis of esophagus to intestinal segment NOS

42.55 Intrathoracic esophageal anastomosis with interposition of colon

42.56 Other intrathoracic esophagocolostomy

Esophagocolostomy NOS

42.58 Intrathoracic esophageal anastomosis with other interposition

Construction of artificial esophagus
Retrosternal formation of reversed gastric tube

DEF: Retrosternal anastomosis of reversed gastric tube: Formation of gastric tube behind breastbone.

42.59 Other intrathoracic anastomosis of esophagus

AHA: 4Q, '88, 11

✓4th **42.6 Antesternal anastomosis of esophagus**

Code also any synchronous:
esophagectomy (42.40-42.42)
gastrostomy (43.1)

42.61 Antesternal esophagoesophagostomy

42.62 Antesternal esophagogastrostomy

42.63 Antesternal esophageal anastomosis with interposition of small bowel

42.64 Other antesternal esophagoenterostomy

Antethoracic:
esophagoenterostomy
esophagoileostomy
esophagojejunostomy

42.65 Antesternal esophageal anastomosis with interposition of colon

DEF: Connection of esophagus with colon segment.

42.66 Other antesternal esophagocolostomy

Antethoracic esophagocolostomy

42.68 Other antesternal esophageal anastomosis with interposition

42.69 Other antesternal anastomosis of esophagus

42.7 Esophagomyotomy

DEF: Division of esophageal muscle, usually distal.

Operations on the Digestive System

42.8–43.99

√4ᵗʰ **42.8**   **Other repair of esophagus**

     42.81   **Insertion of permanent tube into esophagus**
           AHA: 1Q, '97, 15

     42.82   **Suture of laceration of esophagus**

     42.83   **Closure of esophagostomy**

     42.84   **Repair of esophageal fistula, not elsewhere classified**
           EXCLUDES   *repair of fistula:*
                     bronchoesophageal (33.42)
                     esophagopleurocutaneous (34.73)
                     pharyngoesophageal (29.53)
                     tracheoesophageal (31.73)

     42.85   **Repair of esophageal stricture**

     42.86   **Production of subcutaneous tunnel without esophageal anastomosis**
           DEF: Surgical formation of esophageal passage, without cutting, and reconnection.

     42.87   **Other graft of esophagus**
           EXCLUDES   *antesternal esophageal anastomosis with interposition of:*
                     colon (42.65)
                     small bowel (42.63)
                   antesternal esophageal anastomosis with other interposition (42.68)
                   intrathoracic esophageal anastomosis with interposition of:
                     colon (42.55)
                     small bowel (42.53)
                   intrathoracic esophageal anastomosis with other interposition (42.58)

     42.89   **Other repair of esophagus**

√4ᵗʰ **42.9**   **Other operations on esophagus**

     42.91   **Ligation of esophageal varices**
           EXCLUDES   *that by endoscopic approach (42.33)*
           DEF: Destruction of dilated veins by suture strangulation.

     42.92   **Dilation of esophagus**
           Dilation of cardiac sphincter
           EXCLUDES   *intubation of esophagus (96.03, 96.06-96.08)*
           DEF: Passing of balloon or hydrostatic dilators through esophagus to enlarge esophagus and relieve obstruction.

     42.99   **Other**
           EXCLUDES   *insertion of Sengstaken tube (96.06)*
                   intubation of esophagus (96.03, 96.06-96.08)
                   removal of intraluminal foreign body from esophagus without incision (98.02)
                   tamponade of esophagus (96.06)

√3ʳᵈ **43**   **Incision and excision of stomach**
     Code also any application or administration of an adhesion barrier substance (99.77)

     43.0   **Gastrotomy**
           EXCLUDES   *gastrostomy (43.11-43.19)*
                   that for control of hemorrhage (44.49)
           AHA: 3Q, '89, 14

√4ᵗʰ **43.1**   **Gastrostomy**
           AHA: S-O, '85, 5

     43.11   **Percutaneous [endoscopic] gastrostomy [PEG]**
           Percutaneous transabdominal gastrostomy
           DEF: Endoscopic positioning of tube through abdominal wall into stomach.

     43.19   **Other gastrostomy**
           EXCLUDES   *percutaneous [endoscopic] gastrostomy [PEG] (43.11)*
           AHA: ▶2Q, '12, 6;◀ 1Q, '92, 14; 3Q, '89, 14
           TIP: ▶Do not report gastropexy suture of the stomach to the fascia separately when performed as an inherent part of gastrostomy to prevent leakage.◀

     43.3   **Pyloromyotomy**
           DEF: Cutting into longitudinal and circular muscular membrane between stomach and small intestine.

Partial Gastrectomy with Anastomosis to Duodenum

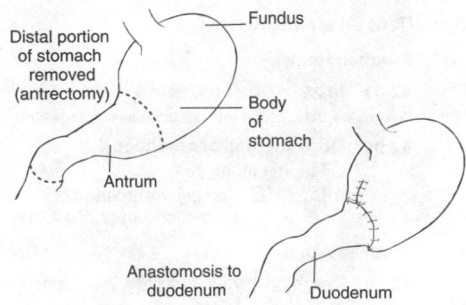

√4ᵗʰ **43.4**   **Local excision or destruction of lesion or tissue of stomach**

     43.41   **Endoscopic excision or destruction of lesion or tissue of stomach**
           Gastric polypectomy by endoscopic approach
           Gastric varices by endoscopic approach
           EXCLUDES   *biopsy of stomach (44.14-44.15)*
                   control of hemorrhage (44.43)
                   open ligation of gastric varices (44.91)
           AHA: 3Q, '96, 10

     43.42   **Local excision of other lesion or tissue of stomach**
           EXCLUDES   *biopsy of stomach (44.14-44.15)*
                   gastric fistulectomy (44.62-44.63)
                   partial gastrectomy (43.5-43.89)

     43.49   **Other destruction of lesion or tissue of stomach**
           EXCLUDES   *that by endoscopic approach (43.41)*
           AHA: N-D, '87, 5; S-O, '85, 6

     43.5   **Partial gastrectomy with anastomosis to esophagus**
           Proximal gastrectomy

     43.6   **Partial gastrectomy with anastomosis to duodenum**
           Billroth I operation   Gastropylorectomy
           Distal gastrectomy

     43.7   **Partial gastrectomy with anastomosis to jejunum**
           Billroth II operation
           AHA: 3Q, '03, 7

√4ᵗʰ **43.8**   **Other partial gastrectomy**

     43.81   **Partial gastrectomy with jejunal transposition**
           Henley jejunal transposition operation
           Code also any synchronous intestinal resection (45.51)

     43.82   **Laparoscopic vertical (sleeve) gastrectomy**
           EXCLUDES   *laparoscopic banding (44.95)*
                   laparoscopic gastric restrictive procedure (44.95)
           DEF: Removal of the majority of the stomach, the greater curvature, resulting in a long vertical shape with preservation of the pyloric valve and nerves of the stomach.
           AHA: 4Q, '11, 178-179
           TIP: This procedure requires no intestinal bypass or artificial device (such as the lap band), thereby reducing risk of dumping syndrome, intestinal obstruction, or other complications.

     43.89   **Open and other partial gastrectomy**
           Partial gastrectomy with bypass gastrogastrostomy
           Sleeve resection of stomach
           EXCLUDES   *laparoscopic sleeve gastrectomy (43.82)*
           AHA: 3Q, '03, 6-8

√4ᵗʰ **43.9**   **Total gastrectomy**

     43.91   **Total gastrectomy with intestinal interposition**

     43.99   **Other total gastrectomy**
           Complete gastroduodenectomy
           Esophagoduodenostomy with complete gastrectomy
           Esophagogastrectomy NOS
           Esophagojejunostomy with complete gastrectomy
           Radical gastrectomy

BI Bilateral Procedure   **NC** Non-covered Procedure   **LC** Limited Coverage Procedure   ▶◀ Revised Text   ● New Code   ▲ Revised Code Title

128 – Volume 3 • February 2013   2014 ICD-9-C

Biliopancreatic Diversion Without Duodenal Switch

Biliopancreatic Diversion with Duodenal Switch

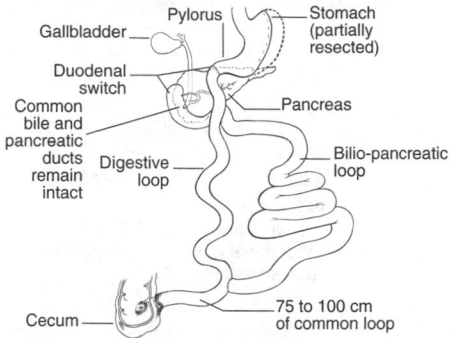

Types of Vagotomy Procedures

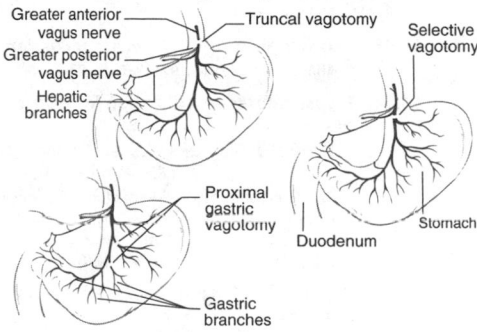

Roux-en-Y Operation (Gastrojejunostomy without gastrectomy)

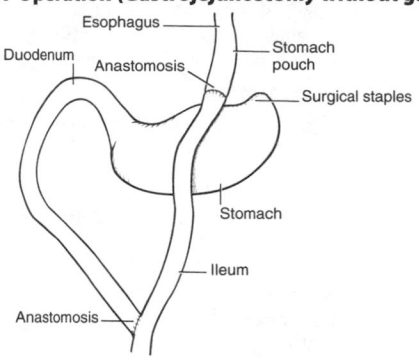

√3ʳᵈ **44   Other operations on stomach**

Code also any application or administration of an adhesion barrier substance (99.77)

√4ᵗʰ **44.0   Vagotomy**

44.00   Vagotomy, not otherwise specified

Division of vagus nerve NOS

DEF: Cutting of vagus nerve to reduce acid production.

44.01   Truncal vagotomy

DEF: Surgical removal of vagus nerve segment near stomach branches.

44.02   Highly selective vagotomy

Parietal cell vagotomy

Selective proximal vagotomy

DEF: Cutting select gastric branches of vagus nerve to reduce acid production and preserve other nerve functions.

44.03   Other selective vagotomy

√4ᵗʰ **44.1   Diagnostic procedures on stomach**

44.11   Transabdominal gastroscopy

Intraoperative gastroscopy

EXCLUDES *that with biopsy (44.14)*

44.12   Gastroscopy through artificial stoma

EXCLUDES *that with biopsy (44.14)*

44.13   Other gastroscopy

EXCLUDES *that with biopsy (44.14)*

AHA: 1Q, '88, 15; N-D, '87, 5

44.14   Closed [endoscopic] biopsy of stomach

Brushing or washing for specimen collection

EXCLUDES *esophagogastroduodenoscopy [EGD] with closed biopsy (45.16)*

AHA: 1Q, '88, 15; N-D, '87, 5

44.15   Open biopsy of stomach

44.19   Other diagnostic procedures on stomach

EXCLUDES *gastric lavage (96.33)*

microscopic examination of specimen from stomach (90.81-90.89)

upper GI series (87.62)

√4ᵗʰ **44.2   Pyloroplasty**

44.21   Dilation of pylorus by incision

DEF: Cutting and suturing pylorus to relieve obstruction.

44.22   Endoscopic dilation of pylorus

Dilation with balloon endoscope

Endoscopic dilation of gastrojejunostomy site

AHA: 2Q, '01, 17

TIP: Assign for stent placement across an extrinsic obstruction of a gastrojejunostomy.

44.29   Other pyloroplasty

Pyloroplasty NOS   Revision of pylorus

AHA: 3Q, '99, 3

√4ᵗʰ **44.3   Gastroenterostomy without gastrectomy**

44.31   High gastric bypass

Printen and Mason gastric bypass

DEF: Connection of middle part of small intestine to upper stomach to divert food passage from upper intestine.

AHA: M J, '85, 17

44.32   Percutaneous (endoscopic) gastrojejunostomy

Bypass: PEGJJ

gastroduodenostomy

EXCLUDES *percutaneous (endoscopic) feeding jejunostomy (46.32)*

DEF: Percutaneous insertion of an endoscopically guided gastrostomy tube that provides an artificial opening into the gastric lumen and portion of the jejunum via the exterior abdominal wall.

44.38   Laparoscopic gastroenterostomy

Bypass:

gastroduodenostomy

gastroenterostomy

gastrogastrostomy

Laparoscopic gastrojejunostomy without gastrectomy NEC

EXCLUDES *gastroenterostomy, open approach (44.39)*

44.39   Other gastroenterostomy

Bypass: Bypass:

gastroduodenostomy   gastrogastrostomy

gastroenterostomy

Gastrojejunostomy without gastrectomy NOS

AHA: 3Q, '03, 6; 1Q, '01, 16, 17

√4ᵗʰ **44.4   Control of hemorrhage and suture of ulcer of stomach or duodenum**

44.40   Suture of peptic ulcer, not otherwise specified

44.41   Suture of gastric ulcer site

EXCLUDES *ligation of gastric varices (44.91)*

Operations on the Digestive System

44.42–45.12

44.42   **Suture of duodenal ulcer site** ◀
AHA: J-F, '87, 11

44.43   **Endoscopic control of gastric or duodenal bleeding**
AHA: 2Q, '04, 12; 2Q, '92, 17; N-D, '87, 4

44.44   **Transcatheter embolization for gastric or duodenal bleeding**
EXCLUDES   *surgical occlusion of abdominal vessels (38.86-38.87)*
DEF: Therapeutic blocking of stomach or upper small intestine blood vessel to stop hemorrhaging; accomplished by introducing various substances using a catheter.
AHA: 2Q, '11, 11; 1Q, '88, 15; N-D, '87, 4

44.49   **Other control of hemorrhage of stomach or duodenum**
That with gastrotomy

44.5   **Revision of gastric anastomosis**
Closure of: Closure of:
   gastric anastomosis   gastrojejunostomy
   gastroduodenostomy   Pantaloon operation

√4ᵗʰ **44.6**   **Other repair of stomach**

44.61   **Suture of laceration of stomach**
EXCLUDES   *that of ulcer site (44.41)*

44.62   **Closure of gastrostomy**

44.63   **Closure of other gastric fistula**
Closure of:
   gastrocolic fistula
   gastrojejunocolic fistula

44.64   **Gastropexy**
DEF: Suturing of stomach into position.
AHA: M-J, '85, 17

44.65   **Esophagogastroplasty**
Belsey operation
Esophagus and stomach cardioplasty
AHA: M-J, '85, 17

44.66   **Other procedures for creation of esophagogastric sphincteric competence**
Fundoplication
Gastric cardioplasty
Nissen's fundoplication
Restoration of cardio-esophageal angle
EXCLUDES   *that by laparoscopy (44.67)*
AHA: ▶3Q, '12, 6;◀ 2Q, '03, 12; 2Q, '01, 3, 5, 6; 3Q, '98, 10; M-J, '85, 17
TIP: ▶Do not assign a separate endoscopy code if performed by endoscopic approach.◀

44.67   **Laparoscopic procedures for creation of esophagogastric sphincteric competence**
Fundoplication
Gastric cardioplasty
Nissen's fundoplication
Restoration of cardio-esophageal angle

44.68   **Laparoscopic gastroplasty**
Banding
Silastic vertical banding
Vertical banded gastroplasty (VBG)
Code also any synchronous laparoscopic gastroenterostomy (44.38)
EXCLUDES   *insertion, laparoscopic adjustable gastric band (restrictive procedure) (44.95)*
other repair of stomach, open approach (44.61-44.65, 44.69)

44.69   **Other**
Inversion of gastric diverticulum
Repair of stomach NOS
DEF: Inversion of gastric diverticulum: Turning stomach inward to repair outpouch of wall.
AHA: 3Q, '03, 8; 2Q, '01, 3; 3Q, '99, 3; M-J, '85, 17; N-D, '84, 13

√4ᵗʰ **44.9**   **Other operations on stomach**

44.91   **Ligation of gastric varices**
EXCLUDES   *that by endoscopic approach (43.41)*
DEF: Destruction of dilated veins by suture or strangulation.

44.92   **Intraoperative manipulation of stomach**
Reduction of gastric volvulus

44.93   **Insertion of gastric bubble (balloon)**   NC

44.94   **Removal of gastric bubble (balloon)**

44.95   **Laparoscopic gastric restrictive procedure**
Adjustable gastric band and port insertion
EXCLUDES   *laparoscopic gastroplasty (44.68)*
other repair of stomach (44.69)

44.96   **Laparoscopic revision of gastric restrictive procedure**
Revision or replacement of:
   adjustable gastric band
   subcutaneous gastric port device

44.97   **Laparoscopic removal of gastric restrictive device(s)**
Removal of either or both:
   adjustable gastric band
   subcutaneous port device
EXCLUDES   *nonoperative removal of gastric restrictive device(s) (97.86)*
open removal of gastric restrictive device(s) (44.99)

44.98   **(Laparoscopic) adjustment of size of adjustable gastric restrictive device**
Infusion of saline for device tightening
Withdrawal of saline for device loosening
Code also any:
   abdominal ultrasound (88.76)
   abdominal wall fluoroscopy (88.09)
   barium swallow (87.61)

44.99   **Other**
EXCLUDES   *change of gastrostomy tube (97.02)*
dilation of cardiac sphincter (42.92)
gastric:
   cooling (96.31)
   freezing (96.32)
   gavage (96.35)
   hypothermia (96.31)
   lavage (96.33)
insertion of nasogastric tube (96.07)
irrigation of gastrostomy (96.36)
irrigation of nasogastric tube (96.34)
removal of:
   gastrostomy tube (97.51)
   intraluminal foreign body from stomach without incision (98.03)
replacement of:
   gastrostomy tube (97.02)
   (naso-)gastric tube (97.01)
AHA: 3Q, '04, 5

√3ʳᵈ **45**   **Incision, excision, and anastomosis of intestine**
Code also any application or administration of an adhesion barrier substance (99.77)

√4ᵗʰ **45.0**   **Enterotomy**
EXCLUDES   *duodenocholedochotomy (51.41-51.42, 51.51)*
that for destruction of lesion (45.30-45.34)
that of exteriorized intestine (46.14, 46.24, 46.31)

45.00   **Incision of intestine, not otherwise specified**

45.01   **Incision of duodenum**

45.02   **Other incision of small intestine**

45.03   **Incision of large intestine**
EXCLUDES   *proctotomy (48.0)*

√4ᵗʰ **45.1**   **Diagnostic procedures on small intestine**
Code also any laparotomy (54.11-54.19)

45.11   **Transabdominal endoscopy of small intestine**
Intraoperative endoscopy of small intestine
EXCLUDES   *that with biopsy (45.14)*
DEF: Endoscopic exam of small intestine through abdominal wall.
DEF: Intraoperative endoscope of small intestine: Endoscopic exam of small intestine during surgery.

45.12   **Endoscopy of small intestine through artificial stoma**
EXCLUDES   *that with biopsy (45.14)*
AHA: M-J, '85, 17

BI Bilateral Procedure   **NC** Non-covered Procedure   **LC** Limited Coverage Procedure   ▶◀ Revised Text   ● New Code   ▲ Revised Code Title

Esophagogastroduodenoscopy

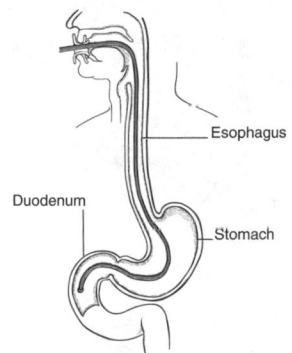

45.13   **Other endoscopy of small intestine**
Esophagogastroduodenoscopy [EGD]
EXCLUDES   *that with biopsy (45.14, 45.16)*
AHA: ▶4Q, '12, 83, 85;◀ 3Q, '04, 5; N-D, '87, 5

45.14   **Closed [endoscopic] biopsy of small intestine**
Brushing or washing for specimen collection
EXCLUDES   *esophagogastroduodenoscopy [EGD] with
closed biopsy (45.16)*

45.15   **Open biopsy of small intestine**
AHA: 2Q, '05, 12

45.16   **Esophagogastroduodenoscopy [EGD] with closed
biopsy**
Biopsy of one or more sites involving esophagus,
stomach, and/or duodenum
AHA: 3Q, '05, 17; 2Q, '01, 9

45.19   **Other diagnostic procedures on small intestine**
EXCLUDES   *microscopic examination of specimen from
small intestine (90.91-90.99)
radioisotope scan (92.04)
ultrasonography (88.74)
x-ray (87.61-87.69)*

√4ᵗʰ **45.2**   **Diagnostic procedures on large intestine**
Code also any laparotomy (54.11-54.19)

45.21   **Transabdominal endoscopy of large intestine**
Intraoperative endoscopy of large intestine
EXCLUDES   *that with biopsy (45.25)*
DEF: Endoscopic exam of large intestine through abdominal
wall.
DEF: Intraoperative endoscopy of large intestine:
Endoscopic exam of large intestine during surgery.

45.22   **Endoscopy of large intestine through artificial
stoma**
EXCLUDES   *that with biopsy (45.25)*
DEF: Endoscopic exam of large intestine lining from rectum
to cecum via colostomy stoma.

45.23   **Colonoscopy**
Flexible fiberoptic colonoscopy
EXCLUDES   *endoscopy of large intestine through
artificial stoma (45.22)
flexible sigmoidoscopy (45.24)
rigid proctosigmoidoscopy (48.23)
transabdominal endoscopy of large intestine
(45.21)*
DEF: Endoscopic exam of descending colon, splenic flexure,
transverse colon, hepatic flexure and cecum.
AHA: ▶3Q, '12, 23;◀ 3Q, '05, 17; S-O, '85, 5

45.24   **Flexible sigmoidoscopy**
Endoscopy of descending colon
EXCLUDES   *rigid proctosigmoidoscopy (48.23)*
DEF: Endoscopic exam of anus, rectum and sigmoid colon.

45.25   **Closed [endoscopic] biopsy of large intestine**
Biopsy, closed, of unspecified intestinal site
Brushing or washing for specimen collection
Colonoscopy with biopsy
EXCLUDES   *proctosigmoidoscopy with biopsy (48.24)*
AHA: 1Q, '03, 10

45.26   **Open biopsy of large intestine**

45.27   **Intestinal biopsy, site unspecified**

45.28   **Other diagnostic procedures on large intestine**

45.29   **Other diagnostic procedures on intestine, site
unspecified**
EXCLUDES   *microscopic examination of specimen
(90.91-90.99)
scan and radioisotope function study (92.04)
ultrasonography (88.74)
x-ray (87.61-87.69)*

√4ᵗʰ **45.3**   **Local excision or destruction of lesion or tissue of small
intestine**

45.30   **Endoscopic excision or destruction of lesion of
duodenum**
EXCLUDES   *biopsy of duodenum (45.14-45.15)
control of hemorrhage (44.43)
fistulectomy (46.72)*
AHA: 2Q, '11, 7

45.31   **Other local excision of lesion of duodenum**
EXCLUDES   *biopsy of duodenum (45.14-45.15)
fistulectomy (46.72)
multiple segmental resection (45.61)
that by endoscopic approach (45.30)*

45.32   **Other destruction of lesion of duodenum**
EXCLUDES   *that by endoscopic approach (45.30)*
AHA: N-D, '87, 5; S-O, '85, 6

45.33   **Local excision of lesion or tissue of small
intestine, except duodenum**
Excision of redundant mucosa of ileostomy
EXCLUDES   *biopsy of small intestine (45.14-45.15)
fistulectomy (46.74)
multiple segmental resection (45.61)*

45.34   **Other destruction of lesion of small
intestine, except duodenum**
AHA: ▶3Q, '12, 12;◀ 2Q, '11, 7
TIP: ▶Assign for endoscopic ablation of lesion of jejunum.◀

√4ᵗʰ **45.4**   **Local excision or destruction of lesion or tissue of large
intestine**
AHA: N-D, '87, 11

45.41   **Excision of lesion or tissue of large intestine**
Excision of redundant mucosa of colostomy
EXCLUDES   *biopsy of large intestine (45.25-45.27)
endoscopic polypectomy of large intestine
(45.42)
fistulectomy (46.76)
multiple segmental resection (17.31, 45.71)
that by endoscopic approach (45.42-45.43)*

45.42   **Endoscopic polypectomy of large intestine**
EXCLUDES   *that by open approach (45.41)*
DEF: Endoscopic removal of polyp from large intestine.
AHA: 2Q, '05, 16; 2Q, '90, 25

45.43   **Endoscopic destruction of other lesion or tissue of
large intestine**
Endoscopic ablation of tumor of large intestine
Endoscopic control of colonic bleeding
EXCLUDES   *endoscopic polypectomy of large intestine
(45.42)*
AHA: 4Q, '02, 61
TIP: Assign for endoscopic treatment of a Dieulafoy lesion of
the large intestine, regardless of technique.

45.49   **Other destruction of lesion of large intestine**
EXCLUDES   *that by endoscopic approach (45.43)*

√4ᵗʰ **45.5**   **Isolation of intestinal segment**
Code also any synchronous:
anastomosis other than end-to-end (45.90-45.94)
enterostomy (46.10-46.39)

45.50   **Isolation of intestinal segment, not
otherwise specified**
Isolation of intestinal pedicle flap
Reversal of intestinal segment
DEF: Isolation of small intestinal pedicle flap: Separation of
intestinal pedicle flap.
DEF: Reversal of intestinal segment: Separation of intestinal
segment.

√3ᵗʰ
√4ᵗʰ   Additional Digit Required   Valid OR Procedure   Non-OR Procedure   Adjunct Code

45.51 **Isolation of segment of small intestine**
Isolation of ileal loop
Resection of small intestine for interposition
AHA: 2Q, '05, 12; 3Q, '03, 6-8; 2Q, '03, 11; 3Q, '00, 7

45.52 **Isolation of segment of large intestine**
Resection of colon for interposition

✓4ᵗʰ **45.6** **Other excision of small intestine**
Code also any synchronous:
anastomosis other than end-to-end (45.90-45.93, 45.95)
colostomy (46.10-46.13)
enterostomy (46.10-46.39)
EXCLUDES *cecectomy (17.32, 45.72)*
enterocolectomy (17.39, 45.79)
gastroduodenectomy (43.6-43.99)
ileocolectomy (17.33, 45.73)
pancreatoduodenectomy (52.51-52.7)

45.61 **Multiple segmental resection of small intestine**
Segmental resection for multiple traumatic lesions of
small intestine

45.62 **Other partial resection of small intestine**
Duodenectomy   Jejunectomy
Ileectomy
EXCLUDES *duodenectomy with synchronous*
pancreatectomy (52.51-52.7)
resection of cecum and terminal ileum
(17.32, 45.72)
AHA: 1Q, '10, 11; 1Q, '04, 10; 1Q, '03, 18

45.63 **Total removal of small intestine**

✓4ᵗʰ **45.7** **Open and other partial excision of large intestine**
Code also any synchronous:
anastomosis other than end-to-end (45.92-45.94)
enterostomy (46.10-46.39)
EXCLUDES *laparoscopic partial excision of large intestine*
(17.31-17.39)
AHA: 4Q, '92, 27

45.71 **Open and other multiple segmental resection
of large intestine**
Segmental resection for multiple traumatic lesions of
large intestine

45.72 **Open and other cecectomy**
Resection of cecum and terminal ileum

45.73 **Open and other right hemicolectomy**
Ileocolectomy
Right radical colectomy
AHA: 1Q, '11, 14; 3Q, '99, 10

45.74 **Open and other resection of transverse colon**

45.75 **Open and other left hemicolectomy**
EXCLUDES *proctosigmoidectomy (48.41-48.69)*
second stage Mikulicz operation (46.04)
DEF: Excision of left descending large intestine.
TIP: Assign for Hartmann procedure, typically involving
resection of the sigmoid colon with the proximal end
terminated as a colostomy and the distal end (rectum)
oversewn. A true Hartmann procedure is done on the left
side only.

45.76 **Open and other sigmoidectomy**
AHA: 3Q, '10, 12; 1Q, '96, 9; 3Q, '89, 15

Colectomy

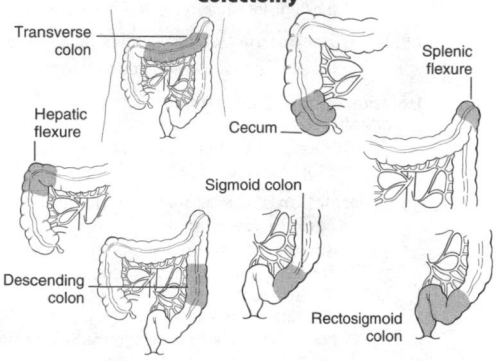

Transverse colon
Hepatic flexure
Splenic flexure
Cecum
Sigmoid colon
Descending colon
Rectosigmoid colon

Intestinal Anastomosis

Area to be excised   End-to-end anastomosis

45.79 **Other and unspecified partial excision of large
intestine**
Enterocolectomy NEC
AHA: 1Q, '09, 5;1Q, '03, 18; 3Q, '97, 9; 2Q, '91, 16

✓4ᵗʰ **45.8** **Total intra-abdominal colectomy**
Excision of cecum, colon, and sigmoid
EXCLUDES *coloproctectomy (48.41-48.69)*
AHA: 4Q, '08, 169-170

45.81 **Laparoscopic total intra-abdominal colectomy**

45.82 **Open total intra-abdominal colectomy**

45.83 **Other and unspecified total intra-abdominal
colectomy**

✓4ᵗʰ **45.9** **Intestinal anastomosis**
Code also any synchronous resection (45.31-45.8,
48.41-48.69)
EXCLUDES *end-to-end anastomosis — omit code*

45.90 **Intestinal anastomosis, not otherwise
specified**

45.91 **Small-to-small intestinal anastomosis**
AHA: 1Q, '10, 11; 3Q, '03, 6-8; M-J, '85, 17

45.92 **Anastomosis of small intestine to rectal stump**
Hampton procedure

45.93 **Other small-to-large intestinal anastomosis**
AHA: 1Q, '03, 18; N-D, '86, 11

45.94 **Large-to-large intestinal anastomosis**
EXCLUDES *rectorectostomy (48.74)*
AHA: 1Q, '09, 5; 3Q, '89, 15

45.95 **Anastomosis to anus**
Formation of endorectal ileal pouch (J-pouch)
(H-pouch) (S-pouch) with anastomosis of small
intestine to anus
AHA: 2Q, '05, 13

✓3ʳᵈ **46** **Other operations on intestine**
Code also any application or administration of an adhesion barrier
substance (99.77)

✓4ᵗʰ **46.0** **Exteriorization of intestine**
INCLUDES loop enterostomy
multiple stage resection of intestine
DEF: Bringing intestinal segment to body surface.

46.01 **Exteriorization of small intestine**
Loop ileostomy

46.02 **Resection of exteriorized segment of small
intestine**

46.03 **Exteriorization of large intestine**
Exteriorization of intestine NOS
First stage Mikulicz exteriorization of intestine
Loop colostomy

46.04 **Resection of exteriorized segment of large
intestine**
Resection of exteriorized segment of intestine NOS
Second stage Mikulicz operation

✓4ᵗʰ **46.1 Colostomy**
Code also any synchronous resection (45.49, 45.71-45.79, 45.8)
> **EXCLUDES** loop colostomy (46.03)
> that with abdominoperineal resection of rectum (48.5)
> that with synchronous anterior rectal resection (48.62)
DEF: Creation of opening from large intestine through abdominal wall to body surface.

46.10 Colostomy, not otherwise specified

46.11 Temporary colostomy

46.13 Permanent colostomy

46.14 Delayed opening of colostomy

✓4ᵗʰ **46.2 Ileostomy**
Code also any synchronous resection (45.34, 45.61-45.63)
> **EXCLUDES** loop ileostomy (46.01)
DEF: Creation of artificial anus by bringing ileum through abdominal wall to body surface.

46.20 Ileostomy, not otherwise specified

46.21 Temporary ileostomy

46.22 Continent ileostomy
DEF: Creation of opening from third part of small intestine through abdominal wall, with pouch outside abdomen.
AHA: M-J, '85, 17

46.23 Other permanent ileostomy

46.24 Delayed opening of ileostomy

✓4ᵗʰ **46.3 Other enterostomy**
Code also any synchronous resection (45.61-45.8)

46.31 Delayed opening of other enterostomy

46.32 Percutaneous (endoscopic) jejunostomy [PEJ]
Endoscopic conversion of gastrostomy to jejunostomy
Percutaneous (endoscopic) feeding enterostomy
> **EXCLUDES** percutaneous [endoscopic] gastrojejunostomy (bypass) (44.32)
DEF: Percutaneous feeding enterostomy: Surgical placement of a (feeding) tube through the midsection of the small intestine through the abdominal wall.
DEF: Conversion of gastrostomy to jejunostomy: Endoscopic advancement of a jejunostomy tube through an existing gastrostomy tube into the proximal jejunum.
AHA: 3Q, '10, 13

46.39 Other
Duodenostomy   Feeding enterostomy
AHA: 3Q, '89, 15

✓4ᵗʰ **46.4 Revision of intestinal stoma**
DEF: Revision of opening surgically created from intestine through abdominal wall, to skin surface.

46.40 Revision of intestinal stoma, not otherwise specified
Plastic enlargement of intestinal stoma
Reconstruction of stoma of intestine
Release of scar tissue of intestinal stoma
> **EXCLUDES** excision of redundant mucosa (45.41)

46.41 Revision of stoma of small intestine
> **EXCLUDES** excision of redundant mucosa (45.33)
AHA: 2Q, '05, 11

46.42 Repair of pericolostomy hernia

46.43 Other revision of stoma of large intestine
> **EXCLUDES** excision of redundant mucosa (45.41)
AHA: 2Q, '02, 9
TIP: Assign for a relocation of a stoma.

✓4ᵗʰ **46.5 Closure of intestinal stoma**
Code also any synchronous resection (45.34, 45.49, 45.61-45.8)

46.50 Closure of intestinal stoma, not otherwise specified

46.51 Closure of stoma of small intestine

46.52 Closure of stoma of large intestine
Closure or take-down of cecostomy
Closure or take-down of colostomy
Closure or take-down of sigmoidostomy
AHA: 1Q, '09, 5; 2Q, '05, 4; 3Q, '97, 9; 2Q, '91, 16; N-D, '87, 8

✓4ᵗʰ **46.6 Fixation of intestine**

46.60 Fixation of intestine, not otherwise specified
Fixation of intestine to abdominal wall

46.61 Fixation of small intestine to abdominal wall
Ileopexy

46.62 Other fixation of small intestine
Noble plication of small intestine
Plication of jejunum
DEF: Noble plication of small intestine: Fixing small intestine into place with tuck in small intestine.
DEF: Plication of jejunum: Fixing small intestine into place with tuck in midsection.

46.63 Fixation of large intestine to abdominal wall
Cecocoloplicopexy   Sigmoidopexy (Moschowitz)

46.64 Other fixation of large intestine
Cecofixation   Colofixation

✓4ᵗʰ **46.7 Other repair of intestine**
> **EXCLUDES** closure of:
> ulcer of duodenum (44.42)
> vesicoenteric fistula (57.83)

46.71 Suture of laceration of duodenum

46.72 Closure of fistula of duodenum

46.73 Suture of laceration of small intestine, except duodenum
AHA: 1Q, '10, 11

46.74 Closure of fistula of small intestine, except duodenum
> **EXCLUDES** closure of:
> artificial stoma (46.51)
> vaginal fistula (70.74)
> repair of gastrojejunocolic fistula (44.63)

46.75 Suture of laceration of large intestine

46.76 Closure of fistula of large intestine
> **EXCLUDES** closure of:
> gastrocolic fistula (44.63)
> rectal fistula (48.73)
> sigmoidovesical fistula (57.83)
> stoma (46.52)
> vaginal fistula (70.72-70.73)
> vesicocolic fistula (57.83)
> vesicosigmoidovaginal fistula (57.83)
AHA: 3Q, '99, 8

46.79 Other repair of intestine
Duodenoplasty
AHA: 3Q, '02, 11
TIP: Assign for duodenoplasty, typically performed for infants with congenital duodenal webs and stenosis.

✓4ᵗʰ **46.8 Dilation and manipulation of intestine**
AHA: 1Q, '03, 14

46.80 Intra-abdominal manipulation of intestine, not otherwise specified
Correction of intestinal   Reduction of:
   malrotation   intestinal volvulus
Reduction of: intussusception
   intestinal torsion
> **EXCLUDES** reduction of intussusception with:
> fluoroscopy (96.29)
> ionizing radiation enema (96.29)
> ultrasonography guidance (96.29)
DEF: Correction of intestinal malrotation: Repair of abnormal rotation.
DEF: Reduction of: Intestinal torsion: Repair of twisted segment. Intestinal volvulus: Repair of a knotted segment. Intussusception: Repair of prolapsed segment.
AHA: 4Q, '98, 82
TIP: Do not assign if the documentation indicates only "running or milking the bowel." This is an integral component of other procedures.

Operations on the Digestive System

46.81–48.34

46.81 Intra-abdominal manipulation of small intestine

46.82 Intra-abdominal manipulation of large intestine

46.85 Dilation of intestine
Dilation (balloon) of duodenum
Dilation (balloon) of jejunum
Endoscopic dilation (balloon) of large intestine
That through rectum or colostomy
EXCLUDES *with insertion of colonic stent (46.86-46.87)*
AHA: 3Q, '07, 5; 3Q, '89, 15

46.86 Endoscopic insertion of colonic stent(s)
Colonoscopy (flexible) (through stoma) with
    transendoscopic stent placement
Combined with fluoroscopic-guided insertion
Stent endoprosthesis of colon
Through the scope [TTS] technique
EXCLUDES *other non-endoscopic insertion of colonic
    stent (46.87)*
AHA: 4Q, '09, 147

46.87 Other insertion of colonic stent(s)
INCLUDES that by:
        fluoroscopic guidance only
        rectal guiding tube
Non-endoscopic insertion
Code also any synchronous diagnostic procedure(s)
EXCLUDES *endoscopic insertion of colonic stent (46.86)*

√4ᵗʰ **46.9 Other operations on intestines**

46.91 Myotomy of sigmoid colon

46.92 Myotomy of other parts of colon

46.93 Revision of anastomosis of small intestine

46.94 Revision of anastomosis of large intestine

46.95 Local perfusion of small intestine
Code also substance perfused (99.21-99.29)

46.96 Local perfusion of large intestine
Code also substance perfused (99.21-99.29)

46.97 Transplant of intestine   LC
NOTE To report donor source — see codes
    00.91-00.93
AHA: 4Q, '00, 66

46.99 Other
Ileoentectomy
EXCLUDES *diagnostic procedures on intestine
    (45.11-45.29)
    dilation of enterostomy stoma (96.24)
    intestinal intubation (96.08)
    removal of:
        intraluminal foreign body from large
            intestine without incision (98.04)
        intraluminal foreign body from small
            intestine without incision (98.03)
        tube from large intestine (97.53)
        tube from small intestine (97.52)
    replacement of:
        large intestine tube or enterostomy device
            (97.04)
        small intestine tube or enterostomy device
            (97.03)*
AHA: 3Q, '99, 11; 1Q, '89, 11

√3ʳᵈ **47 Operations on appendix**
INCLUDES appendiceal stump
Code also any application or administration of an adhesion barrier
    substance (99.77)

√4ᵗʰ **47.0 Appendectomy**
EXCLUDES *incidental appendectomy, so described
    laparoscopic (47.11)
    other (47.19)*
AHA: 4Q, '96, 64; 3Q, '92, 12

47.01 Laparoscopic appendectomy
AHA: 1Q, '01, 15; 4Q, '96, 64

47.09 Other appendectomy
AHA: 4Q, '97, 52

√4ᵗʰ **47.1 Incidental appendectomy**
DEF: Removal of appendix during abdominal surgery as prophylactic
    measure, without significant appendiceal pathology.

47.11 Laparoscopic incidental appendectomy

47.19 Other incidental appendectomy
AHA: 4Q, '96, 65

47.2 Drainage of appendiceal abscess
EXCLUDES *that with appendectomy (47.0)*

√4ᵗʰ **47.9 Other operations on appendix**

47.91 Appendicostomy

47.92 Closure of appendiceal fistula

47.99 Other
Anastomosis of appendix
EXCLUDES *diagnostic procedures on appendix
    (45.21-45.29)*
AHA: 3Q, '01, 16
TIP: Assign for a Malone antegrade continence enema
    procedure, in which the appendix is sutured to the
    abdominal wall, creating an orifice through which the
    patient can administer enemas via a small catheter through
    the appendix and into the cecum.

√3ʳᵈ **48 Operations on rectum, rectosigmoid, and perirectal tissue**
Code also any application or administration of an adhesion barrier
    substance (99.77)

48.0 Proctotomy
Decompression of imperforate anus
Panas' operation [linear proctotomy]
EXCLUDES *incision of perirectal tissue (48.81)*
DEF: Incision into rectal portion of large intestine.
DEF: Decompression of imperforate anus: opening a closed anus by
    means of an incision.
DEF: Panas' operation (linear proctotomy): Linear incision into rectal
    portion of large intestine.
AHA: 3Q, '99, 8

48.1 Proctostomy

√4ᵗʰ **48.2 Diagnostic procedures on rectum, rectosigmoid, and
perirectal tissue**

48.21 Transabdominal proctosigmoidoscopy
Intraoperative proctosigmoidoscopy
EXCLUDES *that with biopsy (48.24)*

48.22 Proctosigmoidoscopy through artificial stoma
EXCLUDES *that with biopsy (48.24)*

48.23 Rigid proctosigmoidoscopy
EXCLUDES *flexible sigmoidoscopy (45.24)*
DEF: Endoscopic exam of anus, rectum and lower sigmoid
    colon.
AHA: 1Q, '01, 8

48.24 Closed [endoscopic] biopsy of rectum
Brushing or washing for specimen collection
Proctosigmoidoscopy with biopsy
AHA: 1Q, '03, 14

48.25 Open biopsy of rectum

48.26 Biopsy of perirectal tissue

**48.29 Other diagnostic procedures on rectum,
rectosigmoid, and perirectal tissue**
EXCLUDES *digital examination of rectum (89.34)
    lower GI series (87.64)
    microscopic examination of specimen from
    rectum (90.91-90.99)*

√4ᵗʰ **48.3 Local excision or destruction of lesion or tissue of rectum**

48.31 Radical electrocoagulation of rectal lesion or tissue
DEF: Destruction of lesion or tissue of rectal part of large
    intestine.

48.32 Other electrocoagulation of rectal lesion or tissue
AHA: 2Q, '98, 18

48.33 Destruction of rectal lesion or tissue by laser

48.34 Destruction of rectal lesion or tissue by cryosurgery

BI Bilateral Procedure   NC Non-covered Procedure   LC Limited Coverage Procedure   ►◄ Revised Text   ● New Code   ▲ Revised Code Title

48.35 Local excision of rectal lesion or tissue
> EXCLUDES biopsy of rectum (48.24-48.25)
> [endoscopic] polypectomy of rectum (48.36)
> excision of perirectal tissue (48.82)
> hemorrhoidectomy (49.46)
> rectal fistulectomy (48.73)

48.36 [Endoscopic] polypectomy of rectum
AHA: 4Q, '95, 65

√4ᵗʰ **48.4 Pull-through resection of rectum**
Code also any synchronous anastomosis other than
end-to-end (45.90, 45.92-45.95)
AHA: 4Q, '08, 169-171

48.40 Pull-through resection of rectum, not otherwise specified
Pull-through resection NOS
> EXCLUDES abdominoperineal pull-through NOS (48.50)

48.41 Soave submucosal resection of rectum
Endorectal pull-through operation
DEF: Soave submucosal resection: Resection of submucosal
rectal part of large intestine by pull-through technique.
DEF: Endorectal pull-through operation: Resection of
interior large intestine by pull-through technique.

48.42 Laparoscopic pull-through resection of rectum

48.43 Open pull-through resection of rectum

48.49 Other pull-through resection of rectum
Abdominoperineal pull-through
Altemeier operation
Swenson proctectomy
> EXCLUDES Duhamel abdominoperineal pull-through
> (48.65)
> laparoscopic pull-through resection of
> rectum (48.42)
> open pull-through resection of rectum
> (48.43)
> pull-through resection of rectum, not
> otherwise specified (48.40)

DEF: Abdominoperineal pull-through: Resection of large
intestine, latter part, by pull-through of abdomen, scrotum
or vulva and anus.
DEF: Swenson proctectomy: Excision of large intestine,
rectal by pull-through and preserving muscles that close
the anus.
AHA: 2Q, '11, 13; 3Q, '01, 8; 2Q, '99, 13

√4ᵗʰ **48.5 Abdominoperineal resection of rectum**
INCLUDES with synchronous colostomy
Combined abdominoendorectal resection
Complete proctectomy
Code also any synchronous anastomosis other than
end-to-end (45.90, 45.92-45.95)
> EXCLUDES Duhamel abdominoperineal pull-through (48.65)
> that as part of pelvic exenteration (68.8)

DEF: Rectal excision through cavities formed by abdomen, anus,
vulva or scrotum.
AHA: 4Q, '08, 169-172; 2Q, '97, 5

48.50 Abdominoperineal resection of the rectum, not otherwise specified

48.51 Laparoscopic abdominoperineal resection of the rectum

48.52 Open abdominoperineal resection of the rectum

48.59 Other abdominoperineal resection of the rectum
> EXCLUDES abdominoperineal resection of the rectum,
> NOS (48.50)
> laparoscopic abdominoperineal resection of
> the rectum (48.51)
> open abdominoperineal resection of the
> rectum (48.52)

√4ᵗʰ **48.6 Other resection of rectum**
Code also any synchronous anastomosis other than
end-to-end (45.90, 45.92-45.95)

48.61 Transsacral rectosigmoidectomy
DEF: Excision through sacral bone area of sigmoid and last
parts of large intestine.

48.62 Anterior resection of rectum with synchronous colostomy
DEF: Resection of front terminal end of large intestine and
creation of colostomy.

48.63 Other anterior resection of rectum
> EXCLUDES that with synchronous colostomy (48.62)
AHA: 1Q, '96, 9

48.64 Posterior resection of rectum

48.65 Duhamel resection of rectum
Duhamel abdominoperineal pull-through

48.69 Other
Partial proctectomy   Rectal resection NOS
AHA: 2Q, '05, 13; J-F, '87, 11; N-D, '86, 11

√4ᵗʰ **48.7 Repair of rectum**
> EXCLUDES repair of:
> current obstetric laceration (75.62)
> vaginal rectocele (70.50, 70.52, 70.53, 70.55)

48.71 Suture of laceration of rectum

48.72 Closure of proctostomy

48.73 Closure of other rectal fistula
> EXCLUDES fistulectomy:
> perirectal (48.93)
> rectourethral (58.43)
> rectovaginal (70.73)
> rectovesical (57.83)
> rectovesicovaginal (57.83)

48.74 Rectorectostomy
Rectal anastomosis NOS
Stapled transanal rectal resection (STARR)
DEF: Rectal anastomosis: Connection of two cut portions of
large intestine, rectal end.

48.75 Abdominal proctopexy
Frickman procedure
Ripstein repair of rectal prolapse
DEF: Fixation of rectum to adjacent abdominal structures.

48.76 Other proctopexy
Delorme repair of prolapsed rectum
Proctosigmoidopexy
Puborectalis sling operation
> EXCLUDES manual reduction of rectal prolapse (96.26)
DEF: Delorme repair of prolapsed rectum: Fixation of rectal
part of collapsed large intestine.
DEF: Proctosigmoidopexy: Suturing rectal part of twisted
large intestine.
DEF: Puborectalis sling operation: Fixation of rectal part of
large intestine by forming puborectalis muscle into sling.

48.79 Other repair of rectum
Repair of old obstetric laceration of rectum
> EXCLUDES anastomosis to:
> large intestine (45.94)
> small intestine (45.92-45.93)
> repair of:
> current obstetrical laceration (75.62)
> vaginal rectocele (70.50, 70.52)

√4ᵗʰ **48.8 Incision or excision of perirectal tissue or lesion**
INCLUDES pelvirectal tissue
rectovaginal septum

48.81 Incision of perirectal tissue
Incision of rectovaginal septum

48.82 Excision of perirectal tissue
> EXCLUDES perirectal biopsy (48.26)
> perirectofistulectomy (48.93)
> rectal fistulectomy (48.73)

√4ᵗʰ **48.9 Other operations on rectum and perirectal tissue**

48.91 Incision of rectal stricture

48.92 Anorectal myectomy
DEF: Excision of anorectal muscle.

48.93 Repair of perirectal fistula
EXCLUDES *that opening into rectum (48.73)*
DEF: Closure of abdominal passage in tissue around rectal part of large intestine.
AHA: 1Q, '07, 13
TIP: Assign for Seton placement, which is a cord or stitch that is passed through the path of the fistula; it generates a fibrous reaction, allowing for tissue ingrowth over a period of time.

48.99 Other
EXCLUDES *digital examination of rectum (89.34)*
dilation of rectum (96.22)
insertion of rectal tube (96.09)
irrigation of rectum (96.38-96.39)
manual reduction of rectal prolapse (96.26)
proctoclysis (96.37)
rectal massage (99.93)
rectal packing (96.19)
removal of:
impacted feces (96.38)
intraluminal foreign body from rectum
without incision (98.05)
rectal packing (97.59)
transanal enema (96.39)

√3ʳᵈ **49 Operations on anus**
Code also any application or administration of an adhesion barrier substance (99.77)

√4ᵗʰ **49.0 Incision or excision of perianal tissue**

49.01 Incision of perianal abscess
AHA: 2Q, '05, 10

49.02 Other incision of perianal tissue
Undercutting of perianal tissue
EXCLUDES *anal fistulotomy (49.11)*

49.03 Excision of perianal skin tags

49.04 Other excision of perianal tissue
EXCLUDES *anal fistulectomy (49.12)*
biopsy of perianal tissue (49.22)
AHA: 1Q, '01, 8

√4ᵗʰ **49.1 Incision or excision of anal fistula**
EXCLUDES *closure of anal fistula (49.73)*

49.11 Anal fistulotomy

49.12 Anal fistulectomy

√4ᵗʰ **49.2 Diagnostic procedures on anus and perianal tissue**

49.21 Anoscopy

49.22 Biopsy of perianal tissue

49.23 Biopsy of anus

49.29 Other diagnostic procedures on anus and perianal tissue
EXCLUDES *microscopic examination of specimen from anus (90.91-90.99)*

√4ᵗʰ **49.3 Local excision or destruction of other lesion or tissue of anus**
Anal cryptotomy
Cauterization of lesion of anus
EXCLUDES *biopsy of anus (49.23)*
control of (postoperative) hemorrhage of anus (49.95)
hemorrhoidectomy (49.46)

49.31 Endoscopic excision or destruction of lesion or tissue of anus

49.39 Other local excision or destruction of lesion or tissue of anus
EXCLUDES *that by endoscopic approach (49.31)*
AHA: 1Q, '01, 8

√4ᵗʰ **49.4 Procedures on hemorrhoids**

49.41 Reduction of hemorrhoids
DEF: Manual manipulation to reduce hemorrhoids.

49.42 Injection of hemorrhoids

49.43 Cauterization of hemorrhoids
Clamp and cautery of hemorrhoids

Dynamic Graciloplasty

Rectum
Generator
Electrodes
Gracilis muscle (transpositional)
Neosphincter
Anal opening

49.44 Destruction of hemorrhoids by cryotherapy

49.45 Ligation of hemorrhoids
AHA: ▶4Q, '12, 81, 82◀

49.46 Excision of hemorrhoids
Hemorrhoidectomy NOS
AHA: 1Q, '07, 13

49.47 Evacuation of thrombosed hemorrhoids
DEF: Removal of clotted material from hemorrhoid.

49.49 Other procedures on hemorrhoids
Lord procedure

√4ᵗʰ **49.5 Division of anal sphincter**

49.51 Left lateral anal sphincterotomy

49.52 Posterior anal sphincterotomy

49.59 Other anal sphincterotomy
Division of sphincter NOS

49.6 Excision of anus

√4ᵗʰ **49.7 Repair of anus**
EXCLUDES *repair of current obstetric laceration (75.62)*

49.71 Suture of laceration of anus

49.72 Anal cerclage
DEF: Encircling anus with ring or sutures.

49.73 Closure of anal fistula
EXCLUDES *excision of anal fistula (49.12)*

49.74 Gracilis muscle transplant for anal incontinence
DEF: Moving pubic attachment of gracilis muscle to restore anal control.

49.75 Implantation or revision of artificial anal sphincter
Removal with subsequent replacement
Replacement during same or subsequent operative episode
AHA: 4Q, '02, 105

49.76 Removal of artificial anal sphincter
Explantation or removal without replacement
EXCLUDES *revision with implantation during same operative episode (49.75)*
AHA: 4Q, '02, 105

49.79 Other repair of anal sphincter
Repair of old obstetric laceration of anus
EXCLUDES *anoplasty with synchronous hemorrhoidectomy (49.46)*
repair of current obstetric laceration (75.62)
AHA: 2Q, '98, 16; 1Q, '97, 9

√4ᵗʰ **49.9 Other operations on anus**
EXCLUDES *dilation of anus (sphincter) (96.23)*

49.91 Incision of anal septum

49.92 Insertion of subcutaneous electrical anal stimulator

49.93 Other incision of anus
Removal of:
foreign body from anus with incision
seton from anus
EXCLUDES *anal fistulotomy (49.11)*
removal of intraluminal foreign body without incision (98.05)

BI Bilateral Procedure   NC Non-covered Procedure   LC Limited Coverage Procedure   ▶◀ Revised Text   ● New Code   ▲ Revised Code Title

136 – Volume 3 • February 2013   2014 ICD-9-CM

49.94　Reduction of anal prolapse
> *EXCLUDES* *manual reduction of rectal prolapse (96.26)*
> DEF: Manipulation of displaced anal tissue to normal position.

49.95　Control of (postoperative) hemorrhage of anus

49.99　Other

√3ʳᵈ 50　Operations on liver
> Code also any application or administration of an adhesion barrier substance (99.77)

50.0　Hepatotomy
> Incision of abscess of liver
> Removal of gallstones from liver
> Stromeyer-Little operation

√4ᵗʰ 50.1　Diagnostic procedures on liver

50.11　Closed (percutaneous) (needle) biopsy of liver
> Diagnostic aspiration of liver
> AHA: 3Q, '05, 24; 4Q, '88, 12
> TIP: When a laparotomy or other open procedure is performed and a needle biopsy of the liver is also performed, assign a separate code for the open procedure and code 50.11 for the needle biopsy.

50.12　Open biopsy of liver
> Wedge biopsy
> AHA: 3Q, '05, 24; 2Q, '05, 13

50.13　Transjugular liver biopsy
> Transvenous liver biopsy
> *EXCLUDES* *closed (percutaneous) [needle] biopsy of liver (50.11)*
> *laparoscopic liver biopsy (50.14)*
> AHA: 4Q, '07, 113

50.14　Laparoscopic liver biopsy
> *EXCLUDES* *closed (percutaneous) [needle] biopsy of liver (50.11)*
> *open biopsy of liver (50.12)*
> *transjugular liver biopsy (50.13)*
> AHA: 4Q, '07, 113

50.19　Other diagnostic procedures on liver
> *EXCLUDES* *laparoscopic liver biopsy (50.14)*
> *liver scan and radioisotope function study (92.02)*
> *microscopic examination of specimen from liver (91.01-91.09)*
> *transjugular liver biopsy (50.13)*

√4ᵗʰ 50.2　Local excision or destruction of liver tissue or lesion

50.21　Marsupialization of lesion of liver
> DEF: Exteriorizing lesion by incision and suturing cut edges to skin to create opening.

50.22　Partial hepatectomy
> Wedge resection of liver
> *EXCLUDES* *biopsy of liver (50.11-50.12)*
> *hepatic lobectomy (50.3)*

50.23　Open ablation of liver lesion or tissue
> AHA: 4Q, '06, 124

Closed Liver Biopsy

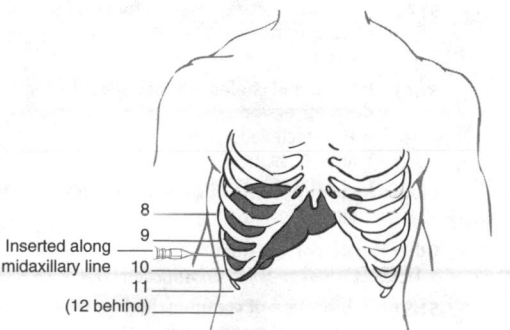

Inserted along midaxillary line
8
9
10
11
(12 behind)

Liver Biopsy (Open, Wedge)

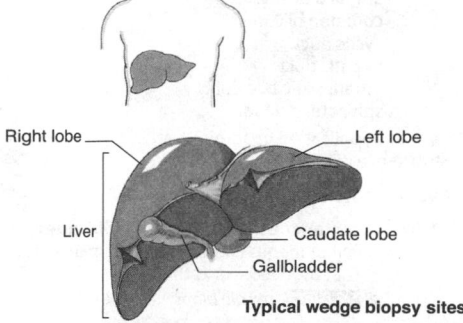

Right lobe — Left lobe
Liver — Caudate lobe
Gallbladder

Typical wedge biopsy sites

50.24　Percutaneous ablation of liver lesion or tissue
> AHA: 4Q, '06, 124

50.25　Laparoscopic ablation of liver lesion or tissue
> AHA: 4Q, '06, 124

50.26　Other and unspecified ablation of liver lesion or tissue
> AHA: 4Q, '06, 124

50.29　Other destruction of lesion of liver
> Cauterization ⎫
> Enucleation ⎬ of hepatic lesion
> Evacuation ⎭
> *EXCLUDES* *ablation of liver lesion or tissue:*
> *laparoscopic (50.25)*
> *open (50.23)*
> *other (50.26)*
> *percutaneous (50.24)*
> *laser interstitial thermal therapy [LITT] of lesion or tissue of liver under guidance (17.63)*
> *percutaneous aspiration of lesion (50.91)*
> AHA: 2Q, '03, 9

50.3　Lobectomy of liver
> Total hepatic lobectomy with partial excision of other lobe

50.4　Total hepatectomy
> AHA: 2Q, '08, 8

√4ᵗʰ 50.5　Liver transplant
> NOTE　To report donor source — see codes 00.91-00.93

50.51　Auxiliary liver transplant　　　NC
> Auxiliary hepatic transplantation leaving patient's own liver in situ

50.59　Other transplant of liver　　　LC
> AHA: 4Q, '08, 120; 2Q, '08, 8

√4ᵗʰ 50.6　Repair of liver

50.61　Closure of laceration of liver

50.69　Other repair of liver
> Hepatopexy

√4ᵗʰ 50.9　Other operations on liver
> *EXCLUDES* *lysis of adhesions (54.5)*

50.91　Percutaneous aspiration of liver
> *EXCLUDES* *percutaneous biopsy (50.11)*
> DEF: Incision into liver through body wall to withdraw fluid.

50.92　Extracorporeal hepatic assistance
> Liver dialysis
> DEF: Devices used outside body to assist liver function.
> AHA: 2Q, '01, 21

50.93　Localized perfusion of liver

50.94　Other injection of therapeutic substance into liver

50.99　Other

Operations on the Digestive System

51–51.59

√3ʳᵈ 51 Operations on gallbladder and biliary tract

     INCLUDES operations on:
         ampulla of Vater
         common bile duct
         cystic duct
         hepatic duct
         intrahepatic bile duct
         sphincter of Oddi

Code also any application or administration of an adhesion barrier substance (99.77)

√4ᵗʰ 51.0 Cholecystotomy and cholecystostomy

51.01 Percutaneous aspiration of gallbladder
Percutaneous cholecystotomy for drainage
That by: needle or catheter
     EXCLUDES *needle biopsy (51.12)*

51.02 Trocar cholecystostomy
DEF: Creating opening in gallbladder with catheter.
AHA: 3Q, '89, 18

51.03 Other cholecystostomy

51.04 Other cholecystotomy
Cholelithotomy NOS

√4ᵗʰ 51.1 Diagnostic procedures on biliary tract
     EXCLUDES *that for endoscopic procedures classifiable to 51.64, 51.84-51.88, 52.14, 52.21, 52.93 -52.94, 52.97-52.98*
AHA: 2Q, '97, 7

51.10 Endoscopic retrograde cholangiopancreatography [ERCP]
     EXCLUDES *endoscopic retrograde:*
         cholangiography [ERC] (51.11)
         pancreatography [ERP] (52.13)
DEF: Endoscopic and radioscopic exam of pancreatic and common bile ducts with contrast material injected through catheter in opposite direction of normal flow.
AHA: 4Q, '03, 118; 3Q, '03, 17; 1Q, '01, 8; 2Q, '99, 13
TIP: Do not assign separately if the ERCP was performed in conjunction with endoscopic sphincterotomy/papillotomy or other therapeutic biliary procedure.

51.11 Endoscopic retrograde cholangiography [ERC]
Laparoscopic exploration of common bile duct
     EXCLUDES *endoscopic retrograde:*
         cholangiopancreatography [ERCP] (51.10)
         pancreatography [ERP] (52.13)
DEF: Endoscopic and radioscopic exam of common bile ducts with contrast material injected through catheter in opposite direction of normal flow.
AHA: 1Q, '96, 12; 3Q, '89, 18; 4Q, '88, 7

51.12 Percutaneous biopsy of gallbladder or bile ducts
Needle biopsy of gallbladder

51.13 Open biopsy of gallbladder or bile ducts

51.14 Other closed [endoscopic] biopsy of biliary duct or sphincter of Oddi
Brushing or washing for specimen collection
Closed biopsy of biliary duct or sphincter of Oddi by procedures classifiable to 51.10-51.11, 52.13
DEF: Endoscopic biopsy of muscle tissue around pancreatic and common bile ducts.

Laparoscopic Cholecystectomy by Laser

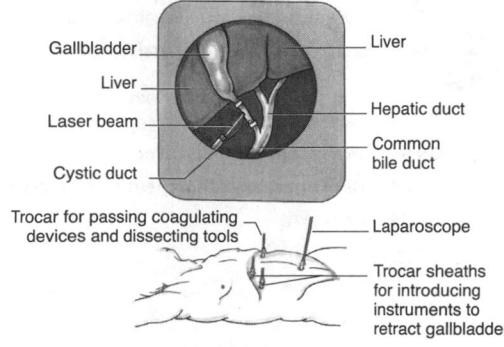

Gallbladder
Liver
Liver
Hepatic duct
Laser beam
Common bile duct
Cystic duct
Trocar for passing coagulating devices and dissecting tools
Laparoscope
Trocar sheaths for introducing instruments to retract gallbladder

51.15 Pressure measurement of sphincter of Oddi
Pressure measurement of sphincter by procedures classifiable to 51.10-51.11, 52.13
DEF: Pressure measurement tests of muscle tissue surrounding pancreatic and common bile ducts.

51.19 Other diagnostic procedures on biliary tract
     EXCLUDES *biliary tract x-ray (87.51-87.59)*
         microscopic examination of specimen from biliary tract (91.01-91.09)

√4ᵗʰ 51.2 Cholecystectomy
AHA: 1Q, '93, 17; 4Q, '91, 26; 3Q, '89, 18

51.21 Other partial cholecystectomy
Revision of prior cholecystectomy
     EXCLUDES *that by laparoscope (51.24)*
AHA: 4Q, '96, 69

51.22 Cholecystectomy
     EXCLUDES *laparoscopic cholecystectomy (51.23)*
AHA: 4Q, '97, 52; 2Q, '91, 16

51.23 Laparoscopic cholecystectomy
That by laser
DEF: Endoscopic removal of gallbladder.
AHA: 4Q, '08, 174; 3Q, '98, 10; 4Q, '97, 52; 1Q, '96, 12; 2Q, '95, 11; 4Q, '91, 26

51.24 Laparoscopic partial cholecystectomy
AHA: 4Q, '96, 69

√4ᵗʰ 51.3 Anastomosis of gallbladder or bile duct
     EXCLUDES *resection with end-to-end anastomosis (51.61-51.69)*

51.31 Anastomosis of gallbladder to hepatic ducts

51.32 Anastomosis of gallbladder to intestine

51.33 Anastomosis of gallbladder to pancreas

51.34 Anastomosis of gallbladder to stomach

51.35 Other gallbladder anastomosis
Gallbladder anastomosis NOS

51.36 Choledochoenterostomy
DEF: Connection of common bile duct to intestine.

51.37 Anastomosis of hepatic duct to gastrointestinal tract
Kasai portoenterostomy
DEF: Kaisi portoenterostomy: A duct to drain bile from the liver is formed by anastomosing the porta hepatis to a loop of bowel.
AHA: 2Q, '02, 12

51.39 Other bile duct anastomosis
Anastomosis of bile duct NOS
Anastomosis of unspecified bile duct to:
     intestine
     liver
     pancreas
     stomach

√4ᵗʰ 51.4 Incision of bile duct for relief of obstruction

51.41 Common duct exploration for removal of calculus
     EXCLUDES *percutaneous extraction (51.96)*
AHA: 1Q, '96, 12; 3Q, '89, 18; 4Q, '88, 7

51.42 Common duct exploration for relief of other obstruction
AHA: 3Q, '89, 18

51.43 Insertion of choledochohepatic tube for decompression
Hepatocholedochostomy
AHA: 3Q, '89, 18; 4Q, '88, 7

51.49 Incision of other bile ducts for relief of obstruction
AHA: 3Q, '89, 18

√4ᵗʰ 51.5 Other incision of bile duct
     EXCLUDES *that for relief of obstruction (51.41-51.49)*

51.51 Exploration of common duct
Incision of common bile duct
AHA: 2Q, '97, 16; 1Q, '96, 12

51.59 Incision of other bile duct
AHA: 2Q, '97, 16; 3Q, '89, 18

BI Bilateral Procedure   **NC** Non-covered Procedure   **LC** Limited Coverage Procedure   ►◄ Revised Text   ● New Code   ▲ Revised Code Title

138 – Volume 3   2014 ICD-9-CM

Operations on the Digestive System

51.6–52.19

✓4ᵗʰ **51.6 Local excision or destruction of lesion or tissue of biliary ducts and sphincter of Oddi**
Code also anastomosis other than end-to-end (51.31, 51.36-51.39)
EXCLUDES *biopsy of bile duct (51.12-51.13)*

51.61 Excision of cystic duct remnant
AHA: 3Q, '89, 18

51.62 Excision of ampulla of Vater (with reimplantation of common duct)

51.63 Other excision of common duct
Choledochectomy
EXCLUDES *fistulectomy (51.72)*

51.64 Endoscopic excision or destruction of lesion of biliary ducts or sphincter of Oddi
Excision or destruction of lesion of biliary duct by procedures classifiable to 51.10-51.11, 52.13

51.69 Excision of other bile duct
Excision of lesion of bile duct NOS
EXCLUDES *fistulectomy (51.79)*

✓4ᵗʰ **51.7 Repair of bile ducts**

51.71 Simple suture of common bile duct

51.72 Choledochoplasty
Repair of fistula of common bile duct

51.79 Repair of other bile ducts
Closure of artificial opening of bile duct NOS
Suture of bile duct NOS
EXCLUDES *operative removal of prosthetic device (51.95)*

✓4ᵗʰ **51.8 Other operations on biliary ducts and sphincter of Oddi**

51.81 Dilation of sphincter of Oddi
Dilation of ampulla of Vater
EXCLUDES *that by endoscopic approach (51.84)*
DEF: Dilation of muscle around common bile and pancreatic ducts; to mitigate constriction obstructing bile flow.

51.82 Pancreatic sphincterotomy
Incision of pancreatic sphincter
Transduodenal ampullary sphincterotomy
EXCLUDES *that by endoscopic approach (51.85)*
DEF: Pancreatic sphincterotomy: Division of muscle around common bile and pancreatic ducts.
DEF: Transduodenal ampullary sphincterotomy: Incision into muscle around common bile and pancreatic ducts, closing approach through first section of small intestine.

51.83 Pancreatic sphincteroplasty

51.84 Endoscopic dilation of ampulla and biliary duct
Dilation of ampulla and biliary duct by procedures classifiable to 51.10-51.11, 52.13

51.85 Endoscopic sphincterotomy and papillotomy
Sphincterotomy and papillotomy by procedures classifiable to 51.10-51.11, 52.13
DEF: Incision of muscle around common bile and pancreatic ducts and closing the duodenal papilla.
AHA: 4Q, '03, 118; 3Q, '03, 17; 2Q, '97, 7

51.86 Endoscopic insertion of nasobiliary drainage tube
Insertion of nasobiliary tube by procedures classifiable to 51.10-51.11, 52.13

51.87 Endoscopic insertion of stent (tube) into bile duct
Endoprosthesis of bile duct
Insertion of stent into bile duct by procedures classifiable to 51.10-51.11, 52.13
EXCLUDES *nasobiliary drainage tube (51.86)*
replacement of stent (tube) (97.05)
AHA: 3Q, '03, 17

51.88 Endoscopic removal of stone(s) from biliary tract
Laparoscopic removal of stone(s) from biliary tract
Removal of biliary tract stone(s) by procedures classifiable to 51.10-51.11, 52.13
EXCLUDES *percutaneous extraction of common duct stones (51.96)*
AHA: 2Q, '00, 11; 2Q, '97, 7

51.89 Other operations on sphincter of Oddi

✓4ᵗʰ **51.9 Other operations on biliary tract**

51.91 Repair of laceration of gallbladder

51.92 Closure of cholecystostomy

51.93 Closure of other biliary fistula
Cholecystogastroenteric fistulectomy

51.94 Revision of anastomosis of biliary tract

51.95 Removal of prosthetic device from bile duct
EXCLUDES *nonoperative removal (97.55)*

51.96 Percutaneous extraction of common duct stones
AHA: 4Q, '88, 7

51.98 Other percutaneous procedures on biliary tract
Percutaneous biliary endoscopy via existing T-tube or other tract for:
dilation of biliary duct stricture
exploration (postoperative)
removal of stone(s) except common duct stone
Percutaneous transhepatic biliary drainage
EXCLUDES *percutaneous aspiration of gallbladder (51.01)*
percutaneous biopsy and/or collection of specimen by brushing or washing (51.12)
percutaneous removal of common duct stone(s) (51.96)
AHA: 1Q, '97, 14; 3Q, '89, 18; N-D, '87, 1

51.99 Other
Insertion or replacement of biliary tract prosthesis
EXCLUDES *biopsy of gallbladder (51.12-51.13)*
irrigation of cholecystostomy and other biliary tube (96.41)
lysis of peritoneal adhesions (54.5)
nonoperative removal of:
cholecystostomy tube (97.54)
tube from biliary tract or liver (97.55)

✓3ʳᵈ **52 Operations on pancreas**
INCLUDES operations on pancreatic duct
Code also any application or administration of an adhesion barrier substance (99.77)

✓4ᵗʰ **52.0 Pancreatotomy**

52.01 Drainage of pancreatic cyst by catheter

52.09 Other pancreatotomy
Pancreatolithotomy
EXCLUDES *drainage by anastomosis (52.4, 52.96)*
incision of pancreatic sphincter (51.82)
marsupialization of cyst (52.3)
DEF: Pancreatolithotomy: Incision into pancreas to remove stones.

✓4ᵗʰ **52.1 Diagnostic procedures on pancreas**

52.11 Closed [aspiration] [needle] [percutaneous] biopsy of pancreas

52.12 Open biopsy of pancreas

52.13 Endoscopic retrograde pancreatography [ERP]
EXCLUDES *endoscopic retrograde:*
cholangiography [ERC] (51.11)
cholangiopancreatography [ERCP] (51.10)
that for procedures classifiable to 51.14-51.15, 51.64, 51.84-51.88, 52.14, 52.21, 52.92-52.94, 52.97-52.98

52.14 Closed [endoscopic] biopsy of pancreatic duct
Closed biopsy of pancreatic duct by procedures classifiable to 51.10-51.11, 52.13

52.19 Other diagnostic procedures on pancreas
EXCLUDES *contrast pancreatogram (87.66)*
endoscopic retrograde pancreatography [ERP] (52.13)
microscopic examination of specimen from pancreas (91.01-91.09)

3ʳᵈ
4ᵗʰ Additional Digit Required   Valid OR Procedure   Non-OR Procedure   Adjunct Code
2014 ICD-9-CM   Volume 3 – 139

Operations on the Digestive System

52.2–52.99

√4ᵗʰ **52.2** **Local excision or destruction of pancreas and pancreatic duct**
    EXCLUDES   *biopsy of pancreas (52.11-52.12, 52.14)*
                pancreatic fistulectomy (52.95)

    52.21 **Endoscopic excision or destruction of lesion or tissue of pancreatic duct**
           Excision or destruction of lesion or tissue of pancreatic duct by procedures classifiable to 51.10-51.11, 52.13

    52.22 **Other excision or destruction of lesion or tissue of pancreas or pancreatic duct**

52.3 **Marsupialization of pancreatic cyst**
    EXCLUDES   *drainage of cyst by catheter (52.01)*
    DEF: Incision into pancreas and suturing edges to form pocket; promotes drainage and healing.

52.4 **Internal drainage of pancreatic cyst**
    Pancreaticocystoduodenostomy
    Pancreaticocystogastrostomy
    Pancreaticocystojejunostomy
    DEF: Withdrawing fluid from pancreatic cyst by draining it through a created passage to another organ.
    DEF: Pancreaticocystoduodenostomy: Creation of passage from pancreatic cyst to first portion of small intestine.
    DEF: Pancreaticocystogastrostomy: Creation of passage from pancreatic cyst to stomach.
    DEF: Pancreaticocystojejunostomy: Creation of passage from pancreatic cyst to midsection of small intestine.

√4ᵗʰ **52.5** **Partial pancreatectomy**
    EXCLUDES   *pancreatic fistulectomy (52.95)*

    52.51 **Proximal pancreatectomy**
           Excision of head of pancreas (with part of body)
           Proximal pancreatectomy with synchronous duodenectomy

    52.52 **Distal pancreatectomy**
           Excision of tail of pancreas (with part of body)

    52.53 **Radical subtotal pancreatectomy**

    52.59 **Other partial pancreatectomy**

52.6 **Total pancreatectomy**
    Pancreatectomy with synchronous duodenectomy
    AHA: 4Q, '96, 71

52.7 **Radical pancreaticoduodenectomy**
    One-stage pancreaticoduodenal resection with choledochojejunal anastomosis, pancreaticojejunal anastomosis, and gastrojejunostomy
    Two-stage pancreaticoduodenal resection (first stage) (second stage)
    Radical resection of the pancreas
    Whipple procedure
    EXCLUDES   *radical subtotal pancreatectomy (52.53)*
    DEF: Whipple procedure: pancreaticoduodenectomy involving the removal of the head of the pancreas and part of the small intestines; pancreaticojejunostomy, choledochojejunal anastomosis, and gastrojejunostomy included in the procedure.
    AHA: 1Q, '01, 13

√4ᵗʰ **52.8** **Transplant of pancreas**
    NOTE To report donor source — see codes 00.91-00.93

    ¹⁰ **52.80** **Pancreatic transplant, not otherwise specified**   NC LC

    52.81 **Reimplantation of pancreatic tissue**

    ¹⁰ **52.82** **Homotransplant of pancreas**   NC LC

    52.83 **Heterotransplant of pancreas**   NC

    52.84 **Autotransplantation of cells of islets of Langerhans**
           Homotransplantation of islet cells of pancreas
           DEF: Transplantation of Islet cells from pancreas to another location of same patient.
           AHA: 4Q, '96, 70, 71

52.85 **Allotransplantation of cells of islets of Langerhans**
    Heterotransplantation of islet cells of pancreas
    DEF: Transplantation of Islet cells from one individual to another.
    AHA: 4Q, '96, 70, 71
    TIP: Assign also code 55.69 Other kidney transplantation, if a renal transplant is performed simultaneously.

52.86 **Transplantation of cells of islets of Langerhans, not otherwise specified**
    AHA: 4Q, '96, 70

√4ᵗʰ **52.9** **Other operations on pancreas**

    52.92 **Cannulation of pancreatic duct**
           EXCLUDES   *that by endoscopic approach (52.93)*
           DEF: Placement of tube into pancreatic duct, without an endoscope.

    52.93 **Endoscopic insertion of stent (tube) into pancreatic duct**
           Insertion of cannula or stent into pancreatic duct by procedures classifiable to 51.10-51.11, 52.13
           EXCLUDES   *endoscopic insertion of nasopancreatic drainage tube (52.97)*
                      replacement of stent (tube) (97.05)
           AHA: 2Q, '97, 7

    52.94 **Endoscopic removal of stone(s) from pancreatic duct**
           Removal of stone(s) from pancreatic duct by procedures classifiable to 51.10-51.11, 52.13

    52.95 **Other repair of pancreas**
           Fistulectomy   } of pancreas
           Simple suture

    52.96 **Anastomosis of pancreas**
           Anastomosis of pancreas (duct) to:
             intestine
             jejunum
             stomach
           EXCLUDES   *anastomosis to:*
                      bile duct (51.39)
                      gallbladder (51.33)

    52.97 **Endoscopic insertion of nasopancreatic drainage tube**
           Insertion of nasopancreatic drainage tube by procedures classifiable to 51.10-51.11, 52.13
           EXCLUDES   *drainage of pancreatic cyst by catheter (52.01)*
                      replacement of stent (tube) (97.05)

    52.98 **Endoscopic dilation of pancreatic duct**
           Dilation of Wirsung's duct by procedures classifiable to 51.10-51.11, 52.13

    52.99 **Other**
           Dilation of pancreatic [Wirsung's] duct   }
                                 } by open approach
           Repair of pancreatic [Wirsung's] duct   }
           EXCLUDES   *irrigation of pancreatic tube (96.42)*
                      removal of pancreatic tube (97.56)

Indirect Repair of Hernia

¹⁰ Noncovered procedure unless reported with code 55.69 or a diagnosis code from 250.x1 or 250.x3, or 251.3.

BI Bilateral Procedure   NC Non-covered Procedure   LC Limited Coverage Procedure   ►◄ Revised Text   ● New Code   ▲ Revised Code Title

140 – Volume 3   **2014 ICD-9-CM**

Indirect Inguinal Hernia

Direct Inguinal Hernia

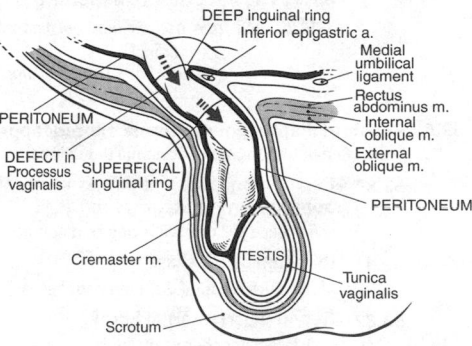

√3rd **53 Repair of hernia**
    INCLUDES hernioplasty
                herniorrhaphy
    Code also any application or administration of an adhesion barrier substance (99.77)
    EXCLUDES manual reduction of hernia (96.27)
    DEF: Repair of hernia: Restoration of abnormally protruding organ or tissue.
    DEF: Herniorrhaphy: Repair of hernia.
    DEF: Herniotomy: Division of constricted, strangulated, irreducible hernia.
    AHA: 3Q, '94, 8

√4th **53.0 Other unilateral repair of inguinal hernia**
    EXCLUDES laparoscopic unilateral repair of inguinal hernia (17.11-17.13)
    AHA: 4Q, '08, 165-167

    53.00 Unilateral repair of inguinal hernia, not otherwise specified
         Inguinal herniorrhaphy NOS
         AHA: 3Q, '03, 10

    53.01 Other and open repair of direct inguinal hernia
         Direct and indirect inguinal hernia
         AHA: 4Q, '96, 66

    53.02 Other and open repair of indirect inguinal hernia

    53.03 Other and open repair of direct inguinal hernia with graft or prosthesis

    53.04 Other and open repair of indirect inguinal hernia with graft or prosthesis

    53.05 Repair of inguinal hernia with graft or prosthesis, not otherwise specified

√4th **53.1 Other bilateral repair of inguinal hernia**
    EXCLUDES laparoscopic bilateral repair of inguinal hernia (17.21-17.24)
    AHA: 4Q, '08, 165-167

    53.10 Bilateral repair of inguinal hernia, not otherwise specified

    53.11 Other and open bilateral repair of direct inguinal hernia

    53.12 Other and open bilateral repair of indirect inguinal hernia

    53.13 Other and open bilateral repair of inguinal hernia, one direct and one indirect

    53.14 Other and open bilateral repair of direct inguinal hernia with graft or prosthesis

    53.15 Other and open bilateral repair of indirect inguinal hernia with graft or prosthesis

    53.16 Other and open bilateral repair of inguinal hernia, one direct and one indirect, with graft or prosthesis

    53.17 Bilateral inguinal hernia repair with graft or prosthesis, not otherwise specified

√4th **53.2 Unilateral repair of femoral hernia**

    53.21 Unilateral repair of femoral hernia with graft or prosthesis

    53.29 Other unilateral femoral herniorrhaphy

√4th **53.3 Bilateral repair of femoral hernia**

    53.31 Bilateral repair of femoral hernia with graft or prosthesis

    53.39 Other bilateral femoral herniorrhaphy

√4th **53.4 Repair of umbilical hernia**
    EXCLUDES repair of gastroschisis (54.71)
    AHA: 4Q, '08, 165-168

    53.41 Other and open repair of umbilical hernia with graft or prosthesis

    53.42 Laparoscopic repair of umbilical hernia with graft or prosthesis

    53.43 Other laparoscopic umbilical herniorrhaphy

    53.49 Other open umbilical herniorrhaphy
        EXCLUDES other laparoscopic umbilical herniorrhaphy (53.43)
                    repair of umbilical hernia with graft or prosthesis (53.41, 53.42)

√4th **53.5 Repair of other hernia of anterior abdominal wall (without graft or prosthesis)**

    53.51 Incisional hernia repair
         AHA: 3Q, '03, 6

    53.59 Repair of other hernia of anterior abdominal wall
         Repair of hernia:
            epigastric
            hypogastric
            spigelian
            ventral
         That by laparoscopic approach
         AHA: 2Q, '06, 10; 3Q, '03, 6; 3Q, '96, 15

√4th **53.6 Repair of other hernia of anterior abdominal wall with graft or prosthesis**
    AHA: 4Q, '08, 165-168

    53.61 Other open incisional hernia repair with graft or prosthesis
        EXCLUDES laparoscopic incisional hernia repair with graft or prosthesis (53.62)
         AHA: 3Q, '03, 11

    53.62 Laparoscopic incisional hernia repair with graft or prosthesis

    53.63 Other laparoscopic repair of other hernia of anterior abdominal wall with graft or prosthesis
         AHA: 2Q, '11, 18

    53.69 Other and open repair of other hernia of anterior abdominal wall with graft or prosthesis
        EXCLUDES other laparoscopic repair of other hernia of anterior abdominal wall with graft or prosthesis (53.63)

√4th **53.7 Repair of diaphragmatic hernia, abdominal approach**
    AHA: 4Q, '08, 165-168

    53.71 Laparoscopic repair of diaphragmatic hernia, abdominal approach

    53.72 Other and open repair of diaphragmatic hernia, abdominal approach

Operations on the Digestive System

53.75–54.3

53.75 Repair of diaphragmatic hernia, abdominal approach, not otherwise specified
> EXCLUDES *laparoscopic repair of diaphragmatic hernia (53.71)*
> *other and open repair of diaphragmatic hernia (53.72)*

☑4th **53.8 Repair of diaphragmatic hernia, thoracic approach**
> DEF: Repair of diaphragmatic hernia though abdomen and thorax.

53.80 Repair of diaphragmatic hernia with thoracic approach, not otherwise specified
> Thoracoabdominal repair of diaphragmatic hernia

53.81 Plication of the diaphragm
> DEF: Tuck repair of diaphragmatic hernia.

53.82 Repair of parasternal hernia
> DEF: Repair of hernia protruding into breastbone area.

53.83 Laparoscopic repair of diaphragmatic hernia, with thoracic approach
> AHA: 4Q, '08, 165-169

53.84 Other and open repair of diaphragmatic hernia, with thoracic approach
> EXCLUDES *repair of diaphragmatic hernia with thoracic approach, NOS, (53.80)*
> AHA: 4Q, '08, 165-169

53.9 Other hernia repair
> Repair of hernia: Repair of hernia:
>   ischiatic   omental
>   ischiorectal   retroperitoneal
>   lumbar   sciatic
>   obturator
> EXCLUDES *relief of strangulated hernia with exteriorization of intestine (46.01, 46.03)*
> *repair of pericolostomy hernia (46.42)*
> *repair of vaginal enterocele (70.92)*

☑3rd **54 Other operations on abdominal region**
> INCLUDES operations on:
>   epigastric region
>   flank
>   groin region
>   hypochondrium
>   inguinal region
>   loin region
>   mesentery
>   omentum
>   pelvic cavity
>   peritoneum
>   retroperitoneal tissue space
> Code also any application or administration of an adhesion barrier substance (99.77)
> EXCLUDES *hernia repair (53.00-53.9)*
> *obliteration of cul-de-sac (70.92)*
> *retroperitoneal tissue dissection (59.00-59.09)*
> *skin and subcutaneous tissue of abdominal wall (86.01-86.99)*

54.0 Incision of abdominal wall
> Drainage of: Drainage of:
>   abdominal wall   retroperitoneal abscess
>   extraperitoneal abscess
> EXCLUDES *incision of peritoneum (54.95)*
> *laparotomy (54.11-54.19)*
> AHA: 2Q, '06, 23; 4Q, '05, 77; 1Q, '97, 11; N-D, '87, 12
> TIP: Assign for incision and drainage (I&D) with debridement of abdominal wall surgical wound postoperative infection. Do not assign a separate debridement code; it's an integral component.

☑4th **54.1 Laparotomy**
> DEF: Incision into abdomen.
> AHA: 1Q, '92, 13

54.11 Exploratory laparotomy
> EXCLUDES *exploration incidental to intra-abdominal surgery — omit code*
> DEF: Exam of peritoneal cavity through incision into abdomen.
> AHA: 3Q, '89, 14; 4Q, '88, 12; J-F, '87, 11
> TIP: An exploratory procedure followed by definitive surgery is coded only to the definitive surgery, except for procedures involving biopsy and/or incidental appendectomy.

54.12 Reopening of recent laparotomy site
> Reopening of recent laparotomy site for:
>   control of hemorrhage
>   exploration
>   incision of hematoma

54.19 Other laparotomy
> Drainage of intraperitoneal abscess or hematoma
> EXCLUDES *culdocentesis (70.0)*
> *drainage of appendiceal abscess (47.2)*
> *exploration incidental to intra-abdominal surgery — omit code*
> *Ladd operation (54.95)*
> *percutaneous drainage of abdomen (54.91)*
> *removal of foreign body (54.92)*
> AHA: 3Q, '03, 17

☑4th **54.2 Diagnostic procedures of abdominal region**

54.21 Laparoscopy
> Peritoneoscopy
> EXCLUDES *laparoscopic cholecystectomy (51.23)*
> *that incidental to destruction of fallopian tubes (66.21-66.29)*
> DEF: Endoscopic exam of peritoneal cavity through abdominal portal.

54.22 Biopsy of abdominal wall or umbilicus

54.23 Biopsy of peritoneum
> Biopsy of: Biopsy of:
>   mesentery   peritoneal implant
>   omentum
> EXCLUDES *closed biopsy of:*
>   *omentum (54.24)*
>   *peritoneum (54.24)*

54.24 Closed [percutaneous] [needle] biopsy of intra-abdominal mass
> Closed biopsy of: Closed biopsy of:
>   omentum   peritoneum
>   peritoneal implant
> EXCLUDES *that of:*
>   *fallopian tube (66.11)*
>   *ovary (65.11)*
>   *uterine ligaments (68.15)*
>   *uterus (68.16)*
> AHA: 4Q, '97, 57

54.25 Peritoneal lavage
> Diagnostic peritoneal lavage
> EXCLUDES *peritoneal dialysis (54.98)*
> DEF: Irrigation of peritoneal cavity with siphoning of liquid contents for analysis.
> AHA: 2Q, '98, 19; 4Q, '93, 28

54.29 Other diagnostic procedures on abdominal region
> EXCLUDES *abdominal lymphangiogram (88.04)*
> *abdominal x-ray NEC (88.19)*
> *angiocardiography of venae cavae (88.51)*
> *C.A.T. scan of abdomen (88.01)*
> *contrast x-ray of abdominal cavity (88.11-88.15)*
> *intra-abdominal arteriography NEC (88.47)*
> *microscopic examination of peritoneal and retroperitoneal specimen (91.11-91.19)*
> *phlebography of:*
>   *intra-abdominal vessels NEC (88.65)*
>   *portal venous system (88.64)*
> *sinogram of abdominal wall (88.03)*
> *soft tissue x-ray of abdominal wall NEC (88.09)*
> *tomography of abdomen NEC (88.02)*
> *ultrasonography of abdomen and retroperitoneum (88.76)*

54.3 Excision or destruction of lesion or tissue of abdominal wall or umbilicus
> Debridement of abdominal wall
> Omphalectomy
> EXCLUDES *biopsy of abdominal wall or umbilicus (54.22)*
> *size reduction operation (86.83)*
> *that of skin of abdominal wall (86.22, 86.26, 86.3)*
> AHA: 1Q, '89, 11

BI Bilateral Procedure   NC Non-covered Procedure   LC Limited Coverage Procedure   ▶◀ Revised Text   ● New Code   ▲ Revised Code Title

54.4 Excision or destruction of peritoneal tissue
Excision of:
    appendices epiploicae
    falciform ligament
    gastrocolic ligament
    lesion of:
        mesentery
        omentum
        peritoneum
    presacral lesion NOS
    retroperitoneal lesion NOS
EXCLUDES *biopsy of peritoneum (54.23)*
        endometrectomy of cul-de-sac (70.32)

√4ᵗʰ **54.5 Lysis of peritoneal adhesions**
Freeing of adhesions of: Freeing of adhesions of:
  biliary tract   peritoneum
  intestines   spleen
  liver   uterus
  pelvic peritoneum
EXCLUDES *lysis of adhesions of:*
        bladder (59.11)
        fallopian tube and ovary (65.81, 65.89)
        kidney (59.02)
        ureter (59.02-59.03)
AHA: 3Q, '94, 8; 4Q, '90, 18
TIP: Code separately only if the documentation specifies that the adhesions were significant, caused symptoms, and/or increased the difficulty of the procedure being performed.

    54.51 Laparoscopic lysis of peritoneal adhesions
        AHA: 2Q, '11, 18; 4Q, '06, 134; 3Q, '03, 6-7; 4Q, '96, 65

    54.59 Other lysis of peritoneal adhesions
        AHA: 1Q, '10, 11; 3Q, '06, 15; 3Q, '03, 11; 1Q, '03, 14;
        4Q, '96, 66

√4ᵗʰ **54.6 Suture of abdominal wall and peritoneum**

    54.61 Reclosure of postoperative disruption of abdominal wall

    54.62 Delayed closure of granulating abdominal wound
        Tertiary subcutaneous wound closure
        DEF: Closure of outer layers of abdominal wound; follows procedure to close initial layers of wound.

    54.63 Other suture of abdominal wall
        Suture of laceration of abdominal wall
        EXCLUDES *closure of operative wound — omit code*

    54.64 Suture of peritoneum
        Secondary suture of peritoneum
        EXCLUDES *closure of operative wound — omit code*

√4ᵗʰ **54.7 Other repair of abdominal wall and peritoneum**

    54.71 Repair of gastroschisis
        DEF: Repair of congenital fistula of abdominal wall.
        AHA: 2Q, '02, 9

    54.72 Other repair of abdominal wall

    54.73 Other repair of peritoneum
        Suture of gastrocolic ligament

    54.74 Other repair of omentum
        Epiplorrhaphy
        Graft of omentum
        Omentopexy
        Reduction of torsion of omentum
        EXCLUDES *cardio-omentopexy (36.39)*
        DEF: Epiplorrhaphy: Suture of abdominal serous membrane.
        DEF: Graft of omentum: Implantation of tissue into abdominal serous membrane.
        DEF: Omentopexy: Anchoring of abdominal serous membrane.
        DEF: Reduction of torsion of omentum: Reduction of twisted abdominal serous membrane.
        AHA: J-F, '87, 11

    54.75 Other repair of mesentery
        Mesenteric plication
        Mesenteropexy
        DEF: Creation of folds in mesentery for shortening.
        DEF: Mesenteriopexy: Fixation of torn, incised mesentery.

√4ᵗʰ **54.9 Other operations of abdominal region**
    EXCLUDES *removal of ectopic pregnancy (74.3)*

    54.91 Percutaneous abdominal drainage
        Paracentesis
        EXCLUDES *creation of cutaneoperitoneal fistula (54.93)*
        DEF: Puncture for removal of fluid.
        AHA: 4Q, '07, 96; 3Q, '99, 9; 2Q, '99, 14; 3Q, '98, 12;
        1Q, '92, 14; 2Q, '90, 25

    54.92 Removal of foreign body from peritoneal cavity
        AHA: 1Q, '89, 11

    54.93 Creation of cutaneoperitoneal fistula
        DEF: Creation of opening between skin and peritoneal cavity.
        AHA: 2Q, '95, 10; N-D, '84, 6

    54.94 Creation of peritoneovascular shunt
        Peritoneovenous shunt
        DEF: Peritoneal vascular shunt: Construction of shunt to connect peritoneal cavity with vascular system.
        DEF: Peritoneovenous shunt: Construction of shunt to connect peritoneal cavity with vein.
        AHA: 1Q, '94, 7; 1Q, '88, 9; S-O, '85, 6
        TIP: Assign for insertion of a Denver shunt if it is described as a peritoneovascular shunt; if it is a Denver pleuroperitoneal shunt, assign instead 34.09.

    54.95 Incision of peritoneum
        Exploration of ventriculoperitoneal shunt at peritoneal site
        Ladd operation
        Revision of distal catheter of ventricular shunt
        Revision of ventriculoperitoneal shunt at peritoneal site
        EXCLUDES *that incidental to laparotomy (54.11-54.19)*
        DEF: Ladd operation: Peritoneal attachment of incompletely rotated cecum, obstructing duodenum.
        AHA: 4Q, '95, 65
        TIP: If a ventriculoperitoneal shunt is explored or revised at the ventricular site, assign instead code 02.41 or 02.42.

    54.96 Injection of air into peritoneal cavity
        Pneumoperitoneum
        EXCLUDES *that for:*
             collapse of lung (33.33)
             radiography (88.12-88.13, 88.15)

    54.97 Injection of locally-acting therapeutic substance into peritoneal cavity
        EXCLUDES *peritoneal dialysis (54.98)*

    54.98 Peritoneal dialysis
        EXCLUDES *peritoneal lavage (diagnostic) (54.25)*
        DEF: Separation of blood elements by diffusion through membrane.
        AHA: 4Q, '93, 28; N-D, '84, 6

    54.99 Other
        EXCLUDES *removal of:*
             abdominal wall sutures (97.83)
             peritoneal drainage device (97.82)
             retroperitoneal drainage device (97.81)
        AHA: 1Q, '99, 4

√3ʳᵈ
√4ᵗʰ   Additional Digit Required   Valid OR Procedure   Non-OR Procedure   Adjunct Code
2014 ICD-9-CM   Volume 3 – 143

10. Operations on the Urinary System (55-59)

✓3ʳᵈ **55　Operations on kidney**
　　INCLUDES operations on renal pelvis
　　Code also any application or administration of an adhesion barrier
　　　substance (99.77)
　　EXCLUDES perirenal tissue (59.00-59.09, 59.21-59.29, 59.91-59.92)

✓4ᵗʰ **55.0　Nephrotomy and nephrostomy**
　　EXCLUDES drainage by:
　　　　　anastomosis (55.86)
　　　　　aspiration (55.92)

55.01　Nephrotomy
　　Evacuation of renal cyst
　　Exploration of kidney
　　Nephrolithotomy
　　DEF: Nephrotomy: Incision into kidney.
　　DEF: Evacuation of renal cyst: Draining contents of cyst.
　　DEF: Exploration of kidney: Exploration through incision.
　　DEF: Nephrolithotomy: Removal of kidney stone through
　　　incision.

55.02　Nephrostomy
　　AHA: 2Q, '97, 4

55.03　Percutaneous nephrostomy without fragmentation
　　Nephrostolithotomy, percutaneous (nephroscopic)
　　Percutaneous removal of kidney stone(s) by:
　　　forceps extraction (nephroscopic)
　　　basket extraction
　　Pyelostolithotomy, percutaneous (nephroscopic)
　　With placement of catheter down ureter
　　EXCLUDES percutaneous removal by fragmentation
　　　　　(55.04)
　　　　　repeat nephroscopic removal during current
　　　　　episode (55.92)
　　DEF: Insertion of tube through abdominal wall without
　　　breaking up stones.
　　DEF: Nephrostolithotomy: Insertion of tube through the
　　　abdominal wall to remove stones.
　　DEF: Basket extraction: Percutaneous removal of stone with
　　　grasping forceps.
　　DEF: Pyelostolithotomy: Percutaneous removal of stones
　　　from funnel-shaped portion of kidney.
　　AHA: 2Q, '96, 5

55.04　Percutaneous nephrostomy with fragmentation
　　Percutaneous nephrostomy with disruption of kidney
　　　stone by ultrasonic energy and extraction
　　　(suction) through endoscope
　　With placement of catheter down ureter
　　With fluoroscopic guidance
　　EXCLUDES repeat fragmentation during current episode
　　　　　(59.95)
　　DEF: Insertion of tube through abdominal wall into kidney
　　　to break up stones.
　　AHA: 1Q, '89, 1; S-O, '86, 11

✓4ᵗʰ **55.1　Pyelotomy and pyelostomy**
　　EXCLUDES drainage by anastomosis (55.86)
　　　　　percutaneous pyelostolithotomy (55.03)
　　　　　removal of calculus without incision (56.0)

55.11　Pyelotomy
　　Exploration of renal pelvis
　　Pyelolithotomy

55.12　Pyelostomy
　　Insertion of drainage tube into renal pelvis

✓4ᵗʰ **55.2　Diagnostic procedures on kidney**

55.21　Nephroscopy
　　DEF: Endoscopic exam of renal pelvis; retrograde through
　　　ureter, percutaneous or open exposure.

55.22　Pyeloscopy
　　DEF: Fluoroscopic exam of kidney pelvis, calyces and
　　　ureters; follows IV or retrograde injection of contrast.

55.23　Closed [percutaneous] [needle] biopsy of kidney
　　Endoscopic biopsy via existing nephrostomy,
　　　nephrotomy, pyelostomy, or pyelotomy

55.24　Open biopsy of kidney

55.29　Other diagnostic procedures on kidney
　　EXCLUDES microscopic examination of specimen from
　　　　　kidney (91.21-91.29)
　　　　pyelogram:
　　　　　intravenous (87.73)
　　　　　percutaneous (87.75)
　　　　　retrograde (87.74)
　　　　radioisotope scan (92.03)
　　　　renal arteriography (88.45)
　　　　tomography:
　　　　　C.A.T scan (87.71)
　　　　　other (87.72)

✓4ᵗʰ **55.3　Local excision or destruction of lesion or tissue of kidney**

55.31　Marsupialization of kidney lesion
　　DEF: Exteriorization of lesion by incising anterior wall and
　　　suturing cut edges to create open pouch.

55.32　Open ablation of renal lesion or tissue
　　AHA: 4Q, '06, 124

55.33　Percutaneous ablation of renal lesion or tissue
　　AHA: 4Q, '06, 124

55.34　Laparoscopic ablation of renal lesion or tissue
　　AHA: 4Q, '06, 124

55.35　Other and unspecified ablation of renal lesion or tissue
　　AHA: 4Q, '06, 124

55.39　Other local destruction or excision of renal lesion or tissue
　　Obliteration of calyceal diverticulum
　　EXCLUDES ablation of renal lesion or tissue:
　　　　　laparoscopic (55.34)
　　　　　open (55.32)
　　　　　other (55.35)
　　　　　percutaneous (55.33)
　　　　biopsy of kidney (55.23-55.24)
　　　　partial nephrectomy (55.4)
　　　　percutaneous aspiration of kidney (55.92)
　　　　wedge resection of kidney (55.4)

55.4　Partial nephrectomy
　　Calycectomy
　　Wedge resection of kidney
　　Code also any synchronous resection of ureter (56.40-56.42)
　　DEF: Surgical removal of a part of the kidney.
　　DEF: Calycectomy: Removal of indentations in kidney.

✓4ᵗʰ **55.5　Complete nephrectomy**
　　Code also any synchronous excision of:
　　　adrenal gland (07.21-07.3)
　　　bladder segment (57.6)
　　　lymph nodes (40.3, 40.52-40.59)

55.51　Nephroureterectomy
　　Nephroureterectomy with bladder cuff
　　Total nephrectomy (unilateral)
　　EXCLUDES removal of transplanted kidney (55.53)
　　DEF: Complete removal of the kidney and all or portion of
　　　the ureter.
　　DEF: Nephroureterectomy with bladder cuff: Removal of
　　　kidney, ureter, and portion of bladder attached to ureter.
　　DEF: Total nephrectomy (unilateral): Complete excision of
　　　one kidney.
　　AHA: 2Q, '05, 4

55.52　Nephrectomy of remaining kidney
　　Removal of solitary kidney
　　EXCLUDES removal of transplanted kidney (55.53)

55.53　Removal of transplanted or rejected kidney
　　AHA: 4Q, 08, 83

55.54　Bilateral nephrectomy
　　EXCLUDES complete nephrectomy NOS (55.51)
　　DEF: Removal of both kidneys same operative session.

BI Bilateral Procedure　　　**NC** Non-covered Procedure　　　**LC** Limited Coverage Procedure　　　▶◀ Revised Text　　　● New Code　　　▲ Revised Code Title

144 – Volume 3　　　　　　　　　　　　　　　　　　　　　　　　　　　　　　　　　　　2014 ICD-9-CM

Symphysiostomy for Horseshoe Kidney

Horseshoe kidney joined at inferior poles

√4ᵗʰ **55.6 Transplant of kidney**

> **NOTE** To report donor source — see codes 00.91-00.93

55.61 Renal autotransplantation

55.69 Other kidney transplantation   LC

> AHA: ▶3Q, '12, 16;◀ 2Q, '11, 6; 4Q, '04, 117; 4Q, '96, 71

55.7 Nephropexy

> Fixation or suspension of movable [floating] kidney

√4ᵗʰ **55.8 Other repair of kidney**

55.81 Suture of laceration of kidney

55.82 Closure of nephrostomy and pyelostomy

> **DEF:** Removal of tube from kidney and closure of site of tube insertion.

55.83 Closure of other fistula of kidney

55.84 Reduction of torsion of renal pedicle

> **DEF:** Restoration of twisted renal pedicle into normal position.

55.85 Symphysiotomy for horseshoe kidney

> **DEF:** Division of congenitally malformed kidney into two parts.

55.86 Anastomosis of kidney

> Nephropyeloureterostomy
> Pyeloureterovesical anastomosis
> Ureterocalyceal anastomosis
> **EXCLUDES** nephrocystanastomosis NOS (56.73)
> **DEF:** Nephropyeloureterostomy: Creation of passage between kidney and ureter.
> **DEF:** Pyeloureterovesical anastomosis: Creation of passage between kidney and bladder.
> **DEF:** Ureterocalyceal anastomosis: Creation of passage between ureter and kidney indentations.

55.87 Correction of ureteropelvic junction

55.89 Other

√4ᵗʰ **55.9 Other operations on kidney**

> **EXCLUDES** lysis of perirenal adhesions (59.02)

55.91 Decapsulation of kidney

> Capsulectomy
> Decortication } of kidney

55.92 Percutaneous aspiration of kidney (pelvis)

> Aspiration of renal cyst
> Renipuncture
> **EXCLUDES** percutaneous biopsy of kidney (55.23)
> **DEF:** Insertion of needle into kidney to withdraw fluid.
> AHA: N-D, '84, 20

55.93 Replacement of nephrostomy tube

55.94 Replacement of pyelostomy tube

55.95 Local perfusion of kidney

> **DEF:** Fluid passage through kidney.

55.96 Other injection of therapeutic substance into kidney

> Injection into renal cyst

55.97 Implantation or replacement of mechanical kidney

55.98 Removal of mechanical kidney

55.99 Other

> **EXCLUDES** removal of pyelostomy or nephrostomy tube (97.61)

√3ʳᵈ **56 Operations on ureter**

> Code also any application or administration of an adhesion barrier substance (99.77)

56.0 Transurethral removal of obstruction from ureter and renal pelvis

> Removal of:
> blood clot
> calculus } from ureter or renal pelvis without incision
> foreign body
> **EXCLUDES** manipulation without removal of obstruction (59.8)
>   that by incision (55.11,56.2)
>   transurethral insertion of ureteral stent for passage of calculus (59.8)
> **DEF:** Removal of obstruction by tube inserted through urethra to ureter.
> AHA: 1Q, '89, 1; S-O, '86, 12
> **TIP:** Assign for laser lithotripsy of the kidney or ureter, unless the documentation specifies extracorporeal shockwave lithotripsy (ESWL), see instead code 98.51.

56.1 Ureteral meatotomy

> **DEF:** Incision into ureteral meatus to enlarge passage.

56.2 Ureterotomy

> Incision of ureter for:
> drainage
> exploration
> removal of calculus
> **EXCLUDES** cutting of ureterovesical orifice (56.1)
>   removal of calculus without incision (56.0)
>   transurethral insertion of ureteral stent for passage of calculus (59.8)
>   urinary diversion (56.51-56.79)
> AHA: S-O, '86, 10

√4ᵗʰ **56.3 Diagnostic procedures on ureter**

56.31 Ureteroscopy

56.32 Closed percutaneous biopsy of ureter

> **EXCLUDES** endoscopic biopsy of ureter (56.33)

56.33 Closed endoscopic biopsy of ureter

> Cystourethroscopy with ureteral biopsy
> Transurethral biopsy of ureter
> Ureteral endoscopy with biopsy through ureterotomy
> Ureteroscopy with biopsy
> **EXCLUDES** percutaneous biopsy of ureter (56.32)

56.34 Open biopsy of ureter

56.35 Endoscopy (cystoscopy) (looposcopy) of ileal conduit

> **DEF:** Endoscopic exam of created opening between ureters and one end of small intestine; other end used to form artificial opening.

56.39 Other diagnostic procedures on ureter

> **EXCLUDES** microscopic examination of specimen from ureter (91.21-91.29)

√4ᵗʰ **56.4 Ureterectomy**

> Code also anastomosis other than end-to-end (56.51-56.79)
> **EXCLUDES** fistulectomy (56.84)
>   nephroureterectomy (55.51-55.54)

56.40 Ureterectomy, not otherwise specified

56.41 Partial ureterotomy

> Excision of lesion of ureter
> Shortening of ureter with reimplantation
> **EXCLUDES** biopsy of ureter (56.32-56.34)

56.42 Total ureterectomy

Operations on the Urinary System

56.5–57.19

√4ᵗʰ **56.5 Cutaneous uretero-ileostomy**

     56.51 Formation of cutaneous uretero-ileostomy
        Construction of ileal conduit
        External ureteral ileostomy
        Formation of open ileal bladder
        Ileal loop operation
        Ileoureterostomy (Bricker's) (ileal bladder)
        Transplantation of ureter into ileum with external diversion

        EXCLUDES *closed ileal bladder (57.87)*
                  replacement of ureteral defect by ileal segment (56.89)

        DEF: Creation of urinary passage by connecting the terminal end of small intestine to ureter, then connecting to opening through abdominal wall.
        DEF: Construction of ileal conduit: Formation of conduit from terminal end of small intestine.

     56.52 Revision of cutaneous uretero-ileostomy
        AHA: 3Q, '96, 15; 4Q, '88, 7

√4ᵗʰ **56.6 Other external urinary diversion**

     56.61 Formation of other cutaneous ureterostomy
        Anastomosis of ureter to skin
        Ureterostomy NOS

     56.62 Revision of other cutaneous ureterostomy
        Revision of ureterostomy stoma
        EXCLUDES *nonoperative removal of ureterostomy tube (97.62)*

√4ᵗʰ **56.7 Other anastomosis or bypass of ureter**
        EXCLUDES *ureteropyelostomy (55.86)*

     56.71 Urinary diversion to intestine
        Anastomosis of ureter to intestine
        Internal urinary diversion NOS

        Code also any synchronous colostomy (46.10–46.13)
        EXCLUDES *external ureteral ileostomy (56.51)*

     56.72 Revision of ureterointestinal anastomosis
        EXCLUDES *revision of external ureteral ileostomy (56.52)*

     56.73 Nephrocystanastomosis, not otherwise specified
        DEF: Connection of kidney to bladder.

     56.74 Ureteroneocystostomy
        Replacement of ureter with bladder flap
        Ureterovesical anastomosis
        DEF: Transfer of ureter to another site in bladder.
        DEF: Ureterovesical anastomosis: Implantation of ureter into bladder.

     56.75 Transureteroureterostomy
        EXCLUDES *ureteroureterostomy associated with partial resection (56.41)*
        DEF: Separating one ureter and joining the ends to the opposite ureter.

     56.79 Other

√4ᵗʰ **56.8 Repair of ureter**

     56.81 Lysis of intraluminal adhesions of ureter
        EXCLUDES *lysis of periureteral adhesions (59.02-59.03)*
                  ureterolysis (59.02-59.03)
        DEF: Destruction of adhesions within ureteral cavity.

     56.82 Suture of laceration of ureter

     56.83 Closure of ureterostomy

     56.84 Closure of other fistula of ureter

     56.85 Ureteropexy

     56.86 Removal of ligature from ureter

     56.89 Other repair of ureter
        Graft of ureter
        Replacement of ureter with ileal segment implanted into bladder
        Ureteroplication
        DEF: Graft of ureter: Tissue from another site for graft replacement or repair of ureter.
        DEF: Replacement of ureter with ileal segment implanted into bladder and ureter replacement with terminal end of small intestine.
        DEF: Ureteroplication: Creation of tucks in ureter.

√4ᵗʰ **56.9 Other operations on ureter**

     56.91 Dilation of ureteral meatus

     56.92 Implantation of electronic ureteral stimulator

     56.93 Replacement of electronic ureteral stimulator

     56.94 Removal of electronic ureteral stimulator
        EXCLUDES *that with synchronous replacement (56.93)*

     56.95 Ligation of ureter

     56.99 Other
        EXCLUDES *removal of ureterostomy tube and ureteral catheter (97.62)*
                  ureteral catheterization (59.8)

√3ʳᵈ **57 Operations on urinary bladder**
     Code also any application or administration of an adhesion barrier substance (99.77)
     EXCLUDES *perivesical tissue (59.11-59.29, 59.91-59.92)*
             ureterovesical orifice (56.0-56.99)

     57.0 Transurethral clearance of bladder
        Drainage of bladder without incision
        Removal of:
            blood clot } from bladder without
            calculus } incision
            foreign body }
        EXCLUDES *that by incision (57.19)*
        AHA: S-O, '86, 11
        DEF: Insertion of device through urethra to cleanse bladder.

√4ᵗʰ **57.1 Cystotomy and cystostomy**
        EXCLUDES *cystotomy and cystostomy as operative approach — omit code*
        DEF: Cystotomy: Incision of bladder.
        DEF: Cystostomy: Creation of opening into bladder.

     57.11 Percutaneous aspiration of bladder

     57.12 Lysis of intraluminal adhesions with incision into bladder
        EXCLUDES *transurethral lysis of intraluminal adhesions (57.41)*
        DEF: Incision into bladder to destroy lesions.

     57.17 Percutaneous cystostomy
        Closed cystostomy
        Percutaneous suprapubic cystostomy
        EXCLUDES *removal of cystostomy tube (97.63)*
                  replacement of cystostomy tube (59.94)
        DEF: Incision through body wall into bladder to insert tube.
        DEF: Percutaneous (closed) suprapubic cystostomy: Incision above pubic arch, through body wall, into the bladder to insert tube.

     57.18 Other suprapubic cystostomy
        EXCLUDES *percutaneous cystostomy (57.17)*
                  removal of cystostomy tube (97.63)
                  replacement of cystostomy tube (59.94)

     57.19 Other cystotomy
        Cystolithotomy
        EXCLUDES *percutaneous cystostomy (57.17)*
                  suprapubic cystostomy (57.18)
        AHA: 4Q, '95, 73; S-O, '86, 11

BI Bilateral Procedure   **NC** Non-covered Procedure   **LC** Limited Coverage Procedure   ►◄ Revised Text   ● New Code   ▲ Revised Code Title

146 – Volume 3   **2014 ICD-9-CM**

Transurethral Cystourethroscopy

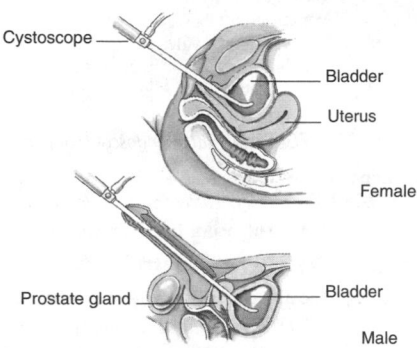

Cystoscope — Bladder

Uterus

Female

Prostate gland — Bladder

Male

☑4ᵗʰ 57.2 Vesicostomy

> **EXCLUDES** *percutaneous cystostomy (57.17)*
> *suprapubic cystostomy (57.18)*

57.21 Vesicostomy

Creation of permanent opening from bladder to skin using a bladder flap

DEF: Creation of permanent opening from the bladder to the skin.

57.22 Revision or closure of vesicostomy

> **EXCLUDES** *closure of cystostomy (57.82)*

☑4ᵗʰ 57.3 Diagnostic procedures on bladder

57.31 Cystoscopy through artificial stoma

57.32 Other cystoscopy

Transurethral cystoscopy

> **EXCLUDES** *cystourethroscopy with ureteral biopsy (56.33)*
> *retrograde pyelogram (87.74)*
> *that for control of hemorrhage (postoperative):*
> *bladder (57.93)*
> *prostate (60.94)*

AHA: 1Q, '11, 25;1Q, '01, 14

57.33 Closed [transurethral] biopsy of bladder

57.34 Open biopsy of bladder

AHA: 2Q, '05, 12

57.39 Other diagnostic procedures on bladder

> **EXCLUDES** *cystogram NEC (87.77)*
> *microscopic examination of specimen from bladder (91.31-91.39)*
> *retrograde cystourethrogram (87.76)*
> *therapeutic distention of bladder (96.25)*

☑4ᵗʰ 57.4 Transurethral excision or destruction of bladder tissue

DEF: Destruction of bladder tissue with instrument inserted into urethra.

57.41 Transurethral lysis of intraluminal adhesions

57.49 Other transurethral excision or destruction of lesion or tissue of bladder

Endoscopic resection of bladder lesion

> **EXCLUDES** *transurethral biopsy of bladder (57.33)*
> *transurethral fistulectomy (57.83-57.84)*

☑4ᵗʰ 57.5 Other excision or destruction of bladder tissue

> **EXCLUDES** *that with transurethral approach (57.41-57.49)*

57.51 Excision of urachus

Excision of urachal sinus of bladder

> **EXCLUDES** *excision of urachal cyst of abdominal wall (54.3)*

57.59 Open excision or destruction of other lesion or tissue of bladder

Endometrectomy of bladder
Suprapubic excision of bladder lesion

> **EXCLUDES** *biopsy of bladder (57.33-57.34)*
> *fistulectomy of bladder (57.83-57.84)*

DEF: Endometrectomy of bladder: Removal of inner lining.
DEF: Suprapubic excision of bladder lesion: Removal of lesion by excision above suprapubic bone arch.

57.6 Partial cystectomy

Excision of bladder domeWedge resection of bladder
Trigonectomy

☑4ᵗʰ 57.7 Total cystectomy

> **INCLUDES** total cystectomy with urethrectomy

57.71 Radical cystectomy

Pelvic exenteration in male
Removal of bladder, prostate, seminal vesicles and fat
Removal of bladder, urethra, and fat in a female

Code also any:
lymph node dissection (40.3, 40.5)
urinary diversion (56.51-56.79)

> **EXCLUDES** *that as part of pelvic exenteration in female (68.8)*

DEF: Radical cystectomy: Removal of bladder and surrounding tissue.
DEF: Pelvic exenteration in male: Excision of bladder, prostate, seminal vessels and fat.

57.79 Other total cystectomy

☑4ᵗʰ 57.8 Other repair of urinary bladder

> **EXCLUDES** *repair of:*
> *current obstetric laceration (75.61)*
> *cystocele (70.50-70.51)*
> *that for stress incontinence (59.3-59.79)*

57.81 Suture of laceration of bladder

57.82 Closure of cystostomy

57.83 Repair of fistula involving bladder and intestine

Rectovesicovaginal
Vesicosigmoidovaginal } fistulectomy

57.84 Repair of other fistula of bladder

Cervicovesical
Urethroperineovesical
Uterovesical
Vaginovesical } fistulectomy

> **EXCLUDES** *vesicoureterovaginal fistulectomy (56.84)*

57.85 Cystourethroplasty and plastic repair of bladder neck

Plication of sphincter of urinary bladder
V-Y plasty of bladder neck

DEF: Cystourethroplasty: Reconstruction of narrowed portion of bladder.
DEF: Plication of sphincter or urinary bladder: Creation of tuck in bladder sphincter.
DEF: V-Y plasty of bladder neck: Surgical reconstruction of the narrowed portion of bladder by V-Y technique.

57.86 Repair of bladder exstrophy

DEF: Surgical correction of a congenital bladder wall defect.

57.87 Reconstruction of urinary bladder

Anastomosis of bladder with isolated segment of ileum
Augmentation of bladder
Replacement of bladder with ileum or sigmoid [closed ileal bladder]

Code also resection of intestine (45.50-45.52)

DEF: Anastomosis of bladder with isolated segment of ileum: Creation of connection between bladder and separated terminal end of small intestine.
AHA: 2Q, '05, 12; 2Q, '03, 11; 3Q, '00, 7
TIP: Assign for closed continent ileovesicostomy, along with code 45.51 Isolation of segment of small intestine, for the continent ileovesicostomy; the ileum and bladder anastomoses are included.

57.88 Other anastomosis of bladder

Anastomosis of bladder to intestine NOS
Cystocolic anastomosis

> **EXCLUDES** *formation of closed ileal bladder (57.87)*

57.89 Other repair of bladder

Bladder suspension, not elsewhere classified
Cystopexy NOS
Repair of old obstetric laceration of bladder

> **EXCLUDES** *repair of current obstetric laceration (75.61)*

Operations on the Urinary System

57.9–58.99

√4ᵗʰ **57.9**   **Other operations on bladder**

     57.91   **Sphincterotomy of bladder**

        Division of bladder neck

        AHA: 2Q, '90, 26

     57.92   **Dilation of bladder neck**

     57.93   **Control of (postoperative) hemorrhage of bladder**

     57.94   **Insertion of indwelling urinary catheter**

     57.95   **Replacement of indwelling urinary catheter**

     57.96   **Implantation of electronic bladder stimulator**   NC

     57.97   **Replacement of electronic bladder stimulator**   NC

     57.98   **Removal of electronic bladder stimulator**

        EXCLUDES   *that with synchronous replacement (57.97)*

     57.99   **Other**

        EXCLUDES   *irrigation of:*

            cystostomy (96.47)

            other indwelling urinary catheter (96.48)

           lysis of external adhesions (59.11)

           removal of:

            cystostomy tube (97.63)

            other urinary drainage device (97.64)

           therapeutic distention of bladder (96.25)

√3ʳᵈ **58**   **Operations on urethra**

     INCLUDES   operations on:

         bulbourethral gland [Cowper's gland]

         periurethral tissue

     Code also any application or administration of an adhesion barrier

       substance (99.77)

     58.0   **Urethrotomy**

        Excision of urethral septum

        Formation of urethrovaginal fistula

        Perineal urethrostomy

        Removal of calculus from urethra by incision

        EXCLUDES   *drainage of bulbourethral gland or periurethral tissue*

            (58.91)

            internal urethral meatotomy (58.5)

            removal of urethral calculus without incision (58.6)

     58.1   **Urethral meatotomy**

        EXCLUDES   *internal urethral meatotomy (58.5)*

        DEF: Incision of urethra to enlarge passage.

√4ᵗʰ **58.2**   **Diagnostic procedures on urethra**

     58.21   **Perineal urethroscopy**

     58.22   **Other urethroscopy**

     58.23   **Biopsy of urethra**

     58.24   **Biopsy of periurethral tissue**

        DEF: Removal of tissue around urethra for biopsy.

     58.29   **Other diagnostic procedures on urethra and periurethral tissue**

        EXCLUDES   *microscopic examination of specimen from*

            urethra (91.31-91.39)

            retrograde cystourethrogram (87.76)

            urethral pressure profile (89.25)

            urethral sphincter electromyogram (89.23)

√4ᵗʰ **58.3**   **Excision or destruction of lesion or tissue of urethra**

     EXCLUDES   *biopsy of urethra (58.23)*

         excision of bulbourethral gland (58.92)

         fistulectomy (58.43)

         urethrectomy as part of:

           complete cystectomy (57.79)

           pelvic evisceration (68.8)

           radical cystectomy (57.71)

     58.31   **Endoscopic excision or destruction of lesion or tissue of urethra**

        Fulguration of urethral lesion

58.39   **Other local excision or destruction of lesion or tissue of urethra**

     Excision of:

        congenital valve ⎤

        lesion   ⎬ of urethra

        stricture   ⎦

     Urethrectomy

     EXCLUDES   *that by endoscopic appoach (58.31)*

√4ᵗʰ **58.4**   **Repair of urethra**

     EXCLUDES   *repair of current obstetric laceration (75.61)*

     58.41   **Suture of laceration of urethra**

     58.42   **Closure of urethrostomy**

     58.43   **Closure of other fistula of urethra**

        EXCLUDES   *repair of urethroperineovesical fistula (57.84*

     58.44   **Reanastomosis of urethra**

        Anastomosis of urethra

        DEF: Repair of severed urethra.

     58.45   **Repair of hypospadias or epispadias**

        AHA: 3Q, '97, 6; 4Q, '96, 35

        DEF: Repair of abnormal urethral opening.

     58.46   **Other reconstruction of urethra**

        Urethral construction

     58.47   **Urethral meatoplasty**

        DEF: Reconstruction of urethral opening.

     58.49   **Other repair of urethra**

        Benenenti rotation of bulbous urethra

        Repair of old obstetric laceration of urethra

        Urethral plication

        EXCLUDES   *repair of:*

            current obstetric laceration (75.61)

            urethrocele (70.50-70.51)

        AHA: 1Q, '09, 15

     58.5   **Release of urethral stricture**

        Cutting of urethral sphincter

        Internal urethral meatotomy

        Urethrolysis

        AHA: 1Q, '97, 13

     58.6   **Dilation of urethra**

        Dilation of urethrovesical junction

        Passage of sounds through urethra

        Removal of calculus from urethra without incision

        EXCLUDES   *urethral calibration (89.29)*

        AHA: 1Q, '11, 25; 1Q, '01, 14; 1Q, '97, 13

√4ᵗʰ **58.9**   **Other operations on urethra and periurethral tissue**

     58.91   **Incision of periurethral tissue**

        Drainage of bulbourethral gland

        DEF: Incision of tissue around urethra.

     58.92   **Excision of periurethral tissue**

        EXCLUDES   *biopsy of periurethral tissue (58.24)*

            lysis of periurethral adhesions (59.11-59.12)

     58.93   **Implantation of artificial urinary sphincter [AUS]**

        Placement of inflatable:

          urethral sphincter

          bladder sphincter

        Removal with replacement of sphincter device [AUS]

        With pump and/or reservoir

     58.99   **Other**

        Repair of inflatable sphincter pump and/or reservoir

        Surgical correction of hydraulic pressure of inflatable

          sphincter device

        Removal of inflatable urinary sphincter without

          replacement

        EXCLUDES   *removal of:*

            intraluminal foreign body from urethra

               without incision (98.19)

            urethral stent (97.65)

        AHA: 1Q, '09, 15

BI   Bilateral Procedure   NC   Non-covered Procedure   LC   Limited Coverage Procedure   ►◄ Revised Text   ● New Code   ▲ Revised Code Title

148 – Volume 3   **2014 ICD-9-CM**

✓3ʳᵈ **59** **Other operations on urinary tract**
Code also any application or administration of an adhesion barrier substance (99.77)

✓4ᵗʰ **59.0** **Dissection of retroperitoneal tissue**

59.00 **Retroperitoneal dissection, not otherwise specified**

59.02 **Other lysis of perirenal or periureteral adhesions**
EXCLUDES that by laparoscope (59.03)

59.03 **Laparoscopic lysis of perirenal or periureteral adhesions**
AHA: 4Q, '06, 134

59.09 **Other incision of perirenal or periureteral tissue**
Exploration of perinephric area
Incision of perirenal abscess
DEF: Exploration of the perinephric area: Exam of tissue around the kidney by incision.
DEF: Incision of perirenal abscess: Incising abscess in tissue around kidney.

✓4ᵗʰ **59.1** **Incision of perivesical tissue**
DEF: Incising tissue around bladder.

59.11 **Other lysis of perivesical adhesions**

59.12 **Laparoscopic lysis of perivesical adhesions**

59.19 **Other incision of perivesical tissue**
Exploration of perivesical tissue
Incision of hematoma of space of Retzius
Retropubic exploration

✓4ᵗʰ **59.2** **Diagnostic procedures on perirenal and perivesical tissue**

59.21 **Biopsy of perirenal or perivesical tissue**

59.29 **Other diagnostic procedures on perirenal tissue, perivesical tissue, and retroperitoneum**
EXCLUDES microscopic examination of specimen from:
perirenal tissue (91.21-91.29)
perivesical tissue (91.31-91.39)
retroperitoneum NEC (91.11-91.19)
retroperitoneal x-ray (88.14-88.16)

59.3 **Plication of urethrovesical junction**
Kelly-Kennedy operation on urethra
Kelly-Stoeckel urethral plication
DEF: Suturing a tuck in tissues around urethra at junction with bladder; changes angle of junction and provides support.

59.4 **Suprapubic sling operation**
Goebel-Frangenheim-Stoeckel urethrovesical suspension
Millin-Read urethrovesical suspension
Oxford operation for urinary incontinence
Urethrocystopexy by suprapubic suspension
DEF: Suspension of urethra from suprapubic periosteum to restore support to bladder and urethra.

59.5 **Retropubic urethral suspension**
Burch procedure
Marshall-Marchetti-Krantz operation
Suture of periurethral tissue to symphysis pubis
Urethral suspension NOS
DEF: Suspension of urethra from pubic bone with suture placed from symphysis pubis to paraurethral tissues; elevates urethrovesical angle, restores urinary continence.
AHA: 1Q, '97, 11

59.6 **Paraurethral suspension**
Pereyra paraurethral suspension
Periurethral suspension
DEF: Suspension of bladder neck from fibrous membranes of anterior abdominal wall; upward traction applied; changes angle of urethra, improves urinary control.

✓4ᵗʰ **59.7** **Other repair of urinary stress incontinence**

59.71 **Levator muscle operation for urethrovesical suspension**
Cystourethropexy with levator muscle sling
Gracilis muscle transplant for urethrovesical suspension
Pubococcygeal sling

59.72 **Injection of implant into urethra and/or bladder neck**
Collagen implant
Endoscopic injection of implant
Fat implant
Polytef implant
DEF: Injection of collagen into submucosal tissues to increase tissue bulk and improve urinary control.
AHA: 4Q, '95, 72, 73

59.79 **Other**
Anterior urethropexy
Repair of stress incontinence NOS
Tudor "rabbit ear" urethropexy
DEF: Pubovaginal sling for treatment of stress incontinence: A strip of fascia is harvested and the vaginal epithelium is mobilized and then sutured to the midline at the urethral level to the rectus muscle to create a sling supporting the bladder.
DEF: Vaginal wall sling with bone anchors for treatment of stress incontinence: A sling for the bladder is formed by a suture attachment of vaginal wall to the abdominal wall. In addition, a suture is run from the vagina to a bone anchor placed in the pubic bone.
DEF: Transvaginal endoscopic bladder neck suspension for treatment of stress incontinence: Endoscopic surgical suturing of the vaginal epithelium and the pubocervical fascia at the bladder neck level on both sides of the urethra. Two supporting sutures are run from the vagina to an anchor placed in the pubic bone on each side.
AHA: 2Q, '01, 20; 1Q, '00, 14, 15, 19

59.8 **Ureteral catheterization**
Drainage of kidney by catheter
Insertion of ureteral stent
Ureterovesical orifice dilation
Code also any ureterotomy (56.2)
EXCLUDES that for:
retrograde pyelogram (87.74)
transurethral removal of calculus or clot from ureter and renal pelvis (56.0)
AHA: 2Q, '05, 12; 2Q, '03, 11; 3Q, '00, 7; 1Q, '89, 1; S-O, '86, 10
TIP: Assign code twice if ureteral stents were placed bilaterally.

✓4ᵗʰ **59.9** **Other operations on urinary system**
EXCLUDES nonoperative removal of therapeutic device (97.61-97.69)

59.91 **Excision of perirenal or perivesical tissue**
EXCLUDES biopsy of perirenal or perivesical tissue (59.21)

59.92 **Other operations on perirenal or perivesical tissue**

59.93 **Replacement of ureterostomy tube**
Change of ureterostomy tube
Reinsertion of ureterostomy tube
EXCLUDES nonoperative removal of ureterostomy tube (97.62)

59.94 **Replacement of cystostomy tube**
EXCLUDES nonoperative removal of cystostomy tube (97.63)

59.95 **Ultrasonic fragmentation of urinary stones**
Shattered urinary stones
EXCLUDES percutaneous nephrostomy with fragmentation (55.04)
shockwave disintegration (98.51)
AHA: 1Q, '89, 1; S-O, '86, 11

59.99 **Other**
EXCLUDES instillation of medication into urinary tract (96.49)
irrigation of urinary tract (96.45-96.48)
AHA: 2Q, '08, 14
TIP: Assign for removal of an infected pubovaginal sling.

Operations on the Urinary System

59–59.99

Operations on the Male Genital Organs

60–60.95

11. Operations on the Male Genital Organs (60-64)

✓3ʳᵈ 60 Operations on prostate and seminal vesicles

    INCLUDES operations on periprostatic tissue

    Code also any application or administration of an adhesion barrier substance (99.77)

    EXCLUDES *that associated with radical cystectomy (57.71)*

60.0 Incision of prostate   ♂

    Drainage of prostatic abscess

    Prostatolithotomy

    EXCLUDES *drainage of periprostatic tissue only (60.81)*

✓4ᵗʰ 60.1 Diagnostic procedures on prostate and seminal vesicles

60.11 Closed [percutaneous] [needle] biopsy of prostate   ♂

    Approach:

      transrectal

      transurethral

    Punch biopsy

    DEF: Excision of prostate tissue by closed technique for biopsy.

60.12 Open biopsy of prostate   ♂

60.13 Closed [percutaneous] biopsy of seminal vesicles   ♂

    Needle biopsy of seminal vesicles

60.14 Open biopsy of seminal vesicles   ♂

60.15 Biopsy of periprostatic tissue   ♂

60.18 Other diagnostic procedures on prostate and periprostatic tissue   ♂

    EXCLUDES *microscopic examination of specimen from prostate (91.31-91.39)*

          x-ray of prostate (87.92)

60.19 Other diagnostic procedures on seminal vesicles   ♂

    EXCLUDES *microscopic examination of specimen from seminal vesicles (91.31-91.39)*

          x-ray:

            contrast seminal vesiculogram (87.91)

            other (87.92)

✓4ᵗʰ 60.2 Transurethral prostatectomy

    EXCLUDES *local excision of lesion of prostate (60.61)*

    AHA: 2Q, '94, 9; 3Q, '92, 13

60.21 Transurethral (ultrasound) guided laser induced prostatectomy [TULIP]   ♂

    Ablation (contact) (noncontact) by laser

    AHA: 4Q, '95, 7

60.29 Other transurethral prostatectomy   ♂

    Excision of median bar by transurethral approach

    Transurethral electrovaporization of prostate (TEVAP)

    Transurethral enucleative procedure

    Transurethral prostatectomy NOS

    Transurethral resection of prostate (TURP)

    DEF: Excision of median bar by transurethral approach: Removal of fibrous structure of prostate.

    DEF: Transurethral enucleative procedure: Transurethral prostatectomy.

    AHA: 3Q, '97, 3

Transurethral Prostatectomy

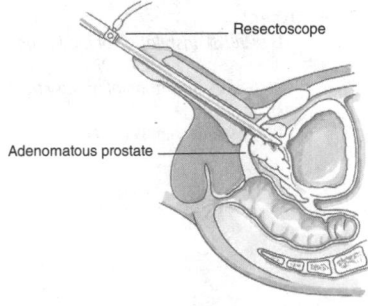

Resectoscope

Adenomatous prostate

60.3 Suprapubic prostatectomy   C

    Transvesical prostatectomy

    EXCLUDES *local excision of lesion of prostate (60.61)*

          radical prostatectomy (60.5)

    DEF: Resection of prostate through incision in abdomen above pubic arch.

60.4 Retropubic prostatectomy   C

    EXCLUDES *local excision of lesion of prostate (60.61)*

          radical prostatectomy (60.5)

    DEF: Removal of the prostate using an abdominal approach with direct cutting into prostatic capsule.

60.5 Radical prostatectomy   C

    Prostatovesiculectomy

    Radical prostatectomy by any approach

    EXCLUDES *cystoprostatectomy (57.71)*

    DEF: Removal of prostate, epididymis and vas ampullae.

    DEF: Prostatovesiculectomy: Removal of prostate and epididymis.

    AHA: 3Q, '93, 12

✓4ᵗʰ 60.6 Other prostatectomy

60.61 Local excision of lesion of prostate   C

    EXCLUDES *biopsy of prostate (60.11-60.12)*

          laser interstitial thermal therapy [LITT] of lesion or tissue of prostate under guidance (17.69)

60.62 Perineal prostatectomy   C

    Cryoablation of prostate

    Cryoprostatectomy

    Cryosurgery of prostate

    Radical cryosurcial ablation of prostate (RCSA)

    EXCLUDES *local excision of lesion of prostate (60.61)*

    DEF: Excision of prostate tissue through incision between scrotum and anus.

    AHA: 4Q, '95, 71

60.69 Other

✓4ᵗʰ 60.7 Operations on seminal vesicles

60.71 Percutaneous aspiration of seminal vesicle   C

    EXCLUDES *needle biopsy of seminal vesicle (60.13)*

60.72 Incision of seminal vesicle   C

60.73 Excision of seminal vesicle   C

    Excision of Müllerian duct cyst

    Spermatocystectomy

    EXCLUDES *biopsy of seminal vesicle (60.13-60.14)*

          prostatovesiculectomy (60.5)

60.79 Other operations on seminal vesicles   C

✓4ᵗʰ 60.8 Incision or excision of periprostatic tissue

60.81 Incision of periprostatic tissue   C

    Drainage of periprostatic abscess

60.82 Excision of periprostatic tissue   C

    Excision of lesion of periprostatic tissue

    EXCLUDES *biopsy of periprostatic tissue (60.15)*

✓4ᵗʰ 60.9 Other operations on prostate

60.91 Percutaneous aspiration of prostate   C

    EXCLUDES *needle biopsy of prostate (60.11)*

60.92 Injection into prostate   C

60.93 Repair of prostate   C

60.94 Control of (postoperative) hemorrhage of prostate   C

    Coagulation of prostatic bed

    Cystoscopy for control of prostatic hemorrhage

60.95 Transurethral balloon dilation of the prostatic urethra   C

    DEF: Insertion and inflation of balloon to stretch the portion of the urethra that passes through the prostate.

    AHA: 4Q, '91, 23

BI Bilateral Procedure   **NC** Non-covered Procedure   **LC** Limited Coverage Procedure   ▶◀ Revised Text   ● New Code   ▲ Revised Code Title

150 – Volume 3   **2014 ICD-9-CM**

60.96 **Transurethral destruction of prostate tissue by microwave thermotherapy**　♂

Transurethral microwave thermotherapy [TUMT] of prostate

EXCLUDES Prostatectomy:
other (60.61-60.69)
radical (60.5)
retropubic (60.4)
suprapubic (60.3)
transurethral (60.21-60.29)

AHA: 4Q, '00, 67

60.97 **Other transurethral destruction of prostate tissue by other thermotherapy**　♂

Radiofrequency thermotherapy
Transurethral needle ablation [TUNA] of prostate

EXCLUDES Prostatectomy:
other (60.61-60.69)
radical (60.5)
retropubic (60.4)
suprapubic (60.3)
transurethral (60.21-60.29)

AHA: 4Q, '00, 67

60.99 **Other**　♂

EXCLUDES prostatic massage (99.94)

AHA: 3Q, '90, 12

√3ʳᵈ 61 Operations on scrotum and tunica vaginalis

61.0 **Incision and drainage of scrotum and tunica vaginalis**　♂

EXCLUDES percutaneous aspiration of hydrocele (61.91)

√4ᵗʰ 61.1 Diagnostic procedures on scrotum and tunica vaginalis

61.11 **Biopsy of scrotum or tunica vaginalis**　♂

61.19 **Other diagnostic procedures on scrotum and tunica vaginalis**　♂

61.2 **Excision of hydrocele (of tunica vaginalis)**　♂

Bottle repair of hydrocele of tunica vaginalis

EXCLUDES percutaneous aspiration of hydrocele (61.91)

DEF: Removal of fluid collected in serous membrane of testes.

61.3 **Excision or destruction of lesion or tissue of scrotum**　♂

Fulguration of lesion
Reduction of elephantiasis } of scrotum
Partial scrotectomy

EXCLUDES biopsy of scrotum (61.11)
scrotal fistulectomy (61.42)

√4ᵗʰ 61.4 Repair of scrotum and tunica vaginalis

61.41 **Suture of laceration of scrotum and tunica vaginalis**　♂

61.42 **Repair of scrotal fistula**　♂

61.49 **Other repair of scrotum and tunica vaginalis**　♂

Reconstruction with rotational or pedicle flaps

√4ᵗʰ 61.9 Other operations on scrotum and tunica vaginalis

61.91 **Percutaneous aspiration of tunica vaginalis**　♂

Aspiration of hydrocele of tunica vaginalis

Hydrocelectomy

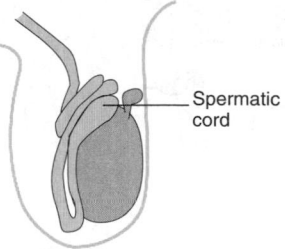

Scrotal skin incised
Sac opened
Fluid-filled sac mobilized
Excess tissue trimmed
Testis
Remaining sacular tissue folded back and sewn to itself to preclude recurrence ("bottle" procedure)

Orchiopexy with Detorsion of Testes

Spermatic cord

Torsion of testis

Testes after correction showing bilateral fixation

61.92 **Excision of lesion of tunica vaginalis other than hydrocele**　♂

Excision of hematocele of tunica vaginalis

DEF: Removal of blood (hematocele) collected in tunica vaginalis.

61.99 **Other**　♂

EXCLUDES removal of foreign body from scrotum without incision (98.24)

√3ʳᵈ 62 Operations on testes

62.0 **Incision of testis**　♂

√4ᵗʰ 62.1 Diagnostic procedures on testes

62.11 **Closed [percutaneous] [needle] biopsy of testis**　♂

62.12 **Open biopsy of testis**

62.19 **Other diagnostic procedures on testes**　♂

62.2 **Excision or destruction of testicular lesion**　♂

Excision of appendix testis
Excision of cyst of Morgagni in the male
Excision of hydatid of Morgagni in the male

EXCLUDES biopsy of testis (62.11-62.12)

62.3 **Unilateral orchiectomy**　♂

Orchidectomy (with epididymectomy) NOS

√4ᵗʰ 62.4 Bilateral orchiectomy

Male castration
Radical bilateral orchiectomy (with epididymectomy)

Code also any synchronous lymph node dissection (40.3, 40.5)

DEF: Removal of both testes.

DEF: Radical bilateral orchiectomy (with epididymectomy): Excision of both testes and structures that store sperm.

62.41 **Removal of both testes at same operative episode**　♂

Bilateral orchidectomy NOS

62.42 **Removal of remaining testis**　♂

Removal of solitary testis

62.5 **Orchiopexy**　♂

Mobilization and replacement of testis in scrotum
Orchiopexy with detorsion of testis
Torek (-Bevan) operation (orchidopexy) (first stage) (second stage)
Transplantation to and fixation of testis in scrotum

DEF: Fixation of testis in scrotum.

DEF: Orchiopexy with detorsion of testis: Fixation and placement of testis in scrotum after correcting angle.

DEF: Torek operation (first stage) (second stage): Transfer of congenitally undescended testis from inguinal canal to scrotum.

DEF: Transplantation to and fixation of testis in scrotum: Transfer of displaced testis to scrotum.

√4ᵗʰ 62.6 Repair of testes

EXCLUDES reduction of torsion (63.52)

62.61 **Suture of laceration of testis**　♂

62.69 **Other repair of testis**　♂

Testicular graft

62.7 **Insertion of testicular prosthesis**　♂

Operations on the Male Genital Organs

Varicocelectomy

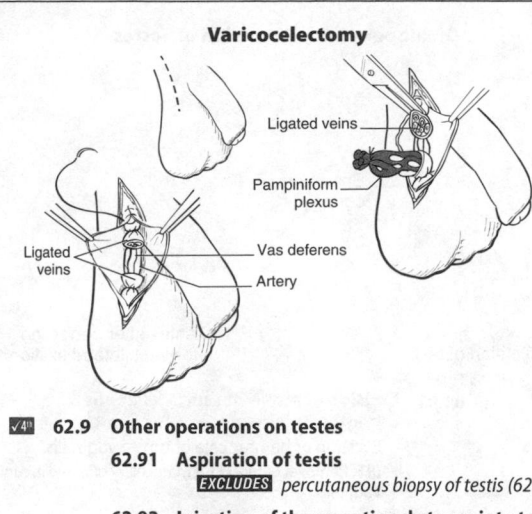

Ligated veins

Pampiniform plexus

Ligated veins

Vas deferens

Artery

√4ᵗʰ **62.9**   **Other operations on testes**

62.91   **Aspiration of testis**   ♂
     EXCLUDES   *percutaneous biopsy of testis (62.11)*

62.92   **Injection of therapeutic substance into testis** ♂

62.99   **Other**   ♂

√3ʳᵈ **63**   **Operations on spermatic cord, epididymis, and vas deferens**

√4ᵗʰ **63.0**   **Diagnostic procedures on spermatic cord, epididymis, and vas deferens**

63.01   **Biopsy of spermatic cord, epididymis, or vas deferens**   ♂

63.09   **Other diagnostic procedures on spermatic cord, epididymis, and vas deferens**   ♂
     EXCLUDES   *contrast epididymogram (87.93)*
                contrast vasogram (87.94)
                other x-ray of epididymis and vas deferens (87.95)

63.1   **Excision of varicocele and hydrocele of spermatic cord**   ♂
High ligation of spermatic vein
Hydrocelectomy of canal of Nuck
DEF: Removal of a swollen vein and collected fluid from spermatic cord.
DEF: High ligation of spermatic vein: Tying off of spermatic vein.
DEF: Hydrocelectomy of canal of Nuck: Removal of fluid collected from serous membrane of inguinal canal.

63.2   **Excision of cyst of epididymis**   ♂
Spermatocelectomy

63.3   **Excision of other lesion or tissue of spermatic cord and epididymis**   ♂
Excision of appendix epididymis
   EXCLUDES   *biopsy of spermatic cord or epididymis (63.01)*

63.4   **Epididymectomy**   ♂
   EXCLUDES   *that synchronous with orchiectomy (62.3-62.42)*

√4ᵗʰ **63.5**   **Repair of spermatic cord and epididymis**

63.51   **Suture of laceration of spermatic cord and epididymis**   ♂

63.52   **Reduction of torsion of testis or spermatic cord**   ♂
     EXCLUDES   *that associated with orchiopexy (62.5)*
     DEF: Correction of twisted testicle or spermatic cord.

63.53   **Transplantation of spermatic cord**   ♂

63.59   **Other repair of spermatic cord and epididymis**   ♂

63.6   **Vasotomy**   ♂
Vasostomy
DEF: Vasotomy: Incision of ducts carrying sperm from testicles.
DEF: Vasostomy: Creation of an opening into duct.

√4ᵗʰ **63.7**   **Vasectomy and ligation of vas deferens**

63.70   **Male sterilization procedure, not otherwise specified**   NC ♂

63.71   **Ligation of vas deferens**   NC ♂
Crushing of vas deferens
Division of vas deferens

63.72   **Ligation of spermatic cord**   NC ♂

63.73   **Vasectomy**   NC ♂
AHA: 2Q, '98, 13

√4ᵗʰ **63.8**   **Repair of vas deferens and epididymis**

63.81   **Suture of laceration of vas deferens and epididymis**

63.82   **Reconstruction of surgically divided vas deferens**

63.83   **Epididymovasostomy**   ♂
DEF: Creation of new connection between vas deferens and epididymis.

63.84   **Removal of ligature from vas deferens**   ♂

63.85   **Removal of valve from vas deferens**   ♂

63.89   **Other repair of vas deferens and epididymis**   ♂

√4ᵗʰ **63.9**   **Other operations on spermatic cord, epididymis, and vas deferens**

63.91   **Aspiration of spermatocele**   ♂
DEF: Puncture of cystic distention of epididymis.

63.92   **Epididymotomy**   ♂
DEF: Incision of epididymis.

63.93   **Incision of spermatic cord**   ♂
DEF: Incision into sperm storage structure.

63.94   **Lysis of adhesions of spermatic cord**   ♂

63.95   **Insertion of valve in vas deferens**   ♂

63.99   **Other**   ♂

√3ʳᵈ **64**   **Operations on penis**
   INCLUDES   operations on:
         corpora cavernosa
         glans penis
         prepuce

64.0   **Circumcision**   ♂
DEF: Removal of penis foreskin.

√4ᵗʰ **64.1**   **Diagnostic procedures on the penis**

64.11   **Biopsy of penis**   ♂

64.19   **Other diagnostic procedures on penis**   ♂

64.2   **Local excision or destruction of lesion of penis**   ♂
   EXCLUDES   *biopsy of penis (64.11)*

64.3   **Amputation of penis**   ♂

√4ᵗʰ **64.4**   **Repair and plastic operation on penis**

64.41   **Suture of laceration of penis**   ♂

64.42   **Release of chordee**   ♂
DEF: Correction of downward displacement of penis.
AHA: 4Q, '96, 34

64.43   **Construction of penis**   ♂

64.44   **Reconstruction of penis**   ♂

64.45   **Replantation of penis**   ♂
Reattachment of amputated penis

64.49   **Other repair of penis**   ♂
     EXCLUDES   *repair of epispadias and hypospadias (58.45)*

64.5   **Operations for sex transformation, not elsewhere classified**   NC ♂

√4ᵗʰ **64.9**   **Other operations on male genital organs**

64.91   **Dorsal or lateral slit of prepuce**   ♂

64.92   **Incision of penis**   ♂

64.93   **Division of penile adhesions**   ♂

64.94   **Fitting of external prosthesis of penis**   ♂
Penile prosthesis NOS

BI   Bilateral Procedure   NC   Non-covered Procedure   LC   Limited Coverage Procedure   ▶◀ Revised Text   ● New Code   ▲ Revised Code Title

64.95 Insertion or replacement of non-inflatable penile prosthesis ♂

Insertion of semi-rigid rod prosthesis into shaft of penis

EXCLUDES *external penile prosthesis (64.94)*
inflatable penile prosthesis (64.97)
plastic repair, penis (64.43-64.49)
that associated with:
construction (64.43)
reconstruction (64.44)

64.96 Removal of internal prosthesis of penis ♂

Removal without replacement of non-inflatable or inflatable penile prosthesis

64.97 Insertion or replacement of inflatable penile prosthesis ♂

Insertion of cylinders into shaft of penis and placement of pump and reservoir

EXCLUDES *external penile prosthesis (64.94)*
non-inflatable penile prosthesis (64.95)
plastic repair, penis (64.43-64.49)

64.98 Other operations on penis ♂

Corpora cavernosa-corpus spongiosum shunt
Corpora-saphenous shunt
Irrigation of corpus cavernosum

EXCLUDES *removal of foreign body:*
intraluminal (98.19)
without incision (98.24)
stretching of foreskin (99.95)

DEF: Corpora cavernosa-corpus spongiosum shunt: Insertion of shunt between erectile tissues of penis.

DEF: Corpora-saphenous shunt: Insertion of shunt between erectile tissue and vein of penis.

DEF: Irrigation of corpus cavernosum: Washing of erectile tissue forming dorsum and side of penis.

AHA: 3Q, '92, 9

TIP: Assign for arterialization of deep dorsal vein of penis, which involves anastomosis of the common femoral artery via a saphenous vein graft to the deep dorsal penile vein.

64.99 Other ♂

EXCLUDES *collection of sperm for artificial insemination (99.96)*

Operations on the Female Genital Organs

65–66.02

12. Operations on the Female Genital Organs (65-71)

√3ʳᵈ **65 Operations on ovary**
Code also any application or administration of an adhesion barrier substance (99.77)

√4ᵗʰ **65.0 Oophorotomy**
Salpingo-oophorotomy
DEF: Incision into ovary.
DEF: Salpingo-oophorotomy: Incision into ovary and the fallopian tube.

65.01 Laparoscopic oophorotomy ♀
65.09 Other oophorotomy ♀

√4ᵗʰ **65.1 Diagnostic procedures on ovaries**

65.11 Aspiration biopsy of ovary ♀
65.12 Other biopsy of ovary ♀
65.13 Laparoscopic biopsy of ovary ♀
AHA: 4Q, '96, 67

65.14 Other laparoscopic diagnostic procedures on ovaries ♀

65.19 Other diagnostic procedures on ovaries ♀
EXCLUDES microscopic examination of specimen from ovary (91.41-91.49)

√4ᵗʰ **65.2 Local excision or destruction of ovarian lesion or tissue**

65.21 Marsupialization of ovarian cyst ♀
EXCLUDES that by laparoscope (65.23)
DEF: Exteriorized cyst to outside by incising anterior wall and suturing cut edges to create open pouch.

65.22 Wedge resection of ovary ♀
EXCLUDES that by laparoscope (65.24)

65.23 Laparoscopic marsupialization of ovarian cyst ♀
65.24 Laparoscopic wedge resection of ovary ♀
65.25 Other laparoscopic local excision or destruction of ovary ♀

65.29 Other local excision or destruction of ovary ♀
Bisection ⎫
Cauterization ⎬ of ovary
Parial excision ⎭
EXCLUDES biopsy of ovary (65.11-65.13)
that by laparoscope (65.25)

√4ᵗʰ **65.3 Unilateral oophorectomy**

65.31 Laparoscopic unilateral oophorectomy ♀
65.39 Other unilateral oophorectomy ♀
EXCLUDES that by laparoscope (65.31)
AHA: 4Q, '96, 66

√4ᵗʰ **65.4 Unilateral salpingo-oophorectomy**

65.41 Laparoscopic unilateral salpingo-oophorectomy ♀
AHA: 4Q, '96, 67

65.49 Other unilateral salpingo-oophorectomy ♀

√4ᵗʰ **65.5 Bilateral oophorectomy**

65.51 Other removal of both ovaries at same operative episode ♀
Female castration
EXCLUDES that by laparoscope (65.53)

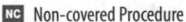
Oophorectomy
Fallopian tube
Fimbria
Ovary
Ovarian cyst

65.52 Other removal of remaining ovary
Removal of solitary ovary
EXCLUDES that by laparoscope (65.54)

65.53 Laparoscopic removal of both ovaries at same operative episode

65.54 Laparoscopic removal of remaining ovary

√4ᵗʰ **65.6 Bilateral salpingo-oophorectomy**

65.61 Other removal of both ovaries and tubes at same operative episode
EXCLUDES that by laparoscope (65.53)
AHA: ▶4Q, '12, 82;◀ 4Q, '96, 65

65.62 Other removal of remaining ovary and tube
Removal of solitary ovary and tube
EXCLUDES that by laparoscope (65.54)

65.63 Laparoscopic removal of both ovaries and tubes at the same operative episode
AHA: 3Q, '09, 5; 4Q, '06, 133, 134; 4Q, '96, 68

65.64 Laparoscopic removal of remaining ovary and tube

√4ᵗʰ **65.7 Repair of ovary**
EXCLUDES salpingo-oophorostomy (66.72)

65.71 Other simple suture of ovary
EXCLUDES that by laparoscope (65.74)

65.72 Other reimplantation of ovary
EXCLUDES that by laparoscope (65.75)
DEF: Grafting and repositioning of ovary at same site.

65.73 Other salpingo-oophoroplasty
EXCLUDES that by laparoscope (65.76)

65.74 Laparoscopic simple suture of ovary
65.75 Laparoscopic reimplantation of ovary
65.76 Laparoscopic salpingo-oophoroplasty

65.79 Other repair of ovary
Oophoropexy

√4ᵗʰ **65.8 Lysis of adhesions of ovary and fallopian tube**

65.81 Laparoscopic lysis of adhesions of ovary and fallopian tube
AHA: 4Q, '96, 67

65.89 Other lysis of adhesions of ovary and fallopian tube
EXCLUDES that by laparoscope (65.81)

√4ᵗʰ **65.9 Other operations on ovary**

65.91 Aspiration of ovary
EXCLUDES aspiration biopsy of ovary (65.11)

65.92 Transplantation of ovary
EXCLUDES reimplantation of ovary (65.72, 65.75)

65.93 Manual rupture of ovarian cyst
DEF: Breaking up an ovarian cyst using manual technique or blunt instruments.

65.94 Ovarian denervation
DEF: Destruction of nerve tracts to ovary.

65.95 Release of torsion of ovary

65.99 Other
Ovarian drilling
AHA: N-D, '86, 9

√3ʳᵈ **66 Operations on fallopian tubes**
Code also any application or administration of an adhesion barrier substance (99.77)

√4ᵗʰ **66.0 Salpingotomy and salpingostomy**

66.01 Salpingotomy
66.02 Salpingostomy

BI Bilateral Procedure   NC Non-covered Procedure   LC Limited Coverage Procedure   ▶◀ Revised Text   ● New Code   ▲ Revised Code Titl●

☑4ᵗʰ **66.1 Diagnostic procedures on fallopian tubes**

     66.11 Biopsy of fallopian tube ♀

     66.19 Other diagnostic procedures on fallopian tubes ♀

        EXCLUDES *microscopic examination of specimen from fallopian tubes (91.41-91.49)*
             radiography of fallopian tubes (87.82-87.83, 87.85)
             Rubin's test (66.8)

☑4ᵗʰ **66.2 Bilateral endoscopic destruction or occlusion of fallopian tubes**

     INCLUDES bilateral endoscopic destruction or occlusion of fallopian tubes by:
          culdoscopy
          endoscopy
          hysteroscopy
          laparoscopy
          peritoneoscopy
       endoscopic destruction of solitary fallopian tube

     DEF: Endoscopic blockage or destruction of both fallopian tubes.
     DEF: Bilateral endoscopic destruction or occlusion of fallopian tubes by:
        Culdoscopy: Endoscopic insertion through posterior structure of vagina.
        Hysteroscopy: Endoscopic insertion through uterus.
        Laparoscopy: Endoscopic insertion through abdomen.
        Peritoneoscopy: Endoscopic insertion through abdominal serous membrane cavity.
        Endoscopic destruction of solitary fallopian tube: Endoscopic destruction of one fallopian tube.

     66.21 Bilateral endoscopic ligation and crushing of fallopian tubes NC ♀

     66.22 Bilateral endoscopic ligation and division of fallopian tubes NC ♀

     66.29 Other bilateral endoscopic destruction or occlusion of fallopian tubes NC ♀

☑4ᵗʰ **66.3 Other bilateral destruction or occlusion of fallopian tubes**

     INCLUDES destruction of solitary fallopian tube
     EXCLUDES *endoscopic destruction or occlusion of fallopian tubes (66.21-66.29)*

     66.31 Other bilateral ligation and crushing of fallopian tubes NC ♀

     66.32 Other bilateral ligation and division of fallopian tubes NC ♀
        Pomeroy operation

     66.39 Other bilateral destruction or occlusion of fallopian tubes NC ♀
        Female sterilization operation NOS

     66.4 Total unilateral salpingectomy ♀

☑4ᵗʰ **66.5 Total bilateral salpingectomy**
     EXCLUDES *bilateral partial salpingectomy for sterilization (66.39)*
             that with oophorectomy (65.61-65.64)

     66.51 Removal of both fallopian tubes at same operative episode ♀

Endoscopic Ligation of Fallopian Tubes

Uterus
Ovary
Ligated fallopian tube
Monitor view
Laparoscopic procedure

66.52 Removal of remaining fallopian tube ♀
     Removal of solitary fallopian tube

☑4ᵗʰ **66.6 Other salpingectomy**
     INCLUDES salpingectomy by:
          cauterization
          coagulation
          electrocoagulation
          excision
     EXCLUDES *fistulectomy (66.73)*

     66.61 Excision or destruction of lesion of fallopian tube ♀
        EXCLUDES *biopsy of fallopian tube (66.11)*

     66.62 Salpingectomy with removal of tubal pregnancy ♀
        Code also any synchronous oophorectomy (65.31, 65.39)
        AHA: 3Q, '95, 15; S-O, '85, 14
        TIP: If salpingectomy is not performed with removal of ectopic pregnancy, assign instead code 74.3 Removal of extratubal ectopic pregnancy.

     66.63 Bilateral partial salpingectomy, not otherwise specified ♀

     66.69 Other partial salpingectomy ♀

☑4ᵗʰ **66.7 Repair of fallopian tube**

     66.71 Simple suture of fallopian tube ♀

     66.72 Salpingo-oophorostomy ♀

     66.73 Salpingo-salpingostomy ♀

     66.74 Salpingo-uterostomy ♀

     66.79 Other repair of fallopian tube ♀
        Graft of fallopian tube
        Reopening of divided fallopian tube
        Salpingoplasty
        DEF: Graft of fallopian: Repair of fallopian tube with implanted graft.
        DEF: Reopening of divided fallopian tube: Reconnection of severed fallopian tube to restore patency.
        DEF: Salpingoplasty: Plastic reconstruction of fallopian tube defect.
        AHA: 2Q, '95, 10
        TIP: When a patient is admitted for tubal ligation reversal, assign this code, along with diagnosis code V26.0 Tuboplasty or vasoplasty after previous sterilization, as the principal diagnosis.

     66.8 Insufflation of fallopian tube ♀
        Insufflation of fallopian tube with:
          air
          dye
          gas
          saline
        Rubin's test
        EXCLUDES *insufflation of therapeutic agent (66.95)*
            that for hysterosalpingography (87.82-87.83)
        DEF: Forceful blowing of gas or liquid into fallopian tubes to test patency.
        DEF: Rubin's test: Introduction of carbon dioxide gas into fallopian tubes to test patency.

☑4ᵗʰ **66.9 Other operations on fallopian tubes**

     66.91 Aspiration of fallopian tube ♀

     66.92 Unilateral destruction or occlusion of fallopian tube ♀
        EXCLUDES *that of solitary tube (66.21-66.39)*

     66.93 Implantation or replacement of prosthesis of fallopian tube ♀

     66.94 Removal of prosthesis of fallopian tube ♀

     66.95 Insufflation of therapeutic agent into fallopian tubes ♀

     66.96 Dilation of fallopian tube ♀

     66.97 Burying of fimbriae in uterine wall ♀
        DEF: Implantation of fringed edges of fallopian tube into uterine wall.

Operations on the Female Genital Organs

66.99–68.19

66.99   **Other**   ♀

EXCLUDES   *lysis of adhesions of ovary and tube (65.81, 65.89)*

AHA: 2Q, '94, 11

√3ʳᵈ **67**   **Operations on cervix**

Code also any application or administration of an adhesion barrier substance (99.77)

67.0   **Dilation of cervical canal**   ♀

EXCLUDES   *dilation and curettage (69.01-69.09)*
that for induction of labor (73.1)

√4ᵗʰ **67.1**   **Diagnostic procedures on cervix**

67.11   **Endocervical biopsy**   ♀

EXCLUDES   *conization of cervix (67.2)*

67.12   **Other cervical biopsy**   ♀

Punch biopsy of cervix NOS

EXCLUDES   *conization of cervix (67.2)*

67.19   **Other diagnostic procedures on cervix**   ♀

EXCLUDES   *microscopic examination of specimen from cervix (91.41-91.49)*

67.2   **Conization of cervix**   ♀

EXCLUDES   *that by:*
cryosurgery (67.33)
electrosurgery (67.32)

DEF: Removal of cone-shaped section from distal cervix; cervical function preserved.

√4ᵗʰ **67.3**   **Other excision or destruction of lesion or tissue of cervix**

67.31   **Marsupialization of cervical cyst**   ♀

DEF: Incision and then suturing open of a cyst in the neck of the uterus.

67.32   **Destruction of lesion of cervix by cauterization**   ♀

Electroconization of cervix
LEEP (loop electrosurgical excision procedure)
LLETZ (large loop excision of the transformation zone)

DEF: Destruction of lesion of uterine neck by applying intense heat.
DEF: Electroconization of cervix: Electrocautery excision of multilayer cone-shaped section from uterine neck.

AHA: 1Q, '98, 3

67.33   **Destruction of lesion of cervix by cryosurgery**   ♀

Cryoconization of cervix

DEF: Destruction of lesion of uterine neck by freezing.
DEF: Cryoconization of cervix: Excision by freezing of multilayer cone-shaped section of abnormal tissue in uterine neck.

67.39   **Other excision or destruction of lesion or tissue of cervix**   ♀

EXCLUDES   *biopsy of cervix (67.11-67.12)*
cervical fistulectomy (67.62)
conization of cervix (67.2)

67.4   **Amputation of cervix**   ♀

Cervicectomy with synchronous colporrhaphy

DEF: Excision of lower uterine neck.
DEF: Cervicectomy with synchronous colporrhaphy: Excision of lower uterine neck with suture of vaginal stump.

√4ᵗʰ **67.5**   **Repair of internal cervical os**

DEF: Repair of cervical opening defect.

AHA: 4Q, '01, 63; 3Q, '00, 11

67.51   **Transabdominal cerclage of cervix**   ♀

67.59   **Other repair of internal cervical os**   ♀

Cerclage of isthmus uteri   Shirodkar operation
McDonald operation   Transvaginal cerclage

EXCLUDES   *laparoscopically assisted supracervical hysterectomy [LASH] (68.31)*
transabdominal cerclage of cervix (67.51)

DEF: Cerclage of isthmus uteri: Placement of encircling suture between neck and body of uterus.
DEF: Shirodkar operation: Placement of purse-string suture in internal cervical opening.

AHA: 4Q, '08, 125

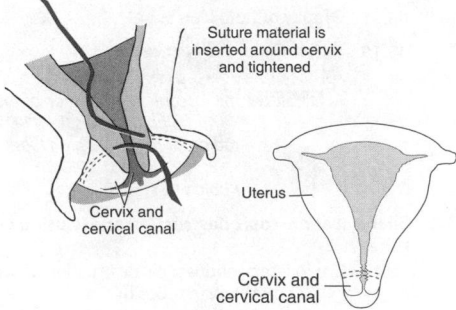

Cerclage of Cervix

Suture material is inserted around cervix and tightened

Cervix and cervical canal

Uterus

Cervix and cervical canal

√4ᵗʰ **67.6**   **Other repair of cervix**

EXCLUDES   *repair of current obstetric laceration (75.51)*

67.61   **Suture of laceration of cervix**   ♀

67.62   **Repair of fistula of cervix**   ♀

Cervicosigmoidal fistulectomy

EXCLUDES   *fistulectomy:*
cervicovesical (57.84)
ureterocervical (56.84)
vesicocervicovaginal (57.84)

DEF: Closure of fistula in lower uterus.
DEF: Cervicosigmoidal fistulectomy: Excision of abnormal passage between uterine neck and torsion of large intestine.

67.69   **Other repair of cervix**   ♀

Repair of old obstetric laceration of cervix

√3ʳᵈ **68**   **Other incision and excision of uterus**

Code also any application or administration of an adhesion barrier substance (99.77)

68.0   **Hysterotomy**   ♀

Hysterotomy with removal of hydatidiform mole

EXCLUDES   *hysterotomy for termination of pregnancy (74.91)*

DEF: Incision into the uterus.

√4ᵗʰ **68.1**   **Diagnostic procedures on uterus and supporting structures**

68.11   **Digital examination of uterus**   ♀

EXCLUDES   *pelvic examination, so described (89.26)*
postpartal manual exploration of uterine cavity (75.7)

68.12   **Hysteroscopy**   ♀

EXCLUDES   *that with biopsy (68.16)*

68.13   **Open biopsy of uterus**   ♀

EXCLUDES   *closed biopsy of uterus (68.16)*

68.14   **Open biopsy of uterine ligaments**   ♀

EXCLUDES   *closed biopsy of uterine ligaments (68.15)*

68.15   **Closed biopsy of uterine ligaments**   ♀

Endoscopic (laparoscopy) biopsy of uterine adnexa, except ovary and fallopian tube

68.16   **Closed biopsy of uterus**   ♀

Endoscopic (laparoscopy) (hysteroscopy) biopsy of uterus

EXCLUDES   *open biopsy of uterus (68.13)*

AHA: ▶2Q, '12, 18◀
TIP: ▶Assign for closed endometrial biopsy via Pipelle suction curette. Code assignment is based on the procedure performed, not the instrumentation.◀

68.19   **Other diagnostic procedures on uterus and supporting structures**   ♀

EXCLUDES   *diagnostic:*
aspiration curettage (69.59)
dilation and curettage (69.09)
microscopic examination of specimen from uterus (91.41-91.49)
pelvic examination (89.26)
radioisotope scan of:
placenta (92.17)
uterus (92.19)
ultrasonography of uterus (88.78-88.79)
x-ray of uterus (87.81-87.89)

BI   Bilateral Procedure   NC   Non-covered Procedure   LC   Limited Coverage Procedure   ▶◀ Revised Text   ● New Code   ▲ Revised Code Title

156 – Volume 3 · February 2013   **2014 ICD-9-CM**

68.2 Excision or destruction of lesion or tissue of uterus

68.21 **Division of endometrial synechiae** ♀
Lysis of intraluminal uterine adhesions
DEF: Separation of uterine adhesions.
DEF: Lysis of intraluminal uterine adhesion: Surgical destruction of adhesive, fibrous structures inside uterine cavity.

68.22 **Incision or excision of congenital septum of uterus** ♀

68.23 **Endometrial ablation** ♀
Dilation and curettage
Hysteroscopic endometrial ablation
DEF: Removal or destruction of uterine lining; usually by electrocautery or loop electrosurgical excision procedure (LEEP).
AHA: 4Q, '96, 68
TIP: The endometrium is ablated by a laser, radiofrequency electromagnetic energy, or electrocoagulation, via a roller ball or a U-shaped wire on the end of the hysteroscope.

68.24 **Uterine artery embolization [UAE] with coils** ♀
EXCLUDES that without coils (68.25)
AHA: 4Q, '11, 179-180
TIP: UAE may be performed for two purposes: to stop severe pelvic bleeding and to obstruct blood flow to uterine fibroids.

68.25 **Uterine artery embolization [UAE] without coils** ♀
Includes that by:
gelatin sponge
gelfoam
microspheres
particulate agent NOS
polyvinyl alcohol [PVA]
spherical embolics
EXCLUDES that with coils (68.24)
AHA: 4Q, '11, 179-180
TIP: UAE may be performed for two purposes: to stop severe pelvic bleeding and to obstruct blood flow to uterine fibroids.

68.29 **Other excision or destruction of lesion of uterus** ♀

Uterine myomectomy
EXCLUDES biopsy of uterus (68.13)
uterine fistulectomy (69.42)
AHA: 3Q, '06, 18; 1Q, '96, 14

68.3 Subtotal abdominal hysterectomy

68.31 **Laparoscopic supracervical hysterectomy [LSH]** ♀

Classic infrafascial SEMM hysterectomy [CISH]
Laparoscopically assisted supracervical hysterectomy [LASH]
DEF: A hysterectomy that spares the cervix and maintains the integrity of the pelvic floor; SEMM version of the supracervical hysterectomy, also called the classic infrafascial SEMM hysterectomy [CISH]; the cardinal ligaments, or lateral cervical ligaments that merge with the pelvic diaphragm remain intact.
AHA: 4Q, '03, 98-99

68.39 **Other and unspecified subtotal abdominal hysterectomy** ♀
Supracervical hysterectomy
EXCLUDES classic infrafascial SEMM hysterectomy [CISH] (68.31)
laparoscopic supracervical hysterectomy [LSH] (68.31)
AHA: 4Q, '03, 98

Vaginal Hysterectomy

Total hysterectomy (uterus only removed)

Total hysterectomy with bilateral salpingectomy (uterus and tubes removed)

Total hysterectomy with bilateral salpingo-oophorectomy (uterus, tubes, and ovaries removed)

68.4 **Total abdominal hysterectomy**
Code also any synchronous removal of tubes and ovaries (65.31-65.64)
EXCLUDES radical abdominal hysterectomy, any approach (68.61-68.69)
DEF: Complete excision of uterus and uterine neck through abdominal approach.
AHA: 4Q, '96, 65

68.41 **Laparoscopic total abdominal hysterectomy** ♀
Total laparoscopic hysterectomy [TLH]
AHA: 3Q, '09, 5; 4Q, '06, 130, 133

68.49 **Other and unspecified total abdominal hysterectomy** ♀
Hysterectomy:
extended
EXCLUDES laparoscopic total abdominal hysterectomy (68.41)
AHA: ▶4Q, '12, 82;◄ 1Q, '12, 3-4; 4Q, '06, 130

68.5 **Vaginal hysterectomy**
Code also any synchronous:
removal of tubes and ovaries (65.31-65.64)
repair of cystocele or rectocele (70.50-70.52)
repair of pelvic floor (70.79)
DEF: Complete excision of the uterus by a vaginal approach.

68.51 **Laparoscopically assisted vaginal hysterectomy [LAVH]** ♀
AHA: 1Q, '12, 3-5; 4Q, '96, 68

68.59 **Other and unspecified vaginal hysterectomy** ♀
EXCLUDES laparoscopically assisted vaginal hysterectomy (68.51)
radical vaginal hysterectomy (68.71-68.79)

68.6 **Radical abdominal hysterectomy**
Code also any synchronous:
lymph gland dissection (40.3, 40.5)
removal of tubes and ovaries (65.31-65.64)
EXCLUDES pelvic evisceration (68.8)
DEF: Excision of uterus, loose connective tissue and smooth muscle around uterus and vagina via abdominal approach.

68.61 **Laparoscopic radical abdominal hysterectomy** ♀
Laparoscopic modified radical hysterectomy
Total laparoscopic radical hysterectomy [TLRH]
AHA: 4Q, '06, 130, 134

68.69 **Other and unspecified radical abdominal hysterectomy** ♀
Modified radical hysterectomy
Wertheim's operation
EXCLUDES laparoscopic radical abdominal hysterectomy (68.61)
laparoscopic total abdominal hysterectomy (68.41)
AHA: 4Q, '06, 130

√4ᵗʰ **68.7** **Radical vaginal hysterectomy**
Code also any synchronous:
lymph gland dissection (40.3, 40.5)
removal of tubes and ovaries (65.31-65.64)
EXCLUDES *abdominal hysterectomy, any approach*
(68.31-68.39, 68.41-68.49, 68.61-68.69, 68.9)
DEF: Excision of uterus, loose connective tissue and smooth muscle
around uterus and vagina via vaginal approach.

68.71 **Laparoscopic radical vaginal**
hysterectomy [LRVH]   ♀
AHA: 4Q, '06, 130

68.79 **Other and unspecified radical vaginal**
hysterectomy   ♀
Hysterocolpectomy
Schauta operation
AHA: 4Q, '06, 130

68.8 **Pelvic evisceration**   ♀
Removal of ovaries, tubes, uterus, vagina, bladder, and
urethra (with removal of sigmoid colon and rectum)
Code also any synchronous:
colostomy (46.10-46.13)
lymph gland dissection (40.3, 40.5)
urinary diversion (56.51-56.79)

68.9 **Other and unspecified hysterectomy**   ♀
Hysterectomy NOS
EXCLUDES *abdominal hysterectomy, any approach*
(68.31-68.39, 68.41-68.49, 68.61-68.69)
vaginal hysterectomy, any approach (68.51-68.59,
68.71-68.79)

√3ʳᵈ **69** **Other operations on uterus and supporting structures**
Code also any application or administration of an adhesion barrier
substance (99.77)

√4ᵗʰ **69.0** **Dilation and curettage of uterus**
EXCLUDES *aspiration curettage of uterus (69.51-69.59)*
DEF: Stretching of uterine neck to scrape tissue from walls.
TIP: If the documentation indicates dilation with both curettage and
suction, assign instead code 69.59.

69.01 **Dilation and curettage for termination of**
pregnancy   ♀
AHA: 1Q, '98, 4

69.02 **Dilation and curettage following**
delivery or abortion   ♀
AHA: 3Q, '93, 6

69.09 **Other dilation and curettage**   ♀
Diagnostic D and C
AHA: 1Q, '98, 4
TIP: Assign for D&C of a blighted ovum, which is not
considered a viable pregnancy.

√4ᵗʰ **69.1** **Excision or destruction of lesion or tissue of uterus and**
supporting structures

69.19 **Other excision or destruction of uterus**
and supporting structures   ♀
EXCLUDES *biopsy of uterine ligament (68.14)*

√4ᵗʰ **69.2** **Repair of uterine supporting structures**

69.21 **Interposition operation**   ♀
Watkins procedure

69.22 **Other uterine suspension**   ♀
Hysteropexy
Manchester operation
Plication of uterine ligament
DEF: Hysteropexy: Fixation or anchoring of uterus.
DEF: Manchester operation: Fixation or anchoring of uterus
with supportive banding tissue of uterine neck and vagina.
DEF: Plication of uterine ligament: Creation of tucks in
suppurative uterine banding tissue.
DEF: Repositioning or realignment of bladder and uterus.

69.23 **Vaginal repair of chronic inversion of uterus** ♀
DEF: Repositioning of inverted uterus via vaginal approach.

69.29 **Other repair of uterus and supporting**
structures   ♀

69.3 **Paracervical uterine denervation**   ♀

Dilation and Curettage

√4ᵗʰ **69.4** **Uterine repair**
EXCLUDES *repair of current obstetric laceration (75.50-75.52)*

69.41 **Suture of laceration of uterus**   ♀

69.42 **Closure of fistula of uterus**   ♀
EXCLUDES *uterovesical fistulectomy (57.84)*

69.49 **Other repair of uterus**   ♀
Repair of old obstetric laceration of uterus

√4ᵗʰ **69.5** **Aspiration curettage of uterus**
EXCLUDES *menstrual extraction (69.6)*

69.51 **Aspiration curettage of uterus for**
termination of pregnancy   ♀
Therapeutic abortion NOS

69.52 **Aspiration curettage following delivery**
or abortion   ♀

69.59 **Other aspiration curettage of uterus**   ♀
AHA: 1Q, '98, 7

69.6 **Menstrual extraction or regulation**   ♀
DEF: Induction of menstruation by low pressure suction.

69.7 **Insertion of intrauterine contraceptive device** ♀

√4ᵗʰ **69.9** **Other operations on uterus, cervix, and**
supporting structures
EXCLUDES *obstetric dilation or incision of cervix (73.1, 73.93)*

69.91 **Insertion of therapeutic device into uterus**   ♀
EXCLUDES *insertion of:*
intrauterine contraceptive device (69.7)
laminaria (69.93)
obstetric insertion of bag, bougie, or pack
(73.1)

69.92 **Artificial insemination**   ♀

69.93 **Insertion of laminaria**   ♀
AHA: 2Q, '10, 6-7
DEF: Placement of laminaria, a sea kelp, in cervical os to
induce labor; applied for six to 12 hours.

69.94 **Manual replacement of inverted uterus**   ♀
EXCLUDES *that in immediate postpartal period (75.94)*

69.95 **Incision of cervix**   ♀
EXCLUDES *that to assist delivery (73.93)*

69.96 **Removal of cerclage material from cervix**   ♀
DEF: Removal of ring inserted to restore uterine neck
competency.

69.97 **Removal of other penetrating foreign**
body from cervix   ♀
EXCLUDES *removal of intraluminal foreign body from*
cervix (98.16)

69.98 **Other operations on supporting**
structures of uterus   ♀
EXCLUDES *biopsy of uterine ligament (68.14)*

69.99 **Other operations on cervix and uterus**   ♀
EXCLUDES *removal of:*
foreign body (98.16)
intrauterine contraceptive device (97.71)
obstetric bag, bougie, or pack (97.72)
packing (97.72)

BI Bilateral Procedure   NC Non-covered Procedure   LC Limited Coverage Procedure   ►◄ Revised Text   ● New Code   ▲ Revised Code Title

158 – Volume 3   **2014 ICD-9-CM**

√3ʳᵈ **70 Operations on vagina and cul-de-sac**

Code also any application or administration of an adhesion barrier substance (99.77)

70.0 Culdocentesis ♀

DEF: Insertion of needle into upper vaginal vault encircling cervix to withdraw fluid.

AHA: 2Q, '90, 26

TIP: Assign for aspiration for sperm antibodies, which involves aspirating fluid from the female peritoneum or cul-de-sac area to check for the presence of sperm antibodies; assign separate codes for any tubal insufflation (66.8), and/or hysteroscopy (68.12).

√4ᵗʰ **70.1 Incision of vagina and cul-de-sac**

70.11 Hymenotomy ♀

70.12 Culdotomy ♀

DEF: Incision into pocket between terminal end of large intestine and posterior uterus.

70.13 Lysis of intraluminal adhesions of vagina ♀

70.14 Other vaginotomy ♀

Division of vaginal septum

Drainage of hematoma of vaginal cuff

DEF: Division of vaginal septum: Incision into partition of vaginal walls.

DEF: Drainage of hematoma of vaginal cuff: Incision into vaginal tissue to drain collected blood.

√4ᵗʰ **70.2 Diagnostic procedures on vagina and cul-de-sac**

70.21 Vaginoscopy ♀

70.22 Culdoscopy ♀

DEF: Endoscopic exam of pelvic viscera through incision in posterior vaginal wall.

70.23 Biopsy of cul-de-sac ♀

70.24 Vaginal biopsy ♀

70.29 Other diagnostic procedures on vagina and cul-de-sac ♀

√4ᵗʰ **70.3 Local excision or destruction of vagina and cul-de-sac**

70.31 Hymenectomy ♀

70.32 Excision or destruction of lesion of cul-de-sac ♀

Endometrectomy of cul-de-sac

EXCLUDES biopsy of cul-de-sac (70.23)

70.33 Excision or destruction of lesion of vagina ♀

EXCLUDES biopsy of vagina (70.24)
vaginal fistulectomy (70.72-70.75)

70.4 Obliteration and total excision of vagina ♀

Vaginectomy

EXCLUDES obliteration of vaginal vault (70.8)

DEF: Vaginectomy: Removal of vagina.

√4ᵗʰ **70.5 Repair of cystocele and rectocele**

70.50 Repair of cystocele and rectocele ♀

EXCLUDES repair of cystocele and rectocele with graft or prosthesis (70.53)

DEF: Repair of anterior and posterior vaginal wall bulges.

70.51 Repair of cystocele ♀

Anterior colporrhaphy (with urethrocele repair)

EXCLUDES repair of cystocele and rectocele with graft or prosthesis (70.53)
repair of cystocele with graft or prosthesis (70.54)

AHA: N-D, '84, 20

70.52 Repair of rectocele ♀

Posterior colporrhaphy

EXCLUDES repair of cystocele and rectocele with graft or prosthesis (70.53)
repair of rectocele with graft or prosthesis (70.55)
STARR procedure (48.74)

AHA: 2Q, '11, 10; 1Q, '06, 12

70.53 Repair of cystocele and rectocele with graft or prosthesis ♀

Use additional code for biological substance (70.94) or synthetic substance (70.95), if known

AHA: 4Q, '07, 114-115

70.54 Repair of cystocele with graft or prosthesis ♀

Anterior colporrhaphy (with urethrocele repair)

Use additional code for biological substance (70.94) or synthetic substance (70.95), if known

AHA: 2Q, '11, 10; 4Q, '07, 114-115

70.55 Repair of rectocele with graft or prosthesis ♀

Posterior colporrhaphy

Use additional code for biological substance (70.94) or synthetic substance (70.95), if known

AHA: 4Q, '07, 114-115

√4ᵗʰ **70.6 Vaginal construction and reconstruction**

70.61 Vaginal construction ♀

AHA: 3Q, '06, 18

70.62 Vaginal reconstruction ♀

AHA: N-D, '84, 20

70.63 Vaginal construction with graft or prosthesis ♀

Use additional code for biological substance (70.94) or synthetic substance (70.95), if known

EXCLUDES vaginal construction (70.61)

AHA: 4Q, '07, 114-115

70.64 Vaginal reconstruction with graft or prosthesis ♀

Use additional code for biological substance (70.94) or synthetic substance (70.95), if known

EXCLUDES vaginal reconstruction (70.62)

AHA: 4Q, '07, 114-115

√4ᵗʰ **70.7 Other repair of vagina**

EXCLUDES lysis of intraluminal adhesions (70.13)
repair of current obstetric laceration (75.69)
that associated with cervical amputation (67.4)

70.71 Suture of laceration of vagina ♀

AHA: N-D, '84, 20

70.72 Repair of colovaginal fistula ♀

DEF: Correction of abnormal opening between midsection of large intestine and vagina.

70.73 Repair of rectovaginal fistula ♀

DEF: Correction of abnormal opening between last section of large intestine and vagina.

70.74 Repair of other vaginoenteric fistula ♀

DEF: Correction of abnormal opening between vagina and intestine other than mid or last sections.

70.75 Repair of other fistula of vagina ♀

EXCLUDES repair of fistula:
rectovesicovaginal (57.83)
ureterovaginal (56.84)
urethrovaginal (58.43)
uterovaginal (69.42)
vesicocervicovaginal (57.84)
vesicosigmoidovaginal (57.83)
vesicoureterovaginal (56.84)
vesicovaginal (57.84)

70.76 Hymenorrhaphy ♀

DEF: Closure of vagina with suture of hymenal ring or hymenal remnant flaps.

70.77 Vaginal suspension and fixation ♀

DEF: Repair of vaginal protrusion, sinking or laxity by suturing vagina into position.

70.78 Vaginal suspension and fixation with graft or prosthesis ♀

Use additional code for biological substance (70.94) or synthetic substance (70.95), if known

AHA: 4Q, '07, 114-115

70.79 Other repair of vagina ♀

Colpoperineoplasty

Repair of old obstetric laceration of vagina

Operations on the Female Genital Organs

70.8   **Obliteration of vaginal vault** ♀
LeFort operation
DEF: LeFort operation: Uniting or sewing together vaginal walls.

✓4th **70.9**   **Other operations on vagina and cul-de-sac**

     70.91   **Other operations on vagina** ♀
EXCLUDES   insertion of:
     diaphragm (96.17)
     mold (96.15)
     pack (96.14)
     pessary (96.18)
     suppository (96.49)
   removal of:
     diaphragm (97.73)
     foreign body (98.17)
     pack (97.75)
     pessary (97.74)
   replacement of:
     diaphragm (97.24)
     pack (97.26)
     pessary (97.25)
   vaginal dilation (96.16)
   vaginal douche (96.44)

     70.92   **Other operations on cul-de-sac** ♀
Obliteration of cul-de-sac
Repair of vaginal enterocele
AHA: 4Q, '94, 54
DEF: Repair of vaginal enterocele: Elimination of herniated cavity within pouch between last part of large intestine and posterior uterus.

     70.93   **Other operations on cul-de-sac with graft or prosthesis** ♀
Repair of vaginal enterocele with graft or prosthesis
Use additional code for biological substance (70.94) or synthetic substance (70.95), if known
AHA: 4Q, '07, 114-115

     70.94   **Insertion of biological graft** ♀
Allogenic material or substance
Allograft
Autograft
Autologous material or substance
Heterograft
Xenogenic material or substance
Code first these procedures when done with graft or prosthesis:
   Other operations on cul-de-sac (70.93)
   Repair of cystocele (70.54)
   Repair of cystocele and rectocele (70.53)
   Repair of rectocele (70.55)
   Vaginal construction (70.63)
   Vaginal reconstruction (70.64)
   Vaginal suspension and fixation (70.78)
AHA: 4Q, '07, 116

     70.95   **Insertion of synthetic graft or prosthesis** ♀
Artificial tissue
Code first these procedures when done with graft or prosthesis:
   Other operations on cul-de-sac (70.93)
   Repair of cystocele (70.54)
   Repair of cystocele and rectocele (70.53)
   Repair of rectocele (70.55)
   Vaginal construction (70.63)
   Vaginal reconstruction (70.64)
   Vaginal suspension and fixation (70.78)
AHA: 4Q, '07, 116

✓3rd **71**   **Operations on vulva and perineum**
Code also any application or administration of an adhesion barrier substance (99.77)

✓4th **71.0**   **Incision of vulva and perineum**

     71.01   **Lysis of vulvar adhesions** ♀

     71.09   **Other incision of vulva and perineum** ♀
Enlargement of introitus NOS
EXCLUDES   removal of foreign body without incision (98.23)

✓4th **71.1**   **Diagnostic procedures on vulva**

     71.11   **Biopsy of vulva** ♀

Marsupialization

Portion of cyst and overlying skin to be excised

Cyst "unroofed"

Cyst walls sutured to skin

     71.19   **Other diagnostic procedures on vulva** ♀

✓4th **71.2**   **Operations on Bartholin's gland**

     71.21   **Percutaneous aspiration of Bartholin's gland (cyst)** ♀

     71.22   **Incision of Bartholin's gland (cyst)** ♀

     71.23   **Marsupialization of Bartholin's gland (cyst)** ♀
DEF: Incision and suturing open a Bartholin's gland cyst.

     71.24   **Excision or other destruction of Bartholin's gland (cyst)** ♀

     71.29 **Other operations on Bartholin's gland** ♀

71.3   **Other local excision or destruction of vulva and perineum** ♀
Division of Skene's gland
EXCLUDES   biopsy of vulva (71.11)
         vulvar fistulectomy (71.72)
AHA: 4Q, '07, 91

71.4   **Operations on clitoris** ♀
Amputation of clitoris   Female circumcision
Clitoridotomy
DEF: Amputation of clitoris: Removal of clitoris.
DEF: Clitoridotomy: Incision into clitoris.
DEF: Female circumcision: Incision of skin fold over clitoris.

71.5   **Radical vulvectomy** ♀
Code also any synchronous lymph gland dissection (40.3, 40.5)
DEF: Removal of over 80 percent of deep tissue from vulva, including tissue of abdomen, groin, labia minora, labia majora, clitoris, mons veneris, and terminal portions of urethra, vagina and other vulvar organs.

✓4th **71.6**   **Other vulvectomy**

     71.61   **Unilateral vulvectomy** ♀
AHA: 2Q, '06, 19
TIP: Assign for a partial radical vulvectomy.

     71.62   **Bilateral vulvectomy** ♀
Vulvectomy NOS

✓4th **71.7**   **Repair of vulva and perineum** ♀
EXCLUDES   repair of current obstetric laceration (75.69)

     71.71   **Suture of laceration of vulva or perineum** ♀

     71.72   **Repair of fistula of vulva or perineum** ♀
EXCLUDES   repair of fistula:
     urethroperineal (58.43)
     urethroperineovesical (57.84)
     vaginoperineal (70.75)

     71.79   **Other repair of vulva and perineum** ♀
Repair of old obstetric laceration of vulva or perineum
AHA: 1Q, '97, 9

71.8   **Other operations on vulva** ♀
EXCLUDES   removal of:
     foreign body without incision (98.23)
     packing (97.75)
     replacement of packing (97.26)

71.9   **Other operations on female genital organs** ♀
AHA: 4Q, '04, 90; 1Q, '03, 13
TIP: Assign for reversal of the type III female circumcision.

BI   Bilateral Procedure   NC   Non-covered Procedure   LC   Limited Coverage Procedure   ►◄ Revised Text   ● New Code   ▲ Revised Code Title

160 – Volume 3   **2014 ICD-9-CM**

Obstetrical Procedures

13. Obstetrical Procedures (72-75)

√3ʳᵈ **72 Forceps, vacuum, and breech delivery**

72.0 Low forceps operation ♀
Outlet forceps operation

72.1 Low forceps operation with episiotomy ♀
Outlet forceps operation with episiotomy

√4ᵗʰ **72.2 Mid forceps operation**

72.21 Mid forceps operation with episiotomy ♀

72.29 Other mid forceps operation ♀

√4ᵗʰ **72.3 High forceps operation**

72.31 High forceps operation with episiotomy ♀

72.39 Other high forceps operation ♀

72.4 Forceps rotation of fetal head ♀
DeLee maneuver Kielland rotation
Key-in-lock rotation Scanzoni's maneuver
Code also any associated forceps extraction (72.0-72.39)

√4ᵗʰ **72.5 Breech extraction**

72.51 Partial breech extraction with forceps to aftercoming head ♀

72.52 Other partial breech extraction ♀

72.53 Total breech extraction with forceps to aftercoming head ♀

72.54 Other total breech extraction ♀

72.6 Forceps application to aftercoming head ♀
Piper forceps operation
EXCLUDES *partial breech extraction with forceps to aftercoming head (72.51)*
total breech extraction with forceps to aftercoming head (72.53)

√4ᵗʰ **72.7 Vacuum extraction**
INCLUDES Malström's extraction

72.71 Vacuum extraction with episiotomy ♀

72.79 Other vacuum extraction ♀
AHA: 2Q, '06, 5
TIP: This code may be assigned with the appropriate code from category 74 Cesarean section and removal of fetus, when a vacuum is applied during cesarean surgery.

72.8 Other specified instrumental delivery ♀

72.9 Unspecified instrumental delivery ♀

√3ʳᵈ **73 Other procedures inducing or assisting delivery**

√4ᵗʰ **73.0 Artificial rupture of membranes**

73.01 Induction of labor by artificial rupture of membranes ♀
Surgical induction NOS
EXCLUDES *artificial rupture of membranes after onset of labor (73.09)*
AHA: 3Q, '00, 5

73.09 Other artificial rupture of membranes ♀
Artificial rupture of membranes at time of delivery

Breech Extraction

Breech presentation
Delivery of legs
Baby rotated for delivery of arms
Umbilicus

73.1 Other surgical induction of labor ♀
Induction by cervical dilation
EXCLUDES *injection for abortion (75.0)*
insertion of suppository for abortion (96.49)

√4ᵗʰ **73.2 Internal and combined version and extraction**

73.21 Internal and combined version without extraction ♀
Version NOS

73.22 Internal and combined version with extraction ♀

73.3 Failed forceps ♀
Application of forceps without delivery Trial forceps

73.4 Medical induction of labor ♀
EXCLUDES *medication to augment active labor — omit code*
AHA: 2Q, '10, 6-7

√4ᵗʰ **73.5 Manually assisted delivery**

73.51 Manual rotation of fetal head ♀

73.59 Other manually assisted delivery ♀
Assisted spontaneous delivery Credé maneuver
AHA: 4Q, '98, 76

73.6 Episiotomy ♀
Episioproctotomy
Episiotomy with subsequent episiorrhaphy
EXCLUDES *that with:*
high forceps (72.31)
low forceps (72.1)
mid forceps (72.21)
outlet forceps (72.1)
vacuum extraction (72.71)
AHA: 4Q, '08, 192; 1Q, '92, 10

73.8 Operations on fetus to facilitate delivery ♀
Clavicotomy on fetus
Destruction of fetus
Needling of hydrocephalic head

√4ᵗʰ **73.9 Other operations assisting delivery**

73.91 External version ♀

73.92 Replacement of prolapsed umbilical cord ♀

73.93 Incision of cervix to assist delivery ♀
Dührssen's incisions

73.94 Pubiotomy to assist delivery ♀
Obstetrical symphysiotomy

73.99 Other ♀
EXCLUDES *dilation of cervix, obstetrical, to induce labor (73.1)*
insertion of bag or bougie to induce labor (73.1)
removal of cerclage material (69.96)

√3ʳᵈ **74 Cesarean section and removal of fetus**
Code also any synchronous:
hysterectomy (68.3-68.4, 68.6, 68.8)
myomectomy (68.29)
sterilization (66.31-66.39, 66.63)
AHA: 2Q, '06, 5

74.0 Classical cesarean section ♀
Transperitoneal classical cesarean section
AHA: 4Q, '11, 133

74.1 Low cervical cesarean section ♀
Lower uterine segment cesarean section
AHA: 1Q, '01, 11

74.2 Extraperitoneal cesarean section ♀
Supravesical cesarean section

74.3 Removal of extratubal ectopic pregnancy ♀
Removal of:
ectopic abdominal pregnancy
fetus from peritoneal or extraperitoneal cavity following uterine or tubal rupture
EXCLUDES *that by salpingostomy (66.02)*
that by salpingotomy (66.01)
that with synchronous salpingectomy (66.62)
AHA: 4Q, '92, 25; 2Q, '90, 25; 2Q, '90, 27; 1Q, '89, 11

72–74.3

Additional Digit Required Valid OR Procedure Non-OR Procedure Adjunct Code

Obstetrical Procedures

74.4–75.99

Amniocentesis

Amniotic sac

Aspiration of amniotic fluid

74.4 **Cesarean section of other specified type** ♀
Peritoneal exclusion cesareansection
Transperitoneal cesarean section NOS
Vaginal cesarean section

√4ᵗʰ **74.9** **Cesarean section of unspecified type**

    74.91 **Hysterotomy to terminate pregnancy** ♀
        Therapeutic abortion by hysterotomy

    74.99 **Other cesarean section of unspecified type** ♀
        Cesarean section NOS
        Obstetrical abdominouterotomy
        Obstetrical hysterotomy

√3ʳᵈ **75** **Other obstetric operations**

  75.0 **Intra-amniotic injection for abortion** ♀
    Injection of:
      prostaglandin
      saline } for induction of abortion
    Termination of pregnancy by intrauterine injection
    EXCLUDES insertion of prostaglandin suppository for abortion (96.49)

  75.1 **Diagnostic amniocentesis** ♀

  75.2 **Intrauterine transfusion** ♀
    Exchange transfusion in utero
    Insertion of catheter into abdomen of fetus for transfusion
    Code also any hysterotomy approach (68.0)

√4ᵗʰ **75.3** **Other intrauterine operations on fetus and amnion**
    Code also any hysterotomy approach (68.0)

    75.31 **Amnioscopy** ♀
        Fetoscopy
        Laparoamnioscopy
        AHA: 3Q, '06, 16-17

    75.32 **Fetal EKG (scalp)** ♀

    75.33 **Fetal blood sampling and biopsy** ♀

    75.34 **Other fetal monitoring** ♀
        Antepartum fetal nonstress test
        Fetal monitoring, not otherwise specified
        EXCLUDES fetal pulse oximetry (75.38)

    75.35 **Other diagnostic procedures on fetus and amnion** ♀
        Intrauterine pressure determination
        EXCLUDES amniocentesis (75.1)
        *   diagnostic procedures on gravid uterus and placenta (87.81, 88.46, 88.78, 92.17)*
        AHA: 3Q, '06, 16-17

75.36 **Correction of fetal defect**

75.37 **Amnioinfusion**
    Code also injection of antibiotic (99.21)
    AHA: 4Q, '98, 76
    TIP: This procedure involves the controlled instillation of sterile normal saline or lactated Ringers solution into the uterine cavity to replace the amniotic fluid.

75.38 **Fetal pulse oximetry**
    Transcervical fetal oxygen saturation monitoring
    Transcervical fetal SpO₂ monitoring
    DEF: Single-use sensor inserted through the birth canal and positioned to rest against the fetal cheek, forehead, or temple; infrared beam of light aimed at the fetal skin is reflected back through the sensor for analysis.
    AHA: 4Q, '01, 64

75.4 **Manual removal of retained placenta**
    EXCLUDES aspiration curettage (69.52)
    *   dilation and curettage (69.02)*
    AHA: 3Q, '06, 11

√4ᵗʰ **75.5** **Repair of current obstetric laceration of uterus**

    75.50 **Repair of current obstetric laceration of uterus, not otherwise specified**

    75.51 **Repair of current obstetric laceration of cervix**

    75.52 **Repair of current obstetric laceration of corpus uteri**
        AHA: 2Q, '08, 8
        TIP: Assign for B-Lynch procedure performed to control intraoperative hemorrhage during a cesarean section.

√4ᵗʰ **75.6** **Repair of other current obstetric laceration**
    Code also episiotomy, if performed (73.6)
    AHA: 1Q, '92, 11

    75.61 **Repair of current obstetric laceration of bladder and urethra**

    75.62 **Repair of current obstetric laceration of rectum and sphincter ani**

    75.69 **Repair of other current obstetric laceration**
        Episioperineorrhaphy   Repair of:
        Repair of: vagina
          pelvic floor   vulva
          perineum   Secondary repair of episiotomy
        AHA: 4Q, '08, 192; 4Q, '07, 12

75.7 **Manual exploration of uterine cavity, postpartum**

75.8 **Obstetric tamponade of uterus or vagina**
    EXCLUDES antepartum tamponade (73.1)

√4ᵗʰ **75.9** **Other obstetric operations**

    75.91 **Evacuation of obstetrical incisional hematoma of perineum**
        Evacuation of hematoma of:
          episiotomy
          perineorrhaphy

    75.92 **Evacuation of other hematoma of vulva or vagina**

    75.93 **Surgical correction of inverted uterus**
        Spintelli operation
        EXCLUDES vaginal repair of chronic inversion of uterus (69.23)

    75.94 **Manual replacement of inverted uterus**

    75.99 **Other**
        AHA: 3Q, '06, 16-17

BI Bilateral Procedure   **NC** Non-covered Procedure   **LC** Limited Coverage Procedure   ▶◀ Revised Text   ● New Code   ▲ Revised Code Title

162 – Volume 3   **2014 ICD-9-CM**

14. Operations on the Musculoskeletal System (76-84)

√3ʳᵈ **76 Operations on facial bones and joints**
> EXCLUDES *accessory sinuses (22.00-22.9)*
> *nasal bones (21.00-21.99)*
> *skull (01.01-02.99)*

√4ᵗʰ **76.0 Incision of facial bone without division**

76.01 Sequestrectomy of facial bone
Removal of necrotic bone chip from facial bone

76.09 Other incision of facial bone
Reopening of osteotomy site of facial bone
> EXCLUDES *osteotomy associated with orthognathic surgery (76.61-76.69)*
> *removal of internal fixation device (76.97)*

√4ᵗʰ **76.1 Diagnostic procedures on facial bones and joints**

76.11 Biopsy of facial bone

76.19 Other diagnostic procedures on facial bones and joints
> EXCLUDES *contrast arthrogram of temporomandibular joint (87.13)*
> *other x-ray (87.11-87.12, 87.14-87.16)*
> AHA: N-D, '87, 12

76.2 Local excision or destruction of lesion of facial bone
> EXCLUDES *biopsy of facial bone (76.11)*
> *excision of odontogenic lesion (24.4)*

√4ᵗʰ **76.3 Partial ostectomy of facial bone**

76.31 Partial mandibulectomy
Hemimandibulectomy
> EXCLUDES *that associated with temporomandibular arthroplasty (76.5)*
> DEF: Partial excision of lower jawbone.
> DEF: Hemimandibulectomy: Excision of one-half of lower jawbone.
> AHA: 2Q, '05, 8
> TIP: Assign for "composite resection," which includes the mandible and floor of the mouth, along with code 27.49 Other excision of mouth.

76.39 Partial ostectomy of other facial bone
Hemimaxillectomy (with bone graft or prosthesis)
> DEF: Partial excision of facial bone other than lower jawbone.
> DEF: Hemimaxillectomy (with bone graft or prosthesis): Excision of one side of upper jawbone and restoration with bone graft or prosthesis.
> AHA: J-F, '87, 14

√4ᵗʰ **76.4 Excision and reconstruction of facial bones**

76.41 Total mandibulectomy with synchronous reconstruction

76.42 Other total mandibulectomy

76.43 Other reconstruction of mandible
> EXCLUDES *genioplasty (76.67-76.68)*
> *that with synchronous total mandibulectomy (76.41)*
> AHA: 2Q, '03, 13

76.44 Total ostectomy of other facial bone with synchronous reconstruction
> DEF: Total facial bone excision with reconstruction during same operative session.
> AHA: 3Q, '93, 6

76.45 Other total ostectomy of other facial bone

76.46 Other reconstruction of other facial bone
> EXCLUDES *that with synchronous total ostectomy (76.44)*

76.5 Temporomandibular arthroplasty
> AHA: 4Q, '99, 20

√4ᵗʰ **76.6 Other facial bone repair and orthognathic surgery**
Code also any synchronous:
bone graft (76.91)
synthetic implant (76.92)
> EXCLUDES *reconstruction of facial bones (76.41-76.46)*

76.61 Closed osteoplasty [osteotomy] of mandibular ramus
Gigli saw osteotomy
> DEF: Reshaping and restoration of lower jawbone projection; closed surgical field, which is a limited "key hole" incision.
> DEF: Gigli saw osteotomy: Plastic repair using a flexible wire with saw teeth.

76.62 Open osteoplasty [osteotomy] of mandibular ramus

76.63 Osteoplasty [osteotomy] of body of mandible

76.64 Other orthognathic surgery on mandible
Mandibular osteoplasty NOS
Segmental or subapical osteotomy
> AHA: 2Q, '04, 9, 10

76.65 Segmental osteoplasty [osteotomy] of maxilla
Maxillary osteoplasty NOS

76.66 Total osteoplasty [osteotomy] of maxilla

76.67 Reduction genioplasty
Reduction mentoplasty
> DEF: Reduction of protruding chin or lower jawbone.

76.68 Augmentation genioplasty
Mentoplasty:
NOS
with graft or implant
> DEF: Extension of the lower jawbone to a functional position by means of plastic surgery.

76.69 Other facial bone repair
Osteoplasty of facial bone NOS

√4ᵗʰ **76.7 Reduction of facial fracture**
> INCLUDES internal fixation
Code also any synchronous:
bone graft (76.91)
synthetic implant (76.92)
> EXCLUDES *that of nasal bones (21.71-21.72)*

76.70 Reduction of facial fracture, not otherwise specified

76.71 Closed reduction of malar and zygomatic fracture

76.72 Open reduction of malar and zygomatic fracture

76.73 Closed reduction of maxillary fracture

76.74 Open reduction of maxillary fracture

76.75 Closed reduction of mandibular fracture

76.76 Open reduction of mandibular fracture

76.77 Open reduction of alveolar fracture
Reduction of alveolar fracture with stabilization of teeth

76.78 Other closed reduction of facial fracture
Closed reduction of orbital fracture
> EXCLUDES *nasal bone (21.71)*

76.79 Other open reduction of facial fracture
Open reduction of orbit rim or wall
> EXCLUDES *nasal bone (21.72)*

√4ᵗʰ **76.9 Other operations on facial bones and joints**

76.91 Bone graft to facial bone
Autogenous
Bone bank } graft to facial bone
Heterogenous

76.92 Insertion of synthetic implant in facial bone
Alloplastic implant to facial bone

76.93 Closed reduction of temporomandibular dislocation

76.94 Open reduction of temporomandibular dislocation

√3ʳᵈ
√4ᵗʰ
Additional Digit Required
2014 ICD-9-CM

Valid OR Procedure

Non-OR Procedure

Adjunct Code

Volume 3 – 163

Operations on the Musculoskeletal System

76.95–77.9

76.95　Other manipulation of temporomandibular joint

76.96　Injection of therapeutic substance into temporomandibular joint

76.97　Removal of internal fixation device from facial bone

　　　　EXCLUDES　removal of:
　　　　　　　dental wiring (97.33)
　　　　　　　external mandibular fixation device NEC (97.36)

76.99　Other

√3rd　77　Incision, excision, and division of other bones

　　　EXCLUDES　laminectomy for decompression (03.09)
　　　　　operations on:
　　　　　　accessory sinuses (22.00-22.9)
　　　　　　ear ossicles (19.0-19.55)
　　　　　　facial bones (76.01-76.99)
　　　　　　joint structures (80.00-81.99)
　　　　　　mastoid (19.9-20.99)
　　　　　　nasal bones (21.00-21.99)
　　　　　　skull (01.01-02.99)

The following fourth-digit subclassification is for use with appropriate categories in section 77 to identify the site. Valid fourth-digit categories are in [brackets] under each code.

　0　unspecified site
　1　scapula, clavicle, and thorax [ribs and sternum]
　2　humerus
　3　radius and ulna
　4　carpals and metacarpals
　5　femur
　6　patella
　7　tibia and fibula
　8　tarsals and metatarsals
　9　other
　　　Pelvic bones
　　　Phalanges (of foot) (of hand)
　　　Vertebrae

§ √4th　77.0　Sequestrectomy
[0-9]　　DEF: Excision and removal of dead bone.

§ √4th　77.1　Other incision of bone without division
[0-9]　　Reopening of osteotomy site
　　　　EXCLUDES　aspiration of bone marrow, (41.31, 41.91)
　　　　　　　removal of internal fixation device (78.60-78.69)
　　　　AHA: For code 77.17: 1Q, '02, 3
　　　　DEF: Incision into bone without division of site.

§ √4th　77.2　Wedge osteotomy
[0-9]　　EXCLUDES　that for hallux valgus (77.51)
　　　　DEF: Removal of wedge-shaped piece of bone.

§ √4th　77.3　Other division of bone
[0-9]　　Osteoarthrotomy
　　　　EXCLUDES　clavicotomy of fetus (73.8)
　　　　　　　laminotomy or incision of vertebra (03.01-03.09)
　　　　　　　pubiotomy to assist delivery (73.94)
　　　　　　　sternotomy incidental to thoracic operation — omit code

§ √4th　77.4　Biopsy of bone
[0-9]　　AHA: For code 77.45: 2Q, '98, 12; For code 77.49: 3Q, '06, 13

√4th　77.5　Excision and repair of bunion and other toe deformities

77.51　Bunionectomy with soft tissue correction and osteotomy of the first metatarsal
　　　　DEF: Incision and removal of big toe bony prominence and reconstruction with soft tissue.

77.52　Bunionectomy with soft tissue correction and arthrodesis
　　　　DEF: Removal of big toe bony prominence and reconstruction with soft tissue and joint fixation.

77.53　Other bunionectomy with soft tissue correction

77.54　Excision or correction of bunionette
　　　　That with osteotomy
　　　　DEF: Resection of fifth metatarsal head via exposure of joint; includes imbrication of capsule.

Repair of Hammer Toe

Corn
Callus
Hammertoe
Hemiphalengectomy
After

77.56　Repair of hammer toe
　　　　Filleting
　　　　Fusion　　　　　} of hammer toe
　　　　Phalangectomy (partial)
　　　　DEF: Repair of clawlike toe defect by joint fusion, or partial removal of toe via traction technique.

77.57　Repair of claw toe
　　　　Capsulotomy
　　　　Fusion
　　　　Phalangectomy (partial)　} of claw toe
　　　　Tendon lengthening
　　　　DEF: Repair of clawlike toe defect by joint fusion, partial removal of toe, joint capsule incision or lengthening of fibrous muscle attachment.

77.58　Other excision, fusion, and repair of toes
　　　　Cockup toe repair
　　　　Overlapping toe repair
　　　　That with use of prosthetic materials

77.59　Other bunionectomy
　　　　Resection of hallux valgus joint with insertion of prosthesis
　　　　DEF: Resection of hallux valgus joint with insertion of prosthesis: Cutting away part of big toe with prosthesis insertion to correct bony prominence.

§ √4th　77.6　Local excision of lesion or tissue of bone
[0-9]　　EXCLUDES　biopsy of bone (77.40-77.49)
　　　　　　　debridement of compound fracture (79.60-79.69)
　　　　AHA: For code 77.61: 4Q, '10, 131 3Q, '01, 9; For code 77.65: 4Q, '04, 128; S-O, '85, 4; For code 77.67: 1Q, '02, 3; 1Q, '99, 8; For code 77.68: ►4Q, '12, 83◄ For code 77.69: 1Q, '08, 4; 2Q, '00, 18
　　　　TIP: Assign for debridement procedures that extend to bone.

§ √4th　77.7　Excision of bone for graft
[0-9]　　AHA: 2Q, '07, 5; 4Q, '99, 11, 13; For code 77.71: 3Q, '03, 19; For code 77.79: 1Q, '08, 5; 2Q, '03, 13; 4Q, '02, 107, 109-110; 2Q, '02, 16; 2Q '00 12, 13; 4Q, '99, 11, 13

§ √4th　77.8　Other partial ostectomy
[0-9]　　Condylectomy
　　　　EXCLUDES　amputation (84.00-84.19, 84.91)
　　　　　　　arthrectomy (80.90-80.99)
　　　　　　　excision of bone ends associated with:
　　　　　　　　arthrodesis (81.00-81.39, 81.62-81.66)
　　　　　　　　arthroplasty (81.40-81.59, 81.71-81.85)
　　　　　　　excision of cartilage (80.5-80.6, 80.80-80.99)
　　　　　　　excision of head of femur with synchronous replacement (00.70-00.73, 81.51-81.53)
　　　　　　　hemilaminectomy (03.01-03.09)
　　　　　　　laminectomy (03.01-03.09)
　　　　　　　ostectomy for hallux valgus (77.51-77.59)
　　　　　　　partial amputation:
　　　　　　　　finger (84.01)
　　　　　　　　thumb (84.02)
　　　　　　　　toe (84.11)
　　　　　　　resection of ribs incidental to thoracic operation — omit code
　　　　　　　that incidental to other operation — omit code
　　　　AHA: For code 77.89: 2Q, '02, 8

§ √4th　77.9　Total ostectomy
[0-9]　　EXCLUDES　amputation of limb (84.00-84.19, 84.91)
　　　　　　　that incidental to other operation — omit code

§　Requires fourth digit. Valid digits are in [brackets] under each code. See category 77 for codes and definitions.

BI　Bilateral Procedure　　　NC　Non-covered Procedure　　　LC　Limited Coverage Procedure　　　►◄ Revised Text　　　● New Code　　　▲ Revised Code Title

√3ʳᵈ **78 Other operations on bones, except facial bones**

    EXCLUDES operations on:
       accessory sinuses (22.00–22.9)
       facial bones (76.01–76.99)
       joint structures (80.00–81.99)
       nasal bones (21.00–21.99)
       skull (01.01–02.99)

The following fourth-digit subclassification is for use with appropriate categories in section 78 to identify the site. Valid fourth-digit categories are in [brackets] under each code.

0 unspecified site	**6 patella**
1 scapula, clavicle, and thorax [ribs and sternum]	**7 tibia and fibula**
	8 tarsals and metatarsals
2 humerus	**9 other**
3 radius and ulna	Pelvic bones
4 carpals and metacarpals	Phalanges (of foot) (of hand)
5 femur	Vertebrae

§ √4ᵗʰ **78.0 Bone graft**
  [0–9]   Bone:
      bank graft
      graft (autogenous) (heterogenous)
    That with debridement of bone graft site (removal of sclerosed, fibrous, or necrotic bone or tissue)
    Transplantation of bone
    Code also any excision of bone for graft (77.70–77.79)
    EXCLUDES that for bone lengthening (78.30–78.39)
    AHA: 2Q, '02, 11; 2Q, '98, 12; 3Q, '94, 10; 1Q, '91, 3;
    For code 78.06: ▶3Q, '12, 11◀
    TIP: Assign a code from this subcategory whether the documentation indicates bone or bone marrow as the grafting material.

§ √4ᵗʰ **78.1 Application of external fixator device**
  [0–9]   Fixator with insertion of pins/wires/screws into bone
    Code also any type of fixator device, if known (84.71–84.73)
    EXCLUDES other immobilization, pressure, and attention to wound (93.51–93.59)
    AHA: 2Q, '94, 4; For code 78.12: 4Q, '05, 129

§ √4ᵗʰ **78.2 Limb shortening procedures**
  [0,2–5,7–9] Epiphyseal stapling
    Open epiphysiodesis
    Percutaneous epiphysiodesis
    Resection/osteotomy

§ √4ᵗʰ **78.3 Limb lengthening procedures**
  [0,2–5,7–9] Bone graft with or without internal fixation devices or osteotomy
    Distraction technique with or without corticotomy/osteotomy
    Code also any application of an external fixation device (78.10–78.19)

§ √4ᵗʰ **78.4 Other repair or plastic operations on bone**
  [0–9]   Other operation on bone NEC
    Repair of malunion or nonunion fracture NEC
    EXCLUDES application of external fixation device (78.10–78.19)
       limb lengthening procedures (78.30–78.39)
       limb shortening procedures (78.20–78.29)
       osteotomy (77.3)
       reconstruction of thumb (82.61–82.69)
       repair of pectus deformity (34.74)
       repair with bone graft (78.00–78.09)
    AHA: 3Q, '91, 20; 4Q, '88, 11; For code 78.41: 2Q, '02, 16; For code 78.47: 3Q, '91, 20; For code 78.49: 3Q, '04, 9; 2Q, '03, 22; 3Q, '02, 12; 2Q, '02, 14, 15; 4Q, '99, 22; 1Q, '97, 5

§ √4ᵗʰ **78.5 Internal fixation of bone without fracture reduction**
  [0–9]   Internal fixation of bone (prophylactic)
    Reinsertion of internal fixation device
    Revision of displaced or broken fixation device
    EXCLUDES arthroplasty and arthrodesis (81.00–81.85)
       bone graft (78.00–78.09)
       insertion of sternal fixation device with rigid plates (84.94)
       limb shortening procedures (78.20–78.29)
       that for fracture reduction (79.10–79.19, 79.30–79.59)
    AHA: 2Q, '99, 11; 2Q, '94, 4; For code 78.52: 2Q, '10, 6; For code 78.55: 2Q, '10, 6; For code 78.59: 3Q, '04, 6; 2Q, '03, 15; 4Q, '99, 13

§ √4ᵗʰ **78.6 Removal of implanted devices from bone**
  [0–9]   External fixator device (invasive)
    Internal fixation device
    Removal of bone growth stimulator (invasive)
    Removal of internal limb lengthening device
    Removal of pedicle screw(s) used in spinal fusion
    EXCLUDES removal of cast, splint, and traction device (Kirschner wire) (Steinmann pin) (97.88)
       removal of posterior spinal motion preservation (facet replacement, pedicle-based dynamic stabilization, interspinous process) device(s) (80.09)
       removal of skull tongs or halo traction device (02.95)
    AHA: 1Q, '00, 15; For code 78.67: 2Q, '03, 14; For code 78.69: 4Q, '02, 110; 2Q, '00, 18

§ √4ᵗʰ **78.7 Osteoclasis**
  [0–9]   DEF: Surgical breaking or rebreaking of bone.

§ √4ᵗʰ **78.8 Diagnostic procedures on bone, not elsewhere classified**
  [0–9]
    EXCLUDES biopsy of bone (77.40–77.49)
       magnetic resonance imaging (88.94)
       microscopic examination of specimen from bone (91.51–91.59)
       radioisotope scan (92.14)
       skeletal x-ray (87.21–87.29, 87.43, 88.21–88.33)
       thermography (88.83)

§ √4ᵗʰ **78.9 Insertion of bone growth stimulator**
  [0–9]   Insertion of:
      bone stimulator (electrical) to aid bone healing
      osteogenic electrodes for bone growth stimulation
      totally implanted device (invasive)
    EXCLUDES non-invasive (transcutaneous) (surface) stimulator (99.86)

√3ʳᵈ **79 Reduction of fracture and dislocation**
    INCLUDES application of cast or splint
       reduction with insertion of traction device (Kirschner wire) (Steinmann pin)
    Code also any:
      application of external fixator device (78.10–78.19)
      type of fixator device, if known (84.71–84.73)
    EXCLUDES external fixation alone for immobilization of fracture (93.51–93.56, 93.59)
       internal fixation without reduction of fracture (78.50–78.59)
       operations on:
         facial bones(76.70–76.79)
         nasal bones (21.71–21.72)
         orbit (76.78–76.79)
         skull (02.02)
         vertebrae (03.53)
       removal of cast or splint (97.88)
       replacement of cast or splint (97.11–97.14)
       traction alone for reduction of fracture (93.41–93.46)

The following fourth-digit subclassification is for use with appropriate categories in section 79 to identify the site. Valid fourth-digit categories are in [brackets] under each code.

0 unspecified site	**5 femur**
1 humerus	**6 tibia and fibula**
2 radius and ulna	Leg NOS
Arm NOS	**7 tarsals and metatarsals**
3 carpals and metacarpals	Foot NOS
Hand NOS	**8 phalanges of foot**
4 phalanges of hand	**9 other specified bone**

§ √4ᵗʰ **79.0 Closed reduction of fracture without internal fixation**
  [0–9]
    EXCLUDES that for separation of epiphysis (79.40–79.49)
    DEF: Manipulative realignment of fracture; without incision or internal fixation.
    AHA: 2Q, '94, 3; 3Q, '89, 17; 4Q, '88, 11; For code 79.01: 4Q, '05, 129; For code 79.05: 3Q, '89, 16

§ √4ᵗʰ **79.1 Closed reduction of fracture with internal fixation**
  [0–9]
    EXCLUDES that for separation of epiphysis (79.40–79.49)
    DEF: Manipulative realignment of fracture; with internal fixation but without incision.
    AHA: 2Q, '94, 4; 4Q, '93, 35; 1Q, '93, 27

§ Requires fourth digit. Valid digits are in [brackets] under each code. See appropriate category for codes and definitions.

√3ʳᵈ √4ᵗʰ Additional Digit Required	Valid OR Procedure	Non-OR Procedure	Adjunct Code

§ ✓4ᵗʰ **79.2** **Open reduction of fracture without internal fixation**
[0-9]   **EXCLUDES** *that for separation of epiphysis (79.50-79.59)*
          AHA: 2Q, '94, 3

§ ✓4ᵗʰ **79.3** **Open reduction of fracture with internal fixation**
[0-9]   **EXCLUDES** *that for separation of epiphysis (79.50-79.59)*
          DEF: Realignment of fracture with incision and internal fixation.
          AHA: 2Q, '98, 12; 3Q, '94, 10; 2Q, '94, 3; 4Q, '93, 35; For code 79.32: 1Q,
          '07, 7; For code 79.35: 1Q, '07, 4; For code 79.36: ▶2Q, '12,11-12◀
          TIP: ▶When arthroscopy assists with visualization of the surgical site,
          do not report the arthroscopy separately.◀

§ ✓4ᵗʰ **79.4** **Closed reduction of separated epiphysis**
[0-2,5,6,9] Reduction with or without internal fixation
          DEF: Manipulative reduction of expanded joint end of long bone to
          normal position without incision.

§ ✓4ᵗʰ **79.5** **Open reduction of separated epiphysis**
[0-2,5,6,9] Reduction with or without internal fixation
          DEF: Reduction of expanded joint end of long bone with incision.

§ ✓4ᵗʰ **79.6** **Debridement of open fracture site**
[0-9]   Debridement of compound fracture
          DEF: Removal of damaged tissue at fracture site.
          AHA: 3Q, '95, 12; 3Q, '89, 16
          TIP: Do not assign a skin/soft tissue debridement procedure code
          (e.g., 86.22) in addition to the open fracture debridement code; all
          debridement is included.

✓4ᵗʰ **79.7** **Closed reduction of dislocation**
          INCLUDES closed reduction (with external traction device)
          EXCLUDES *closed reduction of dislocation of*
                    temporomandibular joint (76.93)
          DEF: Manipulative reduction of displaced joint without incision; with
          or without external traction.

     79.70 **Closed reduction of dislocation of unspecified site**

     79.71 **Closed reduction of dislocation of shoulder**

     79.72 **Closed reduction of dislocation of elbow**

     79.73 **Closed reduction of dislocation of wrist**

     79.74 **Closed reduction of dislocation of hand and finger**

     79.75 **Closed reduction of dislocation of hip**

     79.76 **Closed reduction of dislocation of knee**
                    AHA: N-D, '86, 7

     79.77 **Closed reduction of dislocation of ankle**

     79.78 **Closed reduction of dislocation of foot and toe**

     79.79 **Closed reduction of dislocation of other specified sites**

✓4ᵗʰ **79.8** **Open reduction of dislocation**
          INCLUDES open reduction (with internal and external fixation
                    devices)
          EXCLUDES *open reduction of dislocation of temporomandibular*
                    joint (76.94)
          DEF: Reduction of displaced joint via incision; with or without
          internal and external fixation.

     79.80 **Open reduction of dislocation of unspecified site**

     79.81 **Open reduction of dislocation of shoulder**

     79.82 **Open reduction of dislocation of elbow**

     79.83 **Open reduction of dislocation of wrist**

     79.84 **Open reduction of dislocation of hand and finger**

     79.85 **Open reduction of dislocation of hip**

     79.86 **Open reduction of dislocation of knee**

     79.87 **Open reduction of dislocation of ankle**

     79.88 **Open reduction of dislocation of foot and toe**

     79.89 **Open reduction of dislocation of other specified sites**

§ ✓4ᵗʰ **79.9** **Unspecified operation on bone injury**
[0-9]

✓3ʳᵈ **80** **Incision and excision of joint structures**
          INCLUDES operations on:
                    capsule of joint
                    cartilage
                    condyle
                    ligament
                    meniscus
                    synovial membrane
          EXCLUDES *cartilage of:*
                    ear (18.01-18.9)
                    nose (21.00-21.99)
                    temporomandibular joint (76.01-76.99)

          The following fourth-digit subclassification is for use with appropriate
          categories in section 80 to identify the site:

          0 unspecified site   6 knee
          1 shoulder   7 ankle
          2 elbow   8 foot and toe
          3 wrist   9 other specified sites
          4 hand and finger   Spine
          5 hip

§ ✓4ᵗʰ **80.0** **Arthrotomy for removal of prosthesis,**
[0-9]   **without replacement**
          INCLUDES removal of posterior spinal motion preservation
                    (dynamic stabilization, facet replacement,
                    interspinous process) device(s)
          Code also any:
               insertion of (cement) (joint) (methylmethacrylate) spacer
                    (84.56)
               removal of (cement) (joint) (methylmethacrylate) spacer
                    (84.57)
          EXCLUDES *removal of pedicle screws used in spinal fusion*
                    (78.69)
          DEF: Incision into joint to remove prosthesis.
          AHA: 4Q, '09, 148-149; For code 80.05: ▶3Q, '12, 14;◀ 2Q, '08, 4, 5;
          For code 80.06: ▶3Q, '12, 15;◀ 2Q, '97, 10
          TIP: Assign 80.05 for a Girdlestone procedure, in which an infected
          hip prosthesis is removed without replacement, until the surgical
          site heals.

§ ✓4ᵗʰ **80.1** **Other arthrotomy**
[0-9]   Arthrostomy
          EXCLUDES *that for:*
                    arthrography (88.32)
                    arthroscopy (80.20-80.29)
                    injection of drug (81.92)
                    operative approach — omit code
          DEF: Incision into joint; other than to remove prosthesis.
          DEF: Arthrostomy: Creation of opening into joint.
          AHA: For code 80.15: 3Q, '06, 22-23; For code 80.16: 3Q, '06, 23

§ ✓4ᵗʰ **80.2** **Arthroscopy**
[0-9]   AHA: 3Q, '93, 5; 1Q, '93, 23

§ ✓4ᵗʰ **80.3** **Biopsy of joint structure**
[0-9]   Aspiration biopsy
          AHA: For code 80.39: 3Q, '05, 13-14

§ ✓4ᵗʰ **80.4** **Division of joint capsule, ligament, or cartilage**
[0-9]   Goldner clubfoot release
          Heyman-Herndon(-Strong) correction of metatarsus varus
          Release of:
               adherent or constrictive joint capsule
               joint
               ligament
          EXCLUDES *symphysiotomy to assist delivery (73.94)*
                    that for:
                         carpal tunnel syndrome (04.43)
                         tarsal tunnel syndrome (04.44)
          DEF: Incision and separation of joint tissues, including capsule,
          fibrous bone attachment or cartilage.
          AHA: For code 80.49: 2Q, '02, 16

✓4ᵗʰ **80.5** **Excision, destruction and other repair of intervertebral disc**

     80.50 **Excision, destruction and other repair of intervertebral disc, unspecified**
               Unspecified as to excision or destruction

§   Requires fourth digit. Valid digits are in [brackets] under each code. See appropriate category for codes and definitions.

BI Bilateral Procedure   NC Non-covered Procedure   LC Limited Coverage Procedure   ▶◀ Revised Text   ● New Code   ▲ Revised Code Title

166 – Volume 3 • February 2013   2014 ICD-9-CM

Operations on the Musculoskeletal System

79.2–80.50

80.51 Excision of intervertebral disc

> **NOTE** Requires additional code for any concomitant decompression of spinal nerve root at different level from excision site
>
> Diskectomy
>
> Level:
> > cervical
> > thoracic
> > lumbar (lumbosacral)
>
> Removal of herniated nucleus pulposus
> That by laminotomy or hemilaminectomy
> That with decompression of spinal nerve root at same level
>
> Code also any:
> > concurrent spinal fusion (81.00-81.08)
> > repair of the anulus fibrosus (80.53-80.54)
>
> **EXCLUDES** intervertebral chemonucleolysis (80.52)
> > laminectomy for exploration of intraspinal canal (03.09)
> > laminotomy for decompression of spinal nerve root only (03.09)
> > that for insertion of (non-fusion) spinal disc replacement device (84.60-84.69)
> > that with corpectomy, (vertebral) (80.99)
>
> **DEF:** Discectomy: Removal of intervertebral disc.
> **DEF:** Removal of a herniated nucleus pulposus: Removal of displaced intervertebral disc, central part.
> **AHA:** 2Q, '09, 4-5; 4Q, '08, 184; 2Q, '08, 14; 1Q, '08, 5; 1Q, '07, 9; 1Q, '06, 12; 4Q, '04, 133; 3Q, '03, 12; 1Q, '96, 7; 2Q, '95, 9; 2Q, '90, 27; S-O, '86, 12

80.52 Intervertebral chemonucleolysis

> With aspiration of disc fragments
> With diskography
> Injection of proteolytic enzyme into intervertebral space (chymopapain)
>
> **EXCLUDES** injection of anesthestic substance (03.91)
> > injection of other substances (03.92)
>
> **DEF:** Destruction of intervertebral disc via injection of enzyme.

80.53 Repair of the anulus fibrosus with graft or prosthesis

> **INCLUDES** microsurgical suture repair with fascial autograft
> > soft tissue re-approximation repair with tension bands
> > surgical mesh repair
>
> Anular disc repair
> Closure (sealing) of the anulus fibrosus defect
>
> Code also any:
> > application or administration of adhesion barrier substance, if performed (99.77)
> > intervertebral discectomy, if performed (80.51)
> > locally harvested fascia for graft (83.43)
>
> **DEF:** Adjunct procedure involving closure of defect in annulus fibrosis (ring of cartilage and fibrous tissue surrounding nucleus pulposus of IV disc) following discectomy surgery; prevents later disc herniation.
> **AHA:** 4Q, '08, 183-184

80.54 Other and unspecified repair of the anulus fibrosus

> Anular disc repair
> Closure (sealing) of the anulus fibrosus defect
> Microsurgical suture repair without fascial autograft
> Percutaneous repair of the anulus fibrosus
>
> Code also any:
> > application or administration of adhesion barrier substance, if performed (99.77)
> > intervertebral discectomy, if performed (80.51)
>
> **DEF:** Adjunct procedure involving closure of defect in annulus fibrosis (ring of cartilage and fibrous tissue surrounding nucleus pulposus of IV disc) following discectomy surgery; prevents later disc herniation.
> **AHA:** 4Q, '08, 183-184

80.59 Other destruction of intervertebral disc

> Destruction NEC   That by laser
> **AHA:** 3Q, '02, 10
> **TIP:** Assign for intradiscal electrothermal therapy (IDET), whereby thermal energy (heat) is directed into the outer disc wall (annulus) and inner disc contents (nucleus) via a heating coil, decreasing the pressure inside the disc.

80.6 Excision of semilunar cartilage of knee

> Excision of meniscus of knee
> **AHA:** 2Q, '03, 18; 3Q, '00, 4; 2Q, '96, 3; 1Q, '93, 23

§ ✓4th **80.7 Synovectomy**
[0-9]
> Complete or partial resection of synovial membrane
> **EXCLUDES** excision of Baker's cyst (83.39)
> **DEF:** Excision of inner membrane of joint capsule.

§ ✓4th **80.8 Other local excision or destruction of lesion of joint**
[0-9]
> **AHA:** For code 80.86: 1Q, '08, 7

§ ✓4th **80.9 Other excision of joint**
[0-9]
> **EXCLUDES** cheilectomy of joint (77.80-77.89)
> > excision of bone ends (77.80-77.89)
> **AHA:** For code 80.99: 1Q, '07, 20

✓3rd **81 Repair and plastic operations on joint structures**

✓4th **81.0 Spinal fusion**

> **NOTE** Spinal fusion is classified by the anatomic portion (column) fused and the technique (approach) used to perform the fusion.
>
> For the anterior column, the body (corpus) of adjacent vertebrae are fused (interbody fusion). The anterior column can be fused using an anterior, lateral, or posterior technique.
>
> For the posterior column, posterior structures of adjacent vertebrae are fused (pedicle, lamina, facet, transverse process, or "gutter" fusion). A posterior column fusion can be performed using a posterior, posterolateral, or lateral transverse technique.
>
> **INCLUDES** arthrodesis of spine with:
> > bone graft
> > internal fixation
>
> Code also any:
> > insertion of interbody spinal fusion device (84.51)
> > insertion of recombinant bone morphogenetic protein (84.52)
> > synchronous excision of (locally) harvested bone for graft (77.70-77.79)
> > the total number of vertebrae fused (81.62-81.64)
>
> **EXCLUDES** corrections of pseudarthrosis of spine (81.30-81.39)
> > refusion of spine (81.30-81.39)
>
> **DEF:** Spinal fusion: Immobilization of spinal column.
> **DEF:** Anterior interbody fusion: Arthrodesis by excising disc and cartilage end plates with bone graft insertion between two vertebrae.
> **DEF:** Lateral fusion: Arthrodesis by decorticating and bone grafting lateral surface of zygapophysial joint, pars interarticularis and transverse process.
> **DEF:** Posterior fusion: Arthrodesis by decorticating and bone grafting of neural arches between right and left zygapophysial joints.
> **DEF:** Posterolateral fusion: Arthrodesis by decorticating and bone grafting zygapophysial joint, pars interarticularis and transverse processes.
> **AHA:** 4Q, '10,125-127; 4Q, '03, 99
> **TIP:** Assign also code 03.53 if the fusion was performed for treatment of acute traumatic spinal fracture.

81.00 Spinal fusion, not otherwise specified

81.01 Atlas-axis spinal fusion

> Craniocervical fusion   ⎫ by anterior transoral
> C1–C2 fusion   ⎬ or posterior
> Occiput C2 fusion   ⎭ technique

81.02 Other cervical fusion of the anterior column, anterior technique

> Arthrodesis of C2 level or below:
> > anterior interbody fusion
> > anterolateral technique
> **AHA:** 4Q, '03, 101; 1Q, '01, 6; 1Q, '96, 7

---

§ Requires fourth digit. Valid digits are in [brackets] under each code. See category 80 for codes and definitions.

Operations on the Musculoskeletal System

81.03–81.32

Types of Grafts for Anterior Arthrodesis

Subtalar Joint Arthroereisis

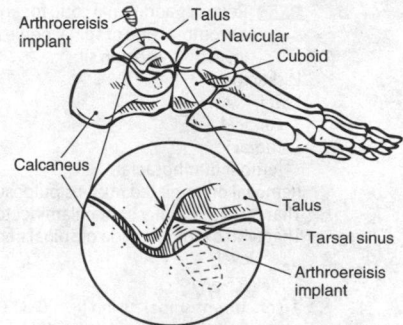

81.03 **Other cervical fusion of the posterior column, posterior technique**

Arthrodesis of C2 level or below, posterolateral technique

81.04 **Dorsal and dorsolumbar fusion of the anterior column, anterior technique**

Arthrodesis of thoracic or thoracolumbar region:
anterior interbody fusion
anterolateral technique
Extracavitary technique
AHA: 3Q, '03, 19

81.05 **Dorsal and dorsolumbar fusion of the posterior column, posterior technique**

Arthrodesis of thoracic or thoracolumbar region,
posterolateral technique
AHA: 2Q, '02, 16; 4Q, '99, 11

81.06 **Lumbar and lumbosacral fusion of the anterior column, anterior technique**

Anterior lumbar interbody fusion [ALIF]
Arthrodesis of lumbar or lumbosacral region:
anterior interbody fusion
anterolateral technique
retroperitoneal
transperitoneal
Direct lateral interbody fusion [DLIF]
Extreme lateral interbody fusion [XLIF]
AHA: 2Q, '08, 14; 1Q, '07, 20; 4Q, '05, 122; 4Q, '02, 107; 4Q, '99, 11

81.07 **Lumbar and lumbosacral fusion of the posterior column, posterior technique**

Facet fusion
Posterolateral technique
Transverse process technique
AHA: 2Q, '11, 10; 2Q, '09, 4; 4Q, '02, 108

81.08 **Lumbar and lumbosacral fusion of the anterior column, posterior technique**

Arthrodesis of lumbar or lumbosacral region,
posterior interbody fusion
Axial lumbar interbody fusion [AxiaLIF]
Posterior lumbar interbody fusion [PLIF]
Transforaminal lumbar interbody fusion [TLIF]
AHA: 2Q, '09, 4-5; 1Q, '08, 5; 1Q, '06, 12, 13; 4Q, '05, 122-123; 4Q, '02, 107, 109; 2Q, '00, 12, 13; 4Q, '99, 13; 2Q, '95, 9

√4ᵗʰ **81.1** **Arthrodesis and arthroereisis of foot and ankle**

INCLUDES arthrodesis of foot and ankle with:
bone graft
external fixation device

DEF: Fixation of foot or ankle joints.

81.11 **Ankle fusion**

Tibiotalar fusion

81.12 **Triple arthrodesis**

Talus to calcaneus and calcaneus to cuboid and navicular

81.13 **Subtalar fusion**

EXCLUDES arthroereisis (81.18)

81.14 **Midtarsal fusion**

81.15 **Tarsometatarsal fusion**

81.16 **Metatarsophalangeal fusion**

81.17 **Other fusion of foot**

81.18 **Subtalar joint arthroereisis**

DEF: Insertion of an endoprosthesis to limit excessive valgu motion of the subtalar joint; nonfusion procedure to prevent pronation.
AHA: 4Q, '05, 124

√4ᵗʰ **81.2** **Arthrodesis of other joint**

INCLUDES arthrodesis with:
bone graft
external fixation device
excision of bone ends and compression

81.20 **Arthrodesis of unspecified joint**

81.21 **Arthrodesis of hip**

81.22 **Arthrodesis of knee**

81.23 **Arthrodesis of shoulder**

81.24 **Arthrodesis of elbow**

81.25 **Carporadial fusion**

81.26 **Metacarpocarpal fusion**

81.27 **Metacarpophalangeal fusion**

81.28 **Interphalangeal fusion**

81.29 **Arthrodesis of other specified joints**

√4ᵗʰ **81.3** **Refusion of spine**

NOTE Spine fusion is classified by the anatomic portion (column) fused and the technique (approach) used to perform the fusion.

For the anterior column, the body (corpus) of adjacent vertebrae are fused (interbody fusion). The anterior column can be fused using an anterior, lateral, or posterior technique.

For the posterior column, posterior structures of adjacent vertebrae are fused (pedicle, lamina, facet, transverse process, or "gutter" fusion). A posterior column fusion can be performed using a posterior, posterolateral, or lateral transverse technique.

INCLUDES arthrodesis of spine with:
bone graft
internal fixation
correction of pseudarthrosis of spine

Code also any:
insertion of interbody spinal fusion device (84.51)
insertion of recombinant bone morphogenetic protein (84.52)
synchronous excision of (locally) harvested bone for graft (77.70-77.79)
the total number of vertebrae fused (81.62-81.64)
AHA: 4Q, '10,125-127; 4Q, '03, 99; 4Q, '01, 64

81.30 **Refusion of spine, not otherwise specified**

81.31 **Refusion of atlas-axis spine**

Craniocervical fusion ⎱ by anterior transoral
C1-C2 fusion   ⎰ or posterior
Occiput C2 fusion   technique

81.32 **Refusion of other cervical spine, anterior column, anterior technique**

Arthrodesis of C2 level or below:
anterior interbody fusion
anterolateral technique

BI Bilateral Procedure   NC Non-covered Procedure   LC Limited Coverage Procedure   ►◄ Revised Text   ● New Code   ▲ Revised Code Title

168 – Volume 3   **2014 ICD-9-CM**

81.33 **Refusion of other cervical spine, posterior column, posterior technique**

Arthrodesis of C2 level or below, posterolateral technique

81.34 **Refusion of dorsal and dorsolumbar spine, anterior column, anterior technique**

Arthrodesis of thoracic or thoracolumbar region:
anterior interbody fusion
anterolateral technique
Extracavitary technique

81.35 **Refusion of dorsal and dorsolumbar spine, posterior column, posterior technique**

Arthrodesis of thoracic or thoracolumbar region, posterolateral technique

81.36 **Refusion of lumbar and lumbosacral spine, anterior column, anterior technique**

Anterior lumbar interbody fusion [ALIF]
Arthrodesis of lumbar or lumbosacral region:
anterior interbody fusion
anterolateral technique
retroperitoneal
transperitoneal
Direct lateral interbody fusion [DLIF]
Extreme lateral interbody fusion [XLIF]
AHA: 4Q, '05, 122-123

81.37 **Refusion of lumbar and lumbosacral spine, posterior column, posterior technique**

Facet fusion
Posterolateral technique
Transverse process technique

81.38 **Refusion of lumbar and lumbosacral spine, anterior column, posterior technique**

Arthrodesis of lumbar or lumbosacral region, posterior interbody fusion
Axial lumbar interbody fusion [AxiaLIF]
Posterior lumbar interbody fusion [PLIF]
Transforaminal lumbar interbody fusion [TLIF]
AHA: 4Q, '05, 122-123; 4Q, '02, 110

81.39 **Refusion of spine, not elsewhere classified**

✓4th **81.4** **Other repair of joint of lower extremity**

INCLUDES arthroplasty of lower extremity with:
external traction or fixation
graft of bone (chips) or cartilage
internal fixation device
AHA: S-O, '85, 4

81.40 **Repair of hip, not elsewhere classified**

81.42 **Five-in-one repair of knee**

Medial meniscectomy, medial collateral ligament repair, vastus medialis advancement, semitendinosus advancement, and pes anserinus transfer

81.43 **Triad knee repair**

Medial meniscectomy with repair of the anterior cruciate ligament and the medial collateral ligament
O'Donoghue procedure

81.44 **Patellar stabilization**

Roux-Goldthwait operation for recurrent dislocation of patella
DEF: Roux-Goldthwait operation: Stabilization of patella via lateral ligament transposed at insertion beneath undisturbed medial insertion; excision of capsule ellipse and medial patella retinaculum; capsule reefed for lateral patella hold.

81.45 **Other repair of the cruciate ligaments**

AHA: M-A, '87, 12

81.46 **Other repair of the collateral ligaments**

81.47 **Other repair of knee**

AHA: 2Q, '06, 13; 2Q, '03, 18; 1Q, '00, 12, 13; 1Q, '96, 3; 3Q, '93, 5
TIP: Assign for Unispacer™ arthroplasty for degenerative arthritis of the knee; the device fits between the natural structures of the knee and helps to stabilize knee alignment.

81.49 **Other repair of ankle**

AHA: 2Q, '01, 15; 3Q, '00, 4

✓4th **81.5** **Joint replacement of lower extremity**

NOTE Removal of prior prothesis — *omit code*
INCLUDES arthroplasty of lower extremity with:
external traction or fixation
graft of bone (chips) or cartilage
internal fixation device or prosthesis
AHA: 4Q, '09, 149; S-O, '85, 4

81.51 **Total hip replacement** BI

Replacement of both femoral head and acetabulum by prosthesis
Total reconstruction of hip
Code also any type of bearing surface, if known (00.74-00.77)
DEF: Repair of both surfaces of hip joint with prosthesis.
AHA: 2Q, '09, 11; 4Q, '04, 113; 2Q, '91, 18

81.52 **Partial hip replacement** BI

Bipolar endoprosthesis
Code also any type of bearing surface, if known (00.74-00.77)
DEF: Repair of single surface of hip joint with prosthesis.
AHA: 2Q, '91, 18

81.53 **Revision of hip replacement, not otherwise specified**

Revision of hip replacement, not specified as to component(s) replaced, (acetabular, femoral or both)
Code also any:
removal of (cement) (joint) spacer (84.57)
type of bearing surface, if known (00.74-00.77)
EXCLUDES *revision of hip replacement, components specified (00.70-00.73)*
AHA: 4Q, '05, 125; 3Q, '97, 12

81.54 **Total knee replacement** BI

Bicompartmental
Partial knee replacement
Tricompartmental
Unicompartmental (hemijoint)
DEF: Repair of a knee joint with prosthetic implant in one, two, or three compartments.

Total Hip Replacement

Damaged femur head ("ball") in degenerated socket (acetabulum)

Cuplike acetabular component of prosthesis fixed into hip bone

Prosthesis anchored into shaft of long bone

Damaged femur head replaced with prosthesis

Partial Hip Replacement

Acetabulum remains intact

Prosthesis

Operations on the Musculoskeletal System

81.33–81.54

Operations on the Musculoskeletal System

81.55–81.85

Total Knee Replacement

Vertebroplasty

Percutaneous Vertebral Augmentation

81.66 **Percutaneous vertebral augmentation**
Arcuplasty
Insertion of inflatable balloon, bone tamp, or other device displacing (removing) (compacting) bone to create a space (cavity) (void) prior to the injection of bone void filler (cement) (polymethylmethacrylate) (PMMA) or other substance
Kyphoplasty
SKyphoplasty
Spineoplasty
EXCLUDES *percutaneous vertebroplasty (81.65)*
AHA: 1Q, '07, 5, 7; 3Q, '06, 13; 4Q, '04, 126
TIP: A vertebral bone biopsy is not integral to this procedure. If performed, report also code 77.49.

81.55 **Revision of knee replacement, not otherwise specified**
Code also any removal of (cement) (joint) spacer (84.57)
EXCLUDES *arthrodesis of knee (81.22)*
revision of knee replacement, components specified (00.80-00.84)
AHA: 4Q, '05, 113; 2Q, '97, 10

81.56 **Total ankle replacement** [BI]

81.57 **Replacement of joint of foot and toe**

81.59 **Revision of joint replacement of lower extremity, not elsewhere classified**

√4ᵗʰ **81.6** **Other procedures on spine**
NOTE Number of vertebrae
The vertebral spine consists of 25 vertebrae in the following order and number:
cervical: C1 (atlas), C2 (axis), C3, C4, C5, C6, C7
thoracic or dorsal: T1, T2, T3, T4, T5, T6, T7, T8, T9, T10, T11, T12
lumbar and sacral: L1, L2, L3, L4, L5, S1
Coders should report only one code from the series 81.62-81.64 to show the total number of vertebrae fused on the patient.
Code also the level and approach of the fusion or refusion (81.00-81.08, 81.30-81.39)
AHA: 4Q, '03, 99

81.62 **Fusion or refusion of 2-3 vertebrae**
AHA: 2Q, '11, 10; 1Q, '10, 23; 2Q, '09, 4-5; 2Q, '08, 14; 1Q, '08, 5; 1Q, '07, 20; 1Q, '06, 12, 13; 4Q, '05, 123; 4Q, '03, 99

81.63 **Fusion or refusion of 4-8 vertebrae**
AHA: 1Q, '10, 23; 4Q, '03, 99-101

81.64 **Fusion or refusion of 9 or more vertebrae**
AHA: 4Q, '03, 99

81.65 **Percutaneous vertebroplasty**
Injection of bone void filler (cement) (polymethylmethacrylate) (PMMA) into the diseased or fractured vertebral body
EXCLUDES *kyphoplasty (81.66)*
percutaneous vertebral augmentation (81.66)
AHA: ▶4Q, '12, 84;◀ 2Q, '08, 15

√4ᵗʰ **81.7** **Arthroplasty and repair of hand, fingers, and wrist**
INCLUDES arthroplasty of hand and finger with:
external traction or fixation
graft of bone (chips) or cartilage
internal fixation device or prosthesis
EXCLUDES *operations on muscle, tendon, and fascia of hand (82.01-82.99)*
DEF: Plastic surgery of hand, fingers and wrist joints.

81.71 **Arthroplasty of metacarpophalangeal and interphalangeal joint with implant**

81.72 **Arthroplasty of metacarpophalangeal and interphalangeal joint without implant**
AHA: 1Q, '93, 28

81.73 **Total wrist replacement**

81.74 **Arthroplasty of carpocarpal or carpometacarpal joint with implant**

81.75 **Arthroplasty of carpocarpal or carpometacarpal joint without implant**
AHA: 3Q, '93, 8

81.79 **Other repair of hand, fingers, and wrist**

√4ᵗʰ **81.8** **Arthroplasty and repair of shoulder and elbow**
INCLUDES arthroplasty of upper limb NEC with:
external traction or fixation
graft of bone (chips) or cartilage
internal fixation device or prosthesis

81.80 **Other total shoulder replacement**
EXCLUDES *reverse total shoulder replacement (81.88)*
AHA: 2Q, '08, 5

81.81 **Partial shoulder replacement**

81.82 **Repair of recurrent dislocation of shoulder**
AHA: 3Q, '95, 15

81.83 **Other repair of shoulder**
AHA: 1Q, '02, 9; 4Q, '01, 51; 2Q, '00, 14; 3Q, '93, 5
TIP: Assign for SLAP (superior labral anterior posterior—glenoid labrum lesion) repair.

81.84 **Total elbow replacement**
Partial elbow replacement

81.85 **Other repair of elbow**

Arthrocentesis

Needle access into fluid filled knee joint

Femur

Patella (kneecap)

Fluid-filled joint capsule

Tibia

81.88 Reverse total shoulder replacement
Reverse ball-and-socket of the shoulder
EXCLUDES *conversion of prior (failed) total shoulder replacement (arthroplasty) to reverse total shoulder replacement (81.97)*
AHA: 4Q, '10, 129-130

√4ᵗʰ **81.9 Other operations on joint structures**

81.91 Arthrocentesis
Joint aspiration
EXCLUDES *that for:*
arthrography (88.32)
biopsy of joint structure (80.30-80.39)
injection of drug (81.92)
DEF: Insertion of needle to withdraw fluid from joint.

81.92 Injection of therapeutic substance into joint or ligament
AHA: 3Q, '10, 14; 2Q, '00, 14; 3Q, '89, 16

81.93 Suture of capsule or ligament of upper extremity
EXCLUDES *that associated with arthroplasty (81.71-81.75, 81.80-81.81, 81.84)*

81.94 Suture of capsule or ligament of ankle and foot
EXCLUDES *that associated with arthroplasty (81.56-81.59)*

81.95 Suture of capsule or ligament of other lower extremity
EXCLUDES *that associated with arthroplasty (81.51-81.55, 81.59)*

81.96 Other repair of joint

81.97 Revision of joint replacement of upper extremity
Partial
Removal of cement spacer
Revision of arthroplasty of shoulder
Total
AHA: 1Q, '04, 12

81.98 Other diagnostic procedures on joint structures
EXCLUDES *arthroscopy (80.20-80.29)*
biopsy of joint structure (80.30-80.39)
microscopic examination of specimen from joint (91.51-91.59)
thermography (88.83)
x-ray (87.21-87.29, 88.21-88.33)

81.99 Other
AHA: 4Q, '05, 124

√3ʳᵈ **82 Operations on muscle, tendon, and fascia of hand**
INCLUDES operations on:
aponeurosis
synovial membrane (tendon sheath)
tendon sheath

√4ᵗʰ **82.0 Incision of muscle, tendon, fascia, and bursa of hand**

82.01 Exploration of tendon sheath of hand
Incision of } tendon sheath of
Removal of rice bodies in } hand
EXCLUDES *division of tendon (82.11)*
DEF: Incision into and exploration of the hand's muscle and its accompanying supportive, connective tissue, bands, and sacs.

82.02 Myotomy of hand
EXCLUDES *myotomy for division (82.19)*
DEF: Incision into hand muscle.

82.03 Bursotomy of hand

82.04 Incision and drainage of palmar or thenar space

82.09 Other incision of soft tissue of hand
EXCLUDES *incision of skin and subcutaneous tissue alone (86.01-86.09)*
AHA: N-D, '87, 10

√4ᵗʰ **82.1 Division of muscle, tendon, and fascia of hand**

82.11 Tenotomy of hand
Division of tendon of hand

82.12 Fasciotomy of hand
Division of fascia of hand

82.19 Other division of soft tissue of hand
Division of muscle of hand

√4ᵗʰ **82.2 Excision of lesion of muscle, tendon, and fascia of hand**

82.21 Excision or lesion of tendon sheath of hand
Ganglionectomy of tendon sheath (wrist)

82.22 Excision of lesion of muscle of hand

82.29 Excision of other lesion of soft tissue of hand
EXCLUDES *excision of lesion of skin and subcutaneous tissue (86.21-86.3)*

√4ᵗʰ **82.3 Other excision of soft tissue of hand**
Code also any skin graft (86.61-86.62, 86.73)
EXCLUDES *excision of skin and subcutaneous tissue (86.21-86.3)*

82.31 Bursectomy of hand

82.32 Excision of tendon of hand for graft
DEF: Resection and excision of fibrous tissue connecting bone to hand muscle for grafting.

82.33 Other tenonectomy of hand
Tenosynovectomy of hand
EXCLUDES *excision of lesion of:*
tendon (82.29)
sheath (82.21)
DEF: Removal of fibrous bands connecting muscle to bone of hand.
DEF: Tenosynovectomy of hand: Excision of fibrous band connecting muscle and bone of hand and removal of coverings.

82.34 Excision of muscle or fascia of hand for graft

82.35 Other fasciectomy of hand
Release of Dupuytren's contracture
EXCLUDES *excision of lesion of fascia (82.29)*
DEF: Excision of fibrous connective tissue; other than for grafting or removing lesion.
DEF: Release of Dupuytren's contracture: Excision of fibrous connective tissue to correct flexion of fingers.

82.36 Other myectomy of hand
EXCLUDES *excision of lesion of muscle (82.22)*

82.39 Other excision of soft tissue of hand
EXCLUDES *excision of skin (86.21-86.3)*
excision of soft tissue lesion (82.29)

√4ᵗʰ **82.4 Suture of muscle, tendon, and fascia of hand**

82.41 Suture of tendon sheath of hand

82.42 Delayed suture of flexor tendon of hand
DEF: Suture of fibrous band between flexor muscle and bone; following initial repair.

82.43 Delayed suture of other tendon of hand

82.44 Other suture of flexor tendon of hand
EXCLUDES *delayed suture of flexor tendon of hand (82.42)*

82.45 Other suture of other tendon of hand
EXCLUDES *delayed suture of other tendon of hand (82.43)*

82.46 Suture of muscle or fascia of hand

Additional Digit Required   Valid OR Procedure   Non-OR Procedure   Adjunct Code

Operations on the Musculoskeletal System

82.5–83.13

√4ᵗʰ **82.5** **Transplantation of muscle and tendon of hand**
AHA: 1Q, '93, 28

82.51 **Advancement of tendon of hand**
DEF: Detachment of fibrous connective muscle band and bone with reattachment at advanced point of hand.

82.52 **Recession of tendon of hand**
DEF: Detachment of fibrous band of muscle and bone with reattachment at drawn-back point of hand.

82.53 **Reattachment of tendon of hand**

82.54 **Reattachment of muscle of hand**

82.55 **Other change in hand muscle or tendon length**

82.56 **Other hand tendon transfer or transplantation**
EXCLUDES pollicization of thumb (82.61)
transfer of finger, except thumb (82.81)
AHA: 2Q, '99, 10; 4Q, '98, 40

82.57 **Other hand tendon transposition**
AHA: 1Q, '93, 28; 3Q, '93, 8

82.58 **Other hand muscle transfer or transplantation**

82.59 **Other hand muscle transposition**

√4ᵗʰ **82.6** **Reconstruction of thumb**
INCLUDES digital transfer to act as thumb
Code also any amputation for digital transfer (84.01, 84.11)

82.61 **Pollicization operation carrying over nerves and blood supply**
DEF: Creation or reconstruction of a thumb with another digit, commonly the index finger.

82.69 **Other reconstruction of thumb**
"Cocked-hat" procedure [skin flap and bone]
Grafts:
bone
skin (pedicle) } to thumb

√4ᵗʰ **82.7** **Plastic operation on hand with graft or implant**

82.71 **Tendon pulley reconstruction**
Reconstruction for opponensplasty
DEF: Reconstruction of fibrous band between muscle and bone of hand.

82.72 **Plastic operation on hand with graft of muscle or fascia**

82.79 **Plastic operation on hand with other graft or implant**
Tendon graft to hand
AHA: J-F, '87, 6

√4ᵗʰ **82.8** **Other plastic operations on hand**

82.81 **Transfer of finger, except thumb**
EXCLUDES pollicization of thumb (82.61)
AHA: 2Q, '05, 7
TIP: Assign this code, along with code 84.11 Amputation of toe, for a procedure in which a toe is transferred to the site of previous traumatic finger amputation.

82.82 **Repair of cleft hand**
DEF: Correction of fissure defect of hand.

82.83 **Repair of macrodactyly**
DEF: Reduction in size of abnormally large fingers.

82.84 **Repair of mallet finger**
DEF: Repair of flexed little finger.

82.85 **Other tenodesis of hand**
Tendon fixation of hand NOS
DEF: Fixation of fibrous connective band between muscle and bone of hand.

82.86 **Other tenoplasty of hand**
Myotenoplasty of hand
DEF: Myotenoplasty of hand: Plastic repair of muscle and fibrous band connecting muscle to bone.

82.89 **Other plastic operations on hand**
Plication of fascia
Repair of fascial hernia
EXCLUDES that with graft or implant (82.71-82.79)

√4ᵗʰ **82.9** **Other operations on muscle, tendon, and fascia of hand**
EXCLUDES diagnostic procedures on soft tissue of hand (83.21-83.29)

82.91 **Lysis of adhesions of hand**
Freeing of adhesions of fascia, muscle, and tendon of hand
EXCLUDES decompression of carpal tunnel (04.43)
that by stretching or manipulation only (93.26)

82.92 **Aspiration of bursa of hand**

82.93 **Aspiration of other soft tissue of hand**
EXCLUDES skin and subcutaneous tissue (86.01)

82.94 **Injection of therapeutic substance into bursa of hand**

82.95 **Injection of therapeutic substance into tendon of hand**

82.96 **Other injection of locally-acting therapeutic substance into soft tissue of hand**
EXCLUDES subcutaneous or intramuscular injection (99.11-99.29)

82.99 **Other operations on muscle, tendon, and fascia of hand**

√3ʳᵈ **83** **Operations on muscle, tendon, fascia, and bursa, except hand**
INCLUDES operations on:
aponeurosis
synovial membrane of bursa and tendon sheaths
tendon sheaths
EXCLUDES diaphragm (34.81-34.89)
hand (82.01-82.99)
muscles of eye (15.01-15.9)

√4ᵗʰ **83.0** **Incision of muscle, tendon, fascia, and bursa**

83.01 **Exploration of tendon sheath**
Incision of tendon sheath
Removal of rice bodies from tendon sheath
DEF: Incision of external covering of fibrous cord for exam.
DEF: Removal of rice bodies from tendon sheath: Incision and removal of small bodies resembling grains of rice.

83.02 **Myotomy**
EXCLUDES cricopharyngeal myotomy (29.31)
AHA: 4Q, '08, 135; 2Q, '89, 18

83.03 **Bursotomy**
Removal of calcareous deposit of bursa
EXCLUDES aspiration of bursa (percutaneous) (83.94)

83.09 **Other incision of soft tissue**
Incision of fascia
EXCLUDES incision of skin and subcutaneous tissue alone (86.01-86.09)
AHA: 1Q, '09, 10

√4ᵗʰ **83.1** **Division of muscle, tendon, and fascia**

83.11 **Achillotenotomy**

83.12 **Adductor tenotomy of hip**
DEF: Incision into fibrous attachment between adductor muscle and hip bone.

83.13 **Other tenotomy**
Aponeurotomy   Tendon transection
Division of tendon   Tenotomy for thoracic
Tendon release   outlet decompression
DEF: Aponeurotomy: Incision and separation of fibrous cords attaching a muscle to bone to aid movement.
DEF: Division of tendon: Separation of fibrous band connecting muscle to bone.
DEF: Tendon release: Surgical detachment of fibrous band from muscle and/or bone.
DEF: Tendon transection: Incision across width of fibrous bands between muscle and bone.
DEF: Tenotomy for thoracic outlet decompression: Incision of fibrous muscle with separation from bone to relieve compressed thoracic outlet.

BI Bilateral Procedure   **NC** Non-covered Procedure   **LC** Limited Coverage Procedure   ▶◀ Revised Text   ● New Code   ▲ Revised Code Title

172 – Volume 3   **2014 ICD-9-CM**

83.14 Fasciotomy
Division of fascia
Division of iliotibial band
Fascia stripping
Release of Volkmann's contracture by fasciotomy
DEF: Division of fascia: Incision to separate fibrous connective tissue.
DEF: Division of iliotibial band: Incision to separate fibrous band connecting tibial bone to muscle in flank.
DEF: Fascia stripping: Incision and lengthwise separation of fibrous connective tissue.
DEF: Release of Volkmann's contracture by fasciotomy: Divisional incision of connective tissue to correct defect in flexion of finger(s).
AHA: 4Q, '06, 102; 3Q, '98, 8
TIP: Assign for all fasciotomy procedures, regardless of whether the approach is open or endoscopic. For fasciotomy of hand, see code 82.12.

83.19 Other division of soft tissue
Division of muscle
Muscle release
Myotomy for thoracic outlet decompression
Myotomy with division
Scalenotomy
Transection of muscle

√4ᵗʰ 83.2 Diagnostic procedures on muscle, tendon, fascia, and bursa, including that of hand

83.21 Open biopsy of soft tissue
EXCLUDES *biopsy of chest wall (34.23)*
closed biopsy of skin and subcutaneous tissue (86.11)

83.29 Other diagnostic procedures on muscle, tendon, fascia, and bursa, including that of hand
EXCLUDES *microscopic examination of specimen (91.51-91.-59)*
soft tissue x-ray (87.09, 87.38-87.39, 88.09, 88.35, 88.37)
thermography of muscle (88.84)

√4ᵗʰ 83.3 Excision of lesion of muscle, tendon, fascia, and bursa
EXCLUDES *biopsy of soft tissue (83.21)*

83.31 Excision of lesion of tendon sheath
Excision of ganglion of tendon sheath, except of hand

83.32 Excision of lesion of muscle
Excision of:
heterotopic bone
muscle scar for release of Volkmann's contracture
myositis ossificans
DEF: Heterotopic bone: Bone lesion in muscle.
DEF: Muscle scar for release of Volkmann's contracture: Scarred muscle tissue interfering with finger flexion.
DEF: Myositis ossificans: Bony deposits in muscle.

83.39 Excision of lesion of other soft tissue
Excision of Baker's cyst
EXCLUDES *bursectomy (83.5)*
excision of lesion of skin and subcutaneous tissue (86.3)
synovectomy (80.70-80.79)
AHA: 3Q, '10, 11; 2Q, '05, 3; 2Q, '97, 6

√4ᵗʰ 83.4 Other excision of muscle, tendon, and fascia

83.41 Excision of tendon for graft

83.42 Other tenonectomy
Excision of:
aponeurosis
tendon sheath
Tenosynovectomy

83.43 Excision of muscle or fascia for graft
AHA: 1Q, '11, 7

83.44 Other fasciectomy
DEF: Excision of fascia; other than for graft.

83.45 Other myectomy
Debridement of muscle NOS
Scalenectomy
DEF: Scalenectomy: Removal of thoracic scaleni muscle tissue.
AHA: 1Q, '99, 8
TIP: Do not assign a skin/soft tissue debridement procedure code (e.g., 86.22) in addition to the muscle debridement (83.45) code; all more superficial debridement is included when multilayer debridement is performed at the same site.

83.49 Other excision of soft tissue

83.5 Bursectomy
AHA: 2Q, '06, 15; 2Q, '99, 11

√4ᵗʰ 83.6 Suture of muscle, tendon, and fascia

83.61 Suture of tendon sheath

83.62 Delayed suture of tendon

83.63 Rotator cuff repair
DEF: Repair of musculomembranous structure around shoulder joint capsule.
AHA: 4Q, '11, 136; 1Q, '06, 6; 2Q, '93, 8

83.64 Other suture of tendon
Achillorrhaphy
Aponeurorrhaphy
EXCLUDES *delayed suture of tendon (83.62)*
DEF: Achillorrhaphy: Suture of fibrous band connecting Achilles tendon to heel bone.
DEF: Aponeurorrhaphy: Suture of fibrous cords connecting muscle to bone.

83.65 Other suture of muscle or fascia
Repair of diastasis recti

√4ᵗʰ 83.7 Reconstruction of muscle and tendon
EXCLUDES *reconstruction of muscle and tendon associated with arthroplasty*

83.71 Advancement of tendon
DEF: Detaching fibrous cord between muscle and bone with reattachment at advanced point.

83.72 Recession of tendon
DEF: Detaching fibrous cord between muscle and bone with reattachment at drawn-back point.

83.73 Reattachment of tendon

83.74 Reattachment of muscle

83.75 Tendon transfer or transplantation

83.76 Other tendon transposition

83.77 Muscle transfer or transplantation
Release of Volkmann's contracture by muscle transplantation

83.79 Other muscle transposition

√4ᵗʰ 83.8 Other plastic operations on muscle, tendon, and fascia
EXCLUDES *plastic operations on muscle, tendon, and fascia associated with arthroplasty*

83.81 Tendon graft
AHA: ▶3Q, '12, 11◀

83.82 Graft of muscle or fascia
AHA: 1Q, '10, 7; 3Q, '01, 9

83.83 Tendon pulley reconstruction
DEF: Reconstruction of fibrous cord between muscle and bone at any site other than hand.

83.84 Release of clubfoot, not elsewhere classified
Evans operation on clubfoot

83.85 Other change in muscle or tendon length
Hamstring lengthening
Heel cord shortening
Plastic achillotenotomy
Tendon plication
DEF: Plastic achillotenotomy: Increase in heel cord length.
DEF: Tendon plication: Surgical tuck of tendon.

83.86 Quadricepsplasty
DEF: Correction of quadriceps femoris muscle.

Operations on the Musculoskeletal System

83.87–84.18

83.87 **Other plastic operations on muscle**
> Musculoplasty
> Myoplasty
> AHA: 1Q, '97, 9

83.88 **Other plastic operations on tendon**
> Myotenoplasty   Tenodesis
> Tendon fixation   Tenoplasty

83.89 **Other plastic operations on fascia**
> Fascia lengthening   Plication of fascia
> Fascioplasty

√4ᵗʰ **83.9** **Other operations on muscle, tendon, fascia, and bursa**
> *EXCLUDES*   nonoperative:
>   *manipulation (93.25-93.29)*
>   *stretching (93.27-93.29)*

83.91 **Lysis of adhesions of muscle, tendon, fascia, and bursa**
> *EXCLUDES*   that for tarsal tunnel syndrome (04.44)
> DEF: Separation of created fibrous structures from muscle, connective tissues, bands and sacs.

83.92 **Insertion or replacement of skeletal muscle stimulator**
> Implantation, insertion, placement, or replacement of skeletal muscle:
>   electrodes
>   stimulator
> AHA: 2Q, '99, 10

83.93 **Removal of skeletal muscle stimulator**

83.94 **Aspiration of bursa**

83.95 **Aspiration of other soft tissue**
> *EXCLUDES*   that of skin and subcutaneous tissue (86.01)

83.96 **Injection of therapeutic substance into bursa**

83.97 **Injection of therapeutic substance into tendon**

83.98 **Injection of locally-acting therapeutic substance into other soft tissue**
> *EXCLUDES*   subcutaneous or intramuscular injection (99.11-99.29)
> AHA: 2Q, '06, 11

83.99 **Other operations on muscle, tendon, fascia, and bursa**
> Suture of bursa

√3ʳᵈ **84** **Other procedures on musculoskeletal system**

√4ᵗʰ **84.0** **Amputation of upper limb**
> *EXCLUDES*   revision of amputation stump (84.3)

84.00 **Upper limb amputation, not otherwise specified**
> Closed flap amputation ⎤
> Kineplastic amputation   ⎥
> Open or guillotine amputation ⎬ of upper limb NOS
> Revision of current traumatic ⎥
>   amputation ⎦
> DEF: Closed flap amputation: Sewing a created skin flap over stump end of upper limb.
> DEF: Kineplastic amputation: Amputation and preparation of stump of upper limb to permit movement.
> DEF: Open or guillotine amputation: Straight incision across upper limb; used when primary closure is contraindicated.
> DEF: Revision of current traumatic amputation: Reconstruction of traumatic amputation of upper limb to enable closure.

84.01 **Amputation and disarticulation of finger**
> *EXCLUDES*   ligation of supernumerary finger (86.26)

84.02 **Amputation and disarticulation of thumb**

84.03 **Amputation through hand**
> Amputation through carpals

84.04 **Disarticulation of wrist**

84.05 **Amputation through forearm**
> Forearm amputation

84.06 **Disarticulation of elbow**
> DEF: Amputation of forearm through elbow joint.

84.07 **Amputation through humerus**
> Upper arm amputation

84.08 **Disarticulation of shoulder**
> DEF: Amputation of arm through shoulder joint.

84.09 **Interthoracoscapular amputation**
> Forequarter amputation
> DEF: Removal of upper arm, shoulder bone and collarbone.

√4ᵗʰ **84.1** **Amputation of lower limb**
> *EXCLUDES*   revision of amputation stump (84.3)

84.10 **Lower limb amputation, not otherwise specified**
> Closed flap amputation   ⎤
> Kineplastic amputation   ⎥ of lower limb
> Open or guillotine amputation ⎬   NOS
> Revision of current traumatic ⎥
>   amputation ⎦
> DEF: Closed flap amputation: Sewing a created skin flap over stump of lower limb.
> DEF: Kineplastic amputation: Amputation and preparation of stump of lower limb to permit movement.
> DEF: Open or guillotine amputation: Straight incision across lower limb; used when primary closure is contraindicated.
> DEF: Revision of current traumatic amputation: Reconstruction of traumatic amputation of lower limb to enable closure.

84.11 **Amputation of toe**
> Amputation through metatarsophalangeal joint
> Disarticulation of toe
> Metatarsal head amputation
> Ray amputation of foot (disarticulation of the metatarsal head of the toe extending across the forefoot, just proximal to the metatarsophalangeal crease)
> *EXCLUDES*   ligation of supernumerary toe (86.26)
> AHA: 2Q, '05, 7; 4Q, '99, 19

84.12 **Amputation through foot**
> Amputation of forefoot
> Amputation through middle of foot
> Chopart's amputation
> Midtarsal amputation
> Transmetatarsal amputation (amputation of the forefoot, including the toes)
> *EXCLUDES*   Ray amputation of foot (84.11)
> DEF: Amputation of forefoot: Removal of foot in front of joint between toes and body of foot.
> DEF: Chopart's amputation: Removal of foot with retention of heel, ankle and other associated ankle bones.
> DEF: Midtarsal amputation: Amputation of foot through tarsals.
> DEF: Transmetatarsal amputation: Amputation of foot through metatarsals.
> AHA: 4Q, '99, 19

84.13 **Disarticulation of ankle**
> DEF: Removal of foot through ankle bone.

84.14 **Amputation of ankle through malleoli of tibia and fibula**

84.15 **Other amputation below knee**
> Amputation of leg through tibia and fibula NOS

84.16 **Disarticulation of knee**
> Batch, Spitler, and McFaddin amputation
> Mazet amputation
> S.P. Roger's amputation
> DEF: Removal of lower leg through knee joint.

84.17 **Amputation above knee**
> Amputation of leg through femur
> Amputation of thigh
> Conversion of below-knee amputation into above-knee amputation
> Supracondylar above-knee amputation
> AHA: 1Q, '05, 16; 1Q, '05, 16; 3Q, '03, 14

84.18 **Disarticulation of hip**
> DEF: Removal of leg through hip joint.

BI Bilateral Procedure   **NC** Non-covered Procedure   **LC** Limited Coverage Procedure   ►◄ Revised Text   ● New Code   ▲ Revised Code Title

174 – Volume 3   **2014 ICD-9-CM**

84.19 Abdominopelvic amputation
Hemipelvectomy
Hindquarter amputation
DEF: Removal of leg and portion of pelvic bone.
DEF: Hemipelvectomy: Removal of leg and lateral pelvis.

✓4th **84.2 Reattachment of extremity**
AHA: 1Q, '95, 8

84.21 Thumb reattachment

84.22 Finger reattachment

84.23 Forearm, wrist, or hand reattachment

84.24 Upper arm reattachment
Reattachment of arm NOS

84.25 Toe reattachment

84.26 Foot reattachment

84.27 Lower leg or ankle reattachment
Reattachment of leg NOS

84.28 Thigh reattachment

84.29 Other reattachment

84.3 Revision of amputation stump
Reamputation
Secondary closure } of stump
Trimming
EXCLUDES revision of current traumatic amputation [revision by
further amputation of current injury]
(84.00-84.19, 84.91)
AHA: 4Q, '99, 15; 2Q, '98, 15; 4Q, '88, 12
TIP: Only assign if the documentation indicates that the amputation
stump revision involves transecting the entire circumference of the
bone.

✓4th **84.4 Implantation or fitting of prosthetic limb device**

**84.40 Implantation or fitting of prosthetic limb
device, not otherwise specified**

84.41 Fitting of prosthesis of upper arm and shoulder

84.42 Fitting of prosthesis of lower arm and hand

84.43 Fitting of prosthesis of arm, not otherwise specified

84.44 Implantation of prosthetic device of arm

84.45 Fitting of prosthesis above knee

84.46 Fitting of prosthesis below knee

84.47 Fitting of prosthesis of leg, not otherwise specified

84.48 Implantation of prosthetic device of leg

✓4th **84.5 Implantation of other musculoskeletal devices and
substances**
EXCLUDES insertion of (non-fusion) spinal disc replacement
device (84.60-84.69)

84.51 Insertion of interbody spinal fusion device
Insertion of:
cages (carbn, ceramic, metal, plastic or titanium)
interbody fusion cage
synthetic cages or spacers
threaded bone dowels
Code also refusion of spine (81.30-81.39)
Code also spinal fusion (81.00-81.08)
AHA: 2Q, '09, 5; 2Q, '08, 14; 1Q, '07, 20; 4Q, '05, 123; 1Q, '04,
21; 4Q, '02, 108-110

**84.52 Insertion of recombinant bone
morphogenetic protein**
rhBMP
That via collagen sponge, coral, ceramic and other
carriers
Code also primary procedure performed:
fracture repair (79.00-79.99)
spinal fusion (81.00-81.08)
spinal refusion (81.30-81.39)
DEF: Surgical implantation of bone morphogenetic proteins
(BMP) and recombinant BMP (rhBMP) to induce new bone
growth formation; clinical applications include delayed
unions and nonunions, fractures, and spinal fusions.
AHA: 2Q, '09, 4-5; 4Q, '02, 110

Spinal Fusion with Metal Cage

Metal cages
support spine
until fusion
occurs

Anterior view

Lateral view

Spinal fusion
with metal cages

Detail

**84.53 Implantation of internal limb lengthening device
with kinetic distraction**
Code also limb lengthening procedure (78.30-78.39)

**84.54 Implantation of other internal limb lengthening
device**
Implantation of internal limb lengthening device, not
otherwise specified (NOS)
Code also limb lengthening procedure (78.30-78.39)

84.55 Insertion of bone void filler
Insertion of:
acrylic cement (PMMA)
bone void cement
calcium based bone void filler
polymethylmethacrylate (PMMA)
EXCLUDES that with percutaneous vertebral
augmentation (81.66)
that with percutaneous vertebroplasty
(81.65)
AHA: 4Q, '04, 128

84.56 Insertion or replacement of (cement) spacer
Insertion or replacement of joint
(methylmethacrylate) spacer
AHA: ►3Q, '12, 14, 15;◄ 2Q, '08, 4; 4Q, '05, 124

84.57 Removal of (cement) spacer
Removal of joint (methylmethacrylate) spacer
AHA: 2Q, '08, 4, 5; 4Q, '05, 113, 124-125

84.59 Insertion of other spinal devices
EXCLUDES initial insertion of pedicle screws with spinal
fusion — omit code
insertion of facet replacement device(s)
(84.84)
insertion of interspinous process device(s)
(84.80)
insertion of pedicle-based dynamic
stabilization device(s) (84.82)
AHA: 1Q, '07, 9, 10

✓4th **84.6 Replacement of spinal disc**
INCLUDES non-fusion arthroplasty of the spine with insertion
of artificial disc prosthesis

**84.60 Insertion of spinal disc prosthesis, not
otherwise specified**
Replacement of spinal disc, NOS
INCLUDES diskectomy (discectomy)

**84.61 Insertion of partial spinal disc prosthesis,
cervical**
Nuclear replacement device, cervical
Partial artificial disc prosthesis (flexible), cervical
Replacement of nuclear disc (nucleus pulposus),
cervical
INCLUDES diskectomy (discectomy)

**84.62 Insertion of total spinal disc prosthesis,
cervical**
Replacement of cervical spinal disc, NOS
Replacement of total spinal disc, cervical
Total artificial disc prosthesis (flexible), cervical
INCLUDES diskectomy (discectomy)

Operations on the Musculoskeletal System

84.63–84.81

84.63 Insertion of spinal disc prosthesis, thoracic

Artificial disc prosthesis (flexible), thoracic
Replacement of thoracic spinal disc, partial or total
INCLUDES diskectomy (discectomy)

84.64 Insertion of partial spinal disc prosthesis, lumbosacral

Nuclear replacement device, lumbar
Partial artificial disc prosthesis (flexible), lumbar
Replacement of nuclear disc (nucleus pulposus), lumbar
INCLUDES diskectomy (discectomy)

[11] **84.65 Insertion of total spinal disc prosthesis, lumbosacral**   **NC**

Replacement of lumbar spinal disc, NOS
Replacement of total spinal disc, lumbar
Total artificial disc prosthesis (flexible), lumbar
INCLUDES diskectomy (discectomy)
AHA: 4Q, '04, 133

84.66 Revision or replacement of artificial spinal disc prosthesis, cervical

Removal of (partial) (total) spinal disc prosthesis with synchronous insertion of new (partial) (total) spinal disc prosthesis, cervical
Repair of previously inserted spinal disc prosthesis, cervical

84.67 Revision or replacement of artificial spinal disc prosthesis, thoracic

Removal of (partial) (total) spinal disc prosthesis with synchronous insertion of new (partial) (total) spinal disc prosthesis, thoracic
Repair of previously inserted spinal disc prosthesis, thoracic

84.68 Revision or replacement of artificial spinal disc prosthesis, lumbosacral

Removal of (partial) (total) spinal disc prosthesis with synchronous insertion of new (partial) (total) spinal disc prosthesis, lumbosacral
Repair of previously inserted spinal disc prosthesis, lumbosacral

84.69 Revision or replacement of artificial spinal disc prosthesis, not otherwise specified

Removal of (partial) (total) spinal disc prosthesis with synchronous insertion of new (partial) (total) spinal disc prosthesis
Repair of previously inserted spinal disc prosthesis

[√4ᵗʰ] **84.7 Adjunct codes for external fixator devices**

Code also any primary procedure performed:
application of external fixator device (78.10, 78.12-78.13, 78.15, 78.17-78.19)
reduction of fracture and dislocation (79.00-79.89)
AHA: 4Q, '05, 127-129

84.71 Application of external fixator device, monoplanar system

EXCLUDES other hybrid device or system (84.73)
ring device or system (84.72)
DEF: Instrumentation that provides percutaneous neutralization, compression, and /or distraction of bone in a single plane by applying force within that plane.
AHA: 4Q, '05, 129

84.72 Application of external fixator device, ring system

Ilizarov type
Sheffield type
EXCLUDES monoplanar device or system (84.71)
other hybrid device or system (84.73)
DEF: Instrumentation that provides percutaneous neutralization, compression, and/or distraction of bone through 360 degrees of force application.

External Fixator Devices

Monoplanar   Ring system   Hybrid

84.73 Application of hybrid external fixator device

Computer (assisted) (dependent) external fixator device
Hybrid system using both ring and monoplanar devices
EXCLUDES monoplanar device or system, when used alone (84.71)
ring device or system, when used alone (84.72)
DEF: Instrumentation that provides percutaneous neutralization, compression, and /or distraction of bone by applying multiple external forces using monoplanar and ring device combinations.

[√4ᵗʰ] **84.8 Insertion, replacement and revision of posterior spinal motion preservation device(s)**

Dynamic spinal stabilization device(s)
INCLUDES any synchronous facetectomy (partial, total) performed at the same level
Code also any synchronous surgical decompression (foraminotomy, laminectomy, laminotomy), if performed (03.09)
EXCLUDES fusion of spine (81.00-81.08, 81.30-81.39)
insertion of artificial disc prosthesis (84.60-84.69)
insertion of interbody spinal fusion device (84.51)
AHA: 4Q, '07, 116-120

84.80 Insertion or replacement of interspinous process device(s)

Interspinous process decompression device(s)
Interspinous process distraction device(s)
EXCLUDES insertion or replacement of facet replacement device (84.84)
insertion or replacement of pedicle-based dynamic stabilization device (84.82)

84.81 Revision of interspinous process device(s)

Repair of previously inserted interspinous process device(s)
EXCLUDES revision of facet replacement device(s) (84.85)
revision of pedicle-based dynamic stabilization device (84.83)

Posterior Spinal Motion Preservation Devices

Interspinous devices   Dynamic stabilization   Facet replacement

---

[11] Noncovered except when patient is 60 years or less.

84.82 **Insertion or replacement of pedicle-based dynamic stabilization device(s)**

> EXCLUDES *initial insertion of pedicle screws with spinal fusion — omit code*
> *insertion or replacement of facet replacement device(s) (84.84)*
> *insertion or replacement of interspinous process device(s) (84.80)*
> *replacement of pedicle screws used in spinal fusion (78.59)*

AHA: 2Q, '11, 10

84.83 **Revision of pedicle-based dynamic stabilization device(s)**

> Repair of previously inserted pedicle-based dynamic stabilization device(s)

> EXCLUDES *removal of pedicle screws used in spinal fusion (78.69)*
> *replacement of pedicle screws used in spinal fusion (78.59)*
> *revision of facet replacement device(s) (84.85)*
> *revision of interspinous process device(s) (84.81)*

84.84 **Insertion or replacement of facet replacement device(s)**

> Facet arthroplasty

> EXCLUDES *initial insertion of pedicle screws with spinal fusion — omit code*
> *insertion or replacement of interspinous process device(s) (84.80)*
> *insertion or replacement of pedicle-based dynamic stabilization device(s) (84.82)*
> *replacement of pedicle screws used in spinal fusion (78.59)*

AHA: 4Q, '07, 120

84.85 **Revision of facet replacement device(s)**

> Repair of previously inserted facet replacement device(s)

> EXCLUDES *removal of pedicle screws used in spinal fusion (78.69)*
> *replacement of pedicle screws used in spinal fusion (78.59)*
> *revision of interspinous process device(s) (84.81)*
> *revision of pedicle-based dynamic stabilization device(s) (84.83)*

√4ᵗʰ **84.9** **Other operations on musculoskeletal system**

> EXCLUDES *nonoperative manipulation (93.25-93.29)*

84.91 **Amputation, not otherwise specified**

84.92 **Separation of equal conjoined twins**

84.93 **Separation of unequal conjoined twins**

> Separation of conjoined twins NOS

84.94 **Insertion of sternal fixation device with rigid plates**

> EXCLUDES *insertion of sternal fixation device for internal fixation of fracture (79.39)*
> *internal fixation of bone without fracture reduction (78.59)*

AHA: 4Q, '10, 130-131

84.99 **Other**

15. Operations on the Integumentary System (85-86)

☑3rd **85 Operations on the breast**

INCLUDES operations on the skin and subcutaneous tissue of:

breast
previous mastectomy site } female or male
revision of previous mastectomy site

85.0 Mastotomy
Incision of breast (skin) Mammotomy
EXCLUDES *aspiration of breast (85.91)*
removal of implant (85.94)
AHA: 1Q, '04, 3; 2Q, '90, 27

☑4th **85.1 Diagnostic procedures on breast**

85.11 Closed [percutaneous] [needle] biopsy of breast
DEF: Mammatome biopsy: Excision of breast tissue using a needle inserted through a small incision, followed by a full cut circle of tissue surrounding the core biopsy to obtain multiple contiguous directional sampling for definitive diagnosis and staging of cancer.
AHA: 2Q, '00, 10; 3Q, '89, 17

85.12 Open biopsy of breast
DEF: Excision of breast tissue for examination.
AHA: 3Q, '89, 17; M-A, '86, 11
TIP: If an entire breast lesion is excised, assign instead code 85.21 Local excision of lesion of breast.

85.19 Other diagnostic procedures on breast
EXCLUDES *mammary ductogram (87.35)*
mammography NEC (87.37)
manual examination (89.36)
microscopic examination of specimen
(91.61-91.69)
thermography (88.85)
ultrasonography (88.73)
xerography (87.36)

☑4th **85.2 Excision or destruction of breast tissue**
EXCLUDES *mastectomy (85.41-85.48)*
reduction mammoplasty (85.31-85.32)

85.20 Excision or destruction of breast tissue, not otherwise specified
EXCLUDES *laser interstitial thermal therapy [LITT] of lesion or tissue of breast under guidance (17.69)*

85.21 Local excision of lesion of breast
Lumpectomy
Removal of area of fibrosis from breast
EXCLUDES *biopsy of breast (85.11-85.12)*
AHA: ▶3Q, '12, 3;◀ 2Q, '90, 27; 3Q, '89, 17; M-A, '86, 11

85.22 Resection of quadrant of breast

85.23 Subtotal mastectomy
EXCLUDES *quadrant resection (85.22)*
DEF: Excision of a large portion of breast tissue.
AHA: 2Q, '92, 7

85.24 Excision of ectopic breast tissue
Excision of accessory nipple
DEF: Excision of breast tissue outside normal breast region.

85.25 Excision of nipple
EXCLUDES *excision of accessory nipple (85.24)*

Mastectomy

Partial mastectomy
(lumpectomy): skin
left intact

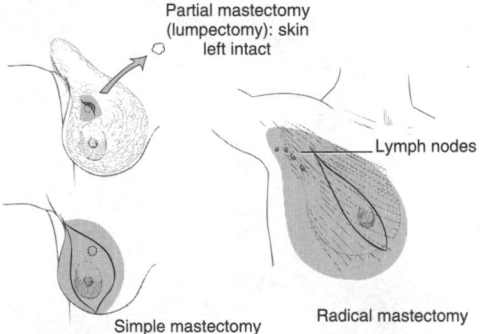

Lymph nodes

Simple mastectomy   Radical mastectomy

☑4th **85.3 Reduction mammoplasty and subcutaneous mammectomy**
AHA: 4Q, '95, 79, 80

85.31 Unilateral reduction mammoplasty
Unilateral:
amputative mammoplasty
size reduction mammoplasty

85.32 Bilateral reduction mammoplasty
Amputative mammoplasty
Biesenberger operation
Reduction mammoplasty (for gynecomastia)

85.33 Unilateral subcutaneous mammectomy with synchronous implant
EXCLUDES *that without synchronous implant (85.34)*
DEF: Removal of mammary tissue, leaving skin and nipple intact with implant of prosthesis.

85.34 Other unilateral subcutaneous mammectomy
Removal of breast tissue with preservation of skin and nipple
Subcutaneous mammectomy NOS
DEF: Excision of mammary tissue, leaving skin and nipple intact.

85.35 Bilateral subcutaneous mammectomy with synchronous implant
EXCLUDES *that without synchronous implant (85.36)*
DEF: Excision of mammary tissue, both breasts, leaving skin and nipples intact; with prostheses.

85.36 Other bilateral subcutaneous mammectomy

☑4th **85.4 Mastectomy**

85.41 Unilateral simple mastectomy
Mastectomy:
NOS
complete
DEF: Removal of one breast.

85.42 Bilateral simple mastectomy
Bilateral complete mastectomy
DEF: Removal of both breasts.
AHA: 2Q, '11, 12

85.43 Unilateral extended simple mastectomy
Extended simple mastectomy NOS
Modified radical mastectomy
Simple mastectomy with excision of regional lymph nodes
DEF: Removal of one breast and lymph nodes under arm.
AHA: ▶2Q, '12, 4;◀ 2Q, '92, 7; 3Q, '91, 24; 2Q, '91, 21
TIP: ▶Modified radical mastectomy includes sentinel node biopsy, a regional axillary lymph resection for staging. Do not report separately.◀

85.44 Bilateral extended simple mastectomy
AHA: 2Q, '92, 7; 3Q, '91, 24; 2Q, '91, 21

85.45 Unilateral radical mastectomy
Excision of breast, pectoral muscles, and regional lymph nodes [axillary, clavicular, supraclavicular]
Radical mastectomy NOS
DEF: Removal of one breast and regional lymph nodes, pectoral muscle and adjacent tissue.
AHA: 2Q, '91, 21
TIP: Do not assign a separate code for lymph node excision (subcategory 40.3 or 40.5); the service is included in the radical mastectomy code.

85.46 Bilateral radical mastectomy
AHA: 2Q, '91, 21

85.47 Unilateral extended radical mastectomy
Excision of breast, muscles, and lymph nodes [axillary, clavicular, supraclavicular, internal mammary, and mediastinal]
Extended radical mastectomy NOS
DEF: Removal of one breast, regional and middle chest lymph nodes, chest muscle and adjacent tissue.

85.48 Bilateral extended radical mastectomy
DEF: Removal of both breasts, regional and middle chest lymph nodes, chest muscle and adjacent tissue.

85.5 **Augmentation mammoplasty**
EXCLUDES *that associated with subcutaneous mammectomy (85.33, 85.35)*
DEF: Plastic surgery to increase breast size.
AHA: 3Q, '97, 12; 4Q, '95, 76, 80

85.50 **Augmentation mammoplasty, not otherwise specified**

85.51 **Unilateral injection into breast for augmentation**
EXCLUDES *injection of fat graft of breast (85.55)*

85.52 **Bilateral injection into breast for augmentation**
Injection into breast for augmentation NOS
EXCLUDES *injection of fat graft of breast (85.55)*

85.53 **Unilateral breast implant**
AHA: 2Q, '00 18; 2Q, '98, 14

85.54 **Bilateral breast implant**
Breast implant NOS

85.55 **Fat graft to breast**
INCLUDES *extraction of fat for autologous graft*
Autologous fat transplantation or transfer
Fat graft to breast NOS
Fat graft to breast with or without use of enriched graft
Micro-fat grafting
EXCLUDES *that with reconstruction of breast (85.70-85.79)*
AHA: 4Q, '10, 132-134

85.6 **Mastopexy**
DEF: Anchoring of pendulous breast.

85.7 **Total reconstruction of breast**
AHA: 4Q, '08, 185-187; 4Q, '95, 77; 1Q, '93, 27
TIP: When a patient is admitted for breast reconstruction following mastectomy, assign diagnosis code V51.0 as the principal or first-listed diagnosis.

85.70 **Total reconstruction of breast, not otherwise specified**
Perforator flap, free

85.71 **Latissimus dorsi myocutaneous flap**
AHA: 2Q, '11, 12

85.72 **Transverse rectus abdominis myocutaneous [TRAM] flap, pedicled**
EXCLUDES *transverse rectus abdominis myocutaneous (TRAM) flap, free (85.73)*

85.73 **Transverse rectus abdominis myocutaneous [TRAM] flap, free**
EXCLUDES *transverse rectus abdominis myocutaneous (TRAM) flap, pedicled (85.72)*
AHA: 4Q, '10, 115

85.74 **Deep inferior epigastric artery perforator [DIEP] flap, free**

85.75 **Superficial inferior epigastric artery [SIEA] flap, free**

85.76 **Gluteal artery perforator [GAP] flap, free**

85.79 **Other total reconstruction of breast**
EXCLUDES *deep inferior epigastric artery perforator [DIEP] flap, free (85.74)*
gluteal artery perforator [GAP] flap, free (85.76)
latissimus dorsi myocutaneous flap (85.71)
perforator flap, free (85.70)
superficial inferior epigastric artery [SIEA] flap, free (85.75)
total reconstruction of breast, not otherwise specified (85.70)
transverse rectus abdominis myocutaneous [TRAM] flap, free (85.73)
transverse rectus abdominis myocutaneous [TRAM] flap, pedicled (85.72)

85.8 **Other repair and plastic operations on breast**
EXCLUDES *that for:*
augmentation (85.50-85.54)
reconstruction (85.70-85.76, 85.79)
reduction (85.31-85.32)
AHA: 4Q, '95, 77

85.81 **Suture of laceration of breast**

85.82 **Split-thickness graft to breast**

85.83 **Full-thickness graft to breast**
AHA: 4Q, '95, 77

85.84 **Pedicle graft to breast**
DEF: Implantation of transferred muscle tissue still connected to vascular source.
AHA: 4Q, '95, 77

85.85 **Muscle flap graft to breast**
AHA: 4Q, '95, 77

85.86 **Transposition of nipple**
DEF: Relocation of nipple.
AHA: 4Q, '95, 78

85.87 **Other repair or reconstruction of nipple**
AHA: 4Q, '95, 78

85.89 **Other mammoplasty**

85.9 **Other operations on the breast**

85.91 **Aspiration of breast**
EXCLUDES *percutaneous biopsy of breast (85.11)*

85.92 **Injection of therapeutic agent into breast**
EXCLUDES *that for augmentation of breast (85.51-85.52, 85.55)*

85.93 **Revision of implant of breast**
AHA: 2Q, '98, 14; 4Q, '95, 76

85.94 **Removal of implant of breast**
AHA: 2Q, '98, 14; 3Q, '92, 4

85.95 **Insertion of breast tissue expander**
Insertion (soft tissue) of tissue expander (one or more) under muscle or platysma to develop skin flaps for donor use
AHA: 2Q, '11, 12

85.96 **Removal of breast tissue expander(s)**
AHA: 2Q, '00, 18; 4Q, '95, 77

85.99 **Other**
AHA: ▶2Q, '12, 8◄

86 **Operations on skin and subcutaneous tissue**
INCLUDES operations on:
hair follicles
male perineum
nails
sebaceous glands
subcutaneous fat pads
sudoriferous glands
superficial fossae
EXCLUDES *those on skin of:*
anus (49.01-49.99)
breast (mastectomy site) (85.0-85.99)
ear (18.01-18.9)
eyebrow (08.01-08.99)
eyelid (08.01-08.99)
female perineum (71.01-71.9)
lips (27.0-27.99)
nose (21.00-21.99)
penis (64.0-64.99)
scrotum (61.0-61.99)
vulva (71.01-71.9)

86.0 **Incision of skin and subcutaneous tissue**

86.01 **Aspiration of skin and subcutaneous tissue**
Aspiration of:
abscess
hematoma } of nail, skin, or subcutaneous tissue
seroma
AHA: 3Q, '89, 16

Additional Digit Required
Valid OR Procedure
Non-OR Procedure
Adjunct Code
2014 ICD-9-CM
February 2013 · Volume 3 – 179

Operations on the Integumentary System

86.02 **Injection or tattooing of skin lesion or defect**
Insertion
Injection } of filling material
Pigmenting of skin
DEF: Pigmenting of skin: Adding color to skin.

86.03 **Incision of pilonidal sinus or cyst**
EXCLUDES marsupialization (86.21)

86.04 **Other incision with drainage of skin and subcutaneous tissue**
EXCLUDES drainage of:
fascial compartments of face and mouth (27.0)
palmar or thenar space (82.04)
pilonidal sinus or cyst (86.03)
AHA: 1Q, '09, 11; 4Q, '04, 76
TIP: If extensive debridement is performed along with the I&D procedure, assign instead code 86.22.

86.05 **Incision with removal of foreign body or device from skin and subcutaneous tissue**
Removal of carotid sinus baroreflex activation device
Removal of loop recorder
Removal of neurostimulator pulse generator (single array, dual array)
Removal of tissue expander(s) from skin or soft tissue other than breast tissue
EXCLUDES removal of foreign body without incision (98.20-98.29)
AHA: 2Q, '96, 15; N-D, '87, 10; N-D, '86, 9

86.06 **Insertion of totally implantable infusion pump**
Code also any associated catheterization
EXCLUDES insertion of totally implantable vascular access device (86.07)
AHA: 2Q, '99, 4; 4Q, '90, 14

86.07 **Insertion of totally implantable vascular access device [VAD]**
Totally implanted port
EXCLUDES insertion of totally implantable infusion pump (86.06)
DEF: Placement of vascular access infusion catheter system under skin to allow for frequent manual infusions into blood vessel.
AHA: 1Q, '01, 13; 1Q, '96, 3; 2Q, '94, 11; 3Q, '91, 13; 4Q, '90, 15

86.09 **Other incision of skin and subcutaneous tissue**
Creation of thalamic stimulator pulse generator pocket, new site
Escharotomy
Exploration:
sinus tract, skin
superficial fossa
Relocation of subcutaneous device pocket NEC
Reopening subcutaneous pocket for device revision without replacement
Undercutting of hair follicle
EXCLUDES creation of loop recorder pocket, new site and insertion/relocation of device (37.79)
creation of pocket for implantable, patient-activated cardiac event recorder and insertion/relocation of device (37.79)
removal of catheter from cranial cavity (01.27)
that for drainage (86.04)
that of:
cardiac pacemaker pocket, new site (37.79)
fascial compartments of face and mouth (27.0)
AHA: 1Q, '05, 17; 2Q, '04, 7, 8; 4Q, '00, 68; 4Q, '99, 21; 4Q, '97, 57; 3Q, '89, 17; N-D, '86, 1; N-D, '84, 6

√4ᵗʰ **86.1** **Diagnostic procedures on skin and subcutaneous tissue**

86.11 **Closed biopsy of skin and subcutaneous tissue**
AHA: 4Q, '08, 99

86.19 **Other diagnostic procedures on skin and subcutaneous tissue**
EXCLUDES microscopic examination of specimen from skin and subcutaneous tissue (91.61-91.79)

√4ᵗʰ **86.2** **Excision or destruction of lesion or tissue of skin and subcutaneous tissue**

86.21 **Excision of pilonidal cyst or sinus**
Marsupialization of cyst
EXCLUDES incision of pilonidal cyst or sinus (86.03)
DEF: Marsupialization of cyst: Incision of cyst and suturing edges to skin to open site.

86.22 **Excisional debridement of wound, infection, or burn**
Removal by excision of:
devitalized tissue
necrosis
slough
EXCLUDES debridement of:
abdominal wall (wound) (54.3)
bone (77.60-77.69)
muscle (83.45)
of hand (82.36)
nail (bed) (fold) (86.27)
nonexcisional debridement of wound, infection, or burn (86.28)
open fracture site (79.60-79.69)
pedicle or flap graft (86.75)
AHA: ▶3Q, '12, 3;◀ 2Q, '11, 11; 3Q, '08, 8; 1Q, '08, 3-4; 3Q, '06, 19; 2Q, '06, 11; 1Q, '05, 14; 4Q, '04, 138; 3Q,'02, 23; 2Q, '00, 9; 1Q, '99, 8; 2Q, '92, 17; 3Q, '91, 18; 3Q, '89, 16; 4Q, '88, 5; N-D, '86, 1
TIP: Assign only if the debridement involves skin and subcutaneous tissues; any deeper structures (e.g., muscle, bone) are coded elsewhere.

86.23 **Removal of nail, nail bed, or nail fold**

86.24 **Chemosurgery of skin**
Chemical peel of skin
DEF: Chemicals applied to destroy skin tissue.
DEF: Chemical peel of skin: Chemicals used to peel skin layers.

86.25 **Dermabrasion**
That with laser
EXCLUDES dermabrasion of wound to remove embedded debris (86.28)
DEF: Removal of wrinkled or scarred skin with fine sandpaper, wire, brushes or laser.

86.26 **Ligation of dermal appendage**
EXCLUDES excision of preauricular appendage (18.29)
DEF: Tying off extra skin.

86.27 **Debridement of nail, nail bed, or nail fold**
Removal of:
necrosis
slough
EXCLUDES removal of nail, nail bed, or nail fold (86.23)

86.28 **Nonexcisional debridement of wound, infection, or burn**
Debridement NOS
Maggot therapy
Removal of devitalized tissue, necrosis, and slough by such methods as:
brushing
irrigation (under pressure)
scrubbing
washing
Ultrasonic debridement
Water scalpel (jet)
DEF: Removal of damaged skin by methods other than excision.
AHA: 4Q, '11, 182; 2Q, '10, 11; 3Q, '09, 13; 1Q, '07, 10, 11; 1Q, '05, 14; 2Q, '04, 5, 6; 4Q, '03, 110; 2Q, '03, 15; 3Q, '02, 23; 2Q, '01, 18; 3Q, '91, 18; 4Q, '88, 5
TIP: Assign for VersaJet debridement, regardless of depth of tissue debrided.

86.3 **Other local excision or destruction of lesion or tissue of skin and subcutaneous tissue**

Destruction of skin by:
  cauterization
  cryosurgery
  fulguration
  laser beam
That with Z-plasty

EXCLUDES *adipectomy (86.83)*
  biopsy of skin (86.11)
  wide or radical excision of skin (86.4)
  Z-plasty without excision (86.84)

AHA: 1Q, '96, 15; 2Q, '90, 27; 1Q, '89, 12; 3Q, '89, 18; 4Q, '88, 7

86.4 **Radical excision of skin lesion**

Wide excision of skin lesion involving underlying or adjacent structure

Code also any lymph node dissection (40.3-40.5)

AHA: 4Q, '09, 74

86.5 **Suture or other closure of skin and subcutaneous tissue**

86.51 **Replantation of scalp**

86.59 **Closure of skin and subcutaneous tissue of other sites**

Adhesives (surgical)(tissue)
Staples
Sutures

EXCLUDES *application of adhesive strips (butterfly) — omit code*

AHA: 4Q, '99, 23

86.6 **Free skin graft**

INCLUDES excision of skin for autogenous graft
EXCLUDES *construction or reconstruction of:*
  penis (64.43-64.44)
  trachea (31.75)
  vagina (70.61-70.64)

DEF: Transplantation of skin to another site.

86.60 **Free skin graft, not otherwise specified**

86.61 **Full-thickness skin graft to hand**

EXCLUDES *heterograft (86.65)*
  homograft (86.66)

86.62 **Other skin graft to hand**

EXCLUDES *heterograft (86.65)*
  homograft (86.66)

86.63 **Full-thickness skin graft to other sites**

EXCLUDES *heterograft (86.65)*
  homograft (86.66)

86.64 **Hair transplant**

EXCLUDES *hair follicle transplant to eyebrow or eyelash (08.63)*

86.65 **Heterograft to skin**

Pigskin graft
Porcine graft

EXCLUDES *application of dressing only (93.57)*

DEF: Implantation of nonhuman tissue.

AHA: 3Q,'02, 23

86.66 **Homograft to skin**

Graft to skin of:
  amnionic membrane ⎱ from donor
  skin ⎰

DEF: Implantation of tissue from human donor.

86.67 **Dermal regenerative graft**

Artificial skin, NOS
Creation of "neodermis"
Decellularized allodermis
Integumentary matrix implants
Prosthetic implant of dermal layer of skin
Regenerate dermal layer of skin

EXCLUDES *heterograft to skin (86.65)*
  homograft to skin (86.66)

DEF: Replacement of dermis and epidermal layer of skin by cultured or regenerated autologous tissue; used to treat full-thickness or deep partial-thickness burns; also called cultured epidermal autograft (CEA).

AHA: 3Q, '10, 7-8; 3Q, '06, 19; 4Q, '98, 76, 79

86.69 **Other skin graft to other sites**

EXCLUDES *heterograft (86.65)*
  homograft (86.66)

AHA: 1Q, '10, 7; 4Q, '99, 15

86.7 **Pedicle grafts or flaps**

EXCLUDES *construction or reconstruction of:*
  penis (64.43-64.44)
  trachea (31.75)
  vagina (70.61-70.64)

DEF: Full thickness skin and subcutaneous tissue partially attached to the body by a narrow strip of tissue so that it retains its blood supply. The unattached portion is sutured to the defect.

86.70 **Pedicle or flap graft, not otherwise specified**

86.71 **Cutting and preparation of pedicle grafts or flaps**

Elevation of pedicle from its bed
Flap design and raising
Partial cutting of pedicle or tube
Pedicle delay

EXCLUDES *pollicization or digital transfer (82.61,82.81)*
  revision of pedicle (86.75)

DEF: Elevation of pedicle from its bed: Separation of tissue implanted from its bed.

DEF: Flap design and raising: Planing and elevation of tissue to be implanted.

DEF: Pedicle delay: Elevation and preparation of tissue still attached to vascular bed; delayed implant.

AHA: 4Q, '01, 66

86.72 **Advancement of pedicle graft**

AHA: 3Q, '99, 9, 10

86.73 **Attachment of pedicle or flap graft to hand**

EXCLUDES *pollicization or digital transfer (82.61, 82.81)*

86.74 **Attachment of pedicle or flap graft to other sites**

Attachment by:
  advanced flap
  double pedicled flap
  pedicle graft
  rotating flap
  sliding flap
  tube graft

DEF: Advanced flap: Sliding tissue implant into new position.

DEF: Double pedicle flap: Implant connected to two vascular beds.

DEF: Pedicle graft: Implant connected to vascular bed.

DEF: Rotating flap: Implant rotated along curved incision.

DEF: Sliding flap: Sliding implant to site.

DEF: Tube graft: Double tissue implant to form tube with base connected to original site.

AHA: 3Q, '99, 9; 1Q, '96, 15

86.75 **Revision of pedicle or flap graft**

Debridement ⎱ of pedicle or flap graft
Defatting ⎰

DEF: Connection of implant still attached to its vascular tissue.

86.8 **Other repair and reconstruction of skin and subcutaneous tissue**

86.81 **Repair for facial weakness**

86.82 **Facial rhytidectomy**

Face lift

EXCLUDES *rhytidectomy of eyelid (08.86-08.87)*

DEF: Revision and tightening of excess, wrinkled facial skin.

Operations on the Integumentary System

86.83–86.99

86.83 Size reduction plastic operation

Liposuction
Reduction of adipose tissue of:
   abdominal wall (pendulous)
   arms (batwing)
   buttock
   thighs (trochanteric lipomatosis)

EXCLUDES *breast (85.31-85.32)*
              liposuction to harvest fat graft (86.90)

DEF: Excision and plastic repair of excess skin and underlying tissue.

AHA: 2Q, '06, 10

TIP: Assign for abdominoplasty or panniculectomy performed after a morbid obesity surgical procedure and significant weight loss.

86.84 Relaxation of scar or web contracture of skin

Z-plasty of skin

EXCLUDES *Z-plasty with excision of lesion (86.3)*

86.85 Correction of syndactyly

DEF: Plastic repair of webbed fingers or toes.

86.86 Onychoplasty

DEF: Plastic repair of nail or nail bed.

86.87 Fat graft of skin and subcutaneous tissue

INCLUDES extraction of fat for autologous graft
Autologous fat transplantation or transfer
Fat graft NOS
Fat graft of skin and subcutaneous tissue with or
    without use of enriched graft
Micro-fat grafting

EXCLUDES *fat graft to breast (85.55)*

86.89 Other repair and reconstruction of skin and subcutaneous tissue

EXCLUDES *mentoplasty (76.67-76.68)*

AHA: 4Q, '02, 107; 1Q, '00, 26; 2Q, '98, 20; 2Q, '93, 11; 2Q, '92, 17

✓4ᵗʰ **86.9 Other operations on skin and subcutaneous tissue**

86.90 Extraction of fat for graft or banking

Harvest of fat for extraction of cells for future use
Liposuction to harvest fat graft

EXCLUDES *that with graft at same operative episode*
           (85.55, 86.87)

86.91 Excision of skin for graft

Excision of skin with closure of donor site

EXCLUDES *that with graft at same operative episode*
           (86.60-86.69)

86.92 Electrolysis and other epilation of skin

EXCLUDES *epilation of eyelid (08.91-08.93)*

86.93 Insertion of tissue expander

Insertion (subcutaneous) (soft tissue) of expander
   (one or more) in scalp (subgaleal space), face,
   neck, trunk except breast, and upper and lower
   extremities for development of skin flaps for
   donor use

EXCLUDES *flap graft preparation (86.71)*
           tissue expander, breast (85.95)

86.94 Insertion or replacement of single array neurostimulator pulse generator, not specified as rechargeable

Pulse generator (single array, single channel, single
   port) for intracranial, spinal, and peripheral
   neurostimulator

Code also any associated lead implantation (02.93,
   03.93, 04.92)

EXCLUDES *cranial implantation or replacement of*
           neurostimulator pulse generator
           (01.20)
           insertion or replacement of single array
              rechargeable neurostimulator pulse
              generator (86.97)

AHA: 4Q, '04, 135

86.95 Insertion or replacement of multiple array neurostimulator pulse generator, not specified as rechargeable

Pulse generator (multiple array, multiple channel,
   multiple port) for intracranial, spinal, and
   peripheral neurostimulator

Code also any associated lead implantation (02.93,
   03.93, 04.92)

EXCLUDES *cranial implantation or replacement of*
           neurostimulator pulse generator
           (01.20)
           insertion or replacement of (multiple array)
              rechargeable neurostimulator pulse
               generator (86.98)

86.96 Insertion or replacement of other neurostimulator pulse generator

Code also any associated lead implantation (02.93,
   03.93, 04.92)

EXCLUDES *cranial implantation or replacement of*
           neurostimulator pulse generator
           (01.20)
           insertion of multiple array neurostimulator
              pulse generator (86.95, 86.98)
           insertion of single array neurostimulator
              pulse generator (86.94, 86.97)

AHA: 2Q, '07, 8; 2Q, '06, 5-6

86.97 Insertion or replacement of single array rechargeable neurostimulator pulse generator

Rechargeable pulse generator (single array, single
   channel, single port) for intracranial, spinal, and
   peripheral neurostimulator

Code also any associated lead implantation (02.93,
   03.93, 04.92)

EXCLUDES *cranial implantation or replacement of*
           neurostimulator pulse generator
           (01.20)

AHA: 4Q, '05, 130

86.98 Insertion or replacement of multiple array (two or more) rechargeable neurostimulator pulse generator

Rechargeable pulse generator (multiple array,
   multiple channel, multiple port) for intracranial,
   spinal, and peripheral neurostimulator

Code also any associated lead implantation (02.93,
   03.93, 04.92)

EXCLUDES *cranial implantation or replacement of*
           neurostimulator pulse generator
           (01.20)

AHA: 4Q, '05, 130

86.99 Other

EXCLUDES *removal of sutures from:*
           abdomen (97.83)
           head and neck (97.38)
           thorax (97.43)
           trunk NEC (97.84)
           wound catheter:
           irrigation (96.58)
           replacement (97.15)

AHA: 4Q, '97, 57; N-D, '86, 1

BI Bilateral Procedure   NC Non-covered Procedure   LC Limited Coverage Procedure   ►◄ Revised Text   ● New Code   ▲ Revised Code Title

182 – Volume 3   2014 ICD-9-CM

16. Miscellaneous Diagnostic and Therapeutic Procedures (87-99)

√3rd **87 Diagnostic radiology**

√4th **87.0 Soft tissue x-ray of face, head, and neck**
EXCLUDES *angiography (88.40-88.68)*

87.01 Pneumoencephalogram
DEF: Radiographic exam of cerebral ventricles and subarachnoid spaces with injection of air or gas for contrast.

87.02 Other contrast radiogram of brain and skull
Pneumocisternogram
Pneumoventriculogram
Posterior fossa myelogram
DEF: Pneumocisternogram: radiographic exam of subarachnoid spaces after injection of gas or contrast.
DEF: Pneumoventriculography: radiographic exam of cerebral ventricles after injection of gas or contrast.
DEF: Posterior fossa myelogram: radiographic exam of posterior channel of spinal cord after injection of gas or contrast.

87.03 Computerized axial tomography of head
C.A.T. scan of head
AHA: 3Q, '05, 12; 3Q, '99, 7

87.04 Other tomography of head

87.05 Contrast dacryocystogram
DEF: Radiographic exam of tear sac after injection of contrast.

87.06 Contrast radiogram of nasopharynx

87.07 Contrast laryngogram

87.08 Cervical lymphangiogram
DEF: Radiographic exam of lymph vessels of neck with or without contrast.

87.09 Other soft tissue x-ray of face, head, and neck
Noncontrast x-ray of:
adenoid
larynx
nasolacrimal duct
nasopharynx
salivary gland
thyroid region
uvula
EXCLUDES *x-ray study of eye (95.14)*

√4th **87.1 Other x-ray of face, head, and neck**
EXCLUDES *angiography (88.40-88.68)*

87.11 Full-mouth x-ray of teeth

87.12 Other dental x-ray
Orthodontic cephalogram or cephalometrics
Panorex examination of mandible
Root canal x-ray

87.13 Temporomandibular contrast arthrogram

87.14 Contrast radiogram of orbit

87.15 Contrast radiogram of sinus

87.16 Other x-ray of facial bones
X-ray of:
frontal area
mandible
maxilla
nasal sinuses
nose
orbit
supraorbital area
symphysis menti
zygomaticomaxillary complex

87.17 Other x-ray of skull
Lateral projection
Sagittal projection } of skull
Tangential projection
DEF: Lateral projection: Side to side view of head.
DEF: Sagittal projection: View of body in plane running midline from front to back.
DEF: Tangential projection: Views from adjacent skull surfaces.

√4th **87.2 X-ray of spine**

87.21 Contrast myelogram
DEF: Radiographic exam of space between middle and outer spinal cord coverings after injection of contrast.

87.22 Other x-ray of cervical spine

87.23 Other x-ray of thoracic spine

87.24 Other x-ray of lumbosacral spine
Sacrococcygeal x-ray

87.29 Other x-ray of spine
Spinal x-ray NOS

√4th **87.3 Soft tissue x-ray of thorax**
EXCLUDES *angiocardiography (88.50-88.58)*
angiography (88.40-88.68)

87.31 Endotracheal bronchogram
DEF: Radiographic exam of main branch of lung with contrast introduced through windpipe.

87.32 Other contrast bronchogram
Transcricoid bronchogram
DEF: Transcricoid bronchogram: Radiographic exam of main branch of lung with contrast introduced through cartilage of neck.

87.33 Mediastinal pneumogram
DEF: Radiographic exam of cavity containing heart, esophagus and adjacent structures.

87.34 Intrathoracic lymphangiogram
DEF: Radiographic exam of lymphatic vessels within chest; with or without contrast.

87.35 Contrast radiogram of mammary ducts
DEF: Radiographic exam of mammary ducts; with contrast.

87.36 Xerography of breast
DEF: Radiographic exam of breast via selenium-coated plates.

87.37 Other mammography
AHA: 3Q, '89, 17; 2Q, '90, 28; N-D, '87, 1
TIP: Assign as an additional code when mammographic localization is performed immediately prior to breast lesion biopsy or excision. Wire localization is included.

87.38 Sinogram of chest wall
Fistulogram of chest wall
DEF: Fistulogram of chest wall: Radiographic exam of abnormal opening in chest.

87.39 Other soft tissue x-ray of chest wall

√4th **87.4 Other x-ray of thorax**
EXCLUDES *angiocardiography (88.50-88.58)*
angiography (88.40-88.68)

87.41 Computerized axial tomography of thorax
C.A.T. scan of heart
C.A.T. scan
Crystal linea scan of x-ray beam
Electronic subtraction } of thorax
Photoelectric response
Tomography with use of computer, x-rays, and camera

87.42 Other tomography of thorax
Cardiac tomogram
EXCLUDES *C.A.T. scan of heart (87.41)*
DEF: Radiographic exam of chest plane.

Miscellaneous Diagnostic and Therapeutic Procedures

87.43–88.14

87.43   **X-ray of ribs, sternum, and clavicle**
Examination for:
   cervical rib
   fracture

87.44   **Routine chest x-ray, so described**
X-ray of chest NOS

87.49   **Other chest x-ray**
X-ray of:
   bronchus NOS
   diaphragm NOS
   heart NOS
   lung NOS
   mediastinum NOS
   trachea NOS

✓4th **87.5**   **Biliary tract x-ray**

87.51   **Percutaneous hepatic cholangiogram**
DEF: Radiographic exam of bile tract of gallbladder; with needle injection of contrast into bile duct of liver.
AHA: 2Q, '90, 28; N-D, '87, 1

87.52   **Intravenous cholangiogram**
DEF: Radiographic exam of bile ducts; with intravenous contrast injection.

87.53   **Intraoperative cholangiogram**
DEF: Radiographic exam of bile ducts with contrast; following gallbladder removal.
AHA: 1Q, '96, 12; 2Q, '90, 28; 3Q, '89, 18; 4Q, '88, 7

87.54   **Other cholangiogram**

87.59   **Other biliary tract x-ray**
Cholecystogram

✓4th **87.6**   **Other x-ray of digestive system**

87.61   **Barium swallow**

87.62   **Upper GI series**

87.63   **Small bowel series**

87.64   **Lower GI series**

87.65   **Other x-ray of intestine**

87.66   **Contrast pancreatogram**

87.69   **Other digestive tract x-ray**

✓4th **87.7**   **X-ray of urinary system**
EXCLUDES   *angiography of renal vessels (88.45, 88.65)*

87.71   **Computerized axial tomography of kidney**
C.A.T. scan of kidney

87.72   **Other nephrotomogram**
DEF: Radiographic exam of kidney plane.

87.73   **Intravenous pyelogram**
Diuretic infusion pyelogram
DEF: Radiographic exam of lower kidney, with intravenous contrast injection.
DEF: Diuretic infusion pyelogram: Radiographic exam of lower kidney with diuretic contrast.

87.74   **Retrograde pyelogram**
TIP: The diagnostic cystoscopy service is included in the retrograde pyelogram code; do not assign 57.32 separately.

87.75   **Percutaneous pyelogram**

87.76   **Retrograde cystourethrogram**
DEF: Radiographic exam of bladder and urethra with contrast injected through catheter into bladder.

87.77   **Other cystogram**

87.78   **Ileal conduitogram**
DEF: Radiographic exam of passage created between ureter and artificial opening into abdomen.
AHA: M-J, '87, 11

87.79   **Other x-ray of the urinary system**
KUB x-ray

Ureteropyelography

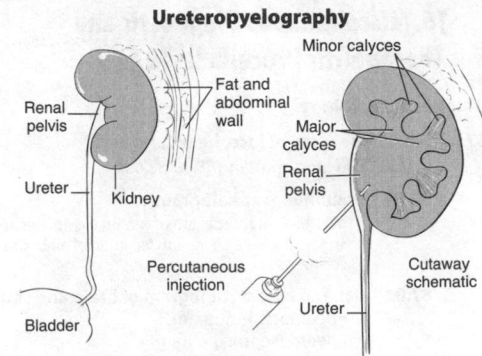

Percutaneous injection

Cutaway schematic

✓4th **87.8**   **X-ray of female genital organs**

87.81   **X-ray of gravid uterus**   ♀
Intrauterine cephalometry by x-ray

87.82   **Gas contrast hysterosalpingogram**   ♀
DEF: Radiographic exam of uterus and fallopian tubes with gas contrast.

87.83   **Opaque dye contrast hysterosalpingogram**   ♀

87.84   **Percutaneous hysterogram**   ♀
DEF: Radiographic exam of uterus with contrast injected through body wall.

87.85   **Other x-ray of fallopian tubes and uterus**   ♀

87.89   **Other x-ray of female genital organs**   ♀

✓4th **87.9**   **X-ray of male genital organs**

87.91   **Contrast seminal vesiculogram**   ♂

87.92   **Other x-ray of prostate and seminal vesicles**   ♂

87.93   **Contrast epididymogram**   ♂

87.94   **Contrast vasogram**   ♂

87.95   **Other x-ray of epididymis and vas deferens**   ♂

87.99   **Other x-ray of male genital organs**   ♂

✓3rd **88**   **Other diagnostic radiology and related techniques**

✓4th **88.0**   **Soft tissue x-ray of abdomen**
EXCLUDES   *angiography (88.40-88.68)*

88.01   **Computerized axial tomography of abdomen**
C.A.T. scan of abdomen
EXCLUDES   *C.A.T. scan of kidney (87.71)*
AHA: 2Q, '98, 13

88.02   **Other abdomen tomography**
EXCLUDES   *nephrotomogram (87.72)*

88.03   **Sinogram of abdominal wall**
Fistulogram of abdominal wall
DEF: Radiographic exam of abnormal abdominal passage.

88.04   **Abdominal lymphangiogram**
DEF: Radiographic exam of abdominal lymphatic vessels with contrast.

88.09   **Other soft tissue x-ray of abdominal wall**

✓4th **88.1**   **Other x-ray of abdomen**

88.11   **Pelvic opaque dye contrast radiography**

88.12   **Pelvic gas contrast radiography**
Pelvic pneumoperitoneum

88.13   **Other peritoneal pneumogram**

88.14   **Retroperitoneal fistulogram**

BI Bilateral Procedure   NC Non-covered Procedure   LC Limited Coverage Procedure   ▶◀ Revised Text   ● New Code   ▲ Revised Code Title

184 – Volume 3   **2014 ICD-9-CM**

88.15 Retroperitoneal pneumogram

88.16 Other retroperitoneal x-ray

88.19 Other x-ray of abdomen
Flat plate of abdomen
AHA: 3Q, '99, 9

√4ᵗʰ 88.2 Skeletal x-ray of extremities and pelvis
EXCLUDES *contrast radiogram of joint (88.32)*

88.21 Skeletal x-ray of shoulder and upper arm

88.22 Skeletal x-ray of elbow and forearm

88.23 Skeletal x-ray of wrist and hand

88.24 Skeletal x-ray of upper limb, not otherwise specified

88.25 Pelvimetry
DEF: Imaging of pelvic bones to measure pelvic capacity.

88.26 Other skeletal x-ray of pelvis and hip

88.27 Skeletal x-ray of thigh, knee, and lower leg

88.28 Skeletal x-ray of ankle and foot

88.29 Skeletal x-ray of lower limb, not otherwise specified

√4ᵗʰ 88.3 Other x-ray

88.31 Skeletal series
X-ray of whole skeleton

88.32 Contrast arthrogram
EXCLUDES *that of temporomandibular joint (87.13)*

88.33 Other skeletal x-ray
EXCLUDES *skeletal x-ray of:*
extremities and pelvis (88.21-88.29)
face, head, and neck (87.11-87.17)
spine (87.21-87.29)
thorax (87.43)

88.34 Lymphangiogram of upper limb

88.35 Other soft tissue x-ray of upper limb

88.36 Lymphangiogram of lower limb

88.37 Other soft tissue x-ray of lower limb
EXCLUDES *femoral angiography (88.48, 88.66)*

88.38 Other computerized axial tomography
C.A.T. scan NOS
EXCLUDES *C.A.T. scan of:*
abdomen (88.01)
head (87.03)
heart (87.41)
kidney (87.71)
thorax (87.41)
AHA: 3Q, '05, 13-14

88.39 X-ray, other and unspecified

√4ᵗʰ 88.4 Arteriography using contrast material
NOTE The fourth-digit subclassification identifies the site to be viewed, not the site of injection.
INCLUDES angiography of arteries
arterial puncture for injection of contrast material
radiography of arteries (by fluoroscopy)
retrograde arteriography
EXCLUDES *arteriography using:*
radioisotopes or radionuclides (92.01-92.19)
ultrasound (88.71-88.79)
fluorescein angiography of eye (95.12)
DEF: Electromagnetic wave photography of arteries with contrast.
AHA: N-D, '85, 14

88.40 Arteriography using contrast material, unspecified site

88.41 Arteriography of cerebral arteries
Angiography of:
basilar artery
carotid (internal)
vertebral artery
posterior cerebral circulation
AHA: 1Q, '00, 16; 1Q, '99, 7; 1Q, '97, 3

88.42 Aortography
Arteriography of aorta and aortic arch
AHA: 2Q, '10, 8-9; 1Q, '99, 17

88.43 Arteriography of pulmonary arteries

88.44 Arteriography of other intrathoracic vessels
EXCLUDES *angiocardiography (88.50-88.58)*
arteriography of coronary arteries (88.55-88.57)

88.45 Arteriography of renal arteries

88.46 Arteriography of placenta   ♀
Placentogram using contrast material

88.47 Arteriography of other intra-abdominal arteries
AHA: 2Q, '09, 7; 1Q, '00, 18; N-D, '87, 4

88.48 Arteriography of femoral and other lower extremity arteries
AHA: 2Q, '06, 23; 3Q, '03, 10; 1Q, '03, 17; 2Q, '96, 6; 2Q, '89, 17

88.49 Arteriography of other specified sites
AHA: 2Q, '10, 8-9

√4ᵗʰ 88.5 Angiocardiography using contrast material
INCLUDES arterial puncture and insertion of arterial catheter for injection of contrast material
cineangiocardiography
selective angiocardiography
Code also synchronous cardiac catheterization (37.21-37.23)
EXCLUDES *angiography of pulmonary vessels (88.43, 88.62)*
DEF: Electromagnetic wave photography of heart and great vessels with contrast.
AHA: 3Q, '08, 18; 3Q, '92, 10; M-J, '87, 11

88.50 Angiocardiography, not otherwise specified

88.51 Angiocardiography of venae cavae
Inferior vena cavography
Phlebography of vena cava (inferior) (superior)

88.52 Angiocardiography of right heart structures
Angiocardiography of:
pulmonary valve
right atrium
right ventricle (outflow tract)
EXCLUDES *intra-operative fluorescence vascular angiography (88.59)*
that combined with left heart angiocardiography (88.54)
AHA: 1Q, '07, 16

88.53 Angiocardiography of left heart structures
Angiocardiography of:
aortic valve
left atrium
left ventricle (outflow tract)
EXCLUDES *intra-operative fluorescence vascular angiography (88.59)*
that combined with right heart angiocardiography (88.54)
AHA: 1Q, '07, 11, 17; 4Q, '05, 71; 3Q, '05, 14; 1Q, '00, 20; 4Q, '88, 4

88.54 Combined right and left heart angiocardiography
EXCLUDES *intra-operative fluorescence vascular angiography (88.59)*

88.55 Coronary arteriography using a single catheter
Coronary arteriography by Sones technique
Direct selective coronary arteriography using a single catheter
EXCLUDES *intra-operative fluorescence vascular angiography (88.59)*
AHA: 2Q, '06, 25-26; 3Q, '02, 20

88.56 Coronary arteriography using two catheters
Coronary arteriography by:
Judkins technique
Ricketts and Abrams technique
Direct selective coronary arteriography using two catheters
EXCLUDES *intra-operative fluorescence vascular angiography (88.59)*
AHA: 3Q, '06, 8; 1Q, '00, 20; 4Q, '88, 4

88.57   **Other and unspecified coronary arteriography**
Coronary arteriography NOS
EXCLUDES   *intra-operative fluorescence vascular angiography (88.59)*
AHA: 1Q, '07, 15; 2Q, '06, 25; 4Q, '05, 71; 3Q, '05, 14; 2Q, '05, 17; 1Q, '00, 21

88.58   **Negative-contrast cardiac roentgenography**
Cardiac roentgenography with injection of carbon dioxide

88.59   **Intra-operative coronary fluorescence vascular angiography**
Intraoperative laser arteriogram (SPY)
SPY arteriogram
SPY arteriography
DEF: Coronary artery bypass grafting (CABG) procedure imaging technology; utilizes dye with high-speed digital infrared photography. Sequence is performed for each graft; provides information on graft patency, vessel size, blood flow velocities.
AHA: 4Q, '10, 114-115; 4Q, '07, 121

√4ᵗʰ   **88.6**   **Phlebography**
NOTE   The fourth-digit subclassification (88.60-88.67) identifies the site to be viewed, not the site of injection.
INCLUDES   angiography of veins
radiography of veins (by fluoroscopy)
retrograde phlebography
venipuncture for injection of contrast material
venography using contrast material
EXCLUDES   *angiography using:*
radioisotopes or radionuclides (92.01-92.19)
ultrasound (88.71-88.79)
fluorescein angiography of eye (95.12)
DEF: Electromagnetic wave photography of veins with contrast.

88.60   **Phlebography using contrast material, unspecified site**

88.61   **Phlebography of veins of head and neck using contrast material**

88.62   **Phlebography of pulmonary veins using contrast material**

88.63   **Phlebography of other intrathoracic veins using contrast material**
AHA: 3Q, '08, 18

88.64   **Phlebography of the portal venous system using contrast material**
Splenoportogram (by splenic arteriography)

88.65   **Phlebography of other intra-abdominal veins using contrast material**

88.66   **Phlebography of femoral and other lower extremity veins using contrast material**
AHA: 2Q, '06, 23

88.67   **Phlebography of other specified sites using contrast material**

88.68   **Impedance phlebography**

√4ᵗʰ   **88.7**   **Diagnostic ultrasound**
INCLUDES   echography
non-invasive ultrasound
ultrasonic angiography
ultrasonography
EXCLUDES   *intravascular imaging (adjunctive) (IVUS) (00.21-00.29)*
that for intraoperative monitoring (00.94)
therapeutic ultrasound (00.01-00.09)
DEF: Graphic recording of anatomical structures via high frequency, sound-wave imaging and computer graphics.
AHA: ▶3Q, '12, 6◀

88.71   **Diagnostic ultrasound of head and neck**
Determination of midline shift of brain
Echoencephalography
EXCLUDES   *eye (95.13)*
AHA: 1Q, '02, 10; 1Q, '92, 11

88.72   **Diagnostic ultrasound of heart**
Echocardiography
Transesophageal echocardiography
EXCLUDES   *echocardiography of heart chambers (37.2...*
intracardiac echocardiography (ICE) (37.28...
intravascular (IVUS) imaging of coronary vessels (00.24)
AHA: 1Q, '07, 11; 3Q, '05, 14; 2Q, '05, 17; 4Q, '04, 121; 1Q, '0... 16; 1Q, '00, 20, 21; 1Q, '99, 6; 3Q, '98, 11
TIP: Assign also code 42.23 Esophagoscopy, NEC, when a transesophageal echocardiogram is performed.

88.73   **Diagnostic ultrasound of other sites of thorax**
Aortic arch
Breast ⎱ ultrasonography
Lung ⎰

88.74   **Diagnostic ultrasound of digestive system**

88.75   **Diagnostic ultrasound of urinary system**

88.76   **Diagnostic ultrasound of abdomen and retroperitoneum**
AHA: 2Q, '99, 14

88.77   **Diagnostic ultrasound of peripheral vascular system**
Deep vein thrombosis ultrasonic scanning
EXCLUDES   *adjunct vascular system procedures (00.40-00.43)*
AHA: 4Q, '99, 17; 1Q, '99, 12; 1Q, '92, 11

88.78   **Diagnostic ultrasound of gravid uterus**
Intrauterine cephalometry:
echo
ultrasonic
Placental localization by ultrasound
AHA: 2Q, '10, 6-7; 4Q, '08, 125

88.79   **Other diagnostic ultrasound**
Ultrasonography of:
multiple sites
nongravid uterus
total body

√4ᵗʰ   **88.8**   **Thermography**
DEF: Infrared photography to determine various body temperature...

88.81   **Cerebral thermography**

88.82   **Ocular thermography**

88.83   **Bone thermography**
Osteoarticular thermography

88.84   **Muscle thermography**

88.85   **Breast thermography**

88.86   **Blood vessel thermography**
Deep vein thermography

88.89   **Thermographay of other sites**
Lymph gland thermography
Thermography NOS

√4ᵗʰ   **88.9**   **Other diagnostic imaging**

88.90   **Diagnostic imaging, not elsewhere classified**
AHA: 2Q, '06, 25-26

88.91   **Magnetic resonance imaging of brain and brain stem**
EXCLUDES   *intraoperative magnetic resonance imagir... (88.96)*
laser interstitial thermal therapy [LITT] of lesion or tissue of brain under guidance (17.61)
real-time magnetic resonance imaging (88.96)

BI Bilateral Procedure   NC Non-covered Procedure   LC Limited Coverage Procedure   ▶◀ Revised Text   ● New Code   ▲ Revised Code Titl...

186 – Volume 3 • February 2013   **2014 ICD-9-...**

88.92   **Magnetic resonance imaging of chest and myocardium**
For evaluation of hilar and mediastinal lymphadenopathy
EXCLUDES *laser interstitial thermal therapy [LITT] of lesion or tissue of breast under guidance (17.69)*
laser interstitial thermal therapy [LITT] of lesion or tissue of lung under guidance (17.69)
AHA: 2Q, '10, 13

88.93   **Magnetic resonance imaging of spinal canal**
Spinal cord levels:
  cervical
  thoracic
  lumbar (lumbosacral)
Spinal cord
Spine

88.94   **Magnetic resonance imaging of musculoskeletal**
Bone marrow blood supply
Extremities (upper) (lower)

88.95   **Magnetic resonance imaging of pelvis, prostate, and bladder**
EXCLUDES *laser interstitial thermal therapy (LITT) of lesion or tissue of prostate under guidance (17.69)*

88.96   **Other intraoperative magnetic resonance imaging**
iMRI
Real-time magnetic resonance imaging
AHA: 4Q, '02, 111

88.97   **Magnetic resonance imaging of other and unspecified sites**
Abdomen
Eye orbit
Face
Neck
EXCLUDES *laser interstitial thermal therapy (LITT) of lesion or tissue of other and unspecified site under guidance (17.69)*

88.98   **Bone mineral density studies**
Dual photon absorptiometry
Quantitative computed tomography (CT) studies
Radiographic densitometry
Single photon absorptiometry
DEF: Dual photon absorptiometry: Measurement of bone mineral density by comparing dissipation of emission from two separate photoelectric energy peaks.
DEF: Quantitative computed tomography (CT) studies: Computer assisted analysis of x-ray absorption through bone to determine density.
DEF: Radiographic densiometry: Measurement of bone mineral density by degree of bone radiopacity.
DEF: Single photon absorptiometry: Measurement of bone mineral density by degree of dissipation of emission from one photoelectric energy peak emitted by gadolinium 153.

89   **Interview, evaluation, consultation, and examination**

89.0   **Diagnostic interview, consultation, and evaluation**
EXCLUDES *psychiatric diagnostic interview (94.11-94.19)*

89.01   **Interview and evaluation, described as brief**
Abbreviated history and evaluation

89.02   **Interview and evaluation, described as limited**
Interval history and evaluation

89.03   **Interview and evaluation, described as comprehensive**
History and evaluation of new problem

89.04   **Other interview and evaluation**

89.05   **Diagnostic interview and evaluation, not otherwise specified**

89.06   **Consultation, described as limited**
Consultation on a single organ system

89.07   **Consultation, described as comprehensive**

89.08   **Other consultation**

89.09   **Consulation, not otherwise specified**

89.1   **Anatomic and physiologic measurements and manual examinations — nervous system and sense organs**
EXCLUDES *ear examination (95.41-95.49)*
eye examination (95.01-95.26)
the listed procedures when done as part of a general physical examination (89.7)

89.10   **Intracarotid amobarbital test**
Wada test
DEF: Amobarbital injections into internal carotid artery to induce hemiparalysis to determine the hemisphere that controls speech and language.

89.11   **Tonometry**
DEF: Pressure measurements inside eye.

89.12   **Nasal function study**
Rhinomanometry
DEF: Rhinomanometry: Measure of degree of nasal cavity obstruction.

89.13   **Neurologic examination**

89.14   **Electroencephalogram**
EXCLUDES *that with polysomnogram (89.17)*
DEF: Recording of electrical currents in brain via electrodes to detect epilepsy, lesions and other encephalopathies.
AHA: 3Q, '05, 12

89.15   **Other nonoperative neurologic function tests**
AHA: 3Q, '95, 5; 2Q, '91, 14; J-F, '87, 16; N-D, '84, 6

89.16   **Transillumination of newborn skull**
DEF: Light passed through newborn skull for diagnostic purposes.

89.17   **Polysomnogram**
Sleep recording
DEF: Graphic studies of sleep patterns.

89.18   **Other sleep disorder function tests**
Multiple sleep latency test [MSLT]

89.19   **Video and radio-telemetered electroencephalographic monitoring**
Radiographic
Video   } EEG Monitoring
EXCLUDES *intraoperative monitoring (00.94)*
AHA: 1Q, '92, 17; 2Q, '90, 27

89.2   **Anatomic and physiologic measurements and manual examinations — genitourinary system**
EXCLUDES *the listed procedures when done as part of a general physical examination (89.7)*
AHA: 1Q, '90, 27

89.21   **Urinary manometry**
Manometry through:
  indwelling ureteral catheter
  nephrostomy
  pyelostomy
  ureterostomy
DEF: Measurement of urinary pressure by:
Indwelling urinary catheter: Semipermanent urinary catheter.
Nephrostomy: Opening into pelvis of kidney.
Pyelostomy: Opening in lower kidney.
Ureterostomy: Opening into ureter.

89.22   **Cystometrogram**
DEF: Pressure recordings at various stages of bladder filling.

89.23   **Urethral sphincter electromyogram**

89.24   **Uroflowmetry [UFR]**
DEF: Continuous recording of urine flow.

89.25   **Urethral pressure profile [UPP]**

89.26   **Gynecological examination**   ♀
Pelvic examination

89.29   **Other nonoperative genitourinary system measurements**
Bioassay of urine
Renal clearance
Urine chemistry
AHA: N-D, '84, 6

Miscellaneous Diagnostic and Therapeutic Procedures *(side tab)*

89.3–89.60 *(side tab)*

✓4ᵗʰ **89.3 Other anatomic and physiologic measurements and manual examinations**

> **EXCLUDES** *the listed procedures when done as part of a general physical examination (89.7)*

89.31 Dental examination
Oral mucosal survey
Periodontal survey

89.32 Esophageal manometry
DEF: Measurement of esophageal fluid and gas pressures.
AHA: 3Q, '96, 13

89.33 Digital examination of enterostomy stoma
Digital examination of colostomy stoma

89.34 Digital examination of rectum

89.35 Transillumination of nasal sinuses

89.36 Manual examination of breast

89.37 Vital capacity determination
> **EXCLUDES** *endoscopic pulmonary airway flow measurement (33.72)*

DEF: Measurement of expelled gas volume after full inhalation.

89.38 Other nonoperative respiratory measurements
Plethysmography for measurement of respiratory function
Thoracic impedance plethysmography
> **EXCLUDES** *endoscopic pulmonary airway flow measurement (33.72)*

DEF: Plethysmography for measurement of respiratory function: Registering changes in respiratory function as noted in blood circulation.
AHA: S-O, '87, 6

89.39 Other nonoperative measurements and examinations
¹⁴C-Urea breath test
Basal metabolic rate [BMR]
Gastric:
  analysis
  function NEC
> **EXCLUDES** *body measurement (93.07)*
> *cardiac tests (89.41-89.69)*
> *fundus photography (95.11)*
> *limb length measurement (93.06)*

AHA: 2Q, '01, 9; 3Q, '00, 9; 3Q, '96, 12; 1Q, '94, 18; N-D, '84, 6
TIP: Assign for Kinevac stimulation of the gallbladder, performed for analysis of function and examination of bile.

✓4ᵗʰ **89.4 Cardiac stress tests, pacemaker and defibrillator checks**

89.41 Cardiovascular stress test using treadmill
AHA: 1Q, '88, 11

89.42 Masters' two-step stress test
AHA: 1Q, '88, 11

89.43 Cardiovascular stress test using bicycle ergometer
DEF: Electrocardiogram during exercise on bicycle with device capable of measuring muscular, metabolic and respiratory effects of exercise.
AHA: 1Q, '88, 11

89.44 Other cardiovascular stress test
Thallium stress test with or without transesophageal pacing

89.45 Artificial pacemaker rate check
Artificial pacemaker function check NOS
Bedside device check of pacemaker or cardiac resynchronization pacemaker [CRT-P]
Interrogation only without arrhythmia induction
> **EXCLUDES** *catheter based invasive electrophysiologic testing (37.26)*
> *non-invasive programmed electrical stimulation [NIPS] (arrhythmia induction) (37.20)*

AHA: 3Q, '10, 9; 1Q, '02, 3

89.46 Artificial pacemaker artifact wave form check

89.47 Artificial pacemaker electrode impedance check

89.48 Artificial pacemaker voltage or amperage threshold check

89.49 Automatic implantable cardioverter/ defibrillator (AICD) check
Bedside check of an AICD or cardiac resynchronization defibrillator [CRT-D]
Checking pacing thresholds of device
Interrogation only without arrhythmia induction
> **EXCLUDES** *catheter based invasive electrophysiologic testing (37.26)*
> *non-invasive programmed electrical stimulation [NIPS] (arrhythmia induction) (37.20)*

AHA: 4Q, '04, 136

✓4ᵗʰ **89.5 Other nonoperative cardiac and vascular diagnostic procedures**
> **EXCLUDES** *fetal EKG (75.32)*

89.50 Ambulatory cardiac monitoring
Analog devices [Holter-type]
AHA: 4Q, '99, 21; 4Q, '91, 23

89.51 Rhythm electrocardiogram
Rhythm EKG (with one to three leads)

89.52 Electrocardiogram
ECG NOS
EKG (with 12 or more leads)
AHA: 1Q, '88, 11; S-O, '87, 6

89.53 Vectorcardiogram (with ECG)

89.54 Electrographic monitoring
Telemetry
> **EXCLUDES** *ambulatory cardiac monitoring (89.50)*
> *electrographic monitoring during surgery — omit code*

DEF: Evaluation of heart electrical activity by continuous screen monitoring.
DEF: Telemetry: Evaluation of heart electrical activity; with radio signals at distance from patient.
AHA: 4Q, '91, 23; 1Q, '88, 11

89.55 Phonocardiogram with ECG lead

89.56 Carotid pulse tracing with ECG lead
> **EXCLUDES** *oculoplethysmography (89.58)*

89.57 Apexcardiogram (with ECG lead)
AHA: J-F, '87, 16

89.58 Plethysmogram
Penile plethysmography with nerve stimulation
> **EXCLUDES** *plethysmography (for):*
> *measurement of respiratory function (89.38)*
> *thoracic impedance (89.38)*

DEF: Determination and recording of blood pressure variations present or passing through an organ.
AHA: S-O, '87, 7

89.59 Other nonoperative cardiac and vascular measurements
AHA: 2Q, '10, 11; 3Q, '05, 21; 3Q, '03, 23; 2Q, '92, 12

✓4ᵗʰ **89.6 Circulatory monitoring**
> **EXCLUDES** *electrocardiographic monitoring during surgery — omit code*
> *implantation or replacement of subcutaneous device for intracardiac hemodynamic monitoring (00.57)*
> *insertion or replacement of implantable pressure sensor (lead) for intracardiac hemodynamic monitoring (00.56)*

AHA: M-J, '87, 11

89.60 Continuous intra-arterial blood gas monitoring
Insertion of blood gas monitoring system and continuous monitoring of blood gases through an intra-arterial sensor
AHA: 4Q, '02, 111

BI Bilateral Procedure   NC Non-covered Procedure   LC Limited Coverage Procedure   ►◄ Revised Text   ● New Code   ▲ Revised Code Title

188 – Volume 3   2014 ICD-9-CM

Central Venous Pressure Monitoring

Subclavian vein

Pressure monitor above right atrium

89.61 Systemic arterial pressure monitoring
 EXCLUDES *intra-aneurysm sac pressure monitoring (intraoperative) (00.58)*
 intravascular pressure measurement of intrathoracic arteries (00.67)
 intravascular pressure measurement of peripheral arteries (00.68)

89.62 Central venous pressure monitoring
 EXCLUDES *intravascular pressure measurement, other specified and unspecified vessels (00.69)*

89.63 Pulmonary artery pressure monitoring
 EXCLUDES *pulmonary artery wedge monitoring (89.64)*

89.64 Pulmonary artery wedge monitoring
 Pulmonary capillary wedge [PCW] monitoring
 Swan-Ganz catheterization
 DEF: Monitoring pulmonary artery pressure via catheter inserted through right lower and upper heart chambers into pulmonary artery and advancing the balloon-tip to wedge it in the distal pulmonary artery branch.

89.65 Measurement of systemic arterial blood gases
 EXCLUDES *continuous intra-arterial blood gas monitoring (89.60)*

89.66 Measurement of mixed venous blood gases

89.67 Monitoring of cardiac output by oxygen consumption technique
 Fick method
 DEF: Fick method: Indirect measure of cardiac output through blood volume flow over pulmonary capillaries; determines oxygen absorption by measurement of arterial oxygen content versus venous oxygen content.

89.68 Monitoring of cardiac output by other technique
 Cardiac output monitor by thermodilution indicator
 DEF: Cardiac output monitor by thermodilution indicator: Injection of ice cold dextrose solution into right lower heart chamber; temperature sensitive catheter monitors disappearance from beat to beat to measure expelled blood volume.

89.69 Monitoring of coronary blood flow
 Coronary blood flow monitoring by coincidence counting technique
 EXCLUDES *intravascular pressure measurement of coronary arteries (00.59)*

89.7 General physical examination

89.8 Autopsy

√3ʳᵈ **90 Microscopic examination - I**
 The following fourth-digit subclassification is for use with categories in section 90 to identify type of examination:
 1 bacterial smear
 2 culture
 3 culture and sensitivity
 4 parasitology
 5 toxicology
 6 cell block and Papanicolaou smear
 9 other microscopic examination

§ √4ᵗʰ **90.0 Microscopic examination of specimen from nervous**
 [1-6,9] **system and of spinal fluid**

§ √4ᵗʰ **90.1 Microscopic examination of specimen from endocrine**
 [1-6,9] **gland, not elsewhere classified**

§ √4ᵗʰ **90.2 Microscopic examination of specimen from eye**
 [1-6,9]

§ √4ᵗʰ **90.3 Microscopic examination of specimen from ear, nose,**
 [1-6,9] **throat, and larynx**

§ √4ᵗʰ **90.4 Microscopic examination of specimen from trachea,**
 [1-6,9] **bronchus, pleura, lung, and other thoracic specimen, and of sputum**

§ √4ᵗʰ **90.5 Microscopic examination of blood**
 [1-6,9]

§ √4ᵗʰ **90.6 Microscopic examination of specimen from spleen and of**
 [1-6,9] **bone marrow**

§ √4ᵗʰ **90.7 Microscopic examination of specimen from lymph node**
 [1-6,9] **and of lymph**

§ √4ᵗʰ **90.8 Microscopic examination of specimen from upper**
 [1-6,9] **gastrointestinal tract and of vomitus**

§ √4ᵗʰ **90.9 Microscopic examination of specimen from lower**
 [1-6,9] **gastrointestinal tract and of stool**

√3ʳᵈ **91 Microscopic examination - II**
 The following fourth-digit subclassification is for use with categories in section 91 to identify type of examination:
 1 bacterial smear
 2 culture
 3 culture and sensitivity
 4 parasitology
 5 toxicology
 6 cell block and Papanicolaou smear
 9 other microscopic examination

§ √4ᵗʰ **91.0 Microscopic examination of specimen from liver, biliary**
 [1-6,9] **tract, and pancreas**

§ √4ᵗʰ **91.1 Microscopic examination of peritoneal and retroperitoneal**
 [1-6,9] **specimen**

§ √4ᵗʰ **91.2 Microscopic examination of specimen from kidney,**
 [1-6,9] **ureter, perirenal and periureteral tissue**

§ √4ᵗʰ **91.3 Microscopic examination of specimen from bladder,**
 [1-6,9] **urethra, prostate, seminal vesicle, perivesical tissue, and of urine and semen**

§ √4ᵗʰ **91.4 Microscopic examination of specimen from female** ♀
 [1-6,9] **genital tract**
 Amnionic sac
 Fetus

§ √4ᵗʰ **91.5 Microscopic examination of specimen from**
 [1-6,9] **musculoskeletal system and of joint fluid**
 Microscopic examination of:
 bone
 bursa
 cartilage
 fascia
 ligament
 muscle
 synovial membrane
 tendon

Requires fourth digit. Valid digits are in [brackets] under each code. See appropriate category for codes and definitions.

Miscellaneous Diagnostic and Therapeutic Procedures

91.6–92.41

§ ✓4ᵗʰ **91.6** **Microscopic examination of specimen from skin and**
[1-6,9] **other integument**
     Microscopic examination of:
       hair
       nails
       skin
     EXCLUDES   *mucous membrane — code to organ site*
            that of operative wound (91.71-91.79)

§ ✓4ᵗʰ **91.7** **Microscopic examination of specimen from operative**
[1-6,9] **wound**

§ ✓4ᵗʰ **91.8** **Microscopic examination of specimen from other site**
[1-6,9]

§ ✓4ᵗʰ **91.9** **Microscopic examination of specimen from unspecified**
[1-6,9] **site**

✓3ʳᵈ **92** **Nuclear medicine**

✓4ᵗʰ **92.0** **Radioisotope scan and function study**

     92.01 **Thyroid scan and radioisotope function studies**
       Iodine-131 uptake
       Protein-bound iodine
       Radio-iodine uptake

     92.02 **Liver scan and radioisotope function study**

     92.03 **Renal scan and radioisotope function study**
       Renal clearance study

     92.04 **Gastrointestinal scan and radioisotope function**
       study
       Radio-cobalt B_{12} Schilling test
       Radio-iodinated triolein study

     92.05 **Cardiovascular and hematopoietic scan and**
       radioisotope function study
       Bone marrow
       Cardiac output
       Circulation time   scan or function
       Radionuclide cardiac   study
         ventriculogram
       Spleen
       AHA: 2Q, '92, 7; 1Q, '88, 11

     92.09 **Other radioisotope function studies**

✓4ᵗʰ **92.1** **Other radioisotope scan**

     92.11 **Cerebral scan**
       Pituitary

     92.12 **Scan of other sites of head**
       EXCLUDES   *eye (95.16)*

     92.13 **Parathyroid scan**

     92.14 **Bone scan**

     92.15 **Pulmonary scan**

     92.16 **Scan of lymphatic system**

     92.17 **Placental scan**   ♀

     92.18 **Total body scan**

     92.19 **Scan of other sites**

✓4ᵗʰ **92.2** **Therapeutic radiology and nuclear medicine**
     EXCLUDES   *that for:*
            ablation of pituitary gland (07.64-07.69)
            destruction of chorioretinal lesion (14.26-14.27)
     DEF: Radiation and nuclear isotope treatment of diseased tissue.
     AHA: 3Q, '92, 5

     92.20 **Infusion of liquid brachytherapy radioisotope**
       I-125 radioisotope
       Intracavitary brachytherapy
       EXCLUDES   *removal of radioisotope*
       AHA: 4Q, '05, 117-118
       TIP: Refer to codes 01.26 and 01.27 for placement or
       removal of balloon catheter used for liquid brachytherapy
       radioisotope infusion.

     92.21 **Superficial radiation**
       Contact radiation [up to 150 KVP]

     92.22 **Orthovoltage radiation**
       Deep radiation [200-300 KVP]

     92.23 **Radioisotopic teleradiotherapy**
       Teleradiotherapy using:
         cobalt-60
         iodine-125
         radioactive cesium

     92.24 **Teleradiotherapy using photons**
       Megavoltage NOS
       Supervoltage NOS
       Use of:
         Betatron
         linear accelerator

     92.25 **Teleradiotherapy using electrons**
       Beta particles
       EXCLUDES   *intra-operative electron radiation therapy*
            (92.41)

     92.26 **Teleradiotherapy of other particulate radiation**
       Neutrons
       Protons NOS

     92.27 **Implantation or insertion of radioactive elements**
       Intravascular brachytherapy
       Code also incision of site
       EXCLUDES   *infusion of liquid brachytherapy radioisotop*
            (92.20)
       AHA: 1Q, '04, 3-4; 1Q, '00, 11, 12; 3Q, '94, 11; 1Q, '88, 4

     92.28 **Injection or instillation of radioisotopes**
       Injection or infusion of radioimmunoconjugate
       Intracavitary injection or instillation
       Intravenous injection or instillation
       Iodine-131 [I-131] tositumomab
       Radioimmunotherapy
       Ytrium-90 [Y-90] ibritumomab tiuxetan
       EXCLUDES   *infusion of liquid brachytherapy radioisotop*
            (92.20)

     92.29 **Other radiotherapeutic procedure**
       AHA: 3Q, '06, 14-15

✓4ᵗʰ **92.3** **Stereotactic radiosurgery**
     Code also stereotactic head frame application (93.59)
     EXCLUDES   *stereotactic biopsy*
     DEF: Ablation of deep intracranial lesions; single procedure;
     placement of head frame for 3-D analysis of lesion, followed by
     radiation treatment from helmet attached to frame.
     AHA: 4Q, '98, 79; 4Q, '95, 70
     TIP: Do not assign when stereotactic technique is used to obtain th
     coordinates for the exact location of a brain tumor, after which ope
     craniotomy is performed. See instead subcategory 01.5.

     92.30 **Stereotactic radiosurgery, not otherwise**
       specified

     92.31 **Single source photon radiosurgery**
       High energy x-rays
       Linear accelerator (LINAC)

     92.32 **Multi-source photon radiosurgery**
       Cobalt 60 radiation
       Gamma irradiation
       AHA: 4Q, '04, 113

     92.33 **Particulate radiosurgery**
       Particle beam radiation (cyclotron)
       Proton accelerator

     92.39 **Stereotactic radiosurgery, not elsewhere**
       classified

✓4ᵗʰ **92.4** **Intra-operative radiation procedures**

     92.41 **Intra-operative electron radiation therapy**
       IOERT
       That using a mobile linear accelerator
       DEF: Use of a mobile linear accelerator unit that delivers
       precision electron radiation beam radiation to highly
       focused anatomic sites, protecting the normal surroundir
       tissues from exposure.
       AHA: 4Q, '07, 122

---

§   Requires fourth digit. Valid digits are in [brackets] under each code. See category 91 for codes and definitions.

BI Bilateral Procedure   **NC** Non-covered Procedure   **LC** Limited Coverage Procedure   ►◄ Revised Text   ● New Code   ▲ Revised Code Tit

190 – Volume 3   **2014 ICD-9-**

✓3ʳᵈ **93** **Physical therapy, respiratory therapy, rehabilitation, and related procedures**

✓4ᵗʰ **93.0** **Diagnostic physical therapy**
        AHA: N-D, '86, 7

    93.01 **Functional evaluation**

    93.02 **Orthotic evaluation**

    93.03 **Prosthetic evaluation**

    93.04 **Manual testing of muscle function**
        AHA: J-F, '87, 16

    93.05 **Range of motion testing**
        AHA: J-F, '87, 16

    93.06 **Measurement of limb length**

    93.07 **Body measurement**
        Girth measurement
        Measurement of skull circumference

    93.08 **Electromyography**
        EXCLUDES *eye EMG (95.25)*
                that for intraoperative monitoring (00.94)
                that with polysomnogram (89.17)
                urethral sphincter EMG (89.23)
        DEF: Graphic recording of electrical activity of muscle.
        AHA: J-F, '87, 16

    93.09 **Other diagnostic physical therapy procedure**

✓4ᵗʰ **93.1** **Physical therapy exercises**
        AHA: J-F, '87, 16; N-D, '86, 7

    93.11 **Assisting exercise**
        EXCLUDES *assisted exercise in pool (93.31)*

    93.12 **Other active musculoskeletal exercise**

    93.13 **Resistive exercise**

    93.14 **Training in joint movements**

    93.15 **Mobilization of spine**

    93.16 **Mobilization of other joints**
        EXCLUDES *manipulation of temporomandibular joint (76.95)*

    93.17 **Other passive musculoskeletal exercise**

    93.18 **Breathing exercise**

    93.19 **Exercise, not elsewhere classified**

✓4ᵗʰ **93.2** **Other physical therapy musculoskeletal manipulation**
        AHA: N-D, '86, 7

    93.21 **Manual and mechanical traction**
        EXCLUDES *skeletal traction (93.43-93.44)*
                skin traction (93.45-93.46)
                spinal traction (93.41-93.42)

    93.22 **Ambulation and gait training**

    93.23 **Fitting of orthotic device**

    93.24 **Training in use of prosthetic or orthotic device**
        Training in crutch walking

    93.25 **Forced extension of limb**

    93.26 **Manual rupture of joint adhesions**
        DEF: Therapeutic application of force to rupture adhesions restricting movement.

    93.27 **Stretching of muscle or tendon**

    93.28 **Stretching of fascia**

    93.29 **Other forcible correction of deformity**
        AHA: N-D, '85, 11

✓4ᵗʰ **93.3** **Other physical therapy therapeutic procedures**

    93.31 **Assisted exercise in pool**

    93.32 **Whirlpool treatment**

    93.33 **Other hydrotherapy**

    93.34 **Diathermy**

    93.35 **Other heat therapy**
        Acupuncture with smouldering moxa
        Hot packs
        Hyperthermia NEC
        Infrared irradiation
        Moxibustion
        Paraffin bath
        EXCLUDES *hyperthermia for treatment of cancer (99.85)*
        DEF: Moxibustion: Igniting moxa, a Chinese plant, for counterirritation of skin.
        DEF: Paraffin bath: Hot wax treatment.

    93.36 **Cardiac retraining**
        DEF: Cardiac rehabilitation regimen following myocardial infarction or coronary bypass graft procedure.

    93.37 **Prenatal training**
        Training for natural childbirth

    93.38 **Combined physical therapy without mention of the components**

    93.39 **Other physical therapy**
        AHA: 2Q, '05, 6; 4Q, '03, 105 -106, 108-110; 3Q, '97, 12; 3Q, '91, 15

✓4ᵗʰ **93.4** **Skeletal traction and other traction**

    93.41 **Spinal traction using skull device**
        Traction using:
          caliper tongs
          Crutchfield tongs
          halo device
          Vinke tongs
        EXCLUDES *insertion of tongs or halo traction device (02.94)*
        DEF: Applying device to head to exert pulling force on spine.
        AHA: 3Q, '01, 8; 3Q, '96, 14; 2Q, '94, 3

    93.42 **Other spinal traction**
        Cotrel's traction
        EXCLUDES *cervical collar (93.52)*
        DEF: Pulling force exerted on spine without skull device.

    93.43 **Intermittent skeletal traction**

    93.44 **Other skeletal traction**
        Bryant's
        Dunlop's   } traction
        Lyman Smith
        Russell's

    93.45 **Thomas' splint traction**
        DEF: Thomas splint: Placement of ring around thigh, attached to rods running length of leg for therapeutic purposes.

    93.46 **Other skin traction of limbs**
        Adhesive tape traction
        Boot traction
        Buck's traction
        Gallows traction

✓4ᵗʰ **93.5** **Other immobilization, pressure, and attention to wound**
        EXCLUDES *external fixator device (84.71-84.73)*
                 wound cleansing (96.58-96.59)

    93.51 **Application of plaster jacket**
        EXCLUDES *Minerva jacket (93.52)*

    93.52 **Application of neck support**
        Application of:
          cervical collar
          Minerva jacket
          molded neck support

    93.53 **Application of other cast**

    93.54 **Application of splint**
        Plaster splint
        Tray splint
        EXCLUDES *periodontal splint (24.7)*

    93.55 **Dental wiring**
        EXCLUDES *that for orthodontia (24.7)*

93.56 **Application of pressure dressing**
Application of:
Gibney bandage
Robert Jones' bandage
Shanz dressing

93.57 **Application of other wound dressing**
Porcine wound dressing
AHA: ▶3Q, '12, 15;◀ 3Q, '02, 23
TIP: ▶Assign for MatriStem (extracellular matrix wound powder) when applied to damaged or amputated skin to facilitate tissue regeneration and promote wound healing.◀

93.58 **Application of pressure trousers**
Application of:
anti-shock trousers
MAST trousers
vasopneumatic device
AHA: 3Q, '96, 13

93.59 **Other immobilization, pressure, and attention to wound**
Elastic stockings
Electronic gaiter
Intermittent pressure device
Oxygenation of wound (hyperbaric)
Stereotactic head frame application
Strapping (non-traction)
Velpeau dressing
AHA: 3Q, '99, 7; 1Q, '99, 12, 13; 1Q, '91, 11; 1Q, '89, 12

☑4ᵗʰ **93.6** **Osteopathic manipulative treatment**

93.61 **Osteopathic manipulative treatment for general mobilization**
General articulatory treatment

93.62 **Osteopathic manipulative treatment using high-velocity, low-amplitude forces**
Thrusting forces

93.63 **Osteopathic manipulative treatment using low-velocity, high-amplitude forces**
Springing forces

93.64 **Osteopathic manipulative treatment using isotonic, isometric forces**

93.65 **Osteopathic manipulative treatment using indirect forces**

93.66 **Osteopathic manipulative treatment to move tissue fluids**
Lymphatic pump

93.67 **Other specified osteopathic manipulative treatment**

☑4ᵗʰ **93.7** **Speech and reading rehabilitation and rehabilitation of the blind**

93.71 **Dyslexia training**

93.72 **Dysphasia training**
DEF: Speech training to coordinate and arrange words in proper sequence.

93.73 **Esophageal speech training**
DEF: Speech training after voice box removal; sound is produced by vibration of air column in esophagus against the cricopharangeal sphincter.

93.74 **Speech defect training**

93.75 **Other speech training and therapy**
AHA: 4Q, '03, 105, 109; 4Q, '97, 36; 3Q, '97, 12

93.76 **Training in use of lead dog for the blind**

93.77 **Training in braille or Moon**

93.78 **Other rehabilitation for the blind**

☑4ᵗʰ **93.8** **Other rehabilitation therapy**

93.81 **Recreational therapy**
Diversional therapy
Play therapy
EXCLUDES *play psychotherapy (94.36)*

93.82 **Educational therapy**
Education of bed-bound children
Special schooling for the handicapped

93.83 **Occupational therapy**
Daily living activities therapy
EXCLUDES *training in activities of daily living for the blind (93.78)*
AHA: 2Q, '05, 6; 4Q, '03, 105-106, 108, 110; 3Q, '97, 12

93.84 **Music therapy**

93.85 **Vocational rehabilitation**
Sheltered employment
Vocational:
assessment
retraining
training

93.89 **Rehabilitation, not elsewhere classified**
AHA: 2Q, '05, 6

☑4ᵗʰ **93.9** **Respiratory therapy**
EXCLUDES *insertion of airway (96.01-96.05)*
other continuous invasive (through endotracheal tube or tracheostomy) mechanical ventilation (96.70-96.72)

93.90 **Non-invasive mechanical ventilation**
NOTE Patients admitted on *non-invasive* mechanical ventilation that subsequently require *invasive* mechanical ventilation; code both types of mechanical ventilation
Bi-level airway pressure
BiPAP without (delivery through) endotracheal tube or tracheostomy
CPAP without (delivery through) endotracheal tube or tracheostomy
Mechanical ventilation NOS
Non-invasive positive pressure (NIPPV)
Non-invasive PPV
NPPV
That delivered by non-invasive interface:
face mask
nasal mask
nasal pillow
oral mouthpiece
oronasal mask
EXCLUDES *invasive (through endotracheal tube or tracheostomy) continuous mechanical ventilation (96.70-96.72)*
DEF: Noninvasive ventilation support system that augments the ability to breathe spontaneously without the insertion of an endotracheal tube or tracheostomy.
AHA: 4Q, '08, 187-189; 1Q, '08, 8-9; 3Q, '04, 3; 1Q, '02, 12, 13; 3Q, '98, 14; 4Q, '91, 21

93.91 **Intermittent positive pressure breathing [IPPB]**
AHA: 4Q, '91, 21

93.93 **Nonmechanical methods of resuscitation**
Artificial respiration
Manual resuscitation
Mouth-to-mouth resuscitition
AHA: 2Q, '03, 17

93.94 **Respiratory medication administered by nebulizer**
Mist therapy

93.95 **Hyperbaric oxygenation**
EXCLUDES *oxygenation of wound (93.59)*

93.96 **Other oxygen enrichment**
Catalytic oxygen therapy
Cytoreductive effect
Oxygenators
Oxygen therapy
EXCLUDES *oxygenation of wound (93.59)*
SuperSaturated oxygen therapy (00.49)

93.97 **Decompression chamber**

93.98 **Other control of atmospheric pressure and composition**
Antigen-free air conditioning
Helium therapy
EXCLUDES *inhaled nitric oxide therapy (INO) (00.12)*
AHA: 1Q, '02, 14

BI Bilateral Procedure   **NC** Non-covered Procedure   **LC** Limited Coverage Procedure   ▶◀ Revised Text   ● New Code   ▲ Revised Code Title

192 – Volume 3 • February 2013   **2014 ICD-9-CM**

93.99 Other respiratory procedures
Continuous negative pressure ventilation [CNP]
Postural drainage
AHA: 4Q, '03, 108; 3Q, '99, 11; 4Q, '91, 22

94 Procedures related to the psyche

94.0 Psychologic evaluation and testing

94.01 Administration of intelligence test
Administration of:
Stanford-Binet
Wechsler Adult Intelligence Scale
Wechsler Intelligence Scale for Children

94.02 Administration of psychologic test
Administration of:
Bender Visual-Motor Gestalt Test
Benton Visual Retention Test
Minnesota Multiphasic Personality Inventory
Wechsler Memory Scale

94.03 Character analysis

94.08 Other psychologic evaluation and testing

94.09 Psychologic mental status determination, not otherwise specified

94.1 Psychiatric interviews, consultations, and evaluations

94.11 Psychiatric mental status determination
Clinical psychiatric mental status determination
Evaluation for criminal responsibility
Evaluation for testamentary capacity
Medicolegal mental status determination
Mental status determination NOS

94.12 Routine psychiatric visit, not otherwise specified

94.13 Psychiatric commitment evaluation
Pre-commitment interview

94.19 Other psychiatric interview and evaluation
Follow-up psychiatric interview NOS

94.2 Psychiatric somatotherapy
DEF: Biological treatment of mental disorders.

94.21 Narcoanalysis
Narcosynthesis

94.22 Lithium therapy

94.23 Neuroleptic therapy

94.24 Chemical shock therapy

94.25 Other psychiatric drug therapy
AHA: S-O, '86, 4

94.26 Subconvulsive electroshock therapy

94.27 Other electroshock therapy
Electroconvulsive therapy (ECT)
EST

94.29 Other psychiatric somatotherapy

94.3 Individual psychotherapy

94.31 Psychoanalysis

94.32 Hypnotherapy
Hypnodrome
Hypnosis

94.33 Behavior therapy
Aversion therapy
Behavior modification
Desensitization therapy
Extinction therapy
Relaxation training
Token economy

94.34 Individual therapy for psychosexual dysfunction
EXCLUDES that performed in group setting (94.41)

94.35 Crisis intervention

94.36 Play psychotherapy

94.37 Exploratory verbal psychotherapy

94.38 Supportive verbal psychotherapy

94.39 Other individual psychotherapy
Biofeedback

94.4 Other psychotherapy and counseling

94.41 Group therapy for psychosexual dysfunction

94.42 Family therapy

94.43 Psychodrama

94.44 Other group therapy

94.45 Drug addiction counseling

94.46 Alcoholism counseling

94.49 Other counseling

94.5 Referral for psychologic rehabilitation

94.51 Referral for psychotherapy

94.52 Referral for psychiatric aftercare
That in:
halfway house
outpatient (clinic) facility

94.53 Referral for alcoholism rehabilitation

94.54 Referral for drug addiction rehabilitation

94.55 Referral for vocational rehabilitation

94.59 Referral for other psychologic rehabilitation

94.6 Alcohol and drug rehabilitation and detoxification
AHA: 2Q, '91, 12

94.61 Alcohol rehabilitation
DEF: Program designed to restore social and physical functioning, free of the dependence of alcohol.

94.62 Alcohol detoxification
DEF: Treatment of physical symptoms during withdrawal from alcohol dependence.

94.63 Alcohol rehabilitation and detoxification

94.64 Drug rehabilitation
DEF: Program designed to restore social and physical functioning, free of the dependence of drugs.

94.65 Drug detoxification
DEF: Treatment of physical symptoms during withdrawal from drug dependence.

94.66 Drug rehabilitation and detoxification

94.67 Combined alcohol and drug rehabilitation

94.68 Combined alcohol and drug detoxification

94.69 Combined alcohol and drug rehabilitation and detoxification

95 Ophthalmologic and otologic diagnosis and treatment

95.0 General and subjective eye examination

95.01 Limited eye examination
Eye examination with prescription of spectacles

95.02 Comprehensive eye examination
Eye examination covering all aspects of the visual system

95.03 Extended ophthalmologic work-up
Examination (for):
glaucoma
neuro-ophthalmology
retinal disease

95.04 Eye examination under anesthesia
Code also type of examination

95.05 Visual field study

95.06 Color vision study

95.07 Dark adaptation study
DEF: Exam of eye's adaption to dark.

95.09 Eye examination, not otherwise specified
Vision check NOS

Miscellaneous Diagnostic and Therapeutic Procedures

95.1–96.25

✓4th **95.1 Examinations of form and structure of eye**

     95.11 Fundus photography

     95.12 Fluorescein angiography or angioscopy of eye

     95.13 Ultrasound study of eye

     95.14 X-ray study of eye

     95.15 Ocular motility study

     95.16 P$_{32}$ and other tracer studies of eye

✓4th **95.2 Objective functional tests of eye**
     EXCLUDES *that with polysomnogram (89.17)*

     95.21 Electroretinogram [ERG]

     95.22 Electro-oculogram [EOG]

     95.23 Visual evoked potential [VEP]
         DEF: Measuring and recording evoked visual responses of body and senses.

     95.24 Electronystagmogram [ENG]
         DEF: Monitoring of brain waves to record induced and spontaneous eye movements.

     95.25 Electromyogram of eye [EMG]

     95.26 Tonography, provocative tests, and other glaucoma testing

✓4th **95.3 Special vision services**

     95.31 Fitting and dispensing of spectacles

     95.32 Prescription, fitting, and dispensing of contact lens

     95.33 Dispensing of other low vision aids

     95.34 Ocular prosthetics

     95.35 Orthoptic training

     95.36 Ophthalmologic counselling and instruction
         Counselling in:
           adaptation to visual loss
           use of low vision aids

✓4th **95.4 Nonoperative procedures related to hearing**

     95.41 Audiometry
         Békésy 5-tone audiometry
         Impedance audiometry
         Stapedial reflex response
         Tympanogram
         Subjective audiometry

     95.42 Clinical test of hearing
         Tuning fork test
         Whispered speech test

     95.43 Audiological evaluation
         Audiological evaluation by:
           Bárány noise machine
           blindfold test
           delayed feedback
           masking
           Weber lateralization

     95.44 Clinical vestibular function tests
         Thermal test of vestibular function

     95.45 Rotation tests
         Bárány chair
         DEF: Irrigation of ear canal with warm or cold water to evaluate vestibular function.

     95.46 Other auditory and vestibular function tests

     95.47 Hearing examination, not otherwise specified

     95.48 Fitting of hearing aid
         EXCLUDES *implantation of electromagnetic hearing device (20.95)*
         AHA: 4Q, '89, 5

     95.49 Other nonoperative procedures related to hearing
         Adjustment (external components) of cochlear prosthetic device

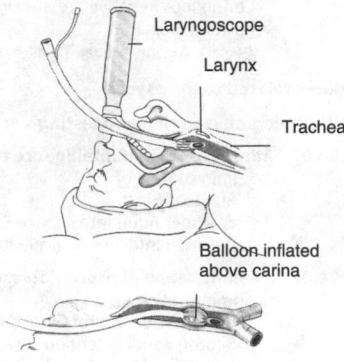

Endotracheal Intubation

Laryngoscope

Larynx

Trachea

Balloon inflated above carina

✓3rd **96 Nonoperative intubation and irrigation**

✓4th **96.0 Nonoperative intubation of gastrointestinal and respiratory tracts**

     96.01 Insertion of nasopharyngeal airway

     96.02 Insertion of oropharyngeal airway

     96.03 Insertion of esophageal obturator airway

     96.04 Insertion of endotracheal tube
         AHA: 4Q, '10, 80; 2Q, '09, 11; 1Q, '07, 11; 2Q, '06, 8; 4Q, '05, 88; 3Q, '05, 10; 2Q, '05, 19

     96.05 Other intubation of respiratory tract
         EXCLUDES *endoscopic insertion or replacement of bronchial device or substance (33.71, 33.79)*
         AHA: 1Q, '97, 14

     96.06 Insertion of Sengstaken tube
         Esophageal tamponade
         DEF: Insertion of Sengstaken tube: Nonsurgical emergency measure to stop esophageal bleeding using compression exerted by inflated balloons; additional tube ports to aspirate blood and clots.

     96.07 Insertion of other (naso-) gastric tube
         Intubation for decompression
         EXCLUDES *that for enteral infusion of nutritional substance (96.6)*
         AHA: 4Q, '08, 139

     96.08 Insertion of (naso-) intestinal tube
         Miller-Abbott tube (for decompression)
         AHA: ▶3Q, '12, 23◀

     96.09 Insertion of rectal tube
         Replacement of rectal tube

✓4th **96.1 Other nonoperative insertion**
     EXCLUDES *nasolacrimal intubation (09.44)*

     96.11 Packing of external auditory canal

     96.14 Vaginal packing

     96.15 Insertion of vaginal mold

     96.16 Other vaginal dilation

     96.17 Insertion of vaginal diaphragm

     96.18 Insertion of other vaginal pessary

     96.19 Rectal packing

✓4th **96.2 Nonoperative dilation and manipulation**

     96.21 Dilation of frontonasal duct

     96.22 Dilation of rectum

     96.23 Dilation of anal sphincter

     96.24 Dilation and manipulation of enterostomy stoma

     96.25 Therapeutic distention of bladder
         Intermittent distention of bladder

BI Bilateral Procedure   **NC** Non-covered Procedure   **LC** Limited Coverage Procedure   ▶◀ Revised Text   ● New Code   ▲ Revised Code Title

194 – Volume 3 • February 2013   **2014 ICD-9-CM**

96.26 Manual reduction of rectal prolapse

96.27 Manual reduction of hernia

96.28 Manual reduction of enterostomy prolapse
AHA: N-D, '87, 11

96.29 Reduction of intussusception of alimentary tract
With:
  fluoroscopy
  ionizing radiation enema
  ultrasonography guidance
Hydrostatic reduction
Pneumatic reduction
EXCLUDES   *intra-abdominal manipulation of intestine,*
             not otherwise specified (46.80)
AHA: 4Q, '98, 82

☑4ᵗʰ 96.3 Nonoperative alimentary tract irrigation, cleaning, and local instillation

96.31 Gastric cooling
Gastric hypothermia
DEF: Reduction of internal stomach temperature.

96.32 Gastric freezing

96.33 Gastric lavage

96.34 Other irrigation of (naso-)gastric tube

96.35 Gastric gavage
DEF: Food forced into stomach.

96.36 Irrigation of gastrostomy or enterostomy

96.37 Proctoclysis
DEF: Slow introduction of large amounts of fluids into lower large intestine.

96.38 Removal of impacted feces
Removal of impaction:
  by flushing manually

96.39 Other transanal enema
Rectal irrigation
EXCLUDES   *reduction of intussusception of alimentary*
             tract by ionizing radiation enema
             (96.29)
AHA: ▶3Q, '12, 23◀

☑4ᵗʰ 96.4 Nonoperative irrigation, cleaning, and local instillation of other digestive and genitourinary organs

96.41 Irrigation of cholecystostomy and other biliary tube

96.42 Irrigation of pancreatic tube

96.43 Digestive tract instillation, except gastric gavage

96.44 Vaginal douche   ♀

96.45 Irrigation of nephrostomy and pyelostomy

96.46 Irrigation of ureterostomy and ureteral catheter

96.47 Irrigation of cystostomy

96.48 Irrigation of other indwelling urinary catheter

96.49 Other genitourinary instillation
Insertion of prostaglandin suppository
AHA: 1Q, '01, 5

☑4ᵗʰ 96.5 Other nonoperative irrigation and cleaning

96.51 Irrigation of eye
Irrigation of cornea
EXCLUDES   *irrigation with removal of foreign body*
             (98.21)

96.52 Irrigation of ear
Irrigation with removal of cerumen

96.53 Irrigation of nasal passages

96.54 Dental scaling, polishing, and debridement
Dental prophylaxis
Plaque removal

96.55 Tracheostomy toilette

96.56 Other lavage of bronchus and trachea
EXCLUDES   *diagnostic bronchoalveolar lavage (BAL)*
             (33.24)
             whole lung lavage (33.99)
AHA: 3Q, '02, 18

96.57 Irrigation of vascular catheter
AHA: 3Q, '93, 5

96.58 Irrigation of wound catheter

96.59 Other irrigation of wound
Wound cleaning NOS
EXCLUDES   *debridement (86.22, 86.27-86.28)*
AHA: ▶3Q, '12, 3;◀ S-O, '85, 7

96.6 Enteral infusion of concentrated-nutritional substances

☑4ᵗʰ 96.7 Other continuous invasive mechanical ventilation
BiPAP delivered through endotracheal tube or tracheostomy (invasive interface)
CPAP delivered through endotracheal tube or tracheostomy (invasive interface)
Endotracheal respiratory assistance
Invasive positive pressure ventilation [IPPV]
Mechanical ventilation through invasive interface
That by tracheostomy
Weaning of an intubated (endotracheal tube) patient
Code also any associated:
  endotracheal tube insertion (96.04)
  tracheostomy (31.1-31.29)
EXCLUDES   *continuous negative pressure ventilation [CNP] (iron lung) (cuirass) (93.99)*
           intermittent positive pressure breathing [IPPB] (93.91)
           non-invasive bi-level positive airway pressure [BiPAP] (93.90)
           non-invasive continuous positive airway pressure [CPAP] (93.90)
           non-invasive positive pressure (NIPPV) (93.90)
           that by face mask (93.90-93.99)
           that by nasal cannula (93.90-93.99)
           that by nasal catheter (93.90-93.99)

NOTE **Endotracheal intubation**
To calculate the number of hours (duration) of continuous mechanical ventilation during a hospitalization, begin the count from the start of the (endotracheal) intubation. The duration ends with (endotracheal) extubation.

If a patient is intubated prior to admission, begin counting the duration from the time of the admission. If a patient is transferred (discharged) while intubated, the duration would end at the time of transfer (discharge).

For patients who begin on (endotracheal) intubation and subsequently have a tracheostomy performed for mechanical ventilation, the duration begins with the (endotracheal) intubation and ends when the mechanical ventilation is turned off (after the weaning period).

NOTE **Tracheostomy**
To calculate the number of hours of continuous mechanical ventilation during a hospitalization, begin counting the duration when mechanical ventilation is started. The duration ends when the mechanical ventilator is turned off (after the weaning period).

If a patient has received a tracheostomy prior to admission and is on mechanical ventilation at the time of admission, begin counting the duration from the time of admission. If a patient is transferred (discharged) while still on mechanical ventilation via tracheostomy, the duration would end at the time of the transfer (discharge).
AHA: 3Q, '10, 3-4; 4Q, '08, 187-190 3Q, '04, 3; 2Q, '92, 13; 4Q, '91, 16; 4Q, '91, 18; 4Q, '91, 21
TIP: Do not assign if the patient is not intubated or does not have a tracheostomy. Refer to subcategory 93.9 for noninvasive mechanical ventilation.

96.70   **Continuous invasive mechanical ventilation of unspecified duration**
Invasive mechanical ventilation NOS

96.71   **Continuous invasive mechanical ventilation for less than 96 consecutive hours**
AHA: 4Q, '10, 80; 2Q, '09, 11; 3Q, '07, 6; 2Q, '06, 8; 3Q, '05, 10; 3Q, '04, 11; 2Q, '02, 19; 1Q, '02, 12; 1Q, '01, 6

[13] **96.72**   **Continuous invasive mechanical ventilation for 96 consecutive hours or more**
AHA: 2Q, '05, 19; 1Q, '04, 23

✓3ʳᵈ **97**   **Replacement and removal of therapeutic appliances**

✓4ᵗʰ **97.0**   **Nonoperative replacement of gastrointestinal appliance**

97.01   **Replacement of (naso-)gastric or esophagostomy tube**

97.02   **Replacement of gastrostomy tube**
AHA: 1Q, '97, 11

97.03   **Replacement of tube or enterostomy device of small intestine**
AHA: 1Q, '03, 10

97.04   **Replacement of tube or enterostomy device of large intestine**

97.05   **Replacement of stent (tube) in biliary or pancreatic duct**
AHA: 2Q, '99, 13

✓4ᵗʰ **97.1**   **Nonoperative replacement of musculoskeletal and integumentary system appliance**

97.11   **Replacement of cast on upper limb**

97.12   **Replacement of cast on lower limb**

97.13   **Replacement of other cast**

97.14   **Replacement of other device for musculoskeletal immobilization**
Splinting
Strapping

97.15   **Replacement of wound catheter**

97.16   **Replacement of wound packing or drain**
EXCLUDES   repacking of:
dental wound (97.22)
vulvar wound (97.26)

✓4ᵗʰ **97.2**   **Other nonoperative replacement**

97.21   **Replacement of nasal packing**

97.22   **Replacement of dental packing**

97.23   **Replacement of tracheostomy tube**
AHA: N-D, '87, 11

97.24   **Replacement and refitting of vagina diaphragm**   ♀

97.25   **Replacement of other vaginal pessary**   ♀

97.26   **Replacement of vaginal or vulvar packing or drain**   ♀

97.29   **Other nonoperative replacements**
AHA: 3Q, '99, 9; 3Q, '98, 12

✓4ᵗʰ **97.3**   **Nonoperative removal of therapeutic device from head and neck**

97.31   **Removal of eye prosthesis**
EXCLUDES   removal of ocular implant (16.71)
removal of orbital implant (16.72)

97.32   **Removal of nasal packing**

97.33   **Removal of dental wiring**

97.34   **Removal of dental packing**

97.35   **Removal of dental prosthesis**

97.36   **Removal of other external mandibular fixation device**

97.37   **Removal of tracheostomy tube**

97.38   **Removal of sutures from head and neck**

Intraaortic Balloon Pump

Transverse aorta
Descending aorta
Aorta
Balloon pump in inflated phase
Thoracic aorta
Femoral artery access
Diaphragm
Abdominal aorta

97.39   **Removal of other therapeutic device from head and neck**
EXCLUDES   removal of skull tongs (02.94)

✓4ᵗʰ **97.4**   **Nonoperative removal of therapeutic device from thorax**

97.41   **Removal of thoracotomy tube or pleural cavity drain**
AHA: 1Q, '99, 10

97.42   **Removal of mediastinal drain**

97.43   **Removal of sutures from thorax**

97.44   **Nonoperative removal of heart assist system**
Explantation [removal] of circulatory assist device
Explantation [removal] of percutaneous external heart assist device
Removal of extrinsic heart assist device
Removal of pVAD
Removal of percutaneous heart assist device
DEF: Non-invasive removal of ventricular assist systems, or intraaortic balloon pump, which is a balloon catheter placed into the descending thoracic aorta and timed to inflate and deflate with the patient's own heart rhythm to aid in blood circulation.
AHA: 4Q, '01, 65

97.49   **Removal of other device from thorax**
EXCLUDES   endoscopic removal of bronchial device(s) or substances (33.78)
AHA: N-D, '86, 9

✓4ᵗʰ **97.5**   **Nonoperative removal of therapeutic device from digestive system**

97.51   **Removal of gastrostomy tube**

97.52   **Removal of tube from small intestine**

97.53   **Removal of tube from large intestine or appendix**

97.54   **Removal of cholecystostomy tube**

97.55   **Removal of T-tube, other bile duct tube, or liver tube**
Removal of bile duct stent
AHA: 1Q, '01, 8
TIP: Assign also code 51.10 if a biliary stent was removed via ERCP guidance.

97.56   **Removal of pancreatic tube or drain**

97.59   **Removal of other device from digestive system**
Removal of rectal packing

✓4ᵗʰ **97.6**   **Nonoperative removal of therapeutic device from urinary system**

97.61   **Removal of pyelostomy and nephrostomy tube**
DEF: Nonsurgical removal of tubes from lower part of kidney.

97.62   **Removal of ureterostomy tube and ureteral catheter**

97.63   **Removal of cystostomy tube**

97.64   **Removal of other urinary drainage device**
Removal of indwelling urinary catheter

97.65   **Removal of urethral stent**

---

[13] LOS must be => 4 days

BI Bilateral Procedure   **NC** Non-covered Procedure   **LC** Limited Coverage Procedure   ►◄ Revised Text   ● New Code   ▲ Revised Code Title

196 – Volume 3   **2014 ICD-9-CM**

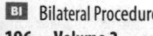

97.69   Removal of other device from urinary system

√4ᵗʰ 97.7 **Nonoperative removal of therapeutic device from genital system**

97.71   Removal of intrauterine contraceptive device ♀

97.72   Removal of intrauterine pack ♀

97.73   Removal of vaginal diaphragm ♀

97.74   Removal of other vaginal pessary ♀

97.75   Removal of vaginal or vulvar packing ♀

97.79   Removal of other device from genital tract
Removal of sutures

√4ᵗʰ 97.8 **Other nonoperative removal of therapeutic device**

97.81   Removal of retroperitoneal drainage device

97.82   Removal of peritoneal drainage device
AHA: 2Q, '90, 28; S-O, '86, 12

97.83   Removal of abdominal wall sutures

97.84   Removal of sutures from trunk, not elsewhere classified

97.85   Removal of packing from trunk, not elsewhere classified

97.86   Removal of other device from abdomen

97.87   Removal of other device from trunk

97.88   Removal of external immobilization device
Removal of:
brace
cast
splint

97.89   Removal of other therapeutic device

√3ʳᵈ 98 **Nonoperative removal of foreign body or calculus**

√4ᵗʰ 98.0 **Removal of intraluminal foreign body from digestive system without incision**
EXCLUDES *removal of therapeutic device (97.51-97.59)*
DEF: Retrieval of foreign body from digestive system lining without incision.

98.01   Removal of intraluminal foreign body from mouth without incision

98.02   Removal of intraluminal foreign body from esophagus without incision

98.03   Removal of intraluminal foreign body from stomach and small intestine without incision

98.04   Removal of intraluminal foreign body from large intestine without incision

98.05   Removal of intraluminal foreign body from rectum and anus without incision

√4ᵗʰ 98.1 **Removal of intraluminal foreign body from other sites without incision**
EXCLUDES *removal of therapeutic device (97.31-97.49, 97.61-97.89)*

98.11   Removal of intraluminal foreign body from ear without incision

98.12   Removal of intraluminal foreign body from nose without incision

98.13   Removal of intraluminal foreign body from pharynx without incision

98.14   Removal of intraluminal foreign body from larynx without incision

98.15   Removal of intraluminal foreign body from trachea and bronchus without incision
EXCLUDES *endoscopic removal of bronchial device(s) or substances (33.78)*

98.16   Removal of intraluminal foreign body from uterus without incision ♀
EXCLUDES *removal of intrauterine contraceptive device (97.71)*

98.17   Removal of intraluminal foreign body from vagina without incision ♀

98.18   Removal of intraluminal foreign body from artificial stoma without incision

98.19   Removal of intraluminal foreign body from urethra without incision

√4ᵗʰ 98.2 **Removal of other foreign body without incision**
EXCLUDES *removal of intraluminal foreign body (98.01-98.19)*

98.20   Removal of foreign body, not otherwise specified

98.21   Removal of superficial foreign body from eye without incision

98.22   Removal of other foreign body without incision from head and neck
Removal of embedded foreign body from eyelid or conjunctiva without incision

98.23   Removal of foreign body from vulva without incision ♀

98.24   Removal of foreign body from scrotum or penis without incision ♂

98.25   Removal of other foreign body without incision from trunk except scrotum, penis, or vulva

98.26   Removal of foreign body from hand without incision
AHA: N-D, '87, 10

98.27   Removal of foreign body without incision from upper limb, except hand

98.28   Removal of foreign body from foot without incision

98.29   Removal of foreign body without incision from lower limb, except foot

√4ᵗʰ 98.5 **Extracorporeal shockwave lithotripsy [ESWL]**
Lithotriptor tank procedure
Disintegration of stones by extracorporeal induced shockwaves
That with insertion of stent
DEF: Breaking of stones with high voltage condenser device synchronized with patient R waves.

98.51   **Extracorporeal shockwave lithotripsy [ESWL] of the kidney, ureter and/or bladder**
AHA: 4Q, '95, 73; 1Q, '89, 2
TIP: If the lithotripsy is documented with an endoscopic approach (e.g., cystoscopic), do not assign 98.51, assign instead 56.0 and 59.95; if by percutaneous nephrostomy, do not assign 98.51, assign instead 55.04.

98.52   **Extracorporeal shockwave lithotripsy [ESWL] of the gallbladder and/or bile duct** NC

98.59   **Extracorporeal shockwave lithotripsy of other sites** NC

Extracorporeal Shock Wave Lithotripsy

Radiographic monitors
Shock wave exit area
Water cushion
Shock wave entry area
Kidney
Lithotripsy unit

Miscellaneous Diagnostic and Therapeutic Procedures

99–99.24

√3ʳᵈ **99　Other nonoperative procedures**

√4ᵗʰ **99.0　Transfusion of blood and blood components**
Use additional code for that done via catheter or cutdown
(38.92-38.94)

99.00　Perioperative autologous transfusion of whole blood or blood components
Intraoperative blood collection
Postoperative blood collection
Salvage
DEF: Salvaging patient blood with reinfusion during perioperative period.
AHA: 4Q, '95, 69

99.01　Exchange transfusion
Transfusion:
exsanguination
replacement
DEF: Repetitive withdrawal of blood, replaced by donor blood.
AHA: 2Q, '89, 15

99.02　Transfusion of previously collected autologous blood
Blood component
DEF: Transfusion with patient's own previously withdrawn and stored blood.
AHA: 4Q, '95, 69; 1Q, '90, 10; J-A, '85, 16

99.03　Other transfusion of whole blood
Transfusion:
blood NOS
hemodilution
NOS

99.04　Transfusion of packed cells
AHA: 4Q, '11, 146; 4Q, '10, 80

99.05　Transfusion of platelets
Transfusion of thrombocytes

99.06　Transfusion of coagulation factors
Transfusion of antihemophilic factor
EXCLUDES ▶infusion of 4-Factor Prothrombin Complex Concentrate (00.96)◀

99.07　Transfusion of other serum
Transfusion of plasma
EXCLUDES injection [transfusion] of:
antivenin (99.16)
gamma globulin (99.14)

99.08　Transfusion of blood expander
Transfusion of Dextran

99.09　Transfusion of other substance
Transfusion of:
blood surrogate
granulocytes
EXCLUDES transplantation [transfusion] of bone marrow (41.00-41.09)
AHA: 1Q, '11, 24

√4ᵗʰ **99.1　Injection or infusion of therapeutic or prophylactic substance**
INCLUDES injection or infusion given:
hypodermically ⎫
intramuscularly ⎬ acting locally or
intravenously ⎭ systemically

99.10　Injection or infusion of thrombolytic agent
Alteplase　　　　Tenecteplase
Anistreplase　　　Tissue plasminogen activator
Reteplase　　　　(TPA)
Streptokinase　　Urokinase
EXCLUDES aspirin — omit code
GP IIb/IIIa platelet inhibitors (99.20)
heparin (99.19)
SuperSaturated oxygen therapy (00.49)
warfarin — omit code
AHA: 4Q, '12, 85; 2Q, '12, 15; 2Q, '11, 4; 3Q, '10, 5; 2Q, '06, 22; 4Q, '05, 101-103; 2Q, '01, 7-9, 23; 4Q, '98, 83
TIP: If a tPA infusion is started in another facility within 24 hours of transferring to the current facility, assign diagnosis code V45.88, whether or not the infusion is continued in the current facility.

99.11　Injection of Rh immune globulin
Injection of:
Anti-D (Rhesus) globulin
RhoGAM

99.12　Immunization for allergy
Desensitization

99.13　Immunization for autoimmune disease

99.14　Injection or infusion of immunoglobulin
Injection of immune sera
Injection or infusion of gamma globulin

99.15　Parenteral infusion of concentrated nutritional substances
Hyperalimentation
Total parenteral nutrition [TPN]
Peripheral parenteral nutrition [PPN]
DEF: Administration of greater than necessary amount of nutrients via other than the alimentary canal (e.g., infusion).
AHA: 4Q, '03, 104

99.16　Injection of antidote
Injection of:
antivenin
heavy metal antagonist

99.17　Injection of insulin

99.18　Injection or infusion of electrolytes

99.19　Injection of anticoagulant
EXCLUDES infusion of drotrecogin alfa (activated) (00.11)

√4ᵗʰ **99.2　Injection or infusion of other therapeutic or prophylactic substance**
INCLUDES injection or infusion given:
hypodermically ⎫
intramuscularly ⎬ acting locally or
intravenously ⎭ systemically
Use additional code for:
injection (into):
breast (85.92)
bursa (82.94, 83.96)
intraperitoneal (cavity) (54.97)
intrathecal (03.92)
joint (76.96, 81.92)
kidney (55.96)
liver (50.94)
orbit (16.91)
other sites — see Alphabetic Index
perfusion:
NOS (39.97)
intestine (46.95, 46.96)
kidney (55.95)
liver (50.93)
total body (39.96)
EXCLUDES SuperSaturated oxygen therapy (00.49)

99.20　Injection or infusion of platelet inhibitor
Glycoprotein IIb/IIIa inhibitor
GP IIb-IIIa inhibitor
GP IIb/IIIa inhibitor
EXCLUDES infusion of heparin (99.19)
injection or infusion of thrombolytic agent (99.10)
AHA: 3Q, '06, 8; 2Q, '04, 3; 4Q, '02, 114; 4Q, '98, 85

99.21　Injection of antibiotic
EXCLUDES injection or infusion of oxazolidinone class of antibiotics (00.14)
AHA: 3Q, '10, 11; 4Q, '98, 76; 2Q, '90, 24; M-A, '87, 9

99.22　Injection of other anti-infective
EXCLUDES injection or infusion of oxazolidinone class of antibiotics (00.14)

99.23　Injection of steroid
Injection of cortisone
Subdermal implantation of progesterone
AHA: 3Q, '00, 15; 1Q, '99, 8; 3Q, '96, 7; 3Q, '92, 9; S-O, '85, 7

99.24　Injection of other hormone
AHA: 1Q, '06, 9

BI Bilateral Procedure　　NC Non-covered Procedure　　LC Limited Coverage Procedure　　▶◀ Revised Text　　● New Code　　▲ Revised Code Title

99.25 Injection or infusion of cancer chemotherapeutic substance
Chemoembolization
Injection or infusion of antineoplastic agent
Use additional code for disruption of blood brain barrier, if performed [BBBD] (00.19)
EXCLUDES   *immunotherapy, antineoplastic (00.15, 99.28)*
implantation of chemotherapeutic agent (00.10)
injection of radioisotope (92.28)
injection or infusion of biological response modifier [BRM] as an antineoplastic agent (99.28)
intravenous infusion of clofarabine (17.70)
AHA: 1Q, '12, 13; 2Q, '11, 4; 4Q, '09, 79; 4Q, '08, 82; 4Q, '07, 104; 2Q, '03, 6, 16; 4Q, '02, 93; 1Q, '99, 4; 1Q, '98, 6; 3Q, '96, 11; 4Q, '95, 67; 2Q, '92, 7; 1Q, '92, 12; 1Q, '88, 8; N-D, '86, 11

99.26 Injection of tranquilizer

99.27 Iontophoresis
DEF: Iontophoresis: Introduction of soluble salts into tissues via electric current.

99.28 Injection or infusion of biological response modifier [BRM] as an antineoplastic agent
Immunotherapy, antineoplastic
Infusion of cintredekin besudotox
Interleukin therapy
Low-dose interleukin-2 [IL-2] therapy
Tumor vaccine
EXCLUDES   *high-dose infusion interleukin-2 [IL-2] (00.15)*
AHA: 4Q, '06, 123; 4Q, '03, 92; 2Q, '99, 8; 2Q, '98, 10; 4Q, '94, 51

99.29 Injection or infusion of other therapeutic or prophylactic substance
EXCLUDES   *administration of neuroprotective agent (99.75)*
immunization (99.31-99.59)
infusion of blood brain barrier disruption substance (00.19)
injection of sclerosing agent into:
     esophageal varices (42.33)
     hemorrhoids (49.42)
     veins (39.92)
injection or infusion of:
     human B-type natriuretic peptide (hBNP) (00.13)
     nesiritide (00.13)
     platelet inhibitor (99.20)
     thrombolytic agent (99.10)
     uterine artery embolization without coils (68.25)
AHA: 4Q, '11, 179-180; 2Q, '10, 4-5, 6-7, 14; 1Q, '10, 21; 1Q, '07, 11; 2Q, '03, 10; 3Q, '02, 19, 24; 1Q, '01, 15; 2Q, '00, 14; 1Q, '00, 8, 18, 23; 4Q, '99, 17; 3Q, '99, 21; 4Q, '98, 83; 2Q, '98, 17, 18, 23, 24; 1Q, '98, 6; 2Q, '97, 11; 1Q, '97, 3; 4Q, '95, 67; 2Q, '95, 12; 4Q, '90, 14; 2Q, '90, 23; 2Q, '89, 17; 1Q, '88, 9; N-D, '87, 4; S-O, '87, 11

√4ᵗʰ **99.3 Prophylactic vaccination and inoculation against certain bacterial diseases**
DEF: Administration of a killed bacteria suspension to produce immunity.

99.31 Vaccination against cholera

99.32 Vaccination against typhoid and paratyphoid fever
Administration of TAB vaccine

99.33 Vaccination against tuberculosis
Administration of BCG vaccine

99.34 Vaccination against plague

99.35 Vaccination against tularemia

99.36 Administration of diphtheria toxoid
EXCLUDES   *administration of:*
     diphtheria antitoxin (99.58)
     diphtheria-tetanus-pertussis, combined (99.39)

99.37 Vaccination against pertussis
EXCLUDES   *administration of diphtheria-tetanus-pertussis, combined (99.39)*

99.38 Administration of tetanus toxoid
EXCLUDES   *administration of:*
     diphtheria-tetanus-pertussis, combined (99.39)
     tetanus antitoxin (99.56)

99.39 Administration of diphtheria-tetanus- pertussis, combined

√4ᵗʰ **99.4 Prophylactic vaccination and inoculation against certain viral diseases**
DEF: Administration of a killed virus suspension to produce immunity.

99.41 Administration of poliomyelitis vaccine

99.42 Vaccination against smallpox

99.43 Vaccination against yellow fever

99.44 Vaccination against rabies

99.45 Vaccination against measles
EXCLUDES   *administration of measles-mumps-rubella vaccine (99.48)*

99.46 Vaccination against mumps
EXCLUDES   *administration of measles-mumps-rubella vaccine (99.48)*

99.47 Vaccination against rubella
EXCLUDES   *administration of measles-mumps-rubella vaccine (99.48)*

99.48 Administration of measles-mumps-rubella vaccine

√4ᵗʰ **99.5 Other vaccination and inoculation**

99.51 Prophylactic vaccination against the common cold

99.52 Prophylactic vaccination against influenza

99.53 Prophylactic vaccination against arthropod-borne viral encephalitis

99.54 Prophylactic vaccination against other arthropod-borne viral diseases

99.55 Prophylactic administration of vaccine against other diseases
Vaccination against:
     anthrax
     brucellosis
     Rocky Mountain spotted fever
     Staphylococcus
     Streptococcus
     typhus
AHA: 2Q, '00, 9; 1Q, '94, 10

99.56 Administration of tetanus antitoxin

99.57 Administration of botulism antitoxin

99.58 Administration of other antitoxins
Administration of:
     diphtheria antitoxin
     gas gangrene antitoxin
     scarlet fever antitoxin

99.59 Other vaccination and inoculation
Vaccination NOS
EXCLUDES   *injection of:*
     gamma globulin (99.14)
     Rh immune globulin (99.11)
immunization for:
     allergy (99.12)
     autoimmune disease (99.13)

√4ᵗʰ **99.6 Conversion of cardiac rhythm**
EXCLUDES   *open chest cardiac:*
     electric stimulation (37.91)
     massage (37.91)
DEF: Correction of cardiac rhythm.

99.60 Cardiopulmonary resuscitation, not otherwise specified
AHA: 1Q, '94, 16

99.61　Atrial cardioversion
DEF: Application of electric shock to upper heart chamber to restore normal heart rhythm.

99.62　Other electric countershock of heart
Cardioversion:
　NOS
　external
Conversion to sinus rhythm
Defibrillation
　External electrode stimulation
AHA: 1Q, '07, 17

99.63　Closed chest cardiac massage
Cardiac massage NOS
Manual external cardiac massage
DEF: Application of alternating manual pressure over breastbone to restore normal heart rhythm.

99.64　Carotid sinus stimulation

99.69　Other conversion of cardiac rhythm
AHA: 4Q, '88, 11

√4ᵗʰ **99.7　Therapeutic apheresis or other injection, administration, or infusion of other therpeutic or prophylactic substance**

99.71　Therapeutic plasmapheresis
EXCLUDES　*extracorporeal immunoadsorption [ECI] (99.76)*

99.72　Therapeutic leukopheresis
Therapeutic leukocytapheresis

99.73　Therapeutic erythrocytapheresis
Therapeutic erythropheresis
AHA: 1Q, '94, 20

99.74　Therapeutic plateletpheresis

99.75　Administration of neuroprotective agent
DEF: Direct application of neuroprotective agent (e.g., nimodipine) to miinimize ischemic injury by inhibiting toxic neurotransmitters, blocking free ions, removing free radicals, and causing vasodilation.
AHA: 4Q, '00, 68

99.76　Extracorporeal immunoadsorption
Removal of antibodies from plasma with protein A columns
AHA: 4Q, '02, 112

99.77　Application or administration of adhesion barrier substance
AHA: 1Q, '10, 11; 4Q, '02, 113

99.78　Aquapheresis
Plasma water removal
Ultrafiltration [for water removal]
EXCLUDES　*hemodiafiltration (39.95)*
　　hemodialysis (39.95)
　　therapeutic plasmapheresis (99.71)

99.79　Other
Apheresis (harvest) of stem cells
AHA: 3Q, '08, 19; 1Q, '06, 12, 13; 1Q, '05, 16; 4Q, '97, 55

√4ᵗʰ **99.8　Miscellaneous physical procedures**

99.81　Hypothermia (central) (local)
EXCLUDES　*gastric cooling (96.31)*
　　gastric freezing (96.32)
　　that incidental to open heart surgery (39.62)
AHA: 3Q, '10, 14

99.82　Ultraviolet light therapy
Actinotherapy

99.83　Other phototherapy
Phototherapy of the newborn
EXCLUDES　*extracorporeal photochemotherapy (99.88)*
　　photocoagulation of retinal lesion (14.23-14.25, 14.33-14.35, 14.53-14.55)
DEF: Treating disease with light rays of various concentrations.
AHA: 2Q, '89, 15

99.84　Isolation
Isolation after contact with infectious disease
Protection of individual from his surroundings
Protection of surroundings from individual

99.85　Hyperthermia for treatment of cancer
Hyperthermia (adjunct therapy) induced by microwave, ultrasound, low energy radio frequency, probes (interstitial), or other means in the treatment of cancer
Code also any concurrent chemotherapy or radiation therapy
AHA: 3Q, '96, 11; 3Q, '89, 17

99.86　Non-invasive placement of bone growth stimulato
Transcutaneous (surface) placement of pads or patches for stimulation to aid bone healing
EXCLUDES　*insertion of invasive or semi-invasive bone growth stimulators (device) (percutaneous electrodes) (78.90-78.99)*

99.88　Therapeutic photopheresis
Extracorporeal photochemotherapy
Extracorporeal photopheresis
EXCLUDES　*other phototherapy (99.83)*
　　ultraviolet light therapy (99.82)
DEF: Extracorporeal photochemotherapy: Treating disease with drugs that react to ultraviolet radiation or sunlight.
AHA: 2Q, '99, 7

√4ᵗʰ **99.9　Other miscellaneous procedures**

99.91　Acupuncture for anesthesia

99.92　Other acupuncture
EXCLUDES　*that with smouldering moxa (93.35)*

99.93　Rectal massage (for levator spasm)

99.94　Prostatic massage

99.95　Stretching of foreskin

99.96　Collection of sperm for artificial insemination

99.97　Fitting of denture

99.98　Extraction of milk from lactating breast

99.99　Other
Leech therapy

BI　Bilateral Procedure　　　NC　Non-covered Procedure　　　LC　Limited Coverage Procedure　　　►◄ Revised Text　　　● New Code　　　▲ Revised Code Titl

200 – Volume 3　　　　　　　　　　　　　　　　　　　　　　　　　　　　　　　　　　　　2014 ICD-9-C

Diagnosis Code/MDC/DRG List

The following list provides the MDC and **Medical** DRG(s) to which the diagnosis code is assigned when listed as the principal diagnosis with the exception of principal diagnosis in combination with secondary diagnosis causing assignment to MDC 24 or the significant HIV related diagnosis causing assignment to MDC 25. Other demographic information may reflect changes in DRG grouping. The resources used to compile this list are the 3M Definitions Manual, Version 30.0, the Medicare Program; Changes to the Hospital Inpatient Prospective Payment System: Proposed Rule *Federal Register*, May 10, 2013.

DX	MDC	DRG
Infectious and Parasitic Diseases		
001.0	06	371-373
001.1	06	371-373
001.9	06	371-373
002.0	18	867-869
002.1	18	867-869
002.2	18	867-869
002.3	18	867-869
002.9	18	867-869
003.0	06	371-373
003.1	18	870-872
003.20	18	867-869
003.21	01	094-096
003.22	04	177-179
003.23	08	548-550
003.24	08	539-541
003.29	18	867-869
003.8	18	867-869
003.9	18	867-869
004.0	06	371-373
004.1	06	371-373
004.2	06	371-373
004.3	06	371-373
004.8	06	371-373
004.9	06	371-373
005.0	06	371-373
005.1	18	867-869
005.2	06	371-373
005.3	06	371-373
005.4	06	371-373
005.81	06	371-373
005.89	06	371-373
005.9	06	391-392
006.0	06	371-373
006.1	06	371-373
006.2	06	371-373
006.3	07	441-443
006.4	04	177-179
006.5	01	097-099
006.6	09	606-607
006.8	18	867-869
006.9	18	867-869
007.0	06	371-373
007.1	06	371-373
007.2	06	371-373
007.3	06	371-373
007.4	06	371-373
007.5	06	371-373
007.8	06	371-373
007.9	06	371-373
008.00	06	371-373
008.01	06	371-373
008.02	06	371-373
008.03	06	371-373
008.04	06	371-373
008.09	06	371-373
008.1	06	371-373
008.2	06	371-373
008.3	06	371-373
008.41	06	371-373
008.42	06	371-373
008.43	06	371-373
008.44	06	371-373
008.45	06	371-373
008.46	06	371-373
008.47	06	371-373
008.49	06	371-373
008.5	06	371-373
008.61	06	391-392
008.62	06	391-392
008.63	06	391-392
008.64	06	391-392
008.65	06	391-392
008.66	06	391-392
008.67	06	391-392
008.69	06	391-392
008.8	06	391-392
009.0	06	391-392
009.1	06	391-392
009.2	06	391-392
009.3	06	391-392
010.00	04	177-179
010.01	04	177-179
010.02	04	177-179
010.03	04	177-179
010.04	04	177-179
010.05	04	177-179
010.06	04	177-179
010.10	04	177-179
010.11	04	177-179
010.12	04	177-179
010.13	04	177-179
010.14	04	177-179
010.15	04	177-179
010.16	04	177-179
010.80	04	177-179
010.81	04	177-179
010.82	04	177-179
010.83	04	177-179
010.84	04	177-179
010.85	04	177-179
010.86	04	177-179
010.90	04	177-179
010.91	04	177-179
010.92	04	177-179
010.93	04	177-179
010.94	04	177-179
010.95	04	177-179
010.96	04	177-179
011.00	04	177-179
011.01	04	177-179
011.02	04	177-179
011.03	04	177-179
011.04	04	177-179
011.05	04	177-179
011.06	04	177-179
011.10	04	177-179
011.11	04	177-179
011.12	04	177-179
011.13	04	177-179
011.14	04	177-179
011.15	04	177-179
011.16	04	177-179
011.20	04	177-179
011.21	04	177-179
011.22	04	177-179
011.23	04	177-179
011.24	04	177-179
011.25	04	177-179
011.26	04	177-179
011.30	04	177-179
011.31	04	177-179
011.32	04	177-179
011.33	04	177-179
011.34	04	177-179
011.35	04	177-179
011.36	04	177-179
011.40	04	177-179
011.41	04	177-179
011.42	04	177-179
011.43	04	177-179
011.44	04	177-179
011.45	04	177-179
011.46	04	177-179
011.50	04	177-179
011.51	04	177-179
011.52	04	177-179
011.53	04	177-179
011.54	04	177-179
011.55	04	177-179
011.56	04	177-179
011.60	04	177-179
011.61	04	177-179
011.62	04	177-179
011.63	04	177-179
011.64	04	177-179
011.65	04	177-179
011.66	04	177-179
011.70	04	177-179
011.71	04	177-179
011.72	04	177-179
011.73	04	177-179
011.74	04	177-179
011.75	04	177-179
011.76	04	177-179
011.80	04	177-179
011.81	04	177-179
011.82	04	177-179
011.83	04	177-179
011.84	04	177-179
011.85	04	177-179
011.86	04	177-179
011.90	04	177-179
011.91	04	177-179
011.92	04	177-179
011.93	04	177-179
011.94	04	177-179
011.95	04	177-179
011.96	04	177-179
012.00	04	177-179
012.01	04	177-179
012.02	04	177-179
012.03	04	177-179
012.04	04	177-179
012.05	04	177-179
012.06	04	177-179
012.10	04	177-179
012.11	04	177-179
012.12	04	177-179
012.13	04	177-179
012.14	04	177-179
012.15	04	177-179
012.16	04	177-179
012.20	04	177-179
012.21	04	177-179
012.22	04	177-179
012.23	04	177-179
012.24	04	177-179
012.25	04	177-179
012.26	04	177-179
012.30	03	154-156
012.31	03	154-156
012.32	03	154-156
012.33	03	154-156
012.34	03	154-156
012.35	03	154-156
012.36	03	154-156
012.80	04	177-179
012.81	04	177-179
012.82	04	177-179
012.83	04	177-179
012.84	04	177-179
012.85	04	177-179
012.86	04	177-179
013.00	01	094-096
013.01	01	094-096
013.02	01	094-096
013.03	01	094-096
013.04	01	094-096
013.05	01	094-096
013.06	01	094-096
013.10	01	094-096
013.11	01	094-096
013.12	01	094-096
013.13	01	094-096
013.14	01	094-096
013.15	01	094-096
013.16	01	094-096
013.20	01	094-096
013.21	01	094-096
013.22	01	094-096
013.23	01	094-096
013.24	01	094-096
013.25	01	094-096
013.26	01	094-096
013.30	01	094-096
013.31	01	094-096
013.32	01	094-096
013.33	01	094-096
013.34	01	094-096
013.35	01	094-096
013.36	01	094-096
013.40	01	094-096
013.41	01	094-096
013.42	01	094-096
013.43	01	094-096
013.44	01	094-096
013.45	01	094-096
013.46	01	094-096
013.50	01	094-096
013.51	01	094-096
013.52	01	094-096
013.53	01	094-096
013.54	01	094-096
013.55	01	094-096
013.56	01	094-096
013.60	01	094-096
013.61	01	094-096
013.62	01	094-096
013.63	01	094-096
013.64	01	094-096
013.65	01	094-096
013.66	01	094-096
013.80	01	094-096
013.81	01	094-096
013.82	01	094-096
013.83	01	094-096
013.84	01	094-096
013.85	01	094-096
013.86	01	094-096
013.90	01	094-096
013.91	01	094-096
013.92	01	094-096
013.93	01	094-096
013.94	01	094-096
013.95	01	094-096
013.96	01	094-096
014.00	06	371-373
014.01	06	371-373
014.02	06	371-373
014.03	06	371-373
014.04	06	371-373
014.05	06	371-373
014.06	06	371-373
014.80	06	371-373
014.81	06	371-373
014.82	06	371-373
014.83	06	371-373
014.84	06	371-373
014.85	06	371-373
014.86	06	371-373
015.00	08	539-541
015.01	08	539-541
015.02	08	539-541
015.03	08	539-541
015.04	08	539-541
015.05	08	539-541
015.06	08	539-541
015.10	08	548-550

DX	MDC	DRG
015.11	08	548-550
015.12	08	548-550
015.13	08	548-550
015.14	08	548-550
015.15	08	548-550
015.16	08	548-550
015.20	08	548-550
015.21	08	548-550
015.22	08	548-550
015.23	08	548-550
015.24	08	548-550
015.25	08	548-550
015.26	08	548-550
015.50	08	539-541
015.51	08	539-541
015.52	08	539-541
015.53	08	539-541
015.54	08	539-541
015.55	08	539-541
015.56	08	539-541
015.60	03	154-156
015.61	03	154-156
015.62	03	154-156
015.63	03	154-156
015.64	03	154-156
015.65	03	154-156
015.66	03	154-156
015.70	08	539-541
015.71	08	539-541
015.72	08	539-541
015.73	08	539-541
015.74	08	539-541
015.75	08	539-541
015.76	08	539-541
015.80	08	548-550
015.81	08	548-550
015.82	08	548-550
015.83	08	548-550
015.84	08	548-550
015.85	08	548-550
015.86	08	548-550
015.90	08	548-550
015.91	08	548-550
015.92	08	548-550
015.93	08	548-550
015.94	08	548-550
015.95	08	548-550
015.96	08	548-550
016.00	11	689-690
016.01	11	689-690
016.02	11	689-690
016.03	11	689-690
016.04	11	689-690
016.05	11	689-690
016.06	11	689-690
016.10	11	689-690
016.11	11	689-690
016.12	11	689-690
016.13	11	689-690
016.14	11	689-690
016.15	11	689-690
016.16	11	689-690
016.20	11	689-690
016.21	11	689-690
016.22	11	689-690
016.23	11	689-690
016.24	11	689-690
016.25	11	689-690
016.26	11	689-690
016.30	11	689-690
016.31	11	689-690
016.32	11	689-690
016.33	11	689-690
016.34	11	689-690
016.35	11	689-690
016.36	11	689-690
016.40	12	727-728
016.41	12	727-728
016.42	12	727-728
016.43	12	727-728
016.44	12	727-728
016.45	12	727-728
016.46	12	727-728
016.50	12	727-728
016.51	12	727-728
016.52	12	727-728
016.53	12	727-728
016.54	12	727-728
016.55	12	727-728
016.56	12	727-728
016.60	13	757-759
016.61	13	757-759
016.62	13	757-759
016.63	13	757-759
016.64	13	757-759
016.65	13	757-759
016.66	13	757-759
016.70	13	757-759
016.71	13	757-759
016.72	13	757-759
016.73	13	757-759
016.74	13	757-759
016.75	13	757-759
016.76	13	757-759
016.90	11	689-690
016.91	11	689-690
016.92	11	689-690
016.93	11	689-690
016.94	11	689-690
016.95	11	689-690
016.96	11	689-690
017.00	09	606-607
017.01	09	606-607
017.02	09	606-607
017.03	09	606-607
017.04	09	606-607
017.05	09	606-607
017.06	09	606-607
017.10	09	595-596
017.11	09	595-596
017.12	09	595-596
017.13	09	595-596
017.14	09	595-596
017.15	09	595-596
017.16	09	595-596
017.20	16	814-816
017.21	16	814-816
017.22	16	814-816
017.23	16	814-816
017.24	16	814-816
017.25	16	814-816
017.26	16	814-816
017.30	02	124-125
017.31	02	124-125
017.32	02	124-125
017.33	02	124-125
017.34	02	124-125
017.35	02	124-125
017.36	02	124-125
017.40	03	154-156
017.41	03	154-156
017.42	03	154-156
017.43	03	154-156
017.44	03	154-156
017.45	03	154-156
017.46	03	154-156
017.50	10	643-645
017.51	10	643-645
017.52	10	643-645
017.53	10	643-645
017.54	10	643-645
017.55	10	643-645
017.56	10	643-645
017.60	10	643-645
017.61	10	643-645
017.62	10	643-645
017.63	10	643-645
017.64	10	643-645
017.65	10	643-645
017.66	10	643-645
017.70	16	814-816
017.71	16	814-816
017.72	16	814-816
017.73	16	814-816
017.74	16	814-816
017.75	16	814-816
017.76	16	814-816
017.80	06	368-370
017.81	06	368-370
017.82	06	368-370
017.83	06	368-370
017.84	06	368-370
017.85	06	368-370
017.86	06	368-370
017.90	18	867-869
017.91	18	867-869
017.92	18	867-869
017.93	18	867-869
017.94	18	867-869
017.95	18	867-869
017.96	18	867-869
018.00	18	867-869
018.01	18	867-869
018.02	18	867-869
018.03	18	867-869
018.04	18	867-869
018.05	18	867-869
018.06	18	867-869
018.80	18	867-869
018.81	18	867-869
018.82	18	867-869
018.83	18	867-869
018.84	18	867-869
018.85	18	867-869
018.86	18	867-869
018.90	18	867-869
018.91	18	867-869
018.92	18	867-869
018.93	18	867-869
018.94	18	867-869
018.95	18	867-869
020.0	18	867-869
020.1	18	867-869
020.2	18	870-872
020.3	04	177-179
020.4	04	177-179
020.5	04	177-179
020.8	18	867-869
020.9	18	867-869
021.0	18	867-869
021.1	06	371-373
021.2	04	177-179
021.3	18	867-869
021.8	18	867-869
021.9	18	867-869
022.0	09	606-607
022.1	04	177-179
022.2	06	371-373
022.3	18	870-872
022.8	18	867-869
022.9	18	867-869
023.0	18	867-869
023.1	18	867-869
023.2	18	867-869
023.3	18	867-869
023.8	18	867-869
023.9	18	867-869
024	18	867-869
025	18	867-869
026.0	18	867-869
026.1	18	867-869
026.9	18	867-869
027.0	18	867-869
027.1	18	867-869
027.2	18	867-869
027.8	18	867-869
027.9	18	867-869
030.0	18	867-869
030.1	18	867-869
030.2	18	867-869
030.3	18	867-869
030.8	18	867-869
030.9	18	867-869
031.0	04	177-179
031.1	09	606-607
031.2	18	867-869
031.8	18	867-869
031.9	18	867-869
032.0	03	154-156
032.1	03	154-156
032.2	03	154-156
032.3	03	154-156
032.81	02	124-125
032.82	05	314-316
032.83	06	371-373
032.84	11	689-690
032.85	09	606-607
032.89	18	867-869
032.9	18	867-869
033.0	04	202-203
033.1	04	202-203
033.8	04	202-203
033.9	04	202-203
034.0	03	152-153
034.1	18	867-869
035	09	602-603
036.0	01	094-096
036.1	01	094-096
036.2	18	870-872
036.3	18	870-872
036.40	05	314-316
036.41	05	314-316
036.42	05	288-290
036.43	05	314-316
036.81	02	123
036.82	08	548-550
036.89	18	870-872
036.9	18	870-872
037	18	867-869
038.0	18	870-872
038.10	18	870-872
038.11	18	870-872
038.12	18	870-872
038.19	18	870-872
038.2	18	870-872
038.3	18	870-872
038.40	18	870-872
038.41	18	870-872
038.42	18	870-872
038.43	18	870-872
038.44	18	870-872
038.49	18	870-872
038.8	18	870-872
038.9	18	870-872
039.0	09	606-607
039.1	04	177-179
039.2	06	371-373
039.3	09	606-607
039.4	09	606-607
039.8	18	867-869
039.9	18	867-869
040.0	18	867-869
040.1	18	867-869
040.2	06	393-395
040.3	18	867-869
040.41	18	867-869
040.42	18	867-869
040.81	08	557-558
040.82	18	867-869
040.89	18	867-869
041.00	18	867-869
041.01	18	867-869
041.02	18	867-869
041.03	18	867-869
041.04	18	867-869
041.05	18	867-869
041.09	18	867-869
041.10	18	867-869
041.11	18	867-869
041.12	18	867-869
041.19	18	867-869
041.2	18	867-869
041.3	18	867-869
041.41	18	867-869
041.42	18	867-869
041.43	18	867-869
041.49	18	867-869
041.5	18	867-869
041.6	18	867-869
041.7	18	867-869
041.81	18	867-869
041.82	18	867-869
041.83	18	867-869
041.84	18	867-869
041.85	18	867-869
041.86	18	867-869
041.89	18	867-869
041.9	18	867-869
042	25	974-977

DX	MDC	DRG	DX	MDC	DRG	DX	MDC	DRG	DX	MDC	DRG	DX	MDC	DRG
045.00	01	097-099	054.11	13	757-759	062.4	01	097-099	074.1	04	193-195	083.2	18	867-869
045.01	01	097-099	054.12	13	757-759	062.5	01	097-099	074.20	05	314-316	083.8	18	867-869
045.02	01	097-099	054.13	12	727-728	062.8	01	097-099	074.21	05	314-316	083.9	18	867-869
045.03	01	097-099	054.19	12	727-728	062.9	01	097-099	074.22	05	306-307	084.0	18	867-869
045.10	01	097-099	054.19	13	757-759	063.0	01	097-099	074.23	05	314-316	084.1	18	867-869
045.11	01	097-099	054.2	03	157-159	063.1	01	097-099	074.3	18	865-866	084.2	18	867-869
045.12	01	097-099	054.3	01	097-099	063.2	01	097-099	074.8	18	865-866	084.3	18	867-869
045.13	01	097-099	054.40	02	124-125	063.8	01	097-099	075	18	865-866	084.4	18	867-869
045.20	18	865-866	054.41	02	124-125	063.9	01	097-099	076.0	02	124-125	084.5	18	867 869
045.21	18	865-866	054.42	02	124-125	064	01	097-099	076.1	02	124-125	084.6	18	867-869
045.22	18	865-866	054.43	02	124-125	065.0	18	865-866	076.9	02	124-125	084.7	18	867-869
045.23	18	865-866	054.44	02	124-125	065.1	18	865-866	077.0	02	124-125	084.8	18	867-869
045.90	01	097-099	054.49	02	124-125	065.2	18	865-866	077.1	02	124-125	084.9	18	867-869
045.91	01	097-099	054.5	18	870-872	065.3	18	865-866	077.2	02	124-125	085.0	18	867-869
045.92	01	097-099	054.6	09	606-607	065.4	18	865-866	077.3	02	124-125	085.1	09	606-607
045.93	01	097-099	054.71	06	393-395	065.8	18	865-866	077.4	02	124-125	085.2	09	606-607
046.0	01	056-057	054.72	01	075-076	065.9	18	865-866	077.8	02	124-125	085.3	09	606-607
046.11	01	056-057	054.73	03	154-156	066.0	18	865-866	077.98	02	124-125	085.4	09	606-607
046.19	01	056-057	054.74	01	097-099	066.1	18	865-866	077.99	02	124-125	085.5	09	606-607
046.2	01	056-057	054.79	18	865-866	066.2	01	097-099	078.0	09	606-607	085.9	18	867-869
046.3	01	056-057	054.8	18	865-866	066.3	18	865-866	078.10	09	606-607	086.0	05	314-316
046.71	01	056-057	054.9	09	606-607	066.40	18	865-866	078.11	09	606-607	086.1	18	867-869
046.72	01	056-057	055.0	01	097-099	066.41	18	865-866	078.12	09	606-607	086.2	18	867-869
046.79	01	056-057	055.1	04	177-179	066.42	18	865-866	078.19	09	606-607	086.3	18	867-869
046.8	01	056-057	055.2	03	152-153	066.49	18	865-866	078.2	18	865-866	086.4	18	867-869
046.9	01	056-057	055.71	02	124-125	066.8	18	865-866	078.3	16	814-816	086.5	18	867-869
047.0	01	075-076	055.79	18	865-866	066.9	18	865-866	078.4	18	865-866	086.9	18	867-869
047.1	01	075-076	055.8	18	865-866	070.0	07	441-443	078.5	18	865-866	087.0	18	867-869
047.8	01	075-076	055.9	18	865-866	070.71	07	441-443	078.6	11	689-690	087.1	18	867-869
047.9	01	075-076	056.00	01	073-074	070.1	07	441-443	078.7	18	865-866	087.9	18	867-869
048	01	075-076	056.01	01	097-099	070.20	07	441-443	078.81	01	091-093	088.0	18	867-869
049.0	01	075-076	056.09	01	097-099	070.21	07	441-443	078.82	06	391-392	088.81	18	867-869
049.1	01	075-076	056.71	08	553-554	070.22	07	441-443	078.88	18	865-866	088.82	18	867-869
049.8	01	097-099	056.79	18	865-866	070.23	07	441-443	078.89	18	865-866	088.89	18	867-869
049.9	01	097-099	056.8	18	865-866	070.30	07	441-443	079.0	18	865-866	088.9	18	867-869
050.1	18	865-866	056.9	18	865-866	070.31	07	441-443	079.1	18	865-866	090.0	18	867-869
050.2	18	865-866	057.0	18	865-866	070.32	07	441-443	079.2	18	865-866	090.1	18	867-869
050.9	18	865-866	057.8	18	865-866	070.33	07	441-443	079.3	18	865-866	090.2	18	867-869
051.01	18	865-866	057.9	18	865-866	070.41	07	441-443	079.4	18	865-866	090.3	02	124-125
051.02	18	865-866	058.10	18	865-866	070.42	07	441-443	079.50	18	865-866	090.40	01	097-099
051.1	09	606-607	058.11	18	865-866	070.43	07	441-443	079.51	18	865-866	090.41	01	097-099
051.2	09	606-607	058.12	18	865-866	070.44	07	441-443	079.52	18	865-866	090.42	01	097-099
051.9	18	865-866	058.21	01	097-099	070.49	07	441-443	079.53	18	865-866	090.49	01	097-099
052.0	01	097-099	058.29	01	097-099	070.51	07	441-443	079.59	18	865-866	090.5	18	867-869
052.1	04	177-179	058.81	09	606-607	070.52	07	441-443	079.6	18	865-866	090.6	18	867-869
052.2	01	097-099	058.82	09	606-607	070.53	07	441-443	079.81	18	865-866	090.7	18	867-869
052.7	18	865-866	058.89	09	606-607	070.54	07	441-443	079.83	18	865-866	090.9	18	867-869
052.8	18	865-866	059.00	18	865-866	070.59	07	441-443	079.88	18	865-866	091.0	12	727-728
052.9	18	865-866	059.01	18	865-866	070.6	07	441-443	079.89	18	865-866	091.0	13	757-759
053.0	01	075-076	059.09	18	865-866	070.70	07	441-443	079.98	18	865-866	091.1	06	393-395
053.10	01	073-074	059.10	18	865,866	070.71	07	441-443	079.99	18	865-866	091.2	18	867-869
053.11	01	073-074	059.11	18	865-866	070.9	07	441-443	080	18	867-869	091.3	09	606-607
053.12	01	073-074	059.12	18	865-866	071	01	097-099	081.0	18	867-869	091.4	16	814-816
053.13	01	073-074	059.19	18	865-866	072.0	12	727-728	081.1	18	867-869	091.50	02	124-125
053.14	01	097-099	059.21	18	865-866	072.1	01	075-076	081.2	18	867-869	091.51	02	124-125
053.19	01	073-074	059.22	18	865-866	072.2	01	097-099	081.9	18	867-869	091.52	02	124-125
053.20	02	124-125	059.29	18	865-866	072.3	07	438-440	082.0	18	867-869	091.61	08	539-541
053.21	02	124-125	059.8	18	865-866	072.71	07	441-443	082.1	18	867-869	091.62	07	441-443
053.22	02	124-125	059.9	18	865-866	072.72	01	073-074	082.2	18	867-869	091.69	06	393-395
053.29	02	124-125	060.0	18	865-866	072.79	18	865-866	082.3	18	867-869	091.7	18	867-869
053.71	03	154-156	060.1	18	865-866	072.8	18	865-866	082.40	18	867-869	091.81	01	097-099
053.79	18	865-866	060.9	18	865-866	072.9	18	865-866	082.41	18	867-869	091.82	09	606-607
053.8	18	865-866	061	18	865-866	073.0	04	177-179	082.49	18	867-869	091.89	18	867-869
053.9	09	595-596	062.0	01	097-099	073.7	18	865-866	082.8	18	867-869	091.9	18	867-869
054.0	09	606-607	062.1	01	097-099	073.8	18	865-866	082.9	18	867-869	092.0	18	867-869
054.10	12	727-728	062.2	01	097-099	073.9	18	865-866	083.0	18	867-869	092.9	18	867-869
054.10	13	757-759	062.3	01	097-099	074.0	03	152-153	083.1	18	867-869	093.0	05	306-307

Diagnosis Code/MDC/DRG List

DX	MDC	DRG	DX	MDC	DRG	DX	MDC	DRG	DX	MDC	DRG	DX	MDC	DRG
093.1	05	306-307	098.51	08	548-550	110.3	09	606-607	120.0	11	689-690	130.3	05	314-316
093.20	05	288-290	098.52	08	548-550	110.4	09	606-607	120.1	07	441-443	130.4	04	177-179
093.21	05	306-307	098.53	08	539-541	110.5	09	606-607	120.2	18	867-869	130.5	07	441-443
093.22	05	306-307	098.59	08	548-550	110.6	09	606-607	120.3	09	606-607	130.7	18	867-869
093.23	05	306-307	098.6	03	152-153	110.8	09	606-607	120.8	18	867-869	130.8	18	867-869
093.24	05	306-307	098.7	06	393-395	110.9	09	606-607	120.9	18	867-869	130.9	18	867-869
093.81	05	314-316	098.81	02	124-125	111.0	09	606-607	121.0	07	441-443	131.00	12	727-728
093.82	05	314-316	098.82	01	094-096	111.1	09	606-607	121.1	07	441-443	131.00	13	757-759
093.89	05	314-316	098.83	05	314-316	111.2	09	606-607	121.2	04	177-179	131.01	13	757-759
093.9	05	314-316	098.84	05	288-290	111.3	09	606-607	121.3	07	441-443	131.02	12	727-728
094.0	01	056-057	098.85	05	314-316	111.8	09	606-607	121.4	07	441-443	131.02	13	757-759
094.1	01	056-057	098.86	06	371-373	111.9	09	606-607	121.5	18	867-869	131.03	12	727-728
094.2	01	097-099	098.89	18	867-869	112.0	03	157-159	121.6	18	867-869	131.09	12	727-728
094.3	01	097-099	099.0	12	727-728	112.1	13	757-759	121.8	18	867-869	131.09	13	757-759
094.81	01	097-099	099.0	13	757-759	112.2	12	727-728	121.9	18	867-869	131.8	18	867-869
094.82	01	056-057	099.1	12	727-728	112.2	13	757-759	122.0	07	441-443	131.9	18	867-869
094.83	02	124-125	099.1	13	757-759	112.3	09	606-607	122.1	04	177-179	132.0	09	606-607
094.84	02	124-125	099.2	12	727-728	112.4	04	177-179	122.2	10	643-645	132.1	09	606-607
094.85	01	056-057	099.2	13	757-759	112.5	18	867-869	122.3	18	867-869	132.2	09	606-607
094.86	03	154-156	099.3	08	545-547	112.81	05	288-290	122.4	18	867-869	132.3	09	606-607
094.87	01	091-093	099.40	12	727-728	112.82	03	154-156	122.5	07	441-443	132.9	09	606-607
094.89	01	056-057	099.40	13	757-759	112.83	01	097-099	122.6	18	867-869	133.0	09	606-607
094.9	01	056-057	099.41	12	727-728	112.84	06	368-370	122.7	18	867-869	133.8	09	606-607
095.0	02	124-125	099.41	13	757-759	112.85	06	391-392	122.8	07	441-443	133.9	09	606-607
095.1	04	177-179	099.49	12	727-728	112.89	18	867-869	122.9	18	867-869	134.0	09	606-607
095.2	06	371-373	099.49	13	757-759	112.9	18	867-869	123.0	06	391-392	134.1	09	606-607
095.3	07	441-443	099.50	12	727-728	114.0	04	177-179	123.1	06	371-373	134.2	09	606-607
095.4	11	689-690	099.50	13	757-759	114.1	09	606-607	123.2	06	391-392	134.8	09	606-607
095.5	08	539-541	099.51	03	152-153	114.2	01	097-099	123.3	06	391-392	134.9	09	606-607
095.6	08	557-558	099.52	06	393-395	114.3	18	867-869	123.4	06	391-392	135	04	196-198
095.7	08	557-558	099.53	12	727-728	114.4	04	177-179	123.5	06	371-373	136.0	18	867-869
095.8	18	867-869	099.53	13	757-759	114.5	04	177-179	123.6	06	371-373	136.1	08	545-547
095.9	18	867-869	099.54	11	689-690	114.9	18	867-869	123.8	06	371-373	136.21	18	867-869
096	18	867-869	099.55	12	727-728	115.00	18	867-869	123.9	06	371-373	136.29	18	867-869
097.0	18	867-869	099.55	13	757-759	115.01	01	097-099	124	18	867-869	136.3	04	177-179
097.1	18	867-869	099.56	06	393-395	115.02	02	124-125	125.0	18	867-869	136.4	18	867-869
097.9	18	867-869	099.59	12	727-728	115.03	05	314-316	125.1	18	867-869	136.5	18	867-869
098.0	12	727-728	099.59	13	757-759	115.04	05	288-290	125.2	18	867-869	136.8	18	867-869
098.0	13	757-759	099.8	12	727-728	115.05	04	177-179	125.3	18	867-869	136.9	18	867-869
098.10	12	727-728	099.8	13	757-759	115.09	18	867-869	125.4	18	867-869	137.0	04	196-198
098.10	13	757-759	099.9	12	727-728	115.10	18	867-869	125.5	18	867-869	137.1	01	091-093
098.11	11	689-690	099.9	13	757-759	115.11	01	097-099	125.6	18	867-869	137.2	11	689-690
098.12	12	727-728	100.0	18	867-869	115.12	02	124-125	125.7	18	867-869	137.3	08	564-566
098.13	12	727-728	100.81	01	097-099	115.13	05	314-316	125.9	18	867-869	137.4	18	867-869
098.14	12	727-728	100.89	01	097-099	115.14	05	288-290	126.0	06	371-373	138	01	091-093
098.15	13	757-759	100.9	18	867-869	115.15	04	177-179	126.1	06	371-373	139.0	01	091-093
098.16	13	757-759	101	03	152-153	115.19	18	867-869	126.2	06	371-373	139.1	02	124-125
098.17	13	757-759	102.0	09	606-607	115.90	18	867-869	126.3	06	371-373	139.8	18	867-869
098.19	12	727-728	102.1	09	606-607	115.91	01	097-099	126.8	06	371-373			
098.19	13	757-759	102.2	09	606-607	115.92	02	124-125	126.9	06	371-373	**Neoplasms**		
098.2	12	727-728	102.3	09	606-607	115.93	05	314-316	127.0	06	391-392	140.0	03	146-148
098.2	13	757-759	102.4	09	606-607	115.94	05	288-290	127.1	06	391-392	140.1	03	146-148
098.30	11	689-690	102.5	03	154-156	115.95	04	177-179	127.2	06	391-392	140.3	03	146-148
098.31	11	689-690	102.6	08	548-550	115.99	18	867-869	127.3	06	391-392	140.4	03	146-148
098.32	12	727-728	102.7	18	867-869	116.0	18	867-869	127.4	06	391-392	140.5	03	146-148
098.33	12	727-728	102.8	18	867-869	116.1	18	867-869	127.5	06	391-392	140.6	03	146-148
098.34	12	727-728	102.9	18	867-869	116.2	18	867-869	127.6	06	391-392	140.8	03	146-148
098.35	13	757-759	103.0	09	606-607	117.0	18	867-869	127.7	06	391-392	140.9	03	146-148
098.36	13	757-759	103.1	09	606-607	117.1	18	867-869	127.8	18	867-869	141.0	03	146-148
098.37	13	757-759	103.2	18	867-869	117.2	18	867-869	127.9	06	391-392	141.1	03	146-148
098.38	12	727-728	103.3	09	606-607	117.3	18	867-869	128.0	18	867-869	141.2	03	146-148
098.39	13	757-759	103.9	18	867-869	117.4	18	867-869	128.1	18	867-869	141.3	03	146-148
098.40	02	124-125	104.0	18	867-869	117.5	18	867-869	128.8	18	867-869	141.4	03	146-148
098.41	02	124-125	104.8	18	867-869	117.6	18	867-869	128.9	18	867-869	141.5	03	146-148
098.42	02	124-125	104.9	18	867-869	117.7	18	867-869	129	06	391-392	141.6	03	146-148
098.43	02	124-125	110.0	09	606-607	117.8	18	867-869	130.0	01	097-099	141.8	03	146-148
098.49	02	124-125	110.1	09	606-607	117.9	18	867-869	130.1	02	124-125	141.9	03	146-148
098.50	08	548-550	110.2	09	606-607	118	18	867-869	130.2	02	124-125	142.0	03	146-148

DX	MDC	DRG	DX	MDC	DRG	DX	MDC	DRG	DX	MDC	DRG	DX	MDC	DRG
142.1	03	146-148	152.3	06	374-376	164.2	04	180-182	173.79	09	606-607	188.4	11	686-688
142.2	03	146-148	152.8	06	374-376	164.3	04	180-182	173.80	09	606-607	188.5	11	686-688
142.8	03	146-148	152.9	06	374-376	164.8	04	180-182	173.81	09	606-607	188.6	11	686-688
142.9	03	146-148	153.0	06	374-376	164.9	04	180-182	173.82	09	606-607	188.7	11	686-688
143.0	03	146-148	153.1	06	374-376	165.0	03	146-148	173.89	09	606-607	188.8	11	686-688
143.1	03	146-148	153.2	06	374-376	165.8	04	180-182	173.90	09	606-607	188.9	11	686-688
143.8	03	146-148	153.3	06	374-376	165.9	04	180-182	173.91	09	606-607	189.0	11	686-688
143.9	03	146-148	153.4	06	374-376	170.0	08	542-544	173.92	09	606-607	189.1	11	686-688
144.0	03	146-148	153.5	06	374-376	170.1	08	542-544	173.99	09	606-607	189.2	11	686-688
144.1	03	146-148	153.6	06	374-376	170.2	08	542-544	174.0	09	597-599	189.3	11	686-688
144.8	03	146-148	153.7	06	374-376	170.3	08	542-544	174.1	09	597-599	189.4	11	686-688
144.9	03	146-148	153.8	06	374-376	170.4	08	542-544	174.2	09	597-599	189.8	11	686-688
145.0	03	146-148	153.9	06	374-376	170.5	08	542-544	174.3	09	597-599	189.9	11	686-688
145.1	03	146-148	154.0	06	374-376	170.6	08	542-544	174.4	09	597-599	190.0	02	124-125
145.2	03	146-148	154.1	06	374-376	170.7	08	542-544	174.5	09	597-599	190.1	02	124-125
145.3	03	146-148	154.2	06	374-376	170.8	08	542-544	174.6	09	597-599	190.2	02	124-125
145.4	03	146-148	154.3	06	374-376	170.9	08	542-544	174.8	09	597-599	190.3	02	124-125
145.5	03	146-148	154.8	06	374-376	171.0	08	542-544	174.9	09	597-599	190.4	02	124-125
145.6	03	146-148	155.0	07	435-437	171.2	08	542-544	175.0	09	597-599	190.5	02	124-125
145.8	03	146-148	155.1	07	435-437	171.3	08	542-544	175.9	09	597-599	190.6	02	124-125
145.9	03	146-148	155.2	07	435-437	171.4	08	542-544	176.0	09	606-607	190.7	02	124-125
146.0	03	146-148	156.0	07	435-437	171.5	08	542-544	176.1	09	606-607	190.8	02	124-125
146.1	03	146-148	156.1	07	435-437	171.6	08	542-544	176.2	03	146-148	190.9	02	124-125
146.2	03	146-148	156.2	07	435-437	171.7	08	542-544	176.3	06	374-376	191.0	01	054-055
146.3	03	146-148	156.8	07	435-437	171.8	08	542-544	176.4	04	180-182	191.1	01	054-055
146.4	03	146-148	156.9	07	435-437	171.9	08	542-544	176.5	17	840-842	191.2	01	054-055
146.5	03	146-148	157.0	07	435-437	172.0	09	595-596	176.8	09	606-607	191.3	01	054-055
146.6	03	146-148	157.1	07	435-437	172.1	02	124-125	176.9	09	606-607	191.4	01	054-055
146.7	03	146-148	157.2	07	435-437	172.2	09	595-596	179	13	754-756	191.5	01	054-055
146.8	03	146-148	157.3	07	435-437	172.3	09	595-596	180.0	13	754-756	191.6	01	054-055
146.9	03	146-148	157.4	07	435-437	172.4	09	595-596	180.1	13	754-756	191.7	01	054-055
147.0	03	146-148	157.8	07	435-437	172.5	09	595-596	180.8	13	754-756	191.8	01	054-055
147.1	03	146-148	157.9	07	435-437	172.6	09	595-596	180.9	13	754-756	191.9	01	054-055
147.2	03	146-148	158.0	17	843-845	172.7	09	595-596	181	13	754-756	192.0	01	054-055
147.3	03	146-148	158.8	06	374-376	172.8	09	595-596	182.0	13	754-756	192.1	01	054-055
147.8	03	146-148	158.9	06	374-376	172.9	09	595-596	182.1	13	754-756	192.2	01	054-055
147.9	03	146-148	159.0	06	374-376	173.00	09	606-607	182.8	13	754-756	192.3	01	054-055
148.0	03	146-148	159.1	17	840-842	173.01	09	606-607	183.0	13	754-756	192.8	01	054-055
148.1	03	146-148	159.8	06	374-376	173.02	09	606-607	183.2	13	754-756	192.9	01	054-055
148.2	03	146-148	159.9	06	374-376	173.09	09	606-607	183.3	13	754-756	193	10	643-645
148.3	03	146-148	160.0	03	146-148	173.10	02	124-125	183.4	13	754-756	194.0	10	643-645
148.8	03	146-148	160.1	03	146-148	173.11	02	124-125	183.5	13	754-756	194.1	10	643-645
148.9	03	146-148	160.2	03	146-148	173.12	02	124-125	183.8	13	754-756	194.3	10	643-645
149.0	03	146-148	160.3	03	146-148	173.19	02	124-125	183.9	13	754-756	194.4	01	054-055
149.1	03	146-148	160.4	03	146-148	173.20	09	606-607	184.0	13	754-756	194.5	01	054-055
149.8	03	146-148	160.5	03	146-148	173.21	09	606-607	184.1	13	754-756	194.6	01	054-055
149.9	03	146-148	160.8	03	146-148	173.22	09	606-607	184.2	13	754-756	194.8	10	643-645
150.0	06	374-376	160.9	03	146-148	173.29	09	606-607	184.3	13	754-756	194.9	10	643-645
150.1	06	374-376	161.0	03	146-148	173.30	09	606-607	184.4	13	754-756	195.0	03	146-148
150.2	06	374-376	161.1	03	146-148	173.31	09	606-607	184.8	13	754-756	195.1	04	180-182
150.3	06	374-376	161.2	03	146-148	173.32	09	606-607	184.9	13	754-756	195.2	06	374-376
150.4	06	374-376	161.3	03	146-148	173.39	09	606-607	185	12	722-724	195.3	12	722-724
150.5	06	374-376	161.8	03	146-148	173.40	09	606-607	186.0	12	722-724	195.3	13	754-756
150.8	06	374-376	161.9	03	146-148	173.41	09	606-607	186.9	12	722-724	195.4	17	843-845
150.9	06	374-376	162.0	04	180-182	173.42	09	606-607	187.1	12	722-724	195.5	17	843-845
151.0	06	374-376	162.2	04	180-182	173.49	09	606-607	187.2	12	722-724	195.8	17	843-845
151.1	06	374-376	162.3	04	180-182	173.50	09	606-607	187.3	12	722-724	196.0	17	840-842
151.2	06	374-376	162.4	04	180-182	173.51	09	606-607	187.4	12	722-724	196.1	17	840-842
151.3	06	374-376	162.5	04	180-182	173.52	09	606-607	187.5	12	722-724	196.2	17	840-842
151.4	06	374-376	162.8	04	180-182	173.59	09	606-607	187.6	12	722-724	196.3	17	840-842
151.5	06	374-376	162.9	04	180-182	173.60	09	606-607	187.7	12	722-724	196.5	17	840-842
151.6	06	374-376	163.0	04	180-182	173.61	09	606-607	187.8	12	722-724	196.6	17	840-842
151.8	06	374-376	163.1	04	180-182	173.62	09	606-607	187.9	12	722-724	196.8	17	840-842
151.9	06	374-376	163.8	04	180-182	173.69	09	606-607	188.0	11	686-688	196.9	17	840-842
152.0	06	374-376	163.9	04	180-182	173.70	09	606-607	188.1	11	686-688	197.0	04	180-182
152.1	06	374-376	164.0	17	843-845	173.71	09	606-607	188.2	11	686-688	197.1	04	180-182
152.2	06	374-376	164.1	05	314-316	173.72	09	606-607	188.3	11	686-688	197.2	04	180-182

Diagnosis Code/MDC/DRG List

DX	MDC	DRG	DX	MDC	DRG	DX	MDC	DRG	DX	MDC	DRG	DX	MDC	DRG
197.3	04	180-182	200.52	17	840-842	201.47	17	840-842	202.33	17	840-842	203.82	17	840-842
197.4	06	374-376	200.53	17	840-842	201.48	17	840-842	202.34	17	840-842	204.00	17	834-836
197.5	06	374-376	200.54	17	840-842	201.50	17	840-842	202.35	17	840-842	204.01	17	834-836
197.6	06	374-376	200.55	17	840-842	201.51	17	840-842	202.36	17	840-842	204.02	17	834-839
197.7	07	435-437	200.56	17	840-842	201.52	17	840-842	202.37	17	840-842	204.10	17	840-842
197.8	06	374-376	200.57	17	840-842	201.53	17	840-842	202.38	17	840-842	204.11	17	840-842
198.0	11	686-688	200.58	17	840-842	201.54	17	840-842	202.40	17	840-842	204.12	17	840-842
198.1	11	686-688	200.60	17	840-842	201.55	17	840-842	202.41	17	840-842	204.20	17	840-842
198.2	09	597-599	200.61	17	840-842	201.56	17	840-842	202.42	17	840-842	204.21	17	840-842
198.3	01	054-055	200.62	17	840-842	201.57	17	840-842	202.43	17	840-842	204.22	17	840-842
198.4	01	054-055	200.63	17	840-842	201.58	17	840-842	202.44	17	840-842	204.80	17	840-842
198.5	08	542-544	200.64	17	840-842	201.60	17	840-842	202.45	17	840-842	204.81	17	840-842
198.6	13	754-756	200.65	17	840-842	201.61	17	840-842	202.46	17	840-842	204.82	17	840-842
198.7	10	643-645	200.66	17	840-842	201.62	17	840-842	202.47	17	840-842	204.90	17	840-842
198.81	09	597-599	200.67	17	840-842	201.63	17	840-842	202.48	17	840-842	204.91	17	840-842
198.82	12	722-724	200.68	17	840-842	201.64	17	840-842	202.50	17	843-845	204.92	17	840-842
198.82	13	754-756	200.70	17	840-842	201.65	17	840-842	202.51	17	843-845	205.00	17	834-836
198.89	17	843-845	200.71	17	840-842	201.66	17	840-842	202.52	17	843-845	205.01	17	834-836
199.0	17	843-845	200.72	17	840-842	201.67	17	840-842	202.53	17	843-845	205.02	17	834-839
199.1	17	843-845	200.73	17	840-842	201.68	17	840-842	202.54	17	843-845	205.10	17	840-842
199.2	17	843-845	200.74	17	840-842	201.70	17	840-842	202.55	17	843-845	205.11	17	840-842
200.00	17	840-842	200.75	17	840-842	201.71	17	840-842	202.56	17	843-845	205.12	17	840-842
200.01	17	840-842	200.76	17	840-842	201.72	17	840-842	202.57	17	843-845	205.20	17	840-842
200.02	17	840-842	200.77	17	840-842	201.73	17	840-842	202.58	17	843-845	205.21	17	840-842
200.03	17	840-842	200.78	17	840-842	201.74	17	840-842	202.60	17	840-842	205.22	17	840-842
200.04	17	840-842	200.80	17	840-842	201.75	17	840-842	202.61	17	840-842	205.30	17	840-842
200.05	17	840-842	200.81	17	840-842	201.76	17	840-842	202.62	17	840-842	205.31	17	840-842
200.06	17	840-842	200.82	17	840-842	201.77	17	840-842	202.63	17	840-842	205.32	17	840-842
200.07	17	840-842	200.83	17	840-842	201.78	17	840-842	202.64	17	840-842	205.80	17	840-842
200.08	17	840-842	200.84	17	840-842	201.90	17	840-842	202.65	17	840-842	205.81	17	840-842
200.10	17	840-842	200.85	17	840-842	201.91	17	840-842	202.66	17	840-842	205.82	17	840-842
200.11	17	840-842	200.86	17	840-842	201.92	17	840-842	202.67	17	840-842	205.90	17	840-842
200.12	17	840-842	200.87	17	840-842	201.93	17	840-842	202.68	17	840-842	205.91	17	840-842
200.13	17	840-842	200.88	17	840-842	201.94	17	840-842	202.70	17	840-842	205.92	17	840-842
200.14	17	840-842	201.00	17	840-842	201.95	17	840-842	202.71	17	840-842	206.00	17	834-836
200.15	17	840-842	201.01	17	840-842	201.96	17	840-842	202.72	17	840-842	206.01	17	834-836
200.16	17	840-842	201.02	17	840-842	201.97	17	840-842	202.73	17	840-842	206.02	17	834-839
200.17	17	840-842	201.03	17	840-842	201.98	17	840-842	202.74	17	840-842	206.10	17	840-842
200.18	17	840-842	201.04	17	840-842	202.00	17	840-842	202.75	17	840-842	206.11	17	840-842
200.20	17	840-842	201.05	17	840-842	202.01	17	840-842	202.76	17	840-842	206.12	17	840-842
200.21	17	840-842	201.06	17	840-842	202.02	17	840-842	202.77	17	840-842	206.20	17	840-842
200.22	17	840-842	201.07	17	840-842	202.03	17	840-842	202.78	17	840-842	206.21	17	840-842
200.23	17	840-842	201.08	17	840-842	202.04	17	840-842	202.80	17	840-842	206.22	17	840-842
200.24	17	840-842	201.10	17	840-842	202.05	17	840-842	202.81	17	840-842	206.80	17	840-842
200.25	17	840-842	201.11	17	840-842	202.06	17	840-842	202.82	17	840-842	206.81	17	840-842
200.26	17	840-842	201.12	17	840-842	202.07	17	840-842	202.83	17	840-842	206.82	17	840-842
200.27	17	840-842	201.13	17	840-842	202.08	17	840-842	202.84	17	840-842	206.90	17	840-842
200.28	17	840-842	201.14	17	840-842	202.10	17	840-842	202.85	17	840-842	206.91	17	840-842
200.30	17	840-842	201.15	17	840-842	202.11	17	840-842	202.86	17	840-842	206.92	17	840-842
200.31	17	840-842	201.16	17	840-842	202.12	17	840-842	202.87	17	840-842	207.00	17	834-836
200.32	17	840-842	201.17	17	840-842	202.13	17	840-842	202.88	17	840-842	207.01	17	834-836
200.33	17	840-842	201.18	17	840-842	202.14	17	840-842	202.90	17	840-842	207.02	17	834-839
200.34	17	840-842	201.20	17	840-842	202.15	17	840-842	202.91	17	840-842	207.10	17	840-842
200.35	17	840-842	201.21	17	840-842	202.16	17	840-842	202.92	17	840-842	207.11	17	840-842
200.36	17	840-842	201.22	17	840-842	202.17	17	840-842	202.93	17	840-842	207.12	17	840-842
200.37	17	840-842	201.23	17	840-842	202.18	17	840-842	202.94	17	840-842	207.20	17	840-842
200.38	17	840-842	201.24	17	840-842	202.20	17	840-842	202.95	17	840-842	207.21	17	840-842
200.30	17	840-842	201.25	17	840-842	202.21	17	840-842	202.96	17	840-842	207.22	17	840-842
200.41	17	840-842	201.26	17	840-842	202.22	17	840-842	202.97	17	840-842	207.80	17	840-842
200.42	17	840-842	201.27	17	840-842	202.23	17	840-842	202.98	17	840-842	207.81	17	840-842
200.43	17	840-842	201.28	17	840-842	202.24	17	840-842	203.00	17	840-842	207.82	17	840-842
200.44	17	840-842	201.40	17	840-842	202.25	17	840-842	203.01	17	840-842	208.00	17	834-836
200.45	17	840-842	201.41	17	840-842	202.26	17	840-842	203.02	17	840-842	208.01	17	834-836
200.46	17	840-842	201.42	17	840-842	202.27	17	840-842	203.10	17	840-842	208.02	17	834-839
200.47	17	840-842	201.43	17	840-842	202.28	17	840-842	203.11	17	840-842	208.10	17	840-842
200.48	17	840-842	201.44	17	840-842	202.30	17	840-842	203.12	17	840-842	208.11	17	840-842
200.50	17	840-842	201.45	17	840-842	202.31	17	840-842	203.80	17	840-842	208.12	17	840-842
200.51	17	840-842	201.46	17	840-842	202.32	17	840-842	203.81	17	840-842	208.20	17	840-842

DX....	MDC.....	DRG	DX....	MDC.....	DRG	DX....	MDC.....	DRG	DX....	MDC.....	DRG	DX....	MDC.....	DRG
208.21	17	840-842	210.3	03	157-159	218.9	13	760-761	230.6	06	374-376	237.9	01	054-055
208.22	17	840-842	210.4	03	157-159	219.0	13	760-761	230.7	06	374-376	238.0	08	542-544
208.80	17	840-842	210.5	03	154-156	219.1	13	760-761	230.8	07	435-437	238.1	08	564-566
208.81	17	840-842	210.6	03	154-156	219.8	13	760-761	230.9	06	374-376	238.2	09	606-607
208.82	17	840-842	210.7	03	154-156	219.9	13	760-761	231.0	03	146-148	238.3	09	597-599
208.90	17	840-842	210.8	03	154-156	220	13	760-761	231.1	04	180-182	238.4	17	840-842
208.91	17	840-842	210.9	03	154-156	221.0	13	760-761	231.2	04	180-182	238.5	17	840-842
208.92	17	840-842	211.0	06	393-395	221.1	13	760-761	231.8	04	180-182	238.6	17	840-842
209.00	06	374-376	211.1	06	393-395	221.2	13	760-761	231.9	04	180-182	238.71	16	814-816
209.01	06	374-376	211.2	06	393-395	221.8	13	760-761	232.0	09	606-607	238.72	16	811-812
209.02	06	374-376	211.3	06	393-395	221.9	13	760-761	232.1	02	124-125	238.73	16	811-812
209.03	06	374-376	211.4	06	393-395	222.0	12	729-730	232.2	09	606-607	238.74	16	811-812
209.10	06	374-376	211.5	07	441-443	222.1	12	729-730	232.3	09	606-607	238.75	16	811-812
209.11	06	374-376	211.6	07	438-440	222.2	12	729-730	232.4	09	606-607	238.76	17	840-842
209.12	06	374-376	211.7	10	643-645	222.3	12	729-730	232.5	09	606-607	238.77	21	919-921
209.13	06	374-376	211.8	06	393-395	222.4	12	729-730	232.6	09	606-607	238.79	17	840-842
209.14	06	374-376	211.9	06	393-395	222.8	12	729-730	232.7	09	606-607	238.8	17	843-845
209.15	06	374-376	212.0	03	154-156	222.9	12	729-730	232.8	09	606-607	238.9	17	843-845
209.16	06	374-376	212.1	03	154-156	223.0	11	686-688	232.9	09	606-607	239.0	06	374-376
209.17	06	374-376	212.2	04	180-182	223.1	11	686-688	233.0	09	597-599	239.1	04	180-182
209.20	17	843-845	212.3	04	180-182	223.2	11	686-688	233.1	13	754-756	239.2	08	564-566
209.21	06	374-376	212.4	04	180-182	223.3	11	686-688	233.2	13	754-756	239.3	09	600-601
209.22	17	843-845	212.5	04	180-182	223.81	11	686-688	233.30	13	754-756	239.4	11	686-688
209.23	06	374-376	212.6	16	814-816	223.89	11	686-688	233.31	13	754-756	239.5	11	686-688
209.24	11	686-688	212.7	05	314-316	223.9	11	686-688	233.32	13	754-756	239.6	01	054-055
209.25	06	374-376	212.8	04	180-182	224.0	02	124-125	233.39	13	754-756	239.7	10	643-645
209.26	06	374-376	212.9	04	180-182	224.1	02	124-125	233.4	12	722-724	239.81	17	843-845
209.27	06	374-376	213.0	08	564-566	224.2	02	124-125	233.5	12	722-724	239.89	17	843-845
209.29	17	843-845	213.1	03	157-159	224.3	02	124-125	233.6	12	722-724	239.9	17	843-845
209.30	17	843-845	213.2	08	564-566	224.4	02	124-125	233.7	11	686-688			
209.31	09	595-596	213.3	04	180-182	224.5	02	124-125	233.9	11	686-688	**Endocrine, Nutritional and**		
209.32	09	595-596	213.4	08	564-566	224.6	02	124-125	234.0	02	124-125	**Metabolic Diseases, and**		
209.33	09	595-596	213.5	08	564-566	224.7	02	124-125	234.8	17	843-845	**Immunity Diseases**		
209.34	09	595-596	213.6	08	564-566	224.8	02	124-125	234.9	17	843-845	240.0	10	643-645
209.35	09	595-596	213.7	08	564-566	224.9	02	124-125	235.0	03	146-148	240.9	10	643-645
209.36	09	595-596	213.8	08	564-566	225.0	01	054-055	235.1	03	146-148	241.0	10	643-645
209.40	06	393-395	213.9	08	564-566	225.1	01	054-055	235.2	06	374-376	241.1	10	643-645
209.41	06	393-395	214.0	09	606-607	225.2	01	054-055	235.3	07	435-437	241.9	10	643-645
209.42	06	393-395	214.1	09	606-607	225.3	01	054-055	235.4	06	374-376	242.00	10	643-645
209.43	06	393-395	214.2	04	180-182	225.4	01	054-055	235.5	06	374-376	242.01	10	643-645
209.50	06	393-395	214.3	06	393-395	225.8	01	054-055	235.6	03	146-148	242.10	10	643-645
209.51	06	393-395	214.4	12	729-730	225.9	01	054-055	235.7	04	180-182	242.11	10	643-645
209.52	06	393-395	214.8	09	606-607	226	10	643-645	235.8	04	180-182	242.20	10	643-645
209.53	06	393-395	214.9	09	606-607	227.0	10	643-645	235.9	04	180-182	242.21	10	643-645
209.54	06	393-395	215.0	08	564-566	227.1	10	643-645	236.0	13	754-756	242.30	10	643-645
209.55	06	393-395	215.2	08	564-566	227.3	10	643-645	236.1	13	754-756	242.31	10	643-645
209.56	06	393-395	215.3	08	564-566	227.4	01	054-055	236.2	13	754-756	242.40	10	643-645
209.57	06	393-395	215.4	08	564-566	227.5	01	054-055	236.3	13	754-756	242.41	10	643-645
209.60	17	843-845	215.5	08	564-566	227.6	01	054-055	234.4	12	722-724	242.80	10	643-645
209.61	04	180-182	215.6	08	564-566	227.8	10	643-645	236.5	12	722-724	242.81	10	643-645
209.62	16	814-816	215.7	08	564-566	227.9	10	643-645	236.6	12	722-724	242.90	10	643-645
209.63	06	393-395	215.8	08	564-566	228.00	05	314-316	236.7	11	686-688	242.91	10	643-645
209.64	11	686-688	215.9	08	564-566	228.01	09	606-607	236.90	11	686-688	243	10	643-645
209.65	06	393-395	216.0	09	606-607	228.02	01	091-093	236.91	11	686-688	244.0	10	643-645
209.66	06	393-395	216.1	02	124-125	228.03	02	124-125	236.99	11	686-688	244.1	10	643-645
209.67	06	393-395	216.2	09	606-607	228.04	06	391-392	237.0	10	643-645	244.2	10	643-645
209.69	17	843-845	216.3	09	606-607	228.09	05	314-316	237.1	01	054-055	244.3	10	643-645
209.70	17	843-845	216.4	09	606-607	228.1	16	814-816	237.2	10	643-645	244.8	10	643-645
209.71	17	840-842	216.5	09	606-607	229.0	16	814-816	237.3	01	054-055	244.9	10	643-645
209.72	07	435-437	216.6	09	606-607	229.8	17	843-845	237.4	10	643-645	245.0	10	643-645
209.73	08	542-544	216.7	09	606-607	229.9	17	843-845	237.5	01	054-055	245.1	10	643-645
209.74	06	374-376	216.8	09	606-607	230.0	03	146-148	237.6	01	054-055	245.2	10	643-645
209.75	17	843-845	216.9	09	606-607	230.1	06	374-376	237.70	01	091-093	245.3	10	643-645
209.79	17	843-845	217	09	606-607	230.2	06	374-376	237.71	01	091-093	245.4	10	643-645
210.0	03	157-159	218.0	13	760-761	230.3	06	374-376	237.72	01	091-093	245.8	10	643-645
210.1	03	157-159	218.1	13	760-761	230.4	06	374-376	237.73	01	091-093	245.9	10	643-645
210.2	03	154-156	218.2	13	760-761	230.5	06	374-376	237.79	01	091-093	246.0	10	643-645
												246.1	10	643-645

Diagnosis Code/MDC/DRG List

DX	MDC	DRG	DX	MDC	DRG	DX	MDC	DRG	DX	MDC	DRG	DX	MDC	DRG
246.2	10	643-645	251.4	10	643-645	260	10	640-641	273.8	17	843-845	278.1	10	640-641
246.3	10	643-645	251.5	06	380-382	261	10	640-641	273.9	17	843-845	278.2	10	640-641
246.8	10	643-645	251.8	10	643-645	262	10	640-641	274.00	08	553-554	278.3	10	640-641
246.9	10	643-645	251.9	10	643-645	263.0	10	640-641	274.01	08	553-554	278.4	10	640-641
249.00	10	637-639	252.00	10	643-645	263.1	10	640-641	274.02	08	553-554	278.8	10	640-641
249.01	10	637-639	252.01	10	643-645	263.2	10	640-641	274.03	08	553-554	279.00	16	814-816
249.10	10	637-639	252.02	10	643-645	263.8	10	640-641	274.10	11	698-700	279.01	16	814-816
249.11	10	637-639	252.08	10	643-645	263.9	10	640-641	274.11	11	691-694	279.02	16	814-816
249.20	10	637-639	252.1	10	643-645	264.0	02	124-125	274.19	11	698-700	279.03	16	814-816
249.21	10	637-639	252.8	10	643-645	264.1	02	124-125	274.81	08	553-554	279.04	16	814-816
249.30	10	637-639	252.9	10	643-645	264.2	02	124-125	274.82	08	553-554	279.05	16	814-816
249.31	10	637-639	253.0	10	643-645	264.3	02	124-125	274.89	08	553-554	279.06	16	814-816
249.40	11	698-700	253.1	10	643-645	264.4	02	124-125	274.9	08	553-554	279.09	16	814-816
249.41	11	698-700	253.2	10	643-645	264.5	02	124-125	275.01	10	642	279.10	16	814-816
249.50	02	124-125	253.3	10	643-645	264.6	02	124-125	275.02	10	642	279.11	16	808-810
249.51	02	124-125	253.4	10	643-645	264.7	02	124-125	275.03	10	642	279.12	16	808-810
249.60	01	073-074	253.5	10	643-645	264.8	10	640-641	275.09	10	642	279.13	16	808-810
249.61	01	073-074	253.6	10	643-645	264.9	10	640-641	275.1	10	642	279.19	16	808-810
249.70	05	299-301	253.7	10	643-645	265.0	10	640-641	275.2	10	640-641	279.2	16	808-810
249.71	05	299-301	253.8	10	643-645	265.1	10	640-641	275.3	10	642	279.3	16	814-816
249.80	10	637-639	253.9	10	643-645	265.2	10	640-641	275.40	10	640-641	279.41	08	545-547
249.81	10	637-639	254.0	16	814-816	266.0	10	640-641	275.41	10	640-641	279.49	08	545-547
249.90	10	637-639	254.1	16	814-816	266.1	10	640-641	275.42	10	640-641	279.50	16	808-810
249.91	10	637-639	254.8	16	814-816	266.2	10	640-641	275.49	10	640-641	279.51	16	808-810
250.00	10	637-639	254.9	16	814-816	266.9	10	640-641	275.5	10	640-641	279.52	16	808-810
250.01	10	637-639	255.0	10	643-645	267	10	640-641	275.8	10	642	279.53	16	808-810
250.02	10	637-639	255.10	10	643-645	268.0	08	553-554	275.9	10	642	279.8	16	814-816
250.03	10	637-639	255.11	10	643-645	268.1	08	553-554	276.0	10	640-641	279.9	16	814-816
250.10	10	637-639	255.12	10	643-645	268.2	08	553-554	276.1	10	640-641			
250.11	10	637-639	255.13	10	643-645	268.9	10	640-641	276.2	10	640-641			
250.12	10	637-639	255.14	10	643-645	269.0	10	640-641	276.3	10	640-641			
250.13	10	637-639	255.2	10	643-645	269.1	10	640-641	276.4	10	640-641			

Diseases of the Blood and Blood Forming Organs

DX	MDC	DRG
250.20	10	637-639
250.21	10	637-639
250.22	10	637-639
250.23	10	637-639
250.30	10	637-639
250.31	10	637-639
250.32	10	637-639
250.33	10	637-639
250.40	11	698-700
250.41	11	698-700
250.42	11	698-700
250.43	11	698-700
250.50	02	124-125
250.51	02	124-125
250.52	02	124-125
250.53	02	124-125
250.60	01	073-074
250.61	01	073-074
250.62	01	073-074
250.63	01	073-074
250.70	05	299-301
250.71	05	299-301
250.72	05	299-301
250.73	05	299-301
250.80	10	637-639
250.81	10	637-639
250.82	10	637-639
250.83	10	637-639
250.90	10	637-639
250.91	10	637-639
250.92	10	637-639
250.93	10	637-639
251.0	10	640-641
251.1	10	643-645
251.2	10	640-641
251.3	10	640-641

DX	MDC	DRG
255.3	10	643-645
255.41	10	643-645
255.42	10	643-645
255.5	10	643-645
255.6	10	643-645
255.8	10	643-645
255.9	10	643-645
256.0	13	760-761
256.1	13	760-761
256.2	13	760-761
256.31	13	760-761
256.39	13	760-761
256.4	13	760-761
256.8	13	760-761
256.9	13	760-761
257.0	10	643-645
257.1	10	643-645
257.2	10	643-645
257.8	10	643-645
257.9	10	643-645
258.01	10	643-645
258.02	10	643-645
258.03	10	643-645
258.1	10	643-645
258.8	10	643-645
258.9	10	643-645
259.0	10	643-645
259.1	10	643-645
259.2	10	643-645
259.3	10	643-645
259.4	10	643-645
259.50	10	643-645
259.51	10	643-645
259.52	10	643-645
259.8	10	643-645
259.9	10	643-645

DX	MDC	DRG
269.2	10	640-641
269.3	10	640-641
269.8	10	640-641
269.9	10	640-641
270.0	10	642
270.1	10	642
270.2	10	642
270.3	10	642
270.4	10	642
270.5	10	642
270.6	10	642
270.7	10	642
270.8	10	642
270.9	10	642
271.0	10	642
271.1	10	642
271.2	06	391-392
271.3	06	391-392
271.4	10	642
271.8	10	642
271.9	10	642
272.0	10	642
272.1	10	642
272.2	10	642
272.3	10	642
272.4	10	642
272.5	10	642
272.6	10	642
272.7	10	642
272.8	10	642
272.9	10	642
273.0	16	814-816
273.1	16	814-816
273.2	17	840-842
273.3	17	840-842
273.4	10	642

DX	MDC	DRG
276.50	10	640-641
276.51	10	640-641
276.52	10	640-641
276.61	10	640-641
276.69	10	640-641
276.7	10	640-641
276.8	10	640-641
276.9	10	640-641
277.00	10	640-641
277.01	15	791, 793
277.02	04	177-179
277.03	06	393-395
277.09	10	640-641
277.1	10	642
277.2	10	642
277.30	08	545-547
277.31	08	545-547
277.39	08	545-547
277.4	07	441-443
277.5	10	642
277.6	10	642
277.7	10	642
277.81	10	642
277.82	10	642
277.83	10	642
277.84	10	642
277.85	10	642
277.86	10	642
277.87	10	642
277.88	11	682-684
277.89	10	642
277.9	10	642
278.00	10	640-641
278.01	10	640-641
278.02	10	640-641
278.03	04	205-206

Column 5 — **Diseases of the Blood and Blood Forming Organs**

DX	MDC	DRG
280.0	16	811-812
280.1	16	811-812
280.8	16	811-812
280.9	16	811-812
281.0	16	811-812
281.1	16	811-812
281.2	16	811-812
281.3	16	811-812
281.4	16	811-812
281.8	16	811-812
281.9	16	811-812
282.0	16	811-812
282.1	16	811-812
282.2	16	811-812
282.3	16	811-812
282.40	16	811-812
282.41	16	811-812
282.42	16	811-812
282.43	16	811-812
282.44	16	811-812
282.45	16	811-812
282.46	16	811-812
282.47	16	811-812
282.49	16	811-812
282.5	16	811-812
282.60	16	811-812
282.61	16	811-812
282.62	16	811-812
282.63	16	811-812
282.64	16	811-812
282.68	16	811-812
282.69	16	811-812
282.7	16	811-812
282.8	16	811-812
282.9	16	811-812
283.0	16	808-810
283.10	16	808-810
283.11	16	811-812

DX	MDC	DRG
283.19	16	808-810
283.2	16	808-810
283.9	16	808-810
284.01	16	808-810
284.09	16	808-810
284.11	16	808-810
284.12	16	808-810
284.19	16	808-810
284.2	17	840-842
284.81	16	808-810
284.89	16	808-810
284.9	16	808-810
285.0	16	811-812
285.1	16	811-812
285.21	16	811-812
285.22	16	811-812
285.29	16	811-812
285.3	16	811-812
285.8	16	811-812
285.9	16	811-812
286.0	16	813
286.1	16	813
286.2	16	813
286.3	16	813
286.4	16	813
286.52	16	813
286.53	16	814-816
286.59	16	813
286.6	16	813
286.7	16	813
286.9	16	813
287.0	16	813
287.1	16	813
287.2	16	813
287.30	16	813
287.31	16	813
287.32	16	813
287.33	16	813
287.39	16	813
287.41	16	813
287.49	16	813
287.5	16	813
287.8	16	813
287.9	16	813
288.00	16	808-810
288.01	16	808-810
288.02	16	808-810
288.03	16	808-810
288.04	16	808-810
288.09	16	808-810
288.1	16	808-810
288.2	16	808-810
288.3	16	814-816
288.4	16	814-816
288.50	16	814-816
288.51	16	814-816
288.59	16	814-816
288.60	16	814-816
288.61	16	814-816
288.62	16	814-816
288.63	16	814-816
288.64	16	814-816
288.65	16	814-816
288.66	16	814-816
288.69	16	814-816
288.8	16	814-816
288.9	16	814-816
289.0	16	814-816
289.1	16	814-816
289.2	06	393-395
289.3	16	814-816
289.4	16	814-816
289.50	16	814-816
289.51	16	814-816
289.52	16	814-816
289.53	16	814-816
289.59	16	814-816
289.6	16	814-816
289.7	16	811-812
289.81	16	814-816
289.82	16	814-816
289.83	17	840-842
289.84	16	813
289.89	16	814-816
289.9	16	814-816

Mental Disorders

DX	MDC	DRG
290.0	19	884
290.10	19	884
290.11	19	884
290.12	19	884
290.13	19	884
290.20	19	884
290.21	19	884
290.3	19	884
290.40	19	884
290.41	19	884
290.42	19	884
290.43	19	884
290.8	19	884
290.9	19	884
291.0	20	894-897
291.1	20	894-897
291.2	20	894-897
291.3	20	894-897
291.4	20	894-897
291.5	20	894-897
291.81	20	894-897
291.82	20	894-897
291.89	20	894-897
291.9	20	894-897
292.0	20	894-897
292.11	20	894-897
292.12	20	894-897
292.2	20	894-897
292.81	20	894-897
292.82	20	894-897
292.83	20	894-897
292.84	20	894-897
292.85	20	894-897
292.89	20	894-897
292.9	20	894-897
293.0	19	880
293.1	19	880
293.81	19	884
293.82	19	884
293.83	19	884
293.84	19	884
293.89	19	884
293.9	19	880
294.10	19	884
294.11	19	884
294.20	19	884
294.21	19	884
294.8	19	884
294.9	19	884
295.00	19	885
295.01	19	885
295.02	19	885
295.03	19	885
295.04	19	885
295.05	19	885
295.10	19	885
295.11	19	885
295.12	19	885
295.13	19	885
295.14	19	885
295.15	19	885
295.20	19	885
295.21	19	885
295.22	19	885
295.23	19	885
295.24	19	885
295.25	19	885
295.30	19	885
295.31	19	885
295.32	19	885
295.33	19	885
295.34	19	885
295.35	19	885
295.40	19	885
295.41	19	885
295.42	19	885
295.43	19	885
295.44	19	885
295.45	19	885
295.50	19	885
295.51	19	885
295.52	19	885
295.53	19	885
295.54	19	885
295.55	19	885
295.60	19	885
295.61	19	885
295.62	19	885
295.63	19	885
295.64	19	885
295.65	19	885
295.70	19	885
295.71	19	885
295.72	19	885
295.73	19	885
295.74	19	885
295.75	19	885
295.80	19	885
295.81	19	885
295.82	19	885
295.83	19	885
295.84	19	885
295.85	19	885
295.90	19	885
295.91	19	885
295.92	19	885
295.93	19	885
295.94	19	885
295.95	19	885
296.00	19	885
296.01	19	885
296.02	19	885
296.03	19	885
296.04	19	885
296.05	19	885
296.06	19	885
296.10	19	885
296.11	19	885
296.12	19	885
296.13	19	885
296.14	19	885
296.15	19	885
296.16	19	885
296.20	19	885
296.21	19	885
296.22	19	885
296.23	19	885
296.24	19	885
296.25	19	885
296.26	19	885
296.30	19	885
296.31	19	885
296.32	19	885
296.33	19	885
296.34	19	885
296.35	19	885
296.36	19	885
296.40	19	885
296.41	19	885
296.42	19	885
296.43	19	885
296.44	19	885
296.45	19	885
296.46	19	885
296.50	19	885
296.51	19	885
296.52	19	885
296.53	19	885
296.54	19	885
296.55	19	885
296.56	19	885
296.60	19	885
296.61	19	885
296.62	19	885
296.63	19	885
296.64	19	885
296.65	19	885
296.66	19	885
296.7	19	885
296.80	19	885
296.81	19	885
296.82	19	885
296.89	19	885
296.90	19	885
296.99	19	885
297.0	19	885
297.1	19	885
297.2	19	885
297.3	19	885
297.8	19	885
297.9	19	885
298.0	19	885
298.1	19	885
298.2	19	887
298.3	19	885
298.4	19	885
298.8	19	885
298.9	19	885
299.00	19	884
299.01	19	884
299.10	19	884
299.11	19	884
299.80	19	885
299.81	19	885
299.90	19	885
299.91	19	885
300.00	19	880
300.01	19	880
300.02	19	880
300.09	19	880
300.10	19	880
300.11	19	880
300.12	19	880
300.13	19	880
300.14	19	883
300.15	19	880
300.16	19	880
300.19	19	880
300.20	19	882
300.21	19	882
300.22	19	882
300.23	19	882
300.29	19	882
300.3	19	882
300.4	19	881
300.5	19	882
300.6	19	882
300.7	19	882
300.81	19	882
300.82	19	882
300.89	19	882
300.9	19	880
301.0	19	883
301.10	19	883
301.11	19	883
301.12	19	881
301.13	19	883
301.20	19	883
301.21	19	883
301.22	19	883
301.3	19	883
301.4	19	883
301.50	19	883
301.51	19	883
301.59	19	883
301.6	19	883
301.7	19	883
301.81	19	883
301.82	19	883
301.83	19	883
301.84	19	883
301.89	19	883
301.9	19	883
302.0	19	887
302.1	19	887
302.2	19	887
302.3	19	887
302.4	19	887
302.50	19	887
302.51	19	887
302.52	19	887
302.53	19	887
302.6	19	887
302.70	19	887
302.71	19	887
302.72	19	887
302.73	19	887
302.74	19	887
302.75	19	887

Diagnosis Code/MDC/DRG List

DX	MDC	DRG	DX	MDC	DRG	DX	MDC	DRG	DX	MDC	DRG	DX	MDC	DRG
302.76	19	887	305.32	20	894-897	307.9	19	884	314.8	19	886	327.09	19	887
302.79	19	887	305.33	20	894-897	308.0	19	880	314.9	19	886	327.10	19	887
302.81	19	887	305.40	20	894-897	308.1	19	880	315.00	19	886	327.11	19	887
302.82	19	887	305.41	20	894-897	308.2	19	880	315.01	19	886	327.12	19	887
302.83	19	887	305.42	20	894-897	308.3	19	880	315.02	19	886	327.13	19	887
302.84	19	887	305.43	20	894-897	308.4	19	880	315.09	19	886	327.14	19	887
302.85	19	887	305.50	20	894-897	308.9	19	880	315.1	19	886	327.15	19	887
302.89	19	887	305.51	20	894-897	309.0	19	881	315.2	19	886	327.19	19	887
302.9	19	887	305.52	20	894-897	309.1	19	881	315.31	19	886	327.20	03	154-156
303.00	20	894-897	305.53	20	894-897	309.21	19	882	315.32	19	886	327.21	01	091-093
303.01	20	894-897	305.60	20	894-897	309.22	19	882	315.34	19	886	327.22	04	204
303.02	20	894-897	305.61	20	894-897	309.23	19	882	315.35	01	091-093	327.23	03	154-156
303.03	20	894-897	305.62	20	894-897	309.24	19	882	315.39	19	886	327.24	03	154-156
303.90	20	894-897	305.63	20	894-897	309.28	19	882	315.4	19	886	327.25	01	091-093
303.91	20	894-897	305.70	20	894-897	309.29	19	882	315.5	19	886	327.26	03	154-156
303.92	20	894-897	305.71	20	894-897	309.3	19	882	315.8	19	886	327.27	01	091-093
303.93	20	894-897	305.72	20	894-897	309.4	19	882	315.9	19	886	327.29	03	154-156
304.00	20	894-897	305.73	20	894-897	309.81	19	882	316	19	884	327.30	01	091-093
304.01	20	894-897	305.80	20	894-897	309.82	19	882	317	19	884	327.31	01	091-093
304.02	20	894-897	305.81	20	894-897	309.83	19	882	318.0	19	884	327.32	01	091-093
304.03	20	894-897	305.82	20	894-897	309.89	19	882	318.1	19	884	327.33	01	091-093
304.10	20	894-897	305.83	20	894-897	309.9	19	882	318.2	19	884	327.34	01	091-093
304.11	20	894-897	305.90	20	894-897	310.0	19	884	319	19	884	327.35	01	091-093
304.12	20	894-897	305.91	20	894-897	310.1	19	884				327.36	01	091-093
304.13	20	894-897	305.92	20	894-897	310.2	01	100-103	**Diseases of the Nervous**			327.37	01	091-093
304.20	20	894-897	305.93	20	894-897	310.81	01	056-057	**System and Sense Organs**			327.39	01	091-093
304.21	20	894-897	306.0	08	557-558	310.89	01	056-057	320.0	01	094-096	327.40	03	154-156
304.22	20	894-897	306.1	04	205-206	310.9	19	884	320.1	01	094-096	327.41	01	091-093
304.23	20	894-897	306.2	05	314-316	311	19	881	320.2	01	094-096	327.42	03	154-156
304.30	20	894-897	306.3	09	606-607	312.00	19	886	320.3	01	094-096	327.43	01	091-093
304.31	20	894-897	306.4	06	391-392	312.01	19	886	320.7	01	094-096	327.44	03	154-156
304.32	20	894-897	306.50	11	698-700	312.02	19	886	320.81	01	094-096	327.49	03	154-156
304.33	20	894-897	306.51	13	760-761	312.03	19	886	320.82	01	094-096	327.51	01	091-093
304.40	20	894-897	306.52	13	760-761	312.10	19	886	320.89	01	094-096	327.52	01	091-093
304.41	20	894-897	306.53	11	698-700	312.11	19	886	320.9	01	094-096	327.53	03	154-156
304.42	20	894-897	306.59	11	698-700	312.12	19	886	321.0	01	097-099	327.59	03	154-156
304.43	20	894-897	306.6	10	643-645	312.13	19	886	321.1	01	097-099	327.8	03	154-156
304.50	20	894-897	306.7	19	882	312.20	19	886	321.2	01	097-099	330.0	01	056-057
304.51	20	894-897	306.8	19	887	312.21	19	886	321.3	01	097-099	330.1	01	056-057
304.52	20	894-897	306.9	19	882	312.22	19	886	321.4	01	097-099	330.2	01	056-057
304.53	20	894-897	307.0	19	887	312.23	19	886	321.8	01	097-099	330.3	01	056-057
304.60	20	894-897	307.1	19	883	312.30	19	886	322.0	01	097-099	330.8	01	056-057
304.61	20	894-897	307.20	01	091-093	312.31	19	883	322.1	01	097-099	330.9	01	056-057
304.62	20	894-897	307.21	01	091-093	312.32	19	883	322.2	01	097-099	331.0	01	056-057
304.63	20	894-897	307.22	01	091-093	312.33	19	886	322.9	01	097-099	331.11	01	056-057
304.70	20	894-897	307.23	01	091-093	312.34	19	883	323.01	01	097-099	331.19	01	056-057
304.71	20	894-897	307.3	19	887	312.35	19	883	323.02	01	097-099	331.2	01	056-057
304.72	20	894-897	307.40	19	887	312.39	19	883	323.1	01	097-099	331.3	01	056-057
304.73	20	894-897	307.41	19	887	312.4	19	886	323.2	01	097-099	331.4	01	056-057
304.80	20	894-897	307.42	19	887	312.81	19	886	323.41	01	097-099	331.5	01	056-057
304.81	20	894-897	307.43	19	887	312.82	19	886	323.42	01	097-099	331.6	01	056-057
304.82	20	894-897	307.44	19	887	312.89	19	886	323.51	01	097-099	331.7	01	056-057
304.83	20	894-897	307.45	19	887	312.9	19	886	323.52	01	097-099	331.81	01	091-093
304.90	20	894-897	307.46	19	887	313.0	19	882	323.61	01	097-099	331.82	01	056-057
304.91	20	894-897	307.47	19	887	313.1	19	882	323.62	01	097-099	331.83	01	056-057
304.92	20	894-897	307.48	19	887	313.21	19	886	323.63	01	097-099	331.89	01	056-057
304.93	20	894-897	307.49	19	887	313.22	19	886	323.71	01	091-093	331.9	01	056-057
305.00	20	894-897	307.50	19	887	313.23	19	886	323.72	01	091-093	332.0	01	056-057
305.01	20	894-897	307.51	19	887	313.3	19	886	323.81	01	097-099	332.1	01	056-057
305.02	20	894-897	307.52	19	886	313.81	19	886	323.82	01	097-099	333.0	01	056-057
305.03	20	894-897	307.53	19	882	313.82	19	886	323.9	01	097-099	333.1	01	091-093
305.1	23	951	307.54	19	882	313.83	19	886	324.0	01	094-096	333.2	01	091-093
305.20	20	894-897	307.59	19	887	313.89	19	886	324.1	01	094-096	333.3	01	091-093
305.21	20	894-897	307.6	19	886	313.9	19	886	324.9	01	094-096	333.4	01	056-057
305.22	20	894-897	307.7	19	886	314.00	19	886	325	01	091-093	333.5	01	056-057
305.23	20	894-897	307.80	19	882	314.01	19	886	326	01	091-093	333.6	01	056-057
305.30	20	894-897	307.81	01	100-103	314.1	19	886	327.00	19	887	333.71	01	056-057
305.31	20	894-897	307.89	19	882	314.2	19	886	327.01	19	887	333.72	01	091-093
									327.02	19	887			

DX	MDC	DRG
333.79	01	091-093
333.81	02	124-125
333.82	01	091-093
333.83	01	091-093
333.84	01	091-093
333.85	01	091-093
333.89	01	091-093
333.90	01	056-057
333.91	01	091-093
333.92	01	091-093
333.93	01	091-093
333.94	01	056-057
333.99	01	056-057
334.0	01	058-060
334.1	01	058-060
334.2	01	058-060
334.3	01	058-060
334.4	01	058-060
334.8	01	058-060
334.9	01	058-060
335.0	01	056-057
335.10	01	056-057
335.11	01	056-057
335.19	01	056-057
335.20	01	056-057
335.21	01	056-057
335.22	01	056-057
335.23	01	056-057
335.24	01	056-057
335.29	01	056-057
335.8	01	056-057
335.9	01	056-057
336.0	01	056-057
336.1	01	091-093
336.2	01	091-093
336.3	01	091-093
336.8	01	091-093
336.9	01	091-093
337.00	01	073-074
337.01	01	073-074
337.09	01	073-074
337.1	01	073-074
337.20	01	073-074
337.21	01	073-074
337.22	01	073-074
337.29	01	073-074
337.3	01	073-074
337.9	01	073-074
338.0	01	091-093
338.11	23	947-948
338.12	23	947-948
338.18	23	947-948
338.19	23	947-948
338.21	01	091-093
338.22	01	091-093
338.28	01	091-093
338.29	01	091-093
338.3	23	947-948
338.4	01	091-093
339.00	01	102-103
339.01	01	102-103
339.02	01	102-103
339.03	01	102-103
339.04	01	102-103
339.05	01	102-103
339.09	01	102-103
339.10	01	102-103
339.11	01	102-103
339.12	01	102-103
339.20	01	102-103
339.21	01	102-103
339.22	01	102-103
339.3	01	102-103
339.41	01	102-103
339.42	01	102-103
339.43	01	102-103
339.44	01	102-103
339.81	01	102-103
339.82	01	102-103
339.83	01	102-103
339.84	01	102-103
339.85	01	102-103
339.89	01	102-103
340	01	058-060
341.0	01	058-060
341.1	01	058-060
341.20	01	097-099
341.21	01	097-099
341.22	01	097-099
341.8	01	058-060
341.9	01	058-060
342.00	01	056-057
342.01	01	056-057
342.02	01	056-057
342.10	01	056-057
342.11	01	056-057
342.12	01	056-057
342.80	01	056-057
342.81	01	056-057
342.82	01	056-057
342.90	01	056-057
342.91	01	056-057
342.92	01	056-057
343.0	01	052-053
343.1	01	052-053
343.2	01	052-053
343.3	01	091-093
343.4	01	052-053
343.8	01	091-093
343.9	01	091-093
344.00	01	052-053
344.01	01	052-053
344.02	01	052-053
344.03	01	052-053
344.04	01	052-053
344.09	01	052-053
344.1	01	052-053
344.2	01	052-053
344.30	01	091-093
344.31	01	091-093
344.32	01	091-093
344.40	01	091-093
344.41	01	091-093
344.42	01	091-093
344.5	01	091-093
344.60	01	073-074
344.61	11	698-700
344.81	01	091-093
344.89	01	091-093
344.9	01	091-093
345.00	01	100-101
345.01	01	100-101
345.10	01	100-101
345.11	01	100-101
345.2	01	100-101
345.3	01	100-101
345.40	01	100-101
345.41	01	100-101
345.50	01	100-101
345.51	01	100-101
345.60	01	100-101
345.61	01	100-101
345.70	01	100-101
345.71	01	100-101
345.80	01	100-101
345.81	01	100-101
345.90	01	100-101
345.91	01	100-101
346.00	01	102-103
346.01	01	102-103
346.02	01	102-103
346.03	01	102-103
346.10	01	102-103
346.11	01	102-103
346.12	01	102-103
346.13	01	102-103
346.20	01	102-103
346.21	01	102-103
346.22	01	102-103
346.23	01	102-103
346.30	01	102-103
346.31	01	102-103
346.32	01	102-103
346.33	01	102-103
346.40	01	102-103
346.41	01	102-103
346.42	01	102-103
346.43	01	102-103
346.50	01	102-103
346.51	01	102-103
346.52	01	102-103
346.53	01	102-103
346.60	01	102-103
346.61	01	102-103
346.62	01	102-103
346.63	01	102-103
346.70	01	102-103
346.71	01	102-103
346.72	01	102-103
346.73	01	102-103
346.80	01	102-103
346.81	01	102-103
346.82	01	102-103
346.83	01	102-103
346.90	01	102-103
346.91	01	102-103
347.00	01	091-093
347.01	01	091-093
347.10	01	091-093
347.11	01	091-093
348.0	01	091-093
348.1	01	091-093
348.2	01	102-103
348.30	01	070-072
348.31	01	070-072
348.39	01	070-072
348.4	01	080-081
348.5	01	080-081
348.81	01	070-072
348.82	01	080-081
348.89	01	070-072
348.9	01	070-072
349.0	01	102-103
349.1	01	091-093
349.2	01	091-093
349.31	21	919-921
349.39	21	919-921
349.81	01	091-093
349.82	01	091-093
349.89	01	070-072
349.9	01	070-072
350.1	01	073-074
350.2	01	073-074
350.8	01	073-074
350.9	01	073-074
351.0	01	073-074
351.1	01	073-074
351.8	01	073-074
351.9	01	073-074
352.0	01	073-074
352.1	01	073-074
352.2	01	073-074
352.3	01	073-074
352.4	01	073-074
352.5	01	073-074
352.6	01	073-074
352.9	01	073-074
353.0	01	073-074
353.1	01	073-074
353.2	01	073-074
353.3	01	073-074
353.4	01	073-074
353.5	01	073-074
353.6	01	073-074
353.8	01	073-074
353.9	01	073-074
354.0	01	073-074
354.1	01	073-074
354.2	01	073-074
354.3	01	073-074
354.4	01	073-074
354.5	01	073-074
354.8	01	073-074
354.9	01	073-074
355.0	01	073-074
355.1	01	073-074
355.2	01	073-074
355.3	01	073-074
355.4	01	073-074
355.5	01	073-074
355.6	01	073-074
355.71	01	073-074
355.79	01	073-074
355.8	01	073-074
355.9	01	073-074
356.0	01	073-074
356.1	01	073-074
356.2	01	073-074
356.3	01	091-093
356.4	01	073-074
356.8	01	073-074
356.9	01	073-074
357.0	01	094-096
357.1	01	073-074
357.2	01	073-074
357.3	01	073-074
357.4	01	073-074
357.5	01	073-074
357.6	01	073-074
357.7	01	073-074
357.81	01	073-074
357.82	01	073-074
357.89	01	073-074
357.9	01	073-074
358.00	01	056-057
358.01	01	056-057
358.1	01	056-057
358.2	01	073-074
358.30	01	056-057
358.31	01	056-057
358.39	01	056-057
358.8	01	073-074
358.9	01	073-074
359.0	01	091-093
359.1	01	091-093
359.21	01	091-093
359.22	01	091-093
359.23	01	091-093
359.24	01	091-093
359.29	01	091-093
359.3	01	091-093
359.4	01	091-093
359.5	01	091-093
359.6	01	091-093
359.71	08	545-547
359.79	08	545-547
359.81	01	091-093
359.89	01	091-093
359.9	01	091-093
360.00	02	121-122
360.01	02	121-122
360.02	02	121-122
360.03	02	124-125
360.04	02	121-122
360.11	02	124-125
360.12	02	124-125
360.13	02	121-122
360.14	02	124-125
360.19	02	121-122
360.20	02	124-125
360.21	02	124-125
360.23	02	124-125
360.24	02	124-125
360.29	02	124-125
360.30	02	124-125
360.31	02	124-125
360.32	02	124-125
360.33	02	124-125
360.34	02	124-125
360.40	02	124-125
360.41	02	124-125
360.42	02	124-125
360.43	02	124-125
360.44	02	124-125
360.50	02	124-125
360.51	02	124-125
360.52	02	124-125
360.53	02	124-125
360.54	02	124-125
360.55	02	124-125
360.59	02	124-125
360.60	02	124-125
360.61	02	124-125
360.62	02	124-125
360.63	02	124-125

DX	MDC	DRG
360.64	02	124-125
360.65	02	124-125
360.69	02	124-125
360.81	02	124-125
360.89	02	124-125
360.9	02	124-125
361.00	02	124-125
361.01	02	124-125
361.02	02	124-125
361.03	02	124-125
361.04	02	124-125
361.05	02	124-125
361.06	02	124-125
361.07	02	124-125
361.10	02	124-125
361.11	02	124-125
361.12	02	124-125
361.13	02	124-125
361.14	02	124-125
361.19	02	124-125
361.2	02	124-125
361.30	02	124-125
361.31	02	124-125
361.32	02	124-125
361.33	02	124-125
361.81	02	124-125
361.89	02	124-125
361.9	02	124-125
362.01	02	124-125
362.02	02	124-125
362.03	02	124-125
362.04	02	124-125
362.05	02	124-125
362.06	02	124-125
362.07	02	124-125
362.10	02	124-125
362.11	02	124-125
362.12	02	124-125
362.13	02	124-125
362.14	02	124-125
362.15	02	124-125
362.16	02	124-125
362.17	02	124-125
362.18	02	124-125
362.20	02	124-125
362.21	02	124-125
362.22	02	124-125
362.23	02	124-125
362.24	02	124-125
362.25	02	124-125
362.26	02	124-125
362.27	02	124-125
362.29	02	124-125
362.30	02	123
362.31	02	123
362.32	02	123
362.33	02	123
362.34	02	123
362.35	02	123
362.36	02	123
362.37	02	123
362.40	02	124-125
362.41	02	124-125
362.42	02	124-125
362.43	02	124-125
362.50	02	124-125
362.51	02	124-125
362.52	02	124-125
362.53	02	124-125
362.54	02	124-125
362.55	02	124-125
362.56	02	124-125
362.57	02	124-125
362.60	02	124-125
362.61	02	124-125
362.62	02	124-125
362.63	02	124-125
362.64	02	124-125
362.65	02	124-125
362.66	02	124-125
362.70	02	124-125
362.71	02	124-125
362.72	02	124-125
362.73	02	124-125
362.74	02	124-125
362.75	02	124-125
362.76	02	124-125
362.77	02	124-125
362.81	02	124-125
362.82	02	124-125
362.83	02	124-125
362.84	02	124-125
362.85	02	124-125
362.89	02	124-125
362.9	02	124-125
363.00	02	124-125
363.01	02	124-125
363.03	02	124-125
363.04	02	124-125
363.05	02	124-125
363.06	02	124-125
363.07	02	124-125
363.08	02	124-125
363.10	02	124-125
363.11	02	124-125
363.12	02	124-125
363.13	02	124-125
363.14	02	124-125
363.15	02	124-125
363.20	02	124-125
363.21	02	124-125
363.22	02	124-125
363.30	02	124-125
363.31	02	124-125
363.32	02	124-125
363.33	02	124-125
363.34	02	124-125
363.35	02	124-125
363.40	02	124-125
363.41	02	124-125
363.42	02	124-125
363.43	02	124-125
363.50	02	124-125
363.51	02	124-125
363.52	02	124-125
363.53	02	124-125
363.54	02	124-125
363.55	02	124-125
363.56	02	124-125
363.57	02	124-125
363.61	02	124-125
363.62	02	124-125
363.63	02	124-125
363.70	02	124-125
363.71	02	124-125
363.72	02	124-125
363.8	02	124-125
363.9	02	124-125
364.00	02	124-125
364.01	02	124-125
364.02	02	124-125
364.03	02	124-125
364.04	02	124-125
364.05	02	124-125
364.10	02	124-125
364.11	02	124-125
364.21	02	124-125
364.22	02	124-125
364.23	02	124-125
364.24	02	124-125
364.3	02	124-125
364.41	02	124-125
364.42	02	124-125
364.51	02	124-125
364.52	02	124-125
364.53	02	124-125
364.54	02	124-125
364.55	02	124-125
364.56	02	124-125
364.57	02	124-125
364.59	02	124-125
364.60	02	124-125
364.61	02	124-125
364.62	02	124-125
364.63	02	124-125
364.64	02	124-125
364.70	02	124-125
364.71	02	124-125
364.72	02	124-125
364.73	02	124-125
364.74	02	124-125
364.75	02	124-125
364.76	02	124-125
364.77	02	124-125
364.81	02	124-125
364.82	02	124-125
364.89	02	124-125
364.9	02	124-125
365.00	02	124-125
365.01	02	124-125
365.02	02	124-125
365.03	02	124-125
365.04	02	124-125
365.05	02	124-125
365.06	02	124-125
365.10	02	124-125
365.11	02	124-125
365.12	02	123
365.13	02	124-125
365.14	02	124-125
365.15	02	124-125
365.20	02	124-125
365.21	02	124-125
365.22	02	124-125
365.23	02	124-125
365.24	02	124-125
365.31	02	124-125
365.32	02	124-125
365.41	02	124-125
365.42	02	124-125
365.43	02	124-125
365.44	02	124-125
365.51	02	124-125
365.52	02	124-125
365.59	02	124-125
365.60	02	124-125
365.61	02	124-125
365.62	02	124-125
365.63	02	124-125
365.64	02	124-125
365.65	02	124-125
365.70	02	124-125
365.71	02	124-125
365.72	02	124-125
365.73	02	124-125
365.74	02	124-125
365.81	02	124-125
365.82	02	124-125
365.83	02	124-125
365.89	02	124-125
365.9	02	124-125
366.00	02	124-125
366.01	02	124-125
366.02	02	124-125
366.03	02	124-125
366.04	02	124-125
366.09	02	124-125
366.10	02	124-125
366.11	02	124-125
366.12	02	124-125
366.13	02	124-125
366.14	02	124-125
366.15	02	124-125
366.16	02	124-125
366.17	02	124-125
366.18	02	124-125
366.19	02	124-125
366.20	02	124-125
366.21	02	124-125
366.22	02	124-125
366.23	02	124-125
366.30	02	124-125
366.31	02	124-125
366.32	02	124-125
366.33	02	124-125
366.34	02	124-125
366.41	02	124-125
366.42	02	124-125
366.43	02	124-125
366.44	02	124-125
366.45	02	124-125
366.46	02	124-125
366.50	02	124-125
366.51	02	124-125
366.52	02	124-125
366.53	02	124-125
366.8	02	124-125
366.9	02	124-125
367.0	02	124-125
367.1	02	124-125
367.20	02	124-125
367.21	02	124-125
367.22	02	124-125
367.31	02	124-125
367.32	02	124-125
367.4	02	124-125
367.51	02	124-125
367.52	02	123
367.53	02	124-125
367.81	02	124-125
367.89	02	124-125
367.9	02	124-125
368.00	02	124-125
368.01	02	124-125
368.02	02	124-125
368.03	02	124-125
368.10	02	124-125
368.11	02	123
368.12	02	123
368.13	02	124-125
368.14	02	124-125
368.15	02	124-125
368.16	02	124-125
368.2	02	123
368.30	02	124-125
368.31	02	124-125
368.32	02	124-125
368.33	02	124-125
368.34	02	124-125
368.40	02	123
368.41	02	123
368.42	02	124-125
368.43	02	123
368.44	02	123
368.45	02	123
368.46	02	123
368.47	02	123
368.51	02	124-125
368.52	02	124-125
368.53	02	124-125
368.54	02	124-125
368.55	02	123
368.59	02	124-125
368.60	02	124-125
368.61	02	124-125
368.62	02	124-125
368.63	02	124-125
368.69	02	124-125
368.8	02	124-125
368.9	02	124-125
369.00	02	124-125
369.01	02	124-125
369.02	02	124-125
369.03	02	124-125
369.04	02	124-125
369.05	02	124-125
369.06	02	124-125
369.07	02	124-125
369.08	02	124-125
369.10	02	124-125
369.11	02	124-125
369.12	02	124-125
369.13	02	124-125
369.14	02	124-125
369.15	02	124-125
369.16	02	124-125
369.17	02	124-125
369.18	02	124-125
369.20	02	124-125
369.21	02	124-125
369.22	02	124-125
369.23	02	124-125
369.24	02	124-125
369.25	02	124-125
369.3	02	124-125
369.4	02	124-125
369.60	02	124-125
369.61	02	124-125
369.62	02	124-125
369.63	02	124-125

DX	MDC	DRG	DX	MDC	DRG	DX	MDC	DRG	DX	MDC	DRG	DX	MDC	DRG
369.64	02	124-125	371.31	02	124-125	372.62	02	124-125	374.9	02	124-125	377.00	01	091-093
369.65	02	124-125	371.32	02	124-125	372.63	02	124-125	375.00	02	124-125	377.01	01	091-093
369.66	02	124-125	371.33	02	124-125	372.64	02	124-125	375.01	02	121-122	377.02	02	124-125
369.67	02	124-125	371.40	02	124-125	372.71	02	124-125	375.02	02	124-125	377.03	02	124-125
369.68	02	124-125	371.41	02	124-125	372.72	02	124-125	375.03	02	124-125	377.04	01	091-093
369.69	02	124-125	371.42	02	124-125	372.73	02	124-125	375.11	02	124-125	377.10	02	123
369.70	02	124-125	371.43	02	124-125	372.74	02	124-125	375.12	02	124-125	377.11	02	123
369.71	02	124-125	371.44	02	124-125	372.75	02	124-125	375.13	02	124-125	377.12	02	123
369.72	02	124-125	371.45	02	124-125	372.81	02	124-125	375.14	02	124-125	377.13	02	124-125
369.73	02	124-125	371.46	02	124-125	327.89	02	124-125	375.15	02	124-125	377.14	02	124-125
369.74	02	124-125	371.48	02	124-125	372.9	02	124-125	375.16	02	124-125	377.15	02	123
369.75	02	124-125	371.49	02	124-125	373.00	02	124-125	375.20	02	124-125	377.16	02	123
369.76	02	124-125	371.50	02	124-125	373.01	02	124-125	375.21	02	124-125	377.21	02	123
369.8	02	124-125	371.51	02	124-125	373.02	02	124-125	375.22	02	124-125	377.22	02	124-125
369.9	02	124-125	371.52	02	124-125	373.11	02	124-125	375.30	02	124-125	377.23	02	124-125
370.00	02	121-122	371.53	02	124-125	373.12	02	124-125	375.31	02	121-122	377.24	02	123
370.01	02	124-125	371.54	02	124-125	373.13	02	124-125	375.32	02	121-122	377.30	02	123
370.02	02	124-125	371.55	02	124-125	373.2	02	124-125	375.33	02	124-125	377.31	02	123
370.03	02	121-122	371.56	02	124-125	373.31	02	124-125	375.41	02	124-125	377.32	02	123
370.04	02	121-122	371.57	02	124-125	373.32	02	124-125	375.42	02	124-125	377.33	02	123
370.05	02	121-122	371.58	02	124-125	373.33	02	124-125	375.43	02	124-125	377.34	02	123
370.06	02	121-122	371.60	02	124-125	373.34	02	124-125	375.51	02	124-125	377.39	02	123
370.07	02	124-125	371.61	02	124-125	373.4	02	124-125	375.52	02	124-125	377.41	02	123
370.20	02	124-125	371.62	02	124-125	373.5	02	124-125	375.53	02	124-125	377.42	02	123
370.21	02	124-125	371.70	02	124-125	373.6	02	124-125	375.54	02	124-125	377.43	02	123
370.22	02	124-125	371.71	02	124-125	373.8	02	124-125	375.55	02	124-125	377.49	02	123
370.23	02	124-125	371.72	02	124-125	373.9	02	124-125	375.56	02	124-125	377.51	01	091-093
370.24	02	124-125	371.73	02	124-125	374.00	02	124-125	375.57	02	124-125	377.52	01	091-093
370.31	02	124-125	371.81	02	124-125	374.01	02	124-125	375.61	02	124-125	377.53	01	091-093
370.32	02	124-125	371.82	02	124-125	374.02	02	124-125	375.69	02	124-125	377.54	01	091-093
370.33	02	124-125	371.89	02	124-125	374.03	02	124-125	375.81	02	124-125	377.61	01	091-093
370.34	02	124-125	371.9	02	124-125	374.04	02	124-125	375.89	02	124-125	377.62	01	091-093
370.35	02	124-125	372.00	02	124-125	374.05	02	124-125	375.9	02	124-125	377.63	01	091-093
370.40	02	124-125	372.01	02	124-125	374.10	02	124-125	376.00	02	124-125	377.71	01	091-093
370.44	02	124-125	372.02	02	124-125	374.11	02	124-125	376.01	02	121-122	377.72	01	091-093
370.49	02	124-125	372.03	02	124-125	374.12	02	124-125	376.02	02	121-122	377.73	01	091-093
370.50	02	124-125	372.04	02	124-125	374.13	02	124-125	376.03	02	121-122	377.75	01	091-093
370.52	02	124-125	372.05	02	124-125	374.14	02	124-125	376.04	02	121-122	377.9	01	091-093
370.54	02	124-125	372.06	02	124-125	374.20	02	124-125	376.10	02	124-125	378.00	02	124-125
370.55	02	121-122	372.10	02	124-125	374.21	02	124-125	376.11	02	124-125	378.01	02	124-125
370.59	02	124-125	372.11	02	124-125	374.22	02	124-125	376.12	02	124-125	378.02	02	124-125
370.60	02	124-125	372.12	02	124-125	374.23	02	124-125	376.13	02	124-125	378.03	02	124-125
370.61	02	124-125	372.13	02	124-125	374.30	02	123	376.21	02	124-125	378.04	02	124-125
370.62	02	124-125	372.14	02	124-125	374.31	02	123	376.22	02	124-125	378.05	02	124-125
370.63	02	124-125	372.15	02	124-125	374.32	02	123	376.30	02	124-125	378.06	02	124-125
370.64	02	124-125	372.20	02	124-125	374.33	02	124-125	376.31	02	124-125	378.07	02	124-125
370.8	02	124-125	372.21	02	124-125	374.34	02	124-125	376.32	02	124-125	378.08	02	124-125
370.9	02	124-125	372.22	02	124-125	374.41	02	124-125	376.33	02	124-125	378.10	02	124-125
371.00	02	124-125	372.30	02	124-125	374.43	02	124-125	376.34	02	123	378.11	02	124-125
371.01	02	124-125	372.31	02	124-125	374.44	02	124-125	376.35	02	123	378.12	02	124-125
371.02	02	124-125	372.33	02	124-125	374.45	02	123	376.36	02	123	378.13	02	124-125
371.03	02	124-125	372.34	02	124-125	374.46	02	124-125	376.40	02	124-125	378.14	02	124-125
371.04	02	124-125	372.39	02	124-125	374.50	02	124-125	376.41	02	124-125	378.15	02	124-125
371.05	02	124-125	372.40	02	124-125	374.51	09	606-607	376.42	02	124-125	378.16	02	124-125
371.10	02	124-125	372.41	02	124-125	374.52	02	124-125	376.43	02	124-125	378.17	02	124-125
371.11	02	124-125	372.42	02	124-125	374.53	02	124-125	376.44	02	124-125	378.18	02	124-125
371.12	02	124-125	372.43	02	124-125	374.54	02	124-125	376.45	02	124-125	378.20	02	124-125
371.13	02	124-125	372.44	02	124-125	374.55	02	124-125	376.46	02	124-125	378.21	02	124-125
371.14	02	124-125	372.45	02	124-125	374.56	02	124-125	376.47	02	124-125	378.22	02	124-125
371.15	02	124-125	372.50	02	124-125	374.81	02	124-125	376.50	02	124-125	378.23	02	124-125
371.16	02	124-125	372.51	02	124-125	374.82	02	124-125	376.51	02	124-125	378.24	02	124-125
371.20	02	124-125	372.52	02	124-125	374.83	02	124-125	376.52	02	124-125	378.30	02	124-125
371.21	02	124-125	372.53	02	124-125	374.84	02	124-125	376.6	02	124-125	378.31	02	124-125
371.22	02	124-125	372.54	02	124-125	374.85	02	124-125	376.81	02	124-125	378.32	02	124-125
371.23	02	124-125	372.55	02	124-125	374.86	02	124-125	376.82	02	123	378.33	02	124-125
371.24	02	124-125	372.56	02	124-125	374.87	02	124-125	376.89	02	124-125	378.34	02	124-125
371.30	02	124-125	372.61	02	124-125	374.89	02	124-125	376.9	02	124-125	378.35	02	124-125

Diagnosis Code/MDC/DRG List

DX	MDC	DRG
378.40	02	124-125
378.41	02	124-125
378.42	02	124-125
378.43	02	124-125
378.44	02	124-125
378.45	02	124-125
378.50	02	123
378.51	02	123
378.52	02	123
378.53	02	123
378.54	02	123
378.55	02	123
378.56	02	123
378.60	02	124-125
378.61	02	124-125
378.62	02	124-125
378.63	02	124-125
378.71	02	124-125
378.72	02	123
378.73	02	123
378.81	02	124-125
378.82	02	124-125
378.83	02	124-125
378.84	02	124-125
378.85	02	124-125
378.86	01	091-093
378.87	02	123
378.9	02	124-125
379.00	02	124-125
379.01	02	124-125
379.02	02	124-125
379.03	02	124-125
379.04	02	124-125
379.05	02	124-125
379.06	02	124-125
379.07	02	124-125
379.09	02	124-125
379.11	02	124-125
379.12	02	124-125
379.13	02	124-125
379.14	02	124-125
379.15	02	124-125
379.16	02	124-125
379.19	02	124-125
379.21	02	124-125
379.22	02	124-125
379.23	02	124-125
379.24	02	124-125
379.25	02	124-125
379.26	02	124-125
379.27	02	124-125
379.29	02	124-125
379.31	02	124-125
379.32	02	124-125
379.33	02	124-125
379.34	02	124-125
379.39	02	124-125
379.40	02	123
379.41	02	123
379.42	02	123
379.43	02	123
379.45	01	056-057
379.46	02	123
379.49	02	123
379.50	02	123
379.51	02	124-125
379.52	02	123
379.53	02	124-125
379.54	02	123
379.55	02	123
379.56	02	124-125
379.57	02	123
379.58	02	123
379.59	02	124-125
379.60	02	124-125
379.61	02	124-125
379.62	02	124-125
379.63	02	124-125
379.8	02	124-125
379.90	02	124-125
379.91	02	124-125
379.92	02	124-125
379.93	02	124-125
379.99	02	124-125
380.00	03	152-153
380.01	08	564-566
380.02	08	564-566
380.03	08	564-566
380.10	03	154-156
380.11	03	154-156
380.12	03	154-156
380.13	03	154-156
380.14	03	154-156
380.15	03	154-156
380.16	03	154-156
380.21	03	154-156
380.22	03	154-156
380.23	03	154-156
380.30	03	154-156
380.31	03	154-156
380.32	03	154-156
380.39	03	154-156
380.4	03	154-156
380.50	03	154-156
380.51	03	154-156
380.52	03	154-156
380.53	03	154-156
380.81	03	154-156
380.89	03	154-156
380.9	03	154-156
381.00	03	152-153
381.01	03	152-153
381.02	03	152-153
381.03	03	152-153
381.04	03	152-153
381.05	03	152-153
381.06	03	152-153
381.10	03	152-153
381.19	03	152-153
381.20	03	152-153
381.29	03	152-153
381.3	03	152-153
381.4	03	152-153
381.50	03	152-153
381.51	03	152-153
381.52	03	152-153
381.60	03	154-156
381.61	03	154-156
381.62	03	154-156
381.63	03	154-156
381.7	03	154-156
381.81	03	154-156
381.89	03	154-156
381.9	03	154-156
382.00	03	152-153
382.01	03	152-153
382.02	03	152-153
382.1	03	152-153
382.2	03	152-153
382.3	03	152-153
382.4	03	152-153
382.9	03	152-153
383.00	03	152-153
383.01	03	152-153
383.02	03	152-153
383.1	03	152-153
383.20	03	152-153
383.21	03	152-153
383.22	03	152-153
383.30	03	154-156
383.31	03	154-156
383.32	03	154-156
383.33	03	154-156
383.81	03	154-156
383.89	03	154-156
383.9	03	152-153
384.00	03	152-153
384.01	03	152-153
384.09	03	152-153
384.1	03	152-153
384.20	03	154-156
384.21	03	154-156
384.22	03	154-156
384.23	03	154-156
384.24	03	154-156
384.25	03	154-156
384.81	03	154-156
384.82	03	154-156
384.9	03	154-156
385.00	03	154-156
385.01	03	154-156
385.02	03	154-156
385.03	03	154-156
385.09	03	154-156
385.10	03	154-156
385.11	03	154-156
385.12	03	154-156
385.13	03	154-156
385.19	03	154-156
385.21	03	154-156
385.22	03	154-156
385.23	03	154-156
385.24	03	154-156
385.30	03	154-156
385.31	03	154-156
385.32	03	154-156
385.33	03	154-156
385.35	03	154-156
385.82	03	154-156
385.83	03	154-156
385.89	03	154-156
385.9	03	154-156
386.00	03	149
386.01	03	149
386.02	03	149
386.03	03	149
386.04	03	149
386.10	03	149
386.11	03	149
386.12	03	149
386.19	03	149
386.2	03	149
386.30	03	149
386.31	03	149
386.32	03	149
386.33	03	149
386.34	03	149
386.35	03	149
386.40	03	154-156
386.41	03	154-156
386.42	03	154-156
386.43	03	154-156
386.48	03	154-156
386.50	03	149
386.51	03	149
386.52	03	149
386.53	03	149
386.54	03	149
386.55	03	149
386.56	03	149
386.58	03	149
386.8	03	149
386.9	03	149
387.0	03	154-156
387.1	03	154-156
387.2	03	154-156
387.8	03	154-156
387.9	03	154-156
388.00	03	154-156
388.01	03	154-156
388.02	03	154-156
388.10	03	154-156
388.11	03	154-156
388.12	03	154-156
388.2	03	154-156
388.30	03	154-156
388.31	03	154-156
388.32	03	154-156
388.40	03	154-156
388.41	03	154-156
388.42	03	154-156
388.43	03	154-156
388.44	03	154-156
388.45	19	886
388.5	03	154-156
388.60	03	154-156
388.61	01	091-093
388.69	03	154-156
388.70	03	154-156
388.71	03	154-156
388.72	03	154-156
388.8	03	154-156
388.9	03	154-156
389.00	03	154-156
389.01	03	154-156
389.02	03	154-156
389.03	03	154-156
389.04	03	154-156
389.05	03	154-156
389.06	03	154-156
389.08	03	154-156
389.10	03	154-156
389.11	03	154-156
389.12	03	154-156
389.13	03	154-156
389.14	03	154-156
389.15	03	154-156
389.16	03	154-156
389.17	03	154-156
389.18	03	154-156
389.20	03	154-156
389.21	03	154-156
389.22	03	154-156
389.7	03	154-156
389.8	03	154-156
389.9	03	154-156

Diseases of the Circulatory System

DX	MDC	DRG
390	08	545-547
391.0	05	314-316
391.1	05	306-307
391.2	05	314-316
391.8	05	314-316
391.9	05	314-316
392.0	05	314-316
392.9	05	314-316
393	05	314-316
394.0	05	306-307
394.1	05	306-307
394.2	05	306-307
394.9	05	306-307
395.0	05	306-307
395.1	05	306-307
395.2	05	306-307
395.9	05	306-307
396.0	05	306-307
396.1	05	306-307
396.2	05	306-307
396.3	05	306-307
396.8	05	306-307
396.9	05	306-307
397.0	05	306-307
397.1	05	306-307
397.9	05	306-307
398.0	05	314-316
398.90	05	314-316
398.91	05	291-293
398.99	05	314-316
401.0	05	304-305
401.1	05	304-305
401.9	05	304-305
402.00	05	304-305
402.01	05	291-293
402.10	05	304-305
402.11	05	291-293
402.90	05	304-305
402.91	05	291-293
403.00	11	682-684
403.01	11	682-684
403.10	11	682-684
403.11	11	682-684
403.90	11	682-684
403.91	11	682-684
404.00	05	304-305
404.01	05	291-293
404.02	11	682-684
404.03	05	291-293
404.10	05	304-305
404.11	05	291-293
404.12	11	682-684
404.13	05	291-293
404.90	05	304-305
404.91	05	291-293
404.92	11	682-684
404.93	05	291-293
405.01	05	304-305
405.09	05	304-305
405.11	05	304-305
405.19	05	304-305
405.91	05	304-305

DX	MDC	DRG	DX	MDC	DRG	DX	MDC	DRG	DX	MDC	DRG	DX	MDC	DRG
405.99	05	304-305	417.1	05	314-316	427.61	05	308-310	437.3	01	091-093	442.82	05	299-301
410.00	05	314-316	417.8	05	314-316	427.69	05	308-310	437.4	01	102-103	442.83	05	299-301
410.01	05	280-285	417.9	05	314-316	427.81	05	308-310	437.5	01	091-093	442.84	05	299-301
410.02	05	314-316	420.0	05	314-316	427.89	05	308-310	437.6	01	091-093	442.89	05	299-301
410.10	05	314-316	420.90	05	314-316	427.9	05	308-310	437.7	01	070-072	442.9	05	299-301
410.11	05	280-285	420.91	05	314-316	428.0	05	291-293	437.8	01	070-072	443.0	08	545-547
410.12	05	314-316	420.99	05	314-316	428.1	05	291-293	437.9	01	070-072	443.1	05	299-301
410.20	05	314-316	421.0	05	288-290	428.9	05	291-293	438.0	01	056-057	443.21	05	299-301
410.21	05	280-285	421.1	05	288-290	428.20	05	291-293	438.10	01	056-057	443.22	05	299-301
410.22	05	314-316	421.9	05	288-290	428.21	05	291-293	438.11	01	056-057	443.23	11	698-700
410.30	05	314-316	422.0	05	314-316	428.22	05	291-293	438.12	01	056-057	443.24	05	299-301
410.31	05	280-285	422.90	05	314-316	428.23	05	291-293	438.13	01	056-057	443.29	05	299-301
410.32	05	314-316	422.91	05	314-316	428.30	05	291-293	438.14	01	056-057	443.81	05	299-301
410.40	05	314-316	422.92	05	314-316	428.31	05	291-293	438.19	01	056-057	443.82	05	299-301
410.41	05	280-285	422.93	05	314-316	428.32	05	291-293	438.20	01	056-057	443.89	05	299-301
410.42	05	314-316	422.99	05	314-316	428.33	05	291-293	438.21	01	056-057	443.9	05	299-301
410.50	05	314-316	423.0	05	314-316	428.40	05	291-293	438.22	01	056-057	444.01	05	299-301
410.51	05	280-285	423.1	05	314-316	428.41	05	291-293	438.30	01	056-057	444.09	05	299-301
410.52	05	314-316	423.2	05	314-316	428.42	05	291-293	438.31	01	056-057	444.1	05	299-301
410.60	05	314-316	423.3	05	314-316	428.43	05	291-293	438.32	01	056-057	444.21	05	299-301
410.61	05	280-285	423.8	05	314-316	428.9	05	291-293	438.40	01	056-057	444.22	05	299-301
410.62	05	314-316	423.9	05	314-316	429.0	05	314-316	438.41	01	056-057	444.81	05	299-301
410.70	05	314-316	424.0	05	306-307	429.1	05	314-316	438.42	01	056-057	444.89	05	299-301
410.71	05	280-285	424.1	05	306-307	429.2	05	302-303	438.50	01	056-057	444.9	05	299-301
410.72	05	314-316	424.2	05	306-307	429.3	05	302-303	438.51	01	056-057	445.01	05	299-301
410.80	05	314-316	424.3	05	306-307	429.4	05	314-316	438.52	01	056-057	445.02	05	299-301
410.81	05	280-285	424.90	05	306-307	429.5	05	306-307	438.53	01	056-057	445.81	11	698-700
410.82	05	314-316	424.91	05	306-307	429.6	05	306-307	438.6	01	056-057	445.89	05	299-301
410.90	05	314-316	424.99	05	306-307	429.71	05	314-316	438.7	01	056-057	446.0	08	545-547
410.91	05	280-285	425.0	05	314-316	429.79	05	314-316	438.81	01	056-057	446.1	08	545-547
410.92	05	314-316	425.11	05	314-316	429.81	05	306-307	438.82	01	056-057	446.20	08	545-547
411.0	05	314-316	425.18	05	314-316	429.82	05	314-316	438.83	01	056-057	446.21	08	545-547
411.1	05	311	425.2	05	314-316	429.83	05	314-316	438.84	01	056-057	446.29	08	545-547
411.81	05	311	425.3	05	314-316	429.89	05	302-303	438.85	01	056-057	446.3	08	542-544
411.89	05	311	425.4	05	314-316	429.9	05	302-303	438.89	01	056-057	446.4	08	542-544
412.	05	302-303	425.5	05	314-316	430	01	064-066	438.9	01	056-057	446.5	08	545-547
413.0	05	311	425.7	05	314-316	431	01	064-066	440.0	05	299-301	446.6	08	545-547
413.1	05	311	425.8	05	314-316	432.0	01	064-066	440.1	11	698-700	446.7	08	545-547
413.9	05	311	425.9	05	314-316	432.1	01	064-066	440.20	05	299-301	447.0	05	299-301
414.00	05	302-303	426.0	05	308-310	432.9	01	064-066	440.21	05	299-301	447.1	05	299-301
414.01	05	302-303	426.10	05	308-310	433.00	01	067-068	440.22	05	299-301	447.2	05	299-301
414.02	05	302-303	426.11	05	308-310	433.01	01	061-066	440.23	05	299-301	447.3	11	698-700
414.03	05	302-303	426.12	05	308-310	433.10	01	067-068	440.24	05	299-301	447.4	06	391-392
414.04	05	302-303	426.13	05	308-310	433.11	01	061-066	440.29	05	299-301	447.5	05	299-301
414.05	05	302-303	426.2	05	308-310	433.20	01	067-068	440.30	05	299-301	447.6	08	545-547
414.06	05	302-303	426.3	05	308-310	433.21	01	061-066	440.31	05	299-301	447.70	05	299-301
414.07	05	302-303	426.4	05	308-310	433.30	01	067-068	440.32	05	299-301	447.71	05	299-301
414.10	05	314-316	426.50	05	308-310	433.31	01	061-066	440.4	05	299-301	447.72	05	299-301
414.11	05	314-316	426.51	05	308-310	433.80	01	067-068	440.8	05	299-301	447.73	05	299-301
414.12	05	314-316	426.52	05	308-310	433.81	01	061-066	440.9	05	299-301	447.8	05	299-301
414.19	05	314-316	426.53	05	308-310	433.90	01	067-068	441.00	05	299-301	447.9	05	299-301
414.2	05	302-303	426.54	05	308-310	433.91	01	061-066	441.01	05	299-301	448.0	05	299-301
414.3	05	302-303	426.6	05	308-310	434.00	01	067-068	441.02	05	299-301	448.1	09	606-607
414.4	05	302-303	426.7	05	308-310	434.01	01	061-066	441.03	05	299-301	448.9	05	299-301
414.8	05	302-303	426.81	05	308-310	434.10	01	067-068	441.1	05	299-301	449	05	299-301
414.9	05	302-303	426.82	05	308-310	434.11	01	061-066	441.2	05	299-301	451.0	05	299-301
415.0	05	314-316	426.89	05	308-310	434.90	01	067-068	441.3	05	299-301	451.11	05	294-295
415.11	04	175-176	426.9	05	308-310	434.91	01	061-066	441.4	05	299-301	451.19	05	294-295
415.12	04	175-176	427.0	05	308-310	435.0	01	069	441.5	05	299-301	451.2	05	294-295
415.13	04	175-176	427.1	05	308-310	435.1	01	069	441.6	05	299-301	451.81	05	294-295
415.19	04	175-176	427.2	05	308-310	435.2	01	069	441.7	05	299-301	451.82	05	299-301
416.0	05	314-316	427.31	05	308-310	435.8	01	069	441.9	05	299-301	451.83	05	299-301
416.1	05	314-316	427.32	05	308-310	435.9	01	069	442.0	05	299-301	451.84	05	299-301
416.2	04	175-176	427.41	05	308-310	436	01	067-068	442.1	11	698-700	451.89	05	299-301
416.8	05	314-316	427.42	05	308-310	437.0	01	070-072	442.2	05	299-301	451.9	05	299-301
416.9	05	314-316	427.5	05	296-298	437.1	01	069	442.3	05	299-301	452	07	441-443
417.0	05	314-316	427.60	05	308-310	437.2	01	077-079	442.81	05	299-301	453.0	07	441-443

DX	MDC	DRG
453.1	05	299-301
453.2	05	294-295
453.3	11	698-700
453.40	05	299-301
453.41	05	299-301
453.42	05	299-301
453.50	05	299-301
453.51	05	299-301
453.52	05	299-301
453.6	05	299-301
453.71	05	299-301
453.72	05	299-301
453.73	05	299-301
453.74	05	299-301
453.75	05	299-301
453.76	05	299-301
453.77	05	299-301
453.79	05	299-301
453.81	05	299-301
453.82	05	299-301
453.83	05	299-301
453.84	05	299-301
453.85	05	299-301
453.86	05	299-301
453.87	05	299-301
453.89	05	299-301
453.9	05	299-301
454.0	05	299-301
454.1	05	299-301
454.2	05	299-301
454.8	05	299-301
454.9	05	299-301
455.0	06	393-395
455.1	06	393-395
455.2	06	393-395
455.3	06	393-395
455.4	06	393-395
455.5	06	393-395
455.6	06	393-395
455.7	06	393-395
455.8	06	393-395
455.9	06	393-395
456.0	06	368-370
456.1	06	368-370
456.20	06	368-370
456.21	06	393-395
456.3	05	299-301
456.4	12	729-730
456.5	12	729-730
456.5	13	760-761
456.6	13	760-761
456.8	05	299-301
457.0	09	600-601
457.1	09	606-607
457.2	09	602-603
457.8	16	814-816
457.9	16	814-816
458.0	05	312
458.1	05	314-316
458.21	05	312
458.29	05	312
458.8	05	314-316
458.9	05	314-316
459.0	05	314-316
459.1	05	299-301
459.2	05	299-301
459.10	05	299-301
459.11	05	299-301
459.12	05	299-301
459.13	05	299-301
459.19	05	299-301
459.30	05	299-301
459.31	05	299-301
459.32	05	299-301
459.33	05	299-301
459.39	05	299-301
459.81	05	299-301
459.89	05	302-303
459.9	05	302-303

Diseases of the Respiratory System

DX	MDC	DRG
460	03	152-153
461.0	03	152-153
461.1	03	152-153
461.2	03	152-153
461.3	03	152-153
461.8	03	152-153
461.9	03	152-153
462	03	152-153
463	03	152-153
464.00	03	152-153
464.01	03	152-153
464.10	04	202-203
464.11	04	202-203
464.20	03	152-153
464.21	03	152-153
464.30	03	152-153
464.31	03	152-153
464.4	03	152-153
464.50	03	152-153
464.51	03	152-153
465.0	03	152-153
465.8	03	152-153
465.9	03	152-153
466.0	04	202-203
466.11	04	202-203
466.19	04	202-203
470	03	154-156
471.0	03	154-156
471.1	03	154-156
471.8	03	154-156
471.9	03	154-156
472.0	03	152-153
472.1	03	152-153
472.2	03	152-153
473.0	03	152-153
473.1	03	152-153
473.2	03	152-153
473.3	03	152-153
473.8	03	152-153
473.9	03	152-153
474.00	03	152-153
474.01	03	152-153
474.02	03	152-153
474.10	03	154-156
474.11	03	154-156
474.12	03	154-156
474.2	03	154-156
474.8	03	154-156
474.9	03	154-156
475	03	152-153
476.0	03	152-153
476.1	03	152-153
477.0	03	152-153
477.1	03	152-153
477.2	03	152-153
477.8	03	152-153
477.9	03	152-153
478.0	03	154-156
478.11	03	154-156
478.19	03	154-156
478.20	03	154-156
478.21	03	152-153
478.22	03	152-153
478.24	03	152-153
478.25	03	154-156
478.26	03	154-156
478.29	03	154-156
478.30	03	154-156
478.31	03	154-156
478.32	03	154-156
478.33	03	154-156
478.34	03	154-156
478.4	03	154-156
478.5	03	154-156
478.6	03	154-156
478.70	03	154-156
478.71	03	152-153
478.74	03	154-156
478.75	03	154-156
478.79	03	154-156
478.8	03	152-153
478.9	03	152-153
480.0	04	193-195
480.1	04	193-195
480.2	04	193-195
480.8	04	193-195
480.9	04	193-195
481	04	193-195
482.0	04	177-179
482.1	04	177-179
482.2	04	193-195
482.30	04	193-195
482.31	04	193-195
482.32	04	193-195
482.39	04	193-195
482.40	04	177-179
482.41	04	177-179
482.42	04	177-179
482.49	04	177-179
482.81	04	177-179
482.82	04	177-179
482.83	04	177-179
482.84	04	177-179
482.89	04	177-179
482.9	04	193-195
483.0	04	193-195
483.1	04	193-195
483.8	04	193-195
484.1	04	177-179
484.3	04	177-179
484.5	04	177-179
484.6	04	177-179
484.7	04	177-179
484.8	04	177-179
485	04	193-195
486	04	193-195
487.0	04	193-195
487.1	03	152-153
487.8	18	865-866
488.01	04	193-195
488.02	04	193-195
488.09	18	865-866
488.11	04	193-195
488.12	04	193-195
488.19	18	865-866
488.81	04	193-195
488.82	04	193-195
488.89	18	865-866
490	04	202-203
491.0	04	202-203
491.1	04	190-192
491.20	04	190-192
491.21	04	190-192
491.22	04	190-192
491.8	04	190-192
491.9	04	190-192
492.0	04	190-192
492.8	04	190-192
493.00	04	202-203
493.01	04	202-203
493.02	04	202-203
493.10	04	202-203
493.11	04	202-203
493.12	04	202-203
493.20	04	190-192
493.21	04	190-192
493.22	04	190-192
493.81	04	202-203
493.82	04	202-203
493.90	04	202-203
493.91	04	202-203
493.92	04	202-203
494.0	04	190-192
494.1	04	190-192
495.0	04	196-198
495.1	04	196-198
495.2	04	196-198
495.3	04	196-198
495.4	04	196-198
495.5	04	196-198
495.6	04	196-198
495.7	04	196-198
495.8	04	196-198
495.9	04	196-198
496	04	190-192
500	04	196-198
501	04	196-198
502	04	196-198
503	04	196-198
504	04	196-198
505	04	196-198
506.0	04	205-206
506.1	04	189
506.2	04	205-206
506.3	04	205-206
506.4	04	190-192
506.9	04	190-192
507.0	04	177-179
507.1	04	177-179
507.8	04	177-179
508.0	04	205-206
508.1	04	196-198
508.2	04	205-206
508.8	04	205-206
508.9	04	205-206
510.0	04	177-179
510.9	04	177-179
511.0	04	193-195
511.1	04	177-179
511.81	04	180-182
511.89	04	186-188
511.9	04	186-188
512.0	04	199-201
512.1	04	199-201
512.2	04	199-201
512.81	04	199-201
512.82	04	199-201
512.83	04	199-201
512.84	04	199-201
512.89	04	199-201
513.0	04	177-179
513.1	04	177-179
514	04	189
515	04	196-198
516.0	04	196-198
516.1	04	196-198
516.2	04	196-198
516.30	04	196-198
516.31	04	196-198
516.32	04	196-198
516.33	04	196-198
516.34	04	196-198
516.35	04	196-198
516.36	04	196-198
516.37	04	196-198
516.4	04	196-198
516.5	04	196-198
516.61	04	196-198
516.62	04	196-198
516.63	04	196-198
516.64	04	196-198
516.69	04	196-198
516.8	04	196-198
516.9	04	196-198
517.1	04	196-198
517.2	04	196-198
517.3	04	196-198
517.8	04	196-198
518.0	04	205-206
518.1	04	199-201
518.2	04	205-206
518.3	04	196-198
518.4	04	189
518.51	04	189
518.52	04	189
518.53	04	189
518.6	04	196-198
518.7	04	205-206
518.81	04	189
518.82	04	204
518.83	04	189
518.84	04	189
518.89	04	205-206
519.00	04	205-206
519.0	04	205-206
519.02	04	205-206
519.09	04	205-206
519.11	04	202-203
519.19	04	202-203
519.2	04	177-179
519.3	04	205-206
519.4	04	205-206
519.8	04	205-206
519.9	04	205-206

Diseases of the Digestive System

DX	MDC	DRG
520.0	03	157-159
520.1	03	157-159
520.2	03	157-159

DX	MDC	DRG	DX	MDC	DRG	DX	MDC	DRG	DX	MDC	DRG	DX	MDC	DRG
520.3	03	157-159	523.33	03	157-159	524.9	03	157-159	528.1	03	157-159	532.31	06	380-382
520.4	03	157-159	523.40	03	157-159	525.0	03	157-159	528.2	03	157-159	532.40	06	377-379
520.5	03	157-159	523.41	03	157-159	525.10	03	157-159	528.3	03	157-159	532.41	06	377-379
520.6	03	157-159	523.42	03	157-159	525.11	03	157-159	528.4	03	157-159	532.50	06	380-382
520.7	03	157-159	523.5	03	157-159	525.12	03	157-159	528.5	03	157-159	532.51	06	380-382
520.8	03	157-159	523.6	03	157-159	525.13	03	157-159	528.6	03	157-159	532.60	06	377-379
520.9	03	157-159	523.8	03	157-159	525.19	03	157-159	528.71	03	157-159	532.61	06	377-379
521.00	03	157-159	523.9	03	157-159	525.20	03	157-159	528.72	03	157-159	532.70	06	383-384
521.01	03	157-159	524.00	03	157-159	525.21	03	157-159	528.79	03	157-159	532.71	06	380-382
521.02	03	157-159	524.01	03	157-159	525.22	03	157-159	528.8	03	157-159	532.90	06	383-384
521.03	03	157-159	524.02	03	157-159	525.23	03	157-159	528.9	03	157-159	532.91	06	380-382
521.04	03	157-159	524.03	03	157-159	525.24	03	157-159	529.0	03	157-159	533.00	06	377-379
521.06	03	157-159	524.04	03	157-159	525.25	03	157-159	529.1	03	157-159	533.01	06	377-379
521.07	03	157-159	524.05	03	157-159	525.26	03	157-159	529.2	03	157-159	533.10	06	380-382
521.08	03	157-159	524.06	03	157-159	525.3	03	157-159	529.3	03	157-159	533.11	06	380-382
521.09	03	157-159	524.07	03	157-159	525.40	03	157-159	529.4	03	157-159	533.20	06	377-379
521.10	03	157-159	524.09	03	157-159	525.41	03	157-159	529.5	03	157-159	533.21	06	377-379
521.11	03	157-159	524.10	03	157-159	525.42	03	157-159	529.6	03	157-159	533.30	06	383-384
521.12	03	157-159	524.11	03	157-159	525.43	03	157-159	529.8	03	157-159	533.31	06	380-382
521.13	03	157-159	524.12	03	157-159	525.44	03	157-159	529.9	03	157-159	533.40	06	377-379
521.14	03	157-159	524.19	03	157-159	525.50	03	157-159	530.0	06	391-392	533.41	06	377-379
521.15	03	157-159	524.20	03	157-159	525.51	03	157-159	530.10	06	391-392	533.50	06	380-382
521.20	03	157-159	524.21	03	157-159	525.52	03	157-159	530.11	06	391-392	533.51	06	380-382
521.21	03	157-159	524.22	03	157-159	525.53	03	157-159	530.12	06	391-392	533.60	06	377-379
521.22	03	157-159	524.23	03	157-159	525.54	03	157-159	530.13	06	391-392	533.61	06	377-379
521.23	03	157-159	524.24	03	157-159	525.60	03	157-159	530.19	06	391-392	533.70	06	383-384
521.24	03	157-159	524.25	03	157-159	525.61	03	157-159	530.20	06	380-382	533.71	06	380-382
521.25	03	157-159	524.26	03	157-159	525.62	03	157-159	530.21	06	380-382	533.90	06	383-384
521.30	03	157-159	524.27	03	157-159	525.63	03	157-159	530.3	06	391-392	533.91	06	380-382
521.31	03	157-159	524.28	03	157-159	525.64	03	157-159	530.4	06	368-370	534.00	06	377-379
521.32	03	157-159	524.29	03	157-159	525.65	03	157-159	530.5	06	391-392	534.01	06	377-379
521.33	03	157-159	524.30	03	157-159	525.66	03	157-159	530.6	06	391-392	534.10	06	380-382
521.34	03	157-159	524.31	03	157-159	525.67	03	157-159	530.7	06	368-370	534.11	06	380-382
521.35	03	157-159	524.32	03	157-159	525.69	03	157-159	530.81	06	391-392	534.20	06	377-379
521.40	03	157-159	524.33	03	157-159	525.71	03	157-159	530.82	06	368-370	534.21	06	377-379
521.41	03	157-159	524.34	03	157-159	525.72	03	157-159	530.83	06	391-392	534.30	06	380-382
521.42	03	157-159	524.35	03	157-159	525.73	03	157-159	530.84	06	368-370	534.31	06	380-382
521.49	03	157-159	524.36	03	157-159	525.79	03	157-159	530.85	06	380-382	534.40	06	377-379
521.5	03	157-159	524.37	03	157-159	525.8	03	157-159	530.86	06	393-395	534.41	06	377-379
521.6	03	157-159	524.39	03	157-159	525.9	03	157-159	530.87	06	393-395	534.50	06	380-382
521.7	03	157-159	524.4	03	157-159	526.0	03	157-159	530.89	06	391-392	534.51	06	380-382
521.81	03	157-159	524.50	03	157-159	526.1	03	157-159	530.9	06	391-392	534.60	06	377-379
521.89	03	157-159	524.51	03	157-159	526.2	03	157-159	531.00	06	377-379	534.61	06	377-379
521.9	03	157-159	524.52	03	157-159	526.3	03	157-159	531.01	06	377-379	534.70	06	380-382
522.0	03	157-159	524.53	03	157-159	526.4	03	157-159	531.10	06	380-382	534.71	06	380-382
522.1	03	157-159	524.54	03	157-159	526.5	03	157-159	531.11	06	380-382	534.90	06	380-382
522.2	03	157-159	524.55	03	157-159	526.61	03	157-159	531.20	06	377-379	534.91	06	380-382
522.3	03	157-159	524.56	03	157-159	526.62	03	157-159	531.21	06	377-379	535.00	06	391-392
522.4	03	157-159	524.57	03	157-159	526.63	03	157-159	531.30	06	383-384	535.01	06	377-379
522.5	03	157-159	524.59	03	157-159	526.69	03	157-159	531.31	06	380-382	535.10	06	391-392
522.6	03	157-159	524.60	03	157-159	526.81	03	157-159	531.40	06	377-379	535.11	06	377-379
522.7	03	157-159	524.61	03	157-159	526.89	03	157-159	531.41	06	377-379	535.20	06	391-392
522.8	03	157-159	524.62	03	157-159	526.9	03	157-159	531.50	06	380-382	535.21	06	377-379
522.9	03	157-159	524.63	03	157-159	527.0	03	154-156	531.51	06	380-382	535.30	06	391-392
523.00	03	157-159	524.64	03	157-159	527.1	03	154-156	531.60	06	377-379	535.31	06	377-379
523.01	03	157-159	524.69	03	157-159	527.2	03	154-156	531.61	06	377-379	535.40	06	391-392
523.10	03	157-159	524.70	03	157-159	527.3	03	154-156	531.70	06	383-384	535.41	06	377-379
523.11	03	157-159	524.71	03	157-159	527.4	03	154-156	531.71	06	380-382	535.50	06	391-392
523.20	03	157-159	524.72	03	157-159	527.5	03	154-156	531.90	06	383-384	535.51	06	377-379
523.21	03	157-159	524.73	03	157-159	527.6	03	154-156	531.91	06	380-382	535.60	06	391-392
523.22	03	157-159	524.74	03	157-159	527.7	03	154-156	532.00	06	377-379	535.61	06	377-379
523.23	03	157-159	524.75	03	157-159	527.8	03	154-156	532.01	06	377-379	535.70	06	391-392
523.24	03	157-159	524.76	03	157-159	527.9	03	154-156	532.10	06	380-382	535.71	06	377-379
523.25	03	157-159	524.79	03	157-159	528.00	03	157-159	532.11	06	380-382	536.0	06	391-392
523.30	03	157-159	524.81	03	157-159	528.01	03	157-159	532.20	06	377-379	536.1	06	391-392
523.31	03	157-159	524.82	03	157-159	528.02	03	157-159	532.21	06	377-379	536.2	06	391-392
523.32	03	157-159	524.89	03	157-159	528.09	03	157-159	532.30	06	383-384	536.3	06	391-392

Diagnosis Code/MDC/DRG List

DX	MDC	DRG
536.40	06	393-395
536.41	06	393-395
536.42	06	393-395
536.49	06	393-395
536.8	06	391-392
536.9	06	391-392
537.0	06	380-382
537.1	06	391-392
537.2	06	391-392
537.3	06	380-382
537.4	06	391-392
537.5	06	391-392
537.6	06	391-392
537.81	06	391-392
537.82	06	391-392
537.83	06	377-379
537.84	06	377-379
537.89	06	391-392
537.9	06	391-392
538	06	391-392
539.01	06	393-395
539.09	06	393-395
539.81	06	393-395
539.89	06	393-395
540.0	06	371-373
540.1	06	371-373
540.9	06	393-395
541	06	393-395
542	06	393-395
543.0	06	393-395
543.9	06	393-395
550.00	06	393-395
550.01	06	393-395
550.02	06	393-395
550.03	06	393-395
550.10	06	393-395
550.11	06	393-395
550.12	06	393-395
550.13	06	393-395
550.90	06	393-395
550.91	06	393-395
550.92	06	393-395
550.93	06	393-395
551.00	06	393-395
551.01	06	393-395
551.02	06	393-395
551.03	06	393-395
551.1	06	393-395
551.20	06	393-395
551.21	06	393-395
551.29	06	393-395
551.3	06	393-395
551.8	06	393-395
551.9	06	393-395
552.00	06	393-395
552.01	06	393-395
552.02	06	393-395
552.03	06	393-395
552.1	06	393-395
552.20	06	393-395
552.21	06	393-395
552.29	06	393-395
552.3	06	391-392
552.8	06	393-395
552.9	06	393-395
553.00	06	393-395
553.01	06	393-395
553.02	06	393-395
553.03	06	393-395
553.1	06	393-395
553.20	06	393-395
553.21	06	393-395
553.29	06	393-395
553.3	06	391-392
553.8	06	393-395
553.9	06	393-395
555.0	06	385-387
555.1	06	385-387
555.2	06	385-387
555.9	06	385-387
556.0	06	385-387
556.1	06	385-387
556.2	06	385-387
556.3	06	385-387
556.4	06	385-387
566.5	06	385-387
566.6	06	385-387
566.8	06	385-387
566.9	06	385-387
557.0	06	393-395
557.1	06	393-395
557.9	06	393-395
558.1	06	393-395
558.2	06	393-395
558.3	06	391-392
558.41	06	391-392
558.42	06	391-392
558.9	06	391-392
560.0	06	388-390
560.1	06	388-390
560.2	06	388-390
560.30	06	388-390
560.31	06	388-390
560.32	06	388-390
560.39	06	388-390
560.81	06	388-390
560.89	06	388-390
560.9	06	388-390
562.00	06	391-392
562.01	06	391-392
562.02	06	377-379
562.03	06	377-379
562.10	06	391-392
562.11	06	391-392
562.12	06	377-379
562.13	06	377-379
564.00	06	391-392
564.01	06	391-392
564.02	06	391-392
564.09	06	391-392
564.1	06	391-392
564.2	06	391-392
564.3	06	391-392
564.4	06	391-392
564.5	06	391-392
564.6	06	391-392
564.7	06	393-395
564.81	06	391-392
564.89	06	391-392
564.9	06	391-392
565.0	06	393-395
565.1	06	393-395
566	06	393-395
567.0	06	371-373
567.1	06	371-373
567.21	06	371-373
567.22	06	371-373
567.23	06	371-373
567.29	06	371-373
567.31	06	371-373
567.38	06	371-373
567.39	06	371-373
567.81	06	393-395
567.82	06	393-395
567.89	06	371-373
567.9	06	371-373
568.0	06	393-395
568.81	06	393-395
568.82	06	393-395
568.89	06	393-395
568.9	06	393-395
569.0	06	393-395
569.1	06	393-395
569.2	06	393-395
569.3	06	377-379
569.41	06	393-395
569.42	06	393-395
569.43	06	393-395
569.44	06	393-395
569.49	06	393-395
569.5	06	371-373
569.60	06	393-395
569.61	06	393-395
569.62	06	393-395
569.69	06	393-395
569.71	06	393-395
569.79	06	393-395
569.81	06	393-395
569.82	06	393-395
569.83	06	393-395
569.84	06	393-395
569.85	06	377-379
569.86	06	393-395
569.87	06	393-395
569.89	06	393-395
569.9	06	393-395
570	07	441-443
571.0	07	441-443
571.1	07	432-434
571.2	07	432-434
571.3	07	432-434
571.40	07	441-443
571.41	07	441-443
571.42	07	441-443
571.49	07	441-443
571.5	07	432-434
571.6	07	432-434
571.8	07	441-443
571.9	07	441-443
572.0	07	441-443
572.1	07	441-443
572.2	07	441-443
572.3	07	441-443
572.4	07	441-443
572.8	07	441-443
573.0	07	441-443
573.1	07	441-443
573.2	07	441-443
573.3	07	441-443
573.4	07	441-443
573.5	04	205-206
573.8	07	441-443
573.9	07	441-443
574.00	07	444-446
574.01	07	444-446
574.10	07	444-446
574.11	07	444-446
574.20	07	444-446
574.21	07	444-446
574.30	07	444-446
574.31	07	444-446
574.40	07	444-446
574.41	07	444-446
574.50	07	444-446
574.51	07	444-446
574.60	07	444-446
574.61	07	444-446
574.70	07	444-446
574.71	07	444-446
574.80	07	444-446
574.81	07	444-446
574.90	07	444-446
574.91	07	444-446
575.0	07	444-446
575.10	07	444-446
575.11	07	444-446
575.12	07	444-446
575.2	07	444-446
575.3	07	444-446
575.4	07	444-446
575.5	07	444-446
575.6	07	444-446
575.8	07	444-446
575.9	07	444-446
576.0	07	444-446
576.1	07	444-446
576.2	07	444-446
576.3	07	444-446
576.4	07	444-446
576.5	07	444-446
576.8	07	444-446
576.9	07	444-446
577.0	07	438-440
577.1	07	438-440
577.2	07	438-440
577.8	07	438-440
577.9	07	438-440
578.0	06	377-379
578.1	06	377-379
578.9	06	377-379
579.0	06	391-392
579.1	06	391-392
579.2	06	391-392
579.3	06	391-392
579.4	06	391-392
579.8	06	391-392
579.9	06	391-392

Diseases of the Genitourinary System

DX	MDC	DRG
580.0	11	698-700
580.4	11	698-700
580.81	11	698-700
580.89	11	698-700
580.9	11	698-700
581.0	11	698-700
581.1	11	698-700
581.2	11	698-700
581.3	11	698-700
581.81	11	698-700
581.89	11	698-700
581.9	11	698-700
582.0	11	698-700
582.1	11	698-700
582.2	11	698-700
582.4	11	698-700
582.81	11	698-700
582.89	11	698-700
582.9	11	698-700
583.0	11	698-700
583.1	11	698-700
583.2	11	698-700
583.4	11	698-700
583.6	11	698-700
583.7	11	698-700
583.81	11	698-700
583.89	11	698-700
583.9	11	698-700
584.5	11	682-684
584.6	11	682-684
584.7	11	682-684
584.8	11	682-684
584.9	11	682-684
585.1	11	682-684
585.2	11	682-684
585.3	11	682-684
585.4	11	682-684
585.5	11	682-684
585.6	11	682-684
585.9	11	682-684
586	11	682-684
587	11	698-700
588.0	11	698-700
588.1	11	698-700
588.81	11	698-700
588.89	11	698-700
588.9	11	698-700
589.0	11	698-700
589.1	11	698-700
589.9	11	698-700
590.00	11	689-690
590.01	11	689-690
590.10	11	689-690
590.11	11	689-690
590.2	11	689-690
590.3	11	689-690
590.80	11	689-690
590.81	11	689-690
590.9	11	689-690
591	11	691-694
592.0	11	691-694
592.1	11	691-694
592.9	11	691-694
593.0	11	698-700
593.1	11	698-700
593.2	11	698-700
593.3	11	689-690
593.4	11	691-694
593.5	11	691-694
593.6	11	698-700
593.70	11	698-700
593.71	11	698-700
593.72	11	698-700
593.73	11	698-700
593.81	11	698-700
593.82	11	698-700
593.89	11	698-700
593.9	11	698-700
594.0	11	698-700
594.1	11	691-694
594.2	11	691-694

DX	MDC	DRG	DX	MDC	DRG	DX	MDC	DRG	DX	MDC	DRG	DX	MDC	DRG
594.8	11	691-694	601.1	12	727-728	611.6	09	600-601	619.8	13	760-761	625.70	13	760-761
594.9	11	691-694	601.2	12	727-728	611.71	09	600-601	619.9	13	760-761	625.71	13	757-759
595.0	11	689-690	601.3	12	727-728	611.72	09	600-601	620.0	13	760-761	625.79	13	760-761
595.1	11	689-690	601.4	12	727-728	611.79	09	600-601	620.1	13	760-761	625.8	13	760-761
595.2	11	689-690	601.8	12	727-728	611.81	09	600-601	620.2	13	760-761	625.9	13	760-761
595.3	11	689-690	601.9	12	727-728	611.82	09	600-601	620.3	13	760-761	626.0	13	760-761
595.4	11	689-690	602.0	12	729-730	611.83	09	600-601	620.4	13	760-761	626.1	13	760-761
595.81	11	689-690	602.1	12	729-730	611.89	09	600-601	620.5	13	760-761	626.2	13	760-761
595.82	11	698-700	602.2	12	729-730	611.9	09	600-601	620.6	13	760-761	626.3	13	760-761
595.89	11	689-690	602.3	12	729-730	612.0	09	600-601	620.7	13	760-761	626.4	13	760-761
595.9	11	689-690	602.8	12	729-730	612.1	09	600-601	620.8	13	760-761	626.5	13	760-761
596.0	11	698-700	602.9	12	729-730	614.0	13	757-759	620.9	13	760-761	626.6	13	760-761
596.1	11	698-700	603.0	12	729-730	614.1	13	757-759	621.0	13	760-761	626.7	13	760-761
596.2	11	698-700	603.1	12	729-730	614.2	13	757-759	621.1	13	760-761	626.8	13	760-761
596.3	11	698-700	603.8	12	729-730	614.3	13	757-759	621.2	13	760-761	626.9	13	760-761
596.4	11	698-700	603.9	12	729-730	614.4	13	757-759	621.30	13	760-761	627.0	13	760-761
596.51	11	698-700	604.0	12	727-728	614.5	13	757-759	621.31	13	760-761	627.1	13	760-761
596.52	11	698-700	604.90	12	727-728	614.6	13	760-761	621.32	13	760-761	627.2	13	760-761
596.53	11	698-700	604.91	12	727-728	614.7	13	757-759	621.33	13	760-761	627.3	13	760-761
596.54	11	698-700	604.99	12	727-728	614.8	13	757-759	621.34	13	760-761	627.4	13	760-761
596.55	11	698-700	605	12	727-728	614.9	13	757-759	621.35	13	760-761	627.8	13	760-761
596.59	11	698-700	606.0	12	729-730	615.0	13	757-759	621.4	13	760-761	627.9	13	760-761
596.6	11	698-700	606.1	12	729-730	615.1	13	757-759	621.5	13	760-761	628.0	13	760-761
596.7	11	698-700	606.8	12	729-730	615.9	13	757-759	621.6	13	760-761	628.1	13	760-761
596.81	11	698-700	606.9	12	729-730	616.0	13	757-759	621.7	13	760-761	628.2	13	760-761
596.82	11	698-700	607.0	12	729-730	616.10	13	757-759	621.8	13	760-761	628.3	13	760-761
596.83	11	698-700	607.1	12	727-728	616.11	13	757-759	621.9	13	760-761	628.4	13	760-761
596.89	11	698-700	607.2	12	727-728	616.2	13	760-761	622.0	13	760-761	628.8	13	760-761
596.9	11	698-700	607.3	12	729-730	616.3	13	757-759	622.10	13	760-761	628.9	13	760-761
597.0	11	689-690	607.81	12	727-728	616.4	13	757-759	622.11	13	760-761	629.0	13	760-761
597.80	11	689-690	607.82	12	729-730	616.50	13	760-761	622.12	13	760-761	629.1	13	760-761
597.81	11	689-690	607.83	12	729-730	616.51	13	760-761	622.2	13	760-761	629.20	13	760-761
597.89	11	689-690	607.84	12	729-730	616.81	13	757-759	622.3	13	760-761	629.21	13	760-761
598.00	11	697	607.85	12	729-730	616.89	13	757-759	622.4	13	760-761	629.22	13	760-761
598.01	11	697	607.89	12	729-730	616.9	13	757-759	622.5	13	760-761	629.23	13	760-761
598.1	11	697	607.9	12	729-730	617.0	13	760-761	622.6	13	760-761	629.29	13	760-761
598.2	11	697	608.0	12	727-728	617.1	13	760-761	622.7	13	760-761	629.31	13	760-761
598.8	11	697	608.1	12	729-730	617.2	13	760-761	622.8	13	760-761	629.32	13	760-761
598.9	11	697	608.20	12	729-730	617.3	13	760-761	622.9	13	760-761	629.81	13	760-761
599.0	11	689-690	608.21	12	729-730	617.4	13	760-761	623.0	13	760-761	629.89	13	760-761
599.1	11	698-700	608.22	12	729-730	617.5	06	391-392	623.1	13	760-761	629.9	13	760-761
599.2	11	698-700	608.23	12	729-730	617.6	09	606-607	623.2	13	760-761			
599.3	11	698-700	608.24	12	729-730	617.8	13	760-761	623.3	13	760-761			
599.4	11	698-700	608.3	12	729-730	617.9	13	760-761	623.4	13	760-761			
599.5	11	698-700	608.4	12	727-728	618.00	13	760-761	623.5	13	760-761			
599.60	11	698-700	608.81	12	729-730	618.01	13	760-761	623.6	13	760-761			
599.69	11	698-700	608.82	12	729-730	618.02	13	760-761	623.7	13	760-761			
599.70	11	695-696	608.83	12	729-730	618.03	13	760-761	623.8	13	760-761			
599.71	11	695-696	608.84	12	729-730	618.04	13	760-761	623.9	13	760-761			
599.72	11	695-696	608.85	12	729-730	618.05	13	760-761	624.01	13	760-761			
599.81	11	698-700	608.86	12	729-730	618.09	13	760-761	624.02	13	760-761			
599.82	11	698-700	608.87	12	729-730	618.1	13	760-761	624.09	13	760-761			
599.83	11	698-700	608.89	12	729-730	618.2	13	760-761	624.1	13	760-761			
599.84	11	698-700	608.9	12	729-730	618.3	13	760-761	624.2	13	760-761			
599.89	11	698-700	610.0	09	600-601	618.4	13	760-761	624.3	13	760-761			
599.9	11	698-700	610.1	09	600-601	618.5	13	760-761	624.4	13	760-761			
600.00	12	725-726	610.2	09	600-601	618.6	13	760-761	624.5	13	760-761			
600.01	12	725-726	610.3	09	600-601	618.7	13	760-761	624.6	13	760-761			
600.10	12	725-726	610.4	09	600-601	618.81	13	760-761	624.8	13	760-761			
600.11	12	725-726	610.8	09	600-601	618.82	13	760-761	624.9	13	760-761			
600.20	12	725-726	610.9	09	600-601	618.83	13	760-761	625.0	13	760-761			
600.21	12	725-726	611.0	09	600-601	618.84	13	760-761	625.1	13	760-761			
600.30	12	725-726	611.1	09	600-601	618.89	13	760-761	625.2	13	760-761			
600.31	12	725-726	611.2	09	600-601	618.9	13	760-761	625.3	13	760-761			
600.90	12	725-726	611.3	09	600-601	619.0	13	760-761	625.4	13	760-761			
600.91	12	725-726	611.4	09	600-601	619.1	06	393-395	625.5	13	760-761			
601.0	12	727-728	611.5	09	600-601	619.2	13	760-761	625.6	13	760-761			

Complications of Pregnancy, Childbirth and the Puerperium

DX	MDC	DRG
630	14	781-782
631.0	14	781-782
631.8	14	781-782
632	14	779
633.00	14	777
633.01	14	777
633.10	14	777
633.11	14	777
633.20	14	777
633.21	14	777
633.80	14	777
633.81	14	777
633.90	14	777
633.91	14	777
634.00	14	779
634.01	14	779
634.02	14	779
634.10	14	779
634.11	14	779
634.12	14	779
634.20	14	779
634.21	14	779
634.22	14	779

Diagnosis Code/MDC/DRG List

DX	MDC	DRG	DX	MDC	DRG	DX	MDC	DRG	DX	MDC	DRG	DX	MDC	DRG
634.30	14	779	636.52	14	779	640.90	14	778	643.03	14	781	647.01	14	774
634.31	14	779	636.60	14	779	640.91	14	774-775	643.10	14	998	647.02	14	774
634.32	14	779	636.61	14	779	640.93	14	778	643.11	14	774-775	647.03	14	781
634.40	14	779	636.62	14	779	641.00	14	998	643.13	14	781	647.04	14	776
634.41	14	779	636.70	14	779	641.01	14	774	643.20	14	998	647.10	14	998
634.42	14	779	636.71	14	779	641.03	14	781-782	643.21	14	774-775	647.11	14	774
634.50	14	779	636.72	14	779	641.10	14	998	643.23	14	781	647.12	14	774
634.51	14	779	636.80	14	779	641.11	14	774	643.80	14	998	647.13	14	781
634.52	14	779	636.81	14	779	641.13	14	781-782	643.81	14	774-775	647.14	14	776
634.60	14	779	636.82	14	779	641.20	14	998	643.83	14	781	647.20	14	998
634.61	14	779	636.90	14	779	641.21	14	774	643.90	14	998	647.21	14	774
634.62	14	779	636.91	14	779	641.23	14	781-782	643.91	14	774-775	647.22	14	774
634.70	14	779	636.92	14	779	641.30	14	998	643.93	14	781	647.23	14	781
634.71	14	779	637.00	14	779	641.31	14	774	644.00	14	778	647.24	14	776
634.72	14	779	637.01	14	779	641.33	14	781	644.03	14	778	647.30	14	998
634.80	14	779	637.02	14	779	641.80	14	998	644.10	14	780	647.31	14	774
634.81	14	779	637.10	14	779	641.81	14	774	644.13	14	780	647.32	14	774
634.82	14	779	637.11	14	779	641.83	14	781-782	644.20	14	781-782	647.33	14	781
634.90	14	779	637.12	14	779	641.90	14	998	644.21	14	774-775	647.34	14	776
634.91	14	779	637.20	14	779	641.91	14	774	645.10	14	998	647.40	14	998
634.92	14	779	637.21	14	779	641.93	14	781-782	645.11	14	774-775	647.41	14	774
635.00	14	779	637.22	14	779	642.00	14	998	645.13	14	781-782	647.42	14	774
635.01	14	779	637.30	14	779	642.01	14	774	645.20	14	998	647.43	14	781
635.02	14	779	637.31	14	779	642.02	14	774	645.21	14	774-775	647.44	14	776
635.10	14	779	637.32	14	779	642.03	14	781	645.23	14	781-782	647.50	14	998
635.11	14	779	637.40	14	779	642.04	14	776	646.00	14	774-775	647.51	14	774
635.12	14	779	637.41	14	779	642.10	14	998	646.01	14	774-775	647.52	14	774
635.20	14	779	637.42	14	779	642.11	14	774	646.03	14	781-782	647.53	14	781
635.21	14	779	637.50	14	779	642.12	14	774	646.10	14	998	647.54	14	776
635.22	14	779	637.51	14	779	642.13	14	781	646.11	14	774-775	647.60	14	998
635.30	14	779	637.52	14	779	642.14	14	776	646.12	14	774-775	647.61	14	774
635.31	14	779	637.60	14	779	642.20	14	998	646.13	14	781	647.62	14	774
635.32	14	779	637.61	14	779	642.21	14	774	646.14	14	776	647.63	14	781
635.40	14	779	637.62	14	779	642.22	14	774	646.20	14	998	647.64	14	776
635.41	14	779	637.70	14	779	642.23	14	781	646.21	14	774-775	647.80	14	998
635.42	14	779	637.71	14	779	642.24	14	776	646.22	14	774-775	647.81	14	774
635.50	14	779	637.72	14	779	642.30	14	998	646.23	14	781	647.82	14	774
635.51	14	779	637.80	14	779	642.31	14	774-775	646.24	14	776	647.83	14	781
635.52	14	779	637.81	14	779	642.32	14	774-775	646.30	14	998	647.84	14	776
635.60	14	779	637.82	14	779	642.33	14	781-782	646.31	14	774-775	647.90	14	998
635.61	14	779	637.90	14	779	642.34	14	776	646.33	14	781-782	647.91	14	774
635.62	14	779	637.91	14	779	642.40	14	998	646.40	14	998	647.92	14	774
635.70	14	779	637.92	14	779	642.41	14	774	646.41	14	774-775	647.93	14	781
635.71	14	779	638.0	14	779	642.42	14	774	646.42	14	774-775	647.94	14	776
635.72	14	779	638.1	14	779	642.43	14	781	646.43	14	781	648.00	14	998
635.80	14	779	638.2	14	779	642.44	14	776	646.44	14	776	648.01	14	774
635.81	14	779	638.3	14	779	642.50	14	998	646.50	14	998	648.02	14	774
635.82	14	779	638.4	14	779	642.51	14	774	646.51	14	774-775	648.03	14	781
635.90	14	779	638.5	14	779	642.52	14	774	646.52	14	774-775	648.04	14	776
635.91	14	779	638.6	14	779	642.53	14	781	646.53	14	781-782	648.10	14	998
635.92	14	779	638.7	14	779	642.54	14	776	646.54	14	776	648.11	14	774-775
636.00	14	779	638.8	14	779	642.60	14	998	646.60	14	998	648.12	14	774-775
636.01	14	779	638.9	14	779	642.61	14	774	646.61	14	774-775	648.13	14	781
636.02	14	779	639.0	14	776	642.62	14	774	646.62	14	774-775	648.14	14	776
636.10	14	779	639.1	14	776	642.63	14	781	646.63	14	781	648.20	14	998
636.11	14	779	639.2	14	776	642.64	14	776	646.64	14	776	648.21	14	774-775
636.12	14	779	639.3	14	776	642.70	14	998	646.70	14	998	648.22	14	774-775
636.20	14	779	639.4	14	776	642.71	14	774	646.71	14	774-775	648.23	14	781
636.21	14	779	639.5	14	776	642.72	14	774	646.73	14	781	648.24	14	776
636.22	14	779	639.6	14	776	642.73	14	781	646.80	14	998	648.30	14	998
636.30	14	779	639.8	14	776	642.74	14	776	646.81	14	774-775	648.31	14	774-775
636.31	14	779	639.9	14	776	642.90	14	998	646.82	14	774-775	648.32	14	774-775
636.32	14	779	640.00	14	778	642.91	14	774	646.83	14	781	648.33	14	781
636.40	14	779	640.01	14	774-775	642.92	14	774	646.84	14	776	648.34	14	776
636.41	14	779	640.03	14	778	642.93	14	781	646.90	14	998	648.40	14	998
636.42	14	779	640.80	14	778	642.94	14	776	646.91	14	774-775	648.41	14	774-775
636.50	14	779	640.81	14	774-775	643.00	14	998	646.93	14	781-782	648.42	14	774-775
636.51	14	779	640.83	14	778	643.01	14	774-775	647.00	14	998	648.43	14	781

DX	MDC	DRG
648.44	14	776
648.50	14	998
648.51	14	774
648.52	14	774
648.53	14	781
648.54	14	776
648.60	14	998
648.61	14	774
648.62	14	774
648.63	14	781
648.64	14	776
648.70	14	998
648.71	14	774-775
648.72	14	774-775
648.73	14	781
648.74	14	776
648.80	14	998
648.81	14	774-775
648.82	14	774-775
648.83	14	781
648.84	14	776
648.90	14	998
648.91	14	774-775
648.92	14	774-775
648.93	14	781
648.94	14	776
649.00	14	998
649.01	14	774-775
649.02	14	774-775
649.03	14	781-782
649.04	14	776
649.10	14	998
649.11	14	774-775
649.12	14	774-775
649.13	14	781-782
649.14	14	776
649.20	14	998
649.21	14	774-775
649.22	14	774-775
649.23	14	781-782
649.24	14	776
649.30	14	998
649.31	14	774-775
649.32	14	774-775
649.33	14	781-782
649.34	14	776
649.40	14	998
649.41	14	774-775
649.42	14	774-775
649.43	14	781-782
649.44	14	776
649.50	14	998
649.51	14	774-775
649.53	14	781-782
649.60	14	998
649.61	14	774-775
649.62	14	774-775
649.63	14	781-782
649.64	14	776
649.70	14	998
649.71	14	774-775
649.73	14	781-782
649.81	14	774-775
649.82	14	774-775
650	14	774-775
651.00	14	998
651.01	14	774-775
651.03	14	781-782
651.10	14	998
651.11	14	774-775
651.13	14	781-782
651.20	14	998
651.21	14	774-775
651.23	14	781-782
651.30	14	998
651.31	14	774-775
651.33	14	781-782
651.40	14	998
651.41	14	774-775
651.43	14	781-782
651.50	14	998
651.51	14	774-775
651.53	14	781-782
651.60	14	998
651.61	14	774-775
651.63	14	781-782
651.70	14	998
651.71	14	774-775
651.73	14	781-782
651.80	14	998
651.81	14	774-775
651.83	14	781-782
651.90	14	998
651.91	14	774-775
651.93	14	781-782
652.00	14	998
652.01	14	774-775
652.03	14	781-782
652.10	14	998
652.11	14	774-775
652.13	14	781-782
652.20	14	998
652.21	14	774-775
652.23	14	781-782
652.30	14	998
652.31	14	774-775
652.33	14	781-782
652.40	14	998
652.41	14	774-775
652.43	14	781-782
652.50	14	998
652.51	14	774-775
652.53	14	781-782
652.60	14	998
652.61	14	774-775
652.63	14	781-782
652.70	14	998
652.71	14	774-775
652.73	14	781-782
652.80	14	998
652.81	14	774-775
652.83	14	781-782
652.90	14	998
652.91	14	774-775
652.93	14	781-782
653.00	14	998
653.01	14	774-775
653.03	14	781-782
653.10	14	998
653.11	14	774-775
653.13	14	781-782
653.20	14	998
653.21	14	774-775
653.23	14	781-782
653.30	14	998
653.31	14	774-775
653.33	14	781-782
653.40	14	998
653.41	14	774-775
653.43	14	781-782
653.50	14	998
653.51	14	774-775
653.53	14	781-782
653.60	14	998
653.61	14	774-775
653.63	14	781-782
653.70	14	998
653.71	14	774-775
653.73	14	781-782
653.80	14	998
653.81	14	774-775
653.83	14	781-782
653.90	14	998
653.91	14	774-775
653.93	14	781-782
654.00	14	998
654.01	14	774-775
654.02	14	774-775
654.03	14	781-782
654.04	14	776
654.10	14	998
654.11	14	774-775
654.12	14	774-775
654.13	14	781-782
654.14	14	776
654.20	14	998
654.21	14	774-775
654.23	14	781-782
654.30	14	998
654.31	14	774-775
654.32	14	774-775
654.33	14	781-782
654.34	14	776
654.40	14	998
654.41	14	774-775
654.42	14	774-775
654.43	14	781-782
654.44	14	776
654.50	14	998
654.51	14	774-775
654.52	14	774-775
654.53	14	781-782
654.54	14	776
654.60	14	998
654.61	14	774-775
654.62	14	774-775
654.63	14	781-782
654.64	14	776
654.70	14	998
654.71	14	774-775
654.72	14	774-775
654.73	14	781-782
654.74	14	776
654.80	14	998
654.81	14	774-775
654.82	14	774-775
654.83	14	781-782
654.84	14	776
654.90	14	998
654.91	14	774-775
654.92	14	774-775
654.93	14	781-782
654.94	14	776
655.00	14	998
655.01	14	774-775
655.03	14	781-782
655.10	14	998
655.11	14	774-775
655.13	14	781-782
655.20	14	998
655.21	14	774-775
655.23	14	781-782
655.30	14	998
655.31	14	774-775
655.33	14	781-782
655.40	14	998
655.41	14	774-775
655.43	14	781-782
655.50	14	998
655.51	14	774-775
655.53	14	781-782
655.60	14	998
655.61	14	774-775
655.63	14	781-782
655.70	14	998
655.71	14	774-775
655.73	14	781-782
655.80	14	998
655.81	14	774-775
655.83	14	781-782
655.90	14	998
655.91	14	774-775
655.93	14	781-782
656.00	14	998
656.01	14	774-775
656.03	14	781-782
656.10	14	998
656.11	14	774-775
656.13	14	781-782
656.20	14	998
656.21	14	774-775
656.23	14	781-782
656.30	14	774-775
656.31	14	774-775
656.33	14	781-782
656.40	14	774-775
656.41	14	774-775
656.43	14	781-782
656.50	14	998
656.51	14	774-775
656.53	14	781-782
656.60	14	998
656.61	14	774-775
656.63	14	781-782
656.70	14	998
656.71	14	774-775
656.73	14	781-782
656.80	14	998
656.81	14	774-775
656.83	14	781-782
656.90	14	998
656.91	14	774-775
656.93	14	781-782
657.00	14	998
657.01	14	774-775
657.03	14	781-782
658.00	14	998
658.01	14	774-775
658.03	14	781-782
658.10	14	774-775
658.11	14	774-775
658.13	14	781-782
658.20	14	774-775
658.21	14	774-775
658.23	14	781-782
658.30	14	774-775
658.31	14	774-775
658.33	14	781-782
658.40	14	774-775
658.41	14	774-775
658.43	14	781-782
658.80	14	998
658.81	14	774-775
658.83	14	781-782
658.90	14	998
658.91	14	774-775
658.93	14	781-782
659.00	14	774-775
659.01	14	774-775
659.03	14	781-782
659.10	14	774-775
659.11	14	774-775
659.13	14	781-782
659.20	14	774-775
659.21	14	774
659.23	14	781-782
659.30	14	774-775
659.31	14	774
659.33	14	781-782
659.40	14	998
659.41	14	774-775
659.43	14	781-782
659.50	14	774-775
659.51	14	774-775
659.53	14	781-782
659.60	14	774-775
659.61	14	774-775
659.63	14	781-782
659.70	14	774-775
659.71	14	774-775
659.73	14	781-782
659.80	14	774-775
659.81	14	774-775
659.83	14	781-782
659.90	14	774-775
659.91	14	774-775
659.93	14	781-782
660.00	14	774-775
660.01	14	774-775
660.03	14	781-782
660.10	14	774-775
660.11	14	774-775
660.13	14	781-782
660.20	14	774-775
660.21	14	774-775
660.23	14	781-782
660.30	14	774-775
660.31	14	774-775
660.33	14	781-782
660.40	14	774-775
660.41	14	774-775
660.43	14	781-782
660.50	14	774-775
660.51	14	774-775
660.53	14	781-782

Diagnosis Code/MDC/DRG List

DX	MDC	DRG	DX	MDC	DRG	DX	MDC	DRG	DX	MDC	DRG	DX	MDC	DRG
660.60	14	774-775	663.93	14	781-782	666.20	14	998	669.82	14	774-775	673.11	14	774
660.61	14	774-775	664.00	14	774-775	666.22	14	774	669.83	14	781-782	673.12	14	774
660.63	14	781-782	664.01	14	774-775	666.24	14	776	669.84	14	776	673.13	14	781-782
660.70	14	774-775	664.04	14	776	666.30	14	998	669.90	14	774-775	673.14	14	776
660.71	14	774-775	664.10	14	774-775	666.32	14	774	669.91	14	774-775	673.20	14	998
660.73	14	781-782	664.11	14	774-775	666.34	14	776	669.92	14	774-775	673.21	14	774
660.80	14	774-775	664.14	14	776	667.00	14	998	669.93	14	781-782	673.22	14	774
660.81	14	774-775	664.20	14	774-775	667.02	14	774	669.94	14	776	673.23	14	781-782
660.83	14	781-782	664.21	14	774-775	667.04	14	776	670.00	14	998	673.24	14	776
660.90	14	774-775	664.24	14	776	667.10	14	998	670.02	14	774	673.30	14	998
660.91	14	774-775	664.30	14	774-775	667.12	14	774	670.04	14	776	673.31	14	774
660.93	14	781-782	664.31	14	774-775	667.14	14	776	670.10	14	998	673.32	14	774
661.00	14	774-775	664.34	14	776	668.00	14	774-775	670.12	14	774	673.33	14	781-782
661.01	14	774-775	664.40	14	774-775	668.01	14	774	670.14	14	776	673.34	14	776
661.03	14	781-782	664.41	14	774-775	668.02	14	774	670.20	14	998	673.80	14	998
661.10	14	774-775	664.44	14	776	668.03	14	781-782	670.22	14	774	673.81	14	774
661.11	14	774-775	664.50	14	774-775	668.04	14	776	670.24	14	776	673.82	14	774
661.13	14	781-782	664.51	14	774-775	668.10	14	774-775	670.30	14	998	673.83	14	781-782
661.20	14	774-775	664.54	14	776	668.11	14	774	670.32	14	774	673.84	14	776
661.21	14	774-775	664.60	14	774-775	668.12	14	774	670.34	14	776	674.00	14	998
661.23	14	781-782	664.61	14	774-775	668.13	14	781-782	670.80	14	998	674.01	14	774
661.30	14	774-775	664.64	14	776	668.14	14	776	670.82	14	774	674.02	14	774
661.31	14	774-775	664.80	14	774-775	668.20	14	774-775	670.84	14	776	674.03	14	781-782
661.33	14	781-782	664.81	14	774-775	668.21	14	774	671.00	14	998	674.04	14	776
661.40	14	774-775	664.84	14	776	668.22	14	774	671.01	14	774-775	674.10	14	998
661.41	14	774-775	664.90	14	774-775	668.23	14	781-782	671.02	14	774-775	674.12	14	774
661.43	14	781-782	664.91	14	774-775	668.24	14	776	671.03	14	781-782	674.14	14	776
661.90	14	774-775	664.94	14	776	668.80	14	774-775	671.04	14	776	674.20	14	998
661.91	14	774-775	665.00	14	774-775	668.81	14	774	671.10	14	998	674.22	14	774
661.93	14	781-782	665.01	14	774-775	668.82	14	774	671.11	14	774-775	674.24	14	776
662.00	14	774-775	665.03	14	781-782	668.83	14	781-782	671.12	14	774-775	674.30	14	998
662.01	14	774-775	665.10	14	774-775	668.84	14	776	671.13	14	781-782	674.32	14	774
662.03	14	781-782	665.11	14	774-775	668.90	14	774-775	671.14	14	776	674.34	14	776
662.10	14	774-775	665.20	14	774-775	668.91	14	774	671.20	14	998	674.40	14	998
662.11	14	774-775	665.22	14	774-775	668.92	14	774	671.21	14	774-775	674.42	14	774-775
662.13	14	781-782	665.24	14	776	668.93	14	781-782	671.22	14	774-775	674.44	14	776
662.20	14	774-775	665.30	14	774-775	668.94	14	776	671.23	14	781-782	674.50	14	998
662.21	14	774-775	665.31	14	774-775	669.00	14	774-775	671.24	14	776	674.51	14	774
662.23	14	781-782	665.34	14	776	669.01	14	774-775	671.30	14	998	674.52	14	774
662.30	14	774-775	665.40	14	774-775	669.02	14	774-775	671.31	14	774	674.53	14	781-782
662.31	14	774-775	665.41	14	774-775	669.03	14	781-782	671.33	14	781-782	674.54	14	776
662.33	14	781-782	665.44	14	776	669.04	14	776	671.40	14	998	674.80	14	998
663.00	14	774-775	665.50	14	774-775	669.10	14	774-775	671.42	14	774	674.82	14	774
663.01	14	774-775	665.51	14	774-775	669.11	14	774	671.44	14	776	674.84	14	776
663.03	14	781-782	665.54	14	776	669.12	14	774	671.50	14	998	674.90	14	998
663.10	14	774-775	665.60	14	774-775	669.13	14	781-782	671.51	14	774	674.92	14	774-775
663.11	14	774-775	665.61	14	774-775	669.14	14	776	671.52	14	774	674.94	14	776
663.13	14	781-782	665.64	14	776	669.20	14	774-775	671.53	14	781-782	675.00	14	998
663.20	14	774-775	665.70	14	774-775	669.21	14	774-775	671.54	14	776	675.01	14	774
663.21	14	774-775	665.71	14	774-775	669.22	14	774-775	671.80	14	998	675.02	14	774
663.23	14	781-782	665.72	14	774-775	669.23	14	781-782	671.81	14	774-775	675.03	14	781-782
663.30	14	774-775	665.74	14	776	669.24	14	776	671.82	14	774-775	675.04	14	776
663.31	14	774-775	665.80	14	774-775	669.30	14	774-775	671.83	14	781-782	675.10	14	998
663.33	14	781-782	665.81	14	774-775	669.32	14	774	671.84	14	776	675.11	14	774
663.40	14	774-775	665.82	14	774-775	669.34	14	776	671.90	14	998	675.12	14	774
663.41	14	774-775	665.83	14	781-782	669.40	14	774-775	671.91	14	774-775	675.13	14	781-782
663.43	14	781-782	665.84	14	776	669.41	14	774	671.92	14	774-775	675.14	14	776
663.50	14	774-775	665.90	14	774-775	669.42	14	774	671.93	14	781-782	675.20	14	998
663.51	14	774-775	665.91	14	774-775	669.43	14	781-782	671.94	14	776	675.21	14	774
663.53	14	781-782	665.92	14	774-775	669.44	14	776	672.00	14	998	675.22	14	774
663.60	14	774-775	665.93	14	781-782	669.50	14	774-775	672.02	14	774	675.23	14	781-782
663.61	14	774-775	665.94	14	776	669.51	14	774-775	672.04	14	776	675.24	14	776
663.63	14	781-782	666.00	14	998	669.60	14	774-775	673.00	14	998	675.80	14	998
663.80	14	774-775	666.02	14	774	669.61	14	774-775	673.01	14	774	675.81	14	774-775
663.81	14	774-775	666.04	14	776	669.70	14	774-775	673.02	14	774	675.82	14	774-775
663.83	14	781-782	666.10	14	998	669.71	14	774-775	673.03	14	781-782	675.83	14	781-782
663.90	14	774-775	666.12	14	774	669.80	14	774-775	673.04	14	776	675.84	14	776
663.91	14	774-775	666.14	14	776	669.81	14	774-775	673.10	14	998	675.90	14	998

DX	MDC	DRG
675.91	14	774-775
675.92	14	774-775
675.93	14	781-782
675.94	14	776
676.00	14	998
676.01	14	774-775
676.02	14	774-775
676.03	14	781-782
676.04	14	776
676.10	14	998
676.11	14	774-775
676.12	14	774-775
676.13	14	781-782
676.14	14	776
676.20	14	998
676.21	14	774-775
676.22	14	774-775
676.23	14	781-782
676.24	14	776
676.30	14	998
676.31	14	774-775
676.32	14	774-775
676.33	14	781-782
676.34	14	776
676.40	14	998
676.41	14	774-775
676.42	14	774-775
676.43	14	781-782
676.44	14	776
676.50	14	998
676.51	14	774-775
676.52	14	774-775
676.53	14	781-782
676.54	14	776
676.60	14	998
676.61	14	774-775
676.62	14	774-775
676.63	14	781-782
676.64	14	776
676.80	14	998
676.81	14	774-775
676.82	14	774-775
676.83	14	781-782
676.84	14	776
676.90	14	998
676.91	14	774-775
676.92	14	774-775
676.93	14	781-782
676.94	14	776
677	14	998
578.00	14	998
578.01	14	774-775
578.03	14	781-782
578.10	14	998
578.11	14	774-775
578.13	14	781,782
579.00	14	774-775
579.01	14	774
579.02	14	774
579.03	14	781-782
579.04	14	776
579.10	14	998
579.11	14	774-775
579.12	14	774-775
579.13	14	781-782
579.14	14	776

Diseases of the Skin and Subcutaneous Tissue

DX	MDC	DRG
680.0	09	602-603
680.1	09	602-603
680.2	09	602-603
680.3	09	602-603
680.4	09	602-603
680.5	09	602-603
680.6	09	602-603
680.7	09	602-603
680.8	09	602-603
680.9	09	602-603
681.00	09	602-603
681.01	09	602-603
681.02	09	602-603
681.10	09	602-603
681.11	09	602-603
681.9	09	602-603
682.0	09	602-603
682.1	09	602-603
682.2	09	602-603
682.3	09	602-603
682.4	09	602-603
682.5	09	602-603
682.6	09	602-603
682.7	09	602-603
682.8	09	602-603
682.9	09	602-603
683	16	814-816
684	09	602-603
685.0	09	602-603
685.1	09	602-603
686.00	09	602-603
686.01	09	602-603
686.09	09	602-603
686.1	09	602-603
686.8	09	602-603
686.9	09	602-603
690.10	09	606-607
690.11	09	606-607
690.12	09	606-607
690.18	09	606-607
690.8	09	606-607
691.0	09	606-607
691.8	09	606-607
692.0	09	606-607
692.1	09	606-607
692.2	09	606-607
692.3	09	606-607
692.4	09	606-607
692.5	09	606-607
692.6	09	606-607
692.70	09	606-607
692.71	09	606-607
692.72	09	606-607
692.73	09	606-607
692.74	09	606-607
692.75	09	606-607
692.76	09	606-607
692.77	09	606-607
692.79	09	606-607
692.81	09	606-607
692.82	09	606-607
692.83	09	606-607
692.84	09	606-607
692.89	09	606-607
692.9	09	606-607
693.0	09	606-607

DX	MDC	DRG
693.1	09	606-607
693.8	09	606-607
693.9	09	606-607
694.0	09	606-607
694.1	09	606-607
694.2	09	606-607
694.3	09	606-607
694.4	09	595-596
694.5	09	595-596
694.60	09	595-596
694.61	02	124-125
694.8	09	595-596
694.9	09	595-596
695.0	09	595-596
695.10	09	595-596
695.11	09	595-596
695.12	09	595-596
695.13	09	595-596
695.14	09	595-596
695.15	09	595-596
695.19	09	595-596
695.2	09	595-596
695.3	09	606-607
695.4	09	595-596
695.50	09	606-607
695.51	09	606-607
695.52	09	606-607
695.53	09	606-607
695.54	09	606-607
695.55	09	606-607
695.56	09	606-607
695.57	09	606-607
695.58	09	606-607
695.59	09	606-607
695.81	09	595-596
695.89	09	606-607
695.9	09	606-607
696.0	08	545-547
696.1	09	595-596
696.2	09	595-596
696.3	09	606-607
696.4	09	606-607
696.5	09	606-607
696.8	09	606-607
697.0	09	606-607
697.1	09	606-607
697.8	09	606-607
697.9	09	606-607
698.0	09	606-607
698.1	12	729-730
698.1	13	757-759
698.2	09	606-607
698.3	09	606-607
698.4	09	606-607
698.8	09	606-607
698.9	09	606-607
700	09	606-607
701.0	09	606-607
701.1	09	606-607
701.2	09	606-607
701.3	09	606-607
701.4	09	606-607
701.5	09	606-607
701.8	09	606-607
701.9	09	606-607
702.0	09	606-607
702.11	09	606-607

DX	MDC	DRG
702.19	09	606-607
702.8	09	606-607
703.0	09	606-607
703.8	09	606-607
703.9	09	606-607
704.00	09	606-607
704.01	09	606-607
704.02	09	606-607
704.09	09	606-607
704.1	09	606-607
704.2	09	606-607
704.3	09	606-607
704.41	09	606-607
704.42	09	606-607
704.8	09	606-607
704.9	09	606-607
705.0	09	606-607
705.1	09	606-607
705.21	09	606-607
705.22	09	606-607
705.81	09	606-607
705.82	09	606-607
705.83	09	606-607
705.89	09	606-607
705.9	09	606-607
706.0	09	606-607
706.1	09	606-607
706.2	09	606-607
706.3	09	606-607
706.8	09	606-607
706.9	09	606-607
707.00	09	592-594
707.01	09	592-594
707.02	09	592-594
707.03	09	592-594
707.04	09	592-594
707.05	09	592-594
707.06	09	592-594
707.07	09	592-594
707.09	09	592-594
707.10	09	592-594
707.11	09	592-594
707.12	09	592-594
707.13	09	592-594
707.14	09	592-594
707.15	09	592-594
707.19	09	592-594
707.20	09	592-594
707.21	09	592-594
707.22	09	592-594
707.23	09	592-594
707.24	09	592-594
707.25	09	592-594
707.8	09	592-594
707.9	09	592-594
708.0	09	606-607
708.1	09	606-607
708.2	09	606-607
708.3	09	606-607
708.4	09	606-607
708.5	09	606-607
708.8	09	606-607
708.9	09	606-607
709.00	09	606-607
709.01	09	606-607
709.09	09	606-607
709.1	09	606-607

DX	MDC	DRG
709.2	09	606-607
709.3	09	606-607
709.4	09	606-607
709.8	09	606-607
709.9	09	606-607

Diseases of the Musculoskeletal System and Connective Tissue

DX	MDC	DRG
710.0	08	545-547
710.1	08	545-547
710.2	08	545-547
710.3	08	545-547
710.4	08	545-547
710.5	08	545-547
710.8	08	545-547
710.9	08	545-547
711.00	08	548-550
711.01	08	548-550
711.02	08	548-550
711.03	08	548-550
711.04	08	548-550
711.05	08	548-550
711.06	08	548-550
711.07	08	548-550
711.08	08	548-550
711.09	08	548-550
711.10	08	545-547
711.11	08	545-547
711.12	08	545-547
711.13	08	545-547
711.14	08	545-547
711.15	08	545-547
711.16	08	545-547
711.17	08	545-547
711.18	08	545-547
711.19	08	545-547
711.20	08	545-547
711.21	08	545-547
711.22	08	545-547
711.23	08	545-547
711.24	08	545-547
711.25	08	545-547
711.26	08	545-547
711.27	08	545-547
711.28	08	545-547
711.29	08	545-547
711.30	08	553-554
711.31	08	553-554
711.32	08	553-554
711.33	08	553-554
711.34	08	553-554
711.35	08	553-554
711.36	08	553-554
711.37	08	553-554
711.38	08	553-554
711.39	08	553-554
711.40	08	548-550
711.41	08	548-550
711.42	08	548-550
711.43	08	548-550
711.44	08	548-550
711.45	08	548-550
711.46	08	548-550
711.47	08	548-550
711.48	08	548-550
711.49	08	548-550
711.50	08	553-554

DX	MDC	DRG	DX	MDC	DRG	DX	MDC	DRG	DX	MDC	DRG	DX	MDC	DRG
711.51	08	553-554	712.29	08	553-554	715.25	08	553-554	716.44	08	553-554	718.04	08	562-563
711.52	08	553-554	712.30	08	553-554	715.26	08	553-554	716.45	08	553-554	718.05	08	564-566
711.53	08	553-554	712.31	08	553-554	715.27	08	553-554	716.46	08	553-554	718.07	08	562-563
711.54	08	553-554	712.32	08	553-554	715.28	08	553-554	716.47	08	553-554	718.08	08	564-566
711.55	08	553-554	712.33	08	553-554	715.30	08	553-554	716.48	08	553-554	718.09	08	564-566
711.56	08	553-554	712.34	08	553-554	715.31	08	553-554	716.49	08	553-554	718.10	08	564-566
711.57	08	553-554	712.35	08	553-554	715.32	08	553-554	716.50	08	553-554	718.11	08	564-566
711.58	08	553-554	712.36	08	553-554	715.33	08	553-554	716.51	08	553-554	718.12	08	564-566
711.59	08	553-554	712.37	08	553-554	715.34	08	553-554	716.52	08	553-554	718.13	08	564-566
711.60	08	548-550	712.38	08	553-554	715.35	08	553-554	716.53	08	553-554	718.14	08	564-566
711.61	08	548-550	712.39	08	553-554	715.36	08	553-554	716.54	08	553-554	718.15	08	564-566
711.62	08	548-550	712.80	08	553-554	715.37	08	553-554	716.55	08	553-554	718.17	08	564-566
711.63	08	548-550	712.81	08	553-554	715.38	08	553-554	716.56	08	553-554	718.18	08	564-566
711.64	08	548-550	712.82	08	553-554	715.80	08	553-554	716.57	08	553-554	718.19	08	564-566
711.65	08	548-550	712.83	08	553-554	715.89	08	553-554	716.58	08	553-554	718.20	08	562-563
711.66	08	548-550	712.84	08	553-554	715.90	08	553-554	716.59	08	553-554	718.21	08	562-563
711.67	08	548-550	712.85	08	553-554	715.91	08	553-554	716.60	08	553-554	718.22	08	562-563
711.68	08	548-550	712.86	08	553-554	715.92	08	553-554	716.61	08	553-554	718.23	08	562-563
711.69	08	548-550	712.87	08	553-554	715.93	08	553-554	716.62	08	553-554	718.24	08	562-563
711.70	08	548-550	712.88	08	553-554	715.94	08	553-554	716.63	08	553-554	718.25	08	564-566
711.71	08	548-550	712.89	08	553-554	715.95	08	553-554	716.64	08	553-554	718.26	08	562-563
711.72	08	548-550	712.90	08	553-554	715.96	08	553-554	716.65	08	553-554	718.27	08	562-563
711.73	08	548-550	712.91	08	553-554	715.97	08	553-554	716.66	08	553-554	718.28	08	564-566
711.74	08	548-550	712.92	08	553-554	715.98	08	553-554	716.67	08	553-554	718.29	08	564-566
711.75	08	548-550	712.93	08	553-554	716.00	08	553-554	716.68	08	553-554	718.30	08	564-566
711.76	08	548-550	712.94	08	553-554	716.01	08	553-554	716.80	08	553-554	718.31	08	562-563
711.77	08	548-550	712.95	08	553-554	716.02	08	553-554	716.81	08	553-554	718.32	08	562-563
711.78	08	548-550	712.96	08	553-554	716.03	08	553-554	716.82	08	553-554	718.33	08	562-563
711.79	08	548-550	712.97	08	553-554	716.04	08	553-554	716.83	08	553-554	718.34	08	562-563
711.80	08	548-550	712.98	08	553-554	716.05	08	553-554	716.84	08	553-554	718.35	08	564-566
711.81	08	548-550	712.99	08	553-554	716.06	08	553-554	716.85	08	553-554	718.36	08	562-563
711.82	08	548-550	713.0	08	553-554	716.07	08	553-554	716.86	08	553-554	718.37	08	562-563
711.83	08	548-550	713.1	08	553-554	716.08	08	553-554	716.87	08	553-554	718.38	08	564-566
711.84	08	548-550	713.2	08	553-554	716.09	08	553-554	716.88	08	553-554	718.39	08	564-566
711.85	08	548-550	713.3	08	553-554	716.10	08	553-554	716.89	08	553-554	718.40	08	564-566
711.86	08	548-550	713.4	08	553-554	716.11	08	553-554	716.90	08	553-554	718.41	08	564-566
711.87	08	548-550	713.5	08	553-554	716.12	08	553-554	716.91	08	553-554	718.42	08	564-566
711.88	08	548-550	713.6	08	553-554	716.13	08	553-554	716.92	08	553-554	718.43	08	564-566
711.89	08	548-550	713.7	08	553-554	716.14	08	553-554	716.93	08	553-554	718.44	08	564-566
711.90	08	548-550	713.8	08	553-554	716.15	08	553-554	716.94	08	553-554	718.45	08	564-566
711.91	08	548-550	714.0	08	545-547	716.16	08	553-554	716.95	08	553-554	718.46	08	564-566
711.92	08	548-550	714.1	08	545-547	716.17	08	553-554	716.96	08	553-554	718.47	08	564-566
711.93	08	548-550	714.2	08	545-547	716.18	08	553-554	716.97	08	553-554	718.48	08	564-566
711.94	08	548-550	714.30	08	545-547	716.19	08	553-554	716.98	08	553-554	718.49	08	564-566
711.95	08	548-550	714.31	08	545-547	716.20	08	553-554	716.99	08	553-554	718.50	08	553-554
711.96	08	548-550	714.32	08	545-547	716.21	08	553-554	717.0	08	562-563	718.51	08	553-554
711.97	08	548-550	714.33	08	545-547	716.22	08	553-554	717.1	08	562-563	718.52	08	553-554
711.98	08	548-550	714.4	08	553-554	716.23	08	553-554	717.2	08	562-563	718.53	08	553-554
711.99	08	548-550	714.81	04	196-198	716.24	08	553-554	717.3	08	562-563	718.54	08	553-554
712.10	08	553-554	714.89	08	545-547	716.25	08	553-554	717.40	08	562-563	718.55	08	553-554
712.11	08	553-554	714.9	08	553-554	716.26	08	553-554	717.41	08	562-563	718.56	08	553-554
712.12	08	553-554	715.00	08	553-554	716.27	08	553-554	717.42	08	562-563	718.57	08	553-554
712.13	08	553-554	715.04	08	553-554	716.28	08	553-554	717.43	08	562-563	718.58	08	553-554
712.14	08	553-554	715.09	08	553-554	716.29	08	553-554	717.49	08	562-563	718.59	08	553-554
712.15	08	553-554	715.10	08	553-554	716.30	08	553-554	717.5	08	562-563	718.65	08	564-566
712.16	08	553-554	715.11	08	553-554	716.31	08	553-554	717.6	08	564-566	718.70	08	564-566
712.17	08	553-554	715.12	08	553-554	716.32	08	553-554	717.7	08	562-563	718.71	08	564-566
712.18	08	553-554	715.13	08	553-554	716.33	08	553-554	717.81	08	562-563	718.72	08	564-566
712.19	08	553-554	715.14	08	553-554	716.34	08	553-554	717.82	08	562-563	718.73	08	564-566
712.20	08	553-554	715.15	08	553-554	716.35	08	553-554	717.83	08	562-563	718.74	08	564-566
712.21	08	553-554	715.16	08	553-554	716.36	08	553-554	717.84	08	562-563	718.75	08	564-566
712.22	08	553-554	715.17	08	553-554	716.37	08	553-554	717.85	08	562-563	718.76	08	564-566
712.23	08	553-554	715.18	08	553-554	716.38	08	553-554	717.89	08	562-563	718.77	08	564-566
712.24	08	553-554	715.20	08	553-554	716.39	08	553-554	717.9	08	562-563	718.78	08	564-566
712.25	08	553-554	715.21	08	553-554	716.40	08	553-554	718.00	08	564-566	718.79	08	564-566
712.26	08	553-554	715.22	08	553-554	716.41	08	553-554	718.01	08	562-563	718.80	08	564-566
712.27	08	553-554	715.23	08	553-554	716.42	08	553-554	718.02	08	562-563	718.81	08	564-566
712.28	08	553-554	715.24	08	553-554	716.43	08	553-554	718.03	08	562-563	718.82	08	564-566

DX	MDC	DRG	DX	MDC	DRG	DX	MDC	DRG	DX	MDC	DRG	DX	MDC	DRG
718.83	08	564-566	719.51	08	555-556	722.51	08	551-552	726.79	08	557-558	729.4	08	557-558
718.84	08	564-566	719.52	08	555-556	722.52	08	551-552	726.8	08	557-558	729.5	08	555-556
718.85	08	564-566	719.53	08	555-556	722.6	08	551-552	726.90	08	557-558	729.6	08	564-566
718.86	08	564-566	719.54	08	555-556	722.70	08	551-552	726.91	08	557-558	729.71	08	557-558
718.87	08	564-566	719.55	08	555-556	722.71	08	551-552	727.00	08	557-558	729.72	08	557-558
718.88	08	564-566	719.56	08	555-556	722.72	08	551-552	727.01	08	557-558	729.73	08	557-558
718.89	08	564-566	719.57	08	555-556	722.73	08	551-552	727.02	08	564-566	729.79	08	557-558
718.90	08	564-566	719.58	08	555-556	722.80	08	551-552	727.03	08	557-558	729.81	08	555-556
718.91	08	564-566	719.59	08	555-556	722.81	08	551-552	727.04	08	557-558	729.82	08	555-556
718.92	08	564-566	719.60	08	555-556	722.82	08	551-552	727.05	08	557-558	729.89	08	555-556
718.93	08	564-566	719.61	08	555-556	722.83	08	551-552	727.06	08	557-558	729.90	08	555-556
718.94	08	564-566	719.62	08	555-556	722.90	08	551-552	727.09	08	557-558	729.91	08	555-556
718.95	08	564-566	719.63	08	555-556	722.91	08	551-552	727.1	08	564-566	729.92	08	555-556
718.97	08	564-566	719.64	08	555-556	722.92	08	551-552	727.2	08	557-558	729.99	08	555-556
718.98	08	564-566	719.65	08	555-556	722.93	08	551-552	727.3	08	557-558	730.00	08	539-541
718.99	08	564-566	719.66	08	555-556	723.0	08	551-552	727.40	08	557-558	730.01	08	539-541
719.00	08	564-566	719.67	08	555-556	723.1	08	551-552	727.41	08	557-558	730.02	08	539-541
719.01	08	564-566	719.68	08	555-556	723.2	01	073-074	727.42	08	557-558	730.03	08	539-541
719.02	08	564-566	719.69	08	555-556	723.3	01	073-074	727.43	08	557-558	730.04	08	539-541
719.03	08	564-566	719.7	08	555-556	723.4	01	073-074	727.49	08	557-558	730.05	08	539-541
719.04	08	564-566	719.80	08	555-556	723.5	08	551-552	727.50	08	557-558	730.06	08	539-541
719.05	08	564-566	719.81	08	555-556	723.6	09	606-607	727.51	08	557-558	730.07	08	539-541
719.06	08	564-566	719.82	08	555-556	723.7	08	551-552	727.59	08	557-558	730.08	08	539-541
719.07	08	564-566	719.83	08	555-556	723.8	08	551-552	727.60	08	557-558	730.09	08	539-541
719.08	08	564-566	719.84	08	555-556	723.9	08	551-552	727.61	08	557-558	730.10	08	539-541
719.09	08	564-566	719.85	08	555-556	724.00	08	551-552	727.62	08	557-558	730.11	08	539-541
719.10	08	553-554	719.86	08	555-556	724.01	08	551-552	727.63	08	557-558	730.12	08	539-541
719.11	08	553-554	719.87	08	555-556	724.02	08	551-552	727.64	08	557-558	730.13	08	539-541
719.12	08	553-554	719.88	08	555-556	724.03	08	551-552	727.65	08	557-558	730.14	08	539-541
719.13	08	553-554	719.89	08	555-556	724.09	08	551-552	727.66	08	557-558	730.15	08	539-541
719.14	08	553-554	719.90	08	555-556	724.1	08	551-552	727.67	08	557-558	730.16	08	539-541
719.15	08	553-554	719.91	08	555-556	724.2	08	551-552	727.68	08	557-558	730.17	08	539-541
719.16	08	553-554	719.92	08	555-556	724.3	08	551-552	727.69	08	557-558	730.18	08	539-541
719.17	08	553-554	719.93	08	555-556	724.4	08	551-552	727.81	08	557-558	730.19	08	539-541
719.18	08	553-554	719.94	08	555-556	724.5	08	551-552	727.82	08	557-558	730.20	08	539-541
719.19	08	553-554	719.95	08	555-556	724.6	08	551-552	727.83	08	557-558	730.21	08	539-541
719.20	08	553-554	719.96	08	555-556	724.70	08	551-552	727.89	08	557-558	730.22	08	539-541
719.21	08	553-554	719.97	08	555-556	724.71	08	551-552	727.9	08	557-558	730.23	08	539-541
719.22	08	553-554	719.98	08	555-556	724.79	08	551-552	728.0	08	557-558	730.24	08	539-541
719.23	08	553-554	719.99	08	555-556	724.8	08	551-552	728.10	08	557-558	730.25	08	539-541
719.24	08	553-554	720.0	08	545-547	724.9	08	551-552	728.11	08	557-558	730.26	08	539-541
719.25	08	553-554	720.1	08	551-552	725	08	545-547	728.12	08	557-558	730.27	08	539-541
719.26	08	553-554	720.2	08	551-552	726.0	08	557-558	728.13	08	557-558	730.28	08	539-541
719.27	08	553-554	720.81	08	551-552	726.10	08	557-558	728.19	08	557-558	730.29	08	539-541
719.28	08	553-554	720.89	08	551-552	726.11	08	557-558	728.2	08	557-558	730.30	08	553-554
719.29	08	553-554	720.9	08	551-552	726.12	08	557-558	728.3	08	557-558	730.31	08	553-554
719.30	08	553-554	721.0	08	551-552	726.13	08	557-558	728.4	08	557-558	730.32	08	553-554
719.31	08	553-554	721.1	08	551-552	726.19	08	557-558	728.5	08	557-558	730.33	08	553-554
719.32	08	553-554	721.2	08	551-552	726.2	08	557-558	728.6	08	557-558	730.34	08	553-554
719.33	08	553-554	721.3	08	551-552	726.30	08	557-558	728.71	08	557-558	730.35	08	553-554
719.34	08	553-554	721.41	08	551-552	726.31	08	557-558	728.79	08	557-558	730.36	08	553-554
719.35	08	553-554	721.42	08	551-552	726.32	08	557-558	728.81	08	557-558	730.37	08	564-566
719.36	08	553-554	721.5	08	551-552	726.33	08	557-558	728.82	08	557-558	730.38	08	564-566
719.37	08	553-554	721.6	08	551-552	726.39	08	557-558	728.83	08	557-558	730.39	08	564-566
719.38	08	553-554	721.7	08	551-552	726.4	08	557-558	728.84	08	557-558	730.70	08	564-566
719.39	08	553-554	721.8	08	551-552	726.5	08	557-558	728.85	08	555-556	730.71	08	564-566
719.40	08	555-556	721.90	08	551-552	726.60	08	557-558	728.86	08	557-558	730.72	08	564-566
719.41	08	555-556	721.91	08	551-552	726.61	08	557-558	728.87	08	555-556	730.73	08	564-566
719.42	08	555-556	722.0	08	551-552	726.62	08	557-558	728.88	08	557-558	730.74	08	564-566
719.43	08	555-556	722.10	08	551-552	726.63	08	557-558	728.89	08	557-558	730.75	08	564-566
719.44	08	555-556	722.11	08	551-552	726.64	08	557-558	728.9	08	557-558	730.76	08	564-566
719.45	08	555-556	722.2	08	551-552	726.65	08	557-558	729.0	08	555-556	730.77	08	564-566
719.46	08	555-556	722.30	08	551-552	726.69	08	557-558	729.1	08	555-556	730.78	08	564-566
719.47	08	555-556	722.31	08	551-552	726.70	08	557-558	729.2	01	073-074	730.79	08	564-566
719.48	08	555-556	722.32	08	551-552	726.71	08	557-558	729.30	09	606-607	730.80	08	539-541
719.49	08	555-556	722.39	08	551-552	726.72	08	557-558	729.31	09	606-607	730.81	08	539-541
719.50	08	555-556	722.4	08	551-552	726.73	08	564-566	729.39	09	606-607	730.82	08	539-541

Diagnosis Code/MDC/DRG List

DX	MDC	DRG
730.83	08	539-541
730.84	08	539-541
730.85	08	539-541
730.86	08	539-541
730.87	08	539-541
730.88	08	539-541
730.89	08	539-541
730.90	08	539-541
730.91	08	539-541
730.92	08	539-541
730.93	08	539-541
730.94	08	539-541
730.95	08	539-541
730.96	08	539-541
730.97	08	539-541
730.98	08	539-541
730.99	08	539-541
731.0	08	553-554
731.1	08	553-554
731.2	08	553-554
731.3	08	553-554
731.8	08	553-554
732.0	08	553-554
732.1	08	553-554
732.2	08	553-554
732.3	08	553-554
732.4	08	553-554
732.5	08	553-554
732.6	08	553-554
732.7	08	553-554
732.8	08	553-554
732.9	08	553-554
733.00	08	553-554
733.01	08	553-554
733.02	08	553-554
733.03	08	553-554
733.09	08	553-554
733.10	08	542-544
733.11	08	542-544
733.12	08	542-544
733.13	08	542-544
733.14	08	542-544
733.15	08	542-544
733.16	08	542-544
733.19	08	542-544
733.20	08	553-554
733.21	08	553-554
733.22	08	553-554
733.29	08	553-554
733.3	08	564-566
733.40	08	553-554
733.41	08	553-554
733.42	08	553-554
733.43	08	553-554
733.44	08	553-554
733.45	08	553-554
733.49	08	553-554
733.5	08	553-554
733.6	04	205-206
733.7	08	564-566
733.81	08	564-566
733.82	08	564-566
733.90	08	564-566
733.91	08	564-566
733.92	08	553-554
733.93	08	542-544
733.94	08	542-544
733.95	08	542-544
733.96	08	542-544
733.97	08	542-544
733.98	08	542-544
733.99	08	564-566
734	08	564-566
735.0	08	564-566
735.1	08	564-566
735.2	08	564-566
735.3	08	564-566
735.4	08	564-566
735.5	08	564-566
735.8	08	564-566
735.9	08	564-566
736.00	08	564-566
736.01	08	564-566
736.02	08	564-566
736.03	08	564-566
736.04	08	564-566
736.05	01	073-074
736.06	01	073-074
736.07	01	073-074
736.09	08	564-566
736.1	08	564-566
736.20	08	564-566
736.21	08	564-566
736.22	08	564-566
736.29	08	564-566
736.30	08	564-566
736.31	08	564-566
736.32	08	564-566
736.39	08	564-566
736.41	08	564-566
736.42	08	564-566
736.5	08	564-566
736.6	08	564-566
736.70	08	564-566
736.71	08	564-566
736.72	08	564-566
736.73	08	564-566
736.74	01	073-074
736.75	08	564-566
736.76	08	564-566
736.79	08	564-566
736.81	08	564-566
736.89	08	564-566
736.9	08	564-566
737.0	08	551-552
737.10	08	551-552
737.11	08	551-552
737.12	08	551-552
737.19	08	551-552
737.20	08	551-552
737.21	08	551-552
737.22	08	551-552
737.29	08	551-552
737.30	08	551-552
737.31	08	551-552
737.32	08	551-552
737.33	08	551-552
737.34	08	551-552
737.39	08	551-552
737.40	08	551-552
737.41	08	551-552
737.42	08	551-552
737.43	08	551-552
737.8	08	551-552
737.9	08	551-552
738.0	03	154-156
738.10	08	564-566
738.11	08	564-566
738.12	08	564-566
738.19	08	564-566
738.2	08	564-566
738.3	08	564-566
738.4	08	551-552
738.5	08	551-552
738.6	08	564-566
738.7	03	154-156
738.8	08	564-566
738.9	08	564-566
739.0	08	555-556
739.1	08	551-552
739.2	08	551-552
739.3	08	551-552
739	08	551-552
739.5	08	555-556
739.6	08	555-556
739.7	08	555-556
739.8	08	555-556
739.9	08	555-556

Congenital Anomalies

DX	MDC	DRG
740.0	01	091-093
740.1	01	091-093
740.2	01	091-093
741.00	01	091-093
741.01	01	091-093
741.02	01	091-093
741.03	01	091-093
741.90	01	091-093
741.91	01	091-093
741.92	01	091-093
741.93	01	091-093
742.0	01	091-093
742.1	01	091-093
742.2	01	091-093
742.3	01	091-093
742.4	01	091-093
742.51	01	091-093
742.53	01	091-093
742.59	01	091-093
742.8	01	091-093
742.9	01	091-093
743.00	02	124-125
743.03	02	124-125
743.06	02	124-125
743.10	02	124-125
743.11	02	124-125
743.12	02	124-125
743.20	02	124-125
743.21	02	124-125
743.22	02	124-125
743.30	02	124-125
743.31	02	124-125
743.32	02	124-125
743.33	02	124-125
743.34	02	124-125
743.35	02	124-125
743.36	02	124-125
743.37	02	124-125
743.39	02	124-125
743.41	02	124-125
743.42	02	124-125
743.43	02	124-125
743.44	02	124-125
743.45	02	124-125
743.46	02	124-125
743.47	02	124-125
743.48	02	124-125
743.49	02	124-125
743.51	02	124-125
743.52	02	124-125
743.53	02	124-125
743.54	02	124-125
743.55	02	124-125
743.56	02	124-125
743.57	02	124-125
743.58	02	124-125
743.59	02	124-125
743.61	02	124-125
743.62	02	124-125
743.63	02	124-125
743.64	02	124-125
743.65	02	124-125
743.66	02	124-125
743.69	02	124-125
743.8	02	124-125
743.9	02	124-125
744.00	03	154-156
744.01	03	154-156
744.02	03	154-156
744.03	03	154-156
744.04	03	154-156
744.05	03	154-156
744.09	03	154-156
744.1	03	154-156
744.21	03	154-156
744.22	03	154-156
744.23	03	154-156
744.24	03	154-156
744.29	03	154-156
744.3	03	154-156
744.41	03	154-156
744.42	03	154-156
744.43	03	154-156
744.46	03	154-156
744.47	03	154-156
744.49	03	154-156
744.5	09	606-607
744.81	03	157-159
744.82	03	157-159
744.83	03	157-159
744.84	03	157-159
744.89	03	154-156
744.9	09	606-607
745.0	05	306-307
745.10	05	306-307
745.11	05	306-307
745.12	05	306-307
745.19	05	306-307
745.2	05	306-307
745.3	05	306-307
745.4	05	306-307
745.5	05	306-307
745.60	05	306-307
745.61	05	306-307
745.69	05	306-307
745.7	05	306-307
745.8	05	306-307
745.9	05	306-307
746.00	05	306-307
746.01	05	306-307
746.02	05	306-307
746.09	05	306-307
746.1	05	306-307
746.2	05	306-307
746.3	05	306-307
746.4	05	306-307
746.5	05	306-307
746.6	05	306-307
746.7	05	306-307
746.81	05	306-307
746.82	05	306-307
746.83	05	306-307
746.84	05	306-307
746.85	05	306-307
746.86	05	308-310
746.87	05	306-307
746.89	05	306-307
746.9	05	306-307
747.0	05	306-307
747.10	05	306-307
747.11	05	306-307
747.20	05	306-307
747.21	05	306-307
747.22	05	306-307
747.29	05	306-307
747.31	05	306-307
747.32	05	306-307
747.39	05	306-307
747.40	05	306-307
747.41	05	306-307
747.42	05	306-307
747.49	05	306-307
747.5	05	299-301
747.60	05	299-301
747.61	05	299-301
747.62	05	299-301
747.63	05	299-301
747.64	05	299-301
747.69	05	299-301
747.81	01	091-093
747.82	01	091-093
747.83	15	791-793
747.89	05	299-301
747.9	05	299-301
748.0	03	154-156
748.1	03	154-156
748.2	03	154-156
748.3	03	154-156
748.4	04	205-206
748.5	04	205-206
748.60	04	205-206
748.61	04	190-192
748.69	04	205-206
748.8	04	205-206
748.9	04	205-206
749.00	03	157-159
749.01	03	157-159
749.02	03	157-159
749.03	03	157-159
749.04	03	157-159
749.10	03	157-159
749.11	03	157-159
749.12	03	157-159
749.13	03	157-159
749.14	03	157-159
749.20	03	157-159
749.21	03	157-159
749.22	03	157-159
749.23	03	157-159
749.24	03	157-159

DX	MDC	DRG
749.25	03	157-159
750.0	03	157-159
750.10	03	157-159
750.11	03	157-159
750.12	03	157-159
750.13	03	157-159
750.15	03	157-159
750.16	03	157-159
750.19	03	157-159
750.21	03	154-156
750.22	03	154-156
750.23	03	154-156
750.24	03	154-156
750.25	03	157-159
750.26	03	157-159
750.27	03	154-156
750.29	03	154-156
750.3	06	368-370
750.4	06	368-370
750.5	06	393-395
750.6	06	393-395
750.7	06	393-395
750.8	06	393-395
750.9	06	393-395
751.0	06	380-382
751.1	06	393-395
751.2	06	393-395
751.3	06	393-395
751.4	06	393-395
751.5	06	393-395
751.60	07	444-446
751.61	07	444-446
751.62	07	441-443
751.69	07	441-443
751.7	07	438-440
751.8	06	393-395
751.9	06	393-395
752.0	13	760-761
752.10	13	760-761
752.11	13	760-761
752.19	13	760-761
752.2	13	760-761
752.31	13	760-761
752.32	13	760-761
752.33	13	760-761
752.34	13	760-761
752.35	13	760-761
752.36	13	760-761
752.39	13	760-761
752.40	13	760-761
752.41	13	760-761
752.42	13	760-761
752.43	13	760-761
752.44	13	760-761
752.45	13	760-761
752.46	13	760-761
752.47	13	760-761
752.49	13	760-761
752.51	12	729-730
752.52	12	729-730
752.61	12	729-730
752.62	12	729-730
752.63	12	729-730
752.64	12	729-730
752.65	12	729-730
752.69	12	729-730
752.7	12	729-730
752.7	13	760-761
752.81	12	729-730
752.89	12	729-730
752.8	13	760-761
752.9	12	729-730
752.9	13	760-761
753.0	11	698-700
753.10	11	698-700
753.11	11	698-700
753.12	11	698-700
753.13	11	698-700
753.14	11	698-700
753.15	11	698-700
753.16	11	698-700
753.17	11	698-700
753.19	11	698-700
753.20	11	698-700
753.21	11	698-700
753.22	11	698-700
753.23	11	698-700
753.29	11	698-700
753.3	11	698-700
753.4	11	698-700
753.5	11	698-700
753.6	11	698-700
753.7	11	698-700
753.8	11	698-700
753.9	11	698-700
754.0	08	564-566
754.1	08	564-566
754.2	08	564-566
754.30	08	564-566
754.31	08	564-566
754.32	08	564-566
754.33	08	564-566
754.35	08	564-566
754.40	08	564-566
754.41	08	562-563
754.42	08	564-566
754.43	08	564-566
754.44	08	564-566
754.50	08	564-566
754.51	08	564-566
754.52	08	564-566
754.53	08	564-566
754.59	08	564-566
754.60	08	564-566
754.61	08	564-566
754.62	08	564-566
754.69	08	564-566
754.70	08	564-566
754.71	08	564-566
754.79	08	564-566
754.81	04	205-206
754.82	04	205-206
754.89	08	564-566
755.00	08	564-566
755.01	08	564-566
755.02	08	564-566
755.10	08	564-566
755.11	08	564-566
755.12	08	564-566
755.13	08	564-566
755.14	08	564-566
755.20	08	564-566
755.21	08	564-566
755.22	08	564-566
755.23	08	564-566
755.24	08	564-566
755.25	08	564-566
755.26	08	564-566
755.27	08	564-566
755.28	08	564-566
755.29	08	564-566
755.30	08	564-566
755.31	08	564-566
755.32	08	564-566
755.33	08	564-566
755.34	08	564-566
755.35	08	564-566
755.36	08	564-566
755.37	08	564-566
755.38	08	564-566
755.39	08	564-566
755.4	08	564-566
755.50	08	564-566
755.51	08	564-566
755.52	08	564-566
755.53	08	564-566
755.54	08	564-566
755.55	08	564-566
755.56	08	564-566
755.57	08	564-566
755.58	08	564-566
755.59	08	564-566
755.60	08	564-566
755.61	08	564-566
755.62	08	564-566
755.63	08	564-566
755.64	08	564-566
755.65	08	564-566
755.66	08	564-566
755.67	08	564-566
755.69	08	564-566
755.8	08	564-566
755.9	08	564-566
756.0	08	564-566
756.10	08	551-552
756.11	08	551-552
756.12	08	551-552
756.13	08	551-552
756.14	08	551-552
756.15	08	551-552
756.16	08	564-566
756.17	01	091-093
756.19	08	551-552
756.2	08	564-566
756.3	04	205-206
756.4	08	564-566
756.50	08	564-566
756.51	08	564-566
756.52	08	564-566
756.53	08	564-566
756.54	08	564-566
756.55	08	564-566
756.56	08	564-566
756.59	08	564-566
756.6	04	205-206
756.70	06	393-395
756.71	06	393-395
756.72	06	393-395
756.73	06	393-395
756.79	06	393-395
756.81	08	564-566
756.82	08	564-566
756.83	08	564-566
756.89	08	564-566
756.9	08	564-566
757.0	09	606-607
757.1	09	606-607
757.2	09	606-607
757.31	09	606-607
757.32	09	606-607
757.33	09	606-607
757.39	09	606-607
757.4	09	606-607
757.5	09	606-607
757.6	09	600-601
757.8	09	606-607
757.9	09	606-607
758.0	19	884
758.1	19	884
758.2	19	884
758.31	19	884
758.32	19	884
758.33	19	884
758.39	19	884
758.4	23	951
758.5	23	951
758.6	12	729-730
758.6	13	760-761
758.7	12	729-730
758.8	12	729-730
758.81	12	729-730
758.81	13	760-761
758.89	12	729-730
758.89	13	760-761
758.9	23	951
759.0	16	814-816
759.1	10	643-645
759.2	10	643-645
759.3	06	393-395
759.4	06	393-395
759.5	01	091-093
759.6	17	843-845
759.7	08	564-566
759.81	08	564-566
759.82	05	306-307
759.83	19	884
759.89	08	564-566
759.9	23	951

Certain Conditions Originating in the Perinatal Period

DX	MDC	DRG
760.0	15	794
760.1	15	794
760.2	15	794
760.3	15	794
760.4	15	794
760.5	15	794
760.61	15	794
760.62	15	794
760.63	15	794
760.64	15	794
760.70	15	794
760.71	15	794
760.72	15	794
760.73	15	794
760.74	15	794
760.75	15	794
760.77	15	794
760.78	15	794
760.79	15	794
760.8	15	794
760.9	15	794
761.0	15	794
761.1	15	794
761.2	15	794
761.3	15	794
761.4	15	794
761.5	15	794
761.6	15	794
761.7	15	794
761.9	15	794
762.0	15	794
762.1	15	794
762.2	15	794
762.3	15	794
762.4	15	795
762.5	15	795
762.6	15	795
762.7	15	794
762.8	15	794
762.9	15	794
763.0	15	795
763.1	15	795
763.2	15	795
763.3	15	795
763.4	15	791, 793
763.5	15	794
763.6	15	795
763.7	15	794
763.81	15	794
763.82	15	794
763.83	15	794
763.84	15	794
763.89	15	794
763.9	15	795
764.00	15	794
764.01	15	794
764.02	15	794
764.03	15	791
764.04	15	794
764.05	15	794
764.06	15	794
764.07	15	794
764.08	15	795
764.09	15	795
764.10	15	794
764.11	15	791, 793
764.12	15	791, 793
764.13	15	791, 793
764.14	15	791, 793
764.15	15	791, 793
764.16	15	791, 793
764.17	15	791, 793
764.18	15	791, 793
764.19	15	794
764.20	15	794
764.21	15	791, 793
764.22	15	791, 793
764.23	15	791, 793
764.24	15	791, 793
764.25	15	791, 793
764.26	15	791, 793
764.27	15	791, 793
764.28	15	791, 793

Diagnosis Code/MDC/DRG List

DX	MDC	DRG
764.29	15	794
764.90	15	794
764.91	15	794
764.92	15	794
764.93	15	794
764.93	15	794
764.94	15	794
764.95	15	794
764.96	15	794
764.97	15	794
764.98	15	795
764.99	15	795
765.00	15	791-792
765.01	15	790
765.02	15	790
765.03	15	790
765.04	15	790
765.05	15	790
765.06	15	791-792
765.07	15	791-792
765.08	15	791-792
765.09	15	999
765.10	15	791-792
765.11	15	791-792
765.12	15	791-792
765.13	15	791-792
765.14	15	791-792
765.15	15	791-792
765.16	15	791-792
765.17	15	791-792
765.18	15	791-792
765.19	15	791-792
765.20	15	795
765.21	15	790
765.22	15	790
765.23	15	790
765.24	15	791-792
765.25	15	791-792
765.26	15	791-792
765.27	15	791-792
765.28	15	791-792
765.29	15	795
766.0	15	795
766.1	15	795
766.21	15	795
766.22	15	795
767.0	15	791, 793
767.11	15	791, 793
767.19	15	795
767.2	15	794
767.3	15	794
767.4	15	791, 793
767.5	15	794
767.6	15	794
767.7	15	791, 793
767.8	15	794
767.9	15	794
768.0	15	794
768.1	15	794
768.2	15	794
768.3	15	794
768.4	15	794
768.5	15	791, 793
768.6	15	795
768.70	15	794
768.71	15	794
768.72	15	791, 793
768.73	15	791, 793

DX	MDC	DRG
768.9	15	794
769	15	790
770.0	15	791, 793
770.10	15	791, 793
770.11	15	791, 793
770.12	15	791, 793
770.13	15	791, 793
770.14	15	791, 793
770.15	15	791, 793
770.16	15	791, 793
770.17	15	791, 793
770.18	15	791, 793
770.2	15	791, 793
770.3	15	791, 793
770.4	15	791, 793
770.5	15	794
770.6	15	794
770.7	04	196-198
770.81	15	794
770.82	15	794
770.83	15	794
770.84	15	791, 793
770.85	15	791, 793
770.86	15	791, 793
770.87	15	794
770.88	15	794
770.89	15	794
770.9	15	794
771.0	15	791, 793
771.1	15	791, 793
771.2	15	791, 793
771.3	15	794
771.4	15	791, 793
771.5	15	791, 793
771.6	15	794
771.7	15	794
771.8	15	791, 793
771.81	15	791, 793
771.82	15	791, 793
771.83	15	791, 793
771.89	15	791, 793
772.0	15	791, 793
772.10	15	791, 793
772.11	15	791, 793
772.12	15	791, 793
772.13	15	791, 793
772.14	15	791, 793
772.2	15	791, 793
772.3	15	794
772.4	15	791, 793
772.5	15	791, 793
772.6	15	795
772.8	15	794
772.9	15	794
773.0	15	794
773.1	15	794
773.2	15	791, 793
773.3	15	791, 793
773.4	15	791, 793
773.5	15	791, 793
774.0	15	794
774.1	15	794
774.2	15	794
774.30	15	795
774.31	15	795
774.39	15	795
774.4	15	791, 793
774.5	15	795

DX	MDC	DRG
774.6	15	795
774.7	15	791, 793
775.0	15	794
775.1	15	791, 793
775.2	15	791, 793
775.3	15	791, 793
775.4	15	791, 793
775.5	15	791, 793
775.6	15	791, 793
775.7	15	791, 793
775.81	15	794
775.89	15	794
775.9	15	794
776.0	15	791, 793
776.1	15	791, 793
776.2	15	791, 793
776.3	15	791, 793
776.4	15	794
776.5	15	794
776.6	15	791, 793
776.7	15	794
776.8	15	794
776.9	15	794
777.1	15	791, 793
777.2	15	791, 793
777.3	15	794
777.4	15	794
777.50	15	791, 793
777.51	15	791, 793
777.52	15	791, 793
777.53	15	791, 793
777.6	15	791, 793
777.8	15	794
777.9	15	794
778.0	15	791, 793
778.1	15	794
778.2	15	794
778.3	15	794
778.4	15	794
778.5	15	794
778.6	15	794
778.7	15	794
778.8	15	795
778.9	15	794
779.0	15	791, 793
779.1	15	791, 793
779.2	15	791, 793
779.31	15	795
779.32	15	791, 793
779.33	15	795
779.34	10	640-641
779.4	15	791, 793
779.5	15	791, 793
779.6	15	794
779.7	01	091-093
779.81	15	794
779.82	15	794
779.83	15	795
779.84	15	794
779.85	15	791, 793
779.89	15	794
779.9	15	794

Symptoms, Signs and Ill-defined Conditions

DX	MDC	DRG
780.01	01	080-081
780.02	19	884
780.03	01	080-081
780.09	01	080-081

DX	MDC	DRG
780.1	19	880
780.2	05	312
780.31	01	100-101
780.32	01	100-101
780.33	01	100-101
780.39	01	100-101
780.4	03	149
780.50	19	887
780.51	03	154-156
780.52	19	887
780.53	03	154-156
780.54	19	887
780.55	19	887
780.56	19	887
780.57	03	154-156
780.58	19	887
780.59	19	887
780.60	18	864
780.61	18	864
780.62	18	864
780.63	18	864
780.64	23	947-948
780.65	23	947-948
780.66	18	864
780.71	23	947-948
780.72	01	052-053
780.79	23	947-948
780.8	09	606-607
780.91	23	947-948
780.92	23	947-948
780.93	23	947-948
780.94	23	947-948
780.95	23	947-948
780.96	23	947-948
780.97	23	947-948
780.99	23	947-948
781.0	01	091-093
781.1	01	091-093
781.2	01	091-093
781.3	01	091-093
781.4	01	091-093
781.5	04	205-206
781.6	01	091-093
781.7	10	640-641
781.8	01	091-093
781.91	01	091-093
781.92	01	091-093
781.93	08	551-552
781.94	01	091-093
781.99	01	091-093
782.0	01	091-093
782.1	09	606-607
782.2	09	606-607
782.3	23	947-948
782.4	07	441-443
782.5	23	947-948
782.61	23	947-948
782.62	23	947-948
782.7	16	813
782.8	09	606-607
782.9	09	606-607
783.0	10	640-641
783.1	10	640-641
783.21	10	640-641
783.22	10	640-641
783.40	10	640-641
783.41	10	640-641
783.42	10	640-641

DX	MDC	DRG
783.43	10	640-641
783.5	10	640-641
783.6	10	640-641
783.7	10	640-641
783.9	10	640-641
784.0	01	102-103
784.1	03	154-156
784.2	09	606-607
784.3	01	091-093
784.40	03	154-156
784.41	03	154-156
784.42	03	154-156
784.43	03	154-156
784.44	03	154-156
784.49	03	154-156
784.51	01	091-093
784.52	01	091-093
784.59	01	091-093
784.60	19	887
784.61	19	886
784.69	19	886
784.7	03	150-151
784.8	03	154-156
784.91	03	154-156
784.92	03	157-159
784.99	03	154-156
785.0	05	308-310
785.1	05	308-310
785.2	05	306-307
785.3	05	314-316
785.4	05	299-301
785.50	05	291-293
785.51	05	291-293
785.52	18	870-872
785.59	18	870-872
785.6	16	814-816
785.9	05	314-316
786.00	04	204
786.01	04	204
786.02	04	204
786.03	04	204
786.04	04	204
786.05	04	204
786.06	04	204
786.07	04	204
786.09	04	204
786.1	04	204
786.2	04	204
786.30	04	204
786.31	04	204
786.39	04	204
786.4	04	204
786.50	05	313
786.51	05	313
786.52	04	204
786.59	05	313
786.6	04	204
786.7	04	204
786.8	04	204
786.9	04	204
787.01	06	391-392
787.02	06	391-392
787.03	06	391-392
787.04	06	391-392
787.1	06	391-392
787.20	06	391-392
787.21	06	391-392
787.22	06	391-392

DX	MDC	DRG
787.23	06	391-392
787.24	06	391-392
787.29	06	391-392
787.3	06	391-392
787.4	06	391-392
787.5	06	391-392
787.60	06	391-392
787.61	06	391-392
787.62	06	391-392
787.63	06	391-392
787.7	06	391-392
787.91	06	391-392
787.99	06	391-392
788.0	11	691-694
788.1	11	695-696
788.20	11	695-696
788.21	11	695-696
788.29	11	695-696
788.30	11	695-696
788.31	11	695-696
788.32	11	695-696
788.33	11	695-696
788.34	11	695-696
788.35	11	695-696
788.36	11	695-696
788.37	11	695-696
788.38	11	695-696
788.39	11	695-696
788.41	11	695-696
788.42	11	695-696
788.43	11	695-696
788.5	11	682-684
788.61	11	695-696
788.62	11	695-696
788.63	11	695-696
788.64	11	695-696
788.65	11	695-696
788.69	11	695-696
788.7	11	695-696
788.8	11	695-696
788.91	11	695-696
788.99	11	695-696
789.00	06	391-392
789.01	06	391-392
789.02	06	391-392
789.03	06	391-392
789.04	06	391-392
789.05	06	391-392
789.06	06	391-392
789.07	06	391-392
789.09	06	391-392
789.1	07	441-443
789.2	16	814-816
789.30	06	391-392
789.31	06	391-392
789.32	06	391-392
789.33	06	391-392
789.34	06	391-392
789.35	06	391-392
789.36	06	391-392
789.37	06	391-392
789.39	06	391-392
789.40	06	393-395
789.41	06	393-395
789.42	06	393-395
789.43	06	393-395
789.44	06	393-395
789.45	06	393-395
789.46	06	393-395
789.47	06	393-395
789.49	06	393-395
789.51	23	947-948
789.59	23	947-948
789.60	06	391-392
789.61	06	391-392
789.62	06	391-392
789.63	06	391-392
789.64	06	391-392
789.65	06	391-392
789.66	06	391-392
789.67	06	391-392
789.69	06	391-392
789.7	06	391-392
789.9	06	391-392
790.01	16	811-812
790.09	16	811-812
790.1	23	947-948
790.21	10	640-641
790.22	10	640-641
790.29	10	640-641
790.3	20	894-897
790.4	23	947-948
790.5	23	947-948
790.6	23	947-948
790.7	18	870-872
790.8	18	865-866
790.91	23	947-948
790.92	23	947-948
790.93	23	947-948
790.94	23	947-948
790.95	23	947-948
790.99	23	947-948
791.0	11	695-696
791.1	11	695-696
791.2	11	695-696
791.3	23	947-948
791.4	07	441-443
791.5	10	637-639
791.6	10	640-641
791.7	11	695-696
791.9	11	695-696
792.0	01	091-093
792.1	06	391-392
792.2	12	729-730
792.3	14	781-782
792.4	03	154-156
792.5	23	947-948
792.9	23	947-948
793.0	01	091-093
793.11	04	205-206
793.19	04	204
793.2	05	302-303
793.3	07	444-446
793.4	06	391-392
793.5	11	695-696
793.6	06	391-392
793.7	08	564-566
793.80	09	600-601
793.81	09	600-601
793.82	09	600-601
793.89	09	600-601
793.91	23	947-948
793.99	23	947-948
794.00	01	091-093
794.01	01	091-093
794.02	01	091-093
794.09	01	091-093
794.10	01	091-093
794.11	02	124-125
794.12	02	124-125
794.13	02	124-125
794.14	02	124-125
794.15	03	154-156
794.16	03	154-156
794.17	08	564-566
794.19	01	091-093
794.2	04	205-206
794.30	05	314-316
794.31	05	314-316
794.39	05	314-316
794.4	11	695-696
794.5	10	643-645
794.6	10	643-645
794.7	10	643-645
794.8	07	441-443
794.9	11	695-696
795.00	13	760-761
795.01	13	760-761
795.02	13	760-761
795.03	13	760-761
795.04	13	760-761
795.05	13	760-761
795.06	13	760-761
795.07	13	760-761
795.08	13	760-761
795.09	13	760-761
795.10	13	760-761
795.11	13	760-761
795.12	13	760-761
795.13	13	760-761
795.14	13	760-761
795.15	13	760-761
795.16	13	760-761
795.18	13	760-761
795.19	13	760-761
795.2	23	951
795.31	18	867-869
795.39	18	867-869
795.4	23	947-948
795.51	04	177-179
795.52	04	177-179
795.6	08	545-547
795.71	16	814-816
795.79	16	814-816
795.81	23	947-948
795.82	23	947-948
795.89	23	947-948
796.0	21	922-923
796.1	01	091-093
796.2	05	314-316
796.3	05	314-316
796.4	23	947-948
796.5	14	781-782
796.6	23	947-948
796.70	06	393-395
796.71	06	393-395
796.72	06	393-395
796.73	06	393-395
796.74	06	393-395
796.75	06	393-395
796.76	06	393-395
796.77	06	393-395
796.78	06	393-395
796.79	06	393-395
796.9	23	947-948
797	19	884
798.0	01	091-093
798.1	05	296-298
798.2	05	296-298
798.9	23	951
799.01	4	205-206
799.02	4	205-206
799.1	04	205-206
799.21	19	880
799.22	19	880
799.23	19	882
799.24	19	883
799.25	19	880
799.29	19	880
799.3	23	947-948
799.4	23	947-948
799.51	19	886
799.52	19	884
799.53	01	091-093
799.54	19	884
799.55	19	884
799.59	19	884
799.81	23	951
799.82	23	951
799.89	23	951
799.9	23	951

Injury and Poisoning

DX	MDC	DRG
800.00	01	082-087
800.01	01	082-087
800.02	01	082-087
800.03	01	082-084
800.04	01	082-084
800.05	01	082-084
800.06	01	082-084
800.09	01	082-087
800.10	01	082-087
800.11	01	082-087
800.12	01	082-087
800.13	01	082-084
800.14	01	082-084
800.15	01	082-084
800.16	01	082-084
800.19	01	082-087
800.20	01	082-087
800.21	01	082-087
800.22	01	082-087
800.23	01	082-084
800.24	01	082-084
800.25	01	082-084
800.26	01	082-084
800.29	01	082-087
800.30	01	082-087
800.31	01	082-087
800.32	01	082-087
800.33	01	082-084
800.34	01	082-084
800.35	01	082-084
800.36	01	082-084
800.39	01	082-087
800.40	01	082-087
800.41	01	082-087
800.42	01	082-087
800.43	01	082-084
800.44	01	082-084
800.45	01	082-084
800.46	01	082-084
800.49	01	082-087
800.50	01	082-087
800.51	01	082-087
800.52	01	082-087
800.53	01	082-084
800.54	01	082-084
800.55	01	082-084
800.56	01	082-084
800.59	01	082-087
800.60	01	082-087
800.61	01	082-087
800.62	01	082-087
800.63	01	082-084
800.64	01	082-084
800.65	01	082-084
800.66	01	082-084
800.69	01	082-087
800.70	01	082-087
800.71	01	082-087
800.72	01	082-087
800.73	01	082-084
800.74	01	082-084
800.75	01	082-084
800.76	01	082-084
800.79	01	082-087
800.80	01	082-087
800.81	01	082-087
800.82	01	082-087
800.83	01	082-084
800.84	01	082-084
800.85	01	082-084
800.86	01	082-084
800.89	01	082-087
800.90	01	082-087
800.91	01	082-087
800.92	01	082-087
800.93	01	082-084
800.94	01	082-084
800.95	01	082-084
800.96	01	082-084
800.99	01	082-087
801.00	01	082-087
801.01	01	082-087
801.02	01	082-087
801.03	01	082-084
801.04	01	082-084
801.05	01	082-084
801.06	01	082-084
801.09	01	082-087
801.10	01	082-087
801.11	01	082-087
801.12	01	082-087
801.13	01	082-084
801.14	01	082-084
801.15	01	082-084
801.16	01	082-084
801.19	01	082-087
801.20	01	082-087
801.21	01	082-087
801.22	01	082-087
801.23	01	082-084
801.24	01	082-084
801.25	01	082-084
801.26	01	082-084

Diagnosis Code/MDC/DRG List

DX	MDC	DRG
801.29	01	082-087
801.30	01	082-087
801.31	01	082-087
801.32	01	082-087
801.33	01	082-084
801.34	01	082-084
801.35	01	082-084
801.36	01	082-084
801.39	01	082-087
801.40	01	082-087
801.41	01	082-087
801.42	01	082-087
801.43	01	082-084
801.44	01	082-084
801.45	01	082-084
801.46	01	082-084
801.49	01	082-087
801.50	01	082-087
801.51	01	082-087
801.52	01	082-087
801.53	01	082-084
801.54	01	082-084
801.55	01	082-084
801.56	01	082-084
801.59	01	082-087
801.60	01	082-087
801.61	01	082-087
801.62	01	082-087
801.63	01	082-084
801.64	01	082-084
801.65	01	082-084
801.66	01	082-084
801.69	01	082-087
801.70	01	082-087
801.71	01	082-087
801.72	01	082-087
801.73	01	082-084
801.74	01	082-084
801.75	01	082-084
801.76	01	082-084
801.79	01	082-087
801.80	01	082-087
801.81	01	082-087
801.82	01	082-087
801.83	01	082-084
801.84	01	082-084
801.85	01	082-084
801.86	01	082-084
801.89	01	082-087
801.90	01	082-087
801.91	01	082-087
801.92	01	082-087
801.93	01	082-084
801.94	01	082-084
801.95	01	082-084
801.96	01	082-084
801.99	01	082-087
802.0	03	154-156
802.1	03	154-156
802.20	03	157-159
802.21	03	157-159
802.22	03	157-159
802.23	03	157-159
802.24	03	157-159
802.25	03	157-159
802.26	03	157-159
802.27	03	157-159
802.28	03	157-159
802.29	03	157-159
802.30	03	157-159
802.31	03	157-159
802.32	03	157-159
802.33	03	157-159
802.34	03	157-159
802.35	03	157-159
802.36	03	157-159
802.37	03	157-159
802.38	03	157-159
802.39	03	157-159
802.4	03	157-159
802.5	03	157-159
802.6	02	124-125
802.7	02	124-125
802.8	08	564-566
802.9	08	564-566
803.00	01	082-087
803.01	01	082-087
803.02	01	082-087
803.03	01	082-084
803.04	01	082-084
803.05	01	082-084
803.06	01	082-084
803.09	01	082-087
803.10	01	082-087
803.11	01	082-087
803.12	01	082-087
803.13	01	082-084
803.14	01	082-084
803.15	01	082-084
803.16	01	082-084
803.19	01	082-087
803.20	01	082-087
803.21	01	082-087
803.22	01	082-087
803.23	01	082-084
803.24	01	082-084
803.25	01	082-084
803.26	01	082-084
803.29	01	082-087
803.30	01	082-087
803.31	01	082-087
803.32	01	082-087
803.33	01	082-084
803.34	01	082-084
803.35	01	082-084
803.36	01	082-084
803.39	01	082-087
803.40	01	082-087
803.41	01	082-087
803.42	01	082-087
803.43	01	082-084
803.44	01	082-084
803.45	01	082-084
803.46	01	082-084
803.49	01	082-087
803.50	01	082-087
803.51	01	082-087
803.52	01	082-087
803.53	01	082-084
803.54	01	082-084
803.55	01	082-084
803.56	01	082-084
803.59	01	082-087
803.60	01	082-087
803.61	01	082-087
803.62	01	082-087
803.63	01	082-084
803.64	01	082-084
803.65	01	082-084
803.66	01	082-084
803.69	01	082-087
803.70	01	082-087
803.71	01	082-087
803.72	01	082-087
803.73	01	082-084
803.74	01	082-084
803.75	01	082-084
803.76	01	082-084
803.79	01	082-087
803.80	01	082-087
803.81	01	082-087
803.82	01	082-087
803.83	01	082-084
803.84	01	082-084
803.85	01	082-084
803.86	01	082-084
803.89	01	082-087
803.90	01	082-087
803.91	01	082-087
803.92	01	082-087
803.93	01	082-084
803.94	01	082-084
803.95	01	082-084
803.96	01	082-084
803.99	01	082-087
804.00	01	082-087
804.01	01	082-087
804.02	01	082-087
804.03	01	082-084
804.04	01	082-084
804.05	01	082-084
804.06	01	082-084
804.09	01	082-087
804.10	01	082-087
804.11	01	082-087
804.12	01	082-087
804.13	01	082-084
804.14	01	082-084
804.15	01	082-084
804.16	01	082-084
804.19	01	082-087
804.20	01	082-087
804.21	01	082-087
804.22	01	082-087
804.23	01	082-084
804.24	01	082-084
804.25	01	082-084
804.26	01	082-084
804.29	01	082-087
804.30	01	082-087
804.31	01	082-087
804.32	01	082-087
804.33	01	082-084
804.34	01	082-084
804.35	01	082-084
804.36	01	082-084
804.39	01	082-087
804.40	01	082-087
804.41	01	082-087
804.42	01	082-087
804.43	01	082-084
804.44	01	082-084
804.45	01	082-084
804.46	01	082-084
804.49	01	082-087
804.50	01	082-087
804.51	01	082-087
804.52	01	082-087
804.53	01	082-084
804.54	01	082-084
804.55	01	082-084
804.56	01	082-084
804.59	01	082-087
804.60	01	082-087
804.61	01	082-087
804.62	01	082-087
804.63	01	082-084
804.64	01	082-084
804.65	01	082-084
804.66	01	082-084
804.69	01	082-087
804.70	01	082-087
804.71	01	082-087
804.72	01	082-087
804.73	01	082-084
804.74	01	082-084
804.75	01	082-084
804.76	01	082-084
804.79	01	082-087
804.80	01	082-087
804.81	01	082-087
804.82	01	082-087
804.83	01	082-084
804.84	01	082-084
804.85	01	082-084
804.86	01	082-084
804.89	01	082-087
804.90	01	082-087
804.91	01	082-087
804.92	01	082-087
804.93	01	082-084
804.94	01	082-084
804.95	01	082-084
804.96	01	082-084
804.99	01	082-087
805.00	08	551-552
805.01	08	551-552
805.02	08	551-552
805.03	08	551-552
805.04	08	551-552
805.05	08	551-552
805.06	08	551-552
805.07	08	551-552
805.08	08	551-552
805.10	08	551-552
805.11	08	551-552
805.12	08	551-552
805.13	08	551-552
805.14	08	551-552
805.15	08	551-552
805.16	08	551-552
805.17	08	551-552
805.18	08	551-552
805.2	08	551-552
805.3	08	551-552
805.4	08	551-552
805.5	08	551-552
805.6	08	551-552
805.7	08	551-552
805.8	08	551-552
805.9	08	551-552
806.00	01	052-053
806.01	01	052-053
806.02	01	052-053
806.03	01	052-053
806.04	01	052-053
806.05	01	052-053
806.06	01	052-053
806.07	01	052-053
806.08	01	052-053
806.09	01	052-053
806.10	01	052-053
806.11	01	052-053
806.12	01	052-053
806.13	01	052-053
806.14	01	052-053
806.15	01	052-053
806.16	01	052-053
806.17	01	052-053
806.18	01	052-053
806.19	01	052-053
806.20	01	052-053
806.21	01	052-053
806.22	01	052-053
806.23	01	052-053
806.24	01	052-053
806.25	01	052-053
806.26	01	052-053
806.27	01	052-053
806.28	01	052-053
806.29	01	052-053
806.30	01	052-053
806.31	01	052-053
806.32	01	052-053
806.33	01	052-053
806.34	01	052-053
806.35	01	052-053
806.36	01	052-053
806.37	01	052-053
806.38	01	052-053
806.39	01	052-053
806.4	01	052-053
806.5	01	052-053
806.60	01	052-053
806.61	01	052-053
806.62	01	052-053
806.69	01	052-053
806.70	01	052-053
806.71	01	052-053
806.72	01	052-053
806.79	01	052-053
806.8	01	052-053
806.9	01	052-053
807.00	04	205-206
807.01	04	205-206
807.02	04	205-206
807.03	04	183-185
807.04	04	183-185
807.05	04	183-185
807.06	04	183-185
807.07	04	183-185
807.08	04	183-185
807.09	04	183-185
807.10	04	183-185
807.11	04	183-185
807.12	04	183-185
807.13	04	183-185
807.14	04	183-185
807.15	04	183-185
807.16	04	183-185

DX	MDC	DRG	DX	MDC	DRG	DX	MDC	DRG	DX	MDC	DRG	DX	MDC	DRG
807.17	04	183-185	812.53	08	562-563	814.17	08	562-563	823.11	08	562-563	832.02	08	562-563
807.18	04	183-185	812.54	08	562-563	814.18	08	562-563	823.12	08	562-563	832.03	08	562-563
807.19	04	183-185	812.59	08	562-563	814.19	08	562-563	823.20	08	562-563	832.04	08	562-563
807.2	04	183-185	813.00	08	562-563	815.00	08	562-563	823.21	08	562-563	832.09	08	562-563
807.3	04	183-185	813.01	08	562-563	815.01	08	562-563	823.22	08	562-563	832.10	08	562-563
807.4	04	183-185	813.02	08	562-563	815.02	08	562-563	823.30	08	562-563	832.11	08	562-563
807.5	03	154-156	813.03	08	562-563	815.03	08	562-563	823.31	08	562-563	832.12	08	562-563
807.6	03	154-156	813.04	08	562-563	815.04	08	562-563	823.32	08	562-563	832.13	08	562-563
808.0	08	535-536	813.05	08	562-563	815.09	08	562-563	823.40	08	562-563	832.14	08	562-563
808.1	08	535-536	813.06	08	562-563	815.10	08	562-563	823.41	08	562-563	832.19	08	562-563
808.2	08	535-536	813.07	08	562-563	815.11	08	562-563	823.42	08	562-563	832.2	08	562-563
808.3	08	535-536	813.08	08	562-563	815.12	08	562-563	823.80	08	562-563	833.00	08	562-563
808.41	08	535-536	813.10	08	562-563	815.13	08	562-563	823.81	08	562-563	833.01	08	562-563
808.42	08	535-536	813.11	08	562-563	815.14	08	562-563	823.82	08	562-563	833.02	08	562-563
808.43	08	535-536	813.12	08	562-563	815.19	08	562-563	823.90	08	562-563	833.03	08	562-563
808.44	08	535-536	813.13	08	562-563	816.00	08	562-563	823.91	08	562-563	833.04	08	562-563
808.49	08	535-536	813.14	08	562-563	816.01	08	562-563	823.92	08	562-563	833.05	08	562-563
808.51	08	535-536	813.15	08	562-563	816.02	08	562-563	824.0	08	562-563	833.09	08	562-563
808.52	08	535-536	813.16	08	562-563	816.03	08	562-563	824.1	08	562-563	833.10	08	562-563
808.53	08	535-536	813.17	08	562-563	816.10	08	562-563	824.2	08	562-563	833.11	08	562-563
808.54	08	535-536	813.18	08	562-563	816.11	08	562-563	824.3	08	562-563	833.12	08	562-563
808.59	08	535-536	813.20	08	562-563	816.12	08	562-563	824.4	08	562-563	833.13	08	562-563
808.8	08	535-536	813.21	08	562-563	816.13	08	562-563	824.5	08	562-563	833.14	08	562-563
808.9	08	535-536	813.22	08	562-563	817.0	08	562-563	824.6	08	562-563	833.15	08	562-563
809.0	08	564-566	813.23	08	562-563	817.1	08	562-563	824.7	08	562-563	833.19	08	562-563
809.1	08	564-566	813.30	08	562-563	818.0	08	562-563	824.8	08	562-563	834.00	08	562-563
810.00	08	562-563	813.31	08	562-563	818.1	08	562-563	824.9	08	562-563	834.01	08	562-563
810.01	08	562-563	813.32	08	562-563	819.0	21	913-914	825.0	08	562-563	834.02	08	562-563
810.02	08	562-563	813.33	08	562-563	819.1	21	913-914	825.1	08	562-563	834.10	08	562-563
810.03	08	562-563	813.40	08	562-563	820.00	08	535-536	825.20	08	562-563	834.11	08	562-563
810.10	08	562-563	813.41	08	562-563	820.01	08	535-536	825.21	08	562-563	834.12	08	562-563
810.11	08	562-563	813.42	08	562-563	820.02	08	535-536	825.22	08	562-563	835.00	08	537-538
810.12	08	562-563	813.43	08	562-563	820.03	08	535-536	825.23	08	562-563	835.01	08	537-538
810.13	08	562-563	813.44	08	562-563	820.09	08	535-536	825.24	08	562-563	835.02	08	537-538
811.00	08	562-563	813.45	08	562-563	820.10	08	535-536	825.25	08	562-563	835.03	08	537-538
811.01	08	562-563	813.46	08	562-563	820.11	08	535-536	825.29	08	562-563	835.10	08	537-538
811.02	08	562-563	813.47	08	562-563	820.12	08	535-536	825.30	08	562-563	835.11	08	537-538
811.03	08	562-563	813.50	08	562-563	820.13	08	535-536	825.31	08	562-563	835.12	08	537-538
811.09	08	564-566	813.51	08	562-563	820.19	08	535-536	825.32	08	562-563	835.13	08	537-538
811.10	08	562-563	813.52	08	562-563	820.20	08	535-536	825.33	08	562-563	836.0	08	562-563
811.11	08	562-563	813.53	08	562-563	820.21	08	535-536	825.34	08	562-563	836.1	08	562-563
811.12	08	562-563	813.54	08	562-563	820.22	08	535-536	825.35	08	562-563	836.2	08	562-563
811.13	04	562-563	813.80	08	562-563	820.30	08	535-536	825.39	08	562-563	836.3	08	562-563
811.19	08	564-566	813.81	08	562-563	820.31	08	535-536	826.0	08	562-563	836.4	08	562-563
812.00	08	562-563	813.82	08	562-563	820.32	08	535-536	826.1	08	562-563	836.50	08	562-563
812.01	08	562-563	813.83	08	562-563	820.8	08	535-536	827.0	08	562-563	836.51	08	562-563
812.02	08	562-563	813.90	08	562-563	820.9	08	535-536	827.1	08	562-563	836.52	08	562-563
812.03	08	562-563	813.91	08	562-563	821.00	08	533-534	828.0	21	913-914	836.53	08	562-563
812.09	08	562-563	813.92	08	562-563	821.01	08	533-534	828.1	21	913-914	836.54	08	562-563
812.10	08	562-563	813.93	08	562-563	821.10	08	533-534	829.0	08	562-563	836.59	08	562-563
812.11	08	562-563	814.00	08	562-563	821.11	08	533-534	829.1	08	562-563	836.60	08	562-563
812.12	08	562-563	814.01	08	562-563	821.20	08	533-534	830.0	03	157-159	836.61	08	562-563
812.13	08	562-563	814.02	08	562-563	821.21	08	533-534	830.1	03	157-159	836.62	08	562-563
812.19	08	562-563	814.03	08	562-563	821.22	08	533-534	831.00	08	562-563	836.63	08	562-563
812.20	08	562-563	814.04	08	562-563	821.23	08	533-534	831.01	08	562-563	836.64	08	562-563
812.21	08	562-563	814.05	08	562-563	821.29	08	533-534	831.02	08	562-563	836.69	08	562-563
812.30	08	562-563	814.06	08	562-563	821.30	08	533-534	831.03	08	562-563	837.0	08	562-563
812.31	08	562-563	814.07	08	562-563	821.31	08	533-534	831.04	08	562-563	837.1	08	562-563
812.40	08	562-563	814.08	08	562-563	821.32	08	533-534	831.09	08	562-563	838.00	08	562-563
812.41	08	562-563	814.09	08	562-563	821.33	08	533-534	831.10	08	562-563	838.01	08	562-563
812.42	08	562-563	814.10	08	562-563	821.39	08	533-534	831.11	08	562-563	838.02	08	562-563
812.43	08	562-563	814.11	08	562-563	822.0	08	562-563	831.12	08	562-563	838.03	08	562-563
812.44	08	562-563	814.12	08	562-563	822.1	08	562-563	831.13	08	562-563	838.04	08	562-563
812.49	08	562-563	814.13	08	562-563	823.00	08	562-563	831.14	08	562-563	838.06	08	562-563
812.50	08	562-563	814.14	08	562-563	823.01	08	562-563	831.19	08	562-563	838.09	08	562-563
812.51	08	562-563	814.15	08	562-563	823.02	08	562-563	832.00	08	562-563	838.10	08	562-563
812.52	08	562-563	814.16	08	562-563	823.10	08	562-563	832.01	08	562-563			

Diagnosis Code/MDC/DRG List

DX	MDC	DRG	DX	MDC	DRG	DX	MDC	DRG	DX	MDC	DRG	DX	MDC	DRG
838.11	08	562-563	843.0	08	537-538	851.21	01	082-087	852.05	01	082-084	854.11	01	082-087
838.12	08	562-563	843.1	08	537-538	851.22	01	082-087	852.06	01	082-084	854.12	01	082-087
838.13	08	562-563	843.8	08	537-538	851.23	01	082-084	852.09	01	082-087	854.13	01	082-084
838.14	08	562-563	843.9	08	537-538	851.24	01	082-084	852.10	01	082-087	854.14	01	082-084
838.15	08	562-563	844.0	08	562-563	851.25	01	082-084	852.11	01	082-087	854.15	01	082-084
838.16	08	562-563	844.1	08	562-563	851.26	01	082-084	852.12	01	082-087	854.16	01	082-084
838.19	08	562-563	844.2	08	562-563	851.29	01	082-087	852.13	01	082-084	854.19	01	082-087
839.00	08	551-552	844.3	08	562-563	851.30	01	082-087	852.14	01	082-084	860.0	04	199-201
839.01	08	551-552	844.8	08	562-563	851.31	01	082-087	852.15	01	082-084	860.1	04	199-201
839.02	08	551-552	844.9	08	562-563	851.32	01	082-087	852.16	01	082-084	860.2	04	199-201
839.03	08	551-552	845.00	08	562-563	851.33	01	082-084	852.19	01	082-087	860.3	04	199-201
839.04	08	551-552	845.01	08	562-563	851.34	01	082-084	852.20	01	082-087	860.4	04	199-201
839.05	08	551-552	845.02	08	562-563	851.35	01	082-084	852.21	01	082-087	860.5	04	199-201
839.06	08	551-552	845.03	08	562-563	851.36	01	082-084	852.22	01	082-087	861.00	05	314-316
839.07	08	551-552	845.09	08	562-563	851.39	01	082-087	852.23	01	082-084	861.01	05	314-316
839.08	08	551-552	845.10	08	562-563	851.40	01	082-087	852.24	01	082-084	861.02	05	314-316
839.10	08	551-552	845.11	08	562-563	851.41	01	082-087	852.25	01	082-084	861.03	05	314-316
839.11	08	551-552	845.12	08	562-563	851.42	01	082-087	852.26	01	082-084	861.10	05	314-316
839.12	08	551-552	845.13	08	562-563	851.43	01	082-084	852.29	01	082-087	861.11	05	314-316
839.13	08	551-552	845.19	08	562-563	851.44	01	082-084	852.30	01	082-087	861.12	05	314-316
839.14	08	551-552	846.0	08	551-552	851.45	01	082-084	852.31	01	082-087	861.13	05	314-316
839.15	08	551-552	846.1	08	551-552	851.46	01	082-084	852.32	01	082-087	861.20	04	205-206
839.16	08	551-552	846.2	08	551-552	851.49	01	082-087	852.33	01	082-084	861.21	04	205-206
839.17	08	551-552	846.3	08	551-552	851.50	01	082-087	852.34	01	082-084	861.22	04	183-185
839.18	08	551-552	846.8	08	551-552	851.51	01	082-087	852.35	01	082-084	861.30	04	205-206
839.20	08	551-552	846.9	08	551-552	851.52	01	082-087	852.36	01	082-084	861.31	04	205-206
839.21	08	551-552	847.0	08	551-552	851.53	01	082-084	852.39	01	082-087	861.32	04	183-185
839.30	08	551-552	847.1	08	551-552	851.54	01	082-084	852.40	01	082-087	862.0	04	183-185
839.31	08	551-552	847.2	08	551-552	851.55	01	082-084	852.41	01	082-087	862.1	04	183-185
839.40	08	551-552	847.3	08	551-552	851.56	01	082-084	852.42	01	082-087	862.21	04	183-185
839.41	08	551-552	847.4	08	551-552	851.59	01	082-087	852.43	01	082-084	862.22	06	368-370
839.42	08	551-552	847.9	08	551-552	851.60	01	082-087	852.44	01	082-084	862.29	04	205-206
839.49	08	551-552	848.0	08	564-566	851.61	01	082-087	852.45	01	082-084	862.31	04	183-185
839.50	08	551-552	848.1	03	157-159	851.62	01	082-087	852.46	01	082-084	862.32	06	393-395
839.51	08	551-552	848.2	08	564-566	851.63	01	082-084	852.49	01	082-087	862.39	04	205-206
839.52	08	551-552	848.3	04	205-206	851.64	01	082-084	852.50	01	082-087	862.8	21	913-914
839.59	08	551-552	848.40	04	205-206	851.65	01	082-084	852.51	01	082-087	862.9	21	913-914
839.61	04	183-185	848.41	04	205-206	851.66	01	082-084	852.52	01	082-087	863.0	06	393-395
839.69	08	562-563	848.42	04	205-206	851.69	01	082-087	852.53	01	082-084	863.1	06	393-395
839.71	04	183-185	848.49	04	205-206	851.70	01	082-087	852.54	01	082-084	863.20	06	393-395
839.79	08	562-563	848.5	08	537-538	851.71	01	082-087	852.55	01	082-084	863.21	06	393-395
839.8	08	562-563	848.8	08	562-563	851.72	01	082-087	852.56	01	082-084	863.29	06	393-395
839.9	08	562-563	848.9	08	562-563	851.73	01	082-084	852.59	01	082-087	863.30	06	393-395
840.0	08	562-563	850.0	01	088-090	851.74	01	082-084	853.00	01	082-087	863.31	06	393-395
840.1	08	562-563	850.11	01	088-090	851.75	01	082-084	853.01	01	082-087	863.39	06	393-395
840.2	08	562-563	850.12	01	088-090	851.76	01	082-084	853.02	01	082-087	863.40	06	393-395
840.3	08	562-563	850.2	01	088-090	851.79	01	082-087	853.03	01	082-084	863.41	06	393-395
840.4	08	562-563	850.3	01	088-090	851.80	01	082-087	853.04	01	082-084	863.42	06	393-395
840.5	08	562-563	850.4	01	088-090	851.81	01	082-087	853.05	01	082-084	863.43	06	393-395
840.6	08	562-563	850.5	01	088-090	851.82	01	082-087	853.06	01	082-084	863.44	06	393-395
840.7	08	562-563	850.9	01	088-090	851.83	01	082-084	853.09	01	082-087	863.45	06	393-395
840.8	08	562-563	851.00	01	082-087	851.84	01	082-084	853.10	01	082-087	863.46	06	393-395
840.9	08	562-563	851.01	01	082-087	851.85	01	082-084	853.11	01	082-087	863.49	06	393-395
841.0	08	562-563	851.02	01	082-087	851.86	01	082-084	853.12	01	082-087	863.50	06	393-395
841.1	08	562-563	851.03	01	082-084	851.89	01	082-087	853.13	01	082-084	863.51	06	393-395
841.2	08	562-563	851.04	01	082-084	851.90	01	082-087	853.14	01	082-084	863.52	06	393-395
841.3	08	562-563	851.05	01	082-084	851.91	01	082-087	853.15	01	082-084	863.53	06	393-395
841.8	08	562-563	851.06	01	082-084	851.92	01	082-087	853.16	01	082-084	863.54	06	393-395
841.9	08	562-563	851.09	01	082-087	851.93	01	082-084	853.19	01	082-087	863.55	06	393-395
842.00	08	562-563	851.10	01	082-087	851.94	01	082-084	854.00	01	082-087	863.56	06	393-395
842.01	08	562-563	851.11	01	082-087	851.95	01	082-084	854.01	01	082-087	863.59	06	393-395
842.02	08	562-563	851.12	01	082-087	851.96	01	082-084	854.02	01	082-087	863.80	06	393-395
842.09	08	562-563	851.13	01	082-084	851.99	01	082-087	854.03	01	082-084	863.81	07	438-440
842.10	08	562-563	851.14	01	082-084	852.00	01	082-087	854.04	01	082-084	863.82	07	438-440
842.11	08	562-563	851.15	01	082-084	852.01	01	082-087	854.05	01	082-084	863.83	07	438-440
842.12	08	562-563	851.16	01	082-084	852.02	01	082-087	854.06	01	082-084	863.84	07	438-440
842.13	08	562-563	851.19	01	082-087	852.03	01	082-084	854.09	01	082-087	863.85	06	393-395
842.19	08	562-563	851.20	01	082-087	852.04	01	082-084	854.10	01	082-087	863.89	06	393-395

DX	MDC	DRG	DX	MDC	DRG	DX	MDC	DRG	DX	MDC	DRG	DX	MDC	DRG
863.90	06	393-395	869.0	21	913-914	873.70	03	157-159	881.10	21	913-914	901.2	21	913-914
863.91	07	438-440	869.1	21	913-914	873.71	03	157-159	881.11	21	913-914	901.3	21	913-914
863.92	07	438-440	870.0	02	124-125	873.72	03	157-159	881.12	21	913-914	901.40	21	913-914
863.93	07	438-440	870.1	02	124-125	873.73	03	157-159	881.20	08	564-566	901.41	21	913-914
863.94	07	438-440	870.2	02	124-125	873.74	03	157-159	881.21	08	564-566	901.42	21	913-914
863.95	06	393-395	870.3	02	124-125	873.75	03	157-159	881.22	08	564-566	901.81	21	913-914
863.99	06	393-395	870.4	02	124-125	873.79	03	157-159	882.0	09	604-605	901.82	21	913-914
864.00	07	441-443	870.8	02	124-125	873.8	09	604-605	882.1	21	913-914	901.83	21	913-914
864.01	07	441-443	870.9	02	124-125	873.9	09	604-605	882.2	08	564-566	901.89	21	913-914
864.02	07	441-443	871.0	02	124-125	874.00	03	154-156	883.0	09	604-605	901.9	21	913-914
864.03	07	441-443	871.1	02	124-125	874.01	03	154-156	883.1	21	913-914	902.0	21	913-914
864.04	07	441-443	871.2	02	124-125	874.02	04	183-185	883.2	08	564-566	902.10	21	913-914
864.05	07	441-443	871.3	02	124-125	874.10	03	154-156	884.0	09	604-605	902.11	21	913-914
864.09	07	441-443	871.4	02	124-125	874.11	03	154-156	884.1	21	913-914	902.19	21	913-914
864.10	07	441-443	871.5	02	124-125	874.12	04	183-185	884.2	08	564-566	902.20	21	913-914
864.11	07	441-443	871.6	02	124-125	874.2	10	643-645	885.0	21	913-914	902.21	21	913-914
864.12	07	441-443	871.7	02	124-125	874.3	10	643-645	885.1	21	913-914	902.22	21	913-914
864.13	07	441-443	871.9	02	124-125	874.4	03	154-156	886.0	21	913-914	902.23	21	913-914
864.14	07	441-443	872.00	03	154-156	874.5	03	154-156	886.1	21	913-914	902.24	21	913-914
864.15	07	441-443	872.01	03	154-156	874.8	09	604-605	887.0	21	913-914	902.25	21	913-914
864.19	07	441-443	872.02	03	154-156	874.9	09	604-605	887.1	21	913-914	902.26	21	913-914
865.00	16	814-816	872.10	03	154-156	875.0	09	604-605	887.2	21	913-914	902.27	21	913-914
865.01	16	814-816	872.11	03	154-156	875.1	21	913-914	887.3	21	913-914	902.29	21	913-914
865.02	16	814-816	872.12	03	154-156	876.0	09	604-605	887.4	21	913-914	902.31	21	913-914
865.03	16	814-816	872.61	03	154-156	876.1	09	604-605	887.5	21	913-914	902.32	21	913-914
865.04	16	814-816	872.62	03	154-156	877.0	09	604-605	887.6	21	913-914	902.33	21	913-914
865.09	16	814-816	872.63	03	154-156	877.1	09	604-605	887.7	21	913-914	902.34	21	913-914
865.10	16	814-816	872.64	03	154-156	878.0	12	729-730	890.0	09	604-605	902.39	21	913-914
865.11	16	814-816	872.69	03	154-156	878.1	12	729-730	890.1	21	913-914	902.40	21	913-914
865.12	16	814-816	872.71	03	154-156	878.2	12	729-730	890.2	08	564-566	902.41	21	913-914
865.13	16	814-816	872.72	03	154-156	878.3	12	729-730	891.0	09	604-605	902.42	21	913-914
865.14	16	814-816	872.73	03	154-156	878.4	13	760-761	891.1	21	913-914	902.49	21	913-914
865.19	16	814-816	872.74	03	154-156	878.5	13	760-761	891.2	08	564-566	902.50	21	913-914
866.00	11	698-700	872.79	03	154-156	878.6	13	760-761	892.0	09	604-605	902.51	21	913-914
866.01	11	698-700	872.8	03	154-156	878.7	13	760-761	892.1	21	913-914	902.52	21	913-914
866.02	11	698-700	872.9	03	154-156	878.8	12	729-730	892.2	08	564-566	902.53	21	913-914
866.03	11	698-700	873.0	09	604-605	878.8	13	760-761	893.0	09	604-605	902.54	21	913-914
866.10	11	698-700	873.1	09	604-605	878.9	12	729-730	893.1	21	913-914	902.55	21	913-914
866.11	11	698-700	873.20	03	154-156	878.9	13	760-761	893.2	08	564-566	902.56	21	913-914
866.12	11	698-700	873.21	03	154-156	879.0	09	604-605	894.0	09	604-605	902.59	21	913-914
866.13	11	698-700	873.22	03	154-156	879.1	09	604-605	894.1	21	913-914	902.81	21	913-914
867.0	11	698-700	873.23	03	154-156	879.2	09	604-605	894.2	08	564-566	902.82	21	913-914
867.1	11	698-700	873.29	03	154-156	879.3	21	913-914	895.0	21	913-914	902.87	21	913-914
867.2	11	698-700	873.30	03	154-156	879.4	09	604-605	895.1	21	913-914	902.89	21	913-914
867.3	11	698-700	873.31	03	154-156	879.5	21	913-914	896.0	21	913-914	902.9	21	913-914
867.4	13	760-761	873.32	03	154-156	879.6	09	604-605	896.1	21	913-914	903.00	21	913-914
867.5	13	760-761	873.33	03	154-156	879.7	21	913-914	896.2	21	913-914	903.01	21	913-914
867.6	12	729-730	873.39	03	154-156	879.8	09	604-605	896.3	21	913-914	903.02	21	913-914
867.6	13	760-761	873.40	09	604-605	879.9	21	913-914	897.0	21	913-914	903.1	21	913-914
867.7	12	729-730	873.41	09	604-605	880.00	09	604-605	897.1	21	913-914	903.2	21	913-914
867.7	13	760-761	873.42	09	604-605	880.01	09	604-605	897.2	21	913-914	903.3	21	913-914
867.8	12	729-730	873.43	03	157-159	880.02	09	604-605	897.3	21	913-914	903.4	21	913-914
867.8	13	760-761	873.44	03	157-159	880.03	09	604-605	897.4	21	913-914	903.5	21	913-914
867.9	12	729-730	873.49	09	604-605	880.09	09	604-605	897.5	21	913-914	903.8	21	913-914
867.9	13	760-761	873.50	09	604-605	880.10	21	913-914	897.6	21	913-914	903.9	21	913-914
868.00	06	393-395	873.51	09	604-605	880.11	21	913-914	897.7	21	913-914	904.0	21	913-914
868.01	10	643-645	873.52	09	604-605	880.12	21	913-914	900.00	21	913-914	904.1	21	913-914
868.02	07	444-446	873.53	03	157-159	880.13	21	913-914	900.01	21	913-914	904.2	21	913-914
868.03	06	393-395	873.54	03	157-159	880.19	21	913-914	900.02	21	913-914	904.3	21	913-914
868.04	11	698-700	873.59	09	604-605	880.20	08	564-566	900.03	21	913-914	904.40	21	913-914
868.09	21	913-914	873.60	03	157-159	880.21	08	564-566	900.1	21	913-914	904.41	21	913-914
868.10	06	393-395	873.61	03	157-159	880.22	08	564-566	900.81	21	913-914	904.42	21	913-914
868.11	10	643-645	873.62	03	157-159	880.23	08	564-566	900.82	21	913-914	904.50	21	913-914
868.12	07	444-446	873.63	03	157-159	880.29	08	564-566	900.89	21	913-914	904.51	21	913-914
868.13	06	393-395	873.64	03	157-159	881.00	09	604-605	900.9	21	913-914	904.52	21	913-914
868.14	11	698-700	873.65	03	157-159	881.01	09	604-605	901.0	21	913-914	904.53	21	913-914
868.19	21	913-914	873.69	03	157-159	881.02	09	604-605	901.1	21	913-914	904.54	21	913-914

Diagnosis Code/MDC/DRG List

DX	MDC	DRG
904.6	21	913-914
904.7	21	913-914
904.8	21	913-914
904.9	21	913-914
905.0	01	091-093
905.1	08	551-552
905.2	08	559-561
905.3	08	559-561
905.4	08	559-561
905.5	08	559-561
905.6	08	562-563
905.7	08	562-563
905.8	08	559-561
905.9	08	559-561
906.0	09	604-605
906.1	09	604-605
906.2	09	604-605
906.3	09	604-605
906.4	09	604-605
906.5	09	604-605
906.6	09	604-605
906.7	09	604-605
906.8	09	604-605
906.9	09	604-605
907.0	01	091-093
907.1	01	091-093
907.2	01	052-053
907.3	01	091-093
907.4	01	091-093
907.5	01	091-093
907.9	01	091-093
908.0	04	205-206
908.1	06	393-395
908.2	12	729-730
908.2	13	760-761
908.3	05	299-301
908.4	05	299-301
908.5	21	913-914
908.6	21	913-914
908.9	21	913-914
909.0	21	922-923
909.1	21	922-923
909.2	21	922-923
909.3	21	922-923
909.4	21	922-923
909.9	21	922-923
910.0	09	604-605
910.1	09	602-603
910.2	09	606-607
910.3	09	606-607
910.4	09	606-607
910.5	09	602-603
910.6	09	604-605
910.7	09	602-603
910.8	09	604-605
910.9	09	602-603
911.0	09	604-605
911.1	09	602-603
911.2	09	606-607
911.3	09	602-603
911.4	09	606-607
911.5	09	602-603
911.6	09	604-605
911.7	09	602-603
911.8	09	604-605
911.9	09	602-603
912.0	09	604-605
912.1	09	602-603
912.2	09	604-605
912.3	09	602-603
912.4	09	606-607
912.5	09	602-603
912.6	09	604-605
912.7	09	602-603
912.8	09	604-605
912.9	09	602-603
913.0	09	604-605
913.1	09	602-603
913.2	09	606-607
913.3	09	602-603
913.4	09	606-607
913.5	09	602-603
913.6	09	604-605
913.7	09	602-603
913.8	09	604-605
913.9	09	602-603
914.0	09	604-605
914.1	09	602-603
914.2	09	606-607
914.3	09	602-603
914.4	09	606-607
914.5	09	602-603
914.6	09	604-605
914.7	09	602-603
914.8	09	604-605
914.9	09	602-603
915.0	09	604-605
915.1	09	602-603
915.2	09	606-607
915.3	09	602-603
915.4	09	606-607
915.5	09	602-603
915.6	09	604-605
915.7	09	602-603
915.8	09	604-605
915.9	09	602-603
916.0	09	604-605
916.1	09	602-603
916.2	09	606-607
916.3	09	602-603
916.4	09	606-607
916.5	09	602-603
916.6	09	604-605
916.7	09	602-603
916.8	09	604-605
916.9	09	602-603
917.0	09	604-605
917.1	09	602-603
917.2	09	606-607
917.3	09	602-603
917.4	09	606-607
917.5	09	602-603
917.6	09	604-605
917.7	09	602-603
917.8	09	604-605
917.9	09	602-603
918.0	02	124-125
918.1	02	124-125
918.2	02	124-125
918.9	02	124-125
919.0	09	604-605
919.1	09	602-603
919.2	09	606-607
919.3	09	602-603
919.4	09	606-607
919.5	09	602-603
919.6	09	604-605
919.7	09	602-603
919.8	09	604-605
919.9	09	602-603
920.	09	604-605
921.0	02	124-125
921.1	02	124-125
921.2	02	124-125
921.3	02	124-125
921.9	02	124-125
922.0	09	604-605
922.1	09	604-605
922.2	09	604-605
922.31	09	604-605
922.32	09	604-605
922.33	09	604-605
922.4	12	729-730
922.4	13	760-761
922.8	09	604-605
922.9	09	604-605
923.00	09	604-605
923.01	09	604-605
923.02	09	604-605
923.03	09	604-605
923.09	09	604-605
923.10	09	604-605
923.11	09	604-605
923.20	09	604-605
923.21	09	604-605
923.3	09	604-605
923.8	09	604-605
923.9	09	604-605
924.00	09	604-605
924.01	09	604-605
924.10	09	604-605
924.11	09	604-605
924.20	09	604-605
924.21	09	604-605
924.3	09	604-605
924.4	09	604-605
924.5	09	604-605
924.8	09	604-605
924.9	09	604-605
925.1	21	913-914
925.2	21	913-914
926.0	12	729-730
926.0	13	760-761
926.11	21	913-914
926.12	21	913-914
926.19	21	913-914
926.8	21	913-914
926.9	21	913-914
927.00	21	913-914
927.01	21	913-914
927.02	21	913-914
927.03	21	913-914
927.09	21	913-914
927.10	21	913-914
927.11	21	913-914
927.20	21	913-914
927.21	21	913-914
927.3	21	913-914
927.8	21	913-914
927.9	21	913-914
928.00	21	913-914
928.01	21	913-914
928.10	21	913-914
928.11	21	913-914
928.20	21	913-914
928.21	21	913-914
928.3	21	913-914
928.8	21	913-914
928.9	21	913-914
929.0	21	913-914
929.9	21	913-914
930.0	02	124-125
930.1	02	124-125
930.2	02	124-125
930.8	02	124-125
930.9	02	124-125
931	03	154-156
932	03	154-156
933.0	03	154-156
933.1	03	154-156
934.0	04	205-206
934.1	04	205-206
934.8	04	205-206
934.9	04	205-206
935.0	03	157-159
935.1	06	393-395
935.2	06	393-395
936	06	393-395
937	06	393-395
938	06	393-395
939.0	11	698-700
939.1	13	760-761
939.2	13	760-761
939.3	12	729-730
939.9	11	698-700
940.0	02	124-125
940.1	02	124-125
940.2	02	124-125
940.3	02	124-125
940.4	02	124-125
940.5	02	124-125
940.9	02	124-125
941.00	22	935
941.01	22	935
941.02	02	124-125
941.03	22	935
941.04	22	935
941.05	22	935
941.06	22	935
941.07	22	935
941.08	22	935
941.09	22	935
941.10	22	935
941.11	22	935
941.12	02	124-125
941.13	22	935
941.14	22	935
941.15	22	935
941.16	22	935
941.17	22	935
941.18	22	935
941.19	22	935
941.20	22	935
941.21	22	935
941.22	02	124-125
941.23	22	935
941.24	22	935
941.25	22	935
941.26	22	935
941.27	22	935
941.28	22	935
941.29	22	935
941.30	22	933-934
941.31	22	933-934
941.32	02	124-125
941.33	22	933-934
941.34	22	933-934
941.35	22	933-934
941.36	22	933-934
941.37	22	933-934
941.38	22	933-934
941.39	22	933-934
941.40	22	933-934
941.41	22	933-934
941.42	02	124-125
941.43	22	933-934
941.44	22	933-934
941.45	22	933-934
941.46	22	933-934
941.47	22	933-934
941.48	22	933-934
941.49	22	933-934
941.50	22	933-934
941.51	22	933-934
941.52	02	124-125
941.53	22	933-934
941.54	22	933-934
941.55	22	933-934
941.56	22	933-934
941.57	22	933-934
941.58	22	933-934
941.59	22	933-934
942.00	22	935
942.01	22	935
942.02	22	935
942.03	22	935
942.04	22	935
942.05	22	935
942.09	22	935
942.10	22	935
942.11	22	935
942.12	22	935
942.13	22	935
942.14	22	935
942.15	22	935
942.19	22	935
942.20	22	935
942.21	22	935
942.22	22	935
942.23	22	935
942.24	22	935
942.25	22	935
942.29	22	935
942.30	22	933-934
942.31	22	933-934
942.32	22	933-934
942.33	22	933-934
942.34	22	933-934
942.35	22	933-934
942.39	22	933-934
942.40	22	933-934
942.41	22	933-934
942.42	22	933-934
942.43	22	933-934
942.44	22	933-934
942.45	22	933-934
942.49	22	933-934
942.50	22	933-934
942.51	22	933-934
942.52	22	933-934

DX	MDC	DRG	DX	MDC	DRG	DX	MDC	DRG	DX	MDC	DRG	DX	MDC	DRG
942.53	22	933-934	944.16	22	935	945.34	22	933-934	948.76	22	933	953.0	01	073-074
942.54	22	933-934	944.17	22	935	945.35	22	933-934	948.77	22	933	953.1	01	073-074
942.55	22	933-934	944.18	22	935	945.36	22	933-934	948.80	22	935	953.2	01	073-074
942.59	22	933-934	944.20	22	935	945.39	22	933-934	948.81	22	933	953.3	01	073-074
943.00	22	935	944.21	22	935	945.40	22	933-934	948.82	22	933	953.4	01	073-074
943.01	22	935	944.22	22	935	945.41	22	933-934	948.83	22	933	953.5	01	073-074
943.02	22	935	944.23	22	935	945.42	22	933-934	948.84	22	933	953.8	01	073-074
943.03	22	935	944.24	22	935	945.43	22	933-934	948.85	22	933	953.9	01	073-074
943.04	22	935	944.25	22	935	945.44	22	933-934	948.86	22	933	954.0	01	073-074
943.05	22	935	944.26	22	935	945.45	22	933-934	948.87	22	933	954.1	01	073-074
943.06	22	935	944.27	22	935	945.46	22	933-934	948.88	22	933	954.8	01	073-074
943.09	22	935	944.28	22	935	945.49	22	933-934	948.90	22	935	954.9	01	073-074
943.10	22	935	944.30	22	933-934	945.50	22	933-934	948.91	22	933	955.0	01	073-074
943.11	22	935	944.31	22	933-934	945.51	22	933-934	948.92	22	933	955.1	01	073-074
943.12	22	935	944.32	22	933-934	945.52	22	933-934	948.93	22	933	955.2	01	073-074
943.13	22	935	944.33	22	933-934	945.53	22	933-934	948.94	22	933	955.3	01	073-074
943.14	22	935	944.34	22	933-934	945.54	22	933-934	948.95	22	933	955.4	01	073-074
943.15	22	935	944.35	22	933-934	945.55	22	933-934	948.96	22	933	955.5	01	073-074
943.16	22	935	944.36	22	933-934	945.56	22	933-934	948.97	22	933	955.6	01	073-074
943.19	22	935	944.37	22	933-934	945.59	22	933-934	948.98	22	933	955.7	01	073-074
943.20	22	935	944.38	22	933-934	946.0	22	935	948.99	22	933	955.8	01	073-074
943.21	22	935	944.40	22	933-934	946.1	22	935	949.0	22	935	955.9	01	073-074
943.22	22	935	944.41	22	933-934	946.2	22	935	949.1	22	935	956.0	01	073-074
943.23	22	935	944.42	22	933-934	946.3	22	933-934	949.2	22	935	956.1	01	073-074
943.24	22	935	944.43	22	933-934	946.4	22	933-934	949.3	22	933-934	956.2	01	073-074
943.25	22	935	944.44	22	933-934	946.5	22	933-934	949.4	22	933-934	956.3	01	073-074
943.26	22	935	944.45	22	933-934	947.0	03	154-156	949.5	22	933-934	956.4	01	073-074
943.29	22	935	944.46	22	933-934	947.1	04	205-206	950.0	02	124-125	956.5	01	073-074
943.30	22	933-934	944.47	22	933-934	947.2	06	368-370	950.1	01	091-093	956.8	01	073-074
943.31	22	933-934	944.48	22	933-934	947.3	06	393-395	950.2	01	091-093	956.9	01	073-074
943.32	22	933-934	944.50	22	933-934	947.4	13	760-761	950.3	01	091-093	957.0	01	073-074
943.33	22	933-934	944.51	22	933-934	947.8	22	935	950.9	01	091-093	957.1	01	073-074
943.34	22	933-934	944.52	22	933-934	947.9	22	935	951.0	01	073-074	957.8	01	073-074
943.35	22	933-934	944.53	22	933-934	948.00	22	935	951.1	01	073-074	957.9	01	073-074
943.36	22	933-934	944.54	22	933-934	948.10	22	935	951.2	01	073-074	958.0	04	175-176
943.39	22	933-934	944.55	22	933-934	948.11	22	933-934	951.3	01	073-074	958.1	04	175-176
943.40	22	933-934	944.56	22	933-934	948.20	22	935	951.4	01	073-074	958.2	21	922-923
943.41	22	933-934	944.57	22	933-934	948.21	22	933	951.5	03	154-156	958.3	18	862-863
943.42	22	933-934	944.58	22	933-934	948.22	22	933	951.6	01	073-074	958.4	21	922-923
943.43	22	933-934	945.00	22	935	948.30	22	935	951.7	01	073-074	958.5	11	682-684
943.44	22	933-934	945.01	22	935	948.31	22	933	951.8	01	073-074	958.6	08	564-566
943.45	22	933-934	945.02	22	935	948.32	22	933	951.9	01	073-074	958.7	04	199-201
943.46	22	933-934	945.03	22	935	948.33	22	933	952.00	01	052-053	958.8	21	922-923
943.49	22	933-934	945.04	22	935	948.40	22	935	952.01	01	052-053	958.90	21	922-923
943.50	22	933-934	945.05	22	935	948.41	22	933	952.02	01	052-053	958.91	21	922-923
943.51	22	933-934	945.06	22	935	948.42	22	933	952.03	01	052-053	958.92	21	922-923
943.52	22	933-934	945.09	22	935	948.43	22	933	952.04	01	052-053	958.93	21	922-923
943.53	22	933-934	945.10	22	935	948.44	22	933	952.05	01	052-053	958.99	21	922-923
943.54	22	933-934	945.11	22	935	948.50	22	935	952.06	01	052-053	959.01	21	913-914
943.55	22	933-934	945.12	22	935	948.51	22	933	952.07	01	052-053	959.09	21	913-914
943.56	22	933-934	945.13	22	935	948.52	22	933	952.08	01	052-053	959.11	21	913-914
943.59	22	933-934	945.14	22	935	948.53	22	933	952.09	01	052-053	959.12	21	913-914
944.00	22	935	945.15	22	935	948.54	22	933	952.10	01	052-053	959.13	21	913-914
944.01	22	935	945.16	22	935	948.55	22	933	952.11	01	052-053	959.14	21	913-914
944.02	22	935	945.19	22	935	948.60	22	935	952.12	01	052-053	959.19	21	913-914
944.03	22	935	945.20	22	935	948.61	22	933	952.13	01	052-053	959.2	21	913-914
944.04	22	935	945.21	22	935	948.62	22	933	952.14	01	052-053	959.3	21	913-914
944.05	22	935	945.22	22	935	948.63	22	933	952.15	01	052-053	959.4	21	913-914
944.06	22	935	945.23	22	935	948.64	22	933	952.16	01	052-053	959.5	21	913-914
944.07	22	935	945.24	22	935	948.65	22	933	952.17	01	052-053	959.6	21	913-914
944.08	22	935	945.25	22	935	948.66	22	933	952.18	01	052-053	959.7	21	913-914
944.10	22	935	945.26	22	935	948.70	22	935	952.19	01	052-053	959.8	21	913-914
944.11	22	935	945.29	22	935	948.71	22	933	952.2	01	052-053	959.9	21	913-914
944.12	22	935	945.30	22	933-934	948.72	22	933	952.3	01	052-053	960.0	21	917-918
944.13	22	935	945.31	22	933-934	948.73	22	933	952.4	01	052-053	960.1	21	917-918
944.14	22	935	945.32	22	933-934	948.74	22	933	952.8	01	052-053	960.2	21	917-918
944.15	22	935	945.33	22	933-934	948.75	22	933	952.9	01	052-053	960.3	21	917-918

Diagnosis Code/MDC/DRG List

DX....	MDC.....	DRG	DX....	MDC.....	DRG	DX....	MDC.....	DRG	DX....	MDC.....	DRG	DX....	MDC.....	DRG
960.4	21	917-918	967.8	21	917-918	975.0	21	917-918	985.3	21	917-918	994.5	21	922-923
960.5	21	917-918	967.9	21	917-918	975.1	21	917-918	985.4	21	917-918	994.6	03	149
960.6	21	917-918	968.0	21	917-918	975.2	21	917-918	985.5	21	917-918	994.7	21	922-923
960.7	21	917-918	968.1	21	917-918	975.3	21	917-918	985.6	21	917-918	994.8	21	922-923
960.8	21	917-918	968.2	21	917-918	975.4	21	917-918	985.8	21	917-918	994.9	21	922-923
960.9	21	917-918	968.3	21	917-918	975.5	21	917-918	985.9	21	917-918	995.0	21	915-916
961.0	21	917-918	968.4	21	917-918	975.6	21	917-918	986	21	917-918	995.1	21	915-916
961.1	21	917-918	968.5	21	917-918	975.7	21	917-918	987.0	21	917-918	995.20	21	917-918
961.2	21	917-918	968.6	21	917-918	975.8	21	917-918	987.1	21	917-918	995.21	21	917-918
961.3	21	917-918	968.7	21	917-918	976.0	21	917-918	987.2	21	917-918	995.22	21	917-918
961.4	21	917-918	968.9	21	917-918	976.1	21	917-918	987.3	21	917-918	995.23	21	917-918
961.5	21	917-918	969.00	21	917-918	976.2	21	917-918	987.4	21	917-918	995.24	21	917-918
961.6	21	917-918	969.01	21	917-918	976.3	21	917-918	987.5	21	917-918	995.27	21	917-918
961.7	21	917-918	969.02	21	917-918	976.4	21	917-918	987.6	21	917-918	995.29	21	917-918
961.8	21	917-918	969.03	21	917-918	976.5	02	124-125	987.7	21	917-918	995.3	21	915-916
961.9	21	917-918	969.04	21	917-918	976.6	21	917-918	987.8	21	917-918	995.4	21	922-923
962.0	21	917-918	969.05	21	917-918	976.7	21	917-918	987.9	21	917-918	995.50	21	922-923
962.1	21	917-918	969.09	21	917-918	976.8	21	917-918	988.0	21	917-918	995.51	21	922-923
962.2	21	917-918	969.1	21	917-918	976.9	21	917-918	988.1	21	917-918	995.52	21	922-923
962.3	21	917-918	969.2	21	917-918	977.0	21	917-918	988.2	21	917-918	995.53	21	922-923
962.4	21	917-918	969.3	21	917-918	977.1	21	917-918	988.8	21	917-918	995.54	21	922-923
962.5	21	917-918	969.4	21	917-918	977.2	21	917-918	988.9	21	917-918	995.55	21	922-923
962.6	21	917-918	969.5	21	917-918	977.3	21	917-918	989.0	21	917-918	995.59	21	922-923
962.7	21	917-918	969.6	21	917-918	977.4	21	917-918	989.1	21	917-918	995.60	21	915-916
962.8	21	917-918	969.70	21	917-918	977.8	21	917-918	989.2	21	917-918	995.61	21	915-916
962.9	21	917-918	969.71	21	917-918	977.9	21	917-918	989.3	21	917-918	995.62	21	915-916
963.0	21	917-918	969.72	21	917-918	978.0	21	917-918	989.4	21	917-918	995.63	21	915-916
963.1	21	917-918	969.73	21	917-918	978.1	21	917-918	989.5	21	917-918	995.64	21	915-916
963.2	21	917-918	969.79	21	917-918	978.2	21	917-918	989.6	21	917-918	995.65	21	915-916
963.3	21	917-918	969.8	21	917-918	978.3	21	917-918	989.7	21	917-918	995.66	21	915-916
963.4	21	917-918	969.9	21	917-918	978.4	21	917-918	989.81	21	917-918	995.67	21	915-916
963.5	21	917-918	970.0	21	917-918	978.5	21	917-918	989.82	21	917-918	995.68	21	915-916
963.8	21	917-918	970.1	21	917-918	978.6	21	917-918	989.83	21	917-918	995.69	21	915-916
963.9	21	917-918	970.81	21	917-918	978.8	21	917-918	989.84	21	917-918	995.7	21	922-923
964.0	21	917-918	970.89	21	917-918	978.9	21	917-918	989.89	21	917-918	995.80	21	922-923
964.1	21	917-918	970.9	21	917-918	979.0	21	917-918	989.9	21	917-918	995.81	21	922-923
964.2	21	917-918	971.0	21	917-918	979.1	21	917-918	990	21	922-923	995.82	21	922-923
964.3	21	917-918	971.1	21	917-918	979.2	21	917-918	991.0	21	922-923	995.83	21	922-923
964.4	21	917-918	971.2	21	917-918	979.3	21	917-918	991.1	21	922-923	995.84	21	922-923
964.5	21	917-918	971.3	21	917-918	979.4	21	917-918	991.2	21	922-923	995.85	21	922-923
964.6	21	917-918	971.9	21	917-918	979.5	21	917-918	991.3	21	922-923	995.86	21	922-923
964.7	21	917-918	972.0	21	917-918	979.6	21	917-918	991.4	21	922-923	995.89	21	922-923
964.8	21	917-918	972.1	21	917-918	979.7	21	917-918	991.5	21	922-923	995.90	18	870-872
964.9	21	917-918	972.2	21	917-918	979.9	21	917-918	991.6	21	922-923	995.91	18	870-872
965.00	21	917-918	972.3	21	917-918	980.0	21	917-918	991.8	21	922-923	995.92	18	870-872
965.01	21	917-918	972.4	21	917-918	980.1	21	917-918	991.9	21	922-923	995.93	18	870-872
965.02	21	917-918	972.5	21	917-918	980.2	21	917-918	992.0	21	922-923	995.94	18	870-872
965.09	21	917-918	972.6	21	917-918	980.3	21	917-918	992.1	21	922-923	996.00	05	314-316
965.1	21	917-918	972.7	21	917-918	980.8	21	917-918	992.2	21	922-923	996.01	05	308-310
965.4	21	917-918	972.8	21	917-918	980.9	21	917-918	992.3	21	922-923	996.02	05	306-307
965.5	21	917-918	972.9	21	917-918	981	21	917-918	992.4	21	922-923	996.03	05	314-316
965.61	21	917-918	973.0	21	917-918	982.0	21	917-918	992.5	21	922-923	996.04	05	308-310
965.69	21	917-918	973.1	21	917-918	982.1	21	917-918	992.6	21	922-923	996.09	05	314-316
965.7	21	917-918	973.2	21	917-918	982.2	21	917-918	992.7	21	922-923	996.1	05	314-316
965.8	21	917-918	973.3	21	917-918	982.3	21	917-918	992.8	21	922-923	996.2	01	091-093
965.9	21	917-918	973.4	21	917-918	982.4	21	917-918	992.9	21	922-923	996.30	11	698-700
966.0	21	917-918	973.5	21	917-918	982.8	21	917-918	993.0	03	152-153	996.31	11	698-700
966.1	21	917-918	973.6	21	917-918	983.0	21	917-918	993.1	03	152-153	996.32	13	760-761
966.2	21	917-918	973.8	21	917-918	983.1	21	917-918	993.2	21	922-923	996.39	11	698-700
966.3	21	917-918	973.9	21	917-918	983.2	21	917-918	993.3	21	922-923	996.40	08	559-561
966.4	21	917-918	974.0	21	917-918	983.9	21	917-918	993.4	21	922-923	996.41	08	559-561
967.0	21	917-918	974.1	21	917-918	984.0	21	917-918	993.8	21	922-923	996.42	08	559-561
967.1	21	917-918	974.2	21	917-918	984.1	21	917-918	993.9	21	922-923	996.43	08	559-561
967.2	21	917-918	974.3	21	917-918	984.8	21	917-918	994.0	21	922-923	996.44	08	559-561
967.3	21	917-918	974.4	21	917-918	984.9	21	917-918	994.1	21	922-923	996.45	08	559-561
967.4	21	917-918	974.5	21	917-918	985.0	21	917-918	994.2	21	922-923	996.46	08	559-561
967.5	21	917-918	974.6	21	917-918	985.1	21	917-918	994.3	21	922-923	996.47	08	559-561
967.6	21	917-918	974.7	21	917-918	985.2	21	917-918	994.4	21	922-923	996.49	08	559-561

DX....	MDC.....	DRG	DX....	MDC.....	DRG	DX....	MDC.....	DRG	DX....	MDC.....	DRG	DX....	MDC.....	DRG
996.51	02	124-125	997.79	05	299-301				V06.2	23	951	V10.63	17	843-845
996.52	21	919-921	997.91	21	919-921	**Supplementary Classification**			V06.3	23	951	V10.69	17	843-845
996.53	02	124-125	997.99	21	919-921	**of Factors Influencing Health**			V06.4	23	951	V10.71	17	843-845
996.54	09	600-601	998.00	21	919-921	**Status and Contact with**			V06.5	23	951	V10.72	17	843-845
996.55	21	919-921	998.01	21	919-921	**Health Services**			V06.6	23	951	V10.79	17	843-845
996.56	21	919-921	998.02	21	919-921	V01.0	23	951	V06.8	23	951	V10.81	17	843-845
996.57	21	919-921	998.09	21	919-921	V01.1	23	951	V06.9	23	951	V10.82	17	843-845
996.59	21	919-921	998.11	21	919-921	V01.2	23	951	V07.0	23	951	V10.83	17	843-845
996.60	21	919-921	998.12	21	919-921	V01.3	23	951	V07.1	23	951	V10.84	17	843-845
996.61	05	314-316	998.13	21	919-921	V01.4	23	951	V07.2	23	951	V10.85	17	843-845
996.62	05	314-316	998.2	21	919-921	V01.5	23	951	V07.31	23	951	V10.86	17	843-845
996.63	01	091-093	998.30	21	919-921	V01.6	23	951	V07.39	23	951	V10.87	17	843-845
996.64	11	698-700	998.31	21	919-921	V01.71	23	951	V07.4	23	951	V10.88	17	843-845
996.65	11	698-700	999.32	05	314-316	V01.79	23	951	V07.51	23	951	V10.89	17	843-845
996.66	08	559-561	999.33	05	314-316	V01.81	15	795	V07.52	23	951	V10.90	17	843-845
996.67	08	559-561	999.34	18	867-869	V01.81	23	951	V07.59	23	951	V10.91	17	843-845
996.68	21	919-921	998.32	21	919-921	V01.83	23	951	V07.8	23	951	V11.0	23	951
996.69	21	919-921	998.33	21	919-921	V01.84	23	951	V07.9	23	951	V11.1	23	951
996.70	21	919-921	998.4	21	919-921	V01.89	23	951	V08	18	865-866	V11.2	23	951
996.71	05	314-316	998.51	18	862-863	V01.9	23	951	V09.0	18	867-869	V11.3	23	951
996.72	05	314-315	998.59	18	862-863	V02.0	23	951	V09.1	18	867-869	V11.4	23	951
996.73	05	314-316	998.6	21	919-921	V02.1	23	951	V09.2	18	867-869	V11.8	23	951
996.74	05	314-316	998.7	21	919-921	V02.2	23	951	V09.3	18	867-869	V11.9	23	951
996.75	01	091-093	998.81	21	919-921	V02.3	23	951	V09.4	18	867-869	V12.00	23	951
996.76	11	698-700	998.82	02	124-125	V02.4	23	951	V09.50	18	867-869	V12.01	23	951
996.77	08	559-561	998.83	21	919-921	V02.51	23	951	V09.51	18	867-869	V12.02	23	951
996.78	08	559-561	998.89	21	919-921	V02.52	23	951	V09.6	18	867-869	V12.03	23	951
996.79	21	919-921	998.9	21	919-921	V02.53	23	951	V09.70	18	867-869	V12.04	23	951
996.80	21	919-921	999.0	18	865-866	V02.54	23	951	V09.71	18	867-869	V12.09	23	951
996.81	11	698-700	999.1	04	175-176	V02.59	23	951	V09.80	18	867-869	V12.1	23	951
996.82	07	441-443	999.2	05	314-316	V02.60	07	441-443	V09.81	18	867-869	V12.21	23	951
996.83	05	314-316	999.31	05	314-316	V02.61	07	441-443	V09.90	18	867-869	V12.29	23	951
996.84	04	205-206	999.32	05	314-316	V02.62	07	441-443	V09.91	18	867-869	V12.3	23	951
996.85	16	808-810	999.33	05	314-316	V02.69	07	441-443	V10.00	17	843-845	V12.40	23	951
996.86	07	438-440	999.34	18	867-869	V02.7	23	951	V10.01	17	843-845	V12.41	23	951
996.87	21	919-921	999.39	18	867-869	V02.8	23	951	V10.02	17	843-845	V12.42	23	951
996.88	21	919-921	999.41	21	915-916	V02.9	23	951	V10.03	17	843-845	V12.49	23	951
996.89	21	919-921	999.42	21	915-916	V03.0	23	951	V10.04	17	843-845	V12.50	23	951
996.90	08	559-561	999.49	21	915-916	V03.1	23	951	V10.05	17	843-845	V12.51	23	951
996.91	08	559-561	999.51	21	915-916	V03.2	23	951	V10.06	17	843-845	V12.52	23	951
996.92	08	559-561	999.52	21	915-916	V03.3	23	951	V10.07	17	843-845	V12.53	23	951
996.93	08	559-561	999.59	21	915-916	V03.4	23	951	V10.09	17	843-845	V12.54	23	951
996.94	08	559-561	999.60	16	811-812	V03.5	23	951	V10.11	17	843-845	V12.55	23	951
996.95	08	559-561	999.61	16	811-812	V03.6	23	951	V10.12	17	843-845	V12.59	23	951
996.96	08	559-561	999.62	16	811-812	V03.7	23	951	V10.20	17	843-845	V12.60	23	951
996.99	08	559-561	999.63	16	811-812	V03.81	23	951	V10.21	17	843-845	V12.61	23	951
997.00	01	091-093	999.69	16	811-812	V03.82	23	951	V10.22	17	843-845	V12.69	23	951
997.01	01	091-093	999.70	16	811-812	V03.89	23	951	V10.29	17	843-845	V12.70	23	951
997.02	01	091-093	999.71	16	811-812	V03.9	23	951	V10.3	17	843-845	V12.71	23	951
997.09	01	091-093	999.72	16	811-812	V04.0	23	951	V10.40	17	843-845	V12.72	23	951
997.1	05	314-316	999.73	16	811-812	V04.1	23	951	V10.41	17	843-845	V12.79	23	951
997.2	05	299-301	999.74	16	811-812	V04.2	23	951	V10.42	17	843-845	V13.00	23	951
997.31	04	205-206	999.75	16	811-812	V04.3	23	951	V10.43	17	843-845	V13.01	23	951
997.32	04	205-206	999.76	16	811-812	V04.4	23	951	V10.44	17	843-845	V13.02	23	951
997.39	04	205-206	999.77	16	811-812	V04.5	23	951	V10.45	17	843-845	V13.03	23	951
997.41	06	393-395	999.78	16	811-812	V04.6	23	951	V10.46	17	843-845	V13.09	23	951
997.49	06	393-395	999.79	16	811-812	V04.7	23	951	V10.47	17	843-845	V13.1	23	951
997.5	11	698-700	999.80	16	811-812	V04.81	23	951	V10.48	17	843-845	V13.21	23	951
997.60	08	564-566	999.81	05	314-316	V04.82	23	951	V10.49	17	843-845	V13.22	17	843-845
997.61	08	564-566	999.82	05	314-316	V04.89	23	951	V10.50	17	843-845	V13.23	23	951
997.62	08	564-566	999.83	16	811-812	V05.0	23	951	V10.51	17	843-845	V13.24	23	951
997.69	08	564-566	999.84	16	811-812	V05.1	23	951	V10.52	17	843-845	V13.29	23	951
997.71	06	393-395	999.85	16	811-812	V05.2	23	951	V10.53	17	843-845	V13.3	23	951
997.72	11	698-700	999.88	05	314-316	V05.3	23	951	V10.59	17	843-845	V13.4	23	951
			999.89	16	811-812	V05.4	23	951	V10.60	17	843-845	V13.51	23	951
			999.9	21	919-920	V05.8	23	951	V10.61	17	843-845	V13.52	23	951
						V05.9	23	951	V10.62	17	843-845	V13.59	23	951
						V06.0	23	951						
						V06.1	23	951						

DX	MDC	DRG	DX	MDC	DRG	DX	MDC	DRG	DX	MDC	DRG	DX	MDC	DRG
V13.61	23	951	V16.59	23	951	V23.82	14	998	V28.82	23	951	V42.7	07	441-443
V13.62	23	951	V16.6	23	951	V23.83	14	998	V28.89	23	951	V42.81	16	814-816
V13.63	23	951	V16.7	23	951	V23.84	14	998	V28.9	23	951	V42.82	16	814-816
V13.64	23	951	V16.8	23	951	V23.85	14	998	V29.0	23	951	V42.83	07	438-440
V13.65	23	951	V16.9	23	951	V23.86	14	998	V29.1	23	951	V42.84	07	951
V13.66	23	951	V17.0	23	951	V23.87	14	998	V29.2	23	951	V42.89	23	951
V13.67	23	951	V17.1	23	951	V23.89	14	998	V29.3	23	951	V42.9	23	951
V13.68	23	951	V17.2	23	951	V23.9	14	998	V29.8	23	951	V43.0	02	124-125
V13.69	23	951	V17.3	23	951	V24.0	14	776	V29.9	23	951	V43.1	02	124-125
V13.7	23	951	V17.41	23	951	V24.1	23	951	V30.00	15	795	V43.21	05	314-316
V13.81	23	951	V17.49	23	951	V24.2	23	951	V30.01	15	795	V43.22	05	314-316
V13.89	23	951	V17.5	23	951	V25.01	23	951	V30.1	15	795	V43.3	05	314-316
V13.9	23	951	V17.6	23	951	V25.02	23	951	V30.2	15	998	V43.4	05	314-316
V14.0	23	951	V17.7	23	951	V25.03	23	951	V31.00	15	795	V43.5	11	698-700
V14.1	23	951	V17.81	23	951	V25.04	23	951	V31.01	15	795	V43.60	08	564-566
V14.2	23	951	V17.89	23	951	V25.09	23	951	V31.1	15	795	V43.61	08	564-566
V14.3	23	951	V18.0	23	951	V25.11	23	951	V31.2	15	998	V43.62	08	564-566
V14.4	23	951	V18.11	23	951	V25.12	23	951	V32.00	15	795	V43.63	08	564-566
V14.5	23	951	V18.19	23	951	V25.13	23	951	V32.01	15	795	V43.64	08	564-566
V14.6	23	951	V18.2	23	951	V25.2	12	729-730	V32.1	15	795	V43.65	08	564-566
V14.7	23	951	V18.3	23	951	V25.2	13	760-761	V32.2	15	998	V43.66	08	564-566
V14.8	23	951	V18.4	23	951	V25.3	13	760-761	V33.00	15	795	V43.69	08	564-566
V14.9	23	951	V18.51	23	951	V25.40	23	951	V33.01	15	795	V43.7	08	564-566
V15.01	23	951	V18.59	23	951	V25.41	23	951	V33.1	15	795	V43.81	23	951
V15.02	23	951	V18.61	23	951	V25.42	23	951	V33.2	15	998	V43.82	23	951
V15.03	23	951	V18.69	23	951	V25.43	23	951	V34.00	15	795	V43.83	23	951
V15.04	23	951	V18.7	23	951	V25.49	23	951	V34.01	15	795	V43.89	23	951
V15.05	23	951	V18.8	23	951	V25.5	23	951	V34.1	15	795	V44.0	23	951
V15.06	23	951	V18.9	23	951	V25.8	23	951	V34.2	15	998	V44.1	23	951
V15.07	23	951	V19.0	23	951	V25.9	23	951	V35.00	15	795	V44.2	23	951
V15.08	23	951	V19.11	23	951	V26.0	12	729-730	V35.01	15	795	V44.3	23	951
V15.09	23	951	V19.19	23	951	V26.0	13	760-761	V35.1	15	795	V44.4	23	951
V15.1	23	951	V19.2	23	951	V26.1	23	951	V35.2	15	998	V44.50	23	951
V15.21	23	951	V19.3	23	951	V26.21	23	951	V36.00	15	795	V44.51	23	951
V15.22	23	951	V19.4	23	951	V26.22	23	951	V36.01	15	795	V44.52	23	951
V15.29	23	951	V19.5	23	951	V26.29	23	951	V36.1	15	795	V44.59	23	951
V15.3	23	951	V19.6	23	951	V26.31	23	951	V36.2	15	998	V44.6	23	951
V15.41	23	951	V19.7	23	951	V26.32	23	951	V37.00	15	795	V44.7	23	951
V15.42	23	951	V19.8	23	951	V26.33	23	951	V37.01	15	795	V44.8	23	951
V15.49	23	951	V20.0	23	951	V26.34	23	951	V37.1	15	795	V44.9	23	951
V15.51	23	951	V20.1	23	951	V26.35	23	951	V37.2	15	998	V45.00	23	951
V15.52	23	951	V20.2	23	951	V26.39	23	951	V39.00	15	795	V45.01	23	951
V15.53	23	951	V20.31	23	951	V26.41	23	951	V39.01	15	795	V45.02	23	951
V15.59	23	951	V20.32	23	951	V26.42	23	951	V39.1	15	795	V45.09	23	951
V15.6	23	951	V21.0	23	951	V26.49	23	951	V39.2	15	998	V45.11	23	951
V15.7	23	951	V21.1	23	951	V26.51	23	951	V40.0	23	951	V45.12	23	951
V15.80	23	951	V21.2	23	951	V26.52	23	951	V40.1	23	951	V45.2	23	951
V15.81	23	951	V21.30	23	951	V26.81	23	951	V40.2	23	951	V45.3	23	951
V15.82	23	951	V21.31	23	951	V26.82	23	951	V40.31	23	951	V45.4	23	951
V15.83	23	951	V21.32	23	951	V26.89	23	951	V40.39	23	951	V45.51	23	951
V15.84	23	951	V21.33	23	951	V26.9	23	951	V40.9	23	951	V45.52	23	951
V15.85	23	951	V21.34	23	951	V27.0	23	951	V41.0	23	951	V45.59	23	951
V15.86	23	951	V21.35	23	951	V27.1	23	951	V41.1	23	951	V45.61	23	951
V15.87	23	951	V21.8	23	951	V27.2	23	951	V41.2	23	951	V45.69	23	951
V15.88	23	951	V21.9	23	951	V27.3	23	951	V41.3	23	951	V45.71	23	951
V15.89	23	951	V22.0	23	951	V27.4	23	951	V41.4	23	951	V45.72	23	951
V15.9	23	951	V22.1	23	951	V27.5	23	951	V41.5	23	951	V45.73	23	951
V16.0	23	951	V22.2	23	951	V27.6	23	951	V41.6	23	951	V45.74	11	698-700
V16.1	23	951	V23.0	14	998	V27.7	23	951	V41.7	23	951	V45.75	23	951
V16.2	23	951	V23.1	14	998	V27.9	23	951	V41.8	23	951	V45.76	04	205-206
V16.3	23	951	V23.2	14	998	V28.0	14	781-782	V41.9	23	951	V45.77	12	729-730
V16.40	23	951	V23.3	14	998	V28.1	14	781-782	V42.0	11	698-700	V45.77	13	760-761
V16.41	23	951	V23.41	14	998	V28.2	14	781-782	V42.1	05	314-316	V45.78	02	124-125
V16.42	23	951	V23.42	14	998	V28.3	23	951	V42.2	05	314-316	V45.79	23	951
V16.43	23	951	V23.49	14	998	V28.4	23	951	V42.3	09	606-607	V45.81	23	951
V16.49	23	951	V23.5	14	998	V28.5	23	951	V42.4	08	564-566	V45.82	23	951
V16.51	23	951	V23.7	14	998	V28.6	23	951	V42.5	02	124-125	V45.83	23	951
V16.52	23	951	V23.81	14	998	V28.81	23	951	V42.6	04	205-206	V45.84	23	951

DX	MDC	DRG
V45.85	23	951
V45.86	23	951
V45.87	23	951
V45.88	23	951
V45.89	23	951
V46.0	23	951
V46.11	23	951
V46.12	23	951
V46.13	23	951
V46.14	23	951
V46.2	23	951
V46.3	23	951
V46.8	23	951
V46.9	23	951
V47.0	23	951
V47.1	23	951
V47.2	23	951
V47.3	23	951
V47.4	23	951
V47.5	23	951
V47.9	23	951
V48.0	23	951
V48.1	23	951
V48.2	23	951
V48.3	23	951
V48.4	23	951
V48.5	23	951
V48.6	23	951
V48.7	23	951
V48.8	23	951
V48.9	23	951
V49.0	23	951
V49.1	23	951
V49.2	23	951
V49.3	23	951
V49.4	23	951
V49.5	23	951
V49.60	23	951
V49.61	23	951
V49.62	23	951
V49.63	23	951
V49.64	23	951
V49.65	23	951
V49.66	23	951
V49.67	23	951
V49.70	23	951
V49.71	23	951
V49.72	23	951
V49.73	23	951
V49.74	23	951
V49.75	23	951
V49.76	23	951
V49.77	23	951
V49.81	23	951
V49.82	23	951
V49.83	23	951
V49.84	23	951
V49.85	23	951
V49.86	23	951
V49.87	23	951
V49.89	23	951
V49.9	23	951
V50.0	09	606-607
V50.1	09	606-607
V50.2	12	727-728
V50.3	23	951
V50.41	9	600-601
V50.42	13	760-761
V50.49	23	951
V50.8	23	951
V50.9	23	951
V51.0	09	606-607
V51.8	09	606-607
V52.0	08	559-561
V52.1	08	559-561
V52.2	23	951
V52.3	23	951
V52.4	23	951
V52.8	23	945-946
V52.9	23	945-946
V53.01	01	091-093
V53.02	01	091-093
V53.09	01	091-093
V53.1	23	951
V53.2	23	951
V53.31	05	314-316
V53.32	05	314-316
V53.39	05	314-316
V53.4	23	951
V53.50	06	393-395
V53.51	06	393-395
V53.59	06	393-395
V53.6	11	698-700
V53.7	08	559-561
V53.8	23	951
V53.90	23	951
V53.91	23	951
V53.99	23	951
V54.01	08	559-561
V54.02	08	559-561
V54.09	08	559-561
V54.10	08	559-561
V54.11	08	559-561
V54.12	08	559-561
V54.13	08	559-561
V54.14	08	559-561
V54.15	08	559-561
V54.16	08	559-561
V54.17	08	559-561
V54.19	08	559-561
V54.20	08	559-561
V54.21	08	559-561
V54.22	08	559-561
V54.23	08	559-561
V54.24	08	559-561
V54.25	08	559-561
V54.26	08	559-561
V54.27	08	559-561
V54.29	08	559-561
V54.81	08	559-561
V54.82	08	559-561
V54.89	08	559-561
V54.9	08	559-561
V55.0	04	205-206
V55.1	06	393-395
V55.2	06	393-395
V55.3	06	393-395
V55.4	06	393-395
V55.5	11	698-700
V55.6	11	698-700
V55.7	13	760-761
V55.8	23	951
V55.9	23	951
V56.0	11	685
V56.1	11	685
V56.2	11	685
V56.31	11	685
V56.32	11	685
V56.8	11	685
V57.0	23	951
V57.1	23	945-946
V57.21	23	945-946
V57.22	23	945-946
V57.3	23	945-946
V57.4	23	945-946
V57.81	23	951
V57.89	23	945-946
V57.9	23	945-946
V58.0	17	849
V58.11	17	837-839, 846-848
V58.12	17	837-839, 846-848
V58.2	23	951
V58.30	23	951
V58.31	23	951
V58.32	23	951
V58.41	23	949-950
V58.42	23	949-950
V58.43	23	949-950
V58.44	23	949-950
V58.49	23	949-950
V58.5	23	949-950
V58.61	23	949-950
V58.62	23	949-950
V58.63	23	949-950
V58.64	23	949-950
V58.65	23	949-950
V58.66	23	949-950
V58.67	23	949-950
V58.68	23	949-950
V58.69	23	949-950
V58.71	23	949-950
V58.72	23	949-950
V58.73	23	949-950
V58.74	23	949-950
V58.75	23	949-950
V58.76	23	949-950
V58.77	23	949-950
V58.78	23	949-950
V58.81	23	949-950
V58.83	23	949-950
V58.82	23	949-950
V58.89	23	949-950
V58.9	23	949-950
V59.01	23	951
V59.02	23	951
V59.09	23	951
V59.1	09	606-607
V59.2	08	564-566
V59.3	23	951
V59.4	11	698-700
V59.5	23	951
V59.6	07	441-443
V59.70	23	951
V59.71	23	951
V59.72	23	951
V59.73	23	951
V59.74	23	951
V59.8	23	951
V59.9	23	951
V60.0	23	951
V60.1	23	951
V60.2	23	951
V60.3	23	951
V60.4	23	951
V60.5	23	951
V60.6	23	951
V60.81	23	951
V60.89	23	951
V60.9	23	951
V61.01	23	951
V61.02	23	951
V61.03	23	951
V61.04	23	951
V61.05	23	951
V61.06	23	951
V61.07	23	951
V61.08	23	951
V61.09	23	951
V61.10	23	951
V61.11	23	951
V61.12	23	951
V61.20	23	951
V61.21	23	951
V61.22	23	951
V61.23	23	951
V61.24	23	951
V61.25	23	951
V61.29	23	951
V61.3	23	951
V61.41	23	951
V61.42	23	951
V61.49	23	951
V61.5	13	760-761
V61.6	14	781-782
V61.7	14	779
V61.8	23	951
V61.9	23	951
V62.0	23	951
V62.1	23	951
V62.21	23	951
V62.22	23	951
V62.29	23	951
V62.3	23	951
V62.4	23	951
V62.5	23	951
V62.6	23	951
V62.81	23	951
V62.82	23	951
V62.83	23	951
V62.84	19	880
V62.85	23	951
V62.89	23	951
V62.9	23	951
V63.0	23	951
V63.1	23	951
V63.2	23	951
V63.8	23	951
V63.9	23	951
V64.00	23	951
V64.01	23	951
V64.02	23	951
V64.03	23	951
V64.04	23	951
V64.05	23	951
V64.06	23	951
V64.07	23	951
V64.08	23	951
V64.09	23	951
V64.1	23	951
V64.2	23	951
V64.3	23	951
V64.41	23	951
V64.42	23	951
V64.43	23	951
V65.0	23	951
V65.11	23	951
V65.19	23	951
V65.2	23	951
V65.3	23	951
V65.40	23	951
V65.41	23	951
V65.42	23	951
V65.43	23	951
V65.44	23	951
V65.45	23	951
V65.46	23	951
V65.49	23	951
V65.5	23	951
V65.8	23	951
V65.9	23	951
V66.0	23	951
V66.1	23	951
V66.2	23	951
V66.3	23	951
V66.4	23	951
V66.5	23	951
V66.6	23	951
V66.7	23	951
V66.9	23	951
V67.00	23	949-950
V67.01	23	949-950
V67.09	23	949-950
V67.1	17	849
V67.2	17	837-839, 846-848
V67.3	23	951
V67.4	23	949-950
V67.51	23	951
V67.59	23	951
V67.6	23	951
V67.9	23	951
V68.01	23	951
V68.09	23	951
V68.1	23	951
V68.2	23	951
V68.81	23	951
V68.89	23	951
V68.9	23	951
V69.0	23	951
V69.2	23	951
V69.3	23	951
V69.4	23	951
V69.5	23	951
V69.8	23	951
V69.9	23	951
V70.0	23	951
V70.1	23	951
V70.2	23	951
V70.3	23	951
V70.4	23	951
V70.5	23	951
V70.6	23	951
V70.7	23	951
V70.8	23	951

Diagnosis Code/MDC/DRG List

DX	MDC	DRG	DX	MDC	DRG	DX	MDC	DRG	DX	MDC	DRG	DX	MDC	DRG
V70.9	23	951	V73.88	23	951	V77.4	23	951	V84.02	23	951	V87.45	23	949-950
V71.01	19	880	V73.89	23	951	V77.5	23	951	V84.03	23	951	V87.46	23	949-950
V71.02	19	880	V73.98	23	951	V77.6	23	951	V84.04	23	951	V87.49	23	949-950
V71.09	19	887	V73.99	23	951	V77.7	23	951	V84.09	23	951	V88.01	13	760-761
V71.1	17	843-845	V74.0	23	951	V77.8	23	951	V84.81	23	951	V88.02	13	760-761
V71.2	04	177-179	V74.1	23	951	V77.91	23	951	V84.89	23	951	V88.03	13	760-761
V71.3	21	922-923	V74.2	23	951	V77.99	23	951	V85.0	23	951	V88.11	23	951
V71.4	21	922-923	V74.3	23	951	V78.0	23	951	V85.1	23	951	V88.12	23	951
V71.5	23	951	V74.4	23	951	V78.1	23	951	V85.21	23	951	V88.21	23	951
V71.6	21	922-923	V74.5	23	951	V78.2	23	951	V85.22	23	951	V88.22	23	951
V71.7	05	313	V74.6	23	951	V78.3	23	951	V85.23	23	951	V88.29	23	951
V71.81	23	951	V74.8	23	951	V78.8	23	951	V85.24	23	951	V89.01	23	951
V71.82	23	951	V74.9	23	951	V78.9	23	951	V85.25	23	951	V89.02	23	951
V71.83	23	951	V75.0	23	951	V79.0	23	951	V85.30	23	951	V89.03	23	951
V71.89	23	951	V75.1	23	951	V79.1	23	951	V85.31	23	951	V89.04	23	951
V71.9	23	951	V75.2	23	951	V79.2	23	951	V85.32	23	951	V89.05	23	951
V72.0	23	951	V75.3	23	951	V79.3	23	951	V85.33	23	951	V89.09	23	951
V72.11	23	951	V75.4	23	951	V79.8	23	951	V85.34	23	951	V90.01	23	951
V72.12	23	951	V75.5	23	951	V79.9	23	951	V85.35	23	951	V90.09	23	951
V72.19	23	951	V75.6	23	951	V80.01	23	951	V85.36	23	951	V90.10	23	951
V72.2	23	951	V75.7	23	951	V80.09	23	951	V85.37	23	951	V90.11	23	951
V72.31	23	951	V75.8	23	951	V80.1	23	951	V85.38	23	951	V90.12	23	951
V72.32	23	951	V75.9	23	951	V80.2	23	951	V85.39	23	951	V90.2	23	951
V72.40	23	951	V76.0	23	951	V80.3	23	951	V85.41	10	640-641	V90.31	23	951
V72.41	23	951	V76.10	23	951	V81.0	23	951	V85.42	10	640-641	V90.32	23	951
V72.42	23	951	V76.11	23	951	V81.1	23	951	V85.43	10	640-641	V90.33	23	951
V72.5	23	951	V76.12	23	951	V81.2	23	951	V85.44	10	640-641	V90.39	23	951
V72.60	23	951	V76.19	23	951	V81.3	23	951	V85.45	10	640-641	V90.81	23	951
V72.61	23	951	V76.2	23	951	V81.4	23	951	V85.51	23	951	V90.83	23	951
V72.62	23	951	V76.3	23	951	V81.5	23	951	V85.52	23	951	V90.89	23	951
V72.63	23	951	V76.41	23	951	V81.6	23	951	V85.53	23	951	V90.9	23	951
V72.69	23	951	V76.42	23	951	V82.0	23	951	V85.54	23	951	V91.00	23	951
V72.7	23	951	V76.43	23	951	V82.1	23	951	V86.0	23	951	V91.01	23	951
V72.81	23	951	V76.44	23	951	V82.2	23	951	V86.1	23	951	V91.02	23	951
V72.82	23	951	V76.45	23	951	V82.3	23	951	V87.01	23	951	V91.03	23	951
V72.83	23	951	V76.46	23	951	V82.4	23	951	V87.02	23	951	V91.09	23	951
V72.84	23	951	V76.47	23	951	V82.5	23	951	V87.09	23	951	V91.10	23	951
V72.85	23	951	V76.49	23	951	V82.6	23	951	V87.11	23	951	V91.11	23	951
V72.86	23	951	V76.50	23	951	V82.71	23	951	V87.12	23	951	V91.12	23	951
V72.9	23	951	V76.51	23	951	V82.79	23	951	V87.19	23	951	V91.19	23	951
V73.0	23	951	V76.52	23	951	V82.81	23	951	V87.2	23	951	V91.20	23	951
V73.1	23	951	V76.81	23	951	V82.89	23	951	V87.31	23	951	V91.21	23	951
V73.2	23	951	V76.89	23	951	V82.9	23	951	V87.32	23	951	V91.22	23	951
V73.3	23	951	V76.9	23	951	V83.01	23	951	V87.39	23	951	V91.29	23	951
V73.4	23	951	V77.0	23	951	V83.02	23	951	V87.41	23	949-950	V91.90	23	951
V73.5	23	951	V77.1	23	951	V83.81	23	951	V87.42	23	949-950	V91.91	23	951
V73.6	23	951	V77.2	23	951	V83.89	23	951	V87.43	23	949-950	V91.92	23	951
V73.81	23	951	V77.3	23	951	V84.01	23	951	V87.44	23	949-950	V91.99	23	951

Major Complication & Comorbidity (MCC) Code List

The following is the standards list of conditions considered to be major complications and comorbidities that when present as a secondary diagnosis may affect DRG assignment under the Medicare Severity DRG (MS-DRG) system version 30.0. An asterisk (*) indicates that a code range is represented.

003.1	098.84	*324	464.31	535.41	638.6	673.31	772.14	
003.21	100.81	325	464.51	535.51	639.3	673.32	772.2	
003.22	112.4	331.81	*480	535.61	639.5	673.33	772.4	
006.3	112.5	333.92	481	537.83	639.6	673.34	773.3	
006.4	112.81	336.1	*482	537.84	641.11	673.81	773.4	
006.5	112.83	343.2	*483	540.0	641.13	673.82	774.4	
*011.6	114.2	*344.0	*484	540.1	641.21	673.83	774.7	
*013.0	115.01	344.81	485	*550.0	641.31	673.84	775.7	
*013.1	115.03	345.2	486	*551.0	641.33	674.01	776.1	
*013.2	115.04	345.3	487.0	551.1	642.11	674.50	776.2	
*013.3	115.05	345.71	488.01	*551.2	642.12	674.51	776.7	
*013.4	115.11	*348.3	488.11	551.3	642.42	674.52	*777.5	
*013.5	115.13	348.4	488.81	551.8	642.51	674.53	777.6	
*013.6	115.14	348.5	506.1	551.9	642.52	674.54	778.0	
*013.8	115.15	348.82	*507	557.0	642.53	707.23	779.0	
*013.9	115.91	358.01	*510	560.2	642.54	707.24	779.2	
*014.0	115.93	410.01	511.1	562.02	642.61	728.86	779.32	
*018.0	115.94	410.11	512.0	562.03	642.62	740.0	779.7	
*018.8	115.95	410.21	513.0	562.12	642.63	740.1	779.85	
*018.9	117.7	410.31	513.1	562.13	642.64	740.2	780.01	
*020	130.0	410.41	516.4	567.0	642.71	742.2	780.72	
022.1	130.3	410.51	*516.6	567.1	642.72	745.0	785.51	
022.3	130.4	410.61	518.4	*567.2	642.73	745.10	785.52	
*036	130.8	410.71	*518.5	*567.3	642.74	745.11	785.59	
037	136.3	410.81	518.81	567.81	644.03	745.19	799.1	
038.0	242.01	410.91	518.84	567.89	644.21	745.2	800.03	
*038.1	242.11	414.12	519.2	567.9	648.01	745.3	800.04	
038.2	242.21	*415	530.21	568.81	648.02	745.7	800.05	
038.3	242.31	421.0	530.4	569.83	654.51	746.01	*800.1	
*038.4	242.41	421.1	530.7	569.85	654.52	746.1	*800.2	
038.8	242.81	421.9	530.82	569.86	654.53	746.2	*800.3	
038.9	242.91	422.0	530.84	570	654.54	746.7	800.43	
040.0	249.10	*422.9	*531.0	572.0	658.41	746.81	800.44	
040.82	249.11	*427.4	*531.1	572.1	658.43	746.82	800.45	
042	249.20	427.5	*531.2	572.2	659.31	746.84	*800.5	
*045.0	249.21	428.21	531.31	572.4	659.33	746.86	*800.6	
*045.1	249.30	428.23	*531.4	573.4	665.01	747.11	*800.7	
052.0	249.31	428.31	*531.5	574.81	665.03	*747.3	*800.8	
052.1	*250.1	428.33	*531.6	575.4	665.11	747.81	*800.9	
052.2	*250.2	428.41	531.71	576.2	669.11	747.83	801.03	
053.0	*250.3	428.43	531.91	576.3	669.12	748.5	801.04	
053.14	260	429.5	*532.0	577.0	669.13	750.3	801.05	
054.3	261	429.6	*532.1	580.0	669.14	751.61	*801.1	
054.5	262	430	*532.2	580.4	669.21	755.55	*801.2	
054.72	277.01	431	532.31	580.81	669.22	756.6	*801.3	
054.74	277.02	432.0	*532.4	580.89	669.32	756.70	801.43	
055.0	277.88	432.1	*532.5	580.9	669.34	756.71	801.44	
055.1	282.42	433.01	*532.6	583.4	670.02	756.72	801.45	
056.01	282.62	433.11	532.71	583.6	670.04	756.73	*801.5	
058.21	282.64	433.21	532.91	584.5	670.22	756.79	*801.6	
058.29	282.69	433.31	*533.0	584.6	670.24	758.32	*801.7	
*062	283.11	433.81	*533.1	584.7	670.32	759.4	*801.8	
*063	284.11	433.91	*533.2	585.6	670.34	767.0	*801.9	
064	284.12	434.01	533.31	590.11	670.80	768.5	803.03	
*066.4	*284.8	434.11	*533.4	590.2	670.82	768.73	803.04	
070.0	286.0	434.91	*533.5	596.6	670.84	769	803.05	
*070.2	286.1	*441.0	*533.6	614.5	671.31	770.0	*803.1	
*070.4	286.6	441.1	533.71	*634.3	671.33	770.12	*803.2	
070.6	*320	441.3	533.91	*634.5	671.42	770.14	*803.3	
070.71	*321	441.5	*534.0	634.61	671.44	770.16	803.43	
072.1	322.0	441.6	*534.1	634.62	673.01	770.18	803.44	
072.2	322.1	*443.2	*534.2	*635.3	673.02	770.2	803.45	
073.0	322.9	444.01	534.31	*635.5	673.03	770.3	*803.5	
084.0	*323.0	446.6	*534.4	*635.6	673.04	770.7	*803.6	
090.41	323.1	452	*534.5	*636.3	673.11	770.84	*803.7	
090.42	323.2	453.0	*534.6	*636.5	673.12	770.86	*803.8	
091.81	*323.4	453.2	534.71	*636.6	673.13	770.87	*803.9	
094.2	*323.5	456.0	534.91	*637.3	673.14	771.1	804.03	
094.81	*323.6	456.20	535.01	*637.5	673.21	771.2	804.04	
094.87	*323.7	464.01	535.11	*637.6	673.22	771.3	804.05	
098.82	*323.8	464.11	535.21	638.3	673.23	771.81	*804.1	
098.83	323.9	464.21	535.31	638.5	673.24	772.13	*804.2	

Major Complication & Comorbidity (MCC) Code List

*804.3	806.9	828.1	*853.0	865.04	901.83	948.51	948.92
804.43	*807.1	835.10	*853.1	*865.1	902.0	948.52	948.93
804.44	807.3	835.11	854.05	866.03	*902.1	948.53	948.94
804.45	807.4	835.12	*854.1	866.10	*902.2	948.54	948.95
804.53	807.5	835.13	860.1	866.11	*902.3	948.55	948.96
804.54	807.6	*839.1	860.2	866.12	*902.4	948.61	948.97
804.55	808.0	*839.3	860.3	866.13	902.50	948.62	948.98
*804.6	808.1	839.50	860.4	867.1	902.51	948.63	948.99
*804.7	808.3	839.59	860.5	867.3	902.52	948.64	*952.0
*804.8	*808.5	839.71	861.02	867.5	902.53	948.65	*952.1
804.93	808.9	850.4	861.03	867.7	902.54	948.66	952.2
804.94	809.1	851.05	*861.1	867.9	902.59	948.71	952.3
804.95	*812.1	*851.1	861.22	*868.1	902.87	948.72	952.4
*805.1	*812.3	*851.2	*861.3	869.1	*903.0	948.73	952.8
805.3	*812.5	*851.3	862.1	*874.0	904.0	948.74	958.0
805.5	*813.1	851.45	862.21	*874.1	904.1	948.75	958.1
805.7	*813.3	*851.5	862.22	887.6	904.2	948.76	958.4
805.9	*813.5	*851.6	*862.3	887.7	*904.4	948.77	958.5
*806.0	*813.9	*851.7	862.9	896.2	948.21	948.81	995.91
*806.1	*820	*851.8	863.1	896.3	948.22	948.82	995.92
*806.2	*821.0	*851.9	*863.3	897.6	948.31	948.83	995.94
*806.3	*821.1	*852.0	*863.5	897.7	948.32	948.84	998.01
806.4	*821.3	*852.1	*863.9	901.0	948.33	948.85	998.02
806.5	*823.1	*852.2	864.03	901.1	948.41	948.86	998.09
*806.6	*823.3	*852.3	864.04	901.2	948.42	948.87	999.1
*806.7	*823.9	*852.4	*864.1	901.3	948.43	948.88	
806.8	828.0	*852.5	865.03	*901.4	948.44	948.91	

Complication and Comorbidity (CC) Code List

The following is the standards list of conditions considered to be complications and comorbidities that when present as a secondary diagnosis may affect DRG assignment under the Medicare Severity DRG (MS-DRG) system version 30.0. An asterisk (*) indicates that a code range is represented.

*001	*017.2	*060	093.23	123.1	*204.0	276.3	295.01
*002	*017.3	061	093.24	123.2	*204.1	276.4	295.02
003.0	*017.4	*065	*093.8	123.3	*204.2	277.00	295.03
003.23	*017.5	066.0	093.9	123.4	*204.8	277.03	295.04
003.24	*017.6	066.1	094.0	123.5	*204.9	277.09	295.10
003.29	*017.7	066.2	094.1	123.6	*205.0	277.1	295.11
003.8	*017.8	066.3	094.3	123.8	*205.1	277.2	295.12
003.9	*017.9	066.8	094.82	124	*205.2	*277.3	295.13
004.0	*021	066.9	094.83	*125	*205.3	277.5	295.14
005.0	022.0	070.1	094.84	*126	*205.8	277.85	295.20
005.1	022.2	070.30	094.85	*127	*205.9	277.86	295.21
005.2	022.8	070.31	094.86	130.1	*206.0	277.87	295.22
005.3	022.9	070.32	094.89	130.2	*206.1	277.89	295.23
005.4	023.8	070.33	094.9	130.5	*206.2	278.03	295.24
005.81	023.9	070.51	095.0	130.7	*206.8	*279.0	295.30
005.89	024	070.52	095.1	130.9	*206.9	*279.1	295.31
006.0	025	070.53	095.2	136.29	*207.0	279.2	295.32
006.1	*026	070.59	095.3	136.4	*207.1	279.3	295.33
006.2	027.0	070.9	095.4	136.5	*207.2	*279.5	295.34
006.8	027.2	071	095.5	*150	*207.8	282.8	295.40
007.1	027.8	072.0	095.6	*151	*208.0	282.9	295.41
007.2	027.9	072.3	095.7	*152	*208.1	283.0	295.42
007.4	*030	*072.7	095.8	*153	*208.2	283.10	295.43
007.5	*031	072.8	095.9	*154	*208.8	283.19	295.44
007.8	*032	073.7	098.0	*155	*208.9	283.9	295.53
007.9	*033	073.8	*098.1	*156	*209.0	*284.0	295.54
*008.0	034.1	073.9	*098.4	*157	*209.1	284.19	295.60
008.1	*036.8	*074.2	*098.5	*158	*209.2	284.2	295.61
008.2	036.9	078.3	098.81	*162	209.30	284.9	295.62
008.3	*039	078.5	098.85	*163	209.71	285.1	295.63
*008.4	040.2	078.6	098.86	*164	209.72	286.2	295.64
008.5	040.3	078.7	098.89	*170	209.73	286.3	295.71
*008.6	040.41	079.51	099.56	*171	209.74	286.4	295.72
009.0	040.42	079.52	100.0	*176	209.79	*286.5	295.73
009.1	040.81	079.53	100.89	183.0	238.5	286.7	295.74
009.2	046.0	*079.8	100.9	*189	238.6	286.9	295.80
009.3	*046.1	080	101	*191	238.73	287.0	295.81
*010.0	046.2	*081	112.0	*192	238.74	287.31	295.82
*010.1	046.3	*082	112.2	*194	238.76	287.32	295.83
*010.8	*046.7	*083	112.82	*196	238.77	287.33	295.84
*010.9	046.8	084.1	112.84	*197	238.79	288.4	295.91
*011.0	046.9	084.2	112.85	*198	245.0	289.7	295.92
*011.1	*047	084.3	112.89	199.0	246.3	289.81	295.93
*011.2	048	084.4	114.0	199.2	251.0	289.82	295.94
*011.3	*049	084.5	114.1	*200.0	251.3	289.83	296.00
*011.4	*050	084.6	114.3	*200.1	253.1	290.11	296.01
*011.5	052.7	084.7	114.4	*200.2	253.2	290.12	296.02
*011.7	052.8	084.8	114.5	*200.3	253.5	290.13	296.03
*011.8	052.9	084.9	114.9	*200.4	253.6	290.20	296.04
*011.9	053.10	*085	115.02	*200.5	254.1	290.21	296.10
*012.0	053.11	*086	115.09	*200.6	255.0	290.3	296.11
*012.1	053.12	*087	115.12	*200.7	255.3	290.41	296.12
*012.2	053.13	088.0	115.19	*200.8	255.41	290.42	296.13
*012.3	053.19	088.81	115.92	*201.0	255.42	290.43	296.14
*012.8	*053.2	088.82	116.0	*201.1	255.5	290.8	296.20
*014.8	053.71	090.0	116.1	*201.2	255.6	290.9	296.21
*015.0	053.79	090.2	117.3	*201.4	259.2	291.0	296.22
*015.1	053.8	090.3	117.4	*201.5	263.0	291.2	296.23
*015.2	054.2	090.40	117.5	*201.6	263.1	291.3	296.24
*015.5	054.40	090.49	117.6	*201.7	263.2	291.81	296.30
*015.6	054.41	090.5	117.8	*201.9	263.8	291.89	296.31
*015.7	054.42	091.3	117.9	*202.0	263.9	291.9	296.32
*015.8	054.43	091.4	118	*202.1	265.0	292.0	296.33
*015.9	054.44	*091.5	*120	*202.2	265.1	*292.1	296.34
*016.0	054.49	*091.6	121.0	*202.3	266.0	292.81	296.40
*016.1	054.71	091.7	121.1	*202.4	268.0	292.82	296.41
*016.2	054.79	091.82	121.2	*202.5	*270	293.0	296.42
*016.3	*055.7	091.89	121.3	*202.6	271.0	293.1	296.43
*016.4	056.00	091.9	121.4	*202.7	271.1	293.81	296.44
*016.5	056.09	093.0	121.5	*202.8	271.8	293.82	296.50
*016.6	*056.7	093.1	121.6	*202.9	274.11	293.9	296.51
*016.7	057.0	093.20	121.8	*203.0	276.0	294.11	296.52
*016.9	059.01	093.21	*122	*203.1	276.1	294.21	296.53
*017.0	059.21	093.22	123.0	*203.8	276.2	295.00	296.54

Complication and Comorbidity (CC) Code List

296.60	349.39	*411	*453.7	536.42	579.3	*636.8	647.81
296.61	349.81	413.0	*453.8	537.0	579.4	*637.0	647.82
296.62	356.3	413.1	453.9	537.3	579.8	*637.2	647.83
296.63	357.0	414.02	454.2	537.4	579.9	*637.4	647.84
296.64	357.81	414.03	456.1	538	581.0	*637.7	647.91
296.89	357.82	414.04	456.21	*539.0	581.1	*637.8	647.92
296.99	358.1	414.06	459.11	*539.8	581.2	638.0	647.93
298.0	*358.3	414.07	459.13	540.9	581.3	638.1	647.94
298.1	359.0	414.10	459.2	550.10	581.81	638.2	648.00
298.3	359.1	414.19	459.31	550.11	581.89	638.4	648.03
298.4	359.4	416.0	459.33	550.12	581.9	638.7	648.04
*299	359.6	416.1	464.30	550.13	*582	638.8	648.31
301.51	359.81	416.2	*466.1	*552.0	583.0	639.0	648.32
304.01	360.00	417.0	475	552.1	583.1	639.1	648.33
304.11	360.01	417.1	478.21	*552.2	583.2	639.2	648.34
304.21	360.02	420.0	478.22	552.3	583.7	639.4	648.51
304.41	360.04	420.90	478.24	552.8	584.8	639.8	648.52
304.51	360.11	420.91	478.34	552.9	584.9	639.9	648.53
304.61	360.12	420.99	478.71	*555	585.4	640.01	648.54
304.71	360.13	*423	488.02	*556	585.5	640.03	648.61
304.81	360.19	*424.9	488.09	557.1	588.1	640.93	648.62
304.91	361.2	*425	491.21	557.9	588.81	641.01	648.63
307.1	*361.8	426.0	491.22	558.1	590.01	641.03	648.64
307.51	361.9	426.12	493.01	558.2	590.10	641.23	648.71
318.1	362.30	426.53	493.02	560.0	590.3	642.01	648.72
318.2	362.31	426.54	493.11	560.1	*590.8	642.02	648.73
322.2	362.32	426.89	493.12	*560.3	591	642.03	648.74
330.0	362.33	427.0	493.21	*560.8	592.1	642.13	*649.3
330.1	362.34	427.1	493.22	560.9	593.4	642.14	649.41
330.2	362.35	427.32	493.91	562.01	593.5	642.31	649.42
330.3	362.40	428.1	493.92	562.11	593.81	642.32	649.43
330.8	362.42	428.20	494.1	564.7	593.82	642.41	649.44
330.9	362.43	428.22	495.7	564.81	595.0	642.43	*649.7
331.3	362.84	428.30	495.8	566	595.82	642.44	651.01
331.4	*363.1	428.32	495.9	567.82	596.1	642.91	651.11
331.5	363.20	428.40	506.0	568.82	596.2	642.92	651.13
332.1	363.63	428.42	508.0	569.3	596.7	642.93	651.21
333.0	*363.7	*429.7	508.1	569.41	596.81	642.94	651.23
333.4	364.00	429.81	*511.8	569.5	596.82	644.13	651.41
333.71	364.01	429.82	511.9	569.61	596.83	644.20	651.43
333.72	364.02	429.83	512.1	569.62	597.0	646.21	651.51
333.79	364.03	432.9	512.2	569.69	599.0	646.22	651.53
333.90	364.22	*435	512.8	569.71	599.1	646.23	651.81
333.91	364.3	436	514	569.79	601.0	646.24	651.83
*334	365.22	437.1	516.0	569.81	601.2	646.31	656.13
*335	368.11	437.2	516.1	569.82	603.1	646.61	656.31
336.0	368.12	437.4	516.2	572.3	604.0	646.62	656.41
336.2	376.01	437.5	516.33	573.1	607.3	646.63	656.43
336.3	376.02	437.6	516.35	573.2	607.82	646.64	656.51
336.8	376.03	*438.2	516.36	574.00	*608.2	646.71	657.01
336.9	377.00	440.24	516.37	574.01	614.0	646.73	658.01
337.1	377.01	440.4	516.5	574.10	614.3	647.01	658.03
*337.2	*377.3	444.09	516.8	574.11	614.7	647.02	658.81
*341	*377.5	444.1	516.9	574.21	615.0	647.03	659.21
*342	*377.6	*444.2	517.1	574.30	616.3	647.04	660.03
343.0	377.71	*444.8	517.2	574.31	616.4	647.11	662.11
343.1	377.72	444.9	517.3	574.40	616.81	647.12	664.21
343.4	377.73	*445.0	518.0	574.41	*619	647.13	664.31
344.1	380.14	*445.8	518.3	574.51	620.5	647.14	664.61
344.2	*383.0	446.0	518.6	574.60	*633	647.21	664.64
344.60	388.61	446.1	518.7	574.61	*634.0	647.22	665.22
344.61	*391	*446.2	518.82	574.70	*634.2	647.23	665.31
345.01	*392	446.3	518.83	574.71	*634.4	647.24	665.41
345.11	393	446.4	*519.0	574.80	634.60	647.31	665.51
345.40	398.0	446.7	522.0	574.91	634.70	647.32	665.61
345.41	398.91	447.2	522.4	575.0	634.71	647.33	665.71
345.50	401.0	447.4	527.3	575.12	634.72	647.34	665.72
345.51	*402.0	447.5	527.4	575.2	634.80	647.41	666.02
345.60	*403.0	449	528.3	575.3	634.81	647.42	666.04
345.61	403.11	451.11	530.12	575.5	634.82	647.43	666.12
345.70	403.91	451.19	530.20	576.1	*635.0	647.44	666.14
345.80	*404.0	451.81	530.86	576.4	*635.2	647.51	666.22
345.81	404.11	451.83	530.87	577.1	*635.4	647.52	666.24
345.91	404.12	451.89	531.30	577.2	*635.7	647.53	666.32
*346.6	404.13	453.1	532.30	578.0	*635.8	647.54	669.24
348.1	404.91	453.3	533.30	578.1	*636.0	647.61	*670.1
348.82	404.92	*453.4	534.30	578.9	*636.2	647.62	670.20
349.1	404.93	*453.5	536.1	579.1	*636.4	647.63	670.30
349.31	*405.0	453.6	*536.41	579.2	*636.7	647.64	671.20

671.21	*733.1	771.5	802.9	*825.3	871.5	*942.3	996.74
671.22	*733.4	771.82	803.00	827.1	871.6	*942.4	996.75
671.23	*733.8	771.83	803.01	830.1	871.9	*942.5	996.76
671.24	*741.0	771.89	803.02	*831.1	872.12	*943.3	996.77
671.30	742.0	772.10	803.06	*832.1	*872.6	*943.4	996.78
671.40	742.4	772.11	803.09	*833.1	*872.7	*943.5	996.79
*671.5	745.12	772.12	803.40	835.00	873.23	*944.3	*996.8
*671.8	745.4	772.5	803.41	835.01	873.33	*944.4	*996.9
671.90	745.5	775.1	803.42	835.02	874.2	*944.5	*997.0
671.91	*745.6	775.2	803.46	835.03	874.3	*945.3	997.1
671.92	746.00	775.3	803.49	836.4	874.4	*945.4	997.2
672.02	746.02	775.4	804.00	*836.6	874.5	*945.5	*997.3
672.04	746.09	775.81	804.01	837.1	875.0	946.3	*997.4
673.30	746.3	775.89	804.02	*839.0	875.1	946.4	997.62
674.02	746.4	776.0	804.06	839.51	*880.2	946.5	*997.7
674.03	746.5	776.3	804.09	839.52	*881.2	947.1	997.99
674.04	746.6	776.5	804.40	839.61	882.2	947.2	998.00
675.11	746.83	776.6	804.41	839.79	883.2	947.3	*998.1
675.12	746.85	777.4	804.42	839.9	884.2	947.4	998.2
*682	746.87	778.1	804.46	850.11	887.0	948.10	*998.3
685.0	747.0	778.5	804.49	850.12	887.1	948.11	998.4
686.01	747.10	779.4	804.50	850.2	887.2	948.20	*998.5
694.4	*747.2	779.5	804.51	850.3	887.3	948.30	998.6
694.5	*747.4	780.03	804.52	850.5	887.4	948.40	998.7
695.0	747.82	780.1	804.56	851.02	887.5	948.50	998.83
695.12	747.89	780.31	804.59	851.03	890.2	948.60	999.0
695.13	747.9	780.32	804.90	851.04	891.2	948.70	999.2
695.14	748.3	780.33	804.91	851.06	892.2	948.80	*999.3
695.15	748.4	781.4	804.92	851.42	893.2	948.90	*999.4
695.53	748.61	781.6	804.96	851.43	894.2	949.3	*999.5
695.54	750.4	781.7	804.99	851.44	896.0	949.4	999.60
695.55	751.1	781.8	*805.0	851.46	896.1	949.5	999.61
695.56	751.2	782.4	805.2	854.02	897.0	*950	999.62
695.57	751.3	784.3	805.4	854.03	897.1	*951	999.63
695.58	751.4	785.4	805.6	854.04	897.2	958.2	999.69
695.59	751.5	785.50	805.8	854.06	897.3	958.3	999.70
707.10	751.60	786.04	*807.0	860.0	897.4	958.7	999.71
707.11	751.62	786.30	807.2	861.00	897.5	*958.9	999.72
707.12	751.69	786.31	808.2	861.01	*900.0	991.0	999.73
707.13	751.7	786.39	*808.4	861.20	900.1	991.1	999.74
707.14	753.0	788.8	808.8	861.21	*900.8	991.2	999.75
707.19	*753.1	*789.5	809.0	862.0	900.9	991.3	999.76
710.3	*753.2	790.01	*810.1	862.29	901.81	991.4	999.77
710.4	753.5	790.7	*811.1	862.8	901.82	992.0	999.78
710.5	753.6	791.1	*812.0	863.0	901.89	993.3	999.79
710.8	754.2	791.3	*812.2	*863.2	901.9	994.1	999.81
*711.0	754.89	799.01	*812.4	*863.4	902.55	994.7	999.82
*711.1	756.13	799.4	*813.2	864.00	902.56	995.0	999.83
*711.2	756.3	800.00	*813.4	864.01	902.81	995.4	999.84
*711.3	756.51	800.01	813.80	864.02	902.82	995.50	999.85
*711.4	756.52	800.02	813.82	864.05	902.89	995.51	V42.0
*711.5	756.83	800.06	813.83	864.09	902.9	995.52	V42.1
*711.6	758.1	800.09	*814.1	865.00	903.1	995.53	V42.6
*711.7	758.2	800.40	*815.1	865.01	903.2	995.54	V42.7
*711.8	758.31	800.41	*816.1	865.02	903.3	995.55	V42.81
*711.9	758.33	800.42	817.1	865.09	903.4	995.59	V42.82
714.31	758.39	800.46	818.1	866.00	903.5	995.80	V42.83
*719.1	759.0	800.49	819.0	866.01	903.8	995.81	V42.84
721.1	759.3	801.00	819.1	866.02	903.9	995.83	*V43.2
*721.4	759.5	801.01	*821.2	867.0	904.3	995.84	*V46.1
721.7	759.6	801.02	822.0	867.2	*904.5	995.85	V55.1
721.91	759.7	801.06	822.1	867.4	904.6	995.86	V62.84
722.71	759.81	801.09	823.00	867.6	904.7	995.90	V85.0
722.72	759.82	801.40	823.02	867.8	904.8	995.93	V85.41
722.73	759.89	801.41	823.20	*868.0	904.9	*996.0	V85.42
728.0	767.11	801.42	823.22	869.0	925.1	996.1	V85.43
728.88	768.70	801.46	823.40	870.2	925.2	996.2	V85.44
729.71	768.71	801.49	823.42	870.3	928.00	996.30	V85.45
729.72	768.72	802.1	823.80	870.4	928.01	996.39	
729.73	770.4	*802.2	823.82	870.8	934.0	*996.4	
729.79	770.5	*802.3	824.1	870.9	934.1	*996.5	
*730.0	770.81	802.4	824.3	871.0	934.8	*996.6	
*730.1	770.83	802.5	824.5	871.1	940.5	996.71	
*730.2	771.0	802.6	824.7	871.2	*941.3	996.72	
*730.8	771.4	802.7	824.9	871.3	*941.4	996.73	
*730.9		802.8	825.1		*941.5		

Pharmacological Listings

Pharmacology Considerations

Medications are listed by classification and brand name for each of the chapters of ICD-9-CM. The list includes many of the common medications and should not be considered exhaustive. The pharmacology considerations that follow are presented as guidance only for the recognition of the link between implication of disease process and treatment.

Infectious and Parasitic Diseases (001-139)

AIDS Related Complex (ARC) Therapeutic Agents

Agenerase	Crixivan
Epivir	Fortovase
Hivid	Intron A
Invirase	Norvir
Pentam	Rescriptor
Retrovir	Rimactane
Roferon-A	Sustiva
Videx	Viracept
Vitravene	Zerit
Ziagen	Zovirax

Antibiotics

Achromycin-V	Amikin
Amoxicillin	Amoxil
Ampicillin	Ancef
Augmentin	Azactam
Bactrim	Bicillin
Biocef	Ceclor
Cefizox[2]	Cefobid
Cefotan	Ceftin
Chloromycetin	Cipro
Claforan	Cleocin
Dificid	Duricef
E-Mycin	ERYC
Erythromycin	Ery-Tab
Factive	Floxin
Fortaz	Garamycin
Levaquin	Macrobid
Maxipime	Mefoxin
Nebcin	Neo-fradin
Minocin	PCE Dispertab
Penicillin G	Penicillin V
Pfizerpen	Pipracil
Primaxin	Proloprim
Septra	Spectrobid
Suprax	Synersid
Tazicef	Tazidime
Terramycin	Tetracycline HCl
Ticar	Timentin
Totacillin	Trimox
Trimpex	Unasyn
Unipen	Vancocin
Vibramycin	Vibra-Tabs
Wycillin	Zefazone
Zinacef	Zithromax
Zosyn	Zymar

Antiparasitics

Antiminth	Aralen
Daraprim	Flagyl
G-well	Helidac
MepronnebuPent	Pentam 300
Penticarinat	Pin-X
Protostat	Vermox

Corticosteroids

Aristocort	Celestone
Cortastat	Cortef
Cortenema	Cortone Acetate
Dalalone	Decadron
Deltasone	Depo-Medrol
Florinef acetate	Hydeltrasol
Hydrocortisone	Hydrocortone
Medralone	Medrol
Orasone	Predalone
Prednisone	Prelone
Protocort	Solu-Cortef

Fungal Medications

Abelcet	AmBisome
Amphocin	Amphotec
Ancobon	Diflucan
Fulvicin P/G	Fungilin
Fungizone	Fungoid
Grifulvin	Grisactin
Gris-PEG	Lamisil
Lotrimin	Lotrisone
Monistat	Mycelex-G
Mycolog	Mycostatin
Nilstst	Nizoral
Spectazole	Sporanox

Tuberculosis Preparations

Capastat	INH Tablets
Lamprene	Laniazid
Myambutol	Mycobutin
Priftin	Pyrazinamide
Rifadin	Rifamate
Rimactane	Seromycin
Sodium P.A.S.	Streptomycin
Trecator-SC	

Viral Agents

Abreva	Agenerase
Combivir	Crixivan
Cytovene	Emtriva
Epivir	Famvir
Flumadine	Fortovase
Foscavir	Fuzeon
Herplex	Hepsera
Hivid	Invirase
Lexiva	Norvir
Relenza	Rescriptor
Retrovir	Reyataz
Sustiva	Symmetrel
Tamiflu	Valtrex
Videx	Viracept
Viramune	Virazole
Vistide	Vitravene
Zerit	Ziagen
Zovirax	

Neoplasms (140-239)

Adjunct

Anzemet	Arrestin
Compazine	Epogen
Ergamisol	Kytril
Leukine	Martinol
Metastron	Neumega
Neupogen	Procrit
Prokine	Quadramet
Reglan	Relcomide
Salagen	Sandostatin
Sylatron	Zinecard
Zofran	

Androgen Inhibitor

Casodex	Eulexin
Lupron	Nilandron
Zoladex	Zytiga

Antibiotic Derivatives

Adriamycin	Blenoxane
Cerubidine	Cosmegen
Doxorubicin	Idamycin
Mutamycin	Mithracin
Nipent	Novantrone
Pacis	Rubex

TheraCys

Antiestrogen

Femara	Nolvadex

Antimetabolites

Adrucil	Cytarabine
Cytosar-U	Droxia
Efudex	Folex
Fludara	Fluoroplex
Fluorouracil	FUDR
Intron A	Leustatin
Methotrexate	Purinethol
Roferon-A	Thioguanine
Xeloda	

Cytotoxic Agents

Adriamycin	BiCNU
CeeNU	Cerubidine
Cytosar-U	Doxorubicin
Gemzar	Hexalen
Hydrea	Intron A
Matulane	Mutamycin
Myleran	Novantrone
Paraplatin	Platinol
Zanosar	

Hormones

Arimidex	Aromasin
Depo-Provera	Eligard
Emcyt	Estinyl
Estradurin	Fareston
Lupron	Megace
Stilphostrol	Teslac
Zoladex	

Monoclonal Antibodies

Avastin	Erbitux
Herceptin	Rituxan
Vectibix	Zevalin

Nitrogen Mustard Derivatives

Alkeran	Cytoxan
Leukeran	Mustargen
Neosar	Thiotepa

Steroids and Combinations

Celestone Soluspan

Other

Afinitor	Camptosar
DTIC-Dome	Elspar
Etopophos	Iressa
Navelbine	Oncaspar
Oncovin	Phosphocol P32
Photofrin	Proleukin
Semzar	Taxol
Taxotere	TICE
Velban	Velcade
VePesid	Vesanoid
Vumon	

Endocrine, Nutritional and Metabolic Diseases and Immunity Disorders (240-279)

Acidifier and Alkalinizers

Ammonium chloride	Citrocarbonate
Sodium bicarbonate	Sodium lactate
Tham	

Antigout Agents

Anturane	Benemid
Colchicine	Probalan
Zyloprim	

Antilipemics

Atorvastatin calcium	Crestor
Fluvastatin sodium	Lescol
Lipitor	Lovastatin
Lovaza	Mevacor
Pravachol	pravastatin sodium
Niaspan	simvastatin
Tricor	Vytorin
Zetia	Zocor

Antioxidants

Aquasol E	Calcium-D
Calcium Health Packs	Carotene-E
Carotene Health Packs	Glutathione
Performance Packs	Pure-E

Appetite Suppressants

Adipex-P	Adipost
Biphetamine	Bontril
Desoxyn	Didrex
Fastin	Ionamin
Mazanor	Meridia
Phentride	Plegine
Pondimin	Prelu-2
Sanorex	Tenuate

Diabetic Agents and Glucagon

Actos	Amaryl
Avandia	DiaBeta
Diabinese	Glucagon
Glucophage	Glucotrol
Glynase	Glyset
Humulin R	Iletin II
Januvia	Lantus
Lispro (Humalog)	Micronase
Novolin	NovoLog
Prandin	Precose
Onglyza	Rezulin
Riomet	Tradjenta
Ultralente	Velosulin
Victoza	

Electrolytes and Replacement Solutions

Calcium acetate	Calcium carbonate
Calcium chloride	Calcium citrate
Calcium gluconate	Calcium lactate
Calcium phosphate, dibasic	Calcium phosphate, tribasic
Dextran	Gendex
Hespan	Magnesium chloride
Magnesium sulfate	Phoslo
Potassium acetate	

Potassium bicarbonate (K+ Care ET, Klor-Con/EF, K-Vescent)

Potassium chloride (Kaochlor, Kaon-Cl, Kato Powder, Kay Ciel, K-Lease, K-Lor, Klor-10%, Klor-Con, Klorvess, Klotrix, K-Lyte/Cl, K-Tab, Micro-K Extencaps,SK-Potassium Chloride, Slow-K, Ten-K)

Potassium gluconate (Glu-K, Kaon, Kayliker, K-G Elixir)

Slow-mag	Ringer's Injection

Hormones

Anadrol-50	Android
A.P.L.	Combipatch
Delatestryl	Depo-Provers
Estrace	Estraderm
Estratab	Estrovis
Factrel	Halotestin
Micronor	Norplant
Ogen	Ortho-Est
Ortho-Novum	Orvette
Pregnyl	premarin
Proscar	Provera
Testoderm	Testred

Parathyroid-like Agents

Aredia	Calcimar
Calderol	Cibacalcin
Didronel	E-Vista
Fosamax	Miacalcin
Osteocalcin	Rocaltrol
Salmonine	

Pituitary Hormones

ACTH	Acthar
Cortrosyn	Diapid
Genotropin	Humatrope
Pegvisomant	Pitressin
Protropin	Somavert
Stimate	

Thyroid Antagonists

Pima	Tapazole

Thyroid Hormones

Cytomel	Euthroid
Levothroid	Levoxine
Levoxyl	Triostat
Synthyroid	Vitamins
Vitamin A	

Vitamin B complex (including cyanocobalamin, hydroxocobalamin, folic acid, leucovorin calcium, niacin, niacinamide, pyridoxine hydrochloride, riboflavin, thiamine hydrochloride)

Vitamin C

Vitamin D (cholecalciferol, ergocalciferol)

Vitamin E

Vitamin K analogs (menadione/menadiol sodium diphosphate, phytonadione, sodium fluoride)

Trace elements (chromium, copper, iodine, manganese, selenium, zinc)

Blood and Blood-Forming Organs (280-289)

Anticoagulants

Abciximab	Aggrastat
Cilostazol	Clopidrogrel bisulfate
Eptifibatide	Integrilin
Plavix	Pletal
Pradaxa	RepPro
Ticlopidine hydrochloride	Ticlid
Tirofiban hydrochloride	

Coagulants

AlphaNine Coagulation Factor
Profilate OSD Antihemophilic Factor
Trasylol

Hematinics

Ferrous fumarate:

Femiron	Feostat
Hemocyte	Ircon
Nephro-Fer	Novofumar
Vitron-C	

Ferrous gluconate:

Fergon	Feratab
Fer-Gen-Sol	

Ferrous sulfate:

ED-IN-SOL	Fe50
Feosol	Fer-In-Sol
Fer-Iron	Slow Fe

HMG-CoA Reductase Inhibitors (Statins):

Crestor	Lipitor
Lovaza	Mevacor
Pravachol	Vytorin
Zocor	

Iron dextran:

DexFerrum	INFeD

Others

Konyne-HT Factor IX Complex Nu-Iron

Monoclate-P Factor VIII:C, Antihemophilic Factor
Promacta: thrombopoeitin receptor antagonist

Mental Disorders (290-319)

Central Nervous System Stimulants

Adderall XR	Atomoxetine HCl
Concerta	Cylert
Desoxyn	Dexedrine
Dopram	Methylin
Provigil	Ritalin
Strattera	Vivarin
Vyvanse	

Cerebral Metabolic Enhancer

Ergostat	Hydergine
Migranal	

Alzheimer's Dementia Agents

Aricept	Cognex
Exelon	Namenda
Reminyl	

Anti-anxiety

Atarax	Ativan
BuSpar	Libritabs
Librium	Miltown
Serax	Tranxene
Valium	Versed
Xanax	

Anti-depressants

Anafranil	Asendin
Aventyl	Celexa
Cymbalta	Desyryl
Effexor	Elavil
Lexapro	Nardil
Norpramin	Pamelor
Parnate	Paxil
Pristiq	Prozac
Remeron	Serzone
Sinequan	Surmontil
Tofranillbutrin	Trialodine
Viibryd	Wellbutrin
Yentreve	Zoloft

Anti-psychotics

Abilify	Clozaril
Etrafon	Haldol
Loxitane	Mellaril
Navane	Orap
Prolixin	Risperdal
Serentil	Seroquel
Serpasil	Stelazine
Thorazine	Triavil
Trilafon	Zyprexa

Sedatives

Ambien	Dalmane
Diprivan	Mebaral
Nembutal	Precedex
ProSom	Restoril
Seconal Sodium	Sonata
Tuinal	Unisom

Other Psychotrophics

Antabuse	Cibalith-S
Eskalith	Lithane
Lithium Carbonate	Lithobid
Luvox	Meridia
Methadone	Zomig
Zyban	

Nervous System and Sense Organs (320-389)

Antibiotics Central Nervous System Agents:

Amikin	Ancef
Cefizox	Fortaz
Garamycin	Kefurox
Nebcin	Rocephin

Tazidime

Anticonvulsants

Banzel	Celontin
Cerebyx	Cholinesterase Inhibitor
Depakene	Depakote
Dilantin	Felbatol
Keppra	Klonopin
Lamictal	Lyrica
Mebaral	Mesantoin
Milontin	Mysoline
Neurontin	Peganone
Phenobarbital	Phenytoin
Phenurone	Rufinamide
Sabril	Tegretol
Tranxene	Tridione
Vimpat	Zarontin

Cholinesterase Inhibitor

Aricept

Dopamine Receptor Agonist

Eldepryl	Mirapex
Parlodel	Permax
Requip	Sinemet
Stalevo	Symmetrel
Tasmar	

Miscellaneous Ophthalmics

Alphagan	Betoptic
Emadine	Iopidine
Lacrisert	Lumigan
Opticrom	OptiPranolol
OPTIVAR	Propine
Restasis	Timoptic
Trusopt	Zaditor

Migraine Agents

Amerge	Cafergot
Depakote	Ergostat
Imitrex	Inderal
Isocom	Maxalt
Midrin	Migranal
Relpax	Sansert
Treximet	Wigraine
Zomig	

Miotics

Carboptic	Miochol-E
Miostat	Pilocar
Pilostat	Phospholine Iodide

Multiple Sclerosis Therapies:

Ampyra	Avonex
Betaseron	Copaxone
Extavia	Prednisone
Rebif	Tysabri

Mydriatics

AK-Dilate	AK-Nefrin
AK-Pentolate	Atropisol
Cyclogyl	Epifrin
Epinal	Eppy/N
Homatropine	Glaucon
Isopto Atropine	Isopto Frin
Isopto Homatropine	Isopto Hyoscine
Minims	Mydfrin
Mydriacyl	

Ophthalmic Antiinfectives

AK-Tracin	Bleph-10 Liqifilm
Chloromycetin	Ciloxan
Garamycin	Ilotycin
Polymyxin B Sulfate	Ocuflox
Sodium Sulamyd	Tobradex
Tobrex	Vigamox
Vira-A	Zymar

Ophthalmic Antiinflammatory Agents

Acular	Decadron Phosphate
Flarex	Fluor-Op
Maxidex	Ocufen
Voltarin	

Otics

Augmentin	Auro-Dri
Cerumex	Chloromycetin Otic
Coly-Mycin S	Cortisporin
Cotrim	LazerSporin-C
Murine Ear	OticTridesilon
PediOtic	Septra

Parasympathomimetics

Duvoid	Evoxac
Mestinon	Prostigmin
Tensilon	Urecholine

Parkinsonism Agents

Akineton	Artane
Benztropine	Cogentin
Comtan	Dopar
Larodopa	Mirapex
Parlodel	Permax
Requip	Sinemet
Symmetrel	

Skeletal Muscle Relaxants

Dantrium	Flexeril
Lioresal	Vanadom
Zaraflex	

Sleep Disorders

Ambien	Baclofen
Clonazepam	Lunesta
Melatonin	Neurontin
Nuvigil	Permax
Provigil	Rozerem
Silenor	Sinemet
Sonata	Strattera

Vertigo Agents

Antivert	Vergon

Circulatory System (390-459)

Alpha Adrenoceptor Agonists

Aldomet	Alpha Receptor
Brilinta	Blocking Agents
Cardura	Catapres
Combipres	Hytrin
Minipress	Regitine
Trandate	Wytensin

Anginal Preparations

Calan	Cardia XT
Cardizem	Dilitrate-SR
Inderal	Isoptin
Isordil	Nitro-Bid
Nitro-Dur	Nitrodisc
Nitrogard	Nitrostat IV
Procardia	Sorbitrate
Transderm-Nitro	

Angiotensin Converting Enzyme Inhibitors

Accupril	Altace
Avapro	Caduet
Capoten	Capozide
Cozaar	Lotensin
Mavik	Monopril
Prinivil	Univasc
Vasotec	Zestril

Antihypertensives

Aldactazide	Aldactone
Aldomet	Apresoline
Atacard	Atenolol
Avapro	Benicar HCT
Calan	Capoten
Cardizem	Cardura
Catapres	Corlopam
Cozaar	Diuril
Edarbi	HydroDIURIL
Hyperstat	Hytrin
Hyzaar	Inderal
Isoptin	Levatol
Lopressor	Minipress

Monopril	Procardia
Renese	Temex
Tenormin	Teveten
Vasotec	Wytensin
Zestric	

Arrhythmia Medications

Betapace	Calan
Cardioquin	Cordarone
Inderal	Isoptin
Mexitil	Multaq
Norpace	Procan
Pronestyl	Quinaglute
Rythmol	Tonocard

Beta Blocking Agents

Blocadren	Cartrol
Coreg	Corgard
Corzide	Inderal
Kerlone	Levatol
Lopressor	Normodyne
Sectral	Tenoretic
Tenormin	Toprol XL
Trandate	Visken
Zebeta	

Calcium Channel Blockers

Adalat	Caduet
Calan	Cardene
Cardiac Glycosides	Cardizem
DynaCirc	Isoptin
Lanoxin (Digoxin)	Norvasc
Posicor	Procardia
Sular	Vascor
Verelan	

Diuretics

Aldactazide	Aldoril
Bumex	Combipres
Demadex	Diuril
Dyazide	Edecrin
Esidrix	Esimil
Furosemide	Lasix
Rauzide	Renese
Zaroxolyn	

Thrombolytic Enzymes

Abbokinase	Activase
Kabikinase	Retavase
Streptase	

Vasodilators, Cerebral

Pavabid

Vasodilators, Coronary

Cardilate	Isordil
Nitro-Bid	Nitro-Dur
Nitrolingual Spray	Nitrostat IV
Pavabid	Peritrate
Sorbitrate	Transderm-Nitro

Vasodilators, Peripheral

Apresoline	Dibenzyline
Esimil	Hyperstat IV
Loniten	Pavabid

Respiratory System (460-519)

Allergy Relief Products

Antihist-1	Benadryl
Brexin	Bromphen
Clarinex	Dristan
Naldecon	Tavist
Trimeton	

Antibiotics

Achromycin	Amikin
Amoxicillin	Amoxil
Ampicillin	Ancef
Augmentin	Azactam
Bactrim	Biaxin
Bicillin	Ceclor

Cefizox	Cefobid
Cefotan	Ceftin
Cipro	Claforan
Duricef	Dynabec
E-Mycin	Ery-Tab
ERYC	Erythromycin
Factive	Floxin
Fortaz	Garamycin
Geocillin	Ilosone
Iotycin	Keflex
Keftab	Kefurox
Levaquin	Mandol
Mefoxin	Meropen
Mezlin	Minocin
Nebcin	Netromycin
PCE Dispertab	Penicillin G
Penicillin V	Pipracil
Primaxin	Raxar
Rocephin	Septra
Spectrobid	Suprax
Tazicef	Tazidime
Tetracycline HCl	Ticar
Timentin	Trovan
Wycillin	Zagam
Zefazone	Zinacef
Zithromax	

Antihistamines

Actifed	Allegra
Allerest	Astepro
Atarax	Benadryl
Bromphen	Chlor-Trimeton
Claritin	Coricidin
Deconamine	Four-Way
Periactin	Tavist
Triaminic	Zyrtec

Asthma Preparations

Accolate	AeroBid
Alupent	Aminophylline
Beclovent	Brethine
Bronkaid	Choledyl SA
Crolom	Dilor
Dulera	Flovent
Intal	Maxair
Metaprel	Primatene
Proventil	Serevent
Singulair	Symbicort
TheoDur	Tilade
Tornalate	Vanceril
Ventolin	Zyflo

Bronchial Dilators

Accolate	Advair Diskus
Alupent	Aminophylline
Arcapta	Asbron G
Atrovent	Brethaire Inhaler
Bricanyl	Bronkephrine
Bronkometer	Combivent
Choledyl	Isuprel
Lufyllin	Marax
Maxair	Medihaler-Iso
Prez-D	Primatene
Proventil	Quadrinal
Quibron	Serevent
Singulair	Slo-bid
Tedral	Theolair
Tornalate	Ventolin
Xolair	Xopenex
Zyflo	

Cold, Cough Preparations and Mucolytics

Calcidrine	Cheracol
Comtrex	Dimetapp
Dimetane	Entex
Guaifed	Humibid
Hycomine	Naldecon
Novahistine	Nucofed
Ornade	Quelidrine

Quibron	Robitussin
Rondec	Ru-Tuss
Rynatan	Rynatuss
Sine-Aid	Triaminic
Tuss-Ornade	Tussi-Organdin
Tussionex	

Corticosteroids

Aristocort	Celestone
Cortone Acetate	Deltasone
Depo-Medrol	Hydeltrasol
Hydrocortone	Prednisone
Solu-Cortef	Solu-Medrol

Nasal Preparations

Adrenalin Chloride	Afrin
Beconase	Decadron Phosphate
Dopram Injectable	Flonase
Nasacort	Nasalide
Nasarel	Nasonex
Omnaris	Otrivin
Privine	Veramyst

Respiratory Stimulants

Rhinocort	Turbinaire
Vancenase	

Respiratory Therapy Agents

Alupent	Arm-a-Med
Survanta	Isoetharine

Digestive System (520-579)

Anorectal Products

Analpram-HC	Proctofoam-HC
Rowasa	

Antacids

Alka-Seltzer	Amphojel
Basaljel	Di-Gel
Gaviscon	Maalox
Mylanta	Polycitra
Riopan	Tums

Antibiotics and Antibacterials

Amikin	Ancef
Azactam	Cefizox
Cefobid	Cefotan
Claforan	Fortaz
Furoxone	Kefzol
Mandol	Mefoxin
Nebcin	Netromycin
Pipracil	Primaxin
Tazicef	Tazidime
Ticar	Unasyn
Vancocin	Zefazone

Antispasmodics and Anticholinergics

Bentyl	Darabid
Donnatal	Levsin
Librax	Prilosec
Pro-Banthine	Quarzan
Reglan	Robinul

Antiulcer

Asacol	cimetidine
esomeprazole magnesium	famotidine
iansoprazole	Nexium
omeprazole	Pepcid AC
Prevacid	Prilosec
ranitidine hydrochloride	Tagamet
Zantac	

Corticosteroids

Alinia	Aristocort
Cortenema	Decadron
Deltasone	Depo-Medrol
Hydeltrasol	Hydrocortone
Prednisone	Solu-Cortef
Solu-Medrol	

Diarrhea Medications

Alinia	Arco-Lase Plus

Charcoal Plus	Donnagel
Furoxone	Kaopectate
Kapectolin	Imodium
Lomotil	Mitrolan
Motofen	Pepto-Bismol

Digestants

Cotazym	Donnazyme
Entozyme	Ku-Zyme
Lactaid	Pancrease
Pancreatin	Ultrase
Viokase	

Flatulence Relief

Flatulex	Gas-X
Kutrase	Mylicon
Phazyme	

Gallstone Dissolution Agent

Actigall Capsules

Gastric Acid Secretion Inhibitor

Axid	Cytotec
Prevacid	Zantac

Gastrointestinal Antigranulomatous Disease

Azulfidine Tablets, EN-tabs	Dipentum Capsules
	Mesasal
Pentasa	Remicade
Rowasa	

Nausea and Vertigo Medications

Aloxi	Anzeme
Anfernet	Antivert
Aprepitant	Bonine
Bucladin-S Softab	Compazine
Dramamine	Emend
Kytril	Marinol
Reglan	Tigan
Torecan	Vergon
Zofran	

Parasympatholytics

Bellergal-S	Bentyl
Cantil	Levsin
Robinul	

Genitourinary System (580-629)

Alpha-adrenergic blockers

Flomax	Rapaflo
Tamsulosin HCL	

Antibiotics

Achromycin	Ancef
Augmentin	Azactam
Azo Gantanol	Azo Gantrisin
Bactrim	Ceclor
Cefizox	Cefobid
Cefotan	Ceftin
Ceptaz	Cipro
Claforan	Duricef
E-Mycin	Ery-tab
Floxin	Fortaz
Garamycin	Keftab
Kefurox	Mefoxin
Mezlin	Monuril
Nebcin	Netromycin
Noroxin	PCE Dispertab
Penetrex	Primaxin
Rocephin	Septra
Sumycin	Suprax
Tazidime	Timentin
Unasyn	Zinacef

Gonadotropin Inhibitors

Antagon	Danocrine Capsules
Synarel Nasal Solution	

Pharmacological Listings

Hormones

Androgen and estrogen combinations:

Estratest	Lybrel
Premarin with	Premphase
Methyltestosterone	Prempro

Estrogens:

Climara	Estrace
Estraderm	Estrofem
Femring	Levolet
Menest	Ogen
Premarin	Seasonale

Gonadotropin:

Lutrepulse	Pregnyl
Profasi	Synarel

Menotropins:

Humegon	Pergonal
Repronex	

Progesterone:

Cycrin	Provera

Progestogen:

Aygestin	Micronor

Urinary Tract Agents

Analgesics:

Pyridium	Rimso-50

Antibacterials:

Bactrim	Cipro
Furadantin	Gantanol
Gantrisin	Macrobid
Macrodantin	NegGram
Neosporin	Noroxin
Proloprim	Septra
Thiosulfil	Trimpex
Uroqid Acid No. 2	

Antispasmodics:

Cystospaz	Levsin
Oxytrol	Toviaz
Urised	Urispas
UroXatral	Vesicare

Vaginal Preparations

Antifungal agents:

Betadine Douche	Femstat
Gyne-Lotrimin	Monistat
Mycelex	Terazol
Vagistat	Yeast-X

Capsules, tablets:

Mycelex-G	Sultrin

Creams:

Amino-Cerv	Estrace
Mycostatin	Nystex
Premarin	SCE-A
Trysul	

Inserts, suppositories:

Terazol	Vagisec Plus

Jellies, ointments:

Aci-Jel	

Pregnancy, Childbirth, Puerperium (630-679)

Antibiotics

Amikin	Ancef
Azactam	Ceclor
Cefizox	Cefobid
Cefotan	Claforan
E-Mycin	Fortaz
Garamycin	Keftab
Kefzol	Mefoxin
Nebcin	PCE Dispertab
Primaxin	Rocephin
Tazidime	Ticar
Timentin	Trobicin

Unasyn	Zefazone
Zolicef	Zyvox

Antihypertensives

Adalat	Aldactazide
Aldactone	Aldomet
Apresoline	Calan
Cardizem	Catapres
Deponit	Diuril
Esidrix	Hydralazine
HydroDIURIL	Hygroton
Hyperstat	Hytrin
Inderal	Isoptin
Levatol	Lopressor
Midamor	Minipress
Minoxidil	Nitrostat
Procardia	Renese
Tenormin	Tridil
Vasotec	Wytensin

Diuretics

Aldactazide	Aldactone
Aldoril	Bumex
Demadex	Diuril
Dyazide	Dyrenium
Edecrin	Esidrix
Esimil	HydroDIURIL
Lasix	Lozol
Maxzide	Rauzide
Renese	Zaroxolyn

Galactokinetic Agents

Syntocinon Nasal Spray

Nausea Medication

Antivert	Arrestin
Bonine	Compazine
Emetrol	Norzine
Tigan	Torecan

Oxytocics

Cervidil	Hemabate
Methergine	Oxytocin
Pitocin	Syntocinon
Uterine Relaxants	Yutopar

Skin and Subcutaneous Tissue (680-709)

Abradants

Ureacin

Acne Preparations

Accutane Tablets	Azelex
Benzac	Benzamycin
Cleocin	Clinda-Derm
Desquam	Emgel
Erycette	Novacet
Persa-Gel	Retin-A
Staticin	Sulfacet-R Acne
Theramycin Z	Xerac

Antibacterials, Antifungals and Combinations

Benzamycin	Fungi-Nail
Loprox	Lotrisone
Neosporin	Nizoral
Sporanox	

Antibiotics

Amikin	Ancef
Azactam	Bactroban
Ceclor	Cefizox
Cefobid	Cefotan
Ceftin	Cipro
Cubicin	Duricef
ERYC	Erythromycin
Floxin	Furacin
Garamycin	Ilosone
Ilotycin	Keflex
Keftab	Kefzol

Mandol	Mefoxin
Mezlin	Netromycin
Pipracil	Primaxin
Rocephin	Silvadene
Spectrobid	Tazidime
Ticar	Timentin
Ultracef	Zefazone
Zinacef	

Antiinflammatory Agents

Aclovate	Aristocort
Cortisporin	Cutivate
Cyclocort	Decadron
Diprolene	Elocon
Halog	Kenalog
Lidex	Lotrisone
Mantadil	NeoDecadron
Nutracort	Synacort
Synalar	Temovate
Topicort	Tridesilon
Ultravate	Westcort

Corticosteroids

Amcort	Celestone
Cortef	Deltasone
Depo-Medrol	Hydeltrasol
Solu-Cortef	Solu-Medrol

Depigmenting Agents

Benoquin Cream	Eldopaque
Eldoquin	

Dermatologicals

Dermatitis Herpetiformis:
Dapsone USP

Dermatitis Relief:

Decaspray	Elidel
Florone	Hytone
Locoid	Mytrex
Psorcon	

Epidermal and Cellular Growth:
Lazer Cream

Fungicides:

Amphotec	Abelcet
BAZA Cream	Clioquinol
Exelderm	Fungoid Creme
Grisactin	Halotex
Lamisil	Loprox
Lotrimin	Lotrisone
Mycelex	Mycolog-11
Mycostatin	Spectazole

Keratolytics:

Adrucil	Fluoroplex
Keralyt Gel	Occlusal-HP

Pruritis Medications:

Alphatrex	Betatrex
Dermoplast	Eldecort
Eurax	Florone
Hytone	Hyzine-50
Locoid	Mytrex
Periactin	Pramosone
Psorcon	Vistaril

Psoriasis Agents:

Amevive	Anthra-Derm
Cormax	Denorex
DHS Tar	Dovonex
Drithocreme	Dritho-Scalp
Enbrel	Hunira
Pentrax	Raptiva
Tazorac	Temovate
Zetar	

Steroids and Combinations:

Neo-Synalar	Psorcon
Synalar	Synemol
Vanoxide-HC	Vytone

Wart Removers:

Compound W	Condylox
LazerFormalyde	Occlusal
Podocon-25	Sal-Acid Plasters
Sal-Plant Gel	Trans-Plantar
Trans-Ver-Sal	Verr-Canth
Verrex	Verrusol
Viranol Gel	

Musculoskeletal System and Connective Tissue (710-739)

Analgesics

Advil	Anacin
Anaprox	Anexsia
Ansaid	Ascriptin
Bufferin	Butazolidin
Clinoril	Darvocet
Darvon	Datril
Disalcid	Dolobid
Easprin	Ecotrin
Empirin/Codeine	Equagesic
Esgic	Exedrin
Feldene	Flexeril
Hydrocodone	Indocin
Lortab/Lorcet	Meclomen
Medipren	Mono-Gesic
Motrin	Nalfon
Naprosyn	Norflex
Norgesic	Orudis
Parafon Forte	Percocet
Percodan	Phenaphen/Codeine
Ponstel	Rufen
Salflex	Sarapin
Synalgos-DC	Talacen
Talwin	Tapentadol
Tolectin	Trilisate
Tylenol	Tylenol/Codeine
Tylox	Vicodin
Wygesic	

Antibiotics (Osteomyelitis Treatments)

Amikin	Ancef
Cefizox	Cefotan
Cipro	Clindamycin
Floxin	Fortaz
Garamycin	Keflex
Keftab	Kefurox
Kefzol	Mandol
Mefoxin	Monocid
Pipracil	Rocephin
Timentin	Vancocin
Zinacef	

Antiinflammatory Agents, Steroids and Combinations

Aristocort	Bextra
Celebrex	Cortone
Decadron	Deltasone
Depo-Medrol	Duexis
Enbrel	Hydeltra-T.B.A.
Hydeltrasol	Hydrocortone
Kenalog	Lodine
Lexiva	Medrol
Relafen	Remicade
Voltren	

Antirheumatic, Disease Modifying Agent

Abatacept	Actemra
Benlysta	Enbrel
Etanercept	Orencia

Calcium Preparations

Calcium-D	Calphosan
Caltrate	Citracal
Dical-D	Neo-Calglucon
Nephro-Calci	Os-Cal
Phos-Ex	Posture

Muscle Relaxants

Actonel	Flexeril
Forteo	Paraflex
Parafon Forte	Robaxin
Robaxisal	Skelaxin
Soma	Valium
Valrelease	

Osteoporosis Preparations

Actonel	Aredia
Boniva	Calcimar
Didronel	Evista
Fosamax	Gerimed
Lexiva	Miacalcin

Congenital Anomalies (740-759)

A pharmacological reference list cannot be presented for this chapter because most conditions listed are treatable only by surgical methods and are not affected by medications.

Conditions in the Perinatal Period (760-779)

Antibiotics

Amoxcillin	Biaxin
Bicillin	Cloxacillin
Dicloxacillin	E-Mycin
Fortaz	Garamycin
Kefzol	Mandol
Mezlin	Nebcin
Rocephin	Spectrobid
Tazicef	Tazidime
Ticar	Vibramycin
Zithromax	

Bronchodilators

Aerolate Jr.	Asbron G
Bronkephrine	Choledyl
Dilor	Proventil
Quadrinal	Somophyllin
Theolair	Ventolin

Corticosteroids

Aristocort	Celeston
Cortone Acetate	Decadron
Deltasone	Depo-Medrol
Hydeltrasol	Prednisone
Solu-Cortef	Solu-Medrol

Electrolytes

Infalyte	Oralyte
Pedialyte	Rehydralyte

Galactokinetics (Milk Flow Stimulants)

Syntocinon Nasal Spray

Galactorrhea (Lactation) Inhibitors

Parlodel

Neonatal Respiratory Distress Syndrome Agents

Exosurf	Survanta

Ophthalmic Ointments, Antibiotics

Ilotycin

Rh Hemolytic Disease-Related Agents

Gamulin Rh
HypRho-D Full Dose (for baby)
HypRho-D Mini-Dose (for mother)
Win Rho-SD

Uterine Contractants

Oxytocin

Vitamins

AquaMEPHYTON

Symptoms, Signs and Ill-Defined Conditions (780-799)

Analgesics

Acetaminophens and combinations:

Acetaminophen	Anacin–Aspirin-Free
Anexsia	Bufferin
Datril	Excedrin
Feverall	Isocom
Midrin	Tylenol

Aspirins:

Easprin	Ecotrin
Forprin	

Aspirin combinations:

Anacin	Ascriptin A/D
Bufferin	Equagesic
Norgesic	

Narcotics, synthetics and combinations:

Alfenta	Anexsia
Astramorph/PF	Azdone
B&O Supprettes	Dalgan
Damason-P	Darvocet-N
Darvon	Demerol
Dilaudid	Dolophine
Duramorph	Esgic
Fioricet	Fiorinal
Hydrocet	Infumorph
Levo-Dromoran	Lortab
Lurline	Mepergan
Methadone-HCl	MS-Contin
MSIR	Nubain
Numorphan	Oralet
Oramorph	Percocet
Percodan	Phenaphen/Codeine
Phrenilin	Roxanol
Roxicodone	Sedapap
Stadol	Sublimaze
Sufenta	Synalgos-DC
Talacen	Talwin-NX
Tylox	Vicodin

Nonsteroidal antiinflammatory drugs (NSAIDs):

Advil	Anaprox
Daypro	Duract
Feldene	Indocin
Lodine	Meclomen
Medipren	Motrin
Nalfon	Naprosyn
Nuprin	Orudis
Ponstel	Rufen
Tolectin	Toradol
Voltaren	

Other:

Alka-Seltzer	Dolobid
Empirin/Codeine	Mono-Gesic
Norflex	Parafon Forte
Salflex	Sarapin
Trilisate	

Antacids

Alka-Seltzer	Amphojel
Basaljel	Maalox
Mylanta	Riopan

Anticonvulsives

Depakane	Depakote
Dilantin	Jabatril
Lamictal	Nurontin
Phenobarbital	Tegretol
Topamax	

Antiflatulents and Antigas Medications

Flatulex	Kutrase
Mylicon	

Antipyretics

Acetaminophen	Ascriptin A/D
Feverall	PediaProfen

Pharmacological Listings

Rufen
Tylenol
Trilisate

Antispasmodics and Anticholinergics
Arco-Lase
Cantil
Donnatal
Kutrase
Levsinex
Prilosec
Quarzan
Valpin-50
Bentyl
Darabid
Kinesed
Levsin
Librax
Pro-Banthine
Robinul

Appetite Suppressants

Amphetamines:
Biphetamine
Dexedrine
Desoxyn
Didrex

Nonamphetamines:
Adipex-P
Fastin
Plegine
Prelu-2
Sanorex
Bontril
Ionamin
Pondimin
Redux
Tenuate

Digestives
Cotazym
Ku-Zyme
Pancreatin
Donnazyme
Pancrease
Viokase

Diuretics
Aldactazide
Bumex
Corzide
Diamox
Diuril
Dyrenium
Enduron
Esidrex
HydroDIURIL
Lasix
Maxzide
Moduretic
Oretic
Rauzide
Saluron
Vaseretic
Aldactone
Capozide
Demadex
Diulo
Dyazide
Edecrin
Enduronyl
Exna
Hydromox
Lozol
Midamor
Naturetin
Prinzide
Renese
Thalitone
Zestoretic

Nausea and Vertigo Agents
Aloxi
Bonine
Emend
Kytril
Phenergan
Torecan
Antivert
Compazine
Emetrol
Norzine
Tigan
Zofran

Sleep Aids
Ambien
Dalmane
Halcion
Restoril
Valmid
Chloral hydrate
Doriden
Lunesta
Rozerem

Hypnotics:
Butisol
Phenobarbital
Mebaral

Sedatives (barbiturates):
Benadryl
Excedrin PM
Mepergan
Tylenol PM
Versed
BufferinAF
Magonate
Phenergan
Unisom

Sedatives (nonbarbiturates):
Eldertonic
Nu-Iron
Niferex

Tonics
Inderal

Tremor Preparations
Eldertonic
Nu-Iron
Niferex
Inderal

Injury and Poisoning (800-999)

Agents Used in Poisonings
Amyl nitrate
Antizole
Benadryl
Digibind
Narcan (Naloxone)
Pralidoxime
Revex
Sodium nitrite
Antilirium
BAL
Desferal
Ipecac Syrup
Penicillamine
Protopam Chloride
Romazicon

Analgesics

Acetaminophens and combinations:
Acetaminophen
Aspirin-Free Anacin
Feverall
Midrin
Tylenol with codeine
Anexsia
Excedrin
Isocom
Tylenol

Aspirins:
Aspirin
Ecotrin
Easprin

Aspirin combinations:
Anacin
Bufferin
Norgesic
Ascriptin A/D
Equagesic

Narcotics, synthetics and combinations:
Alfenta
Astromorph PF
B&O Supprettes
Damason-P
Darvon
Dilaudid
Duramorph
Fioricet
Hydrocet
Levo-Dromoran
Lurline
Methadone HCl
MSIR
Numorphan
Percocet
Phrenilin
Roxicodone
Stadol
Sufenta
Talacen
Tegretol
Vicodin
Zydone
Anexsia
Azdone
Dalgan
Darvocet-N
Demerol
Dolophine
Esgic
Fiorinal
Infumorph
Lortab/Lorcet
Mepergan
MS Contin
Nubain
Oramorph
Percodan
Roxanol
Sedapap
Sublimaze
Synalgos-DC
Talwin
Tylox
Wygesic

Nonsteroidal antiinflammatory drugs (NSAIDs):
Advil
Ansaid
Clinoril
Feldene
Lodine
Medipren
Nalfon
Nuprin
Ponstel
Rufen
Toradol
Anaprox
Cataflam
Daypro
Ibuprofen
Meclamen
Motrin
Naprosyn
Orudis
Relafen
Tolectin
Voltaren

Antibiotics
Achromycin
Amoxicillin
Ancef
Azactam
Cefizox
Cefotan
Claforan
Garamycin
Keftab
Kefzol
Mezlin
Netromycin
Tazidime
Zefazone
Amikin
Amoxil
Augmentin
Ceclor
Cefobid
Cipro
Floxin
Keflex
Kefurox
Mefoxin
Nebcin
Pipracil
Timentin
Zinacef

Anticoagulants
Calciparine
Dicumarol
Heparin Sodium
Organan
Xarelto
Coumadin
Fragmin
Lovenox
Panwarfln

Antihistamines
Allegra
Benadryl
Claritin
Extendryl
Optimine
Tacaryl
Zyrtec
Atarax/Vistaril
Chlor-Trimeton
Dimetap
Hismanal
Seldane
Temaril

Antivertigo Medications
Antivert
Bucladin-S
Vontrol
Bonine
Meclizine

Burn Agents
Americaine
Butesin Picrate
Collagenase Santyl
Eucerin
Panafil
Silvadine
Tronothane
Aquaphor
Chloresium
Dermoplast
Nupercainal
Prophyllin
Sween Cream

Corticosteroids
Aristocort
Decadron
Depo-Medrol
Hydrocortone
Solu-Cortef
Celestone
Deltasone
Hydeltrasol
Prednisone
Solu-Medrol

Detoxifying Agents
Mesnex Injection

Skin Wound Preparations
Betadine
DuoDERM
Debrisan

Wound Dressings
Aquaphor
Critic-Aid
DuoDERM
Lazer
SSD
Chloresium
Debrisan
Granulex
Panafil

Valid Three-digit ICD-9-CM Codes

Three-digit ICD-9-CM codes are used to identify a condition or disease only when a fourth or fifth digit is not available. The following are the only ICD-9-CM codes that are valid without further specificity.

024	Glanders	317	Mild intellectual disabilities	538	Gastrointestinal mucostitis (ulcerative)
025	Melioidosis	319	Unspecified intellectual disabilities	541	Appendicitis, unqualified
035	Erysipelas	325	Phlebitis and thrombophlebitis of intracranial venous sinuses	542	Other appendicitis
037	Tetanus			566	Abscess of anal and rectal regions
042	Human immunodeficiency virus (HIV) disease	326	Late effects of intracranial abscess or pyogenic infection	570	Acute and subacute necrosis of liver
048	Other enterovirus diseases of central nervous system	340	Multiple sclerosis	586	Renal failure, unspecified
		390	Rheumatic fever without mention of heart involvement	587	Renal sclerosis, unspecified
061	Dengue			591	Hydronephrosis
064	Viral encephalitis transmitted by other and unspecified arthropods	393	Chronic rheumatic pericarditis	605	Redundant prepuce and phimosis
		412	Old myocardial infarction	630	Hydatidiform mole
071	Rabies	430	Subarachnoid hemorrhage	632	Missed abortion
075	Infectious mononucleosis	431	Intracerebral hemorrhage	650	Normal delivery
080	Louse-borne [epidemic] typhus	436	Acute, but ill-defined, cerebrovascular disease	677	Late effect of complication of pregnancy, childbirth, and the puerperium
096	Late syphilis, latent	449	Septic arterial embolism		
101	Vincent's angina	452	Portal vein thrombosis	683	Acute lymphadenitis
118	Opportunistic mycoses	460	Acute nasopharyngitis [common cold]	684	Impetigo
124	Trichinosis	462	Acute pharyngitis	700	Corns and callosities
129	Intestinal parasitism, unspecified	463	Acute tonsillitis	725	Polymyalgia rheumatica
135	Sarcoidosis	470	Deviated nasal septum	734	Flat foot
138	Late effects of acute poliomyelitis	475	Peritonsillar abscess	769	Respiratory distress syndrome
179	Malignant neoplasm of uterus, part unspecified	481	Pneumococcal pneumonia [Streptococcus pneumoniae pneumonia]	797	Senility without mention of psychosis
				920	Contusion of face, scalp, and neck except eye(s)
181	Malignant neoplasm of placenta	485	Bronchopneumonia, organism unspecified		
185	Malignant neoplasm of prostate	486	Pneumonia, organism unspecified	931	Foreign body in ear
193	Malignant neoplasm of thyroid gland	490	Bronchitis, not specified as acute or chronic	932	Foreign body in nose
217	Benign neoplasm of breast	496	Chronic airway obstruction, not elsewhere classified	936	Foreign body in intestine and colon
220	Benign neoplasm of ovary			937	Foreign body in anus and rectum
226	Benign neoplasm of thyroid glands	500	Coal workers' pneumoconiosis	938	Foreign body in digestive system, unspecified
243	Congenital hypothyroidism	501	Asbestosis		
260	Kwashiorkor	502	Pneumoconiosis due to other silica or silicates	981	Toxic effect of petroleum products
261	Nutritional marasmus			986	Toxic effect of carbon monoxide
262	Other severe, protein-calorie malnutrition	503	Pneumoconiosis due to other inorganic dust	990	Effects of radiation, unspecified
		504	Pneumonopathy due to inhalation of other dust	V08	Asymptomatic HIV infection status
267	Ascorbic acid deficiency	505	Pneumoconiosis, unspecified		
311	Depressive disorder, not elsewhere classified	514	Pulmonary congestion and hypostasis		
316	Psychic factors associated with diseases classified elsewhere	515	Postinflammatory pulmonary fibrosis		

Present on Admission (POA) Tutorial

Background

The Deficit Reduction Act of 2005 (DRA), section 5001(C), requires that CMS implement Present on Admission (POA) indicators for all diagnoses and external causes of injury on Medicare claims for inpatient acute care discharges beginning October 1, 2007. Critical access hospitals, Maryland waiver hospitals, long term care hospitals, cancer hospitals, and children's inpatient facilities are exempt from this requirement.

Claim Submission Requirements

Beginning October 1, 2007, all inpatient acute care hospital discharges were required to be reported using POA indicators on all diagnoses and external cause of injury codes. The only exception is for a select group of codes that are designated as exempt from the POA regulations. This list of codes may be found at the end of this tutorial. Hospitals that failed to submit claims for discharges on or after April 1, 2008, had claims returned for completion with POA indicators.

CMS is also required to identify at least two conditions will be designated such that when the POA indicator reflects that they developed during the admission, they will not be recognized as major complication/comorbidity (MCC) or complication/comorbidity (CC) conditions under the DRG inpatient prospective payment system (IPPS). These conditions will have met the following criteria:

- high cost and/or high volume
- represent conditions that could have been avoided using evidence-based practice guidelines
- when present with other secondary diagnoses on the claim result in higher DRG payment weight

Effective October 1, 2008 (FY2009), hospitals do not receive additional payment for claims with codes that represent one of the selected conditions when not indicated as present on admission, meaning it developed during the acute care inpatient stay. The regulation effectively deactivates the CC or MCC status of the code, but hospital staff should be aware that other conditions on the case may carry valid CC or MCC status. Refer to page 60 of this tutorial, which provides a list of the 12 conditions that CMS has designated as "Hospital Acquired Conditions" and will be included in the policy for FY2011.

General Guidelines

The POA indicator guidelines are not intended to replace the official ICD-9-CM reporting guidelines. Nor will the POA guidelines supersede the Uniform Hospital Discharge Data Set (UHDDS) definition of principal diagnosis. A principal diagnosis remains defined as the condition established after study to be chiefly responsible for occasioning the admission of the patient to the hospital. The definition of "Other Diagnoses" also remains the same. Coders must report all conditions that coexist at the time of admission, develop subsequently, or that affect the treatment received and/or the length of stay. This has significant impact on the practice of assigning the POA indicators.

Because the POA indicator selection should accurately reflect the patient's conditions upon admission, review of POA guidelines and official coding guidelines is required. Consistent, complete documentation in the medical record is of the utmost importance. Lack of complete documentation may impact DRG case grouping and reimbursement. It is incumbent upon the provider to resolve any documentation issues.

The following is a summary of the basic POA Indicator Guidelines:

- The POA indictor requirement applies only to acute care hospital inpatient admissions or other facilities, as required by regulation for public health reporting.
- A POA condition is defined not only as one that is clearly present at the time of admission, but also those that were clearly present, but not diagnosed until after the time of admission.
- Present on admission is defined as present at the time the order for an inpatient admission is made, regardless of whether the patient's episode of care originated in the emergency department, ambulatory surgery area, or other outpatient area. Conditions that develop during an outpatient encounter are considered present on admission.
- The POA guidelines are not intended to replace any of the other ICD-9-CM Official Guidelines for Coding and Reporting.

Guidelines are not intended to determine whether or not a condition should be coded, but rather how to apply the POA indicator.

The following options should be used to indicate whether a condition was POA:

Y   Yes
N   No
U   Unknown
W   Clinically undetermined

Unreported/not used – (Exempt from POA reporting) – CMS has developed a standard "exempt" list of conditions and external causes. For these codes the POA indicator is left blank, except on the UB-04 form where an indicator of "1" is indicated as the equivalent of a blank. On the UB-04 blanks are undesirable when submitting this data via the 4010A. Beginning on or after January 1, 2011, hospitals were required to begin reporting POA indicators using the 5010 electronic transmittal standards form. The 5010 format eliminates the need to report a POA indicator of "1" for codes that are exempt from POA reporting. The POA field should instead be left blank for codes exempt from POA reporting.

See Appendix 1 of the ICD-9-CM Official Coding Guidelines for Coding and Reporting and the end of this tutorial for the complete list of exempt codes.

When using the options listed above, the following definitions should be used:

Y   present at the time of inpatient admission
N   not present at the time of inpatient admission
U   documentation is insufficient to determine if condition is present on admission
W   Provider is unable to clinically determine whether condition was present on admission or not

Most ICD-9-CM diagnosis codes and E codes require POA indicator assignment. However, there are some diagnoses that are considered exempt from the POA reporting. To view exempt codes, refer to the ICD-9-CM Official Guidelines for Coding and Reporting and the end of this tutorial. The list reflects those conditions that either do not represent a current disease or are always considered POA.

Timeframe for POA Identification and Documentation

There is no specific or required timeframe for which a provider must identify or document a condition to be present on admission. In some clinical situations it may not be possible for a provider to determine whether a condition is POA at the point of admission; review of laboratory or other results may be necessary. A condition may not be recognized or reported by the patient for a period of time after admission, but it does not necessarily mean that the condition was not present on admission. Determination of whether the condition was POA or not should be based on the applicable POA guideline in the *ICD-9-CM Official Guidelines for Coding and Reporting*, or on the provider's best clinical judgment. If it is not clear at the time of coding whether a condition was POA or not, it is appropriate to query the provider for further clarification.

Specific Guidelines

Complete and accurate medical record documentation is a critical aspect of the appropriate assignment of POA indicators. The ICD-9-CM Official Guidelines for Coding and Reporting indicate that to achieve accurate and complete documentation, code assignment, and reporting of diagnoses and procedures, documentation must be a collaborative effort between healthcare provider and the coder. To assist the coder in determining which documentation in the medical record may be used for code selection, an Official Guidelines for Source Documentation Table is provided at the end of this section.

Assignment of POA indicators may be confusing for several types of cases, particularly if the documentation is not clear. The following are examples of POA guidelines and case scenarios illustrating various coding situations:

Note: As always, query the physician for a definitive diagnosis when documentation is inconsistent. The tips are presented as a guide to what information a coder might review in the process of verifying a diagnosis before assigning a POA indicator. The HIM department should work closely with the medical staff to develop a list of criteria for all conditions that are frequently queried.

- **Combination Codes:** Assign "N" if any part of the combination code was not present at the time of admission. If the combination code only identifies the chronic condition and not the associated acute exacerbation, assign "Y."

Example: Obstructive chronic bronchitis with acute exacerbation

Tips: The POA indicator "N" would be assigned if the exacerbation did not happen until after the admission (code 491.21).

Definition of acute exacerbation: the presence of one or more of the following findings are indications of acute exacerbation: increase in sputum purulence, increase in sputum volume, tightening of chest, fluid retention and worsening of dyspnea or shortness of breath and/or wheezing.

Indicators of an acute exacerbation of COPD might be the documentation of either of the following treatments:

- Bronchodilator: Nebulised beta2-agonist or ipratropium bromide. If no response, IV aminophylline or nebulised beta2-agonist and ipratropium bromide in combination

- Oxygen: Given in ambulance or on arrival, 24-28% by mask or 2 ltr/min by nasal prongs.

Source Documents: Laboratory report, physician orders, nursing notes

- **Impending Conditions:** If a threatened or impending condition is present prior to or at the time of admission, report "Y" for the POA indicator.

Example: An impending acute myocardial infarction (code 411.1)

Tips: Impending acute myocardial infarction is also documented as unstable angina. This condition is a type of acute chest pain that occurs when the heart does not get enough oxygen. Patients with atherosclerosis, which is the most common cause of unstable angina, may accelerate to unstable angina. Unstable angina is acute worsening of chest pain.

The chest pain that:

- Occurs without cause

- Lasts longer than 15 to 20 minutes

- Does not go away with nitroglycerine

- May occur along with a drop in blood pressure or significant shortness of breath

Tests to diagnose angina include:

- Blood tests to check the levels of creatine phosphokinase(CPK), myoglobin, and troponin I and T

- Coronary angiography

- ECG (transient ST- or T-wave changes that develop duringa symptomatic episode at rest and resolve when thepatient becomes asymptomatic strongly suggest unstableangina)

- Echocardiography

Drug treatment associated with Impending myocardial infarction:

- Aspirin: 324 mg

- Heparin: 80 units/kg IV bolus with constant IV infusion at18 units/kg/hr titrated to maintain a PTT between 46 and70 seconds

- Nitrates: Sublingual (1-3 tablets); IV (5-100 micro-g/min)

- Beta Blockers: Oral dose appropriate for specific drug: IVmetoprolol (1-5 m slow IV every 5 minutes to 15 mg total);IV propranolol 0.5 to 1.0 mg; IV atenolol 5 mg everyminute to 10 mg total

- Narcotics: Morphine sulfate 2 to 5 mg IV

- Source Documents: Laboratory reports, physician orders, EKG

- **Two or More Contrasting Conditions:** If the symptoms related to the two conditions were present at the time of admission, the POA indicators for both are "Y."

Example: Diverticulitis versus chronic appendicitis (codes 562.11, 542)

Tip: A patient may present with acute abdominal pain but mayimprove clinically and be discharged or transferred before a definitivedetermination of the final diagnosis can be made.

Tests to diagnose diverticulitis include:

- Abdominal palpation, which may indicate left lower quadrant mass

- CT scan may reveal thickening of the inflamed area orbowel spasm if irritable bowel syndrome accompaniesdiverticular disease

- Lab studies may indicate elevated white blood count

Diverticular disease may be diagnosed via barium enema or sigmoidoscopy or colonoscopy services, but these studies are typically not performed if the acute inflamed diverticulitis phase of the disease is present, since these procedures may cause bowel rupture or require strenuous bowel prep.

Tests to diagnose appendicitis include:

- Abdominal palpation, which may indicate right lower quadrant pain, which typically worsens when the patient is asked to cough or upon gentle percussion

- Lab studies may indicate a moderately elevated white blood count, with increased numbers of immature cells

- Enema studies with a contrast agent may be helpful; appendicitis is present if the appendix does not fill with contrast agent

In this example, the POA indicator for codes representing both the diverticulitis and the chronic appendicitis should be "Y," since it was thought that the presenting symptom was caused by one of these conditions.

Source Documents: Radiology reports, laboratory results, physician documentation of abdominal examination findings

- **Symptom Followed by Comparative or Contrasting Conditions:** If a symptom followed by comparative or contrasting conditions is present prior to or at the time of admission, all indicators are reported as "Y."

Example: Chills due to either pneumonia or urinary tract infection. (codes 780.99, 486, 599.0).

Tips: A patient may present with chills but may improve clinically and be discharged or transferred before a definitive determination of the final diagnosis can be made.

A patient presenting with chills is typically worked-up for an infectious disease process. Chest X-rays or other radiological studies may be performed to rule out the presence of pneumonia, but coders should be aware that in some cases, the first chest X-ray may not show any consolidation indicative of pneumonia. After the patient is admitted and hydrated, the follow-up chest X-ray may show signs of pneumonia, but this disease process may have been present at the time of admission. The determination must be made by the physician, who may have documented clinical signs of pneumonia in the initial physical examination.

The search for the underlying cause of an infectious disease process is also typically aided by laboratory studies, which may includes putum or urine cultures. The coder should not assign any diagnosis code based on laboratory findings only, but these findings are clues that help focus the clinical picture for each patient. Coders must also be aware that some cultures may contain contaminated material that does not represent an infectious process. This is particularly problematic with Staphylococcus aureus, which is a bacteria very commonly found on skin surfaces. Culture and sensitivity studies help determine which antibiotics would be most effective in treating the particular infection. Again, the coder may not assign any diagnosis code based on treatment options, but they can provide clues to the type of infectious process that may be present. For example, if a patient presents with fever and chills, is found to have consolidation on chest X-ray and is treated with Sporanox, an antifungal agent, this is indicative of a fungal pneumonia and the physician documentation should specify such.

Source Documents: physical examination, radiology reports, laboratory findings, including urine, sputum or blood cultures, sputum gram stain, biopsy results

In this example, codes for all the presenting diagnoses would be represented with a "Y" POA indicator.

- **Same Diagnosis Code for Two or More Conditions:** When the same ICD-9-CM diagnosis code applies to two or more conditions during the same encounter (e.g. bilateral condition, or two separate conditions classified to the same ICD-9-CM diagnosis code):

- Assign "Y" if all conditions represented by the single ICD-9-CM code were present on admission (e.g. bilateral fracture of the same bone, same site, and both fractures were present on admission)

- Assign "N" if any of the conditions represented by the single ICD-9-CM code was not present on admission (e.g. dehydration with hyponatremia is assigned to code 276.1, but only one of these conditions was present on admission).

- **External Cause of Injury Codes:** If an injury or poisoning occurred prior to or at the time of admission, both the code for the injury/poisoning and the corresponding E code are reported with POA indicator "Y."

Tips: Typically most trauma cases are very straight-forward and it is very clear which injuries were present at the time of admission. However, in cases of multiple trauma, one or several injuries may not be diagnosed initially, but may have been present at the time of admission. For example, if a patient suffers a closed head injury and internal abdominal injuries, a comparatively minor fractured extremity may not be diagnosed or treated initially, during the lifesaving treatment phase. But if the injury was sustained in the original injury, the POA indicator should remain "Y."

Coders should be extremely careful in assigning the appropriate POA indicator if a patient suffers an injury while an inpatient. For example, if a patient falls from the hospital bed and fractures a hip, the codes representing that injury (along with the appropriate E code) should be designated "N" in the corresponding POA indicator assignment.

Source Documents: Emergency Department reports, radiology reports, History and Physical report, consultation reports (particularly orthopedic), physician orders

The following guidelines may be helpful when assigning POA indicators for obstetrical patients.

Coders should also keep in mind that several of the obstetrical related codes (such as code 650, Normal delivery) are found on the POA exemption list and do not require POA indicator assignment.

- **Antepartum Conditions:** If an antepartum condition is present prior to or at the time of the current admission, report "Y" for the POA indicator.

Example: Pregnancy with fetal distress, antepartum (code 656.33).

Tip: Most obstetrical departments in acute care facilities use preprinted forms specifically designed for pregnant patients. These forms should include designations for labor-related conditions that were present at the time the patient was admitted. Other forms are used to detail a patient's course as she progresses from labor through delivery. Although nursing staff document most of the information on these forms, the physician should also document any complication of labor, along with treatment provided.

Source Documents: Obstetrical Intake Record, History & Physical, Labor Record

- **Pre-existing Chronic Conditions:** If a pregnant patient has a chronic condition that was present prior to or at the time of admission, the POA indicator is "Y."

Example: Pregnancy with pre-existing hypertension, delivered (code 642.01).

Tip: The POA guideline related to pre-existing chronic conditions for pregnant patients follows that for other patients. Any pre-existing chronic condition should be coded with POA indicator "Y," denoting that the condition was present before or at the time the patient was admitted. Coders should keep in mind that there may be a specific pregnancy related code for the condition.

Source Documents: Obstetrical Intake Record, History & Physical, Labor Record

- **Acute Conditions:** If a pregnant patient has an acute condition that develops during delivery and it was not present prior to or at the time of admission, the POA indicator is "N."

Example: Second degree perineal laceration, delivered (code 664.11);

Tip: Many of the conditions that are a result of the delivery process itself are, by their very definition, not present on admission. At admission, the pregnant patient has not progressed to the point of delivery or sustained a condition such as a perineal laceration. All conditions that develop as a result of the delivery process itself should be considered not present on admission and designated with POA indicator "N."

Source Documents: Obstetrical Intake Record, History & Physical, Labor Record, Delivery Record, Discharge Summary

- **Co-existing Conditions:** If a patient has a condition that is diagnosed on the current admission but the documentation does not indicate whether it was present at the time of admission, the provider should be queried. If no answer can be determined, the POA indicator is "U."

Example: Pregnant patient delivers and is also found to have a breast nipple abscess (code 675.01).

Tip: In only very limited circumstances should a POA indicator of "U" be assigned, and only if the physician cannot be reached for clarification. Conditions that are pregnancy related should be clearly documented concerning whether they were present at the time of admission. It is typically conditions related to other body systems that may not contain specific enough detail to determine whether they were present at the time of admission. Most acute care facilities have physician query processes in place to address these issues, but in some limited cases, a POA indicator of "U" must be assigned.

Source Documents: Obstetrical Intake Record, History & Physical, Labor Record, Delivery Record, Discharge Summary

One of the most significant challenges to correct POA indicator assignment may be ensuring complete, consistent and appropriate physician documentation at the time of initial coding. While some cases, particularly those for surgical patients admitted for a specific procedure, are very straight-forward and it is clear which conditions were present at the time of admission, many other cases are much more vague. Coders should keep in mind that a patient may present to the hospital with ambiguous signs or symptoms of a disease that could take several days to accurately diagnose. If the presenting signs or symptoms were related to the subsequently diagnosed condition, the POA indicator should be "Y," but only the provider may make this connection and it must be clearly documented in the medical record. The POA Reporting Guidelines include: "Issues related to inconsistent, missing, conflicting or unclear documentation must still be resolved by the provider." This may involve physician queries either during or following the patient encounter; medical record documentation from any provider involved in the care and treatment of the patient may be used to support the determination of whether a condition was present on admission or not. To assist the coder in determining which documentation in the medical record may be used for code selection, the following Official Guidelines for Source Documentation Table was developed. The table includes AHA's *Coding Clinic for ICD-9-CM* official guidelines related to medical record documentation.

CMS staff, in conjunction with representatives from the cooperating parties (AHA, AHIMA, CDC) recently provided clarification on POA assignment for a specific type of case. It involves patients for whom a single diagnosis code captures the fact that the patient was admitted as a result of a head injury and then subsequently lost consciousness after the admission. The POA indicator assigned should be "Y," indicating that the head injury and resulting loss of consciousness occurred prior to (and was present on) admission. This clarification also appears in the 2nd quarter 2010 issue of AHA's *Coding Clinic for ICD-9-CM* in the "Frequently Asked POA Questions" section.

Selected Hospital Acquired Conditions for FY2012

In the IPPS Proposed Rule FY2014 [*Federal Register*, May 10, 2013], CMS did not propose adding or removing any HAC categories from the current list.

For more specific instructions on Medicare POA indicator reporting options, refer to:

> http://www.cms.hhs.gov/HospitalAcqCond/02_Statute_Regulations_Program_Instructions.asp#TopOfPage

Source Documentation Official Guidelines

Issues	Guideline	POA Impact	Coding Clinic Source
Internal Coding Guidelines	A facility's internal guidelines may not conflict with the *Official ICD-9-CM Guidelines for Coding & Reporting* and may not be used in place of actual physician documentation in the medical record used to substantiate code assignment.	A physician must be queried concerning the presence of a diagnosis if there are abnormal lab values or other documentation indicating the possibility of a condition either present on admission or developing later.	2Q, '04, 13-14; 3Q, '00, 6; 1Q, '00, 24
Coding Chronic Conditions	Chronic conditions such as, but not limited to, hypertension, Parkinson's disease, COPD, and diabetes mellitus are chronic systemic diseases that ordinarily should be coded even in the absence of documented intervention or further evaluation. Some chronic conditions affect the patient for the rest of his or her life and almost always require some form of continuous clinical evaluation or monitoring during hospitalization, and therefore should be coded.	If documentation is ambiguous or unclear concerning the presence of a chronic condition, the provider should be queried to determine whether the patient carries the diagnosis. This determination affects the POA indicator, which would be assigned as YES (Y) for most chronic conditions unless initially diagnosed during the present admission.	3Q, '07, 10-11
Information from MD other than attending physician	Code assignment may be based on information documented by another physician as long as it doesn't conflict with that from the attending physician.	Medical record documentation provided by any physician other than the attending physician should be carefully reviewed to ensure that all conditions present and treated are coded appropriately.	1Q, '04, 18-19
Mid-level provider documentation	Codes may be assigned based on documentation by nurse practitioners or physician assistants who provide diagnoses and provide care, if they are considered legally accountable for establishing a diagnosis within the regulations governing the provider and the facility.	Coders should be aware of the admitting and attending regulations for their facility and always review nurse practitioner and physician assistant medical record entries carefully for documentation of codable diagnoses.	4Q, '04, 138
Coding diagnoses from pathology reports (inpatient visits)	When a pathology report reflects a completely different diagnosis than the physician documented (e.g., CA breast vs breast mass), the coder must query the physician for additional clarifying information to resolve the conflict. If the pathology report adds greater detail to a diagnosis made by the attending physician, it may be used for coding purposes.	Coders should ensure that any postoperative diagnosis that is found on a pathology report is also documented elsewhere in the record by the physician. It should also be determined whether the condition in question was actually present on admission, even if the postoperative condition differs from the preoperative condition.	3Q, '08, 11; 1Q, '04, 20-21
Coding diagnoses from autopsy reports (inpatient visits)	The information provided on an autopsy report may be used for coding purposes if it clarifies, or provides greater detail or specificity to the diagnoses provided by the attending physician. The autopsy report is completed by a pathologist, who is a physician.	If an autopsy report is available at the time of coding, the coder must ensure that any diagnoses contained in it are substantiated by the attending physician documentation. Any conflicts should be clarified by the attending physician.	1Q, '01, 5
Anesthesia record diagnosis documentation	An anesthesiologist is a physician and diagnostic information may be coded from the anesthesiology report unless it conflicts with information provided by the attending physician, in which case the attending should be queried.	Anesthesia reports should be regularly reviewed as part of the coding process. This evaluation can also be helpful in determining the onset of various diagnoses, pertinent in the assignment of the POA indicator.	2Q, '00, 15
Diagnoses found in the body of the medical record	Documentation of codable diagnoses is not limited to the final diagnostic statement, discharge summary, H&P or other specific report. If a physician has documented the diagnosis and it does not conflict with diagnostic information listed elsewhere, it may be coded.	Coders should not limit their review to only those medical record reports that most often contain diagnostic information. Codable diagnoses may be found in any area of the record that contains documentation by a physician or other licensed caregiver.	2Q, '00, 17-18
Adding specificity from radiology reports	When a physician has documented a general diagnosis and a radiology report adds specificity to that diagnosis, without any conflicting information concerning the original diagnosis, the specific information may be used in code selection.	Coders should review all diagnostic or therapeutic reports that carry diagnoses by a physician. If the diagnosis does not conflict with that provided by the attending physician, it may be used to aid in code specificity.	1Q, '99, 5
Diagnoses based on physician orders	When a physician orders a prescribed medication for a patient without supporting documentation of a related diagnosis, he or she must be queried concerning the presence of a corresponding diagnosis.	Coders may not assign diagnosis codes based on documentation of physician orders for medications. The query process should include information related to asking the physician to document each condition treated and whether it was a long-standing, chronic or new condition.	3Q, '05, 18-20
Pneumonia coding	While laboratory results can aid in the diagnosis of pneumonia, it is the physician documentation of physical findings, along with supporting information, that substantiates the diagnosis for coding purposes. Coders may not assign a pneumonia code based on laboratory or radiology findings alone, or on treatment by antibiotics or antifungal medications.	Coders must review laboratory, radiology and treatment related documentation and may query the physician based on information contained in these reports. The physician must also document whether the patient had signs or symptoms of the disease process at the time of admission in order to assign the most appropriate POA indicator.	2Q, '98, 3-6
Abnormal lab values	The physician must substantiate that an abnormal lab value represents an actual condition before it may be coded. If the findings are outside the normal range and there is an indication that the physician has ordered further work-up or treatment, the physician should be queried.	No secondary diagnoses should be assigned based on lab values alone. The coder may review the lab and the dates on which the lab studies were performed in order to formulate a physician query to identify whether the patient has a particular condition and whether it was present on admission.	*Official Coding Guidelines* 11/15/06: Section III.B; 2Q, '90, 16

Present on Admission (POA) Tutorial

Issues	Guideline	POA Impact	Coding Clinic Source
Documentation required for reporting body mass index (BMI)	BMI codes may be reported based on documentation by a dietitian's or nurse's note, but the condition must follow UHDDS guidelines for reporting secondary diagnoses. Documentation of the underlying overweight, obesity or morbid obesity condition must be documented by a provider.	Coders should not report codes for BMI alone, without the underlying condition that reflects the clinical significance for the patient encounter.	2Q, '10, 15; 4Q, '08, 191
Using a resident's documentation without attending physician sign-off	Code assignment may be based on other physician documentation (i.e., consultants, residents, etc.) as long as there is no conflicting information from the attending physician. Confirmation of a resident's documentation by the attending physician is dependent on medical staff by-laws, a hospital's internal policies, etc.	Coding management staff should ascertain whether there are specific documentation requirements for residents and their attending physicians and follow those guidelines accordingly.	3Q, '08, 3
Coding based solely on drug administration	It is inappropriate for coders to assign a diagnosis based solely on drug administration without the provider documenting the condition being treated.	When there is a question concerning whether a condition is present, the provider should be queried.	3Q, '08, 14
Clinical information found in *Coding Clinic*	Any clinical information found in *Coding Clinic* does not constitute clinical criteria for establishing a diagnosis, nor does it substitute for the provider's clinical judgment, or eliminate the need for clear and complete physician documentation.	Clinical information presented in *Coding Clinic* is provided as background material to aid the coder's understanding of disease process. When there is a question concerning a specific diagnosis or disease process, the provider should be queried	3Q, '08, 15-16
Required timeframe for physician documentation related to POA	There is no required timeframe concerning when a provider must identify or document a condition to be present on admission.	The coder may use all provider documentation in determining POA indicator assignment, regardless of when it was documented.	3Q, '08, 20
POA indicator requirement for E-codes	Some E-codes are exempt from POA reporting, but others do require POA indicator assignment if they are reported among the secondary diagnoses.	Coders should carefully review the "Categories & Codes Exempt from Diagnosis POA Reporting" section of the most current version of the *ICD-9-CM Official Guidelines for Coding and Reporting*. POA indicators should be assigned for all E-codes not found on the exempt list.	3Q, '08, 21
POA pressure ulcer clarification – multiple stages for one ulcer	A pressure ulcer is only coded and reported once at the highest stage.	If the pressure ulcer is present at the time of admission, the POA indicator is "Y," regardless of whether or not the ulcer progresses to a higher stage during the admission.	1Q, '09, 19
POA pressure ulcer clarification – multiple ulcers of same stage but different POA	ICD-9-CM diagnosis codes may only be reported once on an encounter, so if separate pressure ulcers assigned to the same code have different POA indicators, assign the diagnosis code once, with POA indicator of "N."	Pressure ulcer documentation should be reviewed carefully to ensure that ulcers are differentiated by the 5th digit of subcategory 707.0 if possible. Coders should not attempt to assign the same diagnosis code more than once on an encounter, regardless of POA indicator assignment.	2Q, '10, 17-18
Acute exacerbation of COPD with acute respiratory failure	When a patient is admitted with an acute exacerbation of COPD and subsequently progresses to acute respiratory failure, both conditions are coded separately.	The POA indicator for the acute exacerbation of COPD is "Y." If the documentation is not clear regarding whether the respiratory failure was POA or not, query the provider for clarification. If it developed after admission, assign "N" as the POA indicator. If it cannot be determined, assign "W."	1Q, '10, 18
Respiratory distress progressing to acute respiratory failure	The principal diagnosis is acute respiratory failure since it was the reason for the admission. No additional code is reported for the respiratory distress.	The POA indicator for the acute respiratory failure is "Y" since it developed prior to admission.	1Q, '10, 18
Cancer staging form documentation	Completed cancer staging forms may be used for coding purposes if the attending physician has substantiated and authenticated the final findings.	For oncology cases coders should ensure that a thorough review of the cancer staging form is conducted, particularly if there is a question whether a malignancy existed at the time of surgery or discharge.	2Q, '10, 7-8
Loss of consciousness (LOC) in head injury cases	Regardless of whether a patient loses consciousness before, at, or after admission, the POA indicator for the head injury code is "Y" if the injury occurred prior to admission. LOC is a natural part of the head injury disease process.	While coders must determine total length of loss of consciousness for appropriate head injury coding, if an injury occurred prior to the patient's admission to the hospital, the POA indicator should remain "Y," regardless of the onset of LOC timeframe.	2Q, '10, 17
Radiology report incidental findings	It is not appropriate to assign a diagnosis code for an incidental finding that is unrelated to a sign, symptom or other reason for a radiology exam. The physician of record (ED or attending physician) must indicate that the finding was clinically significant and related to the visit in question.	Coders may use radiology reports to add specificity to another condition already documented by a physician, but should not code incidental conditions based solely on documentation within a radiology report.	3Q, '10, 8-9
Documentation of conditions with up and down arrows	It is not appropriate to assign a diagnosis code based on the presence of up or down arrows along with a condition. The arrows can have variable interpretations and do not necessarily mean "abnormal."	Coders must clarify the significance of the condition with the physician when the documentation includes only up and down arrows, with no actual diagnosis. Abnormal findings are not coded and reported unless the provider indicates their clinical significance.	1Q, '11, 17

Issues	Guideline	POA Impact	Coding Clinic Source
Provider documentation of ICD-9-CM code number instead of a descriptive diagnostic statement	Regulatory and accreditation guidelines require that providers document actual medical terminology to support code assignment. It is not appropriate to list only a code number; ICD-9-CM is a classification system, not a diagnosis system.	Coders may not use solely coded information provided in lieu of an appropriate diagnostic statement for coding and POA determination decisions.	1Q, '12, 6
Borderline diagnoses	"Borderline" diagnoses are coded as confirmed unless the classification provides other instructions. Some conditions require clarification from the provider to determine whether they should be coded.	If a borderline condition has a specific entry, such as "borderline diabetes," that instruction must be followed. If it is unclear, the provider should be queried. Otherwise, all POA guidelines apply; borderline conditions are not uncertain diagnoses.	1Q, '12, 17

POA Examples

The following POA Examples were previously found in the *ICD-9-CM Official Guidelines for Coding and Reporting*, but were deleted from the guidelines for FY 2010. Some coders may find the examples instructional.

General Medical Surgical

1. Patient is admitted for diagnostic work-up for cachexia. The final diagnosis is malignant neoplasm of lung with metastasis.

   Assign "Y" on the POA field for the malignant neoplasm. The malignant neoplasm was clearly present on admission, although it was not diagnosed until after the admission occurred.

2. A patient undergoes outpatient surgery. During the recovery period, the patient develops atrial fibrillation and the patient is subsequently admitted to the hospital as an inpatient.

   Assign "Y" on the POA field for the atrial fibrillation since it developed prior to a written order for inpatient admission.

3. A patient is treated in observation and while in Observation, the patient falls out of bed and breaks a hip. The patient is subsequently admitted as an inpatient to treat the hip fracture.

   Assign "Y" on the POA field for the hip fracture since it developed prior to a written order for inpatient admission.

4. A patient with known congestive heart failure is admitted to the hospital after he develops decompensated congestive heart failure.

   Assign "Y" on the POA field for the congestive heart failure. The ICD-9-CM code identifies the chronic condition and does not specify the acute exacerbation.

5. A patient undergoes inpatient surgery. After surgery, the patient develops fever and is treated aggressively. The physician's final diagnosis documents "possible postoperative infection following surgery."

   Assign "N" on the POA field for the postoperative infection since final diagnoses that contain the terms "possible", "probable", "suspected" or "rule out" and that are based on symptoms or clinical findings that were not present on admission should be reported as "N".

6. A patient with severe cough and difficulty breathing was diagnosed during his hospitalization to have lung cancer.

   Assign "Y" on the POA field for the lung cancer. Even though the cancer was not diagnosed until after admission, it is a chronic condition that was clearly present before the patient's admission.

7. A patient is admitted to the hospital for a coronary artery bypass surgery. Postoperatively he developed a pulmonary embolism.

   Assign "N" on the POA field for the pulmonary embolism. This is an acute condition that was not present on admission.

8. A patient is admitted with a known history of coronary atherosclerosis, status post myocardial infarction five years ago is now admitted for treatment of impending myocardial infarction. The final diagnosis is documented as "impending myocardial infarction."

   Assign "Y" to the impending myocardial infarction because the condition is present on admission.

9. A patient with diabetes mellitus developed uncontrolled diabetes on day 3 of the hospitalization.

   Assign "N" to the diabetes code because the "uncontrolled" component of the code was not present on admission.

10. A patient is admitted with high fever and pneumonia. The patient rapidly deteriorates and becomes septic. The discharge diagnosis lists sepsis and pneumonia. The documentation is unclear as to whether the sepsis was present on admission or developed shortly after admission.

    Query the physician as to whether the sepsis was present on admission, developed shortly after admission, or it cannot be clinically determined as to whether it was present on admission or not.

11. A patient is admitted for repair of an abdominal aneurysm. However, the aneurysm ruptures after hospital admission.

    Assign "N" for the ruptured abdominal aneurysm. Although the aneurysm was present on admission, the "ruptured" component of the code description did not occur until after admission.

12. A patient with viral hepatitis B progresses to hepatic coma after admission.

    Assign "N" for the viral hepatitis B with hepatic coma because part of the code description did not develop until after admission.

13. A patient with a history of varicose veins and ulceration of the left lower extremity strikes the area against the side of his hospital bed during an inpatient hospitalization. It bleeds profusely. The final diagnosis lists varicose veins with ulcer and hemorrhage.

    Assign "Y" for the varicose veins with ulcer. Although the hemorrhage occurred after admission, the code description for varicose veins with ulcer does not mention hemorrhage.

14. The nursing initial assessment upon admission documents the presence of a decubitus ulcer. There is no mention of the decubitus ulcer in the physician documentation until several days after admission.

    Query the physician as to whether the decubitus ulcer was present on admission, or developed after admission. Both diagnosis code assignment and determination of whether a condition was present on admission must be based on provider documentation in the medical record (per the definition of "provider" found at the beginning of these POA guidelines and in the introductory section of the ICD-9-CM Official Guidelines for Coding and Reporting). If it cannot be determined from the provider documentation whether or not a condition was present on admission, the provider should be queried.

15. A urine culture is obtained on admission. The provider documents urinary tract infection when the culture results become available a few days later.

    Assign "Y" to the urinary tract infection since the diagnosis is based on test results from a specimen obtained on admission. It may not be possible for a provider to make a definitive diagnosis for a period of time after admission. There is no required timeframe as to when a provider must identify or document a condition to be present on admission.

16. A patient tested positive for Methicillin resistant Staphylococcus (MRSA) on routine nasal culture on admission to the hospital. During the hospitalization, he underwent insertion of a central venous catheter and later developed an infection and was diagnosed with MRSA sepsis due to central venous catheter infection.

    Assign "Y" to the positive MRSA colonization. Assign "N" for the MRSA sepsis due to central venous catheter infection since the patient did not have a MRSA infection at the time of admission.

Obstetrics

1. A female patient was admitted to the hospital and underwent a normal delivery.

   Leave the "present on admission" (POA) field blank. Code 650, Normal delivery, is on the "exempt from reporting" list.

2. Patient admitted in late pregnancy due to excessive vomiting and dehydration. During admission patient goes into premature labor.

   Assign "Y" for the excessive vomiting and the dehydration. Assign "N" for the premature labor.

3. Patient admitted in active labor. During the stay, a breast abscess is noted when mother attempted to breast feed. Provider is unable to determine whether the abscess was present on admission.

   Assign "W" for the breast abscess.

4. Patient admitted in active labor. After 12 hours of labor it is noted that the infant is in fetal distress and a Cesarean section is performed.

   Assign "N" for the fetal distress.

5. Pregnant female was admitted in labor and fetal nuchal cord entanglement was diagnosed. Physician is queried, but is unable to determine whether the cord entanglement was present on admission or not.

   Assign "W" for the fetal nuchal cord entanglement.

Newborn

1. A single liveborn infant was delivered in the hospital via Cesarean section. The physician documented fetal bradycardia during labor in the final diagnosis in the newborn record.

   Assign " Y" because the bradycardia developed prior to the newborn admission (birth).

2. A newborn developed diarrhea which was believed to be due to the hospital baby formula.

Assign " N" because the diarrhea developed after admission.

3. A newborn born in the hospital, birth complicated by nuchal cord entanglement.

Assign "Y" for the nuchal cord entanglement on the baby's record. Any condition that is present at birth or that developed in utero is considered present at admission, including conditions that occur during delivery.

Categories and Codes Exempt from Diagnosis Present on Admission Requirement

Note: "Diagnosis present on admission" for these code categories are exempt because they represent circumstances regarding the healthcare encounter or factors influencing health status that do not represent a current disease or injury or are always present on admission

Categories & Codes	Description
137-139	Late effects of infectious and parasitic diseases
268.1	Rickets, late effect
326	Late effects of intracranial abscess or pyogenic infection
412	Old myocardial infarction
438	Late effects of cerebrovascular disease
650	Normal delivery
660.7	Failed forceps or vacuum extractor, unspecified
677	Late effect of complication of pregnancy, childbirth, and the puerperium
740-759	Congenital anomalies
905-909	Late effects of injuries, poisonings, toxic effects, and other external causes
V02	Carrier or suspected carrier of infectious diseases
V03	Need for prophylactic vaccination and inoculation against bacterial diseases
V04	Need for prophylactic vaccination and inoculation against certain viral diseases
V05	Need for other prophylactic vaccination and inoculation against single diseases
V06	Need for prophylactic vaccination and inoculation against combinations of diseases
V07	Need for isolation and other prophylactic or treatment measures
V10	Personal history of malignant neoplasm
V11	Personal history of mental disorder
V12	Personal history of certain other diseases
V13	Personal history of other diseases
V14	Personal history of allergy to medicinal agents
V15	Other personal history presenting hazards to health
V16	Family history of malignant neoplasm
V17	Family history of certain chronic disabling diseases
V18	Family history of certain other specific conditions
V19	Family history of other conditions
V20	Health supervision of infant or child
V21	Constitutional states in development
V22	Normal pregnancy
V23	Supervision of high-risk pregnancy
V24	Postpartum care and examination
V25	Encounter for contraceptive management
V26	Procreative management
V27	Outcome of delivery
V28	Antenatal screening
V29	Observation and evaluation of newborns for suspected condition not found

Categories & Codes	Description
V30-V39	Liveborn infants according to type of birth
V42	Organ or tissue replaced by transplant
V43	Organ or tissue replaced by other means
V44	Artificial opening status
V45	Other postprocedural states
V46	Other dependence on machines and devices
V49.60-V49.77	Upper and lower limb amputation status
V49.81-V49.85	Other specified conditions influencing health status
V50	Elective surgery for purposes other than remedying health states
V51	Aftercare involving the use of plastic surgery
V52	Fitting and adjustment of prosthetic device and implant
V53	Fitting and adjustment of other device
V54	Other orthopedic aftercare
V55	Attention to artificial openings
V56	Encounter for dialysis and dialysis catheter care
V57	Care involving use of rehabilitation procedures
V58	Encounter for other and unspecified procedures and after-care
V59	Donors
V60	Housing, household, and economic circumstances
V61	Other family circumstances
V62	Other psychosocial circumstances
V64	Persons encountering health services for specific procedures, not carried out
V65	Other persons seeking consultation
V66	Convalescence and palliative care
V67	Follow-up examination
V68	Encounters for administrative purposes
V69	Problems related to lifestyle
V70	General medical examination
V71	Observation and evaluation for suspected condition not found
V72	Special investigations and examinations
V73	Special screening examination for viral and chlamydial diseases
V74	Special screening examination for bacterial and spirochetal diseases
V75	Special screening examination for other infectious diseases
V76	Special screening for malignant neoplasms
V77	Special screening for endocrine, nutritional, metabolic, and immunity disorders
V78	Special screening for disorders of blood and blood-forming organs
V79	Special screening for mental disorders and developmental handicaps
V80	Special screening for neurological, eye, and ear diseases
V81	Special screening for cardiovascular, respiratory, and genito-urinary diseases
V82	Special screening for other conditions
V83	Genetic carrier status
V84	Genetic susceptibility to disease
V85	Body Mass Index
V86	Estrogen receptor status
V87.32	Contact with and (suspected) exposure to algae bloom
V87.4	Personal history of drug therapy
V88	Acquired absence of other organs and tissue
V89	Suspected maternal and fetal conditions not found
V90	Retained foreign body

Present on Admission (POA) Tutorial

Categories & Codes	Description
V91	Multiple gestation placenta status
E000	External cause status
E001-E030	Activity
E800-E807	Railway accidents
E810-E819	Motor vehicle traffic accidents
E820-E825	Motor vehicle nontraffic accidents
E826-E829	Other road vehicle accidents
E830-E838	Water transport accidents
E840-E845	Air and space transport accidents
E846-E848	Vehicle accidents not elsewhere classifiable
E849.0-E849.6	Place of occurrence
E849.8-E849.9	Place of occurrence
E883.1	Accidental fall into well
E883.2	Accidental fall into storm drain or manhole
E884.0	Fall from playground equipment
E884.1	Fall from cliff
E885.0	Fall from (nonmotorized) scooter
E885.1	Fall from roller skates
E885.2	Fall from skateboard
E885.3	Fall from skis
E885.4	Fall from snowboard
E886.0	Fall on same level from collision, pushing, or shoving, by or with other person, In sports
E890.0-E890.9	Conflagration in private dwelling
E893.0	Accident caused by ignition of clothing, from controlled fire in private dwelling
E893.2	Accident caused by ignition of clothing, from controlled fire not in building or structure
E894	Ignition of highly inflammable material
E895	Accident caused by controlled fire in private dwelling
E897	Accident caused by controlled fire not in building or structure
E917.0	Striking against or struck accidentally by objects or persons, in sports without subsequent fall

Categories & Codes	Description
E917.1	Striking against or struck accidentally by objects or persons, caused by a crowd, by collective fear or panic without subsequent fall
E917.2	Striking against or struck accidentally by objects or persons, in running water without subsequent fall
E917.5	Striking against or struck accidentally by objects or persons, object in sports with subsequent fall
E917.6	Striking against or struck accidentally by objects or persons, caused by a crowd, by collective fear or panic with subsequent fall
E919.0-E919.1	Accidents caused by machinery
E919.3-E919.9	Accidents caused by machinery
E921.0-E921.9	Accident caused by explosion of pressure vessel
E922.0-E922.9	Accident caused by firearm and air gun missile
E926.2	Visible and ultraviolet light sources
E928.0-E928.8	Other and unspecified environmental and accidental causes
E929.0-E929.9	Late effects of accidental injury
E959	Late effects of self-inflicted injury
E970-E978	Legal intervention
E979	Terrorism
E981.0-E981.8	Poisoning by gases in domestic use, undetermined whether accidentally or purposely inflicted
E982.0-E982.9	Poisoning by other gases, undetermined whether accidentally or purposely inflicted
E985.0-E985.7	Injury by firearms air guns and explosives, undetermined whether accidentally or purposely inflicted
E987.0	Falling from high place, undetermined whether accidentally or purposely inflicted, residential premises
E987.2	Falling from high place, undetermined whether accidentally or purposely inflicted, natural sites
E989	Late effects of injury, undetermined whether accidentally or purposely inflicted
E990-E999	Injury resulting from operations of war

10 Steps to Correct Coding

Follow the 10 steps below to correctly code encounters for healthcare services.

Step 1: Identify the reason for the visit or encounter (i.e., a sign, symptom, diagnosis and/or condition).

The medical record documentation should accurately reflect the patient's condition, using terminology that includes specific diagnoses and symptoms, or clearly states the reasons for the encounter.

Choosing the main term that best describes the reason chiefly responsible for the service provided is the most important step in coding. If symptoms are present and documented, but a definitive diagnosis has not yet been determined, code the symptoms. **For outpatient cases, do not code conditions that are referred to as "rule out," "suspected," "probable" or "questionable."** Diagnoses often are not established at the time of the initial encounter/visit. Two or more visits may be necessary to establish the diagnosis. Code only what is documented in the available records and only to the highest degree of certainty known at the time of the patient's visit, unless it is an inpatient medical record, in which case uncertain diagnoses may be reported.

Step 2: After selecting the reason for the encounter, always consult the Alphabetic Index, Volume 2, before verifying code selection in the Tabular section.

The most critical rule is to begin the code selection process in the *Alphabetic Index*. Never turn first to the Tabular List (Volume 1). The Index provides cross references, essential and non-essential modifiers, and inclusion terms not found in the Tabular List. To prevent coding errors, always use both the Alphabetic Index and the Tabular List when locating and assigning a code. Always verify the code found in the Alphabetic Index in the Tabular List. First, the Index does not include the important instructional notes found in the Tabular. Second, the advantage of a classification system is that like items are grouped together. A quick scan of the Tabular might provide coding options for the coder that would have been missed.

Step 3: Locate the main term entry.

The Alphabetic Index is a listing of conditions. Conditions may be expressed as nouns or eponyms, with critical use of adjectives. Some conditions have multiple entries under synonyms. Reasons for encounters may be located under general terms such as admission, encounter, and examination. Other general terms such as history of or status post are used to locate factors influencing health.

Step 4: Read and interpret any notes listed with the main term or the subterm.

Notes such as common fifth-digit references and cross references are identified by italicized type. Always check any cross-references to ensure that all alternative terms are researched.

Step 5: Review entries for modifiers.

Nonessential modifiers are the terms located within parentheses following the main term entry. These parenthetical terms are supplementary words or explanatory information that may either be present or absent in the diagnostic statement and do not affect code selection. The subterms listed under the main term are essential modifiers that do affect coding assignment. Each line of indent represents a more specific code entry.

Step 6: Interpret abbreviations, cross-references, fifth digits, and brackets.

The cross-references used are "see," "see category" and "see also" which indicate alternative term choices for code searches. The abbreviation NEC may follow main terms or subterms. NEC (not elsewhere classified) indicates that there is no specific code for the condition even though the medical documentation may be very specific. Is a fifth digit required? You MUST refer to the Tabular List to discover the correct code. Italicized brackets [ ] enclose a second code that must be used along with the code immediately preceding it, with the bracketed code sequenced as the secondary code. This is a mandatory multiple code situation. Both the underlying condition and the manifestation (code in the slanted bracket) must be reported.

Step 7: Choose a potential code and locate it in the Tabular List.

The coder must follow any Includes, Excludes notes, and other instructional notes, such as "Code first" and "Use additional code," listed in the Tabular for the chapter, category, subcategory, and subclassification level of code selection which direct the coder to use a different or additional code.

Any codes in the Tabular range, 001.0 through 999.9, may be used to identify the diagnostic reason for the encounter. The Tabular encompasses many codes describing disease and injury classifications (e.g., infectious and parasitic diseases, neoplasms, symptoms, signs and ill-defined conditions, etc.).

Codes that describe symptoms and signs, as opposed to definitive diagnoses, should be used for reporting purposes when an established diagnosis has not been made (confirmed) by the physician. Chapter 16 of the ICD-9-CM code book, "Symptoms, Signs, and Ill-Defined Conditions" (codes 780.01-799.9) contains many, but not all, codes for symptoms.

ICD-9-CM classifies encounters with health care providers for circumstances other than a disease or injury using codes in the Supplementary Classification of Factors Influencing Health Status and Contact with Health Services (V01.0-V91.99). There are many occasions when circumstances other than a disease or injury are recorded as chiefly responsible for the encounter.

Step 8: Determine whether the code is at the highest level of specificity.

A code is invalid if it has not been coded to the full number of digits (greatest level of specificity) required. A three-digit code is to be used only if the category is not further subdivided. Assign four-digit codes (subcategory codes) only if there are no five-digit codes for that category. Assign five-digit codes (fifth-digit subclassification codes) for those categories mandating the use of five digits.

Step 9: Assign the code.

Having reviewed all relevant information concerning the possible code choices, assign the code that most completely describes the condition.

Repeat steps one through nine for all additional documented conditions that meet the following criteria:

- Conditions that currently exist at the time of the visit

- Conditions that require or affect patient care, treatment or management.

Step 10: Sequence codes correctly

Sequencing is defined as the order in which the codes are listed on the claim. List first the ICD-9-CM code for the diagnosis, condition, problem or other reason for the encounter/visit, which is shown in the medical record to be chiefly responsible for the services provided. List additional codes that describe any coexisting conditions. Follow the official coding guidelines (See Section II Selection of Principal Diagnosis, Section III Reporting Additional Diagnoses, and Section IV Diagnostic Coding and Reporting Guidelines for Outpatient Services) concerning proper sequencing of codes.

Coding Examples

Diagnosis: Anorexia

- Step 1: The reason for the encounter was the condition, anorexia.

- Step 2: Consult the Index to Diseases.

- Step 3: Locate the main term "Anorexia."

- Step 4: There are no italicized instructional notes to interpret.

- Step 5: Note that there are two possible subterms (essential modifiers), "hysterical" and "nervosa," neither of which is documented in this instance and therefore cannot be used in code selection. The code listed next to the main term is called the default code selection.

- Step 6: There are no abbreviations, cross-references, fifth-digit notations, or brackets.

- Step 7: Turn to code 783.0 in the Tabular List and read the instructional notes. In this case the "Excludes" note indicates that anorexia determined to be of non-organic origin should be coded to Chapter 5. The diagnostic statement does not indicate non-organic origin.

- Step 8: There is no further division of the category past the fourth digit subcategory. Therefore, the subcategory code level is the highest level of specificity.

- Step 9: The default code, 783.0 is the correct code selection.

- Step 10: Since anorexia is listed as the chief reason for the healthcare encounter, the first-listed or principal diagnosis is 783.0.

Diagnosis: Acute bronchitis
- Step 1: The reason for the encounter was the condition, acute bronchitis.

- Step 2. Consult the Index to Diseases.

- Step 3: Locate the main term "Bronchitis."

- Step 4: There are no italicized instructional notes to interpret.

- Step 5: Review entries for modifiers. Since "acute" is not listed as a nonessential modifier, read past the "with" modifier until you find the subterm "acute or subacute" with code 466.0.

- Step 6: There are no abbreviations, cross-references, fifth digit notations, or brackets.

- Step 7: Since there are no more appropriate subterms, turn to code 466.0 in the Tabular List. The Includes note under category 466.0 does refer to possible infective organism, and other alternative terms for acute bronchitis. Note that inclusion term list is not exhaustive, but is only a representative selection of diagnoses that are included in the subcategory. At the beginning of chapter 8, "Diseases of the Respiratory System," you will notice the "use additional code" note that tells you to assign a code to identify the infectious organism. This instructional note applies to the entire chapter.

- Step 8: There is no further division of the category past the fourth- digit subcategory. Therefore, the subcategory code level is the highest level of specificity.

- Step 9: Assign code 466.0.

- Step 10: Repeat steps 1-9 for any additional code assignments.

Diagnosis: Acute bronchitis due to staphylococcus
- Step 1: The reason for the encounter was the condition, acute bronchitis due to staphylococcus.

- Step 2: Follow the steps listed in the above example for the diagnosis of acute bronchitis. You will now start the search for code identifying the underlying infectious organism, which in this case is staphylococcus.

- Step 3. Consult the Index to Diseases.

- Step 4: Locate the main term Staphylococcus, staphylococcal.

- Step 5: The italicized instructional notes states see condition. Locate the main term "Infection, infected, infective".

- Step 6: Review entries for modifiers. Locate the subterm "staphylococcal NEC," where you will find code 041.10 referenced. The abbreviation NEC indicates that a review of the medical record may be necessary to determine if there is documentation concerning the specific type of staphylococcus.

- Step 7: Verify code 041.10 in the Tabular List. The code title is Staphylococcus, unspecified. If there is additional information identifying the organism as aureus or other, assign the appropriate code, 041.11 or 041.19. Otherwise, assign code 041.10, Staphylococcus, unspecified, as an additional code.

- Step 8: There is no further division of the category past the fifth-digit subclassification level. Therefore, the subclassification code level is the highest level of specificity. The final code assignment would be 041.10.

- Step 9: Assign code 041.10.

- Step 10: Sequence codes as directed by the instructional note for category 466. Code first 466.0 and assign code 041.10 as an additional diagnosis.

Diagnosis: Traveler's diarrhea
- Step 1: The reason for the encounter was the condition, traveler's diarrhea.

- Step 2. Consult the Index to Diseases.

- Step 3: Locate the main term "Diarrhea" in the Alphabetic Index.

- Step 4: There are no italicized instructional notes to interpret.

- Step 5: Review entries for modifiers. Note that the nonessential modifiers (in parentheses) after the main term do not include the term "traveler's," which means that the coder should search the subterms for the term "traveler's." The subterm "traveler's" has a possible code selection, 009.2, and includes the subterm "due to specified organism NEC 008.8." The diagnostic statement does not include the infectious agent; therefore, code 008.8 does not apply.

- Step 6: There are no abbreviations, cross-references, fifth-digit notations, or brackets.

- Step 7: Locate code 009.2 in the Tabular List and read all instructional notes under the main category and subcategories. The Includes notes does not list the term "traveler's" under code 009.2. As instructed by the Alphabetic Index, you should code the condition to 009.2. The ICD-9-CM code book implies that "traveler's diarrhea" is the same as infectious diarrhea when it is not attributed to any specified infectious agent.

- Step 8: There is no further division of the category past the fourth-digit subcategory level. Therefore, the subcategory code level is the highest level of specificity. The final code assignment would be 009.2.

- Step 9: Assign code 009.2.

- Step 10: Since infectious diarrhea is listed as the chief reason for the healthcare encounter, the first-listed or principal diagnosis is 009.2.

Diagnosis: Ingrown toenail, infected
- Step 1: The reason for the encounter was the condition, infected ingrown toenail.

- Step 2. Consult the Index to Diseases.

- Step 3: First you must decide what the searchable main term should be. Reminder: search for condition, not anatomical site. The Alphabetic Index helps you determine the main term. Refer to "toenail" in the Alphabetic Index; the closest match is "Toe," which includes the instruction "see condition." Locate the main term "Infection" in the Alphabetic Index. The subterm toe has a subterm "nail" which refers the coder to category 681, Cellulitis and abscess of finger and toe. This does not indicate the condition ingrown toenail. The main term, therefore, is "Ingrown." A review of the Alphabetic Index takes you to "Ingrowing."

- Step 4: There are no italicized instructional notes to interpret.

- Step 5: Review the subterms. The subterm "nail" appears and lists nonessential modifiers (in parentheses) as "finger," "toe" and "infected." These nonessential modifiers complete the diagnostic statement.

- Step 6: There are no abbreviations, cross-references, fifth-digit notations, or brackets.

- Step 7: Verify code 703.0 in the Tabular List Before assigning the code, review all instructional notes under category 703 and under code 703.0. The note, "Excludes: infection, nail NOS (681.9)," can be ignored because the diagnostic statement specifies the infection is due to the ingrowing nail.

- Step 8: Therefore, the subcategory code level is the highest level of specificity. The final code assignment would be 703.0.

- Step 9: The correct code choice is 703.0, Ingrowing nail with infection.

- Step 10: Since infectious infected ingrown toenail is listed as the chief reason for the healthcare encounter, the first-listed or principal diagnosis is 703.0.